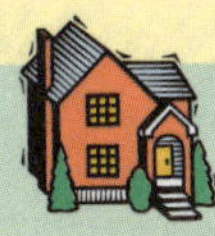

FAMILY HOME CARE BOXES

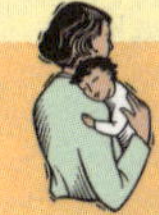

FAMILY FOCUS BOXES

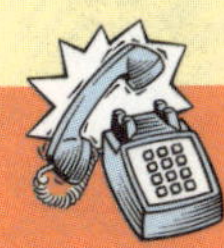

EMERGENCY TREATMENT BOXES

Whaley & Wong's

Nursing Care of Infants and Children

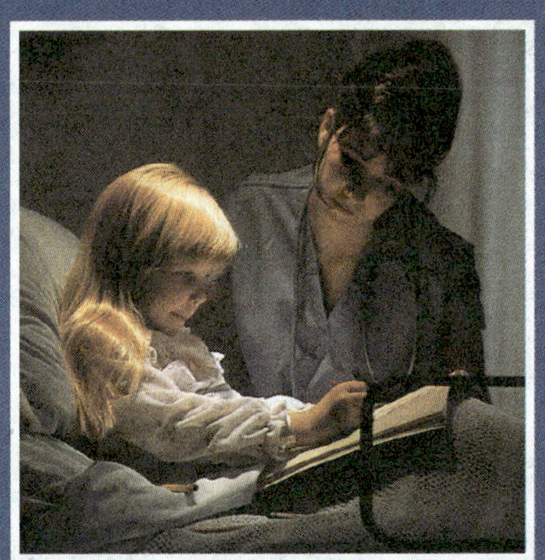

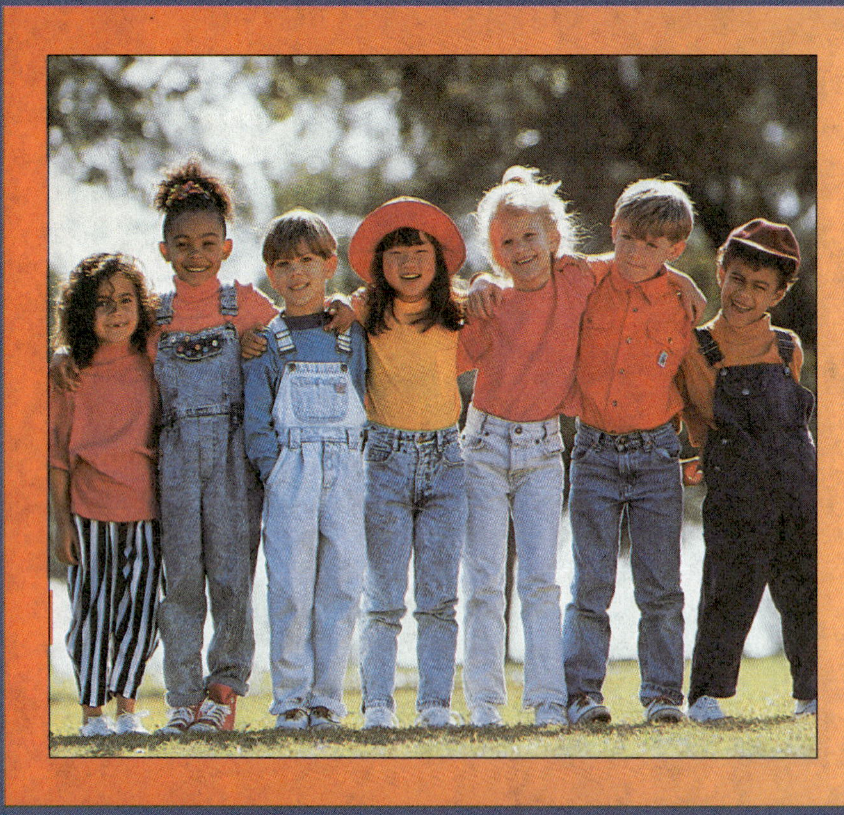

Whaley & Wong's

Nursing Care of Infants and Children

Donna L. Wong, *RN, PhD, PNP, CPN, FAAN*
Nurse Consultant,
Saint Francis Hospital Children's Center;
Adjunct Associate Professor,
Department of Pediatrics,
University of Oklahoma College of Medicine—Tulsa;
Clinical Associate Professor,
University of Oklahoma College of Nursing,
Tulsa, Oklahoma

CONTRIBUTING EDITOR
David Wilson, *RN,C, MS*
Formerly Clinical Instructor,
Eastern Oklahoma Perinatal Center,
Saint Francis Hospital;
Adjunct Faculty,
Anna Vaughn School of Nursing,
Oral Roberts University,
Tulsa, Oklahoma

FIFTH EDITION

with 676 illustrations

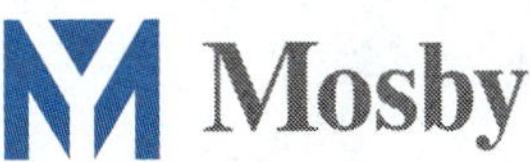

St. Louis Baltimore Boston Carlsbad Chicago Naples New York Philadelphia Portland
London Madrid Mexico City Singapore Sydney Tokyo Toronto Wiesbaden

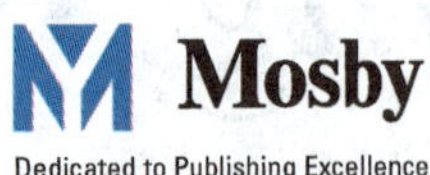

Dedicated to Publishing Excellence

A Times Mirror Company

Publisher: Nancy L. Coon
Editor: Sally Schrefer
Developmental Editor: Janet R. Livingston
Project Manager: Gayle May Morris
Production Editor: Judith Bange
Manufacturing Supervisor: Kathy Grone
Design Manager: Susan Lane
Book Designer: Jeanne Wolfgeher
Cover Photograph: David Leach: Tony Stone Images

A NOTE TO THE READER:

The author and publisher have made every attempt to check dosages and nursing content for accuracy. Because the science of pharmacology is continually advancing, our knowledge base continues to expand. Therefore we recommend that the reader always check product information for changes in dosage or administration before administering any medication. This is particularly important with new or rarely used drugs.

FIFTH EDITION

Printed in the United States of America
Composition by Clarinda Company
Printing/binding by Rand McNally

Mosby–Year Book, Inc.
11830 Westline Industrial Drive
St. Louis, Missouri 63146

Library of Congress Cataloging-in-Publication Data

Wong, Donna L.
Whaley & Wong's nursing care of infants and children / Donna L. Wong ; contributing editor, David Wilson. — 5th ed.
p. cm.
Rev. ed. of: Nursing care of infants and children / Lucille F. Whaley, Donna L. Wong. 4th ed. c1991.
Includes bibliographical references and index.
ISBN 0-8016-7882-X
1. Pediatric nursing. I. Wilson, David. II. Whaley, Lucille F. Nursing care of infants and children. III. Title. IV. Title: Nursing care of infants and children.
[DNLM: 1. Pediatric Nursing. WY 159 W872w 1994]
RJ245.W47 1994
610.73′62—dc20
DNLM/DLC
for Library of Congress 94-39540
CIP

94 95 96 97 98 / 9 8 7 6 5 4 3 2 1

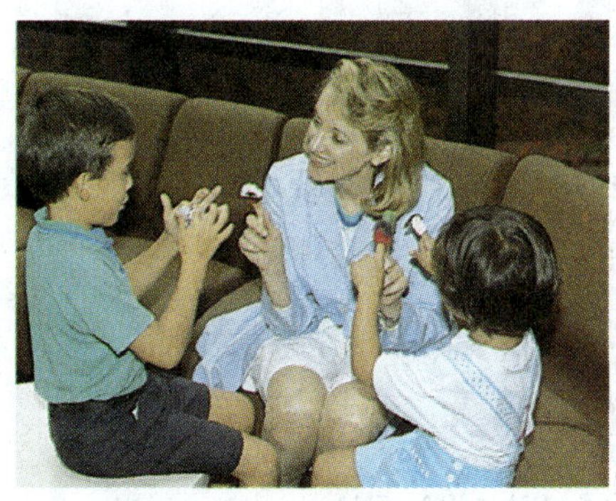

To my husband, ***Ting***
for the unconditional love, intellectual enlightenment, and support that make it all possible

my daughter, ***Nina***
for being my greatest pediatric teacher and the sunshine in my life

my beloved father, ***Rudy***
for being a parent, partner, and friend—I miss you

my mother, ***Madeline***
for making the first typed manuscript a reality and encouraging me through four more

my grandmother, ***Ida***
who at 94 years of age makes finger puppets so we can give atraumatic care

D.L.W.

CONTRIBUTORS

Elizabeth Ahmann, RN, ScD
Consultant, Child and Family Health,
Washington, D.C.;
Section Editor, *Pediatric Nursing,*
Pitman, New Jersey

Annette L. Baker, RN, MSN
Clinical Research Nurse,
Cardiology Department,
Children's Hospital,
Boston, Massachusetts

Linda H. Bearinger, RN, MS, PhD
Assistant Professor and Director,
Adolescent Nursing Graduate and Interdisciplinary Adolescent Health Programs,
School of Nursing and School of Medicine,
University of Minnesota,
Minneapolis, Minnesota

Jeanne T. Boisvert, RN, BSN
Staff Nurse III,
Cardiovascular Nursing Program,
Children's Hospital,
Boston, Massachusetts

Annette C. Bollig, RN, MSN
Director, Critical Care Nursing,
Children's Hospital of Wisconsin,
Milwaukee, Wisconsin

Deborah Brantly, APRN, CNS, MS, LMFT
Author, Consultant, Therapist
Tulsa, Oklahoma

Myra Carmon, RN, EdD, CPNP
Assistant Professor, Parent-Child Nursing,
Georgia State University School of Nursing,
Atlanta, Georgia

Jeanne O'Connor Egan, RN, MSN
Pediatric Clinical Specialist,
Children's Hospital,
Washington, D.C.

Mikel Gray, RN, PhD, PNP, CURN
UroHealth;
Director of Urodynamics,
Suburban Medical Center;
Adjunct Professor,
Lancing School of Nursing,
Bellarmine College,
Louisville, Kentucky

Teresa L. Hall, RN, MS
Nursing Supervisor,
Hathaway Children's Services,
Sylmar, California

Caryn Stoermer Hess, RN, MS
Nursing Consultant,
Englewood, Colorado

Marilyn Hockenberry-Eaton, RN-CS, PhD, PNP, FAAN
Director, Advanced Practitioners,
Texas Children's Hospital,
Houston, Texas

Elizabeth E. Hogue, JD
Attorney in Private Practice,
Burtonsville, Maryland

Marilyn E. Jenkins, RN, MBA, CNA
Director of Nursing,
Shriner's Burns Institute, Cincinnati Unit;
Clinical Faculty,
College of Nursing and Health,
University of Cincinnati,
Cincinnati, Ohio

Ellen Johnsen, RN, BA
Trainer, Consultant,
Community Living Support Center,
Oklahoma State University,
Stillwater, Oklahoma

Stephen Jones, RN,C, MS, PNP
Pediatric Clinical Nurse Specialist,
Pediatric Nurse Practitioner,
Children's Hospital at Albany Medical Center,
Albany, New York

Christina Algiere Kasprisin, RN, MS
University of Vermont College of Nursing,
Burlington, Vermont

Patricia L. King, RN, MS
Director, Patient Care Services,
Shriner's Hospitals for Crippled Children,
Springfield, Massachusetts

Linda M. Kollar, RN, MSN, CPNP
Assistant Director of Nursing,
Division of Adolescent Medicine,
Children's Hospital Medical Center,
Cincinnati, Ohio

William W. Latimer, PhD
Psychology Fellow,
Adolescent Health Program,
Division of General Pediatrics and Adolescent Health,
Department of Pediatrics, School of Medicine,
University of Minnesota,
Minneapolis, Minnesota

Rosemary Liguori, ARNP, MS, CPNP
Assistant Professor,
University of Oklahoma College of Nursing,
Tulsa, Oklahoma

Wendy Low, RN
Vancouver Community College,
Langara Campus—Nursing Program,
Vancouver, British Columbia,
Canada

Kristy Martyn, RN, MSN, CPNP
Director of Family Practitioner Program,
Albany State College School of Nursing,
Albany, Georgia

Lynn E. Mattis, RN, MSN
Clinical Nurse Specialist,
Division of Pediatric Gastroenterology/Nutrition,
Department of Pediatrics,
The Johns Hopkins Hospital,
Baltimore, Maryland

Patricia O'Brien, RN,C, MSN, PNP
Cardiovascular Clinical Nurse Specialist,
Cardiovascular Programs,
Children's Hospital,
Boston, Massachusetts

Kathryn A. Perry, APRN, RN,C, MSN, CNS
Clinical Nurse Specialist for Child Neurology,
Children's Medical Center,
Tulsa, Oklahoma

Margaret Dexheimer Pharris, RN, MS, MPH
Nursing Fellow,
Adolescent Health Program,
Division of General Pediatrics and Adolescent Health,
Department of Pediatrics, School of Medicine,
University of Minnesota,
Minneapolis, Minnesota

Marti Rice, RN, PhD
Assistant Professor,
Georgia State University School of Nursing,
Atlanta, Georgia

Judy Holt Rollins, RN, MS
Consultant, Rollins and Associates;
Adjunct Instructor,
Georgetown University School of Medicine;
Coordinator, Studio G,
Georgetown University Medical Center,
Washington, D.C.;
Associate Editor, *Pediatric Nursing*,
Pitman, New Jersey

Kathleen Rossman, RRT
Special Projects Coordinator,
Eastern Oklahoma Perinatal Center,
Saint Francis Hospital,
Tulsa, Oklahoma

Cindy Hylton Rushton, RN,C, PhD
Clinical Nurse Specialist in Ethics,
The Johns Hopkins Children's Center,
Baltimore, Maryland

Renee Sieving, RN,C, MSN, PNP
Associate Clinical Specialist,
Graduate Studies in Adolescent Nursing,
University of Minnesota School of Nursing,
Minneapolis, Minnesota

Donna Phillips Smith, RN, MS
Genetic Counselor,
H.A. Chapman Institute of Medical Genetics,
Tulsa, Oklahoma

Jamie Stang, RD, MPH
Nutrition Fellow,
Adolescent Health Program,
Division of General Pediatrics and Adolescent Health,
Department of Pediatrics, School of Medicine,
University of Minnesota,
Minneapolis, Minnesota

Amy Verst, RN, MSN, PNP, ATC
Pediatric Nurse Practitioner,
Scottsburg Well Child Clinic;
Clinical Instructor,
Bellarmine College;
Pediatric Nurse Practitioner,
Home of the Innocents;
Certified Athletic Trainer,
Louisville, Kentucky

Judith A. Vessey, RN,C, PhD
Professor, College of Nursing,
University of Arkansas for Medical Sciences;
Research Facilitator,
Arkansas Children's Hospital,
Little Rock, Arkansas

David Wilson, RN,C, MS
Formerly Clinical Instructor,
Eastern Oklahoma Perinatal Center,
Saint Francis Hospital;
Adjunct Faculty,
Anna Vaughn School of Nursing,
Oral Roberts University,
Tulsa, Oklahoma

Janice Marie Wingo, RN, BSN, CPN
Clinical Instructor, Pediatrics,
Saint Francis Hospital Children's Center,
Tulsa, Oklahoma

Marilyn L. Winkelstein, RN, PhD
Assistant Professor,
University of Maryland School of Nursing,
Baltimore, Maryland

Susan B. Zekauskas, RN, MSN, PNP
Assistant Professor of Nursing,
Tulsa Junior College,
Tulsa, Oklahoma

REVIEWERS

Karen Atkins, RN, MSN
Department Director,
Adolescent/Young Unit,
The Children's Hospital of Alabama,
Birmingham, Alabama

Barbara L. Atkinson
Education Specialist,
Automotive Safety for Children Program,
James Whitcomb Riley Hospital for Children,
Indianapolis, Indiana

Johanna Backus, RN,C, BSN
Mary Bridge Children's Hospital,
Tacoma, Washington

Olimpia Banning, RN,C, BSN
Unit Supervisor/Staff Nurse,
Mary Bridge Children's Hospital,
Tacoma, Washington

Pauline C. Beecroft, RN, PhD
Nurse Researcher,
Children's Hospital,
Los Angeles, California;
Senior Research Specialist,
American Association of Critical-Care Nurses,
Aliso Viejo, California

Dorian G. Blevins, RN, MS
Clinican Instructor,
College of Nursing,
University of Utah,
Salt Lake City, Utah

George Blodgett, RN,C
Cardiac Nurse Specialist,
Mary Bridge Children's Hospital,
Tacoma, Washington

Mary Boland, RN, MSN, CPNP
Director, AIDS Program,
Children's Hospital of New Jersey,
Newark, New Jersey;
Director, National Pediatric HIV Resource Center;
Associate in Pediatrics,
University of Medicine and Dentistry,
New Jersey Medical School,
Newark, New Jersey

Marion Broome, RN, PhD
Professor, College of Nursing,
Rush University;
Assistant Chairperson,
Department of Maternal-Child Nursing,
Rush–Presbyterian–St. Luke's Medical Center,
Chicago, Illinois;
Research Consultant,
Children's Memorial Hospital,
Chicago, Illinois

Janet M. Brucker, RN, MS, CNRN
Assistant Director, Nursing,
Texas Children's Hospital,
Houston, Texas

Karen Carlson, RN, PhD
Assistant Professor, College of Nursing,
University of Arkansas for Medical Sciences,
Little Rock, Arkansas

Virginia Clark, RN,C
Mary Bridge Children's Hospital,
Tacoma, Washington

Ellen Rudy Clore, RN, MSN, FNP
Assistant Professor,
University of Florida College of Nursing,
Orlando, Florida

Catherine S. Connell, RN,C, MNSc, RNP, EMT
Instructor,
Baptist School of Nursing—Northwest,
Springdale, Arkansas

Robert J. Connell, EMT-P, EMT-I/C, CFTO
Paramedic/Firefighter,
Certified Fire Training Officer,
Eureka Springs Fire Department,
Eureka Springs, Arkansas

Annette Crew-Gooden, RN, MS
Instructor of Nursing,
Clayton State College,
Morrow, Georgia

Lana K. Davies, RN, MSN
Instructor, Childhood Adaptation,
Research College of Nursing,
Kansas City, Missouri

Elizabeth Edgar, RN,C, BSN
Department Director,
Adolescent Psychiatric Unit,
The Children's Hospital of Alabama,
Birmingham, Alabama

Suzanne L. Feetham, RN, PhD, FAAN
Deputy Director and Chief,
Office of Planning, Analysis, and Evaluation,
National Institute of Nursing Research,
Bethesda, Maryland

Mary Floyd, BS, CLSp(CG)
Genetic Counselor,
H.A. Chapman Institute of Medical Genetics,
Tulsa, Oklahoma

William K. Frankenburg, MD, MSPH
Pediatrics and Preventive Medicine Professor,
University of Colorado Health Sciences Center,
Denver, Colorado

Brenda Geyer, RN,C, MN
Mary Bridge Children's Hospital,
Tacoma, Washington

Nancy Hagelgans, RN, MSN, CETN
Urology Clinical Nurse Specialist,
Denver, Colorado

Connie Hansen
College of Nursing,
Montana State University,
Great Falls, Montana

Rosanne Harrigan, RN, EdD, CPNP, FAAN
Dean and Professor,
School of Nursing,
University of Hawaii at Moana,
Honolulu, Hawaii

Sue Hoffman, RN,C
Staff Nurse Specialist,
Pediatric Orthopaedics,
Mary Bridge Children's Hospital,
Tacoma, Washington

Sharon Holbrook, RN
Nurse Specialist, Physical and Sexual Abuse,
Mary Bridge Children's Hospital,
Tacoma, Washington

Marguerite Jackson, RN, MS, CIC, FAAN
Department of Epidemiology,
University of California—San Diego Medical Center,
San Diego, California

Pat Jamerson, RN,C, MSN, CPCE, CBE
Assistant Professor, Department of Nursing,
William Jewel College,
Liberty, Missouri

Andy Johnson, RN, CPNP
Hemophilia Nurse Practitioner,
Children's Medical Center of Dallas,
Dallas, Texas

Lynn E. Kelly, RN, PhD
Assistant Professor,
Widener University School of Nursing,
Chester, Pennsylvania

Margaret Lamark, RN, BSN
Rochester, New York

Deborah Lammert, APRN, RN,C, MSN, CNS, CCRN-P
Pediatric Cardiovascular Clinical Nurse Specialist,
Saint Francis Hospital Children's Center,
Tulsa, Oklahoma

Norma Liburd, RN,C, MN
Pediatric Clinical Nurse Specialist,
All Children's Hospital,
St. Petersburg, Florida

Rosemary Liguori, ARNP, MS, CPNP
Assistant Professor,
University of Oklahoma College of Nursing,
Tulsa, Oklahoma

Zena Lind, RN,C
Nurse Specialist, Toddler/Preschooler Care,
Mary Bridge Children's Hospital,
Tacoma, Washington

Mary Beth Malloy, RN, MSN
Neonatal Clinical Nurse Specialist,
Loyola University Medical Center,
Maywood, Illinois

Ida Martinson, RN, PhD, FAAN
University of California—San Francisco,
School of Nursing,
Department of Family Health Care Nursing,
San Francisco, California

Mindy Mashburn, RN, MSN, CPNP
Clinical Coordinator of Pediatric Services,
North Texas Community Clinics,
Denton, Texas

Margo McCaffery, RN, MS, FAAN
Consultant in the Nursing Care of Patients with Pain,
Los Angeles, California

Lee McGoodwin, MS, RPH, CSPI
Poison Control Center,
Children's Hospital of Oklahoma,
Oklahoma City, Oklahoma

Carolyn Clavier Mega, RN, MS
Lecturer,
Clemson University School of Nursing;
Staff Nurse,
Greenville Memorial Hospital NICU,
Clemson, South Carolina

Shirley W. Menard, RN, PhD, CPNP, FAAN
Assistant Professor,
University of Texas Health Science Center,
San Antonio, Texas

Caryl E. Mobley, RN, PhD
Assistant Professor,
College of Nursing,
Texas Woman's University,
Dallas, Texas

Becky Morrison, RN, MSN, CPNP
Sickle Cell Nurse Coordinator,
Mesquite, Texas

Dottie Needham, APRN, MSN, CPNP
Pediatric Nurse Practitioner,
Lead Program,
Children's Hospital at Yale–New Haven,
Yale University School of Medicine,
New Haven, Connecticut

Anita Norton, RN, MSN
Chairperson, Department of Nursing;
Instructor, Pediatric Nursing,
Jefferson State Community College,
Birmingham, Alabama

Donna Ortega, RN, MSN
Community College of Denver,
Denver, Colorado

Myung Park, MD
Professor of Pediatrics;
Head, Division of Cardiology,
University of Texas Health Science Center,
San Antonio, Texas

Cathey Pielsticker, RN, MS, CDE
Program Manager,
Diabetes Education Services,
Saint Francis Hospital,
Tulsa, Oklahoma

Ann Pierson, RN,C
Hematology/Oncology Clinic Staff Nurse,
Mary Bridge Children's Health Center,
Tacoma, Washington

Lynda Powers, RN
Pediatric Trauma Nurse Specialist;
Emergency Nursing Pediatric Course Instructor Candidate,
Mary Bridge Children's Hospital,
Emergency Department,
Tacoma, Washington

Jannine Pritchett, RN,C
Intravenous Therapy,
Mary Bridge Children's Hospital,
Tacoma, Washington;
Puyallup Valley Family Practice,
Puyallup, Washington

Marti Rice, RN, PhD
Assistant Professor,
Georgia State University School of Nursing,
Atlanta, Georgia

Julie Robinson, ARNP, MN, CCRN
Mary Bridge Children's Hospital,
Tacoma, Washington

Kathleen Rogacki, RN,C, BSN
Child and Adolescent Certified Nurse;
Nurse Specialist for School-Age Children,
Mary Bridge Children's Hospital,
Tacoma, Washington

Lona Roll, RN, MSN
Clinical Nurse Specialist,
Pediatric Hematology/Oncology,
Santa Rosa's Children's Hospital,
San Antonio, Texas

Amy N. Romanczuk, RN, MSN
Spina Bifida Nurse Coordinator,
Medical University of South Carolina,
Children's Hospital,
Charleston, South Carolina

Jose M. Saavedra, MD
Assistant Professor,
Department of Pediatrics,
The Johns Hopkins Hospital,
Baltimore, Maryland

Nancy Santilli, RN, MSN, PNP, FAAN
Associate Professor/Associate Director,
Comprehensive Epilepsy Program,
Department of Neurology,
University of Virginia Health Sciences Center,
Charlottesville, Virginia

Marilyn C. Savedra, RN, DNSc, FAAN
Professor,
Department of Family Health Care Nursing,
University of California—San Francisco,
San Francisco, California

Nancy Jo Scates, RN,C
Nurse Specialist, Pediatric Gastroenterology;
Nurse Supervisor, GI Clinic,
Mary Bridge Children's Health Center,
Tacoma, Washington

Susie Schulwitz, RN, MS
Clinical Nurse Specialist,
Pediatric Gastroenterology,
Cook–Fort Worth Children's Medical Center,
Fort Worth, Texas

Deborah Scott, RN, DNS
Associate Professor,
University of Louisville School of Nursing,
Louisville, Kentucky

Dianne Fochtman Seleny, RN, MN, CPNP
Pediatric Nurse Practitioner,
Kapiolani Medical Center for Women and Children,
Honolulu, Hawaii

Anne H. Shealy, RN-CS, DSN
Assistant Professor,
Graduate Program,
University of Alabama School of Nursing,
Birmingham, Alabama

Kathleen Simpson, RN,C, MSN
Perinatal Clinical Nurse Specialist,
St. John's Mercy Medical Center,
St. Louis, Missouri

Jane Starn, RN,C, PhD, PNP
Associate Professor, School of Nursing;
Associate Researcher,
Center for Youth Research,
University of Hawaii School of Nursing,
Honolulu, Hawaii

Martin T. Stein, MD
Professor of Pediatrics,
University of California—San Diego,
School of Medicine,
La Jolla, California

Lynn Stover, RN,C, MSN
University of Alabama,
Capstone College of Nursing,
Tuscaloosa, Alabama

Karen Bruner Stroup, PhD
Research Associate,
Automotive Safety for Children Program,
James Whitcomb Riley Hospital for Children,
Indianapolis, Indiana

Judith Talty
Occupant Protection Program Manager,
Automotive Safety for Children Program,
James Whitcomb Riley Hospital for Children,
Indianapolis, Indiana

Mary D. Tesler, RN, MS
Clinical Professor Emeritus,
Department of Family Health Care Nursing,
University of California—San Francisco,
San Francisco, California

Judith A. Vessey, RN,C, PhD
Professor, College of Nursing,
University of Arkansas for Medical Sciences;
Research Facilitator,
Arkansas Children's Hospital,
Little Rock, Arkansas

Sharon Ware, RN, BSN, MA
Nurse Consultant/Sickle Cell Counselor,
ONASCO, Westview Clinic,
Tulsa, Oklahoma

Jo Ellen Welborn, RN, MS
Instructor, Department of Nursing,
East Central University,
Ada, Oklahoma

Kerstin I. West, RN,C, MS
Clinical Research Coordinator,
Eastern Oklahoma Perinatal Center,
Saint Francis Hospital,
Tulsa, Oklahoma

Krena White, RN, MS, MA
Nursing Faculty,
Tulsa Junior College,
Tulsa, Oklahoma

Linda Wildey, RN, MSN
Associate Director of Training and Director of Nursing,
Division of Adolescent Medicine,
Children's Hospital Medical Center,
Cincinnati, Ohio

Marilyn L. Winkelstein, RN, PhD
Assistant Professor,
University of Maryland School of Nursing,
Baltimore, Maryland

Ding-Djung Yang, PhD
Research Associate,
Department of Chemistry,
University of Chicago,
Chicago, Illinois

PREFACE

In offering this fifth edition of *Nursing Care of Infants and Children*, we find ourselves grateful for the support given to the book over the years. The book you are holding has been the leading book in pediatric nursing since it was first published in 1979. Today, it is the most widely used book in nursing education throughout the world. This kind of support places a special responsibility on us to earn your future support again and again, with each new edition. So, with your encouragement and comments, we offer this extensive revision.

While carefully preserving aspects of the book that have met with such universal acceptance—its state-of-the-art, research-based information; its strong, integrated focus on the family; its logical and user-friendly organization; and its easy reading style—we have continued the approach toward revision that began in the fourth edition. We have enlisted the assistance of 40 expert nurse specialists to revise, rewrite, or write portions of the text on areas undergoing rapid and complex change, such as genetics, home care, high-risk newborn care, and adolescent development and health promotion issues. At the same time, we have not compromised the strengths of a text that has been used happily by hundreds of thousands of students and nurses. We carefully supervised each of the revisions and in many cases reorganized and revised the material ourselves, to maintain the consistent organization and writing style that, over the years, have proved so effective in the teaching of pediatric nursing. We remain acutely aware that, in the end, the purpose of the book is to teach.

To that end, we have tried to meet the increasing demands of faculty and students to teach and to learn in an environment characterized by rapid change, enormous amounts of information, fewer clinical facilities, and less time. To help students to quickly locate essential information, most of the features used in the last edition have been retained, and many new ones have been added. Most important, this text encourages students to *think*. The science of nursing and medicine is not black and white. In many instances it includes shades of gray. For example, genetic testing, universal hepatitis B virus vaccination and lead screening, treatment of hyperbilirubinemia, use of acyclovir for chickenpox, and heart transplantation for heart defects represent some of the issues that abound in controversy.

This text also serves as a reference manual for practicing nurses; in essence, the content can be viewed as practice guidelines. Therefore the latest recommendations have been included from authoritative organizations such as the American Academy of Pediatrics, Centers for Disease Control and Prevention, Agency for Health Care Policy and Research, American Nurses' Association, and National Association of Pediatric Nurse Associates and Practitioners. Extensive lists of references and bibliographies have also been provided to substantiate the validity of the information and to encourage additional investigation.

SPECIAL FEATURES

Much effort has been directed toward making this book easy to teach from and, more important, easy to learn from. In this edition the following new features have been added to benefit educators, students, and practitioners.

- A functional and attractive FULL-COLOR DESIGN visually enhances the organization of each chapter, as well as the special features.
- Most of the COLOR PHOTOGRAPHS are new, and anatomic drawings are easy to follow, with color appropriately used to illustrate important aspects, such as saturated and desaturated blood. As an example, the full-color heart illustrations in Chapter 34 clearly depict congenital cardiac defects and associated hemodynamic changes.
- KEY TERMS and CONCEPTS are highlighted throughout each chapter to reinforce student learning.
- FAMILY HOME CARE boxes help nurses and students teach parents about the special needs of their infants and children.
- FAMILY FOCUS boxes present issues of special significance to families who have a child with a particular disorder. This feature is another method of highlighting the needs or concerns of families that should be addressed when family-centered care is provided.
- THINKING CRITICALLY ABOUT . . . boxes replace the Questions and Controversies boxes in the fourth edition. While they continue to present key research information that refutes or questions traditional pediatric nursing practices, the reader is challenged to think critically and improve practice by questioning traditional nursing procedures that are without scientific basis. Such information is valuable to the beginning student, who learns and begins to question before traditional practices become ingrained, and to the practicing nurse, who can refine care based on presented information. These boxes will also help the reader appreciate the complexity of health care and health care reform in a time of expensive technologic advances but shrinking financial resources.
- CRITICAL THINKING EXERCISES describe brief scenarios of child-family-nurse interactions that depict real-life clinical situations. From the synthesis of the topical content and a critical analysis of possible options, the reader chooses the best intervention and learns to make clinical judgments. Immediately following the scenario is the rationale for the correct answer and explanations for not choosing the other options.
- CULTURAL AWARENESS boxes integrate concepts of culturally sensitive care thoughout the text. The emphasis is on the clinical application of the information, whether it focuses on toilet training or on circumcision.

- ATRAUMATIC CARE boxes emphasize the importance of providing competent care without creating undue physical and psychologic distress. Although many of the boxes provide suggestions for managing pain, atraumatic care also considers approaches to promoting self-esteem and preventing embarrassment.
- NURSING CARE PLANS include RATIONALES for nursing interventions that are not immediately evident to the student. This has strengthened the connection between the text and the interventions in the care plans. All care plans have been revised by one contributor, Caryn Hess, to maintain consistency throughout the book and include patient goals (not nursing goals as in previous editions) and the most recent NANDA nursing diagnoses.

Numerous pedagogic devices that enhance student learning have been retained from the previous edition:

- CHAPTER OUTLINES, with page numbers, are at the beginning of each chapter to help readers quickly locate topics of interest.
- RELATED TOPICS, also at the beginning of every chapter, direct the reader to other chapters where pertinent information can be found.
- NURSING ALERTS call the reader's attention to considerations that if ignored could lead to a deteriorating or emergency situation. Key assessment data, risk factors, and danger signs are among the kinds of information included.
- NURSING TIPS present handy information of a nonemergency nature that makes patients more comfortable and the nurse's job a little easier.
- GUIDELINES boxes summarize important interventions for a variety of situations and conditions.
- EMERGENCY TREATMENT boxes are flagged by colored thumb tabs and are listed on the inside front cover, enabling the reader to quickly locate interventions for crisis situations.
- Hundreds of TABLES and BOXES highlight key concepts and nursing interventions.
- KEY POINTS, located at the end of each chapter, help the reader summarize major points, make connections, and synthesize information.
- A highly detailed, cross-referenced INDEX allows readers to quickly access discussions.
- PRINTED ENDPAPERS on the inside front and back covers provide information nurses refer to often, such as vital signs and blood pressure, as well as listings of some of the text's features and their page numbers.

ORGANIZATION OF THE BOOK

The same general approach to the presentation of content has been preserved from the first edition, although much content has been added, condensed, and rearranged within this framework to improve the flow, minimize duplication, and emphasize health care trends, such as home care. The book is divided into two broad parts. **PART I,** sometimes called the "age and stage" approach, considers infancy and childhood in a developmental context. It emphasizes the nurse's role in health promotion and maintenance and in making the family the focus of care. In this developmental context, the care of common health problems is presented, giving readers a sense of the normal problems expected in otherwise healthy children and showing them when in the course of childhood these problems are most likely to be manifested. The remainder of the book, **PART II,** presents the more serious health problems of infancy and childhood that are not peculiar to any particular age-group and that frequently require hospitalization or major medical and nursing intervention.

UNIT I (Chapters 1 through 5) provides a longitudinal view of the child as an individual on a continuum of developmental changes from birth through adolescence and as a member of a family unit maturing within a culture and a community. Chapter 1 includes a discussion of morbidity and mortality in infancy and childhood, including Canadian child mortality, and child health care from a historical perspective. Because of the importance of injuries as the leading cause of death in children, an overview of this topic is included. The nursing process, with emphasis on nursing diagnosis, and the role of the nurse in caring for infants and children are discussed. In addition, there is a new section on Philosophy of Care. This book is about families with children, and to set this tone early, the philosophy of family-centered care is emphasized. This book is also about providing atraumatic care—care that minimizes the psychologic and physical stress that health promotion and illness treatment can inflict. Features such as Family Focus and Atraumatic Care boxes bring these philosophies to life throughout the text. Finally, the philosophy of delivering nursing care is addressed. We believe strongly that children and families need consistent caregivers. To extend this concept of primary care nursing beyond traditional settings, especially into the home, the model of case management is introduced. To elaborate on the development of critical paths or multidisciplinary plans, a sample of an actual plan used at Children's Hospital of Wisconsin—a leader in developing these tools—is included in Chapter 38 for ketodiabetic acidosis. Under Role of the Pediatric Nurse, the therapeutic relationship with the family is explored, including guidelines to help nurses evaluate their relationships and identify overinvolvement or underinvolvement.

The child in the context of family, culture, and community has been elaborated and broadened to emphasize this important influence on development. Chapter 2 provides the opportunity to expand the discussion of social, cultural, and religious influences on child development and health promotion, including socioeconomic factors, customs and folkways, and health beliefs and practices. The content more clearly describes the role of the nurse with such additions as guidelines for culturally sensitive interactions. Cultural Awareness boxes throughout the entire text highlight the influences of culture on children and families. Chapter 3, devoted to the family, further emphasizes the importance of this social group in relation to the health and welfare of children. Family theories establish the tone of the chapter, which includes a variety of parenting situations that reflect contemporary society. An important example is a new section on vulnerable (high-risk) families. Family strengths are addressed, and current findings on adoption, divorce, single-parenting, stepfamilies, and dual-earner families have been incorporated.

The basic overview of child development in Chapter 4 maintains the same general organization and expands on the theoretic approach to personality development and learning. Biologic systems development is deemphasized in this chapter and discussed more fully in relation to major systems dysfunction later in the book. Updates include a discussion of the Food Guide Pyramid and expanded sections on stress and coping.

Chapter 5 focuses on hereditary influences in health promotion. This chapter has been almost completely rewritten, in easy to understand language, to reflect the dramatic and complex changes in our understanding of genetics and genetic testing. Family concerns and ethical issues that arise because of these advances are highlighted throughout the chapter.

UNIT II is concerned with the principles and skills of nursing assessment, including communication and interviewing, observation, physical and behavioral assessment, and health guidance. Chapter 6 contains guidelines for communicating with both children and their families and a detailed description of a health assessment, including an extensive discussion of family assessment and nutritional assessment. Content on communication techniques is now outlined to reduce reading time and provide a concise format for reference. Chapter 7 continues to provide a comprehensive approach to physical examination and developmental assessment, with new material added on temperature measurement and the Denver II, a major revision and restandardization of the Denver Developmental Screening Test.

UNIT III stresses the importance of the neonatal period, the time of greatest risk to child survival, and discusses several health concerns encountered in the vulnerable first month of life. It is the most extensively revised unit in this edition and reflects the outstanding perinatal clinical expertise of David Wilson, this edition's contributing editor. In Chapter 8 several areas have been revised to reflect current issues and developments, especially in terms of the emotional and educational needs of the family during short postpartum admissions. Updates in Chapter 9 more clearly describe dermatologic problems and new thinking regarding hyperbilirubinemia and inborn errors of metabolism.

Chapter 10 stresses the nurse's role in care of the high-risk newborn and the importance of acute observations to the survival of these neonates. Rapid advances in the field of neonatal care have mandated extensive revision with a greater sensitivity to the diverse needs of infants, from those with extremely low birth weight to those of normal gestational age. A discussion of infant stress, including pain and developmental care to reduce stress, is provided. The chapter also includes an updated discussion of cocaine exposure in the neonate.

The discussion of congenital defects in Chapter 11 focuses on important new developments and concerns, such as folic acid supplementation to reduce the risk of neural tube defects and the possibility of latex allergy in children with spina bifida, as well as in health care workers. Because of the diverse group of conditions, five contributors specializing in gastroenterology, neurology, orthopaedics, urology, and surgery revised this content.

UNITS IV through **VII** present the major developmental stages outlined in Unit I, which are expanded to provide a broader concept of these stages and the health problems most often associated with them. Special emphasis is placed on the preventive aspects of care. The chapters on health promotion follow a standard approach that is used consistently for each age-group. New areas and those receiving expanded coverage are development of body image, development of sexuality, sleep problems, alternate child care arrangements, the preschool and kindergarten experience, and dental health. As the book goes to press, major changes in the immunization schedule are current through September 1994.

The chapters on health problems in these units primarily reflect more typical and age-related concerns. The information on many disorders has been rewritten to reflect recent changes. Examples include sudden infant death syndrome, lead poisoning, wound healing, sexual abuse, Lyme disease, attention deficit–hyperactivity disorder, contraception, teenage pregnancy, drug abuse, and suicide. The chapters on adolescence (Chapters 19, 20, and 21) have undergone major revision by a group of well-known nurse, nutrition, and psychology experts. All psychosocial/physiologic conditions in Chapters 18, 20, and 21 include the diagnostic criteria from the *Diagnostic and Statistical Manual of Mental Disorders (DSM-IV)*.

UNIT VIII deals with children who have the same developmental needs as growing children but who, because of congenital or acquired physical, cognitive, or sensory impairment, require alternative interventions to facilitate development. Chapter 22 reflects current trends in the care of families and children with chronic illness or disability such as home care, normalizing children's lives, focusing on developmental needs, enabling and empowering families, and providing early intervention.

The focus in Chapter 23 is primarily on the impact of life-threatening illness and death on the child and family. The sections on hospice and home care, tissue donation, the child's right to die, and the impact of the death on siblings have been expanded. The content in Chapters 24 and 25 of the fourth edition on cognitive, sensory, and communication impairments has been reduced and combined in Chapter 24. Important updates in relation to the definition of mental retardation and the discussion on fragile X syndrome are included. Chapter 25 is now devoted to home care. It presents an overview of home care with specific interventions for the nurse to function successfully in this increasingly important environment. The focus is on building family-nurse partnerships.

Unit IX is concerned with the impact of hospitalization on the child and the family and continues to present a comprehensive overview of the stressors imposed by hospitalization and nursing interventions to prevent or eliminate them. Chapter 26 has greatly expanded discussions of pain assessment and management. The section on discharge planning and home care provides the basic concepts for implementing home care for children with complex health needs and complements Chapter 25. Chapter 27 continues to present information on the safe implementation of procedures with children. We have tried to include as much available research as possible to base the nursing interventions on scientific findings, not traditional practice. A major addition to this important chapter is a section on maintaining healthy skin. It complements the material on wound healing in Chapter 18 and the material on neonatal skin care in Chapter 10. The focus is on prevention of pressure ulcers based on guidelines from the Agency for Health Care Policy and Research. Finally, the material on ostomies has been revised to reflect current practices and devices.

Units X through **XIV** consider serious health problems of infants and children primarily from the biologic systems orientation, which has the practical organizational value of permitting health problems and nursing considerations to relate to specific pathophysiologic disturbances. Important additions and revisions include discussions of venous access devices, including peripherally inserted central catheters (PICC lines); pulse oximetry; respiratory syncytial virus (RSV); tuberculosis; asthma; cystic fibrosis; oral rehydration therapy; short bowel syndrome; gastrointestinal bleeding; seizures; chemotherapy; acquired immunodeficiency syndrome (AIDS); diabetes mellitus; growth disorders; burns; scoliosis; orthotic and prosthetic devices; and the Ilizarov procedure.

Extensive appendixes are also included and contain information on family assessment; developmental assessment; growth measurements, including a complete set of the National Center for Health Statistics growth charts; common laboratory values; NANDA-approved nursing diagnoses; and a new addition, several foreign-language translations of the FACES Pain Rating Scale. All of the appendix material reflects the most current versions of forms, charts, and values.

UNIFYING PRINCIPLES

Several unifying principles have guided the organizational structure of this book since its inception. These principles have been strengthened in the revision to produce a text that is consistent in approach throughout each chapter.

The Family as the Unit of Care

The child is an integral member of the family unit. Nursing care is most effective when it is rendered with the belief that the family is the unit of care. This belief permeates the book. When a child is healthy, the child's health is enhanced when the family is a fully functioning, health-promoting system. The family unit can be manifested in a myriad of structures; each has the potential to provide a caring, supportive environment in which the child can grow, mature, and maximize his or her human potential.

In addition to family-centered care being integrated into every chapter, an entire chapter is devoted to understanding the family as the basic unit in children's lives. Another chapter discusses the social, cultural, and religious influences that impact family beliefs. Separate sections in another chapter deal in depth with family communication and family assessment. The impact of illness, hospitalization, and the death of a child are covered extensively in two additional chapters. The needs of the family are emphasized throughout the text under Nursing Considerations in a separate section on family support. Numerous Family Home Care boxes are included to assist nurses in providing helpful information to families.

An Integrated Approach to Development

Children are whole people. No book on pediatric nursing is complete without extensive coverage of communication, nutrition, play, safety, dental care, sexuality, sleep, self-esteem, and, of course, parenting. Nurses promote the healthy expression of all these dimensions of personhood and need to understand how these functions are expressed by different children at different developmental ages and stages. Effective parenting depends on the parent's knowledge of development, and it is often the nurse's responsibility to provide parents with a developmental awareness of their children's needs. For these reasons, coverage of the many dimensions of childhood are integrated within the growth and development chapters, rather than being presented in separate chapters. Safety concerns, for instance, are much different for a toddler than for an adolescent. Sleep needs change with age, as do nutritional needs. As a result, the units on each age of childhood contain complete information on all these functions as they relate to the specific age. In the unit on the school-age child, for instance, information is presented on nutritional needs; age-appropriate play and its significance; safety concerns characteristic of the age-group; appropriate dental care; sleep characteristics; and means of promoting self-esteem, a particularly significant concern for school-age children. The challenges of being the parent of a school-age child are presented, and interventions are suggested that nurses can use to promote more healthy parenting. Using the integrated approach, students gain an appreciation for the unique characteristics and needs of children at every age and stage.

Focus on Wellness and Illness

In a pediatric nursing text, a focus on illness is expected. Children become ill, and nurses typically are involved in helping children get well. However, it is not sufficient to prepare students to care primarily for sick children. First, health is more than the absence of disease. Being healthy is being whole in mind, body, and spirit. Therefore the majority of the first half of the book is devoted to discussions that promote physical, psychosocial, mental, and spiritual wellness. Much emphasis is placed on anticipatory guidance of parents to prevent injury or illness in the child.

Second, health care is more than ever prevention focused. The objectives set forth in the "Healthy People 2000" report clearly establish a health care agenda in which solutions to medical/social problems lie in preventive strategies, not in more or better treatment.

Third, health care is moving from acute care settings to the community, the home, short-stay centers, and clinics. Nurses must be prepared to function in all areas. To be successful, they must understand the pathophysiology, diagnosis, and treatment of health conditions. Competent nursing care flows from this knowledge and is enhanced by an awareness of childhood development, family dynamics, and communication skill.

Nursing Care

Although the information in this text incorporates information from numerous disciplines (medicine, pathophysiology, pharmacology, nutrition, psychology, sociology), its primary purpose is to provide information on the nursing care of children and families. Discussions of all disorders conclude with a section on Nursing Considerations. In addition, 40 care plans have been included in this fifth edition. Taken together, they provide coverage of the nursing care for virtually every disease, disorder, condition, and crisis of childhood. In a sense, by emphasizing specific health problems through the vehicle of care plans, students gain an intuitive sense of the major health problems of childhood.

The purpose of the care plans, like every other feature of the book, is to teach, to convey information. They include all the current nursing diagnoses approved by NANDA through its Eleventh Conference that have a potential bearing on the health problem. Although the care plans can be individualized for use with a specific patient in a clinical setting, that is not their main purpose. For every diagnosis, appropriate patient goals, extensive possible interventions with rationales, and sample evaluation outcomes are presented. Thus a complete range of nursing care is presented within the context of a care plan and the nursing process.

For almost every health problem for which a care plan is included, the surrounding narrative text is presented according to the nursing process. In these instances specific headings for assessment, nursing diagnoses, planning, implementation, and evaluation, with unifying logos for the five steps, present appropriate information that is then amplified in the care plan, presented in a standard nursing practice context. In keeping with our general purpose of providing practical as well as conceptual information on every page of this book, the care plans provide excellent prototypes for high-quality nursing practice.

The Critical Role of Research

This revision is the product of an exhaustive review of the literature published since the book was last revised. Many readers and researchers have come to rely on the copious bibliographies, so as in previous editions this edition has extensive lists of citations that reflect significant contributions from a broad audience of professionals. So that information is accurate and current, the majority of citations are less than 5 years old, and almost every chapter has entries within 1 year of publication. Examples of current "cutting edge" information are recommendations from the American Academy of Pediatrics on immunizations, asthma, tuberculosis, and sleep position. The section on pain reflects guidelines from the Agency for Health Care Policy and Research (AHCPR) and the American Pain Society. The new discussions on skin care reflect the AHCPR's guidelines on pressure ulcers. The section on nutrition includes the Food Guide Pyramid from the U.S. Department of Agriculture. Lead poisoning has been completely rewritten to reflect the latest Centers for Disease Control and Prevention statements on lead poisoning prevention, diagnosis, and treatment. Cardiopulmonary resuscitation and first aid for choking are based on the 1994 recommendations of the American Heart Association.

The efforts toward updating content have also been extended toward updating the address of every resource listed in the text. Despite this meticulous checking, it is inevitable that some information will change during this edition's publication. Therefore, telephone numbers for each organization are included to facilitate the reader's access to an organization.

CANADIAN CONTENT

The fifth edition of this text includes Canadian statistics regarding infant and child health in Chapter 1 and the latest Canadian immunization schedules in Chapter 12. Throughout the text numerous Canadian resource organizations are also provided. These efforts have been made in an attempt to make the text as valuable as possible to Canadian readers.

TEACHING/LEARNING PACKAGE

For the fifth edition of this text, an extensive number of ancillary products for instructors and students to use in class and clinical settings is offered:

Instructor's Resource Kit. This innovative resource kit for the instructor holds the following components:

Instructor's Manual, with learning objectives, chapter outlines and accompanying teaching strategies, and learning activities.

Test Bank, with 1130 multiple-choice stand-alone test items. An answer key with page-number rationales is included at the end of the test bank.

Pediatric Updates, which describe the very latest research findings, guidelines, or approaches to caring for children and their families. Instructors will receive a new set of *Pediatric Updates* twice a year.

Critical Thinking Exercises, which are in addition to the Critical Thinking Exercises found in the text. Situations and four choices for interventions are described, with the correct answer and rationale provided on the back side of the page.

Case Studies, with the case and related questions on the front side of the page and answers on the back.

Therapeutic Dialogues, which provide examples of how to talk with children or their families when they are in difficult situations.

Overhead Transparencies. Full-color transparency acetates focus on key material in the text, helping instructors to increase student understanding.

Pediatric Quick Reference. The second edition of *Pediatric Quick Reference,* a handy pocket-sized resource, accompanies every copy of the text. The guide features information commonly used, such as assessment data; pain management strategies; fluid requirements; vital sign parameters; emergency interventions, including the 1994 cardiopulmonary resuscitation (CPR) and choking recommendations; laboratory values; and the primary immunization schedule.

Computerized Test Bank. Available in IBM and Macintosh, *CompuTest 3* is the computerized version of the *Test Bank* from the *Instructor's Resource Kit.* Complete with a user's guide, *CompuTest* allows instructors to edit, add, delete, or select questions on the computer.

Study Guide. This comprehensive and challenging study aid presents multiple-choice and matching questions, along with Critical Thinking Case Studies and crossword puzzles based on the key terms used in each chapter in the text. The *Study Guide* includes just the text-page cross-references where answers can be found; the answers are located in the *Instructor's Manual.*

Pediatric Assessment Interactive Videodiscs. Available for purchase, these videodiscs were developed and produced by The Fuld Institute for Technology in Nursing Education. Three case studies help students master the transition from the classroom to the actual practice setting.

■ ■ ■

Just as children and their families bring with them a vast and unique background that affects their role within the health care system, so it is that each nurse brings to each child and family an individual set of characteristics and values that will affect their relationship. Although I have attempted to present a total picture of the child in each age-group both in wellness and in illness, no one child, family, or nurse will be found in this book. I hope that each page, chapter, and unit builds a foundation on which the nurse can begin to construct the ideal of comprehensive, atraumatic, and individualized nursing care for infants, children, adolescents, and their families.

Donna L. Wong

ACKNOWLEDGMENTS

With each edition of *Nursing Care of Infants and Children,* more and more of my colleagues have become involved in the revision of the book. I am grateful to the many nursing faculty members, practitioners, and students who have offered their comments, recommendations, and suggestions. Many of the staff nurses and clinical specialists I work with are the "silent heroes" who teach me so much about the preventive, bedside, and home care that children and families need to maintain health and to recover from illness. I am especially indebted to the outstanding contributors who revised selected chapters of this edition and to the reviewers for their constructive criticism and suggestions.

A very special thanks goes to David Wilson for the major role he assumed as contributing editor. Not only did David revise several chapters, in many cases he reorganized and revised other chapters to maintain the consistent organization and writing style that, over the years, have proved so effective in the teaching of pediatric nursing.

My primary goal in revising this edition has been to present the most current and accurate data available at the time of publication. In reviewing the literature, I have not always been able to locate published updates on certain topics or to use the published data in its existing form. To obtain current and usable data, I contacted several individuals and organizations who generously provided me with what was needed. I am especially grateful to the following people and organizations:

William Frankenburg, MD, shared with me the latest information on the Denver II and granted permission for duplication of the testing form in Appendix B. Hung Shen Lin, MD, secured updated growth charts for Chinese children. Several nurses gave me permission to cite their research findings. For example, Donna Dixon's work on relationships between nurses and parents of hospitalized children is included in Chapter 22, and Sharon Pontious's studies and Marti Rice's research on measurement of temperature are highlighted in Chapter 7. Wendy Lowe kept me informed regarding the Canadian immunization schedule, and the American Academy of Pediatrics kept me updated on the latest developments in several areas of pediatrics, especially immunizations. Deborah Broome from Ross Laboratories and John Huffman from Mead Johnson Nutritionals shared information about infant formulas that is included in Chapter 8.

I especially thank Peggy Cook, librarian at Hillcrest Medical Center, Tulsa, Oklahoma, for the scores of computer searches and hundreds of articles she provided, as well as the many citations she checked for accuracy, that made it possible to update the content through 1994. I also thank Elizabeth Richards, librarian, and Dwight Vance, drug information pharmacist at Saint Francis Hospital, for their efforts in searching the literature, especially regarding pharmaceutical agents.

Not only have numerous individuals helped make the book current and accurate, several people have contributed to making the book attractive with the addition of color photographs. Thanks go to Pat Watson and Ting Wong for the beautiful color photography and to Donald O'Connor for the outstanding color drawings, especially of congenital heart defects in Chapter 34; to David Welborn, Debbie Robinson, Maureen Smith, and Kimberly Kitson at St. Louis Children's Hospital and to Carolyn Duke at St. Louis University School of Nursing Skills Lab for helping coordinate the photography sessions; and to the health professionals, children, and parents who generously allowed us to take photographs.

No book is ever a reality without the dedication and perseverance of the editorial staff, and although it is impossible to list every individual at Mosby who has made exceptional efforts to produce this text, I am especially grateful to Sally Schrefer, Janet Livingston, Shelly Hayden, Judi Bange, Gayle Morris, Susan Lane, Jeanne Wolfgeher, and Bob Boehringer for their support and commitment to excellence. In addition, I wish to thank my typists, Lynne Murtha and Nina Wong, for the superb job they did and for their efforts in meeting very stringent deadlines.

This edition marks a milestone in the publication of this pediatric test, as it is time to bid farewell to Lucille Whaley, my coauthor for the past four editions. After half a century of dedication to nursing, Lucille has retired. I am grateful for the foundation she helped build in writing the original version of the text and for her significant contributions to the next three editions. I learned a great deal about nursing and writing from her and hope that I have continued the tradition of excellence in this edition that our partnership represented in past editions.

Finally, I thank my family—Ting, Nina, and Rudy—for the unselfish love, endless patience, and quiet understanding that allow me to devote such a large part of my life to my career. Truly, without their willingness to assume many of the tasks necessary to produce a textbook and their sacrifices that allowed me the time needed to revise it, this book would never have been completed.

Donna L. Wong

CONTENTS IN BRIEF

PART I
Child Health Promotion and Maintenance

UNIT I
CHILDREN, THEIR FAMILIES, AND THE NURSE

UNIT II
ASSESSMENT OF THE CHILD AND FAMILY

UNIT III
FAMILY-CENTERED CARE OF THE NEWBORN

UNIT IV
FAMILY-CENTERED CARE OF THE INFANT

UNIT V
FAMILY-CENTERED CARE OF THE YOUNG CHILD

UNIT VI
FAMILY-CENTERED CARE OF THE SCHOOL-AGE CHILD

UNIT VII
FAMILY-CENTERED CARE OF THE ADOLESCENT

UNIT VIII
FAMILY-CENTERED CARE OF THE CHILD WITH SPECIAL NEEDS

PART II
Nursing Care of the Ill or Hospitalized Child

UNIT IX
THE CHILD WHO IS HOSPITALIZED

UNIT X
THE CHILD WITH DISTURBANCE OF FLUID AND ELECTROLYTES

UNIT XI
THE CHILD WITH PROBLEMS RELATED TO TRANSFER OF OXYGEN AND NUTRIENTS

UNIT XII
THE CHILD WITH PROBLEMS RELATED TO PRODUCTION AND CIRCULATION OF BLOOD

UNIT XIII
THE CHILD WITH DISTURBANCE OF REGULATORY MECHANISMS

UNIT XIV
THE CHILD WITH A PROBLEM THAT INTERFERES WITH PHYSICAL MOBILITY

APPENDIXES

CONTENTS

PART I
Child Health Promotion and Maintenance

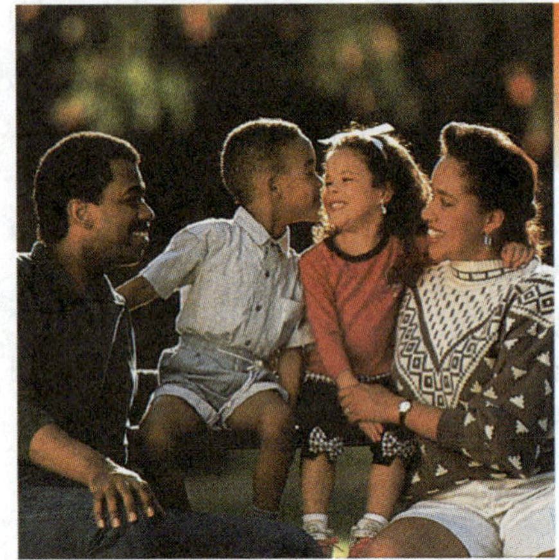

UNIT I
CHILDREN, THEIR FAMILIES, AND THE NURSE

CHAPTER 1
Perspectives of Pediatric Nursing 2

CHAPTER 2
Social, Cultural, and Religious Influences on Child Health Promotion 29

CHAPTER 3
Family Influences on Child Health Promotion 65

CHAPTER 4
Growth and Development of Children 105

CHAPTER 5
Hereditary Influences on Health Promotion of the Child and Family 155

UNIT II

ASSESSMENT OF THE CHILD AND FAMILY

CHAPTER 6
Communication and Health Assessment of the Child and Family 185

CHAPTER 7
Physical and Developmental Assessment of the Child 217

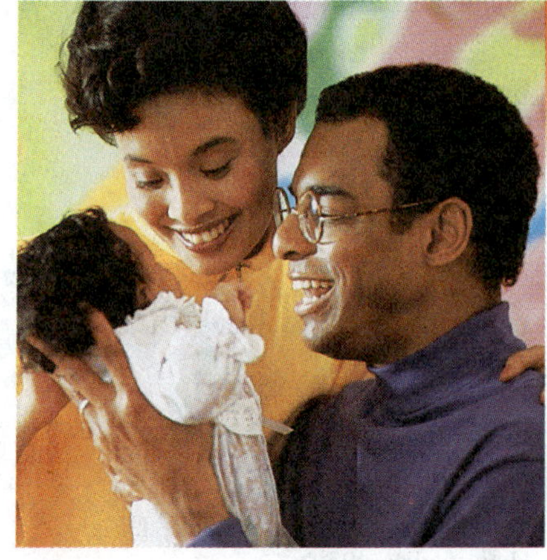

UNIT III

FAMILY-CENTERED CARE OF THE NEWBORN

CHAPTER 8
Health Promotion of the Newborn and Family 287

CHAPTER 9
Health Problems of the Newborn 337

CHAPTER 10
The High-Risk Newborn and Family 365

CHAPTER 11
Conditions Caused by Defects in Physical Development 433

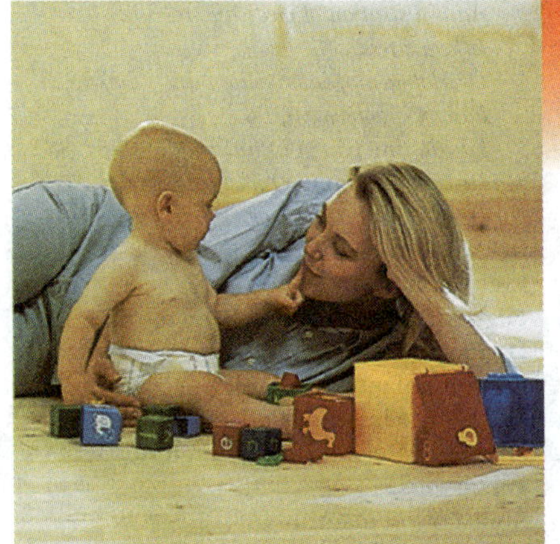

UNIT IV
FAMILY-CENTERED CARE OF THE INFANT

CHAPTER 12
Health Promotion of the Infant and Family 514

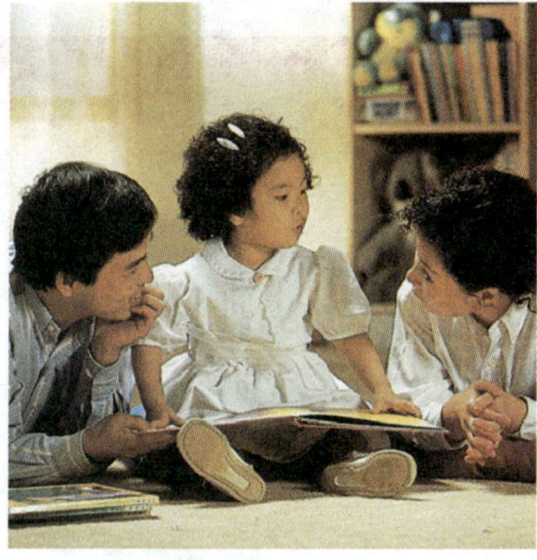

UNIT V
FAMILY-CENTERED CARE OF THE YOUNG CHILD

CHAPTER 16
Health Problems of Early Childhood 667

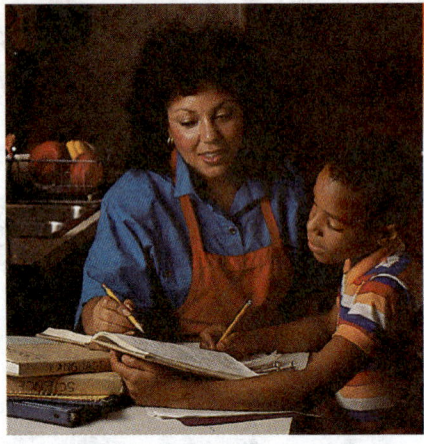

UNIT VI
FAMILY-CENTERED CARE OF THE SCHOOL-AGE CHILD

CHAPTER 17
Health Promotion of the School-Age Child and Family 718

CHAPTER 18
Health Problems of Middle Childhood 761

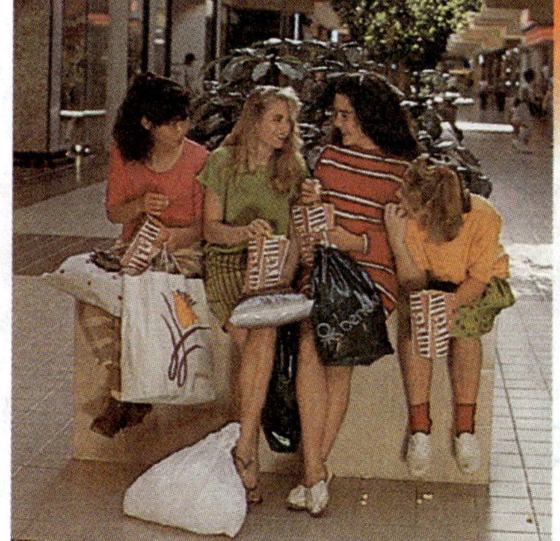

UNIT VII

FAMILY-CENTERED CARE OF THE ADOLESCENT

CHAPTER 19

CHAPTER 20

CHAPTER 21
Behavioral Health Problems of Adolescence 894

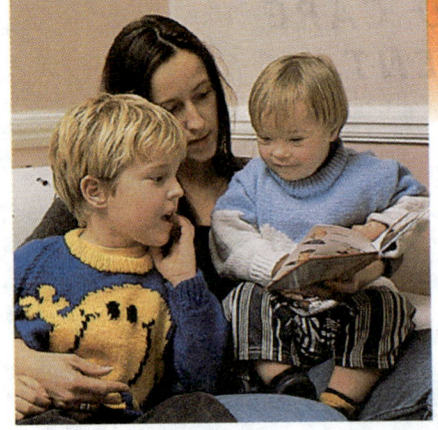

UNIT VIII
FAMILY-CENTERED CARE OF THE CHILD WITH SPECIAL NEEDS

CHAPTER 22
Family-Centered Care of the Child with Chronic Illness or Disability 933

CHAPTER 23
Family-Centered Care of the Child with Life-Threatening Illness 976

PART II

Nursing Care of the Ill or Hospitalized Child

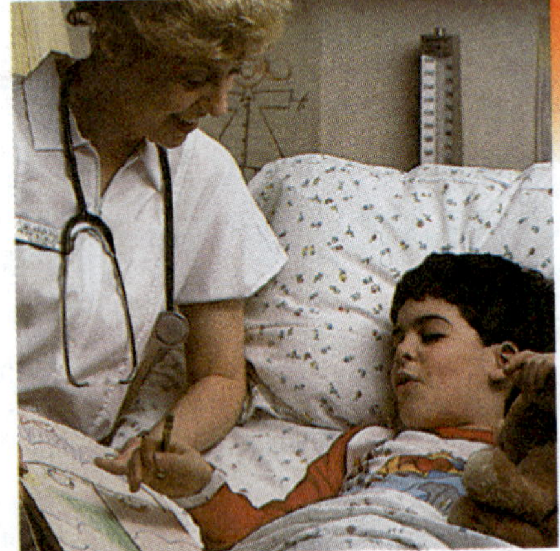

UNIT IX

THE CHILD WHO IS HOSPITALIZED

CHAPTER 26

Family-Centered Care of the Child During Illness and Hospitalization 1064

CHAPTER 27

Pediatric Variations of Nursing Interventions 1132

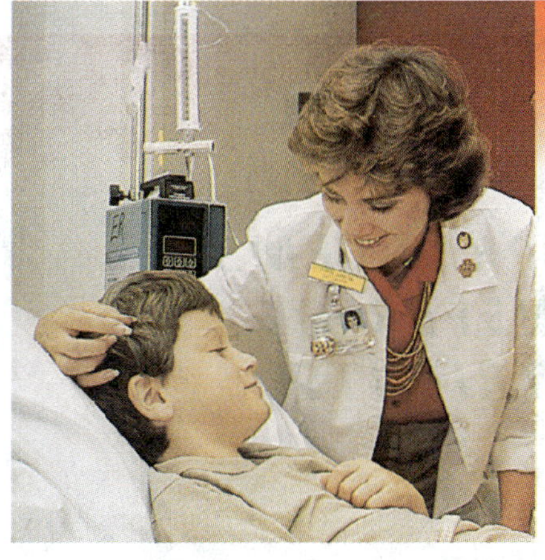

UNIT X

THE CHILD WITH DISTURBANCE OF FLUID AND ELECTROLYTES

CHAPTER 28

Balance and Imbalance of Body Fluids 1203

CHAPTER 29

Conditions That Produce Fluid and Electrolyte Imbalance 1233

CHAPTER 30

The Child with Renal Dysfunction 1282

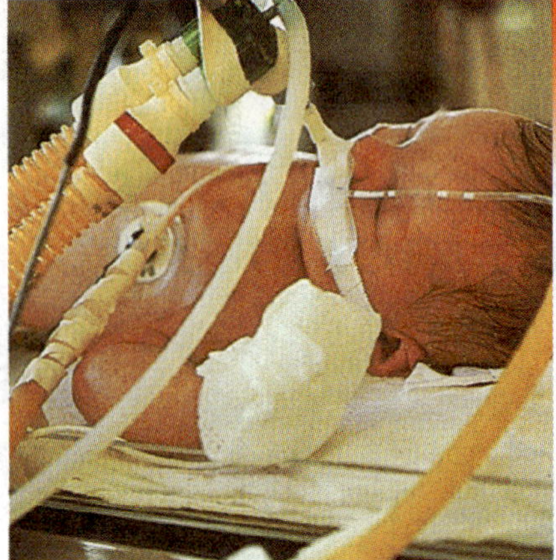

UNIT XI

THE CHILD WITH PROBLEMS RELATED TO TRANSFER OF OXYGEN AND NUTRIENTS

CHAPTER 31
The Child with Disturbance of Oxygen and Carbon Dioxide Exchange 1332

CHAPTER 32
The Child with Respiratory Dysfunction 1372

CHAPTER 33
The Child with Gastrointestinal Dysfunction 1447

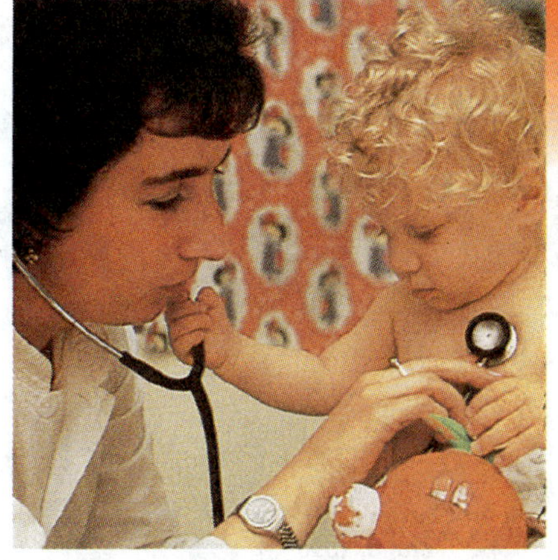

UNIT XII
THE CHILD WITH PROBLEMS RELATED TO PRODUCTION AND CIRCULATION OF BLOOD

CHAPTER 34
The Child with Cardiovascular Dysfunction 1493

CHAPTER 35 The Child with Hematologic or Immunologic Dysfunction 1563

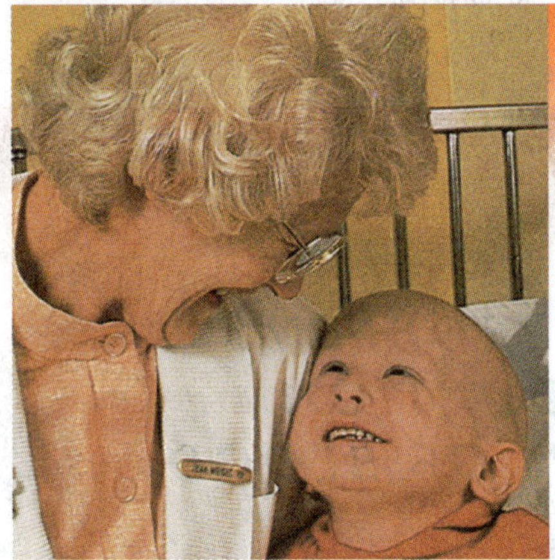

UNIT XIII THE CHILD WITH DISTURBANCE OF REGULATORY MECHANISMS

CHAPTER 36 The Child with Cancer 1611

CHAPTER 37 The Child with Cerebral Dysfunction 1669

CHAPTER 38
The Child with Endocrine Dysfunction 1736

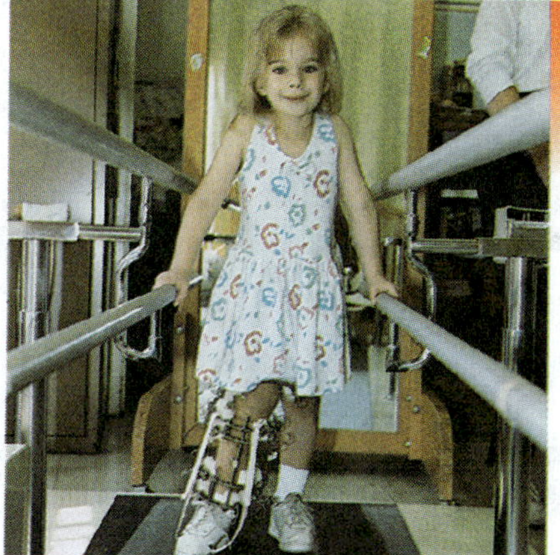

UNIT XIV
THE CHILD WITH A PROBLEM THAT INTERFERES WITH PHYSICAL MOBILITY

CHAPTER 39
The Child with Musculoskeletal or Articular Dysfunction 1793

CHAPTER 40 The Child with Neuromuscular or Muscular Dysfunction 1869

APPENDIXES

PART I

Child Health Promotion and Maintenance

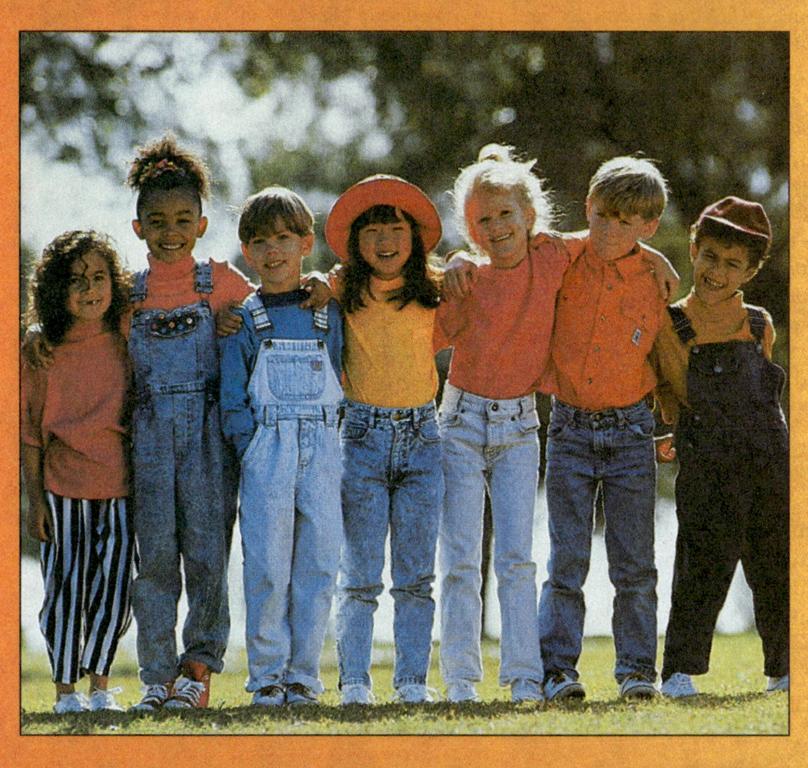

UNIT I

CHILDREN, THEIR FAMILIES, AND THE NURSE

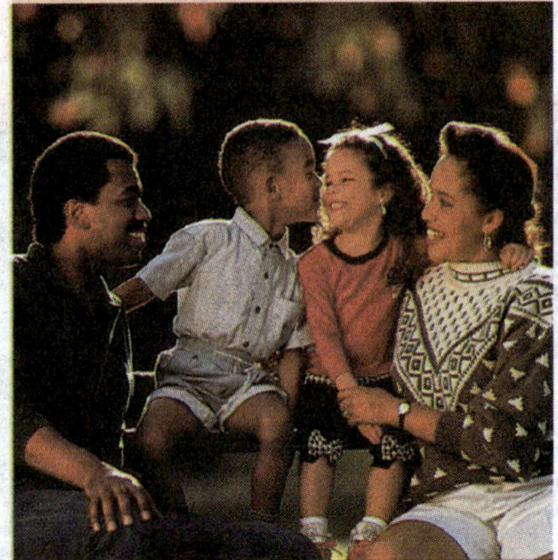

CHAPTER 1 Perspectives of Pediatric Nursing

CHAPTER OUTLINE

RELATED TOPICS

Cancer in children, Ch. 36
Case management, Ch. 25
The child and trauma, Ch. 39
Classification of high-risk newborns, Ch. 10
Cultural/religious influences on health care, Ch. 2
Immunizations, Ch. 12
Injury prevention: infant, Ch. 12; toddler, Ch. 14; preschooler, Ch. 15; school-age child, Ch. 17; adolescent, Ch. 19
Interpersonal relationships, Ch. 4
Preschool and kindergarten experience, Ch. 15
Scope of the problem (chronic illness/disability), Ch. 22
Suicide, Ch. 21
Temperament, Ch. 4

HEALTH DURING CHILDHOOD

Health is a complex phenomenon. The World Health Organization (WHO) has defined ***health*** as "a state of complete physical, mental, and social well-being and not merely the absence of disease." Despite this broad definition, health is traditionally assessed by observing ***mortality*** (death) and ***morbidity*** (illness) rates over a period of time. Therefore the *presence* of disease becomes a prime indicator of health.

Information concerning mortality and morbidity is important to nurses. Such data yield significant information about (1) the causes of death and illness, (2) high-risk age-groups for certain disorders or hazards, (3) advances in treatment and prevention, and (4) specific areas of health counseling. By being aware of such information nurses can better guide their planning and delivery of care.

"HEALTHY PEOPLE 2000"

Although the health of people, including children, in the United States has improved dramatically during the twentieth century, there remains cause for concern. There is a growing awareness that many of the serious domestic problems, such as acquired immunodeficiency syndrome (AIDS), drug abuse, violence, and unwanted pregnancies, have a direct effect on the health of the nation. Most important, the solutions to these problems do not lie in better or more innovative medical treatment, but in *prevention.*

In 1990 "Healthy People 2000" (1991) was issued. It sets the following three broad goals for public health over the 1990s: (1) increase the span of healthy life for Americans, (2) reduce health disparities among Americans, and (3) achieve access to preventive services for all Americans.

Three broad approaches—health promotion, health protection, and preventive services—are employed to achieve the 22 priority areas (see box below), which contain approximately 300 measurable objectives. All health professionals, especially nurses, in any practice setting should be aware of the priority areas and work toward improving the health of U.S. children. Since the main intervention is prevention, many of the strategies nurses use, such as counseling, education, and screening, can be implemented *independently* to help achieve these goals.

"HEALTHY PEOPLE 2000" OBJECTIVES

HEALTH PROMOTION OBJECTIVES

Increase physical activity and fitness.
Improve nutrition.
Reduce tobacco use.
Reduce alcohol and other drug abuse.
Improve family planning.
Improve mental health and reduce mental disorder.
Reduce violent and abusive behavior.
Enhance and expand community-based health promotion programs.

HEALTH PROTECTION OBJECTIVES

Reduce unintentional injuries.
Improve occupational safety and health.
Improve environmental health and reduce human exposure to hazardous substances (i.e., lead).
Ensure safety of food and drugs.
Improve oral health.

PREVENTIVE SERVICES OBJECTIVES

Improve nutritional and infant health.
Reduce heart disease, stroke, and end-stage renal disease.
Prevent and control cancer.
Reduce and control human immunodeficiency virus (HIV) infection.
Prevent sexually transmitted diseases.
Increase immunization and prevent infectious diseases.
Improve clinical preventive services by reducing barriers to health care.

SURVEILLANCE AND DATA SYSTEMS

Improve surveillance and data systems to track progress toward the objectives.

From Mason JO, McGinnis JM: Healthy people 2000: an overview of the national health promotion and disease prevention objectives, *Public Health Rep* 105(5):441-446, 1990.

MORTALITY

Figures describing rates of occurrence for events such as death in children are referred to as ***vital statistics. Mortality statistics*** describe the incidence or number of individuals who have died over a specific period of time. They are usually presented as rates per 100,000 population because of their lower frequency of occurrence than statistics such as infant mortality. Mortality rates are calculated from a sample of death certificates.

In the United States the **National Center for Health Statistics (NCHS),** under the Department of Health and Human Services (DHHS), Public Health Service (PHS), has the responsibility for collection, analysis, and dissemination of data on the health of the American people. Because of the complexity of compiling such data, statistics may vary in different reports and should be interpreted cautiously. For example, figures may be ***estimated*** (from previously collected data), ***provisional*** (from temporary current data), or ***final*** (from complete provisional data). Final statistics are often published 2 or more years after data collection.

Important changes have taken effect in NCHS's reporting of state and race. Since 1991 figures for birth and death are based on the person's state of residence, not on the state where the event occurred. Figures for births and deaths among the states in the United States differ significantly from those published before 1991 (Wegman, 1993).

The tabulation of race for live births (the denominator of infant mortality rates) changed in 1989 from race of child to race of mother. Formerly, to determine the child's race in mixed parentage where one parent was white, the child was assigned the race of the other parent. In general, this change in assignment of race from child to mother results in more white births and fewer nonwhite births. However, infant deaths are recorded by the decedent's race, resulting in a lower infant mortality rate for whites than nonwhites. As a result, infant mortality rates by race after 1989 are not comparable to earlier reports (National Center for Health Statistics, 1993a).

Infant Mortality

The ***infant mortality rate*** is the number of deaths per 1000 live births during the first year of life. It may be further divided into ***neonatal mortality*** (<28 days of life) and ***postneonatal mortality*** (28 days to 1 year). In the United States there has been a dramatic decrease in infant mortality. At the beginning of the twentieth century the rate was about 200 infant deaths per 1000 live births; in 1992 the infant mortality rate dropped to less than 1 in 100 live births, the lowest rate ever recorded in the United States. This decrease has primarily been a result of infectious disease control and nutritional advances during the early 1900s, the advent of antibiotic and antibacterial agents in the middle of the cen

TABLE 1-1 Infant Mortality for 22 Countries with Population over 2.5 Million, 1991 (Rate per 1000 Live Births)

COUNTRY	RATE
Japan	4.4
Singapore	5.5
Finland	5.6*
Sweden	6.2
Hong Kong	6.2
Norway	6.2
Canada	6.4
Netherlands	6.5
Switzerland	6.8
Germany	6.9
Australia	7.1
France	7.2
United Kingdom	7.4
Denmark	7.5
Austria	7.5
Spain	7.7*
Ireland	8.2
Greece	8.2
New Zealand	8.3
Italy	8.3
Belgium	8.4
United States	8.9

From Wegman ME: Annual summary of vital statistics—1992, *Pediatrics* 92(6):743-754, 1993.
*Data for 1990.

tury, and advances in perinatal care during the late 1900s.

However, from a worldwide perspective, the United States lags behind other well-developed countries. In 1987 it ranked last among the 22 countries with the lowest infant mortality rates, with Japan having the lowest rate (Wegman, 1993) (Table 1-1). This is far behind neighboring countries such as Canada, which ranked seventh.

Birth weight is considered the major determinant of neonatal death in technologically developed countries and is closely related to gestational age (Wilcox and Skjaerven, 1992). The relationship between birth weight (and gestational age) and mortality shows that the lower the birth weight, the higher the mortality. The relatively high incidence of low birth weight (LBW) (<2500 g) in the United States is considered a key factor in its higher neonatal mortality rates when compared with other countries. Unfortunately, the percentage of mothers with LBW infants increased in 1991. Almost 20% of mothers less than 15 years of age had little or no prenatal care. Access to and use of high-quality prenatal care is the single most promising preventive strategy to decrease early delivery and infant mortality (Naeye, 1993; Wegman, 1993). Other factors that increase the risk of infant mortality include black race, male sex, short or long gestation, birth order (all but second), maternal age (younger or older), and lower level of maternal education (Centers for Disease Control, 1989; Schoendorf and others, 1992).

While there has been a steady and significant decline in infant mortality, the number of deaths occurring in the first year of life is still proportionately high when compared with

TABLE 1-2 Death Rates by Age, United States, 1992 (Estimated Rates per 100,000 in Specified Group)

AGE	RATE
Under 1 year*	864.5
1-4 years	42.9
5-14 years	22.6
15-24 years	97.4
25-34 years	135.0
35-44 years	233.0
45-54 years	452.2
55-64 years	1,161.0
65-74 years	2,580.1
75-84 years	5,794.2
85 years and over	14,909.1

From National Center for Health Statistics: Annual summary of births, marriages, divorces, and deaths: United States, 1992, *Monthly Vital Statistics Report* 41(13):7, Sept 28, 1993.
*Death rates under 1 year (based on population estimates) differ from infant mortality rates (based on live births).

death rates at other ages (Table 1-2). This is also true of other countries, such as Canada (Table 1-3). In the United States and Canada the death rate for infants under 1 year of age is greater than the rates for individuals ages 1 through 54 years. It is not until age 55 and over that the death rate begins to exceed the rate for infants.

During the first half of the twentieth century, neonatal mortality rates had not shown the remarkable reduction observed in postnatal infant mortality. In the early 1960s attention focused on perinatal health care in an effort to decrease the number of neonatal deaths. The ***perinatal mortality rate*** is commonly defined as the number of deaths in infants under 7 days per 1000 live births and fetal deaths (fetuses of 28 weeks or more gestation), although other definitions exist, such as deaths in infants under 28 days and fetal deaths with a gestation of 20 weeks or more (American Academy of Pediatrics, 1992). As a result of the efforts in perinatal care, the neonatal mortality rate declined from 33 per 1000 live births/fetal deaths in 1950 to an estimated rate of 5.4 in 1992 (National Center for Health Statistics, 1993b). This has largely resulted from better treatment of premature infants and perinatal illnesses, such as respiratory distress syndrome and treatment with surfactant. As Table 1-4 demonstrates, most of the 10 leading causes of death during infancy continue to occur during the perinatal period. The first 4 causes—congenital anomalies, sudden infant death syndrome, disorders relating to short gestation and unspecified LBW, and respiratory distress syndrome—accounted for just over half (54%) of all deaths of infants under 1 year of age in 1991. The next 6 causes accounted for only 15% of all infant deaths (National Center for Health Statistics, 1993a, 1993b).

While a number of perinatal problems have benefited from improved treatment, congenital anomalies continue to be a leading cause of infant mortality, accounting for over 20% of those deaths. The incidence of the majority of birth defects has remained substantially the same. Some, such as heart defects, have been rising, but the increase is

TABLE 1-3 Death Rates for Children, Canada, 1988 (Rates per 100,000 Population)

AGE (YEARS)	RATE		
	TOTAL	MALE	FEMALE
Under 1	717.9	801.6	630.0
1-4	41.4	45.9	36.2
5-9	21.7	26.8	16.4
10-14	24.6	31.0	17.8
15-19	70.8	103.4	36.3
20-24	90.5	138.8	41.1

Data from Canadian Center for Health Information, Statistics Canada, 1988.

the result of enhanced methods of detection, not increased births of affected infants (Khoury and Erickson, 1992). Some defects, specifically anencephaly and spina bifida, are expected to decrease as much as 50% with the current recommendation of folic acid supplementation for all women of childbearing age (American Academy of Pediatrics, 1993a) (see also Defects of Neural Tube Closure, Chapter 11).

Most birth defects are significantly associated with low birth weight; therefore prevention of congenital anomalies depends to a large extent on reducing the number of LBW infants (Mili and others, 1991). Infant mortality from human immunodeficiency virus (HIV) infection has increased only slightly, from a rate of 2.1 per 100,000 live births in 1988 to a rate of 2.2 in 1991 (total of 91 deaths) (Wegman, 1993).

When infant death rates are categorized according to race, a disturbing difference is seen. The infant mortality for whites is considerably lower than for all other races in the United States, with blacks having twice the rate for whites. Although the infant mortality of both groups has declined, the gap has remained fairly constant. Unfortunately, data on minority groups are less readily available. For example, the Hispanic infant mortality rate may be understated and may not represent all Hispanic subgroups, such as Cubans, who have significantly more favorable statistics regarding prenatal care and LBW newborns (Wegman, 1993).

One encouraging note is that the gap in mortality rates between all nonwhite races has been narrowing. Since the Indian Health Service assumed responsibility for the health of Native Americans, infant mortality for Native Americans has declined from 62.7 deaths per 1000 live births in the 1950s to 9.8 in the mid-1980s. This improvement, however, is primarily due to declines in neonatal mortality. The postneonatal death rates for Native Americans remains more than twice as high as in the white race. This suggests that Native American infants leave the hospital healthy but go to unsafe environments, which decreases their chances of survival past the first year (Nakamura and others, 1991). This phenomenon is not unique to the United States; postneonatal mortality for Northwest Ontario Indians is reported to be four times that of the Canadian all-race rate (Honigfeld and Kaplan, 1987).

TABLE 1-4 Leading Causes of Death in Infants Under 1 Year of Age, United States, 1991 (Estimated Rates per 100,000 Live Births)

RANK	CAUSE OF DEATH	RATE
—	All causes	894.4
1	Congenital anomalies	186.9
2	Sudden infant death syndrome	130.1
3	Disorders relating to short gestation and unspecified low birth weight	100.7
4	Respiratory distress syndrome	62.5
5	Newborn affected by maternal complications of pregnancy	37.4
6	Newborn affected by complications of placenta, cord, and membranes	23.4
7	Accidents and adverse effects	23.4
8	Infections specific to the perinatal period	21.4
9	Pneumonia and influenza	14.8
10	Intrauterine hypoxia and birth asphyxia	14.6
—	All other causes	279.2

From National Center for Health Statistics: Advance report of final mortality statistics, 1991, *Monthly Vital Statistics Report* 42(2, suppl):52, DHHS Pub No (PHS) 93-1120, Aug 31, 1993.

TABLE 1-5 Death Rates of Children at Selected Age Intervals According to Sex and Race, United States, 1991 (Rates per 100,000 Population in Specified Group)*

AGE INTERVAL (YEARS)	WHITE		ALL OTHER	
	MALE	FEMALE	MALE	FEMALE
Under 1	860.8	659.2	1586.1	1294.0
1-4	45.5	37.6	76.9	61.9
5-9	22.6	16.9	32.6	24.1
10-14	30.6	17.5	42.3	21.3
15-19	112.2	46.9	196.6	48.8

From National Center for Health Statistics: Advance report of final mortality statistics, 1991, *Monthly Vital Statistics Report* 42(suppl 2):6, DHHS Pub No (PHS) 93:1120, Aug 31, 1993.

*Infant death rates (based on population estimate) may differ from infant mortality rates, (based on live births).

Childhood Mortality

For children older than 1 year of age, death rates have always been less than those for infants, as Table 1-5 shows. Death rates are almost 20 times less for 1- to 4-year-old children and 40 times less for 5- to 14-year-old children as compared with death rates for infants. The school-age years have the lowest rate of death, especially for males. However, a sharp rise occurs during later adolescence primarily from injuries, homicide, and suicide—all potentially preventable conditions. A general trend in racial differences that occurs in infant mortality is also apparent in childhood deaths for all ages and for both sexes. Whites have fewer deaths for all ages, and for both racial groups male deaths outnumber female deaths.

TABLE 1-6 Five Leading Causes of Death in Children at Selected Age Intervals, United States, 1991 (Rates per 100,000)

RANK	AGES 1-4	RATE	AGES 5-14	RATE	AGES 15-24	RATE
	All causes	47.4	All causes	23.6	All causes	100.1*
1	Accidents	17.5	Accidents	10.2	Accidents	42.0
2	Congenital anomalies	5.7	Cancer	3.1	Homicide	22.4*
3	Cancer	3.5	Congenital anomalies	1.4	Suicide	13.1*
4	Homicide	2.8*	Homicide	1.4*	Cancer	5.0
5	Heart disease	2.2	Heart disease	0.8	Heart disease	2.7
	HIV infection† (7)	1.0*	HIV infection (9)	0.3*	HIV infection (6)	1.7*

National Center for Health Statistics: Advance report of final mortality statistics, 1991, *Monthly Vital Statistics Report* 42(suppl 21):21, DHHS Pub No (PHS) 93-1120, Sept 28, 1993.
*Rates increased since 1987.
†Human immunodeficiency virus: rank for each age-group in parentheses if HIV in 10 leading causes of death.

After 1 year of age, there is a dramatic change in the causes of death, with injuries (accidents) being the leading cause until people reach their early forties. Injuries account for about 45% of all childhood deaths from ages 1 to 14 years (Table 1-6). In persons ages 10 to 24, injuries, homicide, and suicide are responsible for about 75% of all deaths (Mortality trends, 1993).

Violent deaths have been steadily increasing among children. From 1979 to 1988 homicide increased by 41% for ages 10 to 14 years and by 13.6% for ages 15 to 19 years. Suicide rates increased even more sharply—75% for ages 10 to 14 years and 34.5% for ages 15 to 19 years (see also Suicide, Chapter 21) (Mortality trends, 1993). Firearm homicide is the leading cause of death among black males ages 15 to 19 years, and the rate of occurrence in metropolitan areas is more than six times that in nonmetropolitan areas (Fingerhut, Ingram, and Feldman, 1992). With the present decline in motor vehicle injuries and increase in firearm fatalities (both intentional and nonintentional), mortality from firearms is expected to become the leading cause of death in persons ages 1 to 44 years by the year 2003 (Deaths, 1994).

A common misconception about violence is that it is interracial. While blacks are overrepresented in the homicide statistics, little violence is actually racially instigated. Eighty percent of homicides occur between members of the same race. The overrepresentation of blacks in violence statistics reflects their increased incidence of living in poverty. When poverty is controlled as an influencing factor, the difference in incidence of violent deaths among blacks and whites disappears (Spivak, Prothrow-Smith, and Hausman, 1988).

The causes of increased violence against children are not fully understood, and the problem of child homicides and suicides is an extremely complex one, involving numerous social, economic, and other influences. Therefore, a multifaceted approach is needed to prevent violent deaths, especially those related to firearms. For example, individuals need to be educated about the risks and benefits of owning a firearm and its safe use and storage. The presence of a gun in a household increases the risk of suicide by about fivefold and the risk of homicide by about threefold. Next, legislative efforts may focus on preventing specific groups, such as felons and children, from having access to firearms. And finally, technologic changes could improve the safety of the firearm, such as a childproof safety device and loading indicator (Deaths, 1994). Nurses can take an active part in these strategies and need to be especially aware of young people who are depressed, engage in high-risk behaviors, are repeatedly in trouble with the criminal justice system, or associate with groups known to be violent (such as gangs).

The major declines in death rates during childhood have been due to decreases in gastrointestinal diseases, infectious diseases, perinatal conditions, neoplasms, and injuries. The absence of infectious diseases as a leading cause of death is testimony to the role antibacterial agents and immunizations have played in the declining mortality rates and the specific causes of death. More effective treatment of severe infections has resulted in other disorders becoming more prominent in the list of leading killers. Most notable among these are the neoplasms. (The incidence of cancer in children is discussed in Chapter 36.)

However, infectious diseases are again playing a prominent role in childhood mortality. Of particular concern is the increasing incidence of HIV infection in children. Among children younger than 15 years of age, 350 deaths were reported in 1991 (National Center for Health Statistics, 1993a; Wegman, 1993). HIV infection is already the seventh, ninth, and sixth leading cause of death among children 1 to 4, 5 to 14, and 15 to 24 years of age, respectively. The greatest increase in the number of reported cases of acquired immunodeficiency syndrome (AIDS) has been among persons ages 13 to 24 years, especially women from heterosexual transmission (Update, 1994).

MORBIDITY

The prevalence of a specific illness in the population at a particular time is known as ***morbidity statistics.*** These are generally presented as rates per 1000 population because of their greater frequency of occurrence. Unlike mortality statistics, morbidity is very difficult to define and may denote acute illness, chronic disease, or disability. The source of data also greatly influences the resulting statistics. Common sources include reasons for visits to physicians, diagnosis for hospital admission, or household interviews, such as the National Health Interview Survey (NHIS), Child Health Supplement. Unlike death rates, which are updated annually, morbidity statistics are revised much less frequently and do not necessarily represent the general population. The following discussion is intended to present an overview of illness in children from a variety of perspectives.

Childhood Morbidity

Acute illness may be defined as symptoms severe enough to limit activity or require medical attention. Respiratory illness accounts for about 50% of all acute conditions; about 11% are caused by infections and parasitic disease, and 15% are caused by injuries. The chief illness of childhood is the common cold (Pless, 1992).

The types of diseases that children contract during childhood vary according to age. For example, upper respiratory tract infection and enuresis tend to decrease with age, whereas other disorders, such as acne and headaches, tend to increase with age. Also, children who have any type of problem are more likely to have that problem again than are children in the general population. Morbidity is not distributed randomly in children. Children from poor families tend to have more health problems than children from nonpoor families. This finding suggests the need for heightened efforts to improve access to health care for low-income children (Newacheck and Starfield, 1988).

Recent concern has focused on groups of children who have increased morbitity—homeless children, children living in poverty, children of LBW, children with chronic illnesses, foreign-born adopted children, and children in daycare centers. A number of different factors account for these at-risk groups. A major cause is barriers to health care, especially for the homeless, the poverty stricken, and those with chronic health problems (see p. 14). Even in regard to LBW, the physical, social, and psychologic environment after birth probably has the largest impact on the health status of these children (Overpeck and others, 1989). Other reasons include improved survival of children with chronic health problems, particularly infants of very LBW. Children residing in certain at-risk environments, especially internationally adopted children, are more likely to have a variety of medical conditions, such as infections (American Academy of Pediatrics, 1991; Hostetter and others, 1991; Johnson and others, 1992).

Injury-related morbidity is also significant. Almost 16 million children are seen in emergency rooms for their injuries—600,000 children are hospitalized, and about 30,000 youngsters suffer permanent disability from injuries each year (Division of Injury Control, 1990).

Probably the most important aspect of morbidity is the degree of disability it produces. ***Disability*** can be measured in days off from school or days confined to bed. It can be a result of an acute or chronic disorder. On an average, a child loses 5.3 days per year because of injury or illness. Of all children under 17 years of age, over 95% are not disabled in any way. About 2% have mild disability, another 2% have moderate disability, and 0.2% are severely disabled (Pless, 1992). (The incidence of chronic conditions is discussed in Chapter 22).

Although childhood is a time of relative health, it is the rare child who never becomes ill. Part of nurses' intervention is education of parents regarding the usual types of childhood illnesses and recognition of those symptoms requiring treatment. Future progress in decreasing childhood morbidity, as in childhood mortality, rests more on parent education than on miraculous discoveries such as antibiotics. Nurses play a vital role in advancing child care through health promotion.

The New Morbidity

In addition to disease and injury, children face other problems that can significantly alter their health. These include behavioral, social (family), and educational problems that are sometimes referred to as the ***new morbidity*** or ***pediatric social illness.*** Many of these are psychosocial problems (such as poverty, violence, aggression, noncompliance, school failure, and adjustment to divorce or bereavement) that are not severe enough to be classified as psychiatric diagnoses but interfere in children's social and academic development.

One of the dilemmas of the new morbidity is its identification in children. For example, the proportion of children with these problems is *greater* than the number of visits children make to health care facilities with a new morbidity diagnosis. Consequently, many children seen at a health center have another primary disorder, usually physical, and are only then diagnosed with a psychosocial or psychosomatic problem. One study found that in half of the health supervision visits, parents or children expressed a total of 30 psychosocial concerns, including conduct/behavior problems; insecurity; family, sibling, or social problems; and learning difficulties (Sharp and others, 1992). There is greater emphasis from health professionals on organic deviations than on mental or social ones, and since insurance companies generally do not reimburse for counseling required in the care of psychosocial problems, there is a distinct disincentive to spend additional time on these issues (American Academy of Pediatrics, 1993b). However, children do have such problems, and those working with children, especially nurses in primary care facilities, need to be aware of their potential existence and to deliberately investigate them. Practitioners who ask directly about specific psychosocial issues, show empathy, provide reassurance, and listen attentively are more likely to learn about social problems from parents (Wissom, Roter, and Wilson, 1994).

Although no conclusive characteristics have been identified for children with new morbidity problems, some findings are significant in terms of defining a high-risk group. These include children (1) from the lowest socioeconomic strata, (2) ages 7 to 14 years, (3) of male gender, (4) from one-parent families, (5) with a presenting complaint of a chronic physical disorder, (6) with reading skills below grade level, and (7) with higher rates of school absenteeism (Goldberg and others, 1984; Gortmaker and others, 1990).

INJURIES—THE LEADING KILLER

Injuries, the leading cause of death in children over age 1 year, cause more deaths and disabilities in children than do all causes of disease combined. As children grow older, the percentage of deaths from injuries increases (Table 1-7). In-

TABLE 1-7 Mortality from Leading Types of Injuries, United States, 1990 (Rates per 100,000 Population in Each Age-Group)

TYPE OF ACCIDENT	AGE (YEARS)			
	UNDER 1	1-4	5-14	15-24
MALES				
All causes	1083.1	52.4	28.5	147.4
Accidents (all types)	25.2	20.8	13.5	65.9
Motor vehicle	5.0 (2)*	6.9 (1)	7.0 (1)	49.5 (1)
Drowning†	2.2 (5)	5.0 (2)	2.1 (2)	4.4 (2)
Fires and burns	2.9 (4)	4.4 (3)	1.0 (3)	1.1 (5)
Firearms	—	—	1.0 (4)	2.4 (3)
Ingestion of food/object	4.6 (3)	0.8 (4)	—	—
Mechanical suffocation	6.7 (1)	0.6 (5)	—	—
Poisoning	—	—	—	1.5 (4)
Accidents as a percent of all deaths	2.3%	40%	47%	45%
FEMALES				
All causes	855.5	41.0	19.3	49.0
Accidents (all types)	21.8	13.7	7.2	20.8
Motor vehicle	4.9 (2)	5.6 (1)	4.7 (1)	17.9 (1)
Drowning†	1.7 (5)	2.6 (3)	0.7 (3)	0.4 (4)
Fires and burns	2.7 (4)	2.9 (2)	0.8 (2)	0.5 (3)
Firearms	—	—	0.1 (4)	0.2 (5)
Ingestion of food/object	3.0 (3)	0.5 (4)	—	—
Mechanical suffocation	5.4 (1)	0.3 (5)	—	—
Poisoning	—	—	—	0.6 (2)
Accidents as a percent of all deaths	2.5%	34%	37%	42%

Modified from National Center for Health Statistics, Public Health Service, U.S. Department of Health and Human Services, as cited in *Accident Facts*, Chicago, 1993, National Safety Council.
*Indicates rank among the leading types of accidents.
†Exclusive of deaths in water transportation.

juries have not shown the dramatic declines seen in other areas of childhood mortality. Some of the reasons include (Committee on Trauma Research, 1985):

1. Injury has traditionally been regarded as an unavoidable accident or a behavioral problem, rather than a health problem. The term ***accident*** suggests a chaotic, random event that is "luck" or "chance"; the term ***injury*** is preferred because it connotes a sense of responsibility and control.
2. Injury control, including research, has not received high priority or sufficient financial support. No central agency coordinates or is responsible for reducing the incidence of injuries.
3. Research on injuries has not been based on a theoretic framework, as has been done with diseases. There is a need to view injuries in terms of ***host,*** the affected person; ***environment,*** the time and place; and ***agent,*** the object that is the direct cause.

Host and Agent

The type of injury and the circumstances surrounding it are closely related to normal growth and developmental behavior (see box on p. 9). As children develop, their innate curiosity impels them to investigate activities and to mimic the behavior of others. This is essential in order to acquire competency as an adult, but it predisposes them to numerous hazards during childhood.

The developmental stage of the child partially determines the types of injuries that are most likely to occur at a specific age and thus helps provide clues to preventive measures. For example, small infants are helpless in any environment, and when they begin to roll over or otherwise propel themselves, they can fall from unprotected surfaces. The crawling infant with a natural tendency to place objects in the mouth is at risk of aspiration or poisoning. The mobile toddler with the instinct to explore and investigate and the ability to run and climb is subject to a variety of injuries, including falls, burns, and collision with objects. As children grow older, their absorption with play often makes them oblivious to environmental hazards such as street traffic or water, and the need to conform and gain acceptance compels older children and adolescents to accept challenges and dares. Although the highest incidence of injury is in children less than 9 years of age, most fatal injuries occur in later childhood and adolescence.

The pattern of deaths caused by injuries, especially from motor vehicles, drowning, and burns, is remarkably consistent in most Western societies, such as Canada. Table 1-7 compares the leading causes of deaths from injuries for each age-group according to sex. The overwhelming cause of death in children over 1 year of age is motor vehicle (MV)–related fatalities, including occupant, pedestrian, bicycle, and motorcycle deaths (Fig. 1-1) (Paulson, 1989). Even though the *percentage* of infants dying from MV-related injuries is small compared with the total number of deaths in that age-group, children under 1 year of age have a high death rate from MV passenger deaths (primarily from failure to be properly restrained).

CHILDHOOD INJURIES: RISK FACTORS

Sex—Preponderance of males; difference mainly due to behavioral characteristics, especially aggression
Temperament—Children with difficult temperament profile (see Chapter 4), especially persistence, high activity, and negative reactions to new situations (Nyman, 1987)
Stress—Predisposes to increased risk taking and self-destructive behavior; general lack of self-protection
Alcohol and drug use—Associated with higher incidence of motor vehicle injuries, drownings, homicides, and suicides
Previous history of injury—Associated with increased likelihood of another injury, especially if initial injury required hospitalization
Developmental characteristics
- Mismatch between child's developmental level and skill required for activity (e.g., all-terrain vehicles)
- Natural curiosity to explore environment
- Desire to assert self and challenge rules
- In older child, desire for peer approval and acceptance

Cognitive characteristics (age specific)
- ***Infancy***—Sensorimotor: explores environment through taste and touch
- ***Young child***
  - Object permanence: actively searches for attractive object
  - Cause and effect: unaware of consequential dangers
  - Transductive reasoning: may fail to learn from experiences; for example, falling from a step is not perceived as same type of danger as climbing a tree
  - Magical and egocentric thinking: cannot comprehend danger to self or others; cannot take place of others to realize danger; if thinking something is safe, believes it to be so
- ***School-age child***—Transitional cognitive processes: unable to fully comprehend causal relationships; attempts dangerous acts without detailed planning regarding consequences
- ***Adolescent***—Formal operations: preoccupied with abstract thinking and loses sight of reality; may lead to feeling of invulnerability

Anatomic characteristics —(especially in young children)
- ***Large head***—Predisposes to cranial injury
- ***Large spleen and liver with wide costal arch***—Predisposes to direct trauma to these organs
- ***Small and light body***—May be thrown easily, especially inside a moving vehicle

Other factors—Poverty, family stress (i.e., maternal illness, recent environmental change), substandard alternative child care, young maternal age, low maternal education, multiple siblings (Scheidt, 1988)

The incidence of vehicular injuries, especially among young children as occupants, has been declining. Mandatory seat belt laws have reduced MV-related deaths and nonfatal injuries in all age-groups, especially young children, but less so among adolescents (Chorba, Reinfurt, and Hulka, 1988; Osberg and DiScala, 1992). Currently, all states in the United States have enacted legislation requiring young children to be properly restrained in motor vehicles. However, seat belt laws vary from state to state in terms of the ages of children covered, types of vehicles affected, penalties for noncompliance, and other special provisions. The usual decline in seat belt use after initiation of the legislation and the high misuse of child restraint systems continue to be major problems (Stewart, 1993). Therefore the effect of mandatory seat belt laws on mortality varies according to different reports.

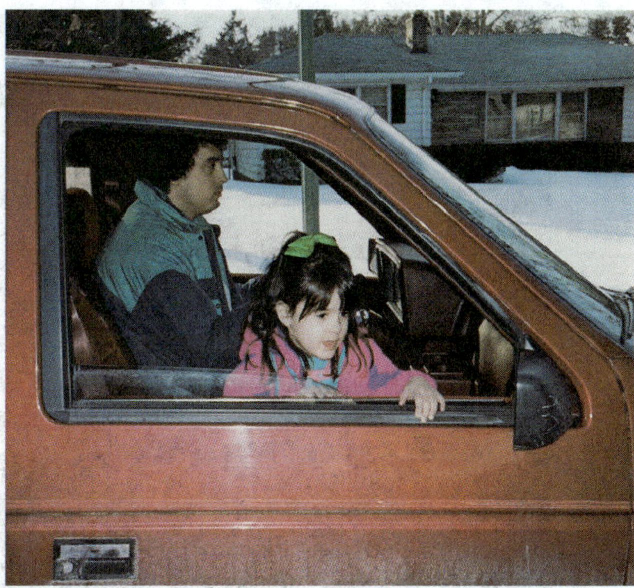

FIG. 1-1 Motor vehicle injuries are the leading cause of death in children over 1 year of age. The majority of fatalities involve occupants who are unrestrained.

Pedestrian injuries in children account for about 35% of MV-related deaths. Most pedestrian injuries occur at midblock, at intersections, in driveways, and in parking lots. Driveway injuries typically involve small children, large vehicles, and backing up (Agran, Winn, and Anderson, 1994). Parents may not be alert to the dangers leading to such injuries and consequently fail to protect their children (Rivara, Bergman, and Drake, 1989).

Bicycle injuries are another important cause of childhood deaths, especially from head injuries (Spence and others, 1993). Although the use of helmets can reduce mortality and morbidity (Sacks and others, 1991), children infrequently wear helmets, and parents are often unaware of their importance (Jones and others, 1993). Both community-wide bicycle helmet campaigns and mandatory-use laws have resulted in significant increases in helmet use (Coté and others, 1992; DiGuiseppi and others, 1989). However, even with a mandatory-use law, issues such as stylishness, comfort, and social acceptability remain important factors in compliance (Gielen and others, 1994). Certainly, nurses can help educate children and families about pedestrian and bicycle safety. In particular, school nurses can promote wearing helmets and encourage peer leaders to act as role models (Wilson and Testani-Dufour, 1993).

When deaths from injuries are compared according to sex and age, the causes differ. Drowning and burns are the second and third leading causes of death in boys ages 1 to 14, but the order is reversed in girls (Fig. 1-2). In addition, improper use of firearms causes more deaths among males than among females (Fig. 1-3). During infancy, more males succumb to death from aspiration or suffocation than do females (Fig. 1-4). More than half of all poisonings occur

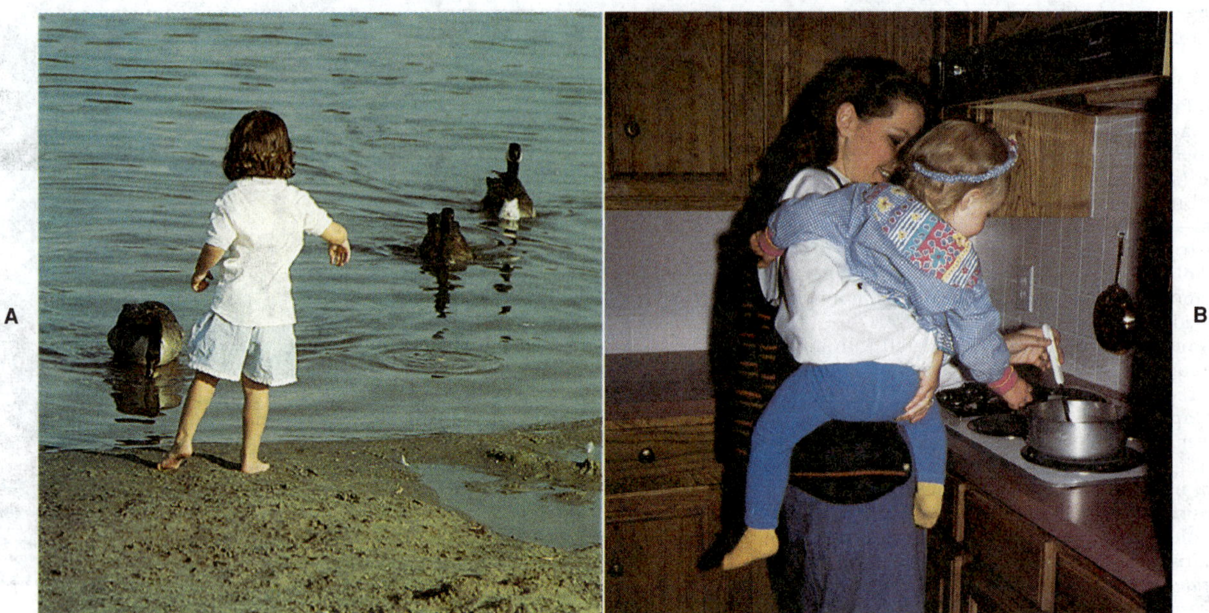

FIG. 1-2 **A,** Drowning is the second leading cause of death from injury in boys and the third in girls ages 1 to 14 years. It remains the second leading cause of death from injury for both sexes ages 15 to 24 years. **B,** Burns are the second leading cause of death from injury in girls and the third in boys ages 1 to 14 years.

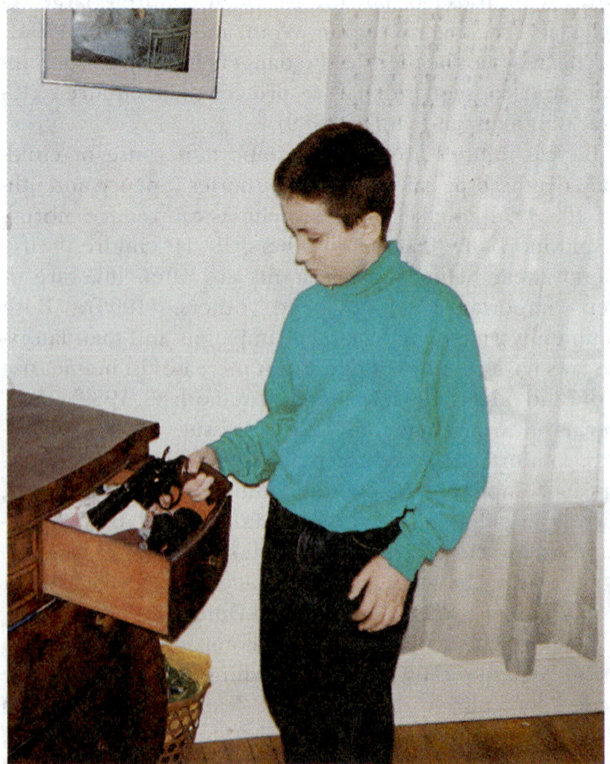

FIG. 1-3 Improper use of firearms is the fourth leading cause of death from injury in boys and girls ages 5 to 14 years and the third cause of death from injury in boys ages 15 to 24 years.

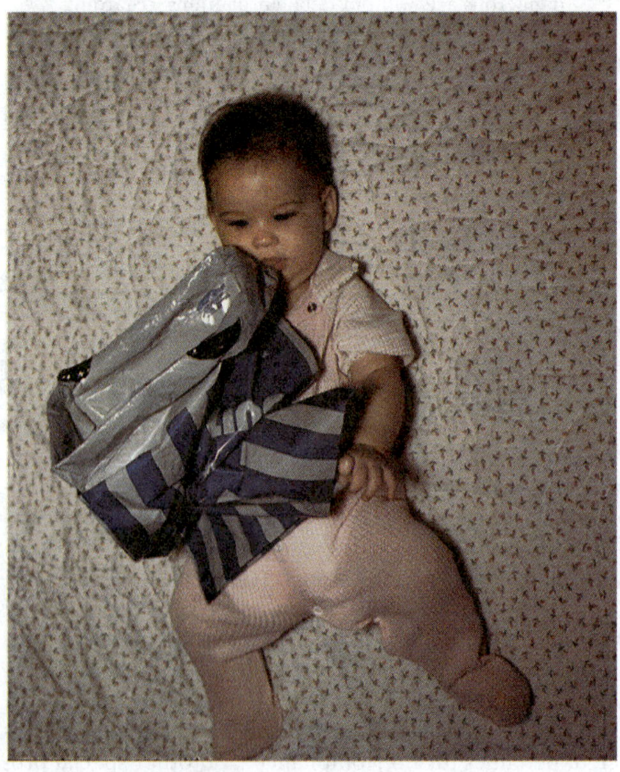

FIG. 1-4 Aspiration/suffocation is often the leading cause of death from injury in infants, especially boys.

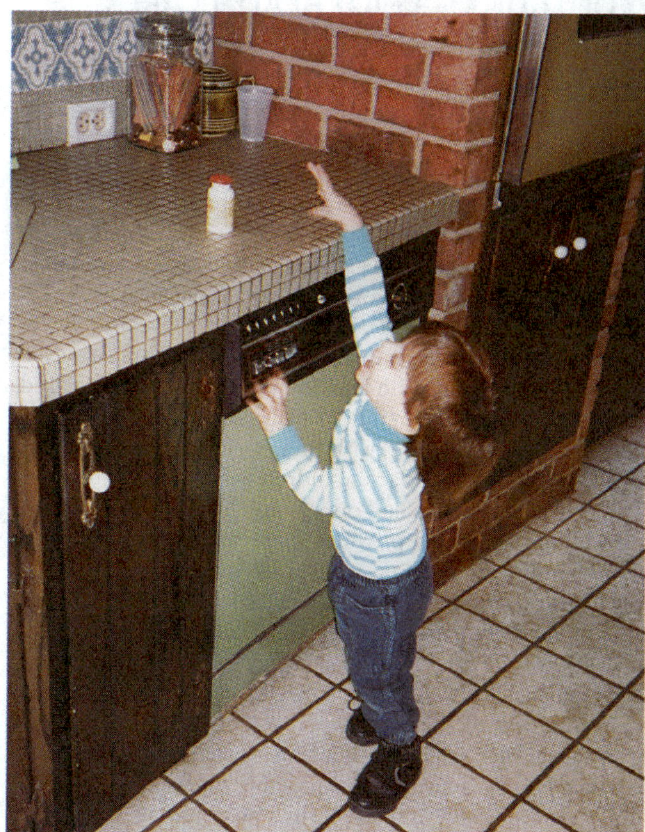

FIG. 1-5 Poisoning causes a considerable number of injuries in children under 4 years of age but is the fourth leading cause of death from injury (usually from suicide) in young people ages 15 to 24 years.

in children under 2 years of age (Fig. 1-5). By age 4 to 5 years, nonintentional poisonings are uncommon. Another increase occurs in the 15- to 24-year age-group, where poisoning is the fourth leading cause of death from injury. Poisoning in this age-group is typically intentional and usually represents death from suicide (especially females) or drug abuse.

Analyzing deaths from specific types of injuries by age and sex is useful in identifying high-risk groups. In a comparison of accidental deaths with other causes of childhood mortality, it is clear that preventing injuries offers the greatest promise for improving survival. Nurses certainly play a major role in providing anticipatory guidance to parents and older children regarding hazards during each age period.

Environment

A number of environmental factors, such as place, time, and equipment, contribute to injuries. The highest number of injuries occurs in the home, especially in children younger than 6 years of age. Older children have almost as many injuries outside the home, especially at school and recreational sites. Among recreational and sports activities, football is one of the most hazardous athletic activities, accounting for 20 injuries per 100,000 participants per year. Serious, potentially fatal injuries result from spinal cord trauma. Among females, gymnastics appears to pose the greatest risks (Runyan and Gerken, 1989). For drowning, the second leading cause of death, the risk factors include living in a warm climate, swimming in undesignated areas, inability to swim, not using or misusing a personal flotation device, and using open boats (Gulaid and others, 1988).

Recent attention has focused on the incidence of deaths and injuries among children and adolescents at work, such as on farms. Injuries occur most frequently among males ages 10 to 19 years and result primarily from farm machinery (tractors, wagons, and trucks) (Dunn and Runyan, 1993; Salmi and others, 1989).

Identification of environmental hazards has in some instances had tremendous influence on reducing the incidence of fatal injuries; for example, placing fences around swimming pools and guards on windows has decreased the incidence of fatal drownings and falls.

Injury Prevention

Theoretically, all injuries are preventable, and one of the chief nursing responsibilities is to anticipate and recognize where safety measures are applicable. Injury prevention necessitates protection, education, and legislation. The two major strategies for injury prevention are:

1. **Passive strategies,** which provide automatic protection by product and environmental design (e.g., the use of automatic seat belts or air bags). Such devices require no active participation by the individual and have the greatest success rate.
2. **Active strategies,** which *persuade* individuals to change their behavior for increased self-protection, such as using seat belts voluntarily, or *require* compliance with safety regulations, such as laws that mandate use of safety restraints in young children. Persuasion through education has been much less effective than legislated change, although it remains a key strategy.

NURSING ALERT Although nurses should play a major role in injury prevention, one study demonstrated that less than 30% of pediatric nurse practitioners routinely gave advice about child car restraints and seat belts, only about 15% offered information about smoke detectors, and 7% or less gave advice about firearms in the home (Jones, 1992). While these statistics may not represent the emphasis placed on injury prevention by all nurses, they are sufficient to highlight the need for improved participation of nurses in this essential area of child health.

The preventive aspects of child care are an ongoing part of health promotion throughout childhood. To protect the child from injury, persons who are responsible for children need to be aware of the normal behavioral characteristics that render children vulnerable to injuries and to be alert to factors in the environment that create a hazard to their safety. Parents and others are often surprisingly unaware of their child's developmental progress and capabilities. Anticipatory guidance regarding developmental expectations serves to alert the parents to the type of injuries that are most likely to occur at any given age and to environmental circumstances that might precipitate an injury (Widome,

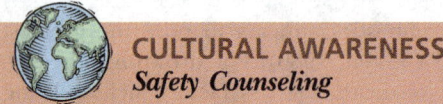

CULTURAL AWARENESS
Safety Counseling

Cultural factors also need to be considered when instituting safety instruction, since noncompliance is one of the major deterrents to injury prevention. For example, cultural characteristics, such as the lack of future orientation and resistance to changing long-standing habits, can interfere with a cultural group's acceptance of injury prevention practices (Foss, 1987). One study found that efforts regarding the use of seat belts among Mexican-American parents were more effective when the dominant decision-making male in the family and the influential older woman, often a grandmother, were included in the educational efforts (Faber, 1986).

1992). For example, infants must not be left where they can fall or roll over, and toddlers must not be given objects or toys with small removable parts or sharp edges or given unsupervised access to places where they can fall, drown, or be burned.

Very early in the parent-child relationship, the parents need to learn how to provide a safe environment for their child, what kinds of behaviors they can expect of the child at various stages in the child's development, and their responsibility for the safety of their child. This is particularly important for first-time parents (see also Cultural Awareness box). Safety responsibility in such areas as purchase of infant equipment, especially a car restraint, should begin *before* the child is born.

It cannot be assumed that parents of one or more children are familiar with all areas of child safety. Moreover, the addition of a new child brings up the issue of sibling rivalry and the unwelcome but realistic possibility that the new child may be at risk from a jealous older sibling. For example, the parents should be cautioned against leaving the infant alone with the older child who feels threatened by the newcomer.

Providing a safe environment for the child involves the combined efforts of family, nurses, and community. At each age level there are environmental attractions that are hazardous to the safety of the child. The specific hazards vary according to the season (drowning, injuries related to winter heating devices), geographic area (water injuries in areas with swimming pools, rivers, or lakes; heater burns in cold climates), and socioeconomic level (lead poisoning and street injuries in slum areas, bicycle injuries in middle-class areas).

Safety should be an intrinsic element of nursing practice. Nurses who themselves practice safety, who are alert to safety needs in the environment, and who recognize the need for safety education contribute to injury reduction. The special problems and preventive measures are discussed as appropriate throughout the book and are related to the various age levels and conditions that predispose to specific hazards.

EVOLUTION OF CHILD HEALTH CARE IN THE UNITED STATES

Children in colonial America were born into a world with many hazards to their health and survival. Epidemics were common, and no control or treatment was known. Physicians were few, and only a small number had any formal training. Midwives also were untrained, basing their practice on past experiences. Books providing information on child care and feeding were scarce and, when available, were useful only to a minority of literate parents.

Medical care by physicians was limited to wealthy European families who lived in or could travel to more developed cities. Children who lived on farms were mainly cared for by another family member or by a competent neighbor. Traveling medicine men, with their various forms of quackery, were common. Black children who were bought as slaves or born to slaves had only as much care as their owner was able or willing to provide (Scott and Winston, 1976). Native American children were treated for disease according to the tradition of each tribe, which was often a mixture of medicine, magic, and religion (Sayre and Sayre, 1976). With the colonization of America, Native Americans were exposed to many new diseases, which were fatal to large numbers of them.

Statistics on childhood mortality during the colonial period are largely unavailable. Epidemic diseases were prevalent, however, and included smallpox, measles, mumps, chickenpox, influenza, diphtheria, yellow fever, cholera, and whooping cough, but the disease that surpassed all others as a cause of childhood death was dysentery. Sometimes entire families succumbed to this illness. Other diseases that were major contributors to childhood illness were the "slow epidemic" of tuberculosis, nutritional diseases, and injuries (Schmidt, 1976).

Although scientific knowledge was accumulating, especially from work done in Europe, there were no organized efforts in the United States to apply that knowledge to the care of the sick. It was not until the Industrial Revolution was well under way in the nineteenth century that the consequences of childhood illness and injury and the effects of child labor, poverty, and neglect became more widely recognized. The end of the nineteenth century is often regarded as the dark ages of pediatrics, and the first half of the twentieth century is regarded as the dawn of improved health care for children (Cone, 1976).

The study of pediatrics began in the last half of the 1800s, particularly under the influence of a Prussian-born physician, ***Abraham Jacobi*** (1830-1919), who is referred to as the ***Father of Pediatrics*** (Leopold, 1957). He was awarded the first professorship in pediatrics in America in 1870, started pediatric departments in several New York hospitals, and was one of the founders of the American Pediatric Society in 1888. With several other physicians he pioneered in the scientific and clinical investigation of childhood diseases. One outstanding achievement was the establishment of "milk stations," where mothers could bring sick children for treatment and learn the importance of pure milk and its proper preparation.

The crusade for pure milk helped bring the dairy industry under legal control and led to the establishment of infant welfare stations. The remarkable decline in infant mortality since 1900 has been achieved through prevention and health-promoting measures such as improved sanitation and pasteurization of milk. Before these regulations existed, the unsanitary milk supply was a chief source of infantile diarrhea and bovine tuberculosis. Cows were often kept in filthy stables and fed garbage and distillery wastes. Milk from cows fed distillery wastes was reported to make infants "tipsy." Some of the cows were so diseased with tuberculosis that they had to be raised on cranes to be milked (Cone, 1976).

At about the same time, increasing concern developed for the social welfare of children, especially those who were homeless or employed as factory laborers. The work of one such reformer, ***Lillian Wald*** (1867-1940), had far-reaching effects on child health and nursing. She founded the Henry Street Settlement in New York City, which eventually provided nursing service, social work, and an organized program of social, cultural, and educational activities. Wald is regarded as the founder of public health or community nursing. She was instrumental in establishing the role of the first full-time school nurse, ***Lina Rogers.*** Soon other nurses were employed to teach parents and children about the prevention or need for treatment of minor skin conditions, malnutrition, and other impairments or illnesses identified in the school. An outgrowth of nursing involvement in school health was the development of pediatric courses and specialized clinical experience in schools of nursing.

As more causes of disease were identified, there was an emphasis on isolation and asepsis. In the early 1900s children with contagious diseases were isolated from adult patients. Parents were prohibited from visiting because they might transmit disease to and from the home. Even toys and personal articles of clothing were kept from the child. It was not until the 1940s and the famous work of Spitz and Robertson on institutionalized children that the effects of isolation and maternal deprivation were recognized. This brought forth a surge of interest in the psychologic health of children and resulted in changes for hospitalized children, such as rooming-in, sibling visitations, child life (play) programs, prehospitalization preparation, parent education, and hospital schooling.

Influenced by social reformers such as Lillian Wald, national leaders began to take action to improve children's living conditions. In 1909 President Theodore Roosevelt called the first ***White House Conference on Children.*** It focused on care of dependent children and attempted to address the deplorable working conditions of youngsters. As a result of this conference, the U.S. Children's Bureau was established under the jurisdiction of the Department of Labor, since at that time laws to regulate child labor were seen as the greatest need. Later, the Bureau was placed under the Department of Health, Education and Welfare (now the ***Department of Health and Human Services***). White House conferences were held approximately every 10 years until 1980 to address the welfare, health, education, social, economic, and psychologic needs of children.

The establishment of the ***Children's Bureau*** in 1912 marked the beginning of a period of studies of economic and social factors related to infant mortality, maternal deaths, and maternal and infant care in rural areas, all of which created the basis for stimulating better standards of care for mothers and children. This helped lead to the first Maternity and Infancy Act (Sheppard-Towner Act) in 1921, which provided grants to states to develop a Division of Maternal and Child Health (MCH) as a unit of the health department. However, this bill eventually lapsed because of opposition from those (especially the American Medical Association [AMA]) who viewed it as a socialist movement.

Still, the passage of the act was a turning point for the creation of the ***American Academy of Pediatrics*** in 1930. The Section on Pediatrics of the AMA supported the bill but were chastised for publicly approving it, inciting the pediatricians to form their own national organization (Hughes, 1993).

With the passage of ***Title V of the Social Security Act (SSA)*** in 1935, a federal-state partnership was established under the administration of the Children's Bureau. Title V included federal grants-in-aid to states, matched by state funds, for three types of work: ***maternal and child health (MCH), Crippled Children's Services (CCS),*** and ***child welfare services.*** The first programs provided by Title V were prenatal, postnatal, and child health clinics and training of personnel. The early emphasis of the CCS Program was on orthopaedic care. With the recognition that a child's ability to function could also be limited by a chronic illness, state CCS programs became involved with children with developmental, behavioral, and educational problems and more recently with home care of children with complex medical conditions. This broadened concept was officially reflected in the 1985 passage of legislation that changed the name of the CCS to the ***Program for Children with Special Health Needs (CSHN).***

Numerous other federal programs have been developed. Some that have had a major impact on maternal and child health include:

Medicaid. In 1965 Medicaid was created under Title XIX of the Social Security Act to reduce financial barriers to health care for the poor. It is the largest maternal-child health program. A major project under Medicaid is the Child Health Assessment Program (CHAP), which provides services for a large number of pregnant women and children. Not all poor children are eligible for Medicaid; financial eligibility varies considerably from state to state.

Aid to Families with Dependent Children (AFDC). AFDC was established by the Social Security Act of 1935 as a cash grant program to enable states to aid needy children without fathers.

MCH Services Block Grant. The MCH Services Block Grant provides health services to mothers and children, particularly those with low income or limited access to health services. Its primary purposes are to reduce infant mortality, reduce the incidence of preventable disease and handicapping conditions among children, and increase the availability of prenatal, delivery, and postpartum care to eligible mothers.

Alcohol, Drug Abuse, and Mental Health Block Grant. Established by the Omnibus Budget Reconciliation Act of 1981, the block grant provides funds to states for (1) projects to support prevention, treatment, and rehabilitation related to substance abuse and (2) grants to community mental health centers for the identification, assessment, and treatment of severely mentally disturbed children and adolescents.

Social Services Block Grant. Established under Title XX of the Social Security Act, this block grant provides states with funds for child daycare, protective and emergency services, counseling, family planning, home-based services, information and referral, and adoption and foster care services.

Women, Infants, and Children (WIC). In 1974 the WIC Special Supplemental Food Program was started. It provides nutritious food and nutrition education to low-income, pregnant, postpartum, and lactating women and to infants and children up to age 5 years. Other nutrition programs include Food Stamps, National School Lunch Program, School Breakfast Program, and Child Care Food Program, which provides financial assistance for nutritious meals to children in daycare centers, family and group daycare homes, and Head Start centers.

Education for All Handicapped Children Act (P.L. 94-142). In 1975 P.L. 94-142 was passed to provide a free appropriate public education to all handicapped children from ages 3 to 21 and to provide for those supportive services (speech, counseling, and so on) that ensure the benefit of special education.

Education of the Handicapped Act Amendments of 1986 (P.L. 99-457). In 1986 P.L. 99-457 was passed to allow for the provision of federal funding to states to develop and implement a statewide, comprehensive, coordinated, and multidisciplinary program of early intervention services for handicapped infants and toddlers and their families.

Family and Medical Leave Act (FMLA). Signed into law in 1993, FMLA allows eligible employees to take up to 12 weeks of unpaid leave from their jobs every year to care for newborn or newly adopted children; to care for children, parents, or spouses who have serious health conditions; or to recover from their own serious health conditions. After the leave, the law entitles employees to return to their previous jobs or to equivalent jobs with the same pay, benefits, and other conditions.

Despite the number of federal and state programs available to assist children and families, there are serious barriers to health care in the United States, including (1) ***financial barriers,*** such as not having insurance or having insurance that does not cover certain services; (2) ***system barriers,*** such as having to travel great distances for health care or state-to-state variations in Medicaid benefits; and (3) ***knowledge barriers,*** such as not knowing about the need or value of prenatal or child health supervision or being unaware of the services that are available. The current thrust in health care initiative is to improve children's and families' access to health care.

One of the most drastic changes in health care delivery has been the establishment of a prospective payment system based on ***diagnosis-related groups (DRGs).*** The DRG categories allow pretreatment (prospective) billing for almost all U.S. hospitals reimbursed by Medicare. With hospitals now financially responsible when Medicare patients exceed the allotted admission stay, more patients are being discharged early. This has created an immense need for home care and other sources of community-based services. The exact impact DRGs will have on pediatric care is uncertain, but because health care cost containment is a national priority, it is inevitable that some form of prospective payment will affect children. Nurses need to be aware of the changing economics and be prepared to meet the challenges.

PEDIATRIC NURSING

PHILOSOPHY OF CARE

Nursing of infants and children is consistent with the ***definition of nursing*** as "the diagnosis and treatment of human responses to actual or potential health problems" (Nursing, 1980). Its goal is to promote the highest possible state of health in each child within the family system. To accomplish this goal, this section focuses on key philosophies of care that guide nursing practice regardless of the child's condition.

Family-Centered Care

The philosophy of ***family-centered care*** recognizes the family as the constant in a child's life and that service systems and personnel must support, respect, encourage, and enhance the strength and competence of the family (Johnson, McGonigel, and Kaufmann, 1989). Families are supported in their natural caregiving and decision-making roles by building on their unique strengths as individuals and families. Patterns of living at home and in the community are promoted. The needs of all family members, not just the child's, are considered (see box below). The philosophy acknowledges diversity among family structures and backgrounds; family goals, dreams, strategies, and actions; and

KEY ELEMENTS OF FAMILY-CENTERED CARE

- Recognizing that the family is the constant in a child's life, whereas the service systems and personnel within those systems fluctuate
- Facilitating parent/professional collaboration at all levels of health care:
  - Care of an individual child
  - Program development, implementation, and evaluation
  - Policy formation
- Honoring the racial, ethnic, cultural, and socioeconomic diversity of families
- Recognizing family strengths and individuality and respecting different methods of coping
- Sharing with parents, on a continuing basis and in a supportive manner, complete and unbiased information
- Encouraging and facilitating family-to-family support and networking
- Understanding and incorporating the developmental needs of infants, children, and adolescents and their families into health care systems
- Implementing comprehensive policies and programs that provide emotional and financial support to meet the needs of families
- Designing accessible health care systems that are flexible, culturally competent, and responsive to family-identified needs

From National Center for Family-Centered Care, Association for the Care of Children's Health, Bethesda, MD, 1990.

family support, service, and information needs (Ahmann, 1994).*

Two basic concepts in this process are enabling and empowerment. Professionals ***enable*** families by creating opportunities and means for all family members to display their present abilities and competencies and to acquire new ones that are necessary to meet the needs of the child and family. ***Empowerment*** describes the interaction of professionals with families in such a way that families maintain or acquire a sense of control over their family lives and attribute positive changes that result from helping behaviors that foster their own strengths, abilities, and actions (Dunst, Trivette, and Deal, 1988).

The ***parent-professional partnership*** is a powerful mechanism for enabling and empowering families. Parents serve as respected equals with professionals† and have the rightful role in deciding what is important for themselves and their family; the professional's role is to support and strengthen the family's ability to nurture and promote its members' development in a way that is both enabling and empowering.

Partnerships imply the belief that partners are capable individuals who become more capable by sharing knowledge, skills, and resources in a manner that benefits all participants. Collaboration is viewed as a continuum. Families have the option of being anywhere along that continuum, depending on the strengths and needs of the child, the family, and the professionals who are involved (Shelton, Jeppson, and Johnson, 1987). The nurse can help *every* family, including those with a previous history of serious personal and/or family problems, to identify their strengths, build on them, and assume a comfortable level of participation (see Thinking Critically About . . . box). Although caring for the family is strongly emphasized throughout the text, it is also highlighted in features such as Cultural Awareness, Family Focus (see p. 24) and Family Home Care boxes.

*Resources on family-centered care are available from the Association for Care of Children's Health, 7910 Woodmont Ave., Suite 300, Bethesda, MD 20814; (301) 654-6549. A facilitator's guide, *Recognizing Family-Centered Care,* and other publications are available from Project Copernicus, 2911 E. Biddle St., Baltimore, MD 21213; (410) 550-9700.

†For information about parent-professional partnerships, a free pamphlet, *Equals in This Partnership,* is available from The National Center for Clinical Infant Programs, 2000 14th St., N., Suite 380, Arlington, VA 22201; (703) 528-4300.

Atraumatic Care

Although tremendous advances have been made in pediatric care, much of what is done to children to cure illness and prolong life is traumatic, painful, upsetting, and frightening. Unfortunately, minimizing the trauma of medical interventions has not kept pace with the technologic advances. With knowledge of the stressors imposed on ill children and their families and armed with interventions shown to be safe and effective in eliminating or reducing the stressors, health professionals must direct their attention to providing care that is as atraumatic as possible.

Atraumatic care is the provision of therapeutic care in settings, by personnel, and through the use of interventions that eliminates or minimizes the psychologic and physical distress experienced by children and their families in the health care system. ***Therapeutic care*** encompasses the prevention, diagnosis, treatment, or palliation of chronic or acute conditions. ***Setting*** refers to whatever place that care

THINKING CRITICALLY ABOUT . . . *Family-Centered Care*

Although professionals readily accept the concept of family-centered care, they have been slow to implement practices that embody the "family as the patient." This lag has occurred in part because family-centered care requires a shift in orientation regarding provisions of services. The philosophy requires stretching beyond clinical practices that have become tradition because of their convenience to the institution and personnel (Ahmann, 1994). Common examples of ***system-based care*** are exclusion policies of not allowing family members to stay with their children during a procedure and restricting visiting hours, as well as numbers and ages of visitors.

On the other hand, family-centered care requires viewing families as the center of care, with their input serving as the major determinant of the interventions provided. For example, exclusion policies are replaced with ***family-based care,*** such as parental and child *choice* regarding separation during procedures, open visiting hours, and no limitations on the ages or numbers of visitors, except per family request (Flint and Walsh, 1988). In fact, should the word "visitors" even by used? Family members certainly are not visitors to their child; nurses and other staff are! (See Thinking Critically About . . . Parental Presence . . . box under Preparation for Procedures, Chapter 27.)

Even ***child-based care*** is not synonymous with family-based care. For example, the hospital dietary service may provide food selections for children but fail to provide inexpensive meals for parents or consider family cultural/religious traditions. Primary nurses may focus on the child's needs but place little emphasis on the family's concerns.

In your practice, what policies can be considered system-, child-, or family-based care? How can those that are not family-based care be changed? What reasons do staff give for preferring system-based care? Compare the agency's policies with its mission statement and purpose. Sadly, you may find what Hostler (1992) reported, that during visits to 30 leading hospitals in the United States, not one single model of excellence in the implementation of family-centered care was found. Fortunately, models of family-centered care, such as the Nursing Mutual Participation Mode (Curley, 1988; Curley and Wallace, 1992), do exist and have documented benefits, such as (Curley and Wallace, 1992; Johnson, Jeppson, and Redburn, 1992):

- Families experience greater feelings of confidence and competence and less stress in caring for their children
- The dependence of families on professional caregivers decreases
- Costs of care decrease
- Professionals experience greater job satisfaction
- Both parents and providers are empowered to develop new skills and expertise

is given—the home, the hospital, or any other health care setting. ***Personnel*** include anyone directly involved in providing therapeutic care. ***Interventions*** range from psychologic approaches, such as preparing children for procedures, to physical interventions, such as providing space for a parent to room in. ***Psychologic distress*** may include anxiety, fear, anger, disappointment, sadness, shame, or guilt. ***Physical distress*** may range from sleeplessness and immobilization to the experience of disturbing sensory stimuli, such as pain, temperature extremes, loud noises, bright lights, or darkness. Simply, atraumatic care is concerned with the who, what, when, where, why, and how of any procedure performed on a child for the purpose of preventing or minimizing psychologic and physical stress (Wong, 1989).

The overriding goal in providing atraumatic care is *first, do no harm.* Three principles provide the framework for achieving this goal: (1) prevent or minimize the child's separation from the family; (2) promote a sense of control; and (3) prevent or minimize bodily injury and pain. Examples of providing atraumatic care include fostering the parent-child relationship during hospitalization, preparing the child before any unfamiliar treatment or procedure, controlling pain, allowing the child privacy, providing play activities for expression of fear and aggression, minimizing loss of control, and respecting cultural differences.

Throughout the text the concept of atraumatic care is an integral part of all discussions of nursing care. Selected examples are highlighted in Atraumatic Care boxes. Many other boxes and tables focusing on culture, family teaching, research, and critical thinking incorporate aspects of providing care as atraumatically as possible. Chapter 26, Family-Centered Care of the Child During Illness and Hospitalization, is organized according to the principles of providing atraumatic care.

Primary Nursing

Part of the trend in nursing practice, particularly in pediatrics, is a deeper commitment to patient accountability. One of the outgrowths of this has been the movement toward ***primary nursing,*** which involves 24-hour responsibility and accountability by one nurse for the care of a small group of patients. The primary nurse becomes the bedside nurse, with few if any duties delegated to other staff. If responsibilities are shared, it is usually with an associate primary nurse who maintains continuity of care when the primary nurse is not working.

One of the traditional problems with primary nursing is providing consistency in scheduling the same nurse and associate. An approach that minimizes this difficulty is to designate one primary nurse and as many associates as are needed to ensure that the same group of nurses care for the child. This group of nurses forms the ***primary core.*** One nurse is assigned to the patient for each shift, and additional nurses are assigned for these individuals' days off. By identifying the primary core for a specific period in advance, all the nurses working with the child can plan care jointly, with the primary nurse maintaining overall responsibility.

The philosophy of primary care is supported throughout the discussion of nursing of children. In some instances the one-to-one relationship between child and nurse is emphasized because of its therapeutic benefit, such as in nonorganic failure to thrive. However, primary nursing is universally a supportive intervention in pediatric nursing because it provides a consistent caregiver for the child and focuses on the family unit as an integral component in the planning and implementation of care.

Case Management*

Nursing case management is an extension of primary nursing (Weinstein, 1991). As a general concept, case management is a care delivery system that balances cost and quality and was created in response to pressure from payers to provide care in a more cost-effective manner. Although the movement to case management began in adult care, it was quickly adapted to pediatric care. Simultaneously, benefits to case management, such as improved patient/family satisfaction, decreased fragmentation of care, and the ability to describe and measure outcomes for a homogenous group of patients, became apparent.

Case management is not a new concept. It has been used in outpatient settings, primarily by assigning a case manager to a particular patient or group of patients. The new model includes a timeline for care as a component of the process. These timelines for care have a variety of names: critical paths, guidelines for care, case management plans, Caremaps,† coordinated care plans, or other titles that are agreed on within a specific agency. Regardless of the name given to the timeline, these are multidisciplinary plans that include all of the components of care for an episode or multiple episodes of illness, as well as the outcomes that are expected as a result of delivering that care. They can be confined to inpatient care or can include the entire continuum of care, including home care (see also Case Management, Chapter 25 and sample multidisciplinary plan under Diabetes Mellitus, Chapter 38).

Variances from the timelines are recorded daily in an effort to determine why there are delays in providing care or why a patient's illness may follow a different course than was expected. Variances are usually categorized as patient, system, caregiver, or community problems. Through a retrospective review process, changes can be made to make care more effective and more efficient. By using case management as a care delivery system, many hospitals have reported dramatic reductions in the length of stay and in the cost of providing care (Thompson, 1994). Improvements in the efficiency of hospital systems and in nurses' job satisfaction have also been reported (Weinstein, 1991).

Concurrent with the movement to provide care in a systematic manner have been efforts by professional and government organizations to develop ***clinical practice guidelines*** for the care of an illness, disease, or related problem. While timelines for care are usually developed within an institution and reflect local practice patterns, clinical guidelines are being developed on a national level that reflect the re-

*Annette C. Bollig, RN, MSN, wrote this section.

†Caremap is a registered trademark of the Center for Case Management, Inc., South Natick, MA.

AHCPR CLINICAL PRACTICE GUIDELINES RELEVANT TO PEDIATRIC PRACTICE

Acute pain management: operative or medical procedures and trauma
Urinary incontinence in adults
Pressure ulcers in adults: prediction and intervention
Treatment of pressure ulcers in adults
Diagnosis and treatment of depressed outpatients in primary care settings
Diagnosis and treatment of sickle cell disease
Initial evaluation and early treatment of the HIV-infected individual
Management of cancer-related pain
Diagnosis and treatment of heart failure
Otitis media in children

Modified from AHCPR. To order guidelines, contact AHCPR Publications Clearinghouse, PO Box 8547, Silver Spring, MD 20907; (800) 358-9295.

search that has been conducted relative to a specific disease or illness. A federal agency that is developing clinical guidelines is the ***Agency for Health Care Policy and Research (AHCPR).*** It was founded in 1989 for the purpose of developing national guidelines and to enhance the quality, appropriateness, and effectiveness of care (Bednar, 1993) (see box above).

As the movement for providing care based on guidelines continues, institutions will be challenged to incorporate clinical guidelines into the timelines for care that are developed locally. The result of this effort will mean that professionally developed clinical guidelines will be integrated into practice at the local level.

Because of the movement to provide care based on clinical guidelines, it is expected that in the future, payment for health care will also be tied to clinical guidelines. This effort will provide encouragement for care to be provided in the most cost-effective manner while ensuring that care is based on guidelines that reflect current research rather than traditional practice.

With the present efforts to improve the health care system in the United States and to provide universal health coverage while controlling costs, managed care has become a key model in health care reform. Nurses should take an active role in being part of the final plan and in creating opportunities for the profession to be a leader, not a follower, in delivery of care (Hemphill and Biester, 1994).

ROLE OF THE PEDIATRIC NURSE

Pediatric nurses are involved in every aspect of a child's and family's growth and development. Nursing functions vary according to regional job structures, individual education and experience, and personal career goals. Just as clients (children and their families) present a vast and unique background, so it is that each nurse brings to the clients an individual set of variables that affects their relationship. No matter where pediatric nurses practice, their primary concern is the welfare of the child and family.

Therapeutic Relationship

The establishment of a therapeutic relationship is the essential foundation for providing quality nursing care (Price, 1993). Pediatric nurses need to be meaningfully related to children and their families and yet separate enough to distinguish their own feelings and needs. In a ***therapeutic relationship,*** caring, well-defined boundaries separate the nurse from the child and family. These boundaries are positive and professional, and promote the family's control over the child's health care (Barnsteiner and Gillis-Donovan, 1990). Both the nurse and the family are empowered, and open communication is maintained. In a ***nontherapeutic relationship,*** these boundaries are blurred, and many of the nurse's actions may serve personal needs, such as a need to feel wanted and involved, rather than the family's needs.

Exploring whether relationships with patients are therapeutic or nontherapeutic can help nurses identify problem areas early in their interactions with children and families (see Guidelines box, p. 18). Although questions for exploring types of involvement can be labeled negative or positive, no one action makes a relationship therapeutic or nontherapeutic. For example, a nurse may spend additional time with the family but still recognize his or her own needs and maintain professional separateness. An important clue to nontherapeutic relationships is the staff's concerns about their peer's actions with the family.

Family Advocacy/Caring

Although the nurse is responsible to self, the profession, and the institution of employment, the primary responsibility is to the consumer of nursing services, the child and family. The nurse must work with members of the family, identifying *their* goals and needs, and plan interventions that best meet the defined problems. As an advocate, the nurse assists children and their families in making informed choices and acting in the child's best interest (Rushton, 1993). Advocacy involves ensuring that families are aware of all available health services, informed adequately of treatments and procedures, involved in the child's care, and encouraged to change or support existing health care practices. The United Nations Declaration of the Rights of the Child (see box on p. 19) provides guidelines for nursing practice to ensure that every child receives optimum care. The nurse uses this knowledge to adapt care for the child's optimum physical and emotional well-being.

As nurses care for children and families, they must demonstrate ***caring,*** expressing compassion and empathy for others. Aspects of caring embody the concept of atraumatic care and the development of a therapeutic relationship with clients. Parents perceive caring as a sign of quality nursing care, which is often focused on the nontechnical needs of the child and family. Parents describe "personable" care as actions by the nurse, including acknowledging the parent's presence, listening, making the parent feel comfortable in the hospital environment, involving the parent and child in the nursing care, showing interest and concern for their welfare, showing affection and sensitivity to the parent and child, communicating with them, and individualizing the nursing care. Parents perceive "personable" nursing care as

GUIDELINES

Exploring Your Relationships with Children and Families

To foster therapeutic relationships with children and families, you must first become aware of your caregiving style, including how effectively you take care of yourself. The following questions should help you understand the therapeutic quality of your professional relationships.

NEGATIVE ACTIONS

Are you overinvolved with children and their families?
- Do you work overtime to care for the family?
- Do you spend off-duty time with children's families either in or out of the hospital?
- Do you call frequently (either the hospital or home) to see how the family is doing?
- Do you show favoritism toward certain patients?
- Do you buy clothes, toys, food, or other items for the child and family?
- Do you compete with other staff members for the affection of certain patients and families?
- Do other staff members comment to you about your closeness to the family?
- Do you attempt to influence families' decisions rather than facilitate their informed decision making?

Are you underinvolved with children and families?
- Do you restrict parent or visitor access to children, using excuses such as the unit is too busy?
- Do you focus on the technical aspects of care and lose sight of the person who is the patient?

Are you overinvolved with children and underinvolved with their parents?
- Do you become critical when parents don't visit their children?
- Do you compete with parents for their children's affection?

POSITIVE ACTIONS

Do you strive to empower families?
- Do you explore families' strengths and needs in an effort to increase family involvement?
- Have you developed teaching skills to instruct families rather than doing everything for them?
- Do you work with families to find ways to decrease their dependence on health care providers?
- Can you separate families' needs from your own needs?

Do you strive to empower yourself?
- Are you aware of your emotional responses to different people and situations?
- Do you seek to understand how your own family experiences influence reactions to patients and families, especially as they affect tendencies toward overinvolvement or underinvolvement?
- Do you have a calming influence, not one that will amplify emotionality?
- Have you developed interpersonal skills in addition to technical skills?
- Have you learned about ethnic and religious family patterns?
- Do you communicate directly with persons with whom you are upset or take issue?
- Are you able to "step back" and withdraw emotionally, if not physically, when emotional overload occurs, yet remain committed?
- Do you take care of yourself and your needs?
- Do you maintain clear, open communication?
- Do you periodically interview family members to determine their current issues (e.g., feelings, attitudes, responses, wishes), communicate these findings to peers, and update records?
- Do you avoid relying on initial interview data, assumptions, or gossip regarding families?
- Do you ask questions if families are not participating in care?
- Do you assess families for feelings of anxiety, fear, intimidation, worry about making a mistake, a perceived lack of competence to care for their child, or fear of health care professionals' overstepping their boundaries into family territory or vice versa?
- Do you explore these issues with family members and provide encouragement and support to enable families to help themselves?
- Do you keep communication channels open among self, family, physicians, and other care providers?
- Do you resolve conflicts and misunderstandings directly with those who are involved?
- Do you clarify information for families or seek the appropriate person to do so?

Do you recognize that from time to time a therapeutic relationship can change to a social relationship or an intimate friendship?
- Are you able to acknowledge the fact when it occurs and understand why it happened?
- Can you ensure that there is someone else who is more objective and can take your place in the therapeutic relationship?

Data from Barnsteiner J, Gillis-Donovan J: Being related and separate: a standard for therapeutic relationships, *MCN* 15(4):223-228, 1990; Fochtman D: Therapeutic relationships, *J Pediatr Oncol Nurs* 8(1):1-2, 1991 (editorial); and Fochtman D: Commitment, *J Pediatr Oncol Nurs* 8(3):103-104, 1991 (editorial).

being integral to establishing a positive relationship (Price, 1993).

The nurse is aware of the needs of children and works with all caregivers to ensure that these fundamental requirements are met. This often necessitates that the nurse expand the boundaries of practice to less traditional settings. The nurse may be involved in education, political/legislative change, rehabilitation, screening, administration, and even engineering and architecture. Regardless of how removed from direct patient care individual nurses become, they continue to foster health care practices that promote the well-being of children by incorporating knowledge of child growth and development into particular roles of practice. For example, as educator the nurse has the primary responsibility of helping others learn about and care for children. Their audience may be other nurses, parents, schoolteachers, other members of the health team, or the general public. In some states nurses are involved in mass media programs for immunization of all children.

Disease Prevention/Health Promotion

The trends toward health care have been prevention of illness and maintenance of health, rather than treatment of disease or disability. Nursing has kept pace with this change,

UNITED NATIONS' DECLARATION OF THE RIGHTS OF THE CHILD

All children need:
- To be free from discrimination
- To develop physically and mentally in freedom and dignity
- To have a name and nationality
- To have adequate nutrition, housing, recreation, and medical services
- To receive special treatment if handicapped
- To receive love, understanding, and material security
- To receive an education and develop his or her abilities
- To be the first to receive protection in disaster
- To be protected from neglect, cruelty, and exploitation
- To be brought up in a spirit of friendship among people

especially in the area of child care. In 1965 specialized ***pediatric nurse practitioner (PNP)*** programs began to develop that have led to several specialized ambulatory or primary care roles for nurses. The thrust of these programs has been to educate nurses beyond the basic preparational stage in areas of child health maintenance so that all children can receive high-quality care (Lancaster and Lancaster, 1993). The practitioner programs have expanded to prepare school nurse, developmental, and oncology pediatric nurse practitioners. Although the curriculum varies, the course content generally includes history taking, physical diagnosis, growth and development, health education, pharmacology, counseling, common childhood problems, and planning care for individuals and groups. Most of these programs are now part of graduate nursing education.

The ***clinical nurse specialist (CNS)*** role has been developed in an attempt to provide expert nursing care. In addition, the CNS serves as a role model for staff's clinical practice, as a researcher to validate nursing observations and interventions, as a change agent within the health care system, and as a consultant/teacher to the health care team (Naylor and Brooten, 1993). The clinical specialist is competent in providing nursing care during all stages of illness or wellness and functions in any of the settings where patients may be found—the hospital, home, community, clinic, or long-term facility. The CNS role has developed within each of the traditional specialty areas and includes subspecialties, such as cardiovascular, oncologic, and neurologic pediatric CNS. The educational preparation includes a graduate degree in nursing. Several graduate programs now combine the PNP and CNS roles. Although the title for the merged roles varies, these nurses are commonly called ***advanced nurse practitioners (ANP*** or ***ARNP)*** (Gleeson and others, 1990; Schroer, 1991).

Every nurse involved with child care must practice preventive health. Regardless of the identified problem, the role of the nurse is to plan care that fosters every aspect of growth and development. Based on a thorough assessment process, problems related to nutrition, immunizations, safety, dental care, development, socialization, discipline, or schooling frequently become obvious. Once the problem is identified, the nurse acts to intervene directly or to refer the family to other health persons or agencies.

The best approach to prevention is education and anticipatory guidance. In this book each chapter on health promotion includes sections on anticipatory guidance. An appreciation of the hazards or conflicts of each developmental period enables the nurse to guide parents regarding childrearing practices aimed at preventing potential problems. One of the most significant examples is safety. Since each age-group is at risk for special types of injuries, preventive teaching can help prevent most injuries, thus significantly lowering permanent disability and mortality from injuries in children.

Prevention also involves less obvious aspects of child care. Besides preventing physical disease or injury, the nurse's role is also to promote mental health. For example, it is not sufficient to administer immunizations without regard for the psychologic trauma associated with the procedure. Optimum health involves the practice of good medicine with a humane approach to health care; the nurse is often the one professional capable of ensuring "humanity."

Health Teaching

Health teaching is inseparable from family advocacy and prevention. Health teaching may be a direct goal of the nurse, such as during parenting classes, or may be indirect, such as helping parents and children understand a diagnosis or medical treatment, encouraging children to ask questions about their bodies, referring families to health-related professional or lay groups, supplying patients with appropriate literature, and providing anticipatory guidance.

Health teaching is often one area in which nurses need preparation and practice with competent role models, because it involves transmitting information at the child and family's level of understanding and desire for information. As an effective educator, the nurse focuses on giving appropriate health teaching with generous feedback and evaluation to promote learning.

Support/Counseling

Attention to emotional needs requires support and sometimes counseling. Frequently the role of child advocate or health teacher is supportive by the very nature of the individualized approach. Support can be offered in many ways, the most common of which include listening, touching, and physical presence. The last two are most helpful with children because they facilitate nonverbal communication.

Counseling involves a mutual exchange of ideas and opinions that provides the basis for mutual problem solving. It involves support, as well as teaching, techniques to foster expression of feelings or thoughts, and approaches to help the family cope with stress. Optimally, counseling not only helps resolve a crisis or problem, but also enables the family to attain a higher level of functioning, greater self-esteem, and closer relationships. Although counseling is often the role of nurses in more specialized areas, counseling techniques are discussed in various sections of the text to help students and nurses cope with immediate crises and refer families for additional professional assistance.

Restorative Role

The most basic of all nursing roles is the restoration of health through caregiving activities. Nurses are intimately involved with meeting the physical and emotional needs of children, including feeding, bathing, toileting, dressing, security, and socialization. Although they are responsible for instituting physicians' orders, they are also held singularly accountable for their own actions and judgments regardless of written orders.

A significant aspect of restoration of health is continual assessment and evaluation of physical status. Indeed, the concentrated focus throughout the text on physical assessment, pathophysiology, and scientific rationale for therapy is to assist the nurse in decision making regarding health status. The nurse must be aware of normal findings in order to intelligently identify and document deviations. In addition, the pediatric nurse never loses sight of the emotional and developmental needs of the individual child, which can significantly influence the course of the disease process.

Coordination/Collaboration

The nurse, as a member of the health team, collaborates and coordinates nursing services with the activities of other professionals. Working in isolation does not serve the child's best interest. First, the concept of "holistic care" can only be realized through a unified interdisciplinary approach. Second, being aware of individual contributions and limitations to the child's care, the nurse must collaborate with other specialists to provide for high-quality health services. Failure to recognize limitations can be nontherapeutic at best and destructive at worst. For example, the nurse who feels competent in counseling but who is really inadequate in this area may not only prevent the child from dealing with a crisis but may also impede future success with a qualified professional.

Even nurses who practice in isolated geographic areas widely separated from other health professionals cannot be considered independent. Every nurse works interdependently with the child and family, collaborating on needs and interventions so that the final care plan is one that truly meets the child's needs. Unfortunately, this is one aspect of collaboration and coordination that is lacking in health care planning. Often numerous disciplines work together to formulate a comprehensive approach without consulting with clients regarding their ideas or preferences. The nurse is in a vital position to include consumers in their care, either directly or indirectly, by communicating their thoughts to the health team.

Ethical Decision Making*

Ethical dilemmas arise when competing moral considerations underlie various alternatives. Parents, nurses, physicians, and other health care team members may reach different but morally defensible decisions by assigning different weight to the competing moral values. These competing moral values may include ***autonomy,*** the patient's right to be self-governing; ***nonmaleficence,*** the obligation to minimize or prevent harm; ***beneficence,*** the obligation to promote the patient's well-being, and ***justice,*** the concept of fairness (Erlen and Burns, 1992). Thus, nurses must determine the most beneficial or least harmful action within the framework of societal mores, professional practice standards, the law, institutional rules, religious traditions, the family's value system, and the nurse's personal values.

When ethical conflicts occur, nurses may experience conflicting loyalties to their profession, colleagues, patients and families, institutions, and society. Moreover, the nurse's role in ethical decision making can be ambiguous. A nurse may be obliged to carry out procedures based on physician orders or hospital policy that are inconsistent with the patient's best interest. At times, members of the health care team do not seek the nurse's input or involvement, leaving the nurse with incomplete information about the clinical situation or without a voice in decision making.

The role of nurses as members of the health care team justifies their participation in collaborative ethical decision making. Nurses routinely use systematic problem-solving skills to resolve clinical problems. Each decision requires the nurse to collect pertinent physiologic and psychosocial data, assess relevant values held by the patient and family, and incorporate those data into a plan of care. Each of these activities is a crucial component of ethical decision making.

Furthermore, since nurses spend the most time directly caring for the child, they are in a unique position to provide insight about the patient's condition and response to therapy. In addition, they assist families in dealing with their grief and stress and often interpret information regarding the child's condition, prognosis, and treatment options to help families make informed decisions. Because of their relationship to families, nurses are often able to represent the child's and parents' values, beliefs, and preferences, thus serving as an important liaison for communication between the family and other health team members.

Participation in ethical decision making requires knowledge of ethical theory and principles, and skills in moral reasoning, communication, and group process. Nurses have an individual responsibility to clarify their personal values and beliefs and to be informed about contemporary ethical thinking; legal, institutional, and public policy; and professional guidelines.

The nurse can also use the professional code of ethics for guidance. A code of ethics provides one means for professional self-regulation. The Code for Nurses by the American Nurses' Association focuses on the nurse's accountability and responsibility to the client and emphasizes the nursing role as an independent professional role that upholds its own legal liability (see box on p. 21).

Nurses must prepare themselves systematically for collaborative ethical decision making. This can be accomplished through formal coursework, continuing education, contemporary literature, and working to establish an environment conducive to ethical discourse. Moreover, nurses must be knowledgeable about mechanisms for dispute resolution, case review by ethics committees, procedural safeguards, state statutes, and case law.

Nurses may face ethical issues regarding patient care,

*Cindy Hylton Rushton, RN,C, PhD, wrote this section.

CODE FOR NURSES

1. The nurse provides services with respect for human dignity and the uniqueness of the client unrestricted by considerations of social or economic status, personal attributes, or the nature of health problems.
2. The nurse safeguards the client's right to privacy by judiciously protecting information of a confidential nature.
3. The nurse acts to safeguard the client and the public when health care and safety are affected by the incompetent, unethical, or illegal practice of any person.
4. The nurse assumes responsibility and accountability for individual nursing judgments and actions.
5. The nurse maintains competence in nursing.
6. The nurse exercises informed judgment and uses individual competence and qualifications as criteria in seeking consultation, accepting responsibilities, and delegating nursing activities to others.
7. The nurse participates in activities that contribute to the ongoing development of the profession's body of knowledge.
8. The nurse participates in the profession's efforts to implement and improve standards of nursing.
9. The nurse participates in the profession's efforts to establish and maintain conditions of employment conducive to high-quality nursing care.
10. The nurse participates in the profession's effort to protect the public from misinformation and misrepresentation and to maintain the integrity of nursing.
11. The nurse collaborates with members of the health professions and other citizens in promoting community and national efforts to meet the health needs of the public.

such as the use of lifesaving measures for very-low-birth-weight newborns or the terminally ill child's right to refuse treatment. They may struggle with questions regarding truthfulness, balancing their rights and their responsibilities in caring for children with AIDS, whistle-blowing, or resource allocation. Throughout the text such dilemmas are addressed in boxes titled Thinking Critically About . . . The conflicting ethical arguments are presented to help nurses clarify their value judgments when confronted with similar sensitive issues.

Research

Practicing nurses should contribute to research, since they are the individuals observing human responses to health and illness. Unfortunately, few nurses systematically record or analyze such observations. For example, pediatric nurses devise innovative methods to encourage children to comply with treatments. Only if these interventions are clinically evaluated and shared with other nurses, especially through publications, can a body of knowledge on nursing practice develop.

Research also implies a questioning of *why* something is effective and *if* there is a better approach. Evaluation is essential to the nursing process, and research is one of the best ways to accomplish this. Therefore nurses need to be more involved in research and in applying research findings to their practice. Throughout the text, research relevant to nursing of children and families is incorporated as appropriate and is also highlighted in the Thinking Critically About . . . boxes. Research findings are presented to encourage nurses to base their practice on theoretic foundations, not tradition, and additional questions may be proposed in the hope of stimulating research in a particular area.

Health Care Planning

Up to this point, the nurse's role has been viewed through the nucleus of a family. However, the nursing role is far more extensive and includes the community or society as a whole. Traditionally nurses have been involved in public health care, on either a continuous or an episodic basis. Rarely, however, have nurses been involved in health care planning, especially on a political or legislative level. Their role must also involve the decision-making body of government. Nursing, as the largest health care profession, needs to have a voice, especially as family/consumer advocate. This does not mean that the nurse must hold public office. Rather, it suggests knowledge and awareness of community needs, interest in government formulation of bills, support of politicians to ensure passage (or rejection) of significant legislation, and active involvement in groups dedicated to the welfare of children, such as professional nursing societies, parent-teacher organizations, parent support groups, religious organizations, and voluntary organizations.

Health care planning involves not only providing new services, but also promoting the highest quality of existing ones. Nursing needs to ensure the excellence of its own profession through each individual member, who practices according to the Code of Nurses and standards of practice. A ***standard of practice*** is the level of performance that is expected of a professional. Pediatric nurses are obligated to follow the Standards of Maternal-Child Health Nursing (see box on p. 22) and specific standards for their specialty, such as pediatric oncology nursing or school nursing.* They should also be involved in making certain their colleagues implement the standards, through education, role modeling, and supervision.

Throughout the text the highest standards of nursing practice are continually reflected in the emphasis on thorough assessment, focus on scientific rationale as the basis for care, summary of nursing care goals and responsibilities, and comprehensive discussion of growth and development. Family-centered principles are continually evident in the consideration of dynamics affecting the child, parents, siblings, and extended members. The nurse is viewed as a vital component of the health care delivery system. Although nursing functions are clearly outlined, nursing responsibilities must be equally emphasized.

*Available from the Association of Pediatric Oncology Nurses, 11512 Allecingie Parkway, Richmond, VA 23235, (804) 379-9150; and the National Association of School Nurses, Lamplighter Lane, P.O. Box 1300, Scarborough, ME 04074, (207) 883-2117.

AMERICAN NURSES' ASSOCIATION STANDARDS OF MATERNAL AND CHILD HEALTH NURSING PRACTICE

Standard I: The nurse helps children and parents attain and maintain optimum health.
Standard II: The nurse assists families to achieve and maintain a balance between the personal growth needs of individual family members and optimum family functioning.
Standard III: The nurse intervenes with vulnerable clients and families at risk to prevent potential developmental and health problems.
Standard IV: The nurse promotes an environment free of hazards to reproduction, growth and development, wellness, and recovery from illness.
Standard V: The nurse detects changes in health status and deviations from optimum development.
Standard VI: The nurse carries out appropriate interventions and treatment to facilitate survival and recovery from illness.
Standard VII: The nurse assists clients and families to understand and cope with developmental and traumatic situations during illness, childbearing, childrearing, and childhood.
Standard VIII: The nurse actively pursues strategies to enhance access to and utilization of adequate health care services.
Standard IX: The nurse improves maternal and child health nursing practice through evaluation of practice, education, and research.

From American Nurses' Association: *Standards of Maternal and Child Health Nursing Practice,* Washington, DC, 1983, The Association. (As of this writing, unrevised and out of print.)

FUTURE TRENDS

The present shift in focus from treatment of disease to promotion of health is likely to further expand nurses' roles in ambulatory care, with prevention and health teaching receiving a major emphasis. As prospective payment becomes a certainty in pediatric care, the need for home care and community health services will necessitate that nurses become more independent and highly skilled beyond the traditional care settings. Both of these trends are illustrated throughout the book, with increased emphasis on prevention through anticipatory guidance, child health and family assessment, and discharge planning and home care.

Technologic advances will also influence pediatric nurses' roles. Increasing technical skills related to patient care, as well as the demand for computer knowledge in the work setting, are inevitable future trends. As more positions are created in the health care system that do not require a nursing background, such as "patient care educator," nurses will be required to continually update their knowledge and prove their unique contribution.

Changing demographics will also impact pediatric nursing. While the actual number of children under age 18 years will increase from 64.3 million in 1990 to an estimated 67.4 million in 2000, their relative importance in terms of proportion of the total population will decrease from 26% to 25%. In other words, the adult population is growing faster than the pediatric population. Accompanying this trend is a decrease in younger children and an increase in older children, as well as a decrease in the white population with an increase in minority groups (Evans, 1989). For example, the fertility rate (per 1000 women ages 15 to 44 years) is 62.8 for non-Hispanic whites, 89.0 for non-Hispanic blacks, and 107.7 for Hispanics (Childbearing patterns, 1993). Such changes will impact the delivery of health care, with problems of adolescents and minority groups taking on more significance. As the elderly make up a larger percentage of the population, health care dollars will be split between the youngest and the oldest groups, with shrinking resources having to meet the needs of both. Nurses will need to keep abreast of developments in adolescent medicine and continually adapt their care to the cultural milieu in which they practice. An ever-present challenge will be cost containment without sacrificing quality care.

PROCESS OF NURSING CHILDREN AND FAMILIES

A systematic thought process is essential to a profession, as it assists the professional in meeting the needs of a client. The ***nursing process*** is the framework for the practice of professional nursing. It is a method of problem identification and problem solving that describes what the nurse actually does. The ***five-step model*** accepted as the nursing process includes assessment, diagnosis (problem identification), planning (with outcome development), implementation, and evaluation.

Assessment

Assessment is a continuous process that is operative at all phases of problem solving and is the foundation for decision making. Derived through multiple nursing skills, it consists of the purposeful collection, classification, and analysis of data from a variety of sources. To ensure an accurate and comprehensive assessment, the nurse must consider information about the patient's biophysical, psychologic, sociocultural, and spiritual background.

Nursing Diagnosis

The second stage of the nursing process is problem identification and nursing diagnosis. At this point the nurse must interpret and make decisions about the data gathered. The nurse then organizes or clusters the data into similar categories to identify significant areas and makes one of the following decisions:

1. No dysfunctional health problems are evident; no interventions are indicated.
2. High risk for dysfunctional health problems exist; interventions are needed to facilitate health promotion.
3. Actual dysfunctional health problems are evident; interventions are needed to facilitate health promotion.

The nursing diagnosis is the naming of the cue clusters that are obtained during the assessment phase. NANDA's currently accepted definition of the term ***nursing diagnosis*** is "a clinical judgment about individual, family, or community responses to actual and potential health problems/life processes. Nursing diagnoses provide the basis for selection

CLASSIFICATION SYSTEMS FOR NURSING DIAGNOSES

HUMAN RESPONSE PATTERNS*

Exchanging—Involves mutual giving and receiving
Communicating—Involves sending messages
Relating—Involves establishing bonds
Valuing—Involves the assigning of relative worth
Choosing—Involves the selection of alternatives
Moving—Involves activity
Perceiving—Involves the reception of information
Knowing—Involves the meaning associated with information
Feeling—Involves the subjective awareness of sensation or affect

FUNCTIONAL HEALTH PATTERNS†

Health perception–health management pattern—Perceptions related to general health management and preventive practices
Nutritional-metabolic pattern—Intake of food and fluids related to metabolic requirements
Elimination pattern—Regularity and control of excretory functions, bowel, bladder, skin, and wastes
Activity-exercise pattern—Activity patterns that require energy expenditure and provide for rest
Sleep-rest pattern—Effectiveness of sleep and rest periods
Cognitive-perceptual pattern—Adequacy of language, cognitive skills, and perception related to required or desired activities; includes pain perception
Self-perception–self-concept pattern—Beliefs and evaluation of self-worth
Role-relationship pattern—Family and social roles, especially parent-child relationships
Sexuality-reproductive pattern—Problems or potential problems with sexuality or reproduction
Coping-stress tolerance pattern—Stress tolerance level and coping patterns, including support systems
Value-belief pattern—Values, goals, or beliefs that influence health-related decisions and actions

*Modified from the North American Nursing Diagnosis Association, Ninth Conference, 1990.
†From Gordon M: *Manual of nursing diagnosis, 1995-1996,* St Louis, 1995, Mosby.

of nursing interventions to achieve outcomes for which the nurse is accountable" (Carroll-Johnson, 1991).

Both NANDA and Marjory Gordon have developed frameworks or classification systems for nursing diagnoses. NANDA bases its framework on 9 human response patterns, and Gordon bases hers on 11 functional health patterns (see box above and Appendix E). Additional research is needed to broaden the list of nursing diagnoses, especially for specialty areas such as pediatrics, and refine a universally accepted taxonomy.

The nursing diagnosis is composed of three components: problem, etiology, and signs and symptoms (often referred to as ***PES***). The first component—the ***problem statement***—describes the child's response to health pattern deficits in the child, family, or community. This is the patient's response to disturbances of life processes, patterns, functions, or development, including those occurring secondary to disease.

Not all children will have actual health problems. Some may have a potential health problem, which is a risk state requiring nursing intervention to prevent the development of an actual problem. Potential health problems indicate the presence of ***risk factors*** (signs indicating a potential health problem), which predispose a child and family to a dysfunctional health pattern and are limited to individuals at greater risk than the population as a whole. Intervention is directed toward reducing risk factors. To differentiate actual from potential health problems, the words "high risk" are included in the nursing diagnosis statement (e.g., "High risk for infection").

The second component, the ***etiology,*** describes the physiologic, situational, and maturational factors that cause the problem or influence its development. The etiology is written using NANDA diagnostic categories (e.g., "Noncompliance related to powerlessness"). In using the PES format, it is important that the nurse not link the problem statement and etiology with words that imply cause and effect. Etiologies are probable causes; using words that imply cause and effect can result in legal or professional difficulties. Although a direct cause-effect relationship may not be involved, the etiology does influence the problem. Therefore the phrase "related to" is used to indicate a relationship between the problem and its etiology.

Differentiating among various etiologies is critically important because *interventions to alter the health problem are directed toward the etiology.* This is a primary concept in understanding the nursing process and the PES format. For example, a problem statement of "Noncompliance in dietary restrictions" could have various etiologies, such as (1) knowledge deficit, (2) denial of illness, (3) low economic resources, or (4) cultural conflict. Interventions for a knowledge deficit would be very different from interventions for low economic resources.

The third component, ***signs and symptoms,*** refers to a cluster of cues and/or defining characteristics that are derived from patient assessment and indicate actual health problems. When a defining characteristic is essential for the diagnosis to be made, it is considered critical. These critical defining characteristics help differentiate between diagnostic categories. For example, in deciding between the diagnostic categories related to family function and coping, the defining characteristics are critical in choosing the most appropriate nursing diagnosis (see Family Focus box, p. 24).

Nursing diagnoses do *not* describe everything that nursing does. Nursing practice consists of three dimensions: dependent, interdependent, and independent activities. The differences reside in the source of authority for the action (Hickey, 1990). ***Dependent activities*** are those areas of nursing practice that hold the nurse accountable for implementing the prescribed medical regimen. ***Interdependent activities*** are those areas of nursing practice in which medical and nursing responsibility and accountability overlap and require collaboration between the two disciplines. ***Independent activities*** are those areas of nursing practice that are the direct responsibility of the nurse.

Throughout the text Nursing Care Plans incorporate nursing diagnoses that relate to the specific condition or disorder. Since nursing diagnoses should only prescribe interventions that nurses can perform independently or interdependently, nursing interventions related to medical management are identified by an asterisk.

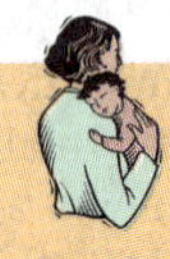

FAMILY FOCUS
Using Defining Characteristics to Select an Appropriate Nursing Diagnosis

An 18-month-old only child is admitted with respiratory distress and a presumptive diagnosis of epiglottitis. Initial nursing actions are focused on the physiologic status of the child. As the condition stabilizes, family assessment data are gathered. The child's immunizations are current, he is clean and well nourished, and his developmental age is appropriate. The parents are present at admission. Both are employed, and the child is cared for by the maternal grandparents. The mother is distraught about the sudden onset of the respiratory distress. She states that earlier just a "runny nose" was present. She asks appropriate questions and seems to understand that epiglottitis is a sudden illness that typically follows symptoms of a cold. She asks what she can do to make her child more comfortable and less fearful, and she is able to implement the suggestions. The father supports both the child and the mother but assumes a more passive, "listening" role.

At least three nursing diagnoses that relate to family/parent situations can be considered. The first step is to review the definition and defining characteristics for each and decide which is most appropriate for this family:

Altered parenting—Inability of nurturing figure to create an environment that promotes optimum growth and development of another human being

Selected defining characteristics:

- Inattentive to infant/child needs
- Inappropriate caretaking behaviors

Family coping: potential for growth—Family member has effectively managed adaptive tasks involved with client's health challenge and is exhibiting desire and readiness for enhanced health and growth in regard to self and in relation to client

Selected defining characteristics:

- Family member attempts to describe growth impact or crisis on own values, priorities, goals, or relationships

Altered family process—Inability of family system (household members) to meet needs of members, carry out family functions, or maintain communication for mutual growth and maturation

Selected defining characteristics:

- Inability of family members to relate to each other for mutual growth and maturation
- Failure to send and receive clear messages
- Inability to accept and receive help

Among these choices, the most appropriate nursing diagnosis is "Family coping: potential for growth." The parents are attentive to the child's needs and appear to have appropriate caregiving skills. The sudden illness of the child has disrupted the family's pattern, but the mother demonstrates effective coping and the ability to learn and implement new comforting skills. The other two diagnoses require some maladaptive feature, which is not found in this situation.

Planning

Once the nursing diagnoses have been identified, a plan of care is developed and outcomes or goals are established. The *outcome* is the projected change in a patient's health status, clinical condition, or behavior that occurs after nursing interventions are instituted. The ultimate goal of nursing care is to convert the nursing diagnoses into a desired health state. The plan must be formulated before the interventions are developed and implemented.

The end point of the planning phase is the development of the nursing plan of care. The care plans in this text provide guidelines for the care of children and families with a particular problem and are standard care plans as opposed to individualized care plans (Table 1-8). ***Standard care plans*** are plans that are sufficiently broad to account for situations that may develop in patients with particular problems. For this reason, the care plans often have numerous nursing diagnoses, both expected and potential. These possible nursing diagnoses guide patient observation and data collection in monitoring the development of adverse reactions.

Individualized care plans are plans that are concerned with only those diagnoses that apply to the particular patient situation. Consequently, in actual practice all the problems presented in a standard care plan may not be relevant. When a standard nursing care plan is used as a guide in developing an individualized plan of care, the problems not pertinent to the situation are eliminated and the outcomes are individualized to the specific situation. To help the reader develop an individualized care plan, the nursing diagnoses in the text are listed in order of priority. In general, potential problems are discussed toward the end of the plan, except in instances where nursing interventions are essential in preventing a potential problem from becoming an actual problem. An example is the nursing diagnosis of high risk for suffocation in the care of a child with epiglottitis, where the intervention of avoiding examination of the throat is essential to prevent complete airway obstruction.

Implementation

The phase of implementation begins when the nurse puts the selected intervention into action and accumulates feedback regarding its effects. The feedback returns in the form of observation and communication and provides a data base on which to evaluate the outcome of the nursing intervention. Throughout the implementation stage, the patient's physical safety and psychologic comfort in terms of atraumatic care are the main concerns.

Evaluation

Evaluation is the last step in the decision-making process. The nurse gathers, sorts, and analyzes data to determine if (1) the goal has been met, (2) the plan requires modification, or (3) another alternative should be considered. Observation guidelines are included in the standard care plans to help the reader identify methods of evaluating whether the goals or outcomes are achieved. The evaluation stage either completes the nursing process or serves as the basis for selection of other alternatives for intervention in solving the specific problem.

Documentation

Although documentation is not one of the five steps of the nursing process, it is essential for evaluation. The nurse can assess and identify problems, plan, and implement without documentation; however, evaluation is best performed with written evidence of progress toward outcomes. The

TABLE 1-8 Characteristics of Standard and Individualized Nursing Care Plans

	STANDARD CARE PLAN*	INDIVIDUALIZED CARE PLAN
Assessment	Information is specific only to problem	Information is specific to identified problem and to child and family
Nursing diagnosis	All probable nursing diagnoses with general etiologic factors are considered	Only nursing diagnoses specific to child and family are considered; cause of disease directs actual plan of care
Planning	Goals are broad and represent patient goals	Goals are specific and reflect patient outcomes
Implementation	Nursing interventions are broad and are applicable to most patients with problem	Nursing interventions are specific and provide direction for nursing care of individual patient
Evaluation	Progress patient is *expected* to make is identified	Progress patient has actually made toward outcome is identified

*Describes format used in care plans in the text; may differ from other types of standardized nursing care plans.

GUIDELINES
Documentation of Nursing Care

Initial assessments and reassessments
Nursing diagnoses and/or patient care needs
Interventions identified to meet the patient's nursing care needs
Nursing care provided
Patient's response to, and the outcomes of, the care provided
Abilities of patient and/or, as appropriate, significant other(s) to manage continuing care needs after discharge

patient's medical record should include evidence of those elements listed in the Guidelines box.

The nursing process has become an integral part of professional practice. The Joint Commission on Accreditation of Healthcare Organizations (JCAHO) has also incorporated the nursing process into the accreditation process. The first standard on which nursing service is evaluated states that individualized, goal-directed nursing care is provided to patients through the use of the nursing process. The JCAHO is actively involved in accrediting many health care providers. Currently, hospitals, nursing homes, ambulatory services, and home health agencies can choose to be accredited by this group.

KEY POINTS

- "Healthy People 2000" sets the health care objectives for the 1990s and focuses on prevention as the method of achieving its goals.
- Although the infant mortality rate in the United States is at an all-time low, the United States lags significantly behind most other major countries, such as Canada.
- Low birth weight, which is closely related to early gestational age, is considered the leading cause of neonatal death in the United States.
- Injuries are the leading cause of death in children over age 1 year, with the majority of injuries being due to motor vehicle injuries.
- Childhood morbidity encompasses acute illness, chronic disease, and disability.
- Eighty percent of childhood illnesses are attributable to infections, with respiratory infections occurring two to three times as often as all other illnesses combined.
- The "new morbidity" refers to behavioral, social, and educational problems that can significantly alter a child's health.
- Children's developmental stage and their environment are important determinants in the prevalence of injuries at a given age and thus help to direct preventive measures.
- Two strategies for injury prevention in children are (1) ***passive,*** which provides automatic protection by product and environmental design; and (2) ***active,*** which persuades people to change their behaviors for increased self-protection.
- During the first half of the 1900s, public health initiatives, such as environmental strategies to control infection and the development of antibiotics, were the major advances leading to decreased childhood deaths.
- During the latter half of the 1900s, the advancement and application of medical knowledge and technology, specifically in care of high-risk and low-birth-weight newborns, lowered the number of deaths in children, especially the neonatal mortality rate.
- The work of Lillian Wald, a social reformer, has had far-reaching effects on child health and nursing. She started visiting nurse services in New York City and was instrumental in establishing the role of the first full-time school nurse.
- Primary nursing involves care and accountability by one nurse for a small patient population. Associate nurses making up the primary core share patient care responsibilities in the absence of the primary nurse.
- The pediatric nurse's roles include a therapeutic relationship, family advocacy, disease prevention/health promotion, health teaching, support-counseling, coordination/collaboration, ethical decision making, research, and health care planning.
- With the shift in focus from treatment of disease to promotion of health, nurses' roles are expanding outside traditional health care facilities, such as in ambulatory care centers, schools, and the family's home.
- The process of nursing children and families includes accurate and comprehensive *assessment,* analysis and synthesis of assessment data to arrive at a ***nursing diagnosis, planning*** of care, ***implementation*** of the plan, and ***evaluation*** of interventions.
- Changing demographics in the United States will result in greater significance of adolescents' and minority groups' problems and decreasing resources for health care.

REFERENCES

Agran PF, Winn DG, Anderson CL: Differences in child pedestrian injury events by location, *Pediatrics* 93(2):284-288, 1994.

Ahmann E: Family-centered care: the time has come, *Pediatr Nurs* 20(1):52-53, 1994.

American Academy of Pediatrics, Committee on Early Childhood, Adoption and Dependent Care: Initial medical evaluation of an adopted child, *Pediatrics* 88(3):642-644, 1991.

American Academy of Pediatrics, Committee on Genetics: Folic acid for the prevention of neural tube defects, *Pediatrics* 92(3):493-494, 1993a.

American Academy of Pediatrics, Committee on Psychosocial Aspects of Child and Family Health: The pediatrician and the "new morbidity," *Pediatrics* 92(5):731-733, 1993b.

American Academy of Pediatrics and American College of Obstetricians and Gynecologists: *Guidelines for perinatal care,* ed 3, Elk Grove Village, IL, 1992, The Academy.

Barnsteiner J, Gillis-Donovan J: Being related and separate: a standard for therapeutic relationships *MCN* 15(4):223-228, 1990.

Bednar B: Developing clinical practice guidelines: an interview with Ada Jacox, *ANNA J* 20(2):121-126, 1993.

Carroll-Johnson RM, editor: *Classification of nursing diagnoses: proceedings of the Ninth Conference,* North American Nursing Diagnosis Association (NANDA), Philadelphia, 1991, JB Lippincott.

Centers for Disease Control: National infant mortality surveillance (NIMS), 1980, *MMWR* 38(SS-3):1-46, 1989.

Childbearing patterns among selected racial/ethnic minority groups—United States, 1990, *MMWR* 42(20):398-403, 1993.

Chorba T, Reinfurt D, Hulka B: Efficacy of mandatory seat-belt use legislation, the North Carolina experience from 1983 through 1987, *JAMA* 260(24):3593-3597, 1988.

Committee on Trauma Research, Commission on Life Sciences, National Research Council, and the Institute of Medicine: *Injury in America: a continuing public health problem,* Washington, DC, 1985, National Academy Press.

Cone TE Jr: Highlights of two centuries of American pediatrics, 1776-1976, *Am J Dis Child* 130:762-775, 1976.

Coté TR and others: Bicycle helmet use among Maryland children: effect of legislation and education, *Pediatrics* 89(6, pt 2):1216-1220, 1992.

Curley M: Effects of the nursing mutual participation model of care on parental stress in the pediatric intensive care unit, *Heart Lung* 17(6):682-688, 1988.

Curley M, Wallace J: Effects of the Nursing Mutual Participation Model of Care on parental stress in the pediatric intensive care unit—a replication, *Pediatr Nurs* 7(6):377-385, 1992.

Deaths resulting from firearm- and motor-vehicle-related injuries—United States, 1968-1991, *MMWR* 43(3):37-42, 1994.

DiGuiseppi CG and others: Bicycle helmet use by children: evaluation of a community-wide helmet campaign, *JAMA* 262:2256-2261, 1989.

Division of Injury Control, Center for Environmental Health and Injury Control, Centers for Disease Control: Childhood injuries in the United States, *Am J Dis Child* 144(6):627-646, 1990.

Dunn KA, Runyan CW: Deaths at work among children and adolescents, *Am J Dis Child* 147(10):1044-1047, 1993.

Dunst C, Trivette C, Deal A: *Enabling and empowering families,* Cambridge, MA, 1988, Brookline Books.

Erlen JA, Burns JA: Demystifying ethical decision making, *Orthop Nurs* 11(1):49-53, 1992.

Evans V: Sociodemographic trends toward the 21st century. In Feeg V, editor: *Pediatric nursing: forum on the future: looking toward the 21st century,* Pitman, NJ, 1989, Anthony J Jannetti.

Faber M: A review of efforts to protect children from injury in car crashes, *Fam Community Health* 9(3):25-41, 1986.

Fingerhut LA, Ingram DD, Feldman JJ: Firearm homicide among black teenage males in metropolitan counties, *JAMA* 267(22):3054-3058, 1992.

Flint NS, Walsh M: Visiting policies in pediatrics: parents' perceptions and preferences, *J Pediatr Nurs* 3(4):237-246, 1988.

Foss R: Sociocultural perspective on child occupant protection, *Pediatrics* 80(6):886-893, 1987.

Gielen AD and others: Psychosocial factors associated with the use of bicycle helmets among children in counties with and without helmet use laws, *J Pediatr* 124(2):204-210, 1994.

Gleeson RM and others: Advanced practice nursing: a model of collaborative care, *MCN* 15(1):9-12, 1990.

Goldberg IR and others: Mental health problems among children seen in pediatric practice: prevalence and management, *Pediatrics* 73(3):278-292, 1984.

Gortmaker S and others: Chronic conditions, socioeconomic risks, and behavioral problems in children and adolescents, *Pediatrics* 85(3):267-276, 1990.

Gulaid J and others: Differences in death rates due to injury among blacks and whites, 1984, *MMWR* 37(SS-3):25-33, 1988.

Healthy people, 2000—national health promotion and disease prevention objectives, GPO 017-001-00474-0, Washington, DC, 1991, US Public Health Service.

Hemphill NP, Biester DJ: Case management in a reformed health care system, *J Pediatr Nurs* 9(2):124-125, 1994.

Hickey PW: *Nursing process handbook,* St Louis, 1990, Mosby.

Honigfeld L, Kaplan D: Native American postneonatal mortality, *Pediatrics* 80(4):575-578, 1987.

Hostetter MK and others: Medical evaluation of internationally adopted children, *N Engl J Med* 325:479-485, 1991.

Hostler S: Personal communication. Cited in Johnson BH, Jeppson ES, Redburn L: *Caring for children and families: guidelines for hospitals,* Bethesda, MD, 1992, Association for the Care of Children's Health.

Hughes JG: Conception and creation of the American Academy of Pediatrics, *Pediatrics* 92(3):469-470, 1993.

Johnson BH, Jeppson ES, Redburn L: *Caring for children and families: guidelines for hospitals,* Bethesda, MD, 1992, Association for the Care of Children's Health.

Johnson BH, McGonigel M, Kaufmann R, editors: *Guidelines and recommended practices for the Individualized Family Service Plan,* Washington, DC, 1989, Association for the Care of Children's Health.

Johnson DE and others: The health of children adopted from Romania, *JAMA* 268(24):3446-3451, 1992.

Jones CS and others: Prevention of bicycle-related injuries in childhood: role of the caregiver, *South Med J* 86(8):859-864, 1993.

Jones NE: Injury prevention: a survey of clinical practice, *J Pediatr Health Care* 6(4):182-186, 1992.

Khoury MJ, Erickson JD: Improved ascertainment of cardiovascular malformations in infants with Down's syndrome, Atlanta, 1968 through 1989: implications for the interpretation of increasing rates of cardiovascular malformations in surveillance systems, *Am J Epidemiol* 136(12):1457-1464, 1992.

Lancaster J, Lancaster W: Nurse practitioners: health care providers whose time has come, *Fam Community Health* 16(2):1-8, 1993.

Leopold J: Abraham Jacobi. In Veeder BS, editor: *Pediatric profiles,* St Louis, 1957, Mosby.

Mili F and others: Prevalance of birth defects among low-birth weight infants, *Am J Dis Child* 145(11):1313-1318, 1991.

Mortality trends and leading causes of death among adolescents and young adults—United States, 1979-1988, *MMWR* 42(23):459-462, 1993.

Naeye RL: Race and infant mortality, *Am J Dis Child* 147(10):1030-1031, 1993.

Nakamura RM and others: Excess infant mortality in an American Indian population, 1940-1990, *JAMA* 266(16):2244-2248, 1991.

National Center for Health Statistics: Advance report of final mortality statistics, 1991, *Monthly Vital Statistics Report* 42(2, suppl), 1993a.

National Center for Health Statistics: Annual summary of births, marriages, divorces, and deaths: United States, 1992, *Monthly Vital Statistics Report* 41(13), 1993b.

Naylor MD, Brooten D: The roles and functions of clinical nurse specialists, *Image J Nurs Sch* 25(1):73-78, 1993.

Newacheck P, Starfield B: Morbidity and use of ambulatory care services among poor and nonpoor children, *Am J Public Health* 78:927-933, 1988.

Nyman G: Infant temperament, childhood accidents, and hospitalization, *Clin Pediatr* 26(8):398-404, 1987.

Nursing: a social policy statement, Kansas City, MO, 1980, American Nurses' Association.

Osberg JS, DiScala D: Morbidity among pediatric motor vehicle crash victims: the effectiveness of seat belts, *Am J Public Health* 82(3):422-425, 1992.

Overpeck M and others: A comparison of the childhood health status of normal birth weight and low birth weight infants, *Public Health Rep* 104(1):58-70, 1989.

Paulson J: Injuries: the leading cause of death in children, *Curr Opin Pediatr* 1(1):192-202, 1989.

Pless I: Morbidity and mortality among the young. In Hoekelman RA and others, editors: *Primary pediatric care,* ed 2, St Louis, 1992, Mosby.

Price PJ: Parents' perceptions of the meaning of quality nursing care, *Adv Nurs Sci* 16(1):33-41, 1993.

Rivara F, Bergman A, Drake C: Parental attitudes and practices toward children as pedestrians, *Pediatrics* 84(6):1017-1021, 1989.

Runyan C, Gerken E: Epidemiology and prevention of adolescent injury: a review and research agenda, *JAMA* 262(16):2273-2279, 1989.

Rushton CH: Child/family advocacy: ethical issues, practical strategies, *Crit Care Med* 21(9):S387, 1993.

Sacks JJ and others: Bicycle-associated head injuries and deaths in the United States from 1984 through 1988: how many are preventable? *JAMA* 266(21):3016-3018, 1991.

Salmi L and others: Fatal farm injuries among young children, *Pediatrics* 83(2):267-271, 1989.

Sayre JW, Sayre RF: American children and the "children of nature," *Am J Dis Child* 130:716-723, 1976.

Scheidt P: Behavioral research toward prevention of childhood injury, *Am J Dis Child* 142(6):612-617, 1988.

Schmidt WM: Health and welfare of colonial American children, *Am J Dis Child* 130:694-701, 1976.

Schoendorf KC and others: Mortality among infants of black as compared with white college-educated parents, *N Engl J Med* 326(23):1522-1526, 1992.

Schroer K: Case management: clinical nurse specialist and nurse practitioner, converging roles, *Clin Nurs Spec* 5(4):189-194, 1991.

Scott R, Winston M: The health and welfare of the black family in the United States, *Am J Dis Child* 130:704-707, 1976.

Sharp L and others: Psychosocial problems during child health supervision visits: eliciting, then what? *Pediatrics* 89(4):619-623, 1992.

Shelton T, Jeppson E, Johnson B: *Family-centered care for children with special health care needs,* Washington, DC, 1987, Association for the Care of Children's Health.

Spence LJ and others: Fatal bicycle accidents in children: a plea for prevention, *J Pediatr Surg* 28(2):214-216, 1993.

Spivak H, Prothrow-Smith D, Hausman A: Dying is no accident, *Pediatr Clin North Am* 35(6):1339-1347, 1988.

Stewart DD: Child passenger safety: current technical issues for advocates and professionals, *Fam Community Health* 15(4):12-27, 1993.

Thompson DG: Critical pathways in the intensive care and intermediate care nurseries, *MCN* 19(1):29-32, 1994.

Update: Impact of the expanded AIDS surveillance case definition for adolescents and adults on case reporting—United States, 1993, *MMWR* 43(9):160-171, 1994.

Wegman ME: Annual summary of vital statistics—1992, *Pediatrics* 92(6):743-754, 1993.

Weinstein R: Hospital case management: the path to empowering nurses, *Pediatr Nurs* 17(3):289-293, 1991.

Widome MD: Injury illiteracy, *Pediatrics* 89(6):1091-1093, 1992.

Wilcox AJ, Skjaerven R: Birth weight and perinatal mortality: the effect of gestational age, *Am J Public Health* 82(3):378-382, 1992.

Wilson PD, Testani-Dufour L: Bicycle safety programs; targeting injury prevention through education, *Pediatr Nurs* 19(4):343-346, 1993.

Wissom LS, Roter DL, Wilson MEH: Pediatrician interview style and mothers' disclosure of psychosocial issues, *Pediatrics* 93(2):289-295, 1994.

Wong D: Principles of atraumatic care. In Feeg V, editor: *Pediatric nursing: forum on the future: looking toward the 21st century,* Pitman, NJ, 1989, Anthony J. Jannetti.

BIBLIOGRAPHY

Mortality and Morbidity

American Academy of Pediatrics, Committeee on Adolescence: Suicide and suicide attempts in adolescents and young adults, *Pediatrics* 81(2):322-324, 1988.

Blum RW and others: American Indian—Alaska native youth health, *JAMA* 267(12):1637-1644, 1992.

Feeg V: New legislative efforts to improve child health and decrease infant mortality, *Pediatr Nurs* 15(2):145-148, 1989.

Fingerhut LA: *Firearm mortality among children, youth, and young adults 1-34 years of age—trends and current status: United States, 1985-90,* Advance data from vital and health statistics, No 231, Hyattsville, Md, 1993, National Center for Health Statistics.

Fingerhut LA, Jones C, Makuc D: *Firearm and Motor vehicle injury mortality—variations by state, race, and ethnicity: United States, 1990-91,* Advance data from vital and health statistics, No 242, Hyattsville, MD, 1994, National Center for Health Statistics.

Healthy people 2000: national health promotion and disease prevention objectives and healthy schools, *J School Health* 61(7):298-328, 1991.

Igoe JB: Healthy people 2000, *Pediatr Nurs* 16(6):584-586, 1990.

Infant mortality—United States, 1991, *MMWR* 42(48):926-930, 1993.

Kliegman RM: Perpetual poverty: child health and the underclass, *Pediatrics* 89(4):710-713, 1992.

Lenaghan P: Healthy people 2000, *J Emerg Nurs* 18(5):480-481, 1992.

Mandelbaum JL: Child survival: what are the issues? *J Pediatr Health Care* 6(3):132-137, 1992.

Mason JO, McGinnis JM: Healthy people 2000: an overview of the national health promotion and disease prevention objectives, *Public Health Rep* 105(5):441-446, 1990.

Report of the National Commission to Prevent Infant Mortality: *Death before life: the tragedy of infant mortality,* Washington, DC, 1988, The Commission.

Rheinstein PH: Healthy people 2000 initiative, *Am Fam Physician* 46(6):1829-1832, 1992.

Simmons SJ: Healthy people 2000: a framework for nursing action, *Orthop Nurs* 10(5):8, 1991.

Sullivan LW: Healthy people 2000, *N Engl J Med* 323(15):1065-1067, 1990.

Urtis J, Clayton D, Jay S: Infant morbidity: a measurement of severity and occurrence of illness in preterm and term infants, *J Pediatr Nurs* 3(2):110-117, 1988.

US Congress, Offices of Technology Assessment: *Healthy children: investing in the future,* OTA-H-345, Washington, DC, Feb 1988, US Government Printing Office.

Wilcox AJ: Infant mortality among blacks and whites, *N Engl J Med* 327(17):1243, 1992 (letter to the editor).

Zadinsky JK, Boettcher JH: Preventability of infant mortality in a rural community, *Nurs Res* 41(4):223-227, 1992.

Injuries

Baker S: Injury science comes of age, *JAMA* 262(16):2284-2285, 1989.

Bass JL and others: Childhood injury prevention counseling in primary care settings: a critical review of the literature, *Pediatrics* 92(4):544-550, 1993.

Betz CL: Injury: our children's greatest health problem, *J Pediatr Nurs* 8(6):353-354, 1993.

Bijur P, Golding J, Haslum M: Persistence of occurrence of injury: can injuries of preschool children predict injuries of school-aged children? *Pediatrics* 82(5):707-712, 1988.

Bourguet C, McArtor R: Unintentional injuries: risk factors in preschool children, *Am J Dis Child* 143(5):556-559, 1989.

Dannenberg AL, Vernick JS: A proposal for the mandatory inclusion of helmets with new children's bicycles, *Am J Public Health* 83(5):644-646, 1993.

Hall JR and others: Traumatic death in urban children, revisited, *Am J Dis Child* 147(1):102-107, 1993.

Jones NE: Childhood injuries: an epidemiologic approach, *Pediatr Nurs* 18(3):235-239, 1992.

Jones NE: Childhood residential injuries, *MCN* 18(3):168-172, 1993.

Landrigan PL and Belville R: The dangers of illegal child labor, *Am J Dis Child* 147(10):1029-1030, 1993.

Lee E, Jacobson J, Levanas V: Stressful life events and accidents at school, *Pediatr Nurs* 15(2):140-142, 1989.

Moore E, and others: Protecting our children through Kid Safe, *Pediatr Nurs* 14(1):32-36, 1988.

Schor E: Unintentional injuries: patterns within families, *Am J Dis Child* 141(12):1280-1284, 1987.

Sewell KH, Gaines SK: A developmental approach to childhood safety education, *Pediatr Nurs* 19(5):464-466, 1993.

US Department of Health and Human Services: A framework for assessing the effectiveness of disease and injury prevention, *MMWR* 41(RR-3):1-13, 1992.

US Department of Health and Human Services: Position papers from the Third National Injury Control Conference: setting the national agenda for injury control in the 1990's, *MMWR* 41(RR-6):entire issue, 1992.

Weesner CL and others: Fatal childhood injury patterns in an urban setting, *Ann Emerg Med* 23(2):231-236, 1994.

Wilson M: Injury prevention: protecting the under-6 set, *Contemp Pediatr* 5(5):19-34, 1988.

Evolution of Child Health Care

Arnold L and others: Lessons from the past, *MCN* 14(2):75-82, 1989.

Burns M, Thornam CB: Broadening the scope of nursing practice: federal programs for children, *Pediatr Nurs* 19(6):546-552, 1993.

Chinn PL, editor: *Health Policy: who cares?* Kansas City, MO, 1991, American Academy of Nursing.

Cone TE, Jr: *History of American pediatrics,* Boston, 1980, Little, Brown.

DeGraw C and others: Public law 99-457: new opportunities to serve young children with special needs, *J Pediatr* 113(6):971-974, 1988.

Donahue MP: *Nursing: the finest art, an illustrated history,* St Louis, 1985, Mosby.

Farel A: Public health in early intervention: historic foundations for contemporary training, *Infants Young Child* 1(1):63-70, 1988.

Gale C: Inadequacy of health care for the nation's chronically ill children, *J Pediatr Health Care* 3(1):20-27, 1989.

Harvey B: New series of essays on pediatric history, *Pediatrics* 92(3):467-468, 1993.

Inglis AD: United States maternal and child health services, *Neonatal Network* 9(8):35-43, 1991.

McMillan JA: What we must do for children in the 1990's, *Contemp Pediatr* 7(7):28-50, 1990.

Murphy M: What price success: can we afford "saved" babies? *J Pediatr Health Care* 3(6):285-286, 1989.

Oberg C: Medically uninsured children in the United States: a challenge to public policy, *Pediatrics* 85(5):824-833, 1990.

Report to Congress and the Secretary by the Task Force on Technology-Dependent Children: fostering home and community-based care for technology-dependent children, vols 1 and 2, US Department of Health and Human Services, Health Care Financing Administration, HCFA Pub No 88-02171, 1988.

Velsor-Friedrich B: The federal government and child health, *J Pediatr Nurs* 5(1):56-58, 1990.

Williams BC, Miller CA: Preventive health care for young children: findings from a 10-country study and directions for United States policy, *Pediatrics* 89(5, suppl):983-998, 1992.

Nursing Process

Alspach J: The revised JCAHO nursing care standards: areas of emphasis, *Crit Care Nurs* 11(8):12-14, 1991.

Carlson JH and others: *Nursing diagnosis: a case study approach,* Philadelphia, 1991, WB Saunders.

Carpenito LJ: *Nursing diagnosis application to clinical practice,* ed 3, Philadelphia, 1991, JB Lippincott.

D'Argenio C: *Implementing nursing diagnosis-based practice,* Gaithersburg, MD, 1991, Aspen.

Fitzpatrick JJ: Conceptual basis for the organization and advancement of nursing knowledge: nursing diagnosis/taxonomy, *Nurs Diagn* 1(3):102-106, 1990.

Gordon M: *Nursing diagnosis: process and application,* ed 3, St Louis, 1994, Mosby.

Guzzetta CE and others: *Clinical assessment tools for use with nursing diagnoses,* St Louis, 1989, Mosby.

Hanna D, Wyman N: Assessment + diagnosis = care planning: a tool for coordination, *Nurs Manage* 18(11):106-109, 1987.

Iyer PW, Camp NH: *Nursing documentation: a nursing process approach,* St Louis, 1991, Mosby.

Jennings BM: Patient outcomes research: seizing the opportunity, *Adv Nurs Sci* 14(2):59-72, 1991.

Levin R and others: Diagnostic content validity of nursing diagnoses, *Image J Nurs Sch* 21(1):40-44, 1989.

Lyons J, Hester N: Research-generated nursing diagnoses for healthy school-age children, *Issues Compr Pediatr Nurs* 10(3):149-159, 1987.

McFarland GK, McFarlane EA: *Nursing diagnosis and intervention: planning for patient care,* ed 2, St Louis, 1993, Mosby.

Mills WC: Nursing diagnosis: the importance of a definition, *Nurs Diagn* 2(1):3-8, 1991.

Mitchell GJ: Nursing diagnosis: an ethical analysis, *Image J Nurs Sch* 23(2):99-104, 1991.

Naylor MD and others: Measuring the effectiveness of nursing practice, *Clin Nurs Spec* 5(4):210-215, 1991.

Pinkley CL: Exploring NANDA's definition of nursing diagnosis: linking diagnostic judgments with the selection of outcomes and interventions, *Nurs Diagn* 2(1):26-32, 1991.

Waltz CF, Sylvia BM: Accountability and outcome measurement: where do we go from here? *Clin Nurs Spec* 5(4):202-203, 1991.

Warren JJ, Hoskins LM: The development of NANDA's nursing diagnosis taxonomy, *Nurs Diagn* 1(4):163-168, 1990.

Pediatric Nursing

Ahmann E: Family-centered care: Shifting orientation, *Pediatr Nurs* 20(2):113-117, 1994.

Bottorff JL: Nursing: a practice science of caring, *Adv Nurs Sci* 14(1):26-39, 1991.

Bru G: Using the revised APON standards of practice, *J Pediatr Oncol Nurs* 7(1):17-21, 1990.

Cipkala-Gaffin, Kane J, Cleveland M: Codependency: is it affecting our nursing practice? *J Pediatr Oncol Nurs* 8(2):62-63, 1991.

Crummette BD, Boatwright DN: Case management in inpatient pediatr nurs, *Pediatr Nurs* 17(5):469-473, 1991.

DePompei PM, Whitford KM, Beam PH: One institution's effort to implement family-centered care, *Pediatr Nurs* 20(2):119-121, 204, 1994.

Dormire SL: Models for moral response in care of seriously ill children, *Image: J Nurs Sch* 21(2):81-84, 1989.

Elder RG, Bullough B: Nurse practitioners and clinical nurse specialists: are the roles merging? *Clin Nurs Spec* 4(2):78-84, 1990.

Ethics in nursing: position statements and guidelines, Washington, DC, 1988, American Nurses' Association.

Feeg V, editor: *Pediatric nursing: forum on the future: looking toward the 21st century,* Pitman, NJ, 1989, Anthony J Jannetti.

Fowler M: Ethical decision making in clinical practice, *Nurs Clin North Am* 24(4):955-965, 1989.

Fry S: Ethical decision making. I. Selecting a framework, *Nurs Outlook* 37(5):248, 1989.

Fry S: Ethics. I. Issues in nursing, *Nurs Clin North Am* 24(2):461-577, 1989.

Hofmann PA: Critical path method: an important tool for coordinating clinical care, *Joint Commission J Quality Improvement* 19(7):235-246, 1993.

Hostler SL: Family-centered care, *Pediatr Clin North Am* 38(6):1545-1560, 1991.

Jerome AM, Ferraro-McDuffie AR: Nurse self-awareness in therapeutic relationships, *Pediatr Nurs* 18(2):153-156, 1992.

Kachoyeanos M and others: Fostering a spirit of inquiry in pediatric staff nurses, *Pediatr Nurs* 17(6):561-565, 1991.

Katz R, editor: Care delivery systems, *AACN Clin Issues Crit Care Nurs* 3(4):entire issue, 1992.

Kaufman J: Case management services for children with special health care needs: a family-centered approach, *J Case Manage* 1(2):53-56, 1992.

Keefe MR: An integrated approach to incorporating research findings into practice, *MCN* 18(2):65-70, 1993.

Keefe MR, Kotzer A: Integrating clinical practice and research: a challenge for the pediatric nurse practitioner, *J Pediatr Health Care* 2(6):275-280, 1988.

Lyons N and others: Too busy for research? Collaboration: an answer, *MCN* 15(2):67-72, 1990.

McVety D: Old-fashioned care still makes the difference, *MCN* 14(2):126-127, 1989.

Miedema F: A practical approach to ethical decisions, *Am J Nurs* 91(12):20-25, 1991.

Namei SK and others: The ethics of role conflict in research, *J Neurosci Nurses* 25(5):326-330, 1993.

Nehring WM: The nurse whose specialty is developmental disabilities, *Pediatr Nurs* 20(1):78-81, 1994.

Nelms B: Child advocacy: the need is great, *J Pediatr Health Care* 3(1):1-2, 1989.

Olsen DP: Empathy as an ethical and philosophical basis for nursing, *Adv Nurs Sci* 14(1):62-75, 1991.

Olson R, Heater B, Becker A: A meta-analysis of the effects of nursing interventions on children and parents, *MCN* 15(2):104-108, 1990.

Owens DK, Nease RF: Development of outcome-based practice guidelines: a method for structuring problems and synthesizing evidence, *Joint Commission J Quality Improvement* 19(7):248-263, 1993.

Raines D: Deciding what to do when the patient can't speak: a preliminary analysis of an ethnographic study of professional nurses in the neonatal intensive care unit, *Neonatal Network* 12(6):43-48, 1993.

Rushton C: Ethical decision-making in critical care. I. The role of the pediatric nurse, *Pediatr Nurs* 14(5):411-412, 1988.

Rushton C: Ethical decision-making in critical care. II. Strategies for nurse preparation, *Pediatr Nurs* 14(6):497-502, 1988.

Rushton C: Ethical unrest: implications for the future. In Feeg V, editor: *Pediatric nursing: forum on the future: looking toward the 21st century,* Pitman, NJ, 1989, Anthony J. Jannetti.

Rushton CH, Hogue EE: Confronting unsafe practice: ethical and legal issues, *Pediatr Nurs* 19(3):284-288, 1993.

Steele S: Nurse and parent collaborative case management in a rural setting, *Pediatr Nurs* 19(6):612-615, 1993.

Thayer MB: Caring: let it begin with me, *Pediatr Nurs* 17(5):504-505, 1991.

Thompson J, Thompson H: Living with ethical decisions with which you disagree, *MCN* 13(4):245-250, 1988.

Weeks LC, Gleason VR, Reiser S: How can a hospital ethics committee help? *Am J Nurs* 89(5):651-654, 1989.

CHAPTER 2

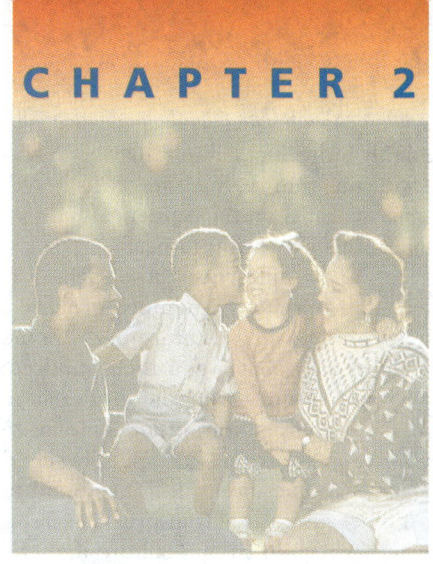

Social, Cultural, and Religious Influences on Child Health Promotion

CHAPTER OUTLINE

RELATED TOPICS

Communicating with families through an interpreter, Ch. 6
Family influences on child health promotion, Ch. 3
Lactose intolerance, Ch. 13
Nutritional assessment, Ch. 6
Sickle cell anemia, Ch. 35
Skin, Ch. 7
Spiritual development: general, Ch. 4; toddler, Ch. 14; preschooler, Ch. 15; school-age child, Ch. 17; adolescent, Ch. 19
Vegetarian diets, Ch. 13

The future of any society depends on its children. If it is to survive, the society must make provision for their care, nurture, and socialization. Cultural survival depends on whether the customs and values of the culture are transmitted from one generation to the next through the medium of the family. The culture into which children are born outlines the roles of their parents, structures their relationships with other people, and determines much of the behavior they acquire. A holistic view of any child requires that nurses develop some understanding of the ways that culture contributes to the development of social and emotional relationships and influences childrearing practices and attitudes toward health. ***Cross-cultural nursing care*** is care provided to individuals, families, or groups that are considered (by self or others) a minority because of race, culture, heritage, or sexual orientation (AAN Expert Panel, 1992). This orientation to cross-cultural nursing includes an awareness of the nurse's own cultural frame of reference and a concerted effort to recognize and appreciate the views and beliefs of the health care recipients to deliver culture-specific and sensitive care.

■ Judy Holt Rollins, RN, MS, coauthored this chapter.

CULTURE

Culture is the sum total of mores, traditions, and beliefs of how people function, and encompasses other products of human works and thoughts specific to members of an intergenerational group, community, or population (Brookins, 1993). Culture differs from both race and ethnicity. ***Race*** generally refers to a group of people with similar physical characteristics, such as skin color, that are transmissible by descent and sufficient to characterize it as a distinct human type. One system of classification includes three recognized types: caucasoid (white), negroid (black), and mongoloid (yellow). ***Ethnicity*** refers to a shared racial, cultural, social, and linguistic heritage (Martinson, 1989). ***Socialization*** is the process by which individuals learn the ways (beliefs, values, and behaviors) of a given society in order to function within that group (Elkin and Handel, 1989).

A culture is composed of individuals who share a set of values, beliefs, practices, and information that is learned, integrative, social, and satisfying. Culture is not a surface veneer that covers a basic outlook shared by all human beings but an ingrained orientation to life that serves as a frame of reference for individual perception and judgment. People from one culture differ from those in other cultures in the ways they think, solve problems, perceive, and structure the world. Culture is, essentially, the way of life of a group of people that incorporates experiences of the past, influences thought and action in the present, and transmits these traditions to future group members. Adaptation is necessary, however, for the culture to survive in an ever-changing world. Consciously and unconsciously, the members abandon, modify, or assume new patterns to meet the needs of the group.

The observable components of a culture, such as material objects (dress, art, utensils, and other artifacts) and actions, are sometimes termed the ***material overt,*** or ***manifest culture; nonmaterial covert culture*** refers to those aspects that cannot be observed directly, such as the ideas, beliefs, customs, and feelings of the culture. Related to the large culture are many ***subcultures,*** each with an identity of its own. Children are socialized into a particular subculture rather than into the culture as a whole. Subcultural influences, such as ethnicity and social class, are discussed in more detail later in this chapter.

The culture in which children are reared determines the type of food they will eat, the language they will speak, the ideals of behavior they will follow, and the way they will conduct themselves in social roles. To be acceptable members of the culture, children must learn how the culture expects them to behave toward others in the group. In turn, they learn how they can expect others to behave toward them.

Cultures and subcultures contribute to the uniqueness of child members in such a subtle way and at such an early age that children grow up to feel that their beliefs, attitudes, values, and practices are the "correct" or "normal" ones; those of other cultures may be viewed as "deviant" or "wrong." A set of values learned in childhood is apt to characterize children's attitudes and behavior for life, guiding their long-range strivings and monitoring their short-range, impulsive inclinations. Thus every ongoing society socializes each succeeding generation to its cultural heritage.

The manner and sequence of the growth and development phenomenon are universal and fundamental features of all children; however, the variations in behavioral responses that children display to similar events are believed to be determined by cultures. Inborn temperament and modes of behavior that prompt children to behave in their own preferred and highly individual manner may be in harmony or in conflict with the culture. Such forces as heredity and maturation impose limits on the influence that parents and other social groups may bring to bear.

The culture fosters and reinforces those behaviors deemed desirable and appropriate; it attempts to depress or extinguish those at conflict with cultural norms. Some cultures encourage aggressive behaviors in their children; others favor amiability and compliance. Some foster individual resourcefulness and competition; others emphasize cooperation and submission to group interest. The child from a culture that values cooperation will not respond to a challenge such as, "I'll bet you can eat your breakfast faster than Johnny can," whereas a child from a culture that emphasizes individual achievement will be stimulated by the challenge.

Cultures may also differ in whether status in the group is based on age or on skill. Even children's play and their types of games are culturally determined. In some cultures children play in groups composed of members of the same sex; in others they play in mixed-sex groups. In some cultures team games predominate; in others most play is limited to individual games.

Standards and norms vary from culture to culture and from location to location; a practice that is accepted in one area may meet with disapproval or create tension in another. The extent to which cultures tolerate divergence from the established norm varies among cultures and subcultural groups. Although conformity provides a degree of security, it is a decided deterrent to change.

SOCIAL ROLES

Much of children's self-concept is derived from their ideas about their social roles. ***Roles*** are cultural creations; therefore the culture prescribes patterns of behavior for persons in a variety of social positions. All persons who hold similar social positions have an obligation to behave in a particular manner. A role prohibits some behaviors and allows for others. Because it delineates and clarifies roles, the culture is a significant influence on the development of children's self-concept (i.e., the attitudes and beliefs they have about themselves).

A social group consists of a system of roles carried out in both primary and secondary groups. A ***primary group*** is characterized by intimate, continued face-to-face contact, mutual support of the members, and the ability to order or constrain a considerable proportion of individual members' behavior. Two such groups are the family and the peer group, both of which exert a great deal of influence on the child. ***Secondary groups*** are groups that have limited, intermittent contact and in which there is generally less concern for members' behavior. These groups offer little in terms of support or pressure toward conformity except in rigidly limited areas. Examples of secondary groups are professional associations and social organizations (also considered in relation to subgroups).

A concept of social role also depends largely on whether

a child is reared in a primary- or secondary-group community. Children are subjected to perceptively different forms of parental training in these two types of environments.

Primary and Secondary Group Influences

Children are reared within a primary-group environment and within a secondary-group environment. The influences, strengths, and limitations of both groups are significant. In a primary-group community (e.g., family, peer group, some contemporary rural, religious, or ethnic communities), all members know each other, most belong to the same subgroups, and all are concerned about each member's behavior. There is a high degree of material and psychologic support among the community members, and since there is one traditional set of values that the entire group agrees on and supports, there is little conflict of values. In a stable community where the members remain within comparatively defined limits and relatives are likely to live close together, young members have ample opportunity to observe and absorb the practices and customs of the culture. Any member of the community feels justified in evaluating and censuring the conduct of another member.

Children reared in relative isolation of secondary-group environmental influences tend to learn that there is only one acceptable way to respond to any given situation. The entire group agrees, and any tendency to deviate is met with collective disapproval. It is the parents' duty to see that the children learn and adhere to social roles and modes of behavior defined and strengthened by the views of the community.

The childrearing orientation in a secondary-group environment, such as urban communities, can differ considerably from that of a primary-group environment. The interaction between primary and secondary groups may serve to reinforce values when both groups endorse that value, or create confusion or conflict when one group rejects a value accepted by the other. An urban community is dynamic and rapidly changing. Many of the traditional behaviors and values may not meet the needs of the changing society. Consequently, parents are often uncertain about what to teach their children. They may wish to rear their children with values consistent with their own, but the differences in experience between the generations are too great. As a result, they often grant their children autonomy in some areas of decision making early in the developmental process, and other secondary groups assume a greater influence. The children are exposed to an assortment of social groups with diverse sets of values and expectations. None of the groups is highly dominant in its influence; therefore the children are exposed to an eclectic set of values, some in agreement and some at conflict with the others. From these they must ultimately select those that they determine to be best for them and adopt them to form a consistent set of roles and behaviors to be incorporated into the self-concept.

Guilt and Shame Orientation

Conditioning children to feel either guilt or shame for misdeeds is a technique used by a culture to control social behavior—to internalize the norms and expectations of others. Some cultural groups value a well-developed conscience (superego) and condition their children to feel guilt following wrongdoing. Offenders get an uncomfortable physical feeling and want to purge themselves. Because guilt is based within the individual, successful conditioning produces self-regulated persons who punish themselves without their being caught in the act of wrongdoing.

In many cultural groups guilt is lacking and social controls are based on the use of shame. Offenders do not want anyone to see them when they have been guilty of wrongful deeds. Sometimes children in these groups learn that anything is acceptable as long as one is not caught; the shame results when the forbidden act is found out by others.

Although both techniques are used by members of both primary- and secondary-group communities, shame is apt to be more successful in a primary-group community because most behaviors are quite public. In secondary-group communities it is less effective; persons are not as apt to be caught and, if caught, can withdraw and join a group that is unaware of the misdeed. Guilt probably has a greater influence on behavior in urban communities, although many authorities believe that the trend in urban America is shifting away from a guilt orientation. Rapid changes in the American culture leave parents unsure of their own values; therefore much of their function is abandoned to the school and peers. Peers are notorious for the use of shame as a disciplinary technique.

SUBCULTURAL INFLUENCES

Except in rare situations, children grow and develop in a blend of cultures and subcultures, those smaller groups within a culture that possess many characteristics of the larger culture while contributing their own particular values. In a large, complex society such as the United States, different groups have their own set of standards, values, and expectations within the collective ways of the large culture. Most were formed when groups of people clustered together by preference, by external pressures from the majority culture, or by geographic isolation. Although many cultural differences are related to geographic boundaries, subcultures are not always restricted by location.

There are even subcultures related to the age stages of development that have traditions, games, loyalties, and rules. Age-related subcultures are easily identified in the behavior of school-age children and adolescents. The culture is handed down by word of mouth from one "generation" to the next, and its rituals and behavior standards are highly resistant to outside influence.

Children's membership in a cultural subgroup is, for the most part, involuntary. They are born into a family with a specific ethnic and/or racial heritage, socioeconomic level, and religious beliefs. Although in the complex American society there are countless subcultures and considerable variation in the way of life, those subcultures that seem to exert the greatest influence on childrearing are ethnicity, social class, and occupational role. In addition, schools and peer-group subcultures are strong influences in the socialization of the child.

Ethnicity

Ethnicity is the classification of or affiliation with any of the basic groups or divisions of mankind or any heterogeneous population differentiated by customs, characteristics, language, or similar distinguishing factors. Ethnic differences extend to many areas and include such manifestations as family structure, language, food preferences, moral codes, and expression of emotion. Some standards of behavior result from the cultural heritage of the specific ethnic group (e.g., the traditional role of the father). Others reflect the interaction between subcultures, most notably between members of the majority culture and a minority subculture.

To establish their place in the group, children learn how to adhere to a mode of behavior that is in accordance with standards distinctive to the group and learn how they can expect others to behave toward them. They take their cues from observing and imitating those to whom they are exposed. For example, children of a racial minority form a perception of their role as a group member by observing the manner in which role models within the subgroup respond to treatment by people outside the subgroup. When they see group members display an attitude of inferiority, they assume this to be the appropriate behavior. These perceptions are then incorporated into their own self-concept.

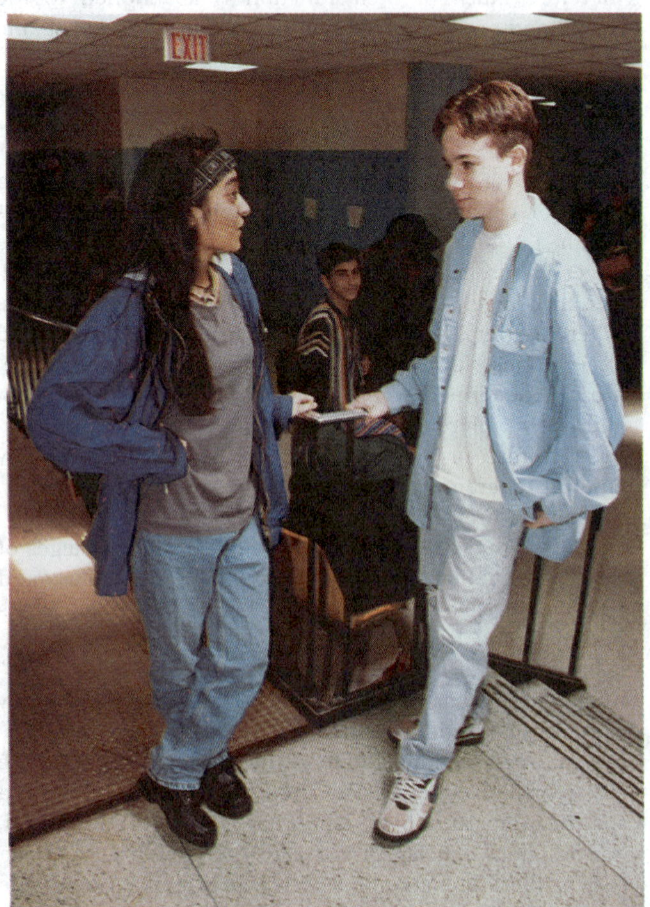

FIG. 2-1 Youngsters from different cultural backgrounds interact within the larger culture.

In the United States the cross-cultural lines are becoming blurred as subcultures are assimilated and blended into the larger culture (Fig. 2-1). Although ethnic differences in childrearing are probably diminishing, they remain important. It is particularly difficult for persons to attempt to maintain an identity with a subculture while living and conforming to the requirements of the larger culture. Universal customs and language of the dominant culture used in commercial and educational systems are different from those of the minority culture. Often the values are in conflict. Consequently, children reared in this environment are confused about roles and values, and they usually adopt those of the more influential or higher-status culture. Youth, in particular, are influenced by the locally dominant group.

Ethnocentrism is the emotional attitude that one's own ethnic group is superior to others, that one's values, beliefs, and perceptions are the correct ones, and that the group's ways of living and behaving are the best way. ***Ethnic stereotyping*** or labeling stems from ethnocentric views of people (Friedman, 1990). Ethnocentrism implies that all other groups are inferior and that their ways are not in the best interests of the group. It is a common attitude among a dominant ethnic group and strongly influences the ability of one person to evaluate the beliefs and behaviors of others objectively. This inherent viewpoint of individuals tends to bias their interpretation and understanding of the behavior of others.

Social Class/Occupation

Although there are exceptions, probably the greatest influence on childrearing practices and their consequences is the social class of the family into which a child is born. Differences in childrearing goals and practices, as well as attitudes toward health, have been found to be greater between social classes than between races or ethnic groups. In North America social class and socioeconomic level are essentially synonymous and are most easily determined by occupation; for example, the upper middle class consists primarily of professional and business people, almost all with a college education. The working class includes employees in manufacturing, trades, and service occupations (such as barbers or hairdressers) who have a high school education. In the lower class the breadwinners are typically unskilled laborers or unemployed families who may or may not be on public assistance (Elkin and Handel, 1989). Since children are reared differently by parents who vary in respect to education, occupation, and income, social class can be expected to produce substantial variation in their upbringing.

Upper-class children live in an enriched environment that provides material comforts and broader opportunities. Although many children from the middle classes enjoy a similar environment, the economic trends of this decade have many parents in the middle class struggling to provide the life-style usually attributed to their class. In reality, some middle-class parents present a life-style to their children at a level more commonly equated with the poor. However, the parents in upper- and middle-class families are usually educated, and other authority figures, such as teachers, with whom the children are routinely in contact are usually from a middle-class background and have activities and expectations for the children that are similar to those of the parents. Parents have occupations that require judgment, creativity, and resourcefulness, and these attributes are fostered in their children.

Because most members of the upper classes, or the power elite, do not participate in studies, information on childrearing practices in these groups is limited. Attitudes toward children appear to be generally permissive; however, much of the actual child care in upper-class families is delegated to surrogates, such as housekeepers, nannies, governesses, or private schools. In middle-class families child care is more likely to consist of daycare, baby-sitters, and nursery school rather than the more expensive alternatives. This in no way implies that a wealthy parent will be detached and uninvolved, or that a middle-class parent will be more involved, because of differing choices of "purchased parent surrogates." Differences in parenting between socioeconomic groups primarily reflect differences in availability of physical and personal resources. For example, the wealthy parent has physical resources available that other classes do not have to the same degree. Affluent parents are more likely to be in a position of being a parent who does not need to work and who therefore has the opportunity to spend more time focused on their children.

Virtually all low-income families and a sizable and growing proportion of middle-income families have been affected by financial stresses, such as rising costs, unemployment, and/or reemployment at lower wages. Parents are working more hours to meet economic demands and therefore have less time to spend with their children (Children's Defense Fund, 1992).

Although differences in parental behavior in different social classes are less marked than they have been in the past, one of the distinctions that has typically been observed in middle classes but not in lower classes is the willingness to delay gratification. Middle-class parents typically have higher educational and occupational aspirations for their children and use long-range planning to meet these goals. The uncertainty of their lives leads some members of the lower classes to take advantage of gratifications when they are available. This characteristic has caused lower classes to be labeled as present oriented, whereas middle classes seem to be future oriented. Better job security through unionization, unemployment compensation, and other welfare features give some segments of the lower classes a sense that life is more predictable. When this perception occurs, people are less apt to seize gratifications lest the opportunity vanish. They are able to develop long-range goals, including an increased interest in education for their children. Unfortunately, recent economic trends have made job security an even less realistic expectation for parents from lower-class families and for increasing numbers of parents from middle-class families. Many families, worrying more about financial considerations, have become increasingly pessimistic regarding their children's future (Children's Defense Fund, 1992).

Intellectual Skills. There appear to be differences in intellectual skills and scholastic achievement between children in the upper and middle classes and those in the lower classes. The more apparent differences lie in the areas of abstract thinking and manipulation. Although the relative merits of testing techniques and standards are a matter of question, there is a higher incidence of academic failure in children from the lower class with its attendant dropout rate. It has been found that parents in the lower classes value the concrete and tangible rather than the abstract and are therefore less inclined to encourage these qualities in their children. Their own educational level discourages these parents from reading to their children and providing other means for learning in the home. There may be no role models in the family to support the value of education, and numerous provisions for intellectual growth are restricted by cost. To compound this, lower-class neighborhoods typically have the poorest schools, and the children are often hampered in their learning by poor health and inadequate nutrition. In addition, children from the lower classes are often penalized within the school because they do not possess the symbols, attitudes, and behaviors characteristically valued by the dominant class group. There is a social class bias in educative influence. Most teachers come from the middle classes, and school board members are from middle and upper classes.

Communication Skills. Any concept that occurs to a person can be expressed in language. However, ease of communication and use of language codes vary among the social classes. Language is much more restricted in the lower classes, and the classes are more easily differentiated by grammar than by pronunciation. Persons in the middle classes use different grammar from those in the lower classes and are able to express more complicated ideas; persons in the lower classes use very simple grammar and are less likely to offer explanations. For example, a middle-class parent may tell a child, "I'd rather you made less noise because I am trying to read a book." A lower-class parent may say, "Shut up" (Elkin and Handel, 1989).

These communication differences are highly significant in relation to school achievement. School is constructed around the elaborate language codes of the middle class; therefore children from the lower classes must learn these language skills, which places them at a decided disadvantage. This is particularly true for bilingual children and children from ethnic groups who have developed a dialect unique to their own group. For example, black English, essentially another language and treated as such, is not spoken by other groups, including middle-class blacks. Many regional dialects and variations in language usage must be taken into consideration when communicating with persons from these groups. English words that sound like another word in a foreign language can cause considerable misunderstanding. For example, when a nurse tried to explain to Spanish parents that their infant died of SIDS (sudden infant death syndrome), the parents thought the nurse said

"SIDA," the Spanish abbreviation for AIDS (acquired immunodeficiency syndrome) (Lawson, 1990).

Aspirations. Middle-class parents typically are positively oriented toward change, whereas parents in the lower classes tend to remain tradition oriented. Consequently, the lower class tends to emphasize conformity to parental values and external regulations, whereas middle-class parents tend to be more concerned with producing self-directed children. This attitude difference reflects the occupation orientation of the different classes. Middle-class occupations tend to involve more self-direction and getting ahead; lower-class occupations tend to be standardized with direct supervision. Middle-class parents encourage their children in activities that foster achievement and that they believe will make them well-rounded, self-directed adults. They involve their children in such activities as dancing lessons, athletics, and scouting. Parents in the lower classes tend to be more concerned that their children grow up to be moral, upright, and religious. Many parents in the lower classes seem less interested in the direction of their children's activities than with their conduct; they are more concerned that their children stay out of trouble.

With few exceptions, parents in all classes love their children and in a broad sense have similar goals regarding childrearing. Differences lie in the parental behavior toward the children in attempting to help them to reach these goals. Parents in the lower classses tend to be more restrictive and rely on coercive techniques in child training. They stress obedience and conformity, and the most frequently used form of discipline for undesirable behavior is physical punishment. Middle-class parents are more apt to make use of manipulative techniques such as reasoning and drawing on the child's sense of guilt. They tend to scold and use isolation rather than physical punishment. There is more concern regarding the *intent* of the act than the *consequence* of the act. Upper middle–class parents tend to be more permissive and foster desirable behavior through more lenient disciplinary methods, such as natural consequences and positive reinforcement. Parents in the lower classes tend to use more restrictive disciplinary methods, such as assertion of authority, deprivation, and punishment. However, these more punitive strategies can be modified with early intervention.

The very poor, who consistently exist on or below the poverty level, live in a perpetual state of despair. Their limited skills give them no bargaining power in the job market, and the education needed to improve their status is beyond them. The poor desire better things for their children but are trapped in a circular pattern that perpetuates their life condition. Their powerlessness to control their fate or condition is a source of fatalism and resignation that is often characteristic of the group in general. Optimism, when it is manifested, is more likely to be expressed in terms of luck or chance. This fatalistic attitude is a significant impediment to occupational and educational aspirations and to seeking health care. It also inhibits them from seeking health care or practicing preventive health care measures. For example, if someone is injured or killed in an automobile accident, it is more likely to be considered bad luck, not something that could have been prevented by wearing a seat belt.

Poverty

A subcultural influence closely related to but different from social class is the condition known as poverty. It is a relative concept and is usually associated with the general standards of a population. An ***absolute standard*** of poverty attempts to delimit some basic set of resources needed for adequate existence; a ***relative standard*** reflects the median standard of living in a society and is the term used in referring to childhood poverty in the United States. That is, what appears to be deprivation in one area may be a standard or norm in another.

In the United States, rates of poverty have changed dramatically—to the detriment of children. Although general poverty rates are basically the same today as they were two decades ago, who is poor has changed. Historically, elderly Americans were more likely to be poor than children. However, federal programs such as Medicare and Social Security reduced their poverty rates. Children in the United States today are nearly twice as likely to be poor as are citizens over 65 years of age (Annie E. Casey Foundation, 1993).

Presently it is estimated that one in five children (21.8%) live in poverty (defined in 1992 as an annual income of $13,950 or less for a family of four [Federal Register, 1992]). This rate is substantially higher than the rate in other comparable countries. Although white children saw their poverty rate increase the most during the 1980s (one in seven are poor), minority children are more likely to be poor. Almost 50% of black children and more than one third of Hispanic children live in families with incomes below the poverty level (Annie E. Casey Foundation, 1993). Large numbers of Native American children also live in poverty, with unemployment rates on one reservation estimated at 80%. Some children on the reservation claim that their main source of food is the school-based free breakfast and lunch program (Rollins, 1993).

Many Americans picture the typical child who is poor as a city dweller with unemployed parents, usually living in a single-parent home. Although chronic poverty is more concentrated in central city areas (Wright, 1993), most of the nation's poor children live in the suburbs or rural areas of the country. Most parents of children who are poor are employed. More than 70% of the increase in the number of poor children that occurred in the early 1980s was due to rising poverty in families with a man present. However, approximately half of all poor children live in households headed by women. The chances of being poor increase substantially when there is only one parent (Annie E. Casey Foundation, 1993).

The character of American poverty is changing. Historically, most of the poor were ***episodically poor*** (i.e., their incomes would fall below the official poverty line from time to time, reflecting short-term fluctuations in household composition or economic circumstances). Today, increasing numbers of families are ***chronically poor*** (i.e., with incomes below the poverty line year after year) (Wright, 1993).

Approximately one fourth of children in families with married parents would be poor if they depended on the father's income alone. Escalating health care costs and unaffordable health insurance premiums, coupled with the unavailability and unaffordability of safe housing, the expense of child care, and low-paying marginal jobs result in families with incomes twice the federal poverty level living in substandard housing, foregoing health care, and eating unbalanced meals and insufficient food (Malloy, 1992). Such factors illustrate the growing inability of the American family to provide economic essentials that all children need.

Homelessness

One of the most pressing problems in the United States is the growing number of homeless families. Homeless individuals are those persons who lack resources and community ties necessary to provide for their own adequate shelter. In the past the homeless population traditionally included single adults, mostly men. Currently, the fastest growing segment of the homeless population consists of families, constituting at least one third of the people without homes throughout the United States (Buckner and others, 1993).

Homeless children have increased in numbers as poverty has become feminized, minorities have become poorer, and low-income housing has become less accessible (Murata and others, 1992). Estimates on the number of homeless children in the United States at any given time range from 68,000 to 100,000. The majority of children are less than 5 years of age and are predominantly from minority groups. Although single mothers with two or three children constitute more than 33% to 50% of the homeless population on the East and West coasts, the homeless family profile reflects a mobile, predominantly white, two-parent family with few children (1.2) in other regions of the country (Page, Ainsworth, and Pett, 1993).

Many families are becoming homeless because of physical abuse, substance abuse, disagreements with the landlord, and poor living conditions (Parker and others, 1991). Other reasons include job layoffs, low income, parental mental illness, domestic conflict, and unexpected family or economic crises. Most families move into homelessness gradually after family members and friends are no longer willing to provide housing (Davidhizar and Frank, 1992).

Another group of homeless children are the "runaway" and "throwaway" adolescents. Nationwide it has been estimated that this group numbers between 250,000 and 500,000. Many runaways are victims of physical and sexual abuse and leave home because of long-term family or school problems. Poor parent-child relationships, extreme family conflict, feelings of alienation from parents, inconsistency in supervision, and unpredictability in discipline are other factors often cited.

Lack of a permanent dwelling deprives children of the most basic necessities for proper growth and development. Homelessness disrupts a child's friendships and schooling (Masten and others, 1993). Homeless children suffer from physical and mental disorders that exceed those found in poor children who have a permanent residence (Bassuk and Rosenberg, 1990), and they are particularly vulnerable for early initiation of and sustained participation in substance-abuse behaviors (Wagner, Melragon, and Menke, 1993).

Migrant Families

One of the most disadvantaged groups is migrant farm workers and their children. Estimates on the size of the migrant and seasonal farm worker population vary (Rust, 1990). However, indications are that in the United States there are between 3 and 5 million migrant and seasonal workers and their dependents, whose average yearly income is well below the poverty level. In addition, most of these families have no health care insurance.

The low position of these families on the economic scale and their rootless, mobile existence subjects them to inadequate sanitation, substandard housing, social isolation, and lack of educational and medical facilities. This life-style is especially deleterious to the children. Schooling and health care are inadequate. Children are apt to live in a number of localities and attend a variety of schools in the course of a year with no continuity in either education or health care. Because both parents work in the fields, children receive little adult supervision; therefore, injury rates are high and meals are erratic. Except where prohibited by law, children are even recruited to work in the fields along with the adults.

Some migrants have a home base to which they return at the end of a growing season; others travel continuously, migrating north in summer and south in winter. With most there is little if any integration into the dominant culture; therefore migrant groups suffer social isolation. Groups who travel together, especially those with the same ethnic background, develop a cohesiveness and form their own set of values and customs. Sometimes a migrant family will leave the migration stream and become a part of a permanent community. However, this involves adaptation to a new environment and life-style that can be stress provoking to these families.

Affluence

On the opposite end of the socioeconomic spectrum are the children of affluent members of society. Although they may live within the warmth of a positive family relationship, some of them appear to be just as deprived as the poverty stricken. Wealth does not provide protection against many of life's problems and disappointments, especially in the area of parent-child relationships. Like their counterparts in the poverty groups, children of the affluent may suffer from social discrimination (too rich or not rich enough to meet different standards), inadequate parenting, lack of discipline, or unsatisfactory role models.

Some children of the wealthy may suffer from lack of parental contact. There may be long separations from loving, caring parents because of social or business interests. Even their places of residence contribute to their isolation and loneliness. In some cases purchased parent surrogates, such as servants, sports professionals (such as tennis or swimming instructors), and private school personnel, provide their adult companionship and authority. Self-indulgent behavior in the rich is often viewed as acceptable.

Many children from wealthy families, just like those from poor families, seem to thrive and flourish, making positive contributions to their families and society. Others grow up to display a lack of motivation or self-discipline and boredom. Some may fail to acquire the necessary skills to handle responsibility and money, especially third-generation rich who are born into wealth and have developed less of the work ethic of earlier generations.

Religion

Probably the most influential factor in shaping the culture of the United States is the Judeo-Christian faith. Many immigrants came to the United States for religious freedom and established a religious and moral atmosphere that persists today. However, there are individual differences that are part of the general culture.

The religious orientation of the family dictates a code of morality, as well as influencing the family's attitudes toward education, male and female role identity, and attitudes regarding their ultimate destiny (Fig. 2-2). It may also determine the school that the children attend, the companions with whom they associate, and often their mate selection. In many cultures the religious beliefs are such an integral part of the culture that it is difficult to distinguish one from the other. In a few instances, such as in the Mennonite and Amish communities, religion is the basis of a common way of life that determines where the children are reared and the life-style. (See also Religious Beliefs, p. 50.)

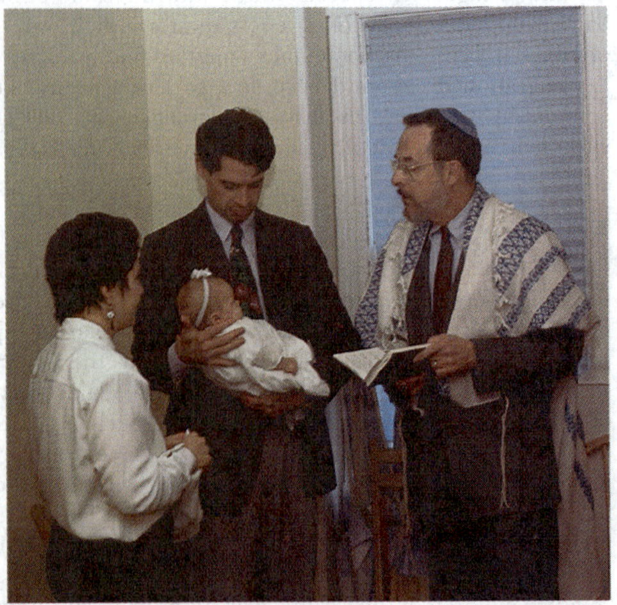

FIG. 2-2 Soon after an infant is born, many families have special religious ceremonies.

Schools

When children enter school, their radius of relationships extends to include a wider variety of peers and a new focus of authority. Although parents continue to exert the major influence on the children, in the school environment teachers have the most significant psychologic impact on their development and socialization. The function of teachers is primarily limited to teaching, but, like parents, they are concerned about the emotional welfare of the children. Both parents and teachers must constrain behavior, and both are in a position to enforce standards of conduct.

Socialization. Next to the family the schools exert the major force in providing continuity between generations by conveying a vast amount of culture from the older members to the young. In this way children are prepared to carry out the traditional social roles they are expected to assume as adults in society. School is the center of "cultural diffusion" wherein the cultural standards of the larger group are mediated to the local community. It governs what is taught and, to a large extent, how it is taught. School rules and regulations regarding attendance, authority relationships, and the system of sanctions and rewards based on achievement transmit to the child the behavioral expectations of the adult world of employment and relationships. School is often the only institution in which children systematically learn about the negative consequences of behaviors that deviate from social expectations. In addition, the school provides an opportunity for some children to participate in the larger society in rewarding ways and often provides avenues for social mobility for both students and teachers. Through education individuals in the lower classes are offered the opportunity for further education and the capacity to move up in the social strata.

Teachers have the responsibility for transmitting the knowledge and values of the dominant culture (i.e., those values on which there is broad consensus). They are expected to stimulate and guide the intellectual development of children and their sense of esthetics and to foster their capacity for creative problem solving.

Traditionally, the socialization process of school began when the child entered kindergarten or the first grade. With over 58% of mothers of children under 6 years of age working outside the home, this socialization process begins much earlier for a significant number of children in a variety of child care settings (National Commission on Children, 1991). Considering that the majority of mothers work because of economic necessity, this trend toward out-of-home care for children will probably continue.

Peer Cultures

Peer groups also have an impact on the socialization of children (Fig. 2-3). Peer relationships become increasingly important and influential as children proceed through school. In school, children have what can be regarded as a culture of their own. It is most apparent in the school and in the unsupervised play group. The play group presents this culture in a much purer form than does the school, in which the culture is partly produced by adults.

During their lives children are exposed to value systems

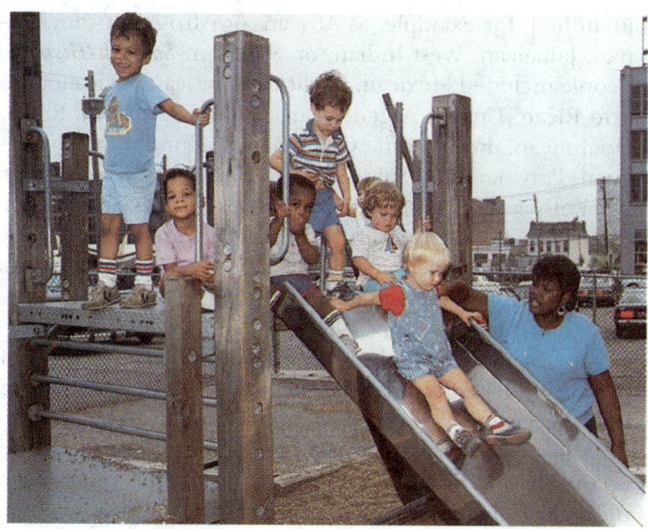

FIG. 2-3 Children from a variety of cultural and ethnic backgrounds begin to socialize in the child care setting.

such as those of the family, ethnic group, and social class. In peer-group interaction they are confronted with a variety of these sets of values. The values imposed by the peer group are especially compelling because children must accept and conform to them in order to be accepted as members of the group. When the peer values are not too different from those of family and teachers, the mild conflict created by these small differences serves to separate children from the adults in their lives and to strengthen the feeling of belonging to the peer group.

The kind of socialization provided by the peer group depends on the special subculture that develops from the background, interests, and capabilities of its members. Some groups support school achievement, others focus on athletic prowess, and still others are decidedly antithetic to educative goals. Scholastic achievement is strongly related to the value system of the peer groups. Many conflicts between teachers and students and between parents and students can be attributed to fear of rejection by peers. There is often a conflict between what is expected from parents regarding academic achievement and what is expected from the peer culture. This is especially pronounced in high school and is discussed further in Chapter 19.

Although it has neither the traditional authority of the parents nor the legal authority of the schools for teaching information, the peer group manages to convey a substantial amount of information to its members, especially about taboo subjects such as sex and drugs. Children's need for the friendship of their peers brings them into an increasingly complex social system. The world of the peer group is different from the adult world, and through peer relationships, children learn ways in which to deal with dominance and hostility and to relate with persons in positions of leadership and authority. Other functions of the peer subculture are to relieve boredom and to provide recognition that individual members do not receive from teachers and other authority figures.

The peer-group culture has secrets, mores, and codes of ethics with which they promote feelings of group solidarity and detachment from adults. They have traditions and folkways that are transferred from "generation to generation" of schoolchildren and that have a great influence over the behavior of all members of the group. There are age-related games and other activities, and as children move from one level to the next, folkways of the younger group are discarded as those of the new are adopted. For example, a school-age child rides a bicycle to school; the high school student prefers a car. As they advance, children are forward oriented only—they look forward with anticipation but may look backward with contempt.

Biculture

Some children are exposed to the values, role relationships, and life-styles of two or more cultures—a virtual "straddling" of cultures. This may occur because the child's parents are from two or more different cultures. In Hawaii, for example, it is common for children to be of four or more cultures. Other children straddle cultures as members of a minority culture within the dominant culture. This biculture is sometimes observed in the play group but usually is not a significant factor until children enter school. Then they must unlearn some of the established practices of one culture in order to become socialized in the other, especially in role relationships. For example, children from Hispanic and Oriental cultures are taught to look away when scolded; in U.S. schools the teacher expects direct eye contact—"Look at me when I speak to you" (Sloat and Matsuura, 1990). Children learn new roles and social behavior more rapidly than their adult counterparts.

This biculture is particularly marked in language differences. The bilingual child is said to be at a disadvantage in school situations of the dominant culture, in which there is controversy over bilingual education. On the one hand those supporting bilingual education adhere to the principle that children will understand more readily and perform more realistically (especially in testing situations) if learning is directed in their own language; others contend that children living in a dominant culture should adopt the ways of that culture, including language. There is less conflict for children when their language and culture are supported by the school, even if the dominant language is used.

Another aspect of biculture occurs when children meld the elements of the dominant culture and the minority culture with the characteristics of a subculture that is uniquely their own.

THE CHILD AND FAMILY IN NORTH AMERICA

America's orientation toward homogenization—"the great melting pot"—is changing. Increased awareness of the growing proportion of ethnic minorities that make up the U.S. population, coupled with a new positive value and emphasis being placed on ethnic diversity, has resulted in a renewed interest in cultural variation (Patterson and Blum, 1993).

The frontier background of the American culture has contributed to the overall orientation to life and childrearing. There has always been a basic optimistic view of the world, a belief that things can be better and that the children can and will be better off than the parents. This hopeful outlook and a general future orientation, together with the possibility of upward social mobility, have created a pervasive overall attitude of optimism. Increasing development of self-confidence and autonomy in children is fostered and encouraged. Children are generally permitted a greater degree of freedom than in more tradition-oriented cultures, where individuals remain in one social class for life.

Family life in America is characterized by increasing geographic and economic mobility. There is less reliance on tradition, families are fragmented, and there is limited opportunity to transmit and acquire the traditional and accepted customs of a culture. Consequently, young adults rely to a greater extent on the professed experts, peers, and the mass media for acquisition of acceptable patterns of behavior, including childrearing practices. Each generation, as it adapts to the new, discards the inadequacies of previous generations. This often constitutes a source of confusion and frustration as parents attempt to adjust to rapid changes; tradition and precedent no longer meet the needs and challenges of rapid change that require new approaches and innovation for problem solving. Competent parents attempt to determine the comparatively stable, essential components of the culture and transmit these to their children. Awareness of changing cultural norms during childrearing helps parents to adapt to the new demands of the culture that are different from those they learned as children.

Minority-Group Membership

The United States has more racial, ethnic, and religious minority groups than any other country. Blacks are the largest minority group, followed closely by Hispanics (Table 2-1).

The definition of various minority groups is not universal. In the 1990 U.S. census form, ***blacks*** included persons identified, for example, as African- or Afro-American, Haitian, Jamaican, West Indian, or Nigerian. ***Spanish/Hispanic*** people included Mexican, Mexican-American, Chicano, Puerto Rican, Cuban, Argentinean, Columbian, Costa Rican, Dominican, Ecuadoran, Guatemalan, Honduran, Nicaraguan, Peruvian, and Salvadoran persons, as well as persons from other Spanish-speaking countries or the Caribbean or Central or South America. ***Mexican-American*** referred only to persons of Mexican origin or ancestry. In some writings the term ***Latino*** refers to individuals from Mexico and Central America (Friedman, 1990).

TABLE 2-1 Number of Children by Race and Spanish Origin

	NUMBER IN MILLIONS		
	1980	1990	2000
Race/Spanish origin			
White	52.2	51.9	53.5
Nonwhite*	11.2	12.4	13.9
Black	9.5	10.3	11.4
Spanish origin	NA	7.1	8.7

Modified from U.S. children and their families: current conditions and recent trends, Select Committee on Children, Youth, and Families, Washington, DC, 1987, US Government Printing Office.

**Nonwhite* refers to all races other than white and includes blacks, Native Americans, Japanese, Chinese, and any other race except white. Blacks comprise the great majority of nonwhites. People of Spanish origin can be of any race.

One of the difficulties with including diverse groups of people under ethnic labels, such as black or Hispanic, is that the groups can differ tremendously in their own cultural heritage. Just as the majority white population differs according to various subcultures, such as socioeconomic status and occupation, so do the minority groups.

NURSING ALERT Any generalization made about an ethnic group may not apply to certain groups or individuals.

When minority groups immigrate to another country, a certain degree of cultural/ethnic blending occurs through the process of ***acculturation,*** those gradual changes produced in a culture by the influence of another culture that cause one or both cultures to be more similar to the other. However, the changes occur to various degrees in different families and groups. Many groups continue to identify with their traditional heritage while adapting to the ill-defined concept of the "American way."

Studies in the past indicate that early in life children become aware of their racial or ethnic status and of the discriminatory attitudes of the majority culture toward their group. The direct effects of discrimination are anger and low self-esteem, which become manifest in a variety of behaviors. Inner conflicts and suppressed hostility that focus children's attention inward may be factors in the failure of many children to achieve in other areas.

Evidence indicates that changes in attitudes are slowly taking place in some groups and in some places. With growing awareness, interest, and understanding by increasing numbers of the majority group, which has accompanied the recent emergence of racial and ethnic pride, minority-group children are becoming more secure and confident in their racial or ethnic identity. Individuals vary in their reactions to membership in a minority group, and much of this variation can be attributed to familial factors. As with all children, the most important influences on development of a positive self-image are warm, understanding parents who take an active interest in fostering their children's growth. Parents who accept their children and react positively and constructively rather than in a negative and self-defeating manner will help their children develop feelings of self-worth, self-esteem, and self-acceptance. The more adequate children feel, the more positive will be their attitudes toward both majority and minority children, the greater will be their ability to withstand prejudice and intolerance, and the less will be their need for counteraggressive behavior.

CULTURAL SHOCK

The term ***cultural shock*** describes the "feelings of helplessness and discomfort and a state of disorientation experienced by an outsider attempting to comprehend or effectively adapt to a different cultural group because of differences in cultural practices, values, and beliefs" (Leininger, 1978). This state occurs with both clients and health care providers who move from one culture to another culture or setting. It can happen to persons who immigrate to a new country (such as the Asian refugees) or to persons from a subcultural group who must adjust to the ways of an unfamiliar subgroup (such as children entering the school subculture or clients who enter the hospital subculture). Cultural shock is characterized by the inability to respond to or function in a new or strange situation.

Numerous factors influence the reactions to a new environment. Language barriers, including dialects and jargon (such as medical language) specific to a subcultural group, inhibit effective communication. Habits and customs (such as different role behaviors or etiquette) and differences in attitudes and beliefs are puzzling to the stranger in the new environment. The outsider experiences an intense sense of isolation and feelings of loneliness and nonrelatedness. Nurses entering an unfamiliar cultural situation can reduce the cultural shock by becoming familiar with the cultural groups with which they work and by learning tolerance of the values, beliefs, and customs of these groups.

Immigrants and refugees from cultures in which children are taught to respect and obey their elders and in which females are considered inferior to males, such as most Asian cultures, may have difficulty dealing with the consequences of Western egalitarianism. When children enter the school system, they learn to question authority and are confronted with the movement for equality of the sexes in all aspects of life. This often creates conflict within the family, especially in families such as the Vietnamese, who consider education highly valuable for their children.

Another source of conflict may arise when children become interpreters for parents or extended family members when interacting with the dominant culture. For example, a child may need to translate messages from school or interpret the health practitioner's instructions during clinic visits. This constitutes a role reversal of child explaining the world to parents. Some children become disrespectful toward their parents for not learning the language and dominant culture. Lynch and Hanson (1992) further add that privacy and confidentiality can be invaded when children must interpret for their parents.

CULTURAL / RELIGIOUS INFLUENCES ON HEALTH CARE

Cultural beliefs and practices are an important part of data gathering in the nursing assessment. Nurses continually encounter beliefs and practices that may facilitate or impede nursing interventions, including attitudes toward family planning, food habits, and folkways that are firmly entrenched in the culture. The language of the client may be different from that of the larger culture, or there may be regional or ethnic peculiarities in the use of basic English. Subcultural influences, such as some religious beliefs and practices, may be in conflict with standard health practices and therapeutic interventions.

SUSCEPTIBILITY TO HEALTH PROBLEMS

Some groups of people are more susceptible and others more resistant to certain illnesses than are persons from other groups. An innate susceptibility is acquired through generations of evolutionary changes that take place within constrained or segregated populations. The proximity to disease, environmental factors, and the general physical status are significant factors associated with health problems.

Hereditary Factors

The genetic constitution of individuals as groups influences the degree to which they are susceptible to a specific disorder. It may be a result of an inherent lack of resistance to a disease organism, a trait that is an advantage in one environment but places the possessor at a disadvantage in another, or it may be the consequence of intermarriage within a relatively narrow range of geographic, ethnic, or religious restrictions.

A geographic constraint is illustrated by the classic example of the common communicable disease rubeola. The rubeola virus, or the populations that were continually exposed to it, became altered in such a way that the disease was considered to be a universal disease of childhood from which the majority of children suffered without ill effects. When other populations (e.g., the inhabitants of the Hawaiian Islands) were exposed to the virus by explorers and missionaries, they experienced a violent response that resulted in high mortality.

Another communicable disease, tuberculosis, appears to be more prevalent in certain ethnic groups such as the Native Americans of the Southwest, Vietnamese immigrants, and Mexican-Americans. In many populations it is difficult to determine how much the increased incidence can be attributed to ethnic factors and how much is related to the life-styles in the lower social strata.

A number of diseases show ethnic or racial differences. For example, Tay-Sachs disease, characterized by early neurologic deterioration and mental retardation, affects primarily Ashkenasi Jewish families, particularly those of Northeastern European origin, whereas Sephardic Jewish families appear to be no more at risk for the disease than other populations. The incidence of cystic fibrosis is highest in whites and almost nonexistent in Orientals, and the rare affected blacks are usually in areas where there is apt to be mixed ancestry. Some selected genetic disorders that are more prevalent in certain populations are listed in Table 2-2. Racial and ethnic differences are further considered in relation to diseases and defects as they are discussed throughout the book.

Other groups appear to have a predisposition for certain diseases. Although sickle cell disease is a classic disorder of blacks, especially Africans, cardiovascular disease, pneumo-

TABLE 2-2 Distribution of Selected Genetic Traits and Disorders by Population or Ethnic Group

ETHNIC OR POPULATION GROUP	GENETIC OR MULTIFACTORIAL DISORDER PRESENT IN RELATIVELY HIGH FREQUENCY
Åland Islanders	Ocular albinism (Forsius-Eriksson type)
Amish	Limb-girdle muscular dystrophy (IN—Adams, Allen counties) Ellis-van Creveld (PA—Lancaster county) Pyruvate kinase deficiency (OH—Mifflin county) Hemophilia B (PA—Holmes county)
Armenians	Familial Mediterranean fever Familial paroxysmal polyserositis
Blacks (African)	Sickle cell disease Hemoglobin C disease Hereditary persistence of hemoglobin F G-6-PD deficiency, African type Lactase deficiency, adult β-Thalassemia
Burmese	Hemoglobin E disease
Chinese	Alpha thalassemia G-6-PD deficiency, Chinese type Lactase deficiency, adult
Costa Rican	Malignant osteopetrosis
English	Cystic fibrosis Hereditary amyloidosis, type III
Eskimos	Congenital adrenal hyperplasia Pseudocholinesterase deficiency Methemoglobinemia
Finns	Congenital nephrosis Generalized amyloidosis syndrome, V Polycystic liver disease Retinoschisis Aspartylglycosaminuria Diastrophic dwarfism
French Canadians (Quebec)	Tyrosinemia Morquio syndrome
Gypsies (Czech)	Congenital glaucoma
Hopi Indians	Tyrosinase-positive albinism
Iceland	Phenylketonuria
Irish	Phenylketonuria Neural tube defects
Japanese	Acatalasemia Cleft lip/palate Oguchi disease
Jews	
Ashkenazi	Tay-Sachs disease (infantile) Niemann-Pick disease (infantile) Gaucher disease (adult type) Familial dysautonomia (Riley-Day syndrome) Bloom syndrome Torsion dystonia Factor XI (PTA) deficiency
Sephardi	Familial Mediterranean fever Ataxia-telangiectasia (Morocco) Cystinuria (Libya) Glycogen storage disease III (Morocco)
Lebanese	Dyggve-Melchoir-Clausen syndrome
Mediterranean people (Italians, Greeks)	G-6-PD deficiency, Mediterranean type β-Thalassemia Familial Mediterranean fever
Navaho Indians	Ear anomalies
Nova Scotia Acadians	Niemann-Pick disease, type D
Middle Eastern people	Dubin-Johnson syndrome (Iran) Ichthyosis vulgaris (Iraq) Werdnig-Hoffman disease (Karaite Jews) G-6-PD deficiency, Mediterranean type Phenylketonuria (Yemen) Metachromatic leukodystrophy (Habbanite Jews, Saudi Arabia)
Polish	Phenylketonuria
Polynesians	Clubfoot
Portugese	Joseph disease
Scandinavians (Norwegians, Swedes, Danes)	Cholestasis-lymphedema (Norwegians) Sjögren-Larsson syndrome (Swedes) Krabbe disease Phenylketonuria
Scots	Phenylketonuria Cystic fibrosis Hereditary amyloidosis, type III
Thai	Lactase deficiency, adult Hemoglobin E disease
Zuni Indians	Tyrosinase-positive albinism

Sources: Cohen, 1984; Damon, 1969; Der Kaloustian, Maffah, and Loiselet, 1980; Ferak, Genčik, and Genčíkova, 1982; Goodman, 1979; McKusick, 1992; Scriver, 1989.

nia, and diabetes are also high among blacks. Hispanics are more likely to suffer from diabetes and infectious/parasitic diseases than their Anglo counterparts, and Native Americans have particularly high rates of tuberculosis, diarrhea, alcoholism, and suicide (Giger and Davidhizar, 1991).

Reactions to certain food items or drugs vary with race. For example, isoniazid, a drug commonly used to treat tuberculosis, is metabolized rapidly by 40% of whites, 60% of blacks, 60% to 90% of Native Americans and Eskimos, and 85% to 90% of Orientals (Giger and Davidhizar, 1991).

The sensitivity to foods containing lactose is a common hereditary characteristic of several cultural groups, especially southern Europeans, Jews, Arabs, blacks, Asians, and Native Americans. Lactose intolerance usually does not become a problem until the child reaches 3 to 5 years of age. However, lactose-intolerant children become uncomfortable with distention, flatus, and diarrhea after ingesting milk or milk products. Unknowing but well-meaning health workers may be responsible for these symptoms in their clients when they prescribe foods containing lactose as sources of nutrients.

An example of resistance to disease, or selective advantage, of a population is found in persons who possess the sickle cell trait. Persons with sickle cell trait are highly resistant to a form of malaria, and in the parts of the world where the organisms are prevalent, there is a high frequency of the trait. However, in an environment where malaria is not a threat, possession of the trait has no advantage and only the negative aspects of the condition remain (risk of sickle cell anemia in offspring).

Physical Characteristics. Among racial groups there are observable differences in physical appearance. The most obvious are skin and hair coloring and texture. Skin color is determined by the amount of melanin pigment present in the skin. Persons from countries located near the equator have darkly pigmented skin, which serves to protect the skin from the year-round exposure to the sun's rays; persons from the northern countries have very light skin, which provides for maximum exposure to the sun's rays (necessary for vitamin D metabolism) during the short daylight hours. There can be wide variations in skin color between these two extremes in terms of geographic origin or from intermixing of dark and light skin color.

As a consequence of the dark pigmentation, the detection of skin color changes can be difficult and requires modification of assessment techniques. For example, vasomotor alterations, cyanosis, and jaundice observable in the skin are not easily recognized in very dark or black skin. Variations in the skin color can alter the appearance of the skin in a given circumstance (see Table 7-9).

Variations in the newborn are often related to racial or ethnic origin. For example, newborn infants of Asian and black parents are smaller than infants of white parentage (David, 1990). Oriental children are usually smaller at all ages. Bluish pigmented areas (mongolian spots) on the sacral region are a common observation on Oriental, black, Native American, and Mexican-American infants.

Socioeconomic Factors

The most overwhelming adverse influence on health is socioeconomic status. A higher percentage of individuals from the lower classes are suffering from some health problem at any one time than are those in any other group. The sum of all aspects of their situation contributes to and compounds health problems; this includes crowded living conditions and poor sanitation, which facilitate transfer of disease, such as tuberculosis. There is a higher incidence of lead poisoning in children from families from the lower classes, where there is more ready access to lead in the environment, such as paint and other lead-containing compounds or utensils, pottery with lead-containing glazes, and burning of lead-containing batteries for heat in winter.

In the lower classes children are less likely to be immunized against preventable diseases than are children in the upper and middle classes. Lack of funds or inaccessibility to health services inhibits treatment for any but severe illness or injury. Sometimes health care is inadequate because of ignorance. In some areas a disorder is so commonplace that it is looked on as unavoidable; it is not recognized as something that requires (or is amenable to) treatment. The parents may not have information regarding causes, treatment, outcome of the illness, or preventive measures. The nurse can use the limited opportunities when the family does come into contact with the health care system to inquire about immunizations, screen for vision problems, provide nutritional information, and offer additional prevention and health promotion resources.

Poverty. A high correlation between poverty and the prevalence of illness has long been observed. Impoverished families suffer from poor nutrition; they have little if any preventive health care, inadequate health maintenance, and very limited access to health services. One of the most significant health problems related to poverty is a high infant mortality rate (Annie E. Casey Foundation, 1993). Health care often ranks low on their list of priorities. Day-to-day needs of food, clothing, and lodging take precedence over health care as long as the ailing person feels able to perform activities of daily living.

Poor families may be denied access to some health institutions for emergency or other hospital care. Frequently they must travel long distances to service centers that are willing to assume their care. In an emergency they must find money for taxi fare, borrow an automobile, or seek other means of transportation. They must find care for dependents, such as other infants and small children, or have them accompany them when taking the ill child for care. Families tend to delay preventive care indefinitely unless health services are relatively accessible. They are more likely to consult folk practitioners or other persons within their community.

Poor nutrition accounts for many health problems in the lower classes. Lack of funds and ignorance result in a diet that may be seriously lacking in essential food substances, especially protein, vitamins, and iron. This inadequate diet often leads to nutritional deficiency disorders and growth retardation in children. In many the total intake is insufficient to support normal growth. Unstructured eating patterns and irregularly scheduled mealtimes can also contribute to erratic food intake and a proportionately larger consumption of nonnourishing snacks, which can result in excessive weight gain.

Because of deficient preventive care, dental problems are more prevalent. Lack of standard immunizations together with reduced resistance from poor nutrition renders the exposed children in poor segments of the population vulnerable to communicable diseases. Poor sanitation and crowded living conditions also contribute to the higher incidence and perpetuation of illness. In general, poor people become ill more frequently and remain ill for longer periods of time than persons in the general population.

Homelessness. Homeless children experience all of the health problems associated with poverty, as well as other types of disorders. Their families have fewer resources with which to control the environment or to promote rehabilitation and prevent disease. Preventive health care, especially immunization and dental care, is seriously lacking. Impaired vision is common among homeless children, perhaps reflecting missed opportunities for vision screening. A high incidence of injuries, burns, and lead toxicity has also been observed (Parker and others, 1991).

Developmental delays, severe depression, anxiety, and learning difficulties have been reported (Bass and others, 1990; Bassuk and Rosenberg, 1990). Masten and others (1993) found more behavior problems, particularly antisocial behavior, among homeless children.

The nutritional status of many homeless families is poor. An inadequate diet can have long-lasting effects on children. Some homeless children exhibit a pattern of stunting without wasting, which is characteristic of poor children experiencing moderate, chronic nutritional stress (Fierman and others, 1991). High rates of iron deficiency among homeless children have been reported (Fierman and others, 1993; Page, Ainsworth, and Pett, 1993). Obesity and hypercholesterolemia have also been noted (Drake, 1992). Lack of adequate food is only part of the problem; homeless families may believe they are meeting nutritional needs, when actually the reverse is true. They may also lack knowledge about how to safely prepare and store food.

The past experiences of runaway adolescents have directly shaped and molded their views of themselves and the world. These experiences, along with a desperate need for money, escape, and sometimes companionship, are often reflected in their high level of risk-taking behavior (Stefanidis and others, 1992). In one study of over 100 homeless and runaway youth, nearly 25% had injected illegal drugs, 20% had shared needles for other purposes, 16% had participated in anal intercourse, 19% had engaged in prostitution, 67% reported having four or more sexual partners, and only 20% reported that they always used condoms (Sugerman and others, 1991). The erratic chaotic life-style of these children increases their vulnerability to any number of physical and psychosocial problems, including child abuse, illicit drug use, and sexually-transmitted diseases.

Migrant Families. Migrants generally suffer more illness, both acute and chronic, than does the general population. They are subject to unhealthy environments, poverty, and insufficient medical care; their health-seeking behavior in general is an illness- or injury-oriented recourse to medical care. Affected persons will postpone seeking care for themselves or their children until physical pain or suffering is almost unbearable.

When medical care is provided to a migrant family, follow-up care is usually impossible because of their transient life-style. Compliance with medical therapies is primarily related to accessibility and availability. For example, medications provided by health workers are more likely to be taken than those that must be obtained at a pharmacy. In addition, medications are often discontinued following self-perceived recovery. Treatment regimens that do not interfere with work or family responsibilities are most likely to be adhered to.

The health problems of migrant children appear to be dental caries, upper respiratory tract infections, otitis media, scabies and lice, intestinal parasites, pesticide exposure, injuries, teenage pregnancy, and growth and development delay (American Academy of Pediatrics, 1989). Other findings indicate that migrant children are significantly more likely to be maltreated than other children (Larson, Doris, and Alvarez, 1990).

Tuberculosis rates among migrant families are high. Farm workers are approximately six times more likely to develop the disease than the general population of employed adults. Drug-resistant tuberculosis is an important consideration among this population; it requires altered treatment regimens, and higher rates of resistance have been found in the ethnic and social groups constituting much of the migrant farm work force (Prevention, 1992).

CUSTOMS AND FOLKWAYS

Nurses need to consider cultural differences in clients when providing health care. An understanding of the various beliefs regarding the causation of illness and disease, as well as traditional health practices, is essential to successful intervention. The more nurses know about the values, beliefs, and customs of other ethnic groups, the better able they are to meet the needs of these families and to gain their cooperation and compliance.

Cultural Relativity

Although clinical characteristics of a disease or condition are essentially the same across cultures, how a child or family interprets or experiences the disease or condition varies. Culture as an influence is one obvious explanation for variance. ***Cultural relativity*** is the concept that any behavior must be judged first in relation to the context of the culture in which it occurs. Nurses must first relate to the family's perceptions and interpretations of experiences from the family's background and cultural belief system before they can intervene effectively.

Some cultures, for example, may view a chronic illness or disability as affecting only particular aspects of a child's life, and the child as a whole is viewed as normal. In contrast, Chinese families more frequently describe the illness as having global effects on many aspects of the child's present and future life (Elfert, Anderson, and Lai, 1991). These contrasting views may result in a difference in the goals and expectations parents have for their children.

In some cultures the child's gender may influence a family's perception of the implications of an illness or disability. For example, in the Arabic and Asian cultures and for some families of Jewish, Italian, Greek, or Indian origin, the male child is held in higher esteem than the female child. The male child may receive better health care and the most food, because this is the child who will take care of his parents in their old age (Issacs, 1989).

Defining disease or signs and symptoms of illness is also influenced by culture. Some cultures, for example, perceive diarrhea as a cleansing of the body that is essential for health maintenance and illness prevention and/or cure. Furthermore, signs or symptoms resulting from diarrhea and ensuing dehydration, such as malaise, fever, anorexia, and irritability, may be viewed as separate illness entities.

Nurses can often recognize a family's health-related cultural perceptions and interpretations through discussion and observation. Implications of these perceptions should be explored and considered when planning effective culturally appropriate interventions.

Relationships with Health Care Providers

The manner of relating with health care providers differs considerably among cultural groups. One area of conflict to some nurses is the attitude toward time and waiting that is part of some cultures. The time orientation of Hispanic and black ethnic groups is in the present. For example, blacks are very flexible in their time orientation; a black family may be late for or miss appointments because other issues take precedence over the appointment and they may not communicate this to the health agency. Hispanics, too, have a very relaxed view of time. Whereas the dominant culture in the United States says that "time flies," the Hispanic says, "time walks." In general, Asian-Americans view the American focus on time as offensive. They spend hours getting to know people and view predetermined, abrupt endings as rude. Introductory small talk is considered good manners (Randall-David, 1989). A Vietnamese family will subordinate time to values considered to be more significant (Stauffer, 1991). For example, they may be late for an appointment because of an overextended visit by a friend in their home. To maintain social harmony, the Vietnamese do not hurry personal visits. Navajo Indians view time on a continuum with no beginning and no end. The present-time orientation may cause a Navajo to eat two meals a day today, four meals tomorrow, no meals the next day, and three meals the day after. This becomes an important nursing consideration if a Navajo is told to take medication with meals to ensure three doses per day (Hanley, 1991).

In many cultural groups the mother assumes the responsibility for health care; in others both parents are involved equally in relationships with health workers. A somewhat different approach is apparent in some of the Oriental cultures. For example, the father in Vietnamese or Filipino families, as unquestioned head of the family, is traditionally the family member who interacts with persons, including health care providers, outside the family unit. Therefore he is the one who represents the family in health matters. In the Hispanic family the father, as head of the house, makes decisions regarding illness and treatment of family members, but the grandmother in the extended family is consulted regarding child care. Usually the family confers with other members before reaching a decision regarding treatment or hospitalization of a child. The Arab family also relies on others to give advice and guidance in a time of crisis. A Japanese father may appear to be passive and uninvolved but actually is involved according to his own cultural standards.

NURSING ALERT In working with families, it is essential for nurses to identify key members—failure to include these significant individuals in teaching can seriously hinder adherence to the plan of care.

Nurses should make themselves aware of any specific attitudes regarding the manner of approach to a child in a given culture. Navajo Indians do not like a stranger near their infants. It is feared that the stranger may "witch" the child and cause the child harm. On the other hand, if a stranger, particularly a woman, lavishes attention on a Hispanic infant but fails to touch the child, the infant will develop symptoms of the "evil eye" (see p. 47). Vietnamese and Korean families may become upset if a newborn is admired at length for fear the evil spirits will overhear and desire the infant.

Some groups, such as the Amish, consider a child's admission to the hospital a family affair, with all members gathering to support and console the child and the parents. In other groups the family is willing to relinquish the care of the child to the hospital authority without interference. Their visits with the child are short, although intense, but this behavior may be misinterpreted by the hospital staff as disinterest or abandonment.

All ethnic groups are proud people who are entitled to be treated with dignity and respect. Family members are addressed by their last names: many groups consider it an affront to be called by their first names. Stereotyping is to be condemned. Persons are individuals who are evaluated in relation to their cultural standards, needs, and preferences (Fig. 2-4).

Nurses who are members of a majority culture may encounter tension and distrust in a child from a minority culture as a result of the child's learned conception or relationships with other persons in the majority group. Based on these perceptions, minority children often suspect that nurses may have hostile feelings toward them and fear ill treatment. When such children are hospitalized, this feeling compounds the feelings of loneliness, helplessness, and retribution that accompany fearful happenings and separation from families. The reverse situation may be encountered by a nurse from a minority culture attempting to meet the needs of a child who has been conditioned to view the nurse's cultural or ethnic group as inferior. Either situation is more likely to occur if the nurse or the child has had little or no personal contact with the other's culture. For example, a child from a minority culture from the inner city who lives in a neighborhood and attends school only with children from his or her minority culture may be more

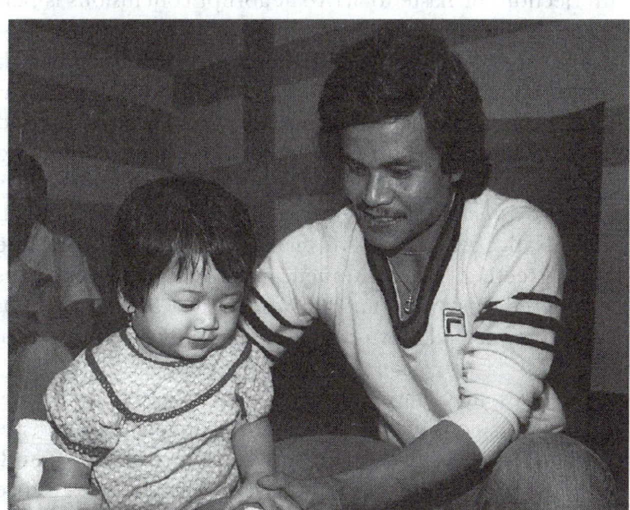

FIG. 2-4 Fathers from many cultures assume an active parenting role.

suspicious of a nurse from a different culture than may be a child from the same minority group who lives in a culturally mixed neighborhood or who attends an integrated school. Taking the opportunity to become familiar with cultures different from one's own and making an effort to get to know each other as individuals can shatter myths and, with time, build the trust needed to establish rewarding relationships between children, their families, and the nurse.

Communication. Communication is basic to all human relationships, but it may be a source of distress and misunderstanding between persons from different ethnic groups, especially if the languages are different. Ideally, conversations with families who are unable to speak the dominant language are best conducted by a health care worker who speaks the language of the family. If this is not possible, it may be necessary to engage the services of an interpreter. However, use of an interpreter can be a source of misunderstanding if the interpreter is unfamiliar with the medical terminology or if there are no corresponding words in the second language to express the ideas and concepts under discussion (see Communicating with Families Through an Interpreter, Chapter 6).

Some persons with poor or limited language comprehension may simply smile and nod in agreement if they do not understand the questions or directives. It is vital that the family fully understand all implications of a child's care and management before they sign permits for special procedures or assume responsibility for the child's care. It is not uncommon for an Oriental family to indicate "yes" when in fact they mean "no" in order to avoid social disharmony. They tend to use indirectness rather than confrontation and may become evasive when direct questioning makes them feel uncomfortable.

Nonverbal communication is a practiced art in many American Indian tribes, and the members are highly sensitive to body language. They emphasize periods of silence to formulate thoughts in preparation for speech and often remain silent after listening to statements by others in order to properly assimilate what has been said. Interruption, interjection, or haste to arrive at abrupt conclusions is perceived as immature behavior.

Eye contact is viewed differently in cultures. Although Anglos are advised to look people straight in the eye, it is not uncommon for persons in some ethnic groups to avoid eye contact and become uncomfortable when conversing with health workers. In non-Western cultures a patient may not look directly into the nurse's eyes as a sign of respect. Some Native Americans will make eye contact during the initial greeting, but continued, unwavering eye contact is considered insulting and disrespectful (Hanley, 1991). Asians may consider eye contact a sign of hostility or impoliteness.

Gestures may have different meanings. For example, some Asians consider pointing with a finger or foot disrespectful. Some Native Americans consider vigorous handshaking a sign of aggression, whereas to Anglos the gesture is a sign of goodwill and strong character.

There may be reluctance on the part of families to question or otherwise initiate contact with health professionals. In the Asian cultures, for example, it is considered a sign of disrespect to question those who are viewed as persons of authority. A Japanese family may wait silently rather than ask or question. They believe that the health professionals know best and will meet their needs without being asked. It is also important to avoid criticism. Criticism can cause the Japanese-American to "lose face," to feel ashamed, which is highly undesirable.

It is necessary to speak slowly and carefully, not loudly, when conversing with families who have poor language comprehension. Many persons are able to read and write English better than they can speak or understand it. Also, the dominant language usually takes over in anxiety-provoking situations, even in persons who are able to communicate satisfactorily under ordinary circumstances.

Terms of address and use of first and last names vary among cultures and can create confusion in institutions. For example, in Asian cultures, the family name is given first in respect for the family and the given names follow. Therefore all siblings in a family have the same first name (in some families it may be the middle names that are the

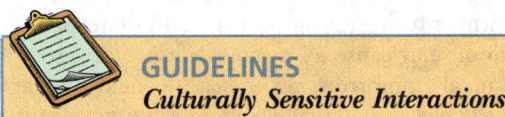

GUIDELINES
Culturally Sensitive Interactions

NONVERBAL STRATEGIES

Invite family members to choose where they would like to sit or stand, allowing them to select a comfortable distance.
Observe interactions with others to determine which body gestures (e.g., shaking hands) are acceptable and appropriate. Ask when in doubt.
Avoid appearing rushed.
Be an active listener.
Observe for cues regarding appropriate eye contact.
Learn appropriate use of pauses or interruptions for different cultures.
Ask for clarification if nonverbal meaning is unclear.

VERBAL STRATEGIES

Learn proper terms of address.
Use a positive tone of voice to convey interest.
Speak slowly and carefully, not loudly, when families have poor language comprehension.
Encourage questions.
Learn basic words and sentences of family's language, if possible.
Avoid professional terms.
When asking questions, tell family why the questions are being asked, the way in which the information they provide will be used, and how it might benefit their child.
Repeat important information more than once.
Always give the reason or purpose for a treatment or prescription.
Use information written in family's language.
Offer the services of an interpreter when necessary (see Chapter 6).
Learn from families and representatives of their culture methods of communicating information without creating discomfort.
Address intergenerational needs (e.g., family's need to consult with others).
Be sincere, open, and honest and, when appropriate, share personal experiences, beliefs, and practices to establish rapport and trust.

same). Ethiopians use no last names but have a very complex system whereby women retain their last names after marriage and the paternal grandfather's name becomes a child's last name. The Mennonites refer to children as sons and daughters of a particular parent, such as "Josiah's son," rather than by the son's name (Elkin and Handel, 1989).

Although all people share the basic emotions, there are decided ethnic variations in the way emotions are expressed. In some cultures (e.g., persons of Italian, Latin, or Jewish background) emotions are expressed openly and members are accustomed to sharing their sorrows and joys with family and friends. Conversely, Nordic and Asian groups are more restrained in expressing emotion.

Nurses caring for persons of another culture will be better able to communicate if they understand the common names used to describe symptoms and diseases: for example, ***miseries*** (pain) and ***locked bowels*** (constipation) in black people and ***caida de la mollera*** (fallen fontanel from dehydration), ***susto*** (fright), ***dolor*** (pain), and ***la diarrhea*** (diarrhea) in Latinos.

Health care providers generally ask questions and use handouts, booklets, and—particularly with children—dolls and pictures as communication aids. This is uncommon in some cultures. For example, Native American healers ask few questions and do not use forms. In some cultures it is considered inappropriate or taboo to look at the inside of the body, even in pictures, or to use dolls or puppets (Malach and Segal, 1990). Nurses need to consider both verbal and nonverbal communication techniques to interact effectively with children and their families from different cultures (see Guidelines box).

Food Customs

Food customs and symbolism of various cultural, ethnic, and religious groups have become an integral part of their lives. Although in a large country such as the United States most persons have adopted the eclectic food habits that have evolved over countless generations, many ethnic and geographic food traditions and preferences are retained. Special holidays, ceremonies, and life experiences such as births, birthdays, weddings, and death are often marked by special food items or feasts. In many cultures specific food practices are followed during pregnancy in the belief that certain foods damage the developing fetus.

The distinctive food customs of ethnic groups are a product of their native environment, determined by availability. Fish is a staple food of persons living near the ocean, such as people from Japan, Polynesia, and Scandinavia. Fruit and vegetable preferences are also directly related to the climate in which these grow naturally or can be cultivated. The types of grain that are ethnically associated are also those that grow best in their native lands. For example, rice is the staple grain of the Orient and Pacific islands. The diet of the Eskimo is predominantly fish and meat, depending on which is the most easily procured in the area. Even in the continental United States there are regional favorites, such as rice, hominy grits, and okra in the southern states. In some cultures food is highly spiced; in others foods tend to be bland. Table 2-3 lists the food items common to most cultures and can be used to select foods that most children know and like. Table 2-4 outlines some of the foods associated with some specific ethnic groups.

It is also of interest that age affects food choices among various cultures. For example, while pizza is a favorite food of Anglo teenagers, pinon nuts are popular with Navajo youth. The fact that a 1993 epidemic on the Navajo reservation associated with pinon nuts affected primarily teenagers and young adults may be related to their food habits (Hantavirus infection, 1993).

There are a number of restrictions related to food items. Some have a physiologic origin, such as lack of dairy foods in the diets of some persons of African or Asian ancestry with lactose intolerance. Others have religious restrictions, such as kosher foods and food preparation of the Orthodox Jewish faith and the vegetarian diet of Seventh Day Adventists (see Vegetarian Diets, Chapter 13).

Children in a strange environment, such as the hospital, feel much more comfortable when they are served familiar foods (Fig. 2-5). Hospital food often tastes strange and bland, especially to children who enjoy the highly seasoned foods of their culture. Also, the family may be concerned that the child is not receiving foods appropriate to their culture and beliefs (see Health Beliefs, p. 47). Where possible, it is advisable to provide children's ethnic foods or allow families to bring favorite foods that are not available on the hospital menu. Concern for differences in food habits and patterns projects an attitude of respect for the family's ethnic or religious heritage.

TABLE 2-3 Foods Common to Most Ethnic Food Patterns

MEAT AND ALTERNATIVES	MILK AND MILK PRODUCTS	GRAIN PRODUCTS	VEGETABLES	FRUITS	OTHERS
Pork*	Milk, fluid	Rice	Carrots	Apples	Fruit juices
Beef	Ice cream	White bread	Cabbage	Bananas	
Chicken		Noodles, macaroni, spaghetti	Green beans	Oranges	
Eggs		Dry cereal	Greens (especially spinach)	Peaches	
			Sweet potatoes or yams	Pears	
			Tomatoes	Tangerines	

From Endres JB, Rockwell RE: *Food, nutrition, and the young child,* St Louis, 1980, Mosby, p 180.
*May be restricted because of religious custom.

TABLE 2-4 Characteristic Food Choices for Six Groups

VEGETABLES	FRUITS	MEATS AND ALTERNATIVES	GRAIN PRODUCTS	OTHERS
BLACK				
Broccoli, corn, greens (mustard, collard, kale, turnips, beet, etc.), lima beans, okra, peas, pumpkin	Grapefruit, grapes, nectarine, plums, watermelon	Sausage, pig's feet, ears, etc., bacon, luncheon meat, organ meats, turkey, catfish, perch, red snapper, tuna, salmon, sardines, shrimp, kidney beans, red beans, black-eyed peas, peanuts, and peanut butter	Corn bread, hominy grits, biscuits, muffins, cooked cereal, crackers	Chitterlings, salt pork, gravies, buttermilk
HISPANIC				
Avocado, chilies, corn, lettuce, peas, potato, prickly pear (cactus leaf called *nopales*), zucchini	Guava, lemon, mango, melons, prickly pear (cactus fruit called *tuna*), zapote (or sapote)	Lamb, tripe, sausage ***(chorizo)***, bologna, bacon, pinto beans, pink beans, garbanzo beans, lentils, peanuts, and peanut butter	Tortillas, corn flour, oatmeal, sweet bread ***(pan dulce)***	Salsa (tomato-pepper, onion relish), chili sauce, guacamole, lard ***(manteca)***, pork cracklings
JAPANESE				
Bamboo shoots, broccoli, burdock root, cauliflower, celery, cucumbers, eggplant, gourd ***(Kampyo)***, mushrooms, napa cabbage, peas, peppers, radishes (daikon or pickles called ***takuwan)***, snow peas, squash, sweet potato, turnips, water chestnuts, yamaimo	Apricot, cherries, grapefruit, grapes, lemon, lime, melons, persimmon, pineapple, pomegranate, plums (dried pickled ***umeboshi***), strawberries	Turkey, raw tuna or sea bass ***(sashimi)***, mackerel, sardines ***(mezashi)***, shrimp, abalone, squid, octopus, soybean curd ***(tofu)***, soybean paste ***(miso)***, soybeans, red beans ***(azuki)***, lima beans, peanuts, almonds, cashews	Rice, rice crackers, noodles (whole-wheat noodle called ***soba*** or ***udon***), oatmeal	Soy sauce, Nori paste (used to season rice), bean thread ***(konyaku)***, ginger ***(shoga;*** dried form called ***denishoga)***
CHINESE				
Bamboo shoots, bean sprouts, bok choy, broccoli, celery, Chinese cabbage, corn, cucumbers, eggplant, greens (collard, Chinese, broccoli, mustard, kale), leeks, lettuce, mushrooms, peppers, scallions, snow peas, taro, water chestnuts, white turnips, white radishes, winter melon	Figs, grapes, kumquats, loquats, mango, melons, persimmon, pineapple, plums, pomegranate	Organ meats, duck, white fish, shrimp, lobster, oyster, sardines, soybeans, tofu, black beans, chestnuts ***(kuri)***	Rice, barley, millet	Soy sauce, sweet and sour sauce, mustard sauce, ginger root, plum sauce, red bean paste
VIETNAMESE*				
Bamboo shoots, bean sprouts, cabbage, carrots, cucumbers, greens, lettuce, mushrooms, onions, peas, spinach, yams	Apple, banana, eggfruit ***(o-ma)***, grapefruit, jackfruit, lychee, mandarin, mango, orange, papaya, pineapple, tangerine, watermelon	Beef, blood, brain, chicken, duck, eggs, fish, goat, kidney, lamb, liver, pork, shellfish, soybeans	French bread, rice, rice noodles, wheat noodles	Fish sauce, fresh herbs, garlic, ginger, lard, MSG, peanut oil, sesame seeds, sesame seed oil, vegetable oil

From Endres JB, Rockwell RE: *Food, nutrition, and the young child,* St Louis, 1980, Mosby, pp 182-183. Modified from *Nutrition during pregnancy and lactation,* California Department of Public Health, revised 1975.
NOTE: Foods common to all ethnic groups have been omitted.
*Information supplied by Hanh-Trang Tran-Viet, Carbondale, Ill.

TABLE 2-4 Characteristic Food Choices for Six Groups—cont'd

VEGETABLES	FRUITS	MEATS AND ALTERNATIVES	GRAIN PRODUCTS	OTHERS
INDIAN *(EAST)*				
Cauliflower, carrots, cucumber, corn-gourds, leeks, egg-plant, beets, radishes, hot pepper, bell pep-per, peas, French beans, okra, pump-kin, red and white cabbage, mung sprouts, bean sprouts, potatoes, tapioca root, sweet potatoes	Oranges, limes, grapes, watermelon, mango, guava, honeydew, chiku, cantaloupe, pineapple, green, yel-low, and red ba-nanas, berries, custard apples	Lamb, beef, duck, chicken, shrimp, cat-fish, buffalo, sunfish, sardines, fresh crab, lobster, peanuts, cashews, almonds, chick-peas, split peas, black-eyed peas, dry mung beans	Rice pancakes, wheat chapati, puri, mixed grain flour bread	Fresh coconut juice, curries, tomato sauce, tamarind sauce, dried grain curries *(pulses)*, yogurt-curry gar-nished with coriander (fresh leaves)

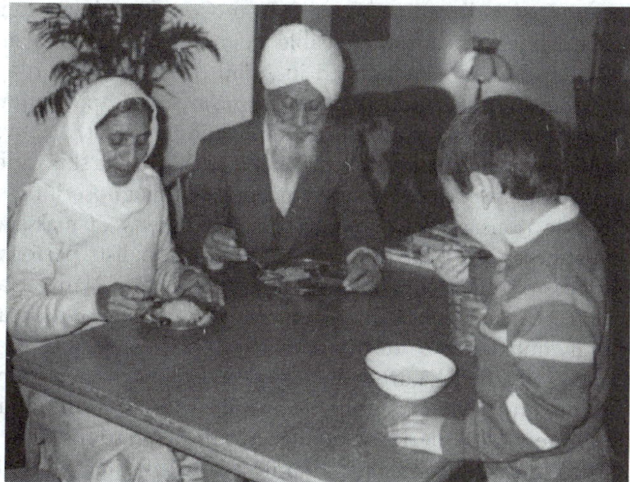

FIG. 2-5 Food customs outside the home can differ significantly from traditional cultural practices.

HEALTH BELIEFS AND PRACTICES

The nurse encounters people of many different racial and ethnic origins in the process of meeting the health needs of children and families. Some of these families have become so enculturated to the majority culture that their health beliefs and practices are consistent with those of the health care system. For many families, however, traditional practices and beliefs are an integral part of their daily lives. Health care workers should be aware that other people may live by different rules and priorities from those of the health care provider, and these rules and priorities decisively influence health-related behavior.

Health Beliefs

The beliefs related to the cause of illness and the maintenance of health are an integral part of the cultural heritage of families. Often inseparable from religious beliefs, they influence the way that families cope with health problems and the way that they respond to health care providers. Predominant among most cultures are beliefs related to natural forces, supernatural forces, and imbalance between forces.

Natural Forces. The most common natural forces held responsible for ill health if the body is not adequately protected include cold air entering the body, impurities in the air, or other natural sources. For example, a Chinese parent may overdress the infant in an effort to keep cold wind from entering the child's body. The Chinese believe that cold weather, rain, or wind is responsible for "cold" conditions. They also believe that an innate energy called ***chi*** enters and leaves the body through the mouth, nose, and ears and flows through the body in definite pathways, or meridians, at specific times and locations. Lack of chi and blood is believed to be a cause of fatigue, low energy, and a variety of ailments.

In the black culture natural phenomena such as phases of the moon, seasons of the year, and planet positions are believed to affect the body and its processes; therefore health maintenance is strongly associated with the ability to read "the signs." Some cultures consider such behavior as overeating, overwork, anxiety, and inadequate food and sleep as natural causes of illness. Most Native Americans consider health to be a state of harmony with nature and the universe.

Supernatural Forces. High on the list of causes of illness are forces beyond comprehension and logical explanation. Evil influences such as voodoo, witchcraft, or evil spirits are viewed in some cultures as causes of adverse health, especially those illnesses that cannot be explained by other means.

A health belief that is common among people from Latin America, Mediterranean, Near East, some Asian, and some African societies is the concept of the "evil eye" (***mal ojo*** is the Hispanic term). It is part of the concept of health as a state of balance; illness is a state of imbalance (see below). Strength and power are associated with the evil eye; therefore, as long as an individual's strength and weakness remain in balance, he or she is unlikely to become a victim of the evil eye. Weaknesses are not necessarily physical. For example, an excess of some emotion, such as envy, can create a weakness. Infants and small children, because of immature development of their internal strength-weakness states, are especially vulnerable to the gaze of the evil eye (Giger and Davidhizar, 1991). Consequently, the evil eye serves to rationalize an inexplicable onset of illness in children who display such symptoms as restlessness, crying, diarrhea, vomiting, and fever.

Although seldom expressed to health care providers, the belief that a witch can cast a spell or curse over others at the request of someone who wishes the person ill or dead is found in Hispanic, African, and Australian aboriginal cultures. The victim is often tortured in effigy by pins driven into a doll at the location where the intended victim is to be hurt. "Voodoo deaths" have occurred from the victim's belief in the curse and may result from dehydration as the victim gives up the will to live and refuses to drink (Chidester, 1990).

Imbalance of Forces. The concept of balance or equilibrium is widespread throughout the world. One of the most common imbalances supported by the Hispanic, Filipino, Chinese, and Arab cultures is that which exists between "hot" and "cold." This belief is reputedly derived from the Hippocratic theory of humoral pathology, which states that illness is caused by an imbalance of the four humors: phlegm, blood, black bile, and yellow bile. Hot and cold describe certain properties and conditions completely unrelated to temperature. Diseases, areas of the body, foods, and illnesses are classified as either "hot" or "cold." In Chinese health belief the forces are termed ***yin*** (cold) and ***yang*** (hot) (Chang, 1991). To maintain health and prevent illness these hot and cold forces must be kept in balance.

Illness is treated by restoring normal balance through the application of appropriate "hot" or "cold" remedies. A "cold" condition such as a respiratory disease is believed to be caused by exposure to cold weather, rain, or cold wind entering the body; it is treated by administration of "hot" foods, herbs, or drugs. Menstruation is considered to be a "hot" condition; therefore women are cautioned against ingesting "hot" foods, which might increase menstrual flow or produce cramping. Ingesting too much of either "hot" or "cold" foods can also be interpreted as a cause of illness.

Health care workers who are aware of this belief are better able to understand why some persons refuse to eat certain foods. It is often useful to discuss the diet with the family to determine their feelings and beliefs regarding food choices. It is possible to help families devise a diet that contains the necessary balance of basic food groups prescribed by the medical subculture while conforming to the beliefs of the ethnic subculture.

The hot-cold food classification may have adverse effects. For example, newborn infants are often started on evaporated milk formulas. Evaporated milk is considered to be a "hot" food, whereas whole milk is viewed as a "cold" food. Infants tend to develop rashes, which are believed to be caused by "hot" foods; in such cases parents may decide to switch to whole milk. However, parents fear that it is dangerous to change too rapidly, so they often feed the child some type of neutralizing substance, which may create additional health problems. Such a problem might be averted if the family's preference is determined before discharge from the hospital and a formula prescribed that is agreeable to both the family and the practitioner.

Health Practices

There are numerous similarities among cultures regarding prevention and treatment of illness. All cultures have some types of home remedies that they apply before seeking help from other persons. Within the ethnic community folk healers who are endowed with the ability to "cure" maladies are sought for special situations and when home remedies are unsuccessful. There is the ***curandero*** (male) or ***curandera*** (female) of the Mexican-American community whose healing powers are believed to be a gift from God. The Asian consults a herbalist, knowledgeable in medicines, and/or an ethnic practitioner practiced in Asian therapies, including ***acupuncture*** (insertion of needles), ***acupressure*** (application of pressure), and ***moxibustion*** (application of heat). Native Americans consult a variety of healers with specific skills and knowledge. Specialized medicine persons diagnose illness, provide nonsacred treatments (usually by way of massage and herbs), and care for souls. Other specialists perform services or affect cures through spiritual means. Native Hawaiins, consult ***kahunas*** and practice ***ho' oponopono*** to heal family imbalance or disputes.

The folk healers are very powerful persons in their community and have the ability to acquire information about an illness without resorting to probing questions. They "speak the language" of the family who seeks help and often combine their rituals and potions with prayer and entreaties to God. They also are able to create an atmosphere conducive to successful management. Furthermore, they exhibit a sincere interest in the family and their problem.

Some folk remedies are compatible with the medical regimen and can be used to reinforce the treatment plan. For example, most of the foods contraindicated for a person with peptic ulcer are "hot" foods and would be avoided by the person's belief system. Also, aspirin (a "hot" medication) is an appropriate therapy for "cold" diseases such as the common cold and arthritis. It is not uncommon to discover that a folk prescription has a scientific basis. However, numerous health remedies or preventive practices have no known scientific basis, such as the use of ***asafetida***, a piece of rotten flesh that looks like a dried sponge and is worn around the neck to prevent contagious diseases, or the wearing of copper or silver bracelets to protect the wearer. Practices that do no harm should be respected.

To overcome the effect of the evil eye usually requires specialized rituals conducted by the appropriate practitioner. For example, the Chicano curandera ascertains that the condition is truly the result of the evil eye by performing an assessment ritual and then, on a confirmed diagno–

CULTURAL PRACTICES POSSIBLY CONSIDERED ABUSIVE BY THE DOMINANT CULTURE

Coining—A Vietnamese practice that may produce weltlike lesions on the child's back when a coin, held on edge, is repeatedly rubbed lengthwise on the oiled skin to rid the body of the disease.

Cupping—An Old World practice (also practiced by the Vietnamese) of placing a container (e.g., tumbler, bottle, jar) containing steam against the skin surface to "draw out the poison" or other evil element. When the heated air within the container cools, a vacuum is created that produces a bruiselike blemish on the skin directly beneath the mouth of the container.

Burning—A practice of some Southeast Asian groups where small areas of skin are burned to treat enuresis and temper tantrums.

Forced kneeling—A child discipline measure of some Caribbean groups where a child is forced to kneel for a long period of time.

Topical garlic application—A practice of Yemenite Jews in which crushed garlic cloves or garlic–petroleum jelly plaster is applied to the wrists to treat infectious disease; the practice can result in blisters or garlic burns.

Traditional remedies that contain lead—***Greta*** and ***azarcon*** (Mexico; used for digestive problems), ***paylooah*** (Southeast Asia; used for rash or fever), and ***surma*** (India; used as a cosmetic to improve eyesight).

sis, performs a curative ritual. Sometimes the faith in the folk practitioner delays obtaining needed medical treatment, although the practitioner will usually suggest medical care if his or her ministrations are unsuccessful.

Health practices of different cultures may also present problems of assessment and interpretation. For example, certain cultural practices or remedies can be misdiagnosed as evidence of "child abuse" by uninformed professionals (see box above).

Other cultural health remedies that are detrimental to health include eating clay or excessive amounts of salt. A mercury compound, ***azogue*** (the Spanish name for quicksilver), is commonly used in Mexico and sometimes sold illegally to low-income Hispanic families in the United States as a "remedy" for diarrhea. Alert health care workers know that the drug can cause permanent central nervous system damage. A careful history can reveal these practices, but it may require the collaboration of a folk healer to convince a user to stop the practice.

Haitian folk medicine considers it essential to rid the newborn of meconium to ensure neonatal survival. The newborn's first food is a ***lok,*** or purgative, prepared by cooking a mixture of castor oil, grated nutmeg, sour orange juice, garlic, unrefined sugar, and water. It may be administered several times until the color of the newborn's bowel movement changes from black to yellow. All other oral intake may be restricted until this occurs, which may result in dehydration (DeSantis, 1988).

Faith healing and religious rituals are closely allied with many folk-healing practices. Wearing of amulets, medals, and other religious relics believed by the culture to protect the individual and facilitate healing is a common practice. It is important for health workers to recognize the value of this practice and keep the items where the family has placed them or nearby. It offers comfort and support and rarely impedes medical and nursing care. If an item must be removed during a procedure, it should be replaced, if possible, when the procedure is completed. The reason for its temporary removal is explained to the family, and they are reassured that their wishes will be respected.

Nurses can be most effective by operating from a multicultural perspective. Adopting a multicultural perspective means using appropriate aspects of each health cultural orientation under consideration to develop culturally acceptable health care interventions.

NURSING ALERT Avoid directly attacking traditional health cultural beliefs and practices as wrong or harmful, or implying that biomedical measures are uniformly correct and effective and the only way to prevent illness or treat sickness. Such attacks usually result in rejection of both biomedical health care practitioners and health teaching based on biomedicine or scientific facts.

Although most subcultures in the large developed countries have become acculturated to the Western medical system, many still maintain faith in traditional healing practices and practitioners. When the folk practices do not interfere with the welfare of the patient, they need not be discouraged. Often a compromise can be reached that accomplishes the goal of the nurse while maintaining the dignity and self-esteem of the client.

Folklore Related to Prenatal Influences

Since ancient times the striking appearance of abnormal human development has been of concern, as evidenced by descriptions in primitive drawings and on clay tablets, and has served as the origin of numerous legendary and mythologic creatures. Consequently, the processes of pregnancy and birth have been surrounded by strongly held beliefs and superstitions that involve taboos and prescriptions for behavior directed toward ensuring the well-being of the unborn child. Even in the face of scientific advances, these superstitions and folkways have survived for generations and may persist in various forms as part of a cultural heritage. The degree to which these beliefs are expressed depends on the strength of the cultural influence, the attitudes of the individual families, and the confidence and credibility engendered by the health care providers.

One of the most universal explanations of defective development has been maternal impressions. It has been a widespread belief that the appearance of the unborn child will be improved if the pregnant woman looks at beautiful people or things. The same concept in reverse has been used to explain birth defects. For example, if a pregnant woman was frightened by a rabbit, it was believed that her child would be born with a cleft ("hare") lip; a microcephalic infant was attributed to the mother's seeing a monkey during pregnancy; and the mother's viewing a person with missing limbs would cause the unborn child to be similarly affected. Activities such as a mother reaching her arms above her head, wearing a lei, walking in circles, or tying knots were believed to cause the umbilical cord to be knotted or twisted around the neck of the fetus. Even the shape of birthmarks and other skin defects is sometimes believed to reflect maternal impressions. For example, eating strawberries by the mother is associated with nevi. Articles of apparel or adornment, food cravings, emotions such as fright and anger, undesirable thoughts, and the time and manner of announcing the pregnancy are all believed to influence the well-being of the unborn child.

Expectant mothers who are able to rationalize the illogical nature of the beliefs will, through a normal fear of having an abnormal infant, conform to the superstitions. In most instances these customs are relatively harmless and are not in conflict with sound health practices. Valuing folkways may decrease the stresses of cultural differences for families (Starn, 1991). However, there are situations when conformity to cultural or subcultural beliefs may compromise the health and well-being of either mother or fetus (e.g., the practice of eating clay, cornstarch, chalk, or other substances). Understanding and judicious management on the part of nurses and other health care workers are required to explore with the mother all the ramifications of the practice without creating undue stress and guilt in the mother.

NURSING ALERT Not all of these beliefs are unfounded. There is evidence that maternal emotions may indeed affect the fetus.

Prolonged stimulation of the autonomic nervous system caused by extreme stress or long-term anxiety produces physiologic changes in the maternal system, such as increased heart rate, vasoconstriction, and decreased gastric motility. In addition to the indirect effect produced by constriction of uterine blood flow, the stress hormones cross the placental membrane to affect the fetus directly. Assisting the expectant mother in dealing with her stresses or securing counseling services for her is part of the nursing considerations.

RELIGIOUS BELIEFS

Religion influences the life-styles of most cultures. Among many groups illness, injury, or death is believed to be sent by God as a punishment for sin. Some may believe that health workers will be unable to help a person whom God is punishing and may express a fatalistic attitude toward treatment, stating that it is "the will of God." Others view it as a test of strength, as the testing of Job in the Bible, and strive to remain faithful and overcome the conflicts.

Religious affiliation has implications for many health-related functions and procedures. It is comforting to the family of an ill child to have this need recognized and respected. Nurses need to determine if there are any special considerations related to spiritual practices that are important to the family. Dietary restrictions are clarified, especially in denominations in which there may be many variations. When specific religious practices do not interfere with the health of the child or the therapy (such as fasting), the wishes of the family are respected. Family members are asked whether they want a clergy member present and whether they prefer hospital staff to call or prefer to do this on their own.

➤ **NURSING TIP** Children will rarely voice a need for spiritual support. Listen closely for indirect references, such as "God doesn't care what happens to people" (Clutter, 1991).

It is important to determine the wishes of the family regarding baptism, rites or practices related to death, and other religious rituals (such as circumcision, communion, or use of amulets or icons). An important role of the nurse is to be aware of spiritual needs of families and convey an attitude of concern for this important element of the child's care. Religion, which offers families understanding and spiritual support, is a valuable asset to health care. Characteristics of selected religions with beliefs that affect health care are outlined in Table 2-5.

In some instances the rights of the family and the responsibility of the state may be in conflict. For example, Jehovah's Witnesses strongly oppose blood transfusions for themselves and for their children. Parents, by law, have the primary obligation to care for and make decisions about their minor children. However, the legal principle of ***parens patriae*** says that the state has an overriding interest in the health and welfare of its citizens. Parents' refusal of medical treatment for their child that is deemed essential can be interpreted as neglect. In addition to advocating for the child and family, the nurse's role may include assuming the role of consultant to the staff and family regarding new, alternative methods to transfusion (Fox, 1990) and, if necessary, coordinating with officials to petition juvenile or family court for temporary guardianship of the child (Quintero, 1993).

IMPORTANCE OF CULTURE AND RELIGION TO NURSES

To begin to understand and to deal effectively with families in a multicultural community or in a unicultural community that is different from one's own, it is most important that nurses be aware of their own attitudes and values regarding a way of life, including health practices. Nurses, too, are a product of their own cultural background and education. They are part of the "nursing culture." Nurses function within the framework of a professional culture with its own values and traditions and, as such, become socialized into their professional culture in their educational program and later in their work environments and professional associations (Friedman, 1990).

Frequently nurses and other health care workers are not aware of their own cultural values and how those values influence their thoughts and actions. Those who are aware of their own culturally founded behavior are more sensitive to cultural behavior in others (see box on p. 55). To recognize that a behavior may be characteristic of a culture rather than an "abnormal" behavior places nurses at an advantage in their relationships with families. When nurses respect the cultural differences of a family, they are better

TABLE 2-5 Religious Beliefs That Affect Nursing Care

BELIEFS ABOUT BIRTH AND DEATH	BELIEFS ABOUT DIET AND FOOD PRACTICES	BELIEFS REGARDING MEDICAL CARE	COMMENTS
ADVENTIST (SEVENTH-DAY ADVENTIST; CHURCH OF GOD)			
Birth: Opposed to infant baptism Baptism in adulthood	Meat prohibited in some groups No alcohol, coffee, or tea	Some believe in divine healing and practice anointing with oil and use of prayer May desire communion or baptism when ill Believe in man's choice and God's sovereignty Some oppose hypnosis as therapy	Sabbath: Saturday for many Accept Bible literally
BAPTIST (27 GROUPS)			
Birth: Opposed to infant baptism Believers baptized by immersion as adults *Death:* Counsel and prayer with clergy, family, patient	Some groups discourage coffee, tea, and alcohol	"Laying on of hands" (some) May encounter some resistance to some therapies, such as abortion Believe God functions through physician Some believe in predestination; may respond passively to care	Fundamentalist and conservative groups accept Bible as inspired word of God
BLACK MUSLIM			
Birth: No baptism *Death:* Carefully prescribed procedure for washing and shrouding dead	Prohibit alcohol, pork, and foods traditional among American blacks (e.g., corn bread, collard greens)	Faith healing unacceptable Always maintain personal habits of cleanliness	General adherence to Moslem tenets overlaid, in many instances, by antagonism to whites, especially Christians and Jews Do not indulge in activities (such as sleeping) more than is necessary to health
BUDDHIST CHURCHES OF AMERICA			
Birth: No infant baptism Infant presentation *Death:* Last rite chanting often practiced at bedside soon after death Priest should be contacted	No requirements or restrictions Some sects are strictly vegetarian Discourage use of alcohol and drugs	Illness believed to be a trial to aid development of soul; illness due to Karmic causes May be reluctant to have surgery or certain treatments on holy days Cleanliness believed to be of great importance Family may request Buddhist priest for counseling	Optimistic outlook; teach ways to overcome fears, anxieties, apprehension
CHURCH OF CHRIST SCIENTIST (CHRISTIAN SCIENCE)			
Birth: No baptism *Death:* No last rites	No requirements or restrictions	Deny the existence of health crisis; see sickness and sin as errors of mind that can be altered by prayer Oppose human intervention with drugs or other therapies; however, accept legally required immunizations Many adhere to belief that disease is a human mental concept that can be dispelled by "spiritual truth" to extent that they refuse all medical treatment	Many desire services of practitioner or reader; will sometimes refuse even emergency treatment until they have consulted a reader Unlikely to donate organs for transplant

Sources: Carpenito, 1992; Conley, 1990; personal communications.

Continued.

TABLE 2-5 Religious Beliefs That Affect Nursing Care—cont'd

BELIEFS ABOUT BIRTH AND DEATH	BELIEFS ABOUT DIET AND FOOD PRACTICES	BELIEFS REGARDING MEDICAL CARE	COMMENTS
CHURCH OF JESUS CHRIST OF LATTER DAY SAINTS (MORMON)			
Birth: No baptism at birth Infant is "blessed" by church official at first opportunity after birth (in church) Baptism by immersion at 8 years *Death:* No special rites but may desire presence of church elders during any acute illness, when condition worsens, when undergoing risky or frightening tests or procedures, when feeling sick enough to die, or when dying	Prohibit tea, coffee, alcohol Some individuals avoid chocolate and other products that contain caffeine Encourage sparing use of meats Fasting for 24 hours on first Sunday each month (from after evening meal Saturday until evening meal Sunday)	Devout adherents believe in divine healing through anointment with oil and "laying on of hands" by church officials (appointed church members) Medical therapy not prohibited	May request Sacrament on Sunday while in hospital Financial support for sick available through well-funded welfare system Discourage cremation Discourage use of tobacco Married adults wear special undergarments
EASTERN ORTHODOX (TURKEY, EGYPT, SYRIA, RUMANIA, BULGARIA, CYPRUS, ALBANIA, ETC.)			
Birth: Most believe in infant baptism by immersion 8 to 40 days after birth *Death:* Last rites obligatory for impending death	Restrictions depend on specific sect	Anointment of the sick No conflict with medical science	Discourage cremation
EPISCOPAL (ANGLICAN)			
Birth: Infant baptism mandatory; urgent if poor prognosis *Death:* Last rites available but not mandatory	Abstain from meat on fast days May fast on Wednesday, Friday, during Lent, and before Christmas Some fast for 6 hours before receiving Holy Communion	Some believe in spiritual healing Rite for anointing sick available but not mandatory	Religious icons very important Communion four times yearly: Christmas, Easter, June 30, and August 15; may be mandatory for some
FRIENDS (QUAKERS)			
Birth: No baptism Infant's name recorded in official book	No requirements or restrictions Most practice moderation Avoid alcohol and illicit drugs	No special rites or restrictions	Believe in plain speech and dress Pacifists
GREEK ORTHODOX			
Birth: Baptism considered important Performed 40 days after birth If not possible to baptize by sprinkling or immersion, church allows child baptism "in the air" by moving child in the form of a cross as appropriate words are said *Death:* Last rites, administration of Sacrament of Holy Communion Should be performed while dying person is still conscious	Church-prescribed fast periods—usually occur on Wednesday, Friday, and during Lent; consist of avoiding meat and (in some cases) dairy products If health compromised, priest may be contacted to convince family to forego fasting	Each health crisis handled by ordained priest; deacon may also serve in some cases Holy Communion administered in hospital Some may desire Sacrament of the Holy Unction performed by priest	Oppose euthanasia Believe every reasonable effort should be made to preserve life until termination by God Discourage autopsies that may cause dismemberment Prefer burial to cremation

TABLE 2-5 Religious Beliefs That Affect Nursing Care—cont'd

BELIEFS ABOUT BIRTH AND DEATH	BELIEFS ABOUT DIET AND FOOD PRACTICES	BELIEFS REGARDING MEDICAL CARE	COMMENTS
HINDU			
Birth: No ritual *Death:* Special prescribed rites Priest pours water into mouth of dead child, ties a thread around neck or wrist to signify blessing (should not be removed) Family washes body and is particular about who touches body	Many dietary restrictions Beef and veal not eaten Some strict vegetarians	Illness or injury believed to represent sins committed in previous life Accept most modern medical practices	Cremation preferred
ISLAM (MUSLIM/MOSLEM)			
Birth: No baptism *Death:* Patient must confess sins and beg forgiveness before death; family should be present Family washes and prepares body, then turns it to face Mecca Only relatives and friends may touch body	Prohibit all pork products and any meat that is not ritually slaughtered Daylight fasting practiced during ninth month of Muhammadan year (Ramadan) Strict Muslims do not use alcohol or mind-altering drugs	Faith healing not acceptable unless psychologic conditions of patient is deteriorating; performed for morale Ritual washing after prayer; prayer takes place five times daily (on rising, midday, afternoon, early evening, and before bed); during prayer, face Mecca and kneel on prayer rug	Older Muslims often have a fatalistic view that may interfere with compliance to therapy May oppose autopsy
JEHOVAH'S WITNESS			
Birth: No baptism *Death:* No last rites	Eat nothing to which blood has been added; can eat animal flesh that has been drained	Adherents are generally absolutely opposed to transfusions of whole blood, packed red blood cells, platelets, and fresh or frozen plasma, including banking of own blood; individuals can sometimes be persuaded in emergencies May be opposed to use of albumin, globulin, factor replacement (hemophilia), vaccines Not opposed to nonblood plasma expanders	Often possible to obtain a court order appointing a hospital official as temporary guardian to consent to a child's transfusion when parents refuse consent Autopsy approved only as required by law No restrictions on giving blood sample
JUDAISM (ORTHODOX AND CONSERVATIVE)			
Birth: No baptism Ritual circumcision of male infants on eighth day; performed by Mohel (ritual circumciser familiar with Jewish law and aseptic technique) Reform Jews favor ritual circumcision, but not as a religious imperative *Death:* Remains are ritually washed by members of the Ritual Burial Society Burial should take place as soon as possible	Numerous dietary kosher laws exist that may be influenced by local practices and family and cultural tradition Allowed only meat from animals that are vegetable eaters, are cloven hoofed, chew their cud, and are ritually slaughtered; fish that have scales and fins Prohibit any combination of meat and milk; milk products served first can be followed by meat in a few minutes, but milk may not be consumed for several hours after eating meat Fasting for 24 hours is part of Yom Kippur observance Matzo replaces leavened bread during Passover week	May resist surgical procedures during Sabbath, which extends from sundown Friday until sundown Saturday Seriously ill and pregnant women are exempt from fasting Illness is grounds for violating dietary laws (e.g., patient with congestive heart failure does not have to use kosher meats, which are high in sodium)	Oppose all forms of mutilation, including autopsy; body parts not donated or removed; amputated limbs, organs, or surgically removed tissues should be made available to family for burial Donation or transplantation of organs requires rabbinical consent May oppose prolongation of life after irreversible brain damage

Continued.

TABLE 2-5 Religious Beliefs That Affect Nursing Care—cont'd

BELIEFS ABOUT BIRTH AND DEATH	BELIEFS ABOUT DIET AND FOOD PRACTICES	BELIEFS REGARDING MEDICAL CARE	COMMENTS
LUTHERAN			
Birth: Baptize only living infants shortly after birth *Death:* Rite for anointing of sick optional Family or patient may request anointing if prognosis is grave	No requirements or restrictions	Church or pastor notified of hospitalization Communion may be given before or after surgery or similar crisis	Accept scientific developments
MENNONITE (SIMILAR TO AMISH)			
Birth: No baptism in infancy Baptism during early or middle teens	No requirements or restrictions	No illness rituals Deep concern for dignity and self-determination of individual that would conflict with shock treatment or medical treatment affecting personality or will	
METHODIST			
Birth: No baptism at birth; performed on children or adults *Death:* No ritual	No requirements or restrictions	Communion may be requested before surgery or similar crisis	Encourage donations of body or body parts to medical science
NAZARENE			
Birth: Baptism optional *Death:* No last rites	No requirements or restrictions Alcohol prohibited	Church official administers communion and laying on of hands Adherents believe in divine healing but not exclusive of medical treatment	Cremation permitted
PENTECOSTAL (ASSEMBLY OF GOD, FOUR-SQUARE)			
Birth: No baptism at birth Baptism by complete immersion after age of accountability *Death:* No last rites	Abstain from alcohol, eating blood, strangled animals, or anything to which blood has been added Some individuals may resist pork	No restrictions regarding medical care Deliverance from sickness is provided for in atonement; may pray for divine intervention in health matters and seek God in prayer for themselves and others when ill	Some insist illness is divine punishment; most consider it an intrusion of Satan Practice glossolalia (speaking in tongues)
ORTHODOX PRESBYTERIAN			
Birth: Infant baptism by sprinkling *Death:* Last rites not a sacramental procedure; scripture reading and prayer	No requirements or restrictions	Communion administered when appropriate and convenient Blood transfusion accepted when advisable Pastor or elder should be called for ill person Believe science should be used for relief of suffering	Full forgiveness granted for any illness connected with a sin
ROMAN CATHOLIC			
Birth: Infant baptism mandatory; especially urgent in poor prognosis, when it may be performed by anyone *Death:* Rite for anointing of sick is mandatory Family or patient may request anointing if prognosis is grave	Fasting (eating only one full meal and no eating between meals) and abstaining from meat mandatory on Ash Wednesday and Good Friday; fasting optional during Lent; no meat on Fridays during Lent as general rule Children and most hospital patients exempt from fasting Some older Catholics may adhere to older rule of no meat on Friday	Encourage anointing of sick, although this may be interpreted by older members of church as equivalent to old terminology "extreme unction" or "last rites"; they may require careful explanation if reluctance is associated with fear of imminent death Traditional church teaching does not approve of contraceptives or abortion	Family may request that major amputated limb be buried in consecreated ground Transplant accepted as long as loss of organ does not deprive donor of life or functional integrity of body Autopsy acceptable Religious articles important

TABLE 2-5 Religious Beliefs That Affect Nursing Care—cont'd

BELIEFS ABOUT BIRTH AND DEATH	BELIEFS ABOUT DIET AND FOOD PRACTICES	BELIEFS REGARDING MEDICAL CARE	COMMENTS
RUSSIAN ORTHODOX			
Birth: Baptism by priest only *Death:* Traditionally after death arms are crossed, fingers set in a cross	No meat or dairy products on Wednesday, Friday, and during Lent	Cross necklace is important and should be removed only when necessary and replaced as soon as possible Adherents believe in divine healing, but not exclusive of medical treatment	Opposed to autopsy, embalming, or cremation
UNITARIAN UNIVERSALIST			
Birth: Some practice infant baptism; most consider it unnecessary *Death:* No ritual	No requirements or restrictions	Most believe in general goodness of their fellow humans and appreciate expression of that goodness by visits from clergy and fellow parishioners during times of illness	Cremation preferred to burial Believe in fully living this life as they know and understand it

able to determine whether the behavior is distinctive to the individual or a characteristic of the culture. What appears to be puzzling behavior may simply be the customary response in the culture (e.g., expression of emotion).

Cultural standards and values, the family structure and function, and past experiences with health care influence a family's feelings and attitudes toward health, their children, and health care delivery systems. It is often difficult for nurses to be nonjudgmental and objective in working with families whose behaviors and attitudes differ from or conflict with their own. To be aware of one's own feelings and attitudes, as well as to respect those of the family, is essential to a helping relationship and achievement of nursing goals. To rely on one's own values and experiences for guidance can result only in frustration and disappointment. It is one thing to know what is needed to deal with a health problem; it is often quite another to implement a fruitful course of action unless nurses work within the cultural and socioeconomic framework of the family.

It is essential to make an effort to adapt ethnic practices to the health needs of the family rather than attempt to change long-standing beliefs. To aid their efforts to understand and respect the cultural beliefs of families, nurses should have a readily available resource file containing pertinent information about the cultural and subcultural characteristics of the community in which they practice (e.g., traditional practices related to infant feeding practices and the time and manner of weaning and toilet training). Bridging cultural gaps in delivery of health care to children requires the establishment of a close relationship with families and other influential persons in the community (such as the local folk healer) and periodic assessment of one's own attitudes and behaviors and those of other health workers toward some of other racial or ethnic origins.

Some characteristics of selected cultures are outlined in Table 2-6. These generalizations are presented to assist nurses in learning the unique beliefs and practices of various groups and are not meant to be stereotypes of any

EXPLORING YOUR CULTURAL HERITAGE

To provide culturally sensitive care to children and their families from cultures that are different from your own you must first become aware of your own cultural values and beliefs and recognize how they influence your attitudes and behaviors. As you begin to understand the values that culture instills, you become better prepared to assess another culture objectively. The following questions have no right or wrong answers. They should help you clarify your attitudes and beliefs and how they influence your ability to work with people from diverse cultural backgrounds.

What ethnic group, socioeconomic class, religion, age-group, and community do you belong to?
- What about these groups do you find embarrassing or would like to change? Why?
- What sociocultural factors in your background might be rejected by members of other cultures?
- What did your parents and significant others say about people who were different from your family?

What do you believe or value?
- How do you define health, disease, illness?
- Are you usually on time? Early? Late?
- How do you feel if others are late? Frustrated? Angry? Not respected?
- What are your views on childhood education?
- Are you comfortable with physical contact (touching, embracing)? How much and with whom?
- What are your religious views and biases? Do you adhere to religious rituals?
- What are your feelings on childrearing practices (including nutrition, discipline, play, roles)?

What experiences have you had with people from ethnic groups, socioeconomic classes, religions, age-groups, or communities different from your own?
- What were those experiences like?
- How did you feel about them?

What personal qualities do you have that will help you establish interpersonal relationships with persons from other cultural groups?

What personal qualities may be detrimental?

Data from Randall-David E: *Strategies for working with culturally diverse communities and clients,* Washington, DC, 1989, Association for the Care of Children's Health; and Niederhauser V: Health care of immigrant children: incorporating culture into practice, *Pediatr Nurs* 15(6):569-574, 1989.

Text continued on p. 60.

TABLE 2-6 Cultural Characteristics Related to Health Care of Children and Families

CULTURAL GROUP	HEALTH BELIEFS	HEALTH PRACTICES
Asians		
Chinese	A healthy body viewed as gift from parents and ancestors and must be cared for Health is one of the results of balance between the forces of *yin* (cold) and *yang* (hot)—energy forces that rule the world Illness caused by imbalance Believe blood is source of life and is not regenerated *Chi* is innate energy Lack of chi and blood results in deficiency that produces fatigue, poor constitution, and long illness	Goal of therapy is to restore balance of yin and yang Acupuncturist applies needles to appropriate meridians identified in terms of yin and yang Acupressure and *tai chi* replacing acupuncture in some areas *Moxibustion* is application of heat to skin over specific meridians Wide use of medicinal herbs procured and applied in prescribed ways Folk healers are herbalist, spiritual healer, temple healer, fortune healer Meals may or may not be planned to balance hot and cold Milk intolerance relatively common Use of condiments (e.g., monosodium glutamate and soy sauce) may create difficulty with some diet regimens (e.g., low-salt diets)
Japanese	Three major belief systems: *Shinto* religious influence Humans inherently good Evil caused by outside spirits Illness caused by contact with polluting agents (e.g., blood, corpses, skin diseases) Chinese and Korean influence Health achieved through harmony and balance between self and society Disease caused by disharmony with society and not caring for body Portuguese influence Upholds germ theory of disease	Believe evil removed by purification Energy restored by means of acupuncture, acupressure, massage, and moxibustion along affected meridians *Kampō* medicine—use of natural herbs Believe in removal of diseased parts Trend is to use both Western and Oriental healing methods Care for disabled viewed as family's responsibility Take pride in child's good health Seek preventive care, medical care for illness May avoid some food combinations (e.g., milk and cherries, watermelon and crab) and believe pickled plums to have special properties
Vietnamese	Good health considered to be balance between yin and yang Believe person's life has been predisposed toward certain phenomena by cosmic forces Health believed to be result of harmony with existing universal order; harmony attained by pleasing good spirits and avoiding evil ones Belief in *am duc,* the amount of good deeds accumulated by ancestors Many use rituals to prevent illness Practice some restrictions to prevent incurring wrath of evil spirits	Family uses all means possible before using outside agencies for health care Fortune-tellers determine event that caused disturbance May visit temple to procure divine instruction Use astrologer to calculate cyclical changes and forces Regard health as family responsibility; outside aid sought when resources run out Certain illnesses considered only temporary (such as pustules, open wounds) and ignored Seek generalist health healers May use special diets to prevent illness and promote health Lactose intolerance prevalent
Filipinos	Believe God's will and supernatural forces govern universe Illness, accidents, and other misfortunes are God's punishment for violations of His will Widely accept "hot" and "cold" balance and imbalance as cause of health and illness	Some use amulets as a shield from witchcraft or as good luck pieces Catholics substitute religious medals and other items

Sources: Anderson and Fenichel, 1989; Clark, 1981; DeSantis, 1988; Geissler, 1994; Giger and Davidhizar, 1991; Holland and Sweeney, 1985; Hollingsworth, Brown, and Brooten, 1980; Orgue, Bloch, and Monrroy, 1983, Randall-David, 1989.

FAMILY RELATIONSHIPS	COMMUNICATION	COMMENTS
Extended family pattern common Strong concept of loyalty of young to old Respect for elders taught at early age—acceptance without questioning or talking back Children's behavior a reflection on family Family and individual honor and "face" important Self-reliance and self-restraint highly valued; self-expression repressed Males valued more highly than females; women submissive to men in family	Open expression of emotions unacceptable Often smile when do not comprehend	Do not react well to painful diagnostic workup; are especially upset by drawing of blood Deep respect for their bodies and believe it best to die with bodies intact; therefore may refuse surgery Believe in reincarnation Older members fear hospitals; often believe hospital is a place to go to die Children sometimes breast-fed for up to 4 or 5 years*
Close intergenerational relationships Family provides anchor Family tends to keep problems to self Value self-control and self-sufficiency Concept of ***haji*** (shame) imposes strong control; unacceptable behavior of children reflects on family Many adopt practices of contemporary middle class Concern for child's missing school may result in sending to school before fully recovered from illness	Issei—born in Japan; usually speak Japanese only Nisei, Sansei, and Yonsei have few language difficulties New immigrants able to read and write English better than able to speak or understand it Make significant use of nonverbal communication with subtle gestures and facial expression Tend to suppress emotions Will often wait silently	Generational categories: *Issei*—1st generation to live in U.S. *Nisei*—2nd generation *Sansei*—3rd generation *Yonsei*—4th generation Issei and Nissei—tolerant and permissive childrearing until 5 or 6, then emphasis on emotional reserve and control Cleanliness highly valued Time considered valuable and used wisely Tendency to practice emotional control may make assessment of pain more difficult
Family is revered institution Multigenerational families Family is chief social network Children highly valued Individual needs and interests are subordinate to those of family group Father is main decision maker Women taught submission to men Parents expect respect and obedience from children	Many immigrants are not proficient in speaking and understanding English May hesitate to ask questions Questioning authority is sign of disrespect; asking questions considered impolite Use indirectness rather than forthrightness in expressing disagreement May avoid eye contact with health professionals as a sign of respect	Consider status more important than money Children taught emotional control Time concept more relaxed—consider punctuality less significant than other values (i.e., propriety) Place high value on social harmony
Family is highly valued, with strong family ties Multigenerational family structure common, often with collateral members as well Personal interests are subordinated to family interests and needs Members avoid any behavior that would bring shame on the family	Immigrants and older persons may not be able to speak or understand English	Tend to have a fatalistic outlook on life Believe time and providence will solve all

*Most Asian cultures consider the child 1 year old at the time of birth. Traditional Chinese custom adds 1 year on January 1 regardless of the birthday—a child born in December is 2 years old the next January.

Continued.

TABLE 2-6 Cultural Characteristics Related to Health Care of Children and Families—cont'd

CULTURAL GROUP	HEALTH BELIEFS	HEALTH PRACTICES
Blacks	Illness classified as: Natural—affected by forces of nature without adequate protection (e.g., cold air, pollution, food and water) Unnatural—evil influences (e.g., witchcraft, voodoo, hoodoo, hex, fix, rootwork); symptoms often associated with eating Believe serious illness sent by God as punishment (e.g., parents punished by illness or death of child) Believe serious illness can be avoided May resist health care because illness is "will of God"	Self-care and folk medicine very prevalent Folk therapies usually religious in origin Attempt home remedies first; poorer people do not seek help until illness serious Usually seek help from: "Old lady"—woman in community with a common knowledge of herbs; consulted regarding pediatric care Spiritualist—has received gift from God for healing incurable diseases or solving personal problems; strongly based in Christianity Priest (voodoo priest/priestess)—most powerful healer Root doctor—meets need for herbs, oils, candles, and ointments Prayer is common means for prevention and treatment
Haitians†	Illnesses have a supernatural or natural origin Supernatural illnesses are caused by angry voodoo spirits, enemies, or the dead, especially deceased ancestors Natural illnesses are based on conceptions of natural causation: Irregularities of blood volume, flow, purity, viscosity, color and/or temperature (hot/cold) Gas *(gaz)* Movement and consistency of mother's milk Hot/cold imbalance in the body Bone displacement Movement of diseases Health is maintained by good dietary and hygienic habits	Health is a personal responsibility Foods have properties of "hot"/"cold" and "light"/"heavy" and must be in harmony with one's life cycle and bodily states Natural illnesses are treated by home remedies first Supernatural illness treated by healers: voodoo priest ***(houngan)*** or priestess ***(mambo),*** midwife ***(fam saj),*** and herbalist or leaf doctor ***(dokte fey)*** Amulets and prayer used to protect against illness due to curses or willed by evil people
Hispanics Mexicans (Latinos, Chicanos, Raza-Latinos)	Health beliefs have strong religious association Believe in body imbalance as a cause of illness, especially imbalance between ***caliente*** (hot) and ***frio*** (cold) or "wet" and "dry" Some maintain good health is a result of "good luck"—a reward for good behavior Illness prevented by performing properly, eating proper foods, and working proper amount of time; accomplished through prayer, wearing religious medals or amulets, and sleeping with relics at home Illness is a punishment from God for wrongdoing, forces of nature, and the supernatural	Seek help from ***curandero*** or ***curandera,*** especially in rural areas Curandero(a) receives his/her position by birth, apprenticeship, or a "calling" via dream or vision Treatments involve use of herbs, rituals, and religious artifacts Practice for severe illness—make promises, visit shrines, offer medals and candles, offer prayers Adhere to "hot" and "cold" food prescriptions and prohibitions for prevention and treatment of illness
Puerto Ricans	Subscribe to the "hot-cold" theory of causation of illness Believe some illness caused by evil spirits and forces	Infrequent use of health care systems Seek folk healers—use of herbs, rituals Consult spiritualist medium for mental disorders ***Santeria*** is system, and practitioners are called ***santeros*** Treatments classified as "hot" or "cold"

†This section was written by Lydia DeSantis, RN, PhD.

FAMILY RELATIONSHIPS	COMMUNICATION	COMMENTS
Strong kinship bonds in extended family; members come to aid of others in crisis Less likely to view illness as a burden Augmented families common (unrelated persons living in same household) Place strong emphasis on work and ambition Sex-role sharing among parents Elderly members respected Maternal grandparent strong influence	Alert to any evidence of discrimination Place importance on nonverbal behavior May use nonstandard English or "black English" Use "testing" behaviors to assess personnel in health care situations before seeking active care Best to use simple, direct, but caring approach	High level of caution and distrust of majority group Social anxiety related to tradition of humiliation, oppression, and loss of dignity Will elect to retain dignity rather than seek care if values are compromised Strong sense of peoplehood High incidence of poverty Black minister a strong influence in black community Visits by family minister are sought, expected, and valued in helping to cope with illness and suffering
Maintenance of family reputation is paramount Lineal authority supreme; children in a subordinate position in family hierarchy Children valued for parental social security in old age and expected to contribute to family welfare at an early age Children viewed as "gifts from god" and treated with indulgence and affection	Recent immigrants and older persons may speak only Haitian creole May prefer family/friends to act as translators and confidants Often smile and nod in agreement when do not understand Quiet and gentle communication style and lack of assertiveness lead health care providers to falsely believe they comprehend health teaching and are compliant Will not ask questions if health care provider is busy or rushed	Will use biomedical and ethnomedical (folk) systems simultaneously Resistant to dietary and work restrictions Adherence to prescribed treatments directly related to perceived severity of illness
Traditionally men considered bread-winners and key decision makers in matters outside the home; women considered homemakers Males considered big and strong ***(macho)*** Strong kinship; extended families include ***compadres*** (godparents) established by ritual kinship Children valued highly and desired, taken everywhere with family Many homes contain shrines with statues and pictures of saints Elderly treated with respect	May use nonstandard English Some bilingual; many only speak Spanish May have a strong preference for native language and revert to it in times of stress May shake hands or engage in introductory embrace Interpret prolonged eye contact as disrespectful	High degree of modesty—often a deterrent to seeking medical care and open discussions of sex Youngsters often reluctant to share communal showers in schools Relaxed concept of time—may be late for appointments More concerned with present than with future and therefore may focus on immediate solutions rather than long-term goals Magicoreligious practices common May view hospital as place to go to die
Family usually large and home centered—the core of existence Father has complete authority in family—family provider and decision maker Wife and children subordinate to father Children valued—seen as a gift from God Children taught to obey and respect parents; corporal punishment to ensure obedience	May use nonstandard English Spanish speaking or bilingual Strong sense of family privacy—may view questions regarding family as impudent	Relaxed sense of time Pay little attention to *exact* time of day Suspicious and fearful of hospitals

Continued.

TABLE 2-6 Cultural Characteristics Related to Health Care of Children and Families

CULTURAL GROUP	HEALTH BELIEFS	HEALTH PRACTICES
Cubans‡	Prevention and good nutrition are related to good health	Diligent users of the medical model Eclectic health-seeking practices, including preventive measures, and, in some instances, folk medicine of both religious and nonreligious origins; home remedies; in many instances seek assistance of santeros and spiritualists to complement medical treatment Nutrition is important; parents show overconcern with eating habits of their children and spend a considerable part of the budget on food; traditional Cuban diet is rich in meat and starch; consumption of fresh vegetables added in U.S.
Native Americans (numerous tribes)	Believe health is state of harmony with nature and universe Respect of bodies through proper management All disorders believed to have aspects of supernatural Violation of a restriction or prohibition thought to cause illness Fear of witchcraft May carry objects believed to guard against witchcraft Theology and medicine strongly interwoven	Medicine persons: Altruistic persons who must use powers in purely positive ways Persons capable of both good and evil—perform negative acts against enemies Diviner-diagnosticians—diagnose but do not have powers or skill to implement medical treatment Specialists—use herbs and curative but nonsacred medical procedures Medicine persons—use herbs and ritual Singers—cure by the power of their song obtained from supernatural beings; effect cures by laying on of hands

‡This section was written by Mercedes Sandaval, PhD.

group. Learning about culture must begin somewhere; Tables 2-5 and 2-6 are presented as beginning frameworks for practicing cross-cultural nursing. Each nurse must assess individuals and families to identify in what ways they are similar to and different from their cultural and religious backgrounds.

KEY POINTS

- Nurses have a responsibility to understand the influence of culture, race, and ethnicity on the development of social and emotional relationships, childrearing practices, and attitudes toward health.
- Culture is the sum total of mores, traditions, and beliefs about how people function and encompasses other products of human works and thoughts specific to members of an intergenerational group, community, or population.
- A child's self-concept evolves from ideas about his or her social roles.
- Primary groups are characterized by intimate contact, mutual support, and behavior constraint among members.
- Secondary groups have limited intermittent contact, little mutual support, and no pressure for conformity.
- Guilt and shame are two behaviors commonly conditioned in children to control social behavior.
- Important subcultural influences on children include ethnicity, social class, occupation, poverty, affluence, religion, schools, peers, and biculture.
- A trend that has significantly influenced the American family is increasing geographic and economic mobility.
- Membership in a minority group presents special challenges for children, although changes in societal attitudes are slowly taking place.
- A child's physical characteristics and susceptibility to health problems are strongly related to ethnic and cultural variations of hereditary and socioeconomic forces.
- Hereditary and socioeconomic forces play an important role in a child's susceptibility to health problems.
- Groups of children suffering from greater physical and mental health problems are those living in poverty who are homeless or have migrant families.
- Drug response, food sensitivity, disease resistance, physical characteristics, and disease states may demonstrate ethnic or cultural variations.
- Because verbal and nonverbal communication is an important culture consideration, nurses need to acknowledge and respect their patient's practices in order for productive interaction to occur.
- Cultural beliefs related to cause of illness and maintenance of health may focus on natural forces, supernatural forces, or imbalance of forces.
- In planning and implementing patient care, nurses need to strive to adapt ethnic practices to the family's health needs rather than attempt to change long-standing beliefs.
- No cultural group is homogeneous; every racial and ethnic group contains great diversity.

FAMILY RELATIONSHIPS	COMMUNICATION	COMMENTS
Strong family ties with mother and father kinships Children supported and assisted by parents long after becoming adults Elderly cared for at home	Most are bilingual (English/Spanish) except for segments of the senior population	In less than 30 years Cubans have been able to obtain a higher standard of living than other Hispanic groups in U.S. Have been able to retain many of their former social institutions: bilingual and private schools, clinics, social clubs, the family as an extended network of support, etc. Many do not feel discriminated against nor harbor feelings of inferiority with respect to Anglo-Americans or "mainstream" population
Extended family structure—usually includes relatives from both sides of family Elder members assume leadership roles	Most continue to speak their Indian language, as well as English Nonverbal communication	Time orientation—present Respect for age Going to hospital associated with illness or disease; therefore may not seek prenatal care, since pregnancy viewed as natural process Tend to take time to form an opinion of professionals Sexual matters not openly discussed with members of opposite sex

REFERENCES

AAN Expert Panel on Culturally Competent Nursing Care: Culturally competent health care, *Nurs Outlook* 40(6):277-284, 1992.

American Academy of Pediatrics: Health care for children of migrant families, *Pediatrics* 84(4):739-740, 1989.

Anderson P, Fenichel D: *Serving culturally diverse families of infants and toddlers with disabilities,* Washington, DC, 1989, National Center for Clinical Infant Programs.

Annie E. Casey Foundation: *Kids count data book: state profiles of child well-being,* Washington, DC, 1993, Center for the Study of Social Policy.

Bass JL and others: Pediatric problems in a suburban shelter for homeless families, *Pediatrics* 85(1):33-38, 1990.

Bassuk EL, Rosenberg L: Psychosocial characteristics of homeless children and children with homes, *Pediatrics* 85(3):257-261, 1990.

Brookins G: Culture, ethnicity, and bicultural competence: implications for children with chronic illness and disability, *Pediatrics* 91(5):1056-1062, 1993.

Buckner J and others: Mental health issues affecting homeless women: implications for intervention, *Am J Orthopsychiatry* 63(3):385-399, 1993.

Carpenito LJ: *Nursing diagnosis: application to clinical practice,* ed 4, Philadelphia, 1992, JB Lippincott.

Chang K: Chinese Americans. In Giger J, Davidhizar R, editors: *Transcultural nursing,* St Louis, 1991, Mosby.

Chidester D: *Patterns of transcendence: religion, death, and dying,* Belmont, CA, 1990, Wadsworth.

Children's Defense Fund: *The state of America's children,* Washington, DC, 1992, CDF.

Clark AL, editor: *Culture and childrearing,* Philadelphia, 1981, FA Davis.

Clutter L: Fostering spiritual care for the child and family. In Smith D, editor: *Comprehensive child and family nursing skills,* St Louis, 1991, Mosby.

Cohen FL: *Clinical genetics in nursing practice,* Philadelphia, 1984, JB Lippincott.

Conley L: Childbearing and childrearing practices in Mormonism, *Neonatal Network* 9(3):41-48, 1990.

Damon A: Race, ethnic group and disease, *Soc Biol* 16:69, 1969.

David R: Race, birthweight, and mortality rates, *J Pediatr* 116(1):101-102, 1990.

Davidhizar R, Frank B: Understanding the physical and psychosocial stressors of the child who is homeless, *Pediatr Nurs* 18(6):559-562, 1992.

Der Kaloustian VM, Maffah J, Loiselet J: Genetic diseases in Lebanon, *Am J Med Genet* 7:187, 1980.

DeSantis L: Cultural factors affecting newborn and infant diarrhea, *J Pediatr Nurs* 3(6):391-398, 1988.

Drake M: The nutritional status and dietary adequacy of single homeless women and their children in shelters, *Public Health Rep* 107(3):312-319, 1992.

Elfert H, Anderson J, Lai M: Parents' perceptions of children with chronic illness: a study of immigrant Chinese families, *J Pediatr Nurs* 6(2):114-120, 1991.

Elkin F, Handel G: *The child and society: the process of socialization,* New York, 1989, Random House, Inc.

Federal Register: (57-FR 5456), Washington, DC, 1992, The Register.

Ferak V, Genčik A, Genčíkova A: Population genetical aspects of primary congenital glaucoma, *Hum Genet* 61:193, 1982.

Fierman A and others: Growth delay in homeless children, *Pediatrics* 88(5):918-925, 1991.

Fierman A and others: Status of immunization and iron nutrition in New York City homeless children, *Clin Pediatr* 32(3):151-155, 1993.

Fox V: Caught between religion and medicine, *AORN J* 52(1):131-134, 138-139, 1990.

Friedman M: Transcultural family nursing: application to Latino and black families, *Pediatr Nurs* 5(3):214-222, 1990.

Geissler EM: *Pocket guide to cultural assessment,* St Louis, 1994, Mosby.

Giger J, Davidhizar R: *Transcultural nursing,* 1991, St Louis, Mosby.

Goodman RM: *Genetic disorders among the Jewish people,* Baltimore, 1979, Johns Hopkins University Press.

Hanley C: Navajo Indians. In Giger J, Davidhizar R, editors: *Transcultural nursing,* 1991, St Louis, Mosby.

Hantavirus infection—Southwestern United States: interim recommendations for risk reduction, *MMWR* 42(RR-11):1-13, 1993.

Issacs P: Growth parameters and blood values in Arabic children, *Pediatr Nurs* 15(6):579-583, 1989.

Larson O, Doris J, Alvarez W: Migrants and maltreatment: comparative evidence from central register data, *Child Abuse Negl* 14(3):375-385, 1990.

Lawson LV: Culturally sensitive support for grieving parents, *MCN* 15(2):76-79, 1990.

Leininger M: *Transcultural nursing,* New York, 1978, John Wiley & Sons.

Lynch E, Hanson M: Developing cross-cultural competence, Baltimore, MD, 1992, Paul H Brookes.

Malach F, Segel N: Perspectives on health care delivery systems for American Indian families, *Child Health Care* 19(4):219-228, 1990.

Malloy C: Children and poverty: America's future at risk, *Pediatr Nurs* 18(6):553-557, 1992.

Martinson IM: The challenge of culturally diverse pediatric clients. In Feeg V, editor: *Pediatric nursing: forum on the future: looking toward the 21st century,* Pitman, NJ, 1989, Anthony J Jannetti.

Masten A and others: Children in homeless families: risks to mental health and development, *J Consult Clin Psychol* 61(2):335-343, 1993.

McKusick V: *Mendelian inheritance in man,* ed 10, Baltimore, 1992, Johns Hopkins University Press.

Murata J and others: Disease patterns in homeless children: a comparison with national data, *J Pediatr Nurs* 7(3):196-204, 1992.

National Commission on Children: *Beyond rhetoric: final report of the National Commission on Children,* Washington, DC, 1991, The Commission.

Orque MS, Bloch B, Monrroy LSA: *Ethnic nursing care,* St Louis, 1983, Mosby.

Page A, Ainsworth A, Pett M: Homeless families and their children's health problems: a Utah urban experience, *West J Med* 158(1):30-35, 1993.

Parker R and others: A survey of the health of homeless children in Philadelphia shelters, *Am J Dis Child* 145(5):520-526, 1991.

Patterson J, Blum R: A conference on culture and chronic illness in childhood: conference summary, *Pediatrics* 91(5):1025-1030, 1993.

Prevention and control of tuberculosis in migrant farm workers, *MMWR* 41(RR-10):1-15, 1992.

Quintero C: Blood administration in pediatric Jehovah's Witnesses, *Pediatr Nurs* 19(1):46-48, 1993.

Randall-David E: *Strategies for working with culturally diverse communities and clients,* Washington, DC, 1989, Association for the Care of Children's Health.

Rollins J: *Project Taking Charge field test site reports: August 1992–March 1993,* Manuscript submitted for publication, 1993.

Rust G: Health status of migrant farmworkers: a literature review and commentary, *Am J Public Health* 80(10):1213-1217, 1990.

Scriver C: *The metabolic basis of inherited disease,* ed 6, New York, 1989, McGraw-Hill.

Sloat A, Matsuura W: Intercultural communication. In Craft M, Denehy J, editors: *Nursing interventions for infants and children,* Philadelphia, 1990, WB Saunders.

Starn J: Cultural childbearing: beliefs and practices, *Int J Childbirth Educ* 6(3):38-39, 1991.

Stauffer R: Vietnamese Americans. In Giger J, Davidhizar R, editors: *Transcultural nursing,* 1991, St Louis, Mosby.

Stefanidis N and others: Runaway and homeless youth: the effects of attachment history on stabilization, *Am J Orthopsychiatry* 62(3):442-446, 1992.

Sugerman S and others: Acquired immunodeficiency syndrome and adolescents: knowledge, attitudes, and behaviors of runaway and homeless youths, *Am J Dis Child* 145(4):431-436, 1991.

Wagner J, Melragon B, Menke E: Homeless children: interdisciplinary drug prevention intervention, *J Child Adolesc Psychiatr Ment Health Nurs* 6(1):22-30, 1993.

Wright J: Homeless children: two years later, *Am J Dis Child* 147(5):518-519, 1993.

BIBLIOGRAPHY

General

Ablon J, Ames GM: Culture and family. In Gilliss CL and others, editors: *Toward a science of family nursing,* Menlo Park, CA, 1989, Addison-Wesley.

Anderson JM: Health care across cultures, *Nurs Outlook* 38(3):136-139, May/June, 1990.

Bauwens EE, Anderson S: Social and cultural influences on health care. In Stanhope M, Lancaster J: *Community health nursing,* ed 3, St Louis, 1992, Mosby.

Betz C: A culturally biased perspective, *J Pediatr Nurs* 7(4):229, 1992.

Bishop S: The mental health of children and families in rural America, *J Child Adolesc Psychiatr Ment Health Nurs* 3(3):77-78, 1990.

Bornstein MH (editor): *Culture approaches to parenting,* Hillsdale, NJ, 1991, Lawrence Erlbaum Associates.

Carpenito LJ: *Nursing diagnosis: application to clinical practice,* ed 4, Philadelphia, 1992, JB Lippincott.

Chan S: Early intervention with culturally diverse families of infants and toddlers with disabilities, *Infants Young Child* 3(2):78-87, 1990.

Choi ES, Hamilton RK: The effects of culture on mother-infant interaction, *JOGNN* 15:256-261, 1986.

Conatser C: Effect of wealth on approach to patient care, *J Assoc Pediatr Oncol Nurses* 3(2):14-19, 1986.

Culture and nursing practice: an applied view, *Holistic Nurs Pract* 6(3): entire issue, 1992.

Evans V: Sociodemographic trends toward the 21st century. In Feeg V, editor: *Pediatric nursing: forum on the future: looking toward the 21st century,* Pitman, NJ, 1989, Anthony J Jannetti.

Fitzgerald FT: Patients from other cultures: how they view you, themselves, and disease, *Consultant* 28(3):65-67, 1988.

Fleming J: Meeting the challenge of culturally diverse populations, *Pediatr Nurs* 15(6):566, 634, 1989 (guest editorial).

Garty B: Garlic burns, *Pediatrics* 91(3):658-659, 1993.

Geber G, Latts E: Race and ethnicity: issues for adolescents with chronic illnesses and disabilities: an annotated bibliography, *Pediatrics* 91(5):1071-1081, 1993.

Groce N, Zola I: Multiculturalism, chronic illness, and disability, *Pediatrics* 91(5):1048-1055, 1993.

Hansen M, Resick L: Health beliefs, health care, and rural Appalachian subcultures from an ethnographic perspective, *Fam Community Health* 13(1):1-10, 1990.

Hayes J, Dreher C: Providing culturally sensitive care. In Smith D, editor: *Comprehensive child and family nursing skills,* St Louis, 1991, Mosby.

LeVine RA, Miller PM, West MM, editors: *Parental behavior in diverse societies,* San Francisco, 1988, Jossey-Bass, Inc.

McCubbin H and others: Culture, ethnicity, and the family: critical factors in childhood chronic illnesses and disabilities, *Pediatrics* 91(5):1063-1070, 1993.

McManus M, Newacheck P: Health insurance differentials among minority children with chronic conditions and the role of federal agencies and private foundations in improving financial access, *Pediatrics* 91(5):1040-1047, 1993.

Newacheck P, Stoddard J, McManus M: Ethnocultural variations in the prevalence and impact of childhood chronic conditions, *Pediatrics* 91(5):1031-1039, 1993.

Olness K: Cultural issues in primary pediatric care. In Hoekelman RA: *Primary pediatric care,* ed 2, St Louis, 1992, Mosby.

Roopnarine JL, Carter DB, editors: *Parent child socialization in diverse cultures: annual advances in applied developmental psychology,* Norwood, NJ, 1992, Ablex.

Spector RE: *Cultural diversity in health and illness,* ed 2, New York, 1985, Appleton-Century-Crofts.

Thiederman SB: Ethnocentrism: a barrier to effective health care, *Nurs Pract* 11(8):52-59, 1986.

Tripp-Reimer T, Afifi LA: Cross-cultural perspectives on patient teaching, *Nurs Clin North Am* 24(3):613-619, 1989.

Tseng W, Hsu J: *Culture and family,* Binghamton, NY, 1990, Haworth Press.

Poverty, Homeless, Migrant

Adams PJ: Effects of poverty and affluence. In Hendee WR: *The health of adolescents,* San Francisco, 1991, Jossey-Bass.

Berne AS and others: A nursing model for addressing the health needs of homeless families, *Image J Nurs Sch* 22(1):8-13, 1990.

Finkelstein J, Parker R: Homeless children in America: taking the next step, *Am J Dis Child* 147(5):520-521, 1993.

Good M: The clinical nurse specialist in the school setting: case management of migrant children with dental disease, *Clin Nurse Spec* 6(2):72-76, 1992.

Hunter L: Sibling play therapy with homeless children: an opportunity in the crisis, *Child Welfare* 72(1):65-75, 1993.

Kaliski D and others: AIDS, runaways, and self-efficacy, *Fam Community Health* 13(1):65-72, 1990.

O'Malley B and others: Infant feeding practices of migrant farm laborers in northern Colorado, *J Am Diet Assoc* 91(9):1084-1087, 1991.

Parker S, Greer S, Zuckerman B: Double jeopardy: the impact of poverty on early child development, *Pediatr Clin North Am* 35(6):1227-1240, 1988.

Rafferty M: Standing up for America's homeless, *Am J Nurs* 89(12):1614-1617, 1989.

Rescoria L, Parker R, Stolley P: Ability, achievement, and adjustment in homeless children, *Am J Orthopsychiatry* 61(2):210-220, 1991.

Rotheram-Borus M and others: AIDS knowledge and beliefs, and sexual behavior of sexually delinquent and non-delinquent (runaway) adolescents, *J Adolesc* 14(3):229-244, 1991.

Shulsinger E: Needs of sheltered homeless children, *J Pediatr Health Care* 4(3):136-140, 1991.

Solar J: Measles statistics inaccurately reported in poverty article, *Pediatr Nurs* 19(3):256, 1993 (letter to editor).

Stricof and others: HIV seroprevalence in a facility for runaway and homeless adolescents, *Am J Public Health* 81(suppl):50-53, 1991.

Velsor-Friedrich B: Poverty: its effects on children and their families, *J Pediatr Nurs* 7(6):412-413, 1992.

Wagner J, Menke E: No place to call home, *The Ohio State University College of Nursing Magazine* 1(10):11-13, 1991.

Wood D: Homeless children: their evaluation and treatment, *J Pediatr Health Care* 3(4):194-199, 1989.

Wood D and others: Health of homeless children and housed, poor children, *Pediatrics* 86(6):858-866, 1990.

Wright J, Weber E: *Homelessness and health,* Washington, DC, 1991, McGraw-Hill.

Young S and others: Family-carried growth records: a tool for providing continuity of care for migrant children, *Public Health Nurs* 7(4):209-214, 1990.

Religion

Abbott DA, Berry M, Meredith WH: Religious beliefs and practice: a potential asset in helping families, *Fam Relations* 39(4):443-448, 1990.

Adams CE and others: The effects of religious beliefs on the health care practices of the Amish, *Nurse Pract* 11(3):58-67, 1986.

Carson V: *Spiritual dimensions of nursing practice,* Philadelphia, 1989, WB Saunders.

Conley L: Childbearing and childrearing practices in Mormonism, *Neonatal Network* 9(3):41-48, 1990.

Gershan JA: Judaic ethical beliefs and customs regarding death and dying, *Crit Care Nurse* 5(1):32-34, 1985.

Lutwak RA, Ney AM, White JE: Maternity nursing and Jewish law, *MCN* 13(1):44-46, 1988.

Masulis K: When parents refuse treatment for their children . . . Jehovah's Witnesses, *J Christ Nurs* 4(2):10-12, 1987.

Nelson M, Joranoric L: Pregnancy, diabetes, and Jewish dietary law, *J Am Diet Assoc* 87(8):1054-1057, 1987.

O'Rouke K: Pain relief: the perspective of Catholic tradition, *J Pain Symptom Manage* 7(8):485-491, 1992.

Roberson MHB: The influence of religious beliefs on health choices of Afro-Americans, *Top Clin Nurs* 7(3):57-63, 1985.

Sodestrom KE, Martinson IM: Patients' spiritual coping strategies: a study of nurse and patient perspectives, *Oncol Nurs Forum* 14(2):41-46, 1987.

Swan R: The law should protect all children . . . children in faith-healing sects, *J Christ Nurs* 4(2):40, 1987.

Thurkauf GE: Understanding the beliefs of Jehovah's Witnesses, *Focus Crit Care* 16(3): 199-204, 1989.

Ethnic Groups: Asian-American

Choi E: Unique aspects of Korean-American mothers, *JOGNN* 15(5):394-400, 1986.

Dung TN: Understanding Asian families: a Vietnamese perspective, *Child Today* 13(2): 1012, 1984.

Handelman L, Menahem S, Eisenbruch IM: Transcultural understanding of a hereditary disorder: mucopolysaccharidosis VI in a Vietnamese family, *Clin Pediatr* 28(10):470-473, 1989.

Leung AK and others: Palpebral fissure length. In Chinese newborn infants: comparison with other ethnic groups, *Clin Pediatr* 29(3):172-174, 1990.

Marrio EB, Hall RR: Asian family traditions and their influence in transcultural health care delivery, *Child Health Care* 15(3):172-177, 1987.

Martinson IM: Impact of childhood cancer on family care in Taiwan, *Pediatr Nurs* 15(6): 636-637, 1989.

Mattson S, Lew L: Culturally sensitive prenatal care for Southeast Asians, *JOGNN* 21(1):48-54, 1992.

Rosenburg JA: Health care for Cambodian children: integrating treatment plans, *Pediatr Nurs* 12:118-125, 1986.

Rosenthal DA, Feldman SS: The acculturation of Chinese immigrants: perceived effects on family functioning of length of residence in two cultural contexts, *J Genet Psychol* 151(4):495-514, 1990.

Stevenson HW, Lee SY: Contexts of achievement: a study of American, Chinese, and Japanese children, *Monogr Soc Res Child Dev* 55(1-2):1-123, 1990.

Yeatman W, Dang V: Coa Gia (coin rubbing), *JAMA* 244:2748-2749, 1980.

Ethnic Groups: Native American

Delisle HF, Ekoe JM: Prevalence of non-insulin-dependent diabetes mellitus and impaired glucose tolerance in two Algonquin communities in Quebec, *Can Med Assoc J* 148(1):41-47, 1993.

Dick RW, Manson SM, Beals J: Alcohol use among male and female Native American adolescents: patterns and correlates of student drinking in a boarding school, *J Stud Alcohol* 54(2):172-177, 1993.

Harrison RL, Davis DW: Caries experience of Native children of British Columbia, Canada, 1980-1988, *Community Dent Oral Epidemiol* 21(2):102-107, 1993.

Inouye DK: Our future is in jeopardy: the mental health of Native American adolescents, *J Health Care Poor Underserved* 4(1):6-8, 1993 (editorial).

Newman WP and others: Atherosclerosis in Alaska Natives and non-natives, *Lancet* 341(8852):1056-1057, 1993.

Olson L and others: Analysis of childhood pedestrian deaths in New Mexico, 1986-1990, *Ann Emerg Med* 22(3):512-516, 1993.

Parker DJ and others: Fire fatalities among New Mexico children, *Ann Emerg Med* 22(3):517-522, 1993.

Satz KJ: Integrating Navajo tradition into maternal-child nursing, *Image* 14:89-91, 1992.

van Breda A: Health issues facing Native American children, *Pediatr Nurs* 15(6):575-577, 1989.

Ethnic Groups: Hispanic American

Charles C: Mental health services for Haitians. In Lefley HP, Pederson PB, editors: *Cross-cultural training for mental health professionals,* Springfield, IL, 1986, Charles C Thomas.

Dawson KA: Comment on Nelson et al: 'Comparative time estimation skills of Hispanic children' *Percept Mot Skills* 74(3 pt 2):1113-1114, 1992 (comment).

de Leon Siantz M: Correlates of maternal depression among Mexican-American migrant farmworker mothers, *Child Adolesc Psychiatr Ment Health Nurs* 3(1):9-13, 1990.

DeSantis L: Childrearing beliefs and practices of Cuban and Haitian parents: implications for nurses. In Carter MA, editor: *Proceedings of the tenth annual conference of the Transcultural Nursing Society,* Salt Lake City, 1985, Transcultural Nursing Society.

DeSantis L: Infant feeding practices of Haitian mothers in South Florida: cultural beliefs and acculturation, *Matern Child Nurs J* 15:77-89, 1986.

DeSantis L: Cuban and Haitian perspectives on child health: a transcultural view. In Wang JF, Simoni PS, Nath CL, editors: *Proceedings of the West Virginia Nurses' Association research symposium,* Charleston, WV, 1988, West Virginia Nurses' Research Conference Group.

Foreman JT: *Susto* and the health needs of the Cuban refugee population, *Top Clin Nurs* 7(3):40-47, 1985.

Guendelman S: At risk: health needs of Hispanic children, *Health Soc Work* 10:183-190, 1985.

Johnson SR and others: The association between hemoglobin and behavior problems in a sample of low-income Hispanic preschool children, *J Dev Behav Pediatr* 13(3): 209-214, 1992.

Kosarchyn C: School nurses' perceptions of the health needs of Hispanic elementary school children, *J School Nurs* 9(1):37-44, 1993.

Mardiros M: A view toward hospitalization: the Mexican American experience, *J Adv Nurs* 9:469-478, 1984.

Munet-Vilaro F, Vessey J: Children's explanation of leukemia: a Hispanic perspective, *J Pediatr Nurs* 5(4):274-282, 1990.

Powell D, Zambrana R, Silva-Palacios V: Designing culturally responsive parent programs: a comparison of low-income Mexican and Mexican-American mothers' preferences, *Fam Relations* 39(3):298-304, 1990.

Shea S and others: Relationships of dietary fat consumption to serum total and low-density lipoprotein cholesterol in Hispanic preschool children, *Prev Med* 20(2):237-249, 1991.

Warrick L and others: Evaluation of a peer health worker prenatal outreach and education program for Hispanic farmworker families, *J Community Health* 17(1):13-26, 1992.

Wood P and others: Hispanic children with asthma: morbidity, *Pediatrics* 91(1):62-69, 1993.

Ethnic Groups: Black American

Brannan JE: Accidental poisoning of children: barriers to resource use in a black, low-income community, *Public Health Nurs* 9(2):81-86, 1992.

Fitzpatrick SB and others: Use of peak flow monitoring among urban black children with asthma, *Natl Med Assoc* 84(6):477-479, 1992 (editorial).

Kalyanpur M, Rao SS: Empowering low-income black families of handicapped children, *Am J Orthopsychiatry* 61(4):523-532, 1991.

Keltner B: Family characteristics of preschool social competence among black children in a Head Start Program, *Child Psychiatry Hum Dev* 21(2):95-108, 1990.

McLoyd VC: The impact of economic hardship on black families and children: psychological distress, parenting, and socioemotional development, *Child Dev* 61(2):311-346, 1990.

Myers HF and others: Parental and family predictors of behavior problems in inner-city black children, *Am J Community Psychol* 20 (5):557-576, 1992.

Nelson-Le Gall S, Jones E: Cognitive-motivational influences on the task-related help-seeking behavior of black children, *Child Dev* 61(2):581-589, 1990.

Porter CP: Social reasons for skin tone preferences of black school-age children, *Am J Orthopsychiatry* 61(1):149-154, 1991.

Rana SR, Sekhsaria S, Castro OL: Hemoglobin S and C traits: contributing causes for decreased mean hematocrit in African-American children, *Pediatrics* 91(4):800-802, 1993.

Roberson MHB: The influence of religious beliefs on health choices of Afro-Americans, *Top Clin Nurs* 7(3):57-73, 1985.

Ryan-Wenger N, Copeland S: Coping strategies used by black school-aged children from low income families, *J Pediatr Nurs* 9(1):33-40, 1994.

Shakoor BH, Chalmers D: Co-victimization of African-American children who witness violence: effects on cognitive, emotional, and behavioral development, *J Natl Med Assoc* 83(3):233-238, 1991.

Slaughter-Defoe DT and others: Toward cultural/ecological perspectives on schooling and achievement of African- and Asian-American children, *Child Dev* 61(2):363-383, 1990.

Tull ES, LaPorte RE: Let's not forget IDDM in African-American children, *Diabetes Care* 14(7):613-614, 1991 (letter).

Unonu JN, Johnson AA: Feeding patterns, food energy, nutrient intakes, and anthropometric measurements of selected black preschool children with Down syndrome, *J Am Diet Assoc* 92(7):856-858, 1992.

Ethnic Groups: Cross-Cultural Comparisons and Other Cultures

Bebout L, Arthur B: Cross-cultural attitudes toward speech disorders, *J Speech Hear Res* 35(1):45-52, 1992.

Burek CL and others: Thyroid autoantibodies in black and in white children and adolescents with type 1 diabetes mellitus and their first degree relatives, *Autoimmunity* 7(2-3):157-167, 1990.

Cornelius LJ: Barriers to medical care for white, black, and Hispanic American children, *J Natl Med Assoc* 85(4):281-288, 1993.

Foucar K and others: Survival of children and adolescents with acute lymphoid leukemia: a study of American Indians and Hispanic and non-Hispanic whites treated in New Mexico (1969 to 1986), *Cancer* 67(8):2125-2130, 1991.

Gayle J, Selik R, Chu SY: Surveillance for AIDS and HIV infection among black and Hispanic children and women of childbearing age, 1981-1989, *MMWR CDC Surveill Summ* 39(3):23-30, 1990.

McGauhey PJ, Starfield B: Child health and the social environment of white and black children, *Soc Sci Med* 136(7):867-874, 1993.

Parkin DM, Stiller CA, Nectoux J: International variations in the incidence of childhood bone tumours, *Int J Cancer* 53(3):371-376, 1993.

Pfefferbaum B, Adams J, Aceves J: The influence of culture on pain in Anglo and Hispanic children with cancer, *J Am Acad Child Adolesc Psychiatry* 29(4):642-647, 1990.

Porter CP, Villarruel AM: Socialization and caring for hospitalized African- and Mexican-American children, *Issues Compr Pediatr Nurs* 14(1):1-16, 1991.

Rotheram-Borus MJ, Phinney JS: Patterns of social expectations among black and Mexican-American children, *Child Dev* 61(2):542-556, 1990.

Rozendal N: Understanding Italian American cultural norms, *J Psychosoc Nurs Ment Health Serv* 25(2):29-35, 1987.

Slaughter-Defoe DT, Kuehne VS, Straker JK: African-American, Anglo-American, and Anglo-Canadian grade 4 children's concepts of old people and of extended family, *Int J Aging Hum Dev* 35(3):161-178, 1992.

Stevenson HW, Chen CS, Uttal DH: Beliefs and achievement: a study of black, white, and Hispanic children, *Child Dev* 61(2):508-523, 1990.

Tripp-Reimer T: Barriers to health care: variations in interpretation of Appalachian client behavior by Appalachian and non-Appalachian health professionals, *West J Nurs Res* 4:179-191, 1982.

Tripp-Reimer T: Retention of a folk-healing practice (matiasma) among four generations of urban Greek immigrants, *Nurs Res* 32:97-101, 1983.

Waldman HB: Differences in the health status of black and white children, *ASDC J Dent Child* 59(5):369-372, 1992.

Webber LS and others: Cardiovascular risk factors in Hispanic, white, and black children: the Brooks County and Bogalusa Heart studies, *Am J Epidemiol* 133(7):704-714, 1991.

Wiggins, LR: Health and illness beliefs and practices among the Old Order Amish, *Health Values* 7(6):24-29, 1983.

CHAPTER 3

Family Influences on Child Health Promotion

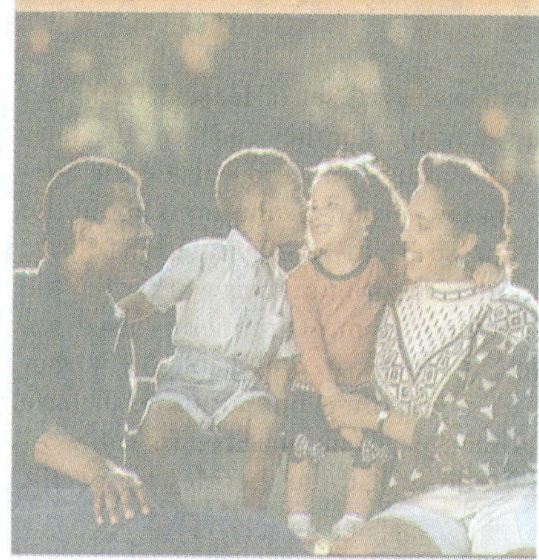

CHAPTER OUTLINE

RELATED TOPICS

Adolescent pregnancy, Ch. 20
Alternate child care arrangements, Ch. 12
Communicating with families, Ch. 6
Family assessment, Ch. 6
Growth and development of children, Ch. 4
Family-centered care of the child with chronic illness or disability, Ch. 22
Preschool and kindergarten experience, Ch. 15
Promotion of parent-infant bonding (attachment), Ch. 8
Sibling rivalry, Ch. 14
Social, cultural, and religious influences on child health promotion, Ch. 2

GENERAL CONCEPTS

DEFINITION OF FAMILY

The term *family* has been defined in a number of ways and for a number of purposes according to the individual's own frame of reference, value judgment, or the discipline. For example, biology describes the family as fulfilling the biologic function of perpetuation of the species. Psychology emphasizes the interpersonal aspects of the family and its responsibility for personality development. Economics views the family as a productive unit providing for material needs, and sociology depicts it as the social unit that reacts with the larger society. Others define family in relation to the persons who make up the family unit: the most common type of relationships are ***consanguineous*** (blood relationships), ***affinal*** (marital relationships), and ***family of origin*** (family unit person is born into).

Earlier definitions emphasized that family members were related by legal ties or genetic relationships and lived in the same household with specific roles. Later definitions have been broadened to reflect both structural and functional changes. Freidman (1992) defines family as "two or more persons who are joined together by bonds of sharing and emotional closeness and who identify themselves as being part of the family."

To further acknowledge the variety of cultural styles, values, and alternative family structures that exist today, an even more inclusive definition of family is sometimes used. This definition allows the individual family to define itself (McGonigel, 1991). In other words, the family decides who they consider "family." These important people in the family's life may be related, unrelated, immediate family, or extended family members.

Traditionally, a family has been conceptualized as a group, with the belief that both a mother and a father are needed to rear a child. Nearly all societies grant a very high rank to the married status, and although this concept has undergone considerable modification, a great deal of emotion has been generated about some of the newer concepts of family—such as communal families, single-parent families, and homosexual families. To accommodate these and other varieties of family styles, the descriptive term ***household*** is being used more frequently. Regardless of the definition chosen, a "family" is whatever the client considers it to be.

Although the concept of household is recognized and appreciated, the term *family* is used throughout this book to indicate the relationships between dependent children and one or more protective adults. It also implies relationships among siblings. Family members share a sense of belonging to their own family that deeply affects their lives.

Nursing of infants and children is intimately involved with care of the child *and* the family. Consequently, nurses must be aware of the functions of the family, various types of family structures, and theories that provide a foundation for understanding the changes within a family and for directing family-oriented interventions.

■ Judy Holt Rollins, RN, MS, revised this chapter.

FAMILY THEORIES

A ***family theory*** can be viewed as a "set of lenses" (Hill and Hansen, 1960) used to describe families and how the family unit responds to events both within and outside the family. Each family theory makes certain assumptions about the family and has inherent strengths and limitations. Most nurses use a combination of theories in their work with children and families. The theories most frequently used are discussed below, as well as summarized in Table 3-1. Other theories that may be used less often but continue to have relevance for nursing practice are summarized in Table 3-1 with examples of applications of these theories to specific family situations.

Family Systems Theory

Family systems theory is derived from general systems theory, a science of "wholeness" that is characterized by interaction among the components of the system and between the system and the environment. ***General systems theory*** expanded scientific thought from a simplistic view of direct cause and effect (*A* causes *B*) to a more complex and interrelated theory (*A* influences *B*, but *B* also affects *A*). In family systems theory the family is viewed as a system that continually interacts with its members and the environment. The emphasis is on the ***interaction*** between the members, such that a change in one family member creates a change in other members, which in turn results in a new change in the original member. Consequently, a problem or dysfunction does not lie in any one member but rather in the type of interactions used by the family. Since it is the interactions, rather than individual members, that are viewed as the source of the problem, the family becomes the patient and the focus of care. Examples of the application of family systems theory to clinical problems are nonorganic failure to thrive and child abuse. According to family systems theory, the problem does not rest solely with the parent or child but exists in the type of interactions between the parent and child, as well as in a host of other factors that affect their relationship.

Understanding family systems theory requires knowledge of numerous basic definitions and concepts that are beyond the focus of this discussion. However, some general concepts that are unique to this theory and have significance to understanding family dynamics are presented.

The family is viewed as a whole that is different from the sum of the individual members. For example, in a household of parents and one child there are not only three individuals, but also four interactive units that characterize the family system. These include three dyads (the marital relationship, the mother-child relationship, and the father-child relationship) and a triangle (the mother-father-child relationship). This concept of ***nonsummativity***—"the whole is greater than the sum of its parts"—implies that, when working with a family, the nurse must be aware of the relationships between family members. To effect positive change in a family, it is necessary to work with and through the several subsystems of the family.

Another important concept, ***adaptability,*** views the family as a highly adaptable unit. When problems exist within

TABLE 3-1 Summary of Family Theories and Applications

ASSUMPTIONS	STRENGTHS	LIMITATIONS	APPLICATIONS
FAMILY SYSTEMS THEORY			
A change in any one part of a family system affects all other parts of the family system (circular causality) Family systems are characterized by periods of rapid growth and change and periods of relative stability Both too little change and too much change are dysfunctional for the family system; therefore a balance between morphogenesis (change) and morphostasis (no change) is necessary Family system can initiate change, as well as react to it	Applicable for family in normal everyday life, as well as for family dysfunction and pathology Useful for families of varying structure and various stages of life cycle	More difficult to determine cause-and-effect relationships because of circular causality	Mate selection, courtship processes, family communication, boundary maintenance, power and control within family, parent-child relationships, adolescent pregnancy and parenthood
FAMILY STRESS THEORY			
Stress is an inevitable part of family life, and any event, even if positive, can be stressful for family Family encounters both normative expected stressors and unexpected situational stressors over life cycle Stress has a cumulative effect on family Families cope and respond to stressors with a wide range of responses and effectiveness	Potential to explain and predict family behavior in response to stressors and to develop effective interventions to promote family adaptation Focuses on positive contribution of resources, coping, and social support to adaptive outcomes Can be used by many disciplines in health field	Relationships between all variables in framework not yet adequately described Do not yet know if certain combinations of resources, coping strategies are applicable to all stressful events	Transition to parenthood and other normative transitions, single-parent families, families experiencing work-related stressors (dual-earner, unemployment), acute or chronic childhood illness or disability, infertility, death of a child, divorce, teenage pregnancy and parenthood
DEVELOPMENTAL THEORY			
Families develop and change over time in similar and consistent ways Family and its members must perform certain time-specific tasks set by themselves and by persons in the broader society Family role performance at one stage of family life cycle influences family's behavioral options at next stage Family tends to be in stage of disequilibrium entering a new life cycle stage and strives toward homeostasis within stages	Provides a dynamic, rather than static, view of family Addresses both changes within family and changes in family as a social system over its life history Anticipates potential stressors that normally accompany transitions to various stages and when problems may peak because of lack of resources	Traditional model more easily applied to two-parent families with children Use of age of oldest child and marital duration as marker of stage transition may be problematic (e.g., in stepfamilies, single-parent families)	Anticipatory guidance, educational strategies, and developing/strengthening family resources for management of transition to parenthood; family adjustment to children entering school, becoming adolescents, leaving home; management of "empty nest" years and retirement
STRUCTURAL-FUNCTIONAL THEORY			
Family performs at least one societal function (e.g., reproduction, socializing children, producing/consuming goods and services) while also meeting family needs Family, as a social system, tends toward stability Family behaviors are largely determined by norms	Considers interplay within family, as well as between family and the larger social system (school, workplace) Views family as both open to outside influence and transactions and as a system that tends to maintain boundaries	Strong emphasis on family stability and maintaining status quo	Dual-career or dual-worker families and management of combined work and family roles and responsibilities Relationships of family unit with schools, other societal institutions

Continued.

TABLE 3-1 Summary of Family Theories and Applications—cont'd

ASSUMPTIONS	STRENGTHS	LIMITATIONS	APPLICATIONS
SYMBOLIC INTERACTIONAL THEORY			
Family is a unit of interacting persons, with each occupying a position within the family to which a number of roles are assigned; family relationships are continually in flux The definition family members make of situations partially determines the effects situations have for them Family members communicate through symbols that have both meaning and value attached to them	More culture- and value-free, less normative and prescriptive Views family as a living social unit and examines both behavior and perceptions	Looks more at family at one point in time Focuses on internal family interactions and processes; less emphasis on family-community/society interactions and relationships Complex framework with many concepts, assumptions	Family communications, decision making, problem solving
EXCHANGE THEORY			
Overall assumption is that humans, families, groups, associations, and even nations seek rewarding statuses, relationships, interactions, and feeling states so that their rewards are maximized and/or their costs are minimized	Breadth and versatility Applicable to various family forms, to families of other cultures and countries Can be applied to individuals, families, groups, organizations, societies	What constitutes a reward or cost is not clear Does not directly address how individuals or families acquire meaning and value in determining what is a reward and/or cost	Rewards and costs associated with paid employment of mothers, decision to have children or be child-free, parenting responsibilities, kin and intergenerational relationships, marital dissolution
CONFLICT THEORY			
Families are viewed as ongoing competitive social systems The conflict inherent in family relationships can be managed by negotiation and problem solving Complete suppression of conflict in a family system is likely to have negative consequences for the family unit and/or its members	Applicable to all family forms and structures Appropriate for examining many situations families are facing in today's society Can see how family conflict changes over time	Can be perceived as having a "negative" focus Can view all conflict as power struggle, which severely limits its use of this theory Needs further use and testing	Divorce, remarriage, stepfamily relationships, conflict over any aspect of family life—relationships with children, in-laws, work-family issues, caretaking of dependent members (children, elders), family violence

the family, change can be effected by altering the interaction or feedback messages that perpetuate disruptive behavior. ***Feedback*** refers to processes within the family that help identify strengths and needs and determine how well goals are being accomplished. Positive feedback initiates change, whereas negative feedback resists change.

When the family system is disrupted, change can occur at any point in the system. Although family systems theorists may pursue the family history in trying to understand current family interaction and problem patterns, the emphasis is on what is occurring now in the family and on intervening to change that pattern. This focus allows for sometimes rapid and dramatic changes.

A major factor that influences a family's adaptability is its ***boundary,*** an imaginary but very real line that exists between the family and its environment. This boundary, or line, may be open or closed. An ***open family*** welcomes input into its system by accepting new ideas, information, resources, and opportunities. This type of family reaches out for help and uses the available support systems. In contrast, a ***closed family*** resists input by viewing change as threatening. The family is suspicious of any available support and strives to maintain the family system by avoiding outside influences. Having knowledge of boundaries is critical when teaching or counseling families. Although open families are receptive to intervention, closed families typically resist assistance and more effort is required to gain their trust and acceptance.

Family Stress Theory

Family stress theory explains how families react to stressful events and suggests factors that promote adaptation to these events. Families encounter ***stressors*** (events that cause stress), including those that are predictable (e.g., parenthood) and those that are unpredictable (e.g., illness or unemployment). These stressors are cumulative, involving simultaneous demands from work, family, and community life. Too many stressful events occurring within a relatively short period of time—usually 1 year—can overwhelm the family's ability to cope, thus placing the family system at risk for breakdown or its members at risk for physical and emotional health problems. When the family experiences too many stressors for it to cope adequately, a state of crisis ensues. For adaptation to occur under these circumstances, a change in family structure and/or interaction is necessary.

Family stress theory also encompasses certain capabilities the family can use to manage a crisis brought on by too many stressors. The ***Typology Model of Adjustment and Adaptation*** (McCubbin and McCubbin, 1989), a comprehensive family stress model, summarizes these capabilities through four components:

1. **Basic attributes** of the family—the family type—that explains how the family typically operates and behaves
2. **Resources** of individual family members, the family unit, and the community, including social support from extended family, friends, neighbors, and health professionals
3. **Perception** of how the family defines the situation, its impact, and their ability to manage
4. **Coping behaviors or strategies** that family members or the family unit can use to keep the family functioning as a unit; decrease an individual member's tension, anxiety, and distress; and increase understanding of the particular situation or problem

The Typology Model of Adjustment and Adaptation helps explain why families differ in their responses to stressors. For example, bringing their child with special needs to a treatment facility for therapy might be considered a crisis by a family without a car or money for public transportation, yet may only be defined as a minor inconvenience by another family with adequate and appropriate resources.

Applying the Typology Model to the desired outcome of family adaptation, the concept of ***fit*** is defined at two levels: the individual family members within the family and the family within the community (McCubbin and McCubbin, 1989; McCubbin and Patterson, 1982). Adaptation occurs over time and is not always a smooth process; Hill (1949) called the process a "roller coaster of family adaptation."

Developmental Theory

Developmental theory is an outgrowth of several theories of development. Foremost among the developers are Duvall (1977), who described eight developmental tasks of the family throughout its life span (see box at right), derived from Erikson's eight stages of man (see Chapter 4), and Rogers (1962), who incorporated role theory into the developmental concept. The family is described as a small group, a semiclosed system of personalities that interacts with the larger cultural social system. As an interrelated system, changes do not occur in one part without a series of changes in other parts.

Developmental theory addresses family change over time by using Duvall's family life cycle stages, based on the predictable changes in the structure, function, and roles of the family, with the age of the oldest child as the marker for stage transition. Thus the arrival of the first child marks the transition from stage I to stage II. As the first child grows and develops, the family enters subsequent stages. In every stage the family is faced with certain developmental tasks. At the same time, each member of the family must achieve individual developmental tasks as part of each family life cycle stage.

Additions to family development theory reflect more inclusive and accurate versions of contemporary family life. For example, should divorce occur, the family life cycle takes a different course (see box on p. 70). New life cycle norms have also been developed for reconstituted families, low-income families, alcoholic families, and dual-career families (Carter and McGoldrick, 1989). Developing norms for gay or lesbian families has been more difficult because of the absence of rituals or markers that typically delineate life cycle stages (Slater and Mencher, 1991).

Developmental theory can be applied to nursing prac-

DUVALL'S DEVELOPMENTAL STAGES OF THE FAMILY

STAGE I: MARRIAGE AND AN INDEPENDENT HOME: THE JOINING OF FAMILIES

Reestablish couple identity.
Realign relationships with extended family.
Make decisions regarding parenthood.

STAGE II: FAMILIES WITH INFANTS

Integrate infants into family unit.
Accommodate to new parenting and grandparenting roles.
Maintain marital bond.

STAGE III: FAMILIES WITH PRESCHOOLERS

Socialize children.
Parents and children adjust to separation.

STAGE IV: FAMILIES WITH SCHOOLCHILDREN

Children develop peer relations.
Parents adjust to their children's peer and school influences.

STAGE V: FAMILIES WITH TEENAGERS

Adolescents develop increasing autonomy.
Parents refocus on midlife marital and career issues.
Parents begin a shift toward concern for older generation.

STAGE VI: FAMILIES AS LAUNCHING CENTERS

Parents and young adults establish independent identities.
Renegotiate marital relationship.

STAGE VII: MIDDLE-AGED FAMILIES

Reinvest in couple identity with concurrent development of independent interests.
Realign relationships to include in-laws and grandchildren.
Deal with disabilities and death of older generation.

STAGE VIII: AGING FAMILIES

Shift from work role to leisure and semiretirement or full retirement.
Maintain couple and individual functioning while adapting to aging process.
Prepare for own death and dealing with loss of spouse and/or siblings and other peers.

Modified from Wright LM, Leahey M: *Nurses and families: a guide to family assessment and intervention,* Philadelphia, 1984, FA Davis.

FAMILY DEVELOPMENT STAGES FOR DIVORCE

STAGE I: DECISION TO DIVORCE
Accept the inability to resolve marital discord.

STAGE II: PLANNING THE BREAKUP
Create viable arrangements for all members of the family.

STAGE III: SEPARATION
Resolve attachment to spouse.
Develop cooperative co-parenting relationship.

STAGE IV: DIVORCE
Resolve the emotional divorce.

STAGE V: SINGLE-PARENT FAMILY OR NONCUSTODIAL SINGLE PARENT
Maintain parental contact with ex-spouse.
Maintain parental contact with children (noncustodial parent).
Maintain relationship with ex-in-laws (custodial parent).
Rebuild a personal social network.

Modified from Danielson C, Hamel-Bissell B, Winstead-Fry P: *Families, health, and illness,* St Louis, 1993, Mosby.

tice in a number of ways. For example, the nurse can assess how well new parents are accomplishing the individual and family developmental tasks associated with transition to parenthood.

Structural-Functional Theory

Structural-functional theory, one of the dominant orientations in modern sociology, has been most systematically applied by Parsons (Rodman, 1965). In analyzing families, this theory focuses less on family change and more on the interrelatedness, interdependence, and integration between family members and all aspects of society and its subcultures, particularly the occupational subsystem. ***Structure*** refers to the arrangement of roles that comprise a social system; ***function*** is the contribution made by an activity or role to the whole and the consequences of the activity for the system. The family is described as a social system with members who have specific roles and functions. The family process is directed toward maintaining an equilibrium between the complementary roles within the family (e.g., husband-wife, father-daughter, mother-son, or wife–mother-in-law).

Internal relationships involve the division of labor between family members and the functions of these divisions for family maintenance. ***Expressive roles*** are seen in integrative or solidifying activities, such as hugging, that bring emotional satisfaction to the family members. ***Instrumental roles*** are activities, such as earning an income, that occur external to the family but that also include satisfactory goal attainment of the family. Traditionally, expressive roles have been assigned to the wife-mother, whereas the husband-father has assumed the instrumental roles. However, the classic breadwinner husband, homemaker wife, and two children now make up only a small proportion of families in developed countries. Both expressive and instrumental roles are becoming less gender-specific.

From a structural-functional viewpoint, the major goal of the family is socialization of its members into society. Families perform certain functions ultimately directed toward this goal. Functions of the family as outlined by Friedman (1992) are:

1. **Affective** to meet the psychologic needs of family members
2. **Socialization** and **social placement** to help children become productive members of society
3. **Reproductive** to ensure family continuity and societal survival
4. **Economic** to provide and allocate sufficient resources for the family
5. **Health care** for the provision of physical necessities, such as food, clothing, shelter, and a high level of wellness

This framework can be applied in nursing practice to assess how well the family is accomplishing these five functions in relation to its overall goal.

Structural-functional theory focuses heavily on the integration of the family within the occupational systems. In many instances occupational roles are segregated from family roles. However, with increasing numbers of women in the work force and greater emphasis on careers, negotiating work-family conflicts in dual-earner families has become a significant facet of family life.

FAMILY NURSING INTERVENTIONS

In working with children, nurses must include family members in their plan of care. In essence, the *patient is the family.* To discover family dynamics and the unit's strengths and weaknesses, a thorough family assessment is needed (see Chapter 6). The interventions nurses use with families depend on their theoretic model of the family. For example, in family systems theory the focus is on the interactions of the members, rather than on an individual member. In this case using group dynamics to involve all members in the intervention process and being a skillful communicator are essential. In the family stress theory crisis intervention strategies are employed, and the chief focus is on helping members cope with the challenging event. In the developmental theory a primary nursing function is to provide anticipatory guidance that prepares members for transition to the next family stage. Nurses are usually most comfortable using teaching strategies. However, education alone may not be sufficient for families to change or cope with a crisis. Several other interventions that nurses can use to constructively help and support family members are listed in the box on p. 71 and are discussed throughout the text.

Just as appropriate strategies differ, the level of assistance a family needs will also depend on the type of crisis, factors affecting family adjustment (see Table 22-2), and the family's level of functioning. Highly functioning families usually need informational interventions. Vulnerable families (see p. 75) benefit from a wider range of supportive and therapeutic interventions. In working with families, nurses must be aware of their degree of professional com-

FAMILY NURSING INTERVENTIONS

Behavior modification
Contracting
Case management/coordination
Collaborative strategies
Counseling, including support, cognitive reappraisal, and reframing
Empowering families through active participation
Environmental modification
Family advocacy
Family crisis intervention
Networking, including use of self-help groups and social support
Providing information and technical expertise
Role modeling
Role supplementation
Teaching strategies, including stress management, life-style modifications, and anticipatory guidance

From Friedman MM: *Family nursing: theory and practice,* ed 3, Norwalk, CT, 1992, Appleton & Lange.

petence in using family nursing interventions. An important nursing role is to recognize situations where referral to more specialized services is required.

FAMILY STRUCTURE AND FUNCTION

FAMILY STRUCTURE

The ***family structure,*** or ***family composition,*** consists of individuals, each with a socially recognized status and position, who interact with one another on a regular, recurring basis in socially sanctioned ways. When members are gained or lost through events (e.g., marriage, divorce, birth, death, abandonment, incarceration), the family composition is altered and roles must be redefined or redistributed.

Traditionally, the family structure refers to either nuclear or extended families. However, family composition has assumed new configurations in recent years, with the single-parent family and stepfamilies becoming prominent forms. In any case, the predominant structural pattern in any society depends to a large extent on the mobility of families as they pursue economic goals and as relationships change. It is not uncommon for children to belong to several different family groups during their lifetime. In general, extended families are associated with agricultural societies, whereas small conjugal units are characteristic of more advanced, industrialized societies.

Nuclear Family

The ***nuclear,*** or ***conjugal, family*** consists of a husband, wife, and their children (natural or adopted) who live in a common household. This is the reproductive unit in which the marital tie (legally or otherwise sanctioned) is the chief binding force. A strongly functional nuclear family is the prototype of human relationships and the basic unit from which more complex familial forms are composed. In some instances one or more additional persons (e.g., a relative, friend, foster child, or others) may reside in the same household. Nuclear families can be combined into larger units in one of two ways: through plural marriage (polygamous families) or through extension of the parent-child relationship (extended family). Some authorities classify childless couples as a nuclear family because the alliance is conjugal with the theoretic potential for reproduction.

The nuclear family is more characteristic of an urban, mobile society. It is highly adaptable, with the ability to adjust and reshape its structure when needed. It is free to move where there is opportunity for higher income with concomitant improvement in other areas, such as social class and prestige. It is not economically bound to a geographic area nor dependent on the cooperative efforts of other members. The family members are employed on an individual basis, and economic resources are in the form of money. The present-day family must purchase the services of specialized individuals and groups, whereas previously these needs and services were met on a cooperative basis by the extended family members.

Although extended families residing in the same household are rapidly disappearing in North American society, the isolated nuclear family without relatives within easy visiting distance is uncommon. This is most often seen where there has been extreme mobility of separate generations, such as wide geographic separations or marriages into different social strata, religious backgrounds, or roles. Most consanguineous family members maintain contact through visits, telephone calls, letters, and gift exchanges. Having no relatives readily available for advice and assistance with child care, as is common in extended families, parents in some nuclear families are more likely to turn to "experts" for childrearing guidance.

The majority of nuclear families in America are associated with an extended kinship network of nuclear families living in separate households but in close geographic proximity. This concept, sometimes referred to as a modified extended family, describes a meaningful aspect of daily existence that is reflected in frequent visiting and the exchange of services and financial aid. This family association meets the members' psychologic needs to a greater extent than do experts, friends, or organizations. It is not uncommon for families to reject the opportunity for social or economic advancement rather than leave such kinship associations.

Affiliative Relationships. Although the nuclear family is predominantly a legally sanctioned institution, there are a number of families in which the attachment is only ***affiliative*** (i.e., nonmarital cohabitation). These families consist primarily of two adults, the "couple households" (Macklin, 1980), but may include children. The mother and father live together, often with children from previous matings, and share family responsibilities. However, the family unit is less stable and relationships are subject to change. Instability of the social environment in the home has been associated with juvenile delinquency, which appears to be related to the number of family constellations (changes in the adult members of the household) experienced during childhood. This is probably a reflection of repeated adjustment to a variety of authority figures (Mednick and Baker, 1980).

Single-Parent Family

The ***single-parent family*** is not a new phenomenon. Throughout history, deaths from disease, childbirth, and wars have resulted in many one-parent families, although frequently remarriage occurs. The contemporary single-parent family, however, has emerged partially as a consequence of women's rights movements wherein more women (and men) have established separate households because of divorce, death, desertion, or illegitimacy. In addition, a more liberal attitude in the courts has made it possible for single persons, both male and female, to adopt children, whereas previously, rigid prerequisites specified that both a father and a mother must be present in the home. Although single-parent families are usually headed by the mother, it is becoming increasingly common for fathers to be awarded custody of dependent children in divorce settlements. A significant number of single-parent families result from a single mother who wishes to have a child but does not choose to have a husband. Also, unmarried mothers often choose to keep and raise their children rather than place them for adoption or marry, and are frequently absorbed into the extended family. With the increased psychologic independence of women as a whole and the increased acceptability of illegitimacy in society, more unmarried women are deliberately choosing mother-child families. The challenges of these single-parent families are discussed on p. 97.

Binuclear Family

The term ***binuclear family*** is used to describe the situation that allows parents to continue the parenting role while terminating the spousal unit (Ahrons, 1979). The degree of cooperation between households and the time the child spends with each can vary. In ***joint custody*** the court assigns divorcing parents equal rights and responsibilities to the minor child or children. These alternate family forms are efforts on the part of those concerned to view divorce as a process of reorganization and redefinition of a family rather than as a family dissolution. Joint custody and co-parenting are discussed further on p. 96 in relation to special parenting situations.

Reconstituted Family

Reconstituted families, also referred to as ***stepfamilies,*** are those in which one or both the married adults have children from a previous marriage residing in the household. The term ***blended families,*** or ***combined families,*** more often refers to families composed of parents and the children each of them brings from a previous marriage. Most reconstituted families involve a mother, her children, and a stepfather. However, 50% of women who marry for the second time while in their childbearing years will give birth after remarrying, usually within 24 months (Wineberg, 1990). Reconstituted families are discussed further on p. 98.

Extended Family

The ***extended family*** is one mode of combining nuclear families into larger units through the parent-child relationship. It consists of the nuclear family plus lineal or collateral relatives. More often it is composed of two or more residential units of three or more generations affiliated through extension of the parent-child relationship (i.e., grandparents, parents, and grandchildren). An extended family can be compounded by either monogamous or polygamous relationships. Broader views recognize the affiliation of collateral relatives as an extended family—not necessarily organized into nuclear families.

Extended family structure is more functional in areas where land is the basis of wealth and sustenance. Today the best examples of extended family units can be found among successful farmers, Native Americans, and certain recent immigrants. Here the family serves as the basic social, educational, and productive unit, providing services and sharing resources. Extended families may form under conditions of either extreme poverty in order to pool resources or extreme wealth in order to consolidate resources. Extended families direct cooperative efforts for common goals; the needs of the individual are sublimated to the welfare of the family enterprise and survival. The children learn early in life to respect their elders, and this value is reinforced through observation of their parents' behavior toward older family members (Fig. 3-1).

In the extended family childrearing is often a shared responsibility. Relatives are always present and available to help young mothers with household chores and child care activities. Daily lives of the children are organized around the needs and requirements of the family, with assigned tasks and obligations. Family ties between the nuclear unit and the main extended family are strong, although there is a high degree of competition between individual nuclear units for acquisition of power and resources.

Polygamous Family

Although it is not legally sanctioned in the United States, sometimes the conjugal unit can be extended by the addition of spouses in polygamous matings. ***Polygamy*** generally refers to either wives ***(polygyny)*** or, very rarely, husbands ***(polyandry).*** Many societies practice polygyny that is further designated as ***sororal,*** in which the wives are sisters, or ***non-***

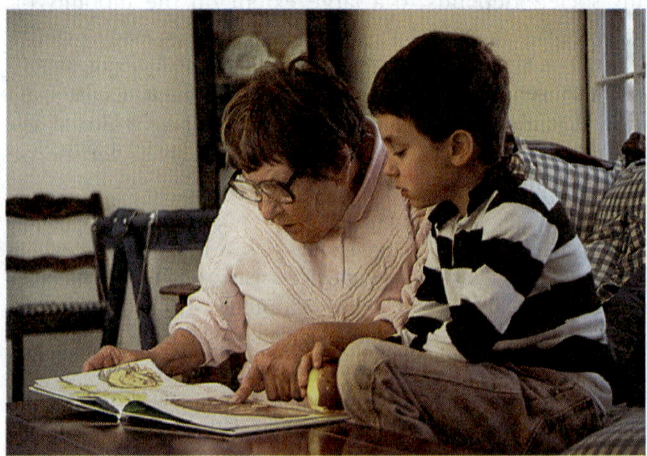

FIG. 3-1 Children benefit from interaction with grandparents even when they do not share the same household.

sororal, in which the wives can be unrelated. Sororal polygyny is widespread throughout the world, and although plural marriages produce problems of adjustment for the members, co-wives who are sisters are more likely to get along with each other and display less jealousy than co-wives who are not. Most often mothers and their children share a husband and father, usually with each mother and her children maintaining a separate household, particularly when the wives are unrelated.

A special form of sororal polygyny is the ***sororate,*** in which a cultural rule specifies that the preferred mate for a widower is the sister of his deceased wife. In a sororate the marriages are successive rather than concurrent.

Where it exists, polygamy is usually accorded a higher status than monogamy. It may be limited to ruling families or to high-status persons and tends to be practiced by a small segment of the population. This is probably a result of economic factors and the unequal sex ratio in some areas at the time of biologic maturity.

Communal Family

The ***communal family*** emerged, as have all previous experimental communities, from a disenchantment with most contemporary life choices. Although communal families may have divergent beliefs, practices, and organization, the basic impetus for formation has been dissatisfaction with social systems and life goals of the larger communities and with the nuclear family structure, in particular, as it exists from either an ideologic or a practical perspective. Relatively uncommon today, communal groups share common ownership of property and goods; in cooperatives there is private ownership of property, but certain goods and services are shared and exchanged cooperatively without monetary consideration. There is strong reliance on group members and material interdependence. Both provide collective security for nonproductive members, share homemaking and childrearing functions, and help overcome the problem of interpersonal isolation or loneliness.

Unlike the traditional extended family, nuclear units in a commune may come and go at will. There is no consanguineous tie between the units. The mother-child tie is strong during infancy and early childhood, but many parents are happy to relinquish older children to the care of others. Although the parents maintain primary responsibility for the health and well-being of the children, the children are free to form close relationships with a number of adults in the commune and are encouraged to do so.

Gay/Lesbian Family

The most common means by which homosexuals acquire children is through legal marriage. Gay men and lesbians marry partners of the opposite sex for a variety of reasons, including love for the spouse, desire for children, family and peer pressure, desire for companionship, and fear of loneliness (Bozett, 1987b, 1988a). Some homosexuals may not be aware of their homosexuality at the time of marriage, whereas others may marry hoping that a heterosexual relationship will abolish their homosexual desires.

Estimates of the number of children of gay or lesbian parents range from 6 to 14 million (Patterson, 1992). While most children in gay/lesbian households are biologic from a former, legal marriage, there are other means by which homosexuals acquire children. For example, they may be foster or adoptive parents (Ricketts and Achtenberg, 1987), lesbian mothers may conceive through artificial fertilization (this is becoming increasingly common) (Pies, 1987), or a gay male couple may become parents through use of a surrogate mother.

Research studies on children reared in lesbian mother households have not found the mother's sexual orientation to be detrimental to the children (Green and others, 1986; Huggins, 1989; Steckel, 1987). In the only reported study of children of gay fathers, Bozett (1987a, 1988b) found that if the children, who ranged in age from 14 to 35 years, had mutual interests and feelings in common with their father and if they believed the father's homosexuality was not outwardly discernible, then the children were more accepting of their father as gay. If there was little mutuality and they thought their father's homosexuality was externally evident, then the children exerted greater control in relation to when, where, and with whom they would be seen in public with their father. Younger children who lived with their father were also more selective in whom they would invite home. However, in no instance did any of "the children express any difficulty with their father in the parental role. . . . even though several of the children thought that homosexuality was immoral, many of them considered their father a friend, confidante, and adviser" (Bozett, 1988b).

In child custody disputes when parental homosexuality is an issue, the courts have expressed concern that the children may become gay, that they may be molested by the parent or the parent's friend, that they will be less psychologically healthy than children from heterosexual homes, and that they may experience difficulties with social relationships (Patterson, 1992). However, according to reported research, children in gay/lesbian households are no more likely to be gay than are children reared in heterosexual households (Bozett, 1989; Gottman, 1990; Huggins, 1989; Paul, 1986); most child molestation is perpetrated by heterosexual men; and the quality of parenting and home life of gay men and lesbians, whether they are single or in a partner relationship, is equivalent to that of nongay parents (Bozett, 1984; Harris and Turner, 1986; Turner, Scadden, and Harris, 1985). It is true that children may be taunted if their peers know their mother or father is homosexual. However, this kind of harassment is similar to that experienced by children in other minority groups, and like other minority parents, gays and lesbians tend to help their children manage these situations constructively as they arise.

Disclosure of parental homosexuality ("coming out") to children may also be a concern. It has been found that generally it is best for children to be told, preferably before adolescence (Patterson, 1992). However, there are a number of factors to consider before telling children: parents should be fairly comfortable with their own gayness before disclosing it to children; it should be discussed with them before they know or suspect; the disclosure should be planned and should take place in a quiet setting where interruptions are unlikely; and children should be assured that the parent's relationship with them will not change as a result of disclosure (Bigner and Bozett, 1990; Miller, 1987; Schulenburg, 1985).

Parents should also be prepared for questions from their children, such as "What does being gay mean?" "What makes a person gay?" "Will I be gay, too?" and "What should I tell my friends about it?" Also, the earlier children are informed, the easier it is for them to deal with the information. Moreover, after disclosure the parent-child relationship may become closer (Schulenburg, 1985; Turner, Scadden, and Harris, 1985). However, even though most children are accepting, during their own sexual awakening in adolescence they may have difficulty dealing with the fact of their parent's homosexuality. In addition, if the parent develops a partner relationship in which the couple live together in a spouselike relationship, the children may develop a resentment toward the partner or have other problems similar to those seen in heterosexual stepparent families (Baptiste, 1987).

Because this family form is more common than most persons may realize, it is important for the nurse to understand that homosexual families are different from the heterosexual family form, not necessarily better or worse. The gay/lesbian family environment can be just as healthy as any other. Nurses need to be nonjudgmental and to learn how to accept differences rather than demonstrate a homophobic prejudice that can have a detrimental effect on the nurse–child/family relationship. Moreover, the more knowledge of the child's family constellation and life-style nurses have, the greater benefit they can be to the gay or lesbian parent and the child.

QUALITIES OF STRONG FAMILIES

1. A belief and sense of ***commitment*** toward promoting the well-being and growth of individual family members, as well as that of the family unit
2. ***Appreciation*** for the small and large things that individual family members do well and ***encouragement*** to do better
3. Concentrated effort to spend ***time*** and do things together, no matter how formal or informal the activity or event
4. A sense of ***purpose*** that permeates the reasons and basis for "going on" in both bad and good times
5. A sense of ***congruence*** among family members regarding the value and importance of assigning time and energy to meet needs
6. The ability to ***communicate*** with one another in a way that emphasizes positive interactions
7. A clear set of ***family rules, values,*** and ***beliefs*** that establishes expectations about acceptable and desired behavior
8. A varied repertoire of ***coping strategies*** that promote positive functioning in dealing with both normative and nonnormative life events
9. The ability to engage in ***problem-solving*** activities designed to evaluate options for meeting needs and procuring resources
10. The ability to be ***positive*** and see the positive in almost all aspects of their lives, including the ability to see crisis and problems as an opportunity to learn and grow
11. ***Flexibility*** and ***adaptability*** in the roles necessary to procure resources to meet needs
12. A ***balance*** between the use of internal and external family resources for coping and adapting to life events and planning for the future

From Dunst C, Trivette C, Deal A: *Enabling and empowering families: principles and guidelines for practice,* Cambridge, MA, 1988, Brookline Books.

FAMILY FUNCTION

Family Strengths and Functioning Style

Family function refers to the interactions of family members, especially the quality of those relationships and interactions. Researchers have become increasingly interested in family characteristics that seem to help families function effectively. Knowledge of these factors guide the nurse at each step of the nursing process. The nurse is better able to predict the ways in which families may cope and respond to a stressful event, provide individualized support that builds on family strengths and unique functioning style, and assist family members in obtaining appropriate resources.

Based on an extensive review of the literature on family strengths, Dunst, Trivette, and Deal (1988) suggest that there are about 12 major, nonmutually exclusive qualities of strong families (see box at right). They caution that not all strong families are characterized by the presence of all 12 qualities, but that a combination of qualities appears to define strong families.

Certain combinations of qualities define ***family-functioning styles*** (unique ways of dealing with life events and promoting growth and development). There are no right or wrong family-functioning styles, but rather differentially effective styles that families are likely to employ in response to different life events and situations (Dunst, Trivette, and Deal, 1988).

Family strengths and unique family-functioning styles are significant resources nurses can employ as one method of meeting families' needs. Building on the very things that make a particular family work well and strengthening the family's reservoir of resources make the family unit even stronger and more capable of negotiating the developmental course of both individual family members and the family unit (Dunst, Trivette, and Deal, 1988).

Vulnerable Families

Certain families lack the supports and security to provide adequately for their children. In some instances social and economic factors have undermined supports for families. For example, incomes of young families have sharply declined in recent years, increasing numbers of families are headed by young single mothers, and gaps in health care coverage continue to grow. Almost half of the infants born in the United States start out at a disadvantage for one or more of the following reasons (Center for the Study of Social Policy, 1993):

EFFECTIVE APPROACHES FOR WORKING WITH VULNERABLE FAMILIES

Emphasize the family unit instead of focusing narrowly on an individual child or other family members.
Build on family strengths instead of emphasizing deficits.
Offer preventive services to avert crises instead of merely reacting to emergencies.
Address family needs comprehensively instead of piecemeal.
Treat families with respect and honor cultural differences.
Offer flexible, responsive services instead of rigid, single-purpose services.

From Children's Defense Fund: *The state of America's children 1992,* Washington, DC, 1994, CDF.

- The mother had not finished high school when she had her first baby.
- The mother and father of the baby were not married at the time of the child's birth.
- The mother was a teenager when her first baby was born and thus still a child herself.

A disadvantaged beginning is only part of the problem. Today's families are more isolated from their neighbors and extended families than in the past, leaving them with fewer informal supports in times of crisis. In addition, the neighborhoods in which many of the most vulnerable families live are increasingly plagued by drugs and violence, and lack necessary services (Children's Defense Fund, 1994).

Most families in crisis do want to be helped to better protect and nurture their children, and most families can change when offered the right kind of help (Fig. 3-2). Effective approaches for helping vulnerable families tend to share certain characteristics (see box above).

In recent years the term ***dysfunctional family,*** which often refers to a continuum of mildly to highly dysfunctional levels, has become increasingly part of both professional and popular literature, imparting a sense of pathology or sickness about the ways in which certain families function. Families are better served when pejorative labels are avoided. *All* families have strengths, as well as vulnerabilities. Nurses who appreciate this fact will strive to develop assessment skills and use assessment tools that help families identify their strengths, as well as needs. With this approach, families can not only survive a critical time, but learn and grow from the experience.

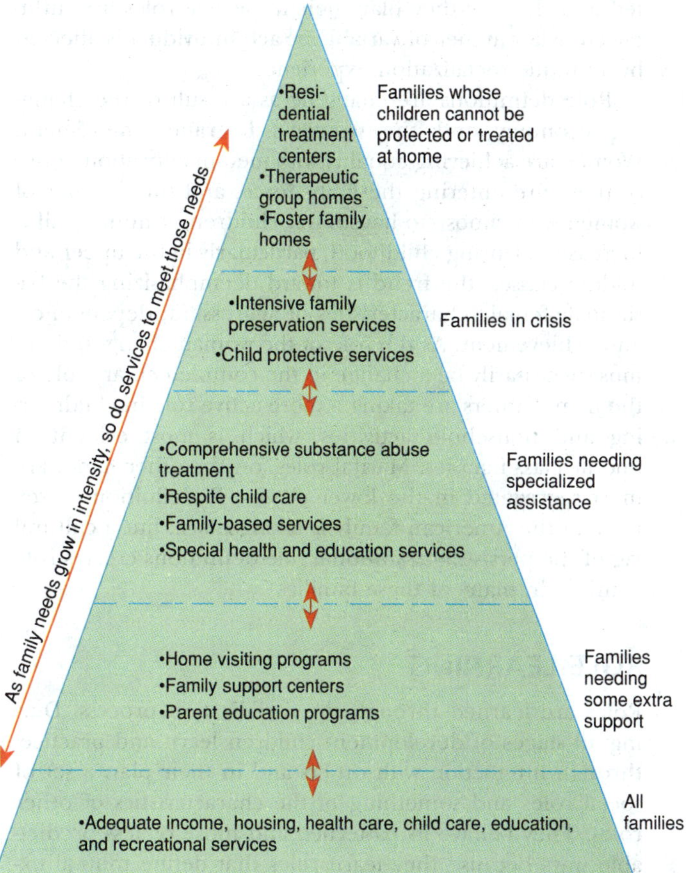

FIG. 3-2 Building a pyramid of services. When communities are able to offer a pyramid of assistance that matches the pyramid of family needs, problems are likely to be solved or alleviated at earlier stages, when they are easier and less costly to address. (From Children's Defense Fund: *The state of America's children 1992,* Washington, DC, 1992, CDF.)

FAMILY ROLES AND RELATIONSHIPS

Each individual has a position, or status, in the family structure, and each occupant of a position plays culturally and socially defined roles in interactions within the group. Within prescribed guidelines for behavior set by the culture, subcultures (including the family group) establish variations in role definition and may specify different requirements for playing the same role. Each family has its own traditions and values and sets its own standards for interaction within and outside the family group. Each determines the experiences the children should have, those they are to be shielded from, and how each of these experiences meets the needs of family members. Conformity to group norms is directly related to the strength and nature of group ties. Where family ties are strong, social control is highly effective, and most members play their roles willingly and with commitment. Conflicts arise when people do not fulfill their roles in ways that meet other family members' expectations, either because they are unaware of the expectations or because they choose not to meet them.

PARENTAL ROLES

In all family groups the socially recognized status of father and mother exists with socially sanctioned roles that prescribe appropriate sexual behavior and childrearing responsibilities. The guides for behavior in these roles serve to control sexual conflict in society and provide for prolonged care of children. The degree to which parents are committed and the way they play their respective roles are influenced by a number of variables. Each individual is affected by a unique socialization experience.

Role definitions are changing as a result of the changing economy and the women's liberation movement. Women are achieving equality with men in education, more of them are entering the labor force, and the number of women who choose to have fewer children or none at all is increasing. During childhood, particularly in the upper and middle classes, the trend is toward deemphasizing the basic male-female characteristics of aggression, dependence, and achievement. As the role of the woman changes, there must necessarily be a change in the complementary role of the man. Fathers are taking a more active role in childrearing and household activities, which is most evident in middle-class families. Marital roles, on the other hand, are most segregated in the lower classes. Redefinition of sex roles in the American family is taking place, but a cultural lag of the persisting traditional role definitions creates role conflicts in many of these families.

ROLE LEARNING

Roles are learned through the socialization process. During all stages of development children learn and practice, through interaction with others and in their play, a set of social roles and something of the characteristics of other roles. They behave in patterned and more or less predictable ways because they learn roles that define mutual expectations in typical and recurring social relationships. Role conceptions are transmitted by socializing agents (parents, peers, authority figures) who use positive and negative sanctions to ensure conformity to their norms. Role behaviors positively reinforced by rewards such as love, affection, friendship, and honors are strengthened. Negative reinforcement takes the form of ridicule, withdrawal of love, expressions of disapproval, or banishment. Types of roles are described in the box at right.

In some cultures the role behavior expected of children conflicts with desirable adult behavior. For example, in the United States children are expected to be submissive in childhood but dominant as adults. This conflict of expectations is known as ***role discontinuity.*** Other cultures value the same behaviors, such as courage and aggression, both in children and adults; this provides ***role continuity.***

Role Structuring in Children

One responsibility of the family is to develop in the children culturally appropriate role behavior. Children learn to perform in expected ways consistent with their position in the family and culture at a very early age. The observed behavior of each child is a single manifestation—a combination of social influences, as well as individual psychologic processes. In this way the uniting of the child's intrapersonal system (the self) with the interpersonal system (the family) is comprehended simultaneously as the conduct of the child.

Role structuring initially takes place within the family unit, where the children fulfill a set of roles and respond to the complementary roles of their parents and other family members. The roles of the children are shaped primarily by the parents, who apply direct or indirect pressures in an attempt to induce or force children into the desired patterns of behavior or direct their efforts toward modification of the role responses of the child on a mutually acceptable basis. Each set of parents has its own techniques, and each will determine the course that the process of socialization is to follow (see Limit-setting and Discipline, p. 85).

Research indicates that birth order influences the role each sibling is assigned within the family (Hoopes and Harper, 1987). When children enter a particular family, they sense the physical, social, and emotional values associated with their own specific role. They then develop characteristic response patterns to fulfill their role. Each sibling position role is created to meet both the family's and the individual's needs. For example, first children learn that their job assignment is to produce outcomes that meet with the family's approval and to enforce explicit family rules. Third children feel especially responsible for balance in the marital relationship. Four sibling patterns are identified, with the position patterns repeating after the fourth sibling (Table 3-2).

TYPES OF ROLES

Ascribed roles are those that are strictly defined by the culture, and very little deviation is allowed in modifying them. Ascribed roles apply to general traits such as sex, age, kinship, social class, and ethnic origin. There are culturally determined behaviors that must be adhered to regarding these roles, and they are expected to be learned in the home. For example, a child who attempts to change an ascribed role (such as sex) will be confronted with serious problems.

Achieved roles are those acquired through effort, and children must do something to attain them. Achieved roles include educational, occupational, religious, and recreational roles. These are based on performance and are acquired through satisfaction of specified requirements. The direction of these role achievements is strongly influenced by values conveyed to the children by their parents. For example, some parents believe that a college education is essential; others encourage children to seek occupational gratification.

Adopted roles are those that are sometimes transient, such as the role of patient or traveler. More often, adopted behavior patterns become fixed into what are known as character roles and apply to the unique behaviors that the child displays in a given situation. Such roles as the leader, the follower, the clown, or the show-off are examples of adopted roles. They are frequently adopted when playing the role meets a need or is the response to a complementary role in another.

Assumed roles are those related to fantasy and are especially important in childhood. This is one of the dominant means for children's adjustment and socialization. Children continually assume roles of persons they observe in their environment. The environment is a primary resource for learning the conduct that befits their position or status. Assumed roles only become a problem if they persist into the world of reality. For example, a child who persistently plays an infantile role is severely hampered in relationships with peers.

TABLE 3-2 Family Role Patterns for Siblings

JOB ASSIGNMENT	INTERPERSONAL RESPONSIBILITIES
THE FIRSTBORN IS RESPONSIBLE FOR:	
Supporting family rules, values, expectations Outcomes, results, products A central place in the family in order to be productive	The individual family members, rather than for the subsystems or the family as a whole One parent (often father) and also responsible *to* the same parent All family members' productivity
THE SECOND-BORN IS RESPONSIBLE FOR:	
Perceiving and supporting the implicit elements in family rules and relationships Opening clogged channels of communication by making the implicit explicit Monitoring the quality of performance Acting out discrepancies between the implicit and explicit to force acknowledgment	Having a unique relationship with everyone in the family One parent (usually mother) and also responsible *to* the same parent The affective state of each family member by supporting their emotional needs Working with, or fighting with, if necessary, the first sibling to flush out discrepancies between implicit and explicit rules
THE THIRD-BORN IS RESPONSIBLE FOR:	
The dynamics and quality of the marital relationship The balance in all dyadic relationships Discovering and enforcing rules about the degree and nature of relationship rules, such as closeness, conflict, dependency, intrusiveness, and loyalty Identifying family issues	Being connected to both mother and father Restoring balance in the marital relationship by connecting with each parent Connecting to all dyadic relationships in the family
THE FOURTH-BORN IS RESPONSIBLE FOR:	
Family unit and harmony Family purposes and goals	Connecting to each family member to ensure unity and harmony All "garbage" in the family because it disrupts unity and harmony Acting out the tensions in relationships; can be quite dramatic

Modified from Hoopes M, Harper J: *Birth order roles and sibling patterns in individual and family therapy,* Rockville, MD, 1987, Aspen.

Children respond to life situations according to behaviors learned in reciprocal transactions. As they acquire important role-taking skills, their relationships with others change. They become proficient at understanding others as they acquire the ability to discriminate their own perspectives from those of others. The children who get along well with others and attain status in the peer group have well-developed role-taking skills (see Role Learning in Children, Chapter 4).

FAMILY SIZE AND CONFIGURATION

The size and composition of the family directly influence child development. No two children grow in exactly the same environment, although identical twins more nearly approximate this. For example, in a nuclear family with two children—even of the same sex—one will live in a family with an older sibling, whereas the other will be reared in a family with a younger sibling. In a family where there is a 10-year age span between the children, one may be born to a 20-year-old mother, the other to a 30-year-old mother. For the child in each situation the environment is different.

Family Size

Parenting practices differ between small and large families. In small families more emphasis is placed on the individual development of the children. Parenting is intensive rather than extensive, and there is constant pressure to measure up to family expectations. Children's development and achievement are measured against that of other children in the neighborhood and social class. In small families there is more democratic participation by the children than in larger families. Adolescents in small families identify more strongly with their parents and rely more on their parents for advice. They have well-developed, autonomous inner controls as contrasted with adolescents from larger families, who rely more on adult authority.

Children in a large family are able to adjust to a variety of changes and crises. There is more emphasis on the group and less on the individual (Fig. 3-3). Cooperation is essential, often because of economic necessity. The large number of persons sharing a limited amount of space requires a greater degree of organization, administration, and authoritarian control. The control is wielded by a dominant family member—a parent or an older child. The number of children reduces the intimate, one-to-one contact between the parent and any individual child. Consequently, children turn to each other for what they cannot get from their parents. The reduced parent-child contact encourages individual children to adopt specialized roles in an attempt to gain recognition in the family.

Discipline is often administered by older siblings in large families. Siblings are usually better attuned to what constitutes misbehavior, and sibling disapproval or ostracism is frequently a more meaningful disciplinary measure than parental interventions. In situations such as death or illness of a parent, an older sibling assumes responsibility for the family at considerable personal sacrifice. Large families seem to generate a sense of security in the children fostered by sibling support and cooperation. However, adolescents from a large family are more peer oriented than family oriented.

Spacing of Children

Age differences between siblings affect the childhood environment, but to a lesser extent than does the sex of the

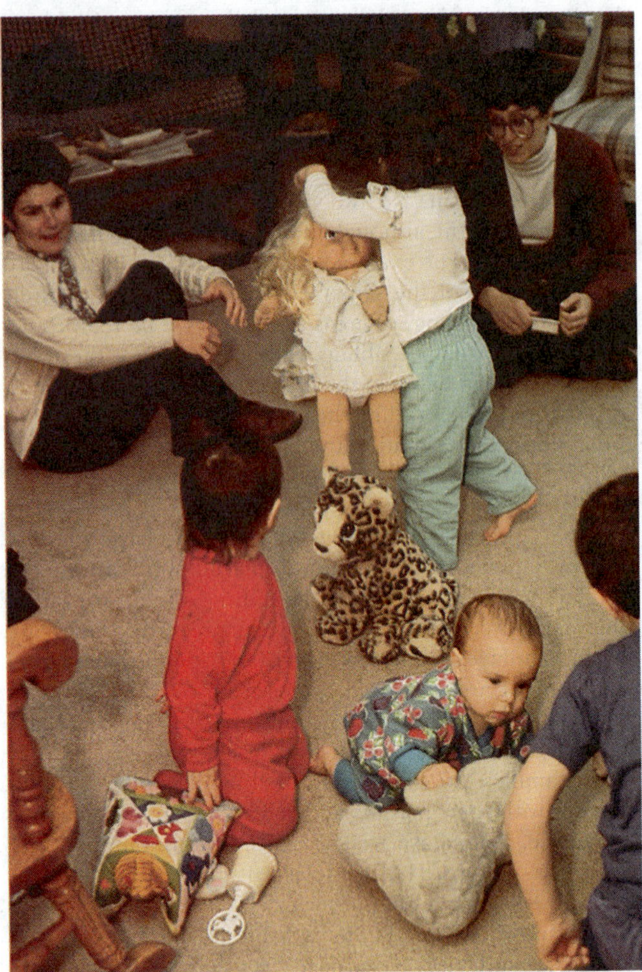

FIG. 3-3 Innumerable relationships and activities are possible in a large family.

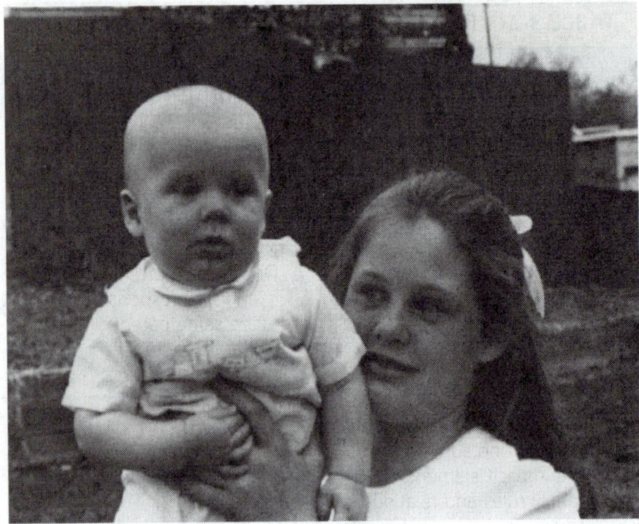

FIG. 3-4 Older school-age children often enjoy taking responsibility for the care of a younger sibling.

siblings. The arrival of a sibling has the greatest impact on the older child, and a 2- to 4-year difference in age appears to be most threatening. When the older child is very young, the self-image is too immature to be threatened. At an older age the child is better able to understand the situation and therefore is less likely to see the newcomer as a threat, although the child does feel the loss of the only-child status. Studies reveal that there is more affection and less rivalry or hostility when children are spaced 4 or more years apart (Lobato, 1990).

In general, the narrower the spacing between siblings, the more the children influence one another, especially in emotional characteristics; the wider the spacing, the greater the influence of the parents. This is not to say that bonds are nonexistent between siblings with large age spans, or that siblings with only a year or two difference in age will always feel a strong bond. However, high accessibility during these developmentally formative years is the almost routine accompaniment of an influential sibling relationship. High-access siblings are generally close in age and the same gender, which promotes access to common life events. They often attend the same school, play with the same friends, date in the same circle, and share a common bedroom and clothing.

Sibling Interaction

Most children have at least one brother or sister. Asked why they chose to have a second child, most parents give as their primary reason the fact that they did not want their firstborn to be an only child (Lobato, 1990). Right or wrong, many people believe that children develop best within the company of other children.

For a number of years, sibling relationships were viewed from a Freudian perspective that emphasizes the concept of sibling rivalry. However, in recent decades researchers have viewed siblings through developmental or ecologic frameworks and have focused on interactions within family systems (Murphy, 1993). Results of these broader perspectives reveal rich and varied sibling interaction (Fig. 3-4).

Perhaps the sibling relationship's most unique feature is its duration. Likely the longest relationship one will share with another human being, the sibling relationship lasts through a lifetime, often 50 to 80 years, as compared with the child-parent relationship of approximately 30 to 50 years. Siblings spend long periods of time together and come to know each other—at their best and worst—extremely well.

Sibling Functions. Siblings exert power, exchange services, and express feelings in reciprocal ways that are often not revealed explicitly in the presence of parents. They see themselves in their brother or sister, experience life vicariously through their sibling's behavior, and begin to expand on their own possibilities. Siblings can also be touchstones for what the other would *not* like to be, and they tend to use each other as yardsticks for comparison. They are sounding boards for one another; they offer a safe forum for experimenting with new behaviors and roles before using either with parents or nonfamily peers.

Brothers and sisters provide each other with tangible services (e.g., lending money, clothing, toys, sports equipment, teaching a skill), help with childhood problems, provide support in dealing with parents or others outside the family, and may provide an introduction to a new friendship group. Children learn to negotiate and bargain, and sometimes to manipulate. Because siblings share approximately equal power, many opportunities arise for conflict and conflict resolution. They learn about sharing, competition, rivalry, and compromise. Siblings can also protect one another from parental-executive abuse of power and can form a coalition to deal with the issues of authority, power, and emotional support. Negotiating with parents is stronger when siblings act together rather than singly.

Siblings interpret the outside world for each other and perform genuine educative functions for the parents. A related function is pioneering, wherein one sibling initiates a process, thereby giving permission to the others to follow accordingly. Patterns may include breaking explicit family rules, taking new developmental pathways (such as leaving the family), or adopting different moral/political codes and life-styles.

Tattling can be an important lever in sibling interactions. On the other hand, there is often a conspiracy of silence among siblings, leaving the parents feeling isolated and excluded. A willingness to make and maintain each other's privacy often serves as a powerful bond of loyalty among the children. It is this loyalty that often distinguishes the relationship between siblings from that between friends.

More Active Sibling Relationships. Sibling relationships vary among cultures. Certain factors, however, may be giving the sibling relationship greater significance in North America than in the past. Shrinking family size, longer life spans, divorce and remarriage, geographic mobility, maternal employment and alternative sources of child care, competitive pressures, stress, and various forms of parental insufficiency may be propelling siblings into greater contact and emotional interdependence than ever before.

For example, siblings often join forces to confront the trauma of divorce. They frequently rely on each other for support when parents remarry. The large number of working mothers means that many young siblings today have large amounts of time when their relationship is not monitored by a personally committed adult. Often an older sibling is required to baby-sit, resulting in children spending more and more time together unsupervised. In a worried, mobile, small-family, high-stress, fast-paced, parent-absent society, children often turn to a brother or sister to meet their need for contact, constancy, and permanency.

Ordinal Position

It has been observed for some time that the birth position of children affects their personalities. Parents treat children differently, and sibling interactions are different depending on the children's position within the family. Also, power is unequally distributed among siblings. Older siblings attempt to dominant younger ones; therefore younger siblings develop interpersonal skills, the ability to negotiate, and an ability to accept unfavorable outcomes to a greater extent than older siblings. Later-born children are obliged to interact with other siblings from birth and seem to be more outgoing and make friends more easily than firstborns (Steelman and Powell, 1985). However, children vary tremendously; these generalizations represent averages and do not apply in all situations. General characteristics of children in the various ordinal positions are presented in the box above.

The Only Child. Being the only child in a family has traditionally been considered to be a disadvantage. Only children have been described as selfish, spoiled, dependent, and lonely. However, a review of 141 research studies indicates that there are no essential personality differences between a child reared alone and one who is reared with one or more siblings (Polit and Falbo, 1987). They display no more evidence of maladjustment or self-centeredness than any other children and tend to strongly resemble firstborn children in such respects as higher educational goals. Only

INFLUENCE OF ORDINAL POSITION ON CHILDREN

FIRSTBORN CHILDREN

Are more achievement oriented
Are more dominant
Receive more physical punishment
Are allowed to show more aggression to siblings
Have stronger consciences, are more self-disciplined and inner directed
Are more socially anxious
Are prone to feelings of guilt
Identify more with parents than with peers
Are more conservative
Are subject to greater parental expectations
Begin to speak earlier in life
Demonstrate higher intellectual achievement
Plan better and experience fewer frustrations
Are likely to be most wanted

MIDDLE CHILDREN

Have more demands made on them for household help
Are praised less often
Receive less of the parents' time
Learn to compromise and be adaptable
Are less stimulated toward achievement
Are more difficult to characterize because of a variety of positions in family

YOUNGEST CHILDREN

Are less dependent than firstborn children
Are less tense, more affectionate, and more good-natured
Tend to identify more with peer group than with parents
Are more flexible in their thinking
Are popular with classmates
Have fewer demands placed on them for household help

ONLY CHILDREN

Resemble firstborn children
Are more mature and cultivated
Experience greater parental pressure for mature behavior and achievement
Demonstrate superiority in language facility
Rarely develop into stereotype of spoiled, selfish child
Often enjoy a rich fantasy life as a result of isolation

children perform better on cognitive tests, are more mature and cultivated, are more socially sensitive, and demonstrate superiority in language facility.

Only children also enjoy the advantage of having parents who, without the distraction of other children, are able to devote more time to them, talk to them, and stimulate them in intellectual activities. However, parents also exert greater pressure for mature behavior at an early age and for achievement. Relative isolation from peers contributes to intellectual pursuits and encourages a rich fantasy life, independence, and originality.

The effects of onliness on personality are questionable. Only children do not have the stereotyped concept of sex-appropriate behavior and often exhibit some characteristics associated with both sexes, but the significant influence is the quality of the parent-child relationship. Because of the wide differences among parents, a typical personality cannot be assigned to the only child. An unusually large number of only children live with a single parent, primarily as a result of divorce.

Multiple Births

A deviation in early development that occurs with variable frequency is multiple births. Twins are not uncommon in the population, but triplets are rare and quadruplets or quintuplets are extremely unusual. In any of these situations the offspring can be of the like or unlike sex (i.e., derived from a single ovum, from multiple ova, or a combination of the two, which can involve one or more cell divisions). The cause of twinning is unknown, and its rate of occurrence has been fairly stable. However, there has been an increase in the number of larger multiples. For example, between 1990 and 1991, the number of triplet and higher-order plural deliveries rose by 10%. As a result, the proportion of multiple births that are twins continued to decline as the proportion of higher-order multiple births (other than twins) increased. Because women in their thirties are almost 2½ times as likely as women in their twenties to have higher-order plural births, the rise in the multiple-birth ratio has been associated with increased childbearing among older women and the expanded use of fertility drugs (National Center for Health Statistics, 1993a).

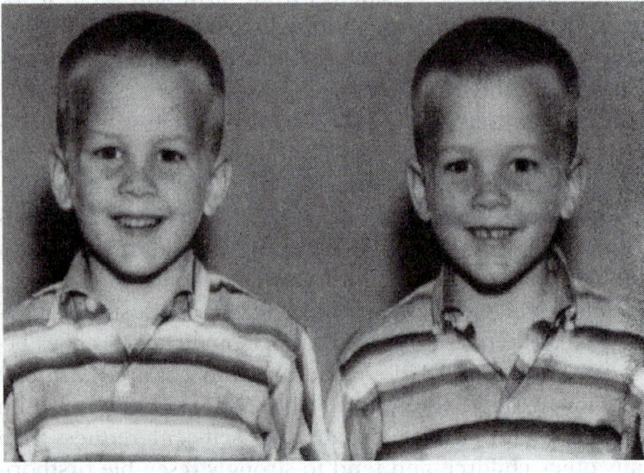

FIG. 3-5 Monozygotic, or identical, twins.

Twins are of two distinct types: identical, or monozygotic (MZ) (Fig. 3-5), and fraternal, or dizygotic (DZ) (see box below). In the United States the overall twinning rate is approximately 1 in 80 pregnancies and consists of one third MZ and two thirds DZ twins.

A special kind of sibling relationship is observed in twins, although getting along with each other and quarreling are not too different from that behavior in any other two siblings, especially if they are different-sex fraternal twins. Twins generally tend to work out a relationship that is reasonably satisfactory to both and demonstrate early independence from parental attention. They develop a remarkable capacity for cooperative play and considerable loyalty and generosity toward each other. It is not uncommon for them to evolve a private language between themselves that may interfere with development of the family language.

In a twinship, one member of the pair, to a greater or lesser extent, is more dominant, outgoing, and assertive than the other, often to the consternation of their parents. However, the seemingly more passive twin is able to accomplish as much and get his or her way as frequently as the more assertive twin.

It has also been observed that there is a difference in behavior between identical and fraternal twins. Whereas there is near unison in the actions of identical twins (although they alternate in assuming the leadership), fraternal twins, even of the same sex, do not display this quality. Sibling rivalry can be quite pronounced in fraternal twins, especially in mixed-sex twins.

CHARACTERISTICS OF TWINS

MONOZYGOTIC (MZ, IDENTICAL TWINS)	DIZYGOTIC (DZ, FRATERNAL TWINS)
Result of one fertilized ovum that became separated early in development	Result of fertilization of two ova
Alike physically and genetically	Differ physically and genetically
Same sex	May be like or opposite sex
Frequency: Occurs uniformly in all populations	Frequency: Varies among races (highest—blacks, lowest—Asians, intermediate—whites)
Unaffected by maternal age	More common with advancing maternal age (maximum at age 35-39, then decreases rapidly)
Tendency unaffected by heredity	Marked familial tendency Expressed only in the female Fathers appear to transmit disposition toward double ovulation to daughters
Similar behavior	Dissimilar behavior; more sibling rivalry

Identical twins also differ in their response to the tendency of some parents to treat twins exactly alike. The present philosophy is to determine the degree to which the children demonstrate an inclination toward togetherness. Some twins thrive best when they are constantly in each other's company; others prefer more individuality and separateness. The conservative approach is to allow the children to follow their natural inclinations. Early years of togetherness are often the basis of the children's security. To separate them too early may produce unnecessary stresses. The tendency is to foster individual differences as they are evidenced in order to ease the process of separation when it becomes advisable.

Parental Adjustment. The entrance of any new member into a household creates a number of stresses, but with multiple births two or more new members must be incorporated into the family at the same time. The problems are obvious. Two infants must be provided with physical care, including feeding, diapering, and all the purchasing and preparation that accompany the care of any infant. Scheduling becomes crucial, and each advancement in development brings new problems and adjustments (e.g., space and sleeping arrangements, selecting a stroller and other equipment). Care must be observed in selecting toys. As play becomes a serious business, some toys that would be safe and appropriate for a single child become weapons when two infants share a playpen. It is a good idea to select different toys for the children as they grow older and encourage sharing.

It is especially important for parents to maintain relationships with each other and other family members. It is doubly important for parents to arrange time together as often as possible. The **National Organization of Mothers of Twins Clubs, Inc.,*** has local chapters throughout the United States to offer information and support to parents of twins and is highly recommended as a resource for all new parents of twins. The **Twins Foundation†**—an organization founded by a group of twins and designed to aid twins and other multiples—is recommended for older children.

Another problem faced by parents of twins occurs at the time of birth. Not only are the parents faced with double the work and care of the newborns, but the process of attachment may also be impeded. The parents first form an attachment to the twins as a unit before they are able to form an attachment to each child individually (see discussion on multiple births and subsequent children under Promote Parent-Infant Bonding [Attachment], Chapter 8). Parents are often surprised that this occurs. Other family members, extended family, and even teachers and baby-sitters will experience the same phenomenon to some extent. As they develop, the children, who are facing the task of differentiating themselves from their environment, must learn to differentiate themselves not only from the parent (usually the mother) but from one another as well.

*12404 Princess Jeanne, N.E., Albuquerque, NM 87112-4640; (505) 275-0955.

†P.O. Box 9487, Providence, RI 02904-9487; (401) 274-8946.

PROMOTING INDIVIDUATION OF TWINS

Select different-sounding names.
Take separate photographs of the children (beginning at birth) so each child will have a picture of "me." Be certain to label each picture.
Avoid dressing children alike.
Use their given names. Avoid referring to them as "the twins."
Take each child on separate short outings occasionally while the other is at home with another family member or a sitter.
Build a one-to-one relationship with each child.
Hold and cuddle each child. Provide frequent body contact with each one.
Play and participate in learning with each child and to the same extent as with a singly born child.
Provide toys according to individual preferences, needs, and interest.
Entertain each as much as feasible. Avoid leaving them to entertain each other for long periods of time.
Provide separate rooms, if possible.
Praise each child individually and, preferably, at different times.
Discipline twins individually.
Provide separate feeding and care schedules according to the needs of the individual child.
Arrange for frequent opportunities for individual contact with other adults.
Encourage play with other children the same age.

Modified from Sater J: Appraising and promoting a sense of self in twins, *MCN* 4:218-226, 1979.

Promoting Individuation. All children proceed through a separation-individuation process as they grow and develop. For twins the process is complicated in a number of ways. Unlike singletons, twins lack a perception of separateness, and the close physical and emotional attachment between them inhibits development of individuality. In addition, twin children are frequently thought of and treated as a unit, and efforts they make in the direction of individuality are often impeded by others (Sater, 1979). There are a number of ways in which parents and others can aid twins in achieving individuation (see box above).

PARENTING

MOTIVATION FOR PARENTHOOD

A dominant characteristic in all societies is that adults are expected to become parents and to be gratified by the experience. Pressures of tradition, sentiment regarding the state of parenthood, and religious exhortations to fulfill divine commands of fertility profoundly influence decision making, since conformity to social-role expectations is a strong influence in family planning.

Although many pregnancies are unplanned, there are numerous reasons why couples decide to initiate a pregnancy. Many consider children a normal part of marriage, others see them as proof of their adulthood, some desire heirs for the family name and fortune, and a few want to fulfill a parent's wish for grandchildren. Having a child in an attempt to save an unstable marriage is a poor reason that usually fails in its goal. However, in most instances the couple sincerely wish to become parents.

Factors that are likely to influence family size are social class, religion, race, financial stability, type of conjugal-role relationships, and the social-psychologic aspects of sexual relations. Of course, how effectively the couple practices contraception may determine whether the family size remains as planned. Also, in the case of divorce and remarriage an individual may decide to have more children with the new spouse.

PREPARATION FOR PARENTHOOD

The basic goals of parenting are to promote the physical survival and health of the children, to foster the skills and abilities necessary to be a self-sustaining adult, and to foster behavioral capabilities for maximizing cultural values and beliefs. However, new parents approach parenthood with meager experience and scant knowledge, although no other task can compare, in overall consequences, with that of rearing a human being. Parents learn by trial and error, committing the same mistakes that have been committed by countless other parents, but they somehow manage to accomplish the task, becoming more skilled with each additional child. Tradition rather than rational planning furnishes the chief norms for childrearing. Experience in having been nurtured as a child is an essential component of successful parenting.

Their own parents are probably the only persons that parents observe intimately in the parental role; this results in a ***generational continuity***—parents rear their own children in much the same way as they themselves were reared. Other essential skills and knowledge parents need in order to feel more comfortable in the parenting role include a basic understanding of childhood growth and development, bathing, feeding, use of play, and interpersonal communication skills. All of this information is integrated throughout this text.

GOALS OF PARENTING

The family, in order to fulfill one of its primary functions, provides for the caregiving, nurturing, and training of children. In the process of childrearing, parents have at least three basic goals for their children:

1. **Survival**—To promote the physical survival and health of their children, thereby ensuring that the children live long enough to produce children of their own
2. **Economic**—To foster the skills and behavioral capacities that the children will need for economic self-maintenance as adults
3. **Self-actualization**—To foster behavioral capabilities for maximizing cultural values and beliefs

PARENTAL DEVELOPMENT

Parents proceed through parental developmental stages as a function of individual adult developmental tasks. In the process of parent-child development, the behavior of each influences the behavior of the other. The ways in which the child and the parents influence one another are discussed in subsequent chapters at greater length in relation to each major stage of child development. Briefly, development of a parental sense can be divided into four phases (Friedman, 1957):

1. **Anticipation.** Looking forward to parenthood, a young couple think about and discuss becoming parents and the way in which they will rear their children. They wonder what changes will develop in their relationship and what kind of parents they will be.
2. **Honeymoon.** This is the early interpersonal adjustment to the infant in which an attachment is formed between the parents and the child and new role learning takes place. The transition in self-image from a nonparent to a parent is made.
3. **Plateau.** The long middle period of parental development parallels child development:
   The child as infant: parents learn to interpret the child's needs.
   The child as toddler: parents learn to accept growth and development.
   The child as preschooler: parents and child learn to separate.
   The child as grade-schooler: parents learn to accept rejection and still be supportive.
   The child as teenager: parents begin to rebuild their lives.
4. **Disengagement.** This phase ends the active parental role, usually at the time of the child's marriage.

TRANSITION TO PARENTHOOD

Although there is disagreement as to whether or not the birth of a couple's first child should be labeled a crisis, the early weeks of an infant's life call for a couple to make drastic adjustments. Although the parents have anticipated and perhaps prepared for the child's arrival, birth means the sudden imposition of totally dependent care 24 hours a day for the new member of the family. It may very well be a crisis if the event is perceived as disturbing old habits and relationships and eliciting new responses. It requires role changes, destroys or significantly modifies former relationships, and means adjusting to new role realignments. Whereas previously the roles of a couple were husband and wife, they now become, in addition, father and mother. It is difficult to adjust to being parents, but it is a normal human experience and a tool for personal growth.

The advent of a new family member requires that the family cope with greater financial responsibilities, a possible loss of income, changes in sleeping habits, and less time for husband and wife to spend with each other (especially if it is a firstborn) and/or with other children. If the events are perceived as aversive, it could well disrupt the couple's bond. Some investigators find that the birth of a first child results in a reduction of the couple's intimacy and affection, whereas others report that the adjustment to parenthood is only mildly stressful.

Parental Factors Affecting Transition to Parenthood

The birth of an infant is a highly significant event that alters the behavior of both mothers and fathers. No amount of preparation can truly and fully prepare prospective parents for the constant and immediate needs of an infant. The importance of early parent-infant interactions is addressed in the discussion of the neonate, especially the attachment process (see Chapter 8). Some of the predominant factors affecting parenting are the age of the parents, the quality of the parental relationship, the amount of previous experience with childrearing, parental support systems, and the effects of stress on parental behavior.

Parental Age. The most satisfactory age for childbearing has been established as the years between 18 and 35. During this time parents are considered to be in optimum health, with a predicted life span that allows sufficient time and vigor to raise a family. However, the age at which parents begin their families has changed over the last few decades in the United States, with a substantial increase in the birth rate for women 30 to 44 years of age and a decline for women ages 20 to 29 years. Recent statistics report that the number of births to women 30 to 34 years of age declined slightly in 1991 for the first time since 1973, when the trend to make up for previously postponed childbearing first began. However, the number of births to women ages 35 to 39 years rose 4% from 1990 to 1991 (National Center for Health Statistics, 1993a).

Reasons for postponing childbearing are related to more women entering career paths, needs of individuals and couples to achieve educational and occupational goals and attain more financial security, and a sense of commitment in a relationship (Soloway and Smith, 1987). Some women who initially decide not to have children change their mind as the "biologic time clock" begins to run out. Although there has been considerable research on the transition to parenthood, the impact of delayed childbearing on the couple, the child, and the family unit has not been fully explored (Koo, Suchindran, and Griffith, 1987).

Father Involvement. Current practices that encourage early father-infant interaction have indicated that fathers appear to be just as intrigued with their newborns as mothers are (see discussion on paternal engrossment under Promote Parent-Infant Bonding [Attachment], Chapter 8). Even fathers who have little initial contact with their neonates will become involved with them over the next few months (Easterbrooks and Goldberg, 1984), although the type of interaction will be different from that of the mother (Fig. 3-6). For example, whereas mothers are likely to hold, soothe, care for, or play quietly with their infants, fathers are more boisterous, engaging in more physically stimulating activities that infants seem to enjoy. However, fathers are more than simply playmates. They are often successful at soothing a distressed infant. Furthermore, a secure attachment to the father can help offset the consequences of an insecure attachment to the mother.

Three types of paternal involvement have been noted (Volling and Belsky, 1991):

1. **Interaction or engagement**—The time that the father spends in direct one-on-one interaction with his infant
2. **Accessibility**—The time spent in proximity to the infant, but not actually interacting
3. **Responsibility**—The extent to which the father takes responsibility for child care and makes arrangements for such things as baby-sitters, doctor's appointments, and child care services

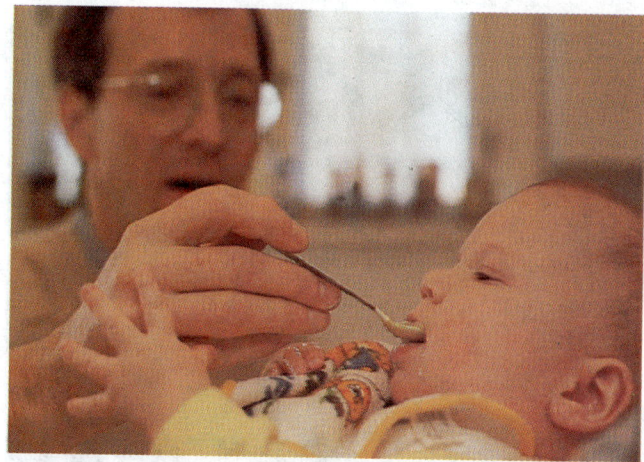

FIG. 3-6 Fathers who assume care of their children may feel more comfortable and successful in their parenting role.

Parenting Education. First-time parents who have had more help preparing themselves to be parents experience less stress in the transition than do those who have not (Gage and Christensen, 1991). Research suggests that programs designed to take place near the time of or during transition are more helpful in easing transitional stress than are those programs designed to take place earlier in life (e.g., high school programs). Age-paced childrearing newsletters have also proved helpful (Riley and others, 1991). (See also Influence of the "Experts," p. 88.)

■ ■ ■

Other factors influencing the transition to the parental role include:

- Parents with previous experience, such as another child, appear to be more relaxed and have less conflict in disciplinary relationships, and they are more aware of normal growth and development expectations.
- The amount of stress experienced by one or both parents may interfere with their ability to exhibit patience and understanding, or otherwise cope with their children's behavior.
- Special characteristics of the infant, such as a temperamentally difficult infant, can cause the parents to lose confidence and doubt their abilities. Also, an infant with special care needs, such as those associated with a disability, can be a significant source of added stress.
- Marital relationships can have a negative effect on parental transition, since marital tension or strife can alter caregiving routines and interfere with enjoyment of the infant. Conversely, parents who support and encourage one another serve as a positive influence on establishing a satisfying parental role. The best single predictor of postpartum marital adjustment is the couple's level of marital adjustment during pregnancy (Wallace and Gotlib, 1990).

Support Systems

Successful adaptation to the stress of transition to parenthood involves at least two types of family resources (McCubbin and Patterson, 1982). First are the ***internal resources*** of

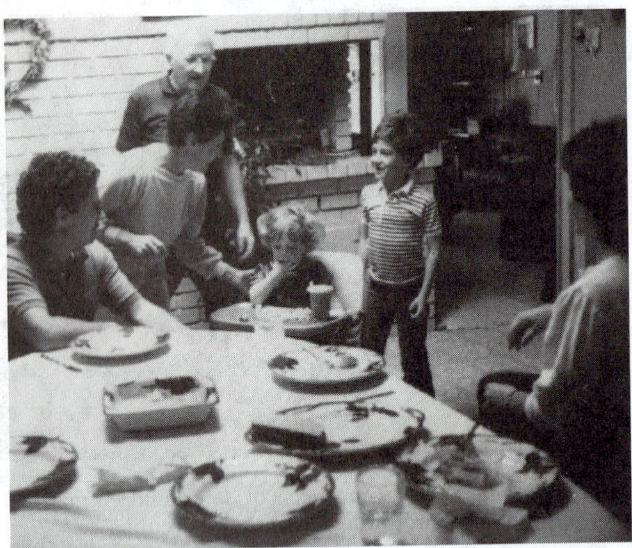

FIG. 3-7 Maintaining relationships with the extended family is important.

the family, such as adaptability and integration. Changing from an orderly, predictable life to a relatively disordered, unpredictable one is a universal adaptation families must make. Rigid schedules are impossible to maintain, and former activities must be curtailed or abandoned. ***Adaptation*** is reflected in learning to be patient, becoming better organized, and becoming more flexible. ***Integration*** involves an attempt of the couple to continue some activities they engaged in before they became parents. In this way couples are able to maintain a sense of continuity and appreciate the importance of the husband-wife relationship.

The second kind of resource for coping with stress is the use of ***coping strategies*** that strengthen the organization and functioning of the family. These include the use of community resources, the use of social support, and the adoption of a future orientation. Interpersonal supports that provide information, advice, and caretaking are derived from friends, relatives, and neighbors. Relationships with family, friends, and community are essential (Fig. 3-7). For fathers, positive work relationships seem to be especially important; for mothers, activities with friends are important (Daniels and Moos, 1988). Arranging for time away from the child or children is also beneficial. Fathers can assume care of the family to allow the mother some time to herself at home or away from the home, even if just for an afternoon or evening. Adoption of a future orientation provides reassurance to parents that things will get better, that they will cope, and that it is realistic to plan for the time when they will be able to engage in self-fulfilling activities.

It is also reassuring to know that others experience ambivalent feelings toward parenthood and share the same difficulties and frustrations. Exchanging ideas and experiences with other parents provides an opportunity to voice concerns and to learn new ways of coping with the multiple problems of childrearing. Whether it is family, friends, or community resources, parents need persons to whom they can turn for advice, comfort, and assistance—persons with whom they can share the joys and difficulties of childrearing.

PARENTING BEHAVIORS

Attitudes Toward Childrearing

There are infinite variations in the way parents rear their children. Some are related to cultural influences; others are related to social class and economic resources. The results of numerous studies suggest that parents differ from one another in two major attitudinal continuums.

Permissiveness-restrictiveness refers to the degree of autonomy that parents allow their children. Some parents exercise close, restrictive control over much of their children's behavior. They limit their children's freedom of expression by imposing many demands and actively surveying their children's behavior to ensure that they comply with rules and regulations. Permissive parents make few demands and allow their children considerable freedom in exploring their environment, expressing their opinions and emotions, and making decisions about their activities. Many find a balance between the two extremes. It is not uncommon to find that many parents become less restrictive as both they and their children mature.

Warmth-hostility refers to how openly or frequently parental affection is expressed and the degree to which affection is mixed with feelings of rejection or hostility. Parents described as warm and nurturant are those who often smile at, praise, and encourage their children while limiting their criticisms, punishments, and signs of disapproval.

Within the wide range of families the amount of affection that parents show their children may vary considerably and be influenced by cultural factors and individual differences in the personality and temperament of both the parents and the children. Children who come from homes in which they are loved and accepted display socially acceptable behavior and are generally good-natured, cheerful, friendly, cooperative, and emotionally stable. Because they are loved and accepted themselves, they are able to form satisfactory relationships with others.

Cool, hostile, or rejecting parents are quick to criticize, belittle, punish, or ignore their children while limiting their expressions of affection or approval. It is important to be aware that these measures of parental warmth or coldness reflect parental behavior in a large number of situations. For example, a parent may be cool and rejecting when a child misbehaves but warm and affectionate in other contexts. Such a parent would be considered high in parental warmth. On the other hand a parent who demonstrates warmth when praising the child but who is critical, punitive, or indifferent in most other situations would be classified as aloof and rejecting. Rejection may be subtle or blatant, and manifestations may be extensive, ranging from neglect and belittling to emotional and physical abuse. Rejecting parents overtly or covertly express feelings of dislike for the child, indicate that the child is unwanted, or state that caring for the child is burdensome.

Children who are rejected develop feelings of insecurity

and inferiority; they believe that if they are unworthy of parental love, they must be of no value. Many develop an avoidant relationship with the rejecting parent(s). Others attempt to win parental affection through attention-getting behaviors that frequently serve only to compound the rejecting behavior of the parents. When these tactics fail, the child may become either hostile and aggressive or withdrawn and submissive. Sometimes rejected children find acceptance through identification with peers or gangs. A persistent pattern of rejection can have pervasive and long-range effects on a child's personality. The problems of disturbed parent-child relationships that are severely damaging to children are discussed in relation to some types of failure-to-thrive syndrome, the abused child, and some of the emotional problems of childhood.

Parental Styles of Control

Although there are variations and degrees in parenting styles, they can generally be described as either authoritarian, permissive, or authoritative. ***Authoritarian,*** or ***dictatorial,*** parents try to control their children's behavior and attitudes through unquestioned mandates. They establish rules and regulations or a standard of conduct that they expect to be followed rigidly and unquestioningly. They value and reward absolute obedience, mute acceptance of their word, and unfailing respect for the family's principles and beliefs. They forcefully punish any behavior that is contrary to parental standards. Parental authority is exercised with little explanation and little involvement of the child in decision making. The message is: "Do it because I say so."

Punishment need not be corporal but may be stern withdrawal of love and approval. The familiar saying—"Children are to be seen, not heard"—typifies this type of childrearing. Careful training often results in rigidly conforming behavior in the children, who tend to be sensitive, shy, self-conscious, retiring, and submissive. They are more apt to be courteous, loyal, honest, and dependable but docile. These behaviors are more typically observed when parental arbitrary power assertion is accompanied by close supervision and a reasonable level of affection. If not, arbitrary power assertion is more likely to be associated with both defiant and antisocial behavior.

Permissive, or ***laissez-faire,*** parents exert little or no control over their children's actions. These well-meaning parents sometimes confuse permissiveness with license. They avoid imposing their own standards of conduct and allow their children to regulate their own activity as much as possible. These parents consider themselves to be resources for the children, not role models. If rules do exist, the parents explain the underlying reason, encourage the children's opinions, and consult them in decision-making processes. They employ lax, inconsistent discipline, do not set sensible limits, and do not prevent the children from upsetting the home routine. The parents rarely punish the children, since most behavior is considered acceptable. Consequently, the children, in effect, control the parents. Children of submissive parents are often disobedient, disrespectful, irresponsible, aggressive, and generally defiant of authority.

Authoritative, or ***democratic,*** parents combine some childrearing practices from both the foregoing extremes. They direct their children's behavior and attitudes by emphasizing the reason for rules and negatively reinforcing deviations. They respect the individuality of each of their children and allow them to voice their objections to family standards or regulations. Parental control is firm and consistent but tempered with encouragement, understanding, and security. Control is focused on the issue, not on withdrawal of love or the fear of punishment. These parents foster "inner-directedness," a conscience that regulates behavior based on feelings of guilt or shame for wrongdoing, not on fear of being caught or punished. Parents' realistic standards and reasonable expectations produce children with high self-esteem who are self-reliant, assertive, inquisitive, content, and highly interactive with other children.

The most successful type of childrearing seems to be the authoritative method. Parents do not set rigid, arbitrary limits but maintain firm control, particularly in areas of parent-child disagreement. Permissiveness is tempered with reasonable and consistent setting of limits. Parental power is shared, and both parents provide leadership but listen to what the children think.

LIMIT-SETTING AND DISCIPLINE

In its broadest sense, ***discipline*** means to teach or refers to a set of rules governing conduct. In a narrower sense, it refers to the action taken to enforce the rules following noncompliance. ***Limit-setting*** refers to establishing the rules or guidelines for behavior. Generally, the clearer the limits that are set and the more consistently they are enforced, the less need there is for disciplinary action.

Therefore the initial goal for the family is for the nurse to help parents establish realistic and concrete "rules." Limit-setting and discipline are positive, necessary components of childrearing and serve several useful functions as they help children:

- Test their limits of control
- Achieve in areas appropriate for mastery at their level
- Channel undesirable feelings into constructive activity
- Protect themselves from danger
- Learn socially acceptable behavior

Children want and need limits. Unrestricted freedom is a tremendous threat to their security and safety. Through testing the limits imposed on them, children learn the extent to which they can manipulate their environment, as well as gain reassurance from knowing that others will be there to protect them from potential harm.

Minimizing Misbehavior

The goals of or reasons for misbehavior may include attention, power, defiance, and a display of inadequacy (the child misses classes because of a fear that he or she is unable to do the work). Children may also misbehave because the rules are not clear or consistently applied. Acting-out behavior, such as a temper tantrum, may represent uncontrolled frustration, anger, depression, or pain.

The best approach is to structure interactions with chil-

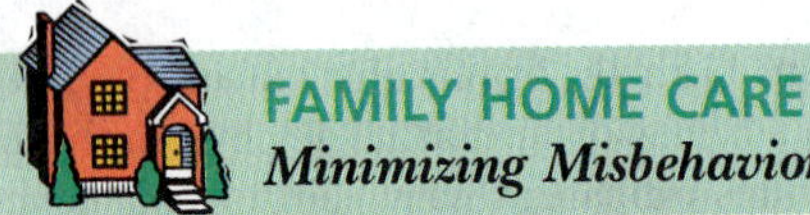

FAMILY HOME CARE
Minimizing Misbehavior

Set realistic goals for acceptable behavior and expected achievements.
Structure opportunities for small successes to lessen feelings of inadequacy.
Praise children for desirable behavior with attention and verbal approval.
Structure the environment to prevent unnecessary difficulties, (e.g., place fragile objects in inaccessible area).
Set clear and reasonable rules; expect the same behavior regardless of the circumstances, and if exceptions are made, clarify that the change is for one time only.
Teach desirable behavior through own example, such as using a quiet, calm voice rather than screaming.
Review expected behavior before special or unusual events, such as visiting a relative or dinner in a restaurant.
Phrase requests for appropriate behavior positively, such as "Put the book down," rather than "Don't touch the book."
Call attention to unacceptable behavior as soon as it begins; use distraction to change the behavior or offer alternatives to annoying actions, such as a quiet toy for one that is excessively noisy.
Give advance notice or "friendly reminders," such as "When the TV program is over, it is time for dinner" or "I'll give you to the count of three and then we have to go."
Be attentive to situations that increase the likelihood of misbehaving, such as overexcitement or fatigue, or decreased personal tolerance to minor infractions.
Offer sympathetic explanations for not granting a request, such as "I am sorry I can't read you a story now, but I have to finish dinner. Then we can spend time together."
Keep any promises made to children.
Avoid outright conflicts; temper discussions with statements such as "Let's talk about it and see what we can decide together" or "I have to think about it first."
Provide children with opportunities for power and control.

dren so that unacceptable behavior is prevented or minimized. While many parents devise strategies that are most effective for their child, general guidelines include those listed in the Family Home Care box.

General Guidelines for Implementing Discipline

Regardless of the type of discipline used, certain principles are essential in ensuring the efficacy of the approach (see Guidelines box). Many strategies, such as behavior modification, can only be implemented effectively when principles of consistency and timing are followed. A pattern of intermittent or occasional enforcement of limits actually prolongs the undesired behavior because children learn that if they are persistent, the behavior is permitted eventually. Delaying punishment weakens its intent, and practices such as telling the child, "Wait until your father comes home," are not only ineffectual, but also convey negative connotations about the other parent.

Types of Discipline

To deal with misbehavior, parents need to implement appropriate disciplinary action. Numerous approaches are available, and some have definite advantages over others.

GUIDELINES
Implementing Discipline

Consistency—Implement disciplinary action exactly as agreed on and for each infraction.
Timing—Initiate discipline as soon as child misbehaves; if delays are necessary, such as to avoid embarrassment, verbally disapprove of the behavior and state that disciplinary action will be implemented.
Commitment—Follow through with the details of the discipline, such as timing of minutes; avoid distractions that may interfere with the plan, such as telephone calls.
Unity—Make certain that all caregivers agree on the plan and are familiar with the details to prevent confusion and alliances between child and one parent.
Flexibility—Choose disciplinary strategies that are appropriate to child's age, temperament, and the severity of the misbehavior.
Planning—Plan discipline strategies in advance and prepare child if feasible, (e.g., explain use of time-out); for unexpected misbehavior, try to discipline when you are calm.
Behavior-orientation—Always disapprove of the behavior, not the child, with such statements as "That was a wrong thing to do. I am unhappy when I see behavior like that."
Privacy—Administer discipline in private, especially with older children who may feel ashamed in front of others.
Termination—Once the discipline is administered, consider child as having a "clean slate" and avoid bringing up the incident or lecturing.

Reasoning involves explaining why an act is wrong and is usually appropriate for older children, especially when moral issues are involved. However, young children cannot be expected to "see the other side" because of their egocentrism. Sometimes children use the "reasoning" as a way of gaining attention. For example, they may misbehave in order for the parents to give them a lengthy explanation of the wrongdoing because negative attention is better than none. When children use this technique, parents may have to end the explanation by stating, "This is the rule, and this is how I expect you to behave. I won't explain it any further."

Unfortunately, reasoning is often combined with ***scolding***, which sometimes takes the form of shame or criticism. For example, the parent may state, "You are a bad boy for hitting your brother." Children take such remarks seriously and personally, believing that *they* are bad.

NURSING ALERT When reprimanding children, focus only on the misbehavior, not on the child. Use of "I" messages rather than "you" messages expresses personal feelings without accusation or ridicule. For example, an "I" message attacks the behavior—"I am upset when Johnny is punched; I don't like to see him hurt"—not the child.

Positive and negative reinforcement is the basis of ***behavior modification*** theory—behavior that is rewarded will be repeated; behavior that is not, will be extinguished. Using ***rewards*** is a positive approach; by encouraging children to behave in specified ways, the tendency to misbehave is lessened. With young children, using paper stars is a very effective method. For older children the "token system" is appropriate, especially if a certain number yields a special reward, such as a trip to the movies or a new book. In planning a reward system, the expected behaviors must be clearly explained to the child and the rewards must be reinforcing. A chart should be used to record the stars or tokens, and every earned reward should be promptly given. Verbal approval should always accompany extrinsic rewards. (A more formal reward system involving a contract, which is appropriate for older children, is discussed in Chapter 27 under Compliance).

Consistently ***ignoring*** behavior will eventually extinguish or minimize the act. Although this approach sounds very simple, it is often difficult to implement consistently. Parents frequently "give in" and resort to previous patterns of discipline. Consequently, the behavior is actually reinforced because the child learns that persistence gains parental approval.

For ignoring to be effective, health professionals must devote a fair amount of time toward (1) explaining the approach in detail, (2) recording behavior before the extinction process is instituted to see if a problem exists and to compare results after ignoring is begun, (3) making certain that the parent's attention is the reinforcer, and (4) warning parents of a phenomenon called "response burst," which refers to an *increase* in the child's behavior soon after the process is initiated because the child is "testing" the parents to see if they are serious about the plan.

The strategy of ***consequences*** involves allowing children to experience the results of their misbehavior and includes three types:

1. **Natural**—Those that occur without any intervention, such as being late and missing dinner
2. **Logical**—Those that are directly related to the rule, such as not being allowed to play with another toy until the used ones are put away
3. **Unrelated**—Those that are imposed deliberately, such as no playing until homework is completed or the use of time-out

Natural or logical consequences are preferred but are effective only when they are meaningful to children. For example, the natural consequence of living in a messy room may do little to encourage cleaning up, but allowing no friends over until the room is neat can be very motivating! Withdrawing privileges is often an unrelated consequence. After the child experiences the consequence, the parent should refrain from any comment, because the usual tendency is for the child to try to place blame for imposing the rule.

Time-out is actually a refinement of the common practice of "sending the child to his or her room" and is a type of unrelated consequence. It is also based on the premise of removing the reinforcer (i.e., the satisfaction or attention the child is receiving from the activity). When placed in an unstimulating and isolated place, children become bored and consequently agree to behave in order to reenter the family group (Fig. 3-8). Time-out avoids many of the problems of other disciplinary approaches because no physical punishment is involved, no reasoning or scolding

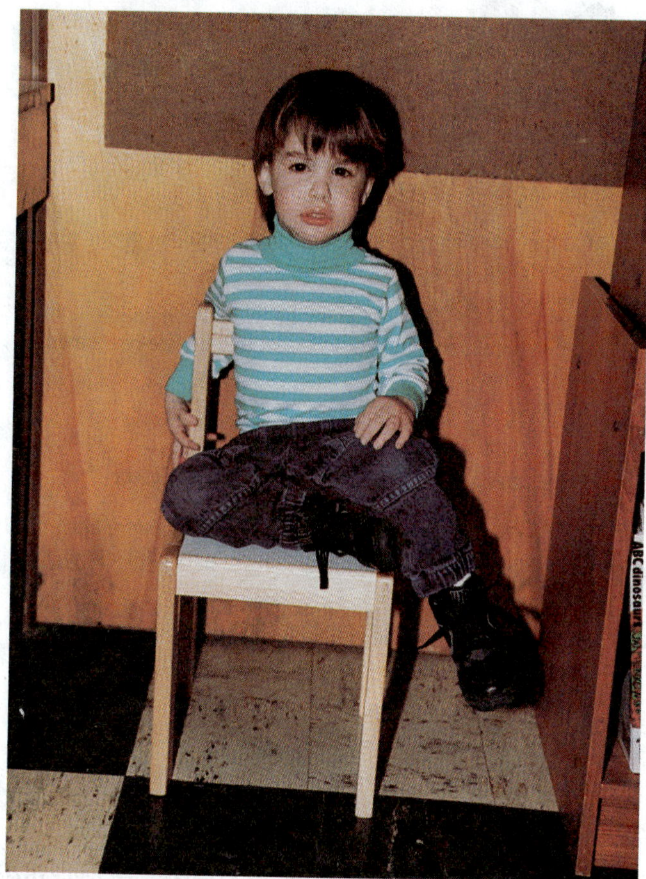

FIG. 3-8 Time-out is an excellent disciplinary strategy for young children.

is given, and the parent is usually not present for all of the time-out, facilitating his or her ability to consistently apply the punishment. It also offers both the child and the parent a "cooling off" time. To be effective, time-out must be planned in advance (see Family Home Care box, p. 88).

Corporal punishment most often takes the form of spanking. Based on the principles of aversive therapy, inflicting pain through spanking causes a dramatic short-term decrease in the behavior. However, there are some serious flaws in this approach: (1) it teaches children that violence is acceptable; (2) many times the spanking is the result of parental rage and may physically harm the child; and (3) children become "accustomed" to spanking, requiring more severe corporal punishment each time. Consequently, parents may use paddles, whips, or other objects, or they may eliminate a spanking because of their unwillingness to "hit the child harder," a practice that may prolong the behavior.

Spanking can result in severe physical injury and even death (Eichelberger, Beal, and May, 1991). Nevertheless, corporal punishment is often exempted from the category of assault, even when it produces specific injuries, which may be treated as "accidental" or "incidental" to discipline (Garbarino and others, 1992).

Even when corporal punishment does not involve serious physical damage to children, the psychologic impact

FAMILY HOME CARE
Using Time-Out

Select an area for time-out that is safe, convenient, and unstimulating, but where the child can be monitored, such as the bathroom, hallway, or laundry room.

Determine what behaviors warrant a time-out.

Make sure children understand the "rules" and how they are expected to behave.

Explain to children the process of time-out:

- When they misbehave, they will be given *one* warning.
- If they do not obey, they will be sent to the place designated for time-out.
- They are to sit there for a specified period of time.
- If they cry, refuse, or display any disruptive behavior, the time-out period will begin *after* they quiet down.
- When they are quiet for the duration of the time, they can then leave the room.

A rule for the length of time-out is *1 minute per year of age;* use a kitchen timer with an audible bell to record the time rather than a watch.

Implement time-out in a public place by selecting a suitable area or explain to children that time-out will be spent immediately on returning home and mark their hand with a felt-tip pen as a reminder.

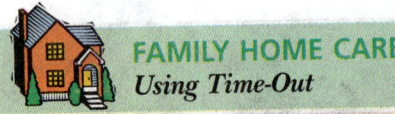

may be great (Hyman and others, 1985). It can also interfere with effective parent-child interaction; children who receive corporal punishment are less likely to learn what they *should* do, because the focus is on what they *should not* do (Nelms, 1993). In addition, when the parent is not around, the misbehavior is likely to occur, for children have not learned to behave well for their own sake. Parental use of corporal punishment has also been found to interfere with the child's development of moral reasoning (Finkelhor and others, 1983).

The use of corporal punishment, a model of violent behavior, has been questioned more of late in conjunction with concern regarding increasing violence in contemporary society. Unfortunately, the practice continues to play a role in the public education of schoolchildren in many parts of the United States (see Chapter 17).

INFLUENCE OF THE "EXPERTS"

Evidence indicates that there have been decided shifts in the overall philosophy of childrearing during the twentieth century. Directions on childrearing, with parental roles and practices defined by the experts, have been transmitted as advice to parents through a steady flow of pamphlets, books, and articles. Recent changes in the opinions of these experts are the result of alterations in the concept of child development and behavior and of research into the effects of parent-child interaction.

The earlier view of child care that advocated rigid scheduling, early weaning and toilet training, and prohibition of devices that provided the child with passive pleasures (such as pacifiers) has been, for the most part, replaced by an easier, warmer, and more relaxed approach toward coping with child behavior that emphasizes "tender loving care" as the basis for satisfactory physical and emotional well-being. Some believe, however, that this approach generates too much permissiveness and produces some undesirable long-term consequences. The current trend in parenting manuals is to reassure parents that they will not be "perfect" parents, that mistakes are allowed, and that while they should keep trying to do a good job of rearing their children, at the same time they should try to be relaxed and spontaneous, and enjoy their children. These manuals attempt to convey the idea that parents are more capable than they think they are.

Parents turn to guidebooks because of an optimistic belief in progress, a faith in the future, and a typical desire to do better—better than they have been doing, better than their own parents, and better than their relatives and neighbors. Through these popular how-to parent books, parents can gain some of the accumulated knowledge of significant researchers in child development that they would be unable to acquire by attempting to read and synthesize the original texts. These guidebooks do not attempt to provide all the answers and are less authoritarian than those of the past. Most are written on the assumption that parents want to raise successful children and need support to view themselves as competent adults whose decisions are valid. Parents must deal with parenting problems on the spot at the same time that they are assimilating helpful advice and new information. They must be made to feel confident in their values and judgment during this process.

In the past, one of the primary deficiencies in how-to books was a disregard for alternate life-styles, cultural variations, or class differences in the population. For example, the working mother was ignored or discouraged, and day-care was seldom mentioned. Fortunately, recent manuals tend to reflect the realities of our more complex society. Some books have also appeared that offer guidelines for single parents, adoptive parents, parents with a child who is disabled, stepparents, and families in the process of divorce. These are primarily authored by individuals who offer help based on their own experiences or by authorities who have made a study of a special problem. Parents can receive some assistance from these supplemental publications to help them cope with the additional stresses imposed by their special circumstances. Since popular parenting manuals vary in their approaches, it is probably best to suggest that parents review some of those that are available and select at least two for use rather than relying on the advice of a single resource.

SPECIAL PARENTING SITUATIONS

Parenting is a demanding task under the most ideal circumstances, but when parents and children are faced with situations that deviate from what is considered to be the norm, the potential for family disruption is increased. Some of the issues that are encountered frequently are divorce, single parenthood, reconstituted families, adoption, and dual-career families. The problems associated with children of alcoholic parents, parents with physical disabilities, homeless parents, or incarcerated parents are ones that are not addressed in the following discussions but may be topics that the reader may wish to investigate.

PARENTING THE ADOPTED CHILD

Adoption establishes the legal relationship of parent and child between persons who are not so related by birth, with the same rights and obligations that exist between children and their biologic parents. In the past the biologic mother alone made the decision to relinquish the rights to her child. In recent years, however, the courts have acknowledged the legal rights of the biologic father regarding this decision. Concerned child advocates have questioned decisions that honor the father's rights when the decision may not be in the best interests of the child. As the rights of the child have become recognized, older children have successfully dissolved their legal bond with their biologic parents to pursue adoption by adults of their choice.

Motivation for Adoption

Persons are motivated to adopt a child for different reasons. Most instances involve an adopting couple who find it impossible to have children of their own. However, many people consider adoption for other reasons. Some feel a responsibility to provide a home for a child who needs one; others are able to have more children of their own but are seriously concerned about overpopulation and elect to increase their family through adoption; many families are finding "room for one more" with whom to share their love; families involved in foster care may pursue adopting the child when parental rights are terminated. In addition, single, divorced, and widowed persons who believe that they have love and security to offer a child are seeking to adopt.

The demand for white infants with no physical or mental problems far exceeds the supply. However, there has been an increase in the number of children with special needs who are finding homes through the adoptive process. These include children with disabilities, older children, children who are of minority or mixed racial ancestry, and children from foreign countries.

The decision to adopt should be a joint one, and various attitudes and feelings must be examined before the couple can assume the responsibility for an adopted child. Most adults assume that they will be able to have children of their own. To discover that they are unable to do so is often accompanied by feelings of inferiority, doubts about masculinity or femininity, and feelings of guilt or blame in relation to the spouse. These feelings and frustrations, superimposed on the anxious waiting for pregnancy, feelings of loss, endless medical procedures to establish the cause of infertility, and failed medical efforts to establish a pregnancy, provide an adoptive couple with their own unique preparation for parenthood.

Whatever motivates a couple to seek adoption as an alternative means to acquire a family, the decision should be based on emotionally healthy needs. The welfare of the child should be the primary consideration in placement, and such motives as the need to strengthen an unstable marriage, to treat emotional problems (including grief over the death of a child), or to treat psychogenic sterility should be carefully explored. Also, when adoption satisfies the needs of only one of the two parents, the outcome is questionable.

Sources of Adoptive Children

In the past the major source of adoptable infants was socially unsanctioned pregnancies, primarily of unwed mothers, since society accords a very high rating to the married status. Although adoption as a means of creating a family is openly acceptable, having children outside the marriage state is generally met with societal disapproval. However, with the widespread use of contraception, more liberalized abortion laws, and more liberal attitudes toward single parents, the number of these children available for adoption has decreased significantly.

Almost half the adoptable children in the United States are adopted by relatives, either extended family members or stepparents. Nonrelative adoptions are primarily arranged through licensed social agencies. A small proportion are arranged independently by individuals such as physicians, lawyers, nurses, and members of the clergy. However, the safest and most satisfactory adoptions are those conducted through a licensed social agency, either public or voluntary. Although adoption through an ***authorized agency*** can be time-consuming, with sometimes frustrating and disappointing delays, the decision to pursue an ***independent adoption*** should be made with caution. While independent adoptions are frequently faster than agency adoptions, independent adoptions sometimes result in serious problems. They are generally more costly, and some are arranged by persons seeking a profit. The child's anonymity may not be guaranteed, and the child's health or legal status may be unclear. Also, since independent contractors frequently do not investigate the adoptive family, unlike adoption agencies, an independent adoption may not always be in the child's best interests.

In recent years the concept of ***open adoption,*** either through an agency or an independent source, has gained greater acceptance. In open adoption, the adoptive parents meet the biologic mother (and sometimes father and other family members) before the birth of the child and mutually agree to the adoption. Arrangements are often made for the child to have contact with the biologic family throughout the child's lifetime.

In a variant form of open adoption, the biologic mother is invited to write an explanatory letter to the child and the adoptive parents, who usually respond with a letter and pictures. It is a voluntary exchange handled through the agency, which keeps all names and addresses confidential. When these exchanges are eventually read by the adopted children, it helps them realize the circumstances of their adoption.

Risks related to agency adoptions are usually less than those encountered in family life. Careful screening of infants can detect all but the more obscure defects, and subsequent development of defects or illnesses is no less predictable than in biologic families. However, inherent emotional difficulties may be intensified in the case of adoption. Common reactions to adoption include anxiety associated with the waiting period until the adoption is legally final, uncertainty regarding whether adoption is the right choice, parents' concerns about their ability to love and parent the child, and coping with the reactions and questions of relatives, other children (if any) in the family, and friends. However, bonding can be as strong and immediate for adoptive parents and children as it is for biologic parents—sometimes even stronger.

Adoptive mothers share many of the same initial feelings for their babies and reactions to becoming parents as birth mothers. Both adoptive and birth mothers react to the first moments with their babies with strong and varied emotions, ranging from happiness to distress. Research indicates that adoptive mothers are likely to develop emotional ties to their babies at much the same time that birth mothers do. Bonding is not hindered by the lack of either a biologic relationship or immediate contact with their babies (Koepke and others, 1991).

Preparation for Adoption

Unlike biologic parents who prepare for their child's birth with prenatal classes and the support of friends and relatives, adoptive parents have few sources of support and preparation for the new addition to their family (Koepke and others, 1991). Nurses who offer services to adoptive parents can provide the information, support, and reassurance needed to reduce parental anxiety regarding the adoptive process and refer them to state parental support groups that provide guidance for adoptive parents. Such sources can be contacted through a state or county welfare office. Prospective parents seeking information on international adoptions can contact **Families Adopting Children Everywhere Inc. (FACE).***

Preadoption counseling should include measures to help parents overcome feelings of inadequacy and make preparations for receiving the child, such as instruction in infant care. Adoptive parents need to prepare for the possibility that the confidentiality or the identity of the biologic parents may not be guaranteed. Some agencies even advise the adoptive parents to maintain an ongoing information store about the natural parents so that they can answer the child's questions and thereby reduce the excessive fantasizing that children may engage in later during identity formation.

Parenting Adopted Children

Most problems faced by adoptive parents are no different from those encountered by natural parents. All parents want to be good parents, but this desire is often intensified in adoptive parents. Adoptive parents have been portrayed as more apprehensive and insecure than biologic parents, and in need of more assistance. However, adoptive parents may feel the need for less assistance than biologic parents. This feeling is probably due to the adoptive parents' completely voluntary decision to become parents, the relatively long time they had to prepare for parenting, and the maturity associated with adopting (Edwards, 1987).

The sooner infants enter their adoptive home, the better for purposes of parent-infant attachment; the more caregivers the infant has had before adoption, the more problems are likely to be encountered in attachment. The infant must break the bond with the previous caregiver and form a new bond with the adoptive parents. The difficulties in forming an attachment will depend on the amount of time the infant has spent with earlier caregivers, such as the birth mother, nurse, or adoption agency personnel.

Siblings, adopted or biologic, who are old enough to understand should be included in decisions regarding the commitment to adopt, with reassurance that they are not being replaced. Ways that the siblings can interact with the adopted child should be stressed (Fig. 3-9).

Acceptance by extended family members and friends may create additional stresses for the family. Parents are encouraged to discuss the issue of adoption with other members of the family, especially the grandparents, whose feelings and attitudes about adoption may not be compatible. This may be a particularly difficult problem when the adopted children are members of different ethnic groups. It should be made clear to everyone that the child is the parents' child, not their "adopted" child.

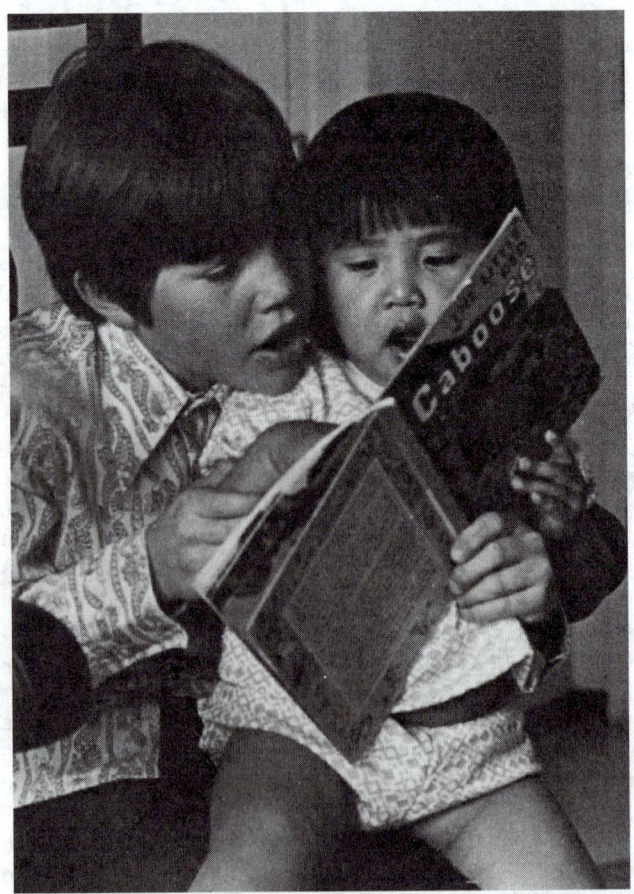

FIG. 3-9 A big brother reads a story to his adopted sister.

*P.O. Box 28058, Northwood Station, Baltimore, MD 21239; (410) 488-2656.

Issues of Origin. The task of telling children that they are adopted is a cause of deep concern and anxiety. There are no clear-cut guidelines for parents to follow in determining precisely when and at what age children are ready for the information, and parents are naturally reluctant to present the children with such unsettling news. However, it is an important aspect of their parental responsibilities, and although they may be tempted to withhold the fact from the child, it is an essential component of the child's identity.

The timing seems to arise naturally as parents become aware of the child's readiness. Most authorities believe that children should be informed at an age young enough so that, as they grow older, they do not remember a time when they did not know that they were adopted. The time must be right for both the parents and the child and is highly individual; it may be when children ask where babies come from, at which time children can also be told the facts of their adoption. If they are told in such a way as to convey the idea that they were active participants in the selection process, they will be less apt to feel that they were abandoned victims in a helpless situation. For example, parents can tell children that their personal qualities drew the parents to them. It is wise for parents who have not previously discussed adoption to tell children that they are adopted before the children enter school to avoid third parties inadvertently telling the children before the parents have the opportunity. Complete honesty between parents and children usually strengthens the relationship (see Thinking Critically About . . . box).

Earlier advice to adoptive parents stressed the need to treat adopted children exactly the same as any biologic siblings and to make them feel no different. This approach, however, denies the differences that adopted children actually feel. At age 5 or 6, children begin to realize that someone had to give them up for them to be "chosen" by the adoptive family. To deny these feelings may actually hurt the child (Brodzinsky, 1988). For both the child and the adoptive parents, it is important to acknowledge the differences in the adoptive situation.

Acknowledging and encouraging discussion of the child's feelings help the child develop a positive self-image. Once the child has been told about the adoption, the child's feelings about it do not end; rather, adjusting to one's own adoption is a continuous process often characterized by a sense of loss and a search for identity throughout childhood and adolescence and even continuing when adopted children become adults and have their own children (Sherry, 1986). Adopted children, however, seem to adapt more easily if the family is comfortable with the adoption, talks about the birth circumstances openly, and has acceptance and support from the extended family, friends, and neighbors. When they are emotionally and developmentally ready, adopted children may benefit from learning about their birth parents and may even decide to contact them, although this is usually recommended only after adolescence in closed adoptions, because of the identity crises and turmoil surrounding the event.

Children should be encouraged to ask questions. Parents can anticipate many of the questions, although children may hesitate to ask about the birth parents, hoping that the adoptive parents will initiate the discussion. This is probably one of the most difficult tasks facing adoptive parents. However, it is not so much what is said to the children but the attitudes and feelings that are communicated. Children should be told about their illegitimacy, if this is an actuality, and the most complete picture possible of the birth parents should be provided.

Parents can anticipate some behavior changes following the disclosure—especially in children who are older. Children may use the fact of their adoption as a weapon to manipulate and threaten parents. There is the inevitable "My real mother would not treat me like this," or "You don't love me as much because I'm adopted." Statements such as these hurt parents and increase their feelings of insecurity, so that as parents they may become over permissive. Adopted children need the same undemanding love, combined with firm discipline and limit-setting, as any other child.

Adoptive parents may experience unwelcomed curiosity and even cruel remarks from others about the child's adoption and appearance. Questions about the child's "real" birth parents, jokes that an infertile mother will now get pregnant, or misguided attempts to match physical charac-

THINKING CRITICALLY ABOUT . . . *Adoption Disclosure*

Although the common wisdom is that adopted children should be told of their adoptive status and be told as early as possible, Donovan (1990) argues that very few supporters of this view can cite any studies or offer any rational argument in support of their position. Donovan's argument poses several questions: Are very young children even capable of understanding the concept "adopted"? Will the fear of losing this new parent or set of parents flow logically from the attempt of the parents or agency to excuse the birth parents by presenting the act of giving up their child as something due to circumstances beyond their control? Is establishing a secure identity through the behavior and attitudes of parents, not by working through issues of origin, the same for adopted children as it is for biologic children? Could the fact that adopted children are significantly more likely to require mental health services be related to negative consequences of prevailing full-disclosure practices? Does the disclosure that one's birth mother "really loved you . . .but" set up a block to attachment? If "love" leads to abandonment, then why should adopted children attach to the new parents who "love" them? Donovan advocates not telling about adoption until asked, telling the truth but only when asked, answering only what is asked, not excusing biologic parents, and not trying to make up for the past.

teristics of the child with the adoptive parents can be distressing. Nurses in contact with adoptive parents can help counter the effects of these thoughtless remarks by affirming the parental role, asking the parents about the child's arrival, and listening to their reports about the child's development and accomplishments.

Adolescence. Adolescence may be an especially trying time for parents of adopted children. The normal confrontations of adolescents and parents may assume more painful aspects in adoptive families. Adolescents may use their adoption as a tool in defying parental authority or as a justification for aberrant behavior. As they attempt to master the task of identity formation, the feeling of abandonment by their biologic parents may come to awareness or may be intensified. Sex differences in reacting to adoption may surface. It has been shown that girls have more difficulty accepting their sexuality, since they may not be able to identify with a nonfertile female parent.

The children fantasize about their parents, and they may feel the need to discover the identity of their biologic parents in order to define themselves and their identity—one of the major tasks of adolescent development. It is important for parents to keep lines of communication open and to reassure the youngsters that they understand the feelings of needing to search for their identities. In some states birth certificates are made legally available to adopted children when they come of age. It is important for parents to be honest with questioning adolescents and to tell them of this possibility (the parents themselves are unable to obtain the birth certificate; it is the children's responsibility if they desire it).

Special Adoptive Situations

The difficulty in finding infants to adopt has created an increased opportunity for adoptive parents to provide homes for children with special needs. The additional burdens of care for children with physical or emotional disabilities are no different from those of biologic children with similar problems, with the possible exception that adoptive parents are aware of the nature of the disabilities before they receive the children. Such children may be eligible for financial assistance from the Federal 4E Adoption Subsidy Program and additional state programs (American Academy of Pediatrics, 1991). However, adoption of older children and/or those of a different racial or ethnic origin poses special considerations for both parents and children.

Older Children. Adopting older children constitutes an emotional experience for everyone concerned—children, parents, siblings (if any), and, often, extended family members. It involves a commitment on the part of both the adopting family and the adopted child. Adoptive families should learn as much as possible about the child before they make a final commitment.

Children awaiting adoption are usually from foster homes, group homes, or institutions. Visits between the potential adoptive family and the child can take place in the child's present home or on some type of outing during which the individuals involved are able to interact, such as on a picnic or a trip to the zoo or a playground. Visits by the child to the home of the adoptive family begin with short excursions such as an afternoon, then a day, followed by a weekend or a week. The number and frequency of visits depend on the needs of the child and the family. During the visits the child and the family determine whether or not they will be able to make a commitment (Brockhaus and Brockhaus, 1982).

One of the difficulties of rearing adopted older children is helping them to deal with having had another set of parents. In addition to their biologic parents, the children may have lost siblings, grandparents, friends, and personal possessions. Often they have lived in several foster homes in which they formed attachments. They need time and assistance in working through the grief process that is an integral part of any loss. At the same time, they must adjust to a new household and relationships. Children who have experienced many losses and disappointments find adjustment more difficult and take a longer period of time to overcome fear of rejection and to develop affectionate ties to the new family. They grieve for those they left behind and may be afraid to love in case they must again move on.

Children who are adopted after age 2 maintain an image of the previous parenting persons that may cause the adopting parents some insecurity. The parents may not feel as close to these children as they would to children adopted in infancy. It is necessary that children who can remember them maintain an image of the biologic parents. As they grow, children are able to clearly distinguish between the parents who loved and cared for them and those who were merely responsible for their birth. Some of the early difficulties of adaptation are related to the change in surroundings, a change that is difficult for all children.

Early in the process of forming lasting relationships, the families alter routines and activities to accommodate the children and avoid conflicts. The children are excited but somewhat frightened that they will be unable to behave in such a way that will ensure acceptance and prevent their being sent away. Eventually the parents and the children are unable to maintain the host-houseguest roles and behaviors and begin a stormy period of adjustment. The children continually test the families, who must repeatedly reassure the children that they are wanted. The children may withdraw or act angry for months. Many conflicts can arise, particularly in the area of parental expectations and discipline. The children's past experiences, good and bad, are brought to the fore, especially during holidays. Although the children are relieved and happy to be in a new home, they often miss the familiar times and relationships. During this time the families may require considerable support and encouragement from sources outside the immediate family unit.

Eventually expectations become more realistic, and family members learn to cope more effectively. The children are increasingly able to integrate past with present. They develop trust and confidence in the parents, and all the members develop into a family unit with autonomy, stability, and identification (Brockhaus and Brockhaus, 1982).

Cross-Racial and International Adoption. Adoption of children of racial backgrounds different from that of the family is relatively commonplace. In addition to the problems faced by adopted children of any age, children of a cross-racial adoption must deal with their differentness. It is advised that parents who adopt such children do everything to preserve the adopted children's racial heritage.

Adoptive parents are urged to investigate the culture of their children's country, maintain their children's family name as a middle name (in some cultures this is a link to the village of their ancestors), and teach children the history and heroes of their native country. Persons from the children's country can provide information about eating and sleeping patterns that will help the family make the adopted children's adaptation easier. Even music, a few words of the native language, and foods from their native country will appeal to the children's senses.

Although the children are full-fledged members of an adopting family and citizens of the adopted country, if they have a foreign appearance or other decided racial characteristics, problems may be encountered outside the family. Bigotry exists that may appear among relatives and friends. Strangers may make thoughtless comments and talk about the children as though they were not members of the family. It is vital that the family make it clear to others that this is their child and a cherished member of the family.

In international adoptions the medical information the parents receive may be quite complete or very sketchy (Hostetter and Johnson, 1989). Many internationally adopted children were born prematurely, and common health problems such as infant diarrhea and malnutrition may delay growth and development. Some children may have serious or multiple health problems, and this can be very stressful for the parents. Many foreign-born children have not been immunized adequately (American Academy of Pediatrics, 1991). Cultural practices, such as constant holding rather than letting the child explore, may further affect the child's progress. On arrival, regardless of age, some internationally adopted children may experience temporary adjustment problems. Sleep disturbances, malaise without fever, abdominal pain, avoidance of school, and preoccupation with food have all been reported (Hostetter and Johnson, 1989). In addition to giving advice on medical management, nurses should provide these parents with opportunities to discuss their feelings and situations.

PARENTING AND DIVORCE

From the mid-1960s to the early 1980s the divorce rate rose significantly, peaking at a rate of 5.3 divorces per 1000 population in 1979 and 1981. The 1989 rate of 4.7 divorces per 1000 population was the lowest rate since 1974. (National Center for Health Statistics, 1990). The divorce rate increased slightly in 1992 (4.8 per 1000 population), continuing a pattern of relatively steady rates in the early 1990s (National Center for Health Statistics, 1993b). More than 1 million children under the age of 18 have been involved in a divorce in every year since 1972. Many of these children are very young, since half of the couples who divorce were married for less than 7 years.

STAGES OF THE DIVORCE PROCESS

ACUTE PHASE

The married couple make the decision to separate. This phase includes the legal steps of filing for dissolution of the marriage and usually, the departure of the father from the home. The duration of this phase lasts from several months to over a year and is accompanied by familial stress and a chaotic atmosphere.

TRANSITIONAL PHASE

The adults and children assume unfamiliar roles and relationships within a new family structure. This phase is often accompanied by a change of residence, a reduced standard of living and altered life-style, a larger share of the economic responsibility being shouldered by the mother, and radically altered parent-child relationships.

STABILIZING PHASE

The postdivorce family reestablishes a stable, functioning family unit. Remarriage frequently occurs, with concomitant changes in all areas of family life.

Modified from Wallerstein JS: Children of divorce: stress and developmental tasks. In Garmezy N, Rutter M, editors: *Stress, coping, and development in children,* New York, 1983, McGraw-Hill.

The process of divorce begins with a period of marital conflict of varying length and intensity, a separation, the actual legal divorce, and the reestablishment of different living arrangements (see box above). Since a function of parenthood is to provide for the security and emotional welfare of children, disruption of the family structure often engenders strong feelings of guilt in the parents.

During a divorce, parents' coping abilities may be compromised. The parents may be much too preoccupied with their own feelings, needs, and life changes to be available and supportive to their children. Newly employed parents, usually mothers, are likely to leave children with new caregivers, in strange settings, or alone after school. The parent may also spend more time away from home, searching for or establishing new relationships. Sometimes, however, the adult feels frightened and alone and begins to depend on the child as a substitute for the absent parent. This dependence places an enormous burden on the child.

Common characteristics in the custodial household following separation and divorce include disorder, coercive types of control, inflammable tempers in both parents and children, reduced parental competence, a greater sense of parental helplessness, poorly enforced discipline, and diminished regularity in enforcing household routines. Noncustodial parents also are seldom prepared for the role of visitor and may not have a residence suitable for children's visits. They may be concerned about maintaining the arrangement over the years to follow.

Impact of Divorce on Children

The results of numerous studies show that divorce has a profound effect on children. Long-term studies indicate that many youngsters suffer for years from psychologic and social difficulties associated with continuing and/or new stresses in the postdivorce family. A main outcome is heightened anxiety about forming enduring relationships as young adults (Wallerstein, 1991). Even when a divorce is amiable and open, children may recall parental separation with the same emotions felt by victims of a natural disaster: loss, grief, and vulnerability to forces beyond their control (Tuttle, 1992).

Family Differences. Family characteristics appear to be more critical to children's well-being than specific child characteristics, such as age or sex. The most important factor is continuing conflict between the divorced parents (Amato and Keith, 1991; Wallerstein and Johnston, 1990). Children cope better when parents adopt an attitude of "together for our child while separate for us" (Leung and Robson, 1990).

High levels of ongoing family conflict are related to problems of social development, emotional stability, and cognitive skills for the child. Greater material conflict before divorce has been found to be predictive of a more problematic parent-child relationship after separation, which is associated with poorer adjustment in the child (Tschann and others, 1990). Conflict, whether in divorced or intact families, leads to lower self-esteem, increased anxiety, and loss of self-control (Slater and Haber, 1984) and reduces the child's attraction to the parents (White, Brinkerhoff, and Booth, 1985).

Support from extended family and friends can help buffer the effects of divorce; grandparents may extend considerable assistance to both their adult child and their grandchildren (Johnson, 1988). On the other hand, relationships with former in-laws tend to deteriorate immediately after separation (Ambert, 1988). Family finances are almost always negatively affected by divorce (Christensen, Dahl, and Retlig, 1990; Weitzman and Adair, 1988). Changes in life-style, financial instability, and loss of status may contribute indirectly to altered childrearing practices and fewer opportunities for children to participate in outside enrichment activities (Demo and Acock, 1988).

Age- and Sex-Related Responses to Divorce. Previously it was believed that divorce had a greater impact on younger children, but more recent observations indicate that divorce constitutes a major disruption for children in all age-groups. However, the responses (behaviors and feelings) can differ (see box below). While young children may fear abandonment, adolescents must deal with the process of emancipation from those they love (Schwartzberg, 1992).

FEELINGS AND BEHAVIORS OF CHILDREN RELATED TO DIVORCE

INFANCY

Effects of reduced mothering or lack of mothering
Increased irritability
Disturbance in eating, sleeping, and elimination
Interference with attachment process

EARLY PRESCHOOL CHILDREN (AGES 2-3 YEARS)

Frightened and confused
Blame themselves for the divorce
Fear of abandonment
Increased irritability, whining, tantrums
Regressive behaviors (e.g., thumb-sucking, loss of elimination control)
Separation anxiety

LATER PRESCHOOL CHILDREN (AGES 3-5 YEARS)

Fear of abandonment
Blame themselves for the divorce; decreased self-esteem
Bewilderment regarding all human relationships
Become more aggressive in relationships with others (e.g., siblings, peers)
Engage in fantasy to seek understanding of the divorce

EARLY SCHOOL-AGE CHILDREN (AGES 5-6 YEARS)

Depression and immature behavior
Loss of appetite and sleep disorders
May be able to verbalize some feelings and understand some divorce-related changes
Increased anxiety and aggression
Feel abandoned by departing parent

MIDDLE SCHOOL-AGE CHILDREN (AGES 6-8 YEARS)

Panic reactions
Feelings of deprivation—loss of parent, attention, money, and secure future
Profound sadness, depression, fear, and insecurity
Feelings of abandonment and rejection
Fear regarding the future
Difficulty expressing anger at parents
Intense desire for reconciliation of parents
Impaired capacity to play and enjoy outside activities
Decline in school performance
Altered peer relationships—become bossy, irritable, demanding, and manipulative
Frequent crying, loss of appetite, sleep disorders
Disturbed routine, forgetfulness

LATER SCHOOL-AGE CHILDREN (AGES 9-12 YEARS)

More realistic understanding of divorce
Intense anger directed at one or both parents
Divided loyalties
Able to express feelings of anger
Ashamed of parental behavior
Feel the need for revenge; may wish to punish the parent they hold responsible
Feel lonely, rejected, and abandoned
Altered peer relationships
Decline in school performance
May develop somatic complaints
May engage in aberrant behavior such as lying, stealing
Temper tantrums
Dictatorial attitude

ADOLESCENTS (AGES 12-18 YEARS)

Able to disengage themselves from parental conflict
Feel a profound sense of loss—of family, childhood
Feelings of anxiety
Worry about themselves, parents, siblings
Express anger, sadness, shame, embarrassment
May withdraw from family and friends
Disturbed concept of sexuality
May engage in acting-out behaviors

Egocentric preschoolers, who see and understand things only in relation to themselves, assume themselves to be the cause of parental distress and interpret the separation as punishment. They feel sadness and strong feelings of responsibility for the loss of the absent parent. Moreover, they consciously fear that they may be abandoned by the remaining parent. Consequently, it is essential to establish some kind of stability for these children; otherwise, they will convert their energies to restabilization efforts rather than to growth and development. They need frequent, repeated, and concrete explanations of what is going to happen to them and how they will be cared for, and assurance that something new will take the place of the old and that they will not be deserted. In order that they do not imagine things, explanations, such as where they will live, who will prepare their meals when the parent is at work, and when they will see the absent parent again, should be specific. They need to focus on reality.

School-age children are able to cope with parental separation better than younger children, even though they feel intense pain, loneliness, and deprivation. Younger children are preoccupied with the departure of one parent, usually the father, and grieve openly and long for his return, fearing replacement. Older children are more likely to perceive one parent as responsible, become angry with both parents, and express this anger with behavior distressing to one parent. School performance may be affected because they are unable to focus on learning; therefore teachers and school counselors should be informed so that they have a better understanding of alterations in the children's behavior and performance. Often children must move to an unfamiliar environment or new neighborhood and form new relationships in addition to coping with the alteration in their family structure. They almost invariably wish for the parents to reunite.

Adolescents may be highly resentful, since their lives are already sufficiently difficult and stressful. Although they are able to comprehend the divorce and are less likely to feel responsibility, adolescents find the divorce of their parents extraordinarily painful. Adolescents' sexual identity is affected by disturbed parental relationships, a precipitous deidealization of both parents, and concern about their own future as a marital partner. They are anxious about the availability of money for future needs. School-age children and adolescents may have lowered self-esteem, poorer academic performance, and greater depression than peers from nondivorced families (Anable, 1991; Brubeck and Beer, 1992). However, the separation of the parents may provide some space in which the older adolescent can develop an emotional detachment from the family and individualization—normal developmental tasks of adolescence.

Although considerable research has looked at sex differences in children's adjustments to divorce, the findings are not conclusive. In general, it appears that boys have more problematic behavior than girls after divorce. Also, postdivorce parenting difficulties tend to be greater with sons than with daughters and typically begin before the divorce (Shaw, Emery, and Tuer, 1993).

Telling the Children. Parents are understandably hesitant to tell children about their decision to divorce. A vast majority of parents neglect to discuss with their preschool children either the divorce or the inevitable changes it brings. Without preparation, even children who remain in the family home are confused by the parental separation, and this confusion seems to overpower any soothing effects remaining in the home may have (Stirtzinger and Cholvat, 1990).

Most likely, the children are already experiencing vague, uneasy feelings that are more difficult to cope with than being told truthfully about the situation. If possible, the initial disclosure should include both parents and siblings, followed by later discussions with each child individually. Ample time should be set aside for the discussions, and they should take place during a period of calm, not after an argument. Parents who physically hold or touch their children provide them with a feeling of warmth that is reassuring. The discussions should include the reason for the divorce—minimizing blame—and reassurance that the divorce is not the fault of the children. Children may feel guilty, as though they have somehow failed or are being punished for misbehavior. They wonder what role they played in the divorce or failure to keep the family together.

Parents need not fear crying in front of the children; it gives the children permission to cry also. Children need to ventilate their feelings. They normally feel anger and resentment and should be allowed to communicate these feelings without punishment. They also have feelings of terror and abandonment and long for consistency and order in their lives. They need to know where they will live, who will take care of them, if they will be with their siblings, and if there will be enough money to live on. The children may also fear that if the parents stopped loving each other, they could stop loving them as well (Rhyne, 1986). Their need for assurance of love is tremendous at this time.

■ ■ ■

Research on the adverse effects of divorce on children should be viewed with some caution and scrutiny. Many of the samples are small, are drawn from one area of the country, or are selected from clinical rather than general populations. The lack of a control group in many studies also limits the conclusions. An area needing further research is the influence of children's temperament and coping abilities on adjustment to divorce.

Although most studies have concentrated on the negative effects of divorce on youngsters, positive outcomes of divorce have been reported. A successful postdivorce family, either as a single-parent or as a reconstituted family, can improve the quality of life for adults and children. Living with conflict is resolved, and a better relationship with one or both parents may result. Children may also have less contact with a disturbed parent. Greater maturity, independence, and commitment to sustaining relationships are also positive outcomes (Wallerstein and Johnston, 1990). However, emotional adjustment is closely associated with the child's personal adjustment before the divorce (Demo and Acock, 1988).

Children's Developmental Tasks Related to Divorce

Most children go through two major phases when adjusting to a divorce: a ***crisis phase,*** which often lasts for a year or longer and is accompanied by an emotional upheaval that affects the relationship with the custodial parent, and an ***adjustment phase,*** in which children settle down and begin to adapt to life in a single-parent home.

Wallerstein and Blakeslee (1989) describe seven developmental tasks in an attempt to conceptualize the responses of children to divorce over a period of time (see box below). The first two must be dealt with immediately, others within the first few months. Successful mastery of the early tasks is linked with maintenance of developmental pace and resumption of schoolwork following an expected period of diminished learning effectiveness and academic performance. Later tasks are associated with a more lesiurely pace and extend over the remainder of the growth period.

Complications sometimes associated with divorce include efforts on the part of one parent to subvert the child's loyalties to the other, abandonment to other caregivers, and adjustment to a stepparent. In the majority of divorce cases the mother receives custody of the child; this has an effect on the male child's identification with a father figure in addition to all the other ramifications of living in a family without a father or in a single-parent family. Many divorced mothers with young children move in with parents, other relatives, or friends in some kind of dependent or sharing arrangement.

Children may feel a sense of shame and embarrassment concerning the family situation. Such feelings cause children to see themselves as different, inferior, or unworthy of love, especially if they feel any responsibility for the family dissolution. Although the social stigma attached to divorce no longer produces the emotions it has in the past, it may still exist in some small towns and can reinforce children's negative self-image. The lasting effects of divorce depend on the children's and the parents' adjustment to the transition from an intact family to a single-parent family and, often, to a reconstituted family.

PSYCHOLOGIC TASKS FOR CHILDREN AFTER DIVORCE

TASK I: UNDERSTANDING THE DIVORCE

Young children: Understand the immediate changes and differentiate fantasy from reality; manage concerns regarding abandonment, placement in foster care, not seeing departed parent again.

Adolescents/young adults: Understand what led to marital failure; evaluate parents' actions; draw useful conclusions for their own lives.

TASK II: STRATEGIC WITHDRAWAL

Acknowledge concern and provide appropriate help to parents and siblings; remove divorce from being their total focus and get back to their own interests, pleasures, activities, peer relationships, etc.

Parents must help children to remain children to complete this task.

TASK III: DEALING WITH LOSS

Deal with loss of intact family and loss of presence of one parent, usually the father.

May be most difficult task.

Deal with feelings of rejection and blame for making one parent leave.

Task is easier if child has good relationship with both parents.

TASK IV: DEALING WITH ANGER

Manage anger at parents for deciding to divorce, yet are aware of parents' needs, anxiety, and loneliness.

Diminished anger and forgiveness come about together.

TASK V: WORKING OUT GUILT

Deal with sense of guilt for causing marital difficulties and driving wedge between parents.

Need to separate guilty ties and get on with their lives.

TASK VI: ACCEPTING PERMANENCE OF DIVORCE

Overcome early denial and fantasies of parents getting back together.

Task may not be completed until parent remarries or child separates from parents and leaves.

TASK VII: TAKING A CHANCE ON LOVE

Most important task for growing children—adolescents and young adults.

Remain open to love, commitment, marriage, fidelity.

Able to turn away from parents' model.

Data from Wallerstein J, Blakeslee S: *Second chances: men, women, and children a decade after divorce,* New York, 1989, Ticknor & Fields.

Custody and Parenting Partnerships

Traditionally when parents separated, the mother was given custody of the children. Now both parents and the courts are seeking alternatives. The present belief is that neither fathers nor mothers should be awarded custody automatically. Rather, custody should be awarded to the parent who is best able to provide for the children's welfare. In certain situations children experience severe stress when living or spending time with a parent. Some recent court decisions have reflected respect for the rights of children by allowing children to legally sever ties with one or both parents.

In most divorce cases the mother still receives custody of the child with visitation agreements for the father. However, more courts are now awarding custody to fathers. Men usually make more money and can offer more material benefits than many women are able to provide. The incidence of delinquent support payments to custodial mothers is a matter of universal knowledge and concern. The single-parent family is commonplace, but many divorced mothers with small children move in with parents, other relatives, or friends in some kind of dependent or sharing arrangement.

Often overlooked are the changes that may occur in the children's relationships with other relatives, especially grandparents. Grandparents on the noncustodial side are often kept from their grandchildren; those on the custodial side may be overwhelmed by their adult child's return to the household with grandchildren.*

**Grandparents,* a newsletter for grandparents in divided families, is published by Scarsdale Family Counseling Service, 405 Harwood Building, Scarsdale NY 10583; (914) 723-3281.

Two less common custody arrangements are divided custody and joint custody. ***Divided,*** or ***split, custody*** means that each parent is awarded custody of one or more of the children, thereby separating siblings. For example, sons might live with the father and daughters with the mother. Joint custody takes one of two forms. In ***joint physical custody*** the parents alternate having the physical care and control of the children on a reasonably equitable basis while maintaining shared parenting responsibilities legally. This type of custody arrangement works well for families who live close to each other and whose occupations allow an active role in the care and rearing of the children. In ***joint legal custody*** the children reside with one parent but both parents are the children's legal guardians and both participate in childrearing (Arditti, 1992).

Co-parenting offers substantial benefits for the family: children can be close to both parents, and life with each parent can be more normal as opposed to the situation of a disciplinarian mother and a recreational father. However, to be successful, the parents must place a high value on the commitment to provide as normal parenting as possible and be able to separate their marital conflicts from the parenting roles (Wallerstein and Johnston, 1990). No matter what type of custody arrangement is awarded, the primary consideration is the welfare of the children.

SINGLE-PARENTING

Single-parent status is acquired by means of divorce, separation, or death, or through birth or adoption of a child by a single person. Although divorce rates have stabilized, the number of single-parent households continues to rise. Today, one child in four lives in a single-parent family, with the majority of single parents being women (Center for the Study of Social Policy, 1993). It is estimated that at least half the children born during the 1980s will spend part of their time in a family headed by a divorced, separated, widowed, or never-married mother (Norton and Glick, 1986). Although some women are single parents by choice, most of these women never planned on being single parents, and many feel pressure to marry or remarry.

Managing shortages of money, time, and energy are major concerns of single parents. Studies repeatedly confirm the financial difficulties of single-parent families, particularly in the case of single mothers. (The average income of single-mother families is 60% that of single-father families; in addition, only 31% of mother-headed households receive any child support or alimony [Center for the Study of Social Policy, 1993].) In fact, the stigma of poverty may be more keenly felt than the discrimination associated with being a single parent (Richards, 1989). In addition, these families are often forced by their financial status to live in communities where inadequate housing and personal safety are concerns. Moreover, single parents may feel guilty about the time spent away from their children. Divorced mothers from marriages where the father assumed the breadwinning role and the mother the householding and parenting roles have been found to have the most difficulty in adjusting to becoming the breadwinner for the family (Fassinger, 1989).

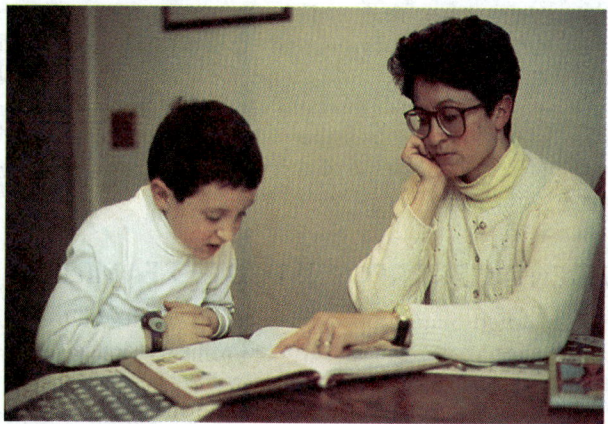

FIG. 3-10 Working mothers must accomplish numerous tasks as part of their busy day.

Many single parents have trouble arranging for adequate child care, and care for sick children is especially difficult to obtain. Single mothers trying to balance work, chores, and child care may frequently give up personal activities, recreation, and even rest.

Although the life of single mothers is often portrayed bleakly, many single mothers do remarkably well and feel contentment in their lives (Fig. 3-10). Many feel they are excellent parents and are proud of their ability to manage their multiple roles effectively (Richards, 1989). These women have a positive attitude and an acceptance of their work status (in and out of the home), and can often count on someone else, such as a boyfriend, relative, or an older child, to help out (Quinn and Allen, 1989).

Supports and resources for single-parent families include health care services that are open evenings and weekends, high-quality child care, respite child care to relieve parental exhaustion and burnout, and parent enhancement centers for advancing education and job skills, providing recreational activities, and offering parenting education. Groups for single-parent fathers and grandparents who are primary caregivers are also important (Strett, 1989). There is a need on the part of the parent for social contacts and a life separate from the children for the emotional growth of both parent and child. The single parent can find support and encouragement from **Parents Without Partners, Inc.,*** an organization designed to meet the needs of this increasingly important group.

Single Fathers

Fathers who have custody of their children have many of the same problems as divorced mothers. They feel overburdened by the responsibility, depressed, and concerned about their ability to cope with the emotional needs of the children, especially the needs of the girls (Hetherington, 1981). The lack of homemaking skills is characteristic of

*International Headquarters, 401 N. Michigan Ave., Chicago, IL 60611-4267; (312) 644-6610.

most fathers. They find it difficult at first to coordinate household tasks, school visits, and other activities associated with managing a household alone. Fathers often demand more assistance with household tasks and more independence from their children than custodial mothers do, and they are likely to make use of alternative caregiving and support systems.

PARENTING IN RECONSTITUTED FAMILIES

In the United States approximately half of all children in homes where parents have divorced will experience yet another major change in their lives within 3 years of a divorce—a return to a nuclear family and the sudden acquisition of a stepparent when the custodial parent remarries (Hetherington, Stanley-Hagen, and Anderson, 1989). The entry of a stepparent into a ready-made family requires adjustments for all the family members. Some obstacles to the role adjustments and family problem solving include disruption of previous life-styles and interaction patterns, complexity in the formation of new ones, and lack of social supports. Despite these problems, most children from divorced families want to live in a two-parent home.

Stepparenting

The term ***parenting coalition*** has been suggested to describe the situation where there are more than two parents for a child, as in stepfamilies (Visher and Visher, 1989). This term implies the need for cooperation rather than competition between the biologic parents and the stepparents. Cooperative parenting relationships can allow more time for each set of parents to be alone to establish their own relationship. Under ideal circumstances, power conflicts between the two households can be reduced, and tension and anxiety can be lessened for all family members. In addition, the children's self-esteem can be increased, and there is a greater likelihood of continued contact with grandparents.

The development of a parenting coalition requires time and corresponds to the stages of stepfamily development described by Papernow (1984): (1) bonding between the couple; (2) recognition that all parenting adults are important to the children's well-being; (3) definition and clarification of acceptable stepparent roles; and (4) ability to share among adults in both households in terms of child-rearing decisions and responsibilities. Flexibility, mutual support, and open communication are critical in successful relationships in stepfamilies and stepparenting situations (Rosen, 1987).

Unfortunately, stepfamilies usually do not seek help to prevent problems from arising. Typically, information and counseling are sought only when problems have surfaced and can no longer be ignored. A preventive rather than remedial approach to stepfamilies and stepparenting is needed (Ganong and Coleman, 1989) (see box above).

TIPS FOR "LIVING IN STEP"

1. Let relationships develop slowly and naturally. Don't expect too much too soon, from the children, from your spouse, or from yourself.
2. Don't criticize or belittle lost (or new) parents, or try to erase or replace them. Stepparents are additional parents.
3. Expect confused feelings, anxieties, competition for attention, bids for loyalty. Decide on standards of discipline and behavior and stick to them.
4. Communicate. Don't pretend everything is fine if it isn't. Look at problems squarely and deal with them openly.
5. If you need help, admit it and get it. Read a book, get counseling, join a support group, call a family meeting.

From Stein B: Yours, mine, and ours: a look at stepfamilies, *Growing Parent* 12(9):1-5, 1984.

Effects on Children

Although there has been a great deal of research on the impact of divorce on children, there is much less data on the outcomes for children in stepfamilies (Hobart, 1988). Becoming a stepchild is often a stressful transition, especially during initial marital rearrangement (Crosbie-Burnett and Skyles, 1989; Hetherington, Stanley-Hagan, and Anderson, 1989; Wallerstein and Blakeslee, 1989). Several transitional factors have been demonstrated to have an effect on children. The relationship with the noncustodial parent usually decreases. Divided loyalties between the two sets of parents may be exacerbated. As time goes on, the entry of new children from the remarriage can cause a stepchild from a previous marriage to have less favored status. In stepfamilies the possibility of a second divorce situation is very critical, since the children have already experienced significant losses in both relationships and environmental and circumstantial changes. Despite these risks and stresses, studies to date have not demonstrated long-term negative effects on children in remarried families (Amato, 1987).

PARENTING IN DUAL-EARNER FAMILIES

No change in family life-style has had more impact than the large numbers of women entering the workplace. As women moved away from the traditional homemaker pattern, the numbers of dual-earner families increased dramatically. In 1993 54% of mothers with children under 3 years of age were in the civilian labor force; 64% of women with children 3 to 5 years of age were employed (Children's Defense Fund, 1994). This trend is unlikely to diminish. As a result, the family is subjected to considerable stress as members attempt to meet the challenge of the often competing demands of occupational needs and those regarded as necessary for a rich family life.

Role definitions are frequently altered to arrange an equitable division of time and labor, as well as to resolve conflicts between earlier and later norms, especially those related to the traditional norms of the culture (Fig. 3-11). Overload is a common source of stress in a dual-earner fam-

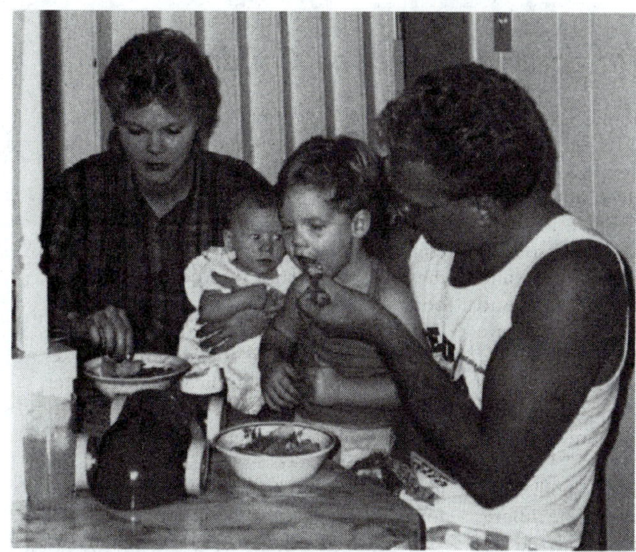

FIG. 3-11 One of the major challenges in dual-earner families is redistributing roles, especially those related to parenting.

ily, and social activities are significantly curtailed. Time demands and scheduling are major problems, and when there are children, the demands can be even more intense; dual-earner couples may increase the strain on themselves in order to avoid creating stress for their children, although there is no evidence to indicate that the dual-earner lifestyle, as such, is stressful to children. However, the stress experienced by the parents may affect the children indirectly.

Working Mothers

Even though working mothers have become the norm in the United States, disapproving attitudes from some health care workers and some child care books, lack of a national policy on child care, and "scripts" from their own childhood of being cared for by an at-home mother contribute to the torn and guilty feelings many working mothers experience (Balk and Christoffel, 1988).

Fathers are taking a more active role in child care. By 1991 one of every five preschool children (under age 5) were cared for by their fathers while their mothers worked outside the home (O'Connell, 1993).

The quality of child care is a persistent concern for all working parents. However, mothers are more likely than fathers to adjust their work schedule to accommodate child care needs. Even in families where the father is the primary caregiver while the mother is at work, 40% of mothers adjusted their work hours to meet child care needs, compared with 6% of fathers (O'Connell, 1993).

The mother's status as a working woman has not been found consistently to have either positive or negative effects on children's development and educational outcomes (Balk and Christoffel, 1988; Bianchi and Spain, 1986). Working women who scored high on measures of emotional well-being, sensitivity to and acceptance of their children, satisfaction with nonwork time, and positive feelings about their marriage were more likely to have securely attached infants, regardless of child care arrangements (Belsky, 1988). One consistent finding is that the "consequences of maternal employment" (mental health, marital satisfaction, children's well-being) are favorable when the woman's employment status is consistent with her and her partner's preferences about it (Spitzke, 1988).

Five characteristics of daycare that are important to the child's development are (1) the timing of entry into care, (2) the amount of time in daycare, (3) the stability of the care, (4) the setting, and (5) the quality of the care (King and MacKinnon, 1988). Any research on the effects of daycare must be examined carefully; the characteristics of the daycare setting and the measures used for child outcomes, such as attachment, must be taken into consideration (see Thinking Critically About . . . box, p. 100).

Nurses play an important role in helping families to find suitable sources of child care and to prepare children for this experience (see Alternate Child Care Arrangements, Chapter 12).

ACCOMMODATING CONTEMPORARY PARENTING SITUATIONS

During recent years both the private and government sectors have noted some of the problems contemporary families face. Many of these issues involve working parents. For example, perhaps one of the greatest stressors for the working single parent or for dual-earner families is when a child becomes ill. Frequency of childhood illness, exclusion practices of most licensed child care programs, and employer's limited sick leave policies are contributing factors (Jordan, 1986). Most agree that a familiar face and familiar place should be goals of sick child care; therefore many argue that the only place for an ill child is at home with a parent or other relative. Other options include (Giebink, 1993):

1. In-home care by a trained provider other than the child's parent
2. Care by a relative
3. On-site care in the child's usual program, either fully integrated with the other children or in a separate "get well" room
4. Care in a separate, specialized group daycare setting for mildly ill children

Sick child care in a group setting is becoming popular in many communities. Although standards and criteria for such settings have been established (Smith, Shillam, and Zimmerman, 1989), research is needed to determine outcomes for children.

Some employers have become more family focused and give parents time off to be with their sick children. Increasing numbers are also more generous in the amount of time they allow parents—fathers as well as mothers—to remain at home after the birth or adoption of a child. More flexible work schedules and family-oriented legislation can also

THINKING CRITICALLY ABOUT . . . *Daycare's Influence on Children*

Although children in daycare settings experience daily separation from their parent(s) and spend a good portion of their day in nonparental child care, the parents and family remain the primary influence on the child's development (Phillips and Howes, 1987). Child care, however, is a collaborative arrangement between the daycare provider and the family. In a review of the research on daycare since 1980, King and MacKinnon (1988) note that the quality of interactions between both the child and parent and the child and caregiver is very important for the child's development, but the latter is very difficult to regulate through licensing requirements.

Regarding cognitive effects, no published study has given support to the fear that young children in daycare are at risk for intellectual decline (Caldwell, 1993). In fact, two major studies have demonstrated that intellectual gains are possible in high-quality daycare settings (Infant Health and Development Program, 1990; Ramey, Brayant, and Suarez, 1985).

Across many socioeconomic levels and from toddlerhood to early school-age, children with daycare experience exceeded home-reared children in social interaction with peers, confidence in social situations, friendliness, and more socially mature behaviors (Schindler, Moley, and Frank, 1987). Some research has found children in daycare to be more aggressive (Haskins, 1985), with different reasoning about rules and transgressions (i.e., not as apt to perceive social misbehavior as needing punishment) (Siegal and Storey, 1985).

Emotional development is usually measured by attachment. Lamb, Sternberg, and Prodromidis (1992) reanalyzed results from 13 studies on associations between the experience, extent, and onset of daycare and attachment security. They found that more infants in exclusively maternal care were rated as securely attached; avoidance occurred more often in daycare children. Insecure attachments were more common in children who entered daycare between 7 and 12 months of age than in those who entered earlier. No differences were noted in attachment distributions in infants receiving more than or less than 20 hours of care per week.

The effects of daycare on infants under age 1 year, remain unclear. This is due to controversy on how to measure attachment in infants and whether the avoidant behavior seen in these infants is really an adaptive behavior of children who routinely separate from the parent (Clarke-Stewart, 1987) or an indication of greater insecurity that will lead to the possibility of social maladjustment in the preschool and school-age years (Belsky, 1988). Longitudinal research involving infants cared for in 10 daycare settings across the United States began in 1991, using an ecologic model that considers the family environment and personal characteristics of the child along with the daycare environment (Caldwell, 1993). Results of this research may more fully answer the question: What are the long-term effects of daycare on the child's development when out-of-home care is started in the first year of life?

ease the burden of managing family and work responsibilities (Arnold and Brecht, 1990). The passage of the Family and Medical Leave Act (FMLA) in 1993 set the stage for a greater focus on the issues that contemporary American families face. The FMLA allows eligible employees to take up to 12 weeks of unpaid leave each year to care for newborn or newly adopted children, parents, or spouses who have serious health conditions, or to recover from their own serious health condition. Federal, state, and local government employees are eligible, as well as employees of private businesses with 50 or more employees within 75 miles of their workplace. A minimum of 1 year's employment and at least 1250 hours during the previous year are required. The law entitles employees to return to their previous job or an equivalent one with the same pay, benefits, and other conditions.

KEY POINTS

- Since there is no agreement about the definition of *family*, a family is what the client considers it to be.
- Three theories that have significant relevance and application to pediatric nursing are family systems theory, family stress theory, and developmental theory.
- Although the traditional family structure has been nuclear or extended, in recent years other forms, such as the single-parent family, have emerged.
- Family size and positioning within the family structure have a strong impact on a child's development.
- Interpersonal skills and a basic understanding of childhood growth and development are two essential areas of focus for parents.
- Parental control tends to be predominantly one of three types: authoritarian, permissive, or authoritative.
- Three areas of special concern to adoptive families include the initial attachment process, the task of telling the children they are adopted, and identify formation during adolescence.
- Marital factors within the home significantly influence a child's development. The impact of divorce on a child depends on the child's age and sex, the outcome, and the quality of the parent-child relationship and parental care following the divorce.
- Single-parenting and stepparenting create adjustment difficulties and add stress to the already-demanding parental role. Significant numbers of children will live in a single-parent or reconstituted family at some point.

REFERENCES

Ahrons CR: The binuclear family: two households, one family, *Altern Lifestyles* 2:499-515, 1979.

Amato PR: Family processes in one-parent, stepparent, and intact families: the child's point of view, *J Marriage Fam* 49:327-337, 1987.

Amato PR, Keith B: Parental divorce and the well-being of children: a meta-analysis, *Psychol Bull* 110(1):26-46, 1991.

Ambert A: Relationships with former in-laws after divorce: a research note, *J Marriage Fam* 50:679-686, 1988.

American Academy of Pediatrics, Committee on Early Childhood, Adoption and Dependent Care: Initial medical evaluation of an adopted child, *Pediatrics* 88(3):642-644, 1991.

Anable KE: Children of divorce: ways to heal the wounds, *Clin Nurse Spec* 5(3):133-137, 1991.

Arditti J: Differences between fathers with joint custody and noncustodial fathers, *Am J Orthopsychiatry* 62(2):186-195, 1992.

Arnold L, Brecht M: Legislative issues affecting parenting: an overview of current policies, *J Perinat Neonat Nurs* 4(2):24-32, 1990.

Balk S, Christoffel K: Advising the working mother, *Contemp Pediatr* 5(9):56-85, 1988.

Baptiste DA: The gay and lesbian stepparent family. In Bozett FW, editor: *Gay and lesbian parents,* New York, 1987, Praeger.

Belsky J: The "effects" of infant day care reconsidered, *Early Childhood Res Q* 3(3):235-272, 1988.

Bianchi S, Spain D: *American women in transition,* New York, 1986, Russell Sage Foundation.

Bigner J, Bozett FW: Parenting by gay fathers. In Bozett FW, Sussman M, editors: *Homosexuality and family relations,* New York, 1990, Harrington Park.

Bozett FW: Parenting concerns of gay fathers, *Top Clin Nurs* 6:60-71, 1984.

Bozett FW: Gay fathers. In Bozett FW, editor: *Gay and lesbian parents,* New York, 1987b, Praeger.

Bozett FW: Children of gay fathers. In Bozett FW, editor: *Gay and lesbian parents,* New York, 1987a, Praeger.

Bozett FW: Gay fatherhood. In Bronstein P, Cowan CP, editors: *Fatherhood today: men's changing role in the family,* New York, 1988a, John Wiley & Sons.

Bozett FW: Social control of identity by children of gay fathers, *West J Nurs Res* 10:550-565, 1988b.

Bozett FW: Gay fathers: a review of the literature. In Bozett FW, editor: *Homosexuality and the family,* New York, 1989, Harrington Park.

Brockhaus JPD, Brockhaus RH: Adopting an older child—the emotional process, *Am J Nurs* 82:288-291, 1982.

Brodzinsky D: As cited in Hering R: Chosen and given, *NY Times Magazine,* Sept 11, 1988.

Brubeck D, Beer J: Depression, self-esteem, suicide ideation, death anxiety, and GPA in high school students of divorced and nondivorced parents, *Psychol Rep* 71(3, pt I):755-763, 1992.

Caldwell B: Impact of day care on children, *Pediatrics* 91(1, pt 2):225-228, 1993.

Carter B, McGoldrick M: *The changing family life cycle: a framework for family therapy,* Needham Heights, MA, 1989, Allyn & Bacon.

Center for the Study of Social Policy: *Kids count,* Washington, DC, 1993, Annie E Casey Foundation.

Children's Defense Fund: *The state of America's children 1992,* Washington DC, 1992, CDF.

Children's Defense Fund: *The State of America's Children 1994,* Washington, DC, 1994, CDF.

Christensen DH, Dahl CM, Rettig KD: Noncustodial mothers and child support: examining the larger context, *Fam Relations* 39(4):388-394, 1990.

Clarke-Stewart L: Predicting child development from day care forms and features: the Chicago study. In Phillips DA, editor: *Quality in child care: what does the research tell us?* Washington, DC, 1987, National Association for the Education of Young Children.

Crosbie-Burnett M, Skyles A: Stepchildren in school and colleges: recommendations for educational policy changes, *Fam Relations* 38:59-64, 1989.

Daniels D, Moos R: Exosystem influences on family and child functioning, *J Soc Behav Pers* 3(4):113-133, 1988.

Demo D, Acock A: The impact of divorce on children, *J Marriage Fam* 50:619-648, 1988.

Donovan D: A contrary view on adoption disclosure, *Child Teens Today* 10(10):4-6, 1990.

Dunst C, Trivette C, Deal A: *Enabling and empowering families: principles and guidelines for practice,* Cambridge, MA, 1988, Brookline Books.

Duvall ER: *Family development,* ed 5, Philadelphia, 1977, JB Lippincott.

Easterbrooks MA, Goldberg WA: Toddler development in the family: impact of father involvement and parenting characteristics, *Child Dev* 55:740-752, 1984.

Edwards J: Perceived needs of adoptive and biologic parents, *Issues Compr Pediatr Nurs* 10:223-234, 1987.

Eichelberger S, Beal D, May R: Hypovolemic shock in a child as a consequence of corporal punishment, *Pediatrics* 87(4):570-571, 1991.

Fassinger P: Becoming the breadwinner: single mothers' reactions to changes in their paid work lives, *Fam Relations* 38:404-411, 1989.

Finkelhor D and others: *The dark side of families: current family violence research,* Newport, CA, 1983, Sage Publications.

Freidman D: Parent development, *Calif Med* 86:25-28, 1957.

Friedman M: *Family nursing: theory and practice,* ed 3, Norwalk, CT, 1992, Appleton-Century-Crofts.

Gage M, Christensen D: Parental role socialization and the transition to parenthood, *Fam Relations* 40(3):332-337, 1991.

Ganong L, Coleman M: Preparing for remarriage: anticipating the issues, seeking solutions, *Fam Relations* 38:28-33, 1989.

Garbarino J and others: *Children in danger: coping with the consequences of community violence,* San Francisco, 1992, Josey-Bass.

Giebink G: Care of the ill child in day-care settings, *Pediatrics* 91(1, pt 2):229-233, 1993.

Gottman J: Children of gay and lesbian parents. In Bozett FW, Sussman M, Editors: *Homosexuality and family relations,* New York, 1990, Harrington Park.

Green R and others: Lesbian mothers and their children: a comparison with solo parent heterosexual mothers and their children, *Arch Sex Behav* 15:167-184, 1986.

Groothuis JR and others: Increased child abuse in families with twins, *Pediatrics* 70(5):769-773, 1982.

Harris MB, Turner PH: Gay and lesbian parents, *J Homosex* 12:103-113, 1986.

Haskins R: Public school aggression among children with varying day care experience, *Child Dev* 56:689-703, 1985.

Hetherington EM: Children and divorce. In Henderson RW, editor: *Parent-child interaction: theory, research, and prospects,* New York, 1981, Academic Press.

Hetherington EM, Stanley-Hagan M, Anderson ER: Marital transitions: a child's perspective, *Am Psychologist* 44(2):303-312, 1989.

Hill R: *Families under stress,* New York, 1949, Harper & Row.

Hill R, Hansen D: The identification of conceptual frameworks utilized in family study, *Marriage Fam Liv* 22:299-311, 1960.

Hobart C: The family system in remarriage: an exploratory study, *J Marriage Fam* 50(3):649-661, 1988.

Hoopes M, Harper J: *Birth order roles and sibling patterns in individual and family therapy,* Rockville, MD, 1987, Aspen.

Hostetter M, Johnson D: International adoption: an introduction for physicians, *Am J Dis Child* 143:325-332, 1989.

Huggins S: A comparative study of self-esteem of adolescent children of divorced lesbian mothers and divorced heterosexual mothers, *J Homosex* 18(1/2):123-135, 1989.

Hyman I and others: *Child abuse in the schools: community and judicial attitudes.* Paper presented at the 62nd annual meeting of the American Orthopsychiatric Association, New York, April 24, 1985.

Infant Health and Development Program: Enhancing the outcome of low-birth-weight premature infants, *JAMA* 263:3035-3040, 1990.

Johnson C: Postdivorce reorganization of relationships between divorcing children and their parents, *J Marriage Fam* 50:221-231, 1988.

Jordan A: The unresolved child care dilemma: care of the acutely ill child, *Rev Infect Dis* 8(4):626-630, 1986.

King D, MacKinnon C: Making difficult choices easier: a review of research on day care and children's development, *Fam Relations* 37:392-398, 1988.

Koepke J and others: Becoming parents: feelings of adoptive mothers, *Pediatr Nurs* 17(4):333-336, 1991.

Koo H, Suchindran C, Griffith J: The completion of childrearing: change and variation in timing, *J Marriage Fam* 49:281-293, 1987.

Lamb M, Sternberg K, Prodromidis M: Nonmaternal care and the security of infant-mother attachment: a reanalysis of the data *Infant Behav Dev* 15:71-83, 1992.

Leung AK, Robson WL: Children of divorce, *J R Soc Health* 110(5):161-163, 1990.

Lobato D: *Brothers, sisters, and special needs,* Baltimore, MD, 1990, Paul H Brookes.

Macklin ED: Nontraditional family forms: a decade of research, *J Marriage Fam* 42:175-192, 1980.

McCubbin HI, Patterson JM: Family adaptation to crisis. In McCubbin HI, Cauble E, Patterson JM, editors: *Family stress, coping, and social support,* Springfield, IL, 1982, Charles C Thomas.

McCubbin M, McCubbin H: Theoretical orientation to family stress and coping. In Figley C, editor: *Treating families under stress,* New York, 1989, Brunner/Mazel.

McGonigel M: Philosophy and conceptual framework. In McGonigel M, Kaufman R, Johnson B, editors: *Guidelines and recommended practices for the Individualized Family Service Plan,* ed 2, Bethesda, MD, 1991, Association for the Care of Children's Health.

Mednick B, Baker R: *Consequences of family structure and maternal state for child and mother's development,* Final report, NICHD (contract N 01-HD-82807), 1980.

Miller B: Counseling gay husbands and fathers. In Bozett FW, editor: *Gay and lesbian parents,* New York, 1987, Praeger.

Murphy S: Siblings and the new baby: changing perspectives, *J Pediatr Nurs* 18(5):277-288, 1993.

National Center for Health Statistics: Annual summary of births, marriages, divorces, and deaths: United States, 1989, *Monthly Vital Statistics Rep* 38(13):5, 1990.

National Center for Health Statistics: Advance report of final natality statistics, 1991, *Monthly Vital Statistics Rep* 42(3, suppl): entire issue, 1993a.

National Center for Health Statistics: Annual summary of births, marriages, divorces, and deaths: United States, 1992, *Monthly Vital Statistic Rep* 41(13):1, 1993b.

Nelms B: Discipline: what do you recommend? *J Pediatr Health Care* 7(1):1-2, 1993.

Norton A, Glick P: One-parent families: a social and economic profile, *Fam Relations* 35:8-17, 1986.

O'Connell M: *Where's papa? Fathers' role in child care,* Washington, DC, 1993, Population Reference Bureau.

Papernow P: The stepfamily cycle: an experimental model of stepfamily development, *Fam Relations* 33:355-363, 1984.

Patterson C: Children of lesbian and gay parents, *Child Dev* 63:1025-1042, 1992.

Paul J: *Growing up with a gay, lesbian, or bisexual parent: an exploratory study of experiences and perceptions,* Unpublished doctoral dissertation, Berkely, CA, 1986, University of California at Berkely.

Phillips D, Howes C: Indicators of quality child care: review of research. In Phillips DA, editor: *Quality in child care: what does the research tell us?* Washington, DC, 1987, National Association for the Education of Young Children.

Pies C: Considering parenthood: psychosocial issues for gay men and lesbians choosing alternative fertilization. In Bozett FW, editor: *Gay and lesbian parents,* New York, 1987, Praeger.

Polit D, Falbo T: Only children and personality development, *J Marriage Fam* 49:309-325, 1987.

Quinn P, Allen K: Facing challenges and making compromises: how single mothers endure, *Fam Relations* 38:390-395, 1989.

Ramey C, Bryant D, Suarez T: Preschool compensatory education and the modifiability of intelligence: a critical review. In Detterman DK, editor: *Current topics in human intelligence,* Norwood, NJ, 1985, Ablex.

Rhyne MC: Understanding and supporting families in the process of divorce, *Nurse Pract* 11(12):37-51, 1986.

Richards L: The precarious survival and hard-won satisfaction of white single-parent families, *Fam Relations* 38:396-403, 1989.

Ricketts W, Achtenberg R: The adoptive and foster gay and lesbian parent. In Bozett FW, editor: *Gay and lesbian parents,* New York, 1987, Praeger.

Riley D and others: How effective are age-paced newsletters for new parents: a replication and extension of earlier studies, *Fam Relations* 40(3):247-253, 1991.

Rodman H: Talcott Parsons' view of the changing American family. In Rodman H, editor: *Marriage, family, and society,* New York, 1965, Random House.

Rogers RH: *Improvement in the construction and analysis of family life cycle categories,* Kalamazoo, MI, 1962, Western Michigan University.

Rosen M: *Stepfathering,* New York, 1987, Ballantine Books.

Sater J: Appraising and promoting a sense of self in twins, *MCN* 4:218-226, 1979.

Schindler P, Morley B, Frank A: Time in day care and social participation of young children, *Dev Psychol* 23:255-261, 1987.

Schulenburg J: *Gay parenting,* New York, 1985, Doubleday.

Schwartzberg AZ: The impact of divorce on adolescents, *Hosp Community Psychiatry* 43(6):634-637, 1992.

Shaw DS, Emery RE, Tuer MD: Parental functioning and children's adjustment in families of divorce: a prospective study, *J Abnormal Child Psychology* 21(1):119-134, 1993.

Sherry S: Helping families adapt to adoption, *Contemp Pediatr* 3:96-111, 1986.

Siegal M, Storey R: Day care and children's conceptions between two theoretical perspectives, *Am Soc Rev* 37:414-424, 1972.

Slater E, Haber J: Adolescent adjustment following divorce as a function of familial conflict, *J Consult Clin Psychol* 52:920-921, 1984.

Slater S, Mencher J: The lesbian family life cycle: a contextual approach, *Am J Orthopsychiatry* 61(3):372-382, 1991.

Smith K, Shillam P, Zimmerman F: Standards and criteria: group child care for sick children, *Pediatr Nurs* 15(6):600-602, 1989.

Soloway N, Smith R: Antecedents of late birth-timing decisions of men and women in dual-career marriages, *Fam Relations* 36:258-262, 1987.

Spitzke G: Women's employment and family relations: a review, *J Marriage Fam* 50(3):595-618, 1988.

Steckel A: Psychosocial development of children of lesbian mothers. In Bozett FW, editor: *Gay and lesbian parents,* New York, 1987, Praeger.

Steelman LC, Powell B: The social and academic consequences of birth order: real, artifactual, or both? *J Marriage Fam* 47:117-124, 1985.

Stirtzinger R, Cholvat L: Preschool age children of divorce: transitional phenomena and the mourning process, *Can J Psychiatry* 35:506-514, 1990.

Strett R: Support services for single parents, *Early Childhood Update* 5:6, winter 1989.

Tschann J and others: Family process and children's functioning during divorce, *J Marriage Fam* 51:431-444, 1990.

Turner PH, Scadden L, Harris MB: *Parenting in gay and lesbian families.* Paper presented at the First Future of Parenting Symposium, Chicago, March 1985.

Tuttle G: Divorce: how are the children coping? *Can Nurse* 88(11):13-16, 1992.

Visher E, Visher J: Parenting coalitions after remarriage: dynamics and therapeutic guidelines, *Fam Relations* 38:65-70, 1989.

Volling B, Belsky J: Multiple determinants of father involvement during infancy in dual-earner and single-earner families, *J Marriage Fam* 53(2):461-474, 1991.

Wallace P, Gotlib I: Marital adjustment during the transition to parenthood: stability and predictors of change, *J Marriage Fam* 52(1):21-29, 1990.

Wallerstein JS: The long-term effects of divorce on children: a review, *J Am Acad Child Adolesc Psychiatry* 30(3):349-360, 1991.

Wallerstein JS, Blakeslee S: *Second chances: men, women, and children a decade after divorce,* New York, 1989, Ticknor & Fields.

Wallerstein JS, Johnston JR: Children of divorce: recent findings regarding long-term effects and recent studies of joint and sole custody, *Pediatr Rev* 11(7):197-204, 1990.

Weitzman M, Adair R: Divorce and children, *Pediatr Clin North Am* 35(6):1313-1323, 1988.

White L, Brinkerhoff DB, Booth A: The effect of marital disruption on child's attachment to parents, *J Fam Issues* 6:5-22, 1985.

Wineberg H: Childbearing after remarriage, *J Marriage Fam* 52(1):31-38, 1990.

World Health Organization: *Health and the family: studies in the demography of family life cycles and their health implication,* Geneva, Switzerland, 1978, The Organization.

BIBLIOGRAPHY

General

Abidin RA, Wilfong E: Parenting stress and its relationship to child health care, *Child Health Care* 18(2):114-116, 1989.

Aldous J: Family development and the life course: two perspectives on family change, *J Marriage Fam* 52(3):571-583, 1990.

Aquilino W: Family structure and home-leaving: a further specification of the relationship, *J Marriage Fam* 53(4):999-1010, 1991.

Atkinson AM: Providers evaluations of the effect of family day care on own family relationships, *Fam Relations* 37(4):399-404, 1988.

Barranti CCR: The grandparent/grandchild relationship: family resource in an era of voluntary bonds, *Fam Relations* 34:343-352, 1985.

Beutler IF and others: The family realm: theoretical contributions for understanding its uniqueness, *J Marriage Fam* 51(3):805-815, 1989.

Brody CJ, Steelman LC: Sibling structure and parental sex-typing of children's household tasks, *J Marriage Fam* 47:265-273, 1985.

Brubaker T, editor: *Family relations,* Newbury Park, CA, 1992, Sage Publications.

Callan VJ: Comparisons of mothers of one child by choice with mothers wanting a second birth, *J Marriage Fam* 47:155-164, 1985.

Clemen-Stone S, Eigsti D, McGuire S: *Comprehensive family and community health nursing,* ed 3, St Louis, 1991, Mosby.

Easley M, Epstein N: Coping with stress in a family with an alcoholic parent, *Fam Relations* 40(2):218-224, 1991.

Felson RB, Zielinski MA: Children's self-esteem and parental support, *J Marriage Fam* 51(3):727-736, 1989.

Frankel F: Sources of family annoyance (SOFA): development, reliability, and validity, *J Pediatr Nurs* 8(3):177-184, 1993.

Fsife BL: A model for predicting the adaptation of families to a medical crisis: an analysis of role integration, *Image* 17:108-112, 1985.

Gilliss CL and others, editors: *Toward a science of family nursing,* Menlo Park, CA, 1989, Addison-Wesley.

Glick PC: Fifty years of family demography: a record of social change, *J Marriage Fam* 50(4):861-873, 1988.

Healy JM Jr, Malley JE, Stewart AJ: Children and their fathers after parental separation, *Am J Orthopsychiatry* 60(4):531-543, 1990.

Kaufman DH: An interview guide for helping children make healthcare decisions, *Pediatr Nurs* 11:365-367, 1985.

Keltner B: Family influences on child health status, *Pediatr Nurs* 18(2):128-131, 1992.

Klaus MH, Kennell JH: *Parent-infant bonding,* ed 2, St Louis, 1982, Mosby.

Lamb ME: Mothers, fathers, and children in a changing world. In Tyson RL, Call J, Galenson E, editors: *Infancy in a changing world,* New York, 1985, Basic Books.

LaRossa R: Fatherhood and social change, *Fam Relations* 37(4):451-457, 1988.

Lavee Y, Olson D: Family types and response to stress, *J Marriage Fam* 53(3):786-788, 1991.

Leahey M, Wright L, editors: *Families and life-threatening illness,* Springhouse, PA, 1987, Springhouse.

Mancini JA, Orthner DK: The context and consequences of family change, *Fam Relations* 37(4):363-366, 1988.

McCubbin HI and others: *Family types and strengths,* Edina, MN, 1988, Burgess International Group.

Melnyk BM: Changes in parent-child relationships following divorce, *Pediatr Nurs* 17(4):337-341, 1991.

Mercer RT, Ferkeoch SL: Predictors of family functioning eight months following birth, *Nurs Res* 39(2):76-82, 1990.

Moriarty HJ: Key issues in the family research process: strategies for nurse researchers, *Adv Nurs Sci* 12(3):1-14, 1990.

Neal AG, Groat HT, Wicks JW: Attitudes about having children: a study of 600 couples in the early years of marriage, *J Marriage Fam* 51(2):313-328, 1989.

Shaw DS: The effects of divorce on children's adjustment: review and implications, *Behav Modif* 15(4):456-485, 1991.

Simon FB, Stierlin H, Wynne LC: *The language of family therapy,* New York, 1985, Family Process Press.

Smoyak SA: Changing American families. In Hoekelman RA and others, editors: *Primary pediatric care,* ed 2, St Louis, 1992, Mosby.

Sprey J: Current theorizing on the family: an appraisal, *J Marriage Fam* 50(4):875-890, 1988.

Tuttle G: How are the children coping? *Can Nurse* 88(11):13-16, 1992.

Wright LM, Leahey M, editors: *Nurses and families: a guide to family assessment and intervention,* Philadelphia, 1984, FA Davis.

Wright L, Leahey M, editors: *Families and chronic illness,* Springhouse, PA, 1987, Springhouse.

Wright L, Leahey M, editors: *Families and psychosocial problems,* Springhouse, PA, 1987, Springhouse Corp.

Family Configuration/Parenting

Bapiste DA: Psychotherapy with gay/lesbian couples and their children in "stepfamilies": a challenge for marriage and family therapists, *J Homosex* 14:223-238, 1987.

Bigner JJ, Jacobsen RB: Parenting behaviors of homosexual and heterosexual fathers, *J Homosex* 18(1/2):173-186, 1989.

Bozett FW: Gay men as fathers. In Hanson SMH, Bozett FW, editors: *Dimensions of fatherhood,* Beverly Hills, CA, 1985, Sage Publications.

Bozett FW, editor: *Gay and lesbian parents,* New York, 1987, Praeger.

Bozett FW: Intervening with gay families with an overweight adolescent. In Leahey M, Wright LM, editors: *Families and chronic illness,* Springhouse, PA, 1987, Springhouse.

Bozett FW: Gay fathers: a review of the literature, *J Homosex* 18(1/2):137-162, 1989.

Cramer D: Gay parents and their children: a review of research and practical implications, *J Counsel Dev* 64(8):504-507, 1986.

Falbo T, Polit-O'Hara DF: Only children: what do we know about them? *Pediatr Nurs* 11:356-360, 1985.

Green GD: Lesbian mothers: mental health considerations. In Bozett FW, editor: *Gay and lesbian parents,* New York, 1987, Praeger.

Green JL: Parenting skills and discipline. In Hoekelman RA and others, editors: *Primary pediatric care,* ed 2, St Louis, 1992, Mosby.

Hall M: Lesbian families: cultural and clinical issues, *Soc Work* 23:380-385, 1987.

Hitchens D, Kirkpatrick M: Lesbian mothers/gay fathers. In Benedek E, editor: *Child psychiatry and the law,* vol 2, New York, 1985, Brunner/Mazel.

Huxley P, Warner R: Primary prevention of parenting dysfunction in high-risk cases, *Am J Orthopsychiatry* 63(4):582-588, 1993.

Matteson DR: The heterosexually married gay and lesbian parent. In Bozett FW, editor: *Gay and lesbian parents,* New York, 1987, Praeger.

McCandlish BM: Against all odds: lesbian mother family dynamics. In Bozett FW, editor: *Gay and lesbian parents,* New York, 1987, Praeger.

Pennington SB: Children of lesbian mothers. In Bozett FW, editor: *Gay and lesbian parents,* New York, 1987, Praeger.

Riley D, Cochran MM: Naturally occurring childrearing advice for fathers: utilization of the personal social network, *J Marriage Fam* 47:275-286, 1985.

Robinson BE, Barret RL: *Fatherhood,* New York, 1986, Guilford.

Simons R and others: Husband and wife differences in determinants of parenting: a social learning/exchange model of parental behavior, *J Marriage Fam* 52(2):375-392, 1990.

Skeen P, Walters L, Robinson B: How parents of gays react to their children's homosexuality and to the threat of AIDS, *J Psychosoc Nurs* 26(12):7-10, 1988.

Wismont JM, Reame NE: The lesbian childbearing experience: assessing developmental tasks, *Image J Nurs Sch* 21(3):137-141, 1989.

Adoption

American Academy of Pediatrics, Committee on Early Childhood, Adoption, and Dependent Care: Health care of foster children, *Pediatrics* 79(4):644-646, 1987.

American Academy of Pediatrics, Task Force on Pediatric AIDS: Infants and children with acquired immunodeficiency syndrome: placement in adoption and foster care, *Pediatrics* 83(4):609-612, 1989.

Hajal F, Rosenberg D: The family life cycle in adoptive families, *Am J Orthopsychiatry* 61(1):78-85, 1991.

Hostetter MK and others: Unsuspected infectious diseases and other medical diagnoses in evaluation of internationally adopted children, *Pediatrics* 83(4):559-564, 1989.

Messer MM, Rasmussen NH: Southeast Asian children in America: the impact of change, *Pediatrics* 78(2):323-329, 1986.

Nickman SL: Adoption and foster care. In Hoekelman RA and others, editors: *Primary pediatric care,* ed 2, St Louis, 1992, Mosby.

Ritchie CW: Adoption: an option often overlooked, *Am J Nurs* 89:1156-1157, 1989.

Rosenwald E, Demi A: A primary prevention group for latency age children dealing with adoption issues, *J Child Adolesc Psychiatr Ment Health Nurs* 6(1):15-21, 1993.

Schor EL: Foster care, *Pediatr Clin North Am* 35(6):1241-1252, 1988.

Smith DW, Sherwen LN: The bonding process of mothers and adopted children, *Top Clin Nurs* 6(3):38-48, 1984.

Divorce

Amato P: The "child of divorce" as a person prototype: bias in the recall of information about children in divorced families, *J Marriage Fam* 53(1):59-69, 1991.

Arditti JA: Noncustodial fathers: an overview of policy and resources, *Fam Relations* 39(4):460-465, 1990.

Bray JH, Berger SH: Noncustodial father and paternal grandparent relationship in stepfamilies, *Fam Relations* 39(4):414-419, 1990.

Depner CE, Bray JH: Modes of participation for noncustodial parents: the challenge for research, policy, practice and education, *Fam Relations* 39(4):378-381, 1990.

Dvoskin AG: Child custody. In Hoekelman RA and others, editors: *Primary pediatric care,* ed 2, St Louis, 1992, Mosby.

Fairchild MW, Zebal BH: Children of divorce. In Hoekelman RA and others, editors: *Primary pediatric care,* ed 2, St Louis, 1992, Mosby.

Ferreiro BW: Presumption of joint custody: a family policy dilemma, *Fam Relations* 39(4):420-426, 1990.

Garvin V, Leber D, Kalter N: Children of divorce: predictors of change following preventive intervention, *Am J Orthopsychiatry* 61(3):438-447, 1991.

Johnston JR: Role diffusion and role reversal: structural variation in divorced families and children's functioning, *Fam Relations* 39(4): 405-413, 1990.

Kimard E, Reinherz H: Effects of marital disruption on children's school aptitude and achievement, *J Marriage Fam* 48:285-293, 1986.

Lebowitz ML: Divorce and the American teenager, *Pediatrics* 76:695-698, 1985.

Lowery CR: Child custody in divorce: parents' decisions and perceptions, *Fam Relations* 34:241-249, 1985.

Lowery CR, Settles SA: Effects of divorce on children: differential impact of custody and visitation patterns, *Fam Relations* 34:455-463, 1985.

Rankin RP, Maneker JS: The duration of marriage in a divorcing population: the impact on children, *J Marriage Fam* 47:43-52, 1985.

Rhyne MC: Understanding and supporting families in the process of divorce, *Nurse Practitioner* 11(12):37-51, 1986.

Wallerstein JS: Children after divorce: wounds that don't heal, *Perspect Psychiatr Care* 24(3/4):107-113, 1987-1988.

Webster-Stratton C: The relationship of marital support, conflict, and divorce to parent perceptions, behaviors, and childhood conduct problems, *J Marriage Fam* 51(2):417-430, 1989.

Single-Parenting

Burns CE: The hospitalization experience and single-parent families: a time of special vulnerability, *Nurs Clin North Am* 19:285-293, 1984.

Grief GL: Children and housework in the single father family, *Fam Relations* 34:353-357, 1985.

Grief GL: Single fathers rearing children, *J Marriage Fam* 47:185-191, 1985.

Kissman K, Allen J: *Single-parent families*, Newbury Park, CA, 1993, Sage Publications.

McLanahan S, Booth K: Mother-only families: problems, prospects, and politics, *J Marriage Fam* 51(3):557-580, 1989.

Rarratt M, Roach M, Colbert K: Single mothers and their infants: factors associated with optimal parenting, *Fam Relations* 40(4):448-454, 1991.

Risman BJ, Park K: Just the two of us: parent-child relationships in single-parent homes, *J Marriage Fam* 50(4):1049-1062, 1988.

Roberts P, Matthews K: Unmarried motherhood, *Can Nurse* 89(4):33-34, 1993.

Weinberg TS: Single fatherhood: how is it different? *Pediatr Nurs* 11:173-175, 1985.

Reconstituted Families

Clawson JF, Sears J: A stepmother in the family, *Pediatr Nurs* 15(3):249-251, 1989.

Coleman M, Ganong L: Stepfamily self-help books: brief annotations and ratings, *Fam Relations* 38(1):90-96, 1989.

Crosbie-Burnett M: Application of family stress theory to remarriage: a model for assessing and helping stepfamilies, *Fam Relations* 38(3):323-331, 1989.

Ganong LH, Coleman M: Do mutual children cement bonds in stepfamilies? *J Marriage Fam* 50(3):687-698, 1988.

Hetherington EM: Coping with family transitions: winners, losers, and survivors, *Child Dev* 60(1):1-14, 1989.

Kurdek L, Fine M: Cognitive correlates of satisfaction for mothers and stepfathers in stepfather families, *J Marriage Fam* 53(3):567-572, 1991.

Peek CW and others: Patterns of functioning in families of remarried and first-married couples, *J Marriage Fam* 50(3):699-708, 1988.

Pill CJ: Stepfamilies: redefining the family, *Fam Relations* 39(2):186-193, 1990.

Pink JET, Wampler KS: Problem areas in stepfamilies: cohesion, adaptability, and the stepfather-adolescent relationship, *Fam Relations* 34:327-335, 1985.

Reuter L, Strang V: Yours, mine, and ours: stepparents and their children, *MCN* 11:264-266, 1986.

Romanczuk AN: Helping the stepparent parent, *MCN* 12:106-110, 1987.

Dual-Earner Family

American Academy of Pediatrics, Committee on Psychosocial Aspects of Child and Family Health: The mother working outside the home, *Pediatrics* 73:874-875, 1984.

Atkinson A: Providers' evaluation of the effect of family day care on own family relationships, *Fam Relations* 37:399-404, 1988.

Benin M, Edwards D: Adolescents' chores: the differences between dual- and single-career families, *J Marriage Fam* 52(2):361-373, 1990.

Brazelton T: *Working and caring*, Reading, MA, 1987, Addison-Wesley.

Brazelton TB: Putting a child in day care: issues for working parents, *Pediatrics* 91(1, pt 2):271-272, 1993.

Bredekamp S: Day-care standards: need and impact, *Pediatrics* 91(1, pt 2): 234-236, 1993.

Caldwell BM: Impact of day care on the child, *Pediatrics* 91 (1, pt 2):225-228, 1993.

Day care for early preschool children: implications for the child and family, *Am J Psychiatry* 150(8):1281-1287, 1993.

Floge L: The dynamics of child-care use and some implications for women's employment, *J Marriage Fam* 47:143-154, 1985.

Hanson S, Ooms T: The economic costs and rewards of two-earner, two-parent families, *J Marriage Fam* 53(3):622-634, 1991.

Kelley SJ, Brant R, Waterman J: Sexual abuse of children in day care centers, *Child Abuse Negl* 17(1):71-89, 1993.

Kuhns CL, Holloway SD: Characteristics of caregivers that promote children's development in day care, *J Pediatr Nurs* 7(4)280-285, 1992.

MacEwen K, Barling J: Effects of maternal employment experiences on children's behavior via mood, cognitive difficulties, and parenting behavior, *J Marriage Fam* 53(3):635-644, 1991.

Menaghan D, Parcel T: Parental employment and family life: research in the 1980s, *J Marriage Fam* 52(4):1079-1098, 1990.

Osterholm MT and others: Infectious diseases and child day care, *Pediatr Infect Dis J* 11(8, suppl):S31-S41, 1992.

Schroeder P, Reder ND: Ensuring quality, affordable child care: mobilizing for action, *Pediatrics* 91(1, pt 2):244-247, 1993.

Thacker SB and others: Infectious diseases and injuries in child day care: opportunities for healthier children, *JAMA* 268(13):1720-1726, 1992.

Thomas VG: Determinant of global life happiness and marital happiness in dual-career black couples, *Fam Relations* 39(2):174-178, 1990.

Tiedje LB, Collins C: Combining employment and motherhood, *MCN* 14:9-14, 1989.

CHAPTER 4

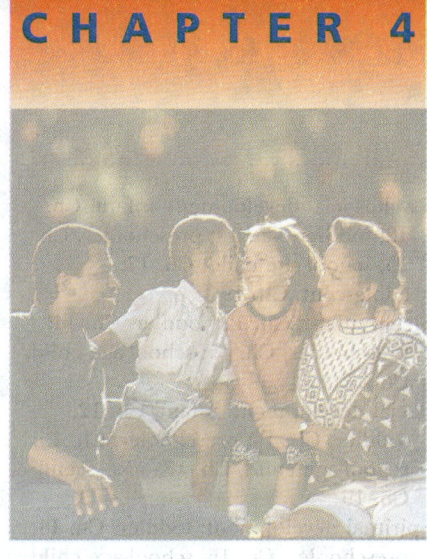

Growth and Development of Children

CHAPTER OUTLINE

RELATED TOPICS

GROWTH AND DEVELOPMENT

FOUNDATIONS OF GROWTH AND DEVELOPMENT

Growth and development, usually referred to as a unit, expresses the sum of the numerous changes that take place during the lifetime of an individual. The entire course is a dynamic process that encompasses several interrelated dimensions: growth, maturation, differentiation, and development. ***Growth*** implies a change in quantity. It results when cells divide and synthesize new proteins. This increase in the number and size of cells is reflected in an increase in the size and weight of the whole or any of its parts.

Maturation, which literally means to ripen, is described as aging or as an increase in competence and adaptability. It is usually used to describe a qualitative change (i.e., a change in the complexity of a structure that makes it possible for that structure to begin functioning or to function at a higher level).

Differentiation is primarily a biologic description of the processes by which early cells and structures are systematically modified and altered to achieve specific and characteristic physical and chemical properties. It is sometimes used to describe one of the trends in development (i.e., mass to specific).

Development is a gradual growth and expansion. It also involves a qualitative change, in this case from a lower to a more advanced stage of complexity. Development is the emerging and expanding of capacities of the individual to provide progressively greater facility in functioning. It is achieved through growth, maturation, and learning.

All of these processes are interrelated. Although they are simultaneous, ongoing processes, none occurs apart from the others. The child's body becomes larger and more complex; the personality simultaneously expands in scope and complexity. Very simply, growth can be viewed as a *quantitative* change, and development as a *qualitative* change.

Stages of Growth and Development

Most authorities in the field of child development conveniently categorize child growth and behavior into approximate age stages or in terms that describe the features of an age-group. The age ranges of these stages are admittedly arbitrary, and since they do not take into account individual differences, they cannot be applied to all children with any degree of precision. However, this categorization affords a convenient means to describe the characteristics associated with the majority of children at periods when distinctive developmental changes appear and specific developmental tasks must be accomplished. It is also significant for nurses to know that there are characteristic health problems peculiar to each major phase of development. The sequence of descriptive age periods and subperiods that is used here and elaborated on in subsequent chapters is listed in the box on p. 107.

Methods of Studying Growth and Development

The early growth period in the human being extends over a longer time than that of any other mammalian species. The long period of childhood allows for more elaborate brain development, body growth, and the development of those characteristics of personality that distinguish humans from lower animals.

■ Judy Holt Rollins, RN, MS, revised this chapter.

DEVELOPMENTAL AGE PERIODS

Prenatal period: Conception to birth
Germinal: Conception to approximately 2 weeks
Embryonic: 2 to 8 weeks
Fetal: 8 to 40 weeks (birth)
A rapid growth rate and total dependency make this one of the most crucial periods in the developmental process. The relationship between maternal health and certain manifestations in the newborn emphasizes the importance of adequate prenatal care to the health and well-being of the infant

Infancy period: Birth to 12 or 18 months
Neonatal: Birth to 28 days
Infancy: 1 to approximately 12 months
The infancy period is one of rapid motor, cognitive, and social development. Through mutuality with the caregiver (parent), the infant establishes a basic trust in the world and the foundation for future interpersonal relationships. The critical first month of life, although part of the infancy period, is often differentiated from the remainder because of the major physical adjustments to extrauterine existence and the psychologic adjustment of the parent.

Early childhood: 1 to 6 years
Toddler: 1 to 3 years
Preschool: 3 to 6 years
This period, which extends from the time the children attain upright locomotion until they enter school, is characterized by intense activity and discovery. It is a time of marked physical and personality development. Motor development advances steadily. Children at this age acquire language and wider social relationships, learn role standards, gain self-control and mastery, develop increasing awareness of dependence and independence, and begin to develop a self-concept.

Middle childhood: 6 to 11 or 12 years
Frequently referred to as the "school age," this period of development is one in which the child is directed away from the family group and is centered around the wider world of peer relationships. There is steady advancement in physical, mental, and social development with emphasis on developing skill competencies. Social cooperation and early moral development take on more importance with relevance for later life stages. This is a critical period in the development of a self-concept.

Later childhood: 11 to 19 years
Prepubertal: 10 to 13 years
Adolescence: 13 to approximately 18 years
The period of rapid maturation and change known as adolescence is considered to be a transitional period that begins at the onset of puberty and extends to the point of entry into the adult world—usually high school graduation. Biologic and personality maturation are accompanied by physical and emotional turmoil, and there is redefining of the self-concept. In the late adolescent period the child begins to internalize all previously learned values and to focus on an individual, rather than a group, identity.

To determine whether growth and development have taken place, the child can be compared with a representative group of children at the same point in time (cross-sectional method), or the same child can be measured and compared at different points in time (longitudinal method). ***Standards*** or ***norms*** regarding the average age for expected parameters to appear, such as height, weight, and motor skills, have been established by these two contrasting methods.

The ***cross-sectional*** method, which tests or measures the characteristics of a number of children representing the various ages or stages of development, is the more common. The observations of children are made at the same point in time. For example, a group of schoolchildren, ages 6 to 12 years, are measured for specific characteristics such as height, weight, mental ability, motor ability, or vocabulary. The data collected and averaged on a group of 6-year-old children, for instance, provide information on the expected achievement of a child in that age-group. This method is especially useful for establishing norms for a given age-group with or without other factors.

The ***longitudinal method*** is often used to determine growth trends and rates. Each child in a group of children is observed and measured periodically over a number of years and through successive stages of growth and development. This approach is also useful in assessing the long-term or delayed effects of an early experience, such as a prolonged illness, malnutrition, or maternal rejection. Although the longitudinal method is more difficult to carry out, the growth and development of a child can be compared at any moment with a representative group of children and can be followed through successive stages to determine the speed and direction of that child's distinctive growth.

Patterns of Growth and Development

There are definite and predictable patterns in growth and development that are continuous, orderly, and progressive. These patterns, sometimes referred to as trends or principles, are universal and basic to all human beings. However, each human being accomplishes these in a manner and time unique to that individual.

Directional Trends. Growth and development proceed in regular, related directions or gradients and reflect the physical development and maturation of neuromuscular functions (Fig. 4-1). The first pattern is the ***cephalocaudal,*** or ***head-to-tail,*** direction. The head end of the organism develops first and is very large and complex, whereas the lower end is small and simple and takes shape at a later period. The physical evidence of this trend is most apparent during the period before birth, but it also applies to postnatal behavioral development. Infants achieve motor control of the head before the trunk and extremities, hold their back erect before they stand, use their eyes before their hands, and gain control of their hands before they have control of their feet.

Second, the ***proximodistal,*** or ***near-to-far,*** trend applies to the midline-to-peripheral concept. A conspicuous illustration is the early embryonic development of limb buds, followed by rudimentary fingers and toes. In the infant, shoulder control precedes mastery of the hands, the whole hand is used as a unit before the fingers can be manipulated, and the central nervous system develops more rapidly than the peripheral nervous system. These trends or patterns are bilateral and appear to be symmetric; each side develops in the same direction and at the same rate as the other.

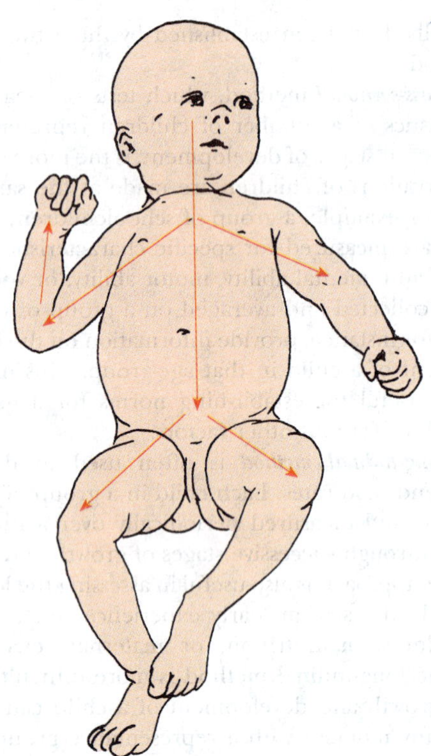

FIG. 4-1 Cephalocaudal describes a "head-to-tail" directional pattern of growth.

The third trend in directional growth, ***differentiation,*** describes development from simple operations to more complex activities and functions. From very broad, global patterns of behavior, more specific, refined patterns emerge. All areas of development (physical, mental, social, emotional) proceed in this direction. Through the processes of development and differentiation, early embryonal cells with vague, undifferentiated functions progress to an immensely complex organism composed of highly specialized and diversified cells, tissues, and organs. Generalized development precedes specific or specialized development; gross, random muscle movements take place before fine muscle control.

Sequential Trends. In all dimensions of growth and development there is a definite, predictable sequence. It is orderly and continuous, with each child normally passing through every stage. New biologic parts and behaviors arise out of and build on those already established. This continuity with the past, or ***epigenesis,*** serves as a foundation for the future and requires interaction with a suitable environment at the proper time. Each stage is affected by those preceding it and affects those that follow. Sequential patterns have been described for motor skills such as locomotion and use of the hands, and for types of behavior such as language and social skills. Children crawl before they stand, and stand before they walk. Children first play alone, then with others in increasing numbers and increasingly complex activities.

Developmental Pace. Although there is a fixed, precise order to development, it does not progress at the same rate or pace in all children. There are periods of accelerated growth and periods of decelerated growth in both total body growth and growth of subsystems. The very rapid growth rate before and after birth gradually levels off throughout early childhood. Relatively slow during middle childhood, the rate increases markedly at the beginning of adolescence and levels off in early adulthood.

Research suggests that normal growth, in particular, height in infants, may occur in brief (possibly even 24-hour) bursts that punctuate long periods in which no measurable growth takes place (Lampl, 1992). Further, findings indicate a stuttering or ***saltatory*** pattern of growth that follows no regular cycle and can occur after "quiet" periods that last as long as 4 weeks. Mothers reported that their children were usually fussy and voraciously hungry a day or two before the growth spurt.

The focus of development and growth shifts at successive stages in development. For instance, the head grows most rapidly before birth, whereas other body parts grow more slowly; after birth other structures grow faster than the head. This growth pattern accounts for shifts in body proportion, facial characteristics, and voice. Similarly, one type of development seems to take precedence over another during various periods of growth. At times of rapid growth, other development may reach a plateau. For example, when children begin to walk, the thrills of upright locomotion take precedence over other activity, such as speech, and they may not learn any new words for 3 to 4 months. Schoolwork may suffer during the early adolescent growth spurt.

Sensitive Periods. There are limited times during the process of growth when children interact with a particular environment in a specific manner. Critical periods, sensitive periods, and vulnerable periods are those times in an organism's lifetime when it is more susceptible to positive or negative influences. Touwen (1989) suggests that ***critical period*** implies the need for specific stimulation, whereas ***sensitive*** and ***vulnerable periods*** of maturation are those during which external conditions may be particularly harmful to specific tissues, organs, or systems.

The quality of interactions during these sensitive periods determines whether the effects on the children will be beneficial or harmful. The character and extent of the interaction's consequences depend on the nature of the environmental influences and the stage of development. For example, physiologic maturation of the central nervous system is influenced by adequacy and timing of contributions from the environment, such as stimulation and nutrition. The first 3 months of prenatal life is a sensitive period for physical growth. During this period of accelerated growth and differentiation, specific organs and systems are most vulnerable to environmental influences; the earlier the impact, the more far-reaching are the effects.

Psychologic development also appears to have sensitive periods when an environmental event has maximum influence on the developing personality. Observers have identified periods in development when behavior patterns are most readily acquired. For example, primary socialization occurs during the first year, when infants make their initial social attachments and establish a basic trust in the world.

At this time a warm, loving relationship with the caregiver is fundamental to a healthy parent-child relationship (see Promote Parent-Infant Bonding [Attachment], Chapter 8).

The sensitive period concept might also be applied to readiness for learning skills such as toilet training or reading. In these instances there appears to be an opportune time when the skill is best learned. However, if the skill is not learned at this time, acquisition at a later time is still possible. The optimum time for school entry has been based on the readiness to acquire the specific types of skills learned in the school setting.

Individual Differences

Each child grows in his or her own unique and personal way. Great individual variation exists in the age at which developmental milestones are reached. The sequence is predictable; the exact timing is not. Rates of growth vary from one individual to another, and measurements are defined in terms of ranges to allow for individual differences among children. In the United States approximately 2 million children are shorter than 98% of their peers; most of these children are healthy, with patterns of growth that are normal variants from other children their age (Henry and Giordano, 1992). Some children are fast growers, others are moderate, and some are slower to reach maturity. For example, periods of fast growth, such as the pubescent growth spurt, may begin earlier or later in some children than in others. Children may grow fast or slow during the spurt and may finish sooner or later than other children. Gender is an influential factor because girls seem to be more advanced in physiologic growth at all ages.

The ***terminal points*** at which growth ceases vary immensely from one child to another. For example, some individuals will grow until reaching a height of over 180 cm (6 feet), and others will cease growing at 150 cm (5 feet); the majority will achieve varying heights between the two. Females as a group reach both height and weight terminal points before males.

There appears to be a tendency for organisms to strive for optimum developmental potential in both structure and function. When environmental factors interfere with normal development for a time (e.g., during periods of inadequate food supply or illness), children's bodies will usually make up for the interrupted period and return to their characteristic pattern of growth. However, if the deprivation is severe or occurs throughout a critical period, development may be permanently impaired.

BIOLOGIC GROWTH AND DEVELOPMENT

As children grow, their external dimensions change. These changes are accompanied by corresponding alterations in structure and function of internal organs and tissues, reflecting the gradual acquisition of physiologic competence. These alterations, although progressive and interdependent, are not a uniform process but are characterized by cycles of accelerated and slow development that vary from organ to organ and system to system. Skeletal muscle growth

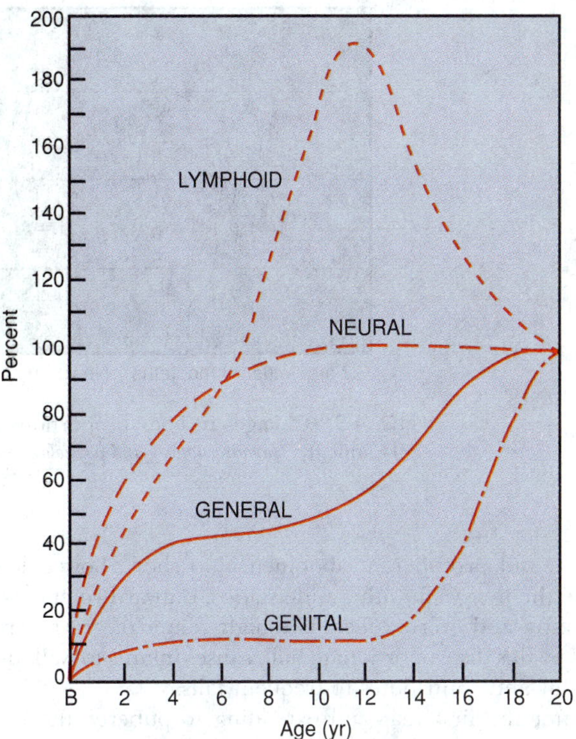

FIG. 4-2 Growth rates for body as a whole and three types of tissues. ***Lymphoid type:*** thymus, lymph nodes, and intestinal lymph masses; ***neural type:*** brain, dura, spinal cord, optic apparatus, and head dimensions; ***general type:*** body as a whole, external dimensions, and respiratory, digestive, renal, circulatory, and musculoskeletal systems. (Modified from Harris JA and others: *The measurement of man,* Minneapolis, 1930, University of Minnesota Press.)

approximates whole body growth; brain, lymphoid, adrenal, and reproductive tissues follow distinct and individual patterns (Fig. 4-2).

External Proportions

Variations in the growth rate of different tissues and organ systems produce significant changes in body proportions during childhood. The cephalocaudal trend of development is most evident in total body growth as indicated by these changes (Fig. 4-3). During fetal development the head is the fastest growing part, and at 2 months of gestation the head constitutes 50% of total body length. During infancy growth of the trunk predominates; the legs are the most rapidly growing part during childhood; then, in adolescence, the trunk once again elongates. In the newborn the lower limbs are one third of the total body length but only 15% of the total body weight; in the adult the lower limbs constitute one half of the total body height and 30% of total body weight. As growth proceeds, the midpoint in head-to-toe measurements gradually descends from a level even with the umbilicus at birth to the level of the symphysis pubis at maturity.

The first year is a period of rapid growth dominated by lengthening of the trunk and accumulation of subcutaneous fat. When infants begin to walk, their large head, heavy

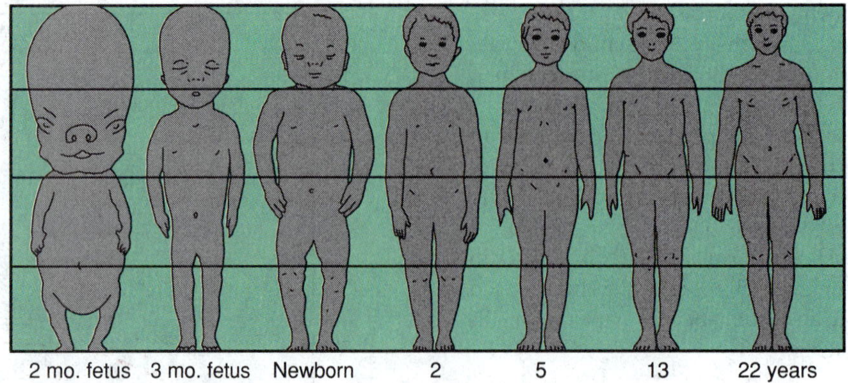

FIG. 4-3 Changes in body proportions from before birth to adulthood. (From Crouch JE, McClintic JR: *Human anatomy and physiology,* ed 2, New York, 1976, John Wiley & Sons.)

trunk, and protuberant abdomen atop short, bowed legs force them to walk with a wide stance, outward rotation of the hips, and everted feet. The high center of gravity created by this disproportionate bulk causes infants to walk unsteadily and contributes to frequent falls.

After the first year and extending to puberty, the legs grow more rapidly than any other part. The bowlegged appearance disappears with locomotion, the abdomen is held in, and the body becomes slender and elongated. Until puberty this slender, long-legged build is characteristic of both sexes; in similar clothes and hairstyle the two sexes are indistinguishable. With the onset of puberty there is a marked alteration in body proportion when all structures show the effects of the pubertal growth spurt. The feet and hands are first to increase in rate of growth; therefore during this transient period they appear large and ungainly in relation to the rest of the body, which is often a source of embarrassment to the adolescent. The trunk again grows faster than the legs, so that a large portion of the increase in height at adolescence is a result of trunk growth.

Since the legs continue to grow until puberty, early-maturing children have shorter than average legs, and the legs of later-maturing children are longer. Inasmuch as the onset of puberty is approximately 2½ years earlier in girls, for a while girls are larger than boys, and girls' legs are shorter than boys' legs. Laterality of growth follows rapid linear growth; both boys and girls proceed to "fill out" during the later stages of adolescent growth.

One of the more outstanding features of changing body proportion is shoulder and hip breadth as a result of hormone secretion from the maturing gonads. Shoulder and hip growth increases in both sexes, but the shoulder width in boys is considerably greater than in girls. The anteroposterior hip diameter increases in girls, and the female pelvis becomes wider, shallower, and roomier than the male pelvis. The differences in deposition of fat produce the distinctive feminine contours in girls, whereas boys lose subcutaneous fat.

Facial proportions show characteristic changes during childhood. In infancy and early childhood the face is small in relation to the skull (Fig. 4-4). The size of the cranial vault reflects the advanced development of the brain. The brain has achieved 25% of its adult size at birth and 50% at the end of 1 year. Over 90% of the growth of the brain cavity has been reached by the end of the fifth year, and 98% has been achieved at age 15 years.

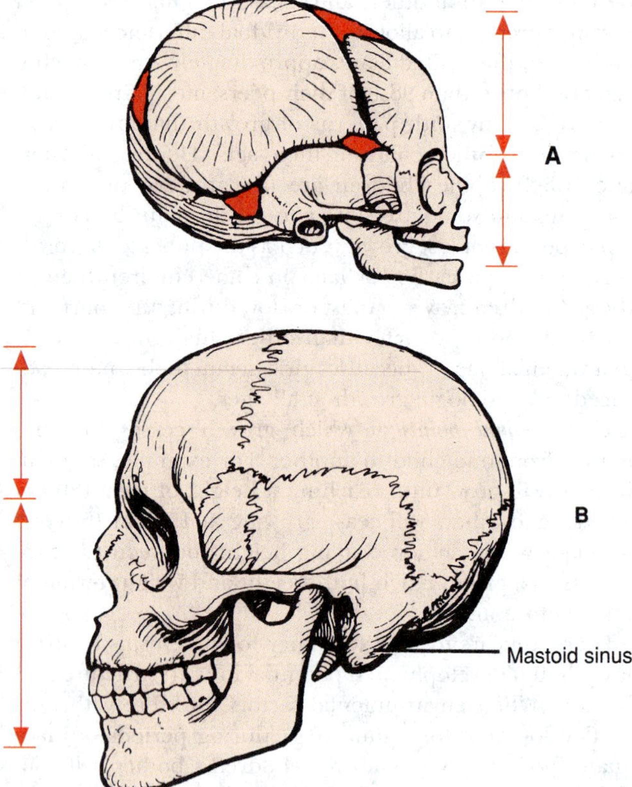

FIG. 4-4 Comparison of face and cranial proportions in, **A,** infant, and, **B,** adult skulls. Note differences in relative size of face and angle of mandible, absence of mastoid sinus in infant, and absence of fontanels *(red)* in adult.

After the first year the facial skeleton grows more rapidly than the brain case. The principal growth occurs in the jaws as they enlarge to accommodate the teeth and in the

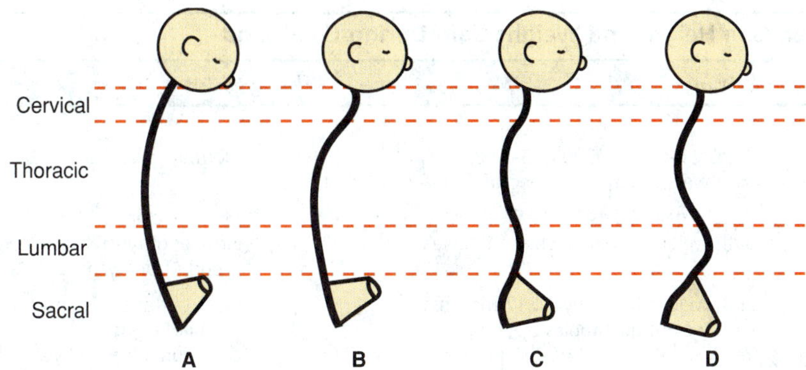

FIG. 4-5 Development of spinal curvatures. **A,** Newborn infant. **B,** Cervical secondary curvature. **C,** Lumbar secondary curvature. **D,** Lordosis.

muscles of mastication as they develop. The face grows first in width and then in length, so that the child's face appears to emerge from underneath the skull, particularly during adolescence.

The size of the face relative to the skull has implications for health in the infant and young child. The large, heavy cranium is the primary site of injury in falls. The changing dimensions of the face alter the diameter and angle of ear structures, particularly the external auditory meatus and the eustachian tube. The latter contributes significantly to the incidence of middle ear infection.

Posture is also altered by growth and maturation of various structures. Within the narrow confines of the uterus the prenatal posture is one of total flexion. The spine curves with the head and extremities bent on the child. The bones in the vertebral column of the newborn form two primary curvatures, one in the thoracic region and one in the sacral region (Fig. 4-5, *A*). Both are forward, concave curvatures that rely largely on the shape of their component bones. The thoracic curve is relatively stable, and movement is limited in scope and amount by thin, intervertebral discs and oblique spinous processes. The sacral curve eventually becomes fused and permanently fixed.

As the infant gains head control, at approximately 3 months of age, a secondary curvature appears in the cervical region (Fig. 4-5, *B*). This curve, unlike the primary curvatures, is convex forward, and its mobility is maintained by thick intervertebral discs and the tension of muscles stretched across its convexity.

To maintain a sitting posture, another secondary curvature develops in the lumbar region (Fig. 4-5, *C*). Like the cervical curve, the lumbar curve is convex and mobile, depends largely on intervertebral discs, and is controlled by the large postural muscles of the spine. When children assume an upright posture in their initial efforts to walk, they compensate for a high center of gravity and the weight of a large liver by an exaggerated lumbar curvature, or ***lordosis*** (Fig. 4-5, *D*). With advancing skill in locomotion there is a gradual progression toward normal upright posture. When situations cause a delay in holding up the head or sitting, the secondary curvatures may fail to develop at the expected time.

Biologic Determinants of Growth

A prominent feature of childhood and adolescence is physical growth. In some tissues growth is continuous (e.g., bone growth and dentition); in others significant alterations occur at specific stages (e.g., appearance of secondary sex characteristics). Satisfactory growth achievement is most commonly judged in terms of an increase in body weight, height, and skeletal growth. Serial measurements taken over time and compared with standardized norms can assess a child's developmental progress with a high degree of confidence. Table 4-1 and Fig. 4-6 indicate the general trends in height and weight gain during childhood.

Linear growth, or ***height,*** occurs almost entirely as a result of skeletal growth and is considered to be a stable measure of general growth. It is not uniform throughout life, but when maturation of the skeleton is complete, linear growth ceases. The maximum growth in length occurs before birth, but the newborn continues to grow at a rapid, though slower, rate. As the months pass, the growth rate rapidly decelerates. By 2 years of age children normally have achieved 50% of their adult height. By age 4 birth length has usually doubled.

At approximately 3 years of age the child begins a relatively stable and steady growth rate of 5 to 6 cm (2 to 2½ inches) per year that continues for the next 9 years. (Occasionally a child will exhibit a transitory midgrowth height increase at age 6 or 7.) This long midgrowth period is ended by a sudden and marked acceleration, the adolescent growth spurt. Although there is wide variation, this increase, which begins about ages 10½ to 11 in girls and 12½ to 13 in boys, lasts approximately 2 to 2½ years. During this time a boy may add 20 cm (8 inches) to his height and a girl 16 cm (6½ inches). Usually, 98% of the terminal height is reached by age 16½ in girls but not until age 17¾ in boys (Table 4-2).

Predictions are of little value until the second year of life. By this time the child has frequently compensated for any deviations related to prematurity or other prenatal influences. However, children with lower birth weights are likely to remain shorter and lighter throughout childhood (Binkin and others, 1988). Variability in the onset of puberty may also alter the predictive value in this age-group.

TABLE 4-1 General Trends in Height and Weight Gain During Childhood

AGE	WEIGHT*	HEIGHT*
Infants		
Birth–6 months	Weekly gain: 140-200 g (5-7 oz) Birth weight doubles by end of first 4-7 months†	Monthly gain: 2.5 cm (1 inch)
6-12 months	Weight gain: 85-140 g (3-5 oz) Birth weight triples by end of first year	Monthly gain: 1.25 cm (½ inch) Birth length increases by approximately 50% by end of first year
Toddlers	Birth weight triples by 14-17 months† Birth weight quadruples by age 2½ Yearly gain: 2-3 kg (4½-6½ lb)	Height at age 2 is approximately 50% of eventual adult height Gain during second year: about 12 cm (4¾ inches) Gain during third year: about 6-8 cm (2⅜-3¼ inches)
Preschoolers	Yearly gain: 2-3 kg (4½-6½ lb)	Birth length doubles by age 4 Yearly gain: 5-7.5 cm (2-3 inches)
School-age children	Yearly gain: 2-3 kg (4½-6½ lb)	Yearly gain after age 7: 5 cm (2 inches) Birth length triples by about age 13
Pubertal growth spurt		
Females—10-14 years	Weight gain: 7-25 kg (15-55 lb) Mean: 17.5 kg (38⅛ lb)	Height gain: 5-25 cm (2-10 inches); approximately 95% of mature height achieved by onset of menarche or skeletal age of 13 Mean: 20.5 cm (8¼ inches)
Males—11-16 years	Weight gain: 7-30 kg (15-65 lb) Mean: 23.7 kg (52⅛ lb)	Height gain: 10-30 cm (4-12 inches); approximately 95% of mature height achieved by skeletal age of 15 years Mean: 27.5 cm (11 inches)

*Yearly height and weight gains for each age-group represent averaged estimates from a variety of sources.
†Jung and Czajka-Narins, 1985.

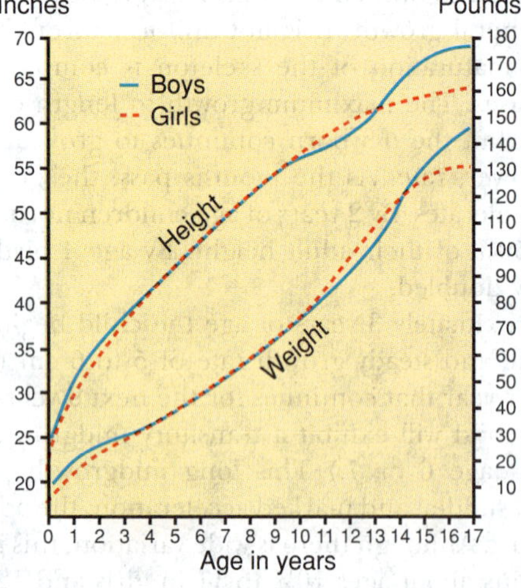

FIG. 4-6 Average height and weight curves for boys and girls. The earlier increase for girls at adolescence is clearly shown. Most girls are larger than boys between ages 11 and 13, probably as a result of earlier influence of sex hormones on physical growth. (From Lowrey GH: *Growth and development of children,* ed 8, St Louis, 1986, Mosby.)

Such predictions are valuable tools to help parents and their slow-maturing children accept the child's unique pattern of growth and to help these puzzled children understand why they are different from their taller age-mates. Predictions are sometimes useful in preventing possible disappointment in the preparation for occupations or careers that have height restrictions and require early beginning physical preparation (e.g., ballet dancing). More important, if parents are satisfied that a child's apparently small size merely reflects the normal expectations based on their own adult size, they will be less likely to make eating an issue, which can result in obesity or food refusal and poor appetite.

TABLE 4-2 Percentage of Mature Height Attained at Different Ages

CHRONOLOGIC AGE (YEARS)	PERCENT OF EVENTUAL HEIGHT	
	BOYS	GIRLS
1	42.2	44.7
2	49.5	52.8
6	65.2	70.3
10	78.0	84.4
11	81.1	88.4
12	84.2	92.9
13	87.3	96.5
14	91.5	98.3
15	96.1	99.1
16	98.3	99.6
17	99.3	100.0
18	99.8	100.0

Modified from Bayley N: Growth curves of height and weight for boys and girls, scaled according to physical maturity, *J Pediatr* 48:187-194, 1956.

At birth, ***weight*** is more variable than height and to a greater extent is a reflection of the intrauterine environment. The rate of weight gain increases rapidly for a short time after birth but soon decreases markedly. After the second year the "normal" rate of weight gain, just like the growth rate in height, assumes a steady annual increase—approximately 2 to 2.75 kg (4½ to 6 pounds) per year—until the adolescent growth spurt. The weight gain usually lags behind the gain in height by about 3 months.

Lifetime weight gain is subject to numerous intrinsic and extrinsic factors that are discussed as they apply to specific situations or conditions. Growth responses become apparent by changes in weight before they appear in other aspects of growth. Weight gain is usually considered to be an indication of satisfactory growth progress in a child and is probably the best index of nutrition and growth. However, it may be difficult to determine if this increase in weight is caused by healthy tissue development or by an unhealthy deposition of fat.

Both ***bone age*** determinations and the state of ***dentition*** are used as indicators of growth (for bone age, see below; see also Chapters 12 and 17 for dentition). Because of its relative regularity, the eruption of teeth is sometimes used as a criterion for developmental assessment, especially the 6-year molar, which seems to be the most universally consistent in timing. However, dental maturation does not correlate well with bone age and is less reliable as an index of biologic age. Retarded eruption is more common than accelerated eruption and may be caused by heredity or may indicate health problems such as endocrine disturbance, nutritional factors, or malposition of teeth.

Skeletal Growth and Maturation

Growth of the skeleton follows a genetically programmed developmental plan that not only furnishes the best indicator of general growth progress but also provides the best estimate of biologic age. Some degree of assessment can be achieved by observation of facial bone development (i.e., nasal bridge height, prominence of malar eminences, and mandibular size), but the most accurate measure of general development is the determination of osseous maturation by radiography (x-ray examination). ***Skeletal,*** or ***bone, age*** appears to correlate more closely with other measures of physiologic maturity (e.g., onset of menarche) than with chronologic age or height. Bone age is determined by comparing the mineralization of ossification centers and advancing bony form to age-related standards. Skeletal maturation begins with the appearance of centers of ossification in the embryo and ends when the last epiphysis is firmly fused to the shaft of its bone. In long bones ossification takes place in two centers. It begins in the ***diaphysis*** (the long central portion of the bone) from a "primary" center and continues in the ***epiphysis*** (the end portions of the bone) at "secondary" centers of ossification. Situated between the diaphysis and the epiphysis, an epiphyseal cartilage plate unites with the diaphysis by columns of spongy tissue, the ***metaphysis.*** At this site the active growth in length takes place, and interference with this growth site by trauma or infection can result in deformity. Under the influence of hormones, principally pituitary growth hormone and thyroid hormone, bones increase in circumference by the formation of new bone tissue beneath the membrane surrounding the bone (periosteum) and in length by proliferation of cartilage.

Over the growth period of approximately 19 to 20 years, this development can be divided into three distinct but overlapping phases: (1) ossification of the diaphysis, (2) ossification of the epiphysis, and (3) invasion and subsequent replacement of growth cartilage plates with bony fusion of epiphysis and diaphysis. These changes do not take place in all bones simultaneously but appear in a specific order and at a specific time. Although the speed of bone growth and amount of maturity at specific ages vary from one child to another, the order of ossification is constant.

The first centers of ossification appear in the 2-month-old embryo, and at birth the number is approximately 400, about half the number at maturity. New centers appear at regular intervals during the growth period and provide the basis for assessment of bone age. Postnatally, at 5 to 6 months of age, the earliest centers to appear are those of the capitate and hamate bones in the wrist. Therefore radiographs of the hand and wrist provide the most useful areas for screening to determine skeletal age, especially before age 6 years (Fig. 4-7). These centers appear earlier in girls than in boys.

Skeletal development advances until maturity through growth of ossification centers and lengthening of long bones at the metaphysis and cartilage plates. Linear growth can continue as long as the epiphysis is separated from the diaphysis by the cartilage plate; when the cartilage disappears, the epiphysis unites with the diaphysis and growth ceases. Epiphyseal fusion also follows an orderly sequence; thus the timing of epiphyseal closure furnishes another medium for measuring skeletal age.

Neurologic Maturation

In contrast to other body tissues, which grow rapidly after birth, the nervous system grows proportionately more rapidly before birth. Two periods of rapid brain cell growth occur during fetal life: a dramatic increase in the number of neurons between 15 and 20 weeks of gestation, and another increase at 30 weeks, which extends to 1 year of age. The rapid growth of infancy continues during early childhood, then slows to a more gradual rate during later childhood and adolescence.

It is believed that no new nerve cells appear after the sixth month of fetal life. Postnatal growth consists of increasing the amount of cytoplasm around the nuclei of existing cells, increasing the number and intricacy of communications with other cells, and advancing their peripheral axions to keep pace with expanding body dimensions. This allows for increasingly complex movement and behavior. Neurophysiologic changes also provide the foundation for language, learning, and behavior development. Neurologic and electroencephalographic development are sometimes used as indicators of maturational age in the early weeks of life.

Growth of the ***brain*** is reflected in head circumference,

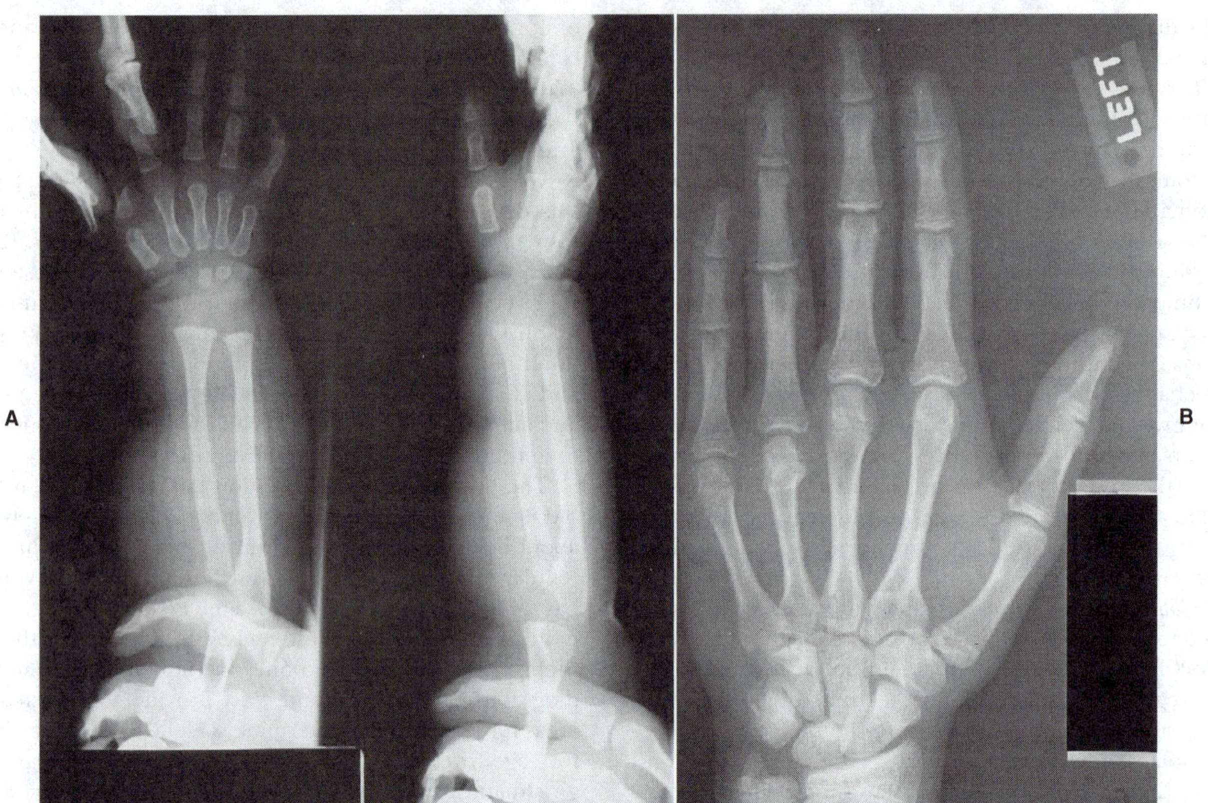

FIG. 4-7 Radiographs illustrating bone age in children. **A,** Eight-month-old (note complete ossification in adult fingers holding child's arm). **B,** Fourteen-year-old, epiphyses visible.

which increases six times as much during the first year as it does in the second year of life (see Appendix C). One half of the postnatal brain growth is achieved by 1 year of age, 75% by age 3, and 90% by age 6. The brain constitutes 12% of the body weight at birth, doubles in weight in the first year, and has tripled by age 5 or 6 years. Thereafter growth slows until the brain is only about 2% of total body weight in adulthood.

Surface configuration also changes with development. The early embryonic brain surface is smooth, but sulci deepen with advancing development throughout childhood. At birth the cortex is only about one half its adult thickness, resulting in very little cortical control over body movements at birth. Movements are guided principally by primitive reflexes (see Chapter 8). With advancing development and maturation the brain, through association pathways, exercises increasing control over much of reflex activity. This allows the growing child to perform progressively complex tasks requiring coordinated movements. Persistence of primitive reflexes may suggest defective cortical development.

Cortical control is closely associated with the acquisition of a myelin coating on the nerves. Although nerve fibers are able to conduct impulses without this myelin sheath, the impulses travel at a slower rate and with more likelihood of diffusion. Myelinization of the various nerve tracts in the central nervous system accelerates rapidly after birth and follows the cephalocaudal and proximodistal sequence, which allows progressively complex neuromotor function. Myelinization begins with spinal cord and cranial nerve fibers, followed by the brainstem and corticospinal tracts. Myelinization accelerates rapidly after birth and follows the cephalocaudal and proximodistal directional sequence, beginning with the spinal and cranial nerve fibers, followed by the brainstem and corticospinal tracts. In general, the pathways concerned with sensation are myelinated before the motor pathways.

The acquisition of motor skills depends on this myelinization and maturation, and no amount of special training or practice will hasten the process. Most of the advancing performance of an infant is a direct result of brain development and depends only indirectly on environmental stimuli.

The ***spinal cord*** also demonstrates alterations relative to the vertebral column during prenatal and early postnatal growth. In the embryo the spinal cord extends the entire length of the vertebral canal. However, because the vertebral column and the cord have different growth rates, the cord in the newborn ends at the level of the third and fourth lumbar vertebrae. As growth continues, the cord becomes higher in relation to the vertebrae until it ends at the level of the first lumbar vertebra in the adult (Fig. 4-8).

The disparity in growth rates also involves the spinal nerves attached to the cord. In the early developing embryo

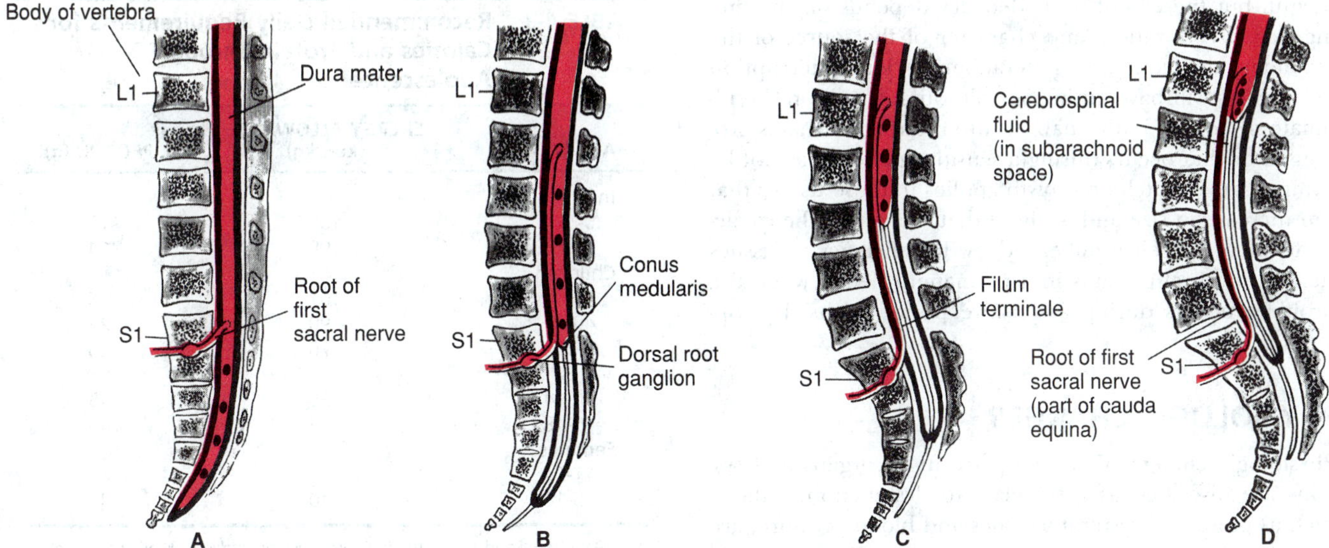

FIG. 4-8 Diagrams showing position of caudal end of spinal cord in relation to vertebral column and meninges at various stages of development. Increasing inclination of root of first sacral nerve is also illustrated. **A,** Eight weeks. **B,** Twenty-four weeks. **C,** Newborn. **D,** Adult. *L1,* First lumbar vertebra; *S1,* first sacral vertebra.

the spinal nerves are directed nearly horizontal to the intervertebral foramina, through which they emerge from the spinal column. At full growth the upper cervical nerves are still directed on a horizontal plane, but lower nerves become directed more and more obliquely downward toward their intervertebral foramina. The sacral and coccygeal nerves are so arranged in relation to one another and in a vertical direction that they resemble the arrangement of hairs on a horse's tail, hence the term ***cauda equina.***

Lymphoid Tissues

Lymphoid tissues contained in the lymph nodes, thymus, spleen, tonsils, adenoids, and blood lymphocytes follow a distinctive growth pattern unlike that of other body tissues. These tissues are small in relation to total body size, but they are well developed at birth. They increase rapidly to reach adult dimensions by 6 years of age and continue to grow. At about age 10 to 12 years the tissues reach a maximum development approximately twice their adult size, followed by a rapid decline to stable adult dimensions by the end of adolescence.

Lymph nodes are large, and the superficially located nodes are often palpable. The tonsils, massive during early childhood, become inconspicuous in the adult. The thymus gland beneath the sternum, a prominent feature in infancy, may be impossible to detect in an adult. The growth pattern of lymphatic tissues parallels the development of immunity and probably reflects the repeated exposure to new infectious agents.

Development of Organ Systems

All tissues and organ systems undergo changes during development. Some are striking; others are more subtle. Many have implications for assessment and care. Since the major importance of these changes relates to their dysfunction, the developmental characteristics of various systems and organs are discussed throughout the book as they relate to these areas. Physical characteristics and function of the body systems are described in relation to assessment (Chapter 7). Physical characteristics and physiologic changes that vary with age are included in age-group descriptions. For example, the relationship of surface area to body mass is of primary importance during very early development; physical characteristics related to hormonal changes are most significant during adolescence and are discussed as they apply to problems associated with this phase.

Catch-Up Growth

When there has been a secondary cause of growth deficiency, such as severe illness or acute malnutrition, recovery from the illness or the establishment of an adequate diet will produce a dramatic acceleration of the growth rate that usually continues until the child's individual growth pattern is resumed. Although the phenomenon has not been satisfactorily explained, during this period the biologic timing mechanism is apparently unaffected. When the problem is corrected, children tend to catch up to the developmental stage at which they would be normally. For example, newborns exhibit a transitory weight loss shortly after birth and then rapidly regain the weight. In addition, during the early months of life the developmental achievements of prematurely born infants lag behind those of full-term infants of the same chronologic age. The deficit in the attainment of developmental landmarks closely corresponds to the degree of prematurity; however, the differences become less conspicuous as the infant matures. Children usually catch up to age-mates by the preschool years.

Catch-up growth involves growth in both length and

weight, but the extent of inadequacy depends on the timing, severity, duration, and character of the source of the secondary deficiency. In general, any serious interruption in progress will have an impact, although small, on the ultimate size of the individual. Growth retardation that is prolonged or that occurs during a sensitive period may not be compensated. Catch-up growth applies to those tissues that can increase in size and to those that still retain the capacity to increase cell numbers. Growth deficiency in tissues such as the brain results in a permanent deficit when the problem occurs during a sensitive period in its development.

PHYSIOLOGIC CHANGES

Physiologic changes that take place in all organs and systems are discussed as they relate to dysfunction. Others, such as pulse and respiratory rates and blood pressure, are an integral part of physical assessment (see Chapter 7). In addition, there are changes in basic functions including metabolism, temperature, and patterns of sleep and rest.

Metabolism

Metabolism—all chemical and energy transformations in the body—is affected by an assortment of intrinsic and extrinsic factors (e.g., body size, age, sex, emotions, exercise, climate, hormones, environmental temperature). Therefore metabolic needs vary among individuals and within each individual. The rate of metabolism when the body is at rest ***(basal metabolic rate,*** or ***BMR)*** demonstrates a distinctive change throughout childhood. Highest in the infant, BMR closely relates to the proportion of surface area to body mass, which changes as the body increases in size. Surface area is considered the best estimate of the amount of functioning protoplasm present in the organism (see Fig. 27-18 for computation of surface area). In both sexes the proportion decreases progressively to maturity. The BMR is slightly higher in boys at all ages and further increases during pubescence over that in girls.

The rate of metabolism determines the caloric requirements of the child. The basal energy requirement of infants is about 108 kcal/kg of body weight and decreases to 40 to 45 kcal/kg at maturity (Table 4-3). Water requirements remain at approximately 1.5 ml per kilocalorie of energy expended throughout life. Children's energy needs vary considerably at different ages and with changing circumstances. The greatest proportion of calories in infancy is used for basal metabolic needs and growth.

The energy requirement to build tissue steadily decreases with age, following the general growth curve; however, exercise needs vary with the individual child and may be considerably more. For short periods (e.g., during strenuous exercise) and more prolonged periods (e.g., illness), the needs can be very high. For example, each degree of fever increases the basal metabolism 10% with a corresponding fluid requirement. A very small portion of ingested calories is lost in stools during normal metabolism, but much more may be lost in this way when the child suffers from conditions that impair digestion or absorption.

TABLE 4-3 Recommended Daily Requirements for Calories and Protein Through Adolescence*

AGE (YEARS)	ENERGY ALLOWANCE (kcal/kg)	PROTEIN (g)
Infants		
0-½	108	13
½-1	98	14
Children		
1-3	102	16
4-6	90	24
7-10	70	28
Males		
11-14	55	45
15-18	45	49
Females		
11-14	47	46
15-18	40	44

*Data from Food and Nutrition Board: *Recommended daily allowances,* ed 10, Washington, DC, 1989, National Academy Press.

Temperature

Body temperature, reflecting metabolism, displays the same decrement from infancy to maturity (see inside back cover). Following the unstable regulatory ability in the neonatal period, heat production steadily declines as the infant grows into childhood. Individual differences of 0.5° to 1° F are normal, and occasionally a child normally displays an unusually high or low temperature. Beginning at approximately 12 years of age, girls display a temperature that remains relatively stable, while the temperature in boys continues to fall for a few years longer. Females maintain a temperature slightly above that of males throughout life.

Even with improved temperature regulation, infants and young children are highly susceptible to temperature fluctuations. Body temperature responds to changes in environmental temperature and is increased with active exercise, crying, and emotional upset. Infections can cause a higher and more rapid temperature increase in infants and young children than in older children. In relation to body weight, an infant produces more heat per unit than children near maturity. Consequently, during active play or when heavily clothed, an infant or small child is likely to become overheated.

Motor Development

Closely allied to biologic development and maturation is the development of basic motor responses. Children's ability to perform motor functions depends on the state of maturation of bones, muscles, and the nervous system and follows the patterns of development described earlier in the chapter. As in all maturation processes motor behavior follows a developmental sequence. ***Reflexive*** or ***rudimentary movements*** are present at birth and form the foundation of all other movements, including sitting, crawling, creeping, reaching, standing, and walking. ***General fundamental skills*** develop during early childhood and include such activities as running, jumping, balancing, catching, and throwing.

There is wide variation in children's abilities to perform these skills. ***Specific skills*** develop during later childhood as general fundamental skills become more refined, fluid, and automatic. There is greater emphasis on form, accuracy, and adaptability, and children begin to apply these skills to sports and other activities that require body movement. ***Specialized skills*** evolve slowly from late childhood through adolescence and depend on training and repetition.

SLEEP AND REST

Sleep, a protective function in all organisms, allows for repair and recovery of tissues following activity. As in most aspects of development, a wide variation exists among individual children and ages of children in the amount and distribution of sleep. As the child matures, not only does a change occur in the quantity of time spent in sleep but also in the quality of that sleep. Also, family influences, social expectations, and cultural variations in sleep patterns must be considered when analyzing sleep problems.

Time and Quality of Sleep

The length of time spent in sleep decreases throughout childhood. Newborns sleep much of the time not occupied with feeding and other aspects of their care. Larger newborns sleep for longer periods than smaller ones because of their larger stomach capacity. As infants mature, the total time spent in sleep gradually decreases, and they remain awake for longer periods and sleep longer at night. During the later part of the first year, most children sleep through the night and take one or two naps during the day. By the time they are 1½ years old, most children have eliminated the second nap. After age 3 years children have usually given up daytime naps, except in those cultures in which an afternoon nap or siesta is customary. From ages 4 to 10 sleep time declines slightly and then increases somewhat during the pubertal growth spurt. The changes in length of sleep in relation to age are illustrated in Fig. 4-9.

Alterations take place in the percentage of sleep time spent in each of the two different identified sleep cycles: (1) ***active sleep,*** characterized by irregular pulse and expirations, many body movements, and short, rapid eye movements ***(REM sleep);*** and (2) ***quiet sleep,*** in which breathing and the heartbeat are regular and body and eye movements are absent ***(non-REM sleep).***

REM sleep is characterized by activity. More oxygen is used, blood flow to the brain is increased, the temperature rises, and brain waves show increased activity. Sensory paths transmit impulses in much the same manner as during waking hours. Later these visual, auditory, and vestibular stimuli are believed to be incorporated by the brain into dream imagery.

During non-REM sleep the heart rate and breathing pattern are regular, and this cycle is believed to provide most of the restorative functions attributed to sleep. Four stages of non-REM sleep are described. ***Stage 1*** consists of drowsiness with decreasing awareness of the external world. Sleep progresses from drowsiness through ***stage 2,*** from which a sleeping person can be easily wakened and, if wakened, may not admit to having been asleep. In ***stage 3,*** sleep becomes increasingly deep, breathing and the heart rate are very stable, the muscles are relaxed, and the brain waves are very slow. ***Stage 4*** is the deepest sleep, from which it is difficult to be roused except by strong stimuli. A child can be moved from one place to another without waking. Making the difficult transition to wakefulness from stage 4 non-REM sleep is significant in some sleep disorders of children.

The sleep of newborns consists of approximately 50% REM sleep, in contrast to approximately 20% in older children. The large amount of active REM sleep in early infancy is believed to serve as an endogenous source of stimulation to the higher brain centers and is important for normal development at a time when exogenous sources are minimal because of the short periods of arousal. REM sleep is probably more important in the early months and may be necessary for development of higher brain centers. The de-

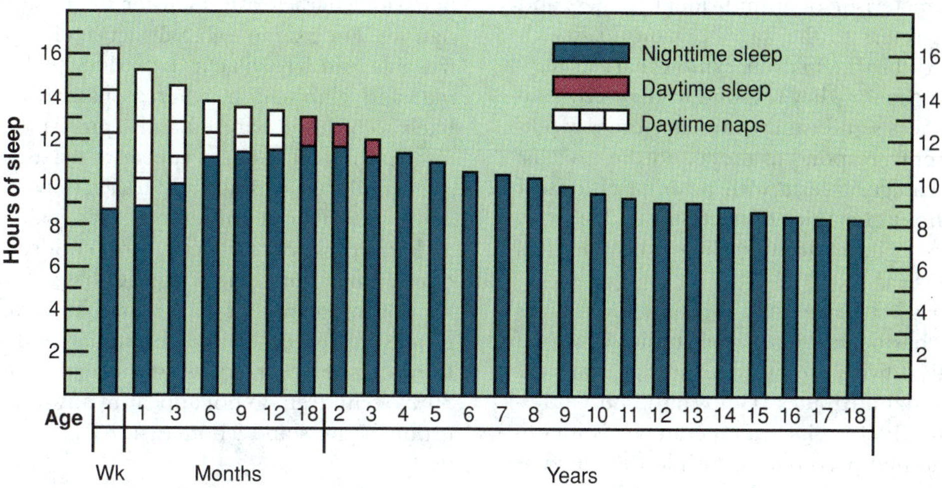

FIG. 4-9 Changes in number of hours of sleep with increasing age. (Modified from Ferber R: *Solve your child's sleep problems,* New York, 1985, Simon & Schuster.)

crease in REM sleep as development progresses may indicate that with longer periods of wakefulness, the more mature brain has less need for this endogenous stimulation. The deep, restful non-REM sleep increases proportionately with age; children who have recently given up napping take a longer time to get into REM sleep during the initial sleep cycle than do either older or younger children, which suggests they are more fatigued.

Sleep Cycles

Once non-REM sleep has developed, a single nighttime sleep period contains all four stages of sleep and is arranged in cycles, which remain constant throughout life. However, the length of the sleep cycles and the amounts of REM and non-REM sleep vary among individuals and developmental ages. The length of a ***sleep cycle*** (time between two consecutive appearances of the same sleep state) increases with age. For example, the length of a sleep cycle in the newborn infant increases from about 50 minutes to about 90 in adolescence. The amount of stage 4 non-REM sleep also decreases but accounts for about 25% of a child's total sleep at all ages.

Partial waking is also characteristic of normal sleep. After about 1 hour of stage 4 sleep the child will arouse for a brief period, which will last a few seconds or up to several minutes. During this waking period the child may exhibit a variety of behaviors. Mild behaviors include rubbing the face, turning over, brief crying, adjusting covers, looking around, and/or unintelligible speech. The child may open the eyes or sit up briefly before returning to sleep. More conspicuous behaviors include sleepwalking, confused threshing, or bed-wetting. Periodic wakenings are normally followed by rapid return to sleep and take place several times during the sleep period. They should not be mistaken for sleeplessness. (See Chapters 12, 15, and 17 for a discussion of sleep problems.)

TEMPERAMENT

Temperament is defined as "the manner of thinking, behaving, or reacting characteristic of an individual" (Chess and Thomas, 1985) and refers to the way a person deals with life. From the time of birth, children exhibit marked individual differences in the way they respond to their environment. These differences significantly influence the way others, particularly parents, respond to them and their needs. Temperament is a categoric term with no implications of good or bad, is without etiologic connections, and, as with other characteristics, is influenced by the environment as development progresses.

A genetic basis has been suggested for some differences in temperament. It has been found from studies of young children that identical twins are more alike than fraternal twins in temperamental attributes (Goldsmith and Gottesman, 1981; Matheny, 1980). Since temperament is identified primarily by parental perceptions, a child described as difficult at one time may be reported as easy at a later time. Parents' perceptions of temperament are both objectively and subjectively determined; both parental characteristics and infant behavior make significant and independent contributions to parents' perceptions (Wolk and others, 1992). Parental relationships with a child can strongly affect behavior. As parental competency increases, the child's behavior may be less difficult or may appear easier to the parent.

ATTRIBUTES OF TEMPERAMENT

Activity—Level of physical motion during activity, such as sleep, eating, play, dressing, and bathing.

Rhythmicity—Regularity in the timing of physiologic functions, such as hunger, sleep, and elimination.

Approach-withdrawal—Nature of initial responses to a new stimulus, such as people, situations, places, foods, toys, and procedures. ***Approach*** responses are positive, displayed by activity or expression; ***withdrawal*** responses are negative expressions or behaviors.

Adaptability—Ease or difficulty with which the child adapts or adjusts to new or altered situations.

Threshold of responsiveness (sensory threshold)—Amount of stimulation, such as sounds or light, required to evoke a response in the child.

Intensity of reaction—Energy level of the child's reactions, regardless of quality or direction.

Mood—Amount of pleasant, happy, friendly behavior compared with unpleasant, unhappy, crying, unfriendly behavior exhibited by the child in various situations.

Distractibility—Ease with which a child's attention or direction of behavior can be diverted by external stimuli.

Attention span and persistence—Length of time a child pursues a given activity ***(attention)*** and the continuation of an activity in spite of obstacles ***(persistence)***.

Characteristics of Temperament

The characteristics of behavioral individuality, derived from parental interviews, were identified, categorized, and rated in the New York Longitudinal Study (NYLS) of child behavior. The temperamental attributes established from analysis of the information are outlined in the box above (Chess and Thomas, 1983).

Categories of Temperament

Further analysis of the NYLS data revealed that most of the behavior characteristics cluster in constellations or combinations. For example, highly active children are frequently irritable and irregular in behaviors such as sleeping, feeding, and elimination, whereas passive children are more likely to be good natured and regular in their habits. These temperamental patterns appear to persist over time and can affect children's adjustment to a variety of settings and situations throughout childhood.

From these observations, most children can be placed in one of three common categories based on their overall pattern of temperamental attributes. However, there are wide ranges in degree of manifestations, and varying combinations can be observed within normal limits. Approximately 30% of children do not appear in any of the following three groups (Chess and Thomas, 1983):

1. **The easy child.** Easygoing children are even-tempered, regular, and predictable in their habits, and they have a positive approach to new stimuli. They are open and adaptable to

change, and they display a mild to moderately intense mood that is typically positive. Approximately 40% of NYLS children fall into this category.

2. **The difficult child.** Difficult children are highly active, irritable, and irregular in their habits. Negative withdrawal responses are typical, and they require a more structured environment. These children adapt slowly to new routines, people, or situations. Mood expressions are usually intense and primarily negative. They exhibit frequent periods of crying, and frustration often produces violent tantrums. This group constitutes about 10% of the NYLS children.
3. **The slow-to-warm-up child.** Slow-to-warm-up children typically react negatively and with mild intensity to new stimuli and, unless pressured, adapt slowly with repeated contact. They respond with only mild but passive resistance to novelty or changes in routine. They are quite inactive and moody but show only moderate irregularity in functions. Fifteen percent of children in the NYLS studies demonstrate this temperament pattern.

Significance of Temperament

Observations indicate that children who display the difficult or slow-to-warm-up patterns of behavior are more vulnerable to the development of behavior problems in early and middle childhood. Any child can develop behavior problems if there is dissonance between the child's temperament and the environment. Demands for change and adaptation that are in conflict with children's capacities can become excessively stressful. However, authorities empha-

TABLE 4-4 Summary of Personality, Cognitive, and Moral Development Theories

STAGE/AGE	PSYCHOSEXUAL STAGES (FREUD)	PSYCHOSOCIAL STAGES (ERIKSON)	RADIUS OF SIGNIFICANT RELATIONSHIPS (SULLIVAN)	COGNITIVE STAGES (PIAGET)	MORAL JUDGMENT STAGES (KOHLBERG)
I Infancy Birth to 1 year	Oral sensory	Trust vs mistrust	Maternal person (unipolar-bipolar)	Sensorimotor (birth to 2 years)	
II Toddlerhood 1-3 years	Anal-urethral	Autonomy vs shame and doubt	Parental persons (tripolar)	Preoperational thought, preconceptual phase (transductive reasoning, e.g., specific to specific) (2-4 years)	Preconventional (premoral) level Punishment and obedience orientation
III Early childhood 3-6 years	Phallic-locomotion	Initiative vs guilt	Basic family	Preoperational thought, intuitive phase (transductive reasoning) (4-7 years)	Preconventional (premoral) level Naive instrumental orientation
IV Middle childhood 6-12 years	Latency	Industry vs inferiority	Neighborhood, school	Concrete operations (inductive reasoning and beginning logic) (7-11 years)	Conventional level Good-boy, nice-girl orientation Law-and-order orientation
V Adolescence 12-19 years	Genitality	Identity and repudiation vs identity confusion	Peer groups and outgroups Models of leadership Partners in friendship, sex, competition, cooperation	Formal operations (deductive and abstract reasoning) (11-15 years)	Postconventional or principled level Social-contract orientation Universal ethical principle orientation (no longer included in revised theory)
VI Early adulthood		Intimacy and solidarity vs isolation	Divided labor and shared household		
VII Young and middle adulthood		Generativity vs self-absorption	Mankind "My kind"		
VIII Later adulthood		Ego integrity vs despair			

size that it is not children's temperament patterns that place them at risk but the degree of "fit" between children and their environment, specifically their parents, that determines the degree of vulnerability. When environmental expectations and demands fit with the individual's style of behavior, potential exists for optimum development. On the other hand, if there is a poor fit, there is greater potential for maladaptive functioning to occur (Johnson, 1992) (See Failure to Thrive, Chapter 13.)

Early identification of temperament provides a useful tool for caregivers in anticipating probable areas of difficulty or risk associated with development. For example, "difficult" children may be prone to colic in infancy, active children require more vigilance to prevent injury, and school entry will require different approaches for children with different temperaments.

Several parental questionnaires have been devised to facilitate assessment of temperament. Nurses who employ these assessment tools are better able to help parents interpret their children's behavior and to provide anticipatory guidance regarding numerous aspects of childrearing. The concept of temperament is also discussed in relation to child development at various ages and coping with the experiences of hospitalization. The most commonly used questionnaires for assessing infant and child temperament are those developed by Carey and McDevitt (Carey and McDevitt, 1978; Fullard, McDevitt, and Carey, 1984; Hegvik, McDevitt, and Carey, 1982).

DEVELOPMENT OF MENTAL FUNCTION AND PERSONALITY

Personality and cognitive skills develop in much the same manner as biologic growth—new accomplishments build on previously mastered skills. Many aspects depend on physical growth and maturation. This is not a comprehensive account of the multiple facets of personality and behavior development. Many aspects are integrated with the child's emotional and social development in later discussion of various age-groups. Table 4-4 summarizes some of the developmental theories.

THEORETIC FOUNDATIONS OF PERSONALITY DEVELOPMENT

According to Freud, all human behavior is energized by psychodynamic forces, and this psychic energy is divided among three components of personality: the id, the ego, and the superego. The ***id,*** the ***unconscious mind,*** is the inborn component that is driven by instincts. The id obeys the pleasure principle of immediate gratification of needs regardless of whether the object or action can actually do so. The ***ego,*** the ***conscious mind,*** serves the reality principle. It functions as the conscious or controlling self that is able to find realistic means for gratifying the instincts while blocking the irrational thinking of the id. The ***superego,*** the ***conscience,*** functions as the moral arbitrator and represents the ideal. It is the mechanism that prevents individuals from expressing undesirable instincts that might threaten the social order.

Psychosexual Development (Freud)

Freud also considered the sexual instincts to be significant in the development of the personality. However, he used the term ***psychosexual*** to describe any ***sensual pleasure.*** Many simple body functions, considered asexual in the usual sense, were viewed as "erotic" activities by Freud, and these activities were thought to be motivated by the general life force he called the ***sex instinct.*** Personality development was viewed as the growth or unfolding of these instincts.

According to Freud's theory, during childhood certain regions of the body assume a prominent psychologic significance as the source of new pleasures, and new conflicts gradually shift from one part of the body to another at particular stages of development. Each stage builds on the previous one, and the maturation of the sex instinct leaves distinct imprints on the developing psyche. Freud believed that children who encounter severe conflicts at any stage may be reluctant to move to the next phase, causing further development to be arrested or impaired. In addition, they may retreat to earlier stages of development if they experience too much anxiety or too many conflicts at a subsequent stage of development.

Although Freud was the first to provide a systematic explanation for human behavior, the theory focuses on a single motive governing behavior—the desire to satisfy biologic needs (dominated by sexual instincts), thereby releasing tensions. The theory, derived from retrospective studies of adults and not from direct observation, is difficult to verify or disconfirm and is of little value in predicting future behaviors.

During the ***oral stage*** (birth to 1 year) the major source of pleasure seeking centers on oral activities such as sucking, biting, chewing, and vocalizing. Children may prefer one of these practices over the others, and the preferred method of oral gratification can provide some indication of the personality they develop. Examples of oral personality traits are pessimism or optimism, determination or submission, gullibility or suspiciousness, admiration or envy, and cockiness or self-belittlement.

Interest during the ***anal stage*** (1 to 3 years) centers on the anal region as sphincter muscles develop and children are able to withhold or expel fecal material at will. At this stage the climate surrounding toilet training can have lasting effects on children's personalities. Examples of anal personality traits are stinginess or overgenerosity, constrictedness or expansiveness, rigid punctuality or tardiness, stubbornness or acquiescence, and orderliness or messiness.

During the ***phallic stage*** (3 to 6 years) the genitals become an interesting and sensitive area of the body. Children recognize differences between the sexes and become curious about the dissimilarities. This is the period associated with the controversial issues of the Oedipus and Electra complexes, penis envy, and castration anxiety. Examples of phallic personality traits are brashness or bashfulness, stylishness or plainness, gaiety or sadness, blind courage or timidity, and gregariousness or isolationism.

During the ***latency period*** (6 to 12 years) children elaborate on previously acquired traits and skills. Physical and psychic energy are channeled into acquisition of knowledge and vigorous play.

The last significant phase, ***genital stage*** (age 12 and over), begins at puberty with maturation of the reproductive system and production of sex hormones. The genital organs become the major source of sexual tensions and pleasures, but energies are also invested in forming friendships and preparation for marriage.

Psychosocial Development (Erikson)

The theory of personality development advanced by Erikson (1963) is the most widely accepted and used. Although built on Freudian theory, it emphasizes a healthy personality as opposed to a pathologic approach. It involves predictable age-related stages during which specific changes are assumed to take place. Erikson also uses the biologic concepts of critical periods and epigenesis, describing key conflicts or core problems the individual strives to master during critical periods in personality development. Successful completion or mastery of each of these core conflicts is built on the satisfactory completion or mastery of the previous core conflict.

At each stage of psychosocial development, children are confronted with a unique problem requiring the integration of personal needs and skills with social demands and cultural expectations. Erikson refers to the individual's efforts to adjust as a ***crisis.*** Crisis in this context implies the normal stresses as opposed to an extraordinary set of events. The tension produced by societal demands must be reduced in order that the favorable outcome can be achieved.

Each psychosocial stage has two components, the favorable and unfavorable aspects of the core conflict, and progress to the next stage depends on resolution of this conflict. No core conflict is ever mastered completely but remains a recurrent problem throughout life. No life situation is ever secure. Each new situation presents the conflict in a new form. For example, when children who have satisfactorily achieved a sense of trust encounter a new experience (e.g., hospitalization), they must again develop a sense of trust in those responsible for their care in order to master the situation.

Erikson's eight stages or "psychosocial crises" are outlined in the following segments. The lasting outcome, or ego quality (Erikson, 1978), of each stage, achieved through a central process (Newman and Newman, 1984), provides the resources for coping. Specific persons in the environment become the key socializing agents in the process (Shaffer, 1984). All eight stages are included, since the later-age stages are important to family functions and have an impact on the development of children.

Although Erikson's theory stresses the rational and adaptive nature of persons, it does not clearly indicate the kinds of experiences needed to cope with and resolve the various crises. There is no concern for individual differences. Regardless of its shortcomings, Erikson's theory provides an excellent framework for explaining children's behaviors in mastering developmental tasks.

The first and most important attribute of a healthy personality to develop is a basic trust. Establishment of basic trust dominates the first year of life and describes all the child's satisfying experiences at this age. Corresponding to Freud's oral stage, the ***trust vs mistrust stage*** (birth to 1 year) is a time of "getting" and "taking in" through all the senses. It exists only in relation to something or someone; therefore, consistent, loving care by a mothering person is essential to the development of trust. Mistrust develops when trust-promoting experiences are deficient or lacking or when basic needs are inconsistently or inadequately met. Shreds of mistrust are sprinkled throughout the personality, but through the process of mutuality with the primary caregiver the individual develops the ego quality of hope, an enduring belief that one can attain one's deep and essential wishes. The result is faith and optimism.

The ***autonomy vs shame and doubt stage*** (1 to 3 years) corresponds to Freud's anal stage, in which the problem of autonomy can be symbolized by the holding on and letting go of the sphincter muscles. The development of autonomy during the toddler period is centered around children's increasing ability to control their bodies, themselves, and their environment. They want to use their powers to do things for themselves, using their newly acquired motor skills of walking, climbing, and manipulating and mental powers of selection and decision making. They also learn to conform to social rules. Negative feelings of doubt and shame arise when children are made to feel unimportant and self-conscious, when their choices are disastrous, when others shame them, or when they are forced to be dependent in areas in which they are capable of assuming control. They come to doubt their abilities. The central process for achieving autonomy is imitation, and the key socializing agents are the parents. The favorable outcomes are self-control and willpower.

The ***initiative vs guilt stage*** (3 to 6 years) corresponds to Freud's phallic stage and is characterized by vigorous, intrusive behavior, enterprise, and a strong imagination. Children explore the physical world with all their senses and powers. They develop a conscience. No longer guided only by outsiders, children respond to an inner voice that warns and threatens. Children sometimes undertake goals or activities that are in conflict with those of parents or others, and being made to feel that their activities or imaginings are bad produces a sense of guilt. Excessive guilt inhibits initiative, but children must learn to retain a sense of initiative without impinging on the rights and privileges of others. The central process is identification, and the key socializing agent is the family. The lasting outcomes are direction and purpose; the courage to imagine and pursue is a valued goal.

The ***industry vs inferiority stage*** (6 to 12 years) correlates with the latency period of Freud. Having achieved the more crucial stages in personality development, children are now ready to be workers and producers. They want to engage in tasks and activities they can carry through to completion; they need and want real achievement. Children learn to compete and to cooperate with others, and they learn the rules. When children succeed in their efforts, they develop a sense of mastery and self-assurance. It is a decisive period in their social relationships with others. Feelings of inadequacy and inferiority may develop if too much is expected of them or if they believe that they cannot measure up to the standards set for them by others. Without experiencing mastery children will shun new activities. The key socializing agents are teachers and peers, and the central process is education. The ego quality developed from a sense of industry is competence, the free exercise of skill and intelligence in the completion of tasks.

The ***identity vs role confusion stage*** (12 to 18 years) corresponds to Freud's genital stage. The development of identity is characterized by rapid and marked physical changes. Previous trust in their bodies shaken, children become overly preoccupied with the way they appear in the eyes of others as compared with their own self-concept. Adolescents struggle to fit the roles they have played and those they hope to play with the current roles and fashions adopted by their peers, to integrate their concepts and values with those of society, and to come to a decision regarding an occupation. Inability to solve the core conflict results in role confusion. The central processes are peer pressure and role experimentation; the key socializing agent is the society of peers. The outcome of successful mastery is devotion and fidelity, the ability to sustain loyalties freely committed in early adolescence to others and loyalties freely pledged in later adolescence to values and ideologies.

The ***intimacy vs isolation stage*** occurs during early adulthood. A sense of intimacy is established on a sense of identity. Intimacy is the capacity to develop an intimate love relationship with another and intimate interpersonal relationships with friends, partners, and other significant persons. Without intimacy the individual feels *isolated* and alone. The central process is mutuality among peers, and the key socializing agents are lovers, spouses, and close friends. The favorable outcome is affiliation and love, the capacity for mutuality that transcends childhood dependency.

Central to the ***generativity vs stagnation stage*** of development in young and middle adulthood is the creation and care of the next generation. The essential element is to nourish and nurture. It may be directed toward one's own children, children of others, or other products of creativity. The individual who fails in this component of personality development becomes self-absorbed and stagnant. The key socializing agents are the spouse, children, and cultural norms, and the central process is person-environment fit and creativity. The favorable outcome is production and care, the commitment to be concerned for what has been generated.

The ***ego integrity vs despair stage*** takes place during old age. A sense of integrity results from satisfaction with life and acceptance of what has been; despair arises from remorse for what might have been. The central process is introspection, and the favorable outcome is renunciation and wisdom, the detached yet active concern with life in the face of death.

Interpersonal Development (Sullivan)

Also built on Freudian theory, the interpersonal development theory by Sullivan (1953) emphasizes the interpersonal relationships in which children engage and the importance of social approval and disapproval in developing a self-concept. What children interpret as unfavorable interactions result in tension and anxiety; the outcome of favorable relationships is a sense of comfort and security. Through repeated interactions children acquire a repertoire of actions and behaviors that produce a feeling of security and avoid anxiety.

The first interactions are those between infants and their "mothering" figure, usually the mother, who gratifies and comforts. This bipolar relationship gradually extends to include others in the family group. Between the ages of 2 and 5, children not only become more outgoing but also direct their social gestures to a wider audience outside but near the home and family, such as relatives and neighborhood children. They engage in peer play, family events, and other aspects of social learning. Observational studies suggest that 2- to 3-year-olds are more likely than older children to remain near an adult and to seek physical affection, while the sociable behaviors of 4- to 5-year-olds normally consist of playful bids for attention or approval that are directed at peers rather than adults.

During the school years children enter into a wider range of relationships with other persons and authority figures at school and in the community. They develop "chumships," the special relationship between two peers—the shared intimacy and common interests of genuine friendships that are lacking in earlier relationships. Personal identity in adolescence is an outgrowth of intimate relationships, first with friends of the same sex, then with friends of the opposite sex.

Although Sullivan's theory recognizes the importance of environment in development and has some predictive value, it does not recognize the biologic maturation process.

THEORETIC FOUNDATIONS OF MENTAL DEVELOPMENT

The term ***cognition*** refers to the process by which developing individuals become acquainted with the world and the objects it contains. Children are born with inherited potentialities for intellectual growth, but they must develop into that potential through interaction with the environment. By assimilating information through the senses, processing it, and acting on it, they come to understand relationships between objects and between themselves and their world. With cognitive development children acquire the ability to reason abstractly, to think in a logical manner, and to organize intellectual functions or performances into higher-order structures.

Cognitive Development (Piaget)

Cognitive development consists of age-related changes that occur in mental activities. The best-known theory regarding children's thinking, and a more comprehensive developmental theory than those already described, has been developed by the Swiss psychologist Jean Piaget (1969). According to Piaget, intelligence enables individuals to make adaptations to the environment that increase the probability of survival, and through their behavior individuals establish and maintain equilibrium with the environment.

Piaget proposes three stages of reasoning: (1) ***intuitive,*** (2) ***concrete operational,*** and (3) ***formal operational.*** When they enter the stage of concrete logical thought at about age 7 years, children are able to make logical inferences, classify, and deal with quantitative relationships about concrete things. Not until adolescence are they able to reason abstractly with any degree of competence.

According to Piaget, children proceed through the stages of mental activity in an orderly and sequential manner. The mechanisms that enable them to adapt to new situations and to move from one stage to the next are assimilation and accommodation. By ***assimilation*** children incorporate new knowledge, skills, ideas, and insights into cognitive schemes (Piaget uses the term ***schema****) already familiar to them. To new situations that do not fit into an established schema, children ***accommodate.*** They change and organize existing schemas to solve more difficult tasks and form new schemas. Children's understanding of a new experience is based on all relevant previous experiences. They achieve equilibrium over and over again by applying schemas already available to them. Thus children achieve an accurate understanding of reality and come to deal with increasingly complex problems in an increasingly effective manner.

One of the most prominent criticisms of Piaget's theory is that it ignores the important concept of unconscious motivation and its impact on behavior. Nor does it account for individual differences and unevenness in cognitive development—some children demonstrate more advanced behavior in one area than in another. Although it emphasizes biologic factors in human development, Piaget's theory provides one of the dominant frameworks for understanding children's thinking. Piaget was very conservative in his descriptions of children's abilities. Recent studies indicate that children, especially preschool children, are capable of more advanced thought than Piaget acknowledged.

Development of Logical Thinking. Piaget believes there are four major stages in the development of logical thinking. Each is derived from and builds on the accomplishments of the previous stage in a continuous, orderly process. The course of intellectual development is both maturational and invariant and is divided into the following periods, subperiods, and stages (ages are approximate).

The ***sensorimotor stage*** of intellectual development (birth to 2 years) consists of six substages (see Chapter 12) that are governed by sensations through which simple learning takes place. Children progress from reflex activity through simple repetitive behaviors to imitative behavior. They develop a sense of "cause and effect" as they direct behavior toward objects and solve problems primarily through trial and error. They display a high level of curiosity, experimentation, and enjoyment of novelty. As a result of interactions with their environment, children begin to develop a sense of self as they are able to differentiate themselves from their environment.

Children become aware that an object has permanence, that it exists even though it is no longer visible. The awareness of ***object permanence*** is extremely important because it is a prerequisite for all other mental activity. All concepts begin with or involve objects in one way or another. Toward the end of the sensorimotor period children begin to use language, and representational thought appears as they imitate the behavior of others, even in the absence of these other persons.

The predominant characteristic of the ***preoperational period*** of intellectual development (2 to 7 years) is ***egocentricity.*** Egocentricity in this sense does not mean selfishness or self-centeredness, but rather the inability to put oneself in the place of another. Children interpret objects and events not in terms of general properties, but in terms of their relationships or their use to them. They are unable to see things from any perspective other than their own; they cannot see another's point of view, nor can they see any reason to do so.

Preoperational thinking is concrete and tangible. Children cannot reason beyond the observable, and they lack the ability to make deductions or generalizations. Thought is dominated by what they see, hear, or otherwise experience. However, they are increasingly able to use language and symbols to represent objects in their environment. Through imaginative play, questioning, and interacting, they begin to elaborate concepts and make simple associations between ideas. One of the most salient features of preoperational thought is lack of conservation or reversibility; children at this stage cannot understand that for every action or operation there is an action or operation that cancels it. For example, children in this age-group are unable to grasp the idea that a ball of clay can be changed and brought back to the original shape. In the latter stage of this period their reasoning is ***intuitive*** (e.g., the stars have to go to bed just as they do), and they are only beginning to deal with problems of weight, length, size, and time.

During the ***concrete operational stage*** (7 to 11 years) thought becomes increasingly logical and coherent. Children are able to classify, sort, order, and otherwise organize facts about the world to use in problem solving. They develop a new concept of permanence—conservation (see Cognitive Development [Piaget], Chapter 17). They realize that volume, weight, and number remain the same even though outward appearances are changed. They are able to deal with a number of different aspects of a situation simultaneously. They do not have the capacity to deal in abstraction; they solve problems in a concrete, systematic fashion based on what they can perceive. Reasoning is inductive. Through progressive changes in thought processes and relationships with others, thought becomes less self-centered. Children can consider points of view other than their own. Thinking has become socialized.

During the ***formal operational stage*** (12 to 15 years) formal operational thought is characterized by adaptability and flexibility. Adolescents can think in abstract terms, use abstract symbols, and draw logical conclusions from a set of observations. They can make hypotheses and test them; they can consider abstract, theoretic, and philosophic matters. Although they may confuse the ideal with the practical, they can deal with and resolve most contradictions in the world.

*A schema is a pattern of action and/or thought.

Moral Development (Kohlberg)

It is theorized that children develop moral reasoning in an invariant developmental sequence. To understand the stages in the development of moral judgment, it is important to be aware of the stages of logical thought and the relationship to cognitive development, as well as to moral behavior. Moral development is based on cognitive developmental theory and consists of three major levels, each with two stages (Kohlberg, 1968).

Kohlberg's theory allows for prediction of behavior but pays little attention to individual differences. Questions arise relative to observed sex differences in attainment of the various sequences of moral development (Holstein, 1976). It has been argued that the theory was derived from interviews with male adults and may not reflect the feminine moral reasoning (Gilligan, 1977).

The ***preconventional level*** of morality parallels the preconceptual level of cognitive development and intuitive thought. At this level morality is external, since children conform to rules imposed by authority figures. Culturally oriented to the labels of good/bad and right/wrong, children integrate these labels in terms of the physical or pleasurable consequences of their actions. The two stages of this level are:

Stage 1: The punishment-and-obedience orientation. Children determine the goodness or badness of an action in terms of its consequences. They avoid punishment and obey unquestioningly those who have the power to determine and enforce the rules and labels. They have no concept of the underlying moral order that supports these consequences.

Stage 2: The instrumental-relativist orientation. The right behavior consists of that which satisfies the child's own needs (and sometimes the needs of others). Although elements of fairness, reciprocity, and equal sharing are evident, they are interpreted in a very practical, concrete manner without the elements of loyalty, gratitude, or justice.

At the ***conventional level*** children are concerned with conformity and loyalty, actively maintaining, supporting, and justifying the social order, as well as personal expectations of those significant in their lives. They value the maintenance of family, group, or national expectations regardless of consequences. This level correlates with the concrete operational stage in cognitive development and consists of two stages:

Stage 3: The interpersonal concordance or "good boy–nice girl" orientation. Behavior that meets with approval and pleases or helps others is viewed as good. Conformity to the norm is the "natural" behavior, and one earns approval by being "nice."

Stage 4: The "law and order" orientation. Obeying the rules, doing one's duty, showing respect for authority, and maintaining the social order is the correct behavior. The rules and authority can be social or religious, depending on which is most valued.

At the ***postconventional, autonomous,*** or ***principled level*** children have reached the cognitive formal operational stage and endeavor to define moral values and principles that are valid and applicable beyond the authority of the groups and persons holding these principles. This level is not associated with the individual's identification with these groups. Level 3 also has two stages, but Stage 6 has been eliminated because Kohlberg determined that it is so rarely attained that it serves no useful purpose in a discussion such as this:

Stage 5: The social-contract, legalistic orientation. Correct behavior tends to be defined in terms of general individual rights and standards that have been examined and agreed on by the entire society. Although procedural rules for reaching consensus become important, with emphasis on the legal point of view, there is also emphasis on the possibility of changing law in terms of societal needs and rational considerations. Agreement and contract outside the legal realm are binding elements of obligation.

Although Kohlberg concludes that the highest stage of moral development is reached only after age 20 and only by a select few, Gilligan (1982) argues that there is a different, equally advanced stage where moral decisions are based on care and concern for others (see Thinking Critically About. . . box). Despite a lack of sophisticated moral reasoning, children can have rich moral values and behavior at any age.

Spiritual Development

Spiritual beliefs are closely related to the moral and ethical portion of children's self-concepts and as such must be considered as part of children's basic needs assessment. Children need to have meaning, purpose, and hope in their lives, and the need for confession and forgiveness is present even in very young children. The research in spiritual de-

THINKING CRITICALLY ABOUT . . .

Kindness and Fairness as the Roots of Moral Behavior

Gilligan (1982) believes that the roots of moral behavior—kindness and fairness—are found in early childhood. Newborns sometimes cry when they hear another infant crying, perhaps demonstrating a capacity to empathize with others. Babies as young as 10 months seem to empathize by whimpering or bursting into tears when faced with a person in distress (Terkel, 1992). Toddlers, seeing someone in distress, will often comfort them by patting or offering a favorite toy (Damon, 1989). Late school-age children begin to empathize with the plight of strangers (e.g., people who are homeless). Feeling empathy for others seems to induce a strong urge to help and behave altruistically (Terkel, 1992). This image of a caring, compassionate person who makes a moral decision by determining how his or her behavior affects other people contrasts sharply with Kohlberg's rational, detached person who bases decisions on moral principles and rules.

velopment is both limited and subject to criticism, particularly in relation to age-stage theories. However, the stage theories provide a useful means for the reader to assess the approximate level of development for any given child. Extending beyond religion (an organized set of beliefs and practices), spirituality affects the whole person: mind, body, and spirit (Clutter, 1991).

Fowler (1974) has identified seven stages in the development of faith, five of which parallel and are closely associated with cognitive and psychosocial development in childhood:

Stage 0: Undifferentiated. This stage of development encompasses the period of infancy when children have no concept of right or wrong, no beliefs, and no convictions to guide their behavior. However, the beginnings of a faith are established with the development of basic trust through their relationships with the primary caregiver.

Stage 1: Intuitive-projective. Toddlerhood is primarily a time of imitating the behavior of others. Children imitate the religious gestures and behaviors of others without comprehending any meaning or significance to the activities. During the preschool years children assimilate some of the values and beliefs of their parents. Parental attitudes toward moral codes and religious beliefs convey to children what they consider good and bad. Children follow parental beliefs as part of their daily lives rather than through an understanding of their basic concepts.

Stage 2: Mythical-literal. Through the school-age years spiritual development parallels cognitive development and is closely related to children's experiences and social interaction. Most children have a strong interest in religion during the school-age years. The existence of a deity is accepted, and petitions to an omnipotent being are important and expected to be answered; good behavior is rewarded, and bad behavior is punished. Children's developing conscience bothers them when they disobey. They have a reverence for many thoughts and matters and are able to articulate their faith. They may even begin to question its validity.

Stage 3: Synthetic-convention. As children approach adolescence, they become increasingly aware of spiritual disappointments. They recognize that prayers are not always answered (at least on their own terms). They begin to reason, to question some of the established parental religious standards, and to drop or modify some religious practices.

Stage 4: Individuating-reflexive. Adolescents become more skeptical and begin to compare the religious standards of their parents with the standards of others. They attempt to determine which to adopt and incorporate into their own set of values. They also begin to compare religious standards with the scientific viewpoint. It is a time of searching rather than reaching. Adolescents are uncertain about many religious ideas but will not achieve profound insights until late adolescence or early adulthood.

THEORETIC FOUNDATIONS OF LANGUAGE DEVELOPMENT

Children learn the complex symbol system of language with astonishing speed. Infants use abstract signifiers (words) to refer to objects and activities before they can walk. They can express hundreds of different messages by age 2 years, and know and use most of the syntactic structures of their native tongue by age 5 years. However, at all stages of language development, children's comprehension vocabulary is greater than their expressed vocabulary, and the acquisition of vocabulary and language keeps pace with cognitive advancement.

Children are born with the mechanism and capacity to develop speech and language skills: intact physiologic function of (1) the respiratory system, (2) speech control centers in the cerebral cortex, and (3) articulation and resonance structures of the mouth and nasal cavities. In addition, acquisition of language requires (1) an intact and discriminating auditory apparatus, (2) intelligence, (3) a need to communicate, and (4) stimulation.

Components of Language

Children first achieve a knowledge of ***phenology,*** referring to the basic units of sound, which are combined to produce words. Each language uses only a portion of all the sounds that humans are capable of generating, and children must learn to hear and to pronounce the speechlike sounds peculiar to their language. Then they learn how to combine these basic sounds into words.

Next children learn the ***semantics*** of language (i.e., that words and sentences convey an expressed meaning). Use of semantics progresses to knowledge of ***syntax,*** the form or structure of a language—the rules that specify how words are combined to form meaningful sentences. The rules of syntax vary considerably from one language to another, but the basic principle is true of all (i.e., individual words in a sentence interact with sentence structure to give the entire sentence a meaning).

Children must also acquire the important component of language, ***pragmatics,*** the principles specifying how language is to be used in different social contexts and situations. Pragmatic abilities and social editing skills evolve gradually over the course of childhood. All children in all cultures go through the same stages of language acquisition regardless of the structure of the language they are learning.

Stages of Language Development

Children proceed through several stages in the development of language. Infants can discriminate speech from other sound patterns and pay particularly close attention to speech from the beginning. By the time they enter school, children have mastered most of the syntactic rules of their native language and can produce a variety of sophisticated, adultlike messages (see box on p. 126).

Theories of Language Development

There are three major theories of language acquisition: learning theory, nativism, and the interactional approach. ***Learning theorists*** believe that language is acquired as children hear and respond to the speech of their companions. However, some disagreement exists among them regarding how children learn to speak. One faction believes that language is learned through operant conditioning as adults reinforce children for their attempts to produce grammatical speech. Others argue that children acquire language by lis-

STAGES IN DEVELOPMENT OF LANGUAGE

Prelinguistic stage—The period before children utter their first meaningful words; develops in steplike fashion over first 10 to 12 months from crying through cooing to babbling.
Holophrastic stage—The period when children's speech consists of one-word utterances, some of which are thought to be holophrases (single-word utterances that represent the meaning of an entire sentence); begins at about 1 year of age.
Telegraphic stage—The period when children's speech consists solely of content words, omitting the less meaningful parts of speech (such as articles, prepositions, and auxiliary verbs); begins at about 18 to 24 months of age.
Preschool period—The period when children begin to produce some very lengthy sentences and speech increases in complexity (ages 30 months to 5 years).
Middle childhood period—The period when children refine their language skills and increase linguistic competence (ages 6 to 14 years). They use bigger words, produce longer and more complex utterances, and learn subtle exceptions to grammatical rules. They begin to understand even the most complex syntactic structures of their native language.

tening to and imitating the speech of their older companions.

Nativists propose that human beings have an inborn linguistic processor, or language acquisition mechanism, that is specialized for language learning. They also believe that there is a critical period for language development and that humans are most proficient at language learning between 2 years of age and puberty.

The ***interactional proponents*** acknowledge that children are biologically prepared to acquire language but suggest that what may be innate is the development and maturation of the nervous system rather than a special linguistic processor. They also recognize the crucial role of environment in language learning, because children must hear simplified versions of adult speech in order to acquire the needed linguistic concepts.

Factors Affecting Language Acquisition

Girls are more advanced in language development than boys. Firstborn children develop language earlier than laterborn children, and children of multiple births (twins, triplets) develop language later than children of single births. Delayed, lack of, or impaired speech can result from a variety of sources, including congenital structural defects of the mouth and nasopharynx, a hearing deficit, neurologic dysfunction (including mental retardation), maternal deprivation, and emotional factors. Some of these factors are discussed in relation to health problems in which impaired speech is a symptom or a consequence. It is also important to note that some of the organ systems and organs on which speech depends, such as the respiratory system for gas exchange and the tongue for eating, are responsible for higher priority functions that take precedence over the lesser important function of communication. During illness or trauma children may direct their limited energy to the more vital functions of these systems: breathing and eating.

THEORETIC FOUNDATIONS OF SOCIAL LEARNING

Learning occurs when behavior changes as a result of experience, and learning theories attempt to explain the ways in which controlled changes in the environment produce predictable changes in behavior. Basically, children acquire new behaviors and produce alterations in existing behaviors through (1) forming associations through conditioning and (2) observing models.

Conditioning (Skinner)

Conditioning is learning by association (i.e., establishing a connection between a stimulus and a response). In ***classical,*** or ***Pavlovian, conditioning*** two events that occur simultaneously or close together in time come to have similar meanings to the child and thus evoke the same response. For example, infants learn very early to associate the sight of the mother's face and the sound of her voice with feeding and other pleasant sensations. Consequently, an infant will cease crying or somehow indicate pleasure when the mother speaks or enters the infant's visual field. This type of learning appears to be the predominant form that takes place during infancy, particularly in the first 6 months, before the development of motor control.

Operant, or ***instrumental, conditioning*** involves the use of rewards or reinforcements to encourage the performance of specific behaviors. Reinforcing desired responses whenever they occur increases the likelihood that they will be repeated. These reinforcements can be inner satisfactions or externally applied reward systems. Behavior that is not in some way reinforced or rewarded will be extinguished. The principles of instrumental conditioning are especially applicable to learning that takes place naturally in toddlers and preschool children. These children can appreciate the significance of rewards and punishments even though they may not be able to conceptualize the context or framework in which they are operating. A substantial proportion of early childhood learning, such as acquisition of motor skills, consists of simple operant conditioning.

Avoidance conditioning discourages undesired behaviors through the use of punishment and fear of punishment. The effectiveness of rewards and punishments depends on the child's subjective assessment of the reward or punishment. Some rewards are not reinforcing, and punishments do not generate fear if they are inappropriate to the developmental level, emotional stage, or value system of the individual child. Punishment is effective in controlling behavior, but it must be correctly timed, brief, appropriate to the child and the undesired behavior, and tempered with love.

Operant conditioning is the basis of behavior-modification procedures that have achieved varying degrees of success in speech therapy and in modifying behavior in overly aggressive and mentally retarded children. Behavior is shaped by reinforcing closer and closer approximations to the behavior being taught.

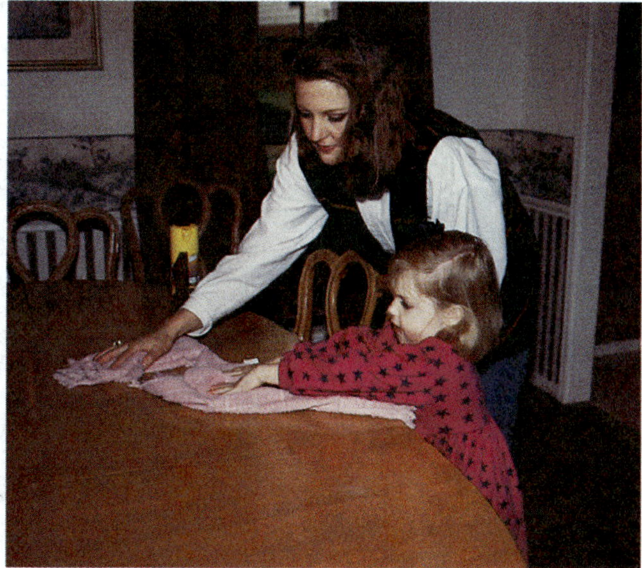

FIG. 4-10 Children learn by imitating the behavior of others.

Modeling or Observational Learning (Bandura)

Much of childhood learning takes place because of children's innate tendency to observe and imitate the behavior of those who are significant in their lives. Children learn many new behaviors from observing parents, siblings, and peers. Learning is immediate, and children can often correctly imitate a behavior on the first attempt. They are more apt to imitate those whom they believe to be prestigious and those whom they see being rewarded for their behavior.

As children gain more complex cognitive skills and the use of language, learning assumes broader dimensions, involving creativity, problem solving, and abstract conceptualization. Modeling requires no reinforcement, although in most situations children imitate a behavior because they are in some way reinforced for doing so. A child may proudly proclaim to be doing something "just like mommy and daddy." Apparently, modeling is its own reward (Fig. 4-10).

Role Learning in Children

A role is a set of duties, rights, obligations, and expected behaviors that accompanies a given position in a social structure. Children are expected to play a variety of roles, such as son or daughter, sister or brother, student, classmate, and playmate. They learn and practice these roles and learn something of the characteristics of other roles through interaction with others and in their play. Children will behave in patterned and more or less predictable ways because they learn roles that define mutual expectations in typical and recurring social relationships (see Chapter 3).

Individuals bring their own unique temperaments, skills, and values to the interpretation and enactment of the roles they play. Because most roles exist independently of the individuals who play them, the functions and norms associated with any given role influence the way persons play the roles and the responses of the people associated with those persons. For example, expectations about the role of teacher affect the behavior of persons playing that role, and those expectations serve as a guide to others in the evaluation of persons in that role.

STAGES OF ROLE TAKING

1. **Egocentric or undifferentiated perspective** (approximately 3 to 6 years). Children are unaware of any perspective other than their own—whatever is right for them is agreeable to others.
2. **Social-informational role taking** (approximately 6 to 8 years). Children recognize that people can have perspectives that differ from their own but only because these persons have received different information. Children are unable to think about the thinking of others and imagine how others will react to an event.
3. **Self-reflective role taking** (approximately 8 to 10 years). Children know that their own and others' viewpoints may conflict even when they receive the same information. They are able to consider another's point of view and recognize that others can place themselves in their shoes. Consequently, children are able to anticipate another's reactions to their behavior but are unable to consider their own and another's perspective at the same time.
4. **Mutual role taking** (approximately 10 to 12 years). Children can consider their own and another's point of view simultaneously and realize that others are able to do the same. They can also assume the perspective of a disinterested child and anticipate the way the active participants (self and other) will react to the viewpoint of either participant.
5. **Social and conventional system role taking** (approximately 12 to 15 years). Young persons now attempt to understand the perspective of another by comparing it with that of the social system in which they operate. They expect others to consider and assume perspectives on events congruent with most persons in their social group.

From Selman RL: The *growth of interpersonal understanding,* New York, 1980, Academic Press.

As their relationships expand, children also become increasingly proficient in understanding other people. They develop the ability to distinguish their own perspectives from those of their companions through role taking. This ability is acquired in a progressive, developmental sequence that parallels the invariant cognitive stages of Piaget (see p. 123). Selman's stages of social role taking are outlined in the box above.

The ability to interact successfully with other people is closely related to role-taking skills. Relationships change as children recognize that others have different motives and intentions. For example, in Selman's stage 1 a friend is someone who not only lives nearby but also does nice things (Fig. 4-11); at stage 2 the term "friend" implies a reciprocal relationship with mutual respect, kindness, and affection (Furman and Bierman, 1983). In adolescence friendship becomes a relationship of common interests and values with a reasonably well-coordinated outlook on life, and a "friend" becomes someone with whom intimate information can be shared (Berndt, 1982). It has also been found that children who are adept in role-taking abilities are bet-

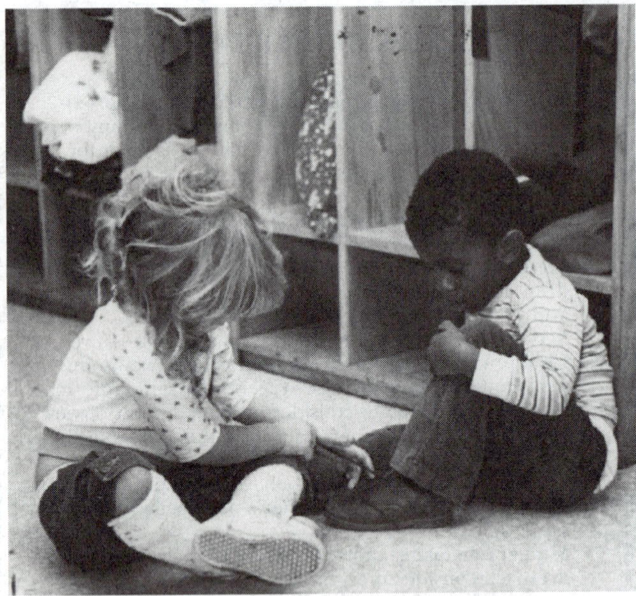

FIG. 4-11 A friend is someone who does nice things.

ter able to establish intimate friendships (McGuire and Weisz, 1982) and are more popular with classmates (Kurdek and Krile, 1982).

DEVELOPMENT OF SELF-CONCEPT

Self-concept comprises all the notions, beliefs, and convictions that constitute children's knowledge of themselves and that influence their relationships with others. It is not present at birth but develops gradually as a result of each child's unique experiences within the self, with significant others, and with the realities of the world (Stuart and Sundeen, 1991). However, the self-concept is subjective and therefore may or may not reflect reality.

The content of the self-concept differs at various stages of development and results from the cognitive capacities and the dominant motives of individuals coming in contact with stage-related cultural expectations. In infancy self-concept is primarily an awareness of one's independent existence learned in part as a result of social contacts and experiences with other people. The process becomes more active during toddlerhood as children explore the limits of their capacities and the nature of their impact on others (Newman and Newman, 1984).

School-age children are more aware of differences in perspectives among people, social norms, and moral imperatives. They are sensitive to social pressures and become preoccupied with issues of self-criticism and self-evaluation. Because school-age children depend on adults for material and emotional resources, the self-concept is likely to be most vulnerable during this time. Little change in self-concept occurs during early adolescence when children anxiously focus on their physical and emotional changes and peer acceptance. Self-concept crystallizes during later adolescence as young people review and evaluate their childhood experiences and organize their self-concept around a set of values, goals, and competencies (Newman and Newman, 1984).

Body Image

Body image, a vital component of the self-concept, is the subjective concepts and attitudes that individuals have toward their own bodies as objects in space. Central to the concept of self, body image is the picture of the body formed in the mind, including feelings about size, function, appearance, and potential. The picture appears to be a learned phenomenon that may be conscious or unconscious and may be cognitive and/or emotional. Body image has physical, psychologic, and social components and includes present and past perceptions. It changes with advancing development and is continually modified by new perceptions and experiences.

The significant others in their lives exert the most important and meaningful impact on children's body image. Labels that are attached to them (such as "skinny," "pretty," or "fat") or body parts (such as "ugly mole," "bug eyes," or "yucky skin") are incorporated into the body image. Because they lack the understanding of deviations from the physical standard or norm, children notice prominent differences in others and unwittingly make rude and often cruel remarks about such minor deviations as large or widely spaced front teeth, large or small eyes, moles, or extreme variations in height.

Development During Growth. Infants receive input about their bodies through self-exploration and sensory stimulation from others. As they begin to manipulate their environment, they become aware of their bodies as being separate from others. Toddlers learn to identify the various parts of their bodies and are able to use symbols to represent objects. Preschoolers become aware of the wholeness of their bodies and discover the genitals. Exploration of the genitals and the discovery of differences between the sexes become important. There is only a vague concept of internal organs and function (Selekman, 1983; Stuart and Sundeen, 1991).

School-age children begin to learn about internal body structure and function and become aware of differences in the body size and configurations of others. They are highly influenced by the cultural norms of society and the fads of the times. Children whose bodies deviate from the norm are often subject to criticism and ridicule.

Adolescence is the age when children become most concerned about the physical self. The familiar body changes and the new physical self must be integrated into the self-concept. Adolescents face conflicts over what they see and what they visualize as the ideal body structure. Body image formation during adolescence is a crucial element in the shaping of an identity, the psychosocial crisis of adolescence.

Self-Esteem

Self-esteem is described as the affective component of the self, and the self-concept is the cognitive component; however, the two are almost indistinguishable, and the terms are often used interchangeably. Self-esteem is a personal,

EVALUATIVE DIMENSIONS OF SELF-ESTEEM

COMPETENCE

How adequate are my cognitive, physical, and social skills?

SENSE OF CONTROL

How well can I complete tasks needed to produce desired actions?

Is someone or something specific versus luck or chance responsible for my successes and failures?

MORAL WORTH

How closely do my actions and behaviors meet moral standards that have been set?

WORTHINESS OF LOVE AND ACCEPTANCE

How worthy am I of love and acceptance from parents, other significant adults, siblings, and peers?

Modified from Sieving R, Zirbel-Donisch S: Development and enhancement of self-esteem in children, *J Pediatr Health Care* 4(6):290-296, 1990.

subjective judgment of one's worthiness derived from and influenced by the social groups in the immediate environment and the individual's perceptions of how he or she is valued by others. Self-esteem is primarily a function of being loved and of gaining the respect of others. Children assess specific dimensions of themselves in forming an overall evaluation of their self-esteem (see box above).

Factors that influence the formation of a child's self-esteem include (1) the child's temperament and personality, (2) abilities and opportunities available to accomplish age-appropriate developmental tasks, (3) significant others, and (4) social roles assumed and the expectations of these roles (Sieving and Zirbel-Donisch, 1990).

Self-esteem is a product of both competence and social acceptance that changes with development. Throughout childhood children experience an increased ability to differentiate components of competence, an increased concern with a variety of significant others who may give or withhold approval, and an increased capacity to experience guilt when internal norms for either competence or social acceptance are violated. ***High self-esteem*** is described as a feeling based on unconditional acceptance of oneself as a worthy and important being (Stuart and Sundeen, 1991).

Highly egocentric toddlers are unaware of any difference between competence and social approval. They are the center of their world, and to them all positive experiences are evidence of their importance and value. Preschool and early school-age children, on the other hand, are increasingly aware of the discrepancy between their competencies and the abilities of more advanced children. They are expected to evaluate a situation and anticipate the consequences of their behavior before they act. The acceptance of adults and peers outside the family group becomes more important to them. Since these valued persons may not be as proud of their achievements or as understanding of their limitations as their families are, their recently acquired capacity for guilt may lead to anxiety over failure, and they will be more vulnerable to feelings of worthlessness and depression. As their competencies increase and they develop meaningful relationships, their self-esteem rises. Their self-esteem is again at risk during early adolescence when they are defining an identity and sense of self in the context of their peer group.

Unless children are continually made to feel incompetent and of little worth, a decrease in self-esteem during vulnerable periods is only temporary. Transitory periods of lowered self-esteem at the stages of development are expected when they must set new goals or when there are very obvious discrepancies in competence. A constant source of anxiety arises from the endless number of separations that occur in the process of acquiring autonomy, independence, and individuality. As an expression of their own urgencies, parents often set overambitious goals for their children and expect them to perform beyond the limits of their capacity. Also, children's attempts at autonomy and achievement are often thwarted by parental overprotection, because either the parents fear the children will be hurt or the parents find it more convenient to do things for them.

To develop and preserve self-esteem, children need to feel that they are worthwhile individuals who are in some way different from, superior to, and more lovable than any other individual in the world. They need recognition for their achievements and the approval of parents and peers. Parents and other authority figures can foster a positive self-concept by providing appropriate encouragement and recognition for achievement and by discouraging inappropriate behaviors. However, when authority figures express disapproval, they must convey to a child that the *behavior* is unacceptable, not the child. Constructive communication, such as the use of "I" messages, conveys feeling and needs without destroying the child's self-esteem.

Children who experience warm, affectionate relationships with their family and who are aware of their parents' acceptance and positive attitudes toward them are more accepting of themselves. Children who have a strong sense of their own worth are confident and able to initiate activities, explore their environment, and take risks in their behavior when confronted with new or novel situations. They approach tasks and relationships with the expectation that they will be well received and successful. Nurses have numerous opportunities to help parents understand their child's self-esteem development and to assist parents in structuring an environment conducive to this development. Methods include exploring with parents their expectations for their children, effective communication techniques, discipline strategies, child-centered guidance, and methods of promoting children's autonomy (Sieving and Zirbel-Donisch, 1990). Such is the focus of nursing—to allow children and their families to grow and to prosper from their experiences in times of both health and illness.

DEVELOPMENT OF SEXUALITY

From the moment of birth, children are treated differently by their families on the basis of their biologic sex. Almost immediately infants are placed in male or female categories with given names that clearly indicate a sex, dressed in pink (girls) or blue (boys), and referred to as either "he" or "she." Thus information regarding a sexual identity is conveyed to children and to the world, and along with these overt messages a set of sex-related attitudes toward them emerges. The outcome of the identification process depends on the characteristics of the parents and other role models, the innate capacities and preferences of the child, and the cultural and familiar value placed on the child's sex.

Families recognize the importance of sex differences and even in infancy treat boys differently from girls. Parental attitudes and expectations regarding sex-appropriate behaviors, acquired from the parents' own upbringing, influence how they react to their children from infancy. These attitudes and expectations are transmitted to infants first in subtle and then in more obvious ways. For example, family members relate to infants differently: little girls are handled more tenderly; little boys are stimulated with boisterous activity and vigorous motor play. Families provide sex-appropriate toys and encourage play consistent with the sex-role expectations of the children.

Four dimensions appear to be involved in the development of sex-role identification. Children (1) learn to apply appropriate gender labels to themselves, (2) acquire sex-appropriate standards of behavior, (3) develop a preference for being the sex that they are, and (4) identify with their parent of the same sex.

Gender Label

The gender label is achieved early and subtly through imitation of the parents' expressions as they refer to children's gender (e.g., "That's a good girl" or "That's a good boy"). Since it is such an important and basic component of children's total identity, the appropriate gender must be assigned as soon as possible in rare cases where the sex of the infant is in doubt (see Abnormal Sexual Development, Chapter 11). The gender orientation has more effect on development than does chromosomal determination of sex.

However, with the increasing number of nontraditional gender roles portrayed on prime time television, children's stereotypical perceptions of men and women may be changing. Children who are familiar with shows that depict men performing traditionally feminine tasks such as cooking, cleaning, and caring for children and women employed outside the home have a more flexible view of sex-related roles (Rosenwasser, Lingenfelter, and Harrington, 1989).

Sex-Role Standards

Beginning when children are toddlers, sex-role standards are differentiated and continuously developed throughout childhood. By the time children are 3 years old, they know whether they are boys or girls, and they have acquired considerable knowledge of and a preference for sex-appropriate behaviors. They can differentiate one sex from the other even before they learn anatomic differences; 2-year-old children can identify others as girls or boys based on external appearances.

Preschool children have definite impressions of masculinity and femininity, and they are reflected in overt play. Most children in this age-group engage in stereotyped sex-appropriate play activities. Little girls are more likely to play at housekeeping, taking care of dolls, dressing up, and cooking; boys choose trucks, blocks, and more physically active play. Boys are generally more aggressive in their play, and in disagreements with peers they are more apt to react with shouting or fighting. Girls tend to be more dependent and introverted in their play.

With the strong women's movement, more liberal views regarding sex-role typing, and the unisex trend in all areas of interaction, these sex-associated characteristics are less apparent than they have been in the past. For example, although boys and younger girls were observed to pay more attention and learn more about objects labeled for their sex, older girls were much more flexible regarding what they considered correct for their sex (Bradbard and others, 1986). However, the United States, like most cultures, still has a strong masculine orientation, with males generally accorded more privileges than females.

Families expect children to learn appropriate sex-role behavior early and to deviate little from it. Each family has its own concept of what constitutes male or female attributes and the types of sex-linked behavior they wish to cultivate in their children. These beliefs are conveyed to the children by a variety of means, and parents exert special efforts to gain compliance with their expectations. Experiences the children are exposed to, toys selected for them, and activities they are encouraged to participate in all reflect some aspect of the family's sex-role conformity to standards of achievement, competition, self-assertiveness, and independence with control of feelings and repression of emotions. With girls the family usually places more emphasis on passive activities and the development of interpersonal sensitivity, docility, interrelatedness with others, and nurturance.

Observing siblings' interaction at play can provide insight into sex-role relationships. Sibling relationships mirror parent relationships within a given family—divorced or intact. For example, older boys from discordant families have been observed to bully their younger sisters (MacKinnon, 1989).

In the case of boys, the prohibition against effeminate behavior is very strong. Boys are rewarded less often for displaying behavior considered appropriate for their sex, but they are discouraged from exhibiting undesirable behavior by negative reinforcement. Parents emphasize the things that boys should *not* do or be (i.e., those things that might label them as "sissies"). Avoidance of the opposite sex-role behavior is a major means of sex-role learning in the American culture, especially for boys. This emphasis seems to be stronger in lower-class families, where sex roles are more clearly defined and segregated. In middle-class homes sex-role differentiation is less clear-cut. Mothers often work outside the home, and male role models are more apt to help with behaviors traditionally assigned to the female, such as housework and baby-sitting.

The family situation may be more influential for sex-role development of girls than of boys, since boys are more apt to learn much of their masculine behaviors from role models outside the home. For example, in lower-class black families in which the father is frequently absent, a male child often associates with gangs to learn a masculine role, whereas a Hispanic youth who has a male model in the home may join such gangs to escape the paternal dominance and be free to express his masculine role.

Girls, on the other hand, are dealt with more leniently in America. Their role is less rigidly defined than that of boys. Girls are permitted to engage in masculine games and activities, to wear pants, and to be a tomboy without strong cultural disapproval. This greater variance may create some confusion in establishing a sex-role identity. A girl's acceptance of a parental role model depends a great deal on whether the role model of her mother is congruent with the girl's concept of a sex role.

Gender Preference

Gender preference for the sex children are born is acquired over a long time and depends on several things. Children will prefer to be a member of their own sex when their behaviors and competence closely approximate the sex-role standards, when they like their parent of the same sex, and when they believe their sex is valued. The sexes are not always valued equally in all cultures or in all families. In cultures where males are more highly valued and are given higher status, boys are likely to develop a firm preference for their sex. However, girls in these cultures may be less certain regarding their gender assignment, even to the point of rejecting their sex group. A deterrent to sex-role preference by children can exist in families where the parents, at a specific birth, had hoped strongly for a child of the opposite sex. The environmental cues within the family will convey to these children that the opposite sex is a preferred one.

Gender Identity

The process by which children style themselves after their parent of the same sex and internalize that parent's values and outlook is ***identification.*** Most children wish to be like their parent of the same sex, and although the motivation for identification is still unsettled, children are more willing to share these parental attributes when they are able to see a degree of similarity between themselves and their parents. Children become aware of the similarity when they perceive actual physical and psychologic similarities, adopt parental behaviors, and are told of similarities by others. Once this identification is formed, it can be strengthened by the continued positive conception of the role model or weakened if the child does not perceive the model as desirable. Identification is not a total, all-or-nothing happening. To some extent children identify with both parents, and as their sphere of social contacts widens, they identify with peers and other adults outside the family.

ROLE OF PLAY IN DEVELOPMENT

Through the universal medium of play children learn what no one can teach them. They learn about their world and about themselves operating within that world—what they can do, how to relate to things and situations, and how to adapt themselves to the demands society makes on them. Play is the *work* of the child. In play children continually practice the complicated, stressful processes of living, communicating, and achieving satisfactory relationships with other people.

CLASSIFICATION OF PLAY

From a developmental point of view, patterns of children's play can be categorized according to content and social character. In both there is an additive effect; each builds on past accomplishments, and some element of each is maintained throughout life. At each stage in development the new predominates.

Content of Play

The content of play involves primarily the physical aspects of play, although social relationships cannot be ignored. The content of play follows the directional trend of the simple to the complex.

Play begins with ***social-affective play,*** wherein infants take pleasure in relationships with people. As adults talk, fondle, nuzzle, and in various ways elicit a response from an infant, the infant soon learns to provoke parental emotions and responses with such behaviors as smiling, cooing, or initiating games and activities. The type and intensity of the adult behavior with children vary among cultures.

Sense-pleasure play is a nonsocial stimulating experience that originates from without. Objects in the environment—light and color, tastes and odors, textures and consistencies—attract children's attention, stimulate their senses, and give pleasure. Pleasurable experiences are derived from handling raw materials (water, sand, food), from body motion (swinging, bouncing, rocking), and from other uses of senses and abilities (smelling, humming) (Fig. 4-12).

Once infants have developed the ability to grasp and manipulate, they persistently demonstrate and exercise their newly acquired abilities through ***skill play,*** repeating an ac-

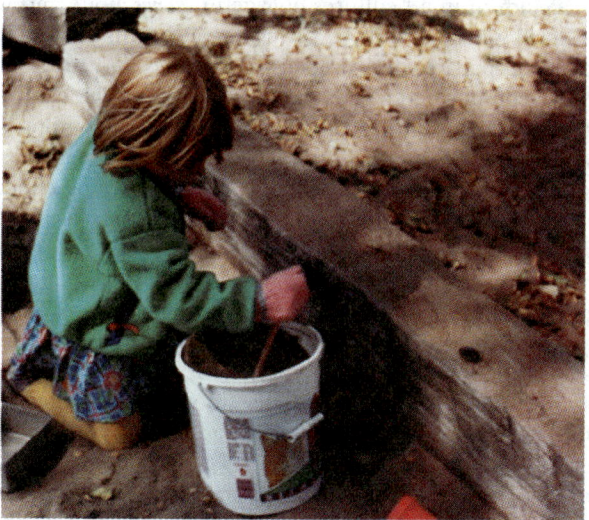

FIG. 4-12 Children derive pleasure from handling raw materials.

tion over and over again. The element of sense-pleasure play is often evident in the practicing of a new ability, but all too frequently the determination to conquer the elusive skill produces pain and frustration (e.g., learning to ride a bicycle).

In ***unoccupied behavior*** children are not playful but focus their attention momentarily on anything that strikes their interest. Children daydream, fiddle with clothes or other objects, or walk aimlessly. This role differs from that of onlookers, who actively observe the activity of others.

One of the vital elements in children's process of identification is ***dramatic play,*** also known as ***symbolic*** or ***pretend play.*** It begins in late infancy (11 to 13 months) as children engage in simple pretending with familiar activities, such as eating, sleeping, or drinking from a cup. In toddlerhood the activities are still primarily those that are familiar. As children enter the preschool stage their play becomes further removed from everyday activities and much more complex. Dramatic play is the predominant form of play in the preschool child.

Once children begin to invest situations and people with meanings and to attribute affective significance to the world, they can pretend and fantasize almost anything. By acting out events of daily life, children learn and practice the roles and identities modeled by the members of their family and society. Pretend play provides a framework within which mature behaviors are tested and assimilated (Connolly, Doyle, and Reznick, 1988).

Children's toys, replicas of the tools of society, provide a medium for learning about adult roles and activities that may be puzzling and frustrating to them. Interacting with the world is one way children get to know it. The simple, imitative, dramatic play of the toddler, such as using the telephone, driving a car, or rocking a doll, evolves into more complex, sustained dramas of the preschooler, which extend beyond common domestic matters to the wider aspects of the world and the society, such as playing policeman, storekeeper, teacher, or nurse. Older children work out elaborate themes, act out stories, and compose plays (Fig. 4-13).

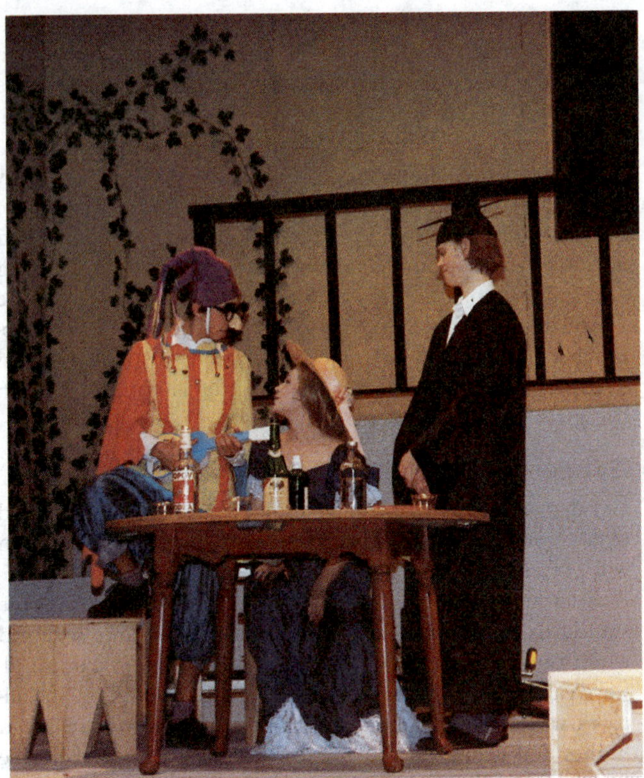

FIG. 4-13 Older children enjoy being in plays.

Children in all cultures engage in ***games*** alone and with others. Solitary activity involving games begins as very small children participate in repetitive activities and progress to more complicated games that challenge their independent skills, such as solving puzzles, solitaire, and computer or video games. When children interact with others, games assume the same developmental trends. Very young children participate in simple, imitative games such as pat-a-cake and peekaboo.

Preschool children learn and enjoy formal games that begin with ritualistic, self-sustaining games, such as ring-around-a-rosy and London Bridge. With the exception of some simple board games, preschool children do not engage in competitive games. They do play competitively but find it difficult not to take competition seriously. Preschoolers hate to lose and will try to cheat, want to change rules, or demand exceptions and opportunities to change their moves. Competitive games are the province of school-age children and adolescents who enjoy a variety of games including cards, checkers, chess, and physically active games such as baseball.

Social Character of Play

The play interactions of infancy are between a child and an adult. Children continue to enjoy the company of an adult but are increasingly able to play alone. As age advances, interaction with age-mates increases in importance and becomes an essential part of the socialization process. Through interaction, highly egocentric infants, unable to tolerate delay or interference, ultimately acquire concern for others and the ability to delay gratification or even to reject gratification at the expense of another. A pair of toddlers engage in considerable combat because their personal needs cannot tolerate delay or compromise. By the time they reach age 5 or 6 years, children are able to arrive at a compromise or make use of arbitration, usually after individual children have attempted but failed to gain their own way. Through continued interaction with peers and the growth of conceptual abilities and social skills, children are able to increase participation with others.

During ***onlooker play*** children watch what other children are doing but make no attempt to enter into the play activity. There is an active interest in observing the interaction of others but no movement toward participating. Watching television is a common example of the onlooker role.

Children who independently play alone are engaging in ***solitary play.*** They may enjoy the presence of other children but make no effort to get close or speak to them. Their interest is centered on their own activity.

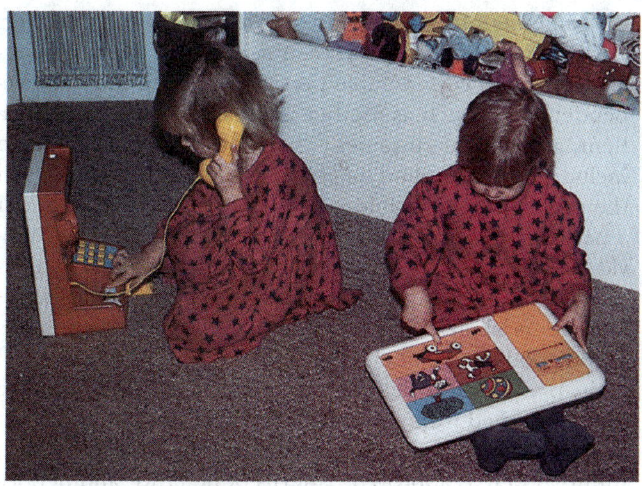

FIG. 4-14 Parallel play.

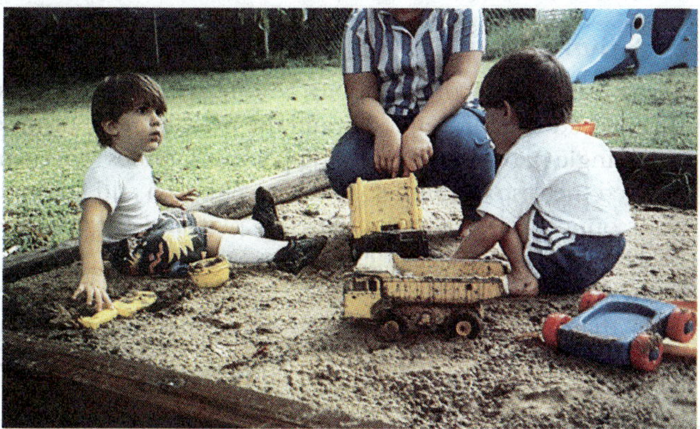

FIG. 4-15 Associative play.

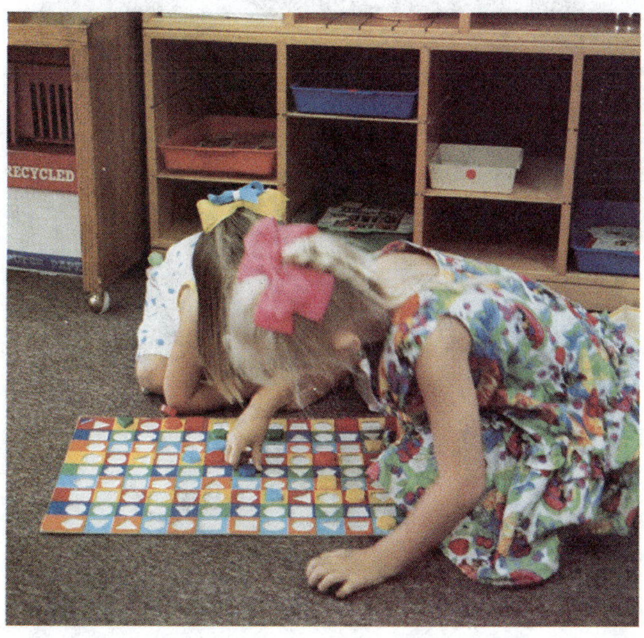

FIG. 4-16 Cooperative play.

During ***parallel play*** children play independently but among other children. They play with toys like those the children around them are using, but as each child sees fit, neither influencing nor being influenced by the other children. Each plays beside, but not with, other children (Fig. 4-14). There is no group association. Parallel play is the characteristic play of toddlers, but it may also occur in other groups of any age. Individuals who are involved in a creative craft with each person separately working on an individual project are engaged in parallel play.

When children play together and are engaged in a similar or even identical activity, but there is no organization, division of labor, leadership assignment, or mutual goal, the play is ***associative.*** Children borrow and lend play materials, follow each other with wagons and tricycles, and sometimes attempt to control who may or may not play in the group. Each child acts according to his or her own wishes; there is no group goal (Fig. 4-15). For example, two children play with dolls, borrowing articles of clothing from each other and engaging in similar conversation, but neither directs the other's actions nor establishes rules regarding the limits of the play session. There is a great deal of behavioral contagion: when one child initiates an activity, the entire group follows the example.

Cooperative play is organized, and the children play in a group *with* other children (Fig. 4-16). The children discuss and plan activities for the purposes of accomplishing an end—to make something, to attain a competitive goal, to dramatize situations of adult or group life, or to play formal games. The group is loosely formed, but there is a marked sense of belonging or not belonging. The goal and its attainment require organization of activities, division of labor, and playing roles. The leader-follower relationship is definitely established, and the activity is controlled by one or two members who assign roles and direct the activity of the others. The activity is organized to allow one child to supplement another's function in order to complete the goal.

FUNCTIONS OF PLAY

The specific values of play or the functions that it serves throughout childhood include sensorimotor development, intellectual development, socialization, creativity, self-awareness, and therapeutic and moral value.

Sensorimotor Development

Sensorimotor activity is a major component of play at all ages and is the predominant form of play in infancy. Active play is essential for muscle development and serves a useful purpose as a release for surplus energy. Through sensorimotor play, children explore the nature of the physical world. Infants gain impressions of themselves and their world through tactile, auditory, visual, and kinesthetic stimulation. Toddlers and preschoolers revel in body movement and exploration of things in space. Children continue to engage in sensorimotor play, although with increasing maturity the play becomes more differentiated and involved. Whereas very young children run for the sheer joy of body movement, older children incorporate or modify the motions into increasingly complex and coordinated activities such as races, games, skating, and bicycle riding.

Intellectual Development

Through exploration and manipulation, children learn colors, shapes, sizes, textures, and the significance of objects (Fig. 4-17). They learn the significance of numbers and how to use them, they learn to associate words with objects, and they develop an understanding of abstract concepts and spatial relationships, such as up, down, under, and over. Activities such as puzzles and games help them develop problem-solving skills. Books, stories, films, and collections expand knowledge and provide enjoyment as well. Play provides a means to practice and expand language skills. Through play children continually rehearse past experiences to assimilate them into new perceptions and relationships. Play helps children comprehend the world in which they live and distinguish between fantasy and reality.

Socialization

From very early infancy children show interest and pleasure in the company of others (Fig. 4-18). Their initial social contact is with the mothering person, but through play with other children they learn to establish social relationships and solve the problems associated with these relationships.

Children pass through four distinct phases in developing social competence in play during their first 5 years. Infants under a year of age investigate other infants in much the same manner as they investigate other objects in their environment. Children between ages 2 and 3 years generally engage in considerable pretend play with mutually dependent roles such as mother and baby, physician and patient, grocer and customer. Their social circle expands to include both short- and long-term friends. When they reach the preschool years, children become increasingly aware of a peer group and can identify stable characteristics of individual playmates. They have one or two favorite playmates with whom they play almost exclusively. They can verbalize judgments about each other and sense a distinction between good friends and mere acquaintances (Howes, 1987).

In play children learn to give and take, which is more readily learned from critical peers than from more tolerant adults. They learn the sex role that society expects them to fulfill, as well as approved patterns of behavior and deportment. Closely associated with socialization is development of moral values and ethics. Children learn right from wrong, the standards of the society, and to assume responsibility for their actions.

Creativity

There is growing concern that the intense academic pressure placed on children today and the prevalence of divorce and single-parent and working-parent families have increased the responsibilities placed on children and lessened their opportunities for spontaneous play and the exercise of imagination (Elkind, 1991).

In no other situation is there more opportunity to be creative than in play. Children can experiment and try out their ideas in play through every medium at their disposal, including raw materials, fantasy, and exploration. Creativity is stifled by pressure toward conformity; therefore striv-

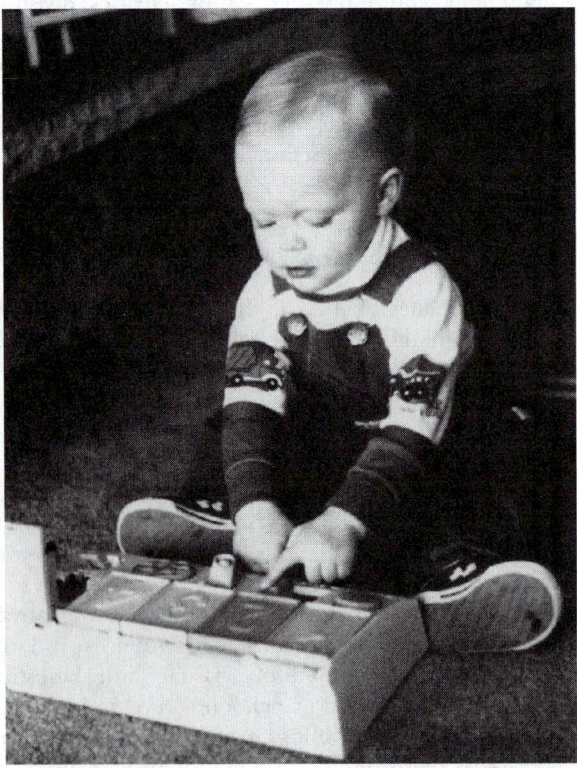

FIG. 4-17 Children learn through exploration with shapes and textures.

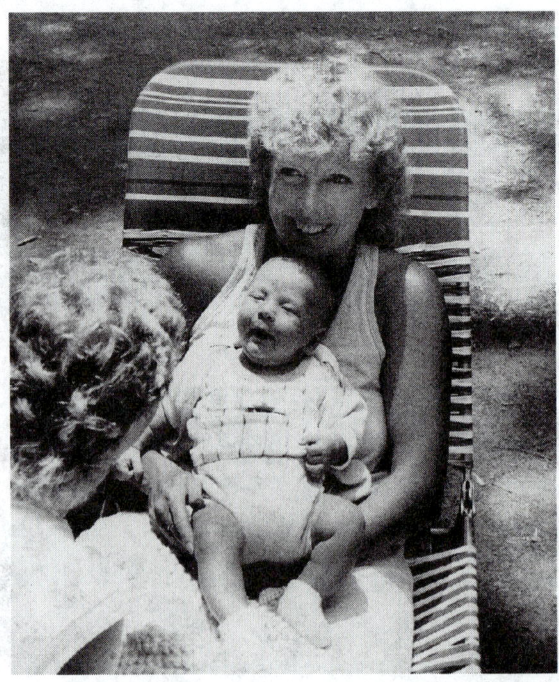

FIG. 4-18 The socialization process begins in early infancy.

ing for peer approval may inhibit creative endeavors in the school-age or adolescent child. Creativity is primarily a product of solitary activity, yet creative thinking is often enhanced in group settings where listening to others' ideas stimulates further exploration of one's own. Once children feel the satisfaction of creating something new and different, they transfer this creative interest to situations outside the world of play.

Self-Awareness

Beginning with active explorations of their bodies and awareness of themselves as separate from the caregiver, the process of self-identity is facilitated through play activities. Children learn who they are and what their place is in the world. They become increasingly able to regulate their own behavior, to learn what their abilities are, and to compare their abilities with those of others. Through play children are able to test their abilities, assume and try out various roles, and learn the effect their behavior has on others.

Therapeutic Value

Play is therapeutic at any age. It provides a means for release from the tension and stress encountered through the environment. In play children can express emotions and release unacceptable impulses in a socially acceptable fashion. Children are able to experiment and test fearful situations and can assume and vicariously master the roles and positions they are unable to perform in the world of reality. Children reveal much about themselves in play. Children are able to communicate to the alert observer through play the needs, fears, and desires they are unable to express with their limited language skills. Throughout their play children need the presence and acceptance of adults to help them control aggression and channel their destructive tendencies.

AGE CHARACTERISTICS OF PLAY

EXPLORATORY STAGE

Age: Approximately 3 to 12 months
Activities: Grasping, holding, and examining articles
Exploration via creeping or crawling

TOY STAGE

Age: 1 to 7 or 8 years
Activities: Imitating adult behavior with replicas of adult tools

PLAY STAGE

Age: 8 to 12 years
Activities: Interest in toys diminishes
Interest in games, sports, and hobbies increases

DAYDREAMING STAGE

Age: Characteristic of older children and pubescents
Activities: Playing the martyr misunderstood and mistreated by everyone or the hero or beauty admired by everyone (Fig. 4-19)

Moral Value

Although children learn at home and at school those behaviors considered right and wrong in the culture, the interaction with peers during play contributes significantly to their moral training. Nowhere is the enforcement of moral standards so rigid as in the play situation. If they are to be acceptable members of the group, children must adhere to the culturally accepted codes of behavior—fairness, honesty, self-control, and consideration for others. Children soon learn that their peers are less tolerant of violations than are adults and that to maintain a place in the play group, they must conform to the standards of the group.

CHARACTERISTICS OF PLAY

There are several aspects of play that display developmental changes and that differentiate children's play from adult play.

Tradition

In general, the play of small children varies little from generation to generation within a culture. Each generation of children imitates the play of the preceding generation; in this way the more satisfying forms of play are perpetuated. Many types of play are characteristic of all cultures (e.g., playing with balls, some form of doll, or some type of walking toy to help children just beginning to walk to maintain balance).

Seasonal changes are accompanied by traditional forms of toys and play activities. Sledding and ice skating are popular in winter; jump rope, bicycling, and in-line skating are spring and summer activities.

Time and Age

The amount of time that children spend in play decreases with age. Older children have less time available for play because of an increase in schoolwork and other responsi-

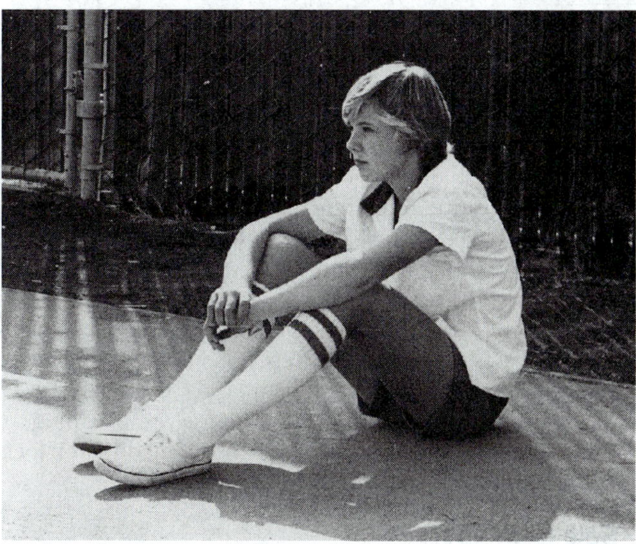

FIG. 4-19 Daydreaming is characteristic of pubescent children.

bilities. With advancing age and development, the number and variety of play activities diminish and play becomes less physically active, but the time spent in specific activities increases as interests narrow and the attention span lengthens. The number of playmates decreases with age as children progress from play with anyone available to play with a few selected and special age-mates.

Children's play can be divided into the following four categories: (1) imitative, (2) exploratory, (3) testing, and (4) model building. At all ages each of these types is evident in children's play, but one type will predominate over the others at specific ages. For example, imitative play can be seen in the infant who mimics the actions of another (pat-a-cake), but it reaches its peak in the dramatic play of preschoolers who play "house," "astronaut," or "school." It can also be observed in circular group singing and rhythmic games such as ring-around-a-rosy.

As children grow older, play activities become less spontaneous, more formal and structured, and increasingly sex appropriate. Whereas infants and small children of both sexes play in much the same way, by the time they enter school, most children engage in activities deemed appropriate for their sex. Despite efforts to break rigid sex role stereotypes, many little boys are clearly aware that they do not play with certain toys, and they avoid their girl playmates.

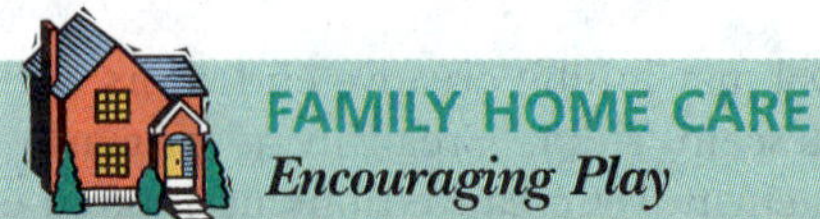

FAMILY HOME CARE
Encouraging Play

Realize that play teaches skills and abilities that are the center of intelligence.
Play with your child.
- Help your child select a play activity.
- Be flexible, creative, and willing to do the unconventional.
- Remain available, giving your child the opportunity to indicate the desired level of adult involvement.
- Offer encouragement by expressing interest and genuine praise in your child's activity.
- Do not turn every play activity into an educational lesson.

Challenge your child from time to time when new skills are learned.
- Present new levels of difficulty.
- Have available a balanced variety of toys encompassing numerous areas of development.

Respect your child's likes and dislikes; remember that learning is best acquired in an enjoyable situation.
Observe your child at play to learn favorite types of toys and activities.
Enroll your child in a play group that meets several times a week, or hire a baby-sitter who can act as a playmate.

From Lewis M, Block JR: Toy play: IQ building, *Mother's Manual,* pp 31-32, Sept/Oct 1982; and Rollins J: Meeting the child's developmental needs through play. In Smith DP and others, editors: *Comprehensive child and family nursing skills,* St Louis, 1991, Mosby.

Patterns of Development

Throughout childhood certain play activities are popular at one age and not at another (see box on p. 135). These activities are so consistent and predictable that childhood is sometimes divided into age stages according to the types of play characteristic of each particular phase of development.

As they grow older, children also use materials in more meaningful ways. For example, an infant or small child first uses a block as something to handle or throw and then as something to represent another object, such as an airplane or car. To older children a block is a building material with which they can construct increasingly complex structures. Instead of representative objects, they require replicas of cars and airplanes. Eventually these materials are discarded altogether.

TOYS

Toys are the inanimate objects with which children interact, and cognitive development appears to be related to the variety and accessibility of objects for children to explore, experiment with, and come to know. Access to playthings, particularly during the earlier years, correlates with the accessibility of caregivers who make objects available, react to children's response to the objects, encourage further exploration, and talk about what is happening. Consequently, although they can be significant in themselves, playthings assume an especially important aspect as a medium of social interchange.

Selecting Toys

The type of toys chosen by and/or provided for children can facilitate learning and development in the areas just described. Toys that are small replicas of the culture and its tools help children assimilate their culture and learn sex and occupational roles. Toys that require pushing, pulling, rolling, and manipulating teach them about the physical properties of the items and help to develop muscles and coordination. Rules and the basic elements of cooperation and organization are learned through board games.

Because they can be employed in a variety of ways, raw materials or multidimensional toys are best for enhancing skills and stimulating the imagination. Through manipulation, playthings such as boxes, clay, and blocks can assume a multitude of symbolic objects and inspire creative impulses. For example, building blocks can be used to construct a variety of things, to count, and to learn shapes and sizes. "Educational" toys are less flexible. There are several ways in which families can encourage children's toy play (see Family Home Care box above).

Play materials need not be expensive or elaborate. Infants and small children derive enjoyment from simple kitchen utensils such as wooden spoons and small plastic plates to bang, pot lids to clang together, and a nest of measuring spoons to rattle. Empty cartons, especially oversized ones used to pack furniture for shipping, can assume the function of clubrooms, hideaways, and other private places. A large mound of dirt (3 to 4 feet high) can become a place for small children to roll toy cars and balls and dig holes during summer and a place for sliding in winter. Paper is a fascinating and versatile raw material for children of any age, and most books on toy materials include recipes for play dough and finger paint.

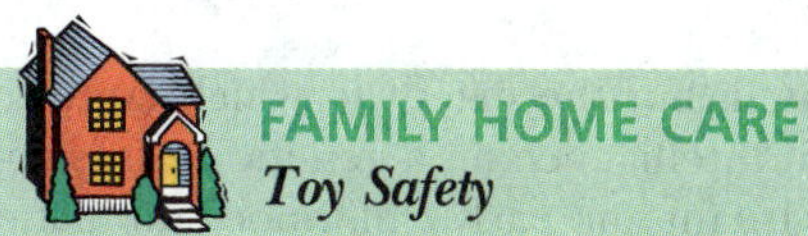

FAMILY HOME CARE
Toy Safety

SELECTION

Select toys that suit the skills, abilities, and interests of children.

Select toys that are safe for the specific child; look for a label that indicates the intended age-group. Toys that are safe for one age may not be safe for another.

- For infants, toddlers, and all children who still mouth objects, avoid toys with small parts that may pose a fatal choking hazard or aspiration hazard. Toys in this category are usually labeled: "Not recommended for children under 3 years."
- For infants avoid toys with strings or cords that are 7 inches or longer, since they may cause strangulation.
- For all children under 8 years, avoid electric toys with heating elements.
- For children under 5 years, avoid arrows or darts.

Check for safety labels such as "flame retardant" or "flame resistant."

Select toys durable enough to survive rough play; look for sturdy construction such as tightly secured eyes, nose, or any small parts.

Select toys light enough that they will not cause harm if one falls on a child.

Look for toys with smooth, rounded edges. Avoid toys with sharp edges that can cut or that have sharp points. Points on the inside of the toy can puncture if the toy is broken.

Avoid toys with any shooting or throwing objects that can injure eyes.

- This includes toys into which other missiles, such as sticks or pebbles, might be used as substitutes for the intended projectiles.
- Arrows and darts used by children should have blunt tips and be manufactured from resilient materials; make certain tips are securely attached.

Make certain that materials in toys are nontoxic.

Avoid toys that make loud noises that might be damaging to a child's hearing.

- Even some squeaking toys are too loud when held close to the ear.
- If selecting caps for cap guns, look for the label required by Federal law to be on boxes or packages of caps that states: "Warning—Do not fire closer than 1 foot to the ear. Do not use indoors."

Make certain that arrows or darts have soft tips, rubber suction cups, or other protective tips. Check to be certain that tips are secure.

If selecting a toy gun, be certain that the barrel or the entire gun is brightly colored to avoid being mistaken as a real gun.

Check toy instructions for clarity. They should be clear to an adult and, when appropriate, to the child.

SUPERVISION

Maintain a safe play environment.

- Remove and discard plastic wrappings on toys immediately; they could suffocate a child.
- Remove large toys, bumper pads, and boxes from playpens; an adventuresome child can use such items as a means of climbing or falling out.

Set "ground rules" for play.

Supervise young children closely during play.

Teach children how to use toys properly and safely.

Instruct older children to keep their toys away from younger brothers, sisters, and friends.

Keep children who are playing with riding toys away from stairs, hills, traffic, and swimming pools.

Establish and enforce rules regarding protective gear.

- Insist that children wear helmets when using bicycles, skateboards, or in-line skates.
- Insist that children wear gloves and wrist, elbow, and knee pads when using skateboards or in-line skates.

Instruct children on electrical safety.

- Teach children the proper way to unplug an electric toy—pull on the plug, not the cord.
- Teach children to beware of electrical appliances and even electrically operated playthings; frequently children are unfamiliar with the hazards of electricity in association with water.

Teach children the safe use of utensils that under certain circumstances can cause injury—scissors, knives, needles, heating elements, or loops, long string, or cord.

MAINTENANCE

Inspect old and new toys regularly for breakage, loose parts, and other potential hazards.

- Look for jagged or sharp edges or broken parts that might constitute a choking hazard.
- Check movable parts to make certain they are attached securely to the toys; sometimes pieces that are safe when attached to the toy become a danger when detached.
- Examine all outdoor toys regularly for rust and weak or sharp parts that could become a danger to a child.
- Check electrical cords and plugs for cracked or fraying parts.

Maintain toys in good repair, without signs of possible hazards such as sharp edges, splinters, weak seams, or rust.

- Make repairs immediately, or discard out of reach of children.
- Sand sharp wooden toys or splintered surfaces smooth.
- Use only paint labeled "nontoxic" to repaint toys, toy boxes, or children's furniture.

STORAGE

Provide a safe place for children to store toys.

Select a toy chest or toy box that is ventilated, is free of self-locking devices that could trap a child inside, and has a lid designed not to pinch a child's fingers or fall on a child's head.

If containers other than toy chests are used for storage purposes, they should be fitted with spring-loaded support devices if they have a hinged lid to avoid entrapment and suffocation.

Teach children to store toys safely in order to prevent accidental injury from stepping, tripping, or falling on a toy.

Playthings meant for older children and adults should be safely stowed away on high shelves, in locked closets, or in other areas unavailable to younger children.

Toy Safety

Selection of toys and play equipment is a joint effort between parents and children, but evaluation of their safety is the responsibility of the adult. Government agencies do not inspect and police all toys on the market. Therefore adults who purchase, supervise purchases, or allow children to use play equipment need to evaluate such equipment for its safety, including toys that are gifts or those purchased by the children themselves. Children need toys and activities that increase their sense of competence but that do not create a threat to their health and safety (see Family Home Care box, p. 137).

SELECTED FACTORS THAT INFLUENCE GROWTH AND DEVELOPMENT

HEREDITY

Inherited characteristics have a profound influence on development. A high correlation exists between parent and child with regard to traits such as height, weight, and rate of growth. The sex of a child, traditionally determined by random selection at the time of conception, directs both the pattern of growth and the behavior of others toward the child. In all cultures, attitudes and expectations are different with respect to the sex of the child. Sex plus other hereditary determinants strongly affects growth rate and the end result of that growth.

Most physical characteristics, including shape and form of features, body build, and physical peculiarities, are inherited and can influence the way children grow and interact with their environment. Children's heritage may cause a deviation from established overall physical standards for growth and development. For example, Japanese children are smaller than average at all ages. Some children are taller and heavier than the average from early childhood and usually achieve their linear growth sooner. Black girls begin the pubertal growth spurt at a slightly earlier age than white girls and for a brief period are slightly taller (Lowrey, 1986).

The relative importance of heredity and environment in molding development has been deliberated by scientists, educators, and health professionals. It is now commonly accepted that the end product is not a result of the *action* of one or the other of these processes but the *interaction* of one with the other. For example, children who receive genes for above-average height can only achieve full potential with an optimum environment, including good diet, love, and freedom from disease. On the other hand, children who inherit genes for less-than-average height will never attain a height greater than their programmed stature even in a superior environment. Children with limited intellectual capability can never excel in a field that requires highly intellectual skills, no matter to what extent they are pushed. But children with superior mentality will be wasted without an environment that stimulates and encourages their innate capacity.

The area that has provoked the greatest controversy is the contribution of heredity and environment to behavior characteristics and intelligence. Intellectual diversity of individuals is undisputed, but the extent to which large human groups differ in intelligence on a genetic basis is continually challenged. Infant and early childhood stimulation programs and innovative educational techniques at all levels of intellectual endowment have substantiated the positive influence of appropriate environmental stimulation on achievement. On the other hand, early childhood deprivation and the alarming effects of inadequate nutrition during critical periods of development are areas of concern to health professionals.

The influences on behavior traits are more difficult to assess. The culture dictates that some hereditary characteristics (e.g., sex) imply conformity to specific behavioral expectations. Many dimensions of personality that appear to be hereditary (e.g., the degree of responsiveness or unresponsiveness, temperament, activity level, extroversion or introversion, the degree of deliberateness or impulsiveness) and various constitutional traits (e.g., beauty, ugliness, physical deformity, sensory handicaps, learning impairment) affect the way others react to children and the interpersonal behavior children display in response. A display of undesirable behavior requires careful evaluation to determine the degree to which the behavior can be attributed to the interpersonal environment or to hereditary influences. This determination can be a significant factor in assessing whether or not such children would profit from therapy or if they should be removed from that environment.

Differences in health and vigor of children may be attributed to hereditary traits. An inherited physical or mental defect or disorder will alter or modify children's physical and/or emotional growth and interactions. The extent to which handicapping conditions interfere with children's growth and well-being are considered in relation to numerous disabilities throughout the remainder of the book.

NEUROENDOCRINE FACTORS

It has been suggested there may be a growth center in the hypothalamic region responsible for maintaining genetically determined growth patterns. It is believed that some functional relationship exists between the hypothalamus and the endocrine system that influences growth. There is also evidence, based on observations of denervated skeletal muscles, that the peripheral nervous system may influence growth, because muscles deprived of nerve supply degenerate. Many of these effects are not sufficiently explained by disuse or diminished blood supply. For example, nail growth on an extremity with a severed nerve will lag behind the nail growth on the corresponding extremity, but the growth returns to normal with regeneration of the nerve. There is no satisfactory explanation for this revived growth rate; the process may involve a chemical substance secreted by nerve cells that modifies the growth and repair processes.

Probably all hormones affect growth in some fashion. Three hormones—growth hormone, thyroid hormone, and androgens—when given to persons deficient in these hormones, stimulate protein anabolism and thereby produce retention of elements essential for building protoplasm and bony tissue. It appears that each of the hormones that has a significant influence on growth manifests its major effect at a different period of growth (see Table 38-1).

GENDER

The sex of the child has some influence on growth and development, although it is not always apparent which differences are related to cultural expectations as opposed to innate characteristics. Extensive research (Jacklin, 1992) indicates there are few actual differences but many myths regarding differences between girls and boys. There is no substantial evidence to indicate that girls are more social and suggestible, lack motivation to achieve, have a lower self-esteem, or are better at learning by rote than boys. Nor is there validity to the myth that boys are more analytic and better at high-level tasks than girls. In most studies boys and girls are equally dependent on caregivers, equally susceptible to persuasive communications, and equally motivated to achieve.

There are sex differences that influence behavior in childhood. In general, boys are more aggressive physically; girls are more aggressive verbally (Archer, Pearson, and Westeman, 1988). Boys also more frequently engage in rough and tumble play and aggressive fantasies. This behavior persists through the college years, although aggression diminishes with age in both sexes. Competitive behavior has been observed more often in boys than in girls in some studies, but there is some question as to the validity of this; other studies find the sexes to be similar in this aspect. Both sexes are alike in their willingness to explore a novel environment.

Studies differ in regard to differences between the activity levels of boys and girls, which may reflect the situations in which the measurements were conducted. The play of both boys and girls is equally organized and planned. Some studies find that boys seem to have more difficulty sitting still, engage in more exploratory behavior, and are stimulated to bursts of high activity in the presence of other boys. Boys exhibit greater impulsiveness and have difficulty resisting distractions, as reflected by the greater incidence of injuries in boys at all ages. However, boys tend to be outside more than girls, and many activities are influenced by motivational factors such as fear, anger, and curiosity.

Both sexes are highly responsive to social situations, although there are some sex differences in social relationships. Boys and girls show interest in confronting social stimuli (e.g., human faces and voices), in imitating models, and in understanding the emotional reactions and needs of others. However, boys have a more extensive sphere of relationships, are highly oriented toward a peer group, and congregate in large groups, whereas girls are more likely to associate in pairs or small groups and become involved in a more intense relationship with a few close friends. Girls appear to be more concerned with the welfare of the group and therefore are more apt to compromise in situations involving conflict.

The sexes are similar in overall self-confidence and self-satisfaction but differ in the areas in which they seem to feel the greatest self-confidence. Boys are apt to view themselves as more powerful and with more control over events. They respond to a challenge, especially when it appeals to their ego or competitive feelings, in order to attain a higher level of achievement. Little difference exists between the sexes regarding motivation to achieve, although some studies find girls to be superior in this respect.

During childhood girls are more likely to comply with adult commands and directions. However, this ready compliance does not extend to relationships with peers. Boys, on the other hand, appear to be more concerned about maintaining status in the peer group, which may render them more vulnerable to pressures and challenges from the group.

Girls have always been considered to demonstrate more nurturant or helping behavior than boys, but this has not been established to the satisfaction of child psychologists. Girls between the ages of 6 and 10 are more often seen behaving in nurturing ways than boys, but many studies of preschool children have not observed this difference. Much of this type of behavior is the result of imitation and modeling; as with other popular beliefs about differences between girls and boys, there is little basis in fact. It may be a result of selective attention of casual observers whose ideas are confirmed or strengthened by behaviors that are consistent with their prior beliefs. Behavior inconsistent with expectations is more likely to go unnoticed, and consequently entrenched ideas are perpetuated.

DISEASE

Altered growth and development is one of the clinical manifestations in a number of hereditary disorders. Growth impairment is particularly marked in skeletal disorders, such as the various forms of dwarfism and at least one of the chromosome anomalies (Turner syndrome). Many of the disorders of metabolism, such as vitamin D–resistant rickets, mucopolysaccharidoses, and the numerous endocrine disorders, interfere with the normal growth pattern. In other disorders the tendency is toward the upper percentile of height (e.g., Klinefelter syndrome and Marfan syndrome).

Many chronic illnesses associated with varying degrees of growth failure are related to congenital cardiac anomalies and respiratory disorders such as cystic fibrosis. Any disorder characterized by the inability to digest and absorb body nutrients will have an adverse effect on growth and development. These include the malabsorption syndromes and defects in digestive enzyme systems. Almost any disease state that persists over an extended period, particularly during a critical period of development, may have a permanent effect on growth. For example, children on long-term corticosteroid therapy exhibit growth retardation.

Children in a prolonged state of disequilibrium caused by illness, such as chronic infections, are under a constant inner stress that inhibits their response to adult demands and contributes to their difficulty in managing stimulating environmental experiences. Behaviors that these children display as they cope with outside stimuli, as well as inner irritations, can be misinterpreted as distractibility and lack of persistence toward a goal. A prolonged illness that occurs in the second year during the phase of rapid acquisition of motor control and autonomy may cause a child to lose the natural impetus peculiar to this stage of development. Such a child may remain passive and require special stimulation to develop the independence that would have developed spontaneously under normal circumstances.

SEASON, CLIMATE, AND OXYGEN CONCENTRATION

There is some evidence that season and climate may have an influence on growth. Growth in height appears to be faster in the spring and summer months, whereas growth in weight proceeds more rapidly during the autumn and winter. These observations have not been satisfactorily explained. This phenomenon may have a hormonal basis, or it may be related to seasonal differences in activity levels.

It was formerly believed that persons living in a warm climate were smaller than those from a cold climate. However, it is much too difficult to separate the effects of climate from other factors such as race, nutrition, or disease. There does seem to be more evidence regarding the effects of hypoxia on growth. Children with disorders that produce a chronic hypoxia are characteristically small as compared with children of the same chronologic age. In addition, children native to high altitudes are smaller than those living at lower altitudes (Yip, Binkin, and Trowbridge, 1988).

PRENATAL INFLUENCES

Certain factors before birth can produce dramatic effects on a child's growth and development and warrant special consideration because of their preventive nature (Pinyerd, 1992). For example, women who smoke past the second trimester of pregnancy are more likely to produce small-size infants.

Infants born with fetal alcohol syndrome (FAS) exhibit prenatal and postnatal growth deficiencies in height and weight. Unfortunately, few of these infants exhibit the usual neonatal catch-up growth observed in small-for-gestational-age newborns and remain growth deficient throughout childhood. Fetal alcohol effect (FAE), although resulting in fewer anomalies, may produce significant central nervous system alterations that may not be obvious until the child is older (Smitherman, 1994).

Fetal exposure to illicit drugs such as marijuana, cocaine, and heroin is often associated with intrauterine growth retardation (IUGR) and prematurity. Cocaine-exposed infants may be at increased risk for inadequate gains in weight and height during the first 2 years of life (Kelley, Walsh, and Thompson, 1991).

The nutritional requirements of childhood are directly related to the rate and direction of growth. During the rapid prenatal growth period, faulty nutrition may negatively influence development from the time of implantation of the ovum until birth. The nutritional needs are met entirely through the maternal system; as a result, maternal deficiencies or abnormalities in the supplementary intrauterine structures will be manifested in fetal development. Although the fetus is usually able to obtain adequate nutrition for prenatal growth unless the mother's nutrition is very poor, severe maternal malnutrition during the period of most rapid brain growth is associated with permanent reduction in the total number of fetal brain cells and has a critical effect on the child's intellectual functioning.

ENVIRONMENTAL HAZARDS

Hazards in the environment are a source of concern to health care providers and others interested in health and safety. No aspect of the potential dangers of daily living has escaped investigation by some group or individual, and more types and sources of environmental pollution are detected as populations and technology expand. Physical injuries are the most prevalent consequences of environmental dangers, and these are discussed extensively throughout the book as they apply in relation to age, specific hazards, and selected physical disabilities. The harmful agents most often associated with health risks are chemicals and radiation. Lead is perhaps the greatest environmental threat to children (see Chapter 16).

The sources and routes of exposure to chemical hazards are surprisingly extensive. Water, air, and food contamination from a variety of origins is well documented and discussed. Newer recognized sources of exposure are substances carried home (usually from the workplace) on clothes or other objects, chemicals secreted in breast milk (especially prescribed drugs and nicotine), and contamination within well-insulated homes (especially from disinfectants or burning of substances that produce toxic fumes) (Rogan, 1980). Passive inhalation of tobacco smoke by infants and children has been found to be a hazard at all stages of development.

The harmful effects of large doses of radiation are unquestioned, although the long-term consequences are still under investigation. The effects of low-dose or short-term radiation are still debatable, as are the safe vs harmful dosage levels. However, the ubiquitous gas radon (and especially its isotopes) has been determined to be an ever-present danger (American Academy of Pediatrics, 1989).

SOCIOECONOMIC LEVEL

The socioeconomic level of children's families apparently has a significant impact on growth and development. At all ages children from upper- and middle-class families are taller than comparative children of families in the lower socioeconomic strata. Girls from upper- and middle-class families also reach menarche up to 3 months earlier than girls from the lower socioeconomic levels. Children with mild to moderate developmental delays who have highly functioning, financially stable families will have better outcomes than similarly at-risk children from impoverished, dysfunctional homes (Curry and Duby, 1994).

The cause of these differences is less definite, although the general health and nutrition of lower socioeconomic levels are probably significant factors. Francis, Williams, and

Yarandi (1993) found that anemia is a serious problem among children from low-income families. Nutritious food sources (especially proteins) are scarce, and other factors (e.g., larger family size and regularity in eating, sleeping, and exercise) may play a role.

Families from lower socioeconomic groups may lack the knowledge or resources needed to provide a safe, stimulating, and enriched environment that fosters optimum development for children. They may be unable to move from unsafe neighborhoods where drug traffic and drive-by shootings are the norm. The effects on the emotional development of children living under these conditions have been compared to those experienced by children living in war zones (Rollins, 1993).

NUTRITION

Probably the single most important influence on growth is nutrition. Dietary factors regulate growth at *all* stages of development, and their effects are exerted in numerous and complex ways. Adequate nutrition provides the essential nutrients in the amount and balance necessary to sustain physiologic needs. These needs vary widely according to age, level of activity, and environmental conditions. Inadequacies in any or all of these essential nutrients will be reflected in altered growth.

During infancy and childhood the demand for calories is relatively great, as evidenced by the rapid increase in both height and weight. Protein and caloric requirements are higher at this time than at almost any period of postnatal development. As the growth rate slows with its concomitant decrease in metabolism, a corresponding reduction in caloric and protein requirements occurs (see Table 4-3). Growth is uneven during the periods of childhood between infancy and adolescence, when there are plateaus and small growth spurts. The child's appetite fluctuates in response to these variations until the turbulent growth spurt of adolescence, when adequate nutrition is extremely important but may be subject to numerous emotional influences. Children's caloric intake must equal their energy output plus that needed for growth. It is estimated that the average child (e.g., the 6- to 10-year-old child) expends 55% of the energy for metabolic maintenance, 25% for physical activity, 8% in fecal loss, and 12% for growth. Sample menus for various age-groups are included in discussions on nutrition in the chapters on health promotion of children in specific age-groups.

Several organizations have published dietary advice for the public; most well-known are the Dietary Guidelines for Americans, which encourage eating a variety of foods, maintaining ideal body weight, consuming adequate starch and fiber, and limiting the intake of fat, cholesterol, sugar, salt, and alcohol. In 1992 the U.S. Department of Agriculture published the Food Guide Pyramid (Fig. 4-20). The pyramid is a visual companion to the Dietary Guidelines for Americans and is intended to help consumers understand more about the food they need, from what food groups, and in what amounts. For example, the pyramid shows that fat, oils, and sweets should be eaten sparingly, whereas cereals and grains should be eaten generously. The Food Guide Pyramid replaces the basic four food groups that traditionally have been used to convey nutrition information to the public and applies to children as young as 2 years of age.

The number of servings and serving sizes are important components of the Food Guide Pyramid. Suggested serving sizes for the five food groups are listed in the box on p. 142. Young children need the same variety of foods as older children but may need less than the 1600 calories provided by the suggested minimum number of servings in each food group. To meet their caloric needs, adjustments are made by using the minimum number of servings and smaller serving sizes. However, it is important that children have the equivalent of at least 2 cups of milk a day. Adolescents, who require increased calories for growth, should have 3 cups of milk a day and may require the maximum number of suggested servings. Current recommendations for fat intake

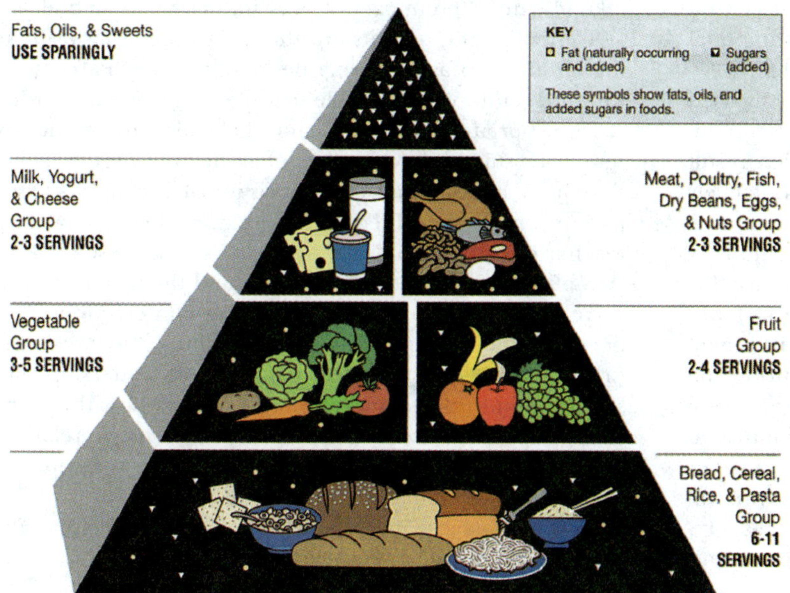

FIG. 4-20 Food Guide Pyramid: a guide to daily food choices. (Courtesy U.S. Department of Agriculture, 1992.)

FOOD GUIDE PYRAMID: SAMPLE SERVING SIZES

BREAD, CEREAL, RICE, AND PASTA GROUP

1 slice of bread
1 ounce of ready-to-eat cereal
½ cup of cooked cereal, rice, or pasta

VEGETABLE GROUP

1 cup of raw leafy vegetable
½ cup of other vegetable, cooked or chopped raw
¾ cup of vegetable juice

FRUIT GROUP

1 medium apple, banana, or orange
½ cup of chopped, cooked, or canned fruit
¾ cup of fruit juice

MILK, YOGURT, AND CHEESE GROUP

1 cup of milk or yogurt
1½ ounces of natural cheese
2 ounces of processed cheese

MEAT, POULTRY, FISH, DRY BEANS, EGGS, AND NUTS GROUP

2-3 ounces of cooked lean meat, poultry, or fish
½ cup of cooked dry beans, 1 egg, or 2 tablespoons of peanut butter count as 1 ounce of lean meat

for children over 2 years of age are that no more than 30% of calories should come from fat and the remainder of calories should come from carbohydrates and protein (see also Hyperlipidemia [Hypercholesterolemia], Chapter 34).

Adequate nutrition is closely related to good health throughout life, and an overall improvement in nourishment is evidenced by the gradual increase in size and early maturation of children in this century. In the growing child, inadequate nutrition is dangerous, particularly during those periods critical for growth. Inadequate nutrition has the greatest impact during the critical periods of rapid cell division. For example, normal development of the central nervous system depends on adequate nutrition during fetal life and throughout the first 2 years of postnatal life.

The term ***malnutrition*** in its strictest sense is usually used to describe undernutrition, primarily that resulting from insufficient caloric intake. However, malnutrition may result from the following: (1) a dietary intake that is quantitatively or qualitatively inadequate, or both, including overnutrition; (2) disease that interferes with appetite, digestion, or absorption while increasing nutritional requirements; (3) excessive physical activity or inadequate rest; or (4) disturbed interpersonal relationships and other environmental or psychologic factors. Severe malnutrition during the critical periods of development, particularly the first 6 months of life, is positively correlated with diminished height, weight, and intelligence scores. The importance of nutrition as a vital aspect of health promotion during all phases of the illness-wellness continuum is included as it relates to developmental phases and specific health problems.

INTERPERSONAL RELATIONSHIPS

Solid interpersonal relationships are essential to psychologic well-being. Relationships with significant others play an important role in development, particularly in emotional, intellectual, and personality development. Not only do the quality and quantity of contacts with other persons exert an influence on growing children, but the widening range of contacts is essential to learning and the development of a healthy personality. During the formative years, culturally determined, age-appropriate behaviors are reinforced and consequently repeated. Thus patterns of reward, punishment, and modeling continually modify children's individuality of character and temperament. Children behave in a manner that elicits rewards from the persons most significant in their lives.

Significant Others

Normal children routinely turn to parents, teachers, and friends for comfort, protection, education, acceptance, and material needs. Parents and caregiving persons are unquestionably the most influential persons during early infancy. They meet the infants' basic needs for food, warmth, comfort, and love; provide stimulation for their senses; and facilitate their expanding capacities. Through these individuals children learn to trust the world and feel secure to venture in increasingly wide relationships. Through constant reinforcement children learn the behaviors that bring satisfaction to the nurturing persons and incorporate these behaviors. Eventually these behaviors become self-motivating. For example, children learn that evacuating the bowel in a proper receptacle produces a positive response from the parents, resulting in a lifetime behavioral pattern.

As they get older, children seek approval from a widening sphere of persons, including other members of their family, their peers, and to a lesser degree other authority figures (e.g., teachers). The increasing importance of the peer group in determining the behavior of school-age children and adolescents is well documented. However, it is the quality of the parent-child relationship that determines to a large extent the impact of peer influence on a child.

Generally, the parents are the most influential in helping children to assume sex-role identification. Parents define and reinforce acceptable sex-role behavior and provide sex-appropriate role models for the children. In the absence of a suitable sex-role model in the family setting, children may adopt some characteristics of the opposite-sex parent or sibling. Frequently children identify with a teacher or other significant person of the same sex.

Siblings are children's first peers, and the way they learn to relate to each other can affect later interactions with peers outside the family group. For example, firstborn children who are accustomed to a position of leadership with siblings tend to assume the same position with peers; younger children are more often followers. Ease in relationships with peers of the same or opposite sex is frequently associated with similar associations in the home.

Pets can play an important role in children's lives (Fig. 4-21). They provide love and affection, as well as close, non-

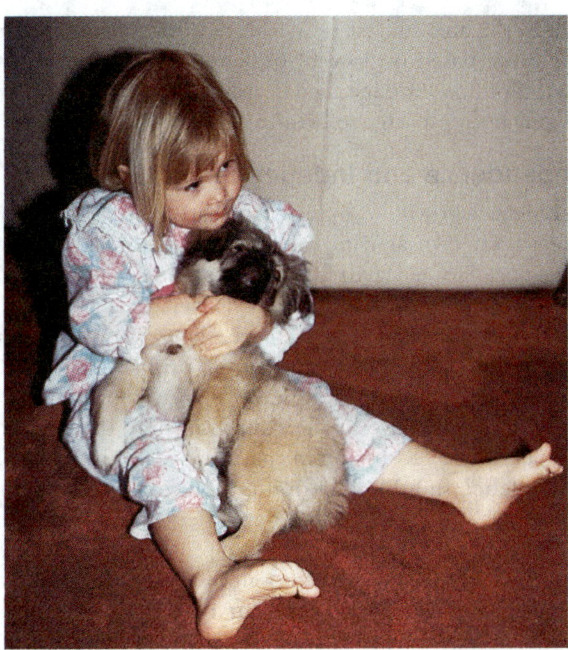

FIG. 4-21 Pets can play an important role in children's lives, providing love and companionship.

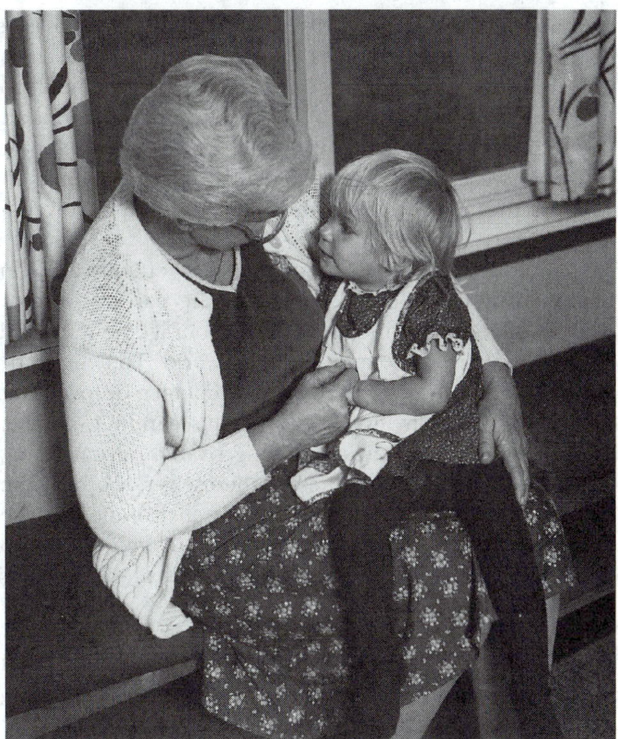

FIG. 4-22 A grandmother is a primary source of unconditional love and comfort.

judgmental companionship, and are on call 24 hours a day. In addition to contact comfort, a pet's noncontingent positive responsiveness is likely to strengthen children's self-concept and self-esteem. By assuming responsibility for helping to care for a pet, children can develop confidence in their abilities and gain respect for a job well done. Benefits for social development include social competence, empathy, and cooperation. Children's relationships with their pets seem to be more important than just the presence of one or more pets in the home; benefits such as greater empathy for other children is associated with strong child-pet bonds (Poresky and Hendrix, 1990).

Love and Affection

The single most important emotional need of children is to be loved and to feel secure in that love. Children strive above all else to gain the love and acceptance of those who are significant in their lives. When they feel secure in this love, they are able to withstand the normal crises associated with growing up and those unexpected crises (e.g., illness or loss) that are superimposed on the anticipated course of development.

Children cannot receive too much love. However, this love must be communicated to them through words and actions that tell them they are loved, not for their actions or achievement, but for what they are or simply *because they are.* Although love is closely associated with discipline, independence, and other factors that influence the child's self-concept, it should be an undemanding, accepting love that is indispensable to the development of a healthy personality. Unconditional love, freely bestowed, helps establish a sense of security and a positive sense of self within children that will persist throughout their lifetime (Fig. 4-22). Children must know they are loved and that whatever happens they can depend on this love. For many children spiritual love is a very significant source of complete, undemanding love. Without the security of loving relationships, children may become tense and insecure and develop undesirable behavior patterns as they attempt to obtain that love or try to compensate for its loss.

The primary source of love, particularly during infancy, is the parent, usually the mother or mothering person. The establishment of this early love attachment (or bonding) profoundly influences subsequent interpersonal relationships. With ever-widening relationships, children need the love and acceptance of others. They need to feel they are wanted, accepted, and belong in whatever relationships are important to them at each stage of development.

Parents may truly love their children but be unable to communicate this love to them. Parents who are insecure in their parenting skills frequently seek advice and reassurance from health professionals. Nurses aware of indications of parental insecurity will be able to provide assistance and reassurance that can preserve and enhance the parent-child relationship and build a sense of confidence in the parent.

Security

Closely allied to the need for love is the need for a sense of security. As they grow and develop in a complex world, children encounter many threats to their sense of security. Indeed, most childhood behavior problems are associated with an element of insecurity. Every change in themselves or their environment creates a feeling of uncertainty. Faced with confusing, conflicting adjustments, young children need the security provided by relatively stable situations and dependable human relationships. The degree to which they can cope with these stresses depends on the patience and support they receive from those most closely involved in their care.

A multitude of factors exists that can generate a feeling of insecurity in children. Ordinarily the parents, who are sources of comfort, guidance, and encouragement, provide a measure of security in an insecure world. To achieve this security, children need the warm acceptance of loving parents, a stable family unit, and judicious handling of stress-provoking situations such as sibling rivalry, relocation to a new neighborhood, and illness in themselves or other members of the family. A disturbed home environment caused by such factors as marital discord, illness of a parent or family member, or death of a family member can shatter their equilibrium.

Infants are disturbed by physical threats, such as hunger, cold, or discomfort. Small children are physiologically disturbed by emotions such as anger, fear, and grief, which they can release only in overt behavior. They can obtain a measure of relief from these feelings by the reassurance that their physical needs will be met, restraints will be placed on their behavior, and expectations that keep pace with their inner controls will be held. Rejection by significant persons, social ineptitude, and physical handicaps often produce insecurity in a child. The number and variety of stressful factors originating within or outside the child are often difficult to determine; therefore those responsible for the child's care must be alert for cues that reveal threats to this sense of security.

Discipline and Authority

Because children live in an organized society, they must be prepared to accept restrictions on their behavior. Discipline is not punishment. Rather, it is the teaching of desirable behavior. Children need to learn the rules governing behavior in the home, the neighborhood, the school, and the community at large. To learn acceptable behavior that permits them to live enjoyably with themselves and others, children need the steady, firm guidance of loving parents and others in authority roles. Good discipline provides children with protection from dangers within and without and relieves them of the burden of decisions they are not prepared to make, yet allows them to develop independence of thought and action within a secure framework.

Children who learn to live within reasonable rules are happier and more secure children. Without the stabilizing influence of controls, children feel uncertain and insecure. Too often, inexperienced and insecure parents fear the loss of a child's love, suffer feelings of guilt over disciplinary action, or even relinquish their authority to the child. To discipline is to teach reality. Sensible, mature parents establish fair rules and regulations in the home and then see that they are carried out. Parents should never exploit children's love for them as a means to control their children. Children's anxiety lest they lose that love is already great. Discipline based on love of the child and carried out with conviction, confidence, and consistency will produce a self-reliant, buoyant, and self-controlled child.

Dependence and Independence

As children grow and mature, they are increasingly able to direct their own activities and to make more independent decisions. However, there are great fluctuations in their ability to function independently. Even with a compelling inner drive to master and achieve, they are not always able to cope with difficult and frustrating problems or conflicts. All children feel the urge to grow up and move toward maturity, but they have at their disposal only those energies not being used to maintain mastery over old conflicts. Independence should be permitted to grow at its own rate.

Periods of regression and dependence not only are normal but are often necessary and helpful. If children feel sufficiently comfortable and content in a situation or relationship and reasonably certain that they can return to this safety and security, they will venture into the untried and untested on their own. If they feel doubtful concerning their abilities to cope, regression to a more comfortable level of competence allows them to replenish their inner resources and prepare to move ahead once again. Independence grows out of dependence; one cannot be considered as distinct from the other.

Children will learn independence of thought and decision making provided the opportunity is not withheld from them. If they are pushed into acting independently before they feel ready, they may withdraw from independence. When they choose not to relinquish the joys of independence and autonomy or to move ahead to new worlds of independence, they will dawdle. Parents, teachers, nurses, and others responsible for the child's care must be able to adjust their expectations and support to meet the child's needs of the moment. It is important to recognize when to help and when not to help children experiment with their immature and imperfect self-control, when to make demands requiring children's utmost ability, and when to allow them to function temporarily on a more immature level. They need these freedoms and controls in the process of becoming mature, self-reliant adults.

Emotional Deprivation

The most prominent feature of emotional deprivation, particularly during the first year, is developmental retardation. Much of the information regarding the adverse effects of interpersonal influences on development has been acquired through retrospective studies of gross deprivation and trauma. The most notable instances involved homeless infants who were placed in institutions for care. These infants, who did not receive consistent caregiving, failed to gain weight even with an adequate diet; they were pale, listless, and immobile, and unresponsive to stimuli that usually elicit a response (such as a smile or cooing) in the normal infant. If the emotional deprivation continues for a sufficient length of time, the child does not survive.

Harlow's classic experiments with infant monkeys illustrate the far-reaching effects of emotional and social deprivation in infancy (Harlow and Harlow, 1962). In these experiments the monkeys were raised by substitute, inanimate "mothers" made of cloth-covered wire from whom they derived nourishment and a measure of comfort but no mothering. These monkeys developed abnormal play and sex behavior. The few who bore offspring were unable to "mother" them. However, those who were allowed peer associations developed normal play and social-sex behavior. Through correlation of these findings with retrospective studies of human infants in comparable age-groups, attempts have been made to explain some of the behaviors observed in these children in later interpersonal relationships.

Although the most remarkable examples of emotional deprivation were first recognized among infants in institutions, the term ***masked deprivation*** has been used to describe children who are reared in homes where there is a distorted parent-child relationship or otherwise disordered home environment. Infants do not thrive if the caregiving person is hostile, fearful of handling them, or indifferent to them and their needs. Such children exhibit poor growth even though they are apparently free of physical disease. Children past the age of infancy who demonstrate physical underdevelopment are also retarded in bone age. These same infants and children display "catch-up" growth in a changed environment.

STRESS IN CHILDHOOD

Stress has been defined and described by numerous authorities from both a physiologic and an emotional point of view. Most discussions are centered on adult responses, but children are frequently among the most affected victims of a wide range of threatening events. Essentially it is "an imbalance between environmental demands and a person's coping resources that . . . disrupts the equilibrium of the person" (Masten and others, 1988).

Most research related to children has been restricted to specific stressors and stress-provoking experiences such as hospitalization, separation and loss, and pain. Studies indicate support for an association between the occurrence of stressful life events and physical and psychologic problems in children (Grey, 1993). A description of all the stressors to which children are exposed is beyond the scope of this section; however, the more common manifestations and stressful events are discussed briefly. Since stress is a normal aspect of life, stressors and some coping strategies are discussed in relation to specific situations throughout the book. For children's response to an intensely stressful event (such as a natural disaster, bombing, or schoolyard shooting) see Posttraumatic Stress Disorder, Chapter 18.

Although children are not strangers to stress, some children appear to be more vulnerable than others. Children's age, temperament, life situation, and state of health affect their vulnerability, reactions, and ability to handle stress. Also, the responses to a stressor can be behavioral, psychologic, or physiologic. It is impossible, unrealistic, and undesirable to protect children from stress, but providing them with interpersonal security helps them develop coping strategies for dealing with stress. The concept of an emotional bank can help parents and caregivers maintain a proper perspective regarding the effects of stress and coping. According to Usdin (1988), children have an emotional bank

WARNING SIGNS: CHILDHOOD STRESS

- Bed-wetting
- Boasts of superiority
- Complaints of feeling afraid or upset without being able to identify the source
- Complaints of neck or back pains
- Complaints of pounding heart
- Complaints of stomach upset, queasiness, or vomiting
- Compulsive cleanliness
- Compulsive ear tugging, hair pulling, or eyebrow plucking
- Cruel behavior toward people or pets
- Decline in school achievement
- Defiance
- Demand for constant perfection
- Depression
- Dirtying pants
- Dislike of school
- Downgrading of self
- Easily startled by unexpected sounds
- Explosive crying
- Extreme nervousness
- Frequent daydreaming and retreats from reality
- Frequent urination or diarrhea
- Headaches
- Hyperactivity, or excessive tension or alertness
- Increased number of minor spills, falls, and other accidents
- Irritability
- Listlessness or lack of enthusiasm
- Loss of interest in activities usually approached with vigor
- Lying
- Nightmares or night terror
- Nervous laughter
- Nervous tics, twitches, or muscle spasms
- Obvious attention-seeking
- Overeating
- Poor concentration
- Poor eating
- Poor sleep
- Psychosomatic illnesses
- Stealing
- Stuttering
- Teeth grinding (sometimes during sleep)
- Thumb-sucking
- Uncontrollable urge to run and hide
- Unusual difficulty in getting along with friends
- Unusual jealousy of close friends and siblings
- Unusual sexual behavior, such as spying or exhibitionism
- Unusual shyness
- Use of alcohol, drugs, or cigarettes
- Withdrawal from usual social activities

From Kuczen B: *Childhood stress: don't let your child be a victim,* New York, 1982, Delacorte Press.

STRESS SCALE FOR CHILDREN

LIFE EVENT	VALUE
1. Death of a parent	100
2. Divorce of parents	73
3. Separation of parents	65
4. Parent's jail term	63
5. Death of a close family member (e.g., grandparent)	63
6. Personal injury or illness	53
7. Parent's remarriage	50
8. Suspension or expulsion from school	47
9. Parent's reconciliation	45
10. Long vacation (summer, etc.)	45
11. Parent or sibling illness	44
12. Mother's pregnancy	40
13. Anxiety over sex	39
14. Birth or adoption of a new baby	39
15. New school or classroom or new teacher	39
16. Money problems at home	38
17. Death or moving away of close friend	37
18. Changes in studies	36
19. More quarrels with parents (or parents quarreling more)	35
20. Change in school responsibilities	29
21. Sibling going away to school	29
22. Family arguments with grandparents	29
23. Winning school or community awards	28
24. Mother or father going to work or stopping work	26
25. School beginning or ending	26
26. Family's living standard changing	25
27. Change in personal habits (e.g., bedtime, homework, etc.)	24
28. Trouble with parents (e.g., lack of communication, hostility, etc.)	23
29. Change in school hours, schedule of courses	23
30. Family's moving	20
31. New sports, hobbies, family recreation activities	20
32. Change in church activities (more involvement or less)	19
33. Change in social activities (e.g., new friends, loss of old ones, peer pressures)	18
34. Change in sleeping habits, giving up naps, etc.	16
35. Change in number of family get-togethers	15
36. Change in eating habits (e.g., going on or off diet, new way of family cooking)	13
37. Vacation	13
38. Christmas	12
39. Breaking home, school, or community rules	11

Add up the points for items that have touched the child's life in the last 12 months.

Score below 150, the child is carrying an average stress load.

Score between 150 and 300, the child has a better-than-average chance of showing some symptoms of stress.

Score over 300, the child's stress load is heavy and there is a strong likelihood for experiencing a serious change in health and/or behavior.

From Saunders A, Remsberg B: *The stress-proof child: a loving parent's guide,* New York, 1984, Holt, Rinehart & Winston.

in which deposits, as well as withdrawals, can be made. "If the child has a good positive balance in the account, he or she can tolerate significant withdrawal experiences. If the child has a low balance, then even a minor withdrawal may bankrupt the account, causing it to be overdrawn."

Parents and other caregivers can try to recognize signs of stress (see box on p. 145) in order to help children deal with stresses before they become overwhelming. If a number of stresses are imposed on children at the same time, the children are more vulnerable. When a succession of stresses produces an excessive stress load, children may experience a serious change in health and/or behavior. An adaptation of the Holmes and Rahe stress scale for adults appears in the box at left, which provides a tool to alert parents or caregivers to situations children experience that are not always viewed by adults as stressful.

It is most important that parents and persons working with children understand the nature of childhood stress and ways it can be recognized or anticipated. Caregivers must *listen* to children so they are aware of children's fears and concerns and must let them know that they are important and that what they say matters. Physical contact is comforting and reassuring to children. Simply holding, touching, or hugging children is both relaxing and comforting and facilitates communication. Spending unhurried time with children, family outings, vacations, and exposing children to positive influences help build children's strength and security. Solid interpersonal relationships are essential to the psychologic well-being of children.

Coping

Coping strategies are the specific ways in which children cope with stressors, as distinguished from ***coping styles,*** which are relatively unchanging personality characteristics or outcomes of coping (Ryan-Wenger, 1992). Coping refers to a special class of individual reactions to stressors—specifically, a reaction to a stressor that resolves, reduces, or replaces the affect state classified as stressful. Children, like adults, respond to everyday stress by trying to change the circumstances (primary control coping) or trying to adjust to circumstances the way they are (secondary control coping) (Band and Weisz, 1988). An example of primary control is via tantrums or aggressive behavior; withdrawal and submission are examples of secondary control.

Coping strategies tend to fall within 1 of 15 categories (see Table 4-5). Any strategy that provides relaxation is effective in reducing stress, and most children have their own natural methods (e.g., withdrawal, physical activity, reading, listening to music, working on a project, or taking a nap). The list is endless. Some turn to parents to solve their problems, or they may develop socially unacceptable strategies such as cheating, stealing, or lying (Kuczen, 1982).

Children can be taught stress-reduction techniques to use in coping. First, they must be helped to recognize signs of tension in themselves and then taught any of a variety of appropriate strategies—special exercises, relaxation and breathing, mental imagery, and numerous other simple activities. Also, parents and other caregivers can anticipate possible stress-provoking events and prepare children for

TABLE 4-5 Children's Coping

CATEGORY	REPRESENTATIVE STRATEGY
Aggressive activities	Yell, argue
Behavioral avoidance	Sleep
Behavioral distraction	Play, watch TV
Cognitive avoidance	Deny that situation exists
Cognitive distraction	Use humor
Cognitive problem solving	Make decision
Cognitive restructuring	Emphasize positive
Emotional expression	Cry
Endurance	Comply/cooperate
Information seeking	Question
Isolating activities	Go to a special place
Self-controlling activities	Relax
Social support	Talk to peers
Spiritual support	Pray
Stressor modification	Propose a compromise

Modified from Ryan-Wenger N: A taxonomy of children's coping strategies: a step toward theory development, *Am J Orthopsychiatry* 62(2):256-263, 1992.

coping by role-playing a scenario or "talking it through" beforehand. Most of the stress-reducing strategies discussed in Chapter 26 in relation to managing pain are effective for any stress situation.

Probably the most useful tool that children can learn is how to solve problems. When children can view any new situation as a problem to be solved and an opportunity to learn, they are not vulnerable to the control of others. It provides them with a sense of mastery over their own lives and reinforces the fact that they have within themselves the ability and information to handle whatever comes their way. Problem-solving skill gives them the confidence to know where and how to seek help when they need it.

Many childhood stressors are related to situations with parents, other family members, teachers, or socioeconomic conditions that are typically outside the children's control. Therefore many stressors are less amenable to change by the children themselves (Ryan-Wenger, 1992).

Childhood Fears

Fear is a normal function, a self-preservation signal that mobilizes the physiologic resources of the organism. Fear and anxiety are often used interchangeably, and the physical reactions to both are almost identical. ***Fear*** is an emotional reaction to a specific real or unreal threat or danger; ***anxiety*** refers to a general uneasiness, apprehension, or feeling of impending doom. Fear is a momentary reaction to danger based on a low estimate of one's own power. Fearful children perceive a threat (person, animal, or situation) as being stronger than themselves and thus capable of harming them. When the balance of power is altered, the fear disappears. For example, children's fears can be alleviated by the presence of an adult whom they perceive as a source of protection; or fear can be overcome by familiarity with the source of the threat, such as a dog or a dark room. Anxiety is general, lasting, and internally generated, and it reflects overall feelings of weakness, ineptitude, and helplessness (Wolman, 1978).

TABLE 4-6 Typical Childhood Fears

AGE	FEARS
Infants	
0-6 months	Loss of support, loud noises, bright lights; sudden movement
7-12 months	Strangers, sudden appearance of unexpected and looming objects (including people), animals, heights
Toddlers	
1-3 years	Separation from parent, the dark, loud or sudden noises, injury, strangers (including strange peers), certain persons (e.g., the doctor), certain situations (e.g., trip to the dentist), animals, large objects or machines, change in environment
Preschoolers	
3-5 years	Separation from parent, supernatural beings such as monsters or ghosts, animals, the dark, noises, "bad" people, injury, death
School-age children	
6-12 years	Supernatural beings, injury, storms, the dark, staying alone, separation from parent, things seen on television or in movies, injury, tests and failure in school, consequences related to unattractive physical appearance, death
Adolescents	Inept social performance, social isolation, sexuality, drugs, war, divorce, crowds, gossip, public speaking, plane and car crashes, death

Modified from Feiner J, Schachter R: When your child is afraid. In Schachter R, McCauley CS: *Why your child is afraid,* New York, 1988, Simon & Schuster.

In childhood the distinction between fear and anxiety is important because childhood fears are specific, and except for the specific fear (or fears), children are happy and active. Childhood fears are limited problems, and most are alleviated with growth and children's increased self-confidence and faith in themselves. Unrealistic fears are abandoned with maturation and learning, to be replaced by realistic fears. As with other stresses, there are individual differences in susceptibility to fear, and certain fears are age related (Table 4-6). Fears that are likely to persist into adulthood are fear of physical danger, death, sickness, bodily injury, physical assault, car accidents, airplane crashes, and war.

Children often come to fear things they did not fear at a younger age because of their lack of awareness (e.g., a busy street), or they may become fearful of familiar things. With the development of imaginative ability, imaginary creatures and situations may become a source of fear. Also, children with superior intelligence are likely to be more aware of real dangers, are less likely to succumb to imaginary fears, and have fewer fears than other children. These observations are probably related to cognitive capacities.

Nurses can help parents learn to recognize fear in their children by explaining that not all children express fear in the same way. Although some children cry and look afraid, others may say "smart" remarks, act silly, bite their nails, suck their thumb, pretend they are not afraid, and/or change their playing, eating, or sleeping patterns.

Coping with fears is the same as coping with other stresses. To help children overcome their fears, parents and others should not shame or show disapproval for their fears, encourage their unreasonable fears, overprotect them, or force them into a situation they fear. For example, throwing a fearful child into deep water will probably increase a fear of water to the point of a lasting phobia. Parents can serve as models by demonstrating strength, decisiveness, and self-confidence. For instance, the parents can take their children by the hand and gently guide them into shallow water or around a dark room. Desensitization by gradually facing the fearsome object or situation is effective with most children. Parents can allow their children to express their fears and encourage them to cope with certain dangers. Most of all, parents need to make their children feel that they will always be loved and will be protected whenever necessary. (See also Posttraumatic Stress Disorder, Chapter 18.)

RESILIENCY

Some children manage to achieve stable personalities and a sense of competence despite adverse conditions and a series of stressful events in their childhood, such as biologic insults, a pathologic family environment, or the negative effects of poverty. This ego-resiliency has been observed in a number of studies (Anthony and Cohler, 1987; Garmezy and Rutter, 1983; Sroufe, 1983; Werner and Smith, 1982). The findings of these observations have determined that resilient children share a number of characteristics in common. They were active, alert, responsive, and sociable as infants, with the ability to elicit positive responses from other people, and acquired a strong sense of autonomy. As children they enjoy school, often using it as a refuge from a disordered home, and are well liked by peers. Although a more recent study of adolescents found similar results, findings also revealed that high-risk adolescents labeled as resilient were significantly more depressed and anxious than were competent children from low-stress backgrounds (Luthar, 1991).

Ego-resilient children use a wide variety of coping strategies, have hobbies and interests that give them a sense of mastery and pride, and have problem-solving and communication skills that they use effectively (Werner, 1987). Central in the histories of all these children, regardless of the type and extent of their adversity, is that they had the opportunity to establish a secure relationship with at least one stable person who accepted them uncritically.

Persons other than the significant other in children's lives can play an enabling role when the person who provides support is unavailable. Other significant persons can promote the competencies of these and other children by assuming a nurturing role and encouraging their independence, teaching them self-help skills, and boosting their self-confidence.

INFLUENCE OF THE MASS MEDIA

There is no doubt that the communications media provide children with a means for extending their knowledge about the world in which they live and have contributed to narrowing the differences between classes. However, there is growing concern regarding the enormous influence the media can have on the developing child.

Linkages have been established between mass media use and risk-taking behaviors in adolescents (Klein and others, 1993). The images of risky behavior presented by the media may serve to establish or reinforce teenagers' perceptions of their social environment. Media content also may directly influence risk perception; media protagonists seldom suffer adverse consequences of their behaviors despite their grossly distorted experience with violence, illness, or crime (Strasburger, 1990).

Children may identify closely with people or characters portrayed in reading materials, movies, videos, and television programming and commercials. While this has always been true of children, recent research indicates that over the past 30 years a greater number of children have selected media figures as their ideal role models, whereas in the past the majority of children chose their parents or parent surrogates as the people they most wanted to be like (Duck, 1990). This trend can be viewed as a grave concern or a magnificent opportunity to promote positive role models and healthy behaviors.

Reading Materials

The oldest form of mass media—books, newspapers, and magazines—contributes to children's competence in almost every direction, as well as providing enjoyment. Recognition of the impact of reading matter used in the schools on the value system and socialization processes prompted reevaluation of textbook content in terms of the biased presentation of male and female role models, the sugar-coated view of life situations, and the unrealistic, biased history of minority groups.

Fairy tales, for generations the mainstay of young children's literature, for a time suffered condemnation as being sexist, overly violent in content, and riddled with unfavorable stereotypes, such as the wicked stepmother, dwarfs, and physical unattractiveness associated with evil. They are now believed to provide an excellent medium for explaining puzzling and important topics such as death, stepparents, and inner feelings and turmoils. To a young child the world is peopled by giants, adults who control their lives and threaten their autonomy, who want children to do something against their will. Children can see these giants overcome. The split view of parents is also portrayed in fairy tales: the "good" parents who give children whatever they want and the "mean" parents who deprive their children of things. Although they do not provide solutions, fairy tales confront children with emotional predicaments and offer suggestions for dealing with them.

Comic books and other pulp reading material have been popular in every generation, usually at the expense of literature provided by schools, libraries, and parents. Many children have nothing else to read. The easy reading, quick action, and adventure in brief episodes seem to fulfill a need for children who are striving to understand both aggression in others and their own impulses. Reading ability, intelligence, and school adjustment apparently have no relationship to the number and type of comic books read. Most comic books appear to be relatively harmless to the majority of children and are in some ways even beneficial. Comic books seem to have only a minor influence on the acquisition of beliefs, values, and behaviors. The popularity of this medium has prompted some educators to encourage translations of literature into comic book form in order to stimulate the interest of students in the classics.

Movies

Movies, not closely bound to reality and often portraying an assortment of socially approved behaviors, perhaps make a contribution to children's value systems, but they do provide opportunities for desirable social learning. On the other hand, children, especially adolescents, flock to the "macho" movies and those whose heroes resort to violent resolution of problems, such as the use of karate techniques and wild automobile chases. The carryover of these influences into daily life and relationships may account in part for the increase in violent behavior of young persons.

A recent concern is the plethora of "slasher" and R-rated movies available to children and teenagers—in theaters and through cable television and videocassettes. The content of movies has changed markedly during the past few years, with mutilation as a major theme. To children who are unable to distinguish between reality and fantasy, these films play on their deepest fears, resulting in bedtime fears, nightmares, and a fearful view of the world (Schmitt, 1989).

Young children can be frightened by some of the movies considered to be safe for family viewing. For example, *Bambi* can be frightening to young children, and the villainous witches in *Snow White* and the *Wizard of Oz* are terrifying figures. Also, some of the classic Disney movies such as *Snow White* and *Cinderella,* which depict stepmothers as evil, destructive persons, can have a deleterious effect on children-stepmother relationships or can be confusing to children who have developed a positive relationship with a stepmother.

Television

The medium that has the most impact on children in America today is television, which has become one of the most significant socializing agents in the life of young children. The content of programs and commercials provides multiple sources for acquiring information, modeling behaviors, and observing value orientations. Besides producing a leveling effect on class differences in general information and vocabulary, TV exposes children to a wider variety of topics and events than they encounter in day-to-day life. Television always has time to talk to children and is a form of access to the adult world. However, research indicates that positive results occur only in cases in which children's television viewing is relatively light (Wilson and Christopher, 1992). Yet the average child in the United States spends more time watching television than in any other activity except sleeping: 25 hours per week for children ages 2 to 5 years, 22 hours for children ages 6 to 12 years, and 23 hours for 12- to 17-year-olds (Fig. 4-23). These figures do not include VCR use (American Academy of Pediatrics, 1990).

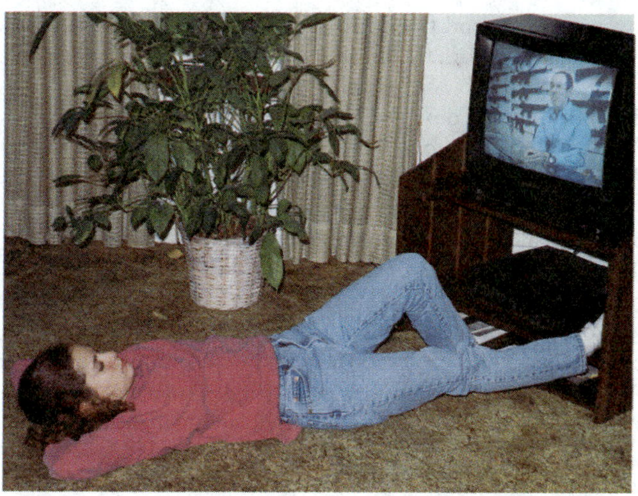

FIG. 4-23 The average child in the United States spends more time watching television than in any other activity except sleeping.

Most researchers have concluded that protracted television viewing can have detrimental effects on children. Increased verbal and physical aggressive behavior, reduced persistence at problem solving, greater sex-role stereotyping, and reduced creativity have been reported repeatedly. In fairness, no one has yet defined the long-term effects of other electronic factors, such as stereo headphones vs conversation, computer games or drills vs active social play, or videotapes vs books. However, it is clear that children in the modern electronic environment are constantly stimulated from outside, which allows them little time to reflect and develop the inner speech that feeds brain development. Television has been accused of robbing children of the chance to develop their own mental pictures that provide the kind of visual imagery helpful in solving math and science problems (Healy, 1990).

Most programs are designed to attract attention by visual jolts; the child establishes the habit of ignoring language in favor of frenetic visual and auditory gimmicks. Even "educational" programming intended to teach children to read does not teach the habits of mind needed to become good readers. The notion of withholding television completely until a child's reading and learning habits are well established has been suggested (Case, 1991).

Excessive television viewing has also been linked to obesity and high blood cholesterol levels in children. This association includes both the onset of obesity and a decrease in the remission of obesity (Gortmaker, Dietz, and Cheung, 1990). In a study of 103 children recruited as preschoolers, investigators found that by the time the less active children entered first grade, they were three times as likely as more active ones to show a gain in fat in the triceps skinfold. Furthermore, by the time the children averaged 7 years of age, they had as a group a 0.8 mm increase in triceps fat for every hour of TV watched per day (Couch potato, 1993).

Researchers in another study aimed at identifying children at risk for heart disease found that more than half of the children with high cholesterol levels watched at least 2 hours or more of television each day. Using a family history of heart disease or high cholesterol as screening indicators for cholesterol testing in children identified only three out of four children with high cholesterol levels. When families were also questioned about the time their children spent watching television, investigators were able to identify 90% of the children (Goldsmith, 1990).

The passive activity of TV viewing is frequently accompanied by eating, in many cases high-caloric snacks. Furthermore, children may expend tremendous mental energy processing the audiovisual messages from TV, which may be very exhausting and make them less likely to engage in physical activity later (Goldsmith, 1990). In a study of the effects of television viewing on resting energy expenditure in obese and normal-weight children, Klesges, Shelton, and Klesges (1993) concluded that television viewing has a fairly profound effect of lowering the metabolic rate and may be a mechanism for the relationship between obesity and the amount of television viewing.

Television programming and advertising, like movies, contain many implicit and explicit messages that promote alcohol consumption, smoking, and promiscuous or unprotected sexual activity. For example, American teenagers see an estimated 14,000 sexual references and innuendoes per year on television, yet only 150 of these references deal with sexual responsibility, abstinence, or contraception (Strasburger, 1989). Although tobacco advertising is banned on television, tobacco products are featured in many televised sports events. In a recent cigarette company–sponsored car race telecast, a tobacco product was seen or mentioned almost 6000 times; its logo was in view during 49% of the broadcast (Blum, 1991). While no clear evidence documents a relationship between television viewing and sexual activity or the use of alcohol or tobacco, the frequency of adolescent pregnancy and sexually transmitted diseases, the prevalence of alcohol-related deaths among adolescents, and the popularity of smoking among youth represent major sources of concern and speculation.

Considerable controversy has been generated and continues regarding the favorable vs deleterious influence of television on child development and behavior. Several factors encourage the learning or performing of TV-influenced behaviors (see box below, left).

Interventions. Many parents are concerned about the effects of TV viewing on their children, and the majority would like information regarding its use (Bernard-Bonnin and others, 1991). Parents need to supervise the amount and type of TV programs their children watch and to teach their children how to watch TV (see Family Home Care box). Recent legislation requiring television stations to meet children's needs for information and education or risk losing their broadcast license is hoped to improve the

FACTORS THAT ENCOURAGE LEARNING OR PERFORMING TV-INFLUENCED BEHAVIORS

Age. Younger children focus on behaviors rather than on motives or consequences. They view alternatives in a concrete manner, and they are unable to differentiate between central and peripheral plot information. Small children remember various assorted items in the program; for example, they remember the *act*, not the motive or consequences.

Identification with characters or situations. Children will more often imitate behaviors of persons and situations similar to those in their own lives.

Reward and punishment syndrome. Children will imitate behaviors they see rewarded or *not* punished when it is expected. They are less likely to repeat an act they see punished; their attention is immediately attracted when they see an act committed that they know should be punished but is not.

Opportunity to reproduce behaviors. Children will imitate behaviors when given the right environment or when violence seems an accepted solution. When children see a situation on television, they will use this information when they encounter a similar situation that requires a solution.

Motivation to reproduce behaviors. Children will imitate behavior when given the appropriate incentives: expectation of reward or lack of punishment. Some children have self-control; others do not.

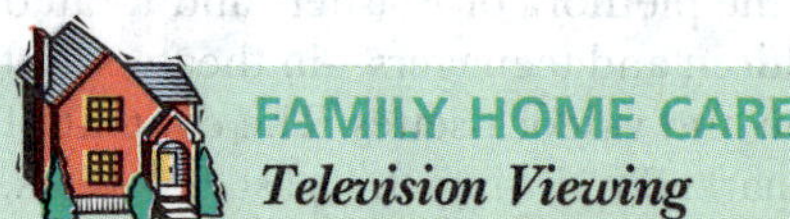

FAMILY HOME CARE
Television Viewing

- Provide a positive role model by developing television substitutes such as reading, athletics, physical conditioning, and hobbies.
- Construct a time chart of child's activities (homework, TV viewing, scheduled outside activities, playing with a friend).
- Discuss with child what both believe to be a balanced set of activities.
- At the beginning of each week select appropriate programs from television schedules.
- Allow child to select programs from this approved list.
- Limit child's viewing to 2 hours or less per day.
- Rule out TV at specific times (e.g., before breakfast or on school nights).
- Make a list of alternative activities (e.g., riding a bicycle, reading a book, or working on a hobby).
- Require that child choose to do something from this list before watching TV.
- Watch programs with child.
- Discuss program and commercial content with child:
  - Distinguish between the real and the unreal.
  - Correlate consequences with actions.
  - Point out subtle messages.
  - Explore alternatives to aggressive conflict resolution.
  - Stress purpose of program (e.g., entertainment, education).
  - Explain likes and dislikes.
- Turn the TV off after the selected program is over.
- Monitor cable and pay TV selections; use a lockbox if necessary.
- Limit use of TV as a safe distraction to potentially stressful times (e.g., keeping the children occupied while the parent gets organized after a difficult day).

quality of children's programming; however, many believe that additional action or legislation may be needed for television and video games.

There may be more subtle and effective ways for parents to mediate their children's viewing habits than discussion, co-viewing, and guidance to programming. Parental attitudes concerning TV, how parents use TV in the home, and the availability of TV may influence the quantity and quality of television children watch. Children seem to watch public broadcast channels more often in homes where parents do not use TV as a form of entertainment, use it often as an educational tool, do not view TV with their child more than half of the time, and allow their child to strongly influence program selection (Taras and others, 1990). When children and parents view TV together, they more frequently watch the commercial channels that the parents prefer. Therefore, encouraging co-viewing without an explanation of purpose may paradoxically decrease the quality of TV content to which the child is exposed. Parental attitude seems to be the factor in the home environment most closely associated with children's viewing habits.

Since children see television as reality, parents can point out to them that what they see on the screen is not reality, that it is people who make the programs. Parents should restrict viewing of violent programs and encourage watching programs with characters who cooperate, help, and care for one another (Murray, 1989). Older children can be encouraged to make short films to illustrate the point.

Parents can help children evaluate TV violence by pointing out the subtleties children miss, such as the aggressor's motives and intentions and the unpleasant consequences the perpetrators suffer as a result of their aggressive acts. Often the consequence is separated from the act by a commercial and children cannot make the correlation. Parents need to point out that conflicts can be resolved without resorting to violent behavior. They can also stress the purpose of the programs—primarily entertainment—and explain why they like or dislike something on TV (e.g., "This show is trying to tell you that crime does not pay and that if one does wrong, one will go to jail"). Explanations and discussions can take place between shows (with the volume turned down), and young children can learn from older children as well as from adults. These discussions can be very effective when begun early and carried out consistently.

It is especially important to identify at-risk children and control their viewing. House rules that specify the type and amount of television help children understand limits, and video-recorded selections of appropriate programs can be substituted for less desirable offerings. Parents need to carefully monitor cable and other pay TV programming, since these popular options present more uncensored programming. Locked boxes are available for cable receivers that allow families to prevent children from viewing programs when unsupervised. The effects of Music Television (MTV) on young viewers has yet to be fully evaluated (Betz, 1994), although one study found that MTV viewing desensitized viewers to violence (Rehman and Reilly, 1985).

Nurses and parents can be powerful forces in influencing the media. They can watch closely for an increase in violence and other undesirable programming and complain to sponsors and TV stations if they believe it is not appropriate. Good programming can be both educational and entertaining.

KEY POINTS

- Growth and development of children are strongly influenced by both genetic and environmental factors.
- The major development phases are the prenatal, infancy, early childhood, middle childhood, and later childhood, or adolescent, phases.
- Information about normal growth and development is derived from both cross-sectional and longitudinal studies.
- Growth and development follow predictable patterns in direction, sequence, and pace.
- Biologic growth is determined by height, weight, bone age, and dentition.
- External proportions and organ systems change with advancing age.
- Critical periods in development are those times when the child is more sensitive to beneficial stimulation or more susceptible to detrimental influences.
- Temperament is a way of thinking, behaving, and reacting to people and situations.
- Temperamental attributes of children can be described as easy, difficult, or slow-to-warm-up.
- According to Freud's psychosexual theory, during childhood certain regions of the body assume a prominent psychologic significance as the source of new pleasures.
- Erikson's psychosocial theory emphasizes the concept of critical periods in personality development when children strive to master core conflicts; each successive stage is built on successful completion of early stages.
- Piaget's theory of cognitive development describes children's progress through stages of mental activity in an orderly, sequential manner that enables them to make adaptations to the environment.
- Moral and spiritual development are accomplished in conjunction with cognitive development.
- Children are born with the capacity for speech and language and master rules of language by the time they enter school.
- According to social learning theory, children learn appropriate behavior through conditioning and observation of role models.
- In the context of the family children learn to apply appropriate sex labels to themselves, acquire sex-appropriate behaviors, develop a preference for their biologic sex, and identify with the parent of the same sex.
- To develop a positive self-concept, children need recognition for their achievements and the approval of others.
- Through play children learn about their world and how to relate to things, people, and situations.
- Play provides a means of development in the areas of sensorimotor and intellectual progress, socialization, creativity, self-awareness, and moral behavior; it serves as a means for release of tension and expression of emotions.
- Growth and development are affected by a variety of conditions and circumstances, including heredity, physiologic function, gender of the child, disease, physical environment, nutrition, and interpersonal relationships.
- Children's vulnerability and reaction to stress depend to a large extent on their age, coping behaviors, and support systems.
- The mass media can be influential in children's learning and behavior.

REFERENCES

American Academy of Pediatrics, Committee on Communications: Children, adolescents and television, *Pediatrics* 85(6):1119-1120, 1990.

American Academy of Pediatrics, Committee on Environmental Hazards: Radon exposure: a hazard to children, *Pediatrics* 83:799-802, 1989.

Anthony EJ, Cohler B, editors: *The invulnerable child,* New York, 1987, Guilford Press.

Archer JA, Pearson NA, Westeman KE: Aggressive behavior of children aged 6-11: gender differences and their magnitude, *Br J Soc Psychol* 27:371-384, 1988.

Band EB, Weisz JR: How to feel better when it feels bad: children's perspectives on coping with everyday stress, *Dev Psychol* 24:247-253, 1988.

Bernard-Bonnin A and others: Television and the 3- to 10-year-old child, *Pediatrics* 88(1):48-54, 1991.

Berndt TJ: The features and effects of friendship in early adolescence, *Child Dev* 53:1447-1460, 1982.

Betz C: The troubled media, *J Pediatr Nurs* 9(1):1, 1994.

Binkin NJ and others: Birth weight and childhood growth, *Pediatrics* 82:828-834, 1988.

Blum A: The Marlboro Grand Prix: circumvention of the television ban on tobacco advertising, *N Engl J Med* 324(13):913-917, 1991.

Bradbard MR and others: Influence of sex stereotypes on children's exploration and memory: a competence versus performance distinction, *Dev Psychol* 22:481-486, 1986.

Carey W, McDevitt S: Revision of the Infant Temperament Questionnaire, *Pediatrics* 61:735-739, 1978.

Case F: Minds at risk, *Washington Post,* C-5, July 29, 1991.

Chess S, Thomas A: Individuality: dynamics of individual behavioral development. In Levine MD and others, editors: *Developmental-behavioral pediatrics,* Philadelphia, 1983, WB Saunders.

Chess S, Thomas A: Temperamental differences: a critical concept in child health care, *Pediatr Nurs* 11:167-171, 1985.

Clutter L: Fostering spiritual care for the child and family. In Smith DP and others, editors: *Comprehensive child and family nursing skills,* St Louis, 1991, Mosby.

Connolly JA, Doyle AB, Reznick E: Social pretend play and social interaction in preschoolers, *J Appl Dev Psychol* 9:301-313, 1988.

Couch potato kids get flabby, *Am J Nurs* 93(11):10, 1993.

Curry D, Duby J: Developmental surveillance by pediatric nurses, *Pediatr Nurs* 20(1):40-44, 1994

Damon W: *The moral child,* New York, 1989, Free Press.

Duck J: Children's ideals: the role of real-life versus media figures, *Aust J Psychol* 42:19-29, 1990.

Elkind D: Postmodern play, *Readings J Rev Commentary Ment Health* 6(2):8-11, 1991.

Erikson EH: *Childhood and society,* ed 2, New York, 1963, WW Norton & Co.

Erikson EH: Reflections on Dr. Borg's life cycle. In Erikson EH, editor: *Adulthood,* New York, 1978, WW Norton & Co.

Fowler JW: Toward a developmental perspective on faith, *Religious Educ* 69:207-219, 1974.

Francis D, Williams D, Yarandi H: Anemia as an indicator of nutrition in children enrolled in a Head Start program, *J Pediatr Health Care* 7:156-160, 1993.

Fullard W, McDevitt S, Carey W: Assessing temperament in one to three year old children, *J Pediatr Psychol* 9:205-217, 1984.

Furman W, Bierman KL: Developmental changes in young children's conception of friendship, *Child Dev* 54:549-556, 1983.

Garmezy N, Rutter M, editors: *Stress, coping, and development in children,* New York, 1983, McGraw-Hill.

Gilligan C: In a different voice: women's conceptions of self and morality, *Harvard Educ Rev* 47:481-517, 1977.

Gilligan C: *Mapping the moral domain,* Cambridge, 1982, Harvard University Press.

Goldsmith HH, Gottesman II: Origins of variation in behavioral style: a longitudinal study of temperament in young twins, *Child Dev* 52:91-103, 1981.

Goldsmith M: Youngsters dialing up cholesterol levels? *JAMA* 264(23):2976, 1990.

Gortmaker S, Dietz W, Cheung L: Inactivity, diet, and the fattening of America, *J Am Diet Assoc* 90(9):1247-1252, 1990.

Grey M: Stressors and children's health, *J Pediatr Nurs* 8(2):85-91, 1993.

Harlow HF, Harlow MK: Social deprivation in monkeys, *Sci Am* 203:136-146, Nov 1962.

Healy J: *Endangered minds: why our children don't think,* New York, 1990, Simon & Schuster.

Hegvik R, McDevitt S, Carey W: The Middle Childhood Temperament Questionnaire, *J Dev Behav Pediatr* 3:197-200, 1982.

Henry J, Giordano B: Introduction—assessment of growth in infants and children: normal and abnormal patterns, *J Pediatr Health Care* 5:289-290, 1992.

Holstein C: Irreversible, stepwise sequence in the development of moral judgment: a longitudinal study of males and females, *Child Dev* 47:51-61, 1976.

Howes C: Social competence with peers in young children: developmental sequences, *Dev Rev* 7:252-272, 1987.

Jacklin CN: Gender. In Levine MD, Carey WB, Crocker AC: *Developmental-behavioral pediatrics,* ed 2, Philadelphia, 1992, WB Saunders.

Johnson J: The tendency for temperament to be "temperamental": conceptual and methodological considerations, *J Pediatr Nurs* 7(5):347-353, 1992.

Jung FE, Czajka-Narins DM: Birth weight doubling and tripling times: an updated look at the effects of birth weight, sex, race and type of feeding, *Am J Clin Nutr* 42:182-189, 1985.

Kelley S, Walsh J, Thompson K: Birth outcomes, health problems, and neglect with prenatal exposure to cocaine, *Pediatr Nurs* 17(2):130-136, 1991.

Klein J and others: Adolescents' risky behavior and mass media use, *Pediatrics* 92(1):24-31, 1993.

Klesges R, Shelton M, Klesges L: Effects of television on metabolic rate: potential implications for childhood obesity, *Pediatrics* 91(2):281-286, 1993.

Kohlberg L: Moral development. In Sills DL, editor: *International encyclopedia of the social sciences,* New York, 1968, Macmillan.

Kuczen B: *Childhood stress,* New York, 1982, Delacorte Press.

Kurdek LA, Krile D: A developmental analysis of the relation between peer acceptance and both interpersonal understanding and perceived social self-competence, *Child Dev* 53:1485-1491, 1982.

Lampl M: Saltation and stasis: a model of human growth, *Science* 258(5083):801-803, 1992.

Lowrey GH: *Growth and development of children,* ed 8, St Louis, 1986, Mosby.

Luthar SS: Vulnerability and resilience: a study of high-risk adolescents, *Child Dev* 62(3):600-616, 1991.

MacKinnon CE: An observational investigation of sibling interactions in married and divorced families, *Dev Psychol* 25:36-44, 1989.

Masten A and others: Competence and stress in school children: moderating effects of individual and family qualities, *J Child Psychol Psychiatry* 29:747-764, 1988.

Matheny AP: Bayley's Infant Behavior Record: behavioral components and twin analysis, *Child Dev* 51:1157-1167, 1980.

McGuire KD, Weisz JR: Social cognition and behavioral correlates of preadolescent chumship, *Child Dev* 53:1478-1484, 1982.

Murray JP: Using TV sensibly, *Child Behav Dev Lett* 5(9):1, 4-5, 1989.

Newman BM, Newman PR: *Development through life: a psychosocial approach,* ed 3, Homewood, IL, 1984, Dorsey Press.

Piaget J: *The theory of stages in cognitive development,* New York, 1969, McGraw-Hill.

Pinyerd B: Assessment of infant growth, *J Pediatr Health Care* 6(5):302-308, 1992.

Poresky R, Hendrix C: Differential effects of pet presence and pet-bonding on young children, *Psychol Rep* 67:51-54, 1990.

Rehman S, Reilly S: Music videos: a dimension of televised violence, *Pa Speech Commun Annu* 41:61-64, 1985.

Rogan WJ: The sources and routes of childhood chemical exposures, *J Pediatr* 97(5):861-865, 1980.

Rollins J: Nurses as gangbusters: a response to gang violence in America, *Pediatr Nurs* 19(6):559-567, 1993.

Rosenwasser SM, Lingenfelter AF, Harrington AF: Nontraditional gender role portrayals on television and children's gender role perceptions, *J Appl Dev Psychol* 10:97-105, 1989.

Ryan-Wenger N: A taxonomy of children's coping strategies: a step toward theory development, *Am J Orthopsychiatry* 62(2):256-263, 1992.

Schmitt BD: Nightmares on main street, *Am J Dis Child* 143:649, 1989 (editorial).

Selekman J: The development of body image in the child: a learned response, *Top Clin Nurs* 5(1):13-21, 1983.

Shaffer DR: *Developmental psychology: theory, research, and applications,* Monterey, CA, 1984, Brooks/Cole.

Sieving R, Zirbel-Donisch S: Development and enhancement of self-esteem in children, *J Pediatr Health Care* 4(6):290-296, 1990.

Smitherman C: The lasting impact of fetal alcohol syndrome and fetal alcohol effect on children and adolescents, *J Pediatr Health Care* 8:121-126, 1994.

Sroufe LA: Infant-caregiving attachment and patterns of adaptation and competence. In Perlmutter M, editor: *Minnesota symposia in child psychology,* vol 16, Hillsdale, NJ, 1983, Lawrence Erlbaum Associates.

Strasburger V: Adolescent sexuality and the media, *Pediatr Clin North Am* 36:747-773, 1989.

Strasburger VC: Television and adolescents: sex, drugs, rock 'n' roll, *Adolesc Med State Art Rev* 1:161-194, 1990.

Stuart GW, Sundeen SJ: *Principles and practice of psychiatric nursing,* ed 4, St Louis, 1991, Mosby.

Sullivan HS: *The interpersonal theory of psychiatry,* New York, 1953, WW Norton & Co.

Taras H and others: Children's television-viewing habits and the family environment, *Am J Dis Child* 144(3):357-359, 1990.

Terkel, S: *Ethics,* New York, 1992, Lodestar.

Touwen BCL: Perspective: critical periods of early brain development, *Infants Young Child* 1:vii-x, 1989.

Usdin G: Investing in the "emotional bank" concept, *Child Teens Today* 8(6):7, 1988.

Werner EE: The roots of resiliency, *Early Childhood Update* 3(4):1-2, 5, 1987.

Werner EE, Smith RS: *Vulnerable but invincible: a longitudinal study of children and youth,* New York, 1982, McGraw-Hill.

Wilson P, Christopher F: The home-television environment: implications for families, *J Home Econ* 84(4):27-31, 1992.

Wolk S and others: Factors affecting parents' perceptions of temperament in early infancy, *Am J Orthopsychiatry* 62(1):71-82, 1992.

Wolman BB: *Children's fears,* New York, 1978, Grosset & Dunlap.

Yip R, Binkin NJ, Trowbridge FL: Altitude and childhood growth, *J Pediatr* 113:486-489, 1988.

BIBLIOGRAPHY

General

Baillargeon R, DeVos J: Object permanence in young infants: further evidence, *Child Dev* 62(6):1227-1246, 1991.

Bradley RH and others: Home environment and cognitive development in the first 3 years of life: a collaborative study involving six sites and three ethnic groups in North America, *Dev Psychol* 25:217-235, 1989.

Brown MS and others: Type A behavior in children: what a pediatric nurse practitioner needs to know, *J Pediatr Health Care* 3:131-136, 1989.

Christopherson ER: Discipline, *Pediatr Clin North Am* 39(3):395-411, 1992.

Dixon SD, Stein MT: *Encounters with children: pediatric behavior and development,* ed 2, St Louis, 1992, Mosby.

Farrar MJ, Raney GE, Boyer ME: Knowledge, concepts, and inferences in childhood, *Child Dev* 63(3):673-691, 1992.

Feehan M and others: Strict and inconsistent discipline in childhood: consequences for adolescent mental health, *Br J Clin Psychol* 30(4):325-331, 1991.

Ferber R: The sleepless child. In Guilleminault C, editor: *Sleep and its disorders in children,* New York, 1987, Raven Press.

Flavell JH, Green FL, Flavell ER: Children's understanding of the stream of consciousness, *Child Dev* 64(2):387-398, 1993.

Guilleminault C, editor: *Sleep and its disorders in children,* New York, 1987, Raven Press.

Harlow HF, Harlow MK: Learning to love, *Am Sci* 54:244-272, 1966.

Hartup WW and others: Conflict and friendship relations in middle childhood: behavior in a closed-field situation, *Child Dev* 64(2):445-454, 1993.

Havighurst RJ: *Developmental tasks and education,* ed 3, New York, 1972, David McKay.

Howes C: Pressuring children to learn versus developmentally appropriate education, *J Pediatr Health Care* 3:181-186, 1989.

Kalish CW, Gelman SA: On wooden pillows: multiple classification and children's category-based inductions, *Child Dev* 63(6):1536-1557, 1992.

Laufer ME: Body image, sexuality and the psychotic core, *Int J Psychoanal* 72(1):63-71, 1991.

Lewis M, Alessandri SM, Sullivan MW: Differences in shame and pride as a function of children's gender and task difficulty, *Child Dev* 63(3):630-638, 1992.

Morrow JD: The eyes have it: visual attention as an index of infant cognition, *J Pediatr Health Care* 7:150-155, 1993.

Parker S, Greer S, Zuckerman B: Double jeopardy: the impact of poverty on early child development, *Pediatr Clin North Am* 35:1227-1240, 1988.

Phillips JL: *The origins of intellect: Piaget's theory,* San Francisco, 1969, WH Freeman & Co.

Rankin WW: Listening with the heart, *J Pediatr Nurs* 3(2):127-129, 1988.

Raymond CL, Benbow CP: Gender differences in mathematics: a function of parental support and student sex typing? *Dev Psychol* 6:808-819, 1986.

Sameroff AJ and others: Stability of intelligence from preschool to adolescence: the influence of social and family risk factors, *Child Dev* 64(1):80-97, 1993.

Seidner B, Stipek DJ, Feshbach ND: A developmental analysis of elementary school-aged children's concepts of pride and embarrassment, *Child Dev* 59:367-377, 1988.

Shapiro CM, Flanigan MJ: Function of sleep, *Br Med J* 306:383-385, 1993.

Strayer J: Children's concordant emotions and cognitions in response to observed emotions, *Child Dev* 64(1):188-201, 1993.

Thomas RM: *Comparing theories of child development,* ed 2, Belmont, CA, 1985, Wadsworth.

Todd AL and others: Antenatal tests of fetal welfare and development at age 2 years, *Am J Obstet Gynecol* 167:66-71, 1992.

Younger B: Understanding category members as "the same sort of thing": explicit categorization in ten-month infants, *Child Dev* 64(1):309-320, 1993.

Temperament

Blackson M and others: Temperament-induced father-son family dysfunction, *Am J Orthopsychiatry* 64(2):280-292, 1994.

Calkins SD, Fox NA: The relations among infant temperament, security of attachment, and behavioral inhibition at twenty-four months, *Child Dev* 63(6):1456-1472, 1992.

Carey WB: Temperament: a tool for coping with problem behavior, *Contemp Pediatr* 6(1):139-153, 1989.

Chess S, Thomas A: *Temperament in clinical practice,* New York, 1986, Guilford Press.

Cowen EI, Wyman PA, Work WC: The relationship between retrospective reports of early child temperament and adjustment at ages 10-12, *J Abnorm Child Psychol* 20(1):39-50, 1992.

Emde RN and others: Temperament, emotion, and cognition at fourteen months: the MacArthur Longitudinal Twin Study, *Child Dev* 63(6):1437-1455, 1992.

Kagan J: Behavior, biology, and the meanings of temperamental constructs, *Pediatrics* 90(3):510-513, 1992.

Kagan J, Snidman N: Temperamental factors in human development, *Am Psychol* 46(8):856-862, 1991.

Kochanska G: Socialization and temperament in the development of guilt and conscience, *Child Dev* 62(6):1379-1392, 1991.

Koniak-Griffin D, Rummell M: Temperament in infancy: stability, change, and correlates, *Matern Child Nurs J* 17(1):25-40, 1988.

Mebert CJ: Dimensions of subjectivity in parents' ratings of infant temperament, *Child Dev* 62(2):352-361, 1991.

Prior M: Childhood temperament, *J Child Psychol Psychiatry* 33(1):249-279, 1992.

Saudino KJ, Eaton WO: Infant temperament and genetics: an objective twin study of motor activity level, *Child Dev* 62(5):1167-1174, 1991.

Turecki S: Temperamentally difficult children, *Feelings Med Signif* 32(1):1-4, 1990.

Wallace MR: Temperament: a variable in children's pain management, *Pediatr Nurs* 15:118-121, 1989.

Worobey J, Blajda VM: Temperament ratings at 2 weeks, 2 months, and 1 year: differential stability of activity and emotionality, *Dev Psychol* 25:257-263, 1989.

Moral and Spiritual Development

Arsenio WF, Kramer R: Victimizers and their victims: children's conceptions of the mixed emotional consequences of moral transgressions, *Child Dev* 63(4):915-927, 1992.

Betz CL: Faith development in children, *Pediatr Nurs* 7(2):22-25, 1981.

Ferszt GG, Taylor PB: When your patient needs spiritual comfort, *Nursing 88,* pp 48-49, April 1988.

Flavell JH and others: Young children's understanding of different types of beliefs, *Child Dev* 63(4):960-977, 1992.

Heyman GD, Dweck CS, Cain KM: Young children's vulnerability to self-blame and helplessness: relationship to beliefs about goodness, *Child Dev* 63(2):401-415, 1992.

Johnson DF, Goldman S: Children's recognition and use of rules of moral conduct in stories, *Am J Psychol* 100:205-224, 1987.

Kahn PH Jr: Children's obligatory and discretionary moral judgments, *Child Dev* 63(2):416-430, 1992.

McCown DE: Moral development in children, *Pediatr Nurs* 10:42-44, 1984.

Rankin WW: Children and morality, *J Pediatr Nurs* 3:412-413, 1988.

Wainryb C: Understanding differences in moral judgments: the role of informational assumptions, *Child Dev* 62(4):840-851, 1991.

Language

Accardo P and others: Toe walking and language development, *Clin Pediatr* 31(3):158-160, 1992.

Activities to encourage speech and language development, *ASHA* 35(2):57-58, 1993.

Castiglia PT: Stuttering, *J Pediatr Health Care* 7:275-277, 1993.

Dunn J, Shatz M: Becoming a conversationalist despite (or because of) having an older sibling, *Child Dev* 60:399-410, 1989.

Echols CH: A perceptually based model of children's earliest productions, *Cognition* 46(3):245-296, 1993.

Holdgrafer GE: Quantity of communicative behavior in children from birth to 30 months, *Percept Mot Skills* 72(3):803-806, 1991.

Hurford JR: The evolution of the critical period for language acquisition, *Cognition* 40(3):159-201, 1991.

Marcus GF and others: Overregularization in language acquisition, *Monogr Soc Res Child Dev* 57(4):1-182, 1992.

Marks JH: Assessment of parent communicative behaviors: an overview, *Clin Commun Disord* 2(3):23-38, 1992.

McCabe AE: Differential language learning styles in young children: the importance of context, *Dev Rev* 9:1-20, 1989.

Nelson K, Hampson J, Shaw LK: Nouns in early lexicons: evidence, explanations and implications, *J Child Lang* 20(1):61-84, 1993.

Rack JP, Hulme C, Snowling MJ: Learning to read: a theoretical synthesis, *Adv Child Dev Behav* 24:99-132, 1993.

Rispoli M: The mosaic acquisition of grammatical relations, *J Child Lang* 18(3):517-551, 1991.

Rose SA, Feldman JF, Wallace IF: Infant information processing in relation to six-year cognitive outcomes, *Child Dev* 63(5):1126-1141, 1992.

Siegel LS: The development of reading, *Adv Child Dev Behav* 24:63-97, 1993.

Play

Bantz DL, Siktberg L: Teaching families to evaluate age-appropriate toys, *J Pediatr Health Care* 7:111-114, 1993.

Bellack JP, Fleming JW: Theoretical practical aspects of play: a universal need. In Fore C, Poster EC, editors: *Meeting psychosocial needs of children and families in health care,* Washington, DC, 1985, Association of Care of Children's Health.

Brown CC, Gottried AW, editors: *Play interactions: the role of toys and parental involvement in children's development,* Skillman, NJ, 1985, Johnson & Johnson Baby Products.

Cohen, D: *The development of play,* New York, 1987, New York University Press.

Lillard AS: Pretend play skills and the child's theory of mind, *Child Dev* 64(2):348-371, 1993.

Marino BL: Assessments of infant play: applications to research and practice, *Issues Compr Pediatr Nurs* 11:227-240, 1988.

Marino BL: Studying infant and toddler play, *J Pediatr Nurs* 6(1):16-20, 1991.

Ogura T: A longitudinal study of the relationship between early language development and play development, *J Child Lang* 18(2):273-294, 1991.

Oppenheim JF: *Buy me! Buy me! The Bank Street guide to choosing toys for children,* New York, 1987, Pantheon Books.

Rollins J: Meeting the child's developmental needs through play. In Smith DP and others, editors: *Comprehensive child and family nursing skills,* St Louis, 1991, Mosby.

Tamis-Le Monda CS, Bornstein MH: Play and its relations to other mental functions in the child, *New Dir Child Dev* 59:17-28, 1993.

von Zuben MV, Crist PA, Mayberry W: A pilot study of differences in play behavior between children of low and middle socioeconomic status, *Am J Occup Ther* 45(2):113-118, 1991.

Nutrition

Allen LH and others: The interactive effects of dietary quality on the growth and attained size of young Mexican children, *Am J Clin Nutr* 56(2):353-364, 1992.

Barness LA and others: Straight talk about feeding young children, *Contemp Pediatr* 5(6):22-55, 1988.

Dwyer J: Promoting good nutrition for today and the year 2000, *Pediatr Clin North Am* 33:799-822, 1986.

Endres JB, Rockwell RE: *Food, nutrition, and the young child,* ed 2, St Louis, 1985, Mosby.

Georgieff MK and others: Effect of neonatal caloric deprivation on head growth and 1-year developmental status in preterm infants, *J Pediatr* 107:581-582, 1985.

Pipes PL: *Nutrition in infancy and childhood,* ed 4, St Louis, 1989, Mosby.

Walker WA, Hendricks KM: *Manual of pediatric nutrition,* Philadelphia, 1985, WB Saunders.

Williams SR: *Nutrition and diet therapy,* ed 5, St Louis, 1985, Mosby.

Stress and Fear

Asendorpf JB: Development of inhibited children's coping with unfamiliarity, *Child Dev* 62(6):1460-1474, 1991.

Atkins FD: Children's perspective of stress and coping: an integrative review, *Issues Ment Health Nurs* 12(2):171-178, 1991.

Berman BD, Boyce WT: Environmental stresses and protective factors in child health and development, *Curr Opin Pediatr* 1:172-175, 1989.

Busen NH: Societal values: a cause of stress in children, *J Pediatr Health Care* 2:300-306, 1988.

Compas BE: Coping with stress during childhood and adolescence, *Psychol Bull* 101:393-403, 1987.

DuBois DL and others: A prospective study of life stress, social support, and adaptation in early adolescence, *Child Dev* 63(3):542-557, 1992.

Dubow EF and others: A two-year longitudinal study of stressful life events, social support, and social problem-solving skills: contributions to children's behavioral and academic adjustment, *Child Dev* 62(3):583-599, 1991.

Fabes RA, Eisenberg N: Young children's coping with interpersonal anger, *Child Dev* 63(1):116-128, 1992.

Garmezy N: Stressors of childhood. In Garmezy N, Rutter M, editors: *Stress, coping, and development in children,* New York, 1983, McGraw-Hill.

Grey M, Hayman LL: Assessing stress in children: research and clinical implications, *J Pediatr Nurs* 2:316-327, 1987.

Hobbie C: Relaxation techniques for children and young people, *J Pediatr Health Care* 3:83-87, 1989.

Honig AS: Research in review: stress and coping in children, part 1, *Young Child* 41(4):50-63, 1986.

Honig AS: Research in review: stress and coping in children, part 2, *Young Child* 41(5):47-59, 1986.

Kagan J: Stress and coping in early development. In Garmezy N, Rutter M, editors: *Stress, coping, and development in children,* New York, 1983, McGraw-Hill.

Langbaum T: What are children worrying about? *Clin Pediatr* 3(12):79, 82, 1986.

Lee MA: Helping children cope with a national disaster, *MCN* 12:87-88, 90, 1987.

Lewis M: Individual differences in response to stress, *Pediatrics* 90(3):487-490, 1992.

Rankin WW: Fear and courage, *J Pediatr Nurs* 3(1):46-47, 1988.

Rutter M: Stress, coping, and development: some issues and some questions. In Garmezy N, Rutter M, editors: *Stress, coping, and development in children,* New York, 1983, McGraw-Hill.

Schor EL: Use of health care services by children and diagnoses received during presumably stressful life transitions, *Pediatrics* 77:834-841, 1986.

Witmer D, Crouthamel CS: Overcoming the common fears of childhood, *Contemp Pediatr* 3(9):76-90, 1986.

Mass Media

Derdeyn A, Strayhorn JM Jr: Debate over effect of horror films on children, *J Am Acad Child Adolesc Psychiatry* 31:165-169, 1992.

Dietz WH, Strasburger VC: Children, adolescents, and television, *Curr Probl Pediatr* 21:8-31, 1991.

Downs A: Children's judgments of televised events: the real versus pretend distinction, *Percept Mot Skills* 70:779-782, 1990.

Lande RG: The video violence debate, *Hosp Community Psychiatry* 44(4):347-351, 1993.

Lorch EP, Bellack DR, Augsbach LH: Young children's memory for televised stories: effects of importance, *Child Dev* 58:453-463, 1987.

Robinson TN and others: Does television viewing increase obesity and reduce physical activity? Cross-sectional and longitudinal analyses among adolescent girls, *Pediatrics* 91:273-280, 1993.

St Peters M and others: Television and families: what do young children watch with their parents? *Child Dev* 62(6):1409-1423, 1991.

Silverman WK, Jaccard J, Burke AE: Children's attitudes toward products and recall of product information over time, *J Exp Child Psychol* 45:365-381, 1988.

Story M, Faulkner P: The prime time diet: a content analysis of eating behavior and food messages in television program content and commercials, *Am J Public Health* 80:738-740, 1990.

Strasburger VC: Children, adolescents, and television, *Pediatr Rev* 13(4):144-151, 1992.

CHAPTER 5

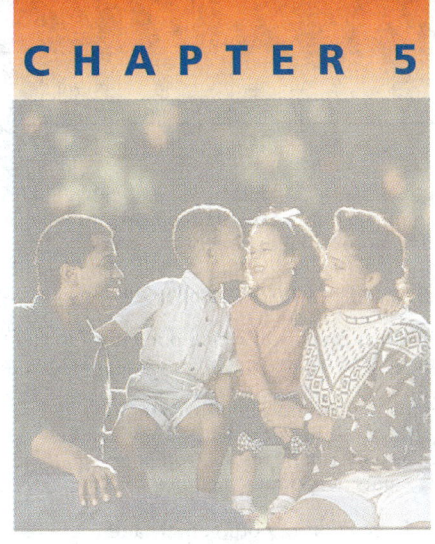

Hereditary Influences on Health Promotion of the Child and Family

CHAPTER OUTLINE

RELATED TOPICS

Abnormal sexual development, Ch. 11
Birth of a child with a physical defect, Ch. 11
Cleft lip and/or cleft palate, Ch. 11
Communicating with families, Ch. 6
Cranial deformities, Ch. 11
Cystic fibrosis, Ch. 32
Defects in physical development, Ch. 11
Down syndrome, Ch. 24
Family-centered care of the child with chronic illness or disability, Ch. 22
Fetal alcohol syndrome, Ch. 11
Fragile X syndrome, Ch. 24
Guidelines for communication and interviewing, Ch. 6
Hypertrophic pyloric stenosis, Ch. 33
Malformations of the central nervous system, Ch. 11
Multiple births, Ch. 3
Muscular dystrophies, Ch. 40
Phenylketonuria, Ch. 9
Retinoblastoma, Ch. 36
Skeletal defects, Ch. 11

GENETIC INFLUENCES ON HEALTH

Hereditary influences on health and disease are assuming increasing importance to persons in the health professions. Medical science has made rapid advances in the control of infectious diseases and nutritional disorders that formerly accounted for the major share of deaths in infancy. At the same time, contributions from the fields of biochemistry and cytology have established a genetic basis and the means for identification of an increasing number of diseases and defects. Consequently, there has been a corresponding increase in the proportion of conditions in which genetic factors are prominent, especially in the pediatric population. In fact, one third of all pediatric hospital admissions are due in part to a genetic cause, although the underlying genetic disorder may not be recognized (Prows, 1992).

To better counsel families and to anticipate probable problems, the nurse needs a fundamental understanding of the principles of genetics and the importance of heredity and the prenatal environment as etiologic factors in dis-

■ Donna Phillips Smith, RN, MS, revised this chapter.

KEY GENETIC TERMS

Allele—Alternative forms of a gene occupying same locus on homologous chromosomes

Association—Nonrandom cluster of malformations without a specific etiology (e.g., CHARGE or VATER association)

Autosome—Chromosome other than a sex (X or Y) chromosome; in normal human cells there are 22 pairs of autosomes and 2 sex chromosomes

Carrier—Person who possesses one copy of affected gene and one copy of unaffected gene and is clinically unaffected; however, may have clinically affected offspring because of expansion of mutation, X-linked expression, or recessive pairing with another

Chromosome aberration—Addition, loss, or structural abnormality of a chromosome; detectable by cytogenetic analysis

Congenital—Condition present at birth, although may not be apparent; causes may be genetic, nongenetic, environmental, or multifactorial

Cytogenetics—Study of relationship of microscopic appearance of chromosomes and their behavior during cell division to genotype and phenotype of individual

Deformation—Fetal abnormalities due to extrinsic factors (e.g., uterine position); may also show subsequent defects

Gamete—One of two cells produced by a gametocyte, male (spermatozoon) and female (ovum), whose union in sexual reproduction initiates development of a new individual

Genes—Genetic material (DNA) responsible for programming body's physiologic functions and characteristics

Genome—Complete genetic information of an organism, usually described as total number of base pairs; human genome contains 3 billion base pairs

Germ cell—Earliest recognizable precursor in embryo of an ovum or spermatozoon

Human Genome Initiative (Project)—Collective name for several projects designed to map and eventually sequence the human genome

Imprinting—Phenomenon in which an allele at a given locus is altered or inactivated, depending on whether it is inherited from mother or father; implies a functional difference in genes inherited from the two parents and explains some variation in expression

Inherited (heritable, hereditary)—Genetic transmission of a particular quality or trait from parent to offspring

Malformation—Morphogenic defect of organ, part of organ, or larger region of the body resulting from intrinsically abnormal developmental process

Major malformation—Structural abnormality with serious medical, surgical, or cosmetic consequences

Minor malformation—Has no serious consequences or is normal variation (e.g., extra nipple or umbilical hernia)

Meiosis—Cell division that results in reproductive cells (gametes) containing a complement of 23 unpaired chromosomes

Mitosis—Cell division resulting in two daughter cells identical to parent cell in chromosome complement (23 pairs) and genetic information

Monogenetic—Genetic disease caused by single-gene mutation

Monosomy—Chromosome abnormality in which one chromosome of a pair is missing; most monosomies are nonviable

Mosaicism—Condition in which an individual harbors two or more genetically distinct cell lines (generally, one cell line is normal and one is abnormal); results from a genetic change after formation of a zygote (i.e., postzygotic event)

Multifactorial—Complex interaction of both genetic and environmental factors that produces an effect on individual

Mutation—Hereditary change in genetic material; can be either change in single gene or change in chromosome characteristics; gene mutations can be passed from parent to offspring or can be new mutation in an individual, which is then heritable in offspring

Nondisjunction—Failure of two chromatids or two homologous chromosomes to separate during cell division, so that both members of a pair pass to new cell, resulting in trisomy of that chromosome pair, or monosomy in cell that does not receive chromosome

Pedigree—Diagram of genetic family tree

Penetrance—Frequency with which a heritable trait is manifested in individuals carrying gene

Phenotype—Clinically exhibited physical or chemical characteristics of individual; produced by interaction of environment with genotype

Polygenic—Inheritance involving many genes at separate loci whose combined, additive effects produce a given phenotype

Proband (index case)—Affected individual (regardless of sex) through whom family comes to attention of investigator

Recessive—Refers to a gene that produces its effect (is expressed) only when it is present in homozygous state

Syndrome—Recognized pattern of malformations with a single, specific etiology (e.g., Down syndrome)

Translocation—Transfer of all or part of a chromosome to a different chromosome following chromosome breakage; can be balanced, producing no phenotypic effects, or unbalanced, producing severe or lethal effects

Trisomy—Condition in which there are three, rather than two, copies of one chromosome in same cell

X inactivation (Lyon hypothesis)—In normal female most of genes on one of X chromosomes are inactivated during early embryonic development, such that alleles on active chromosome are allowed full expression

X-linked—Refers to gene located on X chromosome and to specific mode of inheritance of such genes

Zygote—Conjugation of male and female gametes

eases and disorders of childhood. Key terms for understanding genetics are defined in the box above.

HEREDITY IN HEALTH PROBLEMS

Contained within the nucleus of every somatic cell in the human body are more than 200,000 ***genes,*** the genetic material responsible for programming the body's physiologic process and characteristics. These genes are composed of segments of DNA (deoxyribonucleic acid) and are organized into structures called ***chromosomes,*** which are visible only during certain stages of cell division. Alterations of a whole chromosome, a part of a chromosome, or even a single gene can be manifested as a genetic disorder. Important to this concept is that this alteration may have been passed from the parent and previous generations, or it may be a new alteration in that individual. It is misleading to regard all genetic disorders as having been "passed through the family."

There is probably a genetic component in all disease pro-

TABLE 5-1 Characteristic Age of Onset for Manifestations of Some Genetic Diseases

AGE OF ONSET	CONDITION
Lethal during prenatal life	Some chromosome aberrations Some gross malformations
Birth	Congenital malformations Chromosome aberrations (e.g., Down syndrome) Some forms of adrenogenital syndrome Some forms of deafness
Soon after birth	Phenylketonuria Galactosemia Cystic fibrosis (sometimes)
Infancy	Sickle cell anemia (sometimes later) Tay-Sachs disease Werdnig-Hoffman disease Maple syrup urine disease
Early childhood	Cystic fibrosis Duchenne muscular dystrophy Fragile X syndrome
Near puberty	Limb-girdle muscular dystrophy Some forms of adrenogenital syndrome
Young adulthood	Acute intermittent porphyria Hereditary juvenile glaucoma
Variable onset age	Diabetes mellitus (0 to 80 years) Huntington chorea (15 to 65 years) Myotonic dystrophy (birth to old age)

cesses. In some disorders the genetic defect is known; in others the precise nature of the genetic component is more obscure. In some the disorder is apparent at birth; in others the manifestations do not appear for weeks, months, or years (Table 5-1). Some diseases and disorders are determined by the genetic constitution of the individual, such as muscular dystrophy, Marfan syndrome, and Down syndrome. Other diseases, although genetically determined, do not become clinically apparent until environmental factors precipitate the onset of symptoms. For instance, phenylketonuria is a disorder in which the enzyme to metabolize the protein phenylalanine is lacking. Deleterious effects in the infant are exhibited subsequent to sufficient ingestion of phenylalanine-containing substances, such as milk. Also, the acute symptoms of sickle cell disease are precipitated by certain conditions, such as lowered oxygen tension, infection, or dehydration.

Other disorders result primarily from environmental factors. These include most infectious diseases and trauma. Development of the disease depends on environmental contact with the etiologic agent, but there is strong evidence to indicate a decided genetic element in the susceptibility to most diseases (e.g., tuberculosis, poliomyelitis, and measles in some populations).

Genetic diseases can usually be classified into one of the following three broad categories according to the hereditary factors that produce the observed effect: cytogenetic, monogenetic, and multifactorial. Prenatal environmental influences, such as alcohol exposure and placental abnormalities, are also regarded as being within the realm of genetics, because these effects can produce congenital structural, functional, or growth defects. Although the chromosomes are normal, the anomalies produced can be indistinguishable phenotypically from a genetically determined anomaly. The important difference, however, is that the defects are not inheritable, because they were not caused by a genetic defect.

CONGENITAL MALFORMATIONS

The development of an organism, especially during embryogenesis, is an intricate process in which all parts must be properly integrated to ensure a coordinated whole. The rate must be such that one part is ready when needed by another part; otherwise, either part may cease to grow or may deviate from its normal path. ***Congenital anomalies,*** or ***birth defects,*** can arise at any stage of development and show wide variability in determining factors as well as in type, extent, and frequency of defects. Some defects result when a state, present in one phase of development as a normal condition, persists into another phase as abnormal. For example, a cleft lip is normal in a young embryo, and a patent ductus arteriosus is essential during fetal life. Any agent that interferes with these complex processes will produce a defect in development ranging in severity from an insignificant local anomaly to complete degeneration.

A few congenital defects are clearly caused by a single gene, some are associated with chromosome abnormalities, and others are produced by known intrauterine environmental factors. However many of the more common and severe defects (e.g., pyloric stenosis, central nervous system malformations, cataracts, and congenital heart disease) appear to be consistent with multifactorial inheritance.

The types of malformations that can result from genetic or prenatal environmental causes can be ***major structural abnormalities*** with serious medical, surgical, or quality-of-life consequences, or they can be ***minor anomalies*** or ***normal variants*** with no serious consequences, such as a sacral dimple, an extra nipple, or an umbilical hernia. Malformations can occur in isolation, such as congenital heart defect, or multiple anomalies may be present. A recognized pattern of malformations due to a single specific cause is called a ***syndrome,*** such as Down syndrome or fetal alcohol syndrome. A nonrandom pattern of malformations for which an etiology has not been determined is called an ***association,*** such as ***VATER*** (vertebral defects, imperforate anus, tracheoesophageal fistula and radial/renal defects) association. Neural tube defects, cleft lip and/or cleft palate, deafness, congenital heart defects, and mental retardation are examples of anomalies that can occur in isolation or as part of a syndrome or association and that can be caused by either single-gene or chromosome abnormalities, or prenatal environmental factors.

CHROMOSOME (CYTOGENETIC) DISORDERS

An ***aberration*** is defined as a deviation from that which is normal or typical. ***Chromosome aberrations,*** or ***cytogenetic dis-***

orders, are deviations in either structure or number of a chromosome; the consequences in either situation can be readily observed in the affected individual and are usually severe or even lethal. Although the types of cytogenic disorders are not as varied as those caused by a single gene, the incidence for many of the specific abnormalities is significantly higher than that for any of the single-gene (monogenic) disorders.

A ***structural aberration*** involves loss, addition, rearrangement, or exchange of some of the genes of a chromosome. If there is sufficient remaining genetic material to render the organism viable, structural alterations can produce an endless variety of clinical manifestations. These deviations are usually a result of an error in cell division in that individual, but sometimes the aberration can be inherited from the parent, such as in balanced translocations. Also, fragile, or weak, sites have been identified on both autosomes and on the X chromosome. An X chromosome fragile site has been associated with physical and mental abnormalities termed fragile X syndrome (see Chapter 24).

Deviations in chromosome number involve the gain or loss of a chromosome and are designated with the suffix ***-somy.*** A cell that contains one less than the total number of chromosomes is called a ***monosomy*** because of the loss of one member of a chromosome pair; a cell that contains one more than the total number of chromosomes resulting from the addition of an extra member to a normal pair is called a ***trisomy.*** A number of deviations that are compatible with life occur in humans, especially those involving the sex chromosomes; the more serious outcomes are related to abnormalities of the autosomes. Trisomies are the chromosome aberrations encountered most commonly by health workers. Monosomies may occur as often but are usually nonviable.

The clinical consequences that attend variations in chromosome number frequently consist of discrete, identifiable syndromes, particularly in regard to the trisomies (see Tables 5-2 and 5-3). The chromosome structural anomalies form a more diverse group of reported physical deviations with few recognized syndromes. Some of the chromosome disorders, such as Down syndrome, can be identified on the basis of physical characteristics but require chromosome analysis to rule out rare situations such as translocation Down syndrome.

Causes of Chromosome Defects

There is considerable speculation regarding the precise cause of chromosome errors. Ionizing radiation—especially large doses or from occupational exposure—has been found to be a cause of chromosome breaks, rearrangements, and nondisjunction. Autoimmune diseases appear to have a role in the pathogenesis of nondisjunction during cell division. Viruses have also been implicated, especially in relation to chromosome breakage.

Most of the information regarding factors that cause chromosome errors is related to parental age. The incidence of trisomic births corresponds strongly with increasing maternal age, regardless of the number of pregnancies. For example, the risk for trisomy 21, or Down syndrome, increases dramatically for mothers more than 35 years of age (see Down Syndrome, Chapter 24). There is no positive explanation for this observation. However, throughout a lifetime the germ cells are vulnerable to a variety of exogenous influences and to the normal effects of the aging process. Increasing paternal age is not associated with chromosome abnormalities (Michelena and others, 1993), but it is associated with an increased risk for autosomal dominant disorders, such as skeletal dysplasias.

Errors in Cell Division

The process by which chromosomes are distributed to the daughter cells during cell division is very complex and, therefore, prone to error. These errors can occur during ***gamete formation (meiosis)*** or in early ***postzygotic cell division (mitosis).*** The resulting unequal distribution of genetic material may involve the gain or loss of a whole chromosome or part of a chromosome.

The most common cause of numeric chromosome abnormalities is the process of nondisjunction during cell division. ***Nondisjunction*** is the failure of separation of homologous chromosomes during meiosis I (Fig. 5-1, *A*) or of sister chromosomes during meiosis II (Fig. 5-1, *B*) or mitosis (Fig. 5-1, *C*). The term ***sister chromatid*** refers to the pair of strands that constitute a metaphase (a stage of mitosis) chromosome. This failure to separate can result in one or both members of the pair not passing (segregating) to either daughter cell. Nondisjunction can involve either the autosomes or the sex chromosomes. If nondisjunction takes place at meiosis I, the gamete will contain both the maternally and the paternally derived chromosomes of the pair involved. If it occurs at meiosis II, the gamete will contain a double complement of either the maternal or the paternal chromosome. In either case the resulting gamete will have too many or too few chromosomes. If this gamete is fertilized with a sperm or ovum with a normal chromosome complement, the resulting fetus will be either trisomic (3) or monosomic (1) for the chromosome pair involved. Monosomies are usually not viable, with the exception of monosomy X (Turner syndrome).

Mosaicism is the presence of two or more chromosomally distinct cell lines, usually one normal and one abnormal. This situation occurs when nondisjunction takes place following fertilization (postzygotic cell division). The abnormality may be either numeric or structural, although numeric mosaicism is the most common type seen clinically. Postzygotic mitotic nondisjunction results in a fetus with two or more cell lines. This early cell division following fertilization is the most common cause of mosaicism and usually results in a normal and trisomic cell line, although occasionally a mosaic Turner syndrome (normal and monosomic X cell line) is seen (see Fig. 5-1, *C*). The percentage, or level, of mosaicism depends on the stage of embryonic development in which the cell division error occurs. If it occurs at the first cell division after fertilization, the level of mosaicism may be as high as 50%. If the cell division error occurs in later development, the abnormal cells may be localized to one cell type, such as the brain tissue or germ cell line (ovaries or testes). The extent of clinical manifes-

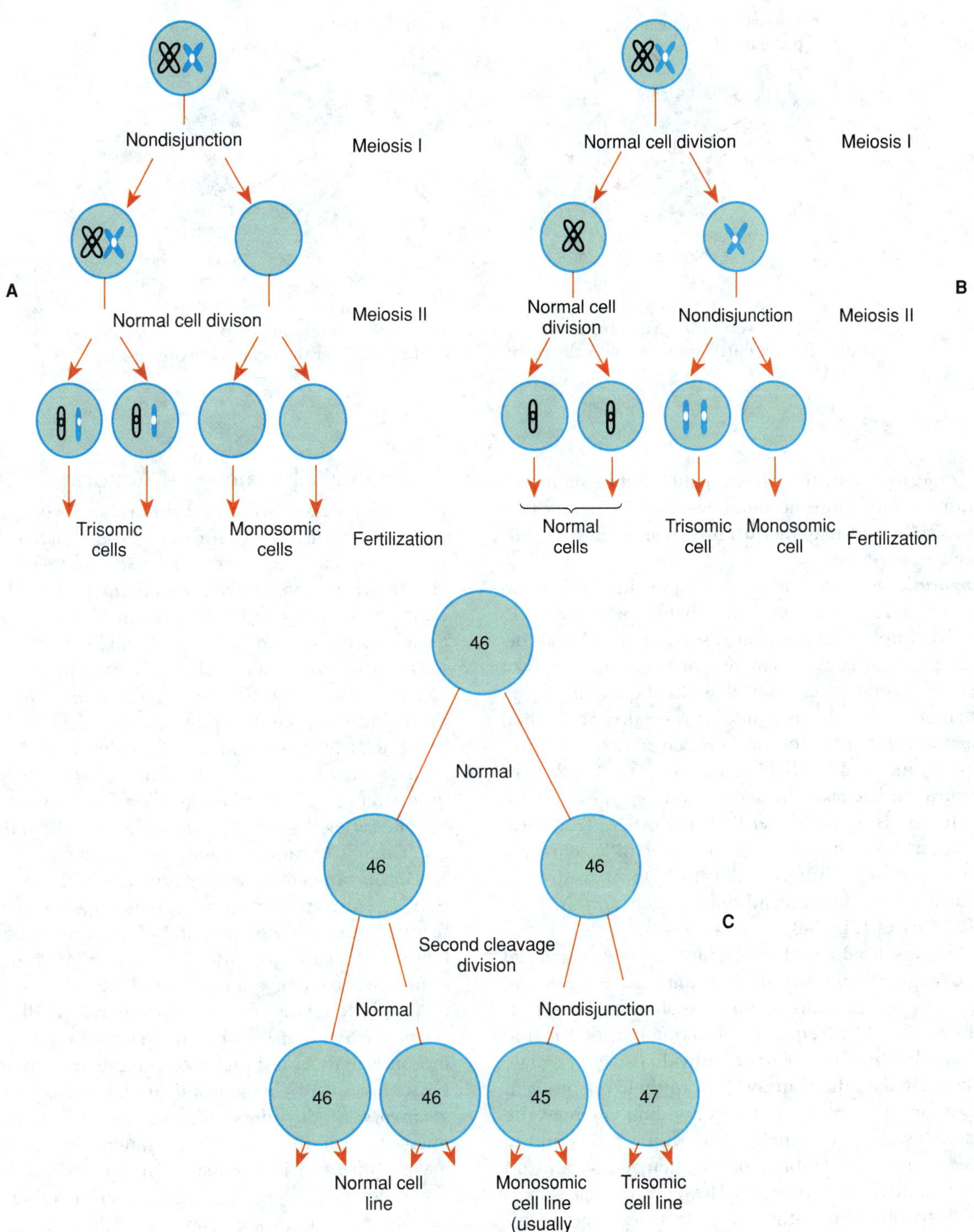

FIG. 5-1 **A,** Nondisjunction during meiosis I. **B,** Nondisjunction during meiosis II. **C,** Nondisjunction following fertilization, during mitosis, resulting in mosaicism.

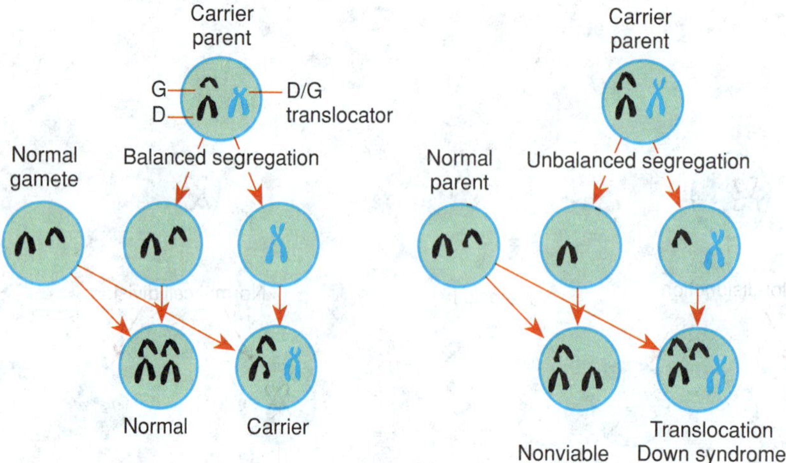

FIG. 5-2 Possible offspring from mating of somatically normal carrier of D/G translocation with genetically and somatically normal individual. *D/G,* Translocated chromosomes D and G.

tations is determined by the type of tissues that contain cells with abnormal chromosome numbers and the percentage of affected cells, and may vary from near normal to a fully manifested syndrome.

A ***translocation*** is a structural abnormality that involves an exchange of genetic material between two or more chromosomes. A simple translocation results when a break occurs in one arm of each of any two nonhomologous (not paired) chromosomes, and the segments below the break points change places. A variation of this occurrence, called a ***robertsonian translocation,*** occurs between acrocentric chromosomes: group D (13, 14, 15) and group G (21, 22). In an ***acrocentric chromosome,*** the centromere is near one end, so that one arm is much longer than the other. Translocations between those groups involving the No. 21 chromosome can result in an inherited form of Down syndrome, called translocation Down syndrome, which accounts for about 5% of cases (Fig. 5-2).

If there is essentially no loss or gain of genetic material in the exchange, the translocation is ***balanced,*** or ***reciprocal.*** Carriers of a balanced translocation are phenotypically normal and occur with a frequency of about 1 in 600 in the general population. These carrier individuals (either male or female) may pass the translocation to their offspring in a balanced or unbalanced form, depending on how the chromosomes segregate to the gametes. If it is passed in the ***unbalanced*** form, the combination is often lethal, and an early spontaneous abortion occurs. However, the risk of having a liveborn offspring with birth defects associated with the unbalanced translocation is 5% to 20%. Approximately 5% of cases of repeated spontaneous abortion (two or more) can be attributed to a balanced translocation carrier parent. Unlike nondisjunction, translocations are not related to increasing maternal age. Translocations, balanced or unbalanced, can be passed from a carrier parent or be ***de novo*** (arising as a new change), which subsequently can be passed to future offspring.

Autosomal Chromosome Abnormalities

Both numeric and structural abnormalities of autosomes account for a variety of syndromes usually characterized by mental deficiencies. A few are associated with a group of characteristics that clearly indicate the precise chromosome anomaly. The first and the most common disorder in which an associated chromosome abnormality was demonstrated is Down syndrome (see Chapter 24). The most viable trisomies are trisomy 21 (Down syndrome), trisomy 18 (Edward syndrome), and trisomy 13. Nurses often note dysmorphic facial features (Table 5-2), behavioral characteristics such as an unusual cry and poor feeding behavior, and other neurologic manifestations such as hypotonia or abnormal reflex responses, which may alert them to these and other major chromosome abnormalities.

Partial chromosome abnormalities involve a missing (deletion) or extra (duplication) segment of a chromosome. The features of classic deletion and contiguous gene (microdeletion and microduplication) syndromes are usually less recognizable at birth. Phenotypic effects of these syndromes may include a cluster of known single-gene disorders. The ***classic deletion syndromes*** can be detected on a routine chromosome analysis and include Cri-du-chat (Table 5-2), Wolf-Hirschhorn, and chromosome 18 deletions. ***Contiguous gene syndromes*** are disorders characterized by microdeletion or microduplication of smaller chromosome segments, which may require special analysis techniques or molecular testing to detect (Greenberg, 1993). Microdeletion syndromes are more common and may have more clinically obvious phenotypic effects than microduplication syndromes. Examples of these syndromes include Prader-Willi, Angelman (see p. 167), DiGeorge, and Beckwith-Wiedemann.

Sex Chromosome Abnormalities

The possible mechanisms by which sex chromosome abnormalities may occur are the same as those previously described (i.e., prefertilization nondisjunction during one of

TABLE 5-2 Common Autosomal Aberrations

SYNDROME	CHROMOSOME ABNORMALITY AND NOMENCLATURE	AVERAGE INCIDENCE (LIVE BIRTH)*	MAJOR CLINICAL MANIFESTATIONS
Cri-du-chat	Deletion of short arm of No. 5 chromosome—46,XY,5p−	1:50,000	Distinctive weak, high-pitched, mewlike cry resembling the cry of a cat; small head; hypertelorism; failure to thrive; severe mental retardation—profound with age
Trisomy 13 (Patau)	Trisomy of No. 13 chromosome—47,XY,+13	1:4000-15,000	Cleft lip and palate (frequently bilateral); ear malformations; microphthalmia; polydactyly; eye defects; cardiac defects; mental retardation; early death
Trisomy 18 (Edward)	Trisomy of No. 18 chromosome—47,XY,+18	1:3500-8000	Deformed and low-set ears; micrognathia; rocker-bottom feet; overlapping (index over third) fingers; prominent occiput; hypertelorism; cardiac defects; mental retardation; failure to thrive; early death
Trisomy 21 (Down)	Trisomy of No. 21 chromosome—47,XY,+21 (trisomy); 46,XY,+(14;21) (translocation); 46,XY/47,XY,+21 (mosaic)	1:700†	Brachycephaly with flat occiput; inner epicanthal folds; small ears, nose, and mouth with protruding tongue; muscular hypotonia; broad, short hands with stubby fingers and transverse palmar crease; broad, stubby feet with wide space between big and second toes; cardiac defects; mental retardation; variable life expectancy

*Data from Nora JJ, Fraser FC: *Medical genetics: principles and practice,* ed 3, Philadelphia, 1989, Lea & Febiger.
†Risk related to maternal age: age 30 years = 1:900; age 35 years = 1:300; age 40 years = 1:100; age 45 years = 1:30.

the meiotic divisions of gametogenesis in either parent or in the early postfertilization divisions of the zygote). An alteration in the number of sex chromosomes does not produce the profound effects that are associated with the autosomal trisomies. Intelligence may be normal or low normal, or the child may have some learning disabilities, but moderate or severe mental retardation is less common.

Turner syndrome, (45, XO) is essentially the only viable monosomy. It is still extremely lethal, with 99% of these fetuses spontaneously aborted. The syndrome should be suspected in the newborn period by the presence of lymphedema of the hands and feet and a low posterior hairline, in childhood by a webbed neck and short stature, and at puberty by delayed development (Table 5-3 and Fig. 5-3). The reason for the growth retardation is unknown. The child's growth is usually normal until 3 years of age and then slows, gradually drifting away from the normal growth curve. There is no prepubertal growth spurt. These girls may have difficulty with peer relationships and understanding social cues. They may exhibit behavioral problems, especially in relation to immature, socially isolated behavior.

Klinefelter syndrome, the most common of all sex chromosome abnormalities, is caused by the presence of one or more additional X chromosomes. The majority of males with this syndrome have a chromosome complement of 47,XXY, but there are numerous variants in the number of extra sex chromosomes. There are no physical characteristics that are helpful in detecting Klinefelter syndrome before the advent of puberty, with the possible exception of mental retardation. Mental impairment of varying degrees is a frequent finding and appears to have a direct relationship to the number of X chromosomes in the cells. The severity of retardation increases with the number of X chromosomes. Characteristic features of the Klinefelter syndrome are listed in Table 5-3 and shown in Fig. 5-4.

The milder physical and mental deficiencies of children with sex chromosome abnormalities compared with children with autosomal abnormalities is due in part to a phenomenom called ***X inactivation*** or ***Lyon hypothesis.*** In all body cells one X chromosome is biologically active; if more than one is present, most (but not all, as previously thought) of the other(s) (Blizzard, 1993) are in some way "switched off," or inactivated, during the very early divisions of the zygote and remain so throughout life. Because of the milder effects of sex chromosome abnormalities, many individuals are phenotypically normal and may remain undiagnosed (Milunsky, 1992). Sex chromosome mosaicism also occurs, which accounts for some variation in phenotype. The aberrant social behavior described as typical of multiple Y chromosome abnormalities is thought to have been exaggerated and more limited to poor impulse control, hyperactivity, and learning disability (Milunsky, 1992).

Multiples of the X and Y chromosome exist, in trisomic or greater numbers (Table 5-3). Regardless of the number of Xs, the presence of a Y appears to be a male determining factor. Therapy of sex chromosome disorders consists primarily of hormone treatment to initiate appropriate pubertal sexual development. Growth hormone therapy may be used in girls with Turner syndrome to increase growth velocity and, hopefully, final height (Rosenthal and others, 1992).

SINGLE-GENE (MONOGENIC) DISORDERS

Disorders that are the result of a defect or mutation of a single gene, rather than a partial or whole chromosome abnormality, are called ***single-gene disorders.*** These disorders, which generally follow a simple, definite inheritance pattern, are rare individually, but collectively they constitute a significant portion of health problems seen in infants and

TABLE 5-3 Common Sex Chromosome Abnormalities

SYNDROME	CHROMOSOME NOMENCLATURE	PHENOTYPE	OCCURRENCE	CLINICAL MANIFESTATIONS
Turner	45,X	Female	1:2500 female births*	Short stature; webbed neck; low posterior hairline; shield-shaped chest with widely spaced nipples; usually sterile (see Fig. 5-3)
Triple X	47,XXX (can also be 48,XXXX or 49,XXXXX)	Female	1:850-1250 female births	Normal female characteristics; usually tall; variable mental capacity and behavior; at risk for impaired language, neuromotor, learning skills, and psychosocial adaptation; fertile
XYY male	47,XYY (can also be 48,XYYY or mosaic)	Male	1:900 male births*	Usually normal sex development; tendency to be tall with long head; poor coordination; may demonstrate aberrant behavior; at risk for learning disabilities
Klinefelter	47,XXY (48,XXYY, 48,XXXY, 49,XXXXY, and so on, mosaics)	Male	1:850 male births*	Tall with long legs; hypogenitalism; sterile; male secondary sex characteristics may be deficient; gynecomastia (30%); poor psychosocial adjustment (see Fig. 5-4)

*Data from Nora JJ, Fraser FC: *Medical genetics: principles and practice,* ed 3, Philadelphia, 1989, Lea & Febiger.

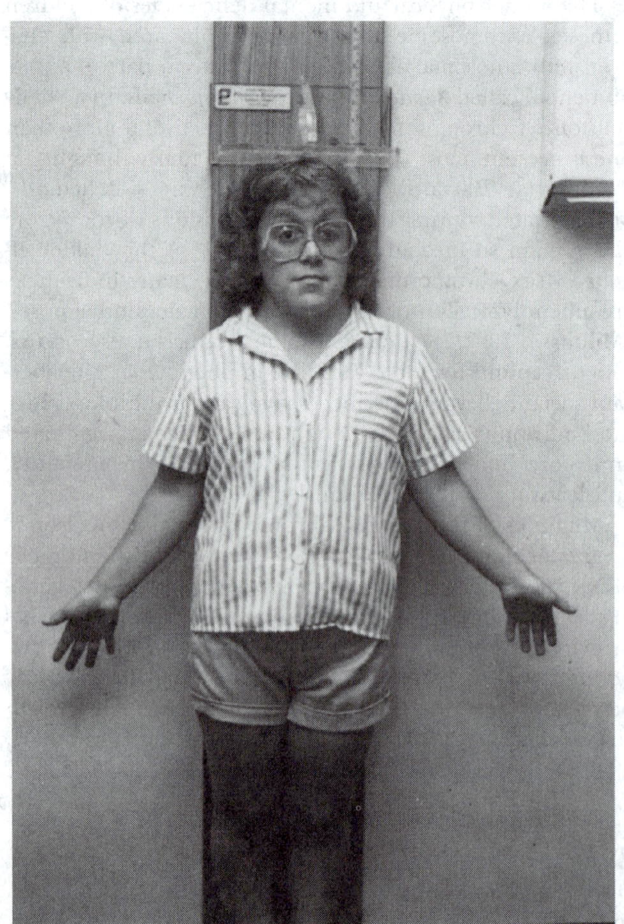

FIG. 5-3 Turner syndrome in 13-year-old girl. Note short stature (126 cm; weight, 37.2 kg), webbed neck, increased abduction or carrying angle of forearms, and broad chest with no breast development.

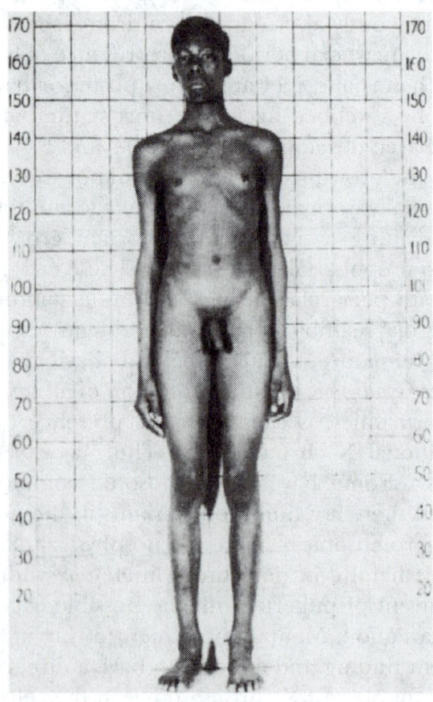

FIG. 5-4 Klinefelter syndrome. (From McKusick VA: *J Chron Dis* 12:1-202, 1960.)

TABLE 5-4 Partial List of Single-Gene Disorders

DISEASE	INHERITANCE	BASIC DEFECT	MANIFESTATIONS	THERAPY
Achondroplasia	Autosomal dominant	Defect in ossification at epiphyseal plate (growth portion of bones)	Very short limbs; large head; lordosis	Supportive
Albinism (ocular)	Autosomal recessive	Deficiency of tyrosinase: failure to convert tyrosine to dopa, and, hence, lack of melanin synthesis	Lack of pigment in skin, hair, and eyes; eye defects	Symptomatic Avoid exposure to sunlight Ophthalmologic care
Cystic fibrosis (Ch. 32)	Autosomal recessive	Defect in pancreatic enzymes	Abnormal secretions, chronic pulmonary disease, malabsorption	Symptomatic, enzyme therapy
Fragile X syndrome (Ch. 24)	Sex-linked dominant	Unknown	Long face, large ears, large testicles, mental retardation	Symptomatic, folic acid therapy
Galactosemia (Ch. 9)	Autosomal recessive	Defect in galactose metabolism	Hypotonia, vomiting, hepatosplenomegaly, cataracts	Galactose-free diet
Hemophilia A (Ch. 35)	Sex-linked recessive	Defect in factor VIII production	Hemorrhage into tissues, joints after injury	Factor VIII replacement therapy
Hypothyroidism (familial)	Autosomal recessive	Deficiency of iodotyrosine deiodinase	Lethargy; stunted growth; mental retardation	Early administration of thyroid hormone
Maple syrup urine disease	Autosomal recessive	Defective metabolism of branched-chain amino acids	Onset in early infancy; neurologic disorders; odor of urine similar to that of maple syrup	Diet low in branched-chain amino acids
Marfan syndrome (arachnodactyly)	Autosomal dominant	Defect in elastic fibers of connective tissues	Tall and thin, with long tapering fingers; poorly developed musculature; associated defects include aortic aneurysm, dislocation of optic lens, winged scapula	Supportive Surgical correction of deformities
Muscular dystrophy (Duchenne) (Ch. 40)	Sex-linked recessive	Protein dystrophin is absent	Muscular atrophy, progressive deterioration of motor function and mental development	Symptomatic
Myotonic dystrophy	Autosomal dominant	Defective calcium metabolism in nerve and muscle cells	Hypotonia, characteristic facial features, respiratory distress, poor feeding, high-arched palate, and cataracts; severe neonatal form leads to early death	Symptomatic
Neurofibromatosis (von Recklinghausen disease) (Ch. 18)	Autosomal dominant	Defect in neural cells—exact mechanism unknown	Café-au-lait spots, multiple fibromas, neurologic and ophthalmologic defects, skeletal anomalies	Symptomatic, surgical removal of tumors
Noonan syndrome	Autosomal dominant	Unknown	Small stature, shield-shaped chest, webbed neck, low posterior hairline, narrow maxilla, low-set ears, ptosis, hypertelorism, cardiac anomalies (pulmonic stenosis)	Correct cardiac anomalies Supportive
Osteogenesis imperfecta (Ch. 39)	Autosomal dominant	Defect in production of type 1 procollagen	Fragile, short, bowed bones, blue sclera, hyperextensible joints, hearing loss	Symptomatic, surgical orthopaedic procedures
Phenylketonuria (Ch. 9)	Autosomal recessive	Defect in phenylalanine metabolism	Eczema, poor feeding, seizures, musty smell to urine, mental retardation	Low phenylalanine diet
Tay-Sachs disease (amaurotic familial idiocy)	Autosomal recessive	Deficiency of hexosaminidase; defect in synthesis of gangliosides	Predominantly in Ashkenazi Jews; progressive neurologic deterioration; blindness, cherry red spot in macula; early death	Supportive
Thalassemias (Ch. 35)	Autosomal recessive	Defect in synthesis of one or more globin chains of hemoglobin	Anemia, hepatosplenomegaly, thinning of bones	Symptomatic, transfusions
Wilson disease	Autosomal recessive	Failure of biliary excretion of copper, leading to copper toxicity	Liver failure, speech abnormalities, tremors, psychiatric and behavioral problems	Anticopper agents, treatment of liver disease

children. They can involve any system in the body. They can be of such minor importance that they have little effect on the child or be so severe as to cause serious disability or to be incompatible with life.

The defective or mutated gene cannot be diagnosed by chromosome analysis, because it is at a more basic level of the chromosome, that of the DNA structure. Diagnosis of a single-gene disorder is presented on p. 168. These disease-producing mutant genes are usually distributed or transmitted in families according to basic mendelian principles of dominant or recessive behavior on the autosomes or sex chromosomes (usually the X). Some generalizations can be applied to dominant and recessive inheritance patterns of the autosomes or sex chromosomes and the resultant diseases and malformations.

Disorders resulting from structural defects seem to be primarily the result of dominant genes; most metabolic defects appear to be caused by recessive genes. Dominant traits are seen more frequently and are usually less severe than are recessive traits. This is probably because of the ***double-dose effect.*** Whereas recessive traits are manifested only when both genes are present, a dominant disorder usually involves a single gene from a heterozygous parent. The presence of a normal gene appears to overcome the effect of a recessive gene.

Codominance occurs when both genes of a heterozygous pair are expressed equally; neither is recessive to the other. This is characteristic of the major blood groups, such as the ABO blood groups, in which both the A and the B antigens are dominant. The O trait, without antigens, behaves as a recessive gene. Codominance is clearly illustrated by type AB blood.

Some examples of single-gene disorders, including the inheritance pattern, basic defect, and manifestations, are outlined in Table 5-4.

A number of variables are observed in many disorders that modify the basic inheritance patterns. In addition, there are genetic phenomena that are not explained by traditional mendelian inheritance. These variations and concepts are discussed following presentation of traditional autosomal dominant, recessive, and sex chromosome X-linked patterns.

Autosomal Inheritance Patterns

Autosomal Dominant Inheritance. Often the first case in a family appears suddenly as a result of new mutation. It is being recognized, however, that in rare cases, especially when a second affected child is born, one parent could have germline mosaicism (i.e., the gene mutation for a disorder is only present in the egg or sperm cells (Thompson, McInnes, and Willard, 1991). Depending on the degree of disability the condition imposes on the individual and the age of onset, it will either die out or continue to be passed on through several generations (Fig. 5-5). For example, Huntington disease, a progressive incapacitating and fatal neuromuscular disease, is usually not manifested until age 40 or later, after the affected person may have passed on the defective gene to offspring. Incomplete penetrance of autosomal dominant disorders is common, and there is wide variability in expression. Regardless of penetrance or variable expression in the parent, there is a 50% risk of passing on the defective gene to offspring, where it may be fully expressed. Other examples of autosomal dominant disorders include achondroplasia, neurofibromatosis, and Marfan syndrome.

Autosomal Recessive Inheritance. Children who display an autosomal recessive disorder will always be homozygous for that trait. The heterozygous person, with only one gene for a rare recessive disorder, remains undetected in the population (Fig. 5-6). It is estimated that each person carries from three to eight genes for such a severe genetic disease. For example, 1 in 20 persons in the United States and Northern European population carry the recessive gene for cystic fibrosis. For phenylketonuria the general population carrier rate is 1 in 50. However, the probability of mating between two persons who carry the same gene is highly unlikely. If they are blood relatives, the likelihood is increased. The chances are also increased if the mating occurs between persons who select a mate because of geographic, ethnic, or religious restrictions or blood relationship ***(consanguinity).*** For example, there is a higher risk that Ashkenazi Jews will be carriers of the gene for Tay-Sachs disease. The age of onset for autosomal recessive disorders is early and because they are usually biochemical defects, heterozygote detection and prenatal diagnosis are often pos-

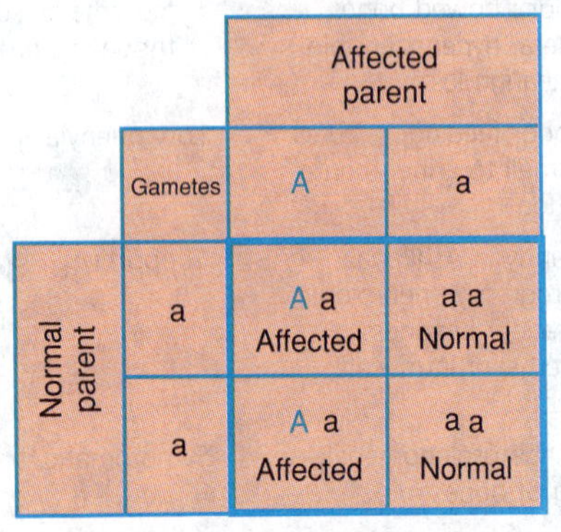

Characteristics of autosomal dominant inheritance

Males and females are affected with equal frequency.
Affected individuals will have an affected parent, although expression may be variable (unless the condition is caused by a new mutation or germline mosaicism).
Children of a heterozygous affected parent have a 50% probability of possessing the defective gene, although it may be nonpenetrant.
Children of affected parents who did not receive the affected gene will have unaffected children.
Traits can be traced vertically through previous generations—a positive family history—unless it is a new mutation, germline mosaicism, or nonpenetrant.

FIG. 5-5 Possible offspring of mating between normal parent and one heterozygous for an autosomal dominant trait.

sible. Other examples of autosomal recessive disorders include the thalassemias, congenital adrenal hyperplasia, and galactosemia.

X-Linked Inheritance Patterns

Genes on the X chromosome differ from those on the Y chromosome; therefore the transmission of traits caused by these genes will vary according to the sex of the individual who carries the gene. The two X chromosomes in the female are alike in gene constitution, with two genes for each trait. Genes on the X chromosome have no counterpart on the Y chromosome; therefore a characteristic determined by a gene on the X chromosome is *always* expressed in the male. One of the most significant aspects of X-linked inheritance is the absence of father-to-son transmission. Although it is essential for development of the male pheno-

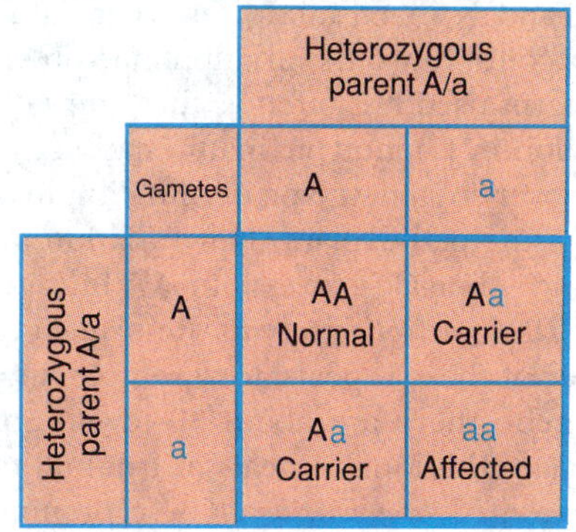

Characteristics of autosomal recessive inheritance

Males and females are affected with equal frequency.
Affected individuals will have unaffected parents who are heterozygous for the trait.
There is a 1 in 4 (25%) chance that any child of two unaffected heterozygous parents will be affected.
Two affected parents will have affected children exclusively.
Affected individuals mated to normal individuals will have normal children, all of whom will be carriers.
There is usually no evidence of the trait in previous generations—a negative family history—unless consanguinity is a factor.

FIG. 5-6 Possible offspring of mating between two parents with a recessive gene on an autosome.

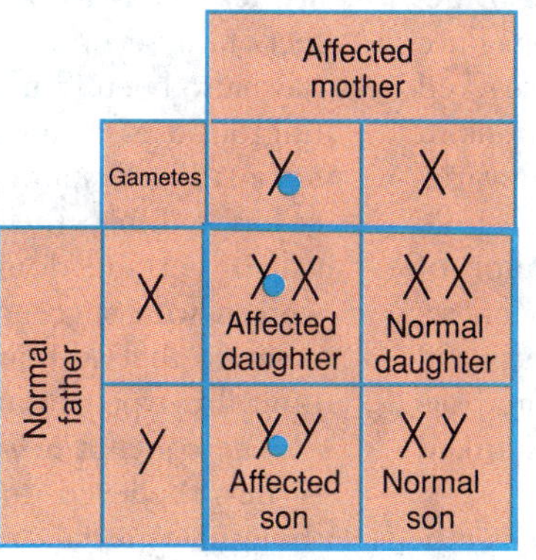

Characteristics of X-linked dominant inheritance

Affected individuals will have an affected parent.
All the daughters but none of the sons of an affected male have the probability of being affected (although usually more mildly).
Half the sons and half the daughters of an affected female will be affected.
Normal children of an affected parent will have normal offspring.
There are no carriers (although expression may vary).
The inheritance pattern shows a positive family history.

FIG. 5-7 Sex differences in offspring ratios in X-linked dominant inheritance. *Solid circle,* Dominant allele on X chromosome.

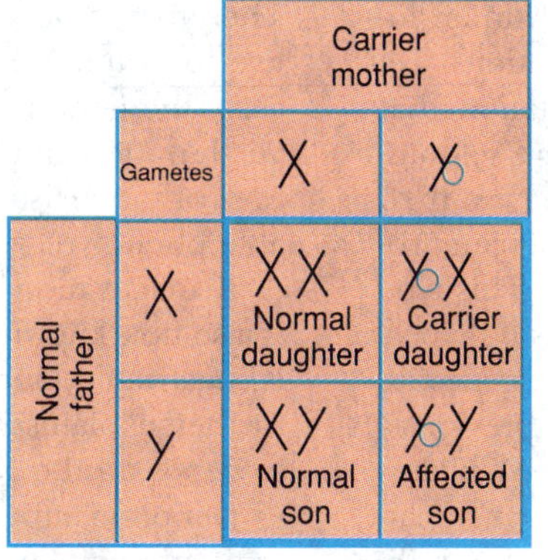

Characteristics of X-linked recessive inheritance

Affected individuals are principally males.
Affected individuals will have unaffected parents (except in the rare possibility that the father is affected and the mother is a carrier).
Half the female siblings of an affected male have the probability of being carriers of the trait.
Unaffected male siblings of an affected male cannot transmit the disorder.
Sons of an affected male are unaffected.
Daughters of an affected male are carriers.
The unaffected male children of a carrier female do not transmit the disorder.

FIG. 5-8 Sex differences in offspring ratios in X-linked recessive inheritance. *Open circle,* Recessive allele on X chromosome.

type, the Y chromosome carries no known medically significant characteristics.

X-Linked Dominant Inheritance. Superficially this pattern resembles an autosomal dominant inheritance pattern (Fig. 5-7). This type of inheritance is relatively uncommon. Examples of X-linked dominant disorders are hypophosphatemic vitamin D–resistant rickets and fragile X syndrome, although the latter exhibits some unusual features of transmission that are discussed in Chapter 24.

X-Linked Recessive Inheritance. The abnormal gene behaves as any recessive gene would; that is, its effect is hidden by a normal dominant gene. Therefore, two recessive genes are usually present if manifestations in the female are seen (Fig. 5-8). This rare situation would require the father to be affected and the mother to be a carrier. However, unequal X inactivation can also produce manifestations in a carrier female. New mutations are not rare. Examples of X-linked recessive disorders include hemophilia types A and B and Duchenne muscular dystrophy.

GENE ACTION VARIATION AND NONTRADITIONAL INHERITANCE

A number of variables have been observed that modify basic inheritance patterns and the effects of chromosome abnormalities. In fact, traditional patterns of inheritance account for only one third of diseases thought to be of genetic origin (Blizzard, 1993). Some of these variations have been recognized for some time; others are newly discovered phenomena that explain some apparent contradictions in the established patterns of inheritance. Some of the variations involve individual genes, and others involve whole chromosome behavior but will still affect manifestation of single-gene disorders. Also, some disorders have been reported to follow more than one inheritance pattern in different families (e.g., a classically recessive disorder may occasionally be reported as following a dominant or X-linked pattern in other families).

The most notable of these gene action variations is mutation. ***Mutation*** is any sudden, usually spontaneous heritable change in the DNA. Defective genes that produce disease are mutations of that gene. A gene mutation may have occurred generations ago and is passed down unchanged until it dies out because an individual does not reproduce, or a new gene mutation can occur spontaneously in an individual. Certain disease-producing gene mutations are known to be "old" mutations, such as the mutation that causes fragile X syndrome, and new mutations are seldom, if ever, identified. Other diseases are known to have a high new mutation rate, such as the 30% to 50% rate for neurofibromatosis and Duchenne muscular dystrophy. This type of definitive determination of a gene mutation is only possible for those single-gene disorders in which the gene site has been located (see p. 161). Some disorders previously described as exhibiting sporadic occurrence (e.g., Williams syndrome) not attributable to a traditional inheritance pattern may be new mutations with effects such that the individual does not reproduce, and the mutation is not passed on to offspring.

Variable expression is an important concept that describes differences in the extent and/or severity of manifestations of genetic diseases. There is a continuum of expression for any affected person from undetectable (mild) to severe clinical manifestation. Therefore a phenotypically normal person may still possess the mutant gene. This situation most often applies to autosomal dominant disorders; for example, a parent of a child with neurofibromatosis may exhibit only a couple of café-au-lait spots. Occasionally, however, it is seen in the other patterns. Genomic imprinting, mosaicism, and X inactivation, discussed later in this section, may account for some variation in expression and penetrance, a term used less often as these new discoveries explain variation in phenotypic manifestation.

The discovery of a new type of mutation in some genetic disorders has helped explain their variation in inheritance patterns and clinical expression. Within genes are sequences of ***DNA nucleotide repeats.*** A normal gene has a certain number of these repeats; for example, in the fragile X syndrome gene there are about 30 to 50. Some persons, however, have additional repeats of from 50 to 200, which have been termed ***premutations.*** These premutations in females are unstable and during meiosis can undergo amplification, expanding to hundreds more repeats, thereby becoming a full mutation and causing the offspring to be affected. Because fragile X is an X-linked disorder, females are less likely to be affected because of the tempering effect of the second X chromosome. These expanding repeats have also been found to occur in myotonic dystrophy, Huntington disease, and spinal muscular atrophy, which are autosomally transmitted disorders. This expanding gene discovery exhibits the old concept of ***genetic anticipation,*** in which certain dominantly inherited disorders tend to worsen with succeeding generations (Randall, 1993). It is believed that additional disorders may be discovered to exhibit this type of mutation (Morell, 1993).

The concept of ***mosaicism*** (see p. 158) is not new, but it is now believed to be more common than previously thought, especially during embryonic development. Placental tissue is commonly found to be mosaic. It is now understood that different cells can have different percentages of mosaicism; for example, a parent's germline cells (which produce the sperm and egg) may be mosaic, but other tissues (e.g., skin, blood [somatic cells]) may be normal. Therefore, a phenotypically normal parent could test negative for a mutation from the DNA of the lymphocytes, yet carry the gene mutation in his or her germ cell line with all the attendant risks of transmission. Different percentages of mosaicism in different tissues can also explain variable phenotypic expression.

X inactivation also produces a functional mosaicism. It is also now known that not all of the second X chromosome is inactivated, and that inactivation is not random, which further explains variable phenotypic expression in regard to genes on the X chromosome.

Genomic imprinting and uniparental disomy are two genetic phenomena that consider the parental origin of genetic information (i.e., maternally or paternally derived). The concept of ***genomic imprinting*** refers to modification, in some instances, of genetic material, resulting in phenotypic differences based on whether the genes/chromosomes were from the mother or the father. Genomic imprinting is exhibited during pregnancy, when paternally derived chromosomes seem to positively influence placental development and maternally derived chromosomes seem to positively influence fetal development. It has also been shown to be a factor in some genetic disorders, most classically Prader-Willi and Angelman syndromes. In both of these disorders about two thirds of affected individuals have a deletion of the same segment of chromosome 15. However, the clinical manifestations of Prader-Willi and Angelman syndromes are markedly different. If the deletion occurs on the paternally derived chromosome 15, the child exhibits Prader-Willi syndrome; if the deletion occurs on the maternally derived chromosome 15, Angelman syndrome is manifested.

Prader-Willi syndrome is characterized by central hypotonia, cognitive dysfunction, dysmorphic appearance, behavioral disturbances, hypothalamic hypogonadism, short stature, and obesity, as well as abnormal low body temperature, an increased tolerance to pain, and diminished salivation (Dimario and others, 1984). In contrast, Angelman syndrome (also called happy puppet syndrome) includes severe mental retardation, characteristic facies, abnormal (puppetlike) gait, and paroxysms of inappropriate laughter.

In some cases both copies of a chromosome pair are determined to have come from one parent, either the mother or the father, instead of one from each, a phenomenon called ***uniparental disomy.*** A child with two maternally derived No. 15 chromosomes exhibits Prader-Willi syndrome, and one with two paternally derived No. 15 chromosomes has Angelman syndrome (Mascari and others, 1992). Another example of uniparental disomy has been reported with cystic fibrosis, in which both chromosomes, each with a mutant recessive gene, came from the carrier mother; the father was not a carrier. In cases that appear to be nonpaternity, uniparental disomy may be a factor. One of the several theories about uniparental disomy is that the chromosome pair was originally a trisomy and the father's chromosome was randomly expelled, leaving two copies of the mother's chromosome. Because the chromosomes appear as a normal "pair," diagnosis of this situation is only possible with molecular (DNA) techniques.

Mitochondrial DNA mutations also account for nontraditional inheritance patterns. ***Mitochondria*** are components of the cell cytoplasm involved in energy production. They contain small circular DNA different from nuclear DNA. Numerous mitochondria are found in the ova, but few are found in sperm cells. Therefore, cell mitochondria are derived from the mother. Male or female offspring can be affected, but only daughters will transmit the mutation to their offspring. Examples of disease-producing mitochondrial DNA mutations include Kearn-Sayre syndrome and Leber hereditary optic atrophy.

CYTOGENETIC AND MOLECULAR GENETIC DIAGNOSIS

Cytogenetic Diagnostic Techniques

Chromosome analysis by ***karyotyping,*** a pictorial representation of the chromosomes matched by size and banding patterns into pairs from 1 to 22 (the 23rd pair are the sex chromosomes) is the basis of genetic diagnosis (Fig. 5-9). Numeric and structural abnormalities such as trisomies are easily seen on chromosome analysis. The cells used to analyze the chromosomes are skin tissue (including fetal skin cells), bone marrow, and, most frequently, blood leukocytes obtained by venipuncture. The chromosomes are cultured and examined during mitosis, when they are most visible. Deletions and translocations of larger segments of genetic material are visible on routine chromosome analysis. How-

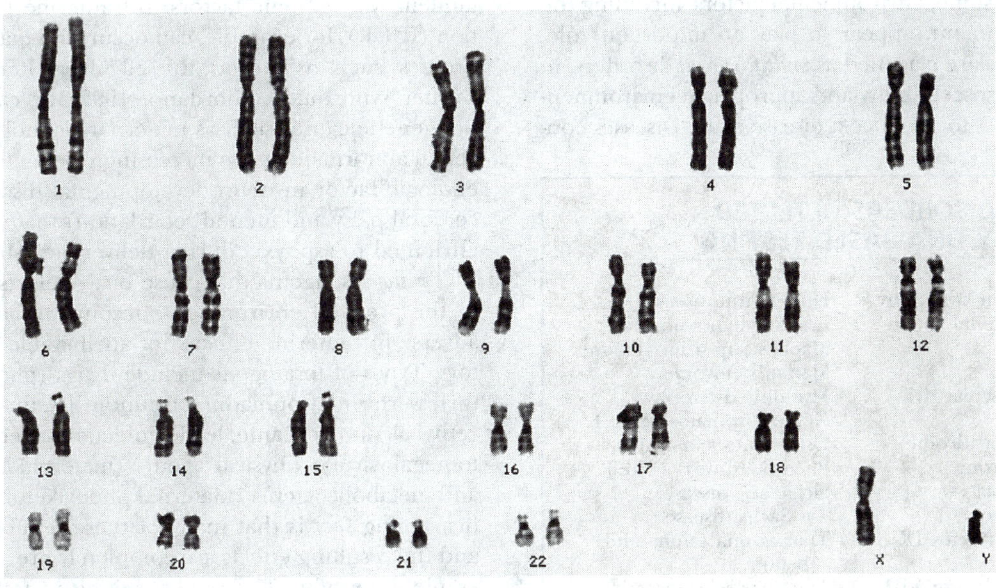

FIG. 5-9 Normal male karyotype. (Courtesy Children's Medical Center, Tulsa, Oklahoma).

ever, microdeletions and fragile sites usually require newer, enhanced resolution techniques that essentially "stretch out" the chromosome, thereby allowing detection of more subtle defects. Another new technique that has enhanced diagnosis of these subtle defects is ***in situ hybridization,*** which uses radioactive or fluorescent probes in a variety of ways to identify chromosome and DNA abnormalities.

Molecular Diagnostic Techniques

Diagnosis of genetic disorders at the gene level has experienced remarkable advances in technique. Identification of single-gene mutations responsible for some genetic disorders is now possible as more and more genes are being ***mapped*** (located on a specific chromosome or segment of a chromosome) through efforts as part of the Human Genome Initiative. In some conditions, such as cystic fibrosis, sickle cell disease, Huntington disease, and fragile X syndrome, the specific gene/DNA mutation is known and can be detected directly. For other disorders, while the exact gene location is not known, the particular chromosome and specific segment is known. By using "linkage" studies and mapping techniques, the likelihood that an individual has inherited the same chromosome segment as a known affected member of the family can be determined. Use of these techniques allows not only diagnosis of an affected individual, but also determination of carrier status and prenatal diagnosis (i.e., whether a fetus is normal, a carrier, or affected). There are about 200 diseases that can be diagnosed by direct or indirect (linkage) DNA testing (see box below).

MULTIFACTORIAL DISORDERS

A number of diseases and defects that are encountered frequently in the population show an increased incidence in some families but have no clear-cut affected-unaffected classification. Although the incidence is higher than would be expected by chance, no specific mode of inheritance can be identified. In some, environmental factors, including the prenatal environment, appear to play an important role. These conditions are classified as ***multifactorial*** disorders, in which a genetic susceptibility and appropriate environmental agents interact to produce a disease state. Diseases considered to be multifactorial (at least in isolation) include neural tube defects, cleft lip and/or cleft palate, congenital hip dislocation, and pyloric stenosis. Determining risks of recurrence is more difficult than for single-gene disorders. For example, anencephaly and/or spina bifida occur in 0.2 to 5 per 1000 births in the general population. The recurrence risk after the first affected child is 3% to 6%. Advances in genetics are enhancing knowledge of multifactorial inheritance to better understand familial risks.

The inherited histocompatibility (tissue) antigens, similar to the blood group antigens, have been implicated in the development of many diseases. These antigens, termed the ***human leukocyte antigen (HLA) system,*** are present on the cell membrane of almost all body cells. They occur in linked pairs and are inherited in the same manner as the blood group antigens. A number of these antigens have been identified and have been classified as follows: class 1—the HLA-A, HLA-B, and HLA-C antigens; class 2—the HLA-D and HLA-DR (D-related) antigens; and class 3—certain complement factors with genes in the HLA region.

A relationship between the HLA system has been shown for several disorders (e.g., insulin-dependent diabetes mellitus, hemochromatosis, psoriasis vulgaris, celiac disease, myasthenia gravis, and several forms of arthritis). Most notable is the striking association between HLA-B27 and idiopathic ankylosing spondylitis in 90% to 95% of affected persons. Although significant associations have been identified in only a few disorders, risk estimates can be determined regarding the frequency with which one of these diseases develops in an individual carrying a specific HLA antigen as compared with the frequency of the disease in persons who do not carry the HLA antigen.

Disorders of the Intrauterine Environment

The prenatal intrauterine environment can have a profound and permanent effect on a developing fetus, even when chromosome or single-gene abnormalities are not present. Sometimes, however, intrauterine effects occur in tandem with genetic factors. Intrauterine growth retardation (IUGR), for example, can occur with many genetic syndromes such as Down, Russell-Silver, Prader-Willi, and Turner syndromes (Giordano, 1992) or can occur from nongenetic causes such as maternal alcohol ingestion. Placental abnormalities are increasingly being found to be the etiologic factor in neurodevelopmental disorders (such as cerebral palsy and mental retardation) that were previously attributed to asphyxia during delivery (Altshuler, 1993).

Teratogens, agents that cause birth defects when present in the prenatal environment, account for the majority of adverse intrauterine effects not attributable to genetic factors. Types of teratogens include drugs (phenytoin [Dilantin], warfarin [Coumadin], tretinoin [Retin-A]); chemicals (ethyl alcohol, cocaine, lead); infectious agents (rubella, cytomegalovirus); physical agents (maternal hyperthermia); and metabolic agents (maternal phenylketonuria). The disheartening fact is that many of these teratogen exposures and the resulting effects are completely preventable; for example, ingestion of alcohol resulting in fetal alcohol syndrome/fetal alcohol effects (FAS/FAE) causes severe birth defects, including mental retardation, and the incidence

DISORDERS DETECTED BY DNA-BASED TESTING

Becker muscular dystrophy
Congenital adrenal hyperplasia
Cystic fibrosis
Duchenne muscular dystrophy
Ehlers-Danlos syndrome
Fragile X syndrome
Friedreich ataxia
Gaucher disease
Hemophilia B (factor IX deficiency)
Hemophilia A (factor VIII deficiency)
Huntington disease
Lesch-Nyhan syndrome
Maple syrup urine disease
Marfan syndrome
Myotonic dystrophy
Neurofibromatosis type I
Osteogenesis imperfecta
Phenylketonuria (PKU)
Sickle cell disease
Tay Sachs disease
Thalassemia (alpha and beta)
Tuberous sclerosis

may be as great as 1 in 300 live births (American Academy of Pediatrics, 1993) (see also Chapter 11).

THERAPEUTIC MANAGEMENT OF GENETIC DISEASE

There is no cure for genetic disease at present, although preventive and corrective therapy is helping to reduce the harmful effects in an increasing number of conditions. Genetic research is making progress in the art of altering the genetic material directly. Meanwhile, the major goal of therapy is modification of the internal or external environment to correct or minimize the effects of the genetic defect.

Therapeutic Modalities

The therapeutic modalities available for genetic disorders are few when compared with the infinite variety of conditions afflicting the population, but with increased understanding of the basic defects and the technical advances being made, an increasing number are becoming amenable to treatment.

Surgical Repair. Surgical repair of structural defects has made it possible to prolong life in a number of multifactorial disorders, such as congenital heart disease and pyloric stenosis. Numerous facial and limb deformities can be altered by plastic and reconstructive techniques. In cases of familial polyposis coli, surgical removal of the colon eliminates the countless polyps that invariably become cancerous. Splenectomy prevents the trapping of abnormal blood cells in that organ in several hereditary disorders of red blood cells. Early diagnosis and enucleation in retinoblastoma have reduced the mortality from this dreaded eye tumor. In the last few years there has been some interest in fetal surgery for some life-threatening anomalies, particularly urinary tract abnormalities.

Diet Modification. For disorders in which an enzyme deficiency causes a toxic accumulation of a substance or its by-products, restricting the intake of foods containing the offending substance often prevents irreversible damage from the improper metabolism of these compounds. Examples include the low-phenylalanine diet prescribed for children with phenylketonuria, elimination of dairy products containing lactose for infants and children with hereditary lactase deficiency, avoidance of foods containing or producing galactose for children with galactosemia, and a diet low in branched-chain amino acids for infants and children with maple syrup urine disease. Women with phenylketonuria must reinstitute a strict low-phenylalanine diet before conception and maintain it throughout pregnancy to prevent a high risk of adverse fetal effects (see Chapter 9).

Product Replacement. In some deficiency diseases, supplying the missing product that cannot be synthesized prevents undesirable effects. For example, thyroid extract is prescribed to prevent the damaging effects of hypothyroidism, and providing the missing blood factors prevents life-threatening and debilitating hemorrhages in the hemophilias. Other examples are insulin for diabetes mellitus, growth hormone for growth hormone deficiency, and corticosteroids for adrenogenital syndrome.

Avoidance of Drugs or Other Substances. In drug-induced disease, such as glucose-6-phosphate dehydrogenase (G-6-PD) deficiency and the porphyrias, avoidance of the drugs that precipitate a reaction provides a simple preventive measure.

Removal of Toxic Substances. Removal of toxic substances that accumulate in vital tissues as a result of a hereditary disease can prevent disabling complications. Some of the deleterious effects of hemochromatosis, a hereditary disorder characterized by an excess accumulation of iron in the liver, heart, and pancreas, can be reduced with the removal of iron by administration of chelating agents.

Immunologic Prevention. The administration of immunoglobulin to Rh-negative mothers following the birth of an Rh-positive infant is effective in preventing Rh-antibody formation that causes hemolytic disease of the newborn in subsequent births.

Transplantation. Replacement of nonfunctioning organs with normal organs is increasing the survival of children with defective organs because the problems of tissue incompatibility are better controlled. Examples of organ transplants include kidneys in hereditary polycystic kidneys, heart in severe cardiac myopathy, liver in hepatic atresia, pancreas in diabetes mellitus, and bone marrow in hereditary hemoglobinopathies, such as thalassemia and sickle cell disease.

Cofactor Administration. Diet supplements can be given when the body is unable to synthesize or effectively use some substances needed as cofactors in metabolism, such as vitamin B_{12} in pernicious anemia, in which absorption of this vitamin is absent.

Recombinant DNA. The transfer of modified genetic material from one organism (a virus) to another causes the viral DNA to become integrated into the cellular DNA of a recipient cell, often a bacteria cell. This recombinant DNA multiplies, producing the missing substance in the host cell. This technology has been applied in growth hormone therapy and factor VIII synthesis.

Gene Transfer. Fragments of DNA from a normal gene can be introduced directly into a recipient cell lacking such a gene. This approach has been attempted in humans with the transfer of normal gene copies of β-hemoglobin into bone marrow cells in an effort to treat a form of β-thalassemia, and has been used in sickle cell disease. Gene transfer has also been successfully used in adenosine deaminase deficiency.

Other Therapies. Other methods such as enzyme repression and competitive inhibition are providing effective treatment in some metabolic disorders. Future therapies include the possibility of replacement or stabilization by injection or oral administration of a substance that the patient lacks.

Environmental Manipulation

Inherited diseases or defects for which there is no therapeutic modality can be modified to enhance the quality of life for the affected individual. Some examples of environmental manipulation include hearing aids for deaf children, glasses or vision enhancers such as enlarged print and books in braille for the visually impaired, mobilizing devices such as braces and wheelchairs for persons with muscle and bone impairment, prosthetic devices for limb deficiencies, and infant stimulation programs to maximize the potential of children who are mentally retarded.

IMPACT OF HEREDITARY DISORDERS ON THE FAMILY

GENETIC SCREENING

Tests to detect the presence of a defective gene are rapidly assuming greater importance in management of genetic disorders as more defects are identified and techniques are developed for easy application. It is probable that with improved technology, mass screening for numerous defects may eventually be a routine procedure. However, to be truly effective, screening programs depend on education of both health professionals and the public regarding these programs. The religious, moral, and ethical issues revolving around screening and prenatal diagnosis are extensive and change over time.

Purposes of Screening

Genetic screening is presumptive identification of an unrecognized genotype in individuals or populations. There are several purposes for this screening: (1) to detect the presence of apparent or nonapparent disease, (2) to provide reproductive information, and (3) to gain information concerning the incidence of a disorder in the population.

Screening for Disease. The rationale for screening for disease in the general population is to discover persons who (1) have the disease, either manifest or incipient, or (2) may, in time or under special circumstances, develop the disease. ***Presymptomatic testing*** refers to this process in high-risk populations (i.e., when there is a family history of genetic disease, especially one of late onset, such as Huntington disease). The purpose of this knowledge in both situations is to anticipate serious consequences and provide the individual with treatment and management that will prevent, reverse, or diminish the adverse effects of the disorder (see Thinking Critically About . . . box). An example is the generalized, systematic screening of newborn infants for phenylketonuria, hypothyroidism, and galactosemia. The mass screening programs have indicated that many of these disorders are more prevalent than formerly believed. Others that are included in some screening programs are congenital adrenal hyperplasia, maple syrup urine disease, sickle cell disease and other hemoglobinopathies, tyrosinemia, adenosine deaminase deficiency, and various other aminoacidurias and urea cycle disorders.

A number of technologies are available for detecting disease—biochemical assays, protein iontophoresis, chromosome analysis, and testing with DNA molecular probes. It has even been suggested that the DNA of an affected child be banked and used to identify markers in other family members at a later date, such as in a subsequent pregnancy.

Screening for Reproductive Information. Screening for heterozygotes (carriers) can detect unaffected persons with certain genes who, when they mate with an individual who carries a similar gene, are at high risk of producing an affected offspring. These individuals are thus provided with the knowledge they need for use in decisions about family planning. Carriers of a number of diseases can be detected by laboratory tests, but because of the rarity of these diseases, mass screening is not feasible except in persons or populations known to be at risk. Persons at risk include close relatives of persons with an inborn error of metabolism or other detectable disorder, or certain ethnic populations known to have a high incidence of a specific disease, such as sickle cell anemia in blacks, Tay-Sachs disease in Ashkenazi Jews, and thalassemia in persons of Mediterranean ancestry.

This type of screening is sometimes controversial. Screening for carrier status for cystic fibrosis (CF) is one such situation that has the potential to create ethical dilemmas (Hulsebus and Williams, 1992). CF is caused by a gene mutation, but there are numerous variations that cause the same phenotypic effect of the disease. Only 85% of these mutations are known, meaning that an individual with a CF-causing gene mutation would not be identified as a carrier 15% of the time. Therefore following screening, a couple may feel safe to proceed with pregnancy, yet still have a child with CF. Other possible dilemmas with carrier status screening include marriage partner selection bias based on carrier status, discovery of nonpaternity or false allegations of nonpaternity (e.g., with uniparental disomy), and misunderstanding of the implications of carrier status (i.e., that

THINKING CRITICALLY ABOUT . . . ***Screening and Presymptomatic Testing for Genetic Diseases***

Advances in genetic testing have resulted in the capability of not only diagnosing a genetic disorder in an individual manifesting symptoms, but also determining if an asymptomatic person will manifest the disease in the future or has the potential to transmit disease-producing genetic material to offspring. This capability has tremendous potential to prevent or *ameliorate* the effects of genetic disease, such as in newborn screening for phenylketonuria or sickle cell disesae. In some cases, however, it also has the power to cause substantial psychologic distress and anxiety for individuals, and may cause them to make life-altering decisions based on a knowledge of the past or the future that they may wish had remained unknown. As such, the ethical and moral responsibilities of genetic screening and presymptomatic testing can be agonizing for health care professionals, in whom it can elicit uncomfortable feelings of "playing God" or "being a psychic with a crystal ball."

individuals are not affected themselves and that there is only potential risk to offspring if the partner is also a carrier). Careful counseling is necessary with carrier screening to ensure that individuals understand the limitations of testing and the implications of results (Asch and others, 1993). Even with careful counseling, there may be significant misunderstanding or misuse of information (Watson and others, 1991).

Presymptomatic testing for individuals at risk of an adult-onset disorder, such as Huntington disease, presents different, but equally weighty, dilemmas. Huntington disease is an autosomal dominant inherited disorder characterized by progressive neuromuscular deterioration and dementia, with eventual complete incapacitation and death. The age of onset is approximately 40 (±12 years) years of age—ironically, after childbearing occurs. Individuals with an affected parent have a theoretic 50% risk of eventually becoming symptomatic. The emotional threat for these individuals as they face an unknown future can be devastating. Now, through DNA testing, with 98% accuracy, it can be determined if they inherited the Huntington gene mutation. For some individuals, the chance that they would find out that they will develop this distressing condition is unbearable, like a delayed death sentence. They would rather not know. Others do want testing in the hope that the news will relieve them of the dread of the unknown and provide direction for their life whether the news is good or bad. Because testing is often of family groups, even those who receive good news may experience survivor guilt if another family member receives bad news (Tibben and others, 1993). An equally devastating situation has occurred with the discovery of a gene defect that causes inherited breast cancer. Women in these cancer-prone families face an 85% risk of developing breast or ovarian cancer. The dread in some women who have had family members die is so great that they will undergo a prophylactic mastectomy. One woman had had this surgery 5 years earlier; then DNA testing revealed she had not inherited the defective gene (Genetic counseling, 1993).

The economic overtones in carrier status screening and presymptomatic testing is also foreboding. Technologic advances have outstripped policy making; therefore discrimination in the workplace and in insurance coverage has occurred on the basis of screening and testing results (Annas, 1993). Maintaining confidentiality of test results while knowing their possible consequences is an additional sobering burden that genetic testing entails (Stephenson 1992-1993, Williams, 1993).

Screening for Epidemiologic Information. Public health officials may use screening as a method of monitoring the incidence of diseases or malformations in a population in order to detect environmental or other causes that might significantly influence the incidence of the disorder. For example, geographic and socioeconomic variations in the incidence of neural tube defects (NTDs) eventually led to research that determined that folic acid supplementation of 0.4 mg per day in women of childbearing age reduces NTD incidence by as much as 50% (American Academy of Pediatrics, 1993).

Significance of Screening to Families

Mass screening programs have received mixed acceptance from health professionals and the general public. The reasons for controversy include lack of knowledge on the part of health professionals about the testing purposes and implications of results, the public cost of testing (if government funded), and the psychologic implications of learning of a carrier status. However, with the success of several well-organized or legislated programs and their significance in the prevention of disease or of the damaging effects of disease, an increasing number of programs are gaining acceptance and support.

Much of family concern regarding screening centers around the issues of informed consent and the use of the screening information. Some states require written consent, some specify the tests to be performed, and some describe the risks, benefits, and the right to be informed of uncertain results, including the process in the event of an abnormal finding. Institutions may provide classes for families to explain the screening program, provide verbal explanation, or distribute written materials. In some areas exemptions from mandated screening are allowed in certain situations, such as objections on religious grounds if there is a conflict with religious practices and beliefs of an established church.

The nature and purposes of the procedure should be clearly explained to clients in language that they can understand. The issue of divulging unexpected findings is subject to debate. If a genetic trait is detected in a child but not in a parent (such as the sickle cell trait), the question of paternity may be raised. It is also important to help families understand the meaning of false-positive and false-negative test results.

Release of information to persons other than the family is also subject to debate. At present the reporting of genetic findings is not mandatory, as it is for certain contagious diseases, and it is questionable whether this would be desirable. A family may not wish for other family members or even the family practitioner to receive the results of screening. Knowledge of screening results by third parties may lead to insurance or employment discrimination. All of these possibilities should be made clear to families in order to provide them with some selective control.

The social stigma attached to the carrier of a defective gene may be a side effect of screening. In some families such knowledge is a source of embarrassment and damaging to the self-esteem of its members. Teenagers are especially vulnerable to the effects of knowing they carry a specific defective gene at a time when identity formation and peer approval are extremely important. Cultural views regarding this knowledge can have profound effects on the members of some ethnic groups. In some cases, social status within the cultural group can be impaired.

Probably the most important area for nursing practice is teaching. Families need an understanding of why the screening is proposed, what the results mean, and how the family can interpret false-positive and false-negative results. Anxiety is greater when families have not received sufficient information about the screening or testing process and its significance for their health. The need for retesting, no matter what the reason, can be extremely stressful to families, and they also have a right to know who assumes the cost of the screening—the family or the state. The nurse is a valuable resource person in ensuring that families are aware of alternatives and in helping them make the best decision for them.

PRENATAL DIAGNOSIS

Advances in technology have greatly increased the spectrum and accuracy of prenatal detection of genetic diseases and defects. Prenatal testing provides the means to detect defects that are best corrected soon after delivery, conditions that may require preterm delivery for early correction, conditions that may require cesarean delivery, conditions that may require medical or surgical treatment before birth, and conditions on which a decision may be based to terminate a pregnancy. In addition, a very important benefit is that normal results provide peace of mind for the expectant family. Risks of prenatal testing vary, depending on the procedure.

A variety of techniques are available for diagnosing a number of diseases and defects in the fetus. Some procedures are considered ***screening tests*** only, meaning that the test only indicates a higher risk than expected in the general population or an age-dependent risk. Other methods are ***diagnostic tests,*** meaning that they determine with a high degree of accuracy the presence or absence of a birth defect or genetic disorder (Table 5-5).

Indications for Prenatal Testing and Types of Procedures

There is approximately a 2% to 5% risk of a major birth defect or genetic disorder with each pregnancy in the general population regardless of other risk factors such as age or family history. Prenatal diagnostic testing of the general pregnancy population is not justified because of the risks, cost, and specificity of diagnostic procedures. Certain general and specific risk factors determine those for whom diagnostic testing, such as amniocentesis, is indicated. Relatively inexpensive and safe screening tests, such as routine ultrasound and maternal serum alpha-fetoprotein (AFP) for

TABLE 5-5 Types of Prenatal Genetic Testing

PURPOSE	ADVANTAGES	DISADVANTAGES	RISKS
MATERNAL SERUM ALPHA-FETOPROTEIN (MS-AFP)			
Screening test for neural tube defects, ventral wall defects, and trisomy pregnancies (e.g., Down syndrome)	Identifies women at higher risk for further testing who would not otherwise receive it	Is not diagnostic; only indicates need for further testing False-positive and false-negative results occur	Venipuncture Minimal risk
ULTRASONOGRAPHY			
Assesses gestational age, fetal growth, placental sufficiency Detects multiple gestation and structural anomalies Screening and diagnostic test	Detects structural anomalies and effects of intrauterine environment that may not be detected by chromosome analysis	Accuracy depends on skill of ultrasonographer, quality of equipment, and size of defect Does not detect biochemical abnormalities	Noninvasive
AMNIOCENTESIS			
Chromosome analysis of fetal cells DNA analysis AFP analysis, other biochemical analyses	Diagnostic for chromosome abnormalities Provides DNA for direct and indirect testing for single-gene disorders High accuracy for detection of neural tube defects by biochemical analysis	Does not detect structural anomalies not caused by chromosome abnormalities except for neural tube or ventral wall defects Usually not performed until second trimester (14-16 weeks) Results are usually available in 2-3 weeks Relatively expensive	Invasive ½% risk of spontaneous abortion Nongrowth of fetal cells requires repeat procedure
CHORIONIC VILLUS SAMPLING (CVS)			
Chromosome analysis of chorionic (fetal) cells DNA analysis	Diagnostic for chromosome abnormalities Provides DNA for direct and indirect testing for single-gene disorders Test is done earlier than amniocentesis (9-12 weeks); therefore results are available earlier	Diagnostic accuracy may be less because of greater risk of maternal cell contamination and false evidence of mosaicism, which may require subsequent amniocentesis	Invasive Risk of spontaneous abortion about 2% Controversial evidence of limb-reduction defects

the remaining population will additionally determine those for whom diagnostic testing is advisable.

Prenatal Screening Tests. It is now accepted practice to offer ***maternal serum alpha-fetoprotein (MS-AFP) testing*** to all pregnant women under the age of 35. AFP, the major protein of early fetal life, is synthesized in the fetal liver and yolk sac. By diffusion across the placenta and the amnion, AFP is present in the maternal circulation. Neural tube defects (NTDs) such as anencephaly and spina bifida, and ventral wall defects (VWDs), such as gastroschisis and omphalocele, are associated with exposed fetal membrane and blood vessel surfaces that increase the leakage of AFP into the amniotic fluid and, consequently, the maternal blood. Therefore an elevated MS-AFP level may indicate the presence of an open NTD or VWD in the fetus.

Certain factors other than NTDs can cause abnormal MS-AFP levels, such as multiple gestation, incorrectly estimated gestational age, fetal hemorrhage and/or fetal death, and placental abnormalities. Other factors affecting results include maternal diabetes, race, and weight. Further diagnostic testing is indicated for abnormal results that cannot be attributed to any of these factors. Even if further testing does not reveal the presence of an NTD or VWD, it was found that 20% to 38% of these "unexplained MS-AFP elevations" were associated with poor pregnancy outcome, such as premature labor, intrauterine growth retardation, and abruptio placenta (Bernstein and others, 1992; Bock, 1992). Subsequent to initiation of MS-AFP testing for NTDs, it was found that a low MS-AFP level was associated with Down syndrome (and occasionally trisomy 13 and trisomy 18) pregnancies, presumably because of a slower rate of protein synthesis. Combining the MS-AFP with other serum markers increases the detection rate significantly, to about 70% to 80% of fetal trisomies. Further diagnostic testing is indicated for abnormal results. Since NTDs and Down syndrome are relatively common birth defects, prenatal screening using a blood specimen at about 15 weeks of gestation is a relatively simple and inexpensive method to identify a population for further testing, in which a birth defect may otherwise be undetected.

Ultrasonography can be a screening or diagnostic technique, depending on the sophistication of the equipment, the skill of the ultrasonographer, and the type of abnormality seen. Ultrasound screening of all pregnant women can potentially detect major or minor findings that indicate a need for further diagnostic testing. Routine ultrasonography is noninvasive and safe, and is standard screening practice in many countries, yet controversy exists in the United States over its actual benefits vs cost (Ewigman and others, 1993). Ultrasound as a diagnostic technique is discussed in the next section.

Prenatal Diagnostic Procedures. There are general, specific, and ethnic risk factors that may be present in any pregnancy that are indicators for diagnostic testing. The specific testing recommended depends on the identified risk. These may be preexisting risks, personal characteristics, or a newly identified risk for this pregnancy (see box at right). General risk factors include age and abnormal MS-AFP screening results. It is a standard recommendation that women 35 years of age or older have amniocentesis, rather than screening, based on an increased risk for Down syndrome with advancing maternal age (D'Alton and DeCherney, 1993). Specific risk factors are usually identified in the family history, previous pregnancy outcomes, or the mother's medical history. Ethnic risk factors are based on a higher carrier rate frequency for certain genetic diseases in selected populations. Indications for prenatal diagnosis when any of these risk factors are present is based on a greater than general population risk that a genetic defect or disorder will occur in this pregnancy. The specific risk is, of course, different for each situation.

Amniocentesis is currently the basis of diagnostic prenatal testing. It is usually performed at 14 to 16 weeks of gestation under ultrasound guidance. Estimated fetal loss following amniocentesis is 0.5%. Amniocentesis provides several types of diagnostic information. First, viable fetal skin cells that have sloughed off and are present in the amniotic fluid are obtained and cultured for chromosome analysis to detect chromosome abnormalities. Chromosome analysis results are obtained in about 10 to 14 days in most facilities and are 99% accurate. Second, DNA may be extracted from the chromosomes for direct DNA and indirect linkage analysis to detect single-gene disorders. Testing for each single-gene disorder is unique; therefore testing of this type

INDICATIONS FOR PRENATAL DIAGNOSIS

GENERAL RISK FACTORS

Maternal age ≥35 years at time of delivery
Elevated or reduced maternal serum alpha-fetoprotein concentration
Results of triple screening: elevated or reduced maternal serum alpha-fetoprotein, human chorionic gonadotropin, and unconjugated estriol concentrations

SPECIFIC RISK FACTORS

Previous child with a structural defect or chromosome abnormality
Previous stillbirth or neonatal death
Structural abnormality in mother or father
Balanced translocation in mother or father
Inherited disorders: cystic fibrosis, metabolic disorders, sex-linked recessive disorders
Medical disease in mother: diabetes mellitus, phenylketonuria
Exposure to a teratogen: ionizing radiation, anticonvulsant medicines, lithium, isotretinoin, alcohol
Infection: rubella, toxoplasmosis, cytomegalovirus
Abnormal ultrasound findings

ETHNIC RISK FACTORS

DISORDER	ETHNIC OR RACIAL GROUP
Tay-Sachs disease	Ashkenazi Jewish, French Canadian
Sickle cell anemia	Black African, Mediterranean, Arab, Indian and Pakistani
α- and β-thalassemia	Mediterranean, Southern and Southeast Asian, Chinese

Modified from D'Alton ME, DeCherney AH: Prenatal diagnosis, *N Engl J Med* 328(2):114-120, 1993.

is done only when a pregnancy is at high risk for a specific disorder, such as cystic fibrosis. The third type of diagnostic information available from amniocentesis is amniotic fluid alpha-fetoprotein levels (AF-AFP). The AFP level in the amniotic fluid is a much more reliable indicator of an NTD or VWD because interfering factors, such as placental diffusion differences, are minimized. Also, an additional test for an enzyme specific to neural tissue acetylcholinesterase (AChE) may be done, which, if positive in the presence of an elevated AF-AFP level, highly suggests an open NTD.

Chorionic-villus sampling (CVS) is a less commonly used procedure to obtain cells for chromosome analysis. An advantage of CVS is that it may be performed between 9 and 12 weeks of gestation, either transcervically or transabdominally. The procedure is somewhat controversial because of a slightly higher rate of fetal loss following the procedure, and some conflicting reports of limb and/or extremity defects. The accuracy of the chromosome analysis may be slightly less than with amniocentesis because of a greater risk for contamination by maternal cells, and if mosaicism is detected, a confirmatory amniocentesis at 14 to 16 weeks is recommended.

High-quality ***ultrasonography*** is an extremely useful noninvasive procedure that can diagnose many conditions prenatally (Lopez, 1989). It is especially useful for detecting birth defects in which the chromosome analysis is most likely normal, such as teratogen exposure; multifactorial conditions, such as isolated congenital heart defect; and anatomic defects, such as skeletal dysplasias and intrauterine growth retardation. Although equipment and ultrasonographer skill may vary, accuracy can be greater than 90% for detecting major neural tube, cardiac, kidney, and bladder anomalies. In addition, sonographic findings may suggest chromosome abnormalities. For example, the presence of duodenal atresia, tracheoesophageal fistula, esophageal atresia, atrioventricular canal defects, ventricular septal defects, atrial septal defects, hypoplasia of the middle quadrant of the fifth digit, or thickened nuchal fold may suggest Down syndrome.

A few additional diagnostic tests are sometimes used. ***Percutaneous umbilical blood sampling*** can be performed after 18 weeks of gestation. This procedure is usually done for prenatal evaluation of fetal hematologic abnormalities, inborn errors of metabolism, fetal infection, and rapid chromosome analysis. The risk of fetal loss from the procedure is 2% (D'Alton and DeCherney, 1993). ***Fetal biopsy*** is an investigational procedure sometimes used to diagnose certain genetic skin disorders and other disorders when DNA studies are unavailable or are uninformative. ***Fetal echocardiography*** may be performed for further diagnosis when a cardiac defect is noted on ultrasound.

Research is underway to improve prenatal diagnostic testing. Early amniocentesis (before 14 weeks) is being investigated but is not yet established practice. The risk of fetal loss may be slightly increased, obtaining amniotic fluid may be more difficult, and AF-AFP concentration standards have not yet been established. More promising in terms of less fetal risk is a new technique under investigation to isolate fetal cells from maternal blood (D'Alton and DeCherney, 1993; Simpson and Elias, 1993). This method would eliminate the need for amniocentesis to obtain fetal cells to test for chromosome abnormalities. Also under investigation are in situ hybridization studies, which use chromosome 21–specific probes. Fetal cells do not have to be cultured; therefore the results would be available in 48 to 72 hours. However, the test is specific only for trisomy 21; therefore other chromosome abnormalities would not be detected.

A new hope for parents at risk of having a child with a genetic disorder is preimplantation genetic diagnosis. Through the technique of in vitro (test tube) fertilization, the embryo can be tested at the six- to eight-cell stage for the presence of the specific genetic disorder. If found to be normal or a carrier but not affected, the embryo is then implanted. This technique has been used for cystic fibrosis and some X-linked disorders (Handyside and others, 1992). For couples who are concerned about termination of a pregnancy for an affected fetus, this new option may be more acceptable.

GENETIC EVALUATION AND COUNSELING

In recent years the significance of genetics as an etiologic agent in disease and disability has assumed a more prominent place in the nursing care of infants and children. The expanded recognition of genetic diseases and defects, as well as an increasingly well-informed public, is creating a justified demand for genetic evaluation and diagnosis, as well as information regarding risks to present and future generations. Unfortunately, however, persons who need expert genetic counseling often make uninformed decisions on their own or are the victims of well-meaning but equally uninformed relatives and acquaintances, or unknowledgeable paraprofessionals. Nurses involved in infant and child care continually encounter genetic diseases and families in which there is a risk that a disorder may be transmitted to an offspring, and children who may have an undiagnosed genetic disorder that needs expert evaluation. It is a responsibility of nurses to be alert to situations in which families could benefit from genetic evaluation and counseling, to become familiar with facilities in their areas where these services are available, and to learn basic genetic principles. In this way, they will be able to direct individuals and families to take advantage of needed services and to be active participants in the genetic evaluation and counseling process. They should be knowledgeable regarding special services that are available to help in the management and support of affected children. Early identification of a genetic disorder allows anticipation of associated conditions and implementation of available preventive measures and therapy to avoid potential complications and actualize or enhance the child's health potential (Prows, 1992).

Genetic counseling is a communication process that deals with the human problems associated with the occurrence, or risk of occurrence, of a genetic disorder in a family. This process involves an attempt by one or more appropriately trained persons to help the individual or family:

- Comprehend the medical facts, including the diagnosis, the probable course of the disorder, and the available management
- Appreciate the way heredity contributes to the disorder, and the risk of recurrence in specified relatives
- Understand the options for dealing with the risk of recurrence
- Choose the course of action that seems appropriate to them in view of their risk and their family goals and act in accordance with that decision
- Make the best possible adjustment to the disorder in an affected family member and/or to the risk of recurrence of that disorder

Clients

The clients, or persons who seek genetic evaluation and counseling, must first be aware that there is a genetic problem or potential problem. They may be referred for genetic services by a family practitioner, a specialist, a nurse, a friend, or a relative, or they may seek counseling as a result of information in the media.

Genetic evaluation for diagnostic purposes may occur at many points along the life span. In the newborn period, birth defects are an obvious reason for referral. Beyond the newborn period, indicators for referral include metabolic disorders, developmental delays, growth delays, behavioral problems, cognitive delays, abnormal or delayed sexual development, and medical problems known to be associated with genetic diseases. For example, a preschooler with hyperactivity and autistic-like behaviors may need evaluation for fragile X syndrome, and a 17-year-old girl with primary amenorrhea should be tested for Turner syndrome. In adulthood an asymptomatic individual with a family history of Huntington disease may desire testing to determine his or her risk of becoming symptomatic in the future.

With so many recent advances in genetic testing, it is not at all unusual to have a child or adult with long-standing medical problems, including mental retardation, be referred for reevaluation of their condition for a genetic disorder that might not have been detected a few years ago, such as microdeletion disorders and single-gene mutations. If a genetic diagnosis is made, the client will usually be referred back to the primary care physician with recommendations for routine management.

Clients may or may not be affected themselves but may request genetic counseling about the heritability of a trait that may be deleterious, beneficial, or merely troublesome. Clients might be a young couple contemplating childbearing who are concerned about a disorder in one of their families or who may seek advice because they are related. A couple who are both members of a population at risk for certain diseases may wish to determine whether they carry the harmful gene (e.g., blacks and sickle cell anemia, Ashkenazi Jews and Tay-Sachs disease, or persons of Mediterranean ancestry and thalassemia). A couple planning adoption might seek counseling regarding a prospective child.

More often, persons who inquire about the possibility of recurrence of a disease or disorder have a child, or had a child who died, with a genetic disease or disorder. They are concerned that they might produce another similarly affected child. This advice might be sought before the couple initiates another pregnancy or after the mother is already pregnant. If prenatal diagnostic testing is not done, the history of a condition in an older sibling, such as galactosemia, alerts health personnel to initiate specific and thorough testing for the condition in a newborn. In this way, early therapy can be initiated when indicated, thus minimizing or eliminating the effects of the disease or defect.

Parents need to know the risk in *their particular situation* and how it relates to the random risk for *any* prospective parents. When families understand the risks involved, they normally make appropriate decisions for them regarding family planning. Parents may also have concerns about risks to unaffected siblings, and reproductive implications for their affected and unaffected offspring. Counseling is also appropriate for prenatal diagnostic testing, so that the couple can make an informed decision about the type of testing recommended based on their individual risk factors. Additional counseling is necessary if abnormal results are obtained and/or for termination of a pregnancy. Couples may also be referred for counseling for infertility or recurrent miscarriages. Occasionally a counselor becomes involved in cases of disputed paternity, questioned maternity (when it is suspected that infants have been substituted for one another at birth), rape, or incestuous matings.

Counseling Services

The most efficient counseling service consists of a group of specialists that may include physicians, geneticists, psychologists, biochemists, cytologists, nurses, social workers, and other auxiliary personnel. The services are most often under the leadership of a physician trained in medical genetics, who assumes responsibility for the medical aspects of the problem. The counseling service may serve only as a referral group, or it may conduct a regular clinic service. Most often it is associated with a large medical center, many of which have extensive outreach programs with satellite clinics throughout adjacent rural areas. There are also numerous specialty clinics that deal with specific genetic disorders (such as cystic fibrosis, muscular dystrophy, hemophilia, or diabetes) and provide their own genetic counseling services. Unfortunately, these units are concentrated in and around large metropolitan areas. As a result, counseling is not always accessible to the large number of persons who would benefit from the service.

Unlike a medical prognosis, which predicts the outcome of a disease, a genetic prognosis directly involves other persons: the affected child, members of the immediate family, other relatives, and future offspring. For genetic evaluation or follow-up, the geneticist and the counselor usually work together to obtain the family history/pedigree and the medical history of the person being evaluated (including pregnancy, labor, and delivery information), perform a physical examination for dysmorphic features, and order appropriate testing such as biochemical and cytogenetic procedures (Hall, 1993). A genetic diagnosis may or may not be made initially. Genetic evaluation is a time-consuming and labor-intensive process. Completing an evaluation on a new family referred for diagnosis requires an average of 7 hours of staff time (Bernhardt and Pyeritz, 1992).

Estimation of Risks

Effective genetic counseling based on a diagnosis or known risk factors requires a thorough evaluation of each situation. Information from which the counselor derives risks of occurrence or recurrence is acquired from a thorough family history, including known genetic information. A careful, detailed family history not only provides a picture of the ***proband*** (the affected person, or ***index case***) in relation to other family members, but also may serve to identify other persons who are similarly affected or who might be presymptomatic or at risk of producing affected children. Analyzing the pattern of affected members of the family can assist in confirming a tentative diagnosis or in determining the level of risk in multifactorial inheritance.

An accurate diagnosis is essential in order to provide specific risk figures. There are over 6000 known inherited disorders, many of which have similar clinical manifestations but totally different modes of inheritance. For example, symptoms in the early stages of severe X-linked muscular dystrophy appear much like those of the milder autosomal recessive and autosomal dominant varieties, autosomal recessive neurogenic muscular atrophies, and nongenetic poliomyelitis. The significance of the risks related to each type of disorder is readily apparent. For disorders with an unknown or multifactorial cause, recurrence risks given are termed ***empiric,*** meaning they are based on observations of recurrence in similar situations, rather than ***theoretic,*** meaning they are based on mendelian inheritance patterns.

The mode of inheritance determines the degree of risk in the major categories of genetic disorders (see box below). In general, the more definite and clear-cut the genetics, the greater the risks; as the causative factors become more obscure, the risk of recurrence is less likely.

ESTIMATION OF GENETIC RISK

HIGH-RISK SITUATIONS

Conditions caused by a factor that segregates during cell division

Recurrence risk: 1:10 or greater
- Can be predicted with high degree of accuracy
- Based on mendelian ratios

Examples: Single-gene disorders, translocated chromosome disorder

MODERATE-RISK SITUATIONS

Conditions that are multifactorial

Recurrence risk: Less than 1:10; usually less than 1:20
- Based on prior experience and observation of the disorder under similar circumstances (empiric)

Examples: Pyloric stenosis, spina bifida, congenital heart defects

RANDOM-RISK SITUATIONS

Conditions caused by environmental agents and not likely to recur in another pregnancy under normal circumstances unless the agent is still operative

Recurrent risk: Approximately 1:30

Examples: Rubella syndrome, fresh mutation, most chromosome aberrations

Interpretation of Risks

When explaining risk estimates, the counselor does not attempt to make recommendations or decisions for clients. The counselor provides appropriate and accurate information about the nature of the disorder, the extent of the risk involved, the probable consequences, and alternative solutions but remains nondirective, leaving the final decision to the persons concerned. In some instances genetic information will increase the family's distress; in others their anxiety will be reduced, depending on their makeup and the meaning that the disorder has for that particular family.

It is helpful to explain risks in different ways and to use examples and working to aid in understanding the meaning of probabilities. Most persons do not have an adequate knowledge of genetics and human biology to fully comprehend these complex concepts. Words and concepts that can be used include "percentages," "chance," "odds," and "likelihood." For example, if a 40-year-old woman has a 1:112 risk of having a child with Down syndrome, other ways to explain it include: "about a 1% chance"; and "Out of 112 women your age having a baby, odds are that 1 of them will have a Down syndrome pregnancy." Games of probability can also be used, such as flipping coins, baseball pools, lotteries, and horse racing.

NURSING ALERT Families may misunderstand probabilities, even when they are fully explained. It is important to impress on them that *each pregnancy is an independent event.* It is not uncommon for parents who are told that a recessive disorder carries a 1:4 risk of recurrence to feel secure with one affected child. They incorrectly reason that because they already have one affected child the next three will be unaffected. Chance has no memory; the risk is 1:4 for each and every pregnancy.

ROLE OF NURSES IN GENETIC COUNSELING AND REFERRAL

Genetic counseling is a professional specialty that requires master's level preparation and board certification because of the crucial nature of the information these professionals provide (Brantly, 1991). The number of board-certified genetic counselors is limited; therefore nurses skilled in counseling techniques are in a unique position to help meet the counseling needs of families in which there is a genetic disease or disorder. Public health nurses work with a family in a close, sustained relationship and earn the family's confidence and trust; genetics nurse specialists,* with advanced preparation in genetic theory, are assuming a prominent position on counseling teams; and practitioners in the specialty areas of maternity and pediatric nursing are constantly involved with families in which there is a genetic defect. New advances in genetic diagnosis have greatly in-

*For additional information contact the International Society of Nurses in Genetics, 3020 Javier Rd., Fairfax, VA 22031; (703) 698-7355.

creased opportunities for, and responsibilities of, nurses in all levels of practice in terms of assessment, referral, education, and counseling (Williams, 1993).

It is a nurse who frequently first identifies a need for counseling and referral by identifying the presence of an inherited disorder in a family history, or by noting physical, mental, or behavioral abnormalities when performing a nursing assessment (see box below). Guidelines for determining individuals who should receive genetic counseling are given in the Guidelines box.

An intake interview is conducted before the primary counseling session or diagnostic workup to assess the needs of the family and attempt to reduce their anxiety; therefore, ample time should be allotted. Ideally, both parents should attend. If possible, child care facilities for other children should be available as part of the counseling service. If this is impossible, some distraction in the form of toys and play equipment can be provided. In the interview the nurse takes a family history for pertinent information and explains the clinic procedures carefully. Many families are concerned about such things as whether they will be required to undress, if blood is to be drawn, if they can accompany the child during the visit, or if they will be told what to do about reproduction. Families who have a relaxed and atraumatic initial discussion are able to gain more from a counseling session.

Taking a Family History

The person taking a family history must allow a liberal amount of time. When possible, it is best to include both parents in the interview in order to elicit information about relatives on both sides of the family. Medical records, birth and death records, family Bibles, and photograph albums are helpful resources, and persons being interviewed should be instructed to bring such items if they are available. It may be necessary to consult other members of the family. The level of education and the degree of understanding vary widely among informants and influence the reliability of the information. There may be reticence on the part of informants, particularly if they view the disorder as something to be ashamed of or in some way threatening. Sometimes true relationships may be concealed, such as illegitimacy or nonpaternity. Nonpaternity is estimated to occur in 3% to 5% of genetic counseling situations (LeRoux and others, 1992).

Skillful interviewing is necessary in order to obtain essential, but often embarrassing or private, information. Since many parents may not be married, parents should be addressed as couples or partners and asked about other unions that may have produced a pregnancy. In eliciting a birth history from the mother and father, the nurse should specifically ask about abortions, miscarriages, and stillbirths, as well as live births. For example, asking, "Have you fathered any other children?" may lead a man to list only live offspring. To identify all members of the family tree, it is best to ask about offspring from even young teenagers. When inquiring about family diseases, it is often necessary to ask the question in different ways. For example, if a client denies any mental retardation in the family, asking other questions, such as about learning problems, being in special education classes, and failing or not completing school, may uncover a family history of cognitive impairment.

The family history is recorded in the form of a ***pedigree chart*** or ***family tree*** (in some disciplines the pedigree chart is termed a ***genogram***), using standard symbols to indicate persons, relationships, and significant details related to them (Fig. 5-10). Construction of a pedigree (see Guidelines box, p. 178) begins with the affected child (proband, index case, original patient) and *all* the mother's pregnancies (Fig. 5-11, *A*). Next, the maternal family history is explored in a similar manner (Fig. 5-11, *B*); then information about relatives on the father's side and any children the fa-

ASSESSMENT CLUES TO GENETIC DISORDERS*

Major or minor birth defects (anomalies) and dysmorphic features—Cardiac defect, ear or eye abnormalities, micrognathia, forehead prominence, hairline low-set on forehead or nape of neck, wide-set eyes, epicanthal folds, low-set ears
Growth abnormalities—Short stature, overgrowth, asymmetric growth, intrauterine growth retardation
Skeletal abnormalities—Limb abnormalities, asymmetry, scoliosis, hyperextensible joints, hypotonic or hypertonic muscle tone, pectus excavatum, finger or joint abnormalities
Vision or hearing problems—Coloboma, cat's eye, hearing loss, vision loss
Metabolic disorders—Unusual odor of breath, urine, or stool
Sexual development abnormalities—Ambiguous genitalia, small penis, delayed onset of puberty, primary amenorrhea, precocious sexual development, large testicles
Skin disorders—Unusual pigmentation, café-au-lait spots, dry and scaly skin, skin tumors
Recurrent infection or immune deficiency—Ear infections, pneumonia
Developmental and speech delays or loss of milestones
Cognitive delays—Learning disabilities, mild to severe mental retardation
Behavioral disorders—Hyperactivity, attention deficit disorder, autistic-like behavior, aggressive behavior

*Suggests genetic etiology if two or more findings are present.

GUIDELINES
Referral Regarding Genetic Counseling

- Individuals with a family history of hereditary diseases or birth defects
- Known balanced translocation carriers or parents who have previously had a fetus or child with a chromosome abnormality
- Couples with a history of multiple miscarriages, stillbirths, or infertility
- Individuals at risk for ethnic-related disorders
- Pregnant women exposed to teratogenic agents
- Pregnant women of advanced maternal age (≥35 years)
- Disorders in which pregnancy could threaten maternal or fetal life or health

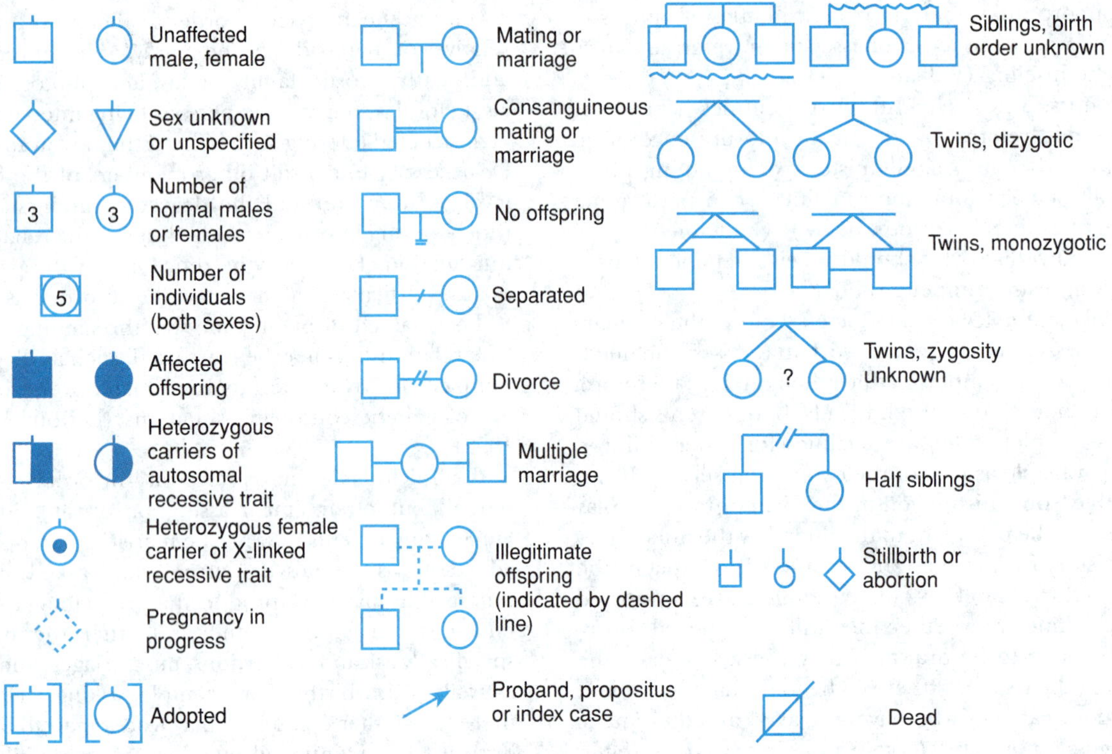

FIG. 5-10 Common pedigree symbols.

GUIDELINES
Pedigree Construction

Begin diagram in the center of a large sheet of paper.
Represent males in a family with a square and females with a circle.
Indicate the proband with an arrow (if the counselee is not the proband, indicate the relationship of the counselee with a "C" under that person's symbol).
Use a horizontal bar to designate a marriage; place the male on the left and the female on the right (use a broken line to indicate an unwed mating and a double bar for a consanguineous mating).
Suspend symbols for outcome of all pregnancies (including offspring, abortions, and stillbirths) vertically from the mating line in order of birth from left to right, regardless of sex and outcome.
Include significant information about all the mother's pregnancies (e.g., bleeding, anemia, radiographs, infectious disease, drugs taken).
Place maternal and paternal relatives in proper relationship to the proband.
Designate generations by Roman numerals, with the earliest generation at the top.
Include at least three generations: parents, siblings, grandparents, aunts, uncles, first cousins, and offspring of proband (if appropriate).
Include name of each person (including maiden names for married women), their date of birth, health problems, and date and cause of death.
Date the pedigree
Make a key for genetic diseases or disorders if more than one is present in a family.

ther may have from previous unions is gathered in the same manner (Fig. 5-11, *C*). It is important at this point to determine whether the couple might be related in any way. Information to be solicited includes not only information about other affected family members, but also information about births—live births, stillbirths, and abortions (especially spontaneous abortions), including gestational age of pregnancy; infertility problems; matings—legally sanctioned, consanguineous, multiple, unwed, and other complex relationships; and health of family members, including any other genetic diseases or disorders or birth defects, and death and causes of death, including early infant deaths. Sometimes the place of birth and ethnic background are significant. For example, the incidence of Tay-Sachs disease is higher in Ashkenazi Jews from eastern Europe than in Jews from other geographic origins. Also, when a pedigree chart is being evaluated, the fact that a sister died in infancy as a "blue baby" might be genetically significant, whereas a healthy sibling who drowned at age 1 year would not. Information concerning first-degree relatives is most important and should be complete.

Follow-Up Care

The success of counseling is measured by the way in which the family uses the information presented to them. Maintaining contact with the family or referral to an agency that can provide a sustained relationship—usually the public health agency in their locality—is one of the most important aspects of the counseling process. Some families do not choose to have follow-up visits, but in most instances these

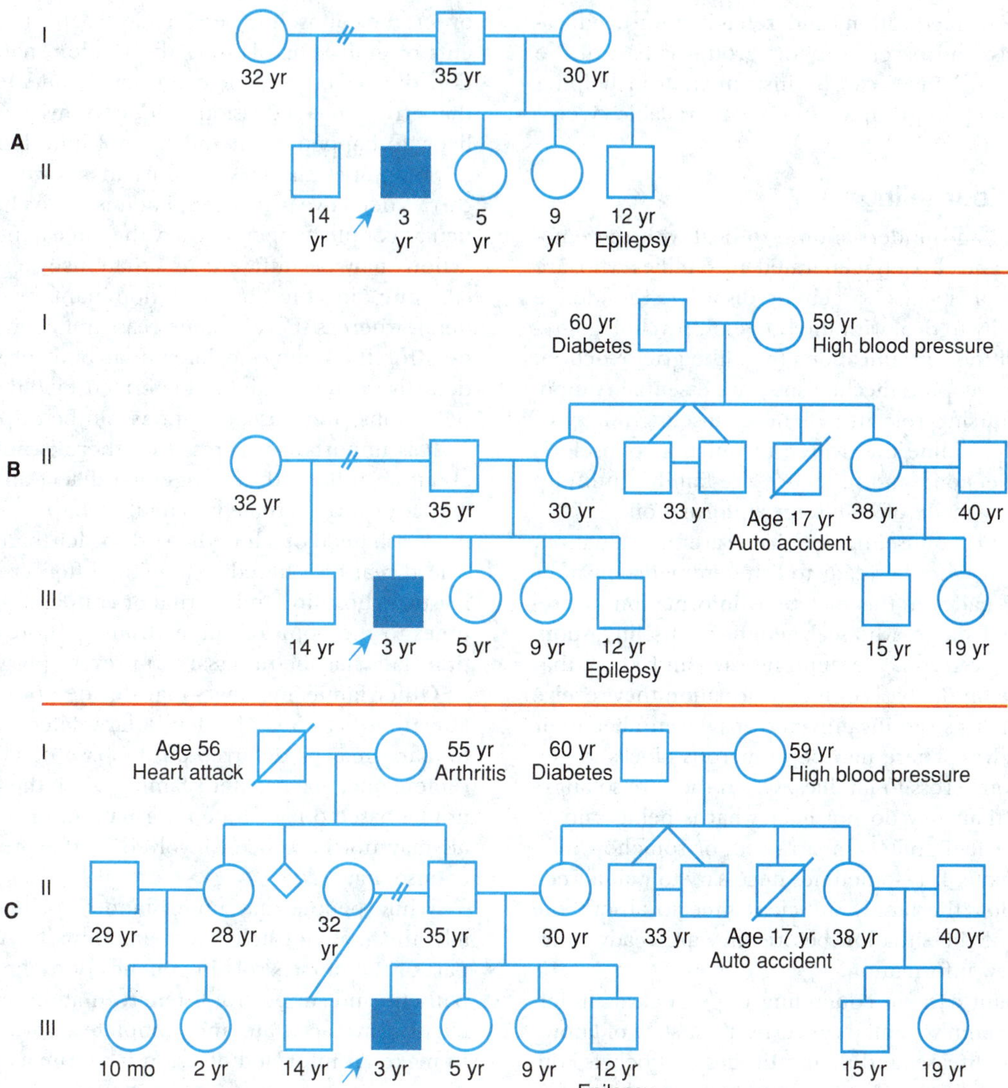

FIG. 5-11 Construction of a pedigree. **A,** Proband, siblings, and parents. **B,** Maternal relatives. **C,** Paternal relatives added.

visits make the family feel that they have not been abandoned and facilitate the process of adjustment to the problem. A summary letter of the interview or counseling session is helpful to review information presented and reinforce recommendations.

Follow-up visits to the counseling service or in the home provide the family with the opportunity to ask questions that they did not ask on previous visits. Often the family members have not really "heard" the information presented to them or have misinterpreted what they have heard, so that it may be necessary to repeat and reinforce counseling. In some disorders a diagnosis in one family member places relatives at risk and is an indication for further screening.

One very important aspect of follow-up care is support and assistance in management of the affected child. For example, a disorder such as phenylketonuria requires conscientious diet management; therefore it is important to make certain that the family understands and follows instructions. Children born subsequently must be carefully observed for early detection of symptoms. Genetic and specialty clinics devote a great deal of their time and efforts in helping families cope with the consequences of genetic disease.

Nurses should be prepared to help families arrive at tentative decisions regarding the future, including family planning, education or institutionalization of a handicapped child, plans for adoption, and many other problems related to their specific situation. Initial and ongoing assessments of the family's coping abilities, resources, and support systems are vital in order to determine their need for additional assistance and support. As with any family with a child with chronic health care needs, nurses must teach the family to become their child's advocate. Also, nurses should be alert for evidence of risk factors that indicate poor adjustment (e.g., child abuse, divorce, or other maladaptive behaviors). Locating agencies and clinics specializing in a specific disorder or its consequences that can provide services (e.g., equipment, medication, and rehabilitation), educational programs, and parent support groups is part of the nurse's resources. Nurses can be instrumental in helping parents start a support group when none is available (Weiss, 1992).

Supportive Counseling

It requires time and understanding to deal with the emotional tension and anxiety generated in families who are faced with the prospect of a genetic disorder. Knowledge of, and the ability to deal with the range of, psychologic responses and all their ramifications (e.g., the grief reaction, guilt, anger, and coping mechanisms) are essential components of the nursing role in genetic counseling. Many of these factors determine the degree to which a counselor's message is understood and influence the family's attitudes and the use they made of counseling information.

Timing of the counseling requires careful evaluation. Some families may not be ready to listen immediately after a diagnosis is made or the first time information is presented to them. Families who seek genetic counseling, spontaneously or by referral, are apprehensive and know that decisions made on the basis of the information they receive may alter their lives significantly and may even alter their view of themselves. There may be numerous blocks to getting information across to families. Often they are so angry or frightened that they do not hear what is being said to them; they may feel guilty, embarrassed, or somehow inferior or inadequate. It is sometimes necessary to wait a week or more to allow the family sufficient time to absorb the initial impact of the situation before they are ready to assimilate any new information.

It is important early in counseling to get a clear understanding of the family's initial concerns, their state of knowledge about the disease, and their attitudes and beliefs concerning the condition, and to determine the kind and amount of information they need or want. Some are not sure they should be at a counseling service. Whether the persons needing help are parents who have given birth to an affected child, relatives of an affected individual, persons who have been identified as carriers of a deleterious gene, or a couple with a higher-risk pregnancy, their feelings, attitudes, and fears must be addressed.

Careful interviewing and assessment will determine the extent and type of information needed and desired by the clients. Misunderstanding of the counseling information is most likely due to the disparity of knowledge between the counselor and the family, and to the heightened emotion surrounding genetic counseling. Information often needs to be repeated several times before the family understands the content and its implications.

Guilt and self-blame are very natural and universal reactions. Nurses must deal with parents' feelings of guilt about carrying "bad genes" or having "made my child sick." For example, the young father of a child with Down syndrome refused to submit to chromosome analysis for fear he might be identified as a carrier of a translocated chromosome and thought he could not endure the guilt this knowledge would generate. Depending on the type of cytogenetic disorder, the counseling person may be able to absolve the parents of guilt by explaining the random nature of segregation during both gamete formation and fertilization and that errors in cell division unique to this pregnancy are not likely to happen again and are not inherited.

Sometimes there is comfort in knowing that everyone carries defective genes and that it is mere chance that a particular couple happen to carry the same abnormal gene. Reactions may be different in situations where one member can pinpoint the "blame" (dominant or X-linked disorders), whereas there is some reassurance in recessive disorders for the couple to know that both of them carry the defective gene. Anxieties generated by old wives' tales, superstitions, and misconceptions can be dispelled.

It is important to stress that there is nothing shameful about an inherited or congenital defect and to emphasize any appropriate remedy. Families have a tendency to be more ashamed of a hereditary disorder than other illnesses. The threat of a hereditary "taint" often creates intrafamilial strife, hostility, and marital or couple disharmony, sometimes to the point of family disintegration. Crisis intervention skills may be necessary to prevent progressive discord.

Other family members may decide not to have children after the diagnosis of a hereditary defect, or the decision to marry may be deferred on the basis of a disorder, even a remote one, in a partner's family. Often these decisions may not be based on accurate information, since these individuals may not have been involved in the proband's family's counseling.

While people may understand the situation intellectually, this may not help them emotionally. A large and vital part of the nurse's role in genetic counseling is that of sympathetic and supportive listener. In addition, ensuring that clients have accurate and complete information on which to make an informed decision is a primary goal.

Burden of Genetic Defect

The way in which members of a family respond to the probability of a genetic disorder will depend a great deal on the nature of the condition and the burden, actual or perceived, that it may place on them. A ***burden*** is considered to be the total amount of distress, economic and emotional, that is placed on persons, their families, and society by the birth of an affected child—the anticipated burden as well as the threat of disability. Various factors that are associated with disorders produce a burden in different ways to determine the total impact on a family. These include severity, chronicity, age of onset, mortality, morbidity, presence or absence of chronic pain, mental retardation, and cosmetic disfigurement.

There is a great deal of variability in the ability of individuals and families to withstand stress, and persons respond differently to probabilities. A degree of risk that is reassuring to one may be threatening or intolerable to another. Also, two individuals will respond differently to a hazard that both perceive as threatening. Some parents will choose to have children even in the face of high risk; others believe that even a moderate risk is too much to take. Some may risk having a child with a disorder that produces a minor defect or even one that causes early death but elect not to risk having a child with a lifelong disability. The longer the duration of the disability, the greater the financial and emotional burden. Having a child with a disability is a grieving process, sometimes called ***chronic sorrow,*** that has delayed resolution while the offspring is alive (Williams, 1993).

In some disorders, such as Down syndrome, the burden of the disease rests primarily on the family rather than on the affected child. In diseases with severe crippling effects, such as muscular dystrophy, the impact of the disease affects both the child and the family.

All of these matters confront a family when they must make a decision about whether to risk a pregnancy that might result in a child with a disability, and nurses should be prepared to explore these probabilities and the availability of prenatal testing with them. If a pregnancy does result in a fetus or child with a genetic defect or disorder and the family does not choose termination, education about the condition and treatment options helps to provide the best outcome possible for the child.

Barriers to Effective Counseling

Obstacles to the use of genetic counseling involve the attitudes of both the family and the counselor. Frequent obstacles to an objective use of information are religious attitudes toward conception and opposition to sterilization and to abortion in situations where there is a high risk of recurrence or where prenatal diagnosis has indicated a defective fetus. Many persons fatalistically accept "the will of God." Another obstacle is the right of the individual—the right of the fetus to come to full term and the right of parents to conceive. A person with a high risk of producing a disabling condition in an offspring may believe that he or she is entitled to the same rights as anyone else, including the right of procreation.

Differences in the ability to comprehend what is said probably interfere most with effective use of counseling information. Clients vary in experiences, education, and intellectual level, and even with careful explanation many are still unable to understand the basic fundamentals of inheritance. They may be able to repeat information but fail to grasp its significance.

Sometimes nurses themselves create barriers with their own biases and personal feelings. There are some diseases that have a special impact on individual nurses, and in such cases it is difficult to be nonjudgmental. The counselor may begin to identify with the client through projection, which interferes with objectivity and may lead to premature closure in the interchange (Kessler, 1992). Families may become defensive if they believe that the nurse is bringing undue pressure to bear on their decision. Others may pressure the nurse to make the decision for them. "What would you do if you were in this situation?" is a common question. In some instances nurses (intentionally or unintentionally) do influence families. They are often tempted to

THINKING CRITICALLY ABOUT . . . *Prenatal Diagnostic Testing*

Prenatal diagnostic testing will identify many fetal abnormalities that would otherwise not be known until birth, late-gestation spontaneous abortion, or fetal death. Many health care professionals and consumers believe that the primary purpose of prenatal diagnosis is to identify fetal anomalies in order to terminate the pregnancy. Therefore, those who for ethical, cultural, and/or religious reasons would not choose abortion may not see any benefit from prenatal screening and testing procedures. While these procedures are only recommended (not mandatory) and are based on individual risk, couples need to be informed of the benefits, as well as the risks, of the procedures regardless of their intentions should a genetic defect or disorder be found.

Since most couples receive normal results from prenatal tests, a significant benefit of prenatal testing in most cases is relief of anxiety and relative peace of mind for the duration of the pregnancy (Clark and DeVore, 1989). In fact, it may be advisable before testing to suggest that a couple concerned with the termination issue postpone decision making, because chances are that no decision will be necessary. If a decision is needed, it is best made in light of the known, not potential, findings.

Should results reveal a fetal abnormality, this information can be provided in a relatively supportive and calm environment, not following the emotion and physical exhaustion of labor and delivery. While this advantage does not eliminate the devastation, it does allow the couple some time to adjust to and cope with the diagnosis, prepare and inform themselves, and make necessary family decisions with the support of the professional counseling team (Lorenz and Kuhn, 1989).

Prior knowledge of a fetal abnormality is advantageous for medical reasons other than pregnancy termination. It permits appropriate pregnancy and delivery management to optimally benefit the fetal outcome. For example, when a fetal abnormality is known, delivery can be planned to take place at a hospital with specialized neonatal facilities. Planned cesarean section has been shown to minimize trauma to a fetus with a spinal defect, and a fetus with a trisomy can be evaluated for the presence of a heart defect that may require intervention soon after birth.

While a couple's religious and/or moral beliefs regarding pregnancy termination may be a very clear-cut issue for them theoretically, when faced with the reality of a fetus with abnormalities, gray areas emerge when the quality of life, pain, suffering, disability, and expected life span are considered. It has been found that couples do consider severity of the condition in their termination decision (Verp and others, 1988). Therefore, while a couple may choose not to undergo prenatal testing, their choice should be an informed one in regard to the advantages, as well as the risks, of testing, regardless of whether or not they would consider termination.

In working with these families, you need to consider your personal beliefs about termination of a pregnancy for fetal abnormalities. Would these beliefs prevent you from providing nonjudgmental, supportive counseling to a couple who must make that decision? In thinking about the pros and cons of prenatal testing, have you considered the benefits discussed above?

direct the decisions of the clients, especially less intelligent persons who may be judged to be less responsible for their actions. In genetic counseling, families should be given all the facts and possible consequences and then be assisted, without coercion, in their problem solving. However, the decision concerning a course of action must be left to them (see Thinking Critically About . . . box, p. 181).

KEY POINTS

- There is a probably a genetic component in all disease processes.
- Genetic diseases are usually classified as those produced by chromosome aberrations, those caused by a single mutant gene, or those resulting from interaction of genetic and environmental factors (multifactorial).
- Environmental teratogens and maternal disease may also disrupt fetal development, leading to birth defects.
- Chromosome aberrations are caused by deviations in either chromosome structure or number.
- Alterations in chromosome number occur as a result of unequal distribution of genetic material during gamete formation or early cell division of the zygote.
- Disorders caused by a single gene are distributed in families according to predictable mendelian principles of inheritance, although there are exceptions based on nontraditional concepts.
- Mutant genes can be dominant or recessive and can be located on an autosome or an X chromosome.
- Variations in gene action include the regularity with which it is manifested (penetrance), the severity or variability of its expression (expressivity), and the different and seemingly unrelated effects associated with the basic defect (pleiotropy).
- Congenital defects, errors or morphogenic development, may arise at any stage of development and demonstrate wide variability in causative factors.
- Although no cure for genetic disease is presently available, various therapeutic measures are used to modify or correct the basic defect.
- The objectives of genetic screening are to detect the presence of disease in individuals, detect unaffected carriers of a disease, and monitor the incidence of disease and/or malformations in a population.
- Prenatal testing includes screening through ultrasound and maternal serum alpha-fetoprotein (MS-AFP) testing, and diagnosis by amniocentesis, ultrasound, chorionic villis sampling (CVS), and DNA testing.
- Genetic counseling is directed toward providing individuals and families with information needed to make decisions about a course of action appropriate to them.
- Nurse's roles in genetic counseling include identifying cases, interviewing families, educating families about their disease and its therapy, and providing follow-up care and support.

REFERENCES

Altshuler G: Some placental considerations related to neurodevelopmental and other disorders, *J Child Neurol* 8:78-94, 1993.

American Academy of Pediatrics, Committee on Genetics: Folic acid for the prevention of neural tube defects, *Pediatrics* 92(3):493-494, 1993.

Annas GJ: Privacy rules for DNA databanks: protecting coded "future diaries," *JAMA* 270(19):2346-2350, 1993.

Asch DA and others: Reporting the results of cystic fibrosis carrier screening, *Am J Obstet Gynecol* 168(1):1-6, 1993.

Bernhardt BA, Pyeritz RE: The organization and delivery of clinical genetic services, *Pediatr Clin North Am* 39(1):1-12, 1992.

Bernstein IM and others: Elevated maternal serum alpha fetoprotein: association with placental sonolucencies, fetomaternal hemorrhage, vaginal bleeding and pregnancy outcome in the absence of fetal anomalies, *Obstet Gynecol* 79(1):71-74, 1992.

Blizzard RM: Genetics and growth: new understanding, *Pediatr Rounds* 2(2):1-4, 1993.

Bock JL: Current issues in maternal serum alpha-fetoprotein screening, *Am J Clin Pathol* 97:541-554, 1992.

Brantly DK: Constructing a family pedigree. In Smith DP and others, editors: *Comprehensive child and family nursing skills,* St Louis, 1991, Mosby.

Clark SL, DeVore GR: Prenatal diagnosis for couples who would not consider abortion, *Obstet Gynecol* 73(6):1035-1037, 1989.

D'Alton ME, DeCherney AH: Prenatal diagnosis, *N Engl J Med* 328(2):114-120, 1993.

DiMario FJ and others: An evaluation of autonomic nervous system function in patients with Prader-Willi syndrome, *Pediatrics* 93:76-81, 1994.

Ewigman BG and others: Effect of prenatal ultrasound screening on perinatal outcome, *N Engl J Med* 329(12):821-872, 1993.

Genetic Counseling: A preview of what's in store, *Science* 259:624, 1993.

Giordano BP: The impact of genetic syndromes on children's growth, *J Pediatr Health Care* 6:309-315, 1992.

Greenberg F: Contiguous gene syndromes, *Growth Genet Horm* 9(3):5-10, 1993.

Hall BD: The state of the art of dysmorphology, *Am J Dis Child* 147:1184-1189, 1993.

Handyside AH and others: Birth of a normal girl after in vitro fertilization and preimplantation diagnostic testing for cystic fibrosis, *N Engl J Med* 327:905-909, 1992.

Hulsebus DR, Williams J: Cystic fibrosis: a new perspective in genetic counseling, *J Pediatr Health Care* 6:338-342, 1992.

Kessler S: Psychological aspects of genetic counseling: suffering and countertransference, *J Genet Counsel* 1(4):303-308, 1992.

LeRoux MG and others: Non-paternity and genetic counselling, *Lancet* 340:607, 1992.

Lopez EI: Prenatal diagnosis by ultrasound, *J Perinat Neonat Nurs* 2(4):34-42, 1989.

Lorenz RP, Kuhn MH: Multidisciplinary team counseling for fetal anomalies, *Am J Obstet Gynecol* 161:263-266, 1989.

Marcari MJ and others: The frequency of uniparental disomy in Prader-Willi syndrome, *N Engl J Med* 326:1599-1607, 1992.

Michelena M and others: Paternal age as a risk factor for Down syndrome, *Am J Med Genet* 45:679-682, 1993.

Milunsky A, editor: *Genetic disorders and the fetus,* ed 3, Baltimore, 1992, Johns Hopkins University Press.

Morell V: The puzzle of the triple repeats, *Science* 260:1422-1423, 1993.

Prows CA: Utilization of genetic knowledge in pediatric nursing practice, *J Pediatr Nurs* 7(1):58-62, 1992.

Randall T: A novel, unstable DNA mutation cracks decades-old clinical enigma, *JAMA* 269(5):557-562, 1993.

Rosenthal RG and others: Six-year results of a randomized prospective trial of human growth hormone and oxandrolone in Turner syndrome, *J Pediatr* 121:49-55, 1992.

Simpson JL, Elias S: Isolating fetal cells from maternal blood, *JAMA* 270(19):2357-2361, 1993.

Stephenson J: A case of discrimination: a family's health insurance is cancelled after fragile X diagnosis, *Natl Fragile X Foundation Newslett,* pp 1-3, fall/winter 1992-1993.

Thompson MW, McInnes RR, Willard HF: *Thompson and Thompson genetics in medicine,* ed 5, Philadelphia, 1991, WB Saunders.

Tibben A and others: On attitudes and appreciation 6 months after predictive DNA testing for Huntington disease in the Dutch program, *Am J Med Genet* 48:103-111, 1993.

Verp MS and others: Parental decision following prenatal diagnosis of fetal chromosome abnormality, *Am J Med Genet* 29:613-622, 1988.

Watson EK and others: Screening for carriers of cystic fibrosis through the primary health care services, *Br Med J* 303:504-507, 1991.

Weiss JO: Support groups for patients with genetic disorders and their families, *Pediatr Clin North Am* 39(1):13-23, 1992.

Williams JK: New genetic discoveries increase counseling opportunities, *MCN* 18:218-222, 1993.

BIBLIOGRAPHY

General

Barch MJ, editor: *The ACT cytogenetics laboratory manual,* ed 2, New York, 1991, Raven Press.

Buyse ML, editor: *Birth defects encyclopedia,* New York, 1990, Alan R Liss.

Cohen FL: *Clinical genetics in nursing practice,* Philadelphia, 1984, JB Lippincott.

Cohen MM, Rosenblum-Vos LS, Prathakar G: Human cytogenetics: a current overview, *Am J Dis Child* 147:1159-1166, 1993.

Cooper DN, Schmidtke J: Diagnosis of genetic disease using recombinant DNA, *Hum Genet* 73:1-14, 1986.

Darras BR, Harper JF, Francke U: Prenatal diagnosis and detection of carriers with DNA probes in Duchenne's muscular dystrophy, *N Engl J Med* 316:985-992, 1987.

Emanuel BS: The use of fluorescence in situ hybridization to identify human chromosome anomalies, *Growth Genet Horm* 9(1):6-12, 1993.

Forsman I: Education of nurses in genetics, *Am J Hum Genet* 43:552-558, 1988.

Frost N: Genetic diagnosis and treatment: ethical considerations, *Am J Dis Child* 147:1190-1195, 1993.

Gilbert-Barness E, Opitz JM, Barness LA: The pathologist's perspective of genetic disease, *Pediatr Clin North Am* 36:163-187, 1989.

Hall JG, editor: Medical genetics, parts I and II, *Pediatr Clin North Am* 39(1-2):entire issues, 1992.

King RA, Rotter JI, Motulsky AG, editors: *The genetic basis of common diseases,* New York, 1992, Oxford University Press.

Levine F, Friedman T: Gene therapy, *Am J Dis Child* 147:1167-1174, 1993.

Levy P, Shapira E: State of the art of biochemical genetics, *Am J Dis Child* 147:1153-1158, 1993.

McKusick VA: Mapping and sequencing the human genome, *N Engl J Med* 320:910-915, 1989.

McKusick VA: Medical genetics: a 40 year perspective on the evolution of a medical specialty from a basic science, *JAMA* 270(19):2351-2356, 1993.

Prows CA: Utilization of genetic knowledge in pediatric nursing practice, *J Pediatr Nurs* 7(1):58-62, 1992.

Robinson A, Linden MG: *Clinical genetics handbook,* ed 2, Boston, 1993, Blackwell Scientific Publications.

Smith DW: *Recognizable patterns of human malformation,* ed 3, Philadelphia, 1982, WB Saunders.

Spence JE and others: Uniparental disomy as a mechanism for human genetic disease, *Am J Hum Genet* 42:217-226, 1988.

Tinley ST: Nurses' and geneticists' role expectations for the genetics nurse clinician, *J Pediatr Nurs* 2:259-264, 1987.

Weiss JO and others: Genetic disorders and birth defects in families and society, *Birth Defects* 20(4):1-8, 1984.

Williams RR: Nature, nurture, and family predisposition, *N Engl J Med* 318:769-770, 1988.

Winter RM: A combined method for grouping cases with multiple malformations, *J Med Genet* 25:119-126, 1988.

Genetic Disorders

Arn PH, Valle DL, Brusilow SW: Inborn errors of metabolism: not rare, not hopeless, *Contemp Pediatr,* pp 47-61, Dec 1988.

Brewer GJ, Yuzbasiyan-Garkan V: Wilson disease, *Medicine* 71(3):139-164, 1992.

Carey JC: Health supervision and anticipatory guidance for children with genetic disorders (including specific recommendations for trisomy 21, trisomy 18, and neurofibromatosis I), *Pediatr Clin North Am* 39(1):25-53, 1992.

Clark LA: Mitochondrial disorders in pediatrics: clinical, biochemical, and genetic implications, *Pediatr Clin North Am* 39(2):319-334, 1992.

Day S, Brunson G, Wang W: A successful education program for parents of infants with newly diagnosed sickle cell disease, *J Pediatr Nurs* 7(1):52-57, 1992.

Fernbach SD, Thomson EJ: Molecular genetic technology in cystic fibrosis: implications for nursing practice, *J Pediatr Nurs* 7(1):20-24, 1992.

Gardner RJ, Sutherland GR: *Chromosome abnormalities and genetic counseling,* New York, 1989, Oxford University Press.

Giordano BP: The impact of genetic syndromes on children's growth, *J Pediatr Health Care* 6:309-315, 1992.

Goldstein H, Nielsen KG: Rates and survival of individuals with trisomy 13 and 18, *Clin Genet* 34:366-372, 1988.

Harvey AS, Leaper PM, Bankier A: CHARGE association: clinical manifestations and developmental outcomes, *Am J Med Genet* 39:48-55, 1991.

Hull C, Hagerman RJ: A study of the physical, behavioral, and medical phenotype, including anthropometric measures of females with fragile X syndrome, *Am J Dis Child* 147:1236-1241, 1993.

Kaback M and others: Tay-Sachs disease: carrier screening, prenatal diagnosis, and the molecular era, *JAMA* 270(19):2307-2315, 1993.

Linden MG and others: 47,XXX: what is the prognosis? *Pediatrics* 82:619-630, 1988.

Lynch M: Special children, special needs: the ectodermal dysplasias, *Pediatr Nurs* 18(3):212-216, 1992.

Marion RW and others: Trisomy 18 score: a rapid, reliable diagnostic test for trisomy 18, *J Pediatr* 113:45-48, 1988.

McKusick VA: *Mendelian inheritance in man,* ed 10, Baltimore, 1992, Johns Hopkins University Press.

Morell J: The puzzle of the triple repeats, *Science* 260:1422-1423, 1993.

Nativio DG, Belz C: Childhood neurofibromatosis, *Pediatr Nurs* 16(6):575-580, 1990.

Powers D, Hiti A: Sickle cell anemia: B^5 gene cluster haplotypes as genetic markers for severe disease expression, *Am J Dis Child* 147:1197-1202, 1993.

Pueschel SM: Growth, thyroid function, and sexual maturation in Down syndrome, *Growth Genet Horm* 6(1):1-5, 1990.

Salbenblat JA and others: Gross and fine motor development in 47,XXY and 47,XYY males, *Pediatrics* 80:240-244, 1987.

Shoffner JM, Wallace DC: Mitochondrial genetics: principles and practice, *Am J Hum Genet* 51:1179-1186, 1992.

Williams JK: School-aged children with Turner's syndrome, *J Pediatr Nurs* 7(1):14-19, 1992.

Multifactorial Disorders and Prenatal Teratogens

American Academy of Pediatrics Committee on Substance Abuse: Fetal alcohol syndrome and fetal alcohol effects, *Pediatrics* 91(5):1004-1005, 1993.

Chiriboga CA: Neurologic complications of drug and alcohol abuse: fetal effects, *Neurol Clin* 11(3):707-727, 1993.

Cohen MM Jr: *The child with multiple birth defects,* New York, 1982, Raven Press.

Czeizel AE, Dudas I: Prevention of the first occurrence of neural tube defect by periconceptual vitamin supplementation, *N Engl J Med* 327:1832-1835, 1992.

Free T and others: A descriptive study of infants and toddlers exposed prenatally to substance abuse, *MCN* 15:245-249, 1990.

Gilbert-Barness E, Opitz JM, Barness LA: The pathologist's perspective of genetic disease: malformations and dysmorphology, *Pediatr Clin North Am* 36:163-187, 1989.

Lippe BM: Short stature in children: evaluation and management, *J Pediatr Health Care* 1:313-322, 1987.

McCabe ER and others: Committee on genetics: maternal phenylketonuria, *Pediatrics* 88(6):1284-1285, 1991.

Mitchell LE, Risch N: The genetics of infantile hypertrophic pyloric stenosis: a reanalysis, *Am J Dis Child* 147:1203-1211, 1993.

Osband BA: Multifactorial inheritance: implications for perinatal and neonatal nurses, *J Perinat Neonat Nurs* 2(4):43-52, 1989.

Pletsch PK: Birth defect prevention: nursing interventions, *JOGNN* 19(6):482-488, 1990.

Pollack RN, Divon MY: Intrauterine growth retardation: definition, classification, and etiology, *Clin Obstet Gynecol* 35(1):99-107, 1992.

Seaver LH, Hoyne HE: Teratology in pediatric practice, *Pediatr Clin North Am* 39(1):111-134, 1992.

Torfs C, Curry C, Roeper P: Gastroschisis, *J Pediatr* 116(1):1-6, 1990.

Vanderwinden JM and others: Nitric oxide synthase activity in infantile hypertrophic pyloric stenosis, *N Engl J Med* 327:511-515, 1992.

Genetic Screening and Prenatal Diagnosis

American Academy of Pediatrics Committee on Genetics: Alpha-fetoprotein screening, *Pediatrics* 88(6):1282-1283, 1991.

American Academy of Pediatrics Committee on Genetics: Newborn screening fact sheets, *Pediatrics* 83:449-464, 1989.

Bernstein IM and others: Elevated maternal serum alpha-fetoprotein: association with placental sonolucencies, fetomaternal hemorrhage, vaginal bleeding, and pregnancy outcome in the absence of fetal anomalies, *Obstet Gynecol* 79(1):71-74, 1992.

Boyd PA: Why might maternal serum AFP be high in pregnancies in which the fetus is normally formed? *Br J Obstet Gynecol* 99:93-95, 1992.

Cobb E and others: What do young people think about screening for cystic fibrosis? *J Med Genet* 28:322-324, 1991.

Cutting GR, Antonarakis SE: Prenatal diagnosis and carrier detection by DNA analysis, *Pediatr Rev* 13(4):138-143, 1992.

DiLiberti JH, Greenstein MA, Rosengren SS: Prenatal diagnosis, *Pediatr Rev* 13(9):334-342, 1992.

Jones SL: Decision making in clinical genetics: ethical implications for perinatal practice, *J Perinat Neonat Nurs* 1:11-23, 1988.

Kaffe S, Hsu LY: Maternal serum alpha fetoprotein screening and fetal chromosome anomalies: is lowering maternal age for amniocentesis preferable? *Am J Med Genet* 42:801-806, 1992.

Lopez EI: Prenatal diagnosis by ultrasound, *J Perinat Neonat Nurs* 2(4):34-42, 1989.

Morgan CD, Elias S: Prenatal diagnosis of genetic disorders, *J Perinat Neonat Nurs* 2(4):1-12, 1989.

National Institutes of Health Consensus Development Conference Statement: *Newborn screening for sickle cell disease and other hemoglobinopathies,* Bethesda, MD, 1987, National Institutes of Health.

Ostrer H: Prenatal diagnosis of genetic disorders by DNA analysis, *Pediatr Ann* 18:701-713, 1989.

Ostrer H, Hejtmancik JF: Prenatal diagnosis and carrier detection of genetic disease by analysis of deoxyribonucleic acid, *J Pediatr* 112:679-687, 1988.

Platt LD, Carlson DE: Prenatal diagnosis—when and how? *N Engl J Med* 327(9):636-638, 1992.

Platt LD and others: The California Maternal Serum Alpha-Fetoprotein Screening Program: the role of ultrasonography in the detection of spina bifida, *Am J Obstet Gynecol* 166:1328-1329, 1992.

Robertson JA: Ethical and legal issues in preimplantation genetic screening, *Fertil Steril* 57(1):1-122, 1992.

Spencer K and others: Free beta human choriogonadotropin in Down's syndrome screening: a multi centre study of its role compared with other biochemical markers, *Ann Clin Biochem* 29:506-518, 1992.

Wenstrom KD and others: Prediction of pregnancy outcome with single versus serial maternal serum alpha fetoprotein tests, *Am J Obstet Gynecol* 167:1529-1533, 1992.

Wertz DC, Fletcher JC: Ethical issues in prenatal diagnosis, *Pediatr Ann* 18:739-749, 1989.

Williams JK: Screening for genetic disorders, *J Pediatr Health Care* 3:115-121, 1989.

Williamson R, Murray JC: Molecular analysis of genetic disorders. In Pitkin RM, Scott J, editors: *Clinical Obstetrics and gynecology,* Philadelphia, 1988, JB Lippincott.

Genetic Counseling

Aylsworth AS: Genetic counseling for patients with birth defects, *Pediatr Clin North Am* 39(2):229-253, 1992.

Clark MH: A pedigree primer, *J Pediatr Nurs* 4:112-118, 1989.

dYdewalle G and others, editors: Experiments on genetic risk perception and decision-making: explorative studies, *Birth Defects* 23(2):209-225, 1987.

Ekwo EE, Kim J, Gosselink CA: Parental perceptions of the burden of genetic diseases, *Am J Med Genet* 28:955-964, 1987.

Farrell CD: Genetic counseling: the emerging reality, *J Perinat Neonat Nurs* 2(4):21-33, 1989.

Fleisher LD: Wrongful births: when is there liability for prenatal injury? *Am J Dis Child* 141:1260-1265, 1987.

Harper PS: *Practical genetic counseling,* London, 1993, Butterworth/Heinemann.

Hildes E and others: Impact of genetic counselling after neonatal screening for Duchenne muscular dystrophy, *J Med Genet* 30:670-674, 1993.

Lin AE, Garver KL: Genetic counseling for congenital heart defects, *J Pediatr* 113:1105-1109, 1988.

Nora JJ, Nora AH: Update on counseling the family with a first-degree relative with a congenital heart defect, *Am J Med Genet* 29:137-142, 1988.

Prows CA: Utilization of genetic knowledge in pediatric nursing practice, *J Pediatr Nurs* 7(1):58-62, 1992.

Reilly PR: Ethical, legal, and social issues in genetics, *Curr Opin Pediatr* 1:448-452, 1989.

Rhodes AM: Minimizing the liability risks of genetic counseling, *MCN* 14:313, 1989.

Rhodes AM: Wrongful birth and wrongful life, *MCN* 14:171, 1989.

Sankaranalayanan K: Prevalence of genetic and partially genetic diseases in man and the estimation of genetic risks of exposure to ionizing radiation, *Am J Hum Genet* 42:651-660, 1988.

Shapiro LR: Pitfalls in genetic counseling for childhood disorders: the pediatrician's role, *Am J Dis Child* 147:1253-1254, 1993.

Somer M, Mustonen H, Norio R: Evaluation of genetic counseling: recall of information, post-counseling reproduction, and attitude of the counselees, *Clin Genet* 34:352-365, 1988.

Weil J: Mother's post counseling beliefs about the causes of their children's genetic disorders, *Am J Hum Genet* 48:145-153, 1991.

Weiss JO: Support groups for patients with genetic disorders and their families, *Pediatr Clin North Am* 39(1):13-23, 1992.

Williams JK: Counseling adolescents about environmental teratogens, *Pediatr Nurs* 12:292-295, 1986.

Williams JK: Genetic counseling in pediatric nursing care, *Pediatr Nurs* 12:287-290, 1986.

Williams JK: New genetic discoveries increase counseling opportunities, *MCN* 18:218-222, 1993.

UNIT II

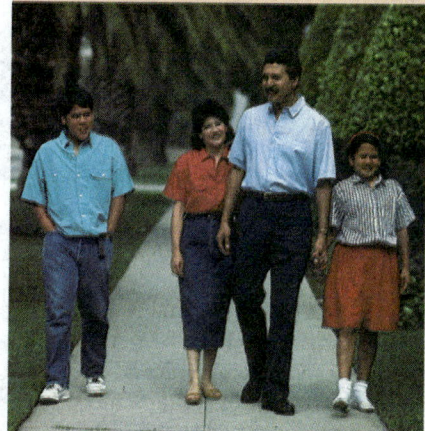

ASSESSMENT OF THE CHILD AND FAMILY

CHAPTER 6 Communication and Health Assessment of the Child and Family

CHAPTER OUTLINE

RELATED TOPICS

Development of self-concept, Ch. 4
Developmental assessment, Ch. 7
Factors affecting the family's adjustment (chronic health conditions), Ch. 22
Family structure and function, Ch. 3
Family theories, Ch. 3
Growth measurements, Ch. 7
Immunizations, Ch. 12
Nutritional disturbances, Ch. 13
Pain assessment, Ch. 26
Preparation for procedures, Ch. 27
Role of play in development, Ch. 4
Sex education, Chs. 15 and 17
Sexually transmitted diseases, Ch. 20
Sleep problems, Chs. 12 and 15
Social, cultural, and religious influences on child health promotion, Ch. 2
Taking a family history, Ch. 5
Use of play in procedures, Ch. 27
Using play/expressive activities to minimize stress, Ch. 26

COMMUNICATION

Communication may be verbal, nonverbal, or abstract. ***Verbal communication*** may involve language and its expression; vocalizations in the form of laughs, moans, and squalls; or the implications of what is not said in light of what has been said. ***Nonverbal communication,*** often called "body language," includes gestures, movements, facial expressions, postures, and reactions. ***Abstract communication*** takes such forms as play, artistic expression, symbols, photographs, and choice of clothing. Because it is possible to exert greater conscious control over verbal communication, it is a less reliable indicator of true feelings, especially with children.

Many factors influence the communication process. To be successful (gratifying), communication must be appropriate to the situation, properly timed, and clearly delivered. This implies that nurses understand and use techniques of effective communication. Verbal and nonverbal messages must be congruous; that is, two or more messages sent via different levels must not be contradictory.

Nurses need to recognize their own feelings and attempt to recognize those of the persons with whom the communicative interchange takes place. Biases and judgments interfere with all aspects of the process. The tendency to approve or disapprove of another's statements inhibits positive reactions. In addition, the transmission and reception of messages may be altered by influences of intimacy or distance, trust and mistrust, security and insecurity, or caring and not caring on the part of the participants. The value of effective communication is increased understanding between the nurse, child, and family. Since nursing of infants and children always involves the inclusion of a caregiver, nurses must be able to communicate not only with children of all ages but with the adults in their lives as well.

VERBAL COMMUNICATION—THE POWER OF WORDS

Words shape reality, and thus they hold tremendous power. A person can change another's perception of reality by the choice of words that are used (Cassell, Coulehan, and Putnam, 1989). For example, if the diagnosis of cancer is always referred to as a tumor, cyst, malignancy, or carcinoma, patients may never really know that they have cancer. Consequently, they may assume less responsibility for their care than if they were aware of the seriousness of the condition. By learning to recognize how patients and health professionals use language to manipulate reality, one can also learn how to change perceptions and communicate more effectively.

Avoidance Language

Probably the most common way people try to alter reality is by avoiding words that truly describe it. For example, euphemisms such as "passed on" are used instead of the word "death." Avoidance language usually indicates that a person wants to hide something, especially feelings. As a rule, accepting a person's use of euphemisms only serves to perpetuate the fears and never helps the person deal with them. In contrast, use of straightforward, precise, descriptive language lends perspective to the situation and allows the person to discuss the fears. Most often, imagined fears are far greater than the actual reality.

Distancing Language

Sometimes people use impersonal words, such as "it" or "others," to shield themselves from the painful reality of a situation. For example, parents may state that they know *someone* with a child who is slow and actually be talking about personal fears regarding *their* child. By realizing that parents need to talk about this difficult subject, the nurse can provide sensitive statements that ease them into discussing their situation.

One of the dangers in supporting distancing language is that the parent may effectively deny that a problem exists. To return to the previous example, if the issue of retardation is never approached directly but is allowed to be "someone else's problem," the parents may not seek appropriate care for their child.

Sometimes distancing is desirable because the topic may be too painful to discuss directly. The use of third-person technique (see box on p. 196) may be very therapeutic in allowing an individual the opportunity to indirectly approach a subject and receive feedback but still remain in control.

NONVERBAL COMMUNICATION—PARALANGUAGE

In addition to the spoken word, messages are relayed through nonverbal means, or ***paralanguage,*** which involves pitch, pause, intonation, rate, volume, and stress in speech (Cassell, Coulehan, and Putnam, 1989). Young children become very adept at understanding paralanguage; long before they know the meaning of words, they sense anxiety or fear by the rise in pitch or the accelerated rate of the parent's voice. By careful attention to the spoken word, nurses can better understand the meaning of another's verbal message and more accurately control their own paralanguage.

Because most people do not exert conscious control over paralanguage, it is a valuable clue to such things as feelings and concerns. For example, ***pausing*** may signify a need to formulate thoughts, recall information, or sometimes fabricate a story. Frequent pauses, however, often make the speaker sound insecure. Long pauses may mean that the individual needs more information.

Rate also sends unspoken messages. Talking too fast usually makes the speaker sound glib and insensitive. Talking slowly with a firm tone and appropriate pauses conveys authority. Therefore a person is much more likely to "hear" instructions if the latter approach is used. Children, in particular, respond attentively to a slow, even, steady voice.

Confirming and Disconfirming Behaviors

People respond to each other through ***confirming behaviors,*** such as nodding the head, using direct eye contact, repeating or requesting clarification, and making appropriate comments, or ***disconfirming behaviors,*** such as tapping fingers or a foot, turning away from the speaker, avoiding eye contact, and interrupting (Heineken and Roberts, 1983). Since there is a reciprocal relationship between such behaviors, nurses need to use confirming behaviors to receive confirmation in return. This "mirroring" effect is particularly evident in children because of their sensitivity to nonverbal cues.

GUIDELINES FOR COMMUNICATION AND INTERVIEWING

The most widely used method of communicating with parents on a professional basis is the interview process. Interviewing, unlike social conversation, is a specific form of goal-directed communication. As nurses converse with children and adults, they focus on individuals to determine the kind of person they are, their usual mode of handling problems, whether help is needed, and the way in which they react to counseling. Developing interviewing skills requires time and practice, but following some guiding principles can facilitate this process.

ESTABLISHING A SETTING FOR COMMUNICATION

Part of the success in interviewing depends on the type of physical and psychological setting the interviewer constructs. Appropriate introduction, role clarification, explanation of the reason for the interview, preliminary acquaintance with the family, and assurance of privacy and confidentiality are prerequisites for establishing a setting that fosters communication.

Appropriate Introduction

Nurses should introduce themselves to, and ask the name of, each family member who is present (see Thinking Critically About . . . box). Address parents or other adults using their appropriate titles, such as "Mr." and "Mrs.," unless they specify a preferred name. Record the preferred name on the medical record (Elizabeth, 1989). Using formal address or their preferred names, rather than using first names or "mom" or "dad," conveys respect and regard for the parents or other caregivers and the critical role they play in the lives of their children (Leff and Walizer, 1992).

At the beginning of the visit, include children in the interaction by asking them their name, age, and other information. Nurses often direct all questions to adults, even when children are old enough to speak for themselves. This serves to terminate one extremely valuable source of information, the patient. When the child is included, follow the general rules for communicating with children (p. 193).

Role Clarification and Explanation of the Interview

During the introduction it is also necessary to clarify the nurse's particular role in the health setting. For example, nurses performing interviews may be pediatric nurse practitioners, inpatient staff nurses, clinical nurses, office nurses, visiting nurses, or school nurses. A parent is much more likely to reveal personal information about the child and family if the relevance and importance of the interview are stressed. If this is not done, parents may refuse to elaborate on certain areas because they feel it has no bearing on the "problem." In addition, since more than one member of the health team may take a history during the course of a hospital admission, it is important to clarify the reason for each interview.

Another reason for role clarification is education of the health consumer. With expanded roles in nursing, it is not unusual for families to think that the examiner is a physician rather than a nurse. Role clarification is especially important because some parents may feel deceived if they later are made aware of the nurse's identity. Since the general consumer acceptance of pediatric nurse practitioners has

THINKING CRITICALLY ABOUT . . . *Nurses' Form of Address*

Language (and dress) convey information about age, class, status, education, role, and professional autonomy. Campbell-Heider and Hart (1993) contend that nurses' use of "Ms.," "Mr.," "Mrs.," "Nurse," or "Doctor" maintains a formality that suggests a professional status. In contrast, when nurses introduce themselves to families by their first names, they encourage a social relationship that is quickly enhanced with informal conversation, especially if it is about the nurse. Nurses may also assume a subordinate position when they address physicians as "Doctor" but the physicians use the nurses' first names. One study's findings suggest that parents' perception of nurses as knowledgeable sources of information was not strong. Parents perceived nurses as "pleasant servants" and relied on physicians for important information about their child's progress (McBurney and Schultz, 1993). Could informal addresses by nurses contribute to this perception of them as "servants?"

With children we might argue that using first names is friendly and less threatening. But consider children's usual forms of address for doctors, teachers, preschool or daycare personnel, coaches, and adult relatives and friends. If first names are used, they are often preceded with "Doctor," "Miss," "Coach," or "Aunt." In many cultures respect for elders must include formal address.

Think about the form of address you use. Is it parallel with forms of address used by other professionals and families? Do nurses with doctorates use the title "Doctor?" Ask for their opinions and experiences regarding using the title. Try using more formal styles of address, such as "Ms." or "Nurse" with your surname, and note the reactions of others. Do you think professionalism and status are influenced by form of address?

been very favorable, it is also important to acknowledge the expertise of the nurse by emphasizing the nurse's role.

Preliminary Acquaintance

To make the family feel at ease and to develop rapport, begin with some general conversation. Comments such as, "How have things been since your last visit?" "Tell me about Johnny," or (to the child) "What do you think is going to happen today?" allow the parent or child to express the main concern in a casual, relaxed atmosphere.

The preliminary acquaintance conversation also reveals how responsive the informant may be to questions. For example, using open-ended statements may lead a person into a lengthy, detailed discussion. In this case direct questions toward specific answers to avoid tangential remarks. At other times a person may respond to open-ended questions with only minimal information; in this case continue to use open-ended questions rather than "yes" or "no" questions.

Assurance of Privacy and Confidentiality

The place where the interview is conducted is almost as important as the interview itself. The physical environment should allow for as much privacy as possible, with distractions, such as interruptions, noise, or other visible activity, kept to a minimum. At times it is necessary to turn off a television or radio. The environment should also have some play provision for young children to keep them occupied during the parent-nurse interview (Fig. 6-1). Parents who are constantly interrupted by their children are unable to concentrate fully and tend to give short, brief answers to terminate the interview as quickly as possible (see Critical Thinking Exercise box).

Confidentiality is also an essential component of the initial phase of the interview. Since the interview is usually shared with other members of the health team or the teacher (as in the case of students), be sure to inform the family of the confidential limits of the conversation. If there is concern regarding confidentiality in a situation, such as talking to a parent suspected of child abuse or a teenager contemplating suicide, deal with this directly and inform the person that in such instances confidentiality cannot be ensured.

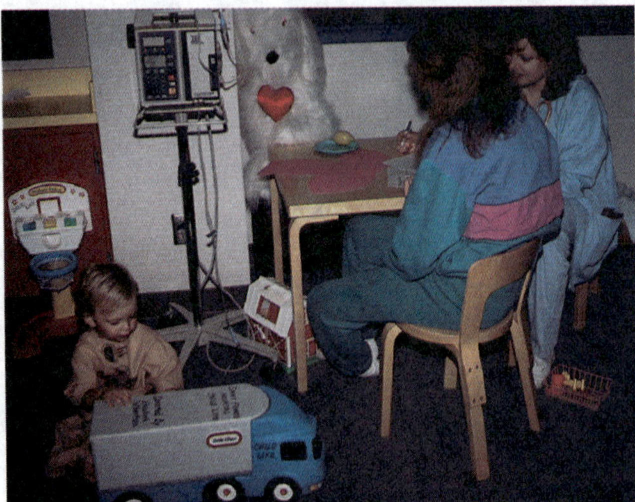

FIG. 6-1 Child plays while nurse interviews parent.

COMMUNICATING WITH FAMILIES

Communicating with the family is a triangular process involving the nurse, parents, and child. Although the following discussion focuses primarily on this triad, in many circumstances significant others, such as siblings, relatives, or other caregivers, may be part of the communication process.

COMMUNICATING WITH PARENTS

Although the parent and child are separate and distinct entities, relationships with the child are frequently mediated via the parent, particularly in the case of younger children. For the most part, information about the child is acquired by direct observation or communicated to the nurse by the parents. Usually it can be assumed that because of the close contact with the child, the parent gives reliable information. Making an assessment of the child requires input from the child (verbal and nonverbal), information from the parent, and the nurse's own observations of the child and interpre-

CRITICAL THINKING EXERCISE

The Interview

During your interview with Ms. Gaines, 2½-year-old Jesse continually interrupts the conversation. Although Ms. Gaines has told her several times to be quiet, the interruptions continue. Frustrated, the mother states firmly, "If you don't be good, the nurse will give you a shot." Jesse begins to cry softly and hugs her mother's legs. Your most appropriate response is to:

1. State: "Ms. Gaines, don't threaten Jesse that way. Her behavior isn't bothering me."
2. Do nothing, because Jesse has become quiet.
3. State: "Jesse, nurses don't give needles because children are not being quiet. Here are paper and crayons to draw some pictures while your mom and I talk."
4. Hug Jesse and give her crayons and paper to draw.

The correct answer is 3. The threat of injections or other painful or frightening procedures should never be used to gain a child's cooperation. You want to reassure Jesse about this, but at the same time reinforce the need for her to be quiet. Providing play materials helps keep her occupied.

Although the other responses may seem appropriate, they fail to remove the threat of a "shot" to Jesse. In particular, the first response can alienate your relationship with the parent. It also dismisses the issue that the interruptions do bother Ms. Gaines and most likely affect the quality of the interview.

tation of the relationship between the child and the parent. Counseling and guidance must be directed to the caregiver of infants and small children; when children are old enough to be active participants in their own health maintenance, the parent becomes a collaborator in health care.

Encouraging the Parent to Talk

Interviewing parents not only offers an opportunity to determine the health and developmental status of the child, but also offers information about all factors that influence the child's life. Whatever the parent sees as a problem should be a concern. These problems are not always easy to identify. Be alert for clues and signals by which a parent communicates worries and anxieties. Careful phrasing with broad open-ended questions such as "What is Jimmy eating now?" provides more information than several single-answer questions such as "Is Jimmy eating what the rest of the family eats?"

Sometimes the parent will take the lead without prompting. At other times it may be necessary to direct another question on the basis of an observation such as "Connie seems unhappy today," or "How do you feel when David cries?" If the parent appears to be tired or distraught, consider asking, "What do you do to relax?" or "What help do you have with the children?" A comment such as "You handle the baby very well. What kinds of experience have you had with babies?" to new mothers who appear comfortable with their first child gives them positive reinforcement and provides an opening for any questions they might have regarding the care of the infant. Often all that is required to keep the parent talking is a nod and saying "yes," or "unhuh."

When attempting to elicit feelings and covert problem areas, avoid closed-ended questions that begin with "Does . . .," "Did . . .," or "Is . . .," which usually require only a single response. In addition, asking questions such as "Does your son have any problems at school?" subtly implies a lack of parental skills and evokes defensiveness. Instead, say, "What . . .," "How . . .," "Tell me about . . .," and encourage elaboration with "You were saying . . .," "You say that . . .," or reflecting back key words or phrases, such as "He was depressed?" Open-ended questions are nonthreatening and encourage description.

Another useful approach is to elicit information about a topic and compare the answer with the person's perception of what "things" should be. For example, after the parent describes what the child is eating, ask, "What do you think your child should be eating?" If there is a discrepancy between the two answers, ask the parent to comment on how important the difference is. This approach allows the parent to discuss areas of concern that may not be disclosed otherwise.

Directing the Focus

The ability to direct the focus of the interview while allowing for maximum freedom of expression is one of the most difficult goals in effective communication. One approach is the use of open-ended or broad questions, followed by guiding statements. For example, if the parent proceeds to list the other children by name, say, "Tell me their ages, too." If the parent continues to describe each child in depth, which is not the purpose of the interview, redirect the focus by stating, "Let's talk about the other children later. You were beginning to tell me about Paul's activities at school." This approach conveys interest in the other children but focuses the assessment on the patient.

In the event that the parent has suggested that a problem exists with one of the other children, reintroduce this subject at the end of the interview to assess the need for further family follow-up. Saying to the parent, "Earlier you were mentioning that your older son is having trouble in school. Tell me what you see as the problem," reintroduces this subject but only in terms of the possible problem.

Listening

Listening is the most important component of effective communication. When listening is truly aimed at understanding the client, it is an active process that requires concentration and attention to all aspects of the conversation—verbal, nonverbal, and abstract. One of the greatest blocks to listening is environmental distraction and premature judgment.

The attitudes and feelings of the nurse are easily injected into an interview. Often nurses' perceptions of a parent's behavior are influenced by their own perceptions, prejudices, and assumptions, which may include racial, religious, and cultural stereotypes. What may be interpreted as passive hostility or disinterest in a parent may be shyness or an expression of anxiety. For example, in Western cultures eye contact and directness are signs of paying attention. However, in many non-Western cultures, including Native Americans, directness, such as looking someone in the eye, is considered rude. Children are taught to avert their gaze and to look down when being addressed by an adult, especially one with authority (Sloat and Matsuura, 1990). Therefore judgments about "listening" need to be made with an appreciation of cultural differences (see Chapter 2).

Although it is necessary to make some preliminary judgments, attempt to listen with as much objectivity as possible by clarifying meanings and attempting to see the situation from the parent's point of view. Effective interviewers use conscious control over their reactions and responses, and the techniques they use.

Use of minimal verbal activity with active listening facilitates parent involvement. It is tempting to spend time explaining, describing, and interpreting health information when the opportunity presents itself. However, it is possible to provide effective health education by properly timing the information and presenting only as much as is necessary at the moment.

Careful listening facilitates the use of clues, verbal leads, or signals from the interviewer to move the interview along. Frequent references to an area of concern, repetition of certain key words, and/or a special emphasis on something or someone serve as cues to the interviewer for the direction of inquiry. Concerns and anxieties are usually mentioned in a casual, offhand manner. Even though they are casual, they are important and deserve more careful scrutiny to identify problem areas. For example, a parent who is concerned about a child's habit of bed-wetting may casually mention that the child's bed was "wet this morning."

Because the interview is almost always triangular—nurse, child, and parent—the parent may wish to convey information in such a way as to prevent the child from hearing it. This requires active listening on the part of the nurse to hear the unspoken message. The following example illustrates this point:

> During a routine health visit the nurse performed a complete history and physical examination on a 4-year-old girl. The child was accompanied by her mother, who appeared to be a reliable, well-informed, and talkative informant. During the child's birth history, the mother gave all the information asked. However, during the family history, the mother stated to the nurse, "I had a hysterectomy 6 years ago." Because the nurse gave no indication of acknowledging the significance of this statement, the mother repeated it, only this time she stressed the "6 years." The nurse, who had not been listening as attentively as she should have, realized that the mother was telling her something very important. The mother raised her eyebrows and gently shook her head "no," warning the nurse not to explore this area too openly. The nurse correctly read the cues and stated, "Let's return to your health history later."
>
> At the completion of the physical examination, the nurse took the child to the Health Center's playroom and then took the opportunity to investigate this contradictory information of a "4-year-old child born to a woman with a hysterectomy 6 years ago." The mother revealed that the child was adopted. The mother was greatly concerned about the fact that the child was unaware of this and requested the nurse's advice.
>
> Fortunately, the nurse had "listened" carefully enough to realize the significance of this woman's concern and allowed her the opportunity to discuss it in private.

Listening is also helpful in assessing reliability. For example, the answers elicited at the beginning of the interview may differ from those at the end, when the parent feels more confident in revealing problems. It is important to identify any discrepancies and reintroduce those topics for further investigation.

Using Silence

Silence as a response is often one of the most difficult interviewing techniques to learn. It requires a sense of confidence and comfort on the part of the interviewer to allow the interviewee space in which to think uninterrupted. Silence permits the interviewee to sort out thoughts and feelings and search for responses to questions. It also allows for sharing of feelings in which two or more people absorb the emotion to its depth.

Sometimes it is necessary to break silence and reopen communication. Do this in a way that encourages the person to continue talking about what is considered important. Breaking a silence by introducing a new topic or by prolonged talking essentially terminates the interviewee's opportunity to use the silence. Suggestions for breaking the silence include statements such as "Is there anything else you wish to say?" "I see you find it difficult to continue; how may I help?" or "I don't know what this silence means. Perhaps there is something you would like to put into words but find difficult to say."

Being Empathic

Empathy is the capacity to understand what another person is experiencing from within that person's frame of reference; it is often described as the ability to put oneself in another's shoes. The essence of empathic interaction is accurately understanding another's feelings (Bellet and Maloney, 1991). Empathy differs from ***sympathy,*** which is *having* feelings or emotions in common with another person, rather than *understanding* those feelings. Sympathy is not therapeutic in the helping relationship, because it leads to feeling emotionally overinvolved and potentially to professional burnout (Holden, 1990).

Of the different types of support, such as empathy, encouragement, or reassurance, empathy is the most beneficial but least used form. Some individuals are naturally empathic; however, empathy can be learned by attending to the verbal and nonverbal language of the interviewee. ***Neurolinguistic programming (NLP)*** is concerned with the *manner* of accessing and understanding information and is an excellent method of increasing empathic communication. Although people may use all of the following sensory modalities to communicate, usually one modality predominates: visual, auditory, or kinesthetic. The specific sensory mode is identified by observing the type of verbs, adjectives, and adverbs the person uses and then using this mode in responding to the individual. For example, if a person using the visual mode states, "I can't *see* why you have to perform these procedures on my child," a response using the same mode is, "What do you see as the reason for them?"

Defining the Problem

To arrive at a solution to a problem or concern, the nurse and the parent must agree that one exists. Sometimes the parent may believe that there is a problem that the nurse is unable to see. For example, a mother was overly concerned about every small sniffle, sneeze, or cough in her infant, who had been carefully examined and found to be healthy with no evidence of a respiratory problem. On careful questioning, the nurse discovered that a previous child had died of pneumonia in infancy. Consequently, the nurse was able to better understand the mother's concern and could help the mother deal with her anxieties about her infant and teach her how to recognize any need for concern.

Occasionally a problem is identified that the parent denies exists. In this case pursue the situation and either find a way to deal with it or enlist the aid of other health team members. For example, the parents of a child with Down syndrome may refuse to believe that their child is different from any other child of the same age. They may say, "He is just a little slow," or "All the child needs to do is to try harder." A child with an obvious behavior problem may be described by the parents as "just stubborn" or "just behaving that way to spite us." Such statements may be clues that the parents have not progressed past the stage of denial in adjusting to the disability.

Solving the Problem

Once the problem is identified and agreed on by parent and nurse, they can begin to arrive at a solution. A parent who is included in the problem-solving process is more apt to follow through with a course of action. Such questions as "What have you tried so far?" or "What have you thought about doing?" provide leads for exploration and give the parents the feeling that their ideas and solutions are worthwhile. These can be followed by "What prevents you from trying that?" "That sounds like a good plan," and "You seem to be stumped. Have you considered trying this?" Such approaches encourage participation and reinforce rather than belittle parents' efforts to solve problems.

Sometimes a parent arrives at a solution that the nurse does not consider to be the best alternative. If it can be ascertained that it will do no harm and the parents are convinced of its merits, it is usually best to allow them to continue with the plan. A course of action is more likely to be carried out when parents can reach their own conclusions. However, when parental decisions may be hazardous, nurses are obligated to discuss the risks with the family and try to reach a more beneficial solution. Whenever possible, decisions should be theirs, with the nurse serving as a *facilitator* in problem solving.

Providing Anticipatory Guidance

The ideal way to handle a situation is to deal with it *before* it becomes a problem. The best preventive measure is anticipatory guidance. Traditionally, anticipatory guidance has focused on providing families with information on normal growth and development, and nurturing childrearing practices. For example, one of the most significant areas in pediatrics is injury prevention. Beginning prenatally, parents need specific instructions on home safety. Because of the child's maturing developmental skills, home safety changes must be implemented early to minimize risks to the child.

Many normal developmental changes can disturb unprepared parents, such as a toddler's diminished appetite, negativism, altered sleeping patterns, and anxiety toward strangers. Such topics are discussed in the chapters on health promotion to provide the nurse with knowledge to counsel parents.

However, anticipatory guidance should extend beyond giving information to empowering families to use the information as a means of building competence in their parenting abilities. To achieve this level of anticipatory guidance (Gorzka and others, 1991):

- Base interventions on needs identified by the family, not by the professional.
- View the family as competent or as having the ability to be competent.
- Provide opportunities for the family to achieve competence.

Avoiding Blocks to Communication

A number of blocks to communication can adversely affect the quality of the helping relationships. Many of these blocks are initiated by the interviewer, such as giving unrestricted advice or forming prejudged conclusions. Another type of block occurs primarily with the interviewees and deals with information overload. When individuals are presented with too much information or information that is overwhelming, they will often demonstrate signals of increasing anxiety or decreasing attention. Such signals should alert the interviewer to give less information or to clarify what has been said. Some of the more common blocks to communication, including signs of information overload, are listed in the box above.

BLOCKS TO COMMUNICATION

Socializing
Giving unrestricted and sometimes unasked-for advice
Offering premature or inappropriate reassurance
Giving overready encouragement
Defending a situation or opinion
Using stereotyped comments or cliches
Limiting expression of emotion by asking directed, closed-ended questions
Interrupting and finishing the person's sentence
Talking more than the interviewee
Forming prejudged conclusions
Deliberately changing the focus

SIGNS OF INFORMATION OVERLOAD

Long periods of silence
Wide eyes and fixed facial expression
Constant fidgeting or attempting to move away
Nervous habits (e.g., tapping, playing with hair)
Sudden disruptions (e.g., asking to go to the bathroom)
Looking around
Yawning, eyes drooping
Frequently looking at a watch or clock
Attempting to change topic of discussion

Communication blocks can be corrected by careful analysis of the interview process. One of the best methods for improving interviewing skills is audiotape and/or videotape feedback. With supervision and guidance, the interviewer can recognize the blocks and consciously avoid them.

Communicating with Families Through an Interpreter

Sometimes communication is impossible because two people speak different languages. In this case it is necessary to obtain information through a third party, the interpreter. When an interpreter is used, the same guidelines for interviewing are used. Specific guidelines for using an adult interpreter are presented in the Guidelines box on p. 192. More detailed information is provided in the article by Buchwald and others (1993).

Communicating with families through an interpreter requires sensitivity to cultural, legal, and ethical considerations. For example, in some cultures using a child as an interpreter is considered an insult to an adult, because children are expected to show respect by not questioning their elders. In some cultures class differences between the interpreter and the family may cause the family to feel intimidated and less inclined to offer information. Therefore, choose the translator carefully and provide time for the interpreter and family to establish rapport (Sloat and Matsuura, 1990).

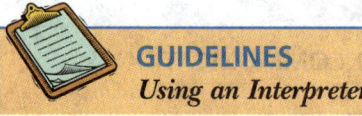

GUIDELINES
Using an Interpreter

Explain to interpreter the reason for the interview and the type of questions that will be asked.
Clarify whether a detailed or brief answer is required and whether the translated response can be general or literal.
Introduce interpreter to family and allow some time before the actual interview so that they can become acquainted.
Communicate directly with family members when asking questions to reinforce interest in them and to observe nonverbal expressions, but do not ignore interpreter.
Pose questions to elicit only one answer at a time, such as "Do you have have pain?" rather than "Do you have any pain, tiredness, or loss of appetite?"
Refrain from interrupting family member and interpreter while they are conversing.
Avoid commenting to interpreter about family members, since they may understand some English.
Be aware that some medical words, such as "allergy," may have no similar word in another language; avoid medical jargon whenever possible.
Respect cultural differences; it is often best to pose questions about sex, marriage, or pregnancy indirectly—ask about "child's father" rather than "mother's husband."
Allow time following the interview for interpreter to share something that he or she felt could not be said earlier; ask about interpreter's impression of nonverbal clues to communication and family members' reliability or ease in revealing information.
Arrange for family to speak with same interpreter on subsequent visits whenever possible.

Issues of legal and ethical concerns may also arise. For example, in obtaining informed consent through an interpreter, it is important that the family be fully informed of all aspects of the particular procedure that they are consenting to. Issues of confidentiality may arise when family members related to another patient are asked to interpret for the family, thus revealing sensitive information that may be shared with other families on the unit.

When no one else is available to translate, children within the family are often asked to assume this role. In this situation it is important to stress *literal* translation of parent responses. To maximize correct translations, it may be necessary to interrupt the parent and ask the child to translate every few sentences. When using children as interpreters, ask questions directed at specific answers and assess the interpreted translation in terms of nonverbal expressions of communication.*

COMMUNICATING WITH CHILDREN

Although the greatest amount of verbal communication may usually be carried out with the parent, do not exclude the child during the interview. Pay attention to infants and younger children through play or by occasionally directing questions or remarks to them. Include older children as active participants.

In communication with children of all ages, the nonverbal components of the communication process convey the most significant messages. It is difficult to disguise feelings, attitudes, and anxiety when relating to children. They are very alert to surroundings and attach meaning to every gesture and move that is made. This is particularly true with very young children.

Active attempts to make friends with children before they have had an opportunity to evaluate an unfamiliar person tend to increase their anxiety. A helpful tactic is to continue to talk to the child and parent but go about activities that do not involve the child directly, thus allowing the child to observe from a safe position. If the child has a special toy or doll, "talk" to the doll first. Ask simple questions such as "Does your teddy bear have a special name?" to ease the child into conversation. Other guidelines for communicating with children are presented in the Guidelines box on p. 193. Specific guidelines for preparing children for procedures, a common nursing function, are discussed in Chapter 27.

Communication Related to Development of Thought Processes

The normal development of language and thought offers a frame of reference in knowing how to communicate with children. Thought processes progress from concrete to functional and finally to abstract, formal operations.

Infancy. Because they are unable to use words, infants primarily use and understand nonverbal communication. Infants communicate their needs and feelings through nonverbal behaviors and vocalizations that can be interpreted by someone who is around them for a sufficient amount of time. Infants smile and coo when content and cry when distressed. Crying is provoked by unpleasant stimuli from inside or outside, such as hunger, pain, body restraint, or loneliness. Adults interpret this to mean that an infant needs something and consequently try to alleviate the discomfort and reduce tension. Crying (or the desire to cry) persists as a part of everyone's communication repertoire.

Infants respond to adults' nonverbal behaviors. They become quiet when they are cuddled, patted, or receive other forms of gentle, physical contact. They derive comfort from the sound of a voice, even though they do not understand the words that are spoken. Until infants reach the age at which they experience stranger anxiety, they readily respond to any firm, gentle handling and quiet, calm speech. Loud, harsh sounds and sudden movements are frightening.

Older infants' attentions are centered on themselves and their parents; therefore any stranger is a potential threat until proved otherwise. Holding out the hands and asking the child to "come" is seldom successful, especially if the infant is with the parent. If infants must be handled, simply pick them up firmly without gestures. Observe the po-

*Interpreting services are also available through American Telephone and Telegraph (AT&T) by calling (800) 628-8486 or (800) 752-6096.

GUIDELINES
Communicating with Children

Allow children time to feel comfortable.
Avoid sudden or rapid advances, broad smiles, extended eye contact, or other gestures that may be seen as threatening.
Talk to the parent if child is initially shy.
Communicate through transition objects such as dolls, puppets, or stuffed animals before questioning a young child directly.
Give older children the opportunity to talk without the parents present.
Assume a position that is at eye level with child (Fig. 6-2).
Speak in a quiet, unhurried, and confident voice.
Speak clearly, be specific, use simple words, and short sentences.
State directions and suggestions *positively*.
Offer a choice only when one exists.
Be honest with children.
Allow them to express their concerns and fears.
Use a variety of communication techniques.

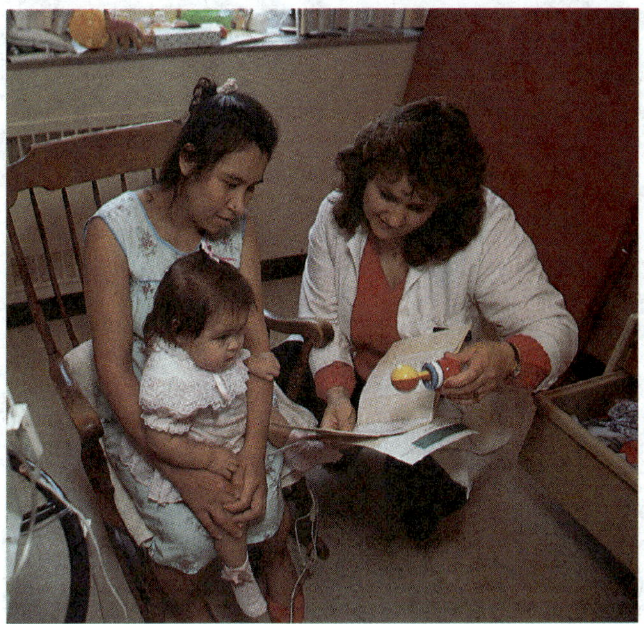

FIG. 6-2 Nurse assumes position at child's level.

sition in which the parent holds the infant. Most infants have learned to prefer a particular position and manner of handling. In general, infants are more at ease upright than horizontal. Also, hold infants so that they can see their parents. Until they have developed the understanding that an object (in this case the parent) removed from sight can still be present, they have no way of knowing that the object is still there.

Early Childhood. Children under 5 years of age are egocentric. They see things only in relation to themselves and from their point of view. Therefore focus communication on *them*. Tell them what they can do or how they will feel. Experiences of others are of no interest to them. It is futile to use another child's experience as an attempt to gain the cooperation of very small children. Allow them to touch and examine articles that will come in contact with them. A stethoscope bell will feel cold; palpating a neck might tickle. Although they have not yet acquired sufficient language skills to express their feelings and wants, toddlers are able to communicate effectively with their hands to transmit ideas without words. They push an unwanted object away, pull another person to show them something, point, and cover the mouth that is saying something they do not wish to hear.

Everything is direct and concrete to small children. They are unable to work with abstractions and interpret words literally. Analogies escape them because they are unable to separate fact from fantasy. For example, they attach literal meaning to such common phrases as "two-faced," "sticky fingers," or "coughing your head off." Children who are told they will get "a little stick in the arm" may not be able to envision an injection (Fig. 6-3). Therefore avoid using a phrase that might be misinterpreted by a small child (see Guidelines box under Preparation for Procedures, Chapter 27).

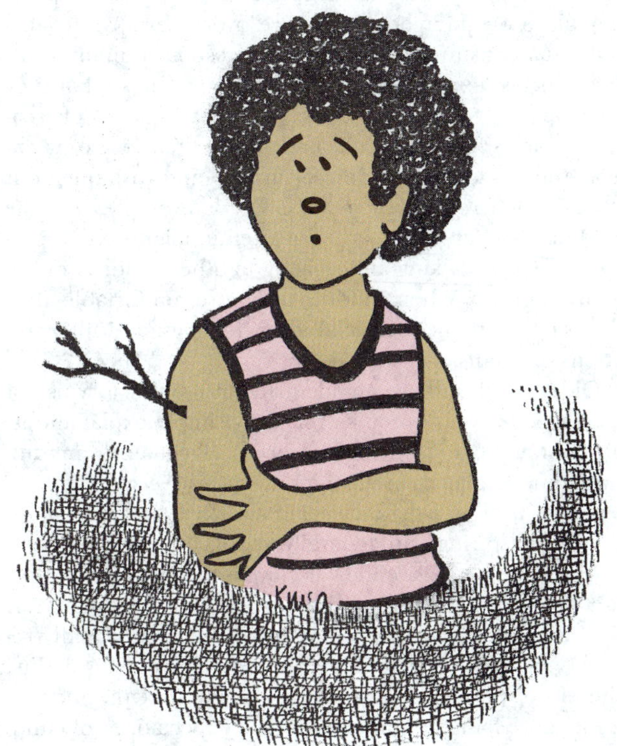

FIG. 6-3 To a young child the expression "a little stick in the arm" is taken literally.

Use language that is consistent with the child's developmental level. For example, in talking with a toddler, use simple, *short* sentences, repeat words that are *familiar* to the child, and limit descriptions to *concrete* explanations. Be certain that nonverbal messages are consistent with words and actions. For example, do not smile while doing something painful; children may think you enjoy hurting them.

Young children assign human attributes to inanimate objects. Consequently, they fear that objects may jump, bite, cut, or pinch all by themselves. Children do not know that these devices are unable to perform without human direction. To minimize their fear, keep unfamiliar equipment out of view until it is needed.

School-Age Years. Younger school-age children rely less on what they see and more on what they know when faced with new problems. They want explanations and reasons for everything but require no verification beyond that. They are interested in the functional aspect of all procedures, objects, and activities. They want to know why an object exists, why it is used, how it works, and the intent and purpose of its user. They need to know what is going to take place and why it is being done to *them* specifically. For example, to explain a procedure such as taking a blood pressure, show the child how squeezing the bulb pushes air into the cuff and makes the "silver" in the tube go up. Let the child operate the bulb. An explanation for the reason might be as simple as "I want to see how far the silver goes up when the cuff squeezes your arm." Consequently, the child becomes an enthusiastic participant.

School-age children have a heightened concern about body integrity. Because of the special importance and value they place on their body, they are overly sensitive to anything that constitutes a threat or suggestion of injury to it. This concern extends to their possessions also, so that they may appear to overreact to loss or threatened loss of treasured objects. Helping children to voice their concerns enables the nurse to provide reassurance and to implement activities that reduce their anxiety. For example, if a shy child dislikes being the center of attention, ignore that particular child by talking and relating to other children in the family or group. When children feel more comfortable, they will usually interject personal ideas, feelings, and interpretations of events.

Older children have an adequate and satisfactory use of language. They still require relatively simple explanations, but their ability to think concretely can facilitate communication and explanation. Commonly they have sufficient experience with health and health workers to understand what is transpiring and generally what is expected of them.

Adolescence. As children move into adolescence, they fluctuate between child and adult thinking and behavior. They are riding a current that is moving them rapidly toward a maturity that may be beyond their coping ability. Therefore, when tensions rise, they may seek the security of the more familiar and comfortable expectations of childhood. Anticipating these shifts in identity allows the nurse to adjust the course of interaction to meet the needs of the moment. No single approach can be relied on consistently, and encountering cooperation, hostility, anger, bravado, and a variety of other behaviors and attitudes can be expected. It is as much a mistake to regard the adolescent as an adult with an adult's wisdom and control as it is to confine to the teenager the concerns and expectations of a child.

Frequently adolescents are more willing to discuss their concerns with an adult outside the family, and they often welcome the opportunity to interact with a nurse. They are accepting of anyone who displays a genuine interest in them. However, adolescents are quick to reject persons who attempt to impose their values on them, whose interest is feigned, or who appear to have little respect for who they are and what they think or say.

As with all children, adolescents need to express their feelings. Generally, they talk quite freely when given an opportunity. However, what adolescents say cannot always be taken at face value. When emotional factors are involved, the feelings that are interjected into words are as significant as the words that are used. To give support, be attentive, try not to interrupt, and avoid comments or expressions that convey disapproval or surprise. Avoid prying and asking embarrassing questions, and resist any impulse to give advice. Frequently adolescents reveal their feelings or a source of concern or ask a question when they are involved in routine matters such as a physical assessment.

Teenagers characteristically have a language and culture all their own that further sets them apart. To avoid misinterpretation, clarify terms frequently. Occasionally adolescents refuse to answer or answer only in monosyllables. Usually this happens when they are opposed to the contact or do not yet feel safe enough to reveal themselves. In this instance confine discussions to irrelevant topics to reduce the element of threat until such time as they feel more secure. Be alert for signals indicating they are ready to talk. The major sources of concern for adolescents are attitudes and feelings toward sex, substance abuse, relationships with parents, peer-group acceptance, and developing a sense of identity.

Interviewing the adolescent presents some special situations. The first may be whether to talk with the adolescent alone, with the adolescent and parents together, or with each individually. Of course, if the adolescent is alone, there is no question, except whether to suggest to the teenager that the parents may be interviewed at another time. If the parents and teenager are together, talking with the adolescent first has the advantage of immediately identifying with the young person, thus fostering the interpersonal relationship. However, talking with the parents initially may provide insight into the family relationship. In either case, give both parties an opportunity to be included in the interview. If time constraints are important, such as during history taking, clarify these at the onset to avoid appearing to "take sides" by talking more with one person than with the other.

Confidentiality is of great important when interviewing adolescents. Explain to parents and teenagers the limits of confidentiality, specifically that young persons' disclosures will not be shared unless they indicate a need for intervention, as in the case of suicidal behavior.

Another dilemma in interviewing adolescents is that two

GUIDELINES
Communicating with Adolescents

BUILD A FOUNDATION

Spend time together.
Encourage expression of ideas and feelings.
Respect their views.
Tolerate differences.
Praise good points.
Respect their privacy.
Set a good example.

COMMUNICATE EFFECTIVELY

Give undivided attention.
Listen, listen, listen.
Be courteous, calm, and open-minded.
Try not to overreact. If you do, take a break.
Avoiding judging or criticizing.
Avoid the "third degree" of continuous questioning.
Choose important issues when taking a stand.
After taking a stand:
Think through all options.
Make expectations clear.

views of a problem frequently exist—the teenager's and the parents'. Clarification of the problem is a major task. However, providing both parties with an opportunity to discuss their perceptions in an open and unbiased atmosphere can, by itself, be therapeutic. Demonstrating positive communication skills can help families communicate more effectively (see Guidelines box).

COMMUNICATION TECHNIQUES

In addition to such conventional interviewing methods as reflection and open-ended questions, a number of techniques encourage family members to express their thoughts and feelings in a less directive and confrontational manner. Several approaches are projective—they present nonspecific material that enables individuals to externalize or project inner aspects of themselves to others.

A variety of verbal techniques can be used to encourage communication. Some of these techniques can be used to pose questions or explore concerns in a less threatening manner. Others can be presented as "word games," which are often well received by children. However, for many children and adults, talking about feelings is difficult and verbal communication may be more stressful than supportive. In such instances several nonverbal techniques can be used to encourage communication.

Both verbal and nonverbal techniques are described in the box on pp. 196-197. Because of the importance of play in communicating with children, play is discussed more extensively below. Any of the verbal or nonverbal techniques can give rise to strong feelings that surface unexpectedly. Be prepared to handle them or to recognize when issues go beyond your ability to deal with them. At that point, consider an appropriate referral.

Play. Play is a universal language of children. It is one of the most important forms of communication and can be an effective technique in relating to ' physical, intellectual, and social dev can often be gleaned from the form . child's play behaviors. Play requires a min. ment or none at all. Therapeutic play is often duce the trauma of illness and hospitalization (Chap. and to prepare children for therapeutic procedures (Cha ter 27).

Because their ability to perceive precedes their ability to transmit, small infants respond to activities that register on their senses. Patting, stroking, and other skin play convey messages. Repetitive actions, such as stretching infants' arms out to the side while they are lying on their back and then folding them across the chest or raising and revolving the legs in a bicycling motion, will elicit pleasurable sounds. Colorful items to catch the eye or interesting sounds such as a ticking clock, chimes, bells, or singing can be used to attract children's attention.

Older infants respond to simple games. The old game of peekaboo is an excellent means of initiating communication with infants while maintaining a "safe," nonthreatening distance. After this intermittent eye-to-eye contact, the nurse is no longer viewed as a stranger but as someone who is a friend. This can be followed by touch games. Clapping an infant's hands together for pat-a-cake or wiggling the toes for "this little piggy" delights an infant or small child. Much of the nursing assessment can be carried out with the use of games and simple play equipment while the infant remains in the safety of the parent's arms or lap. Talking to a foot or other part of the child's body is an effective tactic.

The nurse can capitalize on the natural curiosity of small children by playing games such as "Which hand do you take?" and "Guess what I have in my hand" or by manipulating items such as a flashlight or stethoscope. Finger games are very useful. More elaborate materials, such as puppets and replicas of familiar or unfamiliar items, serve as excellent means to communicate with small children (see Fig. 6-2). The variety and extent are limited only by the nurse's imagination.

Through play children reveal their perceptions of interpersonal relationships with their family, friends, or hospital personnel. Children may also reveal the wide scope of knowledge they have acquired from listening to others around them. For example, through needle play, children may disclose how carefully they have watched each procedure by precisely duplicating the technical skills. They may also reveal how well they remember those who performed procedures. One child who painstakingly reenacted every detail of a tedious medical procedure also played the role of the physician who had repeatedly shouted at her to be still for the long ordeal. Her anger at him was most evident during the play session and revealed the cause for her abrupt withdrawal and passive hostility toward the medical and nursing staff following the test.

Play sessions serve not only as assessment tools for determining children's awareness and perception of their illness but also as methods of intervention and evaluation. In the previous example, when the child revealed anger toward

CREATIVE COMMUNICATION TECHNIQUES WITH CHILDREN

VERBAL TECHNIQUES

"I" Messages

Relate a feeling about a behavior in terms of "I."
Describe effect behavior had on the person.
Avoid use of "you."
"You" messages are judgmental and provoke defensiveness.
Example: "You" message—"You are being very uncooperative about doing your treatments."
Example: "I" message—"I am concerned about how the treatments are going because I want to see you get better."

Third-Person Technique

Involves expressing a feeling in terms of a third person ("he," "she," "they").
Is less threatening than directly asking children how they feel because it gives them an opportunity to agree or disagree without being defensive.
Example: "Sometimes when a person is sick a lot, he feels angry and sad because he cannot do what others can." Either wait silently for a response or encourage a reply with a statement such as "Did you ever feel that way?"
Approach allows children three choices: (1) to agree and, hopefully, express how they feel; (2) to disagree; or (3) to remain silent, in which case they probably have such feelings but are unable to express them at this time.

Facilitative Responding

Involves careful listening and reflecting back to patients the feelings and content of their statements.
Responses are empathic and nonjudgmental, and legitimize the person's feelings.
Formula for facilitative responses: "You feel ____________ because ____________" (Henrich and Bernheim, 1981).
Example: If child states, "I hate coming to the hospital and getting needles," a facilitative response is, "You feel unhappy because of all the things that are done to you."

Storytelling

Uses the language of children to probe into areas of their thinking while bypassing conscious inhibitions or fears.
Simplest technique is asking children to relate a story about an event, such as "being in the hospital."
Other approaches:
Show children a picture of a particular event, such as a child in a hospital with other people in the room, and ask them to describe the scene.
Cut out comic strips, remove words, and have child add statements for scenes (Fig. 6-4).

Mutual Storytelling

Reveals child's thinking and attempts to change child's perceptions or fears by retelling a somewhat different story (more therapeutic approach than storytelling).
Begins by asking child to tell a story about something, followed by another story told by the nurse that is similar to child's tale but with differences that help child in problem areas.
Example: Child's story is about going to the hospital and never seeing his or her parents again. Nurse's story is also about a child (using different names but similar circumstances) in a hospital whose parents visit everyday, but in the evening after work until the child is better and goes home with them.

Bibliotherapy

Uses books in a therapeutic and supportive process.*
Provides children with an opportunity to explore an event that is similar to their own but sufficiently different to allow them to distance self from it and remain in control.
General guidelines for using bibliotherapy are:
Assess child's emotional and cognitive development in terms of readiness to understand the book's message.
Be familiar with the book's content (intended message or purpose) and the age for which it is written.
Read the book to the child if child is unable to read.
Explore the meaning of the book with the child by having child:
Retell the story
Read a special section with the nurse or parent
Draw a picture related to the story and discuss the drawing
Talk about the characters
Summarize the moral or meaning of the story

Dreams

Often reveal unconscious and repressed thoughts and feelings.
Ask child to talk about a dream or nightmare.
Explore with child what meaning dream could have.

"What If" Questions

Encourage child to explore potential situations and to consider different problem-solving options.
Example: "What if you got sick and had to go the hospital?" Children's responses reveal what they know already and what they are curious about; provide opportunity for helping children learn coping skills, especially in potentially dangerous situations.

Three Wishes

Involves asking, "If you could have any three things in the world, what would they be?"
If child answers, "That all my wishes come true," ask child for specific wishes.

Rating Game

Uses some type of rating scale (numbers, sad to happy faces) to rate an event or feeling.
Example: Instead of asking youngsters how they feel, ask how their day has been "on a scale of 1 to 10, with 10 being the best."

Word Association Game

Involves stating key words and asking children to say the first word they think of when they hear the word.
Start with neutral words and then introduce more anxiety-producing words, such as "illness," "needles," "hospitals," and "operation."
Select key words that relate to some event in child's life that is relevant.

Sentence Completion

Involves presenting a partial statement and having child complete it.
Some sample statements are:
The thing I like best (least) about school is ____________.
The best (worst) age to be is ____________.
The most (least) fun thing I ever did was ____________.
The thing I like most (least) about my parents is ________.
The one thing I would change about my family is ________.

*See resources for children's books in Bibliography at end of chapter.

CREATIVE COMMUNICATION TECHNIQUES WITH CHILDREN—cont'd

If I could be anything I wanted, I would be ______.

The thing I like most (least) about myself is ______.

Pros and Cons

Involves selecting a topic, such as "being in the hospital," and having child list "five good things and five bad things" about it.

Is an exceptionally valuable technique when applied to relationships, such as things family members like and dislike about each other.

NONVERBAL TECHNIQUES

Writing

Is an alternative communication approach for older children and adults.

Specific suggestions include:
- Keep a journal or diary.
- Write down feelings or thoughts that are difficult to express.
- Write "letters" that are never mailed (a variation is making up a "pen pal" to write to).
- Keep an account of child's progress from both a physical and an emotional viewpoint.

Drawing

Is one of the most valuable forms of communication—both nonverbal (from looking at the drawing) and verbal (from child's story of the picture).

Children's drawings tell a great deal about them because they are projections of their inner selves.

Spontaneous drawing involves giving child a variety of art supplies and providing the opportunity to draw.

Directed drawing involves a more specific direction, such as "draw a person" or the "three themes" approach (state three things about child and ask child to choose one and draw a picture) (Fig. 6-5).

Guidelines for evaluating drawings

Use spontaneous drawings and evaluate more than one drawing whenever possible.

Interpret drawings in light of other available information about child and family.

Interpret drawings as a whole rather than on specific details of the drawing.

Consider individual elements of the drawing that may be significant:
- ***Sex of figure drawn first***—Usually relates to child's perception of own sex role.
- ***Size of individual figures***—Expresses importance, power, or authority.
- ***Order in which figures are drawn***—Expresses priority in terms of importance.
- ***Child's position in relation to other family members***—Expresses feelings of status or alliance.
- ***Exclusion of a member***—May denote feeling of not belonging or desire to eliminate.
- ***Accentuated parts***—Usually express concern for areas of special importance (e.g., large hands may be a sign of aggression).
- ***Absence of or rudimentary arms and hands***—Suggest timidity, passivity, or intellectual immaturity; tiny, unstable feet may be an expression of insecurity, and hidden hands may mean guilt feelings.
- ***Placement of drawing on the page and type of stroke***—Free use of paper and firm, continuous strokes express security, whereas drawings restricted to a small area and lightly drawn in broken or wavering lines may be a sign of insecurity.
- ***Erasures, shading, or cross-hatching***—Expresses ambivalence, concern, or anxiety with a particular area.

Magic

Uses simple magic tricks to help establish rapport with child, encourage compliance with health interventions, and provide effective distraction during painful procedures.

Although "magician" talks, no verbal response from child is required.

Play

Is universal language and "work" of children.

Tells a great deal about children because they project their inner selves through the activity.

Spontaneous play involves giving child a variety of play materials and providing the opportunity to play.

Directed play involves a more specific direction, such as providing medical equipment or a dollhouse for focused reasons, such as exploring child's fear of injections or exploring family relationships.

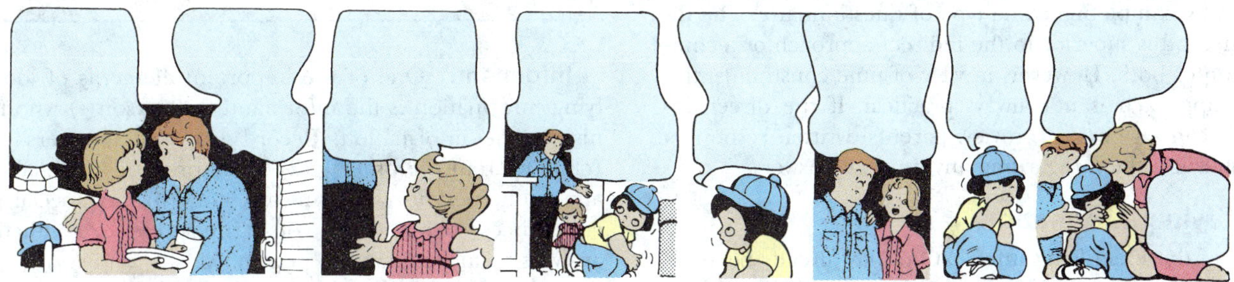

FIG. 6-4 Filling in the blanks on a comic strip is an effective communication technique with older children.

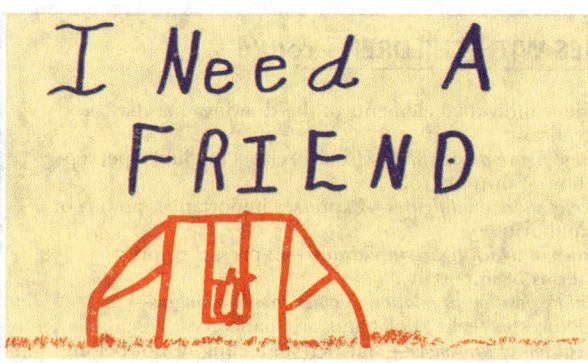

FIG. 6-5 Using the three themes approach, this child chose the theme, "the first day of school." The drawing and title reveal the child's loneliness and insecurity in a new setting.

the physician, the nurse acted the part of the patient but this time did not accept the physician's harsh commands to stay still. Instead the nurse said to the physician all the things the child had wished she could say.

Subsequent play sessions can also be used for evaluation of the child's progress. A change in the type of drawing or the theme of the play may indicate progression toward or away from the ability to deal with anxiety.

HISTORY TAKING

This section deals with interviewing as it relates to the health history. The precise depth and extent of a nursing history vary with its intended purpose. Judgment is used in deciding what data are necessary and relevant for the identification of problems or concerns.

The format used resembles a medical history, but the objective of each assessment area is the identification of nursing diagnoses. The value in following this well-established approach is that it is systematic and familiar to members of the health team. The categories listed in the box on the right encompass children's current and past health status and information about their psychosocial environment.

PERFORMING A HEALTH HISTORY

The format used for history taking may be (1) ***direct***—the nurse asks for information via direct interview with the informant—or (2) ***indirect***—the informant supplies the information by completing some type of questionnaire. The direct method is superior to the indirect approach or a combination of both. However, in view of time constraints, the direct approach is not always practical. If the direct approach cannot be used, review parents' written responses and question them regarding any unusual answers.

Identifying Information

Much of the identifying information may already be available from other recorded sources. However, if the parent and youngster seem anxious, use this opportunity to ask about such information to help them feel more comfortable.

OUTLINE OF A PEDIATRIC HEALTH HISTORY

Identifying information
1. Name
2. Address
3. Telephone
4. Birthdate and place
5. Race/ethnic group
6. Sex
7. Religion
8. Date of interview
9. Informant

Chief complaint (CC)—To establish the major *specific* reason for the child's and parents' seeking professional health attention

Present illness (PA)—To obtain *all* details related to the chief complaint

Past history (PH)—To elicit a profile of the child's previous illnesses, injuries, or operations
1. Birth history (pregnancy, labor, and delivery, perinatal history)
2. Previous illnesses, injuries, or operations
3. Allergies
4. Current medications
5. Immunizations
6. Growth and development
7. Habits

Review of systems (ROS)—To elicit information concerning any potential health problem
1. General
2. Integument
3. Head
4. Eyes
5. Ears
6. Nose
7. Mouth
8. Throat
9. Neck
10. Chest
11. Respiratory
12. Cardiovascular
13. Gastrointestinal
14. Genitourinary
15. Gynecologic
16. Musculoskeletal
17. Neurologic
18. Endocrine

Family medical history—To identify the presence of genetic traits or diseases that have familial tendencies and to assess exposure to a communicable disease in a family member and family habits that may affect the child's health, such as smoking and other chemical use

Psychosocial history—To elicit information about the child's self-concept

Sexual history—To elicit information concerning the child's sexual concerns and/or activities and any pertinent data regarding adults' sexual activity that influence the child

Family history—To develop an understanding of the child as an individual and as a member of a family and a community
1. Family composition
2. Home and community environment
3. Occupation and education of family members
4. Cultural and religious traditions
5. Family function and relationships

Nutritional assessment—To elicit information on the adequacy of the child's nutritional intake and need
1. Dietary intake
2. Clinical examination

Informant. One of the important elements of identifying information is the informant, the person(s) who furnished the information. Record (1) who the person is (child, parent, or other), (2) an impression of reliability and willingness to communicate, and (3) any special circumstances, such as the use of an interpreter or conflicting answers by more than one person.

Assessing reliability is one of the more important judgments to make. A totally reliable informant will always give the same correct answers to questions. Be cautious about accepting vague, confused, or contradictory responses to questions. Ask for clarification as needed and make a note in the written record about the informant, such as "Mother, reliability questionable, answers items with hesitation, speaks primarily Spanish, interpreter (Mrs.________) present for history."

Chief Complaint

The chief complaint is the specific reason for the child's visit to the clinic, office, or hospital. Six guidelines determine appropriate recording of the chief complaint: it should (1) consist of a brief statement, (2) be restricted to one or two symptoms, (3) refer to a concrete complaint, (4) be recorded in the child's or parent's own words, (5) avoid the use of diagnostic terms or translations, and (6) state the duration of the symptoms.

Elicit the chief complaint by asking open-ended, neutral questions, such as "Tell me what seems to be the matter," "How may I help you?" or "Why did you come here today?" Avoid labeling-type questions, such as "How are you sick?" or "What is the problem?" since the reason for the visit may not be an illness or a problem. For example, the visit may be for a routine health assessment, or the chief complaint may be of a nonphysical nature. If the visit is for a well-child examination, ask, "Before we begin, is there anything of particular concern that you would like to discuss?" to encourage the parent (or child) to bring up an issue that may not surface during routine interviewing.

Occasionally it is difficult to isolate one symptom or problem as the chief complaint because the parent may identify many. In this situation be as specific as possible when asking questions. For example, ask parents to identify which *one* problem or symptom caused them to seek help *now.*

Present Illness

The history of the present illness* is a narrative of the chief complaint from its earliest onset through its progression to the present. The four major components are (1) details of *onset,* (2) complete *interval* history (from onset to present), (3) *present* status, and (4) reason for seeking help *now.* The focus of the present illness is on all factors that are relevant to the main problem, even if they have disappeared or changed during the onset, interval, and present status of the complaint.

Analyzing a Symptom. Because pain is often the most characteristic symptom denoting the onset of a physical problem, it is used as an example for analysis of a symptom. Assessment includes (1) type, (2) location, (3) severity, (4) duration, and (5) influencing factors (see Guidelines box; see also Pain Assessment, Chapter 26).

Determining the Reason for Seeking Help. The preceding discussion deals primarily with a description of the problem. However, since most chief complaints have a "duration," it follows that something significant must have occurred to motivate the person to seek help at this time. Such factors may be a change in physical status, a change in behavioral reaction, or a result of social pressure. Eliciting such information may alter the possible nursing diagnosis and plan of care. The following example illustrates the potential significance of determining why a person seeks help at a particular time:

> **Chief complaint:** "I can't control my son. It's always been a problem, but for the past year and a half it has become worse."
>
> **Present history:** Child has had temper tantrums since infancy. He "throws things, hits and kicks people, yells and screams." It occurs whenever he "doesn't get his way." They usually last "a minute or two" and occur almost daily. Mother has responded to them in a variety of ways: hits him, ignores him, takes a special object or privilege away, or insults him. Nothing seems to work. Mother admits that ignoring the behavior is the most difficult approach, and she rarely can do so without eventually hitting or scolding him. Mother is not able to identify why she sought help now.

Further physical history revealed nothing unusual. However, the family history disclosed several significant facts, especially that (1) the father had died 2 months earlier, and (2) he had been ill for 1½ years before his death. The nurse focused the history on events that had occurred since the beginning of the father's illness, which coincided with the son's increased behavior problems. The mother revealed that during her husband's illness she had had too little time to concern herself with her son's behavior, other than real-

GUIDELINES
Analyzing the Symptom: Pain

Type—Be as specific as possible. With young children, asking the parents how they know the child is in pain may help describe its type, location, and severity. For example, a parent may state, "My child must have a severe earache because she pulls at her ears, rolls her head on the floor, and screams. Nothing seems to help." Help older children describe the "hurt" by asking them if it is sharp, throbbing, dull, aching, or stabbing. Record whatever words they use in quotes.

Location—Be specific. "Stomach pains" is too general a description. Children can better localize the pain if they are asked to "point with one finger to where it hurts" or to "point to where Mommy or Daddy would put a Band-Aid." Determine if the pain radiates by asking, "Does the pain stay there or move? Show me with your finger where the pain goes."

Severity—Best determined by finding out how it affects the child's usual behavior. Pain that prevents a child from playing, interacting with others, sleeping, and eating is most often severe. Assess pain intensity using a rating scale, such as a numeric scale or faces scale (see Table 26-2).

Duration—Include the duration, onset, and frequency. Describe this in terms of activity and behavior, such as "pain lasted all night, because child refused to sleep and cried intermittently."

Influencing factors—Include anything that causes a change in the type, location, severity, or duration of the pain: (1) precipitating events (those that cause or increase the pain), (2) relieving events (those that lessen the pain, such as medications), (3) temporal events (times when the pain is relieved or increased), (4) positional events (standing, sitting, lying down), and (5) associated events (meals, stress, coughing).

---

*NOTE: The term *illness* is used in its broadest sense to denote any problem or concern of a physical, emotional, or psychosocial nature. It is actually a history of the chief complaint.

izing that it was a problem. However, after her husband's death she could no longer ignore the severity of her son's behavior or its disruptive effect on the family. As she verbalized these thoughts, she began to identify the specific reason for seeking help now. She stated, "I used to wait for my husband to come home to take the children off my hands. When he was sick, I was too busy worrying about him. But now I am home all alone. When dinnertime comes, there is no one to relieve me."

Although the interventions included several approaches to managing the problem, one of them focused on providing the mother with some freedom from the responsibility of total parenting. Had the nurse not concentrated on uncovering the mother's reason for seeking help at this particular time, a very important clue in planning care might have been missed.

Past History

The past history contains information relating to all previous aspects of the child's health status and concentrates on several areas that are ordinarily deleted in the history of an adult, such as the birth history, a detailed feeding history, immunizations, and growth and development. Since a large amount of data is included in this section, use a combination of open-ended and fact-finding questions. For example, begin interviewing for each section with an open-ended statement, such as "Tell me about your child's birth," to provide informants with the opportunity to relate what they think is most important. Ask fact-finding questions related to specific details whenever necessary to focus the interview on certain topics.

Birth History. The birth history includes all data concerning (1) the mother's health during pregnancy, (2) the labor and delivery, and (3) the infant's condition immediately after birth. The extent of the history depends on the child's age—the younger the child, the more detailed the birth history. With older children, parents may question the relevance of inquiry regarding pregnancy and birth. A response that addresses this concern is, "I will be asking you some questions about your pregnancy and ____________'s (refer to child by name) birth. Your answers will give me a more complete picture of his (her) overall health."

Pregnancy, labor, and delivery. An obstetric history begins with an overview of the pregnancy, preferably by an open-ended question, such as "How was your pregnancy?" This allows the mother to state what she considered most significant. Most important, ask about the use of medications or other remedies that the mother used to relieve physical symptoms.

Basic information in an obstetric history includes maternal age, number of pregnancies (gravida), outcome of pregnancies (parity), length of gestation, and any complications. (For a more detailed obstetric history refer to maternity texts.) Because emotional factors also affect the outcome of pregnancy and the subsequent parent-child relationship, it is important to investigate (1) concurrent crises during pregnancy and (2) prenatal attitudes toward the fetus.

The topic of parental acceptance of pregnancy is best approached through indirect questioning. Asking parents if the pregnancy was planned is a leading statement because they may respond affirmatively for fear of criticism if the pregnancy was unexpected. Rather, encourage parents to disclose their true reactions by referring to specific facts relating to the pregnancy, such as the spacing between offspring, an extended or short interval between marriage and conception, or the concurrent experience of pregnancy and adolescence. The parent can choose to explore such statements with further explanations or, for the moment, may not be able to reveal such feelings. If the parent remains silent, reintroduce this topic later in the interview.

Perinatal history. The perinatal period is the time from birth to 27 days of life, but the primary focus is on the immediate period after birth and during hospitalization. Specific data include (1) weight and length at birth; (2) loss of weight following delivery; (3) time of regaining birth weight; (4) condition of health immediately after birth, such as quality of cry, level of activity (feeble or vigorous), and color of skin; (5) Apgar score (some parents may be aware of this); and (6) possible problems, such as fever, convulsions, hemorrhage, snuffles, skin eruptions, desquamation, paralysis, birth injuries, deformities, or congenital anomalies.

Dietary History. Because parental concerns related to eating are so common and nursing interventions to ensure optimal nutrition so important, the dietary history is discussed separately toward the end of this chapter under Nutritional Assessment.

Previous Illnesses, Injuries, and Surgeries. When inquiring about past illnesses, begin with a general statement, such as "What other illness has your child had?" Since parents are most likely to recall serious health problems, specifically ask about colds, earaches, and common childhood diseases, such as measles, rubella (German measles), chickenpox, mumps, pertussis (whooping cough), diphtheria, scarlet fever, strep throat, tonsillitis, or allergic manifestations. Encourage parents to indicate the onset, symptoms, course, and termination. It is not uncommon for parents to confuse measles with rubella or strep throat with tonsillitis.

In addition to illnesses, ask questions about injuries that required medical intervention, operations, and any other reason for hospitalization, including dates of each incident. It is important to focus on injuries such as falls, poisonings, choking, or burns, since these may be potential areas for parental guidance. While obtaining a history of the injury, inquire about events before the injury (who was the child with, where were the parents, had this ever happened before), as well as the parent's immediate action.

Inquiries about the child's emotional reactions to each experience are important. For example, one mother stated that her 4-year-old daughter had recently been admitted to the hospital for respiratory distress and had become very afraid of medical personnel, procedures, and equipment. The nurse realized from this information that the child needed special preparation for the physical examination.

Allergies. Ask about commonly known allergic disorders, such as hay fever and asthma, as well as unusual reactions to drugs, food, latex products (see section on therapeutic management under Myelomeningocele [Meningomyelocele], Chapter 11) or other contact agents, such as

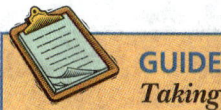

GUIDELINES
Taking a Drug Allergy History

Ask the following questions:
- Are you allergic to any medication? If yes, what is (are) the medication(s) you are allergic to?
- What dosage form did you take?
- What type of reaction did you have?
- How soon after the therapy was started did this occur?
- How long ago did the reaction occur?
- Who told you that it was an allergic reaction?
- Have you taken this drug or other drugs of similar class after this reaction occurred? If yes, did you experience similar problems?

From Pau A, Morgan J, Terlingo A: Drug allergy documentation by physicians, nurses and medical students, *Am J Hosp Pharm* 46(3):570-573, 1989.

poisonous plants, animals, household products, or fabrics. If asked appropriate questions, most people can give reliable information about drug reactions (see Guidelines box).

NURSING ALERT Information about allergic reactions to drugs is essential. Failure to document a serious reaction places the child at risk if the drug is given; misdiagnosing a reaction as a serious allergy may deprive the child of effective treatment.

Current Medications. Inquire about current drug regimens, including vitamins, antipyretics (especially aspirin), antibiotics, antihistamines, decongestants, or antitussives. List all medications, including name, dose, schedule, duration, and reason for administration. Not infrequently parents are unaware of the actual name of the drug. Whenever possible, ask parents to bring the containers with them to the next visit, or ask them for the name of the pharmacy and call for a list of all the child's recent prescription medications. However, this list will not include over-the-counter medications.

Immunizations. A record of all immunizations or "baby shots" is essential. Since many parents are unaware of the exact name and date of each immunization, the most reliable source of information is a hospital, clinic, or private physician's record. List all immunizations and "boosters," stating (1) the name of the specific disease, (2) the number of injections, (3) the dosage, if known (sometimes lesser amounts are given if a reaction is anticipated), (4) the ages when administered, and (5) the occurrence of any reaction following the immunization.

NURSING ALERT Inquire about previous administration of any horse or other foreign serum, recent administration of gamma globulin or blood transfusion, and anaphylactic reactions to neomycin or chicken eggs.

Growth and Development. Questions about growth and development are an essential part of the child's history. The American Academy of Pediatrics recommends developmental appraisal at each health visit (see Recommendations for Health Supervision, Chapter 7). Asking parents about

HABITS TO EXPLORE DURING HEALTH INTERVIEW

- Behavior patterns, such as nail-biting, thumb-sucking, pica (habitual ingestion of nonfood substances), rituals ("security" blanket or toy), and unusual movements (head-banging, rocking, overt masturbation, walking on toes)
- Activities of daily living, such as hour of sleep and arising, duration of nighttime sleep and naps, type and duration of exercise, regularity of stools and urination, age of toilet training, and occurrences of daytime or nighttime bed-wetting
- Unusual disposition, as well as response to frustration
- Use or abuse of alcohol, drugs, coffee, and cigarettes

their perception of the child's development is important because their concerns are good indicators that a problem exists (Glascoe, Altemeier, and MacLean, 1989). Whenever possible, parental responses are compared with existing health records or with current evaluation of actual growth (height, weight, dentition) and developmental performance (screening tests, grades in school, scholastic achievement, play activities, social relationships) (see Development Assessment, Chapter 7).

The most important previous growth patterns to record are (1) approximate weight at 6 months, 1 year, 2 years, and 5 years of age; (2) approximate length at 1 and 4 years; and (3) dentition, including age of onset, number of teeth, and symptoms during teething. Developmental milestones include (1) age of holding up head steadily, (2) age of sitting alone without support, (3) age of walking without assistance, and (4) age of saying first words with meaning.

Use specific and detailed questions when inquiring about developmental milestones. For example, "sitting up" can mean many different activities, such as sitting propped up, sitting in one's lap, sitting with support, sitting up alone but in a hyperflexed position for assisted balance, or sitting up unsupported with the back slightly rounded. The clue to misunderstanding of the requested activity is an unusually early age of achievement.

Probing the area of developmental or intellectual performance can be a delicate one for parents, especially if there is concern for the child's progress. Therefore approach such questioning with broad questions, such as "How is Jimmy doing in school?" rather than with qualifying statements, such as "Does Jimmy do well in school?" If the parents' response is vague and general, follow with questions such as "How does he do in spelling, reading, or math?" Since these questions are appropriate for older children, address them directly to the child, as well as to the parent, for comparison of responses and increased reliability.

Habits. Habits are an important area to explore (see box above). Parents frequently express concerns during this part of the history. Encourage their input by saying, "Please tell me any concerns you have about your child's habits, activities, or development." Investigate further any concerns that are expressed (Glascoe, MacLean, and Stone, 1991).

One of the most common concerns relates to sleep. Many children develop a normal sleep pattern, and all that

GUIDELINES
*Assessing Sleep Problems in Children**

GENERAL HISTORY OF CHIEF COMPLAINT

Ask parents/child to describe sleep problems; record in their words.
Inquire about onset, duration, character, frequency, and consistency of sleep problems:
- Circumstances surrounding onset (birth of sibling, start of toilet training, death of significant other, move from crib to bed)
- Circumstances that aggravate problem, i.e., overtiredness, family conflict, or disrupted routine (visitors)
- Remedies used to correct problem and results of interventions

24-HOUR SLEEP HISTORY

Time and regularity of meals†
- Family members present
  - Activities afterward, especially evening meal

Time of night and day sleep periods
- Hours of sleep and waking
- Hours of being put to bed and taken out of bed
  - How bedtime is decided (when child looks tired or at a time decided by parent; do both parents agree on bedtime?)

Prebedtime or nap rituals (bath, bottle- or breast-feeding, snack, television, active or quiet playing, story)
- Mood before nap or bedtime (wide awake, sleepy, happy, cranky)
- Which parent(s) participates in nap or bedtime rituals?

Nap and bedtime rituals
- Where is child allowed to fall asleep? (own bed or crib, couch, parent's bed, someone's lap, other)
- Is child helped to fall asleep? (rocked, walked, patted, given pacifier or bottle, placed in room with light, television, radio, or tape recorder on, other)
- Are patterns consistent each time, or do they vary?
- Does child awake if sleep aids are changed or taken away (placed in own bed, television turned off, other)?
- Does child verbally insist that parents stay in room?

Child's behaviors if refuses to go to sleep or stay in room
- If child complains of fears, how convincing are the fears?

Sleep environment
- Number of bedrooms
- Location of bedrooms, especially in relation to parent(s)' room
- Sensory features (light on, door open or closed, noise level, temperature)

Night wakings
- Time, frequency, and duration
- Child's behavior (call out, cry, come out of room, appear frightened, confused, or upset)
- Parent(s)' responses (let child cry, go in immediately, take to own bed, feed, pick up, rock, give pacifier, talk, scold, threaten, other)
- Conditions that reestablish sleep
  - Do they always work?
  - How long do the interventions take to work?
  - Which parent intervenes?
  - Do both parents use same or different approach?

Daytime sleepiness
- Occurrence of falling asleep at inappropriate times (circumstances, suddenness and irresistibility of onset, length of sleep, mood on awakening)
- Signs of fatigue (yawning, lying down, as well as overactivity, impulsivity, distractibility, irritability, temper tantrums)

PAST SLEEP HISTORY

Sleep patterns since infancy, especially age when slept during the night, stopped daytime naps, later bedtime
Response to changes in sleep arrangements (crib to bed, different room or house, other)
Sleep behaviors (restlessness, snoring, sleepwalking, nightmares, partial wakings [young child may wake confused, crying, and thrashing, but does not respond to parent; falls asleep with intervention if not excessively disturbed])
Parent(s)' perception of child's sleep habits (good or poor sleeper, light or deep sleeper, needs little sleep)
Family history of sleep problems (sibling behavior imitated by child; some sleep disorders, e.g., narcolepsy and enuresis, tend to recur in families)

Modified from Ferber R: Assessment procedures for diagnosis of sleep disorders in children. In Noshpitz J, editor: *Sleep disorders for the clinician,* London, 1987, Butterworths, pp. 185-193.
*Not all of these areas need to be assessed with every family. For example, if night wakings are not a problem, this section of the interview can be eliminated.
†A convenient point to start the 24-hour history is the evening meal.

is required during the assessment is a general overview of nighttime sleep and nap schedules. However, a number of children also develop sleep problems (see Sleep Problems, Chapters 12 and 15). When sleep problems occur, a more detailed sleep history is required in order to guide appropriate interventions (see Guidelines box).*

Habits related to use of chemicals apply primarily to older children and adolescents. If a youngster admits to smoking, drinking, or drug use, ask about the quantity and frequency. Questions such as "Have you ever had a drinking or drug problem?" or "When was the last time you had a drink or took drugs?" may yield more reliable data than questions such as "How much do you drink?" or "How often do you drink or take drugs?" (Cyr and Wartman, 1988). Clarify that "drinking" includes all types of alcohol, such as beer and wine. When quantities such as a "glass" of wine or a "can" of beer are given, ask about the size of the glass or can.

If older children deny use of chemical substances, inquire about past experimentation. Asking, "You mean you never tried to smoke or drink?" implies that the nurse expects some such activity, and the youngster may be more inclined to answer truthfully. Be aware of the confidential nature of such questioning, the adverse effect that the parents' presence may have on the adolescent's willingness to answer, and that self-report may not be an accurate account of chemical abuse (Zuckerman, Amaro, and Cabral, 1989).

Review of Systems

The review of systems is a specific review of each body system, similar to the order of the physical examination (see

*A sleep chart for the family to record the child's daily sleep and wake activities is available in *Wong and Whaley's Clinical Manual of Pediatric Nursing* (Mosby).

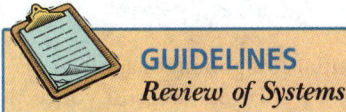

GUIDELINES
Review of Systems

General—Overall state of health, fatigue, recent and/or unexplained weight gain or loss (period of time for either), contributing factors (change of diet, illness, altered appetite), exercise tolerance, fevers (time of day), chills, night sweats (unrelated to climatic conditions), frequent infections, general ability to carry out activities of daily living

Integument—Pruritus, pigment or other color changes, acne, eruptions, rashes (location), tendency to bruising, petechiae, excessive dryness, general texture, disorders or deformities of nails, hair growth or loss, hair color change (for adolescent, use of hair dyes or other potentially toxic substances, such as hair straighteners)

Head—Headaches, dizziness, injury (specific details)

Eyes—Visual problems (ask about behaviors indicative of blurred vision, such as bumping into objects, clumsiness, sitting very close to the television, holding a book close to the face, writing with head near desk, squinting, rubbing the eyes, bending the head in an awkward position), cross-eye (strabismus), eye infections, edema of lids, excessive tearing, use of glasses or contact lenses, date of last optic examination

Nose—Nosebleeds (epistaxis), constant or frequent running or stuffy nose, nasal obstruction (difficulty in breathing), alteration or loss of sense of smell

Ears—Earaches, discharge, evidence of hearing loss (ask about behaviors such as need to repeat requests, loud speech, inattentive behavior), results of any previous auditory testing

Mouth—Mouth-breathing, gum bleeding, toothaches, toothbrushing, use of fluoride, difficulty with teething (symptoms), last visit to dentist (especially if temporary dentition is complete), response to dentist

Throat—Sore throats, difficulty in swallowing, choking (especially when chewing food—may be from poor chewing habits), hoarseness, or other voice irregularities

Neck—Pain, limitation of movement, stiffness, difficulty in holding head straight (torticollis), thyroid enlargement, enlarged nodes or other masses

Chest—Breast enlargement, discharge, masses, enlarged axillary nodes (for adolescent female, ask about breast self-examination)

Respiratory—Chronic cough, frequent colds (number per year), wheezing, shortness of breath at rest or on exertion, difficulty in breathing, sputum production, infections (pneumonia, tuberculosis), date of last chest x-ray examination, and skin reaction from tuberculin testing

Cardiovascular—Cyanosis or fatigue on exertion, history of heart murmur or rheumatic fever, anemia, date of last blood count, blood type, recent transfusion

Gastrointestinal—(Much of this in regard to appetite, food tolerance, and elimination habits has been asked elsewhere), nausea, vomiting (not associated with eating, may be indicative of brain tumor or increased intracranial pressure), jaundice or yellowing skin or sclera, belching, flatulence, recent change in bowel habits (blood in stools, change in color, diarrhea, and constipation)

Genitourinary—Pain on urination, frequency, hesitancy, urgency, hematuria, nocturia, polyuria, unpleasant odor to urine, force of stream, discharge, change in size of scrotum, date of last urinalysis (for adolescent, sexually transmitted disease, type of treatment; for male adolescent, ask about testicular self-examination)

Gynecologic—Menarche, date of last menstrual period, regularity or problems with menstruation, vaginal discharge, pruritus, date and result of last Pap smear (include obstetric history as discussed under birth history when applicable); if sexually active, type of contraception

Musculoskeletal—Weakness, clumsiness, lack of coordination, unusual movements, back or joint stiffness, muscle pains or cramps, abnormal gait, deformity, fractures, serious sprains, activity level

Neurologic—Seizures, tremors, dizziness, loss of memory, general affect, fears, nightmares, speech problems, any unusual habits

Endocrine—Intolerance to weather changes, excessive thirst and urination, excessive sweating, salty taste to skin, signs of early puberty

Guidelines box). Often the history of the present illness provides a complete review of the system involved in the chief complaint. Since asking questions about other body systems may appear unrelated and irrelevant to the parents or child, precede the questioning with an explanation of why the data are needed (similar to the explanation concerning the relevance of the birth history) and reassure the family that the child's main problem has not been forgotten.

Begin the review of a specific system with a broad statement, such as "How has your child's general health been?" or "Has your child had any problems with his eyes?" If the parent states that there have been past problems with some body function, pursue this with an encouraging statement, such as "Tell me more about that." If the parent denies any problems, ask further about specific symptoms, such as "No headaches, bumping into objects, or squinting?" If the parent reconfirms the absence of such symptoms, record positive statements in the history, such as "Mother denies child is having headaches, bumping into objects, or squinting." In this way, anyone who reviews the health history is aware of exactly what symptoms were investigated.

Family Medical History

The family medical history is used primarily for the purpose of discovering the potential existence of hereditary or familial diseases in the parents and child and family habits that may affect the child's health, such as smoking and other chemical use. In general, it is confined to first-degree relatives (parents, siblings, and grandparents and their children) and is more easily recorded using a pedigree chart or genogram (see Fig. 5-11). Information for each family member includes age, marital status, state of health if living, cause of death if deceased, and any evidence of the following conditions: heart disease, hypertension, hyperlipidemia (see Chapter 34), cancer, diabetes mellitus, obesity, congenital anomalies, allergy, asthma, tuberculosis, sickle cell disease, mental retardation, seizures, mental illness such as depression or psychosis, emotional problems, syphilis, or rheumatic fever. In the case of genetic diseases, inquire about the pattern of family transmission of the disorder (see Role of Nurses in Genetic Counseling and Referral, Chapter 5). Confirm the accuracy of the reported disorders by inquiring about the symptoms, course, treatment, and sequelae of each diagnosis.

Geographic Location. One of the important areas to explore when assessing the family health history is geographic location, including birthplace and travel to different areas in or outside of the country for identification of possible exposure to endemic diseases. Although the primary interest focuses on the child's temporary residence in various localities, also inquire about close family members' travel, especially during tours of military service or business trips. Children are especially susceptible to parasitic infestation in areas of poor sanitary conditions and to vector-borne diseases, such as those from mosquitoes or ticks in warm and humid or heavily wooded regions.

Psychosocial History

In the traditional health history a personal and social section is included that concentrates on children's personal status, such as school adjustment and any unusual habits, and on the family and home environment. Since several personal aspects are covered earlier under Growth and Development and under Habits, and the social aspects are discussed in detail under Family Assessment, only those issues related to children's general view of themselves in terms of self-concept are presented here (see Development of Self-Concept, Chapter 4).

Through observation obtain a general idea of how children handle themselves in terms of confidence in dealing with others and ability to answer questions. Watch the parent-child relationship for the types of messages sent to children about their self-worth. Do the parents treat the child with respect, focusing on strengths, or is the interaction one of constant reprimands, with emphasis on the child's weaknesses and faults? Do the parents help the child learn new coping strategies or support the ones the child uses?

Messages about body image are also conveyed through the parent-child interaction. Does the parent label the child and body parts, such as "bad boy," "skinny legs," or "ugly scar?" Look at how the parent touches the child. Is the child handled gently, with soothing touch used to calm an anxious child, or is the child treated roughly, with slaps or restraint used to force compliance? When the child touches certain parts of the body, such as the genitals, does the parent make comments that suggest a negative connotation?

With older children, many of the communication strategies discussed earlier in the chapter are useful in eliciting more definitive information about their self-concept. Children can write down five things they like and dislike about themselves. Sentence completion statements, such as "The thing I like best (or worst) about myself is ________." or "If I could change one thing about myself it would be ________," can be used. Drawing offers numerous possibilities for offering insight. Children can draw a picture of an "ideal person" and then discuss how their characteristics are the same as or different from this portrait. Another activity is to have children make a collage using cutouts from magazines to represent themselves (Winkelstein, 1989). Through play with puppets, dolls, or stuffed animals, children can reveal how they relate to others, often reflecting their own self-image.

Sexual History

The sexual history is an essential component of adolescents' health assessment. The history uncovers areas of concern related to sexual activity, alerts the nurse to circumstances that may indicate screening for sexually transmitted diseases or testing for pregnancy, and provides information related to the need for sexual counseling, such as safe sex practices (Andrist, 1988).

One approach toward initiating a conversation about sexual concerns is to begin with a history of peer interactions. Open-ended statements, such as "Tell me about your social life," or "Who are your closest friends?" generally lead into a discussion of dating and sexual issues. To probe further, include questions about the adolescent's attitudes on such topics as sex education, "going steady," "living together," and premarital sex. Phrase questions to reflect concern and not judgment or criticism of sexual practices.

In any conversation regarding sexual history, be aware of the language that is used in either eliciting or conveying sexual information. Phrases such as "sexually active" have many meanings. For example, one adolescent denied being sexually active despite a positive pregnancy test. When asked again about whether or not she was sexually active, she denied the activity, stating that "I lie perfectly still during intercourse." "Are you having sex with anyone?" is suggested as the most direct and best understood question (Strasburger, 1986).

Other questions to ask adolescents include "Are you using any type of contraception? Why not? Have you discussed this relationship with your parents? If you did, what would their reaction be?" If teenagers deny sexual activity, it is just as important to discuss with them their concerns about not being sexually active as it is to discuss concerns with teenagers who are sexually active. Most teenagers tend to believe "Everyone is doing it but me," and this becomes a major issue for them (Strasburger, 1986). Since homosexual experimentation may occur, all sexual contacts should be referred to in nongender terms, such as "anyone" or "partners," rather than "girlfriends" or "boyfriends."

A detailed account of sexual partners is needed if the patient has a history of, displays any of the symptoms of, or asks for treatment of a sexually transmitted disease. A difficult but necessary part of the interview is to determine the sites of possible infection. Because sexual diseases can be contracted at any of the body orifices, inform the adolescent that a sexually transmitted disease can be acquired without visible signs of disease at nongenital sites, such as the mouth.

The degree of inquiry into the parents' sexual activity depends on many factors. For example, it may be limited to a brief discussion of their plans regarding future children or contraception. In instances in which overt adult sexual activity may be having an adverse effect on the children, a more detailed exploration of this area is warranted. Be sure to make this decision based on facts learned during the interview, since this line of questioning should never be meaningless prying. If parents ask the relevance of revealing such matters, be prepared to offer a sound and logical explanation. It is every person's right to refuse to disclose personal information, especially if not informed of its significance or value.

FAMILY ASSESSMENT

Assessment of the family, both its structure and function, is one of the most important components of the history. Because the quality of the functional relationship between the patient and family members is a major factor in emotional and physical health, family assessment is discussed separately and in greater detail apart from the more traditional health history.

Family assessment is the collection of data about the composition of the family and the relationships among its members. In its broadest sense ***family*** refers to all those individuals who are significant to the nuclear unit, including relatives, friends, and other social groups, such as the school and church (see also Chapter 3). While family assessment should not be confused with family therapy, it can and frequently is therapeutic. Involving family members in discussing family characteristics and activities often stimulates productive discussion and insight into family dynamics and relationships.

Because of the time involved in performing an in-depth family assessment as presented here, selectivity is needed in deciding what aspects to explore. During brief contacts with families a full assessment is not appropriate, and screening with one or two questions from each category may reflect the health of the family system or the potential need for additional assessment. Indications for initiating a comprehensive family assessment are presented in the Guidelines box.

In addition to the discussion of family assessment presented here, assessment issues specific to the family of a child with a chronic illness or disability are included in Chapter 22.

ASSESSMENT OF FAMILY STRUCTURE

Family structure refers to the composition of the family—who lives in the home and those social, cultural, religious, and economic characteristics that influence the child's and family's overall psychobiologic health (see also Chapters 2 and 3). Since the information elicited in this part of the history is often the most personal and confidential, include it toward the end of the interview when rapport is established. The most common method of eliciting information on family structure is interviewing family members (see box on p. 207). The principal areas of concern are (1) family composition, (2) home and community environment, (3) occupation and education of family members, and (4) cultural and religious traditions.

Family composition is primarily concerned with the immediate members of the household but should also include a review of the family's extended support system. For example, in a single-parent family, the household members may consist of the mother and two children, but the mother's parents may be very significant sources of child care and financial support. Although the interview method can be used to collect information about household members—their relationship, ages, and roles within the family, as well as significant individuals outside the family unit—other efficient methods include those discussed below.

In assessing family composition it is sometimes difficult to ascertain the status of the adult relationships. For example, the parent may fail to mention the other parent. In this case ask, "Where is the child's father (or mother)?" Avoid saying "husband" or "wife" because that precludes the existence of nonmarital relationships. If the parent states that the child's father (or mother) is not part of the household, explore this by inquiring about the absent parent's continued relationship with the child and the presence of any other significant male (or female) within the home. Also inquire about previous marriages, separations, death of spouses, or divorces. Ask about the children's reaction to any of these events, which usually have a tremendous effect on their general physical and emotional health.

Several structural assessment tools are valuable in collecting and recording data about family composition and environment. Like the interview method these tools also provide information about relationships, although several additional methods should be used to assess family function.

Tools that involve drawing have several advantages. They:

- Provide an immediate visual presentation of the family tree and extended support systems
- Yield extensive information in a short period of time
- Are easily updated
- May stimulate productive and meaningful communication among family members.

Additional tools involving drawing are discussed on p. 206 under Assessment of Family Function.

The ***genogram*** (family tree, family diagram) uses symbols to diagrammatically record data about family structure. It is a modification of the pedigree chart used in genetics to record the family medical history. Symbols often used in the genogram are presented in Fig. 5-10. Because there is no universal list of pedigree symbols, those used by other health professionals may differ. If in doubt regarding which symbol to use, or if one does not exist, write in the word describing the relationship, such as "foster child." Since the genogram is also concerned with the *strength* of family rela-

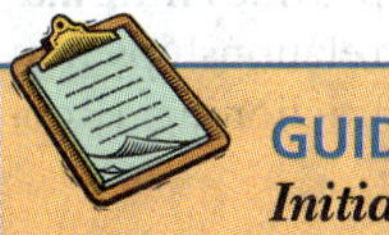

GUIDELINES
Initiating a Comprehensive Family Assessment

Perform a comprehensive assessment on:
- Children receiving comprehensive well-child care
- Children experiencing major stressful life events (e.g., chronic illness, disability, parental divorce, or death of a family member)
- Children requiring extensive home care
- Children with developmental delays
- Children with repeated accidental injuries and those with suspected child abuse
- Children with behavioral or physical problems that suggest family dysfunction as the etiology

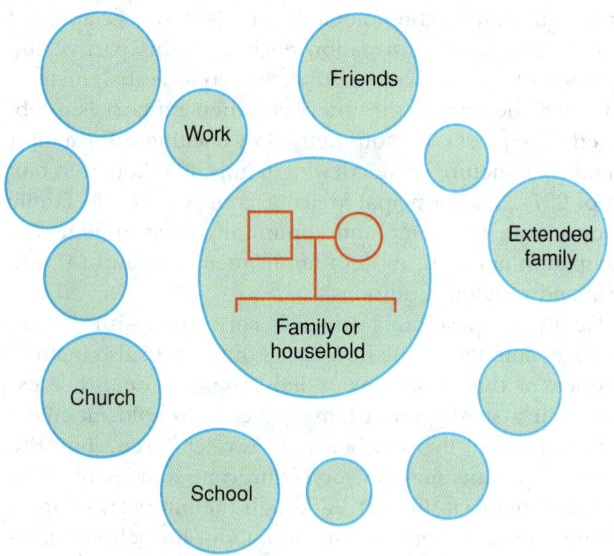

FIG. 6-6 Ecomap. Genogram is completed for immediate family members, and circles are labeled as appropriate. (Modified from Hartman A: *Finding families: an ecological approach to family assessment in adoption,* Newport, CA, 1979, Sage Publications.)

tionships, attachment symbols are often added as additional information on family functioning is obtained (see Fig. 6-7). Because a genogram can become complex, it is helpful to circle the nuclear family on the diagram. Instructions for beginning a genogram are similar to those for a pedigree (see Chapter 5).

The ***ecomap*** is a visual presentation of the family's support system outside the home. It begins with the genogram of the immediate family inside one circle and uses other, smaller circles to represent each member's relationship with other significant people, agencies, or institutions (Hartman, 1979). A blank ecomap is shown is Fig. 6-6. The size of the circles is not important; rather, symbols of attachment (Fig. 6-7) are used to signify the type of relationships, and arrows may be drawn along the connecting lines to denote flow of energy or resources.

ASSESSMENT OF FAMILY FUNCTION

Family function is concerned with how the family behaves toward one another and the quality of the relationships (see also Chapter 3). It is considered the most important component in determining "family health." Assessment of function requires more skill on the part of the interviewer than does assessment of structure and is best approached after structure is assessed. As in assessment of family structure, the more traditional method of eliciting information on family function is interviewing family members. The principal areas of concern are discussed in the box on p. 207.

In addition to observing and interviewing the family to assess family function, both questionnaires and drawings can be used as needed to obtain a comprehensive assessment. The following section discusses selected instruments that are reliable and valid but require little formal training and minimal time to administer. The reader is referred to reviews of other instruments for further information (Dunst, Trivette, and Deal, 1988; McCubbin and Thompson, 1991; Smilkstein, 1984; Speer and Sachs, 1985).

The ***Family APGAR (FAPGAR)*** is a brief screening questionnaire designed to reflect a family member's satisfaction with the functional state of the family (Smilkstein, Ashworth, and Montano, 1982) (see Appendix A). The acronym APGAR is for Adaptation, Partnership, Growth, Affection, and Resolve (commitment). The acronym was chosen because it is familiar to health professionals, but it bears no relationship to the Apgar scoring system for newborns.

The questions in the box on p. 208 can be used in the interview without the APGAR ratings to elicit similar types of information. It can be completed in about 5 minutes, can be used by families with traditional and alternative life-styles and from different cultures, and is appropriate for children age 10 years or older. Separate forms have been designed to assess relationships with friends and fellow workers, since these groups represent other significant sources of support.

The responses to the five questions are scored as follows: "Almost always"—2; "Some of the time"—1; and "Hardly ever"—0. Each score is totaled. Scores of 7 to 10 suggest a highly functional family; 4 to 6, a moderately dysfunctional family; and 0 to 3, a severely dysfunctional family. Also, a low score in any single item could signal family dysfunction. The family APGAR is not recommended for use with individuals from enmeshed (overly close) or "psychosomatic" families. Persons with health problems, such as asthma, atopic dermatitis, or irritable bowel syndrome, may report falsely high scores (Smilkstein, 1993).

The ***Feetham Family Functioning Survey*** provides information about family members' *perception* of relationships that contribute to or are affected by family functioning (Rob-

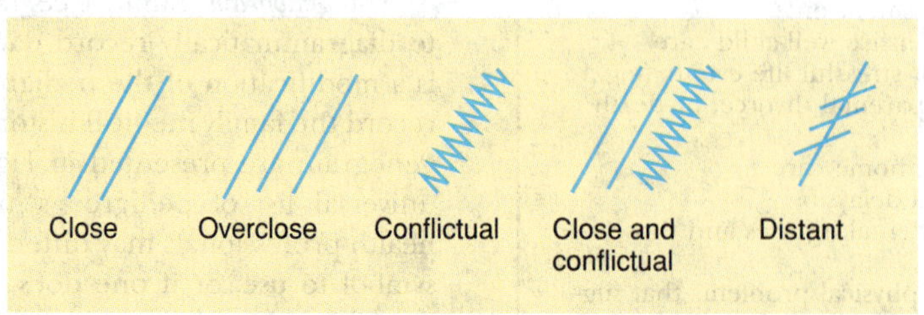

FIG. 6-7 Symbols of attachment or intensity of relationship.

FAMILY ASSESSMENT INTERVIEW

GENERAL GUIDELINES FOR FAMILY INTERVIEW

Schedule the interview with the family at a time that is most convenient for all parties; include as many family members as possible; clearly state the purpose of the interview.
Begin the interview by asking each person's name and their relationship to each other.
Restate the purpose of the interview and the objective.
Keep the initial conversation general to put members at ease and to learn the "big picture" of the family.
Identify major concerns and reflect these back to the family to be certain that all parties perceive the same message.
Terminate the interview with a summary of what was discussed and a plan for additional sessions if needed.

STRUCTURAL ASSESSMENT AREAS

Family Composition

Immediate members of the household (names, ages, and relationships)
Significant extended family members
Previous marriages, separations, death of spouses, or divorces

Home and Community Environment

Type of dwelling/number of rooms/occupants
Sleeping arrangements
Number of floors, accessibility of stairs, elevators
Adequacy of utilities
Safety features (fire escape, smoke detector, guardrails on windows, use of car restraint)
Environmental hazards (e.g., chipped paint, poor sanitation, pollution, heavy street traffic)
Availability and location of health facilities, schools, play areas
Relationship with neighbors
Recent crises or changes in home
Child's reaction/adjustment to recent stresses

Occupation and Education of Family Members

Types of employment
Work schedules
Work satisfaction
Exposure to environmental/industrial hazards
Sources of income and adequacy
Effect of illness on financial status
Highest degree or grade level attained

Cultural and Religious Traditions

Religious beliefs and practices
Cultural/ethnic beliefs and practices
Language spoken in home

Assessment questions include:

Does the family identify with a particular religious/ethnic group? Are both parents from that group?
How is religious/ethnic background part of family life?
What special religious/cultural traditions are practiced in the home (e.g., food choices and preparation)?
Where were family members born, and how long have they lived in this country?
What language does the family speak most frequently?
Do they speak/understand English?
What do they believe causes health or illness?
What religious/ethnic beliefs influence the family's perception of illness and its treatment?
What methods are used to prevent/treat illness?
How does the family know when a health problem needs medical attention?
Who is the person the family contacts when a member is ill?
Does the family rely on cultural/religious healers or remedies? If so, ask them to describe the type of healer or remedy.
Who does the family go to for support (clergy, medical healer, relatives)?
Does the family experience discrimination because of their race, beliefs, or practices? Ask them to describe.

FUNCTIONAL ASSESSMENT AREAS

Family Interactions and Roles

Interactions refer to ways family members relate to each other
Chief concern is amount of intimacy and closeness among the members, especially spouses
Roles refer to behaviors of people as they assume a different status or position

Observations include:

Family members' responses to each other (cordial, hostile, cool, loving, patient, short-tempered)
Obvious roles of leadership vs submission
Support and attention shown to various members

Assessment questions include:

What activities do the family perform together?
Whom do family members talk to when something is bothering them?
What are members' household chores?
Who usually oversees what is happening with the children, such as at school or concerning their health?
How easy or difficult is it for the family to change or accept new responsibilities for household tasks?

Power, Decision Making, and Problem Solving

Power refers to individual member's control over others in family; manifested through family decision making and problem solving
Chief concern is clarity of boundaries of power between parents and children
One method of assessment involves offering a hypothetical conflict or problem, such as a child failing school, and asking family how they would handle this situation

Assessment questions include:

Who usually makes the decisions in the family?
If one parent makes a decision, can the child appeal to the other parent to change it?
What input do children have in making decisions or discussing rules?
Who makes and enforces the rules?
What happens when a rule is broken?

Communication

Concerned with clarity and directness of communication patterns

Observations include:

Who speaks to whom
If one person speaks for another or interrupts
If members appear disinterested when certain individuals speak
If there is agreement between verbal and nonverbal messages
Further assessment includes periodically asking family members if they understood what was just said and to repeat the message

Assessment questions include:

How often do family members wait until others are through talking before "having their say?"
Do parents or older siblings tend to lecture and preach?
Do parents tend to talk "down" to the children?

Expression of Feelings and Individuality

Concerned with personal space and freedom to grow with limits and structure needed for guidance
Observing patterns of communication offers clues to how freely feelings are expressed

Assessment questions include:

Is it OK for family members to get angry or sad?
Who gets angry most of the time? What do they do?
If someone is upset, how do other family members try to comfort this person?
Who comforts specific family members?
When someone wants to do something, such as try out for a new sport or get a job, what is the family's response (offer assistance, discouragement, or no advice)?

FAMILY APGAR

DEFINITION	FUNCTION MEASURED BY THE FAMILY APGAR	RELEVANT OPEN-ENDED QUESTIONS
Adaptation is the use of intrafamilial and extrafamilial resources for problem solving when family equilibrium is stressed during a crisis.	How resources are shared, or the degree to which a member is satisfied with the assistance received when family resources are needed.	How have family members aided each other in time of need? In what way have family members received help or assistance from friends and community agencies?
Partnership is the sharing of decision-making and nurturing responsibilities by family members.	How decisions are shared, or the member's satisfaction with mutuality in family communication and problem-solving.	How do family members communicate with each other about such matters as vacations, finances, medical care, large purchases, and personal problems?
Growth is the physical and emotional maturation and self-fulfillment that is achieved by family members through mutual support and guidance.	How nurturing is shared, or the member's satisfaction with the freedom available within the family to change roles and attain physical and emotional growth or maturation.	How have family members changed during the past years? How has this change been accepted by family members? In what ways have family members aided each other in growing or developing independent life-styles? How have family members reacted to your desires for change?
Affection is the caring or loving relationship that exists among family members.	How emotional experiences are shared, or the member's satisfaction with the intimacy and emotional interaction that exists in the family.	How have members of your family responded to emotional expressions such as affection, love, sorrow, or anger?
Resolve is the commitment to devote time to other members of the family for physical and emotional nurturing. It also usually involves a decision to share wealth and space.	How time (and space and money) is shared, or the member's satisfaction with the time commitment that has been made to the family by its members.	How do members of your family share time, space, and money?

Modified from Smilkstein G: The Family APGAR: a proposal for a family function test and its use by physicians, *J Fam Pract* 6(6):1231-1239, 1978.

erts and Feetham, 1982).* Although recommended primarily as a research instrument, it can be used clinically without scoring the items to identify areas that may be of concern to the family. The survey consists of 25 ratings of family functioning (household tasks; child care; sexual and marital relationships; interaction with family, children, and friends; community involvement; and sources of emotional support) and 2 open-ended questions. Each of the questions on family functioning is rated on three 7-point scales of "How much is there now?" "How much should there be?" and "How important is this to me?" (see box on p. 209). Discrepancy between the first two ratings, together with the rating of importance, contributes to an assessment of the members' perceptions of family functioning. The survey takes less than 10 minutes to complete and can be used with single-parent and two-parent families (Failla and Jones, 1991; Feetham, Perkins, and Carroll, 1993).

Ideally a thorough assessment includes observing the child and family in a variety of settings. Undoubtedly the richest environment for observing a child's development and interactions with family members is the home. Two tools that can be used to assess the child's home environment are the ***Home Observation for Management of the Environment (HOME)**** (Caldwell and Bradley, 1984) and the ***Home Screening Questionnaire (HSQ)*** (Frankenburg and Coons, 1986).† Both are divided into two age-groups—birth to 3 years of age and 3 to 6 years of age (see Appendix A). HOME has an additional inventory for children ages 6 to 10 years; forms are also available for children with moderate to severe disabilities in each of the three age-groups for visual, auditory, orthopaedic, and cognitive impairments.

Some of the HOME items require direct observation, whereas others necessitate questioning of the parents. Each item receives a "yes" or "no" response. The number of "yes" responses correlates with the amount of appropriate environmental stimulation. Any "no" responses indicate possible areas for intervention and counseling. Use of HOME requires about a 1-hour home visit with both the child and the major caregiver.

There is some evidence that the socioeconomic status of

*The survey is available for a fee from Nursing Systems and Research, Children's National Medical Center, 111 Michigan Ave., N.W., Washington, DC 20010; (202) 939-4980.

*The forms and an administration manual are available for a fee from the Center for Research on Teaching and Learning, College of Education, University of Arkansas at Little Rock, 2801 S. University Ave., Little Rock, AK 72204-1099; (501) 569-3422.

†The forms and manual are available for a fee from Denver Developmental Materials, Inc., P.O. Box 6919, Denver, CO 80206-0919; (303) 355-4729.

SAMPLE QUESTION FROM THE FEETHAM FAMILY FUNCTIONING SURVEY

The amount of time you spend with your *spouse.*

a. How much is there now?

LITTLE MUCH
1 2 3 4 5 6 7

b. How much should there be?

LITTLE MUCH
1 2 3 4 5 6 7

c. How important is this to me?

LITTLE MUCH
1 2 3 4 5 6 7

Reproduced with the permission of Suzanne L. Feetham, PhD, RN, FAAN. Developed from research funded by Division of Nursing, HRA, HHS, NU00632, Wayne State University, Detroit, MI, 1977-1980.

the family may influence the results. The HOME may not identify strengths or risks in single-parent families or those in low-income groups (Lotas and others, 1992).

The HSQ was developed using HOME as a guide. The 0- to 3-year form consists of 30 items plus a checklist of toys available to the child in the home. The 3- to 6-year form has 34 items and a similar toy checklist. The questions are written at approximately a third to sixth grade reading level and, unlike the HOME, can be completed by the parents in any setting in about 15 to 20 minutes. Scoring directions are detailed in the manual and are based on credits for different answers. For each age-group there is a minimum score for determining suspect or nonsuspect results.

A ***sociogram*** is a drawing of circles that indicates the significant persons in an individual's life; its use is appropriate for adults and children as young as 5 years of age. Give the person blank paper and a pencil with the instructions: "Draw a circle to represent you. Around the circle draw circles to represent the most significant persons in your life and label each. Draw the circles in proximity to your circle to represent closeness. For example, the person who is most significant is the circle closest to you."

A variation of the sociogram is the ***family circle*** (Thrower, Bruce, and Walton, 1982). The directions differ slightly: "Draw a circle to represent your family. Draw in smaller circles to represent you and the most significant persons in your life. People can be inside or outside the family circle. Draw the circles large or small, depending on their significance to or influence on you." In both the sociogram and the family circle, suggest that family members label the relationships as supportive with a plus sign or negative with a minus sign.

The sociogram or family circle is an immediate portrait of significant persons in the individual's life. Drawing it is also a task that can uncover hidden or repressed relationships. For example, one mother drew a circle inside her circle to represent a child with severe disabilities who was in a residential care facility. She remarked that she had not

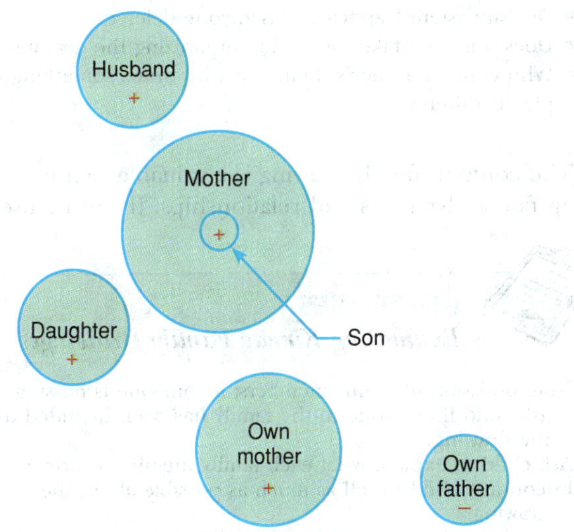

FIG. 6-8 Sociogram of a mother with strong, but unresolved, feelings toward her son in a residential care facility.

realized how unresolved her feelings of attachment to this child were until she had to graphically place him in her life (Fig. 6-8).

After the family completes the sociogram or family circle, encourage them to explore their feelings further with questions such as the following:

- How would you change the circles to improve relationships?
- How do you think you could accomplish these changes?
- If one person in the circle were to change, what effect do you think that would have on others in the circle?

The ***kinetic family drawing (KFD)*** (Burns, 1982; Burns and Kaufman, 1972) involves asking the family member to "Draw your family doing something." In giving directions, offer only a general statement of encouragement to avoid suggesting themes. Drawing the family is appropriate for children over 4 years of age.

The focus of the KFD is not only the family unit but also the activity and interaction of each family member. The drawing describes the person's perspective of family dynamics and his or her place in the family matrix. To evaluate a KFD, either subjective impressions or an objective scoring system may be used (Burns, 1982; Spinetta and others, 1981). Suggestions for evaluating a KFD are listed in the Guidelines box on p. 210.

Another useful technique with children and adults is the ***conjoint family drawing.*** Give the family a large sheet of white paper and a box of colored pencils, pens, or crayons. Ask each member to select a different color pen and not to exchange colors. Instruct them to work together on a drawing but without talking to each other. After the drawing is completed, ask each member to discuss it. Emphasize the process or "how" the drawing took place, rather than the symbolic meaning of each part. Assess the process by looking at:

- Who initiates the drawing?
- Who uses the most or least space?
- Does anyone infringe on another's "space?"

- Do "subsystems" appear, or is anyone deleted?
- Does someone take the lead in organizing the drawing?
- Who copies another's theme, or who draws something completely different?

The conjoint family drawing is a valuable tool in uncovering family dynamics and relationships. It can be used as a learning experience to help "well" families learn more about themselves. When it is used with dysfunctional families, nurses must have sufficient skill in handling issues and feelings that may arise.

GUIDELINES
Evaluating Kinetic Family Drawings

Note omission of family members; if someone is missing, ask child if everyone in the family has been included in the drawing.
Ask child to explain what each family member is doing.
Encourage child to tell as much as possible about the drawing.
Note signs of physical intimacy or distance, such as people close to each other or touching.
Note placement of people in the drawing, such as top or bottom of drawing and proximity to each other.
Note facial expressions, such as happy, sad, blank, or bored.
Note which members are facing each other or turned away from each other and how they are grouped together.

Modified from Burns R: *Self growth in families: kinetic family drawings (KFD)—research and application,* New York, 1982, Brunner/Mazel.

NUTRITIONAL ASSESSMENT

A nutritional assessment is an essential part of a complete health appraisal. Its purpose is to evaluate the child's nutritional status, the state of balance between nutrient intake and nutrient expenditure or need. A thorough nutritional status assessment includes: (1) dietary intake, (2) clinical examination, and (3) biochemical analysis.

DIETARY INTAKE

Knowledge of the child's dietary intake is a useful and practical component of a nutritional assessment. However, it is also one of the most difficult factors to assess. Individuals' recall of food consumption, especially amounts eaten, is frequently unreliable. In addition, people may be hesitant to reveal their eating patterns if they sense criticism from the nurse. People from different cultures may have difficulty adequately describing the types of food they eat. Despite these obstacles, however, a food intake record is essential. Several methods are available.

DIETARY HISTORY

What are the family's usual mealtimes?
Do family members eat together or at separate times?
Who does the family grocery shopping and meal preparation?
How much money is spent to buy food each week?
How are most foods prepared—baked, broiled, fried, other?
How often does the family or your child eat out?
 What kinds of restaurants do you go to?
 What kinds of food does your child typically eat at restaurants?
Does your child eat breakfast regularly?
Where does your child eat lunch?
What are your child's favorite foods, beverages, and snacks?
 What are the average amounts eaten per day?
 What foods are artificially sweetened?
 What are your child's snacking habits?
 When are sweet foods usually eaten?
 What are your child's toothbrushing habits?
What special cultural practices are followed? What ethnic foods are eaten?
What foods and beverages does your child dislike?
How would you describe your child's usual appetite (hearty eater, picky eater)?
What are your child's feeding habits (breast, bottle, cup, spoon, eats by self, needs assistance, any special devices)?
Does your child take vitamins or other supplements? Do they contain iron or fluoride?
Are there any known or suspected food allergies? Is your child on a special diet?
Has your child lost or gained weight recently?
Are there any feeding problems (excessive fussiness, spitting up, colic, difficulty sucking or swallowing)? Are there any dental problems or appliances, such as braces, that affect eating?
What types of exercise does your child do regularly?
Is there a family history of cancer, diabetes, heart disease, high blood pressure, or obesity?

ADDITIONAL QUESTIONS FOR INFANTS

What was the infant's birth weight? When did it double? Triple?
Was the infant premature?
Are you breast-feeding or have you breast-fed your infant? For how long?
If you use a formula, what is the brand?
 How long has the infant been taking it?
 How many ounces does the infant drink a day?
Are you giving the infant cow's milk (whole, low-fat, skimmed)?
 When did you start?
 How many ounces does the infant drink a day?
Do you give your infant extra fluids (water, juice)?
If the infant takes a bottle to bed at nap or nighttime, what is in the bottle?
At what age did you start cereal, vegetables, meat or other protein sources, fruit/juice, finger food, table food?
Do you make your own baby food or use commercial foods, such as infant cereal?
Does the infant take a vitamin/mineral supplement? If so, what type?
Has the infant shown an allergic reaction to any food(s)? If so, list the foods and describe the reaction.
Does the infant spit up frequently, have unusually loose stools, or have hard, dry stools? If so, how often?
How often do you feed your infant?
How would you describe your infant's appetite?

Dietary History

Regardless of the format used in recording food intake, every nutritional assessment should begin with a dietary history. The exact questions used to elicit a dietary history vary with the child's age. In general, the younger the child, the more specific and detailed the history should be. The box on p. 210 provides a sample dietary history for children with additional questions regarding infant feeding.

The broad overview elicited from the dietary history can be helpful in evaluating food frequency records (see box below). It also is concerned with financial and cultural factors that influence food selection and preparation. Because cultural practices are very prevalent in food preparation, it is important to consider carefully the kind of questions that are asked and the judgment made in regard to counseling. For example, some cultures (e.g., Hispanic, black, and Native American) include many vegetables, legumes, and starches in their diet that together provide sufficient essential amino acids, even though the actual amount of meat or dairy protein is low. (See Chapter 2 for cultural food practices.)

The most common and probably easiest method of assessing daily intake is the ***24-hour recall.*** The child or parent recalls every item eaten in the past 24 hours and the approximate amounts. The 24-hour recall is most beneficial when it represents a typical day's intake. Some of the difficulties with a daily recall are the family's inability to remember exactly what was eaten and inaccurate estimation of portion size. To increase accuracy of reporting portion sizes, try using food models and asking additional questions. In general, this method is most useful in providing *qualitative* information about the child's diet.

To improve the reliability of the daily recall, have the family complete a ***food diary*** by recording every food and liquid consumed for a certain number of days. A 3-day record consisting of 2 weekdays and 1 weekend day represents most people's eating patterns. To improve compliance, provide specific charts to record intake and ask the family to record items immediately after eating.

A ***food frequency questionnaire*** or ***record*** provides information about the number of times in a day, week, or month a child consumes items from the four food groups (see box below). In general, it provides more of a qualitative overview but has the advantage of avoiding recall based on a

FOOD FREQUENCY RECORD*

FOOD GROUP	NUMBER OF SERVINGS (DAY, WEEK)	SERVING SIZE (IN CUP, TABLESPOON, OR OUNCE PORTIONS)	FOOD GROUP	NUMBER OF SERVINGS (DAY, WEEK)	SERVING SIZE (IN CUP, TABLESPOON, OR OUNCE PORTIONS)
BREADS/CEREALS/RICE/PASTA Bread, tortilla Cooked pasta, rice, hot cereal Dry cereal (not presweetened) Crackers Muffins Other			**MILK/CHEESE/YOGURT** Milk Cheese Yogurt Pudding Ice cream Other		
VEGETABLES Yellow or orange Green/leafy Other			**OTHER PROTEIN FOODS** Meat Fish Poultry Egg Peanut butter Legumes (dried beans, peas) Nuts Other		
FRUITS/JUICE Citrus (orange, grapefruit, tangerine) Noncitrus Other			**FATS/OILS/SWEETS** Butter, oil, margarine, mayonnaise, salad dressing Soda, punch Cake/cookie, etc. Candy Presweetened cereal		

*For comparison of actual intake with recommended intake, see Food Guide Pyramid, Fig. 4-20.

TABLE 6-1 Clinical Assessment of Nutritional Status

EVIDENCE OF ADEQUATE NUTRITION	EVIDENCE OF DEFICIENT OR EXCESS NUTRITION	DEFICIENCY/EXCESS*
GENERAL GROWTH		
Within 5th and 95th percentiles for height, weight, and head circumference	Below 5th or above 95th percentiles for growth	Protein, calories, fats, and other essential nutrients, especially A, pyridoxine, niacin, calcium, iodine, manganese, zinc
Steady gain with expected growth spurts during infancy and adolescence	Absence of or delayed growth spurts; poor weight gain	
Sexual development appropriate for age	Delayed sexual development	Excess vitamin A, D
SKIN		
Smooth, slightly dry to touch	Hardening and scaling	Vitamin A
Elastic and firm	Seborrheic dermatitis	Excess niacin
Absence of lesions	Dry, rough, petechiae	Riboflavin
Color appropriate to genetic background	Delayed wound healing	Vitamin C
	Scaly dermatitis on exposed surfaces	Riboflavin, vitamin C, zinc
	Wrinkled, flabby	Niacin
	Crusted lesions around orifices, especially nares	Protein and calories Zinc
	Pruritus	Excess vitamin A, riboflavin, niacin
	Poor turgor	Water, sodium
	Edema	Protein, thiamin Excess sodium
	Yellow tinge (jaundice)	Vitamin B_{12} Excess vitamin A, niacin
	Depigmentation	Protein, calories
	Pallor (anemia)	Pyridoxine, folic acid, vitamin B_{12}, C, E (in premature infants), iron Excess vitamin C, zinc
	Paresthesia	Excess riboflavin
HAIR		
Lustrous, silky, strong, elastic	Stringy, friable, dull, dry, thin	Protein, calories
	Alopecia	Protein, calories, zinc
	Depigmentation	Protein, calories, copper
	Raised areas around hair follicles	Vitamin C
HEAD		
Even molding, occipital prominence, symmetric facial features	Softening of cranial bones, prominence of frontal bones, skull flat and depressed toward middle	Vitamin D
Fused sutures after 18 months	Delayed fusion of sutures	Vitamin D
	Hard tender lumps in occiput	Excess vitamin A
	Headache	Excess thiamin
NECK		
Thyroid not visible, palpable in midline	Thyroid enlarged; may be grossly visible	Iodine
EYES		
Clear, bright	Hardening and scaling of cornea and conjunctiva	Vitamin A
Good night vision	Night blindness	
Conjunctiva—Pink, glossy	Burning, itching, photophobia, cataracts, corneal vascularization	Riboflavin
EARS		
Tympanic membrane—Pliable	Calcified (hearing loss)	Excess vitamin D
NOSE		
Smooth, intact nasal angle	Irritation and cracks at nasal angle	Riboflavin Excess vitamin A
MOUTH		
Lips—Smooth, moist, darker color than skin	Fissures and inflammation at corners	Riboflavin Excess vitamin A
Gums—Firm, coral pink color, stippled	Spongy, friable, swollen, bluish red or black color, bleed easily	Vitamin C

*Nutrients listed are deficient unless specified as excess.

TABLE 6-1 Clinical Assessment of Nutritional Status—cont'd

EVIDENCE OF ADEQUATE NUTRITION	EVIDENCE OF DEFICIENT OR EXCESS NUTRITION	DEFICIENCY/EXCESS*
Mucous membranes—Bright pink, smooth, moist	Stomatitis	Niacin
Tongue—Rough texture, no lesions, taste sensation	Glossitis	Niacin, riboflavin, folic acid
	Diminished taste sensation	Zinc
Teeth—Uniform white color, smooth, intact	Brown mottling, pits, fissures	Excess fluoride
	Defective enamel	Vitamin A, C, D, calcium, phosphorus
	Caries	Excess carbohydrates
CHEST		
Infants, shape is almost circular	Depressed lower portion of rib cage	Vitamin D
In children, lateral diameter increases in proportion to anteroposterior diameter	Sharp protrusion of sternum	
Smooth costochondral junctions	Enlarged costochondral junctions	Vitamin C, D
Breast development—Normal for age	Delayed development	See General Growth, above, especially zinc
CARDIOVASCULAR SYSTEM		
Pulse and blood pressure (BP) within normal limits	Palpitations	Thiamin
	Rapid pulse	Potassium
		Excess thiamin
	Arrhythmias	Magnesium, potassium
		Excess niacin, potassium
	Increased BP	Excess sodium
	Decreased BP	Thiamin; excess niacin
ABDOMEN		
In young children, cylindric and prominent	Distended, flabby, poor musculature	Protein, calories
	Prominent, large	Excess calories
In older children, flat	Potbelly, constipation	Vitamin D
Normal bowel habits	Diarrhea	Niacin
		Excess vitamin C
	Constipation	Excess calcium, potassium
MUSCULOSKELETAL SYSTEM		
Muscles—Firm, well-developed, equal strength bilaterally	Flabby, weak, generalized wasting	Protein, calories
	Weakness, pain, cramps	Thiamin, sodium, chloride, potassium, phosphorus, magnesium
		Excess thiamin
	Muscle twitching, tremors	Magnesium
	Muscular paralysis	Excess potassium
Spine—Cervical and lumbar curves (double S curve)	Kyphosis, lordosis, scoliosis	Vitamin D
Extremities—Symmetric; legs straight with minimum bowing	Bowing of extremities, knock-knees	Vitamin D, calcium, phosphorus
	Epiphyseal enlargement	Vitamin A, D
	Bleeding into joints and muscles, joint swelling, pain	Vitamin C
Joints—Flexible, full range of motion, no pain or stiffness	Thickening of cortex of long bones with pain and fragility, hard tender lumps in extremities	Excess vitamin A
	Osteoporosis of long bones	Calcium; excess vitamin D
NEUROLOGIC SYSTEM		
Behavior—Alert, responsive, emotionally stable	Listless, irritable, lethargic, apathetic (sometimes apprehensive, anxious, drowsy, mentally slow, confused)	Thiamin, niacin, pyridoxine, vitamin C, potassium, magnesium, iron, protein, calories
		Excess vitamin A, D, thiamin, folic acid, calcium
	Masklike facial expression, blurred speech, involuntary laughing	Excess manganese
Absence of tetany, convulsions	Convulsions	Thiamin, pyridoxine, vitamin D, calcium, magnesium
		Excess phosphorus (in relation to calcium)
Intact peripheral nervous system	Peripheral nervous system toxicity (unsteady gait, numb feet and hands, fine motor clumsiness)	Excess pyridoxine
Intact reflexes	Diminished or absent tendon reflexes	Thiamin, vitamin E

"typical" day. It is especially useful when verifying a food history or diary.

CLINICAL EXAMINATION

A significant amount of information regarding nutritional adequacy is elicited from a clinical examination, especially from assessing the skin, hair, teeth, gums, lips, tongue, and eyes. The hair, skin, and mouth are vulnerable to nutritional deficiency or excess because of the rapid turnover of epithelial and mucosal tissue. Table 6-1 summarizes clinical signs of possible nutritional deficiency or excess. Few are diagnostic for a specific nutrient, and if suspicious signs are found, they must be confirmed with dietary and biochemical data. Generally, the clinical examination does not reveal children at risk for a deficiency or excess.

An essential parameter of nutritional status is ***anthropometry,*** the measurement of height, weight, head circumference in young children, proportions, skinfold thickness, and arm circumference. Height and head circumference reflect past nutrition, whereas weight, skinfold thickness, and arm circumference reflect present nutritional status, especially of protein and fat reserves. Skinfold thickness measures the body's fat content, since approximately one half of the body's total fat stores are directly beneath the skin. The upper arm muscle circumference correlates with measurements of total muscle mass. Since muscle serves as the body's major protein reserve, this measurement serves as an index of the body's protein stores. Ideally, record growth measurements over a period of time, and compare the *velocity* of growth based on previous and present values. Techniques for anthropomorphic measurement are discussed in Chapter 7 under Growth Measurements.

Numerous biochemical tests are available for assessing nutritional status and include analysis of plasma, blood cells, urine, or tissues from liver, bone, hair, and fingernails. Many of these tests are complicated and are not performed routinely. Common laboratory procedures for nutritional status include measurement of hemoglobin, hematocrit, transferrin, albumin, creatinine, and nitrogen. Laboratory values for these tests and more specific nutrient measurements are given in Appendix D.

EVALUATION OF NUTRITIONAL ASSESSMENT

After collecting the data needed for a thorough nutritional assessment, evaluate the findings to plan appropriate counseling. From the data, assess if the child is (1) malnourished, (2) at risk for becoming malnourished, or (3) well nourished with adequate reserves.

Analyze the daily food diary for the variety and amounts of foods suggested in the Food Guide Pyramid (see Fig. 4-20). For example, if the list includes no vegetables, inquire about this rather than assume that the child dislikes vegetables, because it could be that none were served on that day. Also, evaluate the information in terms of the family's ethnic practices and financial resources. Encouraging increased protein intake with additional meat may be unfeasible for families on a limited budget or in conflict with food practices that use meat sparingly, such as in Asian meal preparation.

Compare findings from clinical examination and anthropometry with the data obtained from the dietary intake. For example, signs of anemia and a dietary record of iron-poor foods suggest laboratory analysis of hemoglobin, hematocrit, and transferrin. Refer any suspicious findings for further evaluation.

KEY POINTS

- Communication, the most important skill nurses must possess in the care of children, has verbal, nonverbal, and abstract components.
- To effectively establish a setting for communication, nurses must make an appropriate introduction, clarify their role and the purpose of the interview, and ensure privacy and confidentiality.
- When communicating with parents, nurses need to encourage parental involvement, listen carefully, use silence, and be empathic.
- Communication with children must reflect their development stage.
- Verbal communication techniques include the third-person technique, use of "I" messages, facilitative responding, storytelling, bibliotherapy, the use of "what if" questions, and other word games.
- Nonverbal communication with children may take the form of writing, drawing, magic, and play.
- The objectives of performing a health history are to identify pertinent information, determine the chief complaint, analyze the present illness, secure the past history, and record a family and sexual history.
- Family assessment is the collection of data about family composition and relationships among members; it focuses on home and community environment, occupation and education, and cultural and religious traditions.
- The family function interview examines interaction and roles, power, decision making, problem solving, communication, and expression of feelings and individuality.
- Nutritional assessment is performed by determination of dietary intake, clinical examination, and biochemical analysis.

REFERENCES

Andrist L: Taking a sexual history and educating clients about safe sex, *Nurs Clin North Am* 23(4):959-973, 1988.

Bellet PS, Maloney MJ: The importance of empathy as an interviewing skill in medicine, *JAMA* 266(13):1831-1832, 1991.

Buchwald D and others: The medical interview across cultures, *Patient Care* 27(7):141-166, 1993.

Burns R: *Self growth in families: kinetic family drawings (KFD)—research and application,* NY, 1982, Brunner/Mazel.

Burns RC, Kaufman SH: *Actions, styles, and symbols in kinetic family drawings (KFD): research and application,* New York, 1972, Brunner/Mazel.

Caldwell B, Bradley R: *Home observation for measurement of the environment,* rev ed, Little Rock, AR, 1984, University of Arkansas.

Campbell-Heider N, Hart CA: Updating the nurse's bedside manner, *Image J Nurs Sch* 25(2):133-139, 1993.
Cassell E, Coulehan J, Putnam S: Making good interview skills better, *Patient Care* 23(6):145-148, 1989.
Cyr M, Wartman S: The effectiveness of routine screening questions in the detection of alcoholism, *JAMA* 1259:51-54, 1988.
Dunst C, Trivette C, Deal A: *Enabling and empowering families: principles and guidelines for practice,* Cambridge, MA, 1988, Brookline Books.
Elizabeth J: Form of address: an addition to history taking? *Br Med J* 298(6668):257, 1989.
Failla S, Jones LC: Families of children with developmental disabilities: an examination of family hardiness, *Res Nurs Health* 14:41-50, 1991.
Feetham S, Perkins M, Carroll R: Exploratory analysis: a technique for analysis of dyadic data in research of families. In Feetham S and others: *Nursing in families: theory/research/education/practice,* Newport, CA, 1993, Sage Publications.
Frankenburg W, Coons C: Home Screening Questionnaire: its validity in assessing home environment, *J Pediatr* 108(4):624-626, 1986.
Glascoe F, Altemeier W, MacLean W: The importance of parents' concerns about their child's development, *Am J Dis Child* 43:955-958, 1989.
Glascoe F, MacLean W, Stone W: The importance of parents' concerns about their children's behavior, *Clin Pediatr* 30(1):8-11, 1991.
Gorzka PA and others: Parenting: categories for anticipatory guidance, *J Child Adolesc Psychiatr Ment Health Nurs* 4(1):16-19, 1991.
Hartman A: *Finding families: an ecological approach to family assessment in adoption,* Newport, CA, 1979, Sage Publications.
Heineken J, Roberts FB: Confirming, not disconfirming: communicating in a more positive manner, *MCN* 8(1):78-80, 1983.
Henrich AP, Bernheim KF: Responding to patients' concerns, *Nurs Outlook* 29(7):428-433, 1981.
Holden RJ: Empathy: the art of emotional knowing in holistic nursing care, *Holistic Nurs Pract* 5(1):70-79, 1990.
Leff P, Walizer E: *Building the healing partnership,* Cambridge, MA, 1992, Brookline Books.
Lotas M and others: The HOME scale: the influence of socioeconomic status on the evaluation of the home environment, *Nurs Res* 41(6):338-341, 1992.
McBurney BH, Schultz C: Defining quality services in a general pediatric unit, *J Nurs Care Qual* 7(3):51-60, 1993.
McCubbin H, Thompson A, editors: *Family assessment inventories for research and practice,* ed 2, Madison, WI, 1991, The University of Wisconsin—Madison.
Roberts CS, Feetham SL: Assessing family functioning across three areas of relationships, *Nurs Res* 31(4):231-235, 1982.
Sloat A, Matsuura W: Intercultural communication. In Craft M, Denehy J, editors: *Nursing interventions for infants and children,* Philadelphia, 1990, WB Saunders.
Smilkstein G: The physician and family function assessment, *Fam Systems Med* 2(3):263-279, 1984.
Smilkstein G: Family APGAR analyzed, *Fam Med* 25(5):293-294, 1993 (letter to the editor).
Smilkstein G, Ashworth C, Montano D: Validity and reliability of the family APGAR as a test of family function, *J Fam Pract* 15(2):303-311, 1982.
Speer J, Sachs B: Selecting the appropriate family assessment tool, *Pediatr Nurs* 11(5):349-355, 1985.
Spinetta J and others: The kinetic family drawing in childhood cancer. In Spinetta J, Deasy-Spinetta P: *Living with childhood cancer,* St Louis, 1981, Mosby.
Strasburger V: The challenge of adolescent medicine in the 1980s, *Child Care Newslett* 5(1):1-3, 1986.
Thrower S, Bruce W, Walton R: The Family Circle Method for integrating family systems concepts in family medicine, *J Fam Pract* 15(3):451-457, 1982.
Winkelstein M: Fostering positive self-concept in the school-age child, *Pediatr Nurs* 15(3):229-233, 1989.
Zuckerman B, Amaro H, Cabral H: Validity of self-reporting of marijuana and cocaine use among pregnant adolescents, *J Pediatr* 115(5, pt 1):812-815, 1989.

BIBLIOGRAPHY

Communication Strategies/Health Interview

Barnsteiner JH, Gillis-Donovan J: Being related and separate: a standard for therapeutic relationships, *MCN* 15:223-228, 1990.
Boyle WE Jr, Hoekelman RA: The pediatric history. In Hoekelman RA and others, editors: *Primary pediatric care,* ed 2, St Louis, 1992, Mosby.
Branch WT, Malik TK: Using "windows of opportunities" in brief interviews to understand patients' concerns, *JAMA* 269(13):1667-1668, 1993.
Brantly D: Communicating with children: age-related techniques. In Smith DP and others, editors: *Comprehensive child and family nursing skills,* St Louis, 1991, Mosby.
Brantly D: Conducting an interview. In Smith DP and others, editors: *Comprehensive child and family nursing skills,* St Louis, 1991, Mosby.
Burr WR: Beyond I-statements in family communication, *Fam Relations* 39(3):266-273, 1990.
Butz A, Alexander C: Use of health diaries with children, *Nurs Res* 40(1):59-61, 1991.
Cameron CO, Juszczak L, Wallace N: Using creative arts to help children cope with altered body image, *Child Health Care* 12(3):108-112, 1984.
Claman L: The squiggle-drawing game in child psychotherapy, *Am J Psychother* 34(3):414-425, 1980.
Crowther D: Metacommunications: a missed opportunity, *J Psychosoc Nurs* 29(4):13-16, 1991.
Denehy J: Communicating with children through drawings. In Craft M, Denehy J, editors: *Nursing interventions for infants and children,* Philadelphia, 1990, WB Saunders.
DiLeo JH: *Interpreting children's drawings,* New York, 1983, Brunner/Mazel.
DiLeo JH: *Children's drawings as diagnostic aids,* New York, 1980, Brunner/Mazel.
Faber A, Mazlish E: *How to talk so kids will listen and listen so kids will talk,* New York, 1980, Avon Books.
Ferber R: Assessment procedures for diagnosis of sleep disorders in children. In Noshpitz J, editor: *Sleep disorders for the clinician,* London, 1987, Butterworths.
Fochtman D: Therapeutic relationships, *J Pediatr Oncol Nurs* 8(1):1-2, 1991.
Fosson A, deQuan MM: Reassuring and talking with hospitalized children, *Child Health Care* 13(1):37-44, 1984.
Foye HR Jr: Anticipatory guidance. In Hoekelman RA and others, editors: *Primary pediatric care,* ed 2, St Louis, 1992, Mosby.
Freeman M: Therapeutic use of storytelling for older children who are critically ill, *Child Health Care* 20(4):208-215, 1991.
Garbarino J and others: *What children can tell us: eliciting, interpreting, and evaluating information from children,* San Francisco, 1989, Jossey-Bass.
Gaynard L, Goldberger J, Laidley L: The use of stuffed, body-outline dolls with hospitalized children and adolescents, *Child Health Care* 20(4):216-224, 1991.
Green M: 20 interview questions that work, *Contemp Pediatr* 9(11):47-71, 1992.
Hahn K: Therapeutic storytelling: helping children learn and cope, *Pediatr Nurs* 13(3):175-178, 1987.
Hart R and others: *Therapeutic play activities for hospitalized children,* St Louis, 1992, Mosby.
Hauck MR: Cognitive abilities of preschool children: implications for nurses working with young children, *J Pediatr Nurs* 6(4):230-245, 1991.
Henderson JA, Thomas GV: Looking ahead: planning for the inclusion of detail affects relative sizes of head and trunk in children's human figure drawings, *Br J Devel Psychol* 8:383-391, 1990.
Hudson C and others: Storytelling: a measure of anxiety in hospitalized children, *Child Health Care* 16(2):118-122, 1987.
Johnson B: Children's drawings as a projective technique, *Pediatr Nurs* 16(1):11-16, 1990.
Kaufman DH: An interview guide for helping children make health-care decisions, *Pediatr Nurs* 11(5):365-367, 1985.
Kemper K: Self-administered questionnaire for structured psychosocial screening in pediatrics, *Pediatrics* 89(3):433-436, 1992.
Kennedy C, Garvin B: Nurse-physician communication, *Appl Nurs Res* 1(3):122-127, 1988.
Koppitz EM: *Psychological evaluation of children's human figure drawings,* New York, 1968, Grune & Stratton.
Krahn G: The use of projective assessment techniques in pediatric settings, *J Pediatr Psychol* 10:179-193, 1985.
Krahn G, Hallum A, Kime C: Are there good ways to give "bad news"? *Pediatrics* 91(3):578-582, 1993.

Kramer N: Comparison of therapeutic touch and casual touch in stress reduction of hospitalized children, *Pediatr Nurs* 16(5):483-485, 1990.

Krietemeyer B, Heiney S: Storytelling as a therapeutic technique in a group for school-aged oncology patients, *Child Health Care* 21(1):14-20, 1992.

Lo W: If you had three wishes . . ., *Contemp Pediatr* 8(5):146, 1991.

Lynn M: Projective technique: a way of getting "hidden" information, part I, *J Pediatr Nurs* 1(6):58-60, 1986.

Marino BL: Studying infant and toddler play, *J Pediatr Nurs* 6(1):16-20, 1991.

McManus IC and others: Teaching communication skills to clinical students, *Br Med J* 306(6888):1322-1327, 1993.

Mellick L, Guy J: Approaching the infant and child in the prehospital arena, *J Emerg Med Serv* 17(3):126-136, 1992.

Messinger R, Davidson PN, Hoekelman RA: Communication with parents and patients. In Hoekelman RA and others, editors: *Primary pediatric care,* ed 2, St Louis, 1992, Mosby.

Olsen DP: Empathy as an ethical and philosophical basis for nursing, *Adv Nurs Sci* 14(1):62-75, 1991.

O'Malley ME, McNamara ST: Children's drawings: a preoperative assessment tool, *AORN J* 57(5):1074-1089, 1993.

Pau A, Morgan J, Terlingo A: Drug allergy documentation by physicians, nurses, and medical students, *Am J Hosp Pharm* 46(3):570-573, 1989.

Pazola K, Gerberg A: Privileged communication—talking with a dying adolescent, *MCN* 15(1):16-23, 1990.

Perlman N, Abramovitch R: Visit to the pediatrician: children's concerns, *J Pediatr* 110(6):988-990, 1987.

Pontious SL: Practical Piaget: helping children understand, *Am J Nurs* 82(1):114-117, 1982.

Rae W: Analyzing drawings of children who are physically ill or hospitalized using the Ipsative method, *Child Health Care* 20(4):198-207, 1991.

Raudsepp E: 7 ways to cure communication breakdowns, *Nursing 90* 20(4):132-142, 1990.

Roller CG: Drawing out young mothers, *MCN* 17(5), 1992.

Rollins J: Childhood cancer: siblings draw and tell, *Pediatr Nurs* 16(1):21-27, 1990.

Sabbeth B: Trial balloons: when families of ill children express needs in veiled ways, *Child Health Care* 17(2):87-92, 1988.

Shiff E: *Experts advise parents: a guide to raising loving, responsible children,* New York, 1988, Delacorte Press.

Smith J, Felice M: Interviewing adolescent patients: some guidelines for the clinician, *Pediatr Ann* 9:238-243, 1980.

Stevens NV: Obtaining a health history. In Smith DP and others, editors: *Comprehensive child and family nursing skills,* St Louis, 1991, Mosby.

Stickler G: Clinical guidelines for the pediatrician, *Pediatrics* 80(1):118-120, 1987.

Sunde ER, Mabe PA, Josephson A: Difficult parents: from adversaries to partners, *Clin Pediatr* 32(4):213-219, 1993.

Thompson SW: Communication techniques for allaying anxiety and providing support for hospitalized children, *J Child Adolesc Psychiatry Ment Health Nurs* 4(3):119-122, 1992.

Tiedman M, Simon K, Clatworthy S: Communicating through therapeutic play. In Craft M, Denehy J, editors: *Nursing interventions for infants and children,* Philadelphia, 1990, WB Saunders.

Vezeau T: Storytelling: a practitioner's tool, *MCN* 18:193-196, 1993.

Walker C: Use of art and play therapy in pediatric oncology, *J Pediatr Oncol Nurs* 6(4):121-126, 1989.

Younger J: Literary works as a mode of knowing, *Image J Nurs Sch* 22(1):39-43, 1990.

Family Assessment

Berkey K, Hanson S: *Pocket guide to family assessment and intervention,* St Louis, 1991, Mosby.

Birenbaum LK: Measurement of family coping, *J Pediatr Oncol Nurs* 8(1):39-42, 1991.

Bradley R, Caldwell B: Using the home inventory to assess the family environment, *Pediatr Nurs* 14(2):97-103, 1988.

Brantly DK: Conducting a psychosocial assessment of the family. In Smith DP and others, editors: *Comprehensive child and family nursing skills,* St Louis, 1991, Mosby.

Clark M, Frankel M, Trowbridge D: A pedigree primer, *J Pediatr Nurs* 4(2):112-118, 1989.

Danielson CB, Hamel-Bissell B, Winstead-Fry P: *Families, health, and illness,* St Louis, 1993, Mosby.

Davis L, Geikie G, Schamess G: The use of genograms in a group for latency age children, *Int J Group Psychother* 38(1):189-210, 1988.

Dobson SM: Genograms and ecomaps, *Nurs Times* 85(51):54-56, 1989.

Donelly E: Family health assessment, *Home Healthc Nurse* 11(2):30-37, 1993.

Fanslow J, Schultz C: Use of the family APGAR in the community setting: a pilot study, *Home Healthc Nurse* 9(5):54-58, 1991.

Gilliss C and others: *Toward a science of family nursing,* Menlo Park, CA, 1989, Addison-Wesley.

Lapp C, Diemert C, Enestvedt R: Family-based practice: discussion of a tool merging assessment with intervention, *Fam Community Health* 12(4):21-28, 1990.

Lipman T: Assessing family strengths to guide plan of care using Hymovich's framework, *J Pediatr Nurs* 4(3):186-196, 1989.

Lynn-McHale D, Smith A: Comprehensive assessment of families of the critically ill, *AACN Clin Issues Crit Care Nurs* 2(2):195-209, 1991.

Roberts C, Feetham S: Assessing family functioning across three areas of relationships, *Nurs Res* 31(4):321-325, 1982.

Rogers J, Holloway R: Completion rate and reliability of the self-administered genogram (SAGE), *Fam Pract* 7(2):149-151, 1990.

Rollins J: Administering a kinetic family drawing. In Smith DP and others, editors: *Comprehensive child and family nursing skills,* St Louis, 1991, Mosby.

Rosenbaum J: A cultural assessment guide: learning cultural sensitivity, *J Can Nurs Assoc* 87(4):32-33, 1991.

Thomas RB: A foundation for clinical family assessment, *Child Health Care* 19(4):244-250, 1990.

Touliatos J, Perlmutter B, Straus M, editors: *Handbook of family measurement techniques,* London, 1990, Sage Publications.

von Bertalanffy L: *General systems theory,* New York, 1968, George Braziller.

Winton P, Bailey D: The family focused interview: a collaborative mechanism for family assessment and goal setting, *J Div Early Childhood* 12(3):195-207, 1988.

Wright L, Leahey M: *Nurses and families: a guide to family assessment and intervention,* Philadelphia, 1984, FA Davis.

Nutritional Assessment

American Academy of Pediatrics, Committee on Nutrition: *Pediatric nutrition handbook,* Elk Grove Village, IL, 1993, The Academy.

Benjamin D: Laboratory tests and nutritional assessment: protein-energy status, *Pediatr Clin North Am* 36(1):139-161, 1989.

Bernstein LH: Monitoring quality of nutrition support: a chemical marker, *Dietetic Curr* 19(2):5-8, 1992.

Buzzard IM, Willet WC, editors: First international conference on dietary assessment methods: assessing diets to improve world health, *Am J Clin Nutr* 59(1, suppl): entire issue, 1994.

Liguori R: Assessing nutritional status. In Smith DP and others, editors: *Comprehensive child and family nursing skills,* St Louis, 1991, Mosby.

Pipes PL, Trahms CM: *Nutrition in infancy and childhood,* ed 5, St Louis, 1993, Mosby.

Simko M, Cowell C, Hreha M: *Practical nutrition: a quick reference for the health care practitioner,* Rockville, MD, 1989, Aspen.

Solomons NW: Assessment of nutritional status: functional indicators of pediatric nutriture, *Pediatr Clin North Am* 32(2):319-334, 1985.

Stuff JE and others: A comparison of dietary methods in nutritional studies, *Am J Clin Nutr* 37:300-306, 1983.

Todd KS, Hudes M, Calloway DH: Food intake measurement: problems and approaches, *Am J Clin Nutr* 37:139-146, 1983.

Sources of Books for Bibliotherapy

Association for the Care of Children's Health: *Books for children and teenagers about hospitalization, illness, and disabling conditions,* Washington, DC, 1987, The Association.

Berg PJ, Devlin MK, Gedaly-Duff V: Bibliotherapy with children experiencing loss, *Issues Compr Pediatr Nurs* 4:37-50, 1980.

Cohen L: "Here's something I want you to read," *RN* 55(10):56-59, 1992.

Cuddigan M, Hanson MB: *Growing pains: helping children deal with everyday problems through reading,* Chicago, 1988, American Library Association.

Dreyer S: *The Bookfinder 4: when kids need books,* Circle Pines, MN, 1989, American Guidance Service.

Fassler J: *Helping children cope: mastering stress through books and stories,* London, 1978, The Free Press.

Fosson A, Husband E: Bibliotherapy for hospitalized children, *South Med J* 77(3):342-346, 1984.

Griffin B: *Special needs bibliography: current books for/about children and young adults regarding social concerns, emotional concerns, the exceptional child,* Dewitt, NY, 1984, The Griffin. (Available from The Griffin, 5390 Gate House Rd., Tully, NY 13159; [315] 696-8813.)

Oppenheim J, Brenner B, Boegehold B: *Choosing books for kids,* NY, 1986, Ballantine Books.

Rubin R: *Bibliotherapy sourcebook,* Phoenix, AZ, 1978, Oryx Press.

Wallace NE: Special books for special children, *Child Health Care* 12(1):34-36, 1983.

CHAPTER 7

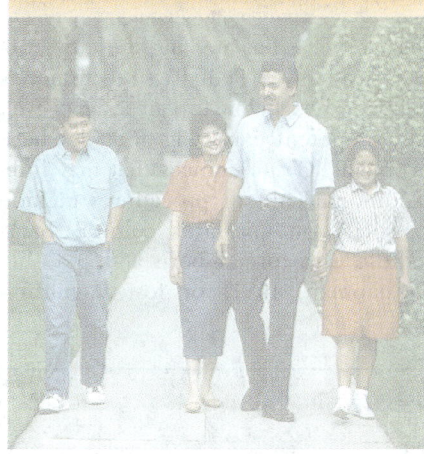

Physical and Developmental Assessment of the Child

CHAPTER OUTLINE

RELATED TOPICS

Altered states of consciousness, Ch. 37
Assessment of cardiac function, Ch. 34
Biologic development: adolescent, Ch. 19
Dental disorders, Ch. 18
Developmental dysplasia of the hip, Ch. 11
Disorders affecting the skin, Ch. 18
Growth and development, Ch. 4
Gynecologic examination, Ch. 20
Hearing impairment; vision impairment, Ch. 24
History taking, Ch. 6
Pain assessment, Ch. 26
Physical assessment: newborn, Ch. 8
Preparation for procedures, Ch. 27
Scoliosis, Ch. 39
Sexually transmitted diseases, Ch. 20
Systemic hypertension, Ch. 34

GENERAL CONCEPTS OF PEDIATRIC PHYSICAL ASSESSMENT

RECOMMENDATIONS FOR HEALTH SUPERVISION

The objectives of pediatric health supervision are maintenance of optimum wellness and prevention of illness. The concept of prevention necessitates an orderly and routine schedule of activities—of which physical examination plays an essential role—that are aimed at meeting these two objectives. The American Academy of Pediatrics recommends the schedule shown in the box below for the care of well children who receive competent parenting and who have no serious health problems. Circumstances that may indicate the need for additional visits or procedures include families of diverse socioeconomic and cultural backgrounds, especially those with foreign-born adopted children (Jenista and Chapman, 1987) or foster children

RECOMMENDATIONS FOR HEALTH SUPERVISION

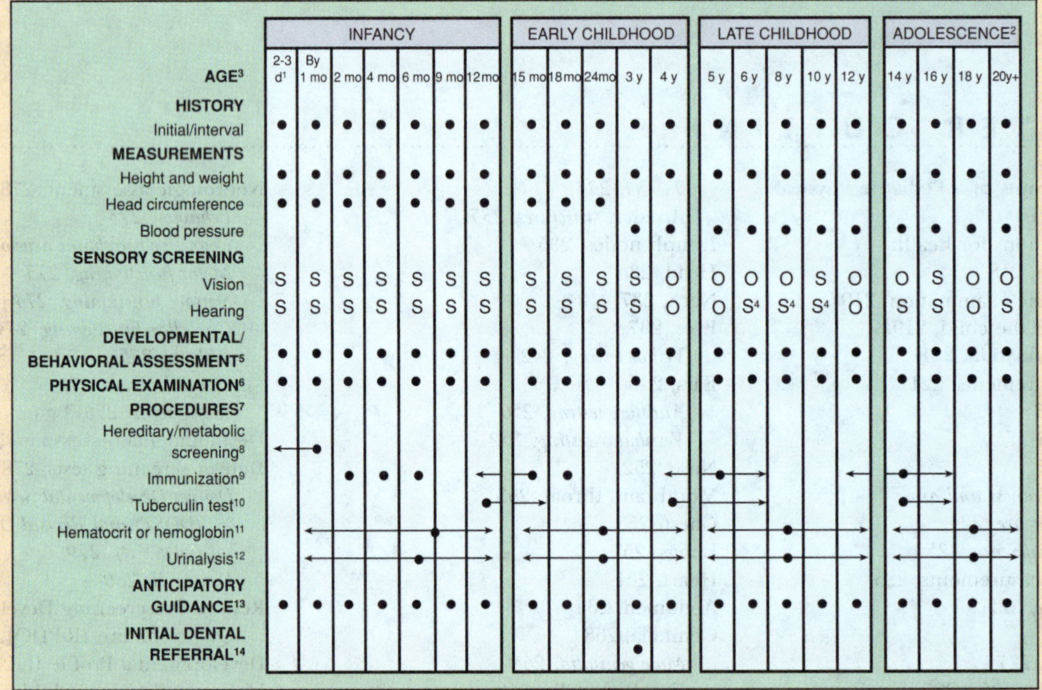

	INFANCY							EARLY CHILDHOOD					LATE CHILDHOOD					ADOLESCENCE[2]			
AGE[3]	2-3 d[1]	By 1 mo	2 mo	4 mo	6 mo	9 mo	12 mo	15 mo	18 mo	24 mo	3 y	4 y	5 y	6 y	8 y	10 y	12 y	14 y	16 y	18 y	20y+
HISTORY																					
Initial/interval	•	•	•	•	•	•	•	•	•	•	•	•	•	•	•	•	•	•	•	•	•
MEASUREMENTS																					
Height and weight	•	•	•	•	•	•	•	•	•	•	•	•	•	•	•	•	•	•	•	•	•
Head circumference	•	•	•	•	•	•	•	•	•	•											
Blood pressure											•	•	•	•	•	•	•	•	•	•	•
SENSORY SCREENING																					
Vision	S	S	S	S	S	S	S	S	S	S	S	O	O	O	O	S	O	O	S	O	O
Hearing	S	S	S	S	S	S	S	S	S	S	S	O	O	S[4]	S[4]	S[4]	O	S	S	O	S
DEVELOPMENTAL/ BEHAVIORAL ASSESSMENT[5]	•	•	•	•	•	•	•	•	•	•	•	•	•	•	•	•	•	•	•	•	•
PHYSICAL EXAMINATION[6]	•	•	•	•	•	•	•	•	•	•	•	•	•	•	•	•	•	•	•	•	•
PROCEDURES[7]																					
Hereditary/metabolic screening[8]	←	•																			
Immunization[9]			•	•	•		←	•	•			←	•	→			←	•	→		
Tuberculin test[10]							•	→				•	—	→				•	→		
Hematocrit or hemoglobin[11]		←	—	—	—	•	→	←	—	•	—	→	←	—	•	—	→	←	—	•	→
Urinalysis[12]		←	—	—	•	—	→	←	—	•	—	→	←	—	•	—	→	←	—	•	→
ANTICIPATORY GUIDANCE[13]	•	•	•	•	•	•	•	•	•	•	•	•	•	•	•	•	•	•	•	•	•
INITIAL DENTAL REFERRAL[14]											•										

1. For newborns discharged in 24 hours or less after delivery.
2. Adolescent-related issues (e.g., psychosocial, emotional, substance usage, and reproductive health) may necessitate more frequent health supervision.
3. If a child comes under care for the first time at any point on the schedule, or if any items are not accomplished at the suggested age, the schedule should be brought up to date at the earliest possible time.
4. At these points, history may suffice: if problem suggested, a standard testing method should be employed.
5. By history and appropriate physical examination: if suspicious, by specific objective developmental testing.
6. At each visit, a complete physical examination is essential, with infant totally unclothed, older child undressed and suitably draped.
7. These may be modified, depending upon entry point into schedule and individual need.
8. Metabolic screening (e.g., thyroid, PKU, galactosemia) should be done according to state law.
9. Schedule(s) per *Report of the Committee on Infectious Diseases,* 1991 Red Book, and current AAP Committee on Infectious Diseases, 1991
10. For high-risk groups, the Committee on Infectious Diseases recommends annual TB skin testing.
11. Present medical evidence suggests the need for reevaluation of the frequency and timing of hemoglobin or hematocrit tests. One determination is therefore suggested during each time period. Performance of additional tests is left to the individual practice experience.
12. Present medical evidence suggests the need for reevaluation of the frequency and timing of urinalyses. One determination is therefore suggested during each time period. Performance of additional tests is left to the individual practice experience.
13. Appropriate discussion and counseling should be an integral part of each visit for care.
14. Subsequent examinations as prescribed by dentist.

From American Academy of Pediatrics: *Policy reference guide,* ed 16, Elk Grove Village, IL, 1993, The Academy, p 608.
Key: • = To be performed; S = subjective, **by history;** O = objective, by a standard **testing method.**
NB: Special chemical, immunologic, and endocrine testing is usually carried out upon specific indications. Testing other than newborn (e.g., inborn errors of metabolism, sickle disease, lead) is discretionary with the physician.
***Author's note:** For more current recommendations see Immunizations, Chapter 12.

(American Academy of Pediatrics, 1987); one-parent families; or those with children who have chronic illnesses or disabilities.

The services required by each child must be individualized by the practitioner. Look for opportunities to review children's previous schedules of health care and institute specific measures or referrals to update the health record. For example, during hospitalization review children's overall record to ensure that they have had sensory screening, appropriate immunizations, and a yearly dental examination.

SEQUENCE OF THE EXAMINATION

Ordinarily the examining sequence follows a head-to-toe direction to provide a general guideline for assessment of each body area in order to minimize omitting segments of the examination. The typical organization of a physical examination is listed in the chapter outline. In examining children, alter the sequence to accommodate the child's developmental needs, but record the findings according to the traditional model. Using developmental and chronologic age as the main criteria for assessing each body system accomplishes several goals:

- Minimizes stress and anxiety associated with assessment of various body parts
- Fosters a trusting nurse-child-parent relationship
- Allows for maximum preparation of the child
- Preserves the essential security of the parent-child relationship, especially with young children
- Maximizes the accuracy and reliability of assessment findings

PREPARATION OF THE CHILD

While the physical examination consists of painless procedures, to a child the use of a tight arm cuff, probes in the ears and mouth, pressing on the abdomen, and listening to the chest with a cold piece of metal can be considerably

GUIDELINES
Performing Pediatric Physical Examination

Perform examination in appropriate, nonthreatening area.
- Have room well lit and decorated with neutral colors.
- Have room temperature comfortably warm.
- Place all strange and potentially frightening equipment out of sight.
- Have some toys, dolls, stuffed animals, and games available for child.
- If possible, have rooms decorated and equipped for different-age children.
- Provide privacy, especially for school-age children and adolescents.

Provide time for play and becoming acquainted.

Observe behaviors that signal child's readiness to cooperate:
- Talking to nurse
- Making eye contact
- Accepting offered equipment
- Allowing physical touching
- Choosing to sit on examining table rather than parent's lap

If signs of readiness are not observed, use the following techniques:
- Talk to parent while essentially "ignoring" child; gradually focus on child or a favorite object, such as a doll.
- Make complimentary remarks about child, such as appearance, dress, or a favorite object.
- Tell a funny story or play a simple magic trick.
- Have a nonthreatening "friend" available, such as a hand puppet to "talk" to child for the nurse (see Fig. 7-31, *A*).

If child refuses to cooperate, use the following techniques:
- Assess reason for uncooperative behavior; consider that a child who is unduly afraid may have had a previous traumatic experience.
- Try to involve child and parent in process.
- Avoid prolonged explanations about examining procedure.
- Use a firm, direct approach regarding expected behavior.
- Perform examination as quickly as possible.
- Have attendant gently restrain child.
- Minimize any disruptions or stimulation.
  - Limit number of people in room.
  - Use isolated room.
  - Use quiet, calm, confident voice.

Begin examination in a nonthreatening manner for young children or children who are fearful:
- Use those activities that can be presented as games, such as test for cranial nerves (see Table 7-17) or parts of developmental screening tests (p. 278).
- Use approaches such as "Simon says" to encourage child to make a face, squeeze a hand, stand on one foot, and so on.
- Use "paper-doll" technique.
  - Lay child supine on an examining table or floor that is covered with a large sheet of paper.
  - Trace around child's body outline.
  - Use body outline to demonstrate what will be examined, such as drawing a heart and listening with the stethoscope before performing the activity on child.

If several children in the family will be examined, begin with the most cooperative child to provide modeling of desired behavior.

Involve child in examination process:
- Provide choices, such as sitting on table or in patient's lap.
- Allow child to handle or hold equipment.
- Encourage child to use equipment on a doll, family member, or examiner.
- Explain each step of the procedure in simple language.

Examine child in a comfortable and secure position:
- Sitting in parent's lap
- Sitting upright if in respiratory distress

Proceed to examine the body in an organized sequence (usually head to toe) with the following exceptions:
- Alter sequence to accommodate needs of different-age children (see Table 7-1).
- Examine painful areas last.
- In emergency situation, examine vital functions (airway, breathing, and circulation) and injured area first.

Reassure child throughout examination, especially about bodily concerns that arise during puberty.

Discuss findings with family at end of examination.

Praise child for cooperation during examination; give reward such as a small toy or sticker.

TABLE 7-1 Age-Specific Approaches to Physical Examination During Childhood

POSITION	SEQUENCE	PREPARATION
INFANT		
Before sits alone: supine or prone, preferably in parent's lap; before 4 to 6 months: can place on examining table After sits alone: use sitting in parent's lap whenever possible If on table, place with parent in full view	If quiet, auscultate heart, lungs, abdomen Record heart and respiratory rates Palpate and percuss same areas Proceed in usual head-to-toe direction Perform traumatic procedures last (eyes, ears, mouth [while crying]) Elicit reflexes as body part examined Elicit Moro reflex last	Completely undress if room temperature permits Leave diaper on male Gain cooperation with distraction, bright objects, rattles, talking Have older infants hold a small block in each hand; until voluntary release develops toward end of the first year, infants will be unable to grasp other objects (e.g., stethoscope, otoscope) (Farber, 1991) Smile at infant; use soft, gentle voice Pacify with bottle of sugar water or feeding Enlist parent's aid for restraining to examine ears, mouth Avoid abrupt, jerky movements
TODDLER		
Sitting or standing on/by parent Prone or supine in parent's lap	Inspect body area through play: "count fingers," "tickle toes" Use minimal physical contact initially Introduce equipment slowly Auscultate, percuss, palpate whenever quiet Perform traumatic procedures last (same as for infant)	Have parent remove outer clothing Remove underwear as body part examined Allow to inspect equipment; demonstrating use of equipment is usually ineffective If uncooperative, perform procedures quickly Use restraint when appropriate; request parent's assistance Talk about examination if cooperative; use short phrases Praise for cooperative behavior
PRESCHOOL CHILD		
Prefer standing or sitting Usually cooperative prone/supine Prefer parent's closeness	If cooperative, proceed in head-to-toe direction If uncooperative, proceed as with toddler	Request self-undressing Allow to wear underpants if shy Offer equipment for inspection; briefly demonstrate use Make up "story" about procedure: "I'm seeing how strong your muscles are" (blood pressure) Use paper-doll technique Give choices when possible Expect cooperation; use positive statements: "Open your mouth"
SCHOOL-AGE CHILD		
Prefer sitting Cooperative in most positions Younger child prefers parent's presence Older child may prefer privacy	Proceed in head-to-toe direction May examine genitalia last in older child Respect need for privacy	Request self-undressing Allow to wear underpants Give gown to wear Explain purpose of equipment and significance of procedure, such as otoscope to see eardrum, which is necessary for hearing Teach about body functioning and care
ADOLESCENT		
Same as for school-age child Offer option of parent's presence	Same as for older school-age child	Allow to undress in private Give gown Expose only area to be examined Respect need for privacy Explain findings during examination: "Your muscles are firm and strong" Matter-of-factly comment about sexual development: "Your breasts are developing as they should be" Emphasize normalcy of development Examine genitalia as any other body part; may leave to end

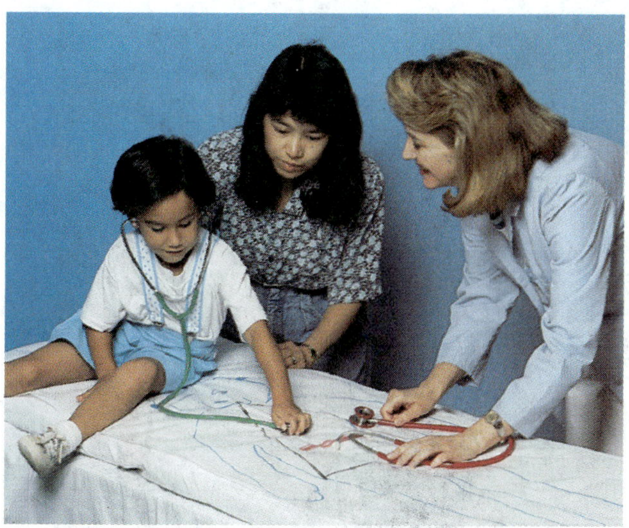

FIG. 7-1 Using paper-doll technique to prepare child for physical examination.

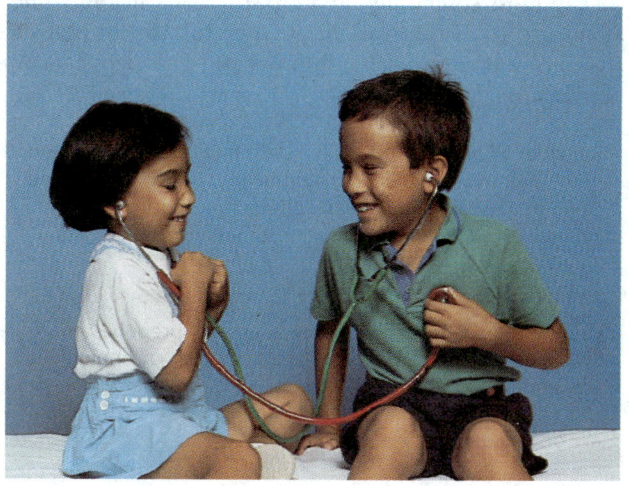

FIG. 7-2 Preparing children for physical examination.

stressful. Therefore the same considerations discussed in Chapter 27 for preparing children for procedures are followed here. In addition to that discussion, general guidelines related to the examining process are presented in the Guidelines box on p. 219. The physical examination should be as pleasant as possible, as well as educational. For example, with preschool and older children, use a detailed drawing or anatomically correct doll to help them learn about their bodies (Vessey, Braithwaite, and Weidmann, 1990). The "paper-doll" technique is a useful approach to teaching children about the part of the body that is being examined (Fig. 7-1). At the conclusion of the visit, the child can take the paper doll home as a memento of the experience.

In most instances children cooperate best when their parents remain with them. There are occasions, however, when older children, particularly adolescents, prefer to be examined alone, such as during the genital examination. Frequently the child being examined is also accompanied by a sibling, who may be disruptive because of boredom. A helpful tactic is to involve the sibling in the examination by allowing the child to hold the stethoscope or a tongue blade and praising the child for the "help" during the assessment.

Table 7-1 summarizes guidelines for positioning, preparing, and examining children at various ages. Since no child fits precisely into one age category, it may be necessary to vary the approach after a preliminary assessment of the child's developmental achievements and needs. Even when the best approach is used, many toddlers are uncooperative and unable to be consoled for much of the physical examination. However, some seem intrigued by the new surroundings and unusual equipment and respond more like preschoolers than toddlers. Likewise, some early preschoolers may require more of the "security measures" employed with younger children, such as continued parent-child contact, and less of the preparatory measures used with preschoolers, such as playing with the equipment before and during the actual examination (Fig. 7-2).

Although the variations in the general approaches are numerous, some of them are discussed here because they are more common. For example, the suggested sequence may change considerably when the child is in pain or when obvious physical defects are present. In either situation examine the affected area last to minimize distress early in the examination and to focus on normal, healthy, or functioning body parts.

Positioning may also be altered because of physical distress. For example, the child who is having difficulty breathing may not be able to lie down; thus perform as much of the physical examination as possible with the child in a sitting or slightly reclining position, or complete the examination at another time.

PHYSICAL EXAMINATION

Although the approach to and sequence of the physical examination differ according to the child's age, the following discussion outlines the traditional model for physical assessment. It emphasizes normal findings, variations from the norm that may cause parents or children concern but that require little or no intervention, and abnormalities that necessitate appropriate referral. The focus here includes all pediatric age-groups; see Chapter 8 for a detailed discussion of a newborn assessment for procedures and findings unique to the neonate.

GROWTH MEASUREMENTS

Measurement of physical growth in children is a key element in evaluation of the health status of children. Physical growth parameters include weight, height (length), skinfold thickness, arm circumference, and head circumference. Values for these growth parameters are plotted on percentile charts, and the child's measurements in percentiles are compared with those of the general population.

The most commonly used growth charts in the United States are from the National Center for Health Statistics (NCHS) and are available for boys and girls ages (see Appendix C):

Birth to 36 months—Records weight by age, recumbent length by age, weight for length, and head circumference by age
Two to 18 years—Records weight by age, stature by age
Prepubescence—Records weight for stature

NURSING ALERT The prepubescent charts are only appropriate for plotting values for prepubescent boys and girls, regardless of chronologic age, and not for any child showing signs of pubescence, such as breast budding, testicular enlargement, or growth of axillary or pubic hair.

Two sets of charts include data for children ages 2 to 3 years; the major difference between the two charts is that one set (for ages birth to 36 months) is based on ***recumbent length*** (length while lying supine), and the other set (for ages 2 to 18 years) uses ***stature*** (height while standing). These two methods of measuring length are not equivalent. Measurements using recumbent length are greater by as much as 2 cm, or nearly 1 inch, in this age-group than measurements obtained using stature. This amount of difference between measurements can lead to an erroneous conclusion of delayed growth if length is plotted during one visit and stature during the next visit on the birth to 36-month chart.

NURSING ALERT Plot only recumbent length on the birth to 36-month NCHS growth chart and stature on the 2- to 18-year growth chart.

The NCHS growth charts use the 5th and 95th percentiles as criteria for determining which children are outside the normal limits for growth. In general, those whose height or weight falls below the 5th percentile are considered underweight or small in stature; those whose measurements are above the 95th percentile are considered overweight or large in stature.

Percentile charts for skinfold thickness and arm circumference are also available and may be used as reference data. However, they should not be considered standards or norms, because values between the 5th and 95th percentile are not ranges of normal.

Overall evaluation of growth requires judgment in interpretation of growth percentiles. Generally, children whose height or weight falls below the 5th percentile or above the 95th percentile should be followed closely. However, small or large size may be genetic (Fig. 7-3). Comparing children's growth trends with those of their parents is essential in evaluating adequate growth. Most children with normal birth weights and heights and normal childhood growth will achieve an adult height within ± 2 inches of the midparental height (MPH). Special charts are available for parent-specific adjustments for evaluation of the child's height (Himes and others, 1985). To calculate the MPH, use the following formula (MacGillivray, 1993).

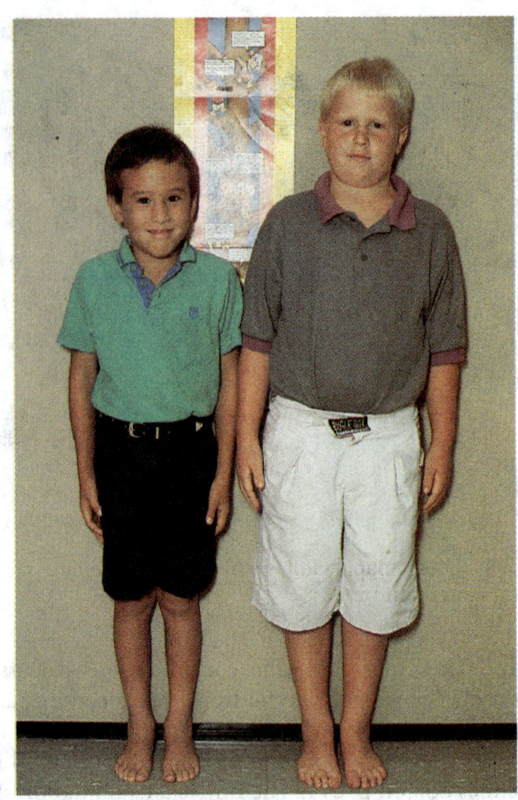

FIG. 7-3 These children of identical age (8 years) are markedly different in size. The child on the left, of Oriental descent, is at the 5th percentile for height and weight. The child on the right is above the 95th percentile for height and weight. However, both children demonstrate normal growth patterns.

For girls:

$$\frac{\text{(Father's height} - \text{13 cm or 5 inches)} + \text{Mother's height}}{2}$$

For boys:

$$\frac{\text{Father's height} + \text{13 cm or 5 inches)} + \text{Mother's height}}{2}$$

A potential concern with the U.S. growth charts is their accuracy in evaluating the growth of children from different ethnic and socioeconomic backgrounds. Growth of Mexican-American children has been found to be less than that of the reference population used for the NCHS growth charts. Mexican-American adolescents are short in stature according to the chart (Martorell, Mendoza, and Castillo, 1989). However, whether the differences for such groups are the result of nutritional factors or genetic background is still unclear. In contrast, accelerated growth of recently immigrated Southeast Asian children is probably the result of improved nutrition and health (Yip, Scanlon, and Trowbridge, 1992).

The type of infant feeding also affects growth. Breast-fed infants grow slower than bottle-fed infants, especially durng 6 to 18 months of age. Typically, this slower growth is

TABLE 7-2 Expected Growth Rates at Various Ages

AGE	EXPECTED GROWTH RATE (cm/yr)
1 to 6 months	18-22
6 to 12 months	14-18
2nd year	11
3rd year	8
4th year	7
5th to 10th years	5-6

From *Human growth and growth disorders: an update,* South San Francisco, 1989, Genentech.

normal, although it may be at or below the 5th percentile (Dewey and others, 1992).

Such findings indicate that these growth charts can serve as a reference guide if they are used from the perspective that different groups of children have varying normal distributions on the growth curves (Vaughan, 1992). The NCHS charts are accurate for U.S. black children because this group was included in the sample population, and for primarily bottle-fed infants.

Children whose growth may be questionable include:

- Children whose height and weight percentiles are widely disparate (e.g., height in the 10th percentile and weight in the 90th percentile, especially with above-average skinfold thickness)
- Children who fail to show the expected growth rates in height and weight, especially during the rapid growth periods of infancy and adolescence (Table 7-2)
- Children who show a sudden increase, except during puberty, or decrease in a previously steady growth pattern
- Since growth is a continuous but uneven process, the most reliable evaluation lies in comparison of growth measurements over a prolonged time.

Length

Length (or recumbent length) refers to measurements taken when children are supine. Until children are 24 months old (36 months if the birth to 36-month chart is used), measure recumbent length. Because of the normally flexed position during infancy, fully extend the body by (1) holding the head in midline, (2) grasping the knees together gently, and (3) pushing down on the knees until the legs are fully extended and flat against the table. If using a measuring board, place the head firmly at the top of the board and the heels of the feet firmly against the footboard.

If such a measuring device is not available, measure length by placing the child on a paper-covered surface, marking the end points of the top of the head and the heels of the feet, and measuring between these two points (Fig. 7-4). For accurate measurement hold the writing utensil at a right angle to the table when marking the cephalic point; position the feet with the toes pointing directly to the ceiling when marking the heel point. Regardless of the method used, have someone assist in holding the child's head in midline while you extend the legs and take the measurements.

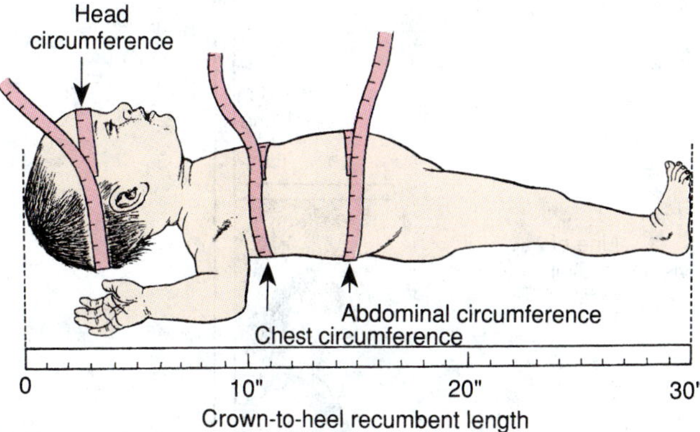

FIG. 7-4 Measurement of head, chest, and abdominal circumference and crown-to-heel (recumbent) length.

Height

Height (or stature) refers to the measurement taken when children are standing upright. Measure height by having the child, with shoes removed, stand as tall and straight as possible, with the head in midline and the line of vision parallel to the ceiling or floor. Be sure the child's back is to the wall or other vertical flat surface, with the heels, buttocks, and back of the shoulders touching the wall and the medial malleoli touching if possible (Fig. 7-5). Check for and correct bending of the knees, slumping of the shoulders, or raising of the heels of the feet.

➤ **NURSING TIP** Normally height is less if measured in the afternoon than in the morning. To minimize this variation, apply modest upward pressure under the jaw or the mastoid processes.

For the most accurate measurement, use a wall-mounted unit (stadiometer). The movable measuring rod of platform scales is accurate only if it maintains a parallel position to the floor and rests securely on the topmost part of the head. To improvise a flat surface for measuring length, attach a paper or metal tape or yardstick to the wall, position the child adjacent to the tape, and place a three-dimensional object, such as a thick book or box, on top of the head. Rest the side of the object firmly against the wall to form a right angle. Measure length or stature to the nearest 1 mm or ⅛ inch.

Occasionally, special length measurements are taken, such as ***sitting height*** or ***crown-to-rump length*** (for newborns see Physical Assessment, Chapter 8). In older infants and children determine sitting height by having the child sit against the wall and measuring between the vertex of the head and the sitting surface. Although not a usual measurement, this method is used for distinguishing children suspected of true growth deficiency from genetic small stature. Normally, sitting height accounts for 70% of total body length at birth, 60% at 2 years, and about 52% at age 10 years.

Weight

Weight is measured with an appropriately sized beam balance scale, which measures weights to the nearest 10 g or

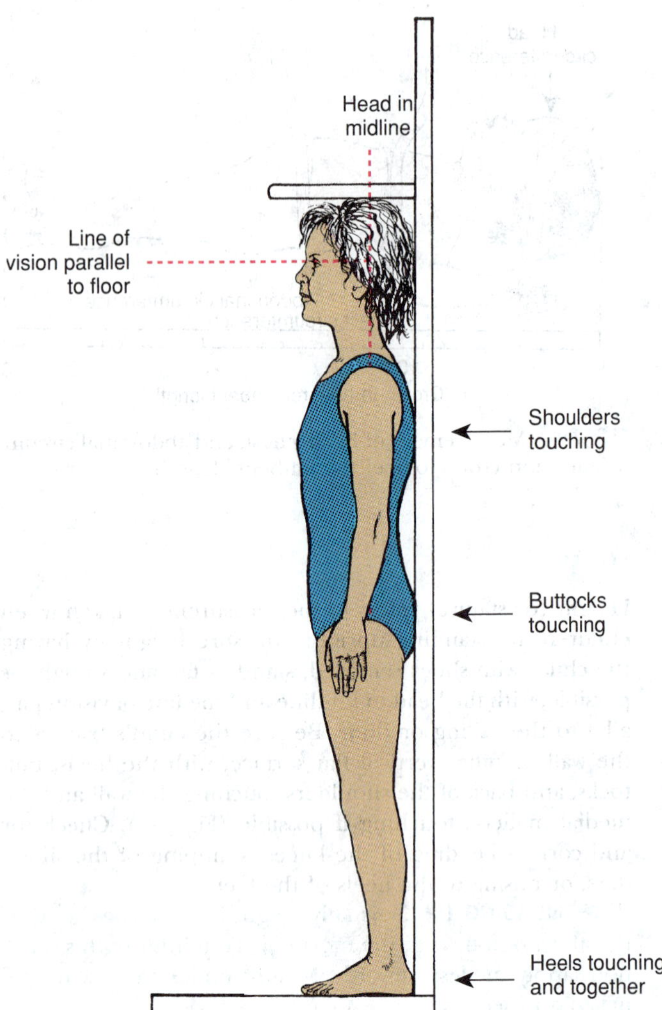

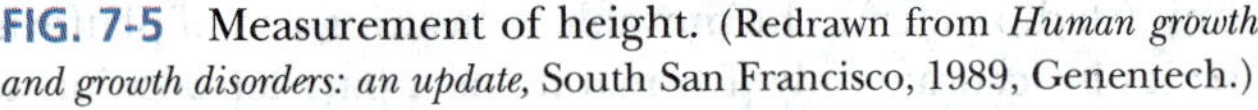

FIG. 7-5 Measurement of height. (Redrawn from *Human growth and growth disorders: an update,* South San Francisco, 1989, Genentech.)

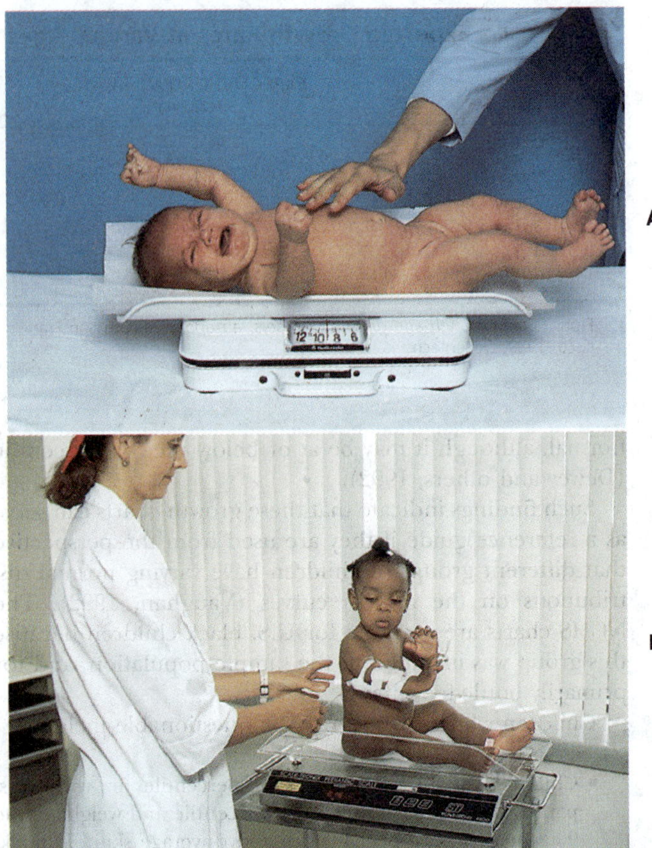

FIG. 7-6 **A,** Infant on scale. **B,** Toddler on scale. Note presence of nurse to prevent falls.

½ ounce for infants and 100 g or ¼ pound for children, or with an electronic digital scale. Before weighing the child, balance the scale by setting it at zero and noting if the balance registers exactly in the middle of the mark. If the end of the balance beam rises to the top or bottom of the mark, add more or less weight, respectively. Some scales are designed to allow for self-correction, but others need to be recalibrated by the manufacturer. Scales vary in their accuracy; infant scales tend to be more accurate than adult platform scales, and newer scales more accurate than older ones, especially at the upper levels of weight measurement. When precise measurements are needed, have a second nurse take the weight independently. If there is a discrepancy, take a third reading (Burke, Roberts, and Maloney, 1988).

Measurements are made in a comfortably warm room. When the birth to 36-month growth chart is used, children should be weighed nude. Older children are usually weighed while wearing their underpants or a light gown. However, with all children, always respect their privacy. If the child must be weighed wearing some article of clothing or some type of special device, such as a prosthesis, note this when recording the weight. Children who are measured for recumbent length are usually weighed on a large platform type of infant scale and placed in a lying-down or sitting position. When weighing infants, place the hand lightly above the body to prevent them from accidentally falling off the scale (Fig. 7-6). Once stature is taken weight can also be measured on an upright platform scale. For maximum asepsis, cover the scale with a clean sheet of paper between each child's measurement.

Skinfold Thickness and Arm Circumference

Measures of relative weight and stature cannot distinguish between adiposity or muscularity. One convenient measure of body fat is skinfold thickness. Skinfold thickness is measured with special calipers, such as the Lange calipers. The most common sites for measuring skinfold thickness are the triceps (most practical for routine clinical use), subscapula, suprailiac, abdomen, and upper thigh. For greatest reliability, follow the exact procedure for measurement and record the average of at least two measurements of one site (see Guidelines box).

Arm circumference is an indirect measure of muscle mass. To measure arm circumference, follow the same pro-

GUIDELINES
Measuring Triceps Skinfold Thickness

With child's right arm flexed 90 degrees at elbow, mark midpoint between acromion and olecranon on posterior aspect of arm.
With arm hanging freely, grasp a fold of skin between thumb and forefinger 1 cm above midpoint.
Gently pull fold away from underlying muscle and continue to hold until measurement is completed.
Place caliper jaws over skinfold at midpoint mark; if a plastic caliper (e.g., Ross Adipometer) is used, apply pressure with thumb to align lines on caliper; follow directions for using other calipers.
Estimate reading to nearest 1.0 mm, 2 to 3 seconds after applying pressure.
Take measurements until duplicates agree within 1 mm.

cedure as for skinfold thickness except measure the midpoint with a paper or steel tape. Place the tape vertically along the posterior aspect of the upper arm to the acromial process and to the olecranon process; half the measured length is the midpoint. Percentiles for triceps skinfold and arm circumference in children are listed in Appendix C and may be used as reference data. However, the percentiles are not standards or norms, because values between the 5th and 95th percentiles are not ranges of normal.

Head Circumference

Measure head circumference in children up to 36 months of age and in any child whose head size is questionable. Measure the head at its greatest circumference, usually slightly above the eyebrows and pinna of the ears and around the occipital prominence at the back of the skull (see Fig. 7-4). Since head shape can affect the location of the maximum circumference, more than one measurement at points above the eyebrows may need to be taken to obtain the most accurate measure. Use a paper or metal tape because a cloth tape can stretch and give a falsely small measurement. For greatest accuracy, use devices with tenths of a centimeter, since the percentile charts have only 0.5 cm increments.

Plot the head size on the appropriate growth chart under head circumference. Generally, head and chest circumferences are equal at about 1 to 2 years of age. During childhood chest circumference exceeds head size by about 5 to 7 cm (2 to 3 in). (For newborns see Physical Assessment, Chapter 8.)

PHYSIOLOGIC MEASUREMENTS

Physiologic measurements, key elements in evaluating physical status of vital functions, include temperature, pulse, respiration, and blood pressure. Compare each physiologic recording with normal values for that age-group (see inside back cover). In addition, compare the values taken on preceding health visits with present recordings. For example, a falsely elevated blood pressure reading may not indicate hypertension if previous recent readings have been

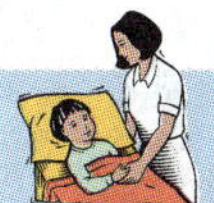

ATRAUMATIC CARE
Reducing Young Children's Fears

Young children, especially preschoolers, fear intrusive procedures because of their poorly defined body boundaries. Therefore avoid invasive procedures, such as measuring rectal temperature, whenever possible. Also, avoid using the word "take" when measuring vital signs, since young children interpret words literally and may think that their temperature or other function will be taken away. Instead, say, "I want to know how warm you are."

within normal limits. The isolated recording may indicate some stressful event in the child's life.

As in most procedures carried out with children, older children and adolescents are treated much the same as are adults. However, special consideration must be given to preschool children (see Atraumatic Care box).

For best results in taking vital signs of infants, count respirations first, before the infant is disturbed, take the pulse next, and measure temperature last. If vital signs cannot be taken without disturbing the child, record the child's behavior (e.g., crying) along with the measurement.

Temperature

Temperature can be measured at several sites in the body via the oral, rectal, axillary, skin, or tympanic membrane route. Recent substitutes for the traditional mercury thermometer are the electronic thermometer, the tympanic membrane sensor, the Tempa-Dot, the plastic strip, and the digital thermometer, which offer the advantages of measuring temperature rapidly and/or avoiding oral or rectal intrusion (see Thinking Critically About . . . box on pp. 226-227 and Table 7-3). Although the accuracy of these instruments differs, accuracy is decreased to a greater extent if correct technique is not used (Pontious and others, 1994b).

➤ **NURSING TIP** When using a tympanic membrane sensor, first use an otoscope to visualize the eardrum. Once the drum is seen, note the type of ear tag and speculum placement in the ear. Use the same procedure for inserting the probe tip.

No universal agreement exists regarding the length of time mercury thermometers should be kept in place. Recommendations based on research are 7 minutes for an oral reading, 4 minutes for a rectal reading, and 5 minutes for an axillary reading. However, these times may vary widely within practice settings and may not represent clinically significant differences from temperature readings taken for shorter intervals.

➤ **NURSING TIP** If in doubt about the optimum length of insertion time, reinsert the mercury thermometer after the first reading for a short time and recheck the scale for a rise. If the value is increased, reinsert the thermometer until the next reading is the same as the previous reading.

Normal body temperature registers 37.0° C (98.6° F) via the oral route. Traditionally it has been assumed that rec-

THINKING CRITICALLY ABOUT . . .

Route of Temperature Measurement in Children

The primary purpose of measuring body temperature is to detect abnormally high or low values. In febrile patients the chief concern is the temperature of the brain, since very high temperatures can cause neural damage. Thus the best sites for measuring temperature are those closest to the brain that reflect central or "core" body heat (Holtzclaw, 1993). The temperature of the mixed venous blood in the pulmonary artery is generally considered the best core value (Erickson and Yount, 1991). Other core sites are the esophagus and bladder. However, these sites involve invasive thermometry and are impractical for routine temperature measurement.

Traditionally, the oral, rectal, and axillary sites have been used in clinical practice. Many clinicians consider the rectal route to be the "gold standard" for routine temperature measurement in children (Freed and Fraley, 1992; Schuman, 1993). However, the accuracy of rectal temperature was challenged as early as 1954 by Gerbrandy, Snell, and Cranston, who found that rectal measurements did not respond quickly to induced heat changes in the body. This slow tracking and the higher rectal temperatures as compared with pulmonary artery temperatures may be due to the relatively poor blood flow to the rectum and the insulating property of the stool (Accuracy, 1991; Terndrup and Milewski, 1991).

Results of studies on the other sites have also yielded conflicting results. Oral temperature assessments are influenced by many factors, such as crying, eating or drinking, smoking, and the location of the thermometer in the mouth. Cole (1993) found that ice water lowered oral temperature in adults, but normal temperature was regained within 15 minutes. Axillary assessments have been found to underestimate core temperature and to be affected by ambient temperature (Martyn, Carmon, and Rice, 1994; Morley and others, 1992; Muma and others, 1991). Thermographs (plastic strip thermometers placed on the skin) have also been found to underestimate core temperature (Lewitt, Marshall, and Salzer, 1982; Martyn, Carmon, and Rice, 1994; Scholefield, Gerber, and Dwyer, 1982) or to produce false-positive findings (afebrile children diagnosed as having fever) (Martyn and others, 1988).

Contributed by Marti Rice, Kristy Martyn, Myra Carmon, and Donna Wong.

Another site that is used for temperature measurement is the tympanic membrane. The ear's proximity to the hypothalamus, the body's temperature-regulating center, makes it a desirable area for reflecting true core temperature. Results of studies using tympanic membrane measurements are conflicting, however. Benzinger and Benzinger (1972) found a higher correlation between tympanic membrane and esophageal measurements than between rectal and esophageal measurements. Ferra-Love (1991) found no significant differences between pulmonary artery and tympanic membrane measurements in adults. Milewski, Ferguson, and Terndrup (1991) found significantly better correlations between rectal and pulmonary artery temperatures than between tympanic membrane and pulmonary artery assessments; at the same time, they found that pulmonary artery and tympanic membrane temperatures were not significantly different, whereas rectal temperatures were significantly warmer. However, another study found that pulmonary artery and tympanic membrane temperatures were highly correlated (r = .91), whereas rectal and ear temperatures were only moderately correlated (r = .52) (Klein and others, 1993). Unfortunately, these studies were all performed on adults; similar research is needed with children.

In comparisons with rectal, oral, or axillary temperature assessments in children, some studies have found tympanic membrane measurements to be fairly insensitive in detecting fevers and recommend caution in use with children less than 3 years of age (Freed and Fraley, 1992; Muma and others, 1991). In contrast, several studies have shown strong positive correlations between tympanic membrane and rectal temperature measurements in children (Chamberlain and others, 1991; Davis, 1993; Kenney and others, 1990; Stewart and Webster, 1992; Talo, Macknin, and Medendrop, 1991). However, Chamberlain and colleagues (1991) and Stewart and Webster (1992) did not obtain the same findings with infants less than 3 months of age, and Davis (1993) found inaccurate readings in children younger than 3 years. Yet others have reported reliable ear measurements in newborns and young infants (Johnson, Bhatian, and Bell, 1991; Weiss, 1991).

Obviously, from a selected review of the literature, it seems that no one routinely used site for temperature assessment provides unequivocal estimates of core body temperature and that similar kinds of comparison studies can yield contradictory results. What factors might influence the discrepancies? One might be the use of the rectal temperature as the "gold standard" for comparison. As some studies have shown, the rectal temperature may change slowly and may not always reflect pulmonary artery values. Some authorities caution that "gold standards" are rarely reached because the subject (like temperature measurement) is changing and improving (Duggan, 1992). Such may be the case with tympanic membrane sensors. The eardrum's anatomic location is superior to the rectal site, and a poor correlation between the two sites may actually indicate more accurate, not less accurate, temperature values from ear thermometry (Terndrup and Milewski, 1991). Perhaps aural temperatures should be considered the "gold standard," and studies showing a poor correlation between ear and rectal temperatures should be used to discourage use of the rectal route (Roscelli, 1993).

Also, most models of ear sensors use "offsets," or internal calculations that transform the ear temperature into supposedly equivalent oral or rectal temperatures. These offsets may be a source of error. For example, each manufacturer uses a different formula to calculate the offset, and the formula (usually based on adult data) is applied to all age-groups (Tourangeau, MacLeod, and Breakwell, 1993). One study found that the actual ear reading, not the offsets, reliably indicated temperature in premature and full-term neonates (Johnson, Bhatia, and Bell, 1991).

In addition, the size of the probe may influence the reading. Many ear probes are too large to be correctly placed in the canal (Treloar and Muma, 1988). A newer infrared ear thermometer, the Ototemp Pedi-Q, features a small (2.5 mm) probe that fits in the infant's ear and gives an actual tympanic membrane temperature (Tourangeau, MacLeod, and Breakwell, 1993).

Also, technique is a very important factor. For the sensor to detect heat from the drum, not from the cooler canals, the ear canal must be straightened, as when using an otoscope. With the ear tugged correctly and the probe tip pointing at the midpoint between the eyebrow and the sideburn on the opposite side of the face, higher temperature readings are obtained (Terndrup and Rajk, 1992).

THINKING CRITICALLY ABOUT . . .

Route of Temperature Measurement in Children—cont'd

Finally, in deciding which route to use, "atraumatic care" should be considered. Children are less upset having their temperature measured via the ear route than via the rectal route (Alexander and Kelly, 1991b; Barber and Kilmon, 1989). Parents may also object to the rectal route. In a British study 37 of 42 parents who were interviewed expressed concers that included a fear of hurting their child, anxieties about being accused of sexual abuse, difficulty comforting their child, and concern for the youngster's feelings (Kai, 1993). For the practitioner, using the tympanic membrane sensor saves time (Alexander and Kelly, 1991a; Barber and Kilmon, 1989).

In considering all the findings for and against different sites of temperature measurement, nurses need to think critically about why the temperature is needed, how clinically significant a small difference in temperature between routes really is, and how much the procedure upsets the child and caregiver. Remember, we are not even sure what normal body temperature is. The "gold standard" of 37° C (98.6° F) in adults has been questioned; the "new" mean oral temperature, reported as 36.8° C (98.2° F), varies among individuals and fluctuates an average of 0.5° C (0.9° F) a day, with a maximum temperature being reached between 4 and 6 PM and a minimum value occurring at 6 AM (Mackowiak Wasserman, and Levine, 1992).

tal temperatures are 1° F higher and axillary temperatures are 1° F lower than oral temperatures. However, it has been demonstrated that this difference is considerably less (Pontious and others, 1994a). Because of these variations, chart the route along with the recorded temperature reading.

Whenever a child feels extra warm to the touch, measure the temperature even if it was normal only a short time before. Other signs of increased body temperature are flushed skin, increased respiratory and heart rate, malaise, and a "glassy look" to the eyes.

Pulse

A satisfactory pulse can be taken radially in children over 2 years of age. However, in infants and young children the apical impulse (heard through a stethoscope held to the chest at the apex of the heart) is more reliable. (See Fig. 7-39 for location of pulses.) Count the pulse for 1 full minute in infants and young children because of possible irregularities in rhythm. However, when frequent apical rates are needed, use shorter counting times (e.g., 15- or 30-second intervals). For greater accuracy, measure the apical rate while the child is asleep; record the child's behavior along with the rate (Margolius, Sneed, and Hollerbach, 1991). Pulses may be graded according to the criteria in Table 7-4. Compare radial and femoral pulses at least once during early childhood to detect the presence of circulatory impairment, such as coarctation of the aorta. (See inside back cover for normal rates for pediatric age-groups.)

Respiration

Count the respiratory rate in the same manner as for the adult patient. However, in infants observe abdominal movements, since respirations are primarily diaphragmatic. Since the movements are irregular, count them for 1 full minute for accuracy (see also p. 257). (See inside back cover for normal respiratory rates in children.)

Blood Pressure (BP)

BP measurement by noninvasive methods is part of a routine vital sign determination. BP should be measured an-

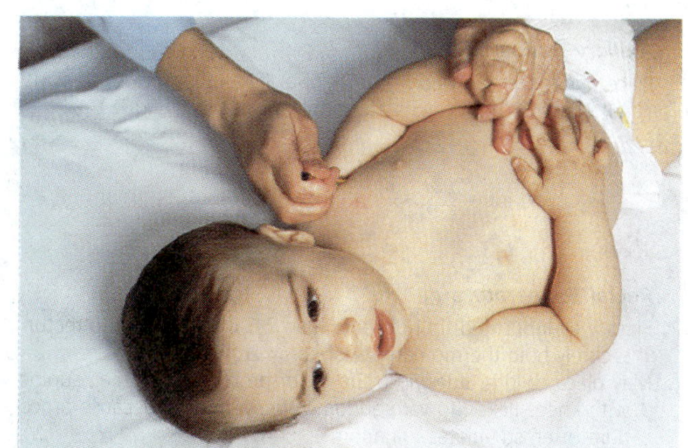

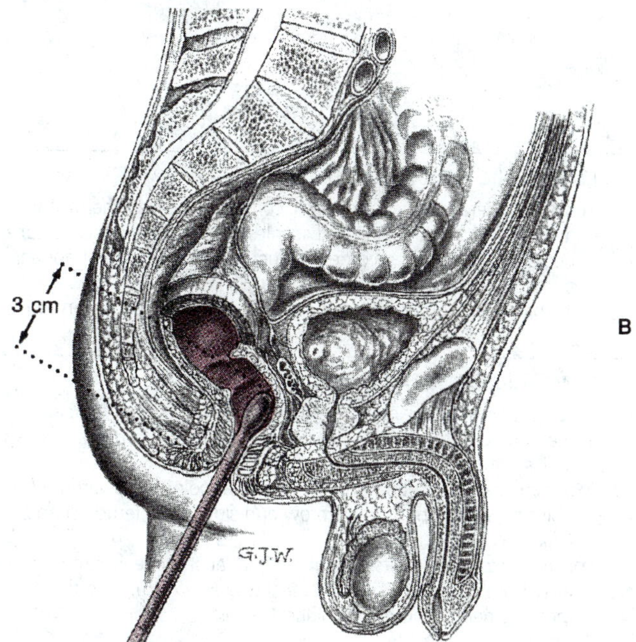

FIG. 7-7 **A,** Position for taking axillary temperature. **B,** Cross-section of rectum illustrates curve at approximately 3 cm from anus, where risk of perforation from thermometer is greatest in infants under 3 months of age.

TABLE 7-3 Comparison of Body Temperature Techniques

DESCRIPTION/PROCEDURE	COMMENTS
MERCURY GLASS THERMOMETER Heat causes mercury to expand and rise in glass tube	Only difference in selection of mercury thermometers is that rectal type has more rounded tip as compared with oral type, which has more slender, elongated tip Appropriate length of time mercury thermometer should remain in place for accurate measurement of temperature is controversial; a general rule is to leave thermometer in place about 3 minutes, or follow agency policy (see also Nursing Tip, p. 225)
Oral Temperature Place under tongue in right or left posterior sublingual pocket, not in front of tongue; have child keep mouth closed without biting on thermometer	Sublingual site indicates rapid changes in core body temperature *better* than rectal site Several factors affect temperature of mouth, such as hot or cold beverages, smoking, open-mouth breathing, and ambient temperature (Neff and others, 1989; Terndrup, Allegra, and Kealy, 1989) Oxygen by mask lowers oral temperature, but clinical significance of difference is questionable (Dressler, Smejkal, and Ruffolo, 1983)
Axillary Temperature Place under arm with tip in center of axilla and kept close to skin, not clothing; hold child's arm firmly against side (Fig. 7-7, *A*)	Recommended for children who object strongly to rectal temperature but for whom an oral temperature is not feasible Has advantage of avoiding intrusive procedure and eliminating risk of rectal perforation and possible peritonitis May be affected by poor peripheral perfusion (lower value) or use of radiant warmers or brown fat in cold-stressed neonates (higher value) (Haddock, Merrow, and Vincent, 1988)
Rectal Temperature Place well-lubricated tip not more than 2.5 cm (1 inch) into rectum; securely hold thermometer close to anus May place child in side-lying, supine, or prone position (i.e., supine with knees flexed toward abdomen); cover penis, because procedure often stimulates urination A small child may be placed prone across parent's lap	Taken only when no other route or device can be used (e.g., in children whose mental age or temperament prevents cooperation and understanding instructions, agitated children, and those who have had oral or axillary injuries or surgery) Not recommended, because core temperature is not obtained unless thermometer is inserted to depth of at least 5 cm, which incurs risk of rectal perforation, especially in neonates less than 3 months of age, since colon curves at depth of 3 cm (Fig. 7-7, *B*); also not recommended in anyone who has had rectal surgery, or in children with diarrhea or those receiving chemotherapy that affects mucosa Accuracy is affected by stool in rectum (higher value)
ELECTRONIC THERMOMETER Senses temperature with electronic component called thermistor mounted at tip of plastic and stainless steel probe, which is connected to electronic recorder, temperature measurement appears on digital display within 60 seconds Place probe in mouth, axilla, or rectum as with mercury thermometer	Idealy suited to pediatric use because plastic sheath is unbreakable, and child's mouth can remain open when oral temperature is taken Accuracy for axillary temperature is supported by some research (Barrus, 1983) but not by other studies (Ogren, 1990)
TYMPANIC MEMBRANE SENSOR Infrared thermometer measures thermal radiation from tympanic membrane; temperature measurement appears on digital display in 1 second Insert covered probe tip gently in ear canal pointing toward midpoint between opposite eyebrow and sideburns (Terndrup and Rajk, 1992) For most accurate results, straighten ear canal for sensor to measure heat from drum, not sides of canal (see Fig. 7-25), take three measurements, and record highest reading	Tympanic membrane is excellent site because both eardrum and hypothalamus (temperature-regulating center) are perfused by same circulation Sensor is unaffected by cerumen; presence of suppurative or nonsuppurative otitis media does not significantly affect measurement (Kenney and others, 1990); warm ambient temperature may increase aural temperature (Zehner and Terndrup, 1991). Procedure is well accepted by infants and children Because of difficulty with correct placement in young infants' ears, accuracy may be affected
PLASTIC STRIP THERMOMETER (THERMOGRAPH) Changes color in response to sensed temperature changes Place strip on forehead until color change occurs; usually takes less than 15 seconds Some strips are used like oral mercury thermometer	Accuracy is variable; best used for screening Advantages for home use include simple instructions and minimal cost

TABLE 7-3 Comparison of Body Temperature Techniques—cont'd

DESCRIPTION/PROCEDURE	COMMENTS
DIGITAL THERMOMETER	
Consists of probe that connects to microprocessor chip, which translates signals into degrees and sends temperature measurement to digital display Used like oral mercury thermometer	More accurate and easier to read, but somewhat more expensive than mercury or plastic strip thermometer
TEMPA-DOT	
Single-use disposable thermometer with specific chemical mixture in each circle that changes color to measure temperature in increments of two tenths of a degree Used like mercury thermometer; kept in mouth (1 minute), axilla (3 minutes), and rectum (3 minutes); color change is read 10-15 seconds after removing thermometer	Found to be accurate and reliable for children with and without fever, especially for temperature below 38° C (100.4° F) (Pontius and others, 1994a, 1994b) Easier to read than mercury or plastic strip thermometer Safer than glass thermometers (disposable and flexible) Read thermometer away from heat source (e.g., radiant warmer) If unused thermometer changes color from storage in warm area (above 35° C [95° F]), place in freezer for 1 hour, then at room temperature for 24 hours before using

TABLE 7-4 Grading of Pulses

GRADE	DESCRIPTION
0	Not palpable
+1	Difficult to palpate, thready, weak, easily obliterated with pressure
+2	Difficult to palpate, may be obliterated with pressure
+3	Easy to palpate, not easily obliterated with pressure (normal)
+4	Strong, bounding, not obliterated with pressure

TABLE 7-5 Commonly Available Blood Pressure Cuffs

CUFF NAME*	BLADDER WIDTH (cm)	BLADDER LENGTH (cm)
Newborn	2.5-4.0	5.0-9.0
Infant	4.0-6.0	11.5-18.0
Child	7.5-9.0	17.0-19.0
Adult	11.5-13.0	22.0-26.0
Large arm	14.0-15.0	30.5-33.0
Thigh	18.0-19.0	36.0-38.0

From Report of the Second Task Force on Blood Pressure Control in Children—1987, *Pediatrics* 79(1):1-25, 1987.
*Cuff name does not guarantee that the cuff will be appropriate size for a child within that age range.

nually in children 3 years of age through adolescence, and in children with symptoms of hypertension, children in emergency rooms and intensive care units, and high-risk infants (Report of the Second Task Force, 1987). Several authorities also recommend routine measurements in low-risk neonates (Seidel, Rosenstein, and Pathak, 1993), although the American Academy of Pediatrics (1993) does not.

Measurement Devices. The most common method of measuring BP uses ***auscultation*** and either a ***mercury-gravity*** or ***aneroid sphygmomanometer.*** Both types are reliable and accurate, but the mercury-gravity manometer does not require recalibration as does the aneroid type.

BP can also be measured using electronic devices that employ oscillometric or Doppler techniques. In ***oscillometry,*** pressure changes are transmitted through the arterial wall to the pressure cuff, and the oscillations are detected by a pressure-sensitive indicator. Oscillometers have digital readouts for systolic, diastolic, and ***mean arterial pressures (MAP),*** and pulse. The MAP is not the same as the mean BP (arithmetic average of systolic and diastolic pressures). Rather, it is a value somewhat lower than the arithmetic mean. BP readings using oscillometry, such as Dinamap, are generally higher and correlate better with direct radial artery values than measurements using auscultation (see Table 7-8) (Park and Menard, 1987). Oscillometry also eliminates common problems found with the auscultation method, such as deflating the cuff too rapidly, not hearing the softest sounds, and rounding numbers for the Korotoff sounds.

The ***Doppler ultrasound*** translates changes in ultrasound frequency caused by blood movement within the artery to audible sound by means of a transducer in the cuff. The Doppler is useful for systolic pressure measurement but is unreliable for diastolic pressure measurement. Oscillometric and Doppler instruments are very useful in measuring BP in infants and have largely replaced the flush method, which reflects only the mean BP, and the auscultatory method.

Selection of Cuff. No matter what type of noninvasive technique is used, the most important factor in accurately measuring BP is the use of an appropriately sized cuff (***cuff size*** refers only to the inner inflatable bladder, not the cloth covering). Unfortunately, authorities disagree on the correct method for determining cuff size. The Report of the Second Task Force (1987) recommends cuff size based on ***limb length*** (Table 7-5):

TABLE 7-6 Recommended Bladder Dimensions for Blood Pressure Cuffs

ARM CIRCUMFERENCE AT MIDPOINT (cm)	CUFF NAME*	BLADDER WIDTH (cm)	BLADDER LENGTH (cm)
5-7.5	Newborn	3	5
7.5-13	Infant	5	8
13-20	Child	8	13
24-32	Adult	13	24
32-42	Wide adult	17	34
42-50	Thigh	20	42

From Frohlich ED and others: Recommendations for human blood pressure determination by sphygmomanometers: report of a special task force appointed by the Steering Committee, American Health Association, *Circulation* 77:501A, 1988.
*Cuff name does not guarantee that the cuff will be appropriate size for a child within that age range.

- Width sufficient to cover approximately 75% of upper arm between top of shoulder and olecranon
- Length sufficient to completely encircle circumference of limb with or without overlapping
- Enough room at antecubital fossa to place bell of stethoscope
- Enough room at upper edge of cuff to prevent obstruction of axilla

The American Heart Association (Frohlich and others 1988) recommends cuff size based on ***limb circumference*** (Table 7-6):

- Width 40% to 50% of limb circumference; measured at upper arm midway between top of shoulder and olecranon
- Length sufficient to completely or nearly completely encircle circumference of limb without overlapping

Using limb length for selecting cuff width may produce satisfactory BP readings in children with average weight for height, but inaccurate readings in children with thick arms. Using limb circumference for selecting cuff width more accurately reflects direct arterial blood pressure than using limb length because this method takes into account the varying thickness of the arm and the amount of pressure required to compress the artery (Park and Guntheroth, 1989). For measurement sites other than the upper arms, use the limb circumference guidelines, although the shape of the limb (i.e., conical shape of the thigh) may prevent appropriate placement of the cuff and result in inaccurate reflection of intraarterial BP.

Cuffs that are either too narrow or too wide affect the accuracy of BP measurements, although wide cuffs tend to affect BP readings less. When the correctly sized cuff is used, the inflated cuff transmits the same pressure on the underlying arterial wall as the pressure registered on the device. If the cuff is too small, the pressure around the artery may be less than that registered on the device, so that the reading is falsely high. If the cuff is too large, the excessive cuff width reduces the kinetic energy of blood flow, resulting in a lower reading. This effect is probably more marked with the auscultatory method than with the oscillometric method (Fig. 7-8) (Park and Guntheroth, 1989).

NURSING ALERT In choosing cuff sizes, use an appropriately sized cuff. When the correct size is not available, use an oversized cuff rather than an undersized one or use another site that more appropriately fits the cuff size. Do not choose a cuff based on the name of the cuff (i.e., an "infant" cuff may be too small for some infants).

When another site is used, BP measurements using noninvasive techniques may differ. Generally, systolic pressure in the lower extremities (thigh or calf) is greater than pressure in the upper extremities, and systolic BP in the calf is higher than that in the thigh. These differences are listed in Table 7-7 and apply to oscillometric measurements taken on the right extremities with the child supine and the cuff size based on the circumference method (Park, Lee, and Johnson, 1993).

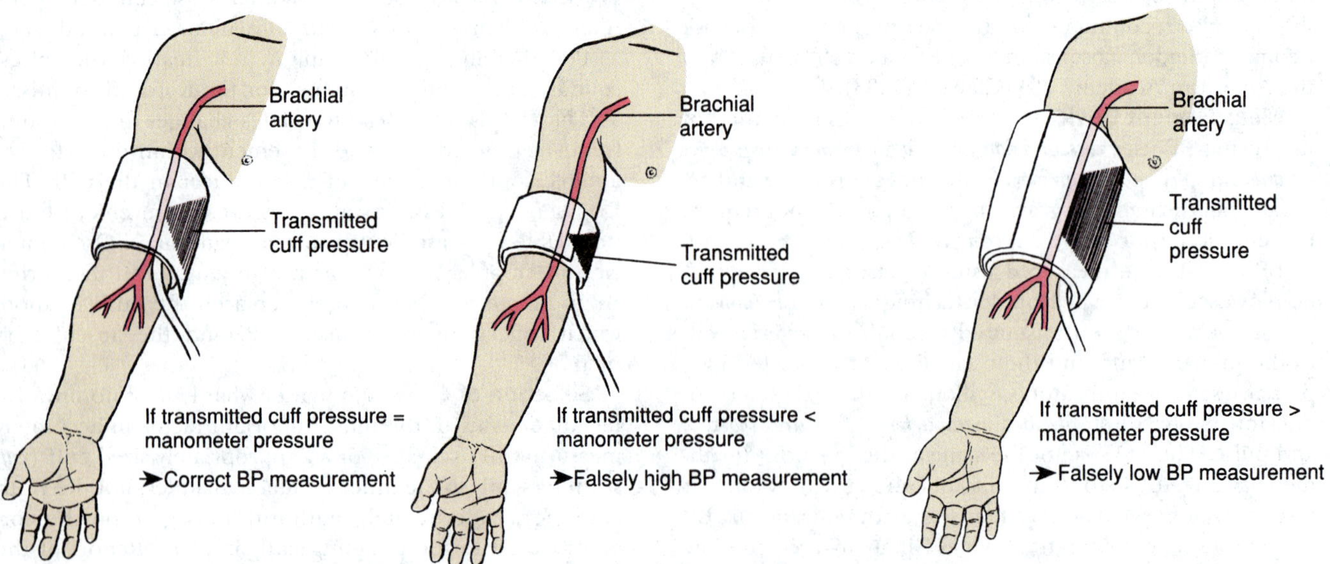

FIG. 7-8 Effect of cuff size on blood pressure measurement.

TABLE 7-7 Differences in Oscillometric Systolic BP Between Arm and Lower Extremity Sites in Normal Children

AGE-GROUP (YEARS)	SYSTOLIC BP × (MEAN ± SD)	
	ARM-THIGH	ARM-CALF
4-8	−7.1±6.8	−9.3± 7.4
9-16	−2.4±7.7	−5.0±26.9

From Park M, Lee D, Johnson GA: Oscillometric blood pressures in the arm, thigh, and calf in healthy children and those with aortic coarctation, *Pediatrics* 91(4):761-765, 1993.

NURSING ALERT Compare BP in the upper and lower extremities at least once to detect abnormalities, such as coarctation of the aorta, in which the lower extremity pressure is less than the upper extremity pressure.

Measurement and Interpretation. Measuring and interpreting BP in infants and children requires additional attention to correct procedure because (1) limb sizes vary and cuff selection must accommodate the circumference; (2) excessive pressure on the antecubital fossa affects the Korotkoff sounds; (3) children easily become anxious, which can elevate BP; and (4) BP values change with age and growth. Larger children, especially in terms of height, have higher normal BPs than smaller children of the same age (de Swiet and others, 1989).

Although the technique of BP measurement in children is generally the same as that used for adults (see Guidelines box), some aspects of the procedure are especially important. Because children are easily upset by unfamiliar procedures, prepare them for BP measurement. For children of preschool age and above, explain each step of the procedure and tell them how the cuff will feel, such as a tight feeling or an arm hug. Use explanations such as "I want to see how strong your muscle is" or "Let's watch the silver rise in the tube."

Since the child should be quiet and relaxed during the procedure, measure BP before performing any anxiety-producing procedures. Infants and small children may be more quiet if the reading is taken while they are sitting in the parent's lap.

Use a pediatric stethoscope and bell for hearing BP sounds in small children and infants. If ausculation is not possible, obtain a systolic reading by palpation; measure the point at which the pulse at the radial or brachial artery reappears as the cuff is deflated.

The average BP readings at various ages throughout childhood using sphygmomanometry are listed on the inside back cover, and readings using oscillometry are listed in Table 7-8.

NURSING ALERT Published norms for BP, such as those on the inside back cover, are valid only if the same method of measurement (auscultation and limb length for cuff size) is used in clinical practice.

GUIDELINES
Measuring Blood Pressure

Use an appropriately sized cuff.
Use same position, preferably sitting, and right arm for brachial artery site (Fig. 7-9, *A*).
Use alternate site as needed to accommodate available cuff sizes:
- Use smaller size on forearm: place cuff above wrist and auscultate radial artery (Fig. 7-9, *B*).
- Use larger size on thigh: place cuff above knee and auscultate popliteal artery (Fig. 7-9, *C*).
- Use larger size on calf: place cuff above malleoli or at midcalf and auscultate posterior tibial or dorsal pedal artery (Fig. 7-9, *D*).

Position limb at level of heart.
Rapidly inflate cuff to about 20 mm Hg above point at which radial pulse disappears.
Release cuff pressure at a rate of about 2 to 3 mm Hg/sec during auscultation of artery.
Read mercury-gravity manometer at eye level.
Record systolic value as onset of a clear tapping sound (first Korotkoff sound).
Record diastolic pressure as:
- Fourth Korotkoff sound (K4) (low-pitched, muffled sound) for children up to age 12 years
- Fifth Korotkoff sound (K5) (disappearance of all sound) for children ages 13 to 18 years

Record also limb, position, cuff size, and method of measurement.
If using electronic monitor, follow manufacturer's instructions and guidelines for correct cuff size.
- With oscillometric device (i.e., Dinamap), can use all four limb sites, but reserve the thigh for last, since it is the most uncomfortable.
- Stabilize limb during cuff deflation, since movement interferes with the device's ability to measure BP accurately.

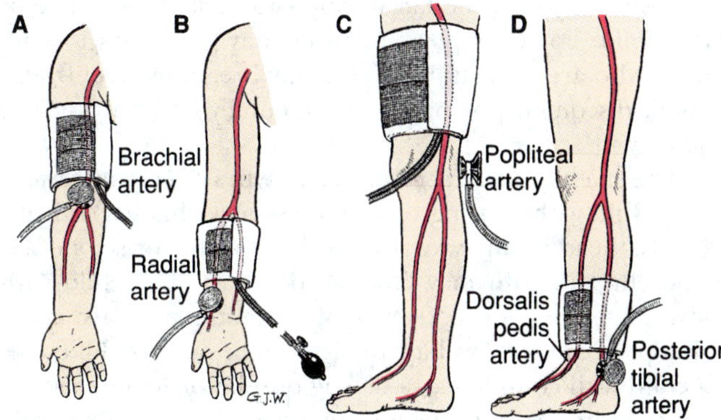

FIG. 7-9 Sites for measuring blood pressure. **A,** Upper arm. **B,** Lower arm or forearm. **C,** Thigh. **D,** Calf or ankle.

➤ **NURSING TIP** Use the following quick formula for normal ***systolic BP*** using auscultation:

1 to 7 years: Age in years + 90
8 to 18 years: (2 × Age in years) + 83

Use the following quick formula for normal ***diastolic BP*** using auscultation:

1 to 5 years: 56
6 to 18 years: Age in years + 52

TABLE 7-8 Normative Oscillometric (Dinamap) BP Values (Systolic/Diastolic, Mean Arterial Pressure in Parentheses)

AGE-GROUP	MEAN	90th PERCENTILE	95th PERCENTILE
Newborn (1-3 days)	65/41 (50)	75/49 (59)	78/52 (62)
1 month to 2 years	95/58 (72)	106/68 (83)	110/71 (86)
2-5 years	101/57 (74)	112/66 (82)	115/68 (85)

From Park M, Menard S: Normative oscillometric blood pressure values in the first 5 years in an office setting, *Am J Dis Child* 143(7):860-864, 1989.

BP values are defined as follows (see also discussion of hypertension in Chapter 34):

Normal blood pressure—Systolic and diastolic BP less than 90th percentile for age and sex

High normal blood pressure—Systolic and diastolic BP between 90th and 95th percentiles for age and sex

High blood pressure—Systolic and diastolic BP at or above 95th percentile for age and sex

GENERAL APPEARANCE

The general appearance of the child is a cumulative, subjective impression of the child's physical appearance, state of nutrition, behavior, personality, interactions with parents and nurse (also siblings if present), posture, development, and speech. Although general appearance is recorded in the beginning of the physical examination, it encompasses all the observations of the child during the interview and physical assessment.

Note the ***facies,*** the facial expression and appearance of the child. For example, the facies may give clues to children who are in pain; have difficulty breathing; feel frightened, discontent, or happy; are mentally deficient; or are acutely ill.

Observe the ***posture, position,*** and types of ***body movement.*** The child with hearing or vision loss may characteristically tilt the head in an awkward position to hear or see better. The child in pain may favor a body part. The child with low self-esteem or a feeling of rejection may assume a slumped, careless, and apathetic pose or posture. Likewise, a child with confidence, a feeling of self-worth, and a sense of security usually demonstrates a tall, straight, well-balanced posture. While observing such "body language," do not interpret too freely but rather record objectively.

Note the child's ***hygiene*** in terms of cleanliness; unusual body odor; the condition of the hair, neck, nails, teeth, and feet; and the condition of the clothing. Such observations are excellent clues to possible instances of neglect, inadequate financial resources, housing difficulties (e.g., no running water), or lack of knowledge concerning children's needs.

General appearance includes an overall impression of the child's state of ***nutrition.*** This impression is more than a statement describing body weight or stature, such as "slender and tall." It is an estimation of the quality, as well as the quantity, of nutritional intake. For example, two children can be of the same height and weight, yet one can appear overweight because of flabby, loose skin, whereas the other child appears strong, robust, and well built because of firm, well-defined musculature. Likewise, a small, slender child may be well nourished with no signs of chronic undernutrition, such as bony prominences, protuberant abdomen, flat buttocks, gaunt facies, and poor muscle tone with evidence of wasting.

Compare your impression of the nutritional state with the parents' history of feeding practices. Discrepancies between the two "impressions" may be a valuable area for nutritional counseling. For example, parents who believe that their child is too thin and eats too little, despite evidence of adequate growth and physical signs of proper nutrition, may find it helpful to keep a daily diary in order to calculate the child's cumulative food intake. Many parents are surprised at the quantity of food ingested, even though the amounts at each meal or snack are small.

Behavior includes the child's personality; level of activity; reaction to stress, requests, or frustration; interactions with others, primarily the parent and nurse; degree of alertness; and response to stimuli. It is one of the most important observations to make during a child's health assessment (see Guidelines box; see also box on p. 273).

GUIDELINES
Observing Behavior

What is the child's overall personality—calm, anxious, tense, content, outgoing, shy, talkative, aggressive, introverted, stable, or moody?
Is the child active, sedentary, fidgety, or restless?
Does the child have a long attention span, or is the child easily distracted?
Does the child sit quietly on the examining table or parent's lap, or does the child climb, run, open doors, and otherwise explore the environment?
How does the child react to commands—with fear or willingness to obey?
How advanced is the child's ability to follow requests? Can the child follow two or three commands in succession without the need for repetition? Is the child attentive to requests, or must they be repeated several times?
Is the child cooperative, belligerent, or argumentative?
What is the child's response to delayed gratification or frustration? Is the child able to withstand momentary discomfort and wait for the requests to be met?
In what tone of voice does the child make requests or talk to the parents?
Does the child seek approval and gain satisfaction from it?
Does the child use eye-to-eye contact during conversation?
Does the child agree with the parent's answers or find reasons to disagree, interrupt, or argue? What is the child's reaction to the nurse—respectful, friendly, reserved, apprehensive, or uninterested?
Is the child interested in the surroundings? Does the child look around the room, ask questions about unfamiliar objects, seem to enjoy exploring them, or attempt to break or destroy them?
Can the child follow directions for using the instruments or imitate their use? Is the child quick or slow to grasp explanations?

Development can be assessed by carefully observing the child, but verify your impressions with screening tests. Various tests for assessing development, speech, vision, and hearing are discussed later in this chapter and in Chapter 24.

Record an overall estimate of the child's speech development, motor skills, degree of coordination, and recent area of achievement under general appearance. For example, the following statement may apply to an 18-month-old child: "Motor development advanced for age; climbs, runs, jumps (most recent motor skill), manipulates small objects with ease; excellent coordination and balance; beginning to name many objects; uses two-word phrases; and enjoys 'talking' to self and others."

SKIN

Skin is assessed for color, texture, temperature, moisture, and turgor. Hair is also inspected for color, texture, quality, distribution, and elasticity. Examination of the skin and its accessory structures primarily involves inspection and palpation.

Factors Influencing Assessment

Physical factors related to the examining environment and the child's skin surface can affect accurate assessment. Since colors such as pink, blue, yellow, or orange cast deceiving glows on the skin, conduct the examination in a well-illuminated room with nonglare lighting and neutral color. The room should also be comfortably warm, since air-conditioning can cause a cold-induced cyanosis and excessive heat can produce flushing. Poor hygiene and artificial paint on nails or lips also mask true determination of color. Sometimes it is necessary to clean the skin with soap and water and to remove cosmetics before beginning inspection. Although not a common situation in pediatrics, remember that such factors can hide signs of ecchymoses, petechiae, pallor, or cyanosis.

Texture, temperature, moisture, and turgor can be subjectively inspected, but palpation must be done for greater accuracy. Clothing always interferes with palpation; thus examine each area of the body nude, either as part of the general overall examination or combined with assessment of each body system. Since texture is affected by climatic exposure, such as cold, sun, and wind, compare the texture of protected areas with that of exposed areas.

Genetic factors influence assessment of color. The normal color in light-skinned children varies from a milky-white and rosy color to a more deeply hued pink color. In general, cyanosis or bluish discolorations are not normal, except in the newborn (see Table 8-3). Dark-skinned children, such as those of American Indian, Hispanic, black, Latin, Mediterranean, or Oriental descent, have inherited various brown, red, yellow, olive-green, and bluish tones in their skin, which can falsely alter assessment. For example, some children of Mediterranean origin normally have bluish-tinged lips, suggestive of cyanosis. Oriental persons, whose skin is normally of a yellow tone, may appear to be jaundiced. Full-blooded black individuals often have normal bluish pigmentation of the gums, buccal cavity, borders of the tongue, and nail beds. The visible portion of their sclera may contain speckled deposits of brown melanin that resemble petechiae.

Physiologic factors also affect assessment of color. Edema increases the amount of interstitial fluid, thereby increasing the distance between the outermost layers of the epidermis and the pigmented and vascular layers. Consequently, edema decreases the intensity of skin color, sometimes producing a false pallor.

In general, the amount of adipose tissue does not markedly affect skin color, because deposition of fat cells is below the pigmented layers of the skin. Overnutrition may not mean adequate nutrition, and pallor that may indicate nutritional iron deficiency is carefully assessed.

Exposure to sunlight stimulates the melanocytes to produce more melanin, thereby increasing the color of the skin. Individuals who are deeply suntanned require as careful observation as those who are genetically dark skinned.

Assess color changes in areas of the body where melanin production is least: sclera, conjunctiva, nail beds, lips, tongue, buccal mucosa, palms, and soles. These areas are rarely affected by edema or the amount of adipose tissue but are sensitive to changes from physical factors, such as use of cosmetics or poor hygiene.

Variations in Skin Color

Many of the specific color changes peculiar to the newborn are described in Table 8-3. Differences in assessment of color changes in ethnic groups are presented in Table 7-9.

The skin receives its pigmented color of yellow, brown, or black from melanin and its shades of red or blue from the color of hemoglobin. Oxygenated hemoglobin in the superficial capillaries of the dermis gives a rosy, pink glow. Reduced (deoxygenated) hemoglobin reflects a bluish tone through the skin, called ***cyanosis,*** which is evident when reduced hemoglobin levels reach 5 mg/dl of blood or more, regardless of the total hemoglobin. In general, the darker the skin pigmentation, the greater the amount of deoxygenated hemoglobin must be for cyanosis to be evident.

Pallor, or paleness, may be a sign of anemia, chronic disease, edema, or shock. However, it may also be a normal complexion characteristic or an indication of indoor living.

Pallor or cyanosis can be compared to the color change normally produced by blanching. For example, in nonpigmented nails, pressing down on the free edge of the nail on the index or middle finger of a child with good skin color produces marked blanching or whitening as compared with the return blood flow. In a child with pallor the difference in color change will be slight. Observe the blanching color change in dark-skinned individuals by gently applying pressure to their lips or gums.

Erythema, or redness of the skin, may be the result of increased temperature from climatic conditions, local inflammation, or infection. It may also appear as a sign of skin irritation, allergy, or other dermatoses. The degree of redness reflects the amount of increased blood flow to the area. Note any reddening and describe the location, size, presence of warmth, itching, type of distribution (e.g., diffuse,

TABLE 7-9 Differences in Color Changes of Racial Groups

COLOR CHANGE	LIGHT SKIN	DARK SKIN
Cyanosis	Bluish tinge, especially in palpebral conjunctiva (lower eyelid), nail beds, earlobes, lips, oral membranes, soles, and palms	Ashen-gray lips and tongue
Pallor	Loss of rosy glow in skin, especially face	Ashen-gray appearance in black skin More yellowish-brown color in brown skin
Erythema	Redness easily seen anywhere on body	Much more difficult to assess; rely on palpation for warmth or edema
Ecchymosis	Purplish to yellow-green areas; may be seen anywhere on skin	Very difficult to see unless in mouth or conjunctiva
Petechiae	Purplish pinpoints most easily seen on buttocks, abdomen, and inner surfaces of arms or legs	Usually invisible except in oral mucosa, conjunctiva of eyelids, and conjunctiva covering eyeball
Jaundice	Yellow staining seen in sclera of eyes, skin, fingernails, soles, palms, and oral mucosa	Most reliably assessed in sclera, hard palate, palms, and soles

clearly circumscribed, parallel to a vein), and presence of characteristic lesions, such as macules, papules, or vesicles (see Chapter 18 for a description of skin lesions).

Plethora is also redness of the skin but is caused by increased numbers of red blood cells as a compensatory response to chronic hypoxia. Intense redness of the lips or cheeks occurs.

Ecchymosis and petechiae are caused by extravasation or hemorrhage of blood into the skin; the only difference between the two is size. ***Ecchymoses*** are large, diffuse areas, usually black and blue in color, and are typically the result of injuries. Since ecchymotic areas may indicate systemic disorders or child maltreatment, always investigate the reported cause of the bruises, especially when they are located in suspicious areas, such as the back or buttocks, rather than on the knees, shins, elbows, or forearms.

Petechiae are small, distinct pinpoint hemorrhages 2 mm or less in size, which can denote some type of blood disorder, such as decreased platelets in leukemia. Because of their size, ecchymoses are more readily observed than are petechiae, which may be visible only in areas of very light-colored skin. Areas of erythema can be distinguished from ecchymosis or petechiae by blanching the skin. Since erythema is a result of increased blood flow *to* the area, exerting pressure will momentarily empty the engorged vessels and produce blanching. Because the other discolorations are produced by blood leaking *into* tissue spaces, blanching will not occur.

Jaundice, a yellow staining of the skin usually caused by bile pigments, is always a significant finding. If a yellow-orange cast is noted in an otherwise healthy child, inquire about the quantity of ingested yellow vegetables, such as carrots, which in excess produce a yellow-orange color from deposits of carotene in the skin, a condition called ***carotenemia.***

Texture

Palpate the skin for texture, noting moisture and temperature. Note any marks or scars that may indicate healed injuries, and inquire about their origin. Normally the skin of young children is smooth, soft, and slightly dry to the touch, not oily or clammy. Note any variations from these findings, because they may indicate common problems of childhood such as cradle cap, eczema, diaper rash, or excessive dryness (xeroderma) all over the body from too frequent bathing, exposure to the weather, or vitamin A deficiency. Excessively moist, clammy skin may indicate serious health problems, particularly heart disease.

Temperature

Evaluate temperature by symmetrically feeling each part of the body and comparing upper areas with lower ones. Note any distinct difference in temperature. Although not a common anomaly, one of the key signs for coarctation of the aorta is warm upper extremities and cool lower ones. Also observe the skin temperature of the dressed child. Young children produce heat rapidly, and they quickly become overheated if dressed too warmly. Many parents do not realize this and fail to change clothing to accommodate climatic variations.

Turgor

Tissue turgor refers to the amount of elasticity in the skin. To assess turgor, grasp the skin on the abdomen between the thumb and index finger, pull it taut, and quickly release it. Elastic tissue immediately assumes its normal position without residual marks or creases. In children with poor skin turgor, the skin remains suspended or tented for a few seconds before slowly falling back on the abdomen. Skin turgor is one of the best estimates of adequate hydration and nutrition.

While evaluating turgor, inspect for signs of ***edema,*** normally evident as swelling or puffiness. Periorbital edema is a sign of several systemic disorders, such as kidney disease, but may normally be evident in children who have been crying or sleeping or who have allergies. Evaluate for change in edema according to position, specific location, and response to pressure. For example, in pitting edema, pressing a finger into the edematous area causes a temporary indentation.

Accessory Structures

Inspection of the accessory structures of the skin, namely the hair, nails, and dermatoglyphics, may be performed while the skin is being examined or when the scalp and extremities are being assessed.

Inspect the ***hair*** for color, texture, quality, distribution, and elasticity. Children's scalp hair is usually lustrous, silky, strong, and elastic. Genetic factors affect the appearance of hair. For example, the hair of black children is usually curlier and coarser than that of white children. Hair that is stringy, dull, brittle, dry, friable, and depigmented may suggest poor nutrition. Note any bald or thinning spots. Although alopecia can be a sign of various skin disorders, such as tinea capitis, loss of hair in infants is often the result of lying in the same position and may be a clue for counseling parents concerning the child's stimulation needs.

Inspect the hair and scalp for cleanliness. Various ethnic groups condition their hair with oils or lubricants, which, if not thoroughly washed from the scalp, clog the sebaceous glands, causing scalp infections. Inspect hair shafts for lice, whose ova appear as grayish translucent flakes. Ova or nits are distinguished from dandruff because the eggs adhere to the hair. If pediculosis capitus is suspected, be careful to guard against self-infestation of the lice by wearing gloves or using tongue blades to inspect the hair, and by handwashing.

Inspect the scalp for ticks, which appear as grayish or brown oval bodies. Although they can be found anywhere on the body, the most common sites are exposed parts, such as the head. Although not all dog or wood ticks transmit serious disease, always record their presence or removal in case symptoms appear.

Unusual hairiness anywhere on the body, such as the arms, legs, trunk, or face, is noted. Tufts of hair anywhere along the spine, especially over the sacrum, are significant because they can mark the site of spina bifida occulta.

In older children who are approaching puberty, look for growth of secondary hair as a sign of normally progressing pubertal changes (see Figs. 19-4 and 19-6). Note precocious or delayed appearance of hair growth because, although not always suggestive of hormonal dysfunction, it may be of great concern to the early- or late-maturing adolescent.

Inspect the ***nails*** for color, shape, texture, and quality. Normally the nails are pink, convex in shape, smooth, and hard but flexible, not brittle. The edges, which are usually white, should extend over the fingers. Dark-skinned individuals may have more deeply pigmented nail beds. Variation in color, such as blueness, suggests cyanosis, and a yellow tint may indicate jaundice. Bluish-black discoloration usually indicates hemorrhage under the nail from trauma. Fungal infections cause the entire nail to become whitish with a pitted surface. Short, ragged nails are typical of habitual biting. Uncut nails with dirt accumulated under the edge sometimes indicate poor hygiene.

Changes in the shape of nails are also significant. For example, concave curves or "spoon nails," called ***koilonychia,*** are sometimes seen in iron deficiency anemia. ***Clubbing*** of the nails is always a significant finding and usually is associated with chronic cyanosis. In clubbing, the base of the nail becomes visibly swollen and feels springy when palpated, rather than firm as in the normal nail (see Fig. 31-7).

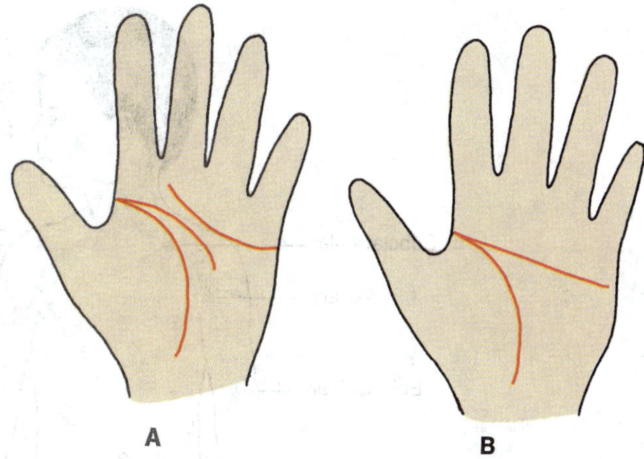

FIG. 7-10 Examples of flexion creases on palm. **A,** Normal. **B,** Transpalmar crease.

Each individual has a distinct set of handprints and footprints. The patterns, or ***dermatoglyphics,*** are unique to the individual and vary a great deal in detail and complexity of patterns. Flexion creases also appear on the palm of the hand and the sole of the foot. The palm normally shows three flexion creases (Figs. 7-10, *A*). In some situations, such as Down syndrome, the two distal horizontal creases are fused to form a single horizontal crease called a ***single palmar crease*** or ***transpalmar crease*** (Fig. 7-10, *B*). If grossly abnormal lines or folds are observed, sketch a picture to describe them and refer the finding to a specialist for further investigation.

LYMPH NODES

Lymph nodes are usually assessed when examining the part of the body where they are located. The usual sites for palpating accessible lymph nodes are shown in Fig. 7-11. The major function of lymph nodes is to collect and filter the lymph of bacteria and other foreign matter as it returns to the circulatory system. Tender, enlarged warm lymph nodes generally indicate infection or inflammation *proximal* to their location. For example, occipital or postauricular adenopathy is often seen in local scalp infection, such as pediculosis, tick bite, or external otitis. Cervical adenopathy usually accompanies acute infections in or around the mouth or throat. In children, however, small, nontender, movable nodes are frequently normal.

Palpate nodes with the distal portion of the fingers by gently but firmly pressing in a circular motion along the regions where nodes are normally present. During assessment of the nodes in the head and neck, tilt the child's head upward slightly but without tensing the sternocleidomastoid or trapezius muscle. This position facilitates palpation of the ***submental, submaxillary, tonsillar,*** and ***cervical nodes.*** Pal-

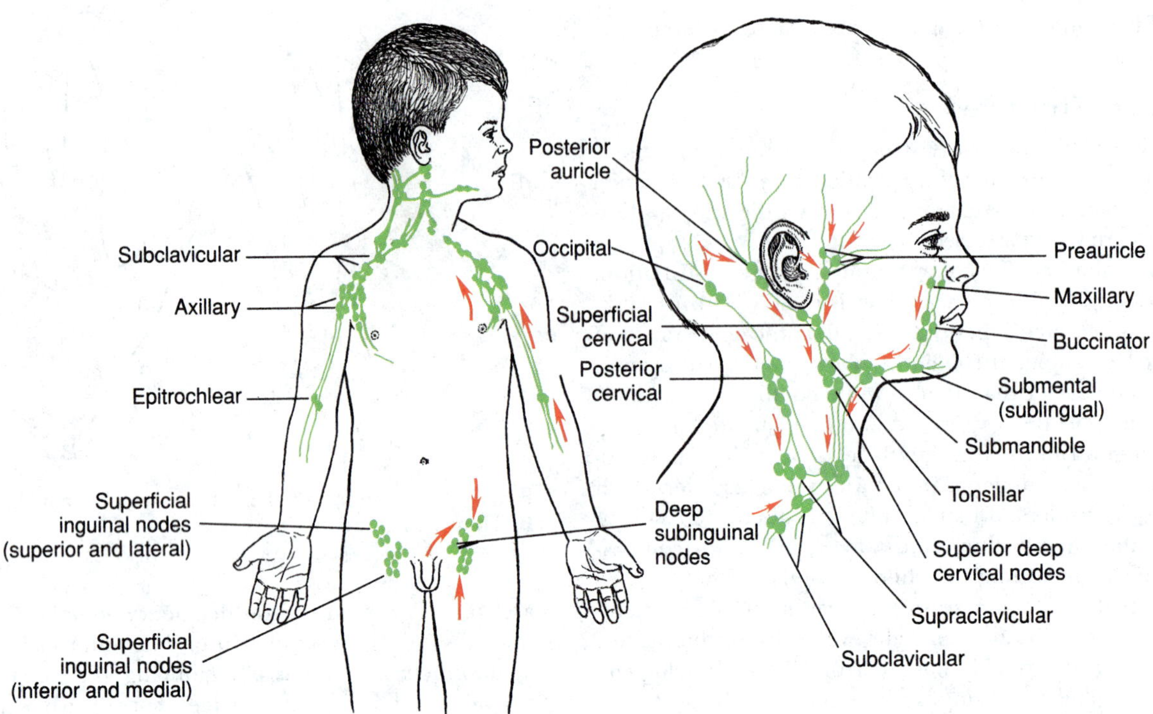

FIG. 7-11 Location of superficial lymph nodes. Arrows indicate directional flow of lymph.

pate the ***axillary nodes*** with the arms relaxed at the side but slightly abducted. Assess the ***inguinal nodes*** with the child supine. Note size, mobility, temperature, and tenderness, as well as the parents' reports of any visible change of enlarged nodes.

HEAD

Observe the head for general ***shape*** and ***symmetry.*** A flattening of one part of the head, such as the occiput, may indicate that the child continually lies in this position. Marked asymmetry is usually abnormal and may indicate premature closure of the sutures (craniosynostosis).

Note ***head control*** in infants and ***head posture*** in older children. Most infants by 4 months of age should be able to hold the head erect and in midline when in a vertical position.

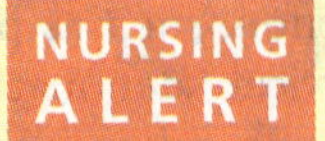

Significant head lag after 6 months of age strongly indicates cerebral injury and is referred for further evaluation.

Evaluate range of motion by asking the older child to look in each direction (to either side, up, and down) or manually putting the younger child through each position. Limited range of motion may indicate ***wryneck,*** or ***torticollis,*** a result of injury to the sternocleidomastoid muscle, in which the child holds the head to one side with the chin pointing toward the opposite side.

NURSING ALERT

Hyperextension of the head (opisthotonos) with pain on flexion is a serious indication of meningeal irritation and is referred for immediate medical evaluation (see also Fig. 7-58 on Brudzinski sign).

Palpate the ***skull*** for patent sutures, fontanels, fractures, and swellings. Normally the posterior fontanel closes by the second month of life and the anterior fontanel fuses between 12 and 18 months of age. Early or late closure is noted, since either may be a sign of a pathologic condition. For a more detailed discussion of the cranial bones, see Chapter 8.

While examining the head, observe the ***face*** for symmetry, movement, and general appearance. Ask the child to "make a face" to assess symmetric movement and disclose any degree of paralysis. Note any unusual facial proportion, such as an unusually high or low forehead, wide- or close-set eyes, or a small, receding chin.

Also note any unusual swellings or sites of edema that may be associated with specific disorders, such as nephrosis or Cushing syndrome, or steroid therapy. Visible and palpable swelling anterior to the earlobe and above the angle of the jaw is characteristic of parotid gland enlargement in mumps, giving the child a characteristic "chipmunk" appearance.

Generally, the head and face are not auscultated or percussed, with the exception of the ***sinuses*** (air cavities within certain bones adjacent to the nasal cavity) (Fig. 7-12). The

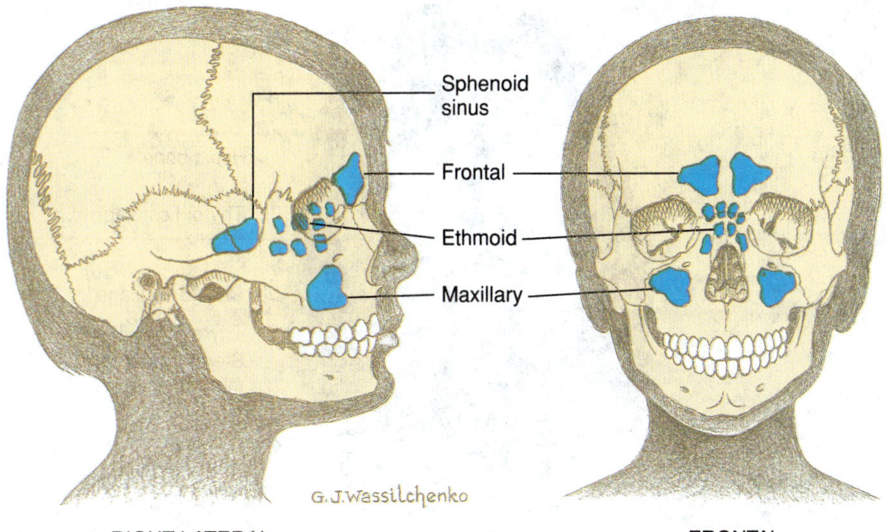

FIG. 7-12 Location of sinuses.

sinuses develop as outpouchings of the nasal airway as the skull bones enlarge throughout infancy and childhood. The maxillary and ethmoid sinuses are present soon after birth (Glasier, Mallory, and Steele, 1989). The frontal and sphenoid sinuses develop later in childhood. Percuss the sinuses for evidence of pain if there are signs of an infection, such as headache and congestion.

NECK

Besides assessing motility of the head and neck, inspect the neck as to size and palpate it for associated structures. The neck is short, with skinfolds between the head and shoulders, during infancy; however, it lengthens during the next 3 to 4 years. A short or webbed neck is associated with various anomalies, such as Turner syndrome. Marked edema of the neck may indicate mumps, local throat or mouth infections, or diphtheria. Distended neck veins often indicate difficulty on expiration, such as in asthma or cystic fibrosis.

Palpate the ***trachea*** by placing the thumb and index finger on each side and sliding them back and forth to note any masses. Normally the trachea is in the midline or slightly to the right of the midline. Note any shift, since it can signify serious lung problems, such as a tumor or foreign body in the lung.

Palpate the ***thyroid gland,*** which is located at the base of the neck. This butterfly-shaped gland straddles the trachea and has two lateral lobes connected by an ***isthmus,*** or band of glandular tissue. The isthmus is the only portion of the thyroid that is usually palpable, because the lobes that curve posteriorly around the trachea are partially covered by the sternocleidomastoid muscle (Fig. 7-13). Normally the thyroid rises as the child swallows. However, palpating the thyroid takes considerable practice and is especially difficult in an infant, whose neck is short and thick. If any masses are detected in the neck, record and report them for further investigation.

EYES

Examination of the eyes involves inspection of all exterior structures for size, symmetry, color, and motility, and inspection of the interior surfaces for examination of retinal structures. To examine each structure accurately requires an understanding of the anatomy of the eyeball (Fig. 7-14). The retinal examination requires the use of an ophthalmoscope and is a highly skilled procedure. Discussion of the funduscopic examination includes the basic normal findings that the nurse should be able to discern with some practice in using the ophthalmoscope. The third part of the examination involves vision testing.

Inspection of External Structures

Observe the eyes for relative placement on the face, symmetry of location, and general slant of the palpebral fissures or lids (Fig. 7-15). If any possible abnormality of placement is observed, measure the interpupillary distance, which is approximately 4.5 to 5.5 cm (1¾ to 2¼ inches), or the inner canthal distance, which averages about 2.5 cm (1 inch) (Laestadius, Aase, and Smith, 1969). Large spacing between the eyes is called ***hypertelorism.*** Although a normal variant in some children, hypertelorism together with other midfacial anomalies may suggest mental retardation.

Epicanthal folds, an excess fold of skin extending from the roof of the nose to the inner termination of the eyebrow and partially or completely overlapping the inner canthus of the eye, are frequently found in Oriental children (Fig. 7-15, *B*). They may be normally present in non-Oriental infants, but they usually disappear as the child grows older.

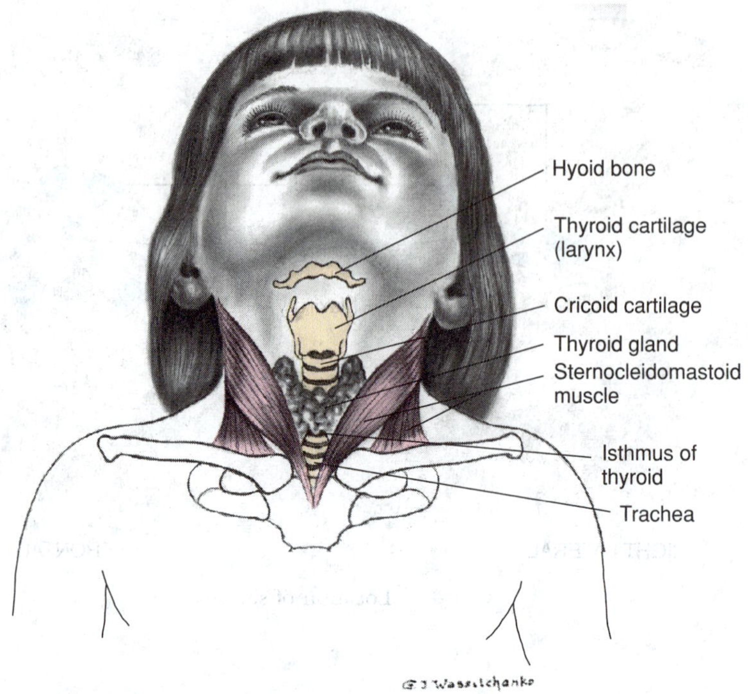

FIG. 7-13 Anterior view of structures in neck.

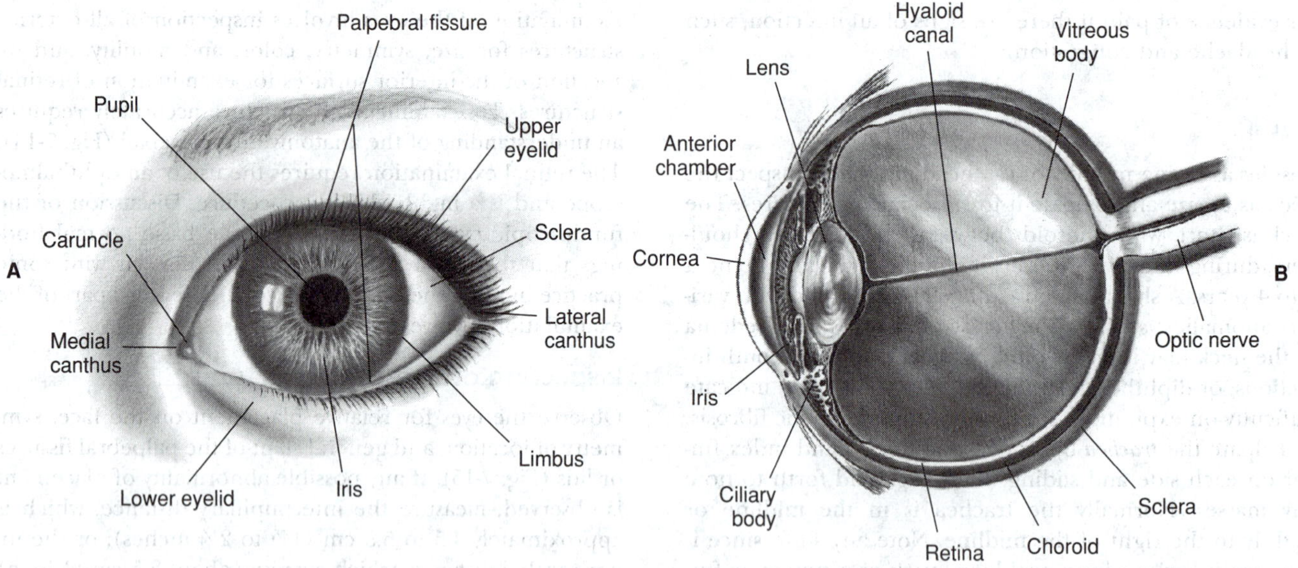

FIG. 7-14 Normal structure of eye. **A**, Anterior view. **B**, Cross-sectional view.

Determine the general slant of the ***palpebral fissures*** or lids by drawing an imaginary line through the two points of the medial canthus and across the outer orbit of the eyes and aligning each eye on the line. Usually the palpebral fissures lie horizontally. However, in Oriental persons the slant is normally upward (Fig. 7-15, *C*). Since eye abnormalities are common in many chromosomal disorders, be careful to observe and record any deviations from the expected. For example, children with Down syndrome characteristically demonstrate hypertelorism, epicanthal folds, and upward palpebral slant.

Inspect the ***lids*** for proper placement on the eye. When the eye is open, the upper lid should fall somewhere between the upper iris and upper rim of the pupil. ***Ptosis*** refers to a lid that covers part of the pupil or the lower part of the iris. The term ***sunset eyes*** or the ***setting-sun sign*** refers

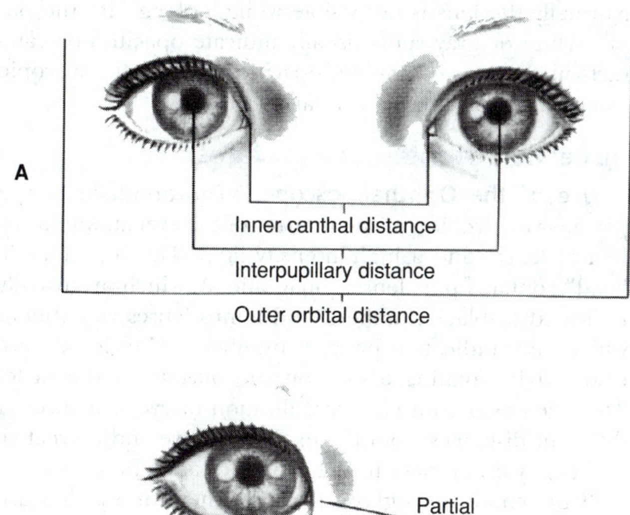

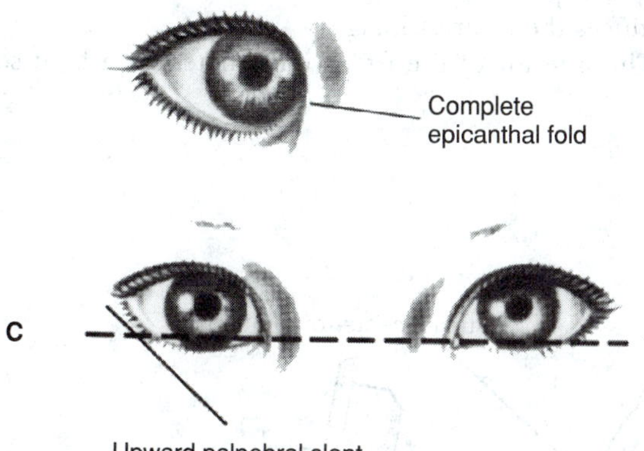

FIG. 7-15 **A,** Anatomic landmarks of eye. **B,** Epicanthal folds. **C,** Upward palpebral slant. (Note imaginary line to determine slant.)

INFLAMMATIONS OF THE EYELID

Hordeolum or **stye**—Inflammation of sebaceous glands near lashes, usually on lower lid; painful, red, swollen areas
Internal stye—Acute inflammation of meibomian glands of upper lid; if upper lid is everted, stye appears as a yellow line across the tarsus (edge of eyelid)
Chalazion—Granulomas or cysts of internal sebaceous glands (meibomian glands); localized, nontender, firm, discrete swellings covered with freely movable skin
Marginal blepharitis—Inflammation of edge of lid; red, scaly, crusted lid edges; may include pustules around base of lashes and pus from meibomian glands
Dacryocystitis—Inflammation and blockage of lacrimal sac or duct; swelling, redness, and pain, below and to nasal side of inner canthus, with purulent discharge

to an upper lid that covers no part of the iris, allowing some of the sclera or "white-of-the-eye" to show. Although either can be a normal variant of lid placement, it can also be a sign of several disorders.

When the eyes are closed, the lids should completely cover the cornea and sclera. Incomplete closure can result in chronic eye irritation and infection. When the lids are opened or closed, no palpebral conjunctiva should be visible. Malposition of the eyelids includes ***ectropion,*** a rolling-out of the lids with exposed conjunctiva, and ***entropion,*** a turning-in of the lid. The latter is normally found in some Oriental children. Check to see if the inturned lid causes irritation of the cornea.

The lids are also observed for color (any sign of hemorrhage), size (any evidence of edema), and mobility. Normally the lids contain the same amount of pigmentation as does the rest of the skin. Inflammation or erythema along the lid is noted. Some of the more common lid disorders are listed in the box above.

Inspect the lining of the lids, the ***palpebral conjunctiva.*** Inspect the lower conjunctival sac by pulling the lid down while the child looks up. To evert the upper lid, hold the upper lashes and gently pull *down* and *forward* while the child looks down. If this is not successful, place the stem of a cotton-tipped applicator 1 cm above the edge of the lid margin and gently push down on the lid with the stick and roll the lid upward. As soon as the lid is everted, use the fingers holding the lashes to keep the lid everted.

Normally the conjunctiva appears pink and glossy. Vertical yellow striations along the edge are the ***meibomian*** or ***sebaceous glands*** near the hair follicle. Located in the inner or medial canthus and situated on the inner edge of the upper and lower lids is a tiny opening called the ***lacrimal punctum.*** Note any excessive tearing or inflammation of the lacrimal apparatus.

Observe the lids for blinking movement. Excessive blinking can indicate eyestrain or a nervous habit. Asymmetric or infrequent blinking can be a sign of paralysis or muscle weakness. Test the ***blink reflex*** by making a quick movement toward the eye.

Inspect the ***eyelashes*** for distribution, direction of growth, and pigmentation. Normally the upper lashes curl upward and the lower lashes curve downward. Lashes that turn inward toward the eyeball can cause conjunctival irritation.

The ***bulbar conjunctiva,*** which covers the eye up to the limbus or junction of the cornea and sclera, should be transparent. Dilation of the blood vessels in the conjunctiva makes it appear red. Although this redness is characteristic of many disorders, it can also indicate eyestrain, irritation, or fatigue.

The ***sclera,*** or white covering of the eyeball, should be clear. Record any yellow staining, since this may indicate jaundice. Tiny black marks in the sclera of heavily pigmented individuals are normal and do not indicate petechiae or the presence of a foreign body. A bluish tone may indicate disorders such as osteogenesis imperfecta or glaucoma.

The ***cornea,*** or covering of the iris and pupil, should be clear and transparent. Record any opacities, since they can be signs of scarring or ulceration, which can interfere with vision. To test for opacities, illuminate the eyeball by shining a light at an angle (obliquely) toward the cornea.

Compare the ***pupils*** for size, shape, and movement. They should be round, clear, and equal. Test their ***reaction to light*** by quickly shining a source of light toward the eye and removing it. As the light approaches, the pupils constrict; as the light fades, the pupils dilate. Test ***accommodation,*** or the focusing ability of the eyes to produce clear vision at different distances, by having the child look at a bright, shiny object at a distance and quickly moving the object toward the face. The pupils constrict as the object is brought near the eye. Normal findings on examination of the pupil may be recorded as ***PERRLA,*** which means "pupil equal, round, reacts to light and accommodation."

Inspect the ***iris*** for size, color, and clarity. The iris should be perfectly round; a cleft or notch at its outer edge is called a ***coloboma.*** Since a visual field defect coincides with the coloboma, report this finding for further ophthalmologic evaluation. Permanent eye color is usually established by 6 to 12 months of age. Lack of usual eye color and a pink glow to the iris are characteristic of ***albinism.*** The pink color is a reflection of the red reflex of the retina. Black-and-white speckling of the iris, known as ***Brushfield spots,*** is seen in Down syndrome.

While inspecting the iris and pupil, also look for the ***lens.*** Normally the lens is not visible while looking into the pupil. White or gray spots usually indicate opacities or cataracts in the lens. Complete opacities prevent funduscopic examination of internal retinal structures.

Inspection of Internal Structures

Use of the Ophthalmoscope. The ophthalmoscope permits visualization of the interior of the eyeball with a system of lenses and a high-intensity light. The "ophthalmic head" contains plus lenses (magnifiers), which are usually indicated by black numbers, and minus lenses (minifiers), which are indicated by red numbers. The lenses are changed by rotating a disk on the outside of the head. These lenses permit clear visualization of eye structures at different distances from the examiner's eye and correct visual acuity differences in the examiner and child.

If the child wears glasses, remove them unless they are worn to correct severe astigmatism, which can cause distortion of the images. The lens of the ophthalmoscope can grossly detect visual acuity problems in the child if the examiner with 20/20 vision (with or without corrective lenses) must use plus or minus lenses to see the retinal structures clearly. With hyperopia, or farsightedness, higher plus or convex lenses are needed; with myopia, or nearsightedness, more minus or concave lenses are used. Use of the ophthalmoscope requires practice to know which lens setting produces the clearest image.

The interior of the eye is illuminated by a light source

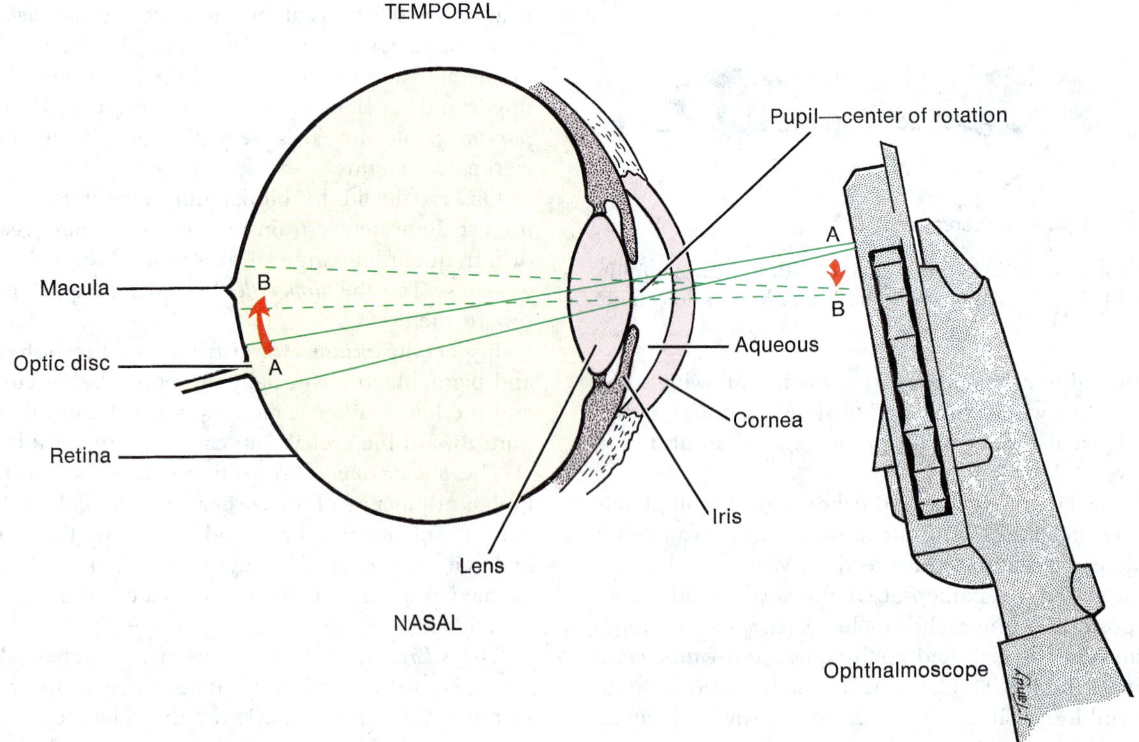

FIG. 7-16 Visual axis through ophthalmoscope. Beam of light *(A)* and its corresponding visual field is usual view when approaching child from side at 15-degree angle. *B* represents a direct visualization with child staring at light.

within the ophthalmic head, which shines through the lens from a small window. There is also a light dial that changes the type of light emitted through the window. For general purposes, the small, white circular light is used for the undilated pupil and the larger white circular light is used for the dilated pupil.

Hold the ophthalmoscope by its body in your dominant hand, and place the instrument lightly against your cheek so that the lens remains directly in front of your eye and the light shines toward the child's eye. With the instrument in position, move toward the child, approaching from the side at a 15-degree angle, not directly toward the eye. When examining the left eye, use your left eye, and vice versa, to prevent eyestrain and to approach the child in the best position. Use your free hand to attract the child's attention away from the instrument's light source and toward a point directly in front of the child to help you move as close as possible to the child. Perform the examination in a dimly lit, but not necessarily dark, room.

From a distance of about 1 foot, begin the examination of the cornea, iris, and lens with a lens setting of +8 to +2. Once near the child's face, change the lens to 0 or −2. Since the light source falls on only part of the retina at a time, systematically move the ophthalmoscope up and down and from side to side to visualize each structure within the fundus (Fig. 7-16).

Preparing the Child. Prepare the child for the ophthalmic examination by showing the child the instrument, demonstrating the light source and how it shines in the eye, and explaining the reason for darkening the room. For infants and young children who do not respond to such explanations, try to use distraction to encourage them to keep their eyes open. Forcibly parting the lids results in an uncooperative, watery-eyed child and a frustrated nurse. Usually, with some practice, you can elicit a red reflex almost instantly while approaching the child and may also gain a momentary inspection of the blood vessels, macula, or optic disc.

Funduscopic Examination. Fig. 7-17 shows the structures of the back of the eyeball, or the ***fundus.*** The fundus is immediately apparent as the ***red reflex.*** The intensity of the color increases in darkly pigmented individuals.

NURSING ALERT A brilliant, uniform red reflex is an important sign because it virtually rules out almost all serious defects of the cornea, aqueous chamber, lens, and vitreous chamber. Record any dark shadows or opacities, because they indicate some abnormality in any of these structures.

As the ophthalmoscope is brought closer to the eye, the most conspicuous feature of the fundus is the ***optic disc,*** the area where the blood vessels and optic nerve fibers enter and exit from the eye. The round or vertically oval disc is creamy pink but lighter than the surrounding fundus and derives its color from the rich capillary network. Its size is important because other structures of the fundus are measured in relationship to the ***disc diameter (DD).*** Most discs have a small, pale depression in their center, called the ***physiologic cup*** or ***depression,*** which represents the blind spot of the retina. It is not always visible but, when large enough to be seen, should not extend to the disc margin. Blurring of the disc margins, loss of the depression, and a bulging

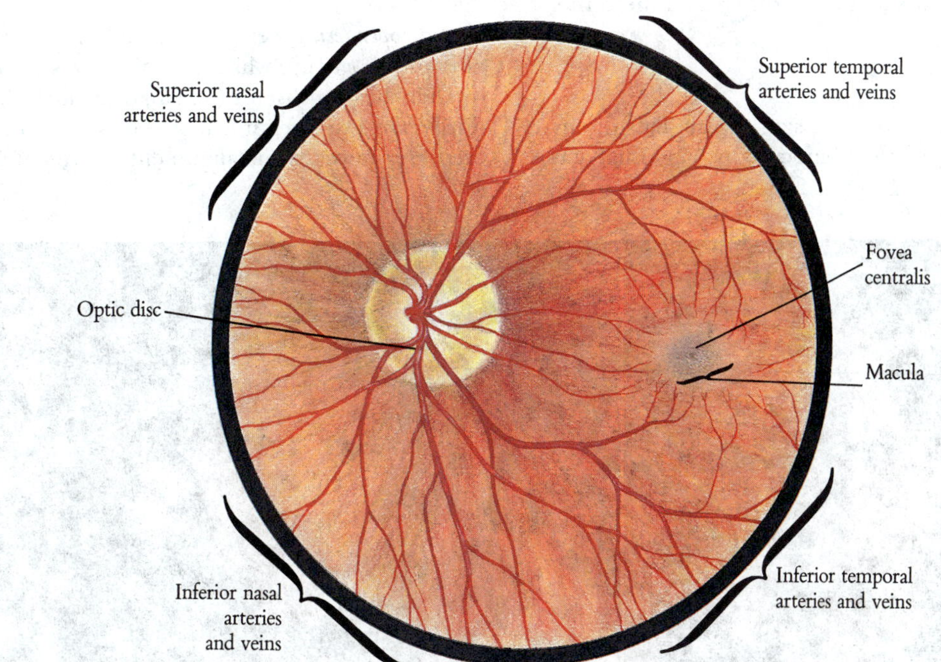

FIG. 7-17 Structures of fundus. Interior circle represents approximate size of area seen with ophthalmoscope. (From Seidel HM and others: *Mosby's guide to physical examination,* ed 3, St Louis, 1994, Mosby.)

disc are important signs of ***papilledema*** or swelling of the optic nerve, which clinically indicates increased intracranial pressure.

After the optic disc is located, inspect the area for blood vessels. The ***central retinal artery and vein*** appear in the depths of the disc and emanate outward with visible branching. The veins are darker in color and about one fourth larger in size than the arteries. A narrow band of light, the ***arteriolar light reflex,*** is reflected from the center of an artery but does not appear in veins. Normally the branches of the arteries and veins cross each other. Observe the pattern of branching for abnormalities such as notching or indenting at the crossings, tortuosity or dilation of the vessels, or small hemorrhages (dark areas) along the branches. Report any of these findings for further investigation.

About 2 DD temporal to the disc is the ***macula,*** the area of the fundus with the greatest concentration of visual receptors. It is about 1 DD in size and darker in color than the fundus (red reflex) or optic disc. The intensity of the color directly correlates with the individual's skin pigmentation; that is, the darker the skin, the darker the color of the macula. In the center of the macula is a minute glistening spot of reflected light called the ***fovea centralis,*** the area of most perfect vision.

Although abnormalities of the macula are usually not apparent unless the eye is dilated, permitting more detailed inspection, at least note its presence. If locating the macula is difficult, ask the child to look directly at the light. As Fig. 7-16 shows, a light shone directly into the eye falls on the fovea. However, since this is the most light-sensitive area of the retina, be careful to focus on the macula only momentarily. Record if direct visualization does *not* cause the light to fall on the center of the fovea, because strabismus may exist when fixation occurs at a point other than the center of the macula.

Vision Testing

Several tests are available for assessing vision. This discussion focuses on four areas: (1) binocularity, (2) visual acuity, (3) peripheral vision, and (4) color vision. Refer to Chapter 24 for behavioral and physical signs that indicate visual impairment.

Binocularity. Normally, by the age of 3 to 4 months, children achieve ***binocularity,*** the ability to fixate on one visual field with both eyes simultaneously. One of the most important tests for binocularity is alignment of the eyes to detect nonbinocular vision, or ***strabismus*** ("cross-eye"), in which one eye deviates from the point of fixation. If the malalignment is constant, the weak eye becomes "lazy" and eventually the brain suppresses the image produced by that eye. If strabismus is not detected and corrected by age 4 to 6 years, a type of blindness known as ***amblyopia*** may result.

Two tests commonly used to detect malalignment are the corneal light reflex and the cover tests. In the ***corneal light reflex test*** (also called ***red reflex gemini test*** or ***Hirschberg test***), a flashlight or the light of the ophthalmoscope is shined directly into the eyes from a distance of about 40.5 cm (16 inches). If the eyes are orthophoric or normal, the light falls symmetrically within each pupil (Fig. 7-18, *A*) or twin red reflexes are observed. If the light falls off center in one eye, the eyes are malaligned. Epicanthal folds may give a false impression of malalignment of the eyes (***pseudostrabismus***) (Fig. 7-18, *B*).

Terms for describing the types of strabismus are:

Estropia or **esophoria**—Inward deviation of the eye (see Fig. 24-7)
Extropia or **exophoria**—Outward deviation of the eye
Phoria—Malalignment that is not obvious until fusion is disrupted
Tropia—Constant or intermittent malalignment of the eyes; more severe and more likely to result in amblyopia than phoria

In the ***cover test,*** cover one eye and observe the movement of the *uncovered* eye while the child gazes on a near (33 cm, or 13 inches) or distant (50 cm, or 20 inches) object. If the uncovered eye does not move, it is aligned. If the uncovered eye moves, a malalignment is present because when

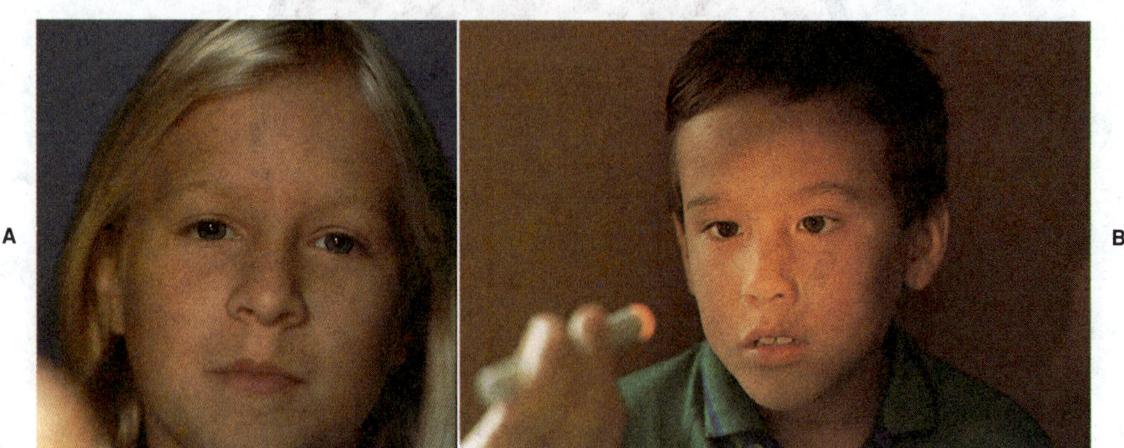

FIG. 7-18 **A,** Corneal light reflex test demonstrating orthophoric eyes. **B,** Pseudostrabismus. Inner epicanthal folds cause eyes to appear malaligned; however, corneal light reflexes fall perfectly symmetrically.

the stronger eye is temporarily covered, the weaker eye attempts to fixate on the object.

In the ***uncover test,*** shift the eye cover back and forth from one eye to the other eye and observe the movement of the *covered* eye while the child is fixating at a point in front of him or her. If normal alignment is present, shifting the cover from one eye to the other eye will not cause movement of the covered eye. If malalignment is present, the covered eye will move from its position when covered to a straight position when uncovered. This test takes more practice than the other cover test because the occluder must be moved back and forth quickly and accurately in order to see the eye move. Since deviations can occur at different ranges, particularly in the case of phorias, it is important to perform the cover tests at both near and far distances.

➤ **NURSING TIP** The cover test is usually easier to perform if you use your hand rather than a card-type occluder (Fig. 7-19). Or try using attractive occluders fashioned like an ice cream cone or happy face lollipop cut from cardboard.

Visual Acuity Testing in Children. ***Visual acuity*** refers to the ability to see near and far objects clearly. The most commonly used test for measuring acuity is the ***Snellen Letter Chart,*** which consists of lines of letters in decreasing size (see Appendix B). Each line is given a value; for example, line 7 is "20."

During testing, children stand 20 feet from the chart (with heels at the 20-foot line) and read each line. If they can read line 7, they have 20/20 vision. This means that at a distance of 20 feet (numerator), they can see the letters 7 mm in height, the accepted standard for normal acuity (Neff, 1991). If they can read only line 2, they have 20/100 vision—they are able to see at a distance of 20 feet what people with 20/20, or normal, eyesight can see at 100 feet. Other letter or symbol screening tests are described in Table 7-10. Many of the tests that are suitable for preschoolers can also be used for difficult-to-test children, such as those with developmental delays. The ***Snellen symbol chart*** is frequently used to screen preschool children (see Appendix B). However, many young children have difficulty because of confusion in identifying the direction of the E, rather than inability to see the symbol clearly. To avoid this problem, the ***Blackbird Preschool Vision Screening System*** was developed by a nurse (Fig. 7-20). The screening system uses a modified E that resembles a bird and a story about the Blackbird to help engage children's attention. Testing is done with flash cards or a wall-mounted chart, and the children are instructed to indicate the direction of the bird's flight. Some have reported a higher percentage of children successfully tested with the Blackbird System than with the Snellen E (Sato-Viacrucis, 1985). The Blackbird System also contains guidelines for vision screening the noncommunicative, nonreaders, or non-English-speaking children to assist screeners with more difficult-to-test populations, and the ***Blackbird Storybook Home Eye Test*** is designed for parents to prescreen young children at home.

Although most chart tests are designed for testing at 20 feet, testing at closer ranges makes it easier to engage children's attention, and the charts require less space for

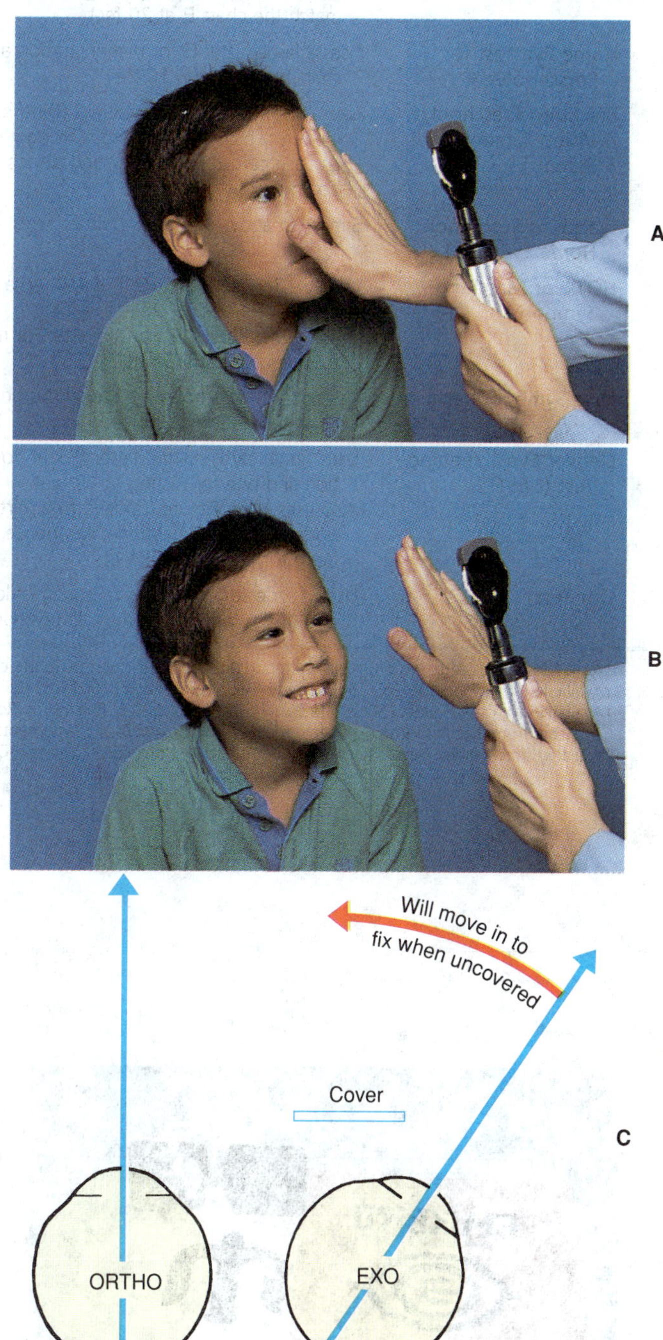

FIG. 7-19 Uncover test for strabismus. **A,** Eye is occluded, child is fixating on light source. **B,** If eye does not move when uncovered, eyes are aligned. **C,** Exophoria. As eye is uncovered, it shifts to fixate on object. (**C** from Prior JA, Silberstein JS, Stang JM: *Physical diagnosis: the history and examination of the patient,* ed 6, St Louis, 1981, Mosby.)

TABLE 7-10 Letter or Symbol Vision Acuity Tests

TEST	DESCRIPTION	COMMENTS*
Snellen Letter†	Uses letters of the English alphabet for testing at 20 feet	For most children above the second grade who are familiar with reading the alphabet
Snellen E†	Uses the capital letter E pointing in four directions; children "read" the chart by showing the direction of the letter E or using a large duplicate E to match the chart E at 20 feet	For illiterate or non-English-speaking people, preschool children, and grade 1 Preschool children often have difficulty with direction despite adequate vision
Home Eye Test for Preschoolers‡	Uses a large letter E for demonstration and an E chart for testing at 10 feet	For use by parents for children ages 3 to 6 years
Blackbird Preschool Vision Screening System§	Uses a modified E to resemble a flying bird; children identify which way the bird is flying Uses flash cards, storytelling, and disposable cardboard eyeglass occluders	For children as young as 3 years Avoids the problem with image reversal and eye-hand coordination that can occur with the letter E
Blackbird Storybook Home Eye Test§	Similar to above	For use by parents for children as young as 2½ years
HOTV or Matching Symbol†	Uses the four letters H, O,T, and V on a chart for testing at 10 or 20 feet Child names the letters on the chart or matches them to a demonstration card	For children as young as 3 years Avoids the problem with image reversal and eye-hand coordination that can occur with the letter E
Faye Symbol Chart§	Use pictures of a house, apple, and umbrella on a chart for testing at 10 feet	For children as young as 27 to 30 months
Denver Eye Screening Test (DEST)‖	Uses single cards for the letter E, one for demonstration and one for testing at 15 feet Also uses Allen Picture Cards (a tree, birthday cake, horse and rider, telephone, car, house, and teddy bear) for testing at 15 feet	For children 2½ years and older May be reliably used with cooperative children from the age of 24 months
Dot Test†	Uses a series of different-sized dots; child points to one of the nine dots randomly positioned on a disk	For children as young as 24 months

*Ages for testing are based on published reports. Proper instruction of young children is essential for successful screening.
†Available from Good-Lite Co., 1540 Hannah Ave., Forest Park, IL 60130; (708) 366-3860.
‡Available from the National Society to Prevent Blindness, 500 E. Remington Rd., Schaumburg, IL 60173; (800) 331-2020.
§Available from Blackbird Vision Screening System, PO Box 277424, Sacramento, CA 95827; (916) 363-6884.
‖Available from Denver Developmental Materials, Inc., PO Box 6919, Denver CO 80206-0919; (303) 355-4729.

the screening lane. Measurements at closer range are converted to the standard 20-foot scale by multiplying the two numbers by the number that converts the first one to 20. For example, 10/25 is equivalent to 20/50. When closer ranges are used, proper positioning of the child (e.g., with heels on the 10-foot mark) is essential. Because young children are active, their tendency to move or lean forward can affect the testing more at close distances than at farther ones (see Critical Thinking Exercise box).

The Snellen charts are usually used for testing far visual acuity to detect ***myopia*** (nearsightedness). However, in school-age children they can also be used to test for ***hyperopia*** (farsightedness). The ***plus lens test for hyperopia*** involves having the child wear a pair of convex or plus lenses. With these lenses the child should be *unable* to read the 20/20 or 20/30 line. Ability to see these lines clearly indicates excessive farsightedness; refer these children for further testing.

Vision performance can also be measured using optical instruments, such as the ***Titmus Vision Tester.**** Three sec-

*Manufactured by Titmus Optical, Inc., Petersburg, VA 23804.

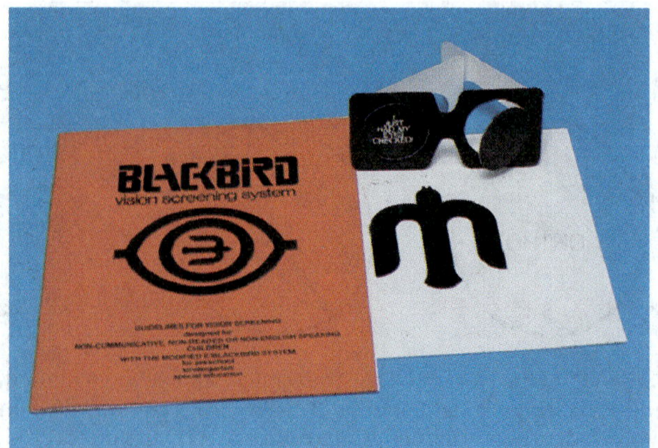

FIG. 7-20 Blackbird Vision Screening System. Note Blackbird symbol and special "eyeglass" occluder.

CRITICAL THINKING EXERCISE
Vision Screening

Your nursing class will be assisting with EPSDT (Early Periodic Screening, Diagnosis, and Treatment) screens for preschoolers. You are responsible for setting up the area for visual screening. You will need all of the following equipment *except:*

1. Snellen acuity charts
2. Pirate patches
3. Penlights
4. A paper or metal tape measure

The correct answer is 1. The Snellen chart is inappropriate because it uses letters, and it cannot be assumed that preschoolers know their alphabet. The "Lazy E" acuity chart is not ideal, because preschoolers may not have the perceptual abilities needed to determine which direction the "legs" of the E are pointing. A picture acuity chart or the Blackbird system should be used with this population. Pirate patches serve as eye occluders and are needed for assessing acuity and alignment. Penlights are needed for assessing corneal light reflex and pupil reactivity. A nonstretchable tape measure is used to determine the correct distance for assessing acuity when using an eye chart.

Contributed by Judith A. Vessey, RN,C, PhD.

tions of tests are available with the Professional Model Titmus Tester:

1. The Michigan Pre-School Test, which tests visual acuity and binocularity using the letter E in children from 3½ years of age through grade 1
2. The Massachusetts Vision Test, which tests visual acuity, hyperopia (plus lens test), and binocularity (both near and far) using the letter E in elementary school children
3. The Adult Series, which tests near and far visual acuity using the standard Snellen letters, binocularity, and color perception in secondary school children and adults

There are no universal criteria for referring children when using the Snellen charts. The American Academy of Pediatrics (1986) recommends the following criteria for vision referral:

1. Children before their fifth birthday who are unable to read the 20/40 line or less
2. Children 5 years and older who are unable to read at the 20/30 line or less
3. A 2-line difference of visual acuity between the eyes, even within the passing range

The National Society to Prevent Blindness (1988) recommends the following criteria for referral of children for a complete eye examination:

1. Three-year-old children with vision in either eye of 20/50 or less (inability to correctly identify one more than half the symbols on the 40-foot line) or a two-line difference in visual acuity between the eyes in the passing range (e.g., 20/20 in one eye and 20/40 in the other eye)
2. All other ages and grades with vision in either eye of 20/40 or less (inability to correctly identify one more than half the symbols on the 30-foot line)
3. All children who consistently show any signs of possible visual disturbances, regardless of visual acuity (see Chapter 24)

Visual Acuity Testing in Infants and Difficult-to-Test Children. In newborns vision is tested mainly by checking for ***light perception*** by shining a light into the eyes and noting responses such as pupillary constriction, blinking, following the light to midline, increased alertness, or refusal to open the eyes after exposure to the light. Although the simple maneuver of checking light perception and eliciting the pupillary light reflex indicates that the anterior half of the visual apparatus is intact, it does not confirm that the infant can see. In other words, this test does not assess whether the brain receives the visual message and interprets the signals.

Another test of visual acuity is the infant's ability to fixate on and follow a target. Although any brightly colored or patterned object can be used, the human face is excellent. Hold the infant upright while moving your face slowly from side to side.

NURSING ALERT If visual fixation and following are not present by 3 to 4 months of age, refer for further ophthalmologic evaluation.

Other signs that may indicate visual loss include fixed pupils, marked strabismus, constant nystagmus, setting-sun sign, and slow lateral movements. Unfortunately, it is very difficult to test each eye separately; the presence of such signs in one eye could indicate unilateral blindness.

Special tests are available for testing infants and other difficult-to-test children to assess acuity and/or confirm blindness. These tests are presented in Table 7-11 with the estimated visual acuity at different ages. The discrepancy between the acuities obtained by the various techniques probably reflects the testing of different responses of the developing infant's brain (Hoyt, Nickel, and Billson, 1982).

Peripheral Vision. In children who are old enough to cooperate, estimate ***peripheral vision,*** or the visual field of each eye, by having children fixate on a specific point directly in front of them as an object, such as a finger or a pencil, is moved from beyond the field of vision into the range of peripheral vision. Check each eye separately and for each quadrant of vision. As soon as children see the object, have them say "stop." At that point measure the angle from the anteroposterior axis of the eye (straight line of vision) to the peripheral axis (point at which the object is first seen). Normally children see about 50 degrees upward, 70 degrees downward, 60 degrees nasalward, and 90 degrees temporally. Limitations in peripheral vision may indicate blindness from damage to structures within the eye or to any of the visual pathways.

Color Vision. Another important test is for color vision. It is estimated that from 8% to 10% of white males and less than half that percentage of black males have inherited the X-linked disorder known as ***color vision deficit*** (less acceptable term, ***color blindness***). From 0.5% to 1% of white females are affected. Although the severity of im-

TABLE 7-11 Special Tests of Visual Acuity and Estimated Visual Acuity at Different Ages

TEST	DESCRIPTION	BIRTH	4 MONTHS	1 YEAR	AGE OF 20/20 VISION
Optokinetic nystagmus	A striped drum is rotated or a striped tape is moved in front of infant's eyes. Presence of nystagmus indicates vision. Acuity is assessed by using progressively smaller stripes.	20/400	20/200	20/60	20-30 months
Forced-choice preferential looking*	Either a homogeneous field or a striped field is presented to infant; an observer monitors the direction of the eyes during presentation of pattern. Acuity is assessed by using progressively smaller striped fields.	20/400	20/200	20/50	18-24 months
Visually evoked potentials	Eyes are stimulated with bright light or pattern, and electrical activity to visual cortex is recorded through scalp electrodes. Acuity is assessed by using progressively smaller patterns.	20/100 to 20/200	20/80	20/40	6-12 months

Data from Hoyt C, Nickel B, Billson F: Ophthalmological examination of the infant: development aspects, *Surv Ophthalmol* 26:177-189, 1982.
*One type of preferential looking test is the ***Teller Acuity Card Test,*** in which a set of rectangular cards containing different black-and-white patterns or grading is presented to the child as an observer looks through a central peephole in the card. The observer, who is hidden from view, observes the variety of visual cues, such as fixation, eye movements, head movements, or pointing. The finest grading the child is judged to be able to see is taken as the acuity estimate. The test is appropriate for children from birth to 24 to 36 months of age (Teller D and others, 1986).

paired perception of color varies considerably, the two most common types are ***protanomaly,*** in which the child confuses gray with pink or pale blue with green, and ***deuteranomaly,*** in which the child confuses gray with pale purple or green.

In most of these individuals, the color vision deficit causes no major problems. However, some of the difficulties encountered by individuals with more severe deficits may be inability to distinguish amber or red traffic lights, failure to see a red brake light on the rear of a car, difficulty in distinguishing green traffic lights from certain types of incandescent street lamps, and a poor sense of color coordination of clothing. For school-age children the greatest difficulty lies in performance of academic skills that use color as a visual aid. Adolescents may be ineligible for certain vocational opportunities, such as electronics, photography, printing, interior decorating, pharmaceuticals, textiles, or police work, and for several types of military service (Kovalesky, 1985).

Tests available for color vision include the ***Ishihara test*** and the ***Hardy-Rand-Rittler (HRR) test.*** Each consists of a series of cards (pseudoisochromatic) on which is printed a color field composed of spots of a certain "confusion" color. Against the field is a number or symbol similarly printed in dots but of a color likely to be confused with the field color by the person with a color vision deficit. As a result, the figure or letter is invisible to an affected individual but is clearly seen by a person with color vision. By using the HRR test, which uses symbols rather than numbers, reliable testing can be done on children as young as 3 years of age (Kovalesky, 1985). Nurses administering the test must be familiar with the testing materials and should be able to inform the parents of the disorder's effects on practical areas of living, its genetic transmission, and its irreversibility.

EARS

Like the eyes, examination of the ears involves inspection of the external auditory structures, visualization of the internal landmarks using the otoscope, and screening for hearing ability.

Inspection of External Structures

The entire external earlobe is called the ***pinna,*** or ***auricle,*** and is located on each side of the head. Measure the height alignment of the pinna by drawing an imaginary line from the outer orbit of the eye to the occiput or most prominent protuberance of the skull. The top of the pinna should meet or cross this line. Low-set ears are commonly associated with renal anomalies or mental retardation. Measure the angle of the pinna by drawing a perpendicular line from the imaginary horizontal line and aligning the pinna next to this mark. Normally the pinna lies within a 10-degree angle of the vertical line (Fig. 7-21). If it falls outside this area, record the deviation and look closely for other anomalies.

Normally the pinna extends slightly outward from the skull. Except in newborn infants, ears that are flat against the head or protruding away from the scalp may indicate problems. For example, a mass or swelling makes the pinna stand forward and may indicate mastoiditis, mumps, or postauricular abscesses. Flattened ears in infants may suggest a frequent side-lying position and may offer a clue to the parents' lack of understanding of the child's stimulation needs.

Fig. 7-22 shows the usual landmarks of the pinna. The ***helix*** is the prominent outer rim of the pinna. The ***antihelix*** is a second curved rim that is adjacent and almost parallel to the helix. The ***concha*** is a deep cavity, within and partly

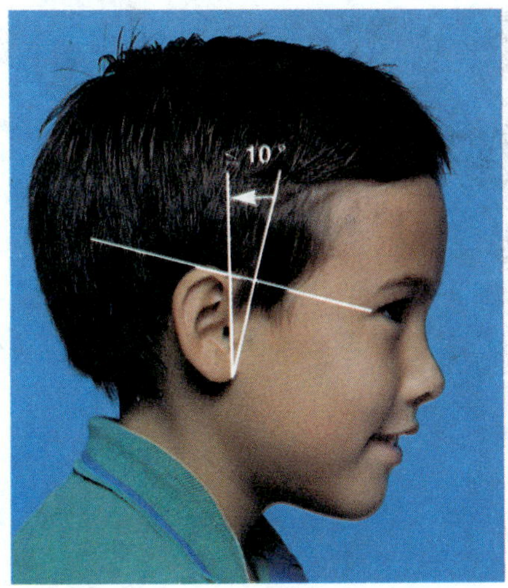

FIG. 7-21 Ear alignment.

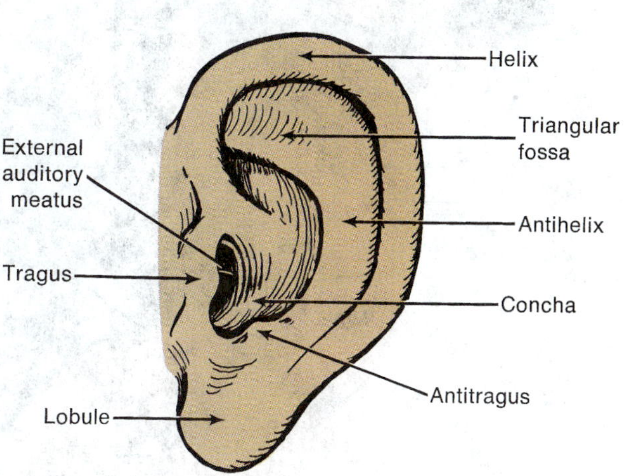

FIG. 7-22 Usual landmarks of pinna.

surrounded by the antihelix, that leads into the external auditory canal. Lying anterior to the concha is a prominent protuberance called the ***tragus,*** and opposite to this is the ***antitragus,*** below which is the ***lobule.*** In some children the lobule is adherent with the helix in an upward and backward slant. An adherent lobule is considered a normal variation. Each of the major projections of the pinna forms corresponding depressions. There is remarkable similarity among external pinnas; note any deviations, because they can be a sign of possible middle ear anomalies and congenital conductive hearing loss.

Inspect the ***skin*** around the ear for small openings, extra tags of skin, or sinuses. If a sinus is found, note this, since it may represent a fistula that drains into some area of the neck or ear. Cutaneous tags represent no pathologic process but may cause parents concern in terms of the child's appearance.

Inspect the ear for general ***hygiene.*** An otoscope is not necessary to look into the external canal to note the presence of ***cerumen,*** a waxy substance produced by the ceruminous glands in the outer portion of the canal. If the ear canal appears totally free of cerumen, ask how the ears are cleaned. Occasionally parents insert cotton-tipped swabs or thin objects, such as bobby pins, into the canal to remove wax. Deep insertion of such objects can damage the drum or walls of the canal, as well as push the wax against the tympanic membrane to form a plug. It is best to question parents about ear cleaning by remarking how clean the ears are and casually asking how they remove the wax. This approach is more likely to yield an honest answer than is direct questioning about the use of specific instruments.

Advise parents or children to clean the ears with a washcloth and, if they use a swab, to gently wipe only the outermost portion of the canal. Caution them against using any sharp, hard object in the ear. If the cerumen is hard and dry (appears dark and crusted, rather than yellow-brown and soft), it can be softened and removed by instilling 2 or 3 drops of mineral oil into the ear for a few days and then rinsing the canal with an ear syringe. Commercial products (Cerumenex, Murine, Debrox) are also available without prescription to aid in removing dried cerumen. If otitis media is suspected, remove the wax by using lukewarm water and a dental irrigation device, large syringe (without needle), or bulb syringe.

NURSING ALERT If using a curette to remove cerumen, use great caution and be certain the child's head is immobilized to avoid traumatizing the canal or puncturing the drum.

Note the presence, color, and odor of any discharge from the aural canal. If discharge is present in one canal, prevent transmitting potentially infectious material to the other ear or to another child through handwashing, using disposable specula, or sterilizing reusable specula between each examination (Overend, Hall, and Godwin, 1992).

Inspection of Internal Structures

Use of the Otoscope. The otic head permits visualization of the tympanic membrane by use of a bright light, a magnifying glass, and a speculum. Some otoscopes have an attachment for a pneumatic device to insert air into the canal to determine membrane compliance (movement). The speculum comes in a variety of sizes (2, 3, 4, and 5 mm) to accommodate different canal widths. The largest speculum that fits comfortably into the ear is used to achieve the greatest area of visualization. The lens or magnifying glass is movable, allowing the examiner to insert an object, such as a curette, into the ear canal through the speculum while still viewing the structures through the lens. The handle is the same as for the ophthalmic head and operates similarly.

Positioning the Child. Before beginning the otoscopic examination, position the child properly and restrain if necessary. Older children usually cooperate and do not need restraint. However, prepare them for the procedure by allowing them to play with the instrument, demonstrating

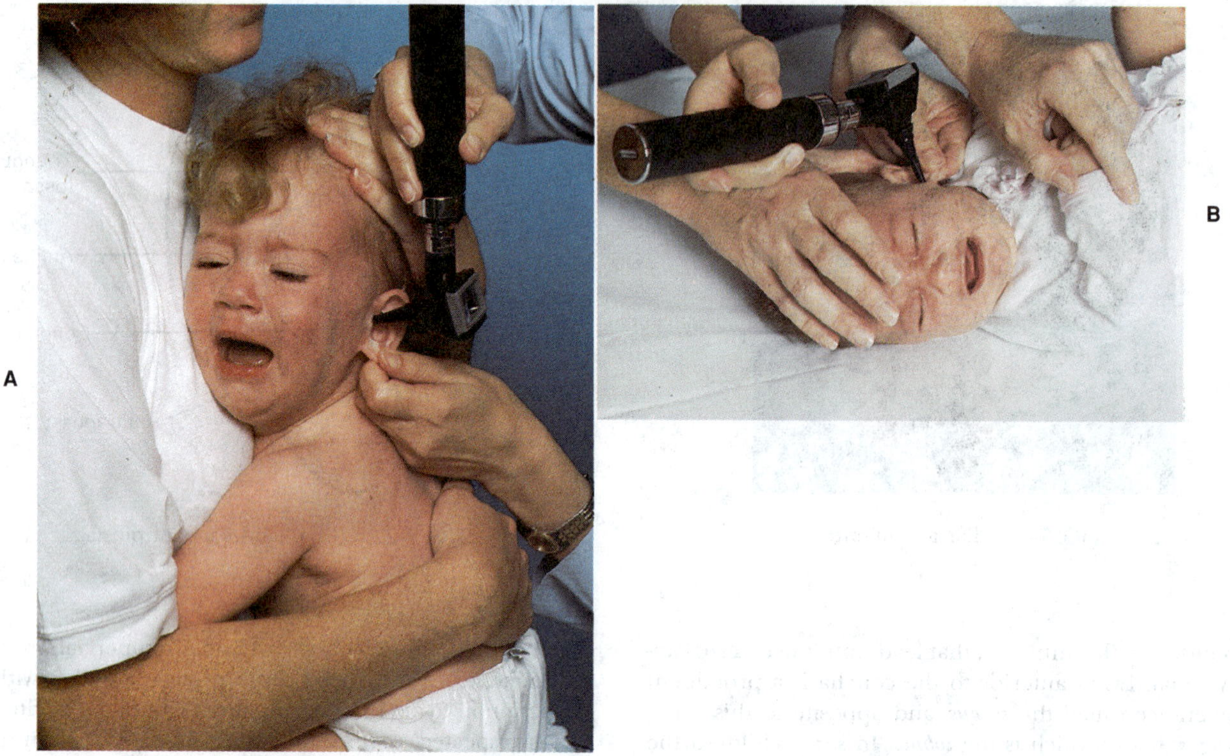

FIG. 7-23 Position for restraining child, **A,** and infant, **B,** during otoscopic examination.

how it works, and stressing the importance of remaining still. A helpful suggestion is to let them observe you examining the parent's ear. Restraint is needed for younger children because the ear examination upsets them (see Atraumatic Care box).

As you insert the speculum into the meatus, move it around the outer rim to accustom the child to the feel of something entering the ear. If examining a painful ear, touch a nonpainful part of the affected ear, then examine the unaffected ear, and finally return to the painful ear. By this time the child is usually less fearful of anything causing discomfort to the ear and will cooperate more.

For their protection and safety, restrain infants and toddlers for the otoscopic examination. There are two general positions of restraint. In one the child sits sideways in the parent's lap with one arm "hugging" the parent and the other arm at the side. The ear to be examined is away from the parent. With one arm the parent holds the child's head firmly against his or her chest, and with the other arm "hugs" the child, thereby securing the child's free arm. Examine the ear using the same procedure for holding the otoscope as described later (Fig. 7-23, *A*).

The other position involves placing the child on the side or abdomen with the arms at the side and the head turned so that the ear to be examined points toward the ceiling. Lean over the child, use the upper part of the body to restrain the arms and upper trunk movements, and use the examining hand to stabilize the head. This position is practical for young infants or for older children who need minimum restraining, but it may not be feasible for other children who protest vigorously. For safety enlist the parent's help in immobilizing the head by firmly placing one hand above the ear and the other on the child's back or side (Fig. 7-23, *B*).

With cooperative children examine the ear with the child in a side-lying, sitting, or standing position. One disadvantage to standing is that the child may "walk away" as the otoscope enters the canal. If the child is standing or sitting, tilt the head slightly toward the child's opposite shoulder to achieve a better view of the drum (Fig. 7-24; see also Nursing Tip, p. 252).

With the thumb and forefinger of the free (usually nondominant) hand, grasp the auricle. For the two positions of restraint, hold the otoscope upside down at the junction of its head and handle with the thumb and index finger. Place the other fingers against the skull to allow the otoscope to move with the child in case of sudden movement. In examining a cooperative child, hold the handle with the otic head upright or upside down. Use the dominant hand to examine both ears or reverse hands for each ear, whichever is more comfortable.

Before using the otoscope, visualize the external ear and the tympanic membrane as being superimposed on a clock (see Fig. 7-27). The numbers become important geographic landmarks. Introduce the speculum into the meatus between the 3 and 9 o'clock positions in a *downward* and *forward* position. Because the canal is curved, the speculum does not permit a panoramic view of the tympanic mem-

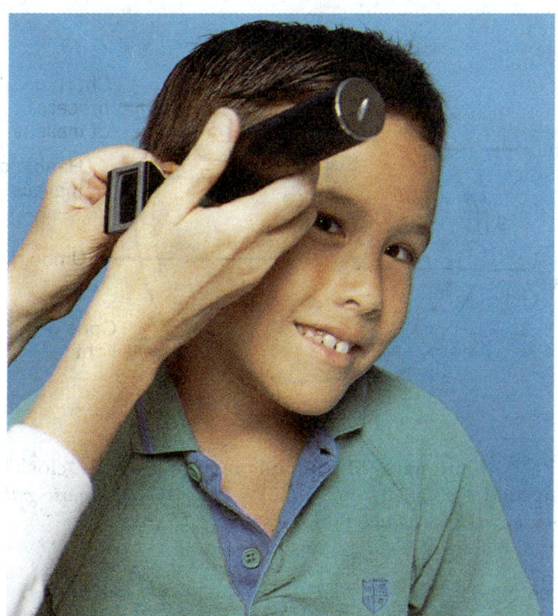

FIG. 7-24 Positioning head by tilting it toward opposite shoulder for better view of tympanic membrane.

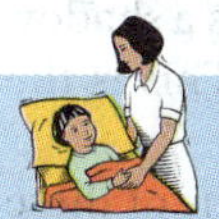

ATRAUMATIC CARE

Reducing Distress from Otoscopy in Young Children

Make examining the ear a game by explaining that you are looking for a "big elephant" in the ear. This kind of "fairy tale" is an absorbing distraction and usually elicits cooperation. After the ear has been examined, clarify that "looking for elephants" was only pretending and thank the child for letting you look in his or her ear.

brane unless the canal is straightened. In infants the canal curves upward. Therefore, pull the pinna *down* and *back* to the 6 to 9 o'clock range to straighten the canal (Fig. 7-25, *A*).

With older children, usually those over 3 years of age, the canal curves downward and forward. Therefore pull the pinna *up* and *back* toward a 10 o'clock position (Fig. 7-25, *B*). If there is difficulty in visualizing the membrane, try repositioning the head, introducing the speculum at a different angle, and pulling the pinna in a slightly different direction.

In neonates and young infants the walls of the canal are pliable and floppy because of the underdeveloped cartilaginous and bony structures. Therefore the very small 2 mm speculum usually needs to be inserted deeper into the canal than in older children. Use great care to avoid damaging the walls or drum. Because the small opening of the speculum permits a limited view, systematically inspect each quadrant of the membrane. In older children do not insert the speculum past the cartilaginous (outermost) portion of the canal, usually a distance of 0.60 to 1.25 cm (¼ to ½ inch). The entire canal is about 2.5 cm (1 inch) long. Insertion of the speculum into the posterior or bony portion of the canal causes pain (Fig. 7-26).

Otoscopic Examination. As you introduce the speculum into the external canal, inspect the walls of the canal, the color of the tympanic membrane, the light reflex, and the usual landmarks of the bony prominences of the middle ear (Fig. 7-27).

The ***walls*** of the external auditory canal are pink, although they are more pigmented in dark-skinned children. Minute hairs are evident in the outermost portion, where cerumen is produced. Note signs of irritation, foreign bodies, or infection.

Foreign bodies in the ear are not uncommon in children and range from erasers to beans. Symptoms may include

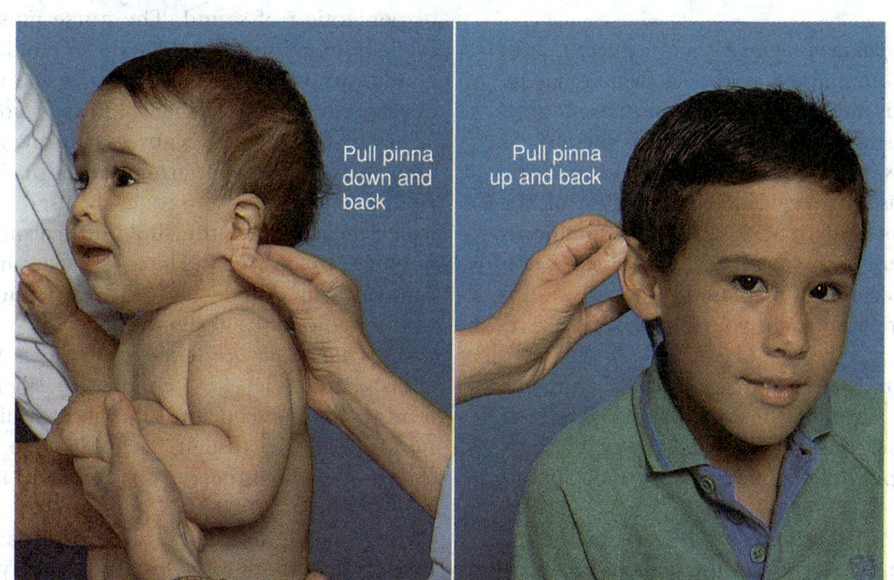

FIG. 7-25 Positioning of eardrum in infant, **A**, and in child over **3** years of age, **B**.

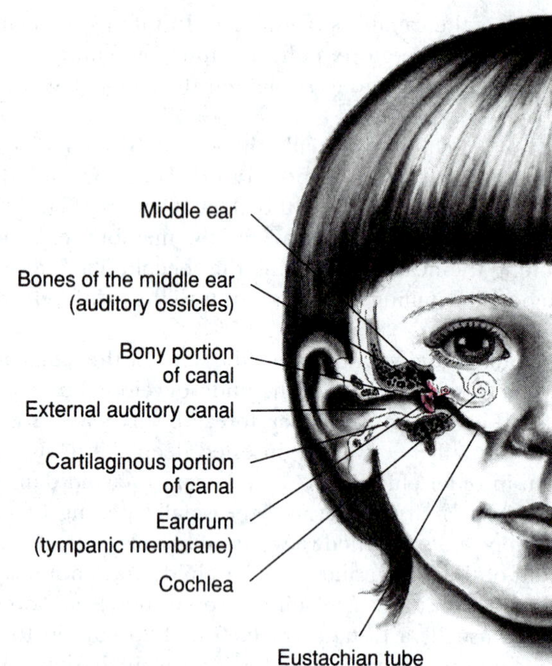

FIG. 7-26 Cross-section of external, middle, and parts of inner ear.

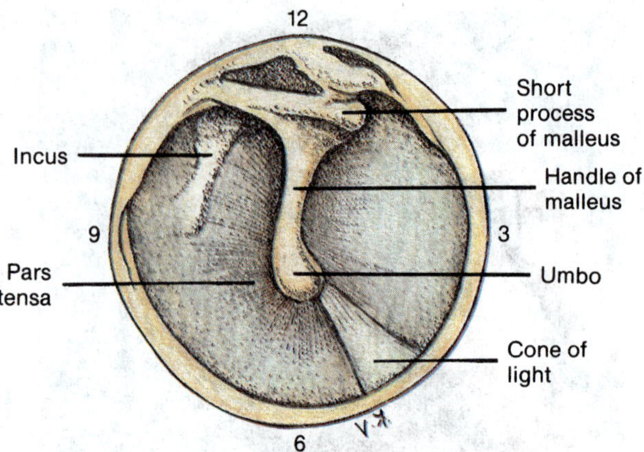

FIG. 7-27 Landmarks of tympanic membrane with "clock" superimposed. (Modified from Potter PA, Perry AG: *Basic nursing: theory and practice*, ed 2, St Louis, 1991, Mosby.)

pain, discharge, and affected hearing. Soft objects, such as paper or insects, can be removed with forceps. Small, hard objects, such as pebbles, can be removed with a suction tip, a hook, or irrigation. However, irrigation is contraindicated if the object is vegetative matter, such as beans or pasta, which swells when in contact with fluid.

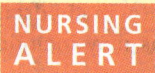

If there is any doubt about the type of object in the ear and the appropriate method to remove it, refer the child to the appropriate practitioner.

The ***color*** of the ***tympanic membrane*** is a translucent, light pearly pink or gray. Note marked erythema (which may indicate suppurative otitis media), a dull nontransparent grayish color (sometimes suggestive of serous otitis media), or ashen-gray areas (signs of scarring from a previous perforation). A black area usually suggests a perforation of the membrane that has not healed; perforations are commonly located at the periphery of the drum. Slight redness is normal in the newborn because of increased vascularity and is often evident in older infants and young children as a result of crying.

The characteristic tenseness and slope of the tympanic membrane cause the light of the otoscope to reflect at about the 5 or 7 o'clock position. The ***light reflex*** is a fairly well-defined cone-shaped reflection, which normally points away from the face.

The ***bony landmarks*** of the drum are formed by the following structures. The ***umbo,*** or tip of the malleus bone, appears as a small, round, opaque concave spot near the center of the drum. The ***manubrium*** (long process or handle) of the malleus appears to be a whitish line extending from the umbo upward to the margin of the membrane. At the upper end of the long process near the 1 o'clock position (in the right ear) is a sharp, knoblike protuberance, representing the ***short process*** of the malleus. Sometimes a shadow is seen at about the 10 or 11 o'clock position. This is the junction of the ***incus*** and the ***stapes*** bones.

Note the absence of the light reflex or loss of any of these landmarks, since it is probably caused by the bulging of the membrane as a result of fluid accumulation in the middle ear. Retraction of the drum with abnormal prominence of the bony landmarks suggests serous otitis media.

Auditory Testing

Several types of hearing tests are available. Some of them, such as audiometric testing, involve specialized equipment that measures the degree of hearing loss. Others, such as tests for the startle reflex in neonates, are rough estimations of perception of sound. The nurse must operate under a high index of suspicion for those children who may have conditions associated with hearing loss and who may have developed behaviors that indicate auditory impairment. Types of hearing loss, causes, clinical manifestations, and appropriate treatment are discussed in Chapter 24.

One of the most frequently used tests is ***audiometry,*** which measures the threshold of hearing for pure-tone frequencies (measured in Hertz [Hz]) at various levels of loudness (measured in decibels [dB]). An audiogram is a record of the audiometric testing.

In a ***threshold acuity test,*** a sound is transmitted to the child's ear at a level the child can easily hear, and then the loudness is reduced until the child indicates the sound is no longer heard (usually by holding up a hand or pushing a button). This procedure is repeated for frequencies between 500 and 8000 Hz. The sounds are usually delivered through headphones that can be compared to a "space helmet." Since the child is listening to very soft sounds, audiometry is best performed in a soundproof room.

Audiometry can also be used as a screening test or "sweep

TABLE 7-12 Selected Hearing and Tympanic Membrane Compliance Tests*

DESCRIPTION	COMMENTS
CLINICAL HEARING TESTS	
In newborns elicit the startle reflex and observe other neonatal responses to loud noises, such as facial grimaces, blinking, gross motor movement, quiet if crying or crying if quiet, opening the eyes, or ceasing sucking activity. During infancy note child's reaction to a noise. Stand about 18 inches away from infant, to the side, and out of child's peripheral field of vision. With the room silent and infant sitting in parent's lap, distracted by some object, make a voice sound such as "ps" or "phth" (high-pitched) or "oo" (low-pitched), ring a bell or a rattle, or rustle tissue paper.	An objective sign of alerting to sound may be an increase in heart rate or respiratory rate. Absence of alerting behaviors suggests hearing loss. Eliciting the startle reflex is used only in infants from birth to 4 months. Test is usually inadequate for children beyond infancy because of their tendency to ignore sounds or be distracted. Compare response of localizing sound to expected age response (see Biologic Development Chapter 12).
CRIB-O-GRAM	
Neonatal screening tool that analyzes hearing responses by comparing the infant's motor activity before, during, and after a sound is introduced. A motion-sensitive transducer is placed beneath the mattress, and a microprocessor "reads" the infant's movements.	Both administration of the test and its scoring are totally automated. The test is repeated several times to increase reliability. A consistent change in activity that coincides with the test sound is scored as a pass. Neonates who are premature or ill may not respond to sound despite adequate hearing.
TYMPANOMETRY	
Measures tympanic membrane compliance (or mobility) and estimates middle ear air pressure. A soft rubber cuff is pressed over the external canal to produce an airtight seal; an automatic reading of air pressure registers on the machine.	Detects middle ear disease and abnormalities but does not indicate the degree of hearing loss or the interpretation of sound. Difficult to perform in young children because of inability to maintain an adequate seal or excessive movement by the child.
CONDUCTION TESTS	
Rinne test—Stem of tuning fork is placed against the mastoid bone until the sound ceases to be audible. Tuning fork is then moved so that the prongs are held near, but not touching, the auditory meatus. Child should again hear the sound ***(Rinne positive).*** If sound is not again audible ***(Rinne negative),*** some abnormality is interfering with the conduction of air through the external and middle chambers.	Requires the cooperation and ability of the child to signal when the sound is no longer audible and when it is again heard. Not useful for most children before preschool age.
Weber test—Stem of tuning fork is held in the midline of the head. Child should hear the sound equally in both ears ***(Weber positive).*** With air conductive loss, child will hear the sound better in the affected ear ***(Weber negative).***	Frequently not suitable for young children because of their difficulty in discriminating between "better, more, or less."
AUDIOMETRY	
Electrical audiometer measures the threshold of hearing for pure-tone frequencies and loudness. A sound is transmitted to the child's ear and reduced until child indicates the sound is no longer heard; this procedure is repeated for several sounds covering the range found in conversation. In an air conduction audiogram the sounds are transmitted through earphones. In a bone conduction audiogram the sounds are passed through a plaque placed over the mastoid bone.	Provides valuable information regarding the severity of the hearing loss, the sound cycles involved, and the possible location of the defect. Requires specialized training of personnel, expensive equipment, and cooperation from the child in terms of confirming the perception of sound. For children ages 24 months to about 5 years, play audiometry can be used; it is based on behavior modification and involves reinforcement for correct response.
EVOKED OTOACOUSTIC EMISSIONS (EOAES)	
Special OAE analyzer delivers a rapid series of clicks to the ear through a probe fitted with a tympanometry tip that is inserted closely in the external auditory canal. The presence of OAEs, defined as sound energy emitted by the cochlea that is believed to be generated by the movement of the outer hairs of the organ of Corti, is usually associated with normal or near-normal cochlear sensitivity; their absence indicates a hearing loss of at least 20-25 dB, provided there is no conductive dysfunction (Abdo, Feghali, and Stapells, 1993)	Preferred method of screening neonates for sensorineural hearing loss (ototoxicity and noise-induced hearing loss). Requires specialized equipment. Minimal training is required. Infants must be in a quiet sleep for testing. Results do not indicate severity of cochlear damage; should be followed by BAER (see below).
BRAINSTEM-AUDITORY EVOKED RESPONSE (BAER)	
Through electrode wires attached to the infant's or child's scalp, electrical or brain wave potentials generated within the auditory system are transmitted to a computer for analysis. Following repetitive acoustic stimulation, the waveforms from a normal sleeping or quiet infant consist of several peaks and valleys that reflect activations of neural structures of the brain.	Requires specialized training of personnel and expensive equipment.

*Any child who is suspected of a hearing loss because of poor performance using screening tests is referred for special audiometric or BAER testing.

check" by presenting several different frequencies at either 20 or 25 dB. The Audioscope incorporates audiometric hearing screening and otoscopy in a single instrument. The Audioscope produces pure tones at 500, 1000, 2000, and 4000 Hz at a fixed hearing level of 25 dB. Failure to respond to any frequency is considered a failure. The instrument is reliable for children 5 years of age and older. Children as young as 3 years of age may be able to respond to the screening if adequately prepared by having a practice session in which they can become acquainted with the directions (Orlando and Frank, 1987). Other hearing tests that may be used in infants and children are described in Table 7-12.

Another test that indirectly provides clues to a potential hearing loss is measurement of tympanic membrane compliance (mobility). Normally the pressure on both sides of the membrane is equal, allowing the drum to move easily when negative or positive pressure is applied. Decreased or low compliance usually indicates middle ear effusion (otitis media), a potential cause of conductive hearing loss. ***Tympanometry,*** a simple, reliable, and easily performed procedure, measures the compliance of the tympanic membrane and middle ear pressure.

Membrane compliance can also be measured by ***pneumatic otoscopy (pneumootoscopy).*** Pressure to the tympanic membrane is applied by means of a bulb attached to the head of the otoscope, and the movement of the drum is observed. A limitation of the test is that the pressures needed to properly assess tympanic membrane mobility and accurately screen for middle ear abnormalities are not known (Cavanaugh, 1989).

➤ **NURSING TIP** Sometimes it takes an extra hand to examine a child's ear—one hand to hold the otoscope, a second hand to straighten the canal, and a third hand to use the bulb (or a curette). The solution is to enlist the child's help (Fig. 7-28). Have the child raise the arm opposite the affected ear up and over the head toward the opposite side. Then ask the child to grasp the upper edge of the earlobe at about the 11 or 1 o'clock position and to pull the lobe gently up and back. With that third "helper" hand, use your hands to manipulate the equipment (Wong, 1992).

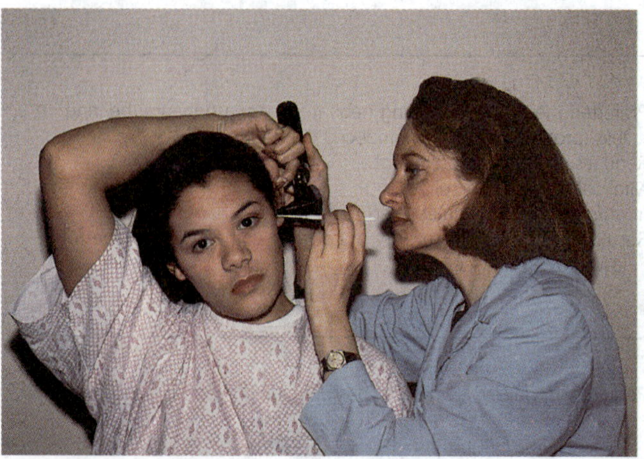

FIG. 7-28 Having the child tug on the ear to straighten the canal leaves both of the nurse's hands available for the otoscopic examination.

Vestibular Testing

Vestibular testing for inner ear function concerning equilibrium is evaluated in young children by holding them at a 30-degree angle and rotating them in a complete circle in each direction. The normal response is nystagmus (movement of the eyes) in the direction of the rotation while being swung and in the opposite direction when the movement stops. For older children use a swivel chair or have them pivot quickly to one side, then the other.

NOSE

The nose marks the beginning of the passageway through the respiratory tract. It is an important organ for filtration, temperature control, and humidification of inspired air, and a sensory organ for olfaction (smell). Each of these functions depends on the patency of the passageways and the mucosal lining of the nasal cavity. Inspection is primarily used for assessing the external and internal structures.

Inspection of External Structures

The nose is located in the middle of the face just below the eyes and above the lips. Compare its placement and alignment by drawing an imaginary vertical line from the center point between the eyes down to the notch of the upper lip. The nose should lie exactly vertical to this line, with each side exactly symmetric. Note its location, any deviation to one side, and asymmetry in overall size and in diameter of the nares (nostrils). The ***bridge*** of the nose is sometimes flat in Oriental and black children. Observe the ***alae nasi*** for any sign of flaring, which indicates respiratory difficulty. Always report any flaring of the alae nasi. Fig. 7-29 illustrates the usual landmarks used in describing the external structures of the nose.

Inspection of Internal Structures

Inspect the ***anterior vestibule*** of the nose is by pushing the tip upward, tilting the head backward, and illuminating the cavity with a flashlight or otoscope without the attached ear speculum. For a deeper view of the inferior and middle turbinates and the middle meatus, use a nasal speculum, such as a 9 mm speculum with a very short barrel that attaches to the otoscope head. Forceps specula are not routinely used in children. Insert the short, wide speculum into the nares, slightly away from the septum, and tilt the otoscope upward to straighten the passageway toward the posterior wall of the cavity. Avoid pushing against the septum, because it causes pain. Generally, inspection is adequate without the speculum, unless a closer examination of the nasal membranes is warranted. If using the nasal speculum, explain the process to the child in a way similar to the preparation given for using the otoscope.

Note the ***color*** of the ***mucosal lining,*** which is normally redder than the oral membranes, as well as any swelling, discharge, dryness, or bleeding. Nasal membranes that are abnormally pale, grayish pink, and swollen suggest nasal al-

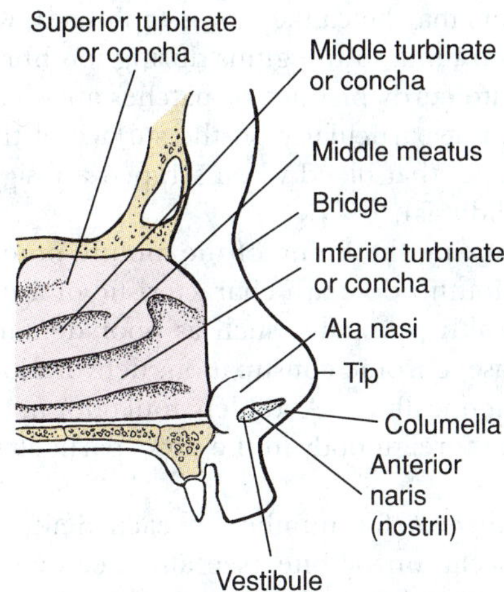

FIG. 7-29 External landmarks and internal structures of nose.

lergies. Red, swollen membranes are usually characteristic of the common cold. These differences in appearance are important diagnostic clues to distinguishing between allergy and cold symptoms.

Normally there should be no discharge from the nose. However, if the child has been crying, a watery discharge is normal. At other times a thin, clear exudate may indicate allergies, chronic rhinitis, or sinusitis. Purulent discharge is caused by infection and can indicate upper respiratory tract infections resulting from either a viral or a bacterial agent. Discharge from one nostril and a foul odor may be caused by a foreign body. If possible, remove the object with forceps (tweezers). If it is deep in the cavity, refer the child to a more experienced practitioner.

Looking deeper into the nose, inspect the ***turbinates,*** or ***concha,*** plates of bone enveloped by mucous membrane that jut into the nasal cavity. The turbinates greatly increase the surface area of the nasal cavity as air is inhaled. The spaces or channels between the turbinates are called the ***meatus*** and correspond to each of the three turbinates. Normally the front end of the inferior and middle turbinate and the middle meatus can be seen. They should be the same color as the lining of the vestibule. Note enlarged, boggy, pale, grayish mucosa. Swollen turbinates greatly occlude the passageways for entry of air.

Also inspect the ***septum,*** which should equally divide the vestibules. Note any deviation, especially if it causes an occlusion of one side of the nose. A perforation may be evident within the septum. If this is suspected, shine the light of the otoscope into one naris and look for light coming through the perforation to the other nostril.

Since olfaction is an important function of the nose, testing for smell may be done at this point or as part of cranial nerve assessment (see Table 7-17).

MOUTH AND THROAT

The mouth is the beginning of the passageway to the digestive tract, but it also functions in the entry or exit of air. The major structure of the exterior of the mouth is the ***lips.***

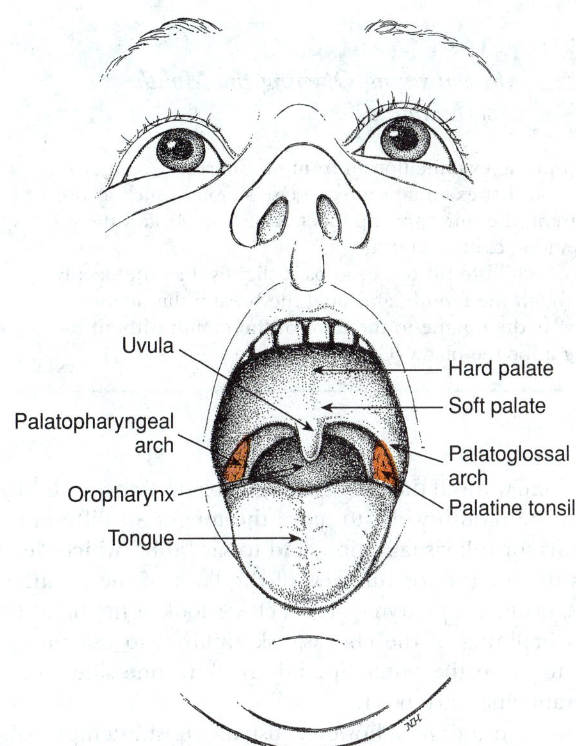

FIG. 7-30 Interior structures of mouth.

Inspection of the lips for color is discussed in the section on skin (p. 233). Note any deviations, such as ***cheilitis,*** the presence of painful, inflamed, and dried cracks or fissures of the lips. Cheilitis may be caused by exposure to harsh climatic conditions, habitual licking or biting of the lips, mouth breathing from respiratory distress, or dehydration, particularly with fever. ***Cheilosis,*** or angular stomatitis, is fissuring at the angles or corners of the lips and may indicate deficiencies of riboflavin or niacin.

Observe for lesions on the lips. The herpes simplex virus produces singular or clusters of vesicular eruptions, often called "cold sores." The lip may also be the site of a primary syphilitic chancre, which appears as a firm nodule that ulcerates and crusts. Whenever potentially infectious lesions are examined, be sure to wear gloves.

Inspection of Internal Structures

The mouth and throat are divided into three areas: (1) the ***oral cavity,*** which extends from the lips to the palatopharyngeal arches; (2) the ***oropharynx,*** which extends from the epiglottis to the lower edge of the adenoids; and (3) the ***nasopharynx,*** which extends from above the lower edge of the adenoids to the nasal cavity. The major structures that are visible on examination within the oral cavity and oropharynx are the mucosal lining of the lips and cheeks, gums or gingiva, teeth, tongue, palate, uvula, tonsils, and posterior oropharynx (Fig. 7-30). Other pharyngeal structures that are not visible on examination are the epiglottis, lingual tonsils, and pharyngeal tonsils or adenoids.

With a cooperative child almost the entire examination

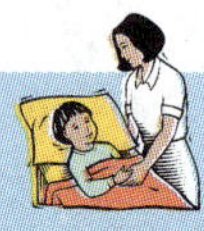

ATRAUMATIC CARE
Encouraging Opening the Mouth for Examination

Perform the examination in front of a mirror.

Let child first examine someone else's mouth, such as the parent, the nurse, or a puppet (Fig. 7-31, *A*) and then examine child's mouth.

Instruct child to tilt the head back slightly, breathe deeply through the mouth, and hold the breath; this action lowers the tongue to the floor of the mouth without using a tongue blade (Greally, 1988).

can be done without the use of a tongue blade. Ask the child to open the mouth wide, to move the tongue in different directions for full visualization, and to say "ahh," which depresses the tongue for full view of the back of the mouth (tonsils, uvula, oropharynx). For a closer look at the buccal mucosa or lining of the cheeks, ask children to use their fingers to move the outer lip and cheek to one side (see also Atraumatic Care box).

Infants and toddlers, however, usually resist attempts to keep the mouth open. Because inspecting the mouth is an upsetting part of the examination, reserve this inspection until last (with examination of the ears) or perform it during episodes of crying. If the child resists opening the mouth, pinch the nostrils closed; this forces the child to open the mouth to breathe. However, use a tongue blade to depress the tongue. Place it along the *side* of the tongue, not the center back area where the gag reflex is elicited. Fig. 7-31, *B*, illustrates proper positioning of the child for oral examination.

Inspect all areas lined with ***mucous membranes*** (inside the lips and cheeks, gingiva, underside of tongue, palate, back of pharynx). The membranes should be bright pink, smooth, glistening, uniform, and moist. Note any deviations, such as color, white patches or ulceration, bleeding, and sensitivity. For example, reddened areas with white ulcerated centers may be canker sores (aphthae), which may be caused by trauma to the gums during toothbrushing or chewing. White curdy plaques or patches anywhere on the oral mucosa, but particularly on the surface of the tongue and hard palate, that bleed when scraped are signs of moniliasis (candidiasis).

While observing the lining of the mouth, note any odor (halitosis). Mouth odors are characteristic of a number of important health problems, such as poor dental hygiene, gingival disease, chronic constipation, dehydration, malnutrition, or systemic illness. A sudden, foul odor in the mouth may indicate a foreign body in the nose, particularly a bean or pea.

Inspect the ***teeth*** for number in each dental arch, hygiene, and occlusion or bite (see also Teething, Chapter 12). Discoloration of tooth enamel with obvious plaque (whitish coating on the surface of the teeth) is a sign of poor dental hygiene and indicates a need for dental counseling. Brown spots in the crevices of the crown of the tooth or between the teeth may be caries (cavities). Chalky white to yellow or brown areas on the enamel may indicate fluorosis (excessive fluoride ingestion). Teeth that appear greenish black may be stained temporarily from ingestion of supplemental iron.

Evaluate malocclusion or poor biting relationship of the teeth in terms of (1) how the jaws relate to each other in vertical, transverse, and anteroposterior directions (e.g., the "bucktoothed" appearance that results when the maxilla is forward in relation to the mandible), (2) how the teeth are aligned, and (3) how the teeth interdigitate when in occlusion. Although parents frequently express concern regarding thumb-sucking and the development of orthodontic problems, thumb-sucking that ceases before the permanent teeth erupt does little harm.

Examine the ***gums*** surrounding the teeth. The color is normally coral pink, and the surface texture is stippled, similar to the appearance of orange peel. In dark-skinned children the gums are more deeply colored and a brownish area is often observed along the gum line. Note if the gums are inflamed; redness, puffiness along the gum line,

A

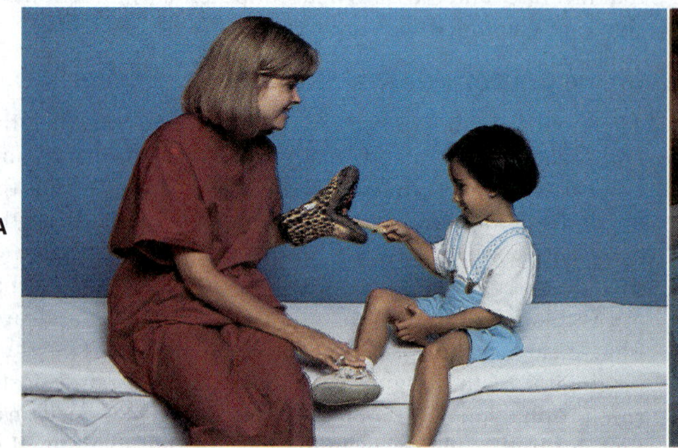

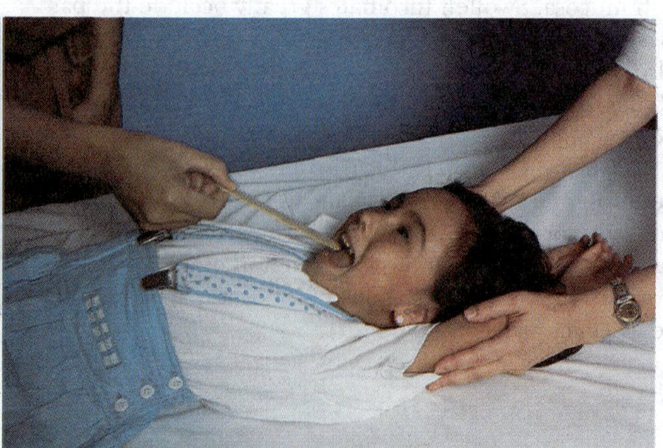

B

FIG. 7-31 **A,** Encouraging child to cooperate. **B,** Positioning child for examination of mouth.

and a tendency to bleed are signs of gingivitis. Counsel the child and family about good dental hygiene, especially flossing.

Inspect the ***tongue*** for the presence of papillae, small projections that contain several taste buds each and give the tongue its characteristic rough appearance. Note changes in the surface texture, such as (1) "geographic tongue," unusual patterns of papillae formation and denuded areas; (2) coated tongue, such as in candidiasis; or (3) an exceptionally beefy red and swollen tongue, which is a sign of various systemic diseases.

Note the size and mobility of the tongue, especially protrusion, which is frequently seen in children with mental retardation. Normally the tip of the tongue extends to the lips. If the child is unable to move the tongue forward to this point, the frenulum, or central band of mucous membrane, which attaches the tongue to the floor of the mouth, may be too short. "Tongue-tie" can result in speech problems.

The roof of the mouth consists of the ***hard palate,*** near the front of the cavity, and the ***soft palate,*** toward the back of the pharynx, which has a small midline protrusion called the ***uvula.*** Inspect both carefully to be sure that they are intact. Sometimes there is a pinpoint cleft in the soft palate that may go undetected unless carefully inspected. Such a cleft is especially important if the uvula is bifid, or separated into two appendages. A submucosal cleft may result in speech problems later on, since air is not effectively trapped for vocalization. The arch of the palate should be dome shaped. A narrow-flat roof or high-arched palate affects the placement of the tongue and can cause feeding and speech problems. Test the movement of the uvula by eliciting a gag reflex, which moves the uvula upward.

While inspecting the recesses of the oropharynx, note the size and color of the ***palatine tonsils.*** They are normally the same color as the surrounding mucosa, glandular rather than smooth in appearance, and barely visible over the edge of the palatoglossal arches. Enlargement, redness, and white patches on the tonsils and surrounding area may indicate suppurative tonsillitis or pharyngitis. Report these findings for further evaluation.

CHEST

Although the thoracic cavity houses two vital organs, the heart and the lungs, the anatomic structures of the chest wall are important sources of information concerning cardiac and pulmonary function, skeletal formation, and secondary sexual development. Inspect the chest for size, shape, symmetry, movement, breast development, and the presence of the bony landmarks formed by the ribs and sternum.

The ***rib cage*** consists of 12 ribs and the sternum, or breast bone, located in the midline of the trunk (Fig. 7-32). The first seven ribs, often called ***true ribs,*** attach directly to the costal cartilages of the sternum at the costochondral junction. The next five ribs are called ***false ribs*** because they do not attach directly to the costal cartilages of the sternum.

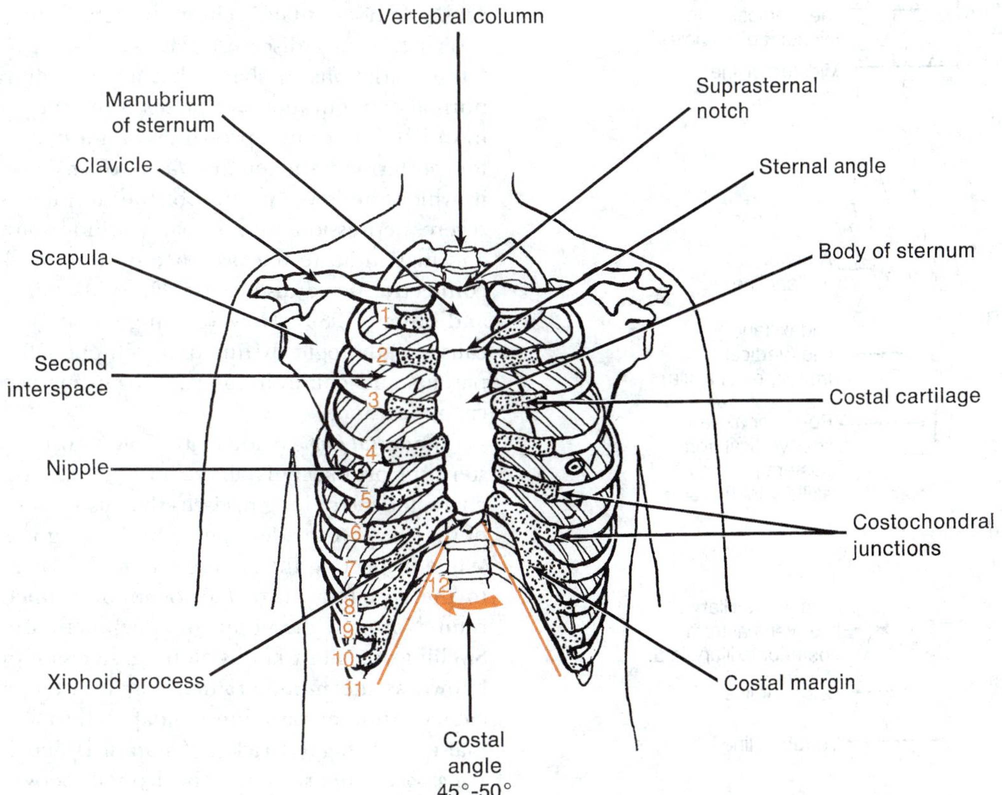

FIG. 7-32 Rib cage.

The eighth, ninth, and tenth ribs attach to the costal cartilages below the seventh rib, and the last two ribs, often called ***floaters,*** have no direct attachment to the sternum or anterior ribs other than their posterior attachment to the vertebral column.

The ***sternum*** is composed of three main parts. The ***manubrium,*** the uppermost portion, can be felt at the base of the neck at the ***suprasternal notch.*** The largest segment of the sternum is the body, which forms the ***sternal angle (angle of Louis)*** as it articulates with the manubrium. At the end of the body is a small, movable process called the ***xiphoid.*** The angle of the costal margin as it attaches to the sternum is called the ***costal angle*** and is normally about 45 to 50 degrees. These bony structures are important landmarks in the location of ribs and intercostal spaces. The first rib attaches directly to the manubrium. The second rib attaches directly to the body of the sternum below the sternal angle. The sternal angle is felt as a ridge a few centimeters below the suprasternal notch. The space immediately below a rib is its corresponding ***intercostal space (ICS).***

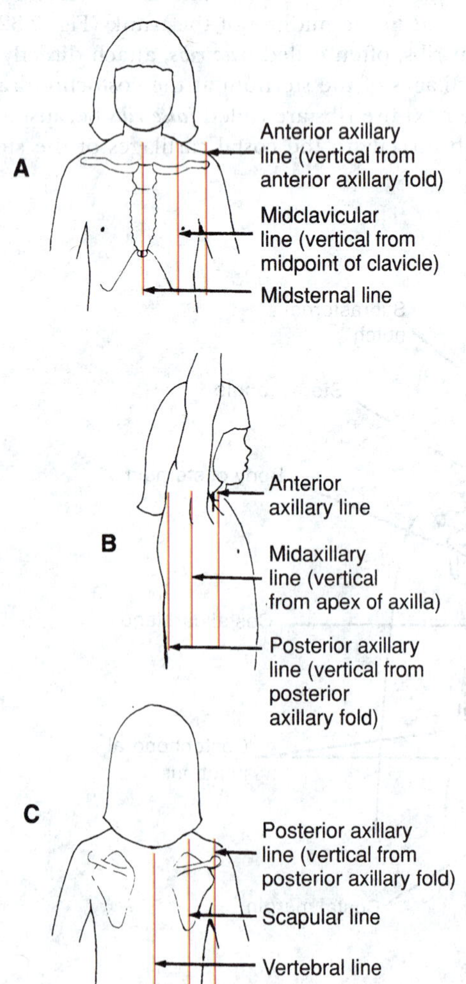

FIG. 7-33 Imaginary landmarks of chest. **A,** Anterior. **B,** Right lateral. **C,** Posterior.

Become familiar with locating and properly numbering each rib, because ribs are geographic landmarks for palpating, percussing, and auscultating underlying organs. Normally all the ribs can be counted by palpating inferiorly from the second rib. The tip of the eleventh rib can be felt laterally, and the tip of the twelfth rib can be felt posteriorly. Other helpful landmarks include the nipples, which are usually located between the fourth and fifth ribs or at the fourth interspace and, posteriorly, the tip of the scapula, which is located at the level of the eighth rib or interspace. In children with thin chest walls, correctly locating the ribs presents little difficulty.

The ***thoracic cavity*** is also divided into segments by drawing imaginary lines on the chest and back. Fig. 7-33 illustrates the anterior, lateral, and posterior divisions.

Measure the ***size*** of the chest by placing the tape around the rib cage at the nipple line (see Fig. 7-34). For greatest accuracy take at least two measurements—one during inspiration and the other during expiration—and record the average. Chest size is important mainly in comparison with its relationship with head circumference, which is discussed on p. 225. Always report marked disporportions, because most are caused by abnormal head growth, although some may be a result of altered chest shape, such as barrel chest or pigeon chest.

During infancy the ***shape*** of the chest is almost circular, with the anteroposterior (front-to-back) diameter equaling the transverse or lateral (side-to-side) diameter. As the child grows, the chest normally increases in the transverse direction, causing the anteroposterior diameter to be less than the lateral diameter. In an older child the characteristic barrel shape of an infant's chest is a significant sign of chronic obstructive lung disease, such as asthma or cystic fibrosis. Other variations in shape that are usually variants of the normal configuration are ***pigeon breast,*** or ***pectus carinatum,*** in which the sternum protrudes outward, increasing the anteroposterior diameter, and ***funnel chest,*** or ***pectus excavatum,*** in which the lower portion of the sternum is depressed. A severe depression may impair cardiorespiratory function and may indicate the presence of an underlying heritable connective tissue disorder, such as Marfan syndrome (Arn and others, 1989). However, in general, neither condition causes pathologic dysfunction, although they often cause parents and children concern regarding acceptable physical appearance.

The ***costal angle*** made by the lower costal margin and the sternum ordinarily is about 45 degrees. A larger angle is characteristic of lung diseases that also cause a barrel shape of the chest. A smaller angle may be a sign of malnutrition. While inspecting the rib cage, note the junction of the ribs to the costal cartilage (costochondral junction) and sternum. Normally the points of attachment are fairly smooth. Swellings or blunt knobs along either side of the sternum, known as the ***rachitic rosary,*** may indicate vitamin D deficiency. Another variation in shape that may either be normal or may suggest rickets (vitamin D deficiency) is ***Harrison groove,*** a depression or horizontal groove where the diaphragm leaves the chest wall. Usually marked flaring of the rib cage below the groove is an abnormal finding.

Body ***symmetry*** is always an important notation during inspection. Asymmetry in the chest may indicate serious underlying problems, such as cardiac enlargement (bulging on left side of rib cage) or pulmonary dysfunction. However, asymmetry is most often a sign of scoliosis, lateral curvature of the spine. Asymmetry warrants further medical investigation.

Movement of the chest wall should be symmetric bilaterally and coordinated with breathing. The chest and abdomen should rise and fall together. During inspiration the chest rises and expands, the diaphragm descends, and the costal angle increases. During expiration the chest falls and decreases in size, the diaphragm rises, and the costal angle narrows (Fig. 7-34). In children under 6 or 7 years of age, respiratory movement is principally abdominal or diaphragmatic. In older children, particularly females, respirations are chiefly thoracic.

Always report any asymmetry of movement. Decreased movement on one side of the chest may indicate pneumonia, pneumothorax, atelectasis, or an obstructive foreign body. Marked ***retraction*** of the muscles either between the ribs (intercostal), above the sternum (suprasternal), or above the clavicles (supraclavicular) is a sign of respiratory difficulty (see Fig. 31-6). Always report this finding as well.

While inspecting the skin surface of the chest, observe the position of the ***nipples,*** as well as any evidence of ***breast development.*** Normally the nipples are located slightly lateral to the midclavicular line between the fourth and fifth ribs. Note symmetry of nipple placement and normal configuration of a darker pigmented areola surrounding a flat nipple in the prepubertal child.

Pubertal breast development usually begins in girls between 10 and 14 years of age (see Fig. 19-3). Record precocious or delayed breast development, as well as evidence of any other secondary sexual characteristics. In males gynecomastia may be caused by hormonal or systemic disorders, but more commonly it is a result of adipose tissue from obesity or a transitory body change during early puberty. In either situation investigate the child's feelings regarding breast enlargement.

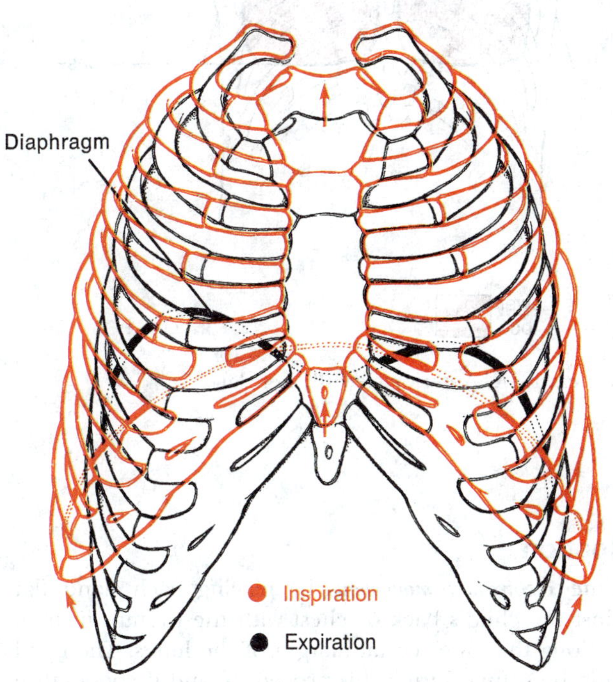

FIG. 7-34 Movement of chest during respiration.

In adolescent females who have achieved sexual maturity, palpate the breasts for evidence of any masses or hard nodules. Use this opportunity to discuss the importance of routine self-breast examination. Although carcinoma of the breast is rare in women under 20 years of age, stress the value of routine self-breast examination so that it becomes a practiced habit during later years. The vast majority of palpable masses are benign (Marks and Fisher, 1987). Emphasize this fact to decrease any fear or concern that results when a mass is felt.

LUNGS

The lungs are situated inside the thoracic cavity, with one lung on each side of the sternum. Each lung is divided into an ***apex,*** which is slightly pointed and rises above the first rib; a ***base,*** which is wide and concave and rides on the dome-shaped diaphragm; and a body, which is divided into ***lobes.*** The right lung has three lobes: the upper, middle, and lower. The left lobe has only two lobes, the upper and lower, because of the space occupied by the heart. The two surfaces of the lung are the ***costal surface,*** which faces the chest wall and backs up to the vertebral column, and the ***mediastinal surface,*** which faces the space lying between the lungs, the mediastinum. The center of the mediastinal surface is called the ***hilus,*** where the bronchus and blood vessels enter the lung (Fig. 7-35, *A*).

Examination of the lungs requires knowledge of their location and their relationship to the rib cage. The trachea bifurcates slightly below the level of the sternal angle. The apex of each lung rises about 2 to 4 cm above the inner third of the clavicles. The lower costal margin crosses the sixth rib at the midclavicular line and the eighth rib at the midaxillary line. The posterior base of the lungs crosses the eleventh rib at the vertebral line. The upper border of the right middle lobe parallels the inferior surface of the fourth rib. Fig. 7-35 illustrates the position of the lobes within the thoracic cavity during relaxation. Respiration causes displacement of the lobes upward (expiration) or downward (inspiration).

Inspection

Inspection of the lungs primarily involves observation of respiratory movements, which are discussed on p. 258. Evaluate respirations for (1) rate (number per minute), (2) rhythm (regular, irregular, or periodic), (3) depth (deep or shallow), and (4) quality (effortless, automatic, difficult, or labored). Also note the character of breath sounds, such as noisy, grunting, snoring, or heavy. Usual terms for describing various patterns of respiration are listed in the box on p. 259.

Always evaluate respiratory rate in relation to general

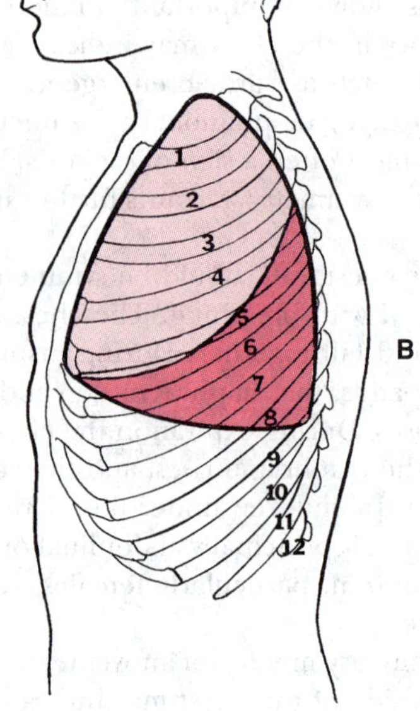

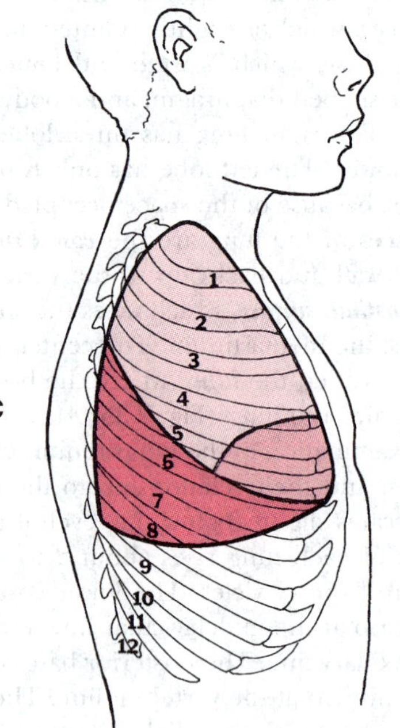

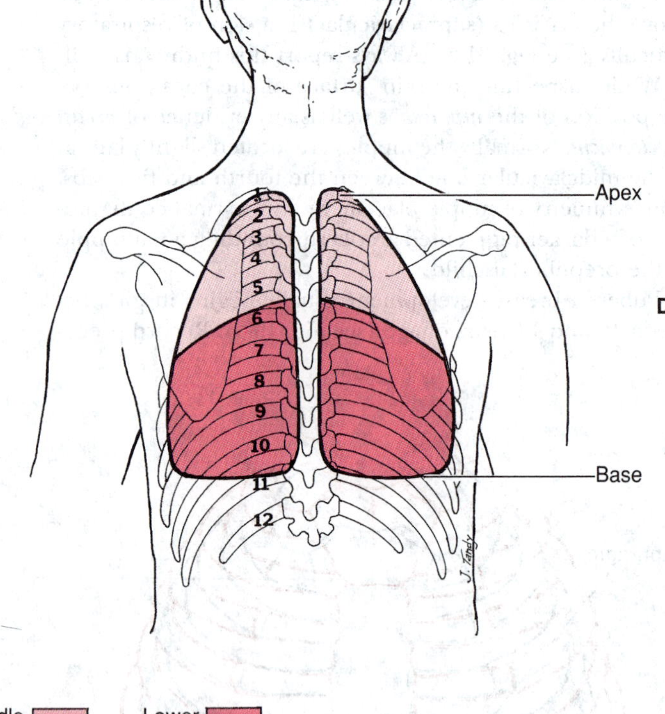

FIG. 7-35 Location of lobes of lungs within thoracic cavity. **A,** Anterior view. **B,** Left lateral view. **C,** Right lateral view. **D,** Posterior view.

physical status. For example, tachypnea is expected with fever, because for every degree Fahrenheit elevation in temperature, the respiratory rate increases four breaths per minute. The usual ratio of breaths to heartbeats is 1:4 (see inside back cover for normal respiratory rates at various ages).

Palpation

Evalute ***respiratory movements*** by placing each hand flat against the child's back or chest with the thumbs in midline along the lower costal margin of the lungs. The child should be sitting during this procedure and if cooperative should take several deep breaths. During respiration the

VARIOUS PATTERNS OF RESPIRATION

Tachypnea—Increased rate
Bradypnea—Decreased rate
Dyspnea—Distress during breathing
Apnea—Cessation of breathing
Hyperpnea—Increased depth
Hypoventilation—Decreased depth (shallow) and irregular rhythm
Hyperventilation—Increased rate and depth
Kussmaul breathing—Hyperventilation, gasping and labored respiration, usually seen in diabetic coma or other states of respiratory acidosis
Cheyne-Stokes respirations—Gradually increasing rate and depth with periods of apnea
Biot breathing—Periods of hyperpnea alternating with apnea (similar to Cheyne-Stokes except that depth remains constant)
Seesaw (paradoxic) respirations—Chest falls on inspiration and rises on expiration
Agonal—Last gasping breaths before death

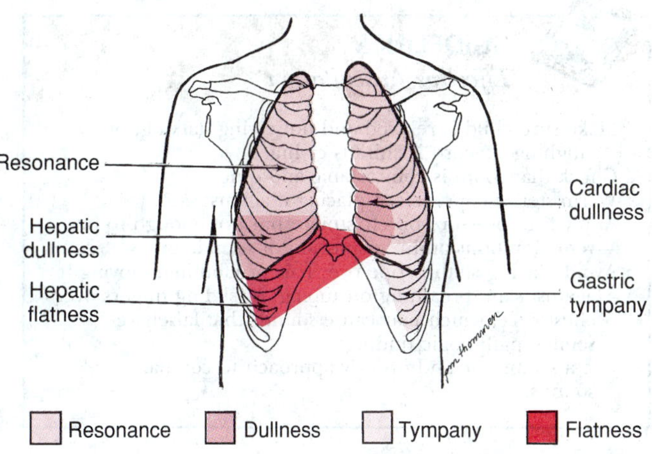

FIG. 7-36 Percussion sounds found in normal thorax.

hands will move with the chest wall. Assess the amount of respiratory excursion and note any asymmetry of movement. Normally in older children the posterior base of the lungs descends 5 to 6 cm (about 2 inches) during a deep inspiration.

Palpate for ***vocal fremitus,*** the conduction of voice sounds through the respiratory tract. With the palmar surfaces of your hands on the child's chest, have the child repeat words, such as "ninety-nine," "one, two, three," or "eee-eee." Feel the vibrations, moving the hands symmetrically on either side of the sternum and vertebral column. In general, vocal fremitus is most intense in the apex and least prominent at the base of the lungs. Decreased vocal fremitus in the upper airway may indicate several gross pulmonary changes. Absence of fremitus usually indicates obstruction of a major bronchus, which may occur as a result of aspiration of a foreign body. Always record and report decreased or absent fremitus for further investigation.

During palpation note other vibrations that indicate pathologic conditions. ***Pleural friction rub,*** which has a grating sensation, is synchronous with respiratory movements and results from opposing surfaces of the inflamed pleural lining rubbing against one another. ***Crepitation,*** a coarse, cracking sensation felt as the hand presses over the affected area, results from air escaping from the lungs into the subcutaneous tissues as a result of injury or surgical intervention. Both pleural friction rubs and crepitation can usually be both heard and felt.

Percussion

The lungs are percussed in order to evaluate the densities of the underlying organs. Fig. 7-36 illustrates the expected percussion sounds within the anterior thorax. ***Resonance*** is heard over all the lobes of the lungs that are not adjacent to other organs. ***Dullness*** is heard beginning at the fifth interspace in the right midclavicular line. Percussing downward to the end of the liver, a ***flat sound*** is heard because the liver no longer overlies the air-filled lung. ***Cardiac dullness*** is felt over the left sternal border from the second to the fifth interspace medially to the midclavicular line. Below the fifth interspace on the left side, ***tympany*** results from the air-filled stomach. Always record and report deviations from these expected sounds.

In percussing the chest, begin over the anterior lung from apex to base, usually with the child supine or sitting. Percuss each side of the chest in sequence in order to compare the sounds, such as the dullness of the liver on the right side with the tympany of the stomach on the left side. When percussing the posterior lung use the same procedure and sequence, although the child should be sitting. Normally only resonance is heard when percussing the posterior thorax from the shoulder to the eighth or tenth rib. At the base of the lungs dullness is heard as the diaphragm is percussed.

Auscultation

Auscultation involves using the stethoscope to evaluate breath and voice sounds. Use both the open bell and the closed diaphragm. The ***open-bell,*** or ***Ford, chestpiece*** conducts sounds with virtually no distortion of pitch and is better for the perception of certain low-pitched sounds. However, it must be placed firmly against the body surface for an airtight seal. Normally the diameter of the bell does not exceed 2.5 cm (1 inch) to achieve a seal that prevents environmental noise from entering. This restriction in size limits the volume of sound heard.

The larger, flatter, and less bulky ***closed-diaphragm,*** or ***Bowles, chestpiece*** is sealed by its own diaphragm. The larger diaphragm admits a greater quantity of sound and is more sensitive to high-pitched sounds. The diaphragm filters out low-frequency vibrations, so that sounds appear to be of higher pitch than when heard through the bell. The self-sealing diaphragm can be placed on a bony or small chest, although a close-fitting seal is still recommended in order to decrease the admittance of environmental sounds. In infants and small children, especially premature infants, use a specially sized pediatric diaphragm to achieve sufficient skin contact and to localize sounds in segmented areas of

GUIDELINES
Effective Auscultation

Make sure child is relaxed and not crying, talking, or laughing. Record if child is crying.
Check that room is comfortable and quiet.
Warm stethoscope before placing it against skin.
Apply firm pressure on chestpiece but not enough to prevent vibrations and transmission of sound.
Avoid placing stethoscope over hair or clothing, moving it against skin, breathing on tubing, or sliding fingers over chestpiece, which may cause sounds that falsely resemble pathologic findings.
Use a symmetric and orderly approach to compare sounds.

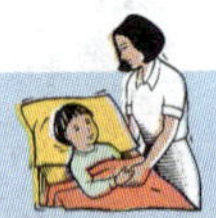

ATRAUMATIC CARE
Encouraging Deep Breaths

Ask child to "blow out" the light on an otoscope or pocket flashlight; discreetly turn off the light on the last try so that the child feels successful (Fig. 7-37).
Place a cotton ball in child's palm; ask child to blow the ball into the air and have parent catch it.
Place a small tissue on the top of a pencil and ask child to blow the tissue off.
Have child blow a pinwheel, a party horn, or bubbles.

CLASSIFICATION OF NORMAL BREATH SOUNDS

VESICULAR BREATH SOUNDS

Heard over entire surface of lungs, with exception of upper intrascapular area and area beneath manubrium.
Inspiration is louder, longer, and higher pitched than expiration.
Sound is soft, swishing noise.

BRONCHOVESICULAR BREATH SOUNDS

Heard over manubrium and in upper intrascapular regions where trachea and bronchi bifurcate.
Inspiration is louder and higher in pitch than in vesicular breathing.

BRONCHIAL BREATH SOUNDS

Heard only over trachea near suprasternal notch.
Inspiratory phase is short, and expiratory phase is long.

the chest. Listen for breath sounds as the child inspires deeply (see Guidelines and Atraumatic Care boxes).

In the lungs breath sounds are classified as vesicular, bronchovesicular, or bronchial (see box above). ***Absent*** or ***diminished breath sounds*** are always an abnormal finding warranting investigation. Fluid, air, or solid masses in the pleural space all interfere with the conduction of breath sounds,

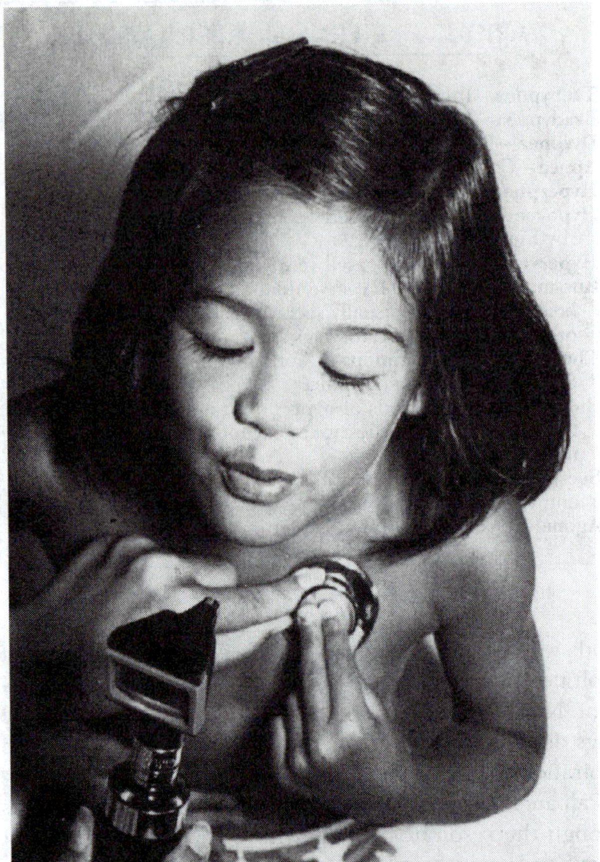

FIG. 7-37 Auscultating lungs while child "blows out" otoscope light.

although in young children breath sounds are easily transmitted through the thin chest wall, so that unilateral breath sounds may not be heard. Diminished breath sounds in certain segments of the lung suggest pulmonary areas that may benefit from postural drainage and percussion. Increased breath sounds following pulmonary therapy indicate improved passage of air through the respiratory tract.

Voice sounds are also part of auscultation of the lung. Normally vocal resonance or voice sounds are heard, but the syllables are indistinct. Elicit them in the same manner as for vocal fremitus, except listen with the stethoscope. Consolidation of lung tissue produces three types of abnormal voice sounds: (1) ***whispered pectoriloquy*** (words are whispered, and syllables are heard; (2) ***bronchophony*** (spoken words are not distinguishable, but the vocal resonance is increased in intensity and clarity); and (3) ***egophony*** ("ee" is heard as the nasal sound "ay" through the stethoscope). Decreased or absent vocal resonance is caused by the same conditions that affect vocal fremitus.

Various pulmonary abnormalities produce ***adventitious sounds*** that are not normally heard over the chest. They are not alterations of normal breath sounds but additional abnormal sounds (Table 7-13). Considerable practice with an experienced tutor is necessary to differentiate the various

TABLE 7-13 Description of Abnormal Lung Sounds

TERM	CHARACTERISTICS	SIMILAR SOUND	CAUSE
Coarse crackle	Discontinuous, interrupted explosive sounds Loud, low in pitch	Agitating a container of moderately heated salt	Air passing through larger airways containing fluid
Fine crackle	Discontinuous, interrupted explosive sounds Less loud than above and of shorter duration; higher in pitch than coarse crackles	Strands of hair rolled between fingers; separating self-adhering fasteners	Air passing through smaller airways containing fluid
Wheeze	Continuous sounds High-pitched; a hissing sound	Two marble plates coated with oil are suddenly separated	Airway narrowed by asthma or partially obstructed by tumor or foreign body
Rhonchus	Continuous sounds Low-pitched; a snoring sound	Cooing of a wood pigeon, croaking of a frog, or snoring	Large upper airway partially obstructed by thick secretions

Data from Ward J: Lung sounds: easy to hear, hard to describe, *Respir Care* 34(1):763-770, 1989; and Murphy R, Holford S: Lung sounds, *Respir Care* 25(7):763-770, 1980.

types of adventitious sounds.* Often it is best to describe the type of sound heard in the lungs rather than trying to label it correctly.

The other important adventitious sound is the pleural friction rub, discussed on p. 259. Its sound can be simulated by cupping one hand to the ear and rubbing a finger of the other hand across the cupped hand. The most common site for a friction rub to be heard is the lower anterolateral chest wall (between the midaxillary and midclavicular lines), the area of greatest thoracic mobility.

HEART

Knowledge of the anatomy and physiology of the normal heart is essential in order to properly evaluate the findings. In addition to the discussion below, the normal circulation of the blood through the heart chambers, major blood vessels, and valves is discussed in Chapter 34.

The heart is situated in the thoracic cavity between the lungs in the mediastinum and above the diaphragm (Fig. 7-38). About two thirds of the heart lies within the left side of the rib cage, with the other third on the right side as it crosses the sternum. Most of the anterior cardiac surface is occupied by the right ventricle. Part of the right atrium and left ventricle also faces anteriorly, whereas the left atrium lies primarily in a posterior position.

The heart is positioned in the thorax like a trapezoid:

Vertically along the right sternal border (RSB) from the second to the fifth rib

Horizontally (long side) from the lower right sternum to the fifth rib at the left midclavicular line (LMCL)

Diagonally from the left sternal border (LSB) at the second rib to the LMCL at the fifth rib

Horizontally (short side) from the RSB and LSB at the second intercostal space (ICS)—base of the heart

*A suggested resource for becoming familiar with normal and abnormal lung sounds is *Lung Sounds: A Practical Guide* (book and audiotape) by R. Wilkins, J. Hodgkin, and B. Lopez (1988, Mosby).

The most important skill in examining the heart is auscultation, which is performed when the child is quiet. Inspection and palpation also yield important information. However, percussion is of little value in assessing cardiac size or function.

Inspection

When examining the chest, note any obvious bulging, especially on the left side, which may indicate cardiac enlargement. Observe the child sitting in a semi-Fowler position and look at the anterior chest wall from an angle, comparing both sides of the rib cage with each other. Normally they are symmetric. In children with thin chest walls, a pulsation may be visible.

Since comprehensive evaluation of cardiac function is not limited to the heart, also consider other findings, such as the presence of all pulses (especially the femoral pulses) (Fig. 7-39), distended neck veins, clubbing of the fingers, peripheral cyanosis, edema, blood pressure, and respiratory status.

Palpation

Use palpation to determine the location of the ***apical impulse (AI)***, the most lateral cardiac impulse that may correspond to the apex. The AI is found:

- Just lateral to the left MCL and fourth ICS in children < 7 years of age
- At the left MCL and fifth ICS in children > 7 years of age

Although the AI gives a general idea of the size of the heart (with enlargement, the apex is lower and more lateral), its normal location is quite variable, making it a rather unreliable indicator of heart size (O'Neill and others, 1989).

The ***point of maximum intensity (PMI)***, as the name implies, is the area of most intense pulsation. Usually, the PMI is located at the same site as the AI, but it can occur elsewhere. For this reason, the two terms should not be used synonymously.

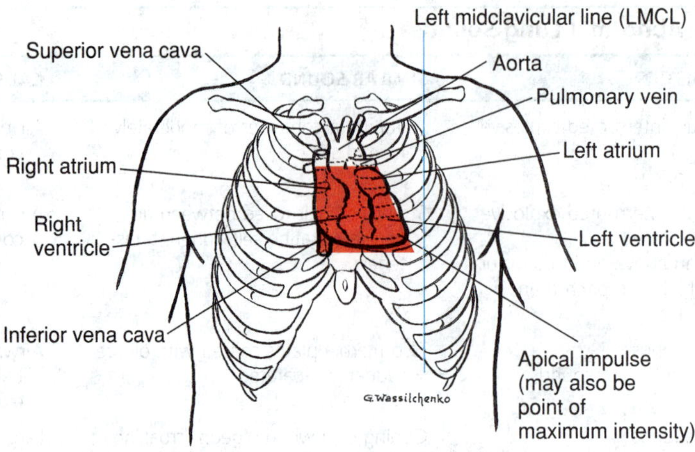

FIG. 7-38 Position of heart within thorax.

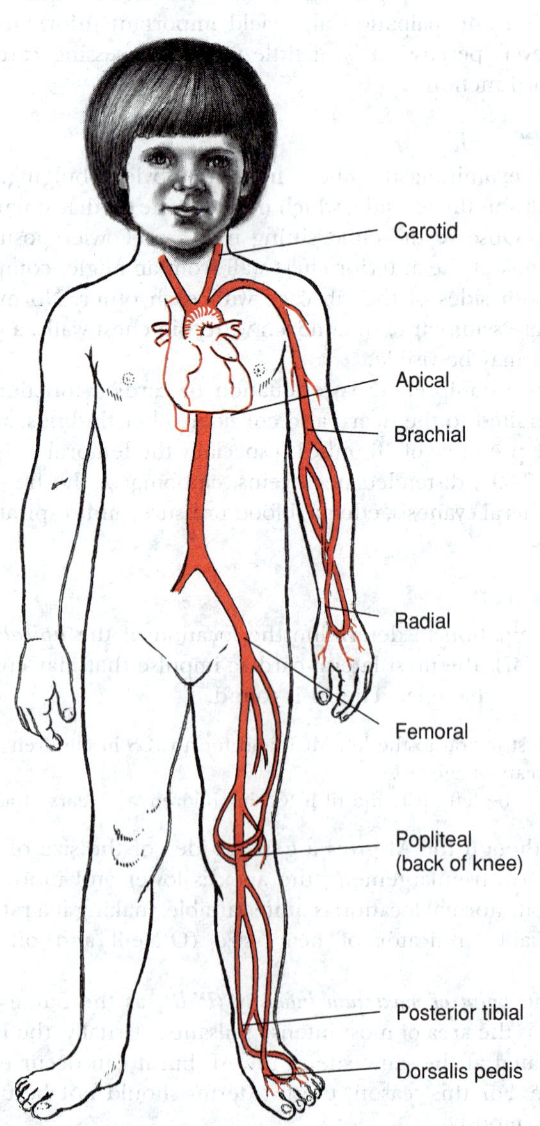

FIG. 7-39 Location of pulses.

Thrills are palpable vibrations most commonly produced by the flow of blood from one chamber of the heart to another through a narrowed or abnormal opening, such as a stenotic valve or a septal defect. They are best felt with the ball of the hand (palmar surface at the base of the fingers) and during expiration. Thrills feel similar to the placing of one's hand on a purring cat.

Pericardial friction rubs are scratchy, high-pitched grating sounds, similar to pleural friction rubs, except that they are not affected by changes in respiration. This is a useful clue in differentiating the two rubs, because the pleural rub will cease if the child holds the breath, but the pericardial rub will not. Both thrills and rubs are abnormal; report them for further evaluation.

During palpation assess ***capillary filling time***—an important test for peripheral circulation. Press the skin lightly on a central site, such as the forehead, or a peripheral site, such as the top of the hand, to produce a slight blanching. The time it takes for the blanched area to return to its original color is the capillary refill time.

NURSING ALERT Capillary refill should be brisk—in less than 2 seconds; prolonged refill is associated with poor systemic perfusion.

Auscultation

Origin of Heart Sounds. The heart sounds are produced by the opening and closing of the valves and the vibration of blood against the walls of the heart and vessels. Normally two sounds—S_1 and S_2—are heard, which correspond respectively to the familiar "lub dub" often used to describe the sounds. ***S_1*** is caused by closure of the ***tricuspid*** and ***mitral valves*** (sometimes called the ***atrioventricular valves***). ***S_2*** is the result of closure of the ***pulmonic*** and ***aortic valves*** (sometimes called ***semilunar valves***). Normally the split of the two sounds in S_2 is distinguishable and widens during inspiration. ***Physiologic splitting*** is a significant normal finding.

NURSING ALERT "Fixed splitting," in which the split in S_2 does not change during inspiration, is an important diagnostic sign of atrial septal defect.

Two other heart sounds—S_3 and S_4—may be produced. ***S_3*** is the result of vibrations produced during ventricular filling. It is normally heard in some children and young adults, but it is considered abnormal in older individuals. ***S_4*** is caused by the recoil of vibrations between the atria and ventricles following atrial contraction at the end of diastole. It is rarely heard as a normal heart sound and indicates the need for further cardiac evaluation.

Another important category of heart sounds is ***murmurs,*** which are produced by vibrations within the heart chambers or in the major arteries from the back-and-forth flow of blood (see Assessment of Cardiac Function, Chapter 34, for a more detailed discussion). Murmurs are classified as:

Innocent—No anatomic or physiologic abnormality exists.
Functional—No anatomic cardiac defect exists but a physiologic abnormality such as anemia is present.
Organic—A cardiac defect with or without a physiologic abnormality exists.

The description and classification of murmurs are skills that require considerable practice and training. In general, recognize murmurs as distinct swishing sounds that occur in addition to the normal heart sounds and record the (1) ***location*** of the area of the heart where the murmur is heard best; (2) ***time*** of the occurrence of the murmur within the S_1S_2 cycle; (3) ***intensity*** (evaluation in relationship to the child's position); and (4) ***loudness.*** The usual subjective method of grading the loudness or intensity of a murmur is listed in Table 7-14. Characteristics of innocent murmurs as opposed to organic murmurs are described in the box above right.

Other abnormal sounds, such as ejection clicks, snaps, gallops, and hums, are beyond the scope of this discussion. The best approach is to become familiar with normal heart sounds and to refer any questionable heart sound for further evaluation.*

Differentiating Normal Heart Sounds. Fig. 7-40 illustrates the approximate anatomic position of the valves within the heart chambers. Note that the anatomic location of the valves does not correspond to the area where the sounds are heard best. The auscultatory sites are located in the direction of the blood flow through the valves.

Normally S_1 is louder at the apex of the heart in the mitral and tricuspid area, and S_2 is louder near the base of the heart in the pulmonic and aortic area. Listen to each sound by inching down the chest (Table 7-15). Also auscultate the following areas for sounds, such as murmurs, which may radiate to these sites: the sternoclavicular area above the clavicles and manubrium, the area along the sternal border, the area along the left midaxillary line, and the area below the scapulae.

*A suggested resource for becoming familiar with normal and abnormal heart sounds is *Heart Sounds and Murmurs: A Practical Guide* (book and audiotape) by B.B. Erickson (1991, Mosby).

CHARACTERISTICS OF INNOCENT MURMURS

Systolic (occur with or after S_1)
Short duration and have no transmission to other areas of the heart
Grade III or less in intensity and do not increase over time
Loudest in the pulmonic area (second or third intercostal space along the left sternal border)
Variable in relationship to position, respiration, and activity (e.g., audible in the supine position but absent in the sitting position; may be louder with exercise, fever, anxiety, or anemia)
Not associated with any physical signs of cardiac disease
Low-pitched, musical, or groaning quality

TABLE 7-14 Grading of the Intensity of Heart Murmurs

GRADE	DESCRIPTION
I	Very faint; frequently not heard if child sits up
II	Usually readily heard; slightly louder than grade I; audible in all positions
III	Loud, but not accompanied by a thrill
IV	Loud, accompanied by a thrill
V	Loud enough to be heard with the stethoscope barely on the chest; accompanied by a thrill
VI	Loud enough to be heard with the stethoscope not touching the chest; often heard with the human ear close to the chest; accompanied by a thrill

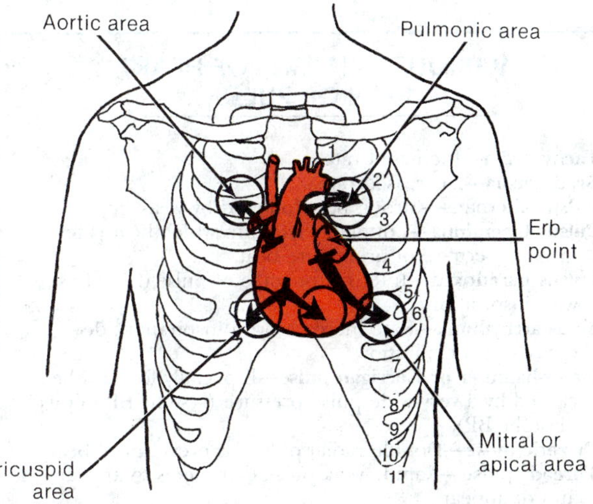

FIG. 7-40 Direction of heart sounds from anatomic valve sites and areas (circled) for auscultation.

TABLE 7-15 Sequence of Auscultating Heart Sounds*

AUSCULTATORY SITE	CHEST LOCATION	CHARACTERISTICS OF HEART SOUNDS
Aortic area	Second right intercostal space close to sternum	S_2 heard louder than S_1; aortic closure heard loudest
Pulmonic area	Second left intercostal space close to sternum	Splitting of S_2 heard best, normally widens on inspiration; pulmonic closure heard best
Erb point	Second and third left intercostal space close to sternum	Frequent site of innocent murmurs and those of aortic or pulmonic origin
Tricuspid area	Fifth right and left intercostal space close to sternum	S_1 heard as louder sound preceding S_2 (S_1 synchronous with carotid pulse)
Mitral or apical area	Fifth intercostal space, left midclavicular line (third to fourth intercostal space and lateral to left midclavicular line in infants)	S_1 heard loudest; splitting of S_1 may be audible because mitral closure is louder than tricuspid closure S_3 heard best at beginning of expiration with child in recumbent or left side-lying position, occurs immediately after S_2, sounds like word S_1 S_2 S_3 "Ken-tuc-ky" S_4 heard best during expiration with child in recumbent position (left side-lying position decreases sound), occurs immediately before S_1, sounds like word S_4 S_1 S_2 "Ten-nes-see"

*Use both diaphragm and bell chestpieces when auscultating heart sounds. Bell chestpiece is necessary for low-pitched sounds of murmurs, S_3, and S_4.

➤ **NURSING TIP** To distinguish between S_1 or S_2 heart sounds, simultaneously palpate the carotid pulse with the index and middle finger and listen to the heart sounds; S_1 is synchronous with the carotid pulse.

Auscultate the heart with the child in at least two positions: sitting and reclining. If adventitious sounds are detected, further evaluate them with the child standing, sitting and leaning forward, and lying on the left side. For example, atrial sounds such as S_4 are heard best with the person in a recumbent position and usually fade if the person sits or stands.

Evaluate for heart sounds (1) ***quality*** (should be clear and distinct, not muffled, diffuse, or distant); (2) ***intensity,*** especially in relation to the location or auscultatory site (should not be weak or pounding); (3) ***rate*** (should be the same as the radial pulse); and (4) ***rhythm*** (should be regular and even). A particular arrhythmia that occurs normally in many children is ***sinus arrhythmia,*** in which the heart rate increases with inspiration and decreases with expiration. Differentiate this rhythm from a truly abnormal arrhythmia by having children hold their breath. In sinus arrhythmia, cessation of breathing causes the heart rate to remain steady. Variations in patterns of heart rate or pulse are listed in the box at left. As with respiratory rate, always evaluate heart rate in relation to general physical status. For example, the pulse rate is usually increased by 8 to 10 beats per minute for each degree Fahrenheit elevation in temperature. Athletic children occasionally have lower heart rates that represent a highly developed and efficient heart muscle (see inside back cover for normal heart rates at various ages).

VARIOUS PATTERNS OF HEART RATE OR PULSE

Tachycardia—Increased rate
Bradycardia—Decreased rate
Pulsus alternans—Strong beat followed by weak beat
Pulsus bigeminus—Coupled rhythm in which beat is felt in pairs because of premature beat
Pulsus paradoxus—Intensity or force of pulse decreases with inspiration
Sinus arrhythmia—Rate increases with inspiration, decreases with expiration
Water-hammer or Corrigan pulse—Especially forceful beat caused by a very wide pulse pressure (systolic BP minus diastolic BP)
Dicrotic pulse—Double radial pulse for every apical beat
Thready pulse—Rapid, weak pulse that seems to appear and disappear

ABDOMEN

Examination of the abdomen involves the usual four skills, except that the order is altered. Start with inspection and then follow with auscultation, percussion, and palpation last because these maneuvers may distort the normal abdominal sounds. The sequence of examination changes according to the age and cooperativeness of the child. Frequently all four types of assessment are performed at different times. For example, auscultate for bowel sounds following evaluation of heart and lung sounds at the beginning of the examination when the child is quiet. Use inspection at any time during the examination. Percuss after lung percussion, and palpate toward the end of the examination when the child is relaxed and more trusting.

Knowledge of the anatomic placement of the abdominal organs is essential to differentiate normal, expected findings from abnormal ones (Fig. 7-41). The ***abdominal cavity*** is the portion of the trunk from directly beneath the dia-

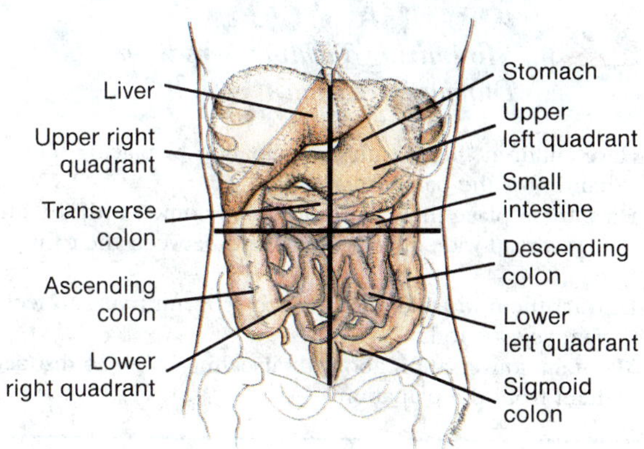

FIG. 7-41 Location of structures in abdomen. Cross rules divide cavity into quadrants. (From Potter PA, Perry AG: *Basic nursing: theory and practice*, ed 2, St Louis, 1991, Mosby.)

phragm and thoracic cavity to the region of the pelvic cavity. For descriptive purposes the abdominal cavity is divided into four quadrants by drawing a vertical line midway from the sternum to the pubic symphysis and a horizontal line across the abdomen through the umbilicus (Fig. 7-41). This method of division actually includes the pelvic cavity. Each section is designated as follows:

- Right upper quadrant (RUQ)
- Right lower quadrant (RLQ)
- Left upper quadrant (LUQ)
- Left lower quadrant (LLQ)

The abdominal cavity contains the major organs of digestion, and the pelvic cavity houses the internal reproductive organs, the lower parts of the digestive tract, and the urinary bladder. However, in infancy the bladder is an abdominal organ.

Inspection

Inspect the ***contour*** of the abdomen while the child is erect and supine. Normally the abdomen of infants and young children is quite cylindric and, in the erect position, fairly prominent because of the physiologic lordosis of the spine. In the supine position the abdomen appears flat. During adolescence the usual male and female contours of the pelvic cavity change the shape of the abdomen to form characteristic adult curves, especially in the female.

The ***size*** and ***tone*** of the abdomen also give some indication of general nutritional status and muscular development. A large, prominent, flabby abdomen is often seen in obese children, whereas a concave abdomen suggests undernutrition. However, carefully note a protruding abdomen, which may indicate pathologic states such as abdominal distention, ascites, tumors, or organomegaly. A protuberant abdomen with spindly extremities and flat, wasted buttocks suggests severe malnutrition that may occur from inadequate protein-energy intake or from diseases such as cystic fibrosis. A midline protrusion from the xiphoid to the umbilicus or pubic symphysis is usually ***diastasis recti,*** or failure of the rectus abdominis muscles to join in utero. In a healthy child a midline protrusion is usually a variation of normal muscular development.

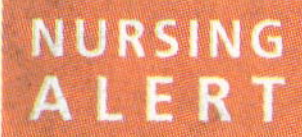

A tense, boardlike abdomen is a serious sign of paralytic ileus and intestinal obstruction.

The ***skin*** covering the abdomen should be uniformly taut, without wrinkles or creases. Sometimes silvery, whitish striae are seen, especially if the skin has been stretched as in obesity or with distention resulting from ascites. Note any scars, ecchymotic areas, excessive hair distribution, or distended veins. Superficial veins may be visible in thin, light-skinned children, but distended veins are an abnormal finding, suggesting vascular or abdominal obstruction or abdominal distention.

Observe ***movement*** of the abdomen. In infants and thin children ***peristaltic waves*** may be visible through the abdominal wall. They are best observed by standing at eye level to and across from the abdomen. Always report this finding, because visible peristaltic waves most often indicate pathologic states, particularly intestinal obstruction such as pyloric stenosis. Abdominal movement in relation to respiration is discussed on p. 266.

Inspect the ***umbilicus*** for herniation, discharge, hygiene, and fistulas, such as a patent ***urachus*** (an abnormal connection between the umbilicus and bladder). If a herniation is present, palpate the sac for abdominal contents and estimate the approximate size of the opening. ***Umbilical hernias*** are common in infants, especially in black children. Since "home remedies" for treatment such as taping coins over the umbilicus or using "belly binders" may be harmful to the skin and actually delay natural closure, ask parents whether such procedures have been used and advise against continuing them. Umbilical hernias normally protrude and expand when the child coughs, cries, or strains.

Hernias may exist elsewhere on the abdominal wall, such as in the inguinal or femoral region (Fig. 7-42). An ***inguinal hernia*** is a protrusion of peritoneum through the abdominal wall in the inguinal canal. It occurs mostly in males, is frequently bilateral, and may be visible as a mass in the scrotum. To locate a hernia, slide the little finger into the external inguinal ring at the base of the scrotum and ask the child to cough. If a hernia is present, it will hit the tip of the finger.

➤ **NURSING TIP** If the child is too young to cough, have the child blow up a balloon or laugh to raise the intraabdominal pressure sufficiently to demonstrate the presence of an inguinal hernia.

A ***femoral hernia,*** which occurs more frequently in girls, is felt or seen as a small mass on the anterior surface of the thigh just below the inguinal ligament in the femoral canal (a potential space medial to the femoral artery). Feel for a hernia by placing the index finger of your right hand on the child's right femoral pulse (left hand for left pulse) and the middle ring finger flat against the skin toward the midline. The ring finger lies over the femoral canal, where the herniation occurs. Palpation of hernias in the pelvic region,

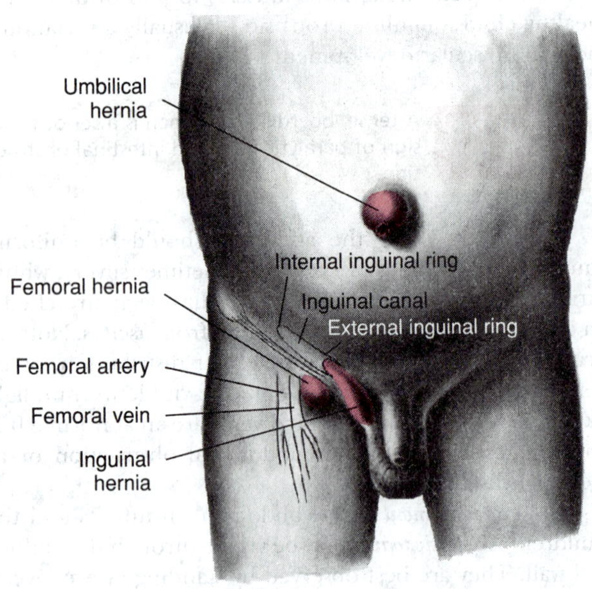

FIG. 7-42 Location of hernias.

particularly inguinal ones, is often part of the examination of genitalia.

Auscultation

Auscultate each of the four quadrants using the diaphragm and bell chestpieces. Unlike listening to the heart or lungs, in which the stethoscope rests gently on the skin, to hear bowel sounds the stethoscope must be pressed firmly against the abdominal surface. With the diaphragm chestpiece this usually presents no difficulty, but with the bell chestpiece, especially one with a short cone, the skin may occlude the opening and prevent transmission of sound.

The most important sound to listen for is ***peristalsis,*** or ***bowel sounds,*** which sound like short metallic clicks and gurgles. Loud grumbling noises, known as ***borborygmi,*** are the familiar "stomach growls," usually denoting hunger. Depending on when the child last ate, a sound may be heard every 10 to 30 seconds; record its frequency per minute. Bowel sounds may be stimulated by stroking the abdominal surface with a fingernail. Always report absence of bowel sounds or hyperperistalsis, since either usually denotes an abdominal disorder.

Various other sounds may be heard in the abdominal cavity. Normally the pulsation of the aorta is heard in the epigastrium. Always refer sounds that resemble murmurs (called ***bruits***), hums, or rubs for further evaluation.

Percussion

Percuss the abdomen in the same manner as in percussion of the lungs (see Fig. 7-36). Normally dullness or flatness is heard on the right side at the lower costal margin because of the location of the liver. Tympany is typically heard over the stomach on the left side and in the rest of the abdomen. An unusually tympanitic sound, like the beating of a tight drum, denotes air in the stomach, which is commonly caused by mouth breathing. However, it can also indicate a pathologic condition such as low intestinal obstruction or paralytic ileus. Lack of tympany may occur normally when the stomach is full after a meal, but in other situations it may signal the presence of fluid or solid masses. Refer variation in percussion tones not explained by normal physiologic processes for further investigation.

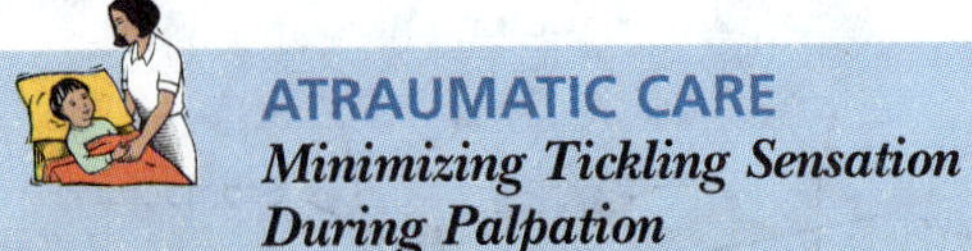

ATRAUMATIC CARE
Minimizing Tickling Sensation During Palpation

Have children "help" with the palpation by placing their hand over the palpating hand.
Have them place their hand on the abdomen with the fingers spread wide apart and palpate between their fingers.
Distract them with statements such as "I am trying to feel what you ate today."
Maintain conversation about their eating habits to distract them from the palpation.

Palpation

Two types of palpation are performed: superficial and deep. For ***superficial palpation*** place the hand lightly against the skin and feel each quadrant, noting any areas of tenderness, muscle tone, and superficial lesions, such as cysts. Also test skin turgor, discussed on p. 234.

Since superficial palpation is often perceived as tickling, use techniques to minimize this sensation (see Atraumatic Care box.) Admonishing the child to stop laughing only draws attention to the sensation and decreases cooperation. Position the child supine with the legs flexed at the hips and knees to relax the abdominal muscles.

Always note tenderness or pain anywhere in the abdomen during superficial palpation. There are two types of abdominal pain:

Visceral, which arises from the viscera or internal organs, such as the intestines, and is usually dull, poorly localized, and difficult for the patient to describe
Somatic, which arises from the walls or linings of the abdominal cavity such as the peritoneum, and is generally sharp, well localized, and more easily described

When assessing abdominal pain, remember that children often respond with an "all-or-none" reaction—either there is no pain or there is great pain. Using a pain measurement scale helps children more specifically rate pain intensity and to distinguish pain from fear (see Pain Assessment, Chapter 26). One approach is to ask children "how thin" and "how fat" they can make themselves. If this produces discomfort, then some degree of peritoneal irritation is probably present.

➤ **NURSING TIP** When a child complains of abdominal pain, observe whether the child's eyes are opened or closed during palpation of the abdomen. The natural reaction of patients with genuine abdominal tenderness is to watch the

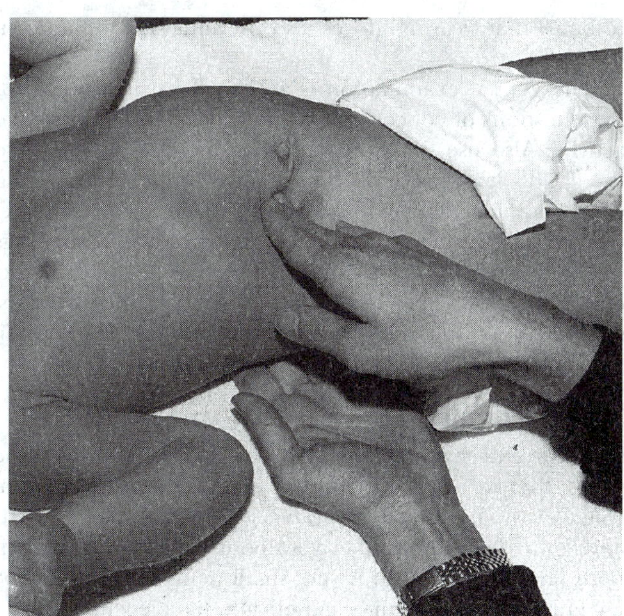

FIG. 7-43 Deep palpation of abdominal organs.

palpating hand carefully to avoid unnecessary pain—the opened eyes sign (Gray, Dixon, and Collin, 1988).

Elicit ***rebound tenderness,*** or ***Blumberg sign,*** if the child complains of abdominal pain. Press firmly over part of the abdomen distal to the area of tenderness and release the pressure suddenly. Rebound tenderness is present if the child feels pain in the original area of tenderness. This response is found only when the peritoneum overlying a diseased organ is inflamed, such as in appendicitis.

Use ***deep palpation*** for palpating organs and large blood vessels and for detecting masses and tenderness not discovered during superficial palpation. If the child complains of abdominal pain, palpate that area of the abdomen *last.* Normally palpation of the midepigastrium causes pain as pressure is exerted over the aorta, but this should not be confused with visceral or somatic tenderness.

Palpate the abdominal organs by pressing them against your free hand, which is placed on the child's back (Fig. 7-43). Begin palpation in the lower quadrants and proceed upward to avoid missing the edge of an enlarged liver or spleen. Except for palpating the liver, successful identification of other organs, such as the spleen, kidney, and part of the colon, requires considerable practice with tutored supervision.

The lower edge of the ***liver*** is sometimes palpable in infants and young children as a superficial mass 1 to 2 cm (⅜ to ¾ inch) below the right costal margin (the distance is sometimes measured in fingerbreadths). Normally the liver descends during inspiration as the diaphragm moves downward. This downward displacement should not be mistaken for a sign of hepatomegaly. In older children the liver frequently is not palpable.

Palpate the ***spleen*** by feeling it between the hand placed against the back and the one palpating the left upper quadrant. The spleen is much smaller than the liver and is positioned behind the fundus of the stomach. The tip of the spleen may be felt during inspiration as it descends within the abdominal cavity. It is sometimes palpable 1 to 2 cm below the left costal margin in infants and young children.

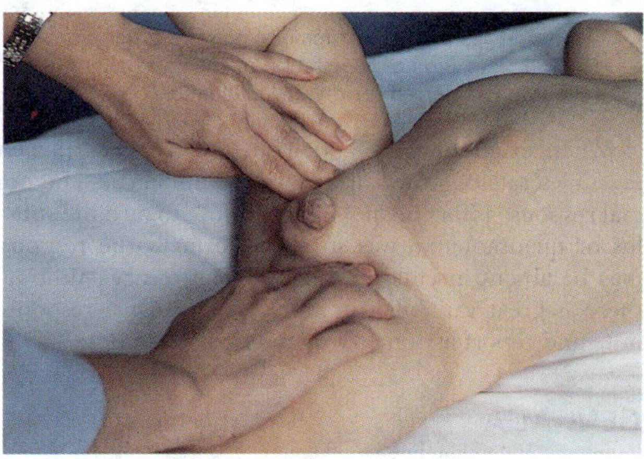

FIG. 7-44 Palpating for femoral pulses.

NURSING ALERT If the liver is palpable 3 cm below the right costal margin or the spleen is palpable more than 2 cm below the left costal margin, these organs are enlarged—a finding that is always reported for further medical investigation.

Other anatomic structures that are sometimes palpable in children include the kidney, bladder, cecum, and sigmoid colon. Palpation of the ***kidney,*** which is discussed in Chapter 8 under assessment of the neonate, is quite difficult because of its deep position within the abdominal cavity. Normally only the tip of the right kidney is palpable because of its lower placement within the cavity, and it is best felt during inspiration. The ***bladder*** may be palpated slightly above the pubic symphysis in infants and young children. It descends deeper into the pelvic cavity during adolescence, when it is not palpable except if distended. Occasionally parts of the colon are palpable. The ***cecum*** is a soft, gas-filled mass in the right lower quadrant. The ***sigmoid colon*** is felt as a sausage-shaped mass that is freely movable over the pelvic brim in the left lower quadrant and is normally tender.

Although most of these structures are not routinely felt, be aware of their relative location and characteristics to avoid mistaking them for abnormal masses that require additional investigation. The most common palpable mass in children is feces, which may be associated with pain in the right lower quadrant from a distended cecum. In sexually active pubescent females a palpable mass in the lower abdomen may be a pregnant uterus.

During palpation of the abdomen locate the ***femoral pulses*** by placing the tips of two or three fingers (index, middle, and/or ring) along the inguinal ligament about midway between the iliac crest and pubic symphysis. Feel both pulses simultaneously to make certain that they are equal and strong (Fig. 7-44).

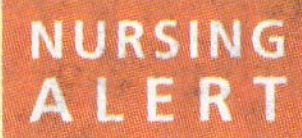

NURSING ALERT Absence of femoral pulses is a significant sign of coarctation of the aorta and is referred for medical evaluation.

When examining the abdomen, test the ***abdominal reflexes*** by scratching the skin toward the umbilicus. The normal response is for the umbilicus to move toward the stimulus or quadrant that was stroked. Normally the response may be absent in children under 1 year of age. Although there is great variability in correctly eliciting a response, note and report asymmetry or absence of response.

GENITALIA

Examination of genitalia conveniently follows assessment of the abdomen while the child is still supine. In adolescents, inspection of the genitalia may be left to the end of the examination. This part of the physical appraisal is usually uneventful for infants or toddlers but begins to be anxiety-producing for older preschoolers, school-age children, and adolescents, mainly because of their concern for modesty and privacy (see Atraumatic Care box).

In examining the genitalia, wear gloves whenever touching body substances. It might be helpful for the adolescent to know that wearing gloves also prevents skin-to-skin contact.

The genital examination is an excellent time for eliciting questions of concern about body functioning or sexual activity. Also use this opportunity to increase or reinforce the child's knowledge of reproductive anatomy by naming each body part and explaining its function. For example, many females are unaware of the existence of two openings within the vulva. They assume that the passage of urine occurs from the vagina. For males, this part of the health assessment is an opportune time to teach self-testicular examination.

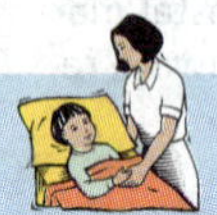

ATRAUMATIC CARE
Examination of Genitalia

Offer older children and adolescents the choice of whether or not they wish to be accomplished by a family member. Whenever possible, the sex of the examiner should also be an option for the teenager. Studies show that some young people feel more comfortable with an examiner of the same sex, although males and females report feeling comfortable with a female examiner (Neinstein and others, 1989; Seymore and others, 1986). For females, the semisitting position is less stressful than the supine position for the pelvic examination (Seymore and others, 1986).

Examine the genitalia matter-of-factly, placing no more emphasis on this part of the assessment than on any other segment. Explain each step of the examination before it is performed, such as checking the scrotum for an inguinal hernia. If male adolescents have an erection during the examination, reassure them that this is a normal involuntary reflex to touch, not a sexual response, and complete the rest of the examination (Church and Baer, 1987). It helps to relieve children's and parents' anxiety by stating the findings (e.g., "Everything looks fine here").

If it is necessary to ask questions about deviations, such as about discharge or difficulty in urinating, respect the child's privacy by covering the lower abdomen with the gown or underpants. To prevent embarrassing interruptions, keep the door or curtain closed and post a "do not disturb" sign. Have a drape ready to cover the genitalia if someone enters the room.

One of the most important factors in successfully performing an atraumatic examination is to recognize any personal fears or anxieties and deal with them. Transfer of anxiety, especially in the beginning practitioner, can increase the child's concern or fear.

Male Genitalia

Note the external appearance of the glans and shaft of the penis, the prepuce, the urethral meatus, and the scrotum (Fig. 7-45). The size of the ***penis*** is generally small in infants and young boys until puberty, when it begins to increase in both length and width. A very small penis may actually be an enlarged clitoris in a genetically female child. In an obese child the penis often looks abnormally small because of the folds of skin partially covering it at the base. An enlarged penis in a young child may denote precocious puberty. Be familiar with normal pubertal growth of the external male genitalia in order to compare the findings with the expected sequence of maturation (see Fig. 19-6).

Examine the ***glans*** (head of the penis) and ***shaft*** (portion between the perineum and prepuce) for signs of swelling, skin lesions, inflammation, or other irregularities. Any of these signs may indicate underlying disorders, especially sexually transmitted diseases. Consider the possibility of sexual abuse, especially in young children, if sexually transmitted disease is present.

If the child is uncircumcised, inspect the ***prepuce*** or ***foreskin*** covering the glans. In infants the prepuce is normally tight and is not retracted for examination, since accidental tearing of the thin membrane may cause scarring and adhesion formation later on. In children *gently* retract the foreskin to examine the glans and the meatus and then replace it. A tight foreskin that cannot be retracted in older boys is called ***phimosis.***

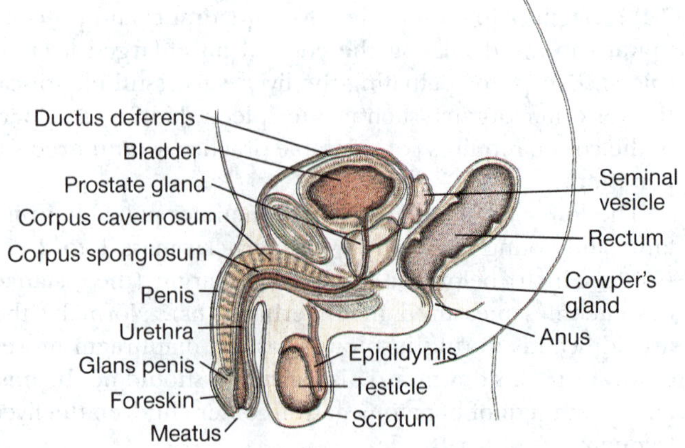

FIG. 7-45 Major structures of genitalia in uncircumcised postpubertal male. (From Potter PA, Perry AG: *Basic nursing: theory and practice*, ed 2, St Louis, 1991, Mosby.)

Carefully inspect the ***urethral meatus*** for location and evidence of discharge. Normally it is centered at the tip of the shaft. It it opens on the ventral, or underneath, side of the glans or shaft, it is called ***hypospadias.*** An opening on the dorsal, or top, part of the penis is termed ***epispadias.*** If the urethral meatus opens into the perineum at the junction of the scrotum, look for signs suggesting ambiguous genitalia. If feasible during inspection, note the strength and direction of the urinary stream during micturition.

Observe the size of the ***scrotum.*** In infants the scrota appear large in relation to the rest of the genitalia. Normally the left scrotum hangs lower than the right and both hang freely from the perineum behind the penis. Note scrota that are small or close to the perineum, or that have any midline separation, which could be enlarged labia. An abnormally large scrotal sac may indicate an inguinal hernia, a hydrocele, or inflammation of the internal reproductive structures, particularly the epididymis.

The skin of the scrotum is usually loose and highly rugated (wrinkled). During early adolescence the skin normally becomes redder and coarser. In dark-skinned children the scrota are more deeply pigmented. Report a smooth, shiny surface with pigmentation that varies markedly from the surrounding skin.

Also note ***hair distribution.*** Normally before puberty no pubic hair is present. Soft downy hair at the base of the penis is an early sign of pubertal maturation. In older adolescent males hair distribution is diamond shaped from the anus to the umbilicus.

While palpating the scrotum, feel for the testes, epididymis, spermatic cords, and, if present, inguinal hernias. The two ***testes*** are felt as small ovoid bodies, about 1.5 to 2 cm (½ to ¾ inch) long—one in each scrotal sac. They do not enlarge until puberty, when they approximately double in size. Normally the testes descend during the last trimester of uterine development, usually by the eighth month of gestation. Therefore undescended testes ***(cryptorchidism)*** is a common finding in premature infants.

Palpating for the presence of the testes requires an understanding of the normal anatomy and physiology of the coverings of the testes and scrotal sac. The scrotum and testes are surrounded by cremasteric fascia, which extends to the cremaster muscle. The muscle attaches to a point in the abdomen and extends downward along the inner surface of the thigh. The muscle or ***cremasteric reflex*** is stimulated by cold, touch, emotional excitement, or exercise. When contracted, the muscle causes the skin of the scrotum to shrink and pulls the testes higher into the pelvic cavity.

Several measures are useful in preventing the cremasteric reflex during palpation of the scrotum. First, warm the hands. Second, if the child is old enough, examine him in a tailor or "Indian" position, which stretches the muscle, preventing its contraction (Fig. 7-46, *A*). Third, block the normal pathway of ascent of the testes by placing the thumb and index finger over the upper part of the scrotal sac along the inguinal canal (Fig. 7-46, *B*). If there is any question concerning the existence of two testes, place the index and middle fingers in a scissors fashion to separate the right and left scrota. If after using these techniques the testes have not been palpated, feel along the inguinal canal and perineum to locate masses that may be undescended testes. Although undescended testes may descend at any time during childhood and are checked at each visit, report failure to palpate testes.

The ***epididymis*** is a vertical ridge of soft nodular tissue behind the testes. The ***spermatic cord*** consists of the blood vessels, nerves, lymphatic glands, and the ductus deferens of the testes. Note and report any masses, swelling, or tenderness.

Female Genitalia

The examination of female genitalia is limited to inspection and palpation of external structures. If a vaginal examination is required, an appropriate referral is made unless the nurse is qualified to perform the procedure. A convenient position for examination of the genitalia involves placing the young child supine on the examining table or in a semireclining position on the parent's lap with the feet supported on your knees as you sit facing the child. Divert the child's attention from the examination by instructing her to try to keep the soles of her feet pressed against each other. Separate the labia majora (see p. 270) with the thumb

A 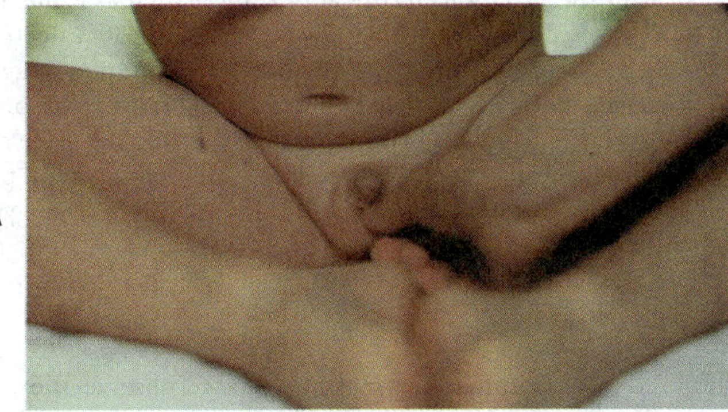

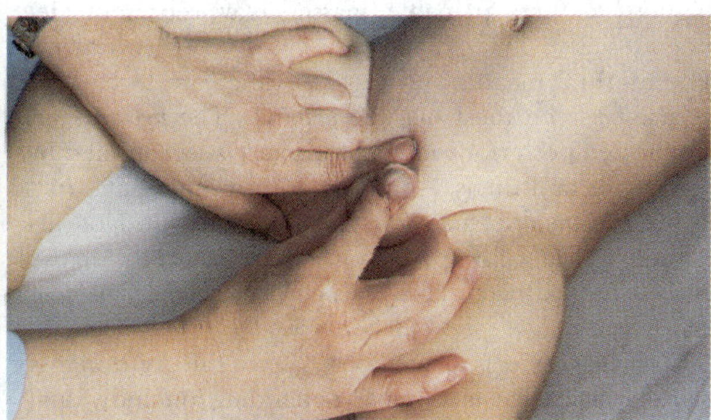 B

FIG. 7-46 **A,** Preventing cremasteric reflex by having child sit in "tailor" position. **B,** Blocking inguinal canal during palpation of scrotum for descended testes.

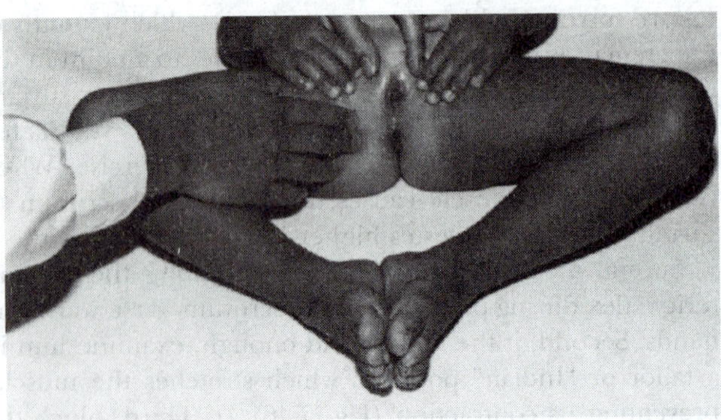

FIG. 7-47 Position for examining genitalia in female child.

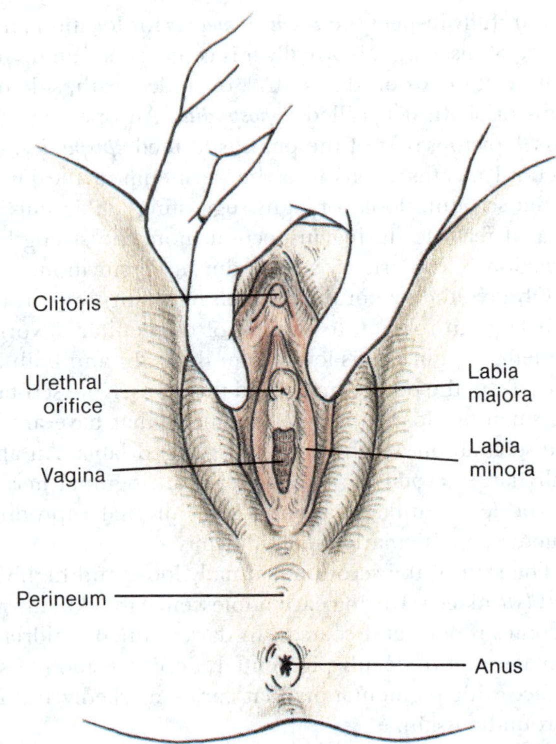

FIG. 7-48 External structures of genitalia in postpubertal female. Labia are spread to reveal deeper structures. (From Potter PA, Perry AG: *Basic nursing: theory and practice*, ed 2, St Louis, 1991, Mosby.)

and index finger to expose the labia minora, urethral meatus, and vaginal orifice. Have the child use her hands "to help" (Fig. 7-47).

Inspect the genitalia for size and location of the structures of the ***vulva*** or ***pudendum*** (area of the external genital organs) (Fig. 7-48). The ***mons pubis*** is a pad of adipose tissue over the symphysis pubis. At puberty the mons is covered with hair, which extends along the labia. The usual pattern of female ***hair distribution*** is an inverted triangle. The appearance of soft downy hair along the labia majora is an early sign of sexual maturation.

The ***clitoris,*** an erectile organ located at the anterior end of the labia minora, is covered by a small flap of skin, the ***prepuce.*** Note its size because, although variable, a large protruding clitoris may represent an underdeveloped phallus.

The ***labia majora*** are two thick folds of skin running posteriorly from the mons to the posterior commissure of the vagina. Internal to the labia majora are two folds of skin, the ***labia minora.*** Although the labia are prominent in the newborn, they gradually atrophy and are almost invisible until their enlargement during puberty.

The inner surface of the labia should be pink and moist. Note any skin lesions such as chancres, blisters, or warts (condylomata acuminata), since they may be sexually transmitted. Observe the size of the labia and any evidence of fusion, which may suggest male scrota. Normally no masses are palpable within the labia. However, in genitalia of an ambiguous nature, palpable masses may represent descended testes.

The urethral meatus and vaginal orifice are located in the space between the labia, the ***vestibule.*** The ***urethral meatus*** is located posterior to the clitoris and is surrounded by Skene glands and ducts. Although not a prominent structure, the meatus appears as a small V-shaped slit. Note its location, especially if it opens from the clitoris or inside the vagina. Gently palpate glands, which are common sites of cysts.

The ***vaginal orifice*** is located posterior to the urethral meatus. Its appearance is variable depending on individual anatomy and sexual activity. Ordinarily examination of the vagina is limited to inspection. However, in the presence of signs suggesting ambiguous genitalia, refer or perform a manual examination to determine if a vaginal vault exists.

In virgins a thin crescent-shaped or circular membrane, called the ***hymen,*** may cover part of the vaginal opening. In some instances, it completely occludes the orifice. After rupture, small rounded pieces of tissue called ***caruncles*** remain. Although an imperforate hymen denotes lack of penile intercourse, a perforate one does not necessarily indicate sexual activity (see also Sexual Abuse, Chapter 16).

Surrounding the vaginal opening are ***Bartholin glands,*** which secrete a clear, mucoid fluid into the vagina for lubrication during intercourse. Palpate the ducts for cysts and note the discharge from the vagina, which is usually clear or whitish. Variations in the appearance, such as white and cheesy or yellow-greenish, and odor may indicate infection. Sudden, foul-smelling, and profuse discharge may suggest a foreign body inside the vaginal vault. The presence of feces or urine from the vagina indicates a fistula from the rectum or urethra. Note any swelling, inflammation, or prolapsed area around the vagina and refer for further gynecologic evaluation.

ANUS

Following examination of the genitalia, observe the anal area, preferably by placing the child on the abdomen. Note the general firmness of the buttocks and symmetry of the gluteal folds. Assess the tone of the anal sphincter by eliciting the ***anal reflex.*** Scratching or gently pricking the anal area results in an obvious quick contraction of the external anal sphincter.

Inspect the sphincter area for ***fissures,*** small cuts or tears in the mucosa that are painful and often lead to constipation as the child refrains from defecating; ***prolapse*** of the rectum, which is evident as a tubelike protrusion that can be retracted manually; ***polyps,*** cherry-red protrusions that often cause bleeding; and ***hemorrhoids,*** dark protrusions of blood vessels. Report any of these findings for further medical investigation. Note any ***mucosal tabs,*** benign protrusions of skin attached to the anal sphincter.

Inspect the skin around the anal area for lesions, the most common of which are caused by diaper rash. If the child complains of perianal itching, testing for pinworms is recommended.

BACK AND EXTREMITIES

Spine

Observe the general ***curvature*** of the spine. Normally the back of a newborn is rounded or C-shaped from the thoracic and pelvic curves. The development of the cervical and lumbar curves approximates development of various motor skills, such as cervical curvature with head control, and gives the older child the typical double-S curve (see Fig. 4-5).

Marked curvatures in posture are abnormal (see Fig. 39-34). ***Scoliosis,*** lateral curvature of the spine, is an important childhood problem, especially in females. Although scoliosis may be palpated by feeling along the spine and noting a sideways displacement, more objective tests include:

1. With the child standing erect, clothed only in underpants (and bra if older girl), observe from behind, noting asymmetry of the shoulders and hips.
2. With the child bending forward so that the back is parallel to the floor, observe from the side, noting asymmetry or prominence of the rib cage.

A slight limp, a crooked hemline, or complaints of a sore back are other signs and symptoms of scoliosis.

Inspect the ***back,*** especially along the spine, for any tufts of hair, dimples, or discoloration. A small dimple (usually with a tuft of hair), called a ***pilonidal cyst,*** may indicate an underlying spina bifida occulta. Palpate the spine to identify each spiny process of the vertebrae or lack of them.

Mobility of the vertebral column is easily assessed in most children because of their propensity for constant motion during the examination. However, to specifically test mobility, ask the child to sit up from a prone position or to do a modified sit-up exercise. Maintaining a rigid straightness when performing these maneuvers is considered abnormal and may indicate central nervous system infection or irritation. However, some individuals who are unable to relax, despite normal skeletal function, may also retain a rigid posture.

Movement of the cervical spine is an important diagnostic sign for neurologic problems, such as meningitis. Normally movement of the head in all directions is effortless.

NURSING ALERT Hyperextension of the neck and spine, called *opisthotonos,* which is accompanied by pain when the head is flexed, is always referred for immediate medical evaluation.

Extremities

Inspect each extremity for symmetry of length and size; refer any deviation for orthopaedic evaluation. Count the fingers and toes to be certain of the normal number. This normalcy is so often taken for granted that an extra digit ***(polydactyly)*** or fusion of digits ***(syndactyly)*** may go unnoticed. Also inspect the fingers and toes for any evidence of clubbing, cyanosis, disorders of the nails (including habitual nail biting), and general hygiene. These are discussed in more detail under assessment of the skin (p. 233). If there is any doubt regarding symmetry of leg length, measure the legs from the anterior iliac spine (felt as the point of the pelvis) to the medial malleolus (ankle bone).

Inspect the arms and legs for ***temperature, color, tenderness,*** and ***masses.*** The temperature in each extremity should be equal, although the feet may normally be colder than the hands. Coolness denotes decreased blood circulation, such as from occlusion of a blood vessel, whereas heat indicates increased blood flow, such as an infection or inflammation. Enlargement of bone, such as from swelling, with redness, heat, and tenderness needs further evaluation. It may signify trauma, infection, or an underlying disease process (e.g., sickle cell disease). A solid mass palpable along a bone with or without pain may be a tumor. Although not all masses are malignant, they must be evaluated further.

Since accidental fractures are common in children, be familiar with assessing orthopaedic injuries. The five main criteria are (1) pain, (2) pulse, (3) paresthesia (abnormal sensation, such as numbness), (4) pallor, and (5) paralysis. Palpation over a possible fractured bone may elicit ***crepitation,*** a grafting sound produced by movement of the broken ends of the bone.

Assess the ***shape*** of bones. Several variations of bone shape may be observed in children. Although many of them cause parents concern, most are benign and require no treatment. ***Bowleg,*** or ***genu varum,*** is lateral bowing of the tibia. It is clinically present when the child stands with the medial malleoli (rounded prominence on either side of the ankle) in apposition and the space between the knees is greater than approximately 5 cm (2 inches) (Fig. 7-49). Toddlers are usually bowlegged after they begin to walk until all their lower back and leg muscles develop. Unilateral or asymmetric bowlegs that are present beyond the age of 2 to 3 years, particularly in black children, may represent pathologic conditions requiring further investigation.

Knock-knee, or ***genu valgum,*** is the opposite of bowleg; the knees are close together but the feet are spread apart. Use the same method of assessment as for genu varum but measure the distance between the malleoli, which should be less than 7.5 cm (3 inches) (Fig. 7-50). Knock-knee is normally present in children from about 2 to 7 years of age. Knock-knee that is excessive (as measured roentgenographically by the tibiofemoral angle), asymmetric, accompanied by short-

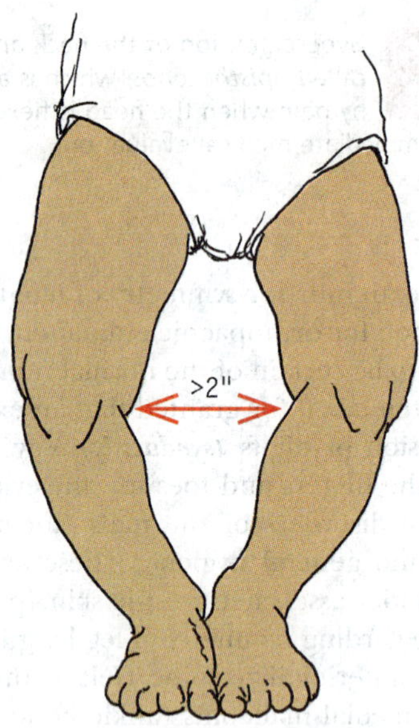

FIG. 7-49 Bowleg.

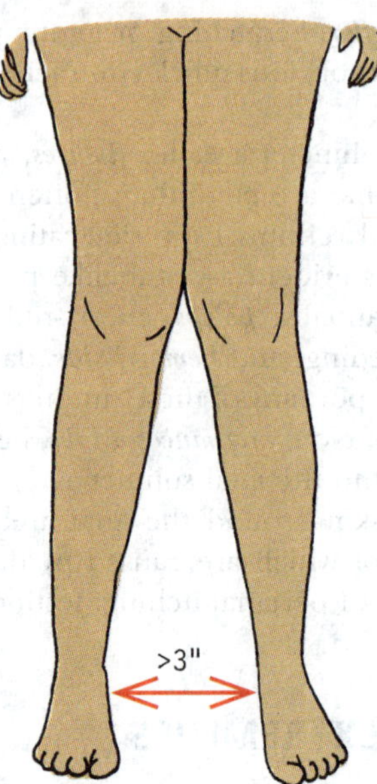

FIG. 7-50. Knock-knee.

ened stature, or evident in a child nearing puberty requires further evaluation.

Observe the ***feet*** for arch development and correct gait. Infants' and toddlers' feet appear flat because the foot is normally wide and the arch is covered by a fat pad. Development of the arch occurs naturally from the action of walking. Normally at birth the feet are held in a valgus (outward) or varus (inward) position. To determine whether a foot deformity at birth is the result of intrauterine position or development, scratch the outer, then inner, side of the sole. If the foot position is self-correctable, it will assume a right angle to the leg.

Assess gait by having the child walk, and estimate the angle of gait, which is the angle between the axis of the foot (imaginary line drawn through center of foot) and the line of progression (Fig. 7-51). Normally the feet turn outward less than 30 degrees and inward less than 10 degrees. Variations in foot positions are described in Chapter 11.

Toddlers have a "toddling" or broad-based gait, which facilitates walking by lowering the center of gravity. As the child reaches preschool age, the legs are brought closer together. By school age the walking posture is much more graceful and balanced.

The most common gait problem in young children is ***pigeon toe,*** or ***toeing in,*** which usually results from torsional deformities, such as internal tibial torsion (abnormal rotation or bowing of the tibia). Tests for tibial torsion include measuring the thigh-foot angle, which requires considerable practice for accuracy.

Observe for walking on the toes. Toe walking, in the absence of neuromuscular disorders, is normal in infants. If it persists longer than 3 months, refer the child for an orthopaedic evaluation. Although there is an association between toe walking and language delay, it does not appear to be clinically significant (Accardo and others, 1992).

Test the ***plantar*** or ***grasp reflex*** while examining the feet.

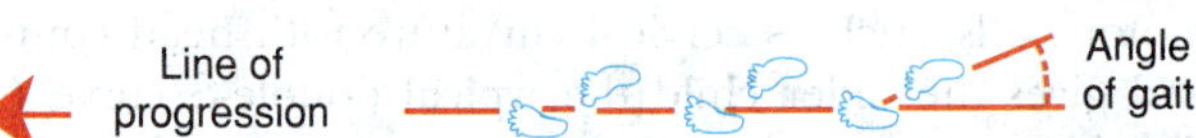

FIG. 7-51 Measurement of angle of gait.

Exert firm but gentle pressure with the tip of the thumb against the lateral sole of the foot from the heel upward to the little toe and then across to the big toe. The normal response in children who are walking is flexion of the toes. ***Babinski sign,*** dorsiflexion of the big toe and fanning of the other toes, is normal during infancy but abnormal after about 1 year or when locomotion begins (see Fig. 8-9, *B*). A positive Babinski sign after age 1 year indicates spinal cord lesions and requires further neurologic examination.

Joints

Evaluate the joints for ***range of motion.*** Normally this requires no specific testing other than observing the child's movements during the examination. However, check the hips for signs of congenital dislocation (see Developmental Dysplasia of the Hip, Chapter 11). Report any evidence of joint immobility or hyperflexibility.

Palpate the joints for ***heat, tenderness,*** and ***swelling.*** These signs, as well as redness over the joint, may indicate infection or any of the collagen diseases and warrant further investigation.

Muscles

Note symmetry and quality of muscle development, tone, and strength. Observe ***development*** by looking at the shape and contour of the body in both a relaxed and a tensed state. Estimate ***tone*** by grasping the muscle and feeling its firmness when it is relaxed and contracted. A common site for testing tone is the biceps muscle of the arm. Children are usually willing to "make a muscle" by clenching their fist.

Estimate ***strength*** by having the child use an extremity to push or pull against resistance, as in the following examples:

Arm strength. Child holds the arms outstretched in front of the body and tries to raise the arms while downward pressure is applied.

Hand strength. Child shakes hands with nurse and squeezes one or two fingers of the nurse's hand.

Leg strength. Child sits on a table or chair with the legs dangling and tries to raise the legs while downward pressure is applied.

Note symmetry of strength in the extremities, hands, and fingers and report any evidence of paresis or weakness.

NEUROLOGIC ASSESSMENT

The assessment of the nervous system is the broadest and most diverse, since every human function, both physical and emotional, is controlled by neurologic impulses. This discussion focuses primarily on a general appraisal of behavior, cognitive-perceptual development, sensory and cerebellar functioning, deep tendon reflexes, the cranial nerves, and "soft" signs.

Behavior

There is no special testing for behavior. Rather, it is an overall impression of the child's personality, affect, level of activity, social interaction, and attention span. Some aspects of assessing behavior are discussed elsewhere (see p. 232). Difficulties at home, at school, and in social situations suggest the need for additional psychologic assessment.

Another approach toward assessing behavior is the use of a behavioral questionnaire, such as the Pediatric Symptom Checklist (see box at right). It is completed by parents of children 6 to 12 years old and focuses on five major areas: mood, play, school, friends, and family relations. Scoring is based on a point system of 0 for "never," 1 for "sometimes," and 2 for "often." The scores are summed; a total score equal to or higher than 28 suggests the need for further evaluation of the child (Jellinek and others, 1988; Murphy and others, 1992). When high scores are found, consider the findings within the overall family context. Parental stress can affect the parent's perception of the child's behavior (Sanger, MacLean, and Van Slyke, 1992).

State of consciousness is a specific area for behavior under neurologic assessment. Hyperirritability, hyporeactivity, lethargy, delirium, stupor, or coma requires immediate referral. Levels of consciousness are described in Chapter 37. Always question parents' perceptions of change in behavior, which usually precedes an altered level of consciousness.

Cognitive-Perceptual Development

Cognitive-perceptual development is best assessed using a standard screening test. Adaptive and speech-comprehension development are significant indicators of

PEDIATRIC SYMPTOM CHECKLIST

1. Complains of aches or pains
2. Spends more time alone
3. Tires easily, little energy
4. Fidgety, unable to sit still
5. Has trouble with a teacher
6. Less interested in school
7. Acts as if driven by a motor
8. Daydreams too much
9. Distracted easily
10. Is afraid of new situations
11. Feels sad, unhappy
12. Is irritable, angry
13. Feels hopeless
14. Has trouble concentrating
15. Less interest in friends
16. Fights with other children
17. Absent from school
18. School grades dropping
19. Is down on himself or herself
20. Visits physician, but physician finds nothing wrong
21. Has trouble with sleeping
22. Worries a lot
23. Wants to be with you more than before
24. Feels he or she is bad
25. Takes unnecessary risks
26. Gets hurt frequently
27. Seems to be having less fun
28. Acts younger than children his or her age
29. Does not listen to rules
30. Does not show feelings
31. Does not understand other people's feelings
32. Teases others
33. Blames others for his or her troubles
34. Takes things that do not belong to him or her
35. Refuses to share

From Jellinek MS and others: Pediatric symptom checklist: screening school-age children for psychosocial dysfunction, *J Pediatr* 112(2):201-209, 1988.

intellectual functioning. If intellectual or perceptual impairment is suspected or learning difficulties exist, refer the child to an appropriate developmental specialist for further evaluation. "Soft" signs that should suggest minimum or borderline brain dysfunction are discussed at the conclusion of assessment of the neurologic system (p. 276).

Motor Functioning

Motor ability primarily involves assessment of voluntary muscle contraction and acquisition of age-specific developmental milestones for gross and fine motor skills (see Developmental Assessment, p. 278). One of the most important milestones in motor development is ***head control.*** Since developmental proceeds in the cephalocaudal direction, head lag suggests early brain damage. Head control is usually acquired by 4 months of age, although, as discussed in Chapter 8, even the newborn demonstrates some head control.

Also observe ***handedness.*** Infants and toddlers may show preference for one hand, but they usually do not display marked preference until the preschool years. Sole use of one hand may indicate paresis on the opposite side. Fail-

TESTS FOR SENSORY DISCRIMINATION

Touch the skin with a pin or piece of cotton and ask child to describe the different sensations.
Place a cold or warm object on the skin (the rubber and metal heads of the reflex hammer work well) and have child differentiate between them.
Touch different parts of the body simultaneously and see if child can localize both points.

TESTS FOR CEREBELLAR FUNCTION

Finger-to-nose test. With child's arm extended, ask child to touch the nose with the index finger with the eyes open and then closed.
Heel-to-shin test. While standing, have child run the heel of one foot down the shin or anterior aspect of the tibia of the other leg, both with the eyes opened and then closed.
Romberg test. With the eyes closed, have child stand with the heels together; falling or leaning to one side is abnormal and is called ***Romberg sign.***

ure to demonstrate handedness by a school-age child suggests failure of the brain to develop dominance, but its diagnostic significance is controversial.

Sensory Functioning

Sensory functioning is mainly assessed in terms of the sensory cranial nerves, in particular, vision and hearing, and peripheral sensation. This discussion is devoted to testing of peripheral sensation. Testing of the cranial nerves is discussed on p. 276, and vision and auditory testing are discussed on pp. 242 and 250, respectively.

Peripheral Sensation. With children old enough to cooperate, assess ***sensory discrimination*** by performing the activities in the box above with the child's eyes closed. Because these tests are similar to playing a game, consider introducing them at the beginning of the examination to decrease the child's anxiety and foster trust.

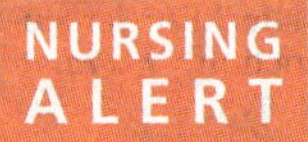

Decreased sensation and hyperesthesia (excessive sensation) are abnormal and must be referred for further neurologic evaluation.

Cerebellar Functioning

The cerebellum mainly controls balance and coordination. Much of the assessment of cerebellar functioning involves observing the child's posture, body movements, gait, and development of fine and gross motor skills. Tests such as balancing on one foot and the heel-to-toe walk in the Denver II also assess balance. Test ***coordination*** by asking the child to reach for a toy, button clothes, tie shoes, or draw a straight line on a piece of paper, provided the child is old enough to accomplish these activities.

Several tests for cerebellar function are described in the box above, right, and can be performed as games. When the Romberg test is done, stay beside the child if there is a possibility that the child may fall.

School-age children should be able to perform these tests, although preschoolers normally can bring the finger only within 5 to 7.5 cm (2 to 3 inches) of their nose. Difficulty in performing these exercises indicates a poor sense of position (especially with the eyes closed) and incoordination (especially with the eyes opened). Coordination can also be tested by any sequence of rapid successive movements, such as quickly touching each finger with the thumb of the same hand. Cerebellar testing is particularly signifi-

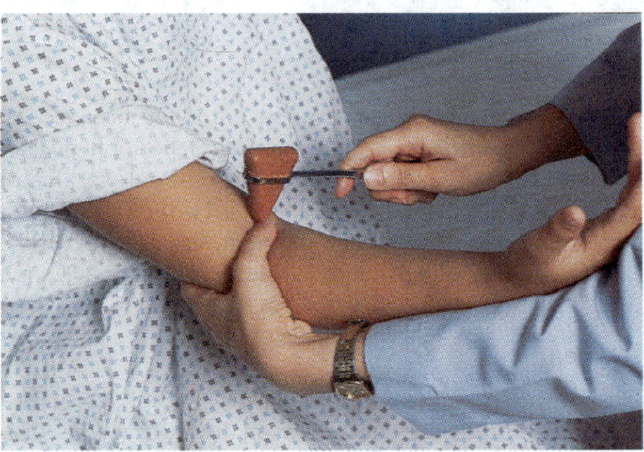

FIG. 7-52 Testing for biceps reflex. Hold child's partially flexed elbow in palm of hand with your thumb over antecubital space. Strike thumbnail with hammer. Normal response is partial flexion of forearm.

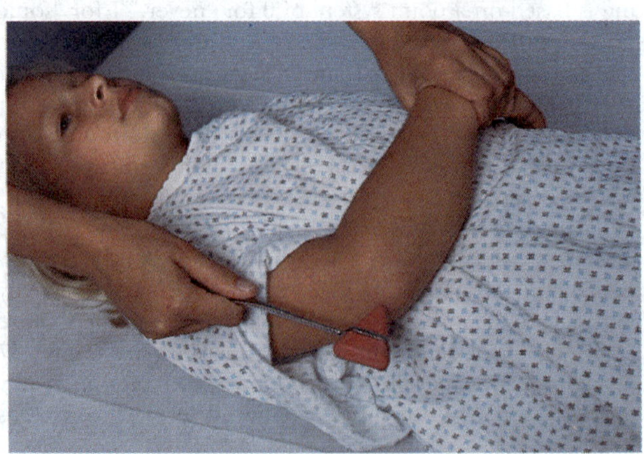

FIG. 7-53 Testing for triceps reflex. Child is placed supine, with forearm resting over chest, and triceps tendon is struck. Alternate procedure: child's arm is abducted, with upper arm supported and forearm allowed to hang freely. Triceps tendon is struck. Normal response is partial extension of forearm.

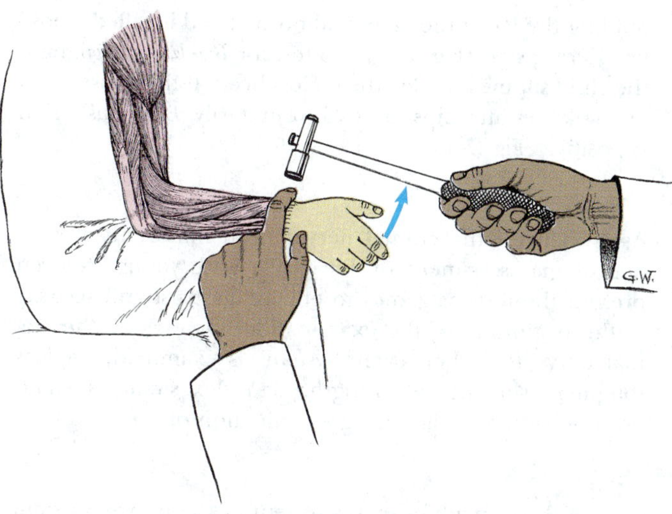

FIG. 7-54 Testing for brachioradialis reflex. Place child's forearm on child's lap (if sitting) or abdomen (if supine) with arm flexed at elbow and palm down. Strike radius about 1 inch (depending on child's size) above wrist. Normal response is flexion of forearm and supination (turning upward) of palm.

cant in children with symptoms of hyperactivity or learning difficulty.

Reflexes

Testing reflexes is an important part of the neurologic examination. Persistence of primitive reflexes, loss of reflexes, or hyperactivity of deep tendon reflexes is usually the result of a cerebral insult. This discussion is primarily concerned with reflexes found in children past infancy. The primitive reflexes of the newborn are discussed in Chapter 8.

Elicit reflexes by using the rubber head of the reflex hammer, flat of the finger, or side of the hand. If the child is easily frightened by equipment, use your hand or finger. Although testing reflexes is a simple procedure to perform, the child may inhibit the reflex by unconsciously tensing the muscle. To avoid tensing, distract younger children with toys or by talking to them. Have older children grasp their two hands in front of them and try to pull them apart.

Several ***superficial reflexes*** are present, such as the abdominal, cremasteric, anal, and plantar. These have been discussed throughout the chapter. ***Deep tendon reflexes*** are stretch reflexes of a muscle. The most common deep tendon reflex is the knee jerk, or patellar reflex (sometimes

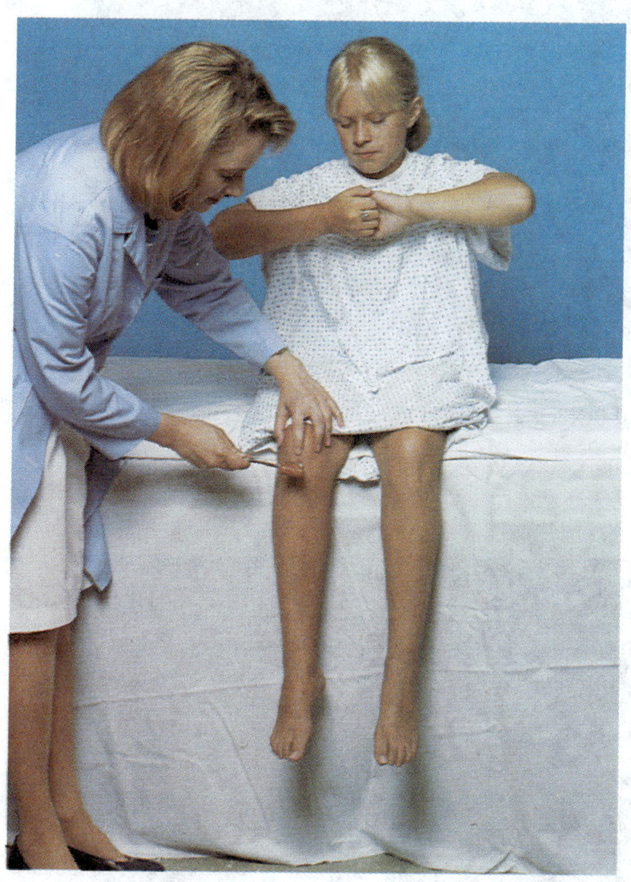

FIG. 7-55 Testing for patellar, or knee jerk, reflex, using distraction. Child sits on edge of examining table (or on parent's lap) with lower legs flexed at knee and dangling freely. Patellar tendon is tapped just below kneecap. Normal response is partial extension of lower leg.

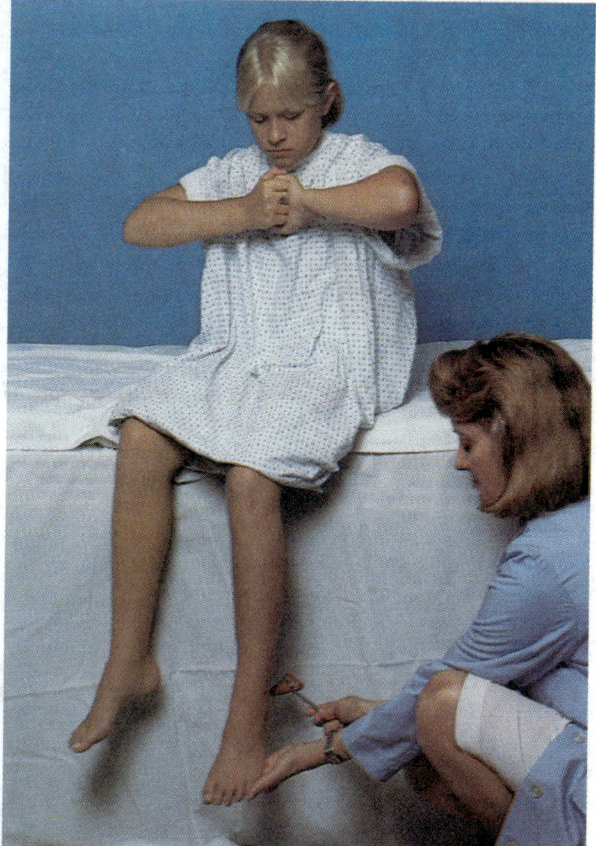

FIG. 7-56 Testing for Achilles reflex. Use same position for eliciting knee jerk reflex. Support foot lightly in your hand and strike Achilles tendon. Normal response is plantar flexion of foot (foot pointing downward, or "planting" toward floor).

called quadriceps reflex). The reflexes normally elicited are described in Figs. 7-52 through 7-56. Use the grading system in Table 7-16 to evaluate reflexes. Report absent or hyperactive reflexes for further evaluation.

Several other reflexes are normally present or absent but are not elicited unless specific indications exist. For example, in the presence of symptoms suggesting meningeal irritation, the Kernig sign and the Brudzinski sign are elicited. To test for ***Kernig sign,*** have the child supine with the leg flexed at the hip and knee. Resistance or pain on extending the leg at the knee is abnormal and is called a positive Kernig sign (Fig. 7-57). To test for ***Brudzinski sign,*** have the child supine and flex the child's head. If this causes pain or the knees and hips to flex involuntarily, Brudzinski sign is positive (Fig. 7-58).

TABLE 7-16 Grading of Reflexes

GRADE	DESCRIPTION
4+	Extremely brisk, hyperactive
3+	Brisker than normal
2+	Average, normal
1+	Diminished
0+	Absent

Cranial Nerves

Assessment of the cranial nerves is an important area of neurologic assessment (Table 7-17). With young children present the tests as games to encourage trust and security at the beginning of the examination. Or include the cranial nerve test when each "system" is examined, such as tongue movement and strength, gag reflex, swallowing, and position of the uvula during examination of the mouth.

"Soft" Signs

One of the difficulties in assessment of the nervous system is differentiating clearly between normal and abnormal findings (sometimes referred to as "hard" signs). There is a gray area called "soft" signs, findings that are normal in a young child but that in the normal course of maturation

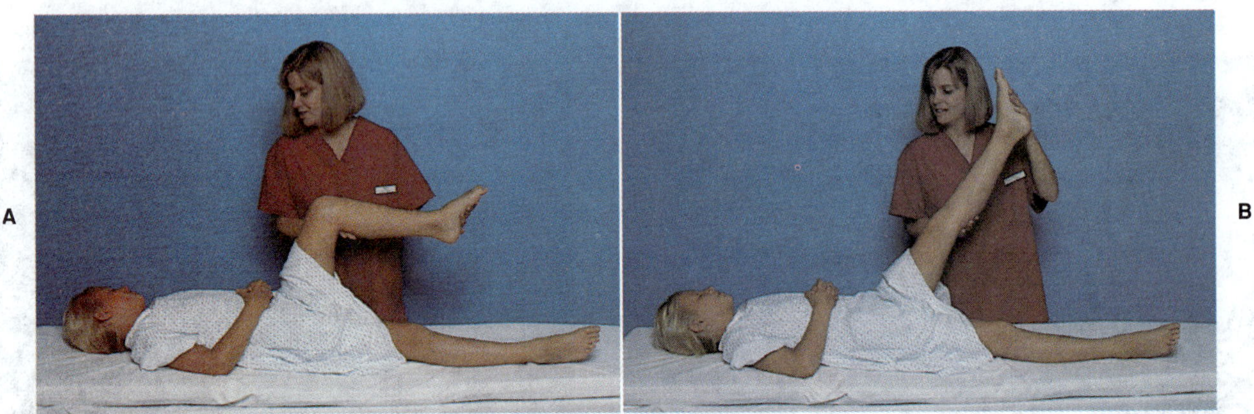

FIG. 7-57 **A,** Testing for Kernig sign. Have child flex leg at hip and knee. **B,** Pain or resistance on extension is abnormal.

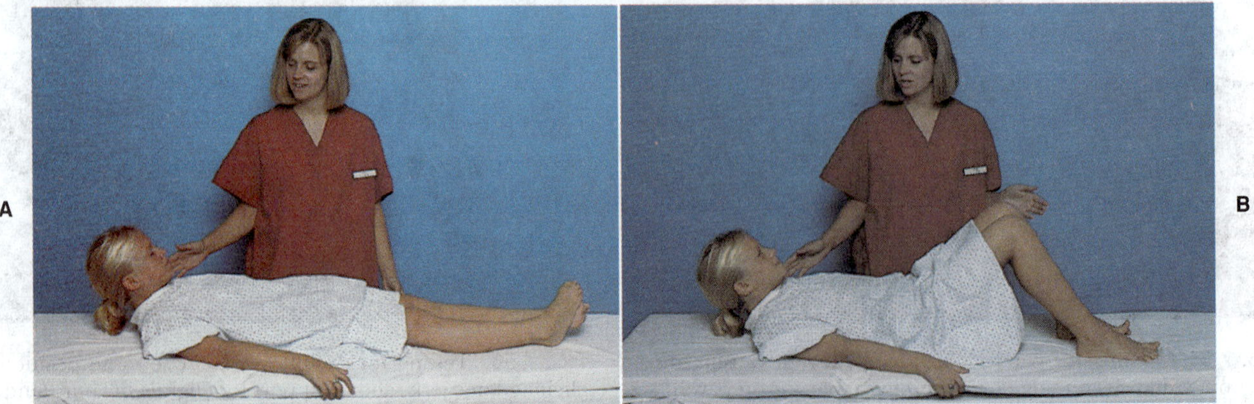

FIG. 7-58 **A,** Testing for Brudzinski sign. Ask child to flex head. **B,** Pain or involuntary flexion of knees and hips is abnormal.

TABLE 7-17 Assessment of Cranial Nerves

DISTRIBUTION/FUNCTION	TEST
I—OLFACTORY NERVE	
Olfactory mucosa of nasal cavity Smell	With eyes closed, have child identify odors such as coffee, alcohol from a swab, or other smells; test each nostril separately
II—OPTIC NERVE	
Rods and cones of retina, optic nerve Vision	Check for perception of light, visual acuity, peripheral vision, color vision, and normal optic disc
III—OCULOMOTOR NERVE	
Extraocular muscles (EOM) of eye: Superior rectus (SR)—moves eyeball up and in Inferior rectus (IR)—moves eyeball down and in Medial rectus (MR)—moves eyeball nasally Inferior oblique (IO)—moves eyeball up and out	Have child follow an object (toy) or light in the six cardinal positions of gaze (see Fig. 7-59)
Pupil constriction and accommodation	Perform PERRLA
Eyelid closing	Check for proper placement of lid
IV—TROCHLEAR NERVE	
Superior oblique muscle (SO)—moves eye down and out	Have child look down and in (see Fig. 7-59)
V—TRIGEMINAL NERVE	
Muscles of mastication	Have child bite down hard and open jaw; test symmetry and strength
Sensory: face, scalp, nasal and buccal mucosa	With child's eyes closed, see if child can detect light touch in the mandibular and maxillary regions Test corneal and blink reflex by touching cornea lightly (approach from the side so that child does not blink before cornea is touched)
VI—ABDUCENS NERVE	
Lateral rectus (LR) muscle—moves eye temporally	Have child look toward temporal side (see Fig. 7-59)
VII—FACIAL NERVE	
Muscles for facial expression	Have child smile, make funny face, or show teeth to see symmetry of expression
Anterior two thirds of tongue (sensory)	Have child identify a sweet or salty solution; place each taste on anterior section and sides of protruding tongue; if child retracts tongue, solution will dissolve toward posterior part of tongue
VIII—AUDITORY, ACOUSTIC, OR VESTIBULOCOCHLEAR NERVE	
Internal ear Hearing/balance	Test hearing; note any loss of equilibrium or presence of vertigo
IX—GLOSSOPHARYNGEAL NERVE	
Pharynx, tongue	Stimulate posterior pharynx with a tongue blade; child should gag
Posterior one third of tongue (sensory)	Test sense of sour or bitter taste on posterior segment of tongue
X—VAGUS NERVE	
Muscles of larynx, pharynx, some organs of gastrointestinal system; sensory fibers of root of tongue, heart, lung, and some organs of gastrointestinal system	Note hoarseness of voice, gag reflex, and ability to swallow Check that uvula is in midline; when stimulated with a tongue blade, should deviate upward and to stimulated side
XI—ACCESSORY NERVE	
Sternocleidomastoid and trapezius muscles of shoulder	Have child shrug shoulders while applying mild pressure; with examiner's hands placed on shoulders, have child turn head against opposing pressure on either side; note symmetry and strength
XII—HYPOGLOSSAL NERVE	
Muscles of tongue	Have child move tongue in all directions; have child protrude tongue as far as possible; note any midline deviation Test strength by placing tongue blade on one side of tongue and having child move it away

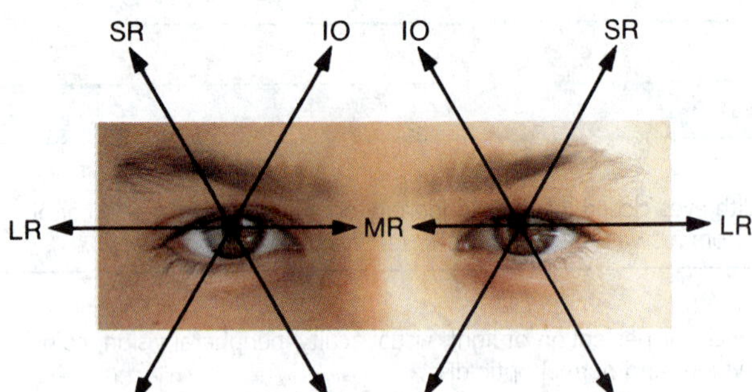

FIG. 7-59 Testing cardinal positions of gaze.

disappear. They represent the persistence of a more primitive form of behavior or response and a failure to perform the age-specific activity. Although the list of soft signs is long and the controversy concerning their significance far from resolved, some of the classic signs are listed in the box at right.

NEUROLOGIC "SOFT" SIGNS

Short attention span
Unusual body movement, such as mirroring
Poor coordination and sense of position
Excessive, sustained, and purposeless movement (hyperactivity)
Hypoactivity
Impulsiveness
Labile emotions
Distractibility
No established handedness
Language and articulation problems
Perceptual deficits (space, form, movement, time)
Problems with learning, especially reading, writing, and arithmetic

DEVELOPMENTAL ASSESSMENT

One of the most essential components of a complete health appraisal is assessment of developmental functioning. ***Screening procedures*** are designed to identify quickly and reliably those children whose developmental level is below normal for their age and who therefore may require further investigation. They also provide a means of recording objective measurements of present developmental functioning for future reference. Since the passage of P.L. 99-457, the Education of the Handicapped Act Amendments of 1986, much greater emphasis has been placed on developmental assessment of children with disabilities, and nurses can play a vital role in providing this service. All of the procedures discussed in this section can be administered in a variety of settings—home, school, daycare center, hospital, practitioner's office, or clinic.

In selecting a screening test, be aware of the instrument's ***validity***—namely, the extent to which it measures what it purports to measure. When screening for a single disease that is diagnosed by a single test, such as anemia, one can use criteria such as sensitivity, specificity, and predictive value of a positive finding. Although these criteria may not be appropriate for developmental tests, such as the Denver II, they are frequently used.

Sensitivity is the percentage of children with true problems who are correctly detected; approximately 80% is preferable. The other 20% of children have problems that are not detected (false-negatives). ***Specificity*** is the percentage of children without problems who are correctly detected. Since there are many more children without problems, 90% is preferable. The other 10% of children without problems are identified as having problems (false-positives). ***Positive predictive value*** is the percentage of children who fail the screening test who have true problems on diagnostic testing—70% or about three of every four referrals is acceptable (Felt and Stancin, 1991; Glascoe and others, 1992; Glascoe, Martin, and Humphrey, 1990).

Validity may also be based on the accuracy with which the ***standard norms*** have been established (e.g., the accuracy of the growth norms used to establish the growth curve). Such norms are most appropriate when screening the child's status, such as growth and development, which are determined by a host of factors, such as genetics, nutritional intake and opportunities to learn. As a result, deviant global measures of growth or development may reflect a variety of conditions, some of which may be pathologic. For instance, a child's language development may be delayed in comparison with that of other children because of a hearing impairment, neglect, mental retardation, or an emotional disorder. Therefore, it is not appropriate to compare the child's development with any one test, since few, if any, currently available diagnostic tests are equally accurate in detecting developmental delays in speech, language, fine and gross motor activities, and emotional and intellectual development (Frankenburg, 1994a).

DENVER SCREENING TESTS

The most widely used developmental screening tests for young children have been the series of tests developed by Dr. William Frankenburg and his colleagues in Denver, Colorado. The oldest and best known, the ***Denver Developmental Screening Test (DDST)***—first published in 1967 and revised in 1981 ***(DDST-R)***—has been standardized in 15 different countries. The test has been substantially revised and restandardized, and has been renamed the ***Denver-II.*** Using the Denver II requires only three new testing materials (a doll, a feeding bottle, and a cup), the new manual, and new forms. Another simplified instrument developed for the parent to complete is the ***Revised Prescreening Developmental Questionnaire (R-PDQ).*** Before administering the Denver II, the examiner should be trained by, and receive a certificate from, a master instructor who has been trained by the Denver faculty. This process helps ensure the validity of the test.*

Although it is not the purpose of this discussion to detail the instruction manual, some points concerning preparation, administration, and interpretation of the Denver II are important to stress. Before beginning the screen, ask if the child was born prematurely and correctly calculate the adjusted age. Up to 24 months of age, allowances are made for infants born prematurely by subtracting the number of weeks of missed gestation from their present age and testing them at the adjusted age. For example, a 16-week-old infant who was born 4 weeks early is tested at a 12-week adjusted age level. Explain to the parents and child, if appropriate, that the screenings are *not* intelligence tests but a method of showing what the child can do at a particular age. Emphasize that the child is *not* expected to perform each item on the test.

Tell the parent before the screening begins that the results of the child's performance will be explained after all the items have been concluded. It is the nurse's responsibility to properly inform parents of any testing or screening procedure before its administration so that they are fully aware of its purpose and intent.

Prepare toddlers and preschoolers for the procedure by presenting it as a game. Frequently the DDST is an excellent way to begin a health appraisal because it is nonthreatening, requires no painful or unfamiliar procedures, and capitalizes on the child's natural activity of play. Since children are easily distracted, perform each item quickly and present only one toy from the kit at a time. After that toy's purpose is concluded, such as building a tower of blocks or identifying its color, replace the toy in the bag and take out another one. Other temporary factors that may interfere with the child's performance include fatigue, illness, fear, hospitalization, separation from the parent, or general unwillingness to perform the activities. In addition, undiagnosed mental retardation, hearing loss, vision loss, neurologic impairment, or a familial pattern of slow development greatly influences the child's performance.

Following completion of the Denver II, ask the parent if the child's performance was typical of behavior at other times. If the parent replies affirmatively and the child's cooperation was satisfactory, explain the results, emphasizing all successful items first, then those items failed but which the child was not expected to pass, and finally those items that were delays. If the parent replies that the child's performance was not typical of usual behavior, it is best to defer any scoring or discussion of results, especially if the refusals yield a suspect score. In this situation reschedule testing for a time when the child is more likely to cooperate.

In explaining a normal score, focus on how well the child performed and reinforce the parents' efforts in satisfactorily stimulating their child. In addition to assessing the child's present developmental level, the Denver II can be used to guide parents toward those activities that are appropriate, although not necessarily expected, for the child's age.* By testing for items to the right of the age line (ones child is not expected to perform), children with advanced development, who may be gifted, can be identified.

In explaining delays, carefully note the parent's response, especially casual acceptance, such as "He'll catch up," or questions, such as "Does this mean my child is retarded?" Be aware of personal anxieties during these situations and refrain from giving glib reassurances, such as "I'm sure he will do better the next time." Rather, respond honestly to parents' questions, yet with appropriate flexibility and concern, stressing the need for further developmental testing.

*Forms and complete instructions are available from Denver Developmental Materials, Inc., P.O. Box 6919, Denver, CO 80206-9019; (303) 355-4729. As of Jan. 1, 1994, the DDST and DDST-R are no longer available, since they have been replaced by the DENVER II.

Denver Developmental Screening Test (DDST) and Revised DDST (DDST-R)

The DDST and DDST-R, as well as the Denver II (see next section), are composed of four major categories: personal-social, fine motor–adaptive, language, and gross motor and are applicable for children from birth through 6 years of age. The age divisions are monthly until 24 months and then every 3 months until 6 years of age. The tests are designed for administration by both professionals and paraprofessionals and take about 15 to 20 minutes to complete. The kits for testing include a red skein of wool, raisins, a small clear bottle with a ⅝-inch opening, a rattle with a narrow handle, eight 1-inch square blocks in red, blue, yellow, and green colors, a small bell, a tennis ball, and a pencil.

The major differences between the DDST and the DDST-R are the arrangement of items on the form and the scoring. On the original form, items are scored as "P" for pass, "F" for fail, or "R" for refusal. On the DDST-R only

*Suggested Denver Developmental Activities are available from Denver Developmental Materials, Inc.

DDST AND DDST-R SCORING

Scoring is based on the number of ***delays,*** defined as failure to perform an item that is passed by 90% of children who are of the same age, or any item that falls completely to the left of the age line.

Abnormal score: Two or more sectors with two or more delays

or

One sector with two or more delays plus one or more sectors with one delay and, in that same sector, no passes through the age line

Questionable score: One sector with two or more delays

or

One or more sectors with one delay and in that same sector no passes through the age line

Untestable score: Number of refusals is large enough to cause the test result to be questionable or abnormal if they were scored as failures

Normal score: Any score that does not meet the above criteria

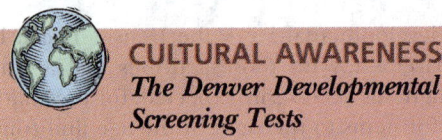

CULTURAL AWARENESS
The Denver Developmental Screening Tests

When administering the DDST, the nurse must consider cultural variations that can erroneously label the child delayed. For example, Southeast Asian children have demonstrated delays in the areas of personal-social development because of lack of familiarity with games such as pat-a-cake and in language because of differences in word usage, such as absence of plurals (Miller, Onotera, and Deinard, 1984). The more protective parental attitude of Southeast Asians toward the young child may also prevent early learning of self-help skills (Fung and Lau, 1985). Several of these variations were noted also in native African children (Olade, 1984). Further research is needed to determine if cultural variations affect screening results with the Denver II.

the items passed are scored (Frankenburg and others, 1981). Each item is designated by a bar that represents the ages at which 25%, 50%, 75%, and 90% of the tested population could perform the particular item. Scoring is based on the number of delays (see box on p. 279).

The DDST and DDST-R have been subjected to several reliability and validity tests and have been found to yield normal, questionable, and abnormal results that correlate fairly well with psychometric tests, such as the Cattell Infant Intelligence Scale and the Revised Bayley Infant Scale. Weaknesses of the DDST include its lack of sensitivity in identifying children with speech and language delays (Borowitz and Glascoe, 1986) and identifying general delays in children of lower socioeconomic groups (Frankenburg, Dick, and Carland, 1975) and from different cultural backgrounds (see Cultural Awareness box).

Denver II

The Denver II, a major revision and a restandardization of the DDST, differs from the DDST in items, test form, interpretation, and referral (see Appendix B). The previous total of 105 items has been increased to 125, including an increase from 21 DDST to 39 Denver II language items. Previous items that were difficult to administer and/or interpret have been either modified or eliminated. Many items that were previously tested by parental report now require observation by the examiner (Frankenburg and others, 1992).

Each item was evaluated to determine if significant differences exist on the basis of sex, ethnic group, maternal education, and place of residence. Items for which clinically significant differences exist were replaced, or if retained, are discussed in the Technical Manual. When evaluating children delayed on one of these items, the examiner can look up norms for the subpopulations to consider if the delay may be due to sociocultural or environmental differences.

The age of the Denver II is similar to the American Academy of Pediatrics' schedule for health supervision (see box on p. 218). The items on the test form are arranged in the same format as the DDST-R. The norms for the distribution bars were updated with the new standardization data but retain the 25th, 50th, 75th, and 90th percentile divisions. The test form contains a place to rate the child's behavioral characteristics (compliance, interest in surroundings, fearfulness, and attention span).

DENVER II SCORING

INTERPRETATION OF DENVER II SCORES

Advanced: Passed an item completely to the *right* of the age line (passed by less than 25% of children at an age older than the child)

OK: Passed, failed, or refused an item intersected by the age line between the 25th and 75th percentiles

Caution: Failed or refused items intersected by the age line on or between the 75th and 90th percentiles

Delay: Failed an item completely to the *left* of the age line; refusals to the left of the age line may also be considered delays, since the reason for the refusal may be inability to perform the task

INTERPRETATION OF TEST

Normal: No delays and a maximum of one caution

Suspect: One or more delays and/or two or more cautions

Untestable: Refusals on one or more items completely to the left of the age line or on more than one item intersected by the age line in the 75% to 90% area

RECOMMENDATIONS FOR REFERRAL FOR SUSPECT AND UNTESTABLE TESTS

Rescreen in 1 to 2 weeks to rule out temporary factors.

If rescreen is suspect or untestable, use clinical judgment based on the following: number of cautions and delays; which items are cautions and delays; rate of past development; clinical examination and history; availability of referral resources.

To determine relative areas of advancement and areas of delay, sufficient items should be administered to establish the basal and ceiling levels in each sector. By scoring appropriate items as "pass," "fail," "refusal," or "no opportunity," and relating such scores to the age of the child, each item can be interpreted as described in the box above. To identify cautions, all items intersected by the age line are administered. To screen solely for developmental delays, only the items located totally to the *left* of the child's age line are administered. Criteria for referral are based on the availability of resources in the community, (also see the box).

Research on the Denver II's validity and accuracy is in its beginning stages. One study found that its sensitivity was acceptable; most children with even subtle developmental problems were identified. However, the test had poor specificity; almost half of the children without developmental problems received suspect scores, resulting in a high rate of overreferrals (Glascoe and others, 1992). However, the results are not universally accepted. Dr. Frankenburg describes the Denver II as presenting norms of development for specific skills, similar to growth charts presenting growth norms. He and other experts maintain that tests of validity that measure how well the results of the Denver II agree with those of standardized tests should not be used, because the Denver II is more a developmental chart or inventory, rather than a screening test (Dworken, 1992). To minimize overreferrals, Frankenburg (1994a) stresses that a decision for referral depends not only on the results of the Denver II, but also on the practitioner's clinical judgment after considering the child's developmental history; general health status; social, cultural, and emotional environment; and the availability of local resources for diagnosis and treatment. (See also Developmental Screening and Interpretation, p. 282.)

REVISED PRESCREENING DEVELOPMENTAL QUESTIONNAIRE (R-PDQ)

The R-PDQ is a revision of the original PDQ (Frankenburg, Fandal, and Thorton, 1987). Advantages of the R-PDQ include the addition and arrangement of items to be more age-appropriate, simplified parent scoring, and easier comparison with Denver Developmental Screening Test (DDST) norms for professionals. The R-PDQ is a parent-answered prescreen consisting of 150 questions from the DDST, although only a subset of questions are asked for each age-group. With less-educated parents, the form may need to be read to the caregiver.

Four different forms are available and are selected based on age: orange (0 to 9 months), purple (9 to 24 months), gold (2 to 4 years), and white (4 to 6 years) (see Appendix B). The caregiver answers the questions until (1) three "NOs" are circled (they do not have to be consecutive) or (2) all of the questions on both sides of the form have been answered. Scoring is based on the number of delays (see box on p. 279). Children who have no delays are considered to be developing normally. If a child has one delay, the caregiver is provided with age-appropriate developmental activities to pursue with the child and a rescreen with the R-PDQ is done 1 month later. If on rescreening, a child has one or more delays, the Denver II is administered as soon as possible. If a child has two or more delays on the first screening with the R-PDQ, the Denver II is administered as soon as possible.

DEVELOPMENTAL PROFILE II

The Developmental Profile II is designed for use with children from birth through a functional age of 9½ years. With normal children it can be used appropriately from birth through age 7 years. The following five scales are included: physical, self-help, social, academic, and communication. Administration time varies from 20 to 40 minutes depending on the child's age and the approach used, either interview, interview and direct testing, or self-interview. The scale tends to have age expectations for some items, especially the academic ones, that are unrealistically late chronologically, giving it a low rate of detection (sensitivity) of children with developmental problems (Glascoe and Byrne, 1993). A detailed self-instructional manual is used for training (Alpern, Boll, and Shearer, 1986).*

MCCARTHY SCALES OF CHILDREN'S ABILITIES (MSCA)

The MSCA is a developmental assessment tool for children 2½ to 8½ years old (McCarthy, 1972). It includes six scales: verbal, perceptual-performance, quantitative, general cognition, memory, and motor. Administration time is from 45 minutes to 1 hour. Eighteen separate tests are administered to the child, and the scores from these tests contribute to one or more of the scores on the six scales. The final score correlates well with intelligence quotients from other standardized tests. It may be used for follow-up when a child fails screening tests or is suspected of having retarded development (Hayes, 1981). A detailed self-instructional manual is used for training.†

WASHINGTON GUIDE TO PROMOTING DEVELOPMENT IN THE YOUNG CHILD

The Washington Guide to Promoting Development in the Young Child provides a framework for developmental assessment based on direct observation of a child's specific behaviors in eight categories: feeding, sleep, play, language, motor activities, discipline, toilet training, and dressing. In each category developmental accomplishments that would be expected for age-groups from birth to 5 years are grouped as "expected tasks," with an accompanying list of "suggested activities" for parental guidance. The Washington Guide differs from other developmental tools in that no score is obtained. It is used to observe the child on a systematic basis, to identify variations in development, and to provide suggestions regarding appropriate childbearing practices (Powell, 1981).

DRAW-A-PERSON (DAP) TEST

Since children's drawings follow a developmental sequence (see discussion on drawing under Gross and Fine Motor Behavior, Chapter 15), tests have been developed to estimate development or intelligence based on elements present in the drawing. Goodenough (1926) constructed her Draw-A-Man Test for children ages 3 to 10 years (see box on p. 282), which was later revised to include a drawing of a woman and a drawing of the self based on nationally representative norms that included ages 3 through 15 years ***(Goodenough-Harris Drawing Test)*** (Harris, 1963). The current form of the test, ***Draw A Person: A Quantitative Scoring System (DAP)***‡ (Naglieri, 1988), is a more recent standardization for children ages 5 to 17 years. The scoring system

*The Developmental Profile II Manual is available from Western Psychological Services, 12031 Wilshire Blvd., Los Angeles, CA 90025; (800) 648-8857.

†The MSCA is available from Psychological Corporation, 555 Academic Ct., San Antonio, TX 78204-2498; (800) 228-0752.

‡The Draw-A-Person Test is available from Psychological Corp., 555 Academic Ct., San Antonio, TX 78204-2498; (800) 228-0752.

METHOD OF SCORING GOODENOUGH DRAW-A-MAN TEST*

1. Head present
2. Legs present
3. Arms present
4. Trunk present
5. Trunk longer than broad
6. Shoulder indicated
7. Both arms and legs attached to trunk
8. Legs and arms attached to trunk at proper level
9. Neck present
10. Outline of neck continuous with that of head or trunk or both
11. Eyes present
12. Nose present
13. Mouth present
14. Both nose and mouth in two dimensions; two lips shown
15. Nostrils indicated
16. Hair shown
17. Hair on more than circumference of head, nontransparent, better than scribble
18. Clothing present
19. Two articles of clothing, nontransparent
20. Entire clothing with sleeves and trousers shown, nontransparent
21. Four or more articles of clothing definitely indicated
22. Costume complete without incongruities
23. Fingers shown
24. Correct number of fingers
25. Fingers in two dimensions, length greater than breadth, angle subtended not greater than 180 degrees
26. Opposite of thumbs shown
27. Hands shown distinct from fingers and arms
28. Arm joints shown (elbows or shoulder or both)
29. Head in proportion
30. Arms in proportion
31. Legs in proportion
32. Feet in proportion
33. Arms and legs in two dimensions
34. Heel shown
35. Lines somewhat controlled
36. Lines well controlled
37. Head outline well controlled
38. Trunk outline well controlled
39. Outline of arms and legs well controlled
40. Outline of features well controlled
41. Ears present
42. Ears present in correct position
43. Eyebrows or lashes present
44. Pupil shown
45. Proportion of eyes correct
46. Glance directed to front in profile drawing
47. Both chin and forehead shown
48. Projection of shin shown
49. Profile with not more than one error
50. Correct profile

*In each item listed give the child 1 point. The number of points multiplied by 3 months plus 3 years equals the mental age.

was changed to be as objective as possible; 64 items are scored for 14 different criteria (e.g., arms, mouth, trunk, attachment of body parts, clothing, and hair). Points are given for the item's presence, detail, and proportion, as well as bonus credit from some items if these three elements are present. Artistic ability is not correlated with scoring, because credit is not given for realism or esthetic quality.

The DAP has several benefits; it is nonverbal, nonthreatening, more culturally unbiased than many other tests, and easy to administer. Since the least number of items and simplest scoring are in the original Goodenough test, nurses may find this version most convenient to use for screening. For accurate testing, the DAP should be used.

Give the child a pencil with an eraser and paper, and simply ask the child to "draw a man or a person." Offer no further directions, other than that the child should draw the best picture of a person that he or she can. Let the child draw as long as needed to finish the picture.

To determine the scoring give 1 point for each item included in the drawing (see box at left). Each point is equal to 3 months. Convert the number of points to months and/or years and add to the base age of 3 years. The final score in months/years is approximately equal to the child's mental age. Calculate the child's intelligence quotient (IQ) by dividing the mental age by the chronologic age and multiplying the result by 100. For example, if a 5-year-old child scores 12 points on the test, he or she has a mental age of 6 years (3 years + [12 × 3 months] = 6 years). Mental age (6 years) divided by actual age (5 years) equals 1.2; 1.2 multiplied by 100 equals an IQ of 120.

DEVELOPMENTAL SCREENING AND INTERPRETATION

Although screening tests are an effective method of applying the knowledge of children's expected rate of development to a large segment of the population, they are only as successful as the individual's expertise in administering them. Since many of the screening tests are devised to be used by paraprofessionals, there are inherent risks in screening if such individuals are not properly trained or supervised. For example, false-positives can label the child as developmentally delayed and cause problems that otherwise might not have existed. False-negative can prevent children with problems from receiving the help they need.

Nurses administering developmental screening or supervising paraprofessionals' testing need to assess the child's "whole picture" and not rely solely on any screening procedure. Development, like growth and health, is a dynamic process. Tests such as the Denver II should be used as part of ***developmental surveillance,*** a continuous comprehensive primary health care approach that includes the parents as partners with professionals (Frankenburg, 1994b). Evaluation of the child's total well-being is the result of evaluating data from a comprehensive health and family history, physical examination, and developmental screening.

KEY POINTS

- The most common approach to examining children follows a head-to-toe sequence.
- Growth measurements during the physical examination focus on length, height, weight, skinfold thickness, and arm

and head circumference. Assessment of growth is measured against standard growth charts to determine a child's status in comparison with other children of the same age.

- Measurements of temperature, pulse, respiration, and blood pressure require accurate assessment techniques to provide useful data.
- The general appearance of a child is a cumulative, subjective impression of physical appearance, state of nutrition, behavior, personality, interactions with parents and nurse, posture, development, and speech.
- Assessment of the skin, which primarily involves inspection and palpation, focuses on color, texture, temperature, moisture, and turgor. The nurse needs to be aware of both physiologic and ethnic factors that may affect these areas.
- In assessment of the lymph nodes, the nurse examines, by palpation, the part of the body in which the glands are located.
- The head is inspected for shape, symmetry, mobility, and head control.
- Assessment of the neck includes palpation of the trachea and thyroid gland.
- Examination of the eyes includes placement and alignment, inspection of external and internal structures, and vision testing.
- Ears are examined for placement and alignment, inspection of external and internal structures, and auditory testing.
- The lungs are examined by methods of inspection, palpation, percussion, and auscultation.
- Auscultation is the most important procedure for examining the heart.
- Heart murmurs are classified as innocent, functional, and organic and should be evaluated for location, time, intensity, and loudness.
- Abdominal assessment follows an orderly sequence of inspection, auscultation, percussion, and palpation, since palpation may distort normal abdominal sounds.
- Examination of the genitalia may be anxiety-provoking in the child, and the nurse must avoid transferring personal anxiety.
- Neurologic assessment addresses behavior, cognitive-perceptual development, motor functioning, sensory and cerebellar functioning, reflexes, cranial nerves, and soft signs.
- The Denver II, a major revision and a restandardization of the DDST, differs from the DDST in items included in the test, the test form, the interpretation of scoring, and referral criteria. Both tests are composed of four categories: personal-social, fine motor–adaptive, language, and gross motor.

REFERENCES

Abdo MH, Feghali JG, Stapells DR: Transient evoked otoacoustic emissions: clinical applications and technical considerations, *Int J Pediatr Otorhinolaryngol* 25:61-71, 1993.

Accardo P and others: Toe walking and language development, *Clin Pediatr* 31(3):158-160, 1992.

Accuracy, correlation and equivalence to adult standards, *Clin Pediatr* 30(4, suppl):17, 1991 (discussion).

Alexander D, Kelly B: Cost effectiveness of tympanic thermometry in the pediatric office setting, *Clin Pediatr* 30(4, suppl):57, 1991a.

Alexander D, Kelly B: Responses of children, parents, and nurses to tympanic thermometry in the pediatric office, *Clin Pediatr* 30(4, suppl):53-56, 1991b.

Alpern G, Boll T, Shearer M: *Developmental Profile II manual,* Los Angeles, CA, 1986, Western Psychological Services.

American Academy of Pediatrics, Committee on Early Childhood, Adoption, and Dependent Care: Health care of foster children, *Pediatrics* 79(4):644-646, 1987.

American Academy of Pediatrics, Committee on Fetus and Newborn: Routine evaluation of blood pressure, hematocrit, and glucose in newborns, *Pediatrics* 92(3):474-476, 1993.

American Academy of Pediatrics, Committee on Practice and Ambulatory Medicine: Vision screening and eye examination in children, *Pediatrics* 77(6):918-919, 1986.

Arn P and others: Outcome of pectus excavatum in patients with Marfan syndrome and in the general population, *J Pediatr* 115(8):954-958, 1989.

Barber N, Kilmon CA: Reactions to tympanic temperature measurement in an ambulatory setting, *Pediatr Nurs* 15(5):477-481, 1989.

Barrus DH: A comparison of rectal and axillary temperatures by electronic thermometer measurement in preschool children, *Pediatr Nurs* 9(6):424-425, 1983.

Benzinger M, Benzinger TH: Tympanic clinical temperature. In *National Bureau of Standards Fifth Symposium on Temperature,* Pittsburgh, 1972, Instrument Society of America.

Borowitz KC, Glascoe FP: Sensitivity of the Denver Developmental Screening Test in speech and language screening, *Pediatrics* 78(6):1075-1078, 1986.

Burke S, Roberts C, Maloney R: Infant and child weights: reliability and validity of scales, *Issues Compr Pediatr Nurs* 11(4):241-249, 1988.

Cavanaugh RM: Pediatricians and the pneumatic otoscope: are we playing it by ear? *Pediatrics* 84(2):362-364, 1989.

Chamberlain JM and others: Comparison of a tympanic thermometer to rectal and oral thermometers in a pediatric emergency room, *Clin Pediatr* 30(suppl 4):24-29, 1991.

Church JL, Baer KJ: Examination of the adolescent: a practical guide, *J Pediatr Health Care* 1(2):65-72, 1987.

Cole FL: Temporal variation in the effects of iced water on oral temperature, *Res Nurs Health* 16(2):107-111, 1993.

Davis K: The accuracy of tympanic temperature measurement in children, *Pediatr Nurs* 19(3):267-272, 1993.

de Swiet M and others: Measurement of blood pressure in children, *Br Med J* 299:107, 1989.

Dewey KG and others: Growth of breast-fed and formula-fed infants from 0 to 18 months: the DARLING study, *Pediatrics* 89(6):1035-1041, 1992.

Dressler DK, Smejkal C, Ruffolo ML: A comparison of oral and rectal temperature measurement on patients receiving oxygen by mask, *Nurs Res* 32(6):373-375, 1983.

Duggan PF: Time to abolish "gold standard," *Br Med J* 304(6841):1568-1569, 1992.

Dworkin PH: Developmental screening: (still) expecting the impossible? *Pediatrics* 89(6):1253-1255, 1992.

Eoff MJ, Joyce B: Temperature measurements in children, *Am J Nurs* 81(5):1010-1011, 1981.

Erickson RS, Yount ST: Comparison of tympanic and oral temperatures in surgical patients, *Nurs Res* 40(2):90-93, 1991.

Farber JM: The invisible handcuffs, *Contemp Pediatr* 8(1):110, 1991.

Felt B, Stancin T: A comparative review of developmental screening tests, *Pediatrics* 88(1):180-182, 1991 (letter to the editor).

Ferra-Love R: A comparison of tympanic and pulmonary artery measures of core temperature, *J Post Anesth Nurs* 6(3):161-164, 1991.

Frankenburg W: Does Denver II produce meaningful results? *Pediatrics* 90(3):478-479, 1992 (reply to the editor).

Frankenburg WK: Preventing developmental delays: is developmental screening sufficient? I. Developmental screening and the Denver II, *Pediatrics,* 93(4):586-589, 1994a.

Frankenburg WK: Preventing developmental delays: is developmental screening sufficient? II. Partners in health care, *Pediatrics* 93(4)589-593, 1994b.

Frankenburg WK, Dick NP, Carland J: Development of preschool-aged children of different social and ethnic groups: implications for developmental screening, *J Pediatr* 87(1):125-132, 1975.

Frankenburg WK, Fandal A, Thornton S: Revision of Denver Prescreening Developmental Quesionnaire, *J Pediatr* 110(4):653-657, 1987.

Frankenburg WK and others: The newly abbreviated and revised Denver Developmental Screening Test, *J Pediatr* 99(6):995-999, 1981.

Frankenburg WK and others: The Denver II: a major revision and restandardization of the Denver Developmental Screening Test, *Pediatrics* 89(1):91-97, 1992.

Freed GL, Fraley JK: Lack of agreement of tympanic membrane temperature assessments with conventional methods in a private practice setting, *Pediatrics* 89(3):384-386, 1992.

Frohlich E and others: Recommendations for human blood pressure determination by sphygmomanometers: report of a special task force appointed by the Stering Committee, American Health Association, *Circulation* 77:501A, 1988.

Fung K, Lau S: Denver Developmental Screening Test: cultural variables, *J Pediatr* 106(2):343, 1985.

Gerbrandy J, Snell ES, Cranston WI: Oral, rectal, and oesophageal temperatures in relation to central temperature control in man, *Clin Sci* 13:615-624, 1954.

Glascoe FP, Byrne KE: The usefulness of the Developmental Profile-II in developmental screening, *Clin Pediatr* 32(4):203-208, 1993.

Glascoe FP, Martin ED, Humphrey S: A comparative review of developmental screening tests, *Pediatrics* 86(4):547-554, 1990.

Glascoe FP and others: Accuracy of the Denver-II in developmental screening, *Pediatrics* 89:1221-1225, 1992.

Glasier C, Mallory G, Steele R: Significance of opacification of the maxillary and ethmoid sinuses in infants, *J Pediatr* 114(1):45-50, 1989.

Goodenough FL: *Measurement of intelligence by drawings,* New York, 1926, World Book.

Gray D, Dixon J, Collin J: The closed eyes sign: an aid to diagnosing non-specific abdominal pain, *Br Med J* 297:837, 1988.

Greally JM: Alternative to "aaah" *Lancet* 1:539, 1988 (letter).

Haddock R, Merrow D, Vincent P: Comparison of rectal and axillary temperatures, *Neonatal Network* 6(5):67-71, 1988.

Haddock R, Vincent P, Merrow D: Axillary and rectal temperatures of full-term neonates: are they different? *Neonatal Network* 5(1):36-40, 1986.

Harris DB: *Children's drawings as measures of intellectual maturity,* San Diego, CA, 1983, Harcourt Brace Jovanovich.

Hayes JS: The McCarthy Scales of Children's Abilities: their usefulness in developmental assessment, *Pediatr Nurs* 7(4):35-37, 1981.

Himes JH and others: Parent-specific adjustments for evaluation of recumbent length and stature of children, *Pediatrics* 75(2):304-313, 1985.

Holtzclaw BJ: Monitoring body temperature, *AACN Clin Issues Crit Care Nurs* 4(1):44-55, 1993.

Hoyt CS, Nickel BL, Billson FA: Ophthalmological examination of the infant: development aspects, *Surv Ophthalmol* 26(4):177-189, 1982.

Jellinek MS and others: Pediatric symptom checklist: screening school-age children for psychosocial dysfunction, *J Pediatr* 112(2):201-209, 1988.

Jenista J, Chapman D: Medical problems of foreign-born adopted children, *Am J Dis Child* 141(3):20-33, 1987.

Johnson KJ, Bhatia P, Bell EF: Infrared thermometry of newborn infants, *Pediatrics* 87(1):34-38, 1991.

Kai J: Parents' perceptions of taking babies' rectal temperature, *Br Med J* 307:660-662, 1993.

Kenney RD and others: Evaluation of an infrared tympanic membrane thermometer in pediatric patients, *Pediatrics* 85(5):854-857, 1990.

Klein DG and others: A comparison of pulmonary artery, rectal, and tympanic membrane temperature measurement in the ICU, *Heart Lung* 22(5):435-441, 1993.

Kovalesky A: *Nurses' guide to children's eyes,* New York, 1985, Grune & Stratton.

Laestadius N, Aase J, Smith D: Normal inner canthal and outer orbital dimensions, *J Pediatr* 74(3):465-468, 1969.

Lewitt EM, Marshall CL, Salzer JE: An evaluation of a plastic strip thermometer, *JAMA* 247(3):321-325, 1982.

MacGillivray MH: The pediatrician's role in identification and management of growth: normal, subnormal, and abnormal patterns, *Pediatr Rounds* 2(1):2-5, 1993.

Mackowiak PA, Wasserman SS, Levine MM: A critical appraisal of 98.6° F, the upper limit of the normal body temperature, and other legacies of Carl Reinhold August Wunderlich, *JAMA* 268(12):1578-1580, 1992.

Margolius FR, Sneed NV, Hollerbach AD: Accuracy of apical pulse rate measurements in young children, *Nurs Res* 40(6):378-380, 1991.

Marks A, Fisher M: Health assessment and screening during adolescence, *Pediatrics* 80(1):135-158, 1987.

Martorell R, Mendoza F, Castillo R: Genetic and environmental determinants of growth in Mexican-Americans, *Pediatrics* 84(5):864-871, 1989.

Martyn K, Carmon M, Rice M: *A comparison of pediatric temperature assessment measures in children,* Manuscript submitted for publication, 1994.

Martyn K and others: Comparison of axillary, rectal, and skin-based temperature assessment in preschoolers, *Nurse Pract* 13(4):31-36, 1988.

McCarthy D: *Manual: McCarthy Scales of Children's Abilities,* New York, 1972, Psychological Corp.

Milewski A, Ferguson KL, Terndrup TE: Comparison of pulmonary artery, rectal, and tympanic membrane temperatures in adult intensive care unit patients, *Clin Pediatr* 30(4, suppl):13-16, 1991.

Miller V, Onotera R, Deinard A: Denver Developmental Screening Test: cultural variations in Southeast Asian children, *J Pediatr* 104(3):481-482, 1984.

Morely CJ and others: Axillary and rectal temperature measurements in infants, *Arch Dis Child* 67(1):122-125, 1992.

Muma BK and others: Comparison of rectal, axillary, and tympanic membrane temperatures in infants and young children, *Ann Emerg Med* 20(1):41-44, 1991.

Murphy JM and others: Screening for psychosocial dysfunction in pediatric practice: a naturalistic study of the pediatric symptom checklist, *Clin Pediatr* 31(11):660-667, 1992.

Naglieri JA: *DAP: Draw A Person, a quantitative scoring system,* San Antonio, TX, 1988, Psychological Corp.

National Society to Prevent Blindness: *Guide to testing distance visual acuity,* Schaumburg, IL, 1988, The Society.

Neff J: Visual acuity testing, *J Emerg Nurs* 17(6):431-436, 1991.

Neff JA and others: Effect of respiratory rate, respiratory depth, and open versus closed mouth breathing on sublingual temperature, *Res Nurs Health* 12(3):195-202, 1989.

Neinstein L and others: Comfort of male adolescents during general and genital examination, *J Pediatr* 115(3):494-497, 1989.

Nichols GA and others: Measuring oral and rectal temperatures of febrile children, *Nurs Res* 21(3):261-264, 1972.

Ogren J: The inaccuracy of axillary temperatures measured with an electronic thermometer, *Am J Dis Child* 144(1):109-111, 1990.

Olade RA: Evaluation of the Denver Developmental Screening Test as applied to African children, *Nurs Res* 33(4):204-207, 1984.

O'Neill T and others: Diagnostic value of the apex beat, *Lancet* 1(8635):410-411, 1989.

Orlando M, Frank T: Audiometer and audioscope hearing screening compared with threshold test in young children, *J Pediatr* 110(2):261-263, 1987.

Overend A, Hall WW, Godwin PGR: Does earwax lose its pathogens on your auriscope overnight? *Br Med J* 305:1571-1573, 1992.

Park JK, Guntheroth WG: Accurate blood pressure measurement in children, *Am J Noninvas Cardiol* 3:297-309, 1989.

Park M: *Pediatric cardiology for the practitioner,* ed 2, St Louis, 1988, Mosby.

Park M, Lee D, Johnson GA: Oscillometric blood pressures in the arm, thigh, and calf in healthy children and those with aortic coarctation, *Pediatrics* 91(4):761-765, 1993.

Park M, Menard S: Accuracy of blood pressure measurement by the Dinamap monitor in infants and children, *Pediatrics* 79(6):907-914, 1987.

Pontious S and others: Accuracy and reliability of temperature measurement in the emergency department by instrument and site in children, *Pediatr Nurs* 20(1):58-63, 1994a.

Pontious S and others: Accuracy and reliability of temperature measurement by instrument and site, *J Pediatr Nurs* 9(2):114-123, 1994b.

Powell ML: *Assessment and management of developmental changes and problems in children,* ed 2, St Louis, 1981, Mosby.

Report of the Second Task Force on blood pressure control in children—1987, *Pediatrics* 79(1):1-25, 1987.

Roscelli JD: Aural, oral, or rectal—does it make any real difference? *Pediatrics* 91(1):166, 1993 (letter to the editor).

Sanger MS, MacLean WE Jr, Van Slyke DA: Relation between maternal characteristics and child behavior ratings: implications for interpreting behavior checklists, *Clin Pediatr* 31(8):461-466, 1992.

Sato-Viacrucis K: The evolution of the Snellen E to the Blackbird, *School Nurse,* pp 18-19, Spring 1985.

Scholefield JH, Gerber MA, Dwyer P: Liquid crystal forehead temperature strips, *Am J Dis Child* 136:198-201, 1982.

Schuman AJ: The accuracy of infrared auditory canal thermometry in infants and children, *Clin Pediatr* 32(6):347-354, 1993.

Seidel HM, Rosenstein BJ, Pathak A: *Care of the full term newborn,* St Louis, 1993, Mosby.

Seymore C and others: Influence of position during examination, and sex of examiner on patient anxiety during pelvic examination, *J Pediatr* 108(2):312-317, 1986.

Stewart JV, Webster D: Re-evaluation of the tympanic thermometer in the emergency department, *Ann Emerg Med* 21(2):158-161, 1992.

Talo H, Macknin ML, Medendrop SV: Tympanic membrane temperatures compared to rectal and oral temperatures, *Clin Pediatr* 30(suppl 4):30-35, 1991.

Teller D and others: Assessment of visual acuity in infants and children: the acuity card procedure, *Dev Med Child Neurol* 28:779-789, 1986.

Terndrup T, Allegra J, Kealy J: A comparison of oral, rectal, and tympanic membrane–derived temperature changes after ingestion of liquids and smoking, *Am J Emerg Med* 7(2):150-154, 1989.

Terndrup TE, Milewski A: The performance of two tympanic thermometers in a pediatric emergency department, *Clin Pediatr* 30(4, suppl):18-23, 1991.

Terndrup TE, Rajk J: Impact of operator technique and device on infrared emission detection tympanic thermometry, *J Emerg Med* 10:683-687, 1992.

Tourangeau A, MacLeod F, Breakwell M: Tap in on ear thermometry, *Can Nurse* 89(8):24-28, 1993.

Treloar D, Muma B: Comparision of axillary, tympanic membrane, and rectal temperatures in young children, *Ann Emerg Med* 17(4):435, 1988.

Vaughan VC: On the utility of growth curves, *JAMA* 267(7):975-976, 1992.

Vessey J, Braithwaite K, Widemann M: Teaching children about their internal bodies, *Pediatr Nurs* 16(1):29-33, 1990.

Weir M, Weir T: Are 'hot' ears really hot? *Am J Dis Child* 143(7):763-764, 1989.

Weiss ME: Tympanic infrared thermometry for full-term and preterm neonates, *Clin Pediatr* 30(4, suppl):42-45, 1991.

Wong DL: Lending a hand to the ear exam, *Contemp Pediatr* 9(7):115, 1992.

Yip R, Scanlon K, Trowbridge F: Improving growth status of Asian refugee children in the United States, *JAMA* 267(7):937-940, 1992.

Zehner WJ, Terndrup TE: The impact of moderate ambient temperature variance on the relationship between oral, rectal, and tympanic membrane temperatures, *Clin Pediatr* 30(4, suppl):61-64, 1991.

BIBLIOGRAPHY

Physical Assessment

Banco L, Jayashekaramurthy S, Graffam J: The inability of a temperature-sensitive pacifier to identify fevers in ill infants, *Am J Dis Child* 142:171-172, 1988.

Barness LA: *Manual of pediatric physical diagnosis,* ed 6, St Louis, 1991, Mosby.

Beach PS, McCormick DP: Editorial comment: clinical applications of ear thermometry, *Clin Pediatr* 30(4, suppl):3-4, 1991.

Betts PR, Voss LD, Bailey BJR: Measuring the heights of very young children, *Br Med J* 304:1351-1352, 1992.

Blondis TA, Snow JH, Accardo PJ: Integration of soft signs in academically normal and academically at-risk children, *Pediatrics* 85:421-425, 1990.

Borders CF: Strabismus/amblyopia: when to refer, *Patient Care* 18:21-52, 1984.

Bowers A, Thompson J: *Clinical manual of health assessment,* ed 4, St Louis, 1992, Mosby.

Brown MS, Murphy MA: *Ambulatory pediatrics for nurses,* ed 2, New York, 1980, McGraw-Hill.

Browning G, Swan I: Sensitivity and specificity of Rinne tuning fork test, *Br Med J* 297(6660):1381-1382, 1988.

Cibis G, Waeltermann J: Rapid strabismus screening for the pediatrician, *Clin Pediatr* 25(6):304-307, 1986.

Combs JT: Two useful tools for exploring the middle ear, *Contemp Pediatr* 10(11):60-75, 1993.

Crouch ER Jr, Crouch ER: Pediatric vision screening: Why? When? What? How? *Contemp Pediatr* 8:9-30, 1991.

Cunningham DR: Auditory screening. In Hoekelman RA and others, editors: *Primary pediatric care,* ed 2, St Louis, 1992, Mosby.

Delancy VL, North C: Skin assessment, *Top Clin Nurs* 5(2):5-10, 1983.

DiChiara E: A sound method for testing children's hearing, *Am J Nurs* 84(9):1104-1106, 1984.

Donham J: Rales and rhonchi: why do we use these terms? *Focus Crit Care* 11(5):20-22, 1984.

Egan D, Brown R: Vision testing of young children in the age range 18 months to 4½ years, *Child Care Health Dev* 10:381-390, 1984.

Elvik SL: Vaginal discharge in the prepubertal girl, *J Pediatr Health Care* 4:181-185, 1990.

Engel J: *Pocket guide to pediatric assessment,* ed 2, St Louis, 1993, Mosby.

Erickson B: *Heart sounds and murmurs: a practical guide,* ed 2, St Louis, 1991, Mosby.

Frary T: Pediatric examination pearls, *J Am Acad Physician Assist* 1(5):389-390, 1988.

Gammon JA: Visual system screening in infants and young children, *Pediatr Rev* 4(3):71-73, 1982.

Gemberling C: The adolescent gynecologic examination: an overview, *J Pediatr Health Care* 1(3):141-151, 1987.

Gershel J and others: Accuracy of the Welch Allyn AudioScope and traditional hearing screening for children with known hearing loss, *J Pediatr* 106(1):15-20, 1985.

Greene J: Making adolescent space in a pediatric office, *Pediatr Nurs* 15(4):402-404, 1989.

Grimes C: Audiologic evaluation in infancy and childhood, *Pediatr Ann* 14(3):210, 1985.

Gundy JH: The pediatric physical examination. In Hoekelman RA and others, editors: *Primary pediatric care,* ed 2, St Louis, 1992, Mosby.

Guo S, Roche A, Moore W: Reference data for head circumference and 1-month increments from 1 to 12 months of age, *J Pediatr* 113(3):490-494, 1988.

Hamill B: Comparing two methods of preschool and kindergarten hearing screening, *J Sch Health* 58(3):95-97, 1988.

Harris JA: Pediatric abdominal assessment, *Pediatr Nurs* 12(5):355-362, 1986.

Heidenreich T, Giuffre M: Postoperative temperature measurement, *Nurs Res* 39(3):153-155, 1990.

Hoekelmann R: An appraisal of the effectiveness of child health supervision, *Curr Opin Pediatr* 1(1):146-155, 1989.

Holte L, Cavanaugh RM Jr, Margolis RH: Ear canal wall mobility and tympanometric shape in young infants, *J Pediatr* 117(1, pt 1):77-80, 1990.

Johnson A, Stayte M, Wortham C: Vision screening at 8 and 18 months, *Br Med J* 299:545-549, 1989.

Killam P: Orthopedic assessment of young children: developmental variations, *Nurse Pract* 14(7):27-28, 1989.

Kirschen D, Rosenbaum A, Ballard E: The dot visual acuity test—a new acuity test for children, *J Am Optom Assoc* 54(12):1055-1059, 1983.

Kresch M: Axillary temperature as a screening test for fever in children, *J Pediatr* 104(4):596-599, 1984.

Kronmiller J: Oral soft tissue abnormalities in children, *Pediatr Nurs,* 13(3):161-165, 1987.

Lieber MT, Taub AS: Common foot deformities and what they mean for parents, *MCN* 13(1):47-50, 1988.

Lilly JR, Bailey WC: Pectus excavatum *Pediatrics* 91(3):677, 1993 (letter to the editor).

Linley JF: Screening children for common orthopedic problems, *Am J Nurs* 87(10):1312-1316, 1987.

MacPhee M, Mori C: Teaching nurses about neuromotor development: an evaluative study, *Pediatr Nurs* 17(5):438-442, 444, 1991.

Marks A, Fisher M: Health assessment and screening during adolescence, *Pediatrics* 80(1):135-158, 1987.

Mason KJ: Pediatric orthopaedics: development norms, *Orthop Nurs* 8(4):45-50, 1989.

McClellan MA: The use of the physical examination to promote development of the preschooler, *Child Health Care* 12(4):174-178, 1984.

Moss JR: Helping young children cope with the physical examination, *Pediatr Nurs* 7(2):17-20, 1981.

Moss JR: Predicting young children's cooperation with the physical examination, *Pediatr Nurs* 9(3):188-190, 1983.

Norton SJ: Application of transient evoked otoacoustic emissions to pediatric populations, *Ear Hear* 14(1):64-73, 1993.

Olk D: Quieting the disruptive sibling, *Contemp Pediatr* 6(10):116, 1989.

Olness K and others: Height and weight status of Indochinese refugee children, *Am J Dis Child* 138:544-547, 1984.

Poets CF and others: Breathing patterns and heart rates at ages 6 weeks and 2 years, *Am J Dis Child* 145:1393-1396, 1991.

Pulmonary terms and symbols: A report of the ACCP-ATS joint committee on pulmonary nonmenclature, *Chest* 67(5):583-593, 1975.

Rieser P: Role of the school nurse in the assessment of linear growth, *Community Nurs Forum* 4(1):1-12, 1987.

Rhoads FA, Grandner J: Assessment of an aural infrared sensor for body temperature measurement in children, *Clin Pediatr* 29(2):112-115, 1990.

Roche A, Guo S, Moore W: Weight and recumbent length from 1 to 12 mo of age: reference data for 1-mo increments, *Am J Clin Nur* 49:599-607, 1989.

Roche A and others: Head circumference reference data: birth to 18 years, *Pediatrics* 79(5):706-712, 1987.

Sackett DL, Rennie D: The science of the art of the clinical examination, *JAMA* 267(19):2650-2652, 1992.

Sane K, Pescovitz OH: The clitoral index: a determination of clitoral size in normal girls and in girls with abnormal sexual development, *J Pediatr* 120(2, pt 1):264-266, 1992.

Sanet R, Ellis G: What is the most effective vision screening tool to use with preschool-age children in early childhood programs? *School Nurse* 6:27-31, 1990.

Schubiner H: Preventive health screening in adolescent patients, *Prim Care* 16(1):211-230, 1989.

Schuman AJ: Taking the pain—and fear—out of office visits, *Contemp Pediatr* 8(4):81-87, 1991.

Seidel H and others: *Mosby's guide to physical examination,* ed 2, St Louis, 1991, Mosby.

Shinozaki T, Deane R, Perkins F: Infrared tympanic thermometer: evaluation of a new clinical thermometer, *Crit Care Med* 16(2):148, 1988.

Solomon J: Physical assessment skills in undergraduate curricula, *Nurs Outlook* 38(4):194-195, 1990.

Stata K: Improving hearing screening programs in the elementary school, *School Nurse* 4(3):16-19, 1988.

Strahlman ER: Vision screening. In Hoekelman RA and others, editors: *Primary pediatric care,* ed 2, St Louis, 1992, Mosby.

Sullivan L: How effective is preschool vision, hearing, and developmental screening? *Pediatr Nurs* 14(3):181-183, 1988.

Szydlo V: Approaching an adolescent about a pelvic exam, *Am J Nurs* 88(11):1502-1506, 1988.

Talbot C: The gynecologic examination of the pediatric patient, *Pediatr Ann* 15(7):501-508, 1986.

Tanner JM, Davies PSW: Clinical longitudinal standards for height and height velocity for North American children, *J Pediatr* 107(3):317-329, 1985.

Thomas I, Gaitantzis Y, Frias J: Palpebral fissure length from 29 weeks gestation to 14 years, *J Pediatr* 111(2):267-268, 1987.

Tolmas HC: Adolescent pelvic examination: an effective practical approach, *Am J Dis Child* 145:1269-1271, 1991.

Wasserman RC: Screening for vision problems in pediatric practice, *Pediatr Rev* 13(1):4-5, 1992.

Westsrate J, Deurenberg P: Body composition in children: proposal for a method for calculating body fat percentage from total body density of skinfold-thickness measurements, *Am J Clin Nutr* 50:1104-1115, 1989.

Wilkins RL, Hodgkin JE, Lopez B: *Lung sounds: a practical guide,* St Louis, 1988, Mosby.

Wong DL: The paper-doll technique, *Pediatr Nurs* 7(6):39-40, 1981.

Yacone-Morton L: Cardiac assessment, *RN* 54(12):28-34, 1991.

Yoos L: A developmental approach to physical assessment, *MCN* 6(3):168-170, 1981.

Developmental Assessment

Adesman AR: Is the Denver II Developmental Test worthwhile? *Pediatrics* 90(6):1009-1010, 1992 (letter to the editor).

Allen MC, Alexander GR: Gross motor milestones in preterm infants: correction for degree of prematurity, *J Pediatr* 116(6):955-959, 1990.

American Academy of Pediatrics, Committee on Children with Disabilities: Screening for developmental disabilities, *Pediatrics* 78(3):526-528, 1986.

Burgess D and others: Parent report as a means of administering the Prescreening Developmental Questionnaire: An evaluation study, *Dev Behav Pediatr* 5(4):195-200, 1984.

Casey PH, Swanson M: A pediatric perspective of developmental screening in 1993, *Clin Pediatr* 32(4):209-212, 1993.

Casey PH and others: Developmental intervention: a pediatric clinical review, *Pediatr Clin North Am* 33(4):899-923, 1986.

Dworkin P: British and American recommendations for developmental monitoring: the role of surveillance, *Pediatrics* 84(6):1000-1010, 1989.

Dworkin P: Developmental screening—expecting the impossible? *Pediatrics* 83(4):619-621, 1989.

Finney JW, Weist MD: Behavioral assessment of children and adolescents, *Pediatr Clin North Am* 39(3):369-378, 1992.

Frankenburg WK, Chen J, Thornton S: Common pitfalls in the evaluation of developmental screening tests, *J Pediatr* 113(5):1110-1113, 1988.

Frankenburg WK, Thornton S: A child development program for a busy office practice, *Contemp Pediatr* 6(2):90-106, 1989.

Glascoe F, Byrne K: Is the Denver II Developmental Test worthwhile? *Pediatrics* 90(6):1010-1011, 1992 (reply to the editor).

Meisels SJ: Uses and abuses of developmental screening and school readiness testing, *Young Child* 42(2):4-9, 1987.

Meisels SJ: Can developmental screening tests identify children who are developmentally at risk? *Pediatrics* 83(4), 1989.

Ouden LD and others: Is it correct to correct? Developmental milestones in 555 "normal" preterm infants compared with term infants, *J Pediatr* 118(3):399-404, 1991.

Sameroff AJ: Environmental context of child development, *J Pediatr* 109(1):192-200, 1986.

Schnelle E: Kindergarten neurodevelopmental screening: the school nurse's role, *School Nurse* 4(3):10-14, 1988.

Simner ML: School readiness and the Draw-A-Man Test: an empirically derived alternative to Harris' scoring system, *J Learn Disabil* 18 (2):77-82, 1985.

Squires JK, Nickel R, Bricker D: Use of parent-completed developmental questionnaires for child-find and screening, *Infants Young Child* 3(2):46-57, 1990.

Steele SM: Assessing developmental delays in preschool children, *J Pediatr Health Care* 2(3):141-145, 1988.

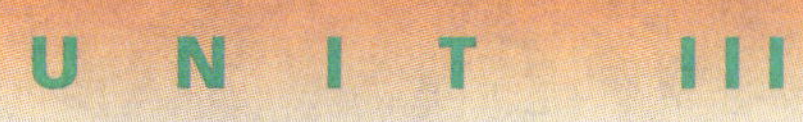

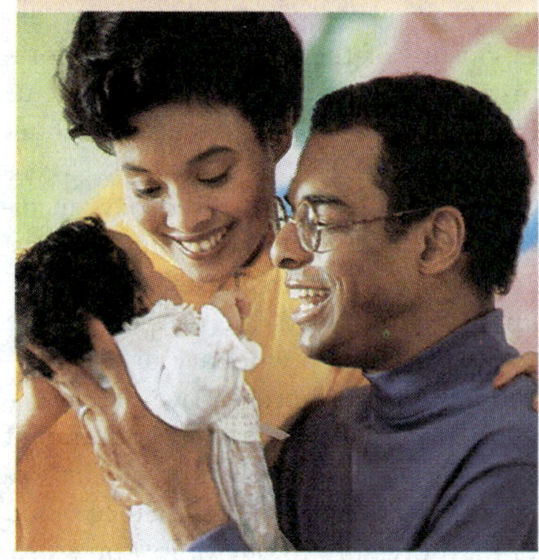

FAMILY-CENTERED CARE OF THE NEWBORN

CHAPTER 8 Health Promotion of the Newborn and Family

CHAPTER OUTLINE

RELATED TOPICS

Abnormal sexual development, Ch. 11
Administration of medication, Ch. 27
Birth injuries, Ch. 9
Blood specimens, Ch. 27
Breast-feeding problems, Ch. 13
Cardiac development and function: embryologic development, Ch. 34
Changes in fluid volume related to growth, Ch. 28
Congenital heart disease, Ch. 34
Dermatologic problems in the newborn, Ch. 9
Diaper dermatitis, Ch. 13
Fluoride, Ch. 14
The high-risk newborn and family, Ch. 10
Motor vehicle injuries, Chs. 12 and 14
Multiple births, Ch. 3
Nutrition, Ch. 12
Physical examination, Ch. 7
Sibling rivalry, Ch. 14
The skin, Ch. 18

ADJUSTMENT TO EXTRAUTERINE LIFE

The most profound physiologic change required of the newborn is transition from fetal or placental circulation to independent respiration. The loss of the placental connection means the loss of complete metabolic support, especially the supply of oxygen and the removal of carbon dioxide. The normal stresses of labor and delivery produce alterations of placental gas exchange patterns, acid-base balance in the blood, and cardiovascular activity in the neonate. Factors that interfere with this normal transition or increase fetal ***asphyxia*** (a condition of hypoxemia, hypercapnia, and acidosis) will affect the fetus's adjustment to extrauterine life.

IMMEDIATE ADJUSTMENTS

Respiratory System

The most critical and immediate physiologic change required of the newborn is the onset of breathing. The stimuli that help initiate the first respiration are primarily chemical and thermal. ***Chemical factors*** in the blood (low oxygen, high carbon dioxide, and low pH) initiate impulses that excite the respiratory center in the medulla. The primary ***thermal stimulus*** is the sudden chilling of the infant who leaves a warm environment and enters a relatively cooler atmosphere. This abrupt change in temperature excites sensory impulses in the skin that are transmitted to the respiratory center.

The significance of ***tactile stimulation*** is questionable. Descent through the birth canal and normal handling during delivery, such as drying the skin, probably have some effect on initiation of respiration. Slapping the neonate's heel or buttocks has no beneficial effect; it can waste precious time in the event of respiratory difficulty and can cause additional damage if cerebral trauma has occurred.

The initial entry of air into the lungs is opposed by the surface tension of the fluid that filled the fetal lungs and alveoli. However, fetal lung fluid is removed by the pulmonary capillaries and lymphatic vessels. Some fluid is also removed during the normal forces of labor and delivery. As the chest emerges from the birth canal, fluid is squeezed from the lungs through the nose and mouth. Following complete emergence of the neonate's chest, a brisk recoil of the thorax occurs. Air enters the upper airway to replace the lost fluid. In cesarean birth the chest is not compressed, and the newborn may need additional respiratory support.

In the alveoli the surface tension of the fluid is reduced by ***surfactant,*** a substance produced by the alveolar epithelium that coats the alveolar surface. The effect of surfactant in facilitating breathing is discussed in relation to respiratory distress syndrome (see Chapter 10).

Circulatory System

Equally important as the initiation of respiration are the circulatory changes that allow blood to flow through the lungs. These changes occur more gradually and are the result of pressure changes in the lungs, heart, and major vessels. The transition from fetal circulation to postnatal circulation involves the functional closure of the fetal shunts: the foramen ovale, the ductus arteriosus, and eventually the ductus venosus. (For a brief review of fetal circulation, see Chapter 34.)

Once the lungs are expanded, the inspired oxygen dilates the pulmonary vessels, which decreases pulmonary vascular resistance and consequently increases pulmonary blood flow. As the lungs receive blood, the pressure in the right atrium, right ventricle, and pulmonary arteries decreases. At the same time there is a progressive rise in systemic vascular resistance from the increased volume of blood through the placenta at cord clamping. This increases the pressure in the left side of the heart. Since blood flows from an area of high pressure to one of low pressure, the circulation of blood through the fetal shunts is reversed (see Fig. 34-2).

The most important factor controlling ductal closure is the increased oxygen concentration of the blood. Secondary factors are the fall in endogenous prostaglandins and acidosis. The foramen ovale closes functionally at or soon after birth from compression of the two portions of the atrial septum. The ductus arteriosus is closed functionally by the fourth day. Anatomic closure from deposition of fibrin and cell products takes considerably longer. Failure of the ducts to close results in various types of congenital heart defects (see Chapter 34).

Because of the reversible flow of blood through the ducts during the early neonatal period, functional murmurs are occasionally heard. In conditions such as crying or straining, the increased pressure shunts unoxygenated blood from the right side of the heart across the ductal opening, causing transient cyanosis.

PHYSIOLOGIC STATUS OF OTHER SYSTEMS

The major life-dependent physiologic changes in the cardiovascular and respiratory systems of the newborn have already been discussed. However, all of the body systems undergo some change, and most systems are immature at birth. Each is observed closely for proper functioning and adjustment to extrauterine life.

Thermoregulation

Next to establishing respiration, heat regulation is most critical to the newborn's survival. Although the newborn's capacity for heat production is adequate, several factors predispose the newborn to excessive heat loss. First, the newborn's large surface area facilitates heat loss to the environment. The normal metabolic rate per unit weight of the newborn is about twice that of the adult, but the neonate's surface area per unit weight is about three times larger than that of the adult. Consequently, the infant produces only two thirds as much heat as an adult but loses twice as much heat per unit area. However, the large body surface is partially compensated for by the newborn's usual position of flexion, which decreases the amount of surface area exposed to the environment.

The second factor that retards the conservation of body heat is the newborn's thin layer of subcutaneous fat. Since core body temperature is approximately 1° F higher than surface body temperature, this temperature gradient (difference) causes a heat transfer from a higher to lower temperature.

A third factor is the newborn's mechanism for producing heat. Unlike the adult, who can increase heat production through shivering, the chilled neonate cannot shiver but produces heat through ***nonshivering thermogenesis (NST).*** NST is produced by stimulating cellular respiration; the resulting oxygen consumption can be three times the amount of any other body tissue (Bliss-Holtz, 1993) (see Thermoregulation, Chapter 10). A thermogenic source unique to the full-term newborn is ***brown adipose tissue (BAT),*** or ***brown fat,*** which owes its name to its larger content of mitochondrial cytochromes. BAT has a greater capacity for heat production through intensified metabolic activity than does ordinary adipose tissue. Heat generated in the brown fat is distributed to other parts of the body by the blood, which is warmed as it flows through the layers of this tissue. Superficial deposits of brown fat are located between the scapulae, around the neck, in the axillae, and behind the sternum. Deeper layers surround the kidneys, trachea, esophagus, some major arteries, and adrenals (Poissonnet, LaVelle, and Burdi, 1988). The location of the brown fat may explain why the nape of the neck often feels warmer than the rest of the body, and brown fat can affect the accuracy of axillary temperature measurement (see p. 302).

Although concern is usually for newborns' ability to conserve heat, they also can have difficulty dissipating heat in an overheated environment. This increases the risk of hyperthermia.

Hemopoietic System

The ***blood volume*** of the newborn depends on the amount of placental transfer of blood. The blood volume of the full-term infant is about 80 to 85 ml/kg of body weight. Immediately after birth the total blood volume averages 300 ml, but, depending on how long the infant is attached to the placenta, as much as 100 ml can be added to the blood volume. The blood values for the newborn are listed in Appendix D.

Fluid and Electrolyte Balance

Changes occur in the ***total body water volume,*** extracellular fluid volume, and intracellular fluid volume during the transition from fetal to postnatal life. Early in gestation the fetus is composed almost entirely of water and at term is 73% fluid, as compared with 58% in the adult. There is a higher level of extracellular fluid than intracellular fluid in the fetus, but this shifts progressively throughout postnatal life, probably because of the growth of cells at the expense of extracellular fluid. The infant has a proportionately higher ratio of extracellular fluid than the adult and consequently has a higher level of total body sodium and chloride and a lower level of potassium, magnesium, and phosphate (see Chapter 28).

A very important aspect of fluid balance is its relationship to other systems. Besides the rate of fluid exchange being seven times greater in the infant than in the adult, the infant's ***rate of metabolism*** is twice as great in relation to body weight. As a result, twice as much acid is formed, leading to more rapid development of acidosis. In addition, the immature kidneys cannot sufficiently concentrate urine to conserve body water. These three factors make the infant more prone to problems of dehydration, acidosis, and possible overhydration.

Gastrointestinal System

The ability of the newborn to digest, absorb, and metabolize foodstuff is adequate but limited in certain functions. ***Enzymes*** are available to catalyze proteins and simple carbohydrates (monosaccharides and disaccharides), but deficient production of pancreatic amylase impairs utilization of complex carbohydrates (polysaccharides). Deficiency of pancreatic lipase limits the absorption of fats, especially with ingestion of foods that have a high saturated fatty acid content, such as cow's milk.

The ***liver*** is the most immature of the gastrointestinal organs. The activity of the enzyme ***glucuronyl transferase*** is reduced, affecting the conjugation of bilirubin with glucuronic acid, which contributes to the physiologic jaundice of the newborn. The liver is also deficient in forming plasma proteins. The decreased plasma protein concentration probably plays a role in the edema usually seen at birth. Prothrombin and other coagulation factors are also low. The liver stores less glycogen at birth than later in life. Consequently, the newborn is prone to hypoglycemia, which may be prevented by early and effective feeding, especially breast-feeding.

Some ***salivary glands*** are functioning at birth, but the majority do not begin to secrete saliva until about age 2 to 3 months, when drooling is common. The stomach capacity is limited to about 90 ml; thus the infant requires frequent

CHANGE IN STOOLING PATTERNS OF NEWBORNS

MECONIUM

Infant's first stool; composed of amniotic fluid and its constituents, intestinal secretions, shed mucosal cells, and possibly blood (ingested maternal blood or minor bleeding of alimentary tract vessels).

Passage of meconium should occur within the first 24 to 48 hours, although it may be delayed up to 7 days in very-low-birth-weight infants (Verma and Dhanireddy, 1993).

TRANSITIONAL STOOLS

Usually appear by third day after initiation of feeding; greenish brown to yellowish brown, thin, and less sticky than meconium; may contain some milk curds.

MILK STOOL

Usually appears by fourth day.

In ***breast-fed infants*** stools are yellow to golden, are pasty in consistency, and have an odor similar to that of sour milk.

In ***formula-fed infants*** stools are pale yellow to light brown, are firmer in consistency, and have a more offensive odor.

small feedings. Since newborns who breast-feed have more frequent feedings, they may have more frequent stools than infants who bottle-feed. However, the pattern may change after the first few weeks.

The infant's ***intestine*** is longer in relation to body size than that in the adult. Therefore there are a larger number of secretory glands and a larger surface area for absorption as compared with the adult's intestine. There are rapid peristaltic waves and simultaneous nonperistaltic waves along the entire esophagus. These waves, combined with an immature relaxed cardiac sphincter, make regurgitation a common occurrence. Progressive changes in the stooling pattern indicate a properly functioning gastrointestinal tract (see box on p. 289).

Renal System

All structural components are present in the renal system, but there is a functional deficiency in the kidney's ability to concentrate urine and to cope with conditions of fluid and electrolyte fluctuations, such as dehydration or a concentrated solute load.

Total volume of urinary output per 24 hours is about 200 to 300 ml by the end of the first week. However, the bladder involuntarily empties when stretched by a volume of 15 ml, resulting in as many as 20 voidings per day. The first voiding should occur within 24 hours. The urine is colorless and odorless and has a specific gravity of approximately 1.020.

Integumentary System

At birth all the structures within the skin are present, but many of the functions of the integument are immature. The two layers of the skin, the ***epidermis*** and ***dermis,*** are loosely bound to each other and are very thin. Slight friction across the epidermis, such as from rapid removal of tape, can cause separation of these layers and blister formation. The transitional zone between the cornified and living layers of the epidermis is effective in preventing fluid from reaching the skin surface.

The ***sebaceous glands*** are very active late in fetal life and in early infancy because of high levels of maternal androgens. They are most densely located on the scalp, face, and genitalia and produce the grayish-white, greasy vernix caseosa that covers the infant at birth. Plugging of the sebaceous glands causes ***milia.***

The ***eccrine glands*** which produce sweat in response to heat or emotional stimuli, are functional at birth, and palmar sweating on crying reaches levels equivalent to those of anxious adults by 3 weeks of age. Observing palmar sweating is helpful in assessing pain (Harpin and Rutter, 1982). The eccrine glands produce sweat in response to higher temperatures than those required in adults, and the retention of sweat may result in miliaria.

The ***apocrine glands,*** sweat glands that develop as attachments to hair follicles, remain small and nonfunctional until puberty.

The growth phases of ***hair follicles*** usually occur simultaneously at birth. During the first few months the synchrony between hair loss and regrowth is disrupted, and there may be overgrowth of hair or temporary alopecia. Boys' hair grows faster than girls' hair, and in both sexes scalp hair growth is slower at the crown.

Because the amount of ***melanin*** is low at birth, newborns are lighter skinned than they will be as children. Consequently, infants are more susceptible to the harmful effects of the sun.

Musculoskeletal System

At birth the ***skeletal system*** contains larger amounts of cartilage than ossified bone, although the process of ossification is fairly rapid during the first year. The nose, for example, is predominantly cartilage at birth and is frequently flattened by the force of delivery. The six skull bones are relatively soft and not yet joined. The sinuses are incompletely formed as well.

Unlike the skeletal system, the ***muscular system*** is almost completely formed at birth. Growth in the size of muscular tissue is caused by hypertrophy, rather than hyperplasia, of cells.

Defenses Against Infection

The infant is born with several defenses against infection. The first line of defense is the ***skin*** and ***mucous membranes,*** which protect the body from invading organisms. The second line of defense is the ***cellular elements*** of the immunologic system, which produces several types of cells capable of attacking a pathogen. The ***neutrophils*** and ***monocytes*** are phagocytes, cells that engulf, ingest, and destroy foreign agents. ***Eosinophils*** also probably have a phagocytic property, since in the presence of foreign protein they increase in number. The ***lymphocytes*** (T- and B-cells) are capable of being converted to other cell types, such as monocytes and antibodies. Although the phagocytic properties of the blood are present in the infant, the inflammatory response of the tissues to localize an infection is immature.

The third line of defense is the formation of specific ***antibodies*** to an antigen. This process requires exposure to various foreign agents for antibody production to occur. Infants are generally not capable of producing their own immunoglobulins (Ig) until the beginning of the second month of life, but they receive considerable passive immunity in the form of IgG from the maternal circulation and from human milk (see pp. 317-318). They are protected against most major childhood diseases, including diphtheria, measles, poliomyelitis, and rubella, for about 3 months, provided the mother has developed antibodies to these illnesses.

Endocrine System

Ordinarily the endocrine system of the newborn is adequately developed, but its functions are immature. For example, the posterior lobe of the pituitary gland produces limited quantities of ***antidiuretic hormone (ADH),*** or ***vasopressin,*** which inhibits diuresis. This renders the newborn highly susceptible to dehydration.

The effect of maternal ***sex hormones*** is particularly evident in the newborn. The labia are hypertrophied, and the breasts in both sexes may be engorged and secrete milk (witch's milk) during the first few days of life to as long as 2 months of age (Madlon-Kay, 1986). Female newborns may have ***pseudomenstruation*** (more often seen as a milky secretion rather than actual blood) from a sudden drop in progesterone and estrogen levels.

Neurologic System

At birth the nervous system is incompletely integrated but sufficiently developed to sustain extrauterine life. Most neurologic functions are ***primitive reflexes.*** The ***autonomic nervous system*** is crucial during transition because it stimulates initial respirations, helps maintain acid-base balance, and partially regulates temperature control.

Myelination of the nervous system follows the cephalocaudal-proximodistal (head-to-toe—center-to-periphery) laws of development and is closely related to the observed mastery of fine and gross motor skills. ***Myelin*** is necessary for rapid and efficient transmission of some, but not all, nerve impulses along the neural pathway. Tracts that develop myelin earliest are the sensory, cerebellar, and extrapyramidal. This accounts for the acute senses of taste, smell, and hearing, as well as the perception of pain, in the newborn. All ***cranial nerves*** are myelinated except the optic and olfactory nerves.

Sensory Functions

The newborn's sensory functions are remarkably well developed and have a significant effect on growth and development, including the attachment process.

Vision. At birth the eye is structurally incomplete. The ***fovea centralis*** is not yet completely differentiated from the macula. The ***ciliary muscles*** are also immature, limiting the ability of the eyes to accommodate and fixate on an object for any length of time. The ***pupils*** react to light, the blink reflex is responsive to a minimal stimulus, and the corneal reflex is activated by a light touch. ***Tear glands*** usually do not begin to function until the infant is 2 to 4 weeks of age.

The newborn has the ability to momentarily fixate on a bright or moving object that is within 20 cm (8 inches) and in the midline of the visual field. In fact, the infant's ability to fixate on coordinate movement is greater during the first hour of life than during the succeeding several days. ***Visual acuity*** is reported to be between 20/100 and 20/400, depending on the vision measurement techniques (see Table 7-11).

The infant also demonstrates visual preferences: medium colors (yellow, green, pink) over dim or bright colors (red, orange, blue); black and white contrasting patterns, especially geometric shapes and checkerboards; large objects with medium complexity rather than small, complex objects; and reflecting objects over dull ones.

Hearing. Once the amniotic fluid has drained from the ears, the infant probably has ***auditory acuity*** similar to that of an adult. The newborn is able to detect a loud sound of about 90 decibels and reacts with a startle reflex. The newborn's response to sounds of low frequency and high frequency differs; the former, such as a heartbeat, metronome, or lullaby, tends to decrease an infant's motor activity and crying, whereas the latter elicits an alerting reaction.

There is an early sensitivity to the sound of human voices and to specific speech sounds. For example, infants younger than 3 days of age can discriminate the mother's voice from that of other females (DeCasper and Fifer, 1980). As early as age 5 days newborns can differentiate between stories repeated to them during the last trimester of pregnancy by their mother and the same stories recited after birth by a different woman (DeCasper and Spence, 1986).

The internal and middle ***ear*** structures are large at birth, but the external canal is small. The mastoid process and the bony part of the external canal have not yet developed. Consequently, the tympanic membrane and facial nerve are very close to the surface and can be easily damaged.

Smell. Newborns react to strong odors such as alcohol or vinegar by turning their heads away. Breast-fed infants are able to smell breast milk and will cry for their mothers when the breasts are engorged and leaking. Infants are also able to differentiate the breast milk of their mother from the breast milk of other women by the smell, and maternal odors are believed to influence the attachment process.

Taste. The newborn can distinguish between tastes, and various types of solutions elicit differing gustofacial reflexes. A tasteless solution elicits no facial expression; a sweet solution elicits an eager suck and a look of satisfaction; a sour solution causes the usual puckering of the lips; and a bitter liquid produces an angry, upset expression. For example, newborns prefer glucose and water to sterile water (Pete, 1989).

Touch. The newborn perceives tactile sensation in any part of the body, although the face (especially the mouth), hands, and soles of the feet seem to be most sensitive. There is increasing documentation that touch and motion are essential to normal growth and development (Gunzenhauser, 1990). Gentle patting of the back or rubbing of the abdomen usually elicits a calming response from the infant. However, painful stimuli, such as a pinprick, elicit an angry, upset response.

NURSING CARE OF THE NEWBORN AND FAMILY

❖ ASSESSMENT

The newborn requires thorough, skilled observation to ensure a satisfactory adjustment to extrauterine life. Physical assessment following delivery can be divided into four phases: (1) the initial assessment using the Apgar scoring system, (2) transitional assessment during the periods of reactivity, (3) assessment of gestational age, and (4) systematic physical examination. In addition, the nurse must be aware of those behaviors that signal successful attachment between the infant and parents. Awareness of the expected normal findings during each assessment process helps the nurse recognize any deviation that may prevent the infant from progressing uneventfully through the early postnatal period. With increasingly shorter labor, delivery, recovery, and postpartum admission, the accomplishment of thorough newborn assessment and parent teaching has become a challenge (see also p. 328).

TABLE 8-1 Infant Evaluation at Birth—Apgar Scoring System

SIGN	0	1	2
Heart rate	Absent	Slow, <100	>100
Respiratory effort	Absent	Irregular, slow	Good, strong cry
Muscle tone	Limp	Some flexion of extremities	Well flexed
Reflex irritability	No response	Grimace	Cry, sneeze
Color	Blue, pale	Body pink, extremities blue	Completely pink

Initial Assessment: Apgar Scoring

The most frequently used method to assess the newborn's immediate adjustment to extrauterine life is the ***Apgar scoring system.*** The score is based on observation of heart rate, respiratory effort, muscle tone, reflex irritability, and color (Table 8-1). Each item is given a score of 0, 1, or 2. Evaluations of all five categories are made 1 and 5 minutes after birth and are repeated until the infant's condition stabilizes. Total scores of 0 to 3 represent severe distress, scores of 4 to 6 signify moderate difficulty, and scores of 7 to 10 indicate absence of difficulty in adjusting to extrauterine life. Many healthy newborns do not achieve a score of 10 because the body is not completely pink. The Apgar score is affected by the degree of prematurity, maternal sedation or analgesia, and neuromuscular disorders (American Academy of Pediatrics, 1986).

The Apgar score reflects the general condition of the infant at 1 and 5 minutes based on the five parameters described above. The Apgar score is not a tool, however, that stands on its own to either interpret past events or predict future events linked to the infant's eventual neurologic or physical status. There has been a considerable amount of discussion and controversy in the past about Apgar scoring because of its misuse as an indicator for the presence or absence of perinatal asphyxia in the medicolegal field (Annotations, 1992). In addition, the Apgar score is not used to determine the newborn's need for resuscitation at birth (American Academy of Pediatrics, 1990a).

Transitional Assessment: Periods of Reactivity

The newborn exhibits behavioral and physiologic characteristics that can at first appear to be signs of stress. However, during the initial 24 hours changes in heart rate, respiration, motor activity, color, mucus production, and bowel activity occur in an orderly, predictable sequence, which is normal and indicates lack of stress. Distressed infants also progress through these stages but at a slower rate.

For 6 to 8 hours after birth the newborn is in the ***first period of reactivity.*** During the first 30 minutes the infant is very alert, cries vigorously, may suck a fist greedily, and appears very interested in the environment. At this time the neonate's eyes are usually open, suggesting that this is an excellent opportunity for mother, father, and child to see each other. Because the newborn has a vigorous suck reflex, this is an opportune time to begin breast-feeding. The newborn usually grasps the nipple quickly, satisfying both mother and child. This is particularly important to remember, since it is likely that after this initially highly active state the infant may be quite sleepy and uninterested in sucking. Physiologically the respiratory rate can be as high as 80 breaths/min, rales may be heard, heart rate may reach 180 beats/min, bowel sounds are active, mucus secretions are increased, and temperature may decrease slightly.

After this initial stage of alertness and activity, the infant enters the ***second stage*** of the first reactive period, which generally lasts 2 to 4 hours. Heart and respiratory rates decrease, temperature continues to fall, mucus production decreases, and urine or stool is usually not passed. The infant is in a state of sleep and relative calm. Any attempt at stimulation usually elicits a minimal response. Because of the decrease in body temperature, avoid undressing or bathing the infant during this time.

The ***second period of reactivity*** begins when the infant awakes from this deep sleep; it lasts about 2 to 5 hours, and provides another excellent opportunity for child and parents to interact. The infant is again alert and responsive, heart and respiratory rates increase, the gag reflex is active, gastric and respiratory secretions are increased, and passage of meconium commonly occurs. This period is usually over when the amount of respiratory mucus has decreased. Following this stage is a period of stabilization of physiologic systems and a vacillating pattern of sleep and activity.

Behavioral Assessment

Another important area of assessment is observation of behavior. Infants' behavior helps shape their environment, and their ability to react to various stimuli affects how others relate to them. The principal areas of behavior for newborns are sleep, wakefulness, and activity, such as crying.

CLUSTERS OF NEONATAL BEHAVIORS IN BRAZELTON NEONATAL BEHAVIORAL ASSESSMENT SCALE

Habituation—Ability to respond to and then inhibit responding to discrete stimulus (light, rattle, bell, pinprick) while asleep
Orientation—Quality of alert states and ability to attend to visual and auditory stimuli while alert
Motor performance—Quality of movement and tone
Range of state—Measure of general arousal level or arousability of infant
Regulation of state—How infant responds when aroused
Autonomic stability—Signs of stress (tremors, startles, skin color) related to homeostatic (self-regulating) adjustment of the nervous system
Reflexes—Assessment of several neonatal reflexes

One method of systematically assessing the infant's behavior is use of the ***Brazelton Neonatal Behavioral Assessment Scale (BNBAS)*** (Brazelton, 1984). The BNBAS is an interactive examination that assesses the infant's response to 28 items organized according to the clusters in the box on p. 292. It is generally used as a research or diagnostic tool and requires special training.

In addition to its use as an initial and ongoing tool to assess neurologic and behavioral responses, the scale can be used as an assessor of initial parent-child relationships, as a preventive instrument that identifies the caregiver as one who may benefit from a role model, and as a guide for parents to help them focus on their infant's individuality and to develop a deeper attachment to their child. Studies have demonstrated that by showing parents the unique characteristics of their infant, a more positive perception of the infant develops, with increased interaction between infant and parent (Beal, 1989)

Patterns of Sleep and Activity. Newborns begin life with a systematic schedule of sleep and activity that is initially evident during the periods of reactivity. For the next 2 to 3 days it is not unusual for infants to sleep almost constantly in order to recover from the exhausting birth process.

The infant's sleep comprises five distinct states; ***state*** refers to an interaction between the infant and the environment in which the infant's behaviors form a continuum from arousal to consciousness (Keefe and others, 1989) (Table 8-2). The cycle of these sleep states is highly variable and is based on the number of hours an infant sleeps per day, which may range anywhere from 10½ to 23 hours (average of 16½ hours). About 50% of total sleep time is spent in irregular or rapid eye movement (REM) sleep. Sleep periods last 20 minutes to 6 hours with little day-night differentiation (Ferber, 1987).

States of sleep and periods of activity are highly influenced by environmental stimuli. As early as the immediate postbirth period, state is influenced by type of care. The sleep of infants in mothers' rooms is significantly more quiet, and they cry less than infants in the nursery (Keefe, 1987). It is especially important for parents to understand these states and the methods effective in altering them. An aware infant exhibits more motor activity before feeding than after. Feeding usually terminates the state of crying when hunger is the cause. Usually swaddling or wrapping an infant snugly in a blanket both promotes sleep and maintains body temperature. Intermittent, vertical rocking promotes more bright-alert behavior, whereas continuous, horizontal rocking induces more drowsy behavior.

Cry. The newborn should begin extrauterine life with a strong, lusty cry. The sounds produced by crying can be described as hunger, anger, pain, and "bid for attention" cries. Discomfort (pain) sounds initially consist of gasps and cries in which the consonant *H* is clearly distinguishable. The duration of crying is as highly variable in each infant as is the duration of sleep patterns. Some newborns may

TABLE 8-2 States of Sleep and Activity

BEHAVIOR	DURATION	IMPLICATIONS FOR PARENTING
REGULAR SLEEP		
Closed eyes Regular breathing No movement except for sudden bodily jerks	4-5 hours/day, 10-20 minutes/sleep cycle	External stimuli do not arouse infant Continue usual house noises Leave infant alone if sudden loud noise awakens infant and child cries
IRREGULAR SLEEP		
Closed eyes Irregular breathing Slight muscular twitching of body	12-15 hours/day, 20-45 minutes/sleep cycle	External stimuli that did not arouse infant during regular sleep may minimally arouse child Periodic groaning or crying is usual; do not interpret as an indication of pain or discomfort
DROWSINESS		
Eyes may be open Irregular breathing Active body movement	Variable	Most stimuli arouse infant Pick infant up during this time rather than leave in crib
ALERT INACTIVITY		
Responds to environment by active body movement and staring at close-range objects	2-3 hours/day	Satisfy infant's needs such as hunger Place infant in area of home where activity is continuous Place toys in crib or playpen Place objects within 17.5-20 cm (7-8 inches) of infant's view
WAKING AND CRYING*		
May begin with whimpering and slight body movement Progresses to strong, angry crying, and uncoordinated thrashing of extremities	1-4 hours/day	Remove intense internal or external stimuli Stimuli that were effective during alert inactivity are usually ineffective Rock and swaddle to decrease crying

*Some classifications divide the fifth state into two states; alert with activity and crying.

cry for as little as 5 minutes or as much as 2 hours or more per day.

Variations in the initial cry can indicate abnormalities. A weak, groaning cry or grunt during expiration usually indicates severe respiratory disturbances. Absent, weak, or constant crying may suggest brain damage. A high-pitched, shrill cry may be a sign of increased intracranial pressure.

Assessment of Attachment Behaviors

One of the most important areas of assessment is careful observation of those behaviors that are thought to indicate the formation of emotional bonds between the newborn and family, especially the mother. Although the words "bonding" and "attachment" are sometimes referred to as separate phenomena, with ***bonding*** representing the development of emotional ties from parent to infant and ***attachment*** representing the emotional ties from infant to parent, in this discussion and in the one on pp. 324-328 the words are used interchangeably to denote both processes.

Unlike physical assessment of the neonate, which has concrete guidelines to follow, assessment of parent-child attachment requires much more skill in terms of observation and interviewing. The assessment process is even more challenging with the trend toward 24-hour delivery and postpartum admissions. However, rooming-in of mother and infant and liberal visiting privileges for father, siblings, and grandparents facilitate recognition of behaviors that demonstrate positive or negative attachment. Guidelines for assessment of bonding behaviors are presented in the Guidelines box.

Talking to the parents uncovers many variables that can affect the development of attachment and parenting (see also Child Maltreatment, Chapter 16). What expectations do they have for this child? In other words, how similar are their predictions of the fantasy child and their realizations about the real child? Encourage them to talk about their relationship with their own parents, since the type of parenting that parents received as a child influences their childrearing practices. Is this a planned birth? How do they see the addition of a dependent family member affecting their life-style? What arrangements have they made in terms of such changes in life-style? What "support system" or significant others are available for assistance? What are their views regarding childrearing?

The labor process also significantly affects the immediate attachment of mothers to their newborn children. Factors such as a long labor, feeling tired or "drugged" after delivery, and problems with breast-feeding can delay the development of initial positive feelings toward the newborn (Pascoe and French, 1989).

During pregnancy, and often even before conception occurs, parents develop an image of the "ideal or fantasy infant." The unborn child has an imagined appearance, pattern of behavior, expected accomplishments, and predetermined effect on the life-style of the family. At birth the fantasy infant becomes the real infant. How closely the dream child resembles the real child influences the bonding process. Assessing such expectations during pregnancy and at the time of the infant's birth allows identification of discrepancies in the parents' view of the fantasy child vs the real child.

The ***Neonatal Perception Inventory (NPI)*** (Broussard, 1979) assessed the mother's perception of her real infant as compared with her image of an "average" infant. It has been hypothesized that for optimum mothering to occur, the mother needs to see her infant as better than an "average" baby. Mothers who do not rate their infants as better than average may be at risk for developing parenting abilities that fail to meet the infant's needs. The NPI II (completed 4 weeks after delivery) accurately predicted later childhood adjustment problems, whereas the NPI I (completed 1 to 2 days after the infant's birth) did not (Broussard, 1976). In follow-up studies over a 19-year period (Broussard, 1984), infants who were negatively perceived had the greatest risk for developing mental disorders.

Since attachment involves a mutually reciprocal interchange, observing the interaction between parent and infant is very important. An excellent opportunity exists during feeding. A useful instrument for systematically describing the parent's and infant's behaviors is the ***Nursing Child Assessment Feeding Scale (NCAFS)*** (Barnard, 1994). It consists of 76 behavioral items; 50 items describe the parent's behavior regarding (1) sensitivity to cues, (2) response to child's distress, (3) social-emotional growth fosterings, and (4) cognitive growth fostering. Twenty-six items focus on the child's behavior in terms of (1) clarity of cues and (2) responsiveness to parent. The results can also be shared with the parent to encourage discussion of feelings about the infant and to highlight behaviors of the dyad that foster successful interaction (Fuller, 1990). The NCAFS is appropriate for use with infants during the first year. Training to become a certificate tester is available through the

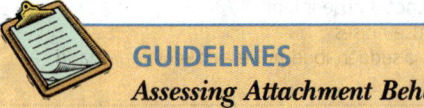

GUIDELINES
Assessing Attachment Behavior

When the infant is brought to the parents, do they reach out for the child and call the child by name?
Do the parents speak about the child in terms of identification—whom the infant looks like; what appears special about their child over other infants?
When parents are holding the infant, what kind of body contact is there—do parents feel at ease in changing the infant's position; are fingertips or whole hands used; are there parts of the body they avoid touching or parts of the body they investigate and scrutinize?
When the infant is awake, what kinds of stimulation do the parents provide—do they talk to the infant, to each other, or to no one; how do they look at the infant—direct visual contact, avoidance of eye contact, or looking at other people or objects?
How comfortable do the parents appear in terms of caring for the infant? Do they express any concern regarding their ability or disgust for certain activities, such as changing diapers?
What type of affection do they demonstrate to the newborn, such as smiling, stroking, kissing, or rocking?
If the infant is fussy, what kinds of comforting techniques do the parents use, such as rocking, swaddling, talking, or stroking?

Nursing Child Assessment Satellite Training (NCAST) program.*

Assessment of Clinical Gestational Age

Assessment of gestational age is an important criterion because perinatal morbidity and mortality are related to gestational age and birth weight. A frequently used method of determining gestational age is the ***Simplified Assessment of Gestational Age*** by Ballard, Novack, and Driver (1979) (Fig. 8-1, *A*). The Ballard scale, an abbreviated version of the ***Dubowitz scale,*** can be used to measure gestational ages of infants between 35 and 42 weeks (Dubowitz and Dubowitz, 1977). It assesses six external physical and six neuromuscular signs. Each sign has a number score, and the cumulative score correlates with a maturity rating of from 26 to 44 weeks of gestation.

The ***New Ballard Scale,*** a revision of the original scale, can be used with newborns as young as 20 weeks of gestation. The tool has the same physical and neuromuscular sections but includes −1 and −2 scores that reflect signs of extremely premature infants, such as fused eyelids; imperceptible breast tissue; sticky friable transparent skin; no lanugo; and square-window (flexion of wrist) angle of greater than 90 degrees (see Fig. 8-1, *A,* and the description of the tests in the box below, left). The examination of infants with a gestational age of 20 weeks or less should be performed at a postnatal age of less than 12 hours. For infants with a gestational age of at least 26 weeks, the examination can be performed up to 96 hours after birth. The scale overestimates gestational age by 2 to 4 days in infants younger than 37 weeks of gestation, especially at gestational ages of 32 to 37 weeks (Ballard and others, 1991).

Weight Related to Gestational Age. The weight of the infant at birth also correlates with the incidence of perinatal morbidity and mortality. Since many infants who weigh less than 2500 g (5½ pounds) are not preterm by gestational age, there is often confusion between the preterm and the small-for-gestational-age infants; fetal growth, gestational age, and fetal maturity are closely related but are not synonymous. Maturity implies functional capacity—the degree to which the neonate's organ systems are able to adapt to the requirements of extrauterine life. Therefore gestational age is more closely related to fetal maturity than is birth weight. Because heredity influences size at birth, it is important to note the size of other family members as part of the assessment process.

Classification of infants at birth by both weight and gestational age provides a more satisfactory method for predicting mortality risks and providing guidelines for management of the neonate. The infant's birth weight, length, and head circumference are plotted on standardized graphs that identify normal values for gestational age (Fig. 8-1, *B*). The infant whose weight is ***appropriate for gestational age (AGA)*** (between 10th and 90th percentile) can be presumed to have grown at a normal rate regardless of the time of birth—preterm, term, or postterm. The infant who is ***large for gestational age (LGA)*** (above 90th percentile) can be presumed to have grown at an accelerated rate during fetal life; the ***small-for-gestational-age (SGA)*** infant (below 10th percentile) can be presumed to have grown at a re-

*For information contact Georgina Sumner, RN, MS, Director, NCAST, University of Washington, NCAST, WJ-10, Seattle, WA 98195; (206) 543-8528.

TESTS USED IN ASSESSING GESTATIONAL AGE

Posture. With infant quiet and in a supine position, observe degree of flexion in arms and legs. Muscle tone and degree of flexion increase with maturity. Full flexion of the arms and legs = 4.

Square window. With thumb supporting back of arm below wrist, apply gentle pressure with index and third fingers on dorsum of hand without rotating infant's wrist. Measure angle between base of thumb and forearm. Full flexion (hand lies flat on ventral surface of forearm) = 4.

Arm recoil. With infant supine, fully flex both forearms on upper arms, hold for 5 seconds; pull down on hands to fully extend and rapidly release arms. Observe rapidity and intensity of recoil to a state of flexion. A brisk return to full flexion = 4.

Popliteal angle. With infant supine and pelvis flat on a firm surface, flex lower leg on thigh and then flex thigh on abdomen. While holding knee with thumb and index finger, extend lower leg with index finger of other hand. Measure degree of angle behind knee (popliteal angle). An angle of less than 90 degrees = 5.

Scarf sign. With infant supine, support head in midline with one hand; use other hand to pull infant's arm across the shoulder so that infant's hand touches shoulder. Determine location of elbow in relation to midline. Elbow does not reach midline = 4.

Heel to ear. With infant supine and pelvis flat on a firm surface, pull foot as far as possible up toward ear on same side. Measure distance of foot from ear and degree of knee flexion (same as popliteal angle). Knees flexed with a popliteal angle of less than 10 degrees = 4.

GUIDELINES
Physical Examination of the Newborn

- Provide a normothermic and nonstimulating examination area
  - Undress only body area examined to prevent heat loss.
- Proceed in an orderly sequence (usually head to toe) with the following exceptions:
  - Perform all procedures that require quiet first, such as auscultating the lungs, heart, and abdomen.
  - Perform disturbing procedures, such as testing reflexes, last.
  - Measure head, chest, and length at same time to compare results.
- Proceed quickly to avoid stressing infant.
  - Check that equipment and supplies are working properly and are accessible.
- Comfort infant during and after examination; involve parent in the following:
  - Talk softly.
  - Hold infant's hands against chest.
  - Swaddle and hold.
  - Give pacifier or gloved finger to suck.

ESTIMATION OF GESTATIONAL AGE BY MATURITY RATING

NEUROMUSCULAR MATURITY

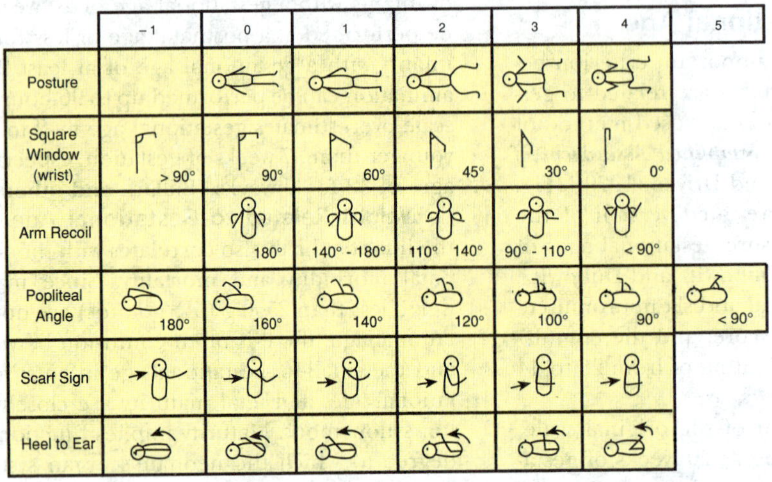

	-1	0	1	2	3	4	5
Posture							
Square Window (wrist)	> 90°	90°	60°	45°	30°	0°	
Arm Recoil		180°	140° - 180°	110° 140°	90° - 110°	< 90°	
Popliteal Angle	180°	160°	140°	120°	100°	90°	< 90°
Scarf Sign							
Heel to Ear							

A PHYSICAL MATURITY

Skin	sticky friable transparent	gelatinous red, translucent	smooth pink, visible veins	superficial peeling &/or rash, few veins	cracking pale areas rare veins	parchment deep cracking no vessels	leathery cracked wrinkled
Lanugo	none	sparse	abundant	thinning	bald areas	mostly bald	
Plantar Surface	heel-toe 40-50 mm: -1 <40 mm: -2	>50 mm no crease	faint red marks	anterior transverse crease only	creases ant. 2/3	creases over entire sole	
Breast	imperceptible	barely perceptible	flat areola no bud	stippled areola 1-2 mm bud	raised areola 3-4 mm bud	full areola 5-10 mm bud	
Eye/Ear	lids fused loosely: -1 tightly: -2	lids open pinna flat stays folded	sl. curved pinna; soft; slow recoil	well-curved pinna; soft but ready recoil	formed & firm instant recoil	thick cartilage ear stiff	
Genitals (male)	scrotum flat, smooth	scrotum empty faint rugae	testes in upper canal rare rugae	testes descending few rugae	testes down good rugae	testes pendulous deep rugae	
Genitals (female)	clitoris prominent labia flat	prominent clitoris small labia minora	prominent clitoris enlarging minora	majora & minora equally prominent	majora large minora small	majora cover clitoris & minora	

MATURITY RATING

score	weeks
-10	20
-5	22
0	24
5	26
10	28
15	30
20	32
25	34
30	36
35	38
40	40
45	42
50	44

FIG. 8-1 **A,** New Ballard Scale for newborn maturity rating. Expanded scale includes extremely premature infants and has been refined to improve accuracy in more mature infants. (**A** from Ballard JL and others: New Ballard Score, expanded to include extremely premature infants, *J Pediatr* 119:418, 1991.)

tarded rate during intrauterine life. Fig. 8-2 illustrates the disparity between birth weights of three preterm infants of the same gestational age and provides their associated risks of mortality. Birth weight and gestational age influence mortality—the lower the birth weight and gestational age, the higher the risk of mortality.

Physical Assessment

The discussion of physical examination focuses on normal findings, variations from the norm that require little or no intervention, and specific potential danger signs that require more careful observation. General guidelines for conducting a physical examination are presented in the Guidelines box on p. 295. Table 8-3 summarizes the physical examination of the newborn. (See also Chapter 7 for further discussion of examination techniques.)

General Measurements. Several important measurements of the newborn are significant when compared with each other as well as when recorded over time on a graph. For the full-term infant, average ***head circumference*** is between 33 and 35.5 cm (13 to 14 inches). Head circumference may be somewhat less immediately after birth because of the molding process that occurs during a normal vaginal delivery. Usually by the second or third day the normal size and contour of the skull have replaced the molded one. ***Chest circumference*** is 30.5 to 33 cm (12 to 13 inches).

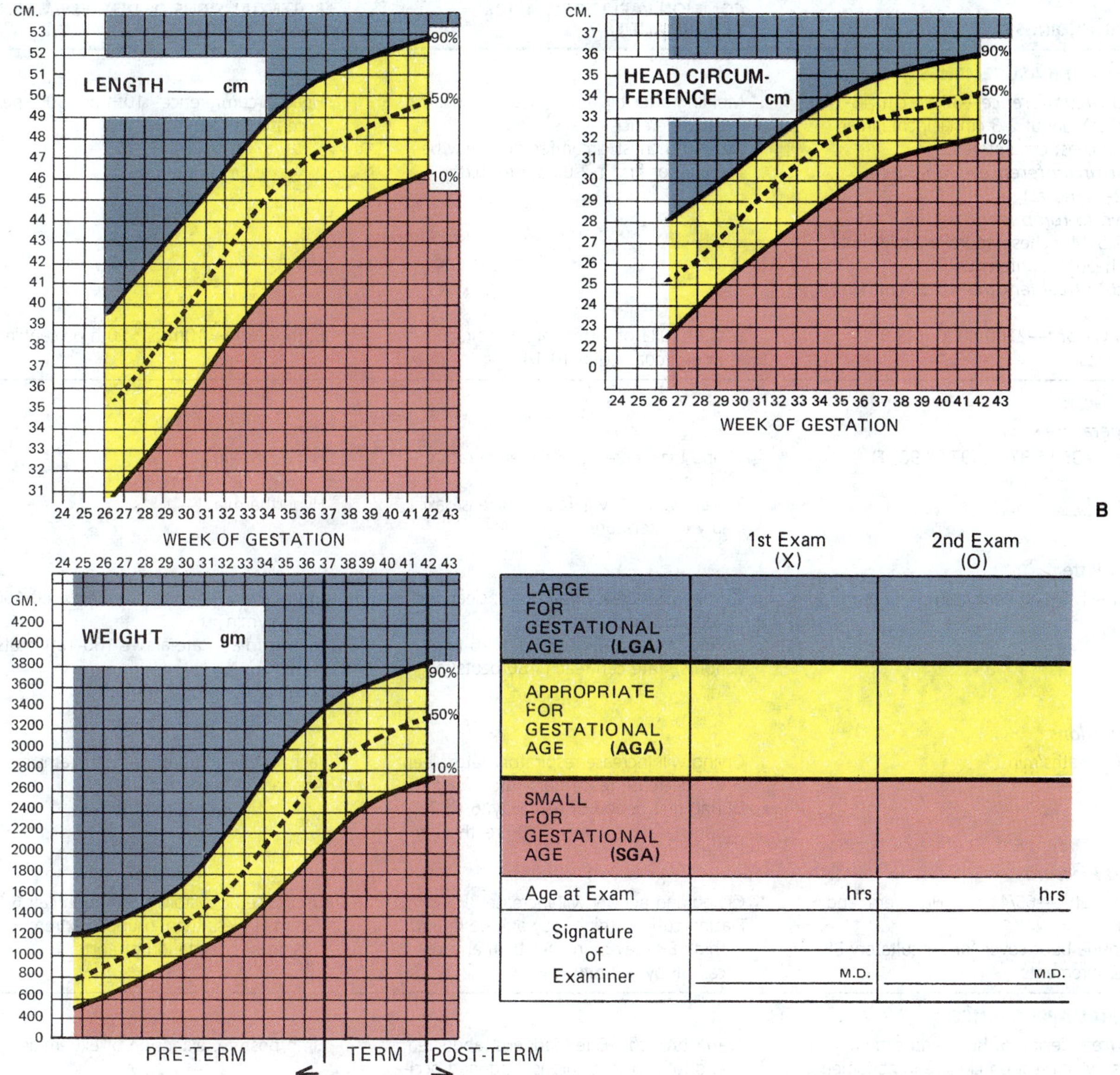

FIG. 8-1, cont'd B, Newborn classification based on maturity and intrauterine growth. (**B** modified from Lubchenko LC, Hansman C, Boyd E: *J Pediatr* 37:403, 1966; and Battaglia FC, Lubchenko LC: *J Pediatr* 71:159, 1967.)

Head circumference is usually about 2 to 3 cm (about 1 inch) greater than chest circumference. Because of the molding of the head during delivery, these measurements may initially appear equal. However, if the head is significantly smaller than the chest, microcephaly or premature closure of the sutures (craniostenosis) is suspected. If the head is more than 4 cm (1¾ inches) larger than the chest in circumference and this relationship remains constant or increases over several days, then hydrocephalus must be considered. Other causes of increased head circumference are caput succedaneum, cephalhematoma, and subdural hematoma. Prematurity and malnutrition cause the head measurement to be significantly larger than the chest circumference, but this is decreased chest size, not increased head circumference.

Compare head circumference with ***crown-to-rump length,*** or ***sitting height***. Crown-to-rump measurements are from 31 to 35 cm (12½ to 14 inches), approximately equal to head circumference. The relationship between the head and crown-to-rump measurements is more reliable than that between the head and chest.

Also measure ***head-to-heel length.*** Because of the usual flexed position of the infant, extend the leg completely when measuring total body length. The average length of-

Text continued on p. 302.

TABLE 8-3 Summary of Physical Assessment of the Newborn

USUAL FINDINGS	COMMON VARIATIONS/MINOR ABNORMALITIES	POTENTIAL SIGNS OF DISTRESS/MAJOR ABNORMALITIES
GENERAL MEASUREMENTS		
Head circumference—33-35 cm (13-14 inches); about 2-3 cm (1 inch) larger than chest circumference *Chest circumference*—30.5-33 cm (12-13 inches) *Crown-to-rump length*—31-35 cm (12.5-14 inches); approximately equal to head circumference *Head-to-heel length*—48-53 cm (19-21 inches)	Molding after birth may decrease head circumference Head and chest circumferences may be equal for first 1-2 days after birth	Head circumference <10th or >90th percentile
Birth weight—2700-4000 g (6-9 pounds)	Loss of 10% of birth weight in first week; regained in 10-14 days	Birth weight <10th or >90th percentile
VITAL SIGNS		
Temperature		
Axillary—36.5°-37° C (97.9°-98° F)	Crying may increase body temperature slightly Radiant warmer will falsely increase axillary temperature	Hypothermia Hyperthermia
Heart Rate		
Apical—120-140 beats/min	Crying will increase heart rate; sleep will decrease heart rate During first period of reactivity (6 to 8 hours), rate can reach 180 beats/min	Bradycardia—Resting rate below 80-100 beats/min Tachycardia—Rate above 160-180 beats/min Irregular rhythm
Respirations		
30-60 breaths/min	Crying will increase respiratory rate; sleep will decrease respiratory rate During first period of reactivity (6 to 8 hours), rate can reach 80 breaths/min	Tachypnea—Rate above 60 breaths/min Apnea >15 seconds
Blood Pressure		
Oscillometric—65/41 mm Hg in arm and calf See inside back cover for auscultatory BP measurements	Crying and activity will increase BP Placing cuff on thigh may agitate infant; thigh BP may be higher than arm or calf BP by 4-8 mm Hg	Oscillometric systolic pressure in calf 6-9 mm Hg less than in upper extremity (sign of coarctation of aorta)
GENERAL APPEARANCE		
Posture—Flexion of head and extremities, which rest on chest and abdomen	*Frank breech*—Extended legs, abducted and fully rotated thighs, flattened occiput, extended neck	Limp posture, extension of extremities
SKIN		
At birth, bright red, puffy, smooth Second to third day, pink, flaky, dry Vernix caseosa Lanugo Edema around eyes, face, legs, dorsa of hands, feet, and scrotum or labia *Acrocyanosis*—Cyanosis of hands and feet *Cutis marmorata*—Transient mottling when infant is exposed to decreased temperature	Neonatal jaundice after first 24 hours Ecchymoses or petechiae caused by birth trauma *Milia*—Distended sebaceous glands that appear as tiny white papules on cheeks, chin, and nose *Miliaria or sudamina*—Distended sweat (eccrine) glands that appear as minute vesicles, especially on face *Erythema toxicum*—Pink papular rash with vesicles superimposed on thorax, back, buttocks, and abdomen; may appear in 24 to 48 hours and resolve after several days *Harlequin color change*—Clearly outlined color change as infant lies on side; lower half of body becomes pink, and upper half is pale	Progressive jaundice, especially in first 24 hours Cracked or peeling skin Generalized cyanosis Pallor Mottling Grayness Plethora Hemorrhage, ecchymoses, or petechiae that persist *Sclerema*—Hard and stiff skin Poor skin turgor Rashes, pustules, or blisters *Café-au-lait spots*—Light brown spots *Nevus flammeus*—Port-wine stain

TABLE 8-3 Summary of Physical Assessment of the Newborn—cont'd

USUAL FINDINGS	COMMON VARIATIONS/MINOR ABNORMALITIES	POTENTIAL SIGNS OF DISTRESS/MAJOR ABNORMALITIES
	Mongolian spots—Irregular areas of deep blue pigmentation, usually in sacral and gluteal regions; seen predominantly in newborns of African, Native American, Asian, or Hispanic descent *Telangiectatic nevi ("stork bites")*—Flat, deep pink localized areas usually seen in back of neck	
HEAD		
Anterior fontanel—Diamond shaped, 2.5-4.0 cm (1-1.75 inches) (see Fig. 8-6) *Posterior fontanel*—Triangular, 0.5-1 cm (0.2-0.4 inch) Fontanels should be flat, soft, and firm Widest part of fontanel measured from bone to bone, not suture to suture	Molding following vaginal delivery Third sagittal (parietal) fontanel Bulging fontanel because of crying or coughing *Caput succedaneum*—Edema of soft scalp tissue *Cephalhematoma* (uncomplicated)—Hematoma between periosteum and skull bone	Fused sutures Bulging or depressed fontanels when quiet Widened sutures and fontanels *Craniotabes*—Snapping sensation along lambdoid suture that resembles indentation of Ping-Pong ball
EYES		
Lids usually edematous Color—Slate gray, dark blue, brown Absence of tears Presence of red reflex Corneal reflex in response to touch Pupillary reflex in response to light Blink reflex in response to light or touch Rudimentary fixation on objects and ability to follow to midline	Epicanthal folds in Oriental infants Searching nystagmus or strabismus *Subconjunctival (scleral) hemorrhages*—Ruptured capillaries, usually at limbus	Pink color of iris Purulent discharge Upward slant in non-Orientals Hypertelorism (3 cm or greater) Hypotelorism Congenital cataracts Constricted or dilated fixed pupil Absence of red reflex Absence of pupillary or corneal reflex Inability to follow object or bright light to midline Blue sclera Yellow sclera
EARS		
Position—Top of pinna on horizontal line with outer canthus of eye Startle reflex elicited by a loud, sudden noise Pinna flexible, cartilage present	Inability to visualize tympanic membrane because of filled aural canals Pinna flat against head Irregular shape or size Pits or skin tags	Low placement of ears Absence of startle reflex in response to loud noise Minor abnormalities may be signs of various syndromes, especially renal
NOSE		
Nasal patency Nasal discharge—Thin white mucus Sneezing	Flattened and bruised	Nonpatent canals Thick, bloody nasal discharge Flaring of nares (alae nasi) Copious nasal secretions or stuffiness (may be minor)
MOUTH AND THROAT		
Intact, high-arched palate Uvula in midline Frenulum of tongue Frenum of upper lip Sucking reflex—Strong and coordinated Rooting reflex Gag reflex Extrusion reflex Absent or minimal salivation Vigorous cry	*Natal teeth*—Teeth present at birth; benign but may be associated with congenital defects *Epstein pearls*—Small, white epithelial cysts along midline of hard palate	Cleft lip Cleft palate Large, protruding tongue or posterior displacement of tongue Profuse salivation or drooling *Candidiasis (thrush)*—White, adherent patches on tongue, palate, and buccal surfaces Inability to pass nasogastric tube Hoarse, high-pitched, weak, absent, or other abnormal cry

Continued.

TABLE 8-3 Summary of Physical Assessment of the Newborn—cont'd

USUAL FINDINGS	COMMON VARIATIONS/MINOR ABNORMALITIES	POTENTIAL SIGNS OF DISTRESS/MAJOR ABNORMALITIES
NECK		
Short, thick, usually surrounded by skinfolds Tonic neck reflex	*Torticollis* (wry neck)—Head held to one side with chin pointing to opposite side	Excessive skinfolds Resistance to flexion Absence of tonic neck reflex Fractured clavicle
CHEST		
Anteroposterior and lateral diameters equal Slight sternal retractions evident during inspiration Xiphoid process evident Breast enlargement	Funnel chest (pectus excavatum) Pigeon chest (pectus carinatum) Supernumerary nipples Secretion of milky substance from breasts ("witch's milk")	Depressed sternum Marked retractions of chest and intercostal spaces during respiration Asymmetric chest expansion Redness and firmness around nipples Wide-spaced nipples
LUNGS		
Respirations chiefly abdominal Cough reflex absent at birth, present by 1-2 days Bilateral equal bronchial breath sounds	Rate and depth of respirations may be irregular, periodic breathing Crackles shortly after birth	Inspiratory stridor Expiratory grunt Retractions Persistent irregular breathing Periodic breathing with repeated apneic spells Seesaw respirations (paradoxical) Unequal breath sounds Persistent fine crackles Wheezing Diminished breath sounds Peristaltic sounds on one side, with diminished breath sounds on same side
HEART		
Apex—Fourth to fifth intercostal space, lateral to left sternal border S_2 slightly sharper and higher in pitch than S_1	*Sinus arrhythmia*—Heart rate increases with inspiration and decreases with expiration Transient cyanosis on crying or straining	*Dextrocardia*—Heart on right side Displacement of apex, muffled Cardiomegaly Abdominal shunts Murmurs Thrills Persistent cyanosis Hyperactive precordium
ABDOMEN		
Cylindric in shape *Liver*—Palpable 2-3 cm below right costal margin *Spleen*—Tip palpable at end of first week of age *Kidneys*—Palpable 1-2 cm above umbilicus *Umbilical cord*—Bluish white at birth with two arteries and one vein *Femoral pulses*—Equal bilaterally	Umbilical hernia *Diastasis recti*—Midline gap between recti muscles *Wharton's jelly*—unusually thick umbilical cord	Abdominal distention Localized bulging Distended veins Absent bowel sounds Enlarged liver and spleen Ascites Visible peristaltic waves Scaphoid or concave abdomen Green umbilical cord Presence of only one artery in cord Urine or stool leaking from cord Palpable bladder distention following scanty voiding Absent femoral pulses Cord bleeding or hematoma
FEMALE GENITALIA		
Labia and clitoris usually edematous Urethral meatus behind clitoris Vernix caseosa between labia Urination within 24 hours	*Pseudomenstruation*—Blood-tinged or mucoid discharge Hymenal tag	Enlarged clitoris with urethral meatus at tip Fused labia Absence of vaginal opening Meconium from vaginal opening No urination within 24 hours Masses in labia Ambiguous genitalia

TABLE 8-3 Summary of Physical Assessment of the Newborn—cont'd

USUAL FINDINGS	COMMON VARIATIONS/MINOR ABNORMALITIES	POTENTIAL SIGNS OF DISTRESS/MAJOR ABNORMALITIES
MALE GENITALIA		
Urethral opening at tip of glans penis Testes palpable in each scrotum Scrotum usually large, edematous, pendulous, and covered with rugae; usually deeply pigmented in dark-skinned ethnic groups Smegma Urination within 24 hours	Urethral opening covered by prepuce Inability to retract foreskin ***Epithelial pearls***—Small, firm, white lesions at tip of prepuce Erection or priapism Testes palpable in inguinal canal Scrotum small	***Hypospadias***—Urethral opening on ventral surface of penis ***Epispadias***—Urethral opening on dorsal surface of penis ***Chordee***—Ventral curvature of penis Testes not palpable in scrotum or inguinal canal No urination within 24 hours Inguinal hernia Hypoplastic scrotum ***Hydrocele***—Fluid in scrotum Masses in scrotum Meconium from scrotum Discoloration of testes Ambiguous genitalia
BACK AND RECTUM		
Spine intact, no openings, masses, or prominent curves Trunk incurvation reflex Anal reflex Patent anal opening Passage of meconium within 48 hours	Green liquid stools in infant under phototherapy Delayed passages of meconium in very-low-birth-weight neonates	Anal fissures or fistulas Imperforate anus Absence of anal reflex No meconium within 36 hours Pilonidal cyst or sinus Tuft of hair along spine Spina bifida (any degree)
EXTREMITIES		
Ten fingers and toes Full range of motion Nail beds pink, with transient cyanosis immediately after birth Creases on anterior two thirds of sole Sole usually flat Symmetry of extremities Equal muscle tone bilaterally, especially resistance to opposing flexion Equal bilateral brachial pulses	Partial syndactyly between second and third toes Second toe overlapping into third toe Wide gap between first (hallux) and second toes Deep crease on plantar surface of foot between first and second toes Asymmetric length of toes Dorsiflexion and shortness of hallux	***Polydactyly***—Extra digits ***Syndactyly***—Fused or webbed digits ***Phocomelia***—Hands or feet attached close to trunk ***Hemimelia***—Absence of distal part of extremity Hyperflexibility of joints Persistent cyanosis of nail beds Yellowing of nail beds Sole covered with creases Transverse palmar (simian) crease Fractures Decreased or absent ROM ***Dislocated or subluxated hip*** Limitation in hip abduction Unequal gluteal or leg folds Unequal knee height (Allis or Galeazzi sign) Audible click on abduction (Ortolani sign) Asymmetry of extremities Unequal muscle tone or range of motion
NEUROMUSCULAR SYSTEM		
Extremities usually maintain some degree of flexion Extension of an extremity followed by previous position of flexion Head lag while sitting, but momentary ability to hold head erect Able to turn head from side to side when prone Able to hold head in horizontal line with back when held prone	Quivering or momentary tremors	***Hypotonia***—Floppy, poor head control, extremities limp ***Hypertonia***—Jittery, arms and hands tightly flexed, legs stiffly extended, startles easily Asymmetric posturing (except tonic neck reflex) ***Opisthotonic posturing***—Arched back Signs of paralysis Tremors, twitches, and myoclonic jerks Marked head lag in all positions

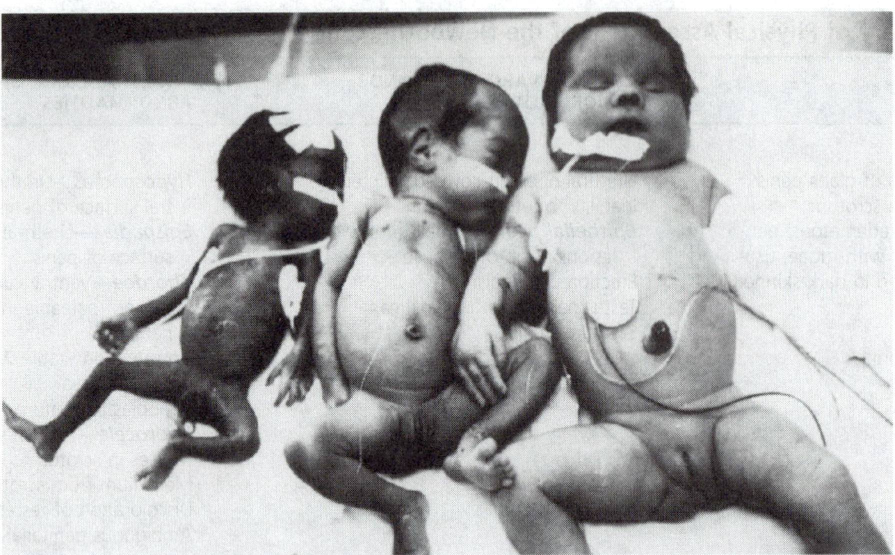

FIG. 8-2 Three babies, same gestational age, weight 600, 1400, and 2750 g, respectively, from left to right. Their associated risks of mortality are over 50%, 10%, and less than 4%, respectively. (From Korones SB: *High-risk newborn infants: the basis for intensive nursing care,* ed 4, St Louis, 1986, Mosby.)

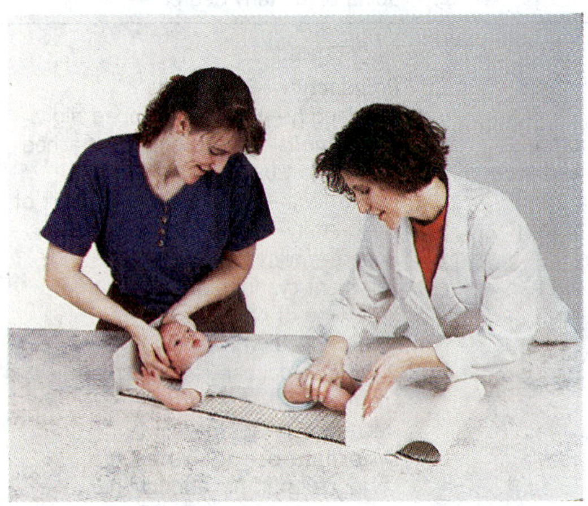

FIG. 8-3 Measurement of infant length. (From Seidel HM and others: *Mosby's guide to physical examination,* ed 3, St Louis, 1995, Mosby.)

the newborn is 48 to 53 cm (19 to 21 inches) (Fig 8-3).

Measure ***body weight*** soon after birth because weight loss occurs fairly rapidly. Normally the newborn loses up to 10% of the birth weight by 3 to 4 days of age because of loss of excessive extracellular fluid and meconium, as well as limited food intake, especially in breast-fed infants (Avoa and Fischer, 1990). The birth weight is regained by the tenth day of life. Most newborns weigh 2700 to 4000 g (6 to 9 pounds), the average weight being about 3400 g (7½ pounds). Accurate birth weights and lengths are important because they provide a baseline for assessment of risk status and future growth.

Another category of measurements is vital signs. Measure ***temperature*** via the axillary route because insertion of a thermometer into the rectum can cause perforation of the mucosa (see Fig. 7-7, *B*). Core (internal) body temperature varies according to the period of reactivity, but should be 36.5° to 37.6° C (97.7° to 99.7° F). In a thermoneutral environment skin temperature is slightly lower than core body temperature. Therefore axillary temperature may be less than rectal or tympanic membrane temperature, although the difference is small (as little as 0.2° F) between axillary and rectal sites (Yetman and others, 1993). Because brown adipose tissue is located in the axillary pocket, axillary readings may be elevated whenever nonshivering thermogenesis (NST) occurs (see p. 289). However, axillary readings may be normal in cold-stressed infants where NST is not triggered or is overwhelmed (Bliss-Holtz, 1993).

There is also controversy regarding the accuracy of tympanic membrane sensors for measuring temperature. (See Thinking Critically About . . . box on p. 226). However, in a comparison of axillary and tympanic membrane temperature measurements in neonates, the use of tempanic membrane readings was helpful in determining the infants' thermal state (Bliss-Holtz, 1993). There is no universal agreement on placement times for glass thermometers, although 3 to 5 minutes is adequate (Bliss-Holtz, 1989; Haddock, Vincent, and Merrow, 1986; Stephen and Sexton, 1987).

Pulse and ***respirations*** vary according to the periods of reactivity and to the infant's behaviors but are usually in the range of 120 to 140 beats/min and 30 to 60 breaths/min, respectively. Both are counted for a full 60 seconds to detect irregularities in rate, rhythm, and quality. Take the heart rate apically with a stethoscope and palpate the femoral arteries for equality of strength or fullness.

Measurement of ***blood pressure (BP)*** provides useful baseline data and may indicate cardiac problems. However, rou-

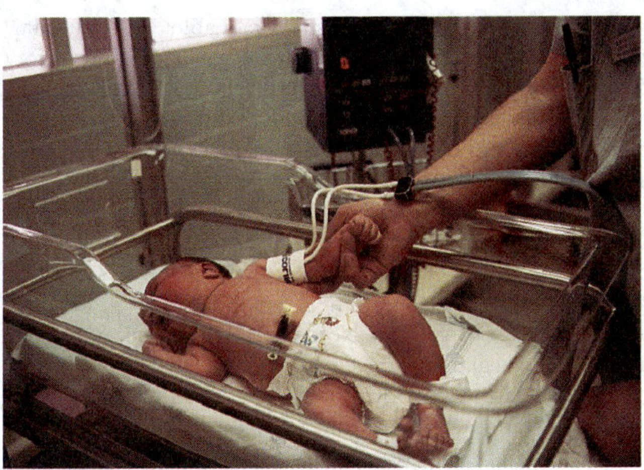

FIG. 8-4 Measurement of blood pressure using oscillometry.

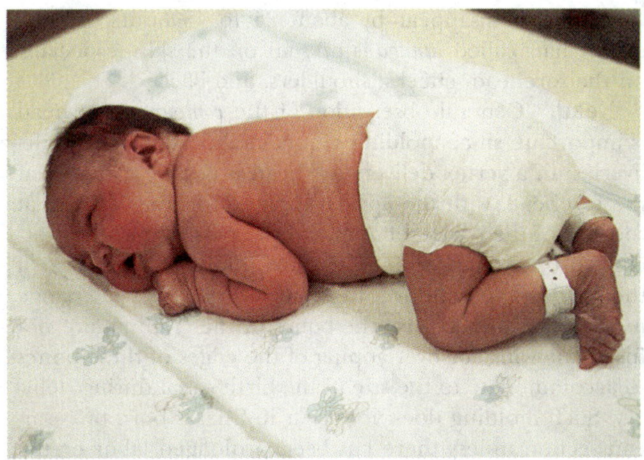

FIG. 8-5 Flexion position of neonate.

tine BP measurement on healthy full-term neonates is not recommended, because it is a poor predictor for hypertension later in life (American Academy of Pediatrics, 1993a). BP is most easily and accurately assessed using oscillometry (Dinamap), although the device is less reliable when the mean arterial BP is below 40 mm Hg (Chia and others, 1990) (Fig. 8-4). The average oscillometric systolic/diastolic BP is 65/41 mm Hg at 1 to 3 days of age (Park and Menard, 1989). Compare BP in the upper and lower extremities, which should be equal.

NURSING ALERT Systolic oscillometric BP in the calf that is 6 to 9 mm Hg less than systolic BP in the upper arm is a sign of coarctation of the aorta and is reported for further evaluation (Park and Lee, 1989).

A suggested schedule for monitoring heart and respiratory rates and temperature is on admission to the nursery and then once every 8 hours until discharge (American Academy of Pediatrics and American College of Obstetrics and Gynecologists, 1992). However, this schedule may vary according to institutional policy. Any change in the infant such as in color, muscle tone, or behavior necessitates more frequent monitoring.

General Appearance. In the full-term newborn the ***posture*** is one of flexion, a result of in utero position (Fig. 8-5). Most infants are born in a vertex (head first) presentation and keep the head flexed, with the chin resting on the upper chest. The arms are flexed at the elbows and rest, folded, on the chest with hands clenched or fisted. The legs are flexed at the knees, the hips are flexed with thighs resting on the abdomen, and the feet are dorsiflexed against the anterior aspect of the legs. The vertebral column is also flexed.

Note any deviation from this very characteristic fetal position. For example, preterm, as well as hypoxic, infants do not assume an attitude of total flexion but rather one of limp extension. Nonvertex presentations also result in variations in posture. In breech presentations the posture will depend on the presenting part; for example, a frank breech presentation results in extended legs, abducted and fully rotated thighs, a flattened head on top, and a neck that appears elongated.

Observe the infant's ***behavior,*** especially the degree of alertness, drowsiness, and irritability, which are common signs of neurologic problems. Mentally ask the following questions when assessing behavior:

- Is the infant awakened easily by a loud noise?
- Is the infant comforted by rocking, sucking, or cuddling?
- Do there seem to be periods of deep and light sleep?
- When awake, does the infant seem satisfied after a feeding?
- What stimuli elicit responses from the infant?
- When disturbed, how much does the infant protest?

Skin. The ***texture*** of the newborn's skin is velvety smooth and puffy, especially about the eyes, the legs, the dorsal aspect of the hands, and feet, and the scrotum or labia.

Skin ***color*** depends on racial and familial background and varies greatly among newborns. In general, the white infant is usually pink to red; the black newborn may appear a pinkish or yellowish brown. Infants of Hispanic descent may have an olive tint or a slight yellow cast to the skin. Infants of Oriental descent may be a rosy or yellowish tan. The color of Native American newborns depends on the tribe and can vary from a light pink to a dark, reddish brown. By the second or third day the skin turns to its more natural tone and is drier and flakier.

Observe the color of the skin in relation to activity, position, and temperature changes. In general, the infant becomes redder when crying and may demonstrate transient periods of cyanosis. Decreased temperature increases the degree of cyanosis because of vasoconstriction. Several other color changes and minor skin blemishes that may be noted on the skin are described in Table 8-3.

At birth the skin is covered with a grayish white, cheeselike substance called ***vernix caseosa,*** a mixture of sebum and desquamating cells. If it is not removed during the bath, it will dry and disappear by about 24 to 48 hours. A fine, downy hair called ***lanugo*** is present on the skin, especially on the forehead, cheeks, shoulders, and back.

Head. General observation of the ***contour*** of the head is important, since molding occurs in almost all vaginal deliveries. In a vertex delivery the head is usually flattened at the forehead, with the apex rising and forming a point at the end of the parietal bones and the posterior skull or occiput dropping abruptly. The usual, more oval contour of the head is apparent by 1 to 2 days after birth. The change in shape occurs because the bones of the cranium are not fused, allowing for overlapping of the edges of these bones to accommodate to the size of the birth canal during delivery. Such molding does not occur in infants born by cesarean section unless there has been prolonged labor or the head has been engaged in the pelvis.

Six bones—the frontal, occipital, two parietals, and two temporals—constitute the cranium. Between the junctions of these bones are bands of connective tissue called ***sutures.*** At the junction of the suture are wider spaces of unossified membranous tissue called ***fontanels.*** The two most prominent fontanels are the ***anterior fontanel,*** formed by the junction of the sagittal, coronal, and frontal sutures, and the ***posterior fontanel,*** formed by the junction of the sagittal and lambdoid sutures (Fig. 8-6, *A*).

➤ **NURSING TIP** The location of the suture is easily remembered because the coronal suture "crowns" the head and the sagittal suture "separates" the head.

Two other fontanels—the ***sphenoidal*** and ***mastoid***—are normally present but are not usually palpable. An additional third fontanel located between the anterior and posterior fontanels along the sagittal suture is found in some normal neonates but is also found in some infants with Down syndrome. Always record the presence of this sagittal or parietal fontanel.

Palpate the skull for all patent sutures and fontanels by using the tip of the index finger and running it along the ends of the bones (Fig. 8-6, *B*). Sutures feel like cracks between the skull bones; fontanels feel like wider "soft spots" at the junction of sutures. Note their size, shape, molding, and any abnormal closure.

The anterior fontanel is diamond shaped and measures 4 to 5 cm (about 2 inches) at its widest point (from bone to bone, rather than from suture to suture). The posterior fontanel is triangular, measuring between 0.5 and 1 cm (less than ½ inch) at its widest part. It is easily located by following the sagittal suture toward the occiput.

The fontanels should feel flat, firm, and well demarcated against the bony edges of the skull. Frequently pulsations are visible at the anterior fontanel. Coughing, crying, or lying down may temporarily cause the fontanels to bulge and become more taut.

NURSING ALERT Always record and report a widened, tense, bulging fontanel (sign of increased intracranial pressure) and a markedly sunken, depressed fontanel (sign of dehydration).

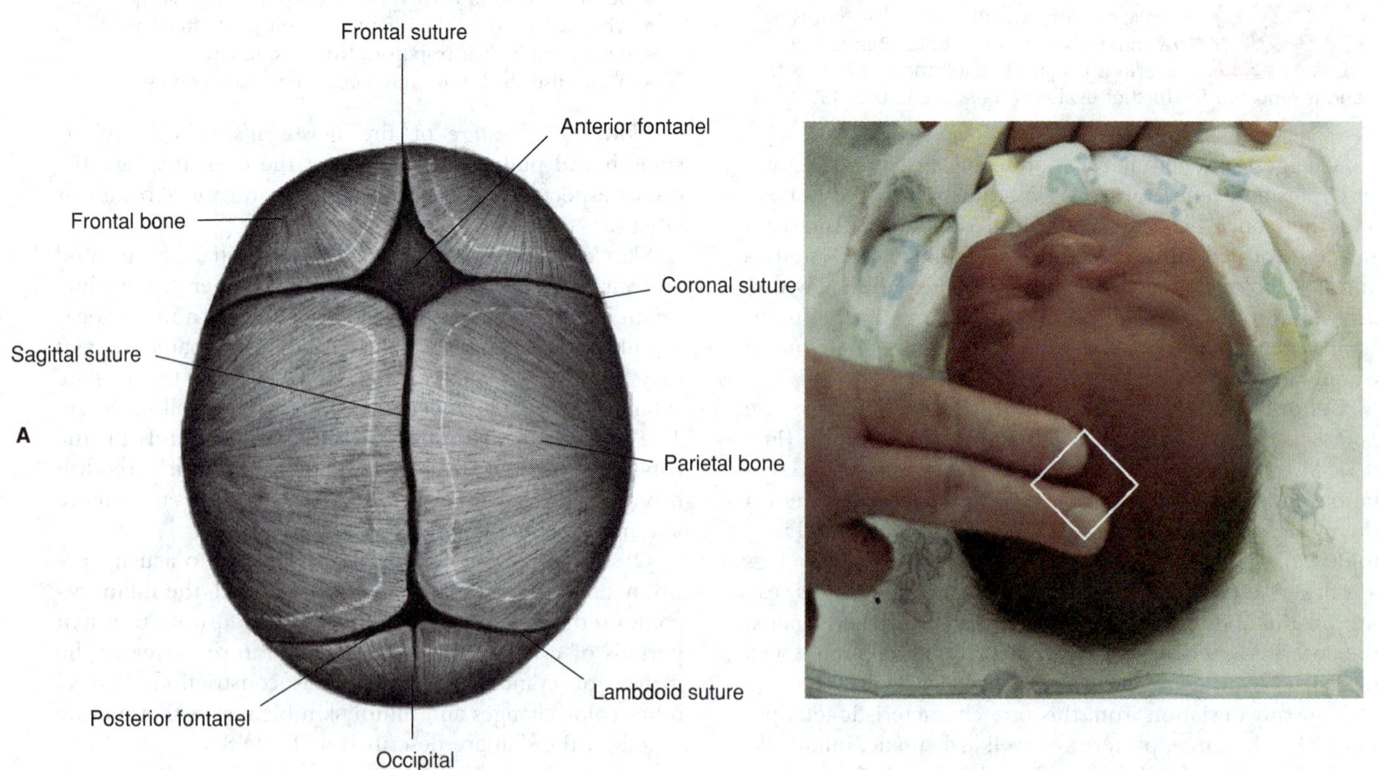

FIG. 8-6 **A,** Location of sutures and fontanels. **B,** Palpating anterior fontanel.

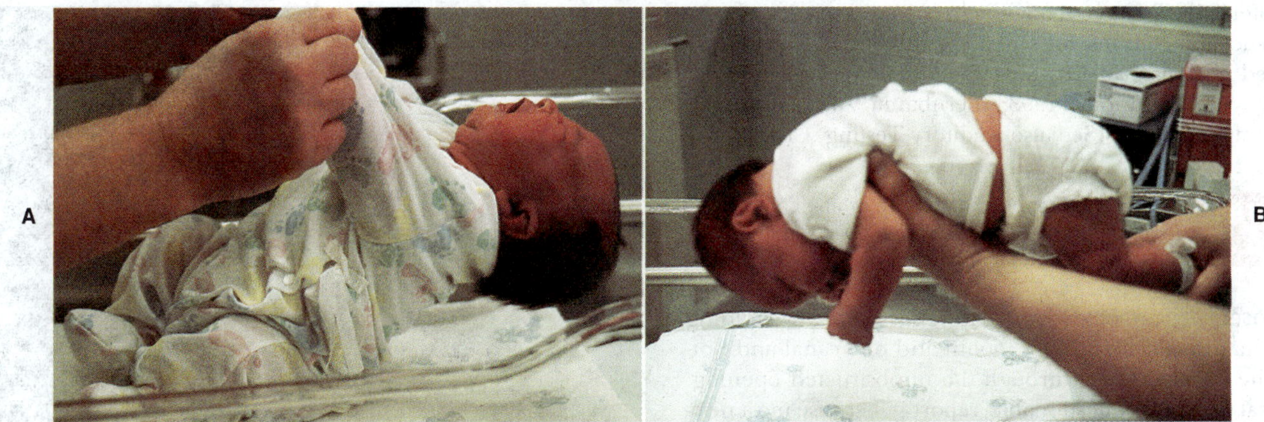

FIG. 8-7 Head control in infant. **A,** Inability to hold head erect when pulled to sitting position. **B,** Ability to hold head erect when placed in ventral suspension.

Palpate the skull for any unusual masses or prominences, particularly those resulting from birth trauma, such as caput succedaneum or cephalhematoma (see Chapter 9). Because of the pliability of the skull, exerting pressure at the margin of the parietal and occipital bones along the lambdoid suture may produce a snapping sensation similar to the indentation of a Ping-Pong ball. This phenomenon, known as ***physiologic craniotabes,*** may be found normally, especially in newborns of breech birth, but also may indicate hydrocephalus or syphilis.

Assess the degree of ***head control.*** Although ***head lag*** is normal, the newborn has some ability to control the head in certain positions. If the supine infant is pulled from the arms into a semi-Fowler position, head lag and hyperextension occur (Fig. 8-7, *A*). However, as infants are brought forward into a sitting position, they attempt to control their heads in an upright position. As the head falls forward onto the chest, many infants attempt to right it into the erect position. If they are held in ventral suspension (i.e., held prone above and parallel to the examining surface) the head is held in a straight line with the spinal column (Fig. 8-7, *B*). When lying on the abdomen, newborns have the ability to lift the head slightly, turning it from side to side. Marked head lag is seen in neonates with Down syndrome, hypoxia, and brain damage.

NURSING ALERT Report evidence of excessive head lag and observe for other signs of neurologic deficit.

Eyes. Since newborns tend to keep their eyes tightly closed, begin the examination of the eyes by observing the lids for edema, which is normally present for the first 2 days after delivery. A lateral upward slope of the eyes with an inner epicanthal fold may indicate Down syndrome. Observe the eyes for symmetry and for hypertelorism, but do not measure the distance between the inner canthi unless there is cause for further investigation. ***Tears*** may be present at birth, but purulent discharge from the eyes shortly after birth is abnormal.

NURSING ALERT Report purulent discharge, which may signify ***ophthalmia neonatorum*** (infectious conjunctivitis of the newborn).

To visualize the surface structures of the eye, hold the infant supine and gently lower the head. The eyes will usually open, similar to the mechanism of a doll's eyes. The ***sclera*** should be white and clear.

Examine the cornea for the presence of any opacities or haziness. The ***corneal reflex*** is present at birth but is generally not elicited unless brain or eye damage is suspected. The pupil usually responds to light by constricting. Absence of the ***pupillary reflex,*** particularly by 3 weeks of age, suggests blindness. A fixed, dilated, or constricted pupil may indicate anoxia or brain damage. A searching ***nystagmus*** is common after birth. ***Strabismus*** is a normal finding because of the lack of binocularity.

Note the color of the ***iris.*** Most light-skinned newborns have slate gray or dark blue eyes, whereas dark-skinned infants have brown eyes. Absence of color is characteristic of albinism.

Although it is difficult to perform a complete funduscopic examination of the retina, always try to elicit a ***red reflex.***

NURSING ALERT Always record and report absence of the red reflex. It may indicate the presence of retinal hemorrhages or congenital cataracts.

Ears. Examine the ears for position, structure, and auditory function. The ***pinna*** is often flattened against the side of the head from pressure in utero. An otoscopic examination is ordinarily not performed, because the canals are filled with vernix caseosa and amniotic fluid, making visualization of the drum difficult.

Assess ***auditory ability*** by making a sharp, loud noise close to the infant's head and noting the presence of the ***startle reflex*** (see Table 8-4) or twitching of the eyelids. Also, be aware of newborns considered at risk for hearing loss so that early testing can be performed (see Hearing Impairment,

Chapter 24). Two recommended tests are the evoked otoacoustic emissions test for screening and brainstem auditory evoked response (BAER) for infants who fail the screening (Early Identification, 1993; Bernbaum and Hoffman-Williamson, 1991). (See also Auditory Testing, Chapter 7.)

NURSING ALERT Always report the absence of any behavioral response to a sudden noise, an indication of congenital deafness.

Nose. Assess patency of the ***nasal canals*** by holding your hand over the infant's mouth and one canal and noting the passage of air through the unobstructed opening. If nasal patency is questionable, report it, because most newborns are obligatory nose breathers and are unable to breathe orally in response to nasal occlusion (Miller and others, 1985).

The ***shape*** of the nose is usually flattened after birth, and bruises are common, especially if forceps were used. Thin white mucus is very common in the newborn, but a thick, bloody nasal discharge without sneezing may suggest the ***snuffles*** of congenital syphilis. ***Sneezing*** is very common.

NURSING ALERT Always report flaring of the nares because it is a serious sign of air hunger from respiratory distress.

Mouth and Throat. The mouth is inspected for its existing structures. The ***palate*** is normally high arched and somewhat narrow. Inspect the hard and soft palates for any clefts, which warrant further investigation. A common finding is ***Epstein pearls***—small, white, epithelial cysts along both sides of the midline of the hard palate. They are insignificant and disappear in several weeks.

The ***frenulum*** of the upper lip is a band of thick, pink tissue that lies under the inner surface of the upper lip and extends to the maxillary alveolar ridge. It usually disappears as the maxilla grows. It is particularly evident when the infant yawns or smiles.

Elicit the ***sucking reflex*** by placing a nipple or gloved finger in the infant's mouth. The infant should exhibit a strong, vigorous suck. To stimulate the ***rooting reflex,*** stroke the cheek and note the infant's response of turning toward the stimulated side and sucking (Fig. 8-8). Assess the ***gag reflex*** when using a tongue blade to visualize the oropharynx.

Inspect the ***uvula*** while the infant is crying and the chin is depressed. However, it may be retracted upward and backward during crying. Tonsillar tissue is generally not seen in the newborn. ***Natal teeth*** (teeth present at birth as opposed to ***neonatal teeth***—teeth that erupt during the first month of life) are seen infrequently and erupt chiefly at the position of the lower central incisors. Report their presence, because natal teeth are frequently found with developmental abnormalities and syndromes, including cleft lip and palate. Most natal teeth are loosely attached, but current thinking suggests preserving them until they exfoliate naturally (Leung, 1989).

Neck. Since the newborn's neck is short and covered

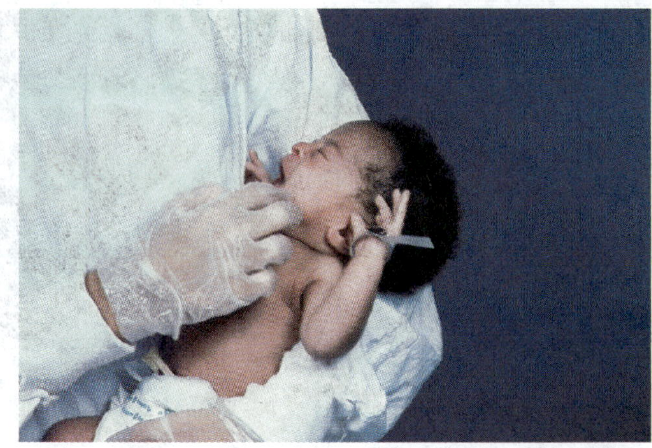

FIG. 8-8 Eliciting rooting reflex. (From Seidel HM and others: *Mosby's guide to physical examination,* ed 3, St Louis, 1995, Mosby.)

with folds of tissue, for adequate assessment allow the head to fall gently backward in slight hyperextension while supporting the back in a slightly raised position. Observe for range of motion, shape, and any abnormal masses and palpate each clavicle for possible fractures (see Fractures, Chapter 9).

Chest. The ***shape*** of the newborn's chest is almost circular because the anteroposterior and lateral diameters are equal. The ribs are very flexible, and slight intercostal retractions are normally seen on inspiration. The xiphoid process is commonly visible as a small protrusion at the end of the sternum. The sternum is generally raised and slightly curved.

Inspect the ***breasts*** for size, shape, and nipple formation, location, and number. Breast enlargement appears in many newborns of either sex by the second or third day and is caused by maternal hormones. Occasionally a milky substance sometimes called ***witch's milk*** is secreted by the infant's breasts. Infrequently, ***supernumerary nipples*** are present; if found, the kidneys should be evaluated because of the association of extra nipples with renal anomalies (Meggyessy and Méhes, 1987).

Lungs. The normal ***respirations*** of the newborn are irregular and abdominal, and the rate is between 30 and 60 breaths/min. Periods of ***apnea*** lasting less than 15 seconds are normal. After the first forceful breaths required to initiate respiration, subsequent breaths should be easy and fairly regular in rhythm. Occasional irregularities occur in relation to crying, sleeping, and feeding.

Perform auscultation when the infant is quiet. Bronchial breath sounds should be equal bilaterally. Report any differences in auscultatory findings between symmetric sites. ***Crackles*** soon after birth indicate areas of atelectasis, which represent the normal transition of the lungs to extrauterine life. However, report persistence of crackles or presence of wheezing.

Heart. ***Heart rate*** may range from 100 to 180 beats/min shortly after birth and, when the infant's condition has stabilized, from 120 to 140 beats/min. Palpate to find the ***point of maximum intensity (PMI),*** which is usually in the fourth to fifth intercostal space, medial to the left midclavicular line. The PMI gives some indication of the location of the heart, which may be displaced in conditions such as diaphragmatic hernia or pneumothorax. If the heart is on the right side of the body, ***dextrocardia*** exists. Report this, since the abdominal organs may also be reversed, with associated circulatory abnormalities.

Auscultation of the specific components of the ***heart sounds*** is difficult because of the rapid rate and effective transmission of respiratory sounds. However, the ***first (S_1)*** and ***second (S_2) sounds*** should be clear and well defined; the second sound is somewhat higher in pitch and sharper than the first. ***Murmurs*** are very frequently heard in the newborn, especially over the base of the heart or at the left sternal border in the third or fourth interspace. Ordinarily they are not associated with specific cardiac defects, since they frequently represent the incomplete functional closure of fetal shunts. (Grading of heart murmurs is discussed in Chapter 7.) However, always record and report any murmur or other unusual sounds.

Abdomen. The normal ***contour*** of the abdomen is cylindric and usually prominent with visible veins. Bowel sounds are heard a few hours after birth. Visible peristaltic waves may be observed in thin newborns but should not be seen in well-nourished infants.

Inspect the ***umbilical cord*** to determine the presence of two arteries, which look like papular structures, and one vein, which has a larger lumen than the arteries and a thinner vessel wall. At birth the cord appears bluish white and moist. After clamping, it begins to dry and appears a dull, yellowish brown. It progressively shrivels in size and turns greenish black.

Palpate after inspecting the abdomen. The ***liver*** is normally palpable 3 cm (about 1 inch) below the right costal margin. The tip of the ***spleen*** can sometimes be felt, but a palpable spleen more than 1 cm below the left costal margin suggests enlargement and warrants further investigation. Palpating the ***kidneys*** requires considerable practice and is best done soon after delivery when muscle tone is least. When felt, the lower half of the right kidney and the tip of the left kidney are 1 to 2 cm above the umbilicus. During examination of the lower abdomen, palpate for ***femoral pulses,*** which should be strong and equal bilaterally.

NURSING ALERT Absence of the femoral pulses may indicate coarctation of the aorta, a congenital heart defect. Always report absent or weak femoral pulses for further evaluation.

Female Genitalia. Normally the ***labia majora*** and ***minora*** (the minora may be more prominent) and ***clitoris*** are edematous, especially following a breech delivery. However, carefully inspect the labia and clitoris to identify any evidence of ambiguous genitalia or other abnormalities. Normally in a female the urethral opening is located behind the clitoris. Any deviation from this may mistakenly suggest that the clitoris is a small penis, which can occur in conditions such as adrenal hyperplasia.

Virtually all female newborns have ***hymens*** (Berenson, 1993). The hymen is often protruding, thick, and vascular. A *hymenal tag* is occasionally visible from the posterior opening of the vagina. It is composed of tissue from the hymen and labia minora. It usually disappears in several weeks. In the posterior vestible (behind the posterior vaginal opening), there may be a white midline streak ***(linea vestibularis)*** or spot ***(partial linea vestibularis)*** (Kellogg and Parra, 1991). The presence of a hymenal tag or vestibular markings is recorded for comparison in case of suspected child abuse. Generally, the vaginal vault is not inspected.

Vaginal discharge may be noted during the first week of life. This pseudomenstruation is a manifestation of the abrupt decrease in maternal hormones and usually disappears by 2 to 4 weeks. ***Fecal discharge*** from the vaginal opening indicates a rectovaginal fistula and is always reported. Vernix caseosa may be present in large amounts between the labia.

Male Genitalia. Inspect the penis for the ***urethral opening,*** which is located at the tip. However, the opening may be totally covered by the ***prepuce,*** or ***foreskin,*** which covers the ***glans penis.*** A tight prepuce is a very common finding in newborns and does not indicate phimosis. Do *not* forcefully retract the prepuce. ***Smegma,*** a white cheesy substance, is commonly found around the glans penis, under the foreskin. An erection is not uncommon in the newborn. Small, white, firm lesions called ***epithelial pearls*** may be seen at the tip of the prepuce.

The ***scrotum*** may be large, edematous, and pendulous in the full-term neonate, especially in the infant born in breech position. It is more deeply pigmented in dark-skinned races. A noncommunicating ***hydrocele*** commonly occurs unilaterally and disappears within a few months. Always palpate the scrotum for the presence of ***testes*** (see Chapter 7). In small newborns, particularly premature infants, the undescended testes may be palpable within the inguinal canal. Absence of the testes may also be a sign of ambiguous genitalia, especially when accompanied by a small scrotum and penis. ***Inguinal hernias*** may or may not be manifested immediately after birth. A hernia is more easily detected when the infant is crying. Palpable ***lymph nodes*** are most commonly found in the inguinal area.

Back and Anus. Inspect the ***spine*** with the infant prone. The shape of the spine is gently rounded, with none of the characteristic S-shaped curves seen later in life. Note any abnormal openings, masses, dimples, or soft areas. A large, protruding sac anywhere along the spine, but most commonly in the sacral area, indicates some type of ***spina bifida.*** A small sinus, which may or may not be communicating with the spine, is a ***pilonidal sinus.*** It is frequently covered with a tuft of hair. Although it may have no pathologic significance, a pilonidal cyst may indicate the existence of spina bifida occulta or be a portal of entry into the spinal column. With the infant still prone, note symmetry of the gluteal folds. Report any evidence of asymmetry; tests for congenital hip dislocation are performed by trained (or skilled) examiners (see Chapter 11).

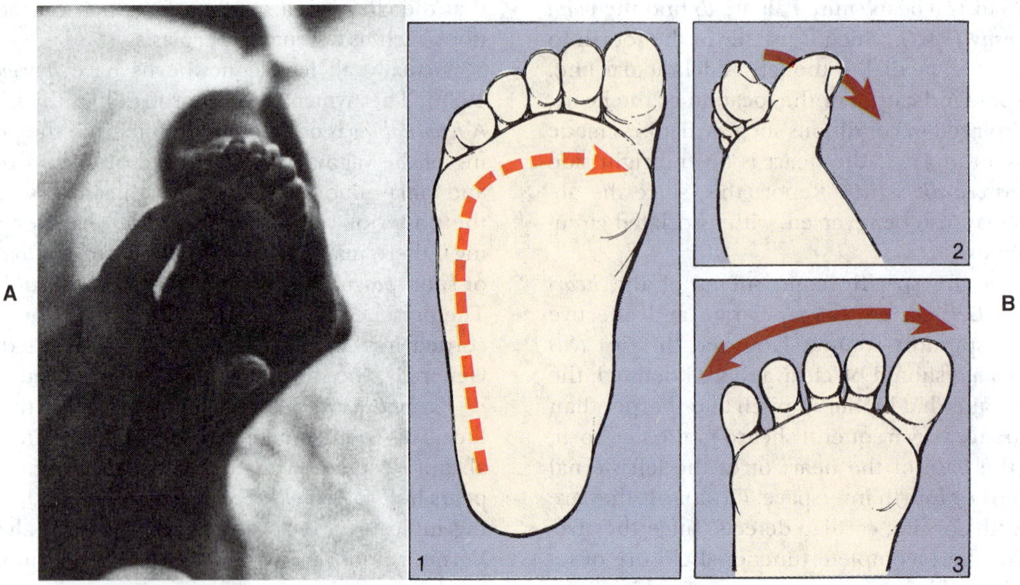

A

B

1 2 3

FIG. 8-9 **A,** Plantar or grasp reflex. **B,** Babinski reflex. *1,* Direction of stroke. *2,* Dorsiflexion of big toe. *3,* Fanning of toes.

Passage of meconium during the first 24 to 48 hours of life indicates ***anal patency.*** If an imperforate anus is suspected and not readily visible, insert a small 5 or 8 French catheter into the anal opening.

> **NURSING ALERT** Do not use a gloved finger or rectal thermometer to test for anal patency because of the risk of mucosal perforation; also, the smaller diameter of the thermometer may pass through even a severely stenotic anus (El Haddad and Corkery, 1985). Always report failure to pass meconium by 48 hours.

With the infant still prone, gently separate the buttocks to inspect the anal area for the presence of ***fissures,*** or small cracks, in the mucosa. Anal fissures are a common cause of constipation, because the infant refuses to strain during defecation in order to avoid pain. Asymmetry of the mucosal folds around the sphincter also suggests fissures.

Extremities. Examine the extremities for symmetry, range of motion, and signs of malformation or trauma. Count the ***fingers*** and ***toes,*** and note supernumerary digits ***(polydactyly)*** or fusion of digits ***(syndactyly).*** A partial syndactyly between the second and third toes is a common variation seen in otherwise normal infants.

Observe range of motion of the ***extremities*** throughout the entire examination. ***Hyperflexibility*** of joints is characteristic of Down syndrome. Elicit the ***scarf sign*** (when negative, elbow brought across chest does not reach midline) to identify abnormal flexion of joints (see Fig. 10-11).

Examine the ***nails;*** the nail beds should be pink, although slight blueness is evident in acrocyanosis. Persistent ***cyanosis*** of the nail beds indicates anoxia or vasoconstriction. ***Yellowing*** of the nail beds may indicate intrauterine distress, postmaturity, or hemolytic disease. ***Short*** or ***absent nails*** are seen in premature infants, whereas ***long nails,*** extending over the ends of the fingers, are characteristic of postmature newborns.

The ***palms*** of the hands should have the usual creases (see Fig. 7-10). A ***transverse palmar crease (simian crease)*** suggests Down syndrome. The full-term newborn usually has creases on the anterior two thirds of the sole of the foot. In postmature infants the sole is covered with deep creases, and in premature infants the creases are absent. The ***soles*** of the feet are flat with prominent fat pads. While examining the feet, elicit the ***grasp*** and ***Babinski reflexes*** (see Table 8-4 and Fig. 8-9). Report any foot abnormalities.

Inspect the extremities for evidence of fractures from birth trauma. The humerus and femur are most commonly involved. Limitation of movement, visible deformity, asymmetry of reflexes, and malposition of the site suggest a fracture.

Also assess ***muscle tone.*** By attempting to extend a flexed extremity, determine if tone is equal bilaterally. Extension of any extremity is usually met with resistance, and when released, the extremity returns to its previous flexed position. ***Hypotonia*** suggests some degree of hypoxia, neurologic disorder, or Down syndrome. ***Asymmetry*** of muscle tone may indicate a degree of paralysis from brain damage or nerve damage. Failure to move the lower limbs suggests a spinal cord lesion or injury. ***Tremors, twitches,*** and ***myoclonic jerks*** characterize neonatal seizures or may indicate neonatal narcotic withdrawal syndrome. Quivering or momentary tremors are usually normal (see Neonatal Seizures, Chapter 10).

Neurologic System. Assessing neurologic status is a critical part of the physical examination of the newborn. Much of the neurologic testing takes place during evaluation of body systems, such as eliciting localized reflexes and observing posture, muscle tone, head control, and move-

TABLE 8-4 Assessment of Reflexes in the Newborn

REFLEXES	EXPECTED BEHAVIORAL RESPONSES
LOCALIZED	
Eyes	
Blinking or corneal reflex	Infant blinks at sudden appearance of a bright light or at approach of an object toward cornea; persists throughout life
Pupillary	Pupil constricts when a bright light shines toward it; persists throughout life
Doll's eye	As head is moved slowly to right or left, eyes lag behind and do not immediately adjust to new position of head; disappears as fixation develops; if persists, indicates neurologic damage
Nose	
Sneeze	Spontaneous response of nasal passages to irritation or obstruction; persists throughout life
Glabellar	Tapping briskly on glabella (bridge of nose) causes eyes to close tightly
Mouth and Throat	
Sucking	Infant begins strong sucking movements of circumoral area in response to stimulation; persists throughout infancy, even without stimulation, such as during sleep
Gag	Stimulation of posterior pharynx by food, suction, or passage of a tube causes infant to gag; persists throughout life
Rooting	Touching or stroking the cheek along side of mouth causes infant to turn head toward that side and begin to suck; should disappear at about age 3-4 months, but may persist for up to 12 months (see Fig. 8-8)
Extrusion	When tongue is touched or depressed, infant responds by forcing it outward; disappears by age 4 months
Yawn	Spontaneous response to decreased oxygen by increasing amount of inspired air; persists throughout life
Cough	Irritation of mucous membranes of larynx or tracheobronchial tree causes coughing; persists throughout life; usually present after first day of birth
Extremities	
Grasp	Touching palms of hands or soles of feet near base of digits causes flexion of hands and toes (see Fig. 8-9, *A*): palmar grasp lessens after age 3 months, to be replaced by voluntary movement; plantar grasp lessens by 8 months of age
Babinski	Stroking outer sole of foot upward from heel and across ball of foot causes toes to hyperextend and hallux to dorsiflex (see Fig. 8-9, *B*); disappears after age 1 year
Ankle clonus	Briskly dorsiflexing foot while supporting knee in partially flexed position results in one to two oscillating movements ("beats"); eventually no beats should be felt
MASS	
Moro	Sudden jarring or change in equilibrium causes sudden extension and abduction of extremities and fanning of fingers, with index finger and thumb forming a C shape, followed by flexion and adduction of extremities; legs may weakly flex; infant may cry (Fig. 8-10); disappears after age 3-4 months, usually strongest during first 2 months
Startle	A sudden loud noise causes abduction of the arms with flexion of elbows; hands remain clenched; disappears by age 4 months
Perez	While infant is prone on a firm surface, thumb is pressed along spine from sacrum to neck; infant responds by crying, flexing extremities, and elevating pelvis and head; lordosis of the spine, as well as defecation and urination, may occur; disappears by age 4-6 months
Asymmetric tonic neck	When infant's head is turned to one side, arm and leg extend on that side, and opposite arm and leg flex (Fig. 8-11); disappears by age 3-4 months, to be replaced by symmetric positioning of both sides of body
Trunk incurvation (Galant) reflex	Stroking infant's back alongside spine causes hips to move toward stimulated side; disappears by age 4 weeks
Dance or step	If infant is held so that sole of foot touches a hard surface, there is a reciprocal flexion and extension of the leg, simulating walking (Fig. 8-12); disappears after age 3-4 weeks, to be replaced by deliberate movement
Crawl	When placed on abdomen, infant makes crawling movements with arms and legs; disappears at about age 6 weeks (Fig. 8-13)
Placing	When infant is held upright under arms and dorsal side of foot is briskly placed against hard object, such as table, leg lifts as if foot is stepping on table; age of disappearance varies

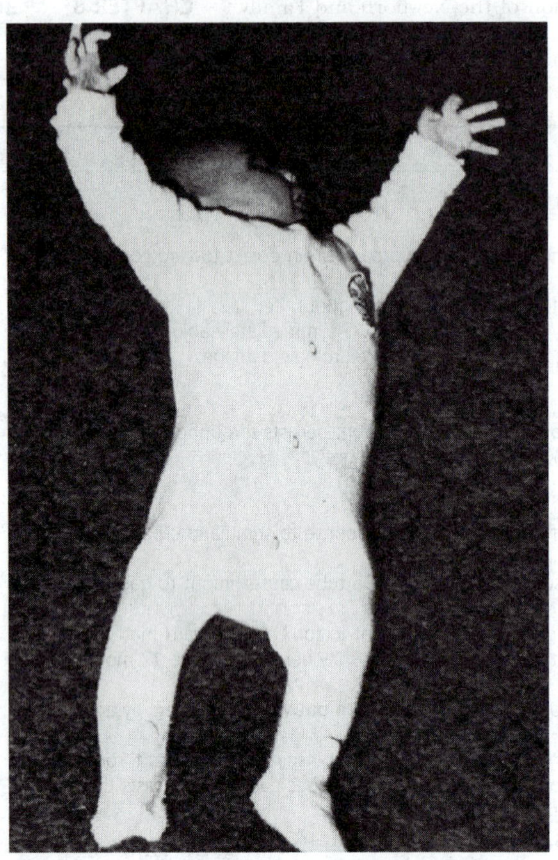

FIG. 8-10 Moro reflex.

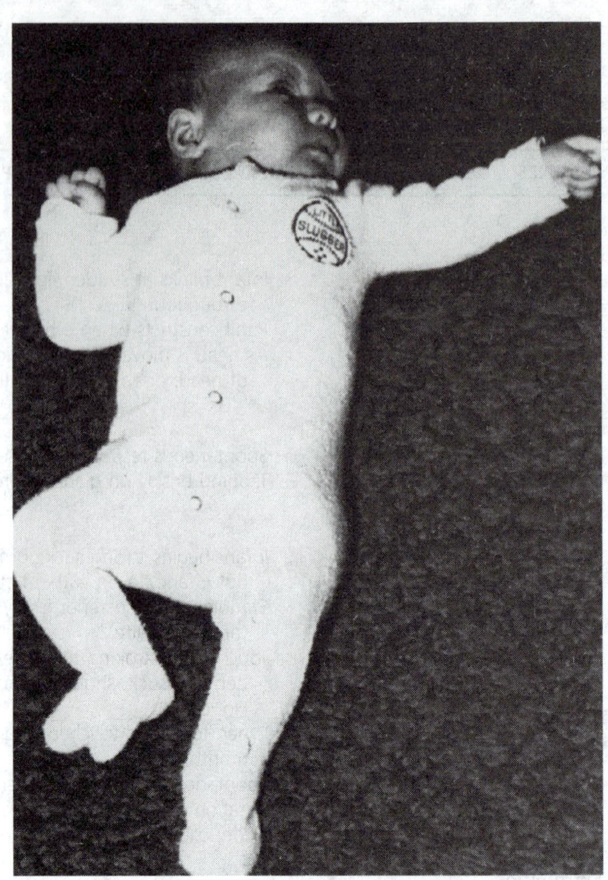

FIG. 8-11 Tonic neck reflex.

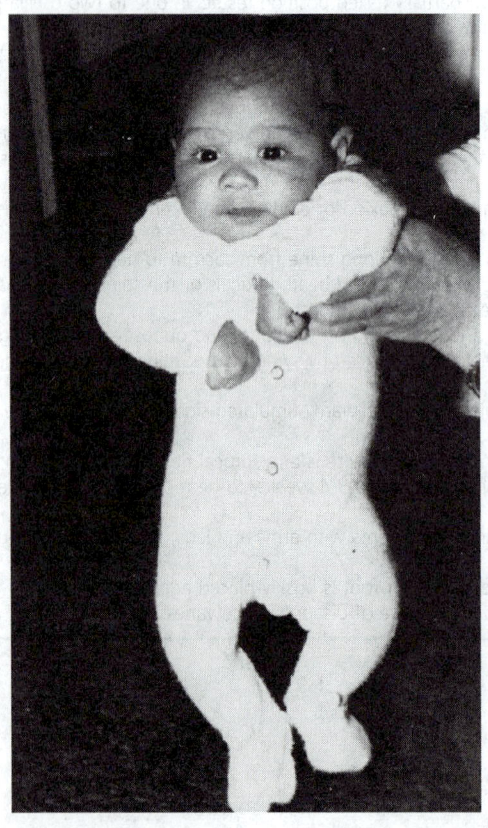

FIG. 8-12 Dance reflex.

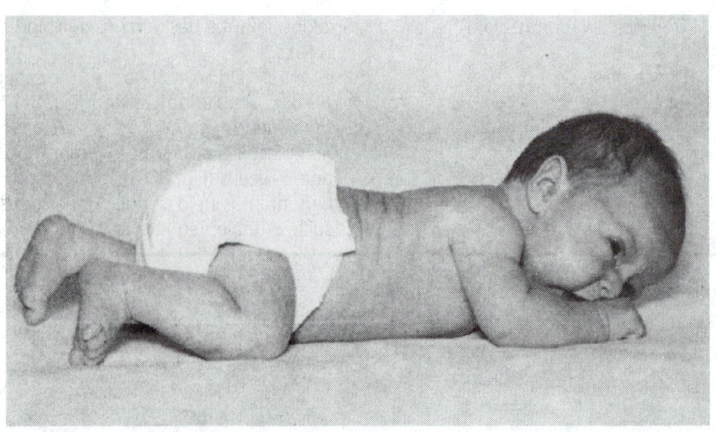

FIG. 8-13 Crawl reflex.

ment. However, several important mass (total body) reflexes also need to be elicited. Test these at the end of the examination, because they may disturb the infant and interfere with auscultation. These reflexes, as well as several local reflexes, are described in Table 8-4. Record and report the absence, asymmetry, persistence, or weakness of a reflex.

❖ Nursing Diagnoses

A number of nursing diagnoses are prominent in the nursing care of the newborn and family, and others specific to individual cases become evident. The most common nursing diagnoses are outlined in the Nursing Care Plan on pp. 329-331.

❖ Planning

The goals for the newborn and family are as follows:

1. Infant will maintain a patent airway.
2. Infant will maintain a stable body temperature.
3. Infant will experience no infections or injuries.
4. Infant will receive optimum nutrition.
5. Family will exhibit attachment behavior.
6. Family will be prepared for discharge and home care.

❖ Implementation

The following discussion on implementing newborn care focuses on nursing care after the infant has been delivered. A more detailed discussion of the birth and immediate care of the neonate can be found in any of the many excellent maternity texts.

Maintain a Patent Airway

Establishing a patent airway, the primary objective in the delivery room, is the responsibility of the attending physicians and nurses. However, maintaining a patent airway continues to be a priority, with attention to proper positioning of the infant to facilitate drainage of secretions, especially after feeding (see Fig. 8-17).

The American Academy of Pediatrics (1992b) recommends the supine or side-lying position during sleep for healthy newborns. Infants with breathing problems or excessive vomiting should sleep prone. This recommendation is based on the possible association between sleeping prone and sudden infant death syndrome (see Chapter 13).

A bulb syringe is kept near the infant and is used if suctioning is required. Used bulb syringes should be replaced every 24 hours in the hospital and boiled for 10 minutes when used in the home to prevent bacterial contamination (Patel and others, 1988).*

NURSING ALERT To avoid aspiration of amniotic fluid or mucus, clear the pharynx first, then the nasal passages. Compress the bulb *before* insertion to prevent forcing secretions into the bronchi.

If more forceful removal of secretions is required, mechanical suction is used. Use of the proper-size catheter and correct suctioning technique is essential in order to prevent mucosal damage and edema. Gentle suctioning is necessary to prevent reflex bradycardia, laryngospasm, and cardiac arrhythmias from vagal stimulation. Suctioning is performed for 5 seconds with sufficient time between each attempt to allow the infant to reoxygenate.

In some nurseries the stomach is routinely emptied (aspirated) to remove amniotic fluid that may cause abdominal distention and interfere with the establishment of respiration. Passing a catheter to the stomach also rules out esophageal atresia. Vital signs are closely monitored, and any indication of respiratory distress is immediately reported.

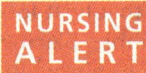

Signs of respiratory distress include tachypnea, grunting, flaring alae nasi, intercostal retractions, stridor, abnormal breath sounds, cyanosis, or pallor.

Maintain a Stable Body Temperature

Conserving the newborn's body heat is an essential nursing goal. At birth a major cause of heat loss is ***evaporation,*** the loss of heat through moisture. The amniotic fluid that bathes the infant's skin favors evaporation, especially when combined with the cool atmosphere of the delivery room. Heat loss through evaporation is minimized by rapidly drying the skin and hair with a warmed towel and placing the infant in a heated environment.

Another source of heat loss is ***radiation,*** the loss of heat to cooler solid objects in the environment that are not in direct contact with the infant. Loss of heat through radiation increases as these solid objects become colder and closer to the infant. The temperature of ambient (surrounding) air in the incubator essentially has no effect on loss of heat through radiation. This is a critical point to remember when attempting to maintain a constant temperature for the infant because, even though the temperature of the ambient air is optimum, the infant can become hypothermic. The use of radiant heating devices such as heat lamps or phototherapy lights with an incubator may cause overheating of the infant, since the neonate cannot effectively dissipate radiant heat through the Plexiglas wall of the incubator. For this same reason, an incubator should not be exposed to direct sunlight (Thomas, 1994).

An example of radiant heat loss is the placement of the incubator close to a cold window or air conditioning unit. The cold from either source will cool the walls of the incubator and subsequently the body of the neonate. To prevent this, the infant is placed as far away as possible from walls, windows, or ventilating units. If heat loss continues to be a problem, a radiant warmer may be placed over the infant or the infant and mother.

Heat loss can also occur through conduction and convection. ***Conduction*** involves loss of heat from the body from direct contact of skin with a cooler solid object; it is minimized by placing the infant on a padded, covered surface rather than directly on a hard table and by providing insulation through clothes and blankets. Placing the newborn very close to the mother, such as in her arms or on her abdomen immediately after delivery, is physically beneficial in

*Home care instructions for using a bulb syringe are available in *Wong and Whaley's Clinical Manual of Pediatric Nursing* (Mosby).

THINKING CRITICALLY ABOUT . . . *Gowning*

A common ritual in many newborn nurseries is the use of cover gowns and "scrub" clothes to prevent infection. However, several studies have shown that this practice is ineffective and costly (Birenbaum and others, 1990; Rush and others, 1990; Thigpen, 1991). Some believe that "gowning" reinforces the use of handwashing; however, research does not support this assumption. Rather, when gowns were used, fewer care providers entered the unit (Donowitz, 1986). One could speculate that the inconvenience of using gowns may even affect care if it discourages staff from visiting patients. What are the gowning policies in your agency and what reasons are given for their use?

terms of conserving heat, as well as fostering maternal attachment.

Convection is similar to conduction, except that heat loss is aided by surrounding air currents. For example, placing the infant in the direct flow of air from a fan or air conditioner vent causes rapid heat loss through convection. Transporting the neonate in a crib with solid sides reduces airflow around the infant.

Protect from Infection and Injury

The most important practice for preventing cross-infection is following universal precautions, especially thorough handwashing of all individuals involved in the infant's care (see Thinking Critically About . . . box above and Infection Control, Chapter 27).

Identification. Proper identification of the newborn is absolutely essential. The nurse must verify that two identifying bands are securely fastened, usually on the wrist and ankle, and verify the information (name, sex, mother's admission number, date, and time of birth) against the birth records and the child's actual sex. Some institutions have more sophisticated methods of infant identification, such as a color photograph kept in the medical record, storage of blood for DNA genotyping, and/or electronic surveillance systems for infant security (Butz and others, 1993). Foot printing or finger printing is *not* currently recommended for newborn identification (American Academy of Pediatrics and American College of Obstetricians and Gynecologists, 1992).

The nurse needs to discuss safety issues with the mother the first time the infant is brought to her. A written copy of the safety instructions should also be given to the parent. Parents are instructed to look at name badges of nurses and hospital personnel who come to take infants and not to relinquish their infants to anyone without proper identification. Some hospitals have systems of color-coded badges or symbols that are changed daily to decrease the likelihood of infant abduction. Mothers are also advised not to leave the infant alone in the crib while they shower; rather, they should ask to have the infant returned to the nursery if a family member is not present in the room. The nurse should document in the chart that these instructions were given.

Eye Care. Prophylactic eye treatment against ***ophthalmia neonatorum,*** infectious conjunctivitis of the newborn, includes the use of (1) silver nitrate (1%) solution, (2) erythromycin (0.5%) ophthalmic ointment or drops, or (3) tetracycline (1%) ophthalmic ointment or drops (preferably in single-dose ampules or tubes) (see Guidelines box). The drug of choice until recently was either erythromycin or tetracycline because both were thought to afford protection against *Chlamydia trachomatis,* the major cause of ophthalmia neonatorum in the United States. Although silver nitrate is effective against gonococcal conjunctivitis, it was thought to be ineffective against *Chlamydia* and can cause a severe chemical conjunctivitis (American Academy of Pediatrics and American College of Obstetricians and Gynecologists, 1992). However, there is accumulating evidence that neither erythromycin nor tetracycline significantly reduces the incidence of chlamydial conjunctivitis and that silver nitrate may be more effective than erythromycin (Zanoni, Isenberg, and Apt, 1992). Although eye prophylaxis is mandatory in the United States, health care facilities are free to choose specific drugs. Effective prophylaxis may be better directed at treating maternal chlamydial infection (Hammerschlag and others, 1989).

Since studies on maternal attachment emphasize that in the first hour of life a newborn has a greater ability to focus on coordinated movement than at any other time during the next several days and since eye contact is very important in the development of maternal-infant bonding, the routine administration of silver nitrate or antibiotics can be postponed for up to 1 hour. However, there must be some kind of checklist to ensure that the drug is given within this time.

Vitamin K Administration. Shortly after birth, vitamin K is administered as a single intramuscular dose of 0.5 to 1 mg to prevent hemorrhagic disease of the newborn (see Chapter 9). Normally vitamin K is synthesized by the intestinal flora. However, since the infant's intestine is sterile at

GUIDELINES
Ophthalmia Neonatorum Prophylaxis

1. Clean the eyelids with sterile cotton and sterile water if needed.
2. Separate lids and apply 2 drops or a 1 to 2 cm (½ inch) ribbon of ointment in each conjunctival sac.
3. Massage lids to ensure spread of the medication.
4. Wipe excess medication from eye with sterile cotton 1 minute after application.
5. Do not rinse eyes with sterile normal saline.

birth and since breast milk contains low levels of vitamin K, the supply is inadequate for at least the first 3 to 4 days. The major function of vitamin K is to catalyze the synthesis of prothrombin in the liver, which is needed for blood clotting and coagulation. The vastus lateralis muscle is the preferred injection site because of the absence of other well-developed muscle masses.

Although only injectable vitamin K is available in the United States, the oral form is used in other countries. However its effectiveness has been questioned. The oral form should be given at birth (2.0 mg) and again at 1 to 2 weeks, with a third dose at 4 weeks to breast-fed infants. If diarrhea occurs in an exclusively breast-fed infant, the dose should be repeated (American Academy of Pediatrics, 1993b).

Hepatitis B (HBV) Vaccine Administration. To decrease the incidence of HBV in children and its serious consequences, cirrhosis and liver cancer, in adulthood, the first of three doses of HBV vaccine is recommended between birth and 2 days of age for uninfected newborns. It is recommended at birth for neonates whose mothers are positive for HBV surface antigen (HBsAg). The injection is given in the vastus lateralis or deltoid muscle (American Academy of Pediatrics, 1992a). (See also Immunizations, Chapter 12.)

Screening for Genetic Disease. A number of genetic disorders can be detected in the newborn period. There is no national policy in the United States; therefore the extent of neonatal screening is determined by state laws and voluntary guidelines. Most states require screening for phenylketonuria (PKU), hypothyroidism, galactosemia, and sickle cell disease (see Chapters 9 and 35). (For information on several diseases that may be included in newborn screening, see American Academy of Pediatrics, 1989a).

The nurse's responsibility is to educate parents regarding the importance of screening and to collect appropriate specimens at the recommended time (after 24 hours of age) (Coody and others, 1993). Accurate screening depends on good-quality blood spots (see Atraumatic Care box) on approved filter paper forms. The blood should completely saturate the filter paper spot on one side only. The paper should not be handled, placed on wet surfaces, or contaminated with substances, such as coffee or tea.

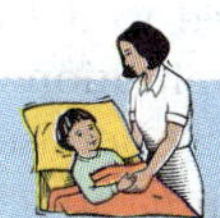

ATRAUMATIC CARE
Heel Punctures

Repeated heel lancing may be needed to obtain sufficient blood for the spot test. The use of automated lancet devices, such as Tenderfoot,* has been found to cause less pain and require fewer punctures than using manual lance blades (Blain-Lewis, 1992; Paes and others, 1993). EMLA, a topical anesthetic, also significantly reduces the pain of heel puncture (Fitzgerald, Millard, and McIntosh, 1989). Giving infants a plain pacifier or a sucrose-flavored pacifier during the procedure decreases the amount of crying (Blass and Hoffmeyer, 1991; Campos, 1993), but less behavioral upset may not indicate less physiologic stress.

*Manufactured by International Technidyne, Inc., Edison, NJ.

Bathing. The bath time can be an opportunity for the nurse to accomplish much more than general hygiene. It is an excellent time for observations of the infant's behavior, such as irritability, state of arousal, alertness, and muscular activity. Bathing is done after the vital signs have stabilized. There is no need to immediately wash a newborn, except to remove blood or vernix caseosa from the face and head. There may be some benefit to leaving the vernix on other parts of the body as a protective covering. Cleansing only grossly soiled areas with soap and water rather than giving a daily bath does not increase infection rates in the hospital (Rush, 1986). As part of infection control, nurses should wear gloves when in contact with body substances such as amniotic fluid or vernix.

The bath time provides an opportunity for the nurse to involve the parents in the care of their child, to teach correct hygiene procedures, and to learn about their infant's individual characteristics (Fig. 8-14). The appropriate types of bathing supplies and the need for safety in terms of water temperature and supervision of the infant at all times during the bath are stressed. For example, if sponges are used, they need to dry thoroughly between each use (may require a clothes dryer) to prevent growth of organisms (Sheth and others, 1986).

Parents are encouraged to examine every finger and toe of their infant during bathing. Frequently normal variations such as Epstein pearls, mongolian spots, or "stork bites" cause parents much worry because they are unaware of the insignificance of such findings. Minor birth injuries may appear as major defects to them. Explaining how these occurred and when they will disappear reassures parents of their infant's normalcy. Common variations are discussed further in Chapter 9.

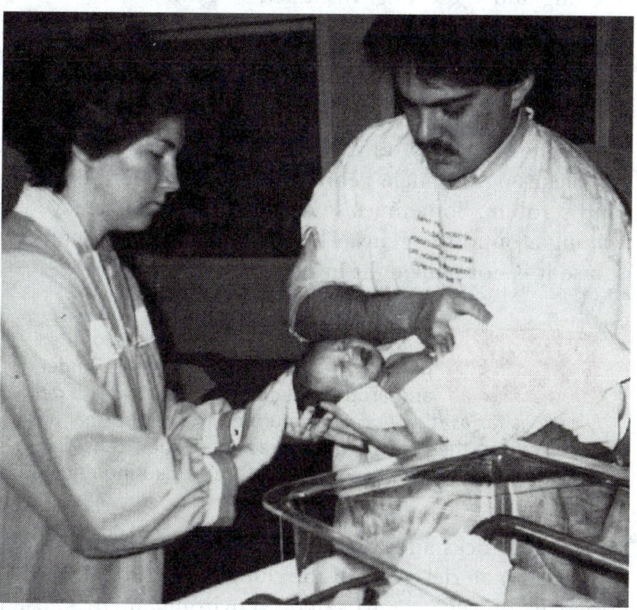

FIG. 8-14 Bath time is an excellent opportunity for parents to learn about their newborn.

One of the most important considerations in skin cleansing is preservation of the skin's "acid mantle," which is formed from the uppermost horny layer of the epidermis, sweat, superficial fat, metabolic products, and external substances such as amniotic fluid, microorganisms, and cosmetics. The infant's skin surface has a pH of about 5 soon after birth, and the bacteriostatic effects of this pH are significant. Consequently, only plain warm water should be used for the bath. If a cleanser is needed, Dove is gentle and effective. Alkaline soaps such as Ivory, oils, powder, and lotions are not used, because they alter the acid mantle, thus providing a medium for bacterial growth. Talcum powder has the added risk of aspiration if it is applied too close to the infant's face. A safer alternative is a cornstarch-based powder (see also Diaper Dermatitis, Chapter 13).

Cleansing proceeds in the cephalocaudal (head-to-toe) direction. A washcloth is used and turned so that a clean part touches the skin with each stroke. The eyes are carefully wiped from the inner to the outer aspect of the lid. The face is cleansed next. The nares are carefully inspected for any crusted secretions. The scalp is usually wiped, although it is sometimes necessary to shampoo the hair. Shampooing is best accomplished by positioning the infant's head over a small basin, lathering the scalp with a mild soap, and rinsing by pouring water from a small vessel over the head into the basin. The rest of the body is kept covered during this procedure. The head is dried quickly in order to prevent heat loss from evaporation. The ears are cleaned with the twisted end of a washcloth, not with a cotton-tipped swab, which, if inserted into the canal, can damage the ear.

The rest of the body is washed in a similar manner. Although the infant's skin requires little rubbing for adequate cleansing, certain areas (e.g., folds of neck, axillae, and creases at joints) need special attention. The area around the neck is especially prone to a rash from regurgitation of feeding and is thoroughly washed and dried.

The genitalia of both sexes require careful cleansing. Cleansing of the vulva is done in a front-to-back direction. The bath is a perfect opportunity to stress this part of hygiene to the mother, for both the infant's and her protection against urinary tract infection.

Cleansing the male genitalia involves washing the penis and scrotum. Sometimes smegma needs to be removed by wiping around the glans. The foreskin is not retracted, because it is normally tight in newborns.

NURSING ALERT If an infant is not to be circumcised, the parents are taught how to cleanse under and around the foreskin by *moving it gently only as far as it will go* and returning it to its normal position. Leaving the prepuce in a retracted position constricts the blood vessels supplying the glans penis, causing edema.

The buttocks and anal area are thoroughly cleansed of any fecal material. As with the rest of the body, the area is dried to prevent a warm, moist environment that fosters growth of bacteria.

Diapers are applied after the bath. They should fit snugly around the thighs and abdomen to prevent urine from leaking. In males cloth diapers are folded with extra thickness in the front to provide greater absorbency. In females the placement of the extra fold depends on whether the infant is prone or supine. Diapers are fastened with the back side overlapping the front side to allow full flexion of the hips.

The nurse should discuss the choice of cloth or disposable diapers with parents.* In the United States the most commonly used diapers are disposable paper diapers and either home-laundered or commercially laundered cloth diapers. A number of factors—cost, convenience, skin care benefits, infection control, and environmental concerns—influence the relative merits of these three diaper types. In general, home-laundered diapers are the least expensive when home labor cost is not included. Once home labor cost is included, the price difference between disposable diapers, diaper service reusable diapers, and home-laundered diapers is quite small, although paper diapers tend to cost the most. Disposable diapers are the most convenient, although a diaper service eliminates the need to shop for replacement diapers.

Disposable diapers with absorbent gelling material (AGM) have benefits related to preserving healthy skin, preventing diaper dermatitis, especially beyond the neonatal period (see Chapter 13), and controlling spread of infection because of their better containment of urine and feces.

The most controversial issue surrounding the discussion of disposable vs cloth diapers has been their effect on the environment. Disposable diapers are discarded as solid waste in landfills, whereas waste from laundered diapers is disposed of as treated sewage. The main differences between solid waste and treated sewage are cost and possibly sanitation, with solid waste being more expensive. However, the manufacture and disposal of cloth and paper diapers affect energy resources and the environment differently. Paper diapers consume more raw materials and generate more solid waste. Cloth diapers, especially home-laundered ones, use more water and energy and create more water and air pollution (Wong and others, 1992).

Care of the Umbilicus. Because the umbilical stump is an excellent medium for bacterial growth, various methods of cord care are practiced. None has proved to be superior, although one study found the topical application of triple dye (a solution of brilliant green, proflavine hemisulfate, and crystal violet) to be more effective than bacitracin ointment (Andrich and Golden, 1984). Also, the use of

---

*Resources for families are *A Matter of Care: An Information Guide for Parents About Diaper Rash* and *Answers to Your Questions About the Environment,* available from The National Association of Pediatric Nurse Associates and Practitioners (NAPNAP), 1101 Kings Highway North, Suite 206, Cherry Hill, NJ 08034, (609) 667-1773; *What's Best for Baby Bottoms,* available from Procter & Gamble, One Procter & Gamble Plaza, Cincinnati, OH 45202, (800) 543-0480; *The Diaper Decision: What to Consider When Making the Choice for Your Baby,* available from American Forest and Paper Association, 1111 19th St., N.W., Suite 800, Washington, DC 20036, (212) 463-2442; and *Making a Decision You Can Trust: The Facts About Diapers and Your Baby,* available from GET REAL, 4204 West Silver Spring Dr., No. 114, Milwaukee, WI 53209, (800) 878-8160.

THINKING CRITICALLY ABOUT . . . *Neonatal Circumcision*

Since 1975 the American Academy of Pediatrics had opposed routine neonatal circumcision on the grounds that there were no valid medical indications for the procedure and that a program of good personal hygiene offered all the advantages of circumcision without the attendant surgical risks. However, in 1989 the American Academy of Pediatrics reversed its position, stating that "newborn circumcision has potential medical benefits and advantages as well as disadvantages and risks." The statement does not recommend the surgical procedure but leaves the decision to the parents after they are "fully informed" of the risks and benefits (American Academy of Pediatrics, 1989b).

Arguments for circumcision include prevention of penile cancer, posthitis (inflammation of prepuce), and balanoposthitis (inflammation of glans and prepuce); decreased incidence of balanitis (inflammation of glans); urinary tract infection (UTI) and some sexually transmitted diseases; and prevention of complications associated with later circumcision (Herzog and Alvarez, 1986; Larsen and Williams, 1990; Maden and others, 1993; Wiswell and Hachey, 1993). However, not all authorities believe that the proposed benefits, especially less UTI during infancy, should dictate the decision to circumcise (Chessare, 1992; Lohr, 1989; Poland, 1990; Winberg and others, 1989). A nonmedical consideration for circumcision is preservation of a male's body image that is consistent with his peers, since circumcision is a common practice in the United States. For many parents the strongest motivating factor for deciding on circumcision for their newborn is the father's circumcision status (Brown and Brown, 1987).

Although neonatal circumcision is a relatively safe procedure when performed by skilled practitioners, it is often delegated to medical students and residents (Cuckow and Mourquand, 1993). Opponents stress the complications: hemorrhage, infection, dehiscence (separation of approximated skin edges), meatitis from loss of protective foreskin, adhesions, concealed penis, urethral fistula, meatal stenosis, amputation, and cosmetic disfigurement.

Most studies have used retrospective methods (chart reviews) to assess the incidence of postoperative complications, with one study reporting a rate of 0.19% (Wiswell and Geschke, 1989). However, the overall complication rate may be considerably higher. When data were collected prospectively (direct observation following the procedure), the overall rate was 7.7% (Infant circumcision, 1989). This difference in reported rates points out the need for more prospective studies, with emphasis on causes for various complications.

Among adverse effects of circumcision is the pain inflicted on the infant. Studies on the use of regional anesthesia document the distress exhibited in unanesthetized infants, such as increased heart rate, behavior changes, prolonged crying, increased cortisol levels, and decreased blood oxygenation (Dixon and others, 1984; Maxwell and others, 1987; Stang and others, 1988). In each of these studies the use of a local dorsal penile nerve block (DPNB) significantly reduced these signs of distress and produced no serious complications. Despite the favorable findings, the American Academy of Pediatrics did not endorse the use of a nerve block or any other type of anesthetic for neonatal circumcision (American Academy of Pediatrics, 1989b). This is in contrast to their earlier statement on neonatal anesthesia, which recommends the use of anesthesia for newborns undergoing surgical procedures (American Academy of Pediatrics, 1987). Unfortunately, the use of nonpharmacologic pain reducers (pacifier, distraction) has not been found to be effective in reducing physiologic distress (Gunnar, Fisch, and Malone, 1984; Marchette, and others, 1991). Preliminary evidence suggests that a sugared pacifier may reduce pain. The study found that infants who sucked on a sugared pacifier, compared with infants who did not, cried less during the circumcision (Blass and Hoffmeyer, 1991). However, the results only showed less behavioral distress.

In view of these arguments for and against circumcision, nurses need to take an active role in ensuring that parents are adequately informed.* What are the consent practices in your facility? Do parents receive unbiased verbal or written information? Do they have choices regarding the infant's pain management and/or their presence during the procedure? Are they given sufficient time to consider the options? Such decisions should be made during the prenatal period when opportunities exist for discussion.

However, during the birth admission, you can also be an advocate for the newborn, especially regarding pain control. Is DPNB or EMLA (eutectic mixture of local anesthetics; see Atraumatic Care box) used? Is there sufficient waiting time for the anesthetic to work (see Atraumatic Care box)? Have you tried a sugared "pacifier," such as a gauze pad moistened with a 24% dextrose solution? Is the infant kept warm during the procedure and released from restraints and comforted as soon as possible after the surgery? Consider strategies to increase use of these comfort measures (e.g., in-service education, written policy, and research to document outcomes of intervention). Factors that have been found to increase physicians' use of DPNB are (1) cooperation of nursery staff (i.e., having equipment available); (2) instruction regarding use of DPNB (i.e., written videotape, lecture, preceptor); (3) belief that DPNB reduces pain; and (4) parents' likelihood of giving consent (Fontaine, 1990).

In many countries, including the United States and Canada, guidelines exist that would not allow a procedure such as circumcision to be performed on a laboratory animal without adequate anesthesia (Council on Scientific Affairs, 1991). Don't human infants warrant as much consideration?

*Information is available from the Circumcision Resource Center, P.O. Box 232, Boston MA 02133; (617) 523-0088.

povidone-iodine increases plasma iodide levels, which may suppress thyroid secretion (Newman, 1989; Ramsey and Svee, 1988). Regardless of the type of treatment, the diaper is placed below the cord to avoid irritation and wetness on the site.

Parents are instructed regarding stump deterioration and proper umbilical care. The stump deteriorates through the process of dry gangrene. Cord separation time is influenced by a number of factors, including type of cord care, type of delivery, and other perinatal events (Gladstone and others, 1988; Novack, Mueller, and Ochs, 1988; Oudesluys-Murphy and DeGroot, 1988):

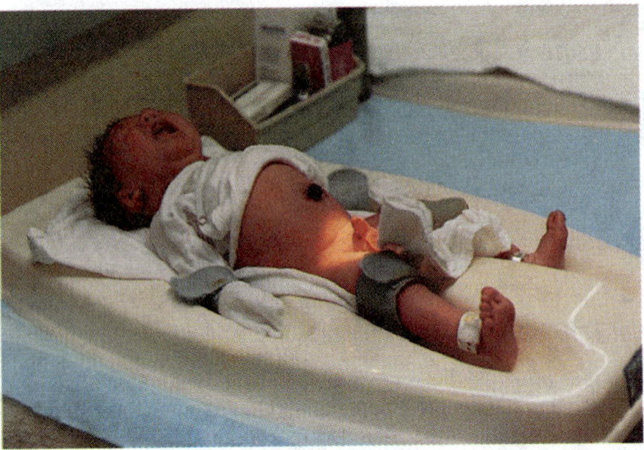

FIG. 8-15 Proper positioning of infant in Circumstraint.

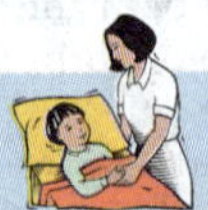

ATRAUMATIC CARE
Anesthesia to the Surgical Site

To reduce the pain of circumcision, a local dorsal penile nerve block (DPNB) can be administered at the base of the penis (Masciello, 1990). For maximum anesthesia, a waiting time of 5 minutes is needed for lidocaine and 3 minutes for chloroprocaine (Spencer and others, 1992). Buffering the lidocaine with 8.4% sodium bicarbonate in a 10:1 ratio and using a 30-gauge needle for the intradermal injection can reduce the pain associated with DPNB (Christoph and others, 1988). EMLA* cream (eutectic mixture of local anesthetics) provides a noninvasive form of local anesthesia (Benini and others, 1993).

*Manufactured by Astra Pharmaceuticals; for product information call (800) 228-EMLA.

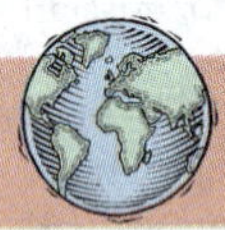

CULTURAL AWARENESS
Circumcision

In the Jewish culture circumcision is performed during a highly significant ceremony called a ***berith,*** or ***brit,*** which takes place on the eighth day of life. A specially trained professional known as a ***mohel*** stretches the prepuce over the glans, pulling it though a slit in a shield (usually a Mogen clamp) and cutting it with a knife. The traditional technique is not sterile, and bleeding is controlled by tight bandaging around the penis (Cohen and others, 1992). Blankets instead of straps are usually used to restrain the infant to a board, and the parents are present (Trochtenberg, 1990).

Female circumcision is also practiced, particularly in Africa, the Middle East, and Southeast Asia—and in immigrants from these countries to the United States, Australia, and Europe. In infants, children, and adolescents, all or part of the genitalia—including the clitoris and labia minora—is removed. The labia majora are scraped, and the vulva is sewn closed, except for a small opening for urine and menses. Anesthesia is used very rarely. In African and Asian cultures, female circumcision is used to prove virginity and to reduce sexual pleasure, thus promoting fidelity. In May 1993 the World Health Organization condemned all forms of female genital mutilation (Female genital mutilation, 1994).

- Average separation time of 14 days using triple dye daily during hospitalization; average time of 10 days using povidone-iodine applied daily until cord separation; average separation time of 7 days using only a dry gauze dressing
- Delayed separation in infants with hyperbilirubinemia and septicemia, in infants delivered by cesarean section, in infants born prematurely, and in the second-born of twins.

It takes a few more weeks for the cord base to heal completely following cord separation. During this time care consists of keeping the cord clean and dry and may include wiping the base with alcohol.

NURSING ALERT Instruct parents to report any signs of cord infection, such as presence of erythema and malodorous, purulent discharge, to their health care professional.

Circumcision. Circumcision, the surgical removal of the foreskin on the glans penis, is usually done in the hospital, although it is not a common practice in most countries. Despite the frequency of the procedure in the United States, there is much controversy regarding the benefits and risks (see Thinking Critically About . . . box, p. 315). In light of these arguments, parents must be allowed an *informed* consent regarding circumcision. Ideally, prospective parents should have an opportunity to examine all the facts and to decide for themselves (including choosing options for pain control and deciding whether or not they observe the procedure) without unnecessary pressure from health care professionals.

Circumcision is usually performed in the nursery. It should not be performed immediately after delivery because of the neonate's unstabilized physiologic status and increased susceptibility to stress. Preoperative nursing care includes allowing the infant nothing by mouth before the procedure to prevent aspiration of vomitus (about 2 hours), checking for a signed consent form, and adequately restraining the infant, usually on a special board (Fig. 8-15). All the equipment used for the procedure, such as gloves, instruments, dressings, and draping towels, must be sterile (see Atraumatic Care box).

The procedure involves freeing the foreskin from the glans penis by using a scalpel, Gomco or Mogen (see Cultural Awareness box) clamp, or Plastibell. In the ***Gomco technique*** the foreskin is clamped and removed; the clamp crushes the nerve endings and blood vessels, promoting hemostasis. In the ***Plastibell procedure*** the foreskin is removed using a plastic ring and a string tied around the foreskin like a tourniquet. The excess foreskin is trimmed. In about 5 to 8 days the plastic ring separates and falls off.

As soon as the procedure is completed, the infant is released from the restraints and comforted. If the parents were not present during the procedure, they are informed of the infant's status and reunited with their son.

Care of the circumcision depends on the type of procedure. If a clamp was used, a petrolatum gauze dressing may be applied loosely to prevent adherence to the diaper. If the Plastibell was applied, no special dressing is required. Since the area is tender, the diaper is applied loosely to prevent friction against the penis; the first void is recorded.

ADVANTAGES OF HUMAN MILK VS COW'S MILK

Contains adequate (not excessive) protein; has greater quantities of certain amino acids, including cystine and taurine
Contains more lactalbumin (produces easily digested curds) than casein (produces large, hard curds)
Contains more lactose, which in the gut stimulates growth of microorganisms, which synthesize some B vitamins and produce organic acids that may retard growth of harmful bacteria
Contains more monounsaturated fatty acids, which enhance absorption of fat and calcium
Contains adequate (not excessive) minerals with exception of fluoride (low in both)
Amounts of iron and zinc are low but more readily absorbed
Contains less calcium and phosphorus but a more favorable ratio of the minerals, which prevents excessive calcium excretion
Contains adequate amounts of vitamins A, B complex, and E; vitamin C content depends on maternal intake; vitamin D is low but more readily absorbed (vitamins C, D, and E are low in cow's milk, but K is higher)
Contains growth modulators that modify growth or maturation
Offers several immunologic benefits: contains various immunoglobulins (Ig), especially IgA; macrophages, granulocytes, T- and B-cell lymphocytes, and other factors that inhibit bacterial growth
Has laxative effect
Is economical, readily available, and sanitary
Has psychologic benefits of close bond between infant and mother during feeding

➤ **NURSING TIP** To check for the first void in disposable diapers made of absorbent gelling material, pinch the crotch of the diaper for a "clumpy, doughy" feeling, because these diapers will feel dry despite voiding.

Normally on the second day a yellowish white exudate forms as part of the granulation process. This is not a sign of infection and is not forcibly removed. As healing progresses, the exudate disappears. Parents are cautioned to report any evidence of bleeding, unusual swelling, or absence of voiding to the practitioner.

Provide Optimum Nutrition

Selection of a feeding method is one of the major decisions faced by parents. In general, there are three acceptable choices: human milk, commercially prepared cow's milk formula, and modified evaporated cow's milk. There are significant nutritional, economic, and psychologic advantages and differences among these methods (see box above). Nurses need to be aware of the types of feeding to help parents choose the method that best meets their needs (see also Chapter 12).

Comparison of Human Milk and Cow's Milk. Although this discussion focuses on the differences between cow's milk and human milk, whole cow's milk is not recommended for infants less than 12 months of age (see Table 8-5). There are significant nutritional differences between human milk and whole cow's milk. Cow's milk contains much more available protein (3.5 g/dl) than human milk (0.7 g/dl), but more than the infant requires. The type of protein also differs. Human milk contains more whey proteins, especially lactalbumin, a more complete protein than casein protein. The higher percentage of casein in cow's milk results in the formation of large, hard curds. Human milk is more easily digested because of the presence of soft, flocculent curds. Therefore, stomach emptying time is more rapid with human milk, necessitating more frequent feedings. Human milk also contains a higher amount of cystine, an amino acid essential during the first few weeks of life, because the enzyme cystathionase, which converts methionine to cystine, is very low in newborns. Taurine, a conditionally essential amino acid (necessary under certain conditions, such as fetal development and early infancy), is also present in larger amounts in human milk. Taurine is involved in fat metabolism, retinal development, and auditory maturation (Gaull, 1989; Tyson and others, 1989).

Cow's milk and human milk both provide 20 kcal/ounce, but human milk contains a higher amount of lactose, a disaccharide that is converted into the monosaccharides glucose and galactose. Galactose is essential for the formation of galactolipids, which are necessary for the growth of the central nervous system.

Although the amount of fat in both types of milk is similar, the type of fat differs. Human milk contains more monounsaturated fatty acids, especially linoleic acid, whereas cow's milk has more polysaturated fatty acids. Human milk has smaller fat globules than cow's milk, which enables the infant to absorb human milk fat more efficiently. In addition, the fat content of human milk varies during the feeding and with time of day. It is highest toward the end of feeding and at midday (Lawrence, 1994).

The mineral content of cow's milk is considerably greater than that of human milk, with the exception of iron and fluoride. Although the amount of iron is low in both types of milk, the iron in human milk is much better absorbed by the infant. Another difference is the amount of calcium and phosphorus, minerals especially needed by the rapidly growing infant. Cow's milk contains more of these minerals but a lower calcium/phosphorus ratio (1.5 to 1). Because of the infant's immature regulatory mechanisms, calcium is excreted, resulting in hypocalcemia, which may cause tetany. Human milk contains a smaller amount but more balanced proportion of these minerals, with a higher calcium/phosphorus ratio (2 to 1). Both types of milk contain adequate amounts of zinc, a mineral identified as essential to the human. However, the zinc in human milk is more readily absorbed. Both types of milk are low in fluoride, and supplementation is recommended (see Fluoride, Chapter 14).

Both human and cow's milk provide adequate amounts of vitamins A and B complex. Vitamin C is low in cow's milk but higher in human milk, provided the mother's intake is adequate. Vitamin D is low in human milk but adequate, depending on the mother's intake and the infant's exposure to sunlight. Cow's milk and its preparations are usually fortified with vitamin D. Human milk contains only one fourth the amount of vitamin K as cow's milk, requiring supplementation at birth.

Although commercial cow's milk formulas are modified to closely resemble the nutritional content of human milk, other significant advantages to human milk exist. The presence of growth modulators, such as epidermal growth factor (EGF), appear to stimulate DNA synthesis and intestinal tract maturation (Lawrence, 1994). Human milk contains high levels of lysozyme activity and immunoglobulin A (IgA) and affords protection against several bacterial and viral diseases, especially those of the respiratory (including otitis media) (Duncan and others, 1993) and gastrointestinal systems. Evidence suggests that human milk protects against development of food allergies and enhances the active immune response to *Haemophilus influenzae* type B vaccine (Pabst and Spady, 1990). In addition, human milk contains numerous other host defense factors, such as macrophages, granulocytes, and T- and B-lymphocytes.

There is preliminary evidence that human milk increases the child's intelligence, especially when fed to premature infants. Human milk may contain factors, such as long-chain lipids and hormones, that influence brain growth and maturation (Lucus and others, 1992). Other physiologic benefits of human milk are its laxative effect and less irritation of the skin from stools. Nonphysiologic advantages are discussed under Breast-Feeding (at right).

NURSING ALERT Do not use microwaving to defrost frozen human milk. High-temperature microwaving (72° C to 98° C [162° to 208° F]) significantly destroys the antiinfective factors. The safety of low-temperature microwaving (20° to 53° C [68° to 127° F]) is questionable (Quan and others, 1992).

Evaporated Milk and Commercially Prepared Formulas. The analysis of human and cow's milk shows that whole cow's milk is unsuitable for infant nutrition. It must be diluted to meet the lowered protein requirement, but when dilute, it does not meet the caloric or fat requirement. Modified evaporated milk or commercially prepared formula is chosen as a substitute.

In the United States a very small percentage of infants are fed ***evaporated milk formula.*** However, it has many advantages over whole milk. It is readily available in cans, needs no refrigeration if unopened, is less expensive than commercial formula, provides a softer, more digestible curd, and contains more lactalbumin and a higher calcium/phosphorus ratio. A common rule for preparing evaporated milk formula is diluting the 13-ounce can of milk with 17 ounces of water and adding 1 to 2 tablespoons of sugar or corn syrup.

Evaporated milk must not be confused with condensed milk, which is a form of evaporated milk with 45% more sugar. Because of its high carbohydrate concentration and disproportionately low fat and protein content, condensed milk is not used for infant feeding. Likewise, skim milk must not be used because it is deficient in caloric concentration, significantly increases the renal solute load and water demands, and deprives the body of essential fatty acids.

Commercially prepared formulas are milk-based formulas that have been modified to closely resemble the nutritional content of human milk (Table 8-5). However, they are not an exact substitute. For example, human milk has more cholesterol and saturated fatty acids than commercial formula. Total cholesterol levels are higher in breast-fed infants, although they decrease once weaning begins. If human milk provides optimum infant nutrition, some have questioned whether the lower cholesterol and higher polyunsaturated fats in commercial formula are sufficient (Kallio and others, 1992).

Commercial formulas are available in three preparations: (1) a ready-to-use form in cans or bottles, (2) a concentrated liquid form that is diluted with an equal amount of water, and (3) a powdered form that must be prepared according to the manufacturer's directions. One consideration in the use of commercially prepared formulas is their cost. Families should do comparison shopping, since one preparation can be considerably more expensive than another.

Breast-Feeding. ***Human milk*** is the preferred form of nutrition for the full-term infant. Unfortunately, the incidence of breast-feeding in the United States has been declining since its peak in 1982, when about 60% of mothers breast-fed their newborns. In 1989 52% of newborns in hospitals were breast-fed, but only 18% were still breast-fed at 6 months of age (Ryan and others, 1991). Although the incidence of breast-feeding decreased among all groups of women, the greatest decline occurred in women who were black, younger in age, low-income, poorly educated, enrolled in the Women and Children (WIC) program, or parents of a low-birth-weight infant. Some believe that the increasingly early discharge of new mothers from hospitals, more aggressive marketing of infant formulas to the public, and more employed mothers have contributed to the decline (Freed, 1993). Some studies have shown that the availability of commercial formula from hospital "discharge packs" may influence mothers to bottle-feed (Frank and others, 1987). However, other studies have found no such effect (Evans, Lyons, and Killien, 1986). Including a manual breast pump in the discharge pack may increase breast-feeding (Dungy and others, 1992).

In addition to the physiologic qualities of human milk, the most outstanding psychologic benefit of breast-feeding is the close maternal-child relationship. The infant is nestled very close to the mother's skin, can hear the rhythm of her heartbeat, feel the warmth of her body, and sense a peaceful security. The mother has a very close feeling of union with her child and feels a sense of accomplishment and satisfaction as the infant sucks milk from her.

Human milk is the most economical form of feeding. It is always available, ready to serve at room temperature, and free of contamination. Although human milk is not sterile, healthy full-term infants can tolerate varying amounts of nonpathogenic and pathogenic organisms (Meier and Wilks, 1987). The protection against infection can provide additional cost savings in terms of fewer medical visits and less time lost from work for the employed mother.

Breast-feeding may also offer protection against obesity and atherosclerosis, although the evidence is inconclusive. Breast-fed infants, especially beyond 2 to 3 months of age,

TABLE 8-5 Normal and Special Infant Formulas*

FORMULA (MANUFACTURER)	PROTEIN SOURCE	CARBOHYDRATE SOURCE	FAT SOURCES	INDICATIONS FOR USE	COMMENTS (NUTRITIONAL CONSIDERATIONS)
HUMAN AND COW'S MILK FORMULAS					
Human breast milk	Mature human milk; whey/casein ratio; 60:40	Lactose	Mature human milk	For all full-term infants except those with galactosemia; may be used with low-birth-weight infants	Recommended sole form of feeding for first 5 to 6 months; nutritionally complete except for fluoride
Evaporated cow's milk formulas	Milk protein; whey/casein ratio: 18:82	Lactose, sucrose	Butterfat	For full-term infants with no special nutritional requirements; use of undiluted cow's milk after 12 months	Supplement with iron and vitamin C; A and D if not fortified; fluoride if fluoridated water is not used for formula preparation
COMMERCIAL INFANT FORMULAS					
Enfamil (Mead Johnson)	Nonfat cow's milk, demineralized whey: whey/casein ratio: 60:40	Lactose	Palm olein, soy, coconut, HOSun† oils	For full-term and premature infants with no special nutritional requirements	Available fortified with iron, 12 mg/L Also available in 24 kcal/oz
Similac (Ross)	Nonfat cow's milk; whey/casein ratio: 18:82	Lactose	Soy, coconut oils	For full-term and premature infants with no special nutritional requirements	Available fortified with iron, 12 mg/L
SMA (Wyeth)	Nonfat cow's milk, reduced-mineral whey: whey/casein ratio: 60:40	Lactose	Oleo, coconut, oleic (safflower), soy oils	For full-term and premature infants with no special nutritional requirements	Supplemented with iron, 12 mg/L
Baby formula (Gerber)	Nonfat cow's milk; whey/casein ratio: 18:82	Lactose	Palm olein, soy, coconut, HOSun oils	For full-term and premature infants with no special nutritional requirements	Available fortified with iron, 11.5 mg/L
Good Start H.A. (Carnation)	Hydrolyzed whey	Lactose, maltodextrin	Palm olein, soy, safflower, coconut oils	For full-term infants	Manufacturer's claim regarding hypoallergenicity has been withdrawn
Good Nature (Carnation)	Nonfat cow's milk	Corn syrup solids	Palm, corn, oleic oils	For feeding older infants	Contains more protein and calcium than "starter" formulas
Similac Natural Care (Ross)	Nonfat cow's milk; whey protein concentrate	Hydrolyzed corn starch, lactose	MCT,‡ coconut, soy oils	For low-birth-weight infants; fed mixed with human milk or fed alternately with human milk; improves vitamin/mineral content of human milk	Protein, 2.7 g/100 ml; osmolality—24 cal/oz—300 mOsm/kg water

*All formulas provide 20 kcal/oz except as noted in product information from the formula manufacturers. For the most current information, consult product-labels or package enclosures.
†HOSun, high-oleic sunflower.
‡MCT, medium-chain triglycerides.
§L-Amino acids include L-cystine, L-tyrosine, and L-tryptophan, which are reduced in hydrolyzed, charcoal-treated casein.
||Ross Laboratories and Mead Johnson manufacture several specialty formulas for metabolic disorders for infants.

Continued.

TABLE 8-5 Normal and Special Infant Formulas*—cont'd

FORMULA (MANUFACTURER)	PROTEIN SOURCE	CARBOHYDRATE SOURCE	FAT SOURCES	INDICATIONS FOR USE	COMMENTS (NUTRITIONAL CONSIDERATIONS)
COMMERCIAL INFANT FORMULAS—cont'd					
Enfamil Human Milk Fortifier (Mead Johnson)	Whey protein concentrate, casein	Corn syrup solids	Trace	For low-birth-weight infants; fed mixed with human milk; increases protein, calories, calcium, phosphorus, and other nutrients	Used only as human milk fortifier, not as separate formula; one packet of powder supplies 3.5 kcal/ml
FOR MILK PROTEIN—SENSITIVE INFANTS ("MILK ALLERGY"), LACTOSE INTOLERANCE					
Prosobee (Mead Johnson)	Soy protein isolate	Corn syrup solids	Palm, soy, coconut, HOSun oils	With milk protein allergy, lactose intolerance, lactase deficiency, galactosemia	Hypoallergenic, zero band antigen; lactose- and sucrose-free
Isomil (Ross)	Soy protein isolate	Corn syrup, sucrose	Soy, coconut oils	With milk protein allergy, lactose intolerance, lactase deficiency, galactosemia	Hypoallergenic; lactose-free
Isomil OF (Ross)	Soy protein isolate	Hydrolyzed corn starch	Soy, coconut oils	For use during diarrhea	Lessens amount and duration of watery stools; contains fiber
Lactofree (Mead Johnson)	Milk protein isolate	Corn syrup solids	Palm olein, soy, HOSun oils	With lactose intolerance, lactase deficiency, galactosemia	Lactose-free
Nursoy (Wyeth)	Soy protein isolate	Sucrose (liquid formula) Corn syrup solids (powdered formula)	Oleo, coconut, soy, HOSun/safflower oils	With milk protein allergy, lactose intolerance, lactase deficiency, galactosemia	Lactose-free
Soyalac (Loma Linda)	Soybean solids	Sucrose, corn syrup	Soy oil	With milk protein allergy, lactose intolerance, lactase deficiency, galactosemia	Lactose-free
I-Soyalac (Loma Linda)	Soy protein isolate	Sucrose tapioca dextrin	Soy oil	With milk protein allergy, lactose intolerance, lactase deficiency, galactosemia	Lactose- and corn-free
FOR INFANTS WITH MALABSORPTION SYNDROMES, MILK ALLERGY (HYDROLYSATE FORMULAS)					
RCF (Ross Carbohydrate Free) (Ross)	Soy protein isolate		Soy, coconut oils	With carbohydrate intolerance	Carbohydrate is added according to amount infant will tolerate
Portagen (Mead Johnson)	Sodium caseinate	Corn syrup solids, sucrose, lactose	MCT (coconut source), corn oil	For impaired fat absorption secondary to pancreatic insufficiency, bile acid deficiency, intestinal resection, lymphatic anomalies	Nutritionally complete

*All formulas provide 20 kcal/oz except as noted in product information from the formula manufacturers. For the most current information, consult product-labels or package enclosures.
†HOSun, high-oleic sunflower.
‡MCT, medium-chain triglycerides.
§L-Amino acids include L-cystine, L-tyrosine, and L-tryptophan, which are reduced in hydrolyzed, charcoal-treated casein.
||Ross Laboratories and Mead Johnson manufacture several specialty formulas for metabolic disorders for infants.

TABLE 8-5 Normal and Special Infant Formulas*—cont'd

FORMULA (MANUFACTURER)	PROTEIN SOURCE	CARBOHYDRATE SOURCE	FAT SOURCES	INDICATIONS FOR USE	COMMENTS (NUTRITIONAL CONSIDERATIONS)
FOR INFANTS WITH MALABSORPTION SYNDROMES, MILK ALLERGY (HYDROLYSATE FORMULAS)—cont'd					
Nutramigen (Mead Johnson)	Casein hydrolysate, L-amino acids§	Corn syrup solids, modified corn starch	Corn, soy oils	For infants and children sensitive to food proteins; use in galactosemic patients	Nutritionally complete; hypoallergenic formula; lactose- and sucrose-free
Pregestimil (Mead Johnson)	Casein hydrolysate, L-amino acids	Corn syrup solids, modified tapioca starch	MCT, soy, HOSun oils	Disaccharidase deficiencies, malabsorption syndromes, cystic fibrosis, intestinal resection	Nutritionally complete; easily digestible protein, carbohydrate, and fat; lactose- and sucrose-free
Alimentum (Ross)	Casein hydrolysate, L-amino acids	Sucrose, modified tapioca starch	MCT, oleic, soy oils	For infants and children sensitive to food proteins or with cystic fibrosis	Nutritionally complete; hypoallergenic formula; lactose-free
SPECIALTY FORMULAS					
Lonalac (Mead Johnson)	Casein	Lactose	Coconut	For children with congestive heart failure, who require reduced sodium intake	For long-term management, additional sodium must be given; supplement with vitamins C and D and iron; Na = 1 mEq/L
Similac PM 60/40 (Ross)	Whey protein concentrate, sodium caseinate (60:40 ratio)	Lactose	Coconut, corn oils	For newborns predisposed to hypocalcemia and infants with impaired renal, digestive, and cardiovascular functions	Low calcium, potassium, and phosphorus; relatively low solute load; Na = 7 mEq/L
DIET MODIFIERS					
Polycose (Ross)		Glucose polymers (corn syrup solids)		Used to increase calorie intake, as in failure-to-thrive infants	Carbohydrate only; a powdered or liquid calorie supplement; powder 23 kcal/tbsp
Moducal (Mead Johnson)		Hydrolyzed corn starch		Used to increase carbohydrate intake	Carbohydrate only; a powdered calorie supplement: 30 kcal/tbsp
Casec (Mead Johnson)	Calcium caseinate			Used to increase protein intake	Protein only; negligible fat and no carbohydrate
MCT Oil (Mead Johnson)			90% MCT (coconut source)	Supplement in fat malabsorption conditions	Fat only; 8.3 kcal/g; 115 kcal/tbsp
FOR INFANTS WITH PHENYLKETONURIA‖					
Lofenalac (Mead Johnson)	Casein hydrolysate, L-amino acids	Corn syrup solids, modified tapioca starch	Corn oil	For infants and children	111 mg phenylalanine per quart of formula (20 cal/qt); must be supplemented with other foods to provide minimal phenylalanine

Continued.

TABLE 8-5 Normal and Special Infant Formulas*—cont'd

FORMULA (MANUFACTURER)	PROTEIN SOURCE	CARBOHYDRATE SOURCE	FAT SOURCES	INDICATIONS FOR USE	COMMENTS (NUTRITIONAL CONSIDERATIONS)
FOR INFANTS WITH PHENYLKETONURIA‖—cont'd					
Phenyl-free (Mead Johnson)	L-Amino acids	Sucrose, corn syrup solids, modified tapioca starch	Corn, coconut oils	For children over 1 year of age	Phenylalanine-free; permits increased supplementation with normal foods
Phenex-1 (Ross)	L-Amino acids	Hydrolyzed corn starch	Soy, coconut, palm oils	For infants	Phenylalanine-free; fortified with L-tyrosine, L-glutamine, L-carnitine, and taurine; contains vitamins, minerals, and trace elements
Phenex-2 (Ross)	L-Amino acids	Hydrolyzed corn starch	Soy, coconut, palm oils	For children and adults	Phenylalanine-free; fortified with L-tyrosine, L-glutamine, L-carnitine, and taurine; contains vitamins, minerals, and trace elements
Pro-Phree (Ross)	None	Hydrolyzed corn starch	Soy, coconut, palm oils	For infants and toddlers requiring reduced protein intake	Must be supplemented with protein; has vitamins, minerals, and trace elements

*All formulas provide 20 kcal/oz except as noted in product information from the formula manufacturers. For the most current information, consult product-labels or package enclosures.
†HOSun, high-oleic sunflower.
‡MCT, medium-chain triglycerides.
§L-Amino acids include L-cystine, L-tyrosine, and L-tryptophan, which are reduced in hydrolyzed, charcoal-treated casein.
‖Ross Laboratories and Mead Johnson manufacture several specialty formulas for metabolic disorders for infants.

tend to grow at a satisfactory but slower rate than bottle-fed infants (Dewey and others, 1991).

Contraindications to breast-feeding include (American Academy of Pediatrics and American College of Obstetricians and Gynecologists 1992; Goldfarb, 1993):

- Serious, debilitating maternal disease, such as heart disorder or advanced cancer
- Cytomegalovirus (CMV)—primary risk is to infants receiving CMV infected donor milk, not to infected mother's infant who already has CMV
- Active tuberculosis
- Human immunodeficiency virus (HIV)—if acceptable feeding substitutes exist
- Galactosemia in the infant

Mastitis is usually not a contraindication if the discomfort is tolerable. Rarely, "breast milk jaundice" may require temporary cessation of breast-feeding (see Chapter 9).

Breast-feeding can also be used with twin births (Sollid and others, 1989). If both twins are full term, they can begin feedings immediately after birth (Fig. 8-16). Simultaneous feeding promotes the rapid production of milk needed for both infants and makes the milk that would normally be lost in the let-down reflex available to one of the twins. When only one infant is hungry, the mother should feed singly. She should also alternate breasts when feeding each infant and avoid favoring one breast for one infant. The sucking patterns of infants vary, and each infant needs the visual stimulation and exercise that alternating breasts provides.

Probably the greatest disadvantage of breast-feeding to many mothers is the perceived inconvenience of loss of freedom and independence. Being committed to feeding the infant every 2 to 3 hours can be overwhelming, especially to women with multiple responsibilities. Many women resume their careers shortly after their pregnancy and prefer to use bottle-feeding. However, breast-feeding and employment are possible, and suggestions for the mother are discussed in Chapter 12. Although breast-feeding is the preferred form of infant feeding, mothers' decisions regarding their preferences must be supported and respected.

Successful breast-feeding probably depends more on the mother's desire to breast-feed, satisfaction with breast-feeding, and available support systems than on any other

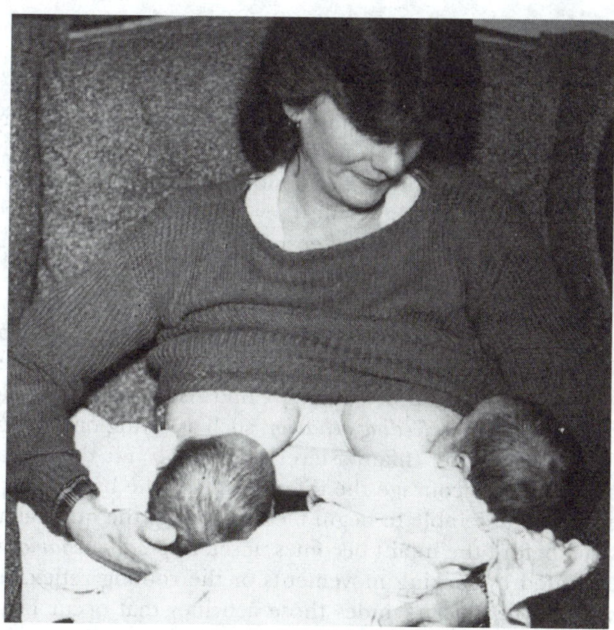

FIG. 8-16 Simultaneous breast-feeding of twins.

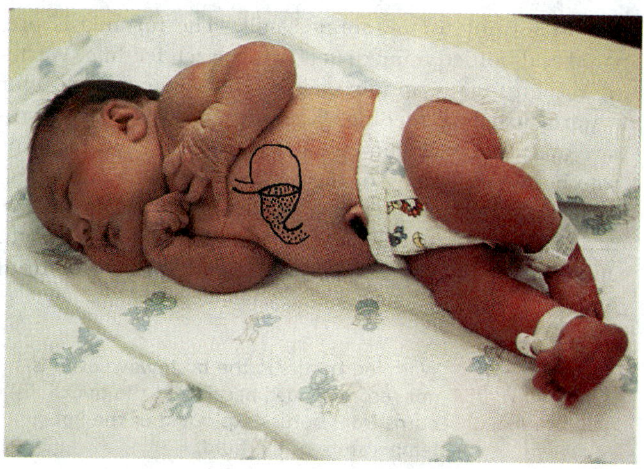

FIG. 8-17 Right-side-lying position after feeding.

factors. Contrary to popular belief, breast-feeding is not instinctive. Mothers need support, encouragement, and assistance during their postpartum hospital stay and at home to enhance their opportunities for success and satisfaction. The following hospital interventions promote breast-feeding (Bernard-Bonnin and others, 1989; Houston and Field, 1988; Kurinij and Shiono, 1991):

- Routines, such as frequent and early breast-feeding, especially during the first hour of life; immediate skin-to-skin contact, rooming-in, feeding on demand, and careful control of drugs
- Direct modeling of the importance of breast-feeding by staff, such as implementing demand nursing with no formula supplementation and decreased emphasis on infant formula products
- Increased information and support to mothers, especially phone follow-up
- Nurses play a very significant role in the breast-feeding decision and must make themselves available to families for guidance and support. Several excellent books (Lawrence, 1994) and organizations, such as ***LaLeche League,**** are available as resources for professionals and breast-feeding mothers.

Bottle-Feeding. Bottle-feeding generally refers to the use of bottles for feeding commercial or evaporated milk formula rather than using the breast, although in some instances human milk may be expressed and fed with a bottle. Bottle-feeding is an acceptable method of feeding. However, nurses should not assume that new parents automatically know how to bottle-feed their infant. These parents also need support and assistance in meeting their infant's needs.

*P.O. Box 1209, Franklin Park, IL 60131-8209; (800) LA-LECHE. In Canada: 495 Main St., Winchester, Ontario, Canada KOC 2K0; (613) 774-2850.

Providing newborns with nutrition is only one aspect of the feeding. Holding them close to the body while rocking or cuddling them helps to ensure the emotional component of feeding. Like breast-fed infants, bottle-fed infants need to be held on either side of the lap to expose them to different stimuli. The feeding should not be hurried. Even though they may suck vigorously for the first 5 minutes and seem to be satisfied, they are allowed to continue sucking. Infants need at least 2 hours of sucking a day. If there are six feedings per day, then about 20 minutes of sucking at each feeding provides for oral gratification.

After feedings infants are positioned on the right side to permit the feeding to flow toward the lower end of the stomach and to allow any swallowed air to rise above the fluid and through the esophagus (Fig. 8-17). This position prevents regurgitation and distention. To maintain the side-lying position, a pillow can be placed snugly behind the back.

Propping the bottle is discouraged for the following reasons:

1. It denies the infant the important component of close human contact.
2. The infant may aspirate formula while sleeping.
3. It may facilitate the development of middle ear infections. As the infant lies flat and sucks, milk that has pooled in the pharynx becomes a suitable medium for bacterial growth. Bacteria then enter the eustachian tube, which leads to the middle ear, causing acute otitis media.
4. It encourages continuous pooling of formula in the mouth, which can lead to bottle caries when the teeth erupt (see Chapter 14).

Preparation of Formula. The two traditional ways of preparing formula are the terminal heat method (all the utensils and formula are boiled together for 25 minutes) and the aseptic method (the equipment is boiled separately, after which the formula is poured into the bottles). Because of improved sanitary conditions in developed countries, neither of these methods is essential. The clean technique is satisfactory, including using a dishwasher. Persons preparing the formula wash their hands well and then wash all the equipment used to prepare the formula, including the cans of formula or evaporated milk. The formula is prepared and bottled immediately before each feeding. Warming the formula is optional, although many parents prefer to warm it before feeding. Warming bottles in the microwave oven is not recommended because of the risk of burns from bottles exploding or the hot temperature of the fluid. Any milk remaining in the bottle after the feeding is discarded, since it is an excellent medium for bacterial growth. Opened cans of formula are covered and refrigerated until the next feeding.

NURSING ALERT Warming bottles in the microwave oven is not recommended because of the risk of burns from bottles exploding or the hot temperature of the fluid.

Recommendations for labeling infant formulas require that the directions for preparation and use of the formula include pictures and symbols for nonreading individuals. In addition, manufacturers are translating the directions into foreign languages, such as Spanish and Vietnamese, to prevent misunderstanding and errors in formula preparation.

NURSING ALERT Impress on families that the proportions *must not be altered*—neither diluted to extend the amount of formula nor concentrated to provide more calories.

Feeding Schedules. Ideally, feeding schedules should be determined by the infant's hunger. ***Demand feedings*** involve feeding infants when they signal readiness. ***Scheduled feedings*** are arranged at predetermined intervals. Some hospitals routinely feed infants every 4 hours. Although this is satisfactory for bottle-fed infants, it hinders the breastfeeding process. Since breast-fed infants tend to be hungry every 2 to 3 hours because of the easy digestibility of the milk, they should be fed on demand.

Supplemental feedings should *not* be offered to breastfed infants before lactation is well established, because they may satiate the infant and may cause nipple preference. Supplemental water is not needed in breast-fed infants, even in hot climates (Sachdev and others, 1991). Satiated infants suck less vigorously at the breast, and milk depends on the breast being emptied at each feeding. If milk is allowed to accumulate in the ducts, causing breast engorgement, ischemia results, suppressing the activity of the acini or milk-secreting cells. Consequently, milk production is reduced. In addition, the process of sucking from a bottle is different from breast-nipple compression. The relatively inflexible rubber nipple prevents the tongue from its usual rhythmic action. Infants learn to put the tongue against the nipple holes to slow down the more rapid flow of fluid. When infants use these same tongue movements during breastfeeding, they may push the human nipple out of the mouth and may not grasp the areola properly (Lawrence, 1989).

Usually by 3 weeks of age, lactation and a feeding schedule are well established. Bottle-fed infants retain about 2 to 3 ounces of formula at each feeding and are fed about six times a day. The quantity of formula consumed is based on the caloric need of 108 kcal/kg; therefore a newborn who weighs 3 kg requires 324 kcal/day. Since commercial formula has 20 kcal/oz, about 16 ounces (480 ml) will provide the daily caloric requirement. Breast-fed infants may feed as frequently as 10 to 12 times a day. Larger infants are able to retain increased amounts because of greater stomach capacity; as a result, they generally sleep through the night sooner than smaller infants or breast-fed infants.

Feeding Behavior. Five fairly distinct behavioral stages occur during successful feeding (O'Grady, 1971). Recognizing these steps can assist nurses in identifying potential feeding problems caused by improper feeding techniques (see also discussion of Nursing Child Assessment Feeding Scale, p. 294). ***Prefeeding behavior,*** such as crying or fussing, demonstrates the infant's level of arousal and degree of hunger. To encourage the infant to grasp the breast properly, it is preferable to begin feeding during the quiet alert state, before the infant becomes upset. ***Approach behavior*** is indicated by sucking movements or the rooting reflex. ***Attachment behavior*** includes those activities that occur from the time the infant receives the nipple and sucks (sometimes more pronounced during initial attempts at breastfeeding). ***Consummatory behavior*** consists of coordinated sucking and swallowing. Persistent gagging might indicate unsuccessful consummatory behavior. ***Satiety behavior*** is observed when infants let the parent know that they are satisfied, usually by falling asleep.

Promote Parent-Infant Bonding (Attachment)

The process of parenting is based on a mutual relationship between parent and infant. As more is learned of the complexity of neonates and of their potential for influencing and shaping their environments, particularly their interaction with significant others, it is apparent that promoting positive parent-child relationships necessitates an understanding of factors involved in identifying behavioral steps in attachment, variables that enhance or hinder this process, and methods of teaching parents ways to develop a stronger relationship with their children, especially by recognizing potential problems. (See also Assessment of Attachment Behaviors, p. 294.)

Infant Behavior. Nurses must appreciate the individuality and uniqueness of each infant. According to the individual temperament, the infant will change and shape the environment, which will undoubtedly influence future development. Obviously, an infant who sleeps 20 hours a day will be exposed to fewer stimuli than one who sleeps 16 hours a day. In turn, each infant will likely effect a different response from parents. The infant who is quiet, undemanding, and passive may receive much less attention than the infant who is responsive, alert, and active. Behavioral characteristics such as irritability and consolability can influence the ease of transition to parenthood and the parent's perception of the infant.

Nurses can positively influence the attachment of parent and child. The first step is recognizing individual differences and explaining to parents that such characteristics are normal. For example, some people believe that infants sleep throughout the day, except for feedings. For some new-

HOW TO MAKE THE INFANT'S WORLD MORE EXCITING*

Infant prefers animated and auditory objects.
Infant enjoys novelty, quickly tires of seeing same objects; mobile should be changed frequently.
Infant prefers to look at medium-intensity colors and contrasting colors, such as black and white.
Infant likes geometric shapes and checkerboards; prefers patterns over straight lines.
Contrasting lights and reflective surfaces such as mirrors are especially interesting.
But most of all, nothing is as fascinating as the human face and voice!

*Objects should be placed about 20 cm (8 inches) away from infant.

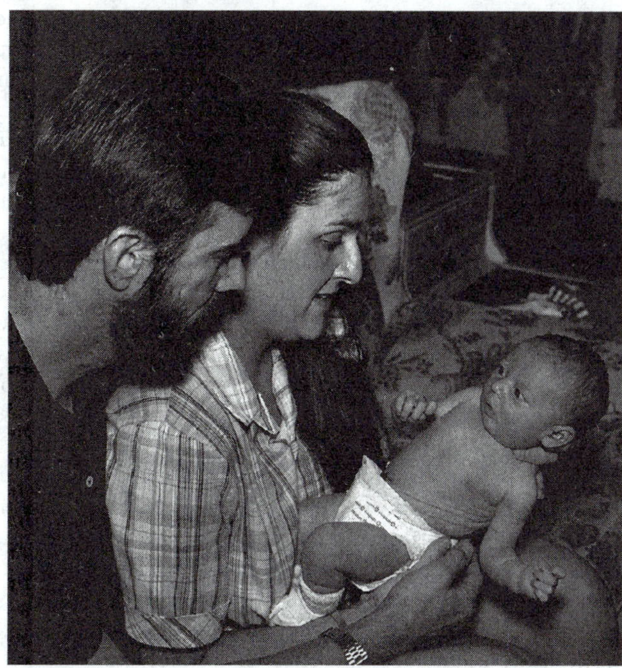

FIG. 8-18 En face position between parents and infant can be significant in attachment process.

borns this may be true, but for many it is not. Understanding that the infant's wakefulness is part of biologic rhythm and not a reflection of inadequate parenting can be crucial in promoting healthy parent-child relationships. Another aspect of helping parents concerns supplying guidelines on how to enhance the infant's development during awake periods. Placing the child in a crib to stare at the same mobile every day is not exciting, but carrying the infant into each room as one does daily chores can be fascinating. A few suggestions can make life more stimulating for the infant and gratifying for the parents (see box above).

Maternal Attachment. Research has suggested that there is a ***maternal sensitive period*** immediately and for a short time after birth when parents have a unique ability to attach to their infants (Klaus and Kennell, 1982). Mothers demonstrate a predictable and orderly pattern of behavior during the development of the attachment process. When mothers are presented with their nude infants, they begin examining the infant with their fingertips, concentrating on touching the extremities, and then proceed to massage and encompass the trunk with their entire hands. Assuming the ***en face position,*** in which the mother's and the infant's eyes meet in visual contact in the same vertical plane, is significant in the formation of affectional ties (Fig. 8-18). Although similar patterns of touching have been observed, additional studies demonstrate different patterns for mothers, as well as the same pattern for nonmaternal persons, such as male and female nurses (Tulman, 1985; Templeton, Edgil, and Douglas, 1988). Consequently, nurses must exercise caution in interpreting behaviors such as touching.

Several studies have attempted to substantiate the long-term benefits of providing parents with opportunities to optimally bond with their infant during the initial postpartum period. Although there has been some evidence that increased parent-child contact encourages prolonged breastfeeding and may minimize the risks of parenting disorders, conclusions about the long-term effects of such early intervention on parenting and child development must be viewed tentatively and cautiously. In addition, some authorities claim that the emphasis on bonding has been unjustified and may lead to guilt and fear in those parents who did not receive early contact with their infant. There is also concern over the literal interpretation of "sensitive" or "critical" to imply that without early contact optimum bonding cannot occur or, conversely, that early contact alone is sufficient to ensure competent parenting (Brown and Hellings, 1989; Lamb, 1982).

Certainly, it should be stressed to parents that while early bonding may be valuable, it does not represent an "all or none" phenomenon. Throughout the child's life there will be multiple opportunities for the development of parent-child attachment. Bonding is a complex process that develops gradually and is influenced by numerous factors, only one of which is the type of initial contact between the newborn and parent.

Another component of successful maternal attachment is the concept of ***reciprocity*** (Brazelton, 1974). As the mother responds to the infant, the infant must respond to the mother by some signal such as sucking, cooing, eye contact, grasping, or molding (conforming to the other's body during close physical contact). The first step is ***initiation,*** in which interaction between infant and parent begins. Next is ***orientation,*** which establishes the partners' expectation of each other during the interaction. Following orientation is ***acceleration*** of the attention cycle to a peak of excitement. The infant reaches out and coos, both arms jerk forward, the head moves backward, the eyes dilate, and the face brightens. After a short time ***deceleration*** of the excitement and ***turning away*** occur, in which the infant's eyes shift away from the mother's and the child grasps his or her shirt. During this cycle of nonattention, repeated verbal or visual attempts to reinitiate the infant's attention are ineffective.

This deceleration and turning away probably prevent the infant from being overwhelmed by excessive stimuli. In a good interaction both partners have synchronized their attention-nonattention cycles. Parents or other caregivers who do not allow the infant to turn away and who continually attempt to maintain visual contact encourage the infant to turn off the attention cycle and thus prolong the nonattention phase.

Although this description of reciprocal interacting behavior is usually observed in the infant by 2 to 3 weeks of age, nurses can use this information to teach parents how to interact with their infant. Recognizing the attention vs nonattention cycles and understanding that the latter is not a rejection of the parent helps parents develop competence in parenting.

Paternal Engrossment. Fathers also show specific attachment behaviors to the newborn. This process of ***paternal engrossment,*** forming a sense of absorption, preoccupation, and interest in the infant, includes (1) visual awareness of the newborn, especially focusing on the beauty of the child, (2) tactile awareness, often expressed in a desire to hold the infant, (3) awareness of distinct characteristics with emphasis on those features of the infant that resemble the father, (4) perception of the infant as perfect, (5) development of a strong feeling of attraction to the child that leads to intense focusing of attention on the infant, (6) experiencing a feeling of extreme elation, and (7) feeling a sense of deep self-esteem and satisfaction. These responses are greatest during the early contacts with the infant and are intensified by the neonate's normal reflex activity, especially the grasp reflex and visual alertness (Greenberg and Morris, 1974). In addition to behavioral reactions, fathers also demonstrate physiologic responses such as increased heart rate and blood pressure during interactions with their newborns (Jones and Thomas, 1989).

The process of engrossment has significant implications for nurses. It is imperative to recognize the importance of early father-infant contact in releasing these behaviors. Fathers need to be encouraged to express their positive feelings, especially if such emotions are contrary to the cultural belief that fathers should remain stoic. If this is not clarified, fathers may feel confused and attempt to suppress the natural sensations of absorption, preoccupation, and interest in order to conform with societal expectations.

Mothers also need to be aware of the responses of the father toward the newborn, especially since one of the consequences of paternal preoccupation with the infant is less overt attention toward the mother. If both parents are able to share their feelings, each can appreciate the process of attachment toward their child and will avoid the unfortunate conflict of being insensitive and unaware of the other's needs. In addition, a father who is encouraged to form a relationship with his newborn is less likely to feel excluded and abandoned once the family returns home and the mother directs her attention toward caring for the infant.

Ideally the process of engrossment should be discussed with parents before the delivery, such as in prenatal classes, to reinforce the father's awareness of his natural feelings toward the expected child. Focusing on the future experience of seeing, touching, and holding one's newborn may also help expectant fathers become more comfortable in accepting their paternal feelings toward the unborn child. This in turn can assist them in being more supportive toward the mother, especially as the labor and delivery event draws near.

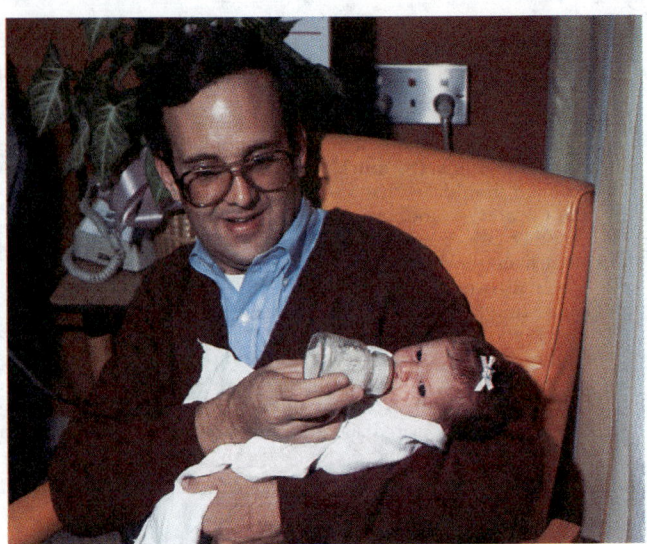

FIG. 8-19 A desire to hold the infant and participate in caregiving activities is an indication of paternal engrossment.

At the infant's birth the nurse can play a vital role in helping the father to release or express engrossment by assessing the neonate in front of the couple; pointing out normal characteristics, especially the grasp reflex, encouraging identification through consistent referral to the child by name; encouraging the father to cuddle, hold, talk to, or feed the infant; and demonstrating whenever necessary the soothing powers of caressing, stroking, and rocking the child (Fig. 8-19). Fathers are encouraged to be with the mother during labor and delivery and to spend time alone with the mother and newborn after delivery. Whenever possible, the father should "room in" with the mother.

The nurse observes for the same indications of affection from the father as those expected in the mother, such as visual contact in the en face position and embracing the infant close to the body. When present, such behaviors are reinforced. If such responses are not obvious, the nurse needs to assess the father's feelings regarding this birth, cultural beliefs that may prevent his expression of emotions, and other factors in order to help him facilitate a positive attachment during this critical period.

Siblings. Although the attachment process has been discussed almost exclusively in terms of the parents and infants, it is essential that nurses be aware of other family members, such as siblings and members of the extended family, who need preparation for the acceptance of this new child. Young children in particular need sensitive preparation for the birth to minimize sibling jealousy.

There is an increasing trend to allow siblings to visit the mother on the postpartum unit and to hold the newborn

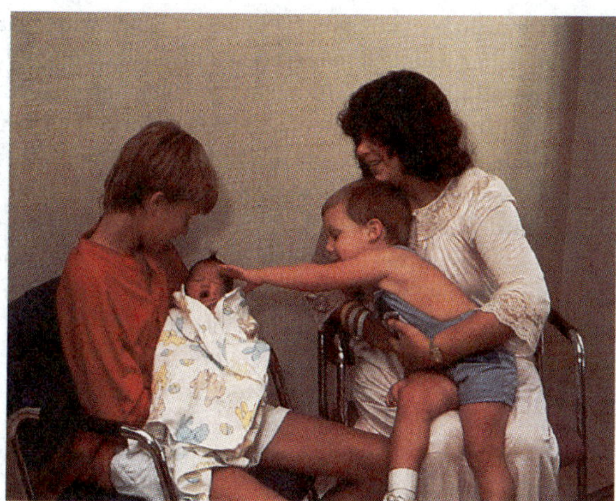

FIG. 8-20 Sibling visitation shortly after birth can be significant in the attachment process.

(Fig. 8-20) (see Thinking Critically About . . . box). Another trend has been siblings witnessing the birth. Unlike sibling visitation, the evidence supporting this practice is much more controversial and conflicting. Children exhibit different degrees of involvement in the birth process. Young children often fall asleep toward the end of delivery. Some reported benefits include children's increased knowledge of the birth process, less regressive behavior following the birth, and more mothering and caregiving behavior toward the infant (Daniels, 1983; Del Giudice, 1986; Trause and Irvin, 1982). Some practitioners add facilitated family bonding and assimilation of the newborn into the family as positive outcomes (Stanford and others, 1992). Parents whose children attended the birth have echoed these same benefits and have expressed their desire to repeat the experience should another pregnancy occur (Krutsky, 1985). Despite these positive findings, opponents believe that allowing children to observe a delivery could lead to emotional difficulties (Sugar, 1991), although there is no research to support this contention. As research mounts, birthing centers that allow siblings at the birth are developing more definitive guidelines, such as an age requirement of at least 4 to 5 years, the presence of a supportive person for the sibling only, and an adequate sequence of preparation in which parents explore all options for preparing their other children (Daniels, 1983).

From observations during sibling visitation there is evidence that sibling attachment occurs. However, the en face position is assumed much less often among the newborn and siblings than between mother and newborn, and when this position is used, it is brief. Siblings focus more on the head or face than on touching or talking to the infant. The siblings' verbalizations are focused less on attracting the infant's attention and more on addressing the mother about the newborn (Marecki and others, 1985). Children who have established a prenatal relationship with the fetus have demonstrated more attachment behaviors, supporting the suggestion of encouraging prenatal acquaintance (Anderberg, 1988). Additional research is needed to establish theories on sibling bonding as have been constructed for parental bonding.

Multiple Births and Subsequent Children. A component of attachment that has special meaning for families with multiple births, ***monotropy*** refers to the principle that a person can become optimally attached to only one individual at a time (Klaus and Kennell, 1982). If a parent can form only one attachment at a time, how can all the siblings of a multiple birth receive optimum emotional care?

Minimal research is available on bonding and multiple births, and even less is known about paternal engrossment and sibling attachment. In regard to maternal-twin bonding, the conclusions of different authors vary. Some report that mothers bond equally to each twin at the time of birth, even if one twin is ill (Abbink, 1982). Others suggest that mothers of twins may take months or even years to form individual attachments to each child and even longer if the twins are identical.

Nurses can be instrumental in promoting bonding of multiple births. The most important principle is to assist the parents in recognizing the individuality of the children, especially in monozygotic (identical) twins. The mother should visit with each newborn, including a sick infant, as much as possible after birth. Rooming-in and breast-feeding are encouraged. Any characteristics that are unique to each

THINKING CRITICALLY ABOUT . . . *Newborn and Sibling Visitation*

Research has demonstrated several benefits of sibling visitation, such as more responsiveness of the sibling to the mother and newborn (Schwab and others, 1983), less regressive behavior after the birth (Kayiatos, Adams, and Gilman, 1984), and no adverse effects, such as increased bacterial infection of neonates (Solheim and Spellacy, 1988). Mothers' opinions of sibling visitation have been very favorable. However, concerns have focused on restrictions in the visiting policy (siblings not allowed in the mother's room or to touch the newborn). Mothers who have not chosen sibling visitation have been primarily worried about the emotional reactions of themselves and their children, especially being upset during and at the end of the visit (Mackey and Miller, 1992).

In light of these findings, health professionals should critically evaluate sibling visitation and birth attendance policies, solicit the family's preferences, support their decision for or against sibling involvement, and prepare the parents for the emotional reaction of young children to visiting the mother.

If the birth experience is a "family event," who has the right to exclude a family member—the institution or the parents? In your community what are the birthing centers' policies? If nurses are to be advocates for families, what could you do to change attitudes and practices? Remember, consumers have powerful voices.

child are emphasized, and each infant is called by name, rather than calling them "the twins." Asking the family questions such as "How do you tell Sally and Amy apart?" and "In what ways are Sally and Amy different and similar?" helps point out their individual characteristics (Anderson and Anderson, 1990). The BNBAS can be used to illustrate these differences and to stress effective strategies for dealing with multiple personalities at the same time. Other strategies for promoting individualism are discussed under Multiple Births in Chapter 3.

Another area of attachment that has received minimal attention is maternal bonding of multiparous mothers. Research suggests that there are several additional tasks to "taking on" a second child. These include (Walz, 1983):

- Promoting acceptance and approval of the second child
- Grieving and resolving the loss of an exclusive dyadic relationship with the first child
- Planning and coordinating family life to include a second child
- Reformulating a relationship with the first child
- Identifying with the second child by comparing with the first child for physical and psychologic characteristics
- Assessing one's affective capabilities in providing sufficient emotional support and nurturance simultaneously to two children

Employed mothers who have a second child report fewer concerns regarding general aspects of separation from their child and the effect of separation on the child, but similar concerns regarding separation due to employment (Pitzer and Hock, 1989). It appears that while experience may decrease some concerns, it may not minimize others.

Prepare for Discharge and Home Care

With increasingly shorter maternity admissions, as well as a trend toward ***mother-infant care,*** also called ***dyad*** or ***couplet care,*** discharge planning, referral, and home visiting have become important components of comprehensive care. First time, as well as "experienced," parents benefit from guidance and assistance with the infant's care, such as breast- or formula feeding, and with the family's integration of a new member, particularly sibling adjustment.

To assess and meet these needs, teaching must begin early, ideally *before the birth.* Not only is the admission time short (typically 24 to 48 hours), but also mothers are in the ***taking-in phase,*** where they demonstrate passive and dependent behaviors. Therefore, on the first postpartum day women may not be able to absorb large amounts of information (Ament, 1990). Rather, this time may be better spent highlighting essential aspects of care, such as infant feeding, rather than teaching infant bathing with a return demonstration. Parents can also be given a list of mother and infant care topics as part of the nursing admission history to choose issues they wish to review. Other topics can be discussed during a follow-up telephone call or home visit. Common concerns focus on newborn feeding patterns, stool cycles, jaundice, and excessive crying (Elmer and Maloni, 1988; Siegel, 1992).

With family structures changing, it is essential that nurses identify the primary caregiver, which may not be the mother but a father, grandparent, or baby-sitter (Carlson, 1993). Also, nurses should not assume that terminology associated with mother-infant care is understood. Words relating to the anatomy (e.g., "meconium," "labia," "edema," and "genitalia") and to breastfeeding (e.g., "areola," "colostrum," and "let-down reflex") may be unfamiliar to mothers. Mothers with other children do not necessarily understand more words, and young age and less education decrease comprehension (DiFlorio, 1991).

An essential area of discharge counseling is the safe transportation of the newborn home from the hospital. Ideally this information should also be provided *before* delivery to allow parents an opportunity to purchase a suitable infant car restraint.

When purchasing a car restraint, parents should consider cost and convenience. The convertible-type seats are more expensive initially but cost less than two separate systems. Convenience is a major factor, because a cumbersome restraint may be used less and improperly. Before buying a restraint, it is best to try out different models. For example, some types are too large for subcompact cars. Asking friends about the advantages and disadvantages of their restraints is helpful, but borrowing their car seat or purchasing a used one can be dangerous. Parents should use only a restraint that has directions for use and a certification label stating that it complies with Federal Motor Vehicle Safety standards (both should be on the seat). They should not use a restraint that has been involved in a crash. Some service clubs and hospitals have loan programs for restraints. Information about approved models and other aspects of car restraints is available from several organizations and sources.*

In the United States and Canada all states and provinces have mandated the use of child restraints (Brady-Fryer and Gent, 1993). Therefore hospitals and birthing centers should have policies regarding the safe discharge of a newborn in a car safety seat and provisions for parents to learn to use the device correctly (American Academy of Pediatrics, 1990b). Parents are more likely to use a restraint correctly and consistently if the proper use of one is demonstrated and its necessity is stressed.

While federal safety standards do not specify the *minimum* weight of an infant and the appropriate type of restraint, newborns weighing 2 kg (4 pounds, 8 ounces) receive relatively good support in convertible seats with a seat back–to–crotch strap height of 14 cm (5½ inches) or less. Rolled blankets and towels may be needed by the crotch to prevent slouching and can be placed along the sides to minimize lateral movements. Seats with shields (large padded surfaces in front of the child) and armrests (found on some other models) are unacceptable because of their proximity to the infant's face and neck (Bull and others, 1989). (For a discussion of appropriate car restraints for prema-

---

***American Academy of Pediatrics,** 141 Northwest Point Blvd., P.O. Box 927, Elk Grove Village, IL 60007, (800) 433-9016; and local division of traffic safety or **National Highway Traffic Safety Administration Auto Safety Hotline,** (800) 424-9393. Guidelines for car seat safety are available in *Wong and Whaley's Clinical Manual of Pediatric Nursing* (Mosby).

NURSING CARE PLAN

The Normal Newborn and Family

Nursing Diagnosis: Ineffective airway clearance related to excess mucus, improper positioning

PATIENT GOAL 1: Will maintain a patent airway

• **NURSING INTERVENTIONS/*RATIONALES***

Suction mouth and nasopharynx with bulb syringe as needed

Compress bulb before insertion and aspirate pharynx, then nose, *to prevent aspiration of fluid*

With mechanical suction, limit each suctioning attempt to 5 seconds with sufficient time between attempts *to allow reoxygenation*

Position infant on right side after feeding *to prevent aspiration*

Position infant prone or on side during sleep as recommended by American Academy of Pediatrics

Perform as few procedures as possible on infant during first hour and have oxygen ready for use if respiratory distress should develop

Take vital signs according to institutional policy and more frequently if necessary

Observe for signs of respiratory distress and report any of the following immediately:

Tachypnea

Grunting, stridor

Abnormal breath sounds

Flaring alae nasi

Cyanosis or pallor

Keep diapers, clothing, and blankets loose enough *to allow maximum lung (abdominal) expansion and to avoid overheating*

Clean nares of any crusted secretions during bath or when necessary

Check for patent nares

• **EXPECTED OUTCOMES**

Airway remains patent

Breathing is regular and unlabored

Respiratory rate is within normal limits (see inside back cover for normal limits)

Nursing Diagnosis: High risk for altered body temperature related to immature temperature control, change in environmental temperature

PATIENT GOAL 1: Will maintain stable body temperature

• **NURSING INTERVENTIONS/*RATIONALES***

Wrap infant snugly in a warmed blanket

Place infant in a preheated environment (under radiant warmer or next to mother)

Place infant on a padded, covered surface

Take infant's temperature on arrival at nursery or mother's room; proceed according to hospital policy regarding method and frequency of monitoring

Maintain room temperature between 24° and 25.5° C (75° to 78° F) and humidity about 40% to 50%

Give initial bath according to hospital policy

Prevent chilling of infant during bath

Postpone bath if there is any question regarding stabilization of body temperature

Dress infant in a shirt and diaper and swaddle in a blanket or cover with blanket

Provide infant with a head covering if heat loss is a problem, *since large surface area of head favors heat loss*

Keep infant away from drafts, air conditioning vents, or fans

Place infant in a recessed cubicle with high-enough walls to *shield from cross-ventilation*

Warm all objects used to examine or cover infant (e.g., place them under radiant warmer)

Uncover only one area of body for examination or procedures

Postpone circumcision until after temperature stabilizes or use radiant warmer during procedure

Be alert to signs of hypothermia or hyperthermia

• **EXPECTED OUTCOME**

Infant's temperature remains at optimum level (36.5° to 37.5° C [97.7° to 99.5° F])

Nursing Diagnosis: High risk for infection or inflammation related to deficient immunologic defenses, environmental factors, maternal disease

PATIENT GOAL 1: Will exhibit no evidence of infection

• **NURSING INTERVENTIONS/*RATIONALES***

Wash hands before and after caring for each infant

Wear gloves when in contact with body secretions

Use of cover gowns is controversial *because studies show they do not decrease infection rates but do increase costs*

Make certain appropriate eye prophylaxis has been carried out

Check eyes daily for evidence of inflammation or discharge

Keep infant from potential sources of infection (e.g., persons with respiratory or skin infections, improperly prepared food sources, other unclean items)

Clean vulva in posterior direction *to prevent fecal contamination of vagina or urethra;* stress this to parents

While cleaning penis, do not retract foreskin; gently wipe away smegma

Maintain asepsis during circumcision

*If infant has been circumcised, cover area with a petrolatum jelly gauze (if ordered)

Check for voiding after circumcision; disposable diaper may feel dry when wet, but crotch area will feel "clumpy" or "doughy" and heavy

Keep umbilical stump clean and dry

Place diapers below umbilical stump

Assess cord daily for odor, color, and drainage

*Apply antibacterial agent and/or alcohol to cord as ordered

*Administer hepatitis B vaccine (HBV) in deltoid muscle

*Dependent nursing action.

Continued.

NURSING CARE PLAN
The Normal Newborn and Family—cont'd

• **EXPECTED OUTCOMES**
Infant exhibits no evidence of infection or inflammation
Eyes remain clear with no evidence of irritation
Genital area is free of irritation
Cord appears dry, surrounding area free of infection
Infant receives HBV vaccine

Nursing Diagnosis: High risk for trauma related to physical helplessness

PATIENT GOAL 1: Will be clearly and correctly identified

• **NURSING INTERVENTIONS/*RATIONALES***
Make certain infant is properly identified *for placement with correct mother*
Ensure that identification (ID) band(s) are properly and securely placed
Check infant's ID band often *to ensure correct infant identity*
Discuss safety issues with parents, especially mother, *to prevent "switching" of infants and possible kidnaping*
Observe staff's ID badge and give infant only to properly identified personnel
Never leave infant alone in crib or room
• **EXPECTED OUTCOMES**
Infant is clearly and correctly identified
Parents observe safety practices
ID band remains in place

PATIENT GOAL 2: Will have no physical injury

• **NURSING INTERVENTIONS/*RATIONALES***
Avoid using rectal thermometer *because of risk of rectal perforation*
Never leave infant unsupervised on a raised surface without sides
Always close diaper pins (if used) and place them away from infant's body
Keep pointed or sharp objects away from infant
Keep own fingernails short and trimmed; avoid jewelry that can scratch infant
Employ appropriate methods of handling and transporting infant

• **EXPECTED OUTCOME**
Infant remains free of physical injury

PATIENT GOAL 3: Will exhibit no evidence of bleeding

• **NURSING INTERVENTIONS/*RATIONALES***
*Administer vitamin K intramuscularly, using vastus lateralis muscle as site of injection
Check circumcision site; assess for any oozing *that may indicate bleeding tendencies*

• **EXPECTED OUTCOME**
Infant exhibits no evidence of bleeding

Nursing Diagnosis: Altered nutrition: less than body requirements (high risk) related to immaturity, parental knowledge deficit

PATIENT GOAL 1: Will receive optimum nutrition

• **NURSING INTERVENTIONS/*RATIONALES***
Assess strength of suck and coordination with swallowing *to identify possible problem affecting feeding*
Offer initial intake according to parent's preference, hospital policy, and practitioner's protocol
Prepare for demand feeding of breast-fed infants; night feedings determined by condition and preferences of mother
Offer bottle-fed infants 2 to 3 ounces of formula every 3 to 4 hours or on demand
Support and assist breast-feeding mothers during initial feedings and more frequently if necessary
Avoid routine water or supplemental feedings for breast-feeding infants because they may *decrease the desire to suck and cause nipple preference*
Encourage father or other support person to remain with mother to help her and infant with positioning, relaxation, and reinforcement
Encourage father or other support person to participate in bottle-feeding
Place infant on right side after feeding *to prevent aspiration*
Observe stool pattern
• **EXPECTED OUTCOMES**
Infant demonstrates strong suck
Infant retains feedings
Infant receives an adequate amount of nutrients (specify amount and frequency of feedings)
Infant loses less than 10% of birth weight

Nursing Diagnosis: Altered family processes related to maturational crisis, birth of term infant, change in family unit

PATIENT (FAMILY) GOAL 1: Will exhibit parent-infant attachment behaviors

• **NURSING INTERVENTIONS/*RATIONALES***
As soon after delivery as possible encourage parents to see and hold infant; place newborn close to face of parents *to establish visual contact*
Ideally, perform eye care after initial meeting of infant and parents, within 1 hour after birth *when infant is alert and most likely to visually relate to parent*
Identify for parents specific behaviors manifested by infant (e.g., alertness, ability to see, vigorous suck, rooting behavior, and attention to human voice)
Discuss with parents their expectations of fantasy child vs real child if indicated
Encourage parents to "talk out" their labor and delivery experience; identify any events that signify loss of control to either parent, especially mother

*Dependent nursing action.

NURSING CARE PLAN
The Normal Newborn and Family—cont'd

• **NURSING INTERVENTIONS/*RATIONALES—cont'd***

Identify behavioral steps in attachment process and evaluate those aspects that could be considered positive and those that may represent inadequate or delayed parenting

Encourage family to call for infant frequently if not rooming-in

Observe and assess reciprocity of cues between infant and parent *to identify behaviors that may need strengthening*

Assist parents in recognizing attention-nonattention cycles and in understanding their significance

Assess variables affecting development of attachment through observing infant and parent and interviewing each parent or other significant caregiver

• **EXPECTED OUTCOMES**

Parents establish contact with infant immediately or soon after birth

Parents demonstrate attachment behaviors, such as touch, eye contact, naming and calling infant by name, talking to infant, participating in caregiving activities

Parents recognize attention-nonattention cycles

PATIENT (SIBLING) GOAL 2: Will demonstrate adjustment/attachment behaviors toward newborn

• **NURSING INTERVENTIONS/*RATIONALES***

Allow to visit and touch newborn when feasible

Explain physical differences in newborn, such as bald head, umbilical stump and clamp, circumcision, *to lessen any fear siblings might have*

Explain to siblings realistic expectations regarding newborn's abilities and needs
- Requires complete care
- Is not a playmate

Encourage siblings to participate in care at home *to make them feel part of the experience*

Encourage parents to spend individual time with other children at home *to reduce feelings of jealousy toward new sibling*

• **EXPECTED OUTCOME**

Siblings express interest in newborn and realistic expectations for their age

PATIENT (FAMILY) GOAL 3: Will be prepared for discharge and home care

• **INTERVENTIONS/*RATIONALES***

Discuss with parents correct preparation of formula
- Stress that proportions must not be altered to dilute or concentrate the formula
- Discourage microwaving of bottles *to avoid burns*

Encourage use of support persons, such as lactation specialist or members of La Leche League, for assistance with breast-feeding

Instruct in other aspects of newborn care
- Bathing
- Umbilical and circumision care
- Recognize states of activity for optimum interaction (see Table 8-2)

Encourage participation in parenting classes, if offered

Discuss importance and proper use of federally approved car restraints
- If infant is small, advise parents to use rolled blankets and towels in crotch area to *prevent slouch and along sides to minimize lateral movement,* but never use padding underneath or behind infant, *since it creates slackness in harness, leading to possible ejection from seal in a crash*
- Refer to organizations that may rent car restraints

If parent-infant attachment is at risk, refer to appropriate agencies (social services, family and child services, at-risk programs)

• **EXPECTED OUTCOMES**

Family demonstrates ability to provide care for infant

Family keeps appointments for follow-up care

Infant rides home in federally approved car restraint

Family members avail themselves of needed services

ture infants see p. 388, and for infants see Motor Vehicle Injuries in Chapters 12 and 14.)

NURSING ALERT Padding is never placed underneath or behind the infant, since it creates slackness in the harness, leading to the possibility of the child's ejection from the seat in the event of a crash. In vehicles with passenger-side air bags, the rear-facing safety seat must be placed in the backseat to avoid injury to the infant from the released air bag forcing the safety seat against the vehicle seat (Passenger air bags, 1994).

❖ EVALUATION

The effectiveness of nursing interventions is determined by continual reassessment and evaluation of care based on the following observational guidelines and expected outcomes:

1. Observe infant's color and respiratory patterns.
2. Monitor axillary temperature regularly; observe for signs of chilling, such as skin mottling.
3. Observe for any evidence of infection, especially at the umbilicus or site of circumcision; check identification bands; check medical record for documentation of prophylactic eye treatment, vitamin K injection, HBV vaccine, and genetic screening test.

4. Monitor daily weight.
5. Observe interactions between infant and family members; interview family regarding their feelings about the newborn.
6. Observe parents' ability to provide care for infant; interview parents regarding any concerns about infant's care at home.
7. Observe parents' correct use of car restraint on discharge.

Expected outcomes:

See Nursing Care Plan, pp. 329-331.

KEY POINTS

- Transition from fetal or placental circulation to independent respiration is the most important physiologic change required of the newborn.
- Chemical and thermal factors help initiate the neonate's first respiration.
- Circulatory changes in the neonate result from shifts in pressure in the heart and major vessels and from functional closures of the fetal shunts.
- The newborn's large surface area, thin layer of subcutaneous fat, and unique mechanism for producing heat predispose the newborn to excessive heat loss.
- The infant's high rate of metabolism is closely correlated with the rate of fluid exchange, which is seven times greater in the infant than in the adult.
- The skin and mucous membranes, the reticuloendothelial system, and antibodies are the first, second, and third lines of defense against infection.
- Apgar scoring, the initial assessment of the newborn, focuses on heart rate, respiratory effort, muscle tone, reflex irritability, and color.
- Physical assessment of the newborn includes assessment of clinical gestational age, general measurements, general appearance, head-to-toe assessment, and parent-infant attachment, or bonding.
- Neurologic assessment focuses on localized reflexes and posture, muscle tone, head control, and movement and is best accomplished during the general physical examination.
- Behavioral assessment of newborns with the Brazelton Neonatal Behavioral Assessment Scale examines responses to seven categories: habituation, orientation, motor performance, range of state, regulation of state, autonomic regulation, and reflexes.
- An instrument for assessing the reciprocal interchange between parent and infant is the Nursing Child Assessment Feeding Scale.
- Physical care for the newborn includes maintaining a patent airway, maintaining a stable body temperature, protecting from infection and injury, and providing optimum nutrition.
- Although the attachment, or bonding, process primarily affects infants and parents, siblings also play an important role.
- With short maternity admissions, teaching needs to begin before birth and continue after discharge with telephone and/or home follow-up.
- An essential aspect of discharge teaching is ensuring the newborn's safe transportation home in a federally approved, backward-facing car restraint.

REFERENCES

Abbink C: Bonding as perceived by mothers of twins, *Pediatr Nurs* 8(6):411-413, 1982.

Ament LA: Maternal tasks of the puerperium reidentified, *JOGNN* 19(4):330-335, 1990.

American Academy of Pediatrics: Neonatal anesthesia, *Pediatrics* 80(3):446, 1987.

American Academy of Pediatrics: *Textbook of Neonatal Resuscitation,* Elk Grove Village, IL, 1990a, The Academy.

American Academy of Pediatrics, Committee on Accident and Poison Prevention: Safe transportation of newborns from the hospital, *Pediatrics* 86(3):486-487, 1990b.

American Academy of Pediatrics, Committee on Drugs: The transfer of drugs and other chemicals into human milk, *Pediatrics* 93(1): 137-150, 1994.

American Academy of Pediatrics, Committee on Fetus and Newborn: Use and abuse of the Apgar score, *Pediatrics* 78(6):1148-1149, 1986.

American Academy of Pediatrics, Committee on Fetus and Newborn: Routine evaluation of blood pressure, hematocrit, and glucose in newborns, *Pediatrics* 92(3):474-476, 1993a.

American Academy of Pediatrics, Committee on Genetics: Newborn screening fact sheets, *Pediatrics* 83(3):449-464, 1989a.

American Academy of Pediatrics, Committee on Infectious Diseases: Universal Hepatitis B immunization, *Pediatrics,* 89(4):795-800, 1992a.

American Academy of Pediatrics, Task Force on Circumcision: Report of the Task Force on Circumcision, *Pediatrics* 84(4):388-391, 1989b.

American Academy of Pediatrics, Task Force on Infant Positioning and SIDS: Positioning and SIDS, *Pediatrics* 89(6):1120-1126, 1992b.

American Academy of Pediatrics, Vitamin K Ad Hoc Task Force: Controversies concerning vitamin K and the newborn, *Pediatrics* 91(5):1001-1003, 1993b.

American Academy of Pediatrics and American College of Obstetricians and Gynecologists: *Guidelines for perinatal care,* ed 3, Elk Grove Village, IL, 1992, The Academy.

Anderberg GJ: Initial acquaintance and attachment behavior of siblings with the newborn, *JOGNN* 17:49-54, 1988.

Anderson A, Anderson B: Toward a substantive theory of mother-twin attachment, *MCN* 15(6):373-377, 1990.

Andrich MP, Golden SM: Umbilical cord care: a study of bacitracin ointment vs. triple dye, *Clin Pediatr* 23:342-344, 1984.

Annotations, *Arch Dis Child* 67:765-766, 1992.

Avoa A, Fischer PR: The influence of perinatal instruction about breastfeeding on neonatal weight loss, *Pediatrics* 86(2):313-315, 1990.

Ballard JL, Novak KK, Driver M: A simplified score for assessment of fetal maturation of newly born infants, *J Pediatr* 95(5):769-774, 1979.

Ballard JL and others: New Ballard Score, expanded to include extremely premature infants, *J Pediatr* 119:417-423, 1991.

Barnard K: *NCAST feeding manual,* Seattle, 1994, University of Washington.

Beal J: The effect on father-infant interaction of demonstrating the Neonatal Behavioral Assessment Scale, *Birth* 16(1):18-22, 1989.

Benini F and others: Topical anesthesia during circumcision in newborn infants, *JAMA* 270(7):850-853, 1993.

Berenson AB: Appearance of the hymen at birth and one year of age: a longitudinal study, *Pediatrics* 91(4):820-825, 1993.

Bernard-Bonnin A and others: Hospital practices and breastfeeding duration: a meta-analysis of controlled trials, *Birth* 16(2):64-66, 1989.

Bernbaum J, Hoffman-Williamson M: *Primary care of the preterm infant,* St Louis, 1991, Mosby.

Birenbaum HJ and others: Gowning on a postpartum ward fails to decrease colonization in the newborn infant, *Am J Dis Child* 144(9):1031-1033, 1990.

Blain-Lewis N: Comparative studies of bruising and healing after heelstick, *Neonatal Intensive Care* 5(5):18-21, 1992.

Blass EM, Hoffmeyer LB: Sucrose as an analgesic for newborn infants, *Pediatrics* 87:215-218, 1991.

Bliss-Holtz J: Comparison of rectal, axillary, and

inguinal temperatures in full-term newborn infants, *Nurs Res* 38(2):85-87, 1989.

Bliss-Holtz J: Determination of thermoregulatory state in full-term infants, *Nurs Res* 42(4):204-207, 1993.

Brady-Fryer B, Gent M: Kids and car seats, *Can Nurse* 89(2):23-25, 1993.

Brazelton TB: Mother-infant reciprocity. In Klaus M and others, editors: *Maternal attachment and mothering disorders,* New Brunswick, NJ, 1974, Johnson & Johnson Baby Products.

Brazelton TB: *Neonatal behavioral assessment scale,* ed 2, Philadelphia, 1984, JB Lippincott.

Broussard ER: Neonatal prediction and outcome at 10/11 years, *Child Psychiatry Hum Dev* 7(2):85-93, 1976.

Broussard ER: Assessment of the adaptive potential of the mother-infant system: the Neonatal Perception Inventories, *Semin Perinatol* 3(1):91-100, 1979.

Broussard ER: The Pittsburgh first borns at age nineteen years. In Call J Calerson E, Tyson R, editors: *Frontiers of infant psychiatry,* vol 2, New York, 1984, Basic Books.

Brown MS, Brown CA: Circumcision decision: prominence and social concerns, *Pediatrics* 80(2):215-219, 1987.

Brown MS, Hellings P: A case study of qualitative versus quantitative reviews: the maternal-infant bonding controversy, *J Pediatr Nurs* 4(2):104-111, 1989.

Bull M and others: Special children, special car seats, *Contemp Pediatr* 6(11):122-136, 1989.

Butz AM and others: Newborn identification: compliance with AAP guidelines for perinatal care, *Clin Pediatr* 32(2):111-113, 1993.

Campos RG: Soothing neonates' response to a stressful procedure, *Neonatal Network* 12(6):93, 1993.

Carlson GE: When grandmothers take care of grandchildren, *MCN* 18(4):206-207, 1993.

Chessare JB: Circumcision: is the risk of urinary tract infection really the pivotal issue? *Clin Pediatr* 31(2):100-104, 1992.

Chia F and others: Reliability of the Dinamap noninvasive monitor in the measurement of blood pressure of ill Asian newborns, *Clin Pediatr* 29(5):262-267, 1990.

Christoph R and others: Pain reduction in local anesthetic administration through pH buffering, *Ann Emerg Med* 17(2):117-120, 1988.

Cohen HA and others: Postcircumcision urinary tract infection, *Clin Pediatr* 31(6):322-324, 1992.

Coody D and others: Early hospital discharge and the timing of newborn metabolic screening, *Clin Pediatr* 32(8):463-466, 1993.

Council on Scientific Affairs, American Medical Association: Council report: use of animals in medical education, *JAMA,* 266:836-837, 1991.

Cuckow P, Mouriquand P: Saving the normal foreksin, *Br Med J* 306(6875):459-460, 1993 (letter to the editor).

Daniels M: The birth experience for the sibling: description and evaluation of a program, *J Nurse Midwife* 28(5):15-22, 1983.

DeCasper AJ, Fifer WP: Of human bonding: newborns prefer their mother's voices, *Science* 208:1174-1176, 1980.

DeCasper AJ, Spence MJ: Prenatal maternal speech influences newborns' perception of speech sounds, *Infant Behav Dev* 9:133-150, 1986.

Del Giudice GT: The relationship between sibling jealousy and presence at the sibling's birth, *Birth* 13(4):250-254, 1986.

Dewey K and others: Adequacy of energy intake among breast-fed infants in the DARLING study: relationships to growth velocity morbidity, and activity levels, J Pediatr 119(4):538-547, 1991.

DiFlorio I: Mothers' comprehension of terminology associated with the care of a newborn baby, *Pediatr Nurs* 17(2):193-196, 1991.

Dixon S and others: Behavioral effects of circumcision with and without anesthesia, *Dev Behav Pediatr* 5(5):246-250, 1984.

Donowitz LG: Failure of the overgown to prevent nosocomial infection in a pediatric intensive care unit, *Pediatrics* 77:35-38, 1986.

Dubowitz LMS, Dubowitz V: *Gestational age of the newborn,* Menlo Park, CA, 1977, Addison-Wesley.

Duncan B and others: Exclusive breast-feeding for at least 4 months protects against otitis media, *Pediatrics* 91(5):867-872, 1993.

Dungy C and others: Effect of discharge samples on duration of breast-feeding, *Pediatrics* 90:233-237, 1992.

Early identification of hearing impairment in infants and young children, *NIH Consens Statement* 11(1):1-24, 1993.

El Haddad M, Corkery JJ: The anus in the newborn, *Pediatrics* 76(6):927-928, 1985.

Elmer E, Maloni JA: Parent support through telephone consultation, *Matern Child Nurs J* 17(1):13-23, 1988.

Evans CJ, Lyons NB, Killien MG: The effect of infant formula samples on breastfeeding practice, *JOGNN* 15(5):401-405, 1986.

Female genital mutilation, *AAP News* 10(2):3, 1994.

Ferber R: Behavioral "insomnia" in the child, *Psychiatr Clin North Am* 10(4):641-653, 1987.

Fitzgerald M, Millard C, McIntosh N: Cutaneous hypersensitivity following peripheral tissue damage in newborn infants and its reversal with topical anaesthesia, *Pain* 39:31-36, 1989.

Fontaine P: Local anesthesia for neonatal circumcisions: are family practice residents likely to use it? *Fam Med* 22(5):371-375, 1990.

Frank DA and others: Commercial discharge packs and breast-feeding counseling: effects on infant-feeding practices in a randomized trial, *Pediatrics* 80(6):845-854, 1987.

Freed GL: Time to teach what we preach, *JAMA* 269(2):243-245, 1993.

Fuller JR: Early patterns of maternal attachment, *Health Care Women Int* 11(4):433-446, 1990.

Gaull G: Taurine in pediatric nutrition: review and update, *Pediatrics* 83(3):433-442, 1989.

Gladstone IM and others: Randomized study of six umbilical cord care regimens, *Clin Pediatr* 27(3):127-129, 1988.

Goldfarb J: Breastfeeding: AIDS and other infectious diseases, *Clin Perinatal* 20(1):225-243, 1993.

Greenberg M, Morris N: Engrossment: the newborn's impact upon the father, *Am J Orthopsychiatry* 44(4):520-531, 1974.

Gunnar MR, Fisch RO, Malone S: The effects of pacifying stimulus on behavioral and adrenocortical responses to circumcision in the newborn, *J Am Acad Child Adolesc Psychiatry* 23(1):34-38, 1984.

Gunzenhauser N, editor: *Advances in touch: new implications in human development,* Skillman, NJ, 1990, Johnson & Johnson Consumer Products.

Haddock B, Vincent P, Merrow D: Axillary and rectal temperatures of full-term neonates: are they different? *Neonatal Network* 5(1):36-40, 1986.

Hammerschlag M and others: Efficacy of neonatal ocular prophylaxis for the prevention of chlamydial and gonococcal conjunctivitis, *N Engl J Med* 320(12):769-772, 1989.

Harpin VA, Rutter N: Development of emotional sweating in the newborn infant, *Arch Dis Child* 57:691-695, 1982.

Herzog LW, Alvarez SR: The frequency of foreskin problems in uncircumcised children, *Am J Dis Child* 140(3):254-256, 1986.

Houston M, Field P: Practices and policies in the initiation of breastfeeding, *JOGNN* 17(6):418-425, 1988.

Infant circumcision: still debatable, *Am J Nurs* 89(10):1268, 1989.

Jones LC, Thomas SA: New fathers' blood pressure and heart rate: relationships to interaction with their newborn infants, *Nurs Res* 38(4):237-241, 1989.

Kallio MJT and others: Exclusive breastfeeding and weaning: effect on serum cholesterol and lipoprotein concentrations in infants during the first year of life, *Pediatrics* 89(4):663-666, 1992.

Kayiatos R, Adams J, Gilman B: The arrival of a rival: maternal perceptions of toddlers' regressive behaviors after the birth of a sibling, *J Nurse Midwife* 29(3):205-213, 1984.

Keefe M: Comparison of neonatal nighttime sleep-wake patterns in nursery versus rooming-in environments, *Nurs Res* 36(3):140-144, 1987.

Keefe M and others: Development of a system for monitoring infant state behavior, *Nurs Res* 38(6):344-347, 1989.

Kellogg ND, Parra JM: Linea vestibularis: a previously undescribed normal genital structure in female neonates, *Pediatrics* 87:926-929, 1991.

Klaus MH, Kennell JH, editors: *Maternal-infant bonding,* ed 2, St Louis, 1982, Mosby.

Krutsky CD: Siblings at birth: impact on parents, *J Nurse Midwife* 30(5):269-276, 1985.

Kurinij N, Shiono P: Early formula supplementation of breast-feeding, *Pediatrics* 88(4):745-750, 1991.

Lamb ME: The bonding of phenomenon: misinterpretations and their implications, *J Pediatr* 101(4):555-557, 1982.

Larsen GL, Williams SD: Postneonatal circumcision: population profile, *Pediatrics* 85(5):808-811, 1990.

Lawrence R: *Breastfeeding: a guide for the medical profession,* ed 4, St Louis, 1994, Mosby.

Leung A: Incidence of natal and neonatal teeth, *J Pediatr* 115(6):1024, 1989.

Lohr J: The foreskin and urinary tract infections, *J Pediatr* 114(3):502-504, 1989.

Lucas A and others: Breast milk and subsequent intelligence quotient in children born preterm, *Lancet* 339(8788):261-264, 1992.

Mackey MC, Miller HM: Women's views of postpartum sibling visitation, *Matern Child Nurs J* 20(1):40-49, 1992.

Maden C and others: History of circumcision, medical conditions, and sexual activity and risk of penile cancer, *J Natl Cancer Inst* 85(1):19-24, 1993.

Madlon-Kay D: "Witch's milk," *Am J Dis Child* 140(3):252-253, 1986.

Marchette L and others: Pain reduction interventions during neonatal circumcision, *Nurs Res* 40(4):241-244, 1991.

Marecki M and others: Early sibling attachment, *JOGNN* 14(5):418-423, 1985.

Masciello AL: Anesthesia for neonatal circumcision: local anesthesia is better than dorsal penile nerve block, *Obstet Gynecol* 75:834-838, 1990.

Maxwell LG and others: Penile nerve block for newborn circumcision, *Obstet Gynecol* 70(3):415-419, 1987.

Meggyessy V, Méhes K: Association of supernumerary nipples with renal anomalies, *J Pediatr* 3:412-413, 1987.

Meier P, Wilks S: The bacteria in expressed mothers' milk, *MCN* 12(6):420-423, 1987.

Miller MJ and others: Oral breathing in newborn infants, *J Pediatr* 107(3):465-469, 1985.

Newman NM: Use of povidone-iodine in umbilical cord care, *Clin Pediatr* 28:37, 1989.

Novack AH, Mueller B, Ochs H: Umbilical cord separation in the normal newborn, *Am J Dis Child* 142:220-223, Feb 1988.

O'Grady R: Feeding behavior in infants, *Am J Nurs* 71(4):736-739, 1971.

Oudesluys-Murphy A, Degroot C: Perinatal factors and separation time of the umbilical cord, *Am J Dis Child* 142(12):1274-1275, 1988.

Pabst HF, Spady DW: Effect of breast-feeding on antibody response to conjugate vaccine, *Lancet* 336(8710):269-270, 1990.

Paes B and others: A comparative study of heel-stick devices for infant blood collection, *Am J Dis Child* 147(3):346-348, 1993.

Park M, Lee D: Normative arm and calf blood pressure values in the newborn, *Pediatrics* 83(2):240-243, 1989.

Park M, Menard S: Normative oscillometric blood pressure values in the first 5 years in an office setting, *Am J Dis Child* 143(7):860-864, 1989.

Pascoe J, French J: Development of positive feelings in primiparous mothers toward their normal newborns, *Clin Pediatr* 28(1):452-456, 1989.

Passenger air bags and infant seats, *AAP News* 10(2):26, 1994.

Patel D and others: Bacterial colonization of plastic bulb syringes, *J Pediatr* 112(3):466-468, 1988.

Pete J: Newborn infants' preference for sterile water versus five-percent glucose and water, *J Pediatr Nurs* 4(4):263-267, 1989.

Pitzer MS, Hock E: Employed mothers' concerns about separation from the first- and second-born child, *Res Nurs Health* 12:123-128, 1989.

Poissonnet C, LaVelle M, Burdi A: Growth and development of adipose tissue, *J Pediatr* 113(1):1-9, 1988.

Poland R: The question of routine neonatal circumcision, *N Engl J Med* 322(18):1312-1315, 1990.

Quan R and others: Effects of microwave radiation on antiinfective factors in human milk, *Pediatrics* 89(4):667-669, 1992.

Ramsey KP, Svee RL: Povidone-iodine cord care, *Pediatrics* 82(6):951, 1988.

Rush J: Does routine newborn bathing reduce *Staphylococcus aureus* colonization rates? A randomized controlled trial, *Birth* 13(3):176-180, 1986.

Rush J and others: A randomized controlled trial of a nursery ritual: wearing cover gowns to care for healthy newborns, *Birth* 17(1):25-30, 1990.

Ryan AS and others: A comparison of breast-feeding data from the national surveys of family growth and the Ross Laboratories Mothers' Survey, *Am J Public Health* 81(8):1049-1052, 1991.

Sachdev H and others: Water supplementation in exclusively breastfed infants during summer in the tropics, *Lancet* 337(8747):929-933, 1991.

Schwab F and others: Sibling visitation in neonatal intensive care unit, *Pediatrics* 71(4):835-838, 1983.

Sheth K and others: *Pseudomonas aeruginosa* otitis externa in an infant associated with a contaminated infant bath sponge, *Pediatrics* 77(6):920-921, 1986.

Siegel SB: Telephone follow-up programs as creative nursing interventions, *Pediatr Nurs* 18(1):86-89, 1992.

Solheim K, Spellacy C: Sibling visitation: effects on newborn infection rates, *JOGNN* 17:43-48, 1988.

Sollid D and others: Breast-feeding multiples, *J Perinat Neonat Nurs* 3(1):46-65, 1989.

Spencer D and others: Dorsal penile nerve block in neonatal circumcision: chloroprocaine versus lidocaine, *Am J Perinatol* 9(3):214-218, 1992.

Stanford J and others: Letting children observe deliveries, *N Engl J Med* 326(16):1085-1086, 1992.

Stang HJ and others: Local anesthesia for neonatal circumcision: effects on distress and cortisol response, *JAMA* 259(10):1507-1511, 1988.

Stephen S, Sexton P: Neonatal axillary temperatures: increases in readings over time, *Neonatal Network* 5(6):25-28, 1987.

Sugar M: Letting children observe deliveries, *N Engl J Med* 325(14):1048, 1991 (letter to the editor).

Templeton J, Edgil A, Douglas A: Reva Rubin revisited, *JOGNN* 17(6):394-399, 1988.

Thigpen JL: Responding to research: realistic use of scrub clothes and cover gowns, *Neonatal Network* 9(5):41-44, 1991.

Thomas K: Thermoregulation in neonates, *Neonatal Network* 13(2):15-22, 1994.

Trause M, Irvin N: Care of the sibling. In Klaus MH, Kennell JH, editors: *Maternal-infant bonding,* ed 2, St Louis, 1982, Mosby.

Trochtenberg DS: Neonatal circumcision, *N Engl J Med* 323(17):1206, 1990 (letter to the editor).

Tulman LJ: Mothers' and unrelated persons' initial handling of newborn infants, *Nurs Res* 34(4):205-210, 1985.

Tyson J and others: Randomized trial of taurine supplementation for infants ≤ 1300-gram birth weight: effect on auditory brainstem-evoked responses, *Pediatrics* 83(3):406-415, 1989.

Verma A, Dhanireddy R: Passage of first stool in very low birth weight infants, *Pediatr Notes* 17(4):1, 1993.

Walz BL: Maternal tasks of taking on a second child in the postpartum period, *Matern Child Nurs J* 12(3):185-216, 1983.

Winberg J and others: The prepuce: a mistake of nature? *Lancet* 1(8638):598-599, 1989.

Wiswell TE, Geschke DW: Risks from circumcision during the first month of life compared with those for uncircumcised boys, *Pediatrics* 83(6):1011-1015, 1989.

Wiswell TE, Hachey W: Urinary tract infections and the uncircumcised state: an update, *Clin Pediatr* 32(4):130-134, 1993.

Wong DL and others: Diapering choices: a critical review of the issues, *Pediatr Nurs* 18(1):41-54, 1992.

Yetman RJ and others: Comparison of temperature measurements by an aural infrared thermometer with measurements by traditional rectal and axillary techniques, *J Pediatr* 122(5):769-773, 1993.

Zanoni D, Isenberg S, Apt L: A comparison of silver nitrate with erythromycin for prophylaxis against ophthalmia neonatorum, *Clin Pediatr* 31(5):295-298, 1992.

BIBLIOGRAPHY

Physiologic Status of the Newborn/ Assessment of the Neonate

Abrams L and others: Effect of peripheral IV infusion on neonatal axillary temperature measurement, *Pediatr Nurs* 15(6):630-632, 1989.

Allen MC, Capute AJ: Tone and reflex development before term, *Pediatrics* 85(suppl):393-399, 1990.

Becker PT, Lederman RP, Lederman E: Neonatal measures of attention and early cognitive status, *Res Nurs Health* 12:381-388, 1989.

Blackburn S: *Assessment of risk in the newborn: neonatal growth and maturity,* ed 2, White Plains, NY, 1990, March of Dimes Birth Defects Foundation.

Catlin EA and others: The Apgar score revisited: influence of gestational age, *J Pediatr* 109:865-868, 1986.

Coen RW and others: A fast, efficient newborn exam, *Patient Care* 22(11):192-197, 200-204, 207, 1988.

Coen RW and others: The detailed newborn examination, *Patient Care* 22(12):93-96, 99, 102, 1988.

Dodman N: Newborn temperature control, *Neonatal Network* 5(6):19-23, 1987.

Fanaroff A, Martin R, editors: *Neonatal-perinatal medicine,* ed 5, St Louis, 1992, Mosby.

Haddock BJ, Merrow DL, Vincent PA: Comparisons of axillary and rectal temperatures in the preterm infant, *Neonatal Network* 6(5):67-71, 1988.

Haith MM: Sensory and perceptual processes in early infancy, *J Pediatr* 109(1):158-171, 1986.

Harpin VA, Rutter N: Barrier properties of the

newborn infant's skin, *J Pediatr* 102(3):419-425, 1983.

Hayes JS, Dreher MC, Nugent JK: Newborn outcomes with maternal marihuana use in Jamaican women, *Pediatr Nurs* 14(2):107-110, 1988.

Hurwitz S: Skin lesions in the first year of life, *Contemp Pediatr* 10(1):110-128, 1993.

Jepson H, Talashek M, Tichy A: The Apgar score: evolution, limitations, and scoring guidelines, *Birth* 18(2):83-92, 1991.

Johnson KJ, Bhatia P, Bell EF: Infared thermometry of newborn infants, *Pediatrics* 87(1):34-38, 1991.

Kellogg ND, Parra JM: Linea vestibularis: a previously undescribed normal genital structure in female neonates, *Pediatrics* 87(6):926-929, 1991.

Kenner C: Measuring neonatal assessment, *Neonatal Network* 9(4):17-22, 1990.

Kunnel MT and others: Comparisons of rectal, femoral, axillary, and skin-to-mattress temperatures in stable neonates, *Nurs Res* 37(3):162-164, 1988.

Lebenthal E, Leung Y: The impact of development of the gut on infant nutrition, *Pediatr Ann* 16(3):211-222, 1987.

Linder N and others: Suckling stimulation test for neonatal tremor, *Arch Dis Child* 64:44-52, 1989.

Lipsitt LP: Learning in infancy: cognitive development in babies, *J Pediatr* 109(1):172-183, 1986.

Medoff-Cooper B, Weininger S, Zukowsky K: Neonatal sucking as a clinical assessment too: preliminary findings, *Nurs Res* 38(3):162-165, 1989.

Moen JE and others: Axillary versus rectal temperatures in preterm infants under radiant warmers, *JOGNN* 16(5):348-352, 1987.

Moss G and others: Routine examination in the neonatal period, *Br Med J* 302(6781):878-879, 1991.

Parker S and others: Jitteriness in full-term neonates: prevalence and correlates, *Pediatrics* 85(1):17-23, 1990.

Ruchala P: The effect of wearing headcoverings on the axillary temperatures of infants, *MCN* 10(4):240, 1985.

Stevens CA and others: Development of human palmar and digital flexion creases, *J Pediatr* 113:128-132, 1988.

Tappero E, Honeyfield M, editors: *Physical assessment of the newborn,* Petaluma, CA, 1993, NICU.

Nursing Care of the Neonate: General

For additional citations on vitamin K supplementation and newborn screening see Chapter 9.

American Academy of Pediatrics, Committee on Genetics: Issues in newborn screening, *Pediatrics* 89(2):345-349, 1992.

Barnes LP: Infant care: teaching the basics, *MCN* 19(1):47, 1994.

Blackburn ST, Loper DL: *Maternal, fetal, and neonatal physiology,* Philadelphia, 1992, WB Saunders.

Cetta F, Lambert G, Ros S: Newborn chemical exposure from over-the-counter skin care products, *Clin Pediatr* 30(5):286-289, 1991.

Coffman S, Levitt MJ, Deets C: Personal and professional support for mothers of NICU and healthy newborns, *JOGNN* 20(5):406-415, 1991.

Dextradeur CC, Godfrey TM: A badge of security, *MCN* 16(3):175-176, 1991.

Hanvey L: Values in maternal and newborn care, *Can Nurse* 86(9):22-24, 1990.

Kendig JW: Care of the normal newborn, *Pediatr Rev* 13(7):262-268, 1992.

Kenner C, Brueggemeyer A, Gunderson LP: *Comprehensive neonatal nursing,* Philadelphia, 1993, WB Saunders.

O'Hara MA: Ophthalmia neonatorum, *Pediatr Clin North Am* 40(4):715-725, 1993.

Seidel HM, Rosenstein BJ, Pathak A: *Primary care of the newborn,* St Louis, 1993, Mosby.

Spadt SK, Sensenig KD: Infant kidnapping: it can happen in any hospital, *MCN* 15(1):52-54, 1990.

Weiss M, Armstrong M: Postpartum mothers; preferences for nighttime care of the neonate, *JOGNN* 29(4):290-295, 1991.

Wilkerson NN, Barrows TL: Synchronizing care with mother-baby rhythms, *MCN* 13(4):264-269, 1988.

Williams JK: Screening for genetic disorders, *J Pediatr Health Care* 3(3):115-121, 1989.

Circumcision

Fergusson DM, Lawton JM, Shannon FT: Neonatal circumcision and penile problems: an 8-year longitudinal study, *Pediatrics* 81(4):537-541, 1988.

Gordon A, Collin J: Save the normal foreskin, *Br Med J* 6869(306):1-2, 1993.

Harris CC: Cultural values and the decision to circumcise, *Image J Nurs Sch* 18(3):98-104, 1986.

Herzog LW: Urinary tract infections and circumcision: a case-control study, *Am J Dis Child* 143(3):348-350, 1989.

Kashani IA, Faraday R: The risk of urinary tract infection in uncircumcised male infants, *Int Pediatr* 4(1):44-45, 1989.

Lindeke L, Iverson S, Fisch R: Neonatal circumcision: a social and medical dilemma, *Matern Child Nurs J* 12(1):31-37, 1986.

Lund MM: Perspectives on newborn male circumcision, *Neonatal Network* 9(3):7-12, 1990.

Myron AV, Maguire DP: Pain perception in the neonate: implications for circumcision, *J Prof Nurs* 7(3):188-195, 1991.

Williams N, Chel J, Kapila L: Why are children referred for circumcision? *Br Med J* 6869(306):28, 1993.

Wiswell TE and others: *Staphylococcus aureus* colonization after neonatal circumcision in relation to device used, *J Pediatr* 119(2):302-304, 1991.

Nutrition

Beckholt AP: Breast milk for infants who cannot breastfeed, *JOGNN* 19(3):216-222, 1990.

Cronenwett L and others: Single daily bottle use in the early weeks postpartum and breast-feeding outcomes, *Pediatrics* 90(5):760-766, 1992.

Danner S: How do we influence the breastfeeding decision? *Birth* 18(4):227-228, 1991.

Dewey K and others: Maternal versus infant factors related to breast milk intake and residual milk volume: the DARLING study, *Pediatrics* 87(6):829-837, 1991.

Dix D: Why women decide not to breastfeed, *Birth* 18(4):222-225, 1991.

Doyle LW and others: Breastfeeding and intelligence, *Lancet* 339(8795):744-745, 1992.

Fomon SJ: *Nutrition of normal infants,* St Louis, 1993, Mosby.

Frantz K: Keep breastfeeding simple, keep it easy, keep it fun, *Birth* 18(4):228-229, 1991.

Freed G, Fraley K, Schanler R: Attitudes of expectant fathers regarding breast-feeding, *Pediatrics* 90(2):224-227, 1992.

Gale R and others: Breast-feeding of term infants: three-hour vs. four-hour non-demand, *Clin Pediatr* 28(10):458-460, 1989.

Gamble D, Morse J: Fathers of breastfed infants: postponing and types of involvement, *JOGNN* 22(4):358-365, 1993.

Grossman LK and others: The effect of postpartum lactation counseling on the duration of breast-feeding in low-income women, *Am J Dis Child* 144(4):471-474, 1990.

Howie PW and others: Protective effect of breast feeding against infection, *Br Med J* 300:11-16, 1990.

Jacobson SW, Jacobson JL: Follow-up on breast-feeding and infant IQ, *Pediatr Alert* 17(9):46, 1992.

Kearney MH: Identifying psychosocial obstacles to breastfeeding success, *JOGNN* 17(2):98-107, 1988.

Kearney MH, Cronenwett L: Breastfeeding and employment, *JOGNN* 20(6):471-480, 1991.

Lucas A and others: Does breast milk increase the IQ of preterm infants? *Pediatr Alert* 17(5):21, 1992.

Maccagno-Smith R, Young M: Breastfeeding the sleepy infant, *Can Nurse* 89(2):20-22, 1993.

Mathew OP: Science of bottle feeding, *J Pediatr* 119(4):511-519, 1991.

Mathew OP, Bhatia J: Sucking and breathing patterns during breast- and bottle-feeding in term neonates, *Am J Dis Child* 143:588-592, 1989.

Minchin MK: Positioning for breastfeeding, *Birth* 16(2):67-73, 1989.

Mok J: HIV-1 infection: breast milk and HIV-1 transmission, *Lancet* 341(8850):930-931, 1993.

Moore E, Bianchi-Gray M, Stephens L: A community hospital–based breastfeeding counseling service, *Pediatr Nurs* 17(4):383-389, 1991.

Nice FJ: Can a breast-feeding mother take medication without harming her infant? *MCN* 14:27-31, 1989.

Nienhuis BJ and others: Is supplemental water necessary for breast-fed babies? *Clin Pediatr* 19(11):669, 1990.

Oberlander T and others: Short-term effects of feed composition on sleeping and crying in newborns, *Pediatrics* 90(5):733-740, 1992.

Page-Goertz S: Discharge planning for the breastfeeding dyad, *Pediatr Nurs* 15(5):543-544, 1989.

Pipes PL: *Nutrition in infancy and childhood,* ed 5, St Louis, 1993, Mosby.

Rentschler DD: Correlates of successful breast-feeding, *Image J Nurs Sch* 23(3):151-154, 1991.

Shrago L, Bocar D: The infant's contribution to breastfeeding, *JOGNN* 19(3):209-215, 1990.

Van de Perre P and others: Infective and anti-infective properties of breastmilk from

HIV-1 infected women, *Lancet* 341(8850): 914-918, 1993.

Walker M: Commentary: another look at positioning for breastfeeding, *Birth* 16(2):74-80, 1989.

Wright AL and others: Breast feeding and lower respiratory tract illness in the first year of life, *Br Med J* 299:946-949, 1989.

Parent-Infant Bonding (Attachment)

American Academy of Pediatrics, Committee on Fetus and Newborn: Postpartum (neonatal) sibling visitation, *Pediatrics* 76(4):650, 1985.

Anderson CJ: Integration of the Brazelton Neonatal Behavioral Assessment Scale into routine neonatal nursing care, *Issues Compr Pediatr Nurs* 9:341-351, 1986.

Beal JA: The Brazelton Neonatal Behavioral Assessment Scale: a tool to enhance parental attachment, *J Pediatr Nurs* 1(3):170-177, 1986.

Beal JA: Methodological issues in conducting research on parent-infant attachment, *J Pediatr Nurs* 6(1):11-15, 1991.

Berland A: Young fathers' support group, *Pediatr Nurs* 13(4):255-257, 1987.

Coffman S: Parent and infant attachment: review of nursing research 1981-1990, *Pediatr Nurs* 18(4):421-425, 1992.

Davis JA: Management of perinatal loss of a twin, *Br Med J* 297(6663):1613, 1988.

Driscoll JW: Maternal parenthood and the grief process, *J Perinat Neonat Nurs* 4(2):1-10, 1990.

Elsters AB, Lamb ME, Kimmerly N: Perceptions of parenthood among adolescent fathers, *Pediatrics* 83(5):758-765, 1989.

Eyer D: *Mother-infant bonding: a scientific fiction,* New Haven, CT, 1992, Yale University Press.

Farel AM and others: Interaction between high-risk infants and their mothers: the NCAST as an assessment tool, *Res Nurs Health* 14(2):109-118, 1991.

Fortier JC and others: Adjustment to a newborn, *JOGNN* 20(1):73-79, 1991.

Fuller JR: Early patterns of maternal attachment, *Health Care Women Int* 11(4):433-446, 1990.

Gaffney KF: New directions in maternal attachment research, *J Pediatr Health Care* 2(4):181-188, 1988.

Gullicks J, Crase S: Sibling behavior with a newborn: parents' expectations and observations, *JOGNN* 22(5):438-446, 1993.

Lobar SL, Phillips S: A clinical assessment strategy for maternal acquaintance-attachment behaviors, *Issues Compr Pediatr Nurs* 15(4): 249-260, 1992.

Mercer RT, Ferketich SL: Predictors of parental attachment during early parenthood, *J Adv Nurs* 15:268-280, 1990.

Novak J, Novak R: Facilitating fathering. In Craft M, Denehy J: *Nursing interventions for infants and children,* Philadelphia, 1990, WB Saunders.

Palkovitz R: Fathers' motives for birth attendance, *Matern Child Nurs J* 16(2):123-129, 1987.

Palkovitz R: Sources of father-infant bonding beliefs: implications for childbirth educators, *Matern Child Nurs J* 17(2):101-113, 1988.

Palkovitz R: Changes in father-infant bonding beliefs across couples' first transition to parenthood, *Matern Child Nurs J* 29(3,4):141-154, 1992.

Porter LS, Sobong LC: Differences in maternal perception of the newborn among adolescents, *Pediatr Nurs* 16(1):101-104, 1990.

Pressler J: Promoting attachment. In Craft M, Denehy J: *Nursing interventions for infants and children,* Philadelphia, 1990, WB Saunders.

Pridham KF: The meaning for mothers of a new infant: relationship to maternal experience, *Matern Child Nurs J* 16(2):103-122, 1987.

Pridham KF, Chang AS: What being the parent of a new baby is like: revision of an instrument, *Res Nurs Health* 12:323-329, 1989.

Tomlinson PS: Fathers' involvement with first-born infants: interpersonal and situational factors, *Pediatr Nurs* 13(2):101-105, 1987.

Tomlinson PS: Verbal behavior associated with indicators of maternal attachment with the neonate, *JOGNN* 19(1):76-77, 1989.

Weingarten CT: Married mothers' perceptions of their premature or term infants and the quality of their relationships with their husbands, *JOGNN* 19(1):64-73, 1990.

Weiss ME, Armstrong M: Postpartum mothers' preferences for nighttime care of the neonate, *JOGNN* 20(4):290-295, 1990.

Wieser MA, Castiglia PT: Assessing early father-infant attachment, *MCN* 9(2):104-106, 1984.

CHAPTER 9

Health Problems of the Newborn

CHAPTER OUTLINE

RELATED TOPICS

Birth of a child with a physical defect, Ch. 11
Blood specimens, Ch. 27
The child with cognitive, sensory, or communication impairment, Ch. 24
Congenital adrenogenital hyperplasia, Ch. 38
Congenital defects caused by prenatal factors, Ch. 11
Diaper dermatitis, Ch. 13
Family-centered care of the child with chronic illness or disability, Ch. 22
Genetic evaluation and counseling, Ch. 5
Genetic screening, Ch. 5
Health promotion of the newborn and family, Ch. 8
The high-risk newborn and family, Ch. 10
Infants of diabetic mothers, Ch. 10

BIRTH INJURIES

Birth injuries are injuries that occur during the birth process. They are most likely to occur when the infant is large, the presentation is breech, forceful extraction is used, or inexperienced practitioners manage the delivery.

Many injuries are minor and resolve spontaneously in a few days; others, although minor, require some degree of intervention. Still others can be serious and even fatal. Part of the nurse's responsibility is to identify such injuries so that appropriate intervention can be initiated as soon as possible. Birth injuries can be classified according to the type of body structure involved (see left-hand box on p. 338).

■ David Wilson, RN,C, MS, revised this chapter.

SOFT TISSUE INJURY

Various types of soft tissue injury may be sustained during the birth process, primarily in the form of bruises and/or abrasions secondary to dystocia. Soft tissue injury usually occurs when there is some degree of disproportion between the presenting part and the maternal pelvis (cephalopelvic disproportion). Common types of soft tissue injury are listed in the right-hand box on p. 338. These traumatic lesions generally fade spontaneously within a few days without treatment. However, petechiae that appear in areas other than the presenting part (during delivery) may be a manifestation of some underlying bleeding disorder and should be evaluated. Petechiae and ecchymoses may also appear on the head, neck, and face of an infant born with a nuchal cord, giving the infant's face a cyanotic appearance.

TYPES OF PHYSICAL INJURIES AT BIRTH

SOFT TISSUE INJURY

Erythema
Abrasion
Petechiae
Ecchymoses
Subcutaneous fat necrosis
Subconjunctival (scleral) hemorrhage
Retinal hemorrhage
Hemorrhage into abdominal organ(s)

HEAD INJURY

Skull molding
Caput succedaneum
Subgaleal hemorrhage
Cephalhematoma
Fracture (depressed or linear)
Intracranial hemorrhage

NEUROLOGIC INJURY

Subdural or epidural hematoma
Facial paralysis
Brachial palsy (Erb-Duchenne paralysis, Klumpke palsy)
Phrenic nerve palsy (diaphragmatic paralysis)
Spinal cord injury

COMMON TYPES OF SOFT TISSUE INJURY

Erythema and abrasions—Usually the result of the application of forceps; discoloration is the same configuration as the instrument.

Petechiae—Nonraised, pinpoint hemorrhages caused by a sudden increase and then release of pressure during passage through the birth canal; may be seen on the chest, face, and head.

Ecchymoses—Small hemorrhagic areas (larger than petechiae) that may occur after traumatic, rapid (or "precipitate"), or breech delivery.

Subcutaneous fat necrosis—Clearly outlined masses located in the subcutaneous tissues that are firm to the overlying skin but movable over the underlying tissue; most likely caused by traumatic manipulation during delivery.

Subconjunctival (scleral) hemorrhages—The result of rupture of capillaries in the sclera from pressure on the fetal head during delivery; most common location is the limbus of the iris.

Retinal hemorrhages—Flame-shaped, irregular, or round areas of bleeding in the retina from excessive pressure on the fetal head during delivery; extensive areas may indicate subdural hematoma or brain trauma.

Nursing Considerations

Nursing care is primarily directed toward assessing the injury, maintaining asepsis of the area to prevent breakdown and infection, and providing an explanation and reassurance to the parents. Accurate descriptions of the injuries are recorded to facilitate subsequent comparative nursing evaluations (e.g., extent of petechiae).

Regardless of how benign the injury, parents are concerned and mourn the loss of the expected "perfect" infant. Explanations of the cause and treatment, if any, need to be thorough and repeated frequently. If the injury is disfiguring, such as extensive facial bruising, nurses can demonstrate acceptance of the child through their example of sensitive, personal care of the infant.

HEAD TRAUMA

Trauma to the head that occurs during the birth process is usually benign but occasionally results in more serious injury. The injuries that produce serious trauma, such as intraventricular hemorrhage and subdural hematoma, are discussed in relation to neurologic disorders in the newborn (see Chapter 10). Skull fractures are discussed in association with other fractures sustained during the birth process. The three most common types of extracranial hemorrhagic injury are caput succedaneum, subgaleal hemorrhage, and cephalhematoma.

Caput Succedaneum

The most commonly observed scalp lesion is caput succedaneum, a vaguely outlined area of edematous tissue situated over the portion of the scalp that presents in a vertex delivery (Fig. 9-1, *A*). The swelling consists of serum and/or blood that has accumulated in the tissues above the bone. Typically the swelling extends beyond the bone margins and may be associated with overlying petechiae or ecchymosis. It is present at or shortly after birth. No specific treatment is needed, and the swelling subsides within a few days.

Subgaleal Hemorrhage

Subgaleal hemorrhage is bleeding into the subgaleal compartment (Fig. 9-1, *B*). The ***subgaleal compartment*** is a potential space that contains loosely arranged connective tissue; it is located beneath the galea aponeurosis, which is the tendinous sheath that connects the frontal and occipital muscles and forms the inner surface of the scalp. The injury occurs as a result of forces that compress and then drag the head through the pelvic outlet (Minarcik and Beachy, 1993). The bleeding extends beyond bone and can continue after birth, with potential for complications. Treatment is usually not needed, but it may be required in the event of blood loss and shock. Resolution of the bleeding may cause hyperbilirubinemia.

Cephalhematoma

Infrequently a cephalhematoma is formed when blood vessels rupture during labor or delivery to produce bleeding into the area between the bone and its periosteum. The injury occurs most often with primiparous women, and it is often associated with forceps delivery. Unlike caput succedaneum, the boundaries of the cephalhematoma are sharply demarcated and do not extend beyond the limits of the bone (Fig. 9-1, *C*). The cephalhematoma may involve one or both parietal bones. Less commonly the occipital and rarely the frontal bones are affected. The swelling is usually minimal at birth and increases in size on the second or third day. Blood loss is not significant.

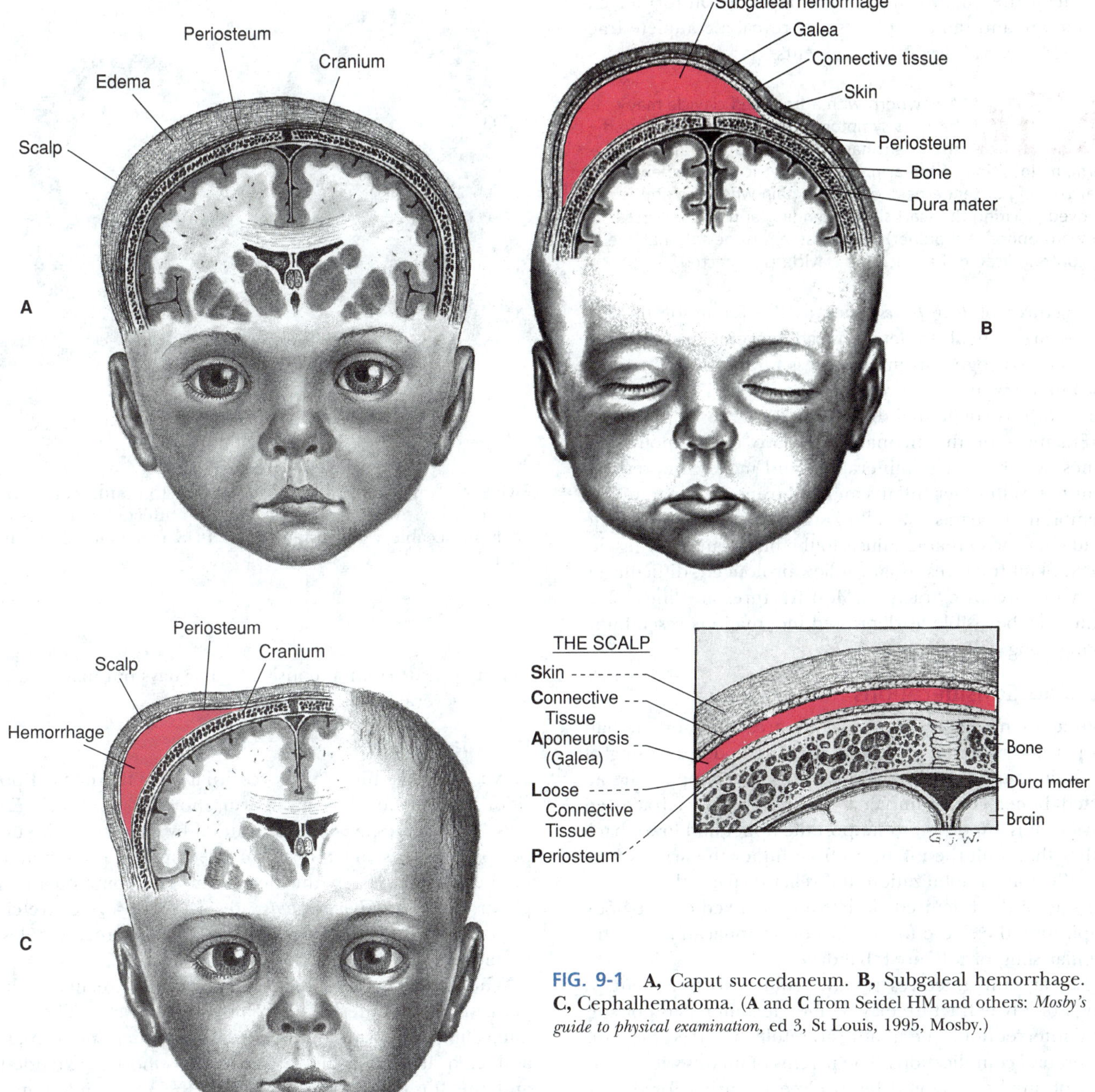

FIG. 9-1 **A,** Caput succedaneum. **B,** Subgaleal hemorrhage. **C,** Cephalhematoma. (**A** and **C** from Seidel HM and others: *Mosby's guide to physical examination,* ed 3, St Louis, 1995, Mosby.)

No treatment is indicated for uncomplicated cephalhematoma. Most lesions are absorbed within 2 weeks to 3 months. Lesions that result in severe blood loss to the area or that involve an underlying fracture require further evaluation. Hyperbilirubinemia may result during resolution of the hematoma. A local infection can develop and is suspected when a sudden increase in swelling occurs.

Nursing Considerations

Nursing care is directed toward assessment and observation of the common scalp injuries and vigilance in observing for possible associated complications such as infection, subdural hematoma, or intraventricular hemorrhage. Because these visible injuries resolve spontaneously, parents need reassurance of their usual benign nature (see also earlier discussion under Soft Tissue Injury).

FRACTURES

Fracture of the ***clavicle,*** or collarbone, is the most frequent birth injury. It is often associated with difficult vertex or breech delivery of infants of greater than average size. ***Crepitus*** (the crackling sound produced by the rubbing together of fractured bone fragments) is often heard and/or felt (especially if the infant is in a prone position) on further examination, and radiographs usually reveal a complete fracture with overriding of the fragments.

NURSING ALERT A newborn with a fractured clavicle may have no symptoms, but suspect a fracture if the infant has limited use of the affected arm, malposition of the arm, an asymmetric Moro reflex, focal swelling or tenderness, or cries in pain when the arm is moved. Eliciting the scarf sign (extending arm across chest toward opposite shoulder) for assessment of gestational age is contraindicated if a fractured clavicle is suspected.

Fractures of ***long bones,*** such as the femur or the humerus, are difficult to detect by radiographic examination. Although osteogenesis imperfecta is a rare finding, a newborn infant with a fracture should be assessed for other evidence of this congenital disorder.

Fractures of the neonatal ***skull*** are uncommon. The bones, which are less mineralized and more compressible than bones in older infants and children, are separated by membranous seams that allow sufficient alteration in the head contour so that it adjusts to the birth canal during delivery. Skull fractures usually follow prolonged, difficult delivery or forceps extraction. Most fractures are linear, but some may be visible as depressed indentations resembling a Ping-Pong ball.

Nursing Considerations

Frequently no intervention may be prescribed other than proper body alignment, careful dressing and undressing of the infant, and handling and carrying that support the affected bone. For example, if the infant has a fractured clavicle, it is important to support the upper and lower back rather than pull the infant up from under the arms. Occasionally, for immobilization and relief of pain, the arm on the side of the fractured clavicle may be fixed on the body by pinning the sleeve to the shirt or by application of a triangular sling or a figure-8 bandage.

Linear skull fractures usually require no treatment. A Ping-Pong type fracture may require decompression by surgical intervention. The infant is carefully observed for signs of cerebral complications. The parents of infants with a fracture of any bone should be involved in caring for the infant during hospitalization as part of discharge planning for care at home.

PARALYSES

Facial Paralysis

Pressure on the facial nerve during delivery may result in injury to cranial nerve VII. Clinical manifestations are primarily loss of movement on the affected side, such as inability to completely close the eye, drooping of the corner of the mouth, and absence of wrinkling of the forehead and nasolabial fold (Fig. 9-2). Paralysis is most noticeable when the infant cries. The mouth is drawn to the unaffected side, the wrinkles are deeper on the normal side, and the eye on the involved side remains open.

No medical intervention is necessary. The paralysis usually disappears spontaneously in a few days but may take as long as several months.

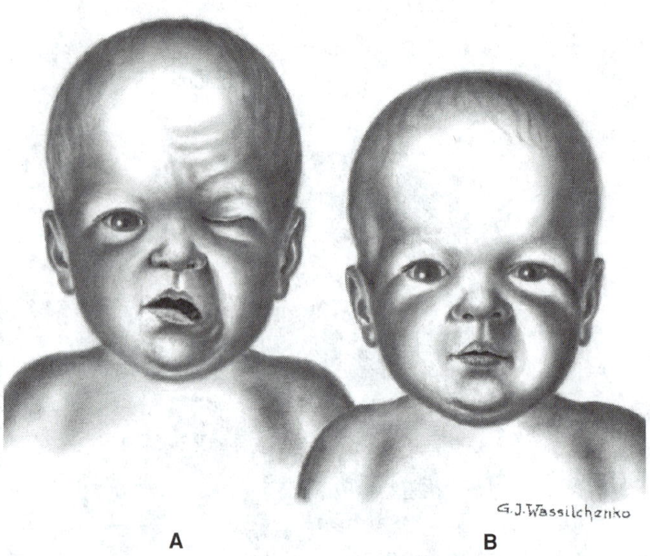

FIG. 9-2 **A,** Paralysis of right side of face 15 minutes after forceps delivery. Absence of movement on affected side is especially noticeable when infant cries. **B,** Same infant 24 hours later.

Brachial Palsy

Plexus injury results from forces that alter the normal position and relationship of the arm, shoulder, and neck. ***Erb palsy (Erb-Duchenne paralysis),*** caused by damage to the upper plexus, is usually a result of stretching or pulling away of the shoulder from the head. The less common lower plexus palsy, or ***Klumpke palsy,*** results from severe stretching of the upper extremity while the trunk is relatively less mobile.

The clinical manifestations of Erb palsy are related to the paralysis of the affected extremity and muscles. The arm hangs limp alongside the body. The shoulder and arm are adducted and internally rotated. The elbow is extended, and the forearm is pronated with the wrist and fingers flexed (Fig. 9-3). In lower plexus palsy the muscles of the hand are paralyzed with consequent wrist drop and relaxed fingers. In severe forms of brachial palsy, the entire arm is paralyzed and hangs limp and motionless at the side.

Treatment of an affected arm is aimed at preventing contractures of the paralyzed muscles and maintaining correct placement of the humeral head within the glenoid fossa of the scapula. Complete recovery from stretched nerves usually takes 3 to 6 months. However, avulsion of the nerves (complete disconnection of the ganglia from the spinal cord that involves both anterior and posterior roots) results in permanent damage. For those injuries that do not improve spontaneously, surgical intervention may be needed to relieve pressure on the nerves or to repair the nerves with grafting. (For an excellent review of care of the child requiring surgery, see Brucker, 1991.)

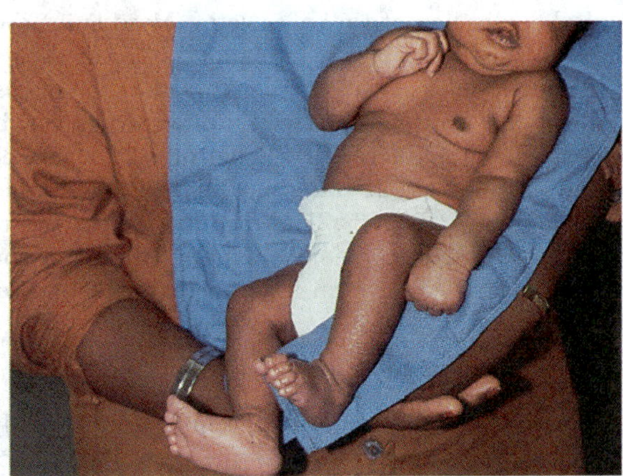

FIG. 9-3 Left-sided brachial plexus (Erb) palsy. Note extended, internally rotated arm and pronated wrist on affected side.

Phrenic Nerve Paralysis

Phrenic nerve paralysis causes diaphragmatic paralysis as demonstrated on radiographic examination by a flattened-appearing diaphragm on the affected side. The injury sometimes occurs in conjunction with brachial palsy. Respiratory distress is the most common and important sign of injury. Because injury to the phrenic nerve is usually unilateral, the lung on the affected side does not expand and respiratory efforts are ineffectual. To facilitate maximum expansion of the uninvolved lung, the infant is positioned on the affected side. Breathing is primarily thoracic, and cyanosis is a prominent sign. Pneumonia is a frequent complication.

Nursing Considerations

Nursing care of the infant with facial nerve paralysis involves aiding the infant in sucking and helping the mother with feeding techniques. Because part of the mouth cannot close tightly around the nipple, the use of a soft rubber nipple with a large hole is often helpful. Sometimes the infant needs to be gavage fed to prevent aspiration. Breast-feeding is not contraindicated, but the mother will need additional assistance in helping the infant to grasp and compress the areolar area.

If the lid of the eye on the affected side does not close completely, artificial tears can be instilled daily to prevent drying of the conjunctiva, sclera, and cornea. The lid is often taped shut to prevent accidental injury. If eye care is needed at home, the parents are taught the procedure for administration of eye drops before the infant's discharge from the nursery (see Chapter 27).

Nursing care of the newborn with brachial palsy is concerned primarily with proper positioning of the affected arm. In upper arm paralysis the arm should be abducted 90 degrees with external rotation at the shoulder, 90-degree flexion at the elbow, full supination of the forearm, and slight extension of the wrist so that the palm of the hand is turned toward the face. The position may be maintained with intermittent splinting. The arm should also receive complete passive range-of-motion exercises several times a day to maintain muscle tone and function.

In dressing the infant, preference is given to the affected arm. Undressing begins with the unaffected arm, and redressing begins with the affected arm to prevent unnecessary manipulation and stress on the paralyzed muscles. Parents are taught to use the "football" position to hold the infant and to avoid picking the child up from under the axillae or by pulling on the arms (Brucker, 1991).

The infant with phrenic nerve paralysis requires the same nursing care as any infant with respiratory distress. As with other birth injuries, emotional needs of the family are similar to those discussed for soft tissue injury (see p. 337). Also, because of the extended length of recovery, follow-up is essential.

DERMATOLOGIC PROBLEMS IN THE NEWBORN

ERYTHEMA TOXICUM NEONATORUM

Erythema toxicum neonatorum, also known as "flea bite dermatitis" or "newborn rash," is a benign, self-limiting eruption that usually appears within the first 2 days of life. The lesions are firm, 1 to 3 mm, pale yellow or white papules or pustules on an erythematous base; they resemble flea bites. The rash appears most commonly on the face, proximal extremities, trunk, and buttocks, but it may be located anywhere on the body except the palms and soles. The rash is more obvious during crying episodes. There are no systemic manifestations, and successive crops of lesions heal without pigmentation. The rash usually lasts about 5 to 7 days.

The etiology is unknown. However, a smear of the pustule will show numerous eosinophils and a relative absence of neutrophils. When the diagnosis is questionable, bacterial, fungal, or viral cultures should be done (Hurwitz, 1993). Although no treatment is necessary, parents are usually concerned about the rash and need to be reassured of its benign and transient nature.

CANDIDIASIS

Candidiasis, also known as moniliasis, is not uncommon in the newborn. *Candida albicans,* the organism usually responsible, may cause disease in any organ system. It is a yeast-like fungus (producing yeast cells and spores) that can be acquired from a maternal vaginal infection during delivery, by person-to-person transmission (especially from poor handwashing technique), or from contaminated hands, bottles, nipples, or other articles. Mucocutaneous, cutaneous, and disseminated candidiasis are all observed in this

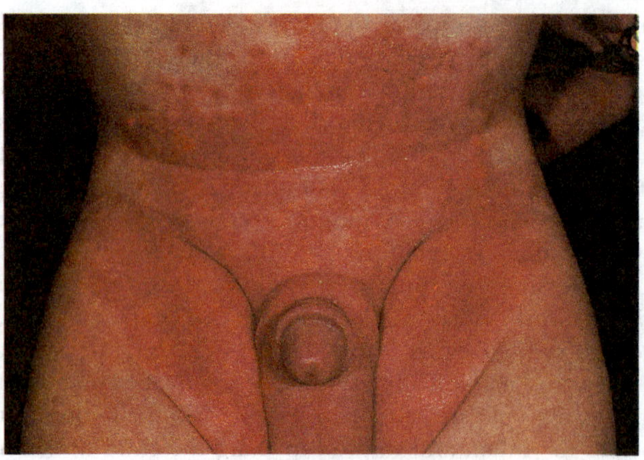

FIG. 9-4 Candida dermatitis. (From Habif TP: *Clinical dermatology: a color guide to diagnosis and therapy,* ed 2, St Louis, 1990, Mosby.)

age-group. It is usually a benign disorder in the neonate, often confined to the oral and diaper regions.

Candidal Diaper Dermatitis

The warm, moist atmosphere created in the diaper area provides an optimum environment for candidal growth. The dermatitis appears in the perianal area, inguinal folds, and lower abdomen. The affected area is intensely erythematous with a sharply demarcated, scalloped edge, frequently with numerous satellite lesions that extend beyond the larger lesion (Fig. 9-4). The usual source of infection is through the gastrointestinal tract when organisms are swallowed from the birth canal during delivery. It may also appear 2 to 3 days after an oral infection.

Therapy consists of applications of an anticandidal ointment, such as nystatin or clotrimazole, with each diaper change (see also Diaper Dermatitis, Chapter 13). Sometimes the infant also is given an oral antifungal preparation to eliminate any gastrointestinal source of infection (see following discussion).

Oral Candidiasis

Oral candidiasis (thrush) is characterized by white adherent patches on the tongue, palate, and inner aspects of the cheeks. It is often difficult to distinguish from coagulated milk. The infant may refuse to suck because of pain in the mouth, but this is uncommon.

NURSING ALERT Candidiasis can be distinguished from coagulated milk when attempts to remove the patches with a tongue blade are unsuccessful, usually resulting in bleeding from the scraped surfaces.

The condition tends to be acute in the newborn and chronic in infants and young children, and it appears when the oral flora are altered as a result of antibiotic therapy. Although the disorder is usually self-limiting, spontaneous resolution may take as long as 2 months, during which time lesions may spread to the larynx, trachea, bronchi, and lungs and along the gastrointestinal tract. The disease is treated with good hygiene, application of a fungicide, and correction of any underlying disturbance. The source of infection, usually the mother, should be treated to prevent reinfection.

Topical application of 1 ml of nystatin (Mycostatin) over the surfaces of the oral cavity four times a day or every 6 hours is usually sufficient to prevent spread of the disease or prolongation of its course. Several other drugs may be used, including amphotericin B (Fungizone), clotrimazole (Lotrimin), or miconazole (Monistat, Micatin), given intravenously or applied topically. These agents have virtually replaced the use of gentian violet solution. Therapy is continued for about 1 week, even if lesions have disappeared within a few days.

Nursing Considerations

Nursing care is directed toward preventing spread of the infection and correct application of the prescribed topical medication. For candidiasis in the diaper area, the caregiver is taught to keep the diaper area clean and to apply the medication to affected areas as prescribed (see also Diaper Dermatitis, Chapter 13).

Oral nystatin is applied after feedings. The medication is distributed over the surface of the oral mucosa and tongue with an applicator, and the remainder of the dose is deposited in the mouth to be swallowed by the infant to treat any gastrointestinal lesions.

Other measures to control thrush, in addition to good hygienic care, include rinsing the infant's mouth with plain water after each feeding before applying the medication and boiling reusable nipples and bottles for at least 20 minutes after thorough washing (spores are heat resistant). Pacifiers should be boiled for at least 20 minutes once daily, and the nipples of breast-feeding mothers should also be treated to prevent reinfection. Infants with candidal diaper dermatitis can introduce the yeast into the mouth from contaminated hands. Therefore placing clothes over the diaper can prevent this cycle of self-infection.

BULLOUS IMPETIGO

Bullous impetigo (impetigo neonatorum) is an infectious skin condition most often caused by various strains of *Staphylococcus aureus.* It is characterized by the eruption of bullous vesicular lesions on previously untraumatized skin. The lesions may appear on any body surface and sometimes become widespread, but the usual distribution involves the buttocks, perineum, trunk, and face. They vary in size from a few millimeters to several centimeters, contain turbid fluid, and are easily ruptured. The bullae rupture in 1 to 2 days, leaving a superficial red, moist, denuded area with very little crusting.

Warm saline compresses are applied to the lesions followed by gentle cleansing and application of a topical antibiotic several times a day. Systemic antibiotics and corticosteroids are sometimes administered to small infants and those with widespread lesions. Recovery is usually rapid and uneventful.

Nursing Considerations

Once the diagnosis is suspected, the infant is isolated until therapy is instituted to prevent spread of the infection to other infants. Persons who have come in contact with the infant are investigated to determine a possible source of the infecting organism. Other infants in the nursery should be scrutinized for early detection of any evidence of infection. Parents and other visitors are instructed regarding precautions for prevention of infection, especially through handwashing (see Infection Control, Chapter 27).

The infant's arms may need to be restrained with elbow restraints or by pulling the undershirt sleeves over the hands and securing the openings with tape or by applying mittens. If restraints of any kind are used, the infant is allowed freedom of movement at supervised times. Rocking, cuddling, and holding during feeding are essential components of care.

"BIRTHMARKS"

Discolorations of the skin are common findings in the newborn infant. (See discussion on skin assessment under Physical Assessment, Chapter 8.) Most, such as mongolian spots or telangiectatic nevi, involve no therapy other than reassurance to parents of the benign nature of these discolorations. Some can be a manifestation of a disease that suggests further examination of the child and other family members (e.g., the multiple flat, light brown ***café-au-lait spots*** that often characterize the autosomal-dominant hereditary disorder neurofibromatosis and are common findings in Albright syndrome).

Darker and/or more extensive lesions demand further scrutiny, and excision of the lesion is recommended when feasible or when excisional biopsy is performed. These lesions include the reddish brown solitary nodule that appears on the face or upper arm and usually represents a spindle and epithelioid cell nevus ***(juvenile melanoma);*** a giant pigmented nevus ***(bathing trunk nevus);*** a dark brown to black irregular plaque that is at risk of transformation to malignant melanoma; and the dark brown or black macules that become more numerous with age ***(junctional*** or ***compound nevi).***

Vascular malformations are permanent lesions that are present at birth. Any vascular structure, capillary, vein, artery, or lymphatics may be involved. The most common vascular malformation is the ***congenital capillary,*** or ***port-wine,*** variety. The lesions are pink, red, or purple "stains" of the skin that often thicken, darken, and proportionately enlarge as the child grows.

Port-wine stains may also be associated with structural malformations, such as glaucoma and/or leptomeningial angiomatosis (tumor of blood or lymph vessels in the pia-arachnoid—***Sturge-Weber syndrome***) or bony and/or muscular overgrowth ***(Klippel-Trenaunay-Weber syndrome).*** Children with port-wine stains on the face (eyelids, forehead, and cheeks) or on extremities should be monitored for these syndromes with periodic ophthalmologic examination, neurologic imaging, and measurement of extremities (Tallman and others, 1991).

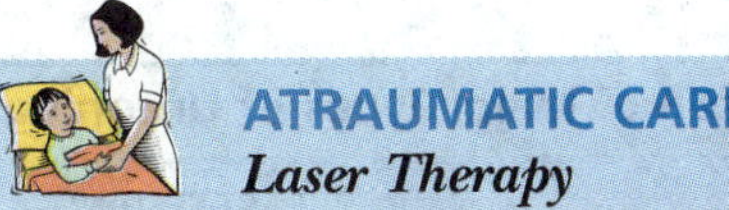

ATRAUMATIC CARE
Laser Therapy

The laser pulse feels like the sharp snap of a rubber band on the skin, and each treatment may involve from 15 to 100 pulses (Strauss and Resnick, 1993). Therefore the child should be given general anesthesia, sedation, and/or a topical anesthetic, such as EMLA (eutectic mixture of local anesthetics [prilocaine 2.5% and lidocaine 2.5%]) (Sherwood, 1993).

The treatment of choice for port-wine stains is the use of the flashlamp-pumped pulsed dye laser. A series of treatments are usually needed (see Atraumatic Care box). The treatments can significantly lighten or completely clear the lesions with almost no scarring or pigment change (Goldman, Fitzpatrick, and Ruiz-Esparza, 1993).

Hemangiomas are tumors that involve only capillaries. They may or may not be visible at birth, enlarge during the first year, and tend to resolve spontaneously. ***Strawberry hemangiomas*** are red, rubbery nodules with a rough surface. Usually no treatment is needed unless they interfere with function, such as breathing, feeding, or vision. Unfortunately, if treatment is needed, surgery usually results in scarring.

Nursing Considerations

Birthmarks, especially those on the face, are upsetting to parents. Families need an explanation of the type of lesion, its significance, and possible treatment. They can benefit from seeing photographs of other infants before and after treatment for port-wine stains or after the passage of time for hemangiomas. If laser therapy is performed, parents are instructed to keep the infant's fingernails trimmed to prevent trauma to the area. The infant should be kept out of the sun for several weeks and then protected with a sunscreen of at least SPF 15. Parents are also cautioned to avoid disturbing (scraping) a hemangioma, since this may cause bleeding and infection at the site.

PROBLEMS RELATED TO PHYSIOLOGIC FACTORS

HYPERBILIRUBINEMIA

The term ***hyperbilirubinemia*** refers to an excessive accumulation of bilirubin in the blood and is characterized by ***jaundice,*** or ***icterus,*** a yellowish discoloration of the skin and other organs. Hyperbilirubinemia is a common finding in the newborn and in most instances is relatively benign. However, it can also indicate a pathologic state.

Hyperbilirubinemia may result from increased unconjugated or conjugated bilirubin. The unconjugated form (Table 9-1) is the type most commonly seen in newborns. The following discussion of hyperbilirubinemia is limited to the unconjugated type.

TABLE 9-1 Comparison of Major Types of Unconjugated Hyperbilirubinemia

	PHYSIOLOGIC JAUNDICE	BREAST-FEEDING—ASSOCIATED JAUNDICE	BREAST MILK JAUNDICE	HEMOLYTIC DISEASE
Cause	Immature hepatic function plus increased bilirubin load from RBC hemolysis	Poor milk intake related to fewer calories consumed by infant before mother's milk is established	Possible factor in breast milk that breaks down bilirubin to a lipid-soluble form, which is reabsorbed from gut Less frequent stooling	Blood antigen incompatibility causes hemolysis of large numbers of RBCs Liver unable to conjugate and excrete excess bilirubin from hemolysis
Onset	After 24 hours (premature infants, prolonged)	2nd-3rd day	4th-5th day	During first 24 hours
Peak	72 hours	2nd-3rd day	10th-15th day	Variable
Duration	Declines on 5th-7th day		May remain jaundiced for weeks	
Therapy	Phototherapy if bilirubin levels increase too rapidly	Frequent breast-feeding Caloric supplements Phototherapy for bilirubin 18-20 mg/dl	Temporary discontinuation of breast-feeding for up to 24 hours to determine cause; if bilirubin levels decrease, breast-feeding can resume May include home phototherapy with uninterrupted breast-feeding	*Postnatal*—Phototherapy; if severe, exchange transfusion *Prenatal*—Transfusion (fetus) Prevent sensitization (Rh incompatibility) of Rh-negative mother with RhoGAM

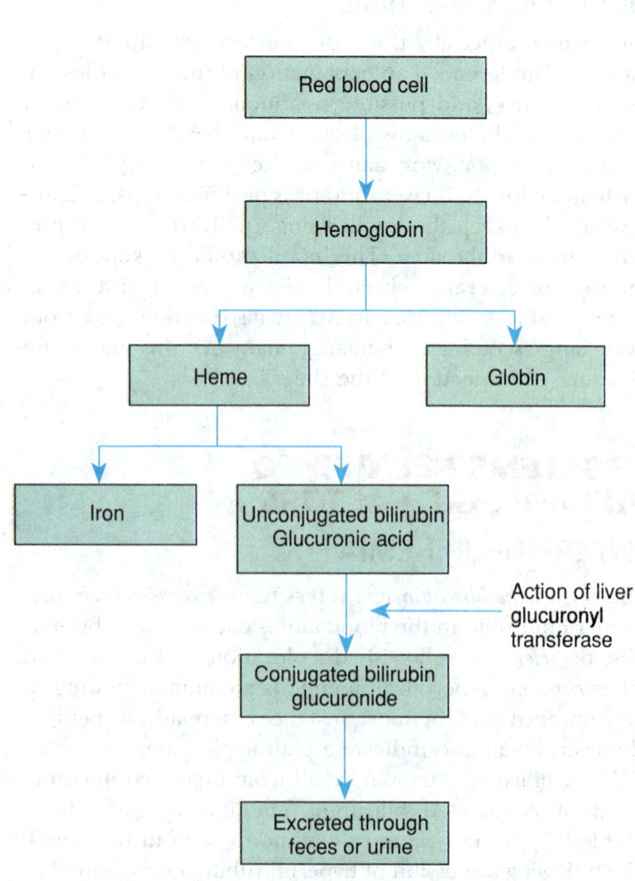

FIG. 9-5 Formation and excretion of bilirubin.

Pathophysiology

Bilirubin is one of the breakdown products of hemoglobin that results from red blood cell (RBC) destruction. When RBCs are destroyed, the breakdown products are released into the circulation, where the hemoglobin splits into two fractions: heme and globin. The globin (protein) portion is used by the body, and the heme portion is converted to ***unconjugated bilirubin,*** an insoluble substance bound to albumin.

In the liver the bilirubin is detached from the plasma protein and, in the presence of the enzyme ***glucuronyl transferase,*** is conjugated with glucuronic acid to produce a highly soluble substance, ***conjugated bilirubin glucuronide,*** which is then excreted into the bile. In the intestine bacterial action reduces the conjugated bilirubin to urobilinogen and stercobilin, the pigment that gives stool its characteristic color. Most of the reduced bilirubin is excreted through the feces; a small amount is eliminated as urobilinogen in the urine (Fig. 9-5).

Normally the body is able to maintain a balance between the destruction of RBCs and the use or excretion of byproducts. However, when developmental limitations or a pathologic process interferes with this balance, bilirubin accumulates in the tissues to produce jaundice. The following are possible causes of hyperbilirubinemia in the newborn:

- Physiologic (developmental) factors (prematurity)
- Association with breast-feeding or breast milk
- Excess production of bilirubin (e.g., hemolytic disease, biochemical defects, bruises)
- Disturbed capacity of the liver to secrete conjugated bilirubin (e.g., enzyme deficiency, bile duct obstruction)
- Combined overproduction and undersecretion (e.g., sepsis)

- Some disease states (e.g., hypothyroidism, galactosemia, infant of a diabetic mother)
- Genetic predisposition to increased production (Native Americans, Asians)

The first two causes are discussed below; the third major cause due to hemolytic disease is presented on p. 351.

Complications. Unconjugated bilirubin is highly toxic to neurons; therefore an infant with severe jaundice is at risk of developing ***bilirubin encephalopathy*** (interchangeably referred to as kernicterus), a syndrome of severe brain damage resulting from the deposition of unconjugated bilirubin in brain cells. ***Kernicterus*** describes the yellow staining of the brain cells that may result in bilirubin encephalopathy (Palmer and Smith, 1990). The damage occurs when the serum concentration reaches toxic levels, regardless of cause. There is evidence that a fraction of unconjugated bilirubin crosses the blood-brain barrier in neonates with physiologic hyperbilirubinemia. When certain pathologic conditions exist in addition to elevated bilirubin levels, there is an increase in the blood-brain barrier's permeability to unconjugated bilirubin and, thus, potential irreversible damage. The exact level of serum bilirubin required to cause damage is as yet unknown (Bratlid, 1990).

Multiple factors contribute to bilirubin neurotoxicity; therefore serum bilirubin levels alone do not predict the risk of brain injury. Factors that enhance the development of bilirubin encephalopathy include metabolic acidosis, lowered albumin levels, free fatty acids, and drugs such as salicylates or sulfonamides that compete for attachment to the plasma protein. In addition, any condition that increases the metabolic demands for oxygen or glucose (such as fetal distress, hypoxia, hypothermia, or hypoglycemia) also increases the risk of brain damage despite lower serum levels of bilirubin.

The signs of bilirubin encephalopathy are those of central nervous system depression or excitation. Generally, the clinical symptoms appear after the peak plasma bilirubin level has been established for several hours. Prodromal symptoms consist of decreased activity, lethargy, irritability, and a loss of interest in feeding. Within several hours these subtle findings are followed by rigid extension of all four extremities, opisthotonos, irritable cry, seizures, and gastric or pulmonary hemorrhage. Those who survive may eventually show evidence of neurologic damage, such as mental retardation, attention deficit disorder, delayed motor development or abnormal motor movement (especially ataxia or athetosis), behavior disorders, perceptual problems, or sensorineural hearing loss.

Physiologic Jaundice

The most common cause of hyperbilirubinemia is the relatively mild and self-limited ***physiologic jaundice,*** or ***icterus neonatorum.*** It is not associated with any pathologic process, as is hemolytic disease of the newborn. Although almost all newborns experience elevated bilirubin levels, only about half demonstrate observable signs of jaundice, which begins after 24 hours, peaks at 72 hours, and declines 5 to 7 days after birth.

Infants of Oriental descent (including Native Americans) have mean bilirubin levels almost twice those seen in whites or blacks; and an increased incidence of hyperbilirubinemia is seen in newborns from certain geographic areas, particularly areas around Greece, who have glucose-6-phosphate dehydrogenase deficiency (G-6-PD), which can cause acute hemolytic anemia. In addition, approximately 1 in 200 breast-fed infants with no evidence of disease develop hyperbilirubinemia. It also develops in a small number of newborns with Crigler-Najjar syndrome, an inherited disorder of absence of glucuronyl transferase.

Mechanisms Involved in Physiologic Jaundice. On average, newborns produce twice as much bilirubin as do adults because of higher concentrations of circulating erythrocytes and a shorter life span of RBCs (only 70 to 90 days, in contrast to 120 days in the older child and the adult). In addition, the ability of the liver to conjugate bilirubin is reduced because of limited glucuronyl transferase production. Newborns also have a lower plasma-binding capacity for bilirubin because of reduced albumin concentrations as compared with older children. Normal changes in hepatic circulation following birth may contribute to excess demands on liver function.

Normally, conjugated bilirubin is reduced to urobilinogen by the intestinal flora and excreted in feces. However, the sterile newborn bowel is initially unable to excrete bilirubin. Consequently, some unconjugated bilirubin is reabsorbed by the intestine and recirculated to the liver (also referred to as enterohepatic shunting). Feeding (1) stimulates peristalsis and produces more rapid passage of meconium, thus diminishing the amount of reabsorption of unconjugated bilirubin, and (2) introduces bacteria to aid in reduction of bilirubin to urobilinogen. Colostrum, a natural cathartic, facilitates meconium evacuation.

Jaundice in Breast-Feeding Infants

Breast-feeding is associated with an increased incidence of jaundice. Two types have been identified. ***Breast-feeding-associated jaundice (early-onset jaundice)*** begins at 2 to 4 days of age and occurs in approximately 10% to 25% of breast-fed newborns. The jaundice is related to the process of breast-feeding, probably from decreased caloric and fluid intake by breast-fed infants before the milk supply is established, since fasting is associated with decreased hepatic clearance of bilirubin.

Breast milk jaundice (late-onset jaundice) begins at age 4 to 5 days and occurs in 2% to 3% of breast-fed infants. Rising levels of bilirubin peak during the third week and then gradually diminish. Despite high levels of bilirubin that may persist for 3 to 12 weeks, these infants are well. The jaundice may be caused by a factor in the breast milk (beta-glucuronidase) that breaks down bilirubin to a lipid-soluble form, which is reabsorbed in the gut. Less frequent stooling by breast-fed infants allows for extended time for reabsorption of bilirubin from stools.

Clinical Manifestations

The most obvious sign of hyperbilirubinemia is jaundice, the yellowish discoloration primarily of the sclera, nails, or skin. As a rule, jaundice that appears within the first 24 hours is caused by hemolytic disease of the newborn, sepsis, or one of the maternally derived diseases, such as diabetes mellitus or infections. Jaundice that appears on the second or third day, peaks on the second to fourth day, and decreases on the fifth to seventh day is usually the result of physiologic jaundice. The intensity of the jaundice is unrelated to the degree of hyperbilirubinemia.

Diagnostic Evaluation

The degree of jaundice is determined by serum bilirubin measurements. Normal values of unconjugated bilirubin are 0.2 to 1.4 mg/dl. In the newborn, levels must exceed 5 mg/dl before jaundice or icterus is observable. Hyperbilirubinemia may be defined as a serum bilirubin value >12.9 mg/dl in full-term infants and >15 mg/dl in preterm infants (Frank, Turner, and Merenstein, 1993). Noninvasive monitoring of bilirubin via cutaneous reflectance measurements ***(transcutaneous bilirubinometry)*** allows for repetitive estimations of bilirubin. These devices work well on dark- and light-skinned infants and correlate fairly well with serum determinations of bilirubin level in full-term infants (Schumacher, 1990). Once phototherapy has been initiated, transcutaneous bilirubinometry is no longer useful as a screening tool.

Therapeutic Management

The primary goals in the treatment of hyperbilirubinemia are to prevent bilirubin encephalopathy and, as in any blood group incompatibility, to reverse the hemolytic process (see p. 351). The main form of treatment involves the use of phototherapy. Exchange transfusion is generally used for reducing dangerously high bilirubin levels that occur with hemolytic disease.

The pharmacologic management of hyperbilirubinemia with phenobarbital has centered primarily on the infant with hemolytic disease and is most effective when given to the mother several days before delivery. Phenobarbital promotes hepatic glucuronyl transferase synthesis (increasing bilirubin conjugation and hepatic clearance of the pigment in bile) and protein synthesis, which may increase albumin for more bilirubin binding sites. The use of phenobarbital in either the antenatal or the postnatal period, however, has not proved to be as effective as other treatments in reducing bilirubin. Bilirubin production in the newborn can be decreased by inhibiting heme oxygenase, an enzyme needed for heme breakdown (to biliverdin), with metalloporphyrins, especially tin-protoporphyrin and tin-mesoporphyrin. The use of heme-oxygenase inhibitors provides a preventive approach to hyperbilirubinemia. Although some studies report good results with metalloporphyrins (Valaes and others, 1994), the procedure is not widely used.

Full-term infants with jaundice may also benefit from early initiation of feedings and frequent breast-feeding. These preventive measures are aimed at promoting increased intestinal motility, decreasing enterohepatic shunting, and establishing normal bacterial flora in the bowel to effectively enhance the excretion of unconjugated bilirubin.

Phototherapy. Phototherapy consists of the application of fluorescent light on the infant's exposed skin. Light promotes bilirubin excretion by ***photoisomerization,*** which alters the structure of bilirubin to a soluble form (lumirubin) for easier excretion.

Studies indicate that blue fluorescent light is more effective in reducing bilirubin. However, because blue light alters the coloration of the infant, the normal light of fluorescent bulbs in the spectrum of 420 to 460 nm is preferred so that the skin of the infant can be better observed for color (jaundice, pallor, cyanosis) or other conditions. For phototherapy to be effective, the infant's skin must be fully exposed to an adequate amount of the light source. The color of the infant's skin does not influence the efficacy of phototherapy. Best results occur within the first 24 to 48 hours of treatment.

An alternative to traditional phototherapy "bililights" is the ***fiberoptic blanket*** or ***panel*** (Wallaby,* Biliblanket†), which consists of a light-generating illuminator, a bundle of plastic fibers affixed to a panel that distributes the energy, and a soft, disposable, light-permeable cover to protect the infant. The blanket delivers therapeutic light consistently and continuously to the infant and achieves the same photoisomerization as conventional phototherapy (Schuman and Karush, 1992). The fiberoptic blanket is especially suited for home phototherapy. The portable blanket permits more infant-parent interaction, as well as better temperature control because the infant can be covered, and eliminates the need for eye patches and placing the lights at the correct distance (Murphy and Oellrich, 1990; Woodall and Karas, 1992).

Much controversy exists regarding if and when to use phototherapy (Commentaries, 1992; Poland, 1993). Consequently, no universally accepted protocols exist. One set of treatment guidelines suggests using phototherapy for well newborns with no signs of hemolysis who have bilirubin levels between 17.5 and 22 mg/dl and for sick infants with possible hemolysis who have bilirubin levels between 13 and 17.5 mg/dl (Newman and Maisels, 1992). Phototherapy has not been found to cause long-term adverse effects. However, its benefit in improving neurologic outcome in full-term infants with serum bilirubin levels of about 15 to 16 mg/dl as compared with no treatment has also not been established (Scheidt and others, 1990). The effectiveness of treatment is determined by a decrease in serum bilirubin. Concurrently, the infant's total physical status is assessed continually because the suppression of jaundice by phototherapy may mask signs of sepsis, hemolytic disease, or hepatitis.

Management of Breast-Feeding Jaundice. Recommendations for prevention and management of early-onset jaundice in breast-fed infants are to encourage frequent breast-feeding, preferably every 2 hours, and avoid supplementation. In late-onset jaundice bilirubin levels are monitored, and breast-feeding may be discontinued for up to 24 hours when bilirubin levels reach 15 mg/dl. Breast-feeding

*Fiberoptic Medical Products, Inc., Allentown, PA.
†Ohmeda, Columbia, MO.

is resumed after a decrease in the bilirubin levels occurs, which rules out other causes of hyperbilirubinemia (Lawrence, 1994). Parents should be offered the option of continuing breast-feeding, since no harmful effects have been found in infants with bilirubin levels of up to 20 mg/dl who continue to consume human milk (Martinez and others, 1993). Home phototherapy and continued breast-feeding is another option for the family (James, Williams, and Osborn, 1993).

Prognosis. Early recognition and treatment of hyperbilirubinemia prevent severe brain damage (bilirubin encephalopathy). Impaired neurologic outcome is directly related to the serum bilirubin concentration (van de Bor and others, 1989). The main handicap is cerebral palsy, but sequelae may include clumsiness, hypotonia, and sensorineural hearing loss (Scheidt and others, 1990, 1991).

Nursing Considerations

❖ Assessment

Part of the routine physical assessment includes observing for evidence of jaundice at regular intervals. Jaundice is most reliably assessed by observing the infant's skin color from head to toe and the color of the sclera and mucous membranes. Applying direct pressure to the skin, especially over bony prominences such as the tip of the nose or the sternum, causes blanching and allows the yellow stain to be more pronounced. For dark-skinned infants, the color of the sclera, conjunctiva, and oral mucosa is the most reliable indicator. Also, bilirubin (especially at high levels) is not uniformly distributed in skin. The nurse observes the infant in natural daylight for a true assessment of color.

NURSING ALERT Evidence of jaundice that appears before the infant is 24 hours of age is an indication for assessing bilirubin levels.

The transcutaneous bilirubin meter is a useful screening device and is used to detect neonatal jaundice in full-term infants. However, phototherapy reduces the accuracy of the instrument; therefore its value is limited to the initial assessment. Institutions in which the device is used set up their own criteria based on their experience with their particular instrument. Blood samples are also taken for measurement of bilirubin in the laboratory.

NURSING ALERT While blood is drawn, the bilirubin lights are turned off, and the blood is transported in a covered tube to avoid a false reading from bilirubin destruction in the test tube.

With short hospital admissions, jaundice may appear after discharge. Therefore a careful history from the parents may reveal significant familial patterns of hyperbilirubinemia (older siblings of the infant). Other considerations in assessment include the ethnic origin of the family (e.g., higher incidence in Oriental infants), type of delivery (e.g., induction of labor), and infant characteristics such as weight loss after birth, gestational age, sex, and presence of any bruising. The method of feeding and frequency of feeding are assessed.

❖ Nursing Diagnoses

After the nursing assessment, a number of nursing diagnoses become evident. The most likely diagnoses are outlined and discussed in the Nursing Care Plan on pp. 350-351. Others may be apparent in individual cases.

❖ Planning

The goals for the infant with hyperbilirubinemia and the family are as follows:

1. Infant will receive appropriate therapy if needed to reduce serum bilirubin levels.
2. Infant will experience no complications from therapy.
3. Family will receive emotional support.
4. Family will be prepared for home phototherapy (if prescribed).

❖ Implementation

Basic nursing care of the child with hyperbilirubinemia differs from that of any newborn infant only in management of specific therapy (see Nursing Care of the Newborn and Family, Chapter 8, and Nursing Care of High-Risk Newborns, Chapter 10).

Prevention of physiologic and breast-feeding jaundice may be possible with early introduction of feedings and frequent nursing. Every effort is made to provide an optimum thermal environment to reduce metabolic needs.

Phototherapy. The infant who receives phototherapy is placed nude under the light source and repositioned frequently to expose all body surface areas to the light. Once phototherapy has been initiated, frequent (every 4 to 12 hours) serum bilirubin levels are necessary, since visual assessment of jaundice is no longer considered valid.

Several precautions are instituted to protect the infant during phototherapy. The infant's eyes are shielded by an opaque mask to prevent exposure to the light (Fig. 9-6).

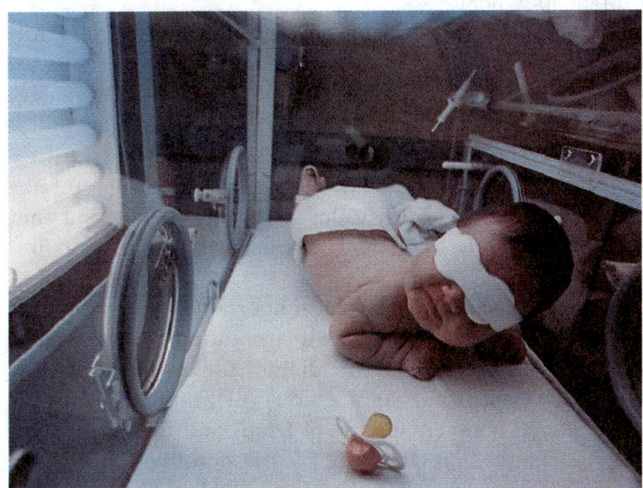

FIG. 9-6 Infant under phototherapy unit. Note that the eyes are shielded and a diaper is used to contain the diarrheal stools.

THINKING CRITICALLY ABOUT . . .
Covering the Genitals During Phototherapy

In the laboratory, exposure of cells to light intensities similar to those used in phototherapy has produced changes in DNA and in sperm and oocytes, as well as abnormal embryo and cleavage patterns, in the American sea urchin. The relationship of these changes to infants receiving phototherapy is unknown (Maisels, 1990). While the chance of gonadal complications is highly unlikely because the period of exposure is relatively brief (Tan, 1991), no long-term studies have been done on gonadal function of males treated with phototherapy at birth.

Consequently, some recommend covering the gonads with a shield, such as a bikini diaper fashioned from a face mask; others believe that this precaution is unnecessary and decreases body surface exposure to the lights. Until a resolution to this controversy is achieved, the best approach is to follow individual institutional protocols. A small diaper may be needed if diarrhea is a problem. Complete exposure and gonadal protection may be achieved if the newborn is placed prone. For home phototherapy, positioning should be discussed with the practitioner, since the recommended sleeping position for healthy infants is supine (American Academy of Pediatrics, 1992; Long and Barron, 1992) (see also Sudden Infant Death Syndrome, Chapter 13).

The eye shield should be properly sized and correctly positioned to cover the eyes completely but prevent any occlusion of the nares. The infant's eyelids are closed before the mask is applied, since the corneas may become excoriated if they come in contact with the dressing. On each nursing shift the eyes are checked for evidence of discharge, excessive pressure on the lids, or corneal irritation. Eye shields are removed during feedings, and this opportunity is taken to provide visual and sensory stimulation. (See also Thinking Critically About . . . box .)

The phototherapy unit may be combined with a radiant heat warmer or servocontrolled incubator to provide an optimum thermal environment. The thermistor should be attached to the infant or covered with opaque tape so that it is not exposed to direct radiation. This may require changing the sensor from the abdomen to the back according to the infant's position. Placing the sensor on the infant's side reduces the need for frequent changes. Vital signs are taken at least every 4 hours to ensure that the infant's body temperature is normothermic. Sometimes it is necessary to regulate the temperature in the incubator to maintain proper body heat.

Infants who are in an open crib must have a protective Plexiglas shield between them and the fluorescent lights to minimize the amount of undesirable ultraviolet light reaching their skin and to protect them from accidental bulb breakage. Their temperature is closely monitored to prevent hyperthermia or hypothermia. Maintaining the infant in a flexed position with rolled blankets placed along the sides of the body helps maintain heat and provides comfort.

Accurate charting is another important nursing responsibility and includes (1) times that phototherapy is started and stopped, (2) proper shielding of the eyes, (3) type of fluorescent lamp (by manufacturer), (4) number of lamps, (5) distance between surface of lamps and infant (should be no less than 18 inches), (6) use of phototherapy in combination with an incubator or open bassinet, (7) photometer measurement of light intensity, and (8) occurrence of side effects.

Side effects of phototherapy. Minor side effects for which the nurse should be alert include loose, greenish stools; transient skin rashes; hyperthermia; increased metabolic rate; dehydration; electrolyte disturbances, such as hypocalcemia; and priapism. To prevent or minimize these effects, the temperature is monitored to detect early signs of hypothermia or hyperthermia and the skin is observed for evidence of dehydration and drying, which can lead to excoriation and breakdown. Oily lubricants or lotions are not used on the skin in order to prevent increased tanning, or a "frying" effect. Full-term infants receiving phototherapy may require additional fluid volume to compensate for insensible and intestinal fluid loss. Because phototherapy enhances the excretion of unconjugated bilirubin through the bowel, loose stools may indicate accelerated bilirubin removal. Frequent stooling can cause perianal irritation; therefore meticulous skin care, especially keeping the skin clean and dry, is essential.

Once phototherapy is permanently discontinued, there is often a subsequent increase in the serum bilirubin level, often called the "rebound effect"; this is usually transient and resolves without resuming therapy.

Another reaction to phototherapy is the ***bronze-baby syndrome,*** in which the serum, urine, and skin turn grayish brown several hours after the infant is placed under the light. This reaction is probably caused by retention of a bilirubin breakdown product of phototherapy (Frank, Turner, and Merenstein, 1993). The syndrome almost always occurs in infants who have elevated conjugated hyperbilirubinemia. The browning generally resolves following discontinuation of phototherapy.

Family Support. Parents need reassurance concerning their infant's progress. All the procedures are explained to familiarize them with the benefits and risks. For example, they need to be reassured that the naked infant who is under the bilirubin light is warm and comfortable. Parents may be concerned about the eye shields, since "blindness" is a frightening experience. Eye shields are removed when the parents are visiting to facilitate the attachment process, and the parents can be reassured that the neonate is accustomed to darkness after months of intrauterine existence and benefits a great deal from auditory and tactile stimulation (see Family Focus box).

One of the most important nursing interventions is rec-

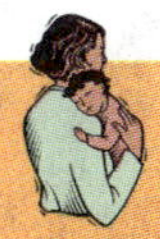

FAMILY FOCUS
Phototherapy and Parent-Infant Interaction

The traditional use of phototherapy has evoked concerns regarding a number of psychobehavioral issues, including parent-infant separation, potential social isolation, decreased sensorineural stimulation, altered biologic rhythms, altered feeding patterns, and activity changes. Parental anxiety is greatly increased, particularly at the sight of the newborn blindfolded and under special lights. The interruption of breast-feeding for phototherapy is a potential deterrant to successful maternal-infant attachment and interaction. Because research has demonstrated that bilirubin catabolism occurs primarily within the first few hours of the initiation of phototherapy, there is increased support for the removal of the infant from treatment for feeding and holding. Intermittent phototherapy may be just as effective as continuous therapy when used correctly. The benefits of stopping phototherapy for parental feeding and holding outweigh concerns related to the clearance of bilirubin (Blackburn and Loper, 1992).

ognition of breast-feeding jaundice. Lack of familiarity among health professionals has caused many newborns prolonged hospitalization, termination of breast-feeding, and unnecessary phototherapy. Care of the new mother may include supporting successful and frequent breast-feeding. Parents also need reassurance of the benign nature of the jaundice and encouragement to resume breast-feeding if temporary cessation is prescribed. Unfortunately, jaundice increases the risk of breast-feeding being discontinued and development of the vulnerable child syndrome, the belief of parents that their child has suffered a "close call" and is vulnerable to serious injury (Kemper, Forsyth, and McCarthy, 1989) (see Critical Thinking Exercise box).

Discharge Planning and Home Care. With short hospital stays, mothers and infants may be discharged before evidence of jaundice is present. It is very important for the nurse to discuss signs of jaundice with the mother, because any clinical symptoms will probably appear at home.

If home phototherapy is instituted, the hospital or home health care nurse is usually responsible for teaching family members and assessing their abilities to implement the treatment safely. General guidelines for home care preparation and education are discussed in Chapters 25 and 26. Written instructions and supervision of care, especially application of eye shields, if needed, are essential. The minor side effects of phototherapy are reviewed, and parents may need instruction in taking axillary temperatures,* and recording times and amounts of feedings and the number of wet diapers and stools. Regardless of how benign the disorder or the therapy, these parents need support and understanding. Siblings also benefit from an explanation of the therapy to allay fears or misconceptions.

In jaundice associated with breast-feeding, follow-up

CRITICAL THINKING EXERCISE
Jaundice

A 10-day-old full-term newborn is brought to the hospital laboratory for a follow-up serum bilirubin measurement. While waiting for laboratory results, the mother becomes tearful and expresses concern that the baby may have a serious illness because of her breast milk and a high bilirubin level. The baby, although quite jaundiced, is well hydrated and alert. The mother says the baby has been breast-feeding every 3 to 4 hours and empties both breasts. In addition, the baby has a normal elimination pattern. The physician has recommended that she interrupt breast-feeding for a few days. The total bilirubin level is 14 mg/dl. Given these facts and the mother's concern, the best intervention is to:

1. Encourage the mother to further verbalize her concerns about having a child with possible brain damage.
2. Encourage the mother to use an automatic breast pump for a couple of days to maintain a steady milk supply.
3. Prepare for an exchange transfusion to decrease the infant's bilirubin level.
4. Suggest that the mother consider stopping breast-feeding to prevent further jaundice.

The correct answer is 2. The age of the baby, health status, and feeding pattern support the concept of hyperbilirubinemia due in part to breast-feeding. Because breast milk jaundice is a normal physiologic occurrence, the mother needs further reassurance that once the bilirubin level starts decreasing (usually within 24 hours of interrupting breast-feeding), she may resume breast-feeding.

The first intervention is not correct because of the infant's healthy, well-nourished status and the fact that kernicterus has not been observed in healthy, full-term, breast-fed infants. An exchange transfusion is not appropriate therapy in this particular situation, and discontinuing breast-feeding is almost always unnecessary.

blood studies are usually required to assess the progress of the jaundice. If temporary cessation of breast-feeding is prescribed, mothers should be taught to pump the breasts every 3 to 4 hours to maintain lactation; the expressed milk is frozen for use after breast-feeding is resumed.

❖ EVALUATION

The effectiveness of nursing interventions is determined by continual reassessment and evaluation of care based on the following observational guidelines and expected outcomes:

1. Observe skin color; review bilirubinometric and/or laboratory findings.
2. Observe for signs of neurologic impairment.
3. Check placement of eye shields; observe skin for signs of dehydration; take temperature.
4. Interview family members and observe parent-infant interactions.

Expected outcomes:

See Nursing Care Plan, pp. 350-351.

*Home care instructions for measuring temperature are available in *Wong and Whaley's Clinical Manual of Pediatric Nursing* (Mosby).

NURSING CARE PLAN
The Newborn with Hyperbilirubinemia

NURSING DIAGNOSIS: High risk for injury from breakdown products of red blood cells in greater numbers than normal and immaturity of liver

PATIENT GOAL 1: Will receive appropriate therapy if needed to accelerate bilirubin excretion

• **NURSING INTERVENTIONS/*RATIONALES***

Initiate early feedings *to enhance excretion of bilirubin in the stool*

Assess skin for evidence of jaundice, *which indicates rising bilirubin levels*

Check bilirubin levels with transcutaneous bilirubinometry *to determine rising levels*

Note time of initial jaundice *to distinguish physiologic jaundice (appears after 24 hours) from jaundice due to hemolytic disease or other causes (appears before 24 hours)*

Assess infant's overall status, especially factors (e.g., hypoxia, hypothermia, hypoglycemia, and metabolic acidosis) *that increase the risk of brain damage from hyperbilirubinemia*

Initiate phototherapy as prescribed

• **EXPECTED OUTCOMES**

Newborn begins feeding soon after birth

Newborn is exposed to prescribed light source

PATIENT GOAL 2: Will experience no complications from phototherapy

• **NURSING INTERVENTIONS/*RATIONALES***

Shield infant's eyes

Make certain that lids are closed before applying shield *to prevent corneal irritation*

Check eyes each shift for drainage or irritation

Place infant nude under light *for maximum skin exposure*

Change position frequently, especially during the first several hours of treatment, *to increase body surface exposure*

Monitor body temperature *to detect hypothermia or hyperthermia*

Check axillary temperature

Chart duration of therapy, type of lights, distance of lights from infant, use of open or closed bassinet, and shielding of infant's eyes *to document correct use of phototherapy*

With increased stooling, cleanse skin frequently *to prevent perianal irritation*

Avoid use of oily applications on skin *to prevent tanning and burning*

Ensure adequate fluid intake *to prevent dehydration*

• **EXPECTED OUTCOME**

Infant displays no evidence of eye irritation, dehydration, temperature instability, or skin breakdown

PATIENT GOAL 3: Will experience no complications from exchange transfusion (if therapy required)

• **NURSING INTERVENTIONS/*RATIONALES***

Give infant nothing by mouth before procedure (usually for 2 to 4 hours) *to prevent aspiration*

Check donor blood for correct blood group and Rh type *to prevent transfusion reaction*

Assist practitioner during procedure; ensure asepsis *to prevent infection*

Keep accurate records of amounts of blood infused and withdrawn *to maintain proper blood volume*

Maintain optimal body temperature of infant during procedure *to prevent hypothermia and cold stress or hyperthermia*

Observe for signs of exchange transfusion reaction (tachycardia or bradycardia, respiratory distress, dramatic change in blood pressure, temperature instability, and rash) *to initiate therapy promptly*

Have resuscitation equipment (supplemental oxygen, airway, manual resuscitation bag, endotracheal tube, and laryngoscope) at bedside *to be prepared for an emergency*

Check umbilical site for bleeding or infection

Monitor vital signs during and following transfusions *to detect complications, such as cardiac dysrhythmias*

• **EXPECTED OUTCOMES**

Infant exhibits no signs of adverse effects from transfusion

Vital signs remain within normal limits (see inside back cover for normal variations)

There is no evidence of infection or bleeding at infusion site

NURSING DIAGNOSIS: Altered family processes related to infant with potentially adverse physiologic response

PATIENT (FAMILY) GOAL 1: Will receive emotional support

• **NURSING INTERVENTIONS/*RATIONALES***

Discontinue phototherapy during family visiting; remove infant's eye shields *to promote family interaction*

Emphasize benign nature of physiologic jaundice *to prevent undue parental concern and potential overprotection of child*

Assure family that skin will regain normal pigmentation

Advise breast-feeding mothers of possibility of prolonged jaundice

Emphasize benign nature of jaundice and benefits of human milk *to prevent early termination of breast-feeding*

• **EXPECTED OUTCOME**

Family demonstrates an understanding of therapy and prognosis

PATIENT (FAMILY) GOAL 2: Will be prepared for home phototherapy (if prescribed)

• **NURSING INTERVENTIONS/*RATIONALES***

Assess family's understanding of jaundice and proposed therapy *to ensure optimum results and safety*

Instruct family regarding:

Placement and care of lamp or fiberoptic unit

*Proper eye care

Apply eye patches

Close lids before applying patches

Be certain patches fit snugly with no possibility of light leaks

*Not required for fiberoptic blanket.

NURSING CARE PLAN
The Newborn with Hyperbilirubinemia—cont'd

Remove patches when light is discontinued—during feeding, bathing, and other caregiving activities, and at least once every 4 to 6 hours
*Proper positioning while under lamp
Rotate to expose all areas of skin
Keep infant nude or dressed in mini-diaper
Providing increased fluid intake
Measuring axillary temperature
Keeping log of time spent under light, infant's color, feeding patterns, amount of feedings, diaper changes
Observing for signs of lethargy, change in sleeping pattern, any difficulty arousing infant, changes in stooling or voiding
Keeping diaper area clean and dry
Importance of bilirubin tests as prescribed

• **EXPECTED OUTCOME**
Family demonstrates ability to provide home phototherapy for infant (specify learning and methods of demonstration)

HEMOLYTIC DISEASE OF THE NEWBORN (HDN)

Hyperbilirubinemia in the first 24 hours of life is most often the result of HDN (erythroblastosis fetalis), an abnormally rapid rate of RBC destruction. Anemia caused by this destruction stimulates the production of RBCs, which, in turn, provides increasing numbers of cells for hemolysis. Major causes of increased erythrocyte destruction are isoimmunization (primarily Rh) and ABO incompatibility.

Blood Incompatibility

The membranes of human blood cells contain a variety of ***antigens,*** also known as ***agglutinogens,*** substances capable of producing an immune response if recognized by the body as a foreign substance. It is the reciprocal relationship between antigens on RBCs and antibodies in the plasma that causes ***agglutination*** (clumping) to take place. In other words, antibodies in the plasma of one blood group (except the AB group, which contains no antibodies) will produce agglutination when mixed with antigens of a different blood group. In the ABO blood group system the antibodies occur naturally. In the Rh system the person must be exposed to the Rh antigen before significant antibody formation takes place to cause a sensitivity response ***(isoimmunization).***

Rh Incompatibility (Isoimmunization). The Rh blood group consists of several antigens, but for simplicity, only the terms ***Rh-positive*** (presence of antigen) and ***Rh-negative*** (absence of antigen) are used in this discussion (see Autosomal Inheritance Patterns, Chapter 5). The presence or absence of the naturally occurring Rh factor determines the blood type.

Ordinarily, no problems are anticipated when the Rh blood types are the same in both mother and fetus or if the mother is Rh-positive and the infant is Rh-negative. Difficulty may arise when the blood of the mother is Rh-negative and that of the infant is Rh-positive. Although the maternal and fetal circulations are separate, sometimes fetal RBCs (with antigens foreign to the mother) gain access to the maternal circulation through minute breaks in the placental vessels. The mother's natural defense mechanism responds to these alien cells by producing anti-Rh antibodies.

Under normal circumstances, this process of isoimmunization has no effect on the fetus during the first pregnancy with an Rh-positive fetus because the initial sensitization to Rh antigens rarely occurs before the onset of labor. However, as larger amounts of fetal blood are transferred to the maternal circulation during placental separation, maternal antibody production is stimulated. During a subsequent pregnancy with an Rh-positive fetus, these previously formed maternal antibodies to Rh-positive blood cells enter the fetal circulation, where they attack and destroy fetal erythrocytes (Fig. 9-7). Since the disease begins in utero, the fetus attempts to compensate for the progressive hemolysis by accelerating the rate of erythropoiesis. As a result, immature RBCs (erythroblasts) appear in the fetal circulation; hence the term ***erythroblastosis fetalis.***

There is wide variability in the development of maternal sensitization to Rh-positive antigens. Sensitization may occur during the first pregnancy if the woman had previously received an Rh-positive blood transfusion. No sensitization may occur in situations in which a strong placental barrier prevents transfer of fetal blood into the maternal circulation. In about 10% to 15% of sensitized mothers there is no hemolytic reaction in the newborn.

In the most severe form of erythroblastosis fetalis, ***hydrops fetalis,*** the progressive hemolysis causes fetal hypoxia, cardiac failure, generalized edema (anasarca), and effusions into the pericardial, pleural, and peritoneal spaces. The fetus may be delivered stillborn or in severe respiratory distress. However, the use of intravascular blood transfusion has improved the outcome of affected fetuses (Vomund and Witter, 1994).

ABO Incompatibility. Hemolytic disease can also occur when the major blood group antigens of the fetus are different from those of the mother. The major blood groups are A, B, AB, and O. The incidence of these blood groups varies according to race and geographic location. In the North American white population, 46% have type O blood, 42% have type A blood, 9% have type B blood, and 3% have type AB blood.

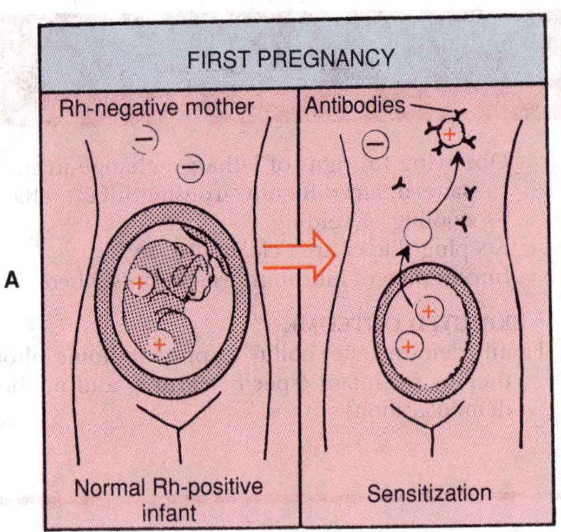

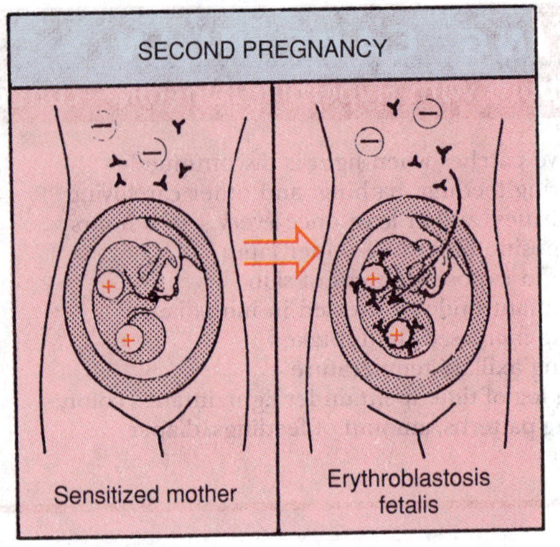

FIG. 9-7 Development of maternal sensitization to Rh antigens. **A,** Fetal Rh-positive erythrocytes enter maternal system. Maternal anti-Rh antibodies are formed. **B,** Anti-Rh antibodies cross placental barrier and attack fetal erythrocytes.

TABLE 9-2 ABO Relationships of Antigens/Antibodies and Donor-Recipient Compatibility

BLOOD GROUP (PHENOTYPE)	GENOTYPE	RBC ANTIGENS	PLASMA ANTIBODIES	RBC COMPATIBILITY	
				AS DONOR TO TYPE	AS RECIPIENT FROM TYPE
A	AA,AO	A	B	AB,A	O,A
B	BB,BO	B	A	AB,B	O,B
AB	AB	A and B	None	AB	O,A,B,AB
O	OO	None	A and B	AB,A,B,O	O

TABLE 9-3 Potential Maternal-Fetal ABO Incompatibilities

MATERNAL BLOOD GROUP	INCOMPATIBLE FETAL BLOOD GROUP
O	A or B
B	A or AB
A	B or AB

The presence or absence of antibodies and antigens determines whether agglutination will occur (Table 9-2). Antibodies in the plasma of one blood group (except the AB group, which contains no antibodies) will produce agglutination or a clumping reaction when mixed with antigens of a different blood group. However, naturally occurring antibodies in the recipient's blood cause agglutination of the donor's RBCs. The agglutinated donor cells become trapped in peripheral blood vessels, where they hemolyze, releasing large amounts of bilirubin into the circulation.

The most common blood group incompatibility in the neonate is between a mother with O blood group and an infant with A or B blood group (see Table 9-3 for possible ABO incompatibilities). Naturally occurring anti-A or anti-B antibodies already present in the maternal circulation cross the placenta and attack the fetal RBCs, causing hemolysis. Usually the hemolytic reaction is less severe than in Rh incompatibility. Although the traditional thinking has been that the number of pregnancies is insignificant in the severity of ABO incompatibility, evidence suggests that the risk of hyperbilirubinemia is greater for subsequent offspring, especially if the first newborn had hyperbilirubinemia (Plotz, 1985).

Clinical Manifestations

Jaundice appears shortly after birth (during the first 24 hours) and serum levels of unconjugated bilirubin rise rapidly. Anemia results from the hemolysis of large numbers of erythrocytes, and hyperbilirubinemia and jaundice result from the liver's inability to conjugate and excrete the excess bilirubin. Most newborns with HDN are not jaundiced at birth. However, hepatosplenomegaly may be evident. If the infant is severely affected, signs of anemia (notably, marked pallor) and hypovolemic shock are apparent.

Diagnostic Evaluation

Diagnosis of isoimmunization before delivery can be made through amniocentesis and analysis of bilirubin levels in amniotic fluid. Increasing bilirubin levels indicate progressive fetal hemolysis and may indicate the need for an intrauterine transfusion or immediate termination of the pregnancy. A new method using polymerase chain reaction determines the RhD genotype of amniotic cells. If the fetus is found to be Rh-negative, no further testing is needed (Bennet and others, 1993). Erythroblastosis fetalis caused by Rh incompatibility can also be assessed by evaluating rising anti-Rh antibody titers in the maternal circulation ***(indirect Coombs test)*** or by testing the optical density of amniotic fluid (delta 00450 test), since bilirubin discolors the fluid (Volmund and Witter, 1994).

The disease in the newborn is suspected on the basis of the timing and appearance of jaundice (see Table 9-1) and can be confirmed postnatally by detecting antibodies attached to the circulating erythrocytes of affected infants ***(direct Coombs test)***. The Coombs test is routinely performed on cord blood samples from infants born to Rh-negative mothers.

Therapeutic Management

The primary aim of therapeutic management of isoimmunization is prevention. Postnatal therapy is usually exchange transfusion. Although phototherapy may control bilirubin levels in mild cases, the hemolytic disease may continue, causing severe anemia.

Prevention of Rh Isoimmunization. The administration of Rho immune globulin (RhIG), a human gamma globulin concentrate of anti-D, to all unsensitized Rh-negative mothers after delivery or abortion of an Rh-positive infant or fetus prevents the development of maternal sensitization to the Rh factor. The injected anti-Rh antibodies are thought to destroy (by subsequent phagocytosis and agglutination) fetal RBCs passing into the maternal circulation before they can be recognized by the mother's immune system. Since the immune response is blocked, anti-D antibodies and memory cells, which produce the primary and secondary immune responses, respectively, are not formed (Blackburn and Loper, 1992; Lott and others, 1993). The inhibition of memory cell formation is especially important because these cells provide long-term immunity by initiating a rapid immune response once the antigen is reintroduced (McCance and Heuther, 1994).

To be effective, RhIG, such as RhoGAM, must be administered to unsensitized mothers within 72 hours (but possibly as long as 3 to 4 weeks) after the first delivery or abortion and repeated after subsequent ones. The administration of RhIG at 26 to 28 weeks of gestation further reduces the risk of Rh immunization. RhIG is not effective against existing Rh-positive antibodies in the maternal circulation.

NURSING ALERT RhIG is administered intramuscularly, not intravenously, only to Rh-negative women with a negative Coombs test—never to the infant or father.

Exchange Transfusion. Exchange transfusion, in which the infant's blood is removed in small amounts (usually 5 to 10 ml at a time) and replaced with compatible blood (such as Rh-negative blood), is a standard mode of therapy for treatment of severe hyperbilirubinemia and the treatment of choice for hyperbilirubinemia caused by Rh incompatibility. Exchange transfusion removes the sensitized erythrocytes, lowers the serum bilirubin level to prevent bilirubin encephalopathy, corrects the anemia, and prevents cardiac failure. Indications for exchange transfusion may include a positive direct Coombs test, hemoglobin concentration of cord blood below 12 g/dl, and a bilirubin level of 20 mg/dl in the full-term infant. However, some authorities advocate delaying exchange transfusions in full-term infants until the bilirubin levels are considerably higher (Newman and Maisels, 1992). An infant born with hydrops fetalis or signs of cardiac failure is a candidate for immediate exchange transfusion with fresh whole blood.

For exchange transfusion, fresh whole blood is typed and cross-matched to the mother's serum. The amount of donor blood used is usually double the blood volume of the infant, which is about 85 ml/kg body weight but is limited to no more than 500 ml. The two-volume exchange transfusion replaces approximately 85% of the neonate's blood.

An exchange transfusion is a sterile surgical procedure. A catheter is inserted into the umbilical vein and threaded into the inferior vena cava. Depending on the infant's weight, 5 to 10 ml of blood is withdrawn within 15 to 20 seconds, and the same volume of donor blood is infused over 60 to 90 seconds. If the blood has been citrated (addition of citrate phosphate dextrose adenine to prevent coagulation), calcium gluconate may be given after infusion of each 100 ml of donor's blood to prevent hypocalcemia.

Intrauterine Transfusion. Infants of mothers already sensitized are sometimes treated by intrauterine transfusion, which consists of infusing blood into the peritoneal cavity or the umbilical vein of the fetus. The need for therapy is based on determinations of the optical density of amniotic fluid (via amniocentesis) as an index of the bilirubin concentration and degree of hemolysis.

Prognosis. The severe anemia of isoimmunization may result in stillbirth, shock, congestive heart failure, poor feeding, or poor weight gain. Hemolytic anemia may result in bilirubin encephalopathy. Complications from exchange transfusion are uncommon. Despite the availability of an effective preventive measure, Rh HDN continues to cause significant morbidity and mortality in the United States (Chavez, Mulinare, and Edmunds, 1991).

Nursing Considerations

The initial nursing responsibility is recognizing hyperbilirubinemia. The possibility of hemolytic disease can be anticipated from the prenatal and perinatal history. Prenatal evidence of incompatibility and a positive Coombs test are cause for increased vigilance for early signs of jaundice in an infant.

If an exchange transfusion is needed, the nurse prepares the infant and the family and assists the practitioner with the procedure. Documentation of blood volumes exchanged, including the amount of blood withdrawn and infused, the time of each procedure, and the cumulative record of the total volume exchanged, are kept. Vital signs, monitored electronically, are evaluated frequently and correlated with removal and infusion of blood. If signs of cardiac or respiratory problems occur, the procedure is stopped temporarily and resumed once the infant's cardiorespiratory function stabilizes. The nurse also observes for signs of transfusion reaction.

NURSING ALERT Signs of exchange transfusion reaction include:
Tachycardia or bradycardia
Respiratory distress
Dramatic change in blood pressure
Temperature instability
Rash

Throughout the procedure the infant requires attention to thermoregulation. Hypothermia increases oxygen and glucose consumption, causing metabolic acidosis. Not only do these consequences hinder the infant's overall physical ability to withstand the long procedure, but they also inhibit the binding capacity of albumin and bilirubin and the hepatic enzymatic reactions, thus increasing the risk of kernicterus. Conversely, hyperthermia damages the donor erythrocytes, elevating the free potassium content and predisposing the infant to cardiac arrest.

The procedure is performed under a radiant warmer. However, the infant is usually covered with sterile drapes that may prevent the radiant heat from sufficiently warming the skin. The blood is also warmed (using specially designed devices, never microwave ovens) before infusion.

After the procedure is completed, the nurse inspects the umbilical site for evidence of bleeding. Usually the catheter remains in place for use during repeated exchanges.

Family Support. Parents frequently feel guilty because they think they have caused the blood incompatibility. Parents should never be made to feel responsible or negligent. They are encouraged to verbalize and express their thoughts. Actions that were taken to prevent any problems, such as frequent antepartum examinations and blood tests, should be referred to and praised.

HYPOGLYCEMIA

Hypoglycemia is present when the infant's blood glucose concentration is significantly lower than that of the majority of infants of the same age and weight. Therefore the determination of an abnormally low blood glucose level varies. In the full-term newborn, hypoglycemia may be defined as plasma glucose concentrations of less than 40 mg/dl in the first 24 hours and 40 to 50 mg/dl thereafter (Cornblath and Schwartz, 1993).

Pathophysiology

After birth the infant must supply nutrients to meet energy requirements for maintaining body temperature, respiration, muscular activity, and regulation of blood glucose. Glucose is primarily derived from glycogen stores deposited in the liver, heart, and skeletal muscles during the last trimester of pregnancy. Under normal circumstances, the full-term infant usually has sufficient sources for the first 2 or 3 days. However, any condition that causes increased energy requirements can rapidly deplete these stores.

Full-term infants who are at a higher risk for developing hypoglycemia shortly after birth include those born of diabetic mothers and infants who are small or large for gestational age (Holtrop, 1993). The types of hypoglycemia include:

Early transitional neonatal—Large or normal-size infants who appear to suffer from hyperinsulinism
Classic transient neonatal—Infants who suffered intrauterine malnutrition that depleted glycogen and fat stores
Secondary—A response to perinatal stresses that increase infant's metabolic needs relative to glycogen stores
Recurrent, severe—Caused by an enzymatic or metabolic-endocrine defect

Clinical Manifestations

The signs of hypoglycemia are usually vague and often indistinguishable from those observed in other newborn conditions, such as hypocalcemia, septicemia, central nervous system disorders, or cardiorespiratory problems. Because the brain depends on glucose for energy, cerebral signs such as jitteriness, tremors, twitching, weak or high-pitched cry, lethargy, limpness, apathy, convulsions, and coma are prominent. Other clinical manifestations are cyanosis, apnea, rapid and irregular respirations, sweating, eye rolling, and refusal to feed. Frequently the symptoms are transient but recurrent.

Diagnostic Evaluation

Diagnosis is confirmed by direct analysis of blood glucose concentration. Two consecutive specimens of blood should be analyzed because of the many factors that can affect correct readings.

NURSING ALERT Proper handling of the specimen is essential, since storage at room temperature increases glycolysis. Accurate readings can be facilitated by storing the blood sample in ice or removing the red blood cells by centrifugation.

Blood sugar level may also be determined with a reagent strip such as Dextrostix or Chemstrip-BG, which may be read either manually or with a glucose reflectance meter. Although simple procedures, the tests are very sensitive and must be performed correctly to prevent false reading. One study found a reflectance meter (AccuChek II) to be accurate in newborns provided blood was collected and transferred to the strip using a capillary tube, and a tissue, not a cotton ball, was used to remove excess blood from the strip (Vitanza, Giacoia, and West, 1988). Color changes that indicate a blood glucose level of less than 40 to 45 mg/dl should be confirmed by a laboratory analysis of whole blood. The American Academy of Pediatrics (1993a) does not recommend universal screening for hypoglycemia in full-term neonates.

Therapeutic Management

Intravenous infusion of glucose is one method of treating hypoglycemia. In full-term infants who are borderline hypoglycemic and clinically asymptomatic, the early institution of formula feeding or breast-feeding may reestablish normoglycemia, thus avoiding the need for intravenous glucose. Infants who are at increased risk for developing hypoglycemia should have their blood glucose measured within 1 hour after birth. The procedure should be repeated every 1 to 2 hours for the first 6 to 8 hours, then every 4 to 6 hours for 2 days.

Oral glucose feedings are ineffective as a treatment for hypoglycemia and in high concentrations can cause gastric irritation and osmotic diarrhea. Hypoglycemia can be prevented in most instances by the initiation of early feeding in normoglycemic newborns. Breast-fed infants should be put to breast as soon as possible after delivery. (See Infants of Diabetic Mothers, Chapter 10, for management of hypoglycemia related to hyperinsulinemia.)

Nursing Considerations

Much of the nursing responsibility for the hypoglycemic infant involves identification of the problem through careful observation of physical status. Another concern is to reduce environmental factors, such as cold stress and respiratory difficulty, that predispose the infant to the development of a decreased blood glucose level. Use of proper feeding techniques with the breast-fed or bottle-fed infant promotes adequate ingestion of nutrients, particularly carbohydrates.

Major nursing objectives also include preventing, anticipating, and recognizing potential dangers of concentrated dextrose infusion. Too-rapid infusion of the hypertonic solution can cause circulatory overload, hyperglycemia, and intracellular dehydration. Maintaining the ordered flow rate with an intravenous pump and checking and charting hourly intake decreases the chance of such hazards. If the intravenous infusion has been temporarily discontinued, the rate is not increased to make up for the fluid lost during the interruption.

The infusion is administered through a large peripheral vein to increase hemodilution of the concentrated solution and to prevent irritation of the vessel walls. Extravasation of the fluid into the surrounding area can cause tissue sloughing. Termination of the glucose solution must be gradual to prevent hypoglycemia caused by hyperinsulinism.

Because hypoglycemia may be a symptom of some other underlying pathophysiologic process, parents are usually very concerned about their infant's progress, particularly since these infants do not feed well or behave responsively. Nurses need to be aware of parents' thoughts, to allow them to express their feelings, and to keep parents aware of the infant's progress.

HYPERGLYCEMIA

Hyperglycemia in the newborn is usually defined as a blood glucose concentration greater than 125 mg/dl in the full-term infant or greater than 150 mg/dl in the preterm infant. Affected infants are usually low-birth-weight infants who are unable to tolerate intravenous glucose infusions at the usual rate. The glucose intolerance is probably related to general immaturity of the usual regulatory mechanisms. Increased blood glucose levels may also occur in infants with sepsis or decreased insulin sensitivity (such as the infant with transient diabetes mellitus), infants receiving methylxanthines, and stressed infants (infants with respiratory distress syndrome, infants undergoing surgical procedures).

Hyperglycemia is usually asymptomatic but detected on routine screening. Most often, hyperglycemia is treated by reducing the infant's glucose intake. Insulin infusion is sometimes administered to very low-birth-weight infants who require but are unable to tolerate IV dextrose solutions with concentrations greater than 5 g/dl.

Nursing Considerations

Blood glucose is monitored frequently, especially in the infant receiving insulin. This requires numerous heel sticks, and sites should be rotated to minimize tissue damage (see Blood Specimens, Chapter 27). Urinary output is carefully measured to detect any evidence of glycosuria and possible osmotic diuresis.

NURSING ALERT Any cerebral signs, such as jitteriness, twitching, seizure activity, or a diminished activity level, are indications for obtaining serum glucose and/or serum calcium levels immediately.

As in care of all infants, parents are given a careful explanation of the therapy and provided with frequent progress reports, as well as support to reduce anxiety (see also Nursing Care of High-Risk Newborns, Chapter 10).

HYPOCALCEMIA

Hypocalcemia, like many conditions in the neonate, is difficult to differentiate from other disorders, and the etiology is ill defined. There are two times during the neonatal period when the incidence is highest. ***Early-onset hypocalcemia,*** which appears within the first 72 hours, is the more common form and typically affects the premature or small-for-gestational-age infant who has experienced perinatal hypoxia. Symptoms include jitteriness, apnea, cyanotic episodes, a high-pitched cry, and abdominal distention.

Late-onset hypocalcemia, which is not apparent until after the first 7 days of life, is commonly referred to as ***cow's milk–induced hypocalcemia*** or ***neonatal tetany.*** It is observed in well-nourished infants who are fed modified cow's milk, such as evaporated milk formula. Cow's milk, which has a high phosphorus content, produces hyperphosphatemia and a resultant hypocalcemia by increasing calcium deposition in the bone and soft tissues, enhancing the hypocalcemia effect of calcitonin, or inhibiting the calcemic response to parathyroid hormone (Demarini and Tsang, 1992). The manifestations of neonatal tetany reflect neuromuscular irritation—twitching, tremors, and focal or generalized convulsive seizures that can be triggered by even minor stimuli and that vary in duration from a few seconds to several minutes. Neonatal tetany is rarely seen in industrialized countries because of the prevalent use of commercial formula or human milk as the newborn's primary source of nutrition.

Diagnostic Evaluation

Diagnosis of hypocalcemia is confirmed with serum electrolyte determinations. Normal serum calcium values are between 8 and 10 mg/dl (4 to 5 mEq/L). In full-term infants hypocalcemia is indicated at total serum calcium levels below 8 mg/dl or ionized calcium levels (the biologically important fraction of calcium) below 4.4 mg/dl (Demarini and Tsang, 1992).

Therapeutic Management

In most instances early-onset hypocalcemia is temporary and resolves in 1 to 3 days. Restoration of a normal calcium level is facilitated by early feedings, physiologic correction of the hypoparathyroidism, and sometimes administration of calcium supplements.

Treatment of hypocalcemia involves intravenous administration of 10% calcium gluconate. The drug is administered slowly over 10 to 30 minutes or as a continuous infusion. Rapid intravenous calcium administration may cause cardiac dysrhythmias and circulatory collapse. The heart rate and blood pressure should be electronically monitored. Care must be taken to ascertain that the needle is positioned within the vein because extravasation into surrounding tissue causes local necrosis, calcification, and sloughing. Intramuscular administration of calcium gluconate is contraindicated because it precipitates in the tissue, causing necrosis. If the infant can tolerate oral fluids, oral doses of calcium are given.

Nursing Considerations

Nursing care of the infant with hypocalcemia is directed toward identifying the cause of the manifestations observed and administration of calcium. The infant is monitored continuously during intravenous infusions. Calcium gluconate can cause tissue necrosis and scar formation; therefore it is recommended that the scalp veins be avoided. Calcium gluconate is also incompatible with a number of drugs, most notably sodium bicarbonate ($NaHCO_3$), which is often given for metabolic acidosis. To prevent tissue necrosis, the infusion site is observed carefully and changed as needed.

The nurse also observes for signs of acute hypercalcemia (vomiting, bradycardia). If such symptoms occur, the injection or infusion is discontinued and the practitioner is notified. Since convulsions are common, seizure precautions are instituted. Minor stimuli, such as picking the infant up for a feeding or a sudden jarring of the crib, can provoke tremors or seizures. During the acute phase, the environment around the infant is manipulated to allow for maximum rest and minimum activity.

The restlessness, irritability, and convulsive activity of the infant are of much concern to the parents. The nurse supports them during the hospitalization and emphasizes that the condition will subside rapidly with no subsequent ill effects. During the acute phase, parents are advised to disturb the infant as little as possible. However, as soon as the calcium level rises, they are encouraged to hold and feed the infant in order to reestablish parent-child attachment.

If the infant is discharged on formula feedings supplemented with calcium salts, the parents are taught the correct procedure for diluting the mineral in the formula and are advised to use only the prescribed formula.

HEMORRHAGIC DISEASE OF THE NEWBORN

Hemorrhagic disease of the newborn is a bleeding disorder that may appear within 1 to 5 days of life as a result of a deficiency of vitamin K. Newborn vitamin K stores are virtually absent, and there is a moderate deficiency of prothrombin activity, which decreases until approximately 72 hours after birth, when it begins to increase. Consequently, vitamin K–dependent coagulation factors (II, VII, IX, X) are significantly reduced. In addition, the newborn's sterile intestinal tract is unable to synthesize the vitamin until feedings have begun. Breast-fed infants are particularly at risk because human milk is a poor source of vitamin K. Hemorrhagic manifestations rarely occur in infants fed fortified cow's milk formula from birth because this is an adequate source of the vitamin.

Signs and symptoms of hemorrhagic disease typically appear 24 to 72 hours after birth and can include oozing from the umbilicus or circumcision site, bloody or black stools, hematuria, ecchymoses on skin and scalp, epistaxis, or bleeding from punctures. Diagnosis can be confirmed in the presence of prolonged prothrombin time (PT) and partial thromboplastin time (PTT) accompanied by normal platelet count and fibrinogen level.

A late form ***(late-onset hemorrhagic disease)*** appears at about 4 to 7 weeks of age. This late-onset disease occurs in totally or predominantly breast-fed infants. It appears to be related to a factor in breast milk that inhibits vitamin K synthesis by the infant's bacterial flora. Manifestations of late-onset disease are evidence of intracranial hemorrhage, deep ecchymoses, bleeding from the gastrointestinal tract, and/or bleeding from mucous membranes, skin punctures, or surgical incisions.

Therapeutic Management

The goal of management is prevention of hemorrhagic disease of the newborn with prophylactic administration of vitamin K. In the United States, intramuscular administration of vitamin K (Aquamephyton, Mephyton) in a dose of 0.5 to 1 mg once during the first 24 hours of life is a standard practice. The use of prophylactic vitamin K is not routinely practiced in all countries, and in some countries oral supplementation is used.

In newborns with the disease, treatment is the same as the preventive measures, except that the vitamin may be given intravenously to prevent a hematoma at an intramuscular site. Bleeding usually ceases within 2 to 4 hours of vitamin K administration.

Nursing Considerations

Nursing care is primarily directed toward prevention and involves careful administration of the vitamin into the vastus lateralis muscle. In instances in which this procedure is not routinely carried out (e.g., home births or emergency deliveries), the nurse observes for signs of the disorder and notifies the practitioner for appropriate diagnosis and treatment. Breast-feeding mothers are encouraged to increase their intake of foods containing vitamin K, primarily vegetables. The best sources are green vegetables, especially broccoli.

INBORN ERRORS OF METABOLISM (IEMs)

IEMs constitute a large number of inherited diseases caused by the absence or deficiency of a substance essential to cellular metabolism, usually an enzyme, and most are characterized by abnormal protein, carbohydrate, or fat metabolism.

All biochemical processes are under genetic control, and each consists of a complex sequence of reactions. Fig. 9-8, *A,* schematically represents a portion of a normal metabolic pathway. A ***substrate*** (the substance on which an enzyme acts) is converted to a product through the action of a specific enzyme. A ***metabolic pathway*** consists of many such reactions, or steps, each depending on the previous reaction and each catalyzed by a specific enzyme.

A specific gene is responsible for production of a specific enzyme in the metabolic pathway. Fig. 9-8, *B,* illustrates how a change in a gene that interferes with the synthesis of an essential enzyme interrupts this process. A block in the normal pathway can produce the following:

1. Accumulation of the substances preceding the block, such as galactose in galactosemia or phenylalanine in phenylketonuria
2. A deficiency in the product, such as thyroxine in familial hypothyroidism
3. An increase in the products of alternate metabolic pathways when these pathways are used, such as the production of phenylketones in phenylketonuria

These effects of defective gene action are observable in the individual as diseases.

The mode of inheritance in IEMs is almost always autosomal recessive. The heterozygote, having one gene with a normal effect, is still able to produce the enzyme in sufficient amounts to carry out the metabolic function under normal circumstances. Therefore the heterozygote does not exhibit symptoms of the disorder. However, the abnormal homozygote, who inherits a defective gene from both parents, has no functioning enzyme and thus is clinically affected.

Individually IEMs are rare; collectively they account for a significant proportion of health problems in children. It is becoming possible to detect and screen for an increasing number of IEMs—to detect the presence of the disease in the heterozygote, the newborn, and the fetus. In many IEMs, early diagnosis and prompt treatment are essential to prevent a relentless course of physical and mental deterioration. Prenatal diagnosis provides for special care of the infant immediately after birth. Neonatal screening is useful in detecting some disorders after a few days of life, but it is less helpful in detecting symptoms early in the neonatal period. Nurses caring for neonates must be certain that screening is performed, especially in infants who are discharged early, are born at home, or are in neonatal intensive care units (Strobel and Keller, 1993). (See also Genetic Screening, Chapter 5.)

Some nonspecific presenting manifestations—including lethargy, persistent vomiting, diarrhea, respiratory distress, hypothermia, coma, and seizures—are observed in a wide variety of both genetic and acquired disorders (Arn, Valle, and Brusilow, 1988). The time of onset may be important. Most IEMs are symptom-free during the first 24 hours of life. Other manifestations that may indicate an IEM include jaundice, hepatomegaly, unusual odor (sweat, urine), abnormal eating patterns (food aversions, vomiting after eating certain foods), coarse facial features, macroglossia, abnormal hair, dysmorphic features, and abnormal eye findings (e.g., cataracts, retinal changes) (Burton, 1987; David-

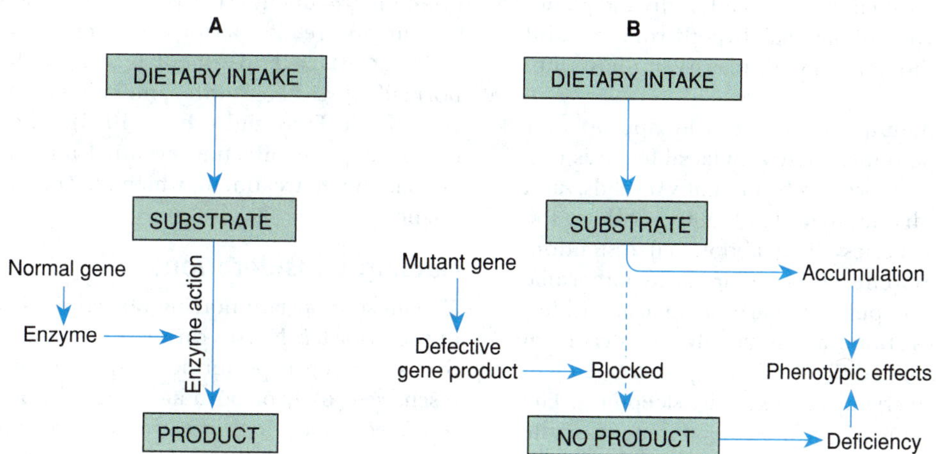

FIG. 9-8 Metabolic pathway. **A,** Normal metabolic pathway. **B,** Effect of defective gene action.

son, 1992). A family history of neonatal deaths (within the same sibling group, in males, or among family members) alerts the observer to the possibility of a genetic disorder. Initial recognition of signs that might indicate an IEM is the responsibility of health professionals, including nurses.

Although there are innumerable IEMs, only three are selected for discussion, because they can be identified in the neonatal period and reasonable success has been achieved with treatment. Some IEMs are also outlined in Table 5-4.

CONGENITAL HYPOTHYROIDISM (CH)

CH (sometimes called by the undesirable term "cretinism") is a deficiency of thyroid hormones believed to be present at birth. Results of screening tests in the United States indicate that CH occurs in approximately 1 of every 4000 newborns (American Academy of Pediatrics, 1993b). Infants with Down syndrome have a much higher rate of either permanent or transient forms of the disorder. Also, a higher incidence of other congenital abnormalities has been observed in infants with CH (New England Congenital Hypothyroidism Collaborative, 1988).

A number of etiologic factors are implicated in hypothyroidism, and the condition may be permanent or transient. ***Permanent CH*** can result from defective thyroid gland development, an enzymatic defect in thyroxine synthesis, or (rarely) pituitary dysfunction. ***Transient hypothyroidism*** results from intrauterine transfer of goiter-inducing substances (such as the antithyroid drugs), which inhibit thyroid secretion. Although self-limiting, this type is potentially fatal because, once the maternal supply is terminated, the infant's thyroid is unable to produce its own hormones. In addition, regardless of etiology, a large goiter in a neonate may cause total obstruction of the airway.

Clinical Manifestations

The severity of the disorder depends on the amount of thyroid tissue present. Usually the newborn does not exhibit obvious signs of hypothyroidism, probably because of the exogenous source of prenatal thyroid hormone supplied by the maternal circulation. Clinical manifestations may be delayed in infants with a functional remnant of thyroid gland, infants with some types of familial hypothyroidism, and breast-fed infants, who may not display symptoms until weaned.

Classic features of untreated CH usually appear after about 6 weeks of life and include typical facial features (depressed nasal bridge, short forehead, puffy eyelids, and large tongue); thick, dry, mottled skin that feels cold to the touch; coarse, dry, lusterless hair; abdominal distention, umbilical hernia, hyporeflexia, bradycardia, hypothermia, hypotension with narrow pulse pressure, anemia, and widely patent cranial sutures. Bone age is greatly retarded from birth. The infant displays difficulty feeding, decreased gastric motility, minimum crying, and excessive sleepiness. The most serious consequence is delayed development of the nervous system, which leads to severe mental retardation. The severity of the intellectual deficit is related to the degree of hypothyroidism and the duration of the condition before treatment. Other nervous system manifestations include slow, awkward movements and abnormal deep tendon reflexes (often referred to as "hung-up" because the relaxation phase after the contraction is slow).

Diagnostic Evaluation

Diagnosis is aimed at early identification of the disorder to prevent the serious effects on mental development resulting from delayed treatment. Neonatal screening consists of an initial filter paper blood spot thyroxine (T_4) measurement followed by measurement of thyroid-stimulating hormone (TSH) in specimens with low T_4 values (American Academy of Pediatrics, 1993b). Tests are routine and mandatory in most areas of the United States. Although a heel-stick blood sample for the spot test is best obtained between 2 and 6 days of age, specimens are usually taken within the first 24 to 48 hours as part of a concurrent screen for other metabolic defects. Early screening can result in overdiagnosis (false-positives) but is preferable to missing the diagnosis.

Screening results that show a low level of T_4 and a high level of TSH indicate CH and the need for further tests to determine the cause of the disease. Additional tests include serum measurement of thyroxine, triiodothyronine (T_3), protein-bound iodine (PBI), and thyrotropin-releasing factor to ascertain the amount of thyroid hormone secreted and the intactness of the homeostatic mechanisms. Tests of thyroid gland function (thyroid scan and uptake) usually involve oral administration of a radioactive isotope of iodine (^{131}I) and measurement of the iodine uptake by the thyroid, usually within 24 hours. In CH, protein-bound iodine, thyroxine, triiodothyronine, and free thyroxine levels are low and thyroid uptake of ^{131}I is decreased. Roentgenography is employed to assess bone age.

Therapeutic Management

Treatment involves lifelong thyroid hormone replacement therapy as soon as possible after diagnosis to abolish all signs of hypothyroidism and reestablish normal physical and mental development. The drug of choice is synthetic levothyroxine sodium (Synthroid or Levothroid). Regular measurement of thyroxine levels is important in ensuring optimum treatment (Heyerdahl, Kase, and Lie, 1991). Bone age surveys are also performed to ensure optimum growth.

Prognosis. If treatment is started shortly after birth, normal physical growth and intelligence are possible (Casado de Frias and others, 1993). The most significant factor adversely affecting eventual intelligence appears to be inadequate treatment, which may be related to noncompliance.

Nursing Considerations

The most important nursing objective is early identification of the disorder. Nurses caring for neonates must be certain that screening is performed, especially in infants who are discharged early or born at home. Although the screening test is very specific, some children may not be identified, and nurses in ambulatory settings for well-infant care need to be aware of the earliest signs of the disorder. Parental remarks about an unusually "quiet and good" baby together with any of the early physical manifestations should lead to a suspicion of hypothyroidism, requiring referral for specific tests. Unfortunately, many parents harbor guilt about their impressions of the infant before the diagnosis because the child's inactivity may not have alerted them to a problem, with the result that treatment is delayed.

Once the diagnosis is confirmed, parents need an explanation of the disorder and the necessity of lifelong treatment. The importance of compliance with the drug regimen must be stressed for the child to achieve normal growth and development (Miculan, Turner, and Paes, 1993). Since the drug is tasteless, it can be crushed and added to formula, water, or food. If a dose is missed, twice the dose should be given the next day (Coody, 1984). Parents also need to be aware of signs indicating overdose, such as rapid pulse, dyspnea, irritability, insomnia, fever, sweating, and weight loss. Ideally they should know how to count the pulse and be instructed to withhold a dose and consult their practitioner if the pulse rate is above a certain value. Signs of inadequate treatment are fatigue, sleepiness, decreased appetite, and constipation.

If the diagnosis was delayed past early infancy, the chance of permanent mental retardation is great. Parents need the same guidance in caring for their child as do others who have an offspring with cognitive impairment (see Chapter 24). They need an opportunity to discuss their feelings regarding late recognition of the disorder. Although treatment will not reverse the intellectual deficit, it may prevent further damage. Genetic counseling is important, especially if the disorder is caused by an inborn error of thyroid hormone synthesis, which is autosomal recessive. (For a discussion of genetic counseling, see Chapter 5.)

PHENYLKETONURIA (PKU)

PKU, a genetic disease inherited as an autosomal-recessive trait, is caused by absence of the enzyme needed to metabolize the essential amino acid, ***phenylalanine.*** The disorder is detected in 1:10,000 to 15,000 live births and primarily affects white children, with the incidence highest in those living in the United States or Northern Europe. It is very rare in the African, Jewish, and Japanese populations.

Classic PKU is at one end of a spectrum of conditions known as ***hyperphenylalaninemia.*** Since rarer forms are the result of a deficiency of other enzymes and are diagnosed and treated differently, the following discussion of PKU is limited to the severe, classic form.

Pathophysiology

In PKU the hepatic enzyme ***phenylalanine hydroxylase,*** which normally controls the conversion of phenylalanine to tyrosine, is absent. This results in the accumulation of phenylalanine in the bloodstream and urinary excretion of abnormal amounts of its metabolites, the phenyl acids (Fig. 9-9). One of these phenyl ketones, ***phenylpyruvic acid,*** gives urine the characteristic musty odor associated with this disease and is responsible for the term ***phenylketonuria.***

Amino acids produced by metabolism of phenylalanine are absent in PKU. One of these, ***tyrosine,*** is needed to form the pigment melanin and the hormones epinephrine and thyroxine. Decreased melanin production results in similar phenotypes of most children with phenylketonuria—blond hair, blue eyes, and fair skin that is particularly susceptible to eczema and other dermatologic problems. Children of genetically darker skin color may be red haired or brunette.

Accumulation of phenylalanine and presumably the decreased levels of the neurotransmitters dopamine and tryptophan affect the normal development of the brain and central nervous system, resulting in defective myelinization, cystic degeneration of the gray and white matter, and disturbances in cortical lamination. Mental retardation occurs *before* the metabolites are detected in the urine and will progress if ingested phenylalanine levels are not lowered.

Clinical Manifestations

Clinical manifestations of PKU include failure to thrive, frequent vomiting, irritability, hyperactivity, and unpredictable, erratic behavior. Bizarre or schizoid behavior patterns are common in older children, such as fright reactions, screaming episodes, head-banging, arm-biting, disorientation, failure to respond to strong stimuli, and catatonia-like positions. Many of the severely retarded children have seizures, and about 80% of untreated persons with PKU demonstrate abnormal electroencephalographs, regardless of whether overt seizures occur. Fortunately, this manifestation is rarely seen because of early detection and treatment.

Diagnostic Evaluation

The objective in diagnosing or treating the disorder is to prevent mental retardation. The most commonly used test for screening newborns is the ***Guthrie blood test,*** a bacterial inhibition assay for phenylalanine in the blood. *Bacillus subtilis,* present in the culture medium, grows if the blood contains an excessive amount of phenylalanine. If properly done, it detects serum phenylalanine levels greater than 4 mg/dl (normal value is 2 mg/dl). Only fresh heel blood, not cord blood, can be used for the test.

The screening test is most reliable if the blood sample is taken after the infant has ingested a source of protein. However, because of early discharge from the hospital, the American Academy of Pediatrics and American College of Obstetricians and Gynecologists (1992) recommend that (1) the test be performed on all newborns before they leave the nursery, regardless of age, and (2) a repeat blood specimen be obtained by the third week of life from all infants in whom the initial specimen was taken within the first 24 hours of life. Special consideration must be given to screening of infants born at home who have no hospital contact.

Because of the possibility of variant forms of hyperphenylalaninemia, a natural protein challenge test is recommended after about 3 months of dietary treatment to confirm the diagnosis of classic PKU.

Therapeutic Management

Treatment of PKU is dietary. Since the genetic enzyme is intracellular, systemic administration of phenylalanine hydroxylase is of no value. Phenylalanine cannot be elimi-

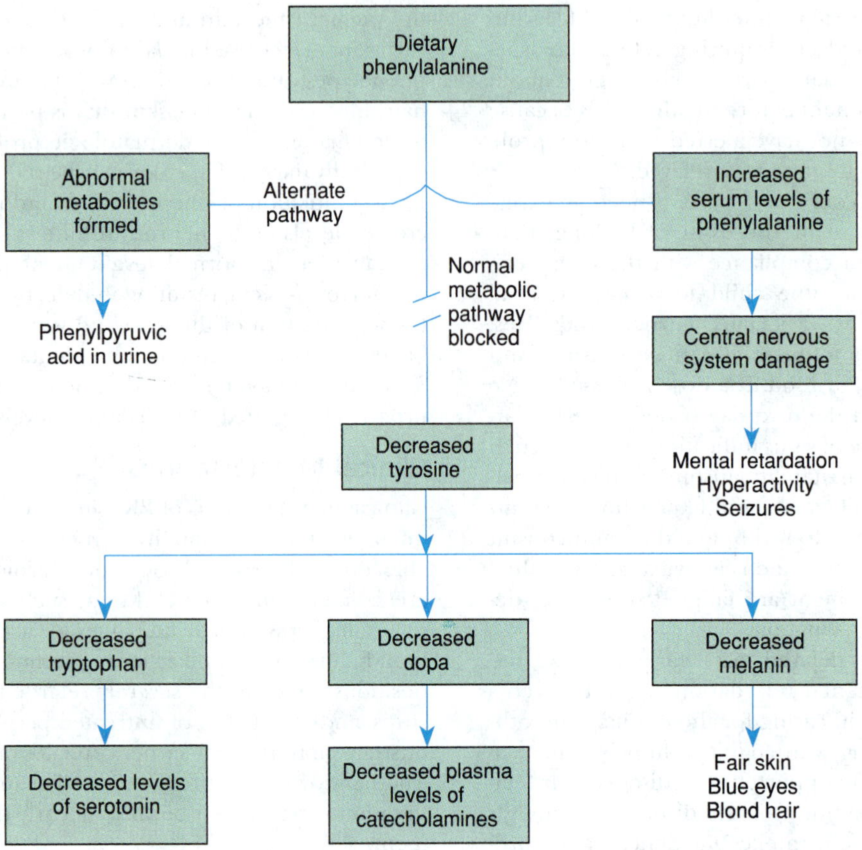

FIG. 9-9 Metabolic errors and consequences in phenylketonuria.

nated, because it is an essential amino acid in tissue growth. Therefore dietary management must meet two criteria: (1) meet the child's nutritional need for optimum growth, and (2) maintain phenylalanine levels within a safe range.

The diet is calculated to allow 20 to 30 mg of phenylalanine per kilogram of body weight per day, which should maintain serum phenylalanine levels between 2 and 8 mg/dl. Significant brain damage usually occurs when levels are greater than 10 to 15 mg/dl. At levels less than 2 mg/dl the body begins to catabolize its protein stores, resulting in growth retardation. The daily amounts are individualized for each child and require frequent changes based on appetite, growth and development, and blood phenylalanine and tyrosine levels.

Since all natural food proteins contain about 15% phenylalanine, specially prepared milk substitutes, such as Lofenalac,* Pro-Phree,† or Phenex-1,† are prescribed for the infant. These products are made from specially treated enzymatic casein hydrolysate, which provides only 0.4% phenylalanine (28.5 mg/8 ounces). They also contain minerals and vitamins to provide a balanced nutritional formula. Tyrosine and several other amino acids are supplied in the formula. Because of the low phenylalanine content of breast milk, total or partial breast-feeding may be possible with close monitoring of phenylalanine levels (Lawrence, 1994). Diet substitutes for older children, such as Phenyl-Free* and Phenex-2,† contain no phenylalanine and allow for greater exchanges with natural low-phenylalanine foods in the diet, leading to a more normal diet.

A low-phenylalanine diet is begun as soon as possible after birth and maintained through adolescence. To evaluate the effectiveness of dietary treatment, frequent monitoring of blood phenylalanine and tyrosine levels is necessary. Since phenylalanine levels greater than or equal to 20 mg/dl in mothers with PKU affect the normal embryologic development of the fetus, the low-phenylalanine diet must be resumed *before* pregnancy in affected women (Koch and others, 1993). These women should also be counseled about the risk that their child might have phenylketonuria (approximately 1/120), and reproductive options should be discussed (American Academy of Pediatrics, 1991).

Prognosis. Although early treatment of infants with PKU greatly improves their chances for achieving normal cognitive development, the outcome is not as favorable as previously thought. Even with adequate dietary control, a high percentage of children exhibit some degree of intellectual impairment. There is evidence of slower language acquisition and, in the school years, a higher frequency of learning and behavior problems, especially hyperactivity, anxiety, and poor concentration (Medical Research Council, 1993).

*Mead Johnson & Co., Evansville, IN.
†Ross Laboratories, Columbus, OH.

Nursing Considerations

The principal nursing considerations involve teaching the family regarding the dietary restrictions. Although the treatment may sound simple, the task of maintaining such a strict dietary regimen is very demanding, especially for older children and adolescents. Foods with low phenylalanine levels, such as vegetables, fruits, juices, and some cereals, breads, and starches, must be measured to provide the prescribed amount of phenylalanine. Most high-protein foods, such as meat and dairy products, are either eliminated or restricted to small amounts. The sweetener aspartame (NutraSweet, Equal) should be avoided because it is converted to phenylalanine in the body. However, small amounts, such as a single 12-ounce serving of diet cola, do not significantly raise phenylalanine levels (Mackey and Berlin, 1992).

During infancy, maintaining the diet presents few problems. Solid foods, such as cereal, fruits, and vegetables, are introduced as usual to the infant. Difficulties arise as the child gets older. Decreased appetite and refusal to eat may reduce intake of the calculated phenylalanine requirement. The child's increasing independence may inhibit absolute control of what he or she eats. Either factor can result in decreased or increased phenylalanine levels. During the school years, peer pressure becomes a major force in deterring the child from eating the prescribed foods or abstaining from high-protein foods such as milkshakes or ice cream. Limitations of this diet are best illustrated by an example: a quarter-pound hamburger may be equal to a 2-day phenylalanine allowance for a school-age child. Illness and growth spurts will increase the body's need for this essential amino acid.

The assistance of a registered nutritionist is essential. Parents need a basic understanding of the disorder and practical suggestions regarding food selection and preparation.* Meal planning is based on an exchange list, and as soon as children are old enough, usually by early preschool, they should be involved in the daily calculation, menu planning, and formula preparation. Using a musical or voice-synthesizer calculator, cards, or colored beads can help children keep track of the daily allowance of phenylalanine foods (Messer, 1985). A system of goal setting, self-monitoring, contracts, and rewards can promote compliance in adolescents (Gleason and others, 1992).

Preparation of the formula can present some difficulties. It tends to be lumpy and has a distinctive odor and taste that has been described as similar to potato but more bitter. A blender or mixer dissolves the powder more easily, but this is inconvenient when traveling. Although the taste is virtually impossible to camouflage, adding orange Tang, fruit-flavored powdered punch, or strawberry or chocolate Quik helps vary the flavor somewhat without greatly altering the phenylalanine content. The chocolate-flavored formula can be heated and served as hot cocoa or frozen into popsicles.

Family Support. In addition to the problem related to a child with a chronic disorder (see Chapter 22), the parents have the burden of knowing that they are carriers of the defect and must make serious decisions regarding future children. Prenatal testing is now available to detect the presence of the defective gene in heterozygotes. Genetic counseling is especially important for an affected child, who theoretically has a 50% chance of bearing an affected offspring (see Genetic Counseling, Chapter 5).

*A helpful resource is *Low-Protein Cookery for Phenylketonuria,* edited by V. Schuett (1988); available from the University of Wisconsin Press, 114 N. Murray St., Madison, WI 53715; (608) 262-8782.

GALACTOSEMIA

Galactosemia is a rare autosomal-recessive disorder affecting approximately 1:50,000 births. It involves an inborn error of carbohydrate metabolism in which the hepatic enzyme ***galactose-1-phosphate uridine transferase (UDP-galactose transferase)*** is absent. The enzyme is one of three needed for the conversion of galactose to glucose (Fig. 9-10). There is considerable genetic variability in enzyme deficiency, with some children having partial transferase activity.

As galactose accumulates in the blood, several organs are affected. Hepatic dysfunction leads to cirrhosis, resulting in jaundice in the infant by the second week of life. The spleen subsequently becomes enlarged as a result of portal hypertension. Cataracts are usually recognizable by 1 or 2 months of age; cerebral damage, manifested by the symptoms of lethargy and hypotonia, is evident soon afterward. Infants with galactosemia appear normal at birth, but within a few days after ingesting milk, which has a high lactose content,

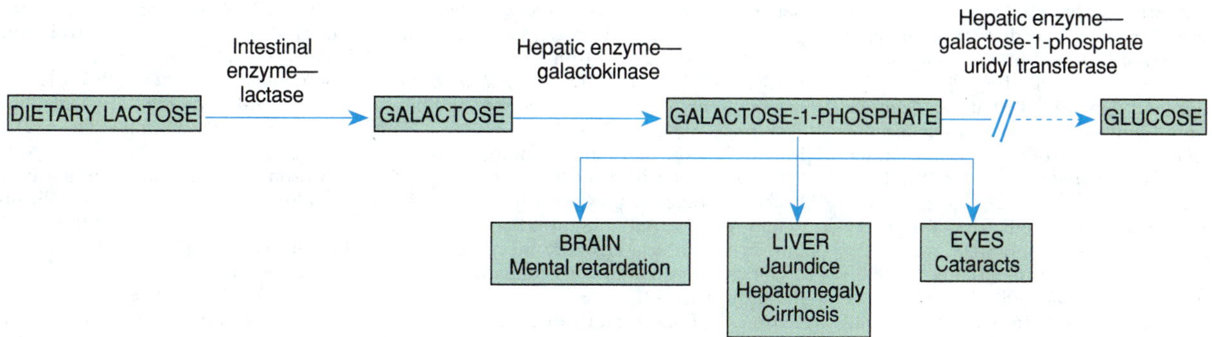

FIG. 9-10 Metabolic errors and consequences in galactosemia.

they begin to vomit and lose weight. Drowsiness, nausea, and diarrhea also occur. Death during the first month of life is not infrequent in untreated infants.

Diagnostic Evaluation

Diagnosis is made on the basis of galactosuria, increased levels of galactose in the blood, or decreased levels of UDP-galactose transferase activity in erythrocytes. Newborn screening for this disease is required in many states. Heterozygotes can also be identified, since heterozygotic individuals have significantly lower levels of the essential enzyme. Although asymptomatic, such individuals have been noted to spontaneously dislike and therefore limit ingestion of galactose-containing foods.

Therapeutic Management

Treatment of galactosemia consists of eliminating all milk and lactose-containing foods, including breast milk. During infancy, lactose-free formulas are used, with soy-protein formula being the feeding of choice.

Prognosis. Follow-up studies of children treated from birth or within the first 2 months of life after symptoms appear have found long-term complications, such as ovarian dysfunction, abnormal speech, cognitive impairment, growth retardation, and motor delay (Waggoner and Buist, 1993). These findings have revealed that eliminating sources of galactose does not significantly improve the outcome. New therapeutic strategies, such as enhancing residual transferase activity, replacing depleted metabolites, or using gene replacement therapy, are needed to improve the prognosis for these children (Segal, 1993).

Nursing Considerations

Nursing interventions are similar to those for PKU, except that dietary restrictions are easier to maintain because many more foods are allowed. However, reading food labels very carefully for the presence of any form of lactose, especially dairy products, is mandatory. Many drugs, such as penicillin, contain lactose as filler and must also be avoided. Unfortunately, lactose is an unlabeled ingredient in pharmaceuticals. (See also Family Support [for PKU], p. 361.)

KEY POINTS

- Problems of the newborn may be attributed to birth injuries, infections, immature physiologic systems, and inborn errors of metabolism.
- The forces of labor and delivery may cause soft tissue injury, head trauma, fractures, and paralysis.
- The most common forms of paralysis in the newborn are facial nerve, brachial plexus, and phrenic nerve palsies.
- Common skin problems of the newborn include erythema toxicum, candidiasis, bullous impetigo, and "birthmarks," especially port-wine stains and hemangiomas.
- Because of immature physiologic status, infants may be predisposed to hyperbilirubinemia, hypoglycemia, hyperglycemia, and hypocalcemia.
- Hyperbilirubinemia is classified according to the two types of bilirubin: unconjugated and conjugated. In the newborn it may result from excess production of bilirubin and/or decreased capacity of the liver to conjugate bilirubin.
- The primary treatment of unconjugated hyperbilirubinemia has been phototherapy. However, much controversy surrounds if and when it should be used.
- Hemolytic disease of the newborn is characterized by abnormally rapid destruction of red blood cells as a result of blood incompatibility between mother and fetus.
- Hypoglycemia can often be prevented with the initiation of early feedings.
- Hemorrhagic disease of the newborn is characterized by oozing from the umbilicus or circumcision site, bloody or black stools, hematuria, ecchymoses on skin and scalp, and epistaxis.
- The most significant inborn errors of metabolism are congenital hypothyroidism, phenylketonuria, and galctosemia.
- Thyroid replacement is required to treat congenital hypothyroidism.
- Dietary control is the treatment of choice for phenylketonuria and galactosemia. However, even with strict control, outcomes for these children are less favorable than previously thought.

REFERENCES

American Academy of Pediatrics, Committee on Fetus and Newborn: Routine evaluation of blood pressure, hematocrit, and glucose in newborns, *Pediatrics* 92(3):474-476, 1993a.

American Academy of Pediatrics, Committee on Genetics: Maternal phenylketonuria, *Pediatrics* 88(6):1284-1285, 1991.

American Academy of Pediatrics, Committee on Genetics: Newborn screening for congenital hypothyroidism: recommended guidelines, *Pediatrics* 91(6):1203-1209, 1993b.

American Academy of Pediatrics, Task Force on Infant Positioning and SIDS: Positioning and SIDS, *Pediatrics* 89(6):1120-1126, 1992.

American Academy of Pediatrics and American College of Obstetricians and Gynecologists: *Guidelines for perinatal care,* ed 3, Evanston, IL, 1992, The Academy.

Arn PH, Valle DL, Brusilow SW: Inborn errors of metabolism: not rare, not hopeless, *Contemp Pediatr* 5(12):47-63, 1988.

Bennett PR and others: Prenatal determination of fetal RhD type by DNA amplification, *N Engl J Med* 329:607-610, 1993.

Blackburn ST, Loper DL: *Maternal, fetal, and neonatal physiology: a clinical perspective,* Philadelphia, 1992, WB Saunders.

Bratlid D: How bilirubin gets into the brain, *Clin Perinatol* 17(2):449-465, 1990.

Brucker J: Brachial plexus birth injury, *J Neurosci Nurs* 23(6):374-380, 1991.

Burton BK: Inborn errors of metabolism: the clinical diagnosis in early infancy, *Pediatrics* 79:359-369, 1987.

Casado de Frias E and others: Evolution of height and bone age in primary congenital hypothyroidism, *Clin Pediatr* 32(7):426-432, 1993.

Chavez GF, Mulinare J, Edmonds LD: Epidemiology of Rh hemolytic disease of the newborn in the United States, *JAMA* 265 (24):3270-3274, 1991.

Coody D: Congenital hypothyroidism, *Pediatr Nurs* 10(5):342-345, 1984.

Commentaries, *Pediatrics* 89(5):819-833, 1992.

Cornblath M, Schwartz R: Hypoglycemia in the neonate, *J Pediatr Endocrinol* 6(2):113-129, 1993.

Davidson A: Management and counseling of children with inherited metabolic disorders, *J Pediatr Health Care* 6(3):146-153, 1992.

Demarini S, Tsang R: Disorders of calcium and magnesium metabolism. In Fanaroff AA, Martin RJ: *Neonatal-perinatal medicine: diseases of the fetus and infant,* ed 5, St Louis, 1992, Mosby.

Frank GG, Turner BS, Merenstein GB: Jaundice. In Merenstein GB, Gardner SL: *Handbook of neonatal intensive care,* ed 3, St Louis, 1993, Mosby.

Gleason LA and others: A treatment program for adolescents with phenylketonuria, *Clin Pediatr* 31(6):331-335, 1992.

Goldman MP, Fitzpatrick RE, Ruiz-Esparza J: Treatment of port-wine stains (capillary malformation) with the flashlamp-pumped pulsed dye laser, *J Pediatr* 122(1):71-77, 1993.

Heyerdahl S, Kase B, Lie S: Intellectual development in congenital hypothyroidism in relation to recommended thyroxine treatment, *J Pediatr* 118(6):850-857, 1991.

Holtrop PC: The frequency of hypoglycemia in full-term large and small for gestational age newborns, *Am J Perinatol* 10(2):150-154, 1993.

Hurwitz S: Skin lesions in the first year of life, *Contemp Pediatr* 10(1):110-128, 1993.

James JM, Williams SC, Osborn LM: Discontinuation of breast-feeding infrequent among jaundiced neonates treated at home, *Pediatrics* 92(1):153-155, 1993.

Kemper K, Forsyth B, McCathy P: Jaundice, terminating breastfeeding, and the vulnerable child, *Pediatrics* 84:773-778, 1989.

Koch R and others: The North American collaborative study of maternal phenylketonuria (PKU), *Int Pediatr* 8(1):89-96, 1993.

Lawrence RA: *Breastfeeding: a guide for the medical profession,* ed 4, St Louis, 1994, Mosby.

Long CA, Barron D: SIDS and infant positioning: implications for critical care, *Pediatr Nurs* 18(5):524-537, 1992.

Lott JW and others: Assessment and management of immunologic dysfunction. In Kenner C, Brueggemeyer A, Gunderson LP: *Comprehensive neonatal nursing: a physiologic perspective,* Philadelphia, 1993, WB Saunders.

Mackey S, Berlin CM: Effect of dietary aspartame on plasma concentrations of phenylalanine and tyrosine in normal and homozygous phenylketonuric patients, *Clin Pediatr* 31:394-399, 1992.

Maisels MJ: Gonad protection for phototherapy, *MCN* 15(4):232, 1990 (letter to editor).

Martinez J and others: Hyperbilirubinemia in the breast-fed newborn: a controlled trial of four interventions, *Pediatrics* 91(2):470-473, 1993.

McCance K, Huether S: *Pathophysiology: the biological basis for disease in infants and children,* ed 2, St Louis, 1994, Mosby.

Medical Research Council Working Party on Phenylketonuria: Phenylketonuria due to phenylalaine hydroxylase deficiency: an unfolding story, *Br Med J* 306(6870):115-119, 1993.

Messer SS: PKU: a mother's perspective, *Pediatr Nurs* 11:121-123, 1985.

Miculan J, Turner S, Paes B: Congenital hypothyroidism: diagnosis and management, *Neonatal Network* 12(6):25-42, 1993.

Minarcik C, Beachy P: Neurologic disorders. In Merenstein GB, Gardner SL: *Handbook of neonatal intensive care,* ed 2, St Louis, 1993, Mosby.

Murphy MR, Oellrich RG: A new method of phototherapy: nursing perspectives, *J Perinatol* 10(3):249-251, 1990.

New England Congenital Hypothyroidism Collaborative: Congenital concomitants of infantile hypothyroidism, *J Pediatr* 112:245-247, 1988.

Newman TB, Maisels MJ: Evaluation and treatment of jaundice in the term newborn: a kinder, gentler approach, *Pediatrics* 89(5):809-818, 1992.

Palmer C, Smith MB: Assessing the risk of kernicterus using nuclear magnetic resonance, *Clin Perinatol* 17(2):307-329, 1990.

Plotz RD: Familial occurrence of hemolytic disease of the newborn due to ABO blood group incompatibility, *Hum Pathol* 16:113-116, 1985.

Poland RL: Home phototherapy: not seeing the light, *Pediatrics* 91(1):147, 1993.

Scheidt PC and others: Phototherapy for neonatal hyperbilirubinemia: six-year follow-up of the National Institute of Child Health and Human Development clinical trial, *Pediatrics* 85(4):455-463, 1990.

Scheidt PC and others: Intelligence at six years in relation to neonatal bilirubin level: follow-up of the National Institute of Child Health and Human Development clinical trial of phototherapy, *Peditrics* 87(6):797-805, 1991.

Schumacher RE: Noninvasive measurements of bilirubin in the newborn, *Clin Perinatol* 17(2):417-435, 1990.

Schuman AJ, Karush G: Fiberoptic vs conventional home phototherapy for neonatal hyperbilirubinemia, *Clin Pediatr* 31(6):345-352, 1992.

Segal S: The challenge of galactosemia, *Int Pediatr* 8(1):125-132, 1993.

Sherwood KA: The use of topical anesthesia in removal of port-wine stains in children, *J Pediatr* 122 (5, pt 2):S36-S41, 1993.

Strauss RP, Resnick SD: Pulsed dye laser therapy for port-wine stains in children: psychosocial and ethical issues, *J Pediatr* 122(4):505-510, 1993.

Strobel SE, Keller CS: Metabolic screening in the NICU population: a proposal for change, *Pediatr Nurs* 19(2):113-117, 1993.

Tallman B and others: Location of port-wine stains and the likelihood of ophthalmic and/or central nervous system complications, *Pediatrics* 87(3):323-327, 1991.

Tan KL: Phototherapy for neonatal jaundice, *Clin Perinatol* 18(3):423-439, 1991.

Valaes T and others: Control of jaundice in preterm newborns by an inhibitor of bilirubin production: studies with tin-mesoporphyrin, *Pediatrics* 93(1):1-11, 1994.

van de Bor M and others: Hyperbilirubinemia in preterm infants and neurodevelopmental outcome at 2 years of age: results of a national collaborative survey, *Pediatrics* 83(6):915-920, 1989.

Vitanza A, Giacoia G, West K: Evaluation of a new glucose reflectance meter for use in the neonatal intensive care unit, *J Perinatol* 8(1):43-45, 1988.

Vomund SL, Witter E: Advanced techniques for the treatment of severe isoimmunization, *MCN* 19(1):18-23, 1994.

Waggoner DD, Buist N: Long-term complications in treated galactosemia, *Int Pediatr* 8(1):97-100, 1993.

Woodall D, Karas JG: A new light on jaundice, *Clin Pediatr* 31(6):353-356, 1992.

BIBLIOGRAPHY

Birth Injuries/Dermatologic Problems

Albright AL, Gartner JC, Wiener ES: Lumbar cutaneous hemangiomas as indicators of tethered spinal cords, *Pediatrics* 83(6):977-980, 1989.

Ashinoff R, Geronemus RG: Effect of the topical anesthetic EMLA on the efficacy of pulsed dye laser treatment of port-wine stains, *J Dermatol Surg Oncol* 16(11):1008-1011, 1990.

Berg FJ, Solomon LM: Erythema neonatorum toxicum, *Arch Dis Child* 62:327-328, 1987.

Butler KM, Baker JB: Candida: an increasingly important pathogen in the nursery, *Pediatr Clin North Am* 35:543-563, 1988.

Eichenfield LF, Honig PJ: Difficult diagnostic and management issues in pediatric dermatology, *Pediatr Clin North Am* 38(3):687-710, 1991.

Esterly NB; Cutaneous hemangiomas, vascular stains, and associated syndromes, *Curr Probl Pediatr* 17:1-69, 1987.

Feigin FD, Adcock LM, Miller DJ: Postnatal bacterial infections. In Fanaroff A, Martin R, editors: *Neonatal-perinatal medicine,* ed 5, St Louis, 1992, Mosby.

Geronemus RG, Ashinoff R: The medical necessity of evaluation and treatment of port-wine stains, *J Dermatol Surg Oncol* 17:76-79, 1991.

Johnstone HA, Marcinak JF: Candidiasis in the breastfeeding mother and infant, *JOGNN* 19(2):171-173, 1990.

Joseph PR, Rosenfeld W: Clavicular fractures in neonates, *Am J Dis Child* 144:165-167, 1990.

Kimble C: Neonatal petechiae: strategies for nursing interventions, *Dermatol Nurs* 8(1):24-28, 1994.

Krusinski PA, Flowers FP: *Handbook of pediatric dermatology,* St Louis, 1990, Mosby.

Mallory SB: Neonatal skin disorders, *Pediatr Clin North Am* 38(4):745-761, 1991.

Mangurten HH: Birth injuries. In Fanaroff A, Martin R, editors: *Neonatal-perinatal medicine,* ed 5, St Louis, 1992, Mosby.

Prendiville J, Esterly NB: When congenital nevi signal underlying disease, *Contemp Pediatr* 4(3):24-52, 1987.

Reese V and others: Association of facial hemangiomas with Dandy-Walker and other posterior fossa malformations, *J Pediatr* 122(3):379-384, 1993.

Silverman RA: Hemangiomas and vascular malformations, *Pediatr Clin North Am* 38(4):811-834, 1991.

Hyperbilirubinemia

Brucker MC, MacMullen NJ: Neonatal jaundice in the home: assessment with a noninvasive device, *JOGNN* 16:355-368, 1987.

Gale R and others: A randomized, controlled application of the Wallaby phototherapy system compared with standard phototherapy, *J Perinatol* 10(3):239-242, 1990.

Haemolytic disease of the newborn, *Lancet* 1(8634):361-362, 1989.

Hill AS, Cochran CK, Dickerson C: Nursing care of the infant with erythroblastosis fetalis, *J Pediatr Nurs* 4:395-402, 1989.

Ives K: Kernicterus in preterm infants; lest we forget (to turn on the lights), *Pediatrics* 90(5):757-759, 1992.

Jones MB: A physiologic approach to identifying neonates at risk for kernicterus, *JOGNN* 19(4):313-318, 1990.

Kemper KJ, Forsyth BW, McCarthy PL: Persistent perceptions of vulnerability following neonatal jaundice, *Am J Dis Child* 144:238-241, 1990.

Lazar L, Litwin A, Merlob P: Phototherapy for neonatal nonhemolytic hyperbilirubinemia, *Clin Pediatr* 32(5):264-266, 1993.

Locklin M: Assessing jaundice in full-term newborns, *Pediatr Nurs* 13:15-19, 1987.

Ludwig MA: Phototherapy in the home setting, *J Pediatr Health Care* 4(6):304-308, 1990.

Meropol SB and others: Home phototherapy: use and attitudes among community pediatricians, *Pediatrics* 91(1):97-100, 1993.

Missiou-Tsagaraki S: Screening for glucose-6-phosphate dehydrogenase deficiency as a preventive measure: prevalence among 1,286,000 Greek newborn infants, *J Pediatr* 119(2):239-299, 1991.

Moderate neonatal hyperbilirubinaemia: hold tight, *Lancet* 338(8777):1242-1243, 1991.

Newman TB, Hope S, Stevenson DK: Direct bilirubin measurements in jaundiced term newborns, *Am J Dis Child* 145(11):1305-1309, 1991.

Newman TB and others: Laboratory evaluation of jaundice in newborns, *Am J Dis Child* 144(3):364-368, 1990.

Page S: RH hemolytic disease of the newborn, *Neonatal Network* 7(6):31-41, 1989.

Rose BS: Phototherapy: all wrapped up? *Pediatr Nurs* 16:57, 1990.

Rosenfeld W, Twist P, Concepcion L: A new device for phototherapy treatment of jaundiced infants, *J Perinatol* 10(3):243-248, 1990.

Stevenson DK, Brown AK: Race, ethnicity, and the propensity for neonatal jaundice, *Clin Pediatr* 31(12):706-707, 1992.

Thornton JG and others: Efficacy and long term effects of antenatal prophylaxis with anti-D immunoglobulin, *Br Med J* 298:1671-1673, 1989.

Watchko JF, Oski FA: Kernicterus in preterm newborns: past, present, and future, *Pediatrics* 90(5):707-715, 1992.

Wilkerson NN: Treating hyperbilirubinemia, *MCN* 14:32-36, 1989.

Metabolic Problems

Amspacher KA: Meeting the challenge of neonatal hyperglycemia, *J Perinat Neonat Nurs* 6(1):43-51, 1992.

Carmen S: Neonatal hypoglycemia in response to maternal glucose infusion before delivery, *JOGNN* 15:319-323, 1986.

Cole MD: New factors associated with the incidence of hypoglycemia: a research study, *Neonatal Network* 10(4):47-50, 1991.

Cornblath M and others: Hypoglycemia in infancy: the need for a rational definition, *Pediatrics* 85(5):834-837, 1990.

Hawdon JM, Ward Platt MP, Aynsley-Green A: Neonatal hypoglycaemia—blood glucose monitoring and baby feeding, *Midwifery* 9:3-6, 1993.

Holtrop PC and others: A comparison of chromogen test strip (Chemstrip bG) and serum glucose values in newborns, *Am J Dis Child* 144(2):183-185, 1990.

Lin HC and others: Accuracy and reliability of glucose reflectance meters in the high-risk neonate, *J Pediatr* 115(6):998-1000, 1989.

Presti B, Kircher T, Reed C: Capillary blood glucose monitor: evaluation in a newborn nursery, *Clin Pediatr* 28(9):412-415, 1989.

Shannon LF: Insulin usage in the neonate, *Neonatal Network* 6(5):31-39, 1988.

Venkataraman PS and others: Pathogenesis of early neonatal hypocalcemia: studies of serum calcitonin, gastrin, and plasma glucagon, *J Pediatr* 110(40):599-603, 1987.

Hemorrhagic Disease of the Newborn

Handel J, Tripp JH: Vitamin K prophylaxis against haemorrhagic disease of the newborn in the United Kingdom, *Br Med J* 303(6810):1109, 1991.

Hilgartner MW: Vitamin K in the newborn, *N Engl J Med* 329:957-958, 1993.

Luban NLC: The new and the old—molecular diagnostics and hemolytic disease of the newborn, *N Engl J Med* 329(9):658-660, 1993.

Matsuda I and others: Late neonatal vitamin K deficiency associated with subclinical liver dysfunction in human milk–fed infants, *J Pediatr* 114(4):602-605, 1989.

McNinch AW, Tripp JH: Haemorrhagic disease of the newborn in the British Isles: two year prospective study, *Br Med J* 303(8610):1105-1109, 1991.

Pramanik AK: Bleeding disorders in neonates, *Pediatr Rev* 13(5):163-173, 1992.

Inborn Errors of Metabolism

Applegarth DA, Dimmick JE, Toone JR: Laboratory detection of metabolic disease, *Pediatr Clin North Am* 36:49-65, 1989.

Irons M: Screening for metabolic disorders: how are we doing? *Pediatr Clin North Am* 40(5):1073-1086, 1993.

Kotzer AM, McCabe ERB: Newborn screening for inherited metabolic disease: principles and practice, *Neonatal Network* 6(4):15-19, 1988.

Schmidt K: A primer to the inborn errors of metabolism for perinatal and neonatal nurses, *J Perinat Neonat Nurs* 2(4):60-71, 1989.

Wright L, Brown A, Davidson-Mundt A: Newborn screening: the miracle and the challenge, *J Pediatr Nurs* 7(1):26-42, 1992.

Congenital Hypothyroidism

Alemzadeh R and others: Is there compensated hypothyroidism in infancy? *Pediatrics* 90(2):207-211, 1992.

Aronson R and others: Growth in children with congenital hypothyroidism detected by neonatal screening, *J Pediatr* 116:33-37, 1990.

Mazzocco M and others: Cognition and thyrosine supplementation among school-aged children with phenylketonuria, *Am J Dis Child* 146(11):1261-1264, 1992.

New England Congenital Hypothyroidism Collaborative: Elementary school performance of children with congenital hypothyroidism, *J Pediatr* 116:27-32, 1990.

Rovet JF: Does breast-feeding protect the hypothyroid infant whose condition is diagnosed by newborn screening? *Am J Dis Child* 144:319-323, 1990.

Rovet JF, Ehrlich RM, Sorbara D: Effect of thyroid hormone level on temperament in infants with congenital hypothyroidism detected by screening of neonates, *J Pediatr* 114(1):63-68, 1989.

Phenylketonuria

Acosta PB, Wright L: Nurses' role in preventing birth defects in offspring of women with phenylketonuria, *JOGNN* 21(4):270-276, 1992.

Berlin CA, Roth KS: All children are special: the child with PKU, *Clin Pediatr* 32(5):316-319, 1993.

Berry HK and others: Valine, isoleucine, and leucine: a new treatment for phenylketonuria, *Am J Dis Child* 144(5):539-543, 1990.

Buist N and others: Towards improving the diet for hyperphenylalaninemia and other metabolic disorders, *Int Pediatr* 8(1):80-88, 1993.

Cockburn F and others: Maternal phenylketonuria: diet, dangers and dilemmas, *Int Pediatr* 7(1):67-74, 1992.

Drogari E and others: Timing of strict diet in relation to fetal damage in maternal phenylketonuria, *Lancet* 927-930, 1987.

Hurst JD, Stullenbarger B: Implementation of a self-care approach in a pediatric interdisciplinary phenylketonuria (PKU) clinic, *J Pediatr Nurs* 1:159-163, 1986.

Kaufman S: An evaluation of the possible neurotoxicity of metabolites of phenylalanine, *J Pediatr* 114(5):895-899, 1989.

Legido A and others: Treatment variables and intellectual outcome in children with classic phenylketonuria, *Clin Pediatr* 32(7):417-432, 1993.

Lehmann WD: Progress in the identification of the heterozygote in phenylketonuria, *J Pediatr* 114(6):915-924, 1989.

Russell FF, Mills BC, Zucconi T: Relationship of parental attitudes and knowledge to treatment adherence in children with PKU, *Pediatr Nurs* 14:514-516, 1988.

Schmidt KA: Phenylketonuria. In Jackson PL, Vessey JA: *Primary care of the child with a chronic condition*, St Louis, 1992, Mosby.

Shriver R: Phenylketonuria—genotypes and phenotypes, *N Engl J Med* 324(18):1280-1281, 1991.

Smith I, Beasley M, Ades A: Intellectual progress and quality of phenylalanine control in early treated children with phenylketonuria, *Int Pediatr* 6(1):52-55, 1991.

Steele S: Phenylketonuria: counseling and teaching functions of the nurse on an interdisciplinary team, *Issues Compr Pediatr Nurs* 12:395-410, 1989.

Galactosemia

Brivet M and others: Effect of lactation in a mother with galactosemia, *J Pediatr* 115(2):280-282, 1989.

Kirkman HN: Galactosemia: recent developments in newborn screening and enzymatic research, *Int Pediatr* 8(1):118-124, 1993.

Segal S: The enigma of galactosemia, *Int Pediatr* 7(1):75-82, 1992.

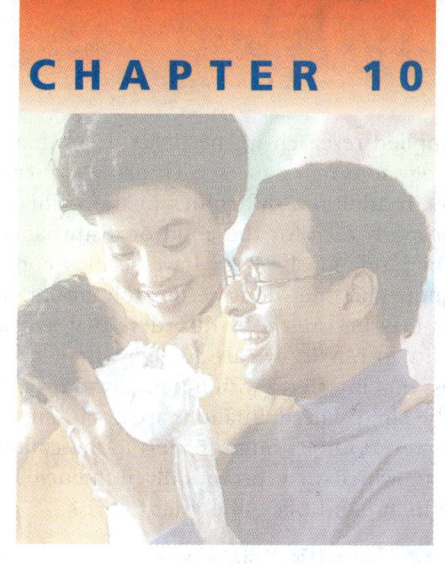

CHAPTER 10

The High-Risk Newborn and Family

CHAPTER OUTLINE

RELATED TOPICS

Administration of medication, Ch. 27
Assessment of clinical gestational age, Ch. 8
Assessment (newborn), Ch. 8
Birth of a child with a physical defect, Ch. 11
Birth injuries, Ch. 9
Bodily injury and pain, Ch. 26
Congenital defects caused by prenatal factors, Ch. 11
Congenital diaphragmatic hernia, Ch. 11
Discharge planning and home care, Ch. 26
Esophageal atresia with tracheoesophageal fistula, Ch. 11
Family-centered home care, Ch. 25
Fetal alcohol syndrome, Ch. 11
Gastroschisis, Ch. 11
Hyperbilirubinemia, Ch. 9
Hypocalcemia, Ch. 9
Hypoglycemia, Ch. 9
Infant mortality, Ch. 1
Malformations of the central nervous system, Ch. 11
Neonatal pain, Ch. 11
Nursing care of the surgical neonate, Ch. 11
Omphalocele, Ch. 11
Pain assessment; pain management, Ch. 26
Promotion of parent-infant bonding (attachment), Ch. 8
Maintaining healthy skin, Ch. 27

GENERAL MANAGEMENT OF HIGH-RISK NEWBORNS

IDENTIFICATION OF HIGH-RISK NEWBORNS

The ***high-risk neonate*** can be defined as a newborn, regardless of gestational age or birth weight, who has a greater than average chance of morbidity or mortality because of conditions or circumstances that are superimposed on the normal course of events associated with birth and the adjustment to extrauterine existence. The high-risk period encompasses human growth and development from the time of viability up to 28 days following birth and includes threats to life and health that occur during the prenatal, perinatal, and postnatal periods.

Assessment and prompt intervention in life-threatening perinatal emergencies often make the difference between a favorable outcome and a lifetime of disability. The nurse in the newborn nursery is familiar with the characteristics of neonates and recognizes the significance of serious deviations from expected observations. When the need for specialized care can be anticipated and planned for, the probability of successful outcome is increased.

Anticipation of Problems

Factors that influence neonatal outcome during this vulnerable period may occur simultaneously. For example, infants born prematurely may suffer from perinatal asphyxia and develop respiratory distress syndrome. The list of factors associated with increased risk in the neonatal period continues to grow as applied research in the fields of perinatology and neonatology adds new data (see Thinking Critically About . . . box). In addition, difficulties in the ability of the mother to properly care for the child or disturbances in the mother-child relationship can have serious consequences—both immediate and long term—for the infant. These difficulties may be caused by disorders that impair the mother's ability to physically care for her infant or by psychologic illness that interferes with her ability to provide proper care for the child. These situations are not discussed in depth here; however, nurses must be alert to indications of these problems, which may profoundly influence the well-being of the infant and place the infant at risk.

■ David Wilson, RN,C, MS, revised this chapter.

Classification of High-Risk Newborns

High-risk infants are most often classified according to birth weight, gestational age, and predominant pathophysiologic problems. The more common problems related to physiologic status are closely associated with the state of maturity of the infant and usually involve chemical disturbances (e.g., hypoglycemia, hypocalcemia) and consequences of immature organs and systems (e.g., hyperbilirubinemia, respiratory distress, hypothermia). Since high-risk factors are common to several specialty areas, particularly obstetrics, pediatrics, and neonatology, specific terminology is needed to describe the developmental status of the newborn (see box on p. 367).

Formerly, weight at birth was considered to reflect a reasonably accurate estimation of gestational age. That is, if infants' birth weights exceeded 2500 g (5½ pounds), they were considered to be mature. However, accumulated data

THINKING CRITICALLY ABOUT . . . *Infant Mortality and Low Birth Weight*

Infant mortality rates may be categorized by the timing of infant deaths: postnatal or neonatal (see box on p. 367). The leading cause of death in the postnatal category is sudden infant death syndrome (SIDS), followed by congenital anomalies, accidents, and infections. The leading cause of death in the neonatal period is associated with infants who are born at low birth weight (<2500 g); these infants are 20 times more likely to die within the first month of life than are newborns who have normal weights. The incidence of death is said to increase 200 fold in very-low-birth-weight (VLBW) (<1500 g) infants (Arnold, 1992). Although infant mortality was decreased by almost 5% from 1991 to 1992, the incidence of death among black infants increased from previous years (Wegman, 1993).

Factors contributing to this relatively high infant mortality rate include a number of intrauterine events that eventually result in a low birth weight. In one study more than 50% of preterm births among black infants were attributed to acute chorioamnionitis and low uteroplacental blood flow (Naeye, 1993). It is highly significant that low birth weight is most closely associated with inadequate prenatal care, especially among younger women and those who live at or below poverty level (Arnold, 1992; Wilcox and Skaerven, 1992). In addition, at least 10% of the U.S. population wherein high rates of infant mortality exist have inadequate or no prenatal care (Wegman, 1993). While survival of extremely-low-birth-weight (ELBW) (<1000 g) and VLBW infants has improved overall, these infants remain at greater risk during childhood years for respiratory problems, neurological deficits, and developmental delays (Hack and others, 1993; Jakobi, Weissman, and Paldi, 1993).

There is little doubt that technologic and research advances (i.e., surfactant extracorporeal membrane oxygenation [ECMO] and high-frequency ventilation [HFV]) have contributed to these increased survival rates. However, given the fact that LBW is a large contributor to infant mortality and morbidity, the challenge for nurses is to decresae events leading to the birth of infants who are at highest risk. Nurses who are at the forefront of community health care are in a position to influence the undesirable outcomes of LBW infants and associated morbidities by identifying mothers at risk, educating them thoroughly regarding the need for preventive health care and prenatal follow-up, and monitoring them for potential complications. Likewise, nurses involved in the care and integration of the family unit are in an excellent position to help the family outline strategies for accessing the available health care resources in order to provide adequate prenatal care and prevent preterm births (Walden, 1994; York and Brooten, 1992). Since the quality of the home environment is also an important factor in these infants' subsequent cognitive development, identification and education of those families most in need of interventions to promote child development are essential (Feingold, 1994).

have shown that intrauterine growth rates are not the same for all infants and that other factors (e.g., heredity, placental insufficiency, and maternal disease) influence intrauterine growth and the birth weight of the infant. From these data a more definitive and meaningful classification system that encompasses birth weight, gestational age, and neonatal outcome has been developed. It has also been determined that the lowest perinatal mortality is found in the full-term infant who weighs between 3000 and 4000 g (Fanaroff and Martin, 1992). (See Fig. 8-2 for size comparison of newborn infants.)

Many perinatal problems can be anticipated before delivery. Prenatal testing and labor monitoring have reduced the incidence of perinatal mortality, and specialized care of the distressed newborn is improving the survival rate. If the infant is likely to require special therapy at or soon after birth, plans can be made for the delivery to take place at a hospital that has the facilities to provide such care. In this way there is no delay in initiating needed care, and some of the hazards associated with transporting the sick newborn are averted. Prenatal evaluation of fetal well-being and advanced surgical techniques have made treatment of certain pathologic conditions in utero possible, thus enhancing the neonate's chances for survival (Collins, 1994; Kenner, Bruggemeyer, and Gunderson, 1993; Vomund and Witter, 1994).

CLASSIFICATION OF HIGH-RISK INFANTS

CLASSIFICATION ACCORDING TO SIZE

Low-birth-weight (LBW) infant—An infant whose birth weight is less than 2500 g regardless of gestational age

Very-very-low-birth-weight (VVLBW) or **extremely-low-birth-weight (ELBW) infant**—An infant whose birth weight is less than 1000 g

Very-low-birth-weight (VLBW) infant—An infant whose birth weight is less than 1500 g

Moderately-low-birth-weight (MLBW)—An infant whose birth weight is 1501 to 2500 g

Appropriate-for-gestational-age (AGA) infant—An infant whose weight falls between the 10th and 90th percentiles on intrauterine growth curves

Small-for-date (SFD) or small-for-gestational-age (SGA) infant—An infant whose rate of intrauterine growth was slowed and whose birth weight falls below the 10th percentile on intrauterine growth curves

Intrauterine growth retardation (IUGR)—Found in infants whose intrauterine growth is retarded (sometimes used as a more descriptive term for the SGA infant)

Large-for-gestational-age (LGA) infant—An infant whose birth weight falls above the 90th percentile on intrauterine growth charts

CLASSIFICATION ACCORDING TO GESTATIONAL AGE

Premature (preterm) infant—An infant born before completion of 37 weeks of gestation, regardless of birth weight

Full-term infant—An infant born between the beginning of the 38 weeks and the completion of the 42 weeks of gestation, regardless of birth weight

Postmature (postterm) infant—An infant born after 42 weeks of gestational age, regardless of birth weight

CLASSIFICATION ACCORDING TO MORTALITY

Live birth—Birth in which the neonate manifests any heartbeat, breathes, or displays voluntary movement, regardless of gestational age

Fetal death—Death of the fetus after 20 weeks of gestation and before delivery, with absence of any signs of life after birth

Neonatal death—Death that occurs in the first 27 days of life; early neonatal death occurs in the first week of life; late neonatal death occurs at 7 to 27 days

Perinatal mortality—Describes the total number of fetal and early neonatal deaths per 1000 live births

Postnatal death—Death that occurs at 28 days to 1 year

INTENSIVE CARE FACILITIES

Awareness of the unique characteristics of perinatal disorders has generated the provision of special care units in major medical facilities. Rapid advances in the understanding of the pathophysiology of the neonate and the increased capacity to apply this knowledge have emphasized the need for appropriate settings in which to care for the seriously ill infant. Advancements in electronics and biochemistry, new methods for monitoring cardiorespiratory function, microtechniques for biochemical determination from minute quantities of blood, noninvasive monitoring, and new methods for assisted ventilation and conservation of body heat have made it possible to effectively manage the newborn with serious illness.

Intensive care of the ill and immature newborn requires specialized knowledge and skill in a number of areas of expertise. Much of the equipment long used in the care of the critically ill adult is unsuited to the singular needs of the very small infant; therefore, commonplace apparatus has been modified to meet these needs. Examples of modifications include respirators that deliver small volumes of oxygen in the proper concentration and pressure, infusion pumps that deliver very small amounts accurately, and crib units that provide a constant source of warmth and at the same time allow maximum access to the infant. Most important, intensive care has created a need for highly skilled personnel trained in the art of neonatal intensive care.

The diversity of special care needs requires that the unit be arranged for graduated care for the infant population. There should be adequate facilities and skilled personnel to provide one-to-one nursing care for each seriously ill infant, in addition to a means for graduation to one-to-three or one-to-four nursing care in a convalescent area where infants require less intensive care until they are ready to leave the unit.

Organization of Services

The most efficient organization of services is a regionalized system consisting of facilities within a designated geographic area. Neonatal intensive care facilities may provide three prescribed levels of care with special equipment, skilled personnel, and ancillary services concentrated in a centralized institution:

Level I facility—Provides management of normal maternal and newborn care but able to identify high-risk pregnancies and/or high-risk neonates early and implement emergency care in the event of complications.

Level II facility—Provides a full range of maternity and newborn care and is equipped to manage the majority of maternal and neonatal complications, depending on the resources available.

Level III facility—Offers the full range of maternal and newborn services of a level II facility and has the capacity to provide care for the most complex neonatal complications; at least one full-time neonatologist is on the staff.

Transporting High-Risk Newborns

When the infant at risk is identified or anticipated, arrangements are made for care in the intensive care facility. There is no question that the uterus is the ideal transport unit for the infant with anticipated difficulties; therefore, whenever possible, the mother is taken where special care is available for her delivery.

Some infants develop difficulties after a seemingly normal pregnancy and uncomplicated labor. Since it is impossible to always predict when infants will require intensive care, a coordinated system is needed to ensure them an optimum opportunity for survival. Each hospital that delivers infants should be able to provide for appropriate neonatal stabilization and arrange for transport to a tertiary care facility. The infant must be kept warm, be adequately oxygenated (including intubation if indicated), have vital signs and oxygen saturation monitored, and, when indicated, receive an intravenous infusion. It may be up to 4 hours before the infant is sufficiently stabilized for transport. The infant is transported in a specially designed incubator unit containing a complete life-support system and other emergency equipment that can be carried by ambulance, van, or helicopter.

The transport team may consist of one or more of the highly trained persons from the NICU: a neonatologist (or a fellow in neonatology), a respiratory therapist, and one or more nurses. The professional assigned to accompany the infant must be constantly alert to every change in the infant's condition and be able to intervene appropriately. The neonate who must be moved from one place to another within the hospital (e.g., to surgery, from delivery room to nursery) is transported in an incubator or radiant warmer accompanied by the necessary personnel and equipment.

NURSING CARE OF HIGH-RISK NEWBORNS

Neonatal intensive care nursing is a highly specialized area of knowledge and practice that requires lengthy supervised experience to reach a level of competence that permits independent functioning. Neonatal intensive care nursing involves an understanding of neonatal physiology and characteristics, a knowledge of the function and management of a number of mechanical devices and apparatus, the ability to recognize very subtle deviations from the expected, and the ability to implement a judicious course of action. Nursing care of the high-risk newborn requires anticipation, intervention, and effective planning strategies for problems encountered with infants who are at risk.

Since the majority of infants who are admitted to intensive care facilities are born before the estimated date of delivery, the major discussion of problems related to the high-risk neonate are directed toward the preterm infant (see p. 397 for a description of the characteristics of preterm infants). The incidence of neonatal complications (e.g., respiratory distress and hypoglycemia) is highest in this group, and often other high-risk factors (e.g., sepsis and congenital malformations) are found in association with prematurity. Nursing problems encountered in the intensive care nursery are discussed, followed by a consideration of common complications. Nursing care of high-risk infants with more serious disorders is examined in relation to specific high-risk conditions.

❖ ASSESSMENT

At birth the newborn is given a cursory, yet thorough, assessment to determine any apparent problems and identify those that demand immediate attention. This examination is primarily concerned with the evaluation of cardiopulmonary and neurologic functions. The assessment includes the assignment of an Apgar score (see Chapter 8) and an evaluation for any obvious congenital anomalies, or evidence of neonatal distress. Delivery rooms are equipped with a special resuscitation area where infants with evidence of distress are stabilized and evaluated before being transported to the NICU for therapy and more extensive assessment (see Assessment of Clinical Gestational Age, Chapter 8).

Maintaining detailed, ongoing records of all activities and observations is an important responsibility of nurses in the intensive care setting. Knowledge about and operation of complex pieces of equipment and mechanical devices are inherent in the care of the ill neonate. However, sophisticated monitoring and life-support systems cannot replace the vigilance and constant scrutiny of the infants by experienced personnel.

Systematic Assessment

A thorough systematic physical assessment (see Guidelines box) is an essential component in the care of the high-risk infant. Subtle changes in feeding behavior, activity, color, or vital signs often indicate an underlying problem. The preterm infant, especially the VLBW infant, is ill equipped to withstand prolonged physiologic stress and may expire within minutes of exhibiting abnormal symptoms if the underlying pathologic process is not corrected. The alert nurse is aware of subtle changes and reacts promptly to implement interventions that will promote optimum functioning in the high-risk neonate. Changes in the infant's status are noted through ongoing observations of the infant's adaptation to the extrauterine environment.

Observational assessments of the high-risk infant are made according to the infant's acuity; the critically ill infant requires close observation and assessment of respiratory function, including continuous pulse oximetry and frequent evaluation of blood gases. Accurate documentation of the infant's status is an integral component of nursing care. With the aid of continuous, sophisticated cardiopulmonary monitoring, nursing assessments and daily care may be coordinanted to allow for minimal handling of the in-

GUIDELINES
Physical Assessment

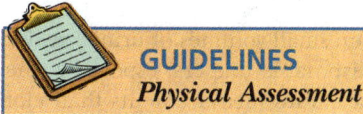

GENERAL ASSESSMENT

Using electronic scale, weigh daily, or more often if ordered.
Measure length and head circumference periodically.
Describe general body shape and size, posture at rest, ease of breathing, presence and location of edema.
Describe any apparent deformities.
Describe any signs of distress: poor color, mouth open, head bobbing, grimace, furrowed brow.

RESPIRATORY ASSESSMENT

Describe shape of chest (barrel, concave), symmetry, presence of incisions, chest tubes, or other deviations.
Describe use of accessory muscles: nasal flaring or substernal, intercostal, or subclavicular retractions.
Determine respiratory rate and regularity.
Auscultate and describe breath sounds: stridor, crackles, wheezing, wet diminished sounds, areas of absence of sound, grunting, diminished air entry, equality of breath sounds.
Determine whether suctioning is needed.
Describe cry if not intubated.
Describe ambient oxygen and method of delivery; if intubated, describe size of tube, type of ventilator and settings, and method of securing tube.
Determine oxygen saturation by pulse oximetry and partial pressure of oxygen and carbon dioxide by transcutaneous oxygen ($tcPo_2$) and transcutaneous carbon dioxide ($tcPco_2$).

CARDIOVASCULAR ASSESSMENT

Determine heart rate and rhythm.
Describe heart sounds, including any murmurs.
Determine the point of maximum intensity (PMI), the point where the heartbeat sounds and palpates loudest (a change in the point of maximum intensity may indicate a mediastinal shift).
Describe infant's color (may be of cardiac, respiratory, or hematopoietic origin): cyanosis, pallor, plethora, jaundice, mottling.
Assess color of nail beds, mucous membranes, lips.
Determine blood pressure. Indicate extremity used and cuff size; check each extremity at least once.
Describe peripheral pulses, capillary refill (<2 to 3 seconds), peripheral perfusion (mottling).
Describe monitors, their parameters, and whether alarms are in "on" position.

GASTROINTESTINAL ASSESSMENT

Determine presence of abdominal distention: increase in circumference, shiny skin, evidence of abdominal wall erythema, visible peristalsis, visible loops of bowel, status of umbilicus.
Determine any signs of regurgitation, and time related to feeding; character and amount of residual if gavage fed; if nasogastric tube in place, describe type of suction, drainage (color, consistency, pH, guaiac).
Described amount, color, consistency, and odor of any emesis.
Palpate liver margin.
Describe amount, color, and consistency of stools; check for occult blood and/or reducing substances if ordered or indicated by appearance of stool.
Describe bowel sounds: presence or absence (must be present if feeding).

GENITOURINARY ASSESSMENT

Describe any abnormalities of genitalia.
Describe amount (as determined by weight), color, pH, labstick findings, and specific gravity of urine (to screen for adequacy of hydration).
Check weight (the most accurate measure for assessment of hydration).

NEUROLOGIC-MUSCULOSKELETAL ASSESSMENT

Describe infant's movements: random, purposeful, jittery, twitching, spontaneous, elicited; level of activity with stimulation; evaluate based on gestational age.
Describe infant's position or attitude: flexed, extended.
Describe reflexes observed: Moro, sucking, Babinski, plantar reflex, and other expected reflexes.
Determine level of response and consolability.
Determine changes in head circumference (if indicated); size and tension of fontanels, suture lines.
Determine pupillary responses in infant >32 weeks of gestation.

TEMPERATURE

Determine skin and axillary temperature.
Determine relationship to environmental temperature.

SKIN ASSESSMENT

Describe any discoloration, reddened area, signs of irritation, blisters, abrasions, or denuded areas, especially where monitoring equipment, infusions, or other apparatus come in contact with skin; also check and note *any* skin preparation used (e.g., povidone-iodine tape).
Determine texture and turgor of skin: dry, smooth, flaky, peeling, etc.
Describe any rash, skin lesion, or birthmarks.
Determine whether intravenous infusion catheter or needle is in place and observe for signs of infiltration.
Describe parenteral infusion lines: location, type (arterial, venous, peripheral, umbilical, central, peripheral central venous); type of infusion (medication, saline, dextrose, electrolyte, lipids, total parenteral nutrition); type of infusion pump and rate of flow; type of needle (butterfly, catheter); appearance of insertion site.

fant (especially the VLBW or ELBW infant) to decrease the effects of environmental stress.

Monitoring Physiologic Data

Most neonates under intensive observation are placed in a controlled thermal environment and monitored for heart rate, respiratory activity, and temperature. The monitoring devices are equipped with an alarm system that indicates when the vital signs are above or below preset limits. However, it is essential to check the heartbeat and compare it with the monitor reading.

The placement of electrodes is a continual nursing problem because of the lack of flat areas on the neonate's chest and the limited space for alternating sites, the size of the electrodes, and irritation from the paste or tape. Electrodes for cardiac monitors can often be applied to the back or the upper arms to provide relief for chest areas; nonadhesive limb electrodes eliminate possible skin irritation from tape. Hydrogel electrodes are gentler to the skin and are easily removed by lifting an edge from the skin and moistening with plain water to release the adhesive. If the same electrode is reapplied to the skin, the hydrogel should be rinsed with plain water to remove accumulated sodium from perspiration, which can eventually irritate the skin. It is important to follow the manufacturer's directions for care and handling of electrodes to avoid malfunction or burns to sensitive skin.

Blood pressure (BP) is monitored routinely in the sick neonate by either internal or external means. Direct recording with arterial catheters is often employed but carries the risks inherent in any procedure in which a catheter is introduced into an artery. An umbilical venous catheter may also be used to monitor the neonate's central venous pressure. Oscillometry (Dinamap) or Doppler transcutaneous apparatus are simple, effective means for detecting alterations in systemic BP (hypotension or hypertension). Normal BP ranges for healthy premature infants are listed in Table 10-1. Infants who are mechanically ventilated and have low Apgar scores have lower pressures. Infants whose mothers are hypertensive have higher BPs (Hegyi and others, 1994).

In the NICU frequent laboratory examinations and their interpretation are integral parts of the ongoing assessment of infants' progress. Accurate intake and output records are kept on all infants. An accurate output can be obtained by collecting urine in a plastic urine collection bag specifically made for premature infants (see Urine Specimens, Chapter 27) or by weighing the diapers, the simplest and least traumatic means of measuring urinary output. The preweighed wet diaper is weighed on a gram scale, and the gram weight of the urine is converted directly to milliliters (e.g., 25 g = 25 ml).

TABLE 10-1 Blood Pressure Ranges in Different Weight Groups of Healthy Premature Infants*

BIRTH WEIGHT (g)	SYSTOLIC (mm Hg)	DIASTOLIC (mm Hg)
501-750	50-62	26-36
751-1000	48-59	23-36
1001-1250	49-61	26-35
1251-1500	46-56	23-33
1501-1750	46-58	23-33
1751-2000	48-61	24-35

Modified from Hegyi T and others: Blood pressure ranges in premature infants. I. The first hours of life, *J Pediatr* 124(4):630, 1994.

*Defined as infants without a history of maternal hypertension, Apgar scores of less than 3 at 1 minute and less than 6 at 5 minutes, pneumothorax, hematorcrit <0.32, serum pH <7.1, use of dopamine, infusion of erythrocytes or colloid, mechanical ventilation, or cardiopulmonary resuscitation.

➤ **NURSING TIP** When small volumes of urine are measured, superabsorbent disposable diapers, especially when kept closed, give more accurate measurements than cloth diapers because they are less affected by evaporative losses (1992).

Plastic collecting devices can be used when it is necessary to collect urine for laboratory examination. Since the volume normally voided is insufficient to float the standard urometer, a refractometer requiring only a single drop of urine is sometimes used. A drop of urine can be aspirated with a syringe from the wet diaper or from cotton balls placed in the diaper.

Blood examinations are a necessary part of the ongoing assessment and monitoring of the sick newborn's progress. The tests most often performed are blood glucose, bilirubin, calcium, hematocrit, and blood gases. Samples may be obtained from the heel, by venipuncture, by arterial puncture, or by an indwelling catheter in an umbilical vein, umbilical artery, or peripheral artery.

➤ **NURSING TIP** Wrapping the foot in a warm, damp washcloth or disposable diaper is a simple way to create adequate vasodilation for a heel stick. Commercial warm packs are also available but should be used with extreme caution in ELBW and VLBW infants to prevent burns.

When numerous blood samples must be drawn, it is important to maintain an accurate record of the amount of blood being removed, especially in ELBW and VLBW infants, who can ill afford to have their blood supply depleted during the acute phase of their illness. To secure frequent samples for monitoring arterial blood gas levels without repeated arterial punctures, pulse oximetry, which measures the saturation of oxygen in the hemoglobin, is typically used. Monitoring of transcutaneous oxygen ($tcPo_2$) and carbon dioxide ($tcPco_2$), which measure the partial pressure of O_2 and CO_2, may also be used. The nurse notes changes in oxygenation (or other aspects being monitored) associated with handling and adjusts the infant's care accordingly (see Infant Stress, p. 382). The frequency of vital signs is determined by the acuity of the infant and by his or her response to handling.

Safety Measures. The proliferation of equipment technology over the past few years has increased the dangers associated with its use, especially performance malfunction and electrical hazards. Malfunction includes such things as inaccurate monitor function, erratic delivery rates in infusion devices, and low or high suction in pumps. Electrical hazards are related to defective equipment, wiring, or grounding, or improper use of equipment.

One of the most effective means for ensuring the safety of infant and staff is the nurse's knowledge, alertness, and education regarding the function of equipment. Electronic monitoring devices are checked to make certain that the alarms are not turned off, which negates their effectiveness. It is important to check equipment for all correct component parts, to remove from use and report equipment that is not performing according to specifications, and to obey the basic rules of electrical safety—handle equipment with care, be alert to signs of trouble, and follow electrical safety guidelines.

Parents need to be instructed regarding safety precautions and observations. They are usually uncomfortable around the equipment and atmosphere of an intensive care unit and therefore appreciate an explanation of the purposes and functions of the devices and pertinent safety aspects. Visiting siblings, especially toddlers, must be supervised closely to avoid their "playing" with the equipment and inadvertently causing harm to the neonate. While most NICUs are closed units, parents must also be educated and informed about specific safety measures designed to prevent neonatal kidnapping. Most institutions have their own protocols for preventing such an occurrence. (See also Protect from Infection and Injury, Chapter 8.)

❖ Nursing Diagnoses

Many nursing diagnoses may be evident after a careful assessment of the infant at risk. Some apply to all infants; others will vary according to the needs and characteristics of individual infants and their families. The nursing diagnoses that represent general guides for nursing intervention are found in the Nursing Care Plan on pp. 391-395. Since a number of health problems accompany the high-risk infant, the nurse is also alert to other conditions and complications discussed later in this chapter and elsewhere in the book.

❖ Planning

The nursing care plan for the high-risk infant depends to a large extent on the diagnosis of the health problem that places the infant at risk. However, the following are basic goals for all high-risk infants and their families:

1. Infant will exhibit adequate oxygenation.
2. Infant will maintain stable body temperature.
3. Infant will exhibit no evidence of nosocomial infection.
4. Infant will receive adequate hydration and nutrition.
5. Infant will maintain skin integrity.
6. Infant will exhibit normal increased intracranial pressure and no evidence of intraventricular hemorrhage (unless pre-existing condition).
7. Infant will experience no pain or a reduction of pain.
8. Infant receives appropriate developmental care.
9. Family receives appropriate support, including preparation for home care or for infant's death.

❖ Implementation

Respiratory Support

The primary objective in the care of high-risk infants is to establish and maintain respiration. Many infants require supplemental oxygen and assisted ventilation. Infants with or without these supportive treatments are positioned to maximize oxygenation. Oxygen therapy is provided on the basis of the infant's requirements and illness (see Respiratory Distress Syndrome, p. 399, and Oxygen Therapy, p. 403).

Thermoregulation

After or concurrent with the establishment of respiration, the most crucial need of the LBW infant is application of external warmth. Prevention of heat loss in the distressed infant is absolutely essential for survival, and maintaining a neutral thermal environment is a challenging aspect of neonatal intensive nursing care. Heat production is a complicated process that involves the cardiovascular, neurologic, and metabolic systems, and the immature neonate has all the problems related to heat production that are faced by the full-term infant (see Thermoregulation, Chapter 8). However, LBW infants are placed at further disadvantage by a number of additional problems. They have an even smaller muscle mass and fewer deposits of brown fat for producing heat, lack insulating subcutaneous fat, and have poor reflex control of skin capillaries.

Pathophysiology. The immature neonate, unable to increase activity and lacking a shivering response, produces heat primarily through increased metabolic processes. Some heat continues to be generated by liver, heart, brain, and skeletal muscles, but the major source of increased production of heat during cold stress is ***nonshivering thermogenesis.*** Norepinephrine, secreted by the sympathetic nerve endings in response to chilling, stimulates fat metabolism in the richly vascularized brown adipose tissue to produce internal heat, which is then conducted through the blood to surface tissues. Significantly, an increase in metabolism requires an increase in oxygen consumption.

The consequences of cold stress that produce additional hazards to the neonate are (1) hypoxia, (2) metabolic acidosis, and (3) hypoglycemia. Increased metabolism in response to chilling creates a compensatory increase in oxygen and calorie consumption. If available oxygen is not increased to accommodate this need, arterial oxygen tension is decreased. This is further complicated by a smaller lung volume in relation to the metabolic rate, which creates diminished oxygen in the blood and concurrent pulmonary disorders. A small advantage is gained by the persistence of fetal hemoglobin (HgF) because its increased capacity to carry oxygen allows the infant to exist for longer periods in conditions of lowered oxygen tension.

Norepinephrine, released in response to cold stress, causes pulmonary vasoconstriction, which further reduces the effectiveness of pulmonary ventilation. This decrease in oxygen diminishes the supply available for glucose metabolism. As a result, glucose is broken down by an alternate, hypoxic pathway (anaerobic glycolysis) that generates increased lactic acid formation. This, together with acid end products of brown fat metabolism, contributes to the acidotic state. Anaerobic metabolism dissipates glycogen at a greatly increased rate over aerobic metabolism, thus precipitating hypoglycemia. This condition is especially marked when glycogen stores are diminished at birth and when there is inadequate caloric intake after birth.

Maintaining Thermoneutrality. To delay or prevent the effects of cold stress, newborns at risk are placed in a heated environment immediately following birth, where they remain until they are able to maintain ***thermal stability,*** the capacity to balance heat production and conservation and heat dissipation. Since overheating produces an increase in oxygen and calorie consumption, the infant is also jeopardized in a hyperthermic environment. A ***neutral thermal environment*** is one that permits the infant to maintain a normal core temperature with minimum oxygen consump-

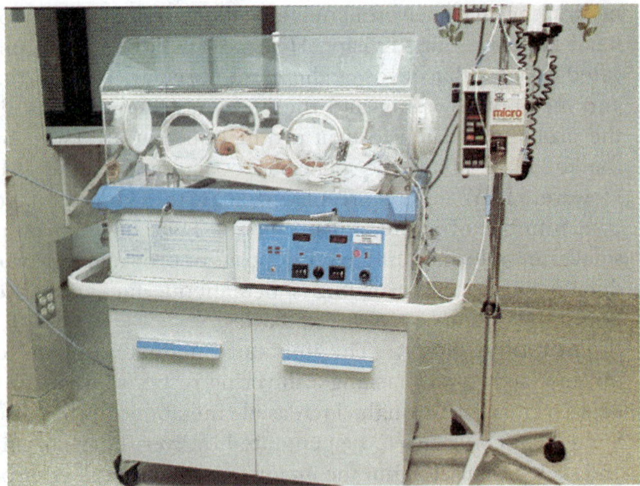

FIG. 10-1 Infant in incubator.

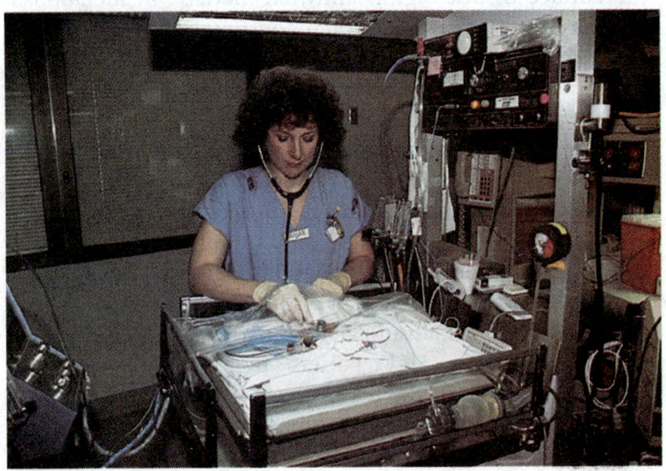

FIG. 10-2 Infant under overhead warming unit.

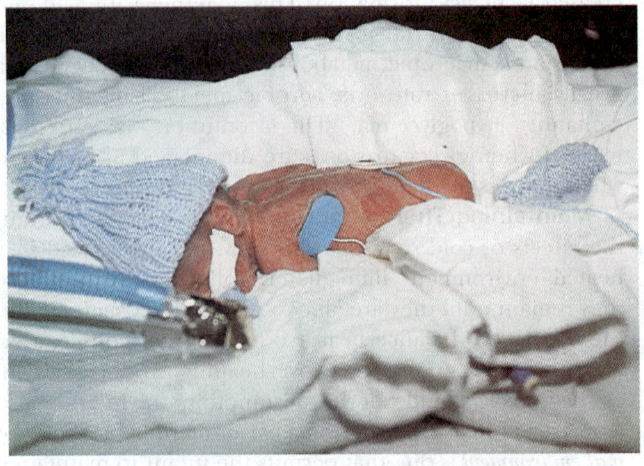

FIG. 10-3 Infant wearing knit cap.

tion and calorie expenditure. Recent studies indicate that optimum thermoneutrality cannot be predicted for every high-risk infant's needs. Guidelines for providing an optimum thermal environment suggest maintaining the infant's axillary temperature within a range of 36.5° to 37.5° C (97.7° to 99.5° F) (Thomas, 1994; Kenner, Brueggemeyer, and Gunderson, 1993; Merenstein and Gardner, 1993).

Thermal regulation in both VLBW and ELBW infants may require air temperature ranges higher than body core temperature. VLBW and ELBW infants, with thin skin and almost no subcutaneous fat, can control body heat loss or gain only within a very limited range of environmental temperatures. In these infants heat loss from radiation, evaporation, and transepidermal water loss is three to five times greater than in larger infants, and a decrease in body temperature is associated with an increase in mortality. A suggested neutral thermal environment for the VLBW infant is that ambient temperature required to maintain the infant's core temperature at rest between 36.7° and 37.3° C (98.1° and 99.1° F), with core and skin temperatures changing less than 0.2° to 0.3° C per hour (Sauer and others, 1984). Further research is needed to define a neutral thermal environment for the ELBW infant (Thomas, 1994).

The three methods for maintaining a neutral thermal environment are by the use of an incubator, a radiant warming panel (Figs. 10-1 and 10-2), and an open bassinet with cotton blankets. The dressed infant under blankets can maintain a temperature within a wider range of environmental temperatures; however, the close observations required by a high-risk infant are best accomplished if the infant remains partially unclothed. The incubator should always be prewarmed before placing an infant in it. The use of ***double-walled incubators*** significantly improves the infant's ability to maintain a desirable temperature and reduce energy expenditure related to heat regulation. The infant is clothed and warmly wrapped in blankets when removed from the warm environment of the incubator for feeding or cuddling. Inside or outside the incubator, head coverings are effective in preventing heat loss (Fig. 10-3). A fabric-insulated cap is more effective than one fashioned from stockinette (Blackburn and Loper, 1992; Greer, 1988).

An effective means for maintaining the desired range of temperature in the infant is by way of a ***manually adjusted*** or ***automatically controlled (servocontrolled) incubator.*** The latter mechanism, when set at the upper and lower limits of the desired circulating air temperature range, adjusts automatically in response to signals from a thermal sensor attached to the abdominal skin. If the infant's temperature drops, the warming device is triggered to increase heat output. The servocontrol is usually set to a desired skin temperature between 36° and 36.5° C (96.8° to 97.7° F) (Merenstein, Gardner, and Blake, 1993). An incubator may be inadequate to maintain thermal stability in the ELBW infant in the immediate postnatal period, thus requiring the use of a radiant warmer (Roncoli and Medoff-Cooper, 1992).

Disadvantages are always inherent in any mechanical device; therefore an important part of nursing assessment is to compare the infant's temperature with the temperature in the incubator. For example, if the infant's temperature fluctuates in response to sepsis, the servocontrolled mechanism would respond by decreasing or increasing the ambient air temperature. Therefore a critical observation could be easily overlooked. A heat-sensing probe attached to the abdomen registers a falsely high temperature when the infant is in the prone position. Either the probe should be moved to the flank area of the back when the infant is placed in the prone position or the infant should remain on the back or side or in a partial side-lying position.

NURSING ALERT When using a servocontrolled incubator, evaluate trends of increased or decreased ambient air temperature in response to fluctuations in the infant's body temperature to rule out sepsis or other dysfunction.

Body temperature regulation can also be influenced by thermal sensors located in the trigeminal area of the face and on the forehead. When the infant's face is exposed to a cool environmental temperature, even though the body is adequately warmed, these temperature-stimulation zones respond as though the infant is cold stressed and may cause heat loss by convection. ***Convective heat loss*** also occurs when infants are exposed to increased air flow velocity and turbulence (e.g., drafts from doors, ventilation system, opening and closing incubator portholes and side panels). The infant being cared for in a radiant warmer will also experience convective heat losses in response to ventilation drafts and traffic flow around the bed; these losses may be partially countered with plastic wrap placed directly on the infant's body or stretched over the side guards of the warmer unit (Blackburn and Loper, 1992) (Fig. 10-4). Oxygen or any source of air, such as an oxygen mask or tube, should not blow directly on the infant's face. Oxygen concentrated around the head, such as that supplied to a hood, must be warmed and humidified.

Radiant heat loss is one of the greatest threats to temperature regulation in the incubator, since the temperature of circulating air within has no influence on heat loss to cooler surfaces without, such as windows, walls, or a lower nursery temperature. Such losses can be effectively reduced with the use of double-walled incubators; the infant will radiate heat to the inner wall, which is surrounded by the warmed incubator air. The use of a dark cloth incubator cover further reduces radiant heat loss and provides some protection from exterior light sources (Nelson, Thomas, and Stein, 1992). Appropriate physiologic monitoring (cardiorespiratory and pulse oximetry) will alert the nurse to any problems the infant may be experiencing while in the darkened environment, which would, of course, warrant visual assessment of the infant's status (see Critical Thinking Exercise box).

A high-humidity atmosphere contributes to body temperature maintenance by reducing ***evaporative heat loss***. Humidity is provided in some incubators by air circulating over a heated water reservoir, which has the additional advantage of decreasing heat loss by convection as the air flows over the infant. Since stagnant, warm water provides an ex-

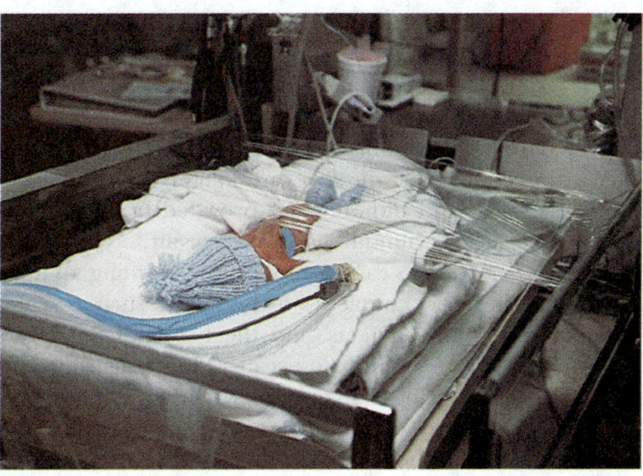

FIG. 10-4 Infant under plastic wrap, which produces a draft-free environment.

CRITICAL THINKING EXERCISE

Thermoregulation

A 24-day-old 3-pound preterm infant in a servocontrolled incubator has consistently lost 30 to 50 g over the last 2 days following 2 weeks of adequate weight gain with gavage feedings. In addition, the environmental temperature in the incubator has steadily increased by 5° C while the infant's axillary temperature has ranged from 36.4° to 36.5° C (97.5° to 97.7° F). The incubator is located near a doorway of the NICU leading to an outer hallway; there is heavy traffic through this doorway. Other vital signs have remained consistently stable, and the incubator has been verified by engineers to be functioning properly. A possible explanation for the infant's increased environmental temperature control and appropriate intervention is:

1. Servocontrol is not effective in maintaining this size infant's temperature; use air temperature control.
2. Air drafts from the doorway traffic and single-walled incubator increase radiant heat loss; a double-walled incubator should be used. An alternative is to use a cloth incubator cover and move the incubator away from the doorway.
3. The infant's larger body surface is creating conductive heat loss; wrap the infant snugly in a cotton blanket inside the incubator.
4. The infant more than likely has suffered damage to the central nervous system, such as an intraventricular hemorrhage, causing subsequent thermal instability; monitor the infant for signs of seizure activity.

The correct answer is 2. Air drafts created by air vents and doors and staff traffic can cause radiant heat loss from the infant's warm body surface to the cooled exterior single wall of the incubator, subsequently increasing the demand for environmental temperature to maintain the infant's core body temperature.

This increased metabolic demand for energy leaves fewer calories available for growth.

Options 1 and 3 are not factual statements. Option 4 is unlikely, primarily because of the infant's age and stable vital signs.

cellent breeding medium for microorganisms, the reservoir is emptied every 8 to 24 hours and replaced with sterile distilled water. The recommended humidity is 50% to 65%; higher humidity and a warmer environment are recommended for VLBW infants. Because of the ever-present danger of infection, most nurseries no longer use water in incubators. Heat and humidity are provided from an external source such as humidified oxygen or air.

Conductive heat loss can be reduced by warming all items that come in direct contact with the infant, such as scales, radiographic film, blankets, and the hands of caregivers. Warming the items before use can reduce this source of heat loss (e.g., storing blankets in a warming unit ready for use and placing a freestanding warming unit or a heat lamp over a scale before weighing an infant).

While the open radiant warmer unit allows easier access to the infant, there is an inherent increase in evaporative water loss (and evaporative heat loss) from the skin, especially in ELBW and VLBW infants. Transepidermal water losses (also called insensible water loss [IWL]) may be increased by as much as 50% to 200%, thus predisposing the infant to dehydration; daily fluid requirements are generally increased to compensate for such losses. The use of plastic wrap over the ELBW or VLBW infant in a radiant warmer will help reduce IWL and convective losses. Plexiglass heat shields are not recommended for use in radiant warmers, since they block radiant heat waves (Blackburn and Loper, 1992).

The infant being cared for in a radiant warmer is kept warm using the servocontrol method; air temperature control is only recommended for brief periods. A reflective aluminum temperature probe cover is used to allow proper function of the servocontrol heating unit. The temperature probe is placed over the liver or between the umbilicus and symphysis pubis; placing the probe over areas of brown fat density and bony prominences will result in inaccurate skin temperature readings. As with incubators used in servocontrol, a dislodged probe or placing the infant prone over the skin probe will cause inaccurate skin temperature readings and subsequently hypothermia or hyperthermia, with either being undesirable. The use of sterile cloth or disposable drapes will also block radiant heat waves in a radiant warmer; during such procedures the use of a warmed blanket under the infant is appropriate. Clothing an infant on servocontrol in an incubator or radiant warmer is not recommended; head covering and foot covering (socks or booties) may be used with discretion.

Prolonged exposure to cold stress in the sick or preterm infant may have disastrous results from which recovery may not be possible, particularly in the ELBW or VLBW infant. Hyperthermia may cause equally untoward effects, since high-risk infants typically have a limited ability to sweat; thus heat dissipation is decreased. In high-risk neonates hyperthermia is usually a result of overheating rather than hypermetabolism. Therefore adequate knowledge of the proper care and use of external heating devices, such as a radiant warmer or an incubator, is as important as the knowledge of the conditions for which they are being used.

There is increasing evidence that ***skin-to-skin (kangaroo) contact*** between the stable preterm infant and parent is a viable option for interaction because of the maintenance of appropriate body temperature by the infant (Merenstein and Gardner, 1993). Other benefits of skin-to-skin contact are discussed later in this chapter.

Protection from Infection

Protection from infection is an integral part of all newborn care, but preterm and sick neonates are particularly susceptible. The protective environment of a regularly cleaned and changed incubator provides effective isolation from airborne infective agents. However, thorough, meticulous, and frequent handwashing is the foundation of a preventive program. This includes *all* persons who come in contact with infants and their equipment. After handling another infant or equipment, no one ever touches an infant without first washing hands.

Personnel with infectious disorders are either barred from the unit until they are no longer infectious or are required to wear suitable shields, such as masks or gloves, to reduce the likelihood of contamination. In some areas annual influenza vaccination is recommended for NICU personnel. Universal precautions as a method of infection control are instituted in all nursery areas to protect the infants and staff (see Chapter 27). In some areas special clothing furnished by the institution is worn by everyone working in the unit. Fresh scrub dresses or suits are put on before entering the unit and are changed any time they become contaminated. When personnel leave the unit, the scrub clothing is protected by a cover gown that is removed and then discarded in the laundry hamper before the wearer reenters the unit. However, the benefit of "gowning" to control infection is not supported by research (American Academy of Pediatrics and American College of Obstetricians and Gynecologists, 1992).

The sources of infection rise in direct relationship to the number of persons and pieces of equipment coming in contact with the infants. Equipment used in the care of infants is cleaned on a regular basis as per the manufacturer's recommendations or institutional protocol; this includes cleaning of cribs, mattresses, incubators, radiant warmers, cardiorespiratory monitors, pulse oximeters, and Dinamap monitors after usage with one infant and before usage with another. Since organisms thrive best in water, plumbing and humidifying equipment are particularly hazardous. Disposable equipment used for water-related therapies, such as nebulizers and plastic oxygen tubing, is changed regularly.

Periodic epidemiologic studies (at least quarterly or monthly is recommended) are carried out in the NICU to evaluate the incidence and types of nosocomial infections, number and types of bacteria colonized from indwelling lines (catheters) and blood, endotracheal tube (ET) secretion, and cerebrospinal (CSF) fluid cultures. Specific trends are monitored and reported to the proper institutional authorities. Readmission of infants from home or admission of unsterile deliveries or infants suspected of having communicable illness are handled per institutional protocol; such infants, however, should be at least physically isolated from other highly susceptible high-risk infants until a diagnosis is established (see American Academy of Pediatrics and American College of Obstetricians and Gynecologists [1992] for further infection control recommendations, including nursery care of infants with specific communicable diseases).

Hydration

It is not uncommon for high-risk infants to receive supplemental parenteral fluids to supply additional calories, electrolytes, and/or water. Adequate hydration is particularly important in preterm infants because their extracellular water content is higher (70% in full-term infants and up to 90% in preterm infants), their body surface is larger, and the capacity for osmotic diuresis is limited in preterm infants' underdeveloped kidneys. Therefore these infants are highly vulnerable to water depletion.

Parenteral fluids may be given to the high-risk neonate via several routes depending on the nature of the illness, the duration and type of fluid therapy, and institutional (or NICU) preference. Common routes of fluid infusion include peripheral, peripherally inserted central venous, surgically inserted central venous or arterial, and, at times, umbilical venous or umbilical arterial catheterization. The preferred sites for intravenous (IV) infusions in neonates are peripheral veins on the dorsal surfaces of hands or feet. Alternative sites are scalp veins and antecubital veins. Special precautions and frequent observations (at least once every hour) must accompany the use of peripheral lines with hypertonic solutions (dextrose 10% to 15%) and hyperalimentation. If peripheral sites are exhausted by long-term therapy, percutaneous central venous lines or a venous cutdown (usually inserted in the saphenous or antecubital vein) may be employed. The increased use of small-gauge percutaneous catheters has reduced the need for the cutdown option.

In most facilities NICU nurses insert peripheral IV catheters, as well as maintain the infusions. IVs must always be delivered by continuous infusion pumps that deliver minute volumes at a preset flow rate. The catheter/needle is secured to the skin with transparent tape, with care taken not to cause undue pressure from the needle hub and tubing. Since ELBW and VLBW infants are highly vulnerable to any fluid shifts, the infusion rates are very carefully regulated and are checked hourly to prevent tissue damage from extravasation, fluid overload, or dehydration. Pulmonary edema, congestive heart failure, patent ductus arteriosus, and intraventricular hemorrhage may occur with fluid overload. Dehydration may cause electrolyte disturbances (particularly Na^+), with potentially serious central nervous system (CNS) effects.

Small, fragile peripheral blood vessels are subject to rupture and subsequent infiltration. This situation is compounded by the use of continuous infusion pumps that continue to infuse fluid into surrounding tissues. Observations are especially important when using hypertonic solutions (calcium, sodium bicarbonate, albumina 25%) and IV drugs (antibiotics and vasoactive drugs such as dopamine and dobutamine), which can cause severe tissue damage. With the increased use of flexible catheters and small armboards, the use of limb restraints has lessened; if used, restraints are checked frequently to ensure that no harm to the patient's extremity occurs and that peripheral circulation is adequate.

➤ **NURSING TIP** A small armboard for the hand may be made by cutting a tongue blade in half (lengthwise) and padding it with gauze.

NURSING ALERT Nurses should be constantly alert for signs of infiltration (such as redness, edema, or color change of tissue, blanching at site) and for signs of overhydration (weight gain over 30 g/24 hr, periorbital edema, tachypnea, tachycardia, and moist crackles on lung auscultation).

Infants who are ELBW, tachypneic, receiving phototherapy, or in a radiant warmer have increased insensible water losses, which require appropriate fluid adjustments. Nurses must monitor fluid status by daily (or more frequent) weights, accurate intake and output of all fluids, including medications and blood products, specific gravity, dipstick measurements of urine, and evaluation of serum electrolyte levels. ELBW infants will often require more frequent monitoring of these parameters because of their inordinate fluid loss, immature renal function, and propensity to dehydration or overhydration. Intolerance of even dextrose 5% is not uncommon in the ELBW infant, with subsequent glycosuria and osmotic diuresis. Alterations in behavior, alertness, and/or activity level in these infants receiving intravenous fluids may signal an electrolyte imbalance, hypoglycemia, or hyperglycemia; the nurse is also observant for tremors or seizures in the VLBW or ELBW infant, since this may be a sign of hyponatremia or hypernatremia.

A common problem observed in infants who have an umbilical catheter in place is vasoconstriction of peripheral vessels that can seriously impair circulation. The response is triggered by arterial vasospasm caused by the presence of the catheter, the infusion of fluids, or injection of medication. Blanching of the buttocks, genitalia, or legs or feet is an indication of vasospasm. The problem is recognized promptly and reported to the practitioner. The nurse must also observe for signs of thrombi in infants with umbilical venous or arterial lines. The precipitation of microthrombi in the vascular bed with the use of such catheters is commonly manifested by a sudden bluish discoloration seen in the toes, called "cath toes." The problem is promptly reported to the practitioner, since failure to alleviate the existing pathology may result in the loss of toes or even a foot or leg.

NURSING ALERT Circulatory effects are observed first in the toes but may extend to include the legs and buttocks. The toes first flush and then turn a mulberry color, and if the condition is not corrected, there may be serious complications involving the loss of a limb. The infant with an umbilical venous or arterial catheter should also be observed closely for catheter dislodging and subsequent bleeding or hemorrhage; urinary output, renal function, and gastrointestinal (GI) function are also evaluated in these infants. While the intent of such catheters is to effectively deliver intravenous fluids (and sometimes medications) and to obtain arterial blood gas samples, they are not without inherent complications.

TABLE 10-2 Characteristics, Problems, and Management Related to Selected Nutrients for the Preterm Infant

CHARACTERISTIC	PROBLEM	MANAGEMENT
Deficiency of proteolytic enzymes	Difficulty digesting casein protein	Feed whey-predominant formula or human milk
Low lactase activity	Poor digestion of lactose, providing substrate for bacterial growth in lower intestinal tract; distention from osmotic effect of lactose	Provide low lactose; feed glucose polymers
Pancreatic lipase; low bile salt levels	Unable to digest and absorb saturated triglycerides	Feed unsaturated medium-chain triglycerides, human milk; provide supplemental vitamin E
Poor sodium conservation	Hyponatremia	Feedings higher in sodium
Rapid bone growth and mineralization	Osteopenia; rickets	Feedings higher in calcium and phosphorus; supplemental vitamin D
Low zinc and copper levels	Skin lesions Related to poor fat absorption	Feed easily digested fats Feedings with adequate zinc and other trace minerals
Low iron	Anemia	Provide supplemental iron
Poor muscle tone of cardiac sphincter	Regurgitation: trigger chemoreceptors (apnea); vagal stimulation (bradycardia)	Semiupright position during feeding; feed small amounts Place prone, with head of bed elevated 30 to 45 degrees after feedings
Limited stomach capacity	Inadequate intake Distention	Small, frequent feedings; continuous gavage feeding Nutrient supplementation Parenteral nutrition
Noncoordination of suck/swallow/gag reflexes	Aspiration Inadequate intake	Alternative feeding methods—gavage Oral exercises
Muscle weakness	Exhaustion	Alternative feeding methods (such as bolus or continuous gavage)

Nutrition

Optimum nutrition is critical in the management of LBW preterm infants, but there are difficulties in providing for their nutritional needs. The various mechanisms for ingestion and digestion of foods are not fully developed, and the more immature the infant, the greater the problem. In addition, the nutritional requirements for this group of infants are not known with certainty. It is known that all preterm infants are at risk because of poor nutritional stores and several physical and developmental characteristics.

Physiologic Characteristics. An infant's need for rapid growth and daily maintenance must be met in the presence of several anatomic and physiologic disabilities. Although some sucking and swallowing activities are demonstrated before birth and in premature infants, coordination of these mechanisms does not occur until approximately 32 to 34 weeks of gestation, and they are not fully synchronized until 36 to 37 weeks. Initial sucking is not accompanied by swallowing, and esophageal contractions are uncoordinated. The gag reflex may not be developed until 36 weeks of gestation. Consequently, infants are highly prone to aspiration and its attendant dangers. As infants mature, the suck-swallow pattern develops but is slow and ineffectual, and these reflexes may also become easily exhausted.

As with most full-term infants, preterm infants have poor muscle tone in the area of the inferior esophageal (cardiac) sphincter. This causes milk in the stomach to be easily regurgitated into the esophagus, where it can trigger the chemoreceptors and cause apnea (vagal stimulation) and bradycardia, and increase the risk of aspiration. The stomach has a very limited capacity in preterm infants and is easily overdistended, further compromising respiration.

Physiologically preterm infants have approximately the same capacity to digest and absorb protein as full-term infants. However, carbohydrates and fats are less well tolerated. The secretion of lactase, a late-developing enzyme, is low in infants born before 34 weeks of gestation; therefore formulas containing lactose may not be well tolerated. Although amylase is deficient in preterm infants, an alternative enzyme (glucoamylase) is able to compensate in most neonates so that they are able to tolerate moderate amounts of starch. Preterm infants are inefficient in digesting and absorbing lipids, especially the saturated triglycerides of cow's milk, because they have low levels of pancreatic lipase and low bile acid. Characteristics and problems related to immaturity are summarized in Table 10-2.

Nutritional Needs. The demand for nutrients in LBW infants is much higher than that in larger infants, and individual infants vary in activity level, ease of achieving basal energy expenditure, thermoneutrality, physical condition, and efficacy of nutrient absorption. The American Academy of Pediatrics, Committee on Nutrition (1985) supports the

TABLE 10-3 Estimated Caloric Requirement in Typical, Growing Premature Infants

CALORIC EXPENDITURE	kcal/kg/day
Resting caloric expenditure	50
Intermittent activity	15
Occasional cold stress	10
Specific dynamic action	8
Fecal loss of calories	12
Growth allowance	25
TOTAL	120

Modified from Committee on Nutrition, American Academy of Pediatrics: Nutritional needs of low-birth-weight infants, *Pediatrics* 75:976-986, 1985.

caloric requirements of preterm infants shown in Table 10-3. Since most of the nutritional stores are accumulated in the final months of gestation, preterm infants are also hampered by low stores of calcium, iron, phosphorus, proteins, and vitamins A and C.

The amount and method of feeding are determined by the size and condition of the infant. Nutrition can be provided by either the parenteral or the enteral route or by a combination of the two. Infants who are ELBW, VLBW, and/or critically ill are often fed exclusively by the parenteral route because of their inability to digest and absorb enteral nutrition. Illness factors resulting in hypoxia and major organ immaturity further preclude the use of enteral feeding until the infant's condition is stabilized; necrotizing enterocolitis has been associated with enteral feedings in acutely ill or distressed infants (see section on necrotizing enterocolitis in this chapter).

Total parenteral nutritional support of acutely ill infants may be accomplished quite successfully with commercially available intravenous solutions specifically designed to meet the infant's nutritional needs, including protein, amino acids, trace minerals, vitamins, carbohydrates (dextrose), and fat (lipid emulsion) (Merenstein and Gardner, 1993). Daily monitoring of weight, electrolytes, renal function, calcium, triglycerides (or lipoprotein), and hydration status is carried out to ensure adequate therapy.

There is still some controversy regarding the type of enteral feeding that best meets the nutritional needs of LBW infants. The predominant view supports the use of milk from an infant's own mother or modified infant formulas. Commercial formulas have been designed specifically to meet the needs of small preterm infants (see Table 8-5) and provide for adequate growth and metabolic stability (studies reported by the American Academy of Pediatrics, Committee on Nutrition, 1985). Prepared formulas have the added advantage of allowing more concentrated feedings.

Evidence indicates that milk produced by mothers whose infants are born before term contains higher concentrations of protein, sodium, and chloride (Anderson, Atkinson, and Bryan, 1981; Gross and others, 1980) and an immunoglobulin A. Thus mothers appear to be the preferred source of milk for their preterm infants. Growth factors, hormones, prolactin, calcitonin, thyroxine, steroids, and taurine, an essential amino acids, are also found in human milk (Merenstein and Gardner, 1993). The milk produced by mothers for their infants changes in content over the first 30 days postnatally, at which time it is similar to full-term human milk (Blackburn and Loper, 1992). Infants fed with their own mother's milk displayed a more rapid rate of growth in all parameters and required a shorter length of time to regain birth weight (Gross, Oehler, and Eckerman, 1983). Human milk supplements are available for infants receiving breast milk who require additional calories and nutrients.

The antiinfectious attributes of human milk provide additional advantages for preterm infants. Secretory immunoglobulin A (IgA) concentration is higher in the milk from mothers of preterm infants than in the milk from mothers of full-term infants. Immunoglobulin A is important in the control of bacteria in the intestinal tract, where it inhibits adherence and proliferation of bacteria at epithelial surfaces (Gross and others, 1981). Additional protection from infection is provided by leukocytes, lactoferrin, and lysozyme, all of which are in human milk. Finally, the psychologic advantages of using the milk from an infant's own mother cannot be overlooked.

The use of donor human milk must be carefully evaluated in reference to transmission of infections such as cytomegalovirus and human immunodeficiency virus (HIV). Pasteurization of donor human milk appears to kill the HIV virus, but it also is harmful to leukocytes, milk lipids, and lactoferrin (Beckholt, 1990).

Although the timing of the first feeding has been a matter of controversy, most authorities now believe that early feeding, usually within 3 to 6 hours after birth (provided that the infant is medically stable), reduces the incidence of complicating factors such as hypoglycemia, dehydration, and the degree of hyperbilirubinemia. The feeding regimen employed varies from institution to institution. The initial enteral feeding is usually not attempted until infants have adapted to extrauterine existence as evidenced by adequate oxygenation, evidence of GI motility, including passage of meconium, and stable cardiopulmonary status.

Nipple Feeding. Vigorous infants can be fed from a nipple with little difficulty, whereas weaker preterm infants will require alternative methods. Sterile water may be offered first. The amount to be fed is determined largely by the infant's weight and tolerance of previous feeding and is increased by small increments until a satisfactory caloric intake is ensured. Sometimes supplementary calories are needed in the form of dietary additives, such as Lipomul* (which provides vegetable fat and carbohydrates), MCT oil† (which provides fat in the form of medium-chain triglycerides), Polycose, and human milk fortifier or formula with increased caloric density.

The rate of increase that is well tolerated varies from one infant to another, and determining this rate is often a nursing responsibility. Preterm infants require more time and patience to feed as compared with full-term infants, and the oral-pharyngeal mechanism may be stressed by an attempt

*Roberts Pharmaceutical Corp., Eatontown, NJ.
†Mead Johnson & Co., Evansville, IN.

CRITICAL THINKING EXERCISE
Infant Feeding

The mother of a 4-pound, 36-week preterm infant who has only recently started nipple feeding expresses concern that the feeding takes 25 to 30 minutes and that the infant has one or two apneic episodes during feedings. The infant is gaining approximately 20 to 30 g per day, and axillary temperature has been 36.6° C (97.9° F) throughout the day. To assist the mother in understanding aspects of feeding a preterm infant, your best response should be to:

1. Suggest that the mother let the experienced nurse feed the infant until the mother learns to feed correctly.
2. Recommend that the mother use a softer, pliable nipple to allow the infant to feed faster.
3. Encourage the mother to continue feeding the infant, with frequent rest periods or pauses.
4. Explain to the mother that the infant will require all feedings to be given by gavage, since the infant is so small and has apnea.

The correct answer is 3. It is not uncommon for preterm infants to experience apnea with nipple feedings. Frequent short breaks in feeding allow for swallowing and breathing to occur.

Option 2 is incorrect—a soft nipple is not desirable, and expediency in feeding is not always the major goal. Since the infant is demonstrating adequate weight gain, there is no reason to gavage feed or suspect pathologic apnea as suggested in Option 4. Option 1 is incorrect because it discounts the mother's involvement in the care of her infant.

to feed too rapidly. It is important not to tire the infants or overtax their capacity to retain the feedings. When infants require a prolonged time period (arbitrarily over 30 to 45 minutes) to complete a feeding, gavage feeding may be considered for the next time (see Critical Thinking Exercise box).

Tolerance related to the infant's ability to nipple feed should be based on an evaluation of respiratory status, heart rate, and oxygen saturation; variations from normal may indicate stress and fatigue (Davis, 1992). The preterm infant will experience difficulty coordinating sucking, swallowing, and breathing, with resultant apnea, bradycardia, and decreased oxygen saturation. The preterm infant's ability to suck on a pacifier does not indicate complete readiness for nipple feeding or ability to coordinate the above-mentioned activities without some degree of stress; a gradual introduction of nippling in the preterm infant is based on careful evaluation of his or her ability to maintain adequate cardiopulmonary functions while nippling (VanderBerg, 1990). When infants are unable to tolerate bottle-feedings, intermittent feedings by gavage are instituted until they gain enough strength and coordination to use the nipple.

NURSING ALERT Poor feeding behaviors such as apnea, bradycardia, cyanosis, pallor, and decreased oxygen saturation in any infant who has previously fed well may indicate an underlying illness.

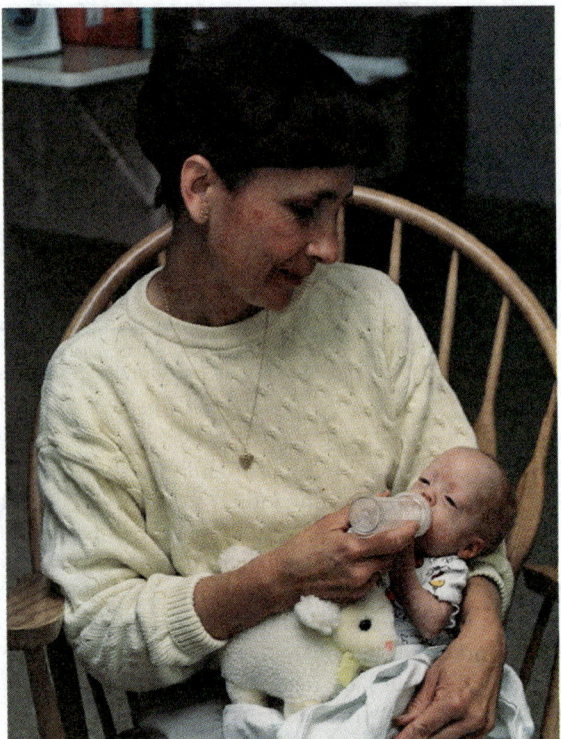

FIG. 10-5 Position for nipple-feeding premature infant.

The nipple used should be relatively firm and stable. A high-flow, pliable nipple, although it requires less energy to use, may provide a flow rate that is too rapid for some preterm infants to manage without risk of aspiration. A firmer nipple facilitates a more "cupped" tongue configuration and allows for a more controlled, manageable flow rate.

The infant is positioned in the feeder's arms or placed semiupright in the lap (Fig. 10-5), and is held with the back curved slightly to simulate the position assumed naturally by most full-term newborns. Stroking the infant's lips, cheeks, and tongue before feeding helps promote oral sensitivity. Inward and upward support to the infant's cheeks and a slightly upward lift to the chin are provided by the fingers to assist nipple compression during feeding (Shaker, 1990).

Bottle-feedings are continued if infants are able to tolerate the feedings and take the required amount. The infant is best fed when fully alert. Drowsy infants feed more slowly, and liquid is more likely to fill the relaxed pharynx before the infant swallows, causing choking (Shaker, 1990). It is believed that many digestive powers require signal stimulation to respond. Some premature infants respond more slowly than full-term infants; therefore the feeding interval, as well as the amount of the feeding, is individualized. Preterm infants are often slow feeders, requiring patience, frequent rest periods, and burping (or bubbling).

NURSING ALERT An increase in gastric residuals, abdominal distention, bilious vomiting, temperature instability, apneic episodes, and bradycardia may indicate early necrotizing enterocolitis (NEC) and should be called to the attention of the practitioner.

Breast-Feeding. Studies indicate that even small preterm infants are able to breast-feed if the infant has adequate sucking and swallowing reflexes and there are no other contraindications, such as respiratory complications, or concurrent illness (Meier and Anderson, 1987; Meier and Pugh, 1985). Mothers who wish to breastfeed their preterm infants are encouraged to pump their breasts until their infants are sufficiently stable to tolerate breast-feeding. Appropriate guidelines for the storage of expressed mother's milk (EMM) should be followed to decrease the risk of milk contamination and destruction of its beneficial properties (Beckholt, 1990). Premature infants are able to breast-feed when they (Gardner, O'Donnell, and Weisman, 1993):

- Experience wakeful periods and awaken before feedings
- Exhibit coordinated suck, swallow, and gag reflexes
- Have supplemental oxygen supplied by flow-by or nasal cannula
- Have adequate thermal support provided by swaddler, hat, or overhead radiant warmer

Time, patience, and dedication on the part of the mother and the nursing staff are needed to help infants with breast-feeding. The process is begun slowly—beginning with one feeding daily and gradually increasing the feedings as the infant tolerates them. Infants should not be placed on an empty breast to feed, since the infant will become exhausted, and nonnutritive sucking (NNS) does not stimulate milk production. The infant will become frustrated and refuse to feed without the reward of milk. Supplementary bottle feeding is inefficient, since the baby expends energy and calories to feed twice. Feeding more often, supplementing by gavage feeding, or using a training nipple is more energy and calorically efficient. Breastfeeding of the preterm infant often requires additional guidance by a lactation consultant; continued support and encouragement by the nursing staff is essential to breastfeeding preterm infants. In addition, postdischarge breastfeeding often requires further guidance, counseling, and support by nursing staff (Davis, 1992; Meier and others, 1993).

Gavage Feeding. Gavage feeding is a safe means of meeting the nutritional requirements of infants who are less than 32 weeks of gestation or infants who weigh less than 1500 g. These infants are usually too weak to suck effectively, are unable to coordinate swallowing, and lack a gag reflex. Gavage feedings may be provided by continuous drip regulated via infusion pump or by intermittent bolus feedings. Recent investigations, however, did show an overall decrease in total milk fat concentration delivery when continuous gavage infusions were administered, suggesting that intermittent gavage of EMM be administered when possible (Brennan-Behm, and others, 1994). For infants learning to nipple feed and who become excessively tired, are listless, or become cyanotic, intermittent gavage feeding is used as an energy-conserving technique.

A 15-inch (37.5 cm) size 5 or 8 French feeding tube is used to instill the formula, and the usual methods for determining correct placement are employed (see Chapter 27 for technique). Although the more relaxed cardiac sphincter makes passage of the tube easier, there may be changes in heart rate and blood pressure in response to vagal stimulation. The procedure is best accomplished when an infant is in a prone or a right side-lying position with the head slightly elevated. It is preferable to insert the tube through the mouth rather than the nares. Nasal insertion obstructs nose breathing and may irritate the delicate nasal mucosa. Passage through the mouth also provides an opportunity to observe the sucking response. However, because of less stimulation of the gag reflex, nasal tube gavage may be used in certain situations, such as in older preterm infants who need supplementation after nipple feeding but who fight, gag, and vomit with oral tube management.

The stomach is aspirated, the contents measured, and the aspirate returned as part of the feeding. The amount of the aspirate depends on the length of time since the previous feeding or concurrent illness. Whether or not the amount of the aspirate is deducted from the total feeding varies among units. Some advocate deducting to avoid overdistending the stomach. For example, if a feeding is 25 ml and the aspirate is 5 ml, the aspirate is returned plus 20 ml of feeding for a total of 25 ml. In other units the amount is determined on an individual basis.

The formula is allowed to flow by gravity, and the length of time varies. This procedure is not used as a timesaving method for the nurse. Complications of indwelling tubes include the obstructed nares, mucous plugs, purulent rhinitis, epistaxis, infection, and possible stomach perforation.

The nurse needs to observe premature infants closely for behaviors that indicate readiness for bottle-feedings. These include (1) a strong, vigorous suck; (2) coordination of sucking and swallowing; (3) a gag reflex; (4) sucking on the gavage tube, hands, or pacifier; and (5) rooting and wakefulness before and sleeping after feedings. When these behaviors are noted, infants can be challenged with nipple feedings introduced slowly.

The infant may be held during gavage feedings by the caregiver or parent (Fig. 10-6). Oxygen may be supplied via nasal cannula to facilitate handling. It is not recommended that the infant be removed from a primary source of oxygen, such as a hood or tent, for feedings, since this decreases oxygen availability. Flow-by oxygen may be given for brief episodes of desaturation, but this is inadequate for the duration of feedings, either by gavage or nipple. Also, NNS on a pacifier helps infants associate the sucking with the feeling of satiety. When compared with other LBW infants, those who are allowed NNS are ready for bottle-feeding earlier, require fewer tube feedings, demonstrate better weight gain, are discharged earlier, and have fewer complications. NNS also increases oxygenation during tube feeding.

Feeding Resistance

Any feeding technique that bypasses the mouth precludes the opportunity for the affected child to "practice sucking and swallowing, or the opportunity to experience normal hunger and satiation cycles." Infants may demonstrate aversion to oral feedings by such behaviors as averting the head to the presentation of the nipple, extruding the nipple by tongue thrust, gagging, or even vomiting.

Developmental delays have been noted in the areas of

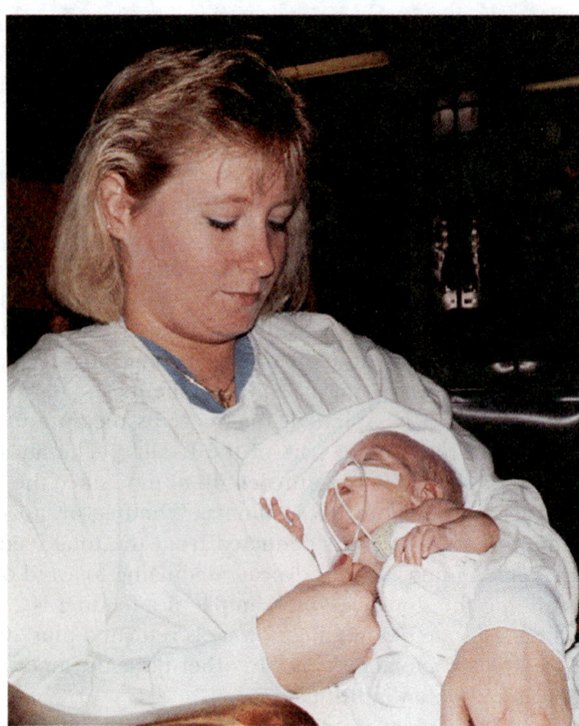

FIG. 10-6 Infant held during gavage feeding. Note oxygen source held in the vicinity of the face.

COMPONENTS OF A CARE PLAN TO OVERCOME FEEDING RESISTANCE

Simulate normal feeding interactions.
- Hold and cuddle infant in "en face" feeding position.
- Engage in eye contact with infant.
- Engage in verbal interaction with infant.

Provide tactile stimulation.
- Begin with torso and progress to head and neck.
- Apply firm, consistent pressure.
- Use palm or hand or textured object (e.g., washcloth).
- Gradually move toward mouth, cheeks, and lips.
- Stroke oral area from cheeks to lips.
- Pace according to child's tolerance.

Overcome oral hypersensitivity (sensitivity to intraoral stimulation).
- Provide oral stimulation as above.
- When external oral stimulation is tolerated, attempt massage of gums and tongue (use finger or soft rubber item).
- Massage gums from center and move toward molar region, and move gradually from anterior to posterior.
- Withdraw stimulus and close child's mouth if child gags.

Encourage oral exploration.
- Assist child in mouthing hands, fingers, toes, or soft rubber toys.
- Play oral games (e.g., blowing a kiss, kissing an object [toy animal]).

Provide oral feedings.
- Introduce small volumes (even 3 to 5 ml) as early as possible.
- Offer feedings consistently (water, formula).
- Avoid force feeding.

Provide feeding stimulation during tube feedings.
- Hold child in feeding position.
- Provide oral stimulation during bolus feedings.
- Give oral feedings before tube feedings.
- Give bolus feedings in response to hunger when possible rather than on predetermined schedule.

Provide nonnutritive sucking to encourage use of oral musculature.

Data from Orr MJ, Allen SS: Optimal oral experiences for infants on long-term total parenteral nutrition, *Nutr Clin Pract* 9:288-295, 1986.

perceptual-motor performance as measured by standard tests, although the area of intellectual function measured within normal limits (O'Connor, Ralston, and Ament, 1988). Other observations include disinterest in or active resistance to oral play, diminished spontaneity and motivation, and shallow interpersonal relationships, probably related to the absence of some early incorporative patterns of normal oral experiences. The longer the period of nonoral feeding, the more severe the feeding problems, especially if this period occurs during the time when the infant progresses from reflexive to learned and voluntary feeding actions (Orr and Allen, 1986). Infancy is the period during which the mouth is the primary instrument for reception of stimulation and pleasure.

Infants who are identified as being at risk for feeding resistance should be provided with regular oral stimulation based on the child's developmental level. Those who exhibit feeding aversion should begin a stimulation program to overcome resistance and acquire the ability to take nourishment by the oral route. Since management requires long-term commitment, successful implementation of a plan for oral stimulation depends on maximum parental involvement and promotion of primary nursing (Orr and Allen, 1986). Key components and interventions are listed in the box above, right.

Energy Conservation

One of the major goals of care for the high-risk infant is conservation of energy. Much of the care described in this section is directed toward this end (e.g., disturbing the infant as little as possible, maintaining a neutral thermal environment, employing gavage feeding, promoting oxygenation, and judiciously implementing any caregiving activities that increase oxygen and caloric consumption). When the infant is not required to expend energy to cope with efforts to breathe, eat, or alter the body temperature, this energy can be used for growth and development. Diminishing environmental noise levels and shading the infant from bright lights also promote rest (See also Infant Stress, p. 382, and Developmental Intervention, p. 382).

The prone position is optimum for most preterm infants and results in improved oxygenation, better-tolerated feedings, and more organized sleep-rest patterns. Infants exhibit less physical activity and energy expenditure when they are placed in the prone position (Fox and Molesky, 1990; Masterson, Zucker, and Schulze, 1987). Others appear to prefer a flexed side-lying posture. Prolonged supine positioning for preterm infants is not desirable, because they appear to lose their sense of equilibrium when supine and use vital energy in attempts to recover balance by postural changes. However, in light of the American Academy of Pediatrics' recommendation for the supine sleeping position, position preferences should be discussed with the practitioner for home care.

Skin Care

The skin of premature infants is characteristically immature relative to that of full-term infants. Because of its increased sensitivity and fragility, no alkaline-based soap is used that might destroy the "acid mantle" of the skin. The increased permeability of the skin facilitates absorption of ingredients. All skin products (e.g., alcohol or povidone-iodine) are used with caution, and the skin is rinsed with water afterward, since these substances may cause severe irritation and chemical burns in LBW infants.

The skin is easily excoriated and denuded; therefore care

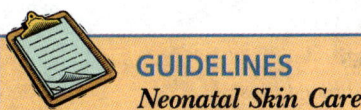

GUIDELINES
Neonatal Skin Care

GENERAL SKIN CARE

Cleanse skin with plain warm water. Use bland, nonalkaline soaps or cleansers only when necessary, such as for removal of stool.

Provide daily cleansing of eye, oral, and diaper areas, and any areas of skin breakdown.

Apply moisturizing agents to skin after cleansing with warm water to retain moisture and rehydrate skin. Cleanse skin gently of any old oil or cream before applying a new layer, except in diaper area (see Diaper Dermatitis, Chapter 13).

When safflower oil is applied, some essential fatty acids may be absorbed in addition to softening skin as a moisturizer.

Use pressure-relieving or reducing mattress to prevent pressure areas (see also Maintaining Healthy Skin, Chapter 27)

USE OF ADHESIVES ON SKIN

Use minimal tape/adhesive. Evaluate need for all tape/adhesive used. Chart amount and placement of all tape used.

Use a protective, pectin-based or hydrocolloid skin barrier between skin and all tape/adhesives. Place on all areas where tape/adhesives are used, such as for securing chest tubes, nasogastric tubes, dressings, extremities to IV board, monitor leads, endotracheal tubes, and temperature probe (cut "keyhole" for temperature probe in barrier or place circular patch of skin barrier over probe).

Place pectin-based or hydrocolloid skin barriers directly over excoriated skin. Leave barrier undisturbed until it begins to peel off. With wet, oozing excoriations, dust site with a small amount of stoma powder (as used in ostomy care), brush excess away, and apply skin barrier. Hold barrier in place for several minutes to allow barrier to soften and mold to the skin surface.

Use transparent elastic film dressings to secure and protect central lines and peripheral arterial line insertion sites, as well as over open skin lesions. Leave dressing in place until it begins to peel off, usually within 5 to 7 days.

Alternate electrode placement and avoid standard adhesive, gelled electrode. Use limb electrodes rather than standard chest electrodes or use hydrogel or synthetic karaya gel electrodes. Assess skin thoroughly underneath electrodes. Remove and rotate electrodes minimally every 24 hours, or more frequently if skin injury is noted.

Remove adhesives with warm water–soaked gauze or a small amount of bland, diluted soap, rather than alcohol or adhesive removers. To remove a skin barrier, slowly and gently peel away from skin, holding barrier in one hand and supporting skin underneath with other hand. If needed, soak off with warm water. Do not use bonding agents such as tincture of benzoin or commercial swabs.

Avoid using scissors to remove tape or dressings to prevent cutting skin or amputating digits.

USE OF SUBSTANCES ON SKIN

Evaluate all substances that come in contact with infant's skin.

Avoid or limit use of the following substances that have potential for percutaneous absorption and systemic effects:

Adhesive removers	Isopropyl alcohol
Boric acid	Neomycin ointment
Chlorhexidene	Povidone iodine
Chlorophenol	Salicylic acid
Epinephrine	Steroids
Estrogen	Tincture of benzoin
Hexachlorophene	Silver sulfadiazine cream
Hydrogen peroxide	

If any of the above agents are used, chart amount and frequency of application.

Before using any topical agent, analyze components of preparation and:
- Use sparingly and only when necessary.
- Confine use to smallest possible area.
- Whenever possible and appropriate, wash off with water.
- Monitor infant carefully for signs of toxicity and systemic effects.

USE OF THERMAL DEVICES

Avoid heat lamps because of increased potential for burns. If needed, measure actual temperature of exposed skin every 15 minutes.

When using heating pads (Aqua-K pads):
- Change infant's position every 15 minutes initially and then every 1 to 2 hours.
- Preset temperature of heating pads <40° C (104° F).

When using preheated transcutaneous electrodes:
- Avoid use on infants <1000 g.
- Set at lowest possible temperature (<44° C [111.2° F]) and secure with plastic wrap.
- Use pulse oximetry rather than transcutaneous monitoring whenever possible.

When prewarming heels before phlebotomy, avoid temperatures >40° C.

Warm ambient humidity, direct away from infant, use aerosolized sterile water, and maintain ambient temperature so as not to exceed 40° C.

Document use of all heating devices.

USE OF FLUID THERAPY/HEMODYNAMIC MONITORING

Be certain fingers or toes are visible whenever extremity is used for IV or arterial line.

Secure catheter or needle with transparent dressing/tape to promote easy visualization of site.

Assess site hourly for signs of ischemia, infiltration, and inadequate perfusion (check capillary refill).

Check that any restraints (e.g., armboards) are secured safely and not restricting circulation or movement (check for pressure areas).

Modified from Malloy MB, Perez-Woods R: Neonatal skin care: prevention of skin breakdown, *Pediatr Nurs* 17(1):41-48, 1991.

must be taken to avoid damage to the delicate structure. The total skin is less thick than that of full-term infants and has fewer elastic fibers; also, there is less cohesion between the thinner skin layers. Adhesives used after heel sticks or to secure monitoring equipment or intravenous infusions may excoriate the skin or adhere to the skin surface so well that the skin can be separated from understructures and pulled away with the tape. The use of skin barriers protects healthy skin and helps excoriated skin heal.

It is unsafe to use scissors to remove dressings or tape from the extremities of very small and immature infants, because it is easy to snip off tiny extremities or nick loosely attached skin. Solvents used to remove tape are avoided because they tend to dry and burn the delicate skin. Guidelines for skin care are listed in the Guidelines box on p. 381.

During skin assessment of preterm infants, nurses are also alert to the subtle signs that indicate zinc deficiency, a common problem in these infants. Breakdown usually occurs in the areas around the mouth, buttocks, fingers, and toes, In VLBW infants it may also occur in the creases of the neck, wrists, ankles, and around wounds. Zinc deficiency is most likely to appear in infants with sepsis, those experiencing nasogastric losses, or those who have had surgery. Any suspicious lesions are reported to the physician so that zinc supplements can be prescribed.

Administration of Medications

Administration of therapeutic agents, such as drugs, ointments, intravenous infusions, and oxygen, requires judicious handling and meticulous attention to details. The computation, preparation, and administration of drugs in minute amounts often require collaboration between nurses to reduce the chance of error. In addition, the immaturity of an infant's detoxification mechanisms and inability to demonstrate symptoms of toxicity (e.g., signs of auditory nerve involvement from ototoxic drugs such as gentamycin) complicate drug therapy and require that nurses be particularly alert for signs of adverse reaction. (See Administration of Medication, Chapter 27.)

Nurses should be aware of the hazards of administering bacteriostatic and hyperosmolar solutions to infants. Benzyl alcohol, a common preservative in bacteriostatic water and saline, has been shown to be toxic to newborns and should not be used to flush intravenous catheters or to dilute or reconstitute medications. It is recommended that medications with preservatives such as benzyl alcohol be avoided whenever possible. Nurses must read labels carefully to detect the presence of preservatives in any medication to be administered to an infant.

Hyperosmolar solutions present a potential danger to preterm infants. Hyperosmolar solutions given orally to infants can produce clinical, physiologic, and morphologic alterations, the most serious of which is necrotizing enterocolitis. Medications (oral or parenteral) should be sufficiently diluted to prevent complications related to hyperosmolality.

Infant Stress

Preterm infants are subject to stress just as other human beings are, but are biologically deficient in their capacity to cope with or adapt to environmental stresses. Stress affects hypothalamus function, causing adverse effects on growth, heat production, and neurologic mechanisms (Gunderson and Kenner, 1987). Interventions designed to reduce stress in premature infants produced improvement in sleeping behavior and growth (see Developmental Intervention and Care, which follows). Nurses can have a profound influence in creating a nonstressful environment by modifying behaviors and environmental factors that produce infant stress in the NICU; for example, gentle handling, correct positioning, and reduction of noxious stimuli (pain relief) help to reduce stress. Alert observation of evidence of stress and providing appropriate intervention help to reduce disorganized behavior (see box above for signs of stress).

SIGNS OF STRESS OR FATIGUE IN NEONATES

AUTONOMIC STRESS

Acrocyanosis
Deep, rapid respirations
Regular, rapid heart rate

CHANGES IN STATE

Dull or sleep states
Crying or fussy
Glassy-eyed or strained alertness

BEHAVIORAL CHANGES

Unfocused and uncoordinated eyes
Limp arms and legs
Flaccid shoulders dropped back
Hiccoughs
Sneezes
Yawning
Straining, having a bowel movement

From Als H: Toward a synactive theory of development: promise for the assessment and support of infant and individuality, *Infant Ment Health J* 3:229-243, 1982.

Developmental Intervention and Care

Much attention has been focused on the effects of early intervention, or its lack, on both normal and preterm infants. Findings indicate that infants are able to respond to a greater variety of stimuli than was previously thought, and that the atmosphere and activities of the NICU are overstimulating. Consequently, infants in the NICU are subjected to *inappropriate* stimulation that may be harmful. For example, the noise level that results from monitoring equipment, alarms, and general unit activity have been correlated with the incidence of intracranial hemorrhage, especially in the ELBW or VLBW infant. Personnel should reduce noise-generating activities, such as closing doors (including incubator portholes), listening to loud radios or talking loudly, and handling equipment (e.g., trash containers). Placing special earmuffs on the infant is also being tried as a method of reducing auditory input. Nursing care activities, such as taking vital signs, changing the infant's position, weighing, and changing diapers, while essential to the care of the high-risk neonate, have been shown to be associated with frequent periods of hypoxia, oxygen desaturation, and elevated intracranial pressure (Peters, 1992). The more im-

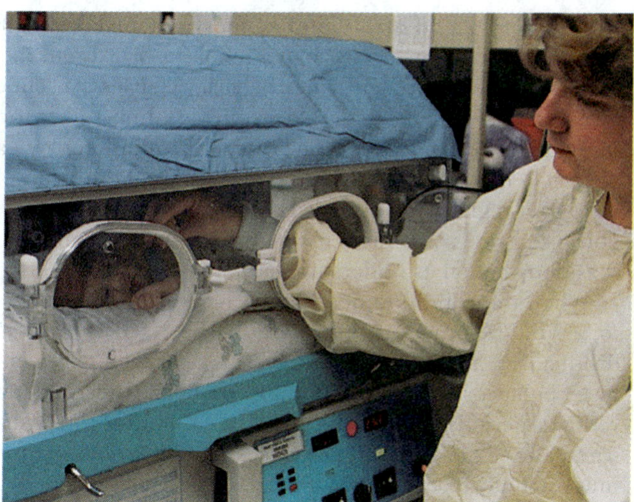

FIG. 10-7 Infant shaded from overhead lights.

BEHAVIORAL MANIFESTATIONS OF DEVELOPMENTAL ORGANIZATION

MOTOR STABILITY BEHAVIORS

Smooth, well-modulated posture and well-modulated tone
Synchronous smooth movements with efficient motoric strategies:
- Hand clasping
- Foot clasping
- Finger folding
- Hand-to-mouth maneuvers
- Grasping
- Suck searching and sucking
- Handholding
- Tucking

STATE STABILITY AND ATTENTION REGULATION BEHAVIORS

Clear, robust sleep states
Rhythmic, robust crying
Good self-quieting or consolability
Robust, focused, shiny-eyed alertness with intent or animated facial expressions, including:
- Frowning
- Cheek softening
- Mouth pursing to "ooh" face
- Cooing
- Attentional smiling

Data from Lawhon G: Management of stress in premature infants. In Angelini DJ, Whelan Knapp CW, Gives KM, editors: *Perinatal/neonatal nursing: a clinical handbook,* Boston, 1986, Blackwell Scientific Publications.

mature the infant, the less able he or she is to habituate to a single procedure, such as taking an oscillometric BP, without becoming overstimulated.

Twenty-four-hour surveillance of sick infants implies maximum visibility and often continuous bright lights. However, many units establish a night-day sleep pattern by either darkening the room, if the infants' conditions allow it, covering cribs with blankets, or placing eye patches over the infant's eyes at night. Infants may have scheduled rest periods during which the lights are dimmed, cribs or incubators are covered with blankets, and the infants are not disturbed for handling of any kind (Strauch, Brandt, and Edwards-Beckett, 1993) (Fig. 10-7).

The present approach to developmental intervention is to tailor the interaction to the developmental level and tolerance of each infant. During the early stages of development (especially before 33 weeks of gestation), stimulation produces uncoordinated, random activity, such as jerky limb extension, hyperflexion, and irregular vital signs. At this stage infants need to have minimum environmental stimulation. They are handled with slow, controlled movements (some infants are unstable if moved abruptly), and their random movements are controlled with limbs held close to their bodies during turning or other position changes. Additional containment measures include support with blanket rolls, when medically feasible. A nest constructed by placing blanket rolls underneath the bed sheet helps infants in maintaining an attitude of flexion when prone or side-lying.

Although it must be individually adjusted, skin contact and short periods of gentle massage can be helpful to reduce stress. Regular passive skin contact (kangaroo care) between parents and LBW infants helps alleviate stress. The parent wears a loose-fitting, open-front top that provides a modified marsupial-like pocket carrier for the infant. The undressed (except for diaper) infant is placed in a vertical position on the parent's bare chest, which permits direct eye contact, skin-to-skin sensations, and close proximity (Affonso, Wahlberg, and Persson, 1989). Skin-to-skin contact between parent and infant, in addition to being a safe and effective method for VLBW infant-parent acquaintance, was perceived in one study as having a positive healing effect for the mother with a high-risk pregnancy. Mothers experienced psychologic healing related to preterm delivery and regained the mothering role through early skin-to-skin contact with their VLBW infants (Affonso and others, 1993). Additional benefits of skin-to-skin care included earlier contact with mechanically ventilated infants, maintenance of neonatal thermal stability, increased feeding vigor, maintenance of organized state, and minimal untoward effects of being held (Gale, Franck, and Lund, 1993; Ludington-Hoe and others, 1994).

When infants have reached sufficient developmental organization and stability (especially between 34 and 36 weeks of gestation) interventions are designed and implemented to support their growing abilities. Nurses become adept at learning to read infants' behavioral clues (see box above) and supplying appropriate interventions. Clues include both approach and avoidance behaviors. Approach behaviors that are supported and enhanced include tongue extension, handclasp, hand-to-mouth movements, sucking, looking, and cooing. Signs of stress or fatigue that signal the infant's need for "time-out" are described in the box on p. 382 and in the Critical Thinking Exercise box on p. 384.

An intervention program for convalescing infants must be individualized and include parents early during the infant's hospitalization; teaching the parents to be responsive to the infant's individual cues is an important function of the NICU nurse (Cusson and Lee, 1994). When infants

CRITICAL THINKING EXERCISE
Developmental Care

You are getting ready to feed a 4-week-old infant born at 28 weeks of gestation. While taking vital signs, you notice that the infant's color is pink but slightly mottled; he is yawning, extending his arms and legs, and splaying his fingers. Oxygen saturation by pulse oximetry indicates a reading within the lower range of normal for this infant. You recognize these behaviors as manifestations of neonatal:

1. Preterm behavior
2. Subtle seizures
3. Stress
4. Onset of infection

The correct answer is 3. Neonates who are preterm may exhibit these signs and others (see box on p. 382) when they are not able to habituate to external stimuli, including routine handling. Alone, these signs do not indicate subtle seizure activity or infection. They are normal preterm behaviors, but only to signal the infant's need for "time out."

are recovering and are free of support systems, medically stable, and on room air or smaller amounts of oxygen, they are assessed to document their behavioral styles. An effective program may be designed to provide limited sensory stimulation involving one or two senses or multisensory experiences that include tactile, visual, auditory, vestibular, olfactory, and gustatory stimuli. The objective of any intervention program is to avoid stressing infants—overstimulation is as detrimental as understimulation.

When the condition of an infant is sufficiently advanced to begin developmental intervention, some activities are individualized according to each infant's cues, temperament, state, behavioral organization, and particular needs. Intervention periods are short (e.g., 1 to 2 minutes of visual stimulation, 2 to 3 minutes of voices, and 5 minutes of quiet music). One type of intervention at a time is applied to document the infant's tolerance and response (see Guidelines box). The types and duration of any stimuli are adjusted on an individual basis, and the parents are involved as early as possible in learning about their infant's particular developmental needs.

Developmental care of the preterm neonate is an ongoing process in the NICU and is incorporated into the daily care given to each infant. The nurse, cognizant of the preterm infant's developmental needs, temperament, and newborn state, as well as environmental conditions that adversely affect the infant, plans nursing care accordingly to enhance optimum physical, psychosocial, and neurologic

GUIDELINES
Developmental Interventions

GENERAL GUIDELINES

Individualize interventions for each infant.
Offer only during periods of alertness.
Begin one type of stimulus at a time.
Provide intervention for short periods.
Space periods according to infant's tolerance.
Continually assess infant's response to developmental interventions.
Titrate interventions according to infant's cues.
Terminate stimulation if infant displays evidence of overstimulation (see box on p. 382)

VISUAL

Place photographs of parents and siblings in visual range (19 to 22 cm) in en face position.
Provide black-and-white mobiles with varied hanging shapes.
Initiate eye contact; repeat as tolerated.
Alternate holding black-and-white pattern still and moving it across infant's visual field.

TACTILE

Stroke skin slowly and gently in head-to-toe direction; begin with trunk and move to more sensitive areas, such as face.
Provide alternate textures (e.g., sheepskin, satin, velvet).
Provide boundaries, foot bracing, blankets.

AUDITORY

Play tape of parents' and siblings' voices.
Softly play classical music, recording of womb sounds, or music box.
Speak with a variety of voice inflections; alternate adult and baby talk.
Call infant by name at each interaction.

VESTIBULAR

Place on water bed with oscillations and waves per minute determined on an individual basis; alternate oscillations with rest periods (may not be acceptable intervention in some units).
Rock in chair.
Place in sling (hammock) and rock.
Provide passive range-of-motion exercises to knee and hip joints.
Close infant's fist around cloth toy.
Lift head to upright position, tip to right and then to left, stopping at midline (only with stable, more mature infants).
Slowly change position during handling.

OLFACTORY

Pass open container of breast milk or formula under nose.
Pass mother's perfume under nose.

GUSTATORY

Place infant's hand or a pacifier in mouth when sucking movements are observed or during gavage feeding.
Place 1 or 2 drops of milk in infant's mouth with each tube feeding.

development. This task is often difficult to accomplish when invasive treatments or interventions are required to essentially stabilize the critically ill neonate.

Family Involvement

Often, professional health workers are so absorbed in the lifesaving physical aspects of care that the emotional needs of infants and their families are ignored. The significance of early parent-child interaction and infant stimulation has been documented by reliable research, and nurses, aware of these infant and family needs, must incorporate activities that facilitate family interaction into the nursing care plan.

The birth of a preterm infant is an unexpected and stressful event for which families are emotionally unprepared. They find themselves simultaneously coping with their own needs, the needs of their infant, and the needs of their families (especially when there are other children). To compound the situation, the precarious nature of their infant's condition engenders an atmosphere of apprehension and uncertainty. They are faced with multiple crises and overwhelming feelings of responsibility, expense, and frustration.

All parents have some anxieties about the outcome of a pregnancy, but following a premature birth the concern is heightened about both the viability and the intactness of their infant. Mothers see their infant only briefly before the newborn is removed to the intensive care unit or even to another hospital, leaving them with just the recollection of the infant's very small size and unusual appearance. They usually feel alone or lost in the maternity ward, belonging neither with mothers who have lost their infants nor with those who delivered healthy, full-term infants. The staff and physicians are often guarded in discussing the infant's condition; mothers are continually expecting to hear that their infant has died, and they are sensitive to the anxieties of other mothers and staff members. Going home without their infant only serves to compound their feelings of disappointment, failure, and deprivation.

When an infant is to be transported from the hospital, the parents need a description of the facility where the infant is going. They need to know the location, reputation, and nature of the facility and the care that the infant is expected to receive. The name of the infant's physician and the telephone number of the nursery should be given to them, and unfamiliar terms, such as "neonatologist," "ventilator," "infusion," and "incubator," should be explained. Explanations are kept simple, and parents are given the opportunity to ask questions. If booklets are available that describe the facility, they are given to the family.

Perhaps most important of all, the parents, especially the mother, should have some contact with the infant before the transport. To be able to see, touch, and (if possible) hold their infant facilitates the attachment process. Often a photograph, or even a videotape, of their infant can serve as a bond until the parents are able to travel to the regional facility. When possible, it is often advisable to transfer the mother to the same institution as her infant.

Parents need to be informed of their infant's progress and reassured that the infant is receiving proper care. They need to understand the smallest aspects of the infant's condition and treatment. Parents need a realistic assessment of the situation that is honest and direct. Using nonmedical terminology, moving at a pace that is comfortable for parents to assimilate the information, and avoiding lengthy technical explanations facilitate communication with family members (Siegel, Gardner, and Merenstein, 1993). Tasks that must be accomplished by parents during their infant's care are presented in the box above.

TASKS OF PARENTS OF A HIGH-RISK INFANT

Work through the events surrounding labor and delivery.
Acknowledge that the infant's life is endangered and that the infant might die, and begin the grief process.
Confront and recognize feelings of inadequacy and guilt in not delivering a healthy child.
Adapt to the neonatal intensive care environment.
Resume parental relationships with infant and initiate the caregiving role, *or*
Adapt to the loss in the event of neonatal death.

Modified from Siegel R, Gardner SL, Merenstein GB: Families in crisis: theoretical and practical considerations. In Merenstein GB, Gardner SL: *Handbook of neonatal intensive care,* ed 3, St Louis, 1993, Mosby.

Facilitating Parent-Infant Relationships

Because of their physiologic instability, infants are separated from their mothers immediately and surrounded by a complex, impenetrable barrier of glass windows, mechanical equipment, and special caregivers. There is increasing evidence to indicate that the emotional separation that accompanies the physical separation of mothers and infants interferes with the normal maternal-infant attachment process discussed in Chapter 8. Maternal attachment is a cumulative process that begins before conception, is strengthened by significant events during pregnancy, and matures through maternal-infant contact during the neonatal period.

When an infant is sick, the necessary physical separation appears to be accompanied by an emotional estrangement on the part of parents that may seriously damage the capacity for parenting their infant. This detachment is further hampered by the tenuous nature of the infant's condition. When survival is in doubt, parents may be reluctant to establish a relationship with their infant. They prepare themselves for the death of the infant while continuing to hope for recovery. This anticipatory grief (Chapter 23) and hesitancy to embark on a relationship are evidenced by behaviors such as delay in giving the infant a name, reluctance in visiting the nursery, or when they do visit, focusing on equipment and treatments rather than on their infant, and hesitancy to touch or handle the infant when they are provided with the opportunity.

Comprehensive management of high-risk newborns includes encouraging and facilitating parental involvement rather than isolating parents from their infant and associated care. This is particularly important in relation to mothers; to reduce the effects of physical separation, mothers are united with their newborn at the earliest opportunity. Preparing the parents to see their infant for the first time is a nursing responsibility.

Before the first visit, the parents should be prepared for their infant's appearance, the equipment that is attached to the child, and some indication of the general atmosphere of the unit. The initial encounter with the intensive care unit is a stressful experience, and the frightening array of people, equipment, and activity is likely to be overwhelming. A book of photographs or pamphlets describing the NICU environment (infants in incubators or under radiant warmers, monitors, mechanical ventilators, and intravenous equipment) provides a useful and nonthreatening introduction to the NICU.

Parents should be encouraged to visit their infant as soon as possible. Even if they saw the infant at the time of transport or shortly after birth, the infant may have changed considerably, especially if there are a number of medical and equipment requirements associated with the infant's hospitalization. At the bedside the nurse should explain the function of each piece of equipment and the role it plays in facilitating recovery. When possible, some items related to therapy can be removed; for example, phototherapy can be temporarily discontinued and eye patches removed to permit eye-to-eye contact.

Parents appreciate the support of a nurse during the initial visit with their infant, but they may also appreciate some time alone with the infant for a short while. It is important during the early visits to emphasize positive aspects of their infant's behavior and development so that parents can focus on their infant as an individual rather than on the equipment that surrounds the child. For example, the nurse may describe the infant's spontaneous behaviors during care, such as grasp, swallowing, and movement, or make comments about the infant's biologic functions. Most institutions have open visiting policies so that parents and siblings may visit their infant as often as they wish.

Parents vary greatly in the degree to which they are able to interact with their infant. Some may wish to touch or hold their infant during the first visit, whereas others may not feel comfortable enough even to enter the nursery. These reactions depend on a variety of prenatal and postnatal factors, such as the parity of the mother and her preparation before birth; the size, condition, and physical appearance of the infant; and the type of treatment the infant is receiving. It is essential to recognize that the individualized pacing and quality of the interactions are more important than early onset of these interactions. Parents may not be receptive to early and extended infant contact, since they need time to adjust to the impact of an infant with birth problems and must be helped to grieve before acceptance of their infant can take place.

The parents' inability to focus on their infant is a clue for the nurse to assist the parents in expressing feelings of guilt, anxiety, helplessness, inadequacy, anger, and ambivalence. Nurses can help parents deal with these distressing feelings and recognize that they are normal responses shared by other parents. It is important to point out and reinforce the positive aspects of parents' behavior and interactions with their infant.

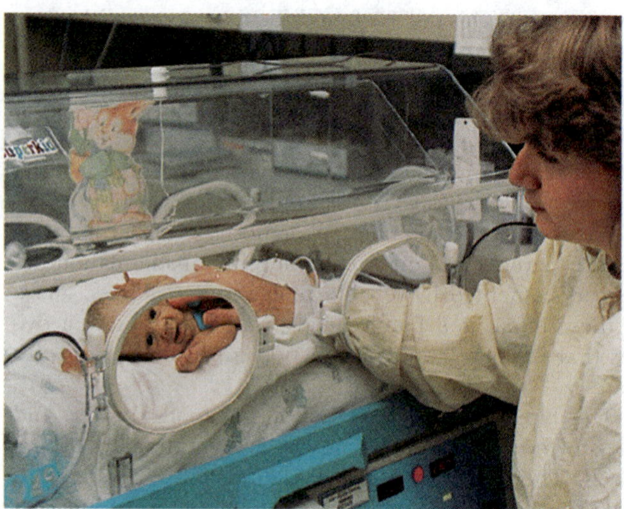

FIG. 10-8 Encouraging interaction of mother and her premature infant in intensive care unit facilitates mother-infant attachment process.

Most parents feel shaky and insecure about initiating interaction with their infant. Nurses can sense parents' level of readiness and offer encouragement in these initial efforts. Parents of premature infants follow the same acquaintance process as do parents of term infants. They may quickly proceed through the process or may require several days or even weeks to complete the process. Parents begin by touching their infant's extremities with their fingertips and poking the infant tenderly, and then proceed to caresses and fondling (Fig. 10-8). Touching is the first act of communication between parents and child. Parents need to be prepared for their infant's exaggerated and generalized startle responses to a touch so that they will not interpret these as negative reactions to their overtures. It may be necessary to limit tactile stimuli when the infant is critically ill and labile, but the nurse can offer other options—speaking softly or sitting at the bedside.

Parents of acutely ill preterm infants may express feelings of helplessness and lack of control. Involving the parent in some type of caregiving activity, no matter how minor it may seem to the nurse, enables the parent to "take on" a more active role. Examples of such caregiving for the acutely ill infant who cannot be held and is seemingly not responding positively include moistening the infant's lips with a small amount of sterile water on a cotton-tipped swab or slipping the diaper from under the infant when it is wet or soiled.

Eventually parents begin to endow their infant with an identity—as part of the family. When an infant no longer appears as a foreign object and begins to take on aspects of family members, such as the father's chin or the sister's nose, nurses can facilitate this incorporation. Parents are encouraged to bring in clothes, a toy, a stuffed animal, or a family snapshot for their infant, and the nurse can help par-

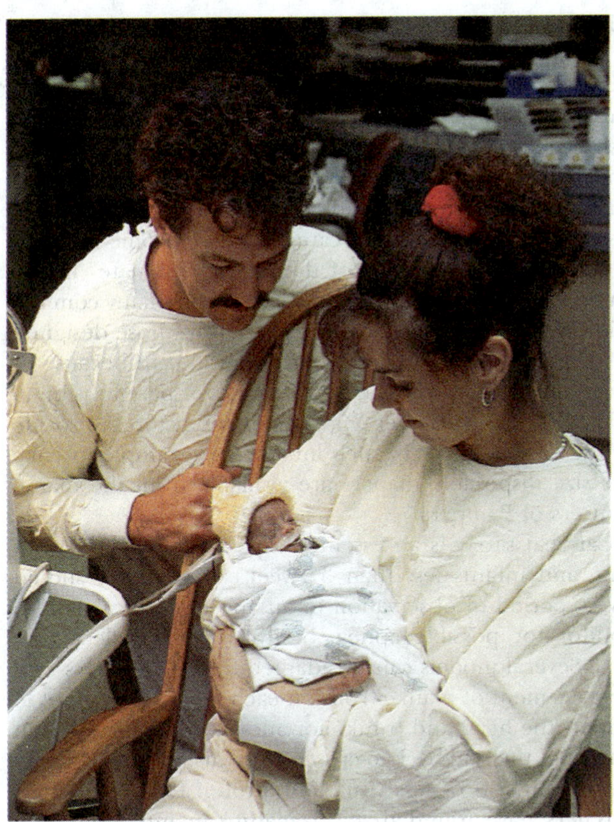

FIG. 10-9 Mother and father visit their newborn infant.

ents set goals for themselves and for the infant. Parents may become involved by reading a children's storybook or nursery rhymes in a soft, soothing voice. Some families tape record the parents' voices telling or reading stories and play the tapes when the infant is able to cope with such stimuli. Feeding schedules are discussed, and parents are encouraged to visit at times when they can become involved in the care of their infant (Fig. 10-9).

Throughout the parental-infant acquaintance process, the nurse listens carefully to what the parents say in order to assess their concerns and their progress toward incorporating their infant into their lives. The manner in which parents refer to their infant and the questions they ask reveal their worries and feelings and can serve as valuable clues to future relationships with the infant. The alert nurse is attuned to these subtle indications of parents' needs that provide guidelines for nursing intervention. Often all that parents need is reassurance that the behaviors about which they are concerned are normal reactions and will disappear as the infant matures (e.g., an exaggerated Moro reflex or inability to coordinate swallowing) and that they will have the support of the nurse during caregiving activities.

Parents need guidance in their relationships with their infant and assistance in their efforts to meet their infant's physical and developmental needs. The nursing staff must help parents understand that their preterm infant offers few behavioral rewards and show them how to accept small rewards from their infant. The infant's reactions and behaviors are explained to parents, who take their infant's jerky, rejective behavior personally. They need reassurance that these behaviors are not a reflection on their parenting skills. Parents are taught to recognize their infant's cues regarding stimulation, handling, and other interaction, especially aversive behaviors that indicate a need for rest. Nurses need to include parents in planning their infant's care and sensory stimulation materials, such as a music box or recording.

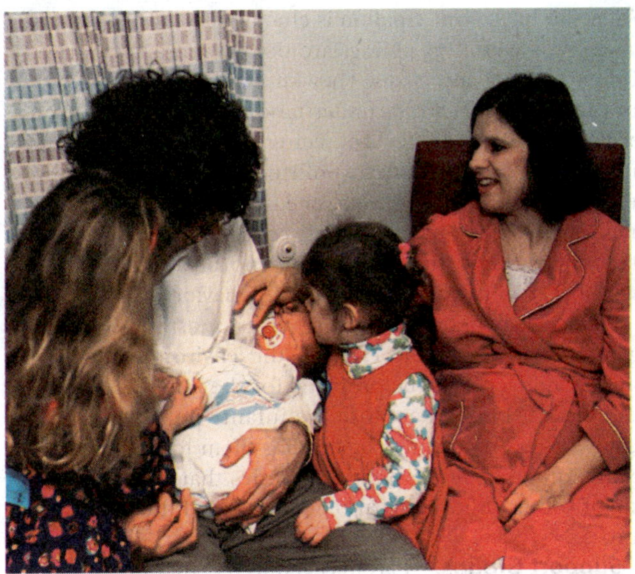

FIG. 10-10 Big sisters get acquainted with the new baby.

Above all, nurses must encourage and reinforce parents during their caregiving activities and interactions with their infant in order to promote healthy parent-child relationships. It is also helpful for the parents to have contact and communication with the infant's primary nurse and associate primary nurse. This decreases the amount of different information given to parents and often instills confidence that while the parents cannot be at their infant's bedside 24 hours a day, there are competent and caring nurses whom they may call to inquire about the infant's status. Periodic parent conferences involving the primary practitioner, primary nurse, and associate primary nurse serve to clarify misunderstandings or problems related to the infant's condition. Other members of the NICU health care team, such as the perinatal social worker or surgeon, may become involved as necessary. The importance of facilitating the parental-infant attachment process cannot be overemphasized, since studies indicate that lack of early attachment in premature infants may contribute to problems such as child abuse later on.

Siblings. In the past, concerns about sibling visitation in the NICU focused on fears of infection and disruption of nursing routines. These fears have not been substantiated, and sibling visits are now part of the normal operation of most NICUs (Fig. 10-10).

The birth of a preterm infant is a difficult time for siblings, who rely on the support of understanding parents.

When the happy anticipation is changed to sadness, worry, and altered routines, siblings are bewildered and deprived of their parents' attention. They know something is wrong, but they have only a dim understanding of what it is. Concern about negative effects of seeing the ill newborn on visiting siblings has not been confirmed. Children have not hesitated to approach or touch the infant, and children less than 5 years of age have been less reluctant than older children; in addition, there have been no measurable differences between previsit and postvisit behaviors.

Potential benefits of sibling visits must be weighed against exposure of the child to the environment of the NICU. Children must be prepared for the unfamiliar NICU atmosphere, but contact with the infant appears to have a positive effect on siblings by helping them to deal with the reality rather than the bizarre fantasies that are characteristic of young children. It also helps to bond the family as a unit.

Support Groups. Parents need to feel that they are not alone. Parent support groups have been of immeasurable value to families of infants in the NICU. Some groups consist of parents who have infants in the hospital who share the same anxieties and concerns. Other groups include parents who have had infants in the NICU and who have dealt with the crisis effectively. The groups are usually under the leadership of a staff person and involve physicians, nurses, and social workers, but it is the parents who can offer other parents something that no one else can provide.

A relatively new national organization evolved from a local parent's group. **Parent Care, Inc.,*** provides information, referrals, and support to parents and professionals concerned with the care of high-risk infants. It also publishes a national newsletter and a resource directory that provide information on items useful to parents, such as "preemie" clothing, and hosts local and national conferences. Information can be obtained by contacting or forming a local group. The **Family Resource Coalition†** is a North American network of family support programs designed to help families of preterm infants.

Discharge Planning and Home Care

Parents become very apprehensive and excited as the time for discharge approaches. They have many concerns and insecurities regarding the care of their infant. They fear the child may still be in danger, that they will be unable to recognize signs of distress or illness in their infant, and that the infant may not yet be ready for discharge. Nurses need to begin early to assist parents in acquiring or increasing their skills in the care of their infant. Appropriate instruction must be provided and sufficient time allowed for the family to assimilate the information and learn the continuing special care requirements. Where rooming-in or other live-in arrangements are available, parents can stay for a few days and nights and assume the care of their infant under the supervision and support of the nursery staff.

There should be appropriate medical and nursing follow-up and referrals to services that can benefit the family, including developmental follow-up. Parents of preterm infants should also be given adequate information about immunizations with other discharge planning information (Langkamp and Langhough, 1993). Public health agencies provide nursing supervision, counseling, and referral for nursing visits. With the trend toward early discharge, many hospital-based home health care agencies become involved in the follow-up and care of the NICU "graduate" in the home. Organized support groups are part of many communities, including those discussed previously, those designed for parents of infants who require special care because of specific defects or disabilities, and those for parents of multiple births (see Chapter 3). Some manufacturers provide for the special needs of such infants. For example, premature size disposable diapers are available from the manufacturers of Pampers.*

Car seat safety is an essential aspect of discharge planning, and infants less than 37 weeks of gestation should have a period of observation in an appropriate car seat to monitor for possible apnea, bradycardia, and decreased SaO_2. Several models can be adapted for small infants with the placement of blanket rolls on each side of the infant to support the head and trunk. For adequate support without slumping, the seat-back-to-crotch strap distance must be 14 cm (5½ inches) or less (Bull and Stroup, 1985). Other researchers have found that "premature infants, both with and without apnea, are at risk for significant hypoxia while placed in a recommended car seat" (Willett and others, 1986, 1989). LBW infants are best transported lying prone in infant-only child safety seats with harnesses designed to fit small bodies (Richards, 1989) or well supported in a car bed restraint (Mini Swinger†) (Bull, Weber, and Stroup, 1988). The American Academy of Pediatrics (1991) has published guidelines for the safe transportation of premature infants. (See Chapter 12 for a discussion of infant car restraints.)

Knowing that members of the staff (especially the primary nurse) are available for telephone or personal contact when the parents take the infant home provides a measure of security to anxious parents. Most NICU facilities maintain a policy of open communication between staff and parents both during the infant's hospitalization and following discharge. It is the responsibility of the NICU staff to make certain that parents are prepared to care for their infant—emotionally and physically.

The term ***vulnerable child syndrome*** is applied to physically healthy children who are perceived by their parents to be at high risk for medical or developmental problems (Culley, Perrin, and Chaberski, 1989). The syndrome has been observed in parents of children who have had an earlier illness or injury from which they had not been expected to recover. The family continues to perceive the child as fragile, vulnerable, "different," and having needs that warrant special status in the family, which adversely affects the

*9041 Colgate St., Indianapolis, IN 46268; (317) 872-9913.
†200 S. Michigan Ave., 16th Floor, Chicago, IL 60604; (312) 341-0900.

*Proctor & Gamble; phone toll free: (800) 543-4932; in Ohio: (800) 582-2623.
†Distributed by Shinn and Associates, 2853 W. Jolly, Okemos, MI 48864; (517) 332-0211.

child's and family's behavior. The parents may lack confidence in their parenting ability persisting beyond the illness. The parents may also become overly indulgent and have difficulty setting limits, resulting in interference with normal development. Consequently, the child becomes dependent, demanding, and out of control (Bernbaum and Hoffman-Williamson, 1986). Overprotection and frequent visits to the health care provider are characteristic.

Problems that may arise in the high-risk newborn include overfeeding, underfeeding, and difficulty separating the child from the parent. To help parents deal with the stress of home care for the infant, nurses can help families to discuss their fears and anxieties, which are exaggerated in parents of preterm infants, and encourage the family to create a normal routine in caring for the infant. Parents need to learn the normal developmental delays expected of premature infants and the importance of setting disciplinary limits and schedules. Continued explanations and clarification of the infant's true health status and ongoing support of the parents' efforts are important aspects of follow-up care.

Developmental Outcome

Some physiologic systems in preterm infants mature earlier than they would have if the infant had remained within the uterus (e.g., the function of some enzyme and immunologic systems and organs, such as the kidneys and gastrointestinal system efficiency); others slow down, such as growth in height and weight; still others keep pace with the development of fetuses still in utero (e.g., reflex behaviors).

Longitudinal studies of infants born prematurely indicate that there are differences in many aspects of development that may be a consequence of the immaturity at birth and related perinatal problems. Preterm infants remain in a lower percentile range for height, weight, and head circumference, although they follow the same general growth pattern as infants born at term. There is a rapid increase in growth during the first 6 months, and growth remains somewhat accelerated until the normal growth curve is reached by age 2 to 3 years (see box below for factors that affect growth and development of preterm infants).

Neurologic impairment (such as intraventricular hemorrhage) and serious sequelae correlate with the size and gestational age of infants at birth and with the severity of neonatal complications. The greater the degree of immaturity, the greater the degree of potential disability. A greater incidence of cerebral palsy, attention deficit disorder, visual-motor deficits, and altered intellectual functioning is observed in preterm than in full-term infants. However, behavioral development can be enhanced when families are provided with support and infants are referred to appropriate services for neurologic and developmental interventions. Parental interest and involvement are very important variables in developmental progress of infants.

All infants at risk seem to benefit from special care, since undesirable sequelae appear to be decreased in infants who receive intensive medical and nursing care as opposed to those whose care is delayed or less than intensive. Although the risk of perinatal complications is highest in ELBW and VLBW infants and the mortality is higher, a positive outcome is believed to be possible even for these survivors of extremely low birth weight.

A concern of personnel in NICUs is the incidence of sensory impairment in surviving premature infants. Retinopathy of prematurity, a complication of oxygen therapy and prematurity, is discussed on p. 416. More difficult to anticipate and detect is a hearing deficit. Because LBW infants show significant visual-motor deficits compared with full-term infants at a later time, many NICUs routinely screen infants for hearing acuity. The brainstem auditory-evoked response (BAER) (also referred to as ABR or auditory brainstem response) monitors stimulus-related changes in the electrical activity of the auditory pathway by way of noninvasive electrodes applied to the scalp. Follow-up testing is a vital part of ongoing care.

FACTORS THAT AFFECT GROWTH AND DEVELOPMENT OF PRETERM INFANTS

Past history
Gestational age at birth
Head circumference, weight, and length at birth
Length of growth delay
Days necessary to regain birth weight
Measurements at term date
Head circumference, weight, length at discharge from hospital
Medical diagnosis, its severity, treatment, and response
Length of hospitalization

Neonatal Loss

The precarious nature of many high-risk infants makes death a very real and ever-present possibility. Although infant mortality has been reduced sharply with improved technology, the mortality rate is still greatest in the neonatal period of life. Nurses in the NICU are the persons who must prepare the parents for an inevitable death and facilitate a family's grieving process after an expected or an unexpected death.

The loss of an infant has special meaning for the grieving parents. It represents a loss of a part of themselves (especially for mothers), a loss of the potential for immortality that offspring represent, and the loss of the dream child that has been fantasized throughout the pregnancy. There is a sense of emptiness and failure. In addition, when an infant has lived for such a short time, there may be few, if any, pleasant memories to serve as a basis for identification and idealization that are part of the resolution of a loss.

To help the parents understand that the death is a reality, it is important that the parents are encouraged to hold their infant before death and if possible be present at the time of death so that their infant can die in their arms if they choose. Many who deny the need to hold the infant later regret the decision (Null, 1989). Parents should be provided with an opportunity to see, touch, hold, caress, examine, and talk to their infant privately after death, and to bathe their infant if they desire as a final act of caring. If parents are hesitant about seeing their dead infant, it is advisable to keep the body in the unit for a few hours, since many parents change their minds after the initial shock of the death.

Parents may need to see and hold the infant more than once: the first time to say "hello" and the last time to say "goodbye." If parents wish to see the infant after the body has been taken to the morgue, the infant should be retrieved, wrapped in a blanket, and taken to the mother's room or other private place. The nurse should stay with the parents and provide them an opportunity for private time alone with their dead infant.

Some units have implemented a hospice approach for families with infants for whom the decision has been made not to prolong life and who are receiving only palliative care. A special "family" room is set aside that contains all supportive equipment needed for the care of the infant and also provides a homelike atmosphere for the family (Landon-Malone, Kirkpatrick, and Stull, 1987). All hospice services are available to the family, and the infant remains under the care and supervision of a primary nurse on the NICU staff. (See Chapter 23 for further discussion of hospice care.)

A photograph of the infant taken before or after death is highly desirable. The parents may not wish to see the photograph at the time of death, but the chance to refer to it later will help make their infant seem more real, which is a part of the normal grief process. A photograph of their infant being held by the hand or touched by an adult offers a more positive image than a morgue type of photograph. Many NICUs have a grief or memory packet made up for the grieving parents, which may include the infant's handprints and footprints, a lock of hair, the bedside name card, and, as appropriate to the family's religious beliefs, a certificate of baptism. In some units special knitted clothing is made by hospital volunteer groups and donated for dressing the infant postmortem. Other tangible remembrances of the child can be provided, such as name tags, armbands, and locks of hair shaved for intravenous insertion or other procedures. Naming the deceased infant is an important step in the grieving process; some parents may hesitate to give the newborn a name that had been chosen during the pregnancy for their special "baby." However, having a tangible person for whom to grieve is an important component of the grieving process (Merenstein and Gardner, 1993).

At least one nurse who is familiar to the family should be present during the discussion about a dead or dying infant. The nurse should talk with parents openly and honestly about funeral arrangements, since few of them have had experience with this aspect of death. Many funeral homes now offer inexpensive arrangements for these special cases. Someone from the NICU should take the responsibility for acquiring this type of information. It is often helpful to parents for the NICU to have a list of local funeral homes, services offered, and a price for the service offered. Families need to be informed of options available, but it is preferable to encourage a funeral because the ritual provides an opportunity for parents to feel the support of friends and relatives. A clergyman of the appropriate faith may be notified if the parents wish. Issues regarding an autopsy or organ donation (when appropriate) are approached in a multidisciplinary fashion (primary practitioner and primary nurse) with respect, tact, and consideration of the family's wishes. (See also Grief and Perinatal Loss in Merenstein and Gardner, 1993.)

Before the parents leave the hospital, they are given the telephone number of the unit (if they do not have it) and invited to call any time they have any further questions. Many intensive care units make it a point to contact the parents following a neonatal death to assess the parents' coping mechanisms, evaluate the grieving process, and provide support as needed. Several organizations are available to offer support and understanding to families who have lost a newborn, including **The Compassionate Friends,*** **SHARE (Source of Help in Airing & Resolving Experiences),**† and **AMEND (Aiding Mothers & Fathers Experiencing Neo-Natal Death).**‡ (See also Chapter 23 for further discussion of the family and the grief process.)

Baptism. Since many Christian parents wish to have their child baptized if death is anticipated or a decided possibility, this becomes a nursing responsibility. Whenever possible, it is most desirable that a representative of the parents' faith (i.e., a Roman Catholic priest or a Protestant minister) perform such a ritual. When death is imminent, a nurse or a physician can perform the baptism by simply pouring water on the infant's forehead (a medicine dropper is a convenient means) while repeating the words, "I baptize you in the name of the Father and the Son and of the Holy Spirit." This includes a birth of any gestational age, particularly when the parents are of the Roman Catholic faith.

When the faith of the parents is uncertain, a conditional baptism can be carried out by saying, "If you are capable of receiving baptism, I baptize you in the name of the Father and of the Son and of the Holy Spirit." The fact of the baptism is recorded in the infant's chart and a notice placed on the crib or incubator. Parents are informed at the first opportunity.

❖ EVALUATION

The effectiveness of nursing interventions is determined by continual reassessment and evaluation of care based on the following observational guidelines and expected outcomes:

1. Take vital signs and perform respiratory assessments at time intervals based on infant's condition and needs; observe infant's respiratory efforts and response to therapy; check functioning of equipment; review laboratory test results.
2. Measure abdominal skin and axillary temperatures at specified intervals.
3. Observe infant's behavior and appearance for evidence of sepsis.

Text continued on p. 395.

*P.O. Box 3696, Oak Brook, IL 60522-3696; (312) 323-5010. In Canada: 685 William Ave., Winnipeg, Canada, R3E 022.

†St. John's Hospital, 800 Carpenter, Springfield, IL 62769; (217) 544-6464, Ext. 5275.

‡Contact Maureen Connelly, 4324 Berrywick Terrace, St. Louis, MO 63128; (314) 487-7582.

NURSING CARE PLAN
The High-Risk Infant*

NURSING DIAGNOSIS: Ineffective breathing pattern related to pulmonary and neuromuscular immaturity, decreased energy, and fatigue

PATIENT GOAL 1: Will exhibit adequate oxygenation

• **NURSING INTERVENTIONS/*RATIONALES***

Position for optimum air exchange
- Place prone when feasible, *since this position results in improved oxygenation, better-tolerated feedings, and more organized sleep-rest patterns*
- Place supine with neck slightly extended and nose pointing to ceiling in "sniffing" position *to prevent any narrowing of airway*

Avoid neck hyperextension *because it reduces diameter of trachea*

Observe for deviations from desired functioning; recognize signs of distress—grunting, cyanosis, nasal flaring, apnea

Suction *to remove accumulated mucus from nasopharynx, trachea, and endotracheal tube*

Suction only as necessary based on assessment (e.g., auscultation of chest, evidence of decreased oxygenation, increased infant irritability)

Never suction routinely, since it *may cause bronchospasm, bradycardia due to vagal nerve stimulation, hypoxia, and increased intracranial pressure [ICP], predisposing infant to intraventricular hemorrhage (IVH)*

Use proper suctioning technique *because improper suctioning can cause infection, airway damage, pneumothoraces, and IVH*

Use two-person suction technique *because assistant can provide immediate hyperoxygenation before and after catheter insertion*

†Carry out percussion, vibration, and postural drainage as prescribed *to facilitate drainage of secretions*

Avoid using Trendelenburg position, *since it can contribute to increased ICP and reduced lung capacity from gravity pushing organs against diaphragms*
- During diaper changes, raise infant slightly under hips and not by raising feet and legs

Use semiprone or side-lying position *to prevent aspiration in infant with excessive mucus or who is being fed*

Observe for signs of respiratory distress—nasal flaring, retractions, tachypnea, apnea, grunting, cyanosis, low oxygenation saturation (Sa_{O_2})

Carry out regimen prescribed for supplemental oxygen therapy (maintain ambient O_2 concentration at minimum FI_{O_2} level based on arterial blood gases, Sa_{O_2}, and transcutaneous oxygen [tcP_{O_2}])

Maintain neutral thermal environment *to conserve utilization of O_2*

Closely monitor blood gas measurements, tcP_{O_2} and Sa_{O_2} readings

Apply and manage monitoring equipment correctly (i.e., cardiac or oxygen)

Demonstrate understanding of function of respiratory support apparatus
- Mechanical ventilation apparatus
- Insufflation bags with masks and/or endotracheal tube adaptor
- Oxygen hoods/tents
- Humidifier warmers

Observe and assess infant's response to ventilation and oxygenation therapy

• **EXPECTED OUTCOMES**

Airway remains patent

Breathing provides adequate oxygenation and CO_2 removal

Respiratory rate and pattern is within appropriate limits for age and weight (specify)

Arterial blood gases and acid-base balance are within normal limits for postconceptional age

Tissue oxygenation is adequate

NURSING DIAGNOSIS: Ineffective thermoregulation related to immature temperature control and decreased subcutaneous body fat

PATIENT GOAL 1: Will maintain stable body temperature

• **NURSING INTERVENTIONS/*RATIONALES***

Place infant in incubator, radiant warmer, or warmly clothed in open crib *to maintain stable body temperature*

Monitor axillary temperature in unstable infants (use skin probe or air temperature control; check function of servocontrolled mechanism when used)

Regulate servocontrolled unit or air temperature control as needed *to maintain skin temperature within accepted thermal range*

Use plastic heat shield as appropriate *to decrease heat loss*

Monitor for signs of hyperthermia—redness, flushing, diaphoresis (rarely)

Check temperature of infant in relation to ambient temperature and temperature of heating unit *to direct radiant heat loss*

Avoid situations that might predispose infant to heat loss, such as exposure to cool air, drafts, bathing, or cold scales

Monitor serum glucose values *to ensure euglycemia*

• **EXPECTED OUTCOME**

Infant's axillary temperature remains within normal range for postconceptional age

NURSING DIAGNOSIS: High risk for infection related to deficient immunologic defenses

PATIENT GOAL 1: Will exhibit no evidence of nosocomial infection

• **NURSING INTERVENTIONS/*RATIONALES***

Ensure that all caregivers wash hands before and after handling infant *to minimize exposure to infective organisms*

---
*Relates primarily to low-birth-weight infant with weight of 1500 to 2500 g.
†Dependent nursing action.

Continued.

NURSING CARE PLAN
The High-Risk Infant—cont'd

Ensure that all equipment in contact with infant is clean or sterile
Prevent personnel with upper respiratory tract or communicable infections from coming into direct contact with infant
Isolate other infants who have infections according to institutional policy
Instruct health care workers and parents in infection control procedures
*Administer antibiotics as ordered
Ensure strict asepsis and/or sterility with invasive procedures and equipment such as peripheral IV therapy, lumbar punctures, and arterial/venous catheter insertion

• **EXPECTED OUTCOME**
Infant exhibits no evidence of nosocomial infection

NURSING DIAGNOSIS: Altered nutrition: less than body requirements (high risk) related to inability to ingest nutrients because of immaturity and/or illness

PATIENT GOAL 1: Will receive adequate nourishment, with caloric intake to maintain positive nitrogen balance, and exhibit appropriate weight gain

• **NURSING INTERVENTIONS/*RATIONALES***
*Maintain parenteral fluid or total parenteral nutrition therapy as ordered
Monitor for signs of intolerance to total parenteral therapy, especially protein and glucose
Assess readiness to nipple feed, especially ability to coordinate swallowing and breathing
Nipple feed infant if strong sucking, swallowing, and gag reflexes are present (usually at gestational age of 34 to 35 weeks) *to minimize risk of aspiration*
Follow unit protocol for advancing volume and concentration of formula *to avoid feeding intolerance*
Use orogastric feeding if infant tires easily or has weak sucking, gag, or swallowing reflexes, *because nipple feeding may result in weight loss*
Assist mothers with expressing breast milk *to establish and maintain lactation until infant can breast-feed*
Assist mothers with breast-feeding when feasible and desirable

• **EXPECTED OUTCOMES**
Infant receives an adequate amount of calories and essential nutrients
Infant demonstrates a steady weight gain (approximately 20 to 30 g/day) once past acute phase of illness

*Dependent nursing action.

NURSING DIAGNOSIS: High risk for fluid volume deficit or excess related to immature physiologic characteristics of preterm infant and/or immaturity or illness

PATIENT GOAL 1: Will exhibit adequate hydration status

• **NURSING INTERVENTIONS/*RATIONALES***
Monitor fluid and electrolytes closely with therapies that increase insensible water loss (IWL) (e.g., phototherapy, radiant warmer)
Implement strategies to minimize IWL such as plastic covering, increased ambient humidity
Ensure adequate parenteral/oral fluid intake
Assess state of hydration (e.g., skin turgor, blood pressure, edema, weight, mucous membranes, urine specific gravity, electrolytes, fontanel)
Regulate parenteral fluids closely *to avoid dehydration, overhydration, or extravasation*
Avoid administering hypertonic fluids (e.g., undiluted medications, concentrated glucose infusions) *to prevent excess solute load on immature kidneys and fragile veins*
Monitor urinary output and laboratory values *for evidence of dehydration or overhydration* (adequate urinary output 1-2 ml/kg/hr)

• **EXPECTED OUTCOME**
Infant exhibits evidence of fluid homeostasis

NURSING DIAGNOSIS: High risk for impaired skin integrity related to immature skin structure, immobility, decreased nutritional state, invasive procedures

PATIENT GOAL 1: Will maintain skin integrity

• **NURSING INTERVENTIONS/*RATIONALES***
See Guidelines box on neonatal skin care, p. 381

• **EXPECTED OUTCOME**
Skin remains clean and intact with no evidence of irritation or injury

NURSING DIAGNOSIS: High-risk for injury from increased intracranial pressure (ICP) related to immature central nervous system and physiologic stress response

PATIENT GOAL 1: Will exhibit normal ICP (unless increased ICP is related to infant's illness) and no evidence of intraventricular hemorrhage (IVH) (unless preexisting condition)

• **NURSING INTERVENTIONS/*RATIONALES***
Decrease environmental stimulation *because stress responses, especially increased blood pressure, increases risk of elevated ICP*

NURSING CARE PLAN
The High-Risk Infant—cont'd

Establish a routine that provides for undisturbed sleep/rest periods *to eliminate or minimize times of stress*
Use minimal handling and handle or disturb infant only when absolutely necessary
Keep extra diapers under buttocks to facilitate changing soiled diapers; raise infant's hips, not feet and legs
Organize (cluster) care during normal waking hours as much as possible *to minimize sleep disruption and frequent intermittent noise*
Close and open drapes and dim lights *to allow for day/night schedule*
Cover incubator with cloth and place "do not disturb" sign nearby *to decrease light and alert others to infant's rest period*
Refrain from loud talking or laughing
Remain calm
Limit number of visitors and staff near infant at one time
Explain meaning of unfamiliar sounds
Keep equipment noise to minimum
Turn alarms as low as safely possible
Attend to alarms and telephones immediately
Place bedside equipment, such as ventilator or IV pump, away from head of bed
Turn outflow valve from ventilator away from infant's ear
Perform treatments requiring equipment at one time
Turn off bedside equipment that is not in use, such as suction and oxygen
Avoid loud, abrupt noises, such as discarding items in trash can, dropping items, placing items on top of incubator, closing doors and drawers, heavy traffic
Turn off any radios or televisions
May place soft earmuffs on infant
Assess and manage pain using pharmacologic and nonpharmacologic methods
Recognize signs of physical stress and overstimulation *to institute appropriate interventions promptly*
Avoid hypertonic medications and solutions *because they increase cerebral blood flow*
Elevate head of bed or mattress between 15 and 20 degrees *to decrease ICP*
Maintain adequate oxygenation *because hypoxia increases cerebral blood flow and ICP* (see interventions under nursing diagnosis of ineffective breathing pattern on p. 391)
Avoid any sudden turning of head to side, *which restricts carotid artery blood flow and adequate oxygenation to brain*

• **EXPECTED OUTCOME**
Infant exhibits no evidence of increased ICP or IVH

NURSING DIAGNOSIS: Pain related to procedures, diagnosis, treatment

PATIENT GOAL 1: Will experience no pain or reduction of pain

• **NURSING INTERVENTIONS/*RATIONALES***
Recognize that infants, regardless of gestational age, feel pain
Differentiate between clinical manifestations of pain (see Chapter 11) and stress/fatigue (see p. 382)
Use nonpharmacologic pain measures appropriate to infant's age and condition: repositioning, swaddling, containment, cuddling, rocking, music, reducing environmental stimulation, tactile comfort measures (stroking, patting), and nonnutritive sucking (pacifier)
Assess effectiveness of nonpharmacologic pain measures *because some measures, (e.g., stroking) may increase premature infant's distress*
Encourage parents to provide comfort measures when possible
Convey an attitude of sensitivity and compassion for infant's discomfort
Discuss with family their concerns about infant's pain
Encourage family to speak with health practitioner about their concerns

• **EXPECTED OUTCOME**
Infant exhibits no or minimal signs of pain

NURSING DIAGNOSIS: Altered growth and development related to preterm birth, unnatural NICU environment, separation from parents

PATIENT GOAL 1: Will attain normal growth and development potential

• **NURSING INTERVENTIONS/*RATIONALES***
Provide optimum nutrition *to ensure steady weight gain and brain growth*
Provide regular periods of undisturbed rest *to decrease unnecessary O_2 use and caloric expenditure*
Provide age-appropriate developmental intervention
Recognize signs of overstimulation (flaccidity, yawning, staring, active averting, irritability, crying) *so that infant is allowed to rest*
Promote parent-infant interaction, *since it is essential for normal growth and development*

• **EXPECTED OUTCOMES**
Infant exhibits a steady weight gain once past the acute phase of illness
Infant is exposed only to appropriate stimuli

Continued.

NURSING CARE PLAN
The High-Risk Infant—con'd

NURSING DIAGNOSIS: Altered family processes related to situational/maturational crisis, knowledge deficit (birth of a preterm and/or ill infant), interruption of parental attachment process

PATIENT (FAMILY) GOAL 1: Will be informed of infant's progress

- **NURSING INTERVENTIONS/*RATIONALES***

Prioritize information *to help parents understand most important aspects of care, signs of improvement, or deterioration in infant's condition*
Encourage parents to ask questions about child's status
Answer questions, facilitate expression of concern regarding care and prognosis
Be honest; respond to questions with correct answers *to establish trust*
Encourage mother and father to visit and/or call unit often *so they are informed of infant's progress*
Emphasize positive aspects of infant's status *to encourage sense of hope*

- **EXPECTED OUTCOME**

Parents express feelings and concerns regarding infant and prognosis, and demonstrate understanding and involvement in care

PATIENT (FAMILY) GOAL 2: Will exhibit positive attachment behaviors

- **NURSING INTERVENTIONS/*RATIONALES***

Encourage parents' visit as soon as possible *so that attachment process is initiated*
Encourage parents to:
  Visit infant frequently
  Touch, hold, and caress infant as appropriate for infant's physical condition
  Become actively involved in infant's care
  Bring clothing to dress infant as soon as condition permits
Reinforce parents' endeavors, *to increase their self-confidence*
Be alert to signs of tension and stress in parents
Enable parents to spend time alone with infant
Help parents interpret infant's responses; comment regarding any positive response and signs of overstimulation or fatigue
Help parents by demonstrating infant care techniques and offer support
Identify resources (e.g., transportation, baby-sitting) *to enable parents to visit*

- **EXPECTED OUTCOMES**

Parents visit infant soon after birth and at frequent intervals
Parents relate positively with infant (e.g., call infant by name, look at and touch infant)
Parents provide care for infant and demonstrate an attitude of comfort in relationships with infant
Parents identify signs of stress or fatigue in infant

PATIENT (SIBLINGS) GOAL 3: Will exhibit positive attachment behaviors

- **NURSING INTERVENTIONS/*RATIONALES***

Encourage siblings to visit infants when feasible
Explain environment, events, appearance of infant, and why infant cannot come home *to prepare them for visiting*
Provide photos of infant or other items if siblings are unable to visit
Encourage siblings to make pictures or bring other small items, such as a letter, for infant and place in incubator or crib

- **EXPECTED OUTCOMES**

Siblings visit infant in NICU or nursery
Siblings exhibit an understanding of explanations (specify)
Siblings receive infant-related items (specify)

PATIENT (FAMILY) GOAL 4: Will be prepared for home care

- **NURSING INTERVENTIONS/*RATIONALES***

Assess readiness of family (especially mother or other primary caregiver) to care for infant in home setting *to facilitate parents' transition to home with infant*
Teach necessary infant care techniques and observations
Encourage parent(s), when possible, to spend one or two nights in a hospital predischarge room before discharge with infant *to foster confidence in caring for infant at home*
Reinforce follow-up medical care
Refer to appropriate agencies or services *so that needed assistance is provided*
Encourage and facilitate involvement with parent support group or refer to appropriate support group(s) *for on-going support*
Offer family opportunity to learn infant cardiopulmonary resuscitation and response to choking incident

- **EXPECTED OUTCOMES**

Family demonstrates ability to provide care for infant
Family members state how and when to contact available services
Family members recognize importance of follow-up medical care

NURSING DIAGNOSIS: Anticipatory grieving related to unexpected birth of high-risk infant, grave prognosis, and/or death of infant

PATIENT (FAMILY) GOAL 1: Will acknowledge possibility of child's death and demonstrate healthy grieving behaviors

- **NURSING INTERVENTIONS/*RATIONALES***

Provide family with the opportunity to hold their infant before death and, if possible, be present at the time of death
Support family's decision for terminating life support

NURSING CARE PLAN
The High-Risk Infant—cont'd

Arrange for or perform appropriate baptism rite for infant

Provide family with the opportunity to see, touch, hold, caress, examine, and talk to their infant privately before and after death

Keep infant's body available for a few hours *to give family members who are hesitant an opportunity to see deceased infant if they change their minds*

Provide photographs taken before and after infant's death for family *to refer to at a later time to make infant real*

Take photograph of infant being held or touched by an adult; avoid morgue-type photograph *because it depersonalizes child*

Provide other tangible remembrances of child's death (e.g., name tags, identification band, lock of hair, footprints, blanket)

Encourage family to name infant if they have not done so

Identify resources to assist with funeral arrangements *to facilitate parental grieving*

• **EXPECTED OUTCOME**

Family discusses the reality of the death and conveys an attitude of realization

PATIENT (FAMILY) GOAL 2: Will receive adequate emotional and physical support

• **NURSING INTERVENTIONS/*RATIONALES***

Be available to family *to provide support*

Provide appropriate religious support (e.g., clergy)

Discuss infant's illness and death with family

Talk with family openly and honestly about funeral arrangements

Have information available regarding inexpensive services in the community

Inform family of all options available *so that they can make informed decisions*

Provide opportunity for family to call the unit if they have any questions regarding infant's illness and death

May contact family after the death *to assess coping and status of grieving process*

Refer family to appropriate support group(s) *for on-going support*

• **EXPECTED OUTCOMES**

Family grieves for infant's death appropriately

Family demonstrates appropriate (culturally and socially influenced) grieving behaviors over infant's death

4. Assess for hydration; assess and measure fluid intake; observe infant during feeding; measure amount of formula or parenteral intake; weigh daily.
5. Observe infant's skin for signs of irritation and breakdown.
6. Observe infant for evidence of increased intracranial pressure or signs of intraventricular hemorrhage.
7. Observe infant's physiologic and behavioral response to pain and to pain-relief interventions.
8. Observe infant's response to developmental care.
9. Observe parental interaction with infant; interview family regarding their feelings, concerns, and readiness for home care.
10. Assess family and observe their behaviors during and after the death of their infant.

Expected outcomes:

See Nursing Care Plan, pp. 391-395.

HIGH-RISK CONDITIONS RELATED TO DYSMATURITY

PRETERM INFANTS

Prematurity accounts for the largest number of admissions to an NICU. Not only does the immaturity place infants at risk for neonatal complications (e.g., hyperbilirubinemia and respiratory distress syndrome, which is highest in the preterm infant), but also for other high-risk factors (e.g., congenital abnormalities in association with prematurity).

Etiology

Most of the aspects concerning high-risk neonates are related to the incidence of prematurity; however, the actual cause of prematurity is not known in most instances. The incidence of prematurity is lowest in the middle to high socioeconomic classes, in which pregnant women are generally in good health, are well nourished, and receive prompt and comprehensive prenatal care; the incidence is highest in the low socioeconomic class, in which a combination of deleterious circumstances is present. Other factors, such as multiple pregnancies, preeclampsia, and placental problems that interrupt the normal course of gestation prior to completion of fetal development, are responsible for a large number of premature births.

The outlook for premature infants is largely, but not entirely, related to the state of physiologic and anatomic immaturity of the various organs and systems at the time of birth. Infants at term have advanced to a state of maturity sufficient to allow a successful transition to the extrauterine environment. Infants born prematurely must make the same adjustments but with functional immaturity proportional to the stage of development reached at the time of birth. The degree to which infants are prepared for extrauterine life can be predicted to some extent by weight and estimated gestational age (see Assessment of Clinical Gestational Age, Chapter 8). An understanding of prenatal development provides some concept of the status of the systems at various stages of development that must cope with functional changes that occur with birth.

CLINICAL EVALUATION

PRETERM | TERM

Posture—The preterm infant lies in a "relaxed attitude," limbs more extended; the body size is small, and the head may appear somewhat larger in proportion to the body size. The term infant has more subcutaneous fat tissue and rests in a more flexed attitude.

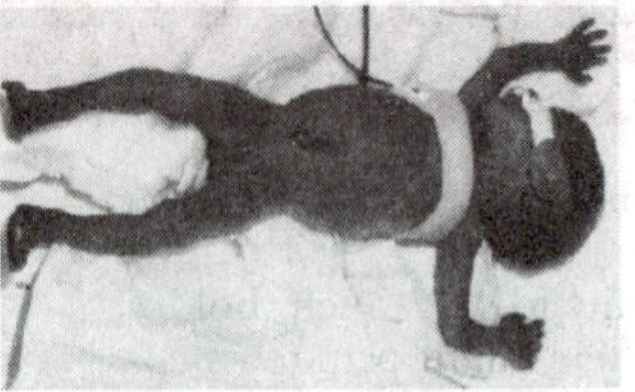

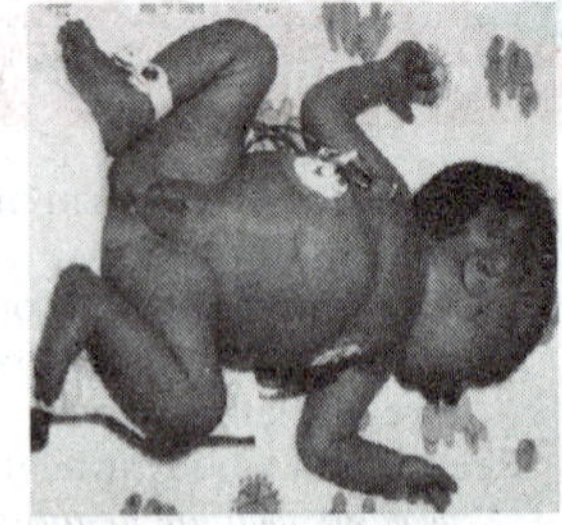

Ear—The preterm infant's ear cartilages are poorly developed, and the ear may fold easily; the hair is fine and feathery, and lanugo may cover the back and face. The mature infant's ear cartilages are well formed, and the hair is more likely to form firm, separate strands.

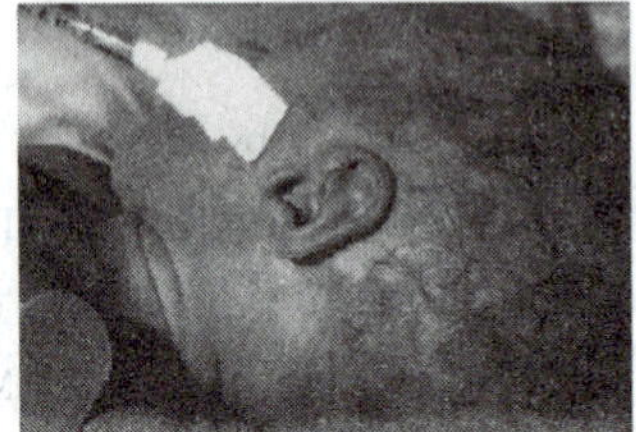

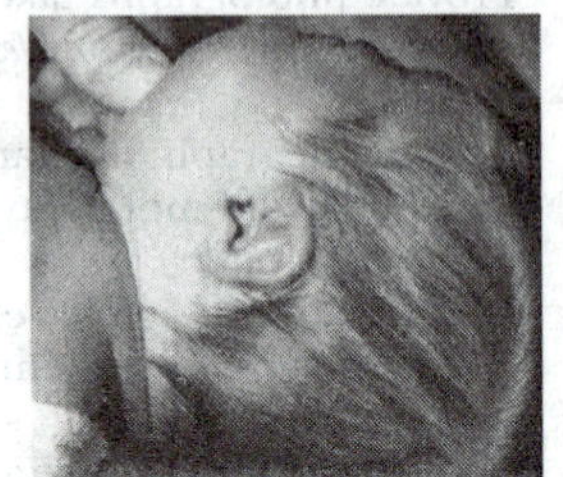

Sole—The sole of the foot of the preterm infant appears more turgid and may have only fine wrinkles. The mature infant's sole (foot) is well and deeply creased.

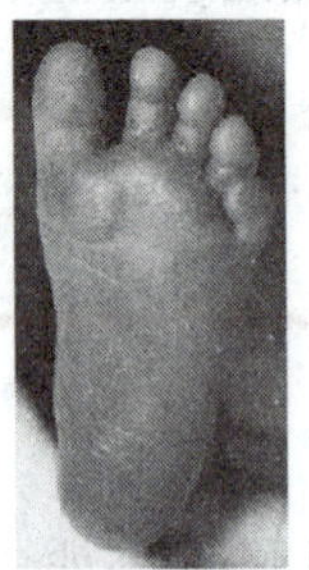

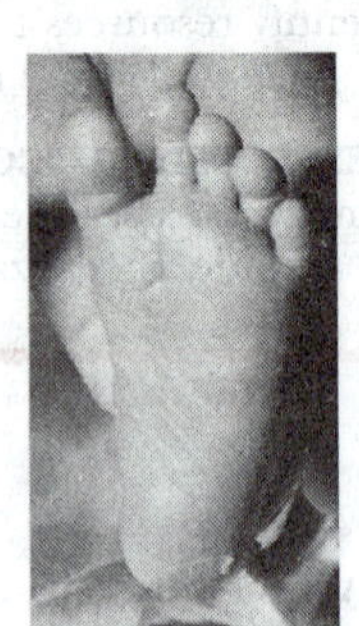

Female genitalia—The preterm female infant's clitoris is prominent, and labia majora are poorly developed and gaping. The mature female infant's labia majora are fully developed, and the clitoris is not as prominent.

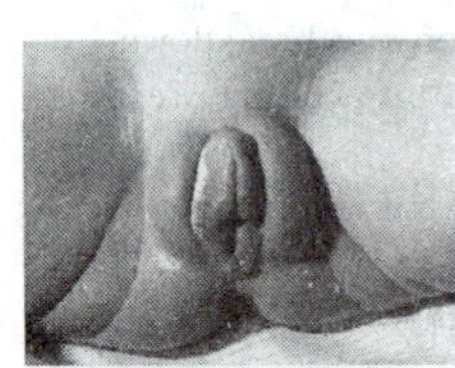

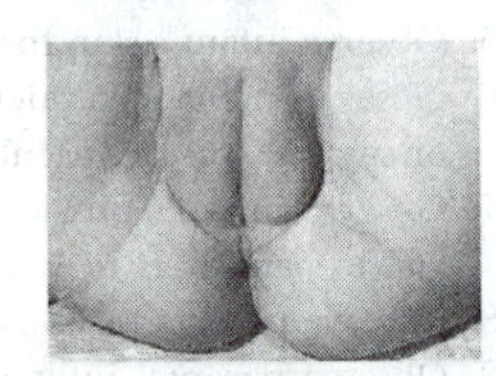

Male genitalia—The preterm male infant's scrotum is undeveloped and not pendulous; minimal rugae are present, and the testes may be in the inguinal canals or in the abdominal cavity. The term male infant's scrotum is well developed, pendulous, and rugated, and the testes are well down in the scrotal sac.

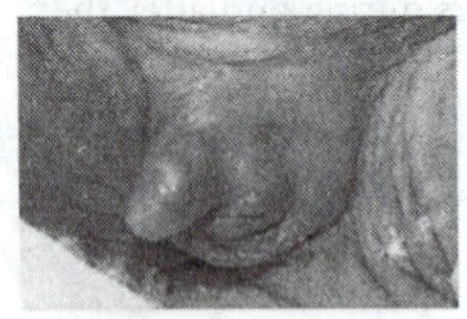

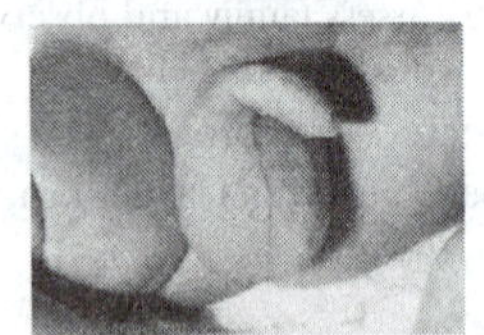

Scarf sign—The preterm infant's elbow may be easily brought across the chest with little or no resistance. The mature infant's elbow may be brought to the midline of the chest, resisting attempts to bring the elbow past the midline.

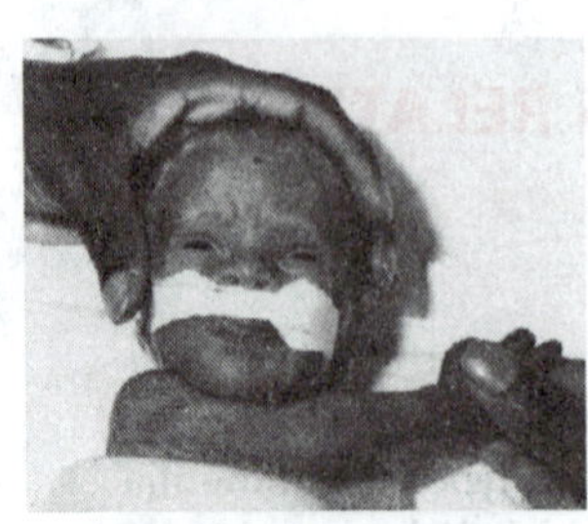

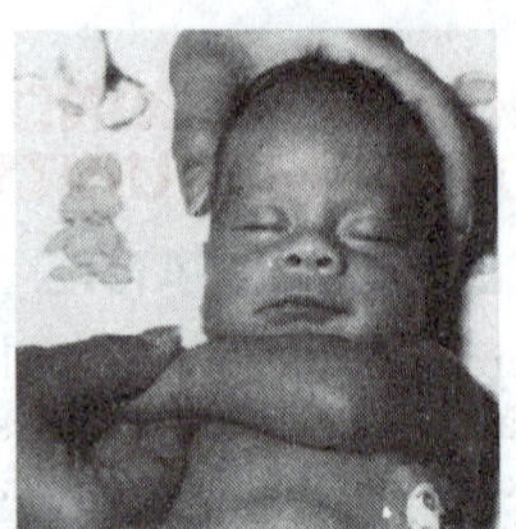

FIG. 10-11 Clinical and neurologic examinations comparing preterm and full-term infants.
(Data from Pierog SH, Ferrara A: *Medical care of the sick newborn,* ed 2, St Louis, 1976, Mosby.)

Characteristics

Preterm infants have a number of characteristics that are distinctive at various stages of development. Identification of these characteristics provides valuable clues to the gestational age and hence to the physiologic capabilities of infants. The general, outward physical appearance changes as the fetus progresses to maturity. Characteristics of skin, general attitude (or posture) when supine, appearance of hair, and amount of subcutaneous fat provide cues to a newborn's physical development. Observation of spontaneous, active movements and response to stimulation and passive movement contributes to the assessment of neurologic status. The appraisal is made as soon as possible after admission to the nursery, since much of the observation and management of infants depends on this information.

On inspection, premature infants are very small and appear scrawny because they lack or have only minimal subcutaneous fat deposits, with a proportionately large head in relation to the body, which reflects the cephalocaudal direction of growth. The skin is bright pink (often translucent, depending on the degree of immaturity), smooth, and shiny (may be edematous), with small blood vessels clearly visible underneath the thin epidermis. The fine lanugo hair is abundant over the body (depending on gestational age) but is sparse, fine, and fuzzy on the head. The ear cartilage is soft and pliable, and the soles and palms have minimal creases, resulting in a smooth appearance. The bones of the skull and the ribs feel soft, and the eyes may be closed. Male infants have few scrotal rugae, and the testes are undescended; the labia and clitoris are prominent in females. (See Fig. 10-11 for a comparison of the features of normal and premature infants.)

In contrast to full-term infants' overall attitude of flexion and continuous activity, premature infants are inactive and listless. The extremities maintain an attitude of extension and remain in any position in which they are placed. Reflex activity is only partially developed—sucking is absent, weak, or ineffectual; swallowing, gag, and cough reflexes are absent or weak; and other neurologic signs are absent or diminished. Physiologically immature, preterm infants are unable to maintain body temperature, have limited ability to excrete solutes in the urine, and have increased susceptibility to infection. A pliable thorax, immature lung tissue, and an immature regulatory center lead to periodic breathing, hypoventilation, and frequent periods of apnea. They are more susceptible to biochemical alterations such as hyperbilirubinemia and hypoglycemia (see Chapter 9), and they have a higher extracellular water content that renders them more vulnerable to fluid and electrolyte derangements. Premature infants will exchange fully half their extracellular fluid volume every 24 hours as compared with one seventh of the volume in adults.

The soft cranium is subject to characteristic nonintentional deformation, or "preemie head," caused by positioning from one side to the other on a mattress. The head looks disproportionately longer from front to back, is flattened on both sides, and lacks the usual convexity seen at the temporal and parietal areas (Budreau, 1987). This positional molding is frequently a concern to parents and may influence the parents' perception of the infant's attractive-

NEUROLOGIC EVALUATION

PRETERM | TERM

Grasp reflex—The preterm infant's grasp is weak; the term infant's grasp is strong, allowing the infant to be lifted up from the mattress.

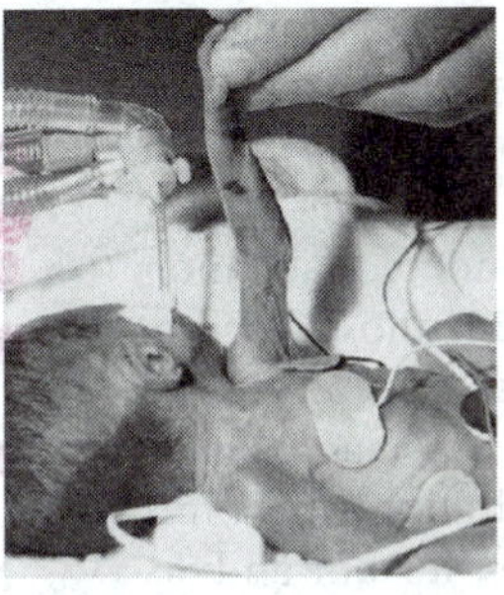

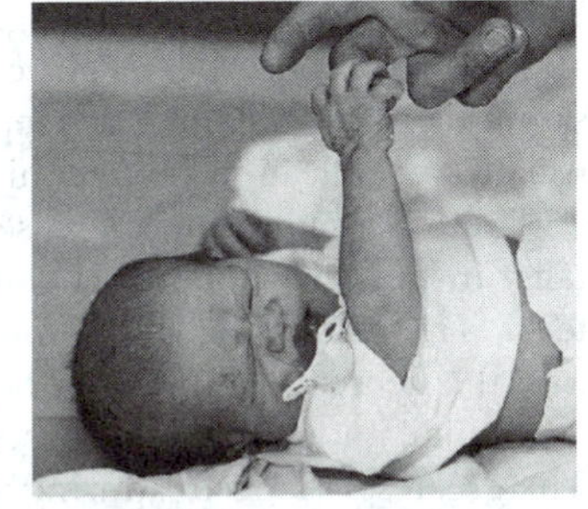

Heel-to-ear maneuver—The preterm infant's he El is easily brought to the ear, meeting with no resistance. This maneuver is not possible in the term infant, since there is considerable resistance at the knee.

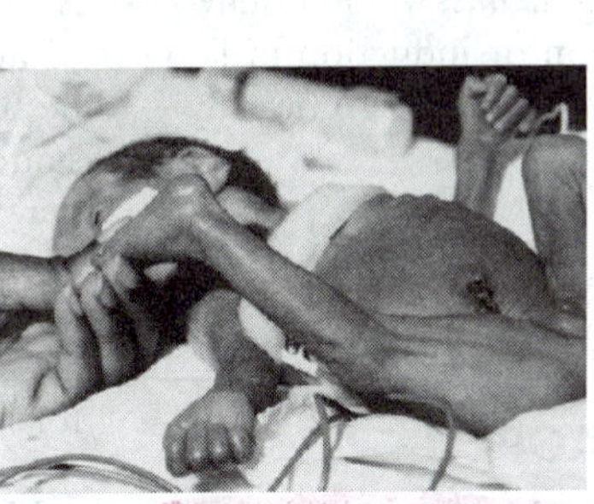

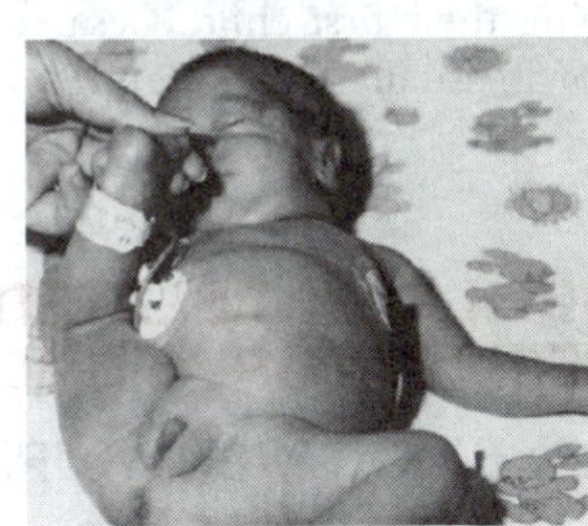

FIG. 10-11, cont'd For legend see opposite page.

ness and their responsiveness to the infant. Positioning the infant on a waterbed mattress can reduce or minimize cranial molding.

Therapeutic Management

When delivery of a preterm infant is anticipated, the intensive care nursery is alerted, and a pediatrician, ideally a neonatologist, is present for the delivery. Infants who do not require resuscitation are transferred immediately to the NICU in a heated incubator where they are weighed, and intravenous lines, oxygen therapy, and other therapeutic interventions are initiated as needed. Resuscitation is conducted in the delivery area until infants can be safely transported to the NICU. Ongoing care is described elsewhere in the chapter and is not repeated in this section.

Nursing Considerations

The nursing care, like the therapeutic management, is individualized for each infant. See appropriate discussions under Nursing Care of High-Risk Newborns for details of care.

POSTMATURE INFANTS

Infants born of a gestation that extends beyond 42 weeks as calculated from the mother's last menstrual period (or by gestational age assessment) are considered to be postmature, or postterm, regardless of birth weight. This constitutes 3.5% to 15% of all pregnancies. The cause of delayed birth is unknown. Some infants are appropriate for gestational age but show the characteristics of progressive placental dysfunction. These infants, often called postmature infants, display the characteristics of infants who are 1 to 3 weeks of age, such as absence of lanugo, little if any vernix caseosa, abundant scalp hair, and long fingernails. Frequently the skin is cracked, parchmentlike, and desquamating. A common finding in postmature infants is a wasted physical appearance that reflects intrauterine deprivation. Depletion of subcutaneous fat gives them a thin, elongated appearance. The little vernix caseosa that remains in the skinfolds may be stained a deep yellow or green, which is usually an indication of meconium in the amniotic fluid.

There is a significant increase in fetal and neonatal mortality in postterm infants as compared with those born at term. They are especially prone to fetal distress associated with the decreasing efficiency of the placenta, macrosomia, congenital anomalies, and meconium aspiration syndrome. The greatest risk occurs during the stresses of labor and delivery, particularly in infants of ***primigravidas,*** women delivering their first child. Cesarean section or induction of labor is usually recommended when infants are significantly overdue.

HIGH RISK RELATED TO DISTURBED RESPIRATORY FUNCTION

APNEA OF PREMATURITY (AOP)

AOP is a common phenomenon in the preterm infant. Rarely observed in full-term infants, the prevalence of apneic spells increases the younger the gestational age. Approximately one third of infants less than 32 weeks of gestation and almost all apparently healthy infants less than 30 weeks of gestation have apneic spells. Characteristically, premature infants are periodic breathers; they have periods of rapid respiration separated by periods of very slow breathing and often short periods during which there are no visible or audible respirations. Apnea is primarily an extension of this periodic breathing and can be defined as a lapse of spontaneous breathing for 20 or more seconds, which may or may not be followed by bradycardia and color change. Apnea of prematurity should not be confused with apnea of infancy (see Chapter 13).

POSSIBLE CAUSES OF NEONATAL APNEA

Airway obstruction with mucus or poor positioning
Anemia, polycythemia
Dehydration
Cooling or overheating
Hypercapnia or hypocapnia
Hypoglycemia
Hypocalcemia
Hyponatremia
Sepsis, meningitis
Seizures
Increased vagal tone (in response to suctioning nasopharynx, gavage tube insertion, reflux of gastric contents, endotracheal intubation)
Periodic breathing
CNS depression from pharmacologic agents
Intraventricular hemorrhage
Patent ductus arteriosus, congestive heart failure
Depression following maternal obstetric sedation
Infants with respiratory distress, pneumonia, inborn errors of metabolism such as hyperammonemia, congenital defects of the upper airways

Pathophysiology

Although the cause of AOP is unknown, it probably reflects the immature and poorly refined neurologic and chemical respiratory control mechanisms. These infants are not as responsive to oxygen and carbon dioxide, and their neurons have fewer dendritic associations than those of the more mature infant. The respiratory reflexes of these infants are significantly more immature, which may be a contributing factor in the etiology. In addition, apnea is characteristically observed during periods of rapid eye movement in sleep.

Clinical Manifestations

A number of factors that appear to promote the incidence of apnea in preterm neonates can be treated. Apnea can be anticipated in infants with any of a variety of circumstances (see box above); conversely, one of these disorders may be suspected in infants with persistent apneic spells. Although apnea is an expected event in preterm neonates, it should not be designated as such until all other causes are ruled out. The observation of apnea is cause to screen for any of the causes listed in the box.

Therapeutic Management

It has been found that administration of methylxanthines (aminophylline, theophylline, or caffeine) is often effective in reducing the frequency of primary apnea-bradycardia spells in newborns. Theophylline and caffeine act as CNS stimulants to breathing. Neonates who receive these drugs have serum drug levels measured regularly and must be closely observed for symptoms of toxicity. Serum drug levels are determined by the size and response of the infant and are maintained within a therapeutic range, such as 5 to 25 mg/ml for caffeine and 2 to 15 mg/ml for theophylline (O'Donnell, 1994).

NURSING ALERT Signs of theophylline or caffeine toxicity are tachycardia (rate greater than 180 to 190 beats/min) at rest, vomiting, irritability, restlessness, diuresis, dysrhythmias, jitteriness, and gastritis (hemorrhagic).

Nursing Considerations

Management of periodic apnea consists of monitoring respiration and heart rate routinely in all small preterm infants and prevention of contributing conditions. Mechanical apnea monitors provide a means to alert the staff to cessation of respiration according to a preset delay time, usually 15 to 20 seconds. Effective monitoring devices do not make alert nursing observation unnecessary. Any mechanical device is subject to malfunction. Without close observation, even of monitored infants, many unidentified episodes of prolonged apnea and severe bradycardia may occur. Nursing observation combined with monitoring is the most effective means of identifying neonatal apnea (Muttitt and others, 1988).

NURSING ALERT When the alarm sounds, infants are first assessed for color and for presence of respiration. If they display the usual color and respirations, the nurse should investigate possible causes of a false alarm, such as faulty lead placement, detached or disconnected leads, improper alarm setting, or mechanical failure.

If it is begun early, gentle tactile stimulation, such as rubbing the back or chest gently or turning the infant over, will stop most apneic spells. If tactile stimulation fails to reinstitute respiration, the nose and oropharynx are suctioned, flow-by 100% oxygen is administered, and if breathing does not begin, the chin is raised gently to open the airway and sufficient pressure is applied with a resuscitation mask and bag to lift the rib cage. The infant is never shaken. After breathing is restored, the infant is assessed for possible precipitating factors, such as temperature, humidity, abdominal distention (if not observed earlier), and oxygen content (if any) being delivered prior to the episode. The use of pulse oximetry monitors has helped in the detection of the onset of an apneic episode. It is important for nurses to document episodes of apnea. A careful record is maintained of the number of apneic spells, the appearance of the infant during and after attacks, and whether the infant self-recovers or whether tactile stimulation is needed to restore breathing. Persistent and repeated periods of apnea may be treated by mechanical ventilation or nasal continuous positive airway pressure (CPAP).

Subsequent investigation into the possible cause of the apneic episode is vital to the care of the preterm infant, since it may be a signal of an underlying condition such as sepsis or intraventricular hemorrhage. Bradycardia may occur with apnea, since there is decreased delivery of oxygen to the myocardium.

Various methods devised to provide an intermittent stimulus for breathing, such as oscillating water beds, have achieved variable success but have decreased in usage with the potential increased risk of intraventricular hemorrhage.

RESPIRATORY DISTRESS SYNDROME (RDS)

Respiratory distress is a name applied to respiratory dysfunction in neonates and is primarily a disease related to developmental delay in lung maturation. The terms ***respiratory distress syndrome (RDS)*** and ***hyaline membrane disease (HMD)*** are most often applied to the severe lung disorder that is not only responsible for more infant deaths than any other disease but also carries the highest risk in terms of long-term respiratory and neurologic complications (see Chapter 32 for a discussion of adult RDS). It is seen almost exclusively in preterm infants. The disorder is rare in infants of narcotic-addicted mothers or infants who have been subjected to chronic intrauterine stress (e.g., maternal preeclampsia or hypertension). Respiratory distress of a nonpulmonary origin in neonates may also be caused by sepsis, exposure to cold, airway obstruction (atresia), intraventricular hemorrhage, hypoglycemia, metabolic acidosis, acute blood loss, and drugs. Pneumonia in the neonatal period is respiratory distress caused by bacterial or viral agents and may occur alone or as a complication of RDS.

Pathophysiology

Preterm infants are born before the lungs are fully prepared to serve as efficient organs for gas exchange. This appears to be a critical factor in the development of RDS. Although the precise cause is still undetermined, several features in the development of the disorder are established, and there are a number of interdependent relationships that complicate the situation.

Before birth there is evidence of fetal respiratory activity. The lungs make feeble respiratory movements, and fluid is excreted through the alveoli. Since the final unfolding of the alveolar septa, which increases the surface area of the lungs, takes place during the last trimester of pregnancy, premature infants are born with numerous underdeveloped and many uninflatable alveoli. There is limited pulmonary blood flow, resulting from the collapsed state of the fetal lungs and from poor vascular development in general and an immature capillary network in particular. Because of the increased pulmonary vascular resistance, the major portion of fetal blood is shunted from the lungs by way of the ductus arteriosus and foramen ovale (see Cardiac Development and Function, Chapter 34).

At the time of birth, infants must initiate breathing and then keep the previously fluid-filled lungs inflated with air. At the same time, the pulmonary capillary blood flow must be increased approximately tenfold to provide for adequate lung perfusion and to alter the intracardiac pressure that closes the fetal cardiac structures. Most full-term infants successfully accomplish these adjustments; preterm infants with respiratory distress are unable to do so. Although numerous factors are involved, most authorities believe that the central factor responsible for this adaptation is normal development of the surfactant system.

Surfactant is a surface-active phospholipid secreted by the alveolar epithelium. Acting much like a detergent, this substance reduces surface tension of fluids that line the alveoli and respiratory passages, resulting in uniform expansion and maintenance of lung expansion at low intraalveolar pressure. Immature development of these functions produces consequences that seriously compromise respiratory efficiency. Deficient surfactant production causes unequal inflation of alveoli on inspiration and collapse of alveoli on end expiration. Without surfactant, infants are unable to keep their lungs inflated and therefore exert a great deal of effort to reexpand the alveoli with each breath. It has been estimated that each breath requires as much negative pressure (60 to 75 cm H_2O) as the initial lung expansion at birth. As a result, infants use more oxygen to expend this energy than they take in, which rapidly leads to exhaustion. With increasing exhaustion they are able to open fewer and fewer alveoli. This inability to maintain lung expansion produces widespread atelectasis.

In the absence of alveolar stability (normal functional residual capacity) and with progressive atelectasis, the pulmonary vascular resistance (PVR) increases, whereas with normal lung expansion it would decrease. Consequently, there is hypoperfusion to the lung tissue with a decrease in effective pulmonary blood flow. The increase in PVR causes partial reversion to the fetal circulation, with a right-to-left shunting of blood through the persisting fetal communications—the ductus arteriosus and foramen ovale.

Inadequate pulmonary perfusion and ventilation produce hypoxemia and hypercapnia. Pulmonary arterioles, with their thick muscular layer, are markedly reactive to diminished oxygen concentration. Thus a decrease in oxygen tension causes vasospasm in the pulmonary arterioles that is further enhanced by a decrease in blood pH. This vasoconstriction contributes to a marked increase in PVR. In normal ventilation with increased oxygen concentration, the ductus arteriosus constricts and the pulmonary vessels dilate to decrease PVR (Fig. 10-12).

Prolonged hypoxemia activates anaerobic glycolysis, which produces increased amounts of lactic acid. An increase in lactic acid causes metabolic acidosis; inability of the atelectatic lungs to blow off excess carbon dioxide produces respiratory acidosis. Lowered pH causes further vasoconstriction. With deficient pulmonary circulation and alveolar perfusion, the Pao_2 continues to fall, the pH falls, and materials needed for surfactant production are not circulated to the alveoli.

Pulmonary edema observed in the early stages of RDS also contributes to impaired gas exchange. Factors believed to facilitate this fluid accumulation in the lungs include renal immaturity or insufficiency resulting from hypoxemia, high fluid intake and patent ductus arteriosus, left ventricular dysfunction associated with papillary muscle necrosis,

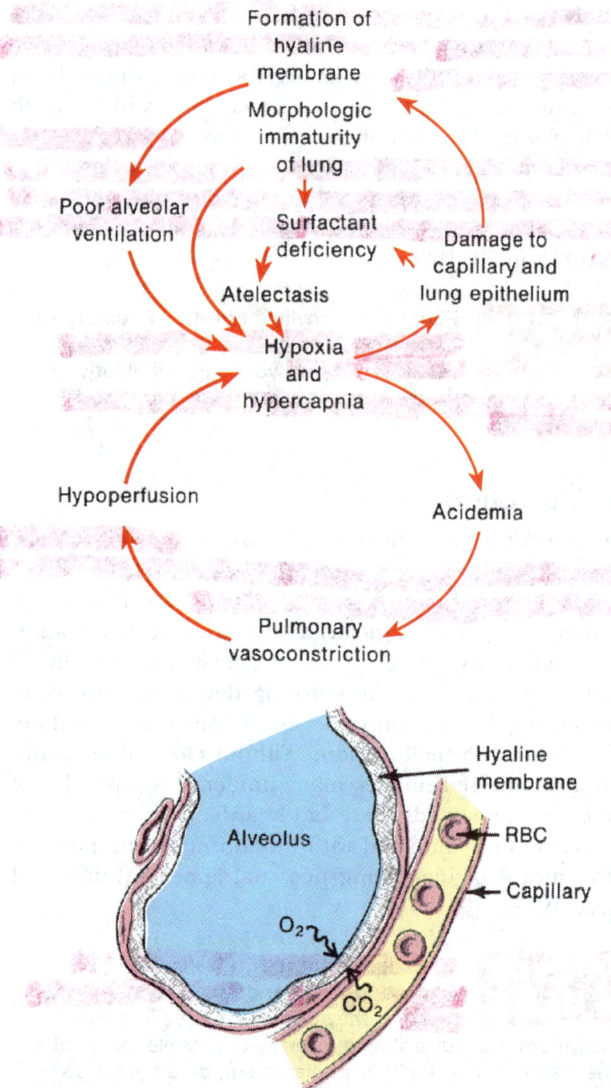

FIG. 10-12 Interdependent relationship of factors involved in pathology of respiratory distress syndrome. (From Pierog SH, Ferrara A: *Medical care of the sick newborn,* ed 2, St Louis, 1976, Mosby.)

low serum protein concentration and low colloid osmotic pressure, increased alveolar surface tension that enhances the shift of interstitial fluid to alveolar spaces, oxygen toxicity, and high plasma vasopressin.

Deficiencies in other systems contribute to respiratory distress. For example, a high threshold of the respiratory center to afferent stimuli and weak gag and cough reflexes reflect the immaturity of the nervous system. In addition, the persistence of fetal hemoglobin, so beneficial in prenatal existence, may place the infant at a disadvantage during respiratory distress. Although the binding power of fetal hemoglobin for oxygen is much greater than in adult hemoglobin, this increased affinity also causes less oxygen to be released to the tissues at normal oxygen tension. In the newborn the arterial oxygen concentration must fall to a lower level for bound oxygen to be released from fetal hemoglobin.

TABLE 10-4 Major Factors in Respiratory Distress

CAUSE	EFFECT
Increased surface tension of alveoli (surfactant deficiency)	Alveolar collapse; atelectasis; increased difficulty of breathing
Impaired gas exchange	Hypoxemia and hypercapnia with respiratory acidosis
Increased pulmonary vascular resistance	Hypoperfusion of pulmonary circulation
Hypoperfusion (with hypoxemia)	Tissue hypoxia and metabolic acidosis
Increased transudation of fluid into lungs	Hyaline membrane formation; impaired gas exchange

A hyaline membrane is formed as hypoxemia and the increased pulmonary vascular pressure cause transudation of fluid into the alveoli. Necrotic cells from damaged alveoli plus the fibrin in the transudate form a membranous layer that lines the alveoli and inhibits gas exchange. Presence of the membrane contributes to respiratory difficulties by greatly diminishing lung distensibility, or ***compliance,*** the elastic quality of lung tissue that permits expansion in response to a given amount of applied pressure during inspiration. Affected lungs are stiffer and require far more pressure than do normal lungs to achieve an equal amount of expansion. The major factors that produce respiratory distress in immature infants are summarized in Table 10-4.

RDS is a self-limiting disease, and following a period of deterioration (approximately 48 hours) and in the absence of complications, affected infants begin to improve by 72 hours. Often heralded by the onset of diuresis, this improvement has been attributed primarily to increased production and greater availability of surface-active material.

Clinical Manifestations

Infants with RDS can develop respiratory distress either acutely or over a period of hours, depending on the acuity of pulmonary immaturity, associated illness factors, and gestational maturity. Usually the observable signs produced by the pulmonary changes begin to appear in infants who apparently achieve normal breathing and color soon after birth. In a matter of a few hours, breathing gradually becomes more rapid (greater than 60 breaths/min). Infants may display retractions—suprasternal or substernal; supracostal, subcostal, or intercostal—which result from a compliant chest wall. Weak chest wall muscles and the highly cartilaginous nature of the rib structure produce an abnormally elastic rib cage. Thus considerable negative pressure is wasted as the infant attempts to produce higher intrathoracic pressure changes. During this early period the infant's color may remain satisfactory and auscultation reveals air entry. Some of the criteria for evaluating respiratory distress in infants are illustrated in Fig. 10-13.

Within a few hours, respiratory distress becomes more obvious. The respiratory rate continues to increase (to 80 to 120 breaths/min), and breathing becomes more labored. It is significant to note that infants will increase the *rate* rather than the *depth* of respiration when in distress. Substernal retractions become more pronounced as the diaphragm works hard in an attempt to fill collapsed air sacs. Fine inspiratory rales can be heard over both lungs, and there is an audible expiratory grunt. This grunting, a useful mechanism observed in the earlier stages of RDS, serves to increase end-expiratory pressure in the lungs, thus maintaining alveolar expansion and allowing gas exchange for an additional brief period. Flaring of the nares is also a sign that accompanies tachypnea, grunting, and retractions in respiratory distress. Central cyanosis (a bluish discoloration of oral mucous membranes and generalized body cyanosis) is a late and serious sign of respiratory distress. Initially cyanosis may be abolished by supplemental oxygen. The use of pulse oximetry and arterial blood gas sampling obviates the necessity for dependence on color to determine oxygen requirements.

At this point the respiratory distress may gradually decrease over 12 to 24 hours, with eventual recovery, or it may increase in severity. In distressed infants cyanosis becomes more marked despite increases in ambient oxygen concentration. Often there is pallor caused by peripheral vasoconstriction, but it is frequently masked by cyanosis. The infants become flaccid and unresponsive and begin to display frequent apneic episodes. Chest auscultation reveals diminished breath sounds. The chances of recovery without assisted ventilation are then very small. Severe RDS is often associated with a shocklike state, as manifested by diminished cardiac inflow and low arterial blood pressure. The ELBW or VLBW infant, as a result of extreme pulmonary immaturity, decreased glycogen stores, and lack of accessory muscles, may have severe RDS at birth, therefore bypassing the aforementioned steps in the development of RDS.

Infants with RDS who survive the first 96 hours have a reasonable chance of recovery. Complications of RDS include those described as complications of oxygen therapy (see Chapter 31), patent ductus arteriosus and congestive heart failure, intraventricular hemorrhage, bronchopulmonary dysplasia, retinopathy of prematurity, necrotizing enterocolitis, and neurologic sequelae.

Diagnostic Evaluation

Laboratory data are nonspecific, and abnormalities observed are identical to those observed in numerous biochemical abnormalities of the newborn (i.e., the findings of hypoxemia, hypercapnia, and acidosis). To determine complicating factors, specific tests are carried out, such as blood, urine, and blood glucose (to test for hypoglycemia), serum calcium (to test for hypocalcemia), blood gas measurements for serum pH (to test for acidosis), and $Pa{O_2}$ (to test for hypoxia). Pulse oximetry is an important component for determining hypoxia. Other special examinations may be employed to diagnose or rule out complications.

Radiographic findings characteristic of RDS include (1) a diffuse granular pattern over both lung fields closely resembling ground glass that represents alveolar atelectasis

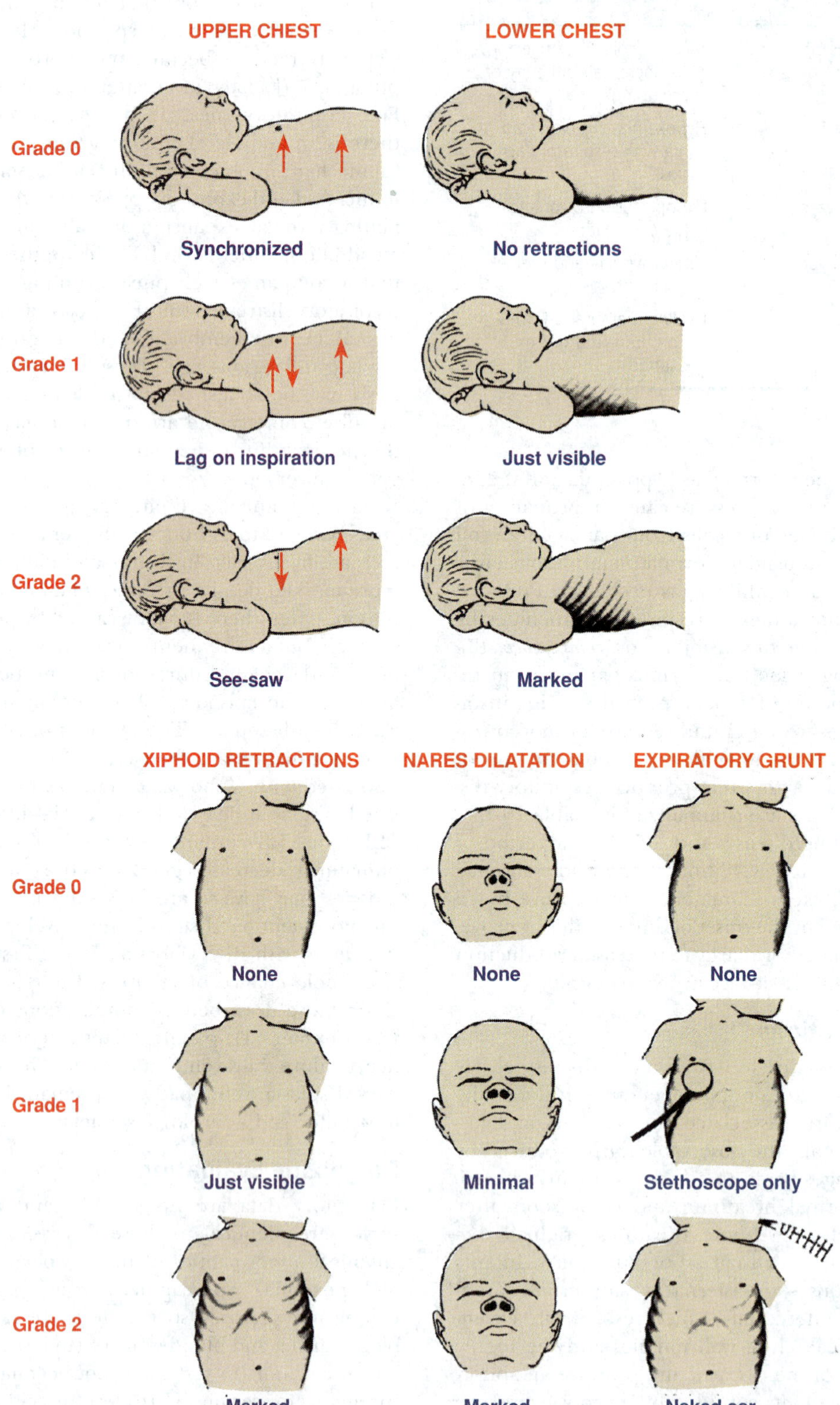

FIG. 10-13 Criteria for evaluating respiratory distress. (Modified from Silvermann WA, Anderson DH: *Pediatrics* 17:1, 1956.)

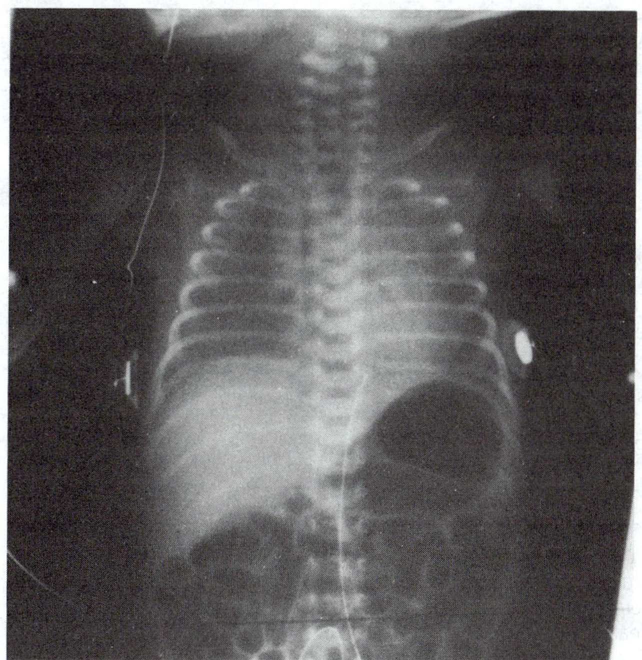

FIG. 10-14 Reticulogranular infiltrate and air bronchogram in hyaline membrane disease. Note air in stomach.

and (2) dark streaks, or bronchograms, within the ground glass areas that represent dilated air-filled bronchioles (Fig. 10-14). It is important to distinguish between RDS and pneumonia in infants with respiratory distress.

Prenatal Diagnosis. Fetal lung maturity depends on gestational age, except in some specific instances that may not be known until the time of labor or delivery. Functional maturity of the fetal lung can be determined by using surfactant phospholipids in amniotic fluid as indicators of maturity. The most commonly tested is the lethicin/sphingomyelin (L/S) ratio, which measures the relationship between these two lipids during gestation. Phospholipids are synthesized by fetal alveolar cells, and the concentrations in amniotic fluid change during gestation. Initially there is more sphingomyelin, but at about 32 to 33 weeks the concentrations become equal, and then sphingomyelin diminishes and lecithin increases significantly until the fetus has developed sufficient surface-active material to maintain alveolar stability at about 35 weeks.

Other key surfactant compounds (also phospholipids) that are needed to stabilize surfactant are phosphatidylcholine (PC) and phosphatidylglycerol (PG). Without these compounds lecithin is not functional as a surfactant. Concentrations of PC parallel those of lecithin, peaking at 35 weeks and then gradually decreasing. At 36 weeks PG appears in amniotic fluid and increases until term. By measuring these phospholipids—L/S ratio, PC, and PG—the maturity of the lungs can be estimated with a high degree of accuracy. Abnormal pregnancies may be associated with acceleration (before 33 weeks) or delay (later than 37 weeks) in fetal lung maturation.

Other, but less frequently employed, methods have been devised to provide rapid, inexpensive, and accurate measures of lung maturity. These include the "shake" or "bubble" test, in which stable foam or bubbles form when amniotic fluid is shaken in the presence of ethanol, and the tap tests, in which abundant bubbles appear in a test tube of amniotic fluid with 6N hydrochloric acid and diethyl ether.

Increasing evidence has shown that certain ***antioxidant enzymes,*** which develop late in gestation, have an important role in protecting alveoli and airway cells from damage by oxygen radicals that appear in hyperoxic states (as in the infant attempting to adapt to an extrauterine existence). The antioxidant system (AOS) has no effect on fetal lung maturity, yet when it is deficient, there is more damage to the already-compromised alveoli and airway cells (Blackburn and Loper, 1992). Another test currently being researched is the TDx Fetal Lung Maturity (FLM) assay, which determines PG levels in amniotic fluid or neonatal tracheal aspirates. The FLM test is quicker than L/S ratio determination (<1 hour vs 4 to 5 hours) and is reported to predict the absence of hyaline membrane disease (or RDS) with greater accuracy; a level of 50 or more is predictive of fetal lung maturity (Ashwood, Palmer, and Lenke, 1992; Steinfeld and others, 1992).

Therapeutic Management

The treatment of RDS is largely supportive and includes all the general measures required for any premature infant, as well as those instituted to correct imbalances. The supportive measures that are most crucial to a favorable outcome are (1) maintain adequate ventilation and oxygenation with either an oxygen hood or mechanical ventilation, (2) maintain acid-base balance, (3) maintain a neutral thermal environment, (4) maintain adequate tissue perfusion and oxygenation, (5) prevent hypotension, and (6) maintain adequate hydration and electrolyte status. Nipple and gavage feedings are contraindicated in any situation that creates a marked increase in respiratory rate because of the greater hazards of aspiration. In addition, administering substrate to the infant with transient hypoxia places the infant at risk for necrotizing enterocolitis. Nutrition is provided by parenteral therapy during the acute stage of the disease.

Oxygen Therapy. The goals of oxygen therapy are to provide adequate oxygen to the tissues, prevent lactic acid accumulation resulting from hypoxia, and at the same time avoid the potentially toxic effects of oxygen barotrauma. Numerous methods have been devised to improve oxygenation (Table 10-5). All require that the gas be warmed and humidified before entering the respiratory tract. If the infant does not require mechanical ventilation, oxygen can be supplied to a plastic hood placed over the infant's head to supply variable concentrations of humidified oxygen (see Oxygen Therapy, Chapter 31). If oxygen saturation of the blood cannot be maintained at a satisfactory level and the carbon dioxide level ($PaCO_2$) rises, infants will require ventilatory assistance.

Continuous positive airway pressure (CPAP) or continuous distending pressure (CDP), the application of 3 to 8 cm of water (positive) pressure to the airway, uses the

TABLE 10-5 Common Methods for Assisted Ventilation in Neonatal Respiratory Distress

METHOD	DESCRIPTION	HOW PROVIDED
COMMON METHODS		
Continuous positive airway pressure (CPAP) or continuous distending pressure (CDP)	Provides constant distending pressure to airway in spontaneously breathing infant	Nasal prongs Nasopharyngeal tubes Endotracheal tube
Positive end-expiratory pressure (PEEP)*	Provides increased end-expiratory pressure during expiration and between mandatory breaths that prevents alveolar collapse; maintains residual airway pressure	Endotracheal intubation and either volume-limited or pressure-limited ventilator
Intermittent mandatory ventilation (IMV)*	Allows infant to breathe spontaneously at own rate but provides mechanical cycled respirations and pressure at regular preset intervals	Endotracheal intubation and ventilator
ALTERNATIVE METHODS		
High-frequency ventilation (HFV)		
High-frequency positive-pressure ventilation (HFPPV)	Low-complaint circuit provides high gas flow through circuit: operates at rates between 60 and 150 breaths/min	Conventional infant ventilators; endotracheal tube
High-frequency oscillation (HFO)	Application of high-frequency, low-volume, sine-wave flow oscillations to airway at rates between 480 to 1200 breaths/min	Variable-speed piston pump (or loudspeaker, fluidic oscillator); endotracheal tube
High-frequency jet ventilation (HFJV)	Uses a separate, parallel, low-complaint circuit and injector port to deliver small pulses or jets of fresh gas deep into airway at rates between 250 and 900 breaths/min	May be used alone or with low-rate IMV; endotracheal tube

*Also referred to as conventional ventilation (vs HFV).

infant's spontaneous respiration to improve oxygenation by helping prevent alveolar collapse and increasing diffusion time. CPAP may be delivered via nasal prongs, an endotracheal tube, a face mask, or a head-enclosing box. Ventilation with CPAP is done entirely by the infant. If oxygenation is not improved and the infant requires assisted ventilation, intermittent mandatory ventilation (IMV) or continuous positive-pressure ventilation (CPPV) is used with positive end-expiratory pressure (PEEP). This allows infants to breathe at their own rate but provides positive pressure at regular preset intervals, with end-expiratory pressure to prevent alveolar collapse and overcome airway resistance. Additional components involved in IMV mechanical ventilation are peak inspiratory pressure (PIP) and rate (number of breaths per minute). The PIP is the maximum amount of positive pressure applied to the infant on inspiration. The total amount of pressure transmitted to the airway throughout an entire respiratory cycle is called the mean airway pressure (MAP). Increasing the MAP in infants with severe RDS correlates positively with improved oxygenation by maintaining functional residual capacity and overcoming the resistive forces of the atelectatic lung (Nugent, 1991). The MAP is affected by changes in the PEEP, PIP, and inspiratory/expiratory (I/E) ratio (Merenstein and Gardner, 1993).

If the PaO_2 cannot be maintained or the $PaCO_2$ level rises, infants may require one of the three high-frequency ventilation (HFV) modalities. HFV delivers gas at very rapid rates to provide adequate minute volumes using lower proximal airway pressures by way of high-frequency positive-pressure ventilation (HFPPV), high-frequency oscillation (HFO), or high-frequency jet ventilation (HFJV). HFV is recommended for intractable respiratory failure, especially for infants with pulmonary air leaks. It is primarily a short-term therapy, and it is believed to reduce the incidence of barotrauma, which frequently complicates oxygen therapy in preterm infants. Barotrauma is believed to be a key factor in the development of bronchopulmonary dysplasia (BPD). However, there is an increased incidence of necrotizing tracheitis, pneumopericardium, and hypotension reported with HFJV. Additional potential advantages of HFV over conventional ventilation are active elimination of carbon dioxide and the ability to ventilate infants with persistent pulmonary hypertension. Both HFJV and HFO have met with varying success for the prevention of BPD and decreased infant mortality rates (Myrer, 1992).

Complications of oxygen therapy. Although lifesaving, oxygen therapy is not without hazards. Positive pressure introduced by mechanical apparatus has caused an increased incidence of air leaks that produce complications, such as pneumothorax and pneumomediastinum (see discussion on p. 408). Other complications directly related to oxygen therapy include retinopathy of prematurity (p. 416), bronchopulmonary dysplasia (p. 409), and various problems associated with intubation, such as nasal, tracheal, or pharyngeal perforation, stenosis, inflammation, palatal grooves,

CRITICAL THINKING EXERCISE
Respiratory Distress Syndrome

A 32-week preterm infant requires mechanical ventilation for the treatment of respiratory distress syndrome as a result of surfactant deficiency. The nurse is aware of problems associated with prematurity and RDS, such as hypoglycemia. Problems for which you are particularly vigilant in light of the use of mechanical ventilation with this infant and the knowledge of pathology include:

1. Meconium aspiration
2. Transient tachypnea
3. Air leaks
4. Persistent pulmonary hypertension

The correct answer is 3. Infants who are preterm and lack adequate surfactant have immature alveoli and increased surface tension that predispose them to the development of air leaks during mechanical ventilation. The other three options are neonatal respiratory conditions usually unrelated to RDS of the type where surfactant deficiency is the major pathology.

subglottic stenosis, tube obstruction, and infection (see Critical Thinking Exercise box).

Medical Therapies. The treatment of the infant with RDS will require the establishment of one or more intravenous lines to maintain hydration and nutrition, to monitor arterial blood gases, and to administer medications. Medications commonly administered during this acute phase include antibiotics for sepsis (see Sepsis) and diuretics such as furosemide (to facilitate renal excretion of water and reduce pulmonary fluid). The administration of pancuronium (for muscle paralysis), phenobarbitol (for sedation), and vitamin E (to decrease oxygen free-radical production) is individualized according to the infant's response to illness. Methylxanthines (theophylline or caffeine) are administered to treat apnea and for weaning from mechanical ventilation (Cusson, 1992). Inotropes such as Dopamine and Dobutamine may be required to support the infant's systemic pressure and maintain effective cardiac output during the acute phase of illness.

It is not uncommon for high-risk neonates, including those with RDS, to receive a blood transfusion (often packed red blood cells) to replace the blood volume lost with frequent sampling. Procedures for properly identifying the blood product, identification of the patient, and administration are found in Chapter 35.

Surfactant. One of the newest (and accepted) additions to the treatment of the infant with RDS is the administration of exogenous surfactant. Exogenous surfactant is derived from a natural source such as human (obtained from donor's amniotic fluid), porcine, or bovine, or from the production of artificial surfactant. Commercially available surfactant products include Exosurf Neonatal* and Survanta,† a natural bovine surfactant. Studies have shown no advantages of either product over another; however, clinical trials with surfactant administration indicate that the infant with RDS benefits from surfactant therapy. Benefits include decreased oxygen requirements and MAP within a matter of hours after administration and an overall decrease in the incidence of pulmonary air leaks. Long-term improvement in the decrease of BPD, intraventricular hemorrhage (IVH), and PDA has not been evidenced in all clinical trials to date; evidence of decreased mortality is positive in most clinical trials (Cusson, 1992).

Complications seen with surfactant administration include pulmonary hemorrhage and patent ductus arteriosus (Pramanik and others, 1993). Additional studies are under investigation for potential benefits of surfactant in infants with meconium aspiration, infectious pneumonia, and congenital diaphragmatic hernia. Surfactant may be administered at birth as a preventive and/or prophylactic treatment of RDS or later on in the course of RDS as a rescue treatment. Surfactant is administered via the endotracheal tube (ET) directly into the infant's trachea; the exact number of doses (single vs multiple) that is most effective has yet to be determined (Pramanik and others, 1993). Nursing responsibilities with surfactant administration include assistance in the delivery of the product, collection and monitoring of arterial blood gases, scrupulous monitoring of oxygenation with pulse oximetry or transcutaneous oxygen ($TcPO_2$), and assessment of the infant's tolerance of the procedure (Cusson, 1992; Grobman and Foley, 1992). Once surfactant is absorbed, there is usually an increase in respiratory compliance requiring adjustment of ventilator settings to decrease MAP and prevent overinflation or hyperoxemia. Suctioning is usually delayed for an hour or so (depending on the type of surfactant and unit protocol) to allow for maximum effects to occur.

Prevention. The most successful approach to prevention of RDS is prevention of premature delivery, especially in elective early delivery and cesarean section. Improved methods for assessing the maturity of the fetal lung by amniocentesis, although not a routine procedure, allow a reasonable prediction of adequate surfactant formation (see Diagnostic Evaluation). Since estimation of a date of delivery can be miscalculated by as much as 1 month, these tests are particularly valuable when scheduling elective cesarean section. An aggressive approach using tocolysis (such as ritadrine and terbutaline administration) to delay delivery and maternal administration of corticosteroids to induce surfactant production appears to reduce the incidence of RDS in preterm infants (Kwong and Egan, 1986; Papageorgiou and others, 1989).

Nursing Considerations

Care of infants with RDS involves all the observations and interventions previously described for high-risk infants. In addition, the nurse is concerned with the complex problems related to respiratory therapy and the constant threat of hypoxemia and acidosis that complicates the care of patients in respiratory difficulty.

The respiratory therapist, an important member of the neonatal intensive care team, is often responsible for the maintenance of respiratory equipment. Although it may be the responsibility of the respiratory therapist to regulate the

*Burroughs Wellcome Co., Research Triangle Park, NC.
†Ross Laboratories, Columbus, OH.

apparatus, nurses should understand the equipment and be able to recognize when it is not functioning correctly. The most essential nursing function is to observe and assess the infant's response to therapy. Since oxygen concentration and ventilation parameters are prescribed according to the infant's blood gas measurements, transcutaneous oxygen ($TcPo_2$) readings, and pulse oximetry readings, and because an infant's status can change rapidly, continuous monitoring and close observation are mandatory.

Changes in oxygen concentration are based on these observations. The amount of oxygen administered, expressed as the fraction of inspired air (Fio_2), is determined on an individual basis according to pulse oximetry and/or direct or indirect measurement of arterial oxygen concentration. Capillary samples, collected from the heel (see Chapter 27 for procedure), are useful for pH and $Paco_2$ determinations but *not* for oxygenation status. Continuous transcutaneous or pulse oximetry readings are recorded at least hourly. Blood sampling is necessary 15 to 30 minutes after ventilator changes for the acutely ill infant and generally ever 2 to 4 hours for sick infants.

In infants with RDS who are acutely ill and/or extremely preterm, an umbilical arterial catheter (UAC) may be used to draw arterial blood for monitoring oxygenation. This method, although initially invasive and therefore performed by the practitioner with sterile precautions, allows for blood sampling without repeated peripheral arterial punctures. The catheter is inserted via one of the umbilical arteries to the premeasured desired position (usually above the level of the diaphragm, T6-T8), resting in the descending aorta. Continuous arterial pressure monitoring may be carried out with an "in-line" transducer. Practices vary regarding medication administration via an umbilical arterial catheter; the nurse, however, is aware of the potential hazards associated with these catheters (infection, hemorrhage, thrombus formation and subsequent vessel occlusion, arterial vasospasm) and implements monitoring and observation strategies to promptly intervene should complications occur (see also Hydration, p. 375). An umbilical venous catheter (UVC) may be used separately or in conjunction with the UAC, depending on the severity of the infant's illness, fluid requirement, and practice. UVCs have historically been associated with more complications than UACs, including hepatic necrosis, intestinal ischemia, and hypertension. When monitored properly, both types of catheters can be used to administer intravenous hyperalimentation to the critically ill neonate with RDS (Merenstein and Gardner, 1993).

Mucus may collect in the respiratory tract as a result of the infant's pulmonary condition. Secretions interfere with gas flow and predispose the infant to obstruction of the passages, including the ET tube. Suctioning should be performed only when necessary, based on individual infant assessment, which includes auscultation of the chest, evidence of decreased oxygenation, excess moisture in the ET tube, or increased infant irritability. The use of preoxygenation and hyperinflation to maintain adequate oxygenation and prevent associated complications is carried out in some centers; further investigation is needed in the neonatal population (Hodge, 1991). Instillation of 0.25 to 0.5 ml of sterile normal saline in the ET tube before insertion of the suction catheter may aid in removing secretions although its value is unproven.

NURSING ALERT Suctioning is not an innocuous procedure (may cause bronchospasm, bradycardia due to vagal nerve stimulation, hypoxia, and increased intracranial pressure [ICP], predisposing the infant to intraventricular hemorrhage) and should *never* be carried out on a routine basis. Improper suctioning technique can also cause infection, airway damage, or even pneumothoraces.

When nasopharyngeal passages, the trachea, or the ET tube is being suctioned, the catheter should be inserted gently but quickly, and then intermittent suction is applied as the catheter is withdrawn. It is imperative that the time the airway is obstructed by the catheter be limited to no more than 5 seconds because continuous suction removes air from the lungs along with the mucus. It is recommended that the "two-person" suctioning procedure be used on infants who are acutely ill and who do not tolerate any procedure without profound decreases in oxygen saturation, decreased BP, and heart rate (Blackburn and Loper, 1992). The object of suctioning an artificial airway is to maintain patency of that airway, not the bronchi. Suction applied beyond the ET tube can cause traumatic lesions of the trachea. The Fio_2 should be increased by 10% before suctioning to compensate for a decrease in Fio_2 during the procedure (see Chapter 31).

NURSING ALERT The oxygenation monitor or pulse oximeter is observed before, during, and after the suctioning to provide an ongoing assessment of oxygenation status and to prevent hypoxemia.

Research indicates that suctioning to a point where the catheter meets resistance and is then withdrawn causes trauma to the tracheobronchial wall. The suction catheter is premeasured and inserted to a predetermined depth to avoid extension beyond the ET tube in order to remove secretions without damage to the tracheobronchial mucosa.

Removal of secretions can be further facilitated by positioning and application of percussion and vibration to the thoracic wall. The technique and positioning for postural drainage, percussion, and vibration are outlined in Chapter 31. However, the Trendelenburg position should not be used with preterm infants, since it can contribute to increased ICP. Percussion and vibration are poorly tolerated in most ELBW and VLBW infants, often resulting in hypoxia, rib fractures, bruising, and further atelectasis. Chest physiotherapy should be carefully evaluated according to the infant's condition and with consideration of benefit/risk factors. Chest percussion and vibration for the removal of secretions may benefit infants with meconium aspiration and bronchopulmonary dysplasia more than preterm infants with RDS.

The most advantageous positions for facilitating an infant's open airway are on the side with the head supported in alignment by a small folded blanket or, when on the back, positioned to keep the neck slightly extended. With the head in the "sniffing" position, the trachea is opened at its maximum; hyperextension reduces the tracheal diameter in neonates. The supported side-lying position can also be used effectively (Bozynski and others, 1988).

Inspection of the skin is part of routine infant assessment. Position changes and use of water pillows are helpful in guarding against skin breakdown.

Mouth care is especially important when infants are receiving nothing by mouth, and the problem is often aggravated by the drying effect of oxygen therapy. Drying and cracking can be prevented by good oral hygiene using sterile water. Irritation to the nares or mouth that occurs from appliances used to administer oxygen may be reduced by the use of a water-soluble ointment. (See also Nursing Care Plan: The Infant with Respiratory Distress Syndrome.*)

The nursing care of an infant with RDS is a demanding role; meticulous attention must be placed on subtle changes in the infant's oxygenation status. The importance of attention to detail cannot be overemphasized, particularly in regard to medication administration.

MECONIUM ASPIRATION SYNDROME (MAS)

Meconium aspiration is a serious condition that accounts for a substantial number of neonatal fatalities. It occurs when fetuses have been subjected to fetal asphyxia or other intrauterine stress that causes increasing peristalsis, relaxing of the anal sphincter, and passage of meconium into the amniotic fluid. The majority of meconium aspiration takes place with the first breath. However, a severely compromised fetus may aspirate in utero. At delivery of the chest and initiation of the first breath, infants inhale fluid and meconium in the nasooropharynx.

Pathophysiology

MAS involves the passage of meconium in utero as a result of hypoxic stress. It occurs primarily in full-term and postterm infants but has been reported in infants less than 37 weeks of gestation. Once the meconium is swallowed or inhaled by the fetus, any gasping activity occurring as a result of intrauterine stress may cause the rather sticky and tenacious product to become aspirated into the lower airways. The net results are partial airway obstruction, air trapping, and hyperinflation distal to the obstruction. A "ball-valve" situation exists wherein gas flows into the lungs on inspiration but is trapped therein on exhalation as a result of the smaller airway diameter. As the infant struggles to take in more air (air hunger), even more meconium may be aspirated. Hyperinflation, hypoxemia, and acidemia result in increased pulmonary vascular resistance. In turn, shunting of blood through the ductus arteriosus (right-to-left) occurs because of increased resistance to blood flow through the pulmonary arteries (and to the lungs), leading to further hypoxemia and acidosis. Ductal shunting increases with hypoxia; some blood may enter the left atrium (LA) from the right atrium (RA) via the foramen ovale, since there is a net decrease in blood returning to the LA via the pulmonary venous system, thus preventing closure of the foramen ovale. This pathologic process is essentially persistence of the fetal circulation, commonly referred to as persistent pulmonary hypertension of the newborn (PPHN), and is discussed later in this chapter. The air trapping of MAS causes overdistention of the alveoli and often air leaks. There is evidence that meconium contributes to the destruction of surfactant, thus increasing surface tension and further predisposing the alveoli to decreased functional capacity.

Clinical Manifestations

Infants who have released meconium in utero for some time before birth are stained from green meconium stools (those with more recent meconium passage may not be stained), tachypneic, hypoxic, and often depressed at birth. They develop expiratory grunting, nasal flaring, and retractions similar to those experienced by infants with RDS. Infants with MAS may initially by cyanotic or pale, as well as tachypneic, and may demonstrate the classic barrel chest from hyperinflation. The infants are often stressed, hypothermic, hypoglycemic, and hypocalcemic. Severe meconium aspiration progresses very rapidly to respiratory failure. These infants will exhibit profound respiratory distress with gasping, ineffective ventilations, marked cyanosis and pallor, and hypotonia.

Diagnostic Evaluation

At birth, meconium can often be visualized via laryngoscopy in the respiratory passages and vocal cords. Chest radiographs show uneven distribution of patchy infiltrates, air trapping, hyperexpansion, and atelectasis. Air leaks may be seen as the illness progresses; oxygenation will be poor, as evidenced by pulse oximetry and arterial blood gases. These infants may quickly develop metabolic and respiratory acidosis. Echocardiography assists in the diagnosis of right-to-left shunting of blood away from the pulmonary system.

Therapeutic Management

Prevention of meconium aspiration includes vigorous suctioning of the hypopharynx before delivery of the shoulders. Suctioning the trachea in infants with thick, particulate meconium is done by direct visualization and laryngoscopy (Wiswell and Bent, 1993). The decision to selectively intubate and visualize the trachea in infants with thin, "pea soup" meconium is primarily a clinical judgment of the practitioner. Resuscitation is initiated and maintained until the infant is stabilized.

Infants with respiratory distress are admitted to the NICU. Management of chemical pneumonitis consists of ventilatory support, intravenous fluids, and chest percussion and postural drainage. Since these infants are prone to develop persistent pulmonary hypertension, they are maintained somewhat hyperoxic and alkalotic as a precautionary measure and may be candidates for extracorporeal membrane oxygenation therapy or high-frequency ventila-

*In *Wong and Whaley's Clinical Manual of Pediatric Nursing* (Mosby).

tion (HFV). Management of the infant with severe MAS may require muscle paralysis with an agent such as pancuronium to effectively mechanically ventilate the hypoxic infant who is struggling (called "fighting the vent") (see Persistent Pulmonary Hypertension of the Newborn, p. 415). Complications are managed symptomatically or as described under the specific disorder.

Nursing Considerations

Nursing considerations are the same as for any high-risk, neonate. See nursing care in oxygen therapy, persistent pulmonary hypertension, and other complications.

EXTRANEOUS AIR SYNDROMES (AIR LEAKS)

Extraneous air syndromes, extraalveolar air accumulation, and air leaks are names applied to various clinically recognized disorders produced as a result of alveolar rupture and subsequent escape of air to tissues in which air is not normally present. Extraneous air collection (1) may occur spontaneously in normal neonates, (2) can result from congenital renal/pulmonary malformations, and (3) often complicates underlying respiratory disease and its therapy (i.e., mechanical ventilation, especially when high distending pressures are required).

Following alveolar rupture, air often vents directly into the pleural space to create a pneumothorax. It may vent into the perivascular interstitium, a condition called pulmonary interstitial emphysema (PIE). PIE may be seen as early as 2 to 3 hours after birth in ELBW and VLBW infants with severe RDS. Localized PIE may resolve by itself; HFV has been reported to improve the outcome in infants with PIE (Merenstein and Gardner, 1993). Air can dissect along the perivascular sheaths to eventually enter the mediastinum and cause pneumomediastinum. More extensive leaks involve the pericardium, manifested as pneumopericardium, or emphysema in the cervical, subcutaneous, or retroperitoneal soft tissues.

Clinical Manifestations

Spontaneous pneumothorax usually occurs during the first few breaths after birth, primarily in full-term or postterm infants, and is evident by the gradual onset of symptoms of respiratory distress after arrival in the nursery. Improper use of positive-pressure ventilation in resuscitation may cause air leaks; conventional mechanical ventilation may contribute to an increase in the incidence of air leaks; however, there are cases, such as in extreme prematurity and meconium aspiration, wherein air leaks may not be altogether preventable. It can be suspected on the basis of respiratory manifestations and a shift in location of maximum intensity of heart sounds and absent or diminished breath sounds (although breath sounds may not be altered because of the small diameter of the chest and auscultation of referred breath sounds). In preterm infants being mechanically ventilated, an air leak may demonstrate hypotension, bradycardia, decreased or absent breath sounds unilaterally, decreased oxygenation (by decreased pulse oximetry), and cyanosis, none of which respond to efforts for oxygenation (a resuscitation bag connected to the ET tube and provision of manual ventilations). An air leak may contribute to an increased incidence of intraventricular hemorrhage in preterm infants. Pneumothorax, predominantly tension pneumothorax, during ventilatory assistance is common. There may also be chest asymmetry, altered cardiac sounds (diminished, shifted, or muffled), palpable liver and spleen, and subcutaneous emphysema. Infants on HFV may demonstrate an air leak by a sudden decrease in systemic pressure or absence of chest movement (due to difficulty in auscultation of the chest with such modalities). The otherwise healthy full-term infant may exhibit only mild to moderate signs of respiratory distress.

NURSING ALERT Early manifestations of pneumothorax include tachypnea, restlessness and irritability, lethargy, grunting, nasal flaring, and retractions. Pneumothorax during ventilatory assistance is evident from abrupt and profound duskiness or cyanosis; significant declines in heart rate, arterial blood pressure, and pulse pressure; and poor peripheral perfusion.

Therapeutic Management

Diagnosis is confirmed by transillumination of the chest with a fiberoptic probe and/or radiographic examination. Treatment is urgent. Evacuation of trapped air is accomplished by chest tube insertion into the pleural space through a small chest incision. The chest tube is then attached to continuous water-seal drainage. A dry suction control drainage system not requiring water is also available (Carroll, 1991). Needle aspiration serves as an emergency measure until a chest tube can be inserted. Pneumomediastinum seldom requires treatment, but pneumopericardium is managed by needle aspiration or pericardial tube drainage. The full-term newborn with a small tension pneumothorax may only require oxygen therapy and intravenous nutrition for a brief period if respiratory distress is not severe. One treatment modality that may be used for these infants is a nitrogen washout. The infant is placed in a hood or tent with 100% oxygen, and a gradient is created in the lungs wherein enhanced absorption of the trapped pleural air is accomplished (Merenstein and Gardner, 1993).

Nursing Considerations

The most important nursing function is close vigilance for the possibility of an air leak in susceptible infants, which is most effective for early detection. Nurses maintain a high level of suspicion in (1) infants with RDS with or without positive-pressure ventilation, (2) infants with meconium-stained amniotic fluid, (3) infants with radiographic evidence of interstitial or lobar emphysema, (4) infants who required resuscitation at birth, or (4) infants receiving CPAP or positive-pressure ventilation. For infants at risk, needle aspiration equipment (30 ml syringe, three-way stopcock, and 23- to 25-gauge butterfly needles) should be at the bedside for emergency use.

The general nursing care of the infant with an exogenous air syndrome is the same as that for all high-risk neonates. Respiratory management is similar to that for infants with RDS. Frequent assessment of breath sounds, monitoring of the efficacy of gas exchange, and regulating oxygen therapy according to the needs of the infants are vital nursing functions. Care of chest tubes is an additional responsibility and is similar to, but not always the same as, that with older children (see Merenstein and Gardner, 1993, pp. 337-338). Attention to pain management with the procedure, however, is vital in these preverbal and significantly stressed infants. (see Bell [1994] for pain management guidelines).

BRONCHOPULMONARY DYSPLASIA (BPD)

BPD, also known as chronic lung disease, is a pathologic process that may develop in the lungs of infants, primarily ELBW and VLBW infants with RDS. BPD may also develop in infants with meconium aspiration syndrome, persistent pulmonary hypertension, pneumonia, and cyanotic heart disease (Blackburn and Loper, 1992). BPD is an iatrogenic disease caused by therapies used to treat lung disease: exposure to high oxygen concentrations, use of positive-pressure ventilation (CPAP or PEEP), and/or endotracheal intubation; prolonged use of these therapies; fluid overload; and patient ductus arteriosus (PDA). The reported incidence of the disorder in survivors of RDS is between 10% and 30%, and the incidence of infants surviving with milder forms of chronic lung disease is much higher (Cusson, 1992). The infants who survive are at risk for frequent hospitalization because of their borderline respiratory reserve, hyperactive airway, and increased susceptibility to respiratory infection (Northway and others, 1990).

Pathophysiology

The pulmonary changes are characterized by interstitial edema and epithelial swelling followed by thickening and fibrotic proliferation of the alveolar walls and squamous metaplasia of the bronchiolar epithelium. Areas of atelectasis and cystlike foci of hyperaeration are visible on radiographs between 10 and 20 days of life and persist for weeks; however, some infants may not demonstrate cystic foci. In addition, ciliary activity is paralyzed by high oxygen concentrations that interfere with the ability to clear the lung of mucus, thus aggravating airway obstruction and atelectasis. As the infant's lungs begin healing, the process is altered, possibly by continuous high oxygenation, inadequate nutrition, or vitamin E deficiency, resulting in decreased surface for O_2 and CO_2 exchange (Blackburn and Loper, 1992). The overall results of this process are hypercarbia, hypoxemia, and subsequent inability to wean successfully from mechanical ventilation.

As survival of immature preterm infants (less than 28 weeks of gestation) increases, the occurrence of BPD also increases. Despite the fact that management of O_2 therapy, barotrauma, fluids, and PDA has improved, BPD is still on the rise in ELBW, VLBW, and early-gestational-age infants (Hagedorn, Gardner, and Abman, 1993).

The marked similarity between BPD and the ***Wilson-Mikity syndrome,*** in which the lungs of premature infants exhibit alveolar thickening and cystlike patterns of hyperventilation, has led some investigators to theorize that the two disorders may be part of a continuous spectrum of the same lung disease. Other diseases associated with similar radiographic findings include congenital heart disease and viral pneumonia caused by cytomegalovirus. There are no laboratory alterations that confirm a diagnosis, which is made on the basis of radiographic findings, a history of mechanical ventilation, tachypnea, auscultatory rales, retractions >38 days, and oxygen therapy >28 days (Blackburn and Loper, 1992).

Therapeutic Management

The first approach to management is prevention of the disorder in susceptible infants. Despite previous theorization that surfactant administration to preterm infants would eradicate BPD, studies so far have failed to show a significant decrease of BPD in infants receiving surfactant for prophylaxis or rescue. There are reported to be many confounding variables involved, and certain institutions report a decreased incidence of BPD in infants given surfactant (Pramanik, 1993). To reduce the risk of barotrauma when mechanical ventilation is being used, the lowest peak inspiratory pressure (PIP) necessary to obtain adequate ventilation is maintained and the lowest level of inspired oxygen is used to maintain adequate oxygenation. Fluid administration is carefully controlled and restricted. Drug or surgical intervention is indicated when there is significant shunting of blood through the PDA.

There is no specific treatment for BPD except to maintain adequate arterial blood gases with the administration of oxygen and to avoid progression of the disease. Some have reported improvement in infants administered dexamethasone (Cusson, 1992; Gladstone, Ehrenkranz, and Jacobs, 1989; Harkavy and others, 1989; Knoppert and Mackanjee, 1994), although infants exhibited significant delay in weight gain, sepsis, necrotizing enterocolitis, pneumonia, hyperglycemia and hypertension (Cusson, 1992). Weaning infants from the ventilator is difficult and must be accomplished gradually. These infants do not tolerate excessive or even normal amounts of fluid well and have a tendency to accumulate interstitial fluid in the lungs, which aggravates the condition.

Oral diuretics are used to control interstitial fluid. Bronchodilators may be effective and promote improvement in infants with chronic lung disease. Theophylline improves lung compliance and reduces expiratory resistance in BPD ventilated infants. Oral electrolyte supplements are given to replace those lost with concurrent oral diuretics and renal water losses.

Growth and development are often delayed in infants with BPD, which is related in part to the difficulties in providing adequate nutrition and in part to the lack of normal sensory stimulation due to prolonged hospitalization. Children with BPD have metabolic needs far greater than those of the average infant (Kurzner and others, 1988). This can create a problem for the caregiver, who must meet the goals of adequate nutrition while avoiding overhydration, especially if the child is ill, eats poorly, or has cardiopulmonary instability (Goldson, 1990). The infant may be further compromised by gastroesophageal reflux, a frequent complication in premature infants (see Chapter 33). There is hope that with the increased knowledge and research in the arena of antioxidants (primarily vitamin E), the incidence of BPD will be decreased (Blackburn and Loper, 1992). (See discussion of antioxidant and oxygen free-radicals under Respiratory Distress Syndrome, p. 399.)

Prognosis. Reports vary regarding the mortality rate for this disorder. The hospital stay is frequently long because of the infant's need for supplemental oxygen, although home oxygen therapy provides selected infants the opportunity for discharge. However, a significant proportion of deaths occur after discharge from the hospital. Use of nasal cannulas provides an acceptable way to administer oxygen for the dependent infant to promote development of motor and social skills (Hagedorn, Gardner, and Abman, 1989).

Nursing Considerations

Infants with BPD expend considerable energy in their efforts to breathe; therefore it is important that they receive plenty of opportunities for rest and additional calories. Growth records provide clues to the need for change in their diets, and some infants require nutritional supplements. Since they tire easily and large quantities of formula might compromise respiration, small, frequent feedings are better tolerated. Reducing environmental stimuli and subsequent hypoxia is an important aspect in the care of these infants. Close attention to the infant's behavioral cues is important in the older infant with BPD, since these may signal CO_2 retention.

Adequate hydration is extremely important because greater amounts of fluid are lost through respiration, and secretions must be thinned sufficiently to facilitate removal by suctioning. However, since BPD increases lung permeability, many infants are subject to pulmonary edema and require fluid restriction.

Because the growing infant with BPD has a restricted fluid intake, has higher caloric requirements than average, and often requires many oral medications, the nurse is challenged by the complexity of care involved. The BPD infant who is aware of hunger yet compromised by not being able to eat fast enough to satiate that hunger because of the increased labor of breathing, may become a difficult or maladaptive feeder. Individualized nursing care aimed at increasing oxygenation needs during feedings, decreasing environmental stimuli, fortifying feedings, and providing more contact with a primary caregiver may serve to facilitate the infant's care (Kenner, Brueggemeyer, and Gunderson, 1993). Feeding schedules should be individualized as much as possible. Oral medications that taste bad to the infant may be given at times separate from feedings to enhance feeding time as a pleasant experience rather than one associated with forced oral administration of medications. Adjustments to overall fluid administration requirements are made, taking into account that the oral medications are also fluids. Regurgitated medications and feedings will need to be dealt with in regard to fluid and caloric needs and the amount of absorption of medication that occurs before emesis.

NURSING ALERT Nurses must be alert to signs of both overhydration and underhydration, such as weight changes, electrolytes, output measurements, urine specific gravity, and signs of edema.

Parents are extremely anxious regarding the prognosis when their infant has BPD. In addition, the lengthy hospitalization interferes with parent-child relationships and deprives the infant of parental stimulation. Nurses should encourage the parents to visit the infant and become involved in the routine care. The parents need to be informed regarding medical care, equipment, and procedures related to their infant and taught procedures, such as suctioning and chest physiotherapy.

Home Care. Since the availability of home cardiac/apnea monitors and home oxygen therapy has increased, many of these infants can be discharged when they are gaining weight, oxygen need is low (less than 1 L/min) and they pass "room air challenge" (i.e., are able to keep O_2 saturation greater than 85% for 20 to 30 minutes in room air). Home care is desirable to promote parent-infant bonding, minimize health care costs, and prevent nosocomial infections. Preparation for home care requires education and considerable reassurance (see Chapter 26). Management of home monitoring equipment and home oxygen therapy is stress provoking, but most families become comfortable with the machinery while their infant is still in the hospital. Families must be reminded about their infant's increased risk of infection and cautioned regarding contact with persons who have respiratory infections. Because of their minimum respiratory reserve, these infants can be threatened by even a minor illness.

Because of the high mortality rate in the first year, parents are taught cardiopulmonary resuscitation* and how to manage any other emergency that might be anticipated for their infant. Helping families cope with their anxieties and reassuring them of their ability to manage the care of their infant are important nursing functions. Parents need follow-up in the home and the comfort of knowing that help is only a telephone call away.

HIGH RISK RELATED TO INFECTIOUS PROCESSES

SEPSIS

Sepsis, or septicemia, refers to a generalized bacterial infection in the bloodstream. Neonates are highly susceptible to infection as a result of diminished nonspecific (inflammatory) and specific (humoral) immunity, such as impaired phagocytosis, delayed chemotactic response, minimal or absent IgA and IgM, and decreased complement levels. Because of the infant's poor response to pathogenic agents,

*Home care instructions are available in *Wong and Whaley's Clinical Manual of Pediatric Nursing* (Mosby).

there is usually no local inflammatory reaction at the portal of entry to signal an infection, and the resulting symptoms tend to be vague and nonspecific. Consequently diagnosis and treatment may be delayed.

Although the mortality from sepsis has diminished, the incidence of septicemia has not diminished. Nursery epidemics are not infrequent, and the high-risk infant has a four times greater chance of developing septicemia than does the normal neonate. The frequency of infection is almost twice as great in male infants as in females and carries a higher mortality for males as well. Other factors increasing the risk of infection are prematurity, invasive procedures such as peripheral IV therapy and endotracheal (ET) tubes, steroid use for lung disease, and nosocomial exposure to a number of pathogens in the NICU. Proper handling of formula and supplies such as syringes and gavage tubes is vital to the prevention of infection.

Breast-feeding has a protective benefit against infection. Colostrum contains agglutinins that are effective against gram-negative bacteria. Human milk contains large quantities of IgA and iron-binding protein that exert a bacteriostatic effect on *Escherichia coli.* Human milk also contains macrophages and lymphocytes that promote a local inflammatory reaction.

Pathophysiology

The premature withdrawal of the placental barrier leaves infants vulnerable to most common viral, bacterial, fungal, and parasitic infections. Normally, immune substances, primarily immunoglobulin G (IgG), are acquired from the maternal system and stored in fetal tissues during the final weeks of gestation to provide newborns with passive immunity to a variety of infectious agents. Early birth interrupts this transplacental transmission; thus preterm infants have a low level of circulating IgG; the concentrations of immune substances directly relate to the length of gestation. Immunoglobulin A (IgA), which plays a role in defense against viral infections, and immunoglobulin M (IgM), with properties that are most efficient in dealing with gram-negative organisms, are not transferred to the fetus, leaving infants highly vulnerable to invasion by these organisms.

Defense mechanisms of neonates are further hampered by a low level of complement, diminished opsonization ability, monocyte dysfunction, and reduced number and inefficient functioning of circulating leukocytes. Furthermore, these leukocytes, with diminished motility and phagocytic capacity, are unable to concentrate their limited numbers selectively at the site of infection. In addition, a hypofunctioning adrenal gland contributes only a meager antiinflammatory response. Consequently, these deficiencies permit rapid invasion, spread, and multiplication of organisms.

Sources of Infection

Sepsis in the neonatal period can be acquired prenatally across the placenta from the maternal bloodstream or during labor from ingestion or aspiration of infected amniotic fluid. Prolonged rupture of the membranes always presents a risk of this type from maternal-fetal transfer of pathogenic organisms. In utero transplacental transfer of organisms and viruses can occur, such as cytomegalovirus, toxoplasmosis, and *Treponema pallidum* (syphilis), which cross the placental barrier during the latter half of pregnancy.

Early sepsis (less than 3 days) is acquired in the perinatal period; infection can occur from direct contact with organisms from the maternal gastrointestinal and genitourinary tracts. The most common infecting organisms are group B streptococcus and *Escherichia coli,* which may be present in the vagina. *E. coli* accounts for about two thirds of all cases of sepsis caused by gram-negative organisms. Group B streptococcus has emerged as an extremely virulent organism in neonates, with a high (50%) death rate in affected infants (Fuller, 1992). Other pathogens that are harbored in the vagina and that may infect the infant include gonococci, *Candida albicans,* herpes simplex virus (type II), *Listeria* organisms, and chlamydia.

Late sepsis (1 to 3 weeks following birth) is primarily nosocomial, and the offending organisms are usually the staphylococci, *Klebsiella,* enterococci, and *Pseudomonas.* Coagulase-negative staphylococcus, considered to be primarily a contaminant in older children and adults, is commonly found to be the cause of septicemia in ELBW and VLBW infants (St. Geme and Harris, 1991). Bacterial invasion can occur through sites such as the umbilical stump; the skin; mucous membranes of the eye, nose, pharynx, and ear; and internal systems such as the respiratory, nervous, urinary, and gastrointestinal systems.

Postnatal infection is acquired by cross-contamination from other infants, personnel, or objects in the environment. Bacteria that are frequently called "water bugs" (because they are able to grow in water) are found in water supplies, humidifying apparatus, sink drains, suction machines, most respiratory equipment, and indwelling venous and arterial catheters used for infusions, blood sampling, and monitoring vital signs. Neonatal sepsis is most common in the infant at risk, particularly the preterm infant or the infant born following a difficult or traumatic labor and delivery, who is least capable of resisting such bacterial invasion. Frequently these organisms are transmitted by the personnel from person to person or object to person by poor handwashing and inadequate housecleaning.

Clinical Manifestations

A few neonatal infections (e.g., pyoderma, conjunctivitis, omphalitis, and mastitis) are easily recognized. However, systemic infections are characterized by subtle, vague, nonspecific, and almost imperceptible physical signs. Often the only complaint concerning an infant's progress is "failure to do well" not looking "right" or nonspecific respiratory distress. Rarely is there any indication of a local inflammatory response, which would suggest the portal of entry into the bloodstream. The presence of some bacteria is indicated by a specific characteristic (e.g., *Pseudomonas* organisms, which produce necrotic purplish skin lesions, or group B β-hemolytic streptococci, which usually result in severe respiratory distress, periods of apnea, and a chest radiograph similar to that with RDS).

All body systems tend to show some indication of sepsis, although often there is little correlation between the manifestations and the etiologic factors involved. For example, convulsions and fever, a universal feature of infection in older children, may be absent in neonates. It is usually nursing observation of subtle changes in the appearance and behavior of infants that leads to the detection of infection. The nonspecific, early signs are hypothermia and change in color, tone, activity, and feeding behavior; in addition, sudden episodes of apnea and unexplained desaturations may signal an infection. Significantly, similar signs may be manifestations of a number of clinical conditions unrelated to sepsis, such as hypoglycemia, hypocalcemia, heroin withdrawal, or CNS disorders. Preterm infants, particularly ELBW and VLBW infants, are highly suspect for early sepsis and pneumonia occurring concurrently with RDS, since preterm delivery has been increasingly shown to be associated with a maternal bacterial pathogen (McCourt, 1994). Since meningitis is a frequent sequela of sepsis, the neonate is evaluated for cerebrospinal fluid (CSF) bacterial growth; clinical signs of neonatal meningitis, particularly in VLBW infants, may not demonstrate typical features of older infants. Clinical signs that may indicate possible neonatal sepsis are listed in the box below.

MANIFESTATIONS OBSERVED IN NEONATAL SEPSIS

GENERAL SIGNS

Infant generally "not doing well"
Poor temperature control—hypothermia, hyperthermia (rare)

CIRCULATORY SYSTEM

Pallor, cyanosis, or mottling
Cold, clammy skin
Hypotension
Edema
Abnormal heartbeat—bradycardia, tachycardia

RESPIRATORY SYSTEM

Irregular respirations, apnea, or tachypnea
Cyanosis
Grunting
Dyspnea
Retractions

CENTRAL NERVOUS SYSTEM

Diminished activity—lethargy, hyporeflexia, coma
Increased activity—irritability, tremors, seizures
Full fontanel
Increased or decreased tone
Abnormal eye movements

GASTROINTESTINAL SYSTEM

Poor feeding
Vomiting
Diarrhea or decreased stooling
Abdominal distention
Hepatomegaly
Hemoccult-positive stools

HEMATOPOIETIC SYSTEM

Jaundice
Pallor
Petechiae, ecchymosis
Splenomegaly

Diagnostic Evaluation

Because sepsis is so easily confused with other neonatal disorders, the diagnosis is established by laboratory and radiographic examination. Isolation of the specific organism is always attempted through cultures of blood, urine, and cerebrospinal fluid. Blood studies may show signs of anemia, leukocytosis, or leukopenia. Leukopenia is usually an ominous sign because of its frequent association with high mortality. An elevated number of immature neutrophils is also suggestive of an infectious process in the neonate (McCourt, 1994).

Therapeutic Management

Early recognition and diagnosis, along with institution of vigorous therapeutic measures, are essential to increase the infant's chance for survival and reduce the likelihood of permanent neurologic damage. Often diagnosis of sepsis is based on suspicion of presenting clinical signs and symptoms, and antibiotic therapy is initiated before laboratory results are available for confirmation and identification of the exact organism. Treatment consists of circulatory support, respiratory support, aggressive administration of antibiotics, and immunotherapy.

Supportive therapy usually involves administration of oxygen if respiratory distress or hypoxia is evident, careful regulation of fluids and correction of electrolyte or acid-base imbalance, and temporary discontinuation of oral feedings. Blood transfusions may be needed to correct anemia and shock, and electronic monitoring of vital signs and regulation of the thermal environment are mandatory.

Antibiotic therapy is continued for 7 to 10 days if cultures are positive, discontinued in 3 days if cultures are negative and the infant is asymptomatic, and most often administered via intravenous infusion. Transfusions with fresh, irradiated granulocytes or polymorphonuclear leukocytes obtained from adult donors by continuous-flow centrifugation leukapheresis have been introduced as therapy for bacterial sepsis. The results have proved to be highly effective in lowering mortality from this disease. Intravenous gammaglobulin has also proved effective as a prophylactic measure against nosocomial infections.

The prognosis is variable. Before the discovery of antibiotics the mortality from bacterial sepsis was 95% to 100%, but early recognition, antibiotics, and supportive therapy have reduced mortality to less than 50%. However, mental sequelae can occur with late diagnosis of meningitis or inadequate length of treatment.

Nursing Considerations

Nursing care of the infant with sepsis involves observation and assessment as outlined for any high-risk infant. Recognition of the existing problem is of paramount importance; it is usually the nurse who observes and assesses infants and who identifies that "something is wrong" with them. Awareness of the potential modes of infection transmission also helps the nurse identify those at risk for developing sepsis. Much of the care of infants with sepsis involves the medical treatment of the illness. Knowledge of the side effects of the specific antibiotic and proper regulation and administration of the drug are vital. Because the volume of fluid required to administer antibiotics via Soluset or Buretrol would seriously compromise a small infant, antibiotics are usually administered via a special injection cap near the infusion site. The medication is administered slowly by mechanical pump.

Prolonged antibiotic therapy poses additional hazards for affected infants. Oral antibiotics, if administered, destroy intestinal flora responsible for synthesis of vitamin K, which can reduce blood coagulability. In addition, antibiotics predispose the infant to growth of resistant organisms and superinfection from fungal or mycotic agents, such as *Candida albicans.* Nurses must be alert for evidence of such complications.

A number of specimens may be needed to help identify the cause and source of the infection. It is recommended that the fully flexed position be avoided for obtaining spinal fluid and that the side-lying position (modified with neck extension) or the sitting position be used for obtaining spinal fluid specimens. Continual cardiorespiratory and pulse oximetry monitoring provides an ongoing assessment of the infant's condition during the procedure.

Part of the total care of infants with sepsis is to decrease any additional physiologic or environmental stress. This includes providing an optimum thermoregulated environment and anticipating potential problems, such as dehydration or hypoxia. Precautions are implemented to prevent spread of infection to other newborns, but to be effective, activities must be carried out by all caregivers. Proper handwashing, use of disposable equipment (e.g., linens, catheters, feeding supplies, and intravenous equipment), disposing of excretions (e.g., vomitus and stool), and adequate housekeeping of the environment and equipment are essential. Since nurses are the most consistent caregivers involved with sick infants, it is usually their responsibility to oversee that all phases of isolation are maintained by everyone.

Another aspect of caring for infants with sepsis involves observation for signs of complications including meningitis and septic shock, a severe complication caused by toxins in the bloodstream.

A number of viral agents, namely cytomegalovirus, herpes, hepatitis, and human immunodeficiency virus (HIV) may also be transmitted to the fetus from the mother. These viruses, when acquired prenatally (congenital), represent a serious threat to the infant's life.

NECROTIZING ENTEROCOLITIS (NEC)

NEC is an acute inflammatory disease of the bowel with increased incidence in preterm and other high-risk infants, but it is most common in those who are preterm. Three factors appear to play an important role in its development: intestinal ischemia, colonization by pathogenic bacteria, and substrate (formula feeding) in the intestinal lumen.

Pathophysiology

The precise cause of the disorder is still uncertain, although it appears to occur in infants whose gastrointestinal tract has suffered vascular compromise. Intestinal ischemia of unknown etiology, immature gastrointestinal host defenses, bacterial proliferation, and feeding substrate are now believed to have a multifactorial role in the etiology of NEC. Prematurity remains the most prominent risk factor in the development of NEC (MacKendrick and Caplan, 1993).

The damage to mucosal cells lining the bowel wall is great—diminished blood supply to these cells causes their death in large numbers; they stop secreting protective, lubricating mucus; and the thin, unprotected bowel wall is attacked by proteolytic enzymes. Thus the bowel wall continues to swell and break down. In addition, it is unable to synthesize protective immunoglobulin M (IgM), and the mucosa is permeable to macromolecules, such as exotoxins, which further hampers intestinal defenses. Gas-forming bacteria invade the damaged areas to produce ***pneumatosis intestinalis,*** the presence of air in the submucosal or subserosal surfaces of the bowel.

A consistent relationship has been observed between the development of NEC and enteric feeding of hypertonic substances (e.g., formula and hyperosmolar medications). It is unclear whether this connection is the result of the formula imposing a stress on an ischemic bowel, serving as a substrate for bacterial growth, or both.

Clinical Manifestations

The prominent clinical signs of NEC are a distended (often shining) abdomen, gastric retention, and blood in the stools. Because NEC closely mimics or resembles septicemia, the infant may have that "not looking well" appearance. Nonspecific signs include lethargy, poor feeding, hypotension, apnea, vomiting (often bile-stained), decreased urine output, and hypothermia. The onset is usually between 4 and 10 days after the initiation of feedings, but signs may be evident as early as 4 hours of age and as late as 30 days. NEC in full-term infants almost always occurs in the first 10 days of life; late-onset NEC is confined primarily to preterm infants and coincides with the onset of feedings after passing through the acute phase of an illness such as RDS.

Diagnostic Evaluation

Radiographic studies show a sausage-shaped dilation of the intestine that progresses to marked distention and the characteristic pneumatosis intestinales—"soapsuds" or bubbly appearance of thickened bowel wall and ultralumina. There may be air in the portal circulation or free air observed in the abdomen, indicating perforation. Laboratory findings may include anemia, leukopenia, leukocytosis, metabolic acidosis, and electrolyte imbalance. In severe cases coagulopathy (disseminated intravascular coagulation [DIC]) and/or thrombocytopenia may be evident. Organisms are often cultured from blood, although bacteremia or septicemia may not be prominent early in the course of the disease.

Therapeutic Management

Treatment of NEC begins with prevention. Oral feedings are withheld for at least 24 to 48 hours from infants who are believed to have suffered birth asphyxia and as long as deemed necessary from ELBW and VLBW infants. Breast milk is the preferred enteral nutrient because it confers some passive immunity (IgA), macrophages, and lysozymes.

Medical treatment of confirmed NEC consists of discontinuation of all oral feedings, institution of abdominal decompression via nasogastric suction, administration of intravenous antibiotics, and correction of extravascular volume depletion, electrolyte abnormalities, acid-base imbalances, and hypoxia. Replacing oral feedings with parenteral fluids decreases the need for oxygen and circulation to the bowel. Serial abdominal radiograph films (every 4 to 6 hours in the acute phase) are taken to monitor for possible progression of the disease to intestinal perforation.

Prognosis. With early recognition and treatment, medical management is increasingly successful. If there is progressive deterioration under medical management or evidence of perforation, surgical resection and anastomosis are done. Extensive involvement may necessitate establishment of an ileostomy, jejunostomy, or colostomy. Sequelae in surviving infants include short-bowel syndrome (see Chapter 33), colonic stricture with obstruction, fat malabsorption, and failure to thrive secondary to intestinal dysfunction.

Nursing Considerations

Nursing responsibilities begin with early recognition. The nurse is a key factor in the prompt recognition of the early warning signs of NEC. Because the signs are similar to those observed in many other disorders of the newborn, nurses must constantly be aware of the possibility of this disease.

NURSING ALERT Observe for indications of early development of NEC by checking the abdomen frequently for distention (measuring abdominal girth, measuring residual gastric contents before feedings, and listening for the presence of bowel sounds) and performing all routine assessments for high-risk neonates.

When the disease is suspected, the nurse assists with diagnostic procedures and implements the therapeutic regimen. Vital signs, including blood pressure, are monitored for changes that might indicate bowel perforation, septicemia, or cardiovascular shock, and measures are instituted to prevent possible transmission to other infants. It is especially important to avoid rectal temperatures because of the increased danger of perforation. To avoid pressure on the distended abdomen and to facilitate continuous observation, infants are frequently left undiapered and positioned supine or on the side.

Conscientious attention to nutritional and hydration needs is essential, and antibiotics are administered as prescribed. The time at which oral feedings are reinstituted varies considerably but is usually at least 7 to 10 days following diagnosis and treatment. Sterile water or electrolyte solution may be given initially and followed by dilute human milk (if available) or elemental predigested formula. The concentration is gradually increased as tolerated until the infant is again taking full-strength feedings.

Since NEC is an infectious disease, one of the most important nursing functions is control of infection. Strict handwashing is the primary barrier to spread, and confirmed multiple cases are isolated. Persons with symptoms of a gastrointestinal disorder should not care for these or any other infants.

The infant who requires surgery requires the same careful attention and observation as any infant with abdominal surgery, including ostomy care (as applicable). This disorder is one of the most frequent reasons for performing ileostomies on newborns. Throughout the medical and surgical management of infants with NEC, the nurse is continually alert to signs of complications, such as septicemia, disseminated intravascular coagulation, hypoglycemia, and other metabolic derangements.

HIGH RISK RELATED TO CARDIOVASCULAR/HEMATOLOGIC COMPLICATIONS

PATENT DUCTUS ARTERIOSUS (PDA)

A common complication of severe respiratory disease in preterm infants is PDA. It occurs in the majority of preterm infants under 1200 g, and the incidence diminishes in direct relationship to increasing birth weight. During fetal life the ductus remains patent through the vasodilatory action of prostaglandins within its tissues. Postnatally the increase in oxygen tension has a constricting effect on the ductus, but it may reopen in these small infants in response to the lowered oxygen tension associated with respiratory impairment.

Clinical Manifestations

Signs of PDA may appear within the first week of life. Early signs of PDA are increased $Paco_2$, decreased Pao_2, increased Fio_2, and recurrent apnea. Other signs include bounding peripheral pulses, wide pulse pressure with decreased diastolic blood pressure, pericardial hyperactivity, cardiomegally, and a systolic or continuous murmur. If the PDA is wide open, a murmur may not be heard. Spontaneous closure usually takes place (usually within 12 weeks), but in infants with severe lung involvement the left-to-right shunting of blood leads to life-threatening pulmonary insufficiency. Confirmation of the diagnosis may be determined by echocardiography.

Therapeutic Management

Therapy consists of careful fluid regulation, respiratory support, and administration of indomethacin, a prostaglandin synthetase inhibitor that has been successful in constricting the ductus in critically ill, preterm infants. However, the drug has been found to inhibit platelet function and affect renal function, and its use has been questioned, especially in the presence of intraventricular hemorrhage. If a ductus reopens following cessation of therapy, reinstitution of the medication may produce a favorable response. Surgical ligation may be necessary if medical therapy is unsuccessful and ductal shunting is perceived as an important contribution to respiratory distress.

Nursing Considerations

Nursing observations are important in the recognition and management of PDA. Assisting in early detection, assessing cardiovascular status carefully, and monitoring for complications following implementation of therapy are nursing responsibilities. The focus of activities related to therapy includes collection of specimens for laboratory examination, continued assessment of renal function (adequate urinary output, any abnormal laboratory findings), and observation for any bleeding tendencies (hematest-positive stools or gastric aspirate, oozing from heel sticks or venipuncture sites, and laboratory evidence of clotting abnormalities).

Other nursing observations and management are the same as for the high-risk infant and the infant with PDA (see Chapter 34).

PERSISTENT PULMONARY HYPERTENSION OF THE NEWBORN (PPHN)

PPHN, formerly known as ***persistent fetal circulation (PFC),*** is a condition in which affected infants display severe pulmonary hypertension, with pulmonary artery pressure levels equal to or greater than systemic pressure, and large right-to-left shunts through both the foramen ovale and the ductus arteriosus. Since full development of pulmonary arterial musculature occurs late in gestation, PPHN is primarily a condition of full-term or postterm infants, many of whom were products of complicated pregnancies or deliveries. The condition is often associated with aspiration (especially meconium aspiration), congenital diaphragmatic hernia with severe respiratory distress, cold stress, respiratory distress (e.g., RDS or pneumonia), and septicemia (group B hemolytic streptococci) and is believed to be precipitated by perinatal factors, such as perinatal asphyxia, that cause or contribute to vasoconstriction of the pulmonary vasculature.

PPHN can be either primary or secondary: primary PPHN occurs when the pulmonary vascular system fails to open with the initial respiration at birth; secondary PPHN results from stress that increases pulmonary vascular resistance and causes a return to fetal cardiopulmonary circulation. PPHN is most frequently observed in infants at 35 to 44 weeks of gestation who have a history of perinatal asphyxia, metabolic acidosis, or sepsis and respiratory distress within the first 24 hours. The infants become hypoxic and display marked cyanosis, tachypnea with grunting and retractions, and decreased peripheral perfusion. A loud pulmonary component of the second heart sound and sometimes a systolic ejection murmur are present.

Diagnosis is established from clinical signs and diagnostic tests, including chest radiography, electrocardiography, and echocardiography.

Therapeutic Management

Treatment includes careful fluid regulation and evaluation of intravascular fluid volume. Supplemental oxygen is administered to reduce hypoxia and decrease pulmonary vasoconstriction. Assisted ventilation may be needed if hypoxia is severe, often by jet hyperventilation (HFV), and is accompanied by paralysis with pancuronium to minimize opposition to the respirator. Vasodilators, such as tolazoline, are sometimes prescribed to decrease PVR, thereby decreasing right-to-left shunting and increasing cardiac output.

Another approach to management of infants with pulmonary complications is the use of ***extracorporeal membrane oxygenation (ECMO)*** with a modified heart-lung machine. Blood is shunted from the right atrium by gravity to a servoregulated roller pump, pumped through a membrane lung and a small heat exchanger, and returned to the systemic circulation via a major artery such as the carotid artery to the aortic arch. A venovenous approach may be used, thus avoiding the need to ligate the carotid artery. ECMO provides oxygen to the circulation and allows the lungs to rest (Kanto, 1994). The goal of ECMO is to "buy time" for the severely injured lung to heal while effectively oxygenating major organ systems, including the brain, heart, kidneys, and lungs (Fig. 10-15). ECMO is very labor intensive and thus expensive. Technical malfunctions may occur, requiring frequent monitoring of the equipment and the patient's response to treatment. Typically, two nurses, one of whom is a perfusionist, are required as minimum staffing for the ECMO patient; more staff, including a respiratory therapist, are required in the acute phase. ECMO requires heparinization of the blood and blood circuit; for this reason it is not used in infants less than 35 weeks of gestation who are prone to intraventricular hemorrhage. Bleeding is one of the major complications associated with ECMO (Cusson, 1992). Innovative treatment modalities such as inhaled nitric oxide and liquid ventilation bear promising results in limited clinical trials for the treatment of PPHN (Finer and others, 1994; Greenspan, 1993; Roberts and Shaul, 1993; Roberts and others, 1992).

Nursing Considerations

The nursing care is the same as for infants with severe respiratory difficulties and infants supported by mechanical respirators. The infant with PPHN is often the sickest in

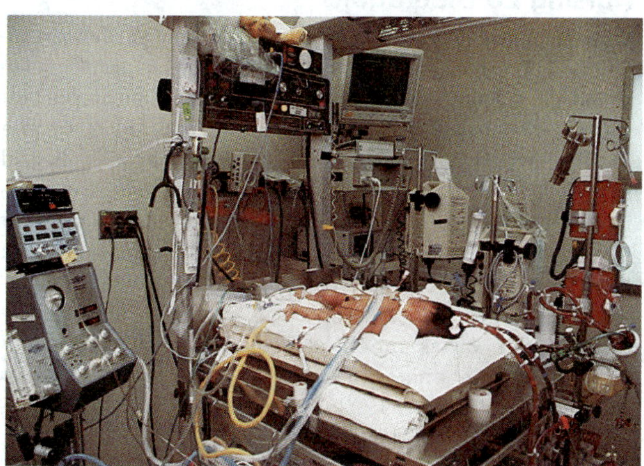

FIG. 10-15 Infant on extracorporeal membrane oxygenation (ECMO).

the unit, depending on the causative factors and reaction to treatment. Because handling for any reason causes a decrease in arterial oxygen concentration, the stresses imposed by routine care must be weighed against the risk of iatrogenic hypoxia. It is important to decrease noxious stimuli that cause crying and struggling and to employ nursing interventions, such as giving pacifiers, that keep nonsedated infants calm. Continuous monitoring of central venous pressure, vital signs, blood pressure, and $tcPCO_2$, and pulse oximetry monitoring of oxygenation decrease the need for physical manipulation and disturbance. Infants are assessed for pulmonary vascular response (e.g., increased PaO_2 and signs of systemic hypotension, gastrointestinal bleeding, or pulmonary hemorrhage).

ANEMIA

Preterm infants tend to develop anemia that is more severe and appears earlier than in more mature infants. It may be a result of hemorrhage during the course of labor and delivery (into brain, liver, spleen, or kidneys), blood disorders (hemolytic disease, thrombocytopenia), or conditions that produce swelling or distention of abdominal organs; or it may be iatrogenic from blood withdrawn in the NICU for laboratory tests. Physiologic characteristics of prematurity tend to contribute to development of anemia (i.e., a drop in the production of hemoglobin and shortened survival time of the red blood cells). This lag in hematopoiesis during continued growth results in physiologic anemia, probably as a consequence of diminished erythropoietin values.

Fortunately, even VLBW infants are able to accommodate the gastrointestinal absorption of iron required for their high needs. Iron is supplied in iron-fortified formulas or iron supplements as both a preventive and therapeutic measure. Transfusions with packed red blood cells are often required for severe anemia, usually for replacement of blood loss resulting from iatrogenic measures. At 4 to 12 weeks of age a "physiologic anemia" reaches a peak, at which time infants sometimes display signs that suggest true anemia.

Nursing Considerations

One of the most common causes of anemia in preterm infants is blood loss associated with frequent sampling for blood gas and metabolic analyses. Therefore an important nursing responsibility is careful monitoring and recording of all blood drawn for tests. It is surprising how easily and rapidly the small total blood volume of premature infants is depleted by repeated withdrawals. However, replacement in light of hepatitis and HIV transmission is less frequent than previously. Investigation into the effectiveness of recombinant human erythropoietin administration is currently under way as a method of increasing red blood cell production in neonates to treat the anemia of prematurity (Carnielli and others, 1992; Messer and others, 1993; Ohls and Christensen, 1991).

Observation for signs of anemia is a vital nursing function. The signs of anemia in the preterm infant are poor feeding, decreased oxygen saturation, systolic murmur, dyspnea, tachycardia, tachypnea, diminished activity, and pallor. However, some infants may not display all of these signs. Poor weight gain may be an indication of a lowered hemoglobin level. Nursing precautions and observations during blood transfusion are discussed in Chapter 35.

POLYCYTHEMIA

The current definition of polycythemia is a venous hematocrit of 65% or more. With a hematocrit above 65%, blood flow becomes increasingly sluggish and hyperviscous, resulting in hypoperfusion of organs. Polycythemia may result from in utero twin-to-twin transfusion and maternal-fetal transfusion, prolonged emptying of placental blood to the infant at birth, or increased red blood cell production after birth. The small-for-gestational-age (SGA) infant is the most at risk for polycythemia; increased red blood cell consumption of glucose further predisposes the infant to hypoglycemia. Among infants with polycythemia a high incidence of cardiopulmonary distress symptoms (persistent fetal circulation, cyanosis, and apnea), seizures, hyperbilirubinemia, and gastrointestinal abnormalities exists.

Appropriate therapy for correcting metabolic disturbances (e.g., hypoxia, hypoglycemia, and hyperbilirubinemia) is implemented, and lowering blood viscosity by partial plasma exchange transfusion may be considered in symptomatic cases.

Nursing Considerations

Nursing care involves watching for signs of polycythemia (e.g., plethora, peripheral cyanosis, respiratory distress, lethargy, jitteriness or seizure activity, hypoglycemia, hyperbilirubinemia) and assisting with diagnostic tests and therapeutic procedures. Care of the infant with hyperbilirubinemia is discussed in Chapter 9.

RETINOPATHY OF PREMATURITY (ROP)

Although often discussed in relation to respiratory dysfunction, ROP is a disorder involving blood vessels. ROP is a term used to describe all phases of retinal changes in the eye observed in preterm infants. The older term, ***retrolental fibroplasia (RLF)***, describes the cicatricial changes that characterize the later stages in the most severely affected infants. ROP is primarily, but not exclusively, a disease of premature infants. The incidence of the disease correlates with the degree of the infant's maturity—the younger the gestational age, the greater the likelihood of the development of ROP.

Numerous factors have been implicated in the cause of ROP in addition to immaturity, including hyperoxemia and hypoxemia, hypercarbia and hypocarbia, patent ductus arteriosus, prostaglandin synthetase inhibitors, apnea, intraventricular hemorrhage, infection, vitamin E deficiency, lactic acidosis, maternal diabetes, prenatal complications, and genetic factors. Previously considered to be an iatrogenic disease related to hyperoxia, ROP is now believed to be a complex disease of prematurity with multiple causes and therefore difficult to completely prevent and manage.

Pathophysiology

The disorder is characterized by severe vascular constriction in the immature retinal vasculature followed by hypoxia in those areas. This appears to stimulate vascular proliferation of retinal capillaries into the hypoxic areas where veins become numerous and dilate. As new vessels proliferate toward the lens, the aqueous humor and then the vitreous humor become turbid. The retina becomes edematous, and hemorrhages separate the retina from its attachment. Advanced scarring occurs from the retina to the lens, destroying the normal architecture of the eye. This extensive retinal detachment and scarring result in irreversible blindness.

Diagnostic Evaluation

A system of classification has been established to describe the location and extent of the developing vasculature involved. Normal vascular growth proceeds in an orderly fashion from the disc toward the ***ora serrata,*** the irregular anterior margin of the retina. The stages of ROP are outlined in the box below. ROP is further classified by location of damage in the retina and by the extent of abnormally developing vascularization (clock hour) (Merenstein and Gardner, 1993; Phelps, 1993).

Therapeutic Management

Although judicious use and careful monitoring of supplemental oxygen have reduced the incidence of ROP, the disease has not been eradicated. Prophylactic administration of vitamin E has been used in some units but is still considered to be an experimental drug; its use is not without complications.

Although prevention is the primary goal of therapeutic management, treatment of retinal pathology is directed toward arresting the proliferation process. Cryotherapy is the best treatment when performed by a pediatric ophthalmologist.

Nursing Considerations

Adherence to the principles of oxygen administration and careful monitoring of oxygenation status are the first lines of defense against development of ROP. In addition, decreasing environmental stimuli and continuous direct lighting may also aid in a decreased incidence of this illness (Lotas, 1992). Constant assessment and vigilance are necessary just as for any high-risk neonate. When the infant suffers partial or complete visual impairment, the parents will need a considerable amount of support and assistance in meeting the special developmental needs of the infant (see Chapter 25).

STAGES OF RETINOPATHY OF PREMATURITY

1. A demarcation line (separates the avascular retina anteriorly from the vascularized retina posteriorly)
2. A ridge (formed from the demarcation line with the height and width, occupies volume, and extends beyond the plane of the retina)
3. A ridge with extraretinal fibrovascular proliferation
4. Retinal detachment

"Plus" disease—increased dilation and tortuosity of peripheral retinal vessels (e.g., Stage 2 plus ROP)

Data from an international classification of retinopathy of prematurity, *Pediatrics* 74:127-133, 1984; Merenstein GB, Gardner SL: *Handbook of neonatal intensive care,* ed 3, St Louis, 1993, Mosby; and Phelps DL: Retinopathy of prematurity, *Pediatr Clin North Am* 40(4):705-714, 1993.

HIGH RISK RELATED TO NEUROLOGIC DISTURBANCE

Neurologic complications are observed with increased frequency in preterm infants and in infants born following a difficult labor and delivery. A disproportionately high incidence of perinatal encephalopathy, or cerebral palsy, and psychomotor retardation is found in the high-risk infant population, especially ELBW and VLBW infants. Preterm infants are also more vulnerable to cerebral insults, such as hypoxia and chemical alterations. In addition, fragility and increased permeability of capillaries and prolonged prothrombin time predispose the brain of the preterm infant to trauma when delicate structures are subjected to increased pressure, such as the forces of labor, high mechanical ventilatory pressures, and seizure activity. All of these factors contribute to intracranial insults, including traumatic bleeding in the newborn, which consists of four major types: intraventricular, subdural, primary subarachnoid, and intracerebellar.

PERINATAL HYPOXIC-ISCHEMIC BRAIN INJURY

Hypoxic-ischemic brain injury, or hypoxic-ischemic encephalopathy, is the most common cause of neurologic impairment observed in infants. The brain damage usually results from asphyxia, either before or during delivery, but it can happen postnatally as well. Ischemia and hypoxemia occur together, although one or the other predominates. The major causes of serious hypoxemia are listed in the left-hand box on p. 418.

Newborns are particularly vulnerable to ischemic injury caused by decreased cerebral blood flow following asphyxia. Infants who have suffered intrauterine oxygen deprivation may be further compromised postnatally, thus compounding an existing problem. It is important to note that hypoxic-ischemic brain damage is extremely variable from infant to infant, causing severe damage in some, whereas others with similar pathologic situations may have little or no residual damage (Pasternak, 1993).

Clinical Manifestations

The neurologic signs that indicate encephalopathy appear within the first hours after the hypoxic episode with manifestations of bilateral cerebral dysfunction. The infant may be stuporous or comatose. Seizures begin after 6 to 12 hours in about 50% of the infants, and they become more frequent and severe by 12 to 24 hours. Between 24 and 72 hours there may be deterioration in the level of conscious-

> **PRIMARY CAUSES OF PERINATAL HYPOXEMIA AND CEREBRAL ISCHEMIA**
>
> **PERINATAL HYPOXEMIA**
> 1. Intrauterine asphyxia with respiratory failure at the time of birth
> 2. Postnatal respiratory insufficiency secondary to severe RDS or recurrent apnea
> 3. Severe cyanotic heart defects (right-to-left shunts) or persistent pulmonary hypertension
>
> **PRIMARY CEREBRAL ISCHEMIA**
> 1. Intrauterine asphyxia with cardiac insufficiency
> 2. Postnatal cardiac insufficiency secondary to severe congenital heart disease or recurrent apnea
> 3. Postnatal cardiovascular collapse secondary to sepsis
>
> Data from Hill A, Volpe JJ: Seizures, hypoxic-ischemic brain injury, and intraventricular hemorrhage in the newborn, *Ann Neurol* 10:109-121, 1981.

ness, and after 72 hours there may be persistent stupor, abnormal tone (usually hypotonia), and evidence of disturbances of sucking and swallowing. Muscular weakness of the hips and shoulders is observed in full-term infants, and lower limb weakness occurs in premature infants. Apneic episodes are seen in approximately 50% of the affected infants.

Improvement in the neurologic deficiencies is highly variable and difficult to predict, although infants who demonstrate the most rapid initial improvement appear to have the best prognosis. Myocardial failure and acute tubular necrosis are frequent complications. The major long-term sequelae of hypoxic-ischemic injury are mental retardation, seizures, and cerebral palsy.

Therapeutic Management

Treatment involves vigorous resuscitation at birth and supportive care to provide adequate ventilation to prevent aggravating the existing hypoxia and measures to maintain cerebral perfusion and prevent cerebral edema. Seizures are managed as described in the discussion on p. 420. Prevention is the most important therapy, however, and every effort should be made to recognize high-risk pregnancies, monitor the fetuses, and initiate appropriate therapy early.

Nursing Considerations

Nursing care is primarily the same as for any high-risk infant: careful assessment and observation for signs that might indicate cerebral hypoxia or ischemia, monitoring of ventilatory and intravenous therapy, observation and management of seizures, and general supportive care to infants and parents, including guidelines for management in the event of cognitive impairment (see Chapter 24). These infants are usually on intravenous alimentation.

PERIVENTRICULAR-INTRAVENTRICULAR HEMORRHAGE (PVH/IVH)

PVH/IVH is known by a variety of terms according to the locus of bleeding: ***periventricular hemorrhage (PVH), intraventricular hemorrhage (IVH), germinal matrix hemorrhage–intraventricular hemorrhage (GMH/IVH),*** and ***subependymal-intraventricular hemorrhage (SE/IVH).*** Most authorities use the term IVH to describe this disorder, which is responsible for a significant percentage of seriously ill infants and neonatal mortality. IVH is extremely common in preterm infants, especially ELBW and VLBW infants less than 32 weeks of gestation; the degree of neonatal immaturity correlates with the incidence of hemorrhage, and subsequent neurologic handicap is not uncommon (Bowen, 1992).

> **CLASSIFICATION OF INTRAVENTRICULAR HEMORRHAGE**
>
> 1—Bleeding into germinal matrix only
> 2—Germinal matrix with blood in the ventricles
> 3—Germinal matrix with blood in the ventricles and ventricular dilation
> 4—Intraventricular and parenchymal bleeding (other than germinal matrix)

Pathophysiology

During the early months of prenatal development there is an extensive but fragile vascular network in the region of the ventricles that receives a disproportionately large amount of cerebral blood flow. Toward term, more blood is directed to the germinal matrix located in the periventricular region near the caudate nuclei of the cerebrum. Therefore premature infants are subject to rupture in this heavily vascularized region, especially during an event that is likely to increase cerebral blood flow, such as hypoxic episodes and the associated increased venous pressure. In IVH the bleeding originates in these capillaries. The blood may rupture through the ependymal lining of the ventricles and fill all or part of the ventricular system. Under pressure the ventricular system can dilate and cause acute hydrocephalus. Eventually, obliterative arachnoiditis may develop and obstruct the flow of cerebrospinal fluid. In severe cases the hemorrhage extends into the cerebral parenchyma. (See box above for the classification of degrees of IVH.)

Several clinical features are associated with IVH, such as birth asphyxia, early gestational age, low birth weight, respiratory distress, metabolic derangements, and hypotension. Posthemorrhagic hydrocephalus and damage to the periventricular white matter of the brain (such as in grade 4) are major determinants in relation to associated chronic problems and prognosis (Bowen, 1992).

Clinical Manifestations

An increase in intracranial pressure (ICP) from hemorrhage is manifested by a deterioration in condition—apnea, bradycardia, cyanosis, hypotonia, drop in hematocrit, full anterior fontanel, increased occipitofrontal circumference (OFC), separated sutures, and neurologic signs, such as twitching, stupor, apnea, and convulsions. Grades 1 and 2 IVH may, however, occur without evidence of symptomatology.

Diagnostic Evaluation

When intracranial hemorrhage is suspected or the infant is at risk, studies of intracranial structures are performed by ultrasonography, computed tomography (CT), or magnetic resonance imaging (MRI). In many NICUs screening with cranial ultrasonography is performed at the bedside (via the anterior fontanel) within 24 to 48 hours of birth and weekly until the infant is at a corrected age of 36 weeks of gestation.

Therapeutic Management

The treatment of IVH is aimed at prevention; prevention of prematurity and any events that may lead to IVH is foremost. The maintenance of oxygenation by decreasing iatrogenic events is the key to maintaining ELBW and VLBW infants neurologically intact. A number of associated factors with prematurity and RDS may predispose the infant to IVH, including acidosis, electrolyte imbalances and rapid fluid shifts (extracellular to intracellular), administration of hyperosmolar solutions (such as $NaHCO_3$), and hypotension followed by rapid volume expansion (such as with tension pneumothorax). Medical treatment with vitamin E, pancuronium (to decrease BP fluctuations), phenobarbitol, indomethacin, and surfactant (for RDS), aimed at preventing IVH, have been used with varying degrees of success (Ment and others, 1994). In the event of an IVH, treatment is both preventive and supportive; prompt detection by clinical signs and/or periodic ultrasonography are key elements in implementing strategies to prevent further damage. Posthemorrhagic hydrocephalus is a common occurrence within a month of the event. In some units serial lumbar punctures are used to decrease CSF and thus decrease ventricular size. Ventricular dilation (grade 3 to grade 4) may be managed with shunting (ventriculoperitoneal) or a temporary external ventricular drainage (EVD) (Kenner, Brueggemeyer, and Gunderson, 1993). In spite of such measures, the long-term outcome is variable and unpredictable.

Nursing Considerations

In addition to the routine observations and management, nursing care is directed toward prevention of fluctuations in cerebral BP. It has been observed that some nursing procedures increase ICP. For example, there is a marked increase in BP during endotracheal suctioning in preterm infants, and head positioning produces measurable changes in ICP. It has been found that ICP is highest when infants are in the dependent position and decreases when the head is in a midline position and elevated 30 degrees.

Cerebral pressure is lower when infants are in a midline position as opposed to a right side-lying position. When the head is turned to the right without body alignment, the resulting venous congestion creates hydrostatic pressure fluctuations that increase ICP. Infants encumbered with tubes and monitoring equipment are more difficult to turn while maintaining head-body alignment.

Other interventions that may reduce the risk of increased ICP include avoiding interventions that cause crying (such as painful procedures). Crying (essentially creating a Valsalva effect) can impede venous return, increase cerebral blood volume, and compromise cerebral oxygenation in LBW infants. Rapid volume expansion following hypotension (primarily in preterms) and administration of hyperosmolar solutions such as $NaHCO_3$ should be avoided. Since air leaks such as pneumothorax produce variable cerebral blood flow, rapid detection and intervention is a key component of nursing care of the high-risk infant. An attitude of minimum handling of infants at high risk is used in many units, since routine nursing care has been shown to cause fluctuations in cerebral blood flow. In addition, research has implicated noxious external stimuli, such as noise, as having a potential role in stimulation that may lead to IVH. Care includes evaluating manipulations and handling, and administering analgesics to reduce discomfort. "Each intervention should be preceded by the questions, 'How stressful will this be for the infant?' and 'Is it necessary?' " (Kling, 1989).

INTRACRANIAL HEMORRHAGE (ICH)

ICH in neonates, although manifested in the same ways as those described in older children, occurs with different frequencies and different degrees of severity.

Subdural Hemorrhage

A subdural hematoma is a life-threatening collection of blood in the subdural space, most often produced by the stretching and tearing of the large veins in the ***tentorium cerebelli,*** the dural membrane that separates the cerebrum from the cerebellum. With improved obstetric care this condition has become relatively uncommon; however, it is especially serious because of the inaccessibility of the hematoma to aspiration by subdural tap. Less frequently, hemorrhage occurs when veins in the subdural space over the surface of the brain are torn (see also Head Injury, Chapter 37).

Subarachnoid Hemorrhage

Subarachnoid hemorrhage, the most common type of intracranial hemorrhage, occurs in term infants as a result of trauma and in preterm infants as a result of the same types of events that cause IVH. Small hemorrhages are the most common. Bleeding is of venous origin, and underlying contusion may also occur.

Intracerebellar Hemorrhage

Intracerebellar hemorrhage is a common finding on postmortem examination of the premature infant and can be a primary hemorrhage in the cerebellum associated with skull compression during abrupt, precipitous delivery, or it may occur secondary to extravasation of blood into the cerebellum from a ventricular hemorrhage. In the full-term infant the bleeding may follow a difficult delivery.

Nursing Considerations

Nursing care is the same as care of the infant with periventricular-intraventricular hemorrhage or with perinatal hypoxic-ischemic brain injury.

NEONATAL SEIZURES

Seizures in the neonatal period are usually the clinical manifestation of a serious underlying disease. The most common cause of seizures in the neonatal period is hypoxic ischemic brain injury (Squires, 1992). Although not life threatening as an isolated entity, seizures constitute a medical emergency because they signal a disease process that may produce irreversible brain damage. Consequently, it is imperative to recognize a seizure and its significance so that the cause, as well as the seizure, can be treated (see box below).

Pathophysiology

The features of neonatal seizures are different from those observed in the older infant or child. For example, the well-organized, generalized tonic-clonic seizures seen in older children are rare in infants, especially preterm infants. The newborn brain, with its immature anatomic and physiologic status and less cortical organization, is insufficient to allow ready development and maintenance of a generalized seizure. The advanced degree of development of limbic structures with connections to the diencephalon and brainstem probably accounts for the higher frequency of seizure manifestations that originate in these structures, such as oral movements, oculomotor deviations, and apnea.

CAUSES OF NEONATAL SEIZURES

METABOLIC

Hypoglycemia; hyperglycemia
Hypocalcemia
Hypomagnesemia
Pyridoxine deficiency
Aminoacidurias (e.g., phenylketonuria, maple syrup urine disease)
Hyperammonemia

TOXIC AND ELECTROLYTE

Hypernatremia; hyponatremia
Narcotic withdrawal
Uremia
Bilirubin encephalopathy (kernicterus)

PRENATAL INFECTIONS

Toxoplasmosis
Syphilis
Cytomegalovirus
Herpes simplex
Hepatitis

POSTNATAL INFECTIONS

Bacterial meningitis
Viral meningoencephalitis
Sepsis
Brain abscess

TRAUMA AT BIRTH

Hypoxic brain injury
Intracranial hemorrhage
Subarachnoid, epidural hemorrhage
Intraventricular hemorrhage of prematurity

MALFORMATIONS

Central nervous system agenesis
Hydroencephalopathy
Parencephalopathy
Tuberous sclerosis

MISCELLANEOUS

Degenerative disease
Benign familial neonatal seizures

Clinical Manifestations

Seizures in newborns may be subtle and barely discernible or grossly apparent. Since most neonatal seizures are subcortical, they do not have the etiologic and prognostic significance of seizures in children. The type of seizure is seldom important, since one may produce any of a variety of manifestations. Neonatal seizures can be divided into four major types. In order of frequency, these classifications are outlined in Table 10-6 and consist of colonic, tonic, myoclonic, and subtle seizures (Volpe, 1989). Clonic, multifocal clonic, and migratory clonic seizures are more common in term infants.

Jitteriness or tremulousness in the newborn is a repetitive shaking of an extremity or extremities that may be observed with crying, may occur with changes in sleeping state, or may be elicited with stimulation. Jitteriness is relatively common in newborns, affecting 44% of healthy full-term newborns in one study (Parker and others, 1990), and in a mild degree may be considered normal during the first 4

TABLE 10-6 Classification of Neonatal Seizures

TYPE	CHARACTERISTICS
Clonic	Rhythmic jerking movements About 1 to 3 per second May migrate randomly from one part of the body to another Simultaneous involvement of separate areas Movements may start at different times and at different rates
Tonic	Extensions of all four limbs (similar to decerebrate rigidity) Upper limbs are maintained in a stiffly flexed position (resembles decorticate rigidity) Appear more frequently in preterm infants Commonly associated with IVH
Myoclonic	Single or multiple flexion jerks of limbs Often indicate a metabolic etiology
Subtle	May develop in either full-term or preterm infants Often overlooked by inexperienced observer Signs: Clonic horizontal eye deviation Repetitive blinking or fluttering of the eyelids, staring Twitching Drooling, sucking, or other oral-buccal-lingual movements Arm movements resemble rowing or swimming Leg movements described as pedaling or bicycling Apnea (common) Signs may appear alone or in combination

days of life. Jitteriness can be distinguished from seizures by several characteristics: jitteriness is not accompanied by ocular movement as are seizures; the dominant movement in jitteriness is tremor, whereas seizure movement is clonic jerking that cannot be stopped by flexion of the affected limb; and jitteriness is highly sensitive to stimulation, whereas seizures are not. If jittery movements persist beyond the fourth day, if the movements are persistent and prolonged after a stimulus, or if they are easily elicited with minimum stimulus, further evaluation is indicated.

A ***tremor*** is defined as repetitive movements of both hands (with or without movement of legs or jaws) at a frequency of 2 to 5 per second and lasting more than 10 minutes (Linder and others, 1989). It is common in newborn infants and has a variety of causes, including neurologic damage, hypoglycemia, and hypocalcemia. In most instances tremors are of no pathologic significance.

Diagnostic Evaluation

Early evaluation and diagnosis of seizures is urgent. In addition to a careful physical examination, the pregnancy and family histories are investigated for familial and prenatal causes. Blood is drawn for glucose and electrolyte examination, and cerebrospinal fluid is obtained for examination for gross blood, cell count, protein, glucose, and culture. Electroencephalography may help identify subtle seizures but is less helpful in establishing a diagnosis. Other diagnostic procedures, such as computed tomography and echoencephalography, may be indicated.

Therapeutic Management

Treatment is directed toward prevention of cerebral damage and involves correction of metabolic derangements, respiratory and cardiovascular support, and suppression of the seizure activity. The underlying cause is treated (e.g., glucose infusion for hypoglycemia, calcium for hypocalcemia, and antibiotics for infection). If needed, respiratory support is provided for hypoxia, and anticonvulsants may be administered, especially when the other measures fail to control the seizures. Phenobarbital is the drug of choice given intravenously or orally and is used if seizures are severe and persistent. Other drugs that may be employed are phenytoin (Dilantin), lorazepam, and diazepam (Valium).

Nursing Considerations

The major nursing responsibilities in the care of infants with seizures are to recognize when the infant is having a seizure so that therapy can be instituted, to carry out the therapeutic regimen, and to observe the response to the therapy and any further evidence of seizures or other symptomatology. Assessment and other aspects of care are the same as for all high-risk infants. Parents need to be informed of their infant's status, and the nurse should reinforce and clarify the explanations of the practitioner. The infant's behaviors need to be interpreted for the parents, and the infant's responses to the treatment must be anticipated and their significance explained. Parents are encouraged to visit their infant and perform the parenting activities consistent with the plan of care. Seizures are a frightening phenomenon and generate a great deal of anxiety and fear, which is easily compounded by the justifiable concern of the staff. Providing support and guidance is an important nursing function.

HIGH RISK RELATED TO MATERNAL CONDITIONS

Conditions in the maternal system can have a significant effect on the fetus that extends into the postnatal period. A number of these conditions that are congenital malformations and disorders and can cause permanent disability are discussed in Chapter 11. Maternal diabetes and drug addiction are presented in the following section.

A number of maternal infections are detrimental to both the mother and the fetus. Some produce permanent physical or mental defects; others cause illness in the newborn period. It is important to be aware of a possible infection in the mother in order to be alert for evidence of the illness in the newborn, and to be aware of signs in the newborn that indicate intrauterine exposure to a maternal infection. (For further discussion see Chapter 11.)

INFANTS OF DIABETIC MOTHERS (IDMs)

Before insulin therapy, few diabetic women were able to conceive; for those who did, the mortality rate for both mother and infant was high. As a result of effective control of maternal diabetes and an increased understanding of fetal disorders, the morbidity and mortality of IDMs have been significantly reduced.

The severity of the maternal diabetes affects infant survival. Severity of maternal diabetes is determined by the duration of the disease before pregnancy, the age of onset, the extent of vascular complications, and abnormalities of the current pregnancy, such as pyelonephritis, diabetic ketoacidosis, pregnancy-induced hypertension, and noncompliance. The single most important factor influencing fetal well-being is the euglycemic status of the mother. It has been found that reasonable metabolic control started before conception and continued during the first weeks of pregnancy can prevent malformations in an IDM.

Effects of Diabetes on the Fetus

Hypoglycemia, defined as a blood sugar level below 40 mg/dl in the first 24 hours and 40 to 50 mg/dl thereafter for all newborns, appears a short time after birth and in IDMs is associated with increased insulin activity in the blood (see also p. 354). It has been demonstrated that IDMs have hypertrophy and hyperplasia of the pancreatic islet cells and that they are actually in a transient state of hyperinsulinism.

It is generally agreed that during fetal life high maternal blood sugar levels provide a continual stimulus to the fetal islet cells for insulin production. This sustained state of hyperglycemia promotes fetal insulin secretion that ultimately leads to excessive growth and deposition of fat, which probably accounts for the infants who are large for gestational age (LGA). When the glucose supply is removed abruptly at the time of birth, the continued production of insulin soon depletes the blood of circulating glucose, creating a state of hyperinsulinism and hypoglycemia within ½ to 4 hours, especially in infants of mothers with class C diabetes or beyond. Precipitous drops in blood glucose levels can cause serious neurologic damage or death.

Tests of fetal well-being are performed routinely on the expectant mother with diabetes during pregnancy. Ultrasonography is performed at 18 to 20 weeks to determine fetal size and to rule out the presence of fetal anomalies. It may be repeated periodically during the course of fetal development. Urinary estriol, protein, and creatinine are measured weekly after 30 weeks of gestation, and nonstress or oxytocin challenge tests for assessment of fetal and placental function are performed after 33 weeks. Before delivery, fetal lung maturation tests via amniocentesis are carried out, including lecithin/sphingomyelin ratio, phosphatidylglycerol, and disaturated phosphatidylcholine measurements.

Some mothers are hospitalized at 36 to 37 weeks of gestation for management. Insulin and dietary alterations are made in accordance with blood glucose determinations. Techniques such as closed- or open-loop continuous insulin infusion devices may be employed to maintain a satisfactory blood glucose concentration in the mother.

Clinical Manifestations

Infants of well-controlled diabetic mothers are essentially no different from other infants, but infants of poorly controlled diabetic mothers have a characteristic appearance. They are usually macrosomic for their gestational age, very plump and full-faced, liberally coated with vernix caseosa, and plethoric. The placenta and umbilical cord are also larger than average. However, infants of mothers with advanced diabetes may be small for gestational age (SGA) or appropriate for gestaitonal age (AGA) because of the maternal vascular involvement. There is an increase in congenital anomalies in this group in addition to a high susceptibility to hypoglycemia, hypocalcemia, hyperbilirubinemia, and RDS. Hyperinsulinemia in an uncontrolled diabetic mother may be a factor in reducing fetal surfactant synthesis, thus contributing to the development of RDS (Blackburn and Loper, 1992). Abnormalities in these infants are the result of exposure to elevated glucose and ketone levels, placental insufficiency, and prematurity. Although they are large, these infants are often prematurely born in an elective early delivery or because of complications.

Therapeutic Management

The most effective management appears to be careful observation of all IDMs, often in the special care nursery. The infants are examined for the presence of any anomalies or birth injuries, and blood studies for initial determinations of glucose, calcium, hematocrit, and bilirubin are obtained on a regular basis.

Since the hypertrophied pancreas is so sensitive to blood glucose concentrations, the administration of oral glucose may trigger a massive insulin release, resulting in rebound hypoglycemia. Therefore feedings of breast milk or formula are begun within the first hour after birth provided that the infant's cardiorespiratory condition is stable (would not feed infant with RDS). Some practitioners prefer early feedings of nonglucose carbohydrates, such as invert sugar or galactose, because they are less insulinogenic. Approximately half of these infants do very well and adjust without complications. Infants born to mothers with uncontrolled diabetes may require intravenous infusions. Oral and intravenous intake may be titrated to maintain adequate blood sugar levels. Frequent blood glucose determinations are needed for the first 2 days of life to assess the degree of hypoglycemia present at any given time. Testing blood taken from the heel with reagent strips is a simple and effective screening evaluation that can then be confirmed by laboratory examinations several times a day.

Nursing Considerations

Because some IDMs are born prematurely, they are subject to the problems discussed in relation to the preterm infant. In addition to the routine care of the newborn, the infants require observation for signs of complications.

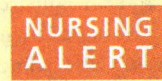

Nurses caring for IDMs are alert to signs of hypoglycemia (Chapter 9), hyperbilirubinemia (Chapter 9), polycythemia (p. 416), and RDS (p. 399).

NARCOTIC-ADDICTED INFANTS

Narcotics, which have a low molecular weight, readily cross the placental membrane and enter the fetal system. When the mother is a habitual user of narcotics, especially heroin or methadone, the unborn child also becomes passively addicted to the drug, which places such infants at risk during the early neonatal period. ***Narcotic abstinence syndrome (NAS)*** is the term used by many to describe the set of behaviors exhibited by the infant exposed to substances in utero causing the withdrawal effect (Merenstein and Gardner, 1993).

Clinical Manifestations

Most passively addicted infants of drug-dependent mothers appear normal at birth but begin to exhibit signs of drug withdrawal within 12 to 24 hours if the mother has been taking heroin by itself. If mothers have been taking methadone, the signs appear somewhat later, anywhere from 1 or 2 days to 2 to 3 weeks or more after birth. The manifestations become most pronounced between 48 and 72 hours of age and may last from 6 days to 8 weeks, depending on the severity of the withdrawal (see box on p. 423).

The clinical manifestations of NAS in neonates, which are predominantly those of autonomic nervous system hyperirritability, may persist for 3 or 4 months. The most common acute signs are tremors, restlessness, hyperactive reflexes, increased muscle tone, sneezing, tachypnea, and a high-pitched, shrill cry. Although these infants suck avidly on fists and display an exaggerated rooting reflex, they are poor feeders with uncoordinated and ineffectual sucking

SIGNS OF NARCOTIC WITHDRAWAL IN THE NEONATE

Irritability	Tachypnea (>60/min)
Tremors	Excoriations (knees, face)
Shrill cry	Frequent sneezing
Hypertonicity of muscles	Frequent yawning
Frantic sucking of hands	Vomiting
Poor feeding	Temperature instability
Hyperactivity	Diarrhea
Little sleeping	Convulsions
Sweating	

and swallowing reflexes. Regurgitation and vomiting after feedings are common, and diarrhea is a later manifestation.

An unusual observation in a large percentage of these infants is generalized sweating, the incidence of which is unusual in newborn infants. It is significant that although passively addicted infants have some tachypnea, cyanosis, and/or apnea, they rarely develop respiratory distress syndrome. Apparently, heroin or stress factors in the intrauterine environment cause accelerated lung maturation even with a high incidence of prematurity.

Not all infants of heroin-addicted mothers will show signs of withdrawal. Because of irregular and varying degrees of drug use, quality of drug, and mixed drug usage by the mother, some infants display mild or variable manifestations. Most manifestations are the vague, nonspecific signs characteristic of all infants in general; therefore it is important to differentiate between drug withdrawal and other disorders before specific therapy is instituted. Often other states (e.g., hypocalcemia, hypoglycemia, or sepsis) coexist with the drug withdrawal.

Infants who do not display the signs of fetal alcohol syndrome but are born to mothers who are also heavy alcohol drinkers have significantly more tremors, hypertonia, restlessness, excessive mouthing movements, crying, and inconsolability than infants of addicted mothers who do not consume alcohol during pregnancy. An added concern regarding narcotic users is that many of the mothers often use other drugs, such as tranquilizers, sedatives, narcotics, amphetamines, phencyclidine (PCP), and other psychotropic agents.

Therapeutic Management

The treatment of the passively addicted infant initially consists of modulating the environment to decrease external stimuli. Drug therapies include parenteral and/or oral administration of phenobarbital, chlorpromazine, diazepam, or paregoric.

Nursing Considerations

When possible, the nursery personnel are alerted to the likelihood of drug-addicted infants. If the mother has had good prenatal care, the practitioner is aware of the problem and therapy has been instituted before delivery. However, a number of mothers deliver their infants without the benefit of adequate care, and the addiction is unknown to health care personnel at the time of delivery. The degree of narcosis or withdrawal is closely related to the amount of drug the mother has habitually taken, the length of time she has been taking of the drug, and the drug level of the mother at the time of delivery. The most severe symptoms are observed in the infants of mothers who have taken large amounts of drugs over a long period. In addition, the nearer to the time of delivery that the mother takes the drug, the longer it takes for the child to develop withdrawal and the more severe are the manifestations. The infant may not exhibit withdrawal symptoms until 7 to 10 days after delivery.

Once the presence of NAS is identified in an infant, nursing care is directed toward reducing the stimuli (such as dimmed lights and decreased noise levels) that might trigger hyperactivity and irritability, providing adequate nutrition and hydration and promoting maternal-infant relationships. Irritable and hyperactive infants have been found to respond to comforting, movement, and close contact. Wrapping infants snugly, as well as rocking and holding them tightly, limits their ability to self-stimulate. Infants who were placed on water beds showed fewer withdrawal symptoms, were released from the hospital sooner, and gained weight more rapidly and earlier when compared with a control group sleeping in conventional bassinets (Oro and Dixon, 1988). Arranging nursing activities to reduce the amount of disturbance helps to decrease exogenous stimulation. Neonatal Abstinence Scoring System, an NAS scoring system, has been developed to monitor infants in an objective manner and evaluate the infant's response to clinical and pharmacologic interventions (Finnegan, 1985).

Loose stools and poor intake and regurgitation following feeding predispose the infants to malnutrition, dehydration, and electrolyte imbalance. Frequent weighing, careful monitoring of intake and output, and supplemental parenteral fluids may be necessary. In addition, the infants burn up energy with continual activity and increase oxygen consumption at the cellular level. It takes considerable time and patience to ensure that they receive a sufficient caloric and fluid intake.

Hyperactive infants must be protected from skin abrasions on the knees, toes, and cheeks that are caused by rubbing on bed linens when lying on their abdomens. Monitoring and recording the activity level and its relationship to other activities, such as feeding and preventing complications, are important nursing functions.

A valuable aid to anticipating problems in newborns is recognizing drug addiction in the mothers. Unless the mothers are enrolled in a methadone rehabilitation program, they seldom risk calling attention to their habit by seeking prenatal care. Consequently, infants and mothers are exposed to the additional hazards of obstetric and medical complications. Moreover, the nature of heroin addiction makes the user susceptible to disorders such as infection (hepatitis, acquired immunodeficiency syndrome [AIDS]), foreign body reaction, and the hazards of inadequate nutrition and premature birth. Methadone treatment does not prevent withdrawal reaction in neonates, but the clinical course may be modified. Also, the intensive psychologic support of mothers is a factor in the treatment and reduction of perinatal mortality. Experience has indicated that mothers are usually anxious and depressed, lack confidence, have poor self-images, and have difficulty with interpersonal relationships. They may have a psychologic need for the pregnancy and an infant.

Initial symptoms or recurrence of withdrawal symptoms may develop after discharge from the hospital; therefore it is important to establish rapport and maintain contact with the family so that they will return for treatment if this occurs. The demands on the caregiver of the narcotic-addicted infant are enormous and nonrewarding in terms of positive feedback. The infants are difficult to comfort and cry for long periods, which can be especially trying for the caregiver following the infant's discharge from the hospital. Long-term follow-up to evaluate the status of the infant and the family is very important. Sudden infant death syndrome (SIDS) and AIDS are observed more frequently in infants born to users of methadone and heroin.

There are many problems in relation to the disposition of infants of drug-dependent mothers. Those who advocate separation of mothers and children argue that the mothers are not capable of assuming responsibility for their infant's care, that child care is frustrating to them, and that their existence is too disorganized and chaotic. Others encourage the maternal-infant bond and recommended a protected environment such as a therapeutic community, a halfway house, or continuous ongoing, supportive services in the home after discharge. Each situation requires careful evaluation and the cooperative efforts of a variety of health professionals, whether the choice is foster home placement or supportive follow-up care of mothers who keep their infants.

COCAINE EXPOSURE

Cocaine, the number one illicit drug used in the United States, has multiple modes of use. However, use of the relatively inexpensive and easily administered "crack" form is increasing alarmingly, especially among women (Hadeed and Siegel, 1989). Because crack vaporizes at relatively low temperatures, it is smoked and absorbed in large quantities through the pulmonary vasculature. The drug readily crosses the placenta, placing the fetus at risk.

Cocaine is a CNS stimulant and peripheral sympathomimetic, and the effects on the fetus are secondary to maternal effects—increased BP, decreased uterine blood flow, and increased vascular resistance. Consequently, the fetus suffers decreased blood flow and oxygenation because of placental and fetal vasoconstriction. The difficulties encountered by cocaine-exposed infants are compounded when the mother is taking the drug in conjunction with other illicit drugs. Also, prenatal exposure to cocaine has been implicated as a risk for SIDS in infancy (Bauchner and others, 1988). Additional findings in infants with prenatal cocaine exposure include cerebral infarcts, renal defects, necrotizing enterocolitis, cardiac anomalies, mild facial dysmorphic features, lower birth weight and length, and a decreased head circumference. Decreased head circumference has been viewed as one of the best predictors of long-term development (Chasnoff and others, 1992).

Clinical Manifestations

Infants born to cocaine users have decreased birth weight, length, and occipitofrontal circumference. Teratogenic effects, possible genitourinary malformations, are less clear and still debated. The infants are jittery, cranky, feed poorly, and often remain intolerant to cuddling and inattentive to cooing and other comforting behaviors. A second and different behavior type seen with prenatal cocaine exposure is the infant who is lethargic, feeds poorly, is hypotonic, and is difficult to arouse (Lester and others, 1991). Scores on the Brazelton Neonatal Assessment Scale have shown infants to be low in responding appropriately to arousal, auditory, and visual stimuli (Lewis, Bennett, and Schmeder, 1989). However, these findings have been refuted in a subsequent study (Mayes and others, 1993).

Therapeutic Management

Treatment of these infants is similar to that for narcotic-addicted infants—reduction of external stimuli, supportive treatment aimed at alleviating symptoms, and, at times, sedation.

Nursing Considerations

Nursing care of cocaine-exposed infants is the same as that for narcotic-addicted infants. Since they have increased flexor tone, these infants respond to swaddling in a semi-flexed position (Schneider, Griffith, and Chasnoff, 1989). Effects of the drug from breast milk (Chasnoff, Lewis, and Squires, 1987) and topical cocaine applications to nipples (Chaney, Franke, and Wadlington, 1988) have been reported; therefore mothers should be cautioned regarding this hazard to their infants.

INFANTS OF MOTHERS WHO SMOKE

Cigarette smoking during pregnancy is clearly associated with significant birth weight deficits up to 440 g in full-term newborns, and there is a definitive dose-response relationship between the number of cigarettes smoked by the mother and these deficits. This dose-related response also affects the Apgar scores—the number of infants with low Apgar scores (whose mothers smoked three packs per day) is nearly four times that of infants whose mothers smoked none or only one pack per day. Also, reviews of large studies indicate that 21% to 39% of the incidence of low birth weight is attributable to maternal cigarette smoking.

The rate of preterm births is increased in mothers who smoke, but the infants are smaller at *all* stages of gestation. They show fetal growth retardation in length, weight, and chest and head circumference, and these deficits are not related to maternal appetite or weight gain. Concentrations of two pharmacologically active substances found in tobacco—nicotine and cotinine—have been found to be higher in newborns of mothers who smoke than in their mothers. In addition, these substances secreted in breast milk have a half-life of 70 to 80 minutes. It has also been

KEY FEATURES OF "FETAL TOBACCO SYNDROME"

1. The mother smoked five or more cigarettes a day throughout pregnancy.
2. The mother had no evidence of hypertension during pregnancy, specifically (a) no preeclampsia and (b) documentation of normal blood pressure at least once after the first trimester.
3. The newborn has symmetric growth retardation at term (up to or greater than 37 weeks), defined as (a) a birth weight less than 2500 g and (b) a ponderal index ([weight in g]/[length in m^3]) greater than 2.32.
4. There is no other obvious cause of intrauterine growth retardation (e.g., congenital infection or anomaly).

Modified from Nieburg P and others: The fetal tobacco syndrome, *JAMA* 253:2998-2999, 1985 (commentary).

shown that cigarette smoking has detrimental effects beyond the neonatal period with deficits in growth, intellectual and emotional development, and behavior. (See also Passive Smoking, Chapter 32.)

The overwhelming evidence of the detrimental effects of maternal cigarette smoking on newborns has led some investigators to suggest the diagnostic term ***fetal tobacco syndrome*** for infants who fit the key features listed in the box above. The purpose of this suggestion is to focus attention on this important health problem that is directly related to maternal behavior.

Nursing Considerations

Nurses are prime candidates for disseminating information to expectant mothers about the risks related to smoking. Mothers who stop or substantially reduce smoking during pregnancy improve the quality of life for their unborn infants. In one study infants of expectant mothers who were given information, support, encouragement, practical guidance, and behavior modification during pregnancy delivered infants with significantly higher birth weights than controls. If mothers continue to smoke while breast-feeding, they should be told to do so *immediately after* breast-feeding to reduce the amount of nicotine and cotinine in the breast milk.

KEY POINTS

- High-risk neonates may be defined as newborns, regardless of gestational age or birth weight, who have a greater than average chance of morbidity or mortality because of conditions or circumstances superimposed on the normal course of events associated with birth and adjustment to extrauterine existence.
- Identification of high-risk newborns may occur during any one of the following stages: preconceptual, prenatal, natal, or postnatal.
- High-risk infants may be classified according to size, gestational age, and morbidity factors.
- Newborn intensive care units are categorized according to the population served and degree of treatment.
- General management of the newborn entails immediate care; protection from infection; monitoring physiologic data, including heart rate, respiratory activity, temperature, and blood pressure; laboratory data; and systematic assessment of the high-risk infant.
- Assessment of the newborn includes a general assessment, respiratory assessment, cardiovascular assessment, gastrointestinal assessment, genitourinary assessment, neurologic-musculoskeletal assessment, skin assessment, and temperature.
- Because their metabolic processes are immature, high-risk newborns are placed in a heated environment to help control thermoneutrality.
- Because of the immature, fragile skin of premature infants, the nurse should use caution when applying topical preparations and, when possible, avoid bandages or dressings.
- Meeting the high-risk infant's nutritional needs requires specific knowledge of physiologic characteristics, the infant's particular needs, and methods of feeding.
- Delayed development in high-risk neonates is a concern; developmental interventions are individualized to ameliorate the effects.
- Parental involvement in the care of high-risk infants is important, and nurses should help to facilitate parent-infant relationships by guiding them to support groups and home health teaching.
- Prematurity accounts for the largest number of admissions to an NICU.
- Several severe respiratory conditions place the infant at high risk: apnea of prematurity, RDS, meconium aspiration syndrome, extraneous air syndromes, and BPD. Therapeutic management of RDS includes oxygen therapy and assisted ventilation.
- Newborns are highly susceptible to infection, particularly septicemia.
- Cardiovascular complications in the high-risk infant may include patent ductus arteriosus and persistent pulmonary hypertension.
- Neurologic disturbances in the high-risk newborn may include perinatal hypoxic-ischemic brain injury, periventricular-intraventricular hemorrhage, intracranial hemorrhage, and neonatal seizures.
- Maternal conditions that pose a threat to the newborn include diabetes and substance abuse.

REFERENCES

Affonso DD, Wahlberg V, Persson B: Exploration of mothers' reactions to the kangaroo method of prematurity care. *Neonatal Network* 7:43-51, 1989.

Affonso D and others: Reconciliation and healing for mothers through skin-to-skin contact provided in an American tertiary level intensive care nursery, *Neonatal Network* 12(3):25-32, 1993.

American Academy of Pediatrics, Committee on Injury and Poison Prevention and Committee on Fetus and Newborn: Safe transportation of premature infants, *Pediatrics* 87(1):120-122, 1991.

American Academy of Pediatrics, Committee on Nutrition: Nutritional needs of low-birth-weight infants, *Pediatrics* 75:976-986, 1985.

American Academy of Pediatrics and American College of Obstetricians and Gynecologists: *Guidelines for perinatal care,* ed 3, Elk Grove Village, IL, 1992, The Academy and College.

Anderson GH, Atkinson SA, Bryan MH: Energy and macronutrient content of human milk during early lactation from mothers giving birth prematurely and at term, *Am J Clin Nutr* 34:258-265, 1981.

Arnold LS: Low birth weight and infant mortality: a health policy perspective, *NAACOG Clin Issues Perinat Womens Health Nurs* 3(1):1-12, 1992.

Ashwood ER, Palmer SE, Lenke RR: Rapid fetal lung maturity testing: commercial versus NBD-phosphatidylcholine assay, *Obstet Gynecol* 80:1048-1053, 1992.

Bauchner H and others: Risk of sudden infant death syndrome among infants with in utero exposure to cocaine, *J Pediatr* 113:831-835, 1988.

Beckholt AP: Breast milk for infants who cannot breastfeed, *JOGNN* 19(3):216-220, 1990.

Bell SG: The national pain management guideline: implications for neonatal intensive care, *Neonatal Network* 13(3):9-17, 1994.

Bernbaum J, Hoffman-Williamson M: Following the NICU graduate, *Contemp Pediatr* 3:22-37, 1986.

Blackburn ST, Loper DL: *Maternal, fetal, and neonatal physiology: a clinical perspective,* Philadelphia, 1992, WB Saunders.

Bowen F: Neurologic evaluation of the preterm infant, *NAACOG Clin Issues Pernat Womens Health Nurs* 3(1):75-95, 1992.

Bozynski MEA and others: Lateral positioning of the stable ventilated very-low-birth-weight infant, *Am J Dis Child* 142:200-202, 1988.

Brennan-Behm M and others: Caloric loss from expressed mother's milk during continuous gavage infusion, *Neonatal Network* 13(2):27-32, 1994.

Brodsky L, Reidy M, Stanievich JF: The effects of suctioning techniques on the distal tracheal mucosa in intubated low birth weight infants, *Int J Pediatr Otorhinolaryngol* 14:1-14, 1987.

Budreau GK: Postnatal cranial modeling and infant attractiveness: implications for nursing, *Neonatal Network* 5(5):13-19, 1987.

Bull MJ, Stroup KB: Premature infants in car seats, *Pediatrics* 75:336-339, 1985.

Bull MJ, Weber K, Stroup KB: Automotive restraint systems for premature infants, *J Pediatr* 112:385-388, 1988.

Carnielli V and others: Effect of high doses of human recombinant erythropoietin on the need for blood transfusions in preterm infants, *J Pediatr* 121(1):98-102, 1992.

Carroll P: Pneumothorax in the newborn, *Neonatal Network* 10(2):27-33, 1991.

Chaney NE, Franke J, Wadlington WB: Cocaine convulsions in a breast-feeding baby, *J Pediatr* 112:134-135, 1988.

Chasnoff IJ, Lewis DE, Squires L: Cocaine intoxication in a breast-fed infant, *Pediatrics* 80:836-838, 1987.

Chasnoff IJ and others: Cocaine/polydrug use in pregnancy: two year follow-up, *Pediatrics* 89:284-289, 1992.

Collaborative Group on Antenatal Steroid Therapy: Effect of antenatal dexamethasone administration on the prevention of respiratory distress syndrome, *Am J Obstet Gynecol* 141:276, 1981.

Collins JE: Fetal surgery: changing the outcome before birth, *JOGNN* 23(2):166-169, 1994.

Culley BS, Perrin EC, Chaberski MJ: Parental perceptions of vulnerability of formerly premature infants, *J Pediatr Health Care* 3:237-245, 1989.

Cusson RM: Innovations in cardiopulmonary care of the low-birth-weight infant, *NAACOG Clin Issues Pernat Womens Health Nurs* 3(1):62-74, 1992.

Cusson RM, Lee AL: Parental interventions and the development of the preterm infant, *JOGNN* 23(1):60-68, 1994.

Davis M: Fluids, electrolytes and nutrition in the low-birth-weight infant, *NAACOG Clin Issues Perinat Womens Health Nurs* 3(1):45-61, 1992.

Fanaroff AA, Martin RJ: *Neonatal-perinatal medicine: diseases of the fetus and infant,* ed 5, St Louis, 1992, Mosby.

Feingold C: Correlates of cognitive development in low-birth-weight infants from low-income families, *J Pediatr Nurs* 9(2):91-97, 1994.

Finer NN and others: Inhaled nitric oxide in infants referred for extracorporeal membrane oxygenation: dose response, *J Pediatr* 124(2):302-308, 1994.

Finnegan LP: Neonatal abstinence. In Nelson N, editor: *Current therapy in neonatal perinatal medicine* 1985-1986, Toronto, 1985, BC Decker.

Fox MD: Measurement of urine output volume: accuracy of diaper weights in neonatal environments, *Neonatal Network* 11(3):11-18, 1992.

Fox MD, Molesky MG: The effects of prone and supine positioning on arterial oxygen pressure, *Neonatal Network* 8:25-29, 1990.

Fuller RA: Group B streptococcal infection in the newborn, *Crit Care Nurs Clin North Am* 4(3):487-493, 1992.

Gale G, Franck L, Lund C: Skin-to-skin (kangaroo) holding of the intubated premature infant, *Neonatal Network* 12(6):49-57, 1993.

Gardner SL, O'Donnell JP, Weisman LE: Breastfeeding the sick neonate. In Merenstein GB, Gardner SL: *Handbook of neonatal intensive care,* ed 3, St Louis, 1993, Mosby.

Gladstone IM, Ehrenkranz RA, Jacobs HC: Pulmonary function tests and fluid balance in neonates with chronic lung disease during dexamethasone treatment, *Pediatrics* 84:1072-1076, 1989.

Goldson E: Bronchopulmonary dysplasia, *Pediatr Ann* 19:13-18, 1990.

Greenspan JS: Liquid ventilation: a developing technology, *Neonatal Network* 12(4):23-28, 1993.

Greer PS: Head coverings for newborns under radiant warmers, *JOGNN* 17(4):265-271, 1988.

Grobman DW, Foley MM: Surfactant replacement therapy in newborns with hyaline membrane disease, *Crit Care Nurs Clin North Am* 4(3):515-520, 1992.

Gross SJ, Oehler JM, Eckerman CO: Head growth and developmental outcome in very low-birth-weight infants, *Pediatrics* 71:70-75, 1983.

Gross SJ and others: Nutritional composition of milk produced by mothers delivering preterm, *J Pediatr* 96:641-644, 1980.

Gross SJ and others: Elevated IgA concentration in milk produced by mothers delivered of preterm infants, *J Pediatr* 99:389-393, 1981.

Gunderson LP, Kenner C: Neonatal stress: physiologic adaptation and nursing implications, *Neonatal Network* 6(1):37-42, 1987.

Hack M and others: Health of very low birth weight children during their first eight years, *J Pediatr* 122(6):887-892, 1993.

Hadeed AJ, Siegel SR: Maternal cocaine use during pregnancy: effect on the newborn infant, *Pediatrics* 84:205-210, 1989.

Hagedorn MI, Gardner SL, Abman SH: Respiratory diseases. In Merenstein GB, Gardner SL: *Handbook of neonatal intensive care,* ed 3, St Louis, 1993, Mosby.

Harkavy KL and others: Dexamethasone therapy for chronic lung disease in ventilator- and oxygen-dependent infants: a controlled trial, *J Pediatr* 115:979-983, 1989.

Hegyi T and others: Blood pressure ranges in premature infants. I. The first hours of life, *J Pediatr* 124(4):627-633, 1994.

Hodge D: Endotracheal suctioning and the infant: a nursing care protocol to decrease complications, *Neonatal Network* 9(5):7-15, 1991.

Jakobi P, Weissman A, Paldi E: The extremely low birthweight infant: the twenty-first century dilemma, *Am J Perinatol* 10(2):155-175, 1993.

Kanto WP Jr: A decade of experience with neonatal extracorporeal membrane oxygenation, *J Pediatr* 124(3):335-345, 1994.

Kenner C, Brueggemeyer A, Gunderson LP: *Comprehensive neonatal nursing: a physiologic perspective,* Philadelphia, 1993, WB Saunders.

Kleiber C, Krutzfield N, Rose EF: Acute histologic changes in the tracheobronchial tree associated with different suction catheter insertion techniques, *Heart Lung* 17(1):10-14, 1988.

Kling P: Nursing interventions to decrease the risk of periventricular-intraventricular hemorrhage, *JOGNN* 18:457-464, 1989.

Knoppert DC, Mackanjee HR: Current strategies in the management of bronchopulmonary dysplasia: the role of corticosteroids, *Neonatal Network* 13(3):53-60, 1994.

Koops B, Abman S, Accurso F: Outpatient management and followup of BPD, *Clin Perinatol* 11:101-122, 1984.

Kurzner SI and others: Growth failure in infants with bronchopulmonary dysplasia: nutrition and elevated resting metabolic expenditure, *Pediatrics* 81:379-384, 1988.

Kwong MS, Egan EA: Reduced incidence of hyaline membrane disease in extremely premature infants following delay of delivery in mother with preterm labor: use of ritodrine and betamethasone, *Pediatrics* 78:767-774, 1986.

Landon-Malone KA, Kirkpatrick JM, Stull SP: Incorporating hospice care in a community hospital NICU, *Neonatal Network* 6(1):13-19, 1987.

Langkamp DL, Langhough R: What do parents of preterm infants know about diphtheria, tetanus, and pertussis immunizations? *Am J Perinatol* 10(3):187, 1993.

Lester BM and others: Neurobehavioral syndromes in cocaine-exposed newborn infants, *Child Dev* 62:694-705, 1991.

Lewis KD, Bennett B, Schmeder NH: The care of infants menaced by cocaine abuse, *MCN* 14:324-329, 1989.

Linder N and others: Suckling stimulation test for neonatal tremor, *Arch Dis Child* 64:44-46, 1989.

Ludington-Hoe SM and others: Kangaroo care: research results, and practice implications and guidelines, *Neonatal Network* 13(1):19-27, 1994.

MacKendrick W, Caplan M: Necrotizing enterocolitis: new thoughts about pathogenesis and potential treatments, *Pediatr Clin North Am* 40(5):1047-1060, 1993.

Masterson J, Zucker C, Schulze K: Prone and supine positioning effects on energy expenditure and behavior of low birth weight neonates, *Pediatrics* 80:689-692, 1987.

Mayes LC and others: Neurobehavioral profiles of neonates exposed to cocaine prenatally, *Pediatrics* 91:778-783, 1993.

McCourt M: At risk for infection: the very-low-birth-weight infant, *J Perinat Neonat Nurs* 7(4):52-64, 1994.

Meier P, Anderson GC: Responses of small preterm infants to bottle- and breast-feeding, *MCN* 12:97-105, 1987.

Meier P, Pugh EJ: Breast-feeding behavior of small preterm infants, *MCN* 10:396-401, 1985.

Meier PP and others: Breastfeeding support services in the neonatal intensive care unit, *JOGNN* 22(4):338-347, 1993.

Ment LR and others: Low-dose indomethacin and prevention of intraventricular hemorrhage: a multicenter randomized trial, *Pediatrics* 93(4):543-550, 1994.

Merenstein GB, Gardner SL: *Handbook of neonatal intensive care,* ed 3, St Louis, 1993, Mosby.

Merenstein GB, Gardner SL, Blake WW: Heat balance. In Merenstein GB, Gardner SL: *Handbook of neonatal intensive care,* ed 3, St Louis, 1993, Mosby.

Messer J and others: Early treatment of premature infants with recombinant human erythropoietin, *Pediatrics* 92(4):519-523, 1993.

Muttitt SC and others: Neonatal apnea: diagnosis by nurse versus computer, *Pediatrics* 82:713-720, 1988.

Myrer ML: New trends in neonatal mechanical ventilation, *Crit Care Nurs Clin North Am* 4(3):507-512, 1992.

Naeye RL: Race and infant mortality, *Am J Dis Child* 147(10):1030-1031, 1993.

Nelson H, Thomas K, Stein M: Thermal effects of hooding incubators, *JOGNN,* 3(1):377-381, Sept/Oct 1992.

Northway WH Jr and others: Late pulmonary sequelae of bronchopulmonary dysplasia, *N Engl J Med* 323(26):1793-1799, 1990.

Nugent J, editor: *Acute respiratory care of the neonate: a self-study course,* Petaluma, CA, 1991, Neonatal Network.

Null S: Nursing care to ease parents' grief, *MCN* 14:84-89, 1989.

O'Connor MJ, Ralston CW, Ament ME: Intellectual and perceptual-motor performance of children receiving prolonged home total parenteral nutrition, *Pediatrics* 81:231-236, 1988.

O'Donnell J: Theophylline misadventures, part 1, *Neonatal Network* 13(2):35-43, 1994.

Ohls RK, Christensen RD: Recombinant erythropoietin compared with erythrocyte transfusion in the treatment of anemia of prematurity, *J Pediatr* 119:781-788, 1991.

Oro AS, Dixon SD: Waterbed care of narcotic-exposed neonates, *Am J Dis Child* 12:186-188, 1988.

Orr MJ, Allen SS: Optimal oral experiences for infants on long-term total parenteral nutrition, *Nutr Clin Pract* 9:288-295, 1986.

Papageorgiou AN and others: Reduction of mortality, morbidity, and respiratory distress syndrome in infants weighing less than 1,000 grams by treatment with betamethasone and ritodrine, *Pediatrics* 83:493-497, 1989.

Parker S and others: Jitteriness in full-term neonates: prevalence and correlates, *Pediatrics* 85:17-23, 1990.

Pasternak JF: Hypoxic-ischemic brain damage in the term infant: lessons from the laboratory, *Pediatr Clin North Am* 40(5):1061-1072, 1993.

Peters KL: Does routine nursing care complicate the physiologic status of the premature neonate with respiratory distress syndrome? *J Perinat Neonat Nurs* 6(2):67-84, 1992.

Phelps DL: Retinopathy of prematurity, *Pediatr Clin North Am* 40(4):705-714, 1993.

Pramanik AK, Holtzman RB, Merritt TA: Surfactant replacement therapy for pulmonary diseases, *Pediatr Clin North Am* 40(5):913-936, 1993.

Richards DD: The challenge of transporting children with special needs, American Academy of Pediatrics, *Safe Ride News,* pp 1-4, spring 1989.

Roberts JD Jr, Shaul PW: Advances in the treatment of persistent pulmonary hypertension of the newborn, *Pediatr Clin North Am* 40(5):983-1004, 1993.

Roberts JD and others: Inhaled nitric oxide in persistent pulmonary hypertension of the newborn, *Lancet* 340:818-819, 1992.

Roncoli M, Medoff-Cooper B: Thermoregulation in low-birth-weight infants, *NAACOG Clin Issues Perinat Womens Health Nurs* 3(1):25-33, 1992.

St Geme JW III, Harris MC: Coagulase-negative staphylococcal infection in the neonate, *Clin Perinatol* 18(2):281-301, 1991.

Schneider JW, Griffith DR, Chasnoff IJ: Infants exposed to cocaine in utero: implications for developmental assessment and intervention, *Infants Young Child* 2(1):25-36, 1989.

Shaker CS: Nipple feeding premature infants: a different perspective, *Neonatal Network* 8(5):9-17, 1990.

Siegel R, Gardner SL, Merenstein GB: Families in crisis: theoretical and practical considerations. In Merenstein GB, Gardner SL: *Handbook of neonatal intensive care,* ed 3, St Louis, 1993, Mosby.

Squires LA: Neonatal seizures, *Crit Care Nurs Clin North Am* 4(3):495-506, 1992.

Steinfeld JD and others: The utility of the TDx test in the assessment of fetal lung maturity, *Obstet Gynecol* 79:460-464, 1992.

Strauch C, Brandt S, Edwards-Beckett J: Implementation of a quiet hour: effect on noise levels and infant sleep states, *Neonatal Network* 12(2):31-35, 1993.

Thomas K: Thermoregulation in neonates, *Neonatal Network* 13(2):15-22, 1994.

VandenBerg KA: Nippling management of the sick neonate in the NICU: the disorganized feeder, *Neonatal Network* 9(1):9-15, 1990.

Volpe JJ: Neonatal seizures: current concepts and revised classification, *Pediatrics* 84:422-428, 1989.

Vomund SL, Witter SE: Advanced techniques for the treatment of severe isoimmunization, *MCN* 19:18-23, 1994.

Walden M: Collaborating with community hospitals for healthier babies through perinatal outreach education, *J Pediatr Nurs* 9(1):59-60, 1994.

Wegman ME: Annual summary of vital statistics—1992, *Pediatrics* 92(6):743-754, 1993.

Wilcox AJ, Skjaerven R: Birth weight and perinatal mortality: the effect of gestational age, *Am J Public Health* 82:378-382, 1992.

Willett LD and others: Risk of hypoventilation in premature infants in car seats, *J Pediatr* 109:245-248, 1986.

Willett LD and others: Ventilatory changes in convalescent infants positioned in car seats, *J Pediatr* 115:451-455, 1989.

Wiswell TE, Bent RC: Meconium staining and the meconium aspiration syndrome: unresolved issues, *Pediatr Clin North Am* 40(5):955-982, 1993.

York R, Brooten D: Prevention of low birth weight, *NAACOG Clin Issues Perinat Womens Health Nurs* 3(1):13-24, 1992.

BIBLIOGRAPHY

General

Abman SH, Groothius JR: Pathophysiology and treatment of bronchopulmonary dysplasia: current issues, *Pediatr Clin North Am* 41(2):277-315, 1994.

Allen MC: The high-risk infant, *Pediatr Clin North Am* 40(3):479-488, 1993.

American Academy of Pediatrics, Committee on Injury and Poison Prevention and Committee on Fetus and Newborn: Safe transportation of premature infants, *Pediatrics* 87(1):120-122, 1991.

Brooke OG and others: Effects on birth weight of smoking, alcohol, caffeine, socioeconomic factors, and psychosocial stress, *Br Med J* 298:795-801, 1989.

Brooten D, editor: Low-birth-weight neonates, *NAACOG Clin Issues Perinat Womens Health Nurs* 3(1), 1992.

Cartlidge PHT, Fox PE, Rutter N: The scars of newborn intensive care, *Early Hum Dev* 21:1-10, 1990.

Chally PS: Moral decision making in neonatal intensive care, *JOGNN* 21(6):475-482, 1992.

Crawford NG, Pruss AM: Preventing neonatal hepatitis B infection during the perinatal period, *JOGNN* 22(6):491-497, 1993.

Cunningham N, Hutchinson S: Neonatal nurses and issues in research ethics, *Neonatal Network* 8(5):29-48, 1990.

Elhassani SB: Preventing neonatal exposure to toxins, *Contemp Pediatr* 6(4):60, 65-70, 79-82, 1989.

Fay MJ: The positive effects of positioning, *Neonatal Network* 6(5):23-28, 1988.

Fonner CJ, Rushton CH, Fletcher AB: Preparation for neonatal emergencies: a neonatal emergency medication sheet, *Pediatr Nurs* 15:527-530, 1989.

Grassi LC: Life, money, quality: the impact of regionalization on perinatal/neonatal intensive care, *Neonatal Network* 6(4):53-58, 1988.

Hack M, Fanaroff AA: Outcomes of extremely low-birth-weight infants between 1982 and 1988, *N Engl J Med* 321(24):1642-1647, 1989.

Hill AS, Rath L: The care and feeding of the low-birth-weight infant, *J Perinat Neonat Nurs* 6(4):56-58, 1993.

Ifft DL and others: Reliability of head circumference measurements for preterm infants, *Neonatal Network* 8(3):41-45, 1989.

Infant mortality—United States, 1991, *MMWR* 42(48):926-930, 1993.

Kitchen WH and others: Health and hospital readmissions of very-low-birth-weight and normal-birth-weight children, *Am J Dis Child* 144:213-218, 1990.

Kresch MJ, Brion LP, Fleischman AR: Delivery room management of meconium-stained neonates, *J Perinatol* 11(1):46-48, 1991.

Letko MD: Detecting and preventing infant hearing loss, *Neonatal Network* 11(5):33-38, 1992.

Lotas MJ: Effects of light and sound in the neonatal intensive care unit environment on the low-birth-weight infant, *NAACOG Clin Issues Perinat Womens Health Nurs* 3(1):34-44, 1992.

MacDonald NE: Minimizing the risks of neonatal HSV, *Emerg Med* 25(7):98-101, 1993.

Marshall RE: Neonatal pain associated with caregiving procedures, *Pediatr Clin North Am* 36:885-903, 1989.

Merenstein GB, Gardner SL: *Handbook of neonatal intensive care,* ed 3, St Louis, 1993, Mosby.

Mitchell SH, Najak ZD: Low-birthweight infants and rehospitalization: what's the incidence? *Neonatal Network* 8(3):27-30, 1989.

Mulligan KS, Webb LZ: Developing an evacuation procedure for a nursery complex, *Neonatal Network* 6(6):47-52, 1988.

Oehler JM, Peter MA, Seyler S: Support groups: are they really helpful in dealing with NICU stress? *Neonatal Network* 8(2):21-25, 1989.

Parry WH, O'Rear GA: Acid-base hemostasis and oxygenation. In Merenstein GB, Gardner SL: *Handbook of neonatal intensive care,* ed 3, St Louis, 1993, Mosby.

Shogan MG, Schumann LL: The effect of environmental lighting on the oxygen saturation of preterm infants in the NICU, *Neonatal Network* 12(5):7-13, 1993.

Thigpen JL: Neonatal mortality: early prediction using a neonatal status score, *Neonatal Network* 6(6):33-39, 1988.

Tobin CR: The Teflon intravenous catheter: incidence of phlebitis and duration of catheter life in the neonatal patient, *JOGNN* 17(1):35-42, 1988.

Tribotti S: Admission to the neonatal intensive care unit: reducing the risks, *Neonatal Network* 8(4):17-22, 1990.

Troiano NH: Applying principles to practice in maternal-fetal transport, *J Perinat Neonat Nurs* 2(3):20-30, 1989.

Urtis JM, Clayton D, Jay SS: Infant morbidity: a measurement of severity and occurrence of illness in preterm and term infants, *J Pediatr Nurs* 3:110-117, 1988.

Wen SW and others: Smoking, maternal age, fetal growth, and gestational age at delivery, *Am J Obstet Gynecol* 162:5-58, 1990.

Wise BV, Lawrence-Nolan L: A risk of blood transfusions for premature infants, *MCN* 15:86-89, 1990.

Zwick MB: Decreasing environmental noise in the NICU through staff education, *Neonatal Intensive Care* 6(2):16-19, 1993.

General Nursing Care

Bass JL, Mehta KA, Camara J: Monitoring premature infants in car seats: implementing the American Academy of Pediatrics policy in a community hospital, *Pediatrics* 91(6): 1137-1141, 1993.

Beachy P, Deacon J, editors: *Core curriculum for neonatal intensive care nursing,* Philadelphia, 1993, WB Saunders.

Blackburn ST, Loper DL: *Maternal, fetal, and neonatal physiology: a clinical perspective,* Philadelphia, 1992, WB Saunders.

Bull MJ, Weber K, Stroup KB: Automotive restraint systems for premature infants, *J Pediatr* 112:385-388, 1988.

Carey BE: Major complications of central lines in neonates, *Neonatal Network* 7(6):17-28, 1989.

Damato EG: Discharge planning from the neonatal intensive care unit, *J Perinat Neonat Nurs* 5(1):43-53, 1991.

DesRosier MB: Taking a baby, *Am J Nurs* 88:67, 1988.

Experience and reason—briefly recorded: urine output measurements in premature infants, *Pediatrics* 83:116-118, 1989.

Gennaro S, Bakewell-Sachs S: Discharge planning and home care for low-birth-weight infants, *NAACOG Clin Issues Perinat Womens Health Nurs* 3(1):29-146, 1992.

Gennaro S, Brooten D, Bakewell-Sachs S: Postdischarge services for low-birth-weight infants, *JOGNN* 20(1):29-36, 1991.

Goldman DJ, Goldman SL: Prematurity. In Jackson PL, Vessey JA: *Primary care of the child with a chronic condition,* St Louis, 1992, Mosby.

Gordin PC: Assessing and managing agitation in a critically ill infant, *MCN* 15:26-32, 1990.

Gunderson LP, Kenner C, editors: *Care of the 24-25 week gestational age infant (small baby protocol),* 1990, Petaluma, CA, Neonatal Network.

Hermansen MC, Buches M: Urine output determination from superabsorbent and regular diapers under radiant heat, *Pediatrics* 81:428-431, 1988.

Kenner C, Brueggemeyer A, Gunderson LP: *Comprehensive neonatal nursing: a physiologic perspective,* Philadelphia, 1993, WB Saunders.

Klaus MH, Fanaroff AA: *Care of the high-risk neonate,* ed 4, Philadelphia, 1993, WB Saunders.

Kunnl MT and others: Comparisons of rectal, femoral, axillary, and skin-to-mattress temperatures in stable neonates, *Nurs Res* 37:162-164, 1988.

Levine AH: Fetal surgery: in utero repair of congenital diaphragmatic hernia, *AORN J* 54(1):16-32, 1991.

Merenstein GB, Gardner SL: *Handbook of neonatal intensive care,* ed 3, St Louis, 1993, Mosby.

Reams PK, Deane DM: Bagged versus diaper urine specimens and laboratory values, *Neonatal Network* 6(6):17-20, 1988.

Thompson CE: Going the distance as a neonatal nurse, *Neonatal Network* 7(3):11, 1988.

Updyke C and others: Positional support for premature infants, *J Occup Ther* 40:712-715, 1986.

Wilson D: Neonatal IVs: practical tips, *Neonatal Network* 11(2):49-53, 1992.

Thermoregulation

Haddock BJ, Merrow DL, Vincent PA: Comparisons of axillary and rectal temperatures in the preterm infant, *Neonatal Network* 6(5):67-71, 1988.

Kaplan M, Eidelman AI: Improved prognosis in severely hypothermic newborn infants treated by rapid rewarming, *J Pediatr* 105:468-469, 1984.

Malin SW, Baumgart S: Optimal thermal management for low birth weight infants nursed under high-powered radiant warmers, *Pediatrics* 79:47-54, 1987.

Marks KH, Nardis EE, Momin MN: Energy metabolism and substrate utilization in low birth weight neonates under radiant warmers, *Pediatrics* 78:465-472, 1986.

Marks KH and others: Thermal head wrap for infants, *J Pediatr* 107:956-959, 1985.

Mayfield SR and others: Temperature measurement in term and preterm neonates, *J Pediatr* 104:271-275, 1984.

Moen JE and others: Axillary versus rectal temperatures in preterm infants under radiant warmers, *JOGNN* 16(5):348-352, 1987.

Ruchala P: The effect of wearing headcoverings on the axillary temperatures of infants, *MCN* 10:240, 1985.

Schiffman RF: Temperature monitoring in the neonate: a comparison of axillary and rectal temperatures, *Nurs Res* 31:274-278, 1982.

Vaughlans B: Early maternal-infant contact and neonatal thermoregulation, *Neonatal Network* 8(5):19-21, 1990.

Feeding and Nutrition

Bier JAB and others: Breast-feeding of very low birth weight infants, *J Pediatr* 123(5):778-778, 1993.

Churella HR, Bachhuber WL, MacLean WC: Survey: methods of feeding low-birth-weight infants, *Pediatrics* 76:243-249, 1985.

Costarino A, Baumgart S: Modern fluid and electrolyte management of the critically ill premature infant, *Pediatr Clin North Am* 33:153-178, 1986.

Feher SDK and others: Increasing breast milk production for premature infants with a relaxation/imagery audiotape, *Pediatrics* 83:57-60, 1989.

Forte A, Mayberry LJ, Ferkeitch S: Breast milk collection and storage practices among mothers of hospitalized neonates, *J Perinatol* 7(1):35-39, 1987.

Gavage tube insertion in the premature infant, *MCN* 12:24-27, 1987.

Gill NE and others: Effect of nonnutritive sucking on behavioral state in preterm infants before feeding, *Nurs Res* 37(5):347-350, 1988.

Hopkinson JM, Schanler RJ, Garza C: Milk production by mothers of premature infants, *Pediatrics* 81:815-820, 1988.

Jain L and others: Energetics and mechanics of nutritive sucking in the preterm and term neonate, *J Pediatr* 111:894-898, 1987.

Kennedy C, Lipsitt L: Temporal characteristics of non-oral feedings and chronic feeding problems in premature infants, *J Perinat Neonat Nurs* 7(3):77-85, 1993.

Kinneer MD, Beachy P: Nipple feeding premature infants in the neonatal intensive-care unit: factors and decisions, *JOGNN* 22(2): 147-155, 1994.

Lebenthal E, Lee PC: Heitlinger LA: Impact of development of the gastrointestinal tract on infant feeding, *J Pediatr* 102:1-9, 1983.

Lebenthal E, Leung YK: Feeding the premature and compromised infant: gastrointestinal considerations, *Pediatr Clin North Am* 35:215-238, 1988.

Lefrak-Okikawa L: Nutritional management of the very low birth weight infant, *J Perinat Neonat Nurs* 2(1):66-77, 1988.

McCoy R and others: Nursing management of breast feeding for preterm infants, *J Perinat Neonat Nurs* 2(1):42-55, 1988.

Measel CP: A practical popular pacifier, *Pediatr Nurs* 8(3):199-200, 1982.

Meier P: Bottle- and breast-feeding: effects on transcutaneous oxygen pressure temperature in preterm infants, *Nurs Res* 37:36-41, 1988.

Meier P, Pugh EJ: Breast-feeding behavior of small preterm infants, *MCN* 10:396-401, 1985.

Meier P, Wilks S: The bacteria in expressed mothers' milk, *MCN* 12:420-423, 1987.

Moore AC: Total parenteral nutrition for infants, *Neonatal Network* 6(2):33-40, 1987.

Moran JR and others: Epidermal growth factor in human milk: daily production and diurnal variation during early lactation in mothers delivering at term and at premature gestation, *J Pediatr* 103:402-405, 1983.

Pereira GR, Barbosa MM: Controversies in neonatal nutrition, *Pediatr Clin North Am* 33:65-89, 1986.

Pete JM: Newborn infants' preference for sterile water versus five-percent glucose and water, *J Pediatr Nurs* 4:263-267, 1989.

Pickler RH, Higgins KE, Crummette BD: The effect of nonnutritive sucking on bottle-feeding stress in preterm infants, *JOGNN* 22(3):230-234, 1992.

Robertson AF, Bhatia J: Feeding premature infants, *Clin Pediatr* 32(1):36-44, 1993.

Saunders RB, Friedman CB, Stramoski PR: Feeding preterm infants: schedule or demand? *JOGNN* 20(3):212-218, 1990.

Tietjen SD: Starting an infant's IV, *Am J Nurs* 90(5):44-47, 1990.

Tsang RC and others, editors: *Nutritional needs of the preterm infant: scientific basis and practical guidelines,* Baltimore, 1993, Williams & Wilkins.

Weaver KA, Anderson GC: Relationship between integrated sucking pressures and first bottle-feeding scores in premature infants, *JOGNN* 17(2):113-120, 1988.

Wilks S, Meier P: Helping mothers express milk suitable for preterm and high-risk infant feeding, *MCN* 13:121-123, 1988.

Wink DM: Better breast milk for preemies? *Am J Nurs* 89:48-50, 1989.

Developmental Outcome

Aylward GP: Environmental influences on the developmental outcome of children at risk, *Infants Young Child* 2:1-9, 1990.

Bauchner H, Brown E, Peskin J: Premature graduates of the newborn intensive care unit: a guide to follow-up, *Pediatr Clin North Am* 35:1207-1226, 1988.

Knutson MG, Biro PJ, Padgett D: Tracking infants at risk: Washington State's high priority infant tracking system, *J Pediatr Health Care* 1:180-189, 1987.

Krywanio ML, Jones LC: Developing an early intervention program for infants at risk, *J Pediatr Nurs* 3:375-382, 1988.

Lawhon G, Melzar A: Developmental care of the very low birth weight infant, *J Perinat Neonat Nurs* 2(1):56-65, 1988.

Rice BR, Feeg VD: First-year developmental outcomes for multiple-risk premature infants, *Pediatr Nurs* 11(1):30-35, 1985.

Saigal S and others: Intellectual and functional status at school entry of children who weighed 1000 grams or less at birth: a regional perspective of births in the 1980s, *J Pediatr* 116:409-416, 1990.

Schraeder BD, Rappaport J, Courtwright L: Preschool development of very low birth-weight infants, *Image J Nurs Sch* 9(4):174-178, 1987.

Slater MA and others: Neurodevelopment of monitored versus nonmonitored very low birth weight infants: the importance of family influences, *J Dev Behav Pediatr* 8(5):278-285, 1988.

Termini L and others: Reasons for acute care visits and rehospitalization in very low-birthweight infants, *Neonatal Network* 8(5): 23-26, 1990.,

Villar J and others: Heterogeneous growth and mental development of intrauterine growth-retarded infants during the first 3 years of life. *Pediatrics* 74:783-791, 1984.

Developmental Intervention and Care

Anderson GC: Skin to skin: kangaroo care in Western Europe, *Am J Nurs* 89:662-666, 1989.

Anderson GC, Marks EA, Wahlberg V: Kangaroo care for premature infants, *Am J Nurs* 86:807-809, 1986.

Barb SA, Lemons PK: The premature infant: toward improving neurodevelopmental outcome, *Neonatal Network* 7(6):7-15, 1989.

Brinker RP and others: Identifying infants from the inner city for early intervention, *Infants Young Child* 2(1):49-58, 1989.

Eyler FD and others: Effects of developmental intervention on heart rate and transcutaneous oxygen levels in low-birthweight infants, *Neonatal Network* 8(3):17-23, 1989.

Field TM and others: Tactile/kinesthetic stimulation effects on preterm neonates, *Pediatrics* 77:654-658, 1986.

Harrison LL: Teaching stimulation strategies to parents of infants at high risk, *MCN* 14:125, 1989.

Heriza CB, Sweeney JK: Effects of NICU intervention on preterm infants. I. Implications for neonatal practice, *Infants Young Child* 2(3):31-47, 1990.

Heriza CB, Sweeney JK: Effects of NICU intervention on preterm infants. II. Implications for movement research, *Infants Young Child* 2(4):29-41, 1990.

Horn MH: Alerting an infant in brightly lit room, *Crit Care Nurs* 6:84, 1986.

Lawhon G, Melzar A: Developmental care of the very low birth weight infant, *J Perinatol Neonat Nurs* 2(1):56-65, 1988.

Long T, Katz K, Pokorni J: Developmental intervention with the chronically ill infant, *Infants Young Child* 1(4):78-88, 1989.

Lott JW: Developmental care of the preterm infant, *Neonatal Network* 7(4):21-28, 1989.

Nelson DB, Clements C: Preterm infant stimulation: the analysis of a concept, *J Pediatr Health Care* 2:79-88, 1988.

Nelson DB, Heitman R, Jennings C: Effects of tactile stimulation on premature infant weight gain, *JOGNN* 15(3):262-267, 1986.

Resnick MB and others: Developmental intervention for low birth weight infants: improved early developmental outcome: *Pediatrics* 80:68-74, 1987.

Robinson J and others: Eyelid opening in preterm neonates, *Arch Dis Child* 64:943-948, 1989.

Rushton CH: Promoting normal growth and development in the hospital environment, *Neonatal Network* 4(6):21-30, 1986.

Thoman EB, Graham SE: Self-regulation of stimulation by premature infants, *Pediatrics* 78:855-860, 1986.

Thomas KA: How the NICU environment sounds to a preterm infant, *MCN* 14:249-251, 1989.

Weibley TT: Inside the incubator, *MCN* 14:96-100, 1989.

Whitelaw A: Kangaroo baby care: just a nice experience or an important advance for preterm infants *Pediatrics* 85:604-605, 1990 (commentary).

Whitelaw G and others: Skin-to-skin contact helps mothers bond with low birth weight babies, *Arch Dis Child* 63:1377-1381, 1988.

White-Traut RC, Nelson MN: Maternally administered tactile, auditory, visual, and vestibular stimulation: relationship to later interactions between mothers and premature infants, *Res Nurs Health* 11:31-39, 1988.

White-Traut RC, Pate CMH: Modulating infant state in premature infants, *J Pediatr Nurs* 2:96-101, 1987.

Family Support

Able-Boone H, Dokecki PR, Smith MS: Parent and health care provider communication and decision making in the intensive care nursery, *Child Health Care* 18:133-141, 1989.

Affleck G and others: Effects of formal support on mothers' adaptation to the hospital-to-home transition of high-risk infants: the benefits and costs of helping, *Child Dev* 60:488-501, 1989.

Anderberg GJ: Initial acquaintance and attachment behavior of siblings with the newborn, *JOGNN* 17(1):49-54, 1988.

Arenson J: Discharge teaching in the NICU: the changing needs of NICU graduates and their families, *Neonatal Network* 6(4):29, 47-51, 1988.

Butts PA and others: Concerns of parents of low birthweight infants following hospital discharge: a report of parent-initiated telephone calls, *Neonatal Network* 7(2):37-42, 1988.

Cagan J: Weaning parents from intensive care unit care, *MCN* 13:275-277, 1988.

Campbell LA: The very low birth weight infant: sensory experience and development, *Top Clin Nurs* 6(4):19-33, 1985.

Censullo M: Home care of the high-risk newborn, *JOGNN* 15:146-153, 1986.

Consolvo CA: Relieving parental anxiety in the care-by-parent unit, *JOGNN* 5:154-159, 1986.

Consolvo CA: Siblings in the NICU, *Neonatal Network* 5(5):7-12, 1987.

Edwards KA, Allen ME: Nursing management of the human response to the premature birth experience, *Neonatal Network* 6(5):82-86, 1988.

Edwards LD, Saunders RB: Symbolic interactionism: a framework for the care of parents of preterm infants, *J Pediatr Nurs* 5:123-128, 1990.

Gottwald SR, Thurman SK: Parent-infant interaction in neonatal intensive care units: implications for research and service delivery, *Infants Young Child* 2(3):1-9, 1990.

Hamelin K, Ramachandran C: Kangaroo care, *Can Nurse* 89(6):15-18, 1993.

Harrison LL, Woods S: Early parental touch and preterm infants, *JOGNN* 20(4):299-306, 1991.

Hayward EA, Janes-Kelly S, Sikora M: Rooming-in: a preventative health care measure in the neonatal intensive care unit, *Neonatal Network* 7(3):29-34, 1988.

Jellinek J and others: Facing tragic decisions with parents in the neonatal intensive care unit: clinical perspectives, *Neonatal Intensive Care* 5(3):24-29, 1992.

Kavanaugh K: Infants weighing less than 500 grams at birth: providing parental support, *J Perinat Neonat Nurs* 2(2):58-66, 1988.

Krahn GL, Hallum A, Kime C: Are there good ways to give "bad news"? *Pediatrics* 91(3):578-582, 1993.

Ladden M: The impact of preterm birth on the family and society. II. Transition to home, *Pediatr Nurs* 16(6):620-622, 626, 1990.

Levy-Shiff R, Sharir H, Mogilner MB: Mother- and father-preterm infant relationships in the hospital preterm nursery, *Child Dev* 60:93-102, 1989.

McBurney BH: The role of the community hospital nurse in supporting parents of transported infants, *Neonatal Network* 6(4):60-64, 1988.

McCain GC: Family functioning 2 to 4 years after preterm birth, *J Pediatr Nurs* 5:97-104, 1990.

McGettigan MC and others: Psychological aspects of parenting critically ill neonates, *Clin Pediatr* 33(1):77-81, 1994.

Montgomery LAV, Williams-Judge S: An anticipatory support program for high-risk parents, *Neonatal Network* 8(3):31-33, 1989.

Murphy KM: Interactional styles of parents following the birth of a high-risk infant, *J Pediatr Nurs* 5:33-41, 1990.

Mussell G and others: Use of live video transmission in the NICU, *Neonatal Network* 8(4):37, 1990.

Oehler JM: The very low-birthweight infant as an early social partner: exploring maternal reactions, expectations, and attitudes, *Neonatal Network* 9(2):79, 1990.

Rivers A, Caron B, Heck M: Experience of families with very low birthweight children with neurologic sequelae, *Clin Pediatr* 26: 223-230, 1987.

Salitros PH: Transitional infant care: a bridge to home for high-risk infants, *Neonatal Network* 4(4):35-41, 1986.

Satariano HJ, Briggs NJ, O'Neal C: Discharges from neonatal intensive care: how satisfied are parents? *Pediatr Nurs* 13:352-353, 1987.

Smith SM: Primary nursing in the NICU: a parent's perspective, *Neonatal Network* 5(4): 25-27, 1987.

Steele KH: Caring for parents of critically ill neonates during hospitalization: strategies for health care professionals, *MCN* 16(1):13-27, 1987.

Thompson DG: Support for the grieving family: a case study, *Neonatal Network* 11(6):73-75, 1992.

Troy P and others: Sibling visiting in the NICU, *Am J Nurs* 88:68-70, 1988.

Whetsell MV, Larrabee MJ: Using guilt constructively in the NICU to affirm parental coping, *Neonatal Network* 7(4):21-27, 1988.

Yoos L: Applying research in practice: parenting the premature infant, *Appl Nurs Res* 2(1):30-34, 1989.

Neonatal Loss

Amadeo DM: A time for tears, *Am J Nurs* 967-969, 1988.

Baird SF: Helping the family through a crisis, *Nursing 87* 17(6):66-67, 1987.

Bright PD: Adolescent pregnancy and loss, *Matern Child Nurs J* 16(1):1-12, 1987.

Brown SE: A case study in death with dignity, *Neonatal Network* 5(2):51-53, 1986.

Eich WF: When is emergency baptism appropriate? *Am J Nurs* 87:1680-1681, 1987.

Evans ML, Englebardt SP: Evaluation of a multidisciplinary perinatal bereavement program, *Neonatal Network* 8(4):31-35, 1990.

Gardner SL, Merenstein GB: Helping families deal with perinatal loss, *Neonatal Network* 5(2):17-22, 1986.

Gardner SL, Merenstein GB: Perinatal grief and loss: an overview, *Neonatal Network* 5(2):7-15, 1986.

Harden M: God bless the child and the keepers, *Am J Nurs* 88:654-655, 1988.

Harrigan R and others: Perinatal grief: response to the loss of an infant, *Neonatal Network* 12(5):25-31, 1993.

Ilse S, Furrh CB: Development of a comprehensive follow-up care plan after perinatal and neonatal loss, *J Perinat Neonat Nurs* 2(2):23-33, 1988.

Johansen L: As birth and death coincide, *MCN* 14:89-92, 1989.

Jost KE, Haase JE: At the time of death: help for the child's parents, *Child Health Care* 18:146-152, 1989.

Krone C, Harris CC: The importance of infant gender and family resemblance with parents' perinatal bereavement process: establishing personhood, *J Perinat Neonat Nurs* 2(2):1-11, 1988.

Leon IG: Perinatal loss: a critique of current hospital practices, *Clin Pediatr* 31(6):366-374, 1992.

Maguire DP, Skoolicas SJ: Developing a bereavement follow-up program, *J Perinat Neonat Nurs* 2(2):67-77, 1988.

Malcolm N, Wooten B: It's hard to say goodbye, *Can Nurse* 83(4):26-28, 1987.

Novak S: In moments of crisis, *MNC* 13:349-351, 1988.

Swanson-Kauffman K: There should have been two: nursing care of parents experiencing the perinatal death of a twin, *J Perinat Neonat Nurs* 2(2):78-86, 1988.

Szgalsky JB: Perinatal death, the family, and the role of the health professional, *Neonatal Network* 8(2):15-19, 1989.

Trouy MB, Ward-Larson C: Sibling grief, *Neonatal Network* 5(4):35-40, 1987.

VanPutte AW: Perinatal bereavement crisis: coping with negative outcomes from prenatal diagnosis, *J Perinat Neonat Nurs* 2(2):12-22, 1988.

Wilson AL and others: Parental responses to perinatal death: mother-father differences, *Am J Dis Child* 139:1235-1241, 1985.

Windau V, Dewitt PJ: Emergency baptism by nurses in an NICU: answering a spiritual need, *Neonatal Network* 7(1):57-62, 1988.

Respiratory Distress Syndrome

Boeckling AC: Exogenous surfactant therapy for premature infants, *J Perinat Neonat Nurs* 6(2):59-66, 1992.

Carroll P: Clinical application of pulse oximetry, *Pediatr Nurs* 19(2):150-151, 1993.

Carter JM and others: High-frequency oscillatory ventilation and extracorporeal membrane oxygenation for the treatment of acute neonatal respiratory failure, *Pediatrics* 85:159-164, 1989.

Cheng M, Williams PD: Oxygenation during

chest physiotherapy of very-low-birth-weight infants: relations among fraction of inspired oxygen levels, number of hand ventilations, and transcutaneous oxygen pressure, *J Pediatr Nurs* 4(6):411-418, 1989.

Clancy GT: Blood gas monitoring and management of neonates with respiratory distress, *J Perinat Neonat Nurs* 1(1):72-83, 1987.

Comer DM: Pulse oximetry: implications for practice, *JOGNN* 21(1):35-41, 1992.

Gunderson LP, Kenner C: Transcutaneous oxygen monitoring: description and clinical application, *Neonatal Network* 6(6):7-14, 1988.

Haney C, Allingham TM: Nursing care of the neonate receiving high-frequency jet ventilation, *JOGNN* 21(3):187-195, 1992.

Harbold LA: A protocol for neonatal use of pulse oximetry, *Neonatal Network* 8(1):41-58, 1989.

Hay WW, Brockway JM, Eyzaguirre M: Neonatal pulse oximetry: accuracy and reliability, *Pediatrics* 83:717-722, 1989.

Hay WW, Thilo E, Curlander JB: Pulse oximetry in neonatal medicine, *Clin Perinatol* 18(3):441-472, 1991.

Horbar JD and others: A multicenter randomized trial comparing two surfactants for the treatment of neonatal respiratory distress syndrome, *J Pediatr* 123(3):757-766, 1993.

Inwood S, Finley GA, Fitzhardinge PM: High-frequency oscillation: a new mode of ventilation for the neonate, *Neonatal Network* 4(5):53-58, 1986.

Karp TB and others: High frequency jet ventilation: a neonatal nursing perspective, *Neonatal Network* 4(5):42-50, 1986.

Klein MD, Whittlesey GC: Extracorporeal membrane oxygenation, *Pediatr Clin North Am* 41(2):365-384, 1994.

Miller EP, Armstrong CL: Surfactant replacement therapy: innovative care for the premature infant, *JOGNN* 19(1):14-17, 1990.

Neumann M: Surfactant administration: an ethical dilemma, *JOGNN* 17(2):80-82, 1988.

Polak MJ, Donnelly WH, Bucciarelli RL: Comparison of airway pathologic lesions after high-frequency jet or conventional ventilation, *Am J Dis Child* 143:228-232, 1989.

Schumacher RE: Extracorporeal membrane oxygenation: will this therapy continue to be as efficacious in the future? *Pediatr Clin North Am* 40(5):1005-1022, 1993.

Respiratory Conditions

American Academy of Pediatrics, Committee on Fetus and Newborn: Recommendations on extracorporeal membrane oxygenation, *Pediatrics* 85:618-619, 1990.

Cunningham AS and others: Tracheal suction and meconium: a proposed standard of care, *J Pediatr* 115:153-154, 1990.

Gregory SEB: Air leak syndromes, *Neonatal Network* 5(4):40-46, 1987.

Kleiber C, Hummel PA: Factors related to spontaneous endotracheal extubation in the neonate, *Pediatr Nurs* 15:347-351, 1989.

Marecki MA: *Chlamydia trachomatis:* a developing perinatal problem, *J Perinat Neonat Nurs* 1(4):1-11, 1988.

Martin RJ, Miller MJ, Carlo WA: Pathogenesis of apnea in preterm infants, *J Pediatr* 109:733-741, 1986.

Murphy JD, Vawter GF, Reid LM: Pulmonary vascular disease in fetal meconium aspiration, *J Pediatr* 104:785-789, 1984.

Russell JC and others: Multicenter evaluation of TDx test for assessing fetal lung maturity, *Clin Chem* 35(6):1005-1010, 1989.

Swaminathan S and others: Long-term pulmonary sequelae of meconium aspiration syndrome, *J Pediatr* 114:356-361, 1989.

Turnage CS: Meconium aspiration syndrome, *J Perinat Neonat Nurs* 3(2):69-80, 1989.

Van Meurs KP and others: Congenital diaphragmatic hernia: long-term outcome in neonates treated with extracorporeal membrane oxygenation, *J Pediatr* 122(6):893-899, 1993.

Weinstein S, Stolar CJH: Newborn surgical emergencies: congenital diaphragmatic hernia and extracorporeal membrane oxygenation, *Pediatr Clin North Am* 40(6):1315, 1993.

Bronchopulmonary Dysplasia

Adams D: Kasey's story, *Neonatal Network* 7(3):19-23, 1988.

Boyzynski MEA: Comprehensive management of the infant with bronchopulmonary dysplasia: a growing challenge, *Infants Young Child* 2(1):14-24, 1989.

Conte VH: Bronchopulmonary dysplasia. In Jackson PL, Vessey JA: *Primary care of the child with a chronic condition,* St Louis, 1992, Mosby.

Frank M: Theophylline: a closer look, *Neonatal Network* 6(2):7-13, 1987.

Hagedorn MI, Gardner SL: Physiologic sequelae of prematurity: the nurse practitioner's role. I. Respiratory issues, *J Pediatr Health Care* 3:288-297, 1989.

Howard-Glenn L: Transition to home: discharge planning for the oxygen-dependent infant with bronchopulmonary dysplasia, *J Perinat Neonat Nurs* 6(2):85-94, 1992.

Lund CH, editor: *Bronchopulmonary dysplasia: strategies for total patient care,* Petaluma, CA, 1990, Neonatal Network.

Martin RJ, Pridham KF: Early experiences of parents feeding their infants with bronchopulmonary dysplasia, *Neonatal Network* 11(3):23-29, 1992.

McElheny JE: Parental adaptation to a child with bronchopulmonary dysplasia, *J Pediatr Nurs* 4:346-352, 1989.

Paulson PR: Nursing considerations for discharging children home on low-flow oxygen, *Issues Compr Pediatr Nurs* 10:109-214, 1987.

Perry MA, Hayes NM: Bronchopulmonary dysplasia: discharge planning and complex home care, *Neonatal Network* 7(3):13-17, 1988.

Pridham KF and others: Parental issues in feeding young children with bronchopulmonary dysplasia, *J Pediatr Nurs* 4:177-185, 1989.

Pridham KF and others: Nipple feeding for preterm infants with bronchopulmonary dysplasia, *JOGNN* 22(2):147-155, 1993.

Sepsis

Amspacher KA: Necrotizing enterocolitis: the never-ending challenge, *J Perinat Neonat Nurs* 3(2):58-68, 1989.

Becker L, Lagomarsino W: Isolation guidelines for perinatal patients: creating a new protocol, *MCN* 12:400-404, 1987.

Cerase PA: Neonatal sepsis, *J Perinat Neonat Nurs* 3(2):48-57, 1989.

Clapp DW and others: Use of intravenously administered immune globulin to prevent nosocomial sepsis in low birth weight infants: report of a pilot study, *J Pediatr* 115:973-978, 1989.

Cohen SP: Bacterial sepsis in the very low birth weight infant, *J Perinat Neonat Nurs* 1(4):66-77, 1988.

Cushing AH: Omphalitis: still potential for disaster, *Contemp Pediatr* 4(5):61-73, 1987.

Gaffney SE, Salinger L: Group B streptococcus: the pregnant woman and her neonate, *JOGNN* 16(2):91-96, 1987.

Gordin PC: Candida infection in the very low birth weight infant, *J Perinat Neonat Nurs* 1(4):47-55, 1988.

Henneberry C: Candida sepsis in the very low birthweight infant, *Neonatal Network* 5(6):39-45, 1987.

Hufnal-Miller CA and others: Enteral theophylline and necrotizing enterocolitis in the low-birthweight infant, *Clin Pediatr* 33(11): 647-653, 1993.

Ittmann PI, Bozynskin ME: Toxic epidermal necrolysis in a newborn infant after exposure to adhesive remover, *J Perinatol* 13(6):476-477, 1993.

Poulsen N: Candidiasis in the premature infant, *Neonatal Network* 8(4):9-14, 1990.

Cardiovascular Conditions

Angeles DM: Pathophysiology and nursing management of persistent pulmonary hypertension of the newborn, *MCN* 17(6):314-321, 1992.

Annibale DJ: Evaluating the strength of medical literature: indomethacin in the neonatal intensive care unit, *Neonatal Intensive Care* 7(3):22-28, 1994.

Fuller R: Cardiac function and the neonatal EKG. I. Introduction to neonatal EKGs, *Neonatal Network* 7(4):47-51, 1989.

Fuller R: Cardiac function and the neonatal EKG. II. Bradycardia, *Neonatal Network* 7(6):61-63, 1989.

Fuller R: Cardiac function and the neonatal EKG. III. Tachycardia, *Neonatal Network* 7(6):65-67, 1989.

Fuller R: Cardiac function and the neonatal EKG. IV. Chamber enlargement and axis determination, *Neonatal Network* 8(1):77-81, 1989.

Goble MM, Rocchini AP: Neonatal hypertension: why it happens, what to do about it, *Contemp Pediatr* 7(2):89-100, 104-108, 113-118, 1990.

Kempley ST and others: Randomized trial of umbilical arterial catheter position: clinical outcome, *Acta Paediatr* 82:173-176, 1993.

Krueger E and others: Prevention of symptomatic patent ductus arteriosus with a single dose of indomethacin, *J Pediatr* 111:749-754, 1987.

Lawson M: Persistent pulmonary hypertension of the newborn: current trends in classification and diagnosis, *Neonatal Network* 6(1):27-35, 1987.

Ment LR and others: Risk factors for early intraventricular hemorrhage in low birth weight infants, *J Pediatr* 121(5):776-783, 1992.

Prullage S, Melichar C: Stabilization and transportation of the infant with PPHN, *Neonatal Network* 12(7):45-51, 1993.

Werner NP: Congestive heart failure: pathophysiology and management throughout infancy, *J Perinat Neonat Nurs* 7(3):59, 1993.

Retinopathy of Prematurity

Bancalari E and others: Influence of transcutaneous oxygen monitoring on the incidence of retinopathy of prematurity, *Pediatrics* 79:663-669, 1987.

Brown DR and others: Retinopathy of prematurity, *Am J Dis Child* 141:154-160, 1987.

Few BJ: Pharmacologic use of vitamin E, *MCN* 13:283, 1988.

Gardner SL, Hagedorn MI: Physiologic sequelae of prematurity: the nurse practitioner's role. II. Retinopathy of prematurity, *J Pediatr Health Care* 4:72-76, 1990.

George DS and others: The latest on retinopathy of prematurity, *MCN* 13:254-258, 1988.

Gracey KM, McLaughlin KL, Smiley MJ: Caring for the infant with retinopathy of prematurity undergoing cryotherapy, *Neonatal Network* 9(7):7-11, 1991.

An international classification of retinopathy of prematurity. II. The classification of retinal detachment, *Pediatrics* 82:37-43, 1988.

Long CA: Cryotherapy: a new treatment for retinopathy of prematurity, *Pediatr Nurs* 15:269-272, 1989.

Multicenter trial of cryotherapy for retinopathy of prematurity: preliminary results, *Pediatrics* 81:697-706, 1988.

Noerr B: Vitamin E (alpha-tocopherol), *Neonatal Network* 9(2):85-87, 1990.

Neurologic Disturbances

Allan WC, Volpe JJ: Periventricular-intraventricular hemorrhage, *Pediatr Clin North Am* 33:47-63, 1986.

Brann AW: Hypoxic ischemic encephalopathy (asphyxia), *Pediatr Clin North Am* 33:451-464, 1986.

Calciolari G, Perlman JM, Volpe JJ: Seizures in the neonatal intensive care unit of the 1980s, *Clin Pediatr* 27:119-123, 1988.

Cunningham M: Intraventricular hemorrhage in the premature, *Dimens Crit Care Nurs* 6:20-27, 1987.

Gilman JT and others: Rapid sequential phenobarbital treatment of neonatal seizures, *Pediatrics* 83:674-678, 1989.

Guzzetta F and others: Periventricular intraparenchymal echodensities in the premature newborn: critical determinant of neurologic outcome, *Pediatrics* 78:995-1006, 1986.

Kuban K, Teele RL: Rationale for grading intracranial hemorrhage in premature infants, *Pediatrics* 74:358-363, 1984.

MacDonald NP: Motor development in premature infants with intracranial hemorrhage, *Pediatr Nurs* 12:263-267, 1986.

Painter MJ, Bergman I, Crumrine P: Neonatal seizures, *Pediatr Clin North Am* 33:91-109, 1986.

Scher MS, Painter MJ: Controversies concerning neonatal seizures, *Pediatr Clin North Am* 36:281-310, 1989.

Torrence C: Neonatal seizures. I. A developmental and clinical understanding, *Neonatal Network* 4(8):9-15, 1985.

Conditions Related to Maternal Conditions

Alexander LL: The pregnant smoker: nursing implications, *JOGNN* 16(3):167-173, 1987.

Barabach LM, Glzaer G, Norris SC: Maternal perception and parent-infant interaction of vulnerable cocaine-exposed couplets, *J Perinat Neonat Nurs* 6(3):76-84, 1992.

Benson MS: Management of infants born to women infected with the human immunodeficiency virus, *J Perinat Neonat Nurs* 7(4):79-89, 1994.

Berk MA and others: Macrosomia in infants of insulin-dependent diabetic mothers, *Pediatrics* 83:1029-1034, 1989.

Brooks-Gunn J, McCarton C, Hawley T: Effects of in utero drug exposure on children's development, *Arch Pediatr Adolesc Med* 148:33-39, 1994.

Dreher M, Nugent K, Hudgins R: Prenatal marijuana exposure and neonatal outcomes in Jamaica: an ethnographic study, *Pediatrics* 93(2):254-260, 1994.

Dusick AM and others: Risk of intracranial hemorrhage and other adverse outcomes after cocaine exposure in a cohort of 323 very low birth weight infants, *J Pediatr* 122(3):438-445, 1993.

Flandermeyer AA: A comparison of the effects of heroin and cocaine abuse upon the neonate, *Neonatal Network* 6(3):42-47, 1987.

Forrest DC: The cocaine-exposed infant. I. Identification and assessment, *J Pediatr Health Care* 6(1):3-7, 1994.

Forrest DC: The cocaine-exposed infant. II. Intervention and teaching, *J Pediatr Health Care* 6(1):7-11, 1994.

Fulroth R, Phillips B, Durand DJ: Perinatal outcome of infants exposed to cocaine and/or heroin in utero, *Am J Dis Child* 143:905-910, 1989.

Griffith DR, Azuma SD, Chasnoff IJ: Three year outcomes of infants exposed prenatally to drugs, *J Am Acad Child Adolesc Psychiatry* (special ed), 1994.

Hayes JS, Dreher MC, Nugent JK: Newborn outcomes with maternal marihuana use in Jamaican women, *Pediatr Nurs* 14:107-110, 1988.

Jorgensen KM: The drug-exposed infant, *Crit Care Nurs Clin North Am* 4(3):481-485, 1992.

Kennard MJ: Cocaine use during pregnancy: fetal and neonatal effects, *J Perinat Neonat Nurs* 3(4):53-63, 1990.

Kuehne EA, Warguska M: Prenatal cocaine exposure. In Jackson PL, Vessey JA: *Primary care of the child with a chronic condition,* St Louis, 1992, Mosby.

Mayes LC and others: Neurobehavioral profiles of neonates exposed to cocaine prenatally, *Pediatrics* 91(4):778-783, 1993.

Rhodes AM: Maternal liability for fetal injury? *MCN* 15:41, 1990.

Samson LF: Infants of diabetic mothers: current perspectives, *J Perinat Neonat Nurs* 6(1):61-70, 1992.

Smith JE, Deitch KV: Cocaine: a maternal, fetal, and neonatal risk, *J Pediatr Health Care* 1:120-124, 1987.

Torrance CR, Horns KM: Appraisal and caregiving for the drug-addicted infant, *Neonatal Network* 8(3):49-59, 1989.

Verklan MT: Safe in the womb? Drug and chemical effects on the fetus and neonate, *Neonatal Network* 8(10):59-65, 1989.

White EE: Developmental abnormalities in the chemically dependent newborn, *Home Healthc Nurs* 5(4):26-31, 1987.

Zaichkin J, Houston RF: The drug-exposed mother and infant: a regional center experience, *Neonatal Network* 12(3):41-49, 1993.

CHAPTER 11

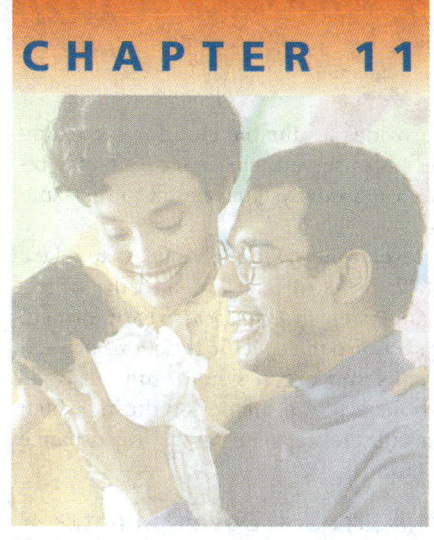

Conditions Caused by Defects in Physical Development

CHAPTER OUTLINE

RELATED TOPICS

Anaphylaxis, Ch. 29
Autosomal inheritance patterns, Ch. 5
Assessment (newborn), Ch. 8
Birth injuries, Ch. 9
"Birthmarks," Ch. 9
Cerebral palsy, Ch. 40
Gastric feeding techniques, Ch. 27
Health promotion of the newborn and family, Ch. 8
The high-risk newborn and family, Ch. 10
Hypertrophic pyloric stenosis, Ch. 33
Multifactorial disorders, Ch. 5
Osteogenesis imperfecta, Ch. 39
Pain assessment; pain management, Ch. 26
Preparation for procedures: surgical procedures, Ch. 27
Promotion of parent-infant bonding (attachment), Ch. 8

DEFECTS IN PHYSICAL DEVELOPMENT

Congenital malformations, also called ***congenital anomalies*** or ***birth defects,*** may be caused by genetic or environmental factors, and not all congenital defects are malformations (e.g., inborn errors of metabolism and mental retardation). However, this chapter is primarily concerned with structural abnormalities and with the impact on the family of the birth of a child with a physical defect. The genetic basis of physical defects is discussed in Chapter 5, and specific disorders are presented as appropriate throughout the book.

PRENATAL DEVELOPMENT

Fetal Growth and Differentiation

Development consists of two distinct but interrelated processes: growth and differentiation. ***Growth*** results when cells divide and synthesize new proteins and is reflected in increased size and weight. It is accomplished by two mechanisms: (1) ***hyperplasia*** (increase in cell number) and (2) ***hypertrophy*** (increase in cell size). Hyperplasia is the predominant form of growth during the embryonic period; although the rate decreases during later stages of gestation, cell division continues in variable degrees throughout childhood. Hypertrophy is more prominent during later periods of growth.

Each organ and tissue has a typical growth pattern, and all organs progress from a stage characterized by increase in cell number to one of growth by increase in cell size. Any interference with this pattern of growth results in a reduction in the size and weight of that organ. However, the consequences of the inhibiting factor depend on whether the insult is inflicted during a period of hyperplasia or during a period of hypertrophy. Interruption of growth during cell enlargement is usually only temporary and can be overcome with proper intervention. Interference with growth during a period of cell proliferation is likely to cause irreversible growth retardation of that organ with permanent deficit in overall cell numbers.

Differentiation is the process by which early cells are systematically modified and specialized to form all the tissues that are necessary to ensure an organized, coordinated individual. Each step in this process depends on successful completion of a previous step. Anything that interferes with one of these steps, such as a mutant gene or environmental agent, will cause an arrest in the development of that particular tissue or organ. Divergence from the normal course of development will result in maldevelopment of a part or, if it occurs at an early age, a sequence of distortions causing more severe or multiple malformations.

There appears to be a relationship between the incidence of one congenital anomaly and the presence of additional anomalies in an affected child. For example, there is an association between malformed ears and kidney abnormalities that reflects a common developmental stage. The knowledge of the stage of development for a variety of organs and systems provides a valuable clue for the examiner. When one defect is observed, closer scrutiny may reveal defects in another organ or system related to the same stage of development.

Extremely rapid development and change take place during the first 8 to 12 weeks of fetal life, and the beginnings of all major organ systems ***(organogenesis)*** are formed. The embryo begins to acquire the specific functions needed to integrate these organs and organ systems into an organized, coordinated whole. It is also the period during which the organism is most vulnerable to structural disturbance from environmental hazards.

Sensitive Periods in Prenatal Development

Every organ, system, and body part goes through a period during which it experiences the most rapid cell division and differentiation. During this time the organism displays a marked susceptibility to injurious influences. These specific stages of crucial developmental advancement are termed ***sensitive,*** or ***critical periods,*** and the major impact of environmental factors on development always coincides with these periods. The origin or method by which prenatal growth processes are disturbed to produce a structural or functional defect is termed ***teratogenesis*** (from the Greek ***teratos,*** monster, and ***genesis,*** production). An agent capable of producing such an effect is a ***teratogen.*** (See Congenital Defects Caused by Prenatal Factors, p. 503.)

The sensitive periods for all organs or parts do not occur simultaneously. A part that is susceptible to adverse influences at one particular time may be resistant to the same influences at other periods of development. At the same time, another part may be highly sensitive at that moment. Susceptibility to environmental influences decreases as organ formation advances—the younger the organism and the fewer the number of cells, the greater the extent of involvement when an adverse influence is applied.

During the period of intensive differentiation most teratogenic agents are highly effective and may produce a variety of deformities. The type of defect that is produced depends on which organ is most susceptible at the time of application. The susceptibility of most tissues to teratogenic influences decreases rapidly in the later periods of development, which are characterized by growth and elaboration of established organs. However, some tissues, particularly the central nervous system, are sensitive to varying degrees throughout fetal life and even beyond. Fig. 11-1 illustrates the approximate times of critical differentiation for some of the major organs and systems.

BIRTH OF A CHILD WITH A PHYSICAL DEFECT

Parental Responses

Part of the preparation for childbirth involves fantasies and images of the expected infant. Normally parents hope for a perfect child, but at the same time they fear that the infant will be abnormal. This fear is often expressed by the expectant parents when they state that their concern is not whether the child is a girl or a boy, just that the infant is

■ David Wilson, RN,C, MS, edited and revised sections of this chapter.

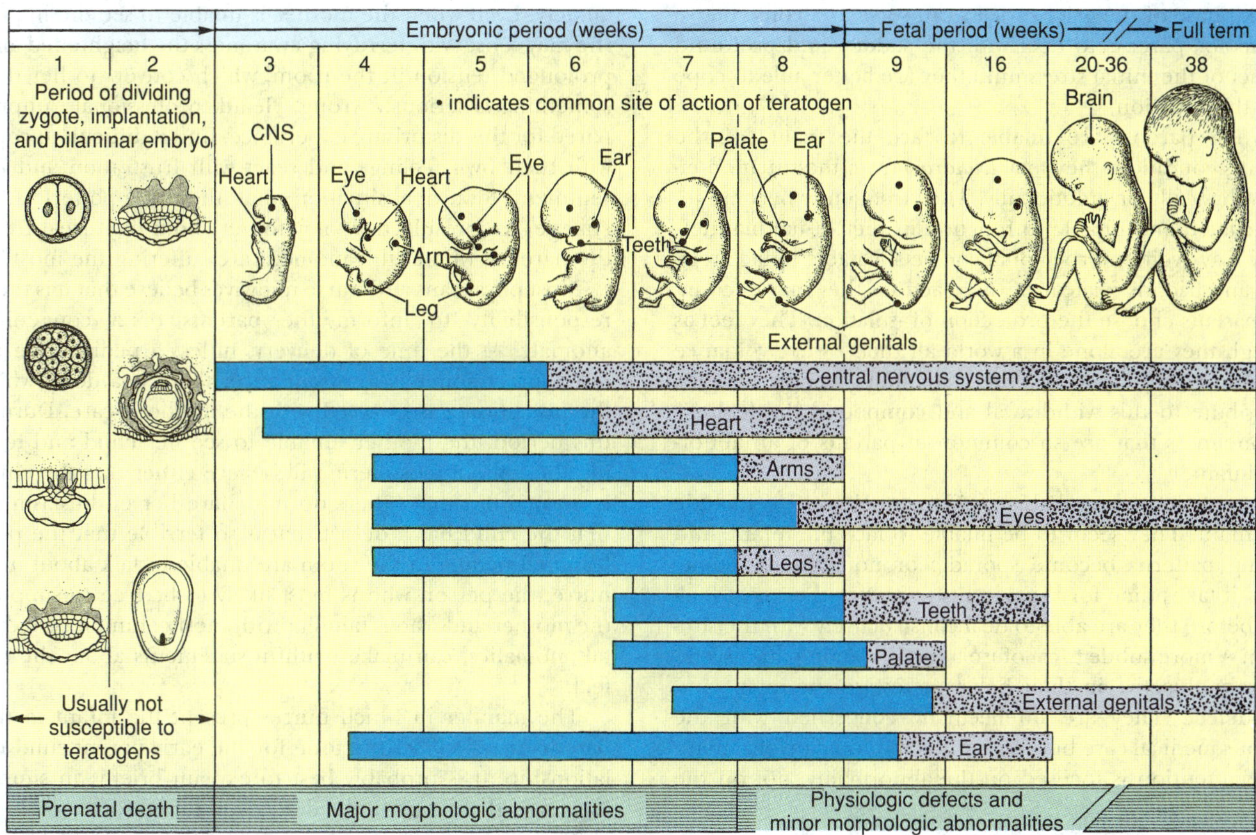

FIG. 11-1 Sensitive, or critical, periods in human development. Solid color denotes highly sensitive periods; stippled color indicates stages when embryo is less sensitive to teratogens. (From Moore KL: *The developing human: clinically oriented embryology,* ed 4, Philadelphia, 1988, WB Saunders.)

healthy. One of the first things the mother wants confirmed at the time of birth is: "Is my baby all right?" In many instances there is some discrepancy between the parents' idealized child and the infant the mother delivers, as, for example, the birth of a boy when they had hoped for a girl. Resolution of this discrepancy is a developmental task of parenthood and is essential to the establishment of a healthy parent-child relationship. If this discrepancy is too great, as with the birth of an infant with a severe defect, or when the wishes of the parents are unrealistic, the resulting emotional stress may be overwhelming.

The more severe the defect, the greater the impact of the experience, especially for the mother. The birth of a child with a physical imperfection abruptly ends the psychologic attachment the mother has formed during pregnancy with the idealized child. She and the father must now deal with loss of the anticipated healthy child while they face meeting the demands of the affected child for care and affection. The birth of an infant with a defect evokes the same psychologic reaction as the death of a child. The need for the parents to grieve for the loss of the expected child while adapting to the care of the child with a disability places overwhelming demands on them at a time when their own psychologic and physiologic resources have been depleted by the birth experience. The impact of this new and unexpected burden inhibits the accomplishment of the grief work that normally follows a loss.

The grief reaction experienced by parents at the birth of a child with a physical disability is the same as the response that follows the loss of any valued or significant object. The parents experience shock, frustration, and anger at what has happened to them, and they ask themselves, "Why? Why me?" Parents may feel shame and embarrassment, often with feelings of personal failure and guilt. Frequently the mother believes that she might have caused harm to the unborn child, and she may associate the condition with wrongdoing or evil thoughts, especially if the pregnancy was unwanted initially. She may believe the defect to be the result of passive or active attempts to terminate the pregnancy, such as deliberate attempts to induce abortion or failure to obtain prenatal care or comply with the practitioner's instructions.

There is a phase of overwhelming ***shock,*** accompanied by weeping and feelings of helplessness. To deal with stress and anxiety, parents use defense mechanisms that have provided protection in the past. A very common response is ***disbelief*** and ***denial,*** which may be short-lived or may last for many months. They do not appear to "hear" what is told to them about their child, and they behave as though nothing is wrong with the child. However, denial during the shock phase of the grief process can serve as a constructive means for parents to deal with the sudden and profound impact of the initial stress until they are better able to cope with the situation.

When parents are unable to face the reality of the infant's condition, they may ***withdraw*** from the situation either physically or emotionally. They frequently become incapacitated and unable to function in their usual manner. They may avoid interpersonal contacts. Unable to face relatives and friends for fear of the reactions they may encounter, parents choose the protection of isolation. They feel as though they are alone in a world all their own. Avoidance behaviors on the part of others, including health workers, contribute to this withdrawal and compound the feelings of loneliness that are so common in parents of an abnormal infant.

Parents may extend this avoidance behavior to include the infant. They seem to be unable to face the infant, and visiting patterns become sporadic or nonexistent. Sometimes it takes time for the parents to master their own feelings before they are able to deal constructively with the situation. A more subtle form of isolation is seen in parents who are very objective in their behavior toward the infant and the defect. They are intellectually concerned with the infant's medical care but display no emotional involvement. Their attention is focused on the abnormality, not on the infant.

Parental reactions may be quite varied, including guilt, anger, anxiety, and sadness, which often extend for years and which depend to a large extent on the type and severity of the defect. A visible anomaly, especially one involving the face, usually elicits a more intense emotional response than one that is less apparent, such as a heart defect. The extent of the impairment cannot be used as a criterion to determine the degree of parental depressive reactions. Because of their limited contact with congenital defects, parents' perception of the abnormality and its implications may be distorted, and much depends on previous feelings they may have experienced with a similar abnormality. Therefore their reactions may seem out of proportion to the actual extent and severity of the impairment as viewed by health professionals.

Nursing Considerations

The attitudes and behaviors of nurses and other health care providers at the birth of a child with a defect significantly influence the effect that the situation has on the parents. During this time parents are particularly sensitive and responsive to the behaviors of those with whom they are in contact. Therefore the reactions of health professionals toward the infant and the parents provide cues to the parents that can affect their feelings toward the infant and themselves. Parents are the persons who exert the greatest influence on the growth and development of the child, and the initial relationship with the child significantly affects the subsequent course of interaction.

Initial Contact. The first indication that all is not well often occurs at the time of delivery. The atmosphere of happy anticipation suddenly changes to one laden with anxiety. Even when the mother is unable to see the infant, she may sense with terrifying awareness the heightened and prolonged tension in the room, which conveys to her that something is seriously wrong. Health professionals, unprepared for this disturbing experience, find it difficult to cope with their own feelings and react with frustration and resentment toward a situation that they are powerless to change. As a result, they may forget about or retreat from the parents, who at this moment are suffering the most.

Most physicians and nurse midwives believe that it is their responsibility to inform the parents of a congenital anomaly. At the time of delivery, unless a pediatrician or nurse practitioner is in attendance, there is a delay while the practitioner is involved with the mother's care. During this period, the mother, unable to see her child and feeling the tense atmosphere, will believe either that the child is normal but that others do not share her enthusiasm or that the child has a defect that is so terrible that the professional people in the room are unable to talk about it. A nurse, the person who is most likely to be free to support the mother and who is familiar with most common congenital anomalies, can make truthful statements about the defect.

The manner in which nurses present the infant to the parents may well set the tone for the early parent-child relationship. It is probably best to explain briefly, in simple language, the nature of the defect and to reinforce and help clarify information given by the practitioner before the infant is shown to them. At this time they are more apt to "hear" what is said. Parents attach a great deal of meaning to the behavior of others during this critical period and will watch the facial expressions of others closely for signs of revulsion or rejection. Presenting the infant as something precious, although incomplete, and emphasizing the well-formed aspects of the infant's body provide some reassurance to parents in this crisis period.

It is important to allow time and opportunity for the parents to express their initial response to the situation. Many issues may surface, such as the importance placed on this particular infant or the cultural significance of one sex over the other. They need to be encouraged to ask questions and to receive honest, straightforward answers without undue optimism or pessimism.

Family Support. Parents must be allowed ample time to grieve for the loss of the expected child before they are able to form an emotional attachment to the child they have. It is a nursing responsibility to help parents with their grief work and to facilitate the formation of a satisfactory adjustment to the child with a defect. They need help to see their infant as a *person,* support in coping with their situation, and guidance in physical care of the child.

Nurses who understand the grief response will be prepared to support the parents through this necessary process. This is particularly important with the birth of a child with a defect, because the parents may not begin to invest any feeling for the child until they are able to talk about and work through their feelings of disappointment, resentment, guilt, and helplessness. Parents need to talk, and the supportive nurse is one who creates and maintains an atmosphere that encourages expression of feelings. Open expression is difficult for many people, and the parent(s) may hesitate to display intense feelings. Containing those feelings expends considerable energy that would be better used later on to develop a relationship with the infant. Nurses, therefore, need to listen closely for cues that indicate areas of discomfort or readiness to talk.

Parents may not be ready to talk about their feelings during the first few days following the birth. Their dream has vanished, and when others avoid them, it is often interpreted as another abandonment. Staying near and available tells them that they are not alone and that someone cares about them and their feelings. What is said to them is also important. Cliches such as "You will be able to have more children" or "It could be a lot worse" are not a comfort to the parents. Such behavior implies that this infant is not important, and this behavior may lose the parents' trust.

Initiating a discussion about matters that were of concern to others in a similar situation may help the parents to know that their feelings are natural. Parents need to be allowed silence and solitude if this is their wish. The parents are likely to be angry and will often direct this anger at anyone at hand—physicians, nurses, friends, and families who have normal children. Serving as a nonjudgmental target for their frustrations helps parents to relieve some of their distress. Nurses must be prepared to accept any or all of the parental reactions and defenses—anger, hostility, rejection, dependency—without anger and without withdrawing from the situation. If nurses make themselves available to the parents for support, they can often find nonthreatening ways to help, comfort, and support. Most important, nurses need to promote communication and understanding within the family and help strengthen family interpersonal relationships.

Care of the Infant. Many parents are very uneasy about handling their infant and require support and encouragement in their caregiving tasks. A longer period of dependency is needed by these parents to regroup their resources for coping. Although they should not feel forced to care for the infant until they are ready for the responsibility, they can be given opportunities to assume care of the infant as soon as possible to help them deal with the reality of the infant's condition. Parents' responses are highly individual and must be evaluated on this premise. However, all parents need sympathetic, patient, and understanding help to gain feelings of adequacy in the care of their child and to facilitate development of a positive relationship with the infant later on. As anxiety and the intensity of emotional responses abate, parents begin to feel more comfortable with the infant and more confident in their ability to provide needed care.

Supplying Information. Parents need to have accurate, up-to-date information given to them early and in language they can understand. Since they do not hear all that is said the first time it is told to them, they want careful explanations about the child's defect, the treatments outlined, and what will be expected of them. Parents often misinterpret information and therefore require repeated explanations. Often the nurse's responsibility is to explain, interpret, and clarify information that has been given by the practitioner and to answer questions. Following basic concepts of interviewing, the nurse determines what the parents know and proceeds from that point. One cannot assume that the parents' failure to ask questions means they understand. Most parents have little or no knowledge of basic anatomy or physiology; therefore pictures and other visual aids can be used effectively to explain both normal and deviant structures.

Teaching the parents to provide the special care that is frequently required for an infant with a physical defect is an important nursing responsibility. Special feeding, holding, and positioning techniques need to be explained and demonstrated. Anticipatory guidance regarding problems that are peculiar to each abnormality reduces apprehension and stimulates the parents to institute preventive measures and to make alert observations.

Numerous agencies and organizations offer services to families of children with congenital defects. Some provide services for a variety of conditions; others are devoted to specific disorders. They help families with ongoing problems and with anticipating problems they will encounter in raising a child with a defect, including financial burdens. Many have local support groups. All have unique and specialized services designed to help support the family and aid parents in their problem solving. Among those that include most types of defects and diseases are the **National Easter Seal Society for Crippled Children and Adults,*** the **March of Dimes–Birth Defects Foundation,**† and the **Association of Birth Defect Children, Inc.,**‡ most of which have branches in all major cities and communities. The state **Program for Children with Special Health Needs** (formerly Crippled Children's Services) is also a prime source of assistance. (See Nursing Care Plan: The Child with Chronic Illness or Disability, Chapter 22).

NURSING CARE OF THE SURGICAL NEONATE

Advances in early detection of defects (including prenatal diagnosis), surgical techniques, and anesthesia have made it possible for correction or amelioration of many physical defects in the newborn period. Some newborns have anomalies that require surgery during the neonatal period, often as emergencies. Fortunately, most malformations are correctable with a high degree of success, even those that are dramatic in their presentation.

Preoperative Care

Most of the problems encountered with the infant undergoing surgery have been discussed in relation to the high-risk infant (e.g., airway maintenance, cardiovascular support, thermoregulation, fluid and electrolyte balance, and nutritional needs). Electronic monitoring of cardiovascular and respiratory status is implemented and maintained, as

*2023 West Ogden Ave., Chicago, IL 60612; (312) 243-8400.
†1275 Mamaroneck Ave., White Plains, NY 10605; (914) 428-7100.
‡827 Irma St., Orlando, FL 32803; (800) 313-ABDC or (407) 245-7035.

well as regular comprehensive assessments (see Systematic Assessment, Chapter 10). Monitoring and assessments are continued in the postoperative period. Some congenital defects are often associated with other anomalies; therefore assessment should include careful observation for evidence of complications related to these.

NURSING ALERT An assessment of the infant's behavior preoperatively is essential, since deviations postoperatively may be a manifestation of pain or unstable condition.

Before surgery the infant will usually require a peripheral intravenous line for fluids and glucose; any electrolyte problems, as well as anemia, are corrected. In some instances a blood product such as packed red blood cells or whole blood is placed on reserve in case blood loss is anticipated. Prophylactic antibiotic administration may begin before surgery, and the infant is observed for any evidence of infection. In addition to routine care, special attention is directed to specific defects, such as abdominal decompression, protection and management of open lesions, and specific measurements (e.g., abdominal girth, head dimensions). (See also discussion of specific defects.)

Compounding the initial shock of having an infant born with a physical defect, the parents are often further traumatized by the prospect of surgery, sometimes shortly after birth. The parents are provided with accurate information regarding the type of surgical procedure anticipated, method of anesthesia, and, most important, what to expect postoperatively. (Parents are sometimes mentally unprepared for the infant's appearance postoperatively; likewise, some may have false hopes or expectations that the infant will be perfect following surgery.) The parents are also assured that the infant's pain management needs will be evaluated and met postoperatively.

When an infant is transported to a tertiary center for surgery shortly after birth, it is helpful for the nurse to stay in contact with the parents, especially the mother, regarding the infant's condition. Snapshots and even videos, when possible, are helpful tools to allay the mother's anxiety; without seeing her infant and without adequate communication, the mother's anxiety and fears about her infant's condition may be far worse than the reality. During this time the father may serve as the vital link of information between the mother, siblings, and the tertiary center where the infant is undergoing surgery.

Postoperative Care

Surgery imposes significant stresses on the neonate, especially the preterm or ill infant. The assessment and observations remain much the same as for preoperative care, with the additional problems related to surgery, such as anesthesia and pain. It is essential to maintain physiologic stability to avoid undesirable consequences (Rushton, 1988). Because the neonate is subject to many adverse effects of stress in all physiologic parameters, continual vigilance is mandatory.

Many of the physiologic problems to which the neonate is vulnerable have been discussed in relation to assessment and nursing care of the normal newborn (Chapter 8) and the high-risk infant (Chapter 10). Optimum ventilation, cardiac function, thermoregulation, fluid regulation, care of the operative site, and control of pain are primary concerns (Table 11-1). Some of the possible reactions, their probable cause, and the nursing responsibilities are further outlined in Table 11-2.

Because of the respiratory characteristics of newborns some compromising responses may be anticipated. The newborn's poor chest wall stability, smaller and more reactive airways, fewer and smaller alveoli, and poorly developed accessory muscles contribute to respiratory dysfunction. Compression by intrapleural fluid, air, or blood or a distended abdomen can further compromise pulmonary efforts. Respiratory distress is a common problem in preterm infants. Most postoperative neonates require mechanical ventilation, which may be further influenced by the type, duration, and urgency of the surgery. Mechanical ventilation may be continued in extensive surgical cases to allow for pain management postoperatively. Neonates are highly subject to acidosis and hypoxia and require continuous monitoring of oxygen and acid-base status. Preterm infants will require close monitoring for respiratory complications from general anesthesia.

Cardiovascular support is of particular importance because the immature sympathetic innervation of the myocardium makes the neonate particularly sensitive to vagal stimulation induced by many postoperative procedures, such as nasogastric (NG) tubes, endotracheal (ET) tubes, and suctioning. Any evidence of early compensation for diminished cardiac output is noted, and interventions are implemented before decompensation occurs.

Careful management of fluid and electrolyte status is vital to neonatal surgical care. The natural tendency for rapid fluid shifts related to characteristics of the neonate (see Chapter 28) may be aggravated by stress and any abnormal losses associated with some surgical procedures. (See also Hydration, Chapter 10.)

NEONATAL PAIN

It has long been believed that the nerve pathways of newborn infants are not sufficiently myelinated to transmit painful stimuli, that the infant does not possess sufficiently integrated cortical function to interpret or recall pain experiences, and that the risk of anesthesia is too great to justify any possible benefit of pain relief (Anand and Hickey, 1987; McLaughlin and others, 1993; Shapiro, 1989). Nurses have been found to hold similar beliefs and to give significantly higher pain intensity ratings to full-term as opposed to preterm neonates (Franck, 1987; Shapiro, 1993). Consequently, invasive procedures (including some types of surgery) are performed on infants without anesthesia.

This traditional view has been refuted by a number of research studies, which indicate that infants, both preterm and full term, perceive and react to pain in much the same manner as children and adults. Evidence indicates that pain pathways, cortical and subcortical centers needed for pain perception, and neurochemical systems associated with

TABLE 11-1 Critical Guidelines for Neonatal Postoperative Care

NURSING RESPONSIBILITIES	RATIONALE
AIRWAY MAINTENANCE*	
Monitor respirations, especially if extubated Monitor oxygenation with pulse oximetry and arterial blood gases, as necessary Monitor and observe color	Effects of anesthetics, surgery, and pain may decrease respiratory effort; alteration in acid-base balance may reflect early respiratory or metabolic response to surgical interventions
CIRCULATION*	
Monitor heart rate Monitor peripheral perfusion—note color and temperature of extremities; capillary refill should be 2 to 3 seconds Monitor blood pressure	A decrease in cardiac output may be seen peripherally before a decrease in blood pressure because of compensatory mechanisms
FLUIDS, ELECTROLYTES, AND GLUCOSE	
Evaluate hydration status (overhydration vs dehydration) by weighing neonate postoperatively	An increase or decrease in fluids given intraoperatively is reflected in weight before external signs of hydration are evident
Monitor electrolytes	A change in electrolyte status often indicates hydration status
Perform bedside glucose monitoring using reagent strips	Stress response to surgery may be evidenced by elevated serum glucose; bedside monitoring is faster than laboratory analysis; physician's order may not be necessary
THERMOREGULATION*	
Maintain a neutral thermal environment Monitor axillary temperature	Effects of anesthesia, exposure to cold, and metabolic response to surgery may decrease body temperature
OPERATIVE SITE	
Observe surgical site/skin status Observe dressings for drainage, bleeding, and amount of output from tubes	Loss of blood may require transfusion; chest tubes, catheters, gastrostomies not draining properly may impair operative site and status
PAIN MANAGEMENT	
Assess need for analgesics (see Neonatal Pain, p. 438) Implement comfort measures	Neonate may not be capable of demonstrating pain response but is capable of perceiving pain
Administer analgesics as needed to prevent pain (see Pain Management, Chapter 26)	Major surgery without adequate anesthesia and analgesia can increase postoperative mortality and morbidity

*Suggested interval for monitoring vital signs postoperatively in neonate: every 15 minutes × 4, every 30 minutes × 2, every 1 hour × 6, then every 2 hours for 24 hours. More frequent monitoring may be needed based on nurse's judgment of infant's status.

pain transmission and modulation are intact and functional in the neonate. Slower conduction speed is offset by shorter interneuron distances traveled by the impulse (Anand and Hickey, 1987; Anand and McGrath, 1993).

Pain perception has both physiologic and psychologic components, and it is accepted that newborns recognize and respond to painful stimuli. However, because pain is a sensation with strong emotional associations, it is difficult to differentiate between pain perception and nociceptive activity in neonates. Consequently, the term ***nociception*** (the perception by nerves of injurious influences or painful stimuli) is frequently used to discuss pain in the neonate.

There is evidence that newborns remember repeated pain experiences by recognizing the activities of the forthcoming event (Barba and others, 1991). They may also develop defensive behaviors, such as pulling away from human touch that typically has caused pain (Penticuff, 1987).

Physiologic responses to painful stimuli have been well documented by numerous studies. The summary of these observations indicates that painful stimuli cause a global stress response in infants undergoing surgery with minimal or no analgesia. This response is evidenced by cardiorespiratory changes (marked increases in heart rate and blood pressure, and decreased $tcPo_2$ or oxygen saturation), palmar sweating, increased intracranial pressure, and hormonal and metabolic changes (release of catecholamines, growth hormone, glucagon, cortisol, other corticosteroids, and aldosterone). Breakdown of carbohydrate and fat stores leads to severe and prolonged hyperglycemia and increases in plasma lactate, pyruvate, ketone bodies, and some fatty acids. Increased protein breakdown has been measured by changes in plasma amino acids and elevated nitrogen excretion (Anand and Hickey, 1987; Anand and McGrath, 1993).

The stress response to surgery was found to be shorter in duration than that observed in adults but was three to five times greater, perhaps as a result of lack of deep anesthesia (Anand, 1986). It was also observed that the response was decreased by appropriate anesthesia, indicating that the nociceptive stimuli of surgery were responsible for the stress response (Anand and Aynsley-Green, 1988; Anand, Sippell, and Aynsley-Green, 1987). Surgical stress due to pain has

TABLE 11-2 Possible Effects of Surgery on Selected Systems

PHYSIOLOGIC RESPONSE	NURSING RESPONSIBILITIES
CARDIOVASCULAR SYSTEM	
Hypotension related to: Large doses of anesthesia Vasodilation (narcotics) Myocardial depression (anesthetic agents) Impaired venous return Hypertension related to: Hypervolemia, pain, hypercarbia Increased intracranial pressure (ICP), vasoconstrictor drugs Tachycardia related to: Compensation for hypovolemia Pain Certain drugs Bradycardia related to: Hypoxemia (most commonly) Vagal stimulation Increased ICP (certain drugs) Vasoconstriction related to: Hypothermia	Observe for signs of low cardiac output: tachycardia, poor perfusion (slow capillary filling; normal is 2-3 seconds in newborn), weak or absent peripheral pulse, decreased intensity of heart sounds, decreased urinary specific gravity Observe for signs of congestive heart failure: tachycardia, increased peripheral vasoconstriction (skin changes such as mottling), pulmonary venous engorgement (respiratory distress) Monitor laboratory data (glucose, electrolytes, hemoglobin, and hematocrit) Administer blood products, vasoactive drugs, cardiotonics as prescribed Monitor and maintain fluid balance, including blood loss Provide ventilatory support as needed
RESPIRATORY SYSTEM	
Increased respiratory rate related to physiologic characteristics Airway obstruction related to: Bronchospasm Laryngeal edema Mucous plugs Compressed lung tissue related to: Air, fluid, or blood in pleural cavities Anatomic defects of diaphragm Intrinsic pulmonary lesions Ventilation/perfusion imbalance related to: Atelectasis Inadequate respiratory effort Pulmonary edema Pneumothorax Hypoventilation related to: Termination of anesthesia Administration of narcotics, hypocarbia, cold stress, lack of surgical stimulus	Observe respiratory rate, symmetry; breath sounds (pitch, intensity, quality, duration, location), color, use of accessory muscles, signs of airway obstruction (decreased breath sounds, decreased Po_2, respiratory distress, improper head alignment), signs of respiratory distress (marked retractions, nasal flaring, grunting, tachypnea, cyanosis), signs of impaired diaphragmatic movement (distended abdomen, constrictive dressings) Monitor oxygenation/ventilation, laboratory data Administer oxygen in amount and manner prescribed Position for optimum ventilation Alleviate any impediment to diaphragmatic excursion
IMMUNE SYSTEM	
Subject to infection related to: Inability to generate rapid and effective immune defenses Effects of anesthesia and surgery may mask assessment data	Observe for evidence of sepsis (bradycardia, temperature instability, poor feeding, change in activity level, irregular respiration or apnea), GI disturbances, evidence of abnormal clotting (bleeding from punctures, surgical sites) Monitor for signs of pulmonary or cardiovascular compromise Monitor fluid administration to maintain vascular volume Administer antibiotics as ordered
ENDOCRINE SYSTEM	
Hypoglycemia related to: Surgical stress Rapid depletion of glycogen stores Decreased gluconeogenesis with stress Hyperglycemia related to: Surgical stress Decreased insulin activity Hypothermia Hypocalcemia related to: Immaturity Stress Decreased parathyroid hormone secretion Hypomagnesemia related to: Hypocalcemia	Observe for apnea, tachypnea, lethargy, pallor, tremors or seizures Monitor serum glucose levels (Dextrosticks/Chemstrips); verify abnormal values Administer supplemental glucose as described Monitor urinary output (1 to 2 ml/kg/hr) Maintain neutral thermal environment Monitor serum calcium levels Observe for lethargy, vital sign instability, apnea, irritability, jitteriness, seizures Administer supplemental calcium if prescribed Observe for neuromuscular excitability (tetany, seizures) Monitor serum magnesium levels in infants with above signs

Data from Rushton CH: The surgical neonate: principles of nursing management, *Pediatr Nurs* 14:141-151, 1988.

TABLE 11-2 Possible Effects of Surgery on Selected Systems—cont'd

PHYSIOLOGIC RESPONSE	NURSING RESPONSIBILITIES
RENAL SYSTEM	
Inability to concentrate urine and excrete waste related to: Immature renal function	Observe for amount and characteristics of urinary output Monitor renal function, drug levels, intravascular volume
GASTROINTESTINAL SYSTEM	
Abdominal distention related to: Hypoactive bowel Obstruction Hypoactivity related to: Bowel surgery Peritonitis Perforation Hyperactivity related to: Obstruction Feeding modification related to: GI surgery (see specific GI surgeries)	Monitor bowel sounds (hyperactivity or hypoactivity) Observe for skin color and integrity (erythema of abdominal wall, prominent veins), abdominal distention (e.g., serial abdominal girth measurements) Palpate abdomen for tenderness Percuss abdomen for organomegaly, evidence of masses Observe frequency, volume, and characteristics of vomiting and vomitus; frequency, volume, and characteristics of stools Delay enteral feedings if prescribed Monitor parenteral feedings and fluid therapy Provide alternative enteral feedings as prescribed (gavage, gastrostomy) Begin and monitor oral feedings as prescribed Provide ostomy care if indicated
NEUROLOGIC SYSTEM	
Hypothermia related to: Immaturity of thermoregulation Seizures related to: Hypoxemia Hypoglycemia Hypocalcemia Unresponsiveness Stress related to: Surgical procedure Pain (see discussion on p. 438)	See Thermoregulation, p. 442 Monitor blood calcium, glucose Observe for any seizure activity, unresponsiveness, evidence of pain (see box on p. 443), signs of hypoglycemia or hypocalcemia (see above) Administer sedatives, analgesics, antiepileptic drugs, glucose, calcium as prescribed
HEMOPOIETIC SYSTEM	
Anemia related to: Blood loss Hyperviscosity related to: Polycythemia Decreased RBC deformability Plasma protein abnormalities due to third-spacing Polycythemia related to: Chronic hypoxia Coagulation defects related to: Inherited coagulation defects Physiologic coagulation factor defects Transitory coagulation disturbances Platelet abnormalities	Monitor any blood loss Monitor laboratory data Administer blood and/or blood products as ordered Observe for complications related to hemopoietic dysfunction and blood administration
FLUID AND ELECTROLYTE DISTURBANCES	
Abnormal fluid losses related to: Blood loss Fluid shifts, e.g., losses to interstitial tissues (third space) Transudated fluid GI, renal, wounds, drains Membrane injury from sepsis or injury Insensible losses from open wounds, exposed viscera	Observe for evidence of dehydration or overhydration (see Chapter 28) Monitor laboratory data Monitor blood pressure, central venous pressure Weigh daily or as ordered Monitor vital signs Monitor fluid and electrolyte administration Administer albumin, electrolytes
ACID-BASE BALANCE	
Acid-base disturbance related to: Cold stress Respiratory embarrassment GI disturbances Infectious processes Surgery Immature buffering mechanisms	Monitor acid-base status Monitor respirations (see above) Administer bicarbonate or other buffer as prescribed Maintain neutral thermal environment (see Thermoregulation, p. 442)

Continued.

TABLE 11-2 Possible Effects of Surgery on Selected Systems—cont'd

PHYSIOLOGIC RESPONSE	NURSING RESPONSIBILITIES
ACID-BASE BALANCE—cont'd	
Acidosis related to:	
Ventilatory insufficiency (respiratory acidosis)	
Ischemic tissue damage	
Cold stress	
THERMOREGULATION	
Hypothermia related to:	Monitor environmental and infant's skin temperatures
Unstable regulatory mechanisms	Maintain optimum thermal environment
Heat loss from large surface area, open wounds, defects	Observe for evidence of hypothermia: peripheral vasoconstriction, apnea, cyanosis, decreased body temperature, respiratory distress, tachycardia
Depletion of glycogen stores and metabolism of brown fat	Minimize heat loss; conserve heat and provide external warmth as needed, including coverings for head and extremities
See Thermoregulation, Chapter 10	Warm any blood and irrigating solutions
	Observe for seizure activity

also been correlated to postoperative clinical outcome; there was an increase in mortality and complications such as hyperglycemia, metabolic acidosis, and sepsis in neonates undergoing cardiac surgery who received a lighter anesthesia and less postoperative analgesia (Anand and Hickey, 1992; Wessel, 1993). The use of opioids for procedure pain has been found to decrease the duration of hypoxemia in newborns with respiratory distress (Pokela, 1994).

It has also been found that neonates release endorphins in response to stress and that the supply may become depleted. It is now recommended that infants receive appropriate analgesia or anesthesia for potentially painful procedures. Relatively safe local or systemic pharmacologic agents are available to permit anesthesia or analgesia to neonates and are indicated for those undergoing surgical procedures (American Academy of Pediatrics, 1987a; Burrows and Berde, 1993; Spear, 1992).

Other effects of pain may include increased wakefulness and irritability, as well as alterations in feeding, vomiting, loss of appetite, and loss of interest in or energy for sucking. Interruptions in sleep-wake patterns, behavioral states, and parent-infant interactions also occur and may interfere with recovery from surgery (Shapiro, 1989).

Pain Assessment

Assessment of pain in the preverbal child is difficult, especially in the neonate, because most evaluative tools and verbal responses do not apply. Evaluation must be based on physiologic changes and behavioral observations. Several studies have been devoted to assessing infant's responses to nociception (Bozzette, 1993; Cote, Morse, and James, 1991; Franck, 1986; Johnston and Strada, 1986; Stevens, Johnston, and Horton, 1993). Although behaviors including vocalizations, facial expressions, body movements, and general state are common to all infants, they vary with different situations. Crying associated with pain is more intense and sustained. Facial expression is the most consistent and specific characteristic, and scales are available to systematically evaluate facial features, such as eye squeeze, brow bulge, and open mouth and taut tongue (Grunau and Craig, 1987; Grunau, Johnston, and Craig, 1990). Most infants respond with increased body movements; however, the infant may be experiencing pain even when lying quietly with eyes closed (Shapiro, 1989). The preterm infant's response to pain may be behaviorally blunted or absent. An infant who receives a muscle-paralyzing agent such as vecuronium during surgery will also be incapable of mounting a behavioral or visible pain response.

Nursing assessment for evidence of pain is indicated any time the infant suffers tissue damage. Observable manifestations identified as indicators of acute pain in neonates are listed in the box on p. 443. In addition, several pain measurement scales attempt to quantify pain by assigning numeric values to categories such as movement, facial expression, cry, vital signs, and state of arousal (Attia and others, 1987; Barrier and others, 1989; Lawrence and others, 1993; Stevens, 1994). Further research on the validity and reliability of such scales is needed to support their clinical use.

NURSING ALERT When in doubt about pain in infants, base your decision on the following rule: Whatever is painful to an adult or child is painful to an infant, unless proved otherwise.

Pain Management

Nonpharmacologic measures used to alleviate pain are discussed extensively in Chapter 26. Those employed to reduce discomfort in the neonatal intensive care unit (NICU) include repositioning, swaddling, containment, cuddling, rocking, music, reducing environmental stimulation, tactile comfort measures, and nonnutritive sucking (Campos, 1989; Franck, 1987; Shapiro, 1989). However, nonpharmacologic measures may not be sufficient to decrease physiologic distress, even if behavioral responses, such as crying, are lessened (Gunnar, Fisch, and Malone, 1984; Marchette and others, 1991). In premature infants, additional stimulation, such as stroking, may *increase* physiologic distress (Brown, 1987).

Morphine is the most widely used narcotic analgesic for

MANIFESTATIONS OF ACUTE PAIN IN THE NEONATE

PHYSIOLOGIC RESPONSES

Vital signs: observe for variations
- Increased heart rate
- Increased blood pressure
- Rapid, shallow respirations

Oxygenation
- Decreased transcutaneous O_2 saturation ($tcPo_2$)
- Decreased arterial O_2 saturation (Sao_2)

Skin: observe color and character
- Pallor or flushing
- Diaphoresis
- Palmar sweating

Other observations
- Increased muscle tone
- Dilated pupils
- Decreased vagal nerve tone
- Increased intracranial pressure
- Laboratory evidence of metabolic or endocrine changes
  - Hyperglycemia
  - Lowered pH
  - Elevated corticosteroids

BEHAVIORAL RESPONSES

Vocalizations: observe quality, timing, and duration
- Crying
- Whimpering
- Groaning

Facial expression: observe characteristics, timing, orientation of eyes and mouth (see Fig. 26-3)
- Grimaces
- Brow furrowed
- Chin quivering
- Eyes tightly closed
- Mouth open and squarish

Body movements and posture: observe type, quality, and amount of movement or lack of movement; relationship to other factors
- Limb withdrawal
- Thrashing
- Rigidity
- Flaccidity
- Fist clenching

Changes in state: observe sleep, appetite, activity level
- Changes in sleep/wake cycles
- Changes in feeding behavior
- Changes in activity level
- Fussiness, irritability
- Listlessness

pharmacologic management of neonatal pain, with fentanyl as an effective alternative (Maguire and Maloney, 1988). Continuous intravenous infusion of opioids provides effective and safe pain control (Farrington and others, 1993). Other methods of relieving pain are with epidural/intrathecal infusion, local and regional nerve blocks, and topical anesthetics (Choonara, 1992; Yaster and others, 1994). (See Pain Management, Chapter 26, for more information on pharmacologic management of pain in the infant.)

Family Support

Parents are universally concerned that their infants are suffering pain during procedures. Nurses need to address these concerns and encourage the parents to speak with the health care professionals involved. Parents have the right to withhold consent for invasive procedures and are entitled to honest answers from those responsible for the infant's care. When permissible, they can also help provide comfort measures for the infant. It is important that parents are aware that nurses are sensitive to the infant's pain and are reassured that the infant will not suffer unduly (Butler, 1988; Shapiro, 1989).

SIGNIFICANT NEURAL TUBE DEFECTS

Cranioschisis—A skull defect through which various tissues protrude

Exancephaly—Brain is totally exposed or extruded through an associated skull defect; fetus usually aborted

Anencephaly—If fetus with exancephaly survives, the brain degenerates to a spongioform mass with no bony covering; incompatible with life usually beyond a few days

Encephalocele—Herniation of brain and meninges through a defect in the skull producing a fluid-filled sac

Rachischisis or spina bifida—Fissure in the spinal column that leaves the meninges and spinal cord exposed

Meningocele—Hernial protrusion of a saclike cyst of meninges filled with spinal fluid (Fig. 11-2, *C*)

Myelomeningocele (meningomyelocele)—Hernial protrusion of a saclike cyst containing meninges, spinal fluid, and a portion of the spinal cord with its nerves (Fig. 11-2, *D*)

MALFORMATIONS OF THE CENTRAL NERVOUS SYSTEM (CNS)*

DEFECTS OF NEURAL TUBE CLOSURE

Abnormalities that are derived from the embryonic neural tube ***(neural tube defects [NTDs])*** constitute the largest group of congenital anomalies that is consistent with multifactorial inheritance. Normally the spinal cord and cauda equina are encased in a protective sheath of bone and meninges (Fig. 11-2, *A*). Failure of neural tube closure produces defects of varying degrees (see box above). They may involve the entire length of the neural tube or may be restricted to a small area.

In the United States rates of NTDs have declined from 1.3 per 1000 births in 1970 to 0.6 per 1000 births in 1989. A partial explanation is the increased use of prenatal diagnostic techniques and termination of pregnancies (Yen and others, 1992).

Etiology

Two of the defects, ***anencephaly*** and ***spinal bifida (SB)***, occur in association with one another more often than would be expected by chance, suggesting a common origin. The CNS defects may alternate in siblings, which also tends to support the theory of a common origin.

Little progress has been made in identifying the etiologies of anencephaly and spina bifida. However, studies have

*Jeanne O'Connor Egan, RN, MSN, revised this section.

shown that women at high risk for having a child with an NTD because they had previously delivered an infant or fetus with spina bifida, anencephaly, or encephalocele significantly reduced the recurrence rate by taking supplements of the ***B vitamin folic acid*** before conception (Mills and others, 1992; MRC, 1991; Recommendations, 1992). ***Folate*** is a generic term for food compounds that have the biologic activity of folic acid, although folates in food are generally not as well absorbed as is folic acid. Other factors possibly involved in the etiology of NTDs include maternal heat exposure (i.e., hot tubs, saunas), valproic acid (an antiepileptic drug), and familial tendency.

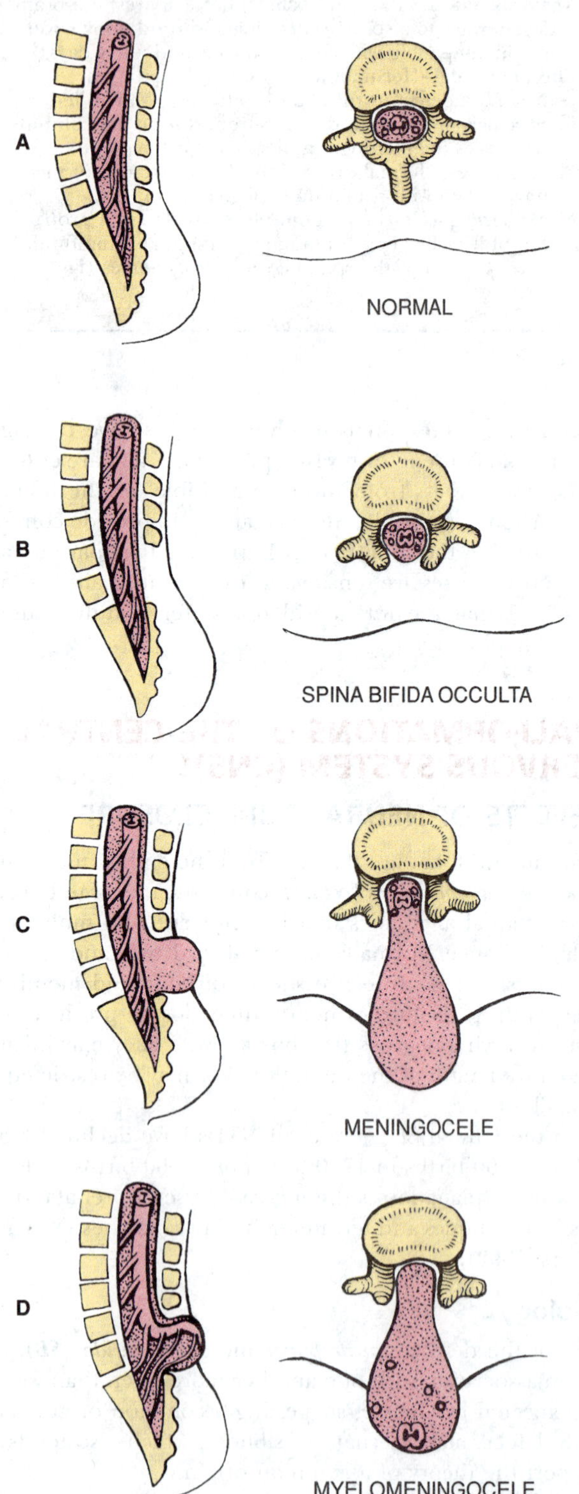

FIG. 11-2 Midline defects of osseous spine with varying degrees of neural herniations. **A,** Normal. **B,** Spina bifida occulta. **C,** Meningocele. **D,** Myelomeningocele.

The American Academy of Pediatrics (1993) recommends daily intake of folic acid for all women of childbearing age. The recommended 0.4 mg daily dose is supplied safely in many multivitamin preparations. Since the greatest risk factor is a previous pregnancy affected by NTDs, women in this category should increase their daily folic acid dose to 4.0 mg, under a practitioner's supervision, beginning 1 month before they plan a pregnancy and during the first trimester, because the neural tube closes about 1 month after conception. A 50% reduction in NTDs is anticipated with folic acid supplementation. As of this writing, the U.S. Food and Drug Administration (FDA) plans to require that folic acid be added to many products made with enriched wheat, corn, or rice, including cereals, bread, farina, and pasta (FDA proposes, 1993).

NURSING ALERT Supplementation of 4.0 mg of folate should not be met through the use of multivitamin preparations alone, because of the risk of excessive ingestion of other vitamins. Excess folate can mask symptoms of vitamin B_{12} deficiency, and excess vitamin A may cause birth defects.

The following discussion of NTDs is limited to the two most common types: anencephaly, a defect incompatible with life, and spina bifida, in particular, myelomeningocele, an abnormality that causes significant disability.

ANENCEPHALY

Anencephaly, the most serious NTD, is a congenital malformation in which both cerebral hemispheres are absent. The condition is incompatible with life, and many affected infants are stillborn. For those who survive, no specific treatment is available. The infants have an intact brainstem and are able to maintain vital functions (such as temperature regulation and cardiac and respiratory function) for a few hours to several weeks but eventually die of respiratory failure (Erlen and Holzman, 1988).

Traditionally these infants have been provided comfort measures, but with no effort at resuscitation. Ethical and moral questions are encountered regarding treatment and withdrawal of support systems (e.g., feedings) if the newborn survives the first few days of life, as well as use of the organs for donor transplants. During this time the family requires emotional support and counseling to cope with the birth of an infant with a fatal defect.

SPINA BIFIDA (SB)/MYELODYSPLASIA

Myelodysplasia refers broadly to any malformation of the spinal canal and cord. Midline defects involving failure of the osseous (bony) spine to close are called ***spina bifida,*** the most common defect of the CNS. SB is categorized into two types: spina bifida occulta and spina bifida cystica.

Spina bifida occulta refers to a defect that is not visible externally. It occurs most commonly in the lumbosacral area (L5 and S1) (Fig. 11-2, *B*). Routine radiographic examinations indicate that the disorder may be seen in as many as 10% to 30% of the general population (Rauen, 1990). However, it may not be apparent unless there are associated cutaneous manifestations or neuromuscular disturbances.

Superficial cutaneous indications include a skin depression or dimple (which may also mark the outlet of a dermal sinus tract that extends to the subarachnoid space), port-wine angiomatous nevi, dark tufts of hair, and soft, subcutaneous lipomas. These signs may be absent, appear singly, or be present in combination.

If associated neurologic involvement is present, the defect is known as ***occult spinal dysraphism.*** The spinal cord or roots can be distorted by fibrous bands and adhesions, intraspinal lipoma (fatty tumor) or subcutaneous lipoma (lipomyelomeningocele), dermoid or epidermoid cyst, diastematomyelia (spinal cord split in two), and tethered cord (Swaiman, 1994). The usual cause is abnormal adhesion, or ***tethering,*** to a bony or fixed structure, resulting in traction on the spinal cord and cauda equina. (See Fig. 4-8 for spinal cord development and Fig. 40-7 for areas innervated by specific spinal nerves.)

Neuromuscular disturbances usually consist of progressive or static changes in gait with foot weakness, foot deformity, and/or bowel and bladder sphincter disturbances. Manifestations may not be evident until the child walks or is toilet trained.

Plain radiography is employed to disclose the precise bony defect in the symptomatic lesion and to establish the diagnosis in the suspected, nonsymptomatic occult variety. Magnetic resonance imaging (MRI) is the most sensitive tool for evaluating the defect. Computed tomography (CT) scan, ultrasound, and myelography are also used to differentiate between SB occulta and other spinal disorders.

Spina bifida cystica refers to a visible defect with an external saclike protrusion. The two major forms of SB cystica are ***meningocele,*** which encases meninges and spinal fluid, but no neural elements (see Fig. 11-2, *C*); and ***myelomeningocele*** (or ***meningomyelocele***), which contains meninges, spinal fluid, and nerves (see Fig. 11-2, *D*). Meningocele is not associated with neurologic deficit, which occurs in varying, often serious, degrees in myelomeningocele. Clinically the term *spina bifida* is used to refer to myelomeningocele.

MYELOMENINGOCELE (MENINGOMYELOCELE)

Myelomeningocele develops during the first 28 days of pregnancy when the neural tube fails to close and fuse at some point along its length. It is detected at birth, accounts for 90% of spinal cord lesions, and may be located at any point along the spinal column. Usually the sac is encased in a fine membrane that is prone to tears through which cerebrospinal fluid (CSF) leaks. In other instances the sac may be covered by dura, meninges, or skin, in which instances there is rapid and spontaneous epithelialization.

The largest number of myelomeningoceles are found in the lumbar or lumbosacral area (Fig. 11-3). The location and magnitude of the defect determine the nature and extent of neurologic impairment. When the defect is located below the second lumbar vertebra, the nerves of the cauda equina are involved, giving rise to symptoms such as flaccid, areflexic partial paralysis of the lower extremities and varying degrees of sensory deficit.

The anomaly most frequently associated with myelomeningocele is hydrocephalus; 90% to 95% of children with

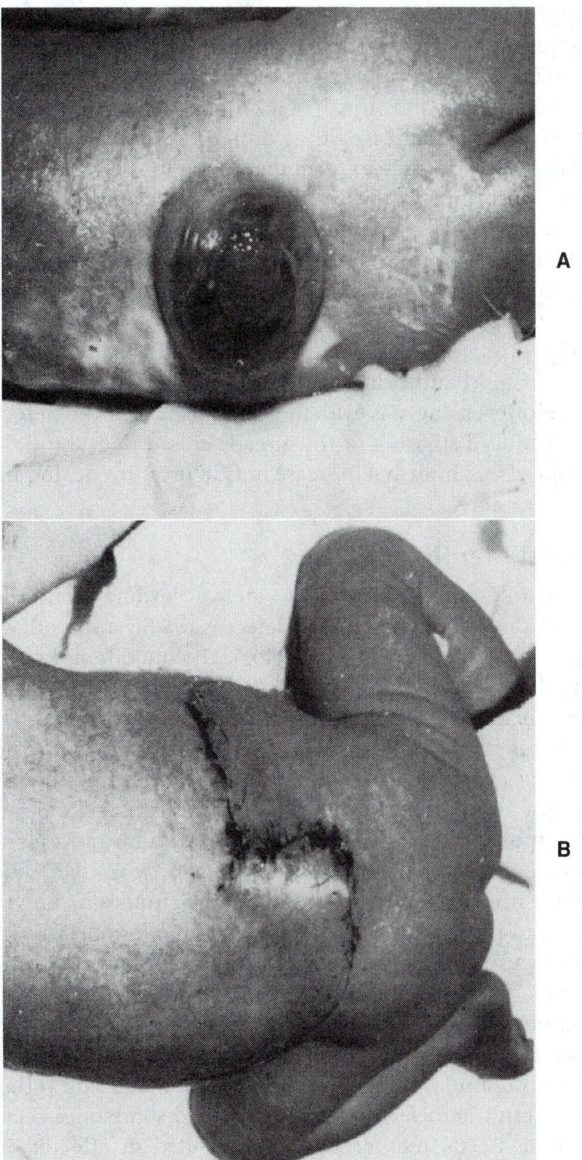

FIG. 11-3 **A,** Meningomyelocele before surgery. (An antibacterial dressing was used.) **B,** Repair of same patient. (Courtesy M.C. Gleason, MD, San Diego, CA. From Ingalls AJ, Salerno MC: *Maternal and child health nursing,* ed 7, St Louis, 1991, Mosby.)

SB have hydrocephalus (Shaer, 1993). Although present at birth, hydrocephalus may not be apparent until shortly thereafter. Careful monitoring of head circumference, fontanel tension, and ventricular size by head ultrasound can indicate its presence. Hydrocephalus can occur because the NTD itself disrupts the flow of CSF. In many cases a ***Chiari malformation*** (type 2) is responsible (see p. 455). Chiari malformation is present, though asymptomatic, in most children with SB. It can, however, adversely affect respiratory function, causing episodic apnea. Other clinical symptoms of problematic Chiari malformation include stridor, hoarse cry from vocal cord paralysis, feeding difficulties, and, in older children, a worsening of upper extremity function.

Pathophysiology

The pathophysiology of SB is best understood when it is related to the normal formative stages of the nervous system. At approximately 20 days of gestation a decided depression, the neural groove, appears in the dorsal ectoderm of the embryo. During the fourth week of gestation the groove deepens rapidly, and its elevated margins develop laterally and then fuse dorsally to form the neural tube. Neural tube formation begins in the cervical region near the center of the embryo and advances in both directions—caudally and cephalically—until by the end of the fourth week of gestation the ends of the neural tube, the anterior and posterior neuropores, are closed.

The primary defect in neural tube malformations is believed by most authorities to be a failure of neural tube closure. However, there is evidence to indicate that the defects are a result of splitting of the already closed neural tube as a result of an abnormal increase in CSF pressure during the first trimester.

Clinical Manifestations

The manifestations of SB vary widely according to the degree of the spinal defect. The defect is readily apparent on inspection. The degree of neurologic dysfunction is directly related to the anatomic level of the defect and thus the nerves involved. Sensory disturbances usually parallel motor dysfunction. The upper level of sensory and motor impairment can be determined by observation of the infant's response to a pinprick over the legs and trunk. The infant will respond to the sensory stimulus with limb movement, arousal, and crying. When withdrawal activity is used to determine the lowest level of spinal cord function, the response to pinprick should begin above the lesion.

Defective nerve supply to the bladder affects both sphincter and detrusor tone, which often causes constant dribbling of urine or produces overflow incontinence in childhood. However, some infants void in a stream. Frequently there is poor anal sphincter tone and poor anal skin reflex, which result in lack of bowel control and sometimes rectal prolapse. Rectal temperatures are avoided in affected infants. If the defect is located below the third sacral vertebra, there is no motor impairment but there may be saddle anesthesia with bladder and anal sphincter paralysis.

Sometimes the denervation to the muscles of the lower extremities will produce joint deformities in utero. These are primarily flexion or extension contractures, talipes valgus or varus contractures, kyphosis, lumbosacral scoliosis, and hip dislocations. The extent and severity of these associated orthopaedic deformities again depend on the degree of nerve involvement. Most flexion deformities result from the pull of stronger, fully innervated muscles acting without the counterpull of their nonfunctioning paralyzed antagonists.

Diagnostic Evaluation

The diagnosis is made on the basis of clinical manifestations and examination of the meningeal sac. Diagnostic measures used to evaluate the brain and spinal cord include MRI, ultrasound, CT, and myelography.

Laboratory examinations are used primarily to determine causative organisms in the major complications of myelomeningocele—meningitis and urinary tract infections. Infants with urinary tract incontinence require urinalysis, culture, and evaluation of blood urea nitrogen (BUN) and creatinine clearance.

Prenatal Detection. It is possible to determine the presence of some major open NTDs prenatally. Ultrasound scanning of the uterus and elevated concentrations of alpha-fetoprotein (AFP), a fetal-specific gamma-1 globulin, in amniotic fluid may indicate the presence of anencephaly or myelomeningocele. The optimum time for performing these diagnostic tests is between 16 and 18 weeks of gestation (American Academy of Pediatrics, 1987b), before AFP concentrations normally diminish and in sufficient time to permit a therapeutic abortion. It is recommended that such diagnostic procedures be considered for all mothers who have borne an affected child, and testing is offered to all pregnant women. In addition, elective prelabor cesarean birth may result in less motor dysfunction.

Therapeutic Management

Management of the child who has a myelomeningocele requires a multidisciplinary approach involving the specialties of neurology, neurosurgery, pediatrics, urology, orthopaedics, rehabilitation, physical therapy, occupational therapy, and social service, as well as intensive nursing care in a variety of specialty areas. The collaborative efforts of these specialists are focused on (1) the myelomeningocele and the problems associated with the defect—hydrocephalus, paralysis, orthopaedic deformities, genitourinary abnormalities; (2) possible acquired problems that may or may not be associated, such as meningitis, hypoxia, and hemorrhage; and (3) other abnormalities, such as cardiac or gastrointestinal malformations.

Initial Care. Care of the newborn involves prevention of infection, neurologic assessment, including observation for associated anomalies, and dealing with the impact of the anomaly on the family. Most authorities believe that early closure, within the first 24 to 72 hours, offers the most favorable outcome, especially in regard to morbidity and mortality from serious infection. Early closure, preferably in the first 12 to 18 hours, not only prevents local infection and trauma to the exposed tissues, but also avoids stretching of other nerve roots, which may occur as the meningeal sac expands during the first 24 hours after birth, thus preventing further motor impairment.

A variety of neurosurgical and plastic surgical procedures are employed for skin closure without disturbing the neural elements or removing any portion of the sac. The objective is satisfactory skin coverage of the lesion and meticulous closure. Wide excision of the large membranous covering may damage functioning neural tissue.

Associated problems are assessed and managed by appropriate surgical and supportive measures. Shunt procedures provide relief from imminent or progressive hydrocephalus (see p. 454). Meningitis, urinary tract infection, and pneumonia are treated with vigorous antibiotic therapy and supportive measures.

Improved surgical techniques do not alter the major physical disability and deformity or chronic urinary tract and pulmonary infections that affect the quality of life for these children. Superimposed on these physical problems are the effects that the disorder has on family life and finances and on school and hospital services.

Orthopaedic Considerations. According to most orthopaedists, musculoskeletal problems that will affect later locomotion should be evaluated early, and treatment, where indicated, should be instituted without delay. Neurologic assessment will determine the neurosegmental level of the lesion, recognition of spasticity and progressive paralysis, the potential for deformity, and functional expectations. Orthopaedic management includes prevention of joint contractures, correction of the deformity, prevention of skin breakdown, and obtaining the best possible locomotor function. The status of the neurologic deficit remains the most important factor in determining the child's ultimate functional abilities.

Great diversity is observed in patterns of musculoskeletal involvement. The hip flexors and adductors are innervated by L1 to L3, whereas extensors and abductors are innervated by L5 to S1. Consequently, there is often an imbalance in muscle pull around a joint. Children with lesions at L2 or above have some hip flexion and are usually confined to a wheelchair for mobility. Children with lesions at L2 to L5 have strong hip flexors and are candidates for crutches and braces, although the majority use a wheelchair most of the time. At levels L3 and L4 there is usually an imbalance between sensory and motor nerve involvement, and hip dislocation is often a problem. Children with sacral lesions are able to walk, but some may require ankle bracing.

Physical therapy and orthopaedic management of children with myelomeningocele is a continuous process to achieve optimum function. Problems such as Arnold-Chiari malformation, hydrocephalus, and tethered spinal cord can complicate expectations. Controversies exist over the orthopaedic management of dislocated hips, scoliosis, and kyphosis.

A variety of devices are available to provide mobility to children with spinal cord lesions, including lightweight braces, special "walking" devices, and custom-built wheelchairs (see also Chapter 39). Corrective procedures, when indicated, are best initiated at an early age so that the child will not lag significantly behind age-mates in developmental progress. Where there is little hope for lower extremity functioning, surgery is seldom recommended.

Management of Genitourinary Function.* Myelomeningocele is one of the most common causes of ***neuropathic (neurogenic) bladder dysfunction*** among children. In infants the goal of treatment is to preserve renal function. In older children the goal is to achieve urinary continence (Fernandes and others, 1994). Urinary incontinence, a chronic, often debilitating problem, commonly arises from the dysfunctional bladder. In addition, neuropathic bladder dysfunction may predispose the child to ***urinary system distress*** (infection, ureterohydronephrosis, and vesicoureteral reflux). The characteristics of bladder dysfunction in children vary according to the level of the lesion and the influence of bony growth and development on the spine. In addition, the presence of hydrocephalus has the potential to affect bladder function, although spinal influences are predominant (Kelalis, King, and Belman, 1992).

During infancy urinary incontinence is physiologic and normal, but urinary system distress may occur. Ongoing urologic monitoring and rapid management of complications are essential for adequate growth and maturation. Ultrasonography of the bladder and ureters, along with routine urine cultures, is used to detect urinary system distress before renal function is compromised. Urodynamic evaluation is ideally completed during the first several months of life. The purpose of this evaluation is to identify bladder dysfunction that may predispose the child to urinary system distress. Specifically, ***high-pressure detrusor hyperreflexia*** (uncontrolled contractions of the detrusor muscle) associated with ***vesicosphincter dyssynergia*** (incoordination of detrusor and sphincter muscles) predisposes the child to urinary system distress.

Infants may have one of several predominant neuropathic bladder disorders. Detrusor contractions associated with vesicosphincter dyssynergia is particularly common. Certain children are able to empty the bladder effectively despite incoordination of the sphincter; others will develop urinary infections or other urinary system distress. Some youngsters will have deficient detrusor contraction strength for complete bladder evacuation. This condition is particularly damaging to the urinary system when it coexists with poor bladder compliance and a high leak point pressure (pressure required to drive urine across the bladder outlet; 40 cm H_2O or greater). A small number of infants will experience detrusor contractions with coordinated response of the sphincter. Effective bladder evacuation is likely and urinary system distress is rare in this group of infants.

As the child grows, detrusor hyperreflexia is often replaced by deficient detrusor contraction strength and stress urinary incontinence (SUI) (leakage produced by physical exertion). The bladder wall is often poorly compliant (producing chronically elevated intravesical pressures), and the bladder outlet, while incompetent, obstructs the outflow of urine. When the leak point pressure exceeds 40 cm H_2O, the child is predisposed to chronic urinary leakage and uri-

*Mikel Gray, RN, PhD, PNP, CURN, wrote this section.

nary distress symptoms, including recurrent urinary tract infections and reflux. When the leak point pressure is lower than 40 cm H_2O, urinary leakage is more severe, although the risk of urinary system distress is lessened. Thus the child with more severe urinary incontinence is less predisposed than the "dryer" child to serious urinary infections.

Conservative management of neuropathic bladder dysfunction in infants typically consists of watchful waiting. The child is allowed to empty the bladder into a diaper, the urine is monitored for infection, and the upper urinary tract is monitored for dilation using ultrasonography. Children who experience urinary system distress or who have significant risk factors identified by urodynamic evaluation, may need ***clean intermittent catheterization (CIC),*** typically with an antispasmodic medication such as oxybutynin or propantheline. Oxybutynin effectively reduces uninhibited contractions and lowers detrusor filling pressure, while CIC allows bladder emptying at low pressures with no measurable side effects (Kasablan and others, 1992). Unfortunately, frequent catheterization (usually every 2 to 3 hours around the clock) is necessary, and compliance to this rigid schedule is difficult for the family. Children with significant urinary system distress (such as vesicoureteral reflux or hydronephrosis) may require temporary urinary diversion to attain adequate urinary outflow. ***Vesicostomy*** is a relatively simple procedure wherein the anterior wall of the bladder is brought to the abdominal wall, creating a small stoma for urinary drainage. The diaper is placed slightly higher to contain urinary leakage. Meticulous skin care is needed, since the skin is exposed to a relatively continuous source of urinary drainage.

Among older children the quest for continence typically begins with a CIC program. The parents are taught the procedure, and the child is taught to self-catheterize as soon as possible, usually by the sixth year of life. The child with detrusor hyperreflexia and dyssynergia often responds well to antispasmodic medications and CIC. In contrast, the child with poor bladder wall compliance and SUI often requires a combination of antispasmodic medications to reduce intravesical filling pressures and an alpha-sympathetic agonist (such as imipramine, pseudoephedrine, or phenylpropanolamine) to enhance sphincter competence. Unfortunately, the combination of medications and CIC is typically only partly effective, and more aggressive interventions are often required to render the neuropathic bladder both continent and free from its predisposition toward producing urinary system distress.

When continence cannot be attained by conservative measures, surgery is considered. ***Augmentation enterocystoplasty*** is a surgical procedure that increases bladder capacity, reverses or halts the deleterious effects of the poorly compliant bladder wall, and reduces harmfully high bladder pressures caused by detrusor hyperreflexia with vesicosphincter dyssynergia (Gray, 1993). A detubularized segment of large or small bowel, as well as a wedge of the fundus of the stomach, has been used to successfully augment bladder capacity. The choice of segment varies according to the surgeon's preference and the status of the patient's urinary and gastrointestinal systems. Large and small bowel segments produce significant volumes of mucus that may clog catheters used for CIC. Augmentation with the stomach produces less mucus, and its acidic secretions may reduce the urinary system's predisposition to infection.

Even though augmentation of the bladder may improve or resolve urinary leakage related to detrusor hyperreflexia, stress urinary incontinence caused by sphincter mechanism deficiency persists. Several procedures may be used to increase sphincter competence. An ***artificial urinary sphincter*** consisting of a urethral cuff, abdominal reservoir, and control pump may be implanted. The cuff is maintained in a closed position until the patient catheterizes or empties the bladder by micturition. Because of the significant risk of infection and mechanical failure requiring reoperation, the popularity of the artificial urinary sphincter has declined.

A ***urethral sling*** offers an alternative to the artificial sphincter. The sling procedure uses a strip of fascia or synthetic material to partially obstruct the proximal urethra. The sling is placed at the proximal one third of the urethra, and the procedure may be completed during bladder augmentation surgery. The surgeon carefully avoids placing excessive tension against the sling to avoid ischemia or other complications. Following augmentation with placement of a urethral sling, the patient can expect to evacuate the bladder with CIC.

Submucosal implantation of a glutaraldehyde (GAX) collagen is a relatively new approach in the treatment of sphincter mechanism deficiency. ***Collagen*** is used to expand the urethral tissue, promoting coaptation (approximation) rather than obstruction. Collagen injection offers several potential advantages to implantation of an artificial urinary sphincter or sling procedure. The procedure does not require open incisional surgery, and collagen is implanted using cystoscopic guidance. In addition, additional injections may be used to improve continence if the first injection fails to completely resolve urinary leakage. The risk for dissipation of the collagen causing recurrence of leakage is a potential disadvantage of the procedure.

Construction of an ***abdominal stoma*** using a specially constructed segment of intussuscepted bowel, ureter, or appendix may be brought to the abdomen and the urethra may be closed when collagen does not successfully resolve SUI.

Uncommonly, children with myelodysplasia may develop severe dysfunction of the bladder that compromises renal function or produces debilitating urinary incontinence that is intractable to other means. ***Urinary diversion,*** typically using a continent neobladder constructed from bowel or stomach, may be required. Whenever feasible, the neobladder is constructed in a way that allows continence, and CIC is used to regularly evacuate urine.

Bowel Control. Some degree of fecal continence can usually be achieved in most children with myelomeningocele with diet modification, regular toilet habits, and prevention of constipation and impaction. It is frequently a lengthy process. Fiber supplements, laxatives, suppositories, and/or enemas aid in producing regular evacuation.

Latex Allergy. Latex allergy was identified as being a serious health hazard when a report linked intraoperative anaphylaxis with latex in children with SB (Slater, 1989). These children are at high risk for developing latex allergy because of repeated exposure to latex products during surgery and from numerous bladder catheterizations (Leger and Meeropol, 1992). Allergic reactions range from urticaria, wheezing, watery eyes, and rashes to anaphylactic shock. More severe reactions tend to occur when latex comes in contact with mucous membranes, wet skin, and the bloodstream and in individuals with atopic disorders. Since casein, a milk protein, is sometimes added to rubber, individuals with a severe allergy to milk may also show signs of an apparent latex reaction (Mäkinen-Kūjnen and others, 1993). The incidence of latex allergy in children with SB ranges from an estimated 18% to 60% (Ellsworth and others, 1993; Young and others, 1992).

The most important goals are prevention of latex allergy and identification of children with a known hypersensitivity (see also p. 450). Allergy testing with the latex extract may be performed with the skin prick test; however, skin testing can cause an allergic reaction. The radioallergosorbent test (RAST) is test the most specific test for IgE antibody (Young and others, 1992). Children who are allergic to latex may be given antihistamines and steroids (dexamethasone) before and after surgery to reduce the possibility of a serious reaction.

Prognosis. The early prognosis for the child with myelomeningocele depends on the neurologic deficit present at birth, including motor ability and bladder innervation and the presence of associated cerebral anomalies. Early surgical repair of the spinal defect, antibiotic therapy to reduce the incidence of total meningitis and ventriculitis, prevention of urinary system dysfunction, and correction of hydrocephalus have significantly increased the survival rate. Based on current medical knowledge and ethical considerations, aggressive management is favored for the child with meningomyelocele.

With the widespread use of folate supplementation during the childbearing years, the incidence of SB should decrease dramatically. Whether folic acid will lessen the severity of the defect in infants born with SB despite supplementation is unknown.

Nursing Considerations

❖ Assessment

At the time of delivery an examination is performed to assess the intactness of the membranous cyst. During transport to the nursery every effort is made to prevent trauma to this protective covering. In addition to the routine assessment of the newborn (see Chapter 8), the infant is assessed for level of neurologic involvement. Movement of extremities or skin response, especially an anal reflex, that might provide clues to the degree of motor or sensory impairment is noted. It is important to observe the infant's behavior in conjunction with the stimulus, since limb movements can be induced in response to spinal cord reflex activity that has no connection with the higher centers. Observation of urinary output, especially if a diaper remains dry, may indicate urinary retention. The head circumference is measured daily (see Chapter 7), and the fontanels are examined for signs of tension or bulging.

❖ Nursing Diagnoses

Following the nursing assessment a number of nursing diagnoses become evident. The most likely diagnoses are outlined and discussed in the Nursing Care Plan on pp. 452-453. Others may be apparent in individual cases.

❖ Planning

The goals for the infant with myelomeningocele and the family include the following:

1. Infant will not experience damage to the myelomeningocele sac.
2. Infant will not experience complications.
3. Family will receive support and education.

❖ Implementation

The basic needs of the infant with a myelomeningocele are essentially the same as for any newborn infant (see Chapter 8). Special needs related to the defect and potential complications are discussed in the following section. As the child matures, the problems increase and involve all aspects of daily living; therefore care is directly related to the child's habilitation at each stage of development.

Care of the Myelomeningocele Sac. The infant is usually placed in an incubator or warmer so that temperature can be maintained without clothing or covers that might irritate the delicate lesion. When an overhead warmer is used, the dressings over the defect require more frequent moistening because of the dehydrating effect of the radiant heat.

Before surgical closure the myelomeningocele is prevented from drying by the application of a sterile, moist, nonadherent dressing over the defect. The moistening solution is usually sterile normal saline (Peterson, 1992). Dressings are changed frequently (every 2 to 4 hours), and the sac is closely inspected for leaks, abrasions, irritation, or any signs of infection. The sac must be carefully cleansed if it becomes soiled or contaminated. Sometimes the sac ruptures during delivery or transport, and any opening in the sac greatly increases the risk of infection to the CNS.

NURSING ALERT Observe for early signs of infection, such as elevated temperature (axillary), irritability, lethargy, and nuchal rigidity, and for signs of increased intracranial pressure (ICP), which might indicate developing hydrocephalus.

➤ **NURSING TIP** To prevent stool contamination of the SB defect preoperatively, obtain a surgical drape (such as Steri Drape*). Cut a portion of the drape to fit the infant's sacrum using nonlatex tape to secure the plastic drape to the sacrum. The rest of the drape is placed loosely over the dressing covering the defect, thus preventing exposure to stool.

Positioning. One of the most difficult, important, and

---

*3M, St. Paul, MN.

challenging aspects of the early care of the infant with myelomeningocele is positioning. Before surgery the infant is kept in the prone position to minimize tension on the sac and the risk of trauma. The prone position allows for optimum positioning of the legs, especially in cases of associated hip dysplasia. A variety of aids, including diaper rolls, pads, small sandbags, or specially designed frames and appliances, can be used to maintain the desired position.

The prone position affects other aspects of the infant's care. For example, in this position the infant is more difficult to keep clean, pressure areas are a constant threat, and feeding becomes a problem. The infant's head is turned to one side for feeding. Fortunately, most defects are repaired early, and the infant can be held for feeding soon after surgery. Physical therapy consultation may be sought for difficult positioning problems.

General Care. Diapering the infant may be contraindicated until the defect has been repaired and healing is well advanced or epithelialization has taken place. The padding beneath the diaper area is changed as needed to keep the skin dry and free of irritation. When urinary retention is detected (the bladder is still an abdominal organ in early infancy), CIC is employed.* Since the bowel sphincter is frequently affected, there is continual passage of stool, often misinterpreted as diarrhea, which is a constant irritant to the skin and a source of infection to the spinal lesion.

Areas of sensory and motor impairment are subject to skin breakdown and therefore require meticulous care. Placing the infant on a pressure-reducing mattress or pad may be needed to prevent pressure on the knees and ankles. Periodic cleansing and gentle massage aid circulation.

Gentle range-of-motion exercises are sometimes carried out to prevent contractures, and stretching of contractures is performed when indicated. However, these exercises may be restricted to the foot, ankle, and knee joint. Where the hip joints are unstable, stretching against tight hip flexors or adductor muscles, which act much like bowstrings, may aggravate a tendency toward subluxation. A physical therapy consultation is usually obtained.

Some infants with unrepaired myelomeningocele are unable to be held in the arms and cuddled as unaffected infants are, so their need for tactile stimulation is met by caressing, stroking, and other comfort measures. To facilitate handling and reduce parental anxiety, the infant can recline on a pillow placed in the parent's lap. Black-and-white drawings or geometric shapes can be placed within the infant's view, and other stimulation usually provided for infants is appropriate. All infants respond to pleasant sounds (see Developmental Intervention, Chapter 10).

Ophthalmic complications occur frequently in children with spina bifida and hydrocephalus. The sudden appearance of a squint, other ocular motility, or papilledema usually denotes uncontrolled hydrocephalus and is reported. Shunt surgery is the first priority but may not restore normal ocular motility and visual function.

*Home care instructions for performing clean intermittant catheterization are available in *Wong and Whaley's Clinical Manual of Pediatric Nursing* (Mosby).

Since children who have SB are prone to develop an allergy to latex, reducing exposure to latex, from birth on, is hoped to decrease the chance of allergy development (Shapiro, 1992; Meeropol, Leger, and Frost, 1993). Latex, a natural product derived from the rubber tree, is used in combination with other chemicals to provide elasticity, strength, and durability to many products.

Avoiding latex products is the most important intervention (Pasquariello and others, 1993). The establishment of a nonlatex environment is being accomplished in many health care facilities where patients (and health care workers) are at high risk.* In addition, there are published lists of products, such as vinyl gloves, that may be substituted for latex (Romanczuk, 1993). Sometimes cloth can be placed between the latex item and the skin, such as cotton gloves under latex gloves or a cloth under a tourniquet or blood pressure cuffs, to reduce contact with the skin (Meeropol, Leger, and Frost, 1993).

The identification of those sensitive to latex is best accomplished through careful screening of *all* patients. (See Guidelines box for questions related to latex allergy.)

NURSING ALERT Ask *all* patients about allergic reactions to latex, not only those at risk, during the health interview with the parent and/or child. Be sure this is a routine part of all preoperative histories.

Children with latex allergy should carry some form of allergy identification, such as a medical bracelet. Education programs regarding latex hypersensitivity are aimed at those who care for high-risk groups, such as children with SB, and may include relatives, school nurses, teachers, child care workers, and baby-sitters. In addition to educating care-

*For additional information contact Ellen Meeropol or Patricia King, Shriner's Hospital, 516 Carew St., Springfield, MA 01104; (413) 787-2015.

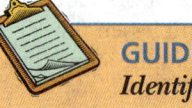

GUIDELINES
Identifying Latex Allergy

Does the child have any symptoms, such as sneezing, coughing, rashes, or wheezing, when handling rubber products (balloons, tennis or Koosh balls, adhesive bandage strips) or when in contact with rubber hospital products, such as gloves or catheters?

Has your child ever had an allergic reaction during surgery?

Does the child have a history of rashes, asthma, or allergic reactions to medication or foods, especially milk, kiwi, bananas, or chestnuts?

How would you identify or recognize an allergic reaction in your child?

What would you do if an allergic reaction occurred?

Has anyone ever discussed latex or rubber allergy or sensitivity with you?

Has the child had any allergy testing?

When did the child last come in contact with any type of rubber product? Were you present?

Modified from Romanczuk A: Latex use with infants and children: it can cause problems, *MCN* 18(4):208-212, 1993.

givers about the child's exposure to medical products that contain latex, nurses need to inform them of common nonmedical latex objects (see box below). Items brought to the hospital, such as floral bouquets, are also screened for latex toys or balloons. Parents should also be given literature explaining signs and symptoms of latex hypersensitivity and appropriate emergency treatment (see Anaphylaxis, Chapter 29).

Postoperative Care. Postoperative care of the infant with myelomeningocele involves the same basic care as that of any postsurgical infant—monitoring vital signs, weight, and intake and output; maintaining body temperature; assessing and relieving pain; providing nourishment, and observing for signs of infection. The wound is managed according to the directions of the surgeon, and general care is continued as preoperatively.

The prone position is maintained after operative closure, although many neurosurgeons allow a side-lying or partial side-lying position unless it aggravates a coexisting hip dysplasia or permits undesirable hip flexion. This offers an opportunity for position changes, which reduces the risk of pressure sores and facilitates feeding. Once the effects of anesthesia have subsided and the infant is alert, feedings may be resumed unless there are other anomalies or associated complications.

Nursing assessments are carried out for implementation of comfort measures in the postoperative period. The infant can be held upright against the body, with care taken to avoid pressure on the operative site. In the case of an unusually large defect, skin grafting may be required for wound closure; the infant must then be kept prone postoperatively with as little movement as possible to prevent tension on the skin graft.

The nurse can assist in determining the extent of neuromuscular involvement. Movement of the extremities or skin response, especially an anal reflex, that might provide cues to the degree of motor or sensory status is noted. The head circumference is measured daily (see Chapter 7), and the fontanels are examined for signs of tension or bulging. The nurse is also alert to early signs of infection, such as elevated or decreased temperature (axillary), irritability, lethargy, and nuchal rigidity, and to signs of increased ICP. Catheterization may be needed for urine retention. Although it may not have been a problem preoperatively, swelling around the operative site may cause transient urine retention, which resolves in 1 to 2 days.

Family Support and Home Care. As soon as the parents are able to cope with the infant's condition, they are encouraged to become involved in care. They need to learn how to continue at home the care that has been initiated in the hospital—positioning, feeding, skin care, and range-of-motion exercises when appropriate. Parents are taught clean catheterization technique when prescribed. The family needs to know the signs of complications and how to reach assistance when needed.

As the child grows and develops, parents need guidance to encourage and stimulate the infant to accomplish age-appropriate developmental tasks within the limits imposed by the disabilities. Upper limb movement can be stimulated early by placing the infant on the floor in a prone position

SELECTED ITEMS POSSIBLY CONTAINING LATEX*

MEDICAL ITEMS

Adhesive bandage strips (Band-Aid brand)
Airways, masks
Anesthesia circuits
Blood pressure cuffs and tubing
Bulb syringe
Catheters
Chux (washable rubber)
Crutches (axillary, hand pads)
Dressings (moleskin, Coban [3M])
Elastic bandages (Ace wrap)
Electrode pads
Endotracheal tubes
Finger cots
Gloves (sterile and examining, surgical and medical)
Intravenous tubing, injection ports, bags, burets
Jobst spandex products
Medication vials
Nasogastric (NG) tubes
Penrose drains
PRN adapter (heparin lock)
Stethoscope tubing
Suction tubing
Syringes
Tape (cloth adhesive, paper)
Theraband strips and tubes
Tourniquet
Urodynamics rectal pressure catheters
Wheelchair cushions, tires

NONMEDICAL ITEMS

Art supplies (paint, markers, glue)
Balloons (not Mylar)
Balls (Koosh, tennis)
Cleaning/kitchen gloves
Condoms
Dental dams and equipment
Diaphragms
Elastic exercisers
Elastic on legs, waist of clothing, rubber pants, possibly disposable diapers
Feeding nipples
Foam rubber lining on splints, braces
Infant toothbrush-massager
Pacifier
Racquet handles
Rubber bands
Water toys, swim, scuba equipment

Modified from Meeropol E, Leger R, Frost J: Latex allergy in patients with myelodysplasia and in health care providers: a double jeopardy, *Urol Nurs* 13(2):39-44, 1993.

*It is very difficult to obtain full and accurate information on the latex content of products, which may vary among companies and product series. Double-checking with suppliers before use with latex-allergic individuals is strongly recommended.

NURSING CARE PLAN

The Infant with Myelomeningocele

NURSING DIAGNOSIS: High risk for infection related to presence of infective organisms, nonepithelialized meningeal sac, paralysis

PATIENT GOAL 1: Will experience minimized risk of central nervous system infection

• **NURSING INTERVENTIONS/*RATIONALES***

Position infant *to prevent contamination from urine and stool*

Cleanse myelomeningocele carefully with sterile normal saline if it becomes soiled or contaminated

*Apply sterile dressings and moisten with sterile solution as ordered (normal saline, antibiotic) *to prevent drying of sac*

*Administer antibiotics as prescribed

Monitor closely for signs of infection (elevated temperature, irritability, lethargy, nuchal rigidity) *to prevent delay in treatment*

Administer similar care to operative site postoperatively

• **EXPECTED OUTCOME**

Meningeal sac remains clean, intact, and exhibits no evidence of infection

PATIENT GOAL 2: Will experience minimized risk of urinary tract infection

• **NURSING INTERVENTIONS/*RATIONALES***

Avoid urethral contamination with stool *to prevent introduction of infective organisms into urinary tract*

Carry out meticulous perineal hygiene *to remove infective organisms*

Monitor urinary output for retention *to minimize risk of infection due to stasis of urine*

*Administer antibiotics as prescribed

*Administer urinary tract antiseptics if prescribed

Ensure adequate fluid intake *to increase urination and prevent bacterial growth*

• **EXPECTED OUTCOME**

Infant exhibits no evidence of urinary tract infection

NURSING DIAGNOSIS: High risk for trauma related to delicate spinal lesion

PATIENT GOAL 1: Will not experience trauma to spinal lesion/surgical site

• **NURSING INTERVENTIONS/*RATIONALES***

Handle infant carefully *to prevent damage to meningeal sac or surgical site*

Place infant in prone position, or side-lying position if permitted, *to minimize tension on the meningeal sac or surgical site*

Apply protective devices around sac (e.g., a surgical plastic drape, cut to fit and taped below the sac by the sacrum and loosely draped over the sac) *to provide a protective shield*

Modify routine nursing activities (e.g., feeding, making bed, comforting activities) *to prevent trauma*

• **EXPECTED OUTCOMES**

Meningeal sac remains intact

Surgical site heals without trauma

NURSING DIAGNOSIS: High risk for impaired skin integrity related to paralysis, continual dribbling of urine, and feces

PATIENT GOAL 1: Will not experience skin irritation

• **NURSING INTERVENTIONS/*RATIONALES***

Change diapers as soon as soiled, if diapered, *to keep skin clean, dry, and free of irritation*

Keep perianal area clean and dry

Place infant on pressure-reducing surface *to reduce pressure on knees and ankles during prone positioning*

Gently massage healthy skin during cleansing and application of lotion *to increase circulation*

• **EXPECTED OUTCOME**

Skin remains clean and dry with no evidence of irritation

NURSING DIAGNOSIS: High risk for trauma related to impaired cerebrospinal fluid circulation

PATIENT GOAL 1: Will not experience increased intracranial pressure

• **NURSING INTERVENTIONS/*RATIONALES***

Measure occipitofrontal circumference daily *to detect increased intracranial pressure and developing hydrocephalus*

Observe for signs of increased intracranial pressure, *which might indicate developing hydrocephalus*

- Irritability
- Lethargy
- Infant
  - Cries when picked up or handled; quiets when lies still
  - Increased occipitofrontal circumference
  - Separated sutures
  - Change in level of consciousness
- Child
  - Headache (especially in morning)
  - Apathy
  - Confusion

• **EXPECTED OUTCOME**

Evidence of increased intracranial pressure and hydrocephalus is detected early, and appropriate interventions are implemented

*Dependent nursing action.

NURSING CARE PLAN
The Infant with Myelomeningocele—cont'd

NURSING DIAGNOSIS: High risk for injury related to repeated exposure to latex products and development of latex allergy

PATIENT GOAL 1: Will experience minimal exposure to latex

• **NURSING INTERVENTIONS/*RATIONALES***

Identify children with latex allergy (see box on p. 450)
Maintain a latex-free environment *to reduce exposure*
Educate family members and other caregivers (i.e., day-care workers, teachers) about
 Risk of latex allergy and items to avoid *to reduce exposure*
 Signs of allergy (from hives, rash, and wheezing to anaphylaxis) *to detect a reaction quickly*
 Emergency treatment, including use of anaphylactic kit and summoning emergency medical services, *to prevent delay in treatment*

• **EXPECTED OUTCOME**

Child does not develop allergic reactions to latex

NURSING DIAGNOSIS: High risk for injury related to neuromuscular impairment

PATIENT GOAL 1: Will experience no or minimized risk of hip and lower extremity deformity

• **NURSING INTERVENTIONS/*RATIONALES***

Carry out passive range-of-motion exercises *to prevent contractures;* do not push past point of resistance *to prevent trauma*
Carry out muscle stretching when indicated *to prevent contractures*
Maintain hips in slight to moderate abduction *to prevent dislocation;* maintain feet in neutral position *to prevent contractures*
Use diaper rolls, pads, small sandbags, or specially designed appliances *to maintain desired position*

• **EXPECTED OUTCOMES**

Lower extremities maintain flexibility
Hips and lower extremities are maintained in correct articulation and alignment

See also:
 Nursing Care Plan: The Child with Chronic Illness or Disability, Chapter 22
 Nursing Care Plan: The Child in the Hospital, Chapter 26
 Nursing Care Plan: The Family of the Ill or Hospitalized Child, Chapter 26

with toys within reach. Activities that encourage body consciousness, such as rolling over and pulling to a sitting position, are encouraged at the appropriate times. Creeping and crawling, even in a limited way, help the child to explore the environment. The parents may need help to modify appliances and activities normally expected of a growing child. For example, the infant who is paraplegic is encouraged to use arms and shoulders as much as possible. When the infant is sitting in an infant seat, stroller, high chair, or feeding table, the hips can be supported, a footrest provided, and hard-soled shoes worn to maintain the feet in correct alignment and to protect the insensitive feet from trauma. A standing table is helpful for a variety of activities, and it is best for the child to begin supported weight bearing and standing as close as possible to the expected time for standing to occur.

It is important for the family to understand the nature of sensory deficit in a child with a spinal defect. The child will be insensitive to pressure or other sources of tissue injury. Therefore the family must be alert to hot or cold items that could cause thermal injury to tissues and to inspect the skin regularly for signs of pressure, especially over bony prominences. Because of sensory impairment, the child is unaware of bladder discomfort; therefore signs of urinary tract infections may be easily overlooked. Urinary tract infection is often considered when the child becomes ill.

The long-range planning with and support of the parents and newborn begin in the hospital and extend throughout childhood. Nurses assume an important role as a central member of the health team. As a coordinator the nurse reviews information with the family, takes responsibility for family teaching, and acts as a liaison between inpatient and outpatient services. The child will need numerous hospitalizations over the years, and each one will be a source of stress to which the younger child is especially vulnerable.

Parents who cope well with their infants may become discouraged later by numerous surgeries, physical therapies, and school adjustments, and ultimately they may not follow the medical plan. This may place parents in an adversarial position with health care providers. Questions may arise over the responsibility of the health care team vs that of the family, and over whether noncompliance constitutes parental neglect (Shaer, 1993).

Changes in functional ability, particularly those in the lower extremities, bowel, or bladder, may indicate the presence of a tethered cord, one that is bound down or restricted in an abnormal position by scar tissue (Storrs and other, 1990). These symptoms usually occur after a growing spurt and can best be detected with MRI. Tethering can be repaired surgically but, unfortunately, may recur.

Habilitation involves solving not only problems of self-help and locomotion but also the most distressing problems of incontinence, which threatens the child's social acceptability. Assistance with preparing the child and the school regarding the special needs of children with disabilities helps provide a better initial adjustment to broader social experiences. It would be difficult to enumerate all that the condition entails in terms of suffering, frustration, family stress, and economic burden. Numerous organizations and agencies are able to offer assistance and support to children and families. The **Spina Bifida Association of America*** provides services and support for families of children with spinal lesions.

The multiple aspects of care of the child with a disability are discussed in Chapter 22 and need not be elaborated on here. Complex problems associated with partial or complete lower extremity paralysis are discussed in Chapters 39 and 40, and include bowel and bladder control, orthopaedic appliances, and the observation and management of complications, especially urinary tract infections (see Chapter 30) and pressure necrosis (see Wounds, Chapter 18).

❖ Evaluation

The effectiveness of nursing interventions is determined by continual reassessment and evaluation of care based on the following observational guidelines and expected outcomes.

1. Inspect the spinal lesion, take appropriate measurements (weight, vital signs, head circumference), observe the child's general health status, and check completed care against the preoperative checklist.
2. Take vital signs, inspect the operative site (or preoperative lesion), inspect skin (especially dependent and pressure areas), measure head circumference, and assess range of motion of lower extremities.
3. Observe parent-infant interactions, behavior of family members, and interview family members regarding their feelings and concerns.

*4590 McArthur, N.W., Washington, DC 20007; (202) 944-3285 or (800) 621-3141.

Expected outcomes:

See Nursing Care Plan, p. 452-453.

HYDROCEPHALUS

Hydrocephalus is a syndrome, or sign, resulting from disturbances in the dynamics of CSF, which may be caused by various diseases. The advent of MRI and CT scanning has provided valuable information about the pathophysiology of hydrocephalus. Although prenatal diagnosis is having an impact on the current prevalence of neural defects at birth, hydrocephalus occurs in 5.8 per 10,000 births (Temporal trends, 1990). The cause is diverse, from either congenital or acquired conditions. Congenital hydrocephalus is usually a result of a maldevelopment or an intrauterine infection. Acquired hydrocephalus can be caused by infection, neoplasm, or hemorrhage (James, 1992).

Pathophysiology

To appreciate the condition, an understanding of the dynamics of CSF and the relationship between the various structures that make up the ventricular and subarachnoid spaces is necessary (Fig. 11-4). The two mechanisms by which CSF is formed include secretion by the choroid plexuses and lymphatic-like drainage by the extracellular fluid of the brain. CSF circulates throughout the ventricular system and is then absorbed within the subarachnoid spaces by a mechanism that is not entirely clear.

Ventricular Circulation. The fluid flows from the lateral ventricles through the ***foramen of Monro*** to the third ventricle, where it combines with fluid secreted into the third ventricle. From there CSF flows through the ***aqueduct of Sylvius*** into the fourth ventricle, where more fluid is formed; it then leaves the fourth ventricle by way of the lateral ***foramen of Luschka*** and the midline ***foramen of Magendie*** into the ***cisterna magna.*** From there CSF flows to the cerebral and cerebellar subarachnoid spaces, where it is absorbed. A large portion is absorbed through the arachnoid villi, but

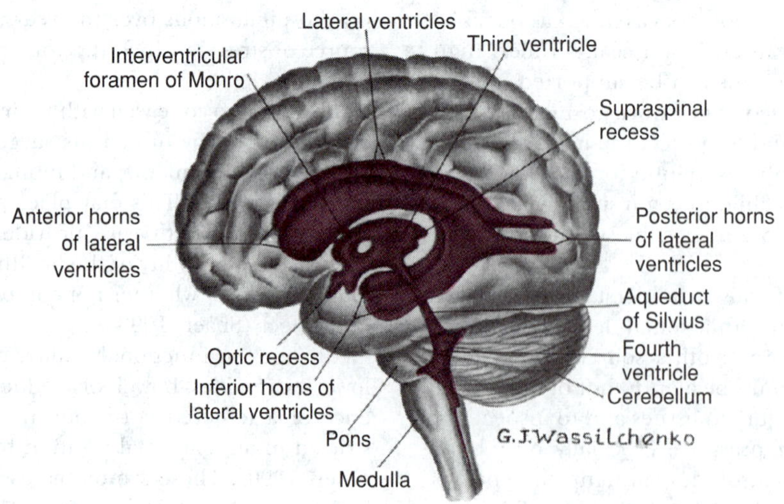

FIG. 11-4 Cerebral ventricular system. (From Thompson JM and others: *Mosby's clinical nursing,* ed 3, St Louis, 1993, Mosby.)

the sinuses, veins, brain substance, and dura also participate in absorption.

Mechanisms of Fluid Imbalance. The causes of hydrocephalus are varied, but the result is either (1) impaired absorption of CSF fluid within the subarachnoid space ***(communicating hydrocephalus)*** or (2) obstruction to the flow of CSF through the ventricular system ***(noncommunicating hydrocephalus).*** Rarely, a tumor of the choroid plexus causes increased CSF secretion. Any imbalance of secretion and absorption causes an increased accumulation of CSF in the ventricles, which become dilated and compress the brain substance against the surrounding rigid bony cranium. When this occurs before fusion of the cranial sutures, it provides enlargement of the skull, as well as dilation of the ventricles. In children under 10 to 12 years of age, previously closed suture lines, especially the sagittal suture, may become diastatic or opened (Swaiman, 1994).

Most cases of noncommunicating hydrocephalus are a result of developmental malformations. Although the defect usually is apparent in early infancy, it may become evident at any time from the prenatal period to late childhood or early adulthood. Other causes include neoplasms, infections, and trauma. An obstruction to the normal flow can occur at any point in the CSF pathway to produce increased pressure and dilation of the pathways proximal to the site of obstruction. Table 11-3 describes the most frequent sites of obstruction and the consequences.

Developmental defects (e.g., Arnold-Chiari malforma-

TABLE 11-3 Sites and Types of Hydrocephalus

SITE AND TYPE	CAUSES AND COMMENTS
NONCOMMUNICATING HYDROCEPHALUS	
Site: Aqueduct of Sylvius *Type:* Stenosis or atresia	Accounts for 20% of hydrocephalus Congenital (X-linked recessive in small number) Insidious onset of symptoms from birth to adulthood
Gliosis	Postinflammatory, usually secondary to perinatal infection or hemorrhage Prenatal maternal infection (toxoplasmosis)
Obstructive	Tumors of third ventricle or midbrain Ependymitis from maternal toxoplasmosis Congenital aneurysm of vein of Galen
Type: Posthemorrhagic	Blood from intraventricular hemorrhage in germinal matrix—seen as most common type of hydrocephalus in preterm infants
Site: Fourth ventricle or subarachnoid pathway	Intraventricular hemorrhage, postinflammatory conditions, or tumors
Type: Posthemorrhagic	Blood from intraventricular hemorrhage in germinal matrix—seen as most common type of hydrocephalus in preterm infants
Site: Fourth ventricle and foramen magnum	Accounts for 50% of all hydrocephalus
Type: Chiari malformations	Accounts for 40% of fourth ventricle obstructions
Type 1	A neural tube defect with herniation of medulla through foramen magnum; may be asymptomatic; similar to type 2, but more mild
Type 2 (Arnold-Chiari malformation)	A more severe defect; downward displacement of brainstem, fourth ventricle, and lower parts of cerebellum through foramen magnum with fixed attachment of spinal cord at site of a myelomeningocele
Type 3	High cervical or occipitocervical myelomeningocele with cervical herniation through body defect
Absence or occlusion of ventricles	Congenital (Dandy-Walker syndrome) caused by obstruction of foramina of Luschka and Magendie Tumors of posterior fossa (e.g., medulloblastoma) cause pressure on surrounding tissues to produce obstruction Less often: subdural hematoma, bacterial or granulomatous meningitis
COMMUNICATING HYDROCEPHALUS	
Site: Arachnoid villi and cisterna magna	Obstruction by thick arachnoid membrane or meninges
Type: Meningitis	Bacterial or granulomatous Acute phase: clumping of purulent fluid in drainage channels Chronic phase: organization of blood and exudate that results in fibrosis of subarachnoid spaces
Prenatal maternal infections	Toxoplasmosis, cytomegalic inclusion disease, mumps
Meningeal malignancy	Secondary to leukemia or lymphoma
Arachnoid cyst	Located in basal cistern or (uncommon) over cerebral cortex
Tuberculosis, fungal, or parasitic infection	More common in children ages 2 to 10 years

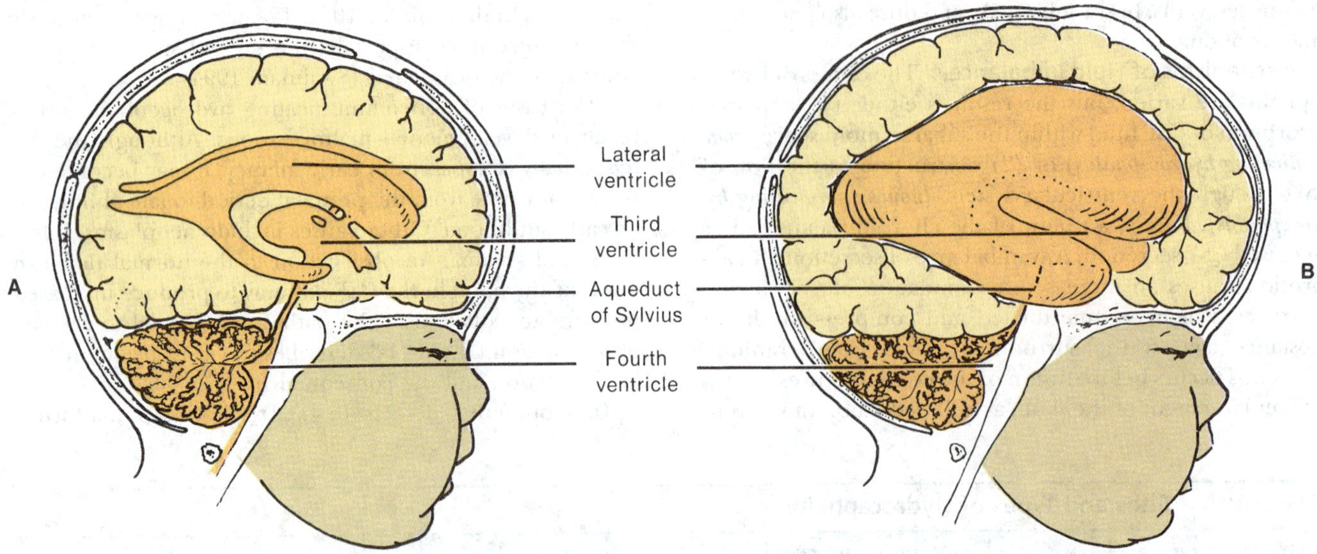

FIG. 11-5 Hydrocephalus: a block in flow of cerebrospinal fluid. **A,** Patent cerebrospinal fluid circulation. **B,** Enlarged lateral and third ventricles caused by obstruction of circulation—stenosis of aqueduct of Sylvius.

tions [see following discussion], aqueduct stenosis, aqueduct gliosis, and atresia of the foramina of Luschcka and Magendie [Dandy-Walker syndrome] account for most cases of hydrocephalus from birth to 2 years of age. ***Dandy-Walker malformation*** represents a disorder of the midline CNS indicative of marked genetic and etiologic factors. A female predominance of 3:1 is noted (Pascual-Castroviejo, 1991). Hydrocephalus is so often associated with myelomeningocele that all such infants should be observed for its development. In the remainder of cases there is a history of intrauterine infection, perinatal hemorrhage (anoxic or traumatic), and neonatal meningoencephalitis (bacterial or viral). In older children hydrocephalus is most often the result of intracranial masses (vascular anomalies, cysts, tumors), preexisting developmental defects, intracranial infections, trauma, or hemorrhage.

Arnold-Chiari Malformations (ACMs). ACM is a brain defect involving posterior fossa contents; the major types are described in Table 11-3. The type 2 malformation, seen almost exclusively with myelomeningocele, is characterized by herniation of a small cerebellum, medulla, pons, and fourth ventricle into the cervical spinal canal through an enlarged foramen magnum. The resulting obstruction of CSF flow causes the hydrocephalus.

Clinical Manifestations

The two factors that influence the clinical picture in hydrocephalus are the acuity of onset and the presence of preexisting structural lesions. In infancy before closure of the cranial sutures, head enlargement is the predominant sign, whereas in older infants and children the lesions responsible for hydrocephalus produce other neurologic signs through pressure on adjacent structures.

Infancy. In infants with hydrocephalus the head grows at an abnormal rate, although the first signs may be bulging fontanels without head enlargement (Fig. 11-5). The anterior fontanel is tense, often bulging, and nonpulsatile. Scalp veins are dilated and markedly so when the infant cries. With the increase in intracranial volume the bones of the skull become thin and the sutures become palpably separated to produce the ***cracked-pot sound (Macewen sign)*** on percussion of the skull. There may be frontal enlargement or ***bossing*** with depressed eyes, and the eyes may be rotated downward, producing a ***setting-sun sign*** (Fig. 11-6), in which the sclera may be visible above the pupil. Pupils are sluggish, with unequal response to light.

The infant is irritable and lethargic, feeds poorly, and may display changes in level of consciousness, opisthotonos (often extreme), and lower extremity spasticity. The infant cries when picked up or rocked and quiets when allowed to lie still. Early infantile reflexes may persist, and normally expected responses may not appear, indicating failure in the development of normal cortical inhibition.

Infants with ACM may exhibit behaviors that reflect cranial nerve dysfunction as a result of brainstem compression, including swallowing difficulties, stridor, apnea, aspiration, respiratory difficulties, and arm weakness. There may be absent or diminished gag reflex (Anderson, 1989).

The preterm infant with posthemorrhagic hydrocephalus may not exhibit any clinical signs and symptoms seen in other conditions. Ventricular dilation is assessed by ultrasonography or CT scanning in preterm infants at high risk for intraventricular hemorrhage (Merenstein and Gardner, 1993).

If hydrocephalus is allowed to progress, development of lower brainstem functions is disrupted, as manifested by difficulty in sucking and feeding and a shrill, brief, high-pitched cry. Eventually the skull becomes enormous and the cortex is destroyed. If the hydrocephalus is rapidly progressive, the infant may display emesis, somnolence, seizures,

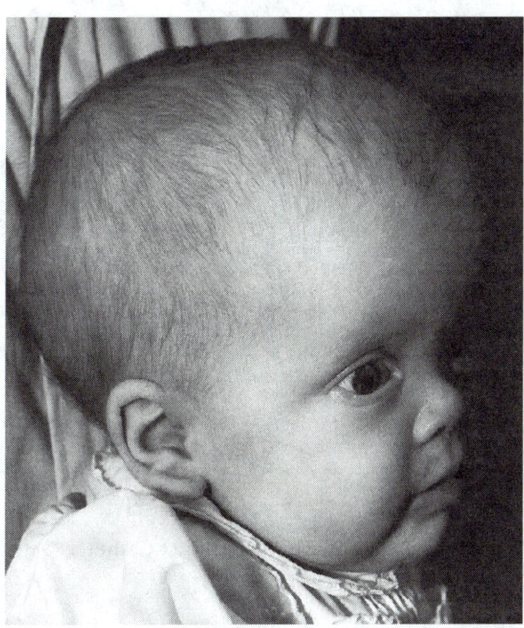

FIG. 11-6 Three-month-old infant with hydrocephalus. The setting-sun sign (forced downward eye deviation) is a neurologic sign unique to hydrocephalus. (From McCullough DC: *Pediatric neurosurgery,* Philadelphia, 1989, WB Saunders.)

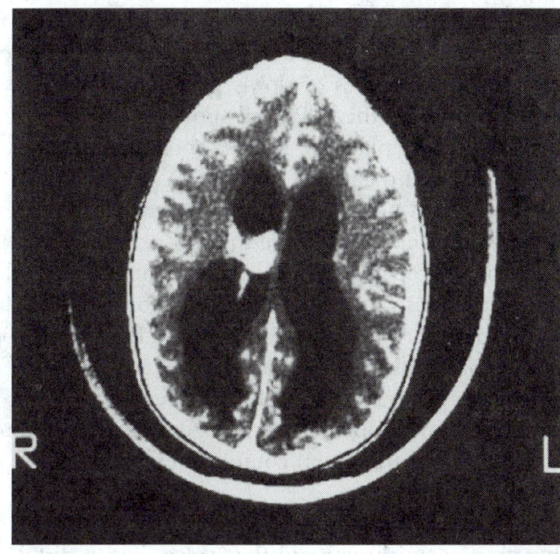

FIG. 11-7 CT scan reveals enlarged ventricles of child with hydrocephalus.

and cardiopulmonary distress. Severely affected infants usually do not survive the neonatal period.

Childhood. The signs and symptoms in early to late childhood are caused by increased ICP, and specific manifestations are related to the focal lesion. Most commonly resulting from posterior fossa neoplasms and aqueduct stenosis, the clinical manifestations are primarily those associated with space-occupying lesions, (i.e., headache on awakening with improvement following emesis or upright posture, papilledema, strabismus, and extrapyramidal tract signs such as ataxia [see Chapter 37]). As with infants, the child will be irritable, lethargic, apathetic, confused, and often incoherent. In one of the congenital defects with later onset, the Dandy-Walker syndrome, characteristic manifestations are bulging occiput, nystagmus, ataxia, and cranial nerve palsies.

Manifestations of ACM in children over 3 years of age are related to spinal cord dysfunction rather than brainstem compression as observed in infants. Commonly seen are scoliosis proximal to the level of the myelomeningocele (usually associated with ACM) and development of upper extremity spasticity, which may progress to weakness and atrophy. Cranial nerve deficits are rare (Anderson, 1989).

Diagnostic Evaluation

In infancy the diagnosis of hydrocephalus is based on head circumference that crosses one or more grid lines on the measurement chart within a period of 2 to 4 weeks and on associated neurologic signs that are present and progressive. However, other diagnostic studies are needed to localize the site of CSF obstruction. Routine daily head circumference measurements are carried out in infants with myelomeningocele, hemorrhage, and intracranial infections. In evaluation of a premature infant, specially adapted head circumference charts are consulted to distinguish abnormal head growth from rapid head growth that takes place normally.

The primary diagnostic tools for detecting hydrocephalus are CT and MRI (Fig. 11-7). Sedation is required, since the child must remain absolutely still for an accurate picture. Diagnostic evaluation of children who have symptoms of hydrocephalus after infancy is similar to that employed in those with a suspected intracranial tumor. In the neonate echoencephalography is useful in comparing the ratio of lateral ventricle to cortex. Sometimes isotope ventriculograms are used to assess the flow and patency of existing shunts and check the size of the ventricles.

Problems in differential diagnosis are related to the child whose head circumference is greater than the 95 percentile but whose head growth parallels the normal growth curve. It is sometimes valuable to measure parental occipitofrontal circumference (OFC) to detect a possible normal familial characteristic (benign familial megalencephaly). (See Table 37-2 for diagnostic tests for neurologic evaluation.)

Therapeutic Management

The treatment of hydrocephalus is directed toward (1) relief of the hydrocephalus, (2) treatment of complications, and (3) management of problems related to the effect of the disorder on psychomotor development. The treatment is, with few exceptions, surgical.

Medical therapy has been largely disappointing. Many newborn infants with progressive cranial enlargement secondary to intracranial hemorrhage demonstrate spontaneous stabilization and resolution. Serial lumbar punctures and medications have been used with varying success. The administration of acetazolamide and isosorbide or furosemide is somewhat beneficial in decreasing the production of CSF in selected cases of slowly progressive disease. The medication reduces the ICP until spontaneous arrest of hydrocephalus takes place or as a temporary measure when surgery is contraindicated.

Surgical Treatment. Improved techniques have established surgical treatment as the therapy of choice in almost all cases of hydrocephalus. This is accomplished by direct removal of an obstruction, such as resection of a neoplasm, cyst, or hematoma or, in rare instances of fluid overproduction, by choroid plexus extirpation (plexectomy or electric coagulation). However, most children require a shunt procedure that provides primary drainage of the CSF from the ventricles to an extracranial compartment, usually the peritoneum.

Most shunt systems consist of a ventricular catheter, a flush pump, a unidirectional flow valve, and a distal catheter. All are radiopaque for easy visualization after placement, and all are tested for accuracy before insertion. A reservoir is frequently added to allow direct access to the ventricular system for administration of medications and removal of fluid. In all models the valves are designed to open at a predetermined intraventricular pressure and close when the pressure falls below that level, thus preventing backflow of fluid. High-pressure valves are used to prevent complications from rapid decompression of the ventricles. Medium-pressure valves are used in most children, especially those with long-standing hydrocephalus. Low-pressure valves are used in small infants. Infants should not be held in a prolonged head-down position, because this interferes with unobstructed flow of CSF.

The preferred procedure is the ***ventriculoperitoneal (VP) shunt,*** especially in neonates and young infants (Fig. 11-8). There is greater allowance for excess tubing, which minimizes the number of revisions needed as the child grows. Since it requires repeated lengthening, the ***ventriculoatrial (VA) shunt*** (ventricle to right atrium) is reserved for older children who have attained most of their somatic growth and children with abdominal pathology. The VA shunt is contraindicated in children with cardiopulmonary disease or elevated CSF protein.

A ***ventricular bypass*** into intracranial channels may be used in older children with noncommunicating hydrocephalus caused by aqueduct stenosis or posterior fossa masses (e.g., medulloblastoma). Technical difficulties preclude its use in infants, since these spaces are poorly developed in the infant. ***Ventriculopleural shunts*** are sometimes used in children over 5 years of age. Other sites that are used occasionally for shunting include the facial vein and the subgaleal or subarachnoid spaces.

The initial shunt is placed when indicated based on individual assessment. There is wide variation in the time of revisions. In most instances revisions are performed when physical signs indicate shunt malfunction (i.e., signs of elevated ICP). Sometimes revisions are planned for specific times during development. In all mechanisms the initial success rate is relatively high; however, shunts are associated with complications that interfere with continued shunt function or that threaten the life of the child.

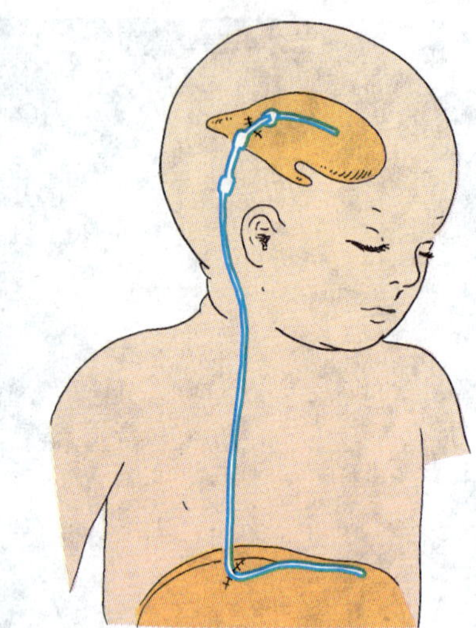

FIG. 11-8 Ventriculoperitoneal shunt. Catheter is threaded beneath the skin.

Complications. The major complications of VP shunts are infection and malfunction. All shunts are subject to mechanical difficulties, such as kinking, plugging, or separation and migration of tubing. Malfunction is most often caused by mechanical obstruction either within the ventricles from particulate matter (tissue or exudate) or at the distal end from thrombosis or displacement as a result of growth. Functional obstruction of a shunt's antisiphon device remains a common complication. The probability of shunt malfunction within 1 year was 40% in one study. (daSilva and Drake, 1992). In another study, disconnections in the system accounted for 15% of the malfunctions (Aldrich and Harmann, 1991). The child with a shunt obstruction often presents as an emergency with clinical manifestations of increased ICP, frequently accompanied by worsening neurologic status.

The most serious complication, shunt infection, can occur at any time, but the period of greatest risk is 1 to 2 months following placement. The infection is generally the result of intercurrent infections at the time of shunt placement. Infections include septicemia, bacterial endocarditis, wound infection, shunt nephritis, meningitis, and ventriculitis. Brain abscess associated with colonic perforation and infection with a gram-negative enteric organism suggests an ascending shunt infection in a child who has a VP shunt. Meningitis and ventriculitis are of greatest concern, since any complicating CNS infection is a significant predictor of intellectual outcome. Infection is treated with massive doses of antibiotics administered intravenously. A persistent infection requires removal of the shunt until the infection is controlled. External ventricular drainage (EVD) is used until CSF is sterile. EVD allows removal of CSF from a tube placed in the child's ventricle that flows by gravity into a collection device.

Another serious shunt-related complication is subdural hematoma caused by too rapid reduction of ICP and size. This usually can be averted by careful assessment of ICP before insertion of the shunt and use of correct valvular pressure. Other complications that may occur include peritonitis, abdominal abscesses, perforation of abdominal organs by catheter or trochar (at time of insertion), fistulas, hernias, and ileus.

Prognosis. The prognosis of children with treated hydrocephalus depends largely on the rate at which hydrocephalus develops, the duration of raised ICP, the frequency of complications, and the cause of the hydrocephalus. For example, malignant tumors may have a high mortality regardless of other complicating factors.

Untreated, hydrocephalus has a 50% to 60% mortality rate caused by the disorder or intercurrent illnesses. In the survivors there is a high incidence of subnormal intellectual capacity, and a large majority have major physical and/or disabling neurologic handicaps such as ataxia, spastic diplegia, poor fine motor coordination, and perceptual deficits. Spontaneous arrest occurs occasionally in approximately 40% of those with near-normal intelligence.

Surgically treated hydrocephalus with continued neurosurgical and medical management has a survival rate of about 80%, with the highest incidence of mortality occurring within the first year of treatment. Of the surviving children approximately one half are intellectually normal. Inattentiveness and hyperactivity are significant behavioral problems in children with both hydrocephalus and mental retardation. The presence of additional medical problems in infancy, including ocular defects, is the most significant variable associated with a high likelihood of mental retardation (Donder, Canady, and Rourke, 1990).

Hydrocephalus in association with myelomeningocele and meningitic complications has a less favorable prognosis. In some children irreversible damage may have been produced by the hydrocephalus or from the original infection; in addition, there are sometimes coincidental cerebral defects. Generally, noninfective hydrocephalus appears to have the best prognosis.

Nursing Considerations

Preoperatively the infant with diagnosed or suspected hydrocephalus is observed carefully for signs of increasing ICP. In infants the head is measured daily at the point of largest measurement—the occipitofrontal circumference (OFC) (see Chapter 7 for technique). To avoid the likelihood of wide discrepancies, the point at which the measurements are taken is indicated on the head with a marking pen. Fontanels and suture lines are gently palpated for size, signs of bulging, tenseness, and separation. An infant with hydrocephalus and normal ICP will display bulging under certain circumstances such as straining or crying; therefore such accompanying behavior is noted. Irritability, lethargy, or seizure activity, as well as altered vital signs and feeding behavior, may indicate advancing pathology.

In older children, who are usually admitted to the hospital for elective or emergency shunt revision, the most valuable indicator of increasing ICP is an alteration in the child's level of consciousness and interaction with the environment. Changes are identified by observing and comparing present behavior with customary behavior, sleep patterns, developmental capabilities, and habits obtained through a detailed history and a baseline assessment. This baseline information serves as a guide for postoperative assessment and evaluation of shunt function.

General nursing care of the infant with hydrocephalus may present special problems. Maintaining adequate nutrition often requires flexible feeding schedules to accommodate diagnostic procedures, since feeding before or after handling can precipitate vomiting. Small feedings at more frequent intervals are often better tolerated than larger ones spaced farther apart. These infants are often difficult to feed and require extra time and innovation.

The nurse is responsible for preparing the child for diagnostic tests such as MRI or a CT scan, and for assisting with procedures such as a ventricular tap, which is often performed to relieve excessive pressure and to obtain CSF during the preoperative period. Sedation is required, since the child must remain absolutely still during diagnostic testing. Drugs commonly used for these procedures include nembutal and chloral hydrate. (See Chapter 27 for preparing children for procedures.) If surgery is anticipated, intravenous infusions should not be placed in a scalp vein.

➤ **NURSING TIP** Oral administration of chloral hydrate, a bitter-tasting liquid, may be given to an infant by the "nipple method." Place the nipple without the bottle in the mouth, add 5 ml of dextrose water to initiate sucking, then add the sedative, and finish with another 5 ml of dextrose water.

Fortunately, almost all children with hydrocephalus are recognized, and treatment is begun early. For those children with significant head enlargement, care must be exercised to see that the head is well supported when the infant is fed or moved to prevent extra strain on the infant's neck, and measures must be taken to prevent development of pressure areas. Not infrequently, infants with irreversible brain damage or with severe developmental defects such as hydroencephaly, in which both cerebral hemispheres fail to develop and are replaced with a membranous sac filled with CSF, are placed in long-term care facilities specially designed for care of these infants.

Postoperative Care. In addition to routine postoperative care and observation, the infant or child is positioned carefully on the unoperated side to prevent pressure on the shunt valve. The child is kept flat to help avert complications resulting from too rapid reduction of intracranial fluid. When the ventricular size is reduced too rapidly, the cerebral cortex may pull away from the dura and tear the small interlacing veins, producing a subdural hematoma. This is not a problem in children with elective shunt revision, since their intraventricular size and pressure have been normal. The surgeon indicates the position to be maintained and the extent of activity allowed. If there is increased ICP, the surgeon will prescribe the head of the bed to be elevated and/or allow the child to sit up to enhance gravity flow through the shunt.

NURSING ALERT Do not pump the shunt to assess function, because this may pull choroid plexuses into the ventricular slits of the shunt tubing. The result may cause blockage, headache by decreasing CSF too rapidly, or obstruction of the peritoneal end of the catheter.

Observation for signs of increased ICP, which indicate obstruction of the shunt, is continued. Neurologic assessment includes pupil dilation (pressure causes compression or stretching of the oculomotor nerve, producing dilation on the same side as the pressure) and blood pressure (hypoxia to the brainstem causes variability in these vital signs). The child is also observed for abdominal distention because CSF may cause peritonitis or a postoperative ileus as a complication of distal catheter placement.

Intake and output are carefully monitored. Children are often placed on fluid restriction with nothing by mouth (NPO) for 24 to 48 hours. The intravenous infusion is closely monitored to prevent fluid overload. Routine feeding is resumed after the prescribed NPO period, but the presence of bowel sounds is determined before feeding children with VP shunts.

Since infection is the greatest hazard of the postoperative period, nurses are continually on the alert for the usual manifestations of CSF infection, which may include elevated vital signs, poor feeding, vomiting, decreased responsiveness, and seizure activity. There may be signs of local inflammation at the operative sites and along the shunt tract. Antibiotics are administered by the intravenous route as ordered, and the nurse may also need to assist with intraventricular instillation. The incision site is inspected for leakage, and any suspected drainage is tested for glucose, an indication of CSF (see Critical Thinking Exercise box).

Meticulous skin care is continued postoperatively, with extra care taken to prevent tissue damage from pressure. Pressure-reducing beds or mattresses may be needed to prevent pressure on prominent areas. The skin is inspected regularly for any signs of pressure, irritation, or infection.

Family Support. Specific needs and concerns of parents during periods of hospitalization are related to the reason for the child's hospitalization (shunt revision, infection, diagnosis) and the diagnostic and/or surgical procedures to which the child must be subjected. Parents may have very little understanding of anatomy; therefore they need further exploration and reinforcement of information that was given to them by the physician and neurosurgeon, as well as information about what they can expect. They are especially frightened of any procedure that involves the brain, and the fear of retardation of brain damage is very real and pervasive. Nurses can allay their anxiety with explanations of the rationale underlying the various nursing and medical activities such as positioning or testing and by simply being available and willing to listen to their concerns.

To prepare for the child's discharge and home care, the parents are instructed on how to recognize signs that indicate shunt malfunction or infection. Active children may have injuries, such as a fall, that can damage the shunt, and the tubing may pull out of the distal insertion site or become disconnected during normal growth.

The management of hydrocephalus in a child is a demanding task for both family and health professionals, and helping the family cope with the child is an important nursing responsibility. Children with hydrocephalus have lifelong special health care needs. The nurse can provide optimum primary health care, including recommended immunizations, treatments for common infectious conditions, or child care and school regulations. The overall aim is to establish realistic goals and an appropriate educational program that will assist the child in achieving the optimum potential. Families can be referred to community agencies for support and guidance. The **National Hydrocephalus Foundation (NHF)*** provides information on the condition for families and assists interested groups in establishing local organizations. Helpful booklets are available from this and other sources.

Anticipatory guidance will prepare parents for possible problems and help them to avoid being overprotective of the child. There need be few restrictions placed on the child's activities (mainly contact sports), and the child is encouraged to live as would any other youngster of the same age and abilities. Parents need support and encouragement in coping with the child and problems the child may encounter in relationships with peers and others. Reactions of other children when the child has a noticeably enlarged head or requires shaving at times of revision are stressful situations for both child and parents (see Chapter 22 for problems and coping with the child with a disability). (See also Nursing Care Plan: The Infant with Hydrocephalus.†)

CRITICAL THINKING EXERCISE

Hydrocephalus

A 3-week-old infant is 8 days postoperative for hydrocephalus that developed following a primary repair of a meningomyelocele. The infant weighs 7.5 pounds and has been taking 90 to 120 ml of formula every 4 hours without problems. Within the last few hours the infant has become agitated and fussy, and only took 15 ml of formula. Given the history and the fact that the infant has a ventriculoperitoneal shunt, the best intervention is to:

1. Request sedation for the infant.
2. Gavage the rest of the feeding to make up the calories and fluids required.
3. Pump the shunt reservoir with the infant in Trendelenburg position.
4. Measure the OFC; observe the shunt site for redness, edema, and drainage; take an axillary temperature; and call the neurosurgeon.

The correct answer is 4. The most common cause of such behavior in infants with shunts is shunt failure. Infection may be a cause of failure; therefore monitoring the temperature and evaluating the shunt site is also important.

Arbitrary pumping of the shunt may cause more problems and should only be done by a physician. Sedation is not indicated in this instance, or at least not until the infant's neurologic status has been evaluated. Gavage feeding may replenish the infant's caloric and fluid requirements but is not the priority; poor feeding often indicates shunt failure and/or subsequent increased ICP. Vomiting, setting-sun sign, and greatly increased OFC may not be seen in newborns with increased ICP.

*Route 1, River Rd., Box 210 A, Joliet, IL 60436; (815) 467-6548.

†In *Wong and Whaley's Clinical Manual of Pediatric Nursing* (Mosby).

CRANIAL DEFORMITIES

In the normal newborn the cranial sutures are separated by membranous seams several millimeters wide. For the first few hours to 1 to 2 days after birth, the cranial bones are highly mobile, which allows the cranial bones to mold and slide over one another, adjusting the circumference of the head to accommodate to the changing shape and character of the birth canal. The principal sutures in the infant's skull are the sagittal, coronal, and lambdoidal sutures, and the major soft areas at the juncture of these sutures are the anterior and posterior fontanels (see Fig. 8-6).

Following birth, growth of the skull bones occurs in a direction *perpendicular* (at right angles) to the line of the suture, and normal closure occurs in a regular and predictable order. Although there are wide variations in the age at which closure takes place in individual children, solid union of all sutures is not completed until very late childhood. Normally sutures and fontanels are ossified by the following ages:

8 weeks—Posterior fontanel closed
6 months—Fibrous union of suture lines and interlocking of serrated edges
18 months—Anterior fontanel closed
10 to 12 years—Sutures unable to be separated by ICP

Closure of a suture before the expected time inhibits the perpendicular growth. Since normal increase in brain volume requires expansion, the skull is forced to grow in a direction *parallel* to the fused suture. This alteration in skull growth always produces a distortion of the head shape when the underlying brain growth is normal. The small head with closed sutures and normal shape is the result of deficient brain growth; the suture closure is secondary to this brain growth failure. Failure of brain growth is not secondary to suture closure.

Various types of cranial deformities are encountered in early infancy. These include the enlarged head with frontal protrusion, or bossing (characteristic of hydrocephalus), the parietal bossing that is seen in chronic subdural hematoma, the small head, and a variety of skull deformities (Fig. 11-9). Some occur during prenatal development; in others, head circumference is usually within normal limits at birth, and the deviation from normal development becomes apparent with advancing age.

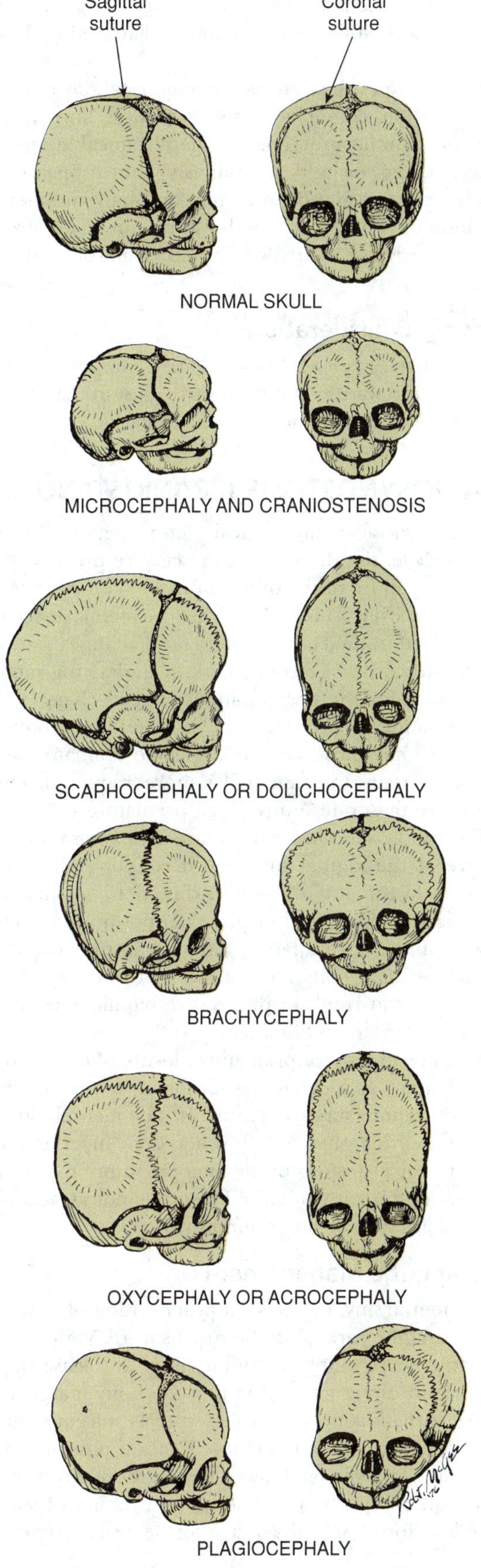

FIG. 11-9 Craniostenosis. Abnormal head configuration resulting from premature closing of cranial sutures.

MICROCEPHALY

Primary microcephaly reflects a small brain and may be caused by an autosomal-recessive disorder, a chromosomal abnormality, or application of a toxic stimulus during the period of induction and major cell migration in prenatal development. These stimuli may be irradiation (especially between 4 and 20 weeks of gestation), maternal infection (notably toxoplasmosis, rubella, or cytomegalovirus), or chemical agents. ***Secondary microcephaly*** can result from a variety of insults that occur during the third trimester of pregnancy, the perinatal period, or early infancy. Infection, trauma, metabolic disorders, and anoxia are all capable of causing decreased brain growth and early closure of cranial sutures. Microcephaly is defined as an OFC greater than 3 standard deviations below the mean (Fanaroff and Martin, 1992).

In both types the neurologic manifestations range from decerebration, complete unresponsiveness, and/or autistic behavior to mild motor impairment, educable mental retardation, and/or mild hyperkinesis. There appears to be a decided relationship between microcephaly and mental retardation of varying degrees; however, not all children with microcephaly are mentally retarded (Fanaroff and Martin, 1992).

Nursing Considerations

There is no treatment. Nursing care is supportive and may be directed toward helping parents adjust to rearing a child with cognitive impairment (see Chapter 24).

CRANIOSYNOSTOSIS (CRANIOSTENOSIS)

In craniosynostosis the clinical picture depends on which sutures close, the duration of the closure process, and the success or failure of the other sutures to compensate by expansion (see Fig. 11-9). Focal hydrodynamic mechanisms are involved in the compensatory skull changes seen in craniosynostosis. Brain atrophy and an underlying motor delay account for the position-induced skull changes (Chadduck, Chadduck, and Boop, 1992). Skull films confirm the type of craniosynostosis; CT is used to evaluate the intracranial contents. Increased ICP is more frequent in children with more than one suture fused prematurely.

The most common form of craniosynostosis is premature closure of the sagittal suture with resulting elongation of the skull in the anteroposterior direction. (A similar head shape is seen as a result of postnatal position maintenance in some premature infants.) Craniosynostosis causes some increase in ICP, which may or may not cause mental retardation but can result in progressive papilledema, optic atrophy, and eventual blindness.

Trigonocephaly, or premature closure of the metopic suture in utero, is a congenital problem that is familial and may not require surgical treatment. The metopic suture occurs where the right and left frontal bone meet on the forehead. Craniosynostosis of the metopic suture may be an autosomal dominantly inherited disorder not associated with functional brain or other abnormalities.

Therapeutic Management

Treatment, if any, involves surgical excision of long bars of bone along or parallel to the fused suture. Various surgical procedures are employed in an effort to release the fused suture and direct growth. Lining the bony margins of the suture with silicone to delay closure is infrequently used. Surgery is performed to achieve the best possible cosmetic effect and, in severe cases, to relieve cerebral pressure symptoms and complications. The advised timing of suture release is before 6 months of age for best cosmetic results.

Nursing Considerations

Nursing care is primarily observation for signs of hemorrhage or infection. Following cranial surgery, pressure bandages are applied and carefully maintained to reduce swelling. Because of the type of bone surgery involved with craniosynostosis, the hematocrit and hemoglobin are carefully monitored. Parents may also wish to provide a compatible blood donor for their infant. Nurses need to inform and guide parents through this blood bank procedure.

Early surgical management of craniosynostosis allows proper expansion of the brain and the creation of an acceptable appearance. Parents require special support and education during this time, especially from other parents whose infants have undergone similar operations. The nurse can serve as a liasion for this type of parental support.

CRANIOFACIAL ABNORMALITIES

Craniofacial abnormalities are those deformities involving the skull and facial bones. They have a low incidence rate in the population, but their effects can be psychologically devastating to affected children and their families. Deformities caused by abnormal growth of cranial bone(s) are listed in the box below.

The disorders are compatible with life; therefore, unless they are corrected or modified, affected children go through their growing period under the burden of a grotesque, freaklike appearance often so severe that parents keep their children away from school, playmates, and sometimes even siblings. Children with Apert syndrome and other craniofacial abnormalities continue to face erroneous assumptions of mental retardation and social stigmatization because of their appearance. For these children to achieve their full potential for intellectual growth, physical competence, and social acceptance, families and health care professionals must play a critical role.

Therapeutic Management

Surgical correction of defects involves peeling the patient's face away from the skull and remolding the understructures. Parts can be brought together, the skull reshaped, and pieces removed. The procedures are performed at various ages, depending on the anomaly, in centers specializ-

CRANIAL ABNORMALITIES CAUSED BY ABNORMAL BONE GROWTH

Hypertelorism—Wide spacing between the eyes
Crouzon disease—Craniofacial dysostosis (abnormal ossification of fetal cartilages) with shallow orbits and underdevelopment of the middle third of the face
Apert syndrome—Craniostenosis resulting in a pointed head; may be extracranial abnormalities, such as syndactyly (webbing) of fingers and toes and cardiac defects
Treacher Collins syndrome—Asymmetric facial deformity including absent cheekbones, underslung jaw, and small chin; there is also downward slant of the eyes and other minor defects
Pierre Robin syndrome—Displacement of the chin as a result of micrognathia (mandibular hypoplasia) or retrognathia (normal-sized mandible positioned posteriorly); there is also glossoptosis with obstruction of the airway, and a cleft palate may be present

ing in this pediatric problem. The timing of surgery is before school entry and is determined on an individual basis to ensure normal growth. Depending on the abnormality, other surgeries are performed, such as mandibular and digit correction. Following surgery, continued growth conforming to the inborn abnormality is unlikely.

Nursing Considerations

Nursing efforts are directed toward preparation for surgery (there may be several surgical procedures over a period of time), postoperative care similar to care of any child with cranial surgery, and support of the child and family. There is frequently adjustment to the unfamiliar body image, which may be as traumatic as the previous deformity. A helmet is worn to protect the operative site and bone grafts for varying lengths of time, from 6 months to 2 years. Follow-up care is very important.

PLAGIOCEPHALY

Plagiocephaly is a rhomboid-shaped deformity that occurs in at least 1 of 300 live births and is rarely caused by brain malformation or unilateral suture stenosis. The rapidly growing infant head is easily molded by continued pressure against a surface, such as the uterine wall or a mattress. As a result, the skull is progressively flattened.

Therapeutic Management

Operative treatment for asymmetric cranioorbital deformity is indicated for functional, aesthetic, and psychosocial reasons. Early operation in infancy (3 to 6 months) is recommended. Plagiocephaly is a subform of premature closure of the craniofacial skeleton that is progressive. A recent innovation for this condition involves application of a helmet constructed of polypropylene shaped normally but large enough to fit the largest diameter of the head. Treatment is begun at 4 to 10 months of age, and the helmet is worn until the head conforms to the shape of the helmet.

Nursing Considerations

An important nursing function is helping to identify children with significant deformity and referring them for evaluation. Nursing care of the surgical patient is the same as that for other children with similar surgery. Care of the child with helmet therapy involves teaching parents the importance of making certain that the child wears the device as prescribed. Mild unpleasant scalp odors that develop are controlled by daily washing of both scalp and helmet.

SKELETAL DEFECTS*

This discussion is limited to those defects in development that are most common, that are amenable to therapy, and that involve nurses to a considerable extent. Less common defects and disorders are listed in Table 11-4.

*Patricia L. King, RN, MS, revised this section.

DEVELOPMENTAL DYSPLASIA OF THE HIP (DDH)

The broad term ***developmental dysplasia of the hip*** describes a group of disorders related to abnormal development of the hip. A change in terminology from congenital hip dysplasia (CHD) and congenital dislocation of the hip (CDH) to DDH more properly reflects a variety of hip abnormalities in which there is a shallow acetabulum, subluxation, or dislocation (Pediatric Orthopaedic Society of North America [POSNA], 1991) (see box on p. 465). DDH has an incidence of 1 to 2 cases per 1000 live births in the United States. It occurs more commonly in females at a ratio of 6:1 (Bennett and MacEwen, 1989). One fifth of the cases involve both hips, and when only one hip is involved, the left hip is affected three times more often than the right.

Etiology and Pathophysiology

The cause of DDH is unknown, but certain factors such as gender, birth order, family history, intrauterine position, delivery type, joint laxity, and postnatal positioning are believed to affect the risk of DDH. A striking relationship exists between the development of dislocation and methods of handling infants. Among the cultures with the highest incidence of dislocation (Navajo Indians and Canadian Eskimos), newly born infants are tightly wrapped in blankets or other swaddling material or are strapped to cradle boards. In cultures where mothers carry infants on their backs or hips in the widely abducted straddle position, such as in the Far East and Africa, the disorder is virtually unknown.

Prenatal factors that are considered to influence development of hip abnormalities are maternal hormone secretion and mechanical factors of intrauterine posture. Toward the end of pregnancy there is increased maternal pelvic laxity mediated by maternal hormone secretion (principally estrogen), which affects the fetal joints as well. All joints are more lax in the newborn period, and the greater incidence of hip dislocation in females may be explained by their greater reactivity to the maternal hormones.

Reliable evidence indicates an association between a higher incidence of developmental hip deformities with breech presentations and cesarean section (often necessitated by abnormal intrauterine position). The position of the legs in frank breech position (i.e., with the hips acutely flexed and knees extended) is an important factor in the etiology of hip dislocation. The larger number of firstborn children may be related to this factor, since the breech position in first deliveries is nearly always a frank breech. Other prenatal factors that contribute to hip dysplasia include twinning and large infant size. A positive family history increases the risk. If one child has DDH, there is a 6% chance that each sibling will also have it. If one parent and one child have DDH, the risk to subsequent children is 36%.

Three degrees of DDH are illustrated in Fig. 11-10 and outlined in the box on p. 465. Also, mounting evidence lends support to the suggestion that there are two types of DDH: the common type due to laxity of the supporting capsule and another type as a result of an abnormality of the

TABLE 11-4 Congenital Defects Involving the Skeleton

DISORDER	DESCRIPTION AND ANATOMIC VARIATION	THERAPY
Achondroplasia	Inherited (autosomal dominant) Defect in ossification at the epiphyseal plate, resulting in very short limbs, large head, and lordosis	None
Osteogenesis imperfecta	Inherited (autosomal dominant, autosomal recessive) Characterized by brittle, fragile, and easily fractured bones Intrauterine fractures may produce congenital deformities	Reduction of fractures Careful handling of extremities See Chapter 39
Pes planus (flatfoot)	Normal finding in infancy May be result of muscular weakness in older child	Rarely indicated Wedge on inner side of heel and sole for persistent or severe cases
Pes valgus	Eversion of entire foot but sole rests on ground	Exercises
Pes varus	Inversion of entire foot but sole rests on ground	Exercises
Metatarsus valgus	Eversion of forefoot while heel remains straight Also called toeing out or duck walk	Passive exercises
Talipes deformities	See p. 469	
Supernumerary digits (polydactyly)	Excessive number of fingers, toes, or both; usually inherited (autosomal dominant)	No treatment, or amputation of extra digits to improve function or for cosmetic reasons
Genu varum (bowleg)	May be congenital, result of rickets, or caused by osteochondrosis of proximal tibial epiphysis	Corrective splinting Osteostomy in severe or neglected cases
Genu recurvatum (back knee)	Congenital, result of prenatal developmental defect or abnormal intrauterine position Developmental, result of postnatal trauma or infection	Repeated corrective casting Exercises
Klippel-Feil syndrome	Absence of one or more cervical vertebrae and two or more fused together Neck short and limited in motion Sometimes kyphosis and scoliosis	Rarely indicated Scapula brought down and fixed if marked deformity or loss of function Bracing of spinal deformities
Arachnodactyly (Marfan syndrome)	Inherited (autosomal dominant) Abnormal length of fingers, toes, and extremities; hypermobility of joints; defects of spine and chest (pigeon breast); other associated abnormalities	Supportive measures
Congenital spine deformities	Kyphosis, scoliosis, lordosis, or a combination of these	Prevention of progression of defect with growth Casting and/or bracing Operative stabilization of affected vertebrae
Arthrogryposis multiplex congenita	Incomplete fibrous ankylosis of many or all joints (except spine and jaw) associated with hypoplasia of attached muscles Contracture deformities—some extension, others flexion	Bracing, splinting, corrective surgery, and rehabilitation efforts

acetabulum. The excessive laxity of the joint may prevent detection in early infancy. The femoral head remains in contact with the acetabulum until additional stress (such as standing) moves it away.

Clinical Manifestations

The diagnosis of DDH should be made in the ***newborn period*** if possible, since treatment initiated before 2 months of age achieves the highest rate of success. In the newborn period dysplasia usually appears as hip joint laxity rather than as outright dislocation. Subluxation and the tendency to dislocate can be demonstrated by the Ortolani or Barlow tests. With the infant relaxed in the supine position and the legs facing the examiner, the hips are flexed at right angles and the knees are flexed. The examiner places the middle finger of each hand over the greater trochanter and the thumbs on the inner side of the thigh at a point opposite the lesser trochanter. The knees are carried to midabduction, and each hip joint in turn is submitted first to forward pressure exerted behind the trochanter and second to backward pressure exerted from the thumbs in front as the opposite joint is held steady. If the femoral head can be felt to slip forward into the acetabulum on pressure from behind, it has been dislocated ***(Ortolani test)*** (Fig. 11-11, *D*).

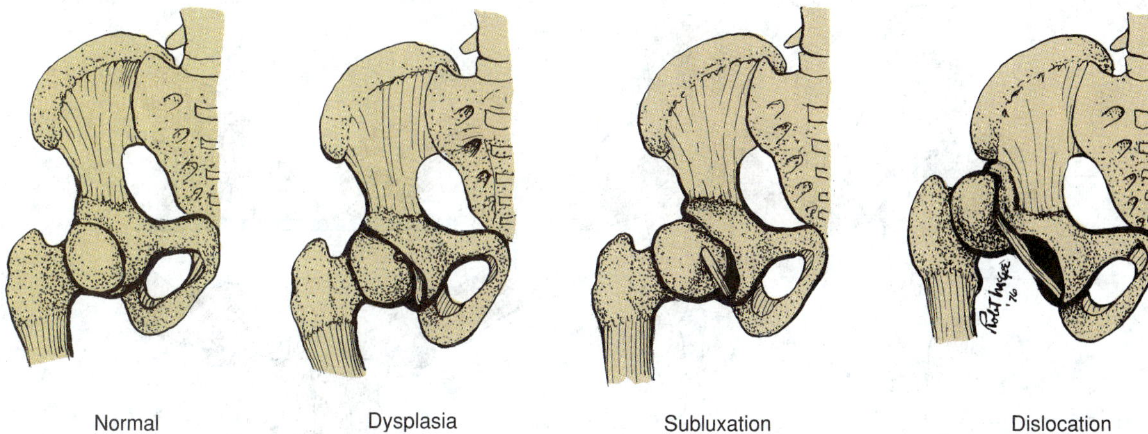

FIG. 11-10 Configuration and relationship of structures in developmental dysplasia of the hip.

DEGREES OF DEVELOPMENTAL DYSPLASIA OF THE HIP

Acetabular dysplasia (or **preluxation**)—The mildest form, in which there is neither subluxation nor dislocation. The dysplasia reflects an apparent delay in acetabular development evidenced by osseous hypoplasia of the acetabular roof, which is oblique and shallow, although the cartilaginous roof is comparatively intact. The femoral head remains in the acetabulum.

Subluxation—Accounts for the largest percentage of congenital hip dysplasias. Subluxation implies incomplete dislocation or disclosable hip and is sometimes regarded as an intermediate state in the development from primary dysplasia to complete dislocation. The femoral head remains in contact with the acetabulum, but a stretched capsule and ligamentum teres cause the head of the femur to be partially displaced. Pressure on the cartilaginous roof inhibits ossification and produces a flattening of the socket.

Dislocation—The femoral head loses contact with the acetabulum and is displaced posteriorly and superiorly over the fibrocartilaginous rim. The ligamentum teres is elongated and taut.

Sometimes an audible click can be heard on exit or entry of the femur out of or into the acetabulum. If, on pressure from the front, the femoral head is felt to slip out over the posterior lip of the acetabulum and immediately slips back in place when pressure is released, the hip is said to be dislocatable or "unstable" ***(Barlow test).***

NURSING ALERT These tests must be performed by experienced operators to prevent fracture or other damage to the hip. If these tests are performed too vigorously in the first 2 days of life, when the hip subluxates freely, persistent dislocation may occur.

The Ortolani and Barlow tests are most reliable from birth to 2 months of age. Adduction contractures develop at about 6 to 10 weeks, and the Ortolani sign disappears. After this time the most sensitive test is limited abduction (Fig. 11-11, *B*). Other signs are shortening of the limb on the affected side ***(Galleazzi sign, Allis sign)*** (Fig. 11-11, *C*), ***asymmetric thigh and gluteal folds*** (Fig. 11-11, *A*), and ***broadening of the perineum*** (in bilateral dislocation). Weight bearing may precipitate a transition from subluxation to dislocation in unrecognized cases. Often the disorder is not apparent at birth.

In the ***older infant*** and ***child*** the affected leg will be shorter than the other with telescoping or piston mobility, that is, the head of the femur can be felt to move up and down in the buttock when the extended thigh is pushed first toward the child's head and then pulled distally. Instability of the hip on weight bearing delays walking and produces a characteristic ***limp.*** When the child stands first on one foot and then on the other (holding onto a chair, rail, or someone's hands), bearing weight on the affected hip, the pelvis tilts downward on the normal side instead of upward as it would with normal stability ***(Trendelenburg sign)*** (Fig. 11-11, *E*). The practitioner should test the child for at least 30 seconds. In both unilateral and bilateral dislocations the greater trochanter is prominent and appears above a line from the anterosuperior iliac spine to the tuberosity of the ischium. The child with bilateral dislocations has marked ***lordosis*** and a peculiar ***waddling gait.***

Diagnostic Evaluation

The primary diagnostic tools in the newborn period are the assessment techniques just described. Although the disorder is usually identified in early infancy, there is also a category that cannot be detected at birth. Therefore ruling out DDH at birth does not provide security, and examination of the hip is carried out at each well-child visit in the event that a late-onset dislocation becomes evident. In older infants and children radiographic examination is useful in confirming the diagnosis. An upward slope in the roof of the acetabulum (the acetabular angle) greater than 40 degrees with upward and outward displacement of the femoral head is a frequent finding in older children. Radiographic examination in early infancy is not reliable, because ossification of the femoral head does not normally take

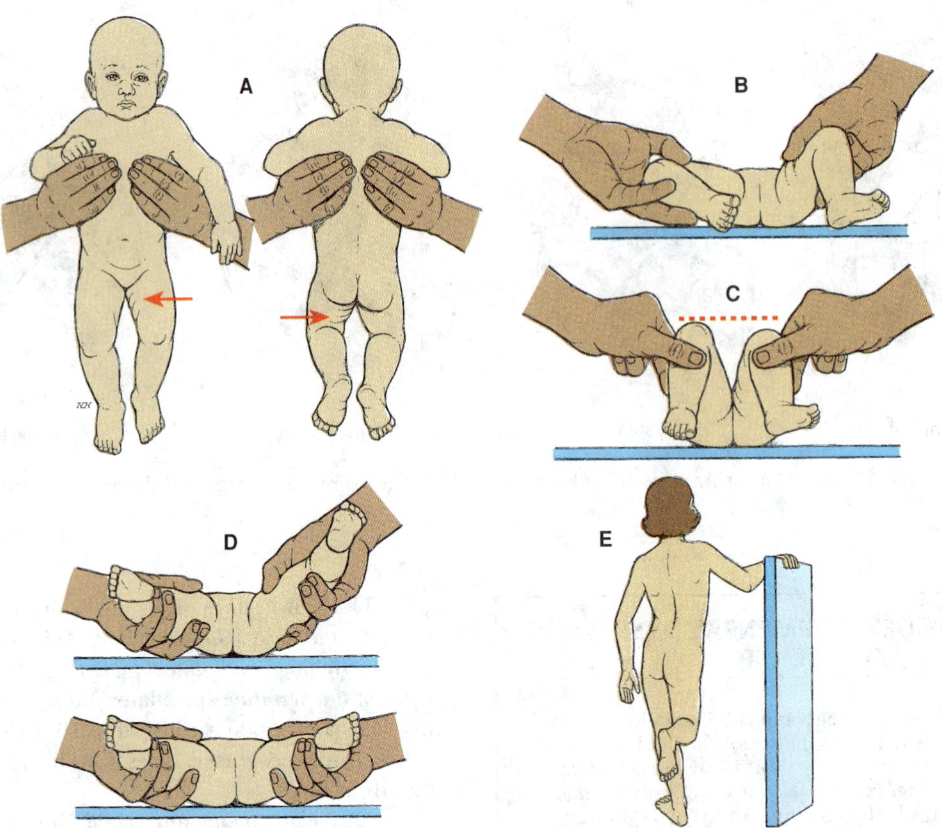

FIG. 11-11 Signs of developmental dysplasia of the hip. **A,** Asymmetry of gluteal and thigh folds. **B,** Limited hip abduction, as seen in flexion. **C,** Apparent shortening of the femur, as indicated by the level of the knees in flexion. **D,** Ortolani click (if infant is under 4 weeks of age). **E,** Positive Trendelenburg sign or gait (if child is weight bearing).

place until the third to sixth month of life. However, the cartilaginous head can be visualized directly with realtime high-resolution ultrasonography. The ultrasound examination can detect slight subluxations and dislocations, as well as monitor progress over time. A CT scan may be useful to assess the position of the femoral head relative to the acetabulum following closed reduction and casting. Arthography can confirm stability and is useful in obtaining and evaluating closed reduction.

Therapeutic Management

Treatment is begun as soon as the condition is recognized, since early intervention is more favorable to the restoration of normal bony architecture and function. The longer treatment is delayed, the more severe the deformity, the more difficult the treatment, and the less favorable the prognosis. The treatment varies with the age of the child and the extent of the dysplasia.

Newborn to Six Months. The hip joint is maintained by dynamic splinting in a safe position with the proximal femur centered in the acetabulum in an attitude of flexion. A variety of abduction devices are available for maintaining the femur in the acetabulum. Of these the ***Pavlik harness*** is the most widely used device, and with time, motion, and gravity the hip works into a more abducted, reduced position (Fig. 11-12). The rate of reduction in infants, when treated between 1 and 8 months, is 80% to 90% (Iwasaki, 1987). The harness is worn continuously until the hip is clinically and radiographically stable, usually about 3 to 6 months. It is highly effective when the device is well constructed, follow-up care is adequate, and the parents follow instructions in its use.

When adduction contracture is present, other devices (such as skin traction) are employed to slowly and gently stretch the hip to full abduction, after which wide abduction is maintained until stability is attained. When there is difficulty in maintaining stable reduction, a hip spica cast is applied and changed periodically to accommodate the child's growth. After 3 to 6 months, sufficient stability is acquired to allow transfer to a removable protective abduction brace. The duration of treatment depends on development of the acetabulum but is usually accomplished within the first year.

Six to Eighteen Months. In this age-group the dislocation is not recognized until the child begins to stand and walk, when attendant shortening of the limb and contractures of hip adductor and flexor muscles become apparent. Gradual reduction by traction is followed by plaster cast immobilization, which is maintained until radiographic examination confirms a stable joint. An individualized home trac-

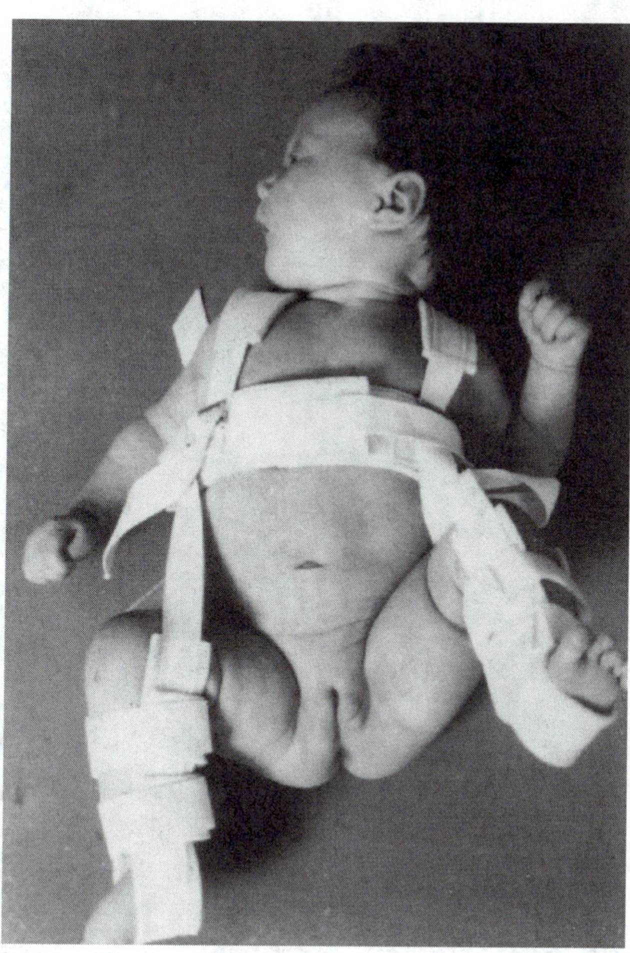

FIG. 11-12 Child in Pavlik harness.

tion program may be developed for the child preoperatively to decrease the length of hospitalization and maintain the home environment. Written directions should be provided to increase compliance with preoperative care.

Often, soft tissue may obstruct and complicate reduction and subsequent joint development. In this case open reduction is performed to remove the obstruction, followed by postoperative spica cast immobilization and, later, replacement with an abduction splint.

Older Child. Correction of the hip deformity in the older child is inherently more difficult than in the preceding age-groups because secondary adaptive changes and other etiologic factors (such as juvenile rheumatoid arthritis or nonambulatory cerebral palsy) complicate the condition. Operative reduction, which may involve preoperative traction, tenotomy of contracted muscles, and any one of several innominate osteotomy procedures designed to construct an acetabular roof, is usually required. After cast removal and before weight bearing is permitted, range-of-motion exercises help restore movement. Next, rehabilitative measures are instituted. Successful reduction and reconstruction become increasingly difficult after the age of 4 years and are usually impossible or inadvisable after age 6 because of severe shortening and contracture of muscles and deformity of the femoral and acetabular structures.

Nursing Considerations

Nurses are in a unique position to detect DDH in the newborn. During the infant assessment process and routine nurturing activities the hips and extremities are inspected for any deviations from normal. Observation for unequal gluteal and thigh folds is routine, and nurses who have been educated to perform the Ortolani and Barlow tests should refer the infant with a positive test to the practitioner. The ambulatory child who displays a limp or an unusual gait is referred for evaluation. This may indicate an orthopaedic or neurologic problem. Nonambulatory children with cerebral palsy are also assessed for evidence of dislocation.

NURSING ALERT Observations during routine care, such as diapering, provide an opportunity to observe the infant for limited movement and a wide perineum, which is an indication to assess for leg shortening, unequal gluteal and thigh folds, and limited abduction.

Care of the Child in a Reduction Device. The major nursing problems in the care of an infant or child in a cast or other device are related to maintenance of the device and adapting nurturing activities to meet the needs of the infant or child. Generally treatment and follow-up care of these children are carried out in a clinic, physician's office, or outpatient unit. Hospitalization may be necessary for cast application or brace fitting but seldom exceeds 24 to 48 hours. Longer hospitalization is required for open reduction.

Family Support and Home Care. The primary nursing goal is teaching parents to apply and maintain the reduction device. The Pavlik harness allows for easy handling of the infant and usually produces less apprehension in the parent than heavy braces and casts. It is important that parents understand the correct use of the appliance, which may or may not allow for its removal during bathing. When the infant has a harness that is not removed, a sponge bath is recommended.

The following instructions for preventing skin breakdown are stressed:

- Always put an undershirt (or a shirt with extensions that close at the crotch) under the chest straps and knee socks under the foot and leg pieces to prevent the straps from rubbing the skin.
- Check frequently (at least two or three times a day) for red areas under the straps and the clothing.
- Gently massage healthy skin under the straps once a day to stimulate circulation. In general, avoid lotions and powders, since they can cake and irritate the skin.
- Always place the diaper *under* the straps.

The parents are permitted to pad shoulder straps at pressure points if desired, but unbuckling or removal is determined on the basis of the family's level of understanding and the degree of deformity in the hip. In general, parents are not encouraged to adjust the harness without supervision. The child should be examined by the practitioner before any adjustment is attempted to ascertain that the hips are in correct placement before the harness is resecured.

Casts and braces offer more challenging nursing problems, since they cannot be removed for routine care, although sometimes the practitioner allows a brace to be removed for bathing. Care of an infant or small child with a cast requires nursing innovation to reduce irritation and to maintain cleanliness of both the child and the cast, particularly in the diaper area. The use of a ***Bradford frame,*** both in the hospital and at home, is helpful to nurses and parents for keeping the cast dry. The importance of spica cast care should be emphasized in providing instructions. The life of the cast should be prolonged so as to hold the legs and hips in proper position postoperatively and prevent an unnecessary cast change.

Cast care and observation are discussed in Chapter 39 and therefore are not elaborated on here. However, inasmuch as DDH is almost the exclusive reason for application of casts in early infancy, some of the problems specific to that age-group are mentioned.

Parents are taught the proper care of the cast (or brace) and are helped to devise means for maintaining cleanliness. A disposable superabsorbent (newborn-size) diaper is tucked beneath the entire perineal opening of the cast. A larger (toddler-size) diaper can be applied and fastened over the small diaper and cast.

For tightly fitting casts, transparent film dressing can be cut into strips as for petalling (see Chapter 39), and one edge can be applied to the cast edge and the other directly to the perineum; this forms a continuous waterproof bridge between the perineum and the cast to prevent leakage. An additional advantage to the use of this dressing material is that it keeps both the skin and the cast dry while allowing for observation of the skin beneath the dressing.

Older infants and small children may stuff bits of food, small toys, or other items under the cast; parents are alerted to this possibility so that suitable preventive measures, such as placing clothing over the cast, can be initiated.

Feeding the infant in a hip spica cast or brace offers problems of positioning. Very young infants can be fed in the supine position with the head elevated, and, with the infant's hips and legs supported on a pillow at the side, the parent can cuddle the infant during feeding. A somewhat similar position can be used for breast-feeding (i.e., with the infant supported on pillows or held in a "football" hold facing the mother with the legs behind her). An alternate position is to hold the infant upright on the mother's lap with the legs of the infant astride the mother's legs.

Infants who are able to sit up can be fed in a feeding table or modified high chair. Parents may be able to fashion a tilt board with padded seat or an adjustable chair. The table or chair provides an excellent place for the child to play in an upright position. The child's car seat is also a vital consideration. Some hospitals have a child passenger safety program. A loan program for the appropriate automotive safety restraint may be offered to the parents, or referral to an agency that provides for this service may be made by the nurse or social worker.* A specially designed car restraint for a young child in a spica cast is shown in Fig. 11-13.

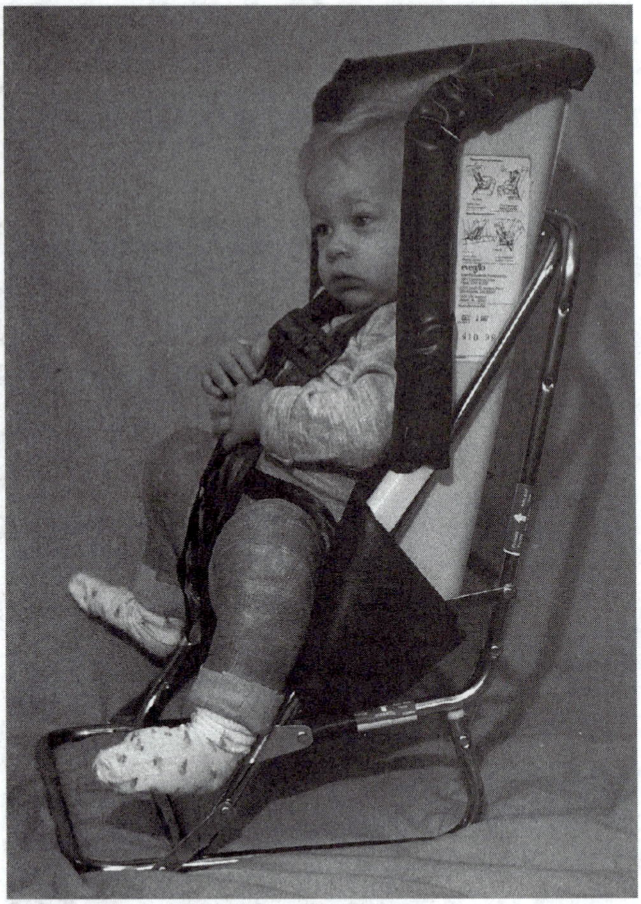

FIG. 11-13 Child in specially designed car restraint (Spelcast).

It is important for nurses, parents, and other caregivers to understand that these children need to be involved in all the activities of any child in the same age-group. Toys are chosen that can be used in a prone position on the floor or in the seats devised for feeding and other activities. Confinement in a cast or appliance should not exclude children from family (or unit) activities. They can be held astride a lap for comfort and transported to areas of activity. The child may be allowed to walk in a cast or brace. An adapted wheelchair or stroller can offer mobility to the older infant or child. (See Chapter 39 for further discussion of care of a child in a spica cast.*)

CONGENITAL CLUBFOOT

Clubfoot is a general term used to describe a common deformity in which the foot is twisted out of its normal shape or position. Any foot deformity involving the ankle is called ***talipes,*** derived from ***talus,*** meaning ankle, and ***pes,*** mean-

*Automobile Safety for Children Program, James Whitcomb Riley Hospital for Children, Indiana School of Medicine, 702 Barnhill Dr., P-121, Indianapolis, IN 46223; (317) 274-2977. In Indiana: 1-800-KID-N-CAR.

*Home care instructions for caring for the child in a cast are available in *Wong and Whaley's Clinical Manual of Pediatric Nursing* (Mosby).

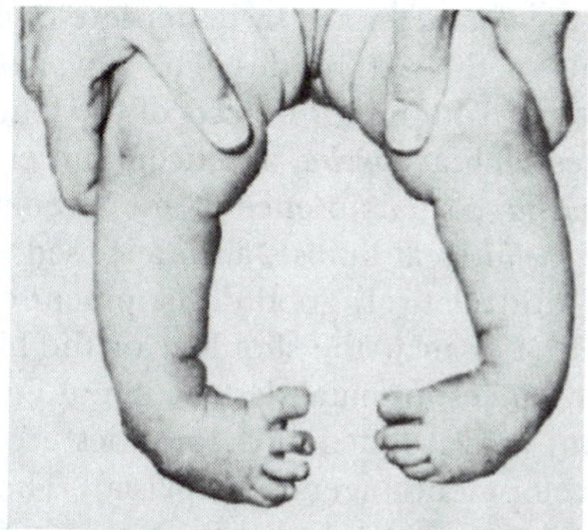

FIG. 11-14 Bilateral congenital talipes equinovarus (congenital clubfoot) in 2-month-old infant. (From Brashear HR Jr, Raney RB: *Handbook of orthopaedic surgery,* ed 10, St Louis, 1986, Mosby.)

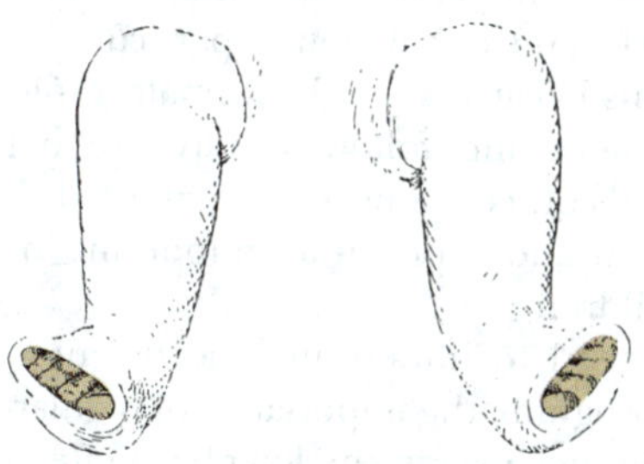

FIG. 11-15 Feet casted for correction of bilateral congenital talipes equinovarus. (From Brashear HR Jr, Raney RB: *Handbook of orthopaedic surgery,* ed 10, St Louis, 1986, Mosby.)

ing foot. Deformities of the foot and ankle are described according to the position of the ankle and foot. The more common talipes deformities involve the following variations:

- **Talipes varus**—An inversion or a bending inward
- **Talipes valgus**—An eversion or bending outward
- **Talipes equinus**—Plantar flexion in which the toes are lower than the heel
- **Talipes calcaneus**—Dorsiflexion, in which the toes are higher than the heel

Most clubfeet are a combination of these positions, and the most frequently occurring type of clubfoot (approximately 95%) is the composite deformity ***talipes equinovarus (TEV),*** in which the foot is pointed downward and inward in varying degrees of severity (Fig. 11-14). Unilateral clubfoot is somewhat more common than bilateral clubfoot and may occur as an isolated defect or in association with other disorders or syndromes, such as chromosomal aberrations, arthrogryposis (a generalized immobility of the joints), cerebral palsy, or spina bifida.

The frequency of clubfoot in the general population is 1:700 to 1:1000 live births, with boys affected twice as often as girls. There is a 35% concordance in monozygotic twins as opposed to a 3% concordance in dizygotic twins, which indicates a hereditary component.

Pathophysiology

The precise cause of clubfoot is unknown. Some authorities attribute the defect to abnormal positioning and restricted movement in utero, although the evidence is not conclusive. Other experts implicate arrested or abnormal embryonic development, since the foot normally goes through flexion and eversion during early development and gradually assumes a normal attitude by the seventh month. Arrested development during this early stage tends to result in a rigid deformity, whereas mechanical pressures from intrauterine position are more likely to be operating in the more flexible deformities.

Diagnostic Evaluation

The deformity is readily apparent and easily detected prenatally through ultrasonography or at birth. However, it must be differentiated from some positional deformities that can be passively corrected or overcorrected. The true clubfoot is fixed, whereas paralytic changes in the lower extremities of children with neuromuscular involvement often produce equinovarus deformity.

Therapeutic Management

The rapid growth during infancy is a potent remodeling force. Treatment is begun as soon as the deformity is recognized and involves three stages: (1) correction of the deformity, (2) maintenance of the correction until normal muscle balance is regained, and (3) follow-up observation to avert possible recurrence of the deformity.

Correction of TEV is most reliably accomplished by manipulation and the application of a series of casts begun immediately or shortly after birth and continued until marked overcorrection is reached (Fig. 11-15). Successive casts allow for gradual stretching of tight structures on the medial side of the foot and gradual contraction of lax structures on the lateral side. Manipulation and casting are repeated frequently (every few days for 1 to 2 weeks, then at 1- to 2-week intervals) to accommodate the rapid growth of early infancy. If manipulation is ineffective, surgical correction is performed to correct bony deformity, release tight ligaments, or lengthen or transplant tendons. The extremity or extremities are casted until the desired result is achieved.

Prognosis. Some feet respond to treatment readily; some respond only to prolonged, vigorous, and sustained efforts; and the improvement in others remains disappointing even with maximum effort on the part of all concerned. Parents should realize that outcomes are not always predictable and depend on the severity of the deformity, age of the child at initial intervention, compliance with treatment protocols, and development of bones, muscles, and nerves. Long-term function is generally good, but studies have shown that in the adult the corrected foot is about one half size smaller than the normal foot and the calf is about 10% smaller (Aronson and Puskarich, 1990).

Nursing Considerations

Nursing care of the child with nonsurgical correction of clubfoot is the same as it is for any child who has a cast (see Chapter 39). The child will spend a considerable time in a corrective device; therefore nursing care plans include both long-term and short-term goals. Conscientious observation of skin and circulation is particularly important in young infants because of their normally rapid growth rate. Since treatment and follow-up care are handled in the orthopaedist's office, clinic, or outpatient department, parent education and support are important in nursing care of these children.

Parents need to understand the diagnosis, the overall treatment program, the importance of regular cast changes, and the role they play in the long-term effectiveness of the therapy. Reinforcing and clarifying the orthopaedic surgeon's explanations and instructions, providing emotional support, teaching parents about care of the cast or appliance (including vigilant observation for potential problems), and encouraging parents to facilitate normal development within the limitations imposed by the deformity or therapy are all part of nursing responsibilities.

METATARSUS ADDUCTUS (VARUS)

Metatarsus adductus, or metatarsus varus, is probably the most common congenital foot deformity. In most instances it is the result of abnormal intrauterine positioning and is usually detected at birth. The deformity is characterized by medial adduction of the toes and forefoot, frequently associated with inversion, and convexity of the lateral border of the (kidney-shaped) foot. Unlike TEV, with which it is often confused, the angulation occurs at the tarsometatarsal joint while the heel and ankle remain in a neutral position. This deformity often causes a pigeon-toed gait in the child.

Management depends on the rigidity of the deformity. Most children under the age of 18 months with mild valgus or varus deformities do not require treatment, because the defect corrects itself in time. When treatment is needed, correction can usually be accomplished by gentle manipulation and passive stretching of the foot, which the parent is taught to perform. Repeated and consistent stretching is continued for the first 6 weeks, after which the treatment is based on the flexibility of the foot. If the child is able to actively overcorrect the deformity voluntarily on stimulation, continued stretching is generally sufficient. If the foot cannot be actively or passively overcorrected, the feet are stretched and manipulated and held with casts and/or orthoses.

Nursing Considerations

The nursing role primarily involves identifying the defect, so that early therapy and instruction of the parents can be instigated. The nurse teaches the parents how to hold the heel firmly and to stretch the forefoot. If casting is needed, the nurse instructs the parents in cast care and observation (see Chapter 39).

SKELETAL LIMB DEFICIENCY

Congenital limb deficiencies, or reduction malformations, are manifested by loss of functional capacity of varying degrees. They are characterized by underdevelopment of skeletal elements of the extremities. The range of malformation can extend from minor defects of the digits to serious abnormalities such as ***amelia***, absence of an entire extremity, or ***meromelia***, partial absence of an extremity, which includes ***phocomelia*** (seal limbs), an interposed deficiency of long bones with relatively good development of hands and feet attached at or near the shoulder or the hips.

In rare instances prenatal destruction of limbs has been reported, but most reduction deformities are primary defects of development (agenesis, aplasia). Therefore, congenital amputations in the literal sense are not amputations, since nonexistent limbs cannot be removed.

Pathophysiology

Limb deficiencies can be attributed to both heredity and environment, and they can originate at any stage of limb development. Formation of limbs may be suppressed at the time of limb bud formation, or there may be interference in later stages of differentiation and growth. Heredity appears to play a prominent role, and prenatal environmental insults have been implicated in a number of cases, such as the well-publicized thalidomide tragedy in the late 1950s and early 1960s, which demonstrated a clear relationship between the time of exposure of the pregnant woman to the antiemetic drug and the presence and type of limb deformity in the newborn. A number of reports suggest that absence or shortening of the digits is associated with chorionic villus sampling, especially if performed before 10 weeks of gestation (Burton, Schulz, and Burd, 1993).

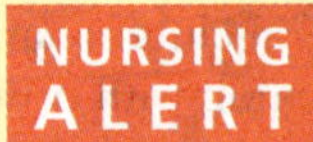

Parents of children with limb deficiencies should be referred for genetic counseling.

Therapeutic Management

Children with congenital limb deficiencies should be fitted with prosthetic devices whenever possible, and a functional replacement should be applied at the earliest possible stage of development in an attempt to match the motor readiness of the infant. This favors natural progression of prosthetic use. For example, an infant with an upper extremity deficiency is fitted with a simple passive device, such as a mitten prosthesis, between 3 and 6 months of age when limb exploration is active, sitting is beginning with the extremities needed for support, and bilateral hand activities are to be encouraged. Lower limb prostheses are applied when the infant is ready to pull to a standing position.

In preparation for prosthetic devices, surgical modification is often necessary to ensure the most favorable use of the device, since severe deformity can interfere with its effective use. Phocomelic digits are preserved for controlling switches of externally powered appliances in upper extremities. Digits (in both upper and lower extremities) provide the child with surfaces for tactile exploration and stimulation. Prostheses are replaced to accommodate growth and increasing capabilities of the child.

Nursing Considerations

Prosthetic application training and habilitation are most successfully carried out in a center that specializes in meeting the special needs of these children, especially very young children and those with multiple amputations. Specialized limb deficiency clinics are most helpful to parents and provide an introduction to support groups for both parents and affected children. Parents must encourage the child in making age-commensurate adjustments to the environment. Although these children need assistance, excessive overprotection may produce overdependency with later maladjustment to school and other situations.

DISORDERS OF THE GASTROINTESTINAL (GI) TRACT*

Congenital defects of the GI tract can involve any portion from the mouth to the anus. Most are apparent at birth or shortly thereafter and are anomalies in which normal growth ceased at a crucial stage of embryonic development, leaving the structure in an embryonic form or only partially completed. The result may be atresia, malposition, nonclosure, or any number of variations.

Atresia is absence of a normal opening or normally patent lumen. Atresia at any point along the length of the GI tract creates an obstruction to the normal progress of nutrients and secretions. The most common anomalies requiring surgical intervention are atresias of the esophagus, intestine, and anus.

Other defects of development of the digestive tract include annular pancreas, malrotation of the intestines, meconium ileus, and Hirschsprung disease. When there is an ***annular pancreas,*** the head of the pancreas surrounds and constricts the second portion of the duodenum, causing obstructive symptoms. ***Malrotation of the small and large intestines*** occurs when there is an abnormal rotation and fixation of the intestines about the axis of the superior mesenteric artery around the tenth week of gestation. Malrotation predisposes to volvulus and obstruction of the small intestine. ***Meconium ileus*** occurs when the intestine becomes obstructed by thick, impacted meconium—the earliest manifestation of cystic fibrosis. ***Hirschsprung disease*** is caused by the congenital absence of ganglion cells in the distal intestine, which leads to abnormal peristalsis and obstruction (see Chapter 33).

The diagnosis and management of most intestinal atresias and obstructions are similar to the diagnosis and management of intestinal obstruction from other factors, most of the which are discussed in Chapter 33. The congenital defects considered in this chapter include abnormalities of the lip and palate, esophagus, and anus. Some malformations of the GI tract are considered here, since they are identified at birth and are cause for considerable parental concern.

*Lynn E. Mattis, RN, MSN, revised this section.

CLEFT LIP (CL) AND/OR CLEFT PALATE (CP)

CL with or without CP is the most common craniofacial malformation and occurs with a frequency of 1 in 800 live births. Isolated CP has an incidence of approximately 1 in 2000 live births. CL with or without CP is more common in

TABLE 11-5 Comparison of Cleft Lip and Cleft Palate

	CLEFT LIP	CLEFT PALATE
Incidence	1:800	1:2000
Inheritance	Multifactorial inheritance Male predominance	Associated with syndromes (chromosomal), environmental factors, or teratogens Female predominance
Anatomy	Unilateral/bilateral May involve external nose, nasal cartilages, nasal septum, maxillary alveolar ridges, and dental anomalies	Soft palate and/or hard palate Midline of posterior palate May involve nostril and absence of nasal septal development (communication with oral and nasal cavity)
Management	Surgical—Z-plasty First few weeks of life if no respiratory, oral, or systemic infections occur	Delayed repair—12-18 months before development of speech
Short-term problems (before repair)	Feeding, possibly	Feeding—aspiration
Special postoperative care	Suture line protection and care Position—right side or upright in infant seat; avoid prone positioning to protect suture line Special feeding—Breck feeder or Asepto syringe, sometimes breast—until suture line heals	May be prone, supine, or side-lying Feeding cup, Breck feeder or Asepto syringe; avoid spoon, fork (also tongue blade, toothbrush, and other objects that could damage suture line)
Long-term problems	Social acceptance (depends on success of repair), orthodontic if associated with CP	Speech, otitis media, possible hearing loss, upper respiratory tract infections Orthodontic Feeding Social acceptance (voice changes, facial appearance if with CL)

males, and CP alone is more common in females. CL appears more often in Orientals and Native Americans and less frequently in Blacks. (See Table 11-5 for a comparison of the two defects.)

CL results from incomplete fusion of the embryonic structures surrounding the primitive oral cavity. The cleft may be unilateral or bilateral and is often associated with abnormal development of the external nose, nasal cartilages, nasal septum, and maxillary alveolar ridges. It may or may not be associated with cleft palate. The extent of the cleft varies greatly from an indentation in the lip to a deep and wide fissure extending to the nostril. In severe clefts the nostril on the affected side is low and the nose is deviated to that side. With bilateral CL the midportion of the upper lip is unattached on either side and may be displaced forward. Dental anomalies, such as missing, malpositioned, or deformed teeth, are common on the side of the cleft.

CP occurs when the primary and secondary palatine plates fail to fuse during embryonic development. CPs vary greatly in degree and may involve only the soft palate or may extend into the hard palate. The cleft may occur only in the midline of the posterior palate but may extend to the nostril on one or both sides. Wide central palatal clefts may be accompanied by partial or complete absence of nasal septal development, resulting in communication between the nasal and oral cavities. Occasionally, small clefts of the soft palate may be difficult to identify.

Etiology

Many factors appear to be involved in the etiology of CL and CP, and evidence indicates that CL with or without CP is developmentally and genetically different from isolated CP. The majority of cases appear to be consistent with the concept of multifactorial inheritance as evidenced by an increased incidence in relatives and a higher concordance in monozygotic twins than in dizygotic twins. Siblings of children with CL with or without CP have an increased risk of the same anomaly but not CP alone, and vice versa (Carey, 1987). There are many recognized syndromes that include CL and CP as a feature. Some of these syndromes are the result of chromosomal abnormalities, and environmental factors or teratogens may be responsible for clefts at a critical point in embryonic development.

Pathophysiology

Development of the primary and secondary palates takes place at different times and involves different developmental processes. CL with or without CP results from failure of the maxillary processes to fuse with the nasal elevations on the frontal prominence, which normally occurs during the sixth week of gestation (Fig. 11-16, *A*). Merging of the upper lip at the midline is completed between the seventh and eighth weeks of gestation. There is evidence, however, that in some cases separation may be a result of rupture subsequent to fusion.

Fusion of the secondary palate (hard and soft palates) takes place later in development, between the seventh and twelfth weeks of gestation (Fig. 11-16, *B* to *D*). At the time the primary palate is completed, the two lateral palatine processes are situated in a vertical position at the side of the tongue. In the process of migrating to a horizontal position, they are, for a short time, separated by the tongue. With development of the neck and jaws, the tongue moves downward, allowing the palatine processes to fuse with each other and with the primary palate to form the roof of the mouth. If there is delay in this movement, or if the tongue fails to descend soon enough, the remainder of development proceeds but the palate never fuses.

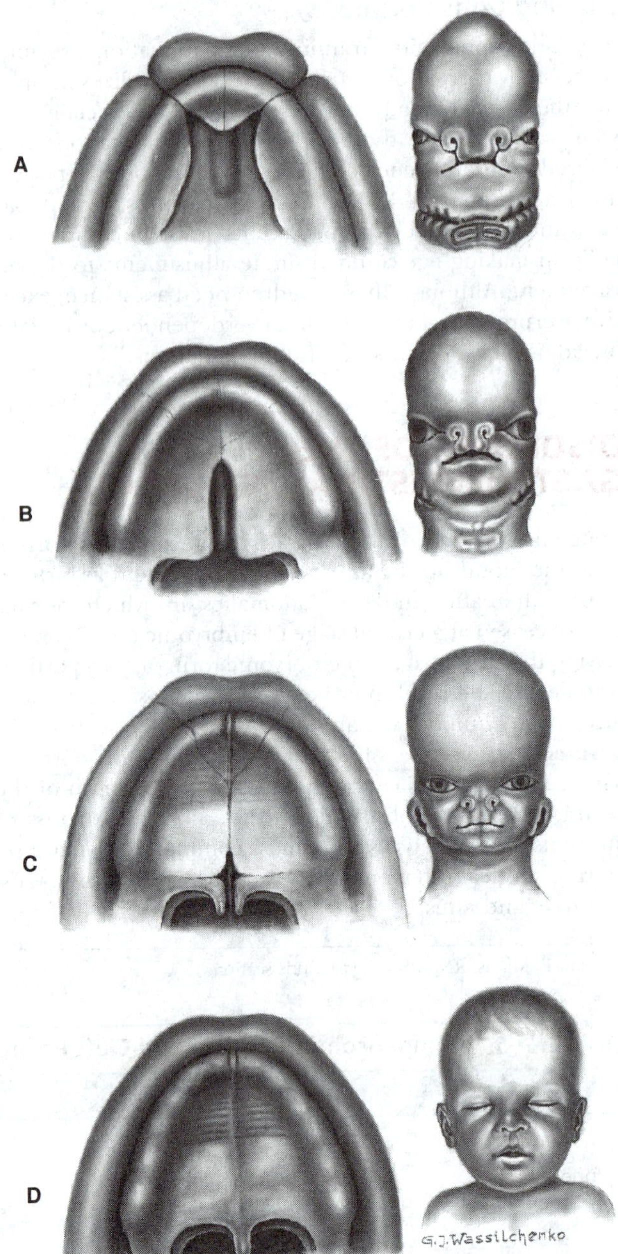

FIG. 11-16 Stages in palatine development.

Diagnostic Evaluation

A cleft that involves the lip with or without CP is readily apparent at birth and is one of the defects that elicits the

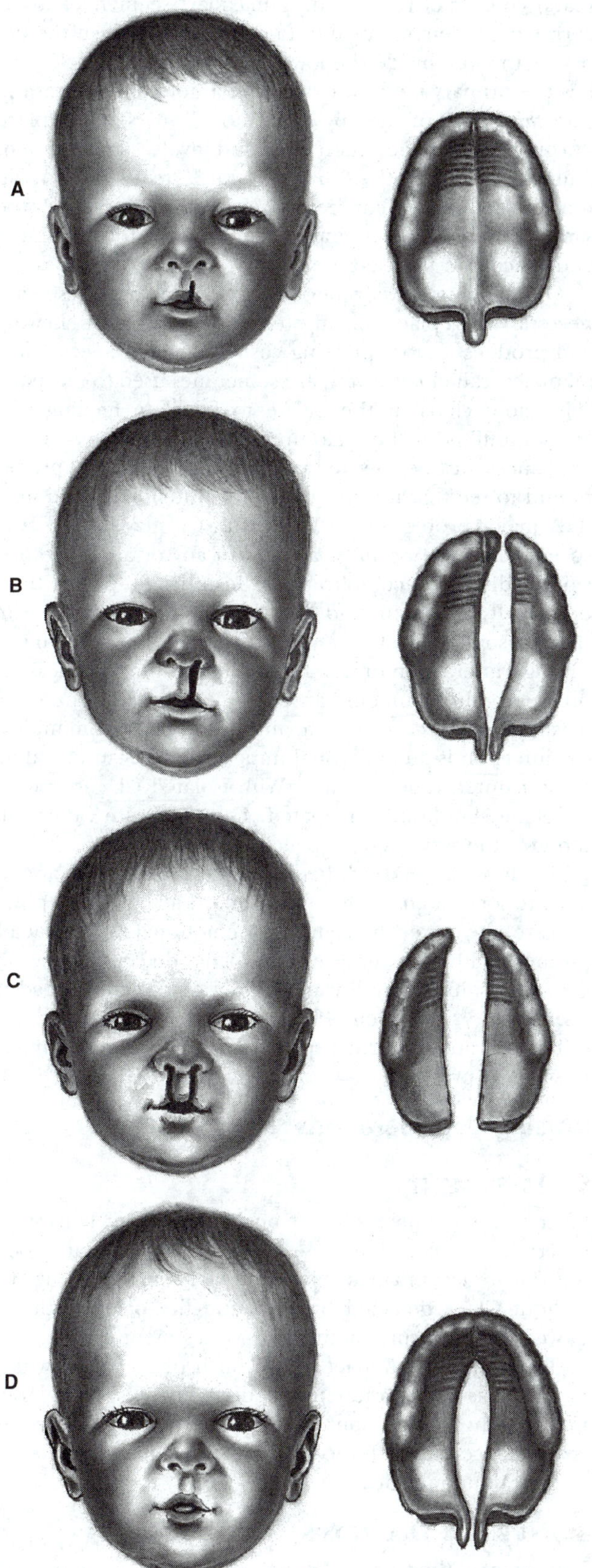

FIG. 11-17 Variations in clefts of lip and palate at birth. **A,** Notch in vermilion border. **B,** Unilateral cleft lip and palate. **C,** Bilateral cleft lip and cleft palate. **D,** Cleft palate.

most severe emotional reactions in parents. An important initial assessment in the diagnostic evaluation is to determine if the defect is isolated or one feature of a broader syndrome. The degree of malformation of the CL or CP can then be evaluated (Fig. 11-17). Clefts of the lip may be unilateral or bilateral, and the extent of the cleft and degree of nasal deformity is variable. CP can occur with CL or as an isolated deformity. As with CL, the degree of deformity varies and may involve only the uvula or may extend through both the soft and hard palates. The severity of the CP has an impact on feeding problems; the infant is unable to generate negative pressure and create suction in the oral cavity. This impairs feeding even though in most cases the infant's ability to swallow is normal.

Therapeutic Management

Treatment of the child with CL is surgical and usually involves no long-term interventions other than possible scar revision. However, management of CP involves the cooperative efforts of a number of disciplines in order to provide optimum results—pediatrics, plastic surgery, orthodontics, otolaryngology, speech/language pathology, audiology, nursing, and social work. Treatment continues over a long time, but even after completion of a program of health care, the child will probably retain defects of speech, facial appearance, or other problems related to the cleft. Management of both defects is directed toward surgical closure of the cleft, prevention of complications, and facilitation of normal growth and development of the child.

Surgical Correction: CL. Closure of the lip defect precedes that of the palate, usually during the first weeks of life, although it is possible to operate earlier. Surgical correction is performed when the infant is free of any oral, respiratory, or systemic infection. The method of repair of the CL involves one of several staggered suture lines (Z-plasty) to minimize notching of the lip from retraction of scar tissue and to lengthen the lip. Surgeons use any of a variety of devices to protect the suture line from trauma, such as a butterfly bandage strip or Logan bow (Fig. 11-18). The arms are restrained at the elbows to prevent the infant's hands from rubbing the incision.

Improved surgical techniques have minimized deformity related to scar retraction, but optimum cosmetic results are difficult to obtain in severe defects. In the absence of infection or trauma, healing takes place with little scar formation. Remaining physical characteristics of the older child are residual nasal deformity, mildly protruding lower lip, and a somewhat flattened lower third of the upper lip, usually with an abnormally shaped red lip margin. Not infrequently, revisions may be required at a later age.

Surgical Correction: CP. CP repair is generally postponed until a later age than repair of the CL in order to take advantage of palatal changes that occur with normal growth. Since clefts vary considerably in size, shape, and degree of deformity, the timing of repair is individualized but is usually performed sometime between 12 and 18 months of age. Most surgeons prefer to close the cleft before the child develops faulty speech habits. Persistent velopharyngeal insufficiency, manifested by nasal regurgitation and na-

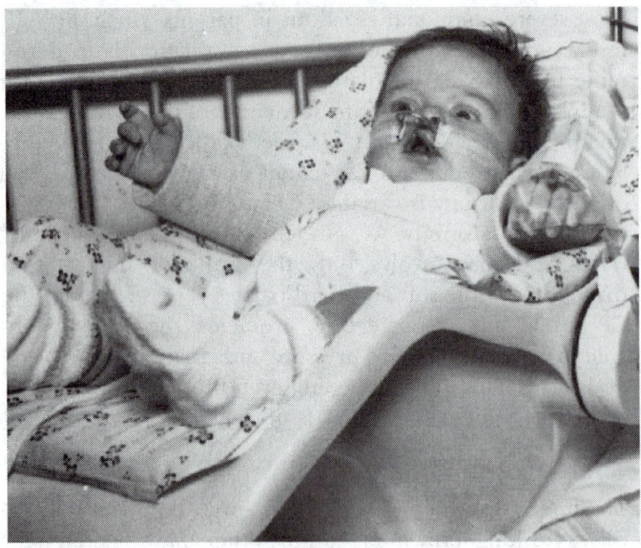

FIG. 11-18 Infant with Logan bow in place to prevent trauma to the suture line. Note elbow restraints.

sal speech, may require a posterior pharyngeal flap procedure or palate bone grafting at a later time.

Long-Term Problems. The care of children with CL and CP often consists of a group of specialists who meet periodically to examine the child and consult with each other and with the parents. Even with adequate anatomic closure, the majority of children with CL and CP have some degree of speech impairment that requires speech therapy. The physical problems are the result of inefficient functioning of the muscles of the soft palate and nasopharynx, improper tooth alignment, and varying degrees of hearing loss.

Improper drainage of the middle ear, as a result of inefficient function of the eustachian tube, causes increased pressure in the middle ear and contributes to recurrent otitis media, which leads to hearing impairment in some children with CP. The problem may be easily overlooked in the infant and young child, thereby contributing to permanent impairment. Upper respiratory tract infections require immediate and meticulous attention, and pressure-equalizing drainage tubes may be inserted to facilitate drainage in chronic serous otitis media.

Extensive orthodontics and prosthodontics are usually needed to correct problems of malposition of the teeth and maxillary arches. There may be missing teeth, or the teeth may be malformed or malpositioned, which can interfere with feeding. In addition, a significant number of these children have an inadequate nasal airway that forces them to breathe through the mouth, which also contributes to oral deformity. Children with both CL and CP often require several stages of orthodontic therapy. The ***first stage*** (at birth to 18 months) is concerned with aligning the maxillary segments into a near-normal relationship. This is frequently done before lip closure in severely expanded segments to facilitate a primary lip closure. The ***second stage*** (at 2 to 5 years) consists of repositioning maxillary segments and/or correcting a dental crossbite (a condition in which the upper teeth close inside the lower teeth) in an attempt to allow the primary teeth to develop in a normal relationship. The ***third stage*** of therapy (at 10 to 11 years) takes place during the mixed-dentition stage and involves correction of faulty occlusion. In the ***fourth stage*** (at 12 to 18 years) treatment of the permanent teeth is accomplished in much the same manner as for any adolescent except for alignment and spacing in the cleft area.

Often temporary or permanent dental prostheses are necessary to replace missing teeth; these assist in chewing and produce a more pleasing cosmetic effect. Special dental plates, called ***obturators,*** are sometimes used to mechanically close clefts in the palate to facilitate feeding and speech until permanent closure is attempted. However, any appliance must be checked periodically to ensure a proper fit and to see that it is performing its intended function.

A major problem for a child with CP may be defective speech. This can occur as a result of any or all of the previously discussed complications: insufficient palate function, faulty dentition, and hearing loss. CP interferes with speech sounds in the mouth that are normally made through interaction of the throat and palatine muscles. Improper tooth alignment can pose a mechanical hazard to development of clear speech, and hearing loss from middle ear infection is an additional impediment because of difficulty in interpreting sounds. With isolated CL, no speech problems should be anticipated. The child with CP usually requires the services of a speech therapist.

Some of the more difficult long-term problems are related to social adjustment of the child. The better the physical care, the better the chance for emotional and social adjustment, although the presence of the defect and the degree of residual disability are not always directly related to a satisfactory adjustment. Physical defects are a threat to the self-image, and abnormal speech quality is an impediment to social expression.

Nursing Considerations

❖ Assessment

Since CL is readily visible at birth, assessment consists of describing the location and extent of the defect and looking for an accompanying palatine cleft during crying. CP without CL is detected by palpating the palate with the gloved finger during the newborn assessment.

The emotional impact of the birth of an infant with a cosmetic, as well as a functional, disability is especially traumatic to the family. Consequently, the nursing assessment is also concerned with the emotional reaction of the family to the infant and the defect.

❖ Nursing Diagnosis

Following a thorough nursing assessment, a number of nursing diagnoses become evident. The most likely diagnoses are outlined and discussed in the Nursing Care Plan on pp. 477-478. Others may be apparent in individual cases.

❖ Planning

The goals of care for the infant with CL and CP are related to preoperative care, short-term postoperative care, and long-term management. The major goals of care for the infant and family include the following:

Preoperative care:
1. Family will cope with the impact of an infant with a defect.
2. Infant will receive optimum nutrition.
3. Infant will be prepared for surgery.

Postoperative care:
1. Infant will experience no trauma and minimal or no pain.
2. Infant will receive optimum nutrition.
3. Infant will experience no complications.
4. Infant and family will receive adequate support.
5. Family will be prepared for care at home and long-term needs of a child with CP.

❖ Implementation

The immediate nursing problems in the care of an infant with CL and CP deformities are related to feeding the infant and dealing with the parental reaction to the defect. Facial deformities are particularly disturbing to parents; CL, especially, is a disfiguring visible defect that may generate a strong negative response in parents. During the initial phase following the birth of an infant with CP and/or CL, it is important for the nurse to place emphasis not only on the infant's physical needs but also on the parents' emotional needs. Parent-infant attachment may be negatively affected by the birth of an infant with an obvious congenital defect (Curtin, 1990). The nurse is in a position to allow for expression of parental grief and fears, which may promote attachment in the preoperative period. It is especially important for nurses to emphasize the positive aspects of the infant's physical appearance and to express optimism regarding surgical correction while acknowledging the parents' concern. The manner of the nurse in handling the infant should convey to the parents that the infant is indeed a precious human being. (See also Birth of a Child with a Physical Defect, p. 434.)

Feeding. Feeding the infant offers a special challenge to nurses. Clefts of the lip or palate reduce the infant's ability to suck, which interferes with compression of the areola and renders breast-feeding and bottle-feeding difficult. Liquid taken into the mouth tends to escape via the cleft palate through the nose. Feeding is best accomplished with the infant's head in an upright position, either held in the caregiver's hand or cradled in the arm. Normal nipples are unsuitable for these infants, who are unable to generate the suction required; therefore, special nipples or other feeding devices are needed. A variety of special "cleft palate" nipples have been devised and used with some success. However, large, soft nipples with large holes, Nursettes, or the long, soft lamb's nipples appear to offer the best means for nipple feeding (Fig. 11-19). The newer "gravity flow" nipple* attached to a squeezable plastic bottle allows formula to be deposited directly into the mouth in much the same manner as with a bulb syringe. Success has also been achieved by the modification of a standard nipple. A single small slit or cross-cut is made in the end of the nipple with a sharp surgical blade or a pair of scissors with sharp, thin blades. This allows the infant to swallow the formula easily, thereby bypassing the suction problem (Richard, 1991). The size of the slit is adjusted to the needs of the infant.

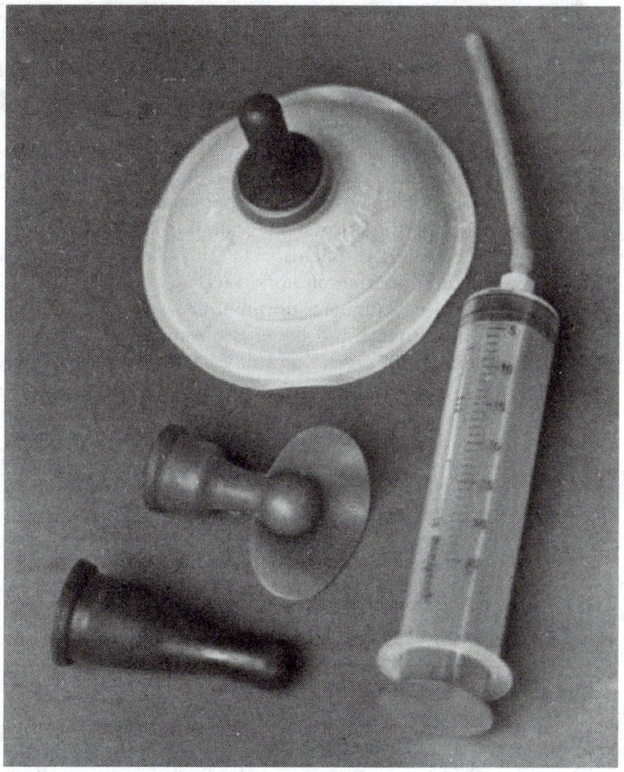

*Ross Laboratories, Columbus, OH 43216.

FIG. 11-19 Some devices used to feed an infant with a cleft lip and palate. *Clockwise:* Lamb's nipple, flanged nipple, special nurser, and syringe with rubber tubing (Breck feeder).

Using these various types of nipples for feeding also has the advantage of helping to meet the infant's sucking needs. Muscle development is especially important for later development of speech. The nipple is positioned in such a way that it is compressed by the infant's tongue and existing palate. If a single-slit nipple is used, the slit is placed vertically so that the infant will be able to produce and stop a flow of milk by alternately opening and closing the opening. No matter which type of nipple is used, gentle, steady pressure on the base of the bottle reduces the chance of choking or coughing, and the person feeding should resist the temptation to remove the nipple because of the noise the infant makes or for fear that the infant will choke. An indication that the infant needs to stop feeding momentarily is the facial signal, which involves elevated eyebrows and a wrinkled forehead; the nipple may be gently removed to allow swallowing of formula in the mouth without upsetting the infant (Richard, 1991). Since these infants have a tendency to swallow excessive amounts of air, they need frequent burping.

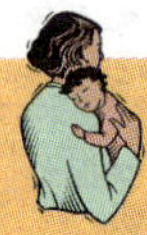

FAMILY FOCUS
Breast-Feeding the Infant with Cleft Lip and/or Cleft Palate

Many health professionals assume that successful breast-feeding is impossible because of the CL and/or CP. On the contrary, breast-feeding is not only possible, it has several benefits, including the normal integration of the infant into the family, decreased problems with otitis media, and passive immunity to upper respiratory tract infections. In addition, breast-feeding enhances normal muscular movements of the mouth and face, and benefits normal speech development (Danner, 1992). In one study infants with CL were breast-fed shortly after surgical repair; there were no complications observed in this group, and they gained weight faster and were discharged sooner than infants with CL repair who were fed by cup (Weatherly-White and others, 1987).

If the mother intended to breast-feed before delivery, she is encouraged and helped to do so as soon as possible after birth. If available, the services of a lactation expert or of La Leche League International, Inc. (see p. 323), should be used.

When the infant has trouble with nipple feeding, a rubber-tipped medicine dropper, Asepto syringe, or Breck feeder (a large syringe with soft rubber tubing) often provides an efficient, safe feeding device. The rubber extension should be sufficiently long to extend well back into the mouth to reduce the likelihood of regurgitation through the nose. The formula is deposited on the back of the tongue, and the flow is controlled by bulb or syringe compression that is adjusted to the infant's needs. With some infants spoon feeding works best, especially if the formula is slightly thickened with cereal. After feeding, the infant is given water to rinse the mouth.

Breast-feeding is also an option. The nipple is positioned and stabilized well back in the oral cavity so that tongue action facilitates milk expression. However, the suction required to stimulate milk may be absent initially; therefore a breast pump may be useful before nursing to stimulate the let-down reflex (see Family Focus box).

Regardless of the feeding method used, the mother should begin to feed the infant as soon as possible, preferably after the initial nursery feeding. In this way she is able to help determine the method best suited to her and the infant and to become adept in the technique before they are discharged from the hospital.

Preoperative Care. In preparation for the surgical repair, the parents are frequently instructed to accustom the infant to some of the needs of the early postoperative period, particularly if surgery is delayed several months. Since it is important for the infant who has a CL repair to avoid the prone position postoperatively, it is helpful to accustom the infant to lying on the back or side to reduce the irritability and resistance associated with any change in routine. It is also helpful to place the infant or child in arm restraints periodically before admission and to feed the infant in the manner to be used postoperatively. No special formula is required, and the infant is usually allowed to eat up to 4 hours preoperatively. Preoperative preparation, including medication, is determined by the surgeon and anesthesiologist.

Postoperative Care: CL. The major efforts in the postoperative period are directed toward protecting the operative site. Following CL repair ***(cheiloplasty)***, a lip protective device may be taped securely to the cheeks to prevent trauma to the suture line. Elbow restraints are applied immediately following surgery to prevent the infant from rubbing the suture line. It is advisable to pin the cuffs of the restraints to the infant's clothing to keep the restraints in place.

An older infant who is able to roll over may require a jacket restraint in addition to arm restraints, to prevent rolling on the abdomen and rubbing the face on the bed. It is important to remove the restraints at regular intervals, such as every 2 hours, to allow for exercising the arms, to provide relief from restrictions, and to observe the skin for signs of irritation. It is advisable to release the restraints one at a time, especially in a very vigorous, active infant or child. Removing restraints also offers an opportunity for cuddling and body contact. Sitting the baby in an infant seat provides a change of position and a different perspective of the environment. Adequate analgesia is recommended to relieve postoperative pain; sedation is sometimes needed for a very restless, anxious infant.

Clear liquids are offered when the infant has fully recovered from the anesthesia, and feeding is usually resumed as tolerated. The Breck feeder is preferred for formula feeding in most cases. The rubber tip should be placed inside from the side of the mouth to avoid the operative area.

The suture line is carefully cleansed of formula or serosanguineous drainage as needed with a cotton-tipped swab dipped in saline. A thin layer of antibiotic ointment may be prescribed for application to the suture line after cleansing. Meticulous care of the suture line is a nursing responsibility, since inflammation or infection will interfere with optimum healing and the ultimate cosmetic effect of the surgical repair.

Gentle aspiration of mouth and nasopharyngeal secretions may be necessary to prevent aspiration and respiratory complications. An upright or infant seat position is helpful for the infant in the immediate postoperative period and for one who has difficulty in handling secretions.

Postoperative Care: CP. The child with a CP repair ***(palatoplasty)*** is allowed to lie on the abdomen, especially immediately postoperatively. The child is often fed a blenderized diet through a cup. Many plastic surgeons will not permit a small spoon to be used, although a wide spoon may be acceptable if the caregiver does not insert the spoon into the mouth, where it might damage the suture line. Oral packing may be secured to the palate following palatoplasty, which is removed after 2 to 3 days.

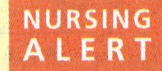

Avoid the use of suction or objects in the mouth such as tongue depressors, thermometers, spoons, or straws.

NURSING CARE PLAN
The Child with Cleft Lip and/or Cleft Palate

Preoperative Care

NURSING DIAGNOSIS: Altered nutrition: less than body requirements related to physical defect

PATIENT GOAL 1: Will consume adequate nourishment

• **NURSING INTERVENTIONS/*RATIONALES***

Administer diet appropriate for age (specify)

Assist mother with breast-feeding if this is mother's preference, because the newborn with either defect can breast-feed

- Position and stabilize nipple well back in oral cavity *so that tongue action facilitates milk expression*
- Stimulate let-down reflex manually or with breast pump before nursing, *since suction required to stimulate milk may be absent initially*

Modify feeding techniques to adjust to defect, *since infant's ability to suck is reduced*

- Hold child in upright (sitting) position *to minimize risk of aspiration*

Use special feeding appliances *that compensate for infant's feeding difficulty*

- Try to nipple feed infant *to meet infant's need for sucking and to promote muscle development for speech*
- Position nipple between infant's tongue and existing palate *to facilitate compression of nipple*
- When using devices without nipples (e.g., Breck feeder, Asepto syringe), deposit formula on back of tongue *to facilitate swallowing* and adjust flow according to infant's swallowing *to prevent aspiration*

Bubble (burp) frequently *because of tendency to swallow excessive amounts of air*

Encourage parents to begin feeding infant as soon as possible *so that they become adept in feeding technique before discharge*

Monitor weight *to assess adequacy of nutritional intake*

• **EXPECTED OUTCOMES**

Infant consumes an adequate amount of nutrients (specify amount)

Infant exhibits appropriate weight gain

NURSING DIAGNOSIS: High risk for altered parenting related to infant with a highly visible physical defect

PATIENT (FAMILY) GOAL 1: Will demonstrate acceptance of infant

• **NURSING INTERVENTIONS/*RATIONALES***

Allow expression of feelings *to encourage family's coping*

Convey attitude of acceptance of infant and family *because parents are sensitive to affective attitudes of others*

Indicate by behavior that child is a valuable human being *to encourage acceptance of infant*

Describe results of surgical correction of defect

- Use photographs of satisfactory results *to encourage feeling of hope*

Arrange meeting with other parents who have experienced a similar situation and coped successfully

• **EXPECTED OUTCOMES**

Family discusses feelings and concerns regarding child's defect, its repair, and future prospects

Family exhibits an attitude of acceptance of infant

See also Nursing Care Plan: The Child Undergoing Surgery, Preoperative Care, Chapter 27

Postoperative Care

NURSING DIAGNOSIS: High risk for trauma of the surgical site related to surgical procedure, dysfunctional swallowing

PATIENT GOAL 1: Will experience no trauma to operative site

• **NURSING INTERVENTIONS/*RATIONALES***

Position on back or side or in infant seat (CL) *to prevent trauma to operative site*

Maintain lip protective device (CL) *to protect the suture line*

Use nontraumatic feeding techniques *to minimize risk of trauma*

Restrain elbows *to prevent access to operative site*

- Use jacket restraints on older infant *to prevent rolling onto abdomen and rubbing face on sheet*
- Avoid placing objects in the mouth following CP repair (suction catheter, tongue depressor, straw, pacifier, small spoon) *to prevent trauma to operative site*
- Prevent vigorous and sustained crying *that can cause tension on sutures*
- Cleanse suture line gently after feeding and as necessary in manner ordered by surgeon (CL) *since inflammation or infection will interfere with healing and the cosmetic effect of surgical repair*

Teach cleansing and restraining procedures, especially when infant will be discharged before suture removal *to minimize complications after discharge*

• **EXPECTED OUTCOME**

Operative site remains undamaged

PATIENT GOAL 2: Will exhibit no evidence of aspiration

• **NURSING INTERVENTIONS/*RATIONALES***

Position *to allow for drainage of mucus* (partial side-lying position, semi-Fowler position) and *to prevent aspiration of formula*

• **EXPECTED OUTCOME**

Child manages secretions and formula without aspiration

Continued.

NURSING CARE PLAN
The Child with Cleft Lip and/or Cleft Palate—cont'd

NURSING DIAGNOSIS: Altered nutrition: less than body requirements related to difficulty eating following surgical procedure

PATIENT GOAL 1: Will consume adequate nourishment

• **NURSING INTERVENTIONS/*RATIONALES***

Monitor IV fluids (if prescribed)

Administer diet appropriate for age and as prescribed for postoperative period (specify)

Involve family in determining best feeding methods, *since family assumes feeding responsibility at home*

Modify feeding techniques *to adjust to defect and surgical repair*

- Feed in sitting position *to minimize risk of aspiration*
- Use special appliances *that compensate for feeding difficulties without causing trauma to operative site*
- Bubble frequently *because of tendency to swallow large amounts of air*
- Assist with breast-feeding if method of choice

Teach feeding and suctioning techniques to family *to ensure optimum home care*

• **EXPECTED OUTCOMES**

Infant consumes an adequate amount of nutrients (specify amounts)

Family demonstrates ability to carry out postoperative care

Infant exhibits appropriate weight gain

NURSING DIAGNOSIS: Pain related to surgical procedure

PATIENT GOAL 1: Will experience optimum comfort level

• **NURSING INTERVENTIONS/*RATIONALES***

Assess behavior and vital signs for evidence of pain

*Administer analgesics and/or sedatives as ordered

Remove restraints periodically while supervised *to exercise arms, provide relief from restrictions, and observe skin for signs of irritation*

Provide cuddling and tactile stimulation and other nonpharmacologic interventions *as needed for optimum comfort*

Involve parents in infant's care *to provide comfort and sense of security*

• **EXPECTED OUTCOME**

Infant appears comfortable and rests quietly

NURSING DIAGNOSIS: Altered family processes related to child with a physical defect, hospitalization

PATIENT (FAMILY) GOAL 1: Will receive adequate support

• **INTERVENTIONS AND EXPECTED OUTCOMES**

See Nursing Care Plan: The Family of the Ill or Hospitalized Child, Chapter 26

Refer family to appropriate agencies and support groups

See also Nursing Care Plan: The Child with Chronic Illness or Disability, Chapter 22

*Dependent nursing action.

Sometimes the infant will have difficulty breathing following surgery, since it is often necessary to alter an established pattern of breathing and adjust to breathing through the nose. This is frustrating but seldom requires more than positioning and support.

The elbows are restrained to keep the hands away from the mouth, and the parents are instructed to maintain this precaution at home until the palate is healed, usually in 4 to 6 weeks. They should be instructed to remove the restraints (usually one at a time) at frequent intervals to allow the child to exercise the arms. The infant should be assessed for pain postoperatively. Opiates may be prescribed for the first 24 to 48 hours postoperatively, or longer if needed, and acetaminophen may be given thereafter.

The older infant is usually discharged on a blenderized or soft diet, which parents are instructed to continue until the surgeon directs them to do otherwise. They should be cautioned against allowing the child to eat hard items such as toast, hard cookies, or potato chips, which could damage the newly repaired palate.

Preparation for Discharge and Home Care. Parents are encouraged to participate in the care of the infant as soon as possible following surgery. They should be taught the proper feeding method with the infant in a sitting position. Parents should also be taught to cleanse the suture line to free any crust that might form and to replace the Logan bow (if used) and elbow restraints. The elbow restraints are usually continued until the suture line is well healed.

Long-Term Family Guidance. The problems of parents in the care of an infant with CP may extend well beyond the initial acceptance and adjustment to the defect and surgical correction. These families need support and encouragement by health professionals and guidance in activities that facilitate the most normal life for the child. With the combined efforts of the family and the health care team, the majority of these infants achieve a satisfactory long-term outcome. Parents need to understand the therapy and the purpose of any appliance. They are taught proper care and placement of the device, and that establishing good mouth care and proper brushing habits is especially important for these children.

Because of the increased risk of middle ear infection, the ears are examined regularly, and hearing tests are scheduled early and repeated periodically throughout childhood. It is particularly important to emphasize the need for an ear examination when the child has symptoms of an upper respiratory tract infection. When treatment can be implemented early, the chances are greater that permanent changes in the ear can be avoided. Parents can be alerted to signs of any hearing impairment in the child in order to obtain needed help and prevent progression of any deficit (see Chapter 24).

The parents are also provided with guidance in helping the child to develop normal speech. They should encourage the child's early attempts to make sounds. Some parents erroneously believe that the child may form poor speech habits if he tries to speak before the palate is repaired. However, attempting to delay speech further hampers this development.

Following surgery, parents can assist palatal function by stimulating the child to use simple words that require coordination of the speech apparatus, encouraging chewing and frequent swallowing to exercise throat and palatine muscles, and engaging in blowing games to help close off the posterior palate. The speech therapist evaluates the individual needs of the child and directs the parents in specific activities to facilitate speech development. The more children are encouraged to use speech, the sooner they will gain self-confidence and assurance in social situations. Some children may require additional surgery to correct defective speech that cannot be managed with speech therapy alone.

Throughout the child's therapy, the ultimate goal should be the development of a healthy personality and self-esteem. Several agencies provide services and information for children with CL and/or CP and their families. These include the **American Cleft Palate Association** and **The Cleft Palate Foundation,*** the **March of Dimes–Birth Defects Foundation,†** and state **Children's Medical Services.**

Evaluation. The effectiveness of nursing interventions is determined by continual reassessment and evaluation of care based on the following observational guidelines:

Preoperative care:

1. Observe and interview family members relative to their understanding, feelings, and concerns regarding the defect and anticipated surgery, and the interactions with the infant.
2. Observe infant during feeding.
3. Complete preoperative checklist.

*1218 Grandview Ave., Pittsburgh, PA 15211; (800) 24-CLEFT or (412) 418-1376.

†1275 Mamaroneck Ave., White Plains, NY 10605; (914) 428-7100. In Canada: **Canadian Cleft Lip and Palate Family Association,** 170 Elizabeth St., Toronto, Ontario, Canada M5G 1E8; and **Aboutface,** 123 Edward St., Suite 1405, Toronto, Ontario, Canada M5G 1E2, (416) 593-1488.

Postoperative care:

1. Inspect operative site, including the protective device.
2. Observe for behavioral and physiologic indicators of pain and response to analgesics.
3. Observe infant during feeding, measure intake and output, and weigh infant daily.
4. Observe operative site for evidence of infection, bleeding, sloughing, or irritation.
5. Observe and interview family regarding their understanding and concerns about the infant, including long-term needs.

Expected outcomes:
See Nursing Care Plan, pp. 477-478.

ESOPHAGEAL ATRESIA (EA) AND TRACHEOESOPHAGEAL FISTULA (TEF)

Congenital EA and TEF are rare malformations that represent a failure of the esophagus to develop as a continuous passage and a failure of the trachea and esophagus to separate into distinct structures. These defects may occur as separate entities or in combination, and without early diagnosis and treatment they pose a serious threat to the infant's well-being.

The incidence is estimated to be from 1 in 3000 to 1 in 3500 live births. There appears to be an equal sex incidence, but the birth weight of most affected infants is significantly lower than average, and there is an unusually high incidence of prematurity in infants with EA. A history of maternal polyhydramnios is common, and approximately half the infants with esophageal defects have associated anomalies, including congenital heart disease, anorectal malformations, and genitourinary anomalies. ***VACTERL syndrome*** describes the combination of vertebral, anorectal, cardiovascular, renal, and limb abnormalities in addition to TEF.

Pathophysiology

The esophagus develops from the first segment of the embryonic gut. During the fourth and fifth weeks of gestation, the foregut normally lengthens and separates longitudinally; each longitudinal portion fuses to form two parallel channels (the esophagus and the trachea) that are joined only at the larynx. Anomalies involving the trachea and esophagus are caused by defective separation, incomplete fusion of the tracheal folds following this separation, or altered cellular growth during embryonic development. The resulting esophageal defect may consist merely of two blind pouches, one at the pharyngeal end and one at the gastric end. More often, one portion ends in a blind pouch and the other is connected to the trachea by way of a fistula.

The most commonly encountered form of EA and TEF (80% to 95% of cases) is one in which the proximal esophageal segment terminates in a blind pouch, and the distal segment is connected to the trachea or primary bronchus by a short fistula at or near the bifurcation (Fig. 11-20, *C*). The second most common type, or "pure" EA (5% to 8%), consists of a blind pouch at each end, widely separated and with no communication to the trachea (Fig. 11-20, *A*). Less frequently, an otherwise normal trachea and esophagus are connected by a fistula (Fig. 11-20, *E*). Extremely rare

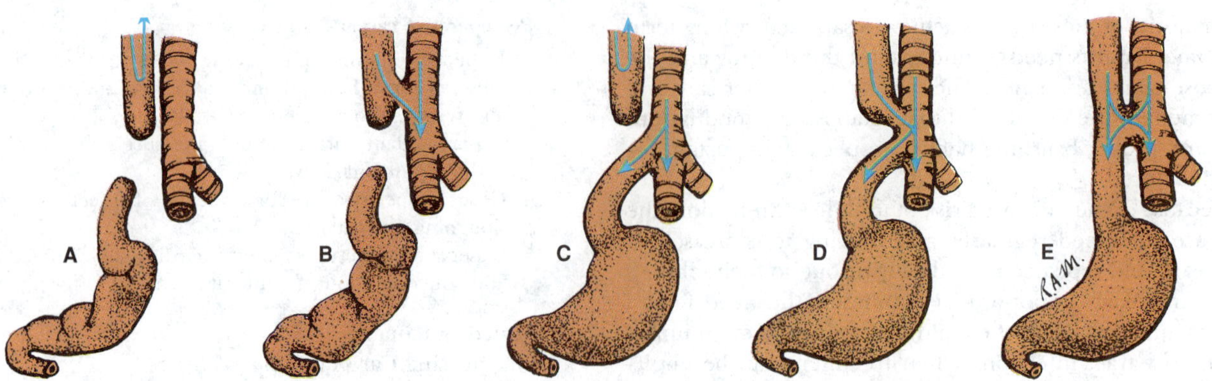

FIG. 11-20 Five most common types of esophageal atresia and tracheoesophageal fistula.

anomalies involve a fistula from the trachea to the upper esophageal segment (Fig. 11-20, *B*) or to both the upper and lower segments (Fig. 11-20, *D*).

Clinical Manifestations

The presence of EA is suspected in an infant with frothy saliva in the mouth and nose and drooling that is frequently accompanied by choking and coughing. If fed, the infant may swallow normally but suddenly coughs and gags; the fluid returns through the nose and mouth. The infant may become cyanotic and stop breathing as the overflow of formula or saliva is aspirated into the trachea or bronchus when there is a proximal esophageal pouch with a TEF.

In the infant who has EA with a distal TEF (type C), the stomach becomes distended with air, and thoracic and abdominal compression (especially during crying) cause the gastric contents to be regurgitated through the fistula and into the trachea, producing a chemical pneumonitis. When the upper segment of the esophagus opens directly into the trachea (types B and D), the infant is in danger of aspirating any swallowed material. Cyanosis or choking during feeding may be the only symptom of type E fistula.

Diagnostic Evaluation

To establish the diagnosis of EA, a radiopaque catheter is gently passed into the esophagus. It will meet with resistance if the lumen is blocked but will pass unobstructed if the lumen is patent. A moderately stiff catheter is used to avoid coiling in the esophageal pouch. Aspiration of stomach contents or auscultation over the stomach as air is introduced through the catheter confirms a patent esophagus.

Although the diagnosis is established on the basis of clinical signs and symptoms, the exact type of anomaly is determined by radiographic studies. A radiopaque catheter is inserted into the hypopharynx and advanced until it encounters an obstruction. Chest films are taken to ascertain esophageal patency or the presence and level of a blind pouch. Films that show air in the stomach indicate a connection between the trachea and the distal esophagus in types C, D, and E. Complete absence of air in the stomach is seen in both types A and B. Occasionally fistulas are not patent, which makes their presence more difficult to diagnose. A careful bronchoscopic examination may be performed to visualize the fistula.

The presence of ***polyhydramnios*** (accumulation of more than 2000 ml of amniotic fluid) prenatally is a clue to the possibility of EA in the unborn infant, especially if the defect is type A, B, or C. Amniotic fluid, normally swallowed by the fetus, is unable to reach the GI tract.

Therapeutic Management

The treatment of EA and TEF includes maintenance of a patent airway, prevention of pneumonia, supportive therapy, and surgical repair of the anomaly. Since type C is the most common, the discussion is directed primarily toward that anomaly.

When EA with a TEF is suspected, the infant is immediately deprived of oral intake, intravenous fluids are initiated, and the infant is positioned to facilitate drainage of secretions and decrease the likelihood of aspiration. Accumulated secretions are suctioned frequently from the mouth and pharynx. A double-lumen catheter should be placed into the upper esophageal pouch and attached to continuous suction. The infant's head is kept in an upright position so that fluid collected in the pouch is easily removed and to prevent aspiration of gastric contents. Since aspiration pneumonia is almost inevitable and appears early, broad-spectrum antibiotic therapy is instituted.

Surgical Correction. Most malformations can be corrected surgically in one operation or staged with two or more procedures. The success depends on early diagnosis before complications occur and on the presence and severity of other associated anomalies. With measures instituted to prevent aspiration pneumonia and to ensure adequate hydration and nutrition, surgery may be postponed to allow for more effective treatment of pneumonia so that the infant can better withstand the complex surgery. The delay also offers an opportunity for further evaluation and assessment to rule out any associated anomalies and to optimize respiratory support.

The surgery consists of a thoracotomy with division and ligation of the TEF and an end-to-end anastomosis of the esophagus. A chest tube is inserted to drain chest fluid. For infants who have multiple anomalies, or who are in very poor condition, a staged operation is preferred that involves gastrostomy, ligation of the TEF, and constant drainage of the esophageal pouch. A delayed esophageal anastomosis is usually attempted after several weeks when the upper pouch elongates and the lower pouch undergoes hypertrophy. The technique of ***bougienage*** (the process whereby a blunt metal instrument is used to dilate a fistula or lengthen membranous tissue) of the upper pouch may be performed to elongate this segment. If an esophageal anastomosis still cannot be accomplished, a ***cervical esophagostomy*** (to allow drainage of saliva) and gastrostomy are performed.

A primary anastomosis cannot be accomplished because of insufficient length of the two segments of esophagus. In these cases an esophageal replacement procedure using a part of the colon or gastric tube interposition may be necessary to bridge the missing esophageal segment. When the stomach is used, a tube is fashioned from the greater curvature of the stomach, tunneled into the chest, and anastomosed to the proximal esophagus. Alternatively, a segment of either the right or the transverse colon is dissected and transplanted, along with its undisturbed blood and nerve supply, through a surgical opening in the diaphragm and ligated to the proximal esophagus, maintaining the proximal-to-distal orientation. Endotracheal intubation may be required, since many of these infants have ***tracheomalacia*** (weakness in the tracheal wall that occurs when a dilated proximal pouch compresses the trachea from early in fetal life or when the trachea does not develop normally because of a loss of intratracheal pressure).

Prognosis. The prognosis for infants with EA or TEF is related to birth weight, associated congenital anomalies, and time of diagnosis. The survival rate is nearly 100% in full-term infants without severe respiratory distress or other anomalies. In premature or low-birth-weight infants with associated anomalies, the incidence of complications is high, with an overall mortality rate of 10% to 15% (Wright, 1990). Potential complications following the surgical repair of esophageal atresia and TEF depend on the type of defect and surgical correction. Complications of an EA and TEF repair include an anastomotic leak, strictures due to tension or ischemia, esophageal motility disorders causing dysphagia, and gastroesophageal reflux.

Nursing Considerations

❖ Assessment

Nursing responsibility for detection of this serious malformation begins immediately after birth. The defect is suspected in any infant who has an excessive amount of frothy saliva in the mouth and unexplained episodes of cyanosis. Cyanosis is usually the result of laryngeal spasm caused by overflow of saliva into the larynx from the proximal esophageal pouch or aspiration, and it normally clears after removal of the secretions from the oral pharynx by suctioning. In addition, a history of maternal polyhydramnios and a small-for-gestational-age infant should alert the nurse to investigate further. The passage of a small-gauge (No. 5 French) orogastric feeding tube via the mouth into the stomach during the initial nursing physical assessment is helpful to rule out TEF and other obstructive defects.

Ideally, the condition is diagnosed before the initial feeding, but often it is not. As mentioned previously, if fed, the infant may swallow normally but suddenly coughs and gags, and the fluid is aspirated or returns through the nose and mouth. For this reason it is customary for the nurse to give the infant the first feeding of plain water or to be present when a parent feeds the child in order to observe the infant's response.

NURSING ALERT Any infant who has an excessive amount of frothy saliva in the mouth or difficulty with secretions and unexplained episodes of cyanosis should be suspected of having a TEF and referred immediately for medical evaluation.

❖ Nursing Diagnoses

Following the initial assessment, a number of nursing diagnoses become evident. The most likely diagnoses are outlined and discussed in the Nursing Care Plan on pp. 483-484. Others may be apparent in individual cases.

❖ Planning

The broad goals for an infant with EA and a TEF and the family are as follows:

1. Infant will experience no respiratory distress.
2. Infant will receive parenteral nutrition.
3. Infant will experience no complications related to airway management.
4. Infant and family will receive adequate support.

❖ Implementation

The infant is placed in an incubator or a radiant warmer, and humidified oxygen is administered to help relieve respiratory distress. Intubation may be necessary if the infant is in respiratory distress.

Preoperative Care. The mouth and nasopharynx are carefully suctioned, and the infant is placed in an optimum position to facilitate drainage and avoid aspiration. The most desirable position for a newborn who is suspected of having the typical EA with a TEF (e.g., type C) is supine or prone with the head elevated on an inclined plane of at least 30 degrees. This positioning serves to minimize the reflux of gastric secretions at the distal esophagus into the trachea and bronchi, especially when intraabdominal pressure is elevated.

It is imperative that any secretions that can be a source of aspiration be removed at once. Until surgery the blind pouch is kept empty by intermittent or continuous suction through an indwelling catheter passed orally or nasally to the end of the pouch. Since the catheter has a tendency to become clogged with secretions, it is irrigated frequently with normal saline and replaced as needed. Sometimes a gastrostomy tube is inserted and left open so that any air entering the stomach through the fistula can escape, thus minimizing the danger of gastric contents being regurgitated into the trachea. The gastrostomy tube is emptied by gravity drainage.

Feedings through the gastrostomy tube and irrigations with fluid are contraindicated before surgery unless a TEF is not present. Nursing interventions include respiratory assessment, thermoregulation, fluid and electrolyte management, and parenteral nutritional support.

Often the infant must be transferred to a hospital with specialized care units. Care is exercised to maintain the desired position and continue suctioning during transport. Specially designed units are equipped for transporting infants to critical care facilities. During transport, the infant may be accompanied by a physician, nurse, or a physician/nurse team. Parents are advised of the infant's condition and provided with necessary support and information.

Postoperative Care. Postoperative care for these infants is the same as for any high-risk newborn. The infant is returned to a radiant warmer, the double-lumen catheter is attached to low suction, parenteral nutrition is provided, and the gastrostomy tube (if a gastrostomy is performed) is returned to gravity drainage until the infant can tolerate feedings, usually on the fifth to seventh postoperative day. Tracheal suction should only be done using a premeasured catheter to avoid injury to the suture line.

Prior to feeding, the gastrostomy tube is elevated and secured at a point above the level of the stomach. This allows gastric secretions to pass to the duodenum, while swallowed air can escape through the open tube. If tolerated, gastrostomy feedings may be initiated and continued until the esophageal anastomosis is healed. Before oral feedings are initiated and the chest tube is removed, a barium swallow is performed to verify the integrity of the esophageal anastomosis.

The initial attempt at oral feeding must be carefully observed to make certain that the infant is able to swallow without choking. Oral feedings are begun with sterile water, followed by frequent small feedings of formula. Until the infant is able to take a sufficient amount by mouth, oral intake may need to be supplemented by bolus or continuous gastrostomy feedings. Ordinarily the infant is not discharged until oral fluids are taken well. The gastrostomy tube may be removed before discharge or maintained for supplemental feedings at home. However, the infant who has undergone palliative surgery will be discharged with the gastrostomy tube in place.

Special Problems. Upper respiratory tract complications are a threat to life in both the preoperative and postoperative periods. In addition to pneumonia, there is a constant danger of respiratory distress resulting from atelectasis, pneumothorax, and laryngeal edema. Any persistent respiratory difficulty after removal of secretions is reported to the surgeon immediately. The infant is monitored for anastomotic leaks as evidenced by purulent chest tube drainage, increased white blood cell count, and temperature instability.

In the infant awaiting esophageal replacement surgery, the upper esophageal segment may be drained by means of a cervical esophagostomy. An esophagostomy is difficult to care for, since the skin may become irritated by moisture from the continued discharge of saliva. Frequent removal of drainage followed by application of a layer of protective ointment or a collection device is usually sufficient treatment. An enterostomal therapist may provide helpful guidance in the prevention and/or treatment of skin breakdown.

For the infant who requires esophageal replacement, nonnutritive sucking is provided by a pacifier. Sometimes small amounts of water or formula are given orally under the guidance of an occupational or speech therapist. In this case, the liquid drains from the esophagostomy but allows the infant to develop mature sucking patterns. The infant who has corrective surgery delayed until 18 to 24 months of age may have a severe problem with eating by mouth after correction. Infants who must remain NPO for an extended period have not been able to go through the process of eating in the normal manner; as a result, they frequently have difficulty with this new task and may develop oral hypersensitivity and food aversion. They require patient, firm guidance in learning the techniques of taking food into the mouth and swallowing after repair (see Feeding Resistance, Chapter 10). A referral to a multidisciplinary feeding behavior program may be necessary.

Family Support, Discharge Planning, and Home Care. One of the difficulties in TEF is the immediate transfer of the sick infant to the intensive care unit and sometimes lengthy hospitalization. The attachment process is facilitated by encouraging parents to visit the infant, participate in his or her care where appropriate, and express their feelings regarding the infant's condition. The nurse in the intensive care unit should assume responsibility for ensuring that the parents are kept fully informed of the infant's progress.

Preparing parents for discharge of their infant involves teaching the techniques that will be continued at home, such as careful suctioning, oral or gastrostomy feeding, and skin care. The parents are taught child or infant behaviors that might be expected after corrective surgery, such as those that indicate that the infant needs to be suctioned, signs of respiratory difficulty, and signs that indicate constriction of the esophagus (poor feeding, dysphagia, drooling, or regurgitating undigested food).

Parents are reminded that it is particularly important to guard against the infant swallowing foreign objects. They are instructed to cut solid food into small pieces, teach the child to chew thoroughly, and avoid foods such as whole hot dogs or large pieces of meat that may become lodged in the esophagus.

Many infants will have some tracheomalacia; therefore parents should be educated regarding signs of respiratory distress. Since many infants with EA and a TEF will develop gastroesophageal reflux, precautions should be initiated (see Gastroesophageal Reflux, Chapter 33).

Discharge planning should include attainment of needed equipment and home nursing services to assist with ongoing assessment of the child and continuity of care.

❖ Evaluation

The effectiveness of nursing interventions is determined by continual reassessment and evaluation of care based on the following observational guidelines:

NURSING CARE PLAN

The Infant with Esophageal Atresia and Tracheoesophageal Fistula

NURSING DIAGNOSIS: Ineffective airway clearance related to abnormal opening between esophagus and trachea or obstruction to swallowing secretions

PATIENT GOAL 1: Will maintain patent airway without aspiration

• **NURSING INTERVENTIONS/*RATIONALES***

Suction as necessary *to remove accumulated secretions from oropharynx*

Position supine with head elevated on an inclined plane (at least 30 degrees) *to decrease pressure against thoracic cavity and to minimize reflux of gastric secretions up distal esophagus and into trachea and bronchi*

Administer oxygen if infant becomes cyanotic *to help relieve respiratory distress*

Do not use positive pressure (e.g., resuscitation bag/mask), *since it may introduce air into stomach and intestines, creating additional pressure in thoracic cavity*

Administer nothing by mouth *to prevent aspiration*

Maintain intermittent or continuous suction of esophageal segment, if ordered preoperatively, *to keep blind pouch empty*

Leave gastrostomy tube, if present, open to gravity drainage *so that air can escape, minimizing risk of regurgitation of gastric contents into trachea*

• **EXPECTED OUTCOMES**

Airway remains patent

Infant does not aspirate secretions

Respirations remain within normal limits

NURSING DIAGNOSIS: Impaired (difficulty) swallowing related to mechanical obstruction

PATIENT GOAL 1: Will receive adequate nourishment

• **NURSING INTERVENTIONS/*RATIONALES***

Administer gastrostomy feedings as prescribed *to provide nourishment until oral feedings are possible*

Progress to oral feedings as prescribed according to infant's condition and surgical correction

Observe closely *to make certain infant is able to swallow without choking*

Monitor intake, output, and weight *to assess adequacy of nutritional intake*

Give infant pacifier *to provide for nonnutritive sucking*

Teach family appropriate feeding techniques *to prepare for discharge*

• **EXPECTED OUTCOME**

Infant receives sufficient nourishment and exhibits a satisfactory weight gain

PATIENT GOAL 2: Patient will learn to take oral feedings (following complete repair)

• **NURSING INTERVENTIONS/*RATIONALES***

Introduce foods one at a time *to evaluate tolerance of food item*

Provide foods with various textures and flavors *to stimulate interest in eating*

Begin with pureed foods and progress to more solid food as child shows readiness

Cut food in small, noncylindrical pieces *to prevent choking*

Avoid foods such as whole hot dogs or large pieces of meat *to decrease risk of choking*

Teach child to chew foods well *to decrease risk of choking*

Refer to speech or occupational therapist, if appropriate, *to facilitate learning*

• **EXPECTED OUTCOME**

Child takes an adequate amount of nourishment and displays no evidence of feeding resistance, malnutrition, or dysphagia

NURSING DIAGNOSIS: High risk for injury related to surgical procedure

PATIENT GOAL 1: Will not experience trauma to surgical site

• **NURSING INTERVENTIONS/*RATIONALE***

Suction only with catheter premeasured to a distance that does not reach to surgical site *to prevent trauma to mucosa*

• **EXPECTED OUTCOME**

Child does not exhibit evidence of injury to surgical site

NURSING DIAGNOSIS: Anxiety related to difficulty swallowing, discomfort from surgery

PATIENT GOAL 1: Will experience a sense of security without discomfort

• **NURSING INTERVENTIONS/*RATIONALES***

Provide tactile stimulation (e.g., cuddling, rocking) *to facilitate optimum development and promote comfort*

Administer mouth care *to keep mouth clean and mucous membranes moist*

Offer pacifier frequently *to provide nonnutritive sucking*

*Administer analgesics as prescribed

Encourage parents to participate in child's care *to provide comfort and security*

• **EXPECTED OUTCOMES**

Infant rests calmly, is alert when awake, and engages in nonnutritive sucking

Mouth remains clean and moist

Child experiences no or minimal pain

Continued.

NURSING CARE PLAN
The Infant with Esophageal Atresia and Tracheoesophageal Fistula—cont'd

NURSING DIAGNOSIS: Altered family processes related to child with a physical defect

PATIENT (FAMILY) GOAL 1: Will be prepared for home care of child

• **NURSING INTERVENTIONS/*RATIONALES***

Teach family skills and observations needed for home care
- Positioning *to prevent aspiration*
- Signs of respiratory distress *to prevent delay in treatment*
- Signs of complications—refusal to eat, dysphagia, increased coughing—*so practitioner can be notified*
- Acquiring needed equipment and services

Care of gastrostomy and esophagostomy when infant has staged surgery, including techniques such as suctioning, feeding, care of operative site and/or ostomies, dressing changes, *to ensure appropriate care after discharge*

• **EXPECTED OUTCOME**

Family demonstrates ability to provide care to infant, an understanding of signs of complications, and appropriate actions

See also:
- Nursing Care Plan: The Family of the Ill or Hospitalized Child, Chapter 26
- Nursing Care Plan: The High-Risk Infant, Chapter 10

1. Monitor infant's respiratory status.
2. Weigh daily; observe infant's eating behavior.
3. Inspect surgical site; observe infant's behavior; monitor vital signs.
4. Observe and interview family members regarding their understanding, feelings, and concerns regarding infant's condition or treatment.

Expected outcomes:

See Nursing Care Plan, pp. 483-484.

ANORECTAL MALFORMATIONS

Anorectal malformations include several forms of imperforate anus (Fig. 11-21). These malformations are among the more common congenital malformations caused by abnormal development, with an incidence of approximately 1 in 500 live births. ***Imperforate anus*** encompasses several forms of malformation without an obvious anal opening, and many have a fistula from the distal rectum to the perineum or genitourinary system. ***Cloacal exstrophy*** is a rare form that includes malformations of the urinary system, genital system, and bowel, which drain into a common channel that communicates with the perineum. Anorectal malformations may occur in isolation or as part of the ***VACTERL syndrome*** (vertebral, anorectal, cardiovascular, tracheoesophageal, renal, and limb abnormalities).

Anorectal anomalies are classified according to sex and level of arrest of rectal descent. The level of rectal descent is determined by the relationship of the termination of bowel to the puborectalis sling of the levator ani musculature. A distinction between the following classifications is important for planning therapy:

Low anomalies—The rectum has descended normally through the puborectalis muscle, the internal and external sphincters are present and well developed with normal function, and there is no connection to the genitourinary tract (Fig. 11-21, *A* or *B*).

Intermediate anomalies—The rectum is at or below the level of the puborectalis muscle; the anal dimple and external sphincter are positioned normally.

High anomalies—The rectum ends above the puborectalis muscle, and there is absence of the internal sphincter. This is usually associated with a genitourinary fistula—rectourethral (male) or rectovaginal (female) (Fig. 11-21, *F*).

Pathophysiology

During embryonic development the cloaca becomes the common channel for the developing urinary, genital, and rectal systems. The cloaca is divided at the sixth week of gestation into an anterior urogenital sinus and a posterior intestinal channel by the urorectal septum. After the lateral folds join the urorectal septum, separation of the urinary and rectal segments takes place. Further differentiation results in the anterior genitourinary system and the posterior anorectal channel. An interruption of this development will lead to incomplete migration of the rectum to its normal perineal position.

Diagnostic Evaluation

Checking for patency of the anus and rectum is a routine part of the newborn assessment and includes observation regarding the passage of meconium. Inspection of the perineal area reveals absence of a normal anus. The appearance of the perineum alone does not accurately predict the level of the lesion. However, complete absence of anal features, a flat perineum, and absence of external sphincter contraction when stimulated generally indicate an intermediate or high lesion. Anomalies associated with anorectal malformation should be considered in the assessment when an anorectal anomaly is noted.

Digital and endoscopic examination identifies constriction or the blind pouch of rectal atresia. Stenosis may not become apparent until 1 year of age or older when the child has a history of difficult defecation, abdominal distention, and ribbonlike stools. Fistulas may not be apparent at birth, but as peristalsis gradually forces the meconium through the fistula, they can be identified by

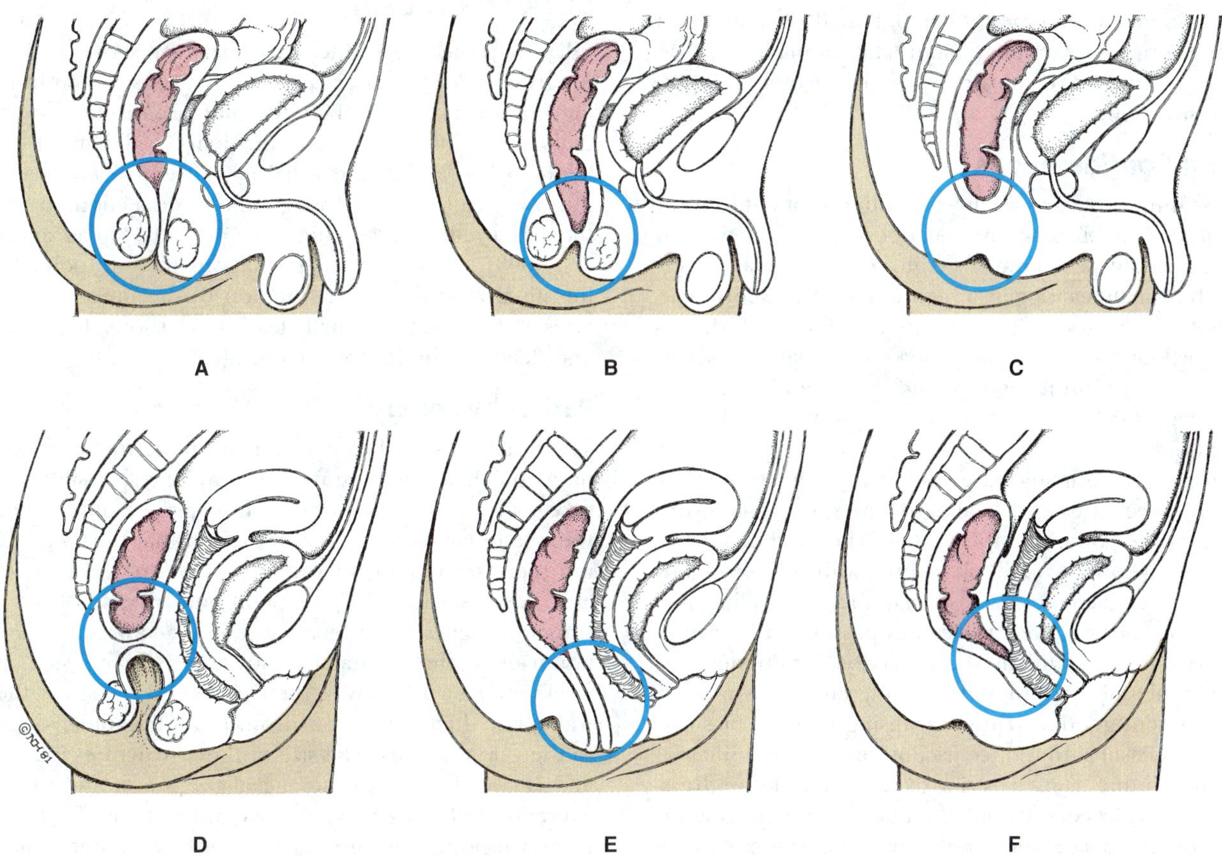

FIG. 11-21 Anorectal stenosis and imperforate anus. **A,** Congenital anal stenosis. **B,** Anal membrane atresia. **C,** Anal agenesis. **D,** Rectal atresia. **E,** Rectoperitoneal fistula. **F,** Rectovaginal fistula.

careful examination. A rectourinary fistula is suspected on the basis of meconium in the urine and confirmed by radiographs of contrast media injected through a tiny catheter into the fistula.

Definitive diagnosis of the extent and location of the high lesion is made by radiographic examination. Abdominal ultrasound is performed to evaluate the infant's anatomic malformation. An intravenous pyelogram and a voiding cystourethrogram are recommended for the infant with a high lesion to identify or rule out the possibility of associated anomalies of the urinary tract. Further examination is also indicated if there is evidence of urinary tract infection or other symptoms. In addition, cardiac evaluation and spinal films may be done to rule out other anomalies.

Therapeutic Management

Successful treatment for a ***low anal stenosis*** is generally accomplished by manual dilations. The procedure, begun by the practitioner, is repeated on a regular basis by the nurses in the hospital and continued at home by the parents after they are carefully instructed in the technique. An imperforate anal membrane is excised and followed by daily anal dilation.

Reconstruction of the anus in the proper position is the goal of the surgical treatment of ***intermediate anorectal malformations.*** The most important consideration in the probable success of reconstruction is the level at which the rectum terminates, especially in its relationship to the puborectalis sling of levator ani muscle. Where the bowel has come through the structure, surgical correction can often be accomplished in the neonatal period by an abdominal pull-through procedure and/or ***anoplasty.***

Infants with ***high anomalies*** require a diverting colostomy in the newborn period. This allows time for the infant to gain weight and for protection of the genitourinary tract from fecal contamination if a fistula is present. Antibiotics are usually administered prophylactically. Final correction of a higher defect is usually postponed for a year. The most prominent procedure is a pull-through procedure or midsagittal ***anorectoplasty.*** The colostomy is closed after the anoplasty has healed and any necessary dilations have been completed.

Prognosis. The prognosis for children with anorectal anomalies depends a great deal on whether the defect is a high or low one. Children with low lesions generally have fewer complications and usually achieve normal bowel continence. Since the internal anal sphincter is absent in most children with high defects, incontinence is a common long-term problem. These children may achieve socially acceptable continence over time. Other potential complications following surgical treatment of anorectal anomalies include strictures, recurrent rectourinary fistula, mucosal prolapse, and constipation.

Nursing Considerations

The first nursing responsibility is assisting in identification of anorectal malformations. A poorly developed anal dimple, a round perineum, a genitourinary fistula, or vertebral abnormalities suggest a high lesion. A newborn who does not pass a stool within 24 hours following birth requires further assessment, and meconium that appears at an inappropriate orifice is reported. Preoperative care includes diagnostic evaluation, GI decompression, and intravenous fluids.

Postoperative nursing care following anorectoplasty is primarily directed toward healing of the surgical site without infection or other complications. When the infant has undergone a pull-through procedure with anoplasty but without a diverting colostomy, special nursing care involves maintaining the anal area as clean as possible with scrupulous perineal care. Initially there may be continuous passage of stool, and a temporary dressing and drain may be used. Frequent gentle perineal cleansing in a tub or small basin and measures to reduce friction on skin are initiated. Protective ointments such as zinc oxide and occlusive dressings such as hydrocolloids will often decrease skin irritation from frequent, loose stools. The preferred position is a side-lying prone position with the hips elevated or a supine position with the legs suspended at a 90-degree angle to the trunk to prevent pressure on perineal sutures.

The infant is given regular feedings when evidence of normal peristalsis returns. In the meantime, there may be an NG tube for abdominal decompression, and intravenous fluids are provided. Care of the infant with a colostomy involves frequent dressing and/or appliance changes, meticulous skin care, and correct application of the collection device (see Chapter 27 for colostomy care).

Family Support, Discharge Planning, and Home Care. Long-term follow-up is essential for children with high lesions. Following the definitive pull-through procedure, toilet training is delayed. Complete continence is seldom achieved at the usual age of 2 to 3 years. Bowel habit training, diet modification, and administration of stool softeners or fiber help children slowly improve bowel management, but optimum results may not be achieved until later childhood or adolescence. Support and reassurance during the slow progression to normal function are essential.

Parents are instructed in perineal and wound care or care of the colostomy as needed. Anal dilations may be necessary for some infants. Parents are advised to observe stooling patterns and to observe for signs of anal stricture or complications. Information on dietary modifications and/or administration of medications is included in counseling. For infants with high lesions, plans for corrective surgery should be discussed. (See Nursing Care Plan: The Infant with Anorectal Malformation.*)

*In *Wong and Whaley's Clinical Manual of Pediatric Nursing* (Mosby).

BILIARY ATRESIA

Biliary atresia, or extrahepatic biliary atresia (EHBA), is a progressive inflammatory process that causes both intrahepatic and extrahepatic bile duct fibrosis, resulting in eventual ductal obstruction. The incidence of biliary atresia is between 1 in 10,000 and 1 in 25,000 live births. There does not seem to be a racial or genetic predilection, although there is a female predominance of 1.4:1 (Karrer and others, 1990). Associated malformations include polysplenia, intestinal atresia, and malrotation of the intestine. Biliary atresia, if untreated, usually leads to cirrhosis, liver failure, and death in the first 2 years of life.

Pathophysiology

The exact cause of biliary atresia is unknown, although immune mechanisms or viral injury may be responsible for the progressive process that results in complete obliteration of the bile ducts. Reports have indicated that biliary atresia is not seen in the fetus or stillborn or newborn infant (Fanaroff and Martin, 1992; Grosfeld and others, 1989). This situation suggests that biliary atresia is acquired late in gestation or in the perinatal period and is manifested a few weeks after birth. Early in the course of the disease, the intrahepatic ducts are patent from the intralobular ductules to the porta hepatis. The size of these structures is variable and is correlated with the age of the infant and with bile excretion following hepatic portoenterostomy. These structures are present in most affected infants under 2 months of age but gradually disappear over the next few months and by 4 months are completely replaced by fibrous tissue.

The degree of involvement of the extrahepatic biliary ducts also is variable. Most commonly the entire extrahepatic system is involved in the obliterative process, but some infants have a patent proximal portion of the extrahepatic duct or patency of the gallbladder, cystic duct, and common bile duct. Microscopic examination of the liver tissue reveals cholestasis with bile duct proliferation and fibrosis.

Clinical Manifestations

Many infants with biliary atresia are full term and appear healthy at birth. If jaundice persists beyond 2 weeks of age, especially if the direct (conjugated) bilirubin is elevated, biliary atresia should be suspected. The urine may be dark, and the stools often become progressively more ***acholic*** or gray, indicating absence of bile pigment. Hepatomegaly is present early in the course of the disease, and the liver is firm on palpation. The serum aminotransferase and alkaline phosphatase levels are usually elevated.

In infants with delayed diagnosis, or in children in whom surgery has failed to provide adequate bile drainage, there is progression of liver disease. Cirrhosis and splenomegaly occur with hypoalbuminemia, ascites, and coagulopathy. Fat malabsorption and malnutrition result in severe failure to thrive. Severe pruritus may also be present as the disease progresses.

Diagnostic Evaluation

The diagnosis of biliary atresia is suspected based on the history, physical findings, and laboratory studies. Laboratory tests include a complete blood count, electrolyte and bilirubin levels, and liver function tests. Additional laboratory analyses, including alpha-1-antitrypsin level, TORCHS titers (see p. 503), hepatitis serology, urine cytomegalovirus, and a sweat test, may be indicated to rule out other conditions that cause persistent cholestasis and jaundice. An abdominal sonogram is usually performed to identify potential causes of extrahepatic obstruction, such as a choledochal cyst. The patency of the extrahepatic biliary system will be demonstrated by a nuclear scintiscan. If there is no evidence of radioactive material excreted into the duodenum, biliary atresia is a possible diagnosis. A percutaneous liver biopsy may establish the diagnosis in many cases of biliary atresia. The definitive diagnosis of biliary atresia is obtained during an exploratory laparotomy and an intraoperative cholangiogram that demonstrates complete obstruction at some level of the biliary tree.

Therapeutic Management

The primary treatment of biliary atresia is ***hepatic portoenterostomy (Kasai procedure).*** This surgical procedure involves dissection of the porta hepatis to expose an area through which bile may drain. A ***roux-en-Y*** jejunal limb is then anastomosed to the porta hepatis (a Y-shaped anastamosis performed to provide bile drainage without reflux). There are several variations of this procedure. In approximately 80% to 90% of infants with biliary atresia who are operated on when younger than 10 weeks of age, bile drainage is achieved (Karrer and others, 1990; Ryckman and others, 1993). However, progressive cirrhosis still occurs in many children, and up to 80% may eventually require liver transplantation (Laurent and others, 1990). Complications following the portoenterostomy procedure include ascending cholangitis, cirrhosis, portal hypertension, and GI bleeding. Prophylactic antibiotics are given following the Kasai procedure to minimize the risk of ascending cholangitis.

Liver transplantation now offers hope for children with a failed Kasai procedure. Liver transplantation is usually restricted to children who do not drain bile after the Kasai procedure and who have late progression of liver disease despite biliary drainage. Even when it is not curative, the Kasai procedure extends survival in the majority of children, thus increasing the chances of finding a suitable donor organ. In addition to orthotopic liver transplantation (patient's liver is not removed), reduced-size liver transplant techniques and living-related donor liver transplantation have improved survival and decreased mortality during the wait for a liver.

Complications following liver transplantation include obstruction and bile leaks at the biliary anastomosis, hemorrhage, infection, and rejection. Immunosuppressive drugs are required following transplantation, including corticosteroids and cyclosporine A. A new immunosuppressive drug, FK-506, is currently being used following liver transplantation in a series of clinical trials.

Medical management of biliary atresia is primarily supportive. It includes nutritional support with infant formulas that contain medium-chain triglycerides and essential fatty acids (Kaufman and others, 1987). Supplementation with fat-soluble vitamins, a multivitamin, and mineral supplements including iron, zinc and selenium are usually required. Aggressive nutritional support in the form of continuous tube feedings or parenteral nutrition may be indicated for severe failure to thrive. Phenobarbital may be prescribed following hepatic portoenterostomy to stimulate bile flow, and ursodeoxycholic acid may be used to decrease cholestasis and the intense pruritus from jaundice. In cases of advanced liver dysfunction, management is the same as in infants with cirrhosis (see Chapter 33).

Prognosis. Untreated biliary atresia results in progressive cirrhosis and death in most children by 2 years of age. The Kasai procedure does improve the prognosis, but it is not a cure. Biliary drainage can be achieved if the surgery is performed before the intrahepatic bile ducts are destroyed, usually by 8 weeks of age; otherwise the prognosis is poor (Karrer and others, 1990). Long-term survival has been reported in children who received the Kasai procedure (Toyosaka and others, 1993). However, even with successful bile drainage, many children ultimately develop liver failure. A cure for pediatric liver disorders is now possible with the success of liver transplantation. The advances in surgical techniques and the development of cyclosporine A and other antirejection drugs have significantly improved the success of transplantation. The 1- to 4-year survival rate of pediatric liver transplantation is now 70% to 88% in most centers (Beath and others, 1993a, 1993b; Ryckman and others, 1993). The major obstacle remains the shortage of suitable donors. Success with segmental size reduction of adult donor livers, living-related donor transplantation, and increased public awareness may improve the availability of donor organs for children in the future.

Nursing Considerations

There are many important nursing interventions for the child with biliary atresia. Education regarding all aspects of the treatment plan and the rationale for therapy should be provided to the family members. In the immediate postoperative period following a hepatic portoenterostomy, nursing care is similar to that following any abdominal surgery. If an interrupted jejunal conduit has been performed, the family will need to be taught how to care for the two stomas and how to refeed the bile following feedings. Teaching includes the proper administration of medications. Administration of nutritional therapy, including special formulas, vitamin and mineral supplements, tube feedings, or parenteral nutrition, is an essential nursing responsibility. The caregivers are taught how to monitor and administer nutritional therapy in the home. Pruritus may be a significant problem that can be relieved by drug therapy or comfort measures such as baths in colloidal oatmeal compounds and trimming of fingernails. The risk of complications of biliary atresia, such as cholangitis, portal hypertension, GI bleeding, and ascites, should be explained to the caregivers.

These children and their families require special psychosocial support. The uncertain prognosis, discomfort, and waiting for transplantation can produce considerable stress (see Cirrhosis, Chapter 33). In addition, extended hospitalizations, as well as pharmacologic and nutritional therapy, can impose significant financial burdens on the family, as with any chronic condition. The expertise of a multidisciplinary health care team including physicians, nurses, nutritionists, pharmacists and social workers is often needed. Parent support groups can be very beneficial. The **Children's Liver Foundation, Inc.,*** provides educational materials, programs, and support systems for parents of children with liver disease.

HERNIAS

A ***hernia*** is a protrusion of a portion of an organ or organs through an abnormal opening. The danger from herniation arises when the organ protruding through the opening is constricted to the extent that circulation is impaired or when the protruding organs encroach on and impair the function of other structures. The herniations of concern in this section are those that protrude through the diaphragm, the abdominal wall, or the inguinal canal. Because inguinal and femoral hernias involve the genitourinary tract, they are discussed in the section regarding defects of the genitourinary tract.

UMBILICAL HERNIA

The umbilical hernia is the most common hernia in infants. It occurs when fusion of the umbilical ring is incomplete at the point where the umbilical vessels exit the abdominal wall. It affects blacks more often than whites and low-birth-weight infants and premature infants more often than full-term infants. An umbilical hernia usually is an isolated defect, but it may be present in association with other congenital anomalies, such as Down syndrome and trisomies 13 and 18. The size of the defect is variable, and it is more prominent when the infant is crying (Fig. 11-22). ***Incarceration,*** in which the hernia is constricted and cannot be reduced manually, is rare; usually the defect spontaneously resolves by 3 to 4 years of age. If the hernia persists beyond this age, it is usually surgically corrected.

*76 South Orange Ave., Suite 202, South Orange, NJ 07079; (201) 761-1111.

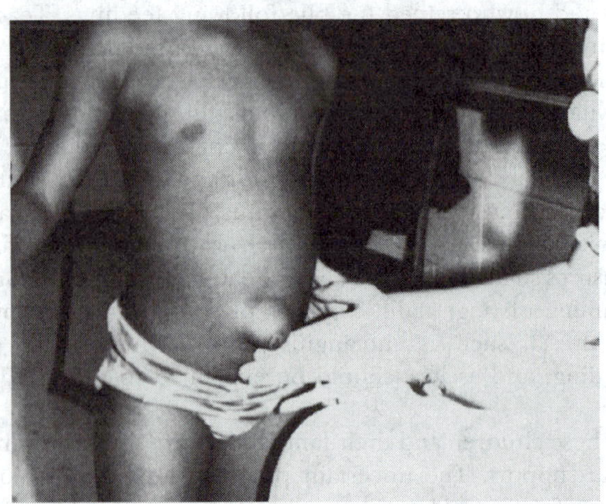

FIG. 11-22 Child with an umbilical hernia.

Nursing Considerations

The appearance of an umbilical hernia may be disconcerting to parents; therefore they need reassurance that the defect usually is not harmful. Taping or strapping the abdomen to flatten the protrusion does not aid in resolution and can produce skin irritation.

CONGENITAL DIAPHRAGMATIC HERNIA (CDH)

CDH results when there is failure of the transverse septum and the pleuroperitoneal folds to completely develop and form the diaphragm. When the posterior part of the diaphragm fails to close, a triangular defect forms the foramen of Bochdalek, the most common type of CDH, which is often asymptomatic. If the diaphragm does not form completely, the intestines and other abdominal structures, such as the liver, can enter the thoracic cavity, compressing the lung. Lung growth may be arrested on the affected side and to a lesser degree on the contralateral side. Respiration is further compromised by hypoplasia and compression of the lung, including the airways and blood vessels. Pulmonary hypoplasia and pulmonary hypertension have also been recently recognized as components in the pathology of CDH in addition to the anatomic defect. This serious defect requires prompt recognition and aggressive treatment to reduce its high mortality.

Clinical Manifestations

The most common manifestation of CDH is acute respiratory distress in the newborn. Entrance of air into the intestines following birth further compromises respiration. Infants with a CDH may be dyspneic and cyanotic, and have a scaphoid abdomen; cardiac output is impaired, and the infant will exhibit signs and symptoms of shock.

Diagnostic Evaluation

Prenatal diagnosis of CDH is possible; the three main features detected by ultrasound confirming the diagnosis are polyhydramnios, mediastinal shift, and the absence of a stomach bubble in the fetus (Moreno and Iovanne, 1993). Fetal surgery for repair of CDH has had mixed success in some medical centers (Levine, 1991). For now, the main advantage of prenatal diagnosis is that it allows for transport to a tertiary medical center, where a multidisciplinary team of neonatologists, neonatal nurses, and pediatric surgeons can intervene early in the acute phase to improve the infant's chances for survival and a positive outcome.

After birth, the diagnosis of CDH may depend on the type of hernia present. In the majority of cases, the diagnosis is suspected on the basis of the clinical manifestations and is confirmed by a chest radiograph. The chest radiograph shows fluid and air-filled loops of intestine in the affected side of the chest. The mediastinum may be shifted to the unaffected side, and auscultation may reveal decreased breath sounds on the affected side.

Therapeutic Management

The infant with a CDH requires immediate respiratory assistance, which includes endotracheal intubation and gastrointestinal decompression with a double-lumen catheter to prevent further respiratory compromise. Positioning the infant with the head and chest elevated higher than the abdomen will facilitate downward displacement of the abdominal organs. In infants with mild respiratory distress, oxygen may be given by hood; however, close attention to the infant's acid-base status is imperative in the management and prevention of pulmonary hypertension. Low ventilatory pressure and the lowest mean airway pressure possible combined with rapid ventilatory rates (80 to 120 breaths per minute) may serve to reduce the incidence of pulmonary leaks from overinflation of the unaffected lung. Bag and mask ventilation is contraindicated to prevent air from entering the stomach and especially the intestines, further compromising pulmonary function.

Intravenous fluids are initiated during the stabilization period. An umbilical arterial catheter may be placed for monitoring arterial blood gases and for provision of adequate glucose. A transcutaneous oxygen pressure monitor or pulse oximeter may be placed preductally (right hand) and postductally (left hand or arm) to monitor the amount of ductal shunting through the patent ductus arteriosus. An umbilical arterial catheter will help monitor postductal arterial oxygen tension (PaO_2). Ductal shunting of deoxygenated blood occurs when pressure in the pulmonary artery is equal to or less than peripheral blood pressure. If pulmonary hypertension is severe, with decreased pulmonary venous return, right atrial pressure will be greater than left atrial pressure, resulting in shunting of blood through the foramen ovale. The net results of these events cause further hypoxia, hypercarbia, and acidosis.

Further preoperative stabilization may include the use of opioids, such as fentanyl, and a paralyzing agent, pancuronium, in infants who are agitated and resisting ventilation. An inotropic drug such as dopamine may be used to support systemic blood pressure. Tolazoline is also used to promote pulmonary vascular vasodilation and decrease the amount of pulmonary hypertension (see Persistent Pulmonary Hypertension of the Newborn, Chapter 10).

Since acidosis increases pulmonary hypertension and consequently shunting of unoxygenated blood away from the lungs, it is imperative to monitor acid-base status closely. Prevention of acidosis may be accomplished with sodium bicarbonate continuous infusion and hyperventilation; tromethamine (THAM) may also be used in the place of sodium bicarbonate. Close attention to the infant's thermoregulation status (maintain neutral thermal environment) and glucose requirements during the acute phase are also a priority of care. The use of high-frequency jet ventilation and/or high-frequency oscillation to manage the infant with a CDH is used in many tertiary centers with varying results; ventilatory management is individualized based on the infant's response and requirements. Some preliminary research studies indicate that nitric oxide given by mechanical ventilation reduces the severity of pulmonary hypertension seen with CDH (Kinsella and others, 1993).

Traditional management has been early surgical repair of the defect. However, increased survival rates have been reported with surgery following a period of preoperative stabilization that may include placing the infant on extracorporeal membrane oxygenation (ECMO) or high-frequency ventilation. Operative treatment involves returning the abdominal organs to the abdomen and repairing the diaphragmatic defect. Postoperative management involves continuation of ventilatory therapy, monitoring of acid-base balance, and even maintaining the infant in a slightly alkalotic state to prevent or decrease the effects of pulmonary hypertension. In addition, gastric decompression, thermoregulation, sedation, and maintenance of adequate cardiac output and peripheral perfusion are continued. Following surgery for CDH, the infant may at first show marked improvement in ventilatory status; the infant may then gradually deteriorate with the combined effects of hypoxemia and pulmonary hypertension. For this reason, close attention to acid-base balance and ventilatory requirements in the postoperative period will help prevent a potentially irreversible poor outcome. If paralysis is continued in the postoperative period, appropriate pain management should not be overlooked. The infant may return from surgery with one or two chest tubes, which will require close monitoring.

Prognosis. The overall mortality rate for infants with CDH remains high (50% to 80%) despite advances in neonatal care (Moreno and Iovanne, 1993). Most deaths are due to severe respiratory distress secondary to hypoplasia of the lung and persistent pulmonary hypertension. Infants

CRITICAL THINKING EXERCISE

Congenital Diaphragmatic Hernia

A prenatal ultrasound examination has revealed the presence of a congenital diaphragmatic hernia in the fetus of a 31-year-old woman who has had two previous cesarean sections. A repeat C-section is carried out, and the newborn is placed under a radiant warmer for stabilization; the weight is approximately 3.5 kg. The newborn is cyanotic, has copious oral secretions, and demonstrates gasping respiratory effort. The most important initial intervention is to:

1. Place the infant in Trendelenburg position to facilitate drainage of secretions
2. Begin bag and mask ventilation with 100% oxygen and a proper-size face mask.
3. Prepare moist, warm saline gauze pads to place over the congenital defect.
4. Suction the oropharynx and prepare a 4 mm endotracheal tube and stylet for immediate intubation.

The correct answer is 4. In most cases the infant with a CDH and respiratory distress will benefit the most from intubation for airway maintenance.

Air from the manual resuscitation bag will enter the stomach and intestines in the chest cavity, further compromising respiratory status. There is no outward defect to cover, and the Trendelenburg position is contraindicated because it increases pressure of organs against lungs.

with severe hypoplasia of the lung often exhibit respiratory distress within the first 24 hours of life. The prognosis also depends on the size of the defect and on pulmonary function of the contralateral side. Ongoing respiratory distress postoperatively due to difficulty reexpanding the hypoplastic lung and associated pulmonary hypertension and right-to-left shunting is not uncommon.

Nursing Considerations

Assessment of the infant at birth is an integral component of nursing care. This is accentuated in life-threatening cases such as CDH, where prompt recognition of neonatal respiratory distress, cyanosis, a scaphoid abdomen, and a possible mediastinal shift would alert the nurse to investigate further. Any one or a combination of these signs may signal the presence of CDH. A newborn in respiratory distress at birth who does not initially respond to resuscitation is further evaluated for CDH; endotracheal intubation is an option for providing adequate oxygenation until CDH is ruled out as a cause of the distress. If CDH is diagnosed prenatally and the infant is in distress, endotracheal intubation is required to prevent further accumulation of air in the stomach and intestines and subsequent respiratory compromise (see Critical Thinking Exercise box, p. 489).

NURSING ALERT Any newborn infant with a scaphoid abdomen, moderate to severe respiratory distress, decreased breath sounds unilaterally, and a history of polyhydramnios should be suspected of having a CDH. Ventilation should not be given with bag and mask to prevent further intestinal air and subsequent respiratory compromise.

Preoperative care involves prompt recognition, resuscitation, and stabilization of the infant, including ventilatory support, blood gas measurements, and administration of intravenous fluids. The stomach is decompressed with a double-lumen tube, and the infant is observed for signs of impaired cardiac output, acidosis, and hypoxemia.

The infant should be positioned on the affected side to take advantage of gravity, which facilitates expansion of the unaffected lung and reduces the likelihood of overexpansion into the unaffected side. Postoperative care includes the routine observations discussed in the care of the high risk infant. Close observation to detect signs of respiratory distress or fluid and electrolyte imbalances is an important nursing function. The infant is closely monitored for signs of mediastinal shift, pulmonary air leak, and infection. Hypovolemia as a result of third-spacing of intravascular fluids may occur; correction with salt-free albumin is one option for treatment of hypovolemia.

Nursing care of the infant with a CDH is also aimed at reducing stimulation either from care activities such as routine suctioning or from environmental factors such as noise and light. Measures that further reduce infant stress should be a routine aspect of care for the infant with a CDH. It is not uncommon for the infant with a CDH to be the sickest and thus the most demanding patient in relation to nursing care.

Because of the serious nature of the condition and the urgency of treatment, the parents are in great need of ongoing support and education regarding postoperative care. The infant with CDH may require long-term hospitalization and care; this further places the infant at risk for delayed acceptance and integration into the family unit. As soon as medically possible, the parents should be involved in the daily care of their child.

HIATAL HERNIA

In hiatal hernia, a subgroup of diaphragmatic hernia, a portion of the stomach herniates through the esophageal hiatus of the diaphragm. These hernias are classified as sliding or paraesophageal hernias. The ***sliding hernia*** is associated with gastroesophageal reflux (GER). The ***paraesophageal hernia*** is more often associated with retrosternal pain and dysphasia, and may cause gastric volvulus and obstruction. Therapeutic management is directed toward treatment of GER, including positioning, pharmacologic treatment, and dietary management. Surgical treatment is required when complications related to GER occur despite medical management (see Gastroesophageal Reflux, Chapter 33).

ABDOMINAL WALL DEFECTS

Gastroschisis and omphalocele are two of the more common forms of congenital abdominal wall defects; gastroschisis occurs in about 1 in 10,000 births, and omphalocele occurs in 2.5 in 10,000 births (Torfs and others, 1990). There is a distinction in terms of embryology that is significant in the determination of prognosis. An ***omphalocele*** occurs when there is herniation of the abdominal contents through the umbilical ring (hernia of the umbilical cord), usually with an intact peritoneal sac, whereas ***gastroschisis*** occurs when the herniation is lateral to the umbilical ring. This herniation is usually to the right of the umbilicus, and there is not a peritoneal sac.

Omphalocele

Omphalocele is related to a true failure of embryonic development. It occurs when there is failure of the caudal or lateral infolding of the abdominal wall at approximately the third week of gestation. With the deficiency in the abdominal wall, the bowel is unable to complete its return to the abdomen between the tenth and twelfth weeks of gestation.

The omphalocele is usually covered only by a translucent peritoneal sac. The sac may contain only a small portion of the bowel or most of the bowel and other abdominal viscera, such as the liver. If the sac ruptures, the abdominal contents become exposed. Omphalocele often is associated with other anomalies, including cardiac defects, imperforate anus, trisomy 18, ileal atresia, and meningocele.

With the increasing frequency of and improvements in prenatal ultrasonography, prenatal diagnosis of some abdominal wall defects is being accomplished. In the past, many centers proceeded with early delivery by cesarean section, but current recommendations are to allow these infants to be delivered by spontaneous vaginal delivery if possible (Meller, Reyes, and Loeff, 1989). The benefits of prenatal ultrasound diagnosis include the ability to transfer the mother to a tertiary care center where pediatric surgeons and a neonatal intensive care unit are available to assist with care following delivery.

Initial management after delivery includes loosely covering the exposed abdominal contents and membranes with saline-soaked pads and a plastic drape to prevent excessive water loss, drying, and temperature instability. Intravenous fluids and antibiotics are administered, and a further evaluation is completed.

Following initial medical management, surgical closure of the omphalocele is made. The sac is resected, and an attempt is made to close the abdominal fascia with sutures. The abdominal wall may need to be stretched. If there is an obvious intestinal atresia, a bowel resection and stoma or primary anastomosis may be performed.

When a primary closure of the defect is not possible because of the small size of the abdominal cavity, a silo is created with a sheet of Silastic material that is sutured to the edges of the skin following removal of the sac. The abdominal contents are placed in the abdomen, and the abdominal wall is stretched before the silo is placed. Following surgery, the silo is suspended using mild tension from the top of the incubator or radiant warmer. Usually the silo is compressed on a daily basis. At the end of approximately 1 week, the infant is returned to the operating room and the silo is removed. The abdominal fascia and skin are then closed with sutures.

Postoperatively these infants often require mechanical ventilation and parenteral nutrition for several days. Postoperative complications include infection, evisceration, intestinal volvulus, obstruction, and development of a ventral hernia.

Gastroschisis

Gastroschisis occurs when the bowel herniates through a defect in the abdominal wall to the right of the umbilical cord and through the rectus muscle. There is no membrane covering the exposed bowel. Controversy exists regarding the etiology of gastroschisis. It has been suggested that at some point between the bowel's stay in the umbilical cord and the completion of fixation, a tear occurs at the base of the umbilical cord, allowing the intestine to herniate (Meller, Reyes, and Loeff, 1989). The gap between the cord and the tear is filled in by skin, giving the appearance of a defect in the abdominal wall to the right of the umbilical cord. The base of the defect is narrow, and the lack of membranes results in thickening and foreshortening of the bowel. Gastroschisis is rarely associated with other major congenital anomalies.

Initial management is similar to that for omphalocele. The exposed bowel is loosely covered in saline-soaked pads, and the abdomen is wrapped in a plastic drape (wrapping around the exposed bowel is contraindicated—if the exposed bowel expands, wrapping could cause pressure necrosis). Intravenous fluids and antibiotics are administered.

The infant with gastroschisis usually requires more urgent surgery because there is no sac covering the exposed bowel. Temperature control and fluid management are extremely important for both gastroschisis and omphalocele. Generally, these infants undergo surgery within several hours following birth. During surgery the abdominal wall is stretched and the mass of bowel is replaced in the abdomen as a whole. If primary closure is not possible, a silo is performed similar to that in an omphalocele (Fig. 11-23). The silo is reduced over several days, at which time, it is removed surgically and the defect is closed.

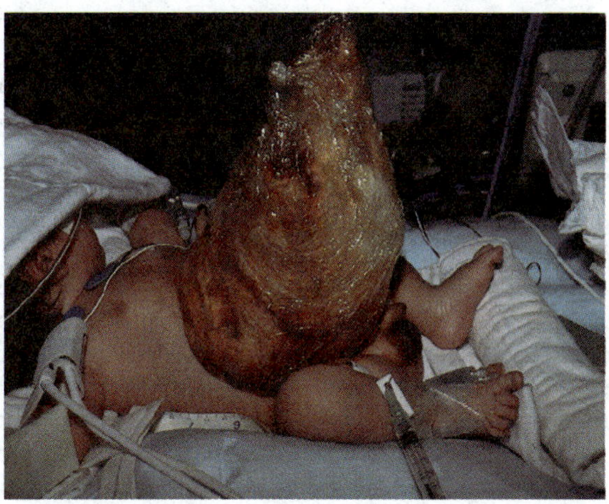

FIG. 11-23 Gastroschisis enclosed in a silo pouch; the bowel is covered with povidone-iodine (Betadine)–soaked gauze and plastic film. Also note infant's gray color, indicating shock, and placement of tape to measure abdominal circumference without disturbing neonate.

Postoperatively most infants require mechanical ventilation and parenteral nutrition. Many of these infants have a prolonged ileus. The advent of parenteral nutrition in the 1960s has been the most significant factor improving the survival in infants with gastroschisis and omphalocele. Respiratory distress may occur postoperatively because of increased abdominal pressure. Other complications include infection, intestinal obstruction, vena cava compression, and subsequent decrease in blood flow to the lower extremities.

Nursing Considerations

Nursing care is similar to that for any high-risk infant. In addition, infection is a constant threat before surgery, and careful positioning and handling are needed to prevent rupture of the omphalocele sac, herniated bowel, or disturbance of the Silastic material used for gradual reduction. Viscera should be protected with saline-soaked pads and plastic drape placed over the defect. Heat and fluid loss from the exposed viscera are major concerns in the preoperative period; therefore thermoregulation is critical. Fluid replacement is vital and must compensate for losses. The gastrointestinal tract is decompressed via an NG tube before surgery to aid in bowel reduction. Postsurgical care includes monitoring for signs of complications and assessment of bowel function. Parenteral nutritional support may be necessary when ileus persists. It may require several weeks for normal bowel function to return before enteral feeding can be initiated.

Family Support, Discharge Planning, and Home Care. Since these abdominal defects are visible and may be shocking to parents, immediate emotional support at the time of birth is essential. The family needs a brief explanation of the defect and reassurance that their child is in no immediate danger (unless circumstances are different). After the parents have had time to interact with their newborn, they should be informed about the surgical treatment and postoperative care (see Critical Thinking Exercise box). At the time of discharge from the hospital, many of these infants are receiving oral feedings, but extended parenteral nutrition may be required if malabsorption and prolonged ileus occur. Oral aversion to feedings is not uncommon after a prolonged period of receiving nothing by mouth; this will require patience and often the involvement of a speech therapist to retrain the infant to suck and swallow (see Feeding Resistance, Chapter 10). Continuity of care may be ensured by a referral to a home health care agency, especially if long-term nutritional support is required.

CRITICAL THINKING EXERCISE
Abdominal Wall Defect

A 2800 g newborn is noted to have a large mass of intestinal contents covering the exterior abdomen and protruding from around the umbilical cord; this event was not anticipated. The mother is 23 years old and single; the father is not involved. The maternal grandmother is present at the delivery and notices the defect. She is visibly shocked. The newborn is not in any respiratory distress. Given these facts, the best intervention at this time is to:

1. Cover the defect with a blanket, show the newborn to the mother, and make no mention of the defect until the pediatrician arrives.
2. Prepare for immediate endotracheal intubation, since this is a life-threatening defect.
3. Allow the mother to hold the newborn briefly while protecting the defect with moist saline gauze.
4. Discuss with the mother surgical options for correction of the defect.

The correct answer is 3. The mother and newborn are not at immediate risk for any health complications that would preclude a short but meaningful time for interaction.

The mother and grandmother need to be reassured that the infant will be completely evaluated on arrival in the nursery (or neonatal intensive care unit) by other health care professionals and that surgical correction is the most probable treatment. Discussing the surgical options immediately after birth is not the best intervention; this discussion may be better received after the mother has had some time to examine the newborn and react to others in the immediate surroundings. The other health care workers' reactions will play an important part in the mother's perception of her newborn in relation to acceptance of the newborn. Covering the baby with a blanket and hiding the defect will only enhance the mother's anxiety and may interfere with her attachment to the infant. There is no need to prepare for intubation at this time, since no respiratory distress is noted.

DEFECTS OF THE GENITOURINARY (GU) TRACT*

External defects of the GU tract are usually obvious at birth. The anatomic location of these defects frequently causes more psychologic concern to parents than does the actual condition or treatment. The timing of medical and surgical procedures for correction of these defects has important implications for children. Surgery involving sexual organs can be particulary disruptive to preschoolers, who fear punishment, retaliation, body mutilation, or castration. Therefore the trend is toward early correction of visible genital defects, preferably without multiple-stage repairs. Renal anomalies, which are typically not obvious at birth, are described in Table 11-6.

PHIMOSIS

Phimosis is a narrowing or stenosis of the preputial opening of the foreskin that prevents retraction of the foreskin over the glans penis. It is a normal finding in infants and young boys and usually disappears as the child grows and the distal prepuce dilates. Occasionally the narrowing obstructs the flow of urine, resulting in a dribbling stream or even ballooning of the foreskin with accumulated urine during voiding.

Inflammation or infection of the phimotic foreskin occurs occasionally and is managed as any other inflammation or infection. Severe phimosis is treated surgically by circumcision.

Nursing Considerations

Proper hygiene of the phimotic foreskin in infants and young boys consists of external cleansing during routine bathing. The foreskin should not be forcibly retracted, because it may create scarring, which can prevent future retraction. Furthermore, retraction of the tight foreskin can result in ***paraphimosis,*** a condition in which the retracted foreskin cannot be replaced in its normal position over the glans. This causes edema and venous congestion created by constriction by the tight band of foreskin—a urologic emergency that requires immediate evaluation.

INGUINAL HERNIA

Inguinal hernias account for approximately 80% of all hernias and occur more frequently in boys (90%) than in girls.

Pathophysiology

Inguinal hernia is derived from persistence of all or part of the processus vaginalis, the tube of peritoneum that precedes the testicle through the inguinal canal into the scro-

*Mikel Gray, RN, PhD, PNP, CURN, revised this section.

TABLE 11-6 Renal Anomalies

ANOMALY	DESCRIPTION AND NURSING IMPLICATIONS
ANOMALIES OF THE KIDNEYS	
Anomalies of Number	
Bilateral agenesis	Fatal anomaly associated with Potter facies and multisystem congenital defects
Unilateral agenesis	Occurs in approximately 1:1500 live births; may be discovered on routine examination; parents and child may be counseled regarding advisability of avoiding contact sports
Supernumerary kidneys	Rare anomaly; intervention indicated if obstruction or infection of anomalous kidney occurs
Anomalies of Rotation	Rotation of kidney from its usual relationship to spine; malrotation is not by itself significant, but it is often associated with clinically significant defects, including renal ectopia or fusion
Anomalies of Ascent	Incomplete ascent of kidney caused by abnormal ureteral bud development; ectopic kidneys are usually located in pelvis; obstruction and infection occasionally occur; abnormally high ascent (intrathoracic kidney) is particularly rare; associated obstruction is rare; crossed renal ectopia occurs when both kidneys ascend on single side of retroperitoneum; renal fusion is possible when crossed ectopia occurs
Anomalies of Fusion	Fusion of kidneys occurs when renal masses meet during embryonic development; horseshoe kidney is union of inferior portions of two kidneys crossing midline; fusion also may occur with crossed renal ectopia
ANOMALIES OF THE RENAL PELVIS AND URETERS	
Bifid renal pelvis	Duplication of renal pelvis; may slightly increase risk of urinary tract infections
Incomplete ureteral duplication	Partial duplication of ureter that opens into single orifice in bladder; peristalsis and evacuation of upper urinary tract may be adversely affected
Complete ureteral duplication	Complete duplication of ureters with separate orifices noted in bladder; reflux of lower ureteral segment is common; upper ureteral segment may be obstructed
Ureteral ectopia	Ureteral orifice opens into a structure rather than bladder base; urethra and vagina are common sites of ectopia; obstruction or continuous urinary incontinence occurs depending on site of ectopic ureteral orifice; defects of associated kidney are common
Ureterocele	Bulging dilation of intravesical ureteral segment; ureterocele may obstruct bladder outlet and is often associated with ureteral duplication

tum during the eighth month of gestation. Following descent of the testicle, the proximal portion of the processus vaginalis normally atrophies and closes, whereas the distal portion forms the tunica vaginalis, which envelops the testicle in the scrotum. When the upper portion fails to atrophy, the abdominal fluid or an abdominal structure can be forced into it, creating a palpable bulge or mass. The persistent sac may end at any point along the inguinal canal; it may stop at the inguinal ring or extend all the way into the scrotum (Fig. 11-24). The hernial sac is present at birth but does not usually become apparent until the infant is able to build up sufficient intraabdominal pressure to open the sac, usually at 2 to 3 months of age. Since the inguinal canal is short, hernias occur relatively early.

Clinical Manifestations

This very common defect is asymptomatic unless the abdominal contents are forced into the patent sac. Most often it appears as a painless inguinal swelling that varies in size. It disappears during periods of rest or is reducible by gentle compression; it appears when the infant cries or strains or when the older child strains, coughs, or stands for a long period. The defect can be palpated as a thickening of the cord in the groin, and the ***silk glove sign*** can be elicited by rubbing together the sides of the empty hernial sac.

Sometimes the herniated loop of intestine becomes partially obstructed, producing variable symptoms that may include fretfulness and irritability, tenderness, anorexia, abdominal distention, and difficulty in defecating. Occasionally the loop of bowel becomes incarcerated (irreducible), with symptoms of complete intestinal obstruction that, left untreated, will progress to strangulation and gangrene. Incarceration occurs more often in infants under 10 months of age and is more common in girls.

Therapeutic Management

The treatment for hernias is prompt, elective surgical repair in healthy infants and children as soon as the defect is diagnosed. Since there is a significant incidence of bilateral involvement, many surgeons advocate exploration of both sides. An irreducible or strangulated hernia should be closely evaluated by the surgeon, since prompt recurrence requiring emergency surgery has been reported in over 50% of patients with incarceration (Stylianos and others, 1993).

Nursing Considerations

Both infants and children tolerate surgery very well, usually on an outpatient basis. Every attempt is made to keep the wound clean and reasonably dry. With infants and small children who are not yet toilet trained, the wound may be

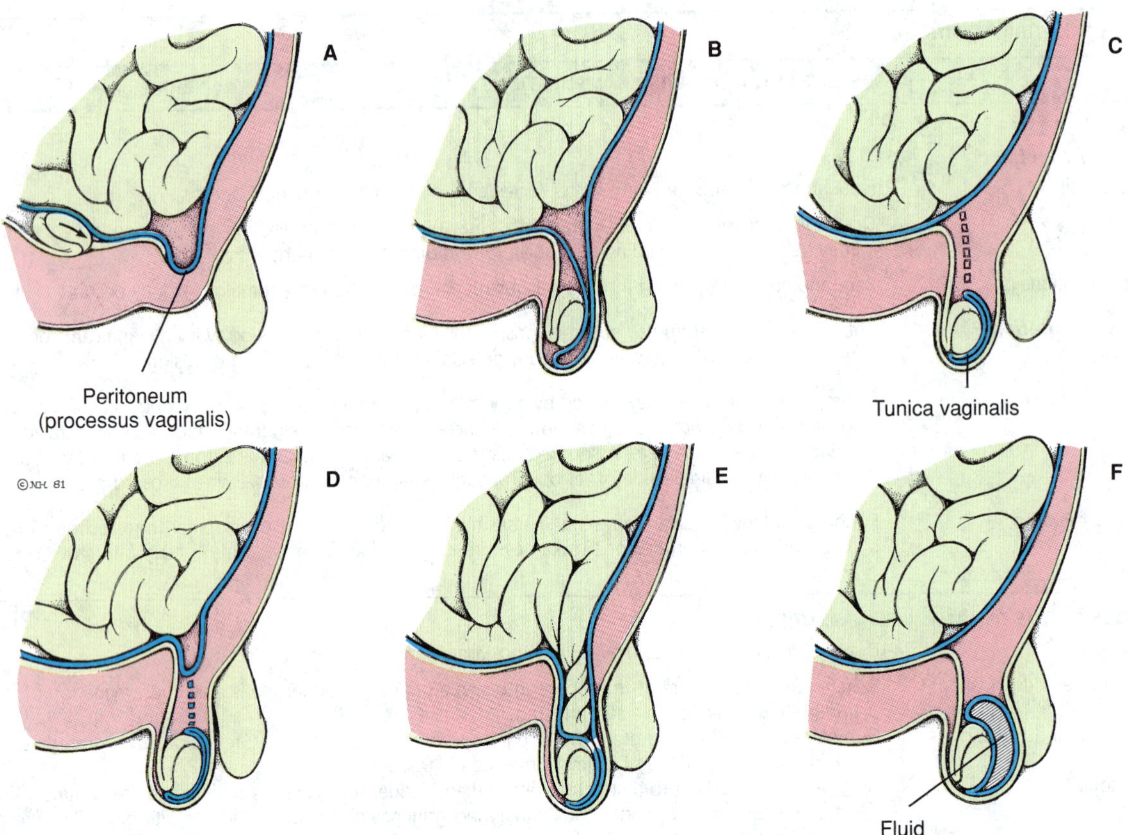

FIG. 11-24 Development of inguinal hernias. **A** and **B,** Prenatal migration of processus vaginalis. **C,** Normal. **D,** Partially obliterated processus vaginalis. **E,** Hernia. **F,** Hydrocele.

covered with an occlusive dressing or left without a dressing. Changing diapers as soon as they become damp helps reduce the chance of irritation or infection of the incision.

Parents are instructed to give the child sponge baths instead of tub baths for 2 to 5 days and to change diapers more frequently than usual during the day and once or twice during the night. There are no restrictions placed on the infant's or toddler's activity, but older children are cautioned against lifting, pushing, wrestling and fighting, bicycle riding, and athletics for about 3 weeks. Schoolchildren are permitted to attend classes as soon as they are comfortable but are excused from physical education activities for the same length of time as specified for restricting physical activity.

If surgery is postponed for some reason, the parents need to be taught the signs of incarcerated hernia, simple measures to reduce it (a warm bath, avoidance of upright positioning, and comfort measures to reduce crying), and where to call for assistance if relief is not obtained in a reasonably short time.

FEMORAL HERNIA

Femoral hernias are rare in children. When they occur, there is a higher incidence in girls than in boys. The disorder is suspected from a swelling in the groin area associated with severe pain. Treatment and management are the same as for inguinal hernia. Strangulation is a frequent complication.

HYDROCELE

Hydrocele is the presence of fluid in the processus vaginalis and is the result of the same developmental process as inguinal hernia (Fig. 11-24, *F*). When the upper segment of the processus vaginalis has been obliterated but the tunica vaginalis still contains peritoneal fluid, this is called a ***noncommunicating hydrocele.*** This type of hydrocele is common in newborns and often subsides spontaneously as fluid is gradually absorbed.

A ***communicating hydrocele*** is one in which the processus vaginalis remains open and into which peritoneal fluid may be forced by intraabdominal pressure and gravity. The length of the hydrocele depends on the length of the processus vaginalis and may extend into the tunica vaginalis within the scrotum. The hydrocele is asymptomatic except for a palpable bulge in the inguinal or scrotal area. Unlike a hernia, the hydrocele may not be reducible and may not be produced by a sudden increase in intraabdominal pressure (such as straining). The scrotum appears to be larger after an active day and smaller in the morning. Since a communicating hydrocele represents a patent processus vaginalis, it can predispose the child to herniation; therefore, surgical repair is indicated if spontaneous resolution does not take place by 1 year of age.

Nursing Considerations

The nursing care of the infant with a hydrocele is essentially the same as that for inguinal hernia. Parents are advised that there is often temporary swelling and discoloration of the scrotum that resolves spontaneously.

CRYPTORCHIDISM (CRYPTORCHISM)

Cryptorchidism is failure of one or both testes to descend normally through the inguinal canal into the scrotum. Absence of testes within the scrotum can be the result of (1) ***undescended (cryptorchid) testes,*** (2) ***retractile testes,*** or (3) ***anorchia*** (absence of testes). Undescended testes can be categorized further according to location:

Abdominal—Proximal to the internal inguinal ring
Canalicular—Between the internal and external inguinal rings
Ectopic—Outside the normal pathways of descent between the abdominal cavity and the scrotum

The incidence of cryptorchidism is 3% to 4% of full-term infants and falls to approximately 1% at age 1 year. The rate does not change in the years that follow (reported in Saggese and others, 1989).

Pathophysiology

Normally the testes descend from the abdomen, where they develop, into the scrotum during the seventh to ninth month of gestation. The progress is aided by the tubernaculum, a mass of tissue containing smooth muscle that is attached to the lower pole of the testes. The process is poorly understood, and the role of hormones in facilitating and/or initiating the descent is also unclear. The testes descend to the scrotum behind the processus vaginalis, a peritoneal outpocketing that retains a communication with the peritoneal cavity and projects down through various muscle and facial planes before the testes enter the inguinal canal (see Fig. 11-24, *A* to *D*).

Normally the upper part of the processus vaginalis atrophies and closes, and the lower part is pinched off to form the tunica vaginalis of the testes. Cryptorchidism occurs when one or both testes fail to descend through the inguinal canal. The descent can be arrested at any point along its normal path. Congenital inguinal hernias frequently accompany the defect. ***Ectopic testis*** is a testis that has progressed normally through the inguinal canal but, after passing through the external inguinal ring, has become lodged in superficial tissue of the abdominal wall, upper thigh, or perineum.

Retractile testes are normally descended testes that are pulled back into the inguinal canal as a result of a hyperactive cremasteric reflex. The ***cremasteric reflex*** is very active after 6 months of age and peaks by 4 to 5 years. This reflex (the drawing up of the scrotum and testicle when the skin over the front and inside of the thigh is stimulated) is particularly sensitive to touch and cold.

Clinical Manifestations

Undescended testes are rarely a cause of discomfort. The entire scrotum, or one side of it, appears smaller than normal and incompletely developed, an observation made by concerned parents who often bring the child for medical evaluation.

Diagnostic Evaluation

It is important to differentiate the true undescended testis from the more common retractile testis. Retractile testes can be "milked" or pushed back into the scrotum, but truly undescended ones cannot. For examination the cremasteric reflex can be obviated by placing the child in a squatting position or by applying firm finger pressure on the external ring before palpating the abdomen or genitalia (see Fig. 7-46).

Undescended testes may be felt along the inguinal canal, but those in the abdominal cavity usually cannot. Ultrasonography, tomography, and laparoscopy are sometimes employed to verify cryptorchidism in children undergoing orchiopexy. Suggestions to employ in diagnostic examination include:

- An undescended testis is usually smaller and softer than its descended mate.
- A well-developed rugous scrotum usually indicates normal testicular descent (may be confused by presence of a hydrocele or inguinal hernia).
- A retractile testis is usually bilateral (the cremasteric reflex is equally brisk on both sides).
- A testicle can usually be distinguished from a lymph node by its elastic nature. A testicle is mobile and can be massaged down into the scrotum, although it will spring back into the canal.
- Application of soap, cornstarch, or talcum powder to the tip of the examiner's fingers facilitates massaging the inguinal canal.

Acquired undescended testes in children who have had normally descended testes are relatively uncommon. Therefore evaluation of the testes should continue to be a part of the routine physical assessment.

Therapeutic Management

A retractile testis that can be manipulated into the scrotum will eventually assume a satisfactory scrotal position without medical or surgical intervention. The diagnosis is not made at a single examination, and parents are asked if they have observed the testes in the scrotum at some time. If so, the anomaly probably represents the retractile variety and the parents can be reassured. By 1 year of age the cryptorchid testes will descend spontaneously in approximately 75% of cases in both full-term and preterm infants (Penny, 1986). In contrast, true undescended testes rarely descend spontaneously after 1 year of age.

A trial with hormone therapy with luteinizing hormone–releasing hormone (nasal spray) and human chorionic gonadotropin (injection) may be attempted (Lala and others, 1993). If the testes do not descend spontaneously, ***orchiopexy*** is performed before the child's second birthday, preferably between 1 and 2 years of age. Surgical repair is done to (1) prevent damage to the undescended testicle by exposure to the higher degree of body heat in the undescended location; (2) decrease the incidence of tumor formation, which is higher in undescended testicles; (3) avoid trauma and torsion; (4) close the processus vaginalis; and (5) prevent the cosmetic and psychologic handicap of an empty scrotum. Because of increased propensity toward neoplastic changes (even after orchiopexy), cryptorchid testes are better observed in the scrotal position, where they can be routinely palpated.

The timing of the surgery is important, as it is in any genital surgery. The repair is not attempted in the first year unless there is an accompanying hernia. Fewer psychologic effects and a higher rate of fertility may be achieved when repair takes place at an early age. Having both testes in the scrotum by school age prevents psychologic problems related to body image and peer-group embarrassment, since the empty scrotum is smaller in size and altered in shape.

In the routine surgical procedure for undescended testes, the testes are brought down into the scrotum and secured in that position without tension or torsion. A simple orchiopexy for a palpable testis can usually be performed in an outpatient surgical unit. Intraabdominal testes require considerable surgical skill because of technical problems resulting from variations in the length of the spermatic cord, and overnight hospitalization may be necessary. In most cases the family can be reassured of normal function in adulthood.

Nursing Considerations

The postoperative nursing care is directed toward prevention of infection and instructing parents in home care of the child. Infection is prevented by carefully cleansing the operative site of stool and urine. Observation of the wound for complications and activity restrictions are discussed. Parents are concerned about the future fertility of the child. Therefore the prognosis for fertility is determined, and the family is counseled regarding this eventuality and the optimum time for discussing the probabilities with the child—ideally as a part of sex education.

HYPOSPADIAS

Hypospadias refers to a condition in which the urethral opening is located below the glans penis or anywhere along the ventral surface (underside) of the penile shaft (Fig. 11-25). In very mild cases the meatus is just below the tip of the penis. In the most severe malformations the meatus is located on the perineum between the halves of the scrotum. ***Chordee,*** or ventral curvature of the penis, results from the replacement of normal skin with a fibrous band of tissue and usually accompanies more severe forms of hypospadias. In addition, the foreskin is usually absent ventrally and, when combined with chordee, gives the organ a hooded and crooked appearance (Fig. 11-26). In severe cases the altered appearance may leave the sex in doubt at birth, since the perineal position of the meatus may be mistaken for a female urethra. Since undescended testes may also be present, the small penis may appear to be an enlarged clitoris. In any case of ambiguous genitalia, further study, such as chromosomal analysis, is essential.

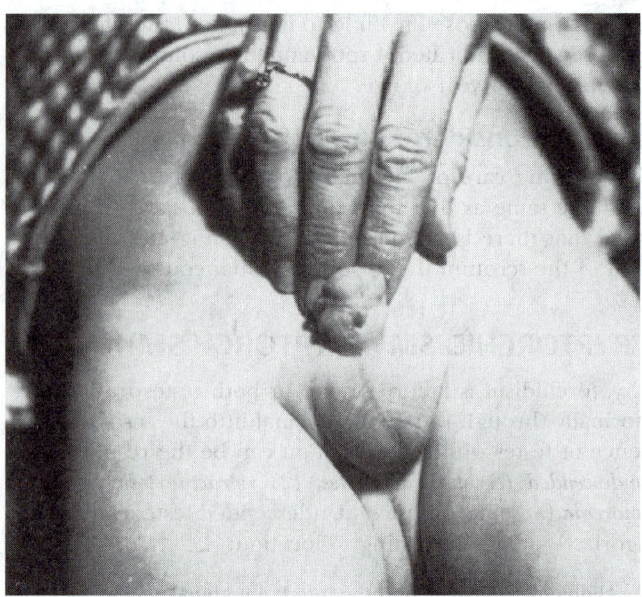

FIG. 11-25 Hypospadias. (Courtesy M.C. Gleason, MD, San Diego, CA. From Ingalls AJ, Salerno MC: *Maternal and child health nursing,* ed 7, St Louis, 1991, Mosby.)

Surgical Correction

The principal objectives of surgical correction are (1) to enhance the child's ability to void in the standing position with a straight stream, (2) to improve the physical appearance of the genitalia for psychologic reasons, and (3) to preserve a sexually adequate organ. Many procedures have been described that accomplish one or more of these goals. The choice of surgical procedure is affected primarily by the severity of the defect and the presence of associated anomalies. ***Glanular hypospadias*** (defect noted at the glans penis) may be corrected by a ***glans approximation procedure (GAP)*** or a ***meatal advancement glanuloplasty (MAGPI)*** procedure. The GAP requires approximation of the nonjoined urethral opening with lengthening of the urethra and deepithelialization of skin at the lateral edges of the defect. While the procedure is relatively simple, the potential for urethrocutaneous fistula is significant. The MAGPI requires a dorsal meatotomy with incision of the tissue between the urethral meatus and the glanular groove. The dorsal epithelium is then advanced distally, and care is taken to avoid disrupting the urethra. The ventral skin is then approximated, redundant tissue is carefully excised, and the defect is closed.

More ***distal hypospadias*** defects typically require alternative approaches. The ***Mathieu procedure*** may be used for distal hypospadias defects when sufficient ventral skin is present. A skin flap is mobilized that is large enough to reach the tip of the penis. The flap is freed with as much subcutaneous tissue attached as feasible. Urethral reconstruction is accomplished by reversing the meatal-based flap distally to the glans penis. Specific strategies are used to provide adequate vascular supply to the mobilized skin grafts

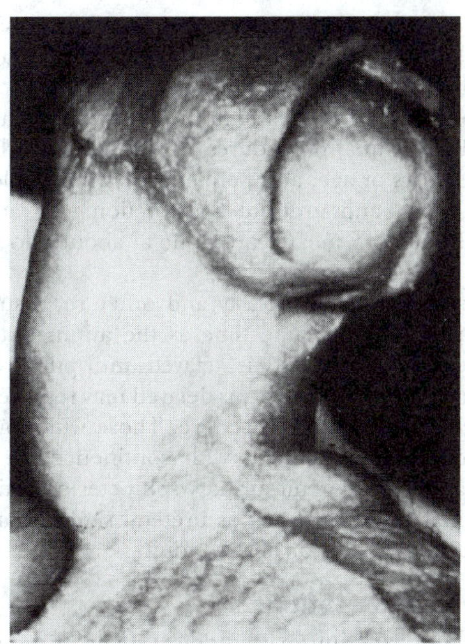

FIG. 11-26 Hypospadias with significant chordee. (From Shirkey HC: *Pediatric therapy,* ed 6, St Louis, 1980, Mosby.)

and to prevent fistula formation. When ventral skin volume is deficient, an ***island flap repair*** may be used. This procedure requires more extensive use of skin grafts to create the new urethra and close the defect.

Commonly, the chordee that often coexists with a hypospadias defect is repaired by release of the ventral skin described previously. When the chordee persists, additional procedures, such as a ***flip-flap procedure, transverse island flap urethroplasty,*** or ***Mustarde procedure,*** may be indicated. Again, more extensive skin flap mobilization is required, and additional reconstruction is used to ensure penile straightening.

Increased surgical experience and improvements in technique have reduced the number of staged procedures applied to hypospadias defects. However, a staged procedure is indicated in particularly severe defects with marked deficits of available skin for mobilization of flaps and in rare cases when scrotal transposition occurs (Belman, 1992).

The preferred time for surgical repair is 6 to 18 months, before the child has developed body image and castration anxiety. Surgical repair of hypospadias as early as 3 months of age has been successful without higher incidence of complications (Sugar and others, 1993). Occasionally a short course of testosterone is administered preoperatively to achieve additional penile size to facilitate the surgery.

Nursing Considerations

Every male newborn should be examined carefully for signs of hypospadias. If the nurse suspects even mild hypospadias, this is reported, because circumcision may be delayed to save the foreskin for repair.

Preparation of parents for the type of procedure to be done and the expected cosmetic result helps avert later problems. Frequently parents are informed of what is to be surgically corrected but are not advised of what to expect as a reasonable consequence. As a result, they are greatly disappointed to see a physically imperfect penis. If children are old enough to understand what is occurring, they are also prepared for the operation and the expected outcome.

Hypospadias repair may require some type of urinary diversion to promote optimum healing and to maintain the position and patency of the newly formed urethra. Following repair of more severe hypospadias, the child is often placed under a bed cradle and immobilized with arm and leg restraints. Restraints can be removed periodically when the child is awake and under supervision, and appropriate diversional activities can be provided. Sedation may be required for the excessively irritable or restless child, and pain is controlled with analgesics. Parental rooming-in is recommended to reduce the child's anxiety.

Parents are taught to care for the indwelling catheter or stent and irrigation technique if indicated. They need to know how to empty the urine bag and how to avoid kinking, twisting, or blockage of the catheter or stent. Often the child is discharged with a catheter or stent dripping directly into the diaper. In older children a urine collection device can be used. Parents are taught how to tape the drainage bag to the leg to allow the child to be mobile and to *never* clamp off a catheter. An extra bag is sent home with the family in case of tears or leakage. The family is advised to encourage the child to increase fluid intake. Twice-daily bathing is recommended, as is loose clothing. Straddle toys, sandboxes, swimming, and rough activities are avoided until allowed by the surgeon.

EPISPADIAS/EXSTROPHY COMPLEX

Bladder exstrophy is a severe defect of the GU system characterized by externalization of the bladder, splaying of the urethra with failure of tubular formation, and diastasis (separation) of the pelvic bone (Fig. 11-27). Epispadias is a defect of the urinary system characterized by failure of urethral canalization similar to that seen in exstrophy. Both of these defects are part of a complex of congenital anomalies of genitourinary development that range from relatively mild defects (such as a glanular epispadias, or a defect on the dorsal surface [topside] of the penile shaft) to severe defects involving multiple organ systems (such as a cloacal exstrophy). Fortunately, the incidence of exstrophy/epispadias complex anomalies is small. Exstrophy is estimated to occur in 3.3 of 100,000 live births (Lancaster, 1987).

Pathophysiology

Exstrophy results from failure of the abdominal wall and underlying structures, including the ventral wall of the bladder, to fuse in utero. As a result, the lower urinary tract is exposed and the everted bladder appears bright red through the abdominal opening. This is accompanied by a constant seepage of urine from the exposed ureteral orifices, making the area malodorous and susceptible to infection. The constant accumulation of urine on the surrounding skin produces tissue ulceration and further infection.

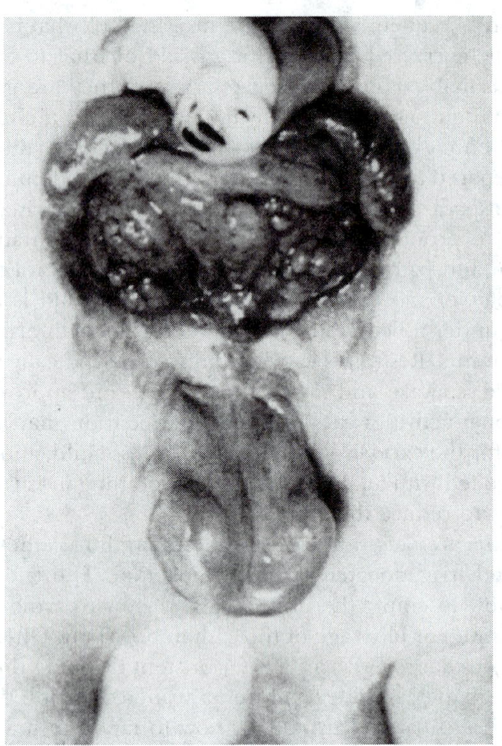

FIG. 11-27 Exstrophy of bladder. (Courtesy E.S. Tank, MD, Division of Urology, University of Oregon Health Sciences Center, Portland, OR.)

Progressive renal damage from infection and obstruction may terminate in renal failure if left untreated.

In males the defect is almost always associated with epispadias and may include other problems, such as undescended testes, a short penis, or inguinal hernia. The sexual handicap in males may be severe because the penis protrudes inadequately. In females the genitalia may be affected, with a cleft or bifid clitoris, completely separated labia, and absent vagina. In either sex, separation of the pubic bones causes difficulty in walking, such as a waddling gait.

Therapeutic Management

The objectives of treatment include (1) preservation of renal function, (2) attainment of urinary control, (3) adequate reconstructive repair for psychologic benefit, and (4) improvement of sexual function, particularly in males. Closure of the bladder is ideally accomplished in the neonatal period. The initial repair is sometimes delayed for several weeks or months, and the parents are instructed in frequent dressing changes. Systemic antibiotics are initiated in the preoperative phase and continued through the postoperative period. Delayed repair usually presents no complications if the parents change the dressings frequently (Kenner and Brueggemeyer, 1993). To promote optimum healing, the infant is usually maintained in traction or elastic external compression for a few weeks until adequate union of the separated pubis takes place.

Final repair is completed before school age. Essentially all patients with exstrophy have vesicoureteral reflux that requires antireflux surgery, usually accompanied by bladder neck reconstruction in an attempt to produce urinary continence. These initial procedures are ordinarily performed at 2½ to 3 years of age, and penile lengthening, release of dorsal chordee, and urethral construction with advancement of the urinary meatus are done at about 4 to 6 years of age.

In females the urethroplasty and other reconstruction are performed at the same time as the antiincontinence procedure, but vaginoplasty is delayed until puberty. Both boys and girls in whom surgery is delayed may require a temporary urinary diversion procedure. Those with complications or continued problems with continence are candidates for an artificial genitourinary sphincter or antirefluxing intestinal diversion, such as ureteral sigmoid implant, bilateral ureterostomy, or ileal conduit.

Nursing Considerations

Physical care of the unrepaired defect includes meticulous hygiene of the bladder area to prevent infection and excoriation of the surrounding tissue. A sterile nonadherent dressing is placed over the exposed bladder area to prevent infection and to keep the diaper from adhering to the mucosa. An ointment may be prescribed for the surrounding skin to protect it from the constantly draining urine. If external compression is used, the skin is inspected periodically for evidence of pressure necrosis.

Other aspects of preoperative care are similar to those for any major abdominal surgery. Since a routine urinalysis is part of most admission procedures, a urine specimen can be obtained by allowing urine to drip into a container by holding the child prone over a basin or by aspirating some urine directly from the bladder area into a medicine dropper or syringe. If a sterile specimen is needed for evaluation of existing infection, the former procedure is preferable, but a sterile container must be used. A mechanical and/or bowel preparation may be required.

Postoperative nursing care following bladder neck reconstruction and antireflux surgery (ureteral reimplantation) includes routine wound care and careful monitoring of urine output from the bladder and/or ureteral drainage tubes. Care following a penile lengthening, chordee release, and urethral reconstruction is similar to care following hypospadias repair.

In addition to routine postsurgical care, nursing following a continent diversion includes wound care, observation of nasogastric suction (surgery requires bowel resection), and measurement and observation of urinary output. In most cases a continent urinary diversion can be surgically created. Clean intermittent catheterization is used to regularly empty the urinary reservoir.

Family Support and Home Care. One of the most devastating aspects of exstrophy of the bladder is its appearance. Although the actual physical care is not difficult, it is not easy for parents to assume responsibility for what to them seems an enormous task because of the emotional impact of the defect.

Parents should be instructed regarding a realistic outcome of surgery, since unrealistic expectations of the cosmetic and functional result may leave them very disappointed and discouraged. When possible, continuous care by one nurse helps the family adjust to all aspects of recovery. As difficult as it was for parents to adjust to the defect at the time of the child's birth, it may be equally disturbing for them to accept the fact that surgical closure does not ensure normal urination and that urinary diversion may be necessary. It is helpful to discuss the long-range advantages of a permanent urinary diversion. A well-fitting ileostomy bag allows the child almost unrestricted freedom in activities enjoyed by other children and results in no major alteration in toileting, except emptying the bag at periodic intervals. This is extremely important to older children and adolescents, who want to be accepted as one of the group and deplore any stigma of being different.

Parents often worry about the child's sexual adjustment, even though they may not voice such thoughts. Part of the nursing admission history is directed toward evaluating the parents' (and child's if appropriate) expectation of the surgical repair, knowledge of the possibility of eventual urinary diversion, and feelings concerning this permanent change in body function.

When the infant is discharged with an unrepaired defect, diapers are placed over the defect and are changed frequently, especially after stooling, to prevent infection, ulceration, and odor. General infant care remains unchanged except for sponge baths rather than immersion in water. A home health referral is an important component of discharge planning, and ideally home visits should begin immediately after the infant's release from the hospital.

Even with improved reconstructive surgery for these patients, substantial psychologic support and guidance are needed to help them adjust to their fears of inadequate penile size, appearance of the genitalia, potential inability to procreate, and rejection by peers, especially the opposite sex. Ongoing discussion groups for parents and children are particularly useful in promoting resolution of these fears and allowing for optimum psychologic adjustment, particularly during adolescence.

OBSTRUCTIVE UROPATHY

Structural or functional abnormalities of the urinary system that obstruct the normal flow of urine can produce renal disorders. When there is interference with urine flow, the collecting system above the obstruction causes ***hydronephrosis*** (the collection of urine in the renal pelvis to the point of cyst formation from the distension), with eventual pressure destruction to renal parenchyma, although the dilating ureters form a reservoir that reduces the effect on the kidneys for a long time.

Obstruction may be congenital or acquired, unilateral or bilateral, complete or incomplete, and the manifestations may be acute or chronic. The obstruction can occur at any level of the upper or lower urinary tract (Fig. 11-28). Partial obstruction may be asymptomatic unless there is a water or solute diuresis. Boys are affected more commonly than girls, and malformations should be suspected when patients have some other congenital defects (e.g., prune belly syndrome, chromosome anomalies, hypospadias, anorectal malformations, and defects of the pinna of the ear).

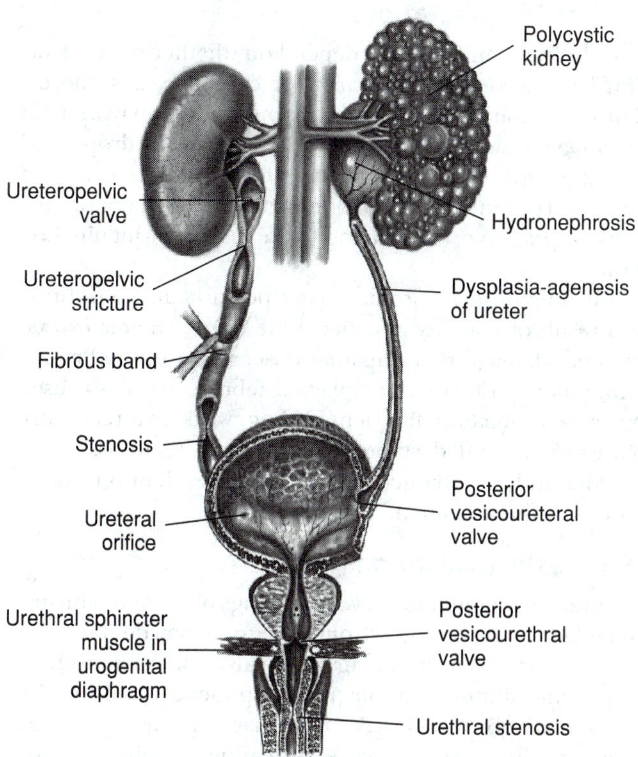

FIG. 11-28 Major sites of urinary tract obstruction.

Pathophysiology

The pathologic changes depend on the location and nature of the defect, the site of obstruction, the duration of the obstruction, and complications such as infection or urinary calculi. With hydronephrosis, glomerular filtration ceases when intrapelvic pressure equals the filtration pressure in glomerular capillaries. However, a pressure gradient usually is established because of some flow beyond the obstruction as a result of periodic relaxation of ureteral wall musculature. There is also an exchange of solutes and water between the pooled urine in the renal pelvis and fluid in the adjoining tissues and fluid compartments (such as interstitial fluid in the pelvic wall and inner kidney medulla), resulting from an intrarenal vascular adjustment caused by a corresponding increase in peritubular capillary pressure.

Damage to distal nephrons in chronic uropathy alters the ability to concentrate urine, contributing to increased urine flow and metabolic acidosis occurring from decreased excretion of acid secondary to impaired ability of the distal nephron to secrete hydrogen ions. Partial obstruction results in progressive loss of renal function as a result of irreversible damage to the nephrons. Pooled urine serves as a medium for bacterial growth; therefore urinary tract infections further increase the extent of renal damage.

Clinical Manifestations

The clinical manifestations depend on whether the obstruction is acute or chronic, partial or complete, and the extent of complications (e.g., infection). There may be pain or ***strangury*** (slow and painful urination, drop by drop), and hematuria (if caused by calculi). The type and location of pain are related to the area of obstruction (e.g., abdominal flank, suprapubic, or radiating to the testicle or inguinal region).

Chronic obstruction may cause polyuria and polydipsia as a result of inability to concentrate urine, anemia caused by renal damage that impairs the secretion of erythropoietin, failure to thrive, unexplained febrile episodes caused by urinary infection, frequent voiding, weak or forceful urinary stream, and daytime and nocturnal enuresis. A full bladder and/or enlarged kidney may be evident on examination of the abdomen.

Diagnostic Evaluation

Laboratory examination reveals findings of acute or chronic renal failure. A voiding cystoureterogram may demonstrate the presence of posterior ureteral valves or vesicoureteral reflux, and ultrasonography may help identify and localize the site of obstruction. Prenatal diagnosis and postnatal screening for urinary tract abnormalities by ultrasonography are being used with increasing frequency. Early identification of affected infants permits early management of abnormalities that otherwise may not be recognized until later in life after irreversible renal damage.

Therapeutic Management

Early diagnosis and surgical correction or bypass procedures, such as ileal conduit or cutaneous ureterostomy, that divert the flow of urine are essential in order to prevent progressive renal damage. Often a percutaneous nephrostomy tube (or tubes) is inserted through the skin and underlying tissues into the renal pelvis to relieve intrarenal pressure until an alternative diversion is established. Medical complications of acute or chronic renal failure and/or infection are managed as described for those disorders.

Prognosis. The prognosis depends on the type of obstruction, the degree of irreversible renal damage, whether renal dysplasia is present, the age at which the diagnosis was established, and the severity of complications. Despite the improvements in corrective surgery, some patients develop renal failure, which may evolve over a highly variable period of time that can extend into adulthood. Renal failure can result from hypoplasia-dysplasia, pyelonephritic scarring, and other proposed mechanisms that cause progressive nephron loss. Careful follow-up of children should extend throughout childhood and adolescence, especially when any degree of renal insufficiency is present.

Nursing Considerations

Nursing goals in urinary tract obstruction include helping to identify cases, assisting with diagnostic procedures, and caring for children with complications (see Chapter 30). Preparing parents and children for procedures is a major nursing responsibility, especially preparation for urinary diversion procedures (see Preparation for Procedures, Chapter 27).

Parents and children need emotional support and counseling during the lengthy management of these disorders. Parents are the primary target during infancy and very early childhood, when most reparative surgery is performed. They will need assistance in managing the apparatus that accompanies many temporary and permanent repair procedures. Many children are discharged with ureteral drainage systems in place that must be protected from damage, and the danger of infection is a constant concern. Parents are taught to care for the equipment and recognize the signs of possible obstruction or infection within the system (see Discharge Planning and Home Care, Chapter 26).

Children with external diversional systems will need psychologic support and guidance, especially as they reach adolescence and body image concerns assume more prominence. Those with progressive renal deterioration may face the prospect of dialysis and/or transplantation and the emotional aspects that accompany these procedures.

ABNORMAL SEXUAL DEVELOPMENT

The birth of a child with ambiguous genitalia is a situation that constitutes a crisis quite different from that of many other congenital anomalies. Uncertain gender is a potential lifetime social tragedy for the child and family. Furthermore, the electrolyte disturbances that accompany conditions such as congenital adrenal hyperplasia can be life-threatening. Thus the identification of appropriate sex must be done quickly and accurately, and requires no less speed and skill than life-threatening anomalies such as tracheoesophageal fistula. Even a brief delay in gender assignment can generate rumors that can be a source of distress to a child and family for years.

Etiology

Genetic sex is determined at the time of conception and depends on whether the ovum is fertilized by a sperm bearing an X chromosome or one bearing a Y chromosome. The phenotypic evidence of sex depends on whether subsequent processes proceed normally: differentiation of primitive gonads, differentiation and development of internal duct systems, and differentiation and development of external genitalia. The normal order of events can be altered by abnormalities of the chromosomal complement, defects of embryogenesis, or biochemical (hormonal) abnormalities. Disturbances in any of these processes will lead to abnormal sexual development evidenced by the presence of ambiguous genitalia at birth.

Normal Sexual Development. For the first 6 weeks of life, the developing embryo is morphologically asexual, neither male nor female. The primitive, bipotential (able to form either a testicle or an ovary) gonad consists of an outer layer (the cortex) and an inner medulla. Differentiation into testes or ovary takes place during the seventh and eighth weeks of gestation. At this time, in the male the medullary portion develops and the cortical zone regresses; in the female the cortex is preserved while the medulla regresses. Active factors from the male testes cause the müllerian duct system to regress. Without these factors the primitive gonad has an inherent tendency to feminize. The embryonic ovary develops in the absence of male hormone stimulation.

The final stage of sexual development is differentiation of the external genitalia, which in the early embryo consists of a urogenital sinus, two lateral labioscrotal swellings, and an anteriorly situated genital tubercle. Depending on the presence or absence of male hormones, the genital tubercle differentiates into a penis or a clitoris. In response to testicular androgens, the labiosacral folds fuse to form a scrotum and ventral skin of the penis; the urethral folds form the perineal and penile urethra. Without the influence of masculinizing secretions, the urethral folds do not fuse and instead become the labia minora, the labiosacral folds remain unfused to separate into the labia majora, and the urogenital sinus differentiates into a lower vagina and the vaginal and urethral openings (Fig. 11-29).

Abnormal Sexual Development. Disturbances in the normal order of events in sex determination will produce abnormal sexual development with the presence of ambiguous or inappropriate external genitalia at birth. Ambiguous genitalia can be variable and may often closely conform to one sex or the other. In some forms the external sexual structures represent those of a perfectly normal male or fe-

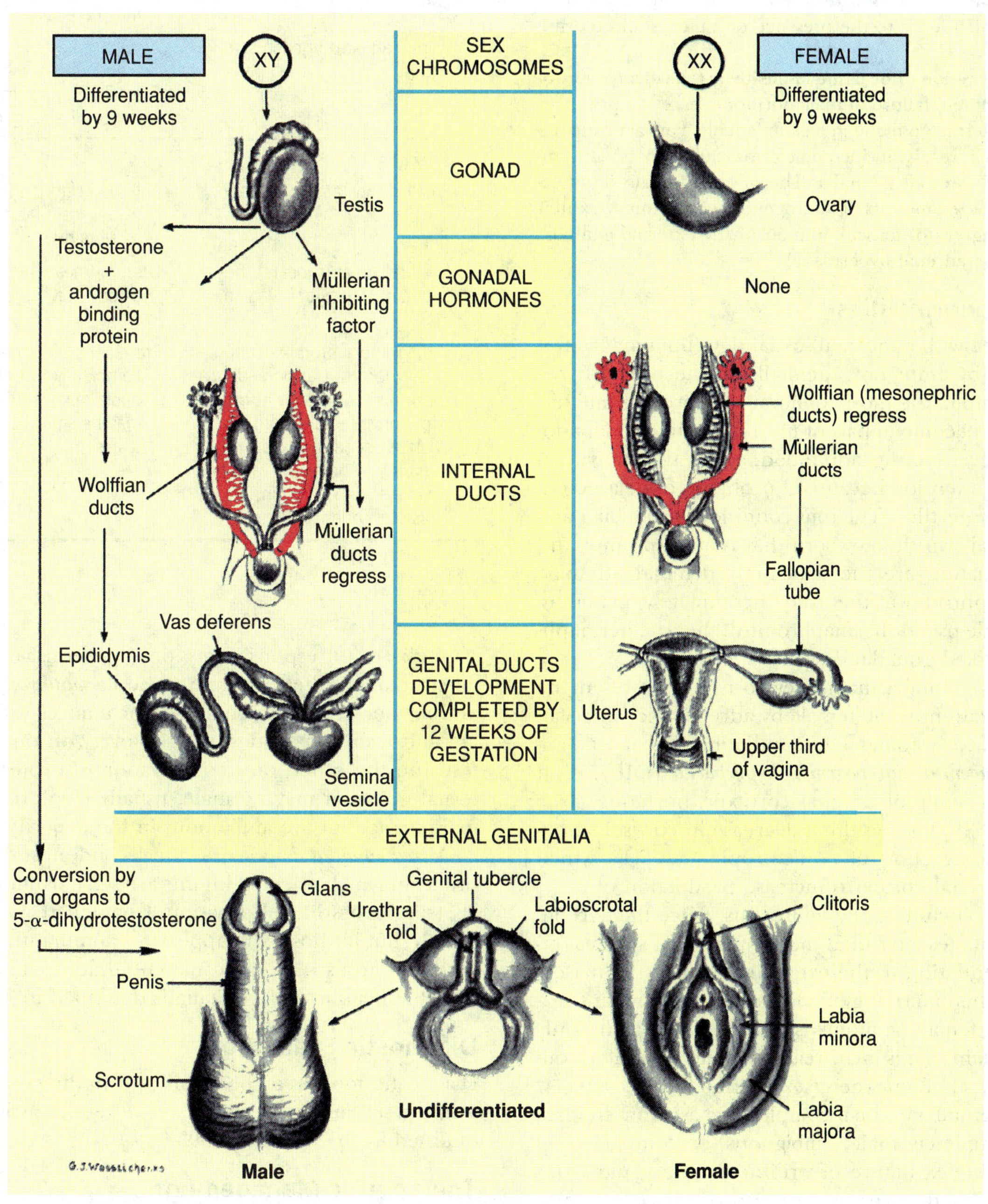

FIG. 11-29 Sex differentiation in male and female. (From Thompson JM and others: *Mosby's manual of clinical nursing,* ed 2, St Louis, 1989, Mosby.)

male, whereas the genetic sex is the direct opposite. A situation in which the phenotypic sex differs from the chromosomal sex is often termed ***intersex.***

A failure or abnormality in any of the four steps of sexual development can lead to abnormal development in subsequent stages. The mechanisms and sites of defective development include:

Abnormal sex determination—Chromosome abnormalities result in disturbance of sexual development (see Chapter 5).

Abnormal differentiation of gonads—When induction of the bipotential gonad fails, sex differentiation proceeds in the direction of the female phenotype, regardless of genetic sex.

Abnormal differentiation of ductal systems—Biologic inactivity of androgenic male organizer substances or insensitivity of ductal tissue to its action results in a persistent female duct system, which leads to the presence of a uterus and uterine tubes.

Abnormal secretion of or tissue insensitivity to testicular androgen—Complete failure of male hormone secretion produces female external genitalia in a genetic male. Partial or incomplete failure results in incomplete masculinization with ambiguity of external genitalia. The genetic female fetus exposed to large amounts of androgenic hormone may exhibit varying degrees of masculinization of the external genitalia (congenital adrenal hyperplasia).

Types of Abnormalities

Some disorders with abnormal sexual development are not characterized by ambiguous genitalia in the newborn period. For example, the most common sex chromosome disorders do not become apparent until later childhood, adolescence, or even young adulthood, when the individual seeks medical attention because of problems of delayed development or infertility. The four conditions producing ambiguous genitalia in the newborn that require prompt and accurate evaluation are the masculinized female (female pseudohermaphrodite), the true incompletely masculinized male (male pseudohermaphrodite), the true hermaphrodite, and mixed gonadal dysgenesis.

Ambiguous genitalia in the newborn is most often the result of virilization in the female by adrenal androgens after the time of early gonadal differentiation. The most common type, ***congenital adrenogenital hyperplasia (CAH),*** is an inherited deficiency of adrenal corticoid hormones (see also Chapter 38). The resulting decrease in cortisol stimulates pituitary secretion of corticotropin (ACTH), which causes the adrenal cortex to increase production of adrenal hormones, including the androgens. Since the adrenal gland differentiates later than the gonadal duct systems but before differentiation of the external genitalia, the masculinization of the external genitalia is the predominant feature. Internal female anatomy is normal. CAH is the only intersex problem that is life-threatening and should be considered in any situation where sex is doubtful.

External genitalia in the incompletely masculinized male may be incompletely male, ambiguous, or completely female. The complex nature of virilization offers numerous opportunities for disturbance in the process. Defects may be a result of deficient production of fetal androgen, deficiency in any of the enzymes needed for testosterone biosynthesis, or unresponsiveness or subresponsiveness of genital structures to testosterone. True ***hermaphrodites*** are rare and may be either genetic males or females with *both* ovarian and testicular tissues, with an ovary on one side and a testis on the other, or a combination of ovotestis. The external genitalia may be male, usually cryptorchid, or normal female, but are ambiguous in the majority of cases.

Mixed gonadal dysgenesis is the second most common disorder, in which affected infants are sex chromosome mosaics (see Errors in Cell Division, Chapter 5). Genitalia vary greatly, but in those who appear predominantly female, the dysplastic testis may cause masculinization at puberty. External appearance of genitalia is described in Table 11-7.

TABLE 11-7 Ambiguous Genitalia

NORMAL FINDINGS	AMBIGUOUS FINDINGS
MALE	
Penile shaft protrudes from perineum and hangs freely	Small penis (less than 2 to 3 cm [0.8 to 1.2 inches] in newborn) may be enlarged clitoris
Urethral meatus centered at tip of glans penis	Urethral meatus anywhere along dorsal or ventral surface of penis, especially on perineum
Two scrotal sacs hang freely, covered with loose, wrinkled skin	Small scrotum with smooth, tight skin and any degree of separation in midline may be enlarged labia
Palpable testes in each scrotum	Absent testes may be undescended; if combined with small scrotum, may be evidence of enlarged labia
FEMALE	
Small clitoris at anterior end of labia	Enlarged clitoris that protrudes from labia may be small penis
Urethral meatus located between clitoris and vagina	Urethral meatus located in clitoris may suggest small penis
Labia minora prominent in newborn but atrophied and almost absent in prepubertal female; completely separated from clitoris to posterior vault of vagina; on palpation, no masses in labia	Prominent labia, partially or completely fused with palpable masses on each side, may be small scrotum with testes

Diagnostic Evaluation

Diagnostic tools and the significant findings that help determine sex and assist in making a gender assignment are outlined in the box on p. 503.

Therapeutic Management

The assignment of a gender sex to the infant whose sex is doubtful constitutes a social emergency. The long-term im-

ASSESSMENT TO DETERMINE A GENDER ASSIGNMENT

History—Previous abortions (may help identify chromosome aberrations); ingestion of steroids; relatives with ambiguous genitalia or who died in the first weeks of life
Physical examination—Presence of palpable gonads strongly suggests a male genotype
Chromosome analysis—Detects chromosome abnormalities and precise genetic sex; results are available in 2 to 3 days
Endoscopy, ultrasonography, and radiographic contrast studies—Reveal presence, absence, or nature of internal genital structures
Biochemical tests—Include 17-ketosteroids, 17-hydroxycorticoids, and urinary pregnanediol; urinary steroid excretion patterns help detect several of the adrenal cortical syndromes
Laparotomy or gonad biopsy—In some instances is the only way to arrive at a definitive diagnosis

plications are such that a hasty decision based on appearance alone may be disastrous, and the optimum sex of rearing may not be the same as the genetic or gonadal sex. *The infant's anatomy rather than genetic sex is the primary criterion on which the choice of gender should be based.* An incomplete female is better able to adjust than is an inadequate male. A functional vagina can be constructed surgically, and with appropriate administration of hormones the anatomically incomplete female can lead a relatively normal life, but it is as yet impossible to construct a satisfactory functional penis from an inadequate phallus for an equally satisfactory adjustment of the incomplete male.

In most instances of ambiguous genitalia it is recommended that the infant be reared as a female. Genetic males with a phallus of adequate size that will respond to testosterone at the time of puberty can be considered for male rearing. Adequate studies should be carried out early to assist in gender selection, even though they may delay final sex assignment for several days or even weeks. Supportive measures, such as appropriate surgical reconstruction techniques that provide normal-appearing external structures, are carried out. Removal of inappropriate internal structures and dysgenic gonads is recommended.

Nursing Considerations

Families need a great deal of support and encouragement from nurses and other members of the health team to cope with this emotionally charged situation. Parents are confused, anxious, and overwhelmed by feelings of guilt and shame. They may pressure for immediate sex assignment because they are concerned about the child and the child's future, and because they must face questioning relatives and friends. The best approach is honesty. The disorder should be treated as any other disorder, and no attempt should be made to camouflage the problem. The sequence of embryologic events leading to the defect can be explained using correct terminology to describe sexual abnormalities. An understanding of the anomaly assists parents in explaining the defect to others, just as with any other physical defect. It requires sympathy and understanding to deal with parental anxiety during this trying period and to guide them throughout the long-term management (see also Chapter 22).

CONGENITAL DEFECTS CAUSED BY PRENATAL FACTORS

DEFECTS CAUSED BY INFECTIOUS AGENTS

The range of pathologic conditions produced by infectious agents is large, and the difference between the maternal and fetal effects caused by any one agent is also great. Some maternal infections, especially during early gestation, can result in fetal loss or malformations because the ability of the fetus to handle infectious organisms is limited and the fetal immunologic system is unable to prevent the dissemination of infectious organisms to the various tissues.

Not all prenatal infections produce teratogenic effects. Further, the clinical picture of disorders caused by transplacental transfer of infectious agents is not always well defined. One group of microbial agents can cause remarkably similar manifestations, and it is not uncommon to test for all when a prenatal infection is suspected. This is the so-called TORCHS complex, an acronym for:

T Toxoplasmosis
O Other (e.g., hepatitis)
R Rubella
C Cytomegalovirus infection
H Herpes simplex
S Syphilis

To determine the causative agent in a symptomatic infant, tests are performed to rule out each of these infections. The "O" category may involve testing for several viral infections (e.g., hepatitis, varicella zoster, measles, mumps, and listeriosis). Bacterial infections are not included in the TORCHS workup, because they are usually identified by clinical manifestations and readily available laboratory tests. Gonococcal conjunctivitis (ophthalmia neonatorum) and chlamydial conjunctivitis have been significantly reduced by prophylactic measures at birth (see Chapter 8). Acquired immunodeficiency syndrome (AIDS), a growing prenatal and postnatal concern, is discussed in Chapter 35. The major maternal infections, their possible teratogenic effects, and specific nursing considerations are outlined in Table 11-8.

Nursing Considerations

One of the major goals in care of infants suspected of having an infectious disease is identification of the causative organism. Until the diagnosis is established, universal precautions are implemented according to institutional policy. In suspected cytomegalovirus and rubella infections, pregnant personnel are cautioned to avoid contact with the infant. Herpes simplex is easily transmitted from one infant to another; therefore risk of cross-contamination is reduced

TABLE 11-8 Infections Acquired from Mother Before, During, or After Birth

FETAL OR NEWBORN EFFECT	COMMENTS AND NURSING CONSIDERATIONS*
ACQUIRED IMMUNODEFICIENCY SYNDROME (AIDS) (HUMAN IMMUNODEFICIENCY VIRUS [HIV])	
No significant difference between infected and uninfected infants at birth in some instances Embryopathy reported by some observers Depressed nasal bridge Mild upward or downward obliquity of eyes Long palpebral fissures with blue sclerae Patulous lips Ocular hypertelorism Prominent upper vermilion border	Transmitted transplacentally; during delivery; in breast milk No treatment currently available other than supportive care IV gamma globulin when diagnosed Average age at diagnosis is 17 months Mandatory HIV testing of mother/newborn not recommended but testing encouraged (American Academy of Pediatrics, 1992)
CHICKENPOX (VARICELLA-ZOSTER VIRUS)	
First trimester exposure—congenital varicella syndrome: limb dysplasia, microcephaly, cortical atrophy, chorioretinitis, cataracts, cutaneous scars, other anomalies, auditory nerve palsy, mental retardation	Transmitted: first trimester (fetal varicella syndrome); intrapartum (infection) Treatment: exposed infants—varicella-zoster immune globulin (VZIG) to infants born to mothers with onset of disease within 5 days before or 2 days after delivery (7 days before and 7 days after in United Kingdom) Isolation precautions 21 days after birth (if hospitalized)
CHLAMYDIA INFECTION *(CHLAMYDIA TRACHOMATIS)*	
Conjunctivitis, pneumonia	Transmitted: last trimester or intrapartum Apply prophylactic medication to eyes at time of birth Treatment: antibiotics
COXSACKIE VIRUS (GROUP B)	
Poor feeding, vomiting, diarrhea, fever; cardiac enlargement, arrhythmias, congestive heart failure; lethargy, seizures, meningeal involvement	Transmitted: first trimester or late in pregnancy
CYTOMEGALIC INCLUSION DISEASE—CID (CYTOMEGALOVIRUS [CMV])	
Growth retardation (small for gestational age) Microcephaly, cerebral calcifications, chorioretinitis Jaundice, hepatosplenomegaly Petechial or purpuric rash Neurologic sequelae: seizure disorders, sensorimotor deafness, mental retardation	Transmitted: throughout pregnancy Affected individuals excrete virus Virus detected in urine by electron microscopy Avoid kissing affected child Pregnant women should avoid close contact with known cases Treatment: antimetabolites, antiviral agent
ERYTHEMA INFECTIOSUM (PARVOVIRUS B19)	
Fetal hydrops and death from anemia and heart failure, early exposure Anemia from later exposure No teratogenic effects established Ordinarily, low risk of ill effect to fetus	Transmitted: transplacentally First-trimester infection most serious effects Pregnant health care workers should not care for patients who might be highly contagious (e.g., aplastic crisis) Routine exclusion of pregnant women from workplace where disease is occurring is not recommended
GONOCOCCAL DISEASE *(NEISSERIA GONORRHOEAE)*	
Ophthalmitis Neonatal gonococcal arthritis, septicemia, meningitis	Transmitted: last trimester or intrapartum Apply prophylactic medication to eyes at time of birth Obtain smears for culture Treatment: penicillin
HEPATITIS B VIRUS (HBV)	
May be asymptomatic Acute hepatitis, changes in liver function	Transmitted: transplacentally, contaminated maternal secretions during delivery, possibly breast-feeding from cracked nipples Treatment: hepatitis B immune globulin to all infants of HBsAG-positive mothers Prevention: universal immunization of all infants with HBV vaccine
HERPES, NEONATAL (HERPES SIMPLEX VIRUS)	
Cutaneous lesions: vesicles at 6 to 10 days of age; may be no lesions Disseminated disease resembles sepsis	History of genital infection in mother/partner in 50% of cases Transmitted: intrapartum either ascending and/or direct contact, especially primary infection

*Isolation precautions depend on institutional policy (see Infection Control, Chapter 27).

TABLE 11-8 Infections Acquired from Mother Before, During, or After Birth—cont'd

FETAL OR NEWBORN EFFECT	COMMENTS AND NURSING CONSIDERATIONS*
Visceral involvement: granulomas Early nonspecific signs: fever, lethargy, poor feeding, irritability, vomiting May include hyperbilirubinemia, seizures, flaccid or spastic paralysis, apneic episodes, respiratory distress, lethargy, or coma (CNS encephalopathy)	Cesarean section sometimes a preventive measure for mothers with active lesions Vaginal delivery of infants of mothers with recurrent infection thought to be at lower risk Suggest infants room-in with mother in private room
LISTERIOSIS *(LISTERIA)*	
Acquired in late pregnancy: stillborn or acutely ill; may die within an hour after birth Late onset: septicemia; meningitis	Transmitted: transplacentally or by aspiration of secretions at birth Segregate infants until cultures are negative
LYME DISEASE *(BORRELIA BURGDORFERI)*	
Stillbirth Congenital defects reported: congenital heart disease, syndactyly, cortical blindness Prematurity Rash	Transmitted: transplacentally Immediate treatment of affected pregnant women with appropriate antibiotic Advise pregnant women to avoid tick exposure in endemic areas
RUBELLA, CONGENITAL (RUBELLA VIRUS)	
Eye defects: cataracts (unilateral or bilateral), microphthalmia, retinitis, glaucoma CNS signs: microcephaly, seizures, severe mental retardation Congenital heart defects: patent ductus arteriosus Auditory: high incidence of delayed hearing loss Intrauterine growth retardation Hyperbilirubinemia, spinal fluid abnormalities, thrombocytopenia, hepatomegaly	Transmitted: first trimester; early second trimester Pregnant women should avoid contact with all affected persons, including infants with rubella syndrome Emphasize vaccination of all unimmunized prepubertal children, susceptible adolescents, and adult females of childbearing age Caution women against pregnancy for at least 3 months after vaccination
SYPHILIS, CONGENITAL *(TREPONEMA PALLIDUM)*	
Copper-colored maculopapular cutaneous lesions (after 7th day), mucous membrane patches, hair loss, nail exfoliation, snuffles (syphilitic rhinitis), profound anemia, poor feeding, pseudoparalysis of one or more limbs, dysmorphic teeth (older child)	Transmitted: transplacentally, usually after 18th week of pregnancy Most severe form of syphilis Strict isolation of infant Treatment: penicillin
TOXOPLASMOSIS *(TOXOPLASMA GONDII)*	
Hydrocephaly, cerebral calcifications, chorioretinitis (classic triad) Microcephaly, seizures, mental retardation, deafness Encephalitis, myocarditis, hepatosplenomegaly, anemia, jaundice, diarrhea, vomiting, purpura	Transmitted: throughout pregnancy Predominant host for organism is cats May be transmitted through cat feces, poorly cooked or raw infected meat Caution pregnant women to avoid contact with cat feces (e.g., emptying cat litter boxes) Treatment: sulfonamides, pyrimethamine

or eliminated by wearing gloves for patient contact. Masks may be required for personnel when caring for infants with an infection such as congenital rubella. The hospital infection control department provides guidelines for the type and duration of precautions. Careful handwashing is the most important nursing intervention in reducing spread of any infection.

Special feeding techniques may need to be implemented for infants with feeding difficulties, and infants subject to seizures are protected from adverse environmental stimuli. Specimens need to be obtained for laboratory examinations, and the infant and parents need to be prepared for diagnostic procedures. When possible, long-term disabilities are prevented by early evaluation and implementation of therapy. The family is taught any special handling techniques needed for the care of their infant and signs of complications or possible sequelae. If sequelae are inevitable, the family will need assistance in determining how they can best cope with the problems, such as assistance with home care, referral to appropriate agencies, or placement in an institution for care.

The major goal of nursing care is prevention of these disorders with provision of adequate prenatal care for the expectant mother and precautions regarding exposure to teratogenic infections.

DEFECTS CAUSED BY CHEMICAL AGENTS

The relationship of the fetal and maternal circulations allows for the interchange of chemical substances across the placental membrane. The limited metabolic capabilities of the fetal liver and its immature enzyme and transport systems render the unborn child ill equipped for maintaining homeostasis when chemical disturbances are imposed by the mother. This includes both substances produced by the mother in response to a disease state (such as diabetes) and exogenous substances ingested or inhaled by the mother.

The teratogenic effect of drugs is not believed to have an effect on developing tissue until day 15 of gestation, when tissue differentiation begins to take place. Before that time drugs usually have little effect, because they are believed to have an insignificant affinity for undifferentiated tissue. Also, until implantation takes place, at approximately 7 days after conception, the embryo is not exposed to maternal blood that contains the drug. However some drugs may affect the uterine lining, making it unsuitable for implantation. Drugs administered between days 15 and 90 may produce an effect if the tissue for which it has an affinity is in the process of differentiation at that time. After 90 days, when differentiation is complete, most fetal tissues are believed to be relatively resistant to teratogenic effects of drugs. However, the impact on ongoing neurologic development is not known.

One drug recognized for its carcinogenic effect is ***diethylstilbestrol.*** Large doses of this hormone given to pregnant women to prevent abortion cause adenocarcinoma of the vagina in a significant proportion of the female offspring when they reach adolescence and early adulthood.

Nursing Considerations

Expectant mothers are cautioned against ingesting any medication without first consulting a practitioner. To help ensure that fewer women will inadvertently take some chemical that might be harmful to the fetus, labels on medications are now required to include information regarding the possible teratogenic effects of the drug. Excessive use of some very commonplace drugs, such as alcohol (see below), valproic acid, and isotretinoin (Accutane), has been shown to produce characteristic malformations in the fetus.

Nurses should be aware of the **Association of Birth Defect Children, Inc.,*** which offers help and information to families with children with defects caused by maternal exposure to drugs, chemicals, radiation, and other environmental agents.

FETAL ALCOHOL SYNDROME (FAS)

Infants and children with FAS have characteristic facial and associated physical features attributed to excessive ingestion of alcohol by the mother during pregnancy. Behavioral problems, cognitive impairment, and psychosocial deficits have also been recognized as originating from alcohol ingestion by the pregnant mother. A number of children and adults who demonstrate cognitive, behavioral, and psychosocial problems without the facial dysmorphia and growth retardation are referred to as having ***fetal alcohol effects (FAE).*** FAS is recognized as the leading cause of mental retardation, outranking Down syndrome and spina bifida (Warren and Bast, 1988). The incidence of FAS cases is on the rise in the United States despite public warnings, including the U.S. Surgeon General's warning that consumption of alcohol during pregnancy may cause mental retardation and other defects. In 1992 the number of reported cases was 3.7 per 10,000 births, as compared with 1979, when the number of reported cases was 1.0 per 10,000 live births (Fetal alcohol syndrome, 1993).

Alcohol (ethanol and ethyl alcohol) interferes with normal pregnancy; the effects on the fetus are permanent; and even moderate use of alcohol during pregnancy may cause long-term postnatal difficulties, including impaired maternal-infant attachment. Since there is no known safe level of alcohol consumption in pregnancy, women who plan to become pregnant should stop consuming alcohol at least 3 months before they plan to conceive.

It is not the degree of alcohol intake in the mother that is related to the presence of abnormalities in the fetus; rather, it is the amount consumed in excess of the liver's ability to detoxify that places the fetus at risk. The liver's capacity to detoxify is limited and inflexible—when the liver receives more alcohol than it is able to handle, the excess is continually recirculated until the organ is able to reduce it to carbon dioxide and water. This circulating alcohol has a special affinity for brain tissue. Other factors that contribute to the teratogenic effects include toxic acetyl aldehyde (a degradation by-product of ethanol) and other substances that may be added to the alcohol. Poor nutritional state, smoking, polydrug intake, and poor prenatal care may further compound the problem when alcohol abuse is observed.

The effects on the fetal brain are reflected in the CNS manifestations of FAS (see box below). Mental retardation,

*827 Irma St., Orlando, FL 32803; (800) 313-ABDC or (407) 245-7035.

MAJOR FEATURES OF FETAL ALCOHOL SYNDROME

FACIAL FEATURES

Short palpebral fissures
Hypoplastic philtrum (vertical ridge in upper lip)
Thinned upper lip
Short, upturned nose
Hypoplastic maxilla
Micrognathia or prognathia in adolescence
Retrognathia in infancy

NEUROLOGIC

Mental retardation
Motor retardation
Microcephaly
Poor coordination
Hypotonia
Hearing disorders

BEHAVIOR

Irritability (infancy)
Hyperactivity (child)

GROWTH

Prenatal growth retardation
Persistent postnatal growth lag, especially in boys

hearing disorders, and a variety of defects in craniofacial development are prominent features (Fig. 11-30). Affected infants display the physical features of the syndrome; the behaviors, however, are nonspecific in newborns and may therefore pass undetected (Fetal alcohol syndrome, 1993). These include difficulty in establishing respirations, irritability, lethargy, seizure activity, tremulousness, poor suck reflex, and abdominal distention. Affected infants frequently develop metabolic problems and have a variety of other birth defects, such as cardiac anomalies, hemangioma, eye and ear anomalies, and neural tube defects (spina bifida).

The initial difficulties in the newborn period are managed by preventing stimulation that might precipitate seizures, sedation and/or anticonvulsant therapy, and general supportive measures. The defects and their effects are irreversible, so the major emphasis must be aimed at prevention in the prenatal period.

Nursing Considerations

The nursing care of affected infants involves the same assessment and observations that are employed for any high-risk infant (see Chapter 10). Poor feeding is characteristic of infants with FAS and can be a significant problem throughout infancy. Special emphasis is placed on monitoring weight gain, analyzing feeding behaviors, and devising strategies to promote nutritional intake.

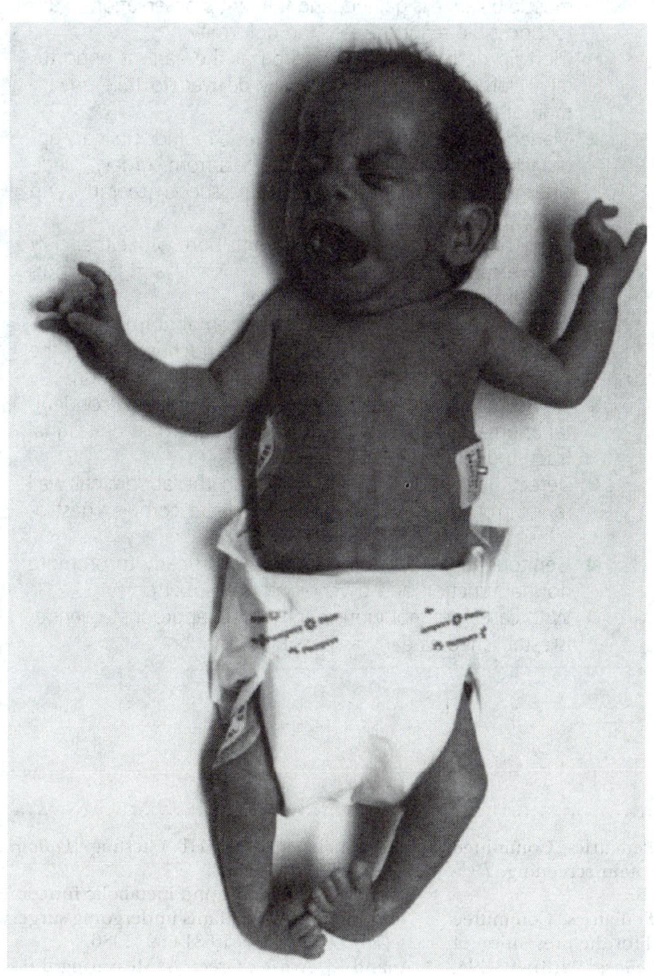

FIG. 11-30 Infant with fetal alcohol syndrome.

The effects of FAS have been identified in adolescents and young adults, primarily in relation to growth deficiencies, delayed motor development, and cognitive impairment. Facial characteristics tend to be more subtle than in infants and children (Streissguth and others, 1991).

The dangers of heavy drinking are known, and women with a history of excessive alcohol ingestion should be counseled regarding the risks to the fetus. It should be emphasized to all women that there is no known "safe" amount of alcohol intake during pregnancy that will preclude either FAS or FAE. Furthermore, FAS/FAE is a *totally preventable* birth defect. A change in drinking habits even as late as the third trimester (when brain growth in the fetus is greatest) is associated with improved fetal outcome (Day and others, 1989).*

RADIATION

Ionizing radiation in large doses has been shown to be both mutagenic and teratogenic in humans. Pelvic irradiation of pregnant women—from natural background radiation that is present everywhere in varying degrees, from occupational exposure, or from diagnostic or therapeutic procedures—is believed to be hazardous to the embryo, although the extent of teratogenicity and the exact dosage required to induce somatic change are still under consideration. Radiation may damage the conceptus at any time during its prenatal existence, and it is known that rapidly dividing and differentiating cells, such as those of the embryo, have increased radiosensitivity. As with other teratogens, the type of effect produced is closely correlated with the stage of development at which the radiation exposure occurs.

Although data are incomplete, there are indications that a larger number of chromosome abnormalities occur in children born to parents who have been exposed to increased preconception radiation. This finding is consistent with the observation that chromosome abnormalities are highest in infants of older mothers, and there is an increased frequency of chromosomally abnormal fetuses born to parents with occupational exposure to radiation. To help prevent the possibility of radiation damage, it is advisable (1) to avoid unnecessary radiation exposure, such as elective radiographs, in women of childbearing age except during the 2 weeks immediately following menstruation, (2) to ask if pregnancy is a possibility, and (3) to advise both men and women who have lower abdominal or pelvic radiographs to avoid conception for several months. Also, the harmful effects of maternal radioactive iodine (RAI) therapy on the fetal thyroid gland have led to the conclusion that termination of pregnancies that occur during RAI therapy should be considered.

*Additional information is available from the **National Organization on Fetal Alcohol Syndrome** (NOFAS), 1815 H St., N.W., Suite 750, Washington, DC 20006; (202) 785-4585.

NUTRITION

The human conceptus has no store of nutrients to sustain vital functions during the prenatal period; therefore it must rely on the mother as its single source of nutrition. A number of related factors, acting alone or in combination, influence fetal access to nutrients. These include reduction of maternal intake of specific nutrients and the general nutritional state of the mother. The chronically malnourished mother has few nutritional reserves available for fetal use, and the accumulated effects of lifetime nutritional deficiency may produce physiologic and anatomic structural defects that impair the mother's ability to support pregnancy and contribute to difficulties during labor. The teenage mother who has special nutritional requirements for meeting her own growth needs may compete with the fetus for available nutrients. Diet fads and restrictive diets, such as the Zen macrobiotic diet, seriously compromise the health of both the mother and the fetus (see Chapter 13).

Current information indicates that the restriction of calories and protein during prenatal development profoundly affects the size, viability, postnatal growth, and behavior of children. The timing and duration of nutritional deprivation appear to be crucial. Of greatest concern are the consequences of dietary restriction at the time the brain is undergoing the most rapid growth and development. Insufficient nutrients to the fetus during the time of rapid brain cell division result in permanent deficiency in brain cell numbers. The long-term consequences of nutritional deficiency may be manifested as cognitive, behavioral, and language retardation. The important role nutrition plays in preventing birth defects is evident in the relationship between folic acid and neural tube defects (see p. 444).

KEY POINTS

- Congenital malformations or anomalies, or "birth defects," are present at birth and are the result of genetic or nongenetic influences.
- Typical reactions of parents to an infant with a physical defect include grief over "loss" of a perfect child, shock, and withdrawal.
- The nurse's primary roles in care of an infant with a physical defect are caregiver, provider of family support, and supplier of information.
- Surgery initiates a number of physiologic responses, including cardiovascular, respiratory, endocrine, renal, gastrointestinal, immune, neurologic, and fluid and electrolyte.
- Nurses must be sensitive to pain in the neonate, be alert for signs of pain, and intervene appropriately.
- One of the largest groups of congenital anomalies includes those associated with the embryonic neural tube, the most common of which are spina bifida occulta and myelomeningocele.
- Folic acid supplementation in women before and during pregnancy prevents many cases of neural tube defects, anencephaly, and spina bifida.
- Care of the infant and child with myelomeningocele requires both immediate and long-term professional supervision. Associated problems include infection, neurologic damage, impaired renal function, musculoskeletal impairment, and latex allergy.
- Hydrocephalus is a symptom of an underlying brain pathology, demonstrated by impaired absorption of cerebrospinal fluid (CSF) or obstruction to the flow of CSF within the ventricles.
- Therapy for hydrocephalus involves relief of the hydrocephalus, treatment of the underlying brain pathology if possible, prevention and/or treatment of complications, and management of problems related to psychomotor development.
- Treatment of developmental dysplasia of the hip involves maintaining the head of the femur correctly positioned in the acetabulum by means of an external device, usually the Pavlik harness.
- Treatment of clubfoot involves manual overcorrection of the deformity, maintenance of the correction until normal muscle balance is gained, and follow-up observation to detect possible recurrence of the deformity.
- Cleft lip deformities are repaired at the earliest opportunity; cleft palate repair is usually delayed to take advantage of growth changes.
- Management of cleft palate involves a multidisciplinary approach to care involving professionals from surgery, medicine, nursing, social work, dentistry, speech therapy, and audiology.
- Major nursing challenges with infants born with either cleft involve feeding. Breast-feeding is possible and is encouraged if this is the mother's choice.
- Tracheosophageal fistula consists of an abnormal connection between the esophagus and the trachea, placing the untreated infant at risk for life-threatening aspiration.
- Anorectal defects are often associated with other congenital anomalies, such as those involving the gastrointestinal tract and kidneys.
- Defects involving herniation through the abdominal wall range from a simple umbilical hernia to complex gastroschisis.
- Genitourinary tract defects are repaired early to promote normal function and psychologic adjustment.
- With cases of ambiguous genitalia, an appropriate gender is established as early as possible

REFERENCES

Aldrich EF, Harmann P: Disconnection as a cause of VP shunt malfunction in multicomponent shunt systems, *Pediatr Neurosurg* 16(6):309-311, 1991.

American Academy of Pediatrics: Committee on Fetus and Newborn, Committee on Drugs, Section on Anethesiology, and Section on Surgery: Neonatal anesthesia, *Pediatrics* 80:446, 1987a.

American Academy of Pediatrics, Committee on Genetics: α-Fetoprotein screening, *Pediatrics* 80:444-445, 1987b.

American Academy of Pediatrics, Committee on Genetics: Folic acid for the prevention of neural tube defects, *Pediatrics* 92(3):493-494, 1993.

American Academy of Pediatrics, Task Force on Pediatric AIDS: Perinatal human immunodeficiency virus (HIV) testing, *Pediatrics* 89(4):791-794, 1992.

Anand KJ: Hormonal and metabolic functions of neonates and infants undergoing surgery, *Curr Opin Cardiol* 1:681-689, 1986.

Anand KJ, Aynsley-Green A: Measuring the severity of surgical stress in newborn infants, *J Pediatr Surg* 23:297-305, 1988.

Anand KJ, Hickey P: Pain and its effects in the

human neonate and fetus, *N Engl J Med* 317:1321-1329, 1987.

Anand K, Hickey P: Halothane-morphine compared with high-dose sufentanil for anesthesia and postoperative analgesia in neonatal cardiac surgery, *N Engl J Med* 326(1):1-9, 1992.

Anand KJ, McGrath PJ: *Pain in neonates,* New York, 1993, Elsevier.

Anand KJ, Sippell WG, Aynsley-Green A: Randomized trial of fentanyl anaesthesia in preterm babies undergoing surgery: effects on the stress response, *Lancet* 31:243-247, 1987.

Anderson SM: Secondary neurologic disability in myelomeningocele, *Infants Young Child* 1(4):9-21, 1989.

Aronson J, Puskarich CL: Deformity and disability from treated clubfoot, *J Pediatr Orthop* 10(1):109-119, 1990.

Attia J and others: Measurement of postoperative pain and narcotic administration in infants using a new clinical scoring system, *Anesthesiology* 67(3A):A532, 1987.

Barba B and others: Pain memory in full-term newborns, *J Pain Symptom Manage* 6:206, 1991.

Barrier G and others: Measurement of postoperative pain and narcotic administration in infants using a new clinical scoring system, *Intensive Care Med* 15:S37-S39, 1989.

Beath S and others: Liver transplantation in babies and children with extrahepatic biliary atresia, *J Pediatr Surg* 28(8):1044-1047, 1993a.

Beath SV and others: Successful liver transplantation in babies under 1 year, *Br Med J* 307:825-828, 1993b.

Belman AB: Hypospadias and other urethral anomalies. In Kelalis PP, King LR, Belman AB, editors: *Clinical pediatric urology,* Philadelphia, 1992, WB Saunders.

Bennett JT, MacEwen GD: Congenital dislocation of the hip, *Clin Orthop* 247:15-21, 1989.

Bozzette M: Observation of pain behavior in the NICU: an exploratory study, *J Perinat Neonat Nurs* 7(1):76-87, 1993.

Brown L: Physiologic responses to cutaneous pain in neonates, *Neonatal Network* 6(3):18-22, 1987.

Burrows FA, Berde CB: Optimal pain relief in infants and children, *Br Med J* 307(6908):815-816, 1993.

Burton BK, Schulz CJ, Burd LI: Spectrum of limb disruption defects associated with chorionic villus sampling, *Pediatrics,* 91:989-993, 1993.

Butler NC: How to raise professional awareness of the need for adequate pain relief for infants, *Birth* 15(1):38-41, 1988.

Carey J: Malformations and syndromes that involve the craniofacies. In Rudolph A, editor: *Pediatrics,* Norwalk, CT, 1987, Appleton & Lange.

Campos RG: Soothing pain-elicited distress in infants with swaddling and pacifiers, *Child Dev* 60:781-792, 1989.

Chadduck WM; Chadduck JB; Boop FA: The subarachnoid spaces in craniosynostosis, *Neurosurgery* 30(6):867-871, 1992.

Choonara I: Management of pain in newborn infants, *Semin Perinatol* 16(1):32-40, 1992.

Côte JJ, Morse JM, James SG: The pain response of the postoperative newborn, *J Adv Nurs* 16:378-387, 1991.

Curtin G: The infant with cleft lip or palate: more than a surgical problem, *J Perinat Neonat Nurs* 3(3):80-89, 1990.

Danner SC: Breastfeeding the infant with a cleft defect, *NAACOGs Clin Issues Perinat Womens Health Nurs* 3(4):634-639, 1992.

daSilva MC, Drake JM: Complications of CSF shunt antisiphon devices, *Pediatr Neurosurg* 17(6):304-309, 1992.

Day NL and others: Prenatal exposure to alcohol: effect on infant growth and morphologic characteristics, *Pediatrics* 84:536-541, 1989.

Deshpande S, Platt MPW, Aynsley-Green A: Patterns of the metabolic and endocrine stress response to surgery and medical illness in infancy and childhood, *Crit Care Med* 21(9, suppl):S359-S360, 1993.

Donder J, Candy AT, Rourke BP: Psychometric intelligence after infantile hydrocephalus: a critical review and reinterpretation, *Childs Nerv Syst* 6(3):148-154, 1990.

Ellsworth PI and others: Evaluation and risk factors of latex allergy in spina bifida patients: is it preventable? *J Urol* 150(2):691-693, 1993.

Erlen JA, Holzman IR: Anencephalic infants: should they be organ donors? *Pediatr Nurs* 14:6-64, 1988.

Fanaroff AA, Martin RJ: Jaundice and liver disease. In Fanaroff AA, Martin RJ, editors: *Neonatal-perinatal medicine: diseases of the fetus and infant,* St Louis, 1992, Mosby.

Farrington EA and others: Continuous intravenous morphine infusion in postoperative newborn infants, *Am J Perinatol* 10(1):84, 1993.

FDA proposes to add folic acid to some foods, *Pediatr Alert* 18(23):136, 1993.

Fernandes ET and others: Neurogenic bladder dysfunction in children: review of pathophysiology and current management, *J Pediatr* 124(1):1-7, 1994.

Fetal alcohol syndrome—United States, 1979-1992, *MMWR* 42(17):338-340, 1993.

Franck LS: A new method to quantitatively describe pain behavior in infants, *Nurs Res* 35:28-31, 1986.

Franck LS: A national survey of the assessment and treatment of pain and agitation in the neonatal intensive care unit, *JOGNN* 16(6):387-393, 1987.

Gray ML: Anatomy related to urinary function. In Broadwell DB, Parrish RS, Saunders RC, editors: *Child health nursing,* Philadelphia, 1993, JB Lippincott.

Grosfeld J and others: The efficacy of hepatoportoenterostomy in biliary atresia, *Surgery* 106(4):692-701, 1989.

Grunau RV, Craig KD: Pain expression in neonates: facial action and cry, *Pain* 28:395-410, 1987.

Grunau RVE, Johnston CC, Craig KD: Neonatal facial and cry responses to invasive and noninvasive procedures, *Pain* 42(3):295-305, 1990.

Gunnar MR, Fisch RO, Malone S: The effects of a pacifying stimulus on behavioral and adrenocortical responses to circumcision in the newborn, *J Am Acad Child Adolesc Psychiatry* 23:34-38, 1984.

Iwasaki K: Management after application of the Pavlik harness in congenital dislocation of the hip, *Arch Orthop Trauma Surg* 106(5):276-280, 1987.

James HE: Hydrocephalus in infancy and childhood, *Am Fam Physician* 45(2):733-742, 1992.

Johnston CC, Strada ME: Acute pain response in infants: a multidimensional description, *Pain* 24:373-382, 1986.

Kanwaljeet S, Anand KS: Relationships between stress responses and clinical outcome in newborns, infants, and children, *Crit Care Med* 21(9, suppl):S358-359, 1993.

Karrer F and others: Congenital biliary tract disease, *Surg Clin North Am* 70(6):1403-1418, 1990.

Kasablan NG and others: The prophylactic value of CIC and anticholinergic medication in infants with myelodysplasia, *Am J Dis Child* 146(7):840-843, 1992.

Kaufman S and others: Nutritional support for the infant with extrahepatic biliary atresia, *J Pediatr* 110(5):679-685, 1987.

Kelalis PP, King LR, Belman AB, editors: *Clin pediatric urology,* Philadelphia, 1992, WB Saunders.

Kenner C, Brueggemeyer: Assessment and management of genitourinary dysfunction. In Kenner C and others: *Comprehensive neonatal nursing: a physiologic perspective,* Philadelphia, 1993, WB Saunders.

Kinsella JP and others: Clinical responses to prolonged treatment of persistent pulmonary hypertension of the newborn with low doses of inhaled nitric oxide, *J Pediatr* 123(1):103-108, 1993.

Lala R and others: Combined therapy with LHRH and HCG in cryptorchid infants, *Eur J Pediatr* 152(suppl 2):531-533, 1993.

Lancaster PAL: Epidemiology of bladder exstrophy, *Teratology* 36:221, 1987.

Laurent J and others: Long-term outcome after surgery for biliary atresia, *Gastroenterology* 99(6):1793-1797, 1990.

Lawrence J and others: The development of a tool to assess neonatal pain, *Neonatal Network* 12(6):59-66, 1993.

Leger RR, Meeropol E: Children at risk: latex allergy and spina bifida *J Pediatr Nurs* 7(6):371-376, 1992.

Levine AH: Fetal surgery: in utero repair of congenital diaphragmatic hernia, *AORN J* 54(1):16-32, 1991.

Maguire DP, Maloney P: A comparison of fentanyl and morphine use in neonates, *Neonatal Network* 7(1):27-32, 1988.

Mäkinen-Kiljunen S and others: Is cows' milk casein an allergen in latex-rubber gloves? *Lancet* 342(8875):863-864, 1993.

Marchette L and others: Pain reduction interventions during neonatal circumcision, *Nurs Res* 40:241-244, 1991.

McLaughlin CR and others: Neonatal pain: a comprehensive survey of attitudes and practices, *J Pain Symptom Manage* 8(1):7-16, 1993.

Meeropol E and others: Allergic reactions to rubber in patients with myelodysplasia, *N Engl J Med* 232(15):1072, 1990.

Meeropol E, Leger R, Frost J: Latex allergy in patients with myelodysplasia and in health care providers: a double jeopardy, *Urol Nurs* 13(2):39-44, 1993.

Meller J, Reyes H, Loeff D: Gastroschisis and omphalocele, *Clin Perinatol* 16(1):113-122, 1989.

Merenstein GB, Gardner SL: *Handbook of neonatal intensive care,* ed 3, St Louis, 1993, Mosby.

Mills JL and others: Maternal vitamin levels during pregnancies producing infants with neural tube defects, *J Pediatr* 120(6):863-871, 1992.-

Moreno CN, Iovanne BA: Congenital diaphragmatic hernia. I. *Neonatal Network* 12(1):19-27, 1993.

MRC Vitamin Study Research Group: Prevention of neural tube defects: results of the Medical Research Council Vitamin Study, *Lancet* 338:131-137, 1991.

Nora JJ, Fraser FC: *Medical genetics: principles and practice,* ed 3, Philadelphia, 1989, Lea & Febiger.

Pascual-Castroviejo I and others: Dandy-Walker malformation: analysis of 38 cases, *Childs Nerv Syst* 7(2):88-97, 1991.

Pasquariello CA and others: Intraoperative anaphylaxis to latex, *Pediatrics* 91(5):983-985, 1993.

Pediatric Orthopaedic Society of North America (POSNA): *Developmental dysplasia of the hip,* Paper presented at the annual meeting, Dallas, 1991.

Penny R: Undescended testes. In Gellis SS, Kagan BM: *Current pediatric therapy 12,* Philadelphia, 1986, WB Saunders.

Penticuff J: Neonatal nursing ethics: toward a consensus, *Neonatal Network* 5:7-16, 1987.

Peterson P: Spina bifida—nursing challenge, *RN* 3:40-47, 1992.

Pokela M: Pain relief can reduce hypoxemia in distressed neonates during routine treatment procedures, *Pediatrics* 93(3):379-383, 1994.

Rauen K: *Guidelines for spina bifida health care services throughout life,* Washington, DC, 1990, Spina Bifida Association of America.

Recommendations for the use of folic acid to reduce the number of cases of spina bifida and other neural tube defects, *MMWR* 41(4):1-7, 1992.

Richard M: Feeding the newborn with cleft lip and/or palate: the enlargement, stimulate, swallow rest (ESSR) method, *J Pediatr Nurs* 6(5):317-321, 1991.

Romanczuk A: Latex use with infants and children: it can cause problems, *MCN* 18(4):208-212, 1993.

Rushton CH: The surgical neonate: principles of nursing management, *Pediatr Nurs* 14:141-151, 1988.

Ryckman F and others: Improved survival in biliary atresia patients in the present era of liver transplantation, *J Pediatr Surg* 28(3):382-386, 1993.

Saggese G and others: Hormonal therapy for cryptorchidism with a combination of human chorionic gonadotropin and follicle-stimulating hormone, *Am J Dis Child* 143:980-982, 1989.

Shaer C: Spina bifida: an overview, *Ethicscope* 1(1):1-3, 1993.

Shapiro C: Pain in the neonate: assessment and intervention, *Neonatal Network* 8(1):7-21, 1989.

Shapiro CR: Nurses' judgments of pain in term and preterm newborns, *JOGNN* 22(1):41-47, 1993.

Shapiro E and others: Complications of latex allergy, *Dialog Pediatr Urol* 15:1-8, 1992.

Slater JE: Rubber anaphylaxis, *N Engl J Med* 320(17):1126-1130, 1989.

Spear RM: Anesthesia for premature and term infants: perioperative implications, *J Pediatr* 120(2):165-176, 1992.

Spina bifida incidence at birth—United States, 1983-1990, *MMWR* 41(27):497-500, 1992.

Stevens BJ: Personal communication, 1994.

Stevens BJ, Johnston CC, Horton L: Multidimensional pain assessment in premature neonates: a pilot study, *JOGNN* 22(6):531-541, 1993.

Storrs B and others: The tethered cord syndrome, *Int Pediatr* 5(2):99-103, 1990.

Streissguth AP and others: Fetal alcohol syndrome in adolescents and adults, *JAMA* 265(15):1961-1967, 1991.

Stylianos S and others: Incarceration of inguinal hernia in infants prior to elective repair, *J Pediatr Surg* 28(4):582-583, 1993.

Sugar EC and others: Pediatric hypospadias surgery: *Pediatr Nurs* 19(6):585-588, 1993.

Swaiman KF: *Pediatric neurology,* ed 2, St Louis, 1994, Mosby.

Temporal trends in the prevalence of congenital malformations, *MMWR* 39:19-23, 1990.

Theorell CJ: Congenital diaphragmatic hernia: a physiologic approach to management, *J Perinat Neonat Nurs* 3(3):66-79, 1990.

Torfs C and others: Gastroschisis, *J Pediatr* 116(1):1-6, 1990.

Toyosaka A and others: Outcome of 21 patients with biliary atresia living more than 10 years, *J Pediatr Surg* 28:1498-1501, 1993.

Warren KR, Bast RJ: Alcohol-related birth defects: an update, *Public Health Rep* 103(6):638-642, 1988.

Weatherly-White RC and others: Early repair and breast-feeding for infants with cleft lip, *Plast Reconstr Surg* 79(6):879-887, 1987.

Wessel DL: Hemodynamic responses to perioperative pain and stress in infants, *Crit Care Med* 21(9, suppl):S361-S362, 1993.

Wright V: The esophagus: congenital anomalies. In Walker W and others, editors: *Pediatric gastrointestinal disease: pathophysiology, diagnosis, management,* St Louis, 1990, Mosby.

Yaster M and others: Local anesthetics in the management of acute pain in children, *J Pediatr* 124(2):165-176, 1994.

Yen IH and others: The changing epidemiology of neural tube defects—United States, 1968-1989, *Am J Dis Child* 146(7):857-861, 1992.

Young MA and others: Latex allergy: a guideline for perioperative nurses, *AORN J* 56(3):485, 488-493, 496-497, 1992.

BIBLIOGRAPHY

The Child with a Physical Defect

Brenner VM: Unilateral pulmonary hypoplasia/agenesis in the neonate: a case report, *Neonatal Network* 6(3):49-57, 1987.

Bucciarelli RL, Eitzman DV: Baby Doe: where we stand now, *Contemp Pediatr* 5(1):116-128, 1988.

Bull MJ and others: Special children, special car seats, *Contemp Pediatr* 6(1):123-134, 1989.

Friedman JM: A practical approach to dysmorphology, *Pediatr Ann* 19:95-101, 1990.

Heller A and others: Birth defects and psychosocial adjustment, *Am J Dis Child* 139:257-263, 1985.

Kilgo JL, Richard N, Noonan MJ: Teaming for the future: integrating transition planning with early intervention services for young children with special needs and their families, *Infants Young Child* 2(2):37-48, 1989.

Lemons PM: Beyond the birth of a defective child, *Neonatal Network* 5(3):13-20, 1986.

Lynch ME: Congenital defects: parental issues and nursing supports, *J Perinat Neonat Nurs* 2(4):53-59, 1989.

Mitchell C, Rutherford PA: The fragile survivor, *Am J Nurs* 87:603-606, 1987.

Ramp JB and others: Conjoined twins: a multidisciplinary approach, *Neonatal Network* 8(1):29-39, 1989.

Shaw N: Common surgical problems in the newborn, *J Perinat Neonat Nurs* 3:50-65, 1990.

Wasserman GA and others: Contributors to attachment in normal and physically handicapped infants, *J Am Acad Child Adolesc Psychiatry* 26(1):9-15, 1987.

Winter RM: A combinational method for grouping cases with multiple malformations, *J Med Genet* 25:118-122, 1988.

Surgery and Pain

Anand KJS, Aynsley-Green A: Measuring the severity of surgical stress in newborn infants, *J Pediatr Surg* 23(4):297-305, 1988.

Anand KJS, Carr DB: The neuroanatomy, neurophysiology, and neurochemistry of pain, stress and analgesia in newborns and children, *Pediatr Clin North Am* 36:795-821, 1989.

Beaver PK: Premature infants' response to touch and pain: can nurses make a difference? *Neonatal Network* 6(3):13-17, 1987.

Bloch EC: Update on anesthesia management for infants and children, *Surg Clin North Am* 72(6):1207-1221, 1992.

Broome M and Tanzillo H: Differentating between pain and agitation in premature neonates, *J Perinat Neonat Nurs* 4(1):53-62, 1990.

Butler NB: The ethical issues involved in the practice of surgery on unanesthetized infants, *AORN J* 46(6):1136-1144, 1987.

Butler NB: How to raise professional awareness of the need for adequate pain relief for infants, *Birth* 15(1):38-41, 1988.

Butler NB: More on neonatal pain, *Perinatal Press* 11(2):19-20, 1988.

Dale JC: A multidisciplinary study of infants' behaviors associated with assumed painful stimuli: phase II, *J Pediatr Health Care* 3(1):34-38, 1989.

Davis D, Calhoon M: Do preterm infants show behavioral responses to painful procedures? In Funk S and others, editors: *Key aspects of comfort,* New York, 1989, Springer.

Dyke RM: Instruments in neonatal research: measuring pain in the preterm infant, *Neonatal Network* 12(6):91-93, 1933.

Filston HC: Fluid and electrolyte management in the pediatric surgical patient, *Surg Clin North Am* 72(6):1189-1206, 1992.

Filston HC, Izant RJ: *The surgical neonate: evaluation and care,* ed 2, 1985, Appleton-Century-Crofts.

Fitzgerald M, Millard C, MacIntosh N: Hyperalgesia in premature infants, *Lancet* 6(8580):292, 1988.

Franck LS: Pain in the nonverbal patient: advocating for the critically ill neonate, *Pediatr Nurs* 15:65, 1989.

Holditch-Davis D: Measuring the behavior of

high-risk infants, *Neonatal Network* 12(3):69-72, 1993.

Holland RM and others: Pediatric surgery. In Merenstein GB, Gardner SL: *Handbook of neonatal intensive care,* ed 3, St Louis, 1993, Mosby.

Jones MA: Identifying signs that nurses interpret as indicating pain in newborns, *Pediatr Nurs* 15:76, 1989.

Kenner C, Harjo J, Brueggemeyer A, editors: *Neonatal surgery: a nusing perspective,* Orlando, FL, 1988, Grune & Stratton.

Kenner C and others: *Comprehensive neonatal nursing: a physiologic perspective,* Philadelphia, 1993, WB Saunders.

Lawson JR: Standards of practice and the pain of premature infants, *Zero to Three* 9:1-5, 1988.

Marshall RE: Neonatal pain associated with caregiving procedures, *Pediatr Clin North Am* 36:885-903, 1989.

Paxton JM: Transport of the surgical neonate, *J Perinat Neonat Nurs* 3(3):43-49, 1990.

Pigeon HM and others: How neonatal nurses report infants' pain, *Am J Nurs* 89:1529-1530, 1989.

Porter FL: Pain in the newborn, *Clin Perinatol* 16(2):549-564, 1989.

Schechter NL: The undertreatment of pain in children: an overview, *Pediatr Clin North Am* 36:781-794, 1989.

Shaw N: Common surgical problems in the newborn, *J Perinat Neonat Nurs* 3(3):50-65, 1990.

Shearer MH: Surgery on the paralyzed, unanesthetized newborn, *Birth* 13(2):79, 1986.

Wise BV, Lawrence-Nolan L: A risk of blood transfusions for premature infants, *MCN* 15:86-89, 1990.

Yaster M: Analgesia and anesthesia in neonates, *J Pediatr* 111:394-396, 1987.

Neurologic Defects

Banta JV: The tethered cord in myelomeningocele: should it be untethered? *Dev Med Child Neurol* 33(2):173-176, 1991.

Barkovich AJ, Edwards MS: Applications of neuroimaging in hydrocephalus, *Pediatr Neurosurg* 18(2):65-83, 1992.

Bartlett SP and others: The operative treatment of craniofacial dysostosis (plagiocephaly), *Plast Reconstr Surg* 85:677-683, 1990.

Brown JP, Reichenbach MA: Screening children with myelodysplasia for readiness to learn self-catheterization, *Rehab Nurs* 14:334-337, 1989.

Brucke JM, Laurent JP: Pediatric craniofacial reconstruction: an overview of perioperative management, *J Neurosci Nurs* 20(3):159-168, 1988.

Bull MJ and others: Safe transportation for infants with severe hydrocephalus, *J Neurosci Nurs* 23(6):347-353, 1991.

Burton BK: Maternal serum α-fetoprotein screening, *Pediatr Ann* 18:687-697, 1989.

Charney EB: Parental attitudes toward management of newborns with myelomeningocele, *Dev Med Child Neurol* 32:14-19, 1990.

Choudhury AR: Avoidable factors that contribute to the complications of ventriculoperitoneal shunt in childhood hydrocephalus, *Childs Nerv Syst* 6(6):346-349, 1990.

Committee Report: Task Force on Allergic Reactions to Latex, *J Allergy Clin Immunol* 92:16-18, 1993.

Farley JA, Dunleavey MJ: Myelodysplasia. In Jackson PL, Vessey JA, editors: *Primary care of the child with a chronic condition,* St Louis, 1992, Mosby.

Fernbach SK, Feinstein KA: Radiologic evaluation of the child with craniosynostosis, *Neurosurg Clin North Am* 2(3):569-585, 1991.

Folate supplements prevent recurrence of neural tube defects, *Nutr Rev* 50(1);22-24, 1992.

French LR, Jackson IT, Melta LJ: A population-based study of craniosynostosis, *J Clin Epidemiol* 43(1):69-73, 1990.

Gaston H: Ophthalmic complications of spina bifida and hydrocephalus, *Eye* 5:279-290, 1991.

Gault ST and others: Craniosynostosis: intracranial pressure and volume, *Plast Reconstruct Surg* 90:377-381, 1992.

Greif L, Miller CL: Shunt lengthening: a descriptive review, *J Neurosci Nurs* 23(2):120-124, 1991.

Holmes LB: Prevention of neural tube defects, *J Pediatr* 12(6):918-919, 1992.

Holzgrene W, Beller FK: Anencephalic infants as organ donors, *Clin Obstet Gynecol* 35(4):821-836, 1992.

Jackson PL: Primary care needs of children with hydrocephalus, *J Pediatr Health Care* 4:59-471, 1990.

Joseph DB and others: Clean, intermittent catheterization of infants with neurogenic bladder, *Pediatrics* 84:78-82, 1989.

Leff P, Walizer E: *Building the healing partnership: parents, professionals and children with chronic illnesses and disabilities,* Cambridge, MA, 1993, Bookline Books.

Loebig M: Mothers' assessment of the impact of children with spina bifida on the family, *Matern Child Nurs J* 19(3):251-264, 1990.

Macedo A, Posel LF: Nursing the family after the birth of a child with spina bifida, *Issues Compr Pediatr Nurs* 10:55-65, 1987.

Mazur JM, Menelaus MB: Neurologic status of spina bifida patients and the orthopedic surgeon, *Clin Orthop* 264:54-64, 1991.

Meeropol E and others: Latex allergy in patients with myelodysplasia and in health care providers: a double jeopardy, *J Urol Nurs* 13:39-44, 1993.

Milunsky A and others: Maternal heat exposure and neural tube defects, *JAMA* 268:882-885, 1992.

Moody BL: Community nursing needs of newborns with myelomeningocele and their families, *Home Health Nurse* 11(1):29-39, 1993.

Myhre CM, Richards T, Johnson J: Maternal serum α-fetorprotein screening: an assessment of fetal well-being, *J Perinat Neonat Nurs* 2(4):13-20, 1989.

Noetzel MJ: Neural tube defects and other congenital and genetic disorders, *Curr Opin Pediatr* 1:308-314, 1989.

Noetzel MJ, Blake JN: Seizures in children with congenital hydrocephalus: long-term outcomes, *Neurology* 42(7):1277-1281, 1992.

Oakley GP: Folic acid—preventable spina bifida and anencephaly, *JAMA* 269(10):1292, 1993.

Oi S and others: Pathophysiology and postnatal outcome of fetal hydrocephalus, *Childs Nerv Syst* 6:338-345, 1990.

Osaenbach RK, Menezes AH: Diagnosis and management of the Dandy-Walker malformation: 30 years experience, *Pediatr Neurosurg* 18(4):179-189, 1992.

Page RB: Hydrocephalus. In Hoekelman RA and others, editors: *Primary pediatric care,* ed 2, St Louis, 1992, Mosby.

Piatt JH: Physical examination of patients with cerebrospinal fluid shunts: is there useful information in pumping the shunt? *Pediatrics* 89(3):470-473, 1992.

Reis JG: Latex sensitivity: controlling health care workers', patients' risks, *AORN J* 59(3):615-621, 1994.

Rothenberg LS: The anencephalic neonate and brain death: an international review, *Transplant Proc* 22(3):1037-1039, 1990.

Rudy DC, Woodside JR: The incontinent myelodysplastic patient, *Urol Clin North Am* 18(2):295-309, 1991.

Scheinblum DT, Hamond M: The treatment of children with shunt infections: extraventricular drainage system care, *Pediatr Nurs* 16:139-143, 1990.

Shesser LK, Kling TF: Practical considerations in caring for a child in a hip spica cast: an evaluation using parental input, *Orthop Nurs* 5(3):11-15, 1986.

Sloan ES: Face value: trends and advances in craniofacial surgery, *Todays OR Nurse* 12:17-22, 1990.

Smith KA: Bowel and bladder management of the child with myelomeningocele in the school setting, *J Pediatr Health Care* 4(4):175-180, 1990.

Spina bifida incidence at birth—United States, 1983-1990, *MMWR* 41(27):497-500, 1992.

Steele S: Young children with meningomyelocele, with special reference to handling, positioning, and child-adult play interactions, *Issues Comp Pediatr Nurs* 11:213-225, 1988.

Steinbok P and others: Long-term outcome and complications of children born with meningomyelocele, *Childs Nerv Syst* 8(2):92-96, 1992.

Terry D, Nisbet K: Nursing care of the child with external ventricular drainage, *J Neurosci Nurs* 23(6):347-353, 1991.

Tilem D, Greenberg CS: Nursing care of the child with a ventriculostomy, *J Pediatr Nurs* 3:188-193, 1988.

Van Cleve L: Parental coping in response to their child's spina bifida, *J Pediatr Nurs* 4:172-176, 1989.

Walters JA, Tunnessen WW: Picture of the month: occult spinal dysraphism, *Am J Dis Child* 146(7):835, 1992.

Willett WC: Folic acid and neural tube defect, *Am J Public Health* 82:666-668, 1992.

Wiswell TE and others: Major congenital neurologic malformations, *Am J Dis Child* 144:61-67, 1990.

Yassin MS and others: Evaluation of latex allergy in patients with meningomyelocele, *Ann Allergy* 69(3):207-211, 1992.

Skeletal Defects

Aiello DH: Congenital dysplasia of the hip, diagnosis, treatment and nursing care, *AORN J* 49:1566-1606, 1989.

Albinana J, Quesada JA, Certucha JA: Children at high risk for congenital dislocation of the hip: late presentation, *J Pediatr Orthop* 13(2):268-269, 1993.

Bull MJ and others: Special children, special car seats, *Contemp Pediatr* 6(1):122-134, 1989.

Castelein RM and others: Natural history of ultrasound, hip abnormalities in clinically normal newborns, *J Pediatr Orthop* 12:423-427, 1992.

Catterall A: A method of assessment of the clubfoot deformity, *Clin Orthop* 264:48-53, 1991.

Edelstein JE, Berger N: Performance comparison among children fitted with myoelectric and body-powered hands, *Arch Phys Med Rehabil* 74(4):376-380, 1993.

Feller N and others: A multidisciplinary approach to developing safe transportation for children with special needs, *Orthop Nurs* 5(5):25-27, 1986.

Garbarino J: Maltreatment of young children with disabilities, *Infants Young Child* 2(2):49-57, 1989.

Hall JG: When a child is born with congenital anomalies, *Contemp Pediatr* 5(8):78-87, 1988.

Krebs DE, Edelstein JE, Thornby MA: Prosthetic management of children with limb deficiencies, *Phys Ther* 71(12):920-934, 1991.

Kyzer SP: Congenital idiopathic clubfoot, *Orthop Nurs* 10(4):11-32, 1991.

Lieber MT, Taub AS: Common foot deformities and what they mean for parents, *MCN* 13:47-50, 1988.

Linley JF: Screening children for common orthopaedic problems, *Am J Nurs* 87:1312-1316, 1987.

Schaming D and others: When babies are born with orthopaedic problems, *RN* 53(4):662-667, 1990.

Shoppe K: Developmental dysplasia of the hip, *Orthop Nurs* 11(5):30-36, 1992.

Short-DeGraff MA, Healey SM: Postpartum depression related to care for the child with special needs, *Infants Young Child* 2(2):24-36, 1989.

Speers A, Speers M: Care of the infant in a Pavlik harness, *Pediatr Nurs* 18(3):229-232, 252, 1992.

Staheli LT: Management of congenital hip dysplasia, *Pediatr Ann* 18:24-32, 1989.

Stout JD, Bull MJ, Stroup KB: Safe transportation for infants and preschoolers with special needs, *Infants Young Child* 2(2):67-73, 1989.

Swagman A: Caring for limb-deficient children and their families, *MCN* 11:46-52, 1986.

Thurman SK, Cornwell JR, Korteland C: The liaison infant family team (LIFT) project: an example of case study evaluation, *Infants Young Child* 2(2):74-82, 1989.

Wenger DR, Leach J: Foot deformities in infants and children, *Pediatr Clin North Am* 33:1411-1427, 1986.

Gastrointestinal Defects/Hernias

Alexander F, Johanningman J, Martin L: Staged repair improves outcome of high-risk premature infants with esophageal atresia and tracheoesophageal fistula, *J Pediatr Surg* 28(2):151-154, 1993.

Beath S and others: Liver transplantation in babies and children with extrahepatic biliary atresia, *J Pediatr Surg* 28(8):1044-1047, 1993.

Beath SV and others: Successful liver transplantation in babies under 1 year, *Br Med J* 307:825-828, 1993.

Brown W and others: Rotavirus 3 and neonatal biliary disease: discussion of divergent results, *Hepatology* 10(4):515-517, 1989.

Buisuttil R and others: Liver transplantation in children, *Ann Surg* 213(1):48-57, 1991.

Chittmittrapap S and others: Oesophageal atresia and associated anomalies, *Arch Dis Child* 64:364-368, 1989.

Curtin G: The infant with cleft lip or palate: more than a surgical problem, *J Perinat Neonat Nurs* 3(3):80-89, 1990.

Dado D: Experience with the functional cleft lip repair, *Plast Reconstr Surg* 86(5):872-881, 1990.

Dienno M: Esophageal atresia, *AORN J* 45(6): 1356-1367, 1987.

Dixon AG: Jeff's story: a unique approach to the care of an infant with esophageal atresia and cervical esophagostomy, *Neonatal Network* 4(6):7-12, 1986.

Eliason MJ: Cleft lip and palate: developmental effects, *J Pediatr Nurs* 6(2):107, 1991.

Fentner S: Abdominal wall defects: omphalocele and gastroschisis, *Neonatal Network* 6(3):29-41, 1987.

Filston HC: Fluid and electrolyte management in the pediatric surgical patient, *Surg Clin North Am* 72(6):1189-1200, 1992.

Howell C and others: Recent experience with diaphragmatic hernia and ECMO, *Ann Surg* 211(6):793-798, 1990.

Jeffs R: Exstrophy, epispadias, and cloacal and urogenital sinus abnormalities, *Pediatr Clin North Am* 34(5):1233-1257, 1987.

Kent PA, Curley MA: Challenges in nursing: infants with congenital diaphragmatic hernia, *Heart Lung* 21(4):381-389, 1992.

Kinsella JP, Abman SH: Inhalation nitric oxide therapy for persistent pulmonary hypertension of the newborn, *Pediatrics* 91(5):997-998, 1992.

Laurent J and others: Long-term outcome after surgery for biliary atresia, *Gastroenterology* 99:1793-1797, 1990.

Levine AH: Fetal surgery: in utero repair of congenital diaphragmatic hernia, *AORN J* 54(1):16, 1991.

MacDonald CA: Biliary atresia, *J Pediatr Nurs* 6(6):374-383, 1991.

Malatack JJ and others: The who, when, and how of liver transplants, *Contemp Pediatr* 5(2):152-160, 1988.

Maxson B and others: Allogeneic bone for secondary alveolar cleft osteoplasty, *J Oral Maxillofac Surg* 48:933-941, 1990.

McNichol J: When eating doesn't come naturally, *MCN* 14:23-26, 1989.

Miel-Vergani G and others: Late referral for biliary atresia: missed opportunities for effective surgery, *Lancet* 1(8635):421-423, 1989.

Millis J and others: Orthotopic liver transplantation for biliary atresia, *Arch Surg* 123:1237-1239, 1988.

Miyano T and others: Current concept of the treatment of biliary atresia, *World J Surg* 17:332-336, 1993.

Moreno CN, Iovanne BA: Congenital diaphragmatic hernia, part I, *Neonatal Network* 12(1):19, 1993.

Nittono H and others: Ursodeoxycholic acid in biliary atresia, *Lancet* 1(8584):528, 1988 (letter).

Oellrich RG, Cusumano MM: Biliary atresia, *Neonatal Network* 5(5):25-32, 1987.

Otte J and others: Size reduction of the donor liver is a safe way to alleviate the shortage of size-matched organs in pediatric liver transplant, *Ann Surg* 211(2):146-157, 1990.

Ozawa K and others: An appraisal of pediatric liver transplantation from living relatives, *Ann Surg* 216(5):547-553, 1991.

Pate CMH: Care of the family following the birth of a child with a cleft lip and/or palate, *Neonatal Network* 5(6):30-37, 1987.

Puntis J and others: Growth and feeding problems after repair of esophageal atresia, *Arch Dis Child* 65:84-88, 1990.

Ricketts R and others: Modern treatment of cloacal exstrophy, *J Pediatr Surg* 26(4):444-450, 1991.

Ryckman F and others: Improved survival in biliary atresia patients in the present era of liver transplantation, *J Pediatr Surg* 28(3): 382-386, 1993.

Skinner M, Grosfeld J: Inguinal and umbilical hernia repair in infants and children, *Surg Clin North Am* 73(3):439-449, 1993.

Sokal E and others: Liver transplantation in children less than 1 year of age, *J Pediatr* 117(2):205-210, 1990.

Strong R and others: Successful liver transplantation from a living donor to her son, *N Engl J Med* 322(21):1501-1507, 1990.

Theorell CJ: Congenital diaphragmatic hernia: a physiologic approach to management, *J Perinat Neonat Nurs* 3(3):66-79, 1990.

Torfs C, Curry C, Roeper P: Gastroschisis, *J Pediatr* 116:1-6, 1990.

Treacy S: Reduced-size liver transplantation for infants and children, *Crit Care Nurs Clin North Am* 4(2);235, 1992.

Ullrich D and others: Treatment with ursodeoxycholic acid renders children with biliary atresia suitable for liver transplantation, *Lancet* 2(8571):1324, 1987 (letter).

Van Meurs K and others: Effect of extracorporeal membrane oxygenation on survival of infants with congenital diaphragmatic hernia, *J Pediatr* 117(6):954-960, 1990.

Genitourinary Defects

American Academy of Pediatrics: Summary of annual meeting of the section on pediatric urology, *Pediatrics* 83:591-596, 1989.

Belman AB: Acquired undescended (ascended) testis: effects of human chorionic gonadotropin, *J Urol* 140:1189-1190, 1988.

Bernhardt J: Percutaneous nephrostomy tubes in the neonate with obstructive uropathy, *Neonatal Network* 4:51-53, 1986.

Castiglia PT: Ambiguous genitalia, *J Pediatr Health Care* 3(6):319-321, 1989.

DiGrande A: The child born with ambiguous genitalia: family assessment and nursing intervention, *Issues Compr Pediatr Nurs* 7:307-318, 1984.

Donahoe PK: The diagnosis and treatment of infants with intersex abnormalities, *Pediatr Clin North Am* 34:1333-1348, 1987.

Gosling J, Chilton C: The anatomy of the bladder urethra and pelvic floor. In Mundy AR, Stephenson TP, Wein AJ, editors: *Urodynamics: principles, practice and application,* London, 1984, Churchill-Livingstone.

Gray ML: *Genitourinary disorders,* St Louis, 1992, Mosby.

Hatch DA: Pediatric urology update, *J Urol Nurs* 10(2):1192-1197, 1991.

Horton HM, Crutchfield P, Garrison C: Hypospadias: when baby boys need surgery, *RN* 53(6):48-51, 1990.

Howe SM, Bates P: The cranberry juice cure: fact or fiction? *Urol Nurs* 8:13-16, 1987.

Huddleston K and others: MIC or foley: comparing gastrostomy tubes, *MCN* 14:20-22, 1989.

Hulbert WC, Duckett JW: Current views on posterior urethral valves, *Pediatr Ann* 17:31-36, 1988.

Jeffs RD: Exstrophy, epispadias, and cloacal and urogenital sinus abnormalities, *Pediatr Clin North Am* 34:1233-1257, 1987.

Kaplan BS and others: Polycystic kidney diseases in childhood, *J Pediatr* 115:867-880, 1989.

Khoury AE, Churchill BM: The artificial urinary sphincter, *Pediatr Clin North Am* 34:1175-1185, 1987.

Kogan SJ: Cryptorchidism: early treatment averts later problems, *Emerg Med* 24(8):137-144, 1992.

Kramer SA: Vesicoureteral reflux. In Kelalis PP, King LR, Belman AB, editors: *Clinical pediatric urology,* Philadelphia, 1992, WB Saunders.

Levitt SB, Reda EF: Hypospadias, *Pediatr Ann* 17:48-57, 1988.

Lobe TE, Schropp KP: Inguinal hernias in pediatrics: initial experience with laparoscopic inguinal exploration of the asymptomatic contralateral side, *J Laparoendosc Surg* 2(3): 135-140, 1992.

Mitchell ME, Rink RC: Pediatric urinary diversion and undiversion, *Pediatr Clin North Am* 34:1319-1332, 1987.

Pagon RA: Diagnostic approach to the newborn with ambiguous genitalia, *Pediatr Clin North Am* 34:1019-1031, 1987.

Pappis CH and others: Unsuspected urological abnormalities in cryptorchid boys, *Pediatr Radiol* 18:51-53, 1988.

Pearson BD, Larson JM: Urine control by elders: non-invasive strategies. In Funk SG and others, editors: *Key aspects of elder care,* New York, 1992, Springer.

Peevy KJ, Speed FA, Hoff CJ: Epidemiology of inguinal hernia in preterm neonates, *Pediatrics* 77:246-247, 1986.

Rajput A, Gauderer MWL, Hack M: Inguinal hernias in very low birth weight infants: incidence and timing of repair, *J Pediatr Surg* 27(10):1322-1324, 1992.

Reinburg YU, Gonzalez Y: Upper urinary tract obstruction in children: current controversies in diagnosis, *Pediatr Clin North Am* 34:1291-1304, 1987.

Rezvani I: Cryptorchidism: a pediatrician's view, *Pediatr Clin North Am* 34:735-746, 1987.

Sheldon CA, Duckett JW: Hypospadias, *Pediatr Clin North Am* 34:1259-1272, 1987.

Stylianos S, Jacir NN, Harris BH: Incarceration of inguinal hernia in infants prior to elective repair, *J Pediatr Surg* 28(4):582-583, 1993.

Tanagho EA: Anatomy of the genitourinary tract. In Tanagho EA, McAnnich JW, editors: *Smith's general urology,* Los Altos, CA, 1992, Lange Medical Books.

Tucker S: Female reproductive system. In Thompson JM and others, editors: *Clinical nursing,* St Louis, 1993, Mosby.

Welsh S, Gatch GC: Imperforate anus: diagnosis and surgical treatment, *AORN J* 42:692-698, 1985.

Prenatal Influences: General

Jankowski CB: Radiation and pregnancy: putting the risks in proportion, *Am J Nurs* 86:260-265, 1986.

Miao CY, Zuberbuhler JS, Zuberbuhler JR: Prevalence of congenital anomalies at high altitude, *J Am Coll Cardiol* 12:224-228, 1988.

Rhodes AM: Legal alternatives for fetal injury, *MCN* 15:111, 1990.

Rivera J, Villar J: Nutritional supplementation during two consecutive pregnancies and the interim lactation period: effect on birth weight, *Pediatrics* 81:51-57, 1988.

Warkany J: Teratogen update: hyperthermia, *Teratology* 33:365-369, 1986.

Yip R: Altitude and birth weight, *J Pediatr* 111:869-876, 1987.

Prenatal Influences: Infectious Agents

For citations on HIV and AIDS, see Chapter 35.

Alkalay AL, Pomerance JJ, Rimoin DL: Fetal varicella syndrome, *J Pediatr* 111:320-323, 1987.

Alpert G, Plotkin SA: A practical guide to the diagnosis of congenital infections in the newborn infant, *Pediatr Clin North Am* 33:465-479, 1986.

American Academy of Pediatrics Committee on Infectious Diseases: Parvovirus B19, erythema infectiosum (fifth disease and pregnancy), *Pediatrics* 85:131-133, 1990.

Bromberg MH, Hsia LSY: Rubella in the perinatal period, *J Perinat Neonat Nurs* 1(4):24-32, 1988.

Brown ZA and others: Effects on infants of a first episode of genital herpes during pregnancy, *N Engl J Med* 317:1246-1251, 1987.

Centers for Disease Control: Prevention of perinatal transmission of hepatitis B virus: prenatal screening of all pregnant women for hepatitis b surface antigen, *MMWR* 37:341-346, 1988.

Centers for Disease Control: Congenital syphilis—New York City, 1986-1988, *MMWR* 38:825-829, 1989.

Centers for Disease Control: Rubella and congenital rubella syndrome–United States, 1985-1988, *MMWR* 38:173-182, 1989.

Conboy TJ and others: Early clinical manifestations and intellectual outcome in children with symptomatic congenital cytomegalovirus infection, *J Pediatr* 111:343-348, 1987.

Griffin MP and others: Cytomegalovirus infection in a neonatal intensive care unit, *Am J Dis Child* 142:1188-1193, 1988.

Hall SM: Congenital toxoplasmosis, *Br Med J* 305:291-297, 1992.

Hutto C and others: Intrauterine herpes simplex virus infections, *J Pediatr* 110:97-101, 1987.

Kaplan KM and others: A profile of mothers giving birth to infants with congenital rubella syndrome, *Am J Dis Child* 1144:118-123, 1990.

Koskiniemi M, Lappalainen M, Hedman K: Toxoplasmosis needs evaluation, *Am J Dis Child* 143:724-728, 1989.

Lin H and others: Transplacental leakage of HBeAg-positive maternal blood as the most likely route in causing intrauterine infection with hepatitis B virus, *J Pediatr* 111:877-881, 1987.

Miller E and others: Outcome in newborn babies given anti-varicella-zoster immunoglobulin after perinatal maternal infection with varicella-zoster virus, *Lancet* 2:371-373, 1989.

Samson LF: Perinatal viral infections and neonates, *J Perinat Neonat Nurs* 1(4):56-65, 1988.

Sever JL and others: Toxoplasmosis: maternal and pediatric findings in 23,000 pregnancies, *Pediatrics* 82:181-192, 1988.

Tedberg AJ and others: Clinical manifestations of epidemic neonatal listeriosis, *Pediatr Infect Dis J* 6:817-820, 1987.

Prenatal Influences: Chemical Agents

Barbour BG: Is fetal alcohol syndrome completely irreversible? *MCN* 14:44-46, 1989.

Chavez CF, Mulinare J, Cordero JF: Maternal cocaine use during early pregnancy as a risk factor for congenital urogenital anomalies, *JAMA* 262:795-798, 1989.

Church MW, Gerkin KP: Hearing disorders in children with fetal alcohol syndrome: findings from case reports, *Pediatrics* 82:147-154, 1988.

Coles CD and others: Persistence over the first month of neurobehavioral differences in infants exposed to alcohol prenatally, *Behav Dev* 10:23-37, 1987.

Committee on Substance Abuse and Committee on Children with Disabilities: Fetal alcohol syndrome and fetal alcohol effects, *Pediatrics* 91(5):1004-1006, 1993.

Eliason MJ, Williams JK: Fetal alcohol syndrome and the neonate, *J Perinat Neonat Nurs* 3(4):64-72, 1990.

Ernhart CB and others: Alcohol teratogenicity in the human: a detailed assessment of specificity, critical period, and threshold, *Am J Obstet Gynecol* 156:33-39, 1987.

Fetal alcohol syndrome—United States, 1979-1992, *MMWR* 42(17):339, 1993.

Graham JM and others: Independent dysmorphology evaluations at birth and 4 years of age for children exposed to varying amounts of alcohol in utero, *Pediatrics* 81:772-778, 1988.

Harnold KC: Teratogenic potential of valproic acid, *JOGNN* 15:111-116, 1986.

Jones KL: The fetal alcohol syndrome, *Growth Genet Horm* 4(1):1, 1988.

Kuller JM: Effects on the fetus and newborn of medications commonly used during pregnancy, *J Perinat Neonat Nurs* 3(4):73-87, 1990.

Little BB and others: Failure to recognize fetal alcohol syndrome in newborn infants, *Am J Dis Child* 144:1142-1146, 1990.

Miller PK: Vitamin A during pregnancy, *Teratology* 35:269-275, 1987.

Mills J, Graubard BI: Is moderate drinking during pregnancy associated with an increased risk for malformations? *Pediatrics* 80:309-314, 1987.

Spohr HL, Willms J, Steinhausen HC: Prenatal alcohol exposure and long-term developmental consequences, *Lancet* 341:907-910, 1993.

Streissguth AP and others: Fetal alcohol syndrome in adolescents and adults, *JAMA* 265(15):1961-1967, 1991.

Verklan MT: Safe in the womb: Drug and chemical effects on the fetus and neonate, *Neonatal Network* 8(10):59-65, 1989.

Warren KR, Bast RJ: Alcohol-related birth defects: an update, *Public Health Rep* 103(6): 638-642, 1988.

Zuckerman B, Bresnahan K: Developmental and behavioral consequences of prenatal drug and alcohol exposure, *Pediatr Clin North Am* 38(6):1387-1406, 1991.

UNIT IV

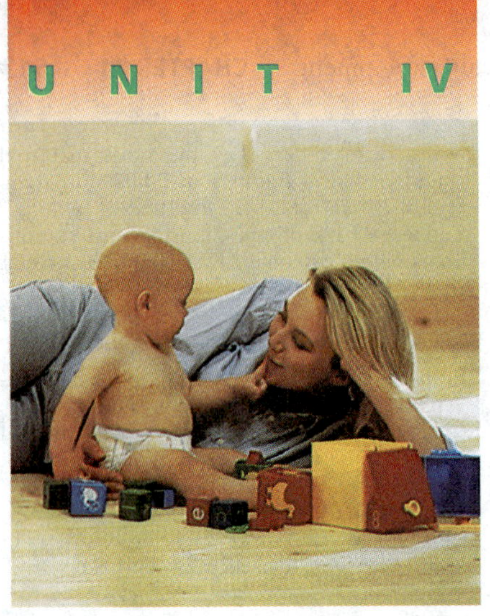

FAMILY-CENTERED CARE OF THE INFANT

CHAPTER 12 Health Promotion of the Infant and Family

CHAPTER OUTLINE

RELATED TOPICS

Animal bites, Ch. 18
Communicable diseases, Ch. 16
Dental health, Ch. 14
Growth and development of children, Ch. 4
Health problems during infancy, Ch. 13
Infant mortality, Ch. 1
Ingestion of injurious agents, Ch. 16
Injuries—the leading killer, Ch. 1
Injury prevention, Ch. 14
Intramuscular administration (of medication), Ch. 27
Limit-setting and discipline, Ch. 3
Paroxysmal abdominal pain (colic), Ch. 13
Preschool and kindergarten experience, Ch. 15
Promotion of parent-infant bonding (attachment), Ch. 8
Provision of optimum nutrition, Ch. 8
Separation anxiety, Ch. 26
Sudden infant death syndrome (SIDS), Ch. 13
Sunburn, Ch. 18
Temperament, Ch. 4

PROMOTING OPTIMUM GROWTH AND DEVELOPMENT

BIOLOGIC DEVELOPMENT

At no other time in life are physical changes and developmental achievements so dramatic as during infancy. All body systems undergo progressive maturation. Concurrent development of skills increasingly allows infants to respond to the environment. Acquisition of these fine and gross motor skills occurs in an orderly head-to-toe and center-to-periphery (cephalocaudal-proximodistal) sequence.

Proportional Changes

During the first year growth is very rapid, especially during the initial 6 months. Infants gain 680 g (1½ pounds) per month until age 5 months, when the birth weight has at least doubled. An average weight for a 6-month-old child is 7.26 kg (16 pounds). Weight gain decreases by half that amount during the second 6 months. By 1 year of age the infant's birth weight has tripled, with an average weight of 9.75 kg (21½ pounds). Infants who are breast-fed beyond 4 to 6 months of age typically gain less weight than those who are bottle-fed (Dewey and others, 1993) (see also p. 591).

Height increases by 2.5 cm (1 inch) per month during the first 6 months and by half that amount monthly during the second 6 months. Increases in length occur in sudden spurts, rather than in a slow, gradual pattern (Lampl, Veldhuis, and Johnson, 1992). Average height is 65 cm (25½ inches) at 6 months and 74 cm (29 inches) at 12 months. By 1 year the birth length has increased by almost 50%. The increase in length occurs mainly in the trunk, rather than in the legs, and contributes to the characteristic physique of the older infant (see Fig. 12-9, *A*).

Head growth is also rapid. During the first 6 months head circumference increases approximately 1.5 cm (½ inch) per month, but decreases to only 0.5 cm (¼ inch) per month during the second 6 months. The average size is 43 cm (17 inches) at 6 months and 46 cm (18 inches) at 12 months. By 1 year head size has increased by almost 33%. Closure of the cranial sutures occurs, with the posterior fontanel fusing by 6 to 8 weeks of age and the anterior fontanel closing by 12 to 18 months of age, with the average age being 14 months (Duc and Largo, 1986).

Expanding head size reflects the growth and differentiation of the nervous system. By the end of the first year the brain has increased in weight about two and one half times. The maturation of the brain is exhibited in the dramatic developmental achievements of infancy (see Table 12-3). The primitive reflexes (see Table 8-4) are replaced by voluntary, purposeful movement, and new reflexes that influence motor development appear (see box below).

The chest assumes a more adult contour, with the lateral diameter becoming larger than the anteroposterior diameter. The chest circumference approximately equals head circumference by the end of the first year. The heart grows less rapidly than does the rest of the body. Its weight is usually doubled by 1 year of age, in comparison with body weight, which triples during the same period. The size of the heart is still large in relation to the chest cavity; its width is about 55% of the width of the chest.

Sensory Changes

During infancy visual acuity gradually improves, and binocular fixation is established. The major developmental characteristics of vision during infancy are listed in the box at left on p. 516.

NEUROLOGIC REFLEXES THAT APPEAR DURING INFANCY

REFLEX	EXPECTED BEHAVIORAL RESPONSE	AGE OF APPEARANCE (MONTHS)
Labyrinth-righting	Infant in prone or supine position is able to raise head	2, strongest at 10
Neck-righting	While infant is supine, head is turned to one side; shoulder, trunk, and finally pelvis will turn toward that side	3, until 24-36
Body-righting	A modification of the neck-righting reflex in which turning hips and shoulders to one side cause all other body parts to follow	6, until 24-36
Otolith-righting	When body of an erect infant is tilted, head is returned to upright, erect position	7-12, persists indefinitely
Landau	When infant is suspended in a horizontal prone position, the head is raised and legs and spine are extended	6-8, until 12-24
Parachute	When infant is suspended in a horizontal prone position and suddenly thrust downward, hand and fingers extend forward as if to protect against falling (see Fig. 12-1)	7-9, persists indefinitely

MAJOR DEVELOPMENTAL CHARACTERISTICS OF VISION

AGE (WEEKS)	DEVELOPMENT
Birth	Visual acuity 20/100-20/400* Pupillary and corneal (blink) reflexes present Able to fixate on moving object in range of 45 degrees when held 20-25 cm (8-10 inches) away Cannot integrate head and eye movements well (doll's eye reflex—eyes lag behind if head is rotated to one side)
4	Can follow in range of 90 degrees Can watch parent intently as he or she speaks to infant Tear glands begin to function Visual acuity is hyperoptic because of less spheric eyeball than in adult
6-12	Has peripheral vision to 180 degrees Binocular vision begins at age 6 weeks, is well established by age 4 months Convergence on near objects begins by age 6 weeks, is well developed by age 3 months Doll's eye reflex disappears
12-20	Recognizes feeding bottle Able to fixate a 1.25 cm (½ inch) block Looks at hand while sitting or lying on back Able to accommodate to near objects
20-28	Adjusts posture to see an object Able to rescue a dropped toy Develops color preference for yellow and red Able to discriminate between simple geometric forms Prefers more complex visual stimuli Develops hand-eye coordination
28-44	Can fixate on very small objects Depth perception begins to develop Lack of binocular vision indicates strabismus
44-52	Visual acuity, 20/40-20/60 Visual loss may develop if strabismus is present Can follow rapidly moving objects

*Measurement of visual acuity differs according to testing procedures (see also Table 7-10)

MAJOR DEVELOPMENTAL CHARACTERISTICS OF HEARING

AGE (WEEKS	DEVELOPMENT
Birth	Responds to loud noise by startle reflex Responds to sound of human voice more readily than to any other sound Low-pitched sounds, such as lullaby, metronome, or heartbeat, have quieting effect
8-12	Turns head to side when sound is made at level of ear
12-16	Locates sound by turning head to side and looking in same direction (Fig. 12-2)
16-24	Locates sound by turning head to side and then looking up or down
24-32	Locates sounds by turning head in a curving arc Responds to own name
32-40	Localizes sounds by turning head diagonally and directly toward sound
40-52	Knows several words and their meaning, such as "no," and names of members of the family Learns to control and adjust own response to sound, such as listening for the sound to occur again

Binocularity, or the fixation of two ocular images into one cerebral picture (fusion), begins to develop by 6 weeks of age and should be well established by age 4 months. Lack of binocular vision results in strabismus and must be detected early to prevent permanent blindness.

Depth perception (stereopsis) begins to develop by age 7 to 9 months but may exist earlier as an innate safety mechanism. Studies have demonstrated that even 2- to 3-month-old infants distinguish depth. At about 7 months the parachute reflex appears, which may be a protective response during a fall (Fig. 12-1 and box on p. 515).

Infants also have a ***visual preference*** for looking at the human face and this preference also has a developmental se-

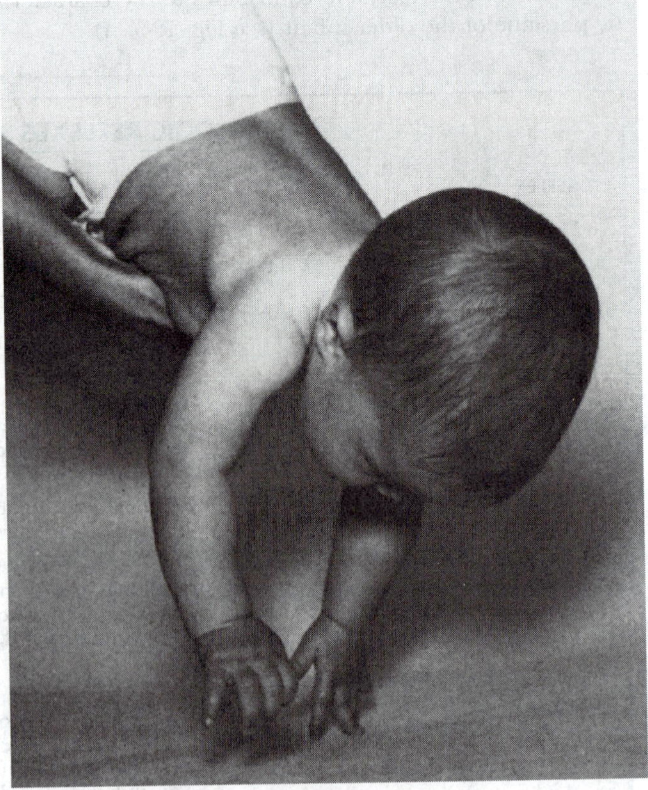

FIG. 12-1 Parachute reflex.

quence. For example, at age 6 weeks they show more interest in a picture of a face with eyes than in one without eyes. By 10 weeks of age a picture with both eyes and eyebrows elicits more response, and by 20 weeks of age the mouth is also necessary. By age 6 months infants respond to facial expressions and can distinguish between familiar and strange faces. This is about the time that stranger anxiety is manifested (see p. 527).

With progressive myelination of the auditory pathway, the specific responses of locating sound replace the generalized response of the neonate (Fig. 12-2). The major developmental characteristics of hearing are listed in the box at right on p. 516. (For further discussion of hearing and the senses of smell, taste, and touch, see Chapter 8.)

Maturation of Systems

Other organ systems also change and grow during infancy. The ***respiratory*** rate slows somewhat (see inside back cover) and is relatively stable. Respiratory movements continue to be abdominal. Several factors predispose the infant to more severe and acute respiratory problems. The close proximity of the trachea to the bronchi and its branching structures rapidly transmits an infectious agent from one anatomic location to another. The short, straight eustachian tube closely communicates with the ear, allowing infection to ascend from the pharynx to the middle ear. In addition, the inability of the immune system to produce immunoglobin (Ig) A in the mucosal lining provides less protection against infection in infancy than during later childhood. The ability of the entire respiratory tract to produce mucus is diminished, decreasing the humidification of the large volume of inspired air.

Although the lumen of the trachea and bronchi enlarges during infancy, it remains small in comparison with the total size of the lung, maintaining high resistance to the volume of air inspired. The small airways are easily blocked by edema, mucus, or a foreign body. The pliant (flexible) rib cage has less elastic recoil, and during respiratory distress the work of breathing is increased. In addition, the volume of dead space, that amount of air needed to fill the respiratory passages with each breath, is large, requiring the infant to breathe about twice as fast as the adult to provide the body with the needed amount of oxygen.

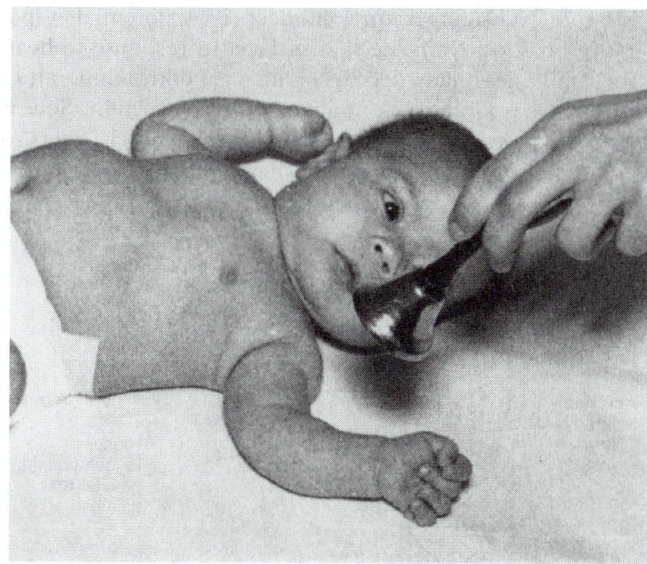

FIG. 12-2 Three-month-old infant locates sound by turning head to side and looking in direction of the sound.

The ***heart*** rate slows (see inside back cover), and the rhythm is frequently ***sinus arrhythmia*** (rate increases with inspiration and decreases with expiration). Blood pressure also changes during infancy (see inside back cover). Systolic pressure rises during the first 2 months as a result of the increasing ability of the left ventricle to pump blood into the systemic circulation. Diastolic pressure decreases during the first 3 months, then gradually rises to values close to those at birth. Fluctuations in blood pressure occur during varying states of activity and emotion.

Significant ***hemopoietic changes*** occur during the first year (see Appendix D). Fetal hemoglobin (HgF) is present for the first 5 months, with adult hemoglobin steadily increasing through the first half of infancy. Fetal hemoglobin results in a shortened survival of red blood cells (RBCs) and thus a decreased number of RBCs. A common result at 2 to 3 months of age is ***physiologic anemia.*** High levels of HgF are thought to depress the production of erythropoietin, a hormone released by the kidney that stimulates RBC production.

Maternal iron stores are present for the first 5 to 6 months and then gradually diminish, which also accounts for lowered hemoglobin levels toward the end of the first 6 months. The occurrence of physiologic anemia is not affected by an adequate supply of iron. However, when erythropoiesis is stimulated, iron supplies are necessary for formation of hemoglobin.

The ***digestive processes*** are immature at birth. Saliva is secreted in small amounts, but the majority of the digestive processes do not begin functioning until age 3 months, when drooling is common because of the poorly coordinated swallowing reflex. The enzyme ***ptyalin*** (also called ***amylase***) is present in small amounts but usually has little effect on the foodstuff because of the small amount of time the food stays in the mouth. Gastric digestion in the stomach consists primarily of the action of hydrochloric acid and rennin, an enzyme that acts specifically on the casein in milk to cause the formation of curds, which are coagulated semisolid particles of milk. The curds cause the milk to be retained in the stomach long enough for digestion to occur.

Digestion also takes place in the duodenum, where pancreatic enzymes and bile begin to break down protein and fat. Secretion of the pancreatic enzyme ***amylase,*** which is needed for digestion of complex carbohydrates, is deficient until about the fourth to sixth month of life. ***Lipase*** is also limited, and infants do not achieve adult levels of fat absorption until 4 to 5 months of age. ***Trypsin*** is secreted in sufficient quantities to catabolize protein into polypeptides and some amino acids.

The immaturity of the digestive processes is evident in the appearance of stools. During infancy solid foods, such as peas, carrots, corn, and raisins, are passed incompletely broken down in the feces. An excess quantity of fiber easily disposes the child to loose, bulky stools.

During infancy the stomach enlarges to accommodate a greater volume of food. By the end of the first year the infant is able to tolerate three meals a day and an evening bottle and may have one or two bowel movements daily. However, with any type of gastric irritation the infant is vulnerable to diarrhea, vomiting, and dehydration (see Chapters 28 and 29).

The liver is the most immature of all the gastrointestinal organs throughout infancy. The ability to conjugate bilirubin and to secrete bile is achieved after the first couple of weeks of life. However, the capacities for gluconeogenesis, formation of plasma protein and ketones, storage of vitamins, and deaminization of amino acids remain relatively immature for the first year of life.

Maturation of suckling, sucking, and swallowing reflexes and the eruption of teeth parallel the changes in the gastrointestinal tract and prepare the infant for the introduction of solid foods. ***Suckling,*** which is first seen at birth, denotes extension and a pulling-in pattern of tongue movements, as in licking. During breast-feeding the lips gently clamp the areola in place as the mandible and tongue thrust forward to grasp the nipple and areola. The sucking fat pads in the cheeks fill the mouth and help maintain negative pressure. The tongue then moves rhythmically forward to the gums and lips and back toward the hard palate to "milk" the collecting ductules. As milk flows from the nipple, it stimulates the swallowing reflex and is ejected into the esophagus.

In bottle-feeding the ***sucking*** action is different. Consequently, breast-fed infants may become confused if given a bottle. The relatively inflexible rubber nipple may prevent the tongue from moving rhythmically forward and backward. In addition, the flow of milk may be too rapid, causing choking. Infants learn to control the stream of milk by pushing the tongue against the rubber nipple holes. When given the breast again, they may use the same action and push the human nipple out of the mouth (Lawrence, 1994).

Swallowing (deglutition) is the ability to collect the food (bolus) and propel it into the esophagus. During the ***infantile (visceral) swallow reflex*** (Fig. 12-3, *A*) food lies in a shallow groove on the top (dorsum) of the tongue. As the tongue is pressed upward toward the palate, the milk flows by gravity down the sloping tongue and along the sides of the mouth in lateral furrows between the tongue, cheek, and gum pads. As the bolus moves downward, the posterior wall of the pharynx comes forward to displace the soft palate (Pipes and Trahms, 1993). This swallowing process is efficient for fluids but not solids.

As the infant grows, the tongue becomes smaller in proportion to the oral cavity and attains greater motility, the orofacial muscles develop, and teeth erupt. Consequently, the ***mature (somatic) swallow reflex*** (Fig. 12-3, *B*) is significantly different. The tongue remains behind the central incisors, and the mandible no longer thrusts forward. The dorsum of the tongue is less concave and remains higher and parallel, not inclined, against the palate, and the lateral furrows are absent because of tooth eruption. Tongue pressure and movement against the hard palate pushes the bolus back into the pharynx. The development of mature sucking is thought to develop after the first 6 months and prepares the infant for ingesting solid foods.

Infants also exhibit a special reflex called the ***Santmyer swallow.*** When a puff of air is directed at the face, the infant has a reflex shallow (Orenstein and others, 1988).

The ***immunologic system*** undergoes numerous changes during the first year. The newborn receives significant amounts of maternal IgG, which confers immunity for about 3 months against antigens to which the mother was exposed. During this time the infant begins to synthesize IgG, and about 40% of adult levels are reached by 1 year of age. Significant amounts of IgM are produced at birth, and adult levels are reached by 9 months of age. The production of IgA, IgD, and IgE is much more gradual, and maximum levels are not attained until early childhood.

During infancy ***thermoregulation*** becomes more efficient; the ability of the skin to contract and of muscles to shiver in response to cold increases. The peripheral capillaries respond to change in ambient temperature to regulate heat loss. In response to cold, the capillaries constrict, conserving core body temperature and decreasing potential evaporative heat loss from the skin surface. In response to heat, the capillaries dilate, decreasing internal body temperature through evaporation, conduction, and convection. Shivering ***(thermogenesis)*** causes the muscles and muscle fibers to contract, generating metabolic heat, which is distributed

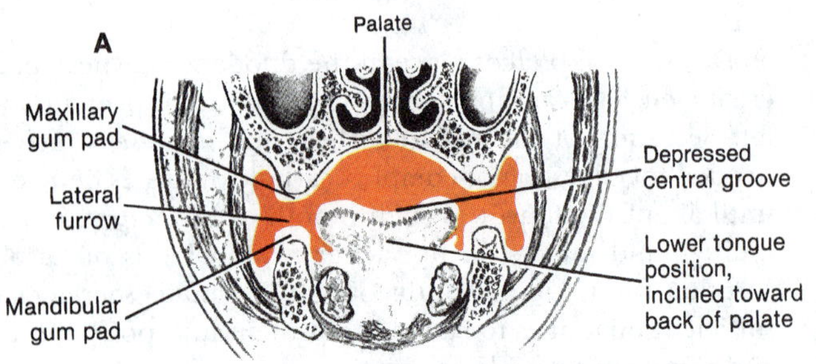

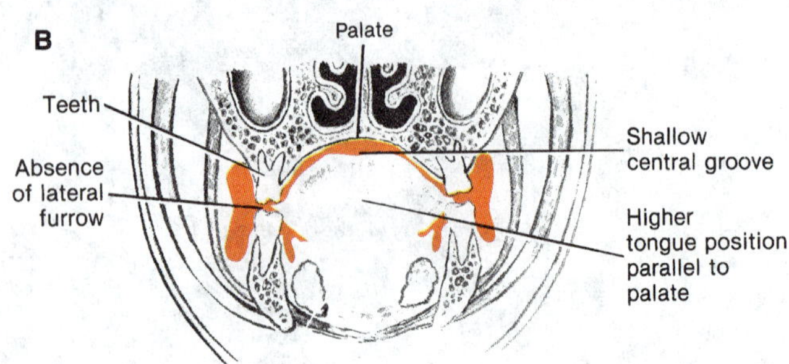

FIG. 12-3 Comparison of, **A,** infantile (visceral) swallow reflex and, **B,** mature (somatic) swallow reflex.

throughout the body. Increased adipose tissue during the first 6 months insulates the body against heat loss.

A shift in the ***total body fluid*** occurs. At birth 75% of the infant's body weight is water and there is an excess of extracellular fluid (ECF). As the percentage of body water decreases, so does the amount of ECF—from 40% at term to 20% in adulthood. The high proportion of ECF, which is composed of blood plasma, interstitial fluid, and lymph, predisposes the infant to a more rapid loss of total body fluid and consequently dehydration.

The immaturity of the ***renal structures*** also predisposes the infant to dehydration. Complete maturity of the kidney occurs during the latter half of the second year, when the cuboidal epithelium of the glomeruli becomes flattened. Before this time the filtration capacity of the glomeruli is reduced. Urine is voided frequently and has a low specific gravity (1.000 to 1.010).

The ***endocrine system*** is adequately developed at birth, but its functions are immature. The interrelatedness of all the endocrine organs has a major effect on the function of any one gland. The lack of homeostatic control because of various functional deficiencies renders the infant especially vulnerable to imbalances in fluid and electrolytes, glucose concentration, and amino acid metabolism.

For example, corticotropin (ACTH) is produced in limited quantities during infancy. ACTH acts on the adrenal cortices to produce their hormones, particularly the glucocorticoids and aldosterone. Because the feedback mechanism between ACTH and the adrenal cortex is immature during infancy, there is much less tolerance for stressful conditions, which affect fluid and electrolytes and the metabolism of fats, proteins, and carbohydrates. In addition, although the islets of Langerhans produce insulin and glucagon during fetal life and early infancy, blood sugar levels tend to remain labile, particularly under conditions of stress.

Fine Motor Development

Fine motor behavior includes the use of the hands and fingers in the prehension (grasp) of an object. Grasping occurs during the first 2 to 3 months as a reflex and gradually becomes voluntary. At 1 month of age the hands are predominantly closed, and by 3 months they are mostly open. By this time infants demonstrate a desire to grasp an object, but they "grasp" it more with the eyes than with the hands. If a rattle is placed in the hand, the infant will actively hold onto it. By 4 months of age the infant regards both a small pellet and the hands and looks from the object to the hands and back again. By 5 months the infant is able to voluntarily grasp an object.

Gradually the palmar grasp (using the whole hand) is replaced with a pincer grasp (using the thumb and index finger). By 8 to 9 months of age the infant uses a crude pincer grasp (Fig. 12-4) but by 11 months has progressed to a neat pincer grasp (Fig. 12-5).

By 6 months of age infants have increased manipulative skill. They hold their bottle, grasp feet and pull them to the mouth, and feed themselves a cracker. By 7 months they transfer objects from one hand to the other, use one hand for grasping, and hold a cube in each hand simultaneously. They enjoy banging objects and will explore the movable parts of a toy.

By 10 months of age the pincer grasp is sufficiently established to enable infants to pick up a raisin and other finger foods. They can deliberately let go of an object and will offer it to someone. By 11 months they put objects into a container and like to remove them. By age 1 year infants try to build a tower of two blocks but fail.

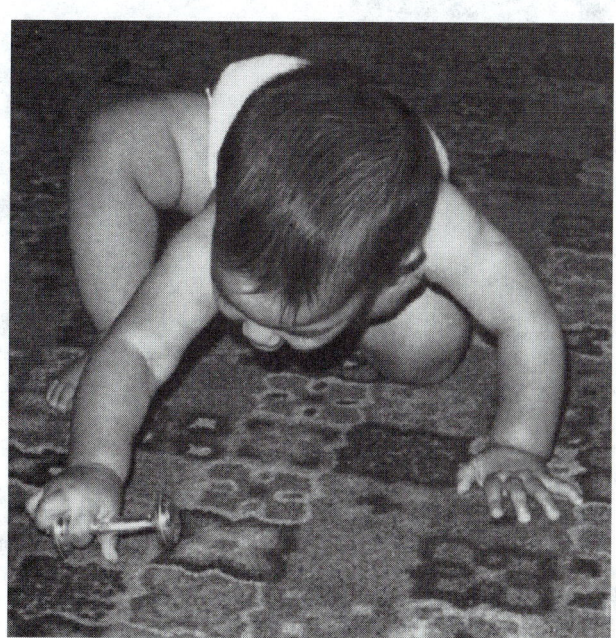

FIG. 12-4 Crude pincer grasp at 8 to 10 months of age.

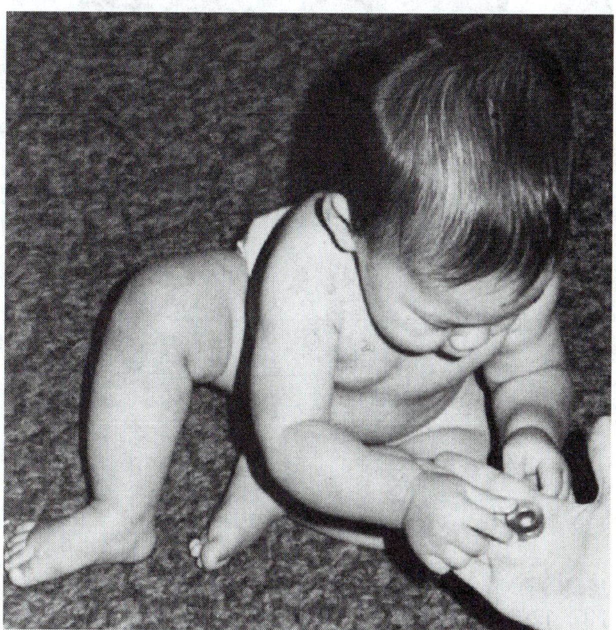

FIG. 12-5 Neat pincer grasp at 10 to 11 months of age.

Gross Motor Development

Gross motor behavior includes developmental maturation in posture, head balance, sitting, creeping, standing, and walking. The full-term neonate is born with some ability to hold the head erect and reflexly assumes the postural tonic neck position when supine. Several of the primitive reflexes have significance in terms of development of later gross motor skills. The ***righting reflexes*** elicit certain postural responses, particularly of flexion or extension. They are responsible for certain motor activities, such as rolling over, assuming the crawl position, and maintaining normal head-trunk-limb alignment during all activities. The neck-righting reflex, which turns the body to the same side as the head, enables the child to roll over from supine to prone. Other reflexes, such as the otolith-righting and labyrinth-righting reflexes, enable the infant to raise the head (see box on p. 515).

The asymmetric tonic neck reflex, which persists from birth to 3 months, prevents the infant from rolling over. The symmetric tonic neck reflex, which is evoked by flexing or extending the neck, helps the infant to assume the crawl position. When the head and neck are extended, the extensor tone of the upper extremities and the flexor tone of the lower extremities increase. The child extends the arms and bends the knees. Because of the strong flexor tone

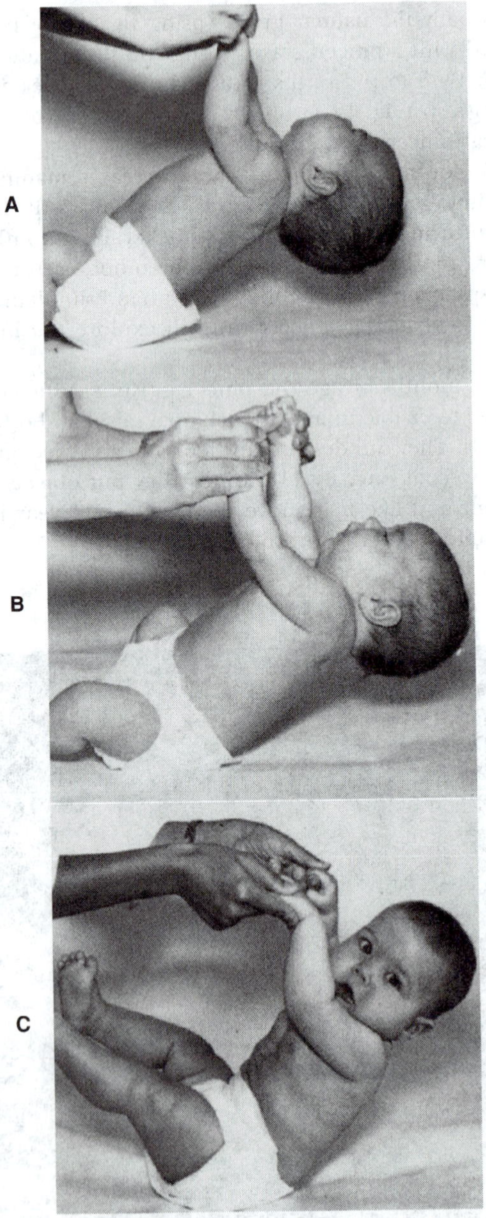

FIG. 12-6 Head control while pulled to sitting position. **A,** Complete head lag at 1 month. **B,** Partial head lag at 2 months. **C,** Almost no head lag at 4 months.

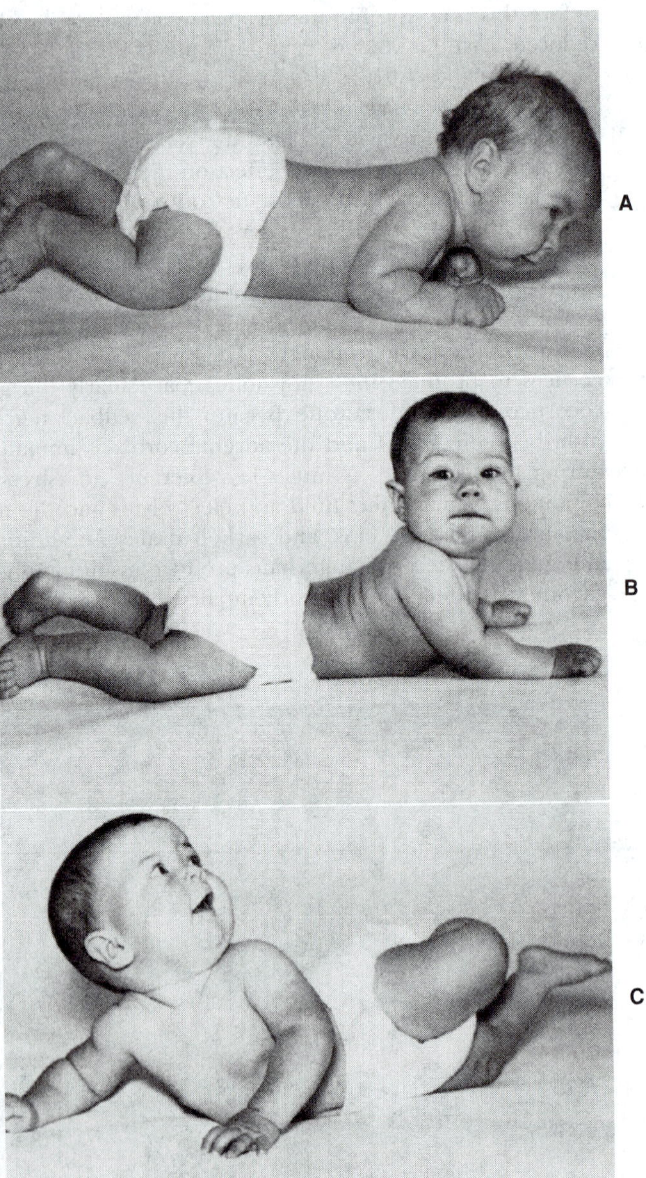

FIG. 12-7 Head control while prone. **A,** Infant momentarily lifts head at 1 month. **B,** Infant lifts head and chest 90 degrees and bears weight on forearms at 4 months. **C,** Infant lifts head, chest, and upper abdomen and can bear weight on hands at 6 months. Note how this position facilitates turning from abdomen to back.

of the lower extremities, the infant may initially crawl backward before crawling forward. This reflex disappears when neurologic maturity allows actual crawling to occur because independent limb movement is required.

Head Control. The full-term newborn can momentarily hold the head in midline and parallel when the body is suspended ventrally and can lift and turn the head from side to side when prone (see Fig. 8-7). This is not the case when the infant is lying prone on a pillow or soft surface; infants do not have the head control to lift their head out of the depression of the object and therefore risk suffocation. However, marked head lag is evident when the infant is pulled from a lying to a sitting position. By 3 months of age infants can hold their head well beyond the plane of the body, and by 4 months of age they can lift the head and front portion of the chest about 90 degrees above the table, bearing their weight on the forearms. Only slight head lag is evident when the infant is pulled from a lying to a sitting position, and by 4 to 6 months head control is well established (Figs 12-6 and 12-7).

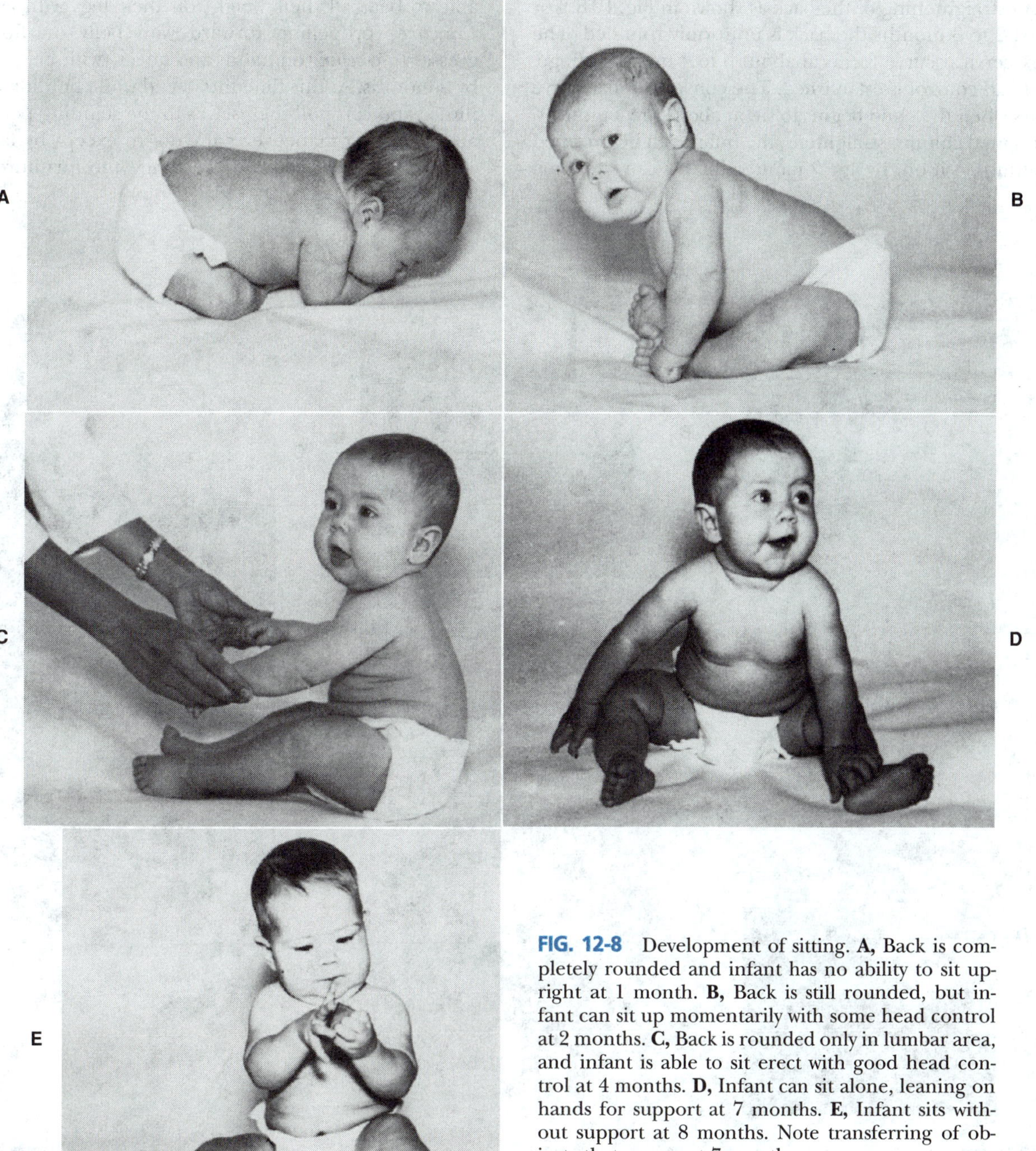

FIG. 12-8 Development of sitting. **A,** Back is completely rounded and infant has no ability to sit upright at 1 month. **B,** Back is still rounded, but infant can sit up momentarily with some head control at 2 months. **C,** Back is rounded only in lumbar area, and infant is able to sit erect with good head control at 4 months. **D,** Infant can sit alone, leaning on hands for support at 7 months. **E,** Infant sits without support at 8 months. Note transferring of objects that occurs at 7 months.

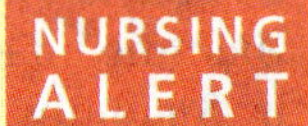

Any child who displays head lag at 6 months of age should have a developmental/neurologic evaluation.

Rolling Over. Newborns may roll over accidentally because of their rounded back. The ability to willfully turn from the abdomen to the back occurs at 5 months, and the ability to turn from the back to the abdomen occurs at 6 months. It is noteworthy that the parachute reflex (see Fig. 12-1), which elicits a protective response to falling, appears at 7 months.

Sitting. The ability to sit follows progressive head control and straightening of the back as shown in Fig. 12-8. For the first 2 to 3 months the back is uniformly rounded. The convex cervical curve forms at about 3 to 4 months of age, when head control is established. The convex lumbar curve appears when the child begins to sit, at about age 4 months. As the spinal column straightens, the infant can be propped in a sitting position. By age 7 months infants can sit alone, leaning forward on their hands for support. By age 8 months they can sit well unsupported and begin to explore their surroundings in this position rather than in a lying position. By 10 months they can maneuver from a prone to a sitting position.

Locomotion. Locomotion involves acquiring the ability to bear weight, propel forward on all four extremities, stand upright with support, and finally walk alone (Fig. 12-9). Following a cephalocaudal pattern, infants 4 to 6 months old have increasing coordination in their arms. Initial locomotion results in infants propelling themselves backward by pushing with the arms. By 6 to 7 months of age infants are able to bear all their weight on their legs with assistance. ***Crawling*** (propelling forward with belly on floor) progresses to ***creeping*** on hands and knees (with belly off floor) by 9 months. At this time they stand while holding onto furniture and can pull themselves to the standing position but are unable to maneuver back down, except by falling. By 11 months they walk while holding onto furniture or with

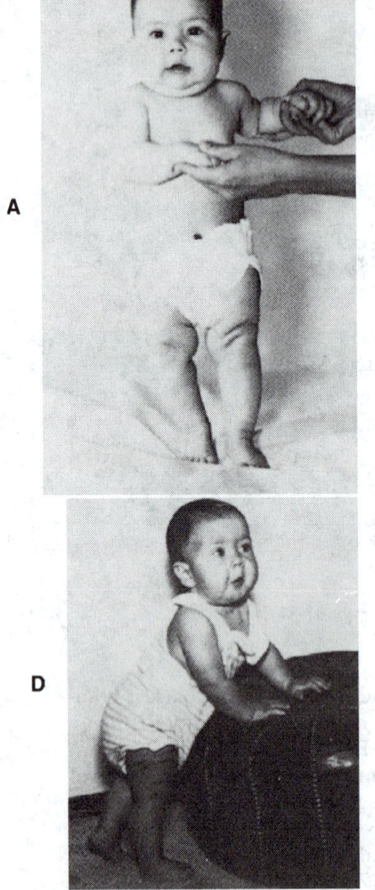

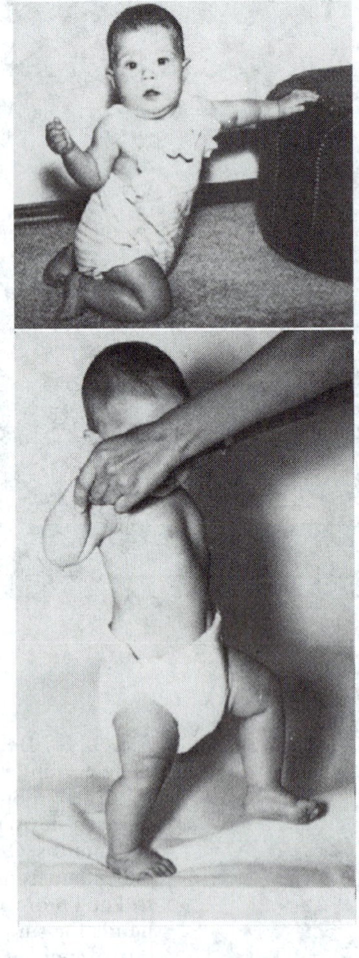

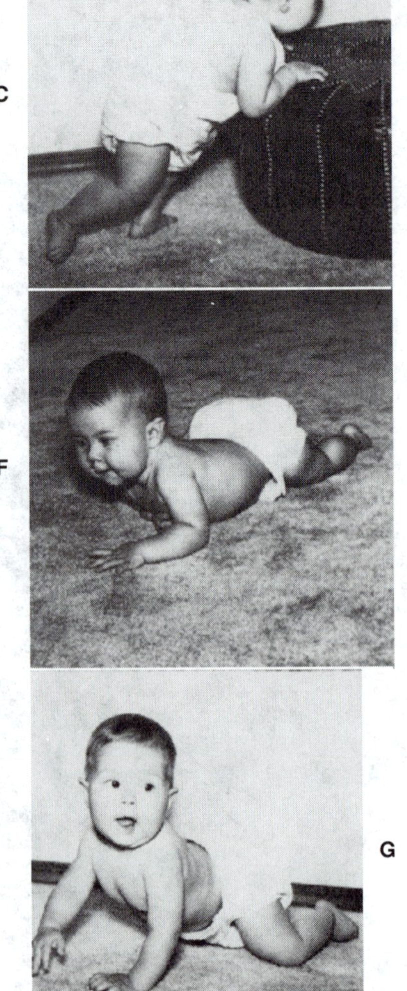

FIG. 12-9 Development of locomotion. **A,** Infant bears full weight on feet by 7 months. **B,** Infant can maneuver from sitting to kneeling position. **C,** Infant can pull self to standing position. **D,** Infant can stand holding onto furniture at 9 months. **E,** While standing, infant takes deliberate step at 10 months. **F,** Infant crawls with abdomen on floor and pulls self forward with hands. **G,** Infant creeps on hands and knees at 9 months.

both hands held, and by age 1 year they may be able to walk with one hand held. A number of infants attempt their first independent steps by their first birthday (Knobloch, Stevens, and Malone, 1980).

Infants' motor age (development) can be assessed by calculating a ***motor quotient (MQ)*** using the following formula:

$$MQ = \frac{\text{Motor age (MA)}}{\text{Chronologic age (CA)}} \times 100$$

For example, if a 12-month-old infant begins to creep, the motor quotient is 9 (MA for this skill) ÷ 12 (CA) × 100, or 75. Values above 80 are considered within normal limits, values below 70 are abnormal, and values between 70 and 80 are borderline (Blasco, 1992).

PSYCHOSOCIAL DEVELOPMENT

Developing a Sense of Trust (Erikson)

Erikson's phase I (birth to 1 year) is concerned with ***acquiring a sense of trust*** while ***overcoming a sense of mistrust.*** Erikson was a neo-Freudian who incorporated much of Freud's theory (see Psychosexual Development [Freud], Chapter 4). The trust that develops is a trust of self, of others, and of the world. Infants "trust" that their feeding, comfort, stimulation, and caring needs will be met. The crucial element for the achievement of this task is the quality of both the parent (caregiver)–child relationship and the care the infant receives. The provision of food, warmth, and shelter by itself is inadequate for the development of a strong sense of self. The infant and parent must jointly learn to satisfactorily meet their needs in order for mutual regulation of frustration to occur. When this synchrony fails to develop, mistrust is the eventual outcome.

Failure to learn "delayed gratification" leads to mistrust. It can result from too much or too little frustration. If parents always meet their children's needs before the children signal their readiness, infants will never learn to test their ability to control the environment. If the delay is prolonged, infants will experience constant frustration and eventually mistrust others in their efforts to satisfy them. Therefore consistency of care is essential.

The trust acquired in infancy is foundational for all the succeeding phases. It allows infants a feeling of physical comfort and security, which assists them in experiencing unfamiliar, unknown situations with a minimum of fear. Erikson has divided the first year of life into two oral/social stages. During the first 3 to 4 months, food intake is the most important social activity in which the infant engages. The newborn can tolerate little frustration or delay of gratification. Primary ***narcissism*** (total concern for oneself) is at its height.

However, as bodily processes such as vision, motor movements, and vocalization are better controlled, infants use more advanced behaviors to interact with others. For example, rather than crying, infants may put their arms up to signify a desire to be held.

The next social modality involves a mode of reaching out to others through ***grasping.*** Initially grasping is reflexive, but even as a reflex it has a powerful social meaning for the parents. The reciprocal response to the infant's grasping is the parents' holding on and touching. There is pleasurable tactile stimulation for both the child and the parents.

Tactile stimulation is extremely important in the total process of acquiring trust. The degree of mothering skill, the quantity of food, or the length of sucking does not determine the quality of the experience. Rather, it is the total nature of the quality of the interpersonal relationship that influences the infant's formulation of trust.

During the second stage, the more active and aggressive modality of ***biting*** occurs. Infants learn that they can hold onto what is their own and can more fully control their environment. During this stage infants may be confronted with one of their first conflicts. If they are breast-feeding, they quickly learn that biting causes withdrawal of the nipple and anxiety in the mother. Yet biting also brings internal relief from teething discomfort and a sense of power or control.

This conflict may be solved in a variety of ways. The mother may wean the infant from the breast and begin bottle-feeding, or the infant may learn to bite substitute "nipples," such as a pacifier, and retain pleasurable breast-feeding. The successful resolution of this conflict strengthens the mother-child relationship because it occurs at a time when infants are recognizing mother as the most significant person in their life.

COGNITIVE DEVELOPMENT

Sensorimotor Phase (Piaget)

The theory most frequently used to explain ***cognition,*** or the ability to know, is that of Piaget. The period from birth to 24 months is termed the sensorimotor phase and is composed of six stages; however, inasmuch as this discussion is concerned with ages birth to 12 months, only the first four stages are discussed (Table 12-1; see Table 14-1 for the stages from 13 to 24 months).

During the sensorimotor phase infants progress from reflex behaviors to simple repetitive acts to imitative activity. Three crucial events take place during this phase. The first event involves ***separation;*** infants learn to separate themselves from other objects in the environment. They realize that others besides themselves control the environment and that certain readjustments must take place for mutual satisfaction to occur. This coincides with Erikson's concept of the formation of trust and mutual regulation of frustration.

The second major accomplishment is achieving the concept of ***object permanence,*** or the realization that objects that leave the visual field still exist. A typical example of the development of object permanence is when infants are able to pursue objects they observe being hidden under a pillow or behind a chair (Fig. 12-10). This skill develops at approximately 9 to 10 months of age, which also corresponds to the time of increased locomotion skills.

The last major intellectual achievement of this period is the ability to use ***symbols,*** or ***mental representation.*** The use of symbols allows the infant to think of an object or situation without actually experiencing it. The recognition of symbols is the beginning of understanding of time and space.

TABLE 12-1 Sensorimotor Phase During Infancy*

STAGE/AGE	COGNITIVE DEVELOPMENT	BEHAVIOR
I. Use of reflexes Birth–1 month	Repetitious use of reflexes establishes a pattern of experiences Totally narcissistic (self-centered) being	Mostly reflexive (sucking, swallowing, rooting, grasping, crying) Little or no tolerance for frustration of delayed gratification
II. Primary circular reactions 1-4 months	Use of reflexes is gradually replaced by voluntary activity Recognition of causality occurs when repetition of events causes one stimulus to produce a consistent response Beginning notion of temporal space of time occurs as infant realizes the progression of an orderly sequence of events Beginning separation of self from others Learns from type of interaction between object or individual rather than from object itself Engages in an activity for the pleasure of the activity more than for its result	Recognizes familiar faces and objects (e.g., bottle) Shows anticipation before feeding Awareness of strange surroundings indicates memory Discovers parts of own body—plays with hands, fingers, feet Becomes bored when left alone Shows no stranger anxiety unless caregiver's skill differs from usual routine
III. Secondary circular reactions 4-8 months	Intentional activity replaces repetitious activity that did not produce a desired result Beginning of object permanence when object is beyond perceptual range Progressive idea of time; awareness of before and after in a sequence of events Able to imitate selective activity from several events Further separation of self from environment Idea of quality and quantity Beginning recognition of symbols as type of communication	Secures objects by pulling on a string Searches for objects that have fallen Shows stranger anxiety Able to tolerate some frustration and delayed gratification Imitates sounds and simple gestures Great interest in mirror image (see Fig. 12-11) Beginning independence in self-feeding Shows displeasure if activity is inhibited Language development; attracts attention by methods other than crying Realizes that parents are present even if not in visual field
IV. Coordination of secondary schemas and their application to new situations 9-12 months	Concept of object permanence advances; beginning of intellectual reasoning Associates symbols with events, but classification is based on own experience Distinguishes objects from the related activity and perceives them as objects Distinguishes end products from their means; attempts to remove barriers to achieve the end	Actively searches for a hidden object (Fig. 12-10) Comprehends meanings of words and simple commands Knows that gestures (bye-bye, kiss) have certain meanings Is able to put objects in a container Works to get toy that is out of reach Ventures away from parent to explore surroundings

*For phases during toddlerhood see Table 14-1.

The first stage, from birth to 1 month, is identified by the infant's ***use of reflexes.*** At birth the infant's individuality and temperament are expressed through the physiologic reflexes of sucking, rooting, grasping, and crying. The repetitious nature of the reflexes is the beginning of associations between an act and a sequential response. When infants cry because they are hungry, a nipple is put in the mouth, and they suck, feel satisfaction, and sleep. They are assimilating this experience while perceiving auditory, tactile, and visual cues. This experience of perceiving certain patterns, or "ordering," is foundational for the subsequent stages.

The second stage, ***primary circular reactions,*** marks the beginning of the replacement of reflexive behavior with voluntary acts. During the period from 1 to 4 months, activities such as sucking or grasping become deliberate acts that elicit certain responses. The beginning of accommodation is evident. Infants incorporate and adapt their reactions to the environment and recognize the stimulus that produced a response. Previously they would cry until the nipple was brought to the mouth. Now they associate the nipple with the sound of the parent's voice. They accommodate this new piece of information and adapt by ceasing to cry when they hear the voice, before receiving the nipple. A realization of causality and a recognition of an orderly sequence of events is taking place. The environment is taken in with all the senses and with whatever motor ability is present.

The ***secondary circular reactions*** stage is a continuation of primary circular reactions and lasts until 8 months of age. In this stage the primary circular reactions are repeated and prolonged for the response that results. Grasping and hold-

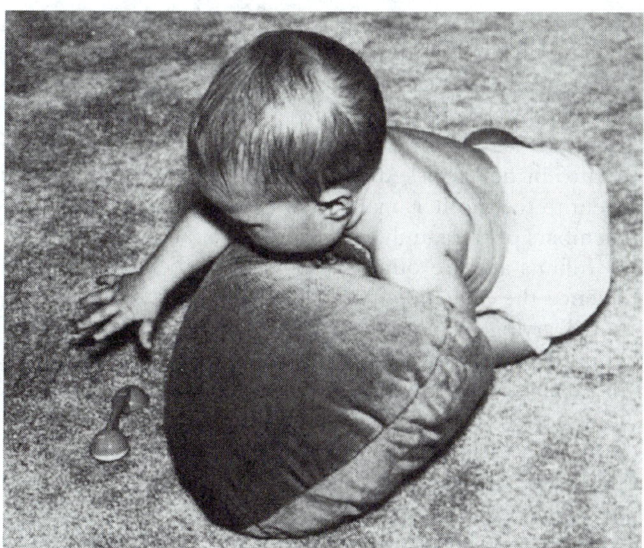

FIG. 12-10 Nine-month-old infant actively searches for object hidden behind pillow.

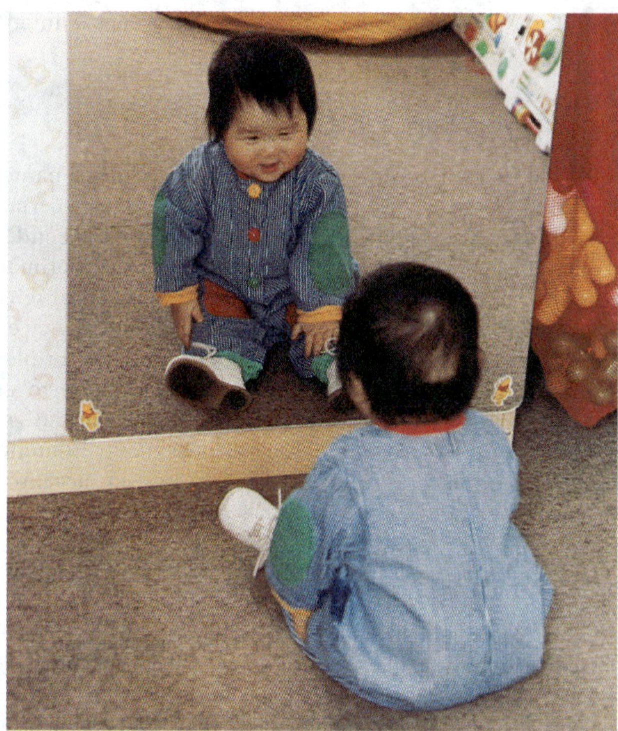

FIG. 12-11 Nine-month-old infant enjoying own image in mirror.

ing now become shaking, banging, and pulling. Shaking is performed to hear a noise, not solely for the pleasure of shaking. Quality and quantity of an act become evident. "More" or "less" shaking produces different responses. Causality, time, deliberate intention, and separateness from the environment begin to develop.

Three new processes of human behavior occur. ***Imitation*** requires the differentiation of selected acts from several events. By the second half of the first year infants can imitate sounds and simple gestures. ***Play*** becomes evident as they take pleasure in performing an act after they have mastered it. Much of infants' waking hours are absorbed in sensorimotor play. ***Affect*** (outward manifestation of emotion and feeling) is seen as infants begin to develop a sense of permanency. During the first 6 months infants believe that an object exists only for as long as they can visually perceive it. In other words, out of sight—out of mind. When the object continues to be present or remembered even though it is beyond the range of perception, affect to external objects is evident. Object permanence is a critical component of parent-child attachment and is seen in the development of stranger anxiety at 6 to 8 months of age (p. 527).

During the fourth sensorimotor stage, ***coordination of secondary schemas and their application to new situations,*** infants use previous behavioral achievements primarily as the foundation for adding new intellectual skills to their expanding repertoire. This stage is largely transitional. Increasing motor skills allow for greater exploration of the environment. They begin to discover that hiding an object does not mean that it is gone but that removing an obstacle will reveal the object. This marks the beginning of intellectual reasoning. Furthermore, they can experience an event by observing it, and they begin to associate symbols with events, such as "bye-bye" with "Daddy goes to work," but the classification is purely their own. Unlike the second stage, where infants learned from the type of interaction between objects or individuals, in this stage they learn from the object itself. Intentionality is further developed in that now they will actively attempt to remove a barrier to the desired (or undesired) action (see Fig. 12-10). If something is in their way, they will attempt to climb over it or push it away. Previously an obstacle would cause them to give up any further attempt to achieve the desired goal.

DEVELOPMENT OF BODY IMAGE

The development of body image parallels sensorimotor development. Infants' kinesthetic and tactile experiences are the first perceptions of their body, and the mouth is the principal area of pleasurable sensations. Other parts of the body are primarily objects of pleasure—the hands and fingers to suck and the feet to play with. As physical needs are met, they feel comfort and satisfaction with their body. Messages conveyed by the caregivers reinforce these feelings. For example, when infants smile, they receive emotional satisfaction from others who smile back.

Achieving the concept of object permanence is basic to the development of self-image. By the end of the first year infants recognize that they are distinct from their parents. At the same time there is increasing interest in their image, especially in the mirror (Fig. 12-11). As motor skills develop, they learn that parts of the body are useful; for example, the hands bring objects to the mouth, and the legs help them move to different locations. All of these achievements transmit message to them about themselves. It is therefore important to transmit positive messages to infants about their bodies.

DEVELOPMENT OF SEXUALITY

A sexual identity begins at birth, when the child is named and significant others, especially the parents, act certain ways toward the infant because of the respective gender. Touch is crucial to infant development and plays a primary role in sexual development. Infants have a great oral sensitivity, manifested through sucking and mouthing. They enjoy skin-to-skin contact and explore their own body for pleasure. Infants are capable of genital self-stimulation to orgasm; erections in male infants are common. Parents' responses to these early manifestations of sexuality influence children's evolving attitude; therefore, a healthy, accepting response by parents is important.

SOCIAL DEVELOPMENT

Infants' social development is initially influenced by their reflexive behavior, such as the grasp, and eventually depends primarily on the interaction between them and the principal caregivers. Attachment to the parent is increasingly evident during the second half of the first year. In addition, tremendous strides are made in communication and personal-social behavior. Play is a major socializing agent and provides stimulation needed to learn from the interaction with the environment.

Attachment

The importance of human physical contact cannot be overemphasized. Parenting is not an instinctual ability but a learned acquired process. The attachment of parent and child, which probably begins before birth and assumes even more importance at birth (see Chapter 8), continues during the first year. In the following discussion of attachment, the word "mother" is used in the broad context of the consistent caregiver with whom the child relates more than anyone else. However, in society's changing social climate and sex role stereotypes, this may very well be the father. Studies on father-child attachment demonstrate that similar stages occur as with mother attachment (Lincoln, 1984) and that fathers are more involved in child care when mothers are employed (although mothers continue to do the majority of infant care) (Jones and Heermann, 1992).

During infancy attachment progresses with the child assuming an increasingly significant role. Two components of cognitive development are required for attachment: (1) the ability to discriminate the mother from other individuals and (2) the achievement of object permanence. Both of these processes prepare the infant for an equally important aspect of attachment—separation from the parent. Separation-individuation should occur as a harmonious, parallel process with emotional attachment.

During the formation of attachment to the parent, the infant progresses through four distinct but overlapping stages. For the first few weeks infants respond indiscriminately to anyone. Beginning at about 8 to 12 weeks of age, they cry, smile, and vocalize more to the mother than to anyone else but continue to respond to mothers, whether familiar or not. At age 6 months or so, infants show a distinct preference for the mother. They follow her more, cry when she leaves, enjoy playing with her more, and feel most secure in her arms. About 1 month after showing attachment to the mother, many infants begin attaching to other members of the family, most often the father.

Infants acquire other developmental behaviors that influence the attachment process. These include (1) differential crying, smiling, and vocalization (more to mother than to anyone else), (2) visual-motor orientation (looking more at mother even if she is not close), (3) crying when mother leaves the room, (4) approach through locomotion (crawling, creeping, or walking), (5) clinging (especially in presence of a stranger), and (6) exploring away from mother while using her as a secure base.

Effects of Prolonged Separation. Attachment is considered so critical to optimum child development that many researchers have documented the effects of prolonged and early separation on infants in the absence of quality mother substitutes. Some of the most famous research on emotional deprivation has been done by John Bowlby, John Robertson, and René Spitz. Bowlby (1969) studied the effects of the infant's separation from the mother and noted severe mental and physical retardation, particularly if emotional deprivation occurred during the first 3 years of life. He observed that the progressive retardation could be arrested or reversed if no further emotional deprivation occurred after the first 2 years but that prolonged, severe deprivation beginning early in the first year and lasting for 3 years led to severe permanent effects. Among these were the inability to form trusting, intimate interpersonal relationships, language impairment, and deficiency in abstract thinking. Robertson (1953) and Bowlby (1969) found typical behavioral reactions of infants who were hospitalized and separated from their mothers (see Separation Anxiety, Chapter 26).

Spitz (1945) studied the effects of emotional deprivation of children raised in foundling homes or institutions. The infants were cared for by one nurse who had responsibility for eight children. Although the caregiver might be a loving, motherly person, she lacked the time necessary to devote individual attention and stimulation to each child. As a result, the children were retarded in physical growth, were more susceptible to disease, and demonstrated decreasing developmental quotients over a 2-year period. Spitz found that children who were given one-to-one attention by a mother substitute developed normally.

Although these studies represent extreme examples of young children reared in environments essentially devoid of quality mothering, rather than temporary separation, such as daycare, the question remains regarding the long-term effects of separation and other stresses on children (see Thinking Critically About . . . box). Based on such findings, nurses need to assess each family with the understanding that stress is not necessarily harmful and that even under adverse conditions children can adapt. Individual risk factors that influence a child's coping ability are evaluated, and tools such as the Infant Temperament Question

THINKING CRITICALLY ABOUT . . . *Stress and Resiliency*

Much of the research on the effects of stress during childhood demonstrates that children have an incredible ability to adapt despite adversity—a concept known as ***resiliency.*** Thomas and Chess (1984) revealed a very high rate of recovery in children with adjustment problems and found that parent separation, divorce, or death did not predict early adult status. Extensive reviews of research regarding the effects of stress on children, such as maternal deprivation, hospitalization, birth of a sibling, and parental death, have confirmed similar findings. Such studies have identified risk factors that increase children's vulnerability to stress, such as "difficult" temperament, lack of "fit" between child and parent, age (especially between 6 months and 5 years), male gender (Pitzer and Hock, 1992), genetics, below-average intelligence, multiple and continuing stresses such as frequent hospital admissions or foster care placements and homes marked by discord or divorce, and lack of social supports.

However, the basic conclusion is that stress alone does not dictate inevitable negative consequences. Rather, emphasis must be placed on individual differences in vulnerability to deprivation and stress. Significant separation or lack of attachment to the mother figure must be viewed in light of other substitutes in the child's life, such as fathers, siblings, relatives, neighbors, and teachers, who also can significantly influence development (Garmezy and Rutter, 1989).

naire (see p. 530) are used to assess "goodness of fit." When parental separation occurs, every effort is made to help the family provide suitable caregiver substitutes for the child. Individuals who are warm, responsive, and interactive with the infant during separation can significantly minimize the physiologic and behavioral effects (Gunnar and others, 1992). The child's plasticity and resiliency to cope are stressed to the family to minimize their feelings of responsibility and guilt (Nelms, 1985).

Separation Anxiety. Between ages 4 and 8 months the infant progresses through the first stage of separation-individuation and begins to have some awareness of self and mother as separate beings. At the same time, object permanence is developing, and the infant is aware that the parent can be absent. Thus, separation anxiety develops and is manifested through a predictable sequence of behaviors.

During the early second half of the first year infants protest when placed in their crib, and a short time later they object when the mother leaves the room. Subsequently, infants may not notice the mother's absence if they are absorbed in an activity. However, when they realize her absence, they protest. From this point onward they become very alert to her activities and whereabouts. By 11 to 12 months they are able to anticipate her imminent departure by watching her behaviors and begin to protest *before* she leaves. At this point many parents learn to postpone alerting the child to their departure until just before leaving.

Stranger Fear. As infants demonstrate attachment to one person, they correspondingly exhibit less friendliness to others. Between ages 6 and 8 months fear of strangers and stranger anxiety become prominent and are related to infants' ability to discriminate between familiar and nonfamiliar people. Such behaviors as clinging to the parent, crying, and turning away from the stranger are common (Fig. 12-12). Suggestions for coping with stranger fear and separation anxiety are discussed on p. 531.

Language Development

The infant's first means of verbal communication is crying. Crying as a biologic sign conveys a message of urgency and signals displeasure, such as hunger. However, crying is also a social event that affects the development of the parent-infant relationship, either by its absence, which usually has a positive effect on parents, or its presence, which may evoke a negative response or persuade parents to minister to the child's physical or emotional needs.

In the first few weeks of life crying has a reflexive quality and is mostly related to physiologic needs. Infants cry for a period of 1 to 1½ hours a day up to 3 weeks of age, then build up to 2, and even 4, hours by 6 weeks. Crying tends to decrease by 12 weeks. It is thought that the increase in crying for no apparent reason during the first few months may be related to the discharge of energy and the maturational changes in the central nervous system. During the end of the first year infants cry for attention, from fear, especially stranger fear, and from frustration, usually in re-

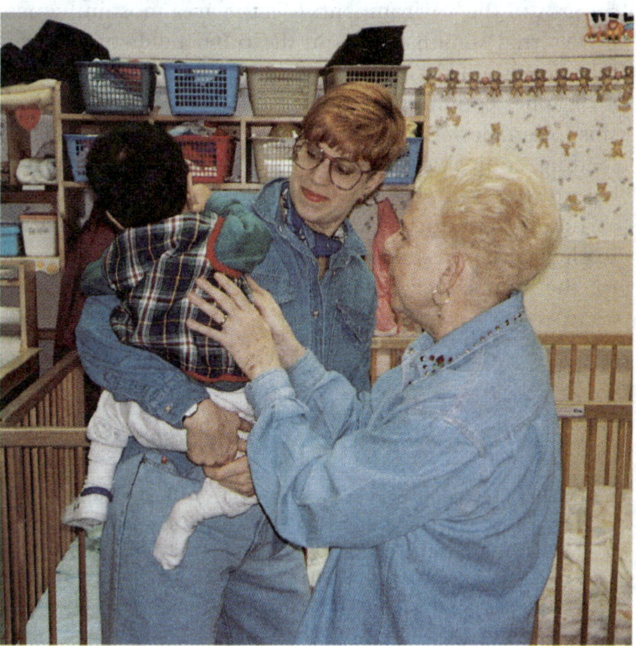

FIG. 12-12 Stranger fear behaviors include clinging to the parent and turning away from a stranger.

sponse to their developing but inadequate motor skills (Brazelton, 1987; Lester, 1985).

Many parents state that they can distinguish between different types of cry and from these messages are able to interpret the infant's needs. However, crying can be a source of acute distress for parents, especially the unconsolable crying of colic (see Chapter 13). Parents benefit from an explanation of the variability of crying among infants and assurance that periods of "unexplained fussiness" are normal. Some parents may need guidance in consoling techniques, such as holding, swaddling, massaging, caressing, rocking, walking, or stimulating sucking.

NURSING ALERT Be alert to parents' reports about maternal postpartum depression and infant crying, because these concerns may indicate a stressed mother-infant relationship (Miller, Barr, and Eaton, 1993).

Vocalizations heard during crying eventually become some syllables and words (e.g., the "mama" heard during vigorous crying). Infants vocalize as early as 5 to 6 weeks of age by making small throaty sounds. By 2 months they make single vowel sounds, such as *ah, eh,* and *uh.* By 3 to 4 months the consonants *n, k, g, p,* and *b* are added, and infants coo, gurgle, and laugh aloud. By 8 months they imitate sounds, add the consonants *t, d,* and *w,* and combine syllables, such as "dada," but they do not ascribe meaning to the word until 10 to 11 months of age (see Family Focus box). By 9 to 10 months they comprehend the meaning of the word "no" and obey simple commands. By age 1 year they can say three to five words with meaning.

Personal-Social Behavior

Personal-social behavior includes the child's personal responses to the environment. It is the area most influenced by external stimuli but, as in the other fields of behavior, follows certain developmental laws. Personal-social behavior implies communication with one's self and with others. It is foundational for the successful mastery of skills such as feeding, control of bodily functions, independence, and cooperativeness in play.

Infants have the ability to shape their environment and to elicit certain responses. Newborns show visual preference for the human face and, as early as 1 week of age, begin to watch the parent intently as he or she speaks to them. As they regard the parent's face, activity diminishes, their head bobs up and down, and their mouth moves, almost as if they were trying to say something.

By 6 to 8 weeks a social smile in response to pleasurable stimuli is present. This has a profound effect on family members and is a tremendous stimulus for evoking continued responses from others. By 3 months infants show considerable interest in the environment: excitement when a toy is presented, refusal to be left alone, recognition of parent, and demonstration of pleasure by squealing. By 4 months they laugh aloud and enjoy strange, novel stimuli.

By 6 months infants are very personable. They play games such as peekaboo when their head is hidden in a towel, they signal their desire to be picked up by extending their arms, and they show displeasure when a toy is removed or their face is washed. There is increasing demonstration of their ability to control the environment. The acquisition of fine and gross motor skills allows much more independence in movement.

By the second half of the first year infants understand simple discipline, such as the meaning of the word "no" or a scolding remark. They comprehend different facial expressions and are sensitive to emotional changes in others. Imitation is developing during this time. By 7 months they imitate actions and noises, by 8 months sounds, and by 10 months games such as pat-a-cake and peekaboo.

From 11 months onward they are increasingly independent. They are learning to feed themselves, using fingers, spoon, and cup (with much spilling), and can help with dressing by putting the foot out for a shoe or pushing the arm through the sleeve. They not only comprehend the meaning of "no," but shake their head to signal understanding. They can follow simple directions and will gladly perform for others to attract and prolong attention.

Play

Play during infancy represents the various social modalities observed during cognitive development. Infants' activity is primarily narcissistic, revolving around their own body. As discussed under development of body image, parts of the body are primarily play and pleasure objects.

During the first year play becomes more sophisticated and interdependent. From birth to 3 months infants' responses to the environment are global and largely undifferentiated. Play is dependent; pleasure is demonstrated by a quieting attitude (1 month), later by a smile (2 months), and then by a squeal (3 months). From 3 to 6 months infants show more discriminate interest in stimuli and begin to play alone with a rattle or soft stuffed toy or to play with someone else. There is much more interaction during play. By 4 months of age they laugh aloud, show preference for certain toys, and become excited when food or a favorite object is brought to them. They recognize an image in a mirror, smile at it, and vocalize to it.

By 6 months to 1 year play involves sensorimotor skills. Actual games are played, such as peekaboo, pat-a-cake, verbal repetition, and imitation of simple gestures in response to demonstration. Play is much more selective, not only in

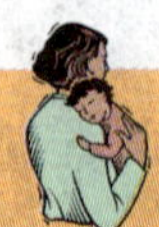

FAMILY FOCUS
Child's Developing Language Skills

During the acquisition of new language skills the child temporarily may give up other recently learned sounds or words. This is often distressing for parents, who have waited in anticipation for the words "dada" or "mama," since these sounds are frequently replaced by other vocalizations and may not be repeated for several weeks. Nurses should reassure parents that the child will again say these special words, and with increased meaning.

TABLE 12-2 Play During Infancy

AGE (MONTHS)	VISUAL STIMULATION	AUDITORY STIMULATION	TACTILE STIMULATION	KINETIC STIMULATION
SUGGESTED ACTIVITIES				
Birth-1	Look at infant at close range Hang bright, shiny object within 20-25 cm (8-10 inches) of infant's face and in midline Hang mobiles with black-and-white designs	Talk to infant; sing in soft voice Play music box, radio, television Have ticking clock or metronome nearby	Hold, caress, cuddle Keep infant warm May like to be swaddled	Rock infant; place in cradle Use carriage for walks
2-3	Provide bright objects Make room bright with pictures or mirrors Take infant to various rooms while doing chores Place infant in infant seat for vertical view of environment	Talk to infant Include in family gatherings Expose to various environmental noises other than those of home Use rattles, wind chimes	Caress infant while bathing, at diaper change Comb hair with a soft brush	Use infant swing Take in car for rides Exercise body by moving extremities in swimming motion Use cradle gym
4-6	Place infant in front of unbreakable mirror Give brightly colored toys to hold (small enough to grasp)	Talk to infant; repeat sounds infant makes Laugh when infant laughs Call infant by name Crinkle different papers by infant's ear Place rattle or bell in hand	Give infant soft squeeze toys of various textures Allow to splash in bath Place nude on soft, furry rug and move extremities	Use swing or stroller Bounce infant in lap while holding in standing position Support infant in sitting position; let infant lean forward to balance self Place infant on floor to crawl, roll over, sit
6-9	Give infant large toys with bright colors, movable parts, and noisemakers Place unbreakable mirror where infant can see self Play peekaboo, especially hiding face in a towel Make funny faces to encourage imitation Give ball of yarn or string to pull apart	Call infant by name Repeat simple words such as "dada," "mama," "bye-bye" Speak clearly Name parts of body, people, and foods Tell infant what you are doing Use "no" only when necessary Give simple commands Show how to clap hands, bang a drum	Let infant play with fabrics of various textures Have bowl with foods of different sizes and textures to feel Let infant "catch" running water Encourage "swimming" in large bathtub or shallow pool Give wad of sticky tape to manipulate	Hold upright to bear weight and bounce Pick up, say "up" Put down, say "down" Place toys out of reach; encourage infant to get them Play pat-a-cake
9-12	Show infant large pictures in books Take infant to places where there are animals, many people, different objects (shopping center) Play ball by rolling it to child, demonstrate "throwing" it back Demonstrate building a two-block tower	Read infant simple nursery rhymes Point to body parts and name each one Imitate sounds of animals	Give infant finger foods of different textures Let infant mess and squash food Let infant feel cold (ice cube) or warm objects; say what temperature each is Let infant feel a breeze (fan blowing)	Give large push-pull toys Place furniture in a circle to encourage cruising Turn in different positions
SUGGESTED TOYS				
Birth-6	Nursery mobiles Unbreakable mirrors See-through crib bumpers Contrasting colored sheets	Music boxes Musical mobiles Crib dangle bells Small-handled clear rattle	Stuffed animals Soft clothes Soft or furry quilt Soft mobiles	Rocking crib/cradle Weighted or suction toy Infant swing
6-12	Various colored blocks Nested boxes or cups Books with rhymes and bright pictures Strings of big beads Simple take-apart toys Large ball Cup and spoon Large puzzles Jack-in-the box	Rattles of different sizes, shapes, tones, and bright colors Squeaky animals and dolls Records with light, rhythmic music	Soft, different-textures animals and dolls Sponge toys, floating toys Squeeze toys Teething toys Books with textures/objects, such as fur and zipper	Activity box for crib Push-pull toys Wind-up swing

terms of specific toys but also in terms of "playmates." Although play is solitary or one-sided, infants choose with whom they will interact. At 6 to 8 months they usually refuse to play with strangers. Parents are definite favorites, and infants know how to attract their attention. At 6 months they extend the arms to be picked up, at 7 months cough to make their presence known, at 10 months pull the parent's clothing, and at 12 months call them by name. This represents a tremendous advance from the newborn who signaled biologic needs by crying to express displeasure.

Stimulation is as important for psychosocial growth as food is for physical growth. Knowledge of developmental milestones allows nurses to guide parents regarding proper play for infants. It is not sufficient to place a mobile over a crib and toys in a playpen for a child's optimum social, emotional, and intellectual development. Play must provide interpersonal contact, as well as recreational and educational stimulation. Infants need to be *played with,* not merely *allowed to play.* Although the type of play infants engage in is called **solitary,** this is only a figurative, not literal, term to denote one-sided play. The kind of toys given to the child is much less important than the quality of personal interaction that occurs.

Table 12-2 lists play activities appropriate for the developmental level of the infant in view of motor, language, and personal-social achievements. Although the activities are grouped according to the major mode of stimulation provided, there is overlap in many instances. In addition, play activities suggested for one age-group may be appropriate for older infants but inappropriate for younger infants.

TEMPERAMENT

The infant's temperament or behavioral style influences the kind of interaction that occurs between the child and parents, and other family members (see general discussion of temperament in Chapter 4). In assessing a child's temperament, it is the parents' perception of the child and the degree of fit between their expectations and the child's actual temperament that are important. The more dissonance or lack of harmony between the child's temperament and the parent's ability to accept and deal with the behavior, the more risk for subsequent parent-child conflicts. (See Thinking Critically About . . . box.)

The ***Infant Temperament Questionnaire (ITQ)*** (Carey and McDevitt, 1978) can be used as a screening tool with parents. The questionnaire focuses on nine temperament variables, but the 95 questions relate specifically to activities such as sleep, feeding, play, diapering, and dressing. The scores from the ITQ help identify the child's temperamental style. Use of the ITQ is well accepted by parents and should be accompanied by an adequate explanation of the results. In discussing the results, it is best to avoid terms such as "difficult" and describe the child in terms of characteristics, such as intense or less predictable.

With knowledge of the infant's temperament, nurses are better able to (1) provide parents with background information that will help them see their child in a better perspective, (2) offer a more organized picture of their child's behavior and possibly reveal distortions in their perceptions of the behavior, and (3) guide parents regarding appropriate childrearing techniques (Chess and Thomas, 1985).

Childrearing Practices Related to Temperament

Most parents realize that their infant is born with unique characteristics, and few parents of difficult infants need to be told of the challenge of caring for them. However, very few parents are aware of the significance of the temperamental characteristics and of constructive approaches to dealing with them. The following are examples of interventions that promote more positive parenting of infants with different temperament styles.*

*Recommended resources for parents are *The Difficult Child* by S. Turecki and L. Tonner (1985, Bantam Books) and *Know Your Child: An Authoritative Guide for Today's Parents* by S. Chess and A. Thomas (1987, Basic Books).

THINKING CRITICALLY ABOUT . . .

Effect of Infant Temperament on Parenting

Although the importance of temperament is generally acknowledged, its influence on parenting is less clear, and studies often report conflicting findings. However, there is evidence that infant temperament does affect parenting, at least in terms of parents' perception of their parenting role.

An "easy" child is apt to make parents feel more thankful and content in their parenting role, whereas a less adaptable and predictable, more fussy infant may cause parents, especially mothers, to be depressed (Mayberry and Alfonso, 1993). Infants who are less predictable in their behavior, such as sleeping, feeding, and general satisfaction, cause parents to feel less competent and to experience less ease in transition to parenthood. Mothers, especially of first-born children, report having major concerns regarding the behavior of "difficult" infants and of having to make large family adjustments because of their infants.

Infants with "difficult" temperaments also tend to have more colic, injuries, and night waking. These children sleep about 2 hours less a night and 1 hour less during the day than the "easy" child. Children's sleep behavior probably influences parental perceptions of their temperament, but exactly what effect these variables have on parenting is unclear (Scher and others, 1992). There is evidence that having a "difficult" child mobilizes parents to provide a more responsive home environment (Houdlin, 1987). One study found that among the various temperament types, the "difficult" group had higher intelligence quotients if the family was of higher socioeconomic status. It might be that in order to deal with the child's negative behaviors, the parents pay greater attention to the child (Maziade and others, 1987). Such findings emphasize the tremendous challenge, as well as the opportunity, that exists in rearing these children.

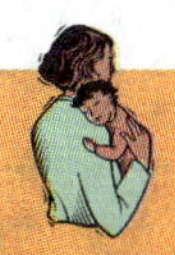

FAMILY FOCUS
Difficult Temperament and Preterm Infants

Parents typically rate preterm, low-birth-weight infants as being more difficult than full-term infants. Parents are often concerned that the difficult temperament is permanent and results from the many negative and painful hospital experiences. The family can be reassured that although these infants may be difficult to parent for the first 6 months of corrected age (chronologic age minus amount of prematurity), no particular perinatal event is responsible. Also, over time the infants tend to become less difficult (Gennaro, Medoff-Cooper, and Lotas, 1992).

"Difficult" children may respond better to scheduled feedings and structured caregiving routines than demand feedings and frequent changes in daily routines. These children sleep less and may need more structured approaches to bedtime to prevent bedtime problems. "Highly distractible children" may require additional soothing measures such as swinging, rocking, or being carried in a pack that the parent wears across the chest or back. Children with "high activity" levels require vigilant watching, and parents need to take extra precautions in safeguarding the home. These children benefit from increased opportunities for gross motor activity to constructively channel their energy.

The child who is "slow to warm up" may demonstrate more stranger fear than other children and may require more gradual and frequent preparation for new situations, such as substitute child care. Even the "easy child" can present problems in that the parents may need reminders to feed the child who sleeps for prolonged intervals and rarely cries. They may have to "retrain" the child because of the ease of developing troublesome habits, such as keeping the child up late or sleeping with the youngster.

Appropriate counseling based on awareness of the child's temperament can greatly enhance the quality of interaction between parents and infant. Even just letting parents know that "difficult" traits are innate can relieve feelings of guilt and incompetence (see Family Focus box).

▪ ▪ ▪

Knowledge of the developmental sequence allows the nurse to assess normal growth and minor or abnormal deviations, helps parents gain realistic expectations of their child's ability, and provides guidelines for suitable play and stimulation. Parents who lack knowledge of child growth and development may set inappropriate behavioral expectations for their children (Kliman and Vukelich, 1985). Emphasizing the child's developmental age rather than chronologic age strengthens the parent-child relationship by fostering trust and lessening frustration. Therefore the importance of a thorough understanding and appreciation of the growth and development of children cannot be overemphasized.

Because of the complexity of the developmental process during the first 12 months, Table 12-3 is presented to help organize and clarify the data already discussed. Although all milestones are important, some represent essential integrative aspects of development that lay the foundation for the achievement of more advanced skills. These essential milestones are designated by a square (▪) in the table. The table represents the *average* monthly age at which various skills are attained. It must be remembered that, although the sequence is the same, the rate will vary among children.

COPING WITH CONCERNS RELATED TO NORMAL GROWTH AND DEVELOPMENT

Separation and Stranger Fear

During infancy a number of fears can appear. However, the fear that causes parents most concern is fear related to strangers and separation. Although erroneously interpreted by some as a sign of undesirable, antisocial behavior, stranger fear and separation anxiety are important components of a strong, healthy parent-child attachment. However, this period can present difficulties for parent and child. Parents may be more confined to the home because baby-sitters are violently protested by the infant. To accustom the infant to new people, parents are encouraged to have close friends or relatives visit often. This provides for other persons with whom the child is comfortable and who can give parents time for themselves.

Infants also need opportunities to safely experience strangers. Usually toward the end of the first year infants begin to venture away from the parent and demonstrate curiosity about strangers. If allowed to explore at their own rate, many infants will eventually "warm up." If parents hold the child away from their face, the infant can observe while maintaining close physical contact.

A number of factors influence the child's intensity of fear of strangers:

- Sex, age, and size of the stranger—female, younger age, and smaller size (including kneeling or sitting rather than standing) being less stressful
- Approach—loud, sudden, intrusive approach causing more distress
- Child's proximity to parent—closer to parent (on parent's lap rather than in infant seat) being less stressful

Consequently, the best approach for the stranger (who may be the nurse) is to talk softly, meet the child at eye level (to appear smaller), maintain a safe distance from the infant, and avoid sudden, intrusive gestures, such as holding the arms out and smiling broadly.

Parents also may wonder whether they should encourage the child's clinging, dependent behavior, especially if there is pressure from others who view this as "spoiling" (see following discussion). Parents need to be reassured that such behavior is healthy, desirable, and necessary for the child's optimum emotional development. If parents can reassure the infant of their presence, the infant will learn to realize that they are still there even if not physically present. Talking to infants when leaving the room, allowing them to hear one's voice on the telephone, and using transitional objects, such as a favorite blanket or toy, reassures them of the parent's continued presence.

Text continued on p. 536.

TABLE 12-3 Growth and Development During Infancy

AGE (MONTHS)	PHYSICAL	GROSS MOTOR	FINE MOTOR
1	Weight gain of 150 to 210 g (5 to 7 ounces) weekly for first 6 months Height gain of 2.5 cm (1 inch) monthly for first 6 months Head circumference increases by 1.5 cm (½ inch) monthly for first 6 months Primitive reflexes present and strong Doll's eye reflexes and dance reflex fading Obligatory nose breathing (most infants)	▪ Assumes flexed position with pelvis high but knees not under abdomen when prone (at birth, knees flexed under abdomen) ▪ Can turn head from side to side when prone; lifts head momentarily from bed (see Fig. 12-7, *A*) Has marked head lag, especially when pulled from lying to sitting position (see Fig. 12-6, *A*) Holds head momentarily parallel and in midline when suspended in prone position Assumes asymmetric tonic neck reflex position when supine When held in standing position, body limp at knees and hips In sitting position back is uniformly rounded, absence of head control (see Fig. 12-8, *A*)	Hands predominantly closed Grasp reflex strong Hand clenches on contact with rattle
2	Posterior fontanel closed Crawling reflex disappears	▪ Assumes less flexed position when prone—hips flat, legs extended, arms flexed, head to side Less head lag when pulled to sitting position (see Fig. 12-6, *B*) Can maintain head in same plane as rest of body when held in ventral suspension When prone, can lift head almost 45 degrees off table When held in sitting position, head is held up but bobs forward (see Fig. 12-8, *B*) Assumes asymmetric tonic neck reflex position intermittently	Hands frequently open Grasp reflex fading
3	Primitive reflexes fading	Able to hold head more erect when sitting, but still bobs forward Has only slight head lag when pulled to sitting position Assumes symmetric body positioning Able to raise head and shoulders from prone position to a 45- to 90-degree angle from table; bears weight on forearms When held in standing position, able to bear slight fraction of weight on legs Regards own hand	▪ Actively holds rattle but will not reach for it Grasp reflex absent Hands kept loosely open Clutches own hand; pulls at blankets and clothes
4	Drooling begins ▪ Moro, tonic neck, and rooting reflexes have disappeared	▪ Has almost no head lag when pulled to sitting position (see Fig. 12-6, *C*) ▪ Balances head well in sitting position (see Fig. 12-8, *C*) Back less rounded, curved only in lumbar area Able to sit erect if propped up Able to raise head and chest off surface to angle of 90 degrees (see Fig. 12-7, *B*) Assumes predominant symmetric position ▪ Rolls from back to side	▪ Inspects and plays with hands; pulls clothing or blanket over face in play Tries to reach objects with hand but overshoots Grasps object with both hands Plays with rattle placed in hand, shakes it, but cannot pick it up if dropped Can carry objects to mouth

▪ Milestones that represent essential integrative aspects of development that lay the foundation for the achievement of more advanced skills.
*Degree of visual acuity varies according to vision measurement procedure used.

SENSORY	VOCALIZATION	SOCIALIZATION/ COGNITION
■ Able to fixate on moving object in range of 45 degrees when held at a distance of 20-25 cm (8-10 inches) Visual acuity approaches 20/100* Follows light to midline Quiets when hears a voice	Cries to express displeasure Makes small, throaty sounds Makes comfort sounds during feeding	Is in sensorimotor phase—stage I, use of reflexes (birth-1 month), and stage II, primary circular reactions (1-4 months) Watches parent's face intently as she or he talks to infant
Binocular fixation and convergence to near objects beginning When supine, follows dangling toy from side to point beyond midline Visually searches to locate sounds Turns head to side when sound is made at level of ear	■ Vocalizes, distinct from crying Crying becomes differentiated Coos Vocalizes to familiar voice	■ Demonstrates social smile in response to various stimuli
■ Follows object to periphery (180 degrees) ■ Locates sound by turning head to side and looking in same direction Begins to have ability to coordinate stimuli from various sense organs	■ Squeals aloud to show pleasure Coos, babbles, chuckles Vocalizes when smiling "Talks" a great deal when spoken to Less crying during periods of wakefulness	Displays considerable interest in surroundings Ceases crying when parent enters room Can recognize familiar faces and objects, such as feeding bottle Shows awareness of strange situations
Able to accommodate to near objects Binocular vision fairly well established Can focus on a 1.25 cm (½-inch) block Beginning eye-hand coordination	Makes consonant sounds *n, k, g, p, b* ■ Laughs aloud Vocalization changes according to mood	Is in stage III, secondary circular reactions Demands attention by fussing; becomes bored if left alone Enjoys social interaction with people Anticipates feeding when sees bottle or mother if breast-feeding Shows excitement with whole body, squeals, breathes heavily Shows interest in strange stimuli Begins to show memory

Continued.

TABLE 12-3 Growth and Development During Infancy—cont'd

AGE (MONTHS)	PHYSICAL	GROSS MOTOR	FINE MOTOR
5	Beginning signs of tooth eruption Birth weight doubles	No head lag when pulled to sitting position When sitting, able to hold head erect and steady Able to sit for longer periods when back is well supported Back straight When prone, assumes symmetric positioning with arms extended ■ Can turn over from abdomen to back When supine, puts feet to mouth	■ Able to grasp objects voluntarily Uses palmar grasp, bidextrous approach Plays with toes Takes objects directly to mouth Holds one cube while regarding a second one
6	Growth rate may begin to decline Weight gain of 90 to 150 g (3 to 5 ounces) weekly for next 6 months Height gain of 1.25 cm (½ inch) monthly for next 6 months ■ Teething may begin with eruption of two lower central incisors ■ Chewing and biting occur	When prone, can lift chest and upper abdomen off table, bearing weight on hands (see Fig. 12-7, *C*) When about to be pulled to a sitting position, lifts head Sits in high chair with back straight Rolls from back to abdomen When held in standing position, bears almost all of weight Hand regard absent	Resecures a dropped object Drops one cube when another is given Grasps and manipulates small objects Holds bottle Grasps feet and pulls to mouth
7	Eruption of upper central incisors	When supine, spontaneously lifts head off table ■ Sits, leaning forward on both hands (see Fig. 12-8, *D*) When prone, bears weight on one hand Sits erect momentarily Bears full weight on feet (see Fig. 12-9, *A*) When held in standing position, bounces actively	■ Transfers objects from one hand to the other (see Fig. 12-8, *E*) Has unidextrous approach and grasp Holds two cubes more than momentarily Bangs cube on table Rakes at a small object
8	Begins to show regular patterns in bladder and bowel elimination Parachute reflex appears (see Fig. 12-1)	■ Sits steadily unsupported (see Fig. 12-8, *E*) Readily bears weight on legs when supported; may stand holding onto furniture Adjusts posture to reach an object	Has beginning pincer grasp using index, fourth, and fifth fingers against lower part of thumb Releases objects at will Rings bell purposely Retains two cubes while regarding third cube Secures an object by pulling on a string Reaches persistently for toys out of reach
9	Eruption of upper lateral incisor may begin	Creeps on hands and knees Sits steadily on floor for prolonged time (10 minutes) Recovers balance when leans forward but cannot do so when leaning sideways ■ Pulls self to standing position and stand holding onto furniture (see Fig. 12-9, *B-D*)	■ Uses thumb and index finger in crude pincer grasp (see Fig. 12-4) Preference for use of dominant hand now evident Grasps third cube Compares two cubes by bringing them together

■ Milestones that represent essential integrative aspects of development that lay the foundation for the achievement of more advanced skills.

SENSORY	VOCALIZATION	SOCIALIZATION/ COGNITION
Visually pursues a dropped object Is able to sustain visual inspection of an object Can localize sounds made below the ear	Squeals Makes vowel cooing sounds interspersed with consonant sounds (e.g., *ah-goo*)	Smiles at mirror image Pats bottle or breast with both hands More enthusiastically playful, but may have rapid mood swings Is able to discriminate strangers from family Vocalizes displeasure when object is taken away Discovers parts of body
Adjusts posture to see an object Prefers more complex visual stimuli Can localize sounds made above the ear Will turn head to the side, then look up or down	▪ Begins to imitate sounds ▪ Babbling resembles one-syllable utterances—*ma, mu, da, di, hi* Vocalizes to toys, mirror image Takes pleasure in hearing own sounds (self-reinforcement)	Recognizes parents; begins to fear strangers Holds arms out to be picked up Has definite likes and dislikes Begins to imitate (cough, protrusion of tongue) Excites on hearing footsteps Laughs when head is hidden in a towel ▪ Briefly searches for a dropped object (object permanence beginning) Frequent mood swings—from crying to laughing with little or no provocation
▪ Can fixate on very small objects Responds to own name Localizes sound by turning head in a curving arch Beginning awareness of depth and space Has taste preferences	▪ Produces vowel sounds and chained syllables—*baba, dada, kaka* Vocalizes four distinct vowel sounds "Talks" when others are talking	▪ Increasing fear of strangers; shows signs of fretfulness when parent disappears Imitates simples acts and noises Tries to attract attention by coughing or snorting Plays peekaboo Demonstrates dislike of food by keeping lips closed Exhibits oral aggressiveness in biting and mouthing Demonstrates expectation in response to repetition of stimuli
	Makes consonant sounds *t, d,* and *w* Listens selectively to familiar words Utterances signal emphasis and emotion Combines syllables, such as *dada,* but does not ascribe meaning to them	Increasing anxiety over loss of parent, particularly mother, and fear of strangers Respond to word "no" Dislikes dressing, diaper change
Localizes sounds by turning head diagonally and directly toward sound Depth perception increasing	Responds to simple verbal commands Comprehends "no-no"	Parent (mother) is increasingly important for own sake Shows increasing interest in pleasing parent Begins to show fears of going to bed and being left alone Puts arms in front of face to avoid having it washed

Continued.

TABLE 12-3 Growth and Development During Infancy—cont'd

AGE (MONTHS)	PHYSICAL	GROSS MOTOR	FINE MOTOR
10	Labyrinth-righting reflex is strongest—when infant is in prone or supine position, is able to raise head	Can change from prone to sitting position Stands while holding onto furniture, sits by falling down Recovers balance easily while sitting While standing, lifts one foot to take a step (see Fig. 12-9, *E*)	Crude release of an object beginning Grasps bell by handle
11	Eruption of lower lateral incisors may begin	When sitting, pivots to reach toward back to pick up an object ■ Cruises or walks holding onto furniture or with both hands held	Explores objects more thoroughly (e.g., clapper inside bell) Has neat pincer grasp (see Fig. 12-5) Drops object deliberately for it to be picked up Puts one object after another into a container (sequential play) Able to manipulate an object to remove it from tight-fitting enclosure
12	■ Birth weight tripled ■ Birth length increased by 50% Head and chest circumference equal (head circumference 46.5 cm [18½ inches]) Has total of six to eight deciduous teeth Anterior fontanel almost closed Landau reflex fading Babinski reflex disappears Lumbar curve develops; lordosis evident during walking	■ Walks with one hand held Cruises well ■ May attempt to stand alone momentarily; may attempt first step alone Can sit down from standing position without help	Releases cube in cup Attempts to build two-block tower but fails Tries to insert a pellet into a narrow-necked bottle but fails Can turn pages in a book, many at a time

■ Milestones that represent essential integrative aspects of development that lay the foundation for the achievement of more advanced skills.

This is a no less trying but necessary time for infants, because parents cannot always be with the child. An excellent example of necessary separation is bedtime. Fear of going to bed or being left alone in the dark commonly occurs during the second half of the first year. Fear at bedtime is only one of the many bedtime problems that can occur in young children, and is discussed on p. 547 and in Chapter 15.

Spoiled Child Syndrome

A common concern of parents is that too much attention can "spoil" a child. Many of the recommendations for promoting attachment, such as attending to the infant's needs to establish trust, accepting fear of strangers and separation from parent, and holding and rocking the crying child, are described by parents as methods of spoiling. However, research on parents' response to crying during early infancy does not support the contention that "picking up a crying baby" leads to spoiling. Ainsworth (1982) found that the amount an infant cried during the first 3 months had no correlation with the frequency of crying during the rest of the first year. However, the degree of maternal responsiveness to crying did. Parents who were less responsive, such as not picking up the infant immediately on crying, had infants who cried *more* than those of parents who responded promptly to crying. Parents of colicky infants less than 3 months old who responded to the crying with increased attention successfully decreased the overall crying time (Taubman, 1984).

If "too much attention" does not cause spoiling in early infancy, parents need to understand what "spoiling" really is and how it differs from normal behavior that may mimic aspects of spoiling. The ***spoiled child syndrome*** has been de-

SENSORY	VOCALIZATION	SOCIALIZATION/ COGNITION
	▪ Says "dada," "mama" with meaning Comprehends "bye-bye" May say one word (e.g., "hi," "bye," "no")	Inhibits behavior to verbal command of "no-no" or own name Imitates facial expressions; waves bye-bye Extends toy to another person but will not release it ▪ Develops object permanence Repeats actions that attract attention and cause laughter Pulls clothes of another to attract attention Plays interactive games such as pat-a-cake Reacts to adult anger; cries when scolded Demonstrates independence in dressing, feeding, locomotive skills, and testing of parents Looks at and follows pictures in a book
	Imitates definite speech sounds	Experiences joy and satisfaction when a task is mastered Reacts to restrictions with frustration Rolls ball to another on request Anticipates body gestures when a familiar nursery rhyme or story is being told (e.g., holds toes and feet in response to "This little piggy went to market") Plays game up-down, "so big," or peekaboo Shakes head for "no"
Discriminates simple geometric forms (e.g., circle) Amblyopia may develop with lack of binocularity Can follow rapidly moving object Controls and adjusts response to sound; listens for sound to recur	▪ Says three to five words besides "dada," "mama" Comprehends meaning of several words (comprehension always precedes verbalization) Recognizes objects by name Imitates animal sounds Understands simple verbal commands (e.g., "Give it to me," "Show me your eyes")	Shows emotions such as jealousy, affection (may give hug or kiss on request), anger, fear Enjoys familiar surroundings and explores away from parent Is fearful in strange situation; clings to parent May develop habit of "security blanket" or favorite toy Has increasing determination to practice locomotor skills ▪ Searches for an object even if it has not been hidden, but searches only where object was last seen

fined as "excessive self-centered and immature behavior, resulting from the failure of parents to enforce consistent, age-appropriate limits" (McIntosh, 1989). Spoiled children demand to have their own way, are inconsiderate of others, and have intrusive, obstructive, and manipulative behavior. Indulging children, combined with clear expectations and limits, does not cause spoiling. But indulgence with failure to provide guidelines for acceptable behavior can result in a "spoiled brat" (McIntosh, 1989).

Several age-related normal behaviors and child characteristics can be mistaken for evidence of spoiling, such as:

- Crying during early infancy that may or may not be associated with colic
- Toddler behaviors such as negativism, persistent exploration, and temper tantrums
- Children with difficult temperaments or attention deficits
- Children experiencing extreme stress from marital discord, abuse, substance abuse, or mental illness in a parent

With anticipatory guidance regarding expected but challenging behaviors and situations that may produce extreme stress in children, parents should feel comfortable in loving their infant without fear of spoiling. However, as the infant gets older, parents need assistance in providing limits that prevent normal, disruptive behaviors, such as temper tantrums, from becoming problems.

Limit-Setting and Discipline

As infants' motor skills advance and mobility increases, parents are faced with the need to set safe limits (see discussion of nurse's role in injury prevention on p. 568). Although there are numerous disciplinary techniques, some are more appropriate for this age than others. Parents can begin discipline using a negative voice and stern eye-to-eye contact. When more definitive measures must be used, one of the most effective approaches is time-out. The basic principles are the same as those discussed in Chapter 3, except that the place for time-out needs to be commensurate with the child's abilities. For example, the playpen is better for most infants than a chair. Although parents may be concerned with instituting discipline during infancy, it is important to stress that the earlier effective disciplinary methods are employed, the easier it is to continue these approaches.

Alternate Child Care Arrangements

For many parents, especially working mothers, the need for locating safe and competent child care facilities for the infant is an increasingly difficult problem—one that is compounded by the number of mothers working outside the home. Over the past 30 years there has been a marked shift in child-care arrangements, with fewer children cared for at home and more children cared for in group centers or other settings.

Types of Child Care. The basic types of care are in-home care, either in the parent's or caregiver's home (family daycare), and center-based care, usually in a daycare center. ***In-home care*** may consist of a full-time baby-sitter who lives in the home, a full-time baby-sitter who comes to the home, cooperative arrangements such as exchange baby-sitting, and family daycare. A licensed ***family daycare home*** typically provides care and protection for up to five children for part of a 24-hour day and does not include informal arrangements such as exchange baby-sitting or caregivers in the child's own home. The five children include the family daycare parents' own children younger than 5 years of age living in the home. Unfortunately, many family daycare homes operate without a license and may care for large numbers of infants without adequate staff and facilities.

Center-based care usually refers to a licensed daycare facility that provides care for six or more children, for 6 or more hours in a 24-hour day. ***Work-based group care*** is another option that is becoming increasingly popular as employers recognize the benefit of quality and convenient child care to their employees. ***Sick-child care*** may also be available for times when the youngster is ill. Such programs are often located in community hospitals (Landis and Chang, 1991).

Guiding Parents in Selecting Child Care. A major nursing responsibility is guiding parents in locating suitable facilities with a well-qualified staff. State licensing agencies can help parents identify daycare centers that accept children of specific age-groups and are convenient to home and work. Their records are available to the public and provide reports from the health, safety, and fire departments, periodic evaluations from the licensing agency, complaints filed against the center, and qualification of the center's employees. State-licensed programs are supposed to abide by established standards, which represent the *minimum* requirements and safeguards. However, enforcement of the standards is sometimes inadequate. Early childhood programs may also belong to a voluntary accreditation system, the National Academy of Early Childhood Programs, which serves as a model for *optimum* care.* References from other parents are also helpful, provided they have investigated the center carefully and have remained involved with the agency's activities.

Other areas for parents to evaluate are the center's daily program, teacher qualifications, nurturing qualities of caregivers, student-to-staff ratio, discipline policy, environmental safety precautions, provision of meals, sanitary conditions, adequate indoor/outdoor space per child, and fee schedule. Although fees vary considerably, a program that charges a minimum fee may also be providing minimum services. In terms of an overall evaluation there is *no substitute for a personal observation of the facility.* Parents should arrange to meet the director and some of the employees, especially those who would be caring for the child. Resources to familiarize parents with characteristics of quality child care and checklists to systematically evaluate the center and make comparisons with other facilities can help parents make successful choices (Green, 1986; Hobbie, 1989; Wong, 1986).†

The same conscientious attention should be applied to locating competent baby-sitters. References from other employers are essential, and there is no substitute for observing the interaction between the individual and the child. Although very young infants need little if any preparation for the introduction of a new caregiver, older infants may benefit from a gradual placement to reduce stranger fear (see Preschool and Kindergarten Experience, Chapter 15). At all times the parent should have the right to visit the child, and regular conferences should be established to review the child's progress.

One of the areas that is increasingly important in selecting child care is the center's health practices. Unfortunately, parents often do not check the center for health and safety features (Rassin and others, 1991). Substantial evidence shows that children, especially those under age 3 years in daycare centers have more illnesses, especially diarrhea, otitis media, respiratory tract infections (especially if the caregiver smokes), hepatitis A, meningitis, and cytomegalovirus, than children cared for in their home (Alho and others, 1993; Hurwitz and others, 1991). The strongest predictor of risk of illness is the number of unrelated children in the room (Bell and others, 1989; Holberg and others, 1993). Parents should inquire about the center's policy regarding attendance and care of sick children (Smith, Shillam, and Zimmerman, 1989).

Another concern is the frequency of injuries in daycare centers and daycare homes. Reports of daycare homes

---

*Information about the accreditation criteria and procedures of the National Academy of Early Childhood Programs is available from the **National Association for the Education of Young Children,** 1834 Connecticut Ave., N.W., Washington, DC 20009; (800) 424-2460 or (202) 232-8777. These criteria are excellent guidelines for evaluating child care facilities.

†Other resources are *Finding the Best Care for Your Infant and Toddler,* available from the National Center for Clinical Infant Programs, 2000 14th St., North Arlington, VA 22201, (703) 528-4300; and *Tips on Selecting the "Right" Day Care Facility,* available from the American Academy of Pediatrics, 141 Northwest Point Blvd., Elk Grove Village, IL 60007, (800) 433-9016 or (708) 228-5005.

found a high rate of safety hazards, even higher than in daycare centers (Turner, Snow, and Poteat, 1993; Wasserman and others, 1989). Other reports indicate that injuries, especially falls on playgrounds, occur frequently in daycare centers (Lee and Bass, 1990; Sacks and others, 1989). What is less clear is whether these risks are greater than those in the child's own home; preliminary data suggest that the risk is not greater (Briss and others, 1994; Rivara and others, 1989). What is clear and distressing is that state regulations for licensed child care have minimal or no criteria for safety, especially in regard to playground, choking, and firearm safety (Runyan and others, 1991).

Nurses play an important role in infection control and injury prevention. Not only can they advise parents regarding the evaluation of a center's sanitary and safety practices, but they can also take an active part in educating staff in measures to minimize transmission of infection and injury. For example, in centers caring for children who are not toilet trained, reducing environmental contamination with urine and feces is an important infection control issue. Studies have shown that disposable superabsorbent diapers contain urine and feces better and result in less environmental contamination than cloth diapers (Kubiak and others, 1993; Van and others, 1991). Nurses can discuss the advantages of disposable versus cloth diapers with staff (Wong and others, 1992). Guidelines for diapering and toileting recently recommended by the American Public Health Association and the American Academy of Pediatrics (1992) include (Fig. 12-13):

1. Handwashing of children and personnel after diaper changing and toileting
2. Use of disposable paper diapers, single-unit reusable cloth diapers with an inner cotton lining attached to an outer waterproof cover, or cloth diapers with a separate overwrap if they are removed as one unit and not reused until cleaned and disinfected
3. Changing diapers as soon as they are soiled
4. Never rinsing cloth diapers, although fecal contents can be flushed down the toilet
5. Sending soiled cloth diapers and clothing home in a sealed plastic bag
6. Cleaning the diaper-changing surface properly and using it only for this purpose

The nurse should also encourage parents to discuss their feelings regarding the child's separation from home, particularly guilt about leaving the child in someone else's care when the parent returns to work. Practical ways of alleviating anxiety and improving the quality of time spent with the child include planning a household schedule that divides major chores into smaller ones, combining household duties with a childcare activity, such as cleaning the bathroom while the child is bathing, and providing time for relaxation and activity with the child.

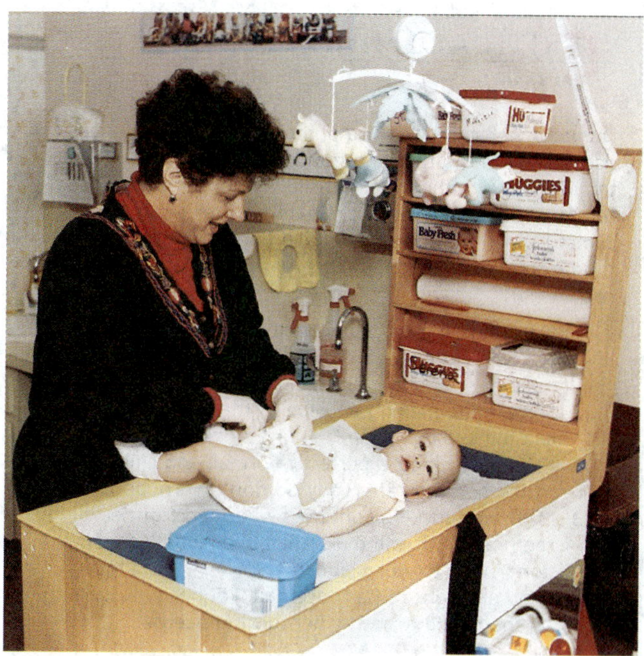

FIG. 12-13 Prevention of urine- and fecal-borne infections requires sanitary practices during diaper changes, such as discarding paper diapers in a covered receptacle, changing paper covers on the diaper-changing surface, and having facilities for handwashing nearby. Soiled cloth diapers and clothing are stored in a plastic bag for transport home.

Thumb-Sucking and Use of Pacifier

Sucking is the infant's chief pleasure, and it may not be satisfied by breast- or bottle-feeding. It is such a strong need that infants who are deprived of sucking, such as those with a cleft lip repair, will suck on their tongue. Some newborns are born with sucking pads on their fingers from in utero sucking activity. Several benefits of nonutritive sucking have been documented, such as increased weight gain in premature infants and decreased crying (Anderson, 1986).

Problems arise when parents are concerned about sucking of fingers, thumb, or pacifier and attempt to restrain this natural tendency. Before giving advice, nurses should investigate the parents' feelings and base guidance on this information (see Critical Thinking Exercise box, p. 540).

During infancy and early childhood there is no need to restrain sucking of fingers or pacifier. Malocclusion may occur if thumb-sucking persists past 4 years of age or when the permanent teeth erupt. There is probably less dental displacement with the use of pacifier than with the use of a hard, rigid finger. Pacifiers may be relinquished earlier than thumbs because they are less readily available. However, there is some evidence that the early introduction of a pacifier (during the first month) may shorten the duration of breast-feeding. Possible explanations include less stimulation of the breasts and less milk production or a sign that breast-feeding difficulties already exist (Victora and others, 1993). The effect of continual use of a pacifier on early speech and language development is unknown, but it is possible that the pacifier may decrease the child's desire to imitate sounds and affect intelligibility. Parents need to be alerted that continual dependency on a pacifier may influence social and speech development (Merrifield and Ryberg, 1985).

Prolonged thumb-sucking in young school-age children may adversely affect their social acceptance. Children ages

CRITICAL THINKING EXERCISE
Thumb-Sucking

During a well-child visit you observe that Mrs. Lopez persistently takes the thumb out of her 10-month-old daughter, Maria's, mouth. You ask if she has concerns about the thumb-sucking. She replies, "Of course. Her teeth are coming in so nice and straight and I don't want the thumb to make them crooked." An appropriate response is:

1. "Sucking on a thumb or pacifier is very common in young children, especially in infants. It satisfies their need to suck and helps them to comfort themselves. Sometimes, making an issue of the sucking can cause it to last longer."
2. "Thumb-sucking is perfectly normal, and children stop when they are ready. So don't worry about it."
3. "If thumb-sucking continues when most of her teeth are in, it will make them crooked. But we don't need to worry about it now."
4. "You are right to be concerned. Let her suck longer on the bottle to satisfy her sucking needs."

The correct answer is 1. The response provides factual information in a nonjudgmental manner that invites further discussion. Options 2 and 3 are partly correct in regard to thumb-sucking but offer premature reassurance. Option 4 is incorrect; at 10 months of age infants should be relying less, not more, on bottle-feeding, which can lead to excessive milk, juice, or other sweetened beverages in place of solid foods and to dental caries (see Weaning, p. 546, and Dental Health, p. 548).

6 to 8 years who viewed slides of children age 7 years who were or were not sucking their thumb rated the thumb-suckers as significantly "less intelligent, happy, attractive, likable, and fun and less desirable as a friend, playmate, seatmate, classmate, and neighbor than when they were in the non-thumb-sucking pose" (Friman and others, 1993).

If the child uses a pacifier, safety considerations in purchasing one must be stressed (see p. 562). To decrease dependence on nonnutritive sucking in young infants, sucking pleasure can be increased by prolonging feeding time. A small-holed, firm nipple causes stronger sucking and slower feeding. Also, the parent's excessive use of the pacifier to calm the child should be explored. It is not unusual for parents to place a pacifier in the infant's mouth as soon as crying begins, thus reinforcing a pattern of distress-relief.

Thumb-sucking reaches its peak at age 18 to 20 months and is most prevalent when the child is hungry or tired. Persistent thumb-sucking in a listless, apathetic child always warrants investigation. It may be a sign of an emotional problem between parent and child or of boredom, isolation, and lack of stimulation.

Treatment for continued sucking of fingers or pacifier in an older child is controversial. Some of the available methods include the use of a bitter substance on the finger (Friman, Barone, and Christopherson, 1986); contracting with the child—using a formal agreement with rewards for meeting a mutually agreed-on goal, (Cipes, Miraglia, and Gaulin-Kremer, 1986); and paradoxical therapy—reframing the situation so that the child finds it unsatisfactory (MacKenzie, 1987).

Teething

One of the more difficult periods in the infant's (and parents') life is the eruption of the deciduous (primary) teeth, often referred to as teething. The age of tooth eruption shows considerable variation among children, but the order of their appearance is fairly regular and predictable (Fig. 12-14). The first primary teeth to erupt are the lower central incisors, which appear at approximately 6 to 8 months of age. These are followed closely by the upper central incisors.

➤ **NURSING TIP** A quick guide to assessment of deciduous teeth during the first 2 years is: *age of the child in months − 6 = number of teeth.* For example: 8 months of age − 6 = 2 teeth at this time.

The exact mechanisms responsible for the eruption of teeth are not fully understood. The growth of the root, dentin, and pulp of the tooth; the pressure exerted against the periodontal tissue; and hormonal control of pituitary growth hormone and thyroid hormone are some of the theories under investigation.

Teething is a physiologic process, and as the crown of the tooth breaks through the periodontal membrane, some discomfort may be experienced. Some children show minimum evidence of teething, such as drooling, increased finger-sucking, or biting on hard objects. Others are very irritable, have difficulty sleeping, and refuse to eat. Generally, signs of illness such as fever, vomiting, or diarrhea are not symptoms of teething but of illness and may warrant further investigation. However, as many parents report, a low-grade temperature is common in the 4- to 19-day period before and on the day of tooth eruption (Jaber, Cohen, and Mor, 1992).

Since teething pain is a result of inflammation, cold is soothing. Giving the child a frozen teething ring or an ice cube wrapped in a washcloth helps relieve the inflammation. Several nonprescription topical anesthetic ointments are available, such as Baby Ora-Jel. The active ingredient in most of them is benzocaine. If these are used, parents are advised to apply them correctly. In the event of persistent irritability that affects sleeping and feeding, systemic analgesics, such as acetaminophen, can be given judiciously. Parents should know that this is a temporary measure.

NURSING ALERT The use of teething powders or procedures such as cutting or rubbing the gums with aspirin are discouraged, because ingestion of the powder, infection or irritation of the tissue, or aspiration of the aspirin can occur.

Infant Shoes

Many parents are unaware of the type of shoes that are appropriate for the older infant and buy expensive infant shoes because of misleading advertising claims. Inflexible shoes that have hard soles can be detrimental by delaying walking, aggravating intoeing and outtoeing, and impeding the development of supportive foot muscles. Therefore counseling parents regarding footwear should begin when

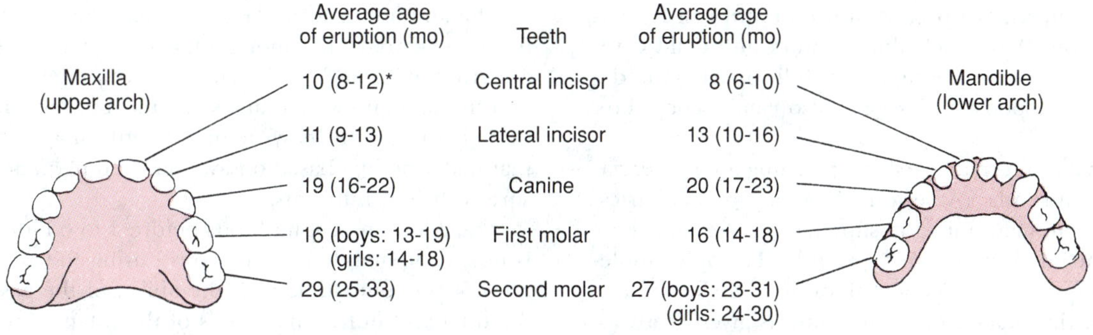

FIG. 12-14 Sequence of eruption of primary teeth. *Range represents ± 1 standard deviation or 67% of subjects studied. (Data from McDonald RE, Avery DR: *Dentistry for the child and adolescent,* ed 6, St Louis, 1994, Mosby.)

infants are 6 months old, well before they are walking (Glendon, 1987).

It is helpful to begin by explaining to parents that changes in the feet occur during infancy and early childhood as locomotion and weight bearing progress. At birth the feet are flat because the arches are protected by fat pads on the soles of the feet. As the bones in the arches develop, the pads disappear and the feet begin to assume a mature shape. A normal arch is determined by proper alignment of all the bones and development of the surrounding musculature, not by the height of the arch.

When children begin walking, the main reason for shoes is *protection.* To provide protection, the shoe should retain its fit, be made of durable material with a smooth interior and few construction seams to irritate the skin, and be soft and flexible, especially in the toe area. A high-top shoe is not necessary for support but may be helpful in keeping the foot in the shoe.

A good shoe conforms to the anatomic shape of the foot, with a rounded toe and sufficient toe room. During weight bearing there should be at least the space of half the width of the thumbnail, or 1.25 cm (½ inch), between the end of the longest toe and the shoe. Roomy and square-toed socks allow for proper growth and alignment. Inexpensive but well-constructed sneakers or soft-leather moccasin-type shoes are suggested as adequate footgear for walking infants.

Even if the shoes are fitted properly, frequent changes are needed to accommodate the infant's rapidly growing feet. Shoe size changes at approximately 3-month intervals between 12 to 36 months; during this time the child's foot should be measured every 3 months (Chong, 1987). Curled toes when shoes are removed and redness and irritation of the skin on the bottom of the toes indicate the need for a larger size.

PROMOTING OPTIMUM HEALTH DURING INFANCY

NUTRITION

Ideally, discussion of optimum nutrition should begin prenatally with the decision to breast- or bottle-feed the infant. The choice for either is highly individual and is discussed in Chapter 8. This section is primarily concerned with infant nutrition during the next 12 months, when growth needs and developmental milestones ready the child for introduction of solid foods. The relatively simple feeding plan for infants, especially during the first 6 months, allows the nurse ample opportunity to educate parents regarding the nutritional needs of their child and to prepare them for the addition of solid foods. This includes education concerning what infants need and do not need.

The First 6 Months

Human milk is the most desirable complete diet for the infant for the first 6 months. The normal infant receiving breast milk from a well-nourished mother needs no specific vitamin and mineral supplements, with the exceptions of fluoride in a dose of 0.25 mg daily (regardless of the fluoride content of the local water supply) and iron by 4 to 6 months of age (when fetal iron stores are depleted) (Calvo, Galindo, and Aspres, 1992; Position statement, 1992). Supplements of 400 IU of vitamin D daily may be indicated if the mother's vitamin D intake is inadequate; some authorities also suggest supplements if the infant does not benefit from adequate ultraviolet light because of dark skin color or little exposure to light (American Academy of Pediatrics, 1993b). However, current concern is focused on too much sun exposure, and some studies provide evidence that vitamin D supplementation may not be necessary (Greer and Marshall, 1989). Even in hot climates, additional fluids are not needed (Brown and others, 1986). Excessive feeding of water may result in water intoxication and failure to thrive.

Employed mothers can continue breast-feeding with guidance and encouragement. Most mothers find that a program of breast-pumping when away from home and bottle-feeding of breast milk, with or without supplemental formula feedings, is successful. Milk can be expressed by hand or pump and safely refrigerated for up to 24 hours. After that time, freezing is suggested (Lawrence, 1994). In addition to efficient breast-pumping, these mothers also cite the need for child care by a trusted agency or individual and support and assistance from significant others (Reifsnider and Myers, 1985). Like all breast-feeding mothers, these women must have proper nutrition and rest for adequate lactation. With a schedule of work and child care, careful planning is required to successfully manage the demands of both responsibilities. (See also Family Focus box on p. 546.)

An acceptable alternative to breast-feeding is commercial iron-fortified formula (American Academy of Pediatrics, 1989b). Like human milk, it supplies all the nutrients needed by the infant for the first 6 months. The only supplementation required is 0.25 mg of fluoride if the local water supply is not fluoridated or if the infant is given ready-to-feed formula, which eliminates the use of fluoridated tap water. Commercially prepared vitamin/iron preparations with or without fluoride are available to meet the specific needs of the infant.

NURSING ALERT If infants are being fed powdered or concentrated formula, they may receive adequate fluoride from tap water but a substantial amount of lead, placing them at risk for lead poisoning. Bottled water is a relatively safe alternative to tap water, but it does not contain fluoride (Shannon and Graef, 1992).

Unmodified whole cow's milk, low-fat cow's milk, and imitation milks are not acceptable as a major source of nutrition for infants because of their altered ability to be digested, increased risk of contamination, and lack of components needed for appropriate growth. Whole milk can cause iron deficiency anemia in infants, presumably from occult gastrointestinal blood loss, although not all research supports this etiology (Fuchs and others, 1993).

NURSING ALERT Whole milk should not be introduced to infants until after 1 year of age (American Academy of Pediatrics, 1993).

TABLE 12-4 Volume of Formula per Feeding and Number of Feedings per Day*

AGE IN MONTHS (MIDPOINT)	FORMULA CONSUMED PER FEEDING (ml)†	(oz)	FEEDINGS PER DAY
1	94.6	3.2	6.6
2	124.2	4.2	6.4
3	162.7	5.5	5.4
4	162.7	5.5	5.5
5	162.7	5.5	4.8
6	177.4	6.0	4.7
7	171.5	5.8	4.4
8	180.4	6.1	4.5
9	168.6	5.7	4.0
10	183.4	6.2	4.0
11	201.1	6.8	4.0
12	174.5	5.9	3.9

From Ross Laboratories, 1989.
*Infants fed human milk or a combination of cow's milk, human milk, and formula are excluded.
†1 fluid ounce = 29.573 ml.

The amount of formula per feeding and the number of feedings per day vary among infants, but general guidelines are given in Table 12-4. Usually infants on demand feeding determine their own feeding schedule, but some infants, especially those with "easy" temperaments, may need a more planned schedule based on average feeding patterns to ensure sufficient nutrients.

The addition of solid foods before 4 to 6 months of age is not recommended. Solid foods during the early months are not yet compatible with the ability of the gastrointestinal tract and nutritional needs of the infant. For example, feeding solids exposes infants to food antigens that may produce food protein allergy.

Developmentally, infants are not ready for solid food. The extrusion (protrusion) reflex is strong and often causes food to be pushed out of the mouth. Infants instinctively suck when given food. Because of their limited motor abilities, infants are unable to deliberately push food away or avoid feeding. Therefore, early introduction of solids is a type of forced feeding that may lead to excessive weight gain (see Thinking Critically About . . . box).

The Second 6 Months

During the second half of the first year human milk or formula continues to be the primary source of nutrition. If breast-feeding is discontinued, commercial iron-fortified formula should be substituted. Formulas specially marked for older infants, such as Good Nature by Carnation Nutritional Products offer no advantages for younger infants and provide excessive protein. Good Nature provides less than the recommended amounts of calories from fat (American Academy of Pediatrics, 1989a; Foeman, Sanders, and Ziegler, 1990).

The major change in feeding habits is the addition of solid foods to the infant's diet. Physiologically and developmentally the infant 4 to 6 months of age is in a transition period. By this time the gastrointestinal tract has matured sufficiently to handle more complex nutrients and is less sensitive to potentially allergenic foods. Tooth eruption is beginning and facilitates biting and chewing. The extrusion reflex has disappeared, and swallowing is more coordinated to allow the infant to easily accept solids. Head control is well developed, permitting infants to sit with support and purposely turn the head away to communicate disinterest in food. Voluntary grasping and improved eye-hand coordination gradually allow infants to pick up finger foods and feed themselves. Their increasing sense of independence is evident in their desire to hold the bottle and try to "help" during feeding. The major developmental milestones associated with feeding are listed in the box on p. 543.

Selection of Foods

The choice of foods to introduce first is variable but should meet the reasons for feeding solids, such as supplying nutrients not found in formula or breast milk. Infant cereal is generally introduced first because of its high iron content (7 mg/3 tablespoons of prepared dry cereal). Commercially prepared ready-to-serve dry cereals include rice, barley, oatmeal, and high-protein cereals, but rice is usually suggested

THINKING CRITICALLY ABOUT . . . *Early Introduction of Solid Foods*

Despite the recommendation to start solid feeding by 4 to 6 months of age, many infants receive solid foods by 2 to 3 months of age. Are they harmed by this practice? To answer this question, Forsyth and others (1993) assessed the relationship between early introduction of solid foods and infant weight gain, gastrointestinal illness, and allergic illnesses during the first 2 years of life. The results were more favorable than those previously reported. Although infants fed solids before 8 to 12 weeks of age were heavier than those introduced to solids at 6 months of age, this difference disappeared at 12 and 24 months. Gastrointestinal disorders were no more frequent in the early-feeding group, although respiratory illness was. In addition the incidence of eczema, an allergy-related dermatitis, was more frequent, but only in the group that was introduced to solids between 8 to 12 weeks of age.

Although more research and a longer follow-up period is needed, these results suggest that a more relaxed approach to early feeding should be considered. Certainly, with all the new adjustment parents have to make, the advice they have to sort out, and the other worries they have, this study brings some balance to the nutritional counseling nurses often do. It is also of interest that when solids are offered at 4 to 6 months of age, infants who are breast-fed are more likely to accept them than infants who are bottle-fed (Sullivan and Birch, 1994).

as an initial food because of its easy digestibility and low allergenic potential. Cereals such as Cream of Farina are not used because infant commercial cereals are a better source of iron. Some of the commercial baby cereals are combined with fruit. There is little nutritional benefit from these preparations, and they are more expensive. Inasmuch as all new foods should be added one at a time, parents should avoid cereal combinations when beginning a new grain.

Infant cereal is mixed with formula until whole milk is given. If the infant is breast-fed, the cereal is mixed with expressed breast milk or water. After 6 months of age, fruit juices can be mixed with the dry cereal; the vitamin C content of the juice enhances the absorption of iron in the cereal. Because of their benefit as a source of iron, infant cereals should be continued until the child is 18 months of age.

Fruit juice can be offered for its rich source of vitamin C and as a substitute for milk for one feeding a day. Large quantities of certain juices, such as apple, pear, prune, sweet cherry, peach, and grape, are avoided because they may cause abdominal pain, diarrhea, or bloating in some children (American Academy of Pediatrics, 1991). Because vitamin C is naturally destroyed by heat, juice is not warmed. Containers of juice are always kept covered and refrigerated to prevent further vitamin loss.

NURSING ALERT Offer fruit juice from a cup, rather than a bottle, to prevent the development of "nursing" caries (see Low-Cariogenic Diet, Chapter 14).

The addition of other foods is arbitrary. A common sequence is strained fruits followed by vegetables and finally meats. If foods are introduced early, citrus fruits, meats, and eggs are still delayed until after 6 months of age because of their potential to result in allergy. At 6 months foods such as a cracker or zwieback can be offered as a type of finger and teething food. By 8 to 9 months junior foods and nutritious finger foods, such as a firmly cooked vegetable, raw pieces of fruit (except grapes), or cheese, can be given. By 1 year well-cooked table foods are served.

Commercially prepared baby foods are the most commonly used types of food served to infants in the United States. They are convenient, contain no added salt or sugar, but are relatively expensive. An alternative is preparing baby foods at home, which is a simple and inexpensive process. Fruits and vegetables can be steamed in a small amount of water and pureed in a blender or food processor. Many of them, such as ripe banana, can be mashed fine with a fork. Fruits such as apples or pears require little or no water in the cooking process. Vegetables such as carrots, potatoes,

DEVELOPMENTAL MILESTONES ASSOCIATED WITH FEEDING

AGE (MONTHS)	BEHAVIOR
Birth	Sucking, rooting, and swallowing reflexes Feels hunger and indicates desire for food by crying; expresses satiety by falling asleep Extrusion reflex is strong
3-4	Extrusion reflex is fading Beginning eye-hand coordination
4-5	Can approximate lips to the rim of a cup
5-6	Can use fingers to feed self a cracker
6-7	Chews and bites May hold own bottle, but may not drink from it (prefers for it to be held)
7-9	Refuses food by keeping lips closed; has preferences Holds a spoon and plays with it during feeding May drink from a straw Drinks from a cup with assistance
9-12	Picks up small morsels of food (finger foods) and feeds self Holds own bottle and drinks from it Drinks from a cup but spills some of the contents Uses a spoon with much spilling

or string beans require additional water in the cooking and blending process.

Preferably, home-prepared infant foods should be fresh or frozen, because canned foods, other than those prepared for infants, may have excessive sodium or sugar or be a source of lead from the container. If sweetening is needed, refined sugar can be used, but honey and corn syrup are avoided because of the risk of infant botulism (Wilkinson and Clore, 1988). There is no evidence that the addition of salt to foods, such as peas, increases the infant's acceptance of the new food (Sullivan and Birch, 1994).

Food Storage

Storage of commercial baby food requires a few simple rules. Unopened jars can remain on the shelf indefinitely. Opened jars are refrigerated and can be used for a couple of days. If the infant does not finish a jar of food at one time, a portion of the food is removed from the jar using a clean spoon. If this is not done, bacteria are introduced, and the salivary enzymes on the feeding spoon begin to digest unused portions of the food. The dried baby foods are prepared in individual portions, thus eliminating storage problems and waste of unused food.

For convenience home-prepared baby foods can be made in advance and frozen in small jars or in special plastic bags that are sealed by heat and can be reheated by being placed in boiling water. If microwave heating is used, the food is mixed thoroughly and checked to ensure a safe temperature before feeding. The temperature of the container may not indicate the heat intensity of the food (resulting in an oral burn). Individual portions of food can be frozen in ice cube trays, transferred to a large container, and individually defrosted as needed. With reasonable care in the preparation and storing of foods there is little need to worry about bacterial contamination.

NURSING ALERT Although microwaving of bottles and baby food is not recommended, it remains a common practice. Guidelines have been developed for microwave heating of refrigerated formula, and these should be given to the family (see Family Home Care box).

Method of Introduction

When the spoon is first introduced, infants often push it away and appear dissatisfied. Some patience and skill are required to overcome this initial response. A small-bowled, straight, long-handled spoon, similar to a demitasse spoon, allows a small portion of food to be placed toward the back of the tongue. If food is placed on the front of the tongue and pushed out, it is simply scooped up and refed. As infants become accustomed to the spoon, they will more eagerly accept the food and eventually open the mouth in anticipation (or keep it closed in dislike). Since the first introduction of food is a new experience, spoon feeding should be attempted after ingestion of some breast milk or formula to associate this activity with a pleasurable and satisfying experience. Trying to introduce a food *after* the entire milk feeding is usually useless because the infant is satiated and has no inclination to try something new.

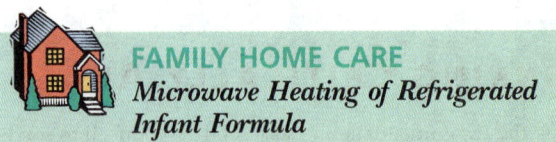

FAMILY HOME CARE
Microwave Heating of Refrigerated Infant Formula

Prior to heating
- Heat only 4 oz or more
- Heat only *refrigerated* formula
- Always *stand* the bottle up
- Always leave bottle top *uncovered* to allow heat to escape

Heating instructions (full power)
- 4-oz bottles
  - Heat for no more than 30 seconds
- 8-oz bottles
  - Heat for no more than 45 seconds

Serving instructions
- Always replace nipple assembly; *invert* 10 times (vigorous shaking is unnecessary)
- Formula should be cool to the touch; formula warm to the touch may be too hot to serve
- Always *test* formula; place several drops on your tongue or on top of the hand (not the inside wrist)

From Sigman-Grant M, Bush G, Anantheswaran R: Microwave heating of infant formula: a dilemma resolved, *Pediatrics* 90(3):414, 1992.

After several spoon feedings, food can be introduced at the beginning of a meal. It is best to introduce many foods during the first year, when the infant is more likely to eat them because of a hearty appetite resulting from a rapid growth rate. During the toddler years eating becomes less of an adventure, and strong food preferences become evident.

One food item is introduced at intervals of 4 to 7 days to allow for identification of food allergies. New foods are fed in small amounts, from 1 teaspoon to a few tablespoons. As the amount of solid food increases, the quantity of milk is decreased to less than 1 L daily to prevent overfeeding.

Because feeding is a learning process as well as a means of nutrition, new foods are given alone to allow the child to learn new tastes and textures. Sometimes it is necessary to camouflage a new food by mixing it with another favorite food to encourage the child to try it, although this should not become a routine. Food should not be mixed in the bottle and fed through a nipple with a large hole. This deprives the child of the pleasure of learning new tastes and developing a discriminating palate. It can also cause problems with poor chewing of food later in life because this experience is lacking. Guidelines for the introduction of new foods are given in the Family Home Care box on p. 545.*

Introducing solid foods can be an exciting time for parent and child. Most infants are good eaters and enjoy eating from a spoon and later feeding themselves. However, the transition from "parent doing it" to "baby doing it" can

*A recommended resource is *Starting Solids: A Guide for Parents and Child Care Providers,* available from the National Association of Pediatric Nurse Associates and Practitioners (NAPNAP), 1101 Kings Highway North, Suite 206, Cherry Hill, NJ 08034-1931.

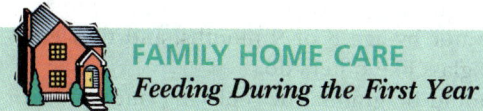

FAMILY HOME CARE
Feeding During the First Year

BIRTH TO 6 MONTHS (BREAST- OR BOTTLE-FEEDING)

Breast-Feeding

Most desirable complete diet for first half of year.*

Requires supplements of fluoride (0.25 mg), regardless of the fluoride content of the local water supply, and iron by 6 months of age.

Requires supplements of vitamin D (400 units) if mother's diet is inadequate.

Formula

Iron-fortified commercial formula is a complete food for the first half of the year.*

Requires fluoride supplements (0.25 mg) when the concentration of fluoride in the drinking water is below 0.3 parts per million (ppm).

Evaporated milk formula requires supplements of vitamin C, iron, and fluoride (in accordance with the fluoride content of the local water supply).

6 TO 12 MONTHS (SOLID FOODS)

May begin to add solids by 5 to 6 months of age.

First foods are strained, pureed, or finely mashed.

Finger foods such as teething crackers, raw fruit, or vegetables can be introduced by 6 to 7 months.

Chopped table food or commercially prepared junior foods can be started by 9 to 12 months.

With the exception of cereal, the order of introducing foods is variable; a recommended sequence is weekly introduction of other foods, beginning with fruit, then vegetables, and then meat.

As the quantity of solids increases, the amount of formula should be limited to approximately 900 ml (30 oz) daily

Method of Introduction:

Introduce solids when infant is hungry.

Begin spoon feeding by pushing food to back of tongue because of infant's natural tendency to thrust tongue forward.

Use small spoon with straight handle; begin with 1 or 2 teaspoons of food; gradually increase to 2 to 3 tablespoons per feeding.

Introduce one food at a time, usually at intervals of 4 to 7 days, to identify food allergies.

As the amount of solid food increases, decrease the quantity of milk to prevent overfeeding.

Never introduce foods by mixing them with the formula in the bottle.

Cereal

Introduce commercially prepared iron-fortified infant cereals and administer daily until 18 months.

Rice cereal is usually introduced first because of its low allergenic potential.

Can discontinue supplemental iron once cereal is given.

Fruits and vegetables

Applesauce, bananas, and pears are usually well tolerated.

Avoid fruits and vegetables marketed in cans that are not specifically designed for infants because of variable and sometimes high lead content and addition of salt, sugar, and/or preservatives.

Offer fruit juice only from a cup, not a bottle, to reduce the development of "nursing caries."

Meat, fish, and poultry

Avoid fatty meats.

Prepare by baking, broiling, steaming, or poaching.

Include organ meats such as liver, which has a high iron, vitamin A, and vitamin B complex content.

If soup is given, be sure all ingredients are familiar to child's diet.

Avoid commercial meat/vegetable combinations because protein is low.

Eggs and cheese

Serve egg yolk hard boiled and mashed, soft cooked, or poached.

Introduce egg white in small quantities (1 tsp) toward end of first year to detect an allergy.

Use cheese as a substitute for meat and as finger food.

*Breast-feeding or commercial formula feeding for up to 12 months of age is recommended. After 1 year whole cow's milk can be given.

be a trying experience, particularly for those who value a clean house or who view cleaning up the mess as a waste of time. The infant's first, second, and often twentieth try at self-feeding or cup feeding is a sloppy experience. Finger foods such as soft fruits or vegetables are just as good playthings as food; they can be squeezed, smeared, squashed, and thoroughly painted on oneself, others, and the surrounding environment. However, all of this is part of learning, and mastery follows many accidents.

If parents find this experience distressing, a few suggestions may prove helpful. The feeding area should have a floor that can be easily wiped and is relatively far from walls, upholstered furniture, or drapes. A hand-held portable vacuum is helpful in cleaning up crumbs. Messes are confined to one area if the child is seated in a high chair rather than allowed to crawl or walk around while drinking or eating. Infants should be expected to get themselves covered with food; therefore a large bib (plastic can be wiped easily but needs to be removed after feeding) should be used, as well as washable clothes that are easily removed. High chairs can be thoroughly cleaned in a shower. Outdoor dining provides an excellent opportunity for practicing with a cup, spoon, or fingers because accidents are simple to hose or sweep away. Children cannot be pressured into eating neatly or developing table manners before manipulative skill is acquired.

If older infants suddenly refuse to eat, the feeding process should be investigated. It is not unusual for an 11-month-old infant to become stubborn, push the spoon away, and refuse to open the mouth. He or she may not be content with having a spoon to play with while someone else does the feeding. Helping parents understand the child's growing need for independence may prevent many temper tantrums and power struggles later on.

Weaning

Defined as the process of giving up one method of feeding for another, ***weaning*** usually refers to relinquishing the breast or bottle for a cup. In Western societies this is generally regarded as a major task for infants and is frequently seen as a potentially traumatic experience. It is psychologically significant because the infant is required to give up a major source of oral pleasure and gratification.

There is no one time for weaning that is best for every child, but generally most infants show signs of readiness during the second half of the first year. They have learned that good things come from a spoon. Their increasing desire for freedom of movement may lessen their desire to be held close for feedings. They are acquiring more control over their actions and can easily manipulate a cup to their lips (even if it is held upside down!). Imitation becomes a powerful motivator by age 8 or 9 months, and they enjoy using a cup or glass like others do.

Weaning should be gradual by replacing one bottle- or breast-feeding at a time. The last feeding to be discontinued is usually the nighttime feeding. It is advisable to never begin allowing a child to take a bottle of milk to bed, because this is a major cause of dental caries in deciduous teeth. If breast-feeding is terminated before 5 or 6 months of age, weaning should be to a bottle to provide for the infant's continued sucking needs. If discontinued later, weaning can be directly to a cup, especially by age 12 to 14 months (Baby bottle, 1993).

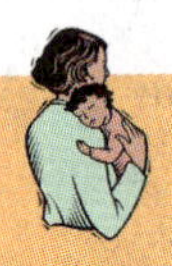

FAMILY FOCUS

Breast-Feeding and Infant Sleep Patterns

Sleep patterns vary greatly among infants, with temperament and type of feeding considered important factors. Typically, bottle-fed infants sleep through the night sooner than breast-fed infants. However, a study by Pinilla and Birch (1993) demonstrated that the sleep pattern of breast-fed infants could be modified to encourage longer nighttime sleep intervals—a possible benefit for the working mother and an incentive to continue breast-feeding. A two-step procedure of behavioral training was used.

The first phase began soon after birth. The parents were instructed to try not to hold, rock, or nurse their infants to sleep; to accentuate differences in environmental cues for day and nighttime hours (e.g., high levels of stimulation during the day but low levels during the night); to feed the infant at a focal feeding time each night (between 10:00 PM and midnight); and to make sure the infant was really complaining before picking him or her up.

When the infant was 3 weeks old, the second phase began. The goal was to "stretch" nighttime feeding intervals by breaking the association between awakening at night (between midnight and 5:00 AM) and being fed. Parents were instructed not to leave the infant alone crying; rather, alternative interventions were encouraged: reswaddling, patting, diapering, or walking the infant in lieu of feeding. If, after these interventions, the infant continued to cry, then a feeding was offered.

The results: by 8 weeks all of the "trained" breast-fed infants slept from midnight to 5:00 AM, compared with 23% of the untrained (control) group. Both groups had similar milk intakes and weight gain. This research indicates that frequent night waking and feeding is not an essential element of breast-feeding. Nurses can offer suggestions to parents to prolong nighttime sleep for the infant and themselves. In fact many of the steps in the training plan help prevent the development of problems associated with nighttime feeding and night crying—regardless of the feeding method.

SLEEP AND ACTIVITY

Sleep patterns vary among infants, and active infants typically sleep less than placid children. Generally, by 3 to 4 months of age most infants have developed a nocturnal pattern of sleep lasting from 9 to 11 hours. The total daily sleep is about 15 hours. The number of naps per day varies, but by the end of a year infants may take one or two naps. Breast-fed infants usually sleep for less prolonged periods, with more frequent waking, especially during the night, than do bottle-fed infants. Because of the trend toward breast-feeding, sleep norms such as those described above, which were based primarily on bottle-fed infants, may not be relevant (Butte, Smith, and Garza, 1990). (See also Family Focus box; for a discussion of sleep position, see Sudden Infant Death Syndrome, Chapter 13.)

Most infants are naturally active and need no encouragement to be mobile. However, problems can arise when devices such as playpens, strollers, commercial swings, and walkers are used excessively. These restrict movement and prevent infants from exploring and developing gross motor skills. Contrary to popular belief, walkers do not enhance coordination and are dangerous if tipped over or placed near stairs (Rieder, Schwartz, and Newman, 1986).

NURSING ALERT Formal infant exercise programs do not provide any long-term benefit to normal infants, and the possibility for damage to the infant's skeletal system exists. For these reasons, such programs are not recommended (American Academy of Pediatrics, 1988).

Sleep Problems

Concerns regarding sleep are common during infancy. Sometimes they are as basic as parents' questioning if the infant needs additional sleep. In this case it is best to investigate the reason for their concern, stressing the individual needs of each child. Infants who are active during wakeful periods and who are growing normally are sleeping a sufficient amount of time.

However, there are a number of more serious concerns that require intervention. Sleep disturbances of physiologic origin are rare with the exception of colic, which is discussed in Chapter 13. The more common sleep disturbances are a learned pattern or developmental characteristic of some infants (Table 12-5). Although many families

TABLE 12-5 Selected Sleep Disturbances During Infancy and Early Childhood

DISORDER/DESCRIPTION	MANAGEMENT
NIGHTTIME FEEDING*	
Child has a prolonged need for middle-of-night bottle- or breast-feeding Child goes to sleep at the breast or with a bottle Awakenings are frequent (may be hourly) Child returns to sleep after feeding; other comfort measures (e.g., rocking or holding) are usually ineffective	Increase daytime feeding intervals to 4 hours or more (may need to be done gradually) Offer last feeding as late as possible at night; may need to gradually reduce amount of formula for length of breast-feeding Offer no bottles in bed Put to bed *awake* When child is crying, check at progressively longer intervals each night; reassure child but do not hold, rock, take to parent's bed, or give bottle or pacifier
DEVELOPMENTAL NIGHT CRYING	
Child age 6-12 months with undisturbed nighttime sleep now awakes abruptly; may be accompanied by nightmares	Reassure parents that this is temporary phase Enter room immediately to check on child but keep reassurances *brief* Avoid feeding, rocking, taking to parent's bed, or any other routine that may initiate trained night crying
TRAINED NIGHT CRYING* (INAPPROPRIATE SLEEP ASSOCIATIONS)	
Child typically falls asleep in place other than own bed (e.g., rocking chair or parent's bed) and is brought to own bed while asleep; on awakening, cries until usual routine is instituted (e.g., rocking)	Put child in own bed when *awake* If possible, arrange separate sleeping area from other family members When child is crying, check at progressively longer intervals each night; reassure child but do not resume usual routine
REFUSAL TO GO TO SLEEP*	
Child resists bedtime and comes out of room repeatedly Nighttime sleep may be continuous, but frequent awakenings and refusal to return to sleep may occur and become a problem if parent allows child to deviate from usual sleep pattern	Evaluate if hour of sleep is too early (child may resist sleep if not tired) Assist parents in establishing consistent before-bedtime routine and enforcing consistent limits regarding child's bedtime behavior If child persists in leaving bedroom, close door for progressively longer periods Use reward system with child to provide motivation
NIGHTTIME FEARS	
Child resists going to bed or wakes during the night because of fears Child seeks parent's physical presence and with parent nearby, falls asleep easily, unless fear is overwhelming	Evaluate if hour of sleep is too early (child may fantasize when nothing to do but think in dark room) Calmly reassure the frightened child; keeping a nightlight on may be helpful Use reward system with child to provide motivation to deal with fears Avoid patterns that can lead to additional problems (e.g., sleeping with child or taking child to parent's room) If child's fear is overwhelming, consider desensitization (e.g., progressively spending longer periods of time alone; consult professional help for protracted fears) Distinguish between nightmares and sleep terrors (confused partial arousals) (see Table 15-3)

Modified from Ferber R: Behavioral "insomnia" in the child, *Psychiatr Clin North Am* 10(4):641-653, 1987.
*Guidelines for parents in dealing with these sleep problems are in *Wong and Whaley's Clinical Manual of Pediatric Nursing* (Mosby).

may report sleep problems that are typical of these patterns, interventions are offered *only* when the pattern is disruptive to the family (see Cultural Awareness box , p. 548).

However, when a sleeping problem is presented, a careful assessment is essential (see box on p. 202 in Chapter 6). Charting sleep habits both before and after interventions is also an important strategy.* Questions regarding the frequency and duration of waking, the usual bedtime routine, the number of nighttime feedings, the perceived problem (e.g., how much disruption the behavior generates), and the attempted interventions are important in planning effective approaches designed for the specific sleep problem. A common suggestion given for any type of sleep problem—"let the child cry until falling asleep"—is very difficult to implement and is inappropriate for certain conditions. Once the parents relent and console the child, they have only reinforced the crying.

*A 2-week sleep record for families is available in *Wong and Whaley's Clinical Manual of Pediatric Nursing* (Mosby).

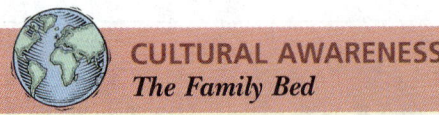

CULTURAL AWARENESS
The Family Bed

Cosleeping, or the "family bed," in which parents allow the children to sleep with them, is a relatively common and accepted practice, especially among black, Hispanic, and Asian families, such as the Japanese (Schachter and others, 1989). Other groups that are adopting cosleeping include (1) single parents, whose need for company may encourage this practice; (2) working parents, who desire the closeness at night that was lost during the day; and (3) parents who have had an issue about sleep or separation in their own past (Brazelton, 1990).

An equally effective and more atraumatic approach to night crying, known as ***graduated extinction,*** is to let the child cry for progressively longer times between *brief* parental interventions that consist only of reassurance, not rocking, holding, or using the bottle or pacifier. For example, the parents may check on the child every 5 minutes during the first night and progressively extend this interval by 5 minutes on successive nights (Ferber, 1985).

Families who cannot tolerate the unexpected crying spells while everyone else is asleep can try the two-step approach. Graduated extinction is used during naps and at bedtime until the parents retire. If the child cries during the night, the parents use comforting measures. However, once the child is partially trained, step 2 is initiated—the use of graduated extinction at all times (Schmitt, 1992).

The best way to prevent sleep problems is to encourage parents to establish bedtime rituals that do not foster problematic patterns. One of the most constructive is placing infants *awake* in their own crib. When infants are accustomed to falling asleep somewhere else, such as in their parent's arms, and then being transferred to their crib, they awaken in unfamiliar surroundings and are unable to fall asleep until the routine is repeated (Anders, Halpern, and Hua, 1992). Also, the bed should be used for sleeping only—not as a playpen. It is advisable not to hang playthings over or on the bed; in this way the child associates the bed with sleep—not with activity. Although these interventions described above and in Table 12-5 are usually successful, it is much easier to prevent the problem with appropriate counseling during the early months of the infant's life.*

DENTAL HEALTH

Good dental hygiene begins as soon as the primary teeth erupt. The teeth and gums are initially cleaned by being wiped with a damp cloth; toothbrushing is too harsh for the tender gingiva. The caregiver can stabilize the infant by cradling the child with one arm and using the free hand to cleanse the teeth. Oral hygiene can be made pleasant by singing or talking to the infant. There are no clear guidelines as to when toothbrushing should begin. However, it is generally recommended that as more teeth erupt and the infant adjusts to the routine of cleaning, a small, soft-bristled toothbrush can be used. Water is preferred to toothpaste, which the infant will swallow (and if the toothpaste is fluoridated, the infant will ingest excessive amounts of fluoride) (Nowak, 1993).

Fluoride, an essential mineral for building caries-resistant teeth, is needed during infancy when unerupted teeth are developing. Fluoride supplements are prescribed as appropriate for:

- All infants 2 weeks of age or older who live in areas with suboptimum levels of fluoride in the local water supply
- Exclusively breast-fed infants, regardless of the fluoride content of the local water supply
- Infants who consume relatively little fluoridated tap water, such as those receiving ready-to-serve formula

Dietary considerations are also important because habits begun during infancy tend to continue into later years. Foods with concentrated sugar are used sparingly (if at all) in the infant's diet. The practice of coating pacifiers with honey or using commercially available hard-candy pacifiers is discouraged. Besides being cariogenic, honey also may cause infant botulism, and parts of the candy pacifier can be aspirated (Ramsey, Goldbach, and Stephenson, 1989) (see p. 562). Parents need to be counseled regarding the detrimental effects of frequent and prolonged bottle- or breast-feeding during sleep, when the sweet milk or other fluid, such as juice, bathes the teeth, producing ***nursing caries.*** (See also Chapter 14 for a more extensive discussion of dental care, including nursing caries.)

IMMUNIZATIONS

One of the most dramatic advances in pediatrics has been the decline of infectious diseases over the past 60 years because of the widespread use of immunization for preventable diseases. Although many of the presently available immunizations can be given to individuals of any age, the recommended primary schedule begins during infancy and, with the exception of boosters, is completed during early childhood. Therefore the discussion of childhood immunizations for diphtheria, tetanus, pertussis or acellular pertussis (DTP or DTaP); polio; measles, mumps, rubella (MMR); *Haemophilus influenzae* type b (Hib); and hepatitis B virus (HBV) is included under health promotion during infancy. Selected vaccines that are generally reserved for children considered at high risk for the disease are discussed here and as appropriate throughout the text. (See also Communicable Diseases, Chapter 16, for a discussion of several of the diseases for which vaccines are available.) All vaccines currently licensed for use in the United States are listed in the box on p. 549.

To facilitate an understanding of immunizations, key terms are defined in the box on p. 550. Although in this discussion the terms *vaccination* and *immunization* are used interchangeably in reference to active immunization, they are not synonymous, because the administration of an immunobiologic cannot automatically be equated with the development of adequate immunity.

*An excellent resource for parents is *Solve Your Child's Sleep Problems* by R. Ferber (1985, Simon & Schuster).

LICENSED VACCINES AND TOXOIDS AVAILABLE IN THE UNITED STATES AND RECOMMENDED ROUTES OF ADMINISTRATION

VACCINE/ROUTE

Adenovirus*/oral
Anthrax/subcutaneous
Bacillus of Calmette and Guérin (BCG)/intradermal or percutaneous
Cholera/subcutaneous or intradermal†
Diphtheria-tetanus-pertussis (DTP)/intramuscular
DTP–*Haemophilus influenzae* type b conjugate (DTP-Hib)/intramuscular
Diphtheria-tetanus-acellular pertussis (DTaP)/intramuscular
Hepatitis B/intramuscular‡
Haemophilus influenzae type b conjugate (Hib)/intramuscular
Influenza/intramuscular
Japanese encephalitis/subcutaneous
Measles/subcutaneous
Measles-mumps-rubella (MMR)/subcutaneous
Meningococcal/subcutaneous
Mumps/subcutaneous
Pertussis/intramuscular
Plague/intramuscular
Pneumococcal/intramuscular or subcutaneous
Poliovirus vaccine, inactivated (IPV)/subcutaneous
Poliovirus vaccine, oral (OPV)
Rabies/intramuscular or intradermal§
Rubella/subcutaneous
Tetanus/intramuscular
Tetanus-diphtheria (Td or DT)/intramuscular
Typhoid (parenteral)/subcutaneous‖
Typhoid (Ty21a)/oral
Varicella/subcutaneous
Yellow fever/subcutaneous

Modified from Centers for Disease Control and Prevention: General recommendations on immunization: recommendations of the Advisory Committee on Immunization Practices (ACIP), *MMWR* 43(RR-1):4, 1994.
*Available only to the U.S. Armed Forces.
†The intradermal dose is lower than the subcutaneous dose.
‡Not administered in dorsogluteal muscle (buttock) because of possible reduced immunization response.
§The intradermal dose of rabies vaccine, human diploid cell (HDCV), is lower than the intramuscular dose and is used only for preexposure vaccination. **Rabies vaccine, adsorbed (RVA) should not be used intradermally.**
‖Booster doses may be administered intradermally unless vaccine that is acetone-killed and dried is used.

Current Status of Immunizations

The routine use of immunizations has dramatically altered the morbidity and mortality from once common and feared childhood diseases. Unfortunately, with success have come both complacency and unwarranted fears that have resulted in unacceptably low immunization rates among children. Although 71% to 96% of children in the United States are *completely* vaccinated before or shortly after starting school, the levels are as low as 11% to 58% in children 2 years of age—the most vulnerable group for developing vaccine-preventable diseases (Zell and others, 1994). The measles epidemic of 1989 to 1991 resulted in over 55,000 reported cases and 132 suspected deaths from measles (Measles, 1993). The cause of the epidemic was attributed to failure to vaccinate children at 12 to 15 months of age (National Vaccine Advisory Committee, 1991). The response to the measles resurgence was a nationwide campaign to immunize all susceptible individuals. This trend was sharply reversed in 1993 when incidences of vaccine-preventable diseases were at or near their lowest reported levels. To emphasize the continuing need to achieve and maintain high vaccination levels among children, particularly those ages birth to 2 years, a comprehensive response to undervaccination in the United States was initiated. The program's goals are (1) to eliminate cases of vaccine-preventable diseases by 1996, (2) to increase all recommended vaccinations among 2-year-olds to at least 90% by 1996, and (3) to establish an effective vaccination-delivery service (Reported vaccine-preventable disease, 1994). To accomplish these goals, the National Vaccine Advisory Committee (NVAC) has developed 18 standards that include (1) improving the quality and quantity of vaccination-delivery services, (2) increasing community participation and education, (3) reducing vaccine costs for consumers, (4) improving surveillance for coverage and disease, and (5) adhering to current recommendations, especially in regard to *true* contraindications (see Table 12-14) (Centers for Disease Control and Prevention, 1993a).

Unfounded fears regarding side effects of vaccines, especially DTP, have also had an impact on immunization rates and vaccine production. Concerns about DTP vaccine causing sudden infant death syndrome (SIDS) and pertussis vaccine resulting in permanent neurologic damage have caused many families to bring lawsuits against vaccine producers, causing a drastic increase in vaccine costs and at one time prompting some manufacturers to stop vaccine production. The Institute of Medicine (IOM) (1993) found no evidence for diphtheria and tetanus toxoids causing encephalopathy, infantile spasms, or SIDS. They did find a relationship between DTP vaccination and acute encephalopathy occurring within 7 days of the vaccination. This association occurs rarely—at a rate of 0 to 10.5/million immunizations—and probably occurs in children with an underlying neurologic disorder.

In response to the concerns of manufactures, practitioners, and parents of children with serious vaccine-associated injuries, the ***National Childhood Vaccine Injury Act (NCVIA)*** of 1986 and the ***Vaccine Compensation Amendments*** of 1987 were passed. Basically, these laws are designed to provide fair compensation for children who are inadvertently injured and provide greater protection from liability for vaccine manufacturers and providers. The NCVIA is concerned with DTP, MMR, and oral and inactivated polio vaccines (IPVs), as well as with selected postvaccine events such as anaphylaxis, encephalopathy, seizures, paralytic poliomyelitis, or death (Golden, 1993; National Childhood Vaccine Injury Act, 1988).

Practitioners are required to fully inform families of the risks and benefits of the vaccines. The U.S. Public Health Service has developed a series of vaccine information pamphlets (VIPs) for the vaccines of concern in the NCVIA. However, the pamphlets are detailed and written

KEY IMMUNIZATION TERMS

Immunization—Inclusive term denoting the process of inducing or providing active or passive immunity *artificially* by administering an immunobiologic

Immunity—An inherited or acquired state in which an individual is resistant to the occurrence or the effects of a specific disease, particularly an infectious agent

Natural immunity—Innate immunity or resistance to infection or toxicity

Acquired immunity—Immunity from exposure to the invading agent, either bacteria, virus, or toxin

Active immunity—Immune bodies are actively formed against specific antigens, either *naturally* by having had the disease clinically or subclinically or *artificially* by introducing the antigen into the individual.

Passive immunity—Temporary immunity by transfusing immune globulins or antitoxins either *artificially* from another human or from an animal that has been actively immunized against an antigen or *naturally* from the mother to the fetus via the placenta

Antibody—A protein, found mostly in serum, that is formed in response to exposure to a specific antigen.

Antigen—A variety of foreign substances, including bacteria, viruses, toxins, and foreign proteins that stimulate the formation of antibodies

Attenuate—Reduce the virulence (infectiousness) of a pathogenic microorganism by such measures as treating it with heat or chemicals or cultivating it on a certain medium

Immunobiologic—Antigenic substances, such as vaccines and toxoids, or antibody-containing preparations, such as globulins and antitoxins, from human or animal donors, used for active or passive immunization or therapy

Vaccine—A suspension of live (usually attenuated) or inactivated microorganisms (e.g., bacteria, viruses, or rickettsiae) or fractions of the microorganism administered to induce immunity and prevent infectious disease or its sequelae

Toxoid—A modified bacterial toxin that has been made nontoxic but retains the ability to stimulate the formation of antitoxin

Antitoxin—A solution of antibodies (e.g., diphtheria antitoxin and botulinum antitoxin) derived from the serum of animals immunized with specific antigens and used to confer passive immunity and for treatment

Immune globulin (IG) or ***intravenous immune globulin (IGIV)***—A sterile solution containing antibodies from large pools of human blood plasma; primarily indicated for routine maintenance of immunity of certain immunodeficient persons and for passive immunization against measles and hepatitis A

Specific immune globulins—Special preparations obtained from blood plasma from donor pools preselected for a high antibody content against a specific antigen (e.g., hepatitis B immune globulin, varicella-zoster immune globulin, rabies immune globulin, tetanus immune globulin, vaccinia immune globulin, and cytomegalovirus immune globulin); like IG and IGIV, do not transmit hepatitis B virus, human immunodeficiency virus (HIV), or other infectious diseases

Vaccination—Originally meant inoculation with vaccinia smallpox virus to make a person immune to smallpox; currently denotes the physical act of administering any vaccine or toxoid

at a higher reading level than is appropriate for many families. Therefore health professionals need to be aware of the importance of providing parents with sufficient time to read the information, discussing the vaccines to determine caregivers' understanding, addressing parents' concerns, and dispelling unfounded fears. Since nurses frequently administer vaccines during health supervision visits, they may have the responsibility for adequately informing parents of the nature, prevalence, and risks of the disease; the type of immunization product to be used; expected benefits; the risk of side effects; and the need for accurate immunization records. Referring to immunizations as "baby shots" and limiting the discussion to vague statements about the vaccines are unacceptable practices.

Strategies that may increase compliance include giving parents vaccine information at the time of the newborn's discharge, mailing reminder cards, making immunization services readily available, removing barriers to vaccination (such as long waiting times and appointment-only systems), and taking every opportunity to immunize children when they enter a health care facility (such as emergency departments, clinics, private offices, and hospitals) (Bell and others, 1994; Houtrouw and Carlson, 1993; Szilagyi and others, 1993).

During the past few years, many new vaccines have been developed and are either being used (highly purified acellular pertussis, HBV, and Hib vaccines) or are being considered for use (hepatitis A and varicella vaccines; see p. 555). The benefits of these advances are now being realized, such as dramatic declines in the incidence of Hib disease, especially epiglottitis and bacterial meningitis, since the vaccine was introduced in 1985 (Gorelick and Baker, 1994; Schoendorf and others, 1994).

However, not all recommendations for vaccines are universally accepted. The controversy over universal infant hepatitis B immunization centers around concerns about the epidemiology of hepatitis B, economic considerations, and doubts regarding long-term immunity. Some critics assert that because the disease is fairly rare in the United States, any immunity gained from the vaccine may very well wear off before exposure occurs; this, they argue, will mean a great deal of expense with little benefit. Those for the vaccine assert that immunizing only high-risk individuals will keep prices high and that avoiding putting the health of any child at risk is the best reason for implementing this schedule until a better alternative is found (McEwen, 1993; Zanga, 1993). The benefit of universal HBV immunization remains to be seen.

Schedule for Immunizations

In the United States two organizations—the **Advisory Committee on Immunization Practices (ACIP)** of the U.S. Public Health Service Centers for Disease Control and Prevention (CDC) and the **Committee on Infectious Diseases of** the American Academy of Pediatrics (AAP)—govern the recommendations for immunization policies and procedures. In Canada, recommendations are from the **National Advisory Committee on Immunization** under the authority of the Minister of National Health and Welfare. Because ACIP is concerned primarily with national health issues and the Committee on Infectious Diseases formulates its recommendations for infants and children who receive regular health care, there are occasionally different perspectives in each group's recommendations. The policies of each committee are recommendations, not rules, and they change as a result of advances in the field of immunology. Nurses need to realize the purpose of each organization, to view immunization practices in light of the needs of an individual child, as well as the community, and to keep informed of the latest advances and changes in policy.

The recommended age for beginning primary immunizations of infants is at birth (Table 12-6). Children born prematurely should receive the *full dose* of each vaccine at the appropriate chronologic age. If the infant is hospitalized, OPV is initiated after discharge to prevent transmission of OPV in the nursery. Recommended schedules for children not immunized during infancy are included in Table 12-7. Tables 12-8 and 12-9 describe immunization schedules for Canadian children. Children who began primary immunization at the recommended age but who fail to receive all the doses do not have to begin the series again, but receive only the missed doses. In situations when there is doubt that the child will return for immunization according to the optimum schedule, HBV, DTP, OPV, MMR, and Hib vaccines can be administered simultaneously. Parenteral vaccines are given in separate syringes in different injection sites (American Academy of Pediatrics, 1994).

Recommendations for Routine Immunizations

Hepatitis B Virus (HBV). HBV, a potentially fatal viral infection that eventually causes cirrhosis or liver cancer during adulthood, is an important pediatric disease, because HBV infections occurring during childhood and adolescence can lead to these consequences. Up to 90% of infants infected perinatally and 25% to 50% of children infected before age 5 years will become HBV carriers. In addition, the incidence of HBV infection increases rapidly during adolescence (American Academy of Pediatrics, 1992). Despite the availability of a safe, effective vaccine, new cases have increased about 50% during the last decade. Past im-

TABLE 12-6 Recommended Schedule for Immunization of Healthy Infants and Children[a] in the United States

RECOMMENDED AGE[b]	IMMUNIZATION(S)[c]	COMMENTS
Birth	HBV[d]	
1-2 months	HBV[d]	
2 months	DTP, Hib,[e] OPV	DTP and OPV can be initiated as early as 4 weeks after birth in areas of high endemicity or during outbreaks
4 months	DTP, Hib,[e] OPV	2-month interval (minimum of 6 weeks) recommended for OPV
6 months	DTP, (Hib,[e,f])	
6-18 months	HBV,[d] OPV	
12-15 months	Hib,[e] MMR	MMR should be given at 12 months of age in high-risk areas; if indicated, tuberculin testing may be done at the same visit
15-18 months	DTaP or DTP	The fourth dose of diphtheria-tetanus-pertussis vaccine should be given 6 to 12 months after the third dose of DTP and may be given as early as 12 months of age, provided that the interval between doses 3 and 4 is at least 6 months and DTP is given; DTaP is not currently licensed for use in children younger than 15 months
4-6 years	DTaP or DTP, OPV	DTaP or DTP and OPV should be given at or before school entry; DTP or DTaP should not be given at or after the seventh birthday
11-12 years	MMR	MMR should be given at entry to middle school or junior high school unless 2 doses were given after the first birthday
14-16 years	Td	Repeat every 10 years throughout life

From American Academy of Pediatrics, Committee on Infectious Diseases: *1994 Red Book: report of the Committee on Infectious Diseases,* ed 23, Elk Grove Village, IL, 1994, The Academy.

[a]Table is not completely consistent with all package inserts. For products used, also consult manufacturer's package insert for instructions on storage, handling, dosage, and administration. Biologics prepared by different manufacturers may vary, and package inserts of the same manufacturer may change from time to time. Therefore the practitioner should be aware of the contents of the current package insert.

[b]These recommended ages should not be construed as absolute. For example, 2 months can be 6 to 10 weeks. However, MMR usually should not be given to children younger than 12 months. If measles vaccination is indicated, monovalent measles vaccine is recommended, and MMR should be given subsequently at 12 to 15 months.

[c]Vaccine abbreviations: *HBV,* hepatitis B virus vaccine; *DTP,* diphtheria and tetanus toxoids and pertussis vaccine; *DTaP,* diphtheria and tetanus toxoids and acellular pertussis vaccine; *Hib, Haemophilus influenzae* type b conjugate vaccine; *OPV,* oral poliovirus vaccine (containing attenuated poliovirus types 1, 2, and 3); *MMR,* live measles, mumps, and rubella viruses vaccine; *Td,* adult tetanus toxoid (full dose) and diphtheria toxoid (reduced dose), for children ≥7 years and adults.

[d]See Table 12-10. An acceptable alternative to minimize the number of visits for immunizing infants of HBsAg-negative mothers is to administer dose 1 at 0 to 2 months, dose 2 at 4 months, and dose 3 at 6 to 18 months.

[e]See text, p. 555.

[f]Hib: dose 3 of Hib is not indicated if the product for doses 1 and 2 was PedvaxHIB (PRP-OMP).

TABLE 12-7 Recommended Immunization Schedules for Children Not Immunized in the First Year of Life in the United States

RECOMMENDED TIME/AGE	IMMUNIZATION(S)[a,b]	COMMENTS
YOUNGER THAN 7 YEARS		
First visit	DTP, Hib,[c] HBV, MMR, OPV	If indicated, tuberculin testing may be done at same visit If child is 5 years of age or older, Hib is not indicated
Interval after first visit:		
1 month	DTP, HBV	OPV may be given if accelerated poliomyelitis vaccination is necessary, such as for travelers to areas where polio is endemic
2 months	DTP, Hib,[c] OPV	Second dose of Hib is indicated only in children whose first dose was received when younger than 15 months
≥8 months	DTP or DTaP,[d] HBV, OPV	OPV is not given if the third dose was given earlier
4-6 years (at or before school entry)	DTP or DTaP,[d] OPV	DTP or DTaP is not necessary if the fourth dose was given after the fourth birthday; OPV is not necessary if the third dose was given after the fourth birthday
11-12 years	MMR	At entry to middle school or junior high school
10 years later	Td	Repeat every 10 years throughout life
7 YEARS AND OLDER[e,f]		
First visit	HBV,[g] OPV, MMR, Td	
Interval after first visit:		
2 months	HBV,[g] OPV, Td	OPV may also be given 1 month after the first visit if accelerated poliomyelitis vaccination is necessary
8-14 months	HBV,[g] OPV, Td	OPV is not given if the third dose was given earlier
11-12 years	MMR	At entry to middle school or junior high
10 years later	Td	Repeat every 10 years throughout life

From American Academy of Pediatrics, Committee on Infectious Diseases: *1994 Red Book: report of the Committee on Infectious Diseases*, ed 23, Elk Grove Village, IL, 1994, The Academy.

[a]Abbreviations for vaccines are explained in the footnotes to Table 12-6. If all needed vaccines cannot be administered simultaneously, priority should be given to protecting the child against those diseases that pose the greatest immediate risk. In the United States these diseases for children younger than 2 years usually are measles and *Haemophilus influenzae* type b infection; for children older than 7 years, they are measles, mumps, and rubella (MMR).

[b]DTP or DTaP, HBV, Hib, MMR, and OPV can be given simultaneously at separate sites if failure of the patient to return for future immunizations is a concern.

[c]See text, p. 555.

[d]DTaP is not currently licensed for use in children younger than 15 months of age and is not recommended for primary immunization (i.e., first 3 doses) at any age.

[e]If person is 18 years or older, routine poliovirus vaccination is not indicated in the United States.

[f]Minimal interval between doses of MMR is 1 month.

[g]Priority should be given to hepatitis B immunization of adolescents.

TABLE 12-8 Routine Primary Immunization Schedule for Infants and Children in Canada

AGE	IMMUNIZATION AGAINST				
2 months	Diphtheria	Pertussis	Tetanus	Poliomyelitis	*Haemophilus influenzae* b[1]
4 months	Diphtheria	Pertussis	Tetanus	Poliomyelitis	*Haemophilus influenzae* b
6 months	Diphtheria	Pertussis	Tetanus	Poliomyelitis[2]	*Haemophilus influenzae* b
12 months	Measles	Mumps	Rubella		
18 months	Diphtheria	Pertussis	Tetanus	Poliomyelitis	*Haemophilus influenzae* b
4-6 years	Diphtheria	Pertussis	Tetanus	Poliomyelitis	
14-16 years	Diphtheria[3]		Tetanus[3]	Poliomyelitis[2]	

From National Advisory Committee on Immunization: *Canadian immunization guide*, ed 4, Canada, 1993, Authority of the Minister of National Health and Welfare, Health Protection Branch, Laboratory Centre for Disease Control.

Notes:

1. Hib schedule shown is for HbOC or PRP-T vaccine. If PRP-OMP is used, give at 2, 4, and 12 months of age.
2. Omit this dose if OPV is used exclusively.
3. Td (tetanus and diphtheria toxoid), a combined adsorbed "adult-type" preparation for use in persons ≥7 years of age, contains less diphtheria toxoid than preparations given to younger children and is less likely to cause reactions in older persons. Repeat every 10 years throughout life.

TABLE 12-9 Routine Immunization Schedules for Children Not Immunized in Early Infancy in Canada

TIMING	IMMUNIZATION AGAINST				
FOR CHILDREN 7 YEARS OF AGE AND YOUNGER					
First visit	Diphtheria	Pertussis	Tetanus	Poliomyelitis	*Haemophilus influenzae* b
	Measles[4]	Mumps[4]	Rubella[4]		
2 months later	Diphtheria	Pertussis	Tetanus	Poliomyelitis	*Haemophilus influenzae* b[5]
2 months later	Diphtheria	Pertussis	Tetanus	Poliomyelitis[2]	
6-12 months later	Diphtheria	Pertussis	Tetanus	Poliomyelitis	*Haemophilus influenzae* b[5]
4-6 years[6]	Diphtheria	Pertussis	Tetanus	Poliomyelitis	
14-16 years	Diphtheria[3]	Tetanus[3]	Poliomyelitis[2]		
FOR CHILDREN 7 YEARS OF AGE AND OLDER					
First visit	Diphtheria[3]		Tetanus[3]	Poliomyelitis	
	Measles	Mumps	Rubella		
2 months later	Diphtheria[3]		Tetanus[3]	Poliomyelitis	
6-12 months later	Diphtheria[3]		Tetanus[3]	Poliomyelitis	
10 years later	Diphtheria[3]		Tetanus[3]		

From National Advisory Committee on Immunization: *Canadian immunization guide,* ed 4, Canada, 1993, Authority of the Minister of National Health and Welfare, Health Protection Branch, Laboratory Centre for Disease Control.
Notes:
1-3 See Table 12-8.
4. Delay until subsequent visit if child is <12 months of age.
5. Recommended schedule and number of doses depend on the product used and the age of the child when vaccination is begun. Not required past age 5.
6. Omit these doses if the previous doses of DPT and polio were given after the fourth birthday.

TABLE 12-10 Recommended Routine Hepatitis B Immunization Schedule for Infants

			VACCINE†			
			RECOMBIVAX HB		ENERGIX-B	
MATERNAL HBsAg STATUS*	DOSE	AGE	μg	(ml)	μg	(ml)
Negative‡	1	0-2 days	2.5	(0.25)	10	(0.5)
	2	1-2 months				
	3	6-18 months				
Positive	1§	0 days	5	(0.5)	10	(0.5)
	2	1 month				
	3	6 months				

Modified from American Academy of Pediatrics, Committee on Infectious Diseases: Universal hepatitis B immunization, *Pediatrics,* 89(4):795-800, 1992.
**HBsAg,* Hepatitis B surface antigen.
†Vaccine dosage is for newborns to children <11 years of age. Children ages 11 to 19 years receive 0.5 ml of Recombivax HB and 1.0 ml of Energix-B. The usual schedule of immunization for older children and adolescents is 0, 1, and 6 months.
‡Alternative schedule: dose one at 1-2 months of age, dose two at 4 months, and dose three at 6-18 months.
§HBIG (hepatitis B immune globulin) should also be administered.

munization strategies targeted several high-risk groups, including health care workers and others in contact with blood and body fluids, recipients of certain blood products (such as those with hemophilia), heterosexuals with multiple partners, sexually active homosexual and bisexual males, intravenous drug abusers, immigrants from countries where HBV is widespread, and children born to mothers who are HBV surface antigen (HBsAg) positive. To improve immunization rates, current recommendations include immunizations for all newborns, as well as several high-risk groups (Centers for Disease Control and Prevention, 1994). The American Academy of Pediatrics (1994) also encourages immunization of all adolescents against HBV.

The vaccine is given intramuscularly in the vastus lateralis or deltoid, including at birth. Regardless of age, the dorsogluteal site is avoided because it has been associated with low antibody seroconversion rates, indicating a reduced immune response (Zuckerman, Cockcroft, and Zuckerman, 1992). It can be safely administered simultaneously at a separate site with DTP, MMR, and Hib vaccines. Dosage depends on the child's age and type of vaccine used (Table 12-10).

Diphtheria. Diphtheria vaccine is commonly administered (1) in combination with tetanus and pertussis vaccines (DTP or DTaP) or DTP and Hib vaccines for children younger than 7 years of age, (2) in a combined vaccine with tetanus (DT) for children younger than 7 years of age who have some contraindication for receiving pertussis vaccine,

TABLE 12-11 Guide to Tetanus Prophylaxis in Routine Wound Management, 1991

HISTORY OF ADSORBED TETANUS TOXOID (DOSES)	CLEAN, MINOR WOUNDS		ALL OTHER WOUNDS*	
	Td†	TIG	Td†	TIG
Unknown or < three	Yes	No	Yes	Yes
≥Three‡	No§	No	No‖	No

From Recommendations of the Immunization Practices Advisory Committee (ACIP): Diphtheria, tetanus, and pertussis: recommendations for vaccine use and other preventive measures, *MMWR* 40(RR-10):1-28, 1991.
*Such as, but not limited to, wounds contaminated with dirt, feces, soil, and saliva; puncture wounds; avulsions; and wounds resulting from missiles, crushing, burns, and frostbite.
†For children <7 years old; DTP (DT, if pertussis vaccine is contraindicated) is preferred to tetanus toxoid alone. For persons ≥7 years of age, Td is preferred to tetanus toxoid alone.
‡If only three doses of *fluid* toxoid have been received, then a fourth dose of toxoid, preferably an adsorbed toxoid, should be given.
§Yes, If >10 years since last dose.
‖Yes, if >5 years since last dose. (More frequent boosters are not needed and can accentuate side effects.)

(3) in smaller doses (15% to 20% of that in DTP or DT) with tetanus vaccine (Td) for use in children age 7 years and older, or (4) as a single antigen when combined antigen preparations are not indicated. Although the diphtheria vaccine does not produce absolute immunity, when given according to the recommended schedule, protective antitoxin persists for 10 years or more.

Tetanus. Three forms of tetanus vaccine—tetanus toxoid, tetanus immune globulin (TIG) (human), and tetanus antitoxin (usually horse serum)—are available. Tetanus toxoid is used for routine primary immunization, usually in one of the combinations listed above, and provides protective antitoxin levels for 10 years or more.

For wound management, passive immunity is available with TIG or animal-source antitoxin. However, because the risk of severe reaction, such as anaphylactic shock or serum sickness, is always greater to the foreign substances of animal serum, the choice is TIG. In persons with a history of two previous doses of tetanus toxoid, a booster dose of the toxoid can be given. When tetanus toxoid and TIG are given concurrently, separate syringes and different sites are used. Table 12-11 presents a summary of the recommended procedure for tetanus prophylaxis in wound management.

Pertussis. Pertussis vaccine is recommended for all children 6 weeks through 6 years of age (up to the seventh birthday) who have no neurologic contraindications to its use. It is not given to children 7 years or older because the risk of receiving the vaccine increases as the incidence, severity and fatality of the disease decrease.

Currently, two forms of pertussis vaccine are available in the United States. The ***whole-cell pertussis vaccine*** is prepared from inactivated cells of *Bordetella pertussis* and contains multiple antigens. In contrast, the ***acellular pertussis vaccine*** contains one or more immunogens derived from the *B. pertussis* organism. The highly purified acellular vaccine is associated with fewer local and systemic reactions than those occuring with the whole-cell vaccine in children of similar age. The whole-cell pertussis vaccine is used for the first three immunizations, usually given at 2, 4, and 6 months of age with diphtheria and tetanus. The acellular vaccine (DTaP [ACEL-IMUNE]) is licensed for use only as the fourth and fifth doses for children who have been immunized previously with at least three doses of the DTP vaccine (American Academy of Pediatrics, 1993a).

Polio. The trivalent form of ***oral poliovirus (OPV)*** (developed by Sabin) is recommended for all children younger than 18 years of age who have no specific contraindications to its use, regardless of the number of administrations of ***inactivated poliovirus vaccine (IPV)*** (developed by Salk) they have received. OPV is used in the United States because the live virus can be shed to contacts, who become immunized through this exposure. However, OPV has caused vaccine-associated paralysis in both recipients and contacts.

Because of the greater risk of vaccine-associated paralysis in children with immunodeficiency diseases, IPV is the vaccine of choice for immunocompromised children and any close contacts because it has no reported history of causing vaccine-associated paralysis. However, IPV has the disadvantage of being given by subcutaneous injection and producing less immunity. In the United States an enhanced potency form of IVP is used.

A recent change in the immunization schedule is that the third dose of polio vaccine can now be given at 6 months, along with the third doses of DTP and *H. influenzae* vaccines. Previously, the third dose was recommended at 18 months of age. This change is hoped to increase polio protection at an earlier age (Marwick, 1993).

Measles. Because of the presence of maternal antibodies, measles (rubeola) virus vaccine was usually delayed until 15 months of age for infants who live in communities where the disease is not prevalent. However, it can now be given at 12 to 15 months of age. During the course of measles outbreaks, the vaccine can be given any time after 6 months of age, followed by a second inoculation after age 12 months.

Because of continued outbreaks of measles among unvaccinated preschool-age children and among vaccinated school-age children and college students, a second measles immunization is recommended. The American Academy of Pediatrics, Committee on Infectious Disease (1994) recommends a second dose of MMR by age 12 years, preferably at entrance to middle school or junior high school. ACIP, however, recommends that the second dose be given before school entry at 4 to 6 years (Centers for Disease Control and Prevention, 1994). Revaccination should include all individuals born after January 1, 1957, who have not received two doses of measles vaccine after 12 months of age. Individuals born before this date are thought to be immune because of exposure to natural measles virus. However, evidence suggests that a significant number of these individuals may be susceptible to measles (Braunstein, Thomas, and Ito, 1990).

Mumps. Mumps virus vaccine is recommended for children at 12 to 15 months of age and is typically given in combination with measles and rubella. It should not be administered to infants younger than 12 months because persisting maternal antibodies can interfere with the immune response.

Because of recent outbreaks of the disease, especially in children 10 to 19 years, mumps immunization is recommended for all individuals born after 1957 who may be susceptible to mumps (i.e., those who have no history of having had the disease or vaccine and when there is no laboratory evidence of immunity).

Rubella. Rubella is a relatively mild infection in children, but in a pregnant woman it presents serious risks to the developing fetus. Therefore the aim of rubella immunization is actually protection of the unborn child rather than the recipient of the immunization.

Rubella immunization is recommended for all children at 12 to 15 months of age and is administered in a combined form with measles and mumps vaccine. Increased emphasis should also be placed on vaccinating all unimmunized prepubertal children and susceptible adolescents and adult women in the childbearing age-group.

Because the live attenuated virus may cross the placenta and present a risk to the developing fetus, rubella vaccine is not given to any pregnant woman. Although this is standard practice, current evidence from women who received the vaccine while pregnant and delivered unaffected offspring indicates that the risk to the fetus is negligible (Centers for Disease Control and Prevention, 1994). In addition, there is no reported danger of administering rubella vaccine to a child if the mother is pregnant.

***Haemophilus Influenzae* Type b (Hib).** Hib conjugate vaccines provide protection against a number of serious infections caused by Hib, especially bacterial meningitis, epiglottitis, bacterial pneumonia, septic arthritis, and sepsis. (Hib is not associated with the viruses that cause influenza, or "flu.")

The following Hib conjugate vaccines are currently available:

- Diphtheria toxoid conjugate (PRP-D) (ProHIBit)
- Diphtheria CRM_{197} protein conjugate (PRP-HbOC) (HibTITER)
- Meningococcal protein conjugate (PRP-OMP) (Pedvax HIB)
- PRP conjugate with tetanus toxoid (PRP-T) (ActHIB and OmniHIB)
- HibTITER is also combined in a vaccine with DTP (Tetramune) (Centers for Disease Control and Prevention, 1994.)

These conjugate vaccines connect Hib to a nontoxic form of another organism, such as meningococcal protein or diphtheria protein. There is *no* antibody response to these nontoxic proteins, but they significantly improve the antibody response to Hib, especially in infants.

HbOC or PRP-T is recommended at 2, 4, and 6 months of age, with a booster at age 12 to 15 months. Only two doses of PRP-OMP are required—at age 2 to 6 months, administered at least 2 months apart with a booster at age 12 to 15 months. PRP-D is not licensed for use in infants under 12 months of age. When possible, the Hib conjugate vaccine used at the first vaccination should be used for all subsequent vaccinations in the primary series. When either a Hib vaccine or Tetramune is used, the vaccine is administered by intramuscular injection (IM) using a separate syringe and at a separate site from any concurrent vaccinations.

Varicella. As of this writing, the universal use of a vaccine for chickenpox (varicella) is under consideration by the U.S. Food and Drug Administration (FDA). If approved, the live virus varicella (Oka/Merck) vaccine is expected to be recommended for all children between 12 and 18 months of age and all older susceptible children, up to age 12 years. The dose will probably be 0.5 ml, given subcutaneously (Watson and others, 1993a, 1993b), with one dose for children 12 months to 12 years and two doses for youngsters after the thirteenth birthday. The vaccine should be kept frozen in the lyophilized form (stable particles that readily go into solution) and used immediately after being reconstituted to ensure maximum response (Watson and others, 1993a).

In clinical trials conducted during the past 15 years, a small number of immunized children subsequently developed chickenpox. However, the disease was mild; children had fewer lesions and less itching, fever, or headache, and more than half had no symptoms other than the rash. The contagiousness of the infection was also significantly reduced (Watson and others, 1993b).

Recommendations for Selected Immunizations

Several additional vaccines are recommended for children at high risk for particular diseases. Most of these children have chronic disorders or impaired immune systems that make them more susceptible to certain infections than the general population. Selected immunizations are presented in Table 12-12. Others, such as the rabies vaccine, are discussed elsewhere in this text.

Reactions

Vaccines for routine immunizations are among the safest and most reliable drugs available. However, minor side effects do occur following many of the immunizations, and rarely a serious reaction may result from the vaccine (Table 12-13).

With inactivated antigens, such as DTP, side effects are most likely to occur within a few hours or days of administration and are usually limited to local tenderness, erythema, and swelling at the injection site; low-grade fever;

TABLE 12-12 Recommendations for Selected Nonmandated Vaccines

DESCRIPTION	ADMINISTRATION/PRECAUTIONS
INFLUENZA VIRUS VACCINE	
Affords protection against strains of influenza Recommended for children age 6 months and older with chronic disorders of cardiovascular or pulmonary systems, including asthma, whose severity warranted regular medical care or hospitalization during preceding year; other eligible children include those with diabetes mellitus, renal dysfunction, anemia, immunosuppression, human immunodeficiency virus (HIV) infection, or those on long-term aspirin therapy (because of risk of developing Reye syndrome after influenza infection)	Administered in fall, preferably November; repeated yearly Intramuscular injection; 2 doses of split vaccine at least 4 weeks apart for children age 12 years or younger; 1 dose of split or whole vaccine for children over 12 years of age Contraindicated in persons with anaphylactic hypersensitivity to eggs May be given simultaneously with other childhood immunizations but at separate site
PNEUMOCOCCAL POLYSACCHARIDE VACCINE (PNEUMOVAX; PNU-IMUNE)	
Affords protection against 23 types of *Streptococcus pneumoniae* Recommended for children age 2 years and older with sickle cell disease, functional or anatomic asplenia, nephrotic syndrome, human immunodeficiency virus (HIV) infection, and Hodgkin disease before beginning cytoreduction therapy	Subcutaneous or intramuscular injection Revaccination is not recommended Should be deferred during pregnancy
MENINGOCOCCAL POLYSACCHARIDE VACCINE (MENOMUNE)	
Affords protection against *Neisseria meningitidis;* sero-groups A, C, Y, and W-135. Recommended for children 2 years and older with terminal complement deficiencies and anatomic or functional asplenia	Subcutaneous injection Duration of protection unknown Safety during pregnancy not established

and behavioral changes (drowsiness, fretfulness, eating less, prolonged or unusual cry) (Long and others, 1990). Local reactions tend to be less severe when the deltoid site is used rather than the vastus lateralis and when a needle of sufficient length to deposit the vaccine in the muscle is used (see Atraumatic Care box on p. 559). Rarely, more severe reactions may occur, especially with pertussis (see Table 12-13). Reactions to DTP tend to be more severe if they occurred with a previous immunization.

Hib vaccine is one of the safest vaccines available but may be associated with low-grade fever and mild local reactions at the site of subcutaneous injection, which resolve rapidly. Fever (temperature more than 38.5° C [101.3° F]) may rarely occur.

Unlike the inactivated antigens, live attenuated virus vaccines such as MMR and OPV multiply for days or weeks, and unfavorable reactions and "vaccine-associated" disorders can occur for a period of 30 to 60 days. However, they are usually mild, although reactions to rubella tend to be more troublesome in older children and adults.

Contraindications/Precautions

Nurses need to be aware of the reasons for withholding immunizations—both for the child's safety in terms of avoiding reactions and for the child's maximum benefit from receiving the vaccine. Unfounded fears and lack of knowledge regarding contraindications can needlessly prevent a child from having protection from life-threatening diseases. The contraindications to the usual childhood vaccines are presented in Table 12-14. A general discussion of specific concerns follows.

NURSING ALERT For several decades pertussis vaccine was considered a rare cause of serious, permanent brain damage or death. After reviewing recent studies, experts have concluded that whole-cell pertussis vaccine has not been proved to cause neurologic damage. Previous contraindications to whole-cell pertussis vaccination are now considered precautions.

The general contraindication for all immunizations is a severe febrile illness. This precaution is to avoid adding the risk of adverse side effects from the vaccine on an already ill child or mistakenly identifying a symptom of the disease as having been caused by the vaccine. The presence of minor illnesses such as the common cold is *not* a contraindication. Live virus vaccines are generally not administered to anyone with an altered immune system, because multiplication of the virus may be enhanced, causing a severe vaccine-induced illness. In addition, household contacts of such children should not receive OPV, because the virus multiplies in the gastrointestinal tract and excreted virus in the stool can be communicated to the immunosuppressed child. Exceptions are made when the risks of contracting the disease outweigh the risks of the immunization, as in children with HIV who should receive MMR, but not OPV.

Another contraindication to live virus vaccines (MMR) is the presence of recently acquired passive immunity through blood transfusions, immunoglobulin, or maternal antibodies. Administration of MMR should be postponed for a *minimum* of 3 months after passive immunization with immunoglobulins and blood transfusions (except washed red blood cells, which do not interfere with the immune response). Suggested intervals between administration of

TABLE 12-13 Possible Side Effects of Recommended Childhood Immunizations and Nursing Responsibilities

IMMUNIZATION	REACTION	NURSING RESPONSIBILITIES
Hepatitis B virus	Well tolerated, few side effects	Explain to parents reason for this immunization Consider that cost for 3 injections may be a factor
Diphtheria	Fever usually within 24-48 hours Soreness, redness, and swelling at injection site Behavioral changes: drowsiness, fretfulness, anorexia, prolonged or unusual crying	Nursing responsibilities for DTP apply to immunizations for diphtheria, tetanus, and pertussis Instruction for DTP: advise parents of possible side effects
Tetanus	Same as for diphtheria but may include urticaria and malaise All may have delayed onset and last several days Lump at injection site may last for weeks, even months, but gradually disappears	Recommend prophylactic use of acetaminophen at time of DTP immunization and every 4-6 hours for a total of 3 doses Advise parents to notify practitioner *immediately* of any unusual side effects, such as those listed under pertussis in Table 12-14
Pertussis	Same as for tetanus but may include loss of consciousness, convulsions, persistent inconsolable crying episodes, generalized or focal neurologic signs, fever (temperature at or above 40.5° C [105° F]), systemic allergic reaction	Before administering next dose of DTP, inquire about reactions, especially those listed under pertussis in Table 12-14
Haemophilus influenzae type b	Mild local reactions (erythema, pain) at injection site Low-grade fever	Advise parents of possible mild side effects
Poliovirus (OPV)	Essentially no immediate side effects Vaccine-associated paralysis rarely occurs within 2 months of immunization (estimated risk 1:7.8 million doses); more likely to occur in close contact than in OPV recipient	Assess presence of family members at risk from trivalent OPV because of immune deficiency states
Measles	Anorexia, malaise, rash, and fever may occur 7 to 10 days after immunization Rarely (estimated risk 1:1 million doses) encephalitis may occur	Advise parents of more common side effects and use of antipyretics for fever If a persistent fever with other obvious signs of illness occurs, have them notify physician immediately
Mumps	Essentially no side effects other than a brief, mild fever	See general comment to parents
Rubella	Fever, lymphadenopathy, or mild rash that lasts 1 or 2 days within a few days after immunization Arthralgia, arthritis, or paresthesia of the hands and fingers may occur about 2 weeks after vaccination and is more common in older children and adults	Advise parents of side effects, especially of time delay before joint swelling and pain; assure them that these symptoms will disappear May recommend use of acetaminophen for pain

immune globulin preparations and MMR depend on the type of immune product and dosage. If the vaccine and immunoglobulin are given simultaneously because of imminent exposure to disease, the two preparations are injected at sites that are far from each other. Vaccination should be repeated after the suggested intervals unless there is serologic evidence of antibody production (Centers for Disease Control and Prevention, 1993b).

Pregnancy is a contraindication to mumps, measles, and rubella vaccines, although the risk of fetal damage is primarily theoretic. Oral poliovirus is also withheld unless there is risk of exposure during an outbreak of the disease. Breast-feeding is not a contraindication for any vaccine.

A final contraindication is a known allergic response to a previously administered vaccine or a substance in the vaccine (see DTP in Table 12-14). Measles, mumps, and rubella virus vaccines contain minute amounts of neomycin, and measles and mumps vaccines, which are grown on chick embryo tissue cultures, may contain substances allergenic to egg-sensitive individuals. However, only a history of anaphylactoid reaction to neomycin or to egg is considered a contraindication to their use. To identify the rare child who may not be able to receive the vaccines, a careful allergy history is taken (see box in Chapter 6 on p. 201). If the child has a history of anaphylaxis, it is reported to the practitioner before administering the vaccine. Although rare, severe

TABLE 12-14 Contraindications and Precautions to Vaccinations[a]

TRUE CONTRAINDICATIONS AND PRECAUTIONS	NOT CONTRAINDICATIONS (VACCINES MAY BE ADMINISTERED)
GENERAL FOR ALL VACCINES (DTP/DTAP, OPV, IPV, MMR, HIB, HEPATITIS B)	
Contraindications	***Not Contraindications***
Anaphylactic reaction to a vaccine contraindicates further doses of that vaccine Anaphylactic reaction to a vaccine constituent contraindicates the use of vaccines containing that substance Moderate or severe illnesses with or without a fever	Mild to moderate local reaction (soreness, redness, swelling) following a dose of an injectable antigen Mild acute illness with or without low-grade fever Current antimicrobial therapy Convalescent phase of illnesses Prematurity (same dosage and indications as for normal, full-term infants) Recent exposure to an infectious disease History of penicillin or other nonspecific allergies or family history of such allergies
DIPHTHERIA, TETANUS, PERTUSSIS OR ACELLULAR PERTUSSIS (DTP/DTAP)	
Contraindications	***Not Contraindications***
Encephalopathy within 7 days of administration of previous dose of DTP	Temperature of <40.5° C (105° F) following a previous dose of DTP Family history of convulsions[c] Family history of sudden infant death syndrome Family history of an adverse event following DTP administration
Precautions[b]	
Fever of ≥40.5° C (105° F) within 48 hours after vaccination with a prior dose of DTP Collapse or shocklike state (hypotonic-hyporesponsive episode) within 48 hours of receiving a prior dose of DTP Seizures within 3 days of receiving a prior dose of DTP[c] Persistent, inconsolable crying lasting ≥3 hours within 48 hours of receiving a prior dose of DTP	
ORAL POLIO (OPV)[d]	
Contraindications	***Not Contraindications***
Infection with HIV or a household contact with HIV Known altered immunodeficiency (hematologic and solid tumors; congenital immunodeficiency; and long-term immunosuppressive therapy) Immunodeficient household contact	Breast-feeding Current antimicrobial therapy Diarrhea
Precaution[b]	
Pregnancy	
INACTIVATED POLIO (IPV)	
Contraindication	
Anaphylactic reaction to neomycin or streptomycin	
Precaution[b]	
Pregnancy	

From Centers for Disease Control and Prevention: General recommendations on immunization: recommendations of the Advisory Committee on Immunization Practices (ACIP), *MMWR* 43(RR-1):24-25, 1994.

[a]This information is based on the recommendations of the Advisory Committee on Immunization Practices (ACIP) and those of the Committee on Infectious Diseases (Red Book Committee) of the American Academy of Pediatrics (AAP). Sometimes these recommendations vary from those contained in the manufacturer's package inserts. For more detailed information, providers should consult the published recommendations of the ACIP, AAP, and the manufacturer's package inserts.

[b]The events or conditions listed as precautions, although not contraindications, should be carefully reviewed. The benefits and risks of administering a specific vaccine to an individual under the circumstances should be considered. If the risks are believed to outweigh the benefits, the vaccination should be withheld; if the benefits are believed to outweigh the risks (e.g., during an outbreak or foreign travel), the vaccination should be administered. Whether and when to administer DTP to children with proven or suspected underlying neurologic disorders should be decided on an individual basis. It is prudent on theoretic grounds to avoid vaccinating pregnant women. However, if immediate protection against poliomyelitis is needed, OPV is preferred, although IPV may be considered if full vaccination can be completed before the anticipated imminent exposure.

[c]Acetaminophen given before administering DTP and thereafter every 4 hours for 24 hours should be considered for children with a personal or family history of convulsions in siblings or parents.

[d]No data exist to substantiate the theoretic risk of a suboptimal immune response from the administration of OPV and MMR within 30 days of each other.

[e]Persons with a history of anaphylactic reactions following egg ingestion should be vaccinated only with caution. Protocols have been developed for vaccinating such persons and should be consulted.

[f]Measles vaccination may temporarily suppress tuberculin reactivity. If testing cannot be done the day of MMR vaccination, the test should be postponed for 4 to 6 weeks.

TABLE 12-14 Contraindications and Precautions to Vaccinations[a]—cont'd

TRUE CONTRAINDICATIONS AND PRECAUTIONS	NOT CONTRAINDICATIONS (VACCINES MAY BE ADMINISTERED)
MEASLES, MUMPS, RUBELLA (MMR)[d]	
Contraindications	***Not Contraindications[d]***
Anaphylactic reactions to egg ingestion and to neomycin[e]	Tuberculosis or positive PPD skin test
Pregnancy	Simultaneous TB skin testing[f]
Known altered immunodeficiency (hematologic and solid tumors, congenital immunodeficiency, and long-term immunosuppressive therapy)	Breast-feeding Pregnancy of mother of recipient Immunodeficient family member or household contact Infection with HIV Nonanaphylactic reactions to eggs or neomycin
Precautions[b]	
Recent immune globulin administration	
Immune globulin products and MMR should not be given simultaneously; if unavoidable, give at different sites and revaccinate or test for seroconversion in 3 months; if IG is given first, MMR should not be given for at least 3-6 months, depending on the dose; if MMR is given first, IG should not be given for 2 weeks	
***HAEMOPHILUS INFLUENZAE* TYPE B (HIB)**	
Contraindication	***Not a Contraindication***
Nonidentified	History of Hib disease
HEPATITIS B VIRUS (HBV)	
Contraindication	***Not a Contraindication***
Anaphylactic reaction to common baker's yeast	Pregnancy

reactions to measles vaccine have occurred in children with egg allergy; as a precaution, such children should be skin tested for sensitivity and, if they react positively, be given incremental doses of vaccine.

Administration

The principal precautions in administering immunizations include proper storage of the vaccine to protect its potency and institution of recommended procedures for injection. The nurse must be familiar with the manufacturer's directions for storage and reconstitution of the vaccine. For example, if the vaccine is to be refrigerated, it should be stored on a center shelf, not on the door where frequent temperature increases from opening the refrigerator can alter the vaccine's potency. For protection against light the vial can be wrapped in aluminum foil. Periodic checks are established to ensure that no vaccine is used after its expiration date.

The DTP vaccines contain the adjuvant alum to retain the antigen at the depot site and prolong the stimulatory effect. Because subcutaneous or intracutaneous injection of the adjuvant can cause local irritation, inflammation, or abscess formation, attention to excellent intramuscular injection technique must be used (see Atraumatic Care box).

The total series requires a number of injections, and every attempt is made to rotate the sites and administer the injections as painlessly as possible (see discussion on intramuscular injections in Chapter 27). When two or more injections are given at separate sites, the order of injections is arbitrary. Some practitioners suggest injecting the less painful one first. Some believe this is DTP, whereas others suggest the MMR or Hib vaccine. Still others advocate in-

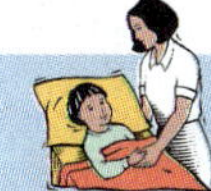

ATRAUMATIC CARE
Immunizations

To minimize local reactions from vaccines:
- Select a needle of adequate length (1 inch in infants) to deposit the antigen deep in the muscle mass (Hick and others, 1989)
- Inject into the vastus lateralis or ventrogluteal muscle; the deltoid may be used in children 18 months or older (Ipp and others, 1989) or in infants receiving HBV vaccine
- Use an air bubble to clear the needle after injecting the vaccine (theoretically beneficial but unproved)

To minimize pain*:
- Apply the topical anesthetic EMLA to the injection site for a minimum of 1 hour, preferably for up to 2 hours for greater penetration (Taddio and others, 1994; Uhari, 1993).
- In preschool children use distraction, such as telling the child to "take a deep breath and blow and blow and blow until I tell you to stop" (French, Painter, and Coury, 1994).

Note: Changing the needle on the syringe after drawing up the vaccine and before injecting it has not be shown to be effective in decreasing local reactions (Salomon and others, 1987).

*See also Pain Management, Chapter 26.

TABLE 12-15 Injury Prevention During Infancy

AGE: BIRTH-4 MONTHS

Major Developmental Accomplishments

Involuntary reflexes, such as the crawling reflex, may propel infant forward or backward and the startle reflex may cause the body to jerk

May roll over

Increasing eye-hand coordination and voluntary grasp reflex

Injury Prevention

Aspiration

Not as great a danger to this age-group, but should begin practicing safeguarding early (see under 4-7 Months)

Never shake baby powder directly on infant; place powder in hand and then on infant's skin; store container closed and out of infant's reach

Hold infant for feeding; do not prop bottle

Know emergency procedures for choking*

Use pacifier with one-piece construction and loop handle

Suffocation/drowning

Keep all plastic bags stored out of infant's reach; discard large plastic garment bags after tying in a knot

Do not cover mattress with plastic

Use a firm mattress and loose blankets; no pillows

Make sure crib design follows federal regulations and mattress fits snugly†

Position crib away from other furniture and away from radiators

Avoid sleeping in bed with infant

Do not tie pacifier on a string around infant's neck

Remove bibs at bedtime

Never leave infant alone in bath

Do not leave infant under 12 months alone on adult or youth mattress

Falls

Always raise crib rails

Never leave infant on a raised, unguarded surface

When in doubt as to where to place child, use the floor

Restrain child in infant seat and never leave child unattended while the seat is resting on a raised surface

Avoid using a high chair until child can sit well with support

Poisoning

Not as great a danger to this age-group, but should begin practicing safeguards early (see under 4-7 Months)

Burns

Install smoke detectors in home

Use caution when warming formula in microwave oven; always check temperature of liquid before feeding

Check bathwater

Do not pour hot liquids when infant is close by, such as sitting on lap

Beware of cigarette ashes that may fall on infant

Do not leave infant in the sun for more than a few minutes; keep exposed areas covered

Wash flame-retardant clothes according to label directions

Use cool-mist vaporizers

Do not leave child in parked car

Check surface heat of car restraint before placing child in seat

Motor vehicles

Transport infant in federally approved, rear-facing car seat*

Do not place infant on the seat or in lap

Do not place child in a carriage or stroller behind a parked car

Bodily damage

Avoid sharp, jagged objects

Keep diaper pins closed and away from infant

AGE: 4-7 MONTHS

Major Developmental Accomplishments

Rolls over

Sits momentarily

Grasps and manipulates small objects

Resecures a dropped object

Has well-developed eye-hand coordination

Can focus on and locate very small objects

Mouthing is very prominent

Can push up on hands and knees

Crawls backward

Injury Prevention

Aspiration

Keep buttons, beads, syringe caps, and other small objects out of infant's reach

Keep floor free of any small objects

Do not feed infant hard candy, nuts, food with pits or seeds, or whole or circular pieces of hot dog

Exercise caution when giving teething biscuits, because large chunks may be broken off and aspirated

Do not feed infant while child is lying down

Inspect toys for removable parts

Keep baby powder, if used, out of reach

Avoid storing large quantities of cleaning fluid, paints, pesticides, and other toxic substances

Discard used containers of poisonous substances

Do not store toxic substances in food containers

Discard used button-sized batteries; store new batteries in safe area

Know telephone number of local poison control center (usually listed in front of telephone directory)

Suffocation

Keep uninflated balloons out of reach

Remove all crib toys that are strung across crib or playpen when child begins to push up on hands or knees or is 5 months old

Falls

Restrain in a high chair

Keep crib rails raised to full height

Poisoning

Make sure that paint for furniture or toys does not contain lead

Place toxic substances on a high shelf or in locked cabinet

Hang plants or place on high surface rather than on floor

*Home care instructions for care of the choking infant and for use of child safety seats are available in *Wong and Whaley's Clinical Manual of Pediatric Nursing* (Mosby).

†Information available from U.S. Consumer Product Safety Commission; (800) 638-CPSC.

TABLE 12-15 Injury Prevention During Infancy—cont'd

Burns Keep faucets out of reach Place hot objects (cigarettes, candles, incense) on high surface Limit exposure to sun; apply sunscreen **Motor vehicles** See under Birth-4 Months	**Bodily damage** Give toys that are smooth and rounded, preferably made of wood or plastic Avoid long, pointed objects as toys Avoid toys that are excessively loud Keep sharp objects out of infant's reach
AGE: 8-12 MONTHS	
Major Developmental Accomplishments	
Crawls/creeps Stands, holding onto furniture Stands alone Cruises around furniture Walks Climbs Pulls on objects	Throws objects Is able to pick up small objects; has pincer grasp Explores by putting objects in mouth Dislikes being restrained Explores away from parent Increasing understanding of simple commands and phrases
Injury Prevention	
Aspiration Keep lint and small objects off floor, furniture, and out of reach of children Take care in feeding solid table food to ensure that very small pieces are given Do not use beanbag toys or allow child to play with dried beans See also under 4-7 Months **Suffocation/drowning** Keep doors of ovens, dishwashers, refrigerators, coolers, and front-loading clothes washers and dryers closed at all times If storing an unused appliance, such as a refrigerator, remove the door Supervise contact with inflated balloons; immediately discard popped balloons and keep uninflated balloons out of reach Fence swimming pools Always supervise when near any source of water, such as cleaning buckets, drainage areas, toilets Keep bathroom doors closed Eliminate unnecessary pools of water Keep one hand on child at all times when in tub	**Falls** Fence stairways at top and bottom if child has access to either end† Dress infant in safe shoes and clothing (soles that do not "catch" on floor, tied shoelaces, pant legs that do not touch floor) Avoid walkers, especially near stairs Ensure that furniture is sturdy enough for child to pull self to standing position and cruise **Poisoning** Administer medications as a drug, not as a candy Do not administer medications unless so prescribed by a practitioner Replace medications and poisons immediately after use; replace caps properly if a child-protector cap is used Have syrup of ipecac in home; use only if advised **Burns** Place guards in front of or around any heating appliance, fireplace, or furnace Keep electrical wires hidden or out of reach Place plastic guards over electrical outlets; place furniture in front of outlets Keep hanging tablecloths out of reach (child may pull down hot liquids or heavy or sharp objects)

jecting at two sites simultaneously (requires two operators). Research is needed to determine which sequence is least painful. Since allergic reactions can occur after injection of vaccines, appropriate precautions are taken (see Nursing Alert under Chemotherapy, Chapter 36).

Another important nursing responsibility is accurate documentation. Each child should have an immunization record for parents to keep, especially for families who move frequently. The following information is documented on the medical record: day, month, and year of administration; manufacturer and lot number of vaccine; and the name, address, and title of the person administering the vaccine. Additional data to record are the site and route of administration and evidence that the parent or legal guardian gave informed consent before the immunization was administered. Any adverse reactions after the administration of any vaccine is reported to the **Vaccine Adverse Event Reporting System (VAERS).***

INJURY PREVENTION

Injuries are a major cause of death during infancy, especially for children 6 to 12 months old. Constant vigilance, awareness, and supervision are essential as the child gains increased locomotor and manipulative skills that are coupled with an insatiable curiosity about the environment. Table 12-15 lists the major developmental achievements of each period during infancy and the appropriate injury prevention plan.

*For information call (800) 822-7967.

Aspiration of Foreign Objects

Asphyxiation by foreign material in the respiratory tract, combined with mechanical suffocation, is the leading cause of fatal injury in children younger than 1 year of age. The size, shape, and consistency of foods or objects are important determinants of fatal obstruction. For example, small spheric or cylindric and pliable objects (less than 3.2 cm, or 1¼ inches) are more likely to completely obstruct the airway. Unfortunately, common household items can be deadly to infants.

As soon as infants have the ability to find their mouth, they are vulnerable to aspiration of small objects, such as those left within reach or removable parts of objects that may on initial inspection appear safe. All **toys** must be carefully inspected for potential danger. Rattles, for example, have small beads in them to produce noise. A broken or cracked rattle can be dangerous because the beads can easily be aspirated while the infant has the toy in the mouth. Stuffed animals are another potentially dangerous toy if any of the parts, such as the eyes or nose, are removable buttons or plastic pieces. An active infant can grab a low-hanging mobile and quickly chew off a small piece. As soon as the infant crawls or plays on the floor, the floor must be kept free of any small articles that can be picked up and swallowed, such as coins.

When infant ***clothes*** are purchased, the type of closure is important. A front button can easily be pulled off and swallowed. Safety pins for diapers are kept closed and away from the dressing table. Even though a young infant may not search for them, practicing this good habit from the beginning prevents future injuries.

Food items are the second most common cause of aspiration, and the most frequent offenders are hot dogs, candy, nuts, and grapes. When new foods are given to the child, nuts, hard candies, marshmallows, large amounts of peanut butter, or fruits with pits or seeds are avoided. When traveling, especially in airplanes, or entertaining, snack foods such as peanuts and popcorn are kept away from young children. If given to young children, hot dogs must be cut into small, irregular pieces rather than served whole or sliced into sections, because their size (diameter), round shape, and consistency allow for complete occlusion of the airway. Perhaps the most dangerous food is dried beans, which, if aspirated, enlarge when they come in contact with the wet mucosa and block the airway.

Pacifiers can also be dangerous because the entire object may be aspirated if it is small or the nipple and shield may become detached from the handle and become lodged in the pharynx. Improvised pacifiers, such as those commonly made in hospitals from a padded nipple, also present dangers. The nipple may separate from the plastic collar and be aspirated (Millunchick and McArtor, 1986). In addition, parents may continue to offer this pacifier to the infant at home. To prevent the hazards of improvised pacifiers, hospitals should use only safe commercial types. Candy pacifiers pose dangers because the candy portion can dislodge from the circular base and be aspirated (Ramsey, Goldbach, and Stephenson, 1989). To be safe, pacifiers should have (Nowak, 1993) (Fig. 12-15):

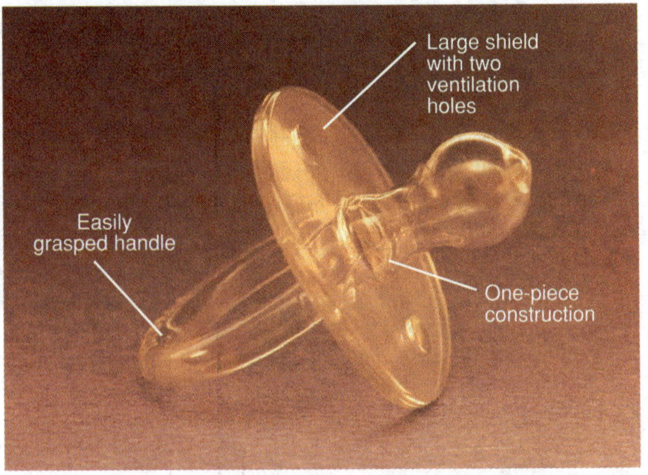

FIG. 12-15 Design of safe pacifier.

- Sturdy, one-piece construction with material that is nontoxic, flexible, and firm but not brittle
- An easily grasped handle
- A mouthguard that cannot be separated from the nipple, has two ventilating holes, and is too large to be aspirated
- No detachable ribbon or string
- A label warning against tying the pacifier around the infant's neck

Using a syringe to accurately measure and dispense oral liquid medications to young children has become common practice. However, the ***syringe cap*** is a potential aspiration hazard (Botash, 1992). As a precaution, keep parts of medication devices out of the reach of children and be certain the cap is removed before dispensing medication.

Even safety devices can be dangerous. To prevent tampering, items (such as baby food jars) may be covered with a plastic oversleeve. The ***tear-down strip*** can be aspirated and is very difficult to locate because it is clear (Livesey and others, 1992).

Another hazardous substance if aspirated is ***baby powder,*** which is usually a mixture of talc (hydrous magnesium silicate) and other silicates. Although the use of talc has been discouraged, it is a common baby care product and can cause severe and often fatal aspiration pneumonia. One of the factors involved in talc aspiration is the similar appearance of baby powder containers and nursing bottles. Talc containers often become favorite playthings and are placed in the mouth. Improper use of powder by sprinkling it directly on the skin creates a cloud of talc dust that is easily inhaled. Parents are advised of the danger of baby powder and are discouraged from using it. If they prefer to use a powder, a cornstarch preparation can be substituted (see Diaper Dermatitis, Chapter 13). Whenever a powder is used, it is placed in the hand and then applied to the skin, never shaken directly from the container to the skin. The container is kept closed and immediately stored in a safe place, especially away from curious toddlers, who often imitate caregiving activities and may accidentally shake it on the infant.

Suffocation

Mechanical suffocation includes suffocation by covering of the airway (i.e., mouth and nose), by pressure on the throat and chest, and by exclusion of air, such as by refrigerator entrapment. Nonfood items cause the majority of deaths in young children. ***Latex balloons,*** whether partially inflated, uninflated, or popped, are the leading cause of pediatric choking deaths from children's products (Holida, 1993). They should be kept away from infants and young children. Even the practice of inflating latex gloves to amuse children in health care settings may pose a danger.

NURSING ALERT
Encourage adults to:
Blow up balloons for children
Supervise their balloon play
Pick up and dispose of broken balloon pieces
Warn older children of dangers of chewing or sucking on balloons
Substitute Mylar balloons for latex balloons

In addition, the accessibility of plastic linings of diapers used on the infant and/or on dolls is especially dangerous to young children.

The ***bed*** or ***crib*** poses a number of hazards. An infant who is placed in a bed under blankets and sheets that are tucked in can be caught under them and be unable to wriggle free. Baby pillows filled with plastic foam beads that make them resemble small bean bags are dangerous; very young infants are suffocated when the pillow contours to the face and blocks the airway (Rollins, 1990). There are potential dangers in adults sleeping with a small infant because of the possibility of their rolling over and smothering the child.

Infant strangulation may occur if the infant's head becomes caught between the crib slats and mattress or objects close to the crib. Suffocation deaths are not confined to cribs; ill-fitting mattresses in adult or youth beds, bunk beds, and waterbeds have also been reported. According to federal regulation the distance between crib slats should not be more than 2⅜ inches (about 6 cm), roughly the width of three adult fingers. Mattresses and bumper pads should fit snugly against the slats. A general rule is that if two adult fingers can be placed between the mattress and crib or bed side, the mattress is too small. A temporary solution is to place large, rolled towels in the space to create a snug fit.

Corner post extensions on cribs are another source of strangulation. Children have died when their clothing caught on raised corner posts as they climbed out of the crib. Voluntary manufacturing standards state the corner post extensions should not exceed 1⁄16 inch. However, the safety of *any* extension is questionable. Decorative extensions need to be removed from cribs. Ideally, information regarding correct crib design should be given prenatally before parents have purchased or borrowed a crib.*

Mesh-sided playpens and cribs can result in death if the sides are left in the lowered position. Infants have suffocated when they fell off the edge of the mattress and the head or chest was compressed between the floorboard and mesh side. Parents should be advised of this danger and encouraged to *always* keep the sides locked securely in the up position whenever the child is in the playpen or crib.

The crib should be positioned away from large furniture, because children who crawl out of the crib may become caught between the two objects. Cribs should also be located away from windows, where drape or blind cords can become wrapped around the infant's neck.

Another cause of suffocation is ***plastic bags.*** Large plastic bags used over garments are very lightweight and can easily and quickly be wrapped around the head of an active infant or pressed against the face. Pillows and mattresses should not be covered with plastic for this reason. Older infants may play with a plastic bag and accidentally pull it over their heads. Because plastic is nonporous, suffocation takes place in a matter of minutes.

Cords either near the infant or tied around the infant's neck can potentially cause strangulation. Bibs are removed at bedtime, and objects such as pacifiers are never hung on a string around the infant's neck. This is a common practice in some cultures that can be remedied by attaching a *short* string tied to a pacifier and pinning the string on the child's shirt.

Toys that have strings attached, such as a telephone, or toys that are tied to cribs or playpens can be hazards because the string can become wrapped around the child's neck or the child can become entrapped in the toy. As a precaution, all cords should be less than 30 cm (12 inches) long. Crib toys should be hung high enough that the infant cannot become entangled in them or should no longer be used once the child is able to reach them.

Restraining straps, if applied too loosely or left unfastened, can be a hazard. For example, a child may slide off a high chair beneath the tray and become strangled on the loose strap. All straps should be fastened securely.

Motor Vehicle Injuries

Automobile injuries are the leading cause of accidental death in children older than 1 year of age. However, a significant number of infants are injured or die from improper restraint within the vehicle, most often from riding on the lap of another occupant (Agran, Winn and Castillo, 1992). All infants must be secured in a federally approved restraint rather than held or placed on the seat of the car. There is no safe alternative.

Infant restraints are designed either as an infant-only model (Fig. 12-16) or as a convertible infant-toddler model. Either restraint is a semi-reclined seat that faces the *rear* of the car. A rear-facing car seat provides the very best protection for the disproportionately heavy head and the weak neck of a young child. This position minimizes the stress on the neck by spreading the forces of a frontal crash over the entire back, neck, and head; the spine is supported by the back of the car seat. If the seat were faced forward, the head would whip forward because of

---

*The booklet *It Hurts When They Cry* gives basic information on hazards, safety features, and proper use of nursery furniture and equipment. It is available at no charge from U.S. Consumer Product Safety Commission, Publication Request, Washington, DC 20207; (800) 638-2772. Additional free information is available from the Danny Foundation, 3158 Danville Blvd, P.O. Box 680, Alamo, CA 94507; (800) 83-DANNY.

the force of the crash, creating enormous stress on the neck.

NURSING ALERT Infants should face the rear from birth to 20 pounds and as close to 1 year of age as possible.

The restraint is anchored to the vehicle with the car seat belt and has a harness system for restraining the infant. Some harness systems require a clip to keep the shoulder straps correctly positioned. Although many infant restraints can be recliners, they are only used in the car in the position specified by the manufacturer.

Generally, the middle of the back seat is considered the safest area of the car. However, an infant restraint may be positioned in the front seat, where the driver can observe the infant without having to turn around, provided that the seatbelt can be locked into position. Parents should check the car's vehicle owner's manual, because additional hardware may be needed.

NURSING ALERT Rear-facing infant safety seats must not be placed in the front seats of cars equipped with an airbag on the passenger side. If an infant seat is placed in the passenger seat with an air bag, the child could be seriously injured if the air bag is released, since rear-facing infant seats extend closer to the dashboard (Health Alert, 1994) (Fig. 12-17).

For restraints to be effective, they must be used properly. Dressing the infant in an outfit with sleeves and legs allows the harness to securely hold the child in the seat. A small blanket or towel rolled tightly can be placed on either side of the head to minimize movement and keep the infant's hips against the back of the seat. Padding between the infant's legs and crotch is added to prevent slouching. Thick, soft padding is not placed under the infant or behind the back because during the impact the padding will compress, leaving the harness straps loose. (For further discussion of restraints see Chapter 14.)

Falls

Falls are most common after 4 months of age when the infant has learned to roll over, but they can occur at any age. Newborns are normally active, assume a flexed position, and have crawling and Moro reflexes that can propel them forward. The best advice is never to place a child unattended on a raised surface that has no type of guardrails. When in doubt, the safest place is the floor. Even though young infants cannot climb over a partially raised crib rail, it is best to form a habit of raising the rail all the way, because someday that infant will be able to climb out. Crib sides should have a latching device that cannot be easily released. The welds attaching the crib corner locks to the corner posts should not be cracked or broken. If the welds are damaged, the bedspring could fall to the floor. Ideally, cribs should be placed on carpeted, not hard, floors.

Another danger area for falling is a ***changing table,*** which is usually high and narrow. Although these tables have a restraining belt, children are never left unattended, even when restrained. The best way to avoid having to leave is to arrange the area with all necessary articles within easy reach so that the child is always in full sight of the caregiver. It only takes a fraction of a second for an infant to fall off. During the latter half of the first year, infants usually resist dressing and diapering and may be difficult to manage. If there is danger that the child is strong enough to resist restraining, the infant should be changed on a safer surface, such as a clean floor.

Infant seats, high chairs, walkers, and ***swings*** present additional opportunities for falls. If the infant seat is placed on a table, the child should never be left unrestrained or unattended. The same rule is essential for other baby equip-

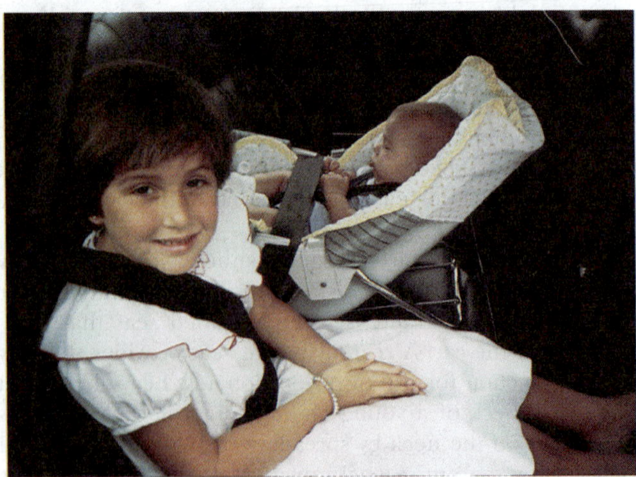

FIG. 12-16 Federally approved infant car restraint. Note placement in middle of back seat and use of car lap/shoulder belt for older child.

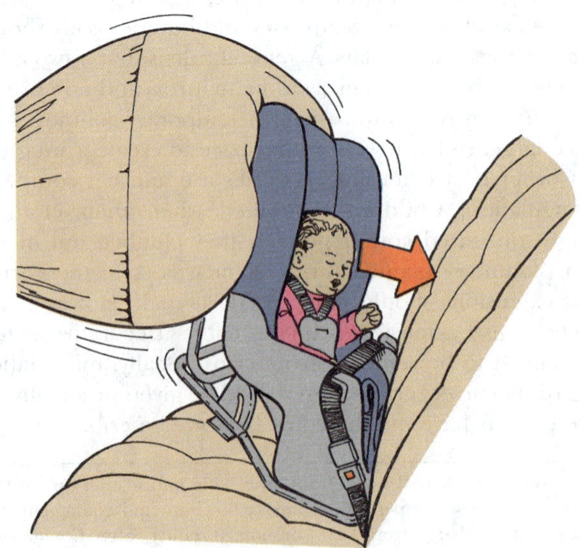

FIG. 12-17 An air bag could strike a child safety seat, seriously injuring the infant. (Redrawn from Health alert, *AAP News* 10(4):22, 1994.)

ment, particularly when the child has learned to crawl and to stand up. Small infants can slip through a high chair if a protective harness is not used. The danger of falls from being unrestrained applies to shopping carts as well (Tully, 1993). High chairs are designed for older infants who can sit well and who are tall enough to have the tray at the level of their chest or abdomen. Walkers are responsible for a number of different types of injuries that occur because the walker tipped over or fell down stairs (Rieder, Schwartz, and Newman, 1986). Parents need to be warned of these dangers and encouraged to keep a constant vigil on their child's activities; the use of walkers should be discouraged.

Once infants are mobile, they should not be allowed to crawl unsupervised on any raised surface, near stairs, or near any water reservoir. Gates should be used at the *bottom* and *top* of ***stairs,*** because both present dangers to the crawling and climbing infant. However, certain types of gates can present hazards. Freestanding enclosures constructed of criss-crossed wood slats that expand and contract can trap the head or neck when children attempt to climb over them. If these types of gates are used, they must be securely fastened to prevent mobility of the slats.

As children begin to pull themselves to a standing position, ***heavy objects,*** such as unsturdy furniture or any free standing item (e.g., wrought iron fish tank stands or concrete birdbath), can be extremely dangerous if pulled down on top of the child. To prevent injury from furniture tipping over, TVs should be placed on lower furniture, as far back as possible. Angle braces or anchors can secure furniture to walls.

Sometimes even when the environment is made safe, infants may literally trip over their own feet from ***clothing.*** Slippery socks; hard, slick soles on shoes or rubber soles that can catch, especially on a carpet; and long pants or pajama bottoms can easily upset a child's balance. Such dangers need to be pointed out to parents, especially when infants are taking their first steps.

Poisoning

Poisoning is one of the major causes of death in children younger than 5 years of age. The highest incidence occurs in those in the 2-year-old group, with the second highest incidence occurring in 1-year-old children. Infants who do not crawl are relatively free from danger of poisonous agents by virtue of immobility. However, once locomotion begins, danger from poisoning is present almost everywhere. There are more than 500 toxic substances in the average home, and about a third of all poisonings occur in the kitchen.

The major reason for ingestion of poisons is ***improper storage.*** To protect the infant, toxic agents should not be placed on a low shelf, table, or floor. Drugs that are kept in a purse pose additional dangers; if the purse is given to infants to play with, they may open it and ingest the drug. Another unrecognized hazard is during diaper changes when infants are near many toxic substances such as ointments, creams, oils, and talc. Parents may even hand infants a potentially poisonous object to quiet them. Such dangers need to be stressed to parents, and toys need to be kept at diapering areas to minimize risks.

Plants are another source of poisoning for infants. Plants are frequently placed on the floor, and the leaves or flowers are attractive and easy to pull off. More than 700 species of plants are known to have caused illness or death.

Another danger is ingestion of ***button-sized batteries*** that are used in devices such as hearing aids, calculators, watches, and cameras. Because they are bright and shiny, they are attractive to children. However, they can cause severe morbidity, even death, if lodged in the esophagus. The strong alkali in a battery can leak and cause a severe caustic burn. As a precaution small batteries must be safely stored and discarded where young children cannot easily retrieve them.

Not all poisonings result from ingestion—***inhalation*** is another possible route, such as inhaling chlorine vapors from household cleaning or pool supplies. Recent concern has addressed passive cocaine toxicity in young children exposed to freebase cocaine ("crack") smoking by adults (Bateman and Heagarty, 1989). Children should be protected from environments where these toxins exist (for a discussion of passive cigarette smoking, see Chapter 32).

The only sure way to prevent poisoning is to remove toxic agents, which means placing them high out of the infant's reach. However, because crawling infants soon become climbing toddlers, it is best to keep all toxic agents, especially drugs, in a locked cabinet. Special plastic hooks can be attached to the inside of cabinet doors to keep them securely closed (see Fig. 12-18). Firm thumb pressure is required to unlatch the hook, and small children are usually unable to manipulate them. Locks are best, but for frequently used cleaning agents, such as those often kept under a kitchen sink, hooks are a practical alternative.

With several hundred toxic substances in each house, locking up all potentially toxic substances could present a problem; however, careful planning can help. A large surplus of cleaning agents, furniture polishes, laundry additives, paints, insecticides, and solvents should be avoided.

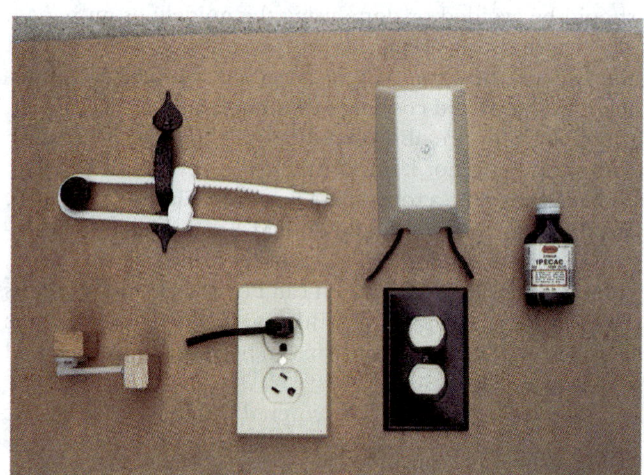

FIG. 12-18 Safety demonstration board. *Clockwise from lower left:* Cabinet latches, shock guard for electrical outlet, syrup of ipecac, and two type of outlet covers (white cover is passive device that automatically covers outlet when plug is removed).

Used poison containers should be promptly discarded and not used to store another poison without adequately marking the package. Any potentially hazardous substance should not be stored in any type of food container. A popular container used to store toxic liquids is a soda bottle. A child who is unaware of the dangerous contents is a vulnerable victim for poisoning. Parents should know the location of local poison control centers and call them in the event of a suspected poisoning. Emergency measures for poisoning are discussed in Chapter 16.

Burns

Burns such as scalding from water that is too hot, excessive sunburn, and burns from house fires, electrical wires, sockets, and heating elements such as radiators, registers, and floor furnaces cause a significant number of deaths and many more injuries in infants. The infant's skin is particularly sensitive to irritation, and the mechanisms for temperature preception are not completely developed. As a general precaution, all homes should have smoke alarms installed near the bedroom areas.

Scald burns from ***hot tap water*** can be prevented by lowering the hot water heater to a safe temperature of 49° C (120° F). In addition, the bathwater should be checked before the infant is immersed. Scalds can also occur from bathing infants in the kitchen sink when the garbage disposal, occluded with debris, causes the draining dishwasher effluent to back up into the sink. The temperature of the effluent from a dishwasher is typically that of the maximum water temperature of the household water heater, but many dishwashers are equipped with heating elements that heat water to a temperature that is even higher (Sheridan, Sheridan, and Tompkins, 1993). As a precaution, instruct caregivers to avoid bathing small children in the kitchen sink while the dishwasher is running. If formula or food is warmed in a ***microwave oven,*** it must be checked before feeding because the container may remain cool while the contents are hot (Smelt and Cawdry, 1989). Another danger is explosion of the bottle from the buildup of steam. Because of these dangers, microwaving infant formula or food should be avoided or done using the guidelines on p. 544. The handles of cooking utensils should be turned toward the back of the stove. When the infant is underfoot, pouring hot liquids and cooking with hot oil are avoided. Hanging tablecloths are also placed out of the infant's reach to prevent pulling hot items off the table.

Sunburn can be a source of a first- or second-degree burn. Exposure to direct sunlight should be avoided. When infants are in the sun, the body, especially the face and head, should be covered. Sunscreen can be used on older infants (see Sunburn, Chapter 18). Although black-skinned infants burn less readily, their thin skin can become sunburned and needs protection.

Electrical outlets should be covered with protective plastic caps that prevent the child from sucking on the outlet or putting objects such as hairpins into it (see Fig. 12-18). Live wires are placed out of reach so that curious infants cannot chew on them and break the rubber coating. Infants should not be allowed to play near television sets, stereo units, or other appliances, whether these units are turned on or off, because infants cannot determine when the appliance is safe.

Any ***heat-producing element*** should have a guard placed in front of it. Fireplaces should be well screened because they are very appealing and within easy access. Small portable heaters should be placed on a high surface. Floor furnaces should have barrier gates to prevent children from crawling or walking over them. Burning cigarettes, candles, and incense are kept out of reach, and infants should not be held by a smoking adult, because falling ashes are a hazard, especially to the eyes. Heated-mist vaporizers are a source of burns and should not be used. If humidity is needed, only cool mist vaporizers are safe.

By law, all infant sleepwear must be flame retardant. Unfortunately, this does not apply to all ***infant clothing.*** Flame-retardant fabric must never be viewed as the ultimate protection against burns. Repeated washing reduces the flame-retardant properties, and the use of soap or bleach destroys the protection. Inasmuch as detergent should be used for washing flame-retardant clothing, infants who are sensitive to such wash agents are unprotected when their clothing is washed even with a mild soap. If sleepwear is home sewn, parents are advised to look for specially treated flame-retardant fabric.

Another type of thermal injury occurs when children are exposed to excessive heat during confinement in poorly ventilated ***vehicles.*** The practice of leaving the windows open a couple of inches is not protective. The nurse should caution parents never to leave children in parked cars, especially when the automobile is in direct sunlight.

Children can also be burned by overheated metal hardware and vinyl seats in cars parked in the sun. As a precaution the surface heat of car restraints should be determined before placing children in them. Covering the restraints and hardware (such as metal latches on seat belts) may be necessary to prevent skin burns. An additional safeguard is buying a light-colored restraint, which absorbs less heat.

Drowning

Drowning in this age-group can occur in only inches of water. Consequently, infants should never be left unsupervised in a bathtub, hot tub, or near a source of water such as a swimming pool, lake, toilet, or bucket. Organized swimming instruction is not recommended for children under 4 years of age, because it may lead to a false sense of security. No infant can be expected to learn the elements of water safety or to react appropriately in an emergency. Therefore all young children need to be considered at risk when near water (American Academy of Pediatrics, Committee on Injury and Poison Prevention, 1993b). Infants and toddlers are also at increased risk of infection and convulsions from swallowing large amounts of water.

Bodily Damage

Injuries can occur in numerous ways. Sharp, jagged-edged objects can cause wounds in the skin. Long-pointed articles, such as the common toothpick or fork, can be poked into the eye or ear, causing serious damage. Such articles should

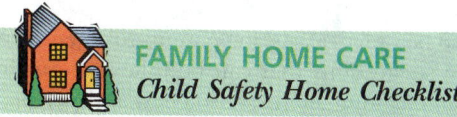

FAMILY HOME CARE
Child Safety Home Checklist

SAFETY: FIRE, ELECTRICAL, BURNS

- ☐ Guards in front of or around any heating appliance, fireplace, or furnace (including floor furnace)*
- ☐ Electrical wires hidden or out of reach*
- ☐ No frayed or broken wires; no overloaded sockets
- ☐ Plastic guards or caps over electrical outlets, furniture in front of outlets*
- ☐ Hanging tablecloths out of reach, away from open fires*
- ☐ Smoke detectors tested and operating properly
- ☐ Kitchen matches stored out of child's reach*
- ☐ Large, deep ashtrays throughout house (if used)
- ☐ Small stoves, heaters, and other hot objects (cigarettes, candles, coffee pots, slow cookers) placed where they cannot be tipped over or reached by children
- ☐ Hot water heater set at 49° C (120° F) or lower
- ☐ Pot handles turned toward back of stove, center of table
- ☐ No loose clothing worn near stove
- ☐ No cooking or eating hot foods or liquids with child standing nearby or sitting in lap
- ☐ All small appliances, such as iron, turned off, disconnected, and placed out of reach when not in use
- ☐ Cool, not hot, mist vaporizer used
- ☐ Fire extinguisher available on each floor and checked periodically
- ☐ Electrical fuse box and gas outlet accessible
- ☐ Family escape plan in case of a fire practiced periodically; fire escape ladder available on upper-level floors
- ☐ Telephone number of fire or rescue squad and address of home with nearest cross street posted near phone

SAFETY: SUFFOCATION AND ASPIRATION

- ☐ Small objects stored out of reach*
- ☐ Toys inspected for small removable parts or long strings*
- ☐ Hanging crib toys and mobiles placed out of reach
- ☐ Plastic bags stored away from young child's reach, large plastic garment bags discarded after tying in knots*
- ☐ Mattress or pillow not covered with plastic or in manner accessible to child*
- ☐ Crib design according to federal regulations with snug-fitting mattress*†
- ☐ Crib positioned away from other furniture or windows*
- ☐ Portable playpen gates up at all times while in use*
- ☐ Accordion-style gates not used*
- ☐ Bathroom doors kept closed and toilet seats down*
- ☐ Faucets turned off firmly*
- ☐ Pool fenced with locked gate
- ☐ Proper safety equipment at poolside
- ☐ Electric garage door openers stored safely and garage door adjusted to rise when door strikes object
- ☐ Doors of ovens, trunks, dishwashers, refrigerators, and front-loading clothes washers and dryers kept closed*
- ☐ Unused appliance, such as a refrigerator, securely closed with lock or doors removed*
- ☐ Food served in small noncylindric pieces*
- ☐ Toy chests without lids or with lids that securely lock in open position*
- ☐ Buckets and wading pools kept empty when not in use*
- ☐ Clothesline above head level
- ☐ At least one member of household trained in basic life support (CPR), including first aid for choking‡

SAFETY: POISONING

- ☐ Toxic substances, including batteries, placed on a high shelf, preferably in locked cabinet
- ☐ Toxic plants hung or placed out of reach*
- ☐ Excess quantities of cleaning fluid, paints, pesticides, drugs, and other toxic substances not stored in home
- ☐ Used containers of poisonous substances discarded where child cannot obtain access
- ☐ Telephone number of local poison control center and address of home with nearest cross street posted near phone
- ☐ Syrup of ipecac in home containing two doses per child
- ☐ Medicines clearly labeled in childproof containers and stored out of reach
- ☐ Household cleaners, disinfectants, and insecticides kept in their original containers, separate from food and out of reach
- ☐ Smoking in areas away from children

SAFETY: FALLS

- ☐ Nonskid mats, strips, or surfaces in tubs and showers
- ☐ Exits, halls, and passageways in rooms kept clear of toys, furniture, boxes, or other items that could be obstructive
- ☐ Stairs and halls well lighted, with switches at both top and bottom
- ☐ Sturdy handrails for all steps and stairways
- ☐ Nothing stored on stairways
- ☐ Treads, risers, and carpeting in good repair
- ☐ Glass doors and walls marked with decals
- ☐ Safety glass used in doors, windows, and walls
- ☐ Gates on top and bottom of staircases and elevated areas, such as porch, fire escape*
- ☐ Guardrails on upstairs windows with locks that limit height of window opening and access to areas such as fire escape*
- ☐ Crib side rails raised to full height; mattress lowered as child grows*
- ☐ Restraints used in high chairs, walkers, or other baby furniture; preferably walkers not used*
- ☐ Scatter rugs secured in place or used with nonskid back
- ☐ Walks, patios, and driveways in good repair

SAFETY: BODILY INJURY

- ☐ Knives, power tools, and unloaded firearms stored safely or placed in locked cabinet
- ☐ Garden tools returned to storage racks after use
- ☐ Pets properly restrained and immunized for rabies
- ☐ Swings, slides, and other outdoor play equipment kept in safe condition
- ☐ Yard free of broken glass, nail-studded boards, other litter
- ☐ Cement birdbaths placed where young child cannot tip them over*

---

*Safety measures are specific for homes with young children. All safety measures should be implemented in homes where children reside and visit frequently, such as those of grandparents or baby-sitters.
†Federal regulations are available from U.S. Consumer Product Safety Commission; (800) 638-CPSC.
‡Home care instructions for infant cardiopulmonary resuscitation and infant/child choking are available in *Wong and Whaley's Clinical Manual of Pediatric Nursing* (Mosby).

be safely stored away from the infant's reach; forks are best avoided for self-feeding until the child has mastered the spoon, usually by age 18 months.

In addition to hazards such as aspiration from toys, small articles can be placed in the ear or nose, and excessive noise from toys can result in sensorineural hearing loss. Although toys with the highest noise levels are model airplanes, air guns, toy cap guns, and firecrackers, even common squeaking toys used by young children may be harmful if placed close to the ear (Axelsson and Jerson, 1985).

Even clothes and hair can present dangers to infants who cannot call attention to the problem. For example, constriction injuries can occur from excessively tight bands on socks, as well as fibers of hair or thread wrapped tightly around appendages, usually toes or fingers (Barton and others, 1988).

Another frequently unrecognized danger to infants is animal attacks. Helpless infants, as newcomers to the home, can provoke jealousy in animals, especially dogs and cats. However, unprovoked attacks by ferrets and roosters have also been reported (Paisley and Lauer, 1988; Prieser and Lavell, 1987). Parents must be constantly vigilant to protect the child from household pets and farm animals (see Animal Bites, Chapter 18).

Nurse's Role In Injury Prevention

When the potential environmental dangers to which infants are vulnerable are considered, the task of preventing these injuries only begins to be appreciated. Nurses must be aware of the possible causes of injury in each age-group in order for *anticipatory* preventive teaching to occur. For example, the guidelines for injury prevention during infancy presented in Table 12-15 should be discussed *before* the child reaches the susceptible age-group. Preventive teaching ideally occurs during pregnancy. Inasmuch as two thirds of all injuries to children occur in the home, the importance of safety cannot be overemphasized. The Family Home Care box summarizes a home safety checklist that can be presented to parents to increase their awareness of danger areas in the home and assist them in implementing safety devices and practices *before* their absence can inflict injury on infants. In addition, displays such as a safety demonstration board (see Fig. 12-18) can be helpful in familiarizing parents with inexpensive, commercial devices that can be used in the home to prevent injuries.

➤ **NURSING TIP** To help parents appreciate the dangers present in their home to young children, suggest that they get eye level with the floor to survey the environment from a child's view.

Injury prevention requires protection of the child and education of the caregiver. Nurses in ambulatory care settings, health maintenance centers, or visiting nurse agencies are in a most favorable position for injury education. This does not exclude nurses in inpatient facilities, who could use visiting times as an excellent opportunity for discussing this topic.

One approach to teaching injury prevention is to relate why children in various age-groups are prone to specific types of injuries. Stressing prevention is just as important as emphasizing the *why* of the injury. However, injury prevention must also be practical. Asking parents for their ideas leads to realistic suggestions that can be followed. For instance, bathroom cleaning agents, cosmetics, and personal care items can be placed on a top shelf in the linen closet, and towels or sheets can be stored on the lower shelves and floor.

If an injury has occurred, the nurse should not be too quick to admonish the parent. Injuries do not always indicate neglect. It is a difficult task to watch children carefully without overprotecting or unnecessarily confining them. Small falls help children learn the dangers of heights. Touching a hot object once can emphasize to the child the pain of a burn. Allowing children to explore while maintaining consistent, age-appropriate limits is sound advice.

Parents need to remember that infants and young children cannot anticipate danger or understand when it is or is not present. A dead electrical wire may present no actual harm, but if the child is allowed to play with it, a poor behavior is enforced and will be practiced when the child encounters a live wire. Although it is always wise to explain why something is dangerous, it must be remembered that small children need to be physically removed from the situation.

It is not easy to teach safety, supervise closely, and refrain from saying "no" a hundred times a day. Parents become acutely aware of this dilemma as soon as the infant learns to crawl. Preventing injuries to children is usually the first reason for limit-setting and discipline, but limits are also set to prevent damage to valuable household objects. When small children are in the home, dangerous objects must be removed or guarded and valuable articles placed out of reach.

When children are taught the meaning of "no," they should also be taught what "yes" means. Children should be praised for playing with suitable toys, their efforts at behaving or listening should be reinforced, and recreational toys that are innovative and creative should be provided for them. Infants love to tear paper and avidly pursue books, magazines, or newspapers left on the floor. Instead of always scolding them for destroying a valued book, child-safe books (such as those constructed of fabric) can be kept available for them to play with. If they enjoy pots and pans, a cabinet can be arranged with safe utensils for them to explore.

One additional factor must be stressed concerning injury prevention and education. Children are imitators; they copy what they see and hear. *Practicing safety teaches safety,* which applies to parents and their children and to nurses and their clients. Saying one thing but doing another confuses children and can lead to difficulties as the child grows older.

ANTICIPATORY GUIDANCE—CARE OF FAMILIES

Childrearing is no easy task; it presents challenges to new parents as well as to "seasoned" parents. With society's changing roles and mores, combined with a highly mobile population, there is little stability for traditional role models and time-honored methods of raising children. As a result, parents look more to professionals for guidance.

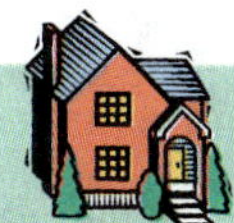

FAMILY HOME CARE
Guidance During Infant's First Year

FIRST 6 MONTHS

Understand each parent's adjustment to newborn, especially mother's postpartal emotional needs.
Teach care of infant and assist parents to understand his or her individual needs and temperament and that the infant expresses wants through crying.
Reassure parents that infant cannot be spoiled by too much attention during the first 4 to 6 months.
Encourage parents to establish a schedule that meets needs of child and themselves.
Help parents understand infant's need for stimulation in environment.
Support parents' pleasure in seeing child's growing friendliness and social response, especially smiling.
Plan anticipatory guidance for safety.
Stress need for immunization.
Prepare for introduction of solid foods.

SECOND 6 MONTHS

Prepare parents for child's "stranger anxiety."
Encourage parents to allow child to cling to them and avoid long separation from either.
Guide parents concerning discipline because of infant's increasing mobility.
Encourage use of negative voice and eye contact rather than physical punishment as a means of discipline.
Encourage showing most attention when infant is behaving well, rather than when infant is crying.
Teach injury prevention because of child's advancing motor skills and curiosity.
Encourage parents to leave child with suitable caregiver to allow some free time.
Discuss readiness for weaning.
Explore parents' feelings regarding infant's sleep patterns.

Nurses are in an advantageous position to render assistance and suggestions. Every phase of a child's life has its particular traumas—toilet training for toddlers, unexplained fears for preschoolers, or identity crises for adolescents. For parents of an infant some challenges center around dependency, discipline, increased mobility, and safety. Major areas for parental guidance during the first year are listed in the Family Home Care box.

KEY POINTS

- Biologic development of the child encompasses proportional changes; sensory changes, including binocularity, depth perception, and visual preference; maturation of biologic systems; fine motor development; and gross motor development.
- Erikson's theory of psychosocial development (birth to 1 year) is concerned with acquiring a sense of trust while overcoming a sense of mistrust.
- Piaget's theory of cognitive development, as it applies to the infant, focuses on the sensorimotor phase, which includes the use of reflexes, primary circular reactions, secondary circular reactions, and coordination of secondary schemata and their application to new situations.
- Development of body image begins in infancy; by 1 year of age infants recognize that they are distinct from their parents.
- Social development of the infant is guided by attachment, language development, personal-social behavior, and participation in play.
- Temperament influences the kind of interaction that occurs between the child and parents and siblings.
- Parents are faced with many concerns, including infant fears, daycare, limit-setting and discipline, thumb-sucking and pacifier use, teething, and choice of infant shoes.
- Breast milk or formula is the most desirable food for the infant during the first 6 months, followed by gradual introduction of solid food during the second 6 months. Whole milk is not recommended until after 12 months.
- Common sleep problems that develop during infancy—and that are easily prevented—are associated with night crying and feeding. Nurses should instruct the parents, after careful assessment, in strategies to deal with the specific problem.
- Fluoride supplements, dietary intake, and cleaning the teeth promote good dental hygiene.
- Recommended routine immunizations include those for hepatitis B virus, diphtheria, tetanus, pertussis, polio, measles, mumps, rubella, and *Haemophilus influenzae* type b.
- Recommended immunizations for selected groups of children are influenza virus, pneumococcal, and meningococcal vaccines.
- Because injuries are a major cause of death during infancy, parents should be alerted to aspiration of foreign objects, suffocation, falls, poisoning, burns, motor vehicle injuries, and bodily damage, as well as preventive actions needed to be taken to make the environment safe for infants.

REFERENCES

Agran PF, Winn DG, Castillo DN: On-lap travel: still a problem in motor vehicles, *Pediatrics* 90(1):27-29, 1992.

Alho OP and others: Control of the temporal aspect when considering risk factors for acute otitis media, *Arch Otolaryngol Head Neck Surg* 119(4):444-449, 1993.

Ainsworth M: Early caregiving and later patterns of attachment. In Klaus M, Robertson M, editors: *Birth, interaction, and attachment,* Skillman NJ, 1982, Johnson & Johnson Baby Products.

American Academy of Pediatrics, Committee on Infectious Diseases: Universal hepatitis B immunization, *Pediatrics* 89(4):795-800, 1992.

American Academy of Pediatrics, Committee on Infectious Diseases: *Haemophilus influenzae* type b conjugate vaccines: recommendations for immunization with recently and previously licensed vaccines, *Pediatrics* 92(3):480-488, 1993a.

American Academy of Pediatrics, Committee on Infectious Diseases: *1994 Red Book: report of the Committee on Infectious Diseases,* ed 23, Elk Grove Village, IL, 1994, The Academy.

American Academy of Pediatrics, Committee on Injury and Poison Prevention: Drowning in infants, children and adolescents, *Pediatrics* 92(2):292-294, 1993.

American Academy of Pediatrics, Committee on Nutrition: Follow-up or weaning formulas, *Pediatrics* 83(6):1067, 1989a.

American Academy of Pediatrics, Committee on Nutrition: Iron-fortified infant fomulas, *Pediatrics* 84(6):1114-1115, 1989b.

American Academy of Pediatrics, Committee on Nutrition: Policy statement: the use of fruit juice in the diets of young children, *AAP News* 7(2):11, 1991.

American Academy of Pediatrics, Committee on Nutrition: *Pediatric nutrition handbook,* ed 3, Elk Grove Village, IL, 1993, The Academy.

American Academy of Pediatrics, Committee on SportsMedicine: Infant exercise programs, *Pediatrics* 82(5):800, 1988.

American Public Health Association and American Academy of Pediatrics: *Caring for our children: national health and safety perfor-*

mance standards: guidelines for out-of-home child care programs, Washington, DC, 1992, The Association.

Anders TF, Halpern LF, Hua J: Sleeping through the night: a developmental perspective, *Pediatrics* 90(4):554-560, 1992.

Anderson G: Pacifiers: the positive side, *MCN* 11(2):122-124, 1986.

Axelsson A, Jerson T: Noisy toys: a possible source of sensorineural hearing loss, *Pediatrics* 76(4):574-578, 1985.

Baby bottle tooth decay, *Pediatr Dent* 15(7):27, 1993 (special issue—reference manual).

Barton D and others: Hair-thread tourniquet syndrome, *Pediatrics* 82(6):925-928, 1988.

Bateman D, Heagarty M: Passive freebase cocaine ("crack") inhalation by infants and toddlers, *Am J Dis Child* 143(1):25-27, 1989.

Bell DM and others: Illness associated with child day care: a study of incidence and cost, *Am J Public Health* 79(4):479-484, 1989.

Bell LM and others: Potential impact of linking an emergency department and hospital-affiliated clinics to immunize preschool-age children, *Pediatrics* 93(1):99-103, 1994.

Blasco PA: Normal and abnormal motor development, *Pediatr Rounds* 1(2):1-6, 1992.

Botash A: Syringe caps: an aspiration hazard, *Pediatrics* 90(1):92-3, 1992.

Bowlby J: *Attachment and loss,* vol 1, New York, 1969, Basic Books.

Braunstein H, Thomas S, Ito R: Immunity to measles in a large population of varying age, *Am J Dis Child* 144(3):296-298, 1990.

Brazelton T: *What every baby knows,* Menlo Park, CA, 1987, Addison-Wesley Publishing.

Brazelton T: Parent-infant cosleeping revisited, *Ab Initio* 2(1):1-7, 1990.

Briss PA and others: A nationwide study of the risk of injury associated with day care center attendance, *Pediatrics* 93(3):364-368, 1994.

Brown K and others: Milk consumption and hydration status of exclusively breast-fed infants in a warm climate, *J Pediatr* 108:677-680, 1986.

Butte N, Smith E, Garza C: Energy utilization of breast-fed and formula-fed infants, *Am J Clin Nutr* 51:350-358, 1990.

Calvo EB, Galindo AC, Aspres NB: Iron status in exclusively breast-fed infants, *Pediatrics* 90(3):375-379, 1992.

Carey WB, McDevitt SC: Revision of the infant temperament questionnaire, *Pediatrics* 61(5):735-739, 1978.

Centers for Disease Control and Prevention: Standards for pediatric immunization practices, *MMWR* 42(RR-5):1-13, 1993a.

Centers for Disease Control and Prevention: Use of vaccines and immune globulin in persons with altered immunocompetence: recommendations of the Advisory Committee on Immunization Practices (ACIP), *MMWR* 42(RR-4):1-18, 1993b.

Centers for Disease Control and Prevention: General recommendations on immunization: recommendations of the Advisory Committee on Immunization Practices (ACIP), *MMWR* 43(RR-1):1-38, 1994.

Chess S, Thomas A: Temperamental differences: a critical concept in child health care, *Pediatr Nurs* 11(3):167-171, 1985.

Chong A: Selecting shoes for children, *Baby Talk* 52(3):40-42, 1987.

Cipes M, Miraglia M, Gaulin-Kremer E: Monitoring and reinforcement to eliminate thumbsucking, *J Pediatr Nurs* 1(5):361, 1986.

Department of Health and Human Services: Reported vaccine-preventable disease—United States, 1993, and the Childhood Immunization Initiative, *MMWR* 43(4):57-60, 1994.

Dewey KG and others: Breast-fed infants are leaner than formula-fed infants at 1 year of age: the DARLING study, *Am J Clin Nutr* 57(2):140-145, 1993.

Duc G, Largo R: Anterior fontanel: size and closure in term and preterm infants, *Pediatrics* 78(5):904-908, 1986.

Ferber R: *Solve your child's sleep problems,* New York, 1985, Simon & Shuster.

Fomon S, Sanders K, Ziegler E: Formulas for older infants, *J Pediatr* 116(5):690-696, 1990.

Forsyth JS and others: Relation between early introduction of solid food to infants and their weight and illnesses during the first two years of life, *Br Med J* 306(6892):1572-1576, 1993.

French GM, Painter EC, Coury DL: Blowing away shot pain: a technique for pain management during immunization, *Pediatrics* 93(3):384-388, 1994.

Friman P, Barone V, Christophersen E: Aversive taste treatment of finger and thumb sucking, *Pediatrics* 78(1):174-176, 1986.

Friman PC and others: Influence of thumb sucking on peer social acceptance in first-grade children, *Pediatrics* 91:784-786, 1993.

Fuchs G and others: Gastrointestinal blood loss in older infants: impact of cow milk versus formula, *J Pediatr Gastroenterol Nutr* 16(1):4-9, 1993.

Garmezy N, Rutter M, editors: *Stress, coping, and development in children,* New York, 1989, McGraw-Hill.

Genarro S, Medoff-Cooper B, Lotas M: Perinatal factors and infant temperament: a collaborative approach . . . common variables of three studies examined, *Nurs Res* 41(6):375-377, 1992.

Glendon M: If the shoe fits . . . wear it, *Pediatr Nurs* 13(4):230-271, 1987.

Golden GS: The national childhood vaccine injury act: an update, *Contemp Pediatr* 10:96-105, 1993.

Gorelick MH, Baker MD: Epiglottitis in children, 1979 through 1992: effects of *Haemophilus influenzae* type b immunization, *Arch Pediatr Adolesc Med* 148(1):47-50, 1994.

Green M: Helping parents make the right child-care choice, *Contemp Pediatr* 3(6):40-49, 1986.

Greer F, Marshall S: Bone mineral content, serum vitamin D metabolite concentrations, and ultraviolet B light exposure in infants fed human milk with and without vitamin D_2 supplements, *J Pediatr* 114(2):203-212, 1989.

Gunnar MR and others: The stressfulness of separation among nine-month-old infants: effects of social context variables and infant temperament, *Child Dev* 63(2):290-303, 1992.

Health alert: Air bag/child seat warning label, *AAP News* 10(4):22, 1994.

Hick J and others: Optimum needle length for diphtheria-tetanus-pertussis inoculation of infants, *Pediatrics* 84(1):136-137, 1989.

Hobbie C: Choosing quality child care programs, *J Pediatr Health Care* 3(5):270-271, 1989.

Holberg CJ and others: Child day care, smoking by caregivers, and lower respiratory tract illness in the first 3 years of life, *Pediatrics* 91(5):885-892, 1993.

Holida DL: Latex balloons: they can take your breath away, *Pediatr Nurs* 19(1):39-43, 68, 1993.

Houldin A: Infant temperament and the quality of the childbearing environment, *Matern Child Nurs J* 16(2):131-143, 1987.

Houtrouw SM, Carlson KL: The relationship between maternal characteristics, maternal vulnerability beliefs, and immunization compliance, *Issues Compr Pediatr Nurs* 16:41-50, 1993.

Hurwitz ES and others: Risk of respiratory illness associated with day-care attendance: a nationwide study, *Pediatrics* 87(1):62-69, 1991.

Institute of Medicine: *Adverse events associated with childhood vaccines,* Washington, DC, 1993, National Academy Press.

Ipp M and others: Adverse reactions to diphtheria, tetanus, pertussis-polio vaccination at 18 months of age: effect of injection site and needle length, *Peditrics* 83(5):679-682, 1989.

Jaber L, Cohen IJ, Mor A: Fever associated with teething, *Arch Dis Child* 67(2):233-234, 1992.

Jones L, Heermann J: Parental division of infant care: contextual influences and infant characteristics, *Nurs Res* 41(4):228-234, 1992.

Kliman DS, Vukelich C: Mothers and fathers: expectations for infants, *Fam Rel* 34:305-313, 1985.

Knobloch H, Stevens F, Malone AF: *Manual of developmental diagnosis,* Hagerstown, PA, 1980, Harper & Row.

Kubiak M and others: Comparison of stool containment in cloth and single-use diapers using a simulated infant feces, *Pediatrics* 91(3):632-636, 1993.

Lampl M, Veldhuis JD, Johnson ML: Saltation and stasis: a model of human growth, *Science* 258(5083):801-803, 1992.

Landis SE, Chang A: Child care options for ill children, *Pediatrics* 88(4):705-718, 1991.

Lawrence RA: *Breast feeding: a guide for the medical profession,* ed 4, St Louis, 1994, Mosby.

Lee EJ, Bass C: Survey of accidents in a university day-care center *J Pediatr Health Care* 4:18-23, 1990.

Lester BM: There's more to crying than meets the ear. In Lester BM, Boukydis CF, editors: *Infant crying,* New York, 1985, Plenum.

Lincoln LM: Fathering and the separation-individuation process, *Matern Child Nurs J* 13(2);103-111, 1984.

Livesey JR: Inhalation injury with a new infant safety device in a child, *Lancet* 340(8816):424-425, 1992 (letter to the editor).

Long SS and others: Longitudinal study of adverse reactions following diphtheria-tetanus-pertussis vaccine in infancy, *Pediatrics* 85(3):294-302, 1990.

MacKenzie E: Thumb-sucking debate, *Pediatrics* 79(3):485-486, 1987.

Marwick C: Simpler vaccine schedules target more tykes, *JAMA* 270(18):2154, 1993.

Mayberry LJ, Affonso DD: Infant temperament and postpartum depression: a review, *Health Care Women Int* 14(2):201-211, 1993.

Maziade M and others: Temperament and intellectual development: a longitudinal study from infancy to four years, *Am J Psychiatry* 144(2):144-150, 1987.

McEwen M: Should there be universal childhood vaccination against hepatitis B? A commentary, *Pediatr Nurs* 19(5):447-452, 1993.

McIntosh B: Spoiled child syndrome, *Pediatrics* 83(1):108-114, 1989.

Measles—United States, 1992, *MMWR* 42(19): 378-381, 1993.

Miller A, Barr R, Eaton W: Crying and motor behavior of six-week-old infants and postpartum maternal mood, *Pediatrics* 92(4):551-558, 1993.

Millunchick E, McArtor R: Fatal aspiration of a makeshift pacifier, *Pediatrics* 77(3):369-370, 1986.

National Childhood Vaccine Injury Act: requirements for permanent vaccination records and for reporting of selected events after vaccination, *NNWR* 37(13):197-200, 1988.

National Vaccine Advisory Committee: The measles epidemic: the problems, barriers, and recommendations, *JAMA* 266:1547-1552, 1991.

Nelms BC: Stress during childhood: long-lasting effects? *Pediatr Nurs* 11(2):95-98, 1985.

Nowak AJ: What pediatricians can do to promote oral health, *Contemp Pediatr* 10(4):90-106, 1993.

Orenstein S and others: The Santmyer swallow: a new and useful infant reflex, *Lancet* 1(8581):345-346, 1988.

Paisley J, Lauer B: Severe facial injuries to infants due to unprovoked attacks by pet ferrets, *JAMA* 259:2005-2006, 1988.

Pinilla T, Birch LL: Help me make it through the night: behavioral entrainment of breast-fed infant's sleep patterns, *Pediatrics* 91(2): 436-444, 1993.

Pipes PL, Trahms CM: *Nutrition in infancy and childhood,* ed 5, St Louis, 1993, Mosby.

Pitzer M Hock E: Infant gender and sibling dyad infuences on maternal separation anxiety, *Matern Child Nurs J* 20(2):65-80, 1992.

Position statement: infant feeding, *Clin Pediatr* 31(8):510, 1992.

Preiser G, Lavell T: Rooster attacks on children, *Pediatrics* 79(3):426-427, 1987.

Ramsey K, Goldbach R, Stephenson S: Near fatal aspiration of a candy pacifier, *Pediatrics* 84(1):126-127, 1989.

Rassin GM and others: Health and safety in day care: parental knowledge, *Clin Pediatr* 30(6):344-349, 1991.

Recommendations for use of *Haemophilus* b conjugate vaccines and a combined diphtheria, tetanus, pertussis, and *Haemophilus* b vaccine: recommendations of the Advisory Committee on Immunization Practices (ACIP), *MMWR* 42(13):1-15, 1993.

Reifsnider E, Myers ST: Employed mothers can breast-feed, too! *MCN* 10:256-259, 1985.

Reported vaccine-preventable disease—United States, 1993, and the Childhood Immunization Initiative, *MMWR* 43(4):57-60, 1994.

Rieder M, Schwartz C, Newman J: Patterns of walker use and walker injury, *Pediatrics* 78(3):488-493, 1986.

Rivara FP and others: Risk of injury to children less than 5 years of age in day care versus home care settings, *Pediatrics* 84(6):1011-1016, 1989.

Robertson J: Some responses of young children to the loss of maternal care, *Nurs Times* 49:382-386, 1953.

Rollins J: Recall of baby pillows likely, *Pediatr Nurs* 16(3):282, 1990.

Runyan CW and others: Analysis of US child care safety regulations, *Am J Public Health* 81(8):981-985, 1991.

Sacks JJ and others: The epidemiology of injuries in Atlanta day-care centers, *JAMA* 266(12):1641-1645, 1989.

Salomon M and others: Evaluation of the two-needle strategy for reducing reactions to DPT vaccination, *Am J Dis Child* 141(7):796-798, 1987.

Schachter F and others: Cosleeping and sleep problems in Hispanic-American urban young children, *Pediatrics* 84(3):522-530, 1989.

Scher A and others: Toddlers' sleep and temperament: reporting bias or a valid link? A research note, *J Child Pyschol Psychiatry* 33(7):1249-1254, 1992.

Schmitt BD: The "two-step" approach to infant sleep problems, *Contemp Pediatr* 9(11):37-38, 1992.

Schoendorf KC and others: National trends in *Haemophilus influenzae* meningitis mortality and hospitalization among children, 1980 through 1991, *Pediatrics* 93(4):663-668, 1994.

Shannon M, Graef J: Lead intoxication in infancy, *Pediatrics* 89(1):87-90, 1992.

Sheridan R, Sheridan M, Tompkins R: Dishwasher effluent burns in infants, *Pediatrics* 91(1):142-143, 1993.

Smelt G, Cawdry H: Burns from fluid heated in a microwave oven, *Br Med J* 298:1452, 1989.

Smith KD, Shillam PJ, Zimmerman FA: Standards and criteria: group child care for sick children, *Pediatr Nurs* 15(6):600-602, 1989.

Spitz RA: Hospitalism: an inquiry into the genesis of psychiatric conditioning in early childhood. In Fenechel D and others, editors: *Psychoanalytic studies of the child,* vol 1, New York, 1945, International University Press.

Sullivan SA, Birch LL: Infant dietary experience and acceptance of solid foods, *Pediatrics* 93(2):271-277, 1994.

Szilagyi PG and others: Missed opportunities for childhood vaccinations in office practices and the effect on vaccination status, *Pediatrics* 91(1):1-7, 1993.

Taddio A and others: Use of lidocaine-prilocaine cream for vaccination pain in infants, *J Pediatr* 124(4):643-648, 1994.

Taubman B: Clinical trial of the treatment of colic by modification of parent-infant interaction, *Pediatrics* 74:998-1003, 1984.

Thacker SB and others: Infectious diseases and injuries in child day care: opportunities for healthier children, *JAMA* 268(13):1720-1726, 1992.

Thomas A, Chess S: Genesis and evolution of behavioral disorders: from infancy to early adult life, *Am J Psychiatry* 141(1):1-9, 1984.

Tully S: Injuries to children in shopping carts, *AAP News* 9(6):11, 1993.

Turner WT, Snow CW, Poteat GM: Accidental injuries among children in day care centers and family day care homes: brief report, *Child Health Care* 22(1):73-79, 1993.

Uhari M: A eutectic mixture of lidocaine and prilocaine for alleviating vaccination pain in infants, *Pediatrics* 92(5):719-721, 1993.

Van R and others: The effect of diaper type and overclothing on fecal contamination in day-care centers, *JAMA* 265(14):1840-1844, 1991.

Victora CG and others: Use of pacifiers and breastfeeding duration, *Lancet* 341(8842): 404-406, 1993.

Wasserman RC and others: Injury hazards in home day care, *J Pediatr* 114(1, pt 1):591-593, 1989.

Watson B and others: The effect of decreasing amounts of live virus, while antigen content remains constant, on immunogenicity of Oka/Merck varicella vaccine, *J Infect Dis* 168(6):1356-1360, 1993a.

Watson BM and others: Modified chickenpox in children immunized with the Oka/Merck varicella vaccine, *Pediatrics* 91(1):17-22, 1993b.

Wilkinson W, Clore E: Infant botulism: a dilemma for nursing, *J Pediatr Nurs* 3(3):164-168, 1988.

Wong DL: Guiding parents in selecting day-care centers, *Pediatr Nurs* 12(3):181-187, 1986.

Wong DL and others: Diapering choices: a critical review of the issues, *Pediatr Nurs* 18(1):41-54, 1992.

Zanga JR: Should there be a universal childhood vaccination against hepatitis B? II. A rebuttal, *Pediatr Nurs* 19(5):451-452, 1993.

Zell ER and others: Low vaccination levels of U.S. preschool and school-age children, *JAMA* 271(11):833-839, 1994.

Zuckerman JN, Cockcroft A, Zuckerman AJ: Site of injection for vaccination, *Br Med J* 305(6862):1158, 1992.

BIBLIOGRAPHY

Growth and Development

Belfer M: Body image: impacts and distortions. In Levine M and others, editors: *Developmental-behavioral pediatrics,* ed 2, Philadelphia, 1992, WB Saunders.

Erikson E: *Childhood and society,* ed 2, New York, 1963, WW Norton.

Friendly DS: Developmental of vision in infants and young children, *Pediatr Clin North Am* 40(4):693-703, 1993.

Knobloch H, Pasamanick B: *Gesell and Amatruda's developmental diagnosis,* New York, 1974, Harper & Row.

Lombardino L and others: Evaluating communicative behaviors in infancy, *J Pediatr Health Care* 1(5):240-246, 1987.

Maier H: *Three theories of child development,* ed 3, New York, 1988, Harper & Row.

Marino B: Assessments of infant play: applications to research and practice, *Issues Compr Pediatr Nurs* 11(4):227-240, 1988.

Piaget J: *The construction of reality in the child,* New York, 1975, Ballantine Books.

Seligman S: Emotional and social development in infancy and early childhood, *Early Child Update* 5(4):1-2, 1989.

Singhi P, Radhika S: Kiss: a developmental milestone or a culture-determined skill? *Am J Dis Child* 146(6):663-664, 1992.

Vaughan III VC: Assessment of growth and development during infancy and early childhood, *Pediatr Rev* 13(3):88-97, 1992.

Zigler E, Lang ME: The emergence of "superbaby": a good thing? *Pediatr Nurs* 11(5): 337-342, 1985.

Attachment/Temperament/Parenting

Barret R, Robinson B: Adolescent fathers: often forgotten parents, *Pediatr Nurs* 12(4): 273-277, 1986.

Belsky J, Rovine M: Nonmaternal care in the first year of life and the security of infant-parent attachment, *Child Dev* 59:157-167, 1988.

Calkins SD, Fox NA: The relations among infant temperament, security of attachment, and behavioral inhibition at twenty-four months, *Child Dev* 63(6):1456-1472, 1992.

Coffman S and others: Temperament and interactive effects: mothers and infants in a teaching situation, *Issues Compr Pediatr Nurs* 15:169-182, 1992.

Graham MV: Parental sensitivity to infant cues: similarities and differences between mothers and fathers, *J Pediatr Nurs* 8(6):376-384, 1993.

Harris E, Weston D, Lieberman A: Quality of mother-infant attachment and pediatric health care use, *Pediatrics* 84(2):248-254, 1989.

Isabella RA: Origins of attachment: maternal interactive behavior across the first year, *Child Dev* 64(2):605-621, 1993.

Koniak-Griffin D, Ludington-Hoe S: Developmental and temperament outcomes of sensory stimulation in healthy infants, *Nurs Res* 37(2):70-76, 1988.

Koniak-Griffin D, Rummell M: Temperament in infancy: stability, change, and correlates, *Matern Child Nurs J* 17(1):25-40, 1988.

Lamb J: The rapproachement subphase of the separation-individuation process, *Matern Child Nurs J* 15(3):129-138, 1986.

Wasserman R and others: Infant temperament and school age behavior: 6-year longitudinal study in the pediatric practice, *Pediatrics* 85(5):801-807, 1990.

Zahr L: Lebanese mother and infant temperaments as determinants of mother-infant interaction, *J Pediatr Nurs* 2(6):418-427, 1987.

Concerns Related to Growth and Development

Castiglia P: Thumb sucking, *J Pediatr Health Care* 2(6):322-323, 1988.

Clutter L: Helping parents prepare for travel and vacations with children, *Pediatr Nurs* 14(3):211-215, 1988.

Friman PC: Concurrent habits: what would Linus do with his blanket if his thumb-sucking were treated? *Am J Dis Child* 144(12):1316-1318, 1990.

Solomon R, Martin K: Can you spoil an infant? A primary care survey, *Am J Dis Child* 144(4):426-427, 1990.

Alternate Child Care Arrangements

American Academy of Pediatrics: *Health in day care: a manual for health professionals,* Elk Grove Village, IL, 1987, The Academy.

American Academy of Pediatrics, Committee on Early Childhood, Adoption, and Dependent Care: The pediatrician's role in promoting the health of patients in early childhood education and/or child care programs, *Pediatrics* 92(3):489-492, 1993.

Bredekamp S: Day-care standards: need and impact, *Pediatrics* 91(1, pt 2):234-236, 1993.

Crowley AA: The child care dilemma: expanding nurse pratitioner involvement, *J Pediatr Health Care* 2(3):128-134, 1988.

Giebink GS: Care of the ill child in day-care settings, *Pediatrics* 91(1, pt 2):229-233, 1993.

Howes C, Phillips DA, Whitebook M: Thresholds of quality: implications for the social development of children in center-based child care, *Child Dev* 63(2):449-460, 1992.

Kuhns CL, Holloway SD: Characteristics of caregivers that promote children's development in day care, *J Pediatr Nurs* 7(4):280-285, 1992.

Novak J, Pecoraro N: Policy and position statement: child care, *J Pediatr Health Care* 3(3):158-159, 1989.

Osterholm MT and others: Infectious diseases and child day care, *Pediatr Infect Dis J* 11(8, suppl):S31-S41, 1992.

Peterson-Sweeney K, Stevens J: Educating child care providers in child health, *Pediatr Nurs* 18(1):37-40, 1992.

Rapp GS, Lloyd SA: The role of "home as haven" ideology in child care use, *Fam Relations* 38:426-430, 1989.

Smith D: Myths about day care: fact or fantasy? *Pediatr Nurs* 10(4):27-280, 1984.

Smith D: Common diseases children contract in day care: patterns and prevention, *Pediatr Nurs* 12(3):175-179, 1986.

Summers K: Establishment of a hospital based children's sick room, *Pediatr Nurs* 14(1):38-39, 1988.

Thompson PJ: Day care for ill children: an employed mothers' dilemma, *Issues Compr Pediatr Nurs* 16:77-89, 1993.

Wilson D, Bess C: Establishing a community-based sick child center, *Pediatr Nurs* 12(6): 439-441, 1986.

Zigler E, Hall NW: Day care and its effect on children: an overview for pediatric health professionals, *J Dev Behav Pediatr* 9:38-46, 1988.

Nutrition

American Academy of Pediatrics: The AAP reexamines its policy on direct advertising of infant formula to the public, *AAP News* 9(4):2, 1993.

Blank D: Relating mothers' anxiety and perception to infant satiety, anxiety, and feeding behavior, *Nurs Res* 35(6):347-351, 1986.

Dusdieker LB and others: Effect of supplemental fluids on human milk production, *J Pediatr* 106(2):207-211, 1985.

Filer L, editor: Assessment of bone mineralization in infants, *J Pediatr* 113(suppl 1, pt 2), 1988.

Finberg L: How good a food for humans is cow's milk? *Am J Dis Child* 146(12):1432, 1992.

Fomon S: Bioavailability of supplemental iron in commercially prepared dry infant cereals, *J Pediatr* 110(4):660-661, 1987.

Fuchs GL and others: Iron status and intake of older infants fed formula vs cow milk with cereal, *Am J Clin Nutr* 58:343-348, 1993.

Hillman L and others: Vitamin D metabolism, mineral homeostasis, and bone mineralization in term infants fed human milk, cow milk-based formula, or soy-based formula, *J Pediatr* 112(5):864-874, 1988.

Katcher AL, Lanese MG: Breast-feeding by employed mothers: a reasonable accommodation in the work place, *Pediatrics* 75(4):664-647, 1985.

Mimouni F and others: Bone mineralizaiton in the first year of life in infants fed human milk, cow-milk formula, or soy-based formula, *J Pediatr* 122(3):348-354, 1993.

Nelson S and others: Lack of adverse reactions to iron-fortified formula, *Pediatrics* 81(3): 360-364, 1988.

Nemethy M, Clore E: Microwave heating of infant formula and breast milk, *J Pediatr Health Care* 4(3):131-135, 1990.

Rogers C, Morris S, Taper L: Weaning from the breast: influences on maternal decisions, *Pediatr Nurs* 13(5):341-345, 1987.

Ryan A, Martinez G, Krieger F: Feeding low-fat milk during infancy, *Am J Phys Anthropol* 73:539-548, 1987.

Schmitt BD: When weaning is delayed, *Contemp Pediatr* 7(6):67-68, 1990.

Sigman-Grant M, Bush G, Anantheswaran R: Microwave heating of infant formula: a dilemma resolved, *Pediatrics* 90(3):412-415, 1992.

Stuff J, Nichols B: Nutrient intake and growth performance of older infants fed human milk, *J Pediatr* 115(6):959-968, 1989.

Sullivan PB: Cows' milk induced intestinal bleeding in infancy, *Arch Dis Child* 68(2):240-245, 1993.

Tsang R, Nichols B, editors: *Nutrition during infancy,* St Louis, 1988, Hanley & Belfus.

Tseng E, Potter S, Picciano M: Dietary protein source and plasma lipid profiles of infants, *Pediatrics* 85(4):548-552, 1990.

Turick-Gibson T: Infant botulism, *Pediatr Nurs* 14(4):280-283, 1988.

Williams K, Morse J: Weaning patterns of first-time mothers, *MCN* 14(3):188-192, 1989.

Worobey J, Lewis M: Behavioral differences in response to stress between breast- and bottle-fed infants, *Top Clin Nutr* 7(3):48-55, 1992.

Sleep and Activity

Alley JM, Rogers CS: Sleep patterns of breast-fed and non-breast-fed infants, *Pediatr Nurs* 12(5):349-351, 1986.

Adair R and others: Reduced night waking in infancy: a primary care intervention, *Pediatrics* 89(4):585-588, 1992.

Adams L, Rickert V: Reducing bedtime tantrums: comparison between positive routines and graduated extinction, *Pediatrics* 84(5):756-761, 1989.

Balsmeyer B: Sleep disturbances of the infant and toddler, *Pediatr Nurs* 16(5):447-452, 1990.

Bardossi K: Getting kids to bed: How tough is too tough? *Contemp Pediatr* 8(1):97-105, 1991.

DeKoninck J, Lorrain D, Gagnon P: Sleep positions and position shifts in five age groups: an ontogenetic picture, *Sleep* 15(2):143-149, 1992.

Edgil AE, Wood KR, Smith DP: Sleep problems of older infants and preschool children, *Pediatr Nurs* 11(2):87-89, 1985.

Ferber R: Sleeplessness, night awakening, and night crying in the infant and toddler, *Pediatr Rev* 9(3);1-14, 1987.

Horne J: Sleep and its disorders in children, *J Child Psychol Psychiatry* 33(3):473-487, 1992.

Jaffa T and others: Sleep disorders in children, *Br Med J* 306(6878):640-643, 1993.

Keener M and others: Infant temperament,

sleep organization, and nighttime parental interventions, *Pediatrics* 81(6):762-771, 1988.

Rickert V, Johnson C: Reducing nocturnal awakening and crying episodes in infants and young children: a comparison between scheduled awakenings and sytematic ignoring, *Pediatrics* 81(2):203-212, 1988.

Schmitt BD: When your child refuses to go to bed, *Contemp Pediatr* 6(7):70-71, 1989.

Schmitt BD: How to help the trained night feeder, *Contemp Pediatr* 9(11):41-49, 1992.

Dental Health

For bibliography, see Chapter 14.

Immunizations

Abbotts B, Osborn LM: Immunization status and reasons for immunization delay among children using public health immunization clinics, *Am J Dis Child* 147:965-968, 1993.

Ad Hoc Working Group for the Development of Standards for Pediatric Immunization Practices: Standards for pediatric immunization practices, *JAMA* 269(14):1817-1822, 1993.

Ada G: The immunological principles of vaccination, *Lancet* 335(8687):523-526, 1990.

Adams WG and others: Decline of childhood *Haemophilus influenzae* type b (Hib) disease in the Hib vaccine era, *JAMA* 269(2):221-226, 1993.

American Academy of Pediatrics, Committee on Infectious Diseases: Acellular pertussis vaccines: recommendations for use as the fourth and fifth doses, *Pediatrics* 90(1):121-123, 1992.

Atkinson WL and others: Measles surveillance—United States, 1991, *MMWR* 41(SS-6):1-12, 1993.

Bernstein HH and others: Comparison of a three-component acellular pertussis vaccine with a whole-cell pertussis vaccine in 15-through 20-month-old infants, *Pediatrics* 93 (4):656-659, 1994.

Blumberg DA and others: Severe reactions associated with diphtheria-tetanus-pertussis vaccine: detailed study of children with seizures, hypotonic-hyporesponsive episodes, high fevers, and persistent crying, *Pediatrics* 91(6):1158-1165, 1993.

Bobo JK and others: Risk factors for delayed immunization in a random sample of 1163 children from Oregon and Washington, *Pediatrics* 91(2):308-314, 1993.

Brown J and others: Missed opportunities in preventive pediatric health care: immunizations or well-child care visits? *Am J Dis Child* 147(10):1081-1084, 1993.

Caulfield M: Hepatitis B: a disease needing a vaccine or a vaccine needing a disease? *Clin Pediatr* 32(7):443-444, 1993.

Cherry JD and others: Pertussis immunization and characteristics related to first seizures in infants and children, *J Pediatr* 122(6):900-903, 1993.

Clayton EW, Hickson GB, Miller CS: Parents' responses to vaccine information pamphlets, *Pediatrics* 93(3):369-372, 1994.

Dixon M, Keeling AW, Kennel S: What pediatric hospital nurses know about immunization, *MCN* 19(2):74-78, 1994.

Edwards KM: Pediatric immunizations, *Curr Probl Pediatr* 23(5):186-209, 1993.

Ellis RW, Douglas RG Jr: New vaccine technologies, *JAMA* 271(12):929-931, 1994.

Engel N: The National Vaccine Injury Compensation Program, *MCN* 15:109, 1990.

Englund JA and others: Acellular and whole-cell pertussis vaccines booster doses: a multicenter study, *Pediatrics* 93(1):37-43, 1994.

Faden H, Duffy L: Effect of concurrent viral infection on systemic and local antibody responses to live attenuated and enhanced-potency inactivated poliovirus vaccines, *Am J Dis Child* 146(11):1320-1323, 1992.

Freed GL and others: Reactions of pediatricians to a new Centers for Disease Control recommendation for universal immunization of infants with hepatitis B vaccine, *Pediatrics* 91(4):699-702, 1993.

Gershon AA: Varicella vaccine: still at the crossroads, *Pediatrics* 90(suppl 1):144-148, 1992.

Givner LB, Woods CR Jr, Abramson JS: The practice of pediatrics in the era of vaccines effective against *Haemophilus influenzae* type b, *Pediatrics* 93(4):680-681, 1994.

Griffin M and others: Risk of seizures and encephalopathy after immunization with the diphtheria-tetanus-pertussis vaccine, *JAMA* 263(12):1641-1645, 1990.

Grimes D, Woolbert L: Measles outbreaks: who are at risk and why, *J Pediatr Health Care* 3(4):187-193, 1989.

Grosheide PM and others: Passive-active immunization of infants of hepatitis Be antigen–positive mothers: comparison of the efficacy of early and delayed active immunization, *Am J Dis Child* 147:1316-1320, 1993.

Hall CB, Halsey NA: Control of hepatitis B: to be or not to be? *Pediatrics* 90(2):274-277, 1992.

Katz S: Poliovirus vaccine policy, *Am J Dis Child* 143(9):1007-1009, 1989.

Kemp A, Van Asperen P, Mukhi A: Measles immunization in children with clinical reactions to egg protein, *Am J Dis Child* 144 (1):33-35, 1990.

Klein N, Morgan K, Wansbrough-Jones M: Parents' beliefs about vaccination: the continuing propagation of false contraindications, *Br Med J* 298:1687, 1989.

Krasinski K, Borkowsky W: Measles and measles immunity in children infected with human immunodeficiency virus, *JAMA* 261 (17):2512-2516, 1989.

Krugman S: Viral hepatitis: A, B, C, D, and E—prevention, *Pediatr Rev* 13(7):245-247, 1992.

Lavi S and others: Administration of measles, mumps, and rubella virus vaccine (live) to egg-allergic children, *JAMA* 263(2):269-271, 1990.

Michaels RH, Ali O: A decline in *Haemophilus influenzae* type b meningitis, *J Pediatr* 122 (3):407-409, 1993.

Murphy TV and others: Declining incidence of *Haemophilus influenzae* type b disease since introduction of vaccination, *JAMA* 269(2): 246-248, 1993.

Peter G: Childhood immunizations, *New Engl J Med* 327(25):1794-1800, 1992.

Progress toward global eradication of poliomyelitis, 1988-1991, *MMWR* 42(25):486-487, 493, 1993.

Puvvada L and others: Systemic reactions to measles-mumps-rubella vaccine skin testing, *Pediatrics* 91(4):835-836, 1993.

Recommendations of the Advisory Committee on Immunization Practices (ACIP): Pertussis vaccination: acellular pertussis vaccine for the fourth and fifth doses of the DTP series, update to supplementary ACIP statement, *MMWR* 41(RR-15):1-5, 1992.

Recommendations of the Immunization Practices Advisory Committee: Pneumococcal polysaccharide vaccine, *MMWR* 38(5):64-76, 1989.

Sharts-Hopko NC: Preventing hepatitis B in infants, *MCN* 17(6):336, 1992.

Sharts-Hopko NC: HIB: a new conjugate and a combination vaccine, *MCN* 19(1):56, 1994.

Vaccination coverage of 2-year-old children—United States, 1991-1992, *MMWR* 42(51& 52):985-989, 1994.

Injury Prevention

For additional citations, see Chapters 1 and 14.

Bass JL and others: Educating parents about injury prevention, *Pediatr Clin North Am* 32(1):233-243, 1985.

Berger LR, Kalishman S: Floor furnace burns to children, *Pediatrics* 71(1):97-99, 1983.

Berger LR and others: Promoting the use of car safety devices for infants: an intensive health education approach, *Pediatrics* 74(1):16-19, 1984.

Children and waterbeds, *Pediatr Nurs* 17(6): 577, 1991 (letter and reply).

Coppens N: Parental responses to children in unsafe situations, *Pediatr Nurs* 16(6):571-574, 1990.

Cotton WH, Davidson PJ: Aspiration of baby powder, *N Engl J Med* 313:1662, 1985.

Gallagher SS, Hunter P, Guyer B: A home injury prevention program for children, *Pediatr Clin North Am* 32(1):95-112, 1985.

Gielen AC, Collins B: Community-based interventions for injury prevention, *Fam Community Health* 15(4):1-11, 1993.

Greensher J, Mofenson HC: Injuries at play, *Pediatric Clin North Am* 32(1):127-139, 1985.

Gunn WJ and others: Injuries and poisonings in out-of-home child care and home care, *Am J Dis Child* 145(7):779-781, 1991.

Johnson G: Aspiration of makeshift pacifier, *Pediatrics* 79(1):170, 1987.

Jones NE: Prevention of childhood injuries. II. Recreational injuries, *Pediatr Nurs* 18(6):619-621, 1992.

Katcher M, Landry G, Shapiro M: Liquid-crystal thermometer use in pediatric office counseling about tap water burn prevention, *Pediatrics* 83(5):766-771, 1989.

Nyman G: Infant temperament, childhood accidents, and hospitalization, *Clin Pediatr* 26(8):398-404, 1987.

Puczynski M, Rademaker D, Gatson RL: Burn injury related to the improper use of a microwave oven, *Pediatrics* 72:714-715, 1983.

Rivera F, Kamitsuka M, Quan L: Injuries to children younger than 1 year of age, *Pediatrics* 81(1):93-97, 1988.

Stewart DD: Child passenger safety: current technical issues for advocates and professionals, *Fam Community Health* 15(4):12-27, 1993.

Temple DM, McNeese MC: Hazards of battery ingestion, *Pediatrics* 71(1):100-103, 1983.

Wagner TJ, Hindi-Alexander M: Hazards of baby powder? *Pediatr Nurs* 10(2):124-125, 1984.

CHAPTER 13

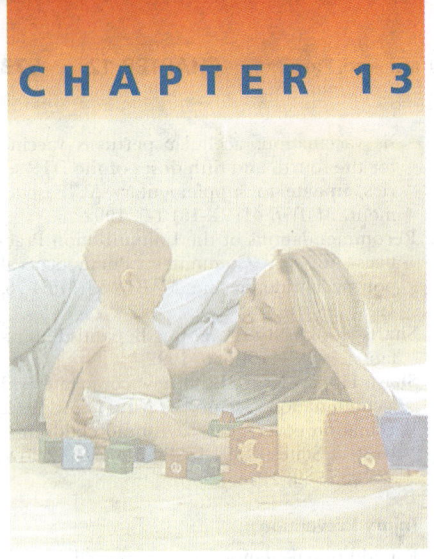

Health Problems During Infancy

CHAPTER OUTLINE

RELATED TOPICS

NUTRITIONAL DISTURBANCES

VITAMIN DISTURBANCES

Vitamins are an essential food element and function in small quantities by regulating specific metabolic activity, usually by acting as ***coenzymes.*** When vitamin coenzymes enter the body, they are combined with a protein ***apoenzyme*** that has been synthesized within the cell to form a ***holoenzyme.*** The quantity of apoenzymes any cell can produce limits the body's ability to make use of excessive vitamins. A deficiency of the vitamin directly affects the metabolic activity it regulates. However, regular ingestion of excessive amounts of vitamins may produce a toxic effect.

True vitamin disturbances are rare in the United States, but subclinical deficiencies are commonly seen, especially in lower socioeconomic groups where proper dietary intake may be unbalanced. It has been reported that in children ages 7 to 18 years, approximately a third of the children and two thirds of adolescent girls consume less than the recommended amount of vitamin B_6. Vitamin D–deficient rickets, once rarely seen because of vitamin D–fortified milk, has increased. Populations at risk include (1) children born of mothers who are vitamin D deficient; (2) individuals who are exposed to minimal sunlight because of their particular clothing, housing in areas of high pollution, or dark skin pigmentation; (3) adherence to vegetarian diets that are low in sources of vitamin D; and (4) use of milk products, such as yogurt or raw cow's milk, that are not supplemented with vitamin D as the primary source of milk. Children may also be at risk secondary to disorders or their treatment. For

Text continued on p. 580.

■ David Wilson, RN, C, MS, revised this chapter.

TABLE 13-1 Vitamins and Their Nutritional Significance

PHYSIOLOGIC FUNCTIONS/ SOURCES	RESULTS OF DEFICIENCY OR EXCESS	NURSING CONSIDERATIONS
VITAMIN A (RETINOL)*		
Functions	***Deficiency***	
Necessary component in formation of pigment rhodopsin (visual purple) Formation and maintenance of epithelial tissue Normal bone growth and tooth development Needed for growth and spermatogenesis Involved in thyroxine formation	Night blindness Keratinization (hardening and scaling) of epithelium Xerophthalmia (hardening and scaling of cornea and conjunctiva) Phrynoderma (toad skin) Drying of respiratory, gastrointestinal, and genitourinary tracts Defective tooth enamel Retarded growth Impaired bone formation Decreased thyroxine formation	Encourage foods rich in vitamin A, such as whole cow's milk As milk consumption decreases, encourage foods rich in vitamin A Ensure adequate intake in preterm infants Advise parents of safe use of supplements in child with measles
Sources	***Excess***	
Natural form—Liver, kidney, fish oils, milk and nonskimmed milk products, egg yolk *Provitamin A (carotene)*—Carrots, sweet potatoes, squash, apricots, spinach, collards, broccoli, cabbage, artichokes	*Early signs*—Irritability, anorexia, pruritus, fissures at corners of nose and lips *Later signs*—Hepatomegaly, jaundice, retarded growth, poor weight gain, thickening of the cortex of long bones with pain and fragility, hard tender lumps in extremities and occiput of the skull May cause birth defects from excessive maternal intake	Emphasize correct use of vitamin supplements and potential hazards of excess Investigate child's dietary habits to calculate approximate intake; if excessive, remove supplemental source (e.g., daily feeding of liver)
	NOTE: Overdose results from ingestion of large quantities of the vitamin only, not the provitamin; large amounts of carotene (carotenemia) cause yellow or orange discoloration of the skin (not the sclera, urine, or feces as in jaundice), but none of the above symptoms	Advise parents of the benign nature of carotenemia; treatment is avoidance of excess pigmented fruits or vegetables, especially carrots; skin color returns to normal in 2 to 6 weeks
VITAMIN B_1 (THIAMINE)†		
Functions	***Deficiency***	Vitamin B complex
Coenzyme (with phosphorus) in carbohydrate metabolism Needed for healthy nervous system	*Gastrointestinal*—Anorexia, constipation, indigestion *Neurologic*—Apathy, fatigue, emotional instability, polyneuritis, tenderness of calf muscles, partial anesthesia, muscle weakness, paresthesia, hyperesthesia, decreased or absent tendon reflexes, convulsions, and coma (in infants) *Cardiovascular*—Palpitations, cardiac failure, peripheral vasodilation, edema	Encourage foods rich in B vitamins Stress proper cooking and storage techniques to preserve potency, such as minimum cooking of vegetables in small amount of liquid; storage of milk in opaque container Advise against fad diets that severely restrict groups of food, such as vegetarianism (vegans or macrobiotics)
Sources	***Excess***	
Pork, beef, liver, legumes, nuts, whole or enriched grains and cereals, green vegetables, fruits, milk, brown rice	Headache Irritability Insomnia Rapid pulse Weakness	Explore need for vitamin supplements when dieting or when using goat milk exclusively for infant feeding (deficient in folic acid) or when the breast-feeding mother is a strict vegetarian (vitamin B_{12}) Emphasize correct use of vitamin supplements and potential hazards of excesses

*Fat soluble.
†Water soluble.
‡Green leafy vegetables include spinach, broccoli, kale, turnip greens, mustard greens, collards, dandelion greens, and beet greens.

Continued.

TABLE 13-1 Vitamins and Their Nutritional Significance—cont'd

PHYSIOLOGIC FUNCTIONS/ SOURCES	RESULTS OF DEFICIENCY OR EXCESS	NURSING CONSIDERATIONS
VITAMIN B_2 (RIBOFLAVIN)†		
Functions Coenzyme (with phosphorus) in carbohydrate, protein, and fat metabolism Maintains healthy skin, especially around mouth, nose, and eyes ***Sources*** Milk and its products, eggs, organ meat (liver, kidney, and heart), enriched cereals, some green leafy vegetables,‡ legumes	***Deficiency*** Ariboflavinosis *Lips*—Cheilosis (fissures at corners of lips), perlèche (inflammation at corners of lips) *Tongue*—Glossitis *Nose*—Irritation and cracks at nasal angle *Eyes*—Burning, itching, tearing, photophobia, corneal vascularization, cataracts *Skin*—Seborrheic dermatitis, delayed wound healing and tissue repair ***Excess*** Paresthesia, pruritus	Same as vitamin B complex
NIACIN (NICOTINIC ACID, NICOTINAMIDE)†		
Functions Coenzyme (with riboflavin) in protein and fat metabolism Needed for healthy nervous system, skin, and normal digestion May lower cholesterol ***Sources*** Meat, poultry, fish, peanuts, beans, peas, whole or enriched grains except corn and rice Milk and its products are sources of tryptophan (60 mg of tryptophan = 1 mg of niacin)	***Deficiency*** Pellagra Oral—Stomatitis, glossitis Cutaneous—Scaly dermatitis on exposed areas Gastrointestinal—Anorexia, weight loss, diarrhea, fatigue Neurologic—Apathy, anxiety, confusion, depression, dementia Death ***Excess*** Release of vasodilator, histamine (flushing, decreased blood pressure, increased cerebral blood flow; aggravates asthma) Dermatologic problems (pruritus, rash, hyperkeratosis, acanthosis nigricans) Increased gastric acidity (aggravates peptic ulcer disease) Hepatotoxicity Increased serum uric acid levels Elevated plasma glucose levels Certain cardiac arrhythmias	Same as vitamin B complex If used as hypolipidemic agent, stress safe dosage to prevent child's accidental ingestion
VITAMIN B_6 (PYRIDOXINE)†		
Functions Coenzyme in protein and fat metabolism Needed for formation of antibodies, hemoglobin Needed for utilization of copper and iron Aids in conversion of tryptophan to niacin ***Sources*** Meats, especially liver and kidney, cereal grains (wheat and corn), yeast, soybeans, peanuts, tuna, chicken, salmon	***Deficiency*** Scaly dermatitis, weight loss, anemia, retarded growth, irritability, convulsions, peripheral neuritis ***Excess*** Peripheral nervous system toxicity (unsteady gait, numb feet and hands, clumsiness of hands, sometimes perioral numbness) May cause peptic ulcer disease or seizures	Same as vitamin B complex Stress proper cooking and storing techniques to preserve potency Cook food covered in small amount of water Do not soak food in water Store in light-resistant container

*Fat soluble.
†Water soluble.
‡Green leafy vegetables include spinach, broccoli, kale, turnip greens, mustard greens, collards, dandelion greens, and beet greens.

TABLE 13-1 Vitamins and Their Nutritional Significance—cont'd

PHYSIOLOGIC FUNCTIONS/ SOURCES	RESULTS OF DEFICIENCY OR EXCESS	NURSING CONSIDERATIONS
FOLIC ACID (FOLACIN; REDUCED FORM IS CALLED FOLINIC ACID OR CITROVORUM FACTOR)†		
Functions	***Deficiency***	
Coenzyme for single-carbon transfer (purines, thymine, hemoglobin) Necessary for formation of red blood cells	Macrocytic anemia, bone marrow depression, glossitis, intestinal malabsorption	Same as vitamin B complex Stress proper cooking and storing techniques to preserve potency Cook food covered in small amount of water Do not soak food in water Store in light-resistant container Women of childbearing age should supplement to prevent neural tube defects
Sources	***Excess***	
Green leafy vegetables,‡ cabbage, asparagus, liver, kidney, nuts, eggs, whole grain cereals, legumes, bananas	Rare because megadoses not available over the counter May cause insomnia and irritability	
VITAMIN B_{12} (COBALAMIN)†		
Functions	***Deficiency***	
Coenzyme in protein synthesis; indirect effect on formation of red blood cells (particularly on formation of nucleic acids and folic acid metabolism) Needed for normal functioning of nervous tissue	Pernicious anemia (One form of deficiency from absence of intrinsic factor in gastric secretions) General signs of severe anemia Lemon-yellow tinge to skin Spinal cord degeneration Delayed brain growth	Same as vitamin B complex
Sources	***Excess***	
Meat, liver, kidney, fish, shellfish, poultry, milk, eggs, cheese, nutritional yeast, sea vegetables	Excess is rare	
BIOTIN		
Functions	***Deficiency***	
Coenzyme in carbohydrate, protein, and fat metabolism Interrelated with functions of other B vitamins	Deficiency is uncommon because synthesized by bacterial flora	Same as vitamin B complex
Sources	***Excess***	
Liver, kidney, egg yolk, tomatoes, legumes, nuts	Unknown	
PANTOTHENIC ACID†		
Functions	***Deficiency***	
Coenzyme in carbohydrate, protein, and fat metabolism Synthesis of amino acids, fatty acids, and steroids	Deficiency is uncommon because of its multiple food sources and synthesis by bacterial flora	Same as vitamin B complex
Sources	***Excess***	
Liver, kidney, heart, salmon, eggs, vegetables, legumes, whole grains	Minimum toxicity (occasional diarrhea and water retention)	
VITAMIN C (ASCORBIC ACID)†		
Functions	***Deficiency***	
Essential for collagen formation Increases absorption of iron for hemoglobin formation Enhances conversion of folic acid to folinic acid Affects cholesterol synthesis and conversion of proline to hydroxyproline	Scurvy *Skin*—Dry, rough, petechiae, perifollicular hyperkeratotic papules (raised areas around hair follicles) *Musculoskeletal*—Bleeding muscles and joints, pseudoparalysis from pain, swelling of joints, costochondral beading (scorbutic rosary)	Encourage foods rich in vitamin C Investigate infant's diet for sources of vitamin, especially when cow's milk is principal source of nutrition Stress proper cooking and storing techniques to preserve potency Wash vegetables quickly; do not soak in water

Continued.

TABLE 13-1 Vitamins and Their Nutritional Significance—cont'd

PHYSIOLOGIC FUNCTIONS/ SOURCES	RESULTS OF DEFICIENCY OR EXCESS	NURSING CONSIDERATIONS
VITAMIN C (ABSORBIC ACID)†—cont'd		
Probably a coenzyme in metabolism of tyrosine and phenylalanine May play role in hydroxylation of adrenal steroids May have stimulating effect on phagocytic activity of leukocytes and formation of antibodies Antioxidant agent (spares other vitamins from oxidation) ***Sources*** Citrus fruits, strawberries, tomatoes, potatoes, melon, cabbage, broccoli, cauliflower, spinach, papaya, mango	*Gums*—Spongy, friable, swollen, bleed easily, bluish red or black color, teeth loosen and fall out *General disposition*—Irritable, anorexic, apprehensive, in pain, refuses to move, assumes semi-froglike position when supine (scorbutic pose) Signs of anemia Decreased wound healing Increased susceptibility to infection ***Excess*** Diarrhea Increased excretion of uric acid and acidification of urine (may cause urate precipitation and formation of oxalate stones) Hemolysis Impaired leukocytosis activity Damage to beta cells of pancreas and decreased insulin production Reproductive failure "Rebound scurvy" from withdrawal of large amounts	Cook vegetables in covered pot with minimum water and for short time; avoid copper or cast iron cookware Do not add baking soda to cooking water Use fresh fruits and vegetables as soon as possible; store in refrigerator Store juice in airtight, opaque container Wrap cut fruit or eat soon after exposing to air In caring for child with scurvy: Position for comfort and rest Handle very gently and minimally Administer analgesics as needed Prevent infection Provide good oral care Provide soft, bland diet Emphasize rapid recovery when vitamin is replaced Emphasize correct use of vitamin supplement and potential hazards of excess Identify groups at risk for vitamin C supplements: those with thalassemia; those on anticoagulant or aminoglycoside antibiotic therapy
VITAMIN D_2 (ERGOCALCIFEROL) AND D_3 (CHOLECALCIFEROL)*		
Functions Absorption of calcium and phosphorus and decreased renal excretion of phosphorus ***Sources*** Direct sunlight Cod liver oil, herring, mackerel, salmon, tuna, sardines *Enriched food sources*—Milk, milk products, enriched cereals, margarine, breads, many breakfast drinks	***Deficiency*** Rickets *Head*—Craniotabes (softening of cranial bones, prominence of frontal bones), deformed shape (skull flat and depressed toward middle), delayed closure of fontanels *Chest*—Rachitic rosary (enlargement of costochondral junction of ribs), Harrison groove (horizontal depression in lower portion of rib cage), pigeon chest (sharp protrusion of sternum) *Spine*—Kyphosis, scoliosis, lordosis *Abdomen*—Potbelly, constipation *Extremities*—Bowing of arms and legs, knock-knee, saber shins, instability of hip joints, pelvic deformity, enlargement of epiphysis at ends of long bones *Teeth*—Delayed calcification, especially of permanent teeth *Rachitic tetany*—Seizures	Encourage foods rich in vitamin D, especially fortified cow's milk In breast-fed infants encourage use of vitamin D supplements if maternal diet inadequate or infant exposed to minimal sunlight In caring for child with rickets: Maintain good body alignment Reposition frequently to prevent decubiti and respiratory infection Handle very gently and minimally Prevent infection Institute seizure precautions Have 10% calcium gluconate available in case of tetany Observe for possibility of overdose from supplements If prescribed, supervise proper use of orthopaedic splints or braces

*Fat soluble.
†Water soluble.
‡Green leafy vegetables include spinach, broccoli, kale, turnip greens, mustard greens, collards, dandelion greens, and beet greens.

TABLE 13-1 Vitamins and Their Nutritional Significance—cont'd

PHYSIOLOGIC FUNCTIONS/ SOURCES	RESULTS OF DEFICIENCY OR EXCESS	NURSING CONSIDERATIONS
	Excess *Acute*—Vomiting, dehydration, fever, abdominal cramps, bone pain, convulsions, and coma *Chronic*—Lassitude, mental slowness, anorexia, failure to thrive, thirst, urinary urgency, polyuria, vomiting, diarrhea, abdominal cramps, bone pain, pathologic fractures *Calcification of soft tissue*—Kidneys, lungs, adrenal glands, vessels (hypertension), heart, gastric lining, tympanic membrane (deafness) Osteoporosis of long bones Elevated serum levels of calcium and phosphorus	Same as vitamin A; may include low-calcium diet during initial therapy
VITAMIN E (TOCOPHEROL)* ***Functions*** Production of red blood cells and protection from hemolysis Muscle and liver integrity Coenzyme factor in tissue respiration Minimizes oxidation of polyunsaturated fatty acids and vitamins A and C in intestinal tract and tissues Possible role in treatment and prevention of bronchopulmonary dysplasia and retinopathy of prematurity is under investigation ***Sources*** Vegetable oils, wheat germ oil, milk, egg yolk, muscle meats, fish, whole grains, nuts, legumes, spinach, broccoli	***Deficiency*** Hemolytic anemia from hemolysis caused by shortened life of red blood cells, especially in premature infants, and focal necrosis of tissues Causes infertility in rats, but not in humans (does *not* increase human male virility or potency) ***Excess*** Little is known: less toxic than other fat-soluble vitamins	Initiate early feeding in premature infants; may need supplementation
VITAMIN K* ***Functions*** Catalyst for production of prothrombin and blood-clotting factors II, VII, IX, and X by the liver ***Sources*** Pork, liver, green leafy vegetables (spinach, kale, cabbage), tomatoes, egg yolk, cheese	***Deficiency*** Hemorrhage ***Excess*** Hemolytic anemia in individuals who are deficient in glucose-6-phosphate dehydrogenase	Administer prophylactically to all newborns Other indications include intestinal disease, lack of bile, prolonged antibiotic therapy; may be used in management of blood-clotting time when anticoagulants such as warfarin (Coumadin) and dicumarol (bishydroxycoumarin), which are vitamin K antagonists, are used

example, vitamin deficiencies of the fat-soluble vitamins A and D may occur in malabsorptive disorders. Children receiving high doses of salicylates, such as for rheumatoid arthritis, may have impaired vitamin C storage. Premature infants may develop rickets in the second month of life as a result of inadequate intake of vitamin D, calcium, and phosphorus (Blackburn and Loper, 1992).

Recent studies indicate that vitamin A deficiency correlates with increased morbidity and mortality in children with measles. Complications from diarrhea and infections were increased, as was morbidity, in infants and children with vitamin A deficiency (Fawzi and others, 1993; Herrera and others, 1992; Udall and Greene, 1992). The American Academy of Pediatrics recommends that vitamin A supplementation be considered in children hospitalized with measles, especially children between the ages of 6 months and 2 years (American Academy of Pediatrics, 1993).

Of equal, if not greater, concern is the overuse of vitamins. An excessive dose of a vitamin is generally defined as 10 or more times the recommended dietary allowance (RDA), although the fat-soluble vitamins, especially A and D, tend to cause toxic reactions at lower doses. With the addition of vitamins to commercially prepared foods, the potential for hypervitaminosis has increased, especially when combined with the injudicious use of vitamin supplements. Hypervitaminosis of A and D presents the greatest problems, because these fat-soluble vitamins are stored in the body. Vitamin D is the most likely of all vitamins to cause toxic reactions in relatively small overdoses. However, there appears to be variance in the tolerance to different vitamin intakes. For example, two children ingesting excessive amounts of vitamin A may not both demonstrate clinical features of intoxication.

It is now well documented that the water-soluble vitamins, primarily niacin, B_6, and C, can also cause toxicity by the following mechanisms:

1. May have direct toxic effects, especially niacin and B_6
2. May lead to dependency states with development of deficiency symptoms when the vitamin is abruptly discontinued, such as ascorbic acid
3. May mask signs of a disease, such as vitamin C and interference with Clinitest results (common dipstick test used to detect glucose or acetone in urine) in diabetes
4. May interact with drugs or other vitamins, such as folic acid's effect on reducing serum phenytoin levels
5. May be combined with high doses of fat-soluble vitamins, such as high-dose multisupplement preparation

Deficiencies and excesses of vitamins A, B complex, C, D, E, and K are summarized in Table 13-1. General nursing considerations are discussed on p. 585, and specific interventions are presented in Table 13-1.

MINERAL DISTURBANCES

A number of minerals are essential nutrients. The ***macrominerals*** refer to those with daily requirements greater than 100 mg and include calcium, phosphorus, magnesium, sodium, potassium, chloride, and sulfur. ***Microminerals,*** or ***trace elements,*** have daily requirements of less than 100 mg and include several essential minerals and those whose exact role in nutrition is still unclear. The greatest concern with minerals is deficiency, especially iron deficiency anemia (see Chapter 35). However, other minerals that may be inadequate in children's diets, even with supplementation, include calcium, phosphorus, magnesium, and zinc (Moss and others, 1989). Low levels of zinc can cause nutritional failure to thrive (Walravens, Hambidge, and Koepfer, 1989).

The regulation of mineral balance in the body is a complex process. Dietary extremes of mineral intake can cause a number of mineral-mineral interactions that could result in unexpected deficiencies or excesses. For example, excessive amounts of one mineral, such as zinc, can result in a deficiency of another mineral, such as copper, even if sufficient amounts of copper are ingested. This is thought to be the result of competition in the process of absorption because of (1) displacement of one mineral by another on the molecule necessary for their uptake from the lumen in the intestinal cell or (2) competition for pathways through the intestinal wall or into the bloodstream. Therefore megadose therapy with one mineral may not cause toxicity from an excess but rather from a deficiency in a competing mineral.

Deficiencies can also occur when various substances in the diet interact with minerals. For example, iron, zinc, and calcium can form insoluble complexes with phytates and/or oxalates (substances found in plant proteins), which impairs the bioavailability of the mineral. This type of interaction is important in vegetarian diets because plant foods, such as soy, are high in phytates (Heaney, Weaver, and Fitzsimmons, 1991). Contrary to popular opinion, spinach is not a rich source of iron or calcium because of its oxylate content.

Deficiencies and excesses of the essential macrominerals and microminerals are summarized in Table 13-2. General nursing considerations are discussed on p. 585, and specific interventions are discussed in the table.

VEGETARIAN DIETS

The importance of vegetarian diets and their relationship to potential nutritional deficiencies in children cannot be overemphasized. The stricter the vegetarian diet, the more difficult it becomes to ensure adequate nutrition for infants and children. The major types of vegetarianism are:

Lacto-ovovegetarians, who exclude meat from their diet but eat milk and eggs and sometimes fish

Lactovegetarians, who exclude meat and eggs but drink milk

Pure vegetarians (vegans), who eliminate any food of animal origin, including milk and eggs

Zen macrobiotics, who are even more restrictive than pure vegetarians in that cereals, especially brown rice, are the mainstay of the diet

Many individuals who are concerned about healthful diets subscribe to vegetarian diets that are not typified by the above categories. Therefore, during nutritional assessment it is necessary to clearly list exactly what the diet includes and excludes.

The lacto-ovovegetarian diet is associated with the least

TABLE 13-2 Minerals and Their Nutritional Significance

PHYSIOLOGIC FUNCTIONS/ SOURCES	RESULTS OF DEFICIENCY OR EXCESS	NURSING CONSIDERATIONS
CALCIUM*		
Functions	***Deficiency***	
Bone and tooth development and maintenance (in combination with phosphorus) Muscle contractions, especially the heart Blood clotting Absorption of vitamin B_{12} Enzyme activation Nerve conduction Integrity of intracellular cement substances and various membranes	Rickets Tetany Impaired growth, especially of bones and teeth	Encourage foods rich in calcium, especially dairy products Caution that oxalates in leafy vegetables (spinach), oxalates in chocolates, and a high phosphorus intake (especially from carbonated beverages) can decrease calcium absorption Discourage use of whole cow's milk in newborns because the phosphorus-to-calcium ratio favors excretion of calcium Advise against fad diets, especially those that restrict dairy products
Sources	***Excess***	
Dairy products, egg yolk, sardines, canned salmon with bones, dark green leafy vegetables (except spinach), soybeans, dried beans, and peas	Drowsiness, extreme lethargy Impaired absorption of other minerals (iron, zinc, manganese) Calcium deposits in tissues (renal failure)	Emphasize correct use of calcium-supplement, especially the possible interaction between megadoses of calcium and resulting deficiency states of other minerals
CHLORIDE*		
Functions	***Deficiency***	
Acid-base and fluid balance Enzyme activation in saliva Component of hydrochloric acid in stomach	Acid-base disturbances (hypochloremic alkalosis, dehydration); occurs mostly in combination with sodium loss	Deficiency and excess are unusual; most diets supply adequate chloride (usually in combination with sodium) Disease states such as excessive vomiting can necessitate chloride replacement
Sources	***Excess***	
Salt, meat, eggs, dairy products, many prepared and preserved foods	Acid-base disturbance	
CHROMIUM†		
Functions	***Deficiency***	
Involved in glucose metabolism and energy production	Possible abnormal glucose metabolism	No specific recommendations are needed
Sources	***Excess***	
Meat, cheese, whole-grain breads and cereals, legumes, peanuts, brewer's yeast, vegetable oils	Unknown	
COPPER†		
Functions	***Deficiency***	
Production of hemoglobin Essential component of several enzyme systems	Anemia, leukopenia, neutropenia	Deficiency from inadequate food sources is less likely than from excess intake of other minerals, especially zinc and possibly iron; therefore emphasize the correct use of any vitamin supplement Caution against cooking acid foods in unlined copper pots, which can lead to chronic and toxic accumulation of copper
Sources	***Excess***	
Organ meats, oysters, nuts, seeds, legumes, corn oil margarine	Severe vomiting and diarrhea Hemolytic anemia	

*Macrominerals—required intake >100 mg/day.
†Microminerals or trace elements—required intake <100 mg/day.

Continued.

TABLE 13-2 Minerals and Their Nutritional Significance—cont'd

PHYSIOLOGIC FUNCTIONS/ SOURCES	RESULTS OF DEFICIENCY OR EXCESS	NURSING CONSIDERATIONS
FLUORINE† ***Functions*** Formation of caries-resistant teeth Strong bone development ***Sources*** Fluoridated water and foods or beverages prepared with fluoridated water; fish, tea, commercially prepared chicken for infants	***Deficiency*** Increased susceptibility to tooth decay ***Excess*** **Fluorosis** (mottling and/or pitting of enamel) Severe bone deformities	In areas with optimally fluoridated water, encourage sufficient intake to supply recommended amount of fluoride (see Chapter 14) In areas of unfluoridated water or when ready-to-use formula, bottled water, or breast milk is used, stress the importance of fluoride supplements In areas with excess fluoride in the water, consider the use of bottled water in drinking and possibly cooking to reduce the fluoride intake to safe levels Fluorine has the narrowest range of safe and adequate intake; therefore stress the importance of storing supplements in a safe area
IODINE† ***Functions*** Production of thyroid hormone Normal reproduction ***Sources*** Seafood, kelp, iodized salt, sea salt, enriched bread, milk (from dairy processing)	***Deficiency*** **Goiter** (enlarged thyroid from decreased thyroxine formation) ***Excess*** Unknown from food sources; may occur from ingestion of iodine preparations, such as saturated solutions of potassium iodide (SSKI)	Encourage use of iodized salt for individuals living far from the sea If iodine preparations are in the home, stress the importance of safe storage
IRON† ***Functions*** Formation of hemoglobin and myoglobin Essential part of several enzymes and proteins	***Deficiency*** **Anemia** (see Chapter 35)	Encourage foods rich in iron Discourage excessive milk consumption, especially more than 1 L per day (milk is a very poor source of iron) If iron supplements are prescribed, teach parents factors that affect absorption (see box below)

FACTORS THAT AFFECT IRON ABSORPTION

Increase
- ***Acidity (low pH)***—Administer iron between meals (gastric hydrochloric acid)
- ***Ascorbic acid (vitamin C)***—Administer iron with juice, fruit, or multivitamin preparation
- Vitamin A
- Calcium
- Tissue need
- Meat, fish, poultry
- Cooking in cast iron pots

Decrease
- ***Alkalinity (high pH)***—Avoid any antacid preparation
- ***Phosphates***—Milk is unfavorable vehicle for iron administration
- ***Phytates***—Found in cereals
- ***Oxalates***—Found in many fruits and vegetables (plums, currants, green beans, spinach, sweet potatoes, tomatoes)
- Tannins—Found in tea, coffee
- Tissue saturation
- Malabsorptive disorders
- Disturbances that cause diarrhea or steatorrhea
- Infection

*Macrominerals—required intake >100 mg/day.
†Microminerals or trace elements—required intake <100 mg/day.

TABLE 13-2 Minerals and Their Nutritional Significance—cont'd

PHYSIOLOGIC FUNCTIONS/ SOURCES	RESULTS OF DEFICIENCY OR EXCESS	NURSING CONSIDERATIONS
Sources Liver, especially pork, followed by calf, beef, and chicken; kidney, red meat, poultry, shellfish, whole grains, iron-enriched infant formula and cereal, enriched cereals and bread, legumes, nuts, seeds, green leafy vegetables (except spinach), dried fruits, potatoes, molasses	***Excess*** Hemosiderosis (excess iron storage in various tissues of the body, especially the spleen, liver, lymph glands, heart, and pancreas) Hemochromatosis (excess iron storage with cellular damage)	Stress the importance of storing iron supplements in a safe area
MAGNESIUM*		
Functions Bone and tooth formation Production of proteins Nerve conduction to muscles Activation of enzymes needed for carbohydrate and protein metabolism	***Deficiency*** Tremors, spasm Irregular heartbeat Muscular weakness Lower extremity cramps Convulsions, delirium	Deficiency and excess are unusual, except in disease states such as prolonged vomiting or diarrhea or kidney dysfunction, where replacement may be needed
Sources Whole grains, nuts, soybeans, meat, green leafy vegetables (uncooked), tea, cocoa, raisins	***Excess*** Nervous system disturbances due to imbalance in calcium-to-magnesium ratio	
MANGANESE†		
Functions Activation of enzymes involved in reproduction, growth, and fat metabolism Normal bone structure Nervous system functioning	***Deficiency*** Unknown ***Excess*** Unknown	No specific recommendations are needed
Sources Nuts, whole grains, legumes, green vegetables, fruit		
MOLYBDENUM†		
Functions Essential component of several oxidative enzymes	***Deficiency*** Very rare; diagnosed in patients on complete total parenteral alimentation	No specific recommendations are needed
Sources Legumes, whole grains, organ meats, some dark green vegetables	***Excess*** Produces secondary copper deficiency (growth failure, anemia, and disturbed bone development)	
PHOSPHORUS*		
Functions Bone and tooth development (in combination with calcium) Involved in numerous chemical reactions, including protein, carbohydrate, and fat metabolism Acid-base balance	***Deficiency*** Weakness, anorexia, malaise, bone pain	Dietary deficiency is uncommon, although prolonged use of antacids can produce deficiency, in which case supplementation is recommended
Sources Dairy products, eggs, meat, poultry, legumes, carbonated beverages	***Excess*** Produces secondary calcium deficiency from disturbed calcium-to-phosphorus ratio	To preserve calcium-to-phosphorus ratio in newborns, discourage use of whole cow's milk

Continued.

TABLE 13-2 Minerals and Their Nutritional Significance—cont'd

PHYSIOLOGIC FUNCTIONS/ SOURCES	RESULTS OF DEFICIENCY OR EXCESS	NURSING CONSIDERATIONS
POTASSIUM* ***Functions*** Acid-base and fluid balance (major extracellular fluid areas) Nerve conduction Muscular contraction, especially the heart Release of energy ***Sources*** Bananas, citrus fruit, dried fruits, meat, fish, bran, legumes, peanut butter, potatoes, coffee, tea, cocoa	***Deficiency*** Cardiac arrhythmias Muscular weakness Lethargy Kidney and respiratory failure Heart failure ***Excess*** Cardiac arrhythmias Respiratory failure Mental confusion Numbness of extremities	Dietary deficiency and excess are unlikely, although disease states such as prolonged nausea and vomiting or the use of diuretics can result in hypokalemia; in such instances encourage replacement with supplements of rich food sources, such as bananas
SELENIUM† ***Functions*** Antioxidant, especially protective of vitamin E Protects against toxicity of heavy metals Associated with fat metabolism ***Sources*** Seafood, organ meats, egg yolk, whole grain; chicken, meat, tomatoes, cabbage, garlic, mushrooms, milk	***Deficiency*** Keshan disease (cardiomyopathy in children; found in China) ***Excess*** Eye, nose, and throat irritation Increased dental caries Liver and kidney degeneration	Deficiency and excess are uncommon in North America, although selenium deficiency can occur in patients on prolonged total parenteral alimentation; in these instances supplementation is required
SODIUM* ***Functions*** Acid-base and fluid balance (major extracellular fluid cation) Cell permeability; absorption of glucose Muscle contraction ***Sources*** Table salt, seafood, meat, poultry, numerous prepared foods	***Deficiency*** Dehydration Hypotension Convulsions Muscle cramps ***Excess*** Edema Hypertension Intracranial hemorrhage	Deficiency intake is very rare, although losses secondary to nausea, vomiting, excessive sweating, and use of diuretics can occur and require replacement Encourage parents to limit excessive use of salt in preparing foods and to limit commercial foods with high sodium content, such as smoked meats
SULFUR* ***Functions*** Essential component of cell protein, especially of hair and skin Enzyme activation Associated with energy metabolism Detoxification of certain chemical reactions ***Sources*** Dairy products, eggs, meat, fish, nuts, legumes	***Deficiency*** Unknown ***Excess*** Unknown	No specific recommendations are needed

*Macrominerals—required intake >100 mg/day.
†Microminerals or trace elements—required intake <100 mg/day.

TABLE 13-2 Minerals and Their Nutritional Significance—cont'd

PHYSIOLOGIC FUNCTIONS/ SOURCES	RESULTS OF DEFICIENCY OR EXCESS	NURSING CONSIDERATIONS
ZINC†		
Functions Component of about 100 enzymes Synthesis of nucleic acids and protein in immune system and coagulation Release of vitamin A from liver Improved wound healing with vitamin C ***Sources*** Seafood (especially oysters), meat, poultry, eggs, wheat, legumes	***Deficiency*** Loss of appetite Diminished taste sensation Delayed healing *Skin lesions*—Erythematous, crusted lesions around body orifices Alopecia Diarrhea Growth failure Retarded sexual maturity	Encourage food sources rich in zinc, especially protein Caution that fiber, phytates, oxalates, tannins (in tea or coffee), iron, and calcium adversely affect zinc absorption Recognize groups at risk for zinc deficiency, such as vegetarians and Mexican-Americans, whose diets may have restricted or low meat content and high fiber, phytate content; and patients with malabsorption syndromes
	Excess Vomiting and diarrhea Malaise, dizziness Anemia, gastric bleeding Impaired absorption of calcium and copper	Emphasize correct use of zinc supplements and the possible interaction with other minerals

deficiencies, although protein intake needs to be monitored. The lactovegetarian diet may also be low in protein, as well as iron. The major deficiencies in the stricter vegetarian diets are inadequate protein for growth, inadequate calories for energy and growth, poor digestibility of many of the natural, unprocessed foods, especially for infants, and deficiencies of vitamin B_{12}, niacin, thiamine, riboflavin, vitamin D, iron, calcium, and zinc. Because vegetarian diets eliminate the major sources of complete proteins (those proteins with all the essential amino acids in amounts needed to support physiologic functions), protein deficiency can occur (see Cultural Awareness box).

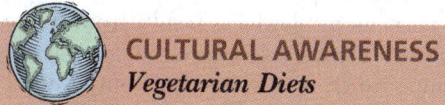

CULTURAL AWARENESS
Vegetarian Diets

In the United States strict vegetarian diets are common among members of Black Muslim or Seventh Day Adventist faiths. Achieving a nutritionally adequate vegetarian diet is not difficult, but it requires careful planning and knowledge of nutrient sources. For children the lacto-ovovegetarian diet is nutritionally adequate; however, the vegan diet requires supplementation with vitamins D and B_{12}, particularly for children ages 2 to 12 years. There have been reported cases of severe neurologic impairment in infants with vitamin B_{12} deficiency whose mothers were on a vegan diet (Graham, Arvela, and Wise, 1992). Infants on a vegan diet should be breast-fed for the first 6 months and preferably for 1 year, fed solid foods after about 4 months, and receive iron-fortified cereal for at least 18 months. The use of vitamin C juices with foods high in iron will further improve iron absorption. If cow's or human milk is not given, fortified soy milk is recommended. Other approaches toward increasing vitamin D and calcium intake in the diet that may be accepted by the macrobiotic teachers are inclusion of fatty fish (herring, salmon, sardines, trout, tuna) and less fiber, since high fiber intake limits mineral absorption by decreasing intestinal transit time and binding calcium, iron, and other minerals (Dagnelie and others, 1990).

NURSING CONSIDERATIONS

Identification of nutrient imbalance is the initial nursing goal and requires assessment based on a dietary history and physical examination for signs of deficiency or excess (see Nutritional Assessment, Chapter 6). Once assessment data are collected, this information is evaluated against standard intakes to identify areas of concern. The most widely used standard is the ***Recommended Dietary Allowances (RDAs)***, developed by the National Academy of Sciences, Food and Nutrition Board. The RDAs are not average requirements but recommendations intended to meet the physiologic needs of almost every healthy person. To meet the needs of those with the highest requirements, the RDAs will exceed most people's requirements. Therefore children consuming less than the RDAs are not necessarily consuming an inadequate diet, but they are more likely at risk for deficiency than those who are consuming nutrients in amounts equal to the RDAs.

Several organizations have published dietary advice for the public. Most well-known are the Dietary Guidelines for Americans, which encourage eating a variety of foods, maintaining ideal body weight, consuming adequate starch and fiber, and limiting intake of fat, cholesterol, sugar, salt, and alcohol. Another source is the Food Guide Pyramid, which replaces the basic four food groups that have traditionally been used to convey nutrition information to the public and applies to children as young as 2 years of age (see Nutrition, Chapter 4).

Since one of the best assurances of nutritional adequacy is eating a variety of foods, families need guidelines for selecting foods that provide essential nutrients without exceeding energy requirements. With a varied diet most children do not need vitamin or mineral supplements. Unfortunately, there are no restrictions on the availability of toxic doses of vitamins or minerals. Nurses need to inform families of the potential dangers from excess vitamins or minerals. The idea that "more is better" is probably best dispelled by a simple explanation of the body's inability to use more than the needed requirement.

Achieving a nutritionally adequate vegetarian diet (with the exception of the strictest diets) is not difficult, but it requires careful planning and knowledge of nutrient sources. For children the lacto-ovovegetarian diet is nutritionally adequate; however, the vegan diet requires supplementation with vitamins D and B_{12} for children ages 2 to 12 years. Infants should be breast-fed for the first 6 months and preferably for 1 year, be fed solid foods after about 4 months, and receive iron-fortified cereal for at least 18 months. The use of vitamin C juices with foods high in iron will further improve iron absorption. However, breast milk from vegetarian mothers can be deficient in vitamin B_{12}; supplementation of both mother and child is advisable. If cow's or human milk or commercial infant formula is not given, fortified soy milk is recommended. A variety of foods should be introduced during the early years to ensure a more well-balanced intake.

NURSING ALERT When solid foods are introduced, the safety and digestibility of the selections must be considered. Raw fruits with seeds, vegetables, and nuts are hazardous for infants and young children because of the danger of aspiration. Beans, grain cereals, and vegetables should be served well cooked and mashed during infancy.

To ensure sufficient protein in the diet, foods with incomplete proteins (those that do not have all the essential amino acids) must be eaten at the same meal with other foods that supply the missing amino acids. The three basic combinations of foods consumed by vegetarians that generally provide the appropriate amounts of essential amino acids are:

Grains (cereal, rice, pasta) and **legumes** (beans, peas, lentils, peanuts)
Grains and **milk products** (milk, cheese, yogurt)
Seeds (sesame, sunflower) and **legumes**

PROTEIN AND ENERGY MALNUTRITION (PEM)

Hunger is one of the world's gravest and most prevalent health problems. It is estimated that at least 40% of the world's children are undernourished and that poor nutritional status may contribute to approximately 60% of all childhood deaths (Mandelbaum, 1992). Children in less technologically developed countries often suffer from the most extreme forms of PEM—marasmus and kwashiorkor.

In the United States milder forms of PEM are seen, although the classic cases of marasmus and kwashiorkor also occur. Unlike developing countries where the main reason for PEM is inadequate food, in the United States PEM occurs despite ample dietary supplies (see Failure to Thrive, p. 595).

Kwashiorkor

Kwashiorkor has been defined in the past as primarily a deficiency of protein with an adequate supply of calories. A diet consisting mainly of starch grains or tubers provides adequate calories in the form of carbohydrates but an inadequate amount of high-quality proteins. There is evidence, however, supporting a multifactorial etiology, including cultural, psychologic, and infective factors that may jointly or singly interact to place the child at risk for kwashiorkor (Jelliffe and Jelliffe, 1992). A mycotoxin mold, ***aflatoxin***, has been implicated in the etiology of this disease; the mold has been found to grow on stored grains and to be present in large numbers in the intestines of children with kwashiorkor (Hendrickse, 1991). Taken from the Ga language (Ghana), the word means "the sickness the older child gets when the next baby is born" and aptly describes the syndrome that develops in the first child, usually between 1 and 4 years of age, when weaned from the breast once the second child is born.

Pathophysiology and Clinical Manifestations. The pathophysiology of kwashiorkor results in part from protein deficiency, both in quantity and quality. Since protein is essential for tissue growth and cell repair, all body systems are affected, but rapidly growing cells, such as those of the epithelium and mucosa, are most severely damaged. The skin is scaly and dry and has areas of depigmentation. Several dermatoses may be evident, partly resulting from the vitamin deficiencies. Permanent blindness results from the severe lack of vitamin A. Immunity is severely affected and is of considerable importance in the development of infections.

Mineral deficiencies are common, especially iron, calcium, and zinc. Acute zinc deficiency is a common complication of severe PEM and results in skin rashes, loss of hair, impaired immune response and susceptibility to infections, digestive problems, night blindness, changes in affective behavior, defective wound healing, and impaired growth. Its depressant effect on appetite further limits food intake.

With kwashiorkor the hair is thin, dry, coarse, and dull. Depigmentation is common, and patchy alopecia may occur. There is loss of weight in conjunction with generalized edema from the hypoalbuminemia. The edema often masks the severe muscular atrophy, making the children appear less debilitated than they actually are (Fig. 13-1). Total body water increases, but total body potassium decreases with retention of sodium, causing signs of hypokalemia and hypernatremia.

Diarrhea frequently occurs from a lowered resistance to infection and further complicates the electrolyte imbalance. Gastrointestinal disturbances occur, such as fatty infiltration of the liver and atrophy of the acini cells of the pancreas. Behavioral changes are evident as the child grows progressively more irritable, lethargic, withdrawn, and apathetic.

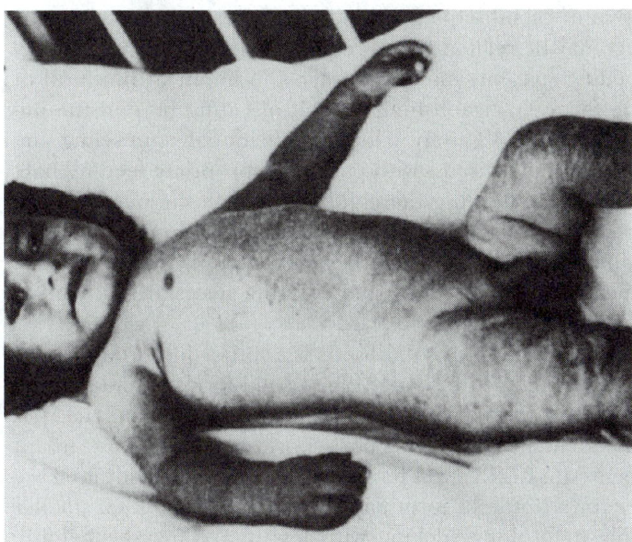

FIG. 13-1 Child with kwashiorkor. Note the edema, which masks muscle wasting. (From Guthrie HA: *Introductory nutrition,* ed 7, St Louis, 1989, Mosby. Courtesy Dr. John Beard, Pennsylvania State University.)

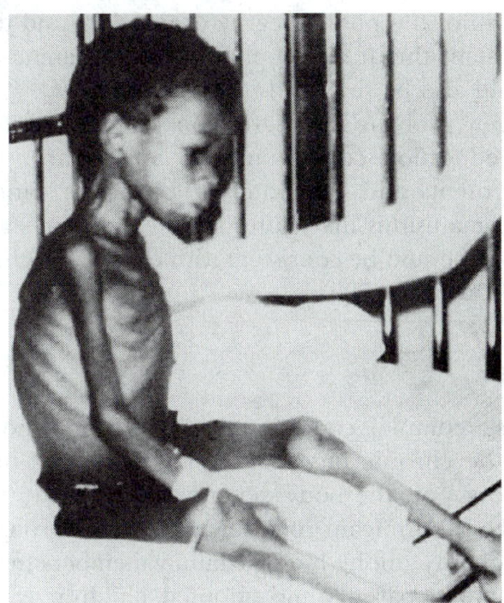

FIG. 13-2 Child with marasmus. (From Dodge PR, Prensky AL, Feigin RD: *Nutrition and the developing nervous system,* St Louis, 1975, Mosby. Courtesy Donald Anderson, M.D., Travis Air Force Base, CA.)

Fatal deterioration may be caused by diarrhea and infection or as the result of circulatory failure.

Marasmus

Marasmus results from general malnutrition of both calories and protein. It is a common occurrence in underdeveloped countries during times of drought, especially in cultures where adults eat first; the remaining food is often insufficient in quality and quantity for the children.

Marasmus is usually a syndrome of physical and emotional deprivation and is not confined to geographic areas where food supplies are inadequate. It may be seen in children with failure to thrive, where the cause is not solely nutritional but primarily emotional. Marasmus may be seen in infants as young as 3 months of age if breast-feeding is not successful and there are no suitable alternatives (Tsang and Nicholas, 1988).

Pathophysiology and Clinical Manifestations. Marasmus is characterized by gradual wasting and atrophy of body tissues, especially subcutaneous fat (Fig. 13-2). Children with the condition appear to be very old; their skin is flabby and wrinkled, unlike children with kwashiorkor, who appear more rounded from the edema. Fat metabolism is less impaired than in kwashiorkor, so that vitamin A deficiency is usually minimal or absent.

In general, the clinical manifestations of marasmus are similar to those seen in kwashiorkor with the following exceptions: with marasmus there is no edema from hypoalbuminemia or sodium retention, which contributes to a severely emaciated appearance; no dermatoses caused by vitamin deficiencies; little or no depigmentation of hair or skin; moderately normal fat metabolism and lipid absorption; and smaller head size and slower recovery following treatment.

As in kwashiorkor, body metabolism is minimal, and maintaining body temperature is complicated by lack of subcutaneous fat. The child is fretful, apathetic, withdrawn, and so lethargic that prostration frequently occurs. Intercurrent infection with debilitating diseases such as tuberculosis, parasitosis, and dysentery is common. Severe, chronic malnutrition in infancy results in decreased brain growth and has implications for the child's future mental capacity.

Therapeutic Management

Treatment of kwashiorkor and marasmus includes providing a diet high in quality proteins and/or carbohydrates, as well as vitamins and minerals. Electrolyte imbalance requires immediate attention, and parenteral fluid replacement may be necessary initially to correct the dehydration and restore renal function. An oral rehydration solution (ORS), recommended by the World Health Organization (WHO), may be used to correct dehydration (Shils, Olson, and Shike, 1994) (see also Diarrhea, Chapter 29). Occasionally, oral fluids are not tolerated, necessitating the use of hyperalimentation. Coexisting problems such as infection, diarrhea, parasitic infestation, and anemia necessitate prompt attention for optimum recovery.

One recommendation is the addition of psychosocial stimulation to the treatment of severely malnourished children. A long-term structured play program involving parents has been shown to result in marked developmental improvements. However, these children continued to be behind in nutritional status and locomotor development.

Nursing Considerations

Provision of essential physiologic needs such as rest, individually tailored activity, and protection from infection is paramount. Since children are usually weak and withdrawn, they depend on others for feeding. Hygiene may be distressing because of the poor integrity of the skin, and decubiti are a constant threat. Appropriate developmental stimulation should also be provided.

A larger problem is prevention of these conditions through education concerning the importance of high-quality proteins and adequate carbohydrates. Since children with marasmus may suffer from emotional starvation as well, care should be consistent with care of the child with failure to thrive (p. 595).

OBESITY

Obesity is a complex condition that may or may not be related to the chronic ingestion of more calories than are needed to supply the body's energy requirement. Genetic factors play a significant role, since there is a strong correlation of obesity among biologic family members that is not evident among parents and adopted children (Stunkard and others, 1990).

Firm evidence links obesity in adolescence to obesity in adulthood (see Obesity, Chapter 21); the evidence for obesity in infancy remaining a risk factor for adult obesity is controversial. Although recent studies have examined the role of infant feeding methods and subsequent overweight, these results are also conflicting. One study found that infants who were breast-fed beyond 6 months of age had slower growth rates than bottle-fed infants during the second half of the first year (Dewey and others, 1989). However, another study found that infants described as vigorous feeders who were breast-fed and had delayed introduction of solid foods were heavier at 6 years of age (Agras and others, 1990). A factor that may influence the effect of breast-feeding on infant weight gain is the mother's attitude—mothers who breast-feed tend to prefer leaner infants than mothers who bottle-feed.

Despite the conflicting data on exactly what causes infant obesity, all authorities agree that prevention holds greater promise than treatment. Besides the physiologic component of increased numbers of fat cells, there are also the psychologic disadvantages of firmly entrenched food habits and dependency on food. Consequently, evaluation of overnutrition early in life is essential, with attention to those factors that may prevent obesity.

Nursing Considerations

The principal nursing goal is prevention of obesity. If infants are overweight for their height, the goal is to slow weight gain, not cause weight loss. During infancy the development of obesity is influenced by parental practices. Therefore intervention involves helping the parent establish appropriate feeding habits for the infant or change inappropriate ones. This involves much more than dietary counseling. Psychologic factors play an important role, particularly the philosophy that a fat baby is a healthy baby, or, more subconsciously, that a fat "healthy" baby is a sign of good mothering (Sherman and Alexander, 1990). Such beliefs are difficult to dispel, and counseling may need to include other family members, such as grandmothers, who can greatly influence the mother's practices (Dietz, 1989).

Although the exact role breast-feeding has on the development of subsequent obesity is unclear, its protective effect may be related to self-regulation of intake. With bottle-feeding, parents may encourage the infant to finish all of the formula, establishing a habit of eating beyond the initial feeling of satiety. During nutritional counseling the nurse should discuss with parents appropriate feeding habits, such as allowing the child to regulate the need for formula and solid food. With proper education parents can come to understand that a "good eater" is not a big eater but one who eats moderately without necessarily "cleaning the plate."

The addition of solid foods is another important aspect of nutritional counseling. When solid foods are added, the quantity of milk should be decreased to less than 1 L per day to maintain the proper caloric balance. If the infant seems unsatisfied with fewer bottle feedings, substituting water for a bottle of formula or using a nipple with a smaller hole to prolong sucking with less intake may be helpful. Substituting skim or low-fat milk for whole milk or formula is unacceptable. Although these alternatives contain a significant reduction in calories, they are not nutritionally sound for infants. Their low fat content deprives the infant of essential fatty acids; significantly increased amounts of solids and electrolytes elevate the renal solute load and water demands; and their vitamin A content is reduced.

The selection of solid foods should also be considered. Approximately 20% of commercial baby foods contain less than 50 kcal/100 g, whereas another 20% contain more than 100 kcal/100 g. Choosing low-calorie foods can significantly lower the daily caloric intake without actually decreasing the total quantity of food. Food charts can be used to familiarize parents with the caloric content of foods, as well as encouraging reading of food labels. Sweet foods are kept to a minimum. This includes not adding additional sugar to the formula or cereal and avoiding finger foods such as cookies. Other foods rich in calories that are restricted in serving size rather than eliminated include butter, cream, ice cream, pudding, and chocolate.

Parents are also encouraged to interpret the infant's signals of discomfort and intervene in ways other than through feeding. Crying, fussiness, or sucking does not necessarily indicate hunger. Rocking, stroking, holding, and offering a pacifier may be more appropriate than automatically responding with food.

Since activity is also an important factor in maintaining appropriate weight, parents are encouraged to promote exercise in their child. Although infants are naturally active, placing them in confined areas, such as cribs or playpens, or in front of a television establishes poor habits. There is a reported direct relationship between time spent viewing television and the tendency toward obesity. However, another study failed to demonstrate a relationship between television viewing, adiposity, and decreased physical activity (Robinson, 1993).

FOOD SENSITIVITY

Food sensitivity is a general term that includes any type of adverse reaction to food or food additives. Food sensitivities can be divided into two broad categories:

Food allergy or **hypersensitivity,** which refers to those reactions involving immunologic mechanisms, usually immunoglobulin E (IgE); the reactions may be immediate or delayed and mild or severe, such as an anaphylactic reaction

Food intolerance, which refers to those reactions involving known or unknown nonimmunologic mechanisms; lactose intolerance is an example of a reaction that looks like allergy but is due to deficiency of the enzyme lactase

However, this classification is not universally accepted; therefore, the terms *food sensitivity, hypersensitivity, allergy,* and *intolerance* are often used interchangeably.

Food allergy is caused by exposure to ***allergens,*** usually proteins (but not the smaller amino acids) that are capable of inducing IgE antibody formation ("sensitization") when ingested. ***Sensitization*** refers to the initial exposure of an individual to an allergen, resulting in an immune response; subsequent exposure induces a much stronger response that is clinically apparent. Consequently, food hypersensitivity typically occurs after the food has been ingested one or more times. In infants an allergic response has been reported to occur with the first ingestion because of transplacental sensitization in utero or because of sensitization to the substance passed through breast milk (Wilson, Self, and Hamburger, 1990). Allergens can also produce an allergic response when inhaled or injected, but these routes rarely apply to food allergens (see also discussion of asthma in Chapter 32). The most common food allergens are eggs, cow's milk, peanuts, soy, wheat, corn, and fish (see box at right).

Food allergies can occur at any time but are common during infancy because the immature intestinal tract is more permeable to proteins than the mature intestinal tract, thus increasing the likelihood of an immune response. Allergies in general demonstrate a genetic component: children who have one parent with allergy have a 50% or greater risk of developing allergy; children who have both parents with allergy have up to a 100% risk of developing allergy. Allergy with a hereditary tendency is referred to as ***atopy.*** Some infants with atopy can be identified at birth from elevated levels of IgE in cord blood.

Deaths have been reported in children who suffered an anaphylactic reaction to food. Onset of the reactions occurred shortly after ingestion (5 to 30 minutes). In most of the children the reactions did not begin with skin signs, such as hives, red rash, and flushing, but rather as an acute asthma attack (Sampson and others, 1992). Parents, teachers, and daycare workers should be educated regarding signs and symptoms of food allergies. Those with food sensitivity should avoid unfamiliar foods, as well as restaurants that do not disclose food ingredients. Hidden ingredients in prepared foods have been implicated as a potential source. In patients with extremely sensitive food allergies the use of medical identification, such as a bracelet, and the rapid injectible epinephrine cartridge can help decrease mortality (Preventing food, 1993).

Although the reason is unknown, many children "outgrow" their food allergies. Children who are allergic to more than one food may develop tolerance to each food at different times. The most common allergens, such as soy, are outgrown less readily than other food allergens. Because of the tendency to lose the hypersensitivity, allergic foods should be reintroduced into the diet after a period of abstinence (usually a year or more) to evaluate if the food can be safely added to the diet (Sampson and Scanlon, 1989).

There is evidence that food allergies can be prevented. The protective role of exclusive breast-feeding and avoidance of hyperallergenic foods is controversial, but most authorities recommend the strategies in the Guidelines box on p. 590 for infants with a family history of atopy.*

HYPERALLERGENIC FOODS/SOURCES

Milk*: Ice cream, butter, margarine (if it contains dairy products), yogurt, cheese, pudding, baked goods, wieners, bologna, canned creamed soups, instant breakfast drinks, powdered milk drinks, milk chocolate

Eggs*: Mayonnaise, creamy salad dressing, baked goods, egg noodles, some cake icing, meringue, custard, pancakes, French toast, root beer

Wheat*: Almost all baked goods, wieners, bologna, pressed or chopped cold cuts, gravy, pasta, some canned soups

Legumes: Peanuts,* peanut butter or oil, beans, peas, lentils

Nuts*: Some chocolates, candy, baked goods, cherry soda (may be flavored with a nut extract), walnut oil

Fish or shellfish*: Cod liver oil, pizza with anchovies, Caesar salad dressing, any food fried in same oil as fish

Soy*: Soy sauce, teriyaki or worcestershire sauce, tofu, baked goods using soy flour or oil, soy nuts, soy infant formulas or milk, soybean paste, tuna packed in vegetable oil, many margarines

Chocolate: Cola beverages, cocoa, chocolate-flavored drinks

Buckwheat: Some cereals, pancakes

Pork, chicken: Bacon, wieners, sausage, pork fat, chicken broth

Strawberries, melon, pineapple: Gelatin, syrups

Corn: Popcorn, cereal, muffins, cornstarch, corn meal, corn bread, corn tortilla

Citrus fruits: Orange, lemon, lime, grapefruit; any of these in drinks, gelatin, juice, or medicines

Tomatoes: Juice, some vegetable soups, spaghetti, pizza sauce, catsup

Spices: Chili, pepper, vinegar, cinnamon

*Most common allergens.

Cow's Milk Allergy

Cow's milk allergy is a multifaceted disorder representing adverse systemic and local gastrointestinal reactions to cow's milk protein. The hypersensitivity may be manifested through a variety of signs and symptoms (see box on p. 590) that may appear within 45 minutes of milk ingestion or after a period of several days (Hill and others, 1989). The diagnosis is initially made from the history, although the practitioner needs to maintain a high index of suspicion, since the timing and diversity of clinical manifestations vary greatly. For example, cow's milk allergy may be manifested

*The pamphlet *Understanding Food Allergy* for parents of infants with food allergies is available from the American Academy of Allergy and Immunology, 611 E. Wells St., Milwaukee, WI 52202; (800) 822-2762.

GUIDELINES
Preventing Atopy in Children

IDENTIFY CHILDREN AT RISK

Family history of allergy
Increased IgE in cord blood and postnatal serum

PRENATAL PRECAUTIONS (LAST TRIMESTER)

Avoid any known food allergens
Avoid milk and other dairy products, peanuts, and eggs
Minimize ingestion of other hyperallergenic foods (see box on p. 589)

POSTNATAL PRECAUTIONS

Breast milk or casein/whey hydrolysate formula (e.g., Nutramigen, Pregestimil, Alimentum) exclusively for at least 6 months
No solid food for 6 months
No cow's milk or soy formula for 12 months
No egg, fish, corn, citrus, peanuts, nuts, or chocolate for 12 months
One new food added at 5-day intervals to identify possible reaction

ENVIRONMENTAL CONTROL

Limited exposure to dust, molds, animals, and cigarette smoke

Data from Johnstone D: Strategy for intervention of food allergy in infants, *Int Pediatr* 4(4):319-325, 1989; and Zeiger R and others: Effectiveness of dietary manipulation in the prevention of food allergy in infants, part 2, *J Allergy Clin Immunol* 78(1, pt 2):224-238, 1986.

as colic (see discussion on p. 593) or sleeplessness in an otherwise healthy infant (Kahn and others, 1989).

Diagnostic Evaluation. A number of diagnostic tests may be performed, including stool analysis for blood (both frank and occult bleeding can occur from the colitis), serum IgE levels, skin-prick testing, and radioallergosorbent test (RAST) (measures IgE antibodies to specific allergens in serum by radioimmunoassay). Both skin testing and RAST help identify the offending food, but the results are not always conclusive.

The most definitive diagnostic strategy is elimination of milk, followed by challenge testing after improvement of symptoms. Challenge testing involves reintroducing small quantities of milk in the diet to detect resurgence of symptoms; at times challenge testing involves the use of a placebo so that the parent is unaware of or "blind" to the timing of allergen ingestion.

NURSING ALERT Careful observation of the child is required during a challenge test because of the possibility of anaphylactic reaction.

Therapeutic Management. Treatment of cow's milk allergy is elimination of all dairy products. For infants fed cow's milk formula, this primarily involves changing the formula to a casein or whey hydrolysate milk formula, in which the protein has been broken down (or "predigested") into its amino acids through enzymatic hydrolysis. Soy-based formula is not recommended, because as many as 20% of these

COMMON CLINICAL MANIFESTATIONS OF COW'S MILK SENSITIVITY

GASTROINTESTINAL	RESPIRATORY	OTHER SIGNS AND SYMPTOMS
Diarrhea	Rhinitis	Eczema
Vomiting	Bronchitis	Excessive crying
Colic	Asthma	Pallor (from anemia secondary to chronic blood loss in gastrointestinal tract)
Abdominal pain	Wheezing	
	Sneezing	
	Coughing	
	Chronic nasal discharge	

infants are also allergic to soy (American Academy of Pediatrics, 1989). Goat's milk is not an acceptable substitute, since it cross-reacts with cow's milk protein and is deficient in folic acid. Infants who are breast-fed but have symptoms of cow's milk hypersensitivity are treated by eliminating all dairy products from the lactating mother's diet. These women need vitamin D and calcium supplementation to prevent deficiency. Infants are maintained on the dairy-free diet for 1 or 2 years, at which time very small quantities of milk are reintroduced.

Nursing Considerations. The principal nursing objectives are identification of potential milk allergy and appropriate counseling of parents regarding substitute formulas. The protein hydrolysate formulas are less palatable than milk-based formulas. Consequently, reluctance to accept the new formula may be a problem. This can be overcome by introducing the formula gradually over a few days using 1 ounce of new formula to 7 ounces of old formula, then 2 to 6 ounces, 3 to 4, and as needed. Parents also need to be reassured that the infant will receive complete nutrition from the new formula and will suffer no ill effects from the absence of cow's milk.

Once solid foods are started, parents need guidance in avoiding all associated milk products (see box on p. 589). Carefully reading all food labels helps avoid ingesting prepared foods containing milk products.

Lactose Intolerance

Lactose intolerance refers to at least two different entities that involve a deficiency of the enzyme ***lactase,*** which is needed for the digestion of lactose. ***Congenital lactose intolerance*** appears soon after birth when the diet contains lactose from milk (infant formula and human). The congenital deficiency is reported to be rare. Causes of lactose intolerance are attributed to disorders such as acquired immunodeficiency syndrome (AIDS) or gastrointestinal infections, such as rotavirus and giardiasis (Castiglia, 1994). ***Late-onset lactose intolerance*** is similar to the congenital type but is manifested later in life. Ethnic groups with a high incidence of lactose intolerance include Orientals, southern Europeans, Arabs, Jews, and blacks. The principal manifestations include diarrhea, abdominal pain, distension, and flatus shortly after ingesting milk products.

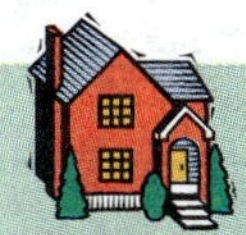

FAMILY HOME CARE
Controlling Symptoms of Lactose Intolerance

In infants substitute soy-based formula for cow's milk formula or human milk.
Limit milk consumption to one glass at a time.
Drink milk with other foods rather than alone.
Eat hard cheese, cottage cheese, or yogurt instead of drinking milk.
Use enzyme tablets (Lactaid, Lactrase, Dairy Ease) to predigest the lactose in milk or supplement the body's own lactase (add tablets to milk or sprinkle on dairy products such as ice cream).
Eat small amounts of dairy foods daily to help colonic bacteria adapt to ingested lactose.

In older children lactose intolerance may be diagnosed on the basis of the history and improvement following a lactose-free diet. In infants and younger children the hydrogen-breath test is frequently used. Undigested carbohydrate, such as lactose, in the colon causes gas production by bacteria. Breath samples are analyzed for the amount of hydrogen.

Treatment of lactose intolerance is elimination of offending dairy products or the use of enzyme replacement. In infants soy-based formula can be substituted for cow's milk formula or human milk. Some children are able to tolerate small amounts of lactose (see Family Home Care box). Pretreated milk (with microbial-derived lactase) is reported to be effective in improving lactose absorption (Castiglia, 1994). Since dairy products are a major source of calcium and vitamin D, supplementation of these nutrients is needed to prevent deficiency. Yogurt contains inactive lactase enzyme, which is activated by the temperature and pH of the duodenum; this lactase activity substitutes for the lack of endogenous lactase. Fresh yogurt may be tolerated better than frozen yogurt.

Nursing Considerations. Nursing care is similar to the interventions discussed for cow's milk allergy: explaining the dietary restrictions to the family; identifying alternate sources of calcium, such as yogurt; explaining the importance of supplementation; and discussing sources of lactose, especially hidden sources, such as its use as a bulk agent in certain medications, and ways of controlling the symptoms. Parents are advised to check with the pharmacist regarding this possibility when obtaining medication.

FEEDING DIFFICULTIES

IMPROPER FEEDING TECHNIQUE

A common cause of feeding problems is improper feeding technique. A satisfactory feeding requires a number of mechanical skills, such as placing the infant to the breast properly (see following section); holding the bottle at an angle that allows fluid, not air, to flow into the nipple; "reading" the infant's cues for burping or satiation; and holding the infant during feeding, rather than propping the bottle. A number of other problems can also occur singly or in combination, such as feeding too much or too little food; feeding too often, especially during the night, or too infrequently; selecting inappropriate foods for the infant's physiologic and motor development; and incorrectly preparing formula. While such feeding problems are more common in inexperienced parents, they can also occur with seasoned parents who are unprepared for an infant with different needs or less clear cues of hunger or satiation.

Most of these feeding problems are easily corrected with guidance and demonstration. Early assessment is essential to prevent complex problems from developing between parent and child at mealtime. Written guidelines for feeding infants can help new parents experience success with their child.

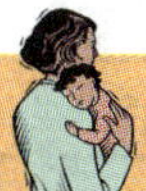

FAMILY FOCUS
Breast-Feeding and Infant Weight Gain

Mothers with breast-fed infants who fail to gain weight according to the standard growth curves are sometimes told that their milk, although nutritionally "good for the baby from an immunologic standpoint," lacks necessary fat for adequate growth. Recent evidence, however, indicates that infants who are exclusively breast-fed grow rapidly during the first 3 months of life but thereafter and up to 18 months demonstrate a slower weight-for-length pattern of growth than formula-fed infants. Breast-fed infants are leaner than formula-fed infants, but growth in head circumference and body length for both groups is equal. In addition, breast-fed infants, even with the introduction of other foods, demonstrate self-regulation in regard to energy intake. Morbidity and activity factors among the same two groups of infants are the same. The conclusions from the studies are that infants who are breast-fed exclusively during the first year of life are at risk of being labeled "growth deficient" when compared with current growth charts based on formula-fed children despite the lack of evidence that they have decreased brain growth or increased morbidity or mortality (Dewey and others, 1992, 1993; Piwoz, Peerson, and Brown, 1992).

Nurses can share these findings with parents to allay fears of an inadequate milk supply, which can discourage mothers from continuing to breast-feed. Also, an evaluation of growth, especially if weight falls below the 5th percentile, must be viewed carefully to avoid the diagnosis of failure to thrive (see p. 595) in infants with no other evidence of inadequate nutrition.

BREAST-FEEDING PROBLEMS

Many mothers have concerns regarding breast-feeding, and with earlier discharge from postpartum units common problems, such as engorgement and painful nipples, may occur after the mother is at home. New mothers are often concerned about their milk supply, and excessive anxiety can affect successful lactation (see Family Focus box).

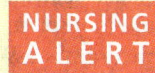

Encourage frequent feedings to increase milk production rather than use of supplemental formula or solid foods.

TABLE 13-3 Common Breast-Feeding Problems

PROBLEM	COMMENTS/INTERVENTIONS
Engorgement	Best intervention is prevention with frequent nursing on both breasts for complete emptying of ducts If engorgement occurs, infant is unable to properly grasp distended areola Interventions: Express manually small amount of milk; electric pump may be beneficial for some Use warm compresses or a warm shower 10-15 minutes before feeding; for severely engorged breasts, cold compresses may be helpful to reduce vascularity after feeding Compress areola with fingers to facilitate infant's grasp (C-hold) Use well-fitting nursing brassiere and wear 24 hours a day For excessive discomfort, take aspirin or acetaminophen 30 minutes before feeding Massage breasts; vary position of infant's mouth on nipple/areola
Painful nipples	Most common causes are poor feeding technique, improper care of breasts, excessive moisture from milk leaking If left untreated, discomfort may cause mother to terminate breast-feeding Interventions for care of breasts: Avoid soaps, oils, or self-prescribed treatments Apply small amount of breast milk to areola after feeding and let dry Air nipples as much as possible; use heat (60-watt bulb placed 18 inches away or hair dryer on low setting) Change breastpads frequently; avoid plastic-backed pads (may trap moisture) Interventions related to feeding: Start let-down reflex before putting infant to breast Begin nursing with less affected breast, then nurse on affected side Position infant properly at breast; check that entire areola is grasped Change infant's position; use football hold For excessive discomfort, take analgesics 30 minutes before feeding; apply ice to nipples after feeding
Let-down reflex	Let-down (ejection) reflex is essential to delivery of milk from alveoli and smaller milk ducts into larger lactiferous ducts and sinuses Controlled primarily by release of prolactin and oxytocin Pain, stress, and anxiety can interfere with reflex Interventions: Provide quiet, relaxing atmosphere for nursing (e.g., soothing music, privacy, pillows for positioning, decreased distractions) Stroke breast gently Apply warmth to breast May need to use oxytocin nasal spray to induce a reflex (used only in newborn period)
Inadequate milk supply	Production of milk depends on supply and demand Rarely is related to organic causes, such as decreased glandular tissue Interventions: Reassure mother that her milk supply will be adequate and depends on frequent nursing Encourage more frequent nursing (at least six to eight times daily, initially at both breasts) Encourage adequate rest, nutrition, and fluids (increased fluids, however, have not been shown to increase milk production) Avoid use of supplemental formula feedings before breast-feeding is well established to prevent nipple preference and satiation (infant will not be hungry enough to breast-feed) Monitor infant's growth; in some cases formula supplementation may be indicated; an alternative to bottle-feeding is use of a supplemental feeding device consisting of a plastic bag or syringe for formula and a thin feeding tube that is placed next to mother's nipple during nursing
Plugged ducts	May occur at any time, especially during first 6 weeks Continue breast-feeding every 2-3 hours Massage breasts before feedings Apply ice compresses to breasts between feedings; remove ice 10-15 minutes before feeding and apply warm compress Alternate feeding positions, positioning infant's chin toward obstructed area.
Mastitis	Inflammation or infection in mammary gland or tissue; results from inadequate emptying of ducts or from cracks in nipple skin Prevention: see Plugged Ducts; if mastitis occurs, current treatment is 10 days of antibiotics Continue breast-feeding during this time to keep breast well drained (unless contraindicated for medical reasons such as systemic illness)

The more common breast-feeding problems and their interventions are summarized in Table 13-3. Most of these problems are easily remedied, provided that the mother receives the attention needed to identify the concern. Assessment includes a detailed history of the complaint, examination of the breasts, and observation of breast-feeding (see Guidelines box).

Many breast-feeding problems respond rapidly to simple interventions, such as correcting the infant's feeding position. However, the mother needs continual reassurance of

GUIDELINES
Observing the Breast-Feeding Couple

Position of mother, her body language, and any possible tension
Position of infant: child's ventral (front) surface should be next to mother's ventral surface with the face directly in front of the breast ("tummy to tummy"); the infant cannot swallow if the head has to turn to the breast
Position of mother's hand on the breast: using two fingers to compress the areola (the C-hold) and support the breast facilitates infant's ability to grasp the areola properly
Position of infant's lips on the areola: the lips should gently clamp the entire areola; the lower lip should not be folded in so that infant sucks the lip
Use of alternate breasts and feeding time on each breast
Technique to break suction: should release suction using fingers between the areola and lips; should not pull infant from the breast abruptly

success and support that allow her the needed rest and relaxation to nurse her infant. Referral to supportive agencies, such as local groups of **La Leche League,*** or a lactation specialist, may be beneficial.

REGURGITATION AND "SPITTING UP"

The return of small amounts of food after a feeding is a common occurrence during infancy. It should not be confused with actual vomiting, which can be associated with a number of disturbances that may be insignificant or serious. It is usually benign, although persistent regurgitation necessitates medical evaluation to rule out gastroesophageal reflux. For clarification the following terms are defined:

Regurgitation—Return of undigested food from the stomach, usually accompanied by burping
Spitting up—Dribbling of unswallowed formula from the infant's mouth immediately after a feeding

The normal occurrence of regurgitation or spitting up should be explained to parents, especially to those who are unduly concerned about it. It can be reduced by some simple measures, such as frequent burping during and after feeding, minimum handling at feeding and after, and positioning the child on the right side with the head slightly elevated after feeding. The inconvenience of spitting up can be managed with the use of absorbent bibs on the infant and protective cloths on the parent.

Sometimes frequent dribbling of formula causes excoriation of the corners of the mouth, chin, and neck. Keeping the area dry promotes healing but can be difficult to maintain. Helpful suggestions include applying a thin film of petrolatum or A and D ointment to the affected areas after cleansing and using absorbent nonplastic-lined terry-cloth bibs, which are changed frequently.

*For information call (800) LA-LECHE.

PAROXYSMAL ABDOMINAL PAIN (COLIC)

Colic is generally described as paroxysmal abdominal pain or cramping that is manifested by loud crying and drawing the legs up to the abdomen. Other definitions include variables such as duration of cry greater than 3 hours a day and parental dissatisfaction with the child's behavior. Some studies report an increase in symptoms (fussiness and crying) in the evening; however, in some infants the onset of symptoms occurs at another time (Hill and others, 1992). Colic is more common in young infants under the age of 3 months than in older infants, and infants with "difficult" temperaments are more likely to be colicky (Barr and others, 1989). Despite the obvious behavioral indications of pain, the child tolerates the formula well, gains weight, and thrives.

Etiology

Among the theories that have been investigated as potential causes are too rapid feeding, overeating, swallowing excessive air, improper feeding technique (especially in positioning and burping), and emotional stress or tension between parent and child. While all of these may occur, there is no evidence that one factor is consistently present. In some infants colic may be a sign of cow's milk allergy or intolerance, and eliminating cow's milk products from the infant's diet and the diet of lactating mothers can reduce the symptoms (Forsyth, 1989; Lothe and Lindberg, 1989). Parental smoking has also been associated with colic.

Some investigators discount the biologic causes of colic and attribute the problem to parents' ineffective responses to the infant's crying or too little carrying of the infant (Hunziker and Barr, 1986; Taubman, 1988). It is of interest that the incidence of colic differs markedly among social classes—with more parents from a higher socioeconomic status reporting colic. A possible explanation may be greater acceptance of an infant's crying behavior among lower social groups (Hide and Guyer, 1982). An increase in crying over the first several weeks is normal and is thought to represent maturation of the nervous system. It may be that some parents are particularly sensitive to crying, especially if it occurs in infants who also demonstrate difficult temperament. One study describes colic as a distinct syndrome involving temperament, crying, and facial activity similar to that of normal infants, yet the mothers of the colicky infants are more concerned about or less tolerant of the crying (Barr and others, 1992).

The biologic theory and the interaction theory present two opposing viewpoints, yet each theory has substantial research to support its tenets. To explain this dichotomy, Geertsma and Hyams (1989) propose that colic has multiple causes and that the intensity of the cry may be significant in distinguishing between them (previous studies have only considered the duration of the cry). They found that infants who passed more flatus cried more intensely and inconsolably than infants with less flatus, who cried less intensely and responded to comforting measures. They suggest that the "high-intensity group" may have pain due to organic causes, such as milk sensitivity, and the "lower-intensity

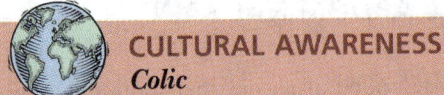

CULTURAL AWARENESS
Colic

Herbal tea containing natural antispasmodic properties is used as a remedy for colic in Israel; according to one study, infants given the herbal tea (vs a placebo) showed significant improvement in relation to irritability and crying associated with colic (Weizman and others, 1993).

group" may have no organic cause but require greater soothing measures than noncolic infants.

Therapeutic Management

Management of colic should begin with an investigation of diagnosable causes, such as cow's milk allergy. If a sensitivity to cow's milk is strongly suspected, a trial substitution of another formula, such as a casein hydrolysate (Nutramigen), is warranted. Soy formulas are avoided because of the possibility of sensitivity to soy protein as well. When no specific inciting agent can be found, the supportive measures discussed under Nursing Considerations are employed.

The use of drugs, including sedatives, antispasmodics, antihistamines, and antiflatulents, is sometimes recommended. The most commonly used sedatives are phenobarbitol and hydroxyzine hydrochloride (Atarax). The antispasmodic dicyclomine hydrochloride (Bentyl) is not recommended for infants under 6 months of age because of rare instances of death (Pinyerd and Zipf, 1989) (see Cultural Awareness box).

Nursing Considerations

The initial step in managing colic is to take a thorough, detailed history of the usual daily events. Areas that should be stressed include (1) diet of the breast-feeding mother; (2) time of day when attacks occur; (3) relationship of the attacks to feeding time; (4) presence of specific family members during attacks and habits, such as smoking by family members; (5) activity of the mother or usual caregiver before, during, and after the crying; (6) characteristics of the cry (duration, intensity); and (7) measures used to relieve the crying and their effectiveness. Of special emphasis is a careful assessment of the feeding process via demonstration by the parent.

If milk sensitivity is suspected, bottle-feeding and breast-feeding mothers should follow a milk-free diet (see box on p. 589) for a minimum of 5 days in an attempt to reduce symptoms in the infant. Mothers need to be cautioned that some nondairy creamers may contain calcium caseinate, a cow's milk protein. If this approach is helpful, lactating mothers may need calcium supplements to meet the body's requirement. Bottle-fed infants may improve with the same dietary modifications as for the child with cow's milk allergy (see p. 590).

More often than not, no change is required in feeding practices. When no cause can be identified, it is preferable to determine the time of the onset of crying and attempt to manipulate the circumstances associated with it. For example, some infants have episodes of colic around the

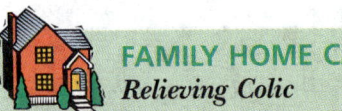

FAMILY HOME CARE
Relieving Colic

Place infant prone over a covered hot-water bottle, heated towel, or covered heating pad.
Massage infant's abdomen.
Respond immediately to the crying.
Change infant's position frequently; walk with child's face down and with body across parent's arm, with parent's hand under infant's abdomen, applying gentle pressure (Fig. 13-3).
Use a front carrier for transporting infant.
Swaddle infant tightly with a soft, stretchy blanket.
Place infant in a wind-up swing.
Take infant for car rides or outside for a change in environment.
Use a commercial device* in the crib that simulates the vibration and sound of a car ride or plays soothing "noise" or in utero sounds.
Provide smaller, frequent feedings; burp infant during and after feedings using the shoulder position, and place infant in an upright seat after feedings.
Introduce a pacifier for added sucking.
In breast-fed infants, mother should avoid all milk products for a trial period.
If household members smoke, avoid smoking near infant; preferably confine smoking activity to outside of home.
If nothing reduces the crying, place infant in crib and allow to cry; periodically hold and comfort child and put down again.

---

*Sweet Dreems, Inc., Sleep Tight Order Department, 4710 E. Walnut St., Westerville, Ohio 43081; (800) NO COLIC ([800] 662-6542).

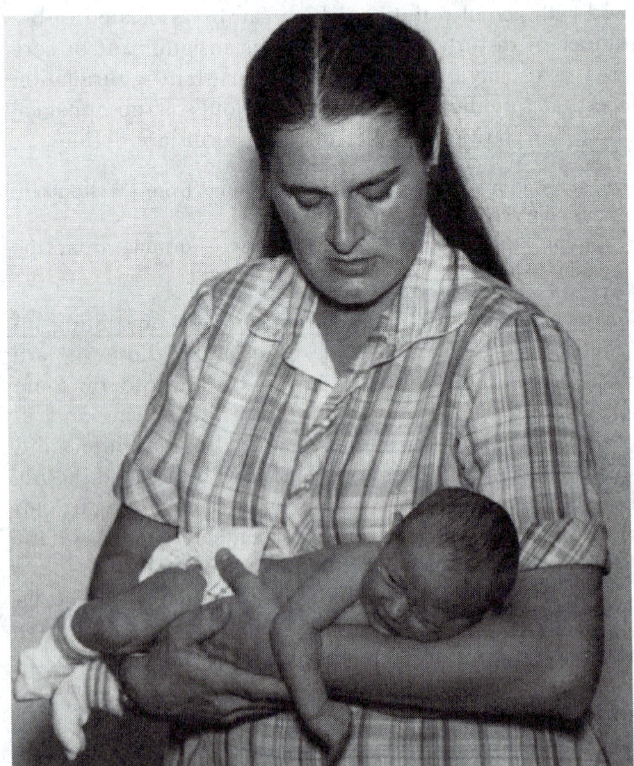

FIG. 13-3 The "colic carry" may be comforting to an infant with colic.

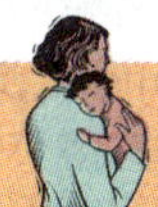

FAMILY FOCUS
Colic

While colic is considered a minor ailment, the presence of a colicky, crying, irritable infant can have an intense emotional impact on parent-child attachment and family relationships. Parents, especially mothers, often relate histories of a daily routine that is laden with feelings of frustration, anger, despair, and helplessness. A vicious circle ensues in which the parent's own anxiety may be transferred to the infant, further increasing the tension, irritability, and crying.

One of the most important areas of nursing concern is the support of parents during the colic period. It should be stressed that despite the crying and obvious pain, the infant is doing well. Colic disappears spontaneously, usually by 3 months of age, although guarantees should never be given, because it may continue for much longer. The parent, especially the mother, should be encouraged to leave the house and arrange for some free time. Most important, it should be emphasized that colic does not indicate poor or inadequate parenting. Parents' negative feelings toward the infant and insecurities regarding their parenting abilities are normal. Parents are encouraged to talk about such feelings, since active listening may do more to relieve the colic syndrome than offering stereotyped advice, remedies, and glib statements such as, "Don't worry about it; your child will eventually outgrow the colicky spells."

CRITICAL THINKING EXERCISE
Colic

During a routine clinic visit you notice that the mother of a 2-month-old infant appears very tired, gets easily confused answering simple questions, and casually mentions that the infant cries much more than her first child did and for no apparent reason. You direct the focus of the interview on the infant's behavior preceding the crying spells; feeding habits, including dietary history; and patterns of sleep. The mother suspects that the infant has colic. The best response to this mother is:

1. "Well, Dr. Smith will be in shortly, and you can discuss this with her."
2. "You must feel a little frustrated about this situation; can you tell me more about your concerns that maybe you have done something wrong with this child?"
3. "Colic is a complex problem for which there are few solutions other than giving the child medications and tolerating the crying the best way possible."
4. "We have some pamphlets on colic in the lobby; after you see the doctor, be sure to pick one up and read it at home."

The correct answer is 2. This allows the mother time to express her feelings about the colicky infant, as well as her own fears about childrearing and possible inadequacies, and opens the door for a discussion of some solutions to the problem. The other options end the discussion and suggest that the mother or another health professional is responsible for a solution.

family's dinner time, when all household members are home and the mother is preoccupied with cooking. The overstimulating, more tense atmosphere may upset the infant. Encouraging someone else to prepare dinner or the mother to prepare dinner earlier in the day and feed the infant in a more quiet area of the house may help reverse the environmental conditions that may have provoked the attack of colic. Other approaches for relieving colic are listed in the Family Home Care box. Parents are encouraged to try as many of these approaches as possible, because not all are effective for every infant (see also the Family Focus and Critical Thinking Exercise boxes).

RUMINATION

Rumination is the active, voluntary return of swallowed food into the mouth. The food is then rechewed, partially or completely reswallowed, or expelled. Technically, this is not a feeding problem, since infant ruminators usually have hearty appetites. However, in some instances rumination may lead to progressive malnutrition and even death, since considerable food and fluid loss can occur.

Rumination differs from regurgitation, which is involuntary. The ruminating infant makes purposeful movements of the mouth, tongue, and stomach in an attempt to force food back into the oropharynx. On successful regurgitation the infant is obviously satisfied with the activity.

Organic causes for rumination are rarely found, although the possibility of gastroesophageal reflux should be investigated in the differential diagnosis. It may also be seen in profoundly retarded children. However it is most often considered a result of a disturbed parent-child relationship. The factors culminating in the disorder may be similar to those described in nonorganic failure to thrive. Some authorities believe rumination is a conditioned behavioral response to an increased need for self-stimulation or parental attention.

Treatment typically involves psychotherapy to improve parenting ability or behavior modification techniques to modify eating patterns. Behavioral approaches vary but may include increased attention, such as holding before, during, and after meals, or the use of time-out.

Nursing Considerations

The primary objective is to terminate the ruminating behavior and restore normal feeding patterns. This is accomplished through a structured feeding plan, such as those used to feed the child with nonorganic failure to thrive (see p. 596). Positive stimulation programs must accompany the feeding plan, since being left alone may trigger ruminating episodes. Parents need to learn how to feed the child, and follow-up after discharge is essential to prevent a recurrence of the behavior.

FAILURE TO THRIVE (FTT)

FTT is a state of inadequate growth resulting from inability to obtain and/or use calories required for growth. FTT has no universal definition, although one of the more common parameters is a weight (and sometimes height) that falls below the 5th percentile for the child's age. Some authorities prefer the 3rd percentile as a criterion, but the widely used National Center for Health Statistics growth charts include only the 5th, not the 3rd, percentile in their measurements. Growth measurements alone are not used to diagnose children with FTT. Rather, the finding of a persistent deviation from an established growth curve is cause for concern.

Three general categories of failure to thrive are:

Organic failure to thrive (OFTT)—Result of a physical cause, such as congenital heart defects, neurologic lesions, microcephaly, chronic urinary tract infection, gastroesophageal reflux, renal insufficiency, malabsorption syndrome, endocrine dysfunction, cystic fibrosis, or AIDS.

Nonorganic failure to thrive (NFTT)—Has a definable cause that is unrelated to disease. NFTT is most often the result of psychosocial factors, such as inadequate nutritional information by the parent; deficiency in maternal care or a disturbance in maternal-child attachment; or a disturbance in the child's ability to separate from the parent, leading to food refusal to maintain attention. NFTT has been described under a variety of less acceptable names, including maternal deprivation, environmental deprivation, and deprivation dwarfism.

Idiopathic failure to thrive—Unexplained by the usual organic and environmental etiologies but may also be classified as NFTT. Both NFTT and idiopathic FTT account for the majority of cases of FTT.

Traditionally the category of NFTT has implied a disturbance in the parent-child interaction. However, this is not always the case. Many other factors can lead to inadequate feeding of the infant, such as the following:

Poverty—Lack of funds to buy sufficient food; may dilute formula to extend available supply

Health beliefs—Use of fad diets, often from excessive concern with preventing conditions such as obesity, hypercholesterolemia, or nursing caries; may involve use of skim milk, diluted formula, or excessive use of fruit juice

Inadequate nutritional knowledge—Cultural confusion of newly arrived immigrants who are unaware of appropriate food selections in American markets; parents with cognitive impairment

Family stress—Overwhelming involvement with another chronically ill child; any number of other stresses (financial, marital, excessive parenting and employment responsibilities, depression, chemical abuse, acute grief)

Feeding resistance—Result of nonoral nutritional therapy early in life

Insufficient breast milk—Result of a number of different causes (fatigue, illness, poor release of milk, insufficient glandular tissue, lack of confidence) (see Family Focus box on p. 591).

In these instances parent education and provision of necessary supports (financial or psychosocial) are successful in correcting the reason for the malnutrition. Dealing with families in which a child has NFTT because of a parent-child disturbance is much more difficult.

Diagnostic Evaluation

Diagnosis is initially made from evidence of growth retardation. If FTT is recent, the weight, but not the height, is below accepted standards (usually the 5th percentile); if FTT is long-standing, both weight and height are depressed, indicating chronic malnutrition. Additional diagnostic procedures include a complete health and dietary history, physical examination for evidence of organic causes, developmental assessment, and a family assessment. Other tests are selected *only* as indicated to rule out organic problems. To prevent the overuse of diagnostic procedures, NFTT should be considered *early* in the differential diagnosis.

Therapeutic Management

Regardless of the cause of FTT, the treatment is directed at reversing the malnutrition. The goal is to provide sufficient calories to support "catch-up" growth—a rate of growth greater than the expected rate for age. Any coexisting medical problems are treated.

In most cases of NFTT a multidisciplinary team of physician, nurse, dietitian, child-life specialist, and social worker or mental health professional is needed to deal with the multiple psychologic problems. Efforts are made to relieve any additional stresses on the family, such as referrals to welfare agencies or supplemental food programs. Involvement of child protective services may be necessary in severe cases.

Prognosis

The prognosis for NFTT is related to the cause. If the parents have simply been ignorant of the infant's needs, teaching may remedy the child's limited caloric intake and permanently reverse the growth failure. Inadequate or decreased feeding periods by the infant's primary caretaker is often observed as the cause of NFTT in conjunction with family disorganization (Blizzard, 1992). When the family dysfunction is extensive, the prognosis is uncertain. Factors related to poor prognosis are severe feeding resistance, lack of awareness in and cooperation from the parent(s), low family income, low maternal educational level, and early age of onset of NFTT. Many of these children are below normal in intellectual development, have poorer language development and less well developed reading skills, attain lower social maturity, and have a higher incidence of behavioral disturbances. Such findings indicate that a long-term plan is needed for the optimum development of these children.

Nursing Considerations

Caring for the child with NFTT presents many nursing challenges, whether treatment takes place in the hospital, clinic, or home. Providing a positive feeding environment, teaching the parent successful feeding strategies, and supporting the child and family are essential components of care.

Nurses play a critical role in the diagnosis of NFTT through their assessment of the child, parents, and family interaction. Knowledge of the characteristics of children with NFTT and their families is essential in helping identify these children and hastening the confirmation of a correct diagnosis. Accurate assessment of initial weight and height and daily weight, as well as recording of all food intake, is mandatory. The feeding behavior of the child is documented, as well as the parent-child interaction during feeding, other caregiving activities, and play. An excellent feeding observation instrument is the Nursing Child Assessment Feeding Scale (NCAFS), which is designed to assess the feeding interaction of infants up to 12 months of age (Barnard and others, 1993).* (See also Nutritional Assessment, Chapter 6.) The approximate developmental age should be assessed on admission by administering an appropriate developmental test. Only after objective measurements are available is a plan of care for stimulation outlined.

The nursing admission history and ongoing assessment should also focus on the following characteristics that have been identified in many of these children and their parents.

The Child. Besides the obvious signs of malnutrition and delayed development, children with NFTT may interact differently from children with OFTT. They may display intense interest in inanimate objects, such as a toy, but much less interest in social interactions. They are often vigilant of people at a distance but become increasingly distressed as they come closer. They may dislike being touched or held and avoid face-to-face contact. However, when held, they protest briefly on being put down and are apathetic when left alone.

Frequently there is a history of difficult feeding, vomiting, sleep disturbance, and excessive irritability. Habit patterns such as crying during feedings, vomiting, hoarding food in the mouth, ruminating after feeding, refusal to switch from liquids to solids, and aversion behavior, such as turning from food or spitting food, become attention-seeking mechanisms to prolong the attention received at mealtime. In addition, chronic reduction in calories can lead to appetite depression, which compounds the problem.

A feature of many children with NFTT is their irregularity (low rhythmicity) in activities of daily living. Some of these children typify the "difficult" temperament pattern. However, another type is the passive, sleepy, lethargic infant who does not wake up for feedings. Parents who have been advised of "demand feeding schedules" may be unsure of whether to wake the child or let the child sleep. Because of their inexperience and lack of guidance, parents may develop a pattern of infrequent feeding that is inadequate to meet the infant's nutritional needs. Such a pattern is particularly detrimental with the breast-feeding infant, in whom frequent nursing is essential to an adequate milk supply. Such characteristics in a child do not necessarily result in NFTT. Rather, a complex set of variables is significant, such as the degree of *fit* between the child's temperament and that of the parents. Since the personalities of infants can have definite effects on the parent-child attachment process, identifying such situations of disharmony may be one approach toward prevention and anticipatory guidance.

The Parents. Some parents are at increased risk for attachment problems because of (1) isolation and social crisis, (2) inadequate support systems, and (3) poor parenting as a child. Other factors that should be considered are lack of education; physical and mental health problems, such as retardation, depression, or drug dependence; immaturity, especially in adolescent parents; and lack of commitment to parenting, such as giving higher priority to career goals. Frequently these parents and their families are under stress and in multiple chronic emotional, social, and financial crises.

▪ ▪ ▪

Planning needs to begin as soon as the problem is identified, whether it is on an outpatient basis or hospitalization is required. The priority nursing goal is providing the infant with sufficient nutrients for growth. More specific nursing care depends on the identified cause of FTT. If an organic etiology is confirmed, care is related primarily to management of the disorder. If the problem is one of inadequate knowledge regarding child feeding, parental education is required. When serious psychosocial factors are involved, hospitalization may be needed and additional interventions are required to meet the needs of both the child and the family.

Since part of the difficulty between parent and child is dissatisfaction and frustration, the child should have a primary core of nurses for all three shifts (Fig. 13-4). Only the same nurse caring for the child over a period of time can learn to perceive the child's cues and reverse the cycle of dissatisfaction, especially in the area of feeding. Since these children are not ill with any physical disorder but are debilitated from general malnutrition, they should be placed in a room with noninfectious children of a similar age.

Since many of these children are responding to stimuli that have led to the negative feeding patterns, the first goal is to structure the feeding environment to encourage eating. Initially staff members may need to feed these children to assess thoroughly the difficulties encountered during the feeding process and to devise strategies that eliminate or

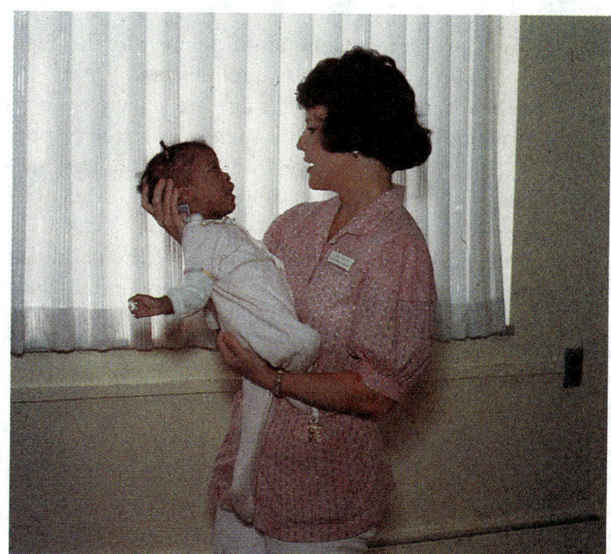

FIG. 13-4 A consistent nurse is important in developing trust with infants with nonorganic failure to thrive.

*Training is required to use the NCAFS, and information on the training program is available from Georgina Sumner, Director, NCAST, WJ-10, University of Washington, Seattle, WA 98195; (206) 543-8526.

GUIDELINES
Feeding Children with Nonorganic Failure to Thrive

Provide a primary core of staff to feed the child. The same nurses are able to learn the child's cues and respond consistently.

Provide a quiet, unstimulating atmosphere. A number of these children are very distractible, and their attention is diverted with minimal stimuli. Older children do well at a feeding table; younger children should always be held.

Maintain a calm, even temperament throughout the meal. Negative outbursts may be commonplace in this child's habit formation. Limits on eating behavior definitely need to be provided, but they should be stated in a firm, calm tone. If the nurse is hurried or anxious, the feeding process will not be optimized.

Talk to the child by giving directions about eating. "Take a bite, Lisa" is appropriate and directive. The more distractible the child, the more directive the nurse should be to refocus attention on feeding. Positive comments about feeding are actively given.

Be persistent. This is perhaps one of the most important guidelines. Parents often give up when the child begins negative feeding behavior. Calm perseverance through 10 to 15 minutes of food refusal will eventually diminish negative behavior. Although forced feeding is avoided, "strictly encouraged" feeding is essential.

Maintain a face-to-face posture with the child when possible. Encourage eye contact and remain with the child throughout the meal.

Introduce new foods slowly. Often these children have been exclusively bottle-fed. If acceptance of solids is a problem, begin with pureed food and, once accepted, advance to junior and regular solid foods.

Follow the child's rhythm of feeding. The child will set a rhythm when the previous conditions are met.

Develop a structured routine. Disruption in their other activities of daily living has great impact on feeding responses, so bathing, sleeping, dressing, and playing, as well as feeding, are structured. The nurse should feed the child in the same way and place as often as possible. The length of the feeding should also be established (usually 30 minutes).

minimize such problems. General guidelines for the feeding process are outlined in the Guidelines box.

Foods appropriate to the child's age are selected. To increase caloric intake, supplements, such as Polycose or powdered milk, can be added to foods, and powdered commercial formula can be prepared to yield 24 cal/oz rather than 20 cal/oz.

Besides attending to the physical needs of the child, the nurse must plan care for appropriate developmental stimulation. Once an approximate developmental age is established, a planned program of play is begun. Ideally a child-life specialist is involved to implement and supervise the stimulation program. Every effort is made to teach the parent how to play and interact with the child.

Nursing care of these children involves a "systems" approach. In other words, for the entire family to become healthy, each member must be helped to change. Care of the parents is aimed at helping them increase their feelings of self-esteem through positive, successful parenting skills. Initially this necessitates providing an environment in which they feel welcomed and accepted. Because these parents are often distrustful of authority figures, it may take some time before they develop any trust toward the nurse. One approach is to emphasize with the parent about the difficulties of childrearing. For example, the nurse may state that many parents find adjusting to parenthood a trying time or that the demands of caring for an infant can become overwhelming.

Teaching infant care techniques to the parents is begun through example and demonstration, not by lecturing. As the nurse perceives the infant's cues, these are emphasized to the parents. For example, during a feeding the nurse might comment that the infant is still hungry because the child sucks vigorously and looks at the nurse. When the infant is satisfied, the nurse points out that the infant is signaling this by releasing the strong suck, closing the eyes, and breathing deeply and more slowly. By example, the child is gently placed in the crib for a nap.

At the same time, the parents are offered an opportunity to care for the infant without having demands made on them. For example, the nurse suggests that at the next feeding one of the parents offer the child the bottle. Whenever the parents participate, they are praised and encouraged to continue caring for the child.

Plans are made to implement these interventions at home. A public health referral is made, and if a foster grandparent was included, this person should also visit the family. Social agencies that can provide financial or housing assistance to lessen the stress of everyday life are also contacted. (See also Nursing Care Plan: The Child with Nonorganic Failure to Thrive.*)

SKIN DISORDERS

DIAPER DERMATITIS

Dermatitis in the diaper area is encountered frequently by nurses in all pediatric settings. Approximately 50% of young children demonstrate some degree of diaper dermatitis, and about 5% have severe rash (intense erythema, scaling, papules, and ulcerations). The peak age for diaper dermatitis is 9 to 12 months and may be associated with decreased frequency of diaper changes and modifications in diet, such as change from breast milk to formula and introduction of solids. The incidence is generally reported as greater in bottle-fed infants than in breast-fed infants (Jordan and others, 1986), although other studies report no difference (Austin and others, 1988; Lane, Rehder, and Helm, 1990).

Pathophysiology and Clinical Manifestations

Diaper dermatitis is caused by prolonged and repetitive contact with an irritant, principally urine, feces, soaps, detergents, ointments, and friction. Although the obvious irritant in the majority of incidences is urine and feces, the specific components that contribute to irritation include a combination of factors (Fig. 13-5).

---

*In *Wong and Whaley's Clinical Manual of Pediatric Nursing* (Mosby).

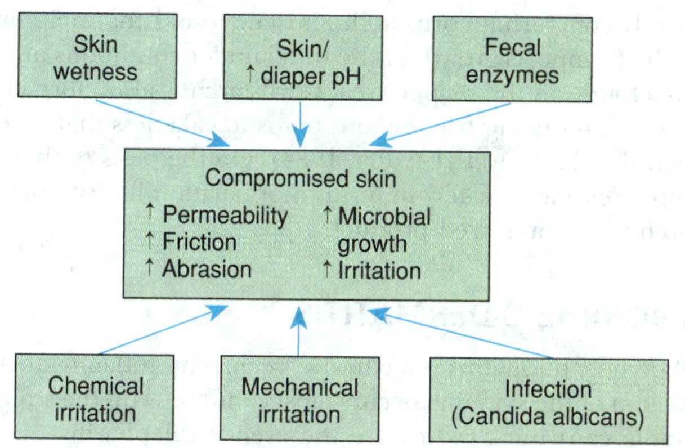

FIG. 13-5 Principal factors involved in development of diaper dermatitis.

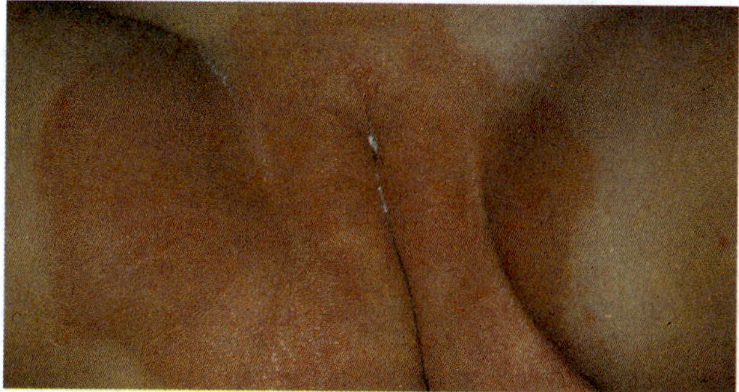

FIG. 13-6 Irritant diaper dermatitis. Note sharply demarcated edges. (From Habif TP: *Clinical dermatology: a color guide to diagnosis and therapy*, ed 2, St Louis, 1990, Mosby.)

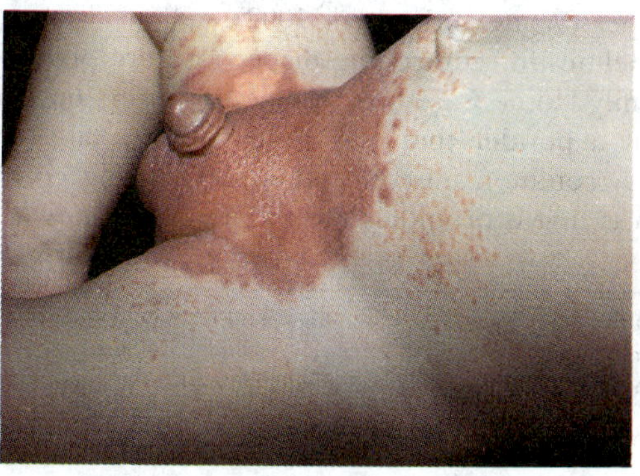

FIG. 13-7 Candidiasis of diaper area. Note beefy red central erythema with satellite pustules. (From Weston WL, Lane AT: *Color textbook of pediatric dermatology*, St Louis, 1991, Mosby.)

Prolonged contact of the skin with diaper wetness affects several skin properties. It produces higher friction, greater abrasion damage, increased transepidermal permeability, and increased microbial counts. Therefore, healthy skin becomes less resistant to potential irritants.

Although ammonia was once thought to cause diaper rash because of the association between the strong odor on diapers and dermatitis, ammonia alone is not sufficient. The important function of urine is related to an increase in pH from the breakdown of urea in the presence of fecal urease. The increased pH promotes the activity of fecal enzymes, principally proteases and lipases, which act as irritants. Fecal enzymes also increase the permeability of skin to bile salts, another potential irritant in feces. The decreased incidence of diaper dermatitis in breast-fed infants is felt to be related to this interaction between pH and fecal enzymes, since feces from breast-fed infants have lower fecal enzyme activity and lower pH (Berg, Buckingham, and Steward, 1986; Buckingham and Berg, 1986).

The eruption of diaper dermatitis can be manifested primarily on convex surfaces or in the folds, and the lesions can represent a variety of types and configurations. Eruptions involving the skin in most intimate contact with the diaper (e.g., the convex surfaces of buttocks, inner thighs, mons pubis, and scrotum) but sparing the folds are likely to be caused by chemical irritants, especially from urine and feces (Fig. 13-6). Other causes are detergents or soaps from inadequately rinsed cloth diapers or the fragrance added to some diapers or disposable wipes.

Perianal involvement is usually the result of chemical irritation from feces, especially diarrheal stools. *Candida albicans* infection produces perianal inflammation with satellite lesions (Fig. 13-7). Whether *C. albicans* initiates or aggravates diaper dermatitis is not known. Risk factors for development of *Candida* infection are an altered immune status and antibiotic therapy (Honig and others, 1988).

Therapeutic Management

Treatment is primarily related to the measures discussed under Nursing Considerations. For stubborn inflammations that do not respond to these interventions, topical glucocorticoid preparations are sometimes required. If steroids are prescribed, their use is generally limited to low-potency preparations such as 1% hydrocortisone cream. Potent fluorinated steroids are avoided because of the potential side effects of striae, epidermal atrophy, suppression of the pituitary-adrenal axis, cessation of longitudinal growth, and frank Cushing syndrome from chronic use. The common use of triamcinolone-containing preparations combined with antiyeast and antibacterial agents such as Mycolog is not recommended, because all of the ingredients may not be needed and certain agents can cause a contact dermatitis.

Candida infections are treated with nystatin ointment. Where *Candida* is the causative agent, oral administration of a fungicide is advised because the gastrointestinal tract is usually the source of infection (see Candidiasis, Chapter 9).

Nursing Considerations

Nursing interventions are aimed at altering the three factors considered to produce dermatitis—wetness, pH, and fecal irritants. The most significant factor amenable to intervention is the moist environment created in the diaper area. Changing the diaper as soon as it becomes wet eliminates a large part of the problem, and removing the diaper to expose healthy skin to air facilitates drying. The use of a hairdryer set on low to dry the skin has been suggested. However, setting the dryer on normal or high can cause burns (Deans, Slater, and Goldfarb, 1990). A dryer or heat lamp is not used on denuded skin, because drying the wound surface delays healing. Instead, occlusive ointments or dressings are applied to provide a moist healing environment for open wounds and to protect the skin from further irritation (see Ostomies, Chapter 27).

Diaper construction has a significant impact on the incidence and severity of diaper dermatitis. Superabsorbent disposable paper diapers have been shown to reduce diaper dermatitis. They contain an absorbent gelling material. The gel binds water tightly to decrease skin wetness, maintains pH control by providing a buffering capacity, and decreases skin irritation by preventing mixing of urine and feces in the diaper (Wong and others, 1992).

Guidelines for controlling diaper rash are presented in the Family Home Care box.* Some caregivers may choose to apply a powder that may contain either talc or cornstarch. A common misconception about using cornstarch on skin is that it promotes the growth of *Candida albicans.* A study comparing cornstarch and talc found that neither product supports growth of the fungi under conditions normally found in the diaper area. Cornstarch is also more effective in reducing friction and tends to cake less than talc when the skin is wet (Leyden, 1984). On the basis of these properties and its safety in terms of inhalation injury, cornstarch is the preferred product.

*A pamphlet describing the development and treatment of diaper rash is *Diaper Rash,* available from the American Academy of Pediatrics, 141 Northwest Point Blvd., P.O. Box 927, Elk Grove Village, IL 60007, (800) 433-9016.

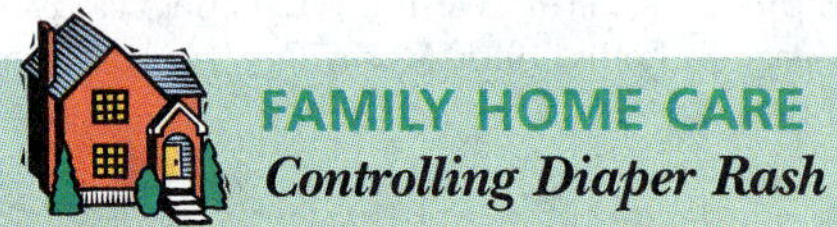

FAMILY HOME CARE

Controlling Diaper Rash

Keep skin dry*
- Use superabsorbent disposable diapers to reduce skin wetness.
- If using cloth diapers, use only overwraps that allow air to circulate; avoid rubber pants.
- Change diapers as soon as soiled, especially with stool, whenever possible, preferably once during the night.
- Expose healthy or only slightly irritated skin to air, not heat, to dry completely.

Apply ointment, such as zinc oxide or petrolatum, to protect skin, especially if skin is very red or has moist, open areas.
- When soiled, wipe off top layer of ointment and reapply.
- To completely remove ointment, especially zinc oxide, use mineral oil; do not wash vigorously.

Avoid overwashing the skin, especially with perfumed soaps or commercial wipes that may be irritating.
- May use a moisturizer or nonsoap cleanser, such as cold cream or Cetaphil, to wipe urine from skin.
- Gently wipe stool from skin using water and mild soap, such as Dove.

*Powder helps keep the skin dry, but talc is very dangerous if breathed into the lungs. Plain cornstarch or cornstarch-based powder is safer. When using any powder product, shake it first into your hand, then apply it to the diaper area. Store the container away from the infant's reach; keep container closed when not in use.

SEBORRHEIC DERMATITIS

Seborrheic dermatitis is a chronic, recurrent, inflammatory reaction of the skin that occurs most commonly on the scalp (cradle cap) but may involve the eyelids (blepharitis), external ear canal (otitis externa), nasolabial folds, and inguinal region. The cause is unknown, although it is more common in early infancy when sebum production is increased. The lesions are characteristically thick, adherent, yellowish, scaly, oily patches that may or may not be mildly pruritic. If pruritus is present, the infant may be irritable. Unlike atopic dermatitis, seborrheic dermatitis is not associated with a positive family history for allergy and is very common in infants shortly after birth and after puberty. Diagnosis is made primarily by the appearance and location of the crusts or scales.

Nursing Considerations

Cradle cap may be prevented with adequate scalp hygiene. Not infrequently parents omit shampooing the infant's hair from fear of damaging the "soft spots" or fontanels. The nurse should discuss how to shampoo the infant's hair and emphasize that the fontanel is like skin anywhere else on the body—it does not puncture or tear with mild pressure.

When seborrheic lesions are present, the treatment is mainly directed at removing the crusts. Parents are taught the appropriate procedure to clean the scalp, which may necessitate a demonstration. Shampooing should be done daily with a mild soap or commercial baby shampoo; medicated shampoos are usually not needed, but an antiseborrheic shampoo containing sulfur and salicylic acid may be used (Hurwitz, 1993). The shampoo is applied to the scalp and allowed to remain on until the crusts are softened, and then the scalp is thoroughly rinsed. Using a fine-tooth comb or a soft facial brush after shampooing helps remove the loosened crusts from the strands of hair.

ATOPIC DERMATITIS (AD) (ECZEMA)

Eczema or eczematous inflammation of the skin refers to a descriptive category of dermatologic diseases and not to a specific etiology. AD is a type of pruritic eczema that usually begins during infancy and is associated with allergy with a hereditary tendency ***(atopy).*** AD presents in three forms based on the age of the child and the distribution of lesions:

1. **Infantile (infantile eczema)**—Usually begins at 2 to 6 months of age and generally undergoes spontaneous remission by 3 years of age.

3. **Childhood**—May follow the infantile form; it occurs at 2 to 3 years of age, and 90% of the children will manifest the disease by age 5 years.
4. **Preadolescent and adolescent**—Begins at about 12 years of age and may continue into the early adult years or indefinitely.

Because the disease occurs predominantly in infancy, this discussion is restricted to the infantile form of atopic dermatitis.

The diagnosis of AD is based on a combination of history and morphologic findings (see box below). Children with the disease have a lower threshold for cutaneous itching, and many authorities believe the dermatologic manifestations appear subsequent to scratching of the intense pruritus. For example, infants will rub their faces against bed linen, and crawling (a form of scratching) results in irritation of knees and elbows. Lesions will disappear if the scratching is stopped.

The majority of children with infantile AD have a family history of eczema, asthma, or allergic rhinitis, which strongly supports a genetic predisposition. The cause is unknown but appears to be related to abnormal function of the skin, including alterations in sweating, peripheral vascular function, and heat tolerance. The disease is better in humid climates and worse in fall and winter, when homes are heated and environmental humidity is lower. The disorder can be controlled but not cured. Recent evidence indicates that house dust mites may play a role in the etiology of AD (Casimir and others, 1993).

CLINICAL MANIFESTATIONS OF ATOPIC DERMATITIS

DISTRIBUTION OF LESIONS

Infantile form—Generalized, especially cheeks, scalp, trunk, and extensor surfaces of extremities (Fig. 13-8)
Childhood form—Flexural areas (antecubital and popliteal fossae, neck), wrists, ankles, and feet
Preadolescent and adolescent form—Face, sides of neck, hands, feet, and antecubital and popliteal fossae (to a lesser extent)

APPEARANCE OF LESIONS

Infantile form
- Erythema
- Vesicles
- Papules
- Weeping
- Oozing
- Crusting
- Scaling
- Often symmetric

Childhood form
- Symmetric involvement
- Clusters of small erythematous or flesh-colored papules or minimally scaling patches
- Dry and may be hyperpigmented
- Lichenification (thickened skin with accentuation of creases)
- Keratosis pilaris (follicular hyperkeratosis) common

Adolescent/adult form
- Same as childhood manifestations
- Dry, thick lesions (lichenified plaques) common
- Confluent papules

OTHER MANIFESTATIONS

Intense itching
Unaffected skin dry and rough
Black children likely to exhibit more papular and/or follicular lesions than white children
May exhibit one or more of the following:
- Lymphadenopathy, especially near affected sites
- Increased palmar creases (many cases)
- Atopic pleats (extra line or groove of lower eyelid)
- Prone to cold hands
- Pityriasis alba (small, poorly defined areas of hypopigmentation)
- Facial pallor (especially around nose, mouth, and ears)
- Bluish discoloration beneath eyes ("allergic shiners")
- Increased susceptibility to unusual cutaneous infections (especially viral)

Therapeutic Management

The major goals of management are to (1) relieve pruritus, (2) hydrate the skin, (3) reduce inflammation, and (4) prevent or control secondary infection. Most of the general measures for managing AD serve to reduce pruritus, as well as other aspects of the disease. General management includes avoiding exposure to skin irritants, avoiding overheating, improving skin hydration, and administration of medications such as antihistamines, topical steroids, and (sometimes) mild sedatives as indicated.

Differing philosophies regarding cleansing and hydrating the skin of the child with AD generally embrace two methods—the wet and the dry methods. In the ***dry method*** baths are infrequent, and skin is cleansed with a nonlipid, hydrophilic agent such as Cetaphil. The ***wet method*** consists of frequent baths (up to four times a day) followed immediately by the application of a lubricant (while the skin is still damp) to trap moisture in the skin. No soap or a very mild, nonperfumed soap (such as Dove, Lowila, or Neutrogena) is used. Some advocate oil or oilated oatmeal baths with light drying so that a protective, oily film remains on the skin. Showers are acceptable as long as a moisturizer is

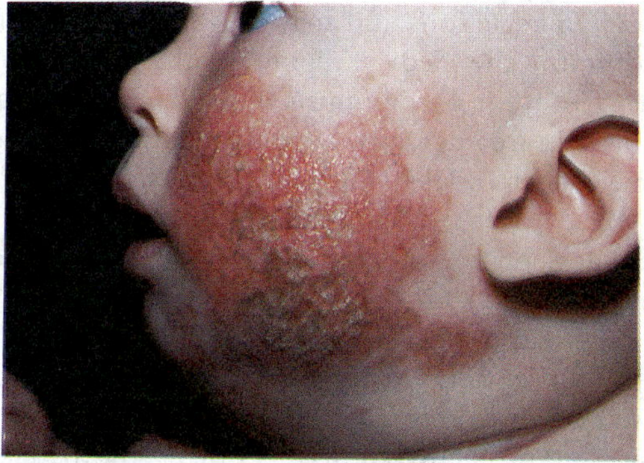

FIG. 13-8 Infantile atopic dermatitis with oozing and crusting of lesions. (From Weston WL, Lane AT: *Color textbook of pediatric dermatology*, St Louis, 1991, Mosby.)

applied within 3 minutes to prevent drying and damaging the skin (Hanifin, 1991).

Enhancing skin hydration can be accomplished by application of preparations that occlude the skin to prevent evaporation and retain moisture in the upper skin layers and/or by replacement of natural moisturizing substances in the skin. A variety of emollients containing petrolatum or lanolin have occlusive properties and are prescribed according to the degree of occlusion desired. For the majority of patients lotions applied twice or three times daily maintain satisfactory hydration. The frequency may be increased if greater hydration is required. Creams or ointments provide more occlusion, and those that contain urea or lactic acid improve the binding of water in the skin, as well as prevent evaporation of moisture.

Sometimes colloid baths, such as the addition of 2 cups of cornstarch to a tub of warm water, provide temporary relief of itching and may help the child sleep if given before bedtime. Cool wet compresses are soothing to the skin and provide antiseptic protection.

Moderate or severe pruritus is usually relieved by administration of oral antihistamine drugs (hydroxyzine [Atarax] or diphenhydramine [Benadryl]), and the amount is tailored to the individual child. Since pruritus increases at night, a mild sedative may be needed.

Occasional flare-ups require the use of topical steroids to diminish inflammation. Low-, moderate-, or high-potency topical corticosteroids are prescribed, depending on the degree of involvement, the area of the body to be treated, the age of the child, and the type of vehicle to be used (e.g., cream, lotion, ointment). Secondary infection is managed with appropriate antibiotic therapy.

There is much controversy regarding prevention of atopic dermatitis by limiting the exposure of high-risk infants to allergens both prenatally and postnatally. Although conclusive evidence for preventive strategies is lacking, the precautions in the Guidelines box on p. 590 may be recommended.

Nursing Considerations

The child with AD presents a nursing challenge. Controlling the intense pruritus is imperative if the disorder is to be successfully managed, since scratching leads to the formation of new lesions and may cause secondary infection. In addition to the medical regimen, other measures can be taken to prevent or minimize the scratching. Fingernails and toenails are cut short, kept clean, and filed frequently to prevent sharp edges. Gloves or cotton stockings may have to be placed over the hands and pinned to shirtsleeves. To prevent any contact with the skin, elbow restraints are sometimes necessary. One-piece outfits with long sleeves and long pants also decrease direct contact with the skin. Whether gloves or elbow restraints are used, the child needs time to be free from such restrictions. An excellent time to remove any protective devices is during the bath or after receiving sedative or antipruritic medication.

Do not remove elbow restraints during sleep because of the likelihood that the child will scratch while asleep.

Conditions that increase itching are eliminated when possible. Woolen clothes or blankets, rough fabrics, and furry stuffed animals are removed. Since heat and humidity cause perspiration, which intensifies the itching, proper dress for climatic conditions is essential. Pruritus is often precipitated by exposure to the irritant effects of certain components of common products such as soaps, detergents, fabric softeners, perfumes, and powders. Most children experience less itching when soft cotton fabrics are worn next to the skin. During cold months, synthetic fabrics (not wool) should be used for overcoats, hats, gloves, and snowsuits. Exposure to latex products, such as gloves and balloons, should also be avoided.

Clothes and sheets are laundered in a mild detergent and rinsed thoroughly in clear water (without fabric softeners and antistatic chemicals). Putting the clothes through a second complete wash cycle without using detergent minimizes the amount of residue remaining in the fabric.

Preventing infection is usually secondary to preventing scratching. Personal hygiene is accomplished as described previously. Baths are given as prescribed, the water is kept tepid, and soaps (except as indicated) and bubble baths are avoided, as well as the use of oils and powders. Skinfolds and diaper areas need frequent cleansing with plain water. A room humidifier or vaporizer may benefit children with extremely dry skin. The lesions are examined for signs of infection, usually the presence of honey-colored crusts with surrounding erythema. Any signs of infection are reported to the practitioner.

NURSING ALERT If the child is being treated with frequent baths for hydration, it is imperative that the emollient preparation be applied immediately following bathing (while the skin is still slightly moist) to prevent drying.

Soaks and compresses are applied, and medications for pruritus or infection are administered as directed. The family is given explicit written instructions on the preparation and use of soaks, special baths, and topical medications, including the order of application if more than one is prescribed. Directions are worded in language the family understands. For example, if a solution is to be diluted in the ratio of 1 to 20 parts of water, it is preferable to express the ratio concretely, such as 1 cup of solution mixed with 20 cups of water. It is important to emphasize that one thick application of a topical medication is *not* equivalent to several thin applications and that excessive use of an agent, particularly steroids, can be hazardous. If children have difficulty remaining still for a 10- or 15-minute soak, bath, or dressing application, these can be carried out at naptime or when the child is engrossed in television, a story, or playing with tub toys.

Since adequate rest is also important for these children, who are usually fretful and irritable, planning meals, baths, medications, and treatments during awake periods is paramount. Sleepy, tired children are normally cranky, and such behavior only intensifies the urge to scratch. During periods of irritability, these children tend to have a poor appetite, which is worsened by restriction of their usual foods.

Diet modification is another source of frustration to parents. When a hypoallergenic diet is prescribed, parents need help in understanding the reason for the diet and guidelines for avoiding hyperallergenic foods (see box on p. 589).

Since hypoallergenic diets take time before visible effects are apparent, parents need reassurance that results may not be seen immediately. If airborne allergens also worsen the eczema, the family is counseled regarding measures to "allergy proof" the home (see Bronchial Asthma, Chapter 32).

Family Support. Parents can be assured that the lesions will not produce scarring (unless secondarily infected) and that the disease is not contagious. However, the child will be subject to repeated exacerbations and remissions. Spontaneous and permanent remission takes place at approximately 2 to 3 years of age in most children with the infantile disorder.

Perhaps it is because the physical problems seem insurmountable during periods of acute exacerbation that the emotional stress becomes so intense for the family members. They need time to discuss negative feelings and to be reassured that these feelings are expected, normal, acceptable, and healthy, provided there is an emotional outlet to dissipate the invested energy. During acute phases, efforts aimed at relieving as much anxiety as possible in both parents and child have a beneficial emotional and physical effect, since stress tends to aggravate the severity of the condition. (See also Nursing Care Plan: The Child with Atopic Dermatitis [Eczema].*)

*In *Wong and Whaley's Clinical Manual of Pediatric Nursing* (Mosby).

TABLE 13-4 Epidemiology of SIDS

FACTORS	OCCURRENCE
Incidence	1.4:1000 live births
Peak age	2 to 4 months; 95% occur by 6 months
Sex	Higher percentage of males affected
Time of death	During sleep
Time of year	Increased incidence in winter; peak in January
Racial	Greater incidence in Native Americans and blacks, followed by whites, Asians, and Hispanics
Socioeconomic	Increased occurrence in lower socioeconomic class
Birth	Higher incidence in: Premature infants, especially infants of low birth weight Multiple births* Neonates with low Apgar scores Infants with central nervous system disturbances and respiratory disorders such as bronchopulmonary dysplasia Increasing birth order (subsequent siblings as opposed to firstborn child) Infants with a recent history of illness
Sleep habits	Prone position; use of polystyrene-filled cushions; overheating (thermal stress)
Feeding habits	Lower incidence in breast-fed infants
Siblings	May have greater incidence
Maternal	Young age; cigarette smoking, especially during pregnancy; substance abuse (heroin, methadone, cocaine)

*Although a rare event, simultaneous death of twins from SIDS can occur.

DISORDERS OF UNKNOWN ETIOLOGY

SUDDEN INFANT DEATH SYNDROME (SIDS)

SIDS, also known by the outdated term "crib death," is defined as the sudden death of an infant under 1 year of age that remains unexplained after a complete postmortem examination, including an investigation of the death scene and a review of the clinical history (Willinger, Hoffman, and Hartford, 1994). It is the leading cause of death in children between the ages of 1 month and 1 year and claims the lives of approximately 7000 infants annually. Table 13-4 summarizes the major epidemiologic characteristics of SIDS.

Etiology

Numerous theories have been proposed regarding the etiology of SIDS; however, the exact cause is yet unknown. The most compelling hypothesis is that SIDS is related to a brainstem abnormality in the neurologic regulation of cardiorespiratory control. Abnormalities include prolonged sleep apnea, increased frequency of brief inspiratory pauses, excessive periodic breathing, and impaired arousal responsiveness to increased carbon dioxide (CO_2) or decreased oxygen. However, sleep apnea is not the cause of SIDS. The vast majority of infants with apnea do not die, and only a minority of SIDS victims have documented apparent life-threatening events (ALTEs) (see Apnea of Infancy, p. 605). A theory that has been disproved associated SIDS with diphtheria, tetanus, and pertussis vaccines (see Immunizations, Chapter 12). The role of maternal smoking during and after pregnancy has also been explored, yet no conclusive evidence has been reached pointing to maternal smoking as a single cause of SIDS (Schoendorf and Kiely, 1992).

Studies from countries other than the United States link sleep habits with an increased risk of SIDS. Sleeping in the prone position may cause oropharyngeal obstruction or affect the thermal balance or arousal state during sleep (Dwyer and others, 1991; Fleming and others, 1990). Another postulated theory is that SIDS may be caused by rebreathing of CO_2. Infants sleeping prone may be unable to move their heads to the side, thus increasing the risk of suffocation and lethal rebreathing. Infant bedding may play an important role in SIDS; rebreathing of exhaled CO_2 was three times higher on softer bedding than on firm bedding (Kemp and others, 1993). The Consumer Product Safety Commission has issued a warning against placing infants to sleep on soft bedding products, such as sheepskins, quilts, comforters, and pillows (Soft bedding, 1994).

The most convincing evidence for advocating nonprone positioning for sleeping comes from Australia, Great Britain, and New Zealand, where the side or supine position for sleeping has been strongly recommended for infants since the late 1980s. In Great Britain alone, the incidence of SIDS decreased by 55% between the years 1991 and 1992 (Bignall, 1993; Willinger, Hoffman, and Hartford, 1994).

In 1992 the American Academy of Pediatrics Task Force on SIDS (1992) issued a statement recommending that healthy infants up to 6 months of age sleep on their side or back. Infants with gastroesophageal reflux, those born prematurely with respiratory distress, and infants with certain upper airway problems may be placed in the prone sleeping position. Following these recommendations, the incidence of SIDS in the United States reportedly dropped 12% in comparison with the same period during the previous year (Spiers and Guntheroth, 1994). In 1994 the American Academy of Pediatrics in conjunction with federal government agencies reaffirmed the side or back position for sleeping infants and also recommended that soft surfaces and gas-trapping objects be avoided in an infant's sleep environment (Infant sleep position, 1994).

There have been no reports of adverse side effects, such as aspiration, ALTEs, or vomiting, from not using the prone position. However, not all authorities are convinced that the prone sleeping position has a direct relationship with SIDS, considering that the epidemiology of SIDS is very complex, involving at least 25 identified significant risk factors (Hunt, 1994).

NURSING ALERT Nurses play an important role in educating parents regarding infant health practices, such as placing the infant on the side or supine on a firm sleep surface, that may prevent the tragedy of SIDS.

Although the etiology is unknown, autopsies reveal consistent pathologic findings, such as pulmonary edema and intrathoracic hemorrhages, that confirm the diagnosis of SIDS. Consequently, autopsies should be performed on infants suspected of dying of SIDS, and these findings should be shared with the parents as soon as possible after the death. Since postmortem findings in SIDS and accidental suffocation are practically the same, and since not all communities have medical examiners to perform autopsies, some deaths may or may not be correctly identified as SIDS. Therefore mortality rates can vary in different regions.

Infants at Risk for SIDS

Certain groups of infants are at increased risk for SIDS. These groups include:

1. Infants with one or more severe ALTEs requiring cardiopulmonary resuscitation (CPR) or vigorous stimulation
2. Preterm infants who continue to have pathologic apnea at the time of hospital discharge
3. Siblings of two or more SIDS victims
4. Infants with certain types of diseases or conditions, such as central hypoventilation

Home monitoring and/or the use of respiratory stimulant drugs is recommended for these groups of children. No diagnostic tests exist to predict which infants, including those in the above groups, will survive or die, and home monitoring is no guarantee of survival. At the present time, strategies to prevent SIDS are best directed at decreasing known or suspected risk factors, such as mothers seeking adequate prenatal care and avoiding cigarette smoking and drug abuse both before and after the child's birth. In addition, adherence to the guidelines for nonprone sleeping in normal infants is a positive step for the prevention of SIDS.

Whether subsequent siblings of the SIDS infant are at increased risk for SIDS is unclear. Even if the increased risk is correct, families have a 99% chance that their subsequent child will *not* die of SIDS. Home monitoring is not recommended for this group of children (National Institutes, 1987).

Nursing Considerations

Loss of a child from SIDS presents several crises with which the parents must cope. In addition to grief and mourning for the death of their child, the parents must face a tragedy that was extremely sudden, unexpected, and unexplained. The psychologic intervention for the family must deal with these additional variables. This discussion focuses primarily on the objectives of care for families experiencing SIDS, rather than on the process of grief and mourning, which is explored in Chapter 23.

One approach toward delineating the nursing care plan for these families is to base it on the usual sequence of events that occur after the infant is found. This approach encompasses the different areas in which nurses may be involved with the family.

Finding the Infant. Usually it is the mother who finds the child dead in the crib. Typically, the child is in a disheveled bed, with blankets over the head, and huddled into a corner. Frothy, blood-tinged fluid fills the mouth and nostrils, and the infant may be lying face down in the secretions, suggesting that he or she bled to death. The diaper is wet and full of stool, which is consistent with a cataclysmic type of death. The hands may be clutching the sheets, as if the child were in distress before death. The initial appearance of the child combined with the shock of such an unexpected event adds to the horror that the parents must face.

Frequently the mother is alone and must deal with her initial shock, panic, grief, questions of the other siblings, and the decision of where to find help. The first persons to arrive may be the police and ambulance attendants. Hopefully, they will handle the situation by asking few questions; giving *no* indication of wrongdoing, abuse, or neglect; making sensitive judgments concerning the resuscitation efforts for the child; and comforting the members of the family as much as possible. These individuals should be properly informed about SIDS in order to recognize its characteristic signs and tell parents that their child probably died of a disease called sudden infant death syndrome, which cannot be predicted or prevented. A compassionate, sensitive approach to the family during the very first few minutes can help spare them some of the overwhelming guilt and anguish that frequently follow this type of death.

Arriving at the Emergency Room. The first contact that nurses typically have with these families is in the emergency room, when the infant is seen by a physician in order to be pronounced dead. Usually there is no attempt at resuscitation. During the time in the emergency room several aspects warrant special consideration. Parents are asked only factual questions, such as when they found the infant, how he or she looked, and who they called for help. Any remarks that may suggest responsibility, such as why didn't they go in earlier, didn't they hear the infant cry out, was the head buried in a blanket, or were the other siblings jealous of this child, are avoided.

The events that took place when help arrived are discussed. If resuscitation was attempted, the infant may have fractured ribs, internal bleeding, and traumatic bruising, which can simulate physical abuse. Also, if statements were made that were misguided, such as "This looks like suffocation," they can be corrected before parents harbor them in their minds as indications of their guilt. The discussion of an autopsy should be presented at this time, emphasizing that a diagnosis cannot be confirmed until the postmortem examination is completed. Instructions about the autopsy and funeral arrangements may need to be repeated or put in writing. If the mother was breast-feeding, she needs information about abrupt discontinuation of lactation (Lawrence, 1994).

Another important aspect of compassionate care for these parents is allowing them to say good-bye to their child. Before they go into the examining room, any blood or emesis is removed from the child, the body is covered partially with a sheet or blanket, and the room is put in order, especially if instruments and equipment were used. These are the parents' last moments with their child, and they should be as quiet, meaningful, peaceful, and undisturbed as possible. The child's belongings are packaged for the parents to take home if they wish. Because the parents leave the hospital without their infant, it is helpful to accompany them to the car or arrange for someone else to take them home (Woolsey, 1988).

Returning Home. When the parents return home, they should be visited by a competent, qualified professional as soon after the death as possible. Printed material that contains excellent information about SIDS (available from the national organizations*) should be provided.

During the initial visit the parents are helped to gain an intellectual understanding of the disease. The nursing objectives are to assess what the parents have been told, what they think happened, and how they have explained this to the other siblings, other family members, and friends.

Some parents are able to discuss their feelings openly, and the nurse supports this coping skill. However, others may be reluctant to express their grief, and the nurse may help these parents bring their feelings out into the open.

The nurse can encourage the expression of emotions by asking about crying and feeling sad, angry, or guilty. It is an attempt to provoke a display of emotion, not just an admission of a feeling. During this session the parents should be helped to explore their usual coping mechanisms and, if these are ineffectual, to investigate new approaches. For example, one parent may refrain from discussing the death for fear of upsetting the other parent, but each may need to hear how the other feels.

The number of visits and plans for subsequent intervention need to be flexible. For example, the siblings may initially appear accepting of the explanation and well adjusted but may later refuse to go to sleep or ask questions about graves or funerals, indicating their need for further help in dealing with the death. Parents facing the question of a subsequent child will need support. Both the birth of a subsequent child and the survival of that child, especially past the age of death of the previous child, are important transitional stages for parents.

Since the mourning process takes at least a year for completion of acceptance and social reorganization, nurses should call on the family periodically to evaluate their progress. Many families receive much solace and support from talking to other parents who have lost a child to SIDS.

*__Sudden Infant Death Syndrome Clearinghouse,__ 8201 Greensboro Dr., Suite 600, McLean, VA 22102, (703) 821-8955; **American Sudden Infant Death Syndrome (SIDS) Institute,** 275 Carpenter Dr., Suite 100, Atlanta, GA 30328, (800) 232-SIDS (in Georgia, [800] 847-SIDS); **The Sudden Infant Death Syndrome Alliance,** 10500 Little Patuxent Parkway, Suite 420, Columbia, MD 21044, (301) 964-8000 or (800) 221-SIDS.

APNEA OF INFANCY (AOI)

AOI generally refers to pathologic apnea in infants of more than 37 weeks of gestation. The clinical presentation of AOI is an ***apparent life-threatening event (ALTE)*** (previously referred to by the inaccurate and misleading expression, "near-miss SIDS") that is described as:

- Frightening to the observer, who fears the child died or would have died without vigorous intervention
- Some combination of:
  Apnea (cessation of breathing for 20 seconds or more; usually central but occasionally obstructive)
  Color change (cyanosis or pallor, but sometimes plethora)
  Marked change in muscle tone (usually extreme limpness)
  Choking or gagging

AOI can be a symptom of many disorders, including sepsis, seizures, upper airway abnormalities, gastroesophageal reflux, hypoglycemia, impaired regulation of breathing during sleep or feeding, or a result of intentional poisoning by a caregiver. However, in about half the cases no cause is identified. Infants with a history of ALTEs are at increased risk for SIDS, but these children constitute less than 7% of all SIDS victims (National Institutes, 1987). A diagnosis of AOI is made when no identifiable cause for the ALTE is found (Keens and Ward, 1993).

Diagnostic Evaluation

The most widely used test is continuous recording of cardiorespiratory patterns (cardiopneumogram or pneumocardiogram). Four-channel pneumocardiograms monitor heart rate, respirations (chest impedance), nasal airflow, and oxygen saturation. A more sophisticated test, polysomnography ("sleep test"), also records brain waves, eye and body movements, esophageal manometry, and end-tidal carbon dioxide measurements. However, none of these tests can predict risk. Some children with normal results may still have subsequent apneic episodes.

Therapeutic Management

Treatment usually involves continuous home monitoring of cardiorespiratory rhythms and/or the use of methylxanthines (respiratory stimulant drugs, such as theophylline or caffeine). Therapeutic levels are typically 6 to 10 or 13 μg/ml theophylline and 10 to 20 μg/ml caffeine. The criteria for discontinuing the monitoring is based on the infant's clinical condition. A general guideline for discontinuation is when infants with ALTEs have gone 2 or 3 months without apneic episodes requiring intervention.

NURSING ALERT The concentration of theophylline required for apnea is less than that required for bronchodilation.

Nursing Considerations

The diagnosis of AOI engenders great anxiety and concern in parents, and the institution of home monitoring presents additional physical and emotional burdens. If monitoring is required, the nurse can be a major source of support to the family in terms of education about the equipment, observation of the infant's status, and immediate intervention during apneic episodes, including cardiopulmonary resuscitation (CPR). To help the family cope with the numerous procedures they must learn, adequate preparation before discharge and written instructions are essential.*

Several types of home monitors are available, and most hospitals select the model that the infant will use at home. Nurses involved in the care at home must become familiar with the equipment, including its advantages and disadvantages (see Family Home Care box). Safety is a major concern, since monitors can cause electrical burns and electrocution. The following precautions are recommended:

1. Remove leads from infant when not attached to monitor.
2. Unplug power cord from electrical outlet when cord is not plugged into monitor.
3. Use safety covers on electrical outlets to discourage children from inserting objects into a socket.

Siblings should also be supervised when near the infant and taught that the monitor is not a play object. Other safety practices include informing local utility and rescue squads of the home monitoring in case of an emergency. Telephone numbers for these services should be posted near all telephones in the home.

Caregivers need detailed information regarding proper attachment of the electrodes to the infant's chest with impedance monitors that detect chest movement. The electrodes are placed in the midaxillary line, at a space one or two fingerbreadths below the nipple (Fig. 13-9). Adhesive electrodes are attached directly to the skin. For home use, electrodes attached to a belt that is placed around the child's trunk are preferred. The belt is positioned so that the electrodes contact the skin in the same area as shown in Fig. 13-9. Newer-technology monitors have memory chips that allow for event recording; this may prove to be an effective tool in evaluating the use of the monitor and reported frequency of alarms (Ahmann, Meny, and Fink, 1992).

*Home care instructions for apnea monitoring and CPR are available in *Wong and Whaley's Clinical Manual of Pediatric Nursing* (Mosby). Educational materials may also be obtained from the American SIDS Institute.

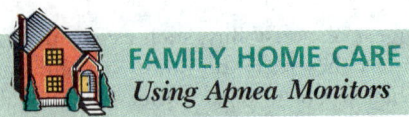

FAMILY HOME CARE
Using Apnea Monitors

Use the monitor as instructed by the practitioner.
Do not adjust the monitor to eliminate false alarms. Adjustments could compromise the monitor's effectiveness.
Place the monitor on a firm surface away from the crib and drapes; plug directly into a wall socket with a three-pronged outlet.
Do not sleep in the same bed as a monitored infant.
Keep pets and children away from the monitor and infant.
Keep the monitor away from possible electrical interferences such as appliances (e.g., electric blankets, televisions, air conditioners, remote telephones).
Check the monitor several times a day to be sure the alarm is working and that it can be heard from room to room. Be sure the caregiver can reach the monitor quickly (in less than 30 seconds).
Periodically check the monitor's breath detection indicator and battery or charger connections.
Be aware that strong signals from nearby radio and television stations, airports, ham radios, or police stations could interfere with the monitor. Check for interference if the monitor is to be operated in these areas.
Read the monitor's user manual carefully; report problems promptly.
Inform local utility and rescue squads of home monitoring as appropriate.
Keep emergency numbers near phones in the home.
Practice safety precautions:
- Remove leads when infant is not attached to the monitor.
- Unplug the power cord from the electrical outlet when the cord is not plugged into the monitor.
- Use safety covers on electrical outlets to prevent children from inserting objects into a socket.

Data primarily from *FDA safety alert: important tips for apnea monitor users,* Department of Health and Human Services, Rockville, MD, 1990.

Monitors are effective only if they are used. They do not prevent death but alert the caregiver to the ALTE in time to intervene. The need to use the monitor and to respond appropriately to alarms must be stressed. Noncompliance can result in the infant's death.

NURSING ALERT If the infant is apneic, gently stimulate the trunk by patting or rubbing it. If the infant is prone, turn to the back and flick the feet. If there is still no response, begin CPR. Never vigorously shake the child. No more than 15 to 30 seconds are spent on stimulation before implementing CPR.

Family Support. Although AOI is not a chronic illness, many of the stresses observed during the monitoring period are characteristic of those of families with chronically ill children. Parents report increased stress, including concern for the child's survival, fear of incompetency in assuming home responsibility, inadequate respite care, social isolation, constant work, and fatigue (Stevens, 1990, 1994). Siblings are affected, as well as the affected child, who may be characterized as "spoiled" and have developmental delays.

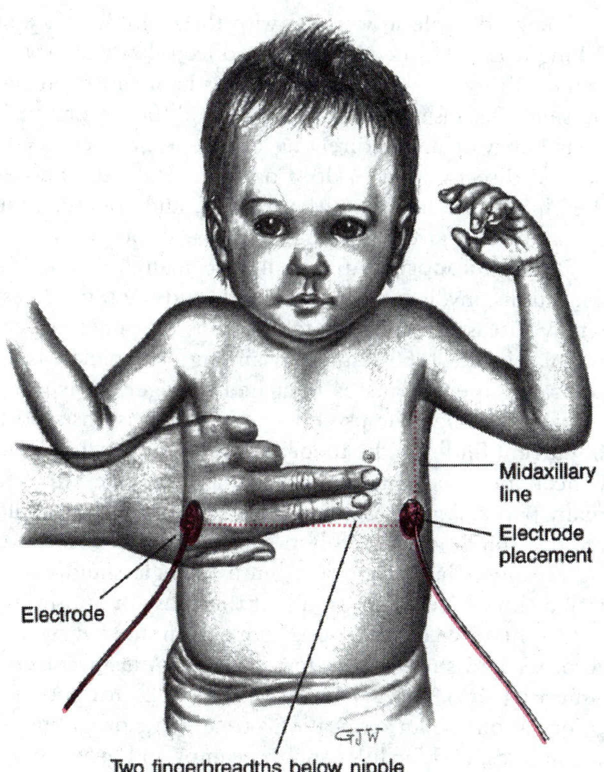

FIG. 13-9 Electrode placement for apnea monitoring. In small infants one fingerbreadth may be used.

> **CLINICAL MANIFESTATIONS OF AUTISM**
>
> **SOCIAL RELATIONS AND BEHAVIOR**
>
> Extreme interpersonal isolation
> Intense, abnormal concern for preservation of sameness
> Unyielding to cuddling and holding
> Do not respond to verbal stimulation
> Bizarre attachment to mechanical objects
> Odd repetitive behaviors, such as flicking a light switch on and off
> Difficult to manage; passive or irritable
> Frequent temper tantrums and/or self-destructive behavior
>
> **DEVELOPMENT**
>
> Mental retardation, usually severe
> May have advanced gross motor skills
> Normal to hyperactive
> May have exceptional ability (e.g., memory)
> Poor suck and feeding responses
>
> **LANGUAGE**
>
> Echolalia or parrot speech (automatic repetition of words spoken to them)
> Pronominal reversal (tendency to use "you" for "I")
> Literal, concrete use of words (e.g., "in" to mean "door")
>
> **SENSORY/PERCEPTUAL PROCESSES**
>
> Sensory deficits even though vision and hearing are intact
> Act as if deaf, yet may be overly sensitive to sound
> Hyposensitive or hypersensitive to pain
> Have aversion to touch

To deal with these potential effects, nurses need to employ the same interventions as those discussed for children with chronic illness (see Chapter 22) and be aware of the need for referral when difficulties are suspected.

To lessen the continuous responsibility of monitoring, other family members, such as grandparents, should be taught how to manipulate the equipment, read and interpret the signals, and administer CPR. They are encouraged to stay with the infant for regular periods to allow parents respite. Support groups of other families who have successfully completed monitoring can also be of benefit. Since baby-sitters are difficult to locate, support group members or nursing students may be potential sources of qualified caregivers.

AUTISM

Autism, a complex developmental disorder accompanied by severe and usually permanent intellectual and behavioral deficits, is manifested during infancy and early childhood. It occurs in 1:2500 children, is about four times more common in males than in females (although females are more severely affected), and is not related to socioeconomic level, race, or religion (Ritvo and others, 1989).

Etiology

The etiology of autism is an unsolved and controversial question. However, considerable evidence supports a biologic cause. Individuals with autism may have abnormal electroencephalograms, seizures, delayed development of hand dominance, persistence of primitive reflexes, metabolic abnormalities (elevated blood serotonin), and cerebellar vermal hypoplasia (part of the brain involved in regulating motion and some aspects of memory) (Volkmar and Cohen, 1988).

There is also strong evidence for a genetic basis that in twins is consistent with an autosomal recessive pattern of inheritance. Twin studies demonstrate a very high concordance (96%) for monozygotic (identical) twins and a 24% concordance for dizygotic (nonidentical) twins. In addition, between 5% and 16% of males with autism are positive for the fragile X chromosome (see Fragile X Syndrome, Chapter 24).

Clinical Manifestations/Diagnostic Evaluation

Children with autism demonstrate several peculiar and bizarre characteristics, primarily in social interactions, communication, and behavior. The clinical manifestations typically seen in children with autism are described in the box above. The majority of children with autism are mentally retarded, with scores typically in the moderate to severe range. More females than males tend to have very low intelligence scores. One study indicated that the following behavioral characteristics be included in the screening of autism for early identification: abnormal social play, poor imitation of others, lack of awareness of others, impaired imaginative play, and deficiencies in nonverbal communication (Stone and others, 1994). Despite relatively severe mental retardation, some children with autism (known as ***savants***) excel in particular areas, such as art, music, memory, mathematic calculation, or perceptual skills, such as puzzle building.

Prognosis

Autism is a severely disabling condition. Only about 1% to 2% of the autistic population ultimately achieve independence, with the majority requiring lifelong supervision. Aggravation of psychiatric symptoms occurs in about half the children during adolescence, with girls having a tendency for continued deterioration. Facilitated communication, which uses another person (the facilitator) to support the affected child's finger (or other body part) pointing to a list of letters, words, or symbols was believed to be a breakthrough in resolving the autistic person's communication problems. However the technique has been met with considerable skepticism by many authorities involved in the care of people with autism (Dillon, 1993; Facilitated communication, 1994; Mulick, Jacobson, and Kobe, 1993). Early recognition of behaviors associated with autism is critical in order to implement appropriate interventions and family involvement (Stone and others, 1994). The prognosis is most favorable for children with communicative speech development by age 6 years and an intelligence quotient above 50 at the time of diagnosis (Gillberg and Steffenburg, 1987).

Nursing Considerations

Therapeutic intervention for the child with autism is a specialized area involving professionals with advanced training. While numerous therapies have been employed, the most promising results have been through highly structured and intensive behavioral modification programs. In general, the objective is to increase social awareness of others, teach verbal communication, and decrease unacceptable behavior. However, the vast majority of these children need assistance and supervision throughout adulthood, although early diagnosis and early educational treatment positively influence the child's future development.

When these children are hospitalized, the parents are essential to planning care and ideally should stay with the child as much as possible. Decreasing stimulation by using a private or semiprivate room, avoiding extraneous auditory and visual distraction, and encouraging the parents to bring in possessions the child is attached to may lessen the disruptiveness of hospitalization. Since physical contact often upsets these children, minimum holding may be necessary to avoid behavioral outbursts.

Care must be taken when performing procedures on, administering medicine to, or feeding these children, since either they are fussy eaters who may willfully starve themselves or gag to prevent eating or they are indiscriminate hoarders, swallowing any available edible or inedible items, such as a thermometer. Their disturbing sleep patterns may also pose problems in a hospital setting. A thorough assessment of the child's usual routine and activities can help maintain an environment that is more manageable and conducive to physical recovery.

A key principle in working with these children is establishing trust. They need to be introduced slowly to new situations, with visits with staff caregivers kept short whenever possible. Because these children have difficulty organizing their behavior and redirecting their energy, they need to be told directly what to do. Communication should be at the child's developmental level, brief, and concrete. Only one request is given at a time, such as "sit on bed."

Family Support. Autism, like so many other chronic conditions, involves the entire family and often becomes "a family disease." Unfortunately, the psychogenetic theory, popular in the 1960s especially among psychoanalysts, had portrayed the parents as detached, refrigerator-type individuals. Although the psychogenetic theory is unsupported by current findings, the theory has caused many public misconceptions about these families and greatly intensified many parents' guilt (Seifert, 1990). Nurses can help alleviate the guilt and shame often associated with this disorder by stressing what is known from a biologic standpoint, as well as how little is known about the cause of autism.

Parents need expert counseling early in the course of the disorder and should be referred to the **Autism Society of America (ASA).*** ASA is the most efficient clearinghouse for information about education, treatment programs and techniques, and facilities such as camps and group homes. There is also a siblings' group called SHARE (Siblings Helping Persons with Autism Through Resources and Energy).

As much as possible, the family is encouraged to care for the child in the home. With the help of family support programs in many states, families are often able to provide home care and assist with the educational services the child needs. As the child approaches adulthood, the family may require assistance in locating a long-term placement facility for the affected adult (see also Chapter 22).

*8601 Georgia Ave., Suite 503, Silver Spring, MD 20910; (301) 565-0433.

KEY POINTS

- Common nutritional disturbances of infancy include vitamin and mineral disturbances, some types of vegetarian diets, protein and calorie malnutrition, obesity, and food intolerance.
- Mineral disturbances may be caused by mineral-mineral interactions and mineral-diet interactions.
- Vegetarians may be classified into four groups: lactoovovegetarians, lactovegetarians, pure vegetarians, and zen macrobiotics.
- Protein and energy malnutrition may occur as a complication of underlying disease, or as a result of fad diets, lack of parental education about infant nutrition, inappropriate management of food allergy, incorrect preparation of formula, or poor food storage and handling.
- Calorie consumption, method of feeding, birth weight, sex, age at introduction of solid foods, and activity level all play a part in infant obesity.
- Food intolerance encompasses food allergies and food sensitivities, the most serious of which are cow's milk allergy and lactose intolerance.

- Common feeding difficulties in the infant include breast-feeding problems, regurgitation and "spitting up," and paroxysmal abdominal pain (colic). Less frequent but serious feeding problems include rumination and failure to thrive.
- Treatment of colic may involve change in feeding practices, correction of a stressful environment, and support of the parent.
- Failure to thrive may be classified as organic, resulting from some physical cause, or nonorganic, resulting from psychosocial factors involving the child and caregiver (e.g., maternal deprivation), environmental causes (e.g., inadequate parental knowledge of child feeding), or unexplained causes.
- Common skin disorders of infancy are diaper dermatitis, seborrheic dermatitis, and atopic dermatitis.
- Sudden infant death syndrome is the leading cause of death in children between the ages of 1 month and 1 year.
- Evidence linking SIDS to the prone sleeping position has led to the recommendation that healthy infants sleep supine or on the side.
- The primary nursing responsibility in care associated with SIDS and other conditions of unknown etiology is emotional support of the family.
- Children with apnea of infancy receive home monitoring to alert the family to an apparent life-threatening event.
- Autism is a severely disabling condition characterized by deficits in social interaction, communication, and behavior.

REFERENCES

Agras W and others: Influence of early feeding style on adiposity at 6 years of age, *J Pediatr* 116(5):805-809, 1990.

Ahmann E, Meny RG, Fink RJ: Use of home apnea monitors, *JOGNN* 21(5):394-399, 1992.

American Academy of Pediatrics, Committee on Infectious Diseases: Vitamin A treatment of measles, *Pediatrics* 91(5):1014-1015, 1993.

American Academy of Pediatrics, Committee on Nutrition: Hypoallergenic infant formulas, *Pediatrics* 83(6):1068-1069, 1989.

American Academy of Pediatrics Task Force on Infant Position and SIDS: Positioning and SIDS, *Pediatrics* 89:1120-1126, 1992.

Austin A and others: A survey of factors associated with diaper dermatitis in thirty-six pediatric practices, *J Pediatr Health Care* 2(6):295-299, 1988.

Barnard K and others: Measurement and meaning of parent-child interaction. In Morrison F, Lord C, Keating D, editors: *Applied developmental psychology,* vol 3, New York, 1993, Academic Press.

Barr R and others: Feeding and temperament as determinants of early infant crying/fussing behavior, *Pediatrics* 84(3):514-521, 1989.

Barr RG and others: The crying of infants with colic: a controlled empirical description, *Pediatrics* 90(1):14-21, 1992.

Berg RW, Buckingham KW, Steward RL: Etiologic factors in diaper dermatitis: the role of urine, *Pediatr Dermatol* 3(2):102-106, 1986.

Bignall J: Decline in sudden infant deaths, *Lancet* 341:887, 1993.

Blackburn ST, Loper DL: *Maternal, fetal, and neonatal physiology: a clinical perspective,* Philadelphia, 1992, WB Saunders.

Blizzard RM: Failure to thrive from emotional deprivation: a historical perspective and what it teaches the physician, *Pediatr Rounds* 1(3):1-8, 1992.

Buckingham KW, Berg RW: Etiologic factors in diaper dermatitis: the role of feces, *Pediatr Dermatol* 3(2):107-112, 1986.

Casimir GJA and others: Atopic dermatitis: role of food and house dust mite allergens, *Pediatrics* 92(2):252-256, 1993.

Castiglia PT: Lactose intolerance, *J Pediatr Health Care* 8(1):36-38, 1994.

Dagnelie P and others: High prevalence of rickets in infants on macrobiotic diets, *Am J Clin Nutr* 51:202-208, 1990.

Deans L, Slater H, Goldfarb I: Bad advice; bad burn: a new problem in burn prevention, *J Burn Care Rehabil* 11(6):563-564, 1990.

Dewey K and others: Infant growth and breast feeding, *Am J Clin Nutr* 50:1116-1118, 1989.

Dewey KG and others: Growth of breast-fed and formula-fed infants from 0 to 18 months: the DARLING study, *Pediatrics* 89(6):1035-1041, 1992.

Dewey KG and others: Breast-fed infants are leaner than formula-fed infants at 1 y of age: the DARLING study, *Am J Clin Nutr* 57(2):140-145, 1993.

Dietz WH Jr: The overweight child: psychosocial effects and treatment, *Feelings Med Signif* 31(1):1-4, 1989.

Dillon KM: Facilitated communication, autism, and ouija, *Skeptical Inquirer* 17(3):281-287, 1993.

Dwyer T and others: Prospective cohort study of prone sleeping position and sudden infant death syndrome, *Lancet* 337(8752):1244-1247, 1991.

Facilitated communication, *AAP News* 10(2):3, 1994.

Fawzi WW and others: Vitamin A supplementation and child mortality: a meta-analysis, *JAMA* 269(7):898-903, 1993.

Fleming PJ and others: Interaction between bedding and sleeping position in the sudden infant death syndrome: a population-based case-controlled study, *Br Med J* 301:85-89, 1990.

Forsyth B: Colic and the effect of changing formulas: a double-blind, multiple-crossover study, *J Pediatr* 115(4):521-526, 1989.

Geertsma M, Hyams J: Colic—a pain syndrome of infancy? *Pediatr Clin North Am* 36(4):905-919, 1989.

Gillberg C, Steffenburg G: Outcome and prognostic factors in infantile autism and similar conditions: a population-based study of 46 cases followed through puberty, *J Autism Dev Disord* 17:273-287, 1987.

Graham SM, Arvela OM, Wise GA: Long-term neurologic consequences of nutritional vitamin B_{12} deficiency in infants, *J Pediatr* 121(5):710-714, 1992.

Hanifin JM: Atopic dermatitis in infants and children, *Pediatr Clin North Am* 38(4):763-790, 1991.

Heaney R, Weaver C, Fitzsimmons M: Soybean phytate content: effect on calcium absorption, *Am J Clin Nutr* 53(3):745-747, 1991.

Hendrickse RG: Kwashiorkor: the hypothesis that incriminates aflatoxins, *Pediatrics* 88(2):376-379, 1991.

Herrera MG and others: Vitamin A supplementation and child survival, *Lancet* 340:267-271, 1992.

Hide DW, Guyer BM: Prevalence of infant colic, *Arch Dis Child* 57:559-560, 1982.

Hill D and others: Recovery from milk allergy in early childhood: antibody studies, *J Pediatr* 114(5):761-766, 1989.

Hill DJ and others: Charting infant distress: an aid to defining colic, *J Pediatr* 121(5):755-758, 1992.

Honig P and others: Amoxicillin and diaper dermatitis, *J Am Acad Dermatol* 19:275-279, 1988.

Hunt CE: Infant sleeping position: back to the bench, *Arch Pediatr Adolesc Med* 148(2):131-133, 1994.

Hunziker U, Barr R: Increased carrying reduces infant crying: a randomized controlled trial, *Pediatrics* 77(5):641-648, 1986.

Hurwitz S: Skin lesions in the first year of life, *Contemp Pediatr* 10(1):110-128, 1993.

Infant sleep position and sudden infant death syndrome (SIDS) in the United States: joint commentary from the American Academy of Pediatrics and selected agencies of the federal government, *Pediatrics* 93(5):820, 1994.

Jelliffe DB, Jelliffe EFP: Causation of kwashiorkor: toward a multifactorial consensus, *Pediatrics* 90(1):110-113, 1992.

Jordan WE, and others: Diaper dermatitis: frequency and severity among a general infant population, *Pediatr Dermatol* 3(3):198-207, 1986.

Kahn A and others: Milk intolerance in children with persistent sleeplessness: a prospective double-blind crossover evaluation, *Pediatrics* 84(4):595-603, 1989.

Keens TG, Ward SLD: Apnea spells, sudden death, and the role of the apnea monitor, *Pediatr Clin North Am* 40(5):897-911, 1993.

Kemp JS and others: Unintentional suffocation by rebreathing: a death scene and physiologic investigation of a possible cause of sudden infant death, *J Pediatr* 122(6):874-880, 1993.

Lane A, Rehder P, Helm K: Evaluations of diapers containing absorbent gelling material with conventional disposable diapers in newborn infants, *Am J Dis Child* 144(3):315-318, 1990.

Lawrence RA: *Breastfeeding: a guide for the medical profession,* ed 4, St Louis, 1994, Mosby.

Leyden JJ: Cornstarch, Candida albicans, and diaper rash, *Pediatr Dermatol* 1(4):322-325, 1984.

Lothe L, Lindberg T: Cow's milk whey protein elicits symptoms of infantile colic in colicky formula-fed infants: a double-blind crossover study, *Pediatrics* 83(2):262-266, 1989.

Mandelbaum JL: Child survival: what are the issues? *J Pediatr Health Care* 6(3):132-137, 1992.

Moss A and others: *Use of vitamin and mineral supplements in the United States: current users, types of products, and nutrients.* Advance data from vital and health statistics, No 174, Hyattsville, MD, 1989, National Center for Health Statistics.

Mulick JA, Jacobson JW, Kobe FH: Anguished silence and helping hands: autism and facilitated communication, *Skeptical Inquirer* 17 (3):270-280, 1993.

National Institutes of Health Consensus Development Conference on Infantile Apnea and Home Monitoring, Sept. 29 to Oct. 1, 1986, *Pediatrics* 79(2):292-299, 1987.

Pinyerd B, Zipf W: Colic: idiopathic, excessive, infant crying, *J Pediatr Nurs* 4(3):147-161, 1989.

Piwoz EG, Peerson JM, Brown KH: Potential for misclassification of infants' growth increments by using existing reference data, *Am J Clin Nutr* 56(1):58-64, 1992.

Preventing food allergy fatalities, *Emerg Med* 25(7):119-123, 1993.

Ritvo E and others: The UCLA–University of Utah epidemiologic survey of autism: prevalence, *Am J Psychiatry* 146(2):194-199, 1989.

Robinson TN: Does television viewing increase obesity and reduce physical activity? Cross-sectional and longitudinal analyses among adolescent girls, *Pediatrics* 91(2):273-280, 1993.

Sampson H, Scanlon S: Natural history of food hypersensitivity in children with atopic dermatitis, *J Pediatr* 115(1):23-27, 1989.

Sampson HA and others: Anaphylactic reactions to foods, *N Engl J Med* 327:380-384, 1992.

Schoendorf KC, Kiely JL: Relationship of sudden infant death syndrome to maternal smoking during and after pregnancy, *Pediatrics* 90(6):905-908, 1992.

Seifert C: *Case studies in autism: a young child and two adolescents,* Lanham, MD, 1990, University Press of America.

Sherman J, Alexander M: Obesity in children: a research update, *J Pediatr Nurs* 5(3):161-167, 1990.

Shils ME, Olson JA, Shike M, editors: *Modern nutrition in health and disease,* ed 8, Philadelphia, 1994, Lea & Febiger.

Soft bedding and suffocation, *AAP News* 10(2): 26, 1994.

Spiers PS, Guntheroth WG: Recommendations to avoid the prone sleeping position and recent statistics for sudden infant death syndrome in the United States, *Arch Pediatr Adolesc Med* 148(2):141-146, 1994.

Stevens MS: A comparison of mothers' and fathers' perceptions of caring for an infant requiring home cardio-respiratory monitoring, *Issues Compr Pediatr Nurs* 13(2):81-95, 1990.

Stevens MS: Parents coping with infants requiring home cardiorespiratory monitoring, *J Pediatr Nurs* 9(1):2-12, 1994.

Stone WL and others: Early recognition of autism: parental reports vs clinical observation, *Arch Pediatr Adolesc Med* 148:174-179, 1994.

Stunkard A and others: The body-mass index of twins who have been reared apart, *N Engl J Med* 322(21):1483-1487, 1990.

Taubman B: Parental counseling compared with elimination of cow's milk or soy milk protein for the treatment of infant colic syndrome: a randomized trial, *Pediatrics* 81(6): 756-761, 1988.

Tsang RC, Nichols BL: *Nutrition during infancy,* St Louis, 1988, Mosby.

Udall JN Jr, Greene HL: Vitamin update, *Pediatr Rev* 13(5):185-194, 1992.

Volkmar F, Cohen D: Neurobiologic aspects of autism, *N Engl J Med* 318(21):1390-1392, 1988.

Walravens P, Hambidge M, Koepfer D: Zinc supplementation in infants with a nutritional pattern of failure to thrive: a double-blind, controlled study, *Pediatrics* 83(4):532-538, 1989.

Weizman Z and others: Efficacy of herbal tea preparation in infantile colic, *J Pediatr* 122(4):650-652, 1993.

Willinger M, Hoffman HJ, Hartford RB: Infant sleep position and risk for sudden infant death syndrome: report of meeting held January 13 and 14, 1994, National Institutes of Health, Bethesda, MD, *Pediatrics* 93(5): 814-819, 1994.

Wilson N, Self T, Hamburger R: Severe cow's milk–induced colitis in an exclusively breast-fed neonate, *Clin Pediatr* 29(2):77-80, 1990.

Wong DL and others: Diapering choices: a critical review of the issues, *Pediatr Nurs* 18(1):41-54, 1992.

Woolsey S: Support after sudden infant death, *Am J Nurs* 88(10):1347-1348, 1988.

BIBLIOGRAPHY

Vitamin and Mineral Disturbances

Benjamin D: Laboratory tests and nutritional assessment: protein-energy status, *Pediatr Clin North Am* 36(1):139-161, 1989.

Butler JC and others: Measles severity and serum retinol (vitamin A) concentration among children in the United States, *Pediatrics* 91(6):1176-1181, 1993.

Chang YT and others: Hypocalcemia in nonwhite breast-fed infants: vitamin D deficiency revisited, *Clin Pediatr* 31(11):695-698, 1992.

Chesney R: Requirements and upper limits of vitamin D intake in the term neonate, infant, and older child, *J Pediatr* 116(2):159-165, 1990.

Cook JD, Dassenko SA, Whittaker P: Calcium supplementation: effect on iron absorption, *Am J Clin Nutr* 53:106-111, 1991.

Council on Scientific Affairs: Vitamin preparations as dietary supplements and as therapeutic agents, *JAMA* 257(14):1929-1936, 1987.

Crombie I and others: Effect of vitamin and mineral supplementation on verbal and non-verbal reasoning of schoolchildren, *Lancet* 355:744-747, 1990.

Dixon A: Think zinc, *Neonatal Network* 5(4):29-33, 1987.

Dwyer J: Promoting good nutrition for today and the year 2000, *Pediatr Clin North Am* 33(4):799-822, 1986.

Erdman J: Nutrient interactions involving vitamins and minerals, *Contemp Nutr* 13(2):1-2, 1988.

Few B: Pharmacologic use of vitamin E, *MCN* 13(4):283, 1988.

Fish W and others: Effect of intramuscular vitamin E on mortality and intracranial hemorrhage in neonates of 1000 grams or less, *Pediatrics* 85(4):578-584, 1990.

Fomon SJ: *Infant nutrition,* St Louis, 1993, Mosby.

Goldstein M: Potential problems with the widespread use of niacin, *Am J Med* 85:881, 1988.

Hathcock JN and others: Evaluation of vitamin A toxicity, *Am J Clin Nutr* 52:183-202, 1990.

Heaney R, Weaver C: Oxalate: effect on calcium absorbability, *Am J Clin Nutr* 50:830-832, 1989.

Holland P and others: Prenatal deficiency of phosphate, phosphate supplementation, and rickets in very-low-birthweight infants, *Lancet* 335:697-701, 1990.

Hurrell R and others: Iron absorption in humans as influenced by bovine milk proteins, *Am J Clin Nutr* 49(3):546-662, 1989.

Johnston CC and others: Calcium supplementation and increases in bone mineral density in children, *N Engl J Med* 327(2):82-87, 1992.

Murphy SP, Subar AF, Block G: Vitamin E intakes and sources in the United States, *Am J Clin Nutr* 52:361-367, 1990.

Nakamura T and others: Mild to moderate zinc deficiency in short children: effect of zinc supplementation on linear growth velocity, *J Pediatr* 123(1):65-69, 1993.

Nestle M: Promoting health and preventing disease: National Nutrition Objectives for 1990 and 2000, *Nutr Today* 23(3):26-30, 1988.

Patel P and others: Intoxication from vitamin A in an asthmatic child, *Can Med Assoc J* 139:755-756, 1988.

Pennington J: The Food and Drug Administration and the dietary guidelines, *Fam Community Health* 12(1):1-13, 1989.

Poland R: Vitamin E for prevention of perinatal intracranial hemorrhage, *Pediatrics* 85(5): 865-867, 1990.

Prestridge L, Shulman R: Vitamin excesses and deficiencies, *Curr Opin Pediatr* 1:397-402, 1989.

Rossouw J: Kwashiorkor in North America, *Am J Clin Nutr* 49:588-592, 1989.

Vrchota K, Oberg C, Harris K: Beriberi in a Southeast Asian adolescent, *Am J Dis Child* 143(3):270-272, 1989.

Williams SR: *Nutrition and diet therapy,* ed 7, St Louis, 1993, Mosby.

Vegetarian Diets

Dagnelie P and others: High prevalence of rickets in infants on macrobiotic diets, *Am J Clin Nutr* 51:202-208, 1990.

Hanning RM, Zlotkin SH: Unconventional eating practices and their health implications, *Pediatr Clin North Am* 32(2):429-445, 1985.

O'Connell J and others: Growth of vegetarian children: the farm study, *Pediatrics* 84(3): 475-481, 1989.

Trahms CM: *Vegetarian diets for children.* In Pipes PL, Trahms CM: *Nutrition in infancy and childhood,* ed 5, St Louis, 1993, Mosby.

Protein and Energy Malnutrition

Benjamin D: Laboratory tests and nutritional assessment: protein-energy status, *Pediatr Clin North Am* 36(1):139-161, 1989.

Graham G, Lembcke J, Morales E: Quality-protein maize as the sole source of dietary protein and fat for rapidly growing young children, *Pediatrics* 85(1):85-91, 1990.

Kulkarni M and others: Age-independent anthropometric criteria in the assessment of PEM, *Am J Dis Child* 142(12):1268-1270, 1988.

McFarlane-Ferreira Y, LeLeiko N: Altered nutritional states: the effects of primary malnutrition, *Curr Opin Pediatr* 1:394-396, 1989.

Obesity

Agras W and others: Does a vigorous feeding style influence early development of adiposity? *J Pediatr* 110(5):799-804, 1987.

Bouchard C and others: The response to long-term overfeeding in identical twins, *N Engl J Med* 322(21):1477-1482, 1990.

Castiglia P: Obesity in infants and toddlers, *J Pediatr Health Care* 1(4):218-220, 1987.

Dietz WH Jr: Prevention of childhood obesity, *Pediatr Clin North Am* 33(4):823-833, 1986.

Griffiths M and others: Metabolic rate and physical development in children at risk of obesity, *Lancet* 336(8707):76-78, 1990.

Korsch B: Childhood obesity, *J Pediatr* 109(2): 299-300, 1986.

Morgan J: Prevention of childhood obesity, *Issues Compr Pediatr Nurs* 9(1):33-38, 1986.

Mossberg H: 40-year follow-up of overweight children, *Lancet* 2(8661):491-493, 1989.

Newmann C: Obesity in childhood. In Levine MD and others, editors: *Developmental-behavioral pediatrics,* ed 2, Philadelphia, 1992, WB Saunders.

Satter E: The feeding relationship, *J Am Diet Assoc* 86(3):352-356, 1986.

Woolston J: Obesity in infancy and early childhood, *J Am Acad Child Adolesc Psychiatry* 26:123-126, 1987.

Food Sensitivity

Berezin S: Gastrointestinal milk intolerance of infancy, *Am J Dis Child* 143(3):361-362, 1989.

Biller J and others: Efficacy of lactase-treated milk for lactose-intolerant pediatric patients, *J Pediatr* 111(1):91-94, 1987.

Brill B: Oral rehydration, food allergy, and specialized nutrition, *Curr Opin Pediatr* 1:384-393, 1989.

Brody JE: *Needless deaths are attributed to food allergy: study of children cites hidden ingredients,* New York, 1992, New York Times.

Institute of Food Technologists' Expert Panel on Food Safety and Nutrition: Food allergies and other food sensitivities, *Contemp Nutr* 10(11):1-2, 1985.

Johnstone D: Strategy for intervention of food allergy in infants, *Int Pediatr* 4(4):319-325, 1989.

Lee B, Geha R, Leung D: IgE response and its regulation in allergic disease, *Pediatr Clin North Am* 35(5):953-967, 1988.

Proujansky R, Winter H, Walker A: Gastrointestinal syndromes associated with food sensitivity, *Adv Pediatr* 35:219-238, 1988.

Savaiano D, Kotz C: Recent advances in the management of lactose intolerance, *Contemp Nutr* 13(9,10):1-4, 1988.

Wytock D, DiPalma J: All yogurts are not created equal, *Am J Clin Nutr* 47(3):454, 1988.

Yunginger J: Allergens: recent advances, *Pediatr Clin North Am* 35(5):981-993, 1988.

Allergy

Arshad SH and others: Effect of allergen avoidance on development of allergic disorders in infancy, *Lancet* 339(8808):1493-1497, 1992.

Burks W: A step-by-step approach to food allergy, *Contemp Pediatr* 13:32-51, 1993.

Sampson HA, Metcalfe DD: Food allergies, *JAMA* 268(20):2840-2844, 1992.

Feeding Difficulties: General

Edgehouse L, Radzyminski G: A device for supplementing breast-feeding, *MCN* 15(1): 34-35, 1990.

Finney J: Preventing common feeding problems in infants and young children, *Pediatr Clin North Am* 33(4):775-788, 1986.

Frappier P, Marino B, Shishmanian E: Nursing assessment of infant feeding problems, *J Pediatr Nurs* 2(1):37-44, 1987.

Heinig MJ and others: Energy and protein intakes of breast-fed and formula-fed infants during the first year of life and their association with growth velocity: the DARLING study, *Am J Clin Nutr* 58:152-161, 1993.

Hill P, Humenick S: Insufficient milk supply, *Image* 21(3):145-148, 1989.

Lierman C and others: Multidisciplinary treatment of feeding disorders in the home, *Pediatr Nurs* 13(4):266-270, 1987.

Riordan J: *Breastfeeding and human lactation,* Boston, 1993, Jones & Bartlett.

Walker M: Functional assessment of infant breast-feeding patterns, *Birth* 16(3):140-147, 1989.

Walker M, Driscoll J: Sore nipples: the new mother's nemesis, *MCN* 14:260-265, 1989.

Failure to Thrive

Bithoney WG, Dubowitz H, Egan H: Failure to thrive/growth deficiency, *Pediatr Rev* 13(12): 453-459, 1992.

Bithoney WG, Newberger EH: Child and family attributes of failure-to-thrive, *Dev Behav Pediatr* 8(1):32-36, 1987.

Bithoney WG, Rathbun J: Failure to thrive. In Levine MD and others, editors: *Developmental-behavioral pediatrics,* ed 2, Philadelphia, 1992, WB Saunders.

Castiglia P: Failure to thrive, *J Pediatr Health Care* 2(1):50-57, 1988.

Endert C, Wooldridge N: Nonorganic failure to thrive, *Diet Curr* 14(1):1-6, 1987.

Handen B, Mandell F, Russo D: Feeding induction in children who refuse to eat, *Am J Dis Child* 140(1):52-54, 1986.

Hilton A: Approaches for feeding the young child with anorexia, *J Pediatr Nurs* 2(1):45-49, 1987.

Kelleher KJ and others: Risk factors and outcomes for failure to thrive in low birth weight preterm infants, *Pediatrics* 91(5):941-948, 1993.

Klein M: The home health nurse clinician's role in the prevention of nonorganic failure to thrive, *J Pediatr Nurs* 5(2):129-135, 1990.

McJunkin J, Bithoney W, McCormick M: Errors in formula concentration in an outpatient population, *J Pediatr* 111(6, pt 1):848-850, 1987.

Pugliese M and others: Parental health beliefs as a cause of nonorganic failure to thrive, *Pediatrics* 80(2):175-182, 1987.

Showers J and others: Nonorganic failure to thrive: identification and intervention, *J Pediatr Nurs* 1(4):240-246, 1986.

Singer L: Long-term hospitalization of failure-to-thrive infants: developmental outcome at three years, *Child Abuse Negl* 10:479-486, 1986.

Singer L: Long-term hospitalization of nonorganic failure-to-thrive infants: patient characteristics and hospital course, *J Dev Behav Pediatr* 8(1):25-31, 1987.

Steele S: Nonorganic failure to thrive: a pediatric social illness, *Issues Compr Pediatr Nurs* 9(1):47-58, 1986.

Sullivan B: Growth-enhancing interventions for nonorganic failure to thrive, *J Pediatr Nurs* 6(4):236-242, 1991.

Wilcox W, Neiburg P, Miller D: Failure to thrive: a continuing problem of definition, *Clin Pediatr* 28(9):391-394, 1989.

Colic

Algranati PS, Dworkin PH: Infancy problem behaviors, *Pediatr Rev* 13(1):16-22, 1992.

Barr R: Infantile colic and lactose intolerance, *J Pediatr* 115(3):501-502, 1989 (letter to the editor).

Carey WB: Colic: exasperating but fascinating and gratifying, *Pediatrics* 84(3):568-569, 1989.

Carey WB: "Colic" or excessive crying in young infants. In Levine MD and others, editors: *Developmental-behavioral pediatrics,* ed 2, Philadelphia, 1992, WB Saunders.

Hartsell M: Sleeptight infant soother and colic, *J Pediatr Nurs* 15(1):59-60, 1990.

Hyams J and others: Colonic hydrogen production in infants with colic, *J Pediatr* 115(4):592-594, 1989.

Loadman W and others: Reducing the symptoms of infant colic by introduction of a vibration/sound-based intervention, *Pediatr Res* 21:182A, 1987.

Miller AR, Barr RG: Infantile colic: is it a gut issue? *Pediatr Clin North Am* 38(6):1407-1423, 1991.

Nacey KA: Pediatric update: infant colic, *J Emerg Nurs* 19(1):65-66, 1993.

Pinyerd BJ: Infant colic and maternal mental health: nursing research and practice concerns, *Issues Compr Pediatr Nurs* 15:155-167, 1992.

Sampson H: Infantile colic and food allergy: fact or fiction? *J Pediatr* 115(4):583-584, 1989.

Schmitt B: When your baby has colic, *Contemp Pediatr* 7(2):85-86, 1990.

Spencer J and others: White noise and sleep induction, *Arch Dis Child* 65(1):135-137, 1990.

Skin Disorders

Antherton D: Controversies in therapeutics: role of diet in treating atopic eczema: elimi-

nation diets can be beneficial, *Br Med J* 297(6661):1458-1460, 1988.
Berg R: Etiology and pathophysiology of diaper dermatitis, *Adv Dermatol* 3:75-98, 1988.
Broadbent J, Sampson H: Food hypersensitivity and atopic dermatitis, *Pediatr Clin North Am* 35(5):1115-1130, 1988.
Burks A and others: Atopic dermatitis: clinical relevance of food hypersensitivity reactions, *J Pediatr* 113(3):447-451, 1988.
Campbell R and others: Effects of diaper types on diaper dermatitis associated with diarrhea and antibiotic use in children in day-care centers, *Pediatr Dermatol* 5(2):83-87, 1988.
Chandra R, Puri S, Hamed A: Influence of maternal diet during lactation and use of formula feeds on development of atopic eczema in high risk infants, *Br Med J* 299:228-230, 1989.
Kramer D, Honig PJ: Diaper dermatitis in the hospitalized child, *J Enterostom Ther* 15(4): 167-170, 1988.
Kramer M: Does breast-feeding help protect against atopic disease? Biology, methodology, and a golden jubilee of controversy, *J Pediatr* 112(2):181-190, 1988.
Krowchuck DP: Practical aspects of the diagnosis and management of atopic dermatitis, *Pediatr Ann* 16:57-66, 1987.
Krusinski P, Flowers F: *Handbook of pediatric dermatology,* St Louis, 1990, Mosby.
Leung D, Kamada M: Developments in allergy, *Curr Opin Pediatr* 1(1):27-34, 1989.
Lucas A and others: Early diet of preterm infants and development of allergic or atopic disease: randomised prospective study, *Br Med J* 300:837-840, 1990.
Mallory SB: Neonatal skin disorders, *Pediatr Clin North Am* 38(4):745-762, 1991.
Nicol NH: Atopic dermatitis: the (wet) wrap-up, *Am J Nurs* 87:1560-1563, 1987.
Novick NL: Diaper rashes, *Pharmacol Times* 57(5):41-47, 1991.
Novotny J: Adolescents, acne, and the side-effects of Accutane, *Pediatr Nurs* 15:247-248, 1989.
Pairaudeau P and others: Inhalation of baby powder: an unappreciated hazard, *Br Med J* 302:1200-1201, 1991.
White KH: Diapering and skin care. In Smith DP and others, editors: *Comprehensive child and family nursing skills,* St Louis, 1991, Mosby.

Apnea

Ahmann E: Family impact of home apnea monitoring: an overview of research and its clinical implications, *Pediatr Nurs* 18(6):611-616, 1992.
Brooks JG: Apparent life-threatening events and apnea of infancy, *Clin Perinatol* 19(4): 809-838, 1992.
Jones SP: Relationship between apnea and GER: what nurses need to know, *Pediatr Nurs* 18(4):413-418, 1992.
Koons AH and others: Neurodevelopmental outcome of infants with apnea of infancy, *Am J Perinatol* 10(3):208-211, 1993.
Muttitt S and others: Neonatal apnea: diagnosis by nurse versus computer, *Pediatrics* 82(5):713-720, 1988.
Norris-Berkemeyer S, Hutchins K: Home apnea monitoring, *Pediatr Nurs* 12(4):259-262, 1986.
Picciano LD, Keller JP: Hospital and home apnea documentation systems: device acquisition and application, *Neonatal Intensive Care* 6(7):28-31, 1993.
Reiterer F, Fox WW: Multichannel polysomnographic recording for evaluation of infant apnea, *Clin Perinatol* 19(4):871-890, 1992.
Saylor C and others: Anxiety in mothers of infants on apnea monitors, *Child Health Care* 18(2):117, 1989.
Spitzer AR, Gibson E: Home monitoring, *Clin Perinatol* 19(4):907-926, 1992.
Toubas P and others: Effects of maternal smoking and caffeine habits on infantile apnea: a retrospective study, *Pediatrics* 78(1):159-163, 1986.

Sudden Infant Death Syndrome

Balarajan R, Raleigh V, Botting B: Sudden infant death syndrome and postneonatal mortality in immigrants in England and Wales, *Br Med J* 298(6675):716-720, 1989.
Bauchner H and others: Risk of sudden infant death syndrome among infants with in utero exposure to cocaine, *J Pediatr* 113(5):831-834, 1988.
Chan M: Sudden infant death syndrome and families at risk, *Pediatr Nurs* 13(3):166-168, 1987.
de Jonge G and others: Cot death and prone sleeping position in the Netherlands, *Br Med J* 298(6675):722, 1989.
Dunne K, Matthews T: Near-miss sudden infant death syndrome: clinical findings and management, *Pediatrics* 79(6):889-893, 1987.
Einspieler C and others: The predictive value of behavioural risk factors for sudden infant death, *Early Hum Dev* 18:101-109, 1988.
Gilbert R and others: Signs of illness preceding sudden unexpected death in infants, *Br Med J* 300(6734):1237-1239, 1990.
Gino C: SIDS research that causes pain, *Am J Nurs* 88(10):1353-1354, 1988.
Goldberg J: The counseling of SIDS parents, *Clin Perinatol* 19(4):927-938, 1992.
Grether J, Schulman J: Sudden infant death syndrome and birth weight, *J Pediatr* 114(4, pt 1):561-567, 1989.
Grether J, Schulman J, Croen L: Sudden infant death syndrome among Asians in California, *J Pediatr* 116(4):525-528, 1990.
Guntheroth WG, Spiers PS: Sleeping prone and the risk of sudden infant death syndrome, *JAMA* 267(17):2359-2362, 1992.
Haglund B, Cnattingius S: Cigarette smoking as a risk factor for sudden infant death syndrome: a population-based study, *Am J Public Health* 80:29-32, 1990.
Herda JA: Nursing interventions aimed at reducing risks of SIDS, *Pediatr Nurs* 18(5):531-534, 1992.
Hoffman HJ, Hillman LS: Epidemiology of the sudden infant death syndrome: maternal, neonatal, and postnatal risk factors, *Clin Perinatol* 19(4):717-738, 1992.
Hunt D, Shannon D: Sudden infant death syndrome and sleeping position, *Pediatrics* 90(1):115-118, 1992.
Jezierski M: Infant death: guidelines for support of parents in the emergency department, *J Emerg Nurs* 15(6):475-476, 1989.
Kahn A and others: Polysomnographic studies of infants who subsequently died of sudden infant death syndrome, *Pediatrics* 82(5):721-727, 1988.
Kahn A and others: Prone or supine body position and sleep characteristics in infants, *Pediatrics* 91(6):1112-1115, 1993.
Kandall SR and others: Relationship of maternal substance abuse to subsequent sudden infant death syndrome in offspring, *J Pediatr* 123(1):120-126, 1993.
Lee N and others: Sudden infant death syndrome in Hong Kong: confirmation of low incidence, *Br Med J* 298(6675):721, 1989.
Long CA, Barron D: SIDS and infant positioning: implications for critical care, *Pediatr Nurs* 18(5):524-527, 1992.
Meny RG and others: Cardiorespiratory recordings from infants dying suddenly and unexpectedly at home, *Pediatrics* 93(1):44-49, 1994.
Nelson E, Taylor B, Weatherall I: Sleeping position and infant bedding may predispose to hyperthermia and the sudden infant death syndrome, *Lancet* 1(8631):199-204, 1989.
Ponsonby A and others: Factors that increase the prone-SIDS association, *N Engl J Med* 329:377-382, 1993.
Poets EF, Southall DP: An editorial view: factors that increase the prone-SIDS association, *N Engl J Med* 329:424-426, 1993.

Autism

Baerg KL: Effective communication with autistic children, *Rehabil Nurs* 16(2):88-90, 1991.
Christian WP: Childhood autism. In Levine M and others, editors: *Developmental-behavioral pediatrics,* ed 2, Philadelphia, 1992, WB Saunders.
Denckla MB, James LS: An update on autism: a developmental disorder, *Pediatrics* 87(5, suppl):751-796, 1991.
Gualtieri C: Fenfluramine and autism: careful reappraisal is in order, *J Pediatr* 108(3):417-419, 1986.
Hays SR: Meeting the challenge of communicating with autistic children, *Rehabil Nurs* 16(2):92-93, 1990.
Kuhn PM: Response to "Effective communication with autistic children," *Rehabil Nurs* 16(2):90-92, 1991.
Lewis M: Gifted or dysfunctional: the child savant, *Pediatr Ann* 14(10):733-742, 1985.
Mundy P, Sheinkopf S: Social behavior and the neurology of autism, *Int Pediatr* 8(2):205-210, 1993.
Ritvo E and others: The UCLA–University of Utah epidemiologic survey of autism: prevalence, *Am J Psychiatry* 146(2):194-199, 1989.
Seifert C: *Holistic interpretation of autism: a theoretical framework,* Lanham MD, 1990, University Press of America.
Seifert C: *Theories of autism,* Lanham MD, 1990, University Press of America.
Stone WL and others: Play and imitation skills in the diagnosis of autism in young children, *Pediatrics* 86(2):267-272, 1990.
Treffert D: An unlikely virtuoso: Leslie Lemke and the story of savant syndrome, *Sciences* 29(1):28-35, 1988.
Tuchman R, Gilman J: Pharmacotherapy of pervasive developmental disorders, *Int Pediatr* 8(2):211-218, 1993.
Zimmerman AW, Frye VH, Potter NT: Immunological aspects of autism, *Int Pediatr* 8(2):199-204, 1993.

UNIT V

FAMILY-CENTERED CARE OF THE YOUNG CHILD

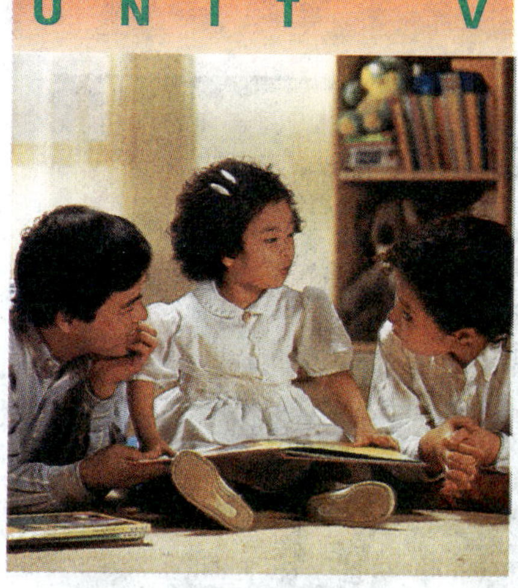

CHAPTER 14 Health Promotion of the Toddler and Family

CHAPTER OUTLINE

RELATED TOPICS

Animal bites, Ch. 18
Attachment, Ch. 12
Dental disorders, Ch. 18
Enuresis, Ch. 18
Family influences on child health promotion, Ch. 3
Fears, Ch. 15
Growth and development of children, Ch. 4
Ingestion of injurious agents, Ch. 16
Injuries—the leading killer, Ch. 1
Injury prevention: infant, Ch. 12; preschooler, 15
Limit-setting and discipline, Ch. 3
Sleep problems, Ch. 12
Social, cultural, and religious influences on child health promotion, Ch. 2
Spiritual development, Ch. 15
Stress in childhood, Ch. 4

PROMOTING OPTIMUM GROWTH AND DEVELOPMENT

The term ***terrible twos*** has often been used to describe the toddler years, the period from 12 to 36 months of age. It is a time of intense exploration of the environment as children attempt to find out how things work, what the word "no" means, and the power of temper tantrums, negativism, and obstinacy. "Getting into things" is their way of learning about their world, especially relationships. Successful mastery of the tasks of this age requires a strong foundation of trust during infancy and frequently necessitates guidance from others when parent and toddler face the struggles of toilet training, limit-setting, and sibling rivalry. Nurses who understand the dynamics of growth and development of the toddler can help families deal effectively with the tasks of this age.

BIOLOGIC DEVELOPMENT

Proportional Changes

Growth slows considerably during toddlerhood. The average ***weight*** at 2 years is 12 kg (27 pounds). The average weight gain is 1.8 to 2.7 kg (4 to 6 pounds) per year. The birth weight is quadrupled by 2½ years of age. The rate of increase in height also slows. The usual increment is an addition of 7.5 cm (3 inches) per year and occurs mainly in elongation of the legs rather than the trunk. The average ***height*** of a 2-year-old is 86.6 cm (34 inches). In general, adult height is about twice the child's height at 2 years of age. Accurate measurement of height and weight during the toddler years should reveal a steady growth curve that is steplike in nature rather than linear (straight), which is characteristic of the growth spurts during the early childhood years.

The rate of increase in ***head circumference*** slows somewhat by the end of infancy, and head circumference is usually equal to chest circumference by 1 to 2 years of age. The usual total increase in head circumference during the second year is 2.5 cm (1 inch). Then the rate of increase slows until age 5 years, when the increase is less than 1.25 cm (½ inch) per year. The anterior fontanel closes between 12 and 18 months of age.

Chest circumference continues to increase in size and exceeds head circumference during the toddler years. Its shape also changes as the transverse or lateral diameter exceeds the anteroposterior diameter. After the second year the chest circumference exceeds the abdominal measurement, which, in addition to the growth of the lower extremities, gives the child a taller, leaner appearance. However, the toddler retains a squat, "pot-bellied" appearance because of the less well developed abdominal musculature and short legs (Fig. 14-1). The legs retain a slightly bowed or curved appearance during the second year from the weight of the relatively large trunk.

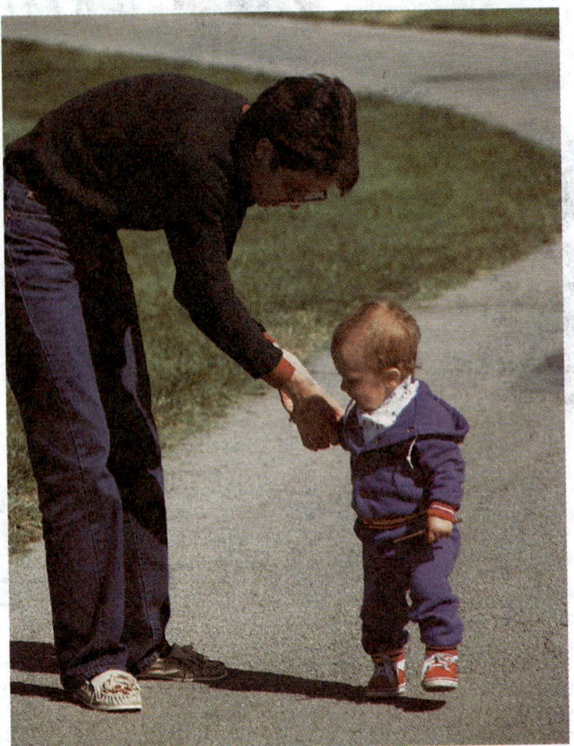

FIG. 14-1 Typical toddling gait.

Sensory Changes

Visual acuity of 20/20 is achieved during the toddler years, although 20/40 is considered acceptable. Full binocular vision is well developed by 12 months of age, and any evidence of persistent strabismus should receive professional attention as early as possible to prevent amblyopia. Depth perception continues to develop but, because of the child's lack of motor coordination, falls from heights remain a persistent danger.

The senses of ***hearing, smell, taste,*** and ***touch*** become increasingly well developed, coordinated with each other, and associated with other experiences. All of the senses are used to explore the environment. Toddlers will visually inspect an object by turning it over; they may taste it, smell it, and touch it several times before they are satisfied with their investigation. They will shake it to see if it makes noise and vigorously test its durability.

Another example of the integrated function of the senses is the toddler's development of specific ***taste preferences.*** The child is much less likely than infants to try a new food because of its appearance or smell, not just its taste. Nonsensory associations with objects also take on significance. For example, if parents refuse a particular food because of their dislike, they will transfer this negative connotation to the child before the child has had an opportunity to taste it. Awareness of these factors is important in several areas of childrearing, such as feeding, teaching socially acceptable habits, and reinforcing appropriate behavioral responses to various situations.

Touch continues to be very important to the toddler. Descending development of the spinal tract is evidenced by increased sensation in the lower extremities, such as tickling the feet. Pleasant tactile sensations soothe and comfort the toddler, especially in times of stress or fatigue.

Maturation of Systems

Most of the physiologic systems are relatively mature by the end of toddlerhood. By the end of the first year all the ***brain*** cells are present but continue to increase in size. Myelination of the spinal cord is almost complete by 2 years of age, which parallels the completion of most of the gross motor skills associated with locomotion. Brain growth is 75% completed by the end of 2 years.

Development of various areas of the brain seem to correspond with the progressive intellectual capacity of the child. Various areas of the cerebral cortex undergo specific changes as developmental progress occurs, such as Broca area for speech and cortical areas for control of the legs, hands, feet, and sphincters. Because this neuromotor organization is so inclusive, complex, and intricate, the child is limited in the ability to attend to any one aspect of behavior for more than a few minutes.

Between 2 and 3 years of age, coordination and consolidation of these voluntary functions allow the toddler to listen better, look longer, and have an extended attention span. Although postural control is increasingly developed as myelination of the spinal cord advances, the immaturity of this control, combined with the child's limited experiences and the lack of visual perception, makes simple acts such as seating oneself in a chair or climbing down stairs difficult tasks.

Volume of the ***respiratory tract*** and growth of associated structures continue to increase during early childhood, lessening some of the factors that predisposed the child to frequent and serious infections during infancy. However, the internal structures of the ear and throat continue to be short and straight, and the lymphoid tissue of the tonsils and adenoids continues to be large. As a result, otitis media, tonsillitis, and upper respiratory tract infections are common. The respiratory and heart rates slow, and the blood pressure increases (see inside back cover). Respirations continue to be abdominal.

The ***digestive processes*** are fairly complete by the beginning of toddlerhood. The acidity of the gastric contents continues to increase and has a protective function, since it is capable of destroying many types of bacteria. Stomach capacity increases to allow for the usual schedule of three meals a day.

One of the more prominent changes of the gastrointestinal system is the voluntary control of elimination. With complete myelination of the spinal cord, control of anal and urethral sphincters is gradually achieved. The physiologic ability to control the sphincters probably occurs somewhere between ages 18 and 24 months. Bladder capacity also increases considerably. By 14 to 18 months of age the child is able to retain urine for up to 2 hours or longer.

The ***skin*** functionally matures during early childhood. The epidermis and dermis are more tightly bound together, increasing their resistance to infection and irritation and creating a more effective barrier against fluid loss. Production of sebum is minimum, which contributes to the development of dry skin. The eccrine glands are functional during early childhood and react to changes in temperature, but they produce very minimal amounts of sweat. Hair grows thicker and coarser and usually darkens and loses some curliness. Fine hair is evident on the lower arms and legs. Production of adipose tissue declines as hyperplasia of muscle cells increases. With the concurrent growth of the lower extremities, the child assumes more adultlike proportions.

Under conditions of moderate variation in temperature, the toddler rarely has the difficulties of the young infant in maintaining ***body temperature.*** The capillaries are able to conserve core body temperature by constricting in response to cold and dilating in response to heat. Shivering, an involuntary act that results in rhythmic muscle contraction, which increases cellular metabolism, producing heat, is much more effective as a source of thermogenesis. The child also learns mechanisms to control body temperature—by putting on clothing when cold or removing it when warm.

The ***defense mechanisms*** of the tissues and blood, particularly phagocytosis, are much more efficient in the toddler than in the infant. The production of antibodies is well established. Immunoglobulin G (IgG), which neutralizes microbial toxins, reaches adult levels by the end of the second year of life. Passive immunity from maternal transfer during fetal life disappears by the beginning of toddlerhood. Immunoglobulin M (IgM), which responds to artificial immunizing techniques and combats serious infection, attains adult levels during late infancy. Immunoglobulins A, D, and E increase gradually, not reaching eventual adult levels until later childhood. Many young children demonstrate a sudden increase in colds and minor infections when entering nursery school because of the exposure to new antigens.

Gross and Fine Motor Development

The major ***gross motor skill*** during the toddler years is the development of locomotion. By 12 to 13 months of age toddlers walk alone, using a wide stance for extra balance; by age 18 months they try to run but fall easily. Between 2 and 3 years of age, refinement of the upright, biped position is evident in improved coordination and equilibrium. By age 2 years, toddlers can walk up and down stairs, and by age 2½ years they jump, using both feet, stand on one foot for a second or two, and manage a few steps on tiptoe. By the end of the second year they stand on one foot, walk on tiptoe, and climb stairs with alternate footing.

Fine motor development is demonstrated in increasingly skillful manual dexterity. Once the pincer grasp is achieved, usually at 9 to 10 months of age, toddlers combine this skill with other developing sensory and cognitive abilities. For example, by age 12 months they are able to grasp a very small object. At age 15 months they can drop a pellet into a narrow-necked bottle. Casting or throwing objects and retrieving them becomes an almost obsessive activity at about 15 months. By 18 months of age they can throw a ball overhand without losing their balance.

Visual perception of geometric shapes is also evident at this time. At age 12 months children selectively look at a round hole in a special form board but are unable to insert a round object. By age 15 months they promptly place the round object in the hole, even if the board is revised or turned upside down. Spatial relations also are evident in their ability to build a tower with blocks; by age 18 months, a tower of three to four blocks; by age 24 months, a tower of six to seven blocks; and by age 30 months, a tower of eight blocks or more.

Fine motor skill and visual ability are demonstrated in toddlers' progressive adeptness in manipulating a pencil or crayon. By age 15 months they will scribble spontaneously and by age 24 months will imitate a circular stroke and a vertical line. By the end of the toddler period, copying a circle and imitating a cross are possible.

Mastery of gross and fine motor skills is evident in all phases of the child's activity, such as play, dressing, language comprehension, response to discipline, social interaction, and proneness to injuries. Activities occur less in isolation and more in conjunction with other physical and mental abilities to produce a purposeful result. For example, the toddler walks to reach a new location, releases a toy to pick it up or to choose a new one, and scribbles to look at the image produced. The possibilities of the exploration, investigation, and manipulation mastery of the environment—and its hazards—are endless.

PSYCHOSOCIAL DEVELOPMENT

Toddlers are faced with the mastery of several important tasks. If the need for basic trust has been satisfied, they are ready to give up dependence for control, independence, and autonomy. Some of the specific tasks include:

- Differentiation of self from others, particularly the mother
- Toleration of separation from parent
- Ability to withstand delayed gratification
- Control over bodily functions
- Acquisition of socially acceptable behavior
- Verbal means of communication
- Ability to interact with others in a less egocentric manner

Mastery of these goals is only begun during late infancy and the toddler years, and such tasks as developing interpersonal relationships with others may not be completed until adolescence. However, crucial foundations for successful completion of such developmental tasks are laid during these early formative years.

Developing a Sense of Autonomy (Erikson)

According to Erikson, the developmental task of toddlerhood is acquiring a sense of ***autonomy*** while overcoming a sense of ***doubt*** and ***shame***. As infants gain trust in the predictability and reliability of their parents, environment, and interaction with others, they begin to discover that their behavior is their own and that it has a predictable, reliable effect on others. However, although they are aware of their will and control over others, they are confronted with the conflict of exerting autonomy and relinquishing the much enjoyed dependence on others. Exerting their will has definite negative consequences, whereas retaining dependent, submissive behavior is generally rewarded with affection and approval. However, continued dependency creates a sense of doubt regarding their potential capacity to control their actions. This doubt is compounded by a sense of shame for feeling this urge to revolt against others' will and a fear that they will exceed their own capacity for manipulating the environment. The latter fear is a basis for instituting limit-setting and consistent discipline at this age. Without appropriate limits on what is acceptable vs nonacceptable behavior, children have no guidelines for establishing the end points of their ability to control.

Just as the infant has the social modalities of grasping and biting, the toddler has the newly gained modality of holding on and letting go. To hold on and let go is evident with the use of the hands, mouth, eyes, and, eventually, the sphincters, when toilet training is begun. These social modalities are expressed constantly in the child's play activities, such as casting or throwing objects; taking objects out of boxes, drawers, or cabinets; holding on tighter when someone says, "No, don't touch"; and spitting out food as taste preferences become very strong.

Several characteristics, especially negativism and ritualism, are typical of toddlers in their quest for autonomy. As toddlers attempt to express their will, they often act with ***negativism***, the persistent negative response to requests. The words "no" or "me do" can be the sole vocabulary. Emotions become very strongly expressed, usually in rapid mood swings. One minute toddlers can be engrossed in an activity, and the next minute they might be violently angry because they were unable to manipulate a toy or open a door. If scolded for doing something wrong, they can have a temper tantrum and almost instantaneously pull at the parent's legs to be picked up and comforted. Often these swift changes are difficult for parents to understand and cope with. Many parents find the negativism exasperating and, instead of dealing constructively with it, give into it, which further threatens children in their search for learning acceptable methods of interacting with others (see p. 628).

In contrast to negativism, which frequently disrupts the environment, ***ritualism***, the need to maintain sameness and reliability, provides a sense of comfort. Toddlers can venture out with security when they know that there still exist familiar people, places, and routines. One can easily understand why change, such as hospitalization, represents such a threat to these children. Without the comfortable rituals, there is little opportunity to exert autonomy. Consequently, dependency and regression occur (see p. 629).

Erikson focuses on the development of the ***ego***, which may be thought of as reason or common sense, during this phase of psychosocial development. There is a struggle as the child deals with the impulses of the ***id*** and attempts to tolerate frustration and learn socially acceptable ways of interacting with the environment. The ego becomes evident as the child is able to tolerate delayed gratification.

There is also a rudimentary beginning of the ***superego***, or conscience, which is the incorporation of the morals of society and the process of acculturation. With the development of the ego, children further differentiate themselves from others and expand their sense of trust within themselves. But as they begin to develop awareness of their own will and capacity to achieve, they also become aware of their ability to fail. This ever-present awareness of potential failure creates doubt and shame. Successful mastery of the task of autonomy necessitates opportunities for self-mastery while withstanding the frustration of necessary limit-setting and delayed gratification. Opportunities for self-mastery are present in appropriate play activities, toilet training, the crisis of sibling rivalry, and successful interactions with significant others.

COGNITIVE DEVELOPMENT

Sensorimotor Phase (Piaget)

The period from 12 to 24 months of age is a continuation of the final two stages of the sensorimotor phase (Table 14-1). During this time the cognitive processes develop rapidly and at times seem similar to mature thinking. However, reasoning skills are still quite primitive and need to be understood to effectively deal with the typical behaviors of this age child. The main cognitive achievement of early childhood is the acquisition of language, which represents mental symbolism.

In the fifth stage, ***tertiary circular reactions*** (from 13 to 18 months of age), the child uses active experimentation to achieve previously unattainable goals. Newly acquired physical skills are increasingly important for the function they serve rather than for the acts themselves. The child incorporates the old learning of secondary circular reactions and

TABLE 14-1 Sensorimotor and Preconceptual Phases During Toddlerhood*

STAGE/AGE	COGNITIVE DEVELOPMENT	BEHAVIOR
SENSORIMOTOR		
V. Tertiary circular reactions 13-18 months	Active experimentation to achieve previously unattainable goals Increased concept of object permanence Differentiation of oneself from objects Early traces of memory Beginning awareness of spatial, causal, and temporal relationships Able to enter into an action at any point without reproducing the entire sequence	Insatiable curiosity about the environment Uses all sensory cues for exploration Ventures away from parent for longer periods Uses physical skills to achieve a particular goal Can find hidden objects, but only in first location Able to insert a round object into a hole Fits smaller objects into each other (nesting) Gestures "up" and "down" Puts objects into a container and takes them out Realizes that "out of sight" is not out of reach; opens doors and drawers to find objects Gains comfort from parent's voice even if the parent is not visually present
VI. Invention of new means through mental combinations 19-24 months	Awareness of object permanence regardless of the number of invisible displacements Can infer a cause while only experiencing the effect Imitation is increasingly smbolic Beginning sense of time in terms of anticipation, memory, and ability to wait Egocentricism in thought and behavior Global organization of thought	Searches for an object through several hiding places Will infer a cause by associating two or more experiences (such as candy missing, sister smiling) Imitates words and sounds of animals Imitates adult behavior (domestic mimicry) Follows directions and understands requests Uses words "up," "down," "come," and "go" with meaning May sit and wait for meals at the table for short period of time Has some sense of time; waits in response to "just a minute"; may use word "now" Refers to self by name Engages in parallel play; demonstrates awareness of ownership Very concerned with ritualistic, routinized schedule
PRECONCEPTUAL		
2-4 years†	Increased use of language as mental symbolization Egocentricism still present in thought, play, and behavior Increased sense of time, space, causality See also box on p. 619	Uses two- to three-word phrases Increased vocabulary Refers to self by pronoun Possessive of own toys, uses word "mine" Begins to use past tense of verbs Uses phrases "going to," "in a minute," "today," "all done" Uses many future-oriented words, such as "tomorrow," "next day," "afternoon," but poor conception of passage of time Follows directions using prepositions—up, behind, under, in back of, and so on

*For the previous four stages during early infancy see Table 12-1.
†Cognitive development and behavior apply primarily to ages 24 to 36 months.

applies the combined knowledge to new situations, with emphasis on the results of the experimentation. In this way there is the beginning of rational judgment and intellectual reasoning. During this stage there is further differentiation of oneself from objects. This is evident in the child's increasing ability to venture away from the parent and to tolerate longer periods of separation.

Awareness of a causal relationship between two events is apparent. After flipping a light switch, toddlers are aware that a reciprocal response occurs. However, they are not able to transfer that knowledge to new situations. Therefore every time they see what appears to be a light switch, they must reinvestigate its function. Such behavior demonstrates the beginning of categorizing data into distinct classes, subclasses, and so on. There are innumerable examples of this type of behavior as toddlers continuously explore the same object each time it appears in a new place. A classic example is their curiosity about electrical outlets. Even if they receive a shock from one of them, they will adamantly poke, taste, and inspect every other outlet. This inability to transfer information leaves toddlers particularly vulnerable to accidents. However, traces of memory are evident because they will usually avoid the outlet where the shock occurred.

Because classification of objects is still rudimentary, the appearance of an object denotes its function. For example, if the child's toys are stored in a paper bag or large container, that toy receptacle is no different than the garbage pail or laundry basket. If allowed to turn over the toy receptacle, the child will just as quickly do the same to other similar objects because, in the child's mind, there is no difference. Expecting toddlers to judge which receptacles are permissible to explore and which are not is inappropriate for this age-group. Instead, the forbidden object, such as the garbage pail, should be placed out of reach.

The discovery of objects as objects leads to the awareness of their spatial relationships. Children are able to recognize different shapes and their relationship to each other. For example, they can fit slightly smaller boxes into each other (nesting) and can place a round object into a hole, even if the board is turned around, upside down, or reversed. However, not until 2 years of age can they do the same thing with a square. Children are also aware of space and the relationship of their body to dimensions such as height. They will stretch, stand on a low stair or stool, and pull a string to reach an object.

Object permanence has also advanced. Although they still cannot find an object that has been invisibly displaced or moved from under one pillow to another pillow without their seeing the change, toddlers are increasingly aware of the existence of objects behind closed doors, in drawers, and under tables. Parents are usually acutely aware of this developmental achievement because they find high places and locked cabinets the only areas inaccessible to toddlers. Parents also experience toddlers' protest behaviors when the parents leave, since toddlers are aware that their parents are absent when they cannot see them.

During ages 19 to 24 months the child is in the final sensorimotor stage, ***invention of new means through mental combinations.*** This stage completes the more primitive, autistic thought processes of infancy and prepares the way for more complex mental operations during the phase of preoperational thought. One of the most dramatic achievements of this stage is in the area of object permanence. Children will now actively search for an object in several potential hiding places. In addition, they can infer a cause when only experiencing the effect. They can infer that an object was hidden in any number of places even if they only saw the original hiding place.

Imitation displays deeper meaning and understanding. Earlier, imitation was very concrete and action oriented. For example, "bye-bye" was a behavioral response more than a conceptual gesture of departure. Now it has a broader meaning, such as Daddy is going to work, it is time for a walk, or something is no longer present. There is greater symbolization to imitation.

One type of symbolic imitation is ***domestic mimicry,*** the imitation of household activity. Toddlers are acutely aware of others' actions and attempt to copy them in gestures and in words. They can imitate the parents' performance of a household task both physically and verbally. Parents often remark how accurately they see themselves in their child when the child engages in domestic mimicry. Such activity is part of the child's learning sex-role behavior.

The conception of time is still embryonic, but children have some sense of timing in terms of anticipation, memory, and the limited ability to wait. They may listen to the command, "Just a minute," and behave appropriately. However, their sense of timing is exaggerated—1 minute can last an hour. Toddlers' limited attention spans also indicate their sense of immediacy and concern for the present.

Egocentrism, or the inability to envision situations from perspectives other than one's own, is evident in all aspects of toddlers' behavior. They see, experience, and live every event in reference to themselves. For example, if a person is positioned between the toddler and another child, the toddler, who is facing the person, will explain that both children can see the middle person's face. The young child is unable to realize that the other person views the middle person from a different perspective, the back. A common example of egocentric behavior is the toddler who takes a toy away from another child. The child is concerned only with playing with the toy and is unable to conceptualize that taking the toy away will make the other child unhappy.

Preconceptual Phase (Piaget)

At approximately 2 years of age the child enters the preconceptual phase of cognitive development, which lasts until about age 4 years. The preconceptual phase is a subdivision of the ***preoperational phase,*** which spans ages 2 to 7 years. The preconceptual phase is primarily one of transition, which bridges the purely self-satisfying behavior of infancy and the rudimentary socialized behavior of latency. The principal characteristics of this stage are egocentric use of language and dependence on perception in problem solving (Thomas, 1985).

During ages 2 to 4 years children learn a variety of words and there is an increasing use of language. In fact, toddlers talk a lot. Speech is primarily of two types—egocentric or socialized. ***Egocentric speech*** consists of repeating words and sounds for the pleasure of hearing oneself and is not intended to communicate. This ***collective monologue*** reflects the child's lingering self-centeredness.

Socialized speech is for communication; however, it is still egocentric in that children communicate about themselves to others. Before age 3 most speech is directed at self-fulfillment or self-reference, such as, "Want drink," or "I do," and is directed mostly to adults. Since children think that everyone else's world is the same as theirs, they expect others to understand their verbal messages even when limited information is conveyed.

Preoperational thinking implies that children cannot think in terms of ***operations***—the ability to manipulate objects in relation to each other in a logical fashion. Rather, toddlers think primarily based on their perception of an event. Problem solving is based on what they see or hear directly rather than on what they recall about objects and events (see box below).

Within the second year the child increasingly uses language symbolically and is concerned with the "why" and "how" of things. For example, a pencil is "something to write with" and food is "something to eat." However, such mental symbolization is closely associated with prelogical reasoning. For instance, a needle is "something that hurts." Such painful experiences take on new significance, since memory is associated with the specific event and fears are likely to develop, such as resistance to people who wear white uniforms or rooms that look like the practitioner's office. Sometimes the child's ability to recall events is underestimated, and little thought is given to the preparation for visits to a hospital or other health facility, resulting in fears that can last a lifetime. Because of the vulnerability of these early years, it is essential to prepare children for new experiences, whether it is a new baby-sitter or a visit to the dentist.

MORAL DEVELOPMENT

Preconventional or Premoral Level (Kohlberg)

Toddlers' development of moral judgment is at the most basic level. There is little, if any, concern for why something is wrong. Young children behave because of the freedom or restriction that is placed on actions. In the ***punishment and obedience orientation,*** whether an action is good or bad depends on whether it results in reward or punishment. If

CHARACTERISTICS OF PREOPERATIONAL THOUGHT

Egocentrism—Inability to envision situations from perspectives other than one's own

Example: If a person is positioned between the toddler and another child, the toddler, who is facing the person, will explain that both children can see the middle person's face. The young child is unable to realize that the other person views the middle person from a different perspective, the back.

Implication: Avoid moralizing about "why" something is wrong if it requires an understanding of someone else's feelings or opinion. Telling a child to stop hitting because hitting hurts the other person is often ineffective because, to the aggressor, it feels good to hit someone else. Instead, emphasize that hitting is not allowed.

Transductive—Reasoning from the particular to the particular

Example: Child refuses to eat a food because something previously eaten did not taste good.

Implication: Accept child's reasoning; offer refused food at different time.

Global organization—Changing any one part of the whole changes the entire whole

Example: Child refuses to sleep in room because location of bed is changed.

Implication: Accept child's reasoning; use same bed position or introduce change slowly.

Centration—Focusing on one aspect rather than considering all possible alternatives

Example: Child refuses to eat a food because of its color, even though its taste and smell are acceptable.

Implication: Accept child's reasoning.

Animism—Attributing lifelike qualities to inanimate objects

Example: Child scolds stairs for making child fall down.

Implication: Join child in the "scolding." Keep frightening objects out of view.

Irreversibility—Inability to undo or reverse the actions initiated physically

Example: When told to stop doing something, such as talking, child is unable to think of opposite activity.

Implication: State requests or instructions *positively* (e.g., "Be quiet").

Magical—Believing that thoughts are all-powerful and can cause events

Example: Child wishes someone died; then if the person dies; child feels at fault because of the "bad" thought that made the death happen.

Calling children "bad" because they did something wrong makes children feel as if they are bad.

Implication: Clarify that thoughts do not make things happen and that child is not responsible.

Use "I" messages rather than "you" messages to communicate thoughts, feelings, expectations, or beliefs without imposing blame or criticism. Emphasize that the act is bad, not the child.

Inability to conserve—Inability to understand the idea that a mass can be changed in size, shape, volume, or length without losing or adding to the original mass (instead, children judge what they see by the immediate perceptual clues given to them)

Example: If two lines of equal length are presented in such a way that one appears longer than the other, child will state that one line is longer even if child measures both lines with a ruler or yardstick and finds that each has the same length.

Implication: Change the most obvious perceptual clue to reorient child's view of what is seen. For example, give medicine in a small medicine cup, rather than a large cup, since child will imagine that the large vessel contains more liquid. If child refuses the medicine in the small cup, pour it into a large cup, because the liquid will appear to be less in a tall, wide container.

Give a large flat cookie rather than a thick small one, or do the reverse with meat or cheese; child will usually eat larger size of favorite food and smaller size of less favorite food.

children are punished for it, the action is bad. If they are not punished, the action is good, regardless of the meaning of the act. For example, if parents allow hitting, the child will perceive that hitting is good because it is not associated with punishment (Thomas, 1985).

The type of discipline also affects children's moral development. When parents use power to control behavior, such as physical punishment or withholding privileges, children receive a negative view of morals, especially toward authority figures, such as law enforcement agencies. When parents withdraw love or attention, children behave primarily because of guilt, rather than from an internalization of morals. However, when parents give explanations for the misbehavior and try to help children change through positive approaches, such as consequences or rewards, children feel less hostility and are more likely to base their actions on an analysis of why an act may be wrong (Schuster and Ashburn, 1986). Of course, the effect of discipline is not limited to the toddler years, and the sole use of explanation is inappropriate. However, parents usually establish discipline techniques at this time, and the use of constructive approaches should begin early (see Limit-Setting and Discipline, Chapter 3).

SPIRITUAL DEVELOPMENT

Because of their immature cognitive processes, toddlers have only a vague idea of God and religious teachings. However, routines, such as saying prayers before meals or at bedtime, can be very important and comforting. Toward the end of toddlerhood, when children are in preoperational thought, there is some advancement of their understanding of God. Religious teachings may influence their behavior, such as reward or fear of punishment (heaven or hell) and moral development (see also discussion in Chapter 15.)

DEVELOPMENT OF BODY IMAGE

As in infancy, the development of body image closely parallels cognitive development. With increasing motor ability toddlers recognize the usefulness of body parts and gradually learn their respective names. They also learn that certain parts of the body have various meanings; for example, during toilet training the genitals become significant and cleanliness is emphasized. By 2 years of age there is recognition of sexual differences and reference to self by name and then by pronoun.

Once they begin preoperational thought, toddlers can use symbols to represent objects, but their thinking may lead to inaccuracies. For example, if someone who is pregnant is called "fat," they will describe all "fat" ladies (sometimes even men!) as having babies. There is a beginning recognition of words used to describe physical appearance, such as "pretty," "handsome," or "big boy." Such expressions eventually influence how children view their own bodies, and such labeling (negative or positive) becomes part of their body image.

Although there has been little research done on body image development in young children, it is evident that body integrity is poorly understood and that intrusive experiences are threatening because they fear their blood and insides will leak out. For example, during a physical assessment toddlers forcefully resist procedures such as examining the ear or mouth and taking a rectal temperature. Toddlers also have unclear body boundaries and may associate nonviable parts, such as feces, with essential body parts. This can be seen in the toddler who is upset by flushing the toilet and watching the stool disappear.

Nurses can assist parents in fostering a positive body image in their child by encouraging them to avoid negative labels, such as "skinny arms" or "chubby legs"—self-perceptions that can last a lifetime. Body parts, especially those related to elimination and reproduction, should be called by their correct names. Respect for the body should be practiced.

DEVELOPMENT OF SEXUALITY

Just as toddlers explore their environment, they also explore their bodies and find that touching certain body parts is pleasurable. Genital fondling (masturbation) can occur and involves manual stimulation, as well as posturing movements (especially in young girls) such as tightening of the thighs or mechanical pressure applied to the pubic or suprapubic area (Fleisher and Morrison, 1990). Other demonstrations of sensual activities include rocking, swinging, and hugging people and toys. Parental reactions to toddlers' sexual behavior will influence the children's own attitudes and should be accepting rather than critical.

Children in this age-group are learning vocabulary associated with anatomy, elimination, and reproduction. Certain associations between words and functions become significant and can influence future sexual attitudes. For example, if parents refer to the genitals as dirty, especially in the context of elimination, the child may transfer this association between "genitals" and "dirty" to sexual functions.

Sex-role differences become obvious to children and are evident in much of their imitative play. Early attitudes are formed about affectional behaviors between adults from observing parental and other adult sexual/sensual activities. (See also Sex Education, Chapter 15.)

SOCIAL DEVELOPMENT

Individuation-Separation

A major task of the toddler period is differentiation of self from significant others, usually the mother. The differentiation process consists of two phases: ***separation,*** the children's emergence from a symbiotic fusion with the mother, and ***individuation,*** those achievements that mark children's assumption of their individual characteristics in the environment (Mahler, Pine, and Bergman, 1975). Although the process begins during the latter half of infancy, the major achievements occur during the toddler years.

Toddlers have an increased understanding and awareness of object permanence and some ability to withstand delayed gratification and tolerate moderate frustration. They begin to lose some of their previous resistance to separation, yet appear to become even more concerned about the parent's whereabouts. They have learned from experience that parents exist when physically absent. Repetition of events such as going to bed without the parents but waking to find them again reinforces the reliability of such brief separations. Consequently, toddlers are able to venture away from their parents for brief periods because of the security of knowing that the parent will be there when they return. Verbal and visual reassurance from the parent gradually replaces some of the previous need to be physically close for comfort.

Toddlers also show less fear of strangers, but only when their parents are present. When left alone with a stranger, they are very fearful and acutely anxious; manifest depressive behavior, such as crying and withdrawal; and may become restless, hyperactive, or passive, reverting to regressive behaviors. Such reactions may be evident when a child is left with a baby-sitter, during the initial days of preschool or daycare, or if the child is hospitalized (see Chapter 26).

These behaviors are not pathologic or harmful if parents realize how desperately their children need them. In fact, indiscriminate friendliness toward strangers and lack of anxiety during separation from parents may be reason for concern. Sensitive, perceptive parents will be aware of the child's need for increased love, affection, and attention when they are together. An attitude such as "They will get used to the baby-sitter" will not help young children positively tolerate separation.

Parents often need help in realizing the necessity of preparing children for an inevitable separation. Particularly with the firstborn, parents tend to overprotect children, shield them from any anxiety-producing experience, and insulate them from less than immediate gratification. Although this is not necessarily harmful, especially if opportunities for independence are allowed later, it does not prepare children for unexpected events. A typical example is the birth of a sibling. The child is faced with the crisis of sibling rivalry, as well as separation from the parent. No wonder the child will not welcome the infant—the intruder caused mother to leave! Allowing children to experience brief periods of separation early during infancy prepares them for such experiences later. Indeed, they may still manifest the typical behaviors of protest, but they will also have learned that mother or father always returns. Therefore it is easy to appreciate the tremendous loss that the death of a parent represents for young children; unlike their other experiences with separation, this time the parent will not return. (For a discussion of the long-term consequences of stressors such as separation, see Thinking Critically About . . . box on p. 527.)

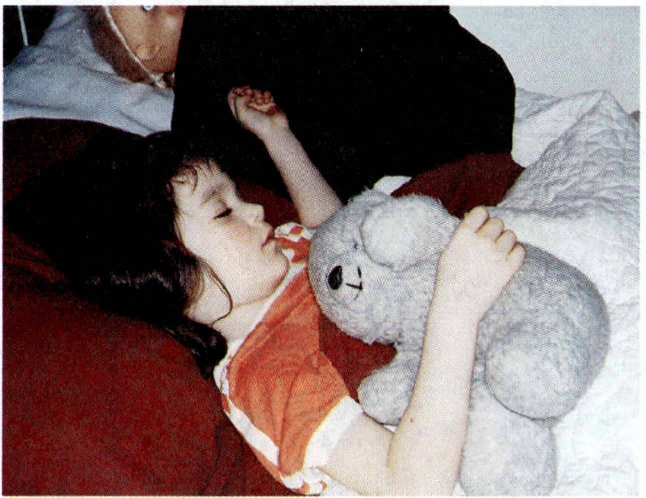

FIG. 14-2 Transitional objects, such as a warm and fuzzy stuffed animal, are sources of security to a toddler.

Transitional objects, such as a favorite blanket or toy, provide security for young children, especially when they are separated from parents, are dealing with a new stress, or are just fatigued (Fig. 14-2). Security objects often become so important to toddlers that they refuse to have them taken away. Such behavior is normal; there is no need to discourage this tendency. During separations, such as daycare, hospitalization, or even staying overnight with a relative, transitional objects should be provided to minimize any feelings of fear or loneliness.

Learning to tolerate and master brief periods of separation is an important developmental task of children in this age-group. In addition, it is a necessary component of parenting, since brief periods of separation from their children allow parents to recoup their energy and patience and to minimize directing their irritations and frustrations at the children.

Language Development

The most striking characteristic of language development during early childhood is the increasing level of comprehension. Although the number of words acquired—from about 4 at 1 year of age to approximately 300 at age 2 years—is notable, *the ability to understand speech is much greater than the number of words the child can say*. This is particularly evident in bilingual families where the vocabulary may be delayed, but comprehension in either language is appropriate.

At age 1 year the child uses one-word sentences or holophrases. The word "up" can mean "pick me up" or "look up there." For the child the one word conveys the meaning of a sentence, but to others it may mean many things or nothing. During this age about 25% of the vocalizations are intelligible. By the age of 2 years the child uses multiword sentences by stringing together two or three words, such as the phrases, "mama go bye-bye" or "all gone," and approximately 65% of the speech is understandable.

Personal-Social Behavior

One of the most dramatic aspects of development in the toddler is personal-social interaction. Parents frequently wonder why their manageable, docile, lovable infant has turned into a determined, strong-willed, volatile-tempered little "tyrant." In addition, the tyrant can swiftly and unpredictably revert back to the adorable infant. All of this is part of "growing up" and is evident in such areas as dressing, feeding, playing, and establishing self-control.

Toddlers are developing skills of independence, which are evident in all areas of behavior. By age 15 months children feed themselves, drink well from a covered cup, and manage a spoon, with considerable spilling. By age 24 months they use a spoon well and by age 36 months may be using a fork. Between ages 2 and 3 years they eat with the family and like to help with chores such as setting the table or removing dishes from the dishwasher, but they lack table manners and may find it difficult to sit through the family's entire meal (see Table 14-4).

In dressing, toddlers also demonstrate strides in independence. The 15-month-old child helps by putting the arm or foot out for dressing and pulls shoes and socks off. The 18-month-old child removes gloves, helps with pullover shirts, and may be able to unzip. By age 2 years the toddler removes most articles of clothing and puts on socks, shoes, and pants without regard for right or left and back or front. Help is still needed to fasten clothes.

Play

Play magnifies toddlers' physical and psychosocial development. Interaction with people becomes increasingly important. The solitary play of infancy progresses to ***parallel play***—the toddler plays alongside, not with, other children. Although sensorimotor play is still prominent, there is much less emphasis on the exclusive use of one sensory modality. The toddler inspects the toy, talks to the toy, tests its strength and durability, and invents several uses for it.

Play assumes many forms and serves several functions (Table 14-2). These youngsters benefit from a wide variety of play interactions (alone, with other children or adults), environments (own home, other children's homes, park), and activities (active, quiet, organized, unstructured).

Imitation is one of the most distinguishing characteristics of play and enriches children's opportunity to engage in fantasy. With less emphasis on sex-stereotyped toys, play objects such as dolls, carriages, dollhouses, dishes, cooking utensils, child-sized furniture, trucks, and dress-up clothes are used by both sexes (Fig. 14-3).

Increased locomotive skills make push-pull toys, stick horses, straddle trucks or cycles, a small, low gym and slide, variously sized balls, and rocking horses appropriate for the energetic toddler. Finger paints, thick crayons, chalk, blackboard, paper, and puzzles with large simple pieces use the child's developing fine motor skills. Interlocking blocks in varied sizes (but large enough to avoid aspiration) and shapes provide hours of fun and, during later years, are useful objects for creative and imaginative play.

Talking is a form of play for the toddler, who enjoys musical toys such as play record players, "talking" dolls and animals, and play telephones. Appropriate children's television programs are excellent for children in this age-group, who learn to associate words with visual images. Toddlers also enjoy "reading" stories from a picture book and imitating the sounds of animals.

Tactile play is also important for the exploring toddler. Water toys, a sandbox with pail and shovel, finger paints, soap bubbles, and clay provide excellent opportunities for creative and manipulative recreation. Parents sometimes forget the fascination of feeling slippery cream, catching airy bubbles, squeezing and reshaping clay, or smearing paints. These types of unstructured activities are as important as educational play to allow children freedom of expression.

Selection of appropriate toys must involve safety factors, especially in relation to size and sturdiness. The oral activ-

TABLE 14-2 Play During Toddlerhood

PHYSICAL DEVELOPMENT	SOCIAL DEVELOPMENT	MENTAL DEVELOPMENT AND CREATIVITY
SUGGESTED ACTIVITIES		
Provide space in which to encourage physical activity Provide sandbox, swing, and other scaled-down playground equipment	Provide replicas of adult tools and equipment for imitative play Permit child to "help" with adult tasks Encourage imitative play Provide toys and activities that allow for expression of feelings Allow child to play with some actual items used in the adult world; for example, let child help wash dishes or play with pots and pans and other utensils (check for safety)	Provide for water play Encourage building, drawing, and coloring Provide various textures in objects for play Provide large boxes and other safe containers for imaginative play Read stories appropriate to age Monitor television viewing
SUGGESTED TOYS		
Push-pull toys Rocking horse, stick horse Riding toy Balls Blocks (unpainted) Pounding board Low gym and slide Pail and shovel Containers Play dough	Music and a record player or tape recorder Purse Housekeeping toys (broom, dishes) Toy telephone Dishes, stove, table and chairs Mirror Puppets, dolls, stuffed animals	Wooden puzzles Cloth picture books Paper, finger paint, thick crayons Blocks Large beads to string Wooden shoe for lacing Appropriate TV programs

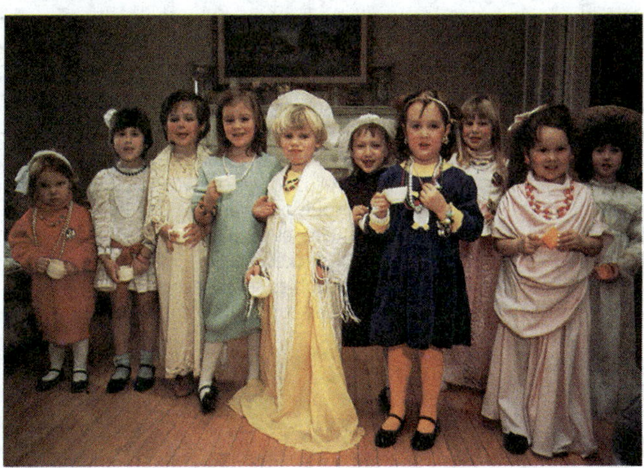

FIG. 14-3 Young children enjoy dressing up.

ity of toddlers makes them at risk for aspirating small objects. Parents need to be especially vigilant of toys played with in other children's homes or those of older siblings. Toys are a potential source of serious bodily damage to toddlers, who may have the physical strength to manipulate them but not the knowledge to appreciate their danger (see Family Home Care box on p. 137).

TEMPERAMENT

Temperamental characteristics of children during infancy tend to predominate during toddlerhood. Most difficult infants remain difficult during early childhood, but the easy infants also become less easy (Carey and McDevitt, 1978). In addition, mothers are more likely to rate children as difficult at ages 1 to 3 years than earlier (McDevitt and Carey, 1981). It is not surprising for parents to see toddlers as more challenging, especially considering the typical negativistic traits of this age-group. Parents of easy infants may be particularly distressed by the behavior change, whereas parents of difficult children may be more prepared, because of a previously troublesome year, or be overwhelmed by the additional behaviors. The use of the ***Toddler Temperament Scale*** can assist in identifying temperamental characteristics that benefit from individualized approaches to childrearing (Fullard, McDevitt, and Carey, 1984). For practitioners in a busy setting, asking parents about their impression of the child's temperament yields reliable data that can help professionals gain a greater understanding of the parent-child interactional process (Houldin, Fullard, and Heverly, 1989).

While temper tantrums are common in toddlers, certain temperament characteristics make some children more prone to such outbursts. Active, intensely responding children are apt to have yelling, screaming, and flinging behavior during tantrums. Parents benefit from forewarning of extreme outbursts and the knowledge that the intensely negative behavior is not abnormal and is tempered by the child's intensely happy moods (Zuckerman and Frank, 1992).

Discipline is also influenced by temperament. Easy children generally respond well to mild forms of discipline, including a stern voice and sustained eye contact. However, difficult children often need more structured types of discipline, such as time-out or rewards, and the effectiveness of one approach may be short-lived. Efforts at preventing misbehavior are especially important with children who have persistent natures (see Limit-Setting and Discipline, Chapter 3). Without "friendly warnings" such children often have difficulty terminating an activity. These children may be punished for behavior that is merely typical of their temperament, and if the unwarranted punishment continues, the pattern can develop into a behavior problem (Chess and Thomas, 1985). Slow-to-warm-up children may also present challenges, especially when combined with toddlers' usual fear of strangers. These children require gradual introduction to new situations, such as daycare and baby-sitters. (See also Temperament, Chapter 4.)

■ ■ ■

Table 14-3 presents a summary of the major features of growth and development for the age-groups of 15, 18, 24, and 30 months. The key developmental ages are 18 and 24 months, although the chronologic ages of 15 and 30 months are also significant. Fifteen months of age is a particularly integrative period of developmental achievement because it represents the completion or fruition of many skills that were unperfected at 1 year of age.

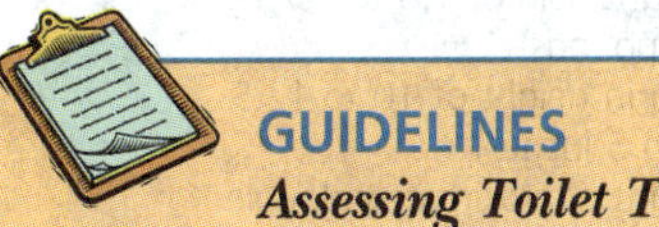

GUIDELINES
Assessing Toilet Training Readiness

PHYSICAL READINESS

Voluntary control of anal and urethral sphincters, usually by ages 18 to 24 months
Ability to stay dry for 2 hours; decreased number of wet diapers; waking dry from nap
Regular bowel movements
Gross motor skills of sitting, walking, and squatting
Fine motor skills to remove clothing

MENTAL READINESS

Recognizes urge to defecate or urinate
Verbal or nonverbal communicative skills to indicate when wet or has urge to defecate or urinate
Cognitive skills to imitate appropriate behavior and follow directions

PSYCHOLOGIC READINESS

Expresses willingness to please parent
Able to sit on toilet for 5 to 10 minutes without fussing or getting off
Curiosity about adults' or older sibling's toilet habits
Impatience with soiled or wet diapers; desire to be changed immediately

PARENTAL READINESS

Recognizes child's level of readiness
Willing to invest the time required for toilet training
Absence of family stress or change, such as a divorce, moving, new sibling, or imminent vacation

TABLE 14-3 Growth and Development During Toddler Years

AGE (MONTHS)	PHYSICAL	GROSS MOTOR	FINE MOTOR
15	Steady growth in height and weight Head circumference 48 cm (19 inches) Weight 11 kg (24 pounds) Height 78.7 cm (31 inches)	Walks without help (usually since age 13 months) Creeps up stairs Kneels without support Cannot walk around corners or stop suddenly without losing balance Assumes standing position without support Cannot throw ball without falling	Constantly casting objects to floor Builds tower of two cubes Holds two cubes in one hand Releases a pellet into a narrow-necked bottle Scribbles spontaneously Uses cup well but rotates spoon
18	Physiologic anorexia from decreased growth needs Anterior fontanel closed Physiologically able to control sphincters	Runs clumsily, falls often Walks up stairs with one hand held Pulls and pushes toys Jumps in place with both feet Seats self on chair Throws ball overhand without falling	Builds tower of three to four cubes Release, prehension, and reach well developed Turns pages in a book two or three at a time In drawing, makes stroke imitatively Manages spoon without rotation
24	Head circumference 49 to 50 cm (19.5 to 20 inches) Chest circumference exceeds head circumference Lateral diameter of chest exceeds anteroposterior diameter Usual weight gain of 1.8 to 2.7 kg (4 to 6 pounds) Usual gain in height of 10 to 12.5 cm (4 to 5 inches) Adult height approximately double height at 2 years May have achieved readiness for beginning daytime control of bowel and bladder Primary dentition of 16 teeth	Goes up and down stairs alone with two feet on each step Runs fairly well, with wide stance Picks up object without falling Kicks ball forward without overbalancing	Builds tower of six to seven cubes Aligns two or more cubes like a train Turns pages of book one at a time In drawing, imitates vertical and circular strokes Turns doorknob, unscrews lid
30	Birth weight quadrupled Primary dentition (20 teeth) completed May have daytime bowel and bladder control	Jumps with both feet Jumps from chair or step Stands on one foot momentarily Takes a few steps on tiptoe	Builds tower of eight cubes Adds chimney to train of cubes Good hand-finger coordination; holds crayon with fingers rather than fist Moves fingers independently In drawing, imitates vertical and horizontal strokes, makes two or more strokes for cross

COPING WITH CONCERNS RELATED TO NORMAL GROWTH AND DEVELOPMENT

Toilet Training

One of the major tasks of toddlerhood is toilet training. The physical ability to control the anal and urethral sphincters is achieved sometime after the child is walking, probably between ages 18 and 24 months. However, complex psychophysiologic factors are also required for readiness. The child must be able to recognize the urge to let go and hold on and be able to communicate this sensation to the parent. In addition, there is probably some necessary motivation in the desire to please the parent by holding on, rather than pleasing oneself by letting go.

Usually physiologic and psychologic readiness is not complete until ages 18 to 24 months. By this time the child has mastered the majority of essential gross motor skills, can communicate intelligibly, is less in conflict with self-assertion and negativism, and is aware of the ability to control the body and please the parent. One of the most im-

SENSORY	VOCALIZATION	SOCIALIZATION
Able to identify geometric forms; places round object into appropriate hole Binocular vision well developed Displays an intense and prolonged interest in pictures	Uses expressive jargon Says four to six words, including names "Asks" for objects by pointing Understands simple commands May use head-shaking gesture to denote "no" Uses "no" even while agreeing to the request	Tolerates some separation from parent Less likely to fear strangers Beginning to imitate parents, such as cleaning house (sweeping, dusting), folding clothes, mowing lawn Feeds self using covered cup with little spilling May discard bottle Manages spoon but rotates it near mouth Kisses and hugs parents, may kiss pictures in a book Expressive of emotions, has temper tantrums
	Says 10 or more words Points to a common object, such as shoe or ball, and to two or three body parts	Great imitator ("domestic mimicry") Manages spoon well Takes off gloves, socks, and shoes and unzips Temper tantrums may be more evident Beginning awareness of ownership ("my toy") May develop dependency on transitional objects, such as "security blanket"
Accommodation well developed In geometric discrimination, able to insert square block into oblong space	Has vocabulary of approximately 300 words Uses two- to three-word phases Uses pronouns "I," "me," "you" Understands directional commands Gives first name; refers to self by name Verbalizes need for toileting, food, or drink Talks incessantly	Stage of parallel play Has sustained attention span Temper tantrums decreasing Pulls people to show them something Increased independence from mother Dresses self in simple clothing
	Gives first and last name Refers to self by appropriate pronoun Uses plurals Name one color	Separates more easily from mother In play, helps put things away, can carry breakable objects, pushes with good steering Begins to notice sex differences; knows own sex May attend to toilet needs without help except for wiping

portant responsibilities of nurses is to help parents identify the readiness signs in their child (see Guidelines box, p. 623).*

In a study of children in the United States, the average age at toilet training (defined as reasonably successful transition from diapers to regular underwear and not necessarily with complete daytime continence) was 2.4 years. Girls were trained significantly earlier (average age 2.25 years) than boys (average age 2.56 years) (Bloom and others, 1993). (See Cultural Awareness box, p. 626.) Although traditionally parents have toilet trained their children, caregivers in alternative care centers are often assuming this task.

A number of techniques can be helpful when initiating training. One is the selection of a potty chair and/or use of the toilet. A freestanding potty chair allows children a feeling of security. Planting the feet firmly on the floor also

*A helpful brochure is *Toilet Training: A Parent's Guide,* available from the American Academy of Pediatrics, 141 Northwest Point Blvd., P.O. Box 927, Elk Grove Village, IL 60009-0927; (800) 433-9016.

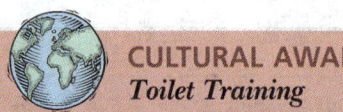

CULTURAL AWARENESS

Toilet Training

The timing, method, and significance of toilet training are influenced by cultural practices. For many families in China, the timing is liberal, the method is unique, and the significance is low. Children are diapered during infancy. Once they are walking, they wear loose pants with a long slit between the legs, and they eliminate on the ground. This practice may continue until the child is 5 years of age. In cold weather, a piece of cloth, like a "curtain," may be inserted. However, the Chinese have a concept that the buttocks are not susceptible to cold, so this is not a common practice.

facilitates defecation (Stadler, 1989). Another option is a portable seat attached to the regular toilet, which may ease the transition from potty chair to regular toilet. Placing a small bench under the feet helps to stabilize the child's position (Fig. 14-4). It is probably best to keep the potty in the bathroom and to let the child observe the excreta being flushed down the toilet to associate these activities with usual practices. If a potty chair is not available, having the child sit *facing* the toilet tank provides added support (Fig. 14-5). Practice sessions should be limited to 5 or 10 minutes, and a parent should stay with the child, practicing sanitary habits after every session. Children should be praised for cooperative behavior and/or successful evacuation. Dressing children in easily removed clothing; using training pants, "pull-on" diapers, or panties; and encouraging imitation by watching others are other helpful suggestions. Forcing children to sit on the potty for long periods, spanking them for having accidents, and other methods of negative control are avoided.

Parents need to give clear instructions to toddlers to encourage elimination. For example, one mother used the phrase "Put pee in potty," when the child sat on the toilet. Several hours later, the child brought the potty to the mother with plastic letters of *P* in it. Also, it may be helpful to stress to children that when they feel the urge to eliminate, they have time to get to the toilet and then urinate or defecate. The entire process of elimination is new to toddlers, and relationships between body functions and habits that adults take for granted may not be clear to children. (See also Fears, Chapter 15.)

Bowel training is usually accomplished before bladder training because of its greater regularity and predictability; however, training may also begin with voiding. There is a stronger sensation for defecation than urination, and the sensation of defecation can be brought to the child's attention. In fact, nighttime bladder training may not be completed until 4 or 5 years of age, and even later training is normal (Fergusson, Horwood, and Shannon, 1986). Limiting fluid intake before the children's hour of sleep and waking them once around midnight may help decrease the incidence of bed-wetting but do not teach voluntary control. Boys may begin toilet training in the stand-up position or by sitting on a potty chair or toilet. Imitating other males is a powerful motivating force.

Daytime accidents are also common, particularly during periods of intense activity. Young children become so engrossed in play activity that if they are not reminded, they will wait until it is too late to reach the bathroom.

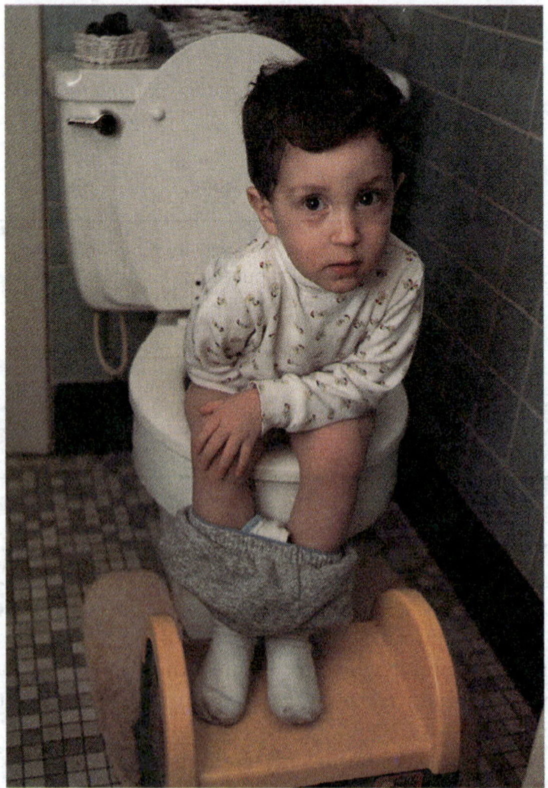

FIG. 14-4 Boys may begin toilet training sitting on a toilet. Note feet on small bench.

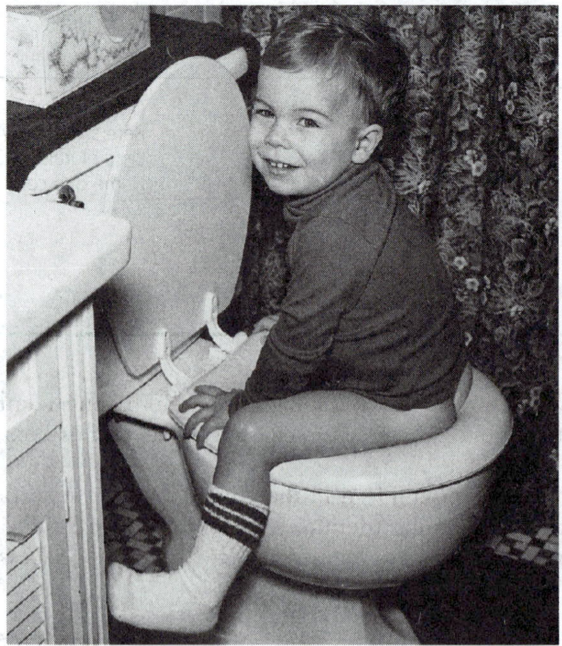

FIG. 14-5 Sitting in reverse fashion on a regular toilet provides additional security to a young child.

Sibling Rivalry

The term ***sibling rivalry*** refers to the natural jealousy and resentment of children to a new child in the family. It typically involves the arrival of a new infant but may be associated with anyone who joins the family. A common example is the merging of stepfamilies. However, the following discussion focuses on the response to a newborn.

Toddlers do not hate or resent the infant but do resent the changes that this additional sibling brings, especially the separation from mother during the birth. The parents now share their love and attention with someone else, the usual routine is disrupted, and toddlers may lose their crib and/or room—all at a time when they thought they were in control of their world. Sibling rivalry tends to be most pronounced in the firstborn, who experiences "dethronement" (loss of sole parental attention). It also seems to be most difficult for young children, particularly in terms of mother-child interaction.

Preparation of children for the birth of a sibling is quite individual, but age dictates some important considerations. Time for toddlers is a vague concept. Preparing children too soon for the birth may lessen their interest by the time the event occurs. A good time to start talking about the new baby is when toddlers become aware of the pregnancy and the changes taking place in the home in anticipation of the new member. Jealousy can develop from feeling left out, and since fantasy dictates reality, fear of the unknown can lead to fear of abandonment, separation anxiety, and insecurity. To avoid additional stresses when the newborn arrives, anticipated changes, such as moving the toddler to a different room or bed, should be done well in advance of the birth.

Toddlers need to have a realistic idea of what the newborn will be like. Telling them that a new playmate will come home soon sets up unrealistic expectations. Rather, parents should stress the activities that will take place when the baby arrives home, such as diapering, bottle- or breast-feeding, bathing, and dressing. At the same time, parents should emphasize which routines will stay the same, such as reading stories or going to the park. If toddlers have had no contact with an infant, it is a good idea to introduce them to one, if feasible. Providing a doll on which toddlers can imitate parental behaviors is another excellent strategy. They can tend to the doll's needs (diapering, feeding) at the same time the parent is performing similar activities for the infant (Fig. 14-6).

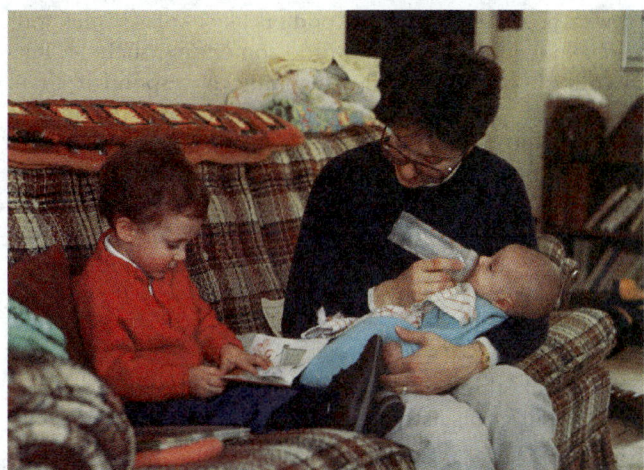

FIG. 14-6 To minimize sibling rivalry, parents should include the toddler during caregiving activities.

Pregnancy is an abstraction for toddlers. They need concrete illustrations of how the baby is growing inside the mother. It is an excellent opportunity for introducing aspects of reproduction and sexuality. Seeing simple pictures of the uterus and fetus and feeling the fetus move help the child feel involved in the experience. Children also benefit from "siblings" classes that may be part of prenatal sessions. They learn about the characteristics of infants and are taught simple tasks of caring for the new baby (Honig, 1986; MacLaughlin and Johnston, 1984; Spadt, Martin, and Thomas, 1990). There is some evidence that participation in a sibling preparation class can decrease sibling rivalry behaviors and help mothers cope better with their children's behaviors (Fortier and others, 1991). Books can also help children prepare for birth and cope with sibling rivalry (Grossman, 1982; Honig, 1986).* (See also Sources of Books for Bibliotherapy at the end of Chapter 6.)

When the new baby arrives, toddlers sense the changed focus of attention. Visitors may initiate problems when they inadvertently favor the infant with attention and presents while neglecting the older child. Parents can minimize this by alerting visitors to the toddler's needs, having small presents on hand for the toddler, and including the child in the visit as much as possible.

How children exhibit jealousy is complex. Some will overtly hit the infant, push the child off the parent's lap, or pull the bottle or breast from the infant's mouth. More often the expressions of hostility and resentment are much more subtle and covert. Toddlers may verbally express a wish that the infant "go back inside mommy," or they will revert to more infantile forms of behavior, such as demanding a bottle, soiling their diaper, clinging for attention, using baby talk, or aggressively acting out toward others. The latter is particularly common in preschoolers who may seem accepting of the new sibling at home but behave poorly in daycare or preschool. This is a form of displacement that says, "I can't let my parents know how I feel, so I will tell you." Encouraging parents to explore how their older child is acting with other caregivers is an important aspect of intervention.

Regardless of how well adjusted and accepting toddlers or preschoolers appear, infants must be protected by supervising the interaction between siblings. Other safety considerations are "baby proofing" the house and instructing children regarding the dangers of small, sharp, or pointed objects to infants. Crib rails should be kept fully raised and the mattress lowered to discourage toddlers from picking up the infant. Infant seats or bassinets should be placed on the floor so that young children cannot pull them off a

*Another excellent book is *The New Baby* by Fred Rogers (1985, GP Putnam's Sons).

raised surface "to see the baby" (MacLaughlin and Johnston, 1984).

The first few weeks at home with a newborn and toddler can be challenging for parents. Assuring them that this period will pass, that the toddler will learn to accept the changes in life-style, and that the newborn will sleep through the night is part of the intervention. Allowing parents to talk about their feelings of ambivalence and frustration and suggesting ways of dealing with the sibling jealousy help all members of the family with this experience. Indeed, sibling rivalry is so common regardless of the children's ages that it is a part of family life. Suggestions, such as spending time with each child, letting children settle their arguments, and accepting angry feelings while teaching children appropriate ways to express hostility, are general guidelines for dealing with the eventual conflicts between brothers and sisters.

Temper Tantrums

As toddlers strive for autonomy, they are confronted with many obstacles, such as the physical inability to complete a task (e.g., attempting to build a tower of blocks) or imposed rules or demands that interfere with their activity (e.g., time to go to sleep after listening to one story). Fatigue may simply lower a child's tolerance to frustration.

As the frustration builds, children may "explode" with activity to release their tension. Typically they may lie down on the floor, kick their feet, and scream. Head-banging, head-rolling, and breath-holding are other behaviors some children use. Although these mannerisms are very disturbing to observe, they usually do not become behavior problems or indicate behaviorally difficult children (Abe, Oda, and Amatomi, 1984; DiMario and Burleson, 1993). Parents should be told that breath-holding and fainting from lack of oxygen cause no physical harm because the accumulation of carbon dioxide stimulates the respiratory control center to initiate breathing. However, head-banging may cause injury, and the child requires protection, such as being held or being placed in a protected environment.

The best approach toward extinguishing attention-seeking behavior is to ignore it (no verbal or eye contact with the child), provided the behavior is not inflicting injury. The parent should remain close by and after the tantrum has subsided offer a toy or a favorite activity to substitute for the ungranted request and to reward the posttantrum behavior. When tantrums occur because the child refuses to comply, the parent can ignore it for a few minutes but may have to physically carry the child if the request must be met, such as getting in the car or going to bed (Schmitt, 1989).

When tantrums do occur, it is important for parents to intervene *immediately* to prevent their buildup of angry feelings and the inability to calmly ignore the behavior. Frequently temper tantrums can be avoided by using an approach for minimizing misbehavior, such as time-out (see Limit-Setting and Discipline, Chapter 3).*

Temper tantrums are common during the toddler years and essentially represent normal developmental behaviors. However, temper tantrums can be signs of serious problems. Nurses should be alert to situations that require further evaluation (see Guidelines box).

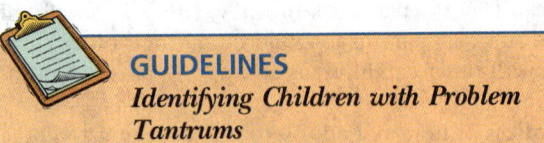

GUIDELINES
Identifying Children with Problem Tantrums

- Parents express concern; feel angry, sad, and helpless; and/or report nothing positive about the child.
- Child is younger than 1 year or older than 4 years.
- Tantrums occur regularly in school.
- Tantrums are associated with aggressive, violent behavior.
- There is a history of other concerns, such as sleep disorders, food refusal, or extreme difficulty with separation.
- Child displays unusual flirtatiousness or extreme modesty (suggests possible sexual abuse).

Modified from Needlman R, Howard B, Zuckerman B: Temper tantrums: when to worry, *Contemp Pediatr* 6(8):12-14, 1989.

Negativism

One of the more difficult aspects of rearing toddlers is related to their persistent negative "no" response to every request. The negativism is not an expression of being stubborn or disrespectful, but a necessary assertion of control. One method of dealing with the negativism is by reducing the opportunities for a "no" answer. Asking the child, "Do you want to go to sleep now?" is almost certain to be met with an emphatic "no." A more appropriate approach is to tell the child when it will be time to go to sleep (preferably within a specific time frame, such as "after reading a story") and proceed accordingly.

In their attempt to exert control, children like to make choices. When confronted with appropriate choices, such as, "You can have a peanut butter and jelly sandwich or chicken noodle soup for lunch," they are more likely to choose one than automatically say no. However, if their response is negative, parents should make the choice for the child. Many of the suggestions for preventing misbehavior in Chapter 3 also help minimize negativism.

Other strategies may also be effective in avoiding or dealing with negative responses. Toddlers like to play games and be challenged. When asked to do something, such as "Put on your shoes," the toddler may quickly respond if challenged with, "I bet I can put my shoes on first." An important rule is to let the child win. Another approach is to use humor, which can get the task done and defuse anger or frustration. If the child refuses to put on the shoes, a humorous response is for the adult to try to squeeze his or her foot in the shoe. Hopefully, the game will end with the child proclaiming, "No, my shoes," and putting them on.

Coping with Stress

Adults rarely think of young children as being exposed to stress or suffering its consequences. However, the normal

*A helpful brochure is *Temper Tantrums: A Normal Part of Growing Up,* available from the American Academy of Pediatrics, 141 Northwest Point Blvd., P.O. Box 927, Elk Grove Village, IL, 60009-0927; (800) 433-9016.

demands of growing up coupled with the usual pressures most families experience mean that few, if any, young children are reared stress-free. Small amounts of stress are beneficial during the early years to help children develop effective coping skills. However, excessive stress is destructive, and young children are especially vulnerable because of their limited ability to cope.

To deal with stress in their children's life, parents must be aware of the signs of stress (see box on p. 145) and be able to identify the source. The normal stresses during toddlerhood are listed in the box below. In addition, any number of other stresses may be imposed on children, such as alternate caregiving arrangements, birth of a sibling, marital discord, relocation, or illness. Watching children at play can identify stressors. For example, one child was seen pounding on a doll, yelling "Go away! Go away!" The parent was quick to observe that the child's recent irritability was probably caused by the stress of a new sibling.

The best approach to dealing with stress is prevention—monitoring the amount of stress in children's lives so that levels exceeding their coping ability do not occur. In many instances this is as simple as increasing the child's rest periods to allow for quiet recovery time. Often it involves adequately preparing the child for change, such as daycare or a new sibling. It also requires helping the child cope with stress. Play is an excellent vehicle for releasing anger or frustration, and toys such as drums, play nails and hammer, clay, and playdough provide alternative methods of dissipating anxiety. They also begin to teach socially acceptable ways of dealing with such feelings. Another approach is the use of relaxation and imagery. Even young children can learn to "let their bodies go limp like a rag doll" or "imagine floating on a cloud."

SOURCES OF STRESS IN TODDLERS

Negativism—Does not like to take orders; may be contrary
Regression—Fears losing newly learned skills; may feel helpless
Rigidity—Wants own way; is upset when rituals are disrupted; dislikes interference
Lack of sociability—Engages in solitary or parallel play but is generally disinterested in socializing
Self-centeredness—Believes the world revolves around her or him; does not want to share; seen with arrival of sibling
Separation anxiety —Fears being separated from parent
Stranger anxiety—Fears strangers; is shy
Toilet training—Especially if begun before the child is ready
Bedtime—Dislikes being ordered to bed; may fear bedwetting or separation from parents; may have terrifying dreams
Tantrums—May revert to temper tantrums or destructive behavior; may hit or bite
Security object—May have a security object that if lost or misplaced, leads to great emotional upset
Overdoing—May become overstimulated or overtired
Fears—In particular, may include animals or anything that makes a loud noise
Illness and hospitalization—Source of many stressors: separation, pain, regression, rigidity, fears, and so on

Modified from Kuczen B: *Childhood stress: don't let your child be a victim,* New York, 1982, Delacorte Press, p 15.

Regression is a retreat from a present pattern of functioning to past levels of behavior. It usually occurs in instances of stress, when one attempts to cope by reverting to patterns of behavior that were successful in earlier stages of development. Regression is common in toddlers because almost any additional stress lessens their ability to master present developmental tasks. Any threat to their autonomy, such as illness, hospitalization, separation, or adjustment to a sibling, represents a need to revert to earlier forms of behavior, such as increased dependency; refusal to use the potty chair; temper tantrums; demand for the bottle, stroller, or crib; and loss of newly learned motor, language, social, and cognitive skills.

At first, such regression appears acceptable and comfortable for children, but on closer inspection it becomes evident that the loss of newly acquired achievements is frightening and threatening, since children are aware of their total helplessness in the recent past. Parents, too, become concerned about regressive behavior and frequently in their efforts to deal with it force the child to cope with an additional source of stress—the pressure to live up to expected standards. Brazelton (1992) suggests that these predictable times of regression, or ***touchpoints,*** are an opportunity to prepare parents for the next step in their child's development.

When regression does occur, the best approach is to ignore it, while praising existing patterns of appropriate behavior. The child is saying, "I can't cope with this present stress and accomplish this new skill as well, but I will eventually if given patience and understanding." For this reason it is advisable not to introduce new areas of learning when an additional crisis is present or expected, such as beginning toilet training shortly before a sibling is born or during a brief period of hospitalization.

Fears are very common during this age and include fear of annihilation, going to sleep, animals, and engines (especially the vacuum cleaner), with the greatest fear continuing to be fear of strangers and separation from parents or other usual caregivers. Because fear of strangers and separation begins in infancy, it is discussed in Chapter 12. The other fears often escalate in the preschool period and consequently are discussed in Chapter 15.

PROMOTING OPTIMUM HEALTH DURING TODDLERHOOD

NUTRITION

During the period from 12 to 18 months of age the growth rate slows, resulting in a slight adjustment from the previous caloric requirement of 108 kcal/kg (50 kcal/pound) of body weight during early infancy to 102 kcal/kg (46 kcal/pound) during the next 2 years. Protein requirements also decrease slightly from 2.2 to 1.5 g/kg for infants to 1.2 g/kg for toddlers but are still higher than at succeeding ages to meet the demands of muscle tissue growth (Food and Nutrition Board, 1989). Fluid needs drop from the infant requirement of approximately 140 ml/kg to the toddler requirement of 115 ml/kg. The reduced fluid requirement represents a decrease in the total body water and an increase in fluid within the cells (intracellular fluid).

The requirements for most vitamins and minerals increase slightly during toddlerhood. The need for minerals such as iron, calcium, and phosphorus may be difficult to meet considering the characteristic food habits of children in this age-group. Milk intake, the chief source of calcium and phosphorus, should average 2 to 3 cups a day. More than a quart of milk consumption daily considerably limits the intake of solid foods, resulting in a deficiency of dietary iron, as well as other nutrients. After 2 years of age children can be given skim or low-fat milk to reduce daily total fat to less than 30% of calories, saturated fatty acids to less than 10% of calories, and cholesterol to less than 300 mg (National Cholesterol Education Program, 1992). Other measures to reduce dietary fat include using lean meats, fat-modified products (such as low-fat cheese), and low-fat cooking. Because less fat in children's diet can also mean fewer calories and nutrients, caregivers must know what kinds of food to choose (Sigman-Grant, Zimmerman, and Kris-Etherton, 1993).

At approximately 18 months of age most toddlers manifest this decreased nutritional need and decreased appetite in a phenomenon known as ***physiologic anorexia.*** They become picky, fussy eaters with strong taste preferences. They may eat voraciously one day and almost nothing the next. They are increasingly aware of the nonnutritive function of food: the pleasure of eating, the social aspect of mealtime, and the control of refusing food. They are influenced by factors other than taste when choosing food. If a family member refuses to eat something, children are likely to imitate that response. If the plate is overfilled, they are likely to push it away, overwhelmed by its size. If food does not appear or smell appetizing, they will probably not try it. Conversely, if food is served attractively and referred to in appealing ways, such as calling an apple slice an "apple cookie" or half a hard-boiled egg a "canoe," children will often try new foods. In essence, mealtime is more closely associated with psychologic components than with nutritional ones, and nutritional counseling must address the characteristics of this age-group.

Nutritional Counseling

Eating habits established in the first 2 or 3 years of life tend to have lasting effects on subsequent years. If food is used as a regard or sign of approval, a child may overeat for nonnutritive reasons. If food is forced and mealtime is consistently unpleasant, the usual pleasure associated with eating may not develop. Mealtimes should be enjoyable rather than times for discipline or family arguments. The social aspect of mealtime may be distracting for young children; therefore an earlier feeding hour may be appropriate. Young children are unable to sit through a long meal and become restless and disruptive. This is particularly common when children are brought to the table just after active play. Calling them in 15 minutes before mealtime allows them ample opportunity to get ready for eating while settling down their active minds and bodies.

For some young children, sitting at the table may be more disruptive than functional. Frequent nutritious snacks can replace a meal. "Grazing"—nibbling and snacking—is a good way to ensure proper nutrition, provided appropriate foods are offered. Between-meal snacks can provide significant nutrition, especially calories, protein, carbohydrate, calcium, and vitamin C.

The method of serving food also takes on more importance during this period. Toddlers need to feel control and achievement in their abilities. Giving them large, adult-size portions contributes to their feeling overwhelmed. In general, what is eaten is much more significant than how much is consumed. Serving sizes need to be appropriate for age.

➤ **NURSING TIP** A general guide to the serving size of food is 1 tablespoon of solid food per year of age or one fourth to one third the adult portion size. Use the tablespoon guide for easily measured foods such as vegetables or rice. Use the fraction guide for milk, or bread, or fruit.

It is often a good idea to offer less than toddlers may eat and let the child ask for more. Young children tend to like less spicy, bland foods, although this is a culturally determined preference. Substitutions should be provided for foods that they do not enjoy, but this practice should be used sparingly to avoid catering to all toddlers' eating requests.

The ritualism of this age also dictates certain principles in feeding practices. Toddlers like the same dish, cup, or

SAMPLE MENU FOR TODDLERS BASED ON FOOD GUIDE PYRAMID*

Breakfast	½ cup dry, unsweetened cereal ½ cup orange juice 4 oz low-fat milk
Snack	½-1 whole banana
Lunch	1 tbsp peanut butter 2 tsp all-fruit preserves 1 slice whole-wheat bread 2 tbsp peas 4 oz low-fat milk
Snack	2 graham crackers 4 oz low-fat milk
Dinner	1 chicken leg, roasted without skin ¼-½ cup macaroni and cheese 2 tbsp green beans, cooked 2 tbsp carrots, cooked 4-6 oz low-fat milk
Snack	½ cup frozen yogurt

TOTAL SERVINGS

Bread, cereal, rice, pasta	6-7
Vegetable	3
Fruit	3-4
Milk, yogurt, cheese	2-3
Meat, poultry, fish, dried beans, eggs, nuts	2

*Use fats, oils, and sweets sparingly. Increase fluids with servings of water. Serving sizes are minimums for nutritional adequacy. Many children eat more.

spoon every time they eat. They may reject a favorite food simply because it is served in a different utensil. If one food touches another, they often refuse to eat it. Mixed foods, such as stews or casseroles, are also rarely favorites. Because toddlers are unpredictable in their table manners, it is best to use plastic dishes and cups, both for economic and for safety reasons. For some children a regular mealtime schedule also contributes to their desire and need for predictability and ritualism.

Appetite and food preferences are sporadic during these years. A child may enjoy one food for 3 days in a row and then suddenly refuse to eat it again for days. Such food fads or "jags" do not ensure a well-balanced diet, but attempts to alter them are met with bitter resentment and unwavering obstinancy. It is preferable to accept such extremes and offer other foods in small portions. Generally, the child will choose another "favorite food" that may compensate for the nutritional inadequacy. Introducing at least three items from the groups in the Food Guide Pyramid at each meal helps develop a variety of taste preferences and well-balanced habits. For snacks, several small pieces of food (carrot sticks, cheese blocks, raisins, crackers, sliced cold meat, apple slices) can be placed in an ice cube tray for a pick-and-choose menu. A sample menu for toddlers is given in the box on p. 630.

Developmentally, most children by 12 months of age are eating the same food prepared for the rest of the family. Some may have mastered using a cup with occasional spilling, although most cannot adeptly use a spoon until 18 months of age or later (Table 14-4) and generally prefer using their fingers. Some children find weaning easy and voluntarily relinquish the bottle by the first birthday. Others are unable to give up that pleasure and require a bottle before bedtime or occasionally during the day (Fig. 14-7). Allowing children to give up the bottle when they are ready is preferable to forcing the issue.

Some toddlers reject all solid food in preference for the bottle, a practice that can be discouraged by gradually diluting the milk with water to make it less satisfying and introducing foods at times when the child is most likely to be hungry, such as on awakening. Occasionally it may be necessary to withhold bottle-feedings, as well as other in-between-meal foods and fluids other than water, until the child is hungry enough to eat solid foods. Forcing the child to eat solid foods usually results in conflicts and does little to establish healthy eating habits.

SLEEP AND ACTIVITY

Total sleep decreases only slightly during the second year and averages about 12 hours. Most children take one nap a day, and by the end of the second or third year many relinquish this habit. The activity level is high, and there is rarely a problem with too little physical exercise, provided inappropriate restrictions are not instituted. With increasing numbers of young children being cared for outside the home, attention to the kinds of activity provided is important. For example, children with high activity levels may benefit from an environment in which outdoor play is encouraged.

Sleep problems, especially going to bed and falling asleep, are common and are probably related to fears of separation. Bedtime rituals (same hour of sleep, snack, quiet activity) are helpful, and transitional objects, such as a favorite stuffed animal or blanket, can ease the insecurity at bedtime. For problems that persist, the interventions outlined in Table 12-5 should be employed.

DENTAL HEALTH

Regular Dental Examinations

Ideally the child should see a dentist (or ***pedodontist,*** a pediatric dentist) soon after the first teeth erupt, usually around 1 year of age, and no later than age 18 months (American Academy of Pediatric Dentistry, 1992). During these visits the dentist can begin to develop a relationship

TABLE 14-4 Developmental Milestones Associated with Feeding

AGE (MONTHS)	DEVELOPMENT
12-18	Drools less Drinks well from cup with lid but may drop it when finished Holds cup with both hands Begins to use a spoon but turns it before reaching mouth
24	Can use a straw and a cup Chews food with mouth closed and shifts food in mouth Distinguishes between finger and spoon foods Uses spoon correctly but with some spilling
36	Spills small amount from spoon Begins to use fork; holds it in fist Uses adult pattern of chewing, which involves rotary action of jaw

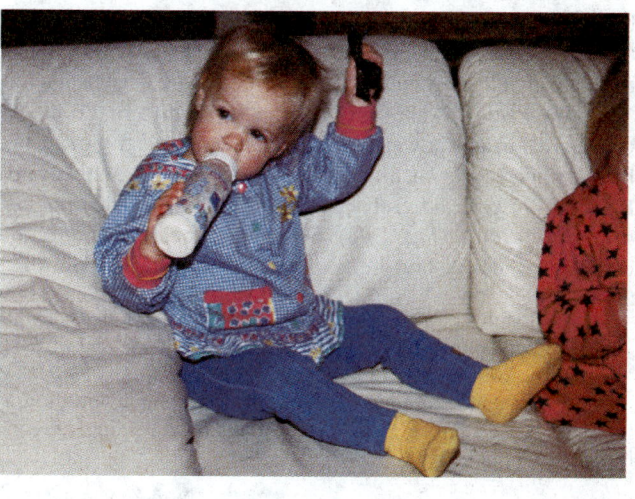

FIG. 14-7 Some children find relinquishing the bottle difficult. Prolonged and frequent bottle feeding can lead to iron deficiency anemia and "bottle-mouth caries."

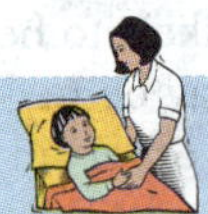

ATRAUMATIC CARE
Dental Visits

Initial visits to the dentist should be nontraumatizing. Because toddlers react negatively to new and potentially frightening experiences, the initial visit can center around meeting the dentist, seeing the equipment, and sitting in the chair. Statements such as "It won't hurt," are avoided because they suggest possible discomfort. If the child is uncooperative, the dentist may just look at the teeth and reserve a more thorough examination for another visit. Modeling can also be effective—the child can observe procedures performed on the parent or a cooperative sibling. This type of conditioning is very important in preparing the child for future experiences.*

*A book to help prepare the child is *When Your Child Goes to the Dentist* by Fred Rogers, available from Family Communications, 4802 Fifth Ave., Pittsburgh, PA 15213; (412) 687-2990.

with the child (see Atraumatic Care box), assess oral health, teach parents correct methods of dental hygiene, and provide nutritional counseling, especially in relation to preventing nursing bottle caries (see p. 634).

Removal of Plaque

The objective of oral hygiene is removal of ***plaque,*** soft bacterial deposits that adhere to the teeth and cause dental ***caries*** (decay) and ***periodontal*** (gum) ***disease.*** The most effective methods for plaque removal are brushing and flossing. Several brushing techniques exist, although there is no universal agreement regarding the best method. One that is suitable for cleaning the primary teeth is the ***scrub method.*** The tips of the bristles are placed firmly at a 45-degree angle against the teeth and gums are moved back and forth in a vibratory motion. The ends of the bristles should be moving gently to avoid damaging the gums and enamel. All the surfaces of the teeth are cleaned in this manner except the lingual (inner or tongue side) surfaces of the front teeth. To clean these surfaces, the toothbrush is placed vertical to the teeth and moved up and down. Only a few teeth are brushed at one time, using six to eight strokes for each section. A systematic approach is used so that all surfaces are thoroughly cleaned.

Young children are only able to brush the mandibular occlusive surface (lower arch, top surface) and the front labial surface (outer or lip side) (Osgasawara, Watanabe, and Kasahara, 1992). Therefore the most effective cleaning is done by parents (Fig. 14-8). Several positions facilitate access to the mouth and help stabilize the head for comfort:

- Stand with child's back toward adult. (When done in front of a bathroom mirror, both child and adult can see what is being done in the mirror.)
- Sit on a couch or bed with child's head resting in adult's lap.
- Sit on the floor or a stool with child's head resting between adult's thighs.

With all positions, one hand is used to cup the chin and the other to brush the teeth.

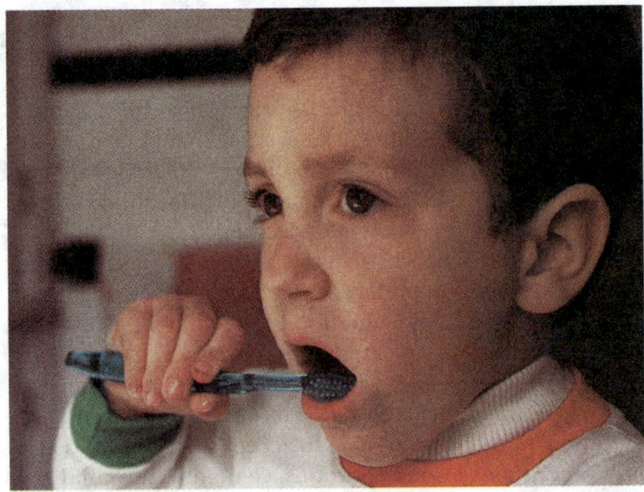

FIG. 14-8 Young children can participate in toothbrushing, but parents need to thoroughly brush all teeth.

➤ **NURSING TIP** To encourage children to open their mouth, ask them to "tweet like a bird" to brush the front teeth and to "roar like a lion" to brush the back teeth. Sing, tell stories, or talk to children during teeth cleaning to prevent boredom.

For effective cleaning, a small toothbrush with soft, rounded, multitufted nylon bristles that are short and uniform in length is recommended. Nylon bristles dry more rapidly after use and retain their shape better than natural bristles. Toothbrushes are replaced as soon as the bristles are frayed or bent. With young children, brushing may be more easily accompanied using only water, since many children dislike the foam from toothpaste and the foam interferes with visibility. There is also the danger of swallowing fluoridated toothpaste (see following discussion under Fluoride). When using toothpaste, children should select the flavor they like to encourage the brushing habit.

After the teeth have been cleaned, flossing removes plaque and debris from between the teeth and below the gum margin where brushing cannot reach. Even if the teeth are widely spaced, flossing is necessary to remove debris below the gum line to prevent ***gingivitis*** (inflammation of the gums). Since young children do not have the dexterity to manipulate the floss, parents are taught the procedure. The type of floss (waxed or unwaxed, fine, and so on) that easily slides between the teeth is chosen. A length of dental floss about 45 cm (18 inches) long can either be tied in a circle or wrapped around the fingers. The circle method may be easier for children to learn. Floss holders are also available and offer the advantage of only one hand being needed for flossing, freeing the other hand to stabilize the child's head.

With about 2.25 cm (1 inch) of floss held tautly against the thumbs, the floss is gently inserted between two teeth, wrapped around the base of the tooth in a C shape, and directed *below* the gingival margin to remove plaque. The floss is then moved toward the occlusal (biting) surface of the tooth to remove plaque between the teeth as well. This

TABLE 14-5 Supplemental Fluoride Dosage Schedule (mg/day*)

AGE	CONCENTRATION OF FLUORIDE IN DRINKING WATER (ppm)		
	<0.3	0.3-0.7	>0.7
2 weeks-2 years	0.25	0	0
2-3 years	0.50	0.25	0
3-16 years	1.00	0.50	0

From American Academy of Pediatrics, Committee on Nutrition: Fluoride supplementation, *Pediatrics* 77(5):758-761, 1986.
*2.2 mg sodium fluoride contains 1 mg fluoride.

sweeping motion is repeated a few times on every tooth surface, using a clean segment of floss.

A disclosing agent used before brushing is helpful in identifying plaque. It also helps motivate children to clean their teeth, because plaque is invisible. After cleaning, the mouth is inspected to ensure that all traces of plaque have been removed. Where plaque remains, the teeth are rebrushed until the red color is gone.

Although it is generally recognized that thorough plaque removal once a day is sufficient, cleaning the teeth more frequently increases the probability of effective cleaning (McDonald and Avery, 1994). Ideally the teeth should be cleaned as soon as possible after each meal and especially before bedtime, and the child should be given nothing to eat or drink except water after the night brushing. At those times when brushing is impractical, the ***swish-and-swallow method*** will remove some debris. With a mouthful of water the child rinses the mouth and swallows, repeating the procedure three or four times.

Fluoride

When adequate amounts of fluoride are ingested before eruption of the teeth and to a lesser extent after tooth eruption, the enamel is more resistant to caries. Fluoride replaces the hydroxyl ion in the calcium hydroxyapatite molecule to form calcium fluorapatite, which alters the crystal of the tooth, making it more resistant to acid solubility. The changes in crystalline structure also affect the anatomy of the tooth—the cusps are shorter and the crevices smaller—thus facilitating plaque removal.

Fluoridation of water is the most cost-effective method of ensuring sufficient intake of the mineral. Before the widespread use of fluoride in beverages, food, dental products, and dietary supplements, children in fluoridated communities experienced about a 60% reduction in caries as compared with youngsters in nonfluoridated communities (fluoride concentration generally below 0.3 ppm). With other fluoride sources available to children living in nonfluoridated areas, this difference has declined to 20% to 40% (Centers for Disease Control, 1991).

In communities where the water fluoride content is below 0.3 to 0.7 ppm, oral fluoride supplements are recommended (Table 14-5). One advantage of supplements is that the child receives a known quantity of fluoride daily. This is in contrast to fluoridated water, where the supply depends on the amount of water consumed. A major disadvantage of supplementation is compliance, cost, and the potential for excessive intake. The supplements are considerably more expensive than community fluoridation, and adhering to a daily administration schedule for 16 years (when the third molar crowns, or "wisdom teeth," are completely calcified) is difficult for many families.

A fluoride dentrifice reduces caries even further when the water supply is fluoridated, because it imparts a topical benefit to the teeth. However, a concern with fluoride toothpaste used in conjunction with other sources of fluoride is excessive flouride ingestion by young children and the possibility of ***fluorosis,*** a condition characterized by an increase in the degree and extent of the enamel's porosity. It can cause staining of the teeth (chalky white to yellow or brown) and, in more severe forms, pitting of the enamel. The prevalence of the moderate to severe form is about 1.3% and is increasing (Centers for Disease Control, 1991). Fluorosis is not a health concern but may be a cosmetic concern for affected children. Fluorosis is directly related to the fluoride dosage and occurs in areas with high levels of natural fluoridation, as well as in unfluoridated areas as a result of ingesting excessive fluoride from additional sources, such as beverages (including bottled water), processed foods, dental products, and supplements. Ingesting excessive fluoride after age 5 or 6 years does not result in fluorosis, because the permanent teeth, except for the third-year molars, are completely calcified.

As a safeguard, the child's use of toothpaste should be supervised to prevent swallowing of excessive amounts. Fluoride rinses, which also offer topical benefits, are not recommended for children under 6 years of age because of the likelihood of their swallowing the liquid (Newbrun, 1992). As with any drug, acute toxicity can occur from ingestion of large quantities of fluoride. A lethal dose for children is estimated to be 32 to 64 mg/kg (Heifetz and Horowitz, 1986). Therefore the same precautions as with any drug must be practiced—store out of reach of children and avoid large supplies in the home (Hess and others, 1984). (See also Guidelines box and Thinking Critically About . . . box, p. 634.)

Low-Cariogenic Diet

Diet is critical to developing good teeth because the carious process depends primarily on fermentable sugars, especially sucrose. Refined table sugar is not the only concentrated sweet food that is cariogenic. Natural foods, including honey, molasses, corn syrup, and dried fruits such as raisins, are highly cariogenic. Complex carbohydrates, such as breads, potato, and pasta, also contribute to caries because they lower the plaque pH (see Dental Disorders, Chapter 18).

Ideally, concentrated sugars and high-carbohydrate snacks should be eliminated. However, since this is impractical, some suggestions can be helpful. The first is that *the frequency with which sugar is consumed is more important than the total amount eaten.* Therefore when sweets are eaten, they are less damaging if consumed immediately after a meal rather than as a snack between meals. When sweets are

GUIDELINES
An Optimum Fluoride Regimen

Base recommendations on the fluoride content of the drinking supply, including bottled or well water, with the exception of breast-feeding infants, who should receive fluoride supplements regardless of the fluoride content of the water supply.

If the water is fluoridated, encourage consumption of tap water either through supplemental feedings to infants or through preparation of concentrated commercial milk-based formula (but not soy formulas, which have a high fluoride content), frozen-concentrated juice, powdered drinks, soup, gelatin, or other foods made with fluoridated water.

If impractical and the child ordinarily drinks little tap water, consider a fluoride supplement; check that dosage is correct.

In areas with excessive fluoride levels, suggest the use of bottled unfluoridated water.

Encourage parents to supervise the young child's toothbrushing, to use a *pea-sized* amount of fluoridated toothpaste or substitute a nonfluoridated brand, and to teach children not to eat toothpaste.

Consider other sources of fluoride in the diet, especially commercial baby food with meat (has high levels from bone particles) and tea.

If the water is unfluoridated, instruct parents in proper administration of supplements:
- Place drops directly on the tongue to allow it to mix with saliva and come in contact with the teeth.
- Encourage older children to chew the tablet and swish it in the mouth for 30 seconds before swallowing.
- Give nothing to eat or drink afterward for 30 minutes.
- Administer supplements on an empty stomach without calcium-rich products, such as milk or formula.

Recommend the daily use of a fluoridated mouthrinse in children 6 years and older and instruct in proper technique:
- Use only the recommended amount.
- Expectorate after a timed 1-minute rinse.
- Avoid food or fluid for 30 minutes afterward.

Advise parents to store fluoridated dentrifices, mouthrinses, and supplements in a safe place away from small children and to keep no more than a 4-month supply of supplements in the home.

Encourage compliance by administering the supplement at the same time each day and posting reminders, such as a fluoride sticker on the bathroom mirror.

Modified from Hess C and others: Fluoride: too much or too little, *Pediatr Nurs* 10(6):397-403, 1984.

served as the dessert, the teeth can be cleaned afterward, decreasing the amount of time the sugar is in the mouth.

The form of sugar is also important. The more cariogenic foods are those that are sticky or hard, since they remain in the mouth longer. Consequently, sucking on lollipops is more cariogenic than eating a chocolate bar.

These suggestions can help parents plan "treats" in a way that is less damaging to the teeth. In addition, parents should be aware of foods that are good snacks and that contribute less to tooth decay (Table 14-6). Some snacks do not contribute to tooth decay and may actually protect against it. Aged cheeses, such as cheddar, may alter the pH and retard bacterial growth. Sugarless gum chewed for about 20 minutes after eating may also protect against cavities by stimulating saliva that neutralizes acid (Jensen and Wefel, 1989). The artificial sweeteners saccharin and aspartame are noncariogenic, and sorbitol has low cariogenic potential (Institute of Food Technologists, 1987).

Likewise, parents should know about hidden sources of sugar, such as numerous prescription and nonprescription drugs, and many popular cereals, including the "all natural" variety (Table 14-7). Reading food labels is *essential* in eliminating sources of sucrose.

A special form of tooth decay in children between 18 months and 3 years of age is ***nursing caries*** (also called ***nursing bottle caries*** or ***bottle-mouth caries***), which occurs when the child is placed in the crib or bed with a bottle of milk, juice, soda pop, or sweetened water at nap or bedtime, or uses the bottle as a pacifier while awake. Frequent nocturnal breast-feeding for prolonged periods also leads to extensive destruction of the teeth (Ripa, 1988). The practice of coating pacifiers in honey can also contribute to caries and may be a potential source of botulism poisoning. Other factors that may contribute to nursing caries include sleep difficulties, a strong-tempered child, single parenting, and less fluoride supplementation or professional counseling (Marino and others, 1989). As the sweet liquid pools in the mouth, the teeth are bathed for several hours in this cariogenic environment. The maxillary (upper) incisors and sometimes molars are affected most, since the mandibular (lower) teeth are thought to be protected by the lower lip, tongue, and saliva (Fig. 14-9). Severely decayed teeth may require

THINKING CRITICALLY ABOUT . . . *Fluoride*

Sources of fluoride include drinking water, dietary supplements, toothpastes, mouthrinses, and professional application. Only about 61% of the population in the United States on central water systems receive optimally fluoridated drinking water (Fluoridation, 1992). The areas least likely to have fluoridated community water systems include rural areas, where the supply may be well water, and the western United States. Only about 15% of children under 2 years of age in 1989 were receiving fluoride supplements, but children living in the West were most likely to receive them (Wagener, Nourjah, and Horowitz, 1992). Two of the objectives named in a report by the U.S. Public Health Service (Healthy people 2000, 1991) were to raise the proportion of people served by optimally fluoridated community water systems to 75% and the proportion of children receiving dietary fluoride supplements but not optimally fluoridated water to 85%.

For these objectives to be met, all health professionals, including nurses, must take an active role in educating the public and ensuring that supplements are used correctly. How knowledgeable are you? Do you know the fluoride content of your local water supply, including well water? Do you know how to obtain this information? In many areas water analysis results can be obtained from dental schools. Do you see the guidelines above being practiced? Are dosages of dietary supplements increased at 2 and 3 years of age and continued until 16 years of age? Are there school fluoridation programs? If the needs of your community are not being met, what strategies could you use?

TABLE 14-6 Lower-Cariogenic Snack Foods

GOOD SNACKS EATEN ALONE	SNACKS BETTER SERVED WITH MEALS
BREADS AND CEREALS	
Popcorn and other seeds	Breads and cereals, pasta, crackers, potato products, pretzels, all sweet baked goods
FRUIT AND VEGETABLES	
All raw, fresh, frozen, or waterpack fruits or vegetables or their juices prepared without addition of sugars*	All items prepared or used with the addition of sugars,* dried fruits such as raisins, catsup, gelatin
MEATS	
Meat of all kinds, including luncheon meats, leftovers, and smoked meat; nuts, peanuts, peanut butter*; bean dips*	Meats prepared with sugars,* candy-coated nuts
DAIRY PRODUCTS	
Milk—whole, low-fat, skim, or buttermilk; cheese, especially cheddar; plain yogurt; dips and spreads*; flavored drinks*; hard boiled eggs	Chocolate milk, malts, shakes, cocoa, ice cream, ice milk, sherbet, other dairy desserts, flavored yogurt

*Check labels for added sugars. Look for (cane, maple, brown) sugar (sucrose), molasses, invert sugar, honey, dextrose (glucose), (modified) corn (sugar, syrup, sweetener, solids), lactose, levulose (fructose), and carob.

TABLE 14-7 Sucrose Content of Selected Cereals

CEREAL (1-OUNCE SERVING)	SUCROSE (GRAMS/1-OUNCE SERVING)
Shredded Wheat	0
Cheerios	1
Cornflakes	2
Total	3
Rice Krispies	3
Raisin Bran (Post)	7
Kellogg's Low-Fat Granola	8
Quaker 100% Natural Cereal	9
Honey Nut Cheerios	10
Frosted Rice	11
Frosted Flakes	12
Froot Loops	13
Apple Jacks	14
Honey Smacks	15
Raisin Bran (Kellogg)	19

the application of stainless steel crowns, with or without white fronts, to preserve the spacing until the permanent teeth erupt.

Prevention involves eliminating the bedtime bottle completely, feeding the last bottle before bedtime, substituting a bottle of water for sweet liquids, not using the bottle as a pacifier, and never coating pacifiers in sweet substances. Juice in bottles, especially commercially available ready-to-use bottles, is discouraged, since the beverage is especially damaging because the sugar is more readily converted to acid. Juice should always be offered in a cup in order to avoid prolonging the bottle-feeding habit.

Nurses are in an excellent position to counsel parents regarding this habit, especially if it occurs during a hospitalization. Although the child may need the comfort of the bottle at this stressful time, parents can be shown photographs depicting the typical tooth destruction and given literature about the condition.* Over an extended hospital stay children can be gradually weaned from the bedtime bottle or given a bottle of water. Health professionals should never contribute to the habit by propping bottles for convenience during feedings. Nurses in clinics or offices should look for children with "companion" or "pacifier" bottles, because these youngsters tend to sleep with their bottle (Kovesi and Levison, 1992).

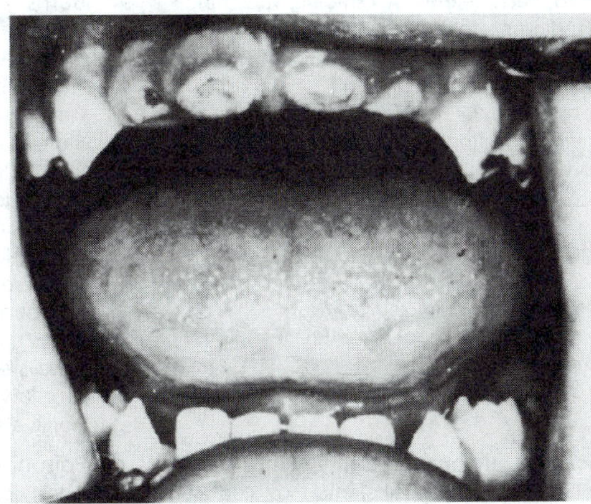

FIG. 14-9 Nursing caries. Note extensive carious involvement of maxillary primary incisors. (From McDonald RE, Avery DR: *Dentistry for the child and adolescent,* ed 6, St Louis, 1994, Mosby.)

INJURY PREVENTION

Injuries cause more deaths in the age-group 4 years and younger than in any other childhood period except adolescence. In addition, the injury death rate has remained relatively unchanged during the past decade, whereas the corresponding rates from all other causes of death combined have declined significantly. Injury's prominence as the leading cause of death among toddlers and preschoolers underscores the need to emphasize safety awareness among parents and other caregivers, such as personnel in alternative

*Sources of information about nursing bottle caries and other aspects of child dental health include **National Institute of Dental Research,** Westwood Building, 5333 Westbard Ave., Bethesda, MD 20816, (301) 496-2883; **American Society of Dentistry for Children,** 211 E. Chicago Ave., Suite 1036, Chicago, IL 60611, (312) 337-2169 or (800) 544-2174 (outside Illinois); **American Dental Association,** 211 E. Chicago Ave., Chicago, IL 60611, (312) 440-2593 or (800) 621-8099 (outside Illinois); and **Canadian Dental Association,** 1815 Alta Vista Dr., Ottawa, Ontario K1G 3Y6, (613) 523-1770. Guidelines for children's dental care are available in *Wong and Whaley's Clinical Manual of Pediatric Nursing* (Mosby).

TABLE 14-8 Injury Prevention During Early Childhood

DEVELOPMENTAL ABILITIES RELATED TO RISK OF INJURY	INJURY PREVENTION
Walks, runs, and climbs Able to open doors and gates Can ride tricycle Can throw ball and other objects	**Motor vehicles** Use federally approved car restraint; if restraint is not available, use lap belt Supervise child while playing outside Do not allow child to play on curb or behind a parked car Do not permit child to play in pile of leaves, snow, or large cardboard container in trafficked area Supervise tricycle riding Lock fences and doors if not directly supervising children Teach child to obey pedestrian safety rules Obey traffic regulations; walk only at crosswalks and when traffic signal indicates it is safe to cross Stand back a step from curb until it is time to cross Look left, right, and left again and check for turning cars before crossing street Use sidewalks; when there is no sidewalk, walk on left, facing traffic Wear light colors at night, and attach fluorescent material to clothing
Able to explore if left unsupervised Has great curiosity Helpless in water; unaware of its danger; depth of water has no significance	**Drowning** Supervise closely when near any source of water, including buckets Keep bathroom doors and lid on toilet closed Have fence around swimming pool and lock gate Teach swimming and water safety (not a substitute for protection)
Able to reach heights by climbing, stretching, standing on toes, and using objects as a ladder Pulls objects Explores any holes or opening Can open drawers and closets Unaware of potential sources of heat or fire Plays with mechanical objects	**Burns** Turn pot handles toward back of stove Place electric appliances, such as coffee maker, frying pan, and popcorn machine, toward back of counter Place guardrails in front of radiators, fireplaces, or other heating elements Store matches and cigarette lighters in locked or inaccessible area; discard carefully Place burning candles, incense, hot foods, ashes, embers, and cigarettes out of reach Do not let tablecloth hang within child's reach Do not let electric cord from iron or other appliance hang within child's reach Cover electrical outlets with protective devices Keep electrical wires hidden or out of reach Do not allow child to play with electrical appliance, wires, or lighters Stress danger of open flames; teach what "hot" means Always check bathwater temperature; adjust hot-water heater temperature to 120° F or lower; do not allow children to play with faucets Apply a sunscreen with SPF 15 or higher when child is exposed to sunlight
Explores by putting objects in mouth Can open drawers, closets, and most containers Climbs Cannot read warning labels Does not know safe dose or amount	**Poisoning** Place all potentially toxic agents in a locked cabinet or out of reach (including plants) Replace medications and poisons immediately; replace child-resistant caps properly Refer to medications as drugs, not as candy Do not store large surplus of toxic agents Promptly discard empty poison containers; never reuse to store a food item or other poison Teach child not to play in trash containers Never remove labels from containers of toxic substances Have syrup of ipecac in home; use only if advised Know number and location of nearest poison control center (usually listed in front of telephone directory)
Able to open doors and some windows Goes up and down stairs Depth perception unrefined	**Falls** Keep screen in window, nail securely, and use guardrail Place gates at top and bottom of stairs Keep doors locked or use child resistant doorknob covers at entry to stairs, high porch, or other elevated area, such as laundry chute Remove unsecured or scatter rugs Apply nonskid mat in bathtub or shower Keep crib rails fully raised and mattress at lowest level Place carpeting under crib and in bathroom Keep large toys and bumper pads out of crib or playpen (child can use these as "stairs" to climb out), then move to youth bed when child is able to crawl out of crib Avoid using walkers, especially near stairs Dress in safe clothing (soles that do not "catch" on floor, tied shoelaces, pant legs that do not hang on floor) Keep child restrained in vehicles; never leave unattended in shopping cart or stroller Supervise at playgrounds; select play areas with soft ground cover and safe equipment (see Guidelines box)

TABLE 14-8 Injury Prevention During Early Childhood—cont

DEVELOPMENTAL ABILITIES RELATED TO RISK OF INJURY	INJURY PREVENTION
Puts things in mouth May swallow hard or nonedible pieces of food	**Choking and suffocation** Avoid large, round chunks of meat, such as whole hot dogs (slice lengthwise into short pieces) Avoid fruit with pits, fish with bones, dried beans, hard candy, chewing gum, nuts, popcorn, grapes, marshmallows Choose large, sturdy toys without sharp edges or small removable parts Discard old refrigerators, ovens, and so on; if storing old appliance, remove doors Keep automatic garage door transmitter in inaccessible place Select safe toy boxes or chests without heavy, hinged lids
Still clumsy in many skills Easily distracted from tasks Unaware of potential danger from strangers or other people	**Bodily damage** Avoid giving sharp or pointed objects—such as knives, scissors, or toothpicks—especially when walking or running Do not allow lollipops or similar objects in mouth when walking or running Teach safety precautions (e.g., to carry fork or scissors with pointed end away from face) Store all dangerous tools, garden equipment, and firearms in locked cabinet Be alert to danger of animals, including household pets Use safety glass and decals on large glassed areas, such as sliding glass doors Teach personal safety Teach name, address, and phone number and to ask for help from appropriate people (cashier, security guard, policeman) if lost; have identification on child (sewn in clothes, inside shoe) Avoid personalized clothing in public places Teach child to never go with a stranger Teach child to tell parents if anyone makes child feel uncomfortable in any way Always listen to child's concerns regarding others' behavior Teach child to say "no" when confronted with uncomfortable situations

care settings, such as daycare facilities. Child protection and adult education are key determinants in injury prevention.

A major factor in the increase of injuries during early childhood is the unrestricted freedom achieved through locomotion combined with an unawareness of danger within the environment. Specific categories of injuries and appropriate prevention are best understood by associating them with the major developmental achievements of young children (Table 14-8). The discussions of injuries in Chapters 1 and 12 are also relevant to safety concerns at this age.

GUIDELINES
Playground Safety

- Be certain play equipment has no sharp edges, corners, or projections.
- Make sure that concrete footings are not exposed.
- Examine area for a safe, resilient surface under equipment, such as sand or wood chips, to reduce the impact from a fall.
- Be certain that size of equipment matches child.
- Make sure there are no holes or other places where fingers, arms, legs, and necks could get caught.
  - The incline of a slide should not exceed 30 degrees and should have evenly spaced rungs for climbing and protective "tunnels."
  - S-hooks on swings must be closed.
- Check for litter, broken glass, exposed wires, electrical outlets, or animal excreta.

Motor Vehicle Injuries

Motor vehicle injuries cause more accidental deaths in all pediatric age-groups after age 1 year than any other type of injury or disease and are responsible for almost one half of all accidental deaths among children ages 1 to 4 years. Many of the deaths are caused by injuries within the car when restraints have not been used or have been used improperly. Approved restraints properly installed and applied can reduce the majority of fatalities and injuries (Osberg and Di-Scala, 1992).

Nurses have a responsibility for educating parents regarding the importance of car restraints and their proper use. Five types of restraints are available: (1) infant-only devices, (2) convertible models for both infants and toddlers, (3) boosters, (4) safety belts, and (5) devices for children with special needs (see Chapter 22). Some cars come equipped with seats that convert to car restraints. The infant-type restraints are discussed in Chapter 12; the convertible restraints and boosters are included here.

The ***convertible restraint*** is suitable for infants in the rearward-facing position and for toddlers in the forward-facing position (Fig. 14-10). The transition point for switching to the forward-facing position is defined by the manufacturer but is generally at a body weight of 7.7 to 9 kg (17 to 20 pounds), with the upper weight limit preferred. The restraint consists of a molded hard plastic or metal frame with energy-absorbing padding and a special harness system designed to hold the child firmly in the seat and distribute the forces to body areas that can withstand the impact.

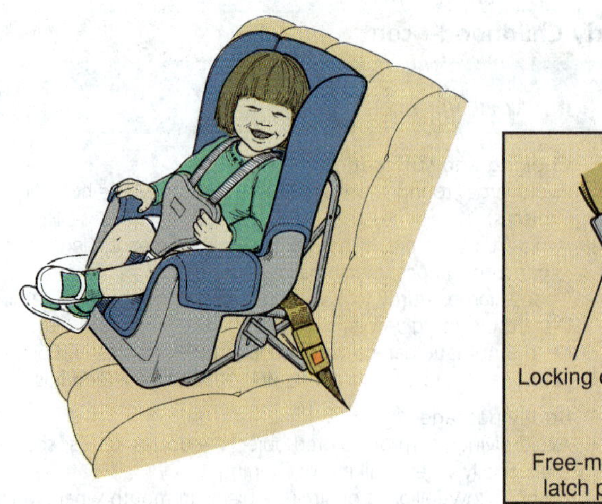

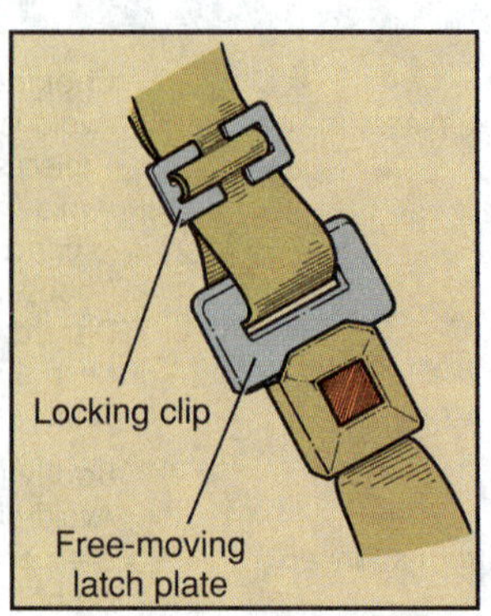

FIG. 14-10 Convertible seat in forward-facing position for older infants and children. *Inset:* Use of locking clip.

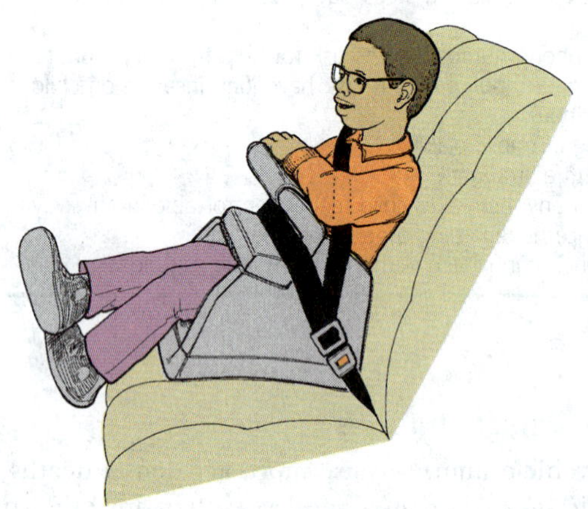

FIG. 14-11 Automobile booster seat. Note placement of shoulder strap (away from neck or face).

Convertible restraints use different types of harness systems: a ***five-point harness*** that consists of a strap over each shoulder, one on each side of the pelvis, and one between the legs (all five come together at a common buckle); a ***padded shield*** that uses shoulder straps attached to a shield that is held in place by a crotch strap; and a ***T-shield*** that has retracting shoulder straps attached to a flat chest shield with a rigid stalk that attaches to a restraint between the legs (Fig. 14-10).

Boosters are not restraint systems like the convertible devices, because they depend on the vehicle belts to hold the child and booster in place. Boosters are of two types: a ***low-shield model*** that primarily uses a lap belt (Fig. 14-11) and a ***belt-positioning model*** that uses a lap/shoulder belt.

Some older model restraints require the use of a top anchor (tether) strap to prevent the child from pitching forward in a crash. If the tether strap is not used, up to 90% of the restraint's protection is lost. Instructions for proper installation of the tether strap and permanent bracket are included with the car restraint. Cars with free-sliding latchplates on the lap/shoulder belt require the use of a metal locking clip to keep the belt in a tight-holding position. The locking clip is threaded onto the belt above the latchplate (see inset, Fig. 14-10). If parents have cars with automatic lap/shoulder belts, they need to have additional lap belts installed to properly secure the restraint.

Children should use car restraints until they have outgrown them. The ***rule of fours*** serves as a guide: if the child either weighs about 40 pounds (18 kg) or is 40 inches (100 cm) tall, then the restraint can be replaced by the car's regular restraint system. Children who outgrow the convertible restraint may still be able to ride safely in a booster seat until the midpoint of the head is higher than the vehicle seat back. If a car safety seat is not available, the lap belt provides more protection than no restraint (except for infants, where there is no safe alternative to approved restraint devices). Shoulder-only automatic belts are designed to protect adults. Children should use the manual shoulder belts in the rear seat. Air bags do not take the place of child safety seats or seat belts (Safety seat guidelines, 1992). The safest area of the car for children is the middle of the back seat.

NURSING ALERT Safety belts should be worn low on the hips, snug, and not on the abdominal area. Children should be taught to sit up straight to allow for proper fit. The shoulder belt is used *only* if it does not cross the child's neck or face.

For any restraint to be effective, it must be used consistently and properly. Examples of misuse include misrouting of the vehicle seat belt through the restraint, failing to use the vehicle seat belt to secure the restraint, failing to use a tether strap, failing to use the restraint's harness system, and incorrectly positioning the child, especially facing infants forward instead of rearward (Bull, Stroup, and Gerhart, 1988; Graham, Kittredge, and Stuemky, 1992). To address these issues, nurses must stress correct use of car restraints and rules that ensure compliance and can emphasize to parents that children riding in car safety seats are

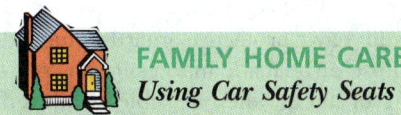

FAMILY HOME CARE
Using Car Safety Seats

Read manufacturer's directions and follow them exactly.
Anchor safety seat securely to car's seat and apply harness snugly to child.
Do not start car until *everyone* is properly restrained.
Always use the restraint, even for short trips.
If child begins to climb out or undo harness, firmly say, "No." It may be necessary to stop the car to reinforce the expected behavior. Use rewards, such as stars or stickers, to encourage cooperative behavior.
Encourage child to help attach buckles, straps, and shields.
Decrease boredom on long trips. Keep special toys in car for quiet play; talk to child; point out objects and teach child about them. Stop periodically. If child wishes to sleep, make sure child stays in restraint.
Insist that others who transport children also follow these safety rules.

generally better behaved than children left unrestrained (see Family Home Care box).*

Injuries may also occur during sudden stops when objects are left unrestrained. On sudden impact, a loose ball becomes a projectile missile. Therefore all items should be secured or stored in the trunk.

Children should never ride in the open back of a truck; the danger of falls can be compounded by another vehicle striking the child. In addition, leaving children unsupervised in a parked vehicle, especially in a private driveway, gives youngsters the opportunity to release the brake or put the car in gear. The child can be injured from a collision or during attempts to jump from the vehicle (Agran, Winn, and Castillo, 1991).

Children over 3 years of age are often involved in pedestrian traffic injuries. Because of their gross motor skills of walking, running, and climbing and their fine motor skills of opening doors and fence gates, they are likely to be in hazardous areas when unsupervised. Unaware of danger and unable to approximate the speed of a car, they are hit by moving vehicles. Running after a ball, playing in a pile of leaves or snow or inside a cardboard box, riding a tricycle, and playing behind a parked car or near the curb are common activities that may result in a vehicular tragedy. A precaution when children are playing in driveways is to attach to the tricycle a pole with a bright flag that is high enough to be visible through an automobile's back window. Another safeguard is the use of a device that beeps when the vehicle is driven in reverse to alert children to the oncoming car, van, or truck.

Preventing vehicular injuries involves protecting and educating children about the danger from moving or parked vehicles. Although preschool children are too young to be trusted to always obey, the parent should emphasize looking for moving vehicles before crossing the street, teach the color of traffic lights for stop and go, and stress the need for following traffic officers signals. Most important, what is preached must be practiced. Children learn through imitation, and consistency reinforces learning.

Drowning

Drowning, not including drowning from water transportation, ranks second among boys and third among girls ages 1 to 4 years as a cause of accidental death. With well-developed skills of locomotion, toddlers are able to reach potentially dangerous areas, such as bathtubs, swimming pools, wading pools, irrigation ditches, post holes, hot tubs, and lakes. Even unlikely sources of water, such as toilets and buckets, are dangerous. As inquisitive toddlers lean over the rim of the receptacle, their large, heavy head, limited strength, and poor coordination make it difficult for them to extricate themselves (Jumbelic and Chambliss, 1990). Therefore water in containers should be removed immediately after use. Toddlers' intense drive for exploration and investigation, combined with an unawareness of the danger of water and their helplessness in water, makes drowning always a threat. Also, death occurs within minutes, diminishing the chance for rescue and survival.

Supervising children when near any source of water is essential; teaching swimming to children under age 4 years does not provide "drown proofing" and may lead to a false sense of security. Four-sided fencing should surround the pool and have a childproof latch. Parents should know cardiopulmonary resuscitation (CPR) and have a telephone and U.S. Coast Guard–approved equipment (life preservers or jackets, or shepherd's crook) at poolside (American Academy of Pediatrics, 1993).

Burns

Burns rank second to motor vehicle injuries among girls and third among boys in this age-group as a cause of accidental death. Toddlers' ability to climb, stretch, and reach objects above their head makes any hot surface a potential source of danger. Scalds from children pulling pots with hot liquids, especially oil and grease, on top of themselves are a major source of burns. As a precaution, pot handles should be turned toward the back of the stove, and electric pots (e.g., coffee maker, frying pan, slow cooker, popcorn maker), including cords, should be placed out of reach. Ideally the knobs for controlling the range burners should be out of reach, not on the front panel where nimble fingers can turn them on and accidentally touch the hot burner. Oven doors should be closed whenever the oven is turned on or when it is cooling. The outside of doors of automatic self-cleaning ovens may become hot and, if touched, could cause a burn. Microwave ovens present much less of a burn hazard to toddlers because the outside remains cool, and they are often inaccessible (Powell and Tanz, 1993).

Other sources of heat, such as radiators, fireplaces, accessible furnaces, kerosene heaters, or wood-burning stoves, should have guards placed in front of them. The tops of some of these heaters are designed to become hot enough to boil water to provide humidity. They are hazardous if touched or if the pan of water is spilled. Portable electric

*More detailed guidelines for car seat safety are available in *Wong and Whaley's Clinical Manual of Pediatric Nursing* (Mosby).

heaters must be placed in a high area, well out of reach of climbing young children.

Hot objects such as candles, incense, hot embers and ashes, cigarettes, pots of tea or coffee, or irons must be placed away from children. The flame of a candle and the smoke of a cigarette invite investigation. Ashtrays with a center well are preferred to prevent the cigarette from falling off the rim, and adults should try not to smoke, cook, or drink hot liquids when children are physically close. If tablecloths are used, the edges should be placed out of reach to prevent injuries from both burns and falling objects. When children are near smoldering fires (campfires, brush fires, fires buried on the beach), wearing shoes can help protect the feet from burns (Riggs and others, 1992).

Flame burns represent one of the most fatal types of burns and commonly occur when children play with matches and accidentally set themselves (and the home) on fire (Fig. 14-12). All matches must be stored safely away from children, and parents need to teach children the dangers of playing with matches. In addition, all homes should have smoke detectors installed to alert the occupants of a fire. A safety plan for immediate escape is also essential.

Electrical burns represent an immediate danger to children. With the ability to manipulate small, thin objects, they are able to insert hairpins or other conductive articles into electrical sockets. Young toddlers may explore outlets and wires by mouthing them. Since water is an excellent conductor, the chance for a severe circumoral electrical burn is great. An unusual electrical burn occurred when a toddler placed a small battery in a wet diaper (Mecrow, 1988).

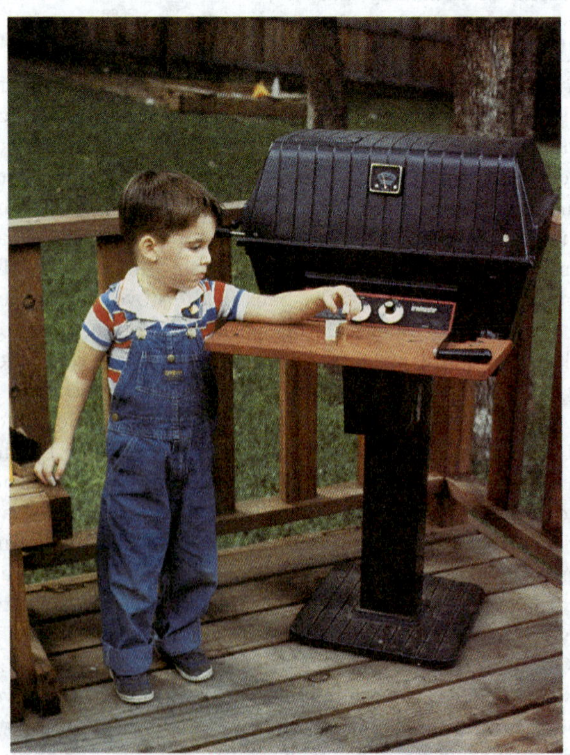

FIG. 14-12 Matches are a potentially deadly hazard for young children.

Electrical outlets should have protective guards plugged into them when not in use or be made inaccessible by placing furniture in front of them when feasible. Children should not be allowed to play with electrical cords, appliances, or batteries, which should be kept out of reach as much as possible.

An example of an appliance that interests children and can present a hazard is an electric popcorn popper. Children can become so excited by the popping that they may inadvertently pull the electric cord and popper off the table, resulting in a burn from contact with the hot oil, corn, or appliance. Steam from a microwaved bag of popcorn (or other foods) can also cause burns.

Scald burns are the most common type of thermal injury in children. A scalding burn is often caused by high-temperature tap water, which children come in contact with either as a result of turning on the hot-water faucet, falling into a bathtub of hot water, or deliberate abuse. Besides the obvious prevention of always supervising youngsters when they are near tap water and checking bathwater temperatures, a recommended passive prevention is to limit household water temperatures to less than 49° C (120° F). At this temperature it takes 10 minutes for exposure to the water to cause a full-thickness burn. Conversely, water temperatures of 54° C (130° F), the usual setting of most water heaters, expose household members to the risk of full-thickness burns within 30 seconds. Nurses can help prevent such burns by advising parents of this common household danger and recommending that they readjust the water heater to a safe temperature. A meat or candy thermometer is a convenient way to measure water temperature. An easy-to-read hot-water gauge that changes color to show water temperatures between 120° and 150° F is available; it shows "hot," "cool," or "OK" water temperature. A special device can also be added to the faucet that reduces the water flow if the set temperature is reached.

Poisoning

Ingestion of toxic agents is common during early childhood. The highest incidence occurs in children in the 2-year-old group. Although in many instances poisoning does not result in mortality, it may cause significant morbidity, such as esophageal stricture from lye ingestion. Mouthing activity increases toddlers' risk of poisoning; exploring objects by tasting them is part of children's curious investigation. Young children's taste is not refined and discriminating. Children under 6 years of age are more likely to eat "disgusting" substances (Rozin and others, 1985). While young children may be able to identify some items as poisonous, they do not understand the toxic effects of ingesting excessive amounts of a familiar drug, such as vitamins. In addition, the apparent safety of such drugs is reinforced by their daily administration (Osborne and Garrettson, 1985). Almost every nonfood substance is potentially harmful, including many house plants, and by 2 years of age toddlers are able to climb most heights, open most drawers or closets, and unscrew most lids. By trial and error younger children also manage to undo tops of bottles, plastic containers, aerosol cans, and jars.

However, they are most likely to ingest substances that are on their level, such as plants, cleaning agents stored under sinks, rat poison, or diaper pail deodorants, especially when stored in the kitchen, bathroom, laundry, or garage. Child-resistant tops are required on some substances, such as prescription drugs, but many young children have opened such "safe" caps. In addition, pharmacists often transfer drugs to regular containers for the elderly, who may have difficulty with child-resistant closures. Newer forms of drugs, such as transdermal patches (Corneli and others, 1989; Reed and Hamburg, 1986) and cough-suppressant lozenges, have created additional dangers, since they are not packaged with safety caps and in the case of lozenges look like candy.

Many potentially toxic substances are not protected with safety caps and must be stored properly. Even common household items, such as mouthwash that contains ethanol (alcohol), can be toxic to young children.

The major reason for poisoning is improper storage (Fig. 14-13). The guidelines suggested in Chapter 12 apply to children in this age-group as well. However, unlike the infant who was unable to reach certain heights or unlatch inventive locks, young children manage to find access to many high-level, tight-security places. For this age-group only a locked cabinet is safe.

Parents should have two doses of ipecac syrup for each child in the home, know its proper use and administration, and have the phone number and location of the nearest poison control center. Emergency and preventive measures for accidental poisoning are discussed in Chapter 16.

Falls

Falls are still a hazard to children in this age-group, although by the later part of early childhood gross and fine motor skills are well developed, decreasing the incidence of falls down stairs or from chairs. However, playground injuries are common (Playground-related injuries, 1988). Children need to be taught safety at play areas, such as no horseplay on high slides or jungle gyms, *sitting* on swings, and staying away from moving swings. Other guidelines for playground safety are listed in the Guidelines box on p. 637).

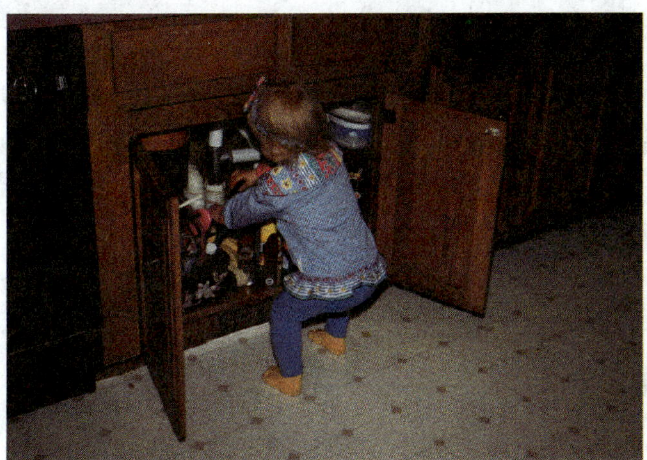

FIG. 14-13 Children are most likely to ingest substances that are on their level, such as cleaning agents stored under sinks, rat poison, plants, or diaper pail deodorants.

The climbing and running activity of the typical toddler is complicated by total neglect for and lack of appreciation of danger, immature coordination, and a high center of gravity. Falling from stairs is a major cause of injury, with more children in this age-group sustaining head injury than older children (Joffe and Ludwig, 1988). Gates must be placed at both ends of stairs. Accessible windows that are left open during warm weather must be screened or guarded with a rail. Falling from open windows is a major cause of accidental death in urban lower socioeconomic groups. Doors leading to stairwells or porches must be locked. A convenient type of lock is a sliding bar or hook that can be attached to the door and frame at a level higher than the child can reach, provided that inventive youngsters do not pull a chair over to unlatch the device.

Another source of falls is from cribs and vehicles. In addition to crib rails being fully raised, the mattress should be kept at the lowest position, and toys or bumper pads that may be used as steps to climb out should be removed. Ideally the floor should be carpeted. Once children reach a height of 89 cm (35 inches), they should sleep in a bed rather than a crib. If a bunk bed is selected, parents should be aware of possible dangers: falls and head entrapment between the mattress and guardrail or between the supporting mattress slats. If the beds are constructed of tubular metal, parents should check for breaks or cracks in the metal and welds, which may lead to collapse and injury (CPSC, 1993). Children who sleep on the top bunk should be 6 years or older.

Children who are unrestrained can fall from high chairs, shopping carts, carriages, and car seats. Therefore proper restraint and adequate supervision are essential.

Clothing can also increase the chance of falling. Slippery shoes or socks, rubber-soled shoes that "catch" on the floor and rug, and loose or cuffed pants can easily make a child fall. Simple safety measures, such as checking clothing and shoes, keeping shoelaces tied with double knots, or using self-adhering closures, can prevent such needless injuries.

Aspiration and Suffocation

Usually by 1 year of age children chew well, but they may have difficulty with large pieces of food such as meat or whole hot dogs and with hard foods such as nuts or dried beans. Young children cannot discard pits from fruit or bones from fish like older children. It takes practice to learn how to chew gum without swallowing it. Therefore the same precautions as discussed for infants regarding food selection must be implemented (see Chapter 12).

Play objects for toddlers must still be chosen with an awareness of the danger of small parts. Large, sturdy toys without sharp edges or removable parts are safest. Coins, paper clips, pull-tabs on cans, thumbtacks, nails, screws, jewelry (especially pierced earrings), and all types of pins are common household objects that can cause significant harm if swallowed or aspirated. Because of the danger of aspiration, parents should be taught emergency procedures for choking (see Airway Obstruction, Chapter 31).*

Another cause of death by traumatic asphyxiation is from electrically operated garage doors. Young children playing in the garage may become trapped under the door. Although the automatic doors should reverse when striking an object, they may not do so when hitting a flexible object or one that is very close to the ground. Precautions include placing controls where they are inaccessible to children, such as high on a wall and in a locked car, and instructing children that the transmitter is not a toy. Periodically the door should be checked to be certain it returns when striking an object.

Suffocation is less frequent from causes seen during infancy but is an ever-present threat from old refrigerators, ovens, and other large appliances. Toddlers can climb inside these appliances and if they close the door behind them will be trapped inside. Discarding old appliances or removing all doors during storage prevents such tragic injuries. Toddlers may also suffocate when toy boxes with heavy, hinged lids accidentally close on their head or neck. Parents should be advised of this danger and encouraged to buy storage chests with lightweight, removable covers.

*Home care instructions on caring for the choking child are available in *Wong and Whaley's Clinical Manual of Pediatric Nursing* (Mosby).

Bodily Damage

Toddlers are still clumsy in many of their skills and can seriously harm themselves when walking while holding a sharp or pointed object or having food or objects such as spoons in their mouths. Preventing such occurrences is the best approach with toddlers. With preschoolers teaching safety is most important. The child should be taught that when walking with a pointed object such as a fork, knife, or scissors, the pointed end is held away from the face. Dangerous garden or workshop equipment and *all firearms* should be stored in a locked cabinet. Power lawn mowers are especially dangerous, and young children should not be allowed in an area where a mower is being used; nor should they be taken for a ride on a mower or allowed to operate the device (American Academy of Pediatrics, 1990). Safety education should include respect for firearms and their proper and appropriate use, including nonpowder guns,

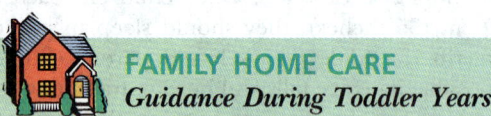

FAMILY HOME CARE
Guidance During Toddler Years

AGES 12 TO 18 MONTHS

Prepare parents for expected behavioral changes of toddler, especially negativism and ritualism.

Assess present feeding habits and encourage gradual weaning from bottle and increased intake of solid foods.

Stress expected feeding changes of physiologic anorexia, presence of food fads and strong taste preferences, need for scheduled routine at mealtimes, inability to sit through an entire meal, and lack of table manners.

Assess sleep patterns at night, particularly habit of a bedtime bottle, which is a major cause of dental caries, and procrastination behaviors that delay hour of sleep.

Prepare parents for potential dangers of the home, particularly motor vehicle, poisoning, and falling injuries; give appropriate suggestions for safeproofing the home.

Discuss need for firm but gentle discipline and ways in which to deal with negativism and temper tantrums; stress positive benefits of appropriate discipline.

Emphasize importance for both child and parents of brief, periodic separations.

Discuss new toys that use developing gross and fine motor, language, cognitive, and social skills.

Emphasize need for dental supervision, types of basic dental hygiene at home, and food habits that predispose to caries; stress importance of supplemental fluoride.

AGES 18 TO 24 MONTHS

Stress importance of peer companionship in play.

Explore need for preparation for additional sibling; stress importance of preparing child for new experiences.

Discuss present discipline methods, their effectiveness, and parents' feelings about child's negativism; stress that negativism is important aspect of developing self-assertion and independence and is not a sign of spoiling.

Discuss signs of readiness for toilet training; emphasize importance of waiting for physical and psychologic readiness.

Discuss development of fears, such as darkness or loud noises, and of habits, such as security blanket or thumb-sucking; stress normalcy of these transient behaviors.

Prepare parents for signs of regression in time of stress.

Assess child's ability to separate easily from parents for brief periods of separation under familiar circumstances.

Allow parents opportunity to express their feelings of weariness, frustration, and exasperation; be aware that it is often difficult to love toddlers at times when they are not asleep!

Point out some of the expected changes of the next year, such as longer attention span, somewhat less negativism, and increased concern for pleasing others.

AGES 24 TO 36 MONTHS

Discuss importance of imitation and domestic mimicry and need to include child in activities.

Discuss approaches toward toilet training, particularly realistic expectations and attitude toward accidents.

Stress uniqueness of toddlers' thought processes, especially through their use of language, poor understanding of time, causal relationships in terms of proximity of events, and inability to see events from another's perspective.

Stress that discipline still must be quite structured and concrete and that relying solely on verbal reasoning and explanation leads to confusion, misunderstanding, and even injuries.

Discuss investigation of preschool or daycare center toward completion of second year.

such as air guns and rifles, which cause serious penetrating injuries (American Academy of Pediatrics, 1987). In addition, the child should be warned of and protected against potential danger from animals (see Bodily Damage, Chapter 12, and Animal Bites, Chapter 18).

Toys can be a source of danger, and safety must be a prime consideration when selecting toys (see Family Home Care box on p. 137). Most toys have age ranges written on them to designate their safety, but this must be tempered with knowledge of the specific child's readiness.

Household safety should be practiced and includes the usual precautions recommended for any age-group (see Family Home Care box on p. 567). An additional safeguard for young children is the use of safety glass in doors, windows, and tabletops and the application of decals on glassed areas to lessen the likelihood of running through glass. Also, children should not be allowed to run, jump, wrestle, or play ball near glass structures (Armstrong and Molyneux, 1992).

ANTICIPATORY GUIDANCE—CARE OF FAMILIES

Understanding toddlers is fundamental to successful childrearing. Nurses, particularly those in ambulatory or child health centers, are in a most favorable position to assist parents in meeting the tasks and needs of children in this age-group. Anticipatory guidance in each of the areas presented in the Family Home Care box can prevent future problems. Advice is sometimes not the sole answer. Actual assistance, such as being available for home visiting or telephone consulting, should be a part of the nurse's flexible repertoire of interventions. Whether parents are experiencing the challenges of rearing a first or a subsequent child, they benefit from sharing their feelings, frustrations, and satisfactions. They need adult companionship, shared childrearing responsibilities, and periodic separations from their children. For single parents such goals can be especially difficult to achieve. Part of a nurse's responsibility is to provide opportunities for parents to express their feelings and meet their emotional and physical needs.

KEY POINTS

- The toddler stage, extending over ages 12 to 36 months, is a period of intense exploration of the environment.
- Biologic development during the toddler years is characterized by the acquisition of fine and gross motor skills that allow children to master a wide variety of activities.
- Although most of the physiologic systems are mature by the end of toddlerhood, development of certain areas of the brain is still occurring, allowing for greater intellectual capacity.
- Locomotion is the major gross motor skill acquired during toddlerhood, followed by increased eye-hand coordination.
- Specific tasks in the psychosocial development of a toddler include differentiating self from others, tolerating separation from parent, coping with delayed gratification, controlling bodily functions, acquiring socially acceptable behavior, verbally communicating, and interacting with others in a less egocentric manner.
- According to Erikson, the major developmental task of toddlerhood is acquiring a sense of autonomy while overcoming a sense of doubt and shame.
- In Piaget's sensorimotor and preconceptual phases of development, the toddler experiments by incorporating the old learning of secondary circular reactions with new skills and applies this knowledge to new situations. There is the beginning of rational judgment, an understanding of causal relationships, and discovery of objects as objects.
- Language is the major cognitive achievement in toddlerhood.
- The most striking characteristic of language development during early childhood is the increasing level of comprehension.
- Preconceptual thought is characterized by centration, global organization of thought processes, animism, and irreversibility.
- Discipline, or a punishment-obedience orientation, aids in children's moral development.
- Development of body image occurs with increasing motor ability, at which point toddlers recognize the importance and capacity of body parts.
- The two phases of differentiation of self from significant others are separation and individuation.
- Parental concerns during the toddler years include toilet training, coping with sibling rivalry, dealing with temper tantrums and negativism, and coping with stress.
- Nutrition is important at this stage because eating habits established in toddlerhood tend to have lasting effects in subsequent years.
- Regular dental examinations, fluoride supplementation, removal of plaque, and provision of a low-cariogenic diet promote optimum dental health.
- Because of increased locomotion, toddlers are at high risk for sustaining injuries. Fatal injuries are primarily the result of motor vehicle accidents, drownings, and burns.

REFERENCES

Abe K, Oda N, Amatomi M: Natural history and predictive significance of head-banging, head-rolling, and breath-holding spells, *Dev Med Child Neurol* 26(5):644-648, 1984.

Agran P, Winn D, Castillo D: Unsupervised children in vehicles: a risk for pediatric trauma, *Pediatrics* 87(1):70-73, 1991.

American Academy of Pediatric Dentistry: *Recommendations for preventive pediatric dental care,* Chicago, The Academy, May 1992.

American Academy of Pediatrics, Committee on Accident and Poison Prevention: Injuries related to "toy" firearms, *Pediatrics* 79(3): 473-474, 1987.

American Academy of Pediatrics, Committee on Accident and Poison Prevention: Ride-on mower injuries in children, *Pediatrics* 86(1): 141-143, 1990.

American Academy of Pediatrics, Committee on Injury and Poison Prevention: Drowning in infants, children, and adolescents, *Pediatrics* 92(2):292-294, 1993.

Armstrong AM, Molyneux E: Glass injuries to children, *Br Med J* 304(6823):360, 1992.

Bloom DA and others: Toilet habits and continence in children: an opportunity sampling in search of normal parameters, *J Urol* 149(5):1087-1090, 1993.

Brazelton TB: *Touchpoints,* Reading, MA, 1992, Addison-Wesley.

Bull MJ, Stroup KB, Gerhart S: Misuse of car safety seats, *Pediatrics* 81(1):98-101, 1988.

Carey WB, McDevitt S: Stability and change in individual temperament diagnoses from infancy to early childhood, *Am Acad Child Psychiatry* 17(2):331-337, 1978.

Centers for Disease Control: Public Health Service report on fluoride benefits and risks, *MMWR* 40(RR-7):1-8, 1991.

Chess S, Thomas A; Temperamental differences: a critical concept in child health care, *Pediatr Nurs* 11(3):167-171, 1985.

Corneli H and others: Toddler eats clonidine patch and nearly quits smoking for life *JAMA* 261:42, 1989, (letter).

SPSC warns that tubular metal bunk beds may collapse, *Safety News,* release No 93-104, US Consumer Product Safety Commission, Washington, DC, Aug 19, 1993.

DiMario FJ, Burleson JA: Behavior profile of children with severe breath-holding spells, *J Pediatr* 122(3):488-491, 1993.

Fergusson DM, Horwood LJ, Shannon FT: Factors related to the age of attainment of nocturnal bladder control: an 8-year longitudinal study, *Pediatrics* 78(5):884-890, 1986.

Fleisher DR, Morrison A: Masturbation mimicking abdominal pain or seizures in young girls, *J Pediatr* 116:810-814, 1990.

Fluoridation of community water systems, *MMWR* 41(21):372-381, 1992.

Food and Nutrition Board, National Research Council: *Recommended Dietary Allowances,* ed 10, Washington, DC, 1989, National Academy Press.

Fortier JC and others: Adjustment to a newborn: sibling preparation makes a difference, *JOGNN* 20(1):73-79, 1991.

Fullard W, McDevitt S, Carey W: Assessing temperament in one- to three-year-old children, *J Pediatr Psychol* 9:205-217, 1984.

Graham CJ, Kittredge O, Stuemky JH: Injuries associated with child safety seat misuse, *Pediatr Emerg Care* 8:351-353, 1992.

Grossman CS: Using children's books to foster acceptance of a new sibling into a one-child family, *Clin Pediatr* 21(8):502, 1982.

Healthy people, 2000—national health promotion and disease prevention objectives, Washington, DC, 1991, US Public Health Service.

Heifetz S, Horowitz H: Amounts of fluoride in self-administered dental products: safety considerations for children, *Pediatrics* 77(6): 876-882, 1986.

Hess CS and others: Fluoride: too much or too little, *Pediatr Nurs* 10(6):397-403, 1984.

Honig JC: Preparing preschool-aged children to be siblings, *MCN* 11(1):37-43, 1986.

Houldin A, Fullard W, Heverly MA: Toddler temperament and quality of child-rearing environment, *Pediatr Nurs* 15(5):491-496, 544, 1989.

The Institute of Food Technologists' Expert Panel on Food Safety and Nutrition: Sweeteners: nutritive and non-nutritive, *Contemp Nutr* 122(9):1-4, 1987.

Jensen ME, Wefel JS: Human plaque pH responses to meals and the effects of chewing gum, *Br Dent J* 167:204-208, 1989.

Joffe M, Ludwig S: Stairway injuries in children, *Pediatrics* 82(3, part 2):457-461, 1988.

Jumbelic MI, Chambliss M: Accidental toddler drowning in 5-gallon buckets, *JAMA* 263: 1952-1953, 1990.

Kovesi T, Levison H: The "companion bottle": a useful predictor of children at risk for the development of nursing bottle caries *Pediatrics* 89(5):976-977, 1992, (letter).

MacLaughlin SM, Johnston KB: The preparation of young children for the birth of a sibling, *J Nurse Midwife* 29(6):371-376, 1984.

Mahler MS, Pine F, Bergman A: *The psychological birth of the human infant: symbiosis and ihndividuation,* New York, 1975, Basic Books.

Marino RV and others: Nursing bottle caries: characteristics of children at risk, *Clin Pediatr* 28(3):129-131, 1989.

McDevitt S, Carey W: Stability of ratings vs. perceptions of temperament from early infancy to 1-3 years, *Am J Orthopsychiatry* 51(2):342-345, 1981.

McDonald RE, Avery DR: *Dentistry for the child and adolescent,* ed. 6, 1994, St Louis, Mosby.

Mecrow IK: Burn to toddler's penis from an electrochemical battery, *Br Med J* 297 (6659):1315, 1988.

National Cholesterol Education Program: Report of the expert panel on blood cholesterol levels in children and adolescents, *Pediatrics* 89(3, pt 2):525-584, 1992.

Newbrun D: Current regulations and recommendations concerning water fluoridation, fluoride supplements, and topical fluoride agents, *J Dent Res* 71(5):1255-1265, 1992.

Ogasawara T, Watanabe T, Kasahara H: Readiness for toothbrushing of young children, *J Dent Child* 59(5):353-359, 1992.

Osberg JS, DiScala C: Morbidity among pediatric motor vehicle crash victims: the effectiveness of seat belts, *Am J Public Health* 82(3):422-425, 1992.

Osborne S, Garrettson L: Perception of toxicity and dose by 3- and 4-year-old children, *Am J Dis Child* 139(8):790-792, 1985.

Playground-related injuries in preschool-aged children—United States, 1983-1987, *MMWR* 37(41):629, 1988.

Powell EC, Tanz RR: Comparison of childhood burns associated with use of microwave ovens and conventional stoves, *Pediatrics* 91(2):344-349, 1993.

Reed M, Hamburg E: Person-to-person transfer of transdermal drug-delivery systems: a case report *N Engl J Med* 314:1120-1121, 1986, (letter).

Riggs D and others: Hot embers and ashes as sources of burns in children, *Am J Dis Child* 146(6):657-658, 1992.

Ripa LW: Nursing caries: a comprehensive review, *Pediatr Dent* 10(4):268-282, 1988.

Rozin P and others: Children's concept of food; the development of contamination sensitivity to disgusting substances, *Dev Psychol* 21(6):1075-1079, 1985.

Safety seat guidelines, *AAP News* 8(12):19, 1992.

Schmitt BD: Parents' guide to behavior problems: how to deal with temper tantrums, *Contemp Pediatr* 6(8):39-40, 1989.

Schuster CS, Ashburn SS: *The process of human development: a holistic approach,* ed 2, Boston, 1986, Little, Brown.

Sigman-Grant M, Simmerman S, Kris-Etherton P: Dietary approaches for reducing fat intake of preschool-age children, *Pediatrics* 91(5):955-960, 1993.

Spadt SK, Martin KR, Thomas AM: Experiential classes for siblings-to-be, *MCN* 15:184-186, 1990.

Stadtler AC: Preventing encopresis, *Pediatr Nurs* 15(3):282-284, 1989.

Thomas RM: *Comparing theories of child development,* ed 2, Belmont, CA, 1985, Wadsworth.

Wagener DK, Nourjah P, Horowitz A: *Trends in childhood use of dental care products containing fluoride: United States, 1983-89.* Advance data from vital and health statistics; No 219, Hyattsville, MD, 1992, National Center for Health Statistics.

Zuckerman BS, Frank DA: Infancy and toddler years. In Levine MD and others, editors: *Developmental-behavioral pediatrics,* ed 2, Philadelphia, 1992, WB Saunders.

BIBLIOGRAPHY

For additional citations relevant to toddlerhood see Chapter 12.

Growth and Development

Ames LB, Ilg FL: *Your two-year old: terrible or tender,* New York, 1979, Delacorte Press.

Dixon SD, Stein MT: *Encounters with children: a practical guide to pediatric behavior and development,* ed 2, St Louis, 1992, Mosby.

Howard BT: Growing together: the toddler years need not be turbulent, *Contemp Pediatr* 7(6):21-40, 1990.

Lamb JM: The rapprochement subphase of the separation-individuation process, *Matern Child Nurs J* 15(3):129-138, 1986.

Larzelere RE, Martin JA, Amberson TG: The toddler behavior checklist: a parent-completed assessment of social-emotional characteristics of young preschoolers, *Fam Relations* 38:418-425, 1989.

Lee J, Fowler MD: Merely child's play? Developmental work and playthings, *J Pediatr Nurs* 1(4):260-270, 1986.

Lincoln LM: Fathering and the separation-individuation process, *Matern Child Nurs J* 13(2):103-111, 1984.

Oberklaid F and others: Assessment of temperament in the toddler age group, *Pediatrics* 85(4):559-566, 1990.

Pontious SL: Practical Piaget: helping children understand, *Am J Nurs* 82(1):114-117, 1982.

Selekman J: The development of body image in the child: a learned response, *Top Clin Nurs* 5(1):12-21, 1983.

Shelly JA and others: *The spiritual needs of children,* Downers Grove, IL, 1982, Inter-Varsity Press.

Toilet Training

The age of mastery: a multi-disciplinary roundtable discussion on toilet training and enuresis, New York, April 14, 1989, Kimberly-Clark.

Berk L, Friman P: Epidemiologic aspects of toilet training, *Clin Pediatr* 29(5):278-282, 1990.

Christophersen ER: Toileting problems in children, *Pediatric Ann* 20(5):240-244, 1991.

Determining reasonable expectations: a multidisciplinary roundtable discussion on special problems in toilet training, New York, April 27, 1990, Kimberly-Clark.

Hauck MR: Mothers' descriptions of the toilet-training process: a phenomenologic study, *J Pediatr Nurs* 6(2):80-86, 1991.

Howe AC, Walker CE: Behavioral management of toilet training, enuresis, and encopresis, *Pediatr Clin North Am* 39(3):413-432, 1992.

Robson WL, Leung AK: Advising parents on toilet training, *Am Fam Physician* 44(4):1263-1266, 1991.

Sibling Rivalry/Temper Tantrums/Discipline

Bhatia MS and others: Temper tantrums: prevalence and etiology, *Clin Pediatr* 29(6): 311-315, 1990.

Castiglia PT: Temper tantrums, *J Pediatr Health Care* 2(5):267-268, 1988.

Castiglia PT: Sibling rivalry, *J Pediatr Health Care* 3(1):52-54, 1989.

Castiglia PT: Jealousy, *J Pediatr Health Care* 6(4):212-213, 1992.

DiMario Jr FJ: Breath-holding spells in childhood, *Am J Dis Child* 146:125-131, 1992.

Faber A, Mazlish E: *Siblings without rivalry: how to help your children live together so you can live too,* New York, 1987, WW Norton.

Hirsch DLO: Behavior therapy. In Levine MD and others, editors: *Developmental-behavioral pediatrics,* ed 2, Philadelphia, 1992, WB Saunders.

Howard BJ: Discipline in early childhood, *Pediatr Clin North Am* 38(6):1351–1369, 1991.

Ivey CL: Effective discipline: gain without pain, *Contemp Pediatr* 8(5):108-115, 1991.

Leung AK, Fagan JE: Temper tantrums, *Am Fam Physician,* 44(2):559-563, 1991.

Leung AK, Robson LM: Sibling rivalry, *Clin Pediatr* 30(5):314-317, 1991.

Needlman R, Howard B, Zuckerman B: Temper tantrums: when to worry, *Contemp Pediatr* 6(8):12-34, 1989.

Pakula LC: Sibling rivalry, *Pediatr Rev* 13(2):72-73, 1992.

Schmitt BD: Sibling rivalry toward a new baby, *Contemp Pediatr* 7(3):111-112, 1990.

Schmitt BD: The stubborn toddler who just says "No," *Contemp Pediatr* 7(4):71-72, 1990.

Schmitt BD: When your child has breath-holding spells, *Contemp Pediatr* 7(5):103, 1990.

Schmitt BD: The child who bites, *Contemp Pediatr* 8(2):99-100, 1991.

Schmitt BD: When siblings quarrel, *Contemp Pediatr* 8(1):73-74, 1991.

Wilford B, Andrews C: Sibling preparation classes for preschool children, *Matern Child Nurs J* 15(3):171-185, 1986.

Stress

Brailey LJ: Stress experienced by mothers of young children, *Health Care Women Int* 11:347-358, 1990.

Garmezy N, Rutter M, editors: *Stress, coping, and development in children,* Baltimore, 1988, Johns Hopkins University Press.

Grey M, Hayman LL: Assessing stress in children: research and clinical implications, *J Pediatr Nurs* 2(5):316-327, 1987.

Kuczen B: *Childhood stress: don't let your child be a victim,* New York, 1982, Delacorte Press.

Lamontagne LL, Mason KR, Hepworth JT: Effects of relaxation on anxiety in children: implications for coping with stress, *Nurs Res* 34:289-292, 1985.

Medeiros DC, Porter BJ, Welch IO: *Children under stress,* Englewood Cliffs, NJ, 1983, Spectrum Books.

Saunders A, Remsberg B: *The stress-proof child: a loving parent's guide,* New York, 1984, Holt, Rinehart & Winston.

Nutrition

American Academy of Pediatrics, Committee on Nutrition: *Pediatric nutrition handbook,* Elk Grove Village, IL, 1993, The Academy.

Lucas B: Nutrition in childhood. In Mahan LK, Arlin MT: *Krause's food, nutrition, and diet therapy,* ed 8, Philadelphia, 1992, WB Saunders.

McCabe EM: Monitoring the fat and cholesterol intake of children and adolescents, *J Pediatr Health Care* 7(2):61-70, 1993.

Pipes P, Trahms CM: *Nutrition in infancy and childhood,* ed 5, St Louis, 1993, Mosby.

Rosenthal SR, Padron CZ: Nutrition assessment of the young child (two through six years). In Simko MD, Cowell C, Hreha MS: *Practical nutrition: a quick reference for the health care practitioner,* Rockville, MD, 1989, Aspen.

Satter E: Developmental guidelines for feeding infants and young children, *Food Nutr News* 56(4):21-26, 1984.

Satter E: *Child of mine: feeding with love and good sense,* Palo Alto, CA, 1986, Bull.

Satter E: *How to get your kid to eat . . . but not too much,* Palo Alto, CA, 1987, Bull.

Schmitt BD: *When your toddler or preschooler won't eat, Contemp Pediatr* 6(9):127-128, 1989.

Schmitt BD: A commonsense approach to sweets, *Contemp Pediatr* 8(9):63-65, 1991.

Dental Health

Alvarez JO, Navia JM: Nutritional status, tooth eruption, and dental caries: a review, *Am J Clin Nutr* 49:417-426, 1989.

American Academy of Pediatrics, Committee on Nutrition: Fluoride supplementation, *Pediatrics* 77(5):758-761, 1986.

Bullen C and others: Improving children's oral hygiene through parental involvement, *J Dent Child* 55(2):125-128, 1988.

Dawes C: Fluorides: mechanisms of action and recommendations for use, *J Can Dent Assoc* 55(9):721-723, 1989.

Felsenfeld AJ, Roberts MA: A report of fluorosis in the United States secondary to drinking well water, *JAMA* 265(4):486-488, 1991.

Griffen AL, Goepferd SJ: Preventive oral health care for the infant, child, and adolescent, *Pediatr Clin North Am* 38(5):1209-1226, 1991.

Johnsen DC: The role of the pediatrician in identifying and treating dental caries, *Pediatr Clin North Am* 38(5):1173-1181, 1991.

Jones KF, Berg JH: Fluoride supplementation, *Am J Dis Child* 146(12):1488-1491, 1992.

Knowledge of the purpose of community water fluoridation—United States, 1990, *MMWR* 41(49):919-927, 1992.

Kronmiller JE, Nirschl RF: Preventive dentistry for children, *Pediatr Nurs* 11:446-449, 1985.

McDermott R, McCormack K: Nursing caries syndrome: implications for children's health care professionals, *Child Health Care* 15(1): 49-54, 1986.

McGuire S: Fluoride content of bottled water, *N Engl J Med* 321(12), 1989.

Nirschl RF, Kronmiller JE: Evaluating oral health needs in preschool children, *Clin Pediatr* 25(7):358-362, 1986.

Nowak AJ: What pediatricians can do to promote oral health, *Contemp Pediatr* 10(4):90-106, 1993.

Schulte JR, Druyan ME, Hagen JC: Early childhood tooth decay, *Clin Pediatr* 31(12):727-730, 1992.

Sheridan PG: NIDR—40 years of research advances in dental health, *Public Health Rep* 103(5):493-499, 1988.

Simard PL and others: Ingestion of fluoride from dentrifices by children aged 12 to 24 months, *Clin Pediatr* 30(11):614-617, 1991.

Stookey GK: Current thoughts on prudent fluoride use, *Ind Dent Assoc J* 72(3):10-14, 1993.

Injury Prevention

Agran P, Winn D, Dunkle D: Injuries among 4- to 9-year-old restrained motor vehicle occupants by seat location and crash impact site, *Am J Dis Child* 143:1317-1321, 1989.

American Academy of Pediatrics, Committee on Accident and Poison Prevention: *Injury control for children and youth,* Elk Grove Village, IL, 1987, The Academy.

American Academy of Pediatrics, Committee on Injury and Poison Prevention: Children in pickup trucks, *Pediatrics* 88(2):393-394, 1991.

Arneson SW, Triplett JL: Riding with Bucklebear: an automobile safety program for preschoolers, *J Pediatr Nurs* 5(2):115-122, 1990.

Becker PG, Turow J: Earring aspiration and other jewelry hazards, *Pediatrics* 78(3):494-496, 1986.

Bull MJ, Stroup KB, Doll JP: A parent guide: selecting and using car safety seats, *Contemp Pediatr* 7(7):113-118, 1990.

Bull MJ and others: Establishing special needs car seat loan program, *Pediatrics* 85(4):540-547, 1990.

Fuchs S and others: Cervical spine fractures sustained by young children in forward-facing car seats, *Pediatrics* 84(2):348-354, 1989.

Gunnip A and others: Car seats: helping parents do it right! *J Pediatr Health Care* 1:190-195, 1987.

Halpern JS: How safe are child safety seats? *J Emerg Nurs* 16(3, pt 1):151-155, 1990.

Jumbelic MI, Chambliss M: Accidental toddler drowning in 5-gallon buckets, *JAMA* 263:1952-1953, 1990.

Killam P, Smith K: Getting kids into car seats, *MCN* 13(2):124-126, 1988.

Okstein CJ, Odal M, Kelly RW: Odontoid fracture in a child occupying a child restraint seat, *Pediatrics* 82(1):117-121, 1988.

Paulson JA: Seat restraint contamination and cleaning, *Pediatrics* 78(1):113-114, 1986.

Ros SP: Lawn mower injuries in children, *Int Pediatr* 4:59-60, 1989.

Schubert W, Ahrenholz DH, Solem LD: Burns from hot oil and grease: a public health hazard, *J Burn Care Rehabil* 11(6):558-562, 1990.

Swartz MK: Playground safety, *J Pediatr Health Care* 6(3):161-162, 1992.

Tong T: Falls from pickup trucks during childhood, *Am J Dis Child* 143:997-998, 1989.

Tron VA, Baldwin VJ, Pirie GE: Hot tub drownings, *Pediatrics* 75:789-790, 1985.

Wilson M: Injury prevention: protecting the under-6 set, *Contemp Pediatr* 5(5):19-34, 1988.

CHAPTER 15

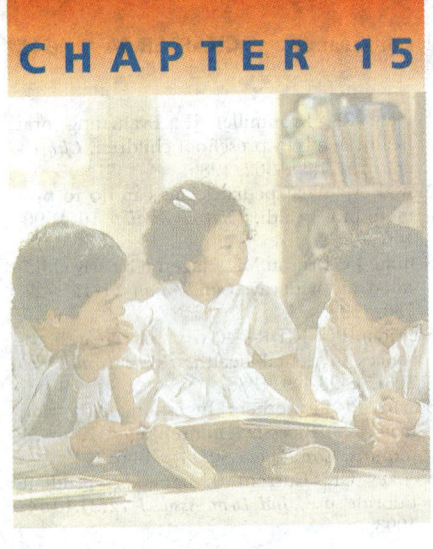

Health Promotion of the Preschooler and Family

CHAPTER OUTLINE

RELATED TOPICS*

Alternate child care arrangements, Ch. 12
Cognitive development, Ch. 14
Dental health, Ch. 14
Drawing, p. 197
Draw-a-Person Test, Ch. 7
Habits (sleep), p. 201
Injury prevention, Ch. 14
Limit-setting and discipline, Ch. 3
School phobia, Ch. 18
Sibling rivalry, Ch. 14
Speech impairment, Ch. 24
Stress in childhood, Ch. 4
Television, Ch. 4
Temper tantrums, Ch. 14
Working mothers, Ch. 3

PROMOTING OPTIMUM GROWTH AND DEVELOPMENT

The combined biologic, psychosocial, cognitive, spiritual, and social achievements during the ***preschool period*** (3 to 5 years of age) prepare preschoolers for their most significant change in lifestyle—entrance into school. Their control of bodily systems, experience of brief and prolonged periods of separation, ability to interact cooperatively with other children and adults, use of language for mental symbolization, and increased attention span and memory ready them for the next major period—the school years. Successful achievement of previous levels of growth and development is essential for preschoolers to refine many of the tasks that were mastered during the toddler years.

BIOLOGIC DEVELOPMENT

The rate of physical growth slows and stabilizes during the preschool years. The average ***weight*** at 3 years is 14.6 kg (32 pounds), at 4 years 16.7 kg (36.75 pounds), and at 5 years 18.7 kg (41.25 pounds). The average weight gain remains about 2.3 kg (5 pounds) per year.

Growth in ***height*** also remains steady at a yearly increase of 6.75 to 7.5 cm (2.5 to 3 inches) and generally occurs in elongation of the legs rather than of the trunk. The aver-

*See also Related Topics in Chapter 14.

age height at 3 years is 95 cm (37.25 inches), at 4 years 103 cm (40.5 inches), and at 5 years 110 cm (43.25 inches).

Physical proportions no longer resemble those of the squat, potbellied toddler. The preschooler is slender but sturdy, graceful, agile, and posturally erect. There is little difference in physical characteristics according to sex, except as dictated by such factors as dress and hairstyle.

Most ***bodily systems*** are mature and stable and can adjust to moderate stress and change. During this period most children are toilet trained. Motor development consists for the most part of increases in strength and refinement of previously learned skills, such as walking, running, and jumping. However, muscle development and bone growth are still far from mature. Excessive activity and overexertion can injure delicate tissues. Good posture, appropriate exercise, and adequate nutrition and rest are essential for optimum development of the musculoskeletal system.

Gross and Fine Motor Behavior

Walking, running, climbing, and jumping are well established by 36 months. Refinement in eye-hand and muscle coordination is evident in several areas. At age 3 the preschooler rides a tricycle, walks on tiptoe, balances on one foot for a few seconds, and broad jumps. By age 4 the child skips and hops proficiently on one foot (Fig. 15-1) and catches a ball reliably. By age 5, the child skips on alternate feet, jumps rope, and begins to skate and swim.

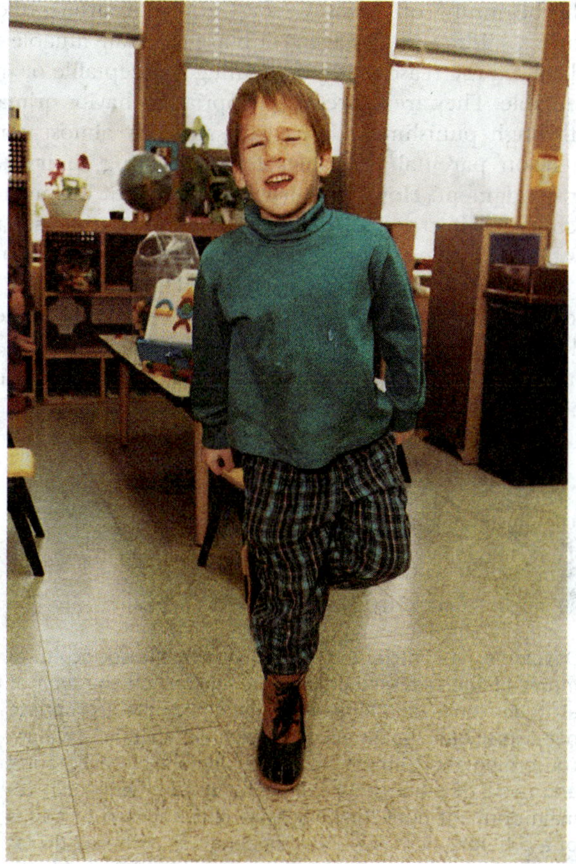

FIG. 15-1 A 4-year-old child has sufficient balance to hop on one foot.

Drawing. Drawing shows several advancements in perception of shape and development of fine muscle coordination. The 3-year-old child copies a circle and imitates a cross and vertical and horizontal lines. The writing instrument is held with the fingers rather than in the fist. The child scribbles or scrawls but names what has been drawn. The 3-year-old is not able to draw a complete stick figure but draws a round circle, later adds facial features, and by age 5 or 6 years can draw several parts (head, arms, legs, body, and facial features). Between 4 and 5 years of age the child can trace a cross and copy a square. The triangle and diamond are usually the last geometric figures to be mastered, sometime between ages 5 and 6.

As children progress from scribbling to picture making, they advance through four distinguishable stages (Kellogg, 1969). In the ***placement stage*** 15-month-old children place their very earliest spontaneous scribblings on the paper in a specific placement pattern, such as in the center, all over, across the lower half, or across the page in a diagonal direction (Fig. 15-2). Approximately 17 different placement patterns appear by age 2 years and once developed are never lost.

By 3 years of age children are in the ***shape stage.*** They draw single-line outline forms, such as rectangles, circles, ovals, crosses, and other odd shapes. As soon as they draw diagrams, they almost immediately progress to the ***design stage,*** in which simple forms are drawn together to make structured designs. When two diagrams are united, the resulting design is called a ***combine.*** Three or more united diagrams produce an ***aggregate.*** Between the ages of 4 and 5 most children enter the ***pictorial stage,*** in which their designs are recognizable as familiar objects. Early pictorial drawings are suggestive of such things as human figures, houses, animals, and trees. Later pictorial drawings are more clearly defined and recognizable; they are not representations of the actual object but esthetically satisfying structures that *resemble* familiar objects. For example, the initial human figure drawing is a circle with arms attached to the head. It is more an aggregate drawing than any attempt to copy a human figure. Drawings of animals follow the human figure drawing but are only a slight modification, such as attaching ears to the top of the head.

Kellogg suggests that uninhibited scribbling and drawing are necessary for children to learn to read and that children who have been free to experiment and produce abstract forms have developed the mental set required for learning symbolic language. Scribbling and drawing also help develop the fine muscle skills and eye-hand coordination eventually required for making precise letters and numbers.

Drawing is also a tool used for assessing intelligence, personality development, and psychosocial adjustment. The precise value of using drawing to measure such concepts is still an inexact science. However, children do reveal thoughts about themselves in their drawings, especially school-age children. It is generally not necessary to have in-depth knowledge of children's drawings to make assumptions about their significance. Being receptive to all the clues, both verbal and nonverbal, is essential in order to un-

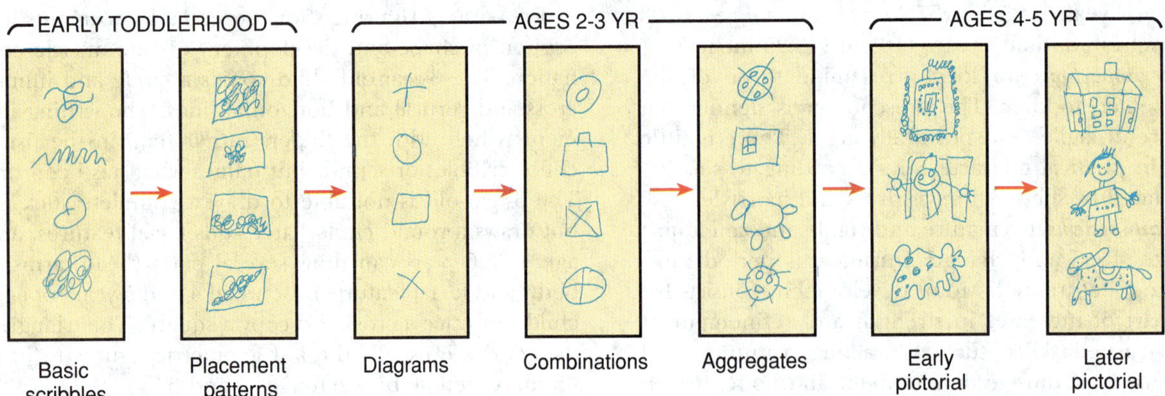

FIG. 15-2 Sequential development in self-taught art. (From Kellogg R: Understanding children's art. In *Readings in Psychology Today*, Del Mar, CA, 1969, Communications/Research/Machine)

derstand how and what children are communicating to others. (See also Cultural Awareness box below and Communication Techniques, Chapter 6.)

PSYCHOSOCIAL DEVELOPMENT

Developing a Sense of Initiative (Erikson)

If preschoolers have mastered the tasks of the toddler period, they are ready to face the developmental endeavors of this stage. Erikson maintains that the chief psychosocial task of the preschool period is acquiring a sense of ***initiative.*** Children are in a stage of energetic learning. They play, work, and live to the fullest and feel a real sense of accomplishment and satisfaction in their activities. Conflict arises when children overstep the limits of their ability and inquiry and experience a sense of ***guilt*** for not having behaved or acted appropriately. Feelings of guilt, anxiety, and fear may also result from thoughts that differ from expected behavior.

A particularly stressful thought is wishing one's parent dead. As a sense of rivalry or competition develops between the same-sex child and parent, the child may think of ways to get rid of the interfering parent. In most situations this contest is resolved when the child strongly identifies with the same-sex parent and peers during the school years. However, if that same-sex parent dies before the identification process is completed, the preschooler can be overwhelmed with feelings of guilt for having wished and therefore causing (in the child's mind) the death. Clarifying for children that wishes cannot make events occur is essential in helping them overcome their guilt and anxiety.

Development of the ***superego,*** or ***conscience,*** starts toward the end of the toddler years and is a major task for preschoolers. Learning right from wrong and good from bad is the beginning of morality (see Cultural Awareness box below). Children in this age-group are generally unable to understand the reasons why something is acceptable or unacceptable. They are aware of appropriate behavior primarily through punishment or reward and rely almost completely on parental principles for developing their own moral judgment. However, verbal enforcement of limits is much more effective. For example, to prevent injuries, parents need to supervise toddlers, keep them fenced in, and tell them not to run into the street. The preschooler is much more aware of danger and can be relied on to listen and obey in most instances. If allowed to disagree and question, they will develop socially acceptable behavior and independence in thought and action.

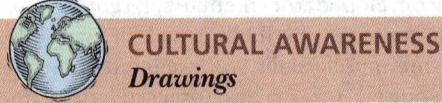

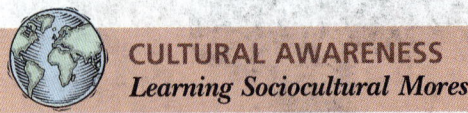

CULTURAL AWARENESS
Drawings

Children's drawings before age 6 are strikingly similar universally, suggesting that some inherent neurologic mechanisms influence the type of self-taught art forms. After age 6 cultural and environmental influence, particularly from parents and teachers, shapes much of what children draw. For example, drawings of physical characteristics (skin color, hair type, facial features), style of dress, type of housing, and scenery may reflect ethnic or geographic variations. Therefore nurses need to consider children's backgrounds when interpreting drawings.

CULTURAL AWARENESS
Learning Sociocultural Mores

Developing a conscience implies learning the sociocultural mores of the family's heritage. Depending on the type of attitudes conveyed, children will learn not only appropriate behaviors, but also tolerant, biased, or prejudicial values concerning their ethnic, religious, and social background and those of other groups. Much of this influence may remain dormant until they associate with children or adults of a different heritage. Then, depending on the particular group, they may be accepted or ostracized for their attitudes.

Oedipal Stage (Freud)

As soon as children comprehend their separateness as persons, they begin to realize that there are categories of objects, such as things, people, males, females, children, and adults. One of the principal goals in further differentiation of oneself from others is learning sex differences and sexually appropriate behavior.

Freud described this goal in psychosexual terms and labeled the period the ***oedipal,*** or ***phallic,*** stage. Conflict arises when the male child realizes that his father is much stronger and more powerful than he. Subconsciously he wishes that his father were dead so he could marry his mother (Oedipus complex). Concurrently he has noticed physical sexual differences, in specific that boys have a penis but that girls do not. In his mind he surmises that girls have lost their penis for some wrongdoing. His guilt regarding his feelings toward his father makes him fear the same punishment of mutilation, resulting in the ***castration complex.*** Girls have similar wishes to marry their father and kill their mother (the ***Electra complex***). However, girls do not fear castration; rather they experience ***penis envy*** (desire to have a penis). The resolution of the Oedipus or Electra complex is identification with the same-sex parent. (See also Development of Sexuality, p. 650.)

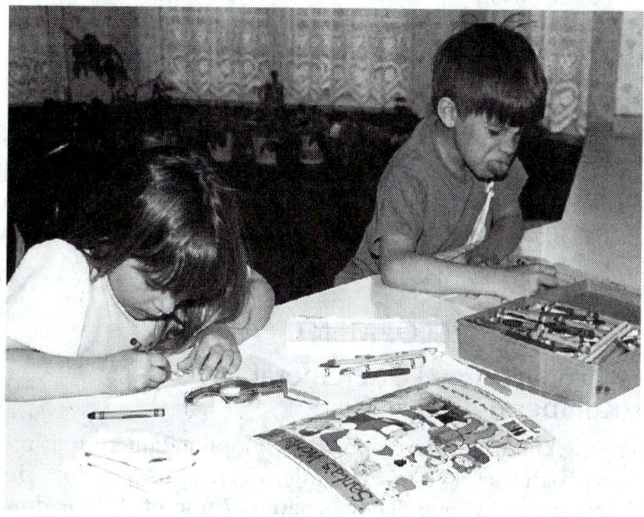

FIG. 15-3 When children play, they express nonverbal messages. One child is absorbed in her drawing, whereas the other child is clearly dissatisfied with his piece of art.

COGNITIVE DEVELOPMENT

One of the tasks related to the preschool period is readiness for school and scholastic learning. Many of the thought processes of this period are crucial for achieving such readiness, and it is intentional that the child begins school between ages 5 and 6 rather than at an earlier age.

Preoperational Phase (Piaget)

Piaget's cognitive theory actually does not include a period specifically for children 3 to 5 years old. The ***preoperational phase*** comprises the age span from 2 to 7 years and is divided into two stages: the ***preconceptual phase,*** ages 2 to 4, and the phase of ***intuitive thought,*** ages 4 to 7.

One of the main transitions during these two phases is the shift from totally egocentric thought to social awareness and the ability to consider other viewpoints. This transition is very closely associated with the development of the superego. Children are able to think and verbalize their mental processes without having to act out their thinking. However, they can only think of one idea at a time. They are unable to think of all parts in terms of the whole. Outside influences or perceptions direct their understanding of a concept. (See box [Characteristics of Preoperational Thought] on p. 619.)

Language continues to develop during the preschool period. Speech remains primarily a vehicle of egocentric communication. Preschoolers assume that everyone thinks as they do and that a brief explanation of their thinking makes them understood by others. Because of this self-referenced, egocentric verbal communication, it is frequently necessary to explore and understand young children's thinking through other, nonverbal approaches. For children in this age-group, the most enlightening and effective method is ***play,*** which becomes the child's way of understanding, adjusting to, and working out life's experiences. Because of children's rich imagination and unlimited ability to invent and imitate, all kinds of play hold therapeutic and communicative value (Fig. 15-3).

Preschoolers increasingly use language without comprehending the meaning of words, particularly concepts of right and left, causality, and time. Children may use the concepts correctly but only in the circumstances in which they have learned them. For example, they may know how to put on shoes by remembering that the buckle is always on the outside of the foot. However, if different shoes have no buckles, they cannot reason which shoe fits which foot. They do not understand the concept of ***right and left.***

Superficially, ***causality*** resembles logical thought. Preschoolers explain a concept as they heard it described by others, but their understanding is limited. An example is the concept of time. Since ***time*** is still incompletely understood, the child interprets it according to his or her own frame of reference, such as "A long time means until Christmas." Consequently, time is best explained in relationship to an event, such as "Your mother will visit you after you finish your lunch." Avoiding words such as "yesterday," "tomorrow," "next week," or "Tuesday" to express when an event is expected to occur and associating time with usual expected daily occurrences help children learn about temporal relationships while increasing their trust in others' predictions.

Preschoolers' thinking is often described as ***magical thinking.*** Because of their egocentrism and transductive reasoning (association of one event with a simultaneous event), they believe that thoughts are all-powerful. Such thinking places them in the vulnerable position of feeling guilty and responsible for bad thoughts, which may coincide with the occurrence of a wished event. A typical example is wishing a new sibling dead. If that sibling does die, young children think their wish caused the death. Their inability to reason the cause and effect of illness or an accident makes it especially difficult for them to understand such events.

Preschoolers believe in the power of words and accept their meaning literally. A significant example of this type of thinking is calling children "bad" because they did something wrong. In their minds telling children that they are bad means that they are bad. For this reason it is better to relate such words to the act by saying, for example, "That was a bad thing to do."

MORAL DEVELOPMENT

Preconventional or Premoral Level (Kohlberg)

Young children's development of moral judgment is at the most basic level. There is little, if any, concern for why something is wrong. They behave because of the freedom or restriction that is placed on actions. In the ***punishment and obedience orientation*** children (ages about 2 to 4 years) judge whether an action is good or bad depending on whether it results in reward or punishment. If children are punished for it, the action is bad. If they are not punished, the action is good, regardless of the meaning of the act. For example, if parents allow hitting, the child will perceive that hitting is good because it is not associated with punishment.

From approximately 4 to 7 years of age children are in the stage of ***naive instrumental orientation,*** in which actions are directed toward satisfying their needs and less frequently the needs of others. There is a very concrete sense of justice. Reciprocity or fairness involves the philosophy of "You scratch my back and I'll scratch yours," with no thought of loyalty or gratitude (Thomas, 1985).

SPIRITUAL DEVELOPMENT

Children's knowledge of faith and religion is learned from significant others in their environment, usually from the parents and their religious practices. However, young children's understanding of spirituality is influenced by their cognitive level. Preschoolers have a concrete conception of a God with physical characteristics who is often like an imaginary friend. They understand simple Bible stories and memorize short prayers, but their understanding of the meaning of these rituals is limited. They benefit from concrete representations of religious practices, such as picture Bible books, and small statues, such as those of the Nativity scene (Shelley and others, 1982).

Development of the conscience is strongly linked to spiritual development. At this age children are learning right from wrong and behave correctly to avoid punishment. Wrongdoing provokes feelings of guilt, and preschoolers often misinterpret illness as a punishment for real or imagined transgressions. It is important that children view God as one who bestows unconditional love, rather than as a judge of good or bad behavior. Praying to God and observing religious traditions (e.g., prayers before meals or bedtime) can help children through stressful periods, such as hospitalization (Clutter, 1991).

DEVELOPMENT OF BODY IMAGE

The preschool years play a significant role in the development of body image. With increasing comprehension of language, preschoolers recognize that individuals have undesirable and desirable appearances. They recognize differences in skin color and racial identity and are vulnerable to learning prejudices and biases. They are aware of the meaning of words such as "pretty" or "ugly," and they reflect the opinions of others regarding their own appearance. By 5 years of age children compare their size with their peers' and can become conscious of being large or short, especially if others refer to them as "so big" or "so little" for their age.

Despite the advances in body image development, preschoolers have poorly defined body boundaries and little knowledge of their internal anatomy. Intrusive experiences are frightening, especially those that disrupt the integrity of the skin, such as injections and surgery. There is a fear that if the skin is "broken" all their blood and "insides" can leak out. Therefore bandages are critical to "keeping everything from coming out."

DEVELOPMENT OF SEXUALITY

Sexual development during these years is a very important phase to a person's overall sexual identity and beliefs. Preschoolers are forming strong attachments to the opposite-sex parent while identifying with the same-sex parent. ***Sex typing,*** or the process by which an individual develops the behavior, personality, attitudes, and beliefs that are appropriate for his or her culture and sex, occurs through several mechanisms during this period. Probably the most powerful are childrearing practices and imitation. The ways in which parents dress, hold, cuddle, caress, discipline, and talk to their child all express some aspect of sexually oriented behavior. Studies increasingly demonstrate that gender identification is not solely biologic or genetic but primarily a result of complex postnatal psychologic factors and that most children are aware of their sex and the expected set of related behaviors by 1½ to 2½ years of age. Although toddlers might be aware of their particular sex, they do not possess the language and cognitive skills to investigate sexual identity as fully as preschoolers.

As sexual identity is developing beyond gender recognition, modesty may become a concern, as well as fears of mutilation. There is sex-role imitation, and "dressing up" like Mommy or Daddy is an important activity. Attitudes and responses of others to role-playing can condition the child to views of self or others. For example, comments such as "Boys shouldn't play with dolls" can influence a boy's self-concept of masculinity. This may be a time when children begin forming images of how they would like to look as adults (Selekman, 1983).

Sexual exploration may be more pronounced now than ever before, particularly in terms of exploring and manipulating the genitals. Questions about sexual reproduction may come to the forefront in the preschooler's search for understanding (see Sex Education, p. 657, and also in Chapters 17 and 19).

SOCIAL DEVELOPMENT

During the preschool period the ***individuation-separation*** process is complete. Preschoolers have overcome much of their anxiety regarding strangers and the fear of separation of earlier years. They relate to unfamiliar people easily and tolerate brief separations from parents with little or no protest. However, they still need parental security, reassurance, guidance, and approval, especially when entering nursery school or elementary school. Prolonged separation, such as that imposed by illness and hospitalization, is difficult, but preschoolers respond very well to anticipatory preparation and concrete explanation. They can cope with changes in daily routine much better than toddlers; however, they may develop more imaginary fears. They gain security and comfort from familiar objects, such as toys, dolls, or photographs of family members. They are able to work through many of their unresolved fears, fantasies, and anxieties through play, especially if guided with appropriate play objects (e.g., dolls or puppets) that represent family members, medical and nursing staff, and other children.

Language

Language during the preschool years is quite sophisticated and complex. Both cognitive ability and environment, particularly consistent role models, influence vocabulary, speech, and comprehension. Language becomes a major mode of communication and social interaction. Vocabulary increases dramatically, from 300 words at age 2 to over 2100 words at the end of 5 years. Sentence structure, grammatical usage, and intelligibility also advance to a more adult level (Lowrey, 1986).

Children between the ages of 3 and 4 form sentences of about three to four words and include only the most essential words to convey a meaning. Such speech is often termed ***telegraphic speech*** for its brevity. Three-year-old children ask many questions and use plurals, correct pronouns, and the past tense of verbs. They name familiar objects, such as animals, parts of the body, relatives, and friends. They can give and follow simple commands. They talk incessantly, regardless of whether anyone is listening or answering them. They enjoy musical or talking toys or dolls and imitate new words proficiently.

From ages 4 to 5 preschoolers use longer sentences of four to five words and use more words to convey a message, such as prepositions, adjectives, and a variety of verbs. They follow simple directional commands, such as "Put the ball on the chair," but can carry out only one request at a time. They answer questions such as "What do you do when you are hungry?" by describing the appropriate action. The pattern of asking questions is at its peak, and children usually repeat the question until they receive an answer.

By the end of age 5 children can use all parts of speech correctly, except for deviations from the rule. They can define simple words by describing their use, shape, or general category of classification, rather than simply describing their outward appearance. For example, they define a ball as "round, something you bounce, or a toy," rather than by its color. They can give some opposites, such as "If Mommy is a woman, Daddy is a man." By the time they are 6 years old, they can describe an object according to its composition, such as "A spoon is made of metal."

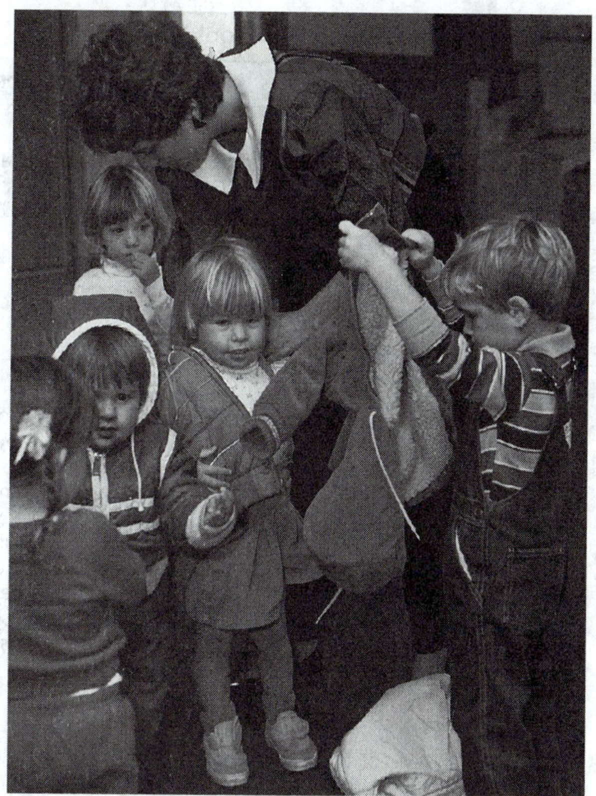

FIG. 15-4 Most preschoolers are able to dress themselves, needing help only for more difficult items of clothing.

Personal-Social Behavior

The pervasive ritualism and negativism of toddlerhood gradually diminish during the preschool years. Although self-assertion is still a major theme, preschoolers demonstrate their sense of autonomy differently. They are able to verbalize their request for independence and perform independently because of their much-refined physical and cognitive development. By 4 or 5 years of age they need little if any assistance with dressing, eating, or toileting (Fig. 15-4). They can also be trusted to obey warnings of danger, although 3- or 4-year-old children may exceed their boundaries at times.

They are also much more sociable and willing to please. They have internalized many of the standards and values of the family and culture. However, by the end of early childhood they begin to question parental values and compare them with those of their peer group and other authority figures; as a result, they may be less willing to abide by the family's code of conduct. Preschoolers become increasingly aware of their position and role within the family. Although this is a more secure age for experiencing the addition of another sibling, relinquishing the position of first or youngest is still difficult and requires appropriate preparation (see Sibling Rivalry, Chapter 14).

TABLE 15-1 Play During Preschool Years

PHYSICAL DEVELOPMENT	SOCIAL DEVELOPMENT	MENTAL DEVELOPMENT AND CREATIVITY
SUGGESTED ACTIVITIES		
Provide space for the child to run, jump, and climb Teach child to swim Teach simple sports and activities	Encourage interaction with neighborhood children Intervene when children become destructive Enroll child in preschool	Encourage creative efforts with raw materials Read stories Monitor television viewing Attend theater and other cultural events appropriate to child's age Take short excursions to park, seashore, museums
SUGGESTED TOYS		
Seesaw Medium-height slide Adjustable swing Vehicles to ride Tricycle Wading pool Wheelbarrow Sled Wagon Roller skates, speed graded to skill	Child-size playhouse Dolls, stuffed toys Dishes, table Ironing board and iron Cash register, toy typewriter Trucks, cars, trains, airplanes Play clothes for dress-up Doll carriage, bed, high chair Doctor and nurse kits Nails, hammer, saw Grooming aids, play makeup or shaving kits	Books Jigsaw puzzles Musical toys (xylophone, toy piano, drum, horns) Picture games Blunt scissors, paper, glue Newsprint, crayons, poster paint, large brushes, easel, finger paint Musical and rhythmic toys Flannel board and pieces of felt in colors and shapes Pregummed geometric shapes (colored) Records, tapes Blackboard and chalk (colored and white) Wooden and plastic construction sets Magnifying glass, magnet

Play

Various types of play are typical of this period, but preschoolers especially enjoy ***associative play***—group play in similar or identical activities but without rigid organization or rules. Play should provide for physical, social, and mental development (Table 15-1).

Play activities for physical growth and refinement of motor skills include jumping, running, and climbing. Tricycles, trucks, wagons, gym and sports equipment, sandboxes, wading pools, and winter sleds can help develop muscles and coordination. Activities such as swimming, ice skating, and skiing teach safety as well as muscle development and coordination.

Manipulative, constructive, creative, and educational toys provide for quiet activities, fine motor development, and self-expression. Easy construction sets, large blocks of various sizes and shapes, a counting frame, alphabet or number flash cards, paints, crayons, simple carpentry tools, musical toys, illustrated books, simple sewing or handicraft sets, large puzzles, and clay are suitable toys. Electronic games and educational computer programs are especially valuable in helping children learn basic skills, such as letters and simple words. Although their attention span is still short, preschoolers are beginning to enjoy crafts, especially with the guidance and assistance of adults. A helpful rule in planning creative activities is one simple project per year of age. For example, 3-year-old children usually have the patience to decorate three eggs but become bored and restless with more.

Probably the most characteristic and pervasive preschooler activity is imitative, imaginative, and dramatic play. Dress-up clothes, dolls, housekeeping toys, dollhouses, playstore toys, telephones, farm animals and equipment, village sets, trains, trucks, cars, planes, hand puppets, and doctor and nurse kits provide hours of self-expression (Fig. 15-5). Probably at no other time is the reproduction of the behavior of significant adults so faithful and absorbing as in

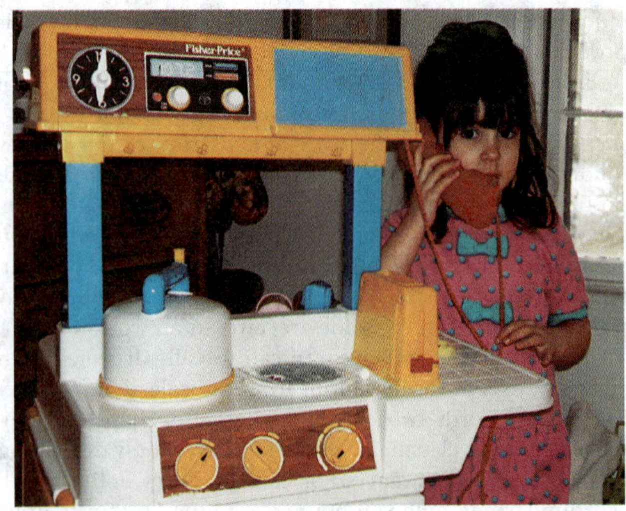

FIG. 15-5 Imaginative and imitative play is typical of preschoolers.

CRITICAL THINKING EXERCISE

Imitative Play

In her bedroom 4-year-old Juanita is playing with her dolls. She pretends one doll is "Mommy" and is talking on the telephone: "Be quiet! Can't you see that I am busy? This is an important call. Go away." She hangs up the phone and chooses another doll, pokes it, and cries, "You're bad. Mommy doesn't like you."

Juanita's mother, Mrs. Ortiz, hears this play conversation and realizes she says similar things to Juanita when she is on the telephone. What advice would you give Mrs. Ortiz:

1. Reassure her that imitation is a normal and healthy activity in 4-year-olds.
2. Suggest that she use a telephone recorder to return calls at more convenient times.
3. Inquire about her reactions to the conversation and discuss possible ways to avoid the situation.
4. Refer the child to a psychologist for further assessment of the apparent child-mother conflict.

The best answer is 3. You want to capitalize on the mother's awareness of the possible messages the child's play has revealed. Your goal is also to empower the parent to find reasonable options that accommodate her lifestyle.

Although a telephone recorder is one option, it may not be the best one. While this play behavior is typical of preschoolers, premature reassurance will not address the issue or solutions. More assessment is needed before suggesting a referral.

4- and 5-year-old children (see Critical Thinking Exercise box). Toward the end of the preschool period, children are less satisfied with make-believe or pretend objects and enjoy actually doing the activity, such as cooking and carpentry.

Television and videotapes also have their places in children's play, although each should only be one part of children's total repertoire of social and recreational activities. Parents and other caregivers should supervise selection of programs, preview programs for appropriateness, and schedule hours for television viewing. Children enjoy and learn from educational children's programs, which are purposely shown before dinner or after meals to provide a quiet activity. Television can become an interactive activity when adults view programs with children and discuss program content (see Television, Chapter 4).

Play is so much a part of the young child's life that reality and fantasy become blurred. The make-believe is reality during play and only becomes fantasy when the toys are put away or the dress-up clothes are removed. It is no wonder that ***imaginary playmates*** are so much a part of this age period.

The appearance of imaginary companions usually occurs between the ages of 2½ and 3 years, and for the most part such playmates are relinquished when the child enters school. There seems to be a relationship between the level of intelligence and the presence of the imaginary companion. The more intelligent children tend to have the most vivid and complex pretend playmates (Fish and Burch, 1985).

Imaginary companions serve many purposes—they become friends in times of loneliness, they accomplish what the child is still attempting, and they experience what the child wants to forget or remember. It is not unusual for the "friend" to have a myriad of vices and to be blamed for wrongdoing. Sometimes the child hopes to escape punishment by saying, "My friend George broke the glass." At other times the preschooler may fantasize that the "companion" misbehaved, and the child plays the role of parent. This becomes a way of assuming control and authority in a safe situation.

Parents often worry about their child having imaginary playmates, not realizing how normal and useful they are. They need to be reassured that children's fantasy is a sign of health that helps them differentiate between make-believe and reality. Parents can acknowledge the presence of imaginary companions by calling them by name and even agreeing to simple requests such as setting an extra place at the table, but they should not allow the child to use the playmate to avoid punishment or responsibility. For example, if the child blames the companion for upsetting the room, the parents need to state clearly that the child is the only person they see and therefore the child is responsible for cleaning up.

TEMPERAMENT

Temperament influences children's social development and interactions. In Chapters 4, 12, and 14 the importance of temperament during early childhood is discussed. Since temperamental characteristics tend to remain stable, the same considerations in terms of childrearing apply during the preschool years.

One major concern in this age-group is the effect of temperament on adjustment in group situations, especially school, and the long-term consequences of temperamental characteristics. In particular, the degree of adaptability to new situations, intensity of response, distractibility, amount of persistence, mood, and activity level may influence a child's chances for success in school (Schor, 1985). There is some evidence that preschoolers born at very low weights are more likely to have temperamental characteristics related to behavior problems and learning skills (Schraeder, Heverly, and Rappaport, 1990), although others have not found this relationship (Oberklaid and others, 1990). Consequently, parents can benefit from suggestions that can promote preschoolers' adjustment. For example, children who are slow to warm up need gradual introduction to new situations and may benefit from the parent's presence until they have settled in. Children with high activity levels tend to adjust better to environments that allow freedom of movement, rather than a structured or regimented classroom. The more awareness parents have of their children's unique behaviors, the better able they are to inform teachers or other caregivers of the children's needs and successful approaches to handling the youngsters.

TABLE 15-2 Growth and Development During Preschool Years

AGE (YEARS)	PHYSICAL	GROSS MOTOR	FINE MOTOR	LANGUAGE
3	Usual weight gain of 1.8 to 2.7 kg (4 to 6 pounds) Average weight of 14.6 kg (32 pounds) Usual gain in height of 7.5 cm (3 inches) Average height of 95 cm (37.25 inches) May have achieved night-time control of bowel and bladder	Rides tricycle Jumps off bottom step Stands on one foot for a few seconds Goes up stairs using alternate feet, may still come down using both feet on step Broad jumps May try to dance, but balance may not be adequate	Builds tower of nine or ten cubes Builds bridge with three cubes Adeptly places small pellets in narrow-necked bottle In drawing, copies a circle, imitates a cross, names what has been drawn, cannot draw stick figure but may make circle with facial features	Has vocabulary of about 900 words Uses primarily "telegraphic" speech Uses complete sentences of three to four words Talks incessantly regardless of whether anyone is paying attention Repeats sentence of six syllables Asks many questions
4	Pulse and respiration rates decrease slightly Growth rate is similar to that of previous year Average weight of 16.7 kg (36.75 pounds) Average height of 103 cm (40.5 inches) Length at birth is doubled Maximum potential for development of amblyopia	Skips and hops on one foot Catches ball reliably Throws ball overhand Walks downstairs using alternate footing	Uses scissors successfully to cut out picture following outline Can lace shoes, but may not be able to tie bow In drawing, copies a square, traces a cross and diamond, adds three parts to stick figure	Has vocabulary of 1500 words or more Uses sentences of four to five words Questioning is at peak Tells exaggerated stories Knows simple songs May be mildly profane if associates with older children Obeys four prepositional phrases, such as "under," "on top of," "beside," "in back of," or "in front of" Names one or more colors Comprehends analogies, such as, "If ice is cold, fire is ______"
5	Pulse and respiration rates decrease slightly Average weight of 18.7 kg (41.25 pounds) Average height of 110 cm (43.25 inches) Eruption of permanent dentition may begin Handedness is established (about 90% are right-handed)	Skips and hops on alternate feet Throws and catches ball well Jumps rope Skates with good balance Walks backward with heel to toe Jumps from height of 12 inches and lands on toes Balances on alternate feet with eyes closed	Ties shoelaces Uses scissors, simple tools, or pencil very well In drawing, copies a diamond and triangle; adds seven to nine parts to stick figure; prints a few letters, numbers, or words, such as first name	Has vocabulary of about 2100 words Uses sentences of six to eight words, with all parts of speech Names coins (e.g., nickel, dime) Names four or more colors Describes drawing or pictures with much comment and enumeration Knows names of days of week, months, and other time-associated words Knows composition of articles, such as, "A shoe is made of ______" Can follow three commands in succession

SOCIALIZATION	COGNITION	FAMILY RELATIONSHIPS
Dresses self almost completely if helped with back buttons and told which shoe is right or left Has increased attention span Feeds self completely Can prepare simple meals, such as cold cereal and milk Can help to set table; can dry dishes without breaking any May have fears, especially of dark and going to bed Knows own sex and sex of others Play is parallel and associative; begins to learn simple games but often follows own rules; begins to share	Is in preconceptual phase Is egocentric in thought and behavior Has beginning understanding of time; uses many time-oriented expressions; talks about past and future as much as about present; pretends to tell time Has improved concept of space as demonstrated in understanding of prepositions and ability to follow directional command Has beginning ability to view concepts from another perspective	Attempts to please parents and conform to their expectations Is less jealous of younger sibling; may be opportune time for birth of additional sibling Is aware of family relationships and sex-role functions Boys tend to identify more with father or other male figure Has increased ability to separate easily and comfortably from parents for short periods
Very independent Tends to be selfish and impatient Aggressive physically as well as verbally Takes pride in accomplishments Has mood swings Shows off dramatically, enjoys entertaining others Tells family tales to others with no restraint Still has many fears Play is associative Imaginary playmates are common Uses dramatic, imaginative, and imitative devices Sexual exploration and curiosity demonstrated through play, such as being "doctor" or "nurse"	Is in phase of intuitive thought Causality is still related to proximity of events Understands time better, especially in terms of sequence of daily events Unable to conserve matter Judges everything according to one dimension, such as height, width, or order Immediate perceptual clues dominate judgment Is beginning to develop less egocentrism and more social awareness May count correctly but has poor mathematic concept of numbers Obeys because parents have set limits, not because of understanding of right and wrong	Rebels if parents expect too much, such as impeccable table manners Takes aggression and frustration out on parents or siblings "Do's" and "don'ts" become important May have rivalry with older or younger siblings; may resent older sibling's privileges and younger sibling's invasion of privacy and possessions May "run away" from home Identifies strongly with parent of opposite sex Is able to run simple errands outside the home
Less rebellious and quarrelsome than at age 4 years More settled and eager to get down to business Not as open and accessible in thoughts and behavior as in earlier years Independent but trustworthy; not foolhardy; more responsible Has fewer fears; relies on outer authority to control world Eager to do things right and to please; tries to "live by the rules" Has better manners Cares for self totally except for teeth, occasionally needing supervision in dress or hygiene Not ready for concentrated close work or small print because of slight farsightedness and still unrefined eye-hand coordination Play is associative; tries to follow rules but may cheat to avoid losing	Begins to question what parents think by comparing them with age-mates and other adults May notice prejudice and bias in outside world Is more able to view other's perspective, but tolerates differences rather than understanding them May begin to show understanding of conservation of numbers through counting objects regardless of arrangement Uses time-oriented words with increased understanding Very curious about factual information regarding world	Gets along well with parents May seek out parent more often than at age 4 years for reassurance and security, especially when entering school Begins to question parents' thinking and principles Strongly identifies with parent of same sex, especially boys with their fathers Enjoys activities such as sports, cooking, shopping with parent of same sex

The ***Behavioral Style Questionnaire*** can be used to identify temperamental characteristics in children who are in the age range of 3 to 7 years (McDevitt and Carey, 1978). Simply asking mothers to rate their child as being either much easier than, easier than, as easy as, more difficult than, or much more difficult than the average child may also be a valuable screening method. Maternal perceptions of their infants as being difficult and having behavior problems (e.g., colic, sleep problems) has significantly predicted behavior problems during the preschool years (Oberklaid and others, 1993).

■ ■ ■

The major developmental achievements for children 3, 4, and 5 years old are summarized in Table 15-2.

COPING WITH CONCERNS RELATED TO NORMAL GROWTH AND DEVELOPMENT

Preschool and Kindergarten Experience

During the preschool years many children attend some type of early childhood program, usually preschool or a daycare center. Group care has become commonplace with the large number of mothers presently employed outside the home (see Alternate Child Care Arrangements, Chapter 12). The effects of early education and stimulation on children have increasingly gained recognition and importance, although recent concern has focused on programs that stress formal academics (Howes, 1989) (for a discussion of the effects of daycare on young children, see Working Mothers, Chapter 3). Since social development widens to include age-mates and other significant adults, preschool provides an excellent vehicle for expanding children's experiences with others.

In preschool or daycare centers children are exposed to opportunities for learning group cooperation, adjusting to various sociocultural differences, and coping with frustration, dissatisfaction, and anger. If activities are tailored to provide mastery and achievement, children increasingly feel success, self-confidence, and personal competence. Whether or not structured learning is imposed is less important than the social climate, type of guidance, and attitude toward the children that is fostered by the teacher or leader. With a teacher who is aware of preschoolers' developmental abilities and needs, the children will learn from the activity that is provided. Most programs incorporate a similar daily schedule of quiet play, active outdoor activity, group activities such as games and projects, creative or free play, and snack and rest periods.

Preschool is particularly beneficial for children who lack a peer-group experience, such as an only child, and for children from impoverished homes. It provides extensive stimulation for language, physical, and social development. It also is an excellent preparation for kindergarten. For a child from a poor home, elementary school can be so overwhelming that all learning is impeded by the sensory overload. Regular school places many more demands on children for prolonged attention, self-disciplined behavior, and demonstrated progress in performance and achievement than does the less-structured atmosphere of preschool.

One of the issues that parents face is the child's readiness for preschool or kindergarten. There are no absolute indicators for school readiness, but children's social maturation, especially attention span, is as important as their academic readiness. Nurses should know the age requirement for school entry in the districts in which their families reside. Children whose birthdate is close to the cut-off date may be less ready for school than their peers, who may be up to 11 months older (American Academy of Pediatrics, 1993). Using a developmental screening tool that addresses cognitive (especially language), social, and physical milestones can identify children who may benefit from diagnostic testing. Developmental screening, which focuses on the potential to learn, differs from readiness testing, which stresses the specific skills the child has acquired (e.g., counts to 10, prints letters of the alphabet, knows days of week, and so on) (Wilson and Knudtson, 1992).

Preparing the Child. Children need preparation for the preschool or kindergarten experience.* The following suggestions are also appropriate for children entering kindergarten. For some children these programs represent a change from their usual home environment, as well as prolonged separation from their parents. Even if children have been cared for by a baby-sitter or in a group setting, preschool and kindergarten differ because the individualized attention may be less, the program may be more structured, and learning may be expected.

The nurse helps parents assess children's readiness in terms of age, physical ability, and cognitive and social development (see Table 15-2). For example, a group experience may be difficult for young children with short attention spans. These children may require a different type of experience that provides for more individualized attention.

Before children begin the experience, the parents should present the idea as exciting and pleasurable. Talking to them about activities such as painting, building with blocks, or enjoying swings and other outdoor equipment allows children to fantasize about the forthcoming event in a positive manner. When the first day of school arrives, the parents should behave confidently. Such behavior requires parents to have resolved their own feelings regarding the experience.

Parents should introduce their child to the teacher and the facility. In some instances it is helpful to remain for at least some part of the first day until the child is comfortable and at ease. If parents do stay, they should be available to the child but inconspicuous. Frequently a full-day routine is too overwhelming for a child and needs to be shortened to a morning or afternoon session. Another action that can facilitate children's adjustment is providing the school with detailed information about the home environment, such as familiar routines, favorite activities, food preferences, names of siblings or pets, and personal habits. Such information helps the child feel familiar in the strange surroundings. When schools automatically request this information, the parent has a valuable clue to evaluating the

*Recommended books for preparing young children for daycare or school include *Going to Day Care* and *When Your Child Goes to School* by Fred Rogers (GP Putnam's Sons).

quality of the program, since it represents the staff's awareness of each child's needs. Transitional objects, such as a favorite toy, may also help the child bridge the gap from home to school.

Sex Education

Preschoolers have experienced a tremendous amount of information during their short lifetimes. Although their thinking may not be mature, they search constantly for explanations and reasons that are logical and reasonable to them. The word "why" seems to supplant the word "no," which was common in toddlerhood. It is only natural that as they learn about "me," they will also want to know such things as "why me," and "how me." Questions such as "Where do babies come from?" are as casual as "Why is the sky blue?" "What makes it rain?" or "Who is that?" It is the *way* in which questions about reproduction are answered that conditions even the youngest children to separate these questions from others about their world. If these questions are answered honestly and as matter-of-factly as any other inquiry, children will continue to search for answers. If they are answered with a "tall tale" or an anxious "You are too young to know about that," children will learn to keep such questions to themselves. Unfortunately, as they harbor these silent mysteries, they are formulating their own theories to explain birth. Since magical thinking need not be based on logic or fact, any fantastic, often terrifying explanation can substitute for truth.

Two rules govern answering sensitive questions about topics such as sex. The first is to *find out what children know and think.* By investigating the theories children have produced as a reasonable explanation, parents can not only give correct information but also help children understand why their explanation is inaccurate. Another reason for ascertaining what the child thinks before offering any information is that the "unasked for" answer may be given. For example, 4-year-old Sally asked her father. "Where did I come from?" Both parents quickly took this inquiry as a clue for offering sex education. After the explanation, Sally exclaimed, "I don't know about all that! All I know is Mary came from New York and I want to know where I was born."

Regardless of whether children are given sex education, they will engage in games of sexual curiosity and exploration. At about 3 years of age children are aware of the anatomic differences between the sexes and are very concerned with how the other "works." This is not really "sexual" curiosity, because many children are still unaware of the reproductive function of the genitals. Their curiosity is for the eliminative function of the anatomy. Little boys wonder how girls can urinate without a penis, so they watch girls go to the bathroom. Since they cannot see anything but the stream of water coming out, they want to observe further for what makes it come out. "Doctor play" is often a game invented for just such investigation. Little girls are no less curious about boys' anatomy. It is very intriguing to have a closer inspection of this "thing" that girls do not have.

One question that parents often have is how to handle such sexual curiosity. A positive approach is to neither condone nor condemn the sexual curiosity but to express that if children have questions they should ask the parents, and then encourage them to engage in some other activity. In this way children can be helped to understand that there are ways that their sexual curiosity can be satisfied other than through playing investigative games. This in no way condemns the act but stresses alternate methods to seek solutions and answers. Allowing children unrestricted permissiveness only intensifies their anxiety and concern, since exploring and searching usually yield little evidence to satisfy their curiosity.

Occasionally parents are faced with special dilemmas (e.g., when children ask to see "how Mommy and Daddy do it" or accidentally witness sexual intercourse). When such events occur, parents must remember that sex education is much more than textbook facts. It is part of a broader concept called ***sexuality;*** two people unite intimately because of the special relationship they have together. Intercourse is not a physical act apart from feeling or emotion but a private act that two people share to express caring and for pleasure. Such an explanation does not deny children's right to be curious; nor does it deny them the request because their wish is bad or dangerous. On the contrary, it teaches appropriate social behavior and in particular stresses the meaningful, intimate relationship between man and woman. When children witness sexual acts, parents should use the opportunity immediately to communicate that sex is healthy and natural. However, to prevent subsequent interruptions, children are cautioned to always knock first, or if they are too young to understand or comply, a lock on the door is appropriate (Goldsmith, 1986).

The second rule for giving information is to *be honest.* It is true that much of the correct information will be forgotten or misunderstood by the preschooler, but what is more important is that the correct information can be restated until the child absorbs and comprehends the facts. Even though the correct anatomic words may be hard to pronounce or even more difficult to remember, they become foundational content for explaining other concepts later on.

Honesty does not imply imparting to children every fact of life or allowing excessive permissiveness in sexual curiosity. When children ask one question, they are looking for one answer. When they are ready, they will ask about the other "unfinished" parts of the story. Sooner or later they will wonder how the "sperm meets the egg" and "how the baby gets out," but it is best to wait until they ask.

Should parents offer too much information, children will simply become bored or end the conversation with an irrelevant question. Parents worry a great deal about whether they can "harm" their children with "too much" information or tell their children things that they will not understand. Generally, knowledge is not harmful. In fact, the experts advise parents to tell their children a bit more than they think their children can understand (Gordon and Snyder, 1989). It does not matter if children do not understand everything parents say. What matters is that parents are approachable.

When children do not ask questions, parents should take advantage of natural opportunities to discuss reproduction, such as talking about someone who is pregnant or discussing a television program or movie about biologic aspects.

Many excellent books on sex education are available for preschool children at public libraries, and the **Sex Information and Education Council of the United States (SIECUS),*** local chapters of **Planned Parenthood Federation of America,†** and the **American Academy of Pediatrics‡** have bibliographies of suggested reading material. *Before* giving or reading any book to a child, parents should read it themselves.

Another concern for some parents is ***masturbation,*** or self-stimulation of the genitals. This occurs at any age for a variety of reasons and, if not excessive, is normal and healthy. It is most common at 4 years of age and during adolescence (Leung and Robson, 1993). For preschoolers it is a part of sexual curiosity and exploration. If parents are concerned about masturbation in their children, it is essential for nurses to investigate the circumstances associated with the activity, because it may be an expression of anxiety, boredom, or unresolved conflicts. For example, a boy who repeatedly touches his penis is not masturbating for pleasure but may be reassuring himself that it is intact. Also, children who openly and publicly masturbate are inviting a reaction, such as discipline, punishment, or criticism. They may be overwhelmed by their sexual feelings and asking others to help them channel them into more constructive outlets. Since masturbation, like other forms of sex play, is a private act, parents should emphasize this to children as part of teaching them socially acceptable behavior.

Gifted Children

The importance of the identification of gifted children and their needs is increasingly being recognized. Although the definition of ***gifted*** varies, the most widely used criterion is superior intelligence—usually defined as an intelligence quotient (IQ) of 130 or above, although this depends on the test. A broader view considers specific academic aptitude, creative or productive thinking, leadership ability, ability in visual or performing arts, and psychomotor ability either singly or in combination as signs of giftedness (Goldsmith and Feldman, 1985; Landesman, 1985). Most children are identified as gifted when they enter school and receive IQ tests; no valid tests exist for predicting giftedness in infancy (Shapiro and others, 1989). However, not all gifted children are identified, and the tragic loss of the opportunity to develop their potential may result. Consequently, nurses who are aware of the behavioral and developmental characteristics of giftedness can assess children's mental and physical capabilities and assist in early identification (see box above, right).

Gifted children can present unique challenges to parents. They often demand increased stimulation as infants and continue to seek a great deal of attention from their parents. Their high energy level and persistence can lead to discipline problems similar to those seen in children with difficult temperaments. Parents may be intimidated by having a child smarter than themselves and be hesitant to set limits. However, gifted children are children first and have the same needs for love, security, and consistent controls as other youngsters. Sometimes children's above-average skills in one area cause adults to exaggerate their abilities in all areas and thus expect excessively mature behavior. Parents may mislabel slower achievement in a particular skill as lack of trying, when it really represents children's natural progression of abilities (McGuffog, 1985). These children benefit from academic settings that provide enrichment and accelerated learning commensurate with their capabilities. Consequently, early identification of giftedness and appropriate parental guidance can be critical to the optimum development of giftedness and the children's emotional adjustment (Mills, 1992).

CHARACTERISTICS OF GIFTED CHILDREN

Birth weight and head circumference above 50th percentile
Early developmental milestones, especially walking
Early development of language and complex usage of speech
Temperamental characteristics of persistence, intensity, extreme self-confidence, sensitivity, and responsiveness to stimulation
Constant questioning and curiosity
Rich fantasy, such as imaginary playmates
Highly developed sense of humor
Strong interest in special areas, such as music, science, or mechanical skills

Modified from Fish L, Burch K: Identifying gifted preschoolers, *Pediatr Nurs* 1(2):125-127, 1985; and Goldsmith LT, Feldman DH: Identifying gifted children: the state of the art, *Pediatr Ann* 14(10):709-716, 1985.

Aggression

The term ***aggression*** refers to behavior that attempts to hurt a person or destroy property. Aggression differs from anger, which is a temporary emotional state, but anger may be expressed through aggression. Hyperaggressive behavior in preschoolers is characterized by unprovoked physical attacks on other children and adults, destruction of others' property, frequent intense temper tantrums, extreme impulsivity, disrespect, and noncompliance (Fig. 15-6) (Landy and Peters, 1990).

Aggression is influenced by a complex set of biologic, sociocultural, and familial variables. There is evidence that gender differences exist and that males are more aggressive than females (Jacklin, 1992). Other factors that tend to increase aggressive behavior are frustration, modeling, and reinforcement.

Frustration, or the continual thwarting of self-satisfaction by parental disapproval, humiliation, punishment, and insults, can lead children to act out against others as a means of release. Especially if they fear their parents, these children will displace their anger on others, particularly peers and other authority figures. This type of aggression fre-

*130 W. 42nd St., Suite 2500, New York, NY 10036; (212) 819-9770.

†National office: 810 7th Ave., New York, NY 10019; (212) 541-7800; (800) 829-7732.

‡AAP Publications, P.O. Box 927, Elk Grove Village, IL 60009-0927; (800) 433-9016.

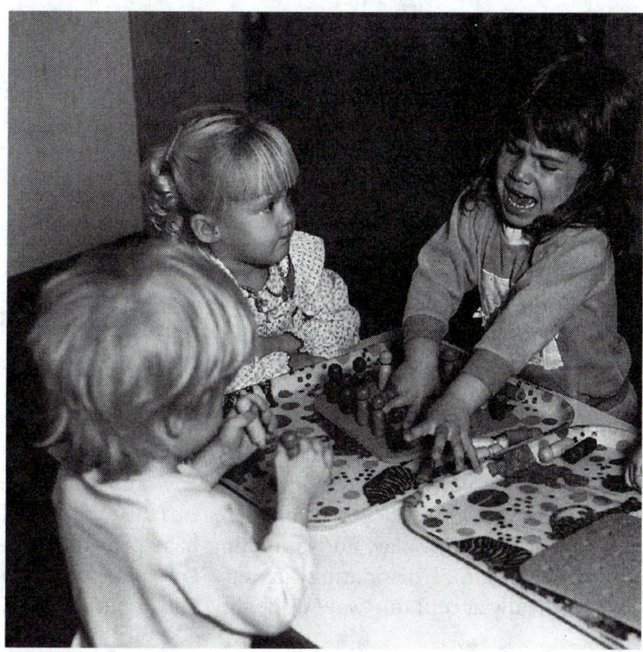

FIG. 15-6 Preschoolers generally direct their aggression toward peers, especially when their desires are frustrated.

quently applies to the "well-behaved child" at home who is a discipline problem at school or a "bully" among playmates.

Modeling, or imitating behavior of significant others, is a powerful influencing force in preschoolers. Children who see their parents fighting, either physically or verbally, are observing behavior that they come to know as acceptable. Also, early harsh discipline may lead to aggressive behavior (Weiss and others, 1992). Another aspect of modeling is establishing a double standard for acceptable conduct. For example, in some families aggression is synonymous with masculinity, and boys are encouraged to defend themselves. Although defending one's rights is to be encouraged for both sexes, at times the principle of "toughness" or "standing up for yourself" is not tempered with judgment, fairness, or equality but becomes an excuse for ruling and dominating others. Such permissive aggression can produce extreme anxiety in children because it makes them feel out of control, even though they outwardly may appear to be the "boss" or "bully."

Another significant source for modeling is television. Numerous studies have found a positive correlation between viewing violent programs and immediate aggression (Singer, 1989). Consequently, parents need encouragement to supervise programming, especially for those children with aggressive tendencies (see discussion under Television, Chapter 4).

Reinforcement can also shape aggressive behavior and is closely associated with modeling "masculine" behavior. Sometimes the reward for aggressive behavior is negative, such as punishment or disapproval, but is reinforcing because it brings attention. For example, children who are ignored by their parents until they hit a sibling learn that such acts are forceful attention mechanisms. In addition, parents who permit aggressive behavior by not interfering communicate silent, implicit approval of such acts.

One of the tasks of preschoolers is learning socially acceptable behavior and the ability to control and redirect aggression toward the appropriate source. Parents can help children by modeling appropriate behavior and encouraging children to express themselves verbally. For example, rather than condoning hitting another child for taking a toy, parents can suggest that the child state how he or she feels, such as "I am angry when you take my ball. Give it back."

Children should not be made to feel guilty or ashamed for being angry or frustrated. When they recognize these feelings, they are better able to channel them into constructive, not destructive, outlets. One of the earliest demonstrations of aggression is temper tantrums (see Chapter 14). If parents handle them constructively by not attending to or reinforcing them and by helping children find control through appropriate play situations, young children will learn to acknowledge such feelings and express them in alternative ways, such as pounding on clay or hitting a punching bag. When children are out of control, they may need to be physically restrained or removed from the scene to prevent them from hurting themselves or others.

Sometimes the type of discipline used to extinguish other forms of unacceptable behavior actually promotes aggressive behavior. For example, if the child is spanked for the act, aggression is used to "teach" a lesson against aggression! Parental permissiveness and lack of discipline, often alternating with extreme punishment, may also foster aggressiveness (Landy and Peters, 1990). The combined use of time-out and reinforcement for solitary play is an effective intervention for aggression. In addition, minimizing anger and frustration can lead to fewer opportunities for acting out behavior (see Family Home Care box on p. 86).

When extreme behaviors, such as aggression, are present in children, parents are often concerned about the need for professional help. Generally, the difference between "normal" and "problematic" behavior is not the actual behavior, but the ***quantity*** (number of occurrences), ***severity*** (interfering with social or cognitive functioning), ***distribution*** (different manifestations), ***onset*** (especially sudden change in behavior), and ***duration*** (at least 4 weeks) of the activity. When aggressive tendencies are evaluated, these factors are assessed to distinguish between behaviors typically seen at various ages and those that may represent an underlying problem. Extreme aggression requires professional treatment and is often difficult to change.

Speech Problems

The most critical period for speech development occurs between 2 and 4 years of age. During this period children are using their rapidly growing vocabulary faster than they can produce the words. This failure to master sensorimotor integrations results in ***stuttering*** or ***stammering*** as children try to say the word they are already thinking about. This dysfluency in speech pattern is a *normal* characteristic of language development. However, when parents or other significant caregivers place undue emphasis or stress on this normal dysfluency, an abnormal speech pattern may develop (Schmitt, 1991).

The best therapy for speech problems is prevention and early detection, especially anticipatory preparation of parents for the expected hesitation in speech during the preschool period (see Speech Impairment, Chapter 24).

Coping with Stress

Although the preschool years generally are less troublesome than toddlerhood for parents, this period of life presents children with many unique stresses. Some are innate and stem from preschoolers' unique understanding of the world, such as fears. Others are imposed, such as beginning school. Although minimum amounts of stress are beneficial during the early years to help children develop effective coping skills, excessive stress is harmful, and young children are especially vulnerable because of their limited capacity to cope.

To help parents deal with stress in their child's life, they must be aware of signs of stress (see Stress in Childhood, Chapter 4) and be helped to identify the source (see box below). In addition, any number of other stresses may be present, such as the birth of a sibling, marital discord, relocation, or illness. The best approach to dealing with stress is prevention—monitoring the amount of stress in children's lives so that levels exceeding their coping ability do not occur. In many instances structuring children's schedules to allow rest and preparing them for change, such as entering school, are sufficient measures.

Because stress is such a constant aspect of daily living, the preschool years are not too young to help children learn to cope with stress. They can learn the meaning of the word "stress" and recognize physical signs of stress reaction, such as rapid pulse, pounding heart, or fatigue. Teaching children relaxation and imagery is very effective. Young children can learn to "let their bodies go limp like a rag doll" or "imagine flying like bird." Parents can use stories to help children imagine pleasurable events. As language skills improve, preschoolers are encouraged to talk about their feelings and to explore other ways of expressing emotions. Play is an excellent vehicle for venting anger or frustration, and toys such as drums, clay, and punching bags provide alternative methods of dissipating anxiety. Toys also begin to teach socially acceptable ways of dealing with such feelings.

Fears

The greatest number and variety of real and imagined fears are present during the preschool years and include fear of the dark, being left alone (especially at bedtime), animals

SOURCES OF STRESS IN PRESCHOOLERS

THREE-YEAR-OLD

Infantile behavior—Reverts to babyish ways; can't completely let go of babyhood
Stubbornness—Although is developing an interest in social relationships and a concept of "we," may lapse into uncooperative behavior
Possessiveness—Guards belongings and may be bossy about them
Jealousy—Particularly when it comes to parents' love
Separation anxiety
Stranger anxiety
Confusion—Can't always discriminate between fantasy and reality
White lies—May result from wishful thinking, fantasy, and desire to please or impress
Imaginary playmate—Often blamed for misdeeds
Fears—May be precipitated by imagination; may also fear dogs or other animals
Speech—May stutter or stumble over words
Activity level—Seems to be in perpetual motion; may exhaust himself or herself
Eating—May forget to eat or lose interest in food
Nap or bedtime—May fear bad dreams, the dark, or missing out on some fun while asleep
Destructiveness—May damage or destroy objects
Questions—Continually asks "why," and is upset if trusted adults do not respond or do not know the answer

FOUR-YEAR-OLD

Insecurity—May develop nervous habits such as nail-biting, facial tic, thumb-sucking, genital manipulation, eye-blinking, or nose-picking; may insist on bringing a familiar item from house to preschool
Exaggerations—May attempt to boost self-image with boasts
Companionship—Enjoys interacting with friends, although there may be many quarrels
Silliness—Tends to engage in rambuctious, silly play; likes words and is fascinated by rhyming syllables or foul language; is disciplined for lack of control
Property rights—Protects belongings; may become bossy
Sex—Interested in the human body; may engage in exhibitionism
Activity level—Enjoys running, jumping, and slamming doors; may be punished for disruptive behavior
Fears—Picks up fears from adults; may fear dark room, snakes and lizards, or anything perceived as "creepy"
Attention—Likes to talk and is frustrated if ignored or put off; whines to get own way

FIVE-YEAR-OLD

Approval—Parents' love and acceptance are vital; seeks praise
School—May have difficulty adjusting to kindergarten
Separation anxiety—Particularly fears loss of mother
Infantile behavior—May occasionally lapse into babyish behavior as a result of realizing that babyhood is ended
Worrying—May develop irrational fears, take information out of context, or fret over a misinterpreted, overheard conversation
Masturbation—Is concerned about being "bad"
Belongings—Protects possessions
Showing off—Performs in order to gain praise
Procrastination—May dillydally now and then
Name calling—Insults others to boost self-image, but is upset when she or he is the victim of mockery

Modified from Kuczen B: *Childhood stress: don't let your child be a victim,* New York, 1982, Delacorte Press, pp 15-17.

(particularly large dogs and snakes), ghosts, sexual matters (castration), and objects or persons associated with pain. The exact cause of children's fears is unknown. Freudians believe that the upsurge of fears during the preschool years results from the anxiety of being injured and mutilated (castration complex). Piaget views fears as a product of the type of thinking in this age-group. Preschoolers are caught between the egocentric thinking of infants, which protects them from imagined fears, and the more logical thought processes of school-age children, which help explain and dispel potential fears. Children in the preconceptual stage still engage in egocentric thought but are now able to imagine an event without actually experiencing it. For example, seeing someone hurt is sufficient for realizing what the hurt must be like and for consequently fearing that hurt. In medical practice this is frequently observed. When watching another child getting an injection, the preschooler may become very upset, almost as if he or she received the injection.

The concept of ***animism*** (ascribing lifelike qualities to inanimate objects) explains why children fear objects. For example, one child refused to move his bowels after watching a television commercial in which the toilet bowl was portrayed as turning into a monster, with the seat cover making a chomping movement. The child was afraid the toilet "would get him" if he sat on it (Pilapil, 1990).

A fear that is peculiar to this age is fear of annihilation. Because of poorly defined body boundaries and improved cognitive abilities, young children develop concerns related to loss of body parts, such as feces being flushed away or their body going down the drain. Since preschool children cannot understand concepts of size, they cannot understand that their body is too large to disappear down the drain.

Preschoolers are also likely to develop parent-induced fears—fears that stem from imitating their parents. When parents demonstrate their fears, the concerns are communicated to the children. Such fears tend to be long-lasting and difficult to dispel.

The best way to help children overcome their fears is by actively involving them in finding practical methods to deal with frightening experiences. This may be as simple as keeping a dim night-light on in the bedroom to assure the child that no monsters lurk in the dark or letting the child bathe a doll or play with toys in a tub of water so that the child can observe that large objects cannot go down the drain. In this way the experience that created the fear in the child can be reconstructed without involving the child directly as the victim. The child is allowed alternative methods to feel in control and powerful while overcoming fear.

Exposing children to the feared object in a safe situation provides a type of conditioning, or ***desensitization.*** For instance, children who are afraid of dogs should never be forced to approach or touch one, but they may be gradually introduced to the experience by watching other children play with a dog. This type of modeling, demonstrating fearlessness in others, can be very effective if children are allowed to progress at their own rate.

Sometimes fears do not subside with simple measures or developmental maturation. When children experience severe fears that disrupt family life, professional help is required. Successful training programs may include (1) muscle relaxation; (2) imagining a pleasant scene; (3) positive self-talk, or reciting brave statements; or (4) thought stopping, or repeating reassuring statements that block fearful thoughts. Rewards or "tokens" may be given for "bravery" and not being afraid. Such interventions can be applied in clinical settings to reduce fears (e.g., of being alone or of painful procedures; see Pain Management, Chapter 26).

PROMOTING OPTIMUM HEALTH DURING THE PRESCHOOL YEARS

A brief discussion of nutrition, sleep, dental health, and injury prevention is presented to emphasize the particular needs or differences of preschoolers vs toddlers. For a more comprehensive understanding the reader is urged to also review the material presented in Chapter 14 under Promoting Optimum Health During Toddlerhood.

NUTRITION

Nutritional requirements for preschoolers are fairly similar to those for toddlers. The requirement for calories per unit of body weight continues to decrease slightly to 90 kcal/kg for an average daily intake of 1800 calories. Fluid requirements may also decrease slightly to about 100 ml/kg daily but depend on activity level, climatic conditions, and state of health. Protein requirements are 1.2 g/kg for an average daily consumption of 24 g (Food and Nutrition Board, 1989).

Some preschoolers still have food habits that are typical of toddlers, such as food fads and strong taste preferences. When children reach 4 years of age, they seem to enter another period of finicky eating, which is generally characteristic of the more rebellious and rowdy behavior of children in this age-group. By age 5 years children are more agreeable to trying new foods, especially if encouraged by an adult who allows the child to help with food preparation or experiments with a new taste or different dish (Fig. 15-7). Mealtimes can become battlegrounds if parents expect excellent table manners. Usually the 5-year-old child is ready for the "social" side of eating, but the 3- or 4-year-old child still has difficulty sitting quietly through a long family meal.

The amount and variety of foods consumed by young children vary greatly from day to day. Consequently, parents sometimes worry about the quantity of food preschoolers consume. In general, the quality is much more important than the quantity, a fact that should be stressed during nutritional counseling. There is some evidence that children self-regulate their caloric intake. If they eat less at one meal, they will compensate at another meal or snack (Birch and others, 1991; Shea and others, 1992). Also, children's likes and dislikes may be related to genetic sensitivity to tastes (Anliker and others, 1991).

One approach toward lessening parental concern is advising parents to keep a weekly record of everything the

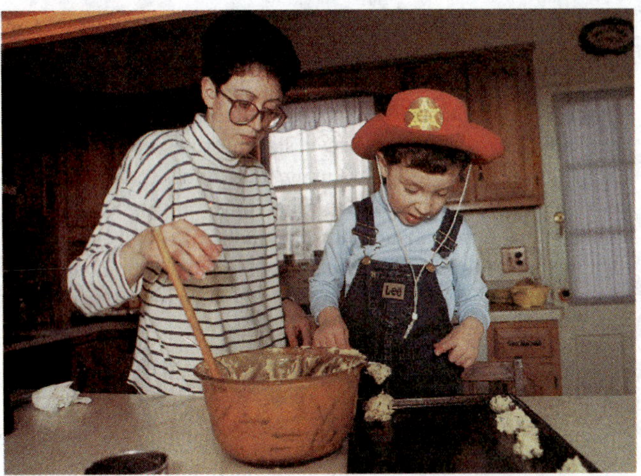

FIG. 15-7 Preschool children enjoy helping adults and are more likely to try new foods if they are included in the preparation.

child eats. In particular, the need for measuring the amount of food, such as setting aside ½ cup of vegetables and serving the child from this premeasured amount, is stressed to provide a more accurate estimate of food intake at each meal. Usually by the end of the week, when they look at the food chart, parents are amazed at how much the child has consumed. In general, preschoolers consume only slightly more than toddlers, or about half of an adult's portion.

SLEEP AND ACTIVITY

Sleep patterns vary widely, but the average preschooler sleeps about 12 hours a night and infrequently takes daytime naps. Children with reported sleep problems sleep less than those without sleeping difficulties (Edgil, Wood, and Smith, 1985).

Motor activity levels continue to be high and allow preschoolers to explore their environment, begin learning physical games and sports, and interact with others. Therefore motor activity is encouraged. Quiet activities, such as television, are increasingly appealing and can become an unhealthy substitute for active play.

Preschoolers' increased gross motor abilities and coordination provide them the opportunity to engage in many sports, if only at a novice level. Whether young children should begin formalized training in an activity at this early age is controversial. The American Academy of Pediatrics (1992) recommends that children's readiness to participate in organized sports should be determined individually. The decision should be based on the child's (not the parent's) motivation and enjoyment. The American Academy of Pediatrics encourages free play, a variety of physical activities, a noncompetitive atmosphere, and emphasis on fun and safety.

Sleep Problems

The preschool years are a prime time for sleep disturbances. Young children sometimes have trouble going to sleep, especially after so much activity and stimulation during the day. Others may develop bedtime fears, wake during the night, or have nightmares or sleep terrors. Still others may prolong the inevitable bedtime through elaborate rituals.

Recommendations for sleep disturbance are offered only after a thorough assessment of the problem has been completed (see Guidelines box on p. 202). Cultural traditions may dictate sleep practices that are contrary to certain well-accepted professional recommendations. Therefore parents' perceptions of a sleep habit may not be considered a problem (see Cultural Awareness box).

Interventions can also differ greatly; for example, nightmares and sleep terrors require very different approaches (Table 15-3). For children who delay going to bed, a recommended approach involves counseling parents about the importance of a consistent bedtime ritual and emphasizing the normalcy of this type of behavior in young children. Attention-seeking behavior is ignored, and the child is not taken into the parents' bed or allowed to stay up past a reasonable hour. Other measures that may be helpful include keeping a light on in the room, providing transitional objects, such as a favorite toy, or leaving a drink of water by the bed.

Helping children slow down before bedtime also contributes to less resistance to going to bed. One approach is to establish limited rituals that signal readiness for bed, such as a bath or story. Parents can reinforce the pattern by stating, "After this story it is bedtime," and consistently carrying through the routine. If extra stimulation such as having visitors arrive at bedtime is disruptive to children's routine, it is advisable to settle children in bed beforehand.

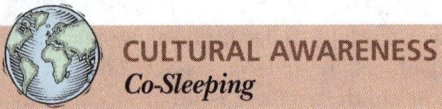

CULTURAL AWARENESS
Co-Sleeping

Although many experts recommend that infants and children be trained to always sleep in their own crib or bed, co-sleeping, or the "family bed" (in which parents allow the children to sleep with them or the siblings to sleep together in one bed), is a relatively common and accepted cultural practice, especially among black, Hispanic, and Asian families, such as the Japanese. Other groups that are adopting co-sleeping include (1) single parents, whose need for company may encourage this practice; (2) working parents, who desire the closeness at night that was lost during the day; and (3) parents who have had an issue about sleep or separation in their own past (Brazelton, 1992).

DENTAL HEALTH

By the beginning of the preschool period, the eruption of the deciduous (primary) teeth is complete. Dental care is essential to preserve these temporary teeth and to teach good dental habits (see Chapter 14). Although preschoolers' fine motor control is improved, they still require assistance and supervision with brushing, and flossing should be done by parents. Professional care and prophylaxis, especially fluoride supplements, should be continued.

TABLE 15-3 Comparison of Nightmares vs Sleep Terrors

NIGHTMARES	SLEEP TERRORS
DESCRIPTION	
A scary dream; takes place with REM sleep and is followed by full waking	A partial arousal from very deep (stage IV, non-REM) nondreaming sleep
TIME OF DISTRESS	
After the dream is over and child wakes and cries or calls; not during the nightmare itself	During the terror itself, as child screams and thrashes; afterward is calm
TIME OF OCCURRENCE	
In the second half of the night, when dreams are most intense	Usually 1 to 4 hours after falling asleep, when nondreaming sleep is deepest
CHILD'S BEHAVIOR	
Crying in younger children, fright in all; these persist even though the child is awake	Initially child may sit up, thrash, or run in a bizarre manner, with eyes bulging, heart racing, and profuse sweating; may cry, scream, talk, or moan; there is apparent fright, anger, and/or obvious confusion, which disappears when child is fully awake
RESPONSIVENESS TO OTHERS	
Child is aware of and reassured by other's presence	Child is not very aware of another's presence, is not comforted, and may push person away and scream and thrash more if held or restrained
RETURN TO SLEEP	
May be considerably delayed because of persistent fear	Usually rapid; often difficult to keep child awake
DESCRIPTION OF DREAM	
Yes (if old enough)	No memory of a dream or of yelling or thrashing
INTERVENTIONS	
Accept dream as real fear Sit with child; offer comfort, assurance, and sense of protection May lie down with child or take to own bed *only* if child is not calmed by other measures and understands this is special occasion Consider professional counseling for recurrent nightmares unresponsive to above approaches	Observe child for a few minutes, *without interfering,* until child becomes calm or wakes fully Intervene only if necessary to protect child from injury Guide child back to bed if needed Stress to parents that sleep terrors are a normal, common phenomenon in preschoolers that requires relatively no intervention

Modified from Ferber R: *Solve your child's sleep problems,* New York, 1985, Simon & Schuster.

If children are cared for away from home, parents are encouraged to monitor the dental care provided by others, including the diet, to keep cariogenic foods to a minimum.

Trauma to teeth during this period is not uncommon, and appropriate care of an evulsed tooth is important (see Chapter 18). Even though the evulsed tooth is not permanent, preservation of the space is necessary for proper eruption of the secondary teeth and prevention of abnormal tongue habits (Greene, Louie, and Wycoff, 1990).

INJURY PREVENTION

Because of improved gross and fine motor skills, coordination, and balance, preschoolers are less prone to falls than toddlers. They tend to be less reckless, listen more to parental rules, and are aware of potential danger, such as hot objects, sharp instruments, and dangerous heights. Putting objects in the mouth as part of exploration has all but ceased, although poisoning is still a danger. Pedestrian motor vehicle injuries increase from activities such as playing in the street, riding tricycles, running after balls, or forgetting safety regulations when crossing streets. In general, the guidelines suggested for injury prevention in Tables 14-8 and 17-2 may apply to children in this age-group as well.

However, emphasis is now on education for safety and potential hazards, in addition to appropriate protection. Because preschoolers are great imitators, it is essential that parents set a good example by "practicing what they preach." Children quickly observe discrepancies in what they are told to do. Establishing habits at this time, such as wearing bicycle helmets with the first bicycle, can create long-term safety behaviors.

ANTICIPATORY GUIDANCE—CARE OF FAMILIES

The preschool years present fewer childrearing difficulties than earlier years, and this stage of development is facili-

FAMILY HOME CARE
Guidance During Preschool Years

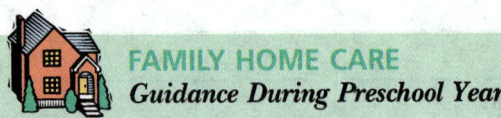

AGE 3 YEARS

Prepare parents for child's increasing interest in widening relationships.
Encourage enrollment in preschool.
Emphasize importance of setting limits.
Prepare parents to expect exaggerated tension-reduction behaviors, such as need for "security blanket."
Encourage parents to offer child choices when child vacillates.
Expect marked changes at 3½ years, when child becomes less coordinated (motor and emotional), becomes insecure, and exhibits emotional extremes.
Prepare parents for normal dysfluency in speech and advise them to avoid focusing on the pattern.
Prepare parents to expect extra demands on their attention as a reflection of child's emotional insecurity and fear of loss of love.
Warn parents that equilibrium of 3-year-old will change to aggressive, out-of-bounds behavior of 4-year-old.
Anticipate more stable appetite with more food selections.
Stress need for protection and education of child to prevent injury (see Injury Prevention, Chapter 14)

AGE 4 YEARS

Prepare for more aggressive behavior, including motor activity and offensive language.
Prepare parents to expect resistance to parental authority.
Explore parental feelings regarding child's behavior.
Suggest some kind of respite for primary caregivers, such as placing child in preschool for part of the day.
Prepare for increasing sexual curiosity.
Emphasize importance of realistic limit-setting on behavior and appropriate discipline techniques.
Prepare parents for highly imaginary 4-year-old who indulges in "tall tales" (to be differentiated from lies) and for child's imaginary playmates.
Expect nightmares or an increase in them and suggest they make sure child is fully awakened from a frightening dream.
Provide reassurance that a period of calm begins at 5 years of age.

AGE 5 YEARS

Expect tranquil period at 5 years.
Prepare child for entrance into school environment.
Make sure immunizations are up to date before entering school.
Suggest that nonemployed mothers (or fathers if appropriate) consider own activities when child begins school.
Suggest swimming lessons.

tated by appropriate anticipatory guidance in the areas already discussed (see Family Home Care box). There is also a shift in childrearing practices from one mainly of protection to one primarily of education, especially in terms of injury prevention.

During this period an emotional transition between parent and child occurs. Although children are still attached to their parents and accept all their values and beliefs, they are nearing the period of life when they will question previous teachings and prefer the companionship of peers. Entry into school marks a separation for parents, as well as for children. Parents need help in adjusting to this change, particularly if the mother has focused her daily activity on home responsibilities. As preschoolers begin preschool or elementary school, mothers may need to seek activities beyond the family, such as community involvement or pursuing a career. In this way all family members are adjusting to change, which is part of the process of growing and developing.

KEY POINTS

- The preschool years comprise the period from 3 to 5 years of age, a time that is considered critical for emotional and psychologic development.
- Biologic development in the preschool period is characterized by mature body systems and refinement in gross and fine motor behavior, as evidenced by participation in activities such as running, riding a tricycle, and drawing.
- According to Erikson, acquiring a sense of initiative is the chief psychosocial task of the preschooler. Development of the superego occurs during this period, and conscience begins to emerge.
- In Freudian theory, preschoolers are in the oedipal stage. Resolution of this stage occurs when children strongly identify with their parent of the same sex.
- According to Piaget, the preschool age is characterized by intuitive or prelogical thinking and a move toward logical thought processes through advanced, complex learning, language, and understanding of causality.
- The seeds of moral development are planted during the preschool period. According to Kohlberg, children are in the stage of naive instrumental orientation, in which they are concerned with satisfying their own needs and, less frequently, the needs of others.
- Social development booms in this period with individuation-separation, more sophisticated language, greater independence, and more complex, imaginative forms of play.
- Four areas of special concern to parents during the preschool period are preschool and kindergarten experience, sex education, speech problems, and stress.
- Nurses can help parents assess a preschooler's readiness for kindergarten by considering the youngster's social maturity, as well as knowledge of specific skills, such as counting to 10 and recognizing letters of the alphabet.
- Two rules that govern answering questions about sex and other sensitive issues are to find out what the child thinks and to be honest.
- Preschool aggression may result from frustration, modeling behavior, and reinforcement.
- Fears constitute a great part of the preschool period; objects, potential annihilation, and parent-induced fears are common sources.
- Health promotion continues to be directed toward proper nutrition, adequate sleep, proper dental care, and injury prevention.

REFERENCES

American Academy of Pediatrics, Committee on School Health: *School health: a guide for health professionals,* ed 5, Elk Grove Village, IL, 1993, The Academy.

American Academy of Pediatrics, Committee on Sports Medicine and Fitness: Fitness, activity, and sports participation in the preschool child, *Pediatrics* 90(6):1002-1004, 1992.

Anliker JA and others: Children's food preferences and genetic sensitivity to the bitter taste of 6-*n*-propylthiouracil (PROP), *Am J Clin Nutr* 54(2):316-320, 1991.

Birch LL and others: The variability of young children's energy intake, *N Engl J Med* 324(4):232-235, 1991.

Brazelton TB: *Touchpoints,* Reading, MA, 1992, Addison-Wesley Company.

Clutter L: Fostering spiritual care for the child and family. In Smith D and others, editors: *Comprehensive child and family nursing skills,* St Louis, 1991, Mosby.

Edgil A, Wood K, Smith D: Sleep problems of older infants and preschool children, *Pediatr Nurs* 11(2):87-89, 1985.

Fish L, Burch K: Identifying gifted preschoolers, *Pediatr Nurs* 1(2):125-127, 1985.

Food and Nutrition Board, National Research Council: *Recommended Dietary Allowances,* ed 10, Washington, DC, 1989, National Academy Press.

Goldsmith LT, Feldman DH: Identifying gifted children: the state of the art, *Pediatr Ann* 14(10):709-716, 1985.

Goldsmith S: *Human sexuality: the family source book,* St Louis, 1986, Mosby.

Gordon S, Snyder CW: *Better sexual health,* Boston, 1989, Allyn & Bacon.

Greene JC, Louie R, Wycoff SJ: Preventive dentistry. II. Periodontal diseases, malocclusion, trauma, and oral cancer. *JAMA* 263(3):421-425, 1990.

Howes C: Pressuring children to learn versus developmentally appropriate education, *J Pediatr Health Care* 3(4):181-186, 1989.

Jacklin C: Gender. In Levine MD, Carey WB, Crocker AC: *Developmental-behavioral pediatrics,* ed 2, Philadelphia, 1992, WB Saunders.

Kellogg R: Understanding children's art. In *Readings in Psychology Today,* Del Mar, CA, 1969, Communications/Research/Machines.

Landesman, S: Defining giftedness, *Pediatr Ann* 14(10):698-706, 1985.

Landy S, Peters R. Identifying and treating aggressive preschoolers, *Infants Young Child* 3(2):24-38, 1990.

Leung A, Robson W: Childhood masturbation, *Clin Pediatr* 32(4):238-241, 1993.

Lowrey G: *Growth and development of children,* ed 8, St Louis, 1986, Mosby.

McDevitt S, Carey W: The measurement of temperament in 3-7 year old children, *J Child Psychol Psychiatry* 19:245-253, 1978.

McGuffog C: Problems of gifted children, *Pediatr Ann* 14(10):719-726, 1985.

Mills CJ: Academically talented children: the case for early identification and nurturance, *Pediatrics* 89(1):156-157, 1992.

Oberklaid F and others: Assessment of temperament in the toddler age group, *Pediatrics* 85:559-566, 1990.

Oberklaid F and others: Predicting preschool behavior problems from temperament and other variables in infancy, *Pediatrics* 91(1):113-120, 1993.

Pilapil V: A horrifying television commercial that led to constipation, *Pediatrics* 85(4):592-593, 1990.

Schmitt BD: Does your child have a stuttering problem? *Contemp Pediatr* 8(3):83-84, 1991.

Schor DP: Temperament and the initial school experience, *Child Health Care* 13(3):129-134, 1985.

Schraeder BD, Heverly MA, Rappaport J: Temperament, behavior problems, and learning skills in very low birth weight preschoolers, *Res Nurs Health* 13:27-34, 1990.

Selekman J: The development of body image in the child: a learned response, *Top Clin Nurs* 5(1):12-21, 1983.

Shapiro BK and others: Giftedness: can it be predicted in infancy? *Clin Pediatr* 28(5):205-209, 1989.

Shea S and others: Variability and self-regulation of energy intake in young children in their everyday environment, *Pediatrics* 90:542-546, 1992.

Shelly J and others: *The spiritual needs of children,* Downer's Grove, IL, 1982, Inter-Varsity Press.

Singer D: Children, adolescents, and television—1989. I. Television violence: a critique, *Pediatrics* 83(3):445-446, 1989.

Thomas RM: *Comparing theories of child development,* ed 2, Belmont, CA, 1985, Wadsworth.

Weiss B and others: Some consequences of early harsh discipline: child aggression and a maladaptive social information processing style, *Child Dev* 63(6):1321-1335, 1992.

Wilson DA, Knudtson MD: Assessing school readiness through the school-entry screening exam, *Nurs Pract* 17(9):24-6, 29-30, 33, 1992.

BIBLIOGRAPHY

Only citations specific to preschoolers are included here; additional references can be found in Chapters 12 and 14.

Growth and Development

Ames LB, Ilg FI: *Your three-year-old: friend or enemy,* New York, 1980, Delacorte Press.

Ames LB, Ilg FI: *Your four-year-old: wild and wonderful,* New York, 1981, Delacorte Press.

Ames LB, Ilg FI: *Your five-year-old: sunny and serene,* New York, 1981, Delacorte Press.

Betz C: Faith development in children, *Pediatr Nurs* 7(2):22-25, 1981.

Dixon SD, Stein MT: *Encounters with children: a practical guide to pediatric behavior and development,* ed 2, St Louis, 1992, Mosby.

Dworkin PH: The preschool child: developmental themes and clinical issues, *Curr Probl Pediatr* 18(2):73-134, 1988.

Forbes GB: Children and food—order amid chaos, *N Engl J Med* 324(4):262-263, 1991.

Garbarino J and others: *What children can tell us,* San Francisco, 1989, Jossey-Bass.

Gelman R, Baillargem R: A review of Piagetian concepts. In Flavell J, Markham E, editors: *Handbook of child psychology,* vol 3, New York, 1984, John Wiley & Sons.

Hauck MR: Cognitive abilities of preschool children: implications for nursing working with young children, *J Pediatr Nurs* 6(4):230-235, 1991.

Howard BJ: Growing together; learning independence in the preschool years, *Contemp Pediatr* 7(7):11-26, 1990.

Kay P: The imaginary companion: review of the literature, *Matern Child Nurs J* 9:8-11, 1980.

Larson CP, Pless B, Miettinen O: Preschool behavior disorders: their prevalence in relation to determinants, *J Pediatr* 113:278-285, 1988.

Lavigne JB and others: Behavioral and emotional problems among preschool children in pediatric primary care: prevalence and pediatricians' recognition, *Pediatrics* 91(3):649-655, 1993.

Lowrey G: *Growth and development of children,* ed 8, St Louis, 1986, Mosby.

Lyytinen P: Developmental trends in children's pretend play, *Child Care Health Dev* 17(1):25, 1991.

Mitchell S: Imaginary companions: friend or foe? *Pediatr Nurs* 6(6):29-30, 1980.

Morrison CD, Bundy AC, Fisher AG: The contribution of motor skills and playfulness to the play performance of preschoolers, *Am J Occup Ther* 45(8):687-694, 1991.

Nicholls AL, Kennedy JM: Drawing development: from similarity of features to direction, *Child Dev* 63(1):227-241, 1992.

Park KA, Waters E: Security of attachment and preschool friendships, *Child Dev* 60:1076-1081, 1989.

Prior M and others: Sex differences in psychological adjustment from infancy to 8 years, *J Am Acad Child Adolesc Psychiatry* 32(2):291-304, 1993.

Rugg HA, Saltarelli LM: Exploratory play with objects: basic cognitive processes and individual differences, *New Dir Child Dev* (59):5-16, 1993.

Schraeder BD, Tobey GY: Preschool temperament of very-low-birth-weight infants, *J Pediatr Nurs* 4(2):119-126, 1989.

Shonkoff JP: Preschool. In Levine MD and others, editors: *Developmental-behavioral pediatrics,* Philadelphia, 1992, WB Saunders.

Sullivan SA, Birch LL: Pass the sugar, pass the salt: experience dictates preference, *Dev Psychol* 26:546-551, 1990.

Thomas A, Chess S: Genesis and evolution of behavioral disorders from infancy to early adult life, *Am J Psychiatry* 141:1-9, 1984.

Preschool and Kindergarten/Gifted Children

Birchfield M: Illnesses and children in a preschool center, *Matern Child Nurs J* 15(3):187-197, 1986.

Casey PH, Evans LD: School readiness: an overview for pediatricians, *Pediatr Rev* 14(1):4-10, 1993.

Karp R and others: Growth and academic achievement in inner-city kindergarten children, *Clin Pediatr* 31(6):336-340, 1992.

Martin S, Ramey C, Ramey S: The prevention of intellectual impairment in children of impoverished families: findings of a randomized trial of educational day care, *Am J Public Health* 80:844-847, 1990.

Palmer DJ and others: An exploratory study of the structure and validity of pediatric examination of educational readiness, *Dev Behav Pediatr* 11(6):317-321, 1990.

Robinson J: *Is your child ready for school?* New York, 1990, Simon & Schuster.

Robinson NM: Educational options for gifted children, *Pediatr Ann* 14(10):745-756, 1985.

Sanson A and others: Risk indicators: assessment of infancy predictors of preschool behavioural maladjustment, *J Child Psychol Psychiatry* 32(4):609-626, 1991.

Sex Education

Aquilino ML, Ely J: Parents and the sexuality of preschool children, *Pediatr Nurs* 11(1):41-46, 1985.

Calderone MS: Sexual health and the child, *Compr Ther* 6(12):3-7, 1980.

Castiglia PT: Masturbation, *J Pediatr Health Care* 2(2):111-112, 1988.

Masters WH, Johnson VE, Kolodny RC: *Human sexuality,* ed 3, Glenview, IL, 1988, Scott, Foresman.

Aggression

Christophersen ER: Oppositional behavior in children, *Pediatr Ann* 20(5):267-270, 1991.

Clore ER, Hibel JA: Overcoming bullying behavior: a challenge to the school nurse, *School Health Watch* 4(1):3-5, 7, 1992-1993.

Gabel S, Shindledecker R: Aggressive behavior in youth: characteristics, outcome, and psychiatric diagnoses, *J Am Acad Child Adolesc Psychiatry* 30(6):982-988, 1991.

Heath E, Kosky R: Are children who steal different from those who are aggressive? *Child Psychiatry Hum Dev* 23(1):9-18, 1992.

Kelso J, Stewart M: Factors which predict the persistence of aggressive conduct disorder, *J Child Psychol Psychiatry* 27(1):77-86, 1986.

Kemph JP and others: Treatment of aggressive children with clonidine: results of an open pilot study, *J Am Acad Child Adolesc Psychiatry* 32(3):577-581, 1993.

Lyons-Ruth K, Alpern L, Repacholi B: Disorganized infant attachment classification and maternal psychosocial problems as predictors of hostile-aggressive behavior in the preschool classroom, *Child Dev* 64(2):572-585, 1993.

Parker JG, Asher SR: Peer relationships and later personal adjustment: are low-accepted children "at risk?" *Psychol Bull* 102:357-389, 1987.

Schmitt BD: When a child hurts other children, *Contemp Pediatr* 7(12):81-82, 1990.

Sleep Problems

Beltramini A, Hertzig M: Sleep and bedtime behavior in preschool-aged children, *Pediatrics* 71(2):153-158, 1983.

Clore ER, Hibel J: The parasomnias of childhood, *J Pediatr Health Care* 7(1):12-16, 1993.

Crawford W, Bennet R, Hewitt K: Sleep problems in pre-school children, *Health Visit* 62(3):79-81, 1989.

Dahl RE: The pharmacologic treatment of sleep disorders, *Psychiatr Clin North Am* 15(1):161-178, 1992.

DiMario F, Enery ES, III: The natural history of night terrors, *Clin Pediatr* 26(10):505-511, 1987.

Edgil A and others: Sleep problems of older infants and preschool children, *Pediatr Nurs* 11(2):87-89, 1985.

Gates D, Morwessel N. Night terrors: strategies for family coping, *J Pediatr Nurs* 4(1):48-53, 1989.

Jimmerson KR: Maternal, environmental, and temperamental characteristics of toddlers with and toddlers without sleep problems *J Pediatr Health Care* 5(2):71-77, 1991.

Leung AK, Robson WL: Nightmares, *J Natl Med Assoc* 85(3):233-235, 1993.

McMenamy C, Katz RC: Brief parent-assisted treatment for children's nighttime fears, *J Dev Behav Pediatr* 10(3):145-148, 1989.

Pagel J: Nightmares, *Am Fam Physician* 39(3): 145-148, 1989.

Rieger I: Sleep disorders in children, *Aust Fam Physician* 18(6):699, 701, 1989.

Stores G: Sleep problems, *Arch Dis Child* 67 (12):1420-1421, 1992.

Fears

Gullone E, King NJ: Psychometric evaluation of a revised fear survey schedule for children and adolescents, *J Child Psychol Psychiatry* 33(6):987-998, 1992.

Vandenberg B: Fears of normal and retarded children, *Psychol Rep* 72(2):473-474, 1993.

CHAPTER 16

Health Problems of Early Childhood

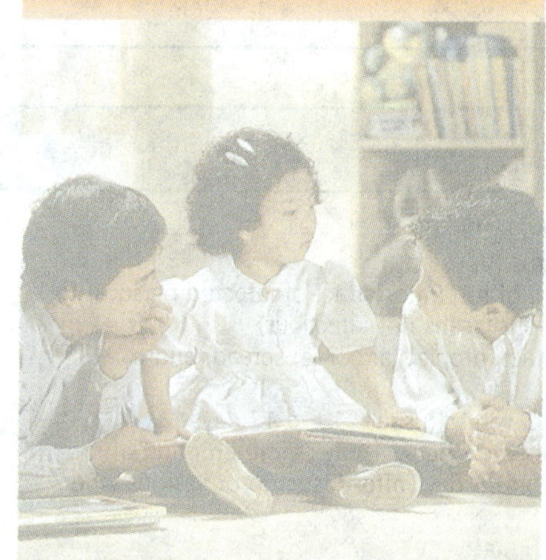

CHAPTER OUTLINE

RELATED TOPICS

INFECTIOUS DISORDERS

COMMUNICABLE DISEASES

The incidence of common childhood communicable diseases has declined greatly since the advent of immunizations. Serious complications resulting from such infections have been further reduced through the use of antibiotics and antitoxins. However, infectious diseases do occur, and nurses must be familiar with the infectious agent in order to recognize the disease and institute appropriate preventive and supportive interventions. To facilitate understanding of communicable diseases, several terms are defined in the box on p. 678.

Nursing Considerations

The more common communicable diseases of childhood, their therapeutic management, and specific nursing care are described in Table 16-1. The following is a general discussion of nursing considerations for communicable diseases. The reader is also referred to Chapter 18 for a discussion of nursing care for dermatologic conditions.

❖ Assessment

Identification of the infectious agent is of primary importance in order to prevent exposure to susceptible individuals. Nurses in ambulatory care settings, such as emergency rooms, health maintenance centers, preschools or regular schools, and practitioners' offices, are often the first persons to see signs of a communicable disease, such as a rash or sore throat. The nurse must operate under a high index of suspicion for common childhood diseases in order to identify potentially infectious cases and to recognize diseases that require medical intervention. An example is the

Text continued on p. 676.

TABLE 16-1 Communicable Diseases of Childhood

DISEASE

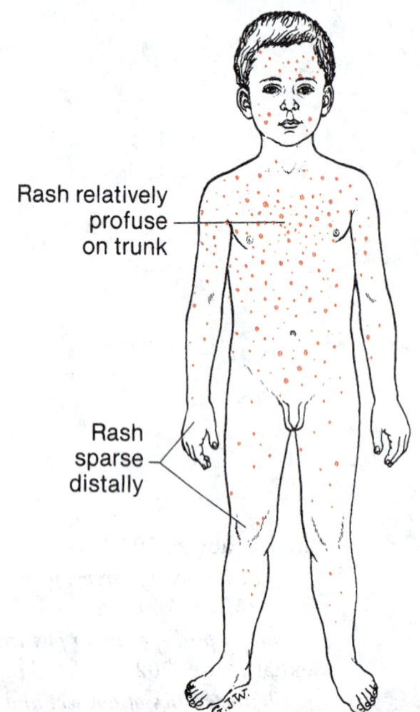

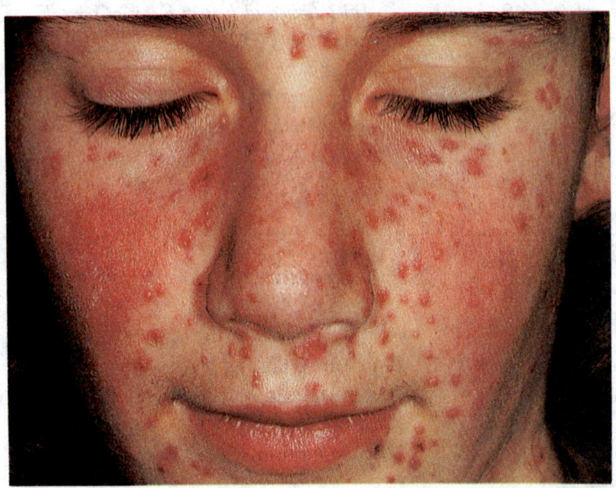

CHICKENPOX (VARICELLA) (Fig. 16-1)

Agent: Varicella zoster virus (VZV)
Source: Primary secretions of respiratory tract of infected persons; to a lesser degree skin lesions (scabs not infectious)
Transmission: Direct contact, droplet (airborne) spread, and contaminated objects
Incubation period: 2 to 3 weeks, usually 13 to 17 days
Period of communicability: Probably 1 day before eruption of lesions (prodromal period) to 6 days after first crop of vesicles when crusts have formed

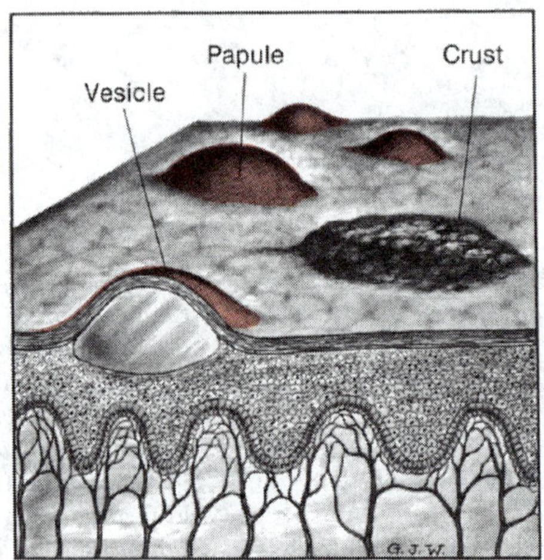

FIG. 16-1 Chickenpox (varicella). (Clinical view from Habif TP: *Clinical dermatology: a color guide to diagnosis and therapy,* ed 2, St Louis, 1990, Mosby.)

DIPHTHERIA

Agent: *Corynebacterium diphtheriae*
Source: Discharges from mucous membranes of nose and nasopharynx, skin, and other lesions of infected person
Transmission: Direct contact with infected person, a carrier, or contaminated articles
Incubation period: Usually 2 to 5 days, possibly longer
Period of communicability: Variable; until virulent bacilli are no longer present (identified by three negative cultures); usually 2 weeks but as long as 4 weeks

CLINICAL MANIFESTATIONS	THERAPEUTIC MANAGEMENT/ COMPLICATIONS	NURSING CONSIDERATIONS
Prodromal stage: Slight fever, malaise, and anorexia for first 24 hours; rash highly pruritic; begins as macule, rapidly progresses to papule and then vesicle (surrounded by erythematous base, becomes umbilicated and cloudy, breaks easily and forms crusts); all three stages (papule, vesicle, crust) present in varying degrees at one time **Distribution:** Centripetal, spreading to face and proximal extremities but sparse on distal limbs and less on areas not exposed to heat (i.e., from clothing or sun) **Constitutional signs and symptoms:** Elevated temperature from lymphadenopathy, irritability from pruritus	**Specific:** Antiviral agent acyclovir (Zovirax) (see text p. 679); varicella-zoster immune globulin (VZIG) after exposure in high-risk children **Supportive:** Diphenhydramine hydrochloride or antihistamines to relieve itching; skin care to prevent secondary bacterial infection **Complications:** Secondary bacterial infections (abscesses, cellulitis, pneumonia, sepsis) Encephalitis Varicella pneumonia Hemorrhagic varicella (tiny hemorrhages in vesicles and numerous petechiae in skin) Chronic or transient thrombocytopenia	Maintain strict isolation in hospital Isolate child in home until vesicles have dried (usually 1 week after onset of disease), and isolate high-risk children from infected children Administer skin care: give bath and change clothes and linens daily; administer topical application of calamine lotion; keep child's fingernails short and clean; apply mittens if child scratches Keep child cool (may decrease number of lesions) Lessen pruritus; keep child occupied Remove loose crusts that rub and irritate skin Teach child to apply pressure to pruritic area rather than scratching it If older child, reason with child regarding danger of scar formation from scratching Avoid use of aspirin; use of acetaminophen controversial (see text, p. 679)
Vary according to anatomic location of pseudomembrane **Nasal:** Resembles common cold, serosanguineous mucopurulent nasal discharge without constitutional symptoms; may be frank epistaxis **Tonsillar/pharyngeal:** Malaise; anorexia; sore throat; low-grade fever; pulse increased above expected for temperature within 24 hours; smooth, adherent, white or gray membrane; lymphadenitis possibly pronounced (bull's neck); in severe cases, toxemia, septic shock, and death within 6 to 10 days **Laryngeal:** Fever, hoarseness, cough, with or without previous signs listed; potential airway obstruction, apprehensive, dyspneic retractions, cyanosis	Antitoxin (usually intravenously); preceded by skin or conjunctival test to rule out sensitivity to horse serum Antibiotics (penicillin or erythromycin) Complete bed rest (prevention of myocarditis) Tracheostomy for airway obstruction Treatment of infected contacts and carriers **Complications:** Myocarditis (second week) Neuritis	Maintain strict isolation in hospital Participate in sensitivity testing; have epinephrine available Administer antibiotics; observe for signs of sensitivity to penicillin Administer complete care to maintain bed rest Use suctioning as needed Observe respirations for signs of obstruction Administer humidified oxygen if prescribed

Continued.

TABLE 16-1 Communicable Diseases of Childhood—cont'd

DISEASE

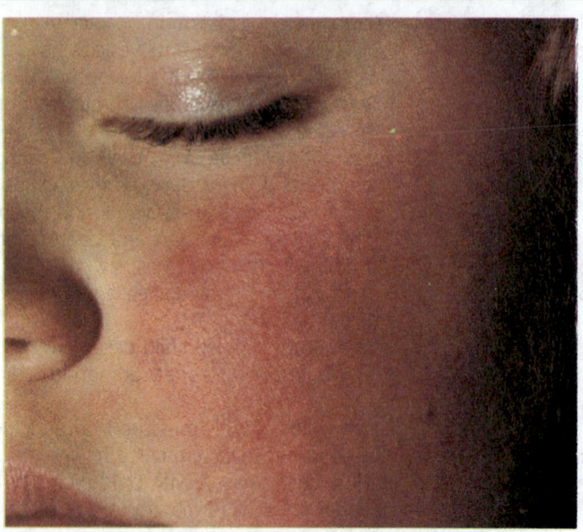

FIG. 16-2 Erythema infectiosum. (From Habif TP: *Clinical dermatology: a color guide to diagnosis and therapy*, ed 2, St Louis, 1990, Mosby.)

ERYTHEMA INFECTIOSUM (FIFTH DISEASE) (Fig. 16-2)

Agent: Human parvovirus B19 (HPV)
Source: Infected persons
Transmission: Unknown; possibly respiratory secretions and blood
Incubation period: 4 to 14 days, may be as long as 20 days
Period of communicability: Uncertain but before onset of symptoms in most children; also for about 1 week after onset of symptoms in children with aplastic crisis

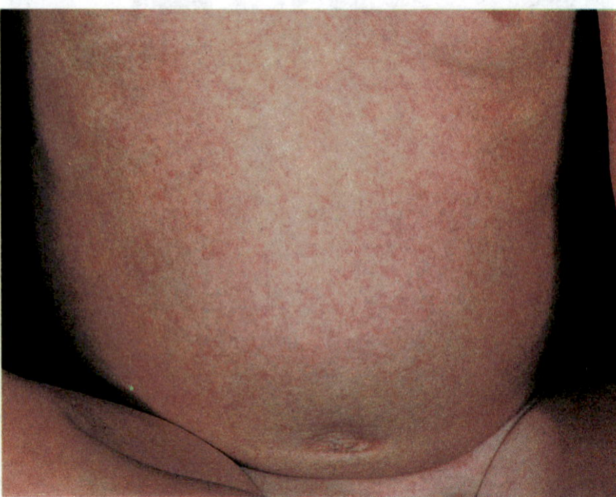

FIG. 16-3 Roseola infantum. (From Habif TP: *Clinical dermatology: a color guide to diagnosis and therapy*, ed 2, St Louis, 1990, Mosby.)

EXANTHEMA SUBITUM (ROSEOLA) (Fig. 16-3)

Agent: Human herpes virus type 6 (HHV-6)
Source: Unknown
Transmission: Unknown (virtually limited to children between 6 months and 2 years of age)
Incubation period: Unknown
Period of communicability: Unknown

CLINICAL MANIFESTATIONS	THERAPEUTIC MANAGEMENT/ COMPLICATIONS	NURSING CONSIDERATIONS
Rash appears in three stages: I—Erythema on face, chiefly on cheeks, "slapped face" appearance; disappears by 1 to 4 days II—About 1 day after rash appears on face, maculopapular red spots appear, symmetrically distributed on upper and lower extremities; rash progresses from proximal to distal surfaces and may last a week or more III—Rash subsides but reappears if skin is irritated or traumatized (sun, heat, cold, friction) In children with aplastic crisis, rash is usually absent and prodromal illness includes fever, myalgia, lethargy, nausea, vomiting, and abdominal pain	**Symptomatic and supportive:** Antipyretics, analgesics, antiinflammatory drugs Possible blood transfusion for transient aplastic anemia **Complications:** Self-limited arthritis and arthralgia (arthritis may become chronic) (Nocton and others, 1993) May result in fetal death if mother infected during pregnancy, but no evidence of congenital anomalies Aplastic crisis in children with hemolytic disease or immune deficiency Myocarditis (rare)	Isolation of child not necessary, except hospitalized child (immunosuppressed or with aplastic crises) suspected of HPV infection is placed on respiratory isolation and universal precautions Pregnant women: need not be excluded from workplace where HPV infection is present; should not care for patients with aplastic crises; explain low risk of fetal death to those in contact with affected children
Persistent high fever for 3 to 4 days in child who appears well Precipitous drop in fever to normal with appearance of rash **Rash:** Discrete rose-pink macules or maculopapules appearing first on trunk, then spreading to neck, face, and extremities; nonpruritic, fades on pressure, lasts 1 to 2 days **Associated signs and symptoms:** Cervical/postauricular lymphadenopathy, injected pharynx, cough, coryza	Nonspecific Antipyretics to control fever **Complications:** Recurrent febrile seizures (possibly from latent infection of central nervous system that is reactivated by fever) Encephalitis (rare)	Teach parents measures for lowering temperature (antipyretic drugs) If child is prone to seizures, discuss appropriate precautions, possibility of recurrent febrile seizures (Kondo and others, 1993)

Continued.

TABLE 16-1 Communicable Diseases of Childhood—cont'd

DISEASE

MEASLES (RUBEOLA) (Fig. 16-4)

Agent: Virus

Source: Respiratory tract secretions, blood, and urine of infected person

Transmission: Usually by direct contact with droplets of infected person

Incubation period: 10 to 20 days

Period of communicability: From 4 days before to 5 days after rash appears but mainly during prodromal (catarrhal) stage

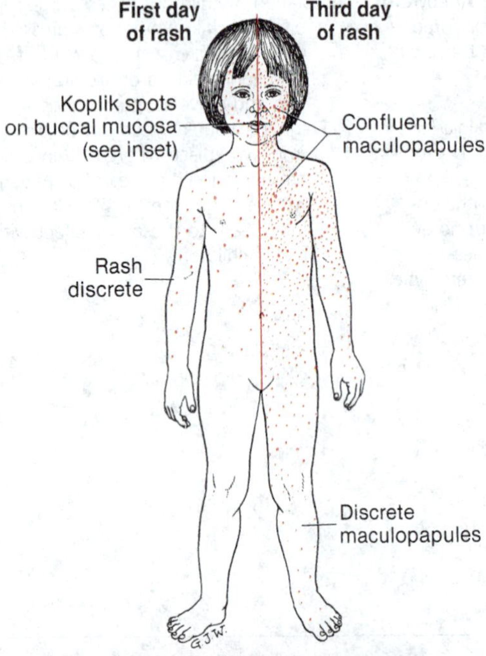

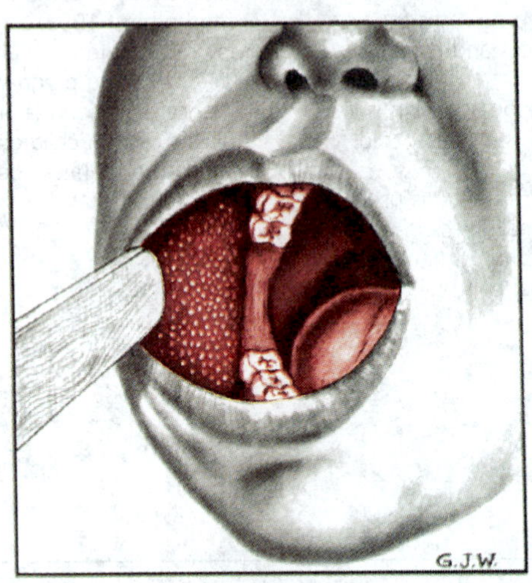

Koplik spots

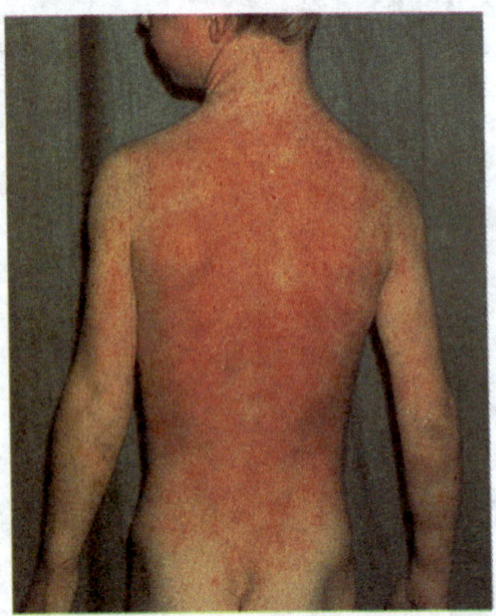

FIG. 16-4 Measles (rubeola). (Clinical view from Seidel HM and others: *Mosby's guide to physical examination,* St Louis, 1991, Mosby.)

MUMPS

Agent: Paramyxovirus

Source: Saliva of infected persons

Transmission: Direct contact with or droplet spread from an infected person

Incubation period: 14 to 21 days

Period of communicability: Most communicable immediately before and after swelling begins

PERTUSSIS (WHOOPING COUGH)

Agent: *Bordetella pertussis*

Source: Discharge from respiratory tract of infected persons

Transmission: Direct contact or droplet spread from infected person; indirect contact with freshly contaminated articles

Incubation period: 5 to 21 days, usually 10

Period of communicability: Greatest during catarrhal stage before onset of paroxysms and may extend to fourth week after onset of paroxysms

CLINICAL MANIFESTATIONS	THERAPEUTIC MANAGEMENT/ COMPLICATIONS	NURSING CONSIDERATIONS
Prodromal (catarrhal) stage: Fever and malaise, followed in 24 hours by coryza, cough, conjunctivitis, Koplik spots (small, irregular red spots with a minute, bluish white center first seen on buccal mucosa opposite molars 2 days before rash); symptoms gradually increase in severity until second day after rash appears, when they begin to subside **Rash:** Appears 3 to 4 days after onset of prodromal stage; begins as erythematous maculopapular eruption on face and gradually spreads downward; more severe in earlier sites (appears confluent) and less intense in later sites (appears discrete); after 3 to 4 days assumes brownish appearance, and fine desquamation occurs over areas of extensive involvement **Constitutional signs and symptoms:** Anorexia, malaise, generalized lymphadenopathy	Vitamin A supplementation (see text p. 679) **Supportive:** Bed rest during febrile period; antipyretics Antibiotics to prevent secondary bacterial infection in high-risk children **Complications:** Otitis media Pneumonia Bronchiolitis Obstructive laryngitis and laryngotracheitis Encephalitis	Isolation until fifth day of rash; if hospitalized, institute respiratory precautions Maintain bed rest during prodromal stage; provide quiet activity **Fever:** Instruct parents to administer antipyretics; avoid chilling; if child is prone to seizures, institute appropriate precautions (fever spikes to 40° C [104° F] between fourth and fifth days) **Eye care:** Dim lights if photophobia present; clean eyelids with warm saline solution to remove secretions or crusts; keep child from rubbing eyes; examine cornea for signs of ulceration **Coryza/cough:** Use cool mist vaporizer; protect skin around nares with layer of petrolatum; encourage fluids and soft, bland foods **Skin care:** Keep skin clean; use tepid baths as necessary
Prodromal stage: Fever, headache, malaise, and anorexia for 24 hours, followed by "earache" that is aggravated by chewing **Parotitis:** By third day, parotid gland(s) (either unilateral or bilateral) enlarges and reaches maximum size in 1 to 3 days; accompanied by pain and tenderness **Other manifestations:** Submaxillary and sublingual infection, orchitis, and meningoencephalitis	**Symptomatic and supportive:** Analgesics for pain and antipyretics for fever Intravenous fluid may be necessary for child who refuses to drink or vomits because of meningoencephalitis **Complications:** Sensorineural deafness Postinfectious encephalitis Myocarditis Arthritis Hepatitis Epididymo-orchitis Sterility (extremely rare in adult males)	Isolation during period of communicability; institute respiratory precautions during hospitalization Maintain bed rest during prodromal phase until swelling subsides Give analgesics for pain; if child is unwilling to chew medication, use elixir form Encourage fluids and soft, bland foods; avoid foods requiring chewing Apply hot or cold compresses to neck, whichever is more comforting To relieve orchitis, provide warmth and local support with tight-fitting underpants (stretch bathing suit works well)
Catarrhal stage: Begins with symptoms of upper respiratory tract infection, such as coryza, sneezing, lacrimation, cough, and low-grade fever; symptoms continue for 1 to 2 weeks, when dry, hacking cough becomes more severe **Paroxysmal stage:** Cough most often occurs at night and consists of short, rapid coughs followed by sudden inspiration associated with a high-pitched crowing sound or "whoop"; during paroxysms cheeks become flushed or cyanotic, eyes bulge, and tongue protrudes; paroxysm may continue until thick mucous plug is dislodged; vomiting frequently follows attack; stage generally lasts 4 to 6 weeks, followed by convalescent stage	Antimicrobial therapy (e.g., erythromycin) Administration of pertussis-immune globulin **Supportive treatment:** Hospitalization required for infants, children who are dehydrated, or those who have complications Bed rest Increased oxygen intake and humidity Adequate fluids Intubation possibly necessary **Complications:** Pneumonia (usual cause of death) Atelectasis Otitis media Convulsions Hemorrhage (subarachnoid, subconjunctival, epistaxis) Weight loss and dehydration Hernia Prolapsed rectum	Isolation during catarrhal stage; if hospitalized, institute respiratory precautions Maintain bed rest as long as fever present Keep child occupied during day (interest in play associated with fewer paroxysms) Reassure parents during frightening episodes of whooping cough Provide restful environment and reduce factors that promote paroxysms (dust, smoke, sudden change in temperature, chilling, activity, excitement); keep room well ventilated Encourage fluids; offer small amount of fluids frequently; refeed child after vomiting Provide high humidity (humidifier or tent); suction gently but often to prevent choking on secretions Observe for signs of airway obstruction (increased restlessness, apprehension, retractions, cyanosis) Involve public health nurse if child cared for at home

Continued.

TABLE 16-1 Communicable Diseases of Childhood—cont'd

DISEASE
POLIOMYELITIS **Agent:** Enteroviruses, three types: type 1—most frequent cause of paralysis, both epidemic and endemic; type 2—least frequently associated with paralysis; type 3—second most frequently associated with paralysis **Source:** Feces and oropharyngeal secretions of infected persons, especially young children **Transmission:** Direct contact with persons with apparent or inapparent active infection; spread is via fecal-oral and pharyngeal-oropharyngeal routes **Incubation period:** Usually 7 to 14 days, with range of 5 to 35 days **Period of communicability:** Not exactly known; virus is present in throat and feces shortly after infection and persists for about 1 week in throat and 4 to 6 weeks in feces
RUBELLA (GERMAN MEASLES) (Fig. 16-5) **Agent:** Rubella virus **Source:** Primarily nasopharyngeal secretions of person with apparent or inapparent infection; virus also present in blood, stool, and urine **Transmission:** Direct contact and spread via infected person; indirectly via articles freshly contaminated with nasopharyngeal secretions, feces, or urine **Incubation period:** 14 to 21 days **Period of communicability:** 7 days before to about 5 days after appearance of rash

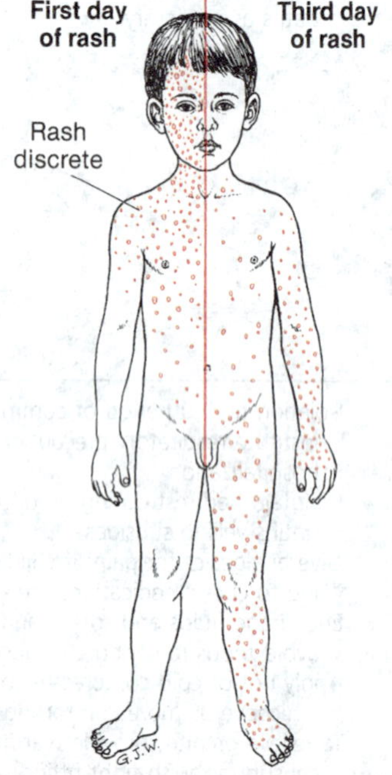

FIG. 16-5 Rubella (German measles). (Clinical view from Habif TP: *Clinical dermatology: a color guide to diagnosis and therapy,* ed 2, St Louis, 1990, Mosby.)

CLINICAL MANIFESTATIONS	THERAPEUTIC MANAGEMENT/ COMPLICATIONS	NURSING CONSIDERATIONS
May be manifested in three different forms: **Abortive or inapparent**—Fever, uneasiness, sore throat, headache, anorexia, vomiting, abdominal pain; lasts a few hours to a few days **Nonparalytic**—Same manifestations as abortive but more severe, with pain and stiffness in neck, back, and legs **Paralytic**—Initial course similar to nonparalytic type, followed by recovery and then signs of central nervous system paralysis	No specific treatment, including antimicrobials or gamma globulin Complete bed rest during acute phase Assisted respiratory ventilation in case of respiratory paralysis Physical therapy for muscles following acute stage **Complications:** Permanent paralysis Respiratory arrest Hypertension Kidney stones from demineralization of bone during prolonged immobility	Maintain complete bed rest Administer mild sedatives as necessary to relieve anxiety and promote rest Participate in physiotherapy procedures (use of moist hot packs and range-of-motion exercises) Position child to maintain body alignment and prevent contractures or decubiti; use footboard Encourage child to move; administer analgesics for maximum comfort during physical activity Observe for respiratory paralysis (difficulty in talking, ineffective cough, inability to hold breath, shallow and rapid respirations); report such signs and symptoms to practitioner; have tracheostomy tray at bedside
Prodromal stage: Absent in children, present in adults and adolescents; consists of low-grade fever, headache, malaise, anorexia, mild conjunctivitis, coryza, sore throat, cough, and lymphadenopathy; lasts for 1 to 5 days, subsides 1 day after appearance of rash **Rash:** First appears on face and rapidly spreads downward to neck, arms, trunk, and legs; by end of first day body is covered with a discrete, pinkish red maculopapular exanthema; disappears in same order as it began and is usually gone by third day **Constitutional signs and symptoms:** Occasionally low-grade fever, headache, malaise, and lymphadenopathy	No treatment necessary other than antipyretics for low-grade fever and analgesics for discomfort **Complications:** Rare (arthritis, encephalitis, or purpura); most benign of all childhood communicable diseases; greatest danger is teratogenic effect on fetus	Reassure parents of benign nature of illness in affected child Employ comfort measures as necessary Isolate child from pregnant women

Continued.

TABLE 16-1 Communicable Diseases of Childhood—cont'd

DISEASE
SCARLET FEVER (Fig. 16-6) **Agent:** Group A β-hemolytic streptococci **Source:** Usually from nasopharyngeal secretions of infected persons and carriers **Transmission:** Direct contact with infected person or droplet spread; indirectly by contact with contaminated articles, ingestion of contaminated milk or other food **Incubation period:** 2 to 4 days, with range of 1 to 7 days **Period of communicability:** During incubation period and clinical illness approximately 10 days; during first 2 weeks of carrier phase, although may persist for months

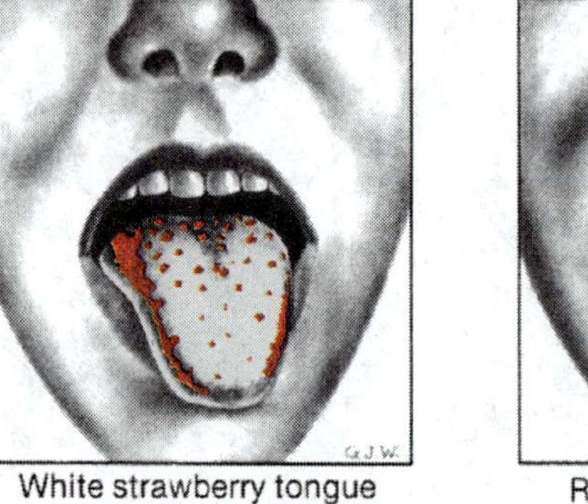

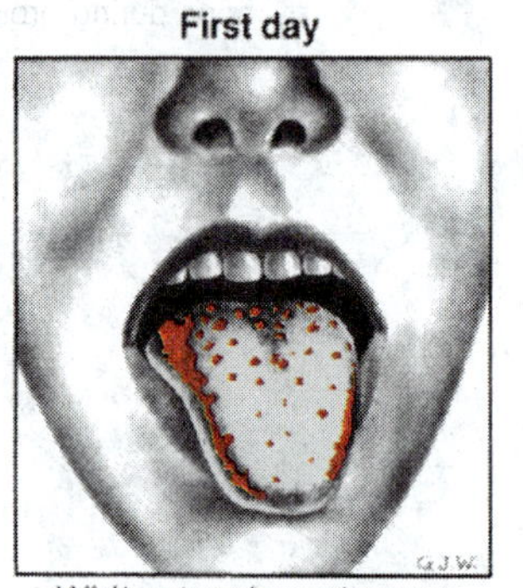

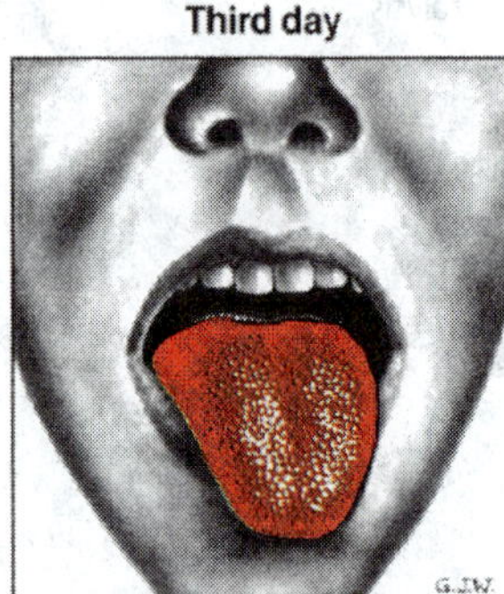

FIG. 16-6 Scarlet fever.

common complaint of a sore throat. Although most often a symptom of a minor viral infection, a sore throat can signal diphtheria or a streptococcal infection, such as scarlet fever. Both of these bacterial conditions require appropriate medical treatment to prevent serious sequelae.

Assessment of the following is helpful in identifying potentially communicable diseases: (1) recent exposure to a known case, (2) prodromal symptoms or evidence of constitutional symptoms, such as a fever or rash (see Table 16-1), (3) immunization history, and (4) history of having the disease. Since immunizations are available for several of the diseases and usually an attack confers lifelong immunity, the possibility of many infectious agents can be eliminated based on these two criteria.

The nurse should also be familiar with tests commonly used to confirm or rule out the diagnosis of infectious diseases. The ***hemagglutination inhibition test*** is used to detect rubella antibodies; a high antibody titer indicates immunity. Specific tests for scarlet fever include a throat culture and the ***anti-streptolysin*** O, which detects rising antibody titer to streptolysin O. A test for diagnosing diphtheria is the ***Schick test,*** which detects a reaction to inoculation with diphtheria toxin. Knowledge of test results allows for appropriate decision making regarding the need for treatment or isolation. For example, rubella is a benign childhood disease that requires no special intervention. Ordinarily the recommendation is to confine the child to the home for about 7 days after the appearance of the rash. However, if the mother is in the first trimester of pregnancy, immediate steps need to be taken to isolate the child from the mother if her antibody titer is low. In addition, any pregnant visitors should avoid close contact with the child.

❖ Nursing Diagnoses

A number of nursing diagnoses are prominent in the care of the child with a communicable disease; others are specific to individual cases. The most common nursing diagnoses are presented in the Nursing Care Plan on pp. 680-681.

❖ Planning

The principal goals in addition to identification of the communicable disease (see Assessment) are as follows:

1. Child will not spread the infection to others.
2. Child will not experience complications.
3. Child will have minimal discomfort.
4. Child and family will receive adequate emotional support.

CLINICAL MANIFESTATIONS	THERAPEUTIC MANAGEMENT/ COMPLICATIONS	NURSING CONSIDERATIONS
Prodromal stage: Abrupt high fever, pulse increased out of proportion to fever, vomiting, headache, chills, malaise, abdominal pain **Enanthema:** Tonsils enlarged, edematous, reddened, and covered with patches of exudate; in severe cases appearance resembles membrane seen in diphtheria; pharynx is edematous and beefy red; during first 1 to 2 days tongue is coated and papillae become red and swollen (white strawberry tongue); by fourth or fifth day white coat sloughs off, leaving prominent papillae (red strawberry tongue); palate is covered with erythematous punctate lesions **Exanthema:** Rash appears within 12 hours after prodromal signs; red pinhead-sized punctate lesions rapidly become generalized but are absent on face, which becomes flushed with striking circumoral pallor; rash is more intense in folds of joints; by end of first week desquamation begins (fine, sandpaper-like on torso; sheet-like sloughing on palms and soles), which may be complete by 3 weeks or longer	Treatment of choice is a full course of penicillin (or erythromycin in penicillin-sensitive children); fever should subside 24 hours after beginning therapy Antibiotic therapy for newly diagnosed carriers (nose or throat cultures positive for streptococci) **Supportive measures:** Bed rest during febrile phase, analgesics for sore throat **Complications:** Otitis media Peritonsillar abscess Sinusitis Glomerulonephritis Carditis, polyarthritis (uncommon)	Institute respiratory precautions until 24 hours after initiation of treatment Ensure compliance with oral antibiotic therapy (intramuscular benzathine penicillin G [Bicillin] may be given if parents' reliability in giving oral drugs is questionable) Maintain bed rest during febrile phase; provide quiet activity during convalescent period Relieve discomfort of sore throat with analgesics, gargles, lozenges, antiseptic throat sprays (Chloraseptic), and inhalation of cool mist Encourage fluids during febrile phase; avoid irritating liquids (citrus juices) or rough foods; when child is able to eat, begin with soft diet Advise parents to consult practitioner if fever persists after beginning therapy Discuss procedures for preventing spread of infection

❖ IMPLEMENTATION

Many of the diseases require only supportive measures until the illness runs its course. Children are usually cared for at home until the disease is no longer communicable and until they feel well enough to resume normal activity.

Prevent Spread. Prevention consists of two components: prevention of the disease and control of its spread to others. Primary prevention rests almost exclusively on immunization (see Immunizations, Chapter 12).

Control measures to prevent spread of the disease include appropriate techniques to reduce risk of cross-transmission of infectious organisms between patients and to protect health care workers from organisms harbored by patients. If the child is hospitalized, the facility's policies for isolation precautions are instituted (see Infection Control, Chapter 27). The most important procedure to stress is handwashing. Persons directly caring for the child or handling contaminated articles must wash their hands before beginning care of another patient. The child is instructed to practice good handwashing technique after toileting and before eating. For those diseases spread by droplets, the nurse instructs the family in measures aimed at reducing airborne transmission. The child who is old enough should use a tissue to cover the face during coughing or sneezing; otherwise the parent should cover the child's mouth with a tissue and then discard it. The usual hygiene measures of not sharing eating and drinking utensils should be stressed to the family.

NURSING ALERT If a child is admitted to the hospital with an undiagnosed exanthema, strict isolation is instituted until a diagnosis is confirmed. Childhood communicable diseases requiring strict isolation are diphtheria and chickenpox. Recent evidence confirms that varicella-zoster virus is spread by aerosol (airborne) transmission (Sawyer and others, 1994).

Prevent Complications. While most youngsters recover without any difficulty, certain groups of children are at risk for serious, even fatal, complications from communicable diseases, especially the viral diseases of chickenpox and erythema infectiosum (EI). Children with an immunodeficiency—those receiving steroid or other immunosuppressive therapy, those with a generalized malignancy such as leukemia or lymphoma, or those with an immunologic disorder—are at risk for viremia from replication of the varicella-zoster virus (VZV) in the blood.

KEY COMMUNICABLE DISEASE TERMS

Communicable disease—An illness caused by a specific infectious agent or its toxic products through a direct or indirect mode of transmission of that agent from a reservoir

Epidemic—A disease occurring in a greater than the expected number of cases in a community

Endemic—A disease occurring regularly within a geographic location

Pandemic—A disease affecting large portions of the population throughout the world

Infectious agent—An organism, such as bacteria or virus, that is capable of producing infection or infectious disease

Reservoir—Environment in which an infectious agent lives and multiplies and on which it depends for survival; humans are the most frequent reservoir of infections that are capable of producing disease in other humans

Host—A person, or other living animal, that affords subsistence or lodgment to an infectious agent under natural conditions

Source of infection—The person, object, or substance from which an infectious agent passes immediately to the host; may be the reservoir (e.g., humans) or any one of the several modes of transmission (e.g., contaminated water)

Carrier—A person or animal that harbors an infectious agent without apparent clinical disease and serves as a potential source of infection

Contact—A person or animal that has been in association with an infected person, animal, or a contaminated environment that might provide an infective agent

Mode of transmission—Mechanism by which an infectious agent is transported from the reservoir to a susceptible human host. Types of transmission include the following:

Direct—Direct and immediate transfer of infectious agents either by direct contact (touching, biting, kissing, or sexual intercourse) or droplet spread usually limited to a distance of about 1 meter or less (sneezing, coughing, spitting, singing, or talking)

Indirect—Contact with contaminated objects or another infected source

Vehicle—Any object serving as an intermediate means by which an infectious agent is transported from the reservoir to the host (usually fomites, water, soil, food, or biologic products such as plasma)

Vector—Arthropods or other invertebrates that transmit infection by inoculation or deposition of infectious agents on skin, food, or other objects

Airborne—Dissemination of microbial aerosols usually into the respiratory tract; may be droplet nuclei or dust (e.g., fungus spores separated from dry soil by wind)

Incubation period—Time interval between infection or exposure to disease and appearance of initial symptoms

Period of communicability—Time or times during which an infectious agent may be transferred directly or indirectly from an infected person to another person

Prodromal period—Interval between the time when early manifestations of disease appear to the time when overt clinical syndrome is evident

Control measures—Methods used to prevent spread of the organism; most common methods are immunizations, health education, medical treatment of infected person, and isolation or quarantine

Isolation—Separation of infected persons from noninfected persons for the period of communicability under conditions that will prevent transmission of the etiologic agent

Quarantine—Restriction of activities of persons who have been exposed to a communicable disease until the incubation period has expired

VZV is so named because it causes two distinct diseases: varicella (chickenpox) and zoster (herpes zoster or shingles). Varicella occurs primarily in children under 15 years of age. However, it leaves the threat of herpes zoster, an intensely painful varicella that is localized to a single dermatome (body area innervated by a particular segment of the spinal cord) (Straus, 1993). Patients who are immunocompromised and healthy infants under 1 year of age (who also have reduced immunity) are at a higher risk for reactivation of VZV, causing herpes zoster, probably as a result of a deficiency in cellular immunity (Terada and others, 1994). (See also Mechanisms Involved in Immunity, Chapter 35.)

Varicella-zoster immune globulin (VZIG) may be given to high-risk children after exposure to chickenpox to prevent the development of varicella. The antiviral agent acyclovir (Zovirax) may also be used to treat varicella infections in children at increased risk for severe varicella or its complications. Other risk groups include otherwise healthy, nonpregnant individuals 13 years of age or older; children older than 12 months with a chronic cutaneous or pulmonary disorder; those receiving long-term salicylate therapy (because of the possible risk of Reye syndrome); and possibly children receiving short, intermittent, or aerosolized courses of corticosteroids. No recommendations have been made for infants age 12 months or younger (American Academy of Pediatries, 1993c). Because long-term effects of acyclovir on the fetus are unknown, it is not recommended for pregnant women with uncomplicated varicella (see Family Focus box). Maternal varicella infection before 20 weeks of gestation is associated with only a small risk of malformations in the fetus (Jones and others, 1994).

When given, oral acyclovir should be administered for 5 days, starting within the first 24 hours of rash onset, at a dose of 20 mg/kg, with a maximum dose of 800 mg four times a day. The recommended dosage for adolescents ages 13 to 18 is 800 mg four times a day for 5 days. The child should take fluids in order to remain well-hydrated (Dennehy, 1993; Farrington, 1992). In children who are immunocompromised, intravenous therapy is recommended.

Children with hemolytic disease, such as sickle cell disease, are at risk for aplastic anemia from EI. The human parvovirus (HPV) infects and lyses red blood cell precursors, thus interrupting the production of red blood cells. Therefore, in patients who need increased red blood cell production to maintain normal cell volumes, the virus may precipitate a severe aplastic crisis (Gowda and others, 1987). Because of dependence on a high rate of red blood cell pro-

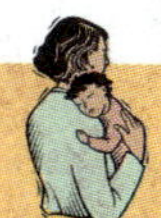

FAMILY FOCUS
Use of Acyclovir for Chickenpox

Acyclovir decreases the number of varicella lesions, speeds healing of lesions, and shortens the duration of fever, itching, lethargy, and anorexia. The drug has little toxicity, and side effects are rare. Despite these benefits, however, the American Academy of Pediatrics (1993c) does not recommend its use in otherwise healthy children with varicella. This group's main argument rests on the cost-benefit ratio.

The annual estimated cost from varicella in the United States is approximately $400 million, with 95% of that attributed to days of work lost by parents caring for their sick children at home. The typical case of varicella in a family results in 8.7 school days and 0.5 parental workdays lost. The cost of a 5-day course of oral acyclovir therapy varies from $50 to $78. If acyclovir were universally used for otherwise normal children with varicella, the cost of the drug would be more than $200 million per year.

Families, however, may view the cost-benefit issue differently. For many parents a sick child at home means loss of more than half a day from work. Caring for an irritable child is also exhausting. Since acyclovir's main advantage is in lessening the severity of the illness, both the child and the parents benefit. With this in mind, nurses should be aware of the issues regarding treatment of chickenpox and discuss the options with the family.* The cost of therapy may be considerably less than the loss of income. Hopefully, with universal varicella vaccination, the incidence of this very common childhood disease will decrease dramatically, making the treatment decision for the family a moot point (see Immunizations, Chapter 12).

*For more information and a parent brochure on the drug, contact Burroughs Wellcome, 3030 Cornwallis Rd., Research Triangle Park, NC 27709; (919) 248-3000.

duction and an immature immune system, the fetus is also vulnerable to severe anemia as a result of maternal HPV infection.

NURSING ALERT High-risk children who have signs of these communicable diseases are referred to the practitioner immediately. School nurses are responsible for warning the parents about recent outbreaks of these communicable diseases to prevent the children's exposure to known cases. In most instances high-risk children are kept out of school until the outbreak is over.

Prevention of complications from diseases such as diphtheria and scarlet fever necessitates parental compliance with antibiotic therapy. Oral preparations are usually prescribed to prevent the trauma of an injection. With oral preparations the need to complete the entire course of therapy is stressed (see Compliance, Chapter 27).

Recent evidence suggests that vitamin A supplementation reduces both morbidity and mortality in measles (Glasziou and MacKerras, 1993). The American Academy of Pediatrics (1993d), based on available data, recommends vitamin A supplementation in the following selected circumstances:

1. Patients 6 months to 2 years of age hospitalized with measles and its complications (e.g., croup, pneumonia, diarrhea)
2. Patients over 6 months of age with measles who have any of the following risk factors (and are not already receiving vitamin A): immunodeficiency; ophthalmologic evidence of vitamin A deficiency; impaired intestinal absorption; moderate to severe malnutrition (including that associated with eating disorders); and recent immigrants from areas with high mortality rates from measles

A single oral dose of 200,000 IU for children at least 1 year old (half that dose for children 6 to 12 months of age) is recommended. The higher dose may be associated with vomiting and headache for a few hours. The dose should be repeated the next day and at 4 weeks for children with ophthalmologic evidence of vitamin A deficiency.

NURSING ALERT Although the risk of vitamin A toxicity from these doses (they are 100 to 200 times the recommended dietary allowance) is very low, nurses should instruct parents on safe storage of the drug. Ideally, vitamin A should be dispensed in the age-appropriate unit dose to prevent excessive administration and possible toxicity.

Provide Comfort. Many of the communicable diseases cause skin manifestations that are bothersome to the child. The chief discomfort from most of the rashes is itching, and measures such as cool baths (usually without soap or with oatmeal preparations) and lotions, such as calamine, are helpful.

NURSING ALERT When lotions with active ingredients such as diphenhydramine in Caladryl are used, they are applied sparingly, especially over open lesions, where excessive absorption can lead to drug toxicity, and in children simultaneously receiving oral diphenhydramine (Schunk and Svendsen, 1988).

To avoid overheating, which increases itching, children should wear lightweight, loose, nonirritating clothing and keep out of the sun. If the child persists in scratching, the nails are kept short and smooth; mittens and clothes with long sleeves or legs may be needed. For severe itching, antipruritic medication, such as diphenhydramine (Benadryl) or hydroxyzine (Atarax), may be required, especially when the child desires to sleep.

An elevated temperature is common, and both antipyretic medicine (acetaminophen) and environmental manipulation are implemented (see Controlling Elevated Temperatures, Chapter 27). The antipyretic is effective in lowering the fever, but evidence suggests that in chickenpox the medication does not significantly reduce the symptoms of itching, anorexia, abdominal pain, fussiness, or vomiting and that it may delay scabbing of the lesions (Doran and others, 1989).

A sore throat, another frequent symptom, is managed with lozenges, saline rinses (if the child is old enough to cooperate), and analgesics. Since most children have a poor appetite during an illness, bland foods and increased liquids (such as broth, juice, gelatin, and flavored ice pops) are usually preferred. During the early stages of the disease

NURSING CARE PLAN
The Child with a Communicable Disease

NURSING DIAGNOSIS: High risk for infection related to susceptible host and infectious agents

PATIENT GOAL 1: Will not become infected

• **INTERVENTIONS/*RATIONALES***

Be highly suspicious of infectious diseases, especially in susceptible children

Identify high-risk children (e.g., those with an immunodeficiency or hemolytic disease) to whom communicable disease may be fatal; in case of an outbreak, advise parents to confine child to the home *to avoid exposure*

Participate in public education and service programs regarding prophylactic immunizations, method of spread of communicable diseases, proper preparation and handling of food and water supplies, control of animal vectors in regard to reservoirs of disease (not a factor in childhood communicable disease but in other infectious illness such as malaria), or screening programs to identify streptococcal infections

• **EXPECTED OUTCOME**

Susceptible children do not contract the disease

PATIENT GOAL 2: Will not spread disease

• **INTERVENTIONS/*RATIONALES***

Institute appropriate infection control practices (see Chapter 27)

Make referral to public health nurse when necessary *to ensure appropriate procedures in the home*

Work with families *to ensure compliance with therapeutic regimens*

Identify close contacts who may require prophylactic treatment (e.g., specific immune globulin or antibiotics)

Report disease to local health department if appropriate

• **EXPECTED OUTCOME**

Infection remains confined to original source

PATIENT GOAL 3: Will exhibit no evidence of complications

• **INTERVENTIONS/*RATIONALES***

Ensure compliance with therapeutic regimen (e.g., bed rest, antiviral therapy, antibiotics, adequate hydration)

Avoid giving aspirin to children with varicella *because of the possible risk of Reye syndrome*

Institute seizure precautions if febrile convulsions are a possibility

Monitor temperature; *unexpected elevations may signal an infection*

Maintain good body hygiene *to reduce risk of secondary infection of lesions*

Offer small, frequent sips of water or favorite drinks *to ensure adequate hydration* and soft, bland foods (gelatin, pudding, ice cream, soups), *since many children are anorectic during an illness;* feed again after vomiting; observe for signs of dehydration

• **EXPECTED OUTCOME**

Child exhibits no evidence of complications such as infection or dehydration

NURSING DIAGNOSIS: Pain related to skin lesions, malaise

PATIENT GOAL 1: Will experience minimal discomfort

• **INTERVENTIONS/*RATIONALES***

Use cool-mist vaporizer, gargles, and lozenges *to keep mucous membranes moist*

Apply petrolatum to chapped lips or nares

Cleanse eyes with physiologic saline solution *to remove secretions or crusts*

Keep skin clean; change bedclothes and linens at least daily

Administer oral hygiene

Keep child cool *because overheating increases itching*

Give cool baths and apply lotion such as calamine *to decrease itching*

Assess need for pain medication (see Chapter 26)

Employ nonpharmacologic pain reduction techniques (see Chapter 26)

*Administer analgesics, antipyretics, and antipruritics as needed

• **EXPECTED OUTCOMES**

Skin and mucous membranes are clean and free of irritants

Child exhibits minimal evidence of discomfort (specify)

NURSING DIAGNOSIS: Impaired social interaction related to isolation from peers

PATIENT GOAL 1: Will have some understanding of reason for isolation

• **INTERVENTIONS/*RATIONALES***

Explain reason for confinement and use of any special precautions *to increase child's understanding of restrictions*

Allow child to play with gloves, mask, and gown (if used) *to facilitate positive coping*

• **EXPECTED OUTCOME**

Child demonstrates understanding of restrictions

PATIENT GOAL 2: Will have opportunity to participate in suitable activities

• **INTERVENTIONS/*RATIONALES***

Always introduce self to child; allow to see face before donning protective clothing, if required

Provide diversionary activity

*Dependent nursing action

NURSING CARE PLAN
The Child with a Communicable Disease—cont'd

Encourage parents to remain with child during hospitalization *to decrease separation and provide companionship*
Encourage contact with friends via telephone (in hospital can use intercom between room and nurse's station)
Prepare child's peers for altered physical appearance, such as with chickenpox, *to encourage peer acceptance*

• **EXPECTED OUTCOMES**
Child engages in suitable activities and interactions
Peers accept child

NURSING DIAGNOSIS: High risk for impaired skin integrity related to scratching from pruritus

PATIENT GOAL 1: Will maintain skin integrity

• **INTERVENTIONS/*RATIONALES***
Keep nails short and clean *to minimize trauma and secondary infection*
Apply mittens or elbow restraints *to prevent scratching*
Dress in lightweight, loose, and nonirritating clothing *because overheating increases itching*
Cover affected areas (long sleeves, pants, one-piece outfit) *to prevent scratching*
Bathe in cool water with no soap or apply cool compresses
Apply soothing lotions (sparingly on open lesions *because absorption of drug is increased*) *to decrease pruritus*
Avoid exposure to heat or sun, *which can aggravate rash* (e.g., chickenpox)

• **EXPECTED OUTCOME**
Skin remains intact

NURSING DIAGNOSIS: Altered family processes related to child with an acute illness

PATIENT (FAMILY) GOAL 1: Will receive adequate emotional support

• **INTERVENTIONS/*RATIONALES***
Inform parents of treatment options, especially acyclovir for varicella
Reinforce family's effort to carry out plan of care
Provide assistance when necessary, such as visiting nurse *to help with home care*
Keep family aware of child's progress *to encourage optimistic attitude*
Stress rapidity of recovery in most cases *to decrease anxiety*

• **EXPECTED OUTCOMES**
Family continues to comply with expectations
Family seeks needed support

children voluntarily curtail their activity, and while bed rest is beneficial, it should not be imposed unless specifically indicated (e.g., in pertussis). During periods of irritability, quiet activity (e.g., reading, music, television, puzzles, coloring) helps distract children from the discomfort.

Support Child and Family. Most communicable diseases are benign, but they produce considerable concern and anxiety for some parents. Often the occurrence of a disease such as chickenpox is the first time the child is acutely uncomfortable. Parents need assistance to cope effectively with manifestations of the illness, such as intense itching. They should be aware of the benefits of acyclovir, especially if child care is an issue. Sometimes a visiting nurse may be beneficial to help the family develop a plan of care and encourage compliance with any treatments.

The family and child need reassurance that recovery from the disease is generally rapid. However, visible signs of the dermatosis may be present for some time after the child is well enough to resume usual activities. For example, children with chickenpox may return to school 6 days after the onset of the rash or sooner if all lesions are crusted (American Academy of Pediatrics, 1994) (see Atraumatic Care box).

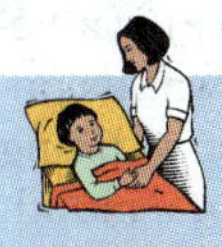

ATRAUMATIC CARE
Returning to School with Visible Skin Lesions

When the disease involves noticeable signs, such as the crusts of chickenpox, the child benefits from preparation before returning to school. For example, the parent can discuss the child's physical appearance with the teacher and/or school nurse and request that they explain the child's condition to classmates.

❖ EVALUATION

The effectiveness of nursing interventions is determined by continual reassessment and evaluation of care based on the following observational guidelines and expected outcomes:

1. Observe or inquire about family members' use of control measures; observe for signs of disease in household contacts.
2. Monitor vital signs, especially temperature; inquire about the identification of high-risk contacts and appropriate isolation of the contact; observe or inquire about compliance with antibiotic therapy.
3. Inquire about effectiveness of comfort measures.
4. Interview family and child regarding their feelings and concerns, especially when child returns to school.

Expected outcomes:
See Nursing Care Plan, pp. 680-681.

CONJUNCTIVITIS

Acute conjunctivitis, inflammation of the conjunctiva, is a common condition in children. It occurs from a variety of causes that are typically age related. In newborns conjunctivitis can occur from infection during birth, most often from *Chlamydia trachomatis* (inclusion conjunctivitis) or *Neisseria gonorrhoeae.* These organisms, as well as herpes simplex virus (HSV), cause serious ocular damage. In infants recurrent conjunctivitis may be a sign of nasolacrimal duct obstruction. In children the usual causes are viral, bacterial, allergic, or related to a foreign body. Bacterial infection accounts for most instances of acute conjunctivitis in children. Diagnosis is made primarily from the clinical manifestations (see box below), although cultures of purulent drainage may be needed to identify the specific infecting agent.

Therapeutic Management

Treatment of conjunctivitis depends on the cause. Allergic, viral, and bacterial forms of conjunctivitis are self-limited. However, because bacterial conjunctivitis is highly contagious, it is usually treated with mild, broad-spectrum topical antibacterial agents such as polymyxin and bacitracin (Polysporin), or trimethoprim and polymyxin (Polytrim) (Donnenfeld, Kaufman, and Schwab, 1993). Drops may be used during the day and an ointment at bedtime because the ointment preparation remains in the eye longer. Ointments are usually not used in the daytime, because they blur vision. Corticosteroids are avoided because they reduce ocular resistance to bacteria. Supportive treatment includes removal of the accumulated secretions. (Prevention of neonatal conjunctivitis, or ophthalmia neonatorum, is discussed in Chapter 8.)

CLINICAL MANIFESTATIONS OF CONJUNCTIVITIS

BACTERIAL CONJUNCTIVITIS ("PINK EYE")

Purulent drainage
Crusting of eyelids, especially on awakening
Inflamed conjunctiva
Swollen lids
Usually both eyes infected

VIRAL CONJUNCTIVITIS

General

Usually occurs with upper respiratory tract infection
Serous (watery) drainage
Inflamed conjunctiva
Swollen lids

Hemorrhagic

Caused by specific virus, enterovirus 70
Severe inflammation
Subconjunctival hemorrhage
Photophobia

ALLERGIC CONJUNCTIVITIS

Itching
Watery to viscous (thick), stringy discharge
Inflamed conjunctiva
Swollen lids
Typically, both eyes affected

CONJUNCTIVITIS CAUSED BY FOREIGN BODY

Tearing
Pain
Inflamed conjunctiva
Usually only one eye affected

Nursing Considerations

Nursing goals include identifying cases of serious conjunctivitis, keeping the eye clean, and properly administering ophthalmic medication. Accumulated secretions are always removed by wiping from the inner canthus downward and outward, away from the opposite eye. Warm, moist compresses, such as a clean washcloth wrung out with hot tap water, are helpful in removing the crusts. Compresses are *not* kept on the eye, because an occlusive covering promotes bacterial growth. Medication is instilled immediately after the eyes have been cleaned and according to correct procedure (see Chapter 27).

NURSING ALERT Signs of serious conjunctivitis include reduction or loss of vision, ocular pain, photophobia, exophthalmos, decreased ocular mobility, corneal ulceration, and unusual patterns of inflammation (e.g., the perilimbal flush associated with iritis or localized inflammation associated with scleritis). If a patient has any of these signs, refer immediately to an ophthalmologist (Donnenfeld, Kaufman, and Schwab, 1993).

Prevention of infection in other family members is an important consideration with bacterial conjunctivitis. The child's washcloth and towel are kept separate from those used by others. Tissues used to clean the eye are disposed of properly. The child should not rub the eyes and is instructed in correct handwashing technique.

STOMATITIS

Stomatitis refers to inflammation of the oral mucosa, which may include the buccal (cheek) and labial (lip) mucosa, tongue, gingiva, palate, and floor of the mouth. It may be due to local or systemic factors. In healthy children aphthous stomatitis and herpetic stomatitis are typically seen. Children with immunosuppression and those receiving chemotherapy or head and neck radiotherapy are at high risk for developing mucosal ulceration and herpetic stomatitis (see Management of Problems Related to Irradiation and Drug Toxicity: Mucosal Ulceration, Chapter 36).

Aphthous stomatitis (aphthous ulcer, canker sore) is a benign but painful condition whose cause is unknown. Its onset is usually associated with mild traumatic injury (biting the cheek, hitting the mucosa with a toothbrush, or a mouth appliance rubbing on the mucosa), allergy, and emotional stress. In some children aphthous stomatitis, fever, and pharyngitis occur periodically (usually at 4- to 6-week intervals), although the children grow normally and exhibit no long-term sequelae (Marshall and others, 1987). The lesions are painful, small, whitish ulcerations surrounded by a red border. They are distinguished from other types of stomatitis by healthy adjacent tissues, absence of vesicles,

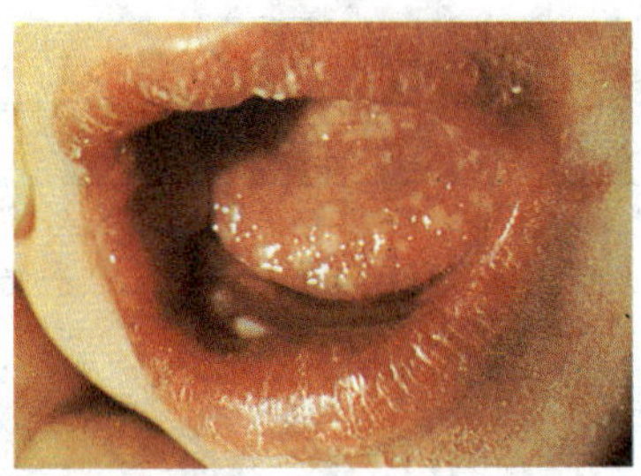

FIG. 16-7 Primary gingivostomatitis. (From Thompson JM and others: *Clinical nursing,* ed 1, 1986, Mosby.)

and no systemic illness. The ulcers persist for 4 to 12 days and heal uneventfully.

Herpetic gingivostomatitis (HGS) is caused by the herpes simplex virus (HSV), most often type 1, and may occur as a primary infection or recur in a less severe form known as recurrent herpes labialis (commonly called "cold sores" or "fever blisters"). The primary infection usually begins with a fever; the pharynx becomes edematous and erythematous; and vesicles erupt on the mucosa, causing severe pain (Fig. 16-7). Cervical lymphadenitis often occurs, and the breath has a distinctly foul odor. The disease can last 5 to 14 days with varying degrees of severity.

In the recurrent form, the vesicles appear on the lips, usually singly or in groups. The precipitating factors for the cold sores include emotional stress, trauma (often related to dental procedures), or exposure to excessive sunlight.

Therapeutic Management

Treatment for both types of stomatitis is aimed at relief of symptoms, primarily pain. Acetaminophen is usually sufficient for mild cases, but with more severe HGS, stronger analgesics such as codeine may be needed. Topical anesthetics are helpful and include over-the-counter preparations, such as Orabase, Anbesol, and Kanka. Lidocaine (Zylocaine Viscous) can be prescribed for the child who can keep 1 teaspoon of the solution in the mouth for 2 to 3 minutes and then expectorate the drug. A mixture of equal parts of diphenhydramine (Benadryl) elixir and Kaopectate provides mild analgesia, antiinflammatory properties, and a protective coating for the lesions (McDonald and Avery, 1994). Specific treatment for children with severe cases of HGS is the use of acyclovir (Zovirax).

Nursing Considerations

The chief nursing goals for children with stomatitis are relief of pain and prevention of spread of the herpes virus. Analgesics and topical anesthetics are used as needed to provide relief, especially before meals to encourage food and fluid intake. Drinking bland fluids through a straw is helpful in avoiding the painful lesions. An oral dressing (Orahesive)* that adheres to the mucosa can provide a barrier over the lesions. Mouth care is encouraged; the use of a very soft-bristled toothbrush or disposable foam-tipped toothbrush provides gentle cleaning near ulcerated areas.

*Manufactured by ConvaTec, Princeton, NJ.

Careful handwashing is essential when caring for children with HGS. Since the infection is autoinoculable, children should keep their fingers out of the mouth; contaminated hands also can infect other body parts. Very young children may need elbow restraints to ensure compliance. All articles placed in the mouth are cleaned thoroughly. Newborns and individuals with immunosuppression should not be exposed to infected children.

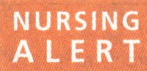

When examining herpetic lesions, wear gloves. The virus easily enters breaks in the skin and can cause herpetic whitlow of the fingers.

Because herpes infection is often associated with sexual transmission, the nurse should explain to parents and older children that HGS is usually caused by type 1 HSV, the type not associated with sexual activity.

INTESTINAL PARASITIC DISEASES

Intestinal parasitic diseases, including helminths (parasitic worms) and protozoa, constitute the most frequent infections in the world. Although many cases are concentrated in the tropical regions, a number of these infections are encountered with relative frequency in the United States. Young children are especially at risk because of typical hand-mouth activity and uncontrolled fecal habits.

Intestinal parasitic infections in humans are caused by various infecting organisms. This discussion is limited to the two most common parasitic infections among children in the United States—giardiasis and pinworms. Table 16-2 describes the outstanding features of other helminths that belong to the family of nematodes. Most nematodes (any organism belonging to the class of tapered cylindric helminths), with the exception of threadworm and *Toxocara,* are effectively treated with mebendazole, pyrantel pamoate, or piperazine citrate (Table 16-3).

GENERAL NURSING CONSIDERATIONS

Nursing responsibilities related to intestinal parasitic infections involve assisting with identification of the parasite, treatment of the infection, and prevention of initial infection or reinfection. Identification of the organism is accomplished by laboratory examination of substances containing the worm, its larvae, or ova. Most are identified by examining feces smears from the stools of persons suspected of harboring the parasite. Fresh specimens are best for revealing parasites or larvae; therefore, collected specimens should be taken directly to the laboratory for examination. If this is not feasible, the specimen is placed in a container with a preservative. Parents need clear instructions on obtaining an adequate sample and the number of samples required (see Collection of Specimens, Chapter 27).

In most parasitic infections examination of other family members, especially children, may be carried out to iden-

TABLE 16-2 Selected Intestinal Parasites

CLINICAL MANIFESTATIONS	COMMENTS
ASCARIASIS—*ASCARIS LUMBRICOIDES* (COMMON ROUNDWORM)	
Light infections: asymptomatic Heavy infections: anorexia, irritability, nervousness, enlarged abdomen, weight loss, fever, intestinal colic Severe infections: intestinal obstruction, appendicitis, perforation of intestine with peritonitis, obstructive jaundice, lung involvement—pneumonitis	Transferred to mouth by way of contaminated food, fingers, or toys Largest of the intestinal helminths Affects principally young children 1-4 years of age Prevalent in warm climates
HOOKWORM DISEASE—*NECATOR AMERICANUS*	
Light infections in well-nourished individuals: no problems Heavier infections: mild to severe anemia, malnutrition May be itching and burning ("ground itch") followed by erythema and a papular eruption in areas to which the organism migrates	Transmitted by discharging eggs on the soil and in turn picking up infection from direct skin contact with contaminated soil Wearing shoes is recommended, although children playing in contaminated soil expose many skin surfaces
STRONGYLOIDIASIS—*STRONGYLOIDES STERCORALIS* (THREADWORM)	
Light infection: asymptomatic Heavy infection: respiratory signs and symptoms; abdominal pain, distention; nausea and vomiting; diarrhea—large, pale stools, often with mucus Threat to life in children with weakened immunologic defenses	Transmission is same as for hookworm except autoinfection common Older children and adults affected more often than young children Severe infections may lead to severe nutritional deficiency
VISCERAL LARVA MIGRANS—*TOXOCARA CANIS* (DOGS); INTESTINAL TOXOCARIASIS—*TOXOCARA CATI* (CATS)	
Depends on reactivity of infected individual May be asymptomatic except for eosinophilia Specific diagnosis difficult	Transmitted by direct contamination of hands from contact with dog, cat, or objects; or ingestion of soil Dogs and cats should be kept away from areas where children play; sandboxes are especially important transmission areas Periodic deworming of diagnosed dogs and cats Control of dog and cat population Continued education and laws to prevent indiscriminate canine and feline defecation
TRICHURIASIS—*TRICHURIS TRICHURA* (WHIPWORM)	
Light infections: asymptomatic Heavy infections: abdominal pain and distention, diarrhea	Transmitted from contaminated soil, vegetables, toys, and other objects Most frequent in warm, moist climates Occurs most often in undernourished children living in unsanitary conditions

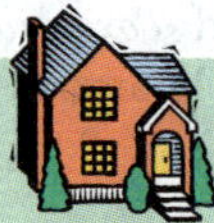

FAMILY HOME CARE

Preventing Intestinal Parasitic Disease

Always wash hands and fingernails with soap and water before eating and handling food and after toileting.
Avoid placing fingers in mouth and biting nails.
Discourage children from scratching bare anal area.
Use superabsorbent disposable diapers to prevent leakage.
Change diapers as soon as soiled and dispose of diapers in closed receptable out of children's reach.
Do not rinse diapers in toilet.
Disinfect toilet seats and diaper-changing areas; use dilute household bleach (10% solution) or Lysol and wipe clean with paper towels.
Drink water that is specially treated, especially if camping.
Wash all raw fruits and vegetables, or food that has fallen on the floor.
Avoid growing foods in soil fertilized with human excreta.
Teach children to defecate only in a toilet, not on the ground.
Keep dogs and cats away from playgrounds or sandboxes.
Avoid swimming in pools frequented by diapered children.
Wear shoes outside.

tify those who are similarly affected. Nurses frequently assume the responsibility for directing and instructing the families in the collection and disposition of specimens. The treatment regimen may need further explanation and reinforcement, particularly when it involves other household members and care of clothing and bed linen. When other members are treated, the family needs to understand the nature of transmission and that in some cases the medication must be repeated in 2 weeks to 1 month to kill organisms hatched since initial treatment.

The nurse's most important function in relation to these parasites is preventive education of children and families regarding good hygiene and health habits. Careful handwashing before eating or handling food and after using the toilet is the most important precautionary method. Other preventive practices are listed in the Family Home Care box.

GIARDIASIS

Giardiasis is caused by the protozoan, *Giardia lamblia* (also called *G. intestinalis, G. duodenalis,* and *Lamblia intestinalis*).

TABLE 16-3 Drugs Used to Treat Intestinal Parasitic Infections

DRUG/PEDIATRIC DOSAGE	SIDE EFFECTS	COMMENTS
Furazolidone (Furoxone) 1.25 mg/kg q.i.d. × 10 days (maximum 100 mg q.i.d.)	Nausea Vomiting Headache Hemolysis possible in glucose-6-phosphate dehydrogenase (G-6-PD) deficiency	Contraindicated during pregnancy
Mebendazole (Vermox) 100 mg b.i.d. × 3 days 100 mg × 1 dose (repeat in 2 weeks for pinworm)	Occasional, transient abdominal pain Diarrhea in massive infection with expulsion of worms	Drug of choice of hookworm, roundworm, pinworm, and whipworm Tablets may be chewed, crushed, or mixed with food Not recommended during pregnancy Recommended for children over 2 years
Metronidazole (Flagyl) 15 mg/kg/day (maximum 750 mg) t.i.d. × 10 days	Nausea Diarrhea Vomiting Metallic taste Abdominal cramps Headache	Drug of choice for giardiasis May be ineffective in children receiving phenobarbital Not recommended during pregnancy, but may be used if initial treatment with paromomycin fails
Piperazine citrate (Antepar) 75 mg/kg/day (maximum 3.5 g) × 2 days (repeat in 2 weeks for pinworm)	Nausea Vomiting Diarrhea Abdominal cramping Urticaria	Side effects are rare with recommended dose May exacerbate seizures in children with seizure disorders
Pyrantel pamoate (Antiminth) 11 mg/kg × 1 dose (maximum 1 g) (repeat in 2 weeks for pinworm)	Nausea Vomiting Diarrhea Abdominal cramps Tenesmus	Side effects are rare with recommended dose Little published data on safety in pregnant women and children under 2 years of age Protect drug from light
Pyrvinium pamoate (Povan) 5 mg/kg × 1 dose (maximum 350 mg) (repeat in 2 weeks for pinworm)	Nausea Vomiting Diarrhea Abdominal cramping	Alternative drug for pinworms Warn parents that drug stains stool and vomitus bright red, as well as clothing or skin if in contact with drug Swallow tablets whole to avoid staining teeth
Quinacrine (Atabrine) 6 mg/kg/day (maximum 300 mg) t.i.d. × 7 days	Nausea Vomiting Temporary yellowish discoloration of skin, sclera, and urine	Highest frequency of side effects Take with meals to decrease gastric upset Advise parents of benign discoloration, which may take 3 months to fade Crush tablets and mix with strong flavoring (e.g., jam) to disguise bitter taste
Thiabendazole (Mintezol) 25 mg/kg b.i.d. (maximum 3 g/day) × 2 days	Drowsiness Dizziness Giddiness Headache Impaired alertness and coordination	Treatment for severe cases of *Toxocara;* also used for threadworm Use with caution in patients with renal or hepatic dysfunction Warn parents of drowsiness and dizziness in child Administer after meals

It is the most common intestinal parasitic pathogen in the United States; its prevalence among children in daycare centers may range from 17% to over 50% during outbreaks (Bartlett and others, 1991). Risk factors for children attending daycare centers include longer duration of total attendance, increased weekly attendance, low family income, and large family size (four or more members) (Novotny and others, 1990). Breast-fed infants exposed to *Giardia* develop much less diarrhea but are not protected from becoming infected (Walterspiel and others, 1994).

Life Cycle, Pathogenesis, and Transmission

Infection begins with ingestion of the cysts, the nonmotile stage of the protozoa. Activated by stomach acid, the cysts pass into the duodenum. Following excystation, trophozoites (parasites in their active feeding stage) emerge and colonize the distal duodenum and proximal jejunum. As the cycle continues, cysts are passed in feces; they are not infective initially but must complete a process of maturation requiring hours to days. Cysts can survive in the environment for months. The mechanism of pathogenesis is not known.

Chief modes of transmission are person-to-person, water (especially mountain lakes, streams, and pools frequented by diapered infants), food, and animals, especially puppies. In children, person-to-person transmission is the most likely cause.

Clinical Manifestations

Although individuals infected with giardiasis may be asymptomatic, young children, especially infants, usually manifest symptoms such as diarrhea, vomiting, anorexia, and failure to thrive. Children over 5 years of age most often complain of abdominal cramps with intermittent loose stools and constipation. The stools may be malodorous, watery, pale, and greasy. Allergic manifestations, such as atopic dermatitis, urticaria, and angioedema, are occasionally present (McKnight and Tietze, 1992). Most infections resolve spontaneously in 4 to 6 weeks, except in rare instances in which the infection becomes chronic and may last for months or years. The chronic form is usually associated with intermittent loose, foul-smelling stools with or without abdominal bloating, flatulence, sulfur-tasting belches, epigastric pain, vomiting, athropathy, headache, or weight loss.

Diagnostic Evaluation

Unlike most other intestinal parasites, *G. lamblia* is not easily diagnosed from stool specimens. Since *Giardia* organisms are excreted in a highly variable pattern, six or more stool specimens collected over several weeks may be necessary to identify the trophozoites or cysts.

Since the organism lives in the upper intestine, aspiration or biopsy of the duodenum or upper jejunum may be performed. The ***string test*** may be used to aspirate duodenal fluid directly. A nylon string is attached to a gelatin capsule, which is swallowed; several hours later the string is withdrawn and the contents are examined microscopically for trophozoites. However, the string test is being used less often because other tests that detect *Giardia* antigen in the stool, such as counterimmunoelectrophoresis (CIE) and enzyme-linked immunosorbent assay (ELISA), are available.

Therapeutic Management

Three drugs are available for treatment of giardiasis (see Table 16-3). The drug of choice is metronidazole because of its efficacy and few side effects. For pregnant women who need treatment, paromomycin may be used first, followed by metronidazole if the initial treatment is unsuccessful (Hill, 1993).

Nursing Considerations

The most important nursing consideration is prevention of giardiasis, especially among children attending daycare centers and the staff. Attention to meticulous sanitary practices, especially during diaper changes, is essential (see Family Home Care box on p. 684). Nurses can play an important role in educating daycare staff regarding appropriate sanitation (see Alternate Child Care Arrangements, Chapter 12.)

Once children are infected, family education regarding administration of the drug is essential.

ENTEROBIASIS (PINWORMS)

Enterobiasis, or pinworms, caused by the nematode *Enterobius vermicularis,* is reported to be the most common helminthic infection in the United States. It is universally present in temperate climatic zones, and may infect about one third of all U.S. children at any one time (Cheng, 1986). Crowded conditions, such as in classrooms and daycare centers, favor transmission.

Life Cycle, Pathogenesis, and Transmission

Infection begins when the eggs are ingested or inhaled. The eggs hatch in the upper intestine, mature in 2 to 4 weeks, and migrate to the cecal area. The females then mate, migrate out the anus, and lay up to 17,000 eggs (Cheng, 1986). The movement of the worms on skin and mucous membrane surfaces causes intense itching, and since the surface of the eggs is durable and adhesive, they easily adhere to almost any surface. As the child scratches, eggs are deposited on the hands and under the fingernails. The typical hand-to-mouth activity of youngsters makes them especially prone to continual reinfection. Pinworm eggs also persist in the environment for up to a week or longer, contaminating anything they contact, such as toilet seats, doorknobs, bed linen, underwear, and food. Since they float in the air, they are also easily inhaled.

Clinical Manifestations

The principal symptom of pinworms is intense perianal itching. However, in young children who have difficulty verbalizing this discomfort, general irritability, restlessness, poor sleep, bed-wetting, distractibility, and short attention span should arouse suspicion that the disorder is present. In females the worms may migrate to the vagina and urethra to cause infection.

Diagnostic Evaluation

The most common test for diagnosing pinworms is the tape test (see Nursing Considerations). The worms may also be identified by using a flashlight to inspect the anal area while the child sleeps. It is best not to place underpants on the child to avoid disturbing the child as much as possible. If worms are found, this can be very upsetting to parents, a fact that should be considered before recommending this procedure.

Therapeutic Management

Four drugs are available for treatment of pinworms (see Table 16-3). The drug of choice is mebendazole, which is safe, effective, convenient, and has few side effects. However, it is not recommended for children under 2 years of age or for pregnant women. Since pinworms are easily transmitted, all household members are treated. Any of the drugs is repeated in 2 weeks to prevent reinfection.

Nursing Considerations

Nursing care is directed at identifying the parasite, eradicating the organism, and preventing reinfection. Parents need clear, detailed instructions for the ***tape test.*** A loop of transparent (not "frosted," or "magic") tape, sticky side out, is placed around the end of a tongue depressor, which is then firmly pressed against the child's perianal area. A convenient commercially prepared tape is also available for this purpose. Pinworm specimens are collected in the morning as soon as the child awakens and *before* the child has a bowel movement or bathes. The procedure may need to be repeated more than once before eggs are collected. Parents are instructed to place the tongue blade in a glass jar or loosely in a plastic bag so that it can be brought in for microscopic examination. For specimens collected in the hospital, practitioner's office, or clinic, the tape is placed smoothly on a glass slide, sticky side down, for examination.

Compliance with the drug regimen is usually excellent because the duration of treatment is typically only one dose. However, the family is reminded of the need to take a second dose in 2 weeks. Posting a reminder on the refrigerator door or bathroom mirror is helpful.

To prevent reinfection, certain cleaning practices, such as washing all clothes and bed linen in hot water and vacuuming the house, may be recommended. However, there is little documentation of their effectiveness, since pinworms survive on so many surfaces. Helpful suggestions include handwashing after toileting and before eating, disposing of diapers in a closed receptacle as soon as they are soiled, and keeping the child's fingernails short to minimize the chance of ova collecting under the nails, dressing children in one-piece pant outfits, and daily showering rather than tub bathing.

INGESTION OF INJURIOUS AGENTS

Since the passage of the Poison Prevention Packaging Act of 1970, which provides that certain potentially hazardous drugs and household products be sold in child-resistant containers, the incidence of poisonings in children has decreased dramatically. However, despite these advances, poisoning remains a significant health concern, with most cases occurring in children under 6 years of age (Unintentional poisoning, 1989). Children are poisoned by a variety of substances, although not all common household items are likely to produce serious problems (see box at right). Many poisonings reflect the ready accessibility of the product in the home, where 90% of poisonings occur. A number take place elsewhere, especially in a grandparent's or friend's home, as well as at unlikely sites such as health care facilities and schools (Litovitz and others, 1993).

NURSING ALERT The following five commonly used and easily available drugs (first four are over-the-counter) can cause serious or fatal consequences if as little as 1/4 teaspoon or 1/2 tablet is ingested: methyl salicylate, camphor, topical imidazolines (sympathomimetics such as those contained in Visine, Afrin, Otrivin, and Clear Eyes), benzocaine, and diphenoxylate-atropine (Lomotil and others). Stress to parents the importance of keeping such drugs away from children. If these agents are ingested, advise parents to seek medical treatment immediately. Emesis is not induced for significant camphor, topical imidazolines, or Lomotil ingestions (Liebelt and Shannon, 1993).

MOST FREQUENTLY REPORTED POISONING IN CHILDREN LESS THAN 6 YEARS OF AGE

SUBSTANCE	TOTAL NUMBER*
NONPHARMACEUTICALS	
Cosmetics/personal care products (perfume, cologne, aftershave)†	126,180
Cleaning products (hypochlorite ["household"] bleach, pine oil disinfectant)	119,219
Plants (nontoxic gastrointestinal irritants, oxalates)	85,291
Foreign bodies/toys/miscellaneous (dessicants, thermometer, bubble-blowing solutions)	48,073
Hydrocarbons (gasoline)	29,353
Insecticides, pesticides	26,725
Arts, crafts, and office supplies (pens, ink)	25,477
Alcohols (rubbing isopropanol alcohol without methyl salicylate)	18,264
Chemicals (alkali)	17,290
Rodenticides	14,349
PHARMACEUTICALS	
Analgesics (pediatric acetaminophen, nonsteroidal antiinflammatory drugs [NSAIDS, excludes aspirin], especially ibuprofen)	85,724
Cough and cold preparations	78,980
Topicals (diaper care products)	54,876
Antimicrobials (antibiotics)	39,333
Vitamins (pediatric and adult multiple vitamins with iron, no fluoride)	35,858
Gastrointestinal preparations (antacids, laxatives)	34,666
Hormones and hormone antagonists (oral contraceptives, corticosteroids)	20,623
Antihistamines (diphenhydramine)	16,593

Data from Litovitz T and others: 1992 annual report of the American Association of Poison Control Centers Toxic Exposure Surveillance System, *Am J Emerg Med* 11(5):494-555, 1993.
*In 1 year; represents categories with more than 14,000 ingestions reported; does not include category Bites and Envenomations.
†Most common substances in each category are in parentheses. Substances ingested are not necessarily most toxic but often represent ready availability.

The developmental characteristics of young children predispose them to poisoning by ingestion. Infants and toddlers explore their environment through oral experimentation. Since the sense of taste is less discriminatory at this age, many unpalatable substances are ingested. In addition, toddlers and preschoolers are developing autonomy and initiative, which increase their curiosity and noncompliant behavior. Imitation is also a powerful motivator, especially when combined with lack of awareness of danger (Brayden and others, 1993a).

This section is primarily concerned with the immediate emergency treatment of ingestion of injurious agents. Specific management of corrosive, hydrocarbon, acetaminophen, salicylate, plant, and iron poisoning is summarized in the box on pp. 688-689. Because of the importance of lead poisoning among young children, ingestion of lead is discussed separately. Appropriate suggestions for poison prevention are discussed on p. 692 and in Chapter 14.

PRINCIPLES OF EMERGENCY TREATMENT

A poisoning may or may not require emergency intervention, but in every instance medical evaluation is necessary

SELECTED POISONINGS IN CHILDREN

CORROSIVES (STRONG ACIDS OR ALKALI)

Drain, toilet, or oven cleaners
Electric dishwasher detergent (liquid, because of higher pH, is more hazardous than granular)
Mildew remover
Batteries
Clinitest tablets
Denture cleaners

Clinical Manifestations

Severe burning pain in mouth, throat and stomach
White, swollen mucous membranes, edema of lips, tongue, and pharynx (respiratory obstruction)
Violent vomiting (hemoptysis)
Drooling and inability to clear secretions
Signs of shock
Anxiety and agitation

Comments

Household bleach is a frequently ingested corrosive but rarely causes serious damage
Liquid preparations cause more damage than granular preparations

Treatment

Inducing emesis is contraindicated (vomiting redamages the mucosa)
Dilute corrosive with water (usually no more than 120 ml [4 oz]), not milk (coats membranes, making assessment difficult) unless vomiting occurs
Provide patent airway if needed
Administer analgesics
Do not allow oral intake
Esophageal stricture may require repeated dilations and/or surgery

HYDROCARBONS

Gasoline
Kerosene
Lamp oil
Mineral seal oil (found in furniture polish)
Lighter fluid
Turpentine
Paint thinner and remover (some types)

Clinical Manifestations

Gagging, choking, and coughing
Nausea
Vomiting
Alterations in sensorium, such as lethargy
Weakness
Respiratory symptoms of pulmonary involvement
- Tachypnea
- Cyanosis
- Retractions
- Grunting

Comments

Immediate danger is aspiration (even small amounts can cause bronchitis and chemical pneumonia)
Gasoline, kerosene, lighter fluid, mineral seal oil, and turpentine cause severe pneumonia

Treatment (Controversial):

Inducing emesis is generally contraindicated
Gastric lavage may be used
Symptomatic treatment of chemical pneumonia includes high humidity, oxygen, hydration, and antibiotics for secondary infection

ACETAMINOPHEN

Clinical Manifestations

Occurs in four stages
1. Initial period (2 to 4 hours after ingestion)
   - Nausea
   - Vomiting
   - Sweating
   - Pallor
2. Latent period (24 to 36 hours)
   - Patient improves
3. Hepatic involvement (may last up to 7 days and be permanent)
   - Pain in right upper quadrant
   - Jaundice
   - Confusion
   - Stupor
   - Coagulation abnormalities
4. Patients who do not die in hepatic stage gradually recover

Comments

Most common drug poisoning in children
Occurs from acute ingestion
Toxic dose is 150 mg/kg or greater in children
Toxicity from chronic therapeutic use is rare but may occur with ingestion of approximately 150 mg/kg/day, or about double the recommended maximum therapeutic dose (90 mg/kg/day) of acetaminophen, for several days (Dovidar, Al-Khalil, and Habersang, 1994; Henretig and others, 1989)

Treatment

Emesis, lavage, activated charcoal
Antidote *N*-acetylcysteine (NAC) is given, usually by nasogastric tube because of the antidote's offensive odor (smells like rotten eggs)
Given as one loading dose and usually 17 maintenance doses in different dosages
May be given intravenously, but use is investigational

ASPIRIN (ASA)

Clinical Manifestations

Acute poisoning
- Nausea
- Disorientation
- Vomiting
- Dehydration
- Diaphoresis
- Hyperpnea
- Hyperpyrexia
- Oliguria
- Tinnitus
- Coma
- Convulsions

Chronic poisoning
- Same as above but subtle onset (often confused with illness being treated)

Dehydration, coma, and seizures may be more severe
Bleeding tendencies

Comments

May be caused by acute ingestion (severe toxicity occurs with 300 to 500 mg/kg [4 to 7 gr/kg])
May be caused by chronic ingestion (i.e., more than 100 mg/kg/day for 2 or more days); can be more serious than acute ingestion
Time to peak serum salicylate can vary with enteric aspirin or the presence of concretions (bezoars)

Treatment

Home use of ipecac for moderate toxicity
Hospitalization for severe toxicity
Emesis, lavage, activated charcoal, and/or cathartic
Lavage will not remove concretions of ASA
Activated charcoal is important early in ASA toxicity
Sodium bicarbonate transfusions to correct metabolic acidosis and urinary alkalinization is effective in enhancing elimination
External cooling for hyperpyrexia
Diazepam for seizures
Oxygen and ventilation for respiratory depression
Vitamin K for bleeding
In extreme cases, hemodialysis (not peritoneal dialysis) may be used

IRON

Mineral supplement or vitamin containing iron

Clinical Manifestations

Occurs in five stages

1. Initial period (½ to 6 hours after ingestion) (if child does not develop gastrointestinal symptoms in 6 hours, toxicity is unlikely)
   Vomiting
   Hematemesis
   Diarrhea
   Hematochezia (bloody stools)
   Gastric pain
2. Latency (2 to 12 hours)
   Patient improves
3. Systemic toxicity (4 to 24 hours after ingestion)
   Metabolic acidosis
   Fever
   Hyperglycemia
   Bleeding
   Shock
   Death (may occur)
4. Hepatic injury (48 to 96 hours)
   Seizures
   Coma
5. Rarely pyloric stenosis develops at 2 to 5 weeks

Comments

Factors related to frequency of iron poisoning include:
- Widespread availability
- Packaging of large quantities in individual containers
- Lack of parental awareness of iron toxicity
- Resemblance of iron tablets to candy (e.g., M & Ms)
- Toxic dose is based on the amount of elemental iron in various salts (sulfate, gluconate, fumarate), which ranges from 20% to 33%; ingestions of 60 mg/kg are considered dangerous

Treatment

Emesis or lavage
Lavage for all chewable tablets or liquids if spontaneous vomiting has not occurred
Chelation therapy with deferoxamine in severe intoxication (turns urine a red to orange color)
If intravenous deferoxamine is given too rapidly, hypotension, facial flushing, rash, urticaria, tachycardia, and shock may occur; stop the infusion, maintain the intravenous line with normal saline, and notify the practitioner immediately.

PLANTS

See box on p. 690

Clinical Manifestations

Depends on type of plant ingested
May cause local irritation of oropharynx and entire gastrointestinal tract
May cause respiratory, renal, and central nervous system symptoms
Topical contact with plants can cause dermatitis

Comments

Some of most frequently ingested substances
Rarely cause serious problems, although some plant ingestions can be fatal
Can also cause choking and allergic reactions

Treatment

Remove plant parts (emesis)
Wash from skin or eyes
Supportive care as needed

to initiate appropriate action. Parents are advised to call the Poison Control Center (PCC) *before* initiating any intervention, since instructions on labels of many household products are not correct treatment measures. The local PCC telephone number (usually listed in the front of the telephone directory*) should be posted near each phone in the house (see Critical Thinking Exercise box, p. 690).

Based on the initial telephone assessment, the PCC counsels the parents to begin treatment at home and/or to bring the child to an emergency facility. When a call is taken, the caller's name and telephone number are recorded to reestablish contact if the connection is interrupted. Since most poisonings are managed outside health care facilities, usually at the patient's home, expert advice is essential in minimizing adverse effects. When the exact quantity or type of ingested toxin is not known, admission to a hospital for laboratory evaluation and surveillance for signs of poisonings (Table 16-4) is critical during the postingestion period.

General guidelines for emergency home treatment of poisoning are listed on p. 691. Selected interventions, especially those that require professional intervention, are discussed next.

Assessment

The first and most important principle in dealing with a poisoning is to treat the child first, not the poison. This necessitates an immediate concern for life support—the ABCs of airway, breathing, and circulation. Vital signs and blood pressure are measured, and respiratory and/or circulatory support is instituted as needed. The victim's condition is

*Also available by calling (800) 555-1212 from any state in the United States.

POISONOUS AND NONPOISONOUS PLANTS

POISONOUS PLANTS	TOXIC PARTS	NONPOISONOUS PLANTS
Apple	Leaves, seeds	African violet
Apricot	Leaves, stem, seed pits	Aluminum plant
Azalea	Foliage and flowers	Asparagus fern
Buttercup	All parts	Begonia
Cherry (wild or cultivated)	Twigs, seeds, foliage	Boston fern
Daffodil	Bulbs	Christmas cactus
Dumb cane, dieffenbachia	All parts	Coleus
Elephant ear	All parts	Gardenia
English ivy	All parts	Grape ivy
Foxglove	Leaves, seeds, flowers	Jade plant
Holly	Berries	Piggyback begonia
Hyacinth	Bulbs	Piggyback plant
Ivy	Leaves	Poinsettia†
Mistletoe*	Berries, leaves	Prayer plant
Oak tree	Acorn, foliage	Rubber tree
Philodendron	All parts	Snake plant
Plum	Pit	Spider plant
Poison ivy, poison oak	Leaves, fruit, stems, smoke from burning plants	Swedish ivy
Pothos	All parts	Wax plant
Rhubarb	Leaves	Weeping fig
Tulip	Bulbs	Zebra plant
Water hemlock	All parts	
Wisteria	Seeds, pods	
Yew	All parts	

*Eating one or two berries or leaves is probably nontoxic.
†Mildly toxic if ingested in massive quantities.

CRITICAL THINKING EXERCISE
Poisoning

Mrs. Berry, a neighbor, calls you. She is very upset because her 2-year-old son has eaten several chewable multivitamins with iron. She asks you if she should give syrup of ipecac. You advise her to:

1. First call the Poison Control Center.
2. Give the antiemetic.
3. Dilute the poison with several glasses of water.
4. Wait to see if the child develops symptoms.

The correct action for the mother is 1, to first call the Poison Control Center, where they will advise her of home treatment, such as using ipecac. The goal is to remove the poison, not dilute it, making option 3 inappropriate. The most toxic ingredient in the drug is iron, which produces symptoms after several hours. Treatment, if needed, should begin long before symptoms appear.

routinely reevaluated. The increased recovery rate from acute poisonings is largely attributable to vigorous use of supportive measures after symptoms appear.

Since shock is a complication of several types of household poisons, particularly corrosives, measures to reduce the effects of shock, such as elevation of legs and head to the level of the heart to promote venous drainage and provision of warmth and rest, are important. Maintenance of respiratory function may require insertion of an airway and/or mechanical ventilation.

The emergency room nurse's responsibility is to be prepared for immediate intervention with any of the necessary equipment. Since time and speed are critical factors in recovery from serious poisonings, anticipation of potential problems and complications may mean the difference between life and death.

Gastric Decontamination

In general, the immediate treatment is to remove the ingested poison by inducing vomiting, counteracting the toxin with activated charcoal, performing gastric lavage, increasing bowel motility (catharsis), or administering an antidote if one exists. Because of the continuing controversy over the use of these measures (except antidotes), each toxic ingestion should be treated individually (Hoffman, 1992). The method typically used in the home is to administer ***ipecac syrup***, an emetic that exerts its action by direct stimulation of the vomiting center and through an irritant effect on the gastric mucosa.

NURSING ALERT The use of an emetic is generally contraindicated in conditions that increase the risk of aspiration and when emesis of the poison, such as a corrosive, redamages the mucosa of the esophagus and pharynx. Emesis is also contraindicated in cases where there is existing or potential for rapid onset of central nervous system depression, dystonias (unusual muscle tone or movements), or seizures.

TABLE 16-4 Common Signs of Poisoning

GENERAL SIGNS	SPECIFIC SIGNS
Gastrointestinal system	**Corrosives**
Abdominal pain	Severe burning pain in mouth, throat, stomach
Vomiting	White, swollen mucous membranes; edema of lips, tongue, pharynx (respiratory obstruction)
Diarrhea	Violent vomiting, hemoptysis
Anorexia	Drooling and inability to clear secretions
Respiratory/circulatory system	Signs of shock
Depressed respirations	Anxiety and agitation
Labored respirations	**Hydrocarbons**
Unexplained cyanosis	Gagging, choking, coughing
Signs of shock: increased, weak pulse; decreased blood pressure; increased, shallow respiration; pallor; cool, clammy skin	Nausea
Central nervous system	Vomiting
Convulsions	Alterations in sensorium (e.g., lethargy)
Overstimulation	Weakness
Sudden loss of consciousness	Respiratory symptoms of pulmonary involvement
Dizziness	Tachypnea
Stupor, lethargy	Cyanosis
Coma	Retractions
	Grunting
	Salicylates
	Nausea
	Disorientation
	Vomiting
	Dehydration
	Diaphoresis
	Hyperpnea
	Hyperpyrexia
	Oliguria
	Tinnitus
	Coma
	Convulsions

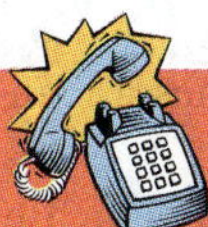

EMERGENCY TREATMENT
Poisoning

1. Assess the victim:
   a. Take vital signs; reevaluate routinely.
   b. Initiate cardiorespiratory support if needed.
   c. Treat other symptoms, such as seizures.
2. Terminate exposure:
   a. Empty mouth of pills, plant parts, or other material.
   b. Flush eyes continuously with normal saline (room-temperature tap water at home) for 15 to 20 minutes.
   c. Flush skin and wash with soap and a soft cloth; remove contaminated clothes, especially if a pesticide, acid, alkali, or hydrocarbon is involved.
   d. Bring victim of an inhalation poisoning into fresh air.
   e. Give one sip of water to dilute ingested poison.
3. Identify the poison:
   a. Question the victim and witnesses.
   b. Look for environmental cues (empty container, nearby spill, odor on breath) and save all evidence of poison (container, vomitus, urine).
   c. Be alert to signs and symptoms of potential poisoning in absence of other evidence, including symptoms of ocular or dermal exposure
   d. Call Poison Control Center or other competent emergency facility for immediate advice regarding treatment.
4. Remove poison and prevent absorption:
   a. Induce vomiting; administer ipecac if ordered:
      —6 to 12 months: 10 ml; do not repeat.*
      —1 to 12 years: 15 ml; repeat dosage *once* if vomiting has not occurred within 20 minutes.
      —Over 12 years: 30 ml; repeat dosage *once* if vomiting has not occurred within 20 minutes.
      —Give 10 to 20 ml/kg of clear fluids after ipecac.
   b. Do not induce vomiting if:
      —Victim is comatose, in severe shock, or convulsing, or has lost the gag reflex.
      —Poison is a low-viscosity hydrocarbon (unless it contains a more toxic substance [e.g., pesticide or heavy metal] or a strong acid or alkali).
   c. Place child in side-lying, sitting, or kneeling position with head below chest to prevent aspiration.
   d. Administer activated charcoal with cathartic (unless used repeatedly; usual dose 1 g/kg unless amount of toxin is known) 30 to 60 minutes *after* vomiting from ipecac, if ordered.

*Emesis of children at home is generally contraindicated between ages 6 to 10 months. Ipecac can only be administered safely in a health care facility because of the high risk of aspiration.

EMERGENCY TREATMENT

Proper administration of ipecac is essential (see Emergency Treatment box). Ipecac is available in 1-ounce (30 ml) vials. However, the label information does not include directions for a second dose if the child fails to vomit after the first dose. Therefore parents need clear instructions for proper use and dose. As a precaution, parents are advised to have full doses of ipecac for *each child* in the home, to carry the emetic when traveling, and to be certain that other caregivers (baby-sitters or relatives) have the emetic available. Because children share activities, it is not uncommon for more than one child to ingest the toxic substance. In an emergency ipecac can be obtained from an all-night pharmacy, convenience store, emergency squad, or emergency department. Ipecac is also inexpensive.

Boehnert and others (1985) found there was no significant difference in time to emesis with out-of-date ipecac. Although out-of-date ipecac may be used in a dire emergency, the family is encouraged to replace the expired bottle. Since neither milk, fluid volume, food, nor activity level alter ipecac's effectiveness (Klein-Schwartz and others, 1991; Rodgers and Matyunas, 1986), the common suggestions of forcing fluids and encouraging movement are unnecessary. If given, clear liquids are preferred for better visualization of white pill fragments. For maximum benefit in removing the poison, ipecac should be administered within 1 hour of a toxic ingestion.

Ipecac's safety has been questioned. One reason is the increased number of drug ingestions for which induced emesis is contraindicated. Medications, such as calcium channel blockers and benzodiazepines, either produce a rapid onset of adverse symptoms (e.g., sedation, seizures, coma) or exaggerate the vagal response induced by gagging, which can lead to significant bradycardia. Under either circumstance, uncontrolled vomiting becomes an undesirable and unsafe event (Shannon, 1993).

Concern also exists over its ready availability, specifically its abuse by individuals with anorexia nervosa and bulimia and by parents who intentionally poison their children with ipecac (Munchausen syndrome by proxy) (McClung and others, 1988; Sutphen and Saulsbury, 1988). In some countries other than the United States, ipecac is available only with a prescription. This practice, however, severely limits its timely use during home management of poisonings.

If the child is admitted to an emergency facility, ***gastric lavage*** may also be done to empty the stomach of the toxic agent. Lavage is indicated for young infants in whom ipecac is contraindicated; if the patient is comatose or convulsing or requires a protected airway; or if the ingested poison is rapidly absorbed (strychnine or cyanide). The use of lavage in petroleum distillate poisoning remains controversial because of the danger of aspiration. When lavage is performed, the largest-diameter tube that can be inserted is used to facilitate passage of gastric contents.

Another method of decontaminating the stomach is the use of ***activated charcoal,*** an odorless, tasteless, fine black powder that absorbs many compounds, creating a stable complex. It is used within 1 hour of the poisoning but *after* giving an emetic, to avoid the charcoal also adsorbing the emetic and minimizing its pharmacologic effect. It is mixed with water or saline cathartic to form a slurry. Slurries are neither gritty nor distasteful but resemble black mud. Sorbitol, an artificial sweetener, is added to a commercial preparation (Actidose) as a flavoring and a cathartic. If the child refuses to take the charcoal, it is given by nasogastric tube.

➤ **NURSING TIP** To increase the child's acceptance of activated charcoal, mix it with flavoring or a sweetener and serve through a straw and in an opaque glass with a cover, such as a disposable coffee cup and lid or an ordinary cup covered with aluminum foil or placed inside a paper bag.

Activated charcoal (without sorbitol) is also used in multiple doses to reduce systemic absorption of many toxic agents, even overdoses of intravenous drugs. After absorption, a toxic substance will reenter the lumen of the gastrointestinal tract by passive diffusion when the concentration of the substance in the gut is lower than that in the blood. Absorption of the toxin by charcoal keeps the concentration gradient high so that diffusion continues (Vale and Proudfoot, 1993).

Some authorities suggest that activated charcoal should replace ipecac as the home remedy. While activated charcoal is safe and highly effective in preventing absorption of many poisons, arguments against its home use include (1) availability—not a stock item in all stores; (2) dosage—should be 10 times the dose of the ingested drug, which is more difficult for parents; (3) compliance—children often refuse to drink the black liquid; and (4) interference with an emetic—if used with ipecac, activated charcoal is given after the emetic, and parents may not remember the correct sequence.

Cathartics, such as sorbitol, magnesium citrate, or magnesium sulfate, may be administered to stimulate evacuation of the bowel, thus decreasing systemic absorption of the poison and aiding in removal of the charcoal. However, the beneficial effects of cathartics are not well established. In addition, excessive amounts of a cathartic, such as sorbitol, can cause severe dehydration in infants from fluid loss in the stool (McCord and Okun, 1987).

In a minority of poisonings specific ***antidotes*** are available to counteract the poison. They are highly effective and should be available in all emergency facilities. The supply of antidotes should be checked routinely and replaced as used or according to expiration dates. Among the more commonly employed antidotes are *N*-acetylcysteine for acetaminophen poisoning, oxygen for carbon monoxide inhalation, naloxone for opioid overdose, flumazenil (Romazicon) for benzodiazepine (Valium, Versed) overdose, Digibind for digoxin toxicity, and antivenin for certain poisonous bites.

Prevention of Recurrence

The ultimate objective is to prevent poisonings from occurring or recurring. One effective counseling method is first to discuss the difficulties of constantly watching and safeguarding young children (see also Family Focus box). With this approach the monumental task of raising children is shared as a common problem, with injury prevention as one part of the parental role, not as the central issue. This approach also incorporates other contributory causes for the incident, such as inadequate support systems, marital discord, discipline techniques (especially use of physical punishment), maternal distress, or any disruption in the family or family activities, such as vacations, moves, visitors, illnesses, or births (Bithoney and others, 1985). A visit to the home, especially after a repeat poisoning situation, is recommended as part of the follow-up care to assess hazards, including family factors, and to evaluate appropriate safeproofing measures. One method of identifying risk areas is to ask specific questions or to have the parent complete a questionnaire designed to isolate factors that predispose children to poisoning.

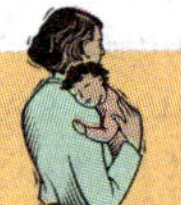

FAMILY FOCUS

Poisoning

A poisoning is more than a physical emergency for the child. It usually represents an emotional crisis for the parents, particularly in terms of guilt, self-reproach, and insecurity in the parenting role. The emergency room is no place to admonish the family for negligence, lack of appropriate supervision, or failure to safe-proof the home. Rather, it is a time to calm and support the child and parents while unaccusingly exploring the circumstances of the injury. If the nurse prematurely attempts to discuss ways of preventing such an incident from recurring, the parents' anxiety will block out any suggestions or offered guidance. Therefore it is preferable for the nurse to delay the discussion until the child's condition is stabilized or, if the child is discharged immediately after emergency treatment, to make a public health referral or send a packet of information (Woolf, Saperstein, and Forjuoh, 1992).

➤ **NURSING TIP** Encourage parents to bend down to the child's eye level and survey the home environment for potential hazards. Have the parents try to open cabinets and reach shelves to access poisons.

The box below is a sample questionnaire of items that may determine what environmental manipulation is needed to "poison-proof" homes. A teaching plan designed to assess parents' preparedness in case of an accidental poisoning and to supply appropriate strategy and instruction where necessary is presented in the box at right. Such tools enable nurses to counsel families systematically and efficiently in the area of injury prevention.

Passive measures (those that do not require active participation) have been the most successful in preventing poisoning and include child-resistant closures and a limited number of tablets in one container. Other preventive methods include the use of warning labels, such as Mr. Yuk or a skull and crossbones, to alert children to potential dangers. Also, some products, such as nail polish remover or furniture polish, are now available with a bittering agent to discourage large ingestions. However, the effectiveness of such measures is questionable (Rodgers and Tenenbein, 1994). One study found that children actually preferred to touch labeled containers after undergoing education incorporating Mr. Yuk stickers (Vernberg, Culver-Dickinson, and Spyker, 1984). Also, skull and crossbones labels may make products look like pirate toys and make them attractive to children.

Since these measures alone are not sufficient to prevent poisoning, ***active measures*** (those that require participation) are essential. Guidelines for preventing the occurrence or recurrence of a poisoning, with emphasis on proper storage of poisonous agents, are listed in the Guidelines box on p. 694.

Even in the busiest health care facilities, poison prevention can be effective. Reminding parents of the telephone number of the local PCC, encouraging them to have ipecac in the home for emergency use, and counseling them on correct use of the emetic can increase their readiness in the event of a poisoning (Woolf and others, 1987).

QUESTIONNAIRE FOR POISON PREVENTION

1. Where do I store cleaning products, medicines, laundry aids, and garden supplies?
2. What do I keep under the sink in the kitchen and bathroom?
3. Do I have any medicines (e.g., pain relievers, tranquilizers, birth control pills, antacids) in my purse?
4. Are all the medicines and household products clearly labeled and in their original container?
5. Do I refer to medicine as candy to encourage my child to take it?
6. Are any medications left on the table or kitchen counter or kept in a purse or diaper bag for handy use?
7. Do I keep drugs prescribed for previous illnesses?
8. Is my child out of sight when I take medicine?
9. When using any medicine or household product, do I keep my eye on it at all times, put it away immediately after use, or put it down where my child cannot get it?
10. Are any of my garden plants or houseplants poisonous?
11. Do all cabinets that store toxic products have a lock on them?
12. What is stored in the garage or basement?
13. Are paints, gasoline, solvents, insecticides, poisons, and fertilizers either on a high shelf or locked in a cabinet?
14. Do I teach my child never to touch any nonfood item without asking me first?

HEAVY METAL POISONING

Heavy metal poisoning can occur from the ingestion of a variety of substances, the most common being lead. Other sources that are important in terms of children are iron (see following section) and mercury. ***Mercury,*** a rare form of

TEACHING STRATEGY FOR PARENT EDUCATION AND PREPARATION FOR ACCIDENTAL POISONING

QUESTION	INTERVENTION
If you suspected that your child had ingested (eaten) a poison, what would you do first?	If answer is correct, ask for more specifics, such as telephone number of local poison control center If answer does not include knowledge of local poison control center, supply information Stress necessity of not wasting time and of saving all evidence of poisoning
Do you have ipecac syrup in your home?	If answer is yes, ask for specific directions concerning its dosage and readministration If answer is no, supply correct information
Should you always make the child vomit?	If answer is no, ask for specific poisons that are treated differently, such as turpentine and drain cleaner If answer is yes, supply correct information Emphasize that instructions on container of household products are minimum and sometimes inaccurate emergency treatment; medical advice should *always* be sought before relying on that information alone
If you suspected that your child had taken a poison, but there were no signs of illness and the child denied doing so, what would you do?	Emphasize need to always seek medical advice rather than waiting for signs or believing the child

GUIDELINES
Poison Prevention

Assess possible contributing factors in occurrence of injury, such as discipline, parent-child relationship, developmental ability, environmental factors, and behavior problems.
Institute anticipatory guidance for possible future injuries based on child's age and maturational level.
Refer to visiting nurse agency to evaluate home environment and need for safe-proofing measures.
Provide assistance with environmental manipulation when necessary, such as lead removal.
Educate parents regarding safe storage of toxic substances (see Family Home Care box on p. 567).
Advise parents to take drugs out of sight of children.
Advise parents to return *immediately* all toxic substances to safe storage.
Teach children the hazards of ingesting nonfood items without supervision.
Advise parents against using plants for teas or medicine.
Discuss problems of discipline and children's noncompliance and offer strategies for effective discipline (see Limit-Setting and Discipline, Chapter 3).
Instruct parents regarding correct administration of drugs for therapeutic purposes and to discontinue drug if there is evidence of mild toxicity.
Have syrup of ipecac available—two doses for each child in the family—but to use only if advised to do so by poison control center or practitioner.
Encourage grandparents or other frequent caregivers to keep syrup of ipecac in home.
Post number of local poison control center with emergency phone list by telephone.
Include by the telephone the home address with nearest cross street in case an ambulance is needed. (In an emergency family members may not remember the house address, and baby-sitters may not be aware of the information.)

heavy metal poisoning, has occurred in children from a variety of sources, such as broken thermometers or thermostats, broken fluorescent lights, and use of interior latex house paint (Mack, 1989; Mercury exposure, 1990). Elemental mercury (also called metallic mercury or quicksilver) is nontoxic if ingested and the gastrointestinal tract is healthy (e.g., has no fistulas). However, mercury is volatile at room temperature and enters the bloodstream after it is inhaled, causing toxicity (tremors, memory loss, insomnia, gingivitis, diarrhea, anorexia, weight loss). The classic form of mercury poisoning is called ***acrodynia*** (or "painful extremities").

NURSING ALERT To prevent inhalation, spilled mercury must be cleaned up quickly, using disposable towels (not an ordinary vacuum cleaner) and rubber gloves and washing the hands well after removing the spill.

Heavy metals have an affinity for certain essential tissue chemicals, which must remain free for adequate cell functioning. When metals are bound to these substances, cellular enzyme systems are inactivated. Treatment involves ***chelation,*** use of a chemical compound that combines with the metal for rapid and safe excretion.

LEAD POISONING

Lead poisoning (sometimes termed ***plumbism***) is a prevalent, significant, and preventable pediatric problem. Although symptomatic lead poisoning, with its associated life-threatening encephalopathy, is rarely seen today, many asymptomatic young children have lead levels sufficiently elevated to cause neurologic and intellectual damage. As the detrimental effects of low levels of lead on the developing central nervous system have been identified, blood lead levels indicating toxicity have decreased. For example, in 1991 the lower level of blood lead concentration was set at <10 μg/dl, a reduction from the 1985 level of <25 μg/dl (American Academy of Pediatrics, 1993b; Centers for Disease Control, 1991).

Although the greatest risk is to poor children under 6 years of age living in urban areas, lead poisoning affects children of all social strata. For example, children of wealthier families living near lead smelters or in old homes in restored urban areas are at risk (Baghurst and others, 1992; Needleman, 1988). The deleading (abatement) process (sanding, scraping, and burning of painted surfaces) contributes significant amounts of ingested and inhaled lead to inhabitants (Amitai and others, 1987; Rey-Alvarez and Menke-Hargrave, 1987).

Factors Related to Lead Absorption

Environmental Factors. The most important contributing factor to lead poisoning is the availability of lead in the environment. Lead enters the system either by ingestion or inhalation. In an unborn fetus lead can enter the body transplacentally if the mother is exposed. The major environmental sources of lead are deteriorating lead-based paint, which contaminates household dust and soil; drinking water contaminated by exposed lead solder or old lead pipes; occupations and hobbies where parents or others in the house bring home lead on clothes, shoes, and skin; and for some children, folk remedies or cosmetics, as well as the use of lead-containing pottery or leaded dishes for food storage. Lead-based paint from old housing remains the most frequent source of lead poisoning in children.

Most lead poisoning results from ingestion of lead dust during normal hand-to-mouth activity. A number of children have been known to actually eat loose lead paint chips. Some children are poisoned during renovation of their home. As mentioned earlier, sanding, scraping, and burning can release large amounts of lead into the air. In 1978 the U.S. Consumer Product Safety Commission banned the addition of lead to paints for residential use, but substantial amounts of lead remain on the painted interior and exterior surfaces of older homes. Although the child's home environment is usually the source of lead, other buildings, such as preschools or daycare centers, as well as a friend or relative's home, can contribute to lead exposure.

Other significant sources of lead in the child's environment are dust, soil, and air that become contaminated by emissions from lead smelters. Fortunately, the use of deleaded gasoline has significantly reduced the level of lead in the air and the incidence of severe lead poisoning in children (Hayes and others, 1994; Piomelli, 1994). Lead-

CULTURAL AWARENESS
Sources of Lead

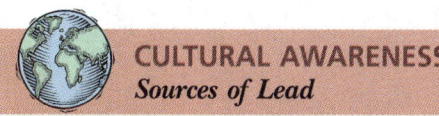

In some cultures the use of traditional ethnic remedies may contain lead and increase children's risk of lead poisoning. These remedies include:

Azarcon (Mexico)—For digestive problems; a bright orange powder; usual dose is ¼ -1 teaspoon, often mixed with oil, milk, or sugar, or sometimes given as a tea; sometimes a pinch is added to a baby bottle or tortilla dough for preventive purposes

Greta (Mexico)—A yellow-orange powder, used in the same way as azarcon

Paylooah (Southeast Asia)—used for rash or fever; an orange-red powder given as ½ teaspoon straight or in a tea

Surma (India)—black powder applied to the inner lower eyelid that is used as a cosmetic to improve eyesight

Unknown ayurvedic (Tibet)—Small, gray-brown balls used to improve slow development; two balls are given orally three times a day.

Modified from Lead poisoning associated with use of traditional ethnic remedies—California, 1991-1992, *MMWR* 42(27):521-524, 1993.

soldered cans for food products, which have been outlawed in the United States, may still be found with imported products. Leaded containers, such as some water fountains and liquids stored in lead crystal, can also contribute to ingested sources of the heavy metal. Use of lead-contaminated water to prepare formula is a major source of poisoning in infants (Shannon and Graef, 1992).

Some sources of lead are related to isolated occupations; for example, lead smelter workers, abatement workers, or urban police officers may bring lead dust home on clothing. Hobbies, such as making leaded glass windows or refinishing old furniture, may also introduce lead into the home (see Cultural Awareness box).

Child Factors. Developmentally, young children are at risk for lead poisoning because of their high level of oral activity. Particularly during late infancy and toddlerhood, children explore their environment by putting objects in their mouth. This normal hand-to-mouth activity contributes to the amount of lead they ingest in dust and dirt. Because of their size, young children inhale air that is closer to the ground, which is more heavily contaminated with lead. In addition, the child who ingests lead often practices ***pica,*** the habitual, purposeful, and compulsive ingestion of nonfood substances (Laraque and others, 1990). Children under the age of 6 are also most at risk for lead poisoning because of their developing nervous systems. In addition, three to five times more lead is absorbed in children than in adults. Diets deficient in iron and calcium and diets high in fats, such as those containing many fried foods, also increase the exposure risk for children living in leaded environments. These conditions make it possible for lead to be more quickly and readily absorbed. The greatest risk appears to be from iron deficiency, even in the absence of anemia (Clark, Royal, and Seeler, 1988; Wasserman and others, 1992).

Pathophysiology and Clinical Manifestations

Normally, ingested lead is very slowly excreted via the kidneys, alimentary tract, and to a small extent, sweat. About 95% of the body burden of lead is stored chiefly in the bones and teeth, where it is inert. However, with chronic ingestion the rate of absorption exceeds the rate of excretion, and excess lead is deposited in the tissues and circulatory system, with about 90% of lead found in the circulating blood attached to the erythrocytes. Even when the chronic ingestion stops, it takes the body twice as long to excrete the stored lead as it did to accumulate it. As a result, several body systems continue to be affected after the environmental removal of the poison (Fig. 16-8).

Central Nervous System. The most serious and irreversible side effects of lead intoxication are on the nervous system. Initially, membrane permeability increases, with a shift of fluid into the interstitial spaces of the brain. As a result, increased intracranial pressure causes cortical atrophy and ***lead encephalopathy*** (convulsions, mental retardation, paralysis, blindness, and ultimately coma and death), which is almost always associated with a blood lead concentration of >100 μg/dl.

However, before lead encephalopathy occurs, low-dose exposure to lead causes neurologic and intellectual deficits that may or may not be reversible. Hyperactivity, aggression, impulsiveness, decreased interest in play, lethargy, irritability, hearing impairment, learning difficulties, short attention span, and distractibility are sometimes seen in low levels of lead poisoning. Studies demonstrate that as prenatal and postnatal lead levels increase, the child's intelligence quotient decreases (Bellinger, Stiles, and Needleman, 1992; Dietrich, Berger, and Succop, 1993). Most children with lead poisoning are asymptomatic, making early identification more difficult.

Hematologic System. Lead is extremely toxic to the biosynthesis of heme, preventing the formation of hemoglobin and causing its precursors, especially erythrocyte protoporphyrin (EP), coproporphyrin, and delta-aminolevulinic acid (ALA), to increase in the body. EP is elevated in the blood when the blood lead concentration is moderately increased but is not a sensitive indicator for low lead exposure. Reduction of the heme molecule in the red blood cell results in anemia. However, with low levels of lead toxicity, anemia may not be present.

Renal System. Lead damages the cells of the proximal tubules, resulting in abnormal excretion of glucose, protein, amino acids, and phosphate and in interference with the synthesis of vitamin D. With adequate treatment, kidney damage is usually reversible. Severe, irreversible lead nephropathy is probably limited to protracted childhood plumbism.

Other Manifestations. Other vague symptoms of plumbism are acute, crampy abdominal pain, vomiting, constipation, anorexia, headache, a loss of developmental progress, and lethargy. Some evidence suggests that in young children lead impairs growth, especially in infants

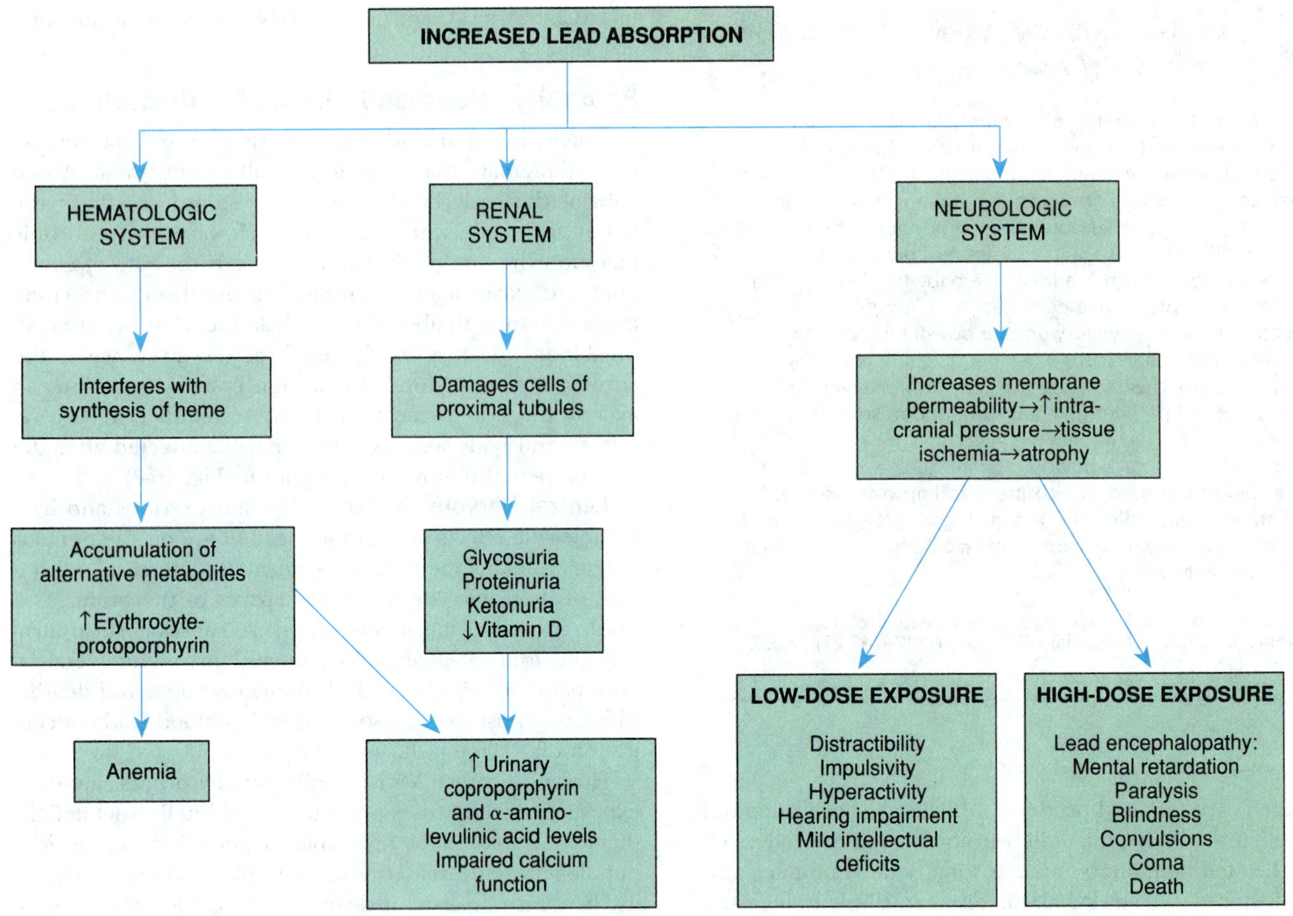

FIG. 16-8 Main effects of lead on body systems.

THINKING CRITICALLY ABOUT . . .

Universal Lead Screening with a Focus on the Family

Although universal lead screening is recommended by the Centers for Disease Control and Prevention (CDC) (1991) and the American Academy of Pediatrics (1993b), it is not universally accepted. The major arguments against this policy include (1) the expense and intensive labor involved in screening, particularly in communities where the risk of lead intoxication is very low; (2) diversion of funds needed for more serious childhood problems and for prevention of lead poisoning in terms of removing lead from dwellings; (3) skepticism about the significance of a lowered intelligence quotient (IQ) of about 5 points, especially in light of coexisting factors, such as poverty and anemia, that can account for the lowered scores; and finally (4) concern for the negative consequences to the child and family, such as the trauma of invasive tests, cost, and anxiety about the diagnosis of "lead-poisoning" for a condition that ranges from a very mild consequence to death (Harvey, 1994; Piomelli, 1994; Schoen, 1993).

Nurses, who are often responsible for screening and testing procedures and educational interventions, need to be aware of the arguments for and against universal lead screening. In particular, they must be sensitive to the potential impact the diagnosis of lead poisoning based on a low lead blood level may have on the family—especially since levels between 10 and 20 μg/dl require no medical intervention.*

*Information for families is available from the National Lead Information Center (National Safety Council), 1019 19th St., N.W., Suite 401, Washington, DC 20036-5105; (800) LEAD-FYI.

with elevated prenatal and postnatal blood lead level (Huseman, Varma, and Angle, 1992; Shukla and others, 1989). However, other researchers have found no effect on stature in young adults who had both low and high levels of lead exposure during childhood (Sachs and Moel, 1989).

Diagnostic Evaluation

Diagnosis is made on measurement of blood lead levels. Since virtually all children are at risk for lead poisoning, universal screening is recommended (see Thinking Critically About . . . box). Priority for screening is given to children ages 6 to 72 months who are at highest risk: (1) those who live in or frequent deteriorated housing or such housing during remodeling, including most homes built before 1960 and many homes built up to 1980; (2) those whose siblings or other close peers have lead poisoning; and (3) those whose household members have lead-related occupations or hobbies, or who live near lead-related industries (Centers for Disease Control, 1991).

Screening tests are usually done on blood collected by finger or heel puncture. The rate of incorrect results is high but can be improved with appropriate skin preparation to reduce lead contamination. Blood collected by venipuncture is needed to confirm the diagnosis. Other tests that may be helpful in determining the presence of lead in the body are (1) radiographs of the abdomen to help detect the presence of lead paint chips; (2) radiographs of the long bones for "lead lines," caused by deposition of lead; (3) blood studies for evidence of anemia; and (4) a lead mobilization test to help predict the amount of lead that may be removed by chelation.

Therapeutic Management

The child's blood lead level determines the degree of risk and the type of intervention (Table 16-5). The objective of treatment is to remove lead in the body and prevent further accumulation of the metal. Therapeutic modalities include removing the source of lead, improving nutrition, and using chelation therapy. With emphasis on early detection of low blood lead levels, removing sources of lead in the environment is the major goal (see Family Home Care box on p. 698).

Chelation therapy is usually reserved for children with high blood lead levels. Drugs that may be used are calcium disodium edetate ($CaNa_2EDTA$ or CaEDTA), dimercaprol (also called BAL [British antilewisite]), and dimercaptosuccinic acid (DSMA) (succimer [Chemet]). Penicillamine (Cuprimine, Depen) is used by some practitioners to chelate children with moderate levels of lead.

The exact course of therapy depends on the severity of the child's condition and the practitioner's preference. Combination therapy with CaEDTA and BAL does not seem to result in a better response but does increase drug toxicity (O'Connor, 1992). $CaNa_2EDTA$ is given preferably intravenously; intramuscular injections are very painful. BAL (prepared in peanut oil) is given only intramuscularly and is also a very painful injection. D-Penicillamine and succimer are administered orally.

TABLE 16-5 Classification of Risk and Treatment for Lead Poisoning

BLOOD LEAD CONCENTRATION (μg/dl)	INTERVENTION
≤9	Child is not considered to be lead poisoned
10-14	Many children with blood lead levels in this range should trigger community-wide childhood lead poisoning prevention activities; children may need to be rescreened more frequently
15-19	Child should receive nutritional and educational interventions and more frequent screening; if blood lead level persists in this range, environmental investigation and intervention should be done
20-44	Child should receive environmental evaluation and remediation and a medical evaluation; may need pharmacologic treatment of lead poisoning
45-69	Child will need both medical and environmental interventions, including chelation therapy
≥70	Child is a medical emergency; medical and environmental management must begin immediately

Modified from Centers for Disease Control: *Preventing lead poisoning in young children,* Atlanta, GA, 1991, Centers for Disease Control.

NURSING ALERT Children with allergy to peanuts or penicillin cannot receive BAL or D-penicillamine, respectively.

Symptomatic treatment during chelation therapy involves observing for and controlling seizures for which the child is at risk and taking measures to reduce the side effects of some of the medications, such as the nausea that can occur with BAL. Depending on the drug being used, serum electrolyte levels should be taken at prescribed intervals, urine specimens analyzed, and fluid intake and output measured. If numerous paint chips are visible in the gastrointestinal tract on radiologic examination, cleansing enemas or a cathartic may be ordered. Every effort is made to prevent infection and maintain adequate hydration. When succimer is given, adequate fluid intake is especially important, as is close monitoring of the absolute neutrophil count. Neutropenia can occur during drug therapy. If nu-

FAMILY HOME CARE
Reducing Blood Lead Levels

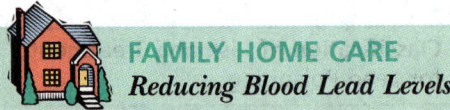

Make sure child does not have access to peeling paint or chewable surfaces painted with lead-based paint, especially window sills and wells.

If a house was built before 1960 (possibly before 1980) and has hard-surface floors, wet mop them at least once a week with a high-phosphate solution (e.g., trisodium phosphate [available in hardware stores]). Wipe other hard surfaces (such as window sills and baseboards) with the same kind of solution. If there are loose paint chips in an area, such as a window well, use a disposable cloth soaked with the high phosphate (5% to 8%) solution to pick up and discard them. Do not vacuum hard-surfaced floors or window sills or wells, since this spreads dust. Use vacuum cleaners with agitators to remove dust from rugs rather than vacuum cleaners with suction only. If a rug is known to contain lead dust and cannot be washed, it should be discarded.

Wash and dry child's hands and face frequently, especially before eating.

Wash toys and pacifiers frequently.

If soil around home is or is likely to be contaminated with lead (e.g., if home was built before 1960 or is near a major highway), plant grass or other ground cover; plant bushes around outside of house so that child cannot play there.

During remodeling of older homes, be sure to follow correct procedures. Be certain children and pregnant women are not in the home, day or night, until process is completed. Following deleading, thoroughly clean house using high-phosphate cleaning solution to damp mop and dust before inhabitants return.

In areas where lead content of water exceeds the drinking water standard, run cold water until it is as cold as it will get before using it for drinking, cooking, and making formula; may use first-flush water for other purposes.

Do not store food in open cans, particularly if cans are imported.

Do not use pottery or ceramic ware that was inadequately fired or is meant for decorative use for food storage or service. Do not store drinks or food in lead crystal.

Avoid folk remedies or cosmetics that contain lead.

Make sure that home exposure is not occurring from parental occupations or hobbies. Household members employed in occupations such as lead smelting should shower and change into clean clothing before leaving work. Construction and abatement workers may also bring home lead contaminants.

Make sure child eats regular meals, since more lead is absorbed on an empty stomach.

Make sure child's diet contains plenty of iron and calcium and not too much fat.

Modified from Centers for Disease Control: *Preventing lead poisoning in young children,* Atlanta, GA, 1991, Centers for Disease Control.

tritional deficiencies coexist, they are treated appropriately, such as with administration of supplemental iron for iron-deficiency anemia. Iron should not be given during chelation, however, especially with BAL because of possible interactive effects.

Prognosis. Although most of the pathophysiologic effects of lead are reversible, the most serious consequences of both high and low lead exposure are the effects on the central nervous system. In children with lead encephalopathy, permanent brain damage can result in mental retardation, behavior changes, possible paralysis, and seizures. However, moderate- to low-dose exposure may also cause permanent neurologic deficits. Young children with blood lead levels averaging 43 μg/dl, when tested as young adults, had more academic problems (reading disabilities, school failures), poor coordination (hand-eye movements, finger tapping), and a higher incidence of minor delinquency than children with lower blood lead levels (Needleman and others, 1990). There is some evidence that treatment of moderate levels of lead poisoning can result in cognitive improvement (Ruff and others, 1993).

Nursing Considerations

The primary nursing goal in lead poisoning is to prevent the child's initial or further exposure to lead. For children with low-level exposure, this often requires identifying the sources of lead in the environment. Careful history taking is one of the most useful and valuable tools and should concentrate on the areas listed in the Guidelines box, especially those related to the home environment (Nordin, Rolnick, and Griffin, 1994) (see Critical Thinking Exercise box). Suggestions for reducing lead in the child's environment are listed in the Family Home Care box.

Children who must undergo chelation therapy are prepared for the injections and allowed to express their pain and anger. Playing with syringes and aggressive play, such as pounding clay or throwing beanbags, provides an excellent outlet for their frustrations. Children also deserve an explanation of the need for the treatment, particularly that it is not punishment. With the more frequent use of home

GUIDELINES
Assessing Potential for Lead Poisoning

Does your child:

1. Live in a house or regularly visit a daycare center, preschool, the home of a babysitter or relative, or other house built before 1960 that has peeling or chipping paint?
2. Live in or regularly visit a house built before 1960 with recent, ongoing, or planned renovation or remodeling?
3. Have a brother or sister, housemate, or playmate being followed up or treated for lead poisoning (i.e., blood level ≥15 mg/dl)?
4. Live with an adult whose job, hobby, or use of ethnic remedies involves exposure to lead?
5. Live near an active lead smelter, battery recycling plant, or other industry likely to release lead?

Modified from Centers for Disease Control: *Preventing lead poisoning in young children,* Atlanta, GA, 1991, Centers for Disease Control.

CRITICAL THINKING EXERCISE

Lead Poisoning

The clinic in which you practice has received funds to begin a program to reduce lead poisoning in children. As a member of the planning committee, which of the following initial projects is effective and easy to implement?

1. Screening for blood lead levels by heel or finger puncture in all children under age 6 years
2. Questioning parents about the age and condition of their home(s) since the child's birth, including recent renovations
3. Screening for blood lead levels by venipuncture in all children under age 6 years who are at risk for lead exposure
4. Questioning parents about hobbies, occupations, and ethnic remedies that may expose the child to lead

The correct answer is 2. Asking about the family's dwelling to identify instances where lead, especially on painted surfaces, could be present is the single most important screening procedure. Although asking about hobbies, occupations, and ethnic remedies should be considered, option 4 is not the priority question. Screening for blood lead levels is expensive and time consuming. Option 3 is incorrect because collection of blood by venipuncture is not a recommended screening procedure, and all children, regardless of risk, should be screened.

oral chelation therapy, parents need to understand the importance of giving the drug as prescribed.

Chelating agents are administered deeply into a large muscle mass. To lessen the pain from $CaNa_2EDTA$, the local anesthetic procaine is injected with the drug. Rotation of sites is essential to prevent the formation of painful areas of fibrotic tissue. Since $CaNa_2EDTA$ and lead are toxic to the kidneys, records are kept of intake and output, and the results of urinalysis are assessed to monitor renal functioning. Because of the risk of seizures, appropriate precautions are instituted at the bedside of children with high blood lead levels.

NURSING ALERT $CaNa_2EDTA$ is never given in the absence of an adequate urinary output. Children receiving the drug intramuscularly must be able to maintain adequate oral intake of fluids.

As in any situational crisis, parents need support and understanding if their child is treated for lead poisoning (see also Thinking Critically About . . . box on p. 696). Many of the families at highest risk for lead poisoning have the fewest resources to comply with measures such as relocation or deleading the home. Appropriate referrals are essential in locating assistance for parents. (See also Nursing Care Plan: The Child with Lead Poisoning.*)

*In *Wong and Whaley's Clinical Manual of Pediatric Nursing* (Mosby).

CHILD MALTREATMENT

The broad term ***child maltreatment*** includes intentional physical abuse or neglect, emotional abuse or neglect, and sexual abuse of children, usually by adults. It is one of the most significant social problems affecting children, and parent-child abuse may be only one type of violence in the family. Violence between parents also often occurs; the abusing parent may also be the abused spouse (McKibben, DeVos, and Newberger, 1989). Family violence also increases the risk of physical and sexual abuse in youngsters who leave the home to avoid maltreatment. Ironically, these "runaways" often encounter continued abuse "on the streets" as they try to survive.

In 1991 about 2.7 million children were reported as victims of child abuse and neglect to child protective services in the United States. However, this does not represent the number of children actually maltreated. Of these reported cases, 33% were found to be substantiated; the rest—67%—were unfounded (considered false) (National Center on Child Abuse and Neglect (1993). (See also Family Focus box on p. 700.) The rate of deaths from child neglect and abuse have decreased somewhat in children 0 to 4 years of age and has remained relatively stable during the 1980s (McClain and others, 1993). Death rates vary by geographic location in the United States—being highest in the South and West and lowest in the Northeast (McClain and others, 1994).

The best available statistics only partially reflect the true incidence of child maltreatment. Some unfounded reports may actually be cases of abuse, and many abuse cases are never reported. According to the National Center on Child Abuse and Neglect (NCCAAN) (1993), the following statistics represent the incidence of child maltreatment in the United States*:

Emotional neglect	3.2 per 1000
Emotional abuse	3.0 per 1000
Educational abuse	4.5 per 1000
Physical neglect	8.1 per 1000
Physical abuse	4.9 per 1000
Sexual abuse	2.1 per 1000

CHILD NEGLECT

Child neglect is the most common form of maltreatment. About one half of all reported cases are associated with deprivation of necessities, and over one third of deaths from maltreatment are in this group. ***Neglect*** is generally defined as the failure of a parent or other person legally responsible for the child's welfare to provide for the child's basic needs and an adequate level of care (Council on Scientific Affairs, 1985).

Little is known about the etiology of neglect, although it appears that many of the risk factors identified in physical abuse apply to neglect as well (see discussion below). Igno-

*Additional information is available from the Clearinghouse on Child Abuse and Neglect Information, P.O. Box 1182, Washington, DC 20013-1182; (703) 385-7565 or (800) FYI-3366.

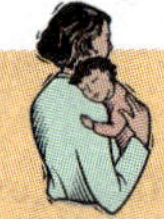

FAMILY FOCUS

False Allegations of Abuse

Although most concern among health professionals is to detect child abuse early and to protect the child from further abuse, prevention of abuse must also include prevention of false allegations of abuse. Although some degree of overreporting is to be expected because the law requires the reporting of suspected maltreatment, the present level of overreporting is considered unreasonably high. Under the present child abuse laws, child protective services have the authority to remove a child from the home solely on the basis of allegations made to an abuse hotline (Radko, 1993). Another reason is the practice of "defensive" medicine—health professionals are legally required to report suspected maltreatment, but there is no penalty for reporting unsubstantiated cases. Therefore playing it "safe" is preferable to failing to report and facing criminal prosecution. A negative effect of the overreporting is that the protective child services are so overburdened with minor cases that children in real danger of serious maltreatment may be poorly investigated (Besharov, 1985).

Despite the fact that more than half of all reports are unfounded, little attention has been directed to the problem of false accusations and its devastating consequences, such as removal of the child from the home, termination of parental rights, public ridicule of the family, loss of employment, and excessive legal fees to regain custody of the child. Nurses play a critical role in carefully documenting all evidence of abuse, giving alleged offenders the opportunity to present their account of the incident, and recognizing diseases or cultural practices that may be confused with abuse (Wong, 1987). In the unfortunate event that a family is wrongly accused of abuse, they may benefit from the services of the National Association of State **VOCAL (Victims of Child Abuse Legislation)** Organizations,* a support group for persons who have experienced false accusations.

Another organization that may be helpful to family members who have been accused of sexual abuse by their adult children is the **False Memory Syndrome (FMS) Foundation.**† The research and educational institution is dedicated to understanding and preventing allegations of abuse based on "false" memories. In recent years adult children, primarily women, claim to suddenly remember childhood sexual abuse, usually by fathers. The abuse is said to have been repressed for many years, but the memory is recovered with the help of a therapist. Once the "victim" remembers the abuse, the revelation is considered a "turning point" and the cause for past problems, such as eating disorders and failed marriages. The recovery is based on confronting the accused, which may involve bringing legal charges against the alleged perpetrator. In many states the statutes of limitation have been extended for allegations of abuse that occurred 40 or 50 years earlier (Coleman, 1992; Gardner, 1992; Wakefield and Underwager, 1992).

*1030 G. St., Suite 200, Sacramento, CA 95814; (916) 448-4730 or (916) 966-4753.
†3508 Market St., Suite 128, Philadelphia, PA 19104, (215) 387-1865.

rance of the child's needs and a lack of resources are important contributing factors. For example, neglectful parents often demonstrate poor parenting skills. They may be unaware that an infant needs to be fed every 3 to 4 hours, may not know what to feed the child, and may have insufficient funds to buy food. The most serious lack of knowledge is failure to recognize emotional nurturing as an essential need of children. (See also Failure to Thrive, Chapter 13.)

Types of Neglect

Neglect takes many forms and can be classified broadly as physical or emotional maltreatment. ***Physical neglect*** involves the deprivation of necessities, such as food, clothing, shelter, supervision, medical care, and education. ***Emotional neglect*** generally refers to failure to meet the child's needs for affection, attention, and emotional nurturance. It may also include lack of intervention for or fostering of maladaptive behavior, such as delinquency or substance abuse. ***Emotional abuse,*** an even more difficult aspect of maltreatment to define, refers to the deliberate attempt to destroy or significantly impair a child's self-esteem or competence. Emotional abuse may take the following forms: rejecting, isolating, terrorizing, ignoring, or corrupting the child (Garbarino, Guttmann, and Seeley, 1986).

PHYSICAL ABUSE

The deliberate infliction of physical injury on a child, usually by the child's caregiver, is termed ***physical abuse.*** Minor physical injury is responsible for more reported cases of maltreatment than major physical injury, but major physical abuse causes more deaths.

As pervasive as the problem is, not one definition of child abuse is universally accepted. Kempe and others (1962) coined the term ***battered child syndrome (BCS)*** to refer to "a clinical condition in young children who have received serious physical abuse, generally from a parent or foster parent." However, this definition restricts abuse to the most severe forms and is less appropriate than broader definitions that include the spectrum of abuse, such as "the nonaccidental injury of a child ranging from minor bruises and lacerations to severe neurologic trauma and death" (Council on Scientific Affairs, 1985). In addition to this definition, each state in the United States defines abuse according to its individual reporting laws.

Munchausen Syndrome by Proxy (MSP)

One of the more unusual and perplexing types of abuse, usually physical, is MSP, which refers to illness that one person fabricates or induces in another person. In children, it is usually the mother who fabricates signs and symptoms of illness in her child, the proxy, to gain attention from the medical staff. Rarely, the father may be the perpetrator (Jones and others, 1993). MSP can take many forms, such as adding maternal blood to the child's urine to simulate hematuria (Salmon and others, 1988), presenting a fictitious medical history (Guandolo, 1985), chronic poisoning of the child (Goebel, Gremse, and Artman, 1993), or suffocating the child to cause apnea and seizures (Jones and others, 1993). Another form of MSP is alleging that the child has been sexually abused by someone else to gain recognition as the child's protector (Rand, 1989).

Such cases are often very difficult to confirm and require a high index of suspicion to protect the children. Warning signs of MSP include:

- Unexplained, prolonged, recurrent, or extremely rare illness
- Discrepancies between clinical findings and history
- Illness unresponsive to treatment
- Signs and symptoms occurring only in parent's presence
- Parent knowledgeable about illness, procedures, and treatments
- Parent very interested in interacting with health team members
- Parent very attentive toward child (refuses to leave hospital)
- Family members with similar symptoms

Consequences for children with MSP can be serious. They often undergo needless and painful medical procedures and treatments. The parent's actions may induce a serious illness in children; one that is fatal in almost 10% of the cases (Wilde and Pedroni, 1993). Children may develop chronic invalidism, accepting the illness story and believing themselves to be ill. Finally, they may develop MSP as an adult (Meadow, 1989). Even when some of these children are removed from the home, they continue to suffer severe psychologic trauma. Other siblings remaining in the home may become substitute victims (McGuire and Feldman, 1989).

Factors Predisposing to Physical Abuse

The exact cause of child abuse is not known, but three major criteria—parental characteristics, characteristics of the child, and environmental characteristics—seem to predispose children to physical injury by their parents or other caregivers. Despite numerous research studies that have attempted to isolate specific attributes of the parent, child, or environment that cause abuse, no single etiologic factor is responsible for abuse. Rather, an ***interaction*** between several variables appears to create a high-risk situation for maltreatment to occur; the greater number of variables, the greater the risk. Different variables may be responsible for certain types of maltreatment. For example, poverty may be more strongly associated with neglect, whereas parental characteristics may be more strongly related to physical abuse.

Parental Characteristics. Extensive research has focused on parental characteristics that distinguish abusive parents from nonabusive parents. Unfortunately, the findings from most of these studies provide conflicting evidence. For example, it is commonly believed that abusive parents were abused as children. However, few studies support this relationship (Widom, 1989).

NURSING ALERT Nurses must be careful to avoid stereotyping parents and children in an attempt to predict or diagnose abuse (Krowchuk, 1989). No test has sufficient sensitivity to predict abuse without falsely accusing many individuals (false positives) and missing some abusers (false negatives).

Although physical punishment tends to occur in abusive parents' childhood, most of the parents were not physically abused as children. However, abusive parents who report that they were severely punished as children are much more likely to injure their own children (Kotelchuck, 1982). If the abuse was not overt physical violence, abusive parents typically recall their punishment as unfair and severe, and they characterize their relationship with their parents as negative. Abusive parents tend to have difficulty controlling aggressive impulses, and the free expression of violence is one of the most consistent qualities of these families (Altemeier and others, 1982).

Another finding is that abusive families are often more socially isolated and have fewer supportive relationships than nonabusive parents. Children of teenage mothers are more at risk of abuse than those from older mothers (Stier and others, 1993). With little or no available support system and the presence of concurrent stresses imposed by the child or environment, these parents are extremely vulnerable to additional crises of any nature and literally strike out at the child as a method of releasing their increasing frustration and anxiety.

Other factors identified in abusive parents include low self-esteem and less adequate maternal functioning. Research findings do not consistently support this belief. However, this does not mean that these parents cannot benefit from learning more constructive ways of rearing their children, especially nonviolent discipline methods.

Characteristics of the Child. The child also unintentionally contributes to the abusive situation. In families of two or more children usually only one child is the victim of abuse. This child's temperament, position in the family, additional physical needs if ill or disabled, activity level, or degree of sensitivity to parental needs all contribute to the potential for physical abuse. For example, one child may not be abused if he or she fits into the "easy-child pattern," whereas another sibling with a difficult temperament may add to the parent's stress sufficiently to precipitate an abusive act. However, temperament alone is not the critical factor; rather, it is the "fit" or compatibility between the child's temperament and the parent's ability to deal with that behavioral style.

Occasionally the abused child is illegitimate, unwanted, brain damaged (especially in situations where the parents cannot accept the retardation), hyperactive, or physically disabled. Sometimes children are abused because they remind the parent of someone the parent dislikes, such as a younger brother or sister who received all the attention from their own parents. Sometimes a difficult pregnancy, labor, or delivery is a predisposing factor in abuse, especially when the infant is born prematurely or with congenital anomalies.

Although one child is usually the victim in an abusive family, removing that child from the home often places the other siblings at risk for abuse. Child maltreatment usually is not confined to one child because of a disturbed parent-child relationship but is a result of a family in distress (Jean-Gilles and Crittenden, 1990). Therefore no child is safe if left in the abusive environment unless the parents can be helped to learn new parenting skills and to meet their needs and release their frustration through outlets other than attacking their children.

Environmental Characteristics. The environment is a significant part of the potential abusive situation. Typically the environment is one of chronic stress, including problems of divorce, poverty, unemployment, poor housing, frequent relocation, alcoholism, and drug addiction. Increased exposure between children and parents, such as that which occurs in crowded living conditions, also increases the likelihood of abuse.

Although most reporting of abuse has been from lower socioeconomic populations, child abuse is by no means a problem of any one societal group. It spans all educational, social, and economic levels. Certainly, stresses imposed by poverty predispose lower socioeconomic families to abusive situations, and abuse in these groups is more apt to be reported. However, concealed crises can also be present in upper-class families. For example, a wealthy family experiencing major life changes, such as rehousing, the birth of an additional child, or marital discord, may have sufficient environmental stressors imposed on them to produce a potentially abusive situation. Wealthy families may be so overinvolved with commitments outside the home that abuse may be inflicted by substitute caregivers. Nurses need to be aware of such factors in order to identify the less obvious examples of child abuse and neglect.

SEXUAL ABUSE

Sexual abuse is one of the most devastating types of child maltreatment, and current estimates indicate that it has increased significantly during the past decade. However, the increased rate of reporting may not reflect a true increase in prevalence of sexual abuse but may be due to changes in legislation and in society's attitudes toward women and children (Feldman and others, 1991). The number of reported occurrences was approximately 15% of all child maltreatment cases in 1991 (Daro and McCurdy, 1992), but many authorities believe that this figure represents only a small percentage of the actual incidence.

As with all forms of child maltreatment, no universal definition for sexual abuse exists. The Child Abuse and Prevention Act (Public Law 100-294) defines ***sexual abuse*** as "the use, persuasion, or coercion of any child to engage in sexually explicit conduct (or any simulation of such conduct) for producing any visual depiction of such conduct, or rape, molestation, prostitution, or incest with children."

To be considered child abuse, these acts have to be committed by a person responsible for the child's care, such as a parent or baby-sitter. If a stranger commits the act, it is considered sexual assault and is handled solely by the police and criminal courts (National Center on Child Abuse and Neglect, 1989). Sexual abuse may include physical abuse, both as part of sexual arousal for the abuser and to force compliance from the child (Hobbs and Wynne, 1990).

Sexual abuse includes several types of sexual maltreatment, including the following (see also Rape, Chapter 20):

Incest—Any physical sexual activity between family members; blood relationship is not required (abusers can include stepparents, nonrelated siblings, grandparents, uncles, and aunts); does not include sexual relations between legally sanctional partners, such as spouses

Molestation—A vague term that includes "indecent liberties," such as touching, fondling, kissing, single or mutual masturbation, or oral-genital contact

Exhibitionism—Indecent exposure, usually exposure of the genitals by an adult male to children or female adults

Child pornography—Arranging and photographing in any media sexual acts involving children, alone or with adults or animals, regardless of consent by the child's legal guardian; also may denote distribution of such material in any form with or without profit

Child prostitution—Involving children in sex acts for profit and usually with changing partners

Pedophilia—Literally means "love of child" and does not denote a type of sexual activity but the preference of an adult for prepubertal children as the means of achieving sexual excitement

Characteristics of Abusers and Victims

Anyone, including siblings and mothers, can be sexual abusers, but a typical abuser is a male that the victim knows. Offenders come from all levels of society. Some are prominent persons in the community, and some, especially in the case of pedophiliacs (also called "child molesters"), are in positions, such as teaching and coaching, where they work closely with children.

Pornography and prostitution may involve strangers, as well as the children's own parents. There are no typical characteristics of these offenders, although the abused children tend to be runaways—young adolescents who engage in these activities to obtain money for food, shelter, drugs, and alcohol. Incestuous relationships between father or stepfather and daughter are generally prolonged, and the victims are usually reluctant to report the situation because of fear of retaliation and fear that they will not be believed. Typically, incestuous relationships begin later than other forms of child abuse, and the average age of the victim is 9 years (Highlights, 1988). The eldest daughter is usually abused, but in her absence another sister is substituted. Sibling incest may also occur (Gilbert, 1992). Sexual abuse by relatives with a strong emotional bond with the victim is the most devastating to the child (Feinauer, 1989).

Boys are also victims of both intrafamilial and extrafamilial abuse. Males are much less likely to report abuse, and they may suffer much greater emotional harm from incestuous relationships, especially between mother and son, than do female victims. Boys are likely to be subjected to anal penetration and oral-genital contact, to have subtle physical findings, and to be abused by a father, stepfather, or mother's boyfriend.

Initiation and Perpetuation of Sexual Abuse

The cycle of sexual abuse often starts innocently, unless it involves an isolated attack, such as rape. Often offenders spend time with the victims to gain their trust before initiating any sexual contact. Most victims are then pressured into being an accessory to the sexual activity through various means (see box below) and may be unaware that sexual activity is part of the offer. Children may not reveal the truth for fear that their parents would not believe them if they told—especially if the offender is a trusted member of the family. Some fear they will be blamed for the situation, and many young children with limited vocabulary have difficulty describing the activity when they do have the courage or opportunity to reveal the abuse.

Seductiveness by the child does not initiate incest. Most young girls experiment in seduction, especially during the preschool years, but the father's response normally differentiates this playfulness from overt sexual invitation. Although the reasons for incest are complicated and can occur in various family types, it does not occur in healthy families. Most incestuous relationships are directly tied to sexual maladjustment and estrangement between husband and wife. Most begin following the cessation of sexual relationships with the usual partner. Most fathers experience little guilt, and many wives at some level are aware of the incestuous affair. The wife may react by tolerating the situation or may resort to use of denial; some remain unaware of the activity. Consequently, the home offers little protection to young victims, since abusers have easy access to their victims and the children feel they cannot reveal their secret to other family members. However, not all incestuous relationships follow this pattern of silence. Currently, reports of father-daughter incest during child custody conflicts have become more common and have raised serious concerns regarding the possibility of false accusation. Rather than tolerating or denying the child's sexual abuse, the other parent (usually the mother) is typically the chief accuser.

METHODS USED TO PRESSURE CHILDREN INTO SEXUAL ACTIVITY

- The child is offered gifts or privileges.
- The adult misrepresents moral standards by telling the child that it is "okay to do."
- Isolated and emotionally and socially impoverished children are enticed by adults who meet their needs for warmth and human contact.
- The successful sex offender pressures the victim into secrecy regarding the activity by describing it as a "secret between us" that other people may take away if they find out.
- The offender plays on the child's fears, including fear of punishment by the offender, fear of repercussions if the child tells, and fear of abandonment or rejection by the family.

NURSING CARE OF THE MALTREATED CHILD

Assessment

One of the most critical responsibilities of all health professionals is identifying abusive situations as early as possible. The characteristics that may predispose members of some families to commit abuse can serve as a framework for assessing vulnerability but do not predict actual abuse. Rather, a thorough physical examination and a careful, detailed history are the diagnostic tools needed to identify abuse. Nurses have a very special role because they may be the first person to see the child and parent and are the consistent caregivers if the child is hospitalized (see Guidelines box).

NURSING ALERT Nurses must be aware of their biases regarding child abuse. Studies show that nurses are less likely to report abuse when the child is female and from a middle-income, as opposed to lower-income, family (Pillitteri and others, 1992) and are significantly less comfortable dealing with sexual abuse, abuse of infants, and fathers as the abusers (Seidl and others, 1993).

Evidence of Maltreatment. Recognition of abuse or neglect necessitates a familiarity with both physical and behavioral signs that suggest maltreatment (see box on p. 704). No one indicator can diagnose maltreatment; rather, it is a pattern or combination of indicators that should arouse suspicion and further investigation. In addition, signs of possible abuse must be coupled with an understanding of diseases, such as bleeding disorders, osteogenesis imperfecta, or sudden infant death syndrome, and cultural practices, such as cupping or coin rubbing (see Health Practices, Chapter 2), that may mimic physical abuse. Unintentional injuries may also be wrongly diagnosed as abuse, such as burns from metal buckles on car seats (Schmitt, Gray, and Britton, 1978), lacerations from seat belts (Baker, 1986), or retinal hemorrhage after cardiopulmonary resuscitation (Goetting and Sowa, 1990). Normal variants, such

GUIDELINES
Talking with Children Who Reveal Abuse

- Provide a private time and place to talk.
- Do not promise not to tell; tell them that you are required by law to report the abuse.
- Do not express shock or criticize their family.
- Use their vocabulary to discuss body parts.
- Avoid using any leading statements that can distort their report.
- Reassure them that they have done the right thing by telling.
- Tell them that the abuse is not their fault, that they are not bad or to blame.
- Determine their immediate need for safety.
- Let the child know what will happen when you report.

CLINICAL MANIFESTATIONS OF POTENTIAL CHILD MALTREATMENT

PHYSICAL NEGLECT

Suggestive Physical Findings

Failure to thrive
Signs of malnutrition, such as thin extremities, abdominal distention, lack of subcutaneous fat
Poor personal hygiene, especially of teeth
Unclean and/or inappropriate dress
Evidence of poor health care, such as nonimmunized status, untreated infections, frequent colds
Frequent injuries from lack of supervision

Suggestive Behaviors

Dull and inactive; excessively passive or sleepy
Self-stimulatory behaviors, such as finger-sucking or rocking
Begging or stealing food; Absenteeism from school; Drug or alcohol addiction; Vandalism or shoplifting } in older child

EMOTIONAL ABUSE AND NEGLECT

Suggestive Physical Findings

Failure to thrive
Feeding disorders, such as rumination
Enuresis
Sleep disorders

Suggestive Behaviors

Self-stimulatory behaviors, such as biting, rocking, sucking
During infancy, lack of social smile and stranger anxiety
Withdrawal
Unusual fearfulness
Antisocial behavior, such as destructiveness, stealing, cruelty
Extremes of behavior, such as overcompliant and passive or aggressive and demanding
Lags in emotional and intellectual development, especially language
Suicide attempts

PHYSICAL ABUSE

Suggestive Physical Findings

Bruises and welts
- On face, lips, mouth, back, buttocks, thighs, or areas of torso
- Regular patterns descriptive of object used, such as belt buckle, hand, wire hanger, chain, wooden spoon, squeeze or pinch marks
- May be present in various stages of healing

Burns
- On soles of feet, palms of hands, back, or buttocks
- Patterns descriptive of object used, such as round cigar or cigarette burns, "glovelike" sharply demarcated areas from immersion in scalding water, rope burns on wrists or ankles from being bound, burns in the shape of an iron, radiator, or electric stove burner
- Absence of "splash" marks and presence of symmetric burns
- Stun gun injury—lesions circular, fairly uniform (up to 0.5 cm), and paired about 5 cm apart (Frechette and Rimsza, 1992).

Fractures and dislocations
- Skull, nose, or facial structures
- Injury may denote type of abuse, such as spiral fracture or dislocation from twisting of an extremity or whiplash from shaking the child
- Multiple new or old fractures in various stages of healing

Lacerations and abrasions
- On backs of arms, legs, torso, face, or external genitalia
- Unusual symptoms, such as abdominal swelling, pain, and vomiting from punching
- Descriptive marks such as from human bites or pulling the hair out

Chemical
- Unexplained repeated poisoning, especially drug overdose
- Unexplained sudden illness, such as hypoglycemia from insulin administration

Suggestive Behaviors

Wary of physical contact with adults
Apparent fear of parents or going home
Lying very still while surveying environment
Inappropriate reaction to injury, such as failure to cry from pain
Lack of reaction to frightening events
Apprehensive when hearing other children cry
Indiscriminate friendliness and displays of affection
Superficial relationships
Acting-out behavior, such as aggression, to seek attention
Withdrawal behavior

SEXUAL ABUSE

Suggestive Physical Findings

Bruises, bleeding, lacerations or irritation of external genitalia, anus, mouth, or throat
Torn, stained, or bloody underclothing
Pain on urination or pain, swelling, and itching of genital area
Penile discharge
Sexually transmitted disease, nonspecific vaginitis, or venereal warts
Difficulty in walking or sitting
Unusual odor in the genital area
Recurrent urinary tract infections
Presence of sperm
Pregnancy in young adolescent

Suggestive Behaviors

Sudden emergence of sexually related problems, including excessive or public masturbation, age-inappropriate sexual play, promiscuity, or overtly seductive behavior
Withdrawn, excessive daydreaming
Preoccupied with fantasies, especially in play
Poor relationships with peers
Sudden changes, such as anxiety, loss or gain of weight, clinging behavior
In incestuous relationships, excessive anger at mother for not protecting daughter
Regressive behavior, such as bed-wetting or thumb-sucking
Sudden onset of phobias or fears, particularly fears of the dark, men, strangers, or particular settings or situations (e.g., undue fear of leaving the house or staying at the daycare center or the baby-sitter's house)
Running away from home
Substance abuse, particularly of alcohol or mood-elevating drugs
Profound and rapid personality changes, especially extreme depression, hostility, and aggression (often accompanied by social withdrawal)
Rapidly declining school performance
Suicidal attempts or ideation

as mongolian spots and congenital anomalies of genitalia, can be mistaken for abuse (Adams and Horton, 1989; Koblenzer, 1989).

Not all forms of physical abuse demonstrate obvious signs. Violent shaking of children, especially infants under 6 months old ***(shaken baby syndrome)***, can cause fatal intracranial trauma without signs of external head injury (American Academy of Pediatrics, 1993a). If MSP is suspected, nurses play an important role in monitoring the parent's activities to identify instances of causing the children's symptoms. Using a hidden video camera to document the parent's behavior is becoming a more common diagnostic procedure, but the parent's right of privacy must be considered (Wilde and Pedroni, 1993).

NURSING ALERT Stress to parents the dangers of shaking infants (can cause "shaken baby syndrome"). Advise against:

- Shaking as a method of burping or waking infant
- Tossing infant in air
- Shaking infant when feeling angry or tense

Neglect and emotional abuse. Neglect from deprivation of necessities is easier to identify than emotional neglect or abuse because physical signs are usually evident. While emotional maltreatment may be readily suspected, it is very difficult to substantiate. Physical signs are often nonspecific, and nurses must rely on behavioral indicators, which range from depression to acting-out behavior, to help identify a possibly abusive situation. Any persistent and unexplained change in the child's behavior is an important clue to possible emotional abuse.

Sexual abuse. Identifying instances of sexual abuse is particularly difficult because frequently few if any obvious physical indications of the activity may exist. Also, many individuals are hesitant to believe children and unwilling to report incidents. Even health professionals are sometimes at fault when they perform cursory physical examinations of the genitalia and ignore behavior or verbal comments that suggest abuse. When sexual abuse is suspected, other children in the family should also be evaluated, since multiple victims are not uncommon.

Unfortunately, there is no typical profile of the victim, and there must be a high index of suspicion to identify these children. Physical signs vary and may include any of those listed for sexual abuse in the box on p. 704. The victim may exhibit various behavioral manifestations. Unfortunately, none of these behaviors is diagnostic of sexual abuse (Legrand, Wakefield, and Underwager, 1989). When abused children exhibit these behaviors, the signs may be incorrectly attributed to the normal stresses of childhood, especially in older school-age children or adolescents. Even those signs considered most predictive of sexual abuse, such as certain genital findings, sexually inappropriate behavior for age, enactment of adult sexual activity, and intense focus on sexual activity (e.g., masturbation), do not always indicate that sexual abuse has occurred (see Thinking Critically About . . . box, p. 706). Conversely, abused children may not demonstrate more knowledge of sexual activity than nonabused children. However, one difference in the abused children's explanation of sexual activity may be unusual affective responses. For example, abused children may relate stories that include fear of going to sleep or of being with a parent (Gordon, Schroeder, and Abrams, 1990).

WARNING SIGNS OF ABUSE

- Physical evidence of abuse and/or neglect, including previous injuries
- Conflicting stories about the "accident" or injury from the parents or others
- Cause of injury blamed on sibling or other party
- An injury inconsistent with the history, such as a concussion and broken arm from falling off a bed
- History inconsistent with child's developmental level; such as a 6-month-old turning on the hot water
- A complaint other than the one associated with signs of abuse (e.g., a chief complaint of a cold when there is evidence of first- and second-degree burns)
- Inappropriate response of caregiver, such as an exaggerated or absent emotional response; refusal to sign for additional tests or agree to necessary treatment; excessive delay in seeking treatment; absence of the parents for questioning
- Inappropriate response of child, such as little or no response to pain; fear of being touched; excessive or lack of separation anxiety; indiscriminate friendliness to strangers
- Child's report of physical or sexual abuse
- Previous reports of abuse in the family
- Repeated visits to emergency facilities with injuries

History Pertaining to the Incident. In addition to observable evidence of abuse, the type of history revealed by the parents or other caregiver, such as the baby-sitter or mother's boyfriend, is a significant factor. Areas of the history that should arouse suspicion of abuse are summarized in the box above.

NURSING ALERT Incompatibility between the history and the injury is probably the most important criterion on which to base the decision to report suspected abuse (Krugman, 1989a, 1989b).

An important point to remember when taking a history is that maltreated children rarely betray their parents by admitting to the abuse they received. If questioned, they will repeat the same story as the parents and try to defend their parents' actions. If the interviewer directly accuses the parents of abuse, the child may accept responsibility for the act in an attempt to vindicate the parents from the accusation. Children may respond in this way for fear of retaliation. However, children also fear losing whatever security and love they have. Between abusive acts children may receive some measure of attention and love from the parents. If they betray the parents, they may lose this and be uncertain or fearful of the consequences, such as foster care. Preserving the present situation may be less frightening than the unknown future.

The ***disclosure of sexual abuse*** can occur in a variety of ways—the act is observed by others, resulting in a direct confrontation; the child tells someone, such as a parent of a

THINKING CRITICALLY ABOUT . . .

Using Findings from the Genital Examination to Diagnose Sexual Abuse in Children

Unlike physical abuse, in which signs of maltreatment are often apparent, little or no evidence of sexual activity may be found in sexual abuse. To help substantiate accusations of molestation, several investigators have attempted to define characteristics of genitalia in males and females that are "diagnostic" of sexual abuse. Of the many findings that have been reported as conclusive or "highly suspect," the following are often considered the most significant: vaginal opening greater than 4 mm (Cantwell, 1983; White, Ingram, and Lyna, 1989), hymenal tears and synechiae (tissue bands) inside the vagina (Emans and others, 1987), reflex anal dilation (Hobbs and Wynne, 1989), and condylomata acuminata (anogenital or venereal warts) (Hanson and others, 1989).

However, most subjects in these studies were children suspected of sexual abuse; without a control group of nonabused children, it is impossible to be certain that the same findings are not present in all children. Even the few studies with control groups found the same genital signs in the nonabused children, although not as often. Surprisingly, little is known about the normal range of genital characteristics in children. What is known casts serious doubt on the diagnostic validity of any of the "highly suspect" signs. McCann and others (1990b) conducted studies on prepubertal children who had been carefully screened to rule out sexual abuse. They found that the size of the vaginal opening varied greatly; an opening greater than 4 mm was not unusual. The size was influenced by the examination position, amount of traction applied to the labia, degree of relaxation during the examination, and the child's age. In examining the anal and vaginal areas, the researchers found that any findings often associated with sexual abuse, including reflex anal dilation (opening of the anal sphincters during knee-chest position), hymenal tears, and vaginal synechiae, also were not unusual in nonabused children (Berenson, Somma-Garcia, and Barnett, 1993; McCann and others, 1989, 1990b). In addition, perianal injuries heal quickly and become less obvious over time (McCann and Voris, 1993).

One of the most controversial issues is the diagnostic importance of finding a sexually transmitted disease in a prepubertal child. For example, the American Academy of Pediatrics (1991) states that for a child with postperinatal condylomata acuminatum, sexual abuse is "probable" and the case should be reported to the community agency for child abuse and neglect. In another statement a confirmed infection with nonperinatal gonorrhea indicates that sexual abuse is "certain." Other reports suggest a different picture. In a study that investigated the likelihood of condylomata acuminata occurring in children who were presumed not to be sexually abused, only 11% of the 73 children (none under 3 years of age) with the warts were judged to be victims of sexual abuse (Cohen, Honig, and Androphy, 1990). However, studies like this one are criticized for using inadequate methods to evaluate possible sexual abuse (Gutman, Herman-Giddens, and Phelps, 1993). Another issue is the possibility of sexual abuse in children with human immunodeficiency virus (HIV) who lack risk factors, such as acquiring the infection perinatally or from transfusions (Gellert and others, 1993).

Obviously, the diagnosis of child sexual abuse is difficult, and *proof* of sexual abuse does not rest on the physical examination. The only definitive physical evidence of sexual assault is presence of sperm (Aiken, 1990). However, presence of sperm in a pubertal girl may not necessarily be there from sexual abuse, but from consent to intercourse (Gardner, 1993). In reviewing cases of sexual abuse with successful conviction of the perpetrator, experts contend that the most important evidence is the quality of the history (including the medical record) and the ability of children to tell their story (De Jong and Rose, 1989).

Nurses who are aware of these recent findings regarding normal genitalia can encourage practitioners to consider their findings on the genital examination very cautiously in terms of diagnosing sexual abuse. The use of a ***colposcope*** can improve the accuracy and reliability of the examination, and nurses are often responsible for assisting the practitioner with the colposcopic examination. The instrument consists of a pair of binoculars mounted on a tripod or a movable mechanical arm. It has a light for better visualization, magnifies the structure from 10 to 20 times, and is equipped with a special camera to take photographs (McCann and others, 1990a).

friend; visible clues of the relationship are observed, such as an accumulation of coins, gifts, or candy; or more obvious clues are seen, such as a child coming home disheveled or becoming pregnant; and physical or behavioral signs and symptoms are observed. Children usually describe the experience in terms of whether it was unpleasant or hurt or was pleasurable (usually a response to hand-genital contact); some indicate no reaction. Young children often feel no guilt or shame because the act is pleasurable and they are unaware of its inappropriateness.

NURSING ALERT When children report potentially sexually abusive experiences, their reports need to be taken seriously, but also cautiously to avoid alarming the child or falsely accusing a person.

Children's reports may vary from contradictory stories to unwavering versions of the experience. While their stories may sound contradictory, this may reflect the child's experiences in several instances of abuse. Also, children who repeatedly tell identical facts may have been prompted to do so. Increasing evidence suggests that the types of interrogation children are exposed to following reports of sexual abuse shape their thinking. In addition, a parent may persuade a child to believe that abuse occurred for a particular purpose, such as gaining custody in a divorce dispute (Yates and Musty, 1988). Consequently, children may falsely accuse individuals of abuse, not because the children are lying but because they are affirming what the interviewer or parent wants to hear. Through the use of leading questions, closed questions (those requiring yes or no answers), intimidation, prodding, and selective reinforcement for certain answers, children begin to tell stories that never occurred. Eventually they may come to consider the fictious experience as reality (Wakefield and Underwager, 1989).

In preparation for an ***interview,*** every effort is made to make the child feel comfortable, with appropriate introductions, and to avoid duplicating the behaviors typically used by offenders, such as touching the child without permission. The interview is conducted in a quiet and private location, preferably a neutral place, such as a school playroom or office, and not where the abuse occurred. Neutral questions are asked first, such as the child's reaction to the hospital (if appropriate). Then the incident is discussed in general terms. The interview should include such nonleading questions as "Do you know why you were brought to the hospital?" "Do you know what will happen here?" or "How do you feel about being here?" Later the question "Can you tell me what happened?" and other questions may then elicit an account of the incident. Sometimes the parents are able to help the child to describe the incident, and questions can then be directed to the circumstances of the assault. Questions should progress chronologically and proceed from the nonsexual to the more sexual content. If the child shows evidence of becoming too upset, the focus is redirected toward more neutral and less emotionally charged areas.

When questioning children who may be victims of abuse, nurses must be very skillful interviewers to avoid biasing the interaction. Courts may allow a hearsay declaration (an out-of-court statement) to be used as legal evidence. Medical records should include verbatim statements made by the child and interviewer that reflect appropriate nonleading questions and statements (Myers, 1986). Nurses should clarify their role in the child abuse investigation process. Some experts suggest that health professionals limit the interview to the child's physical and mental health concerns and leave the topics of the family's social, legal, or other problems to the police or CPS personnel (Koop, 1988).

Children are given the opportunity to ask questions, but if they are reticent, they are never pressured into talking. Young children in particular lack the verbal skills to describe body parts adequately. These children may benefit from play situations that provide opportunities for disclosure, such as drawing or using puppets or anatomically correct dolls and doll houses.

Considerable controversy exists regarding the use of children's ***drawings*** as diagnostic tests for sexual abuse. Two studies that investigated the type of human figure drawings made by allegedly sexually abused and by nonsexually abused children found that those in the abuse group included more details about genitalia than the other group (Hibbard and Hartman, 1990; Hibbard, Roghmann, and Hoekelman, 1987). In these studies it is not known if the interview process with the sexual abuse group influenced the subsequent drawings. Also, in one of these studies the difference between the groups was not statistically significant. The authors caution that the presence of genitalia on a human figure drawing does not prove sexual abuse; the children's description and explanation of the drawing are more relevant than its content. Genitalia on drawings may raise suspicion of abuse but are not diagnostic. The use of drawings as an assessment technique is not supported by scientific research (Conoley and Kramer, 1989; Wakefield and Underwager, 1989).

The controversy regarding the validity of ***anatomically correct dolls*** is of even more concern, because some professionals are using the dolls as diagnostic tools in the investigation of suspected sexual abuse. Research on the dolls' diagnostic value has yielded conflicting results. One study that examined the behavioral responses of abused and nonabused children found no difference between the groups playing with the dolls. The finding that the interviewer could easily influence the children to demonstrate sexual acts with the dolls was a special concern (McIver, Wakefield, and Underwager, 1989). Other researchers who observed only the behavior of nonabused children with the dolls have reported that many of these children's activities were similar to those described by professionals who use the dolls in sexual abuse investigations (Gabriel, 1985). Other studies, however, have shown that the frequency of sexual behavior with the dolls differs among sexually abused and nonsexually abused children. In one study significantly more children who had been sexually abused demonstrated sexual behavior in their play (Jampole and Weber, 1987). While it appears that the use of anatomically correct dolls is not diagnostic of sexual abuse, some professionals believe that the dolls help children communicate what happened and are a useful method of opening up communication, especially with young children (Leventhal and others, 1989). Others maintain that there is no way to use the dolls to obtain reliable evidence about past events (Wakefield and Underwager, 1989).

In interviewing the child, every effort is made to coordinate the number of interviewers and to assign a primary professional to work with the child. Videotaping or audiotaping can be used to limit the number of traumatic events (Wiseman and others, 1992). If nurses are not the primary professional, they can serve as the child's advocate to prevent excessive questioning and embarrassment by others.

Parental Behaviors. Certain behavioral responses of the parents to their child and to the interviewer should alert the nurse to the possibility of maltreatment. Although no one pattern of behaviors is characteristic of these parents, some responses include the following. Abusive parents have difficulty in showing concern toward their child. They are unable to comfort the child and give no indication of realizing how the child may feel, physically or emotionally. Instead they are critical of and angry with the child for being injured. They maintain that the child is responsible for the injury, and, if asked any question regarding their responsibility of protecting or supervising the child, they become hostile and aggressive. They act as if the child's injury is an assault on them. Their entire perception of the incident is in terms of how it affects them, not the child, which is an indication of their preoccupation with their own needs and of their inability to give any support to others.

During the child's hospitalization they may not become involved in the child's care and may show little concern for his or her progress, eventual discharge, or need for follow-up care. However, if they are pressured during interrogation, they immediately demand to take the child home, regardless of the child's readiness for discharge.

Families respond to sexual abuse with a wide variety of emotional reactions, which range from not believing the child to being very supportive. Parents and other family members may display the same type of emotional responses as the victim, such as inability to eat or sleep, and somatic complaints, such as headache. In the acute emotional phase parents have a need to blame someone. The three common targets are the offender, the child, and themselves. The parents commonly express anger at the child for "stupid" behavior and may even restrict the child's privileges as punishment. When the victim is a girl, the parents may question her sexual provocation of the event. Self-blaming parents assume full responsibility, believing that they have been inadequate parents or should not have allowed the child to go out. When a baby-sitter or trusted relative is involved in the assault and the child's complaint has not been believed until gross evidence is presented, the parents are often devastated by guilt.

Child Behaviors. Abused children's responses to their parents or the injury may also support the suspicion of abuse. Although no one pattern is typical, extremes of behavior may be observed. Children may be very unresponsive to the parent or excessively clinging and intolerant of separation. There may be overattachment to the abusive parent, possibly in the hope of preventing any upset that may precipitate anger and another attack. During care of the injury children may be passive and accepting of the discomfort or uncooperative and fearful of any physical contact. Some children maintain a wary watchfulness of all strangers; some shy away from strangers as if frightened; others are unusually affectionate and outgoing.

❖ Nursing Diagnoses

A number of nursing diagnoses are prominent in the nursing care of the maltreated child and family, and others specific to individual cases become evident. The most common nursing diagnoses are outlined in the Nursing Care Plan on pp. 711-712.

❖ Planning

The main goals related to the child who is maltreated and the family are as follows:

1. Child will be protected from further abuse.
2. Child and family will receive adequate support.
3. Hospitalized child and family, including foster parents if appropriate, will be prepared for discharge.
4. Child will not experience any maltreatment.

❖ Implementation

Interventions related to child maltreatment include immediate actions once a child is suspected of being abused, long-range care if the child is placed outside the home, and general strategies that may reduce the occurrence of abuse.

Protect Child from Further Abuse. Initially, identification of instances of suspected abuse or neglect is essential. The nurse may come in contact with abused children in an emergency room, practitioner's office, home, daycare center, or school.

NURSING ALERT The priority is to remove the child from the abusive situation to prevent further injury.

All states and provinces in North America have laws for mandatory reporting of child maltreatment. Suspected child abuse is reported to the local authorities.* Referrals usually come to the Bureau of Child Welfare and are assigned to a caseworker in an agency such as the Child Protective Services (CPS). Once a referral has been made, a caseworker is assigned to investigate the report. Based on the findings, the child is left in the home or temporarily removed.

A court proceeding may be necessary before the child can be placed outside the home or when parental rights are to be terminated. When the courts are involved, they usually require firsthand testimony by the referring parties. Nurses may be subpoenaed to appear in court, or their

*Telephone numbers are usually listed under "Child Abuse" in the business white pages of the local directory, or call the emergency child abuse hotline: (800) 422-4453 ([800] 4-A-CHILD).

GUIDELINES
Recording Assessment Data in Suspected Abuse

HISTORY OF INJURY

1. Date, time, and place of occurrence
2. Sequence of events with recorded times
3. Presence of witnesses, especially person caring for child at time of incident
4. Time lapse between occurrence of injury and initiation of treatment
5. Interview with child when appropriate, including verbal quotations and information from drawing or other play activities
6. Interview with parent, witnesses, or other significant persons, including verbal quotations
7. Description of parent-child interactions (verbal interactions, eye contact, touching, parental concern)
8. Name, age, and condition of other children in home (if possible)

PHYSICAL EXAMINATION

1. Location, size, shape, and color of bruises; approximate location, size, and shape on drawing of body outline
2. Distinguishing characteristics, such as a bruise in the shape of a hand; round burn (possibly caused by cigarette)
3. Symmetry or asymmetry of injury; presence of other injuries
4. Degree of pain; any bone tenderness
5. Evidence of past injuries; general state of health and hygiene
6. Developmental level of child; perform screening test (see Developmental Assessment, Chapter 7)

notes may be introduced as evidence in court hearings. Accurate and factual documentation is essential. A suggested outline for recording pertinent assessment data is presented in the Guidelines box. Behaviors are described, not interpreted, and are recorded daily to establish a progress record. Conversations between the nurse, child, and parent are recorded verbatim as much as possible.

Support Child. Frequently children suspected of abuse are hospitalized for medical management of their injuries. When the sexually abused child has been physically harmed, the care is consistent with that provided a rape victim (see Chapter 20). Regardless of the type of abuse, their needs are the same as those of any hospitalized child. The child should be treated as a child with the usual physical needs, developmental tasks, and play interests—not as a dramatic victim of abuse. The nurse is the child's advocate in this goal. The nurse also encourages the child's relationship with the parents. The nurse does not become a substitute parent to the exclusion of the child's natural parents. Such an intent only intensifies the parents' feelings of inadequacy, worthlessness, and isolation. It in no way helps them understand their child or promotes their trust in health professionals. The goal of the nurse-child relationship is to provide a role model for the parents in helping them to relate positively and constructively to their child and to foster a therapeutic environment for the child in his or her reprieve from the abusing situation.

Support Family. One of the most difficult, yet essential, components of success with abusive parents is the quality of the ***therapeutic relationship.*** It must be one of genuine concern and treatment, not one of accusation and punishment. Nurses must examine their personal feelings toward these parents, particularly when sexual abuse is present. A therapeutic approach is to view the parent as the patient and the child as the victim of abuse. Unless the nurse's attitude is positive, abusive parents will not be motivated to change, since they will not be working with a trusting person who demonstrates the kind of behavior that is being asked of them.

When parental ignorance of childrearing practices has played a part in the abuse, the nurse can educate the parent regarding ***children's physical and emotional needs.*** Because of the parents' own childrearing, they may not be aware of nonviolent methods of discipline, such as time-out or consequences. They may also need help in dealing with their frustration so that they do not vent anger on the child. Since these parents may be sensitive to criticism or domination and already possess a very low self-esteem, teaching is implemented through demonstration and example rather than through lecturing. Any competent parenting abilities they demonstrate are praised to promote their sense of parental adequacy.

Care of the family also depends on the circumstances of the ***sexual abuse.*** With a nonparent offender the family may be more able to support the child than if incest were involved. Family members are encouraged to express their feelings of anger, guilt, shame, and/or embarrassment but are also cautioned to avoid displacing such feelings on the child. For example, it is easy for parents to admonish the child with a statement such as "We told you never to go with strangers," which makes the child feel responsible.

Family members are advised to encourage the child to resume normal activities and to observe the child for signs of distress (see Posttraumatic Stress Disorder, Chapter 18). Children express their feelings primarily through behavior. Parents should be alert for changes in behavior that indicate distress resulting from the incident, such as remaining in the house, refusing to go to school, changes in sleeping patterns, and frequency of dreams and nightmares. Children are encouraged to talk about these feelings and nightmares, since the more they can talk about the experience, the more they are able to gain control over it.

Referral to appropriate agencies is also essential. Most abusive parents tend to live in poverty, and the daily stresses imposed by their life-style are overwhelming. Resources for financial aid, improved housing, and child care should be sought. Self-help groups also provide important services. Such groups as **Parents Anonymous*** (a group for parents who have abused or fear that they may abuse their child, but only in terms of physical abuse, not sexual abuse) and **Parents United International, Inc.**† (a group devoted to helping sexually abused families) are very accepting and nonjudgmental, because everyone has been in the same position.

There is no way to predict which families will be successfully rehabilitated. With father-daughter incest, however, the best results occur when the father accepts full responsibility for the act, the mother acknowledges her role in failing to protect the child, and the child is able to understand and forgive the parents and develop a positive self-image despite the traumatic experience.

Plan for Discharge. Discharge planning should begin as soon as the legal disposition for placement has been decided, which may be temporary foster home placement, return to the parents, or permanent termination of parental rights. The latter is the most drastic solution, but it is necessary in situations of repeated, life-threatening abuse. Whenever children are remanded to a foster home or juvenile institution, they must be allowed an opportunity to express their feelings. No matter how severe the abuse, they usually mourn the loss of their parents. They need help to understand why they must not return home and that this new home is in no way a punishment. Whenever possible, foster parents are encouraged to visit in the hospital, and the nurse should take an active role in helping them understand the child. It is unfortunate that some abused children live in torment as they are sent from one foster home to another, sometimes enduring worse circumstances than those that existed in their original home. Only through constant evaluation of the placement residence and the child's adjustment to a new environment can the vicious circle of abuse, abandonment, and neglect be stopped.

---

*520 S. Lafayette, Park Plaza, Suite 316, Los Angeles, CA 90057; (800) 421-0353.

†P.O. Box 952, San Jose, CA 95108; (408) 453-7616.

Prevent Abuse. Prevention of child maltreatment has been an extremely difficult goal. Programs aimed at identifying potential abusers and instituting supportive intervention before the occurrence of an abusive act have met with variable success. However, nurses have played an important role in such programs. For example, prenatal and infancy home visiting by nurses to primiparas who were either teenagers, unmarried, or of low socioeconomic status resulted in significantly fewer reports of child abuse during the first 2 years (Olds and others, 1986) but a less favorable impact on child abuse during the next 2 years (Olds, Henderson, and Kitzman, 1994). Other community prevention programs have also had disappointing results (Brayden and others, 1993b). The nurses provided information on normal child growth and development and routine health care needs, served as informal support persons, and referred families to appropriate services when a need for assistance was identified.

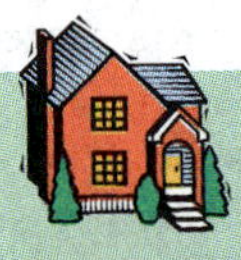

FAMILY HOME CARE
Preventing or Dealing with Sexual Abuse of Children

Sexual assault of children is much more common than most people realize. It may be preventable if children have good preparation. *To provide protection and preparation:*

- Pay careful attention to who is around children. (Unwanted touch *may* come from someone liked and trusted.)
- Back up a child's right to say "no."
- Encourage communication by taking seriously what children say.
- Take a second look at signals of potential danger.
- Refuse to leave children in the company of those not trusted.
- Include information about sexual assault when teaching about safety.
- Provide specific definitions and examples of sexual assault.
- Remind children that even "nice" people sometimes do mean things.
- Urge children to tell about *anybody* who causes them to be uncomfortable.
- Prepare children to deal with bribes and threats, as well as possible physical force.
- Virtually eliminate secrets between children and parents.
- Teach children how to say "no," ask for help, and control who touches them and how.
- Model self-protective and limit-setting behavior for children.

Should it ever become necessary to *help a child recover from a sexual assault:*

- Listen carefully to understand children.
- Support the child for telling by praise, belief, sympathy, and lack of blame.
- Know local resources and choose help carefully.
- Provide opportunities to talk about the assault.
- Provide opportunities for the entire family to go through a recovery process.

Sexual assault affects everyone. *To help deal with this social problem:*

- Provide sympathetic care and support to those who have been victimized.
- Recognize that offenders do not change without intervention.
- Organize neighborhood programs to support each other's efforts to protect children.
- Encourage schools to provide information about sexual assault as a problem of health and safety.
- Organize community groups to support educational treatment, and law enforcement programs.

Modified from Adams C, Fay J: *No more secrets: protecting your child from sexual assault,* San Luis Obispo, CA, 1981, Impact.

Such programs provide models that can be used to reduce factors known to increase the risk of abuse. However, nurses in a variety of settings can implement similar activities. Nurses in prenatal clinics can prepare expectant families for the adjustment of parenthood. Nursery and postpartum nurses can foster the attachment process by encouraging parents to hold and look at their infant. In neonatal intensive care units nurses can minimize the effects of separation by encouraging parents to visit and can help them become comfortable in the child's care. Those in ambulatory settings can teach parents appropriate methods of bathing, feeding, toileting, disciplining, and preventing injuries, while stressing the normal needs and developmental characteristics of children. Nurses need to be sensitive to the parents' needs for attention, reassurance, and reinforcement. Nurses need to know what kinds of community services are available, including self-help groups, and make timely referrals.

Unlike preventive efforts for neglect and physical abuse, which have been aimed at the potential offender, ***prevention of child sexual abuse*** has centered on education of children to protect themselves. Currently there is much controversy regarding the effectiveness of these programs. The main issue is whether young children should be expected to participate in their own protection. Some experts suggest that in the struggle between sexual offender and potential child victim, most factors favor the adult, who has superior knowledge, strength, and skill to overcome most children's efforts at self-protection (Conte, Wolf, and Smith, 1989). Clearly, sexual abuse prevention is more than teaching children to say "no" or to recognize their right not to be touched in "private places." It is equally important to teach children safety in terms of potential risk situations. Several suggestions for parents regarding protecting and educating children against possible molestation are presented in the Family Home Care box.

The nurse is frequently in a position to discuss this topic with parents as part of health maintenance and to provide guidelines. Books are available for parents that describe sexual abuse and its prevention.* Helpful games such as "What if the baby-sitter wants to wrestle and hug but tells you to keep it a secret?" can be used to explore dangerous situations in advance and help children learn the impor-

*Sources of information are the **National Committee for Prevention of Child Abuse,** Publishing Department, 332 S. Michigan Ave., Suite 1600, Chicago, IL 60604-4357, (312) 663-3520; **C. Henry Kempe National Center for the Prevention and Treatment of Child Abuse and Neglect,** 1205 Oneida St., Denver, CO 80220, (303) 321-3963; **American Association for Protecting Children, American Humane Association,** 63 Inverness Dr., E., Englewood, CO 80112, (800) 227-5242 (outside Colorado) or (303) 792-9900; and **National Resource Center on Child Sexual Abuse,** 107 Lincoln St., Huntsville, AL 35801, (800) 543-7006.

NURSING CARE PLAN
The Child Who Is Maltreated

NURSING DIAGNOSIS: High risk for trauma related to characteristics of child, caregiver(s), environment

PATIENT GOAL 1: Will experience no further abuse or neglect

- **NURSING INTERVENTIONS/*RATIONALES***

Implement measures *to prevent abuse:*
- Report suspicions to appropriate authorities
- Assist in removing child from unsafe environment and establishing in a safe environment
- Establish protective measures for the hospitalized child as indicated *to prevent continued abuse in hospital*

Refer family to social agencies for assistance with finances, food, clothing, housing, and health care *to help prevent neglect*

Keep factual, objective records *for documentation,* including:
- Child's physical condition
- Child's behavioral response to parents, others, and environment
- Interviews with family members

Collaborate efforts of multidisciplinary team *to continually evaluate progress of child in foster home or in return to own family*

Be alert for signs of continued abuse or neglect

Help parents identify those circumstances that precipitate an abusive act and alternative ways to deal with the release of anger other than attacking child

Refer for alternative placement when indicated *to prevent further injury or neglect*

- **EXPECTED OUTCOME**

Child experiences no further injury or neglect

NURSING DIAGNOSIS: Fear/anxiety related to negative interpersonal interaction, repeated maltreatment, powerlessness, potential loss of parents

PATIENT GOAL 1: Will experience reduction or relief of anxiety and stress

- **NURSING INTERVENTIONS/*RATIONALES***

Provide consistent caregiver and therapeutic environment during hospitalization *in order to relieve child's stress and to be a role model for family*

Demonstrate acceptance of child while not expecting same in return

Show attention while not reinforcing inappropriate behavior, *since all children have this need*

Plan appropriate activities for attention with nurse, other adults, and other children; use play *to work through relationships*

Praise child's abilities *in order to promote self-esteem*

Treat child as one who has a specific physical problem for hospitalization, not as "abused" victim

Avoid asking too many questions, *since this can upset child and interfere with other professionals' interrogations*

- Use play, especially family or dollhouse activity, *to investigate type of relationships perceived by child*
- Provide one consistent person to whom child relates regarding events of abuse *so that child is not overwhelmed*
- Help child grieve for loss of parents if their rights are terminated *because child may be very attached to parents despite abuse*

Encourage child to talk about feelings toward parents and future placement *to facilitate coping*

Encourage introduction to foster parents before placement if possible *to give child time to adjust*

- **EXPECTED OUTCOMES**

Child exhibits minimal or no evidence of distress
Child engages in positive relationships with caregivers
Child grieves for loss of parent

NURSING DIAGNOSIS: Altered parenting related to child, caregiver, or situational characteristics that precipitate abusive behavior

PATIENT (FAMILY) GOAL 1: Will exhibit evidence of positive interaction with children

- **NURSING INTERVENTIONS/*RATIONALES***

Identify families at risk for potential abuse *so that appropriate intervention is instituted*

Promote parental attachment to child, *since all children have this need*

Emphasize childrearing practices, especially effective methods of discipline, *since parents may lack knowledge about nonviolent discipline methods*

Increase parents' feeling of adequacy and self-esteem

Encourage support systems *that lessen stress and total responsibility of child care on one or both parents*

Teach children to recognize situations that place them at risk for sexual abuse and teach assertive responses *to discourage abuse*

- **EXPECTED OUTCOME**

Families exhibit evidence of positive interaction with children

PATIENT (FAMILY) GOAL 2: Will receive adequate support

- **NURSING INTERVENTIONS/*RATIONALES***

Provide "mothering" by directing attention to parent, taking over child care responsibilities until parent feels ready to participate, and focusing on parent's needs *so that parents can eventually meet child's needs*

Convey an attitude of genuine concern, not one of accusation and punishment, *since this only serves to further alienate family*

Refer parents to special support groups and/or counseling *for long-term support*

Help identify a support group for parents, such as extended family or nearby neighbors; help these significant others understand their important role in also preventing further abuse

Continued.

NURSING CARE PLAN
The Child Who Is Maltreated—cont'd

Refer to social agencies that can provide assistance in areas such as financial support, adequate housing, and employment

• **EXPECTED OUTCOMES**

Parents demonstrate appropriate parenting activities
Parents seek group and individual support
Parents receive assistance with problems

PATIENT (FAMILY) GOAL 3: Will exhibit knowledge of normal growth and development

• **NURSING INTERVENTIONS/*RATIONALES***

Teach realistic expectations of child's behavior and capabilities

Emphasize alternate methods of discipline, such as reward, time-out, consequences, and verbal disapproval, *so that parents learn nonviolent discipline methods*

Suggest methods of handling developmental problems or goals, such as toddler negativism, toilet training, and independence, *since these situations may precipitate abuse*

Teach through demonstration and role modeling, rather than lecture; avoid authoritarian approach, *since family may be sensitive to criticism or domination and lack self-esteem*

• **EXPECTED OUTCOME**

Parents demonstrate an understanding of normal expectations for their child

tance of saying "no." They need reassurance that no matter what the other person says or does, the parents want to know about it and will not punish them. Even if children do participate in the activity before telling the parents, they must be reassured that it was not their fault.

In addition, parents need to be made aware that "nice" people, including friends and relatives, can be offenders; parents should carefully observe how others act toward the child. A sudden change in the child's behavior and a response such as "I don't like Uncle anymore" are clues to investigate the relationship. In the event of any doubt, further solitary encounters with this person and the child should be prevented. It is sometimes to the child's great misfortune that parents do not take certain comments seriously, such as "He hugs me too tight" or "I don't want to go with him." Casual parental statements such as "He just loves you" or "You do whatever adults tell you to do" can place children in jeopardy. Health professionals can alert parents to such dangers and guide them toward an appreciation of the problem, providing concrete guidelines toward child education and protection. (See also Family Home Care box on p. 710.)

❖ EVALUATION

The effectiveness of nursing interventions is determined by continual reassessment and evaluation of care based on the following observational guidelines and expected outcomes:

1. Observe child for additional physical and behavioral evidence of abuse; observe child's reactions to health professionals; if child is hospitalized, check staffing patterns for schedule of consistent group of nurses caring for child.
2. Interview parents regarding their knowledge of children's physical and development needs.
3. Interview child regarding feelings about returning home or placement outside the home.
4. Investigate community programs aimed at preventing child maltreatment.

Expected outcomes:
See Nursing Care Plan, pp. 711-712.

KEY POINTS

- Common disorders during early childhood include communicable diseases, intestinal parasitic infections, conjunctivitis, and stomatitis.
- Nursing goals in the treatment of a communicable disease are identification, provision of comfort, prevention of spread to others, and prevention of complications.
- Intestinal parasitic diseases constitute the most common infections in the world; giardiasis and enterobiasis are the most widespread parasitic infections among children in the United States.
- Although the incidence of poisoning has decreased in the last 30 years as a result of more stringent packaging regulations, childhood poisoning remains a serious health concern.
- The most common accidentally ingested medications are analgesics (acetaminophen and ibuprofen) and cough/cold preparations.
- The major principles of emergency treatment for poisoning are assessment, supportive measures, gastric decontamination, family support, and prevention of recurrence.
- Ipecac is an effective and safe emetic for home use in poisonings but is being used less often. Activated charcoal and gastric lavage are common treatments for many toxic ingestions.
- Parents can reduce the severity of a poisoning by knowing the telephone number of the Poison Control Center, having ipecac in the home (two doses per child), and administering it correctly if prescribed.
- Potential sources of heavy metal poisoning in children are lead, iron, and mercury.
- The most important factor contributing to lead absorption is its availability in the child's environment. Lead-based paint is the most toxic source of lead.
- With increasing awareness of the detrimental effects of low levels of lead on the developing nervous system, acceptable blood lead levels have been decreasing and are now at <10 μg/dl.
- Child maltreatment may take the form of physical abuse or neglect, emotional abuse or neglect, or sexual abuse.

- Parental, child, and environmental characteristics are criteria that may predispose children to maltreatment.
- Identification of abuse entails securing evidence of maltreatment, taking a history pertaining to the incident, and assessing parental and child behaviors.

- The reported incidence of sexual abuse has increased in the last decade; common forms are incest, molestation, rape, exhibitionism, child pornography, child prostitution, and pedophilia.

REFERENCES

Adams J, Horton M: Is it sexual abuse? Confusion caused by a congenital anomaly of the genitalia, *Clin Pediatr* 28(3):146-148, 1989.

Aiken MM: Documenting sexual abuse in prepubertal girls, *MCN* 15:176-177, 1990.

Altemeier WA III and others: Antecedents of child abuse, *J Pediatr* 100(5):823-829, 1982.

American Academy of Pediatrics, Committee on Child Abuse and Neglect: Guidelines for the evaluation of sexual abuse of children, *Pediatrics* 87(2):254-260, 1991.

American Academy of Pediatrics, Committee on Child Abuse and Neglect: Shaken baby syndrome—inflicted cerebral trauma, *Pediatrics* 92(2):872-873, 1993a.

American Academy of Pediatrics, Committee on Environmental Health: Lead poisoning: from screening to primary prevention, *Pediatrics* 92(1):176-183, 1993b.

American Academy of Pediatrics, Committee on Infectious Diseases: The use of oral acyclovir in otherwise healthy children with varicella, *Pediatrics* 91(3):674-676, 1993c.

American Academy of Pediatrics, Committee on Infectious Diseases: Vitamin A treatment of measles, *Pediatrics* 91(5):1014-1015, 1993d.

American Academy of Pediatrics, Committee on Infectious Diseases: *1994 Red Book: report of the Committee on Infectious Diseases,* ed 23, Elk Grove Village, IL, 1994, The Academy.

Amitai Y and others: Hazards of "deleading" homes of children with lead poisoning, *Am J Dis Child* 141(7):758-760, 1987.

Baghurst PA and others: Environmental exposure to lead and children's intelligence at the age of seven years, *N Engl J Med* 327(18):1279-1284, 1992.

Baker RB: Seat belt injury masquerading as sexual abuse, *Pediatrics* 77(3):435, 1986.

Bartlett AV and others: Controlled trial of *Giardia lamblia:* control strategies in day care centers, *Am J Public Health* 81(6):1001-1006, 1991.

Bellinger DC, Stiles KM, Needleman HL: Low-level lead exposure, intelligence and academic achievement: a long-term follow-up study, *Pediatrics* 90(6):855-861, 1992.

Berenson AB, Somma-Garcia A, Barnett S: Perianal findings in infants 18 months of age or younger, *Pediatrics* 91(4):838-840, 1993.

Besharov DJ: "Doing something" about child abuse: the need to narrow the grounds for state intervention, *Harvard J Law Public Policy* 8(3):539-589, 1985.

Bithoney WG and others: Childhood ingestions as symptoms of family distress, *Am J Dis Child* 139(3):456-459, 1985.

Boehnert MT and others: Advances in clinical toxicology, *Pediatr Clin North Am* 32(1):193-211, 1985.

Brayden RM and others: Behavioral antecedents of pediatric poisonings, *Clin Pediatr* 32(1):30-35, 1993a.

Brayden RM and others: A prospective study of secondary prevention of child maltreatment, *J Pediatr* 122(4):511-516, 1993b.

Cantwell HB: Vaginal inspection as it relates to child sexual abuse in girls under thirteen, *Child Abuse Negl* 7:171-176, 1983.

Centers for Disease Control: *Preventing lead poisoning in young children,* Atlanta, GA, 1991, Centers for Disease Control.

Cheng TC: *General parasitology,* Orlando, FL, 1986, Academic Press, College Division.

Clark M, Royal J, Seeler R: Interaction of iron deficiency and lead and the hematologic findings in children with severe lead poisoning, *Pediatrics* 81(2):247-254, 1988.

Cohen BA, Honig P, Androphy E: Anogenital warts in children, *Arch Dermatol* 126:1575-1580, 1990.

Coleman L: Creating "memories" of sexual abuse, *Issues Child Abuse Accus* 4(4):169-176, 1992.

Conoley JC, Kramer JJ, editors: *Tenth mental measurements yearbook,* Lincoln, NB, 1989, University of Nebraska Press.

Conte J, Wolf S, Smith T: What sexual offenders tell us about prevention strategies, *Child Abuse Negl* 13:293-301, 1989.

Council on Scientific Affairs: AMA diagnostic and treatment guidelines concerning child abuse and neglect, *JAMA* 254(6):796-800, 1985.

Daro D, McCurdy K: *Current trends in child abuse reporting and fatalities: results of the 1991 annual 50 state survey,* Chicago, 1992, National Committee for Prevention of Child Abuse.

De Jong A, Rose M: Frequency and significance of physical evidence in legally proven cases of child sexual abuse, *Pediatrics* 84(6):1022-1026, 1989.

Dennehy PH: Should oral acyclovir be used to treat chickenpox in normal children? *Contemp Pediatr* 10(3):31-48, 1993.

Dietrich KN, Berger OG, Succop PA: Lead exposure and the motor developmental status of urban six-year-old children in the Cincinnati prospective study, *Pediatrics* 91(2):301-307, 1993.

Donnenfeld ED, Kaufman HE, Schwab IR: Conjunctivitis: update on diagnosis and treatment, *Patient Care* 27:22-46, 1993.

Doran T and others: Acetaminophen: more harm than good for chickenpox? *J Pediatr* 114(6):1045-1048, 1989.

Douidar SM, Al-Khalil I, Habersang RW: Severe hepatotoxicity, acute renal failure, and pancytopenia in a young child after repeated acetaminophen overdosing, *Clin Pediatr* 33(1):42-45, 1994.

Emans S and others: Genital findings in sexually abused symptomatic and asymptomatic girls, *Pediatrics* 79(5):778-785, 1987.

Farrington E: Acyclovir in the treatment of chickenpox, *Pediatr Nurs* 18(5):499-503, 1992.

Feinauer LL: Comparison of long-term effects of child abuse by type of abuse and by relationship of the offender to the victim, *Am J Fam Ther* 17:48-56, 1989.

Feldman W and others: Is childhood sexual abuse really increasing in prevalence? An analysis of the evidence, *Pediatrics* 88(1):29-33, 1991.

Frechette A, Rimsza ME: Stun gun injury: a new presentation of the battered child syndrome, *Pediatrics* 89(5):898-901, 1992.

Gabriel R: Anatomically correct dolls in the diagnosis of sexual abuse of children, *J Melanie Klein Soc* 3:40-51, 1985.

Garbarino J, Guttmann E, Seeley J: *The psychologically battered child,* San Francisco, 1986, Jossey-Bass, Inc., Publishers.

Gardner RA: Belated realization of child sex abuse by an adult, *Issues Child Abuse Accus* 4(4):177-195, 1992.

Gardner RA: Medical findings and child sexual abuse, *Issues Child Abuse Accus* 5(1):12-23, 1993.

Gellert GA and others: Situational and sociodemographic characteristics of children infected with human immunodeficiency virus from pediatric sexual abuse, *Pediatrics* 91(1):39-44, 1993.

Gilbert CM: Sibling incest: a descriptive study of family dynamics, *J Child Adolesc Psychiatr Ment Health Nurs* 5(1):5-9, 1992.

Glasziou PP, Mackerras DEM: Vitamin A supplementation in infectious diseases: a meta-analysis, *Br Med J* 306(6874):366-370, 1993.

Goebel J, Gremse DA, Artman M: Cardiomyopathy from ipecac administration in Munchausen syndrome by proxy, *Pediatrics* 92:601-603, 1993.

Goetting MG, Sowa B: Retinal hemorrhage after cardiopulmonary resuscitation in children: an etiologic reevaluation, *Pediatrics* 85(4):585-588, 1990.

Gordon B, Schroeder C, Abrams M: Children's knowledge of sexuality: a comparison of sexually abused and nonabused children, *Am J Orthopsychiatry* 60(2):250-257, 1990.

Gowda N and others: Human parvovirus infection in patients with sickle cell disease with and without hypoplastic crisis, *J Pediatr* 110(1):81-84, 1987.

Guandolo VL: Munchausen syndrome by proxy: an outpatient challenge, *Pediatrics* 75(3):526-530, 1985.

Gutman LT, Herman-Giddens ME, Phelps WC: Transmission of human genital papillomavirus disease: comparison of data from adults and children, *Pediatrics* 91(1):31-38, 1993.

Hanson R and others: Anogenital warts in childhood, *Child Abuse Negl* 13:225-233, 1989.

Harvey B: Should blood lead screening recommendations be revised? *Pediatrics* 93:201-204, 1994.

Hayes EB and others: Long-term trends in blood lead levels among children in Chicago: relationship to air lead levels, *Pediatrics* 93:195-200, 1994.

Henretig F and others: Repeated acetaminophen overdosing causing hepatotoxicity in children, *Clin Pediatr* 28(11):525-528, 1989.

Hibbard R, Hartman G: Genitalia in human figure drawings: childrearing practices and child sexual abuse, *J Pediatr* 116(5):822-828, 1990.

Hibbard R, Roghmann K, Hoekelman R: Genitalia in children's drawings: an association with sexual abuse, *Pediatrics* 79(1):129-136, 1987.

Highlights of official child neglect and abuse reporting 1986, Denver, 1988, The American Humane Association.

Hill DR: Giardiasis: issues in diagnosis and management, *Infect Dis Clin North Am* 7(3):503-525, 1993.

Hobbs C, Wynne J: Sexual abuse of English boys and girls: the importance of anal examination, *Child Abuse Negl* 13:195-210, 1989.

Hobbs C, Wynne J: The sexually abused battered child, *Arch Dis Child* 65(4):423-427, 1990.

Hoffman R: Choices in gastric decontamination, *Emerg Med* 24(10)212-224, 1992.

Huseman CA, Varma MM, Angle CR: Neuroendocrine effects of toxic and low blood lead levels in children, *Pediatrics* 90(2):186-189, 1992.

Jampole L, Weber M: An assessment of the behavior of sexually abused and non-sexually abused children with anatomically correct dolls, *Child Abuse Negl* 11:187-192, 1987.

Jean-Gilles M, Crittenden P: Maltreating families: a look at siblings, *Fam Relations* 39(3):232-329, 1990.

Jones KL and others: Offspring of women infected with varicella during pregnancy: a prospective study, *Teratology* 49(1):29-32, 1994.

Jones VF and others: The role of the male caretaker in Munchausen syndrome by proxy, *Clin Pediatr* 32:245-247, 1993.

Kempe CH and others: The battered child syndrome, *JAMA* 181:17-24, 1962.

Klein-Schwartz W and others: The effect of milk on ipecac-induced emesis, *J Toxicol Clin Toxicol* 29(4):505-511, 1991.

Koblenzer PJ: Dermatologic conditions misdiagnosed as evidence of child abuse *JAMA* 261(24):3547-3548, 1989 (letter).

Kondo K and others: Association of human herpesvirus-6 infection of the central nervous system with recurrence of febrile convulsions, *J Infect Dis* 167(5):1197-1200, 1993.

Koop CE: *The surgeon general's letter on child sexual abuse,* Rockville, MD, 1988, US Dept of Health and Human Services, Public Health Service, Health Resources and Services Administration, Bureau of Maternal and Child Health and Resources Development, Office of Maternal and Child Health.

Kotelchuck M: Child abuse and neglect: prediction and misclassification. In Starr RH, editor: *Child abuse prediction policy implications,* Cambridge, MA, 1982, Ballinger.

Krowchuk H: Child abuser stereotypes: consensus among clinicians, *Appl Nurs Res* 2(1):35-39, 1989.

Krugman R: Advances and retreats in the protection of children, *N Engl J Med* 320(8):531-532, 1989a.

Krugman R: New light on a dark area: an update on child abuse and neglect, *Curr Opin Pediatr* 1(1):168-171, 1989b.

Laraque D and others: Blood lead, calcium status, and behavior in preschool children, *Am J Dis Child* 144(2):186-189, 1990.

Legrand R, Wakefield H, Underwager R: Alleged behavioral indicators of sexual abuse, *Issues Child Abuse Accus* 1(2):1-5, 1989.

Leventhal J and others: Anatomically correct dolls used in interviews of young children suspected of having been sexually abused, *Pediatrics* 84(5):900-906, 1989.

Liebelt EL, Shannon MW: Small doses, big problems: a selected review of highly toxic common medications, *Pediatr Emerg Care* 9(5):292-297, 1993.

Litovitz T and others: 1992 annual report of the American Association of Poison Control Centers Toxic Exposure Surveillance System, *Am J Emerg Med* 11(5):494-555, 1993.

Mack R: Mercury—a true healer, a wicked murderer, *Contemp Pediatr* 6(8):139-148, 1989.

Marshall G and others: Syndrome of periodic fever, pharyngitis, and aphthous stomatitis, *J Pediatr* 110(1):43-46, 1987.

McCann J, Voris J: Perianal injuries resulting from sexual abuse: a longitudinal study, *Pediatrics* 91(2):390-397, 1993.

McCann J and others: Perianal findings in prepubertal children selected for nonabuse: a descriptive study, *Child Abuse Negl* 13:179-193, 1989.

McCann J and others: Comparison of genital examination techniques in prepubertal girls, *Pediatrics* 85(2):182-187, 1990a.

McCann J and others: Genital findings in prepubertal girls selected for nonabuse: a descriptive study, *Pediatrics* 86(3):428-439, 1990b.

McClain PW and others: Estimates of fatal child abuse and neglect, United States, 1979 through 1988, *Pediatrics* 91(2):338-343, 1993.

McClain PW and others: Geographic patterns of fatal abuse or neglect in children younger than 5 years old, United States, 1979 to 1988, *Arch Pediatr Adolesc Med* 148:82-86, 1994.

McClung HJ and others: Intentional ipecac poisoning in children, *Am J Dis Child* 142(6):637-639, 1988.

McCord M, Okun A: Toxicity of sorbitol-charcoal suspension, *J Pediatr* 111(2):307-308, 1987.

McDonald RE, Avery DR: *Dentistry for the child and adolescent,* ed 6, St Louis, 1994, Mosby.

McGuire T, Feldman K: Psychologic morbidity of children subjected to Munchausen syndrome by proxy, *Pediatrics* 83(2):289-292, 1989.

McIver W, Wakefield H, Underwager R: Behavior of abused and non-abused children in interviews with anatomically correct dolls, *Issues Child Abuse Accus* 1(1):39-48, 1989.

McKibben L, DeVos E, Newberger E: Victimization of mothers of abused children: a controlled study, *Pediatrics* 84(3):531-535, 1989.

McKnight JT, Tietze PE: Dermatologic manifestations of giardiasis, *J Am Board Fam Pract* 5(4):425-428, 1992.

Meadow R: Munchausen syndrome by proxy, *Br Med J* 299:248-250, 1989.

Mercury exposure from interior latex paint—Michigan, *MMWR* 39(8):125, 1990.

Myers J: Role of physician in preserving verbal evidence of child abuse, *J Pediatr* 109(3):409-411, 1986.

National Center on Child Abuse and Neglect: *Child abuse and neglect: a shared community concern,* Washington, DC, 1989, DHHS Pub No (OHDS) 89-30531.

National Center on Child Abuse and Neglect: *A coordinated response to child abuse and neglect: a basic manual,* Washington, DC, 1993, National Center.

Needleman HL: Why we should worry about lead poisoning, *Contemp Pediatr* 5(3):34-55, 1988.

Needleman H and others: The long-term effects of exposure to low doses of lead in childhood, *N Engl J Med* 322(2):83-88, 1990.

Nocton JJ and others: Human parvovirus-associated arthritis in children, *J Pediatr* 122(2):186-190, 1993.

Nordin JD, Rolnick SJ, Griffin JM: Prevalence of excess lead absorption and associated risk factors in children enrolled in a midwestern health maintenance organization, *Pediatrics* 93:172-177, 1994.

Novotny T and others: Prevalence of *Giardia lamblia* and risk factors for infection among children attending day-care facilities in Denver, *Public Health Rep* 105(1):72-75, 1990.

O'Connor ME: CaEDTA vs CaEDTA plus BAL to treat children with elevated blood lead levels, *Clin Pediatr* 31(7):386-390, 1992.

Olds DL, Henderson CR Jr, Kitzman H: Does prenatal and infancy nurse home visitation have enduring effects on qualities of parental caregiving and child health at 25 to 50 months of life? *Pediatrics* 93(1):89-98, 1994.

Olds DL, and others: Preventing child abuse and neglect: a randomized trial of nurse home visitation, *Pediatrics* 78(1):65-78, 1986.

Pillitteri A and others: Parent gender, victim gender, and family socioeconomic level influences on the potential reporting by nurses of physical child abuse, *Issues Compr Pediatr Nurs* 15:239-247, 1992.

Piomelli S: Childhood lead poisoning in the '90s, *Pediatrics* 93(4):508-510, 1994.

Radko K: Child abuse: guilty until proven innocent or legalized governmental child abuse, *Issues Child Abuse Accus* 5(2):96-101, 1993.

Rand DC: Munchausen syndrome by proxy as a possible factor when abuse is falsely alleged, Issues *Child Abuse Accus* 1(4):32-34, 1989.

Rey-Alvarez S, Menke-Hargrave T: Deleading dilemma: pitfall in the management of childhood lead poisoning, *Pediatrics* 79(2):214-217, 1987.

Rodgers GC Jr, Matyunas NJ: Gastrointestinal decontamination for acute poisoning, *Pediatr Clin North Am* 33(2):261-285, 1986.

Rodgers GC Jr, Tenenbein M: The role of adversive bittering agents in the prevention of pediatric poisonings, *Pediatrics* 93(1):68-69, 1994.

Ruff HA and others: Declining blood lead levels and cognitive changes in moderately lead-poisoned children, *JAMA* 269(13):1641-1646, 1993.

Sachs H, Moel D: Height and weight following lead poisoning in childhood, *Am J Dis Child* 143(7):820-822, 1989.

Salmon R and others: Factitious hematuria with underlying renal abnormalities, *Pediatrics* 82(3):377-379, 1988.

Sawyer MH and others: Detection of varicella-zoster virus DNA in air samples from hospital rooms, *J Infect Dis* 169(1):91-94, 1994.

Schmitt B, Gray J, Britton H: Car seat burns in

infants: avoiding confusion with inflicted burns, *Pediatrics* 62(4):607-609, 1978.
Schoen EJ: AAP lead-screening recommendation ill-advised, *AAP News* 9(11):14, 1993.
Schunk J, Svendsen D: Diphenhydramine toxicity from combined oral and topical use, *Am J Dis Child* 142(10):1020-1021, 1988.
Seidl AH and others: Nurses' attitudes toward the child victims and the perpetrators of emotional, physical, and sexual abuse, *Issues Child Abuse Accus* 5(1):28-38, 1993.
Shannon M: Subject in review: managing toxic ingestions, *Pediatr Alert* 18:125-126, 1993.
Shannon M, Graef J: Lead intoxication in infancy, *Pediatrics* 89(1):87-90, 1992.
Shukla R and others: Fetal and infant lead exposure: effects on growth in stature, *Pediatrics* 84(4):604-612, 1989.
Stier DM and others: Are children born to young mothers at increased risk of maltreatment? *Pediatrics* 91(3):642-648, 1993.
Straus SE: Shingles: sorrows, salves, and solutions, *JAMA* 269(14):1836-1839, 1993.
Sutphen JL, Saulsbury ST: Intentional ipecac poisoning: Munchausen syndrome by proxy, *Pediatrics* 82(3, pt 2):453-456, 1988.
Terada K and others: Varicella-zoster virus (VZV) reactivation is related to the low response of VZV-specific immunity after chickenpox in infancy, *J Infect Dis* 169:650-652, 1994.
Unintentional poisoning mortality—United States, 1980-1986, *MMWR* 38(10):153-157, 1989.
Vale JA, Proudfoot AT: How useful is activated charcoal? *Br Med J* 306(6870):78-79, 1993.
Vernberg K, Culver-Dickinson P, Spyker DA: The deterrent effect of poison-warning stickers, *Am J Dis Child* 138:1018-1020, 1984.
Wakefield H, Underwager R: Interrogation of children, *Issues Child Abuse Accus.* 1(1):14-28, 1989.
Wakefield H, Underwager R: Uncovering memories of alleged sexual abuse: the therapists who do it, *Issues Child Abuse Accus* 4(4):197-213, 1992.
Walterspiel JN and others: Secretory antigiardia lamblia antibodies in human milk: protective effect against diarrhea, *Pediatrics* 93(1):28-31, 1994.
Wasserman G and others: Independent effects of lead exposure and iron deficiency anemia on developmental outcome at age 2 years, *J Pediatr* 121(5):695-703, 1992.
White ST, Ingram DL, Lyna PR: Vaginal introital diameter in the evaluation of sexual abuse, *Child Abuse Negl* 13:217-224, 1989.
Widom CS: Does violence beget violence: a critical examination of the literature, *Psychol Bull* 106(1):3-28, 1989.
Wilde JA, Pedroni AT Jr: Privacy rights in Munchausen syndrome, *Contemp Pediatr* 10(1):83-91, 1993.
Wiseman MR and others: Reliability of videotaped interviews with children suspected of being sexually abused, *Br Med J* 304:1089-1091, 1992.
Wong DL: False allegations of child abuse: the other side of the tragedy, *Pediatr Nurs* 13(5):329-333, 1987.
Woolf AD, Saperstein A, Forjuoh S: Poisoning prevention knowledge and practices of parents after a childhood poisoning incident, *Pediatrics* 90(6):867-870, 1992.
Woolf AD and others: Prevention of childhood poisoning: efficacy of an educational program carried out in an emergency clinic, *Pediatrics* 80(3):359-363, 1987.
Yates A, Musty T: Preschool children's erroneous allegations of sexual molestation, *Am J Psychiatry* 145:989-992, 1988.

BIBLIOGRAPHY

Communicable Diseases

American Academy of Pediatrics, Committee on Infectious Diseases: Parvovirus, erythema infectiosum, and pregnancy, *Pediatrics* 85(1):131-133, 1990.
Asano Y and others: Clinical features of infants with primary human herpesvirus 6 infection (exanthem subitum, roseola infantum), *Pediatrics* 93(1):104-108, 1994.
Asano Y and others: Human herpesvirus type 6 infection (exanthem subitum) without fever, *J Pediatr* 115(2):264-268, 1989.
Bell LM and others: Human parvovirus B19 infection among hospital staff members after contact with infected patients, *N Engl J Med* 321(8):485-491, 1989.
Benenson AS, editor: *Control of communicable diseases in man,* ed 15, Washington, DC, 1990, American Public Health Association.
Chiriboga-Klein S and others: Growth in congenital rubella syndrome and correlation with clinical manifestations, *J Pediatr* 115(2):251-255, 1989.
Controversy about chickenpox, *Lancet* 340(8820):639-640, 1992.
Cromer BA and others: Unrecognized pertussis infection in adolescents, *Am J Dis Child* 147:575-577, 1993.
Dunkle LM and others: A controlled trial of acyclovir for chickenpox in normal children, *N Engl J Med* (325):1539-1544, 1991.
Gratz RR, Boulton P: Health considerations for pregnant child care staff, *J Pediatr Health Care* 8:18-26, 1994.
Gurevich I: Fifth disease and other parvovirus B 19 infections, *Heart Lung* 20(4):342-344, 1991.
Hussey G, Klein M: A randomized, controlled trial of vitamin A in children with severe measles, *N Engl J Med* 323(3):160-164, 1990.
Jones S, Jenista J: Fifth disease: role for nurses in pediatric practice, *Pediatr Nurs* 16(2):148-150, 1990.
Koch W and others: Manifestations and treatment of human parvovirus B19 infection in immunocompromised patients, *J Pediatr* 116(3):355-359, 1990.
Krugman S and others: *Infectious diseases of children,* ed 8, St Louis, 1985, Mosby.
Labson LH: Doctor, I can't stand this itching! *Patient Care* 18(17):89-121, 1984.
Madden EJ: Starting from scratch, *Am J Nurs* 86(7):846, 1986.
McGrath NE: Children with chickenpox: emergency department care and teaching, *J Emerg Nurs* 18(4):353, 1992.
Moffitt J, Feldman S: Chickenpox: new dangers, new therapies, *Contemp Pediatr* 8(11):13-32, 1991.
Moore DA, Hopkins RS: Immunization and infectious diseases, *Am J Epidemiol* 133:1161-1167, 1991.
Rasmussen JE: Recent advances in pediatric dermatology, *Curr Opin Pediatr* 1(1):57-60, 1989.
Relief for that persistent itch, *Patient Care* 18(17):185, 1984.
Risks associated with human parvovirus B19 infection, *MMWR* 38(6):18-20, 1989.
Second opinions: Drug company responds to acyclovir policy and the Committee responds, *AAP News* 9(2):19, 1993.
Suga S and others: Human herpesvirus-6 infection (exanthem subitum) without rash, *Pediatrics* 83(6):1003-1006, 1989.
Ware R: Human parvovirus infection, *J Pediatr* 114(3):343-348, 1989.
Ware R and others: Chronic immune-mediated thrombocytopenia after varicella infection, *J Pediatr* 112(5):742-744, 1988.
Weingarten CT, Gomberg SM: Measles: again an epidemic, *Pediatr Nurs* 18(4):369-384, 1992.

Conjunctivitis/Stomatitis

Bringing pinkeye under control, *Patient Care* 27:47-48, 1993.
Corey L: First-episode, recurrent, and asymptomatic herpes simplex infections, *J Am Acad Dermatol* 18(1, pt 2):169-172, 1988.
Dunlap C, Barker B, Lowe J: 10 oral lesions you should know, *Contemp Pediatr* 8(12):16-28, 1991.
Feldman A, Aretakis D: Herpetic gingivostomatitis in children, *Pediatr Nurs* 12(2):111-113, 1986.
Howes DS: The red eye, *Emerg Med Clin North Am* 6(1):43-56, 1988.
Kovalesky A: *Nurse's guide to children's eyes,* Orlando, FL, 1985, Grune & Stratton.
Lewis L, Glauser T, Joffie M: Gonococcal conjunctivitis in prepubertal children, *Am J Dis Child* 144(5):546-548, 1990.
Lohr JA and others: Comparison of three topical antimicrobials for acute bacterial conjunctivitis, *Pediatr Infect Dis J* 7(9):626-629, 1988.
Reed DB: Viral and bacterial conjunctivitis: prevention of disastrous results, *Postgrad Med* 86(4):103-114, 1989.
Schmitt BD: When your child has an eye infection with pus, *Contemp Pediatr* 10(3):117-118, 1993.
Scully C, Porter S: Recurrent aphthous stomatitis: current concepts of etiology, pathogenesis and management, *J Oral Pathol Med* 18(1):21-27, 1989.
Sheahan SL, Seabolt JP: *Chlamydia trachomatis* infections: a health problem of infants, *J Pediatr Health Care* 3(3):144-149, 1989.
Stanker P and others: Protocol—conjunctivitis, *Sch Nurse* 5(2):34-36, 1989.
Trobe JD: *The physician's guide to eye care,* San Francisco, 1993, American Academy of Ophthalmology.
Weiss A, Brinser JH, Nazar-Stewart V: Acute conjunctivitis in childhood, *J Pediatr* 122(1):10-14, 1993.

Intestinal Parasitic Diseases

Addiss DG, Juranek DD, Spencer HC: Treatment of children with asymptomatic and nondiarrheal *Giardia* infection, *Pediatr Infect Dis J* 10(11):843-846, 1991.

Birkhead G, Vogt R: Epidemiologic surveillance for endemic *Giardia lamblia* infection in Vermont, *Am J Epidemiol* 129(4):762-768, 1989.

Bundy DA and others: Evaluating measures to control intestinal parasitic infections, *World Health Stat Q* 45(2-3):168-179, 1992.

Glickman LT, Magnaval JF: Zoonotic roundworm infections, *Infect Dis Clin North Am* 7(3):717-732, 1993.

Greensmith C and others: Giardiasis associated with the use of a water slide, *Pediatr Infect Dis J* 7:91-94, 1988.

Hood C: *Enterobius vermicularis, Practitioner* 233(1466):503, 1989.

Hotez P: Hookworm disease in children, *Pediatr Infect Dis J* 8(8):516-520, 1989.

Jones JE: Pinworms, *Am Fam Physician* 38(3):159-164, 1988.

Katzman EM: What's the most common helminth infection in the U.S.? *MCN* 14(3):193-195, 1989.

Kubiak M and others: Comparison of stool containment in cloth and single-use diapers using a simulated infant feces, *Pediatrics* 91(3):632-636, 1993.

Kuhls TL: Protozoal infections of the intestinal tract in children, *Adv Pediatr Infect Dis* 8:177-202, 1993.

Pickering L, Engelkirk P: *Giardia lamblia, Pediatr Clin North Am* 35(3):565-577, 1988.

Rauch A and others: Longitudinal study of *Giardia lamblia* infection in a day care center population, *Pediatr Infect Dis J* 9(3):186-189, 1990.

Stehr-Green J and others: Intestinal parasites in pet store puppies in Atlanta, *Public Health Briefs* 77(3):345-346, 1987.

Thompson RC, Reynoldson JA, Mendis AH: Giardia and giardiasis, *Adv Parasitol* 32:71-160, 1993.

Ingestion of Injurious Agents

Birkland P: International update: alternative treatment for common but dangerous acetaminophen overdoses, *J Emerg Nurs* 19(2):32A-33A, 1993.

Edgerton PH: Symptoms of digitalis-like toxicity in a family after accidental ingestion of lily of the valley plant, *J Emerg Nurs* 15(3):220-223, 1989.

Edwards IR: Labelling toxic plants, *NZ Med J* 103(891):275, 1990.

Einhorn A and others: Serious respiratory consequences of detergent ingestions in children, *Pediatrics* 84(3):472-474, 1989.

Fine JS, Goldfrank LR: Update in medical toxicology, *Pediatr Emerg Med* 39(5):1031-1051, 1992.

Grbcich P and others: Effect of fluid volume on ipecac-induced emesis, *J Pediatr* 110(6):970-972, 1987.

Grbcich P and others: Effect of milk on ipecac-induced emesis, *J Pediatr* 110(6):973-975, 1987.

Henretig F and others: Repeated acetaminophen overdosing causing hepatotoxicity in children, *Clin Pediatr* 28(11):525-528, 1989.

Jaimovich DG: Transport management of the patient with acute poisoning, *Pediatr Clin North Am* 40(2):407-430, 1993.

Kulig K: Initial management of ingestions of toxic substances, *N Engl J Med* 326(25):1677-1681, 1992.

Kunkel DB: Plant poisoning in children, *Pediatr Ann* 16(11):927-932, 1987.

Kurt TL: The (internal) dangers of acrylic fingernails, *JAMA* 263(16):2181, 1990.

Lewis RK, Paloucek FP: Assessment and treatment of acetaminophen overdose, *Clin Pharm* 10:765-774, 1991.

Lovejoy FH Jr: Diagnosis of the unknown poison, *Pediatr Rev* 13(7):273-274, 1992.

Mack RB: Dishwasher detergent toxicity—here's looking at you, kid, *Contemp Pediatr* 10(11):49-58, 1993.

Manoguerra AS: Pediatric poisoning, *Emergency* 24(10):19-24, 1992.

Notarianni L: A reassessment of the treatment of salicylate poisoning, *Drug Safety* 7(4):292-303, 1992.

Palatnick W, Tenenbein M: Activated charcoal in the treatment of drug overdose: an update, *Drug Safety* 7(1):3-7, 1992.

Preventing strictures after caustic ingestion, *Emerg Med* 25(6):48, 1993.

Rumack BH: Acetaminophen overdose in children and adolescents, *Pediatr Clin North Am* 33(3):691-701, 1986.

Vertrees J, McWilliams B, Kelly H: Repeated oral administration of activated charcoal for treating aspirin overdose in young children, *Pediatrics* 85(4):594-598, 1990.

Wong D: Dispelling some myths about ipecac, *Am J Nurs* 88(7):952, 1988.

Heavy Metal Poisoning

Banner W Jr, Tong TG: Iron poisoning, *Pediatr Clin North Am* 33(2):393-409, 1986.

Berger O, Gregg D, Succop P: Using unstimulated urinary lead excretion to assess the need for chelation in the treatment of lead poisoning, *J Pediatr* 116(1):46-51, 1990.

Binder S: Childhood lead poisoning: the impact of prevention, *JAMA* 269(13):1679-1681, 1993.

Binns HJ and others: Is there lead in the suburbs? Risk assessment in Chicago suburban pediatric practices, *Pediatrics* 93(2):164-171, 1994.

Bithoney WG, Vandeven AM, Ryan A: Elevated lead levels in reportedly abused children, *J Pediatr* 122(5, pt 1):719-720, 1993.

Brown M, Bellinger D, Matthews J: In utero lead exposure, *MCN* 15(2):94-96, 1990.

Castiglia PT: Pica, *J Pediatr Health Care* 7(4):174-176, 1993.

Cummins SK, Goldman LR: Even advantaged children show cognitive deficits from low-level lead toxicity, *Pediatrics* 90(6):995-997, 1992.

DeRienzo-DeVivio S: Childhood lead poisoning: shifting to primary prevention, *Pediatr Nurs* 18(6):565-567, 1992.

Elemental mercury poisoning in a household—Ohio, 1989, *MMWR* 39(25):424-425, 1990.

Hudson P and others: Elemental mercury exposure among children of thermometer plant workers, *Pediatrics* 79(6):935-938, 1987.

Kimbrough RD, LeVois M, Webb DR: Management of children with slightly elevated blood lead levels, *Pediatrics* 93(2):188-191, 1994.

Klein-Schwartz W and others: Assessment of management guidelines: acute iron ingestion, *Clin Pediatr* 29(6):316-321, 1990.

Liebelt EL, Shannon M, Graef JW: Efficacy of oral meso-2, 3-dimercaptosuccinic acid therapy for low-level childhood plumbism, *J Pediatr* 124:313-317, 1994.

Mahaffey KR: Exposure to lead in childhood: the importance of prevention, *N Engl J Med* 327(18):1308-1309, 1992.

Markowitz M, Rosen J, Bijur P: Effects of iron deficiency on lead excretion in children with moderate lead intoxication, *J Pediatr* 116(3):360-364, 1990.

Mortensen ME, Walson PD: Chelation therapy for childhood lead poisoning: the changing scene in the 1990s, *Clin Pediatr* 32(5):284-291, 1993.

Needleman HL, Jackson RJ: Lead toxicity in the 21st century: will we still be treating it? *Pediatrics* 89(4)678-680, 1992.

Needleman H and others: The long-term effects of exposure to low doses of lead in childhood, *N Engl J Med* 322(2):83-88, 1990.

Rosen JF: Health effects of lead at low exposure levels: expert consensus and rationale for lowering the definition of childhood lead poisoning, *Am J Dis Child* 146(11):1278-1281, 1992.

Sayre JW, Ernhart CB: Control of lead exposure in childhood: are we doing it correctly? *Am J Dis Child* 146(11):1275-1278, 1992.

Schaffer SJ, Szilagyi PG, Weitzman M: Lead poisoning risk determination in an urban population through the use of a standardized questionnaire, *Pediatrics* 93(2):159-164, 1994.

Tejeda DM and others: Do questions about lead exposure predict elevated lead levels? *Pediatrics* 93(2):192-194, 1994.

Tunnessen W, McMahon K, Baser M: Acrodynia: exposure to mercury from fluorescent light bulbs, *Pediatrics* 79(5):786-789, 1987.

Update: iron poisonings—so tragic, so preventable, *Contemp Pediatr* 10(4):123, 1993.

Weitzman M, Glotzer D: Lead poisoning, *Pediatr Rev* 13(12):461-468, 1992.

Weitzman M and others: Lead-contaminated soil abatement and urban children's blood lead levels, *JAMA* 269(13):1647-1654, 1993.

Zelman M and others: Toxicity from vacuumed mercury: a household hazard, *Clin Pediatr* 30(2):121-123, 1991.

Child Maltreatment

Alexander R and others: Incidence of impact trauma with cranial injuries ascribed to shaking, *Am J Dis Child* 144:724-726, 1990.

Alexander R and others: Serial abuse in children who are shaken, *Am J Dis Child* 144(1):58-60, 1990.

American Academy of Pediatrics, Committee on Bioethics: Religious exemptions from child abuse statutes, *Pediatrics* 81(1):169-171, 1988.

American Academy of Pediatrics, Committee on Child Abuse and Neglect and Committee on Community Health Services: Investigation and review of unexpected infant and child deaths, *Pediatrics* 92(5):734-735, 1993.

American Academy of Pediatrics, Committee on Early Childhood, Adoption, and Dependent Care: Developmental issues in foster care for children, *Pediatrics* 91(5):1007-1009, 1993.

American Academy of Pediatrics, Task Force on Child Abuse and Neglect: Public disclosure of private information about victims of abuse, *Pediatrics* 82(3):387, 1988.

Anderson CL: The parenting profile assessment: screening for child abuse, *Appl Nurs Res* 6(1):31-3, 1993.

Andrews AB: Developing community systems for the primary prevention of family violence, *Fam Community Health* 16(4):1-9, 1994.

Baldwin MA: Munchausen syndrome by proxy: neurological manifestations, *J Neurosci Nurs* 26(1):18-23, 1994.

Berenson AB: Appearance of the hymen at birth and one year of age: a longitudinal study, *Pediatrics* 91(4):820-825, 1993.

Berkowitz CD: Child sexual abuse, *Pediatr Rev* 13(12):443-452, 1992.

Besharov DJ: *Recognizing child abuse: a guide for the concerned,* New York, 1990, MacMillan.

Boyd A: Condylomata acuminata in the pediatric population, *Am J Dis Child* 144(7):817-824, 1990.

Brucker JM: Battered child syndrome: educating the pediatric nurse, *J Pediatr Nurs* 6(6):428-429, 1991.

Burgess A, Hartman C, Kelley S: Assessing child abuse: the triads checklist, *J Psychosoc Nurs* 28(4):6-14, 1990.

Ciottone R, Madonna J: Crucial issues in the treatment of a sexually abused latency-aged boy, *Issues Compr Pediatr Nurs* 16:31-40, 1993.

Coleman L: Learning from the McMartin hoax, *Issues Child Abuse Accus* 1(2):68-71, 1989.

Coleman L: Medical examination for sexual abuse: have we been misled? *Issues Child Abuse Accus* 1(3):1-9, 1989.

Courtois CA, Riley CC: Pregnancy and childbirth as triggers for abuse memories: implications for care, *Birth* 19(4):222-223, 1992.

Dubowitz H, Black M, Harrington D: The diagnosis of child sexual abuse, *Am J Dis Child* 146(6):688-693, 1992.

Dubowitz H, Bross DC: The pediatrician's documentation of child maltreatment, *Am J Dis Child* 146(5):596-599, 1992.

Emans SJ: Sexual abuse in girls: what have we learned about genital anatomy? *J Pediatr* 120(2, pt 1):258-260, 1992.

Flaherty E, Weiss H: Medical evaluation of abused and neglected children, *Am J Dis Child* 144(3):330-334, 1990.

Foreman DM, Farsides C: Ethical use of covert videoing techniques in detecting Munchausen syndrome by proxy, *Br Med J* 307(6904):611-613, 1993.

Friedman SR: What is child sexual abuse? *J Clin Psychol* 46(3):372-375, 1990.

Fulginiti V, Krugman R: Cleveland, England: child abuse in the public eye, *Am J Dis Child* 143(6):651-652, 1989.

Gabby T and others: Sexual abuse of children: the detection of semen on skin, *Am J Dis Child* 146:700-703, 1992.

Gage RB: Consequences of children's exposure to spouse abuse, *Pediatr Nurs* 16(3):258-260, 1990.

Gardner RA: Revising the Child Abuse Prevention and Treatment Act: our best hope for dealing with sex-abuse hysteria in the United States, *Issues Child Abuse Accus* 5(1):25-27, 1993.

George J, Quattrone M: Reporting child abuse: duties and dangers, *J Emerg Nurs* 14(1):34-35, 1988.

Goff C and others: Vaginal opening measurement in prepubertal girls, *Am J Dis Child* 143:1366-1368, 1989.

Goldson E: The affective and cognitive sequelae of child maltreatment, *Pediatr Clin North Am* 38(6):1481-1496, 1991.

Grant LJ: Effects of childhood sexual abuse: issues for obstetric caregivers, *Birth* 19(4):220-221, 1992.

Greenfield M: Disclosing incest: the relationships that make it possible, *Psychosoc Nurs* 28(7):20-23, 1990.

Gutman LT: Sexual abuse and human papillomavirus infection, *J Pediatr* 116(3):495-496, 1990.

Gutman LT and others: Evaluation of sexually abused and nonabused young girls for intravaginal human papillomavirus infection, *Am J Dis Child* 146:694-699, 1992.

Heger A, Emans S: Introital diameter as the criterion for sexual abuse, *Pediatrics* 85(2):222-223, 1990.

Herman-Giddens ME: Vaginal foreign bodies and child sexual abuse, *Arch Pediatr Adolesc Med* 148(2):195-200, 1994.

Herman-Giddens M, Berson N: Harmful genital care practices in children: a type of child abuse, *JAMA* 261(4):577-579, 1989.

Hibbard R, Hartman G: Genitalia in human figure drawings: childrearing practices and child sexual abuse, *J Pediatr* 116(5):822-828, 1990.

Horsham P: Child sexual abuse: what parents need to know, *Can Nurse* 88(8):32-35, 1992.

Hyden PW, Gallagher TA: Child abuse intervention in the emergency room, *Pediatr Emerg Med* 39(5):1053-1081, 1992.

Ifudu O, Kolasinski SL, Friedman EA: Brief report: kidney-related Munchausen's syndrome, *N Engl J Med* 327(6):388-389, 1992.

Irons TG: Documenting sexual abuse of a child, *Emerg Med* 25(6):57-75, 1993.

Jaudes PK, Martone M: Interdisciplinary evaluations of alleged sexual abuse cases, *Pediatrics* 89(6):1164-1168, 1992.

Johnson CF: Symbolic scarring and tattooing: unusual manifestations of child abuse, *Clin Pediatr* 34(1):46-49, 1994.

Johnson C, Kaufman K, Callendar C: The hand as a target organ in child abuse, *Clin Pediatr* 29(2):66-72, 1990.

Kelley SJ: Parental stress response to sexual abuse and ritualistic abuse of children in day-care centers, *Nurs Res* 39(1):25-29, 1990.

Kelley SJ: Methodological issues in child sexual abuse research, *J Pediatr Nurs* 6(1):21-29, 1991.

Kerns DL, Ritter ML, Thomas RG: Concave hymenal variations in suspected child sexual abuse victims, *Pediatrics* 90(2):265-272, 1992.

Kharasch S, Vinci R, Reece R: Esophagitis, epiglottitis and cocaine alkaloid ("crack"): "accidental" poisoning or child abuse? *Pediatrics* 86(1):117-119, 1990.

Kiefer L: Defense considerations in the child as witness in allegations of sexual abuse. II. The child witness: legal competency, *Issues Child Abuse Accus* 1(2):48-57, 1989.

Kivlahan C, Kruse R, Furnell D: Sexual assault examinations in children: the role of a statewide network of health care providers, *Am J Dis Child* 146(11):1365-1370, 1992.

Krivacska JJ: Primary prevention of child sexual abuse: alternative, non-child directed approaches, *Issues Child Abuse Accus* 1(4):1-9, 1989.

Lesniak LP: Penetrating the conspiracy of silence: identifying the family at risk for incest, *Fam Community Health* 16(2):66-76, 1993.

Leventhal JM and others: Fractures in young children: distinguishing child abuse from unintentional injuries, *Am J Dis Child* 147(1):87-92, 1993.

Lewin L: Establishing a therapeutic relationship with an abused child, *Pediatr Nurs* 16(3):263-264, 1990.

Lipscomb GH and others: Male victims of sexual assault, *JAMA* 267(22):3064-3066, 1992.

Lyons TJ, Oates RK: Falling out of bed: a relatively benign occurrence, *Pediatrics* 92(1):125-127, 1993.

McCann J and others: Comparison of genital examination techniques in prepubertal girls, *Pediatrics* 85(2):182-187, 1990.

McCann J and others: Genital findings in prepubertal girls selected for nonabuse: a descriptive study, *Pediatrics* 86(3):428-439, 1990.

Monteleone JA: *Recognition of child abuse for the mandated reporter,* St Louis, 1994, GW Medical/Mosby.

Monteleone JA, Brodeur AE: *Child maltreatment: a clinical guide and reference,* St Louis, 1994, GW Medical/Mosby.

Monteleone JA, Brodeur AE: *Child maltreatment: a color atlas,* St Louis, 1994, GW Medical/Mosby.

O'Brien C: Medical and forensic examination by a sexual assault nurse examiner of a 7-year-old victim of sexual assault, *J Emerg Nurs* 18(3):199-204, 1992.

Pagel JR, Pagel PR: Participants' perceptions of a mandated training course in the identification and reporting of child abuse, *Pediatr Nurs* 19(6):554-558, 1993.

Position statement: Sexual abuse allegations in child custody cases: the role of the pediatrician, *Clin Pediatr* 31(6):375, 1992.

Post CA: Play therapy with an abused child: a case study, *Child Adolesc Psychiatr Ment Health Nurs* 3(1):34-36, 1990.

Rand DC: Munchausen syndrome by proxy: integration of classic and contemporary types, *Issues Child Abuse Accus* 2(2):83-89, 1990.

Reece RM: Fatal child abuse and sudden infant death syndrome: a critical diagnostic decision, *Pediatrics* 91(2):423-429, 1993.

Riggs S, Alario A, McHorney C: Health risk behaviors and attempted suicide in adolescents who report prior maltreatment, *J Pediatr* 116(5):815-821, 1990.

Senner A, Ott M: Munchausen syndrome by proxy, *Issues Compr Pediatr Nurs* 12(4):345-357, 1989.

Simkin P: Overcoming the legacy of childhood sexual abuse: the role of caregivers and childbirth educators, *Birth* 19(4):224-225, 1992.

Southall DP, Samuels MP: Ethical use of covert videoing for potentially life threatening child abuse: a response to Drs Foreman and Farsides, *Br Med J* 307(6904):613-614, 1993.

Stahler G, DuCette J, Povich E: Using mediation to prevent child maltreatment: an exploratory study, *Fam Relations* 39(3):317-322, 1990.

Underwager R, Wakefield H: *The real world of child interrogations,* Springfield, IL, 1990, Charles C Thomas.

Welldon EV: Women who sexually abuse children, *Br Med J* 300:1527-1528, 1990.

Wong DL: The "evidence" is shaky at best, *Am J Nurs* 9(2):18, 1991.

Yates A, Terr L: Anatomically correct dolls: should they be used as the basis for expert testimony? *J Am Acad Child Adolesc Psychiatry* 27(3):387-388, 1988.

UNIT VI

FAMILY-CENTERED CARE OF THE SCHOOL-AGE CHILD

CHAPTER 17 Health Promotion of the School-Age Child and Family

CHAPTER OUTLINE

RELATED TOPICS

Dental health, Ch. 14
Eating problems/disorders, Ch. 21
Growth and development of children, Ch. 4
Guidelines: Assessing sleep problems in children, p. 202
Health problems of middle childhood, Ch. 18
Injuries—the leading killer, Ch. 1
Limit-setting and discipline, Ch. 3
Nutrition, Ch. 4
Physical and developmental assessment of the child, Ch. 7
Psychosocial history, Ch. 6
Injuries and health problems related to sports participation, Ch. 39
Sleep problems, Chs. 12 and 15
Television, Ch. 4

PROMOTING OPTIMUM GROWTH AND DEVELOPMENT

The segment of the life span that extends from age 6 to approximately age 12 has a variety of labels, each of which describes an important characteristic of the period. The middle years are most often referred to as ***school-age*** or the ***school years.*** Psychosocially this period begins with entrance into the wider sphere of influence represented by the school environment, which has a significant impact on development and relationships.

Physiologically the middle years begin with shedding the first deciduous tooth and end at puberty with the acquisition of final permanent teeth (with the exception of the wisdom teeth). During the preceding 5 to 6 years, children have progressed from helpless infants to sturdy, complicated individuals with the capacity to communicate, conceptualize in a limited way, and become involved in complex social and motor behavior. Physical growth has been equally rapid. In contrast, the period of middle childhood, between the rapid growth of early childhood and the turmoil of the prepubescent growth spurt, is a time of gradual growth and development, with steadier and more even progress in both its physical and emotional aspects.

BIOLOGIC DEVELOPMENT

During middle childhood, growth in height and weight assumes a slower but steady pace as compared with the earlier years and the years immediately ahead. Between ages 6 and 12, children will grow an average of 5 cm (2 inches) per year to gain 30 to 60 cm (1 to 2 feet) in height and will almost double in weight, increasing 2 to 3 kg (4½ to 6½ pounds) per year. The average 6-year-old child is about 116 cm (45 inches) tall and weighs about 21 kg (46 pounds); the average 12-year-old child stands about 150 cm (59 inches) tall and weighs approximately 40 kg (88 pounds). During this age period girls and boys differ very little in size, although boys tend to be slightly taller and somewhat heavier than girls. Toward the end of the school-age years both boys and girls begin to increase in size, although most girls begin to surpass boys in both height and weight, to the acute discomfort of both.

Proportional Changes

School-age children are more graceful than they were as preschoolers, and they are steadier on their feet. Their body proportions take on a slimmer look with longer legs, varying body proportion, and a lower center of gravity. Posture improves over that of the preschool period to facilitate locomotion and efficiency in using the arms and trunk. These proportions make climbing, bicycle riding, and other activities much easier. Fat gradually diminishes, and its distribution patterns change, contributing to the thinner appearance of children during the middle years.

Accompanying the skeletal lengthening and fat diminution is an increase in the percentage of body weight represented by muscle tissue. By the end of this age period both boys and girls will double their strength and physical capabilities, and their steady and relatively consistent acquisition of refined coordination will increase their poise and skill. However, this increased strength can be misleading. Although strength increases, muscles are still functionally immature as compared with those of the adolescent and are more readily damaged by muscular injury caused by overuse.

The most pronounced changes and those that seem best to indicate increasing maturity in children are a decrease in head circumference in relation to standing height, a decrease in waist circumference in relation to height, and an increase in leg length related to height. These observations often provide a clue to a child's degree of maturity that has proved useful in predicting readiness for meeting the demands of school. There appears to be a correlation between physical indications of maturity and success in school.

Facial Changes. Certain physiologic and anatomic characteristics are typical of children in the middle childhood years. Facial proportions change as the face grows faster in relation to the remainder of the cranium. The skull and brain grow very slowly during this period and increase little in size thereafter. Since all of the primary (deciduous) teeth are lost during this age span, middle childhood is sometimes known as the ***age of the loose tooth*** (Fig. 17-1) and the early years of middle childhood are known as the ***ugly duckling stage,*** when the new secondary (permanent) teeth appear to be much too large for the smaller face.

Maturation of Systems

Maturity of the ***gastrointestinal system*** is reflected in fewer stomach upsets, better maintenance of blood sugar levels, and an increased stomach capacity, which permits retention of food for longer periods. The school-age child does not

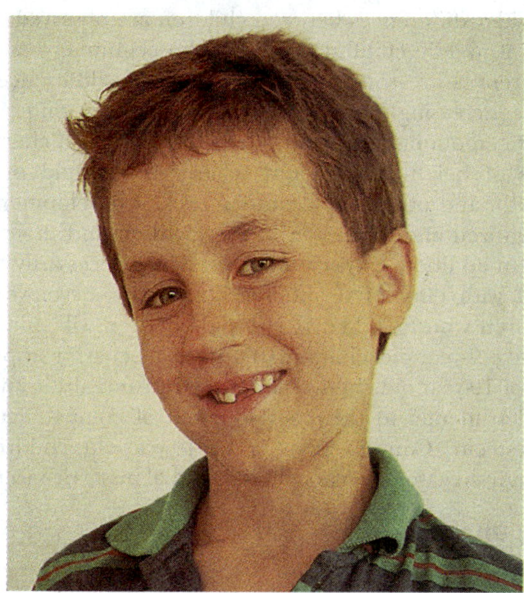

FIG. 17-1 Middle childhood is the stage of development when deciduous teeth are shed.

■ Marilyn L. Winkelstein, RN, PhD, revised this chapter.

need to be fed as carefully, as promptly, or as frequently as before. Caloric needs in relation to stomach size are less than they were in the preschool years and less than they will be during the coming adolescent growth spurt.

Physical maturation is evidenced in other body tissues and organs. ***Bladder capacity,*** although differing widely among individual children, is generally greater in girls than in boys. There are individual variations in frequency of urination and differences in the same child according to circumstances such as temperature, humidity, time of day, amount of fluids ingested, and emotional state.

The ***heart*** grows more slowly during the middle years and is smaller in relation to the rest of the body than at any other period of life. Consequently, many believe that strongly competitive sports with prolonged, intense physical exertion may be damaging to school-age children. Heart and respiratory rates steadily decrease, and blood pressure increases during ages 6 to 12 (see inside back cover).

The ***immune system*** becomes more competent in its ability to localize infections and to produce an antibody-antigen response. Although children have several infections in the first 1 to 2 years of school because of increased exposure to other children, immunity to a wide variety of pathogenic microorganisms develops (Miller, 1989).

Bones continue to ossify throughout childhood, but, since mineralization is not completed until maturity, children's bones resist pressure and muscle pull less than mature bones. Consequently, care must be taken to prevent alterations in bone structure, and children should be provided with well-fitted shoes, chairs, and desks that allow correct sitting posture with the feet able to reach the floor and the hips able to fit well back in the seat. Children should have ample opportunity to move around and should observe appropriate caution in carrying heavy loads. For example, they should shift books and/or tote bags from one arm to the other. Back packs distribute weight more evenly.

Wider differences between children are observed at the end of middle childhood than at the beginning—and the differences are sometimes striking. These differences become increasingly apparent and, if extreme or unique, may create emotional problems unless the associated characteristics of height and weight relationships, rapid or slow growth, and other important features of development are recognized and explained to the children and their families. In addition, physical maturity is not necessarily correlated with emotional and social maturity. Seven-year-old children who look like 10-year-old children will think and act like 7-year-old children. To expect behavior appropriate for 10-year-old children from them is unrealistic and can be detrimental to their development of competence and self-esteem. Conversely, to treat 10-year-old children as though they were 7 years old is an equal disservice to them.

Prepubescence

Preadolescence is the period that begins toward the end of middle childhood and ends with the thirteenth birthday. Since puberty signals the beginning of the development of secondary sex characteristics, ***prepubescence,*** the 2-year period that precedes puberty, typically occurs during preadolescence.

Toward the end of middle childhood the discrepancies in growth and maturation between boys and girls begin to be apparent. On the average, there is a difference of approximately 2 years between girls and boys in the age at which observable signs of pubescence appear. Preadolescence is, for some, a period of rapid growth, especially for girls; for others, mostly boys, it is generally a period of continued steady growth in height and weight. On the whole it is a healthy period of childhood—the period between childhood diseases and the diseases of adulthood.

There is no universal age at which children assume the characteristics of preadolescence. The first physiologic signs begin to appear at about 9 years (particularly in girls) and are usually clearly evident in 11- to 12-year-old children. Although preadolescent children do not want to be different, at this age the variability in physical growth and physiologic changes between children of the same sex, between the two sexes, and even within each individual child is often striking. This variability, especially in relation to the onset of secondary sex characteristics, is of utmost concern to the preadolescent. Either early or late appearance of these characteristics is a source of embarrassment and uneasiness to both sexes. Early appearance of secondary sex characteristics in girls may be associated with dissatisfaction with physical appearance, greater general unhappiness, and lower self-esteem. Late-developing boys often have a negative self-concept. Both early appearance of physical characteristics in girls and late appearance in boys have been linked to participation in such risk-taking behaviors as early sexual activity in girls and substance use and reckless vehicle use in boys (Irwin and Millstein, 1992).

Preadolescence is a time when there is considerable overlapping of developmental characteristics with elements of both middle childhood and early adolescence. However, there are sufficient unique characteristics to set this period apart as an age category, even with the wide range of variability in ages 11 and 12 (or even 9 to 13) in some children. Generally, the earliest age at which puberty begins is 10 years in girls and 12 years in boys, although there has been an increase in the number of girls reaching puberty at age 9. The average age of puberty in girls is 12, and in boys it is 14. Boys experience little sexual maturation during preadolescence.

PSYCHOSOCIAL DEVELOPMENT

Middle childhood is the period in psychosexual development that Freud has described as the ***latency period,*** which has been considered to be a time of sexual tranquility between the oedipal phase of early childhood and the eroticism of adolescence. It is during this time that children experience the intimacy of relationships with same-sex peers following the indifference of earlier years and preceding the heterosexual fascination that accompanies the changes of puberty. However, the concept of sexual latency is now being questioned in the light of early sexual exploration and the exploitation of sex in the media.

Developing a Sense of Industry (Erikson)

Successful mastery of Erikson's first three stages of psychosocial development is probably the most important accomplishment in terms of development of a healthy personality (Erikson, 1963). With a foundation of trust, autonomy, and initiative, children are fairly certain to progress through subsequent stages with relative ease. Successful completion of these stages implies confidence in an environment of loving relationships within a stable family unit that has prepared the child to engage in experiences and relationships beyond these intimate groups. It has been suggested that the individual's fundamental attitude toward work is established during middle childhood. It is during this time that children receive the systematic instruction prescribed by their individual cultures and develop the skills needed to become useful, contributing members of their social communities.

A sense of industry, for which a more descriptive term is the ***stage of accomplishment,*** is achieved somewhere between age 6 and adolescence. The goal of this stage of development is to achieve a sense of personal and interpersonal competence by the acquisition of technologic and social skills. School-age children are eager to build skills and participate in meaningful and socially useful work. Interests expand in the middle years, and, with a growing sense of independence, children want to engage in tasks that can be carried through to completion (Fig. 17-2). Failure to develop a sense of accomplishment results in a sense of ***inferiority.***

There are many attributes of industry that contribute to the child's sense of competence and mastery. Intrinsic motivation is associated with increased competence in mastering new skills and assuming new responsibilities. Children gain a great deal of satisfaction from independent behavior in exploring and manipulating their environment and from interaction with peers. Extrinsic sources of reinforcement in the form of grades, material rewards, additional privileges, and recognition provide encouragement and stimulation. Often the acquisition of skills is a means for achieving success in special activities such as athletics or social organizations such as scouting. Peer approval is a strong motivating power.

The danger inherent in this period of personality development is the imposition of situations that might result in a sense of inadequacy or inferiority. This may happen if the previous stages have not been successfully achieved or if a child is incapable of or unprepared for assuming the responsibilities associated with developing a sense of accomplishment. Feelings of inferiority or lack of worth can be derived from children themselves or from the social environment. Children with physical or mental limitations are at a disadvantage for acquisition of certain skills, and, when the reward structure is based on evidence of mastery, children who are incapable of developing these skills are bound to feel inadequate and inferior.

Even children without chronic disabilities represent such a wide range of individual differences in capabilities and preferences that they will experience feelings of inadequacy in some areas. No child is able to do well in everything, and children must learn that they will not be able to master each skill that they attempt. All children, even children who in most instances have positive attitudes toward work and their own capabilities, will feel some degree of inferiority in regard to a specific skill that they cannot master.

To some extent, success or aptitude in one area may compensate for failure or ineptitude in another. However, the differences in reinforcement provided for success in various areas have a very significant effect on feelings of adequacy. For example, in the United States reading proficiency is more highly rewarded than mechanical aptitude such as tinkering with broken automobile engines. A higher social value is placed on success in team sports than on suc-

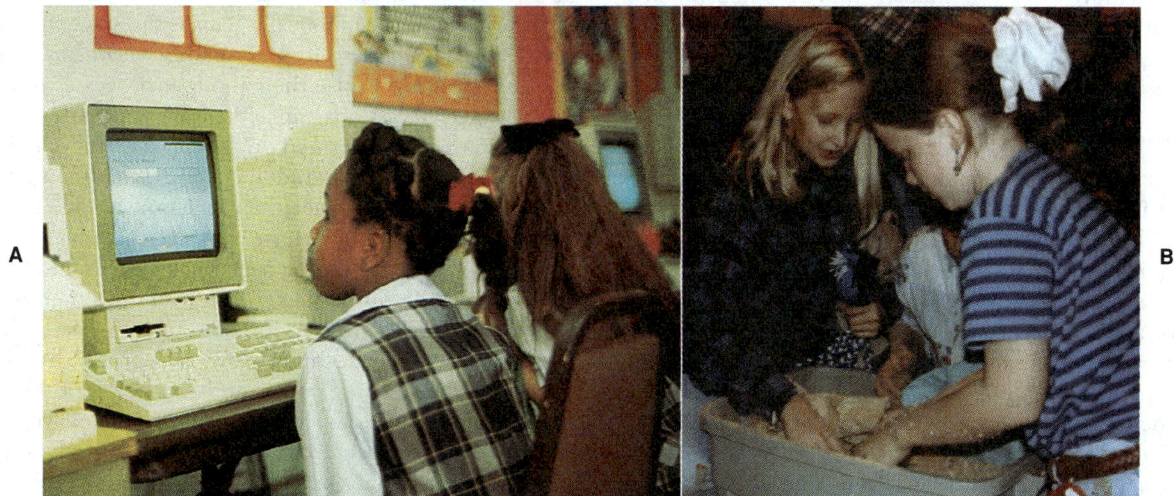

FIG. 17-2 School-age children are motivated to complete tasks. **A,** Working alone. **B,** Working with others.

cess in operating a ham radio. However, compensating for the inability to excel in more socially valued skills through mastery of other less valued skills is difficult for the child. Also, as a corollary to this, the social environment places a negative value on any kind of failure, and this serves to further stimulate feelings of inferiority in the less capable child. Repeated failures often generate such strong feelings in the child that eventually the child is reluctant to attempt any new task that may bring failure or is fearful of not being able to perform as well as his or her peers. Thus intrinsic motivation toward engaging in a task for the pleasure of the challenge conflicts with the external forces that cause feelings of doubt and inferiority. Consequently, the child may no longer try.

Much depends on the child's concept of success or failure. Children who aspire for more than they are capable of will usually experience failure. In contrast, children who set their aspirations lower than their level of achievement are more likely to experience success. Most accomplishments during the school years are very public. Success or failure in school is known to family, teachers, peers, and others. In the social environment of school and sometimes at home, feelings of inferiority may be produced through comparison with others, suggesting that the child is not as good as some peer, sibling, or another subcultural group. This inadequacy becomes a source of embarrassment. The child may even be shamed for the failure. These earlier conflicts of doubt and guilt are very closely associated with feelings of inferiority.

A sense of accomplishment also involves the ability to cooperate and to compete with others—to cope more effectively with people. Middle childhood is the time when children learn the value of doing things alongside and with others and the benefits derived from division of labor in the accomplishment of goals. Children need and want real achievement. When they have access to tasks that need to be done, that they are able to do well despite individual differences in their innate capacities and emotional development, and that they are suitably rewarded for, children will be able to achieve a sense of industry and accomplishment that prepares them for establishing a stable identity later in life.

TEMPERAMENT

The enduring reactivity patterns or temperamental traits identified in infancy continue to be important in middle childhood as determinants of some aspects of behavior. Analyzing behavioral patterns observed in past situations can provide clues to the way that a child may react to new situations, although long-range projections are not always successful. Through interaction with environment, experiences, motives, and abilities, many children change. Major temperamental characteristics persist into adolescence in many children; in others they do not.

Parents and teachers are persons who are in the best position to assess a child's behavioral style and try to make their demands and expectations consonant with the individual child's temperamental characteristics. With easy children this rarely poses a problem. They adapt readily to almost any childrearing program and new situation. School entry or other experiences are usually smooth and accomplished with minimal stress. Difficulties arise with difficult, slow-to-warm-up children and children who are easily distracted.

Slow-to-warm-up children who usually exhibit discomfort when introduced to new situations need time to become accustomed to a new environment, authority figures, and expectations. These children may respond with tears, somatic complaints, or other maneuvers to avoid the event. They should be encouraged to try new experiences but also should be allowed to adapt to their surroundings at their own speed. Pressure to move quickly into new situations only strengthens the tendency to withdraw. Even afterschool activities can be cause for reaction, but attending with a friend or contracting for permission to withdraw after a trial of a specified number of times may provide them with sufficient incentive to try.

Difficult or easily distracted children may benefit from "practice" sessions in which they are prepared for the event by role-playing, visiting the site, stories, or other methods of getting them acquainted with what to expect. Children who are very persistent need to know when they are expected to stop what they are doing so that the signal to stop will not come as a surprise, thus triggering a reaction. Children with difficult temperaments need to be handled with exceptional patience, firmness, and understanding so that they can learn appropriate behavior in their interactions with others. It is important for teachers to be matched to the temperament of children whenever possible to ensure a "good fit." Although teachers should be sensitive and understanding of children with all temperaments, there are some who are better able to cope with difficult children.

COGNITIVE DEVELOPMENT (PIAGET)

Somewhere around the beginning of the school years, children begin to acquire the ability to relate a series of events and actions to mental representations that can be expressed both verbally and symbolically. This is the stage in development that Piaget describes as ***concrete operations,*** wherein children are able to use their thought processes to experience events and actions. Since the word "operation" implies an action that is performed on an object or set of objects, a ***mental operation*** is an alteration or transformation that is carried out in thought rather than in action. Toddlers or preschool children can perform acts that involve ordering, such as correctly arranging a graduated set of circles from largest to smallest on a stick, or they can find their way to a friend's house, but they are unable to verbalize the action or actions involved in the process. School-age children are able to articulate the process and can perform the action mentally without the need to carry out the behaviors.

As children move from the preschool years into the world of wider relationships, their conceptual abilities become increasingly more flexible. During the ***concrete-operational period*** children rapidly acquire cognitive operations and apply these new skills when thinking about objects, situations, and events. Their rigid, egocentric outlook is replaced by thought processes that allow them to see things from the point of view of another. They become aware of a variety of perspectives and become more sensitive to the fact that others do not always perceive events exactly as they do. They are able to delay an action until they have evaluated alternative responses to situations, and their steady reduction in egocentricity helps form the basis for logical thought and the development and maturation of morality.

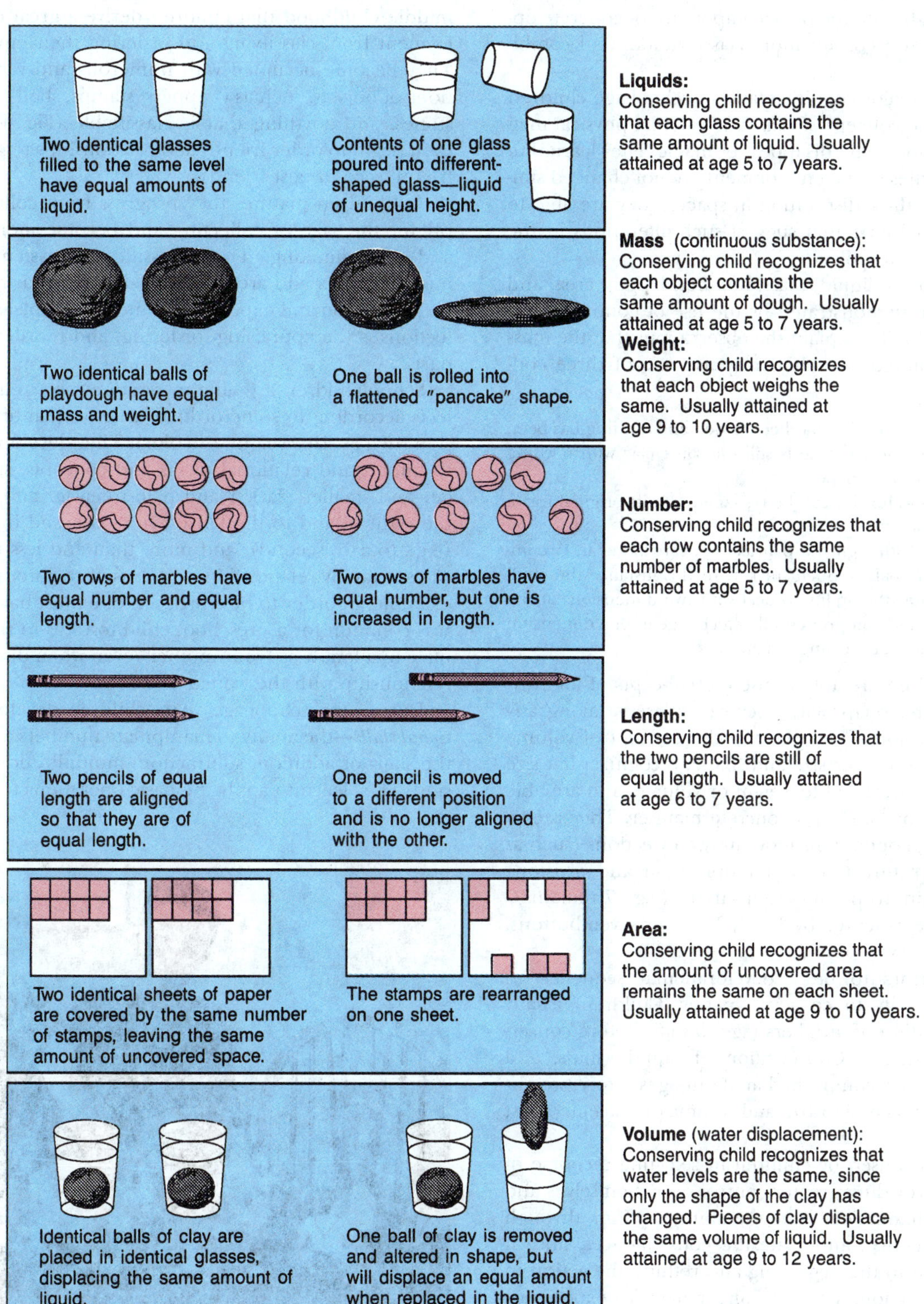

FIG. 17-3 Common methods for testing the child's ability to conserve.

The concrete-operational stage takes place between the years 7 and 11. During this stage children develop an understanding and use for relationships between things and ideas. They progress from making judgments based on what they see ***(perceptual thinking)*** to making judgments based on what they reason ***(conceptual thinking)***. They are increasingly able to master symbols and to use their memory store of past experiences in evaluating and interpreting the present. They gain insight into the basic components of concrete operational thought: conservation, classification, and combinational skills.

One of the major cognitive tasks of school-age children is mastering the concept of ***conservation***—that physical matter does not appear and disappear by magic. They learn that certain properties of the environment are not changed simply by altering their disposition in space. They are able to resist perceptual cues that suggest such alterations in the physical state of an object.

Conservation of liquid, mass, number, length, area, and volume can be demonstrated by the use of commonplace items (Fig. 17-3). To explain the observations that the mass has been unaltered, the child may use one of three concepts:

Identity—Since nothing has been added and nothing has been taken away, the pancake is still the same clay with nothing changed but the shape.

Reversibility—The clay can be reshaped into its original form, that of a ball.

Reciprocity—Although the pancake appears larger in circumference, the ball is much thicker. In this instance the child demonstrates the ability to deal with two dimensions at the same time and comprehend that a change in one dimension compensates for a change in another.

When children are able to use the concepts of identity, reversibility, and reciprocity, they can conserve along any physical dimension. They perceive the concept of volume in relation to container size and shape, recognize that size is not necessarily related to weight or volume, and are able to manipulate or "see" in a concrete manner. They recognize that logical operations move in two directions (such as addition and subtraction or multiplication and division) and that certain properties are invariant (e.g., 7 remains 7 whether it is represented by 3 + 4, 2 + 5, or seven buttons, seven stars, or seven boys).

There appears to be a developmental sequence in children's capacity to conserve matter. Children usually grasp conservation of numbers (ages 5 to 6) before conservation of substance. Conservation of liquids, mass, and length usually is accomplished at about ages 6 to 7, weight sometime later (ages 9 to 10), and volume displacement last (ages 9 to 12).

Reversibility is used by children in selecting a course of action, thus providing greater control over themselves and their environment. They have the ability to think through an action sequence, anticipate the consequences, and, if needed, return to the beginning and rethink the action in a different direction. They no longer need to experience an action before they can anticipate the results. Reversibility allows mental action and provides children with the ability to disassemble and reassemble certain kinds of things in their thoughts.

Classification skills involve the ability to group objects according to the attributes that they share in common. School-age children now have the ability to place things in a sensible and logical order, to group and sort, and, in doing so, to hold a concept in their minds while they make decisions based on that concept. It is characteristic of middle childhood that children derive a great deal of enjoyment from classifying and ordering their environment. They become occupied with numerous and varied collections of objects, such as wrappers, stamps, shells, dolls, cars, stones, and anything that is classifiable (Fig. 17-4). They even begin to order friends and relationships (e.g., first best friend, second best friend).

As children mature, they progress from collecting simply for the sake of collecting and become more selective and discriminating. Their classification systems become more complex and are based on abstract ideas rather than on perception and experience. Much of the pleasure of collections is the appraising, ordering, and reordering of the parts.

Schoolchildren are able to ***serialize*** (i.e., to arrange objects according to some ordinal scale or quantified dimension such as size, weight, or color). They develop the ability to understand relational terms and concepts, such as bigger and smaller; darker and paler; heavier and lighter; to the right of and to the left of; first, last, and intermediate (e.g., fourth, second); and more than and less than. They can see family relationships in terms of reciprocal roles; for example, in order to be a brother, one must have a sibling. It is common for a preschool child to refer to the adult female in a family as "your mother" even when discussing the relationship with the woman's husband.

During the school-age years children develop ***combinational skills***—the ability to manipulate numbers and to learn the skills of addition, subtraction, multiplication, and division. They learn to apply the basic operations to any object

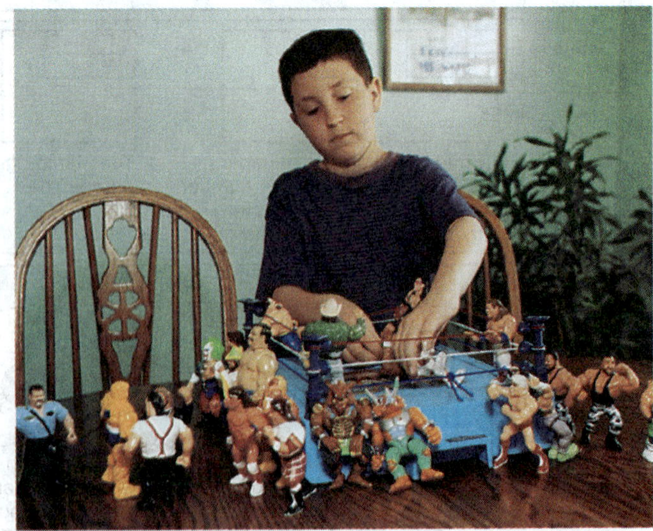

FIG. 17-4 School-age children are often avid collectors.

or quantity. They learn the alphabet and the ever-widening world of symbols called words that can be arranged in terms of structure and their relationship to the alphabet. They learn to tell time, to see the relationship of events in time (history) and places in space (geography), and to combine time and space relationships (geology and astronomy).

The most significant skill, the ***ability to read,*** is acquired during the school years and becomes the most valuable tool for independent inquiry. Children's capacity for exploration, imagination, and expansion of knowledge is enhanced with the ability to read as they progress from the repetition and confusion of early efforts to increasing facility and comprehension. Formal academic learning begins at ages 5 to 6 years, when children's intellectual capabilities and cognitive processes are ready to assume appropriate intellectual achievements.

MORAL DEVELOPMENT (KOHLBERG)

As children move from egocentrism to more logical patterns of thought, they also move through stages in development of conscience and moral standards. Growth in moral thought and judgment progresses between ages 6 and 12. Young children do not believe that standards of behavior come from within themselves but that rules are established and set down by others. At first, rules are perceived as definite, covering limited situations, and requiring no reason or explanation. Children learn the standards for acceptable behavior, act according to these standards, and feel guilty when they violate the standards. Although children 6 or 7 years old know the rules and what they are supposed to do, they do not understand the reasons behind them. Young children usually judge an act by its consequences. Rewards and punishment guide their judgment; a "bad act" is one that breaks a rule or does harm. When a child and an adult differ in judging an act, the adult is right. Children may believe that what other people tell them to do is right and that what they think themselves is wrong. Consequently, children 6 or 7 years old are more likely to interpret accidents and misfortunes as punishment for misdeeds or "bad" acts.

Older school-age children are able to judge an act by the intentions that prompted it rather than just by the consequences. Rules and judgments become less absolute and authoritarian and begin to be founded more on the needs and desires of others. Rules of conduct are more readily considered in terms of mutual agreement and are based on cooperation and respect for others. For older children a rule violation is apt to be viewed in relation to the total context in which it appears; reactions are influenced by the situation, as well as by the morality of the rule itself. However, it is not until adolescence or beyond that children are able to view morality on an abstract basis with sound reasoning and principled thinking. Whereas a younger child can judge an act only according to whether it is right or wrong, older children will take into account a different point of view to make a judgment. They are able to understand and accept the concept of doing as they would have others do to them.

SPIRITUAL DEVELOPMENT

Children at this age think in very concrete terms but are avid learners and have a great desire to learn about their God. They picture God as human and tend to describe him in terms of character traits such as loving and helping. He is a very important person in the lives of many children. They are fascinated by heaven and hell and, with a developing conscience and concern about rules, they fear going to hell for misbehavior. School-age children want and expect to be punished for misbehavior but, if given the option, tend to choose a punishment that "fits the crime." Often they view illness or injury as a punishment for a real or imagined misdeed. The beliefs and ideals of family and religious personages are more influential than their peers in matters of faith.

School-age children begin to learn the difference between the natural and the supernatural but have difficulty understanding symbols. Consequently, religious concepts must be presented to them in concrete terms. They try to relate phenomena in the world in a logical, systematic manner, which is at once both satisfying and occasionally disheartening. Religion affords a means whereby children can relate themselves to their deity in a direct and personal way.

Children are comforted by prayer or other religious rituals, and if these activities are a part of their daily lives, they can help children cope with threatening situations (Fig. 17-5). Their petitions to their God in prayers tend to be for

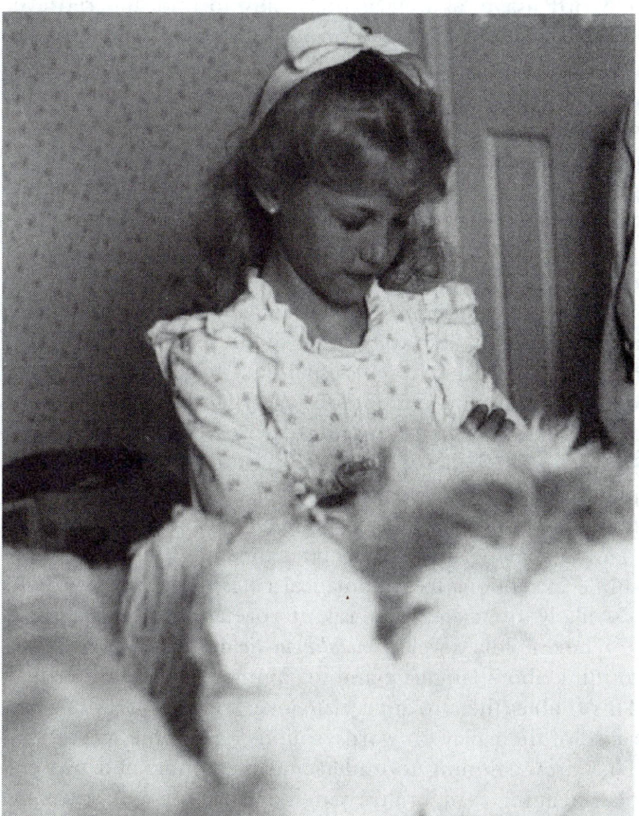

FIG. 17-5 Children are comforted by prayer or other religious rituals.

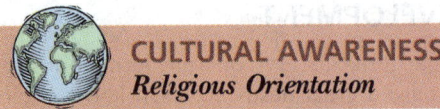

CULTURAL AWARENESS
Religious Orientation

Many schools and communities have a Judeo-Christian orientation toward prayer, holidays, and values. This may result in conflict and discomfort for children of other religious/ethnic groups. Sensitivity must be exercised so as not to offend and confuse children from other religious backgrounds, such as the Buddhist, Hindu, and Muslim faiths.

very tangible rewards. Although younger children expect their prayers to be answered, as they get older they begin to recognize that this does not always occur and become less concerned when prayers are not answered. They are able to discuss their feelings about their faith and how it relates to their lives (see Cultural Awareness box).

LANGUAGE DEVELOPMENT

Children enter middle childhood with remarkably efficient language skills, but they will achieve many important linguistic accomplishments during the school-age years. During the elementary school years they learn to correct previous syntactic errors and begin to use more complex grammatical forms, such as correct past tenses for irregular verbs, correct plurals for irregular nouns, and correct use of personal pronouns.

Word usage, as well as the ability to find and retrieve words quickly when called on to produce what they know in a relatively short period of time, grows considerably during the school years. Children learn to apply the minimum distance principle—the rule that the subject of a verb in an active sentence is the noun or pronoun that immediately precedes it. For example, a 6-year-old child will understand the sentence "Ask Mary her last name" but until age 9 or 10 years will be confused by the sentence "Ask Mary what to bring to the party."

Narrative skills improve markedly. School-age children are increasingly able to provide directives that others can correctly interpret without visual data (e.g., explaining directions over the telephone). By age 10 to 12 years the child should be able to use factive words (such as "know," "think," and "believe") and complex pronouns and conjunctions, and be able to form grammatically correct sentences. School-age children gradually become more proficient at making inferences about meanings and learn the subtle exceptions to grammatical rules, which make them less likely to engage in literal interpretation of messages.

They rapidly develop ***metalinguistic awareness***—an ability to think about language and to comment on its properties. This enables them to appreciate jokes, riddles, and puns because of their play on words, sounds, or double meanings. They are beginning to understand metaphors and proverbial meaning to figurative statements such as, "A stitch in time saves nine." The acquisition of cognitive skills enables them to think about the quality of their own and others' speech and to evaluate and clarify messages.

SOCIAL DEVELOPMENT

Children at the beginning of the middle childhood years normally enter a period of less intense emotions, secure in their dependency on their parents and family and with self-confidence tempered by a more realistic perspective. Their energies are now available to explore the environment beyond the family, to gradually increase the scope of interpersonal interactions, and to invest their curiosity in a greater understanding of the world.

Identification with peers appears to be a strong influence in children's gaining independence from parents. The aid and support of the group provide children with enough security to risk the moderate parental rejection brought about by each small victory in their development of independence.

Questions of masculinity and femininity take on importance as sex-role learning assumes more prominence. Boys associate with boys, and girls with girls, each pursuing their own interests, with communication between the sexes confined to that which is necessary. Much of the child's concept of the appropriate sex role is acquired through relationships with peers. During the early school years there is little difference relative to sex in the play experiences of children. Games and many other activities are shared by both girls and boys. However, in the later school years the differences become marked. Boys and girls grow more intolerant of each other, especially on the surface.

Social Relationships and Cooperation

Daily relationships with age-mates provide the most important social interactions in the life of school-age children. For the first time, children are able to join in group activities with unrestrained enthusiasm and steady participation, when formerly interactions had been limited to short periods under considerable adult supervision. With increased skills and wider opportunities, children are able to become involved with one or several peer groups in which they can gain status as respected members.

There are valuable lessons to be learned from daily interaction with age-mates. First, children learn to appreciate the numerous and varied points of view that are represented in the peer group. As they play together, children discover that there are numerous occupations for fathers and mothers, perhaps more than one version of the same song, different rules for the same game, and different customs for celebrating the same holiday. As children interact with peers who see the world in ways that are somewhat different from the way they see it, they become aware of the limits of their own point of view. Because age-mates are peers and are not forced to accept one another's ideas as they are expected to accept those of adults, other children have a significant influence on decreasing the egocentric outlook of the individual child. Consequently, they learn to argue, persuade, bargain, cooperate, and compromise in order to maintain friendships.

Second, children become increasingly sensitive to the social norms and pressures of the peer group. The peer group establishes standards for acceptance and rejection, and children may be willing to modify their behavior in order to

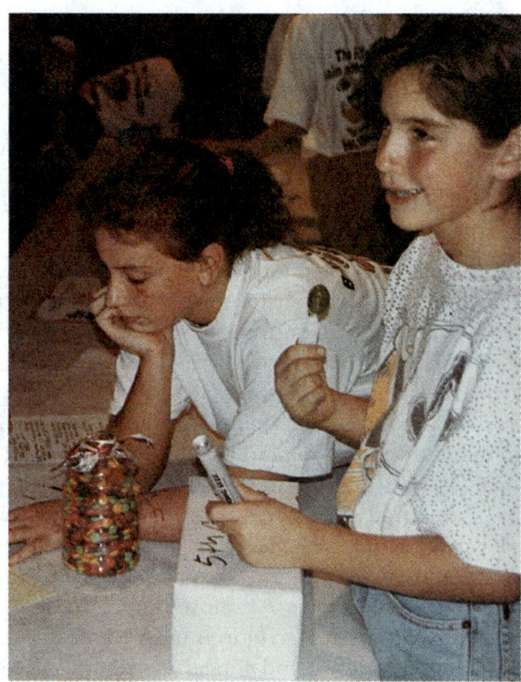

FIG. 17-6 School-age children enjoy engaging in activities with a "best friend."

be accepted by the group. They are judged by the physical impression they convey, the skills they can perform, and other abilities they can demonstrate. This need for peer approval becomes a powerful influence toward conformity. The child learns to dress, talk, and otherwise behave in a manner acceptable to the group. A variety of roles, such as class joker or class hero, may be assumed by the individual child in order to gain approval from the group. However, no child will be able to adapt perfectly to all the requirements made by the peer group. If some children find that the discrepancies between the values of the peer group and the values of their families are too great, they may be forced to relinquish the pleasure of interaction with the group in order to abide by the regulations established in the home. Thus, to diminish conflict within the family, some children may be forced into a position outside the peer group.

Third, the interaction among peers leads to the formation of intimate friendships between same-sex peers (Fig. 17-6). School age is the time when children have "best friends" with whom they share secrets, private jokes, and adventures and come to one another's aid in times of trouble. In the course of these friendships children also fight, threaten, break up, and reunite. These dyadic relationships, in which children experience love and closeness for a peer, seem to be important as a foundation for heterosexual relationships in adulthood. The conflicts encountered in the relationship are usually resolved in terms that the children are able to control. Since neither child has authority over the other, as in an adult-child relationship, the children must work through their differences within the framework of their commitment to each other. Friendships between children of different races are common during early childhood but tend to decline in preadolescence (Sandler, 1989).

Clubs and Peer Groups. One of the outstanding characteristics of middle childhood is the formation of formalized groups or clubs. Initially, children in the early middle years merely hang around the periphery of the formalized group, watching, learning, practicing various skills, and participating in group activities whenever the members of the gang allow them to do so. In a year or two, as they advance in age, children eventually take their places as full-fledged participating members. The process is facilitated if they have a buddy.

One of the prominent features of middle childhood groups is the code of rigid rules imposed on the members. There is an exclusiveness in the selection of persons who have the privilege of joining. They often adopt a "uniform" and special words that signify membership in the group. Acceptance in the group is often determined on a pass-fail basis that is based on social or behavioral criteria. Conformity is the core of the group structure. There are often secret codes, shared interests, and special modes of dress, and each child must abide by a standard of behavior established by the group. Understanding of and conformity to the rules provide children with feelings of security and relieve them of the responsibility of making decisions.

Membership in the group provides children with a comfortable place in society. Many of the values of the group, such as physical strength, daring, ingenuity, and comradeship, have not been stressed in the family, but these, too, are worthy values and contribute to an individual child's total personality. By merging their identities with that of their peers, children are able to move from the family group to an outside group as a step toward seeking further independence. They substitute conformity to a peer-group pattern for conformity to a family pattern while they are still too shaky and insecure to function independently.

During the early school years the groups are rather small and loosely organized, with changing membership and little formal structure. They do not demonstrate the elements of give-and-take, cooperation, and order that are seen in groups of older children. As a rule, girls' groups are less formalized than boys' groups, and although there may be a mixture of both sexes in the earlier school years, the groups of later school years are composed predominantly of children of the same sex. Common interests are a frequent basis around which a group is structured.

Children's strong desire not to be different creates problems for those who are, for various reasons, unable to meet the accepted standards of the peer group. Children with disabilities or those who are in some way so deprived that they are unable to compete have a difficult time. Self-consciousness results when children are unable to dress as other children dress, do not have spending money like other children, or appear different from other children, such as the child who has numerous freckles, red hair, or minor physical defects such as strabismus. Any of these differences will set a child apart from the group and often make the child a target for the criticism and ridicule of the peer group.

Poor relationships with peers and a lack of group identification can also contribute to bullying behavior. ***Bullying*** is defined as one or more individuals inflicting physical, verbal, or emotional abuse on another. Bullying can also involve the threat of bodily harm, weapon possession, gang activity, and assault and battery.* Bullying behavior occurs frequently in school-age children who lack appropriate academic or social skills and often represents an attempt to act out anger and resentment about poor peer relationships.

Although peer-group identification and association are essential to a child's emergence into the world, there can be dangers inherent in strong peer-group attachment. Peer pressures may force children into taking risks, even against their better judgment. Minor infractions and immoralities, such as stealing apples from the neighbor's tree, smoking, or sexual exposure, are disturbing to adults but seem to be a normal part of peer-group activity. However, peer-group activities that result in unacceptable, unlawful or criminal gang violence are increasing in the United States and represent a significant challenge for health professionals and teachers who work with children (Rollins, 1993).

Relationships with Families

Although the peer group is highly influential and necessary to normal child development, parents are still the primary influence in shaping children's personalities, setting standards for behavior, and establishing value systems. It is the family values that usually predominate when parental and peer value systems come into conflict. Although children may appear to reject parental values while testing the new values of the peer group, ultimately they will retain and incorporate into their own value systems the parental values they have found to be of worth. Peer associations seem to remain within the social class system, and not infrequently there may be discriminate membership on the basis of ethnic or racial origin.

As children move into the wider world of peer-group relationships, parents are faced with the task of relinquishing their hold. They may find it difficult to face the rejection that is demonstrated as their children stand solidly with the peer group. During this time children will want to spend more time in the company of their peers and may seem eager to leave the house; they will often prefer activities of the group to family activities. This can be very disturbing to parents. During this time parents can best serve the interests of their children through tolerant understanding and support even when there may be intolerance and criticism of the parents and their ways when those ways deviate from those of the group. In the child's eyes the parents no longer assume the stature they previously enjoyed. Children discover that parents can be wrong, and they begin to question the knowledge and authority of the parents who previously were considered to be all-knowing and all-powerful.

Although increased independence is the goal of middle childhood, children are not yet prepared to reject parental control. Children need and want restrictions placed on their behavior; they are not yet prepared to cope with all the problems of their expanding environment. They feel more secure knowing that there is an authority greater than themselves to implement such controls and restrictions. Children may complain loudly about the restrictions and try their best to break down parental barriers, but they are uneasy if they can succeed in doing so. Children feel secure with reasonable, consistent controls. They respect the adults on whom they can rely to prevent them from acting on each and every urge. Children sense in this behavior an expression of love and concern for their welfare.

Children also need their parents as adults, not as pals. Sometimes parents, hurt at their children's rejection, attempt to maintain their love and gratitude by assuming the role of "pals." Children need the stable, secure strength provided by mature adults to whom they can turn during troubled relationships with peers or stressful changes in their world. During a disruption in their lives, such as times of failure, periods of illness, or a move that separates them from the security of friends, children need the firm, secure anchor of parental interest and concern. With a secure base in a loving family, children are able to develop confidence in themselves and gain the maturity needed to break loose from the group and stand independently.

Children's relationships with siblings change during the middle years (Vandell, Minnett, and Santrock, 1987). With age, siblings become more equal in power and status. Whereas in earlier years older siblings were influential in the younger siblings' learning, the previous instruction/help relationship becomes one of companionship. Positive emotional tone increases, but sibling conflict increases as the siblings get older. The researchers believe that middle childhood is a period of transition for sibling relationships, a juncture between the open bickering of early childhood and the supportive relationship observed in adult siblings.

DEVELOPMENT OF SELF-CONCEPT

Closely associated with developing a sense of industry is developing a concept of one's value and worth. With the emphasis on skill building and broadened social relationships, children are continually occupied in the process of self-evaluation. Children's self-concepts are composed of their own critical self-assessment plus what they interpret as the opinions of family members and outside social contacts—the mental picture they have of themselves, including their bodies. Although each child is different and unique, some aspects of the self-concept are common to others.

Body Image

Body image is the thoughts children entertain about their bodies. School-age children are quite knowledgeable about the human body, and social development during this period focuses to a large extent on the body and its capabilities. School-age children are able to draw a recognizable human figure, although individually their portrayal of body parts may vary considerably. They are acutely aware of bodies—their own, those of their peers, and those of adults. It

*See Clore ER, Hibel JA: Overcoming bullying behavior: a challenge to the school nurse, *School Healthwatch* 4:3-7, 1992-1993; available from F&M Projects, 276 5th Ave., Suite 902, New York, NY 10001.

is important that children know body functions and that adults correct misinformation children may have about the body (e.g., what is fat).

Social development during the school years, with emphasis on peer relationships, prescribes that children conform to group norms. They evaluate themselves to determine how their physical appearance, body configuration, and coordination compare to those of their peers. The head is the most noticeable and, to them, important part of the body. They also model themselves after their parents and compare themselves to favored peers and images observed in the media.

Children are acutely aware of physical disabilities in others, and it is not unusual for them to believe that their own bodies are not all right, are not the right size or the right shape, or are in some way defective. They respond to such concerns in a variety of ways. For example, they will conceal perceived shortcomings of body or performance, such as the obese child who refrains from going swimming, the child who conveniently forgets a gym suit, the child who conceals an imagined defect, or the child with enuresis who declines invitations to slumber parties. Children seldom express these concerns to families. However, they need to be reassured about both the uniqueness and the sameness of their bodies while their privacy is respected and they are allowed appropriate protective strategies. Children who are different become acutely aware of the differences and may find themselves excluded from the group. When children are teased or criticized about being different, the effect will be lasting. They remember the teasing well into adulthood.

Self-Esteem

Self-esteem is children's picture of their individual worth and consists of both positive and negative qualities. Children actively strive to achieve internalized goals or levels of attainment. At the same time, they continually receive feedback on the quality of their performance from those whom they consider to be authorities. By the time they reach school age, children have already received messages regarding the extent to which they are able to accomplish tasks that have been delegated to them. For example, one child may have been given prestigious responsibilities at home or at school or received special commendation for an achievement. On the other hand, another child may have been sent to a special class for slow learners or may have been the last person chosen when children choose up sides for a game. These and other signs serve as clues to social evaluation that children then incorporate as part of their self-evaluation.

Children approach the process of self-evaluation from a framework of either self-confidence or self-doubt. Children who during the preschool years have mastered the maturational crises of autonomy and initiative are able to face the world with feelings of pride rather than shame. At first, children's self-concepts are formed exclusively from what they perceive to be their parents' evaluation of them. During middle childhood the opinions of peers and teachers further complicate the process. Criticisms and peer approval are sources of data for evaluation. Parents and other adults are no longer the only persons who respond to their skills, talents, and abilities. Peers also identify skills and capabilities, and each child soon begins to internalize these outside opinions. If children regard themselves as worthwhile or satisfactory persons, they are considered to have high self-esteem, self-confidence, or a positive self-concept. If they view themselves as worthless, they are said to have poor or low self-esteem.

Pets have also been observed to influence a child's self-esteem. Pets can be important in making a child feel loved, accepted, and secure (Davis, 1985). It has been found that children who "bond" with a pet before the age of 6 years or after the age of 10 years score higher on tests of self-concept than children who acquire animals in middle childhood (Poresky and others, 1988).

The difficulty that children encounter in the attempt to assess their own abilities is their inclination to rely on their own expectations or on the expectations expressed by others regarding their performance. They depend almost entirely on external evidence of worth, such as school grades, teachers' comments, and parental and peer approval. Children do not yet have the capacity to develop their own, independent criteria by which they can evaluate their own accomplishments, and it is especially difficult for them to assess their achievement in abstract skills.

Nothing succeeds like success. The significant adults in children's lives can often manage, unseen, to manipulate their environment so that they meet with success. Each small success increases a child's self-image a little. The more positive children feel about themselves, the more confident they feel in trying again for success. All children profit from feelings that they are in some ways special to significant adults. A positive self-image makes them feel likable and worthwhile, and that they are persons with a valuable contribution to make in their world. Such feelings lead to self-respect, self-confidence, and a general feeling of happiness. Parents can assist their school-age children in developing self-esteem by helping to increase their self-confidence, by being honest, providing opportunities for creativity, helping them succeed in activities, and providing positive reinforcement. Nurses can enhance self-esteem by fostering supportive relationships between children and members of their families and by emphasizing children's strengths and positive aspects of their behavior (Winkelstein, 1989).

DEVELOPMENT OF SEXUALITY

Evidence indicates that many children experience some form of sex play during or before preadolescence as a response to normal curiosity, not as a result of love or sexual urge. Children are experimentalists by nature, and this play is incidental and transitory. Any adverse emotional consequences or guilt feelings depend on how the behavior is managed by the parents, if it is discovered, or whether children view their actions as wrong in the eyes of significant persons, particularly the parents (Levine, 1992).

Much of children's attitude toward sex that is acquired indirectly at a very early age affects the way in which they respond to sexual information presented at a later time.

Many parents discourage sex exploration either through subtle substitution of activities that divert their children's attention from the genitalia or by expressions of anger or disgust at their behavior. These tactics clearly communicate to children that they should not engage in such activities or ask questions about sex or their genitals, which limits the children's sources of information.

In addition, parents seldom teach young children the correct terminology for sexual organs or sexual feeling; therefore the only vocabulary available to them is the one that identifies sexual organs with excretory functions. Thus these parental attitudes influence the children's perception of the cleanliness of their genitalia. If they learn that excretory organs and functions are dirty, they may associate the "dirtiness' with the reproductive organs and functions. If children learn the correct terminology for the organs and their functions, this association should be reduced or eliminated.

Sex Education

Because parents often either repress or avoid their children's sexual curiosity, the sexual information that they receive in childhood is acquired almost entirely from their peers. When peers are the primary source of sexual information, it is transmitted and exchanged in secret, clandestine conversation and contains a large amount of misinformation. The context in which these communications take place creates anxiety in children and barriers to trust; therefore, they continue to keep sexuality a secret. These reactions inhibit spontaneous expressions or questioning of the parents.

The subject of where sex education should be taught and by whom arouses a good deal of controversy. Many individuals and groups are unconditionally opposed to the inclusion of sex education in the schools. Others believe that sex information should not be taught separately from other information but should be presented as naturally as information about other body functions and natural phenomena such as the solar system, the changing seasons, and the migratory habits of birds. Children's questions about sex should be answered to the same extent as their questions about any other topic—honestly and at their level of understanding. During the preschool years children will be satisfied with simple answers, but as they gain more knowledge and understanding of the world, their curiosity about everything will be deeper. When sex is treated as though it is a normal part of growth and development and questions are answered matter-of-factly, parental responses are less apt to contain overtones of guilt and anxiety that in turn produce anxiety in children.

Middle childhood appears to be an ideal time for formal sex education, and many authorities believe that the topic is best presented from a life-span approach. Initial curiosity about differences in body structure between boys and girls and between children and adults occurs in the preschool years, and the next stage, adolescence, arouses both anxiety and excitement about sexual encounters. Information about sexual maturation and the process of reproduction presented during middle childhood helps to minimize a child's uncertainty, embarrassment, and feelings of isolation that often accompany the events of puberty.

Although sex education programs are not universally a part of the elementary school curriculum, some progressive educators have successfully incorporated sex education into a number of school programs. Because of the natural social orientation of this period of development, structured group learning situations can be successfully used for discussion of sexuality. Children are more comfortable if boys and girls are segregated for discussions, but each needs information about both sexes.

An approach that has been advanced suggests that sexuality can best be presented in the context of its central role as a biologic mechanism for the survival of the culture. Children can learn that sexual maturation and reproduction are each individual's contribution to the natural order of things. This approach provides a natural entry into discussion of sexuality as a basis for family units, marriage, and attitudes toward children, as well as an entry into a presentation of the biologic facts of sexuality. More difficult, but equally important, is for children to view sexual intimacy as a close, personal relationship and a means of conveying love, as well as a means for ensuring the survival of the species.

Preadolescents need more precise information. They are interested in concrete information, such as "What if I start my period in the middle of class?" or "How can I keep people from telling I have an erection?" It is important to tell them what they want to know and what they can expect to happen as they become mature sexually.

Nurse's Role in Sex Education

No matter where nurses practice, they can provide information on human sexuality to both parents and children. Nurses can help parents by first becoming knowledgeable about human sexuality themselves, including the common myths and misconceptions associated with sex and the reproductive process. They need to know their own attitudes and feelings toward sexuality and to feel comfortable with these feelings.

During encounters with parents, nurses can be open and available for questions and discussion. They can set an example by the language they use in discussing body parts and their function and by the way in which they deal with problems that have emotional overtones, such as exploratory sex play and masturbation. Parents need to be helped to understand normal behaviors and to view sexual curiosity in their children as a part of the developmental process. Assessing the parents' level of knowledge and understanding of sexuality provides cues to their need for supplemental information that will better prepare them for the increasingly complex explanations that will be needed as their children grow older.

Sometimes short classes or group discussions for parents are helpful for discussing disturbing behaviors and anticipating the questions and forthcoming learning needs of the children. When possible, it is wise to include both parents. Sex education in the home should be assumed by both parents so that the children will not acquire a distorted view of either the male or the female role that may alter relationships with the opposite sex in later life. Most important, nurses should take an active role in encouraging, developing, and providing sex education to children at all levels as an integral part of their learning.

PLAY

As children enter the school years, their play takes on new dimensions that reflect a new stage of development. Not only does play involve increased physical skill, intellectual ability, and fantasy, but as they form groups and cliques, children begin to evolve a sense of team or club. To belong to a group is of vital importance. Each individual child must abide by the rules of the group, which may be extremely rigid, and energy is devoted to team success, as well as personal success.

Rules and Rituals

The need for conformity in middle childhood is strongly manifested in the activities and games so important in the life of school-age children. Up to this point they have either played games they have invented themselves or have played in the company of a friend or an adult, and rules more or less evolved with the game. Now they begin to see the need for rules, and the games they play have fixed and unvarying rules that may be bizarre and extraordinarily rigid (especially those made up by the group). But part of the enjoyment of the game is to know the rules, since knowing means belonging. Once the rules are established and agreed on, the demand for conformity is vigorous (Fig. 17-7).

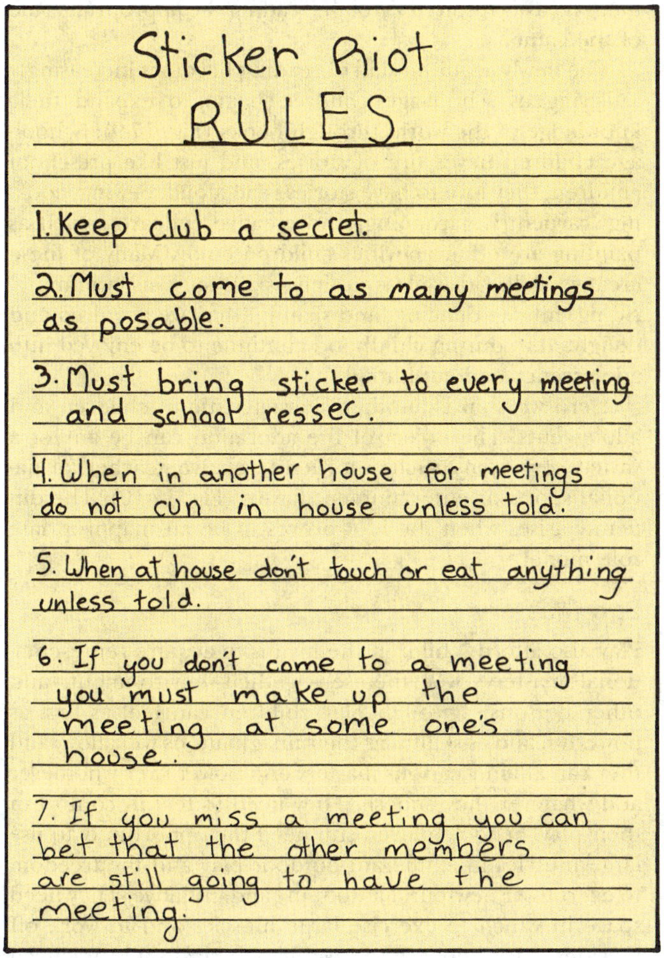

Sticker Riot
RULES

1. Keep club a secret.

2. Must come to as many meetings as posable.

3. Must bring sticker to every meeting and school ressec.

4. When in another house for meetings do not cun in house unless told.

5. When at house don't touch or eat anything unless told.

6. If you don't come to a meeting you must make up the meeting at some one's house.

7. If you miss a meeting you can bet that the other members are still going to have the meeting.

FIG. 17-7 A list of club rules compiled by a group of 9-year-old children.

Conformity and ritual permeate the play of school-age children. Not only do they dominate in games, but they are also evident in much of the children's behavior and language. Childhood is full of chants and taunts such as, "Eeny, meeny, miney, mo," "Johnny's mad and I'm glad," "Last one is a rotten egg," and "Step on a crack, break your mother's back." Children derive a great deal of pleasure from such sayings that have been handed down with few changes through generation after generation of children. Sometimes these sayings are elaborated on with particular variations to meet the special attributes of a particular group. The undeviating ritual frequently is invested with some magical quality that serves to give the children involved a sense of power over the unconquerable world about them.

Team Play. A more complex form of group play that evolves from group games is the team game and those sports that form part of the life of the early school years. The rules of such games may even require the presence of a referee, umpire, or person of authority in order that they can be followed more accurately. Team membership has three significant characteristics that promote child development during the middle years (Newman and Newman, 1991).

First, children learn to subordinate personal goals to group goals. Team membership means that each child is accountable to the other team members and carries with it the responsibility that each member's acts may affect the success or failure of the entire group. Each member's behavior is open to public evaluation, and children risk ostracism or ridicule if they contribute to a team loss. Team accomplishments reflect on all the players. Although individual skills are recognized, team successes and failures are shared by all members—the best and the poorest alike. In this way children learn the concept of interdependence, that all players must rely on one another. Unfortunately instead of the better members helping the weaker members to improve, all too often the poorer members are scorned and scapegoated, especially when the team loses.

Second, children learn about division of labor as an effective strategy for the attainment of a goal. They learn that each position on a team has a specific function and that the team has a greater chance of winning if each person performs a specific function instead of the work of all the other members. Once children learn this concept in team play, they can transfer the knowledge to other aspects of life. Once they learn that certain goals are best accomplished by dividing tasks among several individuals, they begin to see a relationship to principles of organization in other social structures. A corollary to this is the concept that some children are best equipped to perform one part of the task, whereas other children are best suited to another aspect of the task.

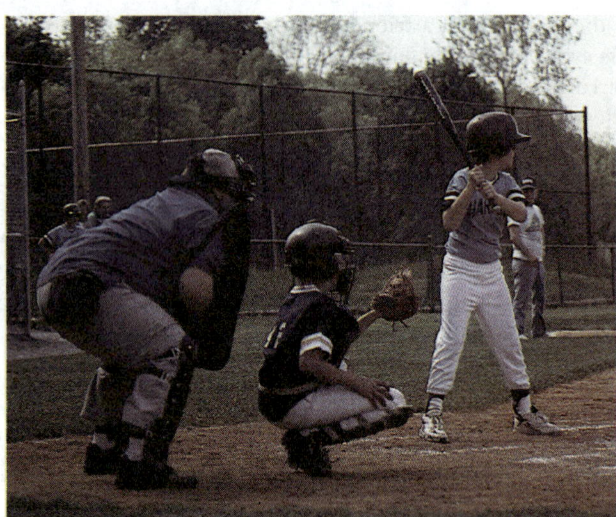

FIG. 17-8 Activities engaged in by school-age children, such as Little League baseball, vary according to the child's interest and opportunity.

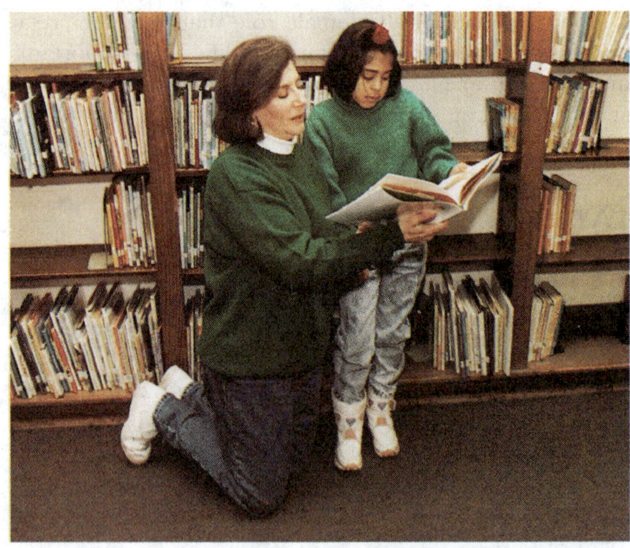

FIG. 17-9 Selecting a book with the assistance of an adult.

Third, team play helps children to learn about the nature of competition and the importance of winning—an attribute highly valued in the United States. In all team play there is a winning and losing side. Since losing is often interpreted as failure, children will go to great lengths to avoid the public embarrassment and personal shame that accompany failure. The more a child identifies with the team and values membership in the group, the more distasteful losing becomes. Fear of losing and the failure it implies are strong incentives for group commitment. The importance of winning is not universally valued, however. Some cultures and subcultures place emphasis on the game and consideration for one's companion rather than on the outcome.

Team play can also contribute to children's social, intellectual, and skill growth. Children will work hard to develop the skills needed to become members of a team, to improve their contribution to the group effort, and to anticipate the consequences of their behavior for the group. Team play helps stimulate cognitive growth, as children are called on to learn many complex rules, make judgments about those rules, plan strategies, and assess the strengths and weaknesses of members of their own team and the opposing team (Fig. 17-8).

Quiet Games and Activities

Although the play of school-age children is highly active, they also enjoy many quiet and solitary activities. The middle childhood years are the time for collections, which constitute another ritual. Young school-age children's collections are an odd assortment of unrelated objects in messy, disorganized piles. Collections of later years are more orderly and selective, and they are organized neatly in scrapbooks, on shelves, or in boxes.

School-age children become fascinated with increasingly complex board or card games, such as Monopoly and rummy, that they can play with a best friend or a group. As in all games, their adherence to rules is fanatic. There is usually much discussion and argument, but the disagreement is easily resolved through reading the appropriate rule of the game.

The newly acquired skill of reading becomes increasingly satisfying as school-age children begin to expand their knowledge of the world through books (Fig. 17-9). School-age children never tire of stories, and just like preschool children, they love to have stories read aloud. Sewing, cooking, carpentry, gardening, and creative endeavors such as painting are other activities children enjoy. Many of these creative skills, as well as athletic skills such as swimming, riding, hiking, dancing, and skating, that are acquired and delighted in during childhood continue to be enjoyed into adolescence and adulthood.

Hero worship is another characteristic of children and adolescents. The object of the adoration can be any of a variety of persons, such as a friend, relative, teacher, or national sports or entertainment figure (Fig. 17-10). The difficulty arises when the idol proves to be an inappropriate role model.

Ego Mastery

Play also affords children the means to acquire representational mastery over themselves, their environment, and other persons. Through play children can feel as big, as powerful, and as skillful as their imaginations will allow, and they can attain vicarious mastery and power over whomever and whatever they choose. They need to feel in control in their play. Schoolchildren still need the opportunity to use large muscles in exuberant outdoor play and the freedom to exert their newfound autonomy and initiative. They need space in which to exercise large muscles and to work off tensions, frustrations, and hostility. Physical skills practiced and mastered in play help them develop a feeling of personal competence, which contributes to a sense of accom-

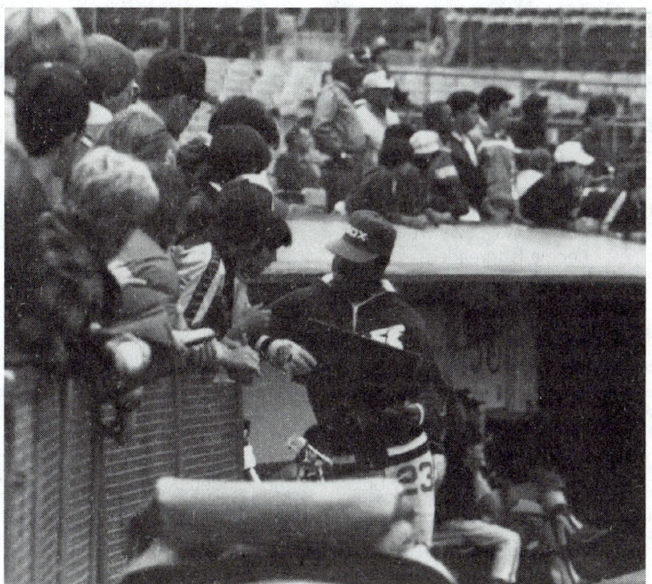

FIG. 17-10 Hero worship is a characteristic of middle childhood.

plishment and helps provide a place of status in the peer group.

■ ■ ■

A summary of growth and development in middle childhood is presented in Table 17-1. Since each child has a unique developmental pattern, any attempt to describe the typical child of any age-group can only represent an average and should not be considered as absolute criteria for any given child.

COPING WITH CONCERNS RELATED TO NORMAL GROWTH AND DEVELOPMENT

SCHOOL EXPERIENCE

The school serves as the agent for transmitting the values of the society to each succeeding generation of children and as the setting for much of their relationship with peers. As a socializing agent second only to the family, the school exerts a profound influence on the social development of children.

School entrance causes a sharp break in the structure of a child's world. For some children it is their first experience in conforming to a group pattern imposed by an adult who is not a parent and who has responsibility for too many children to be constantly aware of each child as an individual. Children want to go to school and usually adapt to the new condition with little difficulty. Successful adjustment is directly related to the child's physical and emotional maturity and the parent's readiness to accept the separation associated with school entrance. Cooperation among parents and support for the child are successful ways of coping with school entry stress (Elizur, 1986). Unfortunately, some parents express their unconscious attempts to delay their child's maturity by clinging behavior, particularly with their youngest child.

Anticipatory Socialization

By the time they enter school, the majority of children have a fairly realistic concept of what school involves. They receive information regarding the role of pupil from parents, playmates, and the communication media. In addition, most children have had some experience with daycare or preschool, and kindergarten.

Children's attitudes toward school and the extent of their adjustment are strongly influenced by the attitudes of their parents. Middle-class children have fewer adjustments to make and less to learn about expected behavior, since the school tends to reflect middle-class customs and values, although this may be tempered by the school's location and predominant teachers and student body. Parents who view school as a place that they have helped to create and support and that is directed toward the same objectives for socialization as their own usually prepare their children with useful anticipatory socialization and furnish them with confidence to meet the challenge. Parents who view the school as an agency of an alien culture and one that they have little, if any, power to affect may unknowingly teach their children to be fearful of school, even though they agree with its purposes and objectives.

Anticipatory socialization is also provided by television, the power of which cannot be overestimated in the acquisition of information and attitudes. Whether programming has socialization as the primary objective (such as the children's program, "Sesame Street") or general entertainment (including commercials), television viewing increases a child's vocabulary, extends the child's horizons, and paves the way for the school experience. Despite its tremendous potential for educating, television relies heavily on images to convey information. Consequently, difficult complex issues are often not adequately explored by the medium. Extensive television viewing may also encourage children to seek simple answers to tough problems and to believe that violence is the most effective and quick solution to conflict (American Academy of Pediatrics, 1991a).

Although most children have had some experience with schooling before they enter first grade, the extent to which early childhood education prepares children for primary school varies. Some preschool programs merely provide custodial care; others emphasize emotional, social, and intellectual development as well. The type of early childhood programming that stresses a cognitive over a social emphasis appears to be more effective in facilitating later academic performance, particularly in children from low-income families.

Role of the Teacher

To facilitate transition from home to school, educators select teachers with personality characteristics that allow them to deal with potential problems of young children. Because they react to the teacher on the basis of past experience,

TABLE 17-1 Growth and Development During School-Age Years

AGE (YEARS)	PHYSICAL AND MOTOR	MENTAL	ADAPTIVE	PERSONAL-SOCIAL
6	Growth and weight gain continues slowly Weight: 16-23.6 kg (35½-58 pounds); height: 106.6-123.5 cm (42-48 inches) Central mandibular incisors erupt Loses first tooth Gradual increase in dexterity Activity age; constant activity Often returns to finger feeding More aware of hand as a tool Likes to draw, print, and color Vision reaches maturity	Develops concept of numbers Counts 13 pennies Knows whether it is morning or afternoon Defines common objects such as fork and chair in terms of their use Obeys triple commands in succession Knows right and left hands Says which is pretty and which is ugly of a series of drawings of faces Describes the objects in a picture rather than simply enumerating them Attends first grade	At table, uses knife to spread butter or jam on bread At play, cuts, folds, pastes paper toys, sews crudely if needle is threaded Takes bath without supervision; performs bedtime activities alone Reads from memory; enjoys oral spelling game Likes table games, checkers, simple card games Giggles a lot Sometimes steals money or attractive items Has difficulty owning up to misdeeds Tries out own abilities	Can share and cooperate better Has great need for children of own age Will cheat to win Often engages in rough play Often jealous of younger brother or sister Does what adults are seen doing May have occasional temper tantrums Is a boaster Is more independent, probably influence of school Has own way of doing things Increases socialization
7	Begins to grow at least 2 inches a year Weight: 17.7-30 kg (39-66½ pounds); height: 111.8-129.7 cm (44-51 inches) Maxillary central incisors and lateral mandibular incisors erupt More cautious in approaches to new performances Repeats performances to master them Jaw begins to expand to accommodate permanent teeth	Notices that certain parts are missing from pictures Can copy a diamond Repeats three numbers backward Develops concept of time; reads ordinary clock or watch correctly to nearest quarter hour; uses clock for practical purposes Attends the second grade More mechanical in reading; often does not stop at the end of a sentence, skips words such as "it," "the," and "he"	Uses table knife for cutting meat; may need help with tough or difficult pieces Brushes and combs hair acceptably without help May steal Likes to help and have a choice Is less resistant and stubborn	Is becoming a real member of the family group Takes part in group play Boys prefer playing with boys; girls prefer playing with girls Spends a lot of time alone; does not require a lot of companionship
8-9	Continues to grow at 5 cm (2 inches) a year Weight: 19.6-39.6 kg (43-87 pounds); height: 117-141.8 cm (46-56 inches) Lateral incisors (maxillary) and mandibular cuspids erupt Movement fluid: often graceful and poised Always on the go; jumps, chases, skips Increased smoothness and speed in fine motor control; uses cursive writing Dresses self completely Likely to overdo; hard to quiet down after recess More limber; bones grow faster than ligaments	Gives similarities and differences between two things from memory Counts backward from 20 to 1; understands concept of reversibility Repeats days of the week and months in order; knows the date Describes common objects in detail, not merely their use Makes change out of a quarter Attends third and fourth grades Reads more; may plan to wake up early just to read Reads classic books, but also enjoys comics More aware of time; can be relied on to get to school on time Can grasp concepts of parts and whole (fractions) Understands concepts of space, cause and effect, nesting (puzzles), conservation (permanence of mass and volume)	Makes use of common tools such as hammer, saw, or screwdriver Uses household and sewing utensils Helps with routine household tasks such as dusting, sweeping Assumes responsibility for share of household chores Looks after all of own needs at table Buys useful articles; exercises some choice in making purchases Runs useful errands Likes pictorial magazines Likes school; wants to answer all the questions Is afraid of failing a grade; is ashamed of bad grades Is more critical of self Takes music and sport lessons	Is easy to get along with at home Likes the reward system Dramatizes Is more sociable Is better behaved Is interested in boy-girl relationships but will not admit it Goes about home and community freely, alone or with friends Likes to compete and play games Shows preference in friends and groups Plays mostly with groups of own sex but is beginning to mix Develops modesty Compares self with others Enjoys Scouts, group sports

TABLE 17-1 Growth and Development During School-Age Years—cont'd

AGE (YEARS)	PHYSICAL AND MOTOR	MENTAL	ADAPTIVE	PERSONAL-SOCIAL
		Classifies objects by more than one quality; has collections Produces simple paintings or drawings		
10-12	*Boys:* Slow growth in height and rapid weight gain; may become obese in this period Weight: 24.3-58 kg (54-128 pounds); height: 127.5-162.3 cm (50-64 inches) Posture is more similar to an adult's; will overcome lordosis *Girls:* pubescent changes may begin to appear; body lines soften and round out Remainder of teeth will erupt and tend toward full development (except wisdom teeth)	Writes brief stories Attends fifth to seventh grades Writes occasional short letters to friends or relatives on own initiative Uses telephone for practical purposes Responds to magazine, radio, or other advertising Reads for practical information or own enjoyment—stories or library books of adventure or romance, or animal stories	Makes useful articles or does easy repair work Cooks or sews in small way Raises pets Washes and dries own hair Is responsible for a thorough job of cleaning hair, but may need reminding to do so Is sometimes left alone at home for an hour or so Is successful in looking after own needs or those of other children left in his or her care	Is fond of friends Chooses friends more selectively; may have a "best friend" Loves conversation Develops beginning interest in opposite sex Is more diplomatic Likes family; family really has meaning Likes mother and wants to please her in many ways Demonstrates affection Likes dad, too; he is adored and idolized Respects parents Loves friends; talks about them constantly

children respond best to teachers with attributes that they would desire in a warm, loving parent. As a parent surrogate, the teacher in the early grades performs many of the activities formerly assumed by the parents (usually the mother), such as recognizing the children's personal needs (such as a need to go to the bathroom or for help with clothing) and helping to develop their social behavior (such as manners).

Teachers, like parents, are concerned about the psychologic and emotional welfare of children. Although the functions of teachers and parents differ, both place constraints on behavior, and both are in a position to enforce standards of conduct. However, the teacher's primary responsibility is stimulating and guiding children's intellectual development, as opposed to providing for their physical welfare beyond the school setting.

Teachers share the parental influence in shaping a child's attitudes and values. They serve as models with whom children can identify and whom they try to emulate. Teacher approval is sought; teacher disapproval is avoided. The teacher is a very significant person in the life of a child during the early school years, and hero worship of a teacher may extend into late childhood and preadolescence. It is not uncommon for the first or second grader to be heartbroken and tearful at leaving a familiar teacher at the end of the school term or to be upset when faced with a substitute teacher for even a short period.

Children's interest in school and learning and much of their social interaction and self-concept are related to interactions with the teacher (Fig. 17-11). The differential systems of reward and punishment administered by the teachers affect the emotional adjustment and self-concept of children, as well as how they respond to school in general (see also Thinking Critically About . . . box on corporal punishment in school, p. 738). The interaction between the teacher and individual pupils affects the pupil's acceptance by other children, which in turn affects the child's self-concept. Behaviors praised by the teacher usually acquire a positive value, whereas those viewed negatively by the teacher are similarly devalued by the children. In this way

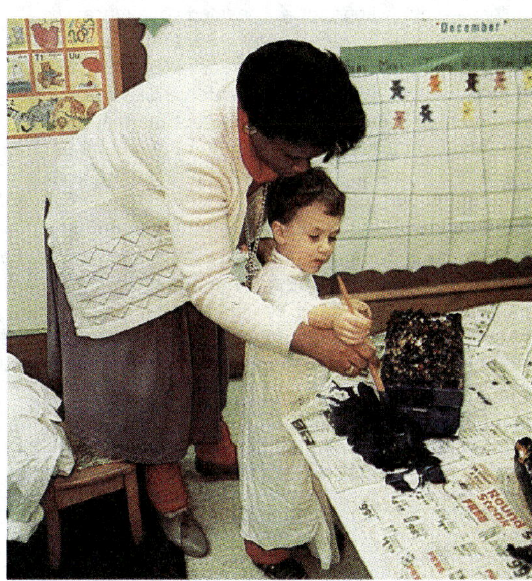

FIG. 17-11 School represents an important change in a child's life, and teachers exert a significant influence on the child.

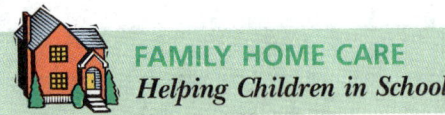

FAMILY HOME CARE
Helping Children in School

GENERAL GUIDELINES

Be supportive—through companionship share ideas and thoughts.
Be positive—every child should experience some success each day.
Share an interest in reading—use the library, discuss books they are reading.
Support and encourage activity rather than passivity.
Encourage originality—help children make their own projects from discarded articles or other available materials.
Foster the development of hobbies and collections.
Encourage children to wonder and reflect during free time.
Encourage family experiences and trips to places of interest.
Encourage questions—help children discover sources for information or places in which to explore and investigate.
Stimulate creative thinking and problem solving—help children try out new solutions to problems without fear of making mistakes.
Use rewards rather than punishment.

SPECIFIC GUIDELINES

Meet the teacher at the beginning of school and plan to visit the school to see what is taught and expected.
Send the child to school every day—teachers are concerned when parents make other plans for their children; it conveys the impression that school is unimportant.
Demonstrate an interest in what the child is learning.
Demonstrate an interest in content and growth more than in grades.
Make it clear to the child that schoolwork is between the child and the teacher; teacher and child should set goals for better school performance to allow the child to feel responsible for school successes and failures.
Take advantage of situations that support and reinforce school learning.
Share information with teachers that will help them understand the child better.
Communicate with the teacher if there appears to be a problem—avoid waiting for a scheduled conference.
Provide a quiet, well-lighted area for study that is safe from interruption; do not allow television or radio.
Avoid dictating a study time, but do enforce rules, such a no television until homework is done; accept the child's word that work is complete.
Help with homework should focus on explaining the question, not giving the answer.
Teach the child to break large tasks (such as a report) into smaller manageable tasks spread over the allotted time rather than attempt the entire project the night before it is to be completed.
Limit home tutoring to special circumstances, such as when the teacher requests parental assistance after a child's prolonged absence.
Request special help for children with learning problems.
Support the school staff by showing respect for both the school system and the teacher, at least in the child's presence.

the teacher exerts considerable influence in a number of areas, such as attitudes toward minority groups, the disabled, or less favorably endowed children. Teacher approval of and self-acceptance in children are very closely related.

The teacher sets the emotional tone of the classroom. Those who are able to establish a positive social climate are usually concerned about the mental health and social dynamics of the children. Feeling a responsibility for personality development in their pupils, they are alert and sensitive to a child's anxieties, peer-group relationships, self-concepts, and general attitudes toward school. Learner-centered behaviors, such as supportive statements that reassure or commend children, accepting and clarifying statements that help them refine ideas and feelings to provide a sense of being understood, and constructive assistance that aids them with their own problem solving, all contribute to the expansion and development of a positive self-concept.

Role of the Parents

Parents share responsibility within the schools for helping children achieve their maximum potential. There are numerous ways in which parents can supplement the school program (see Family Home Care box). Cultivating responsibility is the goal of parental assistance. Being responsible for schoolwork helps children learn to keep promises, meet deadlines, and succeed at their jobs as adults. Responsible children may occasionally ask for help (e.g., with a spelling list), but usually they like to think through their work by themselves. Excessive pressure or lack of encouragement from parents may inhibit the development of these desirable traits (Schmitt, 1990).

LIMIT-SETTING AND DISCIPLINE

Numerous factors influence the amount and manner of discipline and limit-setting imposed on school-age children: the psychosocial maturity of the parents, childhood child-rearing experiences of the parents, temperament of the children, context of the children's misconduct, and response of the children to rewards and punishments. The purpose of discipline is (1) to help the child interrupt or inhibit a forbidden action; (2) to point out a more acceptable form of behavior so that the child knows what is right in a future situation; (3) to provide some reason, understandable to the child, that explains why one action is inappropriate and another action is more desirable; and (4) to stimulate the child's ability to empathize with the victim of a misdeed (Newman and Newman, 1991).

As children are increasingly able to see a situation from the point of view of another, they are able to understand the effects of their reactions on others and themselves. Disciplinary techniques should help children control their own behavior. Reasoning is an effective technique for this age-group. With advancing cognitive skills they are able to benefit from more complex types of disciplinary strategies. For example, withholding privileges, requiring recompense, imposing penalties, and contracting can be used with great success. Problem solving is the best approach to limit-setting, and children themselves can be included in the process of determining appropriate disciplinary measures.

Dishonest Behavior

During middle childhood it is not uncommon for children to engage in what is considered to be antisocial behavior. Lying, stealing, and cheating may become manifest in previously well-behaved children. It is especially disturbing to parents who may have difficulty coping with this behavior.

Lying can occur for a number of reasons. Preschool children often have difficulty distinguishing between fact and fantasy. They do not as yet have the cognitive capacity to deliberately mislead. Sometimes they misperceive or fail to remember an event. By the time they reach school age they still tell stories but can distinguish between what is real and what is make-believe. If not, they need to be taught to distinguish between fantasy and reality. Often children will exaggerate a story or situation as a means to impress their family or friends.

Young children will lie to escape punishment or get out of some difficulty, even when the evidence of their misbehavior is before their eyes. Lying is more common in families in which punishment is severe. Also, the honesty and veracity modeled by the parents is repeated in the children. If parents lie, the children will emulate their behavior. Older children may lie in order to meet expectations set by others to which they have been unable to measure up. They may lie because of a low self-esteem, as a means for getting ahead or acquiring something with little effort, or for a variety of other reasons. However, most children are very concerned with the wrongfulness of lying and cheating—especially in their friends. They are quick to tell on others when they catch them in the act of cheating.

Parents need to be reassured that all children lie sometimes and that they often have difficulty separating fantasy from reality. Parents should be helped to understand the importance of their own behavior as role models and of being truthful in their relationships with children. The issue can be discussed with the children directly to impress on them how much of their own security and respect is lost when they are not believed.

Cheating is most common in young children, ages 5 to 6. They find it difficult to lose at a game or contest and cheat in order to win. They have not yet acquired the full realization of the wrongfulness of this behavior and do it almost automatically. It usually disappears as they mature. However, when children observe parental behaviors, such as boasting about cheating on income taxes or some transaction, they assume this to be appropriate behavior. Parents need to be aware of the types of behaviors they model for their children. When they set examples of honesty, children are more likely to conform to these standards.

Like other ethically related behavior, ***stealing*** is not an unexpected event in the younger child. Between ages 5 and 8 years, children's sense of property rights is limited, and they tend to take something simply because they are attracted to it, or they take money for what it will buy. They are equally likely to give away something valuable that belongs to them. When young children are caught and punished, they are penitent—"didn't mean to," and promise "never to do it again," but it is quite likely that they will repeat the performance the following day. Often they not only steal, but will lie about it as well or attempt to justify the act with excuses. It is seldom helpful to trap children into admission by asking directly if they did the offensive thing. Children do not take on such responsibility until nearer the end of middle childhood.

There are several reasons why children steal: lack of a sense of property rights, trying to acquire the means with which to bribe favors from other children, a strong desire to own the coveted item, or as a means for revenge in order to "get back at someone" (usually a parent) for what they consider to be unfair treatment. Older children may steal to supplement an inadequate income from other sources. Sometimes stealing is an indication that something is seriously wrong or lacking in the child's life. For example, a child may steal to make up for love or another satisfaction that he feels is lacking.

In some settings where living arrangements are crowded and children have little privacy and much of the family property is communal, children may fail to develop a sense of property rights. Also, sometimes parents unintentionally confuse children with seemingly conflicting values. In the attempt to teach unselfishness, they may force children to share belongings with others, with the result that the children fail to develop a true sense of property rights.

If children are told not to take money from their mother's purse or their father's pocket, but observe the parents doing the same thing, they receive conflicting messages. Parents may go through a child's pockets or other private areas at night and even discard, without explanation, items of which they do not approve. Children should have some place that is private to them alone and is respected by other family members. If children's personal rights are respected, they are more likely to respect the rights of others.

It is difficult for many parents to cope with stealing by their children. However, in most situations it is best not to attempt to find a hidden or deep meaning to the stealing. An admonition, together with an appropriate and reasonable punishment, such as having the older child pay back the money or return the stolen items, will take care of the majority of cases. Most children can be taught to respect the property rights of others with little difficulty, despite the temptations and opportunities presented to them. Some children simply need more time to learn the importance of the culture's rules regarding private property.

COPING WITH STRESS

Children of today are under a tremendous amount of stress, and they are pressured from a variety of directions. It is impossible to describe all the stressors to which children are subjected. Some are discussed elsewhere in this book under specific types of stresses, especially those in which nurses assume a major role, such as hospitalization, illness, abuse, crippling injuries, and death or the threat of death.

In the normal course of growing up, children are pressured by their peers to identify with their friends; to eat, dress, and look like their friends; to talk about the same things that their friends talk about; to engage in the same activities as their friends and yet to compete with them. They are pressured by parents to excel in school, in athletics, or other activities and socially at ever younger ages. Children in middle-class America today face more stresses in their effort to live up to greater expectations than have children in previous generations. They are overprogrammed with activities such as ballet lessons, music lessons, athletics, and other activities until the cumulative effect is overwhelming.

Although children receive better treatment than in earlier times when beatings and child labor were commonplace, their physical and emotional well-being is threatened by different stresses. Children are stressed by conflict within the home. An assessment of quality of life in school-age children indicated that hearing parents quarrel was high on the list of things that worry children the most (Neff and Dale, 1990). The high divorce rate and the number of single-parent families results in altered relationships and increasing responsibilities for children. Increasing violence within the family, the school, and the community also serves as a major stressor for many children. At least 3.3 million children are at risk for witnessing domestic violence or parental abuse each year (Jaffee, Wolfe, and Wilson, 1990). A survey of public and private school-age children in California revealed that 52% of fourth, fifth, and sixth grade students feared getting stabbed (Winton, 1992). Seventy-two percent of inner-city children know someone who was shot or murdered (Hechinger, 1992). Exposure to violence in the family, school, or community affects children's ability to concentrate and function (Groves and others, 1993). Garbarino and colleagues (1992) noted that children exposed to violence often display symptoms associated with posttraumatic stress disorder, such as poor performance in school, nightmares, flashbacks, and a fatalistic orientation to the future.

The school environment is often a stressful experience for some children and a threat to their self-image. A report by Krugman and Krugman (1984) describes a number of children who were emotionally abused by an elementary school teacher whose behavior included harassment, labeling ("stupid"), screaming at the children until they cried, inappropriate threats to obtain class control, unrealistic academic goals, fear-inducing techniques, and physical punishments (see Thinking Critically About . . . box). The students displayed behaviors noticeably different from those of previous school years, symptoms of stress, expressions of excessive worry about school, change from positive to negative self-perception, and verbalizations of fear of physical harm from the teacher. Although parents and nurses should be cautious in attempts to interpret such behaviors (they are in many ways similar to school phobia; see Chapter 18), a high degree of suspicion might be justified if the symptoms are not explained by other factors or represent a marked change from previous patterns.

Children are also being encouraged to feel, think, and behave at a level of maturity far beyond what could reasonably be expected of persons their age (Elkind, 1981). They are expected to take on many adult-type responsibilities, to make decisions they are not really able to make, and to achieve more. They have little time for being *children.*

THINKING CRITICALLY ABOUT . . . *Corporal Punishment in School*

Although school should provide a safe environment for fostering education and self-esteem, it may also be a violent and stressful environment. As of this writing, 23 states in the United States allow corporal punishment in schools. The use of punishment such as paddling, slapping, pinching, or forcing the child to eat noxious substances (such as soap) or assume tiring positions for long periods of time is often based on religious beliefs and the philosophy that it is a teacher's right to preserve a disciplined classroom. It is ironic that teachers, by law, must report abuse inflicted by parents by these same methods, but teachers are permitted by law in many states to inflict the same abuse. Isn't this sanctioned child abuse (Nelms, 1988)?

Corporal punishment by teachers (or anyone else) can result in significant physical injuries, such as a fractured coccyx, ruptured kidney, broken bones and consequent fat emboli, subdural hematoma, internal hemorrhage, and damage to the sciatic nerve. In addition, it can cause intense psychologic stress from humiliation, degradation, a desire to retaliate, internalization of resentment and hatred, and the potential for more violence. Studies show that when corporal punishment in school is abolished, attendance, scholastic performance, and morale improve.

Health professionals can contribute to the abolishment of corporal punishment in schools. Several organizations, such as the National Association of Pediatric Nurse Associates and Practitioners (1993), the American Academy of Pediatrics (1991b), and the Society for Adolescent Medicine (1992), have issued statements promoting the legal prohibition of such punishment in schools and the use of alternative methods of managing student behavior.

Do you know about the school board policies and relevant state laws regarding corporal punishment? What are your views about the use of physical punishment as a disciplinary method? Certainly, the use of atraumatic care in any setting speaks strongly against the use of physical violence on children. (See also Limit-Setting and Discipline in Chapter 3 and Atraumatic Care in Chapter 1.)

From Liguori R: Abolishing corporal punishment in the school: role of the school nurse, *School Healthwatch* 2(2):3-7, 1994. Available from F&M Projects, 276 5th Ave., Suite 902, New York, NY 10001.

Children need time for the spontaneous activities of childhood.

The sources of such problems can be categorized as (1) inner feelings, such as being angry, embarrassed, feeling jealous, or being unable to fall asleep; (2) the behavior of others, such as fights with friends, being teased, being ignored, not being listened to, parents traveling or fighting, or teachers getting angry; and (3) objective situations, such as school, moving, hospitalization, auditions, sports, or being left alone (Saunders and Remsberg, 1984). The responses are those observed in any stress situation: doing nothing, acting impulsively, or problem solving. Potential sources of stress are listed in the box below.

Many variables contribute to children's ability to cope with stress. Masten and others (1988) found that children ages 8 to 13 with low IQs, low socioeconomic status, and poor family relationships displayed disruptive behavior in school when faced with a stressful life event (e.g., parental separation or a death in the family). Under similar circumstances, more advantaged children did not exhibit such behavior, although they were less interested in school than nonstressed peers. Boys appeared to be more susceptible than girls. It was speculated that boys experienced less social support at school than did girls.

POTENTIAL SOURCES OF STRESS IN MIDDLE CHILDHOOD

SOURCES OF STRESS FOR THE SIX-YEAR-OLD

Expectations—Parents, teachers, and other adults begin to demand more

School—First grade introduces the child to the more formal, academic setting; it may be the child's first experience away from home all day

Activity level—May find it difficult to sit still for long periods of time; may have frequent accidents, such as spilling milk

Competition—The child wants to be "first" or best

Shyness—May initially be shy in a new situation but usually recovers quickly

Aggression—May become hostile or aggressive; temper tantrums peak

Sensitivity—Begins to read body language or facial expressions and becomes upset when disapproval is sensed

Teasing—Engages in teasing, but becomes upset when on the receiving end

Decisions—Has difficulty coping with increasing independence

Jealousy—Sibling rivalry is common

Fears—Usually center around newly found independence and might include fear of getting lost or fear of making an embarrassing social blunder

SOURCES OF STRESS FOR THE SEVEN-YEAR-OLD

Moodiness—Is often moody, unhappy, or pensive

Approval—Continues to need praise and approval from peer group and parents

Modesty—Demands privacy when in the bathroom or dressing

Organization—Is comfortable with rules, regulations, routines, and order; becomes upset when they are disrupted

Interruptions—Hates to be disturbed when intensely involved in an activity

Idols—Has a desire to be more like an admired idol

Friendship—Becomes more selective about playmates

SOURCES OF STRESS FOR THE EIGHT-YEAR-OLD

Self-criticism—Is very critical of personal ability and performance

Parental authority—Is beginning to resent parental authority

Loneliness—Likes frequent interaction with friends; may hate to miss school

Praise—Continues to seek approval but can identify when praise is not genuine

Independence—Many begin to stay alone for brief periods of time while parents run errands, with resulting feelings of uneasiness

SOURCES OF STRESS FOR THE NINE-YEAR-OLD

Rebelliousness—Occasionally tests independence by rebelling

Opposite sex—Engages in sex-segregated play; expresses an aversion to the opposite sex

Fair play—Has a keen sense of what is fair and is vehement in demanding personal rights when a situation is perceived as unfair

Interruptions—Continues to dislike interruptions but will usually resume an activity after an interruption

Propriety—Has a sense of propriety and will often be upset if siblings or parents offend the child's notion of decorum or dignity

SOURCES OF STRESS FOR THE TEN- TO TWELVE-YEAR-OLD

Sexual maturation—Girls, in particular, may become self-conscious regarding obvious signs of development

Social issues—A new level of awareness can generate concern regarding pressing societal problems

Size—Both boys and girls may be upset by the fact that the girls are taller; the extremely small or extremely large child may be concerned about his or her size

Shyness—If the child already has a problem in this area, it is likely to become more pronounced at this stage

Opposite sex—May become interested, yet shy, around members of the opposite sex

Confusion—Too much freedom can cause the child to flounder

Health—It is not uncommon for a child to become a hypochondriac during this period of development

Money—Child is anxious to earn and handle money, but often uses poor judgment

Competition—Continues to be highly competitive and looks to peer group for prestige

Burnout—Child may become vigorously involved in so many activities that he or she finally becomes exhausted

Self-concept—May engage in teasing, scapegoating, or vicious attacks to temporarily boost his or her self-image; guilt often ensues; may be self-conscious about attempting a new skill

Parents—Often becomes highly critical or intolerant of parents

Idols—Continues hero worshipping

Fair play—Continues to have a highly developed sense of fair play

Drugs and sex—May be tempted to experiment with drugs or sex because everyone is doing it

Peer pressure—Becomes a powerful motivating force

Self-criticism—Child may be highly critical of personal performance

From Kuczen B: *Childhood stress: don't let your child be a victim,* New York, 1982, Delacorte Press.

NURSING ALERT The nurse who observes the following signs of stress in a child should explore the situation further:

Stomach pains or headache
Sleep problems
Bed-wetting
Changes in eating habits
Aggressive or stubborn behavior
Reluctance to participate
Regression to earlier behaviors (e.g., thumb-sucking)

To help children cope with the stresses in their lives, the parent, teacher, or health worker must be able to recognize signs that indicate a child is undergoing stress (see box on p. 145) and identify the source promptly. Children need to be taught how to recognize signs of stress in themselves, such as a pounding heart, rapid breathing, or butterflies in the stomach. Once they are able to recognize that they are stressed, they can employ techniques for managing their stress. Probably the most useful technique is to help them plan a means for dealing with any stress through problem solving (Kuczen, 1982).

First, they need to learn relaxation techniques such as deep-breathing exercises, progressive relaxation of muscle groups, and positive imagery. Encouraging them to "blow off steam" through physical activity reduces tension and anxiety. Second, they must identify the problem. Those involving situations or actions of others are relatively simple to identify. Feelings within themselves are sometimes more difficult. Third, alternative actions must be explored. Children should list all possibilities, including those that they know will not work. Fourth, they need to examine what might happen as a consequence of each alternative they have listed. By this time they are relaxed and ready for the final step, to select what they perceive to be the best option. It is sometimes helpful to have children model their behavior after someone they know who has successfully coped with a similar problem. When children are assisted with the process a few times, they are able to apply problem solving automatically.

Fears

A wide variety and degree of anxiety symptoms, including fear of the dark, excessive worry about past behavior, self-consciousness, social withdrawal, and an excessive need for reassurance, are considered normal developmental events for children (Bell-Dolan, Last, and Strauss, 1990). School-age children are less fearful of body safety than they were as preschoolers, although they still fear being hurt, kidnapped, or having to undergo surgery. They also fear death and are fascinated by all the aspects of death and dying. There is a lessening of the fear of noises, darkness, storms, and dogs. Most of the new fears that trouble school-age children are related to school and family (e.g., fear of failing, fear of teachers and bullies) and fear of something bad happening to their parents.

Parents and other persons involved with children should discuss children's fears with them individually or through group activities. Their viewpoints must be respected, and their need to communicate their concerns recognized. Sometimes children of this age are often inclined to hide their fears to avoid being ridiculed or labeled "a baby" or "chicken." Hiding fears does not end them; therefore children who are afraid to communicate them may develop displaced fears, or phobias. Children need to know that their concerns are listened to and understood. Parents who convey this to their children without becoming overprotective will help them feel less lonely and, therefore, less frightened.

Latchkey Children

The term ***latchkey children*** is used to describe children who are left to care for themselves or whose care arrangements are so loose that they are ineffective (Berman and others, 1992) (Fig. 17-12). The increasing numbers of single-parent families and working mothers, together with a lack of available child care, has created a stress-provoking situation for millions of school-age children in the United States.

Inadequate adult supervision after school leaves children at greater risk for injury and delinquent behavior. Latchkey children feel more lonely, isolated, and fearful than children who have someone to care for them. To cope with their fears and anxieties while alone, these children devise several strategies—hiding (in a bathroom, closet, shower, or under a bed), playing the television at loud volume as a distraction to drown out noises and indicate that someone was at home, and using pets as a comfort.

Many communities and persons concerned about their welfare are trying to help children and their parents deal

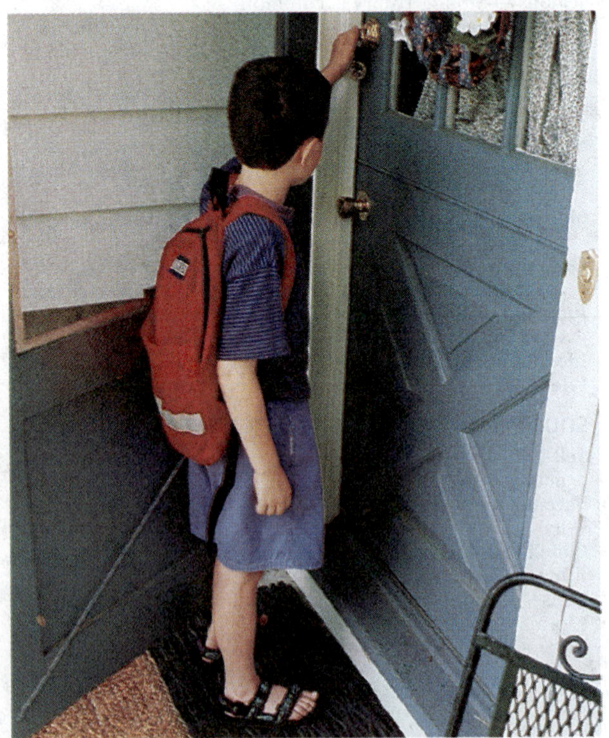

FIG. 17-12 A child unlocks the door to let himself into his home after school.

with this potentially serious problem. School-age care programs have been implemented by some communities and employers. Some guidelines appropriate for presentation to parents and/or children to help alleviate their stress and increase the children's safety are listed in the Family Home Care box. Other types of programs include those designed to teach self-help skills to children and those that provide telephone check-in and reassurance programs for children. One such program involves soliciting the assistance of volunteer "grandmas" (Ehrman, 1986), a hotline program that links latchkey children to reassuring older persons.

Nurses should be aware of services in their communities designed to meet the needs of latchkey children and include this information in anticipatory guidance of school-age children and their families. It is vital that children have adequate supervision and companionship. Services for latchkey children should be part of every pediatric nurse's resources so they can provide parents with information on programs available in the community, other possible care arrangements, and call-in services.

PROMOTING OPTIMUM HEALTH DURING THE SCHOOL YEARS

HEALTH BEHAVIORS

Children should begin to learn good health practices at an early age and be able to actively and responsibly participate in their health care. It is during the early years that lifelong habits and beliefs are established. With increased cognitive skills children are capable of making decisions about what health behaviors they will pursue and selecting from alternatives. By the end of middle childhood, children should be able to assume personal responsibility for self-care in the areas of hygiene, nutrition, exercise and recreation, sleep, and safety. Competence involves the ability to make decisions based on evaluation of internal strengths and weaknesses and external environmental influences.

Studies on causal beliefs of children about illness and wellness have determined that they rank self-controlled or self-initiated actions (such as eating and exercise) ahead of

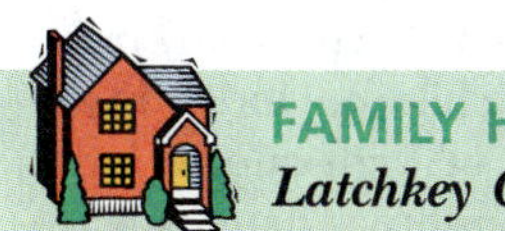

FAMILY HOME CARE
Latchkey Children

SAFETY

Teach child not to display keys and to always lock doors.
Tell child not to enter the house after school if the door is ajar, a window is open, or anything appears unusual.
Walk through the after-school routine with the child.
Consult with public safety officials about burglar-proofing and fireproofing the home.
Teach child first-aid procedures.
Teach safety rules to the child who is expected to cook (microwave ovens are safest).
Emphasize fire safety rules and conduct practice fire drills.
Teach and reinforce traffic and bicycle safety.
Teach child weather-related safety (e.g., stay inside but do not take a bath during an electrical storm; go to and stay in a storm cellar during a tornado warning).
Teach and reinforce water safety practices (e.g., do not go swimming alone; caution about safe bathing methods and keeping the toilet lid down when infants or toddlers are in their care).
Keep firearms securely locked away and teach child that they are for adult use only.
Teach child not to open the door to anyone.

TELEPHONE USE

Be certain that child knows home telephone number, address, and parents' names.
Teach child to tell callers that parents are "busy"; do not tell a caller that parents are not at home.
Teach child not to tell casual callers the home address. Tell the caller that the parent is not able to come to the phone right now and to call back later.
Keep a list of emergency numbers by the telephone. Make certain that child knows how to report emergencies.
Have a list of telephone numbers of friends or neighbors who will be at home and available for help with emergencies.
Ask public safety officials to offer classes about when and how to call them.
If a "telephone hotline" for latchkey children exists, teach child how to use it.

AFTER-SCHOOL ACTIVITIES

Arrange for child to spend some afternoons with friends.
Provide structured activities for the child.
Have the child attend a public library–sponsored activity rather than watch television at home.
Discuss with child things to do after school
Emphasize positive aspects of independence and resourcefulness but do not demand too much from child.
Help child feel successful in self-care.
Counsel parents to consider the potential problems of an older child assuming care of younger ones before the child is developmentally ready.

LONELINESS

Help child talk about experiences and feelings about being alone after school.
Consider a pet to help comfort and provide company for the child.
Be punctual in arriving home. A child's anxiety level accelerates when parents are not home when expected.
Call child if there is to be a delay in arriving home.
Leave a tape-recorded message for the child to play on arrival home from school.
Form a group of parents with flex-time so that their children can be cared for by one of the group after school.

Modified from McClellan MA: On their own: latchkey children, *Pediatr Nurs* 10:198-202, 1983.

uncontrollable elements (such as germs and bad weather) as causes of illness. Older but not younger school-age children are able to understand health and illness as reciprocal aspects of the wellness concept (Green and Bird, 1986).

Little is known about how school-age children acquire positive health behaviors. However, both boys and girls view themselves as healthy and manage their own care in the areas of seat belt use, exercise, emergency situations, and dental health. There are few differences in health perceptions and behaviors between girls and boys except that boys report more dental visits than girls (Graham and Uphold, 1992).

Health education is a primary component of comprehensive health care, and programs should be designed to promote desired health behavior through guided learning and modeling. An optimum program should help children learn about their bodies and how their behavior affects their health.

Children can be taught to take a more active role in relationships with health care providers. If asked what they would like to ask the practitioner, most children have specific questions related to the reason for their visit (Igoe, 1989). At least one program has been successful in teaching assertive and participatory behavior. The behaviors encouraged in the children were (1) asking questions, (2) telling about themselves, (3) listening and learning about new ways to take care of themselves, (4) helping decide what to do, and (5) doing those things that promote health (Igoe, 1988). (See also Health Education, p. 749).

NUTRITION

Although calorie needs are diminished in relation to body size during middle childhood, resources are being laid down for the increased growth needs of the adolescent period. It is important to impress on children and their parents the value of a diet balanced to promote growth (see box on p. 743). When children enter school, they develop an eating style that is increasingly independent of parental influence and scrutiny. Parents do not know what their children eat when they are away from home. A parent may pack a lunch to be eaten at school but be unaware of how much is eaten, traded, sold, or thrown away.

Mealtime continues to be a central issue in many families. Although it should be a pleasant part of a child's day, parents' concern and emphasis on manners often make it a battleground. Likes and dislikes established at an early age continue in middle childhood, although the propensity for single food preferences begins to end and children acquire a taste for an increasing variety of foods. Since children usually eat as the family does, the quality of their diet depends to a large extent on their family's pattern of eating. Other interests and participation in outside activities often compete with mealtime.

Outside Influences

Influenced by the mass media and the temptation of an immense variety of "junk food," it is all too easy for children to fill up on empty calories—foods that do not promote growth, such as sugars, starches, and excess fats. They have more freedom to move without parental supervision and often have small amounts of money to spend on candy, soft drinks, and other easily accessible treats. Midafternoon snacks are common, and it is wise to encourage fruit, nuts, and other wholesome finger foods to meet this need. Nutrition is a joint responsibility of both the child and the family.

The popularity of fast-food restaurants has aroused the interest of nutritionists and other health professionals concerned with children's nutrition. The restaurants are fast, relatively inexpensive, and appealing to children, and their convenience is attractive to busy parents as an alternative to eating at home. Because the nutritional content of fast-foods is usually known, it is easier for nutrition-conscious parents to help children select appropriate items from the available menu. Nurses can support consumer groups and parents in advocating more of these restaurants to offer items higher in nutritional value (such as skimmed milk, broiled meats, and fresh fruits and vegetables) and listing ingredients on the menu as required for packaged foods. Some publications, such as a report by the Massachusetts Medical Society Committee on Nutrition (1989), offer consumer guidelines for fast-foods.

The threat of childhood obesity is an increasingly prevalent health problem in school-age children today in the United States. The easy availability of high-calorie foods, combined with the tendency toward more sedentary activities (such as watching television) and the trend away from walking or cycling and toward transportation by automobile and bus, have reduced caloric expenditure. The consumption of a high-fat diet may also contribute to obesity. A comparative study of children in Seventh-Day Adventist schools and those in public schools revealed that the Seventh-Day Adventist children consumed a diet with less meat, dairy products, eggs, and junk food than the public school children. Although the Seventh-Day Adventist children were comparable in height, they were leaner than the public school children (Sabate and others, 1990). The problem of childhood obesity is discussed further in Chapter 21. Given the threat of obesity and a diet-conscious society, however, many school-age children attempt to diet in an effort to either prevent obesity or to lose weight because of imagined overweight or to conform to peer behaviors and pressures. Children need to be educated about food selection and the importance of body-building nutrients as opposed to empty caloric intake.

School Programs

Working parents who assume their children to be sufficiently mature frequently leave the responsibility of meal preparation to them. Although most older school-age children are capable of preparing simple fare, all too often breakfast and/or lunch may be inadequate, makeshift, or nonexistent. In recognition of this problem, the federal government has established the National School Lunch Program (NSLP) and the School Breakfast Program (SBP) in many areas. These meals must meet specified nutritional requirements and furnish one third of the daily recom-

ACTIVITIES FOR NUTRITION TEACHING OF SCHOOL-AGE CHILDREN

- Have children collect pictures of snack foods from magazines and categorize as good, sometimes good, or not good (can be made into a poster for display).
- Collect articles about nutrition issues related to health and disease prevention.
- Conduct nutrition discussions, helping children brainstorm and express what they know about topics such as:
  - Vitamins
  - Sugar
  - Cholesterol
  - Proteins
  - Exercise
  - Basic food groups
  - Minerals
  - Fiber
  - Sodium
  - Fast foods
  - Reading labels
- Ask each child to keep a record of foods eaten for a 24-hour period; then have the children discuss the records either in pairs or in small groups.
- Ask each child to keep an exercise diary to become aware of how active or inactive they are.
- Bring and/or have children bring labels from grocery items and discuss the contents of the product, including the ingredients and percentages of each ingredient.
- Take a walk or field trip to a local produce market (or department of supermarket). Ask the manager to show children how to select fresh, ripe items and introduce them to new or less popular fruits and vegetables with which they may be unfamiliar.
- Show films or film strips available through state and local health departments.
- Arrange for someone to speak on a selected topic related to nutrition. This may be someone from a local hospital, college, health department, or a parent.
- Help children assemble recipes for health snacks and prepare a booklet to be presented to parents, teachers, or others.
- Bring, or have children bring, items with which to assemble a chef's salad, a healthy drink, or other nutritious item.
- Teach awareness of media messages by having children:
  - Note television commercial advertisements
  - Bring pictures from magazines
  - Discuss the ways in which the advertisers entice viewers or readers to buy the product
- Have children devise a commercial for a healthy snack or meal, using the tactics they observed and discussed.

Data from Loschiavo JP: Modifying the eating behavior of young children, *School Nurse* 3(6):30-35, 1987.

mended dietary allowance for children in the United States. Most schools subscribe to the programs, and, although it is difficult to measure directly, it is believed that these school feeding programs positively influence the behavior and learning capacity of children. Improvement in comprehensive tests of basic skills was documented in a study by Meyers and others (1989). However, the average school lunch may also exceed the recommended dietary guidelines for saturated and total fat (Whitaker and others, 1993). In addition, children who purchase school lunches often select only the items they want, or, if they must take all the items in the lunch, no one insists that they eat them.

Nutrition Education. Nutrition education can and should be integrated throughout a child's school years as part of classroom learning. In school daily food choices, serving sizes, and the elements of a wholesome diet can be taught using the U.S. Department of Agriculture Food Guide Pyramid (see Nutrition, Chapter 4). Children should be encouraged to limit their intake of total and saturated fats and to increase their intake of complex carbohydrates, fruits, and vegetables. Some learning activities appropriate to school-age children are outlined in the box above. The school nurse can take an active role in nutrition education by working with teachers to plan and implement units of nutrition instruction and with parents and children to give nutritional guidance (see box at right).

SAMPLE MENU FOR SCHOOL-AGE CHILDREN BASED ON FOOD GUIDE PYRAMID*

Breakfast	2 four-inch waffles 2 tbsp syrup ½ cup orange juice
Lunch	1 four-once cheese-burger and bun ½ cup raw carrot sticks ¾ cup apple juice
Snack	1 cup frozen yogurt *or* 1 cup unsweetened cereal with lowfat milk
Dinner	1 cup spaghetti with tomato sauce 1 piece garlic bread Green salad with romaine lettuce and dressing ½ cup broccoli 1 banana 1 cup low-fat milk
Snack	2 cups plain popcorn

TOTAL SERVINGS

Bread, cereal, rice, pasta	6-7
Vegetable	3
Fruit	3
Milk, yogurt, cheese	3
Meat, poultry, fish, dried beans, nuts	2

*Use fats, oils, and sweets sparingly. Increase fluids with servings of water.
Serving sizes are minimums for nutritional adequacy. Many children eat more.

SLEEP AND REST

The amount of sleep and rest required during middle childhood is a highly individual matter. There is no specific amount needed by a child at any given age. The amount depends rather on the child's age, activity level, and other factors such as health status. The growth rate has slowed; therefore, less energy is expended in growth than was expended during the preceding periods and than will be required during the adolescent growth spurt.

During the school years children usually do not require a nap, but they spend 8 to 9.5 hours in bed and sleep approximately 95% of that time (Coble and others, 1987). Fewer bedtime problems are observed with advancing years, but occasional difficulties are still associated with the necessary bedtime ritual. Usually there is little problem for children 6 and 7 years old, and the task of going to bed can be facilitated by encouraging quiet activity before bedtime, such as coloring and reading. For many children bedtime is improved considerably by allowing them a small radio to which they can listen for a specified time.

Although most children in middle childhood must frequently be reminded to go to bed, 8- to 9-year-old children and 11-year-old children are particularly resistant. Often children are unaware that they are tired; if they are allowed to remain up later than usual, they are fatigued the following day. Sometimes bedtime resistance can be resolved by allowing a later bedtime in deference to their advancing age. However, it should be made clear that this privilege depends on compliance—going to bed without stalling and without complaints. A firm approach to bedtime is usually the most successful. Parents can help children by giving them a little advance warning, but children should realize that when the final bedtime is announced, the parents really mean it. Twelve-year-old children usually offer no difficulty in relation to bedtime. Some even retire early in order to enjoy slow preparations for bed, to read, or to listen to music.

Sleep Problems

During middle childhood there is a marked reduction in the need for sleep initiation and maintenance. The child is in control of sleep associations, and the major causes of sleep disturbances of younger children are not present. Nighttime sleep is usually continuous, and the child has developed a repertoire of tactics (such as reading or playing quietly without involving the parents) to deal with occasional difficulties in falling asleep. If a child's sleep problem concerns the family, a thorough assessment is needed to plan appropriate interventions (see box on p. 202).

The cause of ***bedtime resistance*** is not always clear. For some children it is related to normal fears of their age, such as fear of the dark, strange noises, intruders, or other imagined phenomena. Children who are subject to frightening dreams are hesitant to retire, and their sleep is more apt to be disturbed following emotional stimulation before bedtime. Sometimes children are loath to give up some exciting or interesting activity in which they are involved, or they are reluctant to leave the protective social circle of the family. Another factor associated with time for retirement is related to status. For example, older children are given the privilege of a later bedtime than younger children. Promotion to a later bedtime is highly prestigious, and age-mates compare their bedtimes. This may explain why parental decisions are often strongly contested by children who believe that playmates enjoy a more privileged position in this area. In some situations going to bed is used as a method of control. When going to bed early is imposed as a punishment or staying up a little longer is a reward, children may view bedtime as punitive or status-degrading.

Some children resort to multiple "curtain calls," such as wanting a drink of water, one more story, needing to go to the bathroom, or wanting to watch television. Often children persist in coming out of their rooms repeatedly after being put back to bed. Some voice fears, such as someone outside their window. The parents may have difficulty determining whether the fear is legitimate or whether the behavior is a bid for attention. Consistent reassurance and limit-setting usually resolve the problem. Children feel tense and insecure when limits are applied inconsistently, such as granting permission one night and punishing the next for the same behavior.

The night terrors of preschool children may be replaced by sleepwalking and sleeptalking. Like night terrors, ***sleepwalking (somnambulism)*** is associated with transition from stage 4 to stage 1 of non-REM sleep and occurs approximately 90 to 120 minutes following the onset of sleep. The phenomenon is more common in boys than in girls, and there is evidence to indicate that there may be a hereditary basis to its occurrence (Guilleminault, 1987).

The episodes are characterized by a lack of responsiveness to the environment, automatic actions, and retrograde amnesia of variable severity (Guilleminault, 1987). The episodes begin when the child sits up abruptly and walks. During sleepwalking, movements are clumsy and repetitive; finger and hand movements are often observed. Most commonly, children move about restlessly, then lie down and return to sleep. However, they may get out of bed and engage in nonpurposeful walking. They rarely perform purposeful acts during sleepwalking. Any attempts to communicate with a child elicit only mumbled and slurred responses. ***Sleeptalking,*** like sleepwalking, is not purposeful, and speech is usually incomprehensible and monosyllabic.

The best approach is to leave sleepwalking children alone unless they are in danger or may endanger others. However, clumsiness and stereotyped movements can make sleepwalking very dangerous. If the environment is not safe, a child can get hurt. Usually children complete their mission and return quietly to bed. If they must be wakened, it is best to call them by name slowly and softly, orient them to where they are, explain that they were walking in their sleep, and assure them that it will not happen when they are more relaxed. Preventive measures include avoiding overfatigue, getting adequate rest, employing relaxation techniques, and relieving any stress the children may be experiencing.

Sleepwalking is usually self-limiting and requires no treatment. More troublesome cases may require low-dose sedation, such as diazepam, before retiring. Persistent sleepwalking occurs in some older children and adolescents who are well-behaved and tend to repress strong emotions, such as anger. They may benefit from learning to express their feelings and from doing self-relaxation before bedtime (Ferber, 1992).

Nightmares are a part of the normal developmental process, although they are less common in children ages 6 to 12 than the bad dreams of younger children. However, nightmares at this more tranquil age may indicate a specific underlying conflict that strongly influences the child's behavior and thought (Terr, 1987). Children have numerous worries, and nightmares are not an unusual accompaniment to daytime worries. Resolving worries will frequently reduce nightmares.

A traumatic event will often produce ***posttraumatic nightmares,*** which are anxiety provoking and literal in their depiction of the trauma. As time goes on, the dreams of affected children may consist of "modified repetitions"; that is, they may add more current material to the recurrent dreams (e.g., involving others who were not a part of the traumatic event). Some even believe these dreams are predictive. Current external stresses, movies, or stories may also precipitate a nightmare by reactivating old traumas (Terr, 1987). For a comparison of nightmares and night terrors see Table 15-3.

PHYSICAL ACTIVITY

Exercise is essential for developmental progress in a number of areas, including muscle development and tone, refinement of balance and coordination, gaining strength and endurance, and stimulating body functions and metabolic processes. Throughout middle childhood children's increasing capabilities and adaptability permit greater speed and effort in motor activities; and larger, stronger muscles with greater efficiency and skill permit longer and increasingly strenuous play without exhaustion. During this period children acquire the necessary coordination, timing, and concentration that are required to participate in adult-type activities, even though they may lack the strength, stamina, and control of the adolescent and adult. Consequently, a larger amount of physical activity is expected and encouraged during the school years.

Children should be afforded opportunities that provide satisfying experiences to meet individual likes and dislikes. Children need ample space in which to run, jump, skip, and climb, as well as safe facilities and equipment to use both inside and outside. Appropriate activities that promote coordination and development during the school-age years include running, skipping rope, swimming, roller skating, ice skating, and bicycle riding. Positive reinforcement achieved by experiencing increasingly smooth, rhythmic, and efficient use of the body conditions the child toward regular physical activity. However, it must be kept in mind that although school-age children are large and appear to be strong, they may not be prepared yet for strenuous competitive athletics.

Most children need little encouragement to engage in physical activity. They have so much energy that they seldom know when to stop. However, children with disabilities or those who hesitate to become involved in active play, such as obese children, require special assessment and help in determining activities that will appeal to them, that are compatible with their limitations, and that at the same time meet their developmental needs. Also, parents need to limit television viewing to encourage outside activities.

Physical Fitness

In the past, physical fitness has been considered to be the physical prowess needed to engage in competitive sports. Today the term is applied to optimum functioning of all physical systems of the body and includes five components: muscle strength, endurance, flexibility, body composition, and cardiorespiratory endurance (American Academy of Pediatrics, 1987d). Enhanced cardiorespiratory endurance can be achieved by engaging in aerobic activities that maintain the heart rate at 75% of maximum for 20 to 25 minutes and are performed three times a week. Suitable activities include swimming, running, bicycling, field hockey, aerobic dancing, and fast walking.

Concern has been generated by the diminishing level of physical fitness in school-age children, the decrease in funding for school physical education programs, and the decreased amount of time spent in moderate to vigorous activity in physical education classes (Simons-Morton and others, 1993). In addition, the perception that aerobic activities are not pleasurable and the increasing attraction of television as a spare-time activity are believed to contribute to the lack of motivation in children to acquire a lifelong habit of maintaining physical fitness. Nurses can support efforts to include physical fitness as an integral part of school programs and encourage children in finding and engaging in activities they find both pleasurable and beneficial. Nurses should help children develop an enjoyment of activities that have the potential to contribute to lifelong fitness.

Sports. A great deal of controversy has surrounded the trend toward earlier participation in competitive athletics and determining the amount and type of competitive sports that are appropriate for children in the elementary grades. The current view is that virtually every child is suited for some type of sport, and authorities do not discourage participation if children are matched to the type of sport appropriate to their abilities and to their physical and emotional constitution. School-age children enjoy competition, and when teachers, parents, and coaches understand each child's physical limitations and teach them the proper techniques and safety to avoid injury to developing bones and muscles, a safe and appropriate sport can be found for even the most unskilled and nonaggressive child.

During middle childhood girls have the same basic structure as boys and thus have a similar response to systematic exercise training. At puberty, when boys become larger and have more muscle mass, it is usually recommended that girls compete only against other girls. Before puberty there is no essential difference in strength and size between girls and boys, making these precautions unnecessary (Metcalf and Roberts, 1993).

Enjoyment of sports and fitness in childhood can be encouraged by well-organized extracurricular sports programs based in the community or school (see box on p. 746). The

GOALS OF ORGANIZED ATHLETICS FOR PREADOLESCENT CHILDREN

Organized extracurricular athletic programs for preadolescent children should focus on assisting children to develop:

- Enjoyment of sports and fitness that will be sustained through adulthood
- Physical fitness
- Basic motor skills
- A positive self-image
- A balanced perspective on sports in relation to the child's school and community life
- A commitment to the values of teamwork, fair play, and sportsmanship

Modified from American Academy of Pediatrics, Committee on Sports Medicine and Committee on School Health: Organized athletics for preadolescent children, *Pediatrics* 84:583-584, 1989.

SAFEGUARDS FOR ATHLETIC PROGRAMS

Every athletic program should require the following:

- Participation physical examinations at least every 2 years
- Warm-up procedures
- The availability of a medically trained person who is competent in recognizing significant injuries during practices and games of contact sports
- The establishment of policies for first aid, referral of injured participants, treatment, rehabilitation, and certification for return to participation
- Suitable and well-maintained sports facilities
- Appropriate protective equipment
- Strict enforcement of rules concerning safety
- A formal surveillance method to ensure that goals are met

Modified from American Academy of Pediatrics, Committee on Sports Medicine and Committee on School Health: Organized athletics for preadolescent children, *Pediatrics* 84:583-584, 1989.

American Academy of Pediatrics (1989b) recommends the preadolescent years as a time to teach fundamental motor skills, develop fitness in a practical, safe, and gradual manner, and promote desired attitudes and values. Activities should include practice sessions and unstructured play; the actual game or event should be managed in a manner that stresses mastery of the sport and enhancing self-image rather than winning or pleasing others. All children should have an opportunity to participate; and special ceremonies should recognize all participants rather than individuals.

In addition to ensuring the interest, suitability, and safety (see box above, right) of the sport, parents must make certain that coaches (if involved in the sport) are skillful in managing children and do not engage in abusive types of behavior. Coaches, parents, and others involved in children's sports play critical roles in shaping children's self-esteem (American Academy of Pediatrics, 1989b). Any sport for children should emphasize the pleasure of the activity, which more often involves individual rather than team sports. It is wise to expose children to a variety of individual sports. The overall emphasis of both team and individual sports should be on playing and learning. Parents who pressure their children to perform beyond their capabilities run the risk of the child being injured, developing a distaste for the activity, and developing a lowered self-image.

The same principles described in the preceding paragraphs apply to children with chronic illnesses such as diabetes, epilepsy, asthma, or allergies if the disorder is mild and can be controlled with medication. Children with mental retardation need not be excluded from sports competition if they are matched evenly against other children of equal abilities and provided with skilled supervision and coaching. Sometimes the activities need to be modified to accommodate the limitations of these children.

Acquisition of Skills

School-age children also demonstrate increasing capacity in fine muscle facility and complex artistic skills. Handedness is well established by the beginning of the school years, and the child makes great strides in writing and drawing during this age period. It is a period of energetic and vibrant creative productivity. With the tools of language and reading, children can create poems, stories, and plays. With more advanced fine motor skills, they are able to master an unlimited variety of handicrafts, such as ceramics, needlework, wood carving, and beadwork. They avidly pursue these skills in solitude, with a friend, or in programs offered through organizations such as boys' or girls' clubs, scouting, or the YWCA and YMCA, which use crafts as a means to occupy, entertain, and educate children.

Music is a favorite form of expression in middle childhood (Fig. 17-13). School-age children are stimulated and invigorated by music. They can sing in harmony, play instruments in orchestras and bands, and manage music at a more complex level. They can compose original songs, learn lyrics almost effortlessly, and turn any empty moment into an occasion for singing, as any family, bus driver, or group leader can attest to.

School-age children are capable of assuming responsibility for their own needs, although their distaste for soap and water and "dress" clothes is legendary. School-age children can and want to assume their share of household tasks, which usually are related to the male and females roles that have been defined by their culture, and many assume responsibility for tasks outside the home, such as baby-sitting, yard work, or paper routes (Fig. 17-14).

Television and Video Games

For some time, child development specialists and parents have been concerned about the effect that television has on child development and behavior. There is no doubt that children learn from television, but the values and attitudes are not always realistically displayed and often conflict with those they have been taught. School-age children are better able to distinguish fantasy from reality, and some have had sufficient life experience to be able to view much of television fare with skepticism. However, television rarely depicts the reality of day-to-day situations that confront chil-

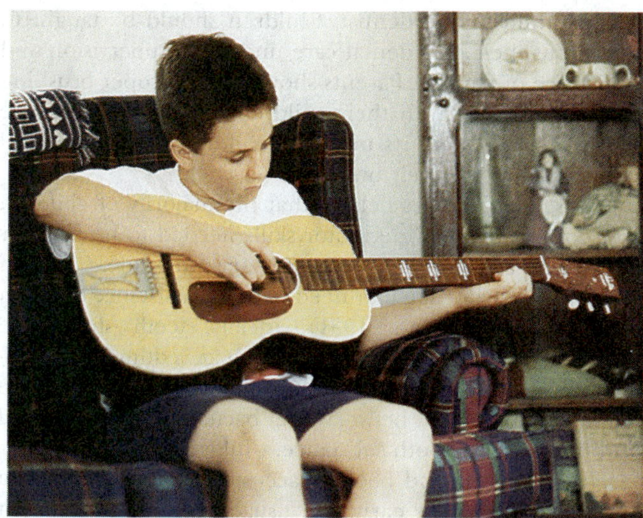

FIG. 17-13 Music is a favorite form of expression for school-age children.

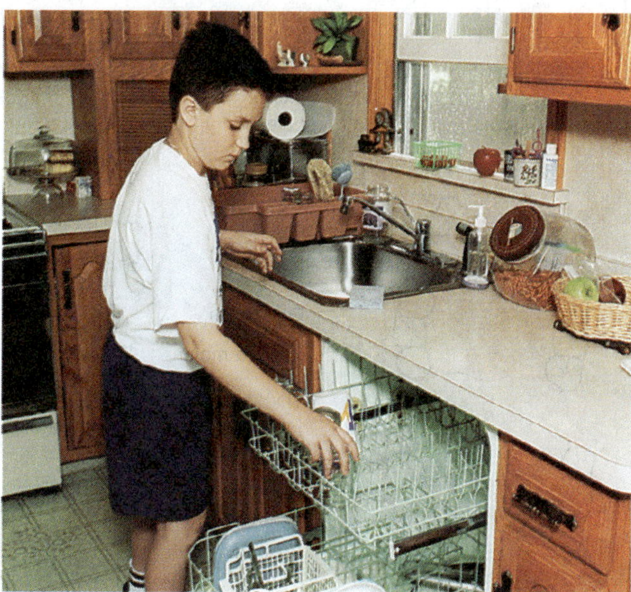

FIG. 17-14 Children can assume responsibility for a variety of household tasks.

dren. In addition, many children watch extensive amounts of violence on television (Bernard-Bonnin and others, 1991). To reduce exposure to violence and to maximize the beneficial effects of television, the American Academy of Pediatrics (1991a) recommends parental monitoring of program selection, coviewing with children, and discussions of program content. (See Chapter 4 for a more in-depth discussion of children and television.)

Video games have been criticized and supported in relation to their effect on children and adolescents. They have been reputed to keep children from school and to cause tension, sleeplessness, and violence. Others support the activity as a means for improving eye-hand coordination and as a substitute for the inactivity of passive television viewing. Other benefits include development of inductive reasoning (drawing generalizations from specific observations), improving spatial perception, and learning to handle multiple variables that interact simultaneously.

Research suggests that video games may affect physical and psychologic functioning. Physical effects may include triggering of epileptic seizures (Maeda and others, 1990) (see Seizure Disorders, Chapter 37). Laboratory research suggests a short-term relationship between playing violent games and increased aggressive fantasies and behavior (Funk, 1992; Graybill and others, 1985). Positive and creative applications of video games have been used in physical rehabilitation (Adriaenssens and others, 1988), among pediatric oncology patients (Kolko and Rickard-Figuero, 1985), and in education (Schwartz, 1988).

A study of the frequency of video game playing by seventh and eight graders indicated that girls spent 1 to 2 hours per week playing the games, whereas boys averaged 4 hours per week. A small number of children spent 15 hours or more per week in this activity; for these children there is some concern that video game playing could become habitual and addictive (Griffiths, 1991). Half of the children in the study preferred video games with violent themes, whereas only 2% chose educational games.

Although there is no clear evidence that violent video games cause increased aggressive behavior, for some children repeated exposure to violent themes may influence future behavior. Parent and teacher education relating to video games should include recommendations to limit playing time, monitor game selection and content, and increase access to games that are educational (Funk, 1993).

DENTAL HEALTH

The first permanent (secondary) teeth erupt at about 6 years of age. Before their appearance they have been developing in the jaw beneath the deciduous (primary) teeth. Meanwhile, the roots of the latter are gradually being absorbed, so that at the time a deciduous tooth is shed, only the crown remains. At 6 years of age all the primary teeth are present, and those of the secondary dentition are relatively well formed. At this time eruption of the permanent teeth begins, usually starting with the 6-year molar, which erupts posterior to the deciduous molars. The others appear in approximately the same order as eruption of the primary teeth and follow shedding of the deciduous teeth (Fig. 17-15).

The pattern of shedding primary teeth and the eruption of secondary teeth are subject to wide variation among children. To allow the larger permanent teeth to occupy the limited space left by shed primary teeth, a series of complicated changes must take place in the jaws. It is at this time that many of the difficulties created by crowding of teeth become apparent. With the appearance of the second permanent (12-year) molars, most of the permanent teeth are present. The third permanent molars, or wisdom teeth, may

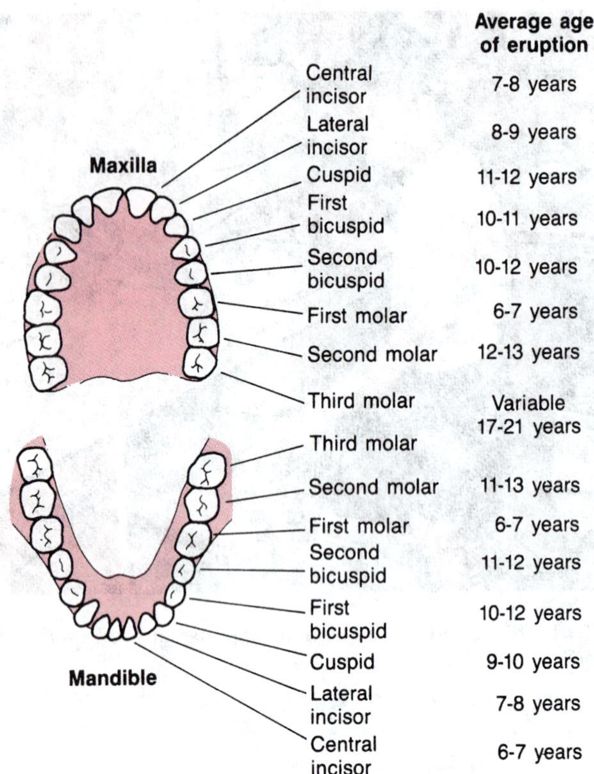

FIG. 17-15 Sequence of eruption of secondary teeth. (Data from McDonald RE, Avery DR: *Dentistry for the child and adolescent,* ed 6, St Louis, 1994, Mosby.)

erupt from 18 to 25 years of age or later. Permanent dentition is somewhat more advanced in girls than in boys.

Since it is during the school-age years that the permanent teeth erupt, good dental hygiene and regular attention to dental caries are a vital part of health supervision during this period. Children of this age tend to become lax about oral hygiene unless they are carefully supervised. Children are assuming more responsibility for their own care but are not sufficiently motivated by improved appearance and odor, as they will be during adolescence. School nurses should be alert for opportunities to teach correct brushing and flossing techniques, to reinforce avoidance of fermentable carbohydrates and sticky sweets, and to be alert for problems of malocclusion, toothache, and mouth infections (Scanlan, 1991).

Comprehensive dental supervision is as essential as regular medical supervision and should be an integral part of the overall health maintenance program. Regular dental prophylaxis (teeth cleaning) by a dentist or dental hygienist is an important aspect of dental care. Fluoride application should be continued to decrease the susceptibility of the tooth enamel to acid breakdown. (See Chapter 14 for a discussion of fluoride and other aspects of dental care.)

Brushing

One of the most effective means of preventing dental caries is a regimen of proper oral hygiene tailored to the individual child by the dentist. Children should be taught to carry out their own dental care under the supervision and guidance of parents. Parents should learn proper brushing technique along with their children and should supervise their children's efforts until the children can assume full responsibility for their own care.

Most practitioners believe that the majority of children do not possess the fine motor skills needed to brush their teeth properly until approximately second grade. Children under 10 years of age may need parental assistance to brush back teeth (Scanlan, 1991). Ideally, teeth should be brushed after meals, after snacks, and at bedtime. The bedtime brushing is especially important because there is more time for interaction between oral bacteria and unremoved substrate on the tooth substance. Children who brush their teeth frequently and become accustomed to the feel of a clean mouth at an early age usually maintain the habit throughout life.

The thoroughness of plaque removal (cleaning) can be checked using a plaque-disclosing agent that stains any remaining plaque red. The child should inspect the teeth closely with the aid of a mirror and under adequate light. The teeth are again cleansed with a fluoridated dentifrice to remove the remaining plaque and provide further protection. This procedure may be carried out regularly or occasionally, according to instructions from the child's dentist. Toothpastes recommended by the American Dental Association Council on Dental Therapeutics carry a seal of approval, easily identified on the package. They have been submitted to testing and demonstrate the ability to reduce the incidence of dental caries when used correctly.

For school-age children with mixed and permanent dentition the best toothbrush is one of a soft nylon bristles with an overall length of about 21 cm (6 inches). Many dental supply companies provide brushes to schools at minimal cost (Scanlan, 1991). Numerous methods of brushing the teeth have been described and recommended for children, but there is no conclusive evidence that one method is superior over another. The thoroughness of the cleaning is more important than the specific technique used. The dentist will assess all factors, such as manipulative skills and special needs of a child, and suggest the most appropriate brushing technique and regimen. Brushing is followed by flossing. Flossing is done by the parents until children acquire the manual dexterity needed. Most children are not able to floss properly until about 8 or 9 years of age.

SCHOOL HEALTH

Child health maintenance is ultimately the responsibility of parents; however, public schools and health departments in the United States have contributed to the improvement of child health by providing a healthful school environment, health services, and health education functions that emphasize sound health practices. Most of these constitute major components of community health services and involve large amounts of public funds and large numbers of health professionals, including nurses, on either a full-time or part-time basis.

FACTORS THAT CONTRIBUTE TO HEALTHFUL SCHOOL LIVING

A clean, safe, and wholesome school and classroom environment that provides suitable lighting, seating, heating, ventilation, furniture, equipment, and a safe play area
A health program that is concerned about the physical and mental health of children, teachers, and other staff members involved in the school operation
A schedule of activities that is suited to the capabilities and maturational level of each child
A regular physical education program
A planned food service program that provides both meal services and an example of good nutrition practices

CONTENT OF SCHOOL HEALTH SERVICES

Health appraisal—Screening tests (vision, hearing), measurements (height, weight), and medical, dental, and psychologic examinations
Emergency care and safety—Emergency treatment (first aid), notification of parents, and transportation of the ill or injured child to home or hospital
Communicable disease control—Detection and exclusion of affected children and policies for readmission and attendance at school (immunizations required in most states before school entry)
Counseling and guidance—Health guidance, referral, and follow-up for parents and children with special health needs
Adjustment to individual student needs

RECOMMENDATIONS FOR SCHOOL HEALTH PROGRAMS

Health education is a subject that should be taught as part of basic education and deserves the same priority in the curriculum as traditional subjects.
Planned integrated programs of comprehensive health education should be a requirement for students from kindergarten through grade 12 and should be taught by specially qualified teachers or those certified to teach health education.
Health education should include the active participation of students for the most effective learning of sound health concepts.
Financial support for health education programs must be ensured. Proper funding is critical to the development of effective programs, and the agencies responsible must be convinced to continue or increase funding.
Comprehensive health education programs should be directed by qualified health educators who function in consultation and cooperation with school personnel and administrators.
The programs should be monitored by a well-organized school health committee composed of representative parents, students, pediatricians, and health agencies (e.g., public health nurses) in the community.
Health education should be a part of every elementary school and secondary school teachers' training program.
School districts, other public agencies, the medical community, and private agencies should intensify their health education program for adults as part of a coordinated community health education effort, and pediatricians should make health education a regular component of the child health supervision and routine illness visits.
Research studies to evaluate the impact of such programs on students must be carried out at local and national levels.

From American Academy of Pediatrics, Committee on School Health: Health education and schools, *Pediatrics* 75:1160-1165, 1985.

A safe and healthful school environment is the first essential element of any school health program. Conditions within the school setting should make a positive contribution to the physical, mental, and social development of the children. (See boxes above for factors that contribute to healthful school living and the characteristics of an ongoing school health program of health maintenance through assessment, screening, and referral activities.)

Health Education

Health education of schoolchildren is primarily directed toward providing knowledge of health and influencing habits, attitudes, and conduct in relation to health and accident prevention. The Committee on School Health of the American Academy of Pediatrics believes that community health programs can be instrumental in changing poor health practices and makes the recommendations outlined in the box above, right (American Academy of Pediatrics, 1985).

A viable health education program is based on sound health concepts but should be adjusted to meet specific local needs, objectives, and legal requirements. Parents must understand and approve the health education curriculum so that its teaching will be reinforced at home. A comprehensive approach to health education is more successful in developing positive health practices than one in which the subjects are taught in isolation. A recent survey of school administrators, school nurses, and informed parents of children attending public schools identified a need for education in the following areas: drug education, sex education, and AIDS education (Attala and others, 1993). However, many of these topics are associated with differing social and cultural attitudes and should be presented accurately but with sensitivity to those attitudes.

Health education concerning Acquired Immunodeficiency Syndrome (AIDS) is a specific example. Most authorities agree that AIDS education needs to begin in the elementary grades to prevent high-risk behaviors. However, educational programs concerning AIDS must be developmentally appropriate and to be effective must be implemented with parental and community support. Young children need information on how the AIDS virus is transmitted in simple, accurate terms without elaborate, unnecessary discussions of sex. Misconceptions that increase children's anxiety about contracting the virus should be corrected. Although many children have heard that sex and drugs cause AIDS, some children believe that AIDS can be contracted by standing near a drug dealer (Schonfeld and others, 1993). Children need information on how AIDS is transmitted through infected blood on shared drug needles and that the virus is not spread through common forms of expressing affection such as hugging and holding hands (Schonfeld and others, 1993).

School Nursing Services

School nurses assume a major role in the school health program. Working in collaboration with others in the school and community, their service consists of three interrelated aspects of child health care: health supervision, health counseling, and health education. These functions are not necessarily limited to the confines of the school environment but extend into the community in which the students live. As a health practitioner, the school nurse is in a position to promote and evaluate health services throughout the community as they affect children and to collaborate with agencies in planning for health and safety. For some children, especially those in poverty, the school nurse may be the only contact with illness prevention and health promotion (Jones and Clark, 1993).

Traditionally, school nurses have been viewed from a limited perspective that placed them in the role of disease detector, applier of bandages, and official caregiver in cases of illness and injury. Although these are still important functions, this traditional role has acquired much broader dimensions. Many health care reformers propose that the role of school health service be enlarged into family health centers. These centers should be located in the schools or in school-linked settings (Igoe, 1993). Within these centers, the school nurse practitioner will provide primary health care that includes assessment of physical, psychomedical, psychoeducational, behavioral, and learning disorder problems, as well as comprehensive well-child care. The school nurse practitioner will also develop, implement, and evaluate health care plans and programs.

Some school districts have hired paraprofessionals (health aides, licensed vocational nurses) to meet the needs of students and staff. These paraprofessionals are trained to assist a professional and are not equipped to "recognize, assess, manage, or make appropriate referrals for the myriad health problems now being handled in schools" (American Academy of Pediatrics, 1987c). The competence of the paraprofessional must be determined and documented by the health practitioner, and the paraprofessional must be provided with regular supervision, preferably direct supervision, by a licensed professional school nurse.

Since the passage of Public Laws 94-142 and 99-457, which require the integration of children with chronic illness or disability into the regular classrooms, school nurses are responsible for the medical and nursing needs of these children in the school setting. School nurses assess and monitor all health problems that come into the school and compile a health care list of all such problems and their associated therapies. Nurses usually call the parent of the child and arrange for a visit to the home, made by either themselves or a public health nurse, where they gather information and determine if a nursing care plan is needed at the school. They collaborate with the family, including their suggestions in the care plan. The plan is discussed with the child's teachers, and any needed education is provided. School nurses are the only ones in the school system qualified to deal with medical problems.

Sometimes all that is required is an assessment and making the teacher aware that the child has a health problem. In other cases more complex teaching is needed, such as how to observe for certain signs (e.g., insulin reaction), techniques that must be learned (e.g., tracheostomy suctioning, gastrostomy or nasogastric tube feedings), and management of emergencies (care of a child during a seizure). School nurses instruct teachers in the necessary procedures and review their performance approximately every 4 weeks. Most teachers are required to demonstrate competence in cardiopulmonary resuscitation (CPR). The American Academy of Pediatrics (1993a) also recommends that high school students receive training in basic life support as part of their health education program.

Children who must take medications at school need written authorization from the child's attending physician and/or written permission from the parents allowing the nurse to administer or supervise the administration of the medication. The medication must be brought to the school in a container appropriately labeled by the pharmacist or physician (American Academy of Pediatrics, 1993b). Medications are kept locked up in the nurse's office; the child is not allowed to carry them at school. This may vary in some school districts or situations involving children who usually have the responsibility for taking their own medications. The children are allowed to do so provided the physician and a parent provide the required authorization. Guidelines for administration of medications in schools can also be obtained from the **National Association of School Nurses, Inc.***

The preparation, qualifications, and utilization of school nurses and school nurse practitioners vary throughout the United States. Some communities consider the school nurse an essential member of the school organization with a full-time school commitment; in other communities school health practice is merely a part of the total community health program assumed by the health department. The relative merits of the two types of services are a matter of controversy.

INJURY PREVENTION

Because school-age children have developed more refined muscular coordination and control and can apply their cognitive capacities to a more judicious course of action, the incidence of unintentional injury is diminished in children in this age-group as compared with the incidence in early childhood. School-age children have a wider environment and more environments in which they need protection; they acquire skills and interests that expose them to new perils;

*Lamplighter Lane, P.O. Box 1300, Scarborough, ME 04074; (207) 883-2117.

TABLE 17-2 Injury Prevention During School-Age Years

DEVELOPMENTAL ABILITIES RELATED TO RISK OF INJURY	INJURY PREVENTION
Is increasingly involved in activities away from home Is excited by speed and motion Is easily distracted by environment Can be reasoned with	**Motor vehicles** Educate child regarding proper use of seat belts while a passenger in a vehicle Maintain discipline while a passenger in a vehicle (e.g., keep arms inside, do not lean against doors or interfere with driver) Emphasize safe pedestrian behavior Insist on wearing safety apparel (e.g., helmet) where applicable, such as riding bicycle, motorcycle, moped
Is apt to overdo May work hard to perfect a skill Has cautious, but not fearful, gross motor actions Likes swimming	**Drowning** Teach child to swim Teach basic rules of water safety Select safe and supervised places to swim Check sufficient water depth for diving Swim with a companion Use an approved flotation device in water or boat Advocate for legislation requiring fencing around pools Learn CPR
Has increasing independence Is adventuresome Enjoys trying new things	**Burns** Instruct child in behavior in areas involving contact with potential burn hazards (e.g., gasoline, matches, bonfires or barbecues, lighter fluid, firecrackers, cigarette lighters, cooking utensils, chemistry sets); avoid climbing or flying kites around high-tension wires Instruct child in proper behavior in the event of fire (e.g., fire drills at home, school, and so on) (see Chapter 29) Teach child safe cooking (use low heat, avoid any frying, be careful of steam burns, scalds, or exploding foods, especially from microwaving)
Adheres to group rules May be easily influenced by peers Strong allegiance to friends	**Poisoning** Educate child regarding hazards of taking nonprescription drugs and chemicals, including aspirin and alcohol Teach child to say "no" if offered illegal or dangerous drugs or alcohol Keep potentially dangerous products in properly labeled receptacles—preferably out of reach
Has increased physical skills Needs strenuous physical activity Is interested in acquiring new skills and perfecting attained skills Is daring and adventurous, especially with peers Frequently plays in hazardous places Confidence often exceeds physical capacity Desires group loyalty and has strong need for friends' approval Attempts hazardous feats Accompanies friends to potentially hazardous facilities Delights in physical activity Is likely to overdo Growth in height exceeds muscular growth and coordination	**Bodily damage** Help provide facilities for supervised activities Encourage playing in safe places Keep firearms safely locked up except during adult supervision Teach proper care of, use of, and respect for devices with potential danger (power tools, firecrackers, and so on) Teach children not to tease or surprise dogs, invade their territory, take dogs' toys, or interfere with dogs' feeding Stress eye, ear, or mouth protection when using potentially hazardous objects or devices or when engaged in potentially hazardous sports Teach safety regarding use of corrective devices (glasses); if child wears contact lenses, monitor duration of wear to prevent corneal damage Stress careful selection and maintenance of sports and recreation equipment Emphasize proper conditioning, safe practices, and use of safety equipment for sports or recreational activities Caution against engaging in hazardous sports, such as those involving trampolines Use safety glass and decals on large glassed areas, such as sliding glass doors Teach name, address, and phone number and to ask for help from appropriate people (cashier, security guard, policeman) if lost; have identification on child (sewn in clothes, inside shoe) Teach stranger safety: Avoid personalized clothing in public places Never go with a stranger Tell parents if anyone makes child feel uncomfortable in any way Always listen to child's concerns regarding others' behavior Teach child to say "no" when confronted with uncomfortable situations

they have less supervision; and they take more responsibility and begin to participate in the adult world.

As previously described, the type of injuries most prevalent in children in any age-group largely reflects the child's developmental stage. Table 17-2 outlines some of the developmental characteristics and accomplishments of middle childhood that predispose such children to physical injury and guidelines for injury prevention.

The incidence of injury during middle childhood is significantly higher in school-age boys than in school-age girls, and their death rate is twice that of girls (see Chapter 1). Most injuries occur in or near the home or school. The prevalence of injury depends on the dangers present in the environment, protection offered by adults, and the behavior patterns of the children. Also, school-age children, although conscious of rules and frequently imposing them in relationships with peers, tend to challenge established rules. It is often difficult to maintain a balance between the level of supervision and restriction needed by children and the children's need for freedom and independence.

The incidence of transportation-related injuries in school-age children is higher than that of younger children, and the incidence of non–motor vehicle–involved bicycle injury is higher than that of teenagers and preschool children. The incidence of injuries from burns and poisonings is lowest in school-age children. However, physically active school-age children are highly susceptible to cuts and abrasions, and the incidence of childhood fractures, strains, and sprains is impressive.

Risk-Taking Behavior

Achieving social acceptance is a primary objective for school-age children, and they will often attempt dangerous acts (sometimes extreme behaviors) to prove themselves worthy of acceptance and improve their status in the peer group (Levine, 1992). Peer pressure is a normal part of psychologic development, but at the same time it is a major contributor to risk-taking behaviors. Peer challenges often encourage problem behaviors that place children at risk for injury or hazardous habits. School-age children are in the process of moving from preoperational to concrete operational thinking and are only beginning to understand causal relationships. Therefore they may attempt certain activities without planning or evaluating the consequences.

Risk takers often are persons with inadequate self-regulatory behavior. They are "impulsive rather than constrained, uninhibited rather than shy: they flout rules from an early age, and they covet adoration from their peers" (Lipsitt, 1988). These children need to learn the motivation or the incentives for such behavior and to visualize the consequences if the risk-taking behavior ends in a tragic outcome.

Motor Vehicle Injury

As in all other age-groups, the most common cause of severe accidental injury and death in school-age children is motor vehicle accidents—either as pedestrian or as passenger. Pedestrian fatalities are two and a half times more frequent than occupant deaths in school-age children, and the peak incidence is in the 5- to 9-year-old age-group (Dunne, Asher, and Rivara, 1992). Most of the injuries are caused by children who misinterpret traffic signs or disobey common traffic safety regulations, cross the street against a red light, cross in other than designated crosswalks, dart into the street, and walk in the same direction as the traffic. Parents consistently overestimate the street-crossing skills of young children ages 5 to 6 years and need education about their children's developmental abilities and competence as pedestrians (Dunne, Asher, and Rivara, 1992). Nurses can help parents to develop more realistic expectations of their children's behavior and teach them to model safe street-crossing behaviors through pedestrian skills training programs.

Use of restraint systems, door-lock mechanisms, and appropriate passenger seating and behavior are simple but effective measures for eliminating noncrash injuries and reducing the severity of crash injuries. The importance of emphasizing the correct use of seat restraints cannot be overemphasized. Children in this age-group do not usually require special car seats, and, despite evidence that safety belt use saves life and injury, estimates of seat belt use in children ages 5 to 13 are still discouragingly low (Agran, Winn, and Dunkle, 1989).

Injuries to children ages 5 to 9 years restrained in adult-type seat belts are related to anatomic differences between adults and children. Although booster seats are available for these children, low usage has been reported (Agran, Winn, and Dunkle, 1989). Children's sitting height is less than the adult's, and the center of gravity is located above the level of the lap belt. Consequently, the greater proportion of body mass above the belt may cause more forward motion and jackknifing over the belt, increasing the risk of head injury from impact with interior vehicle parts. Lap/shoulder belts may lie over the face and neck of a small-sized child. The child's smaller and less developed iliac crests are not suited to serve as an anchor for belts designed to restrain adults, and their intraabdominal organs are less protected by the bony pelvis (Agran, Winn, and Dunkle, 1989). The natural behavior of children (such as readjusting the seating position, moving about, and otherwise altering the fits of the restraint) influences the effectiveness of the restraint.

Studies support the effectiveness of education in increasing compliance with seat belt use (Roberts and Fanurik, 1986; Roberts and Turner, 1986). Parents should make certain that the restraints are fitted to their children and fastened correctly. To reduce the risk of sliding beneath the standard seat belt during a collision, children should sit up straight and well back in the seat, and the seat should be moved forward until the feet fit firmly against the toe board. Children should be cautioned against assuming alternate seating positions, such as tailor fashion, while riding in the car. In addition to using lap/shoulder belts, parents should advocate for equipping all cars with air bags (Evans, 1990). (See Chapter 14 for a comprehensive discussion of safety restraints.) Although it has been established that seat belts reduce motor vehicle injuries, most school buses are not

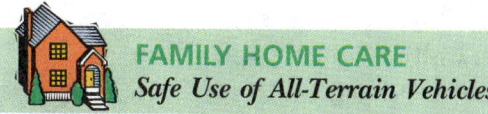

FAMILY HOME CARE
Safe Use of All-Terrain Vehicles

Vehicles should be sturdy and stable; quality construction is essential.
Riders should receive instruction from a mature, experienced cyclist.
Riding should be supervised and allowed only after the rider has demonstrated competence in handling the machine on familiar terrain (preferably require licensing).
Riders should wear approved helmets and protective clothing (e.g., trousers, boots, gloves).
Riders should avoid public roadways.
Riding should be restricted to familiar terrain.
Nighttime riding should not be allowed.
Vehicle should not carry more than one person.

Based on and modified from American Academy of Pediatrics, Committee on Accident and Poison Prevention: All-terrain vehicles: two-, three, and four-wheeled unlicensed motorized vehicles, *Pediatrics* 79:306-308, 1987.

equipped with seat restraints. Advocates argue that seat belts in buses would serve two purposes: (1) reduce the risk of injury, and (2) serve to teach and reinforce the importance of seat belt use while riding in any motor vehicle (Spital, Spital, and Spital, 1986). Seat belts specifically designed for school buses can also keep children from being ejected from their seats and colliding with hard interior surfaces (Widome, 1988).

All-terrain vehicles (ATVs), designed for off-road use by children and adolescents, are becoming increasingly popular with children under 16 years of age but are responsible for a significant number of childhood injuries. The two- and four-wheeled motorized vehicles are unlicensed and require no advanced training. They all have a short wheelbase and low profile, which makes them relatively unstable and unable to be seen easily. The vehicles can also achieve substantial speed. Most injuries occur when the driver loses control of the vehicle, is thrown from the vehicle, or collides with fixed objects or other vehicles (American Academy of Pediatrics, 1987a). Immature judgment and/or motor skills are the most common factors contributing to injury (Dolan, Knapp, and Andres, 1989). The Committee on Accident and Poison Prevention of the American Academy of Pediatrics (1987a) views ATVs as a major hazard to the health of children, opposes their use by children, and states that "the safe use of these vehicles requires skill, judgment, and experience." However, for parents who allow their use, the Committee provides safety guidelines (see Family Home Care box).

Bicycle Injury

The majority of school-age children have bicycles, and their penchant for riding them increases the risk of injury on streets and byways. Bicycle injuries account for approximately 600,000 emergency room visits and more than 1200 deaths annually (Weiss, 1992). Most childhood bicycle injuries (approximately 480,000 per year) occur in children ages 5 to 14 (Hancock, 1987). Deaths are usually caused by head injuries and almost always are the result of bicycle/motor vehicle collision (Spence and others, 1993).

One study found that most collisions between motor vehicles and bicycles occurred during afternoon rush hour (4 PM to 6 PM), and all bicycle injuries, whether or not a car was involved, occurred between 4 PM and 8 PM (Selbst, Alexander, and Ruddy, 1987). Many injuries are related to violations of traffic laws by the bicyclist, including wrong-way riding (facing traffic), failure to yield the right-of-way, and turning violations. Others have been related to road conditions described as hazardous—bumps, potholes, and gravel (Selbst, Alexander, and Ruddy, 1987). There is no difference in the number, severity, or distribution of injuries among young children using their bicycles for play in their own neighborhood and older children using their bicycles for transportation on streets with heavy traffic (Agran and Winn, 1993).

In addition to major injuries, cuts and bruises from falls and collisions account for a large number of injuries. Other injuries include trauma to internal organs from bicycle handlebars (Sparnon and Ford, 1986). These injuries initially seem to be trivial, but injured children develop serious symptoms (e.g., pain, vomiting, or collapse) hours later. Hematuria has also been reported as a result of improperly fitted bicycle seats (Nichols, 1984).

Many of the difficulties of school-age children can be attributed to their developmentally related limited range of vision and their inability to process perceptions of road situations sufficiently well and quickly enough to ride safely in traffic. Other important factors are lack of instruction in use of the equipment, lack of safety equipment, and riders who are unfamiliar with the bicycle (e.g., having ridden their bicycle for less than a month).

To prevent bicycle injuries, both parents and children should learn and periodically review bicycle safety. Children need bicycles that are suited to their size and age—they should be able to stand with the balls of both feet on the ground when seated on the bicycle, be able to place both feet flat on the ground when straddling the center bar, and be able to grasp the brake lever comfortably and easily enough to apply sufficient pressure to brake the bicycle (American Academy of Pediatrics, 1989a). Parents should be discouraged from buying their child a bicycle that the child can "grow into."

Since head injury is the major cause of bicycle-related fatalities (Cushman and others, 1991), probably the single most important aspect of bicycle safety is to encourage the rider to wear a protective helmet (Fig. 17-16). Hard-shelled helmets lined with expanded polystyrene (Styrofoam) provide the best head protection. The helmet should be one that can be adjusted to the individual child's head, fits securely, and does not limit the child's vision or hearing. A brightly colored helmet improves visibility. The helmet should carry the seal indicating it has passed the safety standards of the American National Standards Institute. Since children's head sizes have nearly reached adult size before their full skeletal height is reached, a helmet purchased at

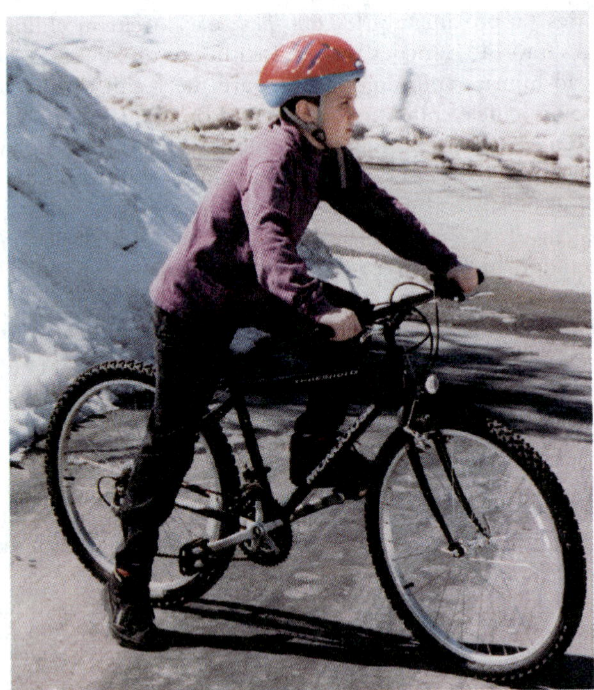

FIG. 17-16 The right-size bike is important; the child should be able to sit on the bike and place the balls of both feet on the ground. The foot should comfortably reach and manipulate the pedal in the down position. Wearing a protective helmet is mandatory for safe cycling.

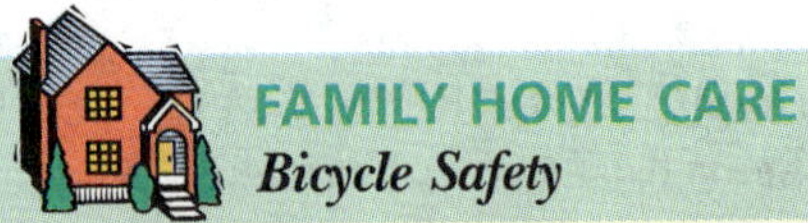

FAMILY HOME CARE
Bicycle Safety

Ride bicycles with traffic and away from parked cars.
Ride single file.
Walk bicycles through busy intersections only at crosswalks.
Give hand signals well in advance of turning or stopping.
Keep as close to the curb as practical.
Watch for drain grates, potholes, soft shoulders, and loose dirt or gravel.
Keep both hands on handlebars, except with signaling.
Never ride double on a bicycle.
Do not carry packages that interfere with vision or control; do not drag objects behind bike.
Watch for and yield to pedestrians.
Watch for cars backing up or pulling out of driveways; be especially careful at intersections.
Look left, right, then left before turning into traffic or roadway.
Never hitch a ride on a truck or other vehicle.
Learn rules of the road and respect for traffic officers.
Obey all local ordinances.
Wear well-fitted helmet.
Wear shoes that fit securely while riding.
Wear light colors at night and attach fluorescent material to clothing and bicycle.
Be certain the bicycle is the correct size for rider.
Equip bicycle with proper lights and reflectors.
Have the bicycle inspected to ensure good mechanical condition.

age 7 or 8 may be worn through adolescence with a few alterations in the fitting pads.

In a study of serious head injuries in bicycle riders, only 4% wore helmets (Thompson, Rivara, and Thompson, 1989). Although most young riders acknowledge that wearing a helmet is important for safety, reasons for not wearing them include because they forgot, because their friends do not wear them, and because they find the helmets uncomfortable (DiGuiseppi, Rivara, and Koepsell, 1990). For many it is primarily one of personal appearance. Taunts of schoolmates are powerful deterrents, and some children who are not allowed to ride a bicycle without a helmet choose to walk rather than incur the ridicule of age-mates (Howland and others, 1989).

Parental attitudes and behaviors also influence children's use of bicycle helmets. Parental nonuse of a helmet is strongly associated with lack of intention to require the children to use helmets. In contrast, sibling helmet ownership correlates highly with children's helmet use (Pendergast and others, 1992). Parents who had not purchased helmets for their children gave the following reasons: they had never thought of it, helmets are too expensive, and their children would not wear helmets if they had them (DiGuiseppi, Rivara, and Koepsell, 1990). Parents, as well as children, need to be educated on safety. The American Academy of Pediatrics (1990) recommends that (1) parents be informed of the dangers of riding without a helmet, (2) retail outlets carry inexpensive helmets available at the time of bicycle purchase, (3) the Consumer Product Safety Commission develop mandatory standards for helmets, (4) parents and community-based programs promote bicycle safety and helmet use, and (5) the media depict helmet use in all programs and promotional materials.

Numerous bicycle helmet promotion programs have been developed by schools, hospital emergency rooms, and communities (Cushman and others, 1991; Parkin and others, 1993; Scheidt, Wilson, and Stern, 1992; Wilson and Testani-Dufour, 1993). Programs that are most successful are those that address the cost of helmets and peer pressure and combine multimedia public education announcements with the support of community organizations.

Guidelines for bicycle safety are listed in the Family Home Care box (see also Critical Thinking Exercise box).

Other Vehicles

After a short period of decline, ***skateboards*** are again assuming popularity, with an accompanying resurgence of related injuries. Although severe injuries are uncommon and moderate injuries are reported frequently, the severity of injuries increases with the decreasing age of the children (Retsky, Jaffe, and Christoffel, 1987). School-age children often use their skateboards on streets and highways, increasing the likelihood of high-speed collisions with objects or vehicles. Recommendations for safe skateboard use are listed in the Family Home Care box on p. 755.

Like skateboard injuries, ***roller skate*** or ***in-line skate injuries*** involve predominantly the upper extremities (especially the wrist and forearm) as children attempt to break the fall

CRITICAL THINKING EXERCISE
Bicycle Helmets

During the past month in your school district, one child died and another sustained a serious head injury from bicycle-vehicle collisions. Neither child wore a bicycle helmet. As a school nurse, you are considering effective approaches to increase the students' use of bicycle helmets. Which of the following is most likely to achieve your goal?

1. Send home to every family an educational packet of material about bicycle safety.
2. Ask the local television station to report the details of the victims' injuries and the families' grief.
3. Invite local athletes engaged in sports, such as football, that require protective headgear to discuss being safe and acting "cool."
4. Organize other school nurses, faculty, and parents to petition the state legislature for mandatory bicycle helmet laws.

All the options are constructive ones, but the one most likely to influence the schoolchildren immediately is 3. Issues of stylishness, comfort, and social acceptability are major determinants of compliance (Gielen and others, 1994). Education by respected athletes provides a strong incentive for youngsters to wear helmets.

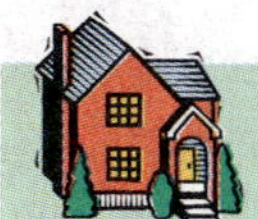

FAMILY HOME CARE
Skateboard Safety

Children younger than 5 years of age should not use skateboards. They are not developmentally prepared to protect themselves from injury.

Children who ride skateboards should wear helmets and protective padding, especially on knees and elbows, to prevent injury.

Skateboards should never be ridden near traffic. Their use should be prohibited on streets and highways. Activities that bring skateboards together (e.g., "catching a ride") are especially dangerous.

Some types of use, such as riding homemade ramps on hard surfaces, may be particularly hazardous.

Modified from American Academy of Pediatrics, Committee on Accident and Poison Prevention: Skateboard injuries, *Pediatrics* 83:1070-1071, 1989.

with outstretched arms. Safety measures are basically the same as for skateboards. The skill level of the child should be carefully evaluated before the child is allowed to use these conveyances. Younger children sustain injuries more frequently than older children. Some authorities believe that children should not be encouraged to engage in these activities until their bone strength and skills are sufficiently mature to decrease the risk of fracture—in most cases this occurs between 9 and 10 years of age (Inkelis and others, 1988).

Twenty-five percent of the 19,100 ***ride-on mower injuries*** and 30% of the deaths reported by the Consumer Product Safety Commission (Smith, 1988) were children. The children were either run over or backed over by another driver or fell either from the mower on which they were riding or from a trailer being pulled by a mower. Fourteen percent of the injuries were sustained by children between the ages of 5 and 16 who were operating the mower. Similar injuries and problems can be attributed to snowmobiles.

Injuries at School

The risk of injury at school is relatively low, despite the amount of time children spend in that environment. The injuries occur in the gyms, shops, and laboratories, as well as on the playground and playing fields. Most injuries occur on the way to and from school. Many are related to sports activities (see Chapter 39). Persons concerned for child safety should be alert to hazards in the school environment and should become involved in efforts to make the environment safe from every aspect—physical facilities, equipment, training practices, and supervision.

Farm Injuries

Many school-age children are involved in farm activities and play in the farm environment. They may be children of migrant workers, and as such, they constitute a significant proportion of agricultural workers. Most injuries take place during the summer when children are home from school and in the autumn when farming activity is brisk (Swanson and others, 1987). Health facilities are also more scattered and less accessible for emergency treatment than they are in urban areas.

Health workers need to be aware of the problems and to emphasize to the farm family the hazards related to their environment and ways to prevent injuries, especially when children are present. Rural schools should provide safety awareness for children regarding machinery operating, safety procedures, and injury prevention (Salmi and others, 1989; Swanson and others, 1987). Nurses in rural areas can be advocates for farm safety programs and for revision of the current farm safety legislation.

Other Injuries

Falls are still a source of injury but less so than in preschool children and toddlers. "Flipping," a popular activity in which children jump from an elevated surface and perform an aerial flip with the idea of landing upright, has resulted in several serious injuries to the face and head and places children at risk for back and spinal cord injury (Goepp and others, 1993). Seasonal injuries such as sledding accidents are common and more likely to occur when children sled ride without adult supervision and in streets as opposed to parks (Shugerman and others, 1992). Horseback riding injuries are another source of concern for parents of school-age children. The most common cause of death from horseback riding activities is head injury, followed by injuries to the chest and abdomen (Bixby-Hammett, 1992). Before enrolling children for riding lessons, parents should determine the instructor's safety record with students and whether the instructor is certified by a recognized organization. Injuries at public playgrounds and amusement parks (especially water slides), as well as around the home (power tools, ladders, fireworks), are ongoing concerns of parents and health care providers.

Injuries to eyes and teeth are a constant threat to school-age children involved in rough play (see Chapter 24 [eyes] and Chapter 18 [teeth]). The normally shallow bony orbit of children in this age-group makes them particularly vulnerable to eye trauma, especially during contact sports or activities, such as baseball or softball. Wearing protective eye and mouth gear is essential.

Injuries have been reported for a variety of toys (slingshots, water balloons, lawn darts, chemistry sets) and household equipment (mowers, lawn trimmers). Gunshot wounds, previously a major problem in older children, has become a significant problem during the past few years, particularly in the inner city. In a survey of 242 families it was found that 10% owned guns and 79% of these families kept the gun loaded, unlocked, and within a child's reach (Wiley and Casey, 1993). Also, the so-called "toy" forearms (air guns and air rifles) cause frequent firearm injuries to children, many less than 12 years of age (American Academy of Pediatrics, 1987b).

Nurse's Role in Injury Prevention

Nurses are primary advocates for preventive care and guidance. Safety education can be incorporated in all aspects of nursing care, and anticipatory guidance for both parents and school-age children is part of nursing interventions. The most effective means of prevention is education of the child and family regarding the hazards of risk-taking behavior and improper use of equipment. No piece of equipment is safe unless a child is physically and mentally equipped to use it. A careful history and a knowledge of normal growth and development serve as guidelines for both planned and impromptu consultation.

It is especially important for nurses to be conscientious regarding preventive teaching and guidance. Parents are often unaware of hazards to their children at various ages, especially those related to normal developmental progress. Susceptibility to injuries and understanding of safety issues are influenced by children's developmental level. Nurses who understand the growth and development of school-age children will be able to provide effective safety education to parents and children and to correct misconceptions before injuries occur.

A major function of school nurses is preventive education and safety. They should be alert to hazards in the school and instrumental in evaluating safety risks and implementing safety programs. Preventive education for children, parents, and school personnel is an ongoing part of the school nurse's responsibility. Characteristics of the school-age child and preventive measures are listed in Table 17-2.

ANTICIPATORY GUIDANCE—CARE OF FAMILIES

The parents of the school-age child find themselves in the position of sharing their child's time and interests with the

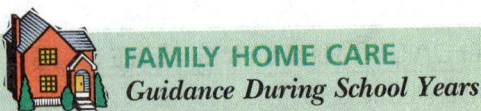

FAMILY HOME CARE
Guidance During School Years

AGE 6 YEARS

Prepare parents to expect strong food preferences and frequent refusal of specific food items.
Prepare parents to expect increasingly ravenous appetite.
Prepare parents for emotionality as child experiences erratic mood changes.
Help parents anticipate continued susceptibility to illness.
Teach injury prevention and safety, especially bicycle safety.
Encourage parents to respect child's need for privacy and to provide a separate bedroom for child, if possible.
Prepare parents for child's increasing interests outside the home.
Help parents understand the need to encourage child's interactions with peers.

AGES 7 TO 10 YEARS

Prepare parents to expect improvement in health with fewer illnesses, but warn them that allergies may increase or become apparent.
Prepare parents to expect an increase in minor injuries.
Emphasize caution in selecting and maintaining sports equipment and reemphasize safety.
Prepare parents to expect increased involvement with peers and interest in activities outside the home.
Emphasize the need to encourage independence while maintaining limit-setting and discipline.
Prepare mothers to expect more demands at 8 years.
Prepare fathers to expect increasing admiration at 10 years; encourage father-child activities.
Prepare parents for prepubescent changes in girls.

AGES 11 TO 12 YEARS

Help parents prepare child for body changes if pubescence.
Prepare parents to expect a growth spurt in girls.
Make certain child's sex education is adequate with accurate information.
Prepare parents to expect energetic but stormy behavior at 11, to become more even tempered at 12.
Encourage parents to support child's desire to "grow up" but to allow regressive behavior when needed.
Prepare parents to expect an increase in masturbation.
Instruct parents that the amount of rest child needs may increase.
Help parents educate child regarding experimentation with potentially harmful activities.

HEALTH GUIDANCE

Help parents understand the importance of regular health and dental care for child.
Encourage parents to teach and model sound health practices—including diet, rest, activity, and exercise.
Stress the need to encourage children to engage in appropriate physical activities.
Emphasize providing a safe physical and emotional environment.
Encourage parents to teach and model safety practices.

increasingly important peer group. As a child feels the need to fit into a peer group and gain a sense of industry through individual and cooperative production and performance, he or she moves away from the close, familiar relationships of the family group. It is through these early peer relationships that children begin to prepare for moving from narrow, sheltered family relationships to a broader world of relationships and increased independence. Parents must learn to provide support as unobtrusively as possible without feeling rejected, hurt, or angry. The nurse can help parents of the school-age child by providing anticipatory guidance and reassurance throughout this period of child development and maturation (see Family Home Care box).

KEY POINTS

- Middle childhood, also known as the school years, is a comfortable period of life that extends from 6 to 12 years of age.
- Although slower than previous years, there is a steady gain in height and weight with maturation of body systems; primary teeth are lost and replaced by permanent teeth.
- Skeletal lengthening, a higher ratio of muscle mass to fat, and maturation of the gastrointestinal system are major components in biologic development during middle childhood.
- Developing a sense of industry or accomplishment is a major task during the middle years (Erikson).
- Piaget's theory of concrete operations refers to the school-age period, when children are able to use their thought processes to experience events and actions and make judgments based on what they reason.
- Through identity, reversibility, and reciprocity, children master the cognitive task of conservation.
- The child develops a conscience and is able to understand and adhere to rules and standards set by others.
- Spiritual development entails a curiosity about deities, a knowledge of the difference between the natural and the supernatural, and reliance on prayers or other religious rituals.
- Entertaining different points of view, becoming sensitive to social norms of peers, and forming peer friendships are the most important features of social development in the middle years.
- Children develop a self-concept from their own self-assessment and feedback from others.
- Increased socialization, earlier pubertal development, and constant media exposure make the school years an ideal time for sex education.
- Cooperative play, team activities, and acquisition of skills are prime elements of play during the school years; rules and rituals assume greater importance.
- Optimum nutrition is often hampered by an affinity for and availability of junk foods, irregular family meals, and schedules of working parents.
- Typical parental concerns during middle childhood include dishonest behavior, lying, cheating, stealing, and school-related stress.
- The school years are an ideal time for children to begin to take responsibility for their own health.
- School health ideally offers programs that include health appraisal, emergency care, safety education, communicable disease control, counseling, guidance, and health education, with adjustment to individual student needs.
- The major sources of accidental injury during middle childhood involve a variety of conveyances, including motor vehicles, bicycles, skateboards, and in-line skates.
- Injury prevention is directed toward safety education, provision of safe play areas and equipment, and well-supervised sports activities.

REFERENCES

Adriaenssens EE and others: The video invasion of rehabilitation, *Burns* 14:417-419, 1988.

Agran PF, Winn DG: The bicycle: a developmental toy versus a vehicle, *Pediatrics* 91:752-755, 1993.

Agran PF, Winn DG, Dunkle D: Injuries among 4- to 9-year-old restrained motor vehicle occupants by seat location and crash impact site, *Am J Dis Child* 143:1317-1321, 1989.

American Academy of Pediatrics: *The injury prevention program,* Elk Grove Village, IL, 1989a, The Academy.

American Academy of Pediatrics: *Guidelines for parents: television and the family,* Elk Grove Village, IL, 1991a, The Academy.

American Academy of Pediatrics, Committee on Accident and Poison Prevention: All-terrain vehicles: two-, three-, and four-wheeled unlicensed motorized vehicles, *Pediatrics* 79:306-308, 1987a.

American Academy of Pediatrics, Committee on Accident and Poison Prevention: Injuries related to "toy" firearms, *Pediatrics* 79:473-474, 1987b.

American Academy of Pediatrics, Committee on Accident and Poison Prevention: Bicycle helmets, *Pediatrics* 85:229-230, 1990.

American Academy of Pediatrics, Committee on School Health: Health education and schools, *Pediatrics* 75:1160-1161, 1985.

American Academy of Pediatrics, Committee on School Health: Qualifications and utilization of nursing personnel delivering health services in schools, *Pediatrics* 79:647-648, 1987c.

American Academy of Pediatrics, Committee on School Health: Corporal punishment in schools, *Pediatrics* 88(1):173, 1991b.

American Academy of Pediatrics, Committee on School Health: Basic life support training in school, *Pediatrics* 91:158-159, 1993a.

American Academy of Pediatrics, Committee on School Health: Guidelines for the administration of medication in school, *Pediatrics* 92:499-500, 1993b.

American Academy of Pediatrics, Committee on Sports Medicine and Committee on School Health: Physical fitness and the schools, *Pediatrics* 80:449-450, 1987d.

American Academy of Pediatrics, Committee on Sports Medicine and Committee on School Health: Organized athletics for preadolescent children, *Pediatrics* 84:583-584, 1989b.

Attala JM and others: Health needs of school-age children in two midwestern counties, *Issues Compr Pediatr Nurs* 16:51-60, 1993.

Bell-Dolan D, Last C, Strauss C: Symptoms of anxiety disorders in normal children, *J Am Acad Child Adolesc Psychiatry* 29:759-765, 1990.

Berman BD and others: After-school child care and self-esteem in school-age children, *Pediatrics* 89:654-659, 1992.

Bernard-Bonnin A and others: Television and the 3- to 10-year-old child, *Pediatrics* 88:48-54, 1991.

Bixby-Hammett DM: Pediatric equestrian injuries, *Pediatrics* 89:1173-1176, 1992.

Coble PA and others: EEG sleep of healthy children 6 to 12 years of age. In Guilleminault C, editor: *Sleep and its disorders in children,* New York, 1987, Raven Press.

Cushman R and others: Helmet promotion in the emergency room following a bicycle injury: a randomized trial, *Pediatrics* 88:43-47, 1991.

Davis JH: Children and pets: a therapeutic connection, *Pediatr Nurs* 11:377-379, 1985.

DiGuiseppi CG, Rivara FP, Koepsell TD: Attitudes toward bicycle helmet ownership and use by school-age children, *Am J Dis Child* 144:83-86, 1990.

Dolan MA, Knapp JF, Andres J: Three-wheel and four-wheel all-terrain vehicle injuries in children, *Pediatrics* 84:694-698, 1989.

Dunne RG, Asher KN, Rivara FP: Behavior and parental expectations of child pedestrians, *Pediatrics* 89:486-490, 1992.

Ehrman D: Hotline provides latchkey children phone link to retirees, *Child Teens Today* 7(4):5, 1986.

Elizur J: The stress of school entry: parent coping behaviors and children's adjustment to school, *J Child Psychol Psychiatry* 27:625-638, 1986.

Elkind D: *The hurried child, growing up too fast too soon,* Menlo Park, CA, 1981, Addison-Wesley.

Erikson EH: *Childhood and society,* ed 2, New York, 1963, WW Norton.

Evans L: Restraint effectiveness, occupant ejection from cars, and fatality reduction, *Accid Anal Prev* 22:167-75, 1990.

Ferber R: Sleep disorders. In Levine, MD and others: *Developmental-behavioral pediatrics,* ed 2, Philadelphia, 1992, WB Saunders.

Funk JB: Reevaluating the impact of video games, *Clin Pediatr* 32:86-90, 1993.

Garbarino J and others: *Children in danger: coping with the consequences of community violence,* San Francisco, 1992, Jossey-Bass.

Gielen AC and others: Psychosocial factors associated with the use of bicycle helmets among children with and without helmet use laws, *J Pediatr* 124(2):204-210, 1994.

Goepp JG and others: Injuries sustained during flipping—a new fad activity, *Pediatr Emerg Care* 9:95-97, 1993.

Graham MV, Uphold CR: Health perceptions and behaviors of school-aged boys and girls, *J Community Health Nurs* 9:77-86, 1992.

Graybill D and others: Effects of playing violent versus nonviolent video games on the aggressive ideation of aggressive and nonaggressive children, *Child Study J* 15:199-205, 1985.

Green KE, Bird JE: The structure of children's beliefs about health and illness, *J Sch Health* 56:325-328, 1986.

Griffiths M: Amusement machine playing in childhood and adolescence: a comparative analysis of video games and fruit machines, *J Adolesc* 14:53-73, 1991.

Groves BM and others: Silent victims: children who witness violence, *JAMA* 269:262-264, 1993.

Guilleminault C: Disorders of arousal in children: somnambulism and night terrors. In Guilleminault C, editor: *Sleep and its disorders in children,* New York, 1987, Raven Press.

Hancock LA: Safe biking—a bike helmet, *J Pediatr Health Care* 1:334-335, 1987.

Hechinger FM: *Fateful choices: healthy youth for the 21st century,* New York, 1992, Hill and Wong.

Howland J and others: Barriers to bicycle helmet use among children, *Am J Dis Child* 143:741-744, 1989.

Igoe JB: Healthy long-term attitudes on personal health can be developed in school-age children, *Pediatrician* 15:127-136, 1988.

Igoe JB: HealthPACT helps youngsters to be more active in their health care, *Child Behav Dev Lett* 5(4):1-2, 1989.

Igoe JB: School-linked family health centers in health care reform, *Pediatr Nurs* 19:67-68, 1993.

Inkelis DH and others: Roller skating injuries in children, *Pediat Emerg Care* 4:127-132, 1988.

Irwin CE, Millstein SG: Risk-taking behaviors and biopsychosocial development during adolescence. In Susman EJ, Feagans LV, Ray WJ: *Emotion, cognition, health and development in children and adolescents,* Hillsdale, NJ, 1992, Lawrence Erlbaum Associates.

Jaffe PG, Wolfe DA, Wilson SK: *Children of battered women,* Newbury Park, CA, 1990, Sage Press.

Jones ME, Clark D: What school nurses really do: a study of school nurse utilization, *J Sch Nurs* 9:10-17, 1993.

Kolko DJ, Rickard-Figuero JL: Effects of video games on the adverse corollaries of chemotherapy in pediatric oncology patients: a single-case analysis, *J Consult Clin Psychol* 53:223-228, 1985.

Krugman RD, Krugman MK: Emotional abuse in the classroom, *Am J Dis Child* 138:284-286, 1984.

Kuczen B: *Childhood stress,* New York, 1982, Delacorte Press.

Levine MD: Middle childhood. In Levine MD and others: *Developmental-behavioral prediatrics,* ed 2, Philadelphia, 1992, WB Saunders.

Lipsitt LP: On teaching skills to risk takers, *Child Behav Dev Lett* 5(5):8, 1988 (editoral).

Maeda Y and others: Electroclinical study of video game epilepsy, *Dev Med Child Neurol* 32:493-500, 1990.

Massachusetts Medical Society Committee on Nutrition: Fast-food fare: consumer guidelines, *N Engl J Med* 321:752-756, 1989.

Masten AS and others: Many variables determine the effects of stress, *J Child Psychol Psychiatry* 29:745-762, 1988.

Metcalf JA, Roberts SO: Strength training and the immature athlete: an overview, *Pediatr Nurs* 19:325-332, 1993.

Meyers AF and others: School breakfast program and school performance, *Am J Dis Child* 143:1234-1239, 1989.

Miller ME: Immunodeficiency of immaturity. In Stiehm R: *Immunologic disorders in infants and children,* Philadelphia, 1989, WB Saunders.

National Association of Pediatric Nurse Associates and Practitioners: Policy statement on corporal punishment. *J Pediatr Health Care* 7:90, 1993.

Neff EJ, Dale JC: Assessment of quality of life in school-aged children: a method—phase I, *Matern Child Nurs J* 19:313-330, 1990.

Nelms BC: Corporal punishment in the schools: sanctioned abuse? *J Pediatr Health Care* 3:219-220, 1988 (editorial).

Newman BM, Newman PR: *Development through life: a psychosocial approach,* ed 5, Pacific Grove, CA, 1991, Brookes-Cole.

Nichols TW, Jr: Bicycle-seat hematuria *N Engl J Med* 311:1128, 1984 (letter).

Parkin PC and others: Evaluation of a promotional strategy to increase bicycle helmet use by children, *Pediatrics* 91:772-777, 1993.

Pendergast RA and others: Correlates of children's bicycle helmet use and short-term failure of school-level interventions, *Pediatrics* 90:354-358, 1992.

Poresky RH and others: Pets influence self-concept, *J Psychol* 122:463-469, 1988.

Retsky J, Jaffe D, Christoffel KK: Child injuries due to skateboards: recurrence in the 1980s *Clin Res* 35:915A, 1987 (abstract).

Roberts M, Fanurik D: Rewarding elementary school children for their use of safety belts, *Health Psychol* 5:185-196, 1986.

Roberts M, Turner D: Rewarding parents for their children's use of safety seats, *J Pediatr Psychol* 11:25-36, 1986.

Rollins JA: Nurses as gangbusters: a response to gang violence in America, *Pediatr Nurs* 19:559-567, 1993.

Sabate J and others: Anthropometric parameters of schoolchildren with different lifestyles, *Am J Dis Child* 144:1159-1163, 1990.

Salmi LR and others: Fatal farm injuries among young children, *Pediatrics* 83:267-271, 1989.

Sandler A: Social development in middle childhood, *Pediatr Ann* 18:380-387, 1989.

Saunders A, Remsberg B: *The stress-proof child,* New York, 1984, Holt, Rinehart, & Winston.

Scanlan BJ: An holistic approach to school dental health, *J Sch Nurs* 7:12-15, 1991.

Scheidt PC, Wilson MH, Stern MS: Bicycle helmet law for children: a case study of activism in injury control, *Pediatrics* 89:1248-1250, 1992.

Schmitt B: Preventing problems with schoolwork, *Contemp Pediatr* 7(9):31-32, 1990.

Schonfeld DJ and others: Understanding of acquired immunodeficiency syndrome by elementary school children—a developmental survey, *Pediatrics* 92:389-395, 1993.

Schwartz S: A comparison of componential and traditional approaches to training reading skills, *Appl Cognitive Psychol* 2:189-201, 1988.

Selbst SM, Alexander D, Ruddy R: Bicycle-related injuries, *Am J Dis Child* 141:140-144, 1987.

Shugerman RP and others: Risk factors for childhood sledding injuries: a case-control study, *Pediatr Emerg Care* 8:283-286, 1992.

Simons-Morton BG and others: The physical activity of fifth-grade students during physical education classes, *Am J Public Health* 83:262-264, 1993.

Smith EV: *Hazard analysis of ride-on mowers,* Consumer Product Safety Commission, May 1988.

Society for Adolescent Medicine, Ad Hoc Corporal Punishment Committee: Corporal punishment in schools, *J Adolesc Health* 13:240-246, 1992.

Sparnon AL, Ford WDA: Handlebar injuries in children, *J Pediatr Surg* 21:118-119, 1986.

Spence LJ and others: Fatal bicycle accidents in children: a plea for prevention *J Pediatr Surg* 28:214-216, 1993.

Spital M, Spital A, Spital R: The compelling case for seat belts on school buses, *Pediatrics* 78:928-932, 1986.

Swanson JA and others: Accidental farm injuries in children, *Am J Dis Child* 141:1276-1279, 1987.

Terr LC: Nightmares in children. In Guilleminault C, editor: *Sleep and its disorders in children,* New York, 1987, Raven Press.

Thompson RS, Rivara FP, Thompson DC: A

case-control study of the effectiveness of bicycle safety helmets, *N Engl J Med* 320:1361-1367, 1989.

Vandell D, Minnett A, Santrock J: Sibling relationships change during middle childhood, *J Appl Dev Psychol* 8:247-257, 1987.

Weiss BD: Trends in bicycle helmet use by children: 1985 to 1990, *Pediatrics* 89:78-80, 1992.

Whitaker RC and others: School lunch: a comparison of the fat and cholesterol content with dietary guidelines, *J Pediatr* 123:857-862, 1993.

Widome MD: School bus seat belts? *Pediatrics* 82:134-135, 1988 (letter).

Wiley CC, Casey R: Family experiences, attitudes, and household safety practices regarding firearms, *Clin Pediatr* 32:71-76, 1993.

Wilson PD, Testani-Dufour LT: Bicycle safety programs: targeting injury prevention through education, *Pediatr Nurs* 19:343-346, 1993.

Winkelstein ML: Fostering positive self-concept in the school-age child, *Pediatr Nurs* 15:229-233, 1989.

Winton R: Pupils versed in violence, survey shows, *The Los Angeles Times,* pp J1, J6, Oct 25, 1992.

BIBLIOGRAPHY

General

Adger H, DeAngelis C: Sexuality education: our schools can do better, *Contemp Pediatr* 6(10):56-67, 1989.

Brooks RB: Self-esteem during the school years: its normal development and hazardous decline, *Pediatr Clin North Am* 39:537-549, 1992.

Carey WB: Temperament issues in the school-aged child, *Pediatr Clin North Am* 39:569-584, 1992.

Castiglia P: Nightmares, *J Pediatr Health Care* 7(3):125-126, 1993.

Dixon SD, Stein MT: *Encounters with children: pediatric behavior and development,* ed 2, St Louis, 1992, Mosby.

Dworkin PH: Behavior during middle childhood: developmental themes and clinical issues, *Pediatr Ann* 18:347-355, 1989.

Feldman H: The development of thinking skills in school-age children, *Pediatr Ann* 18:356-362, 1989.

Ferber R: Sleep schedule-dependent causes of insomnia and sleepiness in middle childhood and adolescence, *Pediatrician* 17:13-20, 1990.

Flavell JH: *Cognitive development,* ed 2, Englewood Cliffs, NJ, 1985, Prentice-Hall, Inc.

Landman GB: Language development from six to twelve, *Pediatr Ann* 18:373-379, 1989.

Maccoby EE: *Social development: psychological growth and the parent-child relationship,* New York, 1980, Harcourt Brace Jovanovich, Inc.

Mahowald MW, Rosen GM: Parasomnias in children, *Pediatrician* 17:21-31, 1990.

Mason KJ: Pediatric orthopaedics: developmental norms, *Orthop Nurs* 8(4):45-50, 1989.

Riesch S and others: Effects of communication training on parents and young adolescents, *Nurs Res* 42:10-16, 1993.

Shelly JA: *The spiritual needs of children,* Downers Grove, IL, 1982, InterVarsity Press.

Sieving RE, Zirbel-Donisch ST: Development and enhancement of self-esteem in children, *J Pediatr Health Care* 4:290-296, 1990.

Stone JL, Church J: *Childhood and adolescence,* ed 5, New York, 1983, Random House.

Weir R, Rideout E, Crook J: Pediatric use of emergency departments, *J Pediatr Nurs* 3:204-210, 1989.

Melnyk BM: Changes in parent child relationships following divorce, *Pediatr Nurs* 17:337-341, 1991.

Minde KK: Effect of social change on the behavior of school-age children, *Pediatrician* 15:170-175, 1988.

Nelms BC: Children feel the pressure too, *J Pediatr Health Care* 3:229, 1989 (editorial).

Nowicki S, Oxenford C: The relation of hostile nonverbal communication styles to popularity in preadolescent children, *J Genet Psychol* 150:39-44, 1989.

Rowland BH, Robinson BE, Coleman M: A survey of parents' perceptions regarding latchkey children, *Pediatr Nurs* 12:278-283, 1986.

Ryan-Wenger NM, Copeland SG: Coping strategies used by black school-age children from low-income families, *J Pediatr Nurs* 9:33-40, 1994.

Williams RL, Fosarelli PD: Telephone call-in services for children in self-care, *Am J Dis Child* 141:965-968, 1987.

Stress and Coping

Birgenheier PS: Parents and children, war and separation, *Pediatr Nurs* 19:471-476, 1993.

Gage RB: Consequences of children's exposure to spouse abuse, *Pediatr Nurs* 16:258-260, 1990.

Humphreys J: Children of battered women: worries about their mothers, *Pediatr Nurs* 17:342-345, 354, 1991.

Health Promotion

American Academy of Pediatrics, Committee on School Health: *School health: a guide for health professionals,* Elk Grove Village, IL, 1987, American Academy of Pediatrics.

American Academy of Pediatrics, Committee on School Health: Prevention of hepatitis B virus infection in school settings, *Pediatrics* 91:848-850, 1993.

Bailey-Britton AM: The relationship between health and academic performance in school-age children, *Issues Compre Pediatr Nurs* 10:273-289, 1987.

Baldwin J, Davis LL: Assessing parents as health educators, *Pediatr Nurs* 15:453-462, 1989.

Bausell RB: A national survey assessing pediatric preventive behaviors, *Pediatr Nurs* 11:438-444, 1985.

Carmon M and others: Cardiovascular screening programs: implications for school nurses, *Pediatr Nurs* 16:509-511, 1990.

Clore E, Hibel J: The parasomnias of childhood, *J Pediatr Health Care* 7(1):12-16, 1993.

Cowell JM and others: School health services: a hub of services to children and their families, *Pediatr Nurs* 17:86-88, 1991.

Cox CL and others: The health self-determinism index for children, *Res Nurs Health* 13:267-271, 1990.

Eiden H, Thomas M, Fosarelli P: A teaching tool for children in self-care, *J Pediatr Health Care* 1:292-297, 1987.

Farrand LL, Cox CL: Determinants of positive health behavior in middle childhood, *Nurs Res* 42:208-213, 1993.

Farren M, McKevitt RK: Nursing roles in school health. In Hoekelman RA and others, editors: *Primary pediatric care* ed 2, St Louis, 1992, Mosby.

Giordana BP, Igoe JB: Health promotion: the new frontier, *Pediatr Nurs* 17:490-492, 1991.

Hester ND: Health concerns of school-age children, *Issues Compr Pediatr Nurs* 10:251-262, 1987.

Igoe JB: Beyond green beans and oat bran: a health agenda for the 1990s for school-age youth, *Pediatr Nurs* 16:289-292, 1990.

Igoe JB: Healthy people 2000, *Pediatr Nurs* 16:584-586, 1990.

Igoe JB: An update on student health fairs, *Pediatr Nurs* 17:170-172, 1991.

Kornguth ML: School illnesses: who's absent and why? *Pediatr Nurs* 16:95-99, 1990.

Lear JG: Building a health/education partnership: the role of school-based health centers, *Pediatr Nurs* 18(2):172-173, 1992.

Lyons JF, Hester NO: Research-generated nursing diagnoses for healthy school-age children, *Issues Compr Pediatr Nurs* 10:149-150, 1987.

Maheady DC: Camp nursing practice in review, *Pediatr Nurs* 17:247-250, 1991.

McCarthy B: A partnership to save children's lives: the school nurse/medic alert kids program, *J Sch Nurs* 9:23-25, 1993.

Moore JB: Determining the relationship of autonomy to self-care agency of locus of control in school-age children, *Matern Child Nurs J* 16(1):47-60, 1987.

O'Brien RW, Bush PJ, Parcel GS: Stability in a measure of children's health locus of control, *J Sch Health* 59(4):161-164, 1989.

Resnicow K and others: A three-year evaluation of the Know Your Body program in inner-city school children, *Health Educ Q* 19:463-480, 1992.

Rose DA, Chen SC, Souter CM: Development of an in-service education program by school nurses, *J Community Health Nurs* 4(3):171-178, 1987.

Vessey JA, Braithwaite KB, Wiedmann M: Teaching children about their internal bodies, *Pediatr Nurs* 16:29-33, 1990.

Vessey JA, Swanson MN: School-based clinics and the pediatric nurse: an interview with Surgeon General Designee M. Joycelyn Elders, *Pediatr Nurs* 19:359-362, 1993.

Nutrition

American Academy of Pediatrics, Committee on Nutrition: Indications for cholesterol testing in children, *Pediatrics* 83:141-142, 1989.

Berenson G and others: Cardiovascular health promotion for elementary school children: the Heart Smart Program, *Ann NY Acad Sci* 623:299-313, 1991.

Gates DM, McClure MJ: Forestalling the progress of heart disease, *MCN* 14:174-178, 1989.

McCabe E: Monitoring the fat and cholesterol intake of children and adolescents, *J Pediatr Health Care* 7(2):61-70, 1993.

Mistretta E, Stroud S: Hypercholesterolemia in children: risk and management, *Pediatr Nurs* 16:152-154, 1990.

Nicklas T and others: Nutrient adequacy of low-fat intakes for children: the Bogalusa Heart Study, *Pediatrics* 89:221-228, 1992.

Nolan R: Childhood hypercholesterolemia: implications for nurse practitioners, *Pediatr Nurs* 20:46-50, 1994.

Pipes PL, Trahms CM: *Nutrition in infancy and childhood,* ed 5, St Louis, 1993, Mosby.

Williams SR: *Nutrition and diet therapy,* ed 7, St Louis, 1993, Mosby.

Injury Prevention

American Academy of Pediatrics, Committee on Injury and Poison Prevention: Children and fireworks, *Pediatrics* 88:652-653, 1991.

American Academy of Pediatrics, Committee on Injury and Poison Prevention: Drowning in infants, children and adolescents, *Pediatrics* 92:292-294, 1993.

Avner JR, Baker MD: Dog bites in urban children, *Pediatrics* 88:55-57, 1991.

Christoffel KK: Child passenger safety, *Am J Dis Child* 143:1271-1272, 1989.

Coppens NM: Parental responses to children in unsafe situations, *Pediatr Nurs* 16:571-574, 1990.

Grossman DC, Rivara FP: Injury control in childhood, *Pediatr Clin North Am* 39:471-485, 1992.

Jones NE: Childhood injuries: an epidemiologic approach, *Pediatr Nurs* 18:235-239, 1992.

Jones NE: Prevention of childhood injuries. I. Motor vehicle injuries, *Pediatr Nurs* 18:380-382, 1992.

Jones NE: Prevention of childhood injuries. II. Recreational injuries, *Pediatr Nurs* 18:619-621, 1992.

Nakayama DK, Pasieka KB, Gardner MJ: How bicycle-related injuries change bicycling practices in children, *Am J Dis Child* 144:928-929, 1990.

Ostrum GA: Sports-related injuries in youths: prevention is the key—and nurses can help! *Pediatr Nurs* 19:333-342, 1993.

Pless I, Arsenault A: The role of health education in the prevention of injuries to children, *J Soc Issues* 43:87-103, 1987.

Pless IB, Verreault R, Tenina S: A case-control study of pedestrian and bicyclist injuries in childhood, *Am J Public Health* 79:995-998, 1989.

Powell EC, Tanz RR: Comparison of childhood burns associated with use of microwave ovens and conventional stoves, *Pediatrics* 91:344-349, 1993.

Ridenour MV: Elementary school playgrounds: safe play areas or inherent dangers, *Percept Mot Skills* 64:447-451, 1987.

Rivara FP and others: Attitudes and practices toward children as pedestrians, *Pediatrics* 84:1017-1021, 1989.

Scheidt PC: Behavioral research toward prevention of childhood injury, *Am J Dis Child* 142:612-617, 1988.

Senturia YD, Christoffel KK, Donovan AA: Children's household exposure to guns: a pediatric practice-based survey, *Pediatrics* 93(3):469-475, 1994.

Sewell KH, Gaines SK: A developmental approach to childhood safety education, *Pediatr Nurs* 19:464-466, 1993.

Solis GR: Evaluation of a children's safety fair, *Pediatr Nurs* 17:255-258, 1991.

Widner-Kolberg MR: The nurse's role in pediatric injury prevention, *Crit Care Nurs Clin North Am* 3:391-197, 1991.

Wilson MH: Preventing injury in the "middle years," *Contemp Pediatr* 6(6):20-54, 1989.

CHAPTER 18

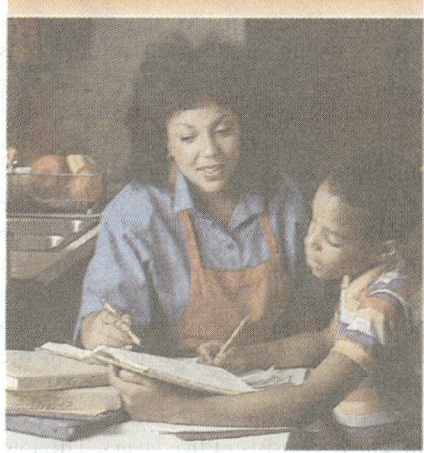

Health Problems of Middle Childhood

CHAPTER OUTLINE

RELATED TOPICS

Acne, Ch. 20
Autism, Ch. 13
"Birthmarks," Ch. 9
Bullous impetigo, Ch. 9
Burns, Ch. 29
Candidiasis, Ch. 9
Communicable diseases, Ch. 16
Dental health: infant, Ch. 12; toddler, Ch. 14; preschooler, Ch. 15; school-age child, Ch. 17
Maintaining healthy skin, Ch. 27
Pain assessment; pain management, Ch. 26
Physical assessment: newborn, Ch. 8
Physical examination: skin, Ch. 7
Preparation for procedures, Ch. 27
Restraints, Ch. 27
Sexually transmitted diseases, Ch. 20
Skin disorders: infancy, Ch. 13
Suicide, Ch. 21

DISORDERS AFFECTING THE SKIN

THE SKIN

The skin and its component and associated structures constitute the integumentary system. The largest organ in the body, the skin is a thin structure (only about 1 mm thick at birth, increasing to approximately twice that thickness at maturity) that serves primarily as an insulator, not as an organ of exchange.

Anatomically and physiologically the skin differs markedly in various areas of the body, and each variation is adapted to meet special stresses. Regions such as the soles of the feet, the eyelids, and the back vary in skin thickness and looseness and in the kinds and quantities of appendages they contain, such as sweat glands and hair follicles. These variations are the basis for the localization of many disorders to specific areas and for the distribution of certain eruptions in characteristic patterns.

Purposes of the Skin

This functionally simple but morphologically complex structure serves several physical functions essential to life.

Protection. The skin serves as a protection against trauma, including mechanical, thermal, chemical, and radiant. The intact tough outer layer is a mechanical barrier. Organisms and chemicals penetrate it with difficulty, and it is further protected by the oily and slightly acid secretions of its sebaceous glands, which limit the growth of bacteria.

Impermeability. Very few substances are able to penetrate the skin with ease. It seals the body from the environment. The outer side of the upper layer, with its low water content, is in equilibrium with the viable cells underneath. It protects against loss of essential body constituents to the environment. The effectiveness of this impermeable membrane is demonstrated by the profuse fluid loss that follows damage to the epidermis by superficial burns, injury, poison ivy, or other agents. Loss of water and some electrolytes takes place only through pores in this effective barrier.

Heat Regulation. The skin also adjusts heat loss to heat production to maintain the thermal balance of the body. This is accomplished primarily through functioning of cutaneous blood vessels and sweat glands. The vascular supply to the skin, much more extensive than needed for tissue nourishment, is regulated by way of central and local neural and hormonal processes.

Sensation. As a sensory organ, perceptions (touch, pain, heat, and cold) are registered through the nerves that permeate the skin. To some extent, skin is also an organ of expression that betrays strong feelings: blushing (shame or embarrassment), redness (anger), blanching (fear), and sweating (anxiety).

Skin Structure

The skin consists of two layers: the epidermis and the corium or dermis. Under the dermis is the subcutaneous tissue or hypodermis that is composed primarily of fatty tissue of varying thickness. The activity of the skin is controlled by the autonomic nervous system and the endocrine glands (Fig. 18-1).

The efficiency with which the skin layers prevent evaporative loss of water (independent of sweat) increases with development. A transitional zone between the epidermal layers allows more of the larger fluid content (70%) of the lower layers to enter the outer, drier layers (15% water), where it is lost in greater or lesser amounts, depending on environmental temperature and humidity. In the young child the transitional zone is less effective than that in an older child or adult. The fluid loss is most marked in the prematurely born infant.

Epidermis. The epidermis, the outermost portion of relatively uniform thickness, consists of five layers. The lowest, the ***stratum germinativum,*** or "basal layer," is composed of specialized cells called ***keratinocytes*** or ***basal cells*** that are continually replacing the cell population. As they multiply, the older cells are displaced outwardly by the constant stream of new cells. The older cells progressively flatten and alter until they form dead, scalelike, or horny flakes with no cellular details and that are composed of ***keratin.*** These flakes are constantly sloughed off the surface of the body. This continual epidermal renewal is nourished by fluid from blood vessels in the dermis. The intact epidermis provides a relatively impenetrable barrier to the loss of body contents and the entrance of environmental hazards.

All layers of the epidermis consist of peaks and valleys, but the basal layer has the most dramatic arrangement. The peaks that protrude downward into the dermis are called ***rete pegs*** or ***rete ridges.*** They help anchor the epidermis to the dermis (Wysocki, 1992). Elaborating the epidermis are specialized cellular invaginations of epidermal origin, the glandular appendages and hair follicles. Although they are situated mainly in the dermis, these structures are lined with epithelial cells and are derived from the epithelial skin layer. This has significance when a large area of epidermis is damaged. It is from the cells lining these structures that new epithelium is derived.

Diseases of the skin focus sharply on the epidermis, which is the site of many distinctive patterns, ranging from the vesiculation of contact dermatitis to common superficial tumors. Clearly visible, these morphologic changes produce the varied patterns on which a dermatologic diagnosis is made.

Dermis. The dermis, or ***corium,*** constitutes the bulk of the skin. It is a firm, fibrous, and elastic connective tissue network containing an elaborate system of blood vessels, lymphatics, and nerves and varies throughout the body from 1 to 4 mm in thickness. In addition, it is invaded by the epidermal downgrowth of hair follicles and glands. Functionally the corium has a major protective role for these varied essential components of the skin.

More hidden than the epidermis, changes in the dermis are more difficult to interpret on inspection. Biopsy and histologic studies are more often needed to confirm a diagnosis based on manifestations in the corium. Since it is composed predominantly of connective tissue, the dermis frequently permits an awareness and observation of many dif-

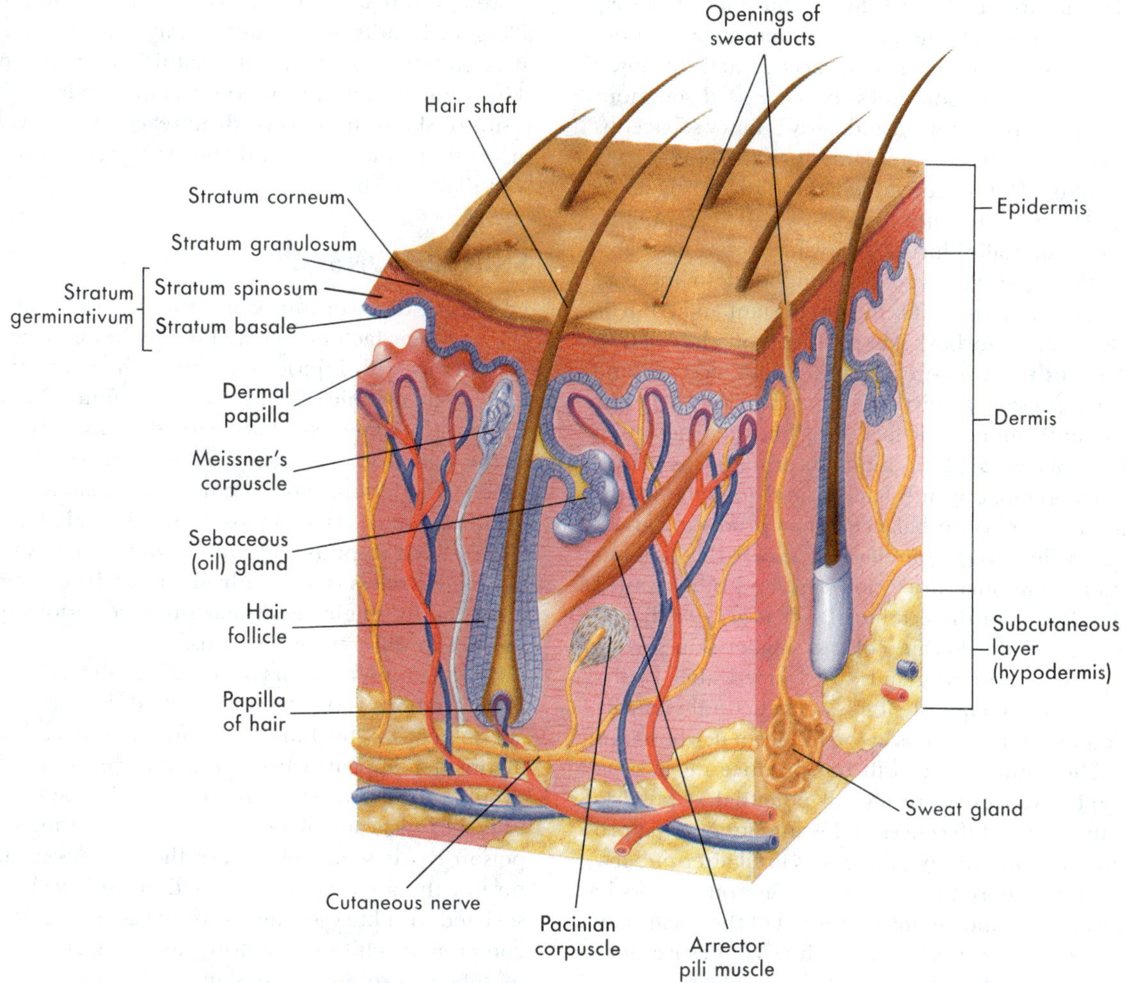

FIG. 18-1 Microscopic diagram of the skin. The epidermis, shown in longitudinal section, is raised at one corner to reveal the ridges in the dermis. (From Thibodeau GA, Patton KT: *Anatomy and physiology*, ed 2, St Louis, 1993, Mosby.)

fuse systemic disorders of connective tissue—the "collagen" diseases.

Subcutaneous Tissue. A thick layer of subcutaneous tissue lies beneath the dermis and is composed of a looser type of connective tissue that varies greatly in extent in various parts of the body. In addition to larger blood vessels, lymph channels, and nerve trunks, the subcutaneous tissue serves as a depot for the storage of fat that acts as a cushion, insulates the body against cold, and largely determines its contours.

Hair. The various skin appendages develop at different times and at different rates. An extensive growth of fine body hair, lanugo, begins to appear at the end of the second intrauterine month, reaches its maximum development between the seventh and eighth months of fetal life, and begins to decrease before birth. It continues to regress steadily during early infancy and is replaced by a less extensive distribution of hair. Hair follicles are fully developed at birth, but the amount and texture of scalp hair vary among individual infants. The scalp hair is lost during the first few months after birth and then is slowly replaced by permanent hair, which gradually thickens and often darkens as the child grows.

At puberty the secretion of androgenic hormones stimulates an increase in the thickening and darkening of scalp hair, the growth of hair in the axilla and pubic regions of both sexes, and the growth of facial hair in boys. Late in adolescence some boys acquire additional amounts and distribution of body hair, such as on the chest.

Sebaceous Glands. The sebaceous glands form in connection with hair follicles. Their function is to produce a fatty secretion called ***sebum*** that helps keep the skin supple by decreasing water loss. The sebaceous activity is maintained at a relatively constant rate by the secretion of androgens; an increase in androgens causes an increase in sebum production. Sebaceous glands have a regional distribution and are most abundant on the scalp, the face, and the genitals; are less numerous on the trunk; are sparse on the extremities; and do not appear on the palms and soles.

Sebaceous glands begin to form during the fifth month

of fetal life and are very active during the month before birth, when they produce the protective vernix caseosa observed on newborn infants. The sebaceous activity slowly subsides after birth and continues to decrease throughout infancy. In the newborn period and early infancy sebaceous secretion may cause minor problems such as "cradle cap" in some infants. The secretion remains low during early childhood, which contributes to dryness and susceptibility to chapping, especially during the winter months. Sebaceous secretion gradually rises in childhood to increase markedly at puberty, where it remains constant and contributes greatly to the disturbing skin problems of adolescence.

Sweat Glands. The sweat glands, both eccrine and apocrine, are present at birth. They appear between the fifth and seventh months of fetal life, but their activity is scant. The ***eccrine sweat glands*** function primarily as part of the body heat–regulating mechanism and to some extent in maintaining electrolyte balance. They produce a transparent, watery liquid ***(perspiration*** or ***sweat)*** that is composed of salts, ammonia, uric acid, urea, and other wastes. At birth the density of the eccrine glands is greater than at any other time of life (because of the smaller skin surface area and because no new glands are formed after birth). The sweat glands are equivalent in size, structural maturity, and position within the dermis in the full-term newborn and the adult. They function at birth but produce more sweat as childhood advances, to reach full potential at puberty. There are individual differences in the amount of sweat produced, and there are no sex differences until after puberty, when males sweat more than females. Numerous factors influence the amount and chemical content of the sweat (e.g., emotions and some disease states such as congestive heart failure in infancy and cystic fibrosis).

Apocrine sweat glands, located primarily in the axilla, areola of the breast, and anal area, are inactive throughout infancy and childhood and mature during puberty. They are much larger than eccrine glands and are connected with hair follicles. When the secretions from these glands are acted on by bacteria, they cause the unpleasant odor associated with sweating.

Skin of Younger Children

The major skin layers arise from different embryologic origins. Early in the embryonic period, a single layer of epithelium forms from the ectoderm, while simultaneously the corium develops from the mesenchyme. In the infant and small child the epidermis is still loosely bound to the dermis, partly because the rete pegs are flat. This poor adherence causes the layers to separate readily during an inflammatory process to form blisters. This is especially true in preterm infants, who have an even greater propensity to blister formation and separation during careless handling (such as removal of adhesive tape). The skin is thinner than in older children, and the cells of all strata are more compressed.

Several characteristics influence skin responses in infants and young children. Their skin is far more susceptible to superficial bacterial infection. They are more likely to have associated systemic symptoms with some infections and are more apt to react to a primary irritant than to a sensitizing allergen. Infants and young children are more frequently affected by chronic atopic dermatitis (eczema). The infant's skin is much more prone to develop a toxic erythema as a result of skin eruptions or drug reactions and is subject to maceration, infection, and the sweat retention associated with diaper rash.

SKIN LESIONS

Lesions of the skin can be a result of a wide variety of specific etiologic factors. In general, skin lesions originate from (1) contact with injurious agents such as infectious organisms, toxic chemicals, and physical trauma; (2) hereditary factors; (3) some external factor that produces a reaction in the skin (e.g., allergens); or (4) or a systemic disease of which the lesions are a cutaneous manifestation (e.g., measles, lupus erythematosus, nutritional deficiency diseases). Such responses are highly individual. An agent that may be harmless to one individual may be damaging to another, and a single agent may produce various types of responses in different individuals.

Among other factors involved in the etiology of skin manifestations is the age of the child. For example, infants are subject to "birthmark" malformations and atopic dermatitis that appears early in life; the school-age child is susceptible to ringworm of the scalp; and acne is a characteristic skin disorder of puberty. Contact dermatitis, such as poison ivy, is seen only where the noxious agent is a feature of the area. Similarly, reactions to insect bites are associated with life-cycle and seasonal activities. Although less common in children, tension and anxiety may produce, modify, or prolong many skin conditions.

Pathophysiology of Dermatitis

Over half of dermatologic problems are various forms of dermatitis. This implies a sequence of inflammatory changes in the skin that are grossly and microscopically similar but diverse in course and causation. Acute responses produce intercellular and intracellular edema, the formation of intradermal vesicles, and an initial minimum infiltration of inflammatory cells into the epidermis. In the dermis there is edema, vascular dilation, and early perivascular cellular infiltration. The location and manner of these reactions produce the lesions characteristic of each disorder. The changes are reversible, and the skin ordinarily recovers without blemish and completely intact unless complicating factors such as ulceration from the primary irritant, scratching, and infection are introduced or underlying vascular disease develops. In chronic conditions permanent effects are seen that vary according to the disorder, the general condition of the affected individual, and available therapy.

Clinical Manifestations and Diagnostic Evaluation

Although the history and subjective symptoms are explored first, objective findings are often noted simultaneously. One of the more advantageous aspects of skin lesions is that often the diagnosis is readily established after simple, careful inspection.

History and Subjective Symptoms. Many cutaneous lesions are associated with local symptoms, the most common of which is itching ***(pruritus)*** that varies in kind and intensity. Pain or tenderness often accompanies some skin lesions, and other sensations may be described as burning, prickling, stinging, or crawling. Alterations in local feeling or sensation include absence of sensation ***(anesthesia),*** excessive sensitiveness ***(hyperesthesia),*** diminished sensation ***(hypesthesia*** or ***hypoesthesia),*** or abnormal sensation, such as burning or prickling ***(paresthesia).*** These symptoms may remain localized or may migrate, may be constant or intermittent, and may be aggravated by a specific activity or circumstance, such as exposure to sunlight.

It is also important to determine whether the child has had an allergic condition such as asthma or hay fever or has had previous skin disease. Atopic dermatitis, often associated with allergies, frequently begins in infancy. It should be determined when the lesion or symptom first became apparent, as well as whether it is related to ingestion of a food or other substance, including any medication the child might be taking. It should be kept in mind that the condition may be related to an activity such as contact with plants, insects, or chemicals.

Objective Findings. Much can be determined by the distribution, size, morphology, and arrangement of the lesions. Extrinsic causes usually result from physical, chemical, or allergic irritants or from an infectious agent such as bacteria, fungi, viruses, or animal parasites. Skin manifestations can be produced by such intrinsic causes as a specific infection (such as measles or chickenpox), drug sensitization, or other allergic phenomena. Other diagnostic tools are subjective symptoms, the history, and medical and laboratory studies.

Lesion. According to the nature of the pathologic process, lesions assume more or less distinct characteristics. Names that have been applied to these lesions are important for descriptive purposes in the processes of record keeping and communication. Nurses should also become familiar with the more common terms used to describe skin lesions seen in dermatologic conditions:

Erythema—A reddened area caused by increased amounts of oxygenated blood in the dermal vasculature

Ecchymoses (bruises)—Localized red or purple discolorations caused by extravasation of blood into dermis and subcutaneous tissues

Petechiae—Pinpoint, tiny, and, sharp circumscribed spots in the superficial layers of the epidermis

Primary lesions—Skin changes produced by some causative fac-

Macule—flat; nonpalpable; circumscribed; less than 1 cm in diameter; brown, red, purple, white, or tan in color
Examples: Freckles; flat moles; rubella; rubeola

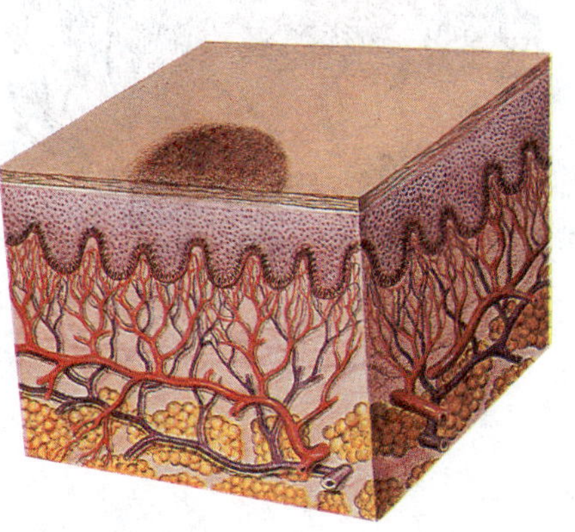

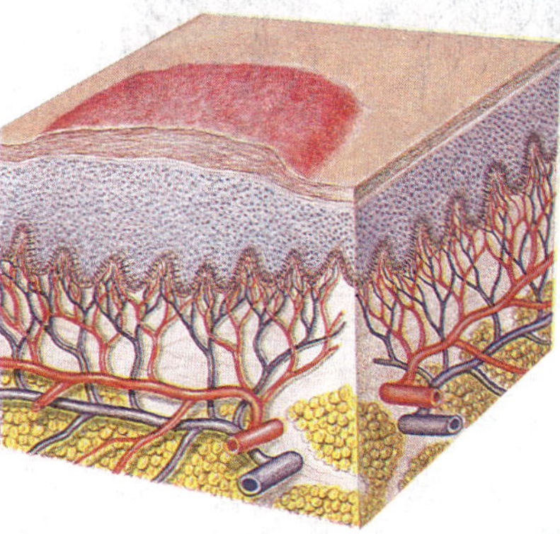

Plaque—elevated; flat topped; firm; rough; superficial papule greater than 1 cm in diameter; may be coalesced papules
Examples: Psoriasis; seborrheic and actinic keratoses

Patch—flat; nonpalpable; irregular in shape; macule that is greater than 1 cm in diameter
Examples: Vitiligo; port-wine marks

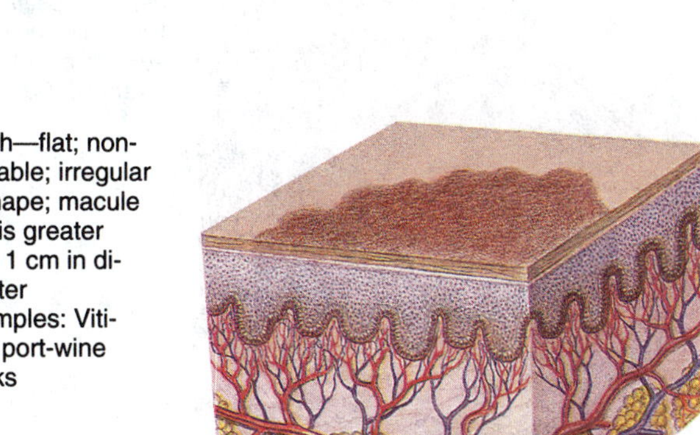

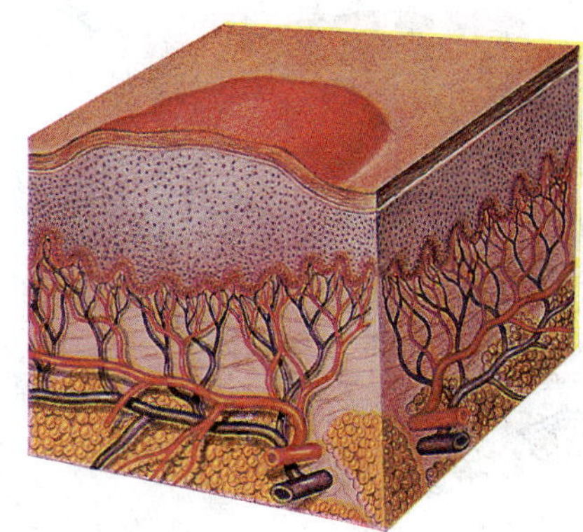

Wheal—elevated, irregular-shaped area of cutaneous edema; solid, transient, changing, variable diameter; pale pink with lighter center
Examples: Urticaria; insect bites

FIG. 18-2 Primary skin lesions. (From Seidel HM and others: *Mosby's guide to physical examination,* ed 3, St Louis, 1995, Mosby.)

Continued.

Papule—elevated; palpable; firm; circumscribed; less than 1 cm in diameter; brown, red, pink, tan, or bluish red in color
Examples: Warts; drug-related eruptions; pigmented nevi

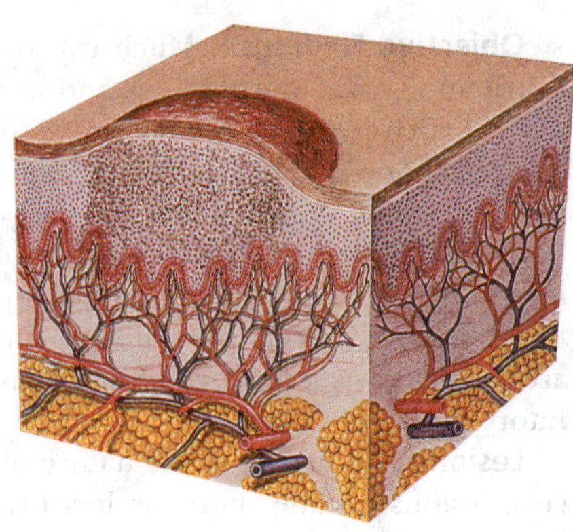

Nodule—elevated; firm; circumscribed; palpable; deeper in dermis than papule; 1 to 2 cm in diameter
Examples: Erythema nodosum; lipomas

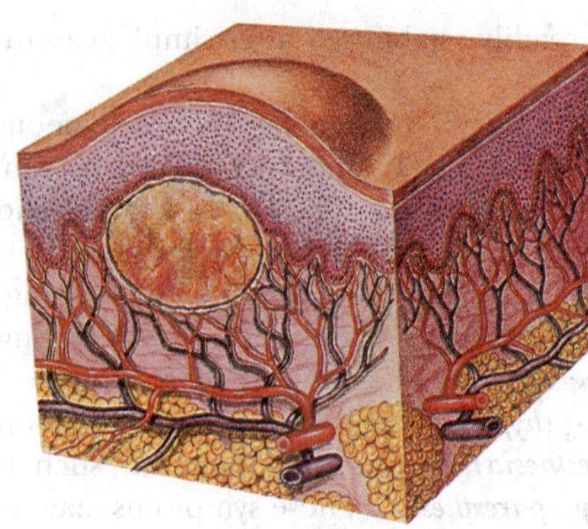

Vesicle—elevated; circumscribed; superficial; filled with serous fluid; less than 1 cm in diameter
Examples: Blister; varicella

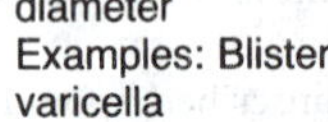

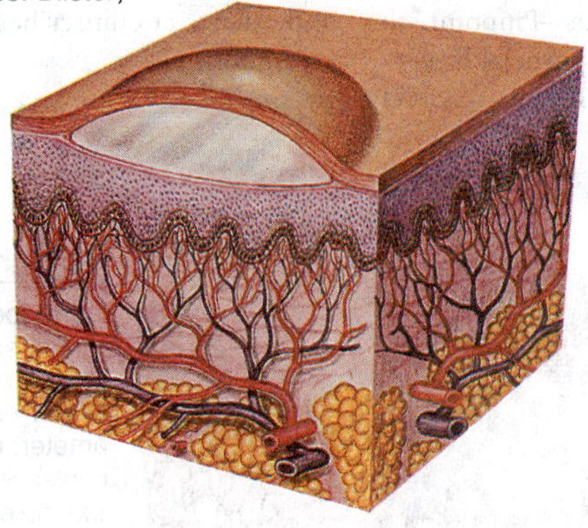

Pustule—elevated; superficial; similar to vesicle but filled with purulent fluid
Examples: Impetigo; acne; variola

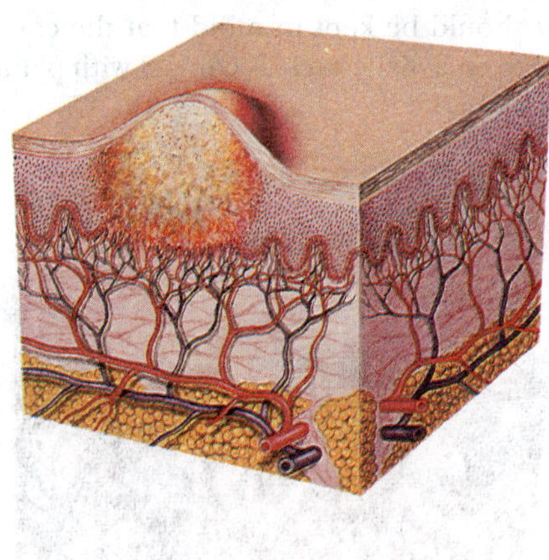

Bulla—vesicle greater than 1 cm in diameter
Examples: Blister; pemphigus vulgaris

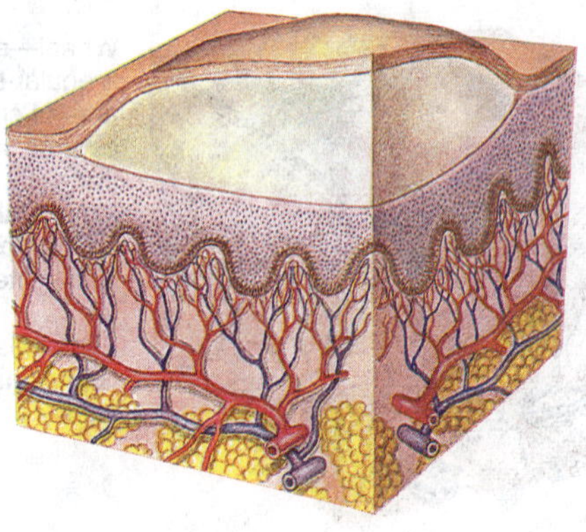

Cyst—elevated; circumscribed; palpable; encapsulated; filled with liquid or semisolid material
Example: Sebaceous cyst

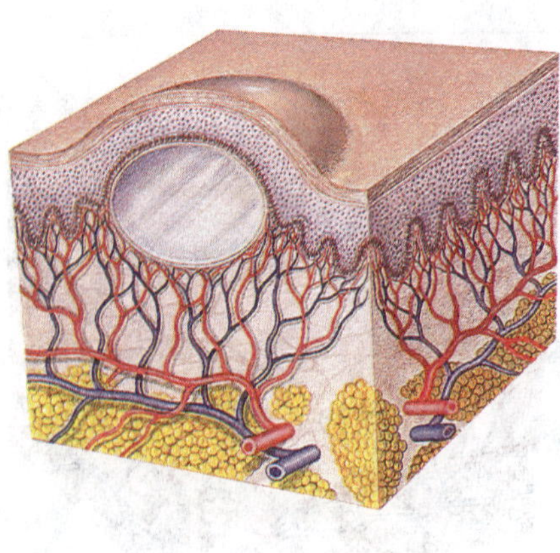

FIG. 18-2, cont'd Primary skin lesions. (From Seidel HM and others: *Mosby's guide to physical examination*, ed 3, St Louis, 1995, Mosby.)

tor (Fig. 18-2); common primary lesions in pediatric skin disorders are macules, papules, and vesicles

Secondary lesions—Changes that result from alteration in the primary lesions, such as those caused by rubbing, scratching, medication, or involution and healing (Fig. 18-3)

Distribution pattern—The pattern in which lesions are distributed over the body, whether local or generalized, and specific areas associated with the lesions

Configuration and arrangement—The size, shape, and arrangement of a lesion or groups of lesions (e.g., ***discrete*** [individually distinct], ***clustered*** [appear close together], ***diffuse*** [scattered], ***confluent*** [running together], or ***annular*** [ringed] or ***arciform*** lesions).

Laboratory Studies. When it is suspected that a skin problem might be related to a systemic disease, such as one of the collagen diseases or immunodeficiency disease, studies are needed to rule out these possibilities. Diagnostic modalities include microscopic examination, cultures, skin scrapings or biopsy, cytodiagnosis, patch testing, and Wood light examination. Allergic skin testing and various other laboratory tests (blood count, sedimentation rate) are used when indicated.

WOUNDS

Wounds are structural or physiologic disruptions of the integument that call for normal or abnormal tissue repair responses. All wounds can be classified as acute or chronic. ***Acute wounds*** are those that heal uneventfully within the usual time frame. ***Chronic wounds*** are those that do not heal in the expected time frame or are associated with many complications. In children most wounds are acute and can be prevented from becoming chronic wounds through appropriate nursing care. Wounds are classified in the same manner as burns: partial-thickness, full-thickness, and complex wounds that include muscle and/or bone (see Burns, Chapter 29, and Maintaining Healthy Skin, Chapter 27). Wounds that often become chronic skin injuries are burns and ***pressure ulcers,*** localized areas of cellular necrosis that develop when soft tissue is compressed between a bony prominence and a firm surface (Hagelgans, 1993).

Some types of acute wounds include:

Abrasion—Removal of the superficial layers of skin by rubbing or scraping

Evulsion—Forcible pulling out or extraction of tissue

Laceration—Torn or jagged wound; accidental cut wound

Incision—Division of the skin made with a sharp object; cut

Penetrating wound—Disruption of the skin surface that extends into underlying tissue or into a body cavity

Puncture—Wound with relatively small opening compared with the depth

Process of Wound Healing

Epidermal Injuries. Abrasions are the most common epidermal wounds of childhood, usually in the form of a skinned knee or elbow. In most injuries the margins of the abraded area are superficial, involving only the outer layers of epidermis, although the central portion may extend into the dermis. Initially the defect is filled by a blood clot and necrotic debris, which subsequently dehydrate to form a scab. Epithelial tissue is composed of ***labile cells,*** which are constantly destroyed and replaced throughout life. Injury to these tissues is accomplished by ***regeneration*** (i.e., rapid replacement by similar cells).

The epithelial wound heals by migration and proliferation of epithelial cells from the wound margin and from cells surviving in transected skin appendages. This response begins within 24 to 48 hours after the wound is incurred.

Crust—dried serum, blood, or purulent exudate; slightly elevated; size varies; brown, red, black, tan, or straw in color
Examples: Scab on abrasion; eczema

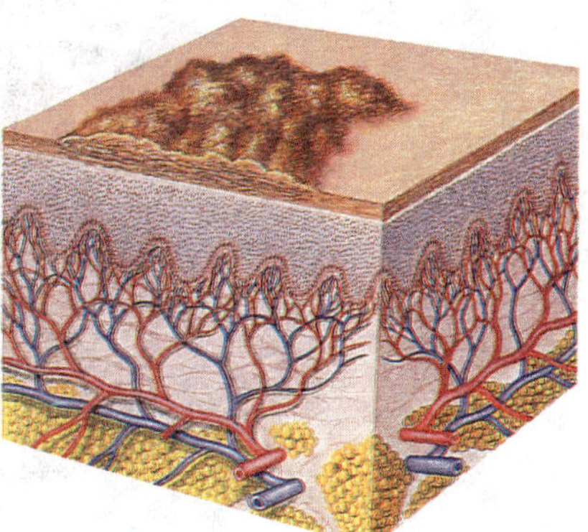

Scale—heaped-up keratinized cells; flaky exfoliation; irregular; thick or thin; dry or oily; varied size; silver, white, or tan in color
Examples: Psoriasis; exfoliative dermatitis

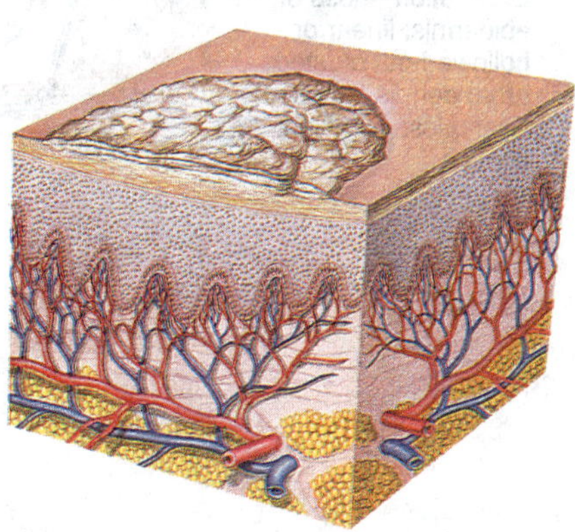

Lichenification—rough, thickened epidermis; accentuated skin markings caused by rubbing or irritation; often involves flexor aspect of extremity
Example: Chronic dermatitis

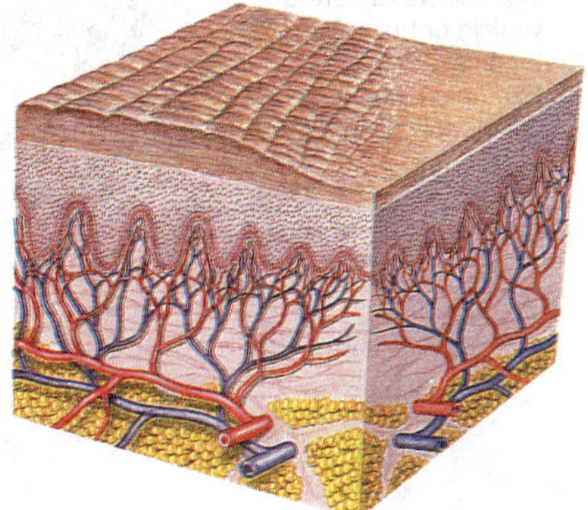

FIG. 18-3 Secondary skin lesions. (From Seidel HM and others: *Mosby's guide to physical examination,* ed 3, St Louis, 1995, Mosby.)

Continued.

Scar—thin to thick fibrous tissue replacing injured dermis; irregular; pink, red, or white in color; may be atrophic or hypertrophic
Example: Healed wound or surgical incision

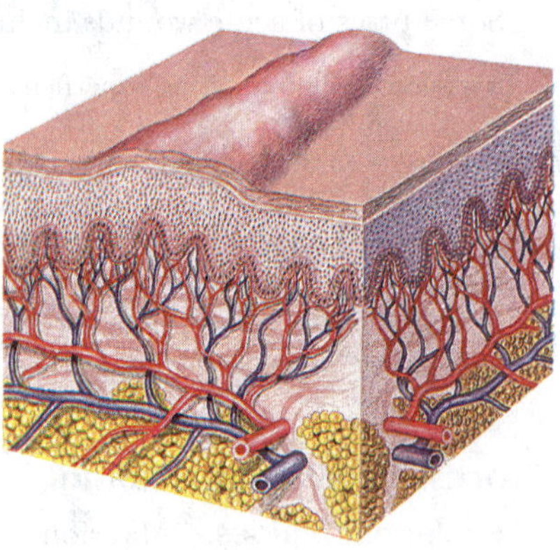

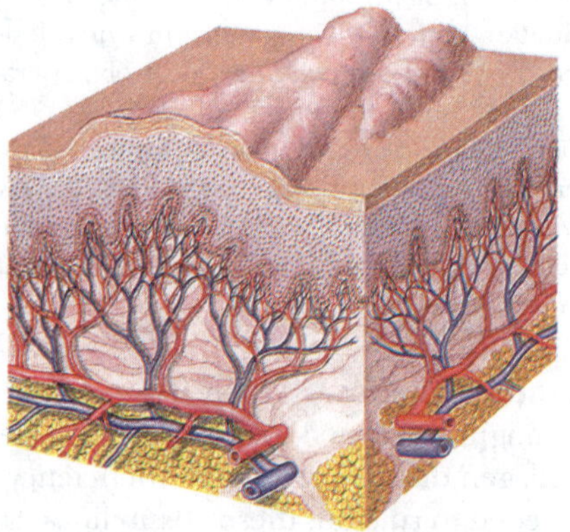

Keloid—irregularly shaped, elevated, progressively enlarging scar; grows beyond boundaries of wound; caused by excessive collagen formation during healing
Example: Keloid from ear piercing or burn scar

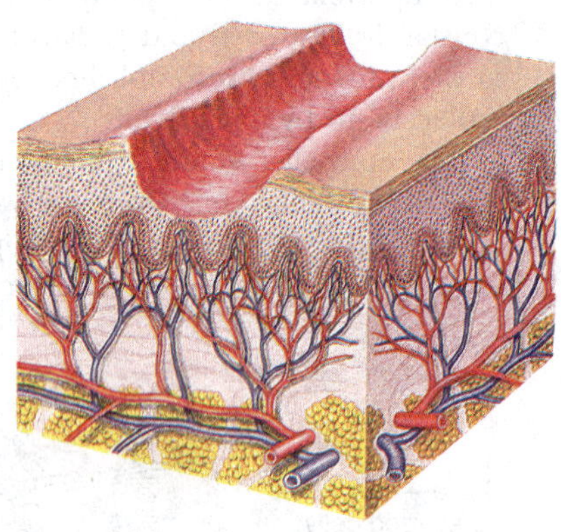

Excoriation—loss of epidermis; linear or hollowed-out crusted area; dermis exposed
Examples: Abrasion; scratch

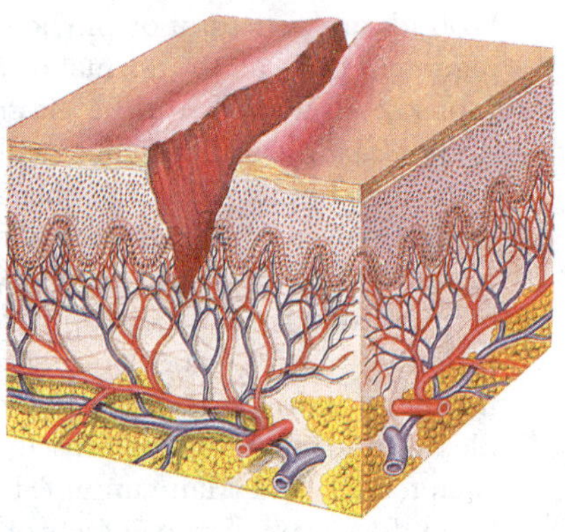

Fissure—linear crack or break from epidermis to dermis; small; deep; red
Examples: Athlete's foot: cheilosis

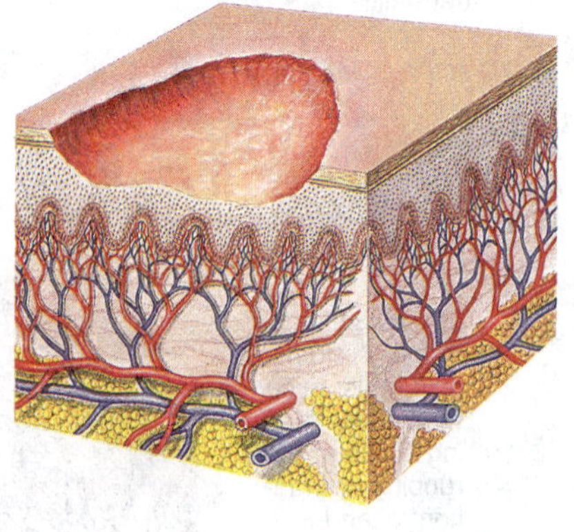

Erosion—loss of all or part of epidermis; depressed; moist; glistening; follows rupture of vesicle or bulla; larger than fissure
Examples: Varicella; variola following rupture

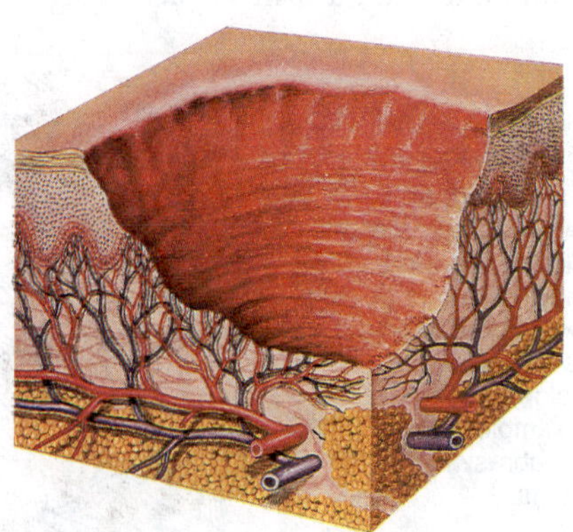

Ulcer—loss of epidermis and dermis; concave; varies in size; exudative; red or reddish blue
Examples: Decubiti; stasis ulcers

FIG. 18-3, cont'd Secondary skin lesions. (From Seidel HM and others: *Mosby's guide to physical examination,* ed 3, St Louis, 1995, Mosby.)

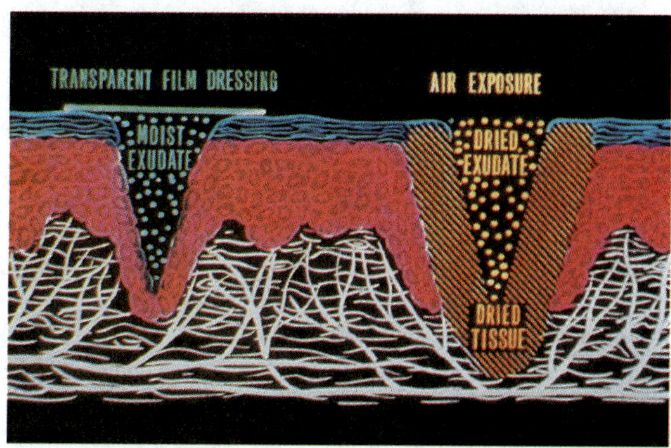

FIG. 18-4 Process of epithelialization is facilitated by maintaining a moist environment as opposed to a dry, open environment. In a moist environment, epithelial cells freely migrate across the wound surface. (Courtesy ConvaTec, Princeton, NJ.)

Cell migration ceases when migrating cells make contact with epithelial cells migrating from all other sites. Fixed basal cells adjacent to the wound edge and in skin appendages begin to divide rapidly to replace the migrated cells. As resurfacing is accomplished, the migrated cells begin to divide and thicken the new epithelial layer.

Epithelial cells advance over the wound surface by "flowing." The first cell advances, anchors, and then moves no more. Instead, a cell from behind advances over it, anchors, and subsequently is overridden by other cells that advance over both the primary cells—similar to a leapfrog movement. Epithelial cells move most rapidly in moist environments, such as those covered with a transparent or other occlusive-type dressing, and the rate of epithelization depends on a variety of elements, particularly the amount of oxygen supplied to the wound (Hunt, 1990). Allowing the skin to dry and form an ***eschar*** or crust (scab) impedes the migration of epithelial cells (Fig. 18-4). In addition, fluid may collect and infection may occur under the eschar.

Injury to Deeper Tissues. Tissues composed of ***permanent cells,*** such as muscle and nerve cells, are unable to regenerate. Therefore these tissues repair themselves by substituting fibrous connective tissue for the injured tissue. This fibrous tissue, or ***scar,*** serves as a patch to preserve or restore the continuity of the tissue. Wounds involving permanent cells include surgical incisions, lacerations, ulcers, evulsions, and full-thickness burns. Injured cells of glandular organs and bones, composed of ***stable*** cells, multiply less vigorously and heal more slowly (see Bone Healing and Remodeling, Chapter 39).

Phases of Wound Healing. The nonspecific repair mechanism of wound healing with scar formation involves the processes of inflammation, fibroplasia, contraction, and scar maturation (Table 18-1). The initial response at the site of injury is ***inflammation,*** a vascular and cellular response, which prepares the tissues for the subsequent repair process. There is a transient constriction of transected blood vessels, lasting 5 to 10 minutes, followed by active vasodilation of all local small vessels and increased blood flow to the area. This is accompanied by increased permeability of small venules, allowing plasma to leak into surrounding tissues ***(edema).*** A blood clot is formed along wound edges, forming a framework for future growth of capillaries ***(angiogenesis)*** and epithelial cells.

At the same time, vessel walls become lined with leukocytes, primarily neutrophils, which pass through the walls and concentrate at the injured site, where they ingest bacteria and debris ***(phagocytosis).*** The presence of neutrophils is superseded by macrophages, which continue phagocytosis, and also by growth factors needed for skin repair and angiogenesis. Fibroblasts attracted to the area from blood

TABLE 18-1 Summary of Wound Healing Process

PHASE	ACTIVITY	COMMENTS
1. **Inflammation** (3 to 5 days)	Clot formation as meshwork for capillary growth Inflammation with phagocytosis; wound debris removed Epithelial cell migration	Wound weakest during this phase
2. **Fibroplasia** (5 days to 4 weeks)	Granulation tissue formed Migration of fibroblasts Secretion of collagen Abundant capillary buds	Wound fragile Granulation tissue bleeds profusely if disturbed
3. **Scar contracture** (1 to 6 weeks)	Continued deposition of collagen Further organization and remodeling Blood vessels compressed Healing area contracts Blood flow across wound gradually ceases	Appears as broad, pinkish, raised scar Heavy use of any affected muscles is discouraged
4. **Scar maturation** (several months)	Formation of mature scar Shrinkage of wound Contracture deformity can occur if wound is near a joint	Scar is acellular and avascular tissue Pale in color Does not tan when exposed to sunlight Will not sweat or produce hair May cause itching

vessels deposit fibrin throughout the clot. Adjacent capillaries begin to form buds that stretch across the supporting fibrin threads, and epithelial cells secrete a fibrolytic enzyme that allows their advancement across the wound. This initial phase of wound healing takes place during the first 3 to 5 days following injury.

Fibroplasia (granulation or ***proliferation),*** the second phase of healing, lasts from 5 days to 4 weeks. Fibroblasts, immature connective tissue cells, migrate to the healing site and begin to secrete collagen into the meshwork spaces. Granulation tissue is highly vascular, "beefy" red, and shiny connective tissue that organizes and restructures, forming thicker, stronger fibers arranged in orderly layers. A thin layer of epithelial tissue is regenerated over the surface of the wound, and leukocytes gradually disappear from the area.

During ***contraction*** and ***maturation,*** the third and fourth phases of wound healing, collagen continues to be deposited and organized into layers, compressing the new blood vessels and gradually ceasing blood flow across the wound. Fibroblasts disappear as the wound becomes stronger. Fibroblast movement causes contraction of the healing area, helping to bring wound edges closer together. A mature scar is then formed. The maturation process may continue for years, and the extent to which the scar remodels and matures varies among individuals.

Children heal aggressively with abundant scar tissue, especially during growth spurts. The highly elastic quality of children's skin pulls on wounds, which defend against the pull by aggressive scarring. Consequently, the child's skin heals with more scar tissue than the less elastic skin of the adult.

Types of Wound Healing. Repair healing takes place in one of three ways: by primary, secondary, or tertiary intention (Fig. 18-5). ***Primary intention*** healing takes place when all layers of the wound (skin, subcutaneous tissue, and muscle) margins are neatly approximated, as in a surgical incision. Unless infection interferes or the wound edges separate, these wounds heal with a minimum of scarring.

Repair by ***secondary intention*** takes place in wounds that occur from ulceration and lacerations in which the edges cannot be approximated, such as an evulsion or a third-degree burn. The inflammatory reaction may be greater, and the chance of infection increased. Often debris, cells, and exudate must be cleaned away (debrided) before healing can take place. Healing takes place from the edges inward and from the bottom of the wound upward until the defect is filled. More granulation tissue and a larger scar are formed than in healing by primary intention.

Repair by ***tertiary intention*** takes place when suturing is delayed after injury or the wound later breaks down and is sutured or resutured when granulation is present. More granulation tissue is formed than in healing by primary intention, and there is greater chance of microorganisms invading the wound. Frequently, suturing a contaminated wound is deliberately delayed to afford better removal of infection before closing. Wounds healed by tertiary intention result in a larger and deeper scar than those healed by primary intention.

First intention (clean incision)

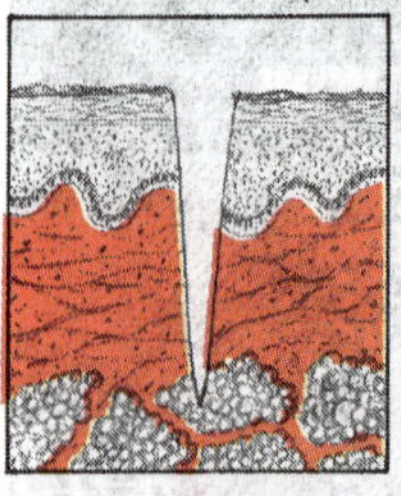
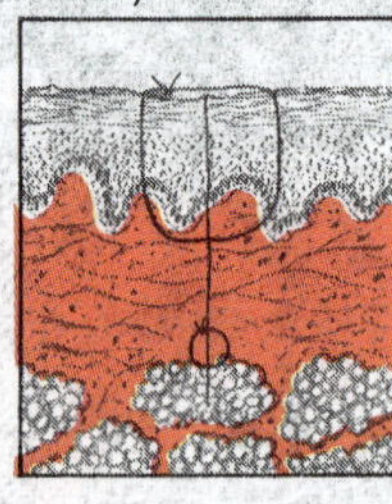
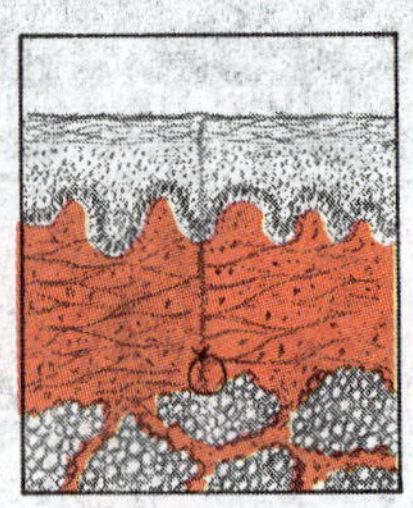

Second intention (wide, irregular wound)

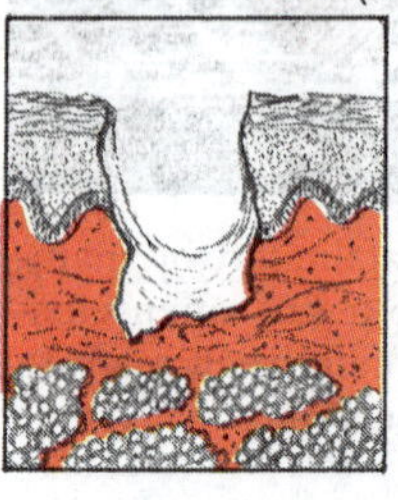
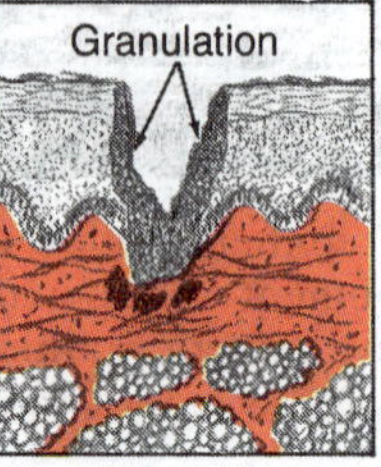

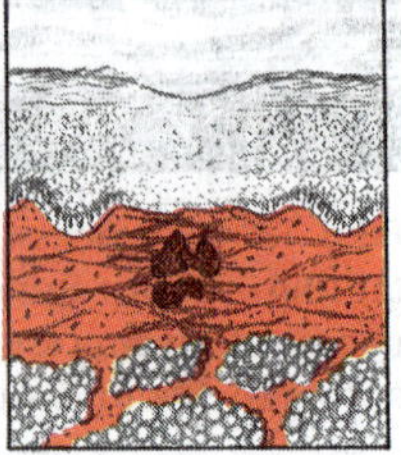

Third intention (puncture wound)

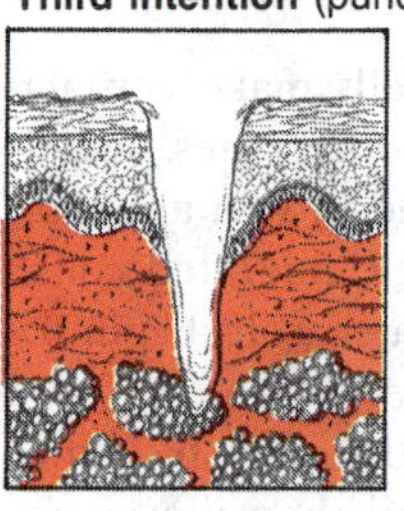
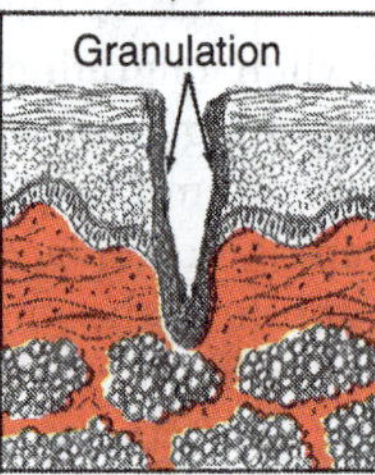

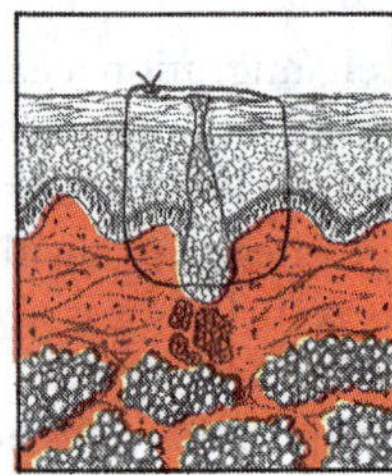

FIG. 18-5 Types of wound healing.

Factors That Influence Healing

During the last two decades understanding of wound healing has revolutionized the interventions used to promote healing. Emphasis has shifted from interventions directed at maintaining a dry environment that promoted eschar formation to those that promote a moist, crust-free environment that enhances the migration of epithelial cells across the wound and facilitates resurfacing.

An acute full-thickness wound kept in a moist environment usually reepithelializes in 12 to 15 days, whereas the same wound when kept open to the air heals in approximately 25 to 30 days (Alvarez, Rozint, and Meehan, 1990). A superficial wound covered with an occlusive dressing, rather than the typical adhesive bandage strip, heals faster and results in a better cosmetic appearance (Woodley and Kim, 1992) (see Fig. 18-4).

Eschar (thick, fibrin-containing necrotic tissue) also interferes with healing by preventing wound contraction. In most situations it is best to remove eschar and other dead tissue from the wound. Repeated application of occlusive dressings mobilizes the body's own enzymes to lyse the eschar, a process known as ***autolysis.***

Adequate nutrition is essential for wound healing. In particular, sufficient protein, calories, vitamin C, and zinc are needed for extensive wounds, such as burns; supplemental nutrition is an integral aspect of severe wound treatment.

TABLE 18-2 Factors That Delay Wound Healing

FACTOR	EFFECT ON HEALING
Dry wound environment	Allows epithelial cells to dry out and die; impairs migration of epithelial cells across wound surface
Nutritional deficiencies	
Vitamin C	Inhibits formation of collagen fibers and capillary development
Protein	Reduces supply of amino acids for tissue repair
Zinc	Impairs epithelialization
Impaired circulation	Reduces supply of nutrients to wound area Inhibits inflammatory response and removal of debris from wound area
Stress (pain, poor sleep)	Releases catecholamines that cause vasoconstriction
Antiseptics	
Hydrogen peroxide	Toxic to fibroblasts; can cause subcutaneous gas formation (mimics gas-forming infection)
Povidone-iodine	Toxic to white and red blood cells and fibroblasts
Chlorhexidine	Toxic to white blood cells
Corticosteroids	Impair phagocytosis Inhibit fibroblast proliferation Depress formation of granulation tissue Inhibit wound contraction
Foreign bodies	Inhibit wound closure Increase inflammatory response
Infection	Increases inflammatory response Increases tissue destruction
Mechanical friction	Damages or destroys granulation tissue
Fluid accumulation	Accumulation in area inhibits tissues from approximating
Radiation	Inhibits fibroblastic activity and capillary formation May cause tissue necrosis
Diseases	
Diabetes mellitus	Inhibits collagen synthesis Impairs circulation and capillary growth Hyperglycemia impairs phagocytosis
Anemia	Reduces oxygen supply to tissues

Much research is being done to find new methods of promoting wound healing. Some research has indicated that a topical application of epidermal growth factor (EGF) significantly accelerated the rate of wound healing (Brown and others, 1989).

Numerous factors have been identified that delay healing (Table 18-2). Many traditional practices, such as the application of antiseptics (hydrogen peroxide and povidone-iodine [Betadine] solutions) to wounds, have only a minimal disinfectant effect, may have a cytotoxic effect on healthy cells, and, in the case of povidone-iodine, may be absorbed through the skin, especially in neonates and young children (LeVeen, LeVeen, and LeVeen, 1993). Povidone-iodine should be used cautiously in anyone with thyroid or renal disorders (Welch, 1992).

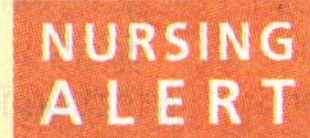

Do not put anything in a wound that one would not put in the eye. The safest solution is normal saline.

GENERAL THERAPEUTIC MANAGEMENT

The human body tends to heal; therefore treatment is directed toward eliminating or ameliorating influences that interfere with normal healing processes. Some disorders may demand aggressive therapy, but by and large the major aim of any treatment is to prevent further damage, eliminate the cause, prevent complications, and provide relief from discomfort while tissues undergo healing. Factors that contribute to the dermatitis and prolong the course of the disease must be eliminated when possible. The most common offenders in pediatrics are environmental factors (such as soaps, bubble baths, shampoos, rough or tight clothing, wet diapers, blankets, and toys) and the natural elements (such as dirt, sand, heat, cold, moisture, and wind). Dermatitis can also be aggravated by home remedies and medications.

Dressings

Dressings are frequently applied to skin lesions and are universally used for wound management. Dressings serve several useful functions: (1) provide a moist healing environment, (2) protect the wound from infection and trauma, (3) provide compression in the event of anticipated bleeding or swelling, (4) apply medication, (5) absorb drainage, (6) debride necrotic tissue, (7) reduce pain, and (8) control odor. To provide a moist environment, open wounds are covered with an occlusive ointment or dressing (Table 18-3). No one dressing meets the needs of all types of wounds. The traditional gauze dressing should not be used on open wounds because it allows the wound surface to dry, does little to prevent bacterial invasion, and adheres to the dried scab so that removal disturbs the newly regenerating epithelial cells.

Topical Therapy

A variety of agents and methods are available for treatment of dermatologic problems. In selecting a therapeutic program the practitioner considers (1) a choice of active ingredient, (2) a proper vehicle or base, (3) the cosmetic effect, (4) the cost, and (5) instructions for its use. In addition, several basic concepts are kept in mind. Overtreatment is avoided. For example, when the dermatitis is acute, the applications should be mild and bland to avoid further irritation. Broken or inflamed skin, especially in children, is more absorbent than intact skin, and chemicals that are nonirritating to intact skin may be quite irritating to inflamed skin.

Topical applications may be applied to treat the disor-

TABLE 18-3 Properties of Commonly Used Occlusive Dressings

EXAMPLES	INDICATIONS	ADVANTAGES	DISADVANTAGES	CONSIDERATIONS
POLYURETHANE FILMS				
Op-Site, Tegaderm, Bio-clusive, Blister-film, Ensure-it, Accuderm, Uniflex, Opraflex	Protection of partial-thickness red wounds Cover dressing for hydrophilic preparations and hydrogels	Transparent; good adhesion; waterproof; reduces pain, minimizes friction forces to wound; time-saving; easy to store	Adhesive injury to intact and new skin; nonabsorbent; some products difficult to apply; variable barrier function; can promote wound infection	Protect wound margins; avoid in wounds with infection, copious drainage, or tracts; change only if dressing leaks
HYDROCOLLOIDS				
DuoDerm, J&J, Ulcer Dr., Comfeel, Restore, Intact, Intrasite, Tegasorb	Protection of superficial and small, deep red wounds Autolytic debridement of small, noninfected yellow wounds*	Absorbent; nonadhesive to healing tissue; good barrier; waterproof; reduces pain; easy to apply; time saving; easy to store	Nontransparent; may soften and lose shape with heat or friction; odor and brown drainage on removal (melted dressing material)	Frequency of changes will depend on amount of exudate (change as needed for leakage); avoid in wounds with infection
HYDROGEL SHEETS				
Vigilon, Geliperm, Elastogel, Cutinova	Protection of superficial and moderately deep red wounds Autolytic debridement of small, noninfected yellow or black wounds* Delivery system for topical antimicrobial creams (increases penetration)	Absorbent; nonadhesive; reduces pain; compatible with topicals; good conformity; easy to store	Poor barrier; semitransparent; requires cover dressing to secure; can promote growth of *Pseudomonas* and yeast; expensive	Avoid in infected wounds; change every 8 hr or as needed for leakage

Slightly modified from Cuzzell JZ: Choosing a wound dressing: a systematic approach, *AACN Clin Issues Crit Care Nurs* 1(3):566-577, 1990.
*NOTE: Users should read package inserts for any contraindications to the use of these products. Some dressings, such as Duoderm CGF, have recently been approved for application to infected wounds, provided that the wound is cultured and treated for the infection. However, Duoderm CGF should not be used on third-degree burns.

der, reduce the itching associated with many diseases, decrease external stimuli, or apply external heat or cold. The emollient action of soaks, baths, and lotions provides a soothing film over the skin surface that reduces external stimuli. Ordinarily lukewarm, tepid, or cool applications offer the greatest relief.

NURSING ALERT Application of heat tends to aggravate most conditions, and its use is usually reserved for reducing specific inflammatory processes, such as folliculitis and cellulitis.

Topical Corticosteroid Therapy. The glucocorticoids are the therapeutic agents used most widely for skin disorders. Their local antiinflammatory effects are merely palliative so that the medication must be applied until the disease state undergoes a remission or the causative agent is eliminated. Corticosteroids are applied directly to the affected area, and, because they are essentially nonsensitizing and have only minor side effects, they can be applied over prolonged periods with continuing effectiveness. As with the use of any steroids, their use in large amounts may mask signs of infection, and symptoms may be exacerbated following termination of the drug. Families are cautioned that the medication cannot be used for all skin disorders. The concentrations available without prescription are not adequate for some stubborn conditions (e.g., psoriasis) and may cause worsening of inflammation caused by fungus or bacteria. It has also been found that users apply too much topical hydrocortisone; therefore they should be counseled that it is both effective and economical to apply only a thin film and massage it into the skin.

Other Topical Therapies. Other topical treatments include chemical cautery (especially useful for warts), cryosurgery, electrodesiccation (chiefly used for warts, granulomas, and nevi), ultraviolet therapy (primarily used in psoriasis and acne), laser therapy, and special acne therapies such as dermabrasion and acne "surgery."

Systemic Therapy

Therapeutic agents are often used as an adjunct to topical therapy in dermatologic disorders, and those most frequently used therapeutically are the corticosteroids and the antibiotics. The corticosteroid hormones, with their capacity to inhibit inflammatory and allergic reactions, are valuable in the treatment of severe skin disorders. Dosage is carefully adjusted and gradually tapered to the minimum that is effective and tolerated. In infants and children, dosage is larger than is usually calculated from body-weight ratios. However, prolonged use may temporarily suppress growth.

Antibiotics, which interfere with the growth of microorganisms, are used in severe or widespread skin infections. However, because they tend to produce a hypersensitivity in the patient, they are used with caution. Antifungal agents are the only means for treating systemic fungal infections.

NURSING CARE OF THE CHILD WITH A SKIN DISORDER

❖ ASSESSMENT

To help establish a diagnosis, it is important for nurses to accurately describe any deviation in the character of the skin, using both inspection and palpation. The color, shape, and distribution of the lesions or wounds are noted. The individual lesions are described according to the accepted terminology and may involve more than one type, such as a maculopapular rash. Wounds are assessed for depth of tissue damage, evidence of healing, and signs of infection.

NURSING ALERT Signs of wound infection are:

Increased erythema, especially beyond wound margin
Edema
Purulent exudate
Pain
Increased temperature

To confirm or amplify the findings made by inspection, the skin is gently palpated to detect characteristics such as temperature, moisture, texture, elasticity, and the presence of edema. It should be indicated whether the findings are restricted to the area of the lesion(s) or are generalized.

The child's subjective symptoms provide additional information. Older children are able to describe the condition as painful, itching, or tingling or in other descriptive terms. However, much can be determined by observing the younger child's behavior and the parents' account of these reactions. Does the child scratch? Is the child restless or irritable? Does the child favor or avoid using a body part? A careful history may provide clues. Has the child had access to chemicals or been in the woods or around a woodpile? Has the child eaten a new food? Is the child taking medication? Has the child any known allergy? Do any playmates have a similar lesion? A doubtful diagnosis is frequently confirmed on the basis of history.

❖ NURSING DIAGNOSES

Nursing diagnoses are determined following an assessment of the child and the skin lesions. The major diagnoses identified for the child with a skin disorder are outlined in the Nursing Care Plan.

❖ PLANNING

The goals for the child with a skin condition and the family are as follows:

1. Child will exhibit signs of wound healing.
2. Child will not experience secondary damage, such as from infection, to the lesion.
3. Child will demonstrate acceptable level of comfort, especially if pain or itching exist.
4. Child and family will receive appropriate education and support.

❖ IMPLEMENTATION

Therapeutic programs are usually designed to provide general measures, such as rest, protection, and relief of discomfort, and specific treatments, such as a definitive medication or physical technique. Since only a few skin diseases are contagious, it is usually not necessary to isolate the affected child unless there is a danger of acquiring a secondary infection (e.g., the child who is receiving large doses of corticosteroids or other immunosuppressant drugs or the child with an immunologic deficiency disorder). If the skin manifestation is caused by a viral exanthem, such as measles or chickenpox, the child is prevented from exposing other susceptible children.

Wound Care. Small wounds to the skin are managed by the parents at home. The parents are instructed to wash their hands and then wash the wound gently with mild soap and water for several minutes, followed by thorough rinsing. To prevent possible tattooing, an abrasion from which the dirt cannot be removed will require abrading with the patient under topical anesthesia, and those covering a very large area (over 15% of the body) will need medical attention (see Atraumatic Care box). Open wounds are covered with a dressing, such as a commercial adhesive bandage, although larger wounds may benefit from the use of occlusive dressings (see Table 18-3). If occlusive dressings are applied, instruct the parents on their correct application and removal. For example, hydrocolloid dressings adhere best if a wide margin is left around the wound and the dressing is pressed against intact skin until it adheres.* The edges of the dressing can be secured to the skin with waterproof tape. The dressings are removed if leakage occurs or after a specific time interval, usually 7 days. Dressings are removed carefully to protect intact skin from damage and the epithelial surface of the wound.

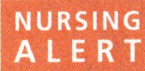

➤ **NURSING TIP** To remove transparent or hydrocolloid dressings, raise one edge of the dressing and pull *parallel* to the skin to loosen the adhesive. The longer the dressings are left on, the easier they are to remove.

NURSING ALERT Advise parents that the yellow gel forming under hydrocolloid dressings may look like pus and has a distinct odor (somewhat fruity) but is normal leakage.

Lacerations present a special challenge. The injured child and family are usually very distressed by the bleeding and are in variable degrees of shock; parental guilt usually accompanies the injury. Because scalp lacerations bleed so profusely, they are especially frightening. The initial nurs-

*Information on the use of the hydrocolloid dressing Duoderm is available from ConvaTec Professional Services, (800) 422-8811.

ing intervention is to apply pressure to the area and attempt to calm the child before further examination. Unless there is bleeding from a severed artery, the wound can be cleansed with a forced jet of sterile tepid water or saline (via syringe) and examined for extent, depth, and presence of foreign material such as dirt, glass, or fabric fragments.

NURSING ALERT Hydrogen peroxide and povidone-iodine are contraindicated for cleaning fresh open wounds. Hydrogen peroxide can cause formation of subcutaneous gas when applied under pressure (Schneider and Hebert, 1987).

The location of the wound also dictates assessment. For example, wounds over bony areas may contain bone chips, and clear fluid seeping from severe head wounds may indicate cerebrospinal fluid. A pressure dressing is applied for transfer to medical care; the child in a medical facility is prepared for suturing (see Atraumatic Care box).

Puncture wounds that do not require a tetanus booster are soaked in hot water and soap for several minutes. Causing the wound to rebleed may be helpful. An adhesive bandage can be applied if desired. Puncture wounds of the head, chest, or abdomen or those that could still contain a portion of the puncturing object must be evaluated.

Parents are cautioned against opening blisters or kissing a wound "to make it better." The wound can easily become contaminated from germs in the human mouth. If scabs form, they are allowed to slough off without assistance; picking or early removal may cause scarring. Parents are advised to seek medical help if there is evidence of infection.

Relief of Symptoms. Most of the therapeutic regimens are directed toward relief of pruritus, the most common subjective complaint. Itching is believed to result from stimulation of C fibers at the dermoepidermal junction. These fibers are similar to but distinct from pain fibers. Substances released within the skin, histamine and endopeptidases, also elicit itching, although their release triggers are unknown (Barnett, 1987).

Cooling the affected area and increasing the skin pH make conditions for enzymatic action less favorable (Madden, 1986). Such measures include cool baths or compresses to reduce external stimuli to the area and alkaline applications, such as baking soda baths, to increase skin pH. Maintenance of cleanliness and good aeration improve comfort. Clothing and bed linen should be soft and lightweight to decrease the irritation from friction and stimulation.

During any type of treatment, both affected and unaffected skin is protected from damage and secondary infection. Preventing scratching is of primary importance. Older children will usually cooperate, although they may need to be reminded to stop scratching or rubbing; but in smaller and uncooperative children the use of techniques and devices such as mittens, (especially during sleep) or special coverings is required. Keeping fingernails short, well trimmed, and clean helps reduce the chance of secondary infection.

Antipruritic medications, especially hydroxyzine (Atarax), may be prescribed for severe itching, especially if it disturbs the child's rest. Pain and discomfort are usually managed with nonpharmacologic measures and mild analgesia; severe pain may require more potent medication. Occlusive dressings over wounds reduce pain. For suturing wounds a topical anesthetic or intradermal buffered lidocaine can be used. (See Pain Management, Chapter 26.)

Topical Therapy. Therapy usually involves some type of topical treatment, and the mode of application depends on the nature and location of the lesion being treated. For example, soothing lotions, creams, and intermittent wet dressings or soaks help cool and dry; ointments, lotions, and creams soften and lubricate dry, scaling areas. Nurses and parents are responsible for the application of topical therapeutic agents and the administration of systemic medications.

It is especially important to wash the hands before and after application of topical therapies. The skin is assessed before the treatment or application of medication and reassessed after the treatment is completed. Any observed changes are noted and described.

Wet compresses. Wet compresses or dressings cool the skin by evaporation, relieve itching and inflammation, and cleanse the area by loosening and removing crusts and debris. Any of a variety of ingredients, such as plain water or Burow solution (available without a prescription), can be applied on Kerlix gauze, plain gauze, or (preferably) soft cotton cloths such as freshly laundered handkerchiefs or strips from diaper, sheeting, or pillowcase material.

Dressings immersed in the desired solution are wrung out slightly and applied to the affected area wet but not dripping. They are applied flat and smooth and in such a way that motion is not totally restricted—fingers are wrapped separately, and arms and legs are wrapped so that elbows and knees can bend. Dressings are kept in place by Kerlix or other cotton wrap, tubular stockinette, mittens, or socks (two pair—one to hold the dressings in place, the other to take up movement) but are left uncovered. When evaporation begins to dry them, the dressings are removed, rewet in the solution, and reapplied to the area using aseptic technique. The solution is not poured or syringed directly over the dressings. As fluid evaporates, the solution becomes increasingly concentrated and thus stronger, which may be damaging to sensitive lesions.

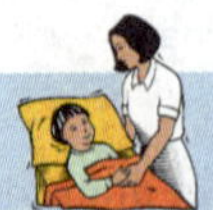

ATRAUMATIC CARE
Painless Suturing and Wound Cleansing

The topical application of tetracaine, adrenaline, and cocaine (TAC) or AC (without tetracaine) gel to wounds, especially on the head, scalp, and face, provides anesthesia in 10 to 15 minutes. If further anesthesia is required or if TAC is not available, using *buffered* lidocaine reduces the stinging and burning of the injection (see Pain Management, Chapter 26).

Fresh solution at room temperature is applied at 2-, 3-, or 4-hour intervals and is allowed to remain on the lesion from 30 minutes to 1½ hours. Wet dressings are seldom continued after about 48 hours. The child must be guarded against chilling during treatment, and no more than 20% of the body should be covered at one time to avoid the risk of hypothermia. After treatment, the skin is dried thoroughly by patting with a towel. Application of lotion or other medication may be ordered at this time.

Soaks. When children are uncooperative in the use of wet dressings, soaks are often used for removal of crusts and for their mild astringent action, with the same solution as

TABLE 18-4 Topical Preparations

DESCRIPTION	CHARACTERISTICS	APPLICATION	COMMENTS
LOTIONS			
Powder suspended in solution	Liquid evaporates, cools the skin Provides a coating of soothing, lubricating, protective, drying powder	Apply evenly over skin with hands or gauze "Paint" on with brush or cotton ball	Not applied to oozing surfaces Ordinarily not washed off between applications Removed by soaking with solution used for soaks or dressings
CREAMS AND GELS			
Thick liquid or soft solid	Contain oil with a high melting point (cream) Tend to disappear when rubbed into skin	Place a teaspoonful in palm of hand and rub briskly between hands until thin and smooth Apply to skin area	Less occlusive than other preparations Esthetically more pleasing Nongreasy, easily applied Readily removed with soap and water
OINTMENT			
Oil is main constituent: animal (lanolin), petrolatum, vegetable oil	Those with high water content disappear on application Water-repellent ointments retain heat for increased absorption of medication Can cause maceration when used with occlusive dressings Absorbent ointments contain no water but absorb water	Not applied to hairy, intertriginous, or macerated areas	Greasy sensation Difficult to remove with water (except those with high water content) Absorbent ointments are more lubricating than water-in-oil
PASTES			
Powders mixed with ointment base	Medications incorporated into pastes are released more slowly than from creams and ointments More porous and less occlusive than ointments	Apply with a tongue depressor and "butter" on	More difficult to apply Must be removed with mineral oil
POWDERS			
Chemically inert	Soothing Absorb moisture Reduce friction Chiefly prophylactic Applied to intertriginous areas	Apply in fine film to prevent caking and lumping when wet Sprinkle powder in palm, then apply to skin	Use is controversial in pediatrics Exert care to prevent inhalation by child
SPRAYS AND AEROSOLS			
Active agents suspended in alcohol-base spray	Alternative method of delivering a solution to skin	Shake container thoroughly before application Shield child's face from spray to avoid inhalation	Useful when direct application is difficult or uncomfortable for the child
SOAPS AND SHAMPOOS			
Bacterial agents	Effective in eliminating common pathogens and parasites	Bathe or shampoo as usual	Useful adjunctive treatment Those containing lindane used with caution
SUNSCREEN AGENTS			
See p. 791			

NURSING CARE PLAN
The Child with a Skin Disorder

NURSING DIAGNOSIS: Impaired skin integrity related to environmental agents, somatic factors, immunologic deficit

PATIENT GOAL 1: Will exhibit signs of skin healing

• **NURSING INTERVENTIONS/*RATIONALES***

Carry out therapeutic regimens as prescribed or support and assist parents in carrying out treatment plan *to promote skin healing*

Provide moist environment (dressing or ointment) *for optimum wound healing*

*Administer topical treatments and applications

*Administer systemic medications, if ordered

Prevent secondary infection and autoinoculation, *since these delay healing*

Reduce external stimuli that aggravate condition, *causing delay in healing*

Encourage rest *to support body's natural defenses*

Encourage well-balanced diet *to support body's natural defenses*

Administer skin care and general hygiene measures *to promote skin healing*

• **EXPECTED OUTCOME**

Affected area exhibits signs of healing

NURSING DIAGNOSIS: High risk for impaired skin integrity related to mechanical trauma, body secretions, increased susceptibility to infection

PATIENT GOAL 1: Will maintain skin integrity

• **NURSING INTERVENTIONS/*RATIONALES***

Keep intact skin clean and dry; cleanse skin at least once daily *to minimize risk of infection*

Inspect total skin area frequently for evidence of irritation or breakdown *so that appropriate therapy can be initiated*

Protect skinfolds and surfaces that rub together *to prevent mechanical trauma to skin*

Keep clothing and linen clean and dry *to prevent excoriation and infection of skin*

Apply protective lotion to anal and perineal areas, knees, elbows, ankles, and chin, *since excoriation is most likely to occur in these areas*

Carry out good perineal care under urine collection device when applicable *to prevent impaired skin integrity*

Remove adhesives and occlusive dressings carefully *to prevent skin trauma*

• **EXPECTED OUTCOME**

Skin remains clean, dry, and free of irritation

PATIENT GOAL 2: Will exhibit no evidence of secondary infection

• **NURSING INTERVENTIONS/*RATIONALES***

Maintain careful handwashing before handling affected child *to prevent infection*

Wear surgical gloves when handling or dressing affected parts if indicated by nature of lesion *to prevent contamination of lesion(s)*

Teach child and family hygienic care and medical asepsis *to prevent secondary infection*

Devise methods to prevent secondary infection of lesion in small or uncooperative children

- Keep nails short and clean *to minimize trauma and secondary infection*
- Apply mittens or elbow restraints *to prevent child from reaching skin lesion(s)*
- Dress in one-piece outfit with long sleeves and legs *to keep lesion(s) covered and out of child's reach*

Observe skin lesions for signs of infection (increased erythema, edema, purulent exudate, pain, increased temperature) *so that appropriate therapy can be initiated*

• **EXPECTED OUTCOMES**

Skin lesions remain confined to primary sites

Skin lesions exhibit no signs of secondary infection

PATIENT GOAL 3: Will maintain integrity of healthy skin

• **NURSING INTERVENTIONS/*RATIONALES***

Teach and impress on child importance of keeping hands away from lesion(s) *to prevent spreading lesion(s) and secondary infection*

Help child determine ways of preventing autoinoculation *to increase compliance*

Devise means for keeping small or uncooperative children from spreading infection to other areas

Keep healthy skin dry *to prevent maceration*

• **EXPECTED OUTCOMES**

Healthy skin remains clean and intact

Skin lesions remain confined to primary sites

NURSING DIAGNOSIS: High risk for infection related to presence of infective organisms

PATIENT GOAL 1: Will not spread infection to self or others

• **NURSING INTERVENTIONS/*RATIONALES***

Implement universal precautions *to prevent spread of infection*

Isolate affected child from susceptible individuals if indicated *to prevent spread of infection*

Maintain careful handwashing after caring for child *to remove infective organisms*

Avoid unnecessary close contact with affected child during infective stage of disease

Use correct technique for disposal of dressings, solutions, and other fomites in contact with lesion(s) *to safely dispose of infective organisms*

Teach and reinforce positive habits of hygienic care *to decrease risk of infection*

• **EXPECTED OUTCOMES**

Infection remains confined to primary site

Child and family comply with preventive measures

---

*Dependent nursing action.

NURSING CARE PLAN

The Child with a Skin Disorder—cont'd

NURSING DIAGNOSIS: High risk for impaired skin integrity related to allergenic factors

PATIENT GOAL 1: Will experience no occurrence or recurrence of skin lesion(s)

- **NURSING INTERVENTIONS/*RATIONALES***

Avoid or reduce contact with agents or circumstances known to precipitate skin reaction *to prevent occurrence or recurrence of lesion(s)*

Teach child to recognize agents or circumstances that produce reaction *to prevent occurrence or recurrence of lesion(s)*

- **EXPECTED OUTCOME**

Child avoids precipitating agents

NURSING DIAGNOSIS: Pain related to skin lesions, pruritus

PATIENT GOAL 1: Will exhibit optimum comfort level

- **NURSING INTERVENTIONS/*RATIONALES***

Avoid or reduce external stimuli that aggravate discomfort, such as clothing and bed linen

Implement other appropriate nonpharmacologic pain reduction techniques (see Chapter 26)

*Apply soothing treatments and topical applications as ordered *to relieve pain or pruritus*

*Administer medications *to relieve discomfort and/or restlessness and irritability*

Advocate for child regarding appropriate anesthesia for wound suturing *to prevent unnecessary pain and emotional trauma*

- **EXPECTED OUTCOME**

Child remains calm and exhibits no evidence of discomfort or pruritus

NURSING DIAGNOSIS: Body image disturbance related to perception of appearance

PATIENT GOAL : Will demonstrate positive self-image

- **NURSING INTERVENTIONS/*RATIONALES***

Encourage child to express feelings about personal appearance and perceived reactions of others *to facilitate coping*

Discuss with child improvement in skin condition *to instill hope*

- **EXPECTED OUTCOME**

Child verbalizes feelings and concerns

PATIENT GOAL 2: Will receive tactile contact

- **NURSING INTERVENTIONS/*RATIONALES***

Hold child; remember that there is no substitute for the stimulation and comfort of human contact

Touch and caress unaffected area *to provide tactile contact without risk of spreading infection*

- **EXPECTED OUTCOMES**

Child exhibits signs of comfort

Child responds positively to tactile stimulation

PATIENT GOAL 3: Will receive adequate support

- **NURSING INTERVENTIONS/*RATIONALES***

Teach self-care where appropriate *to encourage sense of adequacy*

Involve child in planning treatment schedules *to give child some control*

Support and encourage child in efforts to deal with multiple problems that may be associated with disorder, including discomfort, rejection, discouragement, and feelings of self-revulsion *to facilitate coping*

Encourage child to maintain usual activities *so that child experiences normalcy in situation*

Help child improve appearance (e.g., attractive clothing) *to promote positive self-image*

- **EXPECTED OUTCOMES**

Child collaborates in determining means for improving appearance

Child maintains customary activities and relationships

Child participates in own care and treatment

NURSING DIAGNOSIS: Altered family processes related to having a child with a severe skin condition (e.g., eczema, psoriasis, ichthyosis)

PATIENT (FAMILY) GOAL 1: Will receive adequate support

- **NURSING INTERVENTIONS/*RATIONALES***

Teach family skills needed *to carry out therapeutic program*

Provide written instructions *to increase compliance*

Inform family of expected and unexpected results of therapy and a course of action to follow

Help devise special techniques to carry out therapy *to increase compliance and cooperation*

Be aware of overprotectiveness and restrictiveness, *to prevent stifling child's emotional growth*

Allow and encourage family members, particularly the one who cares for the child most of the time, to express negative feelings, such as anger, frustration, and perhaps guilt, *to facilitate coping*

Stress that negative feelings are normal, acceptable, and expected but that they must have an outlet if family members are to remain healthy

Encourage family in efforts to carry out plan of care *to provide support*

Provide assistance when appropriate

Refer to agencies and services that assist with social, financial, and medical problems *to provide ongoing support*

- **EXPECTED OUTCOME**

Family demonstrates necessary skills (specify)

*Dependent nursing action.

for wet compresses. Gaining young children's cooperation for hand or foot soaks is difficult unless the procedure is made attractive to them through play.

➤ **NURSING TIP** Older infants and toddlers delight in playing with brightly colored objects or poker chips scattered over the bottom of the receptacle, and preschoolers can be challenged to hold a floating item beneath the water's surface. These activities require supervision; infants and small children will often place items in their mouths, and children can easily lose control with water play. Washing dishes, cars, dolls, or doll clothes will occupy many children for quite some time.

The older child is able to cooperate but may need something to do during the procedure such as listening to music, a story, or watching television.

➤ **NURSING TIP** A single extremity (a foot or a hand) can be easily soaked by placing the solution and the extremity in a plastic sealable bag. The closure is then zipped snugly around the limb.

Baths. Baths are especially useful in the treatment of widespread dermatitis by evenly distributing the soothing antipruritic and antiinflammatory effects of the solution, usually oatmeal or mineral oil preparations. The solution is added to a tub of lukewarm water. The temperature of the bath is tepid, and the treatment usually lasts 15 to 30 minutes. Therapeutic baths are always more interesting when the child is accompanied by toy boats or other items for water play.

Topical applications. Various applications are applied to skin lesions to ease discomfort, prevent further injury, and facilitate healing (Table 18-4). Most preparations are placed directly on the skin and left uncovered; others may be applied under an occlusive dressing. A thin application of the ointment or cream is covered with plastic film and anchored with adhesive or covered with a commercial transparent dressing. Occlusive dressings promote moisture retention and nonevaporation of the preparation, all of which increase the penetration of the medication. Regardless of the type of preparation used, parents need detailed information on how to apply it and how long the preparation should remain on the skin or under an occlusive dressing.

➤ **NURSING TIP** Apply topical applications systematically with the contour of the body surface (not simply up and down). Children love to be "painted." Therefore lotion applications can be fun when an ordinary paintbrush is used.

NURSING ALERT Provide written instructions and demonstrate to parents the correct amount of topical medication to apply (e.g., size of a pea; thin film to cover). If more than one preparation is applied, mark the containers 1 and 2 for parents to remember the correct order. Stress that more is not necessarily better with some medications, such as steroids.

Home Care and Family Support. Dermatologic conditions always involve the family. Since few situations require hospitalization and children who are hospitalized will complete a therapy program at home, the family must carry out the treatment plan; therefore their cooperation is essential. Regimens that are simple to accomplish in the hospital or office may be frustrating and baffling at home. The family often needs assistance in adapting equipment available in the home to the therapy.

It is important that the child and family be given as detailed explanations as possible about both the expected and the unexpected results of treatment, including any ill effects that might occur. If unexplained reactions do develop, the family is directed to discontinue treatment and report the reactions to the appropriate person(s). The use of over-the-counter medicines is discouraged unless they have first been discussed with the attending practitioner and received approval.

Since the skin is the most visible portion of the body, defects in its surface that alter its appearance are sometimes a source of distress to the child and of revulsion and rejection by others. Parents of other children may fear that their children will "catch" the disorder. Occasionally the affected child's own family members will reduce their interaction with him or her, especially close physical contact, or otherwise demonstrate a distaste for the condition, which the child may interpret as rejection. This is seldom a difficulty with dermatitis of short duration, but chronic conditions can create problems in development of a positive self-concept.

❖ EVALUATION

The effectiveness of nursing interventions is determined by continual reassessment and evaluation of care based on the following observational guidelines and expected outcomes:

1. Observe if reasonable care is used in performing nursing activities, and observe lesions and child's reactions to therapies.
2. Observe signs of wound healing.
3. Use assessment techniques to identify relief of discomfort as described in Chapter 26.
4. Reassess skin lesions; observe and interview child and family regarding compliance with therapy.

Expected outcomes:

See Nursing Care Plan, pp. 776-777.

INFECTIONS OF THE SKIN

BACTERIAL INFECTIONS

Normally, the skin harbors a variety of bacterial flora, including the major pathogenic varieties of staphylococci and streptococci. The degree of their pathogenicity depends on the invasiveness and toxigenicity of the specific organism, the integrity of the skin, the barrier of the host, and the immune and cellular defenses of the host. Children with immunodeficiency, such as infants, children with congenital immune deficiency disorders, children in a debilitated condition, those on immunosuppressive therapy, and those with a generalized malignancy such as leukemia or lymphoma, are at risk for developing bacterial infections.

Because of the characteristic "walling-off" process of the inflammatory reaction (abscess formation), staphylococci are more difficult to attack, and the local infected area is

TABLE 18-5 Bacterial Infections

DISORDER/ORGANISM	MANIFESTATIONS	MANAGEMENT	COMMENTS
Impetigo contagiosa (Fig. 18-6)—*Staphylococcus*	Begins as a reddish macule Becomes vesicular Ruptures easily, leaving superficial, moist erosion Tends to spread peripherally in sharply marginated irregular outlines Exudate dries to form heavy, honey-colored crusts Pruritus common Systemic effects: minimal or asymptomatic	Careful removal of undermined skin, crusts, and debris by softening with 1:20 Burow solution compresses Topical application of bactericidal ointment Systemic administration of oral or parenteral antibiotics (penicillin) in severe or extensive lesions	Tends to heal without scarring unless secondary infection Autoinoculable and contagious Very common in toddler, preschooler
Pyoderma—*Staphylococcus, Streptococcus*	Deeper extension of infection into dermis Tissue reaction more severe Systemic effects: fever, lymphangitis	Soap and water cleansing Wet compresses Bathing with antibacterial soap as prescribed	Autoinoculable and contagious May heal with or without scarring
Folliculitis (pimple), furuncle (boil), carbuncle (multiple boils)—*Staphylococcus aureus*	Folliculitis: infection of hair follicle Furuncle: larger lesion with more redness and swelling at a single follicle Carbuncle: more extensive lesion with widespread inflammation and "pointing" at several follicular orifices Systemic effects: malaise, if severe	Skin cleanliness Local warm, moist compresses Topical application of antibiotic agents Systemic antibiotics in severe cases Incision and drainage of severe lesions, followed by wound irrigations with antibiotics or suitable drain implantation	Autoinoculable and contagious Furuncle and carbuncle tend to heal with scar formation A lesion should *never* be squeezed
Cellulitis—*Streptococcus, Staphylococcus, Haemophilus influenzae* (Fig. 18-7)	Inflammation of skin and subcutaneous tissues with intense redness, swelling, and firm infiltration Lymphangitis "streaking" frequently seen Involvement of regional lymph nodes common May progress to abscess formation Systemic effects: fever, malaise	Oral or parenteral antibiotics Rest and immobilization of both affected area and child Hot moist compresses to area	Hospitalization may be necessary for child with systemic symptoms Otitis media may be associated with facial cellulitis
Staphylococcal scalded skin syndrome—*S. aureus*	Macular erythema with "sandpaper" texture of involved skin Epidermis becomes wrinkled (in 2 days or less), and large bullae appear	Systemic administration of antibiotics Gentle cleansing with saline, Burow solution, or 0.25% silver nitrate compresses	Infant subject to fluid loss, impaired body temperature regulation, and secondary infection, such as pneumonia, cellulitis, and septicemia Heals without scarring

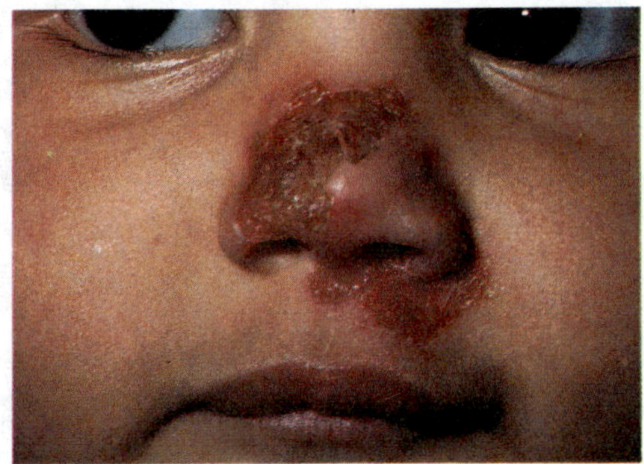

FIG. 18-6 Impetigo contagiosa. (From Weston WL, Lane AT: *Color textbook of pediatric dermatology,* St Louis, 1991, Mosby.)

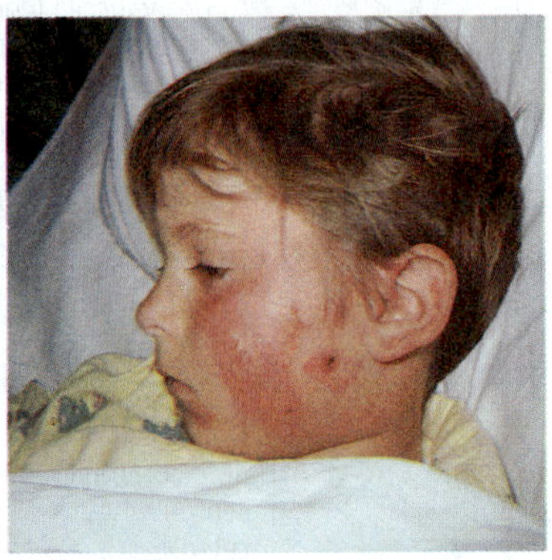

FIG. 18-7 Cellulitis of cheek from puncture wound. (From Weston WL, Lane AT: *Color textbook of pediatric dermatology,* St Louis, 1991, Mosby.)

associated with an increase in numbers of bacteria all over the skin surface that serve as a source of continuing infection. Staphylococcal infections occur most often in children in the younger age-groups, and the incidence decreases with advancing age. All of these factors emphasize the importance of careful handwashing and cleanliness when caring for infected children and their lesions to prevent spread of the infection and as an essential prophylactic measure when caring for infants and small children. Common bacterial skin disorders are outlined in Table 18-5.

Nursing Considerations

The major nursing functions related to bacterial skin infections are to prevent the spread of infection and to prevent complications. Handwashing is mandatory before and after contact with an affected child. Handwashing is also emphasized to both the child and the family, and the child should be provided with towels separate from those of other family members. Impetigo contagiosa is easily spread by self-inoculation; therefore the child must be cautioned against touching the involved area. This is difficult to accomplish;

TABLE 18-6 Viral Infections

DISEASE	MANIFESTATIONS	MANAGEMENT	COMMENTS
Verruca (warts) Cause: human papillomavirus (various types)	Small, benign tumors Usually well-circumscribed, gray or brown, elevated firm papules with a roughened, finely papillomatous texture Occur anywhere, but usually appear on exposed areas such as fingers, hands, face, and soles May be single or multiple Asymptomatic	Not uniformly successful Local destructive therapy, individualized according to location, type, and number—surgical removal, electrocautery, curettage, cryotherapy (liquid nitrogen), caustic solutions (lactic acid and salicyclic acid in flexible collodion, retinoic acid, salicyclic acid plasters), x-ray treatment Hypnotherapy may be effective	Common in children Tend to disappear spontaneously Course unpredictable Most destructive techniques tend to leave scars Autoinoculable Repeated irritation will cause to enlarge
Verruca plantaris (plantar wart)	Located on plantar surface of feet and, because of pressure, are practically flat; may be surrounded by a collar of hyperkeratosis	Apply caustic solution to wart, wear foam insole with hole cut to relieve pressure on wart; soak 20 min after 2-3 days; repeat until wart comes out	Destructive techniques tend to leave scars, which may cause problems with walking
Herpes simplex virus Type I (cold sore, fever blister) Type II (genital)	Grouped, burning, and itching vesicles on inflammatory base, usually on or near mucocutaneous junctions (lips, nose, genitals, buttocks) Vesicles dry, forming a crust, followed by exfoliation and spontaneous healing in 8-10 days May be accompanied by regional lymphadenopathy	Avoidance of secondary infection Burow solution compresses during weeping stages Topical therapy has proved to have effect on recurrences Oral antiviral (Acyclovir) for initial infection or to reduce severity in recurrence	Heal without scarring unless secondary infection Aggravated by corticosteroids Positive psychologic effect from treatment May be fatal in children with depressed immunity
Varicella zoster virus (herpes zoster; shingles)	Caused by same virus that causes varicella (chickenpox) Virus has affinity for posterior root ganglia, posterior horn of spinal cord, and skin; crops of vesicles usually confined to dermatome following along course of affected nerve Usually preceded by neuralgic pain, hyperesthesias, or itching May be accompanied by constitutional symptoms	Symptomatic Analgesics for pain Mild sedation sometimes helpful Local moist compresses Drying lotions may be helpful Ophthalmic variety: systemic corticotropin (ACTH) and/or corticosteroids Acyclovir	Pain in children usually minimal Postherpetic pain does not occur in children Chickenpox may follow exposure; isolate affected child from other children in a hospital or school May occur in children with depressed immunity; can be fatal
Molluscum contagiosum Cause: pox virus	Flesh-colored papules with a central caseous plug (umbilicated) Usually asymptomatic	Cases in well children resolve spontaneously in about 18 months Treatment reserved for troublesome cases Curettage or cryotherapy	Common in school-age children Spread by skin-to-skin contact, including autoinoculation and fomite-to-skin contact

distraction or reminders are useful but are not helpful when the child is alone, such as at bedtime.

Children and parents are often tempted to squeeze follicular lesions. They must be warned that squeezing will not hasten the resolution of the infection and that there is a risk of making the lesion worse or spreading the infection. No attempt should be made to puncture the surface of the pustule with a needle or sharp instrument. A child with a sty may waken with the eyelids of the affected eye sealed shut with exudate. The child or the parents are instructed to gently wipe the lid with clear warm water and a clean washcloth until the exudate has been removed.

The child with limited cellulitis of an extremity is usually managed at home on a regimen of oral antibiotics and warm compresses. The parents are taught the procedures and instructed in administration of the medication. Children with more extensive cellulitis, especially around a joint with lymphadenitis or on the face, are usually admitted to the hospital for parenteral antibiotics. Nurses are responsible for administering the medication, applying compresses, and maintaining the intravenous infusion.

VIRAL INFECTIONS

Viruses are intracellular parasites that produce their effect by using the intracellular substances of the host cells. Composed of only a DNA or RNA core enclosed in an antigenic protein shell, viruses are unable to provide for their own metabolic needs or to reproduce themselves. After a virus penetrates a cell of the host organism, it sheds the outer shell and disappears within the cell, where the nucleic acid core stimulates the host cell to form more virus material from its intracellular substance. In a viral infection the epidermal cells react with inflammation and vesiculation (as in herpes simplex) or by proliferating to form growths (warts).

Most of the communicable diseases of childhood are associated with rashes, and each rash is characteristic. The type of lesion and the configuration of the viral exanthems of rubeola, rubella, and chickenpox are described in Table 16-1. Other common viral disorders of the skin are outlined in Table 18-6.

DERMATOPHYTOSES (FUNGAL INFECTIONS)

The dermatophytoses (ringworm) are infections caused by a group of closely related filamentous fungi that invade primarily the stratum corneum, hair, and nails. These are superficial infections that live on, not in, the skin. They are confined to the dead keratin layers and are unable to survive in the deeper layers. Since the keratin is being desquamated constantly, the fungus must multiply at a rate that equals the rate of keratin production to maintain itself; otherwise the infection would be shed with the discarded skin cells. Common dermatophytoses are outlined in Table 18-7.

Three principal types of fungi are responsible for dermatophyte infections: *Trichophyton, Microsporum,* and *Epidermophyton.* They are designated by the Latin word *tinea,* with further designation related to the area of the body where they are found, for example, tinea capitis (ringworm of the scalp) (see Fig. 18-8, *A*). Dermatophyte infections are most often transmitted from one person to another or from infected animals to humans. Atopic individuals are more susceptible to dermatophyte infections. Fungi exert their effect by means of an enzyme that digests and hydrolyzes the keratin of hair, nails, and the stratum corneum. Dissolved hair breaks off to produce the bald spots characteristic of tinea capitis. In the annular lesions the fungi are found principally in the edge of the inflamed border as they move outward from the inflammation. Diagnosis is made from microscopic examination of scrapings taken from the advancing periphery of the lesion, which almost always produces scale.

Nursing Considerations

When teaching families regarding the care of children with ringworm, it is important to emphasize good health and hygiene. Because of the infectious nature of the disease, sev-

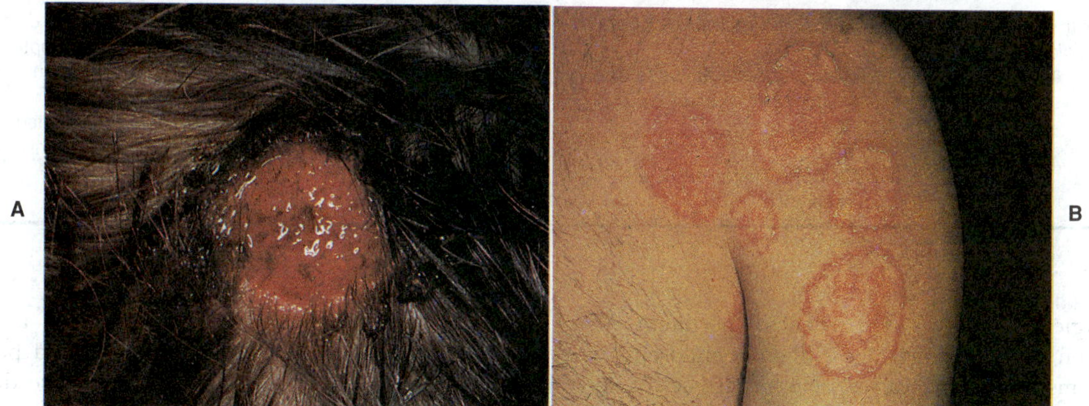

FIG. 18-8 A, Tinea capitis. **B,** Tinea corporis. Both infections are caused by *Microsporum canis,* the "kitten" or "puppy" fungus. (From Habif TP: *Clinical dermatology: a color guide to diagnosis and therapy,* ed 2, St Louis, 1990, Mosby.)

TABLE 18-7 Dermatophytoses (Fungal Infections)

DISEASE/ORGANISM	MANIFESTATIONS	MANAGEMENT	COMMENTS
Tinea capitis—*Trichophyton tonsurans, Microsporum audouini, Microsporum canis* (Fig. 18-8, *A*)	Lesions in scalp but may extend to hairline or neck Characteristic configuration of scaly, circumscribed patches and/or patchy, scaling areas of alopecia Generally asymptomatic, but severe, deep inflammatory reaction may occur that manifests as boggy, encrusted lesions (kerions) Pruritic Microscopic examination of scales is diagnostic	Oral griseofulvin Oral ketoconazole for difficult cases Selenium sulfide shampoos Topical antifungal agents (e.g., clotrimazole, haloprogin, miconazole)	Person-to-person transmission Animal-to-person transmission Rarely, permanent loss of hair *M. audouini* transmitted from one human being to another directly or from personal items; *M. canis* usually contracted from household pets, especially cats Atopic individuals more susceptible
Tinea corporis—*Trichophyton rubrum, Trichophyton mentagrophytes, M. canis, Epidermophyton* (Fig. 18-8, *B*)	Generally round or oval, erythematous scaling patch that spreads peripherally and clears centrally; may involve nails (tinea unguium) Diagnosis: direct microscopic examination of scales Usually unilateral	Oral griseofulvin Local application of antifungal preparation such as tolnaftate, haloprogin, miconazole, clotrimazole; apply 1 inch beyond periphery of lesion; continual application 1 to 2 weeks after no sign of lesion	Usually of animal origin from infected pets Majority of infections in children caused by *M. canis* and *M. audouini*
Tinea cruris ("jock itch")—*Epidermophyton floccosum, T. rubrum, T. mentagrophytes*	Skin response similar to tinea corporis Localized to medial proximal aspect of thigh and crural fold; may involve scrotum in males Pruritic Diagnosis: same as for tinea corporis	Local application of tolnaftate liquid Wet compresses or sitz baths may be soothing	Rare in preadolescent children Health education regarding personal hygiene
Tinea pedis ("athlete's foot")—*T. rubrum, Trichophyton interdigitale, E. floccosum*	On intertriginous areas between toes or on plantar surface of feet Lesions vary: Maceration and fissuring between toes Patches with pinhead-sized vesicles on plantar surface Pruritic Diagnosis: direct microscopic examination of scrapings	Oral griseofulvin Local applications of tolnaftate liquid and antifungal powder containing tolnaftate Acute infections: compresses or soaks followed by application of glucocorticoid cream Elimination of conditions of heat and perspiration by clean, light socks and well-ventilated shoes; avoidance of occlusive shoes	Most frequent in adolescents and adults; rare in children, but occurrence increases with wearing of plastic shoes Transmission to other individuals rare despite general opinion to contrary Ointments not successful
Candidiasis (moniliasis)—*Candida albicans*	Grows in chronically moist areas Inflamed areas with white exudate, peeling, and easy bleeding Pruritic Diagnosis: characteristic appearance	Amphotericin B, nystatin ointment, or other antifungal preparations to affected areas	Common form of diaper dermatitis (see Chapter 13) Oral form common in infants (see Chapter 9) May be disseminated in immunosuppressed children

eral basic hygienic measures are particularly pertinent. Affected children are not to exchange with other children any grooming items, headgear, scarves, or other articles of apparel that have been in proximity to the infected area. Affected children are provided with their own towel and directed to wear a protective cap at night to avoid transmitting the fungus to bedding, especially if they sleep with another person. Since the infection can be acquired by animal-to-human transmission, all household pets should be examined for the presence of the disorder. Other sources of infection are seats with headrests, such as theater seats or seats in public transportation.

Treatment with the drug griseofulvin frequently continues for weeks or months, and because subjective symptoms

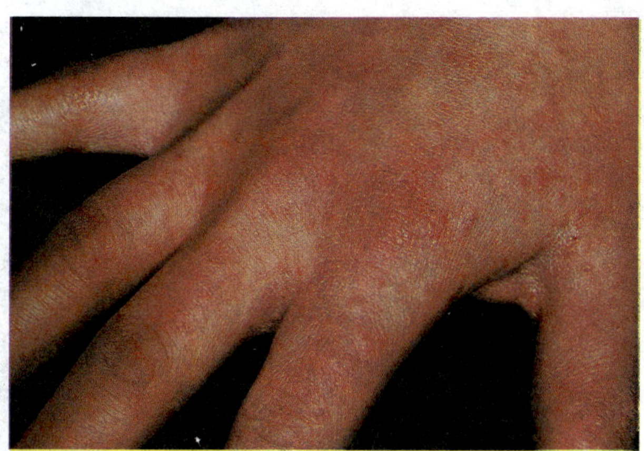

FIG. 18-9 Scabies. (From Habif TP: *Clinical dermatology: a color guide to diagnosis and therapy,* ed 2, St Louis, 1990, Mosby.)

subside, children or parent may be tempted to decrease or discontinue the drug. The nurse should impress on members of the family the importance of maintaining the prescribed dosage schedule. They are also instructed regarding the possibility of side effects from the drug such as headache, gastrointestinal upset, fatigue, insomnia, and photosensitivity. For children who take the drug over many months, periodic testing is required to monitor leukopenia and assess liver and renal function.

SCABIES

Scabies is an endemic infestation caused by the scabies mite, *Sarcoptes scabiei.* Lesions are created as the impregnated female scabies mite burrows into the stratum corneum of the epidermis (never into living tissue), where she deposits her eggs and fecal material. These burrows form minute, linear, grayish brown, threadlike lesions that are often difficult to see.

Clinical Manifestations

The reaction causes intense pruritus that leads to punctate discrete excoriations secondary to the itching. Maculopapular lesions are characteristically distributed in intertriginous areas: interdigital surfaces (Fig. 18-9), axillary-cubital area, popliteal folds, and inguinal region. However, there is large variability in the type of lesions. Infants often develop an eczematous eruption; therefore the observer must look for discrete papules, burrows, or vesicles. A mite is identified as a black dot at the end of a burrow. In children over 2 years of age, the largest percentage of eruptions are found in the hands and wrists, and in children less than 2 years, on feet and ankles. Children with Down syndrome may not complain of itching; therefore they can get a severe infestation before it is recognized.

The inflammatory response and itching occur after the host becomes sensitized to the mite, approximately 30 to 60 days following initial contact. (In persons previously sensitized to the mite, the inflammatory response occurs within 48 hours after exposure.) After this time, anywhere the mite has traveled will begin to itch and develop the characteristic eruption. Consequently, mites will not necessarily be located at all sites of eruption. Also, a person needs prolonged contact with the mite to become infested. Since it takes about 45 minutes for the mite to burrow under the skin, transient body contact is less likely to cause transfer of the mite. The diagnosis is made by microscopic identification from scrapings of the burrow.

Therapeutic Management

The treatment of scabies is the application of a scabicide, usually 1% lindane (Kwell, Scavene) in a vanishing cream base. Permethrin 5% cream (Elimite) is safer and more effective than lindane and is becoming the preferred treatment (Taplin and others, 1990). Because of the length of time between infestation and physical symptoms (30 to 60 days), all persons who were in close contact with the affected child will need treatment. This may include persons such as boyfriends or girlfriends, baby-sitters, and grandparents, as well as immediate family members. The objective is to treat as thoroughly as possible the first time. Enough medication for the entire family should be prescribed, allowing 2 ounces for adults and 1 ounce for each child.

Nursing Considerations

Nurses instructing families in use of the scabicide should emphasize the importance of following the directions accurately. Lindane lotion is applied to cool, dry skin—not following a hot bath. It is applied over the entire cutaneous surface from the neck down and left on for the recommended time, usually 4 hours for infants and 6 hours for older children and adults. Since it is a superficial skin disorder, penetration need not be promoted. One liberal application is sufficient.

Touching and holding the affected child should be minimized until treatment is completed, and hands should be washed carefully after contact is made. Nurses in hospitals are to wear gloves when caring for an affected child. Following treatment, freshly laundered bed linen and underclothing are used, and previously worn clothing is washed in very hot water and ironed. Families need to know that although the mite will be killed, the rash and the itch will not be eliminated until the stratum corneum is replaced, which takes approximately 2 to 3 weeks. Soothing ointments or lotions can be used for itching. Antibiotics may be given for secondary infection.

PEDICULOSIS CAPITIS

Pediculosis capitis (head lice, or "cooties") is an infestation of the scalp by *Pediculus humanus capitis,* a very common parasite, especially in school-age children. These lice infestations are not a major health threat, but they are highly communicable and create embarrassment and a panic reaction in the family and community. They can also cause a child to be ridiculed by other children.

The ***louse*** is a blood-sucking organism that requires approximately five meals a day. The adult louse lives only about 48 hours when away from a human host, and the life

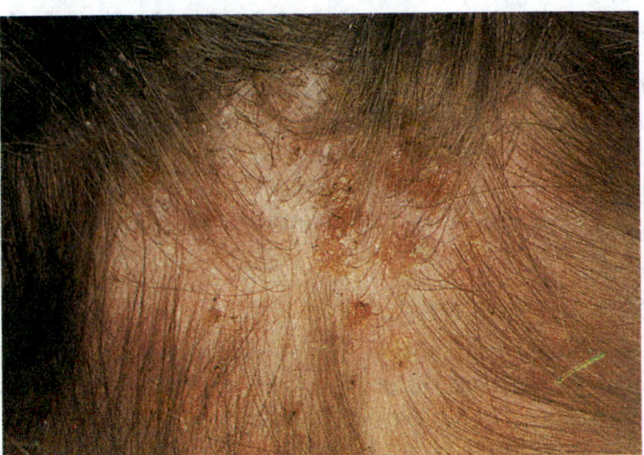

FIG. 18-10 Pediculosis capitis. (From Habif TP: *Clinical dermatology: a color guide to diagnosis and therapy,* ed 2, St Louis, 1990, Mosby.)

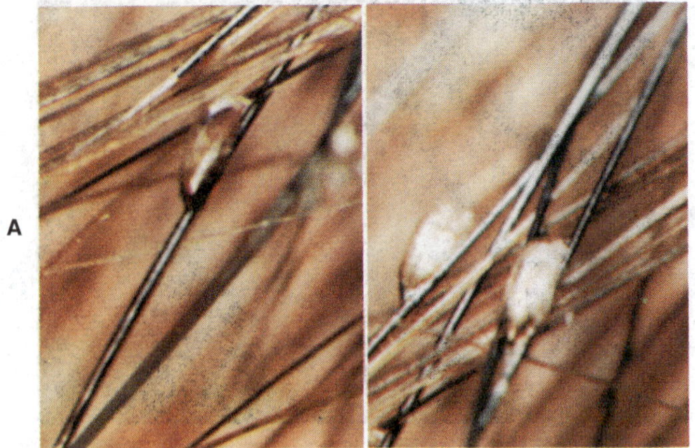

FIG. 18-11 **A,** Empty nit case. **B,** Viable nits. (From *The contemporary approach to the control of head lice in schools and communities,* Pittsburgh, 1991, SmithKline Beecham.)

span of the average female is only 1 month. The female lays her eggs at night at the junction of a hair shaft and close to the skin because the eggs need a warm environment. The ***nits,*** or eggs, hatch in approximately 7 to 10 days.

Clinical Manifestations and Diagnostic Evaluation

Itching, caused by the crawling insect and insect saliva on the skin, is usually the only symptom. The most common sites of involvement are the occipital area, behind the ears, at the nape of the neck, and (occasionally) the eyebrows and eyelashes. Diagnosis is made by observation of the white eggs (nits) firmly attached to the hair shafts. Because of their brief life span and mobility, adult lice are more difficult to locate. Nits must be differentiated from dandruff, lint, hair spray, and other items of similar size and shape. On inspection nits are attached to the hair shaft. Scratch marks and/or inflammatory papules caused by secondary infection may also be found on the scalp in the vulnerable areas (Fig. 18-10).

Therapeutic Management

Treatment consists of the application of pediculicides and manual removal of nit cases. A number of highly effective products are available. A prescription drug, 1% lindane shampoo (gamma benzene hexachloride—Kwell, Scabene), is applied as directed and repeated in 7 to 10 days to kill the hatching nymphs. However, lindane is not effective against nits and, if not used properly, is potentially toxic. It is not recommended for children under 2 years of age. Therefore other products are preferred. Permethrin 1% creme rinse (Nix) kills both lice and nits after one application. This product and preparations of pyrethrin with piperonyl butoxide (RID or A-200 pyrinate) can be obtained without a prescription and are more effective and safer than lindane. In fact, in a study comparing these pediculicides and other products, as well as their nit-removal combs, Nix (and its comb) was found to be the most effective product (Clore and Longyear, 1993).

Nursing Considerations

Nurses should be aware of several things to successfully manage or assist parents in coping with pediculosis. It should be emphasized that *anyone* can get pediculosis; it has no respect for age, socioeconomic level, or cleanliness. The louse does not jump or fly, but it can be transmitted from one person to another on personal items. Therefore children are cautioned against sharing combs, hats, caps, scarves, coats, and other items used on or near the hair. Children who share lockers are more likely to contract an infestation, and slumber parties place children at risk. Lice are not carried or transmitted by pets.

Nurses or parents should carefully inspect the head of a child who scratches the head more than usual for bite marks, redness, and nits. The hair is systematically spread with two flat-sided sticks or tongue depressors, and the scalp observed for any movement that indicates a louse. Nurses should wear gloves when examining the hair of an individual child, but changing gloves between each child may be unrealistic when nurses screen large numbers of children. In this case new sticks should be used for each child (Clore, 1994).

Lice are small and grayish tan, have no wings, and are visible to the naked eye. The nits, or eggs, appear as tiny whitish oval specks adhering to the hair shaft about ¼ inch (but may be farther) from the scalp. The adherent nature of the nits distinguishes them from dandruff, which falls off readily. ***Empty nit cases,*** indicating hatched lice, are translucent rather than white and are located more than ¼ inch from the scalp (Fig. 18-11).

If evidence of infestation is found, it is important to perform the treatment according to the directions described on the label of the pediculicide. Parents are advised to read the directions carefully before beginning treatment. Instructions on the labels indicate that dead lice and remaining nits are removed with an extra-fine-tooth comb. Most

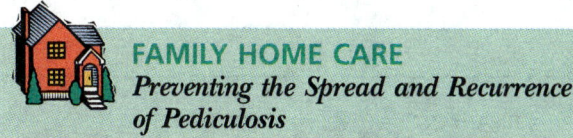

FAMILY HOME CARE
Preventing the Spread and Recurrence of Pediculosis

Machine wash all washable clothing, towels, and bed linens in hot water and dry in a hot dryer for at least 20 minutes. Dry-clean nonwashable items.
Thoroughly vacuum carpets, car seats, pillows, stuffed animals, rugs, mattresses, and upholstered furniture.
Seal nonwashable items in plastic bags for 14 days if unable to dry-clean or vacuum.
Soak combs, brushes, and hair accessories in lice-killing products for 1 hour or in boiling water for 10 minutes.

From Clore ER: Dispelling the common myths about pediculosis, *J Pediatr Health Care* 3:28-33, 1989.

preparations include a comb to dislodge the firmly adhered nits. Commercial products (Step 2 or Clear) may be used to loosen attached nits for removal. However, if the comb is ineffective in removing the nit cases, they must be removed with tweezers or between the fingernails.

The child is made as comfortable as possible during the application process, because the pediculicide must remain on the scalp and hair for several minutes. If eye irritation occurs, the eyes must be flushed well with tepid water.

➤ **NURSING TIP** Playing "beauty parlor" during the shampoo is a useful strategy. The child lies supine, with the head over a sink or basin, and covers the eyes with a dry towel or washcloth. This prevents medication, which can cause chemical conjunctivitis, from splashing into the eyes.

Live lice survive for up to 48 hours away from the host, but nits are shed into the environment and are capable of hatching in 7 to 10 days. Therefore measures must be taken to prevent further infestation (see Family Home Care box). Spraying with insecticide is not recommended because of the danger to children and animals. Families should also be advised that the pediculicide is relatively costly, especially when several members of the household require treatment.

The psychologic effects of lice infestations can be highly stressful to children. They are influenced by the reactions of others, including their parents, and may be made to feel ashamed or guilty. Parents are strongly cautioned against cutting a child's hair or, worse, shaving a child's head. Lice infest short hair as readily as long hair, and these actions only compound the child's distress and serve as a continual reminder to peers, who are always ready to taunt another with something out of the ordinary.

Prevention. The increasing incidence of pediculosis in schoolchildren has become a serious concern for school nurses, parents, and community health agencies. School nurses usually coordinate school-community prevention control programs for pediculosis. The **National Pediculosis Association*** offers education and advocates a "no nits" policy for treated children's reentry into school.

*P.O. Box 149, Newton, MA 02161; (617) 449-6487 or (800) 446-4NPA.

SYSTEMIC DISORDERS RELATED TO SKIN LESIONS

SYSTEMIC MYCOTIC (FUNGAL) INFECTIONS

Mycotic (systemic or deep fungal) infections have the capacity to invade the viscera, as well as the skin. The best known of these are primarily lung diseases, which are usually acquired by inhalation. They produce a variable spectrum of disease, and some are quite common in certain geographic areas. They are not transmitted from person to person but appear to reside in the soil, from which their spores are airborne. The cutaneous lesions are granulomatous and appear as ulcers, plaques, nodules, fungating masses, and abscesses. The course of deep fungal diseases is chronic, with slow progression that favors sensitization (Table 18-8).

RICKETTSIAL INFECTIONS

Rickettsiae are intracellular parasites, similar in size to bacteria, that inhabit the alimentary tract of a wide range of natural hosts. With the exception of Q fever, mammals become infected only through the bites of infected insects (lice and fleas) or arachnids (ticks and mites), which serve as both infectors and reservoirs. Rickettsial diseases are more common in temperate and tropical climates and in areas where humans live in association with arthropods. Infection in humans is incidental (except epidemic typhus) and not necessary for the survival of the rickettsial species. However, once the organism invades a human, it causes a disease that varies in intensity from a benign self-limiting illness to a fulminating and frequently fatal one. Some rickettsial infections are outlined in Table 18-9.

LYME DISEASE

Lyme disease is the most common tick-borne disorder in the United States. Although the disease is being reported with increasing frequency, the exact incidence is unknown.

Etiology

Lyme disease is caused by the spirochete, *Borrelia burgdorferi,* which enters the skin and bloodstream through the saliva and feces of ticks. The most commonly known vectors of the disease are the deer tick *Ixodes dammini* (also known as *Ixodes scapularis*) in the Midwest and Northeast and *Ixodes pacificus* in the Pacific Northwest regions of the United States. The ticks are clear to light brown and are very small, 2 to 4 mm in length (the size of a poppy seed), making detection difficult. The preferred hosts of *I. dammini* are white-tailed deer and white-footed mice.

Clinical Manifestations

The disease may present in any of three stages, which may be distinct or isolated, overlapping, or absent. Exacerbations and remission are common. The symptoms (with or without the rash) are flulike in nature.

Stage 1 consists of the tick bite at the time of inoculation, followed in 3 to 32 days by the development of ***erythema chronicum migrans (ECM)*** at the site of the bite. The

TABLE 18-8 Systemic Mycoses

DISORDER/ORGANISM	SKIN MANIFESTATIONS	SYSTEMIC MANIFESTATIONS	TREATMENT	COMMENTS
North American blastomycosis—*Blastomyces dermatitidis*	Chronic granulomatous lesions and microabscesses in any part of body Initial lesion is a papule; undergoes ulceration and peripheral spread	Pulmonary symptoms, such as cough, chest pain, weakness, and weight loss May have skeletal involvement, with bone destruction and formation of cutaneous abscesses	Intravenous administration of amphotericin B	Usual portal of entry is lungs Source of infection unknown Noninfectious Pulmonary infections may be mild and self-limiting and require treatment Progressive disease often fatal
Cryptococcosis—*Cryptococcus neoformans (Torula histolytica)*	Usually on face; acneiform, firm, nodular, painless eruption	Central nervous system (CNS) manifestations; headache, dizziness, stiff neck, and signs of increased intracranial pressure Low-grade fever, mild cough, lung infiltration	Intravenous amphotericin B; may be administered intrathecally for CNS involvement 5-Flurocytosine for meningitis Excision and drainage of local lesions	Acquired by inhalation of dust but may enter through skin Prognosis serious Noninfectious Increased incidence in persons receiving corticosteroids with lymphoreticular malignancies, or with type II diabetes
Histoplasmosis—*Histoplasma capsulatum*	Not distinctive or uniform but most appear as punched-out or granulomatous ulcers	General systemic symptoms may include pallor, diarrhea, vomiting, irregular spiking temperature, hepatosplenomegaly, and pulmonary symptoms Any tissue of body may be involved with related symptoms	Intravenous amphotericin B for severe cases Oral ketoconazole	Organism cultured from soil, especially where contaminated with fowl droppings Fungus enters through skin or mucous membranes of mouth and respiratory tract Endemic in Mississippi and Ohio River valleys Disseminated diseases most common in infants and children
Coccidioidomycosis (valley fever)—*Coccidioides immitis*	Erythema nodosum Erythema multiforme Erythematous maculopapular rash	Primary lung disease usually asymptomatic May be sign of acute febrile illness Disseminated disease is very serious	Intravenous amphotericin B Intravenous miconazole (synthetic imidazole) Intraventricular miconazole plus oral ketoconazole for CNS involvement Surgical resection of persistent pulmonary cavities	Inhalation of aerospores from soil Endemic in southwestern United States Usually resolves spontaneously Increased incidence in dark-skinned races (Filipino, black, Mexican, Asian)

lesion begins as a small erythematous papule that enlarges radially over a period of days to weeks, resulting in a large circumferential ring with a raised, edematous doughnutlike border (Fig. 18-12). The thigh, groin, and axilla are common sites. The lesion is described as "burning," feels warm to the touch, and occasionally is pruritic.

Many patients develop multiple, smaller secondary annular lesions without the indurated center. They may occur anywhere, except on the palms and soles, and in untreated patients they disappear in 3 to 4 weeks. Constitutional symptoms, including headache, malaise, fatigue, anorexia, stiff neck, generalized lymphadenopathy, splenomegaly, conjunctivitis, sore throat, abdominal pain, and cough, are often observed.

Stage 2, the most serious stage of the disease, is characterized by systemic involvement of neurologic, cardiac, and musculoskeletal systems that appears 2 to 11 weeks after the cutaneous phase is completed. Headache is the most frequent symptom, but in early stages it is not associated with neurologic abnormalities. Later neurologic features include meningoencephalitis, cranial nerve palsies, and peripheral radiculoneuritis.

Cardiac complications, which may appear in a smaller number of persons 4 to 5 weeks after ECM, are commonly

TABLE 18-9 Eruptions Caused by Rickettsiae

DISORDER/ORGANISM/HOST	MANIFESTATIONS	MANAGEMENT	COMMENTS
Rocky Mountain spotted fever—*R. rickettsii* Arthropod: tick Transmission: tick Mammal source: wild rodents; dogs	Gradual onset: fever, malaise, anorexia, myalgia Abrupt onset: rapid temperature elevation, chills, vomiting, myalgia, severe headache Maculopapular or petechial rash primarily on extremities (ankles and wrists) but may spread to other areas, characteristically on palms and soles	Control: protection from tick bite by proper wearing apparel, tick repellent Tetracycline or chloramphenicol Vigorous supportive therapy	Usually self-limited in children Onset in children may resemble any infectious disease Severe disease rare in children Children and dogs should be inspected regularly if they play in wooded areas See Table 18-12 for management of ticks
Epidemic typhus—*R. prowazekii* Arthropod: body louse Transmission: infected feces into broken skin Mammal source: humans	Abrupt onset of chills, fever, diffuse myalgia, headache, malaise Maculopapular rash becomes petechial 4 to 7 days later, spreading from trunk outward	Control: immediate destruction of vectors Tetracycline or chloramphenicol	Patient should be isolated until deloused See discussion on p. 784 for management of pediculosis Excreta from infected lice also in dust—disinfect patient's clothing, bedding, and possessions and wash in hot water
Endemic typhus—*R. typhi* Arthropod: rat fleas, or lice Transmission: flea bite; inhaling or ingesting flea excreta Mammal source: rats	Headache, arthralgia, backache followed by fever; may last 9-14 days Maculopapular rash after 1-8 days of fever; begins in trunk and spreads to periphery; rarely involves face, palms, soles	Control; eliminate rat reservoir, insect vectors, or both Supportive treatment: tetracycline or chloramphicol	Fairly common in United States Shorter duration than epidemic typhus A mild, seldom fatal illness Difficult to distinguish from epidemic typhus
Rickettsialpox—*R. akari* Arthropod: mouse mite Transmission: mite Mammal source: house mouse	Maculopapular rash following primary lesion and eschar at site of bite, fever, chills, headache	Control: eradication of rodent reservoir and mite vector Tetracycline or chloramphenicol Supportive treatment	Self-limited, nonfatal disease Endemic in New York City Found in many cities in United States

atrioventricular conduction abnormalities and may result in severe heart block. Patients may be asymptomatic but can develop syncope, palpitations, dyspnea, chest pain, and severe bradycardia.

Stage 3, or the late stage, may develop months or years later. Musculoskeletal pains that involve the tendons, bursae, muscles, and synovia may develop. Arthritis may occur and even become chronic. In children the arthritis is characterized by intermittently painful swollen joints (primarily the knees), with spontaneous remissions and exacerbations. Late neurologic problems may include deafness, chronic encephalopathy, and keratitis.

Diagnostic Evaluation

The diagnosis is based primarily on the history, observation of the lesion, and development of subsequent manifestations. Many persons do not remember a tick bite or the rash. Laboratory diagnosis is usually established in later stages through serologic testing, either by indirect immunofluorescence (IFA) or enzyme immunoassay (EIA). However, these tests are not yet standardized, and false-negative and false-positive results may occur.

Therapeutic Management

At the time the rash appears or shortly thereafter, children over 9 years of age are treated with oral doxycycline or amoxicillin, and children under 9 years of age are given amoxicillin or penicillin. The length of treatment depends on the clinical response and other disease manifestations but is usually from 10 to 14 days (American Academy of Pediatrics, Committee on Infectious Diseases, 1994). The treatment is effective in preventing second-stage manifestations in most cases. Neurologic, cardiac, and arthritic manifestations are managed with intravenous antibiotics, such as ceftriaxone or penicillin G. Follow-up care is important in ensuring that treatment is initated or terminated as needed.

Nursing Considerations

The major thrust of nursing care, especially in endemic areas, is prevention. Prevention of the disorder involves educating parents to protect their children from exposure to ticks with simple measures (see p. 799). In endemic areas tick habitats can include yards and parks, as well as wooded areas.

Parents or other caregivers should examine their chil-

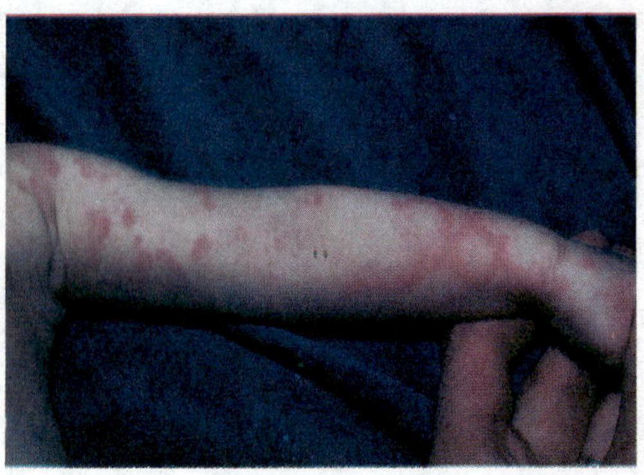

FIG. 18-12 Lyme disease. Note annular red rings in erythema chronicum migrans. (From Weston WL, Lane AT: *Color textbook of pediatric dermatology,* St Louis, 1991, Mosby.)

dren carefully for ticks if they have been in areas where ticks are likely to be found and remove them promptly (see Table 18-12). Parents should also be alert for signs of the skin lesion, especially if their children are known to have been exposed to the tick vector.

The use of insect repellents such as those containing diethyltoluamide (DEET) can protect against insects. Parents should be advised to use them judiciously. DEET is absorbed through the skin; therefore, repeated, heavy applications may cause toxicity in infants and children.

Information about Lyme disease, especially Lyme disease during pregnancy, can be obtained from the **National Lyme Borreliosis Foundation.*** Information is also available from the Lyme disease hotline.†

CAT SCRATCH DISEASE (CSD)

CSD is a subacute regional adenitis that follows the scratch or bite of an animal, especially a cat (99% of cases). Most cases are probably caused by *Rochalimaea henselae,* a rickettsia (Margileth and Hayden, 1993). The disease is usually a benign, self-limiting illness that resolves spontaneously in about 2 to 4 months.

The usual manifestations are a painless, nonpruritic erythematous papule at the site of inoculation, followed by regional lymphadenitis. The disease may persist for several months before gradual resolution. In some children the adenitis progresses to suppuration, and a few children may be very ill with various symptoms, including a prolonged high temperature. The diagnosis is made on the basis of three of the following: (1) contact (usually a kitten) and regional inoculation lesion, (2) lymphadenopathy, (3) a positive CSD skin test, and (4) biopsy of lymph node with histopathology compatible with CSD (Margileth and Hadfield, 1990). A new test, the indirect fluorescent antibody test for *R. henselae,* is also available (Zangwill and others, 1993). The disease may persist for several months before gradual resolution. In some children, especially those who are immunocompromised, the adenitis may progress to suppuration and serious complications.

The treatment is primarily supportive. Antibiotics do not appear to shorten the duration or prevent progression to suppuration, although some have reported improvement with administration of trimethoprim-sulfamethoxazole (Collip, 1992; Flessner, 1989). Activity is limited to prevent trauma to the large lymph nodes, and bed rest is indicated for children who have fevers. Analgesics may be needed for discomfort and fever. Most children can continue normal activities during the course of the disease. The animals are not ill during the time they transmit the disease, and most authorities do not recommend disposal of a cherished pet.

SKIN DISORDERS RELATED TO CHEMICAL OR PHYSICAL CONTACTS

CONTACT DERMATITIS

Contact dermatitis is an inflammatory reaction of the skin to chemical substances, natural or synthetic, that evoke a hypersensitivity response or to those agents that cause direct irritation. The initial reaction occurs in an exposed region, most commonly the face and neck, backs of the hands, forearms, male genitalia, and lower legs. There is characteristically a sharp delineation between inflamed and normal skin early in the reaction that ranges from a faint, transient erythema to massive bullae on an erythematous swollen base. Itching is a constant symptom.

The cause may be a primary irritant or a sensitizing agent. A ***primary irritant*** is one that irritates any skin. A ***sensitizing agent*** produces an irritation on those who have met the irritant or something chemically related to it, have undergone an immunologic change, and have become sensitized. Prior exposure is not a necessarily factor in the reaction. A sensitizer irritates in relatively low concentrations only persons who are allergic to it.

The clinical course is relatively short (1 to 4 weeks) if the causative agent is eliminated, and whether or not there are complications from secondary invasion or reactions to topical therapy depends on the severity of the original reaction.

Sensitizing reactions are acquired by repeated or prolonged exposure, and the sensitizing capacity of different substances varies widely. Strong sensitizers require only one or two exposures and occur in a higher percentage of individuals; weak sensitizers require numerous exposures, and a smaller percentage of those exposed will be sensitized. The length of time from exposure to development of sensitivity varies considerably and may be as short as a week or much longer. Sometimes with repeated exposure and reactions the skin loses its capacity to return to normal, or secondary factors become predominant to produce a chronic inflammatory process.

The major goal in treatment is to prevent further exposure of the skin to the offending substance. Provided there is no further irritation, the normal recuperative powers of the skin will produce satisfactory results without treatment. The most frequent offenders are plant and animal irritants, the prototype of which is poison ivy (see p. 789).

The most common contact dermatitis in infants occurs on the convex surfaces of the diaper area as a result of

*Box 462, Tolland, CT 06084; (203) 871-2900 or (203) 872-6346.
†(914) 285-LYME.

chemical irritation from ammonia, putrefactive enzymes acting on urinary amino acids, or, less often, laundry products (see Diaper Dermatitis, Chapter 13). Other agents that frequently produce dermatologic responses from contact are animal irritants such as wool, feathers, and furs; vegetable irritants such as oleoresins, oils, and turpentine; and chemicals of all kinds, including synthetic fabrics (e.g., shoe components), dyes, metals, cosmetics, perfumes, and soaps (including bubble baths). The list is endless.

Several cosmetic products advertised as safe for children may be responsible for skin irritation in children. These include a cream hair relaxer marketed especially for children that contains lye and must be used with extreme care. Because children's hair is more resistant to artificial curling or straightening, pediatric preparations contain chemicals as strong as or stronger than those intended for use on adults.

Nursing Considerations

Nurses frequently detect evidence of contact dermatitis during routine physical assessments. Skin manifestations in specific areas suggest limited contact, such as around the eyes (mascara), areas of the body covered by clothing but not protected by undergarments (wool), or areas of the body not covered by clothing (ultraviolet injury). Generalized involvement is more likely to be caused by bubble bath or soap. Often nurses are able to elicit the offending agent and counsel families regarding management. If the lesions persist, are extensive, or show evidence of infection, medical evaluation is indicated.

POISON IVY, OAK, AND SUMAC

Contact with the dry or succulent portions of any of three poisonous plants produces localized, streaked or spotty, oozing, and painful impetiginous lesions. Poison ivy grows almost everywhere east of the Rockies, poison oak is mainly found west of the Rockies, and poison sumac is usually restricted to swamp areas of the Southeast. Only Nevada, Hawaii, and Alaska (and regions above 4000 feet) appear to be free of the plants (Fig. 18-13).

The offending substance in these plants is an oil, ***urushiol,*** that is extremely potent. Sensitivity to urushiol is not inborn but is developed after one or two exposures and may change over a lifetime. Repeated exposures appear to lower the reaction; exposure after long periods away from it may elicit a heightened response. Some highly sensitive persons may suddenly become resistant, and vice versa. All parts of the plants contain urushiol; thus dried leaves and stems contain the irritant. Even smoke from burning brush piles can produce a reaction. There is widespread contact with the skin from the smoke of burning plants, and lung reactions from smoke inhalation can be life-threatening.

Animals do not seem to be affected by the oil; dogs or other animals who have run or played in the plants may carry the sap on their fur, and animals who eat the plants can transfer the oil in saliva. Shoes, tools, and toys can transfer the oil. Golf balls that have been in the rough are sources of contact.

Clinical Manifestations

The substance begins to take effect as soon as it touches the skin. It penetrates through the epidermis and bonds with the dermal layer, where it initiates an immune response. The full-blown reaction is evident after about 2 days, with redness, swelling, and itching at the site of contact. Several days later, streaked or spotty blisters oozing serum from damaged cells produce the characteristic impetiginous lesions (Fig. 18-14). The lesions dry and heal spontaneously, and itching stops by 10 to 14 days.

Therapeutic Management

Treatment of the lesions includes calamine lotion, soothing Burow solution compresses, and/or Aveeno baths to relieve discomfort. Topical corticosteroid gel is very effective for prevention or relief of inflammation, especially when applied before formation of blisters. Oral corticosteroids may be needed for several reactions, and a sedative such as diphenhydramine (Benadryl) may be ordered.

Nursing Considerations

When it is known that the child has made contact with the plant, the area is immediately flushed (preferably within 15

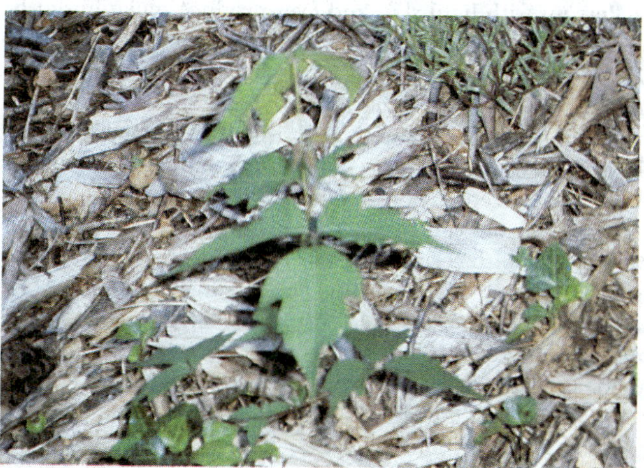

FIG. 18-13 Poison ivy.

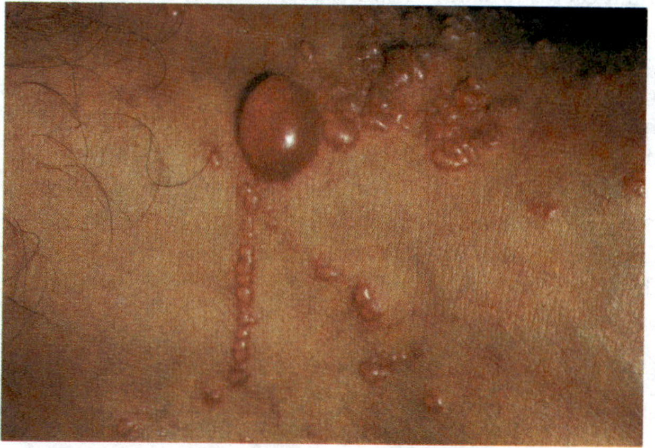

FIG. 18-14 Poison ivy; note "streaked" blisters surrounding one large blister. (From Habif TP: *Clinical dermatology: a color guide to diagnosis and therapy,* ed 2, St Louis, 1990, Mosby.)

minutes) with *cold* running water to neutralize the urushiol not yet bonded to the skin. The best thing to wash with is an organic solvent, such as alcohol. If there is a stream nearby, an effective method is to have the child enter the water (clothes and all) and allow the water to rinse the oil from both skin and clothing. Using *mild* soap may be helpful but is not critical. Harsh soap and water are contraindicated because they remove protective skin oils and dilute the urushiol, allowing it to spread, and hard scrubbing irritates the skin (Mackreth, 1991). All clothing that has come in contact with the plant is removed with care and thoroughly laundered in hot water and detergent. Every effort should be made to prevent the child from scratching the lesions. Although the lesions do not spread by contact with the blister serum or from scratching, the lesions can become secondarily infected.

Prevention. Prevention is best accomplished by avoidance of contact and removal of the plant from the environment when feasible. All children, especially those known to be sensitive, should be taught to recognize the plant. Information regarding means for destroying plants can be obtained from an expert nursery or the U.S. Departments of Agriculture or Forestry.

FOREIGN BODIES

Small wooden splinters can be removed by parents with a needle and tweezers that have been sterilized with alcohol or a flame. The area around the sliver is washed with soap and water before removal is attempted. The sliver is exposed with the needle and then grasped firmly by the tweezers and pulled in the same direction in which it entered. Some foreign bodies should have medical evaluation; these include a fishhook, a deeply imbedded object such as a needle in a foot or near a joint, glass splinters, or other difficult-to-see objects. A small hand vacuum cleaner is effective in removing loose items such as glass splinters, gravel, dirt, or leaves from the surface of the skin before they become imbedded. This is especially valuable for trauma victims.

Cactus Spines

Small cactus prickles or spines are often troublesome to remove, and attempts are distressing to the child and family. Large spines or clumps can be removed with tweezers. To remove very fine spines, a number of options are available. In a study using a variety of methods on animal models, Martinez and others (1987) found that the most effective method involved an application of a thin layer of water-soluble household glue covered with a single layer of gauze. The application was allowed to dry and then removed. Other methods reported as highly successful include the following:

- Apply hair removal wax, let dry, and remove (Hennes, 1988). Takes less time to dry than glue.
- Place cellophane tape, sticky side down, over the spines and lift off (Cooper, 1988).
- Drop wax from a lighted candle over the affected area (from a sufficient height to avoid burning the skin), then cool by immersing in cold water and lift off.
- Apply facial beauty mask gel (Gelbard, 1984; Putnam and Lawton, 1985).

SUNBURN

Sunburn is a very common skin injury caused by overexposure to ultraviolet (UV) light waves—either sunlight or artificial light in the ultraviolet range. The sun emits a continuous spectrum of visible and nonvisible light rays that range in length from very short to very long. The shorter, higher-frequency waves are more damaging than longer wavelengths, but much of the light is filtered out as it travels through the atmosphere. Of the light that does filter through, ***ultraviolet A (UVA) waves*** are the longest and cause only minimum burning but play a significant role in photosensitive and photoallergic reactions. They are also responsible for premature aging of the skin and potentiate the effects of UVB. ***Ultraviolet B (UVB)*** waves are shorter and responsible for tanning, burning, and most of the harmful effects attributed to sunlight, especially skin cancer.

Numerous factors influence the amount of UVB exposure. Radiation is strongest at midday (10 AM to 3 PM), when the distance from the sun to a given spot on the earth is shortest. Solar intensity also varies with the seasons, time zones, and altitude. Exposure is greater at higher altitudes and less when the sky is hazy (although its effect is easily underestimated). Window glass effectively screens out UVB but not UVA. Fresh snow and water reflect ultraviolet rays, especially when the sun is directly overhead; some are reflected by sand.

Some persons are more susceptible to sunburn than others. Protection from effects of the sun is provided by the fibrous keratin of the outer epidermis and the pigment melanin, produced by the melanocytes of the innermost, or basal, layer of the epidermis. Areas of the body with thick keratin layers (palms and soles) offer the greatest protection. The protective pigment layer decreases the intensity of all ultraviolet light by physically blocking and scattering the radiation. Ultraviolet rays stimulate the melanocytes to produce more melanin, turning the skin darker. After several days of exposure, the dark melanin is able to absorb most of the incoming ultraviolet radiation before the rays can cause further damage.

Persons with light skin and eyes produce melanin slowly and are more prone to burn, whereas very dark-skinned people are able to tolerate more rays without damage. A high altitude increases the risk of burning; the sun becomes stronger near the equator; and sunlight is reflected from the surfaces of sand, snow, and water. Sunlight penetrates the atmosphere even on hazy days.

Other factors can play a role in sensitivity to ultraviolet rays. People with certain diseases (e.g., porphyria, lupus erythematosus) are more sensitive to the sun's rays. Some substances increase the skin's sensitivity, including numerous medications (e.g., barbiturates, oral contraceptives, sulfonamides, anticonvulsants), topical products (e.g., retinoic acid [Retin-A], antiseptic soap, after-shave lotions, colognes), and certain foods containing photosensitizing chemicals (e.g., carrots, parsley, limes).

The ultraviolet rays penetrate the skin surface, where

they precipitate a chemical change in the cell molecules, producing toxic by-products that irritate surrounding tissues. The result is redness, tissue swelling, increased capillary permeability, and the tenderness characteristic of superficial (first-degree) burns and the coagulation, necrosis, and blistering of partial-thickness (second-degree) burns (see Burns, Chapter 29). Sunburned skin is exquisitely sensitive, and severe sunburn may be accompanied by nausea, chills, fever, abdominal cramping, and headache. Dehydration may occur.

Excessive or long-term exposure to the sun causes permanent damage to the skin. Ninety percent of skin cancers occur in areas that are exposed to sunlight, and rates of skin cancers are higher in parts of the world where sunlight is more intense. Studies have also shown that childhood is a crucial time for sun exposure. Children who immigrate to sunny climates after 10 years of age develop cancer at lower rates than native-born children. In general, children receive three times as much sun exposure as adults, and teenagers, with their emphasis on the desirability of a tanned skin (Hurwitz, 1989), are a high-risk group.

Nursing Considerations

Treatment involves stopping the burning process, decreasing the inflammatory response, and rehydrating the skin. Local application of cool tap water soaks or immersion in a tepid water bath for 20 minutes or until the skin is cool limits tissue destruction and relieves the discomfort. After the cool applications, a bland oil-in-water moisturizing lotion can be applied, but petrolatum-based products that trap radiant heat in the tissues are avoided. Acetaminophen is recommended for relief of discomfort. Partial-thickness burns are treated the same as those from any heat source.

Prevention. Protection from sunburn is the major goal of management, and the harmful effects of the sun on the delicate skin of infants and children are receiving increased attention. Protection can be achieved by physical means (i.e., protective clothing and a hat) or by chemical means. Two types of products are available for sun protection: ***topical sunscreens,*** which partially absorb ultraviolet light, and ***sun blockers,*** which block out ultraviolet rays by reflecting sunlight. The most frequently recommended sun blockers are zinc oxide and titanium dioxide ointments.

Some chemicals have the capacity to absorb certain wavelengths of light and thus provide protection to the cutaneous surface when applied to the skin. Sunscreens are products containing a ***sun protective factor (SPF)*** based on evaluation of effectiveness against ultraviolet rays. The SPF is indicated by a number, such as 15, which indicates that if individuals normally burn in 10 minutes without a sunscreen, use of a sunscreen with an SPF of 15 will allow them to remain in the sun for 15 times 10, or 150 minutes (2½ hours) before acquiring the same degree of erythema or burn.

Most chemical sunscreens are available with an SPF ranging from 2 to over 30; the higher the number, the greater the protection. The American Academy of Pediatrics recommends waterproof sunscreens with a minimum SPF of 15. The SPF provides information primarily in relation to the effects of UVB, not UVA. Claims such as "broad-spectrum" or "UVA-UVB sunblock" are usually unsubstantiated. One product that affords protection against UVA is Parsol 1789, found in Photoplex and UVA Guard.

There is disagreement regarding the frequency of application. One opinion is that reapplication of sunscreen does not extend the period of protection; the protection will remain the same no matter how many times it is reapplied (Nicol, 1989). However, the predominant view is that sunscreen should be applied 15 to 20 minutes before exposure (so that the protective chemicals can penetrate the upper skin layers) and reapplied frequently and liberally (Hurwitz, 1989).

The most effective sunscreens are those containing ***p-aminobenzoic acid (PABA)*** and ***PABA-esters,*** which are effective against UVB. PABA is more effective, penetrates the outer layer of skin, and may accumulate with repeated use, thus providing protection even when the child is swimming or sweating. PABA may stain clothing; PABA-esters are less likely to stain clothing but are less effective than PABA. However, PABA can cause an allergenic response in sensitive persons, manifested as redness and itching 24 hours after application. ***Benzophenones*** also offer protection against UVA but are less effective than the PABA preparations and wash off easily. For best results, the sunscreen should be effective against both UVA and UVB.

The range of sunscreens available offer the consumer access to a type and combination to meet any need. Preparations made specifically for children are marketed especially for infants and children (Nicol, 1989). Sunscreens are applied evenly to all exposed areas, with special attention given to skinfolds and areas that might become exposed as clothing shifts. Parents are directed to read labels of sunscreen products carefully for the SPF and follow the manufacturer's directions for application.

NURSING ALERT Sunscreens are not recommended for infants under 6 months of age. Infants should be kept out of the sun or physically shaded from it. Fabric with a tight weave, such as cotton, offers good protection.

It is wise to avoid direct sun exposure when solar radiation is assumed to be of maximum intensity. The strongest radiation occurs when the sun is at its highest (directly overhead). Earlier or later in the day with the sun at a 45-degree angle, the earth's atmosphere provides protection equivalent to a SPF of 2.4 (Holloway, 1990).

➤ **NURSING TIP** Observe the length of one's shadow to assess the time when the sun's rays are most damaging. Seek protection from the sun when the shadow is shorter than one's height (Holloway, 1990).

Persons who care for or work with children, such as teachers, daycare workers, coaches, youth group leaders, and relatives, should be made aware of sun safety for children. Sun damage is cumulative. Although most long-term effects (cancer, wrinkling) are not evident until adulthood, skin care must begin in childhood. It should be the goal of every nurse to teach skin care as a basic practice that be-

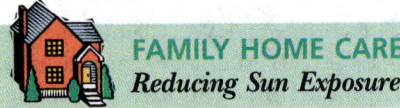

FAMILY HOME CARE
Reducing Sun Exposure

Remember that tanning indicates sun injury and risks of skin cancer begin in childhood.
Keep infants and children out of the sun as much as possible.
  Use carriage with hood when taking infants outdoors.
  Use canopy on stroller for older infants.
Schedule child's activities to avoid sun exposure between 10 AM and 3 PM whenever possible.
Take increased precautions when living or vacationing in the mountains or the tropics.
Protect child when outdoors with clothing (sun hat, long-sleeved shirt, long pants).
Apply sunscreen with SPF of at least 15.
Apply sunscreen to exposed areas:
  Before every exposure
  On cloudy as well as sunny days
  Even when child plays in shade; sun reflects from sand, snow, cement, and water
Reapply liberally every 2 to 3 hours and whenever child goes in the water or sweats heavily.
Check with child's practitioner regarding any medications the child is taking and observe for any evidence of side effects (rash, redness, swelling).
Examine skin regularly for signs of any change in pigmented nevi (rapid growth, crusting, ulceration, bleeding, change in pigmentation, development of inflamed satellite lesions, loss of normal skin lines) or subjective symptoms (tenderness, pain, itching).
Prohibit child from using sun lamps or tanning parlors.
Set a good example by following the above guidelines.

Modified from *For every child under the sun,* New York, The Skin Cancer Foundation.

comes a routine part of a child's life, much the same as tooth care (see Family Home Care box).

COLD INJURY

Cold injuries are most commonly seen in very cold regions. The nature of the heat-regulating mechanisms of the body are such that the inner portion of the body, or core, produces heat and the periphery, or outer area, conserves or dissipates the heat. When the body attempts to conserve heat, the outer tissues are subjected to low temperatures, and local trauma may result.

Chilblain, redness and swelling of the skin, occurs when extremities, usually the hands, are exposed intermittently to temperatures of 30° to 60° F. The response may vary but is characterized by intense vasodilation that increases the temperature of involved tissues above unaffected tissue and produces edematous, reddish blue patches that itch and burn. As warming takes place, the sensations become more intense but ordinarily subside in a few days.

Frostbite is the term used to describe tissue damage caused when excessive heat loss to local tissues allows ice crystals to form in tissues. The mechanisms of slow and rapid freezing differ. Slow freezing causes ice crystals to form in the extracellular fluid, leading to increased osmolality and movement of water from the cells. This causes cellular dehydration and destruction. Rapid freezing produces both extracellular and intracellular freezing and immediate cellular destruction. Rapid freezing takes place at high altitudes or with high conductivity from cold water immersion.

When frozen tissues thaw, the tissue damage is like that from a high-temperature burn—red blood cell aggregation, stasis, venous thrombosis, tissue edema and ischemic damage, increased tissue pressure, and death and necrosis of surrounding tissues. The frostbitten part appears white or blanched, feels solid, and is without sensation.

Rapid rewarming is associated with less tissue necrosis than slow thawing. It restores blood flow and shortens the period of cellular damage. Rewarming produces a flush (sometimes deep purple) and a return of sensation, which is extremely painful. Large blisters may appear 24 to 48 hours after rewarming and begin to reabsorb within 5 to 10 days, followed by formation of a hard black eschar. Superficial injury often heals satisfactorily.

Therapeutic Management

Rewarming is accomplished by immersing the part in well-agitated water at 100° to 108° F, and discomfort is managed with analgesics and sedatives. Care of blistered skin is similar to that described for burns. It is seldom possible to estimate the extent of tissue loss until new skin layers are revealed after the eschar layer separates; therefore amputation of extremities is usually delayed for 60 to 90 days unless there is evidence of gangrene.

Nursing Considerations

The frostbite victim should be transferred to the nearest emergency treatment center; the injured parts are protected from trauma. The injured areas are handled gently, and the patient is prevented from ambulating on injured feet. Rubbing injured tissues is contraindicated and can cause damage by rupture of crystallized cells. After rewarming, a loose dressing is applied. Dry heat is not applied. (See Burns, Chapter 29, and Pain Management, Chapter 26.)

HYPOTHERMIA

Hypothermia is defined as the cooling of the body's core temperature (pulmonary artery or esophageal) to injurious levels, usually identified as below 35° C (95° F). Hypothermia occurs in environmental settings when heat production by exercise and metabolism is less than heat lost by convection, conduction, or radiation. There is a 6% drop in blood flow for each 1° C decrease in core temperature (Coln and Emmrich, 1989). Very young children with a large surface area relative to body mass, and thin persons are at the greatest risk for hypothermia.

The body in positive heat balance attempts to conserve heat by alternate vasoconstriction and vasodilation in extremities. Threat of prolonged or severe cold exposure causes the body to conserve core temperature at the expense of the extremities by shunting warm blood to the core

TABLE 18-10 Physical Effects of Hypothermia

TEMPERATURE	CHARACTERISTICS
35° C (95° F)	Increased respiratory rate, decreased intestinal motility; vigorous shivering; may be conscious and alert; task performance often impaired
32° C (90° F)	May continue uncontrollable shivering or may begin to show muscular rigidity; decreased respiratory rate; atrial fibrillation; may still be conscious but sensorium changes evident; impaired cognition, reasoning, and speech; loss of manual skills and dexterity; brief vasodilation that causes flushes and warm sensation and possible confusion
30° C (86° F)	Decreased cerebral blood flow; may show increased blood pressure (may be difficult to obtain), tachycardia, and tachypnea; may have supraventricular arrhythmia, PCVs, and T-wave inversion; usually conscious, but a loss of consciousness is preceded by irritability
27° C (80° F)	Bradycardia and slowed respiratory rate; metabolic rate decreased by 50%; decreased oxygen uptake, CO_2 production; ventricular fibrillation; rigid extremities
25° C (77° F)	Hypotension; glomerular filtration and blood flow to kidneys reduced by 30%
20° C (68° F)	Unconscious; nonfunctioning reflexes; unresponsive pupils; respirations barely detectable or undetectable; extremities and trunk cold to touch; abnormal ECG; pulse may decrease to 4 per minute, progressing to cardiac standstill; flat EEG; dead appearance
18° C (65° F)	Injury to peripheral tissue

after passing through the muscles of the extremities. Shivering contributes to warming by raising the metabolic rate to increase the heat of blood before it returns to the core (Coln and Emmrich, 1989). Clinical manifestations related to degree of hypothermia are outlined in Table 18-10.

Therapeutic Management

Rewarming is the major objective of therapy. For mild hypothermia (30° to 35° C [86° to 95° F]) only external application of heat lamps or immersion in water (38° to 42° C [100.4° to 107.6° F]) is necessary to restore core temperature with little risk of complications. Lower temperatures require core rewarming by any of several modalities—warm humidified oxygen, intravenous fluids, rectal lavage, peritoneal lavage (dialysis) with warm fluids, hemodialysis, application of external warmth to core circulation areas (groin, axilla, posterior neck region), and/or extracorporeal blood rewarming.

Supportive therapy includes maintenance of ventilation, cardiac monitoring, monitoring renal function, and correcting fluid and acid-base imbalances. Prognosis is directly correlated with the degree of hypothermia, method of rewarming, and presence of underlying medical conditions.

Nursing Considerations

Nursing care consists of monitoring vital functions and assisting with therapies. Obtaining a history from family or other observers, including outside environmental temperature, length of exposure to elements, location of exposure site (e.g., outside or inside a vehicle or structure), and any care that may have been given, is essential (McGuire, 1987). If trauma is associated with the hypothermia, the mechanism and circumstances of injury are ascertained.

Prevention. Anticipation of cold conditions and knowledge of cold survival techniques are the basis of prevention. Children living in cold climates should have adequate protection when outdoors. Multiple layers of warm clothing are more effective than a single heavy layer for reducing the rate of heat loss, although they do not prevent it. Families living in cold climates should take precautions against unexpected prolonged exposure to cold (e.g., store extra blankets, food rations, and other equipment in their vehicles in the event of an unexpected mechanical breakdown).

Loss of central core temperature can be reduced by 50% when an individual assumes the fetal position. A person suspected of hypothermia should be moved to a sheltered area, and wet clothing should be removed and replaced with dry, warm garments. Warm, high-calorie liquids are important if the person is conscious.

SKIN DISORDERS RELATED TO DRUG SENSITIVITY

DRUG REACTIONS

Although any drug is capable of producing almost any form of reaction in the susceptible individual, some have a tendency to produce a particular reaction consistently, and some are more likely than others to produce an untoward effect. Many are allergenic responses following a prior administration of the drug, even a topical application. Other factors influence a drug response in a particular individual. For example, drug eruptions occur with less frequency in children than in adults; the incidence increases with the number of drugs being given; climate may be a factor when light sensitivity produces a response on sun-exposed surfaces; and it is well known that genetic factors affect the way in which some individuals are able to metabolize specific drugs.

Manifestations of drug reactions may be delayed or immediate. Seven days are usually required for a child to develop sensitivity to a drug that has never been administered previously. With prior sensitivity the manifestations appear almost immediately. Rashes are the most common manifestation of adverse drug reactions in children—exanthematous, urticarial, or eczematoid. However, individual drug reactions may vary from a single lesion to extensive, generalized epidermal necrosis. Cutaneous manifestations can resemble almost any skin disease and can be seen in almost any degree of severity. With few exceptions, the distribution of a drug eruption is widespread, since it results from a circulating agent, appears as an inflammatory response with itching, is sudden in onset, and may be associated with constitutional symptoms such as fever, malaise, gastrointestinal upsets, anemia, or liver and kidney damage.

Drug reactions are also related to the amount of drug administered and the route of administration. For example, larger amounts precipitate a more severe response than a small amount, and drugs taken orally are less sensitizing than those administered intravenously. Another common response is a fixed eruption, (i.e., a recurrent eruption at the same site with each readministration of the drug). The lesion, a purplish red round or oval plaque with a sharp border seen most frequently on the extremities, disappears slowly, and the pigmentation deepens with each episode.

In most cases treatment for simple cutaneous reactions consists of discontinuation of the drug. Sometimes a decision is made to continue the drug (such as an antibiotic in an infant or small child) until the cause of the rash is clearly indicated. In urticarial-type eruptions antihistamines may be ordered, and for widespread and severe lesions corticosteroids are beneficial. Severe anaphylactic reactions are a medical emergency (see Anaphylaxis, Chapter 29).

Nursing Considerations

The most effective means of a management is prevention. Parents always remember a severe response. A careful history will elicit evidence of a previous drug reaction. The history should include the name of the drug, nature of the reaction, drug dose, and how soon after administration the reaction occurred (see Past History, Chapter 6).

Nurses who suspect that a rash is caused by a medication should withhold any further dose and report the eruption to the practitioner. The most frequent offenders in drug reactions are penicillin and sulfonamides, and nurses must be alert to this possibility. However, even commonplace drugs, including aspirin, barbiturates, chemical agents in a number of foods, flavoring agents, and preservatives, are capable of producing an undesired response. Persons who have severe reactions are reminded to obtain and wear an identification bracelet or chain in case of emergency or inadvertent administration of the offending drug.

ERYTHEMA MULTIFORME

Erythema multiforme is an acute, cutaneous disorder most often resulting from infections (usually viruses) or drug reactions. The characteristic lesion consists of an urticarial plaque with a dusky or vesicular center, which appears primarily on the palms, soles, and extensor surfaces.

Treatment involves discontinuing the drug, applying wet compresses for erosive lesions, and administering analgesics for discomfort. Antihistamines may be prescribed for pruritus.

ERYTHEMA MULTIFORME EXUDATIVUM (STEVENS-JOHNSON SYNDROME) (SJS)

SJS is the severe form of erythema multiforme and is characterized by lesions of the skin and mucous membranes, fever, and multiple systemic symptoms. The disease is presumed to be primarily a hypersensitivity reaction to certain drugs, although the reaction may follow an upper respiratory tract infection. The disorder is relatively rare, occurs at any age, and is more common in males than in females.

The syndrome usually begins with flulike symptoms—malaise, sore throat, fever, and severe headache. Balanitis, conjunctivitis, or stomatitis appears next, followed in a few days by an erythematous papular rash. The lesions can involve any cutaneous surface, including the palms and soles, but usually spare the scalp. They can be scattered or confluent. The initial lesions enlarge by peripheral expansion with a vesicular center that often becomes bullous. Mucous membrane ulceration often becomes severe enough to interfere with eating, and many patients have pulmonary involvement.

Mild disease requires only symptomatic treatment. However, severe disease requires hospitalization. Fluid and nutritional requirements are high, and most patients respond well to viscous lidocaine to relieve ulcer pain and to a liquid diet. Intravenous feedings may be needed for extensive oral involvement. Meticulous mouth care is important, and skin care frequently requires management in a burn unit (see Stomatitis, Chapter 16). Daily ophthalmologic examination is advised. Dry eyes are a problem, as well as risk of chronic mild symblepharon (adhesion of lids to the eyeball). Antibiotics are administered to patients with positive cultures, but the use of corticosteroids is controversial, and its efficacy unproved.

The mortality is estimated to be from 10% to 15% during the acute phase, especially in patients with pulmonary involvement. The disease is self-limiting, and the skin lesions gradually disappear without scarring in 2 to 3 weeks but may recur on reexposure to an offending drug. Since these patients are usually managed in a burn unit, the nursing care is the same as for a burned child. The family needs emotional support to cope with the life-threatening nature of the disease.

TOXIC EPIDERMAL NECROLYSIS (TEN) (LYELL DISEASE)

TEN is a drug-induced injury to the skin characterized by a generalized erythematous rash that rapidly evolves into bullae and peeling. It appears to be a hypersensitivity reaction with precipitating factors similar to those responsible for erythema multiforme. The more common offending drugs are phenobarbital, phenytoin, allopurinol, sulfonamides, and penicillin. The clinical appearance is the same as that seen in the more common (in children) ***staphylococcal scalded skin syndrome (SSSS).***

The disease begins with a prodromal period of fever and malaise and a generalized erythematous rash that rapidly evolves into bullae and extensive epidermal peeling. Oral lesions are similar to those observed in SJS. Treatment consists of withdrawal of the offending drug, fluid and electrolyte replacement, and skin management as for severe burns. The disease can be protracted, and the mortality rate can range from 25% to 50%. It is essential that families of children receiving anticonvulsants or sulfonamides be informed of the significance of a rash and the importance of reporting it to their health professional promptly.

MISCELLANEOUS SKIN PROBLEMS

CONGENITAL SKIN DISORDERS

There are a number of congenital skin disorders, usually inherited as autosomal dominant traits. Psoriasis in children less than 16 years of age is uncommon (Table 18-11), and photosensitivity eruptions associated with other inherited diseases appear early in childhood. Ichthyoses are a heterogeneous group of disorders characterized by scaling that create a challenging problem in treatment. Because of wide variability, these disorders are not discussed in detail.

TABLE 18-11 Miscellaneous Skin Disorders

DISEASE/CAUSATIVE AGENT	LOCAL MANIFESTATIONS	MANAGEMENT	COMMENTS
Urticaria—Usually allergic response to drugs or infection	Development of wheals Vary in size and configuration and tend to appear quickly, spread irregularly, and fade within a few hours May be constant or intermittent, sparse or profuse, small or large, discrete or confluent May be acute, chronic, or recurrent in acute attacks	Local soothing and antipruritic applications Antihistamines Epinephrine or ephedrine Cortisone or corticotropin (ACTH) in severe cases Severe upper respiratory involvement may require tracheostomy	Known etiologic agents should be avoided May be accompanied by malaise, fever, lymphadenopathy Severe cases may involve mucous membranes, internal organs, and joints Obstruction to air passages constitutes medical emergency (see Chapter 31)
Intertrigo—Mechanical trauma and aggravating factors of excessive heat, moisture, and sweat retention	Red, inflamed, moist, partially denuded, marginated areas, the shape of which is determined by location Appears where opposing skin surfaces rub together, such as intergluteal folds, groin, neck, and axilla Excessive moisture and obesity are often factors	Affected areas kept clean and dry Skinfolds kept separated with a generous supply of nonmedicated powder Exposure to air and light Removal of excess clothing	A form of diaper irritation Prevent recurrence by keeping susceptible areas clean and dry Frequently associated with overheating from too much clothing
Psoriasis—Unknown; hereditary predisposition; may be triggered by stress	Round, thick, dry, reddish patches covered with coarse, silvery scales over trunk and extremities; first lesions commonly appear in scalp; facial lesions more common in children than adults Affected cells proliferate at a much more rapid rate than normal cells	Exposure to sunlight, ultraviolet light Topical corticosteroids Tar derivatives Trihydroxyanthracine Keratolytic agents (salicylic acid) Psoralin—ultraviolet A (PUVA)* Emollients may provide relief	Uncommon in children under age 6 years Persons are otherwise healthy individuals Coal tar and psoralin act synergistically with ultraviolet light Keratolytic agents enhance absorption of corticosteroids Humidifiers may help in winter
Alopecia			
Alopecia areata	Sudden onset of asymptomatic, noninflammatory, round, bald patches in hairy parts of body	Psychologic support Inducement of allergic contact dermatitis to stimulate growth of hair Minoxidil (peripheral vasodilator)	Family history in 10%-26% of cases Some concern regarding drug therapy safety Refer to support groups†
Traumatic alopecia	Traction alopecia around scalp margins from tight hair styles (e.g., braids, pony tails, corn rows)	Counseling regarding hair styling, use of hair cosmetics, hot combs, rollers	More prevalent in black children and adolescents Prolonged traction can produce fibrosis of hair root and permanent loss
Trichotillomania	Compulsive hair pulling	Determine and treat cause	Chronic hair pulling may require psychologic therapy
Tinea capitis	See Table 18-7	See Table 18-7	See Table 18-7

*Still considered investigational.
†**National Alopecia Areata Foundation,** 710 C St, Suite 11, San Rafael, CA 94901; (415) 456-4644.

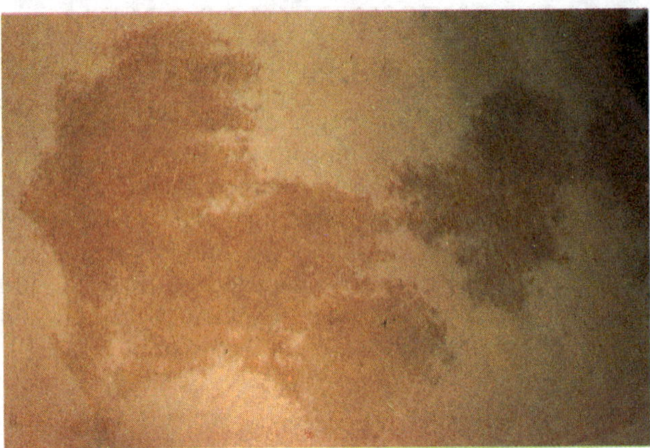

FIG. 18-15 Café-au-lait patches. (From Seidel HM and others: *Mosby's guide to physical examination,* ed 3, St Louis, 1995, Mosby.)

CRITERIA FOR DIAGNOSIS OF NEUROFIBROMATOSIS-1

An individual with two or more of the following clinical signs meets the criteria for NF1:
- Six or more café-au-lait spots larger than 5 mm in diameter in prepubertal children and larger than 15 mm in postpubertal individual
- Two or more neurofibromas of any type or one plexiform neurofibroma
- Freckling in the axillary or inguinal region
- Optic glioma
- Two or more Lisch nodules
- A distinctive osseous lesion (e.g., sphenoid dysplasia or thinning of long bone cortex with or without pseudoarthrosis)
- A first-degree relative with NF1 according to the criteria listed above

NEUROFIBROMATOSIS-1 (NF1)

NF1, or von Recklinghausen disease, is a relatively common genetic disorder with an autosomal dominant inheritance pattern. It occurs in 1:3000 persons and has one of the highest mutation rates known. The manifestations are highly variable and appear to result from some defect that alters peripheral nerve differentiation and growth.

There is marked clinical variability in manifestations, which first appear as small, discrete, flat, pigmented skin lesions with smooth edges (***café-au-lait spots, pigmented nevi;*** Fig. 18-15) and/or axillary or inguinal freckling that develops in early infancy or childhood. Slow-growing cutaneous and subcutaneous neurofibromas that grow along the course of a peripheral nerve may appear in later childhood or adolescence and increase in number with age. ***Lisch nodules,*** dome-shaped clear–to–yellow or brown elevations on the iris surface, develop before puberty in most affected individuals. ***Elephantiasis*** (thickening and enfolding of the skin) occurs in some individuals.

Other characteristics may include developmental delay or retardation, seizures, scoliosis or kyphosis, short stature, macrocephaly, speech defects, learning disabilities, or a variety of congenital malformations. The severity varies considerably and can vary within the same family. One family member may have only café-au-lait spots or axillary freckling, whereas another has more severe manifestations.

The diagnosis is established by physical findings based on National Institutes of Health (NIH) Consensus Conference guidelines (see box above, right). In doubtful cases nodule biopsy may be performed. A family history is elicited to determine if the specific case is inherited or if it represents a new mutation. Risk for transmitting the disorder to offspring is 50%. Therapy is limited to excision of tumors that produce pain or impair function and symptomatic management of other manifestations.

Nursing Considerations

Nursing care is primarily recognition of signs that indicate a possibility of the disease, referral for diagnosis, and family counseling and support. It is important that a diagnosis be made, even when the only manifestations are a few café-au-lait spots. The family will need to know the genetic implications and be alert for signs that indicate the child is developing any of the more serious characteristics at a later time. Cancer occurs to excess in patients with the disorder, although the rates vary widely. Other members of the family should be assessed for possible evidence of the disorder.

Families can be referred to the **National Neurofibromatosis Foundation, Inc.,*** an organization with the purpose of increasing public awareness of NF1 to provide help and support to families affected by the disorder and stimulating research. Professionals involved with persons with the disease can get recent information and technical help in treatment, lists of meetings, and funding sources from a new computerized telecommunications network, NFORMATION.

BITES AND STINGS

ARTHROPOD BITES AND STINGS

Bites and stings account for a significant incidence of mild to moderate discomfort, and most are managed by simple symptomatic measures, such as compresses, calamine lotion, and prevention of secondary infection.

Arthropods include insects and arachnids, such as mites, ticks, spiders, and scorpions. The major offending creatures, their manifestations, and management are outlined in Table 18-12.

Some proteins in insect venom are species specific, others are common to a number of species; therefore crossover reactivity is common. The usual local response to a sting is sharp pain, a local wheal (less than 2 inches in diameter), and erythema accompanied by intense itching at the site, lasting less than 24 hours. The reaction is produced by enzymes, cytotoxic proteins, and vasoactive compounds, primarily histamine and kinins (Schuberth, 1989).

Systemic reactions can occur, and, although a rare occurrence, in some instances can be life-threatening. Non-

*141 5th Ave., Suite 7-S, New York, NY 10010; (800) 323-7938, (212) 460-8980.

TABLE 18-12 Skin Lesions Caused by Arthropods

MECHANISM/CHARACTERISTICS	MANIFESTATIONS	MANAGEMENT
INSECT BITES—FLIES, GNATS, MOSQUITOES, FLEAS		
Mechanism: Foreign protein in insects' saliva introduced when skin is penetrated for a blood-sucking meal Distribution: Almost everywhere—fleas, mosquitoes, ants Suburbs and rural areas—bees Urban areas—hornets, wasps, yellow jackets	Hypersensitivity reaction Papular urticaria Firm papules; may be capped by vesicles or excoriated Little or no reaction in nonsensitized person	Treatment: Use antipruritic agents and baths Administer antihistamines Prevent secondary infection Prevention: Avoid contact Remove focus, such as treating furniture, mattresses, carpets, and pets, where insects may live Apply insect repellent when exposure is anticipated
CHIGGERS—HARVEST MITE		
Mechanism: Creeps into skin pores and hair follicles to feed Manifestations: Erythematous papules Intense itching	Same as insect bites Favor warm areas of body, especially intertriginous areas and areas covered with clothing	Avoid contact, especially in areas of tall grass and underbrush Apply insect repellent when exposure is anticipated May require systemic steroids for extensive bites
HYMENOPTERAN STINGS—BEES, WASPS, HORNETS, YELLOW JACKETS, FIRE ANTS		
Mechanism: Injection of venom through stinging apparatus Venom contains histamine, allergenic proteins, and often a spreading factor, hyaluronidase Severe reactions caused by hypersensitivity and/or multiple stings	Local reaction: small red area, wheal, itching, and heat Systemic reactions: may be mild to severe, including generalized edema, pain, nausea and vomiting, confusion, respiratory embarrassment, and shock	Treatment: Carefully scrape off stinger if present Cleanse with soap and water Apply cool compresses Apply common household product (e.g., lemon juice, paste made with aspirin, baking soda, or Adolph's Meat Tenderizer) Administer antihistamines Severe reactions: administer epinephrine, corticosteroids; treat for shock Prevention: Teach child to wear shoes, to avoid wearing bright clothing, flowery prints, shiny jewelry, or perfumed grooming products (cologne, scented hairspray) that might attract the insect, and to avoid places where the insect may be contacted Hypersensitive children should wear identifying tag to indicate allergy and therapy needed; family should keep emergency medication and be taught its administration
BLACK WIDOW SPIDER		
Mechanism: Venom injected through a clawlike appendage; has neurotoxic action Characteristics: Spider is shiny black, with a body about 1.25 cm (0.5 inches) long and a red or orange hourglass-shaped marking on underside Avoids light and bites in self-defense	Mild sting at time of bite Area becomes swollen, painful, and erythematous Dizziness, weakness, and abdominal pain May produce delirium, paralysis, convulsions, and (if large amount of venom absorbed) death	Treatment: Cleanse wound with antiseptic Apply cool compresses Administer antivenin Administer muscle relaxant, such as calcium gluconate; analgesics and/or sedatives; hydrocortisone or diazepam IV Prevention: Teach children to avoid places that harbor the spider (e.g., woodpiles)

Continued.

TABLE 18-12 Skin Lesions Caused by Arthropods—cont'd

MECHANISM/CHARACTERISTICS	MANIFESTATIONS	MANAGEMENT
BROWN RECLUSE SPIDER		
Mechanism: Venom injected via fangs Venom contains powerful necrotoxin Characteristics: Spider is slender, long-legged, with body length of 1 to 2 cm; color is fawn to dark brown; recognized by fiddle-shaped mark on head Shy; bites only when annoyed or surprised Prefers dark areas where seldom disturbed	Mild sting at time of bite Transient erythema followed by bleb or blister; mild to severe pain in 2-8 hours; purple, star-shaped area in 3-4 days; necrotic ulceration in 7-14 days (Fig. 18-16) Systemic reactions may include fever, malaise, restlessness, nausea and vomiting, and joint pain Generalized petechial eruption Wounds heal with scar formation	Treatment: Apply cool compresses locally Administer antibiotics, corticosteroids Relieve pain Wound may require skin graft Prevention: Teach children to avoid possible nesting sites
SCORPIONS		
Mechanism: Sting by means of a hooked caudal stinger that discharges venom Venom of more venomous species contains hemolysins, endotheliolysins, and neurotoxins Characteristics: Usual habitat is southwestern United States	Intense local pain, erythema, numbness, burning, restlessness, vomiting Ascending motor paralysis with convulsions, weakness, rapid pulse, excessive salivation, thirst, dysuria, pulmonary edema, coma, and death Some species produce only local tissue reaction with swelling at puncture site (distinctive) Symptoms subside in a few hours Deaths occur among children under 4 years of age, usually in first 24 hours	Treatment: Delay absorption of venom by keeping child quiet; place involved area in dependent position Administer antivenin Relieve pain Admit to PICU for surveillance Prevention: Teach children to avoid possible nesting sites
TICKS		
Mechanism: In process of sucking blood, head and mouth parts are buried in skin Characteristics: Feed on blood of mammals Significant in humans because of pathologic organism carried May be vectors of various infectious diseases, such as Rocky Mountain spotted fever, Q fever, tularemia, relapsing fever, Lyme disease, tick paralysis Must attach and feed 1-2 hours to transmit disease Usual habitat is very wooded area	Tick usually attached to skin, head embedded Produce firm, discrete, intensely pruritic nodules at site of attachment May cause urticaria or persistent localized edema	Treatment: Grasp tick with tweezers (forceps) as close as possible to point of attachment Pull straight up with steady, even pressure; if bare hands touch tick during removal, wash hands thoroughly with soap and water Remove any remaining part (e.g., head) with sterile needle Cleanse wounds with soap and disinfectant Prevention: Teach children to avoid areas where prevalent Inspect skin (especially scalp) after being in wooded areas

life-threatening systemic reactions begin several minutes to several hours after the sting and consist of simple urticaria, erythema, pruritus, and angioedema. Serious, life-threatening reactions usually begin within 5 to 10 minutes after the sting and can include airway obstruction secondary to laryngeal edema, bronchospasm, hypotension, and cardiovascular collapse (Schuberth, 1989).

To prevent contact with stinging and biting insects, children are taught behaviors that reduce the likelihood of injury. In addition, topical insect repellents are generally believed to provide safe and effective protection for several hours. The best all-purpose repellents contain the active ingredient ***diethyltoluamide (DEET),*** which is effective for a variety of insects, including mosquitoes, chiggers, ticks, fleas, deerflies, and sand flies. Protection can last from 1 to several hours, but the effectiveness is affected by the concentration of active ingredients and the product must be reapplied after sweating, swimming, wiping, or exposure to rain. Since some adverse effects have been reported in young children and because long-term effects of DEET are unknown, caution is advised against excessive application or prolonged use, especially of those products with high concentrations of DEET. There is evidence that concentrations above 30% to 35% have little added benefit. The insect repellent should not be applied to children's hands, since it may be rubbed in the eyes. It should be removed with soap

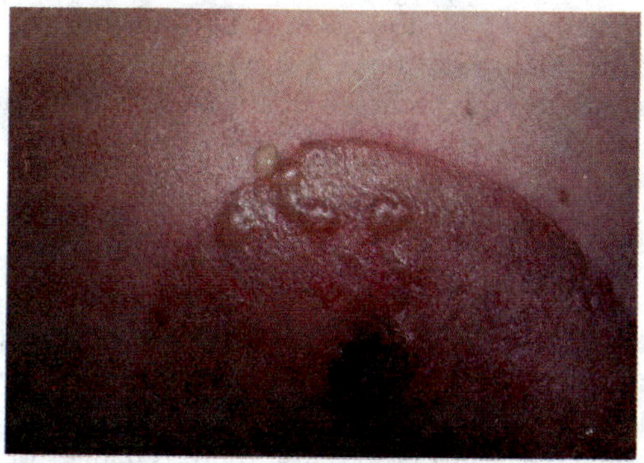

FIG. 18-16 Brown recluse spider bite; note central necrosis surrounded by purplish area and blisters. (From Weston WL, Lane AT: *Color textbook of pediatric dermatology,* St Louis, 1991, Mosby.)

and water when the child is brought inside (Shannon, 1994).

Most bites are managed by simple symptomatic measures such as cool compresses, calamine lotion, and prevention of secondary infection. The emergency treatment or specific suggestions for some bites and stings are discussed briefly. Often treatment consists of application of a substance that relieves the swelling and discomfort and can be made from common household products.

Hymenoptera Stings

When an insect stings, its stinger often remains imbedded in the skin. Since bees have barbed stingers that penetrate the skin, any pressure on the venom sac at the tip of the barb pushes more venom into the skin. The best approach is to flick the stinger off with the fingernail or knife blade—the area should never be squeezed. Another method is to cover the area with transparent tape and then peel the tape off. The stinger should come off with the tape.

Children are taught to avoid contact with bees and to recognize the insect (e.g., it is not part of the flower). For those who have become sensitized to hymenoptera bites and demonstrate a severe life-threatening systemic response, intramuscular administration of epinephrine provides immediate relief and must be available for emergency use. For hypersensitive children a kit must be available that contains epinephrine, a hypodermic syringe, and perhaps ephedrine and an antihistamine preparation (a tourniquet is included in the kit, but its use is not recommended). Hypersensitive children should wear medical identification, such as a bracelet, and the families are reminded to check the expiration date on the kit and replace an outdated one. Families should determine if a school nurse is available at the school; if not, someone at the school should be designated to inject the epinephrine in case of an emergency.

Children with a history of generalized reactivity to an insect sting should undergo skin testing with the radioallergosorbent test (RAST), and possibly immunotherapy with venous extract (desensitization) to prevent serious or fatal reactions. In the United States venous extracts are available for the honeybee, yellow jacket, yellow hornet, and wasp (Stafford, Moffitt, and Yates, 1992).

Arachnid Bites

Most arachnids in the United States, including tarantulas, are relatively harmless. All spiders produce venom that is injected via fangs. Some are able to pierce skin; in others the venom is insufficiently toxic. There is a local tissue reaction that is relieved by cool compresses or the methods described for hymenoptera stings.

Only scorpions and two spiders—the brown recluse and black widow—inject venom deadly enough to require immediate attention. Children bitten by any of these arachnids must receive medical attention as soon as possible.

Ticks

Ticks are troublesome creatures because they become partially imbedded in the skin as they feed. Numerous methods have been suggested for their removal, but the only really effective method is to grasp the tick with curved forceps as close as possible to the point of attachment and pull straight up with a steady, even pressure (Needham, 1985). If a portion of the body (e.g., the head) remains, it can be removed with a sterile needle in the same manner as a sliver. The bite is cleansed with soap and a disinfectant after removal. If the hands have touched the tick, they are washed thoroughly with soap and water.

To avoid ticks, children should wear long pants tucked into the socks and a long-sleeved shirt when walking in infested areas, especially in the spring and summer. Whenever possible, children should avoid grass and shrubbery where ticks may be lurking. Ticks can also be picked up by dogs and other household pets. Parents are advised to check their children carefully for the organisms when their children have been in areas where they might be acquired. Light clothing makes ticks more visible.

ANIMAL BITES

Animal bites are common injuries and include both wild and domestic animals. Wild animal bites are discussed in relation to rabies, and the local wounds are treated the same as bites of domestic animals, such as dogs, cats, hamsters, and mice; therefore this discussion is directed primarily toward dog bites.

Over half the victims of dog bites are less than 4 years of age, and boys are bitten more frequently than girls. Contrary to accepted belief, stray dogs are seldom involved in the attacks; most of the dogs are owned by the family of the victim or a neighbor. Most dog attacks occur in or adjacent to the owners' yards, and the attack is usually preceded by verbal or physical contact with the animal. The problem is unlikely to diminish, since the animal population is increasing rapidly, and there is a growing trend to acquire large, aggressive guard dogs (Baker, 1989). For example, the proportion of deaths resulting from attacks by pit bull dogs increased from 20% to 62% from the late 1970s to the late 1980s (Sacks, Sattin, and Bonzo, 1989).

About 90% of animal bites are caused by dogs, and less than 10% are caused by cats (Esposito and Adams, 1989). However, cat scratches are extremely common (see Cat Scratch Disease, p. 788). Most dog or cat injuries are to the upper extremities. Small children are more likely to receive bites or scratches to the head, face, and neck because of their tendency to put their heads near the animal's head and flail their arms rather than protecting their heads.

Deaths from dog bite–related injuries in the United States from the late 1970s to the late 1980s were predominantly in the pediatric age-group (Sacks, Sattin, and Bonzo, 1989). Of reported cases 70% were in children less than 10 years of age and, where the breed of dog was known, pit bulls were implicated almost three times as often as German shepherds, previously reported as the most dangerous breed. Also, pit bull attacks were almost twice as likely to be caused by strays.

Animal bites are potentially serious because of the likelihood of significant infection—5% of dog bites and 20% to 50% of cat bites (Baker, 1989). Injuries vary in intensity from small puncture wounds to complete evulsion of tissue that can be associated with significant crush injury. Dog bites generally present as lacerations or evulsions; cats exert less biting force, but their sharp teeth penetrate more deeply, inoculating organisms deep into tissues.

The location of a bite influences the incidence of infection. Injuries to the arm and hand tend to become infected more often than those on the legs, scalp, and face. Redness, swelling, and tenderness develop around the site of injury, often accompanied by purulent or serosanguineous drainage. It may be difficult to assess hand infection, since most lymphatic drainage is contained in the dorsal subcutaneous space, and swelling occurs in this area when the injury may be elsewhere.

Therapeutic Management

General wound care consists of rinsing the wound with copious amounts of saline or Ringer's lactate delivered under pressure via a large syringe and of washing the surrounding skin with mild soap. A clean pressure dressing is applied, and the extremity is elevated if the wound is bleeding. Medical evaluation is advised because there is danger of tetanus and rabies, although dogs in most urban areas are required to be immunized against rabies. Bites from wild animals, such as squirrels, bats, and raccoons, are potentially dangerous (see Rabies, Chapter 37).

Prophylactic antibiotics are indicated for puncture wounds and wounds in areas that may prove to be cosmetically or functionally impaired if infected. Extensive lacerations are debrided and loosely sutured to allow for drainage in the event of infection. Primary closure of jagged irregular wounds with associated crush injury and devitalized tissue is contraindicated, except for facial wounds because of cosmetic reasons (Avery and First, 1989). Tetanus toxoid is administered according to standard guidelines (see Chapter 12), and rabies protocol is followed. Injuries to

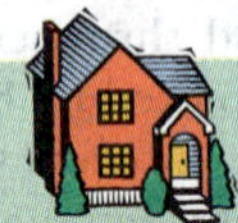

FAMILY HOME CARE
Animal Safety

- Avoid all strange animals, especially wild, sick, or injured ones. The same techniques employed in teaching children not to talk to strangers should be used to teach them not to approach strange animals.
- Notify the Health Department or police of any wild, sick, or injured animals.
- Never permit a child to break up an animal fight, even when his own pet is involved. Use a rake, broom, or garden hose to separate the animals.
- Become aware, and make children aware, of the danger of mistreating or teasing pets. Pets are not toys, but living creatures who will bite if mauled, annoyed, or frightened.
- Alert your child to dangerous and nervous animals in your neighborhood and do not permit him to enter yards or houses that harbor them.
- Do not allow a child to disturb an animal that is eating or sleeping. Set a good example by your own behavior.
- Do not let your pet come into indiscriminate contact with other animals.
- Avoid the indiscriminate contact between your pet and human beings.
- Do *not* purchase or obtain pets for your children until such time as they demonstrate their maturity and ability to handle and care for the pets. This ability is rare in a child under 4 years of age and unusual in a child under 6. Factors to be considered at any age are the maturity and disposition of the child and the animal. Some people never develop this maturity.
- Stress to children the importance of avoiding routes, when riding bicycles or tricycles, where dogs are known to chase vehicles.
- Teach children that each animal has the right to a free existence and freedom from man-inflicted pain. Set a good example by your own behavior.
- Under your supervision or that of some other adult, have children make friends with pets, in the immediate neighborhood, with which the children will be in contact.
- Never hold your face close to an animal.
- Do not permit a child or young person to lead a large dog.
- Never tease, pull the tail, or take away food, bone, or toy with which an animal is playing.
- Do not run, ride a bicycle, or skate in front of a dog. It will startle the dog.
- Do not touch a dog while the dog is asleep or unaware of your presence. Always speak to any dog that has not seen you approach so that the dog becomes aware of your presence and will not be startled.
- Avoid all unnecessary contact with wild animals—now an important spreader of rabies.
- Do not overexcite an animal, even in play.
- Do not keep animals confined with short ropes or chains. This may make them aggressive and vicious, especially when teased.
- Have children avoid dogs raised in a home without children. Such animals may resent children.
- Do not allow an inexperienced child or adult to feed a dog. Such persons may pull back when the animal moves to take the food, frightening the animal. This practice is dangerous.

From Mofenson HC, Greensher J, Teitelbaum H: How to avoid animal bites, *Med Times* 100:92, 1972.

poorly vascularized areas such as the hands are more likely to become infected than those in more vascularized areas such as the face; puncture wounds are more apt to become infected than lacerations.

Nursing Considerations

The most important aspect related to animal bites is prevention. It is important that children understand animal behavior and develop an honest respect for all animals. It is vital that they learn how to treat animals and how to react to them (see Family Home Care box). Parents should monitor their children's behavior with a dog and instruct them not to tease or surprise a dog, invade its territory, interfere with its feeding or sleeping, take its toy, or interact with a sick or injured dog or a dog with pups (Riegger and Guntzelman, 1990). Meeting a strange dog can be both frightening and a danger to a child. The child should remain calm and follow the suggestions outlined in the box.

Parents who are considering getting a pet, especially a dog, for themselves or their children should receive some advice about choosing the dog that is least likely to be a danger to their children. The level of sociability with children is the key to a selection, and dogs range from dangerous, bad, and unsuitable to tolerant of children to exceptionally good with children—some under certain conditions. For example, dogs that are too clumsy, impetuous, or vigorous are not suitable for small children, and some dogs must be raised with the children. A categorization of dogs related to their potential interaction with children can be found in the publication *The Right Dog for You.**

SNAKEBITES

Most snakes in the United States are harmless, and few poisonous snakebites are reported each year. Of the estimated 8000 bites from poisonous snakes, fewer than 20 are fatal (Avery and First, 1989), or 0.25%. Asian and African snakes are far more dangerous than those in the United States and Europe. The major species in the United States are the *Crotilidae* (pit vipers), which include rattlesnakes, copperheads, and cottonmouths, and the *Elapidae,* which include coral snakes and cobras. Almost all bites are attributed to the *Crotilidae.*

The manifestations and morbidity are highly variable and depend on the species and size of the snake, the amount of venom injected, the time of year, the age and size of the child, and the location of the bite. Also, injection of venom is not an invariable consequence of a bite; 20% to 25% of all bites by poisonous snakes are not associated with injection of venom (Ginsburg and Gädeke, 1989).

The initial action after snakebite is to move the victim away from the area, to attempt to calm the child, and to place the child at rest. A *loose* tourniquet applied proximal to the bite delays the flow of lymph, which can carry the venom to the systemic circulation. It should not be tight enough to occlude circulation; a pulse distal to the bite should be palpable. Any constricting items of clothing or jewelry should be removed from the affected limb. A splint should be applied to immobilize the limb, and the victim should be transported to the nearest medical facility.

NURSING ALERT Do not apply ice to the snake bite, because doing so decreases the blood supply to the envenomated site, thereby allowing the venom to work more destruction while decreasing the effect of antivenom on the natural immune mechanisms.

If the child has been bitten by a large snake, if less than 30 minutes (some authorities say 5 minutes) have elapsed since the child was bitten, and if medical help is more than 30 minutes away, suction may be beneficial. Suction should be applied by a suction device such as the Sawyer Extractor, which is very effective if used within 3 minutes.

If possible, the dead snake should be transported with the patient for identification. If there is any possibility that a child has been bitten by a coral snake, aggressive use of antivenom is indicated, because once symptoms occur, it is next to impossible to stop the respiratory paralysis and death.

HUMAN BITES

Children often acquire lacerations from the teeth of other humans in rough play, during fights, or as victims of child abuse. Many preschool children bite others out of frustration or anger. Most childhood bites by humans are superficial and rarely become infected when the child receives early treatment (Esposito and Adams, 1989). Because human dental plaque and gingiva harbor pathogenic bacteria, all human bites should receive attention. Also, delayed treatment increases the risk of infection.

If the laceration is less than ¼ inch in length, the wound can be treated at home. The wound is washed vigorously with soap and water, and a pressure dressing is applied to stop bleeding. Ice applications minimize discomfort and swelling. Increased pain or redness at the wound site is an indication that the child should receive medical attention for antibiotic therapy. Tetanus toxoid is needed if more than 5 years has elapsed since the last immunization. Wounds greater than ¼ inch should receive medical attention.

DENTAL DISORDERS

DENTAL CARIES

Dental caries (cavities) is one of the most common chronic diseases that affect individuals at all ages. Although 100% preventable, dental caries is the principal oral problem in children and adolescents. Although the overall incidence of dental caries in children has decreased since the introduction of fluoridation, it is still an important health problem. Reducing the incidence and consequences of the disorder is of primary importance in childhood because dental caries, if untreated, results in total destruction of involved teeth. The ages of greatest vulnerability are 4 to 8 years for the primary dentition and 12 to 18 years for the

*By D.F. Tortora (1980, Simon & Schuster).

secondary or permanent dentition (see Figs. 12-14 and 17-15 for sequence of tooth eruption).

Pathophysiology

Dental caries is a multifactorial disease. The incidence of lesions and the likelihood of progressive invasion vary considerably and depend on a number of factors being present in the right combination: (1) the host, (2) microorganisms, (3) substrate, and (4) time.

Host. The prevalence of caries is directly related to the tooth size and morphology and to the consistency, composition, and amount of saliva. Improperly developed, crowded, or deeply fissured teeth increase the incidence of caries. The areas most subject to attack by bacteria are (in order of difficulty of complete cleansing) grooves and fissures, interdermal areas, gum margins, and other smooth surfaces. Newly erupted teeth that have not yet acquired sufficient surface minerals are more susceptible to decay than those that have been erupted for 2 or more years. Undoubtedly hereditary factors influence resistance and susceptibility, since similar patterns and anatomic characteristics are seen in successive generations. Salivary flow can mechanically clean away bacteria and food debris. It also contains buffering systems, lysozymes, peroxidases, and immunoglobulins that influence the development of caries.

Microorganisms. Certain types of microflora that produce different effects contribute to the formation of dental caries. ***Acidogenic bacteria*** act on fermentable carbohydrates in dental plaque to produce organic acids that decalcify hard surface tooth enamel. With the inner organic matrix exposed, proteolytic organisms and acids digest and destroy the inner tooth structure. These destructive organisms are harbored and protected in a gelatinous plaque formed on the tooth surface by still another group of bacteria that are thought to play no primary role in production of decay.

Substrates. Caries formation is strongly influenced by the two concurrent processes that continually operate on enamel surfaces—***acid production*** and ***acid neutralization*** by saliva. The material on which the acid-forming bacteria act consists essentially of carbohydrates. Among the fermentable carbohydrates, sucrose has been consistently implicated as the most cariogenic. Sucrose-containing substances, especially in tenacious forms that cling (such as chewy candy) or that promote prolonged contact with the teeth (such as hard candy and lollipops), when ingested between meals, contribute markedly to the development of dental caries. Saliva, some foods, and chewing gum after a meal tend to help neutralize much of the acid formed from sucrose.

Time and Other Factors. Bacterial enzymes act on salivary glycoproteins to produce a tenacious protein matrix on the tooth surface. This substance, along with the microorganisms, forms ***dental plaque.*** If plaque removal is inadequate or nonexistent for a significant length of time (a few days), the plaque is metabolized by the bacteria to form acid, which initiates the demineralization of enamel.

Other factors that contribute to caries formation are heredity, the amount of fluoride in drinking water, lack of or ineffectual oral hygiene, and the child's general state of health. Hereditary factors appear to influence both resistance and susceptibility to dental caries. For example, structural defects, such as deep fissures on occlusive surfaces, predispose the teeth to decay, and persons in whom acid formation exceeds neutralization are more prone to caries. The effectiveness of the buffering action of saliva is highly variable among individuals.

Fluoride incorporated into the crystallites of the surface enamel increases the resistance to acid dissolution. Poor oral hygiene that permits the accumulation of food debris on tooth surfaces provides for proliferation of acid-forming bacteria that thrive in this environment. Removal of food particles and bacteria-laden plaque inhibits destructive acid formation.

The susceptibility to dental decay may be influenced by the general health of the child. Children who suffer from chronic debilitating disease show increased caries activity, as do children with systemic conditions that alter the quality and quantity of saliva produced.

Diagnostic Evaluation

Because the permanent teeth erupt during middle childhood, children are more susceptible to development of dental caries during this time than at any other age. Caries penetrate the vulnerable teeth rapidly at this age, as opposed to the slower, intermittent activity characteristic at later ages.

Caries on visible surfaces are easily detected by oral inspection. Large, extensive caries are apparent even to the untrained eye, but small, beginning lesions are best identified by trained professionals. Caries between the teeth may not be located without x-ray examination. The most common site of decay is the fissures of the molars (Griffen and Goepferd, 1991).

Therapeutic Management

Well-informed health care professionals can provide dental information and make periodic dental assessments. However, dentists are best prepared to provide both of these services and are the only ones qualified to treat most dental problems. Prophylaxis is the major thrust of dental therapy, including hygiene and fluoride treatment (see Chapter 14). ***Plasticized sealant,*** applied to deep fissures and grooves of healthy teeth, is effective in blocking cavity formation. Ismail (1989) reported 46% fewer cavities in sealed teeth than in unsealed teeth 4 years after application.

Treatment of dental caries involves removal of all carious portions of teeth as soon as detected, preparation of a retentive cavity, and replacement of the lost portion of the tooth with a material that is durable in the mouth environment. This restoration of involved teeth not only prevents progression of established caries, but also reduces the number of bacteria in the oral cavity to decrease the danger to uninvolved teeth.

Nursing Considerations

Oral inspection is an integral part of the nursing assessment of the child in any setting. If there is any evidence of dental caries or other unhealthy state, the child is referred for dental services. The family may have a family dentist or a pedodontist who can provide needed care. An alarming number of children do not receive regular dental supervision, and a significant number reach adulthood without having been examined or treated by a dentist. Nurses can be active members of preventive educational programs and serve as counselors to families regarding the importance of regular dental care, oral hygiene, and dietary management.

Nurses can encourage good oral hygiene by teaching correct tooth cleaning to both children and their parents. The random brushing allowed during the early childhood years should be replaced by more careful and methodic cleansing techniques. Children are taught to brush the teeth according to the method recommended by their dentist and the proper use of dental floss (see Chapter 14). The importance of regular administration of fluoride is emphasized (see Chapter 14). This includes the knowledge of the fluoride content of the drinking water, including bottled water if this is the family practice. School-age children can usually manage the chewable tablets, which have both a topical and a systemic effect. It is often difficult for parents to give medications on a daily basis over a period of years; therefore the children are taught to assume responsibility for taking fluoride as part of their daily dental hygiene.

Restriction of cariogenic foods is also important in the preventive management of dental caries, but this should be viewed as an activity in which all family members are involved and not simply a directive for the child to obey. It should not be communicated in such a way that the child interprets the withholding of sweets as a punishment.

Concern has been generated about the sugar content of children's pharmaceutical products, especially since children with chronic conditions, such as seizure disorders, asthma, and recurrent urinary tract or ear infections, must take medications over a period of years. Evidence indicates a significant association between intake of sucrose-based medications and an increased incidence of dental caries (Shaw and Glenwright, 1989). Children with chronic illness who regularly take medications containing sugar are cautioned to brush their teeth after taking the medication, just as they would after eating any carbohydrate substance. Also, children taking tricyclic antidepressants are more prone to develop dental caries.

Sometimes the greatest task for nurses is not teaching dental care but counseling children and families to be motivated to develop sound dental hygiene and nutritional practices. School nurses have an excellent opportunity to engage in detection of dental needs, educating children in dental hygiene and preventing dental problems, making referrals, and motivating children to comply with prophylaxis and treatment.

Children should be prepared for dental services in such a way that visits to the dentist are a positive experience. Keeping appointments and following through on recommended treatments and practices are habits that extend beyond childhood.

PERIODONTAL DISEASE

Periodontal disease, inflammatory and degenerative conditions involving the gums and tissues supporting the teeth, often begins in childhood and accounts for a significant amount of tooth loss in adulthood. The more common periodontal problems are ***gingivitis*** (simple inflammation of the gums) and ***periodontitis*** (inflammation of the gums and loss of connective tissue and bone in the supporting structures of the teeth). An uncommon condition is ***acute necrotizing ulcerative gingivitis*** ("trench mouth").

The most prevalent periodontal disease, gingivitis, is a reversible inflammatory disease that begins very early in many children and is most often associated with the buildup of plaque on the teeth. Changes take place in the plaque bacteria, in both type and number of organisms, causing them to release a variety of destructive exotoxins, enzymes, and other noxious agents. They act to produce an inflammatory reaction in the gingival tissues, causing the gums to become red, edematous, tender, and subject to bleeding at the slightest irritation.

Management is directed toward prevention by conscientious brushing and flossing and by depriving the bacteria of the substrates required to produce the disease. The implementation and maintenance of preventive dental practice, including the use of fluoride, plus good dental hygiene are effective in preventing both caries and periodontal disease.

Nursing Considerations

Nursing care of the child with periodontal disease is primarily supportive and preventive; it includes education regarding dental hygiene and regular inspection of the gingival tissues for signs of early inflammation. The child should be directed to see the dentist at any sign of inflammation or irritation.

Nurses caring for teenagers should observe for evidence of chewing tobacco use. The easily detectable clinical lesions appear as tooth erosion, periodontal destruction, and red or white mucosal alterations. The primary site of lesions is the anterior mandibular mucobuccal fold region.

MALOCCLUSION

When teeth of the upper and lower dental arches approximate in the proper relationships, the physiologic function of mastication is more effective, and the cosmetic effect is more pleasing. Teeth that are uneven, crowded, or overlapping, or that otherwise interfere with their ability to meet their opponents in the opposite jaw in the appropriate relationships, many be predisposed to dental disease (Fig. 18-17). More than half of children 12 to 17 years of age suffer from malocclusions that could be corrected.

The most common cause of malocclusion is hereditary factors, but abnormal growth and habits such as thumb-sucking and tongue thrusting also contribute to the disordered alignment and occlusion of the teeth. The important aspects in treatment of malocclusion are elimination of habits that aggravate the deformity and corrective therapy at the optimum time. Orthodontic treatment is usually most successful when it is started in the later school-age years or the early adolescent years, after the last primary teeth have been shed and before growth ceases. However, the trend is toward early correction to prevent problems if the irregularity interferes with normal function and speech; therefore

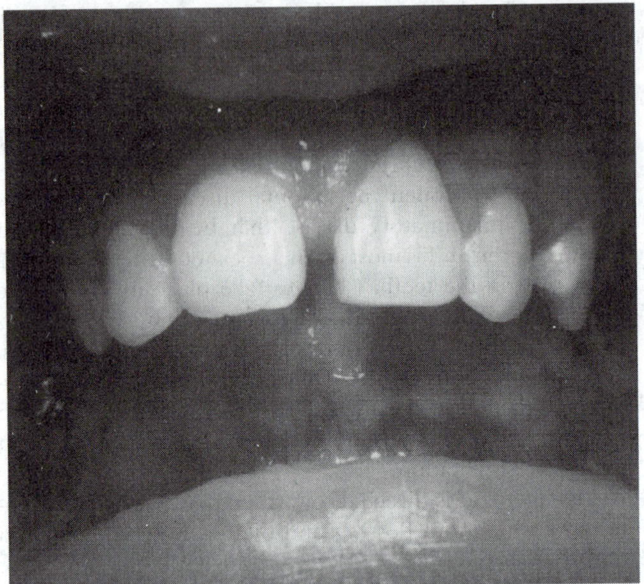

FIG. 18-17 Malocclusion in a school-age child.

referral should be made as soon as malocclusion is evident. For example, removal of extra teeth, impacted teeth, or prosthetic replacement of missing teeth can prevent problems from developing.

Nursing Considerations

The nurse who detects evidence of malocclusion in a child is obligated to recommend that the teeth be examined by a dentist for possible orthodontia. With the trend toward earlier correction, the sooner the child is evaluated, the better will be the chance for receiving needed treatment. Dealing with habits that predispose to malocclusion, such as thumb- or finger-sucking, is more difficult to manage.

Although orofacial appearance is a subjective phenomenon, there may be a risk of adverse effect on a child's self-esteem and body image. Poorly aligned teeth can be a source of psychologic as well as physical stress to affected children. Many children with malocclusion suffer from teasing from peers or siblings if the irregularities are severe enough. However, it is usually the parents who initiate an orthodontic examination.

After fixed appliances, or braces, have been applied, the child is advised that there will be some discomfort for a few days. During the orthodontic treatments, which average 18 to 30 months, proper oral hygiene is vital. Although the bands or brackets protect the teeth they cover, plaque can collect on the unprotected surfaces or under loose-fitting bands. The teeth are to be brushed with a fluoride toothpaste after every meal and snack and at bedtime, using the method recommended by the dentist. Some orthodontists recommend using an oral irrigating device to remove food from between the teeth and around the braces. However, the device does not remove plaque and is not a substitute for thorough brushing. The orthodontist cautions the child about foods that should not be eaten. Some can damage the braces; others may be difficult to remove from the teeth during cleaning. Forbidden items include chewing gum, ice, nuts, toffee, hard candy, corn-on-the-cob, uncut apples, hard taco shells, nachos, and popcorn.

> **PERIODS FOR INCREASED FREQUENCY OF DENTAL TRAUMA**
>
> **Preschool** (1 to 3 years)—Injury usually secondary to falls or child abuse
> **School age** (7 to 10 years)—Injury more often following bicycle and playground accidents
> **Adolescence** (16 to 18 years)—Injury generally sustained secondary to fights, athletic injury, and automobile accidents
>
> Data from Berkowitz R, Ludwig S, Johnson R: Dental trauma in children and adolescents, *J Pediatr* 19:166-171, 1980.

Occasionally tooth movement or poking at braces with a pencil or other object may cause an arch wire to break or protrude. If this happens the child is instructed to cover the broken portion with a special wax provided by the dentist and schedule an appointment as soon as possible. Regular visits are usually scheduled every 3 to 6 weeks.

Sometimes children need considerable reinforcement for orthodontic compliance. It may be difficult for some to relate the present barriers of discomfort, inconvenience, and embarrassment with the future reinforcers of improved appearance and dental health. Teenagers with a heightened awareness of body image and physical attractiveness are especially at risk for noncompliance (see Chapter 27 for a discussion of compliance).

TRAUMA

Injury to the teeth is not an uncommon occurrence in childhood (see box above). This includes fractures of varying degrees of severity, chipping, dislocation, or evulsion. All tooth injuries require prompt treatment by a competent dentist to prevent permanent displacement or loss. Delayed examination and diagnosis of tooth damage all too frequently result in infection or pulp involvement that could have been avoided by early attention. Also, because it can affect the remaining teeth, loss of a permanent tooth requires professional attention to maintain normal alignment and position of teeth.

Boys experience injury to permanent teeth much more frequently than girls, although this observation is not supported in all studies. Trauma usually involves the maxillary incisors, and children with protruding teeth, craniofacial abnormalities, or neuromuscular disorders are more likely to sustain dental injuries. A tooth that is ***avulsed*** (evulsed, exarticulated, or "knocked out") can be reimplanted and retained permanently if replaced without delay (Krasner, 1990).

Nursing Considerations: Tooth Evulsion

A permanent tooth that is avulsed should be replanted by the child, parent, or nurse and stabilized as soon as possible so that the blood supply to the tooth can be reestablished and the tooth kept alive (see Emergency Treatment box). If the tooth is replaced within 30 minutes, there is a 70% chance that it will become reattached and roots will not resorb or the crown exfoliate. Evulsed primary teeth are usually not reimplanted.

Before reimplantation it is important to carefully rinse a dirty tooth in milk, saline solution, or under running water to avoid disturbing the adhering periodontal membrane, which is essential to the success of the reimplantation. The tooth is held by the crown, not the root, while rinsing, with the drain plugged. The tooth is then fit back into its socket the best way possible, even if it means placing it backward or at an angle (Kochman, 1989). If the tooth is reimplanted almost immediately, excessive pressure is not needed; however, it becomes extremely difficult after clot formation (in approximately 10 minutes). The tooth is held in place by the child during transportation to a dentist. Care is taken to avoid sudden stops or turns that might cause the child to swallow or aspirate the loose tooth.

If the child or parents are reluctant to reimplant the tooth, the next best alternative is to place the tooth in cold milk, contact lens solution, or saline for transport to the dentist. Cold milk has precisely the osmolality needed to maintain fluid balance within the tissues surrounding the tooth. Tap water is not recommended (Kochman, 1989).* The third alternative for transport is to place the tooth under the child's tongue, or under the parent's tongue if the child is too young or too anxious. After implantation, the tooth will usually become firmly attached, although endodontic therapy is often required. If reimplantation is not permanent, the tooth may be retained anywhere from 6 months to 12 years and serves to facilitate normal development and occlusion, since loss of teeth during the period of permanent tooth eruption may adversely affect such development.

As with all mouth trauma, an evulsed tooth causes a large amount of bleeding, which is most distressing to the child. Bleeding is frightening to children and their families; therefore the nurse or anyone who is faced with dental trauma should be prepared to cope with the emotionality that accompanies a tooth evulsion. Using a calm approach and providing gentle reassurance to the child requires only a moment and goes a long way toward reducing anxiety.

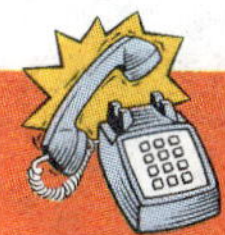

EMERGENCY TREATMENT
Evulsed Tooth

Recover tooth.
Hold tooth by crown; avoid touching root area.
If tooth is dirty, rinse it gently under running water or saline; be sure to insert stopper in sink or basin (to avoid tooth loss).
Insert tooth into socket.
Have child maintain tooth in place.
Transport child to dentist immediately.
Avoid sudden stops or sharp turns to prevent dislodging tooth.

IF RELUCTANT TO REIMPLANT TOOTH:

Place evulsed tooth in suitable medium for transport:
a. Cold milk
b. Saliva—under child's or parent's tongue
If child is holding tooth in the mouth, avoid sudden stops to prevent swallowing tooth.
DON'T FORGET TO TAKE TOOTH

EMERGENCY TREATMENT

DISORDERS OF CONTINENCE

ENURESIS*

Enuresis (bed-wetting) is a common and troublesome disorder that is defined as repeated voiding of urine during the day or at night into bed or clothes. Most often this is involuntary, but occasionally it may be intentional. To qualify for a diagnosis of enuresis, the voiding of urine must occur at least twice a week for at least 3 months or else must cause clinically significant distress or impairment in social, academic (occupational), or other important areas of functioning. The individual must have reached an age at which continence is expected; the chronologic or developmental age of the child must be at least 5 years (see Cultural Awareness box, p. 806). In addition, the urinary incontinence is not due exclusively to the direct physiologic effects of a substance (e.g., diuretics) or a general medical condition (e.g., diabetes mellitus or insipidus, spina bifida, seizure disorder, or sickle cell disease) (American Psychiatric Association, 1994).

Enuresis can also be defined as ***primary*** (bed-wetting in children who have never been dry for extended periods) or ***secondary*** (the onset of wetting after a period of established urinary continence). The passage of urine may occur only during nighttime sleep (nocturnal), only during the waking hours (diurnal), or during both times of the day. The nocturnal type is most common.

The prevalence of enuresis at age 5 years is 7% for males and 3% for females; at age 10 years the prevalence is 3% for males and 2% for females. At age 18 years the prevalence is 1% for males and less for females (American Psychiatric Association, 1994). It affects some 5 million children in the United States (Houts, 1991).

Although most children with enuresis do not have a coexisting mental disorder, the prevalence of coexisting mental and other developmental disorders is higher than in the general population. It can also cause serious psychologic problems. The degree of impairment is related to the condition's effect on the child's social life, such as not being able to attend overnight camps, and its effect on others, who may ostracize or ridicule the youngster. Talking with these children is enlightening. Adolescents with enuresis have described themselves as tense, having difficulty sleeping, and having bad dreams. Children state they are embarrassed about the disorder and are often hesitant to sleep at other children's homes. Avoiding overnight excur-

*A commercial preparation, Save-A-Tooth, is available from Biological Rescue Products, Conshohocken, PA 19428; (800) 882-0505.

*Deborah Brantly, APRN, CNS, MS, LMFT, revised this section.

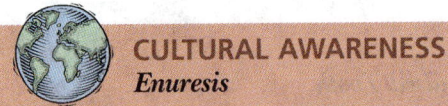

CULTURAL AWARENESS
Enuresis

The age at which children attain urinary continence varies widely. For example, white children in the United States tend to achieve continence earlier than African-American children. In addition, children in Great Britain and Sweden appear to attain continence slightly earlier than children in the United States, and in the extreme, the East African Digos often achieve bladder control by the age of 12 months. Therefore practitioners must be sensitive to the differences among groups before labeling a child enuretic (Rappaport, 1992).

sions can impede normal socialization or self-esteem. Self-esteem can be further assaulted if parental response to the disorder is harsh or punitive. Behavioral problems can be associated with these psychologic effects. However, research suggests that adults treated for enuresis as children show normal psychologic profiles (Stromgren and Thomsen, 1990); they differ from adults who did not experience childhood enuresis only by a moderately lower socialization score and a slightly higher paranoid score, both of which produced no significant differences in their overall socialization and adult functioning.

Etiology and Pathophysiology

No clear etiology for enuresis has been determined. However, predictive factors have been noted, including longer duration of sleep in infancy, a positive family history, and a slower rate of physical development in children up to 3 years of age. There is a high concordance rate of enuresis in monozygotic twins and an even higher one in dizygotic twins, suggesting more than a pure genetic link in the disorder. However, generally, family studies indicate that the closer the familial relationship, the greater the concordance of enuresis (Friman and Warzak, 1990). Approximately 75% of all children with functional enuresis have a first-degree relative who has, or has had, the disorder (American Psychiatric Association, 1994).

Enuresis is primarily an alteration of neuromuscular bladder functioning and as such is benign and self-limiting. The symptom can result from other situations. Some children exhibit temporary regressive behavior resulting in enuresis after the birth of a sibling or other trauma. Others have occasional "accidents" when they become so involved in play that they are unaware of a full bladder or "forget" to empty their bladder. In other children enuresis may be caused by problems with toilet training that are related to the age at which training began, the emotional atmosphere that surrounds the training situation, or an excessive amount of emotional dependence on the parent, usually the mother. Occasionally enuresis can be one behavioral manifestation of a personality disorder.

Although several theories have been proposed, no one theory thoroughly explains enuresis. The ***sleep theory*** stems from the observation of many parents that these children are difficult to arouse from sleep. Recent research suggests, however, that depth of sleep as measured by electroencephalography is not the cause of nocturnal enuresis (Rappaport, 1993). However, this "theory" continues to prevail in many treatment regimens.

Another theory relates to ***functional bladder capacity,*** the volume of urine voided after maximum delay of micturition. Although there is evidence that some children with enuresis have a smaller bladder capacity than nonaffected children, evidence suggests that this is not the cause. For example, children without enuresis but with a smaller bladder capacity awaken during the night to void, as opposed to children with enuresis who do not awaken.

The ***nocturnal polyuria theory*** currently offers the most promising etiology of nocturnal enuresis. It suggests that the kidneys of these children fail to concentrate urine during sleep because of insufficient ***antidiuretic hormone (ADH).*** One study showed that serum levels of ADH and urine osmolality were higher at night in children without enuresis than in children with enuresis (Rittig and others, 1989). The ADH circadian rhythm may thus be a significant biologic marker in enuresis, but additional research must be conducted to further clarify its role.

The ***dysfunctional detrussor activity theory*** suggests that an unstable bladder detrussor muscle spontaneously contracts, producing bed-wetting, either by abnormal innervation or other unknown reasons. Studies of this theory have been contradictory and inconclusive; more research is needed to clarify these contradictions and to determine if there may be a relationship between ADH production and detrussor activity.

Clinical Manifestations

The predominant symptom of enuresis is urgency that is immediate and accompanied by acute discomfort, restlessness, and sometimes urinary frequency. With nocturnal enuresis, the child may or may not feel urgency. If awareness of the urgency is present, the child often reports difficulty awakening to urinate. Spontaneous voiding during sleep occurs, usually resulting in multiple nightly incidents. Spontaneous remission of nocturnal enuresis occurs in approximately 15% of cases, which, if left untreated, can continue into adolescence and adulthood.

Diagnostic Evaluation

During initial phases of evaluation, a routine physical examination is performed to rule out known physical etiologies, such as urinary tract infection, structural disorders, major neurologic deficits, nocturnal epilepsy, disorders that increase the normal output of urine (such as diabetes mellitus and diabetes insipidus), and disorders that impair the concentrating ability of the kidneys (such as chronic renal failure or sickle cell disease). The examination may include diagnostic evaluation of functional bladder capacity. This is determined by having the children hold off voiding until they feel the strongest urgency, at which time they void into a measured container. A bladder volume of 300 to 350 ml is sufficient to hold a night's urine.

If other psychologic difficulties are evident or a primary etiology of personality disorder is suspected, a routine psychiatric evaluation may be sought.

A history of wetting behavior is gathered, including information about the toilet-training process and parental attempts at coping with the bed-wetting behavior. Parental attitudes are usually easily assessed during this time by listening and asking parents how they have attempted to cope with the wetting. An important feature of assessment is a baseline count of enuretic incidents and the times of day each occurs. This is necessary not only to establish diagnostic reliability, but also to establish outcome success after treatment. This baseline is gathered for 1 to 2 weeks by the child and family. It usually consists of a chart or calendar given to the family on which they indicate the date of the incident, the time of the incident, and the approximate size of the enuretic episode.

Therapeutic Management

Enuresis not resulting from known organic causes has been treated in several ways. No method has achieved universal endorsement; however, the more successful outcomes are becoming clearer. Frequently, more than one technique is employed. Programs have defined successful treatment as a specified period of dry nights, varying from 7 to 28 consecutive dry nights.

Conditioning therapy involves training the child to awaken to urinate after a stimulus is given, especially with a urine alarm. The device consists of a wire pad that is placed inside the underpants and is attached to a bell or buzzer that is moisture sensitive. When the system detects urine, the bell or buzzer sounds, which fully awakens the child. The child is thus conditioned to awaken at the initiation of micturition or to the stimulus of the bell or buzzer and eventually learns to continue voiding in the toilet. The success rate of the urine alarm is higher than that of other methods; it is consistently approximately 75%, with a lower relapse rate of approximately 41% (Friman and Warzak, 1990). Relapse is addressed by reinstituting the alarm during sleep, many times producing longer-lasting results. Some studies have shown that using an intermittent alarm schedule can reduce the relapse rate to as low as 17% (Friman and Warzak, 1990) and that coupling alarm use with other behavioral procedures can reduce the relapse rate to 15% to 25% (Houts, 1991). This method is inexpensive compared with drug therapy and has no side effects.

Retention control training (RCT) was initiated after the observation of reduced functional bladder capacity in children who were bed-wetters. The child drinks fluids and delays urination as long as can be tolerated in order to stretch the bladder to accommodate increasingly larger volumes of urine. It has been documented to be maximally effective 50% of the time (Friman and Warzak, 1990). The use of Kegel, or pelvic muscle, exercises may also promote continence (Schneider, King, and Surwit, 1994).

With the ***waking schedule*** treatment, the child is awakened during the night at intervals to void. It has been found to reduce incidents, but it has not been successful in eliminating the incidents (Friman and Warzak, 1990).

Drug therapy is increasingly being prescribed to treat enuresis. Three types of drugs are commonly used: tricyclic antidepressants, antidiuretics, and antispasmotics. The selection depends on the interpretation of the cause. The drug used most frequently is the tricyclic antidepressant drug imipramine (Tofranil), which exerts an anticholinergic action in the bladder to inhibit urination. The dosage and time of administration are individualized, and the drug is given in amounts sufficient to lighten sleep but not to cause wakefulness. The suggested length of treatment is 6 to 8 weeks, followed by gradual withdrawal over 4 weeks. Since this drug is dangerous in overdosage, parents must be cautioned about judicious use and keeping supplies of the drug far from the reach of younger siblings.

Anticholinergic drugs, especially oxybutynin, reduce uninhibited bladder contractions and may be helpful for children with daytime urinary frequency. Success has also been achieved with desmopressin (DDAVP) nasal spray, an analog of vasopressin, which reduces nighttime urinary output to a volume less than functional bladder capacity. Typically, the child receives two sprays before bedtime. The medication is generally well tolerated but may cause nasal irritation or rare headaches or nausea.

One of the challenges of using the drug therapeutically is the difficulty simulating the normal circadian rhythm of ADH secretion. Another concern for some families is the cost of the treatment. DDAVP may cost from $120 to $240 a month for daily doses of 20 to 40 μg (Fitzwater and Macknin, 1992). Some children have been successfully treated with daily doses of 10 μg or less (Key, Bloom, and Sanvordenker, 1992). Although DDAVP is very effective in reducing the number of wet nights, only about 25% of children may become completely dry. Information on the long-term effects of the drug are not known (Moffatt and others, 1993).

Several other therapies/treatment options are available, but their outcomes are not well researched. These include stream interruption, paired associations, overlearning, reinforcement systems, and self-monitoring (motivation therapy). Frequently one or more of these therapies are coupled with other treatment modalities. Counseling may be beneficial in helping the child, and sometimes the family, adjust to the bed-wetting.

Nursing Considerations

No matter which of the various techniques are used, the nurse can help both children and parents to understand the problem of enuresis, the treatment plan, and the probable difficulties they may encounter in the process. Essential to the success of any method is the supportive management of parents and their children. Both need encouragement and patience. The problem is discussed with the parents, and, since any treatment involves and requires the child's active participation, children are included as well. In some treatment interventions, the child is in charge of the intervention; therefore parents must be taught to support the child to follow through rather than intervene themselves. The most important predictor for the outcome of treatment is family difficulties. Family disturbances influence the initial arrest of the enuresis, the relapse rate, and the long-term success rate.

Many parents believe that enuresis is caused by an emotional disturbance and fear that they have somehow produced the situation by improper childrearing practices.

They need reassurance that the bed-wetting is not a manifestation of emotional disturbance nor does it represent willful misbehavior. They need to understand that enuresis is a medical disorder and that scolding, shaming, threatening, and punishing a child are contraindicated because of their negative emotional impact and limited success in reducing the behavior. The parents are encouraged to be patient and understanding, communicating love and that the child has value.

Communication with children is directed toward eliminating the emotional impact of the problem by relieving them of feelings of shame, guilt, and the burden of parental disapproval and toward building up their self-confidence and motivating them toward independent control. More important, the nurse can provide consistent support and encouragement to help sustain them through the inconsistent and unpredictable treatment process. Children need to believe that they are helping themselves and to sustain feelings of confidence and hope. Children who have mastered bed-wetting demonstrate an improvement in self-concept (Moffatt, Kato, and Pless, 1987).

ENCOPRESIS

According to the American Psychiatric Association (1994), encopresis is repeated involuntary or intentional passage of feces into inappropriate places (e.g., clothing or floor). The event must occur at least once a month for at least 3 months, and the chronologic or developmental age of the child must be at least 4 years. The fecal incontinence must not be due exclusively to the direct physiologic effects of a substance (e.g., laxatives) or a general medical condition except through a mechanism involving constipation. The consistency of the stool may vary from normal or near-normal consistency to liquid, especially in individuals who have overflow incontinence secondary to fecal retention.

A child who has never achieved fecal continence by 4 years of age is said to have ***primary encopresis.*** This type is more frequently observed as a result of neglect, lax training methods, mental subnormalities, and familial causes. ***Secondary encopresis*** is fecal incontinence occurring in a child over 4 years of age after a period of established fecal continence (American Psychiatric Association, 1994). The disorder is more common in males than in females.

Etiology

One of the most common causes of encopresis is constipation, which may be precipitated by environmental change, such as the birth of a new sibling, moving to a new house, changing schools, or even having to use new or unfamiliar toilet facilities. Voluntary retention usually follows a painful incident with voluntary suppression of defecation (e.g., a child with anal fissures). Involuntary retention may be produced by emotional problems caused by the encopresis that sets up a fear-pain cycle and results in a learned process of abnormal defecation patterns. Psychogenic encopresis, in which the soiling is caused by the emotional problems, is often related to a disturbed mother-child relationship.

Normally children and adolescents have one or two soft-formed stools per day. Children with soiling problems tend to form large-bore stools, which are painful to excrete. Therefore they tend to avoid defecation and withhold stooling. Stool held in the rectum and sigmoid colon loses water and progressively hardens, causing successively more painful bowel movements. Thus a pain-retention-pain cycle is established. Many children have diarrhea or loose leakage in their clothing and pass small amounts of hard stool, suggesting leakage around an impaction (Stroh, Stern, and McCarthy, 1989).

During school years children may experience exacerbations at the transition to school. Some of the reasons for developing retentive tendencies at this time are fear of using school bathrooms, a busy schedule, and the interruption of an established time schedule for bowel evacuation. Children at any age may react to stress with bowel dysfunction.

Clinical Manifestations

The manifestation of simple constipation is painful expulsion of hard, pelletlike stools. Voluntary retention is usually temporary, and there is a history of a painful precipitating episode and blood-streaked stools. Involuntary retention is associated with a history of abdominal pain, distention, moodiness, poor appetite, and accumulation of stools with periodic passage of voluminous stools. Children display a characteristic posturing during suppression of colonic signals to defecate—stiffening, standing in a corner with straight legs and a bright-red face, "doing a little dance," "crawling," or hiding behind furniture or a tree when playing outdoors. They typically hide soiled underwear. It is not unusual for soiling to take place after bathing because of reflex stimulation.

The child with encopresis often feels ashamed and may wish to avoid situations (e.g., camp or school) that might lead to embarrassment. The amount of impairment is a function of the effect on the child's self-esteem, the degree of social ostracism by peers, and the anger, punishment, and rejection on the part of caregivers (American Psychiatric Association, 1994). School performance and attendance are affected as the child's offensive odor becomes a target for scorn and derision from classmates. The child is not well liked by peers because of it and may be severely rejected by the parents as a result of the symptom. The rejection by peers and parents causes further withdrawal and other behavioral manifestations.

Therapeutic Management

Treatment is directed toward the cause of the soiling. Diet, lubricants, and a toilet ritual that encourages the child to establish normal defecation are used. Fecal impaction is relieved by catharsis, suppositories, and/or mineral oil. Customary dosages are usually insufficient. Dietary changes may be helpful, such as elimination of milk and dairy products and increased amounts of high-fiber foods, such as fruits, vegetables, and cereals, as well as increased fluids. Behavior therapy may be indicated to eliminate any fear that has developed as a result of painful defecation. Frequently, psychotherapeutic intervention with the child and the family becomes necessary.

Nursing Considerations

A thorough history of the soiling is essential—when soiling began, how often it occurs, under what circumstances, and if the child uses the toilet successfully at all (Stroh, Stern, and McCarthy, 1989). Since parents and child are reluctant to volunteer information, direct questioning about the soiling is more successful. Following the history, a complete physical assessment is performed.

Education regarding the physiology of normal defecation, toilet training as a developmental process, and the treatment outlined for the particular family is prerequisite to a successful outcome. The regimen prescribed for stimulating elimination is explained to parents. Sitting the child on the toilet at routine intervals is not recommended, because it may intensify parent-child conflict and result in a power play. Enemas may be needed for impactions, but long-term use prevents the child from assuming responsibility for defecation. Initially lubricants are given liberally, but stimulant cathartics often cause abdominal cramps that can be a frightening experience for a child.

Family counseling is directed toward reassurance that most problems resolve successfully, although the child may have relapses during periods of stress, such as vacation or illness. If encopresis persists beyond occasional relapses, the condition will need to be reevaluated. Behavior modification techniques are explained, and the family is assisted with a plan suited to their particular situation (see Family Focus box).

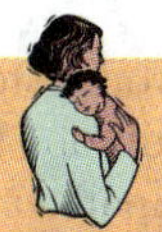

FAMILY FOCUS

Helping Families Understand Encopresis

The prevailing attitude of nurses toward the family of a child with encopresis is one of no-fault, thus relieving the guilt of both parents and child. Since parents and children are often reluctant to volunteer information, direct questioning about the soiling is more successful. Parents are usually relieved to know that other parents share this problem and are surprised to know that functional changes that take place as the condition develops make control of seepage impossible. Many parents complain that their children soil because they do not take time from play for a bowel movement. Actually, the children may be unaware of a prior sensation and unable to control the urge once it begins. They may be so accustomed to bowel accidents that they are unable to smell or feel it and even deny soiling when it occurs (Stroh, Stern, and McCarthy, 1989).

DISORDERS WITH BEHAVIORAL COMPONENTS*

ATTENTION DEFICIT–HYPERACTIVITY DISORDER (ADHD)

ADHD is the latest term applied to a persistent pattern of inattention and/or hyperactivity-impulsivity that is more frequent and severe than is typically observed in individuals at a comparable level of development. Some hyperactive-impulsive or inattentive symptoms that cause impairment must have been present before age 7 years, although many individuals are diagnosed after the symptoms have been present for a number of years. The syndrome of manifestations affects 3% to 5% of school-age children and is almost 10 times more frequent in boys than in girls. The difficulties are most often school related, behavioral or academic, and difficulties with social relationships in general are often manifested by aggressive behavior and mood lability that interferes with peer relationships and makes disciplining difficult.

Early identification of affected children is needed, since the characteristics of the disorder significantly interfere with the normal course of emotional and psychologic development. In an attempt to cope with attention deficit, many of these children develop maladaptive behavior patterns that are a deterrent to psychosocial adjustment. Their behavior evokes negative responses from others, and repeated exposure to negative feedback adversely affects the child's self-concept, especially in boys (Harris and others, 1992). About half of the children with ADHD also have learning disabilities (see p. 813). Most children with ADHD have average or above-average intelligence and are often very creative children. These children may have various strengths that are not evident in a typical classroom structure.

Etiology

The etiology of ADHD is uncertain, obscure, and often speculative. As the definition implies, it may be related to virtually any illness or trauma affecting the brain that occurs at any stage of development—before, during, or after birth. Multiple causes, including psychosocial factors, are probably involved.

Behavioral and learning disorders have been noted in children with some of the ***sex chromosome abnormalities.*** For example, in girls with Turner syndrome there is a high incidence of impaired spatial abilities and right-left directional sense, and a large number of boys with Klinefelter syndrome have learning, behavioral, or peer problems. A sex-linked factor may be operating, because the disorder is much more common in boys than in girls.

A popular theory is the concept of a ***developmental lag.*** Distractibility, short attention span, and impulsiveness are all normal characteristics of children at a much younger developmental level. However, current research indicates that symptoms of ADHD do not diminish with age. Symptoms, such as inattentiveness and impulsivity, last into adolescence

*Definitions of attention deficit–hyperactivity disorder, learning disorders, and posttraumatic stress disorder are modified from the American Psychiatric Association: *Diagnostic and statistical manual of mental disorders,* ed 4 (DSM-IV), Washington, DC, 1994, American Psychiatric Association.

and young adulthood in 50% to 60% of affected youngsters (Kelly and Aylward, 1992; Rostain, 1991). In addition, hyperactivity may be merely a normal variant of innate temperament in some children who represent the extreme end of the normal distribution curve for activity.

Support for a ***biochemical etiology*** is suggested by the way in which a majority of hyperactive children respond to central nervous system stimulant drugs. In these hyperactive children there appears to be an absence or insufficiency of norepinephrine, a neurotransmitter that normally appears in high concentrations in areas of the brain that have much to do with activity level, mood, and awareness. Another theory suggests some alteration in the reticular activating system of the midbrain, a key area for controlling consciousness and attention, that interferes with its function of filtering out extraneous stimuli. Consequently, these children are unable to focus on one stimulus but are compelled to respond to every stimulus in the environment. Central nervous system stimulants that increase the level of norepinephrine and/or activate the reticular activating system cause a reduction in the undesired behavior. The fact that these children show few, if any, symptoms in a stress situation (such as in the clinician's or principal's office) provides additional support to this hypothesis, because stress increases the level of norepinephrine. In a study of adults who were hyperactive as children, there was reduced cerebral glucose metabolism, especially in the areas of the brain involved in the control of attention and motor activity (Zametkin and others, 1990).

Interest in diet as a factor in hyperactivity continues to generate controversies. There are those who believe that the observed behavioral patterns are related to an innate sensitivity to certain food items and/or food additives. Although this theory does not have wholehearted support, some children do show improvement when certain foods are eliminated from their diet, particularly those that cause more hyperallergic reactions, such as chocolate, cow's milk, and eggs (Egger, Stolla, and McEwen, 1992). Others may have adverse effects from sucrose or aspartame (the artificial sweetener Nutrasweet) (Shaywitz and others, 1994; Wolraich and others, 1994).

Clinical Manifestations

The behaviors exhibited by the child with ADHD are not unusual aspects of child behavior. The difference lies in the quality of motor activity and developmentally inappropriate inattention, impulsivity, and hyperactivity the child displays. The manifestations may be numerous or few, mild or severe, and will vary with the developmental level of the child. Any given child will not have every manifestation that is characteristic of a syndrome, and the degree of severity is highly variable. Mild manifestations of the symptoms may not be apparent in a good educational and family environment, whereas severe symptomatology will be recognizable even in the most healthy and accommodating environment. Every dysfunctional child is, in some respects, different from all other children with ADHD (see box on p. 811).

Most behavioral manifestations are apparent at an early age, but the learning disabilities may not become evident until the child enters school. The disorder is unpredictable; it may remit spontaneously at any age, and the number of years a child will require treatment is unknown.

Another major clinical manifestation is distractability. The stimuli may be from external sources or internal sources relative to the child. Children frequently demonstrate immaturity relative to chronologic age. Selective attention is often seen, in which the child has difficulty attending to "nonpreferred" tasks, such as completing chores, finishing homework, etc. The child usually does not consider the consequences of behavior and therefore tends to take excessive physical risks (often beginning early in life) and demonstrates inappropriate or lack of social skills.

Children may demonstrate one of three subtypes of ADHD (American Psychiatric Association, 1994):

1. **Combined type**—Six (or more) symptoms of inattention and six (or more) symptoms of hyperactivity-impulsivity have persisted for at least 6 months. Most children and adolescents with the disorder have the combined type. It is not known whether the same is true of adults with the disorder.
2. **Predominantly inattentive type**—Six (or more) symptoms of inattention (but fewer than six symptoms of hyperactivity-impulsivity) have persisted for at least 6 months.
3. **Predominantly hyperactive-impulsive type**—Six (or more) symptoms of hyperactivity-impulsivity (but fewer than six symptoms of inattention) have persisted for at least 6 months. Inattention may often still be a significant clinical feature in such cases.

Course of ADHD. In the majority of affected children the disorder is relatively stable through early adolescence. In most individuals, symptoms diminish during late adolescence and adulthood, although a minority experience the full complement of symptoms of ADHD into middle adulthood. Other adults may no longer have the full disorder but still retain some symptoms that cause functional impairment (American Psychiatric Association, 1994).

Diagnostic Evaluation

The basic characteristics outlined in the box on p. 811 are the basis for establishing a diagnosis of ADHD. It is important to emphasize the need for a complete and thorough multidisciplinary evaluation of the child, incorporating the efforts of the pediatrician, often a developmental pediatrician or pediatric neurologist, psychologist, pediatric nurse, classroom teacher, reading/math specialist, special education teacher, possibly a speech therapist, and the child's parents. The clinicians and professionals must first determine whether the child's behavior is age-appropriate or truly problematic.

A history, both medical and developmental, and description of the child's behavior should be obtained from as many observers of the child as possible, especially parents and teachers, along with the observations of the health professionals involved. It should include descriptions of the child's behavior in home and school situations. In obtaining descriptive material, the interviewer must question the observers carefully, because some persons, especially parents, may be so concerned with gross behaviors that they overlook less distressing but equally important symptoms.

DIAGNOSTIC CRITERIA FOR ATTENTION-DEFICIT/HYPERACTIVITY DISORDER

A. Either (1) or (2):
(1) Six (or more) of the following symptoms of **inattention** have persisted for at least 6 months to a degree that is maladaptive and inconsistent with developmental level:
Inattention
(a) Often fails to give close attention to details or makes careless mistakes in schoolwork, work, or other activities
(b) Often has difficulty sustaining attention in tasks or play activities
(c) Often does not seem to listen when spoken to directly
(d) Often does not follow through on instructions and fails to finish schoolwork, chores, or duties in the workplace (not due to oppositional behavior or failure to understand instructions)
(e) Often has difficulty organizing tasks and activities
(f) Often avoids, dislikes, or is reluctant to engage in tasks that require sustained mental effort (such as schoolwork or homework)
(g) Often loses things necessary for tasks or activities (e.g., toys, school assignments, pencils, books, or tools)
(h) Is often easily distracted by extraneous stimuli
(i) Is often forgetful in daily activities
(2) Six (or more) of the following symptoms of **hyperactivity-impulsivity** have persisted for at least 6 months to a degree that is maladaptive and inconsistent with developmental level:
Hyperactivity
(a) Often fidgets with hands or feet or squirms in seat
(b) Often leaves seat in classroom or in other situations in which remaining seated is expected
(c) Often runs about or climbs excessively in situations in which it is inappropriate (in adolescents or adults, may be limited to subjective feelings of restlessness)
(d) Often has difficulty playing or engaging in leisure activities quietly
(e) Is often "on the go" or often acts as if "driven by a motor"
(f) Often talks excessively
Impulsivity
(g) Often blurts out answers before questions have been completed
(h) Often has difficulty awaiting turn
(i) Often interrupts or intrudes on others (e.g., butts into conversations or games)

B. Some hyperactive-impulsive or inattentive symptoms that caused impairment were present before age 7 years.
C. Some impairment from the symptoms is present in two or more settings (e.g., at school [or work] and at home).
D. There must be clear evidence of clinically significant impairment in social, academic, or occupational functioning.
E. The symptoms do not occur exclusively during the course of a pervasive developmental disorder, schizophrenia, or other psychotic disorder and are not better accounted for by another mental disorder (e.g., mood disorder, anxiety disorder, dissociative disorder, or a personality disorder).

Code based on type:
314.01 Attention-Deficit/Hyperactivity Disorder, Combined Type: if both Criteria A1 and A2 are met for the past 6 months
314.00 Attention-Deficit/Hyperactivity Disorder, Predominantly Inattentive Type: if Criterion A1 is met but Criterion A2 is not met for the past 6 months
314.01 Attention-Deficit/Hyperactivity Disorder, Predominantly Hyperactive-Impulsive Type: if Criterion A2 is met but Criterion A1 is not met for the past 6 months

Coding note: For individuals (especially adolescents and adults) who currently have symptoms that no longer meet full criteria, "in partial remission" should be specified.

From American Psychiatric Association: *Diagnostic and statistical manual of mental disorders (DSM-IV)*, ed 4, Washington, DC, 1994, The Association.

For example, parents may report a "colicky" infant, a child who began to run as soon as he walked, a toddler who is compelled to touch everything in sight, and a child who resists sleep until exhausted. A history of delayed or atypical language development is associated with specific learning disabilities. A pregnancy and birth history may provide clues to a situation that might have produced an episode of hypoxia.

A physical examination, including a detailed neurologic evaluation, will help rule out any severe neurologic disorders. Psychologic testing, especially projective tests, is valuable in determining visual-perceptual difficulties, problems with spatial organization, and other phenomena that suggest cortical or diencephalic involvement, and it helps to identify the child's intelligence and achievement levels. Psychiatric and other disorders, as well as traumatic experiences, are ruled out, including lead poisoning, seizures, partial hearing loss, psychosis, and witnessing sexual activity and/or violence.

Therapeutic Management

Management of the child with ADHD usually involves a multiple approach that includes family education and counseling, medication, proper classroom placement, environmental manipulation, and sometimes psychotherapy for the child. Medication is prescribed only if appropriate for the individual child. Diet modification is not often seen as a treatment option.

Behavioral Therapy and Psychotherapy. Behavioral therapy is an important component of the treatment plan for children with ADHD. The prevention of undesired behavior is emphasized. Because of maturation and learning, successful contingencies for identified behaviors do not remain as effective as they once were. It is often a challenge to identify new appropriate continencies and reward systems to meet the child's developing needs. Families who participate in therapy can be instructed in and role-play effective parenting skills, such as positive reinforcement, rewarding small increments of desired behaviors, and age-appropriate consequences (e.g., time-out, response-cost, etc.). Through collaborative team work, parents can learn techniques to help the child become more successful at home and in school, such as the use of organization charts for completing self-care activities and using a word processor instead of manually writing out assignments. Therapy with a knowledgeable counselor or psychologist can reinforce behavioral goals, assist with family support, and help children gain increased self-esteem and work through situations that are problematic for them.

Pharmacologic Therapy. Many drugs have been advocated for management of the symptoms of ADHD. The most frequently prescribed medications are the sympathomimetic amines methylphenidate (Ritalin) or dextroamphetamine (Dexedrine). They produce strong effects on central nervous system dopamine and norepinephrine. Methylphenidate is preferred because of its less marked effect on prolactin and growth hormone. The child is begun on a small dose that is gradually increased until the desired response is achieved. Other drugs are magnesium pemoline (Cylert) and the tricyclic antidepressants. Pemoline is a mild central nervous system stimulant with a slower onset, and its effect appears less marked. Tricyclic antidepressants, principally imipramine (Tofranil) and desipramine (Norpramin), have proved to be effective in some children, but cardiac side effects must be monitored.

Regularly scheduled reevaluation of the child is essential to determine medication effectiveness, detect and evaluate any side effects, monitor development and health status (such as blood pressure), and assess family interaction. Medications may be prescribed to assist the child in self-regulating his or her behaviors that may be counterproductive to effective problem solving and socialization.

Nursing Considerations

Nurses, especially school nurses, are active participants in all aspects of management of the child with ADHD. Nurses in the community setting work with families in the home on a long-term basis to help plan and implement therapeutic regimens and to evaluate the effectiveness of therapy. They are in the best position to coordinate services and serve as a liaison between other health and education professionals directly involved in the child's therapy program. School nurses have an understanding of the child's special needs and work with teachers. The nurse in any setting (community, school, hospital, practitioner's office) can provide support and guidance to children and families during the difficult tasks associated with growing up with a disabling condition.

The management of the child with ADHD begins with an explanation to the parents and the child about the diagnosis, including the nature of the problem and the practitioner's concept of the underlying central nervous system basis for the disorder. Most parents are confused and feel some measure of guilt. To some it is confirmation of the fear that the child may be "crazy" or has some irreversible, serious disease; to others it is a relief. They need the opportunity to vent their feelings and suspicions. A common complaint of parents is that health professionals have not listened to what they have to say about their child.

The parents need information about the prognosis and an understanding of the treatment plan. The greater their understanding of the disorder and its effects, the more likely they will be to carry out the recommended program of therapy. It is important that they understand that the therapy is not necessarily a panacea and that it will extend over a long period. This has particular significance for changes they need to make in environmental management. Reading material to help the child and family can be obtained from a variety of sources.

Medication. Parents are reminded that some medications (pemoline) require 2 to 3 weeks to achieve an effect. Others are begun at low dosage and increased until the desired effect is attained. When evaluating the child's response to the medication, it is helpful to obtain reports from the teacher, as well as from the parents, since the parents may see the child when the effects of the drug are wearing off. Observing the child's behavior through visits to the home and school is useful for assessing attention span, interactional patterns with others at school, and behaviors with academic tasks. The nurse can consult with the teacher about the child's behavior in general. This information provides data needed to regulate dosage based on recorded, systematic observations of the child's behaviors in at least two settings.

Parents need to be informed of the possible side effects of the medication—anorexia, blurred vision, and sleeplessness—which usually disappear after several weeks. If anorexia is a concern with methylphenidate, encouraging nutritious snacks in the evening as the effects of the medication are decreasing and serving frequent small meals with healthy "on the go" snacks are often helpful suggestions. A common complaint is that the child becomes quiet and very sensitive, crying at the slightest provocation. Sleeplessness is reduced by administering the medication early in the day. It has also been found that the absorption of methylphenidate is accelerated when administered with meals and impeded when given before meals. Another troublesome side effect is depressed growth, probably caused by interference with the release of growth hormone; therefore the practitioner may sometimes discontinue the drug on weekends or on vacations to allow for some catch-up growth, although some believe there is no theoretic or practical advantage to the practice (Brown, 1986).

Children on tricyclic antidepressants display a dramatic increase in the incidence of dental caries. The marked anticholinergic action of the drugs increases saliva viscosity and produces a dry mouth. Emphasis on rigorous dental hygiene, conscientious home fluoride treatment, regular visits to the dentist, limited intake of refined carbohydrates, and artificial saliva is an important nursing function. The child should be kept well hydrated.

Parents may express concern that the child may become addicted to antidepressant drugs. There is always the possibility of abuse, including suicide attempts; however, usually the child is no longer interested in the drug once the need is past—particularly since the effect of the drug in these children is opposite that produced in normal individuals. However, parents are cautioned to keep the drugs safely stored away from children who may inadvertently ingest them.

Environmental Manipulation. Families are encouraged to learn how to modify the environment to allow the child to be more successful. Consistency is always an important parenting skill and is even more so for those whose child has difficult behavior. It is also important to have consistency between families and teachers in terms of reinforcing the same goals. Fostering improved organizational skills necessitates a much more highly structured environment than most children require. The child should be encouraged to make more appropriate choices and to take responsibility for actions.

Other helpful interventions include teaching parents how to make organization charts (e.g., listing all activities preceding leaving for school), decreasing distractions in the environment while completing homework (e.g., television off, having a consistent study area equipped with needed supplies, etc.), helping parents to understand ways to model positive behaviors and problem solving, etc. The list of interventions is probably endless, but the focus is on strategies to help the child be successful and cope with deficits while emphasizing strengths (Comfort, 1992).

Appropriate Classroom Placement. The philosophy of providing the "least restrictive environment" encourages mainstreaming children in the classroom as much as possible. If learning disabilities exist, special training activities may be accomplished in self-contained classes with a limit of six to eight children, special resource rooms with equipment and teaching teams, mobile consultants who move from room to room to provide assistance to teachers and children, and special first grade programs in which high-risk children receive special attention to prevent or reduce the need for services as they progress. The purpose of programs for children with special learning disabilities is to assist them toward more successful achievement, personal adjustment, and eventual retention in the regular classroom. However, because a true perceptual problem exists, improvement is noted by an increased attention span, allowing the child to focus on one stimulus while blocking out others; refinement of fine motor control; and advancement in other areas of disability.

Psychiatric, Psychologic, and Social Therapies. Counseling or therapy can be very helpful for children who demonstrate signs of anxiety or depression. Therapy can help the child to develop a healthier self-esteem and practice problem-solving strategies. The adolescent may benefit from group work focusing on social skill development. Therapy is also indicated for members of dysfunctional families.

LEARNING DISORDERS

Learning disorders exist when the individual's achievement on individually administered, standardized tests in reading, mathematics, or written expression is substantially below that expected for age, schooling, and level of intelligence. The learning problems significantly interfere with academic achievement or activities of daily living that require reading, mathematic, or writing skills (American Psychiatric Association, 1994). They do not include learning problems that result primarily from visual, hearing, or motor disabilities; mental retardation; emotional disturbances; or environmental disadvantage. The types of disabilities include ***dyslexia*** (difficulty with reading), ***dysgraphia*** (difficulty with writing), ***dyscalculia*** (difficulty with calculation), right-left confusion, and short attention span.

A comprehensive battery of tests is needed to confirm a learning disability. These include intelligence tests (these children tend to have normal or above-average IQs), hand-eye coordination tests, and measurements of auditory and visual perception, comprehension, and memory. Often there is a wide gap between verbal and performance scores on IQ tests.

Therapeutic Management

Special training activities in the schools are designed to offer assistance in such areas of deficit as visual perception, auditory perception, and other areas involving integration and coordination. The purpose of programs for children with special learning disabilities is to assist them toward more successful achievement, personal adjustment, and eventual retention in the regular classroom. However, according to Public Law 94-142, The Education for All Handicapped Children's Act, children with learning disorders must receive free public education in the least restrictive environment (see Chapters 1 and 22).

Nurses must understand which type of learning disability a child has in order to best provide direction for the child, parents, and teachers. Children with an auditory perceptual deficit appear unable to follow directions or to comprehend large amounts of verbal teaching. These children need to be taught with diagrams, pictures, demonstration, and written lists. Children with a visual perceptual deficit may have difficulty reading, lining up numbers for mathematic operations, or judging distance. These children may have dyslexia (letter reversals) and do better with demonstration and a verbal approach. Children with an integrative deficit may have difficulty sequencing data or storing and retrieving sensory data. Multisensory techniques should be used, and comprehension should be checked frequently throughout instruction. Children with motor deficits may need to use typewriters in the classroom, since their handwriting will *not* improve. They may need to find alternatives to physical competition that requires coordination of movement (Selekman, 1991). The **Association for Children and Adults with Learning Disabilities*** provides information and support to families with a child with a learning disability.

Children with learning disorders grow up to be adults with learning disorders. The goal is to help them identify their area of weakness and to compensate for it.

---

*4156 Library Rd., Pittsburgh, PA 15234; (412) 341-1515.

TABLE 18-13 Spectrum of Tic Disorders

	MILD ⟵⟶		CHRONIC
Duration	Acute	Subacute	Chronic
Motor tics	Simple Few	Complex	Obscene gestures Multiple
Vocal tics	None	Noises	Coprolalia
Suppressible	Yes		No

TIC DISORDERS

A *tic* is an involuntary, recurrent, random, rapid, highly stereotyped movement or vocalization, occurring in 10% to 35% of all children (Table 18-13). Tics can be simple or complex and involve motor movements, eye movements, or vocalizations (see box above, right). Tics decrease during concentration, are markedly diminished during sleep, and become more exaggerated when the affected children are experiencing stress or excitement. Obsessive-compulsive behaviors, in the form of ritualistic activities, also may be present and can occur in individuals free of tics. No major psychologic components are evident (Golden, 1987). A number of medications can precipitate tics.

Almost all mild transient tic disorders of childhood are self-limited and disappear within a few months, usually less than a year. The most common tics involve the eyes, head, and face, and treatment does not affect recovery. Tic disorders can begin at any time during childhood. Boys are affected at least three times as often as girls, and in over 50% of cases, tics are observed in other family members (Avery and First, 1989).

Tic disorders that persist beyond 1 year are considered to be chronic and consist of one form of either motor or vocal manifestations but not both (Erenberg, 1988). The most severe of the chronic tics is Gilles de la Tourette's syndrome. Diagnosis of a tic disorder is based on clinical observations.

Most tic disorders resolve by late childhood or adolescence without treatment and cause no physical harm to the child. Therapeutic management consists primarily of support to the child and family, reassurance about the prognosis, and education regarding expectations (of the child) for control. Although the child is able to suppress the manifestations to some degree, persistent pressure for control constitutes an additional stress to an affected child. Haloperidol or pimozide may provide relief of symptoms of chronic tics, and genetic counseling is also advised for families of children with chronic tics.

TYPES OF TICS

Simple motor—Eye blinking, grimacing, neck jerking, shoulder jerking

Complex motor—Jumping, squatting, stamping the foot, thrusting out an arm, hitting or biting self, ritualistic movements (smelling an object, touching own or another's body, obsessive or compulsive patterns of behavior), grooming behaviors

Simple vocal—Throat clearing, sniffing, grunting, coughing, snorting, lip noises

Complex vocal—Echolalia (repeating last-heard sound, word, or phrase of another), palilalia (repeating own sounds or words), coprolalia (use of socially unacceptable words, often obscene), shouting words out of context

TOURETTE SYNDROME (TS)

TS is the most complex and severe of the tic disorders. It begins between ages 2 and 16, persists throughout life, and is characterized by rapidly repetitive multiple motor and vocal movements. The etiology is uncertain, although most theories implicate abnormalities of various neurotransmitters. Support for a genetic origin, based on family studies, suggests that the disorder is inherited as a autosomal-dominant, sex-influenced trait (Calderon-Gonzalez and Calderon-Sepulveda, 1993).

The manifestations of TS wax and wane in intensity and exhibit a continuing pattern of change in which old tics disappear and new tics develop (see box below). The onset is usually mild, and the initial tic of brief duration. The minor tics then come and go, becoming more intense and lasting longer (Erenberg, 1988). Some tics may be severe from the onset, often with no symptom-free periods. Diagnosis is based on clinical observations, especially if other family members are affected. The tics do not lead to physical deterioration or affect the child's life expectancy.

Therapeutic Management

Treatment of TS is primarily symptomatic and consists of child and family education and support. Children with more severe tics sometimes obtain symptomatic relief from medications. Haloperidol, a dopamine-blocking agent, is

DIAGNOSTIC CRITERIA FOR TOURETTE DISORDER

A. Both multiple motor and one or more vocal tics have been present at some time during the illness, although not necessarily concurrently. (A *tic* is a sudden, rapid, recurrent, nonrhythmic, stereotyped motor movement or vocalization.)
B. The tics occur many times a day (usually in bouts) nearly every day or intermittently throughout a period of more than 1 year, and during this period there was never a tic-free period of more than 3 consecutive months.
C. The disturbance causes marked distress or significant impairment in social, occupational, or other important areas of functioning.
D. The onset is before age 18 years.
E. The disturbance is not due to the direct physiologic effects of a substance (e.g., stimulants) or a general medical condition (e.g., Huntington disease or postviral encephalitis).

From *Diagnostic and statistical manual of mental disorders*, ed 4 (DSM-IV), Washington, DC, 1994, American Psychiatric Association.

the most widely prescribed drug. Pimozide (Orap) and fluphenazine, with similar action to haloperidol, or clonidine, an alpha-2-adrenergic drug, may also be prescribed. Genetic counseling is advised.

Nursing Considerations

Nurses are important in the management of TS. Education of children, families, teachers, and others involved in children's everyday life is a major aspect of therapy. Punishment for the behaviors is inappropriate, since they are involuntary. Affected children are often quick to anger, have a low frustration tolerance, and may engage in temper tantrums. These children need to be guided toward acceptable substitute behaviors in order to develop normally, socially and emotionally (Comings and Comings, 1985). For example, suggest a child retire to a quiet area to gain control of emotions or provide a pillow, stuffed toy, or punching bag on which to vent feelings.

Influential persons in the children's lives must help foster feelings of self-esteem. Children with TS demonstrate a constant, ongoing battle over the control of their impulses, which becomes more difficult with controlling behaviors of parents. Children with TS are more likely to be well-adjusted if they perceive parental relationships as positive (Edell and Motta, 1989). A child's self-concept can be damaged if parents react to the disability with guilt or anger, which they usually manifest as hostility.

Nurses may assist families engaged in long-term monitoring of symptoms, which includes establishing the waxing and waning and whether or not they interfere with development and adaptation in an important way, requiring more intense therapy. Families of children on medication need to be alert to possible side effects, including lethargy, personality change, increased appetite and overweight, depression, parkinsonian symptoms (tremor, muscle rigidity, shuffling gait, hypokinesia, and difficulty chewing, swallowing, and speaking), and anticholinergic symptoms (confusion, excitement, dilated pupils, blurred vision, dry mouth, and dysphagia).

The family may benefit from referral to health agencies such as the local health departments, social services, and parent groups. The **Tourette Syndrome Association*** is active in research and education and provides services to affected children and their families.

POSTTRAUMATIC STRESS DISORDER (PTSD)

PTSD refers to the development of characteristic symptoms following exposure to an extreme traumatic stressor involving direct personal experience of an event that involves actual or threatened death or serious injury, or other threat to one's physical integrity; or witnessing an event that involves death, injury, or a threat to the physical integrity of another person; or learning about unexpected or violent death, serious harm, or threat of death or injury experienced by a family member or other close associate. The person's response to the event must involve intense fear, helplessness, or horror (or in children, the response must involve disorganized or agitated behavior). The characteristic symptoms resulting from the exposure to the extreme trauma include persistent reexperiencing of the traumatic event, persistent avoidance of stimuli associated with the trauma and numbing of general responsiveness, and persistent symptoms of increased arousal. The full symptom picture must be present for more than 1 month, and the disturbance must cause clinically significant distress or impairment in social, educational, occupational, or other important areas of functioning (American Psychiatric Association, 1994).

The response to the event takes place in a sequence of three stages. The ***initial response*** to the stressor is intense arousal, which usually lasts for a few minutes to 1 or 2 hours, depending on the stressor and the individual. The stress hormones are at the maximum as the individual prepares for "fight" or "flight." A prolonged arousal phase may indicate psychosis.

The ***second phase,*** which lasts approximately 2 weeks, is one in which defense mechanisms are mobilized. It is a period of quiescence in which the event appears to have produced no impression. The victims feel numb, and stress hormone secretion is absent. The reaction is outside their awareness, not well controlled, and involves some type of behavioral pattern. Defense mechanisms are less adaptive to specific situations and may not be what the situation demands. Denial that anything is wrong is a frequently observed defense mechanism.

The ***third phase*** is one of coping, which normally extends over 2 to 3 months. It is one of consciously directed inquiry. The victims want to know what happened and appear to be getting worse, when actually they are getting better. Numerous psychologic symptoms may be apparent, such as depression, repetitive phenomenon, phobic symptoms, anxiety symptoms, and conversion reactions. Children frequently display repetitive actions. They play out the situation over and over again in an attempt to come to terms with their fear. Flashbacks are common. This phase can be self-perpetuating, and a prolonged reaction can develop into an obsession with the traumatic event. Some traumatic effects remain indefinitely (Terr, 1989). Researchers have also found that children with PTSD have impaired startle inhibition, indicating long-lasting alteration in the brainstem circuits that help startle modulation (Ornitz and Pynoos, 1989).

Nursing Considerations

Children need to deal with any traumatic event; much depends on the intensity of the event and their reaction to it. Their reactions depend heavily on their social environment and the way in which their caretaking adults react to the event. Children usually react in much the same manner as their caregivers (contagious pathology); therefore it is important to be aware of these reactions also. In the second, or defense, phase of the PTSD the appropriateness of the defense mechanism must be assessed, and children must be assisted in application of their defense. If children do not engage in some catharsis or if their defense phase is pro-

*42-40 Bell Blvd., Bayside, NY 11361; (718) 224-2999.

longed, they may need referral for special psychologic help.

Coping is a learned response, and children in the third phase can be helped to use their coping strategies to deal with their fear. Children usually are willing to accept reasoning. Those who are assisted in their catharsis and allowed expression will survive without serious lasting effects. They should be encouraged to play out the stress and/or discuss their feelings about the event. If they are unable to do this, they may become obsessed with the traumatic event and need professional help. Conversion reactions are common obsessive behaviors in children.

Children need professional help if any of the phases of PTSD are prolonged. Boys tend to have a prolonged defense phase more often than girls. Occasionally the event will be unrecognized, and the affected child will engage in what is considered to be unusual behavior. In the case of any sudden change in behavior, the child needs to be assessed for a traumatic event—"Did something happen?" When the change in behavior is determined to be a traumatic event, treatment can be implemented.

SCHOOL PHOBIA

Children, other than beginning students, who resist going to school because of dread of the school situation, concerns with leaving home, or both, are said to have school phobia. As a rule, children below the age of 13 who fear school tend to be separation-anxious—children who are afraid of leaving the people they love. For these children the term "school refuser" is rapidly replacing "school phobia," which is more accurate after the age of 13 years. By this time children have worked through immature separation fears (Last and others, 1987).

Anxiety that frequently verges on panic is a constant manifestation, and children can develop symptoms as a protective mechanism to keep them from facing the situation that distresses them. Physical symptoms are prominent and may affect any part of the body—anorexia, nausea, vomiting, diarrhea, dizziness, headache, leg pains, or abdominal pains, to name a few. They may even develop a low-grade fever. A striking feature of school phobia is the prompt subsiding of symptoms when it is evident that the child can remain at home. Another significant observation is absence of symptoms on weekends and holidays, unless they are related to other places such as Sunday school or parties. Occasional mild reluctance is not uncommon among schoolchildren, but if the fear continues for longer than a few days, it must be considered a serious problem—a warning of an important personality problem.

Unlike most other behavior problems of children, school phobia is more common in girls than in boys; there is no relationship to socioeconomic status, ethnic origin, or other subcultural affiliation; and no particular age predominates. The onset is usually sudden and precipitated by a school-related incident. A poor attendance record for trivial reasons can be elicited by a careful history.

Etiology

School phobia can be caused by a number of factors. Sometimes the complaints can be related to a transient, specific cause such as fear of a mismatched or overcritical teacher, fear of failing an examination or giving an oral recitation for a painfully shy child, or discrimination based on race, dress, or physical defect. Sometimes it may be related to a school bully or threatening gang. An insecure home situation in which the child fears that he may be deserted by a parent while he is gone may be the basis of anxiety, especially if the parent has previously threatened to leave for some reason.

A frequent source of fear is separation anxiety based on a strong dependent relationship between the mother and child in which the child is reluctant to leave the mother and she is equally reluctant (even though this may be unconscious) to have the child leave her. The intense need for closeness between mother and child is normal in infancy, but the persistence of this type of relationship into childhood is totally inappropriate. Characteristically, these children are not afraid to go to school, but rather they are afraid to leave home. They fear something dreadful might happen while they are separated from their families. No event is required to trigger the associated behaviors. However, symptoms may be precipitated by a situation that intensifies the mutual dependency between the mother and the child, such as illness, arrival of a new baby, a move to a strange neighborhood or a new school, or parental discord.

In some instances children have an unrealistic, exaggerated view of their abilities and achievements. When they feel threatened by incidents that challenge their estimate of themselves, such as a minor episode that leads to embarrassment, return to school after an absence, transfer to another class, or even imagined social or academic failure, they become anxious and withdraw, frequently seeking proximity to the mother. Sometimes the step-up in expectations at school or change of important personnel at school (e.g., teacher or principal) is a contributing factor. Occasionally the child may be suffering from an undiagnosed learning disability.

Therapeutic Management

The treatment for school phobia depends on the cause. The children really *want* to go to school but just cannot force themselves to do so; they are not delinquent children. They are anxious, tense, and distressed because they are unable to muster enough courage to attend school. If the cause of the problem is an examination, relationship with a bully, or a mismatch between teacher and child, it can be dealt with accordingly. When the child is helped to understand and cope with the fear, the symptoms usually disappear. In severe cases when returning to school is unsuccessful, professional psychiatric consultation is usually desirable to help identify possible distorted family relationships or a personality disturbance in the child and to help both child and family understand the sources of the problem.

Nursing Considerations

The primary goal for the child with school phobia is to *return the child to school.* The longer the child is permitted to stay out of school, the more difficult it is to reenter. Well-meaning parents or others who permit the child to stay away from school and support any efforts with written excuses only confirm the child's feelings of worthlessness and inability to cope. Parents must be convinced gently but firmly that *immediate* return is essential and that they, the parents, are the ones who must insist on the child's return for it to be effective.

Some modifications in school attendance might be necessary for the child with severe symptoms. The child who is unable to return to regular classes may be allowed to go to school on a part-time basis, spending the time in the counselor's office or nurse's office and getting homework from the teacher after class. It may be necessary to transport the child to and from school or even have a parent attend class with the child. However, this practice is not allowed to continue for an unlimited time, and the time limit should be agreed on beforehand. The essential factor is that the child must return to school right away, maintain the pattern of going, and remain there even while a solution is being worked out. The school nurse can provide both teacher and parents with support in carrying out this plan.

Prevention. Prevention of school phobia, as well as other dependency problems, can be developed by the encouragement of independence at appropriate times during infancy and early childhood. For example, by 6 months of age children are left with a baby-sitter during a parents' night out. Two-year-olds can be left home (while awake) with a sitter. By 3 years of age children should experience being left somewhere other than their home (e.g., grandparents' home). As soon as they are able, they are allowed to feed, dress, and wash themselves. By 3 to 4 years of age children can be allowed to play in the yard by themselves, and later they should be allowed to play in the neighborhood by themselves.

Certain clues indicate that a child may be subject to first-time fear; thus children can be helped to adjust to it. Extra preparation may be needed for children who are very fearful, have trouble adjusting to new situations, or are very clinging (Last and others, 1987). Many individuals continue to manifest some form of fear throughout their school careers. When the problem is identified early and effectively treated, and negative emotions surrounding school are minimized, a child is less likely to carry residual fears throughout life.

For most first-time school fears, as for any new and potentially frightening experience, simple reassurances and a little advance preparation are all that is needed. Direct contact with the school and teachers is an excellent means of allaying anticipatory anxiety. Parents can take children to visit the school about a month before school starts, introduce them to the teacher, and let them experience the classroom firsthand.

Bedtime, when the family is usually relaxed, is an excellent time to help children resolve first-day jitters. Bedtime stories and books suited to the occasion are available from bookstores and libraries. Another option is a tape entitled "I Can Take Care of Myself,"* one of a series designed to help children cope with a variety of common fears (dark, nightmares, baby-sitters, doctors, dentists, monsters).

Parents who suspect that their child may be especially frightened may want to accompany the child to school and wait outside the classroom the first day. A gradual breakaway over succeeding days should relieve their child's and their own anxiety. If the distress extends beyond 2 weeks, professional help may be needed (Last and others, 1987).

RECURRENT ABDOMINAL PAIN (RAP)

RAP is one of the somatic complaints of childhood that is almost always attributed to a psychogenic etiology, although it can be a symptom of either psychosomatic or organic disease. RAP is traditionally defined as three or more separate episodes of abdominal pain during a 3-month period. Similar to the "spastic" or "irritable colon syndrome" of adulthood, the disorder affects 10% to 20% of school-age children at some time in their childhood. It is rarely seen in children less than 5 years of age; its peak incidence is in children ages 10 to 12 years. Girls are affected slightly more often than boys (Coleman and Levine, 1986).

Etiology and Pathophysiology

Only a minority of youngsters with RAP have an organic basis for their pain, which includes inflammatory bowel disease, peptic ulcer disease, lactose intolerance, pelvic inflammatory disease, urinary bladder infection, and pancreatitis. Psychiatric disorders such as depression and school avoidance account for a small number of these cases. In 90% to 95% of cases no organic cause can be found (Farrell, 1984; Poole, 1984). The bulk of children with RAP suffer from functional abdominal pain, which is ill defined and often misinterpreted to mean fictitious or imagined pain (Olson, 1987).

The most plausible etiologic theories describe functional abdominal pain as dyskinesia (Davidson, 1986) or dysmotility (Coleman and Levine, 1986) and as multifactorial (Levine and Rappaport, 1984). Normally, intestinal contents arrive at the distal portion of the intestine with a relatively high fluid content, where fluid is extracted to a greater degree in the distal colon and rectum. In dysmotility (dyskinesia) the normally relaxed distal intestine fails to relax, preventing the flow of its contents toward the rectum. The resulting excessive distention in the proximal bowel and spasms of the distal intestinal musculature produce the dysmotility. Pressure on nerve endings causes pain.

The basis for a multifactorial etiology describes both causative and predisposing factors: (1) somatic predisposition, dysfunction, or disorder; (2) life-style and habit, including routines, diet, and life tempo; (3) temperament and learned response patterns, such as the child's behavior style, personality, and learned coping skills; and (4) milieu and critical events (i.e., the child's intimate surroundings [familial, social, and cultural norms] and unexpected sources of stress or gratification) (Coleman and Levine, 1986).

Children at risk for RAP tend to be high achievers who have great personal goals or whose parents have unusually high expectations. They are described as being more mature and sensitive than others or as worriers. At risk are children who are overly concerned about what others think

**Happy Heart Tapes* by J. Thomas can be obtained from the Center for Attitude Modification, P.O Box 2886, Del Mar, CA 92014; (619) 453-7310.

about them but have difficulty meeting the expectations of parents, teachers, and others. They are uncomfortable with expressions of anger or argument, especially in those persons who are significant in their lives. School attendance is adversely affected, and these children generally exhibit poor learning performance. It is not uncommon for symptoms to be aggravated during school days.

Clinical Manifestations

Children with RAP have real pain that the child usually locates in the periumbilical and/or epigastric area. However, on palpation the pain is more likely to be experienced in the epigastric area or in the lower right or left quadrant and is accompanied by vague tenderness without muscle guarding. Other symptoms that may accompany the abdominal pain are headache, flushing, pallor, dizziness, and fatigue. Nausea, vomiting, and diarrhea are sometimes part of the syndrome. The symptoms reflect the heightened intensity of response to stimulation of the autonomic bowel sites. The loose stools are the result of the exaggerated propulsive motility, and the pain is caused by the sharply increased mechanical tension in the gut.

Diagnostic Evaluation

Diagnosis consists of a complete family history and the child's health history, physical examination, and laboratory tests. The family history may provide evidence of a hereditary disorder or mimicry of adult symptoms. The child is evaluated for evidence of an organic basis for symptoms such as pain that radiates to the back, pain that awakens the child from sleep, recurrent fever, and weight loss. The pain is assessed for location, quality, frequency, duration, any associated symptoms, alleviating factors, and exacerbating factors (Olson, 1987).

Therapeutic Management

Treatment is difficult. Hospitalization may be necessary, and the child frequently shows improvement in the hospital environment. Initial efforts are directed toward ruling out organic causes of the pain, relieving discomfort, and attempting to determine the situations that precipitate attacks.

Most authorities recommend a high-fiber diet (including fiber-containing cookies), psyllium bulk agents, and lubricants such as mineral oil to help colonic emptying. If these measures are not effective, they are discontinued. Bowel training to establish regular bowel habits is encouraged. When simple measures are ineffective, an antispasmodic drug such as propantheline bromide may be prescribed to relieve the muscle spasm.

Nursing Considerations

The nurse can be instrumental in assessment and management of recurrent abdominal pain in children. Many of the techniques used in a routine assessment can elicit information that might help identify those factors that contribute to the child's symptomatology. The child's social and psychologic adjustment should be evaluated, and details of the pain should be obtained directly from the child when possible.

Questions that provide clues to parent-child relationships and how the family deals with angry feelings provide useful information for diagnosis and management. Relationships with peers, school problems, and other concerns of the child need to be explored, and any evidence of depression should be noted. It is also significant that psychogenic somatic symptoms generally do not awaken the child from sleep.

Once the diagnosis has been established, the parents and the child need an explanation of the pain, which can be compared to a skeletal muscle cramp or "charley horse" for easier comprehension. Reassurance that the symptoms are not unique to their child and that the pain can be expected to subside is helpful in relieving parental fears and anxieties.

A high-fiber diet is discussed with the child and family (see Chapter 33), and bowel training is emphasized. The child is encouraged to establish a pattern of sitting on the toilet for 10 to 15 minutes immediately after breakfast to take advantage of the increased colonic activity following meals. If necessary, stimulatory suppositories can be used to induce early morning defecation.

When parents are reassured that there is no organic cause of the pain, they will need some guidance regarding what they can do during a pain episode. All too often they feel helpless and anxious, which tends to compound the child's distress. The simple expedient of putting the child at rest by having him or her lie down in a peaceful, quiet environment and providing comfort will often relieve the symptoms in a short time. A heating pad may also help ease the discomfort. (See also Nonpharmacologic [Pain] Management, Chapter 26.) If pain is not relieved by these simple measures, the parents are taught how to administer antispasmodics. For example, if pain is precipitated by meals, having the child take the medication 20 to 30 minutes before mealtime may prevent an episode.

The most valuable assistance that the nurse can provide is support and reassurance to the family. One of the most difficult aspects of therapy is helping parents and child understand the cause of the pain. When open communication is established and families are able to see a relationship between stress-provoking situations and the child's symptoms, the chance for remedial action is enhanced. Follow-up care and continued support are essential because the symptoms tend to remit and exacerbate; therefore the availability of a supportive health professional can be a source of comfort to the child and family.

CONVERSION REACTION

Conversion reaction, also known as hysteria, hysterical conversion reaction, conversion symptoms, and childhood hysteria, is a psychophysiologic disorder with a sudden onset that can usually be traced to a precipitating environmental event. The manifestations involve primarily the voluntary musculature and special senses and include abdominal pain, fainting, pseudoseizures, paralysis, headaches, and visual field restriction. Once considered rare in childhood, the diagnosis occurs more frequently than has generally been acknowledged. In childhood the disorder is observed with equal frequency in both sexes, but girls outnumber boys during adolescence. The most commonly observed symptom is seizure activity, which can be differentiated from symptoms of neurogenic origin by formal tests, the most useful of which is the finding of a normal electroencephalogram.

It has been observed that nearly all children with conversion reaction have experienced a major family crisis before the onset of symptoms. Particularly traumatic is an unresolved grief reaction in the child, such as loss of a parent or other significant person through death, divorce, or moving (Maloney, 1980). It is not uncommon for the child to exhibit symptoms of the lost person. The families of children with conversion reaction characteristically display problems in communication, and depression or hypochondriasis in a parent is a common finding.

Educating the child and family regarding the cause underlying emotional stresses or feelings and alternative approaches to coping with stress may alleviate the child's symptoms, although families are not always receptive to the intervention. If deep personality problems are evident, psychiatric consultation is usually indicated. Nursing care is similar to that for the child with récurrent abdominal pain.

CHILDHOOD DEPRESSION

Depression in childhood is often difficult to detect because children may be unable to express their feelings and tend to act out their problems and concerns. Authorities agree that childhood depression exists but they do not agree whether or not it is the same as adult depression. The characteristics of depression are largely determined by parallel developments in symbolism, language, and cognitive development. Younger children demonstrate a more cause-and-effect relationship between the stressors and the depressive manifestations, which are primarily the biologic deprivation syndromes. As children develop, the relationships between stressful events and depression are less clear. Their reactions are less physiologic and more cognitively complex, and the observed behaviors tend to be age specific. Depressed children exhibit a distinctive style of thinking characterized by low self-esteem, hopelessness, and a tendency to explain negative events in terms of personal shortcomings (McCauley and others, 1988).

Some states of depression are of a temporary nature (e.g., acute depression precipitated by a traumatic event). This might include a period of hospitalization, loss of a parent through death or separation, or loss of a significant relationship with something (a pet), someone (a friend or family member), or a place (move from a familiar home, neighborhood, or city). The easily identified manifestations include a sad, downcast face, tearfulness, irritability, and withdrawal from previously enjoyed activities and relationships. The child tends to spend more time in solitary activities, especially television viewing, and schoolwork is impaired. Some children become more dependent and clinging; others become more aggressive and disruptive. Sleeplessness and/or loss of appetite are not common reactions. Responses are not sustained and can be modified with social and family support.

CRITERIA FOR MAJOR DEPRESSIVE EPISODE

A. Five (or more) of the following symptoms have been present during the same 2-week period and represent a change from previous functioning; at least one of the symptoms is either (1) depressed mood or (2) loss of interest or pleasure.
   Note: Do not include symptoms that are clearly due to a general medical condition, or mood-incongruent delusions or hallucinations.
   (1) Depressed mood most of the day, nearly every day, as indicated by either subjective report (e.g., feels sad or empty) or observation made by others (e.g., appears tearful). **Note:** In children and adolescents, can be irritable mood.
   (2) Markedly diminished interest or pleasure in all, or almost all, activities most of the day, nearly every day (as indicated by either subjective account or observation made by others)
   (3) Significant weight loss when not dieting or weight gain (e.g., a change of more than 5% of body weight in a month), or decrease or increase in appetite nearly every day. **Note:** In children, consider failure to make expected weight gains.
   (4) Insomnia or hypersomnia nearly every day
   (5) Psychomotor agitation or retardation nearly every day (observable by others, not merely subjective feelings of restlessness or being slowed down)
   (6) Fatigue or loss of energy nearly every day
   (7) Feelings of worthlessness or excessive or inappropriate guilt (which may be delusional) nearly every day (not merely self-reproach or guilt about being sick)
   (8) Diminished ability to think or concentrate, or indecisiveness, nearly every day (either by subjective account or as observed by others)
   (9) Recurrent thoughts of death (not just fear of dying), recurrent suicidal ideation without a specific plan, or a suicide attempt or a specific plan for committing suicide

B. The symptoms do not meet criteria for a mixed episode, which includes symptoms of a manic episode, such as rapidly alternating moods (sadness, irritability, euphoria).

C. The symptoms cause clinically significant distress or impairment in social, occupational, or other important areas of functioning.

D. The symptoms are not due to the direct physiologic effects of a substance (e.g., a drug of abuse, a medication) or a general medical condition (e.g., hypothyroidism).

E. The symptoms are not better accounted for by bereavement; i.e., after the loss of a loved one, the symptoms persist for longer than 2 months or are characterized by marked functional impairment, morbid preoccupation with worthlessness, suicidal ideation, psychotic symptoms, or psychomotor retardation.

Slightly modified from American Psychiatric Association: *Diagnostic and statistical manual of mental disorders (DSM-IV)*, ed 4, Washington, DC, 1994, The Association.

More serious and less common are depressive responses to more chronic stress and loss; these are frequently observed in children with chronic illness or disability. There is no apparent precipitating event, but there is often a history of frequent disruptions in important relationships. Commonly there is also a history of depressive illness in one or both parents during the child's lifetime. The manifestations are similar to responses to acute reactions. Some of the primary and associated symptoms that are observed in depressed children and the DSM-IV criteria currently used for establishing a diagnosis of major depression are outlined in the box on p. 819. There are a number of similarities among major depressive disorders in childhood and several other psychologic disorders.

Therapeutic Management

Depressed children are managed by a health team especially prepared in the care of children with mental disorders. Treatment of depression should be undertaken in the least constrictive environment, usually outpatient management. Suicidal children are admitted to the hospital for protection if the family is unable to provide constant monitoring. For children with associated disruptive behavior, such as fighting with peers or family, hospitalization may be advised. Most therapeutic regimens focus on counseling and/or pharmacotherapy with tricyclic antidepressants and serotonergic-reuptake inhibitors (fluoxetine [Prozac], trazodone [Desyrel]) (Hodgman and others, 1993).

Nursing Considerations

The management of childhood depression is usually psychotherapeutic and highly individualized. Nurses should be aware that depression is a problem that can easily be overlooked in the school-age child and one that can interrupt normal growth and development. Recognizing depression and making appropriate referrals is an important nursing function. Identification of the depressed child requires a careful history (health, growth and development, social, and family health), interviews with the child, and observations by the nurse, parents, and teachers. If the child is placed on antidepressants, the child and family need to be instructed to monitor the child for side effects of the specific drug prescribed. See Chapter 21 for a more definitive discussion of suicide, because suicidal ideation is common during depression.

CHILDHOOD SCHIZOPHRENIA

Childhood schizophrenia refers to severe deviations in ego functioning and is generally reserved for psychotic disorders that appear after the first 4 or 5 years of life. Schizophrenia in adults occurs with relative frequency, and although childhood psychosis is not as common, it is by no means rare.

The cause of schizophrenia is unknown, but three risk factors have been identified: genetic characteristics, gestational and birth complications, and winter birth. Biologic relatives of affected individuals have an increased chance of developing the disorder. For example, the risk for the children if both parents are afflicted is 40%. The rate of concordance is 10% for dizygotic (nonidentical) twins and 40% to 50% for monozygotic (identical) twins. Current thinking supports the etiology being related to altered development of the central nervous system. Psychosocial theories, especially in regard to the parent-child relationship, have not been supported, but certain social and environmental factors may play a role in a child's vulnerability to developing schizophrenia (Carpenter and Buchanan, 1994).

SOME CHARACTERISTICS OF CHILDHOOD SCHIZOPHRENIA

- Bizarre behavioral patterns and stereotyped movements such as robotlike walking, whirling, or graceful gyrations
- Periods of hypoactivity alternating with periods of hyperactivity
- Inappropriate affect that ranges from flatness to explosiveness
- Common occurrences of temper tantrums
- Language disturbances such as speaking in fragmented sentences, parrotlike repetition of words, development of a private language, and altered tone of voice; some schizophrenic children are mute or will only utter a single word on rare occasions
- Distorted time orientation with a blending of past, present, and future
- Distorted sense of and use of their bodies
- Apparent denial of the human quality in people, such as attempting to use a person as a step stool to reach an object
- Conveying a nonhuman identity by action, sounds, or posture, such as barking or calling self a vacuum cleaner
- Frequent occurrences of compulsive behavior and phobias

Childhood schizophrenia is characterized by a gradual onset of neurotic symptoms that show wide variation according to each affected child's developmental level, the age of onset, the nature of early childhood experiences, and the type of defense mechanisms used. However, the basic core disturbance is a lack of contact with reality and the subsequent development of a world of the child's own. Secondary characteristics represent impairment in a wide number of areas of development, including cognition, perception, emotion, language, and physical motor control. The most common manifestations involve language disturbances, impaired interpersonal relationships, and inappropriate affect (outward expression of emotion) (see box above).

Treatment involves management of the symptoms, the prevention of a relapse, and the social and occupational rehabilitation of the young person. Antipsychotic drugs that may be used include haloperidol and clozapine.

Nursing Considerations

Nursing of psychotic children is a highly specialized area, but since these problems are being recognized with increasing frequency, nurses should be alert to the possibility. A child who consistently demonstrates abnormal behavior should be referred for evaluation.

KEY POINTS

- Middle childhood is a relatively healthy period and most problems encountered are not considered serious.
- The skin serves several important functions: protection, prevention of loss of body fluids, heat regulation, and sensation.
- It is important for nurses to be able to describe skin lesions accurately.
- The stages of wound healing consist of inflammation, fibroplasia, scar contraction, and scar maturation.
- Wound healing occurs by primary, secondary, or tertiary intention.
- Bacterial, viral, and fungal infections are common in childhood.
- Prevention of infection or reinfection is the primary goal in management of pediculosis.
- Contact dermatitis may involve a reaction to a primary irritant or sensitization.
- Teaching prevention of thermal injury, especially sunburn, is an important nursing function.
- Adverse reactions to drugs occur more often in the skin than in any other organ.
- Dental care continues to be important; most frequent problems that arise are dental caries and malocclusion.
- The behavioral disorders of childhood are primarily attention deficit–hyperactivity disorder and tic disorders.
- Other major behavioral or mental disorders involving school-age children include school phobia, recurrent abdominal pain, conversion reaction, depression, and schizophrenia.

REFERENCES

Alvarez O, Rozint J, Meehan M: Principles of moist wound healing: indications for chronic wounds. In Krasner D, editor: *Chronic wound care: a clinical source book for health care professionals,* King of Prussia, PA, 1990, Health Management.

American Academy of Pediatrics, Committee on Infectious Diseases: *Red book: Report of the Committee on Infectious Disease,* ed 23, Elk Grove Village, IL, 1994, American Academy of Pediatrics.

American Psychiatric Association: *Diagnostic and statistical manual of mental disorders,* ed 4 (DSM-IV), Washington, DC, 1994, American Psychiatric Association.

Avery ME, First LR, editors: *Pediatric medicine,* Baltimore, 1989, Williams & Wilkins.

Baker MD: Bites and scratches: when pets fight back, *Contemp Pediatr* 6(6):76-84, 1989.

Barnett NK: Pruritus. In Hoekelman RA, editor-in-chief: *Primary pediatric care,* St Louis, 1987, Mosby.

Brown G and others: Enhancement of wound healing by topical treatment with epidermal growth factor, *N Engl J Med* 321:76-79, 1989.

Brown GL: Attention deficit disorder. In Gellis SS, Kagan BM: *Current pediatric therapy 12,* Philadelphia, 1986, WB Saunders.

Calderon-Gonzalez R, Calderon-Sepulveda RF: Tourette syndrome: current concepts, *Int Pediatr* 8(2):176-188, 1993.

Carpenter WT, Buchanan RW: Medical progress: schizophrenia, *N Engl J Med* 330(10)681-690, 1994.

Clore ER: Head-lice screening, Sch Health Watch 5(2):2, 1994.

Clore ER, Longyear LA: A comparative study of seven pediculides and their packaged nit removal combs, *J Pediatr Health Care* 7(2):55-60, 1993.

Coleman WL, Levine MD: Recurrent abdominal pain: the cost of the aches and the aches of the cost, *Pediatr Rev* 8:143-151, 1986.

Collipp PJ: Cat-scratch disease: therapy with trimethoprim-sulfamethoxazole, *Am J Dis Child* 146(4):397-399, 1992.

Coln D, Emmrich P: Hypothermia and frostbite. In Eichenwald HF, Ströder J, editors: *Current therapy in pediatrics—2,* Toronto, 1989, BC Decker.

Comfort RL: Living with an unconventional child, *J Pediatr Health Care* 6(3):114-120, 1992.

Comings DE, Comings BG: Tourette syndrome: clinical and psychological aspects of 250 cases, *Am J Genet* 37:435-450, 1985.

Cooper LI: Removing cactus spines, *Am J Dis Child* 142:1140, 1988 (letter).

Davidson M: Recurrent abdominal pain: look to dyskinesia as the culprit, *Contemp Pediatr* 3(12):16-42, 1986.

Edell BH, Motta RW: The emotional adjustment of children with Tourette's syndrome, *J Psychol* 123:51-57, 1989.

Egger J, Stolla A, McEwen LM: Controlled trial of hyposensitisation in children with food-induced hyperkinetic syndrome, *Lancet* 339(8802):1150-1153, 1992.

Erenberg G: Identification and management of patients with tics/Tourette syndrome, *Feelings* 30:21-24, 1988.

Esposito AL, Adams D: Infection of skin and subcutaneous tissue. In Eichenwald, HF, Ströder J, editors: *Current therapy in pediatrics—2,* Toronto, 1989, BC Decker.

Farrell MK: Abdominal pain, *Pediatrics* 74(suppl):955-957, 1984.

Fitzwater D, Macknin M: Risk/benefit ratio in enuresis therapy, *Clin Pediatr* 31(5):308-310, 1992.

Flessner MF: A tough diagnosis in a neutropenic patient: it's cat-scratch disease, *JAMA* 261:991, 1989.

Friman P, Warzak W: Nocturnal enuresis: a prevalent, persistent, yet curable parasomnia, *Pediatrician* 17:38-45, 1990.

Gelbard MK: Removal of small cactus spines from the skin, *JAMA* 252:3368, 1984.

Ginsburg CM, Gädeke R: Snakebites. In Eichenwald HF, Ströder J, editors: *Current therapy in pediatrics—2,* Toronto, 1989, BC Decker.

Golden GS: Movement disorders: sorting the benign from the serious, *Contemp Pediatr* 4(5):77-92, 1987.

Griffen AL, Goepferd SJ: Preventive oral health care for the infant, child, and adolescent, *Pediatr Clin North Am* 38(5):1209-1226, 1991.

Hagelgans NA: Pediatric skin care issues for the home care nurse, *Pediatr Nurs* 19(5):499-507, 1993.

Harris M and others: Self-fulfilling effects of stigmatizing information on children's social interactions, *J Personality Soc Psychol* 63(1):41-50, 1992.

Hennes H: Removal of cactus spines from the skin, *Am J Dis Child* 142:587, 1988.

Hodgman C and others: Managing depression in children, *Patient Care* 27(10):51-60, 1993.

Holloway L: Shadow method for sun protection, *Lancet* 335:484, 1990 (letter).

Houts AC: Nocturnal enuresis as a biobehavioral problem, *Behav Ther* 22(2):133-151, 1991.

Hunt TK: Basic principles of wound healing, *J Trauma* 30(12, suppl):S122-S128, 1990.

Hurwitz S: There's no such thing as "a good tan," *Contemp Pediatr* 5(5):55-66, 1989.

Ismail AI and others: Effect of sealants to children's teeth, *J Public Health Dent* 49:206-211, 1989.

Kelly DP, Aylward GP: Attention deficits in school-aged children and adolescents: current issues and practice, *Pediatr Clin North Am* 39:487-512, 1992.

Key DW, Bloom DA, Sanvordenker J: Low-dose DDAVP in nocturnal enuresis, *Clin Pediatr* 31(5):299-300, 1992.

Kochman D: What to do about facial trauma, *Contemp Pediatr* 6(7):72-83, 1989.

Krasner PR: The treatment of avulsed teeth, *J Pediatr Health Care* 4:86-90, 1990.

Last CG and others: Separation anxiety and school phobia: a comparison using DSM-III criteria, *Am J Psychiatry* 144:653-657, 1987.

LeVeen HH, LeVeen RF, LeVeen EG: The mythology of povidone-iodine and the development of self-sterilizing plastics, *Surg Gynecol Obstet* 176(2):183-190, 1993.

Levine MD, Rappaport LA: Recurrent abdominal pain in school children: the loneliness of the long-distance physician, *Pediatr Clin North Am* 31:969-991, 1984.

Mackreth B: Poison ivy, don't rub it the wrong way, *Patient Care* 16(8):21-25, 1991.

Madden EJA: Itch, *J Pain Symptom Manage* 1(2):97-99, 1986.

Maloney MJ: Diagnosing hysterical conversion reactions in children, *J Pediatr* 97:1016-1020, 1980.

Margileth A, Hadfield T: A new look at old cat-scratch, *Contemp Pediatr* 7(12):25-48, 1990.
Margileth AM, Hayden GF: Cat scratch disease: from feline affection to human infection, *N Engl J Med* 329(1):53-54, 1993.
Martinez TT and others: Removal of cactus spines from the skin, *Am J Dis Child* 141:1291-1292, 1987.
McCauley E and others: Cognitive attributes of depression in children and adolescents, *J Consult Clin Psychol* 56:903-908, 1988.
McGuire MA: Think hypothermia, *Point of View* 24(3):12-14, 1987.
Moffatt MEK, Kato C, Pless TB: Improvements in self-concept after treatment of nocturnal enuresis: randomized controlled trial, *J Pediatr* 110:647-652, 1987.
Moffatt MEK and others: Desmopressin acetate and nocturnal enuresis: how much do we know? *Pediatrics* 92(3):420-425, 1993.
Needham GR: Evaluation of five popular methods for tick removal, *Pediatrics* 75:997-1002, 1985.
Nicol NH: What's new with sunscreens? Choices—choices—choices, *Pediatr Nurs* 15:417-418, 1989.
Olson A: Recurrent abdominal pain: an approach to diagnosis and management, *Pediatr Ann* 16:834-842, 1987.
Ornitz EM, Pynoos RS: Startle modulation in children with posttraumatic stress disorder, *Am J Psychiatry* 146:866-869, 1989.
Poole SR: Recurrent abdominal pain in childhood and adolescence, *Am Fam Physician* 30:131-137, 1984.
Putnam MH, Lawton MB: Resourceful women unmask cactus spines, *JAMA* 253:2830, 1985.
Rappaport LA: Enuresis. In Levine M and others: *Developmental-behavioral pediatrics,* ed 2, 1992, WB Saunders.
Rappaport LA: The treatment of nocturnal enuresis—where are we now, *Pediatrics* 92(3):465-466, 1993.
Riegger M, Guntzelman J: Prevention and amelioration of stress and consequences of interaction between children and dogs, *JAMA* 196(11):1781-1785, 1990.
Rittig S and others: Abnormal diurnal rhythm of plasma vasopressin and urinary output in patients with enuresis, *Am J Physiol* 256(4, pt2):F664-671, 1989.
Rostain AL: Attention deficit disorders in children and adolescents, *Pediatr Clin North Am* 38(3):607-635, 1991.
Sacks JJ, Sattin RW, Bonzo SE: Dog bite–related fatalities from 1979 through 1988, *JAMA* 262:1489-1492, 1989.
Schneider D, Hebert L: Subcutaneous gas from hydrogen peroxide administration under pressure, *Am J Dis Child* 141:10-11, 1987.
Schneider S, King LR, Surwit RS: Kegel exercise and childhood incontinence: a new role for an old treatment, *J Pediatr* 124:91-92, 1994.
Schuberth KC: How dangerous are insect stings? *Contemp Pediatr* 6(5):69-88, 1989.
Selekman J: Primary care of the child with a learning disability. In Jackson P, Vessey J: *Primary care of children with chronic conditions,* St Louis, 1991, Mosby.
Shannon M: Mosquitoes, ticks, and deet, *Pediatr Alert* 19(20):67, 1994.
Shaw L, Glenwright HD: The role of medications in dental caries formation: need for sugar-free medications for children, *Pediatrician* 16:153-155, 1989.
Shaywitz BA and others: Aspartame, behavior, and cognitive function in children with attention deficit disorder, *Pediatrics* 93(1):70-75, 1994.
Stafford CT, Moffitt JE, Yates AB: Insect sting anaphylaxis referral is imperative, *Emerg Med* 24(11):230-231, 1992.
Stroh SE, Stern HP, McCarthy SG: Fecal incontinence in children: a clinical update, *AACN* 14(4):252-254, 1989.
Stromgren A, Thomsen PH: Personality traits in young adults with a history of conditioning-treated childhood enuresis, *Acta Psychiatr Scand* 81:538-541, 1990.
Taplin D and others: Comparison of crotamiton 10% cream (Eurax) and permethrin 5% cream (Elimite) for the treatment of scabies in children, *Pediatr Dermatol* 7(1):67-73, 1990.
Terr L: Traumatic events in childhood have lasting effects, *AAP News* 5(5):1, 1989.
Welch JS: Efficacy and safety of povidone-iodine underscored, *J Emerg Nurs* 18(3):191-192, 1992.
Wolraich ML and others: Effects of diets high in sucrose or aspartame on the behavior and cognitive performance of children, *N Engl J Med* 330(5):301-307, 1994.
Woodley DT, Kim YH: A double-blind comparison of adhesive bandages with the use of uniform suction blister wounds, *Arch Dermatol* 128(10):1354-1357, 1992.
Wysocki A: Skin structure. In Bryant RA, editor: *Acute and chronic wounds: nursing management,* St Louis, 1992, Mosby.
Zametkin AJ and others: Cerebral glucose metabolism in adults with hyperactivity of childhood onset, *N Engl J Med* 323(20):1361-1366, 1990.
Zangwill KM and others: Cat-scratch disease in Connecticut: epidemiology, risk factors, and evaluation of a new diagnostic test, *N Engl J Med* 329:8-13, 1993.

BIBLIOGRAPHY

Skin Disorders: General

Bolton L, Rijswijk LV: Wound dressings: meeting clinical and biological needs, *Dermatol Nurs* 3(1):146-161, 1991.
Bryant R: *Acute and chronic wounds: nursing management,* St Louis, 1992, Mosby.
Chauvin VG: Common skin rashes in children and adolescents, *Sch Nurse* 5(1):23-38, 1989.
Ching D, Mell D: Use of adhesive dressings in skin care: DuoDerm Extra Thin, *J Pediatr Health Care* 4(3):155-156, 1990.
Connell S: A two-part quality assurance project addressing infection rates of wounds sutured in the emergency department, *J Emerg Nurs* 17:212-214, 1991.
Cuzzell JZ, Stotts NA: Trial and error yields to knowledge, *Am J Nurs* 90(10):53-63, 1990.
Engebo DA: Safe and effective use of tetracaine, adrenaline, and cocaine (TAC) solution anesthetic for anesthetizing of lacerations, *J Emerg Nurs* 16:100-101, 1990.
Garvin G: Wound healing in pediatrics, *Nurs Clin North Am* 25(1):181-192, 1990.
Gries M, Gladfelter K: Caring for the patient with an alteration in skin integrity, *Adv Clin Care* 6(3):34-37, 1991.
Hurwitz S: *Clinical pediatric dermatology: a textbook of skin disorders of childhood and adolescence,* ed 2, Philadelphia, 1993, WB Saunders.
Inaba AS: The rusty nail—and other puncture wounds of the foot, *Contemp Pediatr* 10(3):138-156, 1993.
Krasner D: *Chronic wound care: a clinical source book for healthcare professionals,* King of Prussia, PA, 1990, Health Management Publications.

Infections

Brady M: Common viral skin problems of childhood: warts and molluscum, *J Pediatr Health Care* 2:208-210, 1988.
Caputo RV: Fungal infections in children, *Dermatol Clin North Am* 4:137-150, 1986.
Coskey RJ, Coskey LA: Diagnosis and treatment of impetigo, *J Am Acad Dermatol* 17:62-63, 1987.
Frieden IJ: Diagnosis and management of tinea capitis, *Pediatr Ann* 16:39-48, 1987.
Gellis SE: Warts and molluscum contagiosum in children, *Pediatr Ann* 16:69-76, 1987.
Goldberg GN: An individualized approach to wart therapy, *Contemp Pediatr* 3(11):123-133, 1986.
Guess HA and others: Epidemiology of herpes zoster in children and adolescents: a population-based study, *Pediatrics* 76:512-517, 1985.
Krugman S and others: Infectious diseases of children, ed 9, St Louis, 1992, Mosby.
Putman CD, Reynolds MS: Mupirocin: a new topical therapy for impetigo, *J Pediatr Health Care* 3(4):224-227, 1989.
Rasmussen JE: Cutaneous fungus infections in children, *Pediatr Rev* 13(4):152-156, 1992.
Rasmussen JE: Impetigo: changing bacteria, changing therapies, *Contemp Pediatr* 9(2):14-22, 1992.

Scabies and Pediculosis

Bowerman JG and others: Comparative study of permethrin 1% creme rinse and lindane shampoo for the treatment of head lice, *Pediatr Infect Dis J* 6:252-255, 1987.
Brimhall CL, Esterly NB: Uninvited guests: skin infestations of childhood, *Contemp Pediatr* 7(1):18-57, 1990.
Brozena SJ: Scabies: update on diagnosis and treatment, *J Sch Nurs* 8(4):15-19, 1992.
Hubbard TW, Triquet MD: Brush-culture methods for diagnosing tinea capitis, *Pediatrics* 9(3):416-418, 1992.
Molinaro F: Treatment of pediculosis and scabies, *Pediatr Nurs* 18(6):600-602, 1992.
Park BR, Smith D: Treatment of head lice and scabies in children, *Pediatr Nurs* 15:522-524, 1989.
Sanford-Driscoll M: Pharmacotherapy of head lice in children: an update, *J Pediatr Health Care* 1:284-287, 1987.
Vargo K, Cohen BA: Prevalence of undetected tinea capitis in household members of children with disease, *Pediatrics* 92(1):155-157, 1993.

Systemic Disorders

Agre F, Schwartz R: The value of early treatment of deer tick bites for the prevention of Lyme disease, *Am J Dis Child* 147:945-947, 1993.

Distinguishing Lyme disease from its lookalikes, *Emerg Med* 24(11):28-50, 1992.

Koehler JE: Progress in cat scratch disease, *JAMA* 271:531, 1994.

Lee BC: Be ready for Lyme disease in your own backyard, *RN* 52(4):26-29, 1989.

Magid D and others: Prevention of Lyme disease after tick bites: a cost effectiveness analysis, *N Engl J Med* 327(8):534-541, 1992.

Malatack JJ, Jaffe R: Granulomatous hepatitis in three children due to cat-scratch disease without peripheral adenopathy, *Am J Dis Child* 147:949-953, 1994.

Maran JN, Crispell KA: Lyme disease: an elusive diagnosis, *J Pediatr Health Care* 3:60-66, 1989.

Matuschka FR, Spielman A: Risk of infection from and treatment of tick bite, *Lancet* 342:529-530, 1993.

Nocton JJ and others: Detection of *Borrelia burgdorferi* DNA by polymerase chain reaction in synovial fluid from patients with Lyme arthritis, *N Engl J Med* 330(4):229-234, 1994.

Perkins BA: Cat scratch disease; *A. felis* vs. *R. henselae, N Engl J Med* 327:1599-1601, 1992.

Piesman J: Dynamics of *Borrelia burgdorferi* transmission by nymphal *Ixodes dammini* ticks, *J Infect Dis* 167:1082-1085, 1993.

Rahn DW: Lyme disease—where's the bug? *N Engl J Med* 330(4):282-283, 1994.

Salazar JC, Gerber MA, Goff CW: Long-term outcome of Lyme disease in children given early treatment, *J Pediatr* 122(4):591-593, 1993.

Shapiro ED and others: A controlled trial of antimicrobial prophylaxis for Lyme disease after deer-tick bites, *N Engl J Med* 327(25): 1992.

Slota M, O'Connor K: Recognizing and treating cat scratch disease with encephalopathy in children, *Crit Care Nurse* 12(6):39-42, 1992.

Steere AC and others: The overdiagnosis of Lyme disease, *JAMA* 269(14):1812-1816, 1993.

Chemical and Physical Injuries

Bargoil SC, Erdman LK: Safe tan, an oxymoron, *Cancer Nurs* 16(2):139-144, 1993.

Beyea SC: What people expect you to know about poison ivy, *RN* 52(8):23-25, 1989.

Guin JD, Kligman AM, Maibach HI: Managing the poison-plant rashes, *Patient Care* 26(8): 63-66, 70-72, 1992.

Hurwitz S, Rhodes A, Wiley H: *For every child under the sun: a guide to sensible sun protection,* New York, 1986, The Skin Cancer Foundation.

Jarrett P, Sharp C, McLelland J: Protection of children by their mothers against sunburn, *Br Med J* 306(6890):1448, 1993.

Leach J: How to recognize photosensitivity disorders, *Contemp Pediatr* 6(6):56-74, 1989.

Lewis RM, Fischer RG: Sunscreen agents, *Pediatr Nurs* 13:200, 1987.

Parker F: The skin and the elements: sun, plants, and stinging and biting organisms, *Emerg Care Q* 4(3):21-31, 1988.

Protecting yourself from poison ivy, oak, and sumac, *Patient Care* 26(8):77-78, 1992.

Rumsfield J: Sunscreen: what you and your patients should know, *Dermatol Nurs* 2(3):139-147, 1990.

Sullivan SA: How severe is this frostbite? *Am J Nurs* 93(2):59-64, 1993.

Weinstock MA and others: Nonfamilial cutaneous melanoma incidence in women associated with sun exposure before 20 years of age, *Pediatrics* 84:199-204, 1989.

Miscellaneous Skin Disorders

Blum NJ and others: Trichotillomania, *Pediatrics* 91:993, 1993.

Dunn ML, Cockerline EB, Rice MR: Treatment options for psoriasis, *Am J Nurs* 88:1082-1087, 1988.

Eldridge R and others: Neurofibromatosis type 1 (Recklinghausen's disease), *Am J Dis Child* 143:833-837, 1989.

Hofman KJ and others: Neurofibromatosis type 1: the cognitive phenotype, *J Pediatr* 124(4):S1-S8, 1994.

Kaminester LH: The many guises of psoriasis, *J Emerg Med* 25(7):27-41, 1993.

Korf BR: Diagnostic outcome in children with multiple café au lait spots, *Pediatrics* 90(6): 924-927, 1992.

Nigro JF, Esterly NB: Psoriasis—chronic but controllable, *Contemp Pediatr* 10(10):114-128, 1993.

Obringer AC, Meadows AT, Zackai EH: The diagnosis of neurofibromatosis-1 in the child under the age of 6 years, *Am J Dis Child* 143:717-721, 1989.

Pau AK and others: Drug allergy documentation by physicians, nurses, and medical students, *Am J Hosp Pharm* 46:558-560, 1989.

Prendiville JS and others: Management of Stevens-Johnson syndrome and toxic epidermal necrolysis in children, *J Pediatr* 115:881-887, 1989.

Swedo SE and others: Trichotillomania: a profile of the disorder from infancy through adulthood, *Int Pediatr* 7(2):144-150, 1992.

Taylor JA and others: Toxic epidermal necrolysis, *Clin Pediatr* 28:404-407, 1989.

Bites and Stings

Adamski DB: Assessment and treatment of allergic response to stinging insects, *J Emerg Nurs* 16:77-80, 1990.

Cardoni AA: Meat tenderizer and bee stings, *Pediatrics* 74:447, 1984 (letter).

Eitzen EM, Seward PLN: Arthropod envenomations in children, *Pediatr Emerg Care* 4:266-270, 1988.

Graft DF and others: A prospective study of the natural history of large local reactions after hymenoptera stings in children, *J Pediatr* 104:664-668, 1984.

Hibel JA, Clore ER: Prevention and primary care treatment of stings from imported fire ants, *Nurse Practitioner* 17(6):65-71, 1992.

Hoff GL and others: Bats, cats and rabies in an urban community, *South Med J* 86(10): 1115-1118, 1993.

Sofer S, Shahak E, Gueron M: Scorpion envenomation and antivenom therapy, *J Pediatr* 124:973-978, 1994.

Dental Problems

Bimstein E: Periodontal health and disease in children and adolescents, *Pediatr Clin North Am* 38(5):1183-1207, 1991.

Centers for Disease Control and Prevention: Recommended infection-control practices for dentistry, 1993, *MMWR* 42(RR-8):1-12, 1993.

Crall JJ: Promotion of oral health and prevention of common pediatric dental problems, *Pediatr Clin North Am* 33:887-898, 1986.

Feldman AL, Aretakis DA: Herpetic gingivostomatitis in children, *Pediatr Nurs* 12:111-113, 1986.

Herrmann HJ, Roberts MW: Preventive dental care: the role of the pediatrician, *Pediatrics* 80:107-110, 1987.

Krasner P, Person P: Preserving avulsed teeth for replantation, *J Am Dent Assoc* 123(11):80-88, 1992.

Kronmiller JE: Oral soft tissue abnormalities in children, *Pediatr Nurs* 13:161-165, 1987.

Lewis DL and others: Cross-contamination potential with dental equipment, *Lancet* 340(8830):1252-1254, 1992.

McDonald RE, Avery DR: Dentistry for the child and adolescent, ed 6, St Louis, 1994, Mosby.

McGuire S: Fluoride content of bottled water, *N Engl J Med* 321:836-837, 1989.

Robertson JS, Maddux JE: Compliance in pediatric orthodontic treatment: current research and issues, *Child Health Care* 15:40-48, 1986.

Starr RM, Gravitz RF: Pit and fissure sealants in the prevention of tooth decay, *Pediatr Nurs* 11:289-291, 1985.

Weinstein LB, Abrams RA, Ayers CS: Increasing awareness of sugar ingestion among children, *Pediatr Nurs* 14:277-279, 1988.

Elimination Disorders

Castiglia PT: Encopresis, *J Pediatr Health Care* 1:335-337, 1987.

Castiglia PT: Nocturnal enuresis, *J Pediatr Health Care* 1:280-282, 1987.

Egger J and others: Effect of diet treatment in enuresis in children with migraine or hyperkinetic behavior, *Clin Pediatr* 31(5):302-307, 1992.

Feldman PC and others: Use of play with clay to treat children with intractable encopresis, *J Pediatr* 122(3):483-488, 1993.

Gibson LY: Bedwetting: a family's recurrent nightmare, *MCN* 14:270-272, 1989.

Hamburger B: Treating nocturnal enuresis, *Can Nurse* 89(4):26-28, 1993.

Marcovitch H: Treating bed wetting, *Br Med J* 306(6877):536, 1993.

McClung HJ and others: Is combination therapy for encopresis nutritionally safe? *Pediatrics* 91(3):591-594, 1993.

Miller K: Concomitant nonpharmacologic therapy in the treatment of primary nocturnal enuresis, *Clin Pediatr* 32(special ed):32-37, 1993.

Murray RD and others: Cisapride for intractable constipation in children: observations from an open trial, *J Pediatr Gastroenterol Nutr* 11(4):503-508, 1990.

Nørgaard JP, Djurhuus JC: The pathophysiology of enuresis in children and young adults, *Clin Pediatr* 32(special ed):5-9, 1993.

Novello AC, Novello JR: Enuresis, *Pediatr Clin North Am* 34:719-733, 1987.

O'Regan S and others: Constipation: a commonly unrecognized cause of enuresis, *Am J Dis Child* 140:260-261, 1986.

Schmitt BD: If your child is constipated and soils his underwear, *Patient Care* 26(13):232, 1992.

Schmitt BD, Mauro RD: Encopresis: 20 management mistakes, *Patient Care* 26(13):221-331, 1992.

Sprague-McRae J and others: Encopresis: a study of treatment alternatives and historical and behavioral characteristics, *Nurse Practitioner* 18(10):52-63, 1993.

Stadtler AC: Preventing encopresis, *Pediatr Nurs* 15:282-284, 1989.

Stenberg A, Lackgren G: Treatment with oral desmopressin in adolescents with primary nocturnal enuresis, *Clin Pediatr* 32(special ed):25-27, 1993.

Warzak WJ: Psychosocial implications of nocturnal enuresis, *Clin Pediatr* 32(special ed):38-40, 1993.

Attention Deficit–Hyperactivity Disorder/Learning Disorders

Ahmann PA and others: Placebo-controlled evaluation of Ritalin side effects, *Pediatrics* 91(6):1101-1106, 1993.

American Academy of Pediatrics: Learning disabilities, dyslexia, and vision, *Pediatrics* 90(1):124-126, 1992.

Brinckerhoff LC: Self-advocacy: a critical skill for college students with learning disabilities, *Fam Community Health* 16(3):23-33, 1993.

Calderon-Gonzalez R: Attention deficit disorders spectrum: neurological and neuropsychological basis, *Int Pediatr* 8(2):189-197, 1993.

Cantwell DP, Baker L: Attention-deficit disorders in children: the role of the nurse practitioner, *Nurse Practitioner* 12(7):38-52, 1987.

Coleman WL, Lindsay RL: Interpersonal disabilities: social skill deficits in older children and adolescents, *Pediatr Clin North Am* 39(3):551-567, 1992.

Cowell JM: Dilemmas in assessing the health status of children with learning disabilities, *J Pediatr Health Care* 4:24-31, 1990.

Funk JB and others: Attention deficit hyperactivity disorder, creativity, and the effects of methylphenidate, *Pediatrics* 91(4):816-819, 1993.

Hammil DD: A timely definition of learning disabilities, *Fam Community Health* 16(3):1-8, 1993.

Kelly DP, Aylward GP: Attention deficits in school-aged children and adolescents, *Pediatr Clin North Am* 39(3):487-512, 1992.

Keys MP: The pediatrician's role in reading disorders, *Pediatr Clin North Am* 40(4):869-879, 1993.

Lewis-Abney K: Correlates of family functioning when a child has attention deficit disorder, *Issues Compr Pediatr Nurs* 16(3):175-190, 1993.

Mann EM and others: Cross-cultural differences in rating hyperactive-disruptive behaviors in children, *Am J Psychiatry* 149:1539-1542, 1992.

Mercugliano M: Psychopharmacology in children with development disabilities, *Pediatr Clin North Am* 40(3):593-616, 1993.

Nass R: Development dyslexia: an update, *Pediatr Rev* 13(6):231-235, 1992.

Parrish JM: Behavior management in the child with developmental disabilities, *Pediatr Clin North Am* 40(3):617-628, 1993.

Pelham WE and others: Relative efficacy of long-acting stimulants on children with attention deficit-hyperactivity disorder: a comparison of standard methylphenidate, sustained-release methylphenidate, sustained tained-release dextroamphetamine, and pemoline, *Pediatrics* 86(2):226-237, 1990.

Purvis P, Whelan RJ: Collaborative planning between pediatricians and special educators, *Pediatr Clin North Am* 39(3):451-469, 1992.

Rosner J: Helping children overcome learning disabilities, *Except Parent* 23(8):36-38, 1993.

Rumsey JM: The biology of development dyslexia, *JAMA* 268(7):912-915, 1992.

Schmitt BD: The child with a short attention span (ADD), *Contemp Pediatr* 10(1):57-61, 1993.

Shapiro BK, Gallico RP: Learning disabilities, *Pediatr Clin North Am* 40(3):491-505, 1993.

Shaywitz SE and others: Prevalence of reading disability in boys and girls, *JAMA* 264(8):998-1002, 1990.

Silver LB: ADHD: *Attention deficit–hyperactivity disorder and learning disabilities: booklet for parents,* Summit, NJ, 1989, CIBA-Geigy.

Silver LB: ADHD: *Attention deficit–hyperactivity disorder and learning disabilities: booklet for the classroom teacher,* Summit, NJ, 1990, CIBA-Geigy.

Smitherman CH: A drug to ease attention deficit–hyperactivity disorder, *MCN* 15:365-, 1990.

Tirosh E and others: Effects of methylphenidate on sleep in children with attention-deficit hyperactivity disorder, *Am J Dis Child* 147:1313-1315, 1993.

Vatz RE, Weinberg LS: Treatment of attention-deficit hyperactivity disorder, *JAMA* 269 (18):2368, 1993.

Wolraich ML and others: Stimulant medication use by primary care physicians in the treatment of attention deficit hyperactivity disorder, *Pediatrics* 86(1):95-101, 1990.

Behavior Disorders

Adkins AS: Helping your patient cope with Tourette syndrome, *Pediatr Nurs* 15:135-137, 1989.

Barabas G: Tourette's syndrome: an overview, *Pediatr Ann* 17:391-393, 1988.

Brooks RB: Self-esteem during the school years, its normal development and hazardous decline, *Pediatr Clin North Am* 39(3):537-551, 1992.

Castiglia P: School phobias/school avoidance, *J Pediatr Health Care* 7(5):229-232, 1993.

Coleman WL, Lindsay RL: Interpersonal disabilities: social skill deficits in older children and adolescents, *Pediatr Clin North Am* 39:551-567, 1992.

Costello EJ, Shugart MA: Above and below the threshold: severity of psychiatric symptoms and functional impairment in a pediatric sample, *Pediatrics* 90:359-368, 1992.

Dolgan JI: Depression in children, *Pediatr Ann* 19:45-50, 1990.

Epstein M, Cullinan D: Depression in children, *J Sch Health* 56:10-12, 1986.

Erenberg G, Cruse RP, Rothner AD: The natural history of Tourette syndrome: a follow-up study, *Ann Neurol* 22:383-385, 1987.

Finney JW, Weist MD: Behavioral assessment of children and adolescents, *Pediatr Clin North Am* 39:369-378, 1992.

Garrison WT and others: Interactions between parents and pediatric primary care physicians about children's mental health, *Hosp Community Psychiatry* 43:489-493, May 1992.

Gartner JC: Recurrent abdominal pain—who needs a workup? *Contemp Pediatr* 6(9):62-82, 1989.

Gottlieb SE, Friedman SB: Conduct disorders in children and adolescents, *Pediatr Rev* 12(7):218-223, 1991.

Greenbaum S, Turner B, Stephens RD: *Set straight on bullies,* Malibu, CA, 1989, National School Safety Center.

Kenealy P: Children's strategies for coping with depression, *Behav Ther* 27:27-34, 1989.

Maisami M, Freeman JM: Conversion reactions in children as body language: a combined child psychiatry/neurology team approach to the management of functional neurologic disorders in children, *Pediatrics* 80:46-52, 1987.

McGrath PJ, Feldman W: Clinical approach to recurrent abdominal pain in children, *J Dev Behav Pediatr* 7:56-60, 1986.

Mitchell J, Varley C, McCauley E: Depression in children and adolescents, *Child Health Care* 16:290-293, 1988.

Nelms BC: Assessing childhood depression: do parents and children agree? *Pediatr Nurs* 12:23-26, 1986.

Niebuhr VN, Smith KE: Simple tests to assess behavior problems, *Contemp Pediatr* 7(1):117-138, 1990.

Page-Goertz S: Recurrent abdominal pain in children, *Issues Compr Pediatr Nurs* 11:179-191, 1988.

Pineiro-Carrero VM and others: Abnormal gastroduodenal motility in children and adolescents with recurrent functional abdominal pain, *J Pediatr* 113:820-825, 1988.

Porter E: The school nurse's role in school phobia, *Sch Nurse* 3(4):8-11, 1987.

Promoting emotional health—role of the nurse practitioner, *J Pediatr Health Care* 2:1-2, 1988.

Roddy SM: Bad habit, simple tic, or Tourette syndrome? *Contemp Pediatr* 6(11):22-36, 1989.

Sadler LS: Depression in adolescents: context, manifestations, and clinical management, *Nurs Clin North Am* 26(3):559-571, 1991.

Sadler LS: Adolescent depression, *J Sch Nurs* 9(1):12-19, 1993.

Sandler SB: What psychotropic drugs can—and can't—do for your patients, *Contemp Pediatr* 10(3):120-136, 1993.

Schmitt BD: School refusal, *Pediatr Rev* 8:99-101, 1986.

Simmons JE: When to refer to a child psychiatrist, *Contemp Pediatr* 4(2):77-94, 1987.

Solomon SD and others: Efficacy of treatment for posttraumatic stress disorder, *JAMA* 268(5):633-638, 1992.

Wyllie R, Kay M: Causes of recurrent abdominal pain, *Clin Pediatr* 32(6):369-371, 1993.

UNIT VII

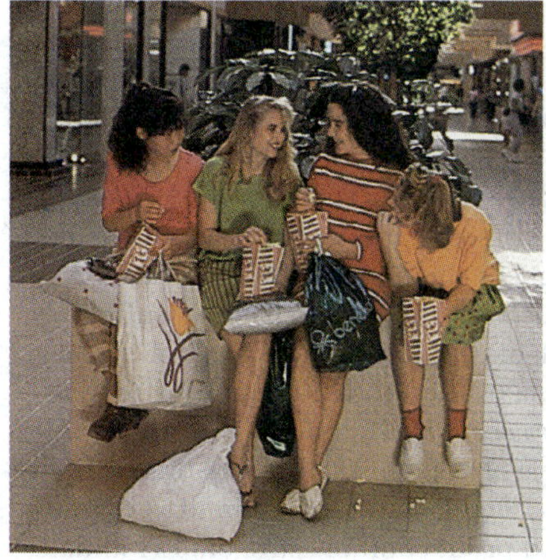

FAMILY-CENTERED CARE OF THE ADOLESCENT

CHAPTER 19 Health Promotion of the Adolescent and Family

CHAPTER OUTLINE

RELATED TOPICS

PROMOTING OPTIMUM GROWTH AND DEVELOPMENT

Adolescence is a period of transition between childhood and adulthood, a time of profound biologic, intellectual, psychosocial, and economic change. During this period individuals reach physical and sexual maturity, develop more sophisticated reasoning abilities, and make educational and occupational decisions that will shape their adult careers. The changes of adolescence have important implications for understanding the kinds of health risks to which young people are exposed, the health-enhancing and risk-taking behaviors in which they engage, and the major opportunities for health promotion among this population.

In the process of examining widely accepted theories of adolescent development, researchers have challenged many popular notions. For example, the belief was commonly held that teenagers' behaviors are overwhelmingly determined by "raging hormones" and that adolescence is a period when abnormal behavior is the norm. Both notions are misguided; furthermore, these misconceptions are not benign. They may have detrimental effects on attitudes and interactions with individual adolescents and on policy and program development of youth (U.S. Congress, 1991a). Although current research supports a more positive view of this life period, it also confirms that adolescence involves a complex interplay of biologic, cognitive, psychologic, and social change, *perhaps more so than at any other time of life.* Unfortunately, the United States as a society has provided little help to individuals as they try to cope with the normal changes of adolescence (U.S. Congress, 1991a).

Change during adolescence occurs on multiple levels. Individual level changes include biologic maturation, cognitive development, and psychologic development. Change also occurs in the social contexts of adolescents' families, peer groups, schools, and workplaces. Adolescence can be thought of as involving three distinct subphases: ***early adolescence*** (ages 11 to 14), ***middle adolescence*** (ages 15 to 17), and ***late adolescence*** (ages 18 to 20). The changes, opportunities, pressures, skills, and resources available to young people differ during these subphases. For example, early adolescence is characterized primarily by the changes of puberty and responses to those changes. Middle adolescence is characterized by transition to a dominant peer orientation, with all the stereotypical adolescent preoccupations of music, dress and appearance, language, and behavior. Late adolescence involves transitions into adulthood, including taking on adult work roles and developing adult relationships (Crockett and Petersen, 1993).

BIOLOGIC DEVELOPMENT

Neuroendocrine Events of Puberty

The fundamental biologic changes of adolescence are collectively referred to as ***puberty.*** Puberty involves a predictable sequence of hormonal and physical changes that occur universally over a defined period of time. It encompasses both sexual maturation and physical growth. It is generally accepted that the events of puberty are triggered by hormonal influences and are controlled by the anterior pituitary gland in response to a stimulus from the hypothalamus. Puberty begins as some not completely understood cluster of events triggers the production of ***gonadotropin-releasing hormone (GnRH)*** by the hypothalamus. GnRH travels through a network of capillaries to the anterior pituitary gland, where it stimulates the production and secretion of ***follicle-stimulating hormone (FSH)*** and ***lutenizing hormone (LH).*** Increasing levels of FSH and LH in the blood stimulate gonadal response. For females, FSH stimulates growth of ovarian follicles and production of estrogen. LH initiates ovulation, the formation of the corpus luteum, and progesterone production. For males, LH acts on testicular Leydig cells, prompting maturation of the testicles and testosterone production. FSH, acting with LH, stimulates sperm production. The sex steroids—estrogen, progesterone, testosterone and other androgens—are released from the gonads and effect biologic changes in various organs, including muscles, bones, skin, and hair follicles. Increasing serum levels of sex steroids also provide feedback to the hypothalamus, causing decreases in GnRH secretion. When serum sex hormone levels decrease, the hypothalamus is stimulated to increase GnRH secretion, again initiating the sequence that produces the appropriate gonadal responses (Fig. 19-1).

Initiation of Puberty. The precise mechanism that institutes the changes at puberty is not completely understood. Although the pituitary gland and gonads are capable of mature function and can respond to stimuli at any age, the ***hypothalamic-pituitary-gonadal system*** is maintained in a dormant state throughout childhood by some central ner-

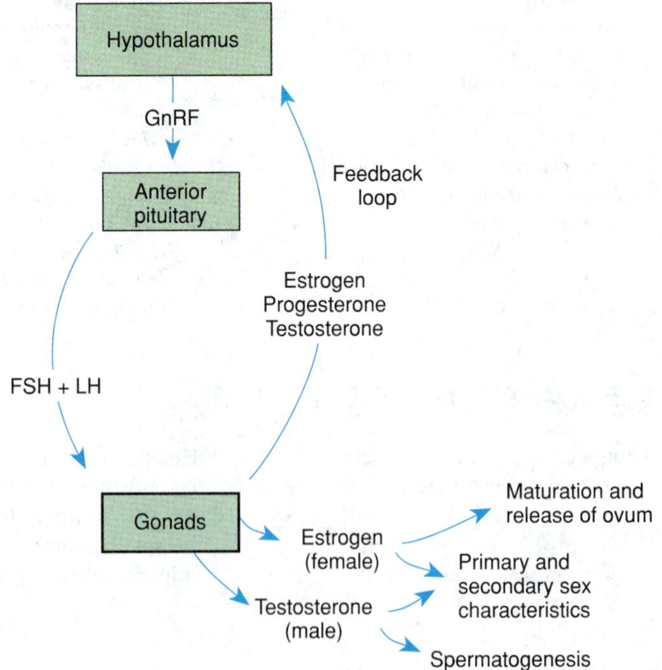

FIG. 19-1 Hormonal interaction between hypothalamus, pituitary, and gonads.

■ Renee E. Sieving, RN,C, MSN, PNP, assisted by Linda H. Bearinger, RN, MS, PhD, wrote this chapter.

vous system inhibitory mechanism in the region of the hypothalamus. It is believed that the receptor sites in the hypothalamus are so highly sensitive that the most minute quantities of circulating sex hormones are sufficient to inhibit the secretion of GnRH during childhood. The hypothalamus loses this negative sensitivity at puberty, which allows the hypothalamic-pituitary-gonadal mechanism to attain full secretory function. As puberty progresses, the pituitary and gonads become increasingly sensitive to positive hormonal stimulation (Comerci, 1987).

Changes in Reproductive Hormones

Females. The primary sex characteristic in females is the development and release of an egg, or ***ovum,*** from the ovaries approximately every 28 days. Beginning in ***early puberty,*** FSH stimulates estrogen production by the ovaries. However, concentrations of estrogen do not reach levels high enough to cause ovulation. By the time girls reach ***midpuberty,*** estrogen is generally produced in larger amounts. This quantity of estrogen production results in the building of an endometrial lining of the uterus and first menstruation, or ***menarche.*** At menarche, ova still do not generally mature enough to be released. However, as puberty continues to progress, one ovarian follicle becomes dominant during each menstrual cycle and produces increasing amounts of estrogen during the early-cycle, follicular phase. This follicle releases an ovum, a process termed ***ovulation,*** around day 14 of the menstrual cycle. After ovulation the follicle involutes and its estrogen production decreases; this leads to a drop in serum estrogen and progesterone. The pituitary gland responds to the drop in these hormone levels with increased production of FSH, initiating the start of a new menstrual cycle.

By direct action, estrogens cause growth and development of the vagina, uterus, and fallopian tubes. The skin of the labia majora, as well as that of the breast areola and nipples, grows and darkens under the influence of estrogen. Estrogen is responsible for breast enlargement. Estrogen also promotes the growth of pubic and axillary hair, pigmentation of genital skin, and widening of the hips. At low levels estrogen tends to stimulate skeletal growth in both boys and girls, but at higher levels it inhibits growth.

Males. The primary male sex characteristic is the development of viable sperm. During puberty FSH acts on testicular cells, which stimulates the production of viable sperm. FSH and LH also act on a different group of testicular cells, resulting in increased production and secretion of testosterone. In this process of sexual development, boys do not experience a discrete event analogous to menstruation or ovulation in girls. However, just as the production of a mature ovum tends to occur 1 year or more after menarche in girls, the production of viable sperm tends to follow boys' first ejaculations. The capacity to ejaculate appears relatively early in boys' sexual development, approximately 1 year after initial testicular enlargement and the appearance of pubic hair. From a clinical perspective, however, an adolescent should be considered potentially fertile with a first menstrual period or first ejaculation.

Testosterone and other androgens have a direct impact on growth of the penis, scrotum, prostate, and seminal vesicles of the testicles. The tremendous growth-promoting properties of these hormones also result in rapid increases in muscle mass, skeletal growth, bone age, and bone density. In both sexes androgens are responsible for the development of pubic, axillary, facial, and body hair. Clinically, increased activity of androgens is associated with pubertal conditions such as acne, body odor, deepening of the voice, a spurt in height, and an increase in red blood cell levels.

Pubertal Sexual Maturation

Increases in reproductive hormones are responsible for dramatic changes in secondary sexual characteristics that occur during puberty. As with general growth, development of secondary sexual characteristics occurs in a predictable sequence. This sequence has been divided into a series of five phases termed the ***Tanner stages*** (Figs. 19-2 through 19-6). While the sequence of sexual development is predictable, the ages at which these changes occur and the rate of developmental progression vary considerably among individuals. Over the course of pubescence, many young people have questions about the timing, rate, and normalcy of their body changes. These concerns provide nurses with a prime opportunity to discuss health-related topics such as puberty, sexuality, nutrition, exercise, and safe methods of weight control.

Sexual Maturation in Girls. In 4 out of 5 girls, changes in the nipple and areola and development of a small bud of breast tissue ***(thelarche)*** are the earliest, most easily visible changes of puberty. The average age of thelarche is 11 years, with a range of 9 to 13.5 years. The appearance of pubic hair ***(adrenarche)*** usually follows initial breast development by about 2 to 6 months; however, in a minority of normally developing girls, pubic hair may precede breast development. Early in puberty there is often an increase in normal vaginal discharge ***(physiologic leukor-***

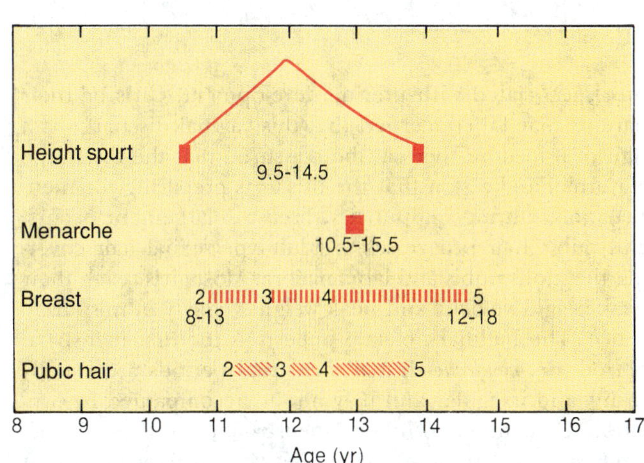

FIG. 19-2 Approximate timing of developmental changes in girls. Number indicates stages of development. Range of ages during which some of the changes occur is indicated by inclusive numbers below them. See Figs. 19-3 and 19-4 for explanation. (From Marshall WA, Tanner JM: *Arch Dis Child* 44:291, 1969.)

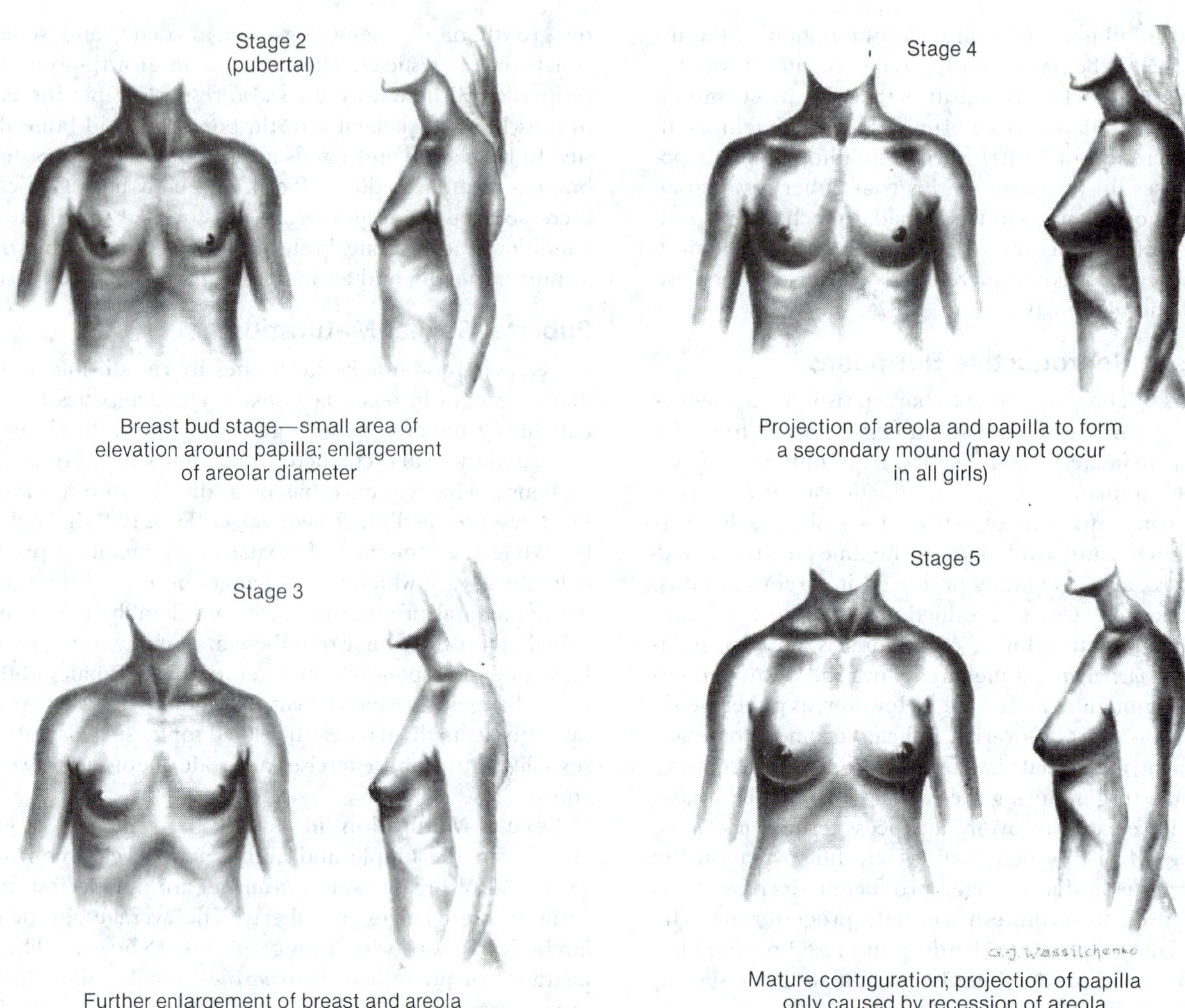

Stage 2
(pubertal)
Breast bud stage—small area of elevation around papilla; enlargement of areolar diameter
Stage 3
Further enlargement of breast and areola with no separation of their contours
Stage 4
Projection of areola and papilla to form a secondary mound (may not occur in all girls)
Stage 5
Mature configuration; projection of papilla only caused by recession of areola into general contour

FIG. 19-3 Development of the breast in girls—average age span, 11 to 13 years. Stage I (prepubertal—elevation of papilla only) is not shown. (Modified from Marshall WA, Tanner JM: *Arch Dis Child* 44:291, 1969; and Daniel WA, Paulshock BZ: *Patient Care*, pp 122-124, May 13, 1979.)

rhea), associated with uterine development. Girls or their parents may be concerned that this vaginal discharge is a sign of infection; they can be reassured that the discharge is normal and a sign that the uterus is preparing for menstruation. During midpuberty, breast enlargement occurs, and pubic hair progresses to adult-type sexual hair covering the mons pubis and labia majora. Most girls reach their peak height velocity and peak weight velocity in mispubescence. The hallmark of late puberty is the first menstrual period, or ***menarche.*** Initial menstrual periods are usually scanty and irregular and may not be accompanied by ovulation. Ovulation and regular menstrual periods usually begin 6 to 14 months after menarche. Menarche occurs about 2 years after the appearance of breast buds, approximately 9 months after attainment of peak height velocity and 3 months after attainment of peak weight velocity. The mean age of menarche in the United States is 12.8 years, with a normal age range of 10.5 to 15 years. Menarche has been related to a critical gain in body fat content, although this is controversial (Garn, LaVelle, and Pilkington, 1983). Girls may be considered to have ***pubertal delay*** if breast development has not occurred by age 13 or if menarche has not occurred within 4 years of the onset of breast development.

In the United States the mean age of menarche has gradually decreased over the past century, corresponding to population improvements in nutrition, sanitation, and control of infectious diseases. This decline in average age of menarche appears to have leveled off in recent years (Neinstein, 1991). Internationally, a decline in average age at first menses has not been seen in countries where individuals are more likely to be malnourished and suffer from chronic illness (Steinberg, 1989a).

Sexual maturation influences young peoples' satisfaction with their appearance, with the effects appearing to differ for girls and boys (Crockett and Petersen, 1993). For girls, physical maturation can lead to greater dissatisfaction with

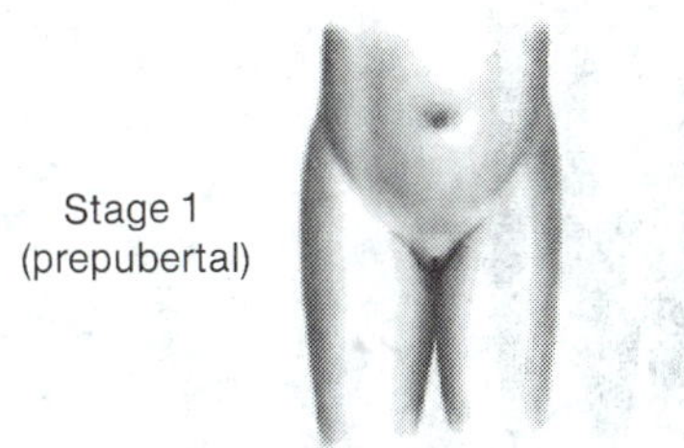

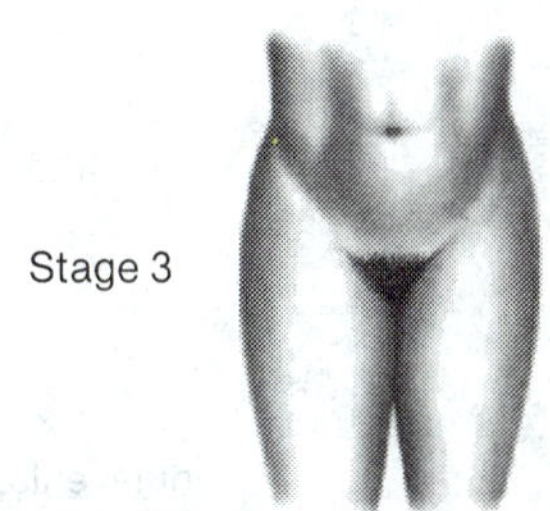

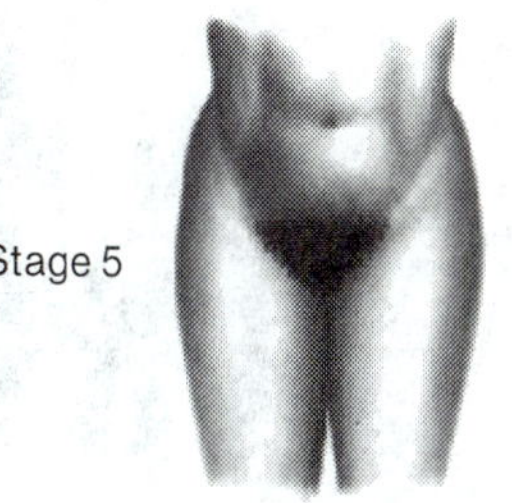

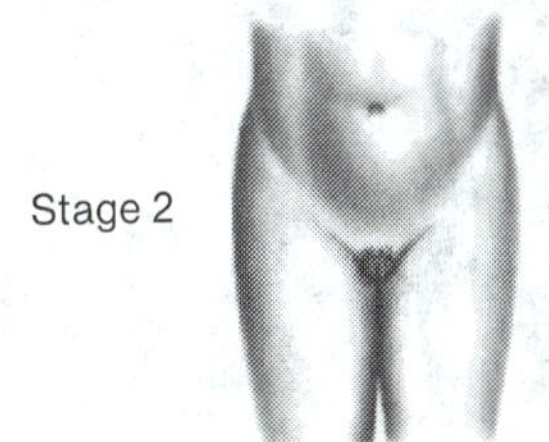

No pubic hair; essentially the same as during childhood; no distinction between hair on pubis and over the abdomen

Stage 2
Sparse growth of long, straight, downy, and slightly pigmented hair extending along labia; between stages 2 and 3 begins to appear on pubis

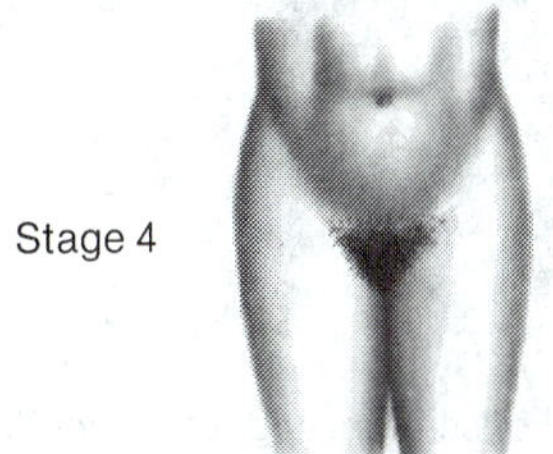

Stage 4
Pubic hair denser, curled, and adult in distribution but less abundant and restricted to the pubic area

FIG. 19-4 Growth in pubic hair in girls—average age span for stages 2 through 5, 11 to 14 years. (Modified from Marshall WA, Tanner JM: *Arch Dis Child* 44:291, 1969; and Daniel WA, Paulshock BZ: *Patient Care,* pp 122-124, May 13, 1979.)

their appearance (Dorn, Crockett, and Petersen, 1988). For example, one recent student found that one fourth of seventh through twelfth grade girls reported being satisfied with their weight as compared with one half of boys (Blum and others, 1989). Normal increases in weight and fat deposition that accompany puberty among girls conflict with cultural norms that emphasize a slender look (Faust, 1983). Early-maturing girls suffer most because they begin to develop at a time when their age-mates still exemplify prepubertal slimness (Crockett and Petersen, 1993). Unfortunately, an all-too-common response to changes in body shape among teenage girls is to engage in extensive dieting at a time when nutritional requirements are at a peak. For some, the focus on slimness and dieting may trigger the development of eating disorders (Attie, Brooks-Gunn, and Petersen, 1990; see Chapter 21). Consequently, health promotion efforts related to pubertal growth, eating behaviors, and body image are important for adolescent girls, especially early-maturing girls.

Sexual Maturation in Boys. The first pubescent changes in boys are testicular enlargement accompanied by thinning, reddening, and increased looseness of the scrotum. These events usually occur between 9.5 and 14 years of age. Early puberty is also characterized by the initial appearance of pubic hair. Penile enlargement begins, and testicular enlargement and pubic hair growth continue throughout midpuberty. During this period there is also increasing muscularity, early voice changes, and development of early facial hair. Temporary breast enlargement and ten-

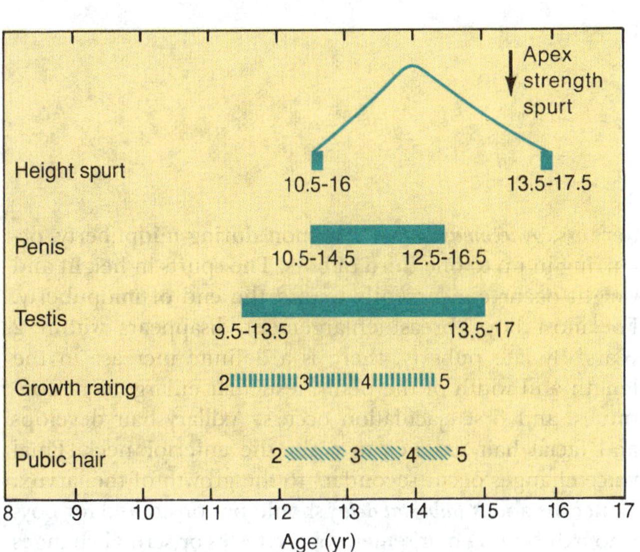

FIG. 19-5 Approximate timing of developmental changes in boys. Numbers indicate stages of development. Range of ages during which some of the changes occur is indicated by inclusive numbers below them. (See Fig. 19-6 for explanation. (From Marshall WA, Tanner JM: *Arch Dis Child* 45:13, 1970.)

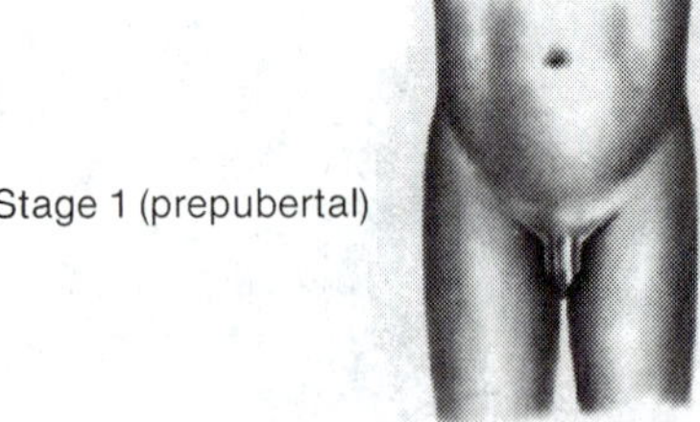

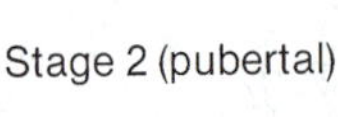
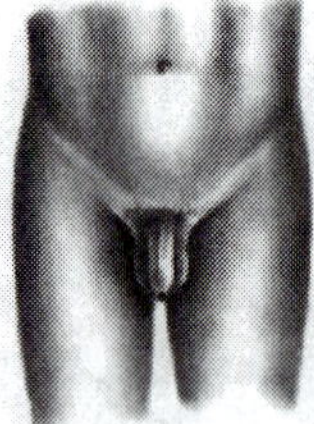

No pubic hair; essentially the same as during childhood; no distinction between hair on pubis and over the abdomen

Stage 2 (pubertal)
Initial enlargement of scrotum and testes; reddening and textural changes of scrotal skin; sparse growth of long, straight, downy, and slightly pigmented hair at base of penis
Stage 3
Initial enlargement of penis, mainly in length; testes and scrotum further enlarged; hair darker, coarser, and curly and spread sparsely over entire pubis

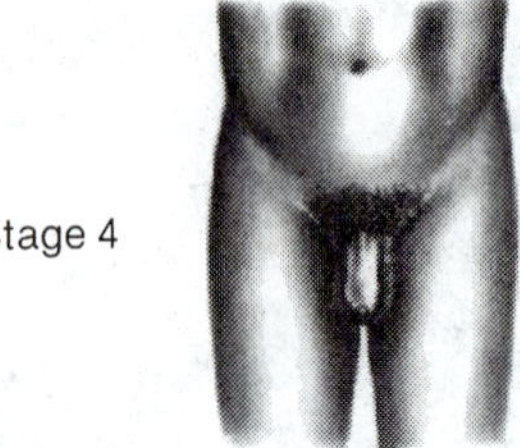

Stage 4
Increased size of penis with growth in diameter and development of glans; glans larger and broader; scrotum darker; pubic hair more abundant with curling but restricted to pubic area

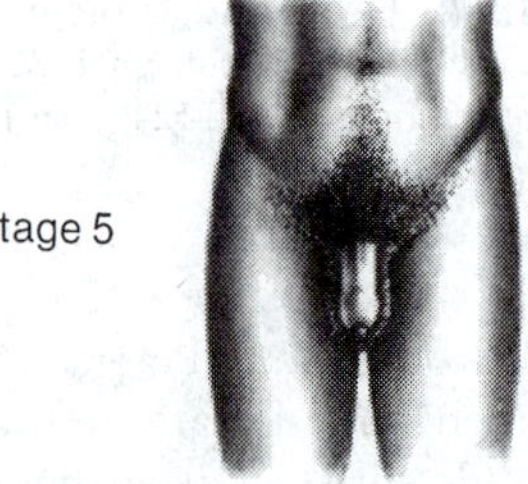

Stage 5
Testes, scrotum, and penis adult in size and shape; hair adult in quantity and type with spread to inner surface of thighs

FIG. 19-6 Developmental stages of secondary sex characteristics and genital development in boys—average age span, 12 to 16 years. (Modified from Marshall WA, Tanner JM: *Arch Dis Child* 45:13, 1970; and Daniel WA, Paulshock BZ: *Patient Care,* pp 122-124, May 13, 1979.)

derness, ***gynecomastia,*** are common during midpuberty, occurring in up to one third of boys. The spurts in height and weight occur concurrently toward the end of midpuberty. For most boys, breast enlargement disappears within 2 years. By late puberty, there is a definite increase in the length and width of the penis, testicular enlargement continues, and first ejaculation occurs. Axillary hair develops and facial hair extends to cover the anterior neck. Final voice changes occur secondary to the growth of the larynx. Concerns about ***pubertal delay*** should be considered for boys who exhibit no enlargement of the testes or scrotal changes by ages 13.5 to 14, or if genital growth is not complete 4 years after the testicles begin to enlarge.

Changes in the size and shape of the penis and testicles and changes in genital functioning can be areas of great concern for adolescent boys. Although the ability for penile erection is present at birth, only with pubertal maturation do boys have seminal emissions. Ejaculation may occur spontaneously as a nocturnal emission or "wet dream," as a result of self-stimulation, or during sexual activity with others. Unless they are prepared in advance, spontaneous ejaculations are frequently puzzling, troublesome, and embarrassing events for boys. Pubertal changes and related concerns create important opportunities for health promotion among young teenage boys. Health care professionals can be a resource for boys and provide appropriate information and guidance around issues related to sexual maturation.

Physical Growth During Puberty

Along with increases in reproductive hormones and sexual maturation, major changes in skeletal and lean body mass occur during puberty. The final 20% to 25% of linear growth is achieved during puberty, and up to 50% of ideal adult body weight is gained during this time as well. The pubertal ***growth spurt*** refers to the general increase in growth of the skeleton, muscles, and internal organs, which reaches a peak rate at about 12 years of age in girls and at about 14 years of age in boys. Although accelerated growth occurs in all adolescents, the age of onset, duration, and

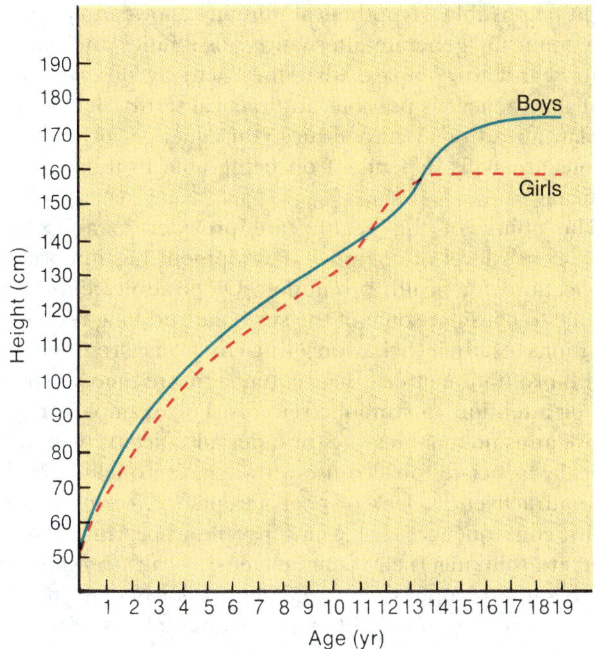

FIG. 19-7 Linear growth throughout childhood. (From Tanner JM, Whitehouse RH, Takaishi M: *Arch Dis Child* 41:454-471, 1966.)

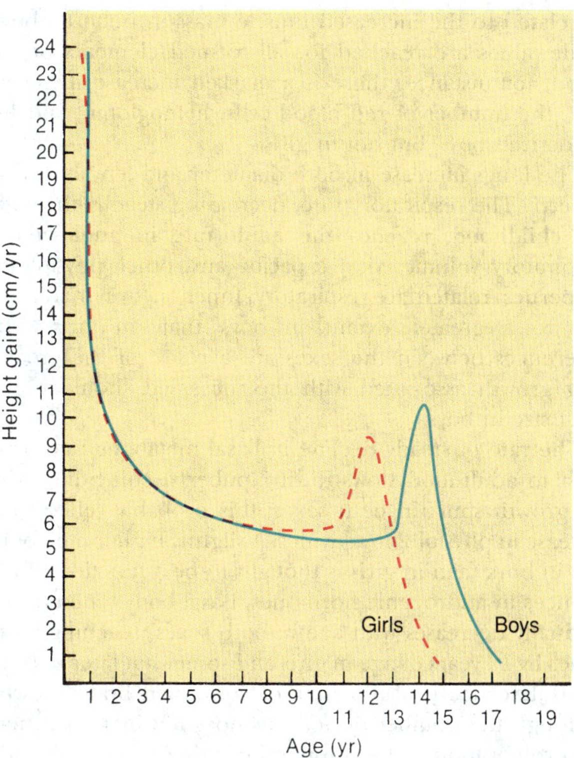

FIG. 19-8 Linear growth in centimeters per year. (From Tanner JM, Whitehouse RH, Takaishi M: *Arch Dis Child* 41:454-471, 1966.)

extent vary among individuals. Genetic endowment is the most important determinant of the onset, rate, and duration of pubertal growth.

Normal Patterns of Growth. Once the process of growth begins, the sequence of changes is progressive and usually predictable. Awareness of this sequence is not only important for reassuring concerned adolescents and parents, but it is also useful in diagnosing conditions associated with abnormal growth. In general, girls begin puberty and reach maturity about 1½ to 2 years earlier than boys. The pubertal growth spurt begins as early as 9½ years or as late as 14½ years in girls, and as early as 10½ years and as late as 16 years in boys.

General growth includes accumulation of body mass, along with increases in height and weight. ***Lean body mass,*** primarily muscle mass, increases in both girls and boys during early puberty. For girls, the rate of muscle mass growth peaks at menarche and then slows. For boys, muscle mass continues to increase throughout puberty, resulting in the attainment of significantly higher lean body mass in boys than in girls. In girls, gain in ***fat mass*** increases markedly early in puberty and continues to increase following menarche. In boys, there is a peak deceleration in the rate of fat mass accumulation at the time of their growth spurt, and thereafter a slower and much less dramatic increase than in girls.

The rate of ***linear growth*** (height) (Figs. 19-7 and 19-8) begins to increase in girls during early puberty, while in boys the rate does not increase until midpuberty. ***Peak height velocity (PHV)*** occurs at about 12 years of age in girls, around 6 to 12 months before menarche. PHV is used as a predictor of menarche; height at menarche is a predictor of ultimate adult height. Very few girls grow more than 2 inches in height following menarche. Growth in girls' height usually ceases 2 to 2½ years after menarche. Boys typically reach peak height velocity at about 14 years of age, following growth of the testicles and penis and the appearance of axillary and mature pubic hair. Among most boys, growth in height ceases at 18 or 20 years of age. Increases in leg length tend to precede growth of the trunk by about 6 to 9 months and that of the shoulders and chest by about 1 year. In short, teenagers tend to follow a linear growth pattern in which they outgrow their shoes first, then their pants, and finally their shirts. ***Peak weight velocity*** occurs about 6 months after PHV in girls. In contrast, weight and height spurts occur simultaneously for boys. On average, girls will gain 5 to 20 cm (2 to 8 inches) in height and 7 to 25 kg (15 to 55 pounds) in weight during adolescence, and boys will gain 10 to 30 cm (4 to 12 inches) in height and 7 to 30 kg (15 to 65 pounds) in weight during adolescence.

Other Physiologic Changes

In addition to the characteristic changes of puberty already discussed, numerous others occur. The size and strength of the heart, blood volume, and systolic blood pressure increase, whereas the heart rate decreases. Consistent with the general developmental timetable, these changes appear earlier in girls, who establish a slightly higher pulse rate and a slightly lower systolic blood pressure than boys. Blood volume, which has increased steadily during childhood, reaches higher levels in boys than in girls, a fact that may be related to the increased muscle mass in pubertal boys. Adult values are reached for all formed elements of the blood; for instance, there is a marked increase in serum iron, the number of red blood cells, hemoglobin, and hematocrit in boys, but not in girls.

The lungs increase in both diameter and length during puberty. The respiratory rate, decreasing steadily throughout childhood, reaches the adult rate in adolescence. Respiratory volume, vital capacity, and other physiologic properties related to respiratory function are increased, and to a greater extent in boys than in girls. The differences between the sexes are a result of the greater lung growth associated with the increased shoulder and chest size in boys.

The rate of steady decline in basal metabolic rate from birth to adulthood slows during puberty, coinciding with the growth spurt in both sexes; this probably reflects the increase in physiologic activities. A slightly higher metabolic rate in boys than in girls is thought to be a function of differences in androgenic hormones. Basal body temperature gradually decreases with age in both sexes, reaching adult values by 12 years of age in girls and somewhat later in boys.

Adolescence is also a time of continued brain growth. Although the number of neurons does not increase, there is a proliferation of the support cells that brace and nourish the neurons. In addition, the growth of the myelin sheath around the nerve cells continues at least until puberty, enabling faster neural processing. This "fine tuning" of the neural system coincides with development of the more advanced cognitive capacities of youth (Graber and Petersen, 1991).

COGNITIVE DEVELOPMENT

Emergence of Formal Operational Thought (Piaget)

Jean Piaget (1972) described the shift from childhood to adolescence as a movement from concrete to formal operational thought. Children's thinking is oriented to things and events that they can observe directly. Unable to think in terms of abstract possibilities, they process information based on what is directly observable. For most young people, emergence of ***formal operational thinking*** occurs between the ages of 11 and 14. Formal operational thought includes being able to think in abstract terms, think about possibilities, and think through hypotheses. Youth become able to think about abstractions; thus they can symbolically associate behaviors with abstract concepts such as attractiveness, adult status, or happiness (Steinberg, 1991). Adolescents also become capable of using a future time perspective rather than being tied to the here-and-now thinking of childhood (Greene, 1986). They are able to imagine possibilities, such as a sequence of future events that might occur, including college or occupational opportunities, or how current situations, such as relationships with parents or friends, could change to meet an imagined ideal. Hypothetical reasoning is aligned with thinking about possibilities. To think through hypotheses, one needs to see beyond what is directly observable and reason in terms of what might be possible. Hypothetical thinking allows adolescents to systemically generate alternative possibilities and explanations and to compare what they actually observe with what they believe is possible. In practical terms, being able to plan ahead or identify future consequences of possible actions are skills dependent on being able to think hypothetically.

The ability of the health care provider to assess an adolescent's level of cognitive development has important implications for health promotion. Older adolescents may be able to consider some of the symbolic and long-term implications of their behaviors; thus they may respond to health promotion efforts that require a future time perspective or attention to symbolic rewards. For example, an effective antismoking message for older adolescents may symbolically associate tobacco use with negative qualities such as unattractiveness, lack of peer acceptance, or long-term health consequences. For young people who primarily use concrete thinking (i.e., younger teens), health promotion efforts should emphasize immediate risks or benefits of the behavior. For example, although younger adolescents may be unable to comprehend the long-range consequences of smoking, they can appreciate some of the short-term consequences of cigarette use, including resulting bad breath or the cost of purchasing cigarettes.

Along with cognitive development, decision-making abilities increase over the adolescent period. Young people develop the ability to consider hypothetical risks and benefits of possible behaviors, along with potential consequences of such behaviors. In addition, the likelihood of teenagers consulting with adult experts, mentors, and role models increases over the junior and senior high school years (Lewis, 1981). By middle adolescence, most teenagers are able to reason as well as adults; likewise, they demonstrate reasoning flaws similar to those of adults (Kuhn, Amsel, and O'Loughlin, 1988). Health promotion efforts, especially those aimed at younger adolescents, should offer learning strategies that enhance decision-making skills. Such efforts might include discussions emphasizing health-promoting norms for behavior among young people and alternatives to unhealthy behaviors, as well as practicing skills necessary to resist unhealthy behaviors (Perry and Kelder, 1992).

Even with the best framework for health promotion, persons who are capable of formal operational thought and reasoned decision making do not use these processes all the time. In the face of time pressures, overriding personal stress, or overwhelming peer pressures, young people are more likely to abandon rational thought processes (Keating and Clark, 1986). Thoughts about unfamiliar or emotionally arousing topics also tend to be less sophisticated and more vulnerable to the effects of stresses and pressures (Linn, 1983). Unfortunately, many of the health-related decisions adolescents confront, such as those related to substance use or sexual behavior, involve issues that are personally stressful, emotion laden, or new (Hamburg, 1986). Under such conditions, people, including those who typically use advanced decision-making skills, tend not to use their capacities for abstract formal reasoning.

Adolescent Conceptions of Self

With development of formal operational thought, adolescents become able to describe the self more abstractly. Compared with children, they are more psychologic in their self-descriptions, focusing on personal and interpersonal characteristics, beliefs, and emotional states. They also develop a more differentiated self-concept, recognizing that their behavior and performance vary from setting to setting. With time, they become able to integrate these disparate observation of self into abstract personal characterizations (e.g., "I am a sensitive person") (Harter, 1990).

Psychologist David Elkind (1978) points out that the intellectual advances of adolescence may occasionally result in problems for young people, particularly before they adjust to having such powerful cognitive tools. Being able to think about one's own thoughts and emotions may lead to periods of extreme self-absorption—a form of ***adolescent egocentrism.*** Adolescent egocentrism leads to two patterns of thinking that help to explain some of the health-related beliefs and behaviors of youth. The first, the ***imaginary audience,*** involves having such a heightened sense of self-consciousness that an adolescent imagines that everyone is focused on his or her behavior. For example, a teen who is diabetic may worry about injecting insulin at school because "everybody will notice." The second pattern of thinking, called the ***personal fable,*** is the belief that one's feelings and experiences are completely unique. For example, a sexually active adolescent may choose not to use condoms, truly believing that "other people can get sexually transmitted diseases, but not me," or an adolescent who has been drinking may choose to drive home after a party, believing that he or she could never be involved in a car crash.

Changes in Social Cognition

Gains in cognitive abilities also have an impact on perspective-taking capacities of young people. Adolescents are better able than children to "step into the shoes" of others. During elementary school, children begin to realize that other people have thoughts and feelings; however, they have difficulty understanding that what affects their own thoughts and feelings can also influence the thoughts and feelings of others. Preadolescents develop limited perspective-taking skills, first learning to step into the shoes of best friends, then peers and family members, and finally people of other ages and backgrounds. However, perspective-taking capacities develop further during adolescence. According to Robert Selman (1976), an adolescent becomes able to engage in ***mutual role taking.*** In other words, teens can both understand the perspectives of others and see how the thoughts or actions of one person can influence those of others. Role-taking capabilities continue to expand throughout adolescence. Older teens are able to understand that people's perspectives are influenced by their social roles, as well as by their cultural and ethnic backgrounds. They are able to discuss various issues highlighting points of importance to people in various social roles (e.g., "From a parent's perspective, having a curfew is important because . . ."). Older adolescents also realize that the perspectives people hold are complicated in that they are influenced by a range of intrapersonal, interpersonal, and sociocultural factors. Ultimately, gains in perspective-taking skills that take place during adolescence lead to increased capacity to learn from the experiences of others. Older adolescents are able to consider the choices, behaviors, and outcomes experienced by others in making their own health-related choices. This newfound capacity significantly expands the opportunities to learn health-promoting behaviors, in that once perspective-taking skills reach this point, young people can learn from their own experiences, as well as from the life experiences of others.

DEVELOPMENT OF VALUE AUTONOMY

With advances in cognitive development, adolescents' beliefs become more abstract and increasingly rooted in general ideologic principles. At the same time, young people are gaining increasing emotional independence from parents, relying less on their parents' beliefs and values than they did as children. Adolescents also progress toward greater behavioral independence, encountering situations and decisions they have not previously experienced. With these new capacities and experiences, young people face a variety of cognitive conflicts caused by having to compare the advice of parents and friends and having to deal with competing pressures to behave in given ways. These conflicts may prompt young people to consider, in serious and thoughtful terms, what it is that they themselves really believe. Whereas earlier in life they may have merely accepted the decisions or points of view of adults, adolescents begin to substitute a set of values distinct from those of significant adults in their lives. This struggle to clarify values, created in part by an expanded behavioral independence, is a large part of the process of developing a sense of what has been termed ***value autonomy*** (Steinberg, 1989b). The development of a personal value system is a gradual process, with evidence that value autonomy occurs relatively late in adolescence, between the ages of 18 and 20 (Steinberg, 1989b). Moral reasoning and religious beliefs represent two important aspects of value autonomy that evolve during adolescence.

Moral Development

Moral development parallels advances in reasoning and social cognition. With the attainment of abstract thought and the realization that people's perspectives and opinions may differ, the ways adolescents approach moral issues change. According to one theory of moral development (Kohlberg and Gilligan, 1972), older children and young adolescents function at a ***conventional level of moral reasoning*** in which absolute moral guidelines are seen to emanate from authorities such as parents or teachers. Thus judgments of right and wrong are made according to a set of concrete rules. A major concern is to act or behave in ways that will gain or maintain the approval of others. The correctness of society's rules is not questioned—one "does one's duty" by upholding and respecting the social order.

Elements of ***principled moral reasoning*** emerge during adolescence. With this level of reasoning, absolutes and rules come to be questioned as moral standards are seen as subjective and based on points of view that are subject to disagreement. One may have a moral duty to abide by social standards for behavior—but only insofar as those standards support and serve human ends. Thus occasions arise in which social conventions ought to be questioned and when principles such as justice, caring, or quality of life take precedence over established social norms. Empirical research on Kohlberg's theory has demonstrated that aspects of both conventional and principled reasoning are present during adolescence, and different levels of reasoning are used at different times and in different situations (Steinberg, 1989a). James Rest and his colleagues (1978) have shown that the use of principled moral reasoning increases over the course of adolescence, whereas the use of conventional reasoning decreases. During the high school years the proportion of principled responses given by subjects in their studies increased from about 25% to about 33%, and in late adolescence and early adulthood to about 45%.

Kohlberg's scheme of moral development focuses on an orientation to justice. This orientation holds as its ideal a morality based on reciprocity and equal respect. From this orientation the most important consideration in making moral decisions would be whether the individuals involved were treated "fairly" by the ultimate decision. Gilligan (1982) proposes that an equally valid alternative to the justice orientation is one that emphasizes caring. From this perspective, the ideal is a morality of attention to others and responses to human need. As opposed to the justice orientation, which assumes that moral decisions are best made from a detached position of "objectivity," the caring orientation is rooted in the belief that our moral decisions should be shaped by our attachments and our responsiveness to others. Studies (Gilligan, 1986; Walker, de Vries, and Trevethan, 1987) have found that while both men and women are capable of approaching moral problems from the perspectives of justice and caring, women may be more likely to give caring-oriented responses before justice-oriented ones, whereas men are more likely to follow the opposite pattern.

Spiritual Development

Religious beliefs also become more abstract and principled during the adolescent years. Specifically, adolescents' beliefs become more oriented toward spiritual and ideologic matters and less oriented toward rituals, practice, and the strict observance of religious customs (Wuthnow and Glock, 1973). For example, although 87% of all adolescents pray and 95% believe in God, 60% report that organized religion does not play a very important role in their lives (Farel, 1982). Compared with children, adolescents place more emphasis on the internal aspects of religious commitment, such as what a person believes, and less on the external manifestations, such as whether an individual goes to church (Elkind, 1978).

Generally speaking, the stated importance of participation in organized religion declines somewhat during the adolescent years. More high school students than post–secondary school young people attend church regularly; and, not surprisingly, the younger the adolescents, the more likely they are to view religion as being important to them. Among older adolescents there is more decline in the importance of organized religion among college students than among young people not in college. Late adolescence appears to be a time when individuals reexamine and reevaluate many of the beliefs and values of their childhood. Consistent with developmental changes in the value autonomy, the religious beliefs of young people are likely to become more personalized and less bound to the traditional religious practices they may have been exposed to when they were younger (Steinberg, 1989a).

Although religious cults and dramatic religious conversion have attracted a great deal of attention in the popular media, they remain rare phenomena among American adolescents and often reflect nonreligious concerns. Membership in a religious cult is often associated with a preceding period of psychologic stress, identity diffusion, rootlessness, and dissatisfaction with mainstream societal values (Conger, 1977).

PSYCHOSOCIAL DEVELOPMENT

Identity Development

The task of identity formation is to develop a stable, coherent picture of oneself that includes integrating one's past and present experiences with a sense of where one is headed in the future. Before adolescence the child's identity is like pieces of a puzzle scattered about on a table. Both cognitive development and social situations encountered during adolescence push individuals to combine puzzle pieces—to reflect on their place in society, on the way others view them, and on their options for the future (Steinberg, 1989a). For most individuals, puzzle pieces first form a coherent whole sometime during late adolescence and early adulthood. Erik Erikson, one of the most influential theorists in the area of psychosocial development, describes identity achievement as one of the main psychosocial tasks of the adolescent years. According to Erikson (1968), "from among all possible and imaginable relations (the adolescent) must make a series of ever-narrowing selections of personal, occupational, sexual, and ideological commitments."

Social forces play a large role in shaping an adolescent's sense of self. Erikson (1968) argues that the key to identity achievement lies in adolescents' interactions with others. The people with whom a young person interacts serve as mirrors that reflect information back to the adolescent about who she or he is and who she or he ought to be. During the period of identity formation, adolescents also learn from others what it is they ought to keep doing and what it is they ought not to do. Society also plays an important role in determining the range of available alternatives open to young people involved in identity formation. Optimally, adolescents have opportunities to explore a range of possible options related to ideologic, occupational, and interpersonal roles before having to make identity commitments (Crockett and Petersen, 1993).

Progress toward identity achievement can be measured by the status of personal commitments in occupational, social, and ideologic domains. The status of personal commitments has four proposed levels: achievement, moratorium, foreclosure, and diffusion (Marcia, 1966). Individuals who demonstrate ***identity achievement*** have established a coherent identity after actively exploring possible alternatives; individuals currently engaged in this exploration are in ***moratorium. Foreclosure*** refers to making identity commitments without a period of exploration or experimentation, and identity ***diffusion*** refers to a lack of firm identity commitments, along with a lack of effort to make those commitments. Research suggests that individuals progress from diffusion to moratorium to identity achievement, or alternatively from diffusion to foreclosure, during the adolescent years (Crockett and Petersen, 1993).

As suggested above, the experiences and opportunities within one's social environment can impact both the content of identity and progression toward identity achievement (Ianni, 1989). Research on identity development among minority adolescents has shown that identity foreclosure is more common among these adolescents than among teenagers from the majority culture, perhaps because of restricted opportunities to explore alternative roles. Identity diffusion also appears to be more common among minority males than among other groups. Spencer and Markstrom-Adams (1990) suggest several barriers to identity formation among minority youth. These include conflicting values between the minority reference group and the broader society, a lack of adult role models who exemplify positive ethnic identity, and inadequate preparation for the stereotyping and prejudice that are frequently experienced.

Development of Autonomy

Becoming an autonomous, self-governing person is another of the fundamental psychosocial tasks of adolescence. Autonomy includes emotional, cognitive, and behavioral components. Cognitive, or value, autonomy is discussed earlier in this chapter. The following discussion focuses on ***emotional autonomy,*** that aspect of independence related to changes in an individual's close relationships, and ***behavioral autonomy,*** the capacity to make independent decisions and follow through with them. Generally, emotional and behavioral autonomy are likely to surface as psychosocial concerns somewhat earlier during adolescence than value autonomy, which usually does not become a prominent concern until middle or late adolescence.

Individuals generally begin the process of emotional autonomy during early adolescence by becoming more emotionally independent from their parents but less separate from their friends (Steinberg and Silverberg, 1986). In the process of separating from their parents, younger adolescents often shift a portion of their emotional ties to other adults, often developing "crushes" on teachers, coaches, nationally known media figures, or the parent of a best friend. By the end of adolescence, individuals are far less emotionally dependent on their parents than they were as children. This emotional autonomy can be seen in several ways. First, older adolescents do not generally rush to their parents when they are worried or upset. Second, they no longer see their parents as all-knowing or all-powerful. Third, teenagers often have increasing amounts of emotional energy invested in relationships outside of their families. Finally, older adolescents are able to see and interact with their parents as people—not just as their parents (Steinberg, 1989b).

As adolescents increasingly find themselves in situations where adults are not present and where they must make decisions and take responsibility for their own actions, the extent to which they are capable of independent decision making and autonomous behavior takes on added importance. An individual who is behaviorally autonomous is able to turn to others for advice when it is appropriate, weigh alternative courses of action based on his or her own judgment and the suggestions of others, and reach an independent conclusion about how to behave (Hill and Holmbeck, 1986). Behavioral autonomy includes the ability to make independent decisions based on one's own choices rather than conforming to the opinions of others. Decision-making abilities improve over the adolescent years, with older adolescents being more likely than younger adolescents to be aware of risks involved with a particular decision, consider future consequences, turn to "experts" for advice, and realize when vested interests may influence the advice of others (Lewis, 1981). Conformity to parents' opinions declines during early adolescence; however, conformity to peer influence increases during this time, peaking at around age 14 (Steinberg and Silverberg, 1986). During middle and late adolescence, conformity to *both* parents and peers declines, allowing for genuine behavioral autonomy (Steinberg, 1989b). Subjective feelings of self-reliance increase steadily over the adolescent years, and, contrary to popular notion, adolescent girls consistently report feeling more self-reliant than adolescent boys (Steinberg and Silverberg, 1986).

Also, in contrast to popular stereotypes, the development of autonomy during adolescence does not typically involve rebellion, nor is it usually accompanied by strained or tense family relationships. Especially in households where guidelines for adolescent behavior are clear and consistently enforced, where changes in guidelines are open to discussion, and where an atmosphere of interpersonal warmth, concern, and fairness exists, family relationships nurture a gradual and smooth maturational process over the course of the adolescent years. Problems in the development of autonomy are often understandable reactions to excessively controlling circumstances or to growing up in the absence of clear standards (Baumrind, 1991). In addition to dispelling the myths that major parent-child conflicts and adolescent rebellion are essential to the development of autonomy, research has shown that parent and peer influences are not necessarily opposing forces but can play complementary roles in the development of a healthy degree of individual independence.

Achievement

Another set of psychosocial tasks encountered during adolescence centers around achievement. Broadly speaking, achievement concerns the development of motives, capabilities, interests, and behaviors related to performance in evaluative situations. The study of the development of achievement during adolescence has focused almost exclusively on young people's performance in educational settings and on the development and implementation of plans for future scholastic and occupational careers. A variety of theories have attempted to explain why some young people, more than others, achieve at higher levels in school (Steinberg, 1989a). Some have focused on differences in individuals' motivations to succeed. Others have examined young people's beliefs about success and failure. Still others have pointed to differences in adolescents' opportunities for success and to the roles of important adults and peers in their lives. Various indicators of achievement are highly interrelated. For example, success in school during the early elementary years leads to later success in school; doing well in school generally leads to higher levels of educational attainment, which in turn lead to more challenging forms of employment with greater earning power.

Although there are distinct differences, the actual process leading toward occupational achievement can be a lengthy one in contemporary society. Because, for many, career options have expanded and changed so dramatically, and because increasing numbers of individuals enter college after completing high school, many adolescents do not decide on a career until well into early adulthood.

An extensive literature (e.g., Conger, 1977) documents the relationship between social class and both educational and occupational achievement. One of the most significant problems facing those interested in promoting achievement during adolescence concerns socioeconomic disparities in educational and occupational achievement. Beginning in early childhood, through no action of their own, many individuals find themselves on an educational course that directs them toward low levels of academic achievement, curtailed schooling, and limited occupational mobility. They reach adulthood with little hope and few dreams for their future. Understanding how this course is set in motion and identifying factors that help individuals from economically disadvantaged backgrounds to succeed despite tremendous odds are necessary steps in building interventions that promote the development and health of young people from lower socioeconomic populations (Schorr and Schorr, 1988).

Sexuality

Human sexuality involves a combination of genital sex and sexual behavior, as well as physical, cognitive, emotional, and spiritual aspects of personality that contribute to communication, relationships, self-help, and pleasuring skills (Greydanus, Demarest, and Sears, 1985). Adolescence represents a critical time in the development of sexuality. Hormonal, physical, cognitive, and social changes that occur during adolescence all have an impact on sexual development.

Of all the developmental changes that affect adolescent sexuality, perhaps none is more obvious than the impact of puberty. Adolescents must come to terms with hormonal influences, physiologic manifestations such as menstruation and ejaculation, and physical changes such as breast and genital development. All of these changes have a profound impact on the way teenagers perceive their bodies (i.e., ***body image***). In addition to transitions in body image, increasing levels of pubertal hormones have been shown to contribute to increased levels of sexual motivation among both boys and girls (Udry and Billy, 1987; Udry and others, 1985). Higher hormone levels have also been associated with sexual behavior among boys (Udry and others, 1985). Evidence also suggests that early development of secondary sex characteristics is associated with early sexual activity. For example, studies have shown that early-maturing girls begin dating earlier and initiate sexual intercourse at younger ages than same-age peers (Simmons and others, 1979). Even when physical development occurs at an average onset and pace, the degree to which adolescents feel comfortable with their bodies may affect sexual behaviors (Grant and Demetriou, 1988).

Changes in sexual motivations and feelings, happening at the same time as shifts in cognitive skills, contribute to painful conjectures ("Is what I'm feeling normal?"), self-conscious concern ("Am I good-looking enough?"), and hypothetical thinking ("What if she wants to have sex?"). The emergence of formal operational thinking also increases adolescents' decision-making capabilities around sexual issues. As they mature, teens become better able to think through potential risks and benefits of sexual behaviors before they engage in any behavior. Older adolescents may also be able to conceptualize more long-term consequences of present behaviors. One of the important tasks of adolescence is to incorporate sexuality successfully into close, intimate relationships (Sullivan, 1953). This task is made possible by the advanced cognitive abilities that emerge over the course of adolescence.

Part of adolescent identity formation involves the development of ***sexual identity***. As they begin to integrate changes involved with puberty, young adolescents also develop emotional and social identities separate from their families. For young adolescents, the process of sexual identity development usually involves forming close friendships with same-sex peers with whom they may experiment sexually, often to satisfy curiosity. Sexual activity among young teens varies by gender. Masturbation provides an opportunity for sexual self-exploration; participation in this behavior is influenced by learned cultural attitudes, as well as sex-role expectations. Boys typically begin masturbating during early adolescence, the age of first masturbation is extremely variable for girls. Although some girls begin masturbating during early adolescence, many do not masturbate until after they have had intercourse. Relationships with members of the opposite sex often occur at a distance. About one third of males and one fourth of females have had sexual intercourse by age 15; these young people are at high risk for sexually transmitted diseases and behavior problems (Seidman and Rieder, 1994).

Many teens begin to make a shift from relationships with same-sex peers to intimate relationships with members of the opposite sex during middle adolescence (Fig. 19-9). Opposite-sex relationships typically begin with peer activities involving both boys and girls. Pairing off as couples be-

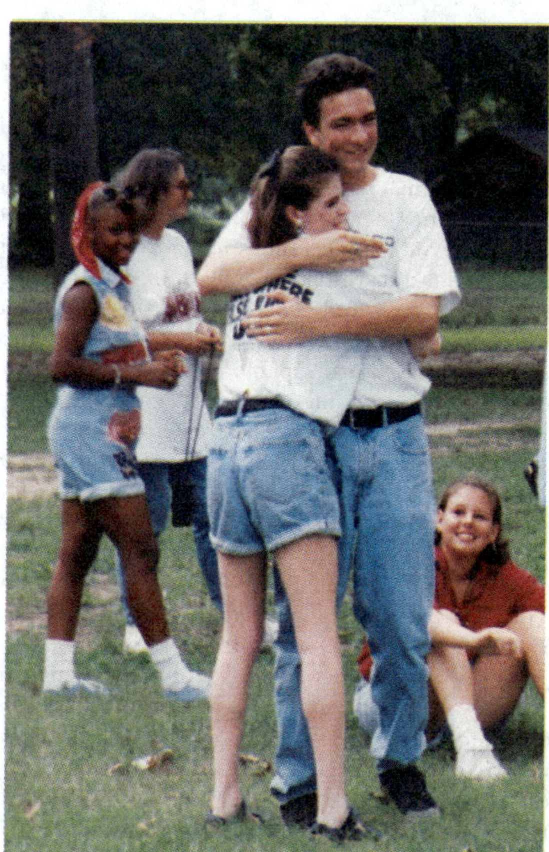

FIG. 19-9 Heterosexual relationships are an important part of adolescence.

comes more common as middle adolescence progresses (Kaluger and Kaluger, 1988). The type and degree of seriousness of partner relationships vary. Initial relationships are usually noncommittal, extremely mobile, and seldom characterized by any deep romantic attachments. Sexual activity becomes more common during middle adolescence. Nationally, approximately 53% of tenth grade males and 43% of females report having had sexual intercourse. By twelfth grade, 76% of males and 67% of females report having had intercourse (CDC, 1992). The relationship between love and sexual expression is brought into focus during middle adolescence. Most young people oppose exploitation, pressure, or force in sex and sex solely for the sake of physical enjoyment without a personal relationship. Adolescents find it hard to believe that sex can exist without love; therefore each relationship is viewed as real love.

An integrated sexual identity often emerges during late adolescence as individuals incorporate sexual experiences, feelings, and cognitions. For most, this identity is consistent with their own physical and mental capacities and with societal limits and expectations. Most older adolescents identify themselves as being predominantly heterosexual or homosexual, with a smaller number self-identifying as bisexual and an even smaller group still unsure of their sexual orientation (Remafedi and others, 1992). Whatever their sexual orientation, most older teens possess the capacity to have intimate relationships that satisfy the emotional and sexual needs of both partners.

The meanings and implications of sexual activity as it affects psychosocial development may be quite different for adolescent boys and girls, that is, sexual socialization differs for males and females in our society. Typically, adolescent boys' first sexual experiences are in early adolescence through masturbation. Before adolescent boys begin dating, they have generally already experienced orgasm and know how to arouse themselves sexually. For males, the development of sexuality during adolescence revolves around efforts to integrate the forming of close relationships into an already existing sense of sexual capability. Girls' first sexual experiences are likely to be very different and to carry very different meanings. Masturbation is a less prevalent activity among girls, and it is less regularly practiced. The adolescent girl, in contrast to the adolescent boy, is more likely to experience sex for the first time in a perceived close relationship. For girls, the development of sexuality involves the integration of sexual activity into an existing capacity for emotional involvement (Steinberg, 1989a).

Sexual orientation represents an important aspect of sexual identity. Sexual orientation is defined as a pattern of sexual arousal toward persons of the same and/or opposite sex, encompassing sexual attractions, fantasies, sexual behavior, and group affiliation. The relative heterosexual or homosexual intensity for each of the factors encompassing sexual arousal may be inconsistent with another, thereby defying dichotomous classification of individuals (Remafedi and others, 1992). For instance, individuals may engage in homosexual activity or have same-sex attractions but not identify themselves as homosexual or maintain an enduring preference for sexual activity with people of the same sex. In a study of seventh through twelfth grade students, 4.5% of students reported homosexual attractions, 2.6% reported same-sex fantasies, and 1% reported same-sex experiences, but only 0.4% labeled themselves as homosexual and 0.7% as bisexual (Remafedi and others, 1992).

Adolescence is a period during which individuals commonly question their own sexual orientation. Uncertainty about sexual orientation may diminish over the course of the adolescent years. Although many children and adolescents experiment sexually with both same-sex and opposite-sex peers, by the end of adolescence over 9 out of 10 people report an exclusive preference for heterosexual relationships.

Although data collected by Kinsey in the 1930s and 1940s suggested that 4% of adult men and 2% of adult women were exclusively homosexual, the current prevalence of homosexual behavior and identity among adolescents is unknown (American Academy of Pediatrics, 1993).

In addition to all the normal tasks of adolescence, teens who have identified themselves as lesbian, gay, or bisexual have unique issues related to the development of sexual orientation that they are addressing. This developmental process occurs over a prolonged period of time and can be thought of as a sequence of four stages (Taylor and Remafedi, 1993, Troiden, 1988). Initially, during preadolescence or adolescence, individuals become ***sensitized*** to feeling different in relation to stereotypic gender activities (e.g., "all boys play sports" and "girls are always feminine") but often do not believe homosexuality to be relevant to themselves. This is in part because the socially created categories of homosexual, heterosexual, and bisexual hold little or no meaning for children. Although a majority of gay males and lesbians do not recall being gender inappropriate as children, most perceived themselves as different (Troiden, 1988). Often during adolescence, a stage of ***identity confusion*** marks the experience of lesbian girls and gay boys as they begin to consider the possibility that their feelings or behaviors could be regarded as homosexual. These thoughts can lead to states of inner confusion, anxiety, or guilt, since they may differ from earlier self-perceptions or societal expectations. Cognitive coping strategies to deal with identity confusion include ***denial*** of homosexual feelings; ***repair,*** which involves vigorous attempts to find a "cure"; ***avoidance*** of situations that might confirm a homosexual identity; ***redefinition*** of behavior as being temporary (e.g., "this is only a phase" or "only with this specific person"); or ***acceptance,*** involving acknowledgment of same-sex behavior, feelings, or fantasies. Coping strategies such as denial and redefinition may be sustained for extended time periods—as long as individuals' social environments, relationships, and level of sexual desire support and maintain them. The third stage, ***identity assumption,*** is considered the beginning of the "coming out" process. During this stage, individuals acknowledge and accept a homosexual or bisexual identity and begin to share it with others. They may associate regularly with others who are gay or lesbian, experiment with sexual expression, and learn more about homosexual subcultures. Identity assumption usually occurs during the early to mid-twenties. The last stage of homosexual identity development involves ***commitment,*** or adopting homosexuality or bisexuality as a way of life. Entering a same-sex love relationship often marks the onset of this stage. With commitment, it becomes easier and more attractive to remain a homosexual than to try to function as a heterosexual. Progression from one stage of this process to another has been described as "a tentative and to-and-fro movement, rather than a steady, self-assured march" (Coleman and Remafedi, 1989).

Intimacy

Intimate relationships are emotional attachments between two people characterized by concern for each other's well-being; a willingness to disclose private, possibly sensitive topics; and a sharing of common interests and activities. Intimate relationships are distinct from sexual relationships. It is possible for individuals to have close relationships without becoming sexually involved. At the same time, people can be involved in sexual relationships that are not particularly intimate.

It is not until adolescence—a time characterized by pubertal changes, advances in social cognitive abilities, and broadening of social worlds—that truly intimate relationships first emerge. Although children have important friendships, these relationships are activity oriented. To a child, a friend is someone who likes to do the same things he or she does. Adolescents' close friendships are more likely to include a strong emotional foundation in which individuals understand and care about each other. The development of intimacy during adolescence involves changes in the adolescent's needs for intimacy, as well as changes in the capacity and opportunities to have intimate friendships. Puberty and its resultant changes in sexual impulses often raise new issues and concerns requiring serious, intimate discussions. Over the course of the adolescent years, individuals become more capable of emotional closeness, and they become more interested in seeking it in their relationships with other people. The greater degree of behavioral independence often accompanying the transition into adolescence provides more opportunities for teens to be alone with friends and to come into meaningful contact with adults outside of their families (Steinberg, 1989a). Although research on intimacy during adolescence has focused on peer friendships, intimate relationships are by no means limited to peers. In addition to forming close friendships with peers, teens may also have intimate relationships with parents, siblings, and adults who are not part of their immediate families.

Harry Stack Sullivan (1953) was among the first to describe the developmental course of intimacy. Usually adolescents develop the capacity for intimacy through preadolescent and early adolescent relationships with same-sex peers. Intimate relationships with opposite-sex peers develop relatively late during adolescence. Opposite-sex friendships may play a more important role in the development of intimacy among boys than among girls, who may develop and experience intimacy earlier during the course of adolescence with same-sex peers (Buhrmester and Furman, 1987).

More recently, Kathleen White and her colleagues (1987) have described a series of qualitative stages individuals move through in their close relationships with others. Children most often function at a ***self-focused*** level with friends, still wrapped up in their own needs and perspectives. They tend to react to friends' actions in simplistic ways—either by trying to hold on to the friendship at all costs or by trying to flee from it. During adolescence, many individuals move into ***role-focused*** friendships, behaving in ways that are dominated by conventional norms. In their close relationships, individuals at this level attempt to keep things nice, avoid controversy, and control their emotions. Role-focused persons are generally more concerned with conforming with the appropriate roles and norms in a relationship (e.g., what the "good" girlfriend does) than with a friend as an individual. It may not be until later in adolescence that people develop the capacity for having ***individuated-connected*** friendships. With this level of friendship, individuals are able to form close intimate relationships with others that acknowledge the complexity and contradictions in close relationships. Differences in outlook between individuals are not only tolerated but encouraged as part of what makes the relationship vital.

Although teens may begin dating during early adolescence, these early dating relationships are not usually very psychosocially intimate. Early dating relationships typically follow highly ritualized "scripts," in which adolescents are more likely to play stereotypic roles than to really be themselves. There is some evidence to suggest that participating in mixed-sex group activities—such as going to parties or other events—may have a positive impact on the well-being of young teens, especially girls, whereas serious dating in couples may have a more negative effect (Simmons and Blyth, 1987; Tobin-Richards, 1985). All in all, a moderate degree of dating with serious relationships delayed until late adolescence may be the most ideal pattern of interpersonal involvement (Steinberg, 1989a).

SOCIAL ENVIRONMENTS

Although all adolescents experience similar biologic and cognitive changes and face similar psychosocial tasks, the health-related effects of these changes are not the same for all people. Why aren't individuals affected in the same ways by puberty, by changes in thinking patterns, and by changes in social and legal status? The answer lies in the fact that biologic, cognitive, and social changes of adolescence are shaped by the social environment in which the changes take place (Bronfenbrenner, 1979). The social environment provides the opportunities, barriers, role models, and support for individuals' development and health. Thus systems within the social environment, including family, peers, schools, community, and the larger society, all contribute uniquely to an adolescent's development and health (O'Keefe and Reid-Nash, 1987).

An ***ecologic model*** can be used as a way of understanding adolescents' social environments (Bronfenbrenner, 1979). According to this model, the social environment may be divided into proximal and more distal systems. Bronfenbrenner (1979) refers to these parts of the social environment as microsystems, mesosystems, exosystems, and macrosystems. ***Microsystems*** are the most proximal social contexts in which adolescents participate directly, such as family, peer groups, school, and the workplace. All of these contexts have substantial influences on the development and health-related behaviors of adolescents (Perry, Kelder, and Komro, 1993). The next layer of social environment, ***mesosystems,*** is formed by linkages between microsystems. The extent to which individuals in one microsystem are involved in other systems determines the strength or "richness" of the mesosystem. For example, regular interactions between family members and school personnel, which have positive effects on student achievement and school performance (Entwisle, 1990), reflect a rich mesosystem. The third layer of social environment, ***exosystems,*** consists of settings that influence adolescent behavior and development but in which they do not directly participate. Many community-level influences fall within this layer. These include opportunities within a community for health-enhancing or health-compromising behaviors, such as the availability of age-appropriate activities for young people that do not include alcohol or the availability of cigarette vending machines. The most distal social environment, the ***macrosystem,*** consists of culturally based belief systems, as well as economic and political systems. These systems can have profound effects on young people's health-related behaviors and development, mostly through their influences on more proximal systems. Bronfenbrenner's model points out that social systems are embedded within each other and that what happens within one system can influence what happens in others. To have the most impact on adolescent health promotion, interventions must address multiple environmental systems (Perry, Kelder, and Komro, 1993; Schorr and Schorr, 1988).

Families

Over the past several decades, changes that have taken place within the family microsystem have important implications for adolescent health. High rates of divorce, increasing numbers of single-parent families, and greater percentages of working mothers have become characteristic of contemporary U.S. society. The "ideal" family consisting of an employed father, an at-home mother, and two or more school-aged children now accounts for less than 10% of American households, as compared with 60% of households in 1955 (Hill, 1987). Higher rates of divorce and the decisions of single women to have children have resulted in over half of U.S. children spending part of their childhood in a single-parent family (Stipek and McCroskey, 1989). Correspondingly, many young people find themselves in reconstituted families, thus developing relationships with stepparents during their adolescent years. Changes in family structure have been accompanied by changes in parent work patterns, with the percentage of mothers who work outside the home doubling since 1970 (Hoffman, 1989).

Changes in family structure and parent employment have resulted in young people having more time unsupervised by adults. The result is increased time alone or with peers (Bearinger, 1990). Although for mature adolescents there may be little risk involved with minimal supervision, for less competent teens, decreased adult supervision may result in more risk-taking behaviors, such as substance use and sexual intercourse. Poorly monitored teenagers are also more likely to socialize with deviant peers (Patterson and Stouthamer-Loeber, 1984). Lack of adult supervision also decreases adolescents' opportunities for communication and intimacy with a parent or other supportive adults. Although quantity of time does not guarantee quality, sufficient quantity is necessary for communication and the development of intimate relationships. Consistently, adolescents who feel close to their parents show more positive psychosocial development and behavioral competence, less susceptibility to negative peer pressure, and lower tendencies to be involved in risk-taking behaviors (Blum and others, 1989; Steinberg, 1986, 1989b). In many situations lack of direct adult supervision may be counterbalanced by parent monitoring and communication about adolescents' activities during parental absence. However, spending greater amounts of time with parents may compromise the health of teens in dysfunctional or abusive families. In these situations the type and content of communication may be the critical important factors to address (Perry, Kelder, and Komro, 1993).

In addition to adult supervision, overall parenting style

also affects adolescent development. Clearly, both effective conflict resolution within families and family cohesion create conducive environments for healthy adolescent development. These two characteristics, along with parent expectations for mature behavior on the part of the adolescent, and the practice of setting and enforcing reasonable limits for behavior are thought to form the basis of effective parenting (Maccoby and Martin, 1983). This parenting style, termed ***authoritative parenting***, is related to greater psychosocial maturity and school performance (Steinberg, Elman, and Mounts, 1989), along with less substance abuse among young people (Baumrind, 1991).

Adolescents from low-income households spend less supervised time with adults; they are more likely to have parents working at more than one job; they are more likely to drop out of high school; and they are more likely to experience violence in their homes and communities (Perry, Kelder, and Komro, 1993). While disorder within their larger social environments often creates a need for a buffer that could include spending quality time with adults, poor adolescents often experience fewer of these types of health-enhancing activities (Garmezy, 1991).

Peer Groups

One hallmark of adolescence is the increasing value young people place on friendships and relationships with peers (Fig. 19-10). In short, adolescents spend more time with their peers than do children. Compared with children, their peer groups are more autonomous and are more likely to include peers of the opposite sex (Brown, 1990). Given the changes that have taken place within family systems in contemporary society, peer groups have come to play an even more significant role in the socialization of adolescents.

Peers serve as credible sources of information, role models of new social behaviors, sources of social reinforcement, and bridges to alternative life-styles. Close and supportive peer friendships appear to have beneficial effects for young people (Savin-Williams and Berndt, 1989). However, adolescents with greater peer identification than parental identification, especially when peers model and support problem behaviors, are more prone to deviant and health-compromising behaviors. Thus the transition to greater peer involvement, like other developmental transitions of adolescence, is a process requiring guidance, skills, and, to be accomplished optimally, a prolonged time to complete the transitions. At a time when they are developing interpersonal skills to deal with peer pressure, young adolescents who lack adult supervision and opportunities for communication with adults may be more susceptible to peer influences and at a higher risk for poor peer-group selection than teens who have close relationships with caring adults (Perry, Kelder, and Komro, 1993).

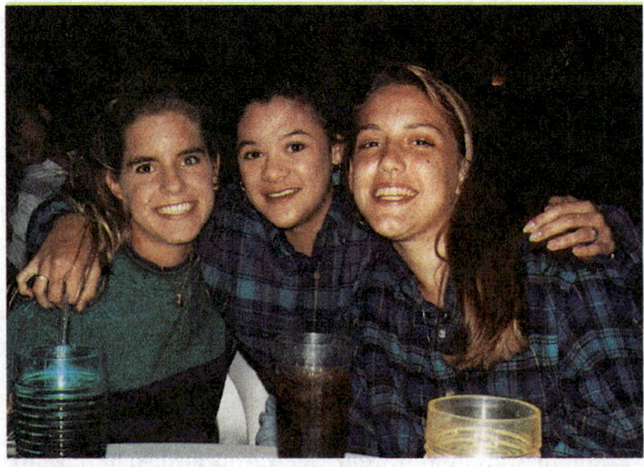

FIG. 19-10 The peer group is a major influence in adolescent development.

The heightened value placed on adolescent peer relationships leads to questions about the quality and nature of peer influence. Rather than thinking of all peer influence as being either good or bad, it is important to recognize that the influence of peers varies from one adolescent to another, from one peer group to another, and across different societies and cultures. Adolescents' selection of peer groups seems to be most strongly influenced by sociodemographic factors and by common patterns of behavior including, for example, substance use, school achievement, and religious participation. Peers can have either positive or negative effects on adolescent behavior. Negative effects might include increased substance use, gang membership, and violent behaviors. Examples of positive effects are outcomes for adolescents who share an orientation supporting academic achievement, an environmental commitment, or a commitment to religious youth groups (Perry, Kelder, and Komro, 1993). Peers can be also be a positive force in health promotion among teens. Same-age and older adolescents can encourage healthy behavior by serving as positive role models and promoting prohealth norms in the peer group (Klepp, Halper, and Perry, 1986; Perry and Sieving, 1991). For most adolescents, prosocial pressures from peers are greater than antisocial ones, and adolescents report being more swayed by prosocial or neutral pressures than by pressures toward misconduct (Crockett and Petersen, 1993).

Schools

In contemporary society, schools have come to play an increasingly important role in preparing young people for adulthood (Fig. 19-11). Schooling is now essential for a successful future for both boys and girls. Failure to complete high school reduces employment opportunities and the probability of earning an adequate income. Yet, there is ample evidence that schools in the United States are not meeting the developmental needs of all young people. Adolescents of color seem to fare especially poorly in the current system. For example, the percentage of 13-year-olds who are at least one grade behind ranges from 22% for white girls to 47% for Hispanic boys, with the rates for blacks falling between those of Hispanics and whites (U.S. Bureau of the Census, 1988). Dropout rates are highest among Hispanic and American Indian adolescents (Blum and others, 1992; U.S. Congress, 1991a).

Ranked as one of the most important problems is the lack of parental involvement in schools. Research has shown

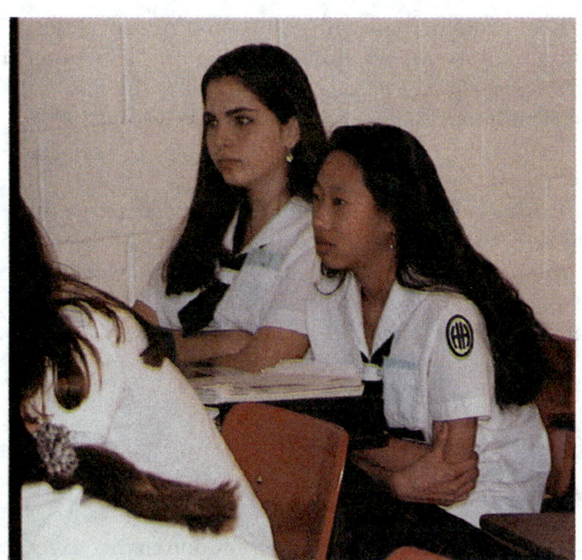

FIG. 19-11 School is an important part of adolescents' life.

that involving parents increases the effectiveness of school at all levels (Epstein, 1987). It is likely that with the larger number of single-parent and two-parent working families, parents have less time for involvement in schools. Young people who are living in single-parent families generally have lower grade point averages and are less likely to complete high school, even when the family income and mother's education level are taken into account (McLanahan and Bumpass, 1988).

There is also evidence that the transition from elementary school can have negative effects on youth. The timing of school transitions is critical, especially in cases where the school environment is not appropriate to the developmental needs of the adolescent. In particular, the transition into a junior high school at age 12 or 13 typically occurs at the same time as the rapid physical changes of puberty. A comparison of seventh graders in a junior high school to seventh graders in a kindergarten–to–eighth grade (K-8) school revealed that the attitudes of the junior high school seventh graders were more negative, self-esteem and leadership declined for girls, and participation in extracurricular activities, grade point averages, and math scores were lower. Among the boys, junior high seventh graders were more likely to be victims of robbery, beatings, or threats (Simmons, 1987). Relatively few K-8 schools exist in the United States, and the trend is toward earlier rather than later transitions out of primary school. Earlier transition may be advantageous if it precedes the changes of puberty. It would enable young adolescents to become accustomed to the change in school environment before having to cope with pubertal events (Simmons, 1987).

Another characteristic of school that may have negative effects is a system of grading that acknowledges few young people for their academic successes. Teenagers whose grades fall below average may spend a high proportion of their time in environments in which they perceive negative evaluations by adult authorities. Students' reactions to such environments may include alienation from school; then, subgroups of adolescents may unite and develop countercultures or exhibit antisocial behavior. This process may be most intense for young people from poorer families who attend schools that include students from a broad range of socioeconomic classes (Simmons, 1987). In addition, students with below-average grades are more likely to be engaged in health-compromising behaviors such as tobacco and alcohol use, unprotected sexual intercourse, and suicide attempts (Blum, 1987).

The social environment of schools also has an impact on student outcomes. Small classroom and school size are both related to higher-quality social environments within schools. Relatively small high schools enhance personal development and prosocial behavior of students (Entwisle, 1990). Teachers from high schools with low enrollments report better control over classroom and school practices, greater cooperation among staff, better-behaved students, greater agreement on school goals, and higher morale (Pallas, 1988).

Research findings on school practices and conditions that lead to better student outcomes has prompted the Carnegie Council on Adolescent Development (1989) to develop recommendations for improving school environments. These include (1) creating small learning communities within schools; (2) implementing practices that foster achievement rather than those, such as tracking, that isolate some students, leading to failure and dropping out; (3) implementing practices that foster health and fitness; (4) encouraging involvement of families; and (5) strengthening connections between schools and communities. (Crockett and Petersen, 1993).

Work

For the majority of young people in the United States, the workplace becomes a fourth microsystem. Most teens are employed in a relatively restricted array of jobs: restaurant workers, cashiers, sales clerks, clerical assistants, and unskilled laborers. The jobs tend to be monotonous, require little initiative or decision making, and rarely use skills learned in school; furthermore, some are highly stressful, requiring work under extreme time pressure (Greenberger and Steinberg, 1986). Adolescent work as it exists today may negatively affect development. The typical teenager's job neither provides continuity to adult employment nor links teens to adults who could serve as vocational mentors. In addition, the monotonous nature of many adolescent jobs is neither intellectually stimulating nor related to role experimentation involved in identity development. Rather, involvement in work may take time away from other activities that could contribute to identity development. Greater involvement in work can also lead to fatigue, decreased interest in school, reduced extracurricular involvement, and poorer grades (Steinberg and others, 1982). Detrimental effects are especially likely for adolescents who work more than 20 hours a week. Although much work done by teens may not contribute to healthy development, jobs that allow young people to develop intellectual and social skills, to have some autonomy, or to feel that their contributions matter can prove to be positive experiences. Jobs that provide adolescents with experiences relevant to future employment or that link them to adults who can serve as vocational mentors may be especially valuable (Hamilton, 1990).

Community and Society

Society influences adolescent health and development indirectly through the structures of social institutions, division of economic wealth, and construction and implementation of public policies. Society also provides a dominant set of values and expectations for behavior to which adolescents are exposed. These values and expectations are transmitted through the mass media, as well as through local institutions and social networks.

In the United States, adolescence is a time during which individuals are expected to make the transition from childhood to adulthood. Adolescents are given more autonomy than children and are also expected to show more responsible behavior. Young people are given more personal control over health-related behaviors but often fail to receive necessary guidance, support, or access to positive adult role models. At the same time, society seeks to limit adolescents' involvement in some risk-taking behaviors that may convey adult status, such as alcohol and tobacco use or sexual intercourse. Many of these same behaviors are glamorized through media programming and advertising campaigns directed at teens. For some teens faced with societal expectations to "grow up," risk-taking behaviors take on specific functional meanings. Behaviors such as substance use or unsafe sex may offer adolescents opportunities to challenge social authority, demonstrate autonomy, or gain social approval (Perry and Kelder, 1992).

Local communities, as part of the broader societal context, also influence adolescents' capacity for healthy development. The local community has a more proximal influence on adolescents' motivations and opportunities to engage in health-enhancing or risk-taking behaviors. For example, adults within the community serve as direct role models, affecting youth expectations concerning their likely roles and activities as adults (Ianni, 1989). Communities with a high proportion of employed, well-educated, financially successful adults provide a different array of models than impoverished neighborhoods where poor households predominate, as well as chronic illness and drug abuse, and the financially successful adults are those involved in illicit activities. Such environmental characteristics affect young people's expectations for the future, their perceptions of how current behavior could jeopardize future chances, and, consequently, their motivation to avoid high-risk behavior (Dryfoos, 1991).

A community's economic resources play a significant role in the health and well-being of young people. Resources affect opportunities for health promotion (e.g., by influencing the quality of local schools and health-related services). Schools in wealthy areas can provide high-quality education that will enhance students' interest in school and their chances of future success. Wealthy communities also provide opportunities for alternative, health-enhancing activities through community clubs and organizations. Thus community resources influence the type and number of health risks young people face, as well as the local capacity for health promotion (Crockett and Petersen, 1993).

■ ■ ■

During adolescence, young people experience biologic changes associated with puberty, changes in their abilities to think abstractly and to imagine possibilities, and changes in their social roles and environments. These transitions, summarized in Table 19-1, are encountered during early adolescence, middle adolescence, and late adolescence.

PROMOTING OPTIMUM HEALTH DURING ADOLESCENCE

What do we mean by health promotion? What exactly is it that we are trying to promote? From a broad perspective, health includes physical health, psychologic well-being, and social role functioning (Perry and Jessor, 1985). From this perspective of health, health promotion involves empowering individuals, families, and communities to take developmentally and contextually appropriate actions toward realizing their potential; it includes physical, cognitive, emotional, and social dimensions (Irwin and Vaughan, 1988). For adolescents, health promotion involves helping youth acquire the power (including knowledge, attitudes, and skills), authority (permission to use their power), and opportunities to make choices that increase the likelihood of their creating positive expression of health for themselves in their contexts (Igoe, 1991).

A comprehensive approach to health promotion combines activities aimed at individuals, with interventions focused on changing norms, attitudes, and behaviors of peer groups, families, communities, and society at large (National Institute of Nursing Research, 1993). For example, prevention of tobacco use involves more than a teacher's lecture on the consequences of cigarette and smokeless tobacco use, a ban on tobacco use in schools, a parent's admonition not to smoke, or a nurse's question to an adolescent about smoking history. In reality, it requires all these pieces and more. Effective health promotion requires enlisting the support of the many individuals and institutions that affect the lives of adolescents (Millstein, Petersen, and Nightingale, 1993).

Are adolescents in need of health promotion? By some measures, adolescents are a relatively healthy group. If health is limited to physical illness, adolescents fare quite well. However, if the definition of health includes physical fitness, psychologic health, and social well-being, unmet needs of this age-group become apparent. These needs were recognized by the U.S. Department of Health and Human Services (1991). In the agenda-setting document, *Healthy People 2000,* goals were specifically targeted at adolescents for special risk reduction efforts in the areas of mental health, substance use, sexual behavior, violence, unintentional injury, nutrition, physical activity and fitness, and oral health.

TABLE 19-1 Growth and Development During Adolescence

EARLY ADOLESCENCE (11-14 YEARS)	MIDDLE ADOLESCENCE (14-17 YEARS)	LATE ADOLESCENCE (17-20 YEARS)
GROWTH		
Rapidly accelerating growth Reaches peak velocity Secondary sex characteristics appear	Growth decelerating in girls Stature reaches 95% of adult height Secondary sex characteristics well advanced	Physically mature Structure and reproductive growth almost complete
COGNITION		
Explores newfound ability for limited abstract thought Clumsy groping for new values and energies Comparison of "normality" with peers of same sex	Developing capacity for abstract thinking Enjoys intellectual powers, often in idealistic terms Concern with philosophic, political, and social problems	Established abstract thought Can perceive and act on long range operations Able to view problems comprehensively Intellectual and functional identity established
IDENTITY		
Preoccupied with rapid body changes Trying out of various roles Measurement of attractiveness by acceptance or rejection of peers Conformity to group norms	Modifies body image Very self-centered; increased narcissism Tendency toward inner experience and self-discovery Has a rich fantasy life Idealistic Able to perceive future implications of current behavior and decisions; variable application	Body image and gender role definition nearly secured Mature sexual identity Phase of consolidation of identity Stability of self-esteem Comfortable with physical growth Social roles defined and articulated
RELATIONSHIPS WITH PARENTS		
Defining independence-dependence boundaries Strong desire to remain dependent on parents while trying to detach No major conflicts over parental control	Major conflicts over independence and control Low point in parent-child relationship Greatest push for emancipation; disengagement Final and irreversible emotional detachment from parents; mourning	Emotional and physical separation from parents completed Independence from family with less conflict Emancipation nearly secured
RELATIONSHIPS WITH PEERS		
Seeks peer affiliations to counter instability generated by rapid change Upsurge of close idealized friendships with members of the same sex Struggle for mastery takes place within peer group	Strong need for identity to affirm self-image Behavioral standards set by peer group Acceptance by peers extremely important—fear of rejection Exploration of ability to attract the opposite sex	Peer group recedes in importance in favor of individual friendship Testing of male-female relationships against possibility of permanent alliance Relationships characterized by giving and sharing
SEXUALITY		
Self-exploration and evaluation Limited dating, usually group Limited intimacy	Multiple plural relationships Decisive turn toward heterosexuality (if is homosexual, knows by this time) Exploration of "self appeal" Feeling of "being in love" Tentative establishment of relationships	Forms stable relationships and attachment to another Growing capacity for mutuality and reciprocity Dating as a male-female pair Intimacy involves commitment rather than exploration and romanticism
PSYCHOLOGIC HEALTH		
Wide mood swings Intense daydreaming Anger outwardly expressed with moodiness, temper outbursts, and verbal insults and name-calling	Tendency toward inner experiences; more introspective Tendency to withdraw when upset or feelings are hurt Vascillation of emotions in time and range Feelings of inadequacy common; difficulty in asking for help	More constancy of emotion Anger more apt to be concealed

The rationale for focusing on these particular health issues becomes obvious when one examines the major sources of mortality and morbidity during adolescence and later in life. Overall, the three primary causes of mortality during adolescence are injuries, homicide, and suicide; together they are responsible for 75% of all adolescent deaths. Major causes of adolescent morbidity include injury and disability associated with the use of motor and recreational vehicles, consequences of sexual activity such as pregnancy and sexually transmitted diseases, and the outcomes of substance use. Mental disorders, chronic illness, eating disorders, and oral health problems are other important sources of morbidity (Bearinger and Blum, 1994; Irwin and others, 1991; Millstein, Petersen, and Nightingale, 1993; U.S. Congress, 1991a, 1991b). Chapters 20 and 21 provide further information about many of the major threats to adolescent health and well-being.

The goals in *Healthy People 2000* also target selected subgroups in order to address inequities in health status that exist among subsets of the U.S. population; adolescents are targeted as one of the subgroups experiencing health inequities. For example, a substantial gap in life expectancy exists between black and white adolescents. African-American and American Indian males have a higher risk of premature mortality than any other racial/ethnic group. Male adolescents die at a rate more than twice that of females. Mortality rates increase by more than 200% between early and late adolescence. There are also age differences in the causes of death, with a shift toward more violent deaths occurring in late adolescence. Among white adolescents a dramatic increase in suicide occurs during later adolescence, making it the second leading cause of death in this group. For older black adolescents a different picture emerges, but one that also points to increases in violence, with homicide ranking as the most likely cause of death among this group. Similar to mortality, patterns of morbidity also vary within the adolescent population. For example, rates of vehicular injury are high among males, whereas for females morbidities associated with "quietly disturbed" behaviors such as eating disorders and emotional distress are common (Bearinger and Blum, 1994; Millstein, Petersen, and Nightingale, 1993).

ADOLESCENTS' PERSPECTIVES ON HEALTH

To be most effective, adolescent health promotion efforts must incorporate adolescents' perspectives on what health means. It also must focus on their concerns and priorities related to health and health care services. From a positive perspective, adolescents' developmentally based sense of curiosity and movement toward autonomy provide opportunities for health promotion that should not be wasted (Millstein, 1993).

One 13-year-old girl, when asked what health meant to her, responded: "You want to do things . . . to live . . . to get out, have fun, be active. You have to be healthy to work hard . . . to survive in this world. If you're not, you might as well be put out on a mountain like they used to do to babies in the ancient myths and let the wolves eat you 'cause you're not going to get anywhere" (Irwin, 1976). Adolescents define health in much the same way as adults: health means being able to live up to one's potential; being able to function physically, mentally, and socially; and experiencing positive emotional states. The content of their definitions often goes beyond an "absence of illness" perspective; it includes ideas of what can be done to maintain and enhance health (Millstein and Irwin, 1987).

Adolescents' health-related interests and concerns include stress and anxiety, relationships with adults and peers, weight, acne, and feeling down or depressed (Bearinger and Blum, 1994). Health concerns are often consistent with the immediate developmental tasks that teens face. For example, younger adolescents—in the midst of the physical changes of puberty—often have particular interest in issues related to growth and development. In the process of making transitions from middle or junior high school to senior high school, middle adolescents often have questions and concerns related to peer-group acceptance, relationships with friends, and physical appearance. Older adolescents' concerns focus increasingly on school performance, as well as on future career/employment plans and emotional health issues (Millstein, 1993).

Among the behaviors that adolescents view as risky are substance use, sexual activity, and risks related to the use of recreational and motor vehicles. Adolescents also identify health threats that primarily involve psychologic issues such as clinical depression and eating/weight problems. Another set of perceived health threats are in their environment, including broad threats such as violence and pollution, as well as threats within the more immediate social environment, including school problems and conflicts with parents, teachers, and friends. When adolescents are asked about general threats to youth, they respond differently than if asked about how their own personal behaviors produce certain risks. Like adults, adolescents tend to underestimate the potentially negative consequences of their own behaviors (Millstein, 1993).

Although young people identify health risks and concerns that are primarily social and psychologic in nature, many are reluctant to seek health services for problems they do not consider to be organic in nature, despite the fact that they indicate they would like help with these problems (Bearinger and Blum, 1994). An adolescent's reluctance to seek health care is influenced by many factors, including perceived availability of confidential services, characteristics of health care providers, geographic access, and financial limitations.

The availability of confidential services is particularly important to adolescents, especially when they have concerns related to sensitive issues such as sexual or substance use behaviors. Many report that they are unwilling to seek health care related to sensitive topics if their parents will know about the visit (Resnick, Littman, and Blum, 1992). Although many states have provisions for confidential care related to problems such as substance abuse and sexual health, adolescents demonstrate significant misperceptions about whether and where they can receive confidential health care (American School Health Association, 1989).

Adolescents may be more likely to participate in health care services when they are delivered by caring, respectful providers. Characteristics of providers that teenagers identify as desirable include compassion, warmth, understanding, an ability to communicate with the adolescent, a willingness to be straightforward and honest, and competence. On the other hand, adolescents report disliking providers who treat them in a patronizing manner and who appear unfriendly or impersonal. Adolescents appear to view providers in adolescent-oriented settings as being more attuned to them, whereas in traditional settings providers are viewed as cold, aloof, and inconsiderate of adolescent patients (Resnick and Bearinger, 1986).

In the United States 1 out of 7 adolescents is without access to health insurance (U.S. Congress, 1991a); in 1988 these numbers translated into almost 5 million uninsured teens. Minority and poor adolescents are overrepresented among the uninsured. Black teens are almost twice as likely as white teens to not have health insurance; Hispanic adolescents are three times more likely to be uninsured than their non-Hispanic counterparts. Among adolescents living in families below the poverty level, less than 40% are covered by Medicaid (Bearinger and Blum, 1994). Although research has shown clear links between poverty and poor health outcomes, poor and near-poor adolescents continue to make fewer health care visits, experience significantly longer intervals between visits, and receive less preventive care than is warranted by their health status (Newacheck and McManus, 1989). One mechanism to reduce financial barriers to health promotion is through the development of state and federal policies that ensure universal coverage for preventive services.

FACTORS THAT PROMOTE ADOLESCENT HEALTH AND WELL-BEING

Chapters 20 and 21 focus on a variety of health problems of youth, as well as on factors that put individuals at risk for these problems. Research has also identified adolescents who—despite being exposed to risk factors such as poverty, high rates of neighborhood violence, parental abuse or neglect, or parent divorce—develop into competent, healthy adults. Psychologist Michael Rutter and others have stressed the importance of understanding how this group of young people succeed despite odds against them. Rutter (1979) states: "The potential for prevention surely lies in increasing our understanding of the reasons why some children are not damaged by deprivation." Important questions for nurses and other professionals involved in health promotion are "Who doesn't experience adverse health outcomes (e.g. teen pregnancy, sexually transmitted diseases, school failure, delinquency, depression, suicide, and substance abuse)?" and "Why?" Answers to these questions lead to identification of personal and environmental factors that protect adolescents from experiencing high-risk health outcomes. Future health promotion efforts with adolescents can focus on nurturing such protective factors.

Researchers (Garmezy, 1991; U.S. Congress, 1991a; Werner, 1989) have identified three sets of factors that characterize children and youth who cope successfully when faced with adverse life situations such as poverty, parental alcoholism or psychopathology, or poor relationships between parents. These protective factors include individual personal attributes, attributes of families, and attributes of the larger social environment. Protective personal factors include the ability to adapt to new persons and situations, possessing at least average intelligence, and having competence in language and reading skills. Adolescents who cope successfully in the midst of adverse circumstances are often supported by caring, cohesive families in which the parents are concerned with the well-being of their children. This "family" support can also be provided by some other caring adult—such as a grandparent—in the absence of a supportive parent. Protective factors within the community include connections with adults outside the family, the school, or a church group. For example, health care providers who are able to connect with adolescents help to support successful coping. Schools that are small, comfortable, safe, and intellectually engaging can make a difference in the health and well-being of young people. Involvement with healthy peer groups, guided by caring and culturally appropriate adults, have also been shown to prevent poor outcomes such as delinquent behavior (U.S. Congress, 1991a).

Evidence about the potential positive impact of social interactions suggests guidelines for making changes in adolescent environments that support overall health and well-being (U.S. Congress, 1991a). Nurses involved with adolescents can develop interventions that shift the balance for young people from vulnerability to resilience, either by decreasing exposures to health risks or stressful life events (such as the impact of parental alcoholism or the threats of violence) or by increasing the number of protective factors (such as communication and problem-solving skills, or sources of emotional support) available to them.

Contexts for Adolescent Health Promotion

There is a growing consensus that the most effective adolescent health promotion efforts involve multiple systems and address multiple issues. Research suggests that interventions integrating programs and expertise from health care, school, and community-based settings can effectively increase adolescents' prevention skills, improve their access to health care services, build adult motivation and support for adolescent prevention practices, and change physical environments and social norms to support healthy behavior (Pentz, 1993; Dryfoos, 1991). Such a comprehensive approach to health promotion requires a great deal of cooperation and coordination on the part of complex institutions. On the other hand, by not limiting the responsibility for adolescent health to one person or one setting, multiple opportunities for health promotion occur (Bearinger and McAnarney, 1988). Individual efforts serve to reinforce important themes, thus becoming an integral part of an overall health promotion strategy (Millstein, Petersen, and Nightingale, 1993). For example, a plan for smoking cessation devised by a teenager with the help of a nurse is most likely to be successful if the teen is encouraged by peers and family members to abstain, and if use and access to tobacco products are discouraged through policy interventions such as "smoke-free" schools and bans on cigarette vending machines.

Parent Involvement

Many parents are interested, concerned, and involved in the lives of their adolescent children. Furthermore, research has shown that having parents who are appropriately involved can be a significant protective factor in the lives of adolescents. Thus efforts to exclude parents from adolescent health services are both unrealistic and unwise. What must be sought in providing health care is a balance between the individual adolescent's growing autonomy and the parents' diminishing control over, and responsibility for, the adolescent. The American Medical Association (1992) recommends that parents be offered health guidance at least once during their child's early adolescence, once during middle adolescence, and once during late adolescence. Such guidance can include information about normative adolescent development, along with signs and symptoms of troubled adolescents. Parents can be engaged in discussion of parenting behaviors that promote healthy adolescent adjustment, including maintaining open communication, employing age-appropriate limit-setting, monitoring their child's social and recreational activities, and acting as role models for health-enhancing behaviors. Parents should be encouraged to discuss health-related behaviors with their adolescents. Kreipe (1991) offers a set of principles that can be used to guide office counseling with parents of adolescents.

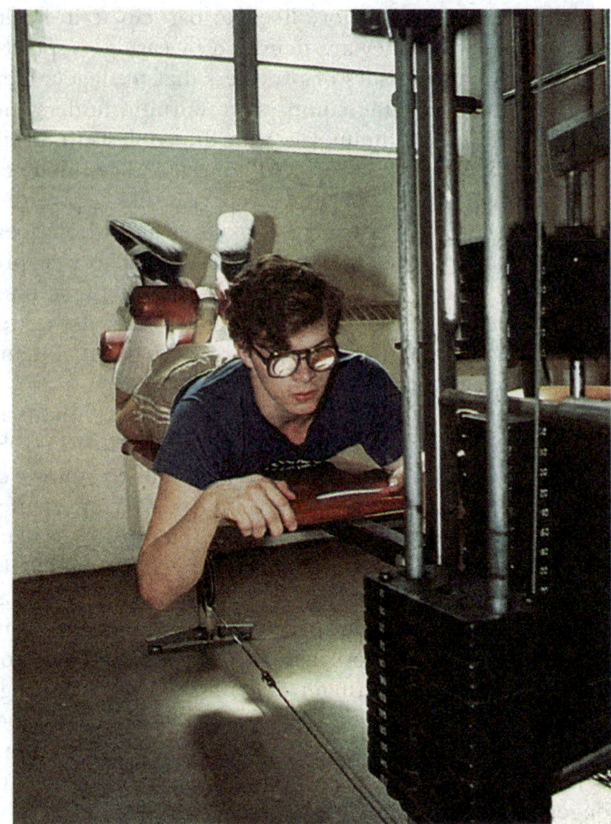

FIG. 19-12 Adolescents should be encouraged to participate in activities that contribute to lifelong physical fitness.

Schools

Schools continue to be a primary site for adolescent health promotion and disease prevention (National Institute of Nursing Research, 1993). Schools offer unique opportunities for health promotion. Large numbers of young people can be affected by school-based health promotion efforts, since virtually all teens attend school at least through the early adolescent years. Group interventions offer adolescents a sense of anonymity, which they may prefer when obtaining information about sensitive topics (Millstein, 1993). School personnel often have special expertise and experience with health education. Through daily contact, school staff are able to develop supportive relationships with a limited number of students. Parent-teacher associations and school boards also link schools to the larger community in ways that can be used to expand the scope of adolescent health promotion efforts (Elster, Panzarine, and Holt, 1993).

School-based health promotion interventions include both classroom health education and school-level policies and environmental changes. Classroom programs often include components that focus on building students' knowledge and skills and establishing peer support for health-enhancing behaviors. Programs have effectively used classroom peer leaders as positive role models and social support for healthy behaviors (Perry and Kelder, 1992). Out-of class assignments often involve parents or other admired adults, emphasizing the roles that adults can play as resources regarding health issues. Classroom programs have been designed to address health-related issues, including healthy eating and exercise habits (Fig. 19-12), nonviolent conflict resolution, substance use and abuse prevention, and promotion of responsible sexual behavior. Other school-level interventions involve changing the school environment itself. Examples of this type of intervention include efforts to improve physical education and food service programs or to adopt tobacco-free school policies. School-wide environmental changes may serve to reinforce classroom programs aimed at promoting health-enhancing behavior.

School-Based and School-Linked Health Services

Another promising avenue for health promotion connected with schools is school-based and school-linked clinics. School-based clinics (SBCs) are located on school grounds and serve adolescents within a specific school. School-linked clinics (SLCs) may be located off school grounds or on school campuses but serve more than one school. Originally designed to address issues related to adolescent pregnancy, SBCs and SLCs have expanded to include services that address a broad range of health problems and psychosocial issues of students. In combination, school-linked health services and traditional school-based health promotion efforts provide a comprehensive approach to health promotion that integrates health care, education, and environmental support.

Several private foundations, states, and local governments have provided considerable resources to initiate school-linked health services in which adolescents are offered confidential services at minimal cost. Parental consent for services is usually obtained on a blanket basis before adolescents seek services. These services have been found to increase adolescents' access to preventive and primary care services (Kirby and others, 1993), a fact that may be related to their highly visible locations, convenient hours, affordability, and ability to provide confidential care. SLCs have made a concerted effort to provide the services of a multidisciplinary team of health professionals—which may include nurses, nurse practitioners, health educators, medical assistants, physicians, psychologists, nutritionists, and social workers—skilled in meeting both the mental and physical health needs of adolescents (U.S. Congress, 1991a). Research shows that adolescents are receptive to services offered by SLCs, especially when emotionally charged tissues such as depression are involved (Millstein, 1993).

Among the potential barriers to the use of schools as sites for health promotion are a lack of resources and community-level resistance to program implementation. Some schools may be reluctant to commit resources to health promotion activities that may decrease the time available to pursue more traditional educational goals. Other schools may be faced with vocal groups of parents or community members who express concern for schools becoming involved in issues that they consider should be taught at home. Barriers, including inadequate funding, community and provider resistance, limitations in the numbers of trained personnel, and lack of systematic data on effectiveness, have interfered with the successful implementation of SLCs in some communities (U.S. Congress, 1991a). Political influences and variations in the resources available within any particular community result in a lack of uniformity in the scope, depth, and quality of health education and health services offered to students across school systems (Elster, Panzarine, and Holt, 1993).

Communities

Community-level approaches to adolescent health promotion, involving both media campaigns and initiatives on the part of community groups, offer the advantage of reaching a broad audience. Specifically, community-based approaches can reach adolescents who may not attend school or have no source of preventive health care. This type of approach directly addresses changing social environments where risk behaviors occur. For example, violence prevention may be more effectively addressed by changing community-wide standards related to issues such as conflict resolution than by focusing on the individual. Community-level approaches have the potential to be most effective when they involve various sectors of the community (including adolescents) and include persons representing a variety of youth-serving agencies (Dexheimer Pharris, 1994). With the involvement of multiple sectors, adolescents have opportunities to hear consistent health messages across a variety of their social contexts. Bracht and Tsouros (1990) provide a framework for understanding strategies for involving communities in health promotion.

The mass media is one vehicle commonly used in community-level health promotion efforts. Adolescents report obtaining a great deal of their health information from media sources such television, radio, and magazines (Price and others, 1988). Therefore, media campaigns can be an effective way to reach adolescents with health promotion messages. Messages can also be targeted to appeal to parents and other adults who have an impact on health-related behavior of youth. Information delivered by mass media campaigns uses brief images and therefore provides short, superficial coverage of specific issues. Typically, the goal of mass media campaigns involves increasing knowledge and changing attitudes around a single issue. Used alone, media campaigns have little direct influence on changing health behaviors (National Institute for Nursing Research, 1993).

The goal of initiatives launched by parent and community groups is to build climates within communities that support health-enhancing behaviors. Such initiatives aim to create social contexts in which teenagers encounter more health-promoting messages and norms. An example of a community-level initiative is a task force developed to address issues related to adolescent alcohol use. Goals of this task force may include educating community members about the extent and consequences of adolescent alcohol use, developing strategies that decrease the availability of alcohol to young people within the community (such as better enforcement of age-of-alcohol-sales laws), and sponsoring alcohol-free social events for community youth.

Health Care Settings

Consistent, supportive, one-on-one interactions between adolescents and members of the health care team provide significant opportunities for health promotion. These relationships can create "safe environments" in which adolescents can disclose sensitive information related to health risk. This information can be incorporated into preventive interventions specific to individual adolescent needs (Elster, Panzarine, and Holt, 1993).

Health care settings offer the advantage of being able to provide confidential services. This is particularly essential in sensitive situations such as those involving substance use, sexual concerns, or abuse (Millstein, 1993). However, interventions provided through health care settings can, when appropriate, include parents, with the young person being clearly aware of what will remain confidential and what will be discussed with parents. Another advantage of health promotion efforts within health care settings is the resources available to address various components of health—including physical, emotional, and social needs (Elster, Panzarine, and Holt, 1993).

There are limitations of health promotion interventions provided in health care settings, as well as advantages. Individual care is time-intensive, thereby limiting the number of adolescents who can be reached through one-on-one encounters. While one-on-one interventions can foster health-enhancing attitudes and behaviors of individual adolescents, they do not address changes in social environments, such as peer groups and communities, that may be necessary to support these attitudes and behaviors (Elster, Panzarine, and Holt, 1993).

To be effective, health care services for adolescents must be accessible and appropriate. To be ***accessible,*** services must be available, affordable, and approachable. Services must include outreach to adolescents and their parents, informing them of the availability of services. Mechanisms for low- or no-cost services must be developed, since cost is a major barrier to adolescents receiving appropriate care. Locating health care services in places such as schools, youth services centers, shopping malls, and detention facilities, as well as offering convenient clinical hours, are two strategies that improve access for teens who may not use traditional services. To be ***appropriate,*** services must take into consideration the cultural contexts, as well as adolescents' needs for confidential, developmentally appropriate care. For example, the constellation of appropriate health services for urban Latino teens may be very different from services for a rural population of white teens. Finally, to provide appropriate services, professionals must be prepared to address the common health concerns of adolescents (i.e., to be well educated in adolescent health issues [Bearinger and Gephart, 1993; U.S. Congress, 1991a]).

Health-Screening Interview

One vehicle for health promotion used by nurses and other professionals in health care settings is the health-screening interview. Through information gained during an interview, both assets and threats to the adolescent's well-being can be identified. The health interview also offers an opportunity for health professionals to build trusting relationships with adolescents. This sense of trust may be critical if adolescents are going to act on information, attitudes, and skills shared by health providers that will help teens successfully negotiate particular stressors.

Interview Process

The development of trust between the adolescent and the health professional is vital to a health-screening interview. Ensuring confidentiality is one of the most essential ingredients for establishing a trusting relationship. In general, adolescents do have the right to confidential communication with providers unless a life-threatening situation arises. Health care providers need to become familiar with the legal rights of adolescent patients in their state, as well as their obligations to adolescent patients and families (English, 1990).

The boundaries around confidentiality and privacy should be established at the beginning of the interview so that adolescents feel that they can discuss sensitive topics. A brief, clear explanation of confidentiality should acknowledge that (1) most things discussed during the interview will not be shared with others and (2) life-threatening issues that need to be shared with parents or other adults (e.g., report of ongoing abuse, suicidal or homicidal plans) will not be done without the adolescent's prior knowledge. To allow for private conversation, most of the health-screening interview can be completed with parents out of the room (Fig. 19-13).

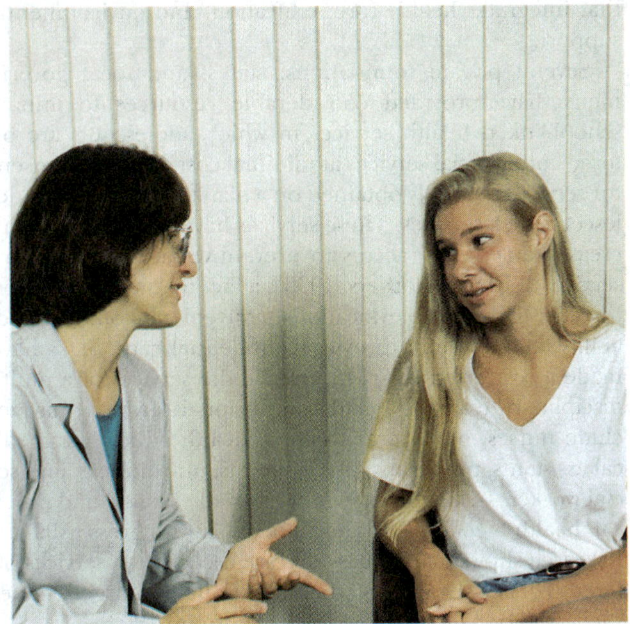

FIG. 19-13 Most of the health screening interview with the adolescent can be completed with parents out of the room. (From Barkauskas VH and others: *Health and physical assessment,* St Louis, 1994, Mosby.)

The Guidelines box lists several useful guidelines for interviewing adolescents. To convey an interest in adolescents' perspectives, nurses should begin by asking teens to explain their reasons for the visit. At the beginning of the interview, adolescents should be given a nonthreatening explanation of why questions are asked. One way of clarifying this is: "I'll be asking you questions, including ones that some people find personal or even embarrassing, so that I can better understand your health." To increase adolescents' comfort in disclosing sensitive information, nurses should avoid lectures and questions that convey judgmental attitudes. Asking open-ended questions and avoiding assumptions (e.g., all teens have supportive families, all teens are heterosexual) also give adolescents opportunities to share more of their psychosocial contexts. Any medical language used during the interview should be clarified, and adolescents should be asked to explain any terms they use that are unfamiliar. Restating issues a teenager verbalizes during an interview allows for a mutual understanding of their concerns.

Interview Content

In reviewing the major morbidities and moralities of youth, it becomes clear that many of the threats to adolescent health are psychosocial and behavioral in nature. Therefore, in the limited time available with adolescent clients, emphasis should be placed on assessment of high-risk psychosocial behaviors (Schubiner, 1989). This type of screen-

GUIDELINES
Interviewing Adolescents

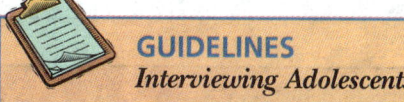

Ensure confidentiality and privacy; interview adolescent without parents.

Show concern for adolescent's perspective: "First, I'd like to talk about your main concerns" and "I'd like to know what you think is happening."

Offer a nonthreatening explanation for the questions you ask: "I'm going to ask a number of questions to help me better understand your health."

Maintain objectivity; avoid assumptions, judgments, and lectures.

Ask open-ended questions when possible; move to more directive questions if necessary.

Begin with less sensitive issues and proceed to more sensitive ones.

Use language that both the adolescent and you understand.

Restate: reflect back to adolescents what they have said, along with feelings that may be associated with their descriptions.

ing will help to identify the majority of adolescents who are coping well, those who require simple health information and/or counseling, and those who have significant psychosocial problems and need referral to appropriate resources.

After obtaining information on the adolescent's major concerns, the mnemonic device ***SAFE TIMES*** can be used as a guide for other routine health-screening questions (Schubiner, 1989). As shown in the box at right, each letter of this mnemonic device represents an important issue or set of issues in preventive care. The less sensitive issues are toward the bottom (i.e., safety, education). It is best to begin the interview with less sensitive topics, ending with more sensitive areas such as sexuality. Routine health screening using the SAFE TIMES format usually takes about 10 to 15 minutes (Schubiner, 1989).

In the following section, the SAFE TIMES areas are discussed to provide an overview of trends related to each set of health-related issues. Suggestions for screening questions, laboratory testing, and preventive interventions within each area follow guidelines put forth by the American Medical Association (1992) and the U.S. Preventive Services Task Force (1990).

HEALTH CONCERNS OF ADOLESCENCE

Safety (Injury Prevention)

Unintentional injuries kill more adolescents than any other single cause of death in the United States. Motor vehicle crashes are the single greatest cause of death, accounting for nearly two thirds of fatal injuries among young people (Bearinger and Blum, 1994). The majority of fatal and nonfatal motor vehicle crashes involve alcohol (Regale, 1988). Homicide, a form of intentional injury, is the second leading cause of death among all U.S. adolescents (Schubiner, 1989); for black teens it is the most likely cause of death (Millstein, Petersen, and Nightingale, 1993). In the United States over half of all homicides occur among friends or

SAFE TIMES: A METHOD FOR HEALTH-SCREENING INTERVIEWS WITH ADOLESCENTS

S SEXUALITY

a. Pubertal development, menstrual history (girls)
b. Extent of sexual activity, type of relationships, symptoms of STDs
c. Pregnancy and STD prevention methods
d. Orientation issues (attractions, behaviors)
e. History of sexual abuse

A AFFECT

a. Symptoms of depression ("feeling down or blue") or hopelessness ("discouraged about the future")

ABUSE

a. Use of tobacco, alcohol, marijuana, cocaine, other drugs

F FAMILY

a. Who the patient lives with and if there are any family conflicts or problems
b. Family history—medical, psychiatric

E EXAMINATION

a. Self-breast or self-testicular examination (middle to late adolescence)
b. Explain pelvic examination (if indicated)

T TIMING OF DEVELOPMENT

a. For younger adolescents—"Is your development going too fast, too slow, or at about the right speed?" and "Do you feel too tall, too short, or about the right height?"
b. For all, "Do you feel too thin, too heavy, or about the right weight?"

I IMMUNIZATION

a. Tetanus-diphtheria (Td) needed every 10 years
b. Measles-mumps-rubella (MMR) unless two vaccines given during childhood or pregnancy
c. Hepatitis B if engaging in risk behavior
d. PPD yearly for high-risk groups
e. Pneumovax, influenza if chronic disease

M MINERALS

a. Iron—supplementation required if less than two servings of meats daily or low hemoglobin
b. Calcium—supplementation required (especially in females) for those who drink less than 2 to 3 glasses of milk daily (e.g., Tums, 3 to 4 tablets daily)
c. Cholesterol—intake of fats, lipid levels

E EDUCATION, EMPLOYMENT

a. If in school, what grades attained; any problems?
b. Work history and future plans

S SAFETY

a. Especially car safety, use of seat belts, drinking and driving, or accepting rides from drivers using drugs
b. Motorcycles, mopeds, all-terrain vehicles
c. Handguns in the home, handgun availability

Note: In clinical interviewing, SAFE TIMES is best used in reverse disorder.

Modified from Schubiner H: Preventive health screening in adolescent patients, Prim Care 16:211-230, 1989.

TABLE 19-2 Injury Prevention During Adolescence

DEVELOPMENTAL ABILITIES RELATED TO RISK OF INJURY	INJURY PREVENTION
Need for independence and freedom Testing independence Age permitted to drive a motor vehicle (varies) Inclination for risk taking Feeling of indestructibility Need for discharging energy, often at expense of logical thinking and other control mechanisms Strong need for peer approval May attempt hazardous feats Peak incidence for practice and participation in sports Access to more complex tools, objects, and locations Can assume responsibility for own actions	**Motor/nonmotor vehicles** *Pedestrian*—Emphasize and encourage safe pedestrian behavior *Passenger*—Promote appropriate behavior while riding in a motor vehicle *Driver*—Provide competent driver education; encourage judicious use of vehicle, discourage drag racing, "playing chicken"; maintain vehicle in proper condition (brakes, tires, etc.) Teach and promote safety and maintenance of two-wheeled vehicles Promote and encourage wearing of safety apparel such as helmet, long trousers Reinforce the dangers of drugs, including alcohol, when operating a motor vehicle **Drowning** Teach nonswimmer to swim Teach basic rules of water safety Judicious selection of place to swim Sufficient water depth for driving Swimming with companion **Burns** Reinforce proper behavior in areas involving contact with burn hazards (gasoline, electric wires, fires) Advise regarding excessive exposure to natural or artificial sunlight (ultraviolet burn) Discourage smoking Encourage use of sunscreen **Poisoning** Educate in hazards of drug use, including alcohol **Falls** Teach and encourage general safety measures in all activities **Bodily damage** Promote acquisition of proper instruction in sports and use of sports equipment Instruct in safe use of and respect for firearms and other devices with potential danger (e.g., power tools, firecrackers) Provide and encourage use of protective equipment when using potentially hazardous devices Promote access to and/or provision of safe sports and recreational facilities Be alert for signs of depression (potential suicide) Discourage use of and/or availability of hazardous sports equipment (trampoline, surfboards) Instruct regarding proper use of corrective devices such as glasses, contact lenses, hearing aids Encourage and foster judicious application of safety principles and prevention

family members (Rosenberg and Mercy, 1991); firearms are involved in 70% of teen homicides (Fingerhut and others, 1991). In addition to being the leading cause of death, injuries also account for substantial morbidity among youth. The leading causes of injury-related morbidity include vehicular crashes, firearms, drownings, poisonings, burns, and falls (Bearinger and Blum, 1994) (Table 19-2).

During an interview, the time available for safety issues should focus on injuries related to motor vehicle crashes and firearm use. One might initially ask how the adolescent "gets around town." Further questions and health education might focus on seat belt and/or helmet use and the practice of drinking and driving or riding with drivers who have been drinking. Adolescents should be asked whether they have access to firearms, including access at home, whether they carry a gun, and whether they ever use alcohol in combination with handling guns. Stringham and Weitzman (1988) and the American Medical Association (1992) describe health education strategies to prevent violence-related injuries, including counseling on nonviolent ways to resolve conflicts and discouraging the possession and use of weapons.

Education and Employment

In 1990 over 30% of U.S. youth dropped out of school before completing high school. The dropout rate varies considerably by ethnicity; in 1990 only 42% of Hispanic teens graduated from high school by age 19, compared with 61% of African-American teens and 73% of white teens (Annie E. Casey Foundation, 1993). The graduation rate for American Indian teens is lower than that of any other racial/ethnic group (Blum and others, 1992). School problems can be a marker for other difficulties, such as learning disabilities, language barriers, alcohol or other drug use, family problems, lack of supportive relationships at school, and employment needs (American Medical Association, 1992; Schubiner, 1989). In contemporary U.S. society a good education is critical to economic self-sufficiency. Teens who drop out of high school can expect to earn approximately one-third less income each year than those who graduate (Annie E. Casey Foundation, 1993).

Specific questions about recent grades, school absences, transfers and suspensions can be used to screen for school-related problems. Specific management plans for youth who note school problems should be coordinated with school personnel and with the adolescent's parents or caregivers if possible.

Minerals (Nutrition)

Nutrition screening is another essential area of an adolescent health assessment. Puberty marks the beginning of accelerated physical growth, which can as much as double adolescents' nutritional requirements for iron, calcium, zinc, and protein for 1.5 to 2 years (Schubiner, 1989). At the same time, growing independence, the need for peer acceptability, concern with physical appearance, and an active life-style may affect eating habits, food choices, nutrient intake, and thus nutritional status (Story, Heald, and Dwyer, 1991). Although problems related to overt nutritional deficiencies (excluding iron deficiencies) have decreased since the 1940s, they have been replaced by problems of dietary imbalances and excesses. Excess intake of calories, sugar, fat, cholesterol, and sodium are common among adolescents and are found in all income and racial/ethnic groups and both genders (Fig. 19-14). Inadequate intake of certain vitamins (folic acid, vitamin B_6, vitamin A) and minerals (iron, calcium, zinc) is also evident, particularly among girls and teens of low socioeconomic status. In combination with other factors, these dietary patterns could result in increased risk for chronic diseases such as heart disease, osteoporosis, and some types of cancer later in life (Story, Heald, and Dwyer, 1991)

Routine nutrition screening should include questions about meal patterns, dieting behaviors, consumption of high-fat and high-salt foods, and recent changes in weight. In terms of laboratory screening, the American Medical Association (1992) recommends annual weight and height determinations and screening for hypertension. A screening hemoglobin and/or hematocrit is recommended for adolescent girls at their first health-screening visit and at the end of pubertal development (Neinstein, 1991). Adolescents whose parents have a serum cholesterol level greater than 240 mg/dl and adolescents who are over 19 years of age should be screened for total blood cholesterol at least once during the teen years (American Medical Association, 1992). Healthy dietary habits should be discussed with all adolescents, including the benefits of a healthy diet; ways to consume healthy foods, including those rich in calcium, iron, and other vitamins and minerals; and safe weight management (American Medical Association, 1992).

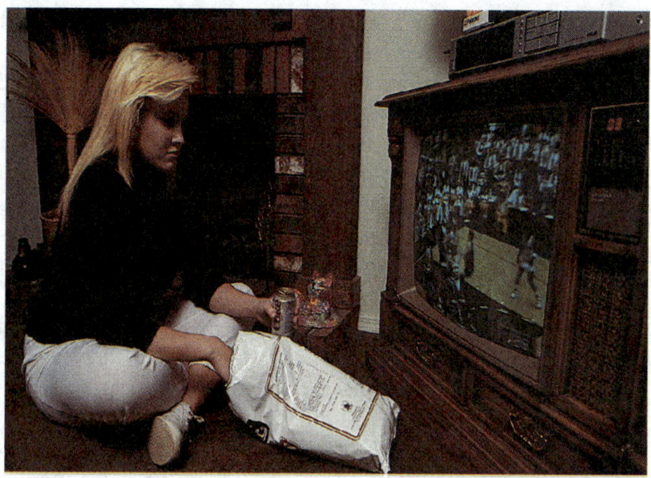

FIG. 19-14 Snacking on empty calories is common among adolescents, especially during inactivity.

Immunizations

An immunization update is an important part of adolescent preventive care. Obtaining a record of the teen's prior immunizations is important. Adolescents should receive a tetanus-diphtheria (Td) vaccine 10 years after their most recent childhood diphtheria-pertussis-tetanus (DPT) vaccination. With the exception of pregnant teens, all adolescents should receive a second measles-mumps-rubella (MMR) vaccine unless they have documentation of two MMR vaccinations during childhood but not before 12 months of age. Susceptible adolescents who engage in risk-taking behaviors should also be vaccinated against hepatitis B virus. This includes adolescents who have had more than one sexual partner during the previous 6 months, have exchanged sex for drugs or money, are males who have had sex with other males, or have been injecting drugs or sexually partnered with a drug user who injects. Widespread use of the hepatitis B vaccine is encouraged because risk factors are often not easily identifiable among adolescents (American Medical Association, 1992) (see Immunizations, Chapter 12).

Young people should receive a tuberculin skin test if they have been exposed to active tuberculosis (TB), have lived in a homeless shelter, have been incarcerated, have lived in or come from an area with a high prevalence of tuberculosis, or currently work in a health care setting. The frequency of TB testing depends on risk factors of the individual adolescents (American Medical Association, 1992) (see Tuberculosis, Chapter 32).

Timing of Development

The physical changes of pubertal development may be a cause of concern or question for many young adolescents.

Early-maturing girls and late-maturing boys, being out of synch with their age-mates' growth patterns, may have special concerns. Questions such as "Do you feel that you are developing too fast, too slow, or at about the right speed?" and "Do you feel too tall, too short, or about the right height for someone your age?" allow adolescents a chance to discuss their concerns related to physical development.

Adolescent obesity poses a risk for both immediate problems (such as social and psychologic problems in large part resulting from negative social attitudes) and long-term consequences (such as adult obesity and its attendant medical risks). National survey data indicate that 15% to 25% of American adolescents are significantly overweight (U.S. Department of Health and Human Services, 1988). Adolescent girls have a higher rate of obesity (26%) than adolescent boys (18%) (Gortmaker, Dietz, and Sobal, 1987). Eating disorders (i.e., anorexia nervosa and bulimia nervosa) commonly are manifested during the adolescent and young adult years. Up to 5% of young women have anorexia, and nearly 1 in 5 have bulimia, although definitions and rates vary in different surveys (Schubiner, 1989). These disorders, like obesity, can lead to considerable morbidity and mortality if left untreated (Story, Heald, and Dwyer, 1991). Chapter 21 provides further information on eating disorders commonly seen among adolescents.

"Do you feel too heavy, too thin, or about the right weight?" is a question that can serve as a simple screen, along with height and weight measurements, for obesity and other eating disorders. Adolescents whose body mass index (weight/height^2) is over the 85th percentile—those at highest risk for obesity—should be provided with an appropriate referral for nutrition and exercise counseling (see Story, Heald, and Dwyer, 1991, for a comprehensive approach to management of adolescent obesity). Adolescents should be referred for further assessment for organic disease, anorexia nervosa, or bulimia if any of the following factors are present: weight loss greater than 10% of previous weight; recurrent dieting when not overweight; use of self-induced emesis, laxatives, starvation, or diuretics to lose weight; distorted body image; or body mass index (BMI) below the 5th percentile.

Examination

Although at times adolescents may have high levels of self-concern, they often understand little about their bodies. Discussing and teaching self-examination of the breasts or testicles as part of the physical examination may be a useful way to defuse some of the anxiety that comes with the invasion of the adolescent's privacy. Although breast cancer is very rare in this age-group, teaching breast self-examination (BSE) to middle and older adolescent girls may encourage them to develop a lifelong habit. Unlike the lower incidence of breast cancer in young women, testicular cancer is the most common solid tumor in young men (Murphey, 1983). Review of the normal structures of the scrotum with instruction on self-examination can be done as part of health promotion for middle to older adolescent boys (Schubiner, 1989).

Family

Having family members who are emotionally available and appropriately involved in their lives has proved to be a key factor in the well-being of adolescents (U.S. Congress, 1991a). On the other hand, family dysfunction can be a strong contributor to a multitude of adolescent problems, including depression, alcohol and other drug abuse, eating disorders, and school failure. A wide variety of family disorders, including parental discord, alcohol or drug abuse, mental illness, or family violence, can lead to additional stresses in coping with the tasks of adolescence.

Questions such as "How are things going at home?" and "How easy is it for you to talk to your parents?" help to give a general sense of family relationships. More directed questions such as "Are you currently having conflicts with your family?" and "How does your family generally solve disagreements?" also give insight into family functioning.

Generally, if an adolescent is doing well in school, relates well to peers, and is able to resolve areas of conflict with family members, family intervention is not necessary. Nurses can support positive conflict resolution around minor issues such as curfew hours and appropriate limit-setting among adolescents and their families. Families dealing with major conflicts or dysfunctional relationships should be referred to a family therapist or other mental health professional.

Abuse

By twelfth grade, 89.5% of U.S. students have used alcohol, 64.4% have tried smoking, and 40.7% have tried marijuana (Johnston, O'Malley, and Bachman, 1991). Furthermore, in U.S. society, tobacco, alcohol, and marijuana use may be viewed by young people as functional behavior—offering an opportunity to challenge authority, to demonstrate autonomy, to gain entry into a peer group, or simply to relieve the stresses of growing up (Perry and Kelder, 1992). Although chemical use may be extensive among U.S. teens, there have been substantive, documented consequences of early experimentation with alcohol, tobacco, and other drugs. Automobile accidents caused by drinking and driving are the leading cause of death among teenagers (Fell and Nash, 1989). Persons who begin smoking at younger ages are more likely to become heavier smokers and are at increased risk for illness and death attributable to smoking (Schultz, 1991; Taioli and Wynder, 1991). Substance use has also been implicated with other problem behaviors such as delinquency, absenteeism, dropping out of school, lower academic achievement, and precocious sexual behavior (Newcomb and Bentler, 1989).

Adolescents can be asked if they or their friends have ever tried tobacco, alcohol, or other drugs. They should also be asked about their own current use as well as current use patterns among peers. Practices of drinking and driving or riding with someone who has been drinking should be assessed. If answers to these initial questions indicate some level of problem use, the adolescents should be asked about the amount and frequency of use; the frequency of getting "bombed" or "high"; use in relation to sexual activity; and getting into difficulties with peers, school, parents, and/or the law in relation to use.

Young people who have begun experimenting or who engage in low-level use need to be made aware of other options that can help them achieve the same goals and of the risks of higher-level use. Furthermore, they need to know the short-term effects of alcohol, tobacco, or other drugs, particularly in relation to driving and school or work performance (Schubiner, 1989). Cessation plans should be discussed with adolescents who use tobacco products. Adolescents whose substance use patterns endanger their health should be referred to an appropriate mental health provider (American Medical Association, Substance Abuse: see Overview, Chapter 21).

Affect

A national survey of eighth and tenth graders found that 34% of girls and 15% of boys reported feeling "sad and hopeless" during the previous month; 18% of girls and 9% of boys reported that they often felt that they had nothing to look forward to (American School Health Association, 1989) (Fig. 19-15). Diagnosable mental health disorders, ranging from anxiety and depression to schizophrenia, are experienced by 18% to 22% of adolescents (U.S. Congress, 1991a). In 1987, 15% of tenth graders reported having made a suicide attempt (American School Health Association, 1989).

A brief psychologic screening is warranted during the course of adolescents' routine health visits. Screening for depression or suicidal risk should be done with adolescents who note declining school grades, chronic melancholy, family dysfunction, alcohol or other drug use, sexual orientation issues/concerns, a history of abuse, or previous suicidal attempts. Most adolescents who are depressed will respond affirmatively to the question "Have you been feeling down or blue lately?" although they may not necessarily "look" depressed (Mitchell and Rothenberg, 1984). Nonsuicidal adolescents who report commonly feeling "blue," "down," or "depressed" should be referred to a psychologist, psychiatrist, or other mental health professional who works with young people.

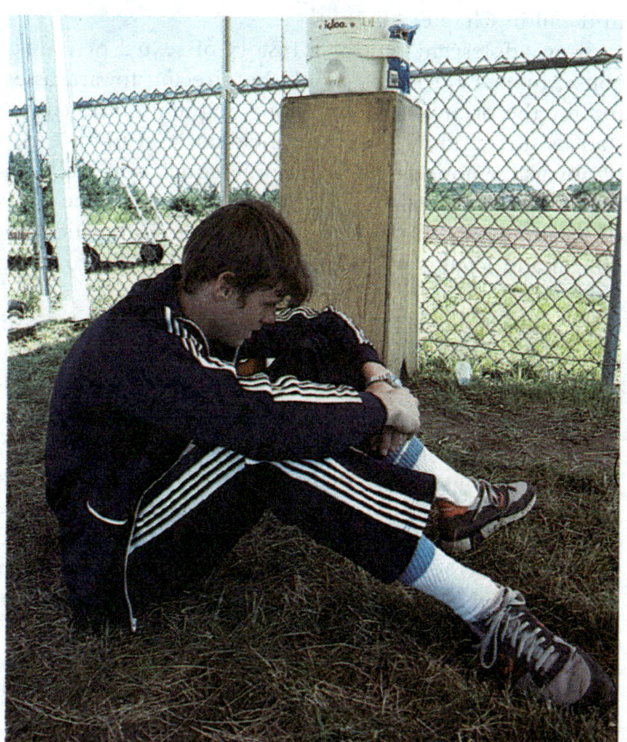

FIG. 19-15 Adolescents use being alone as a method of coping with stress.

It is crucial to explore thoughts about and possible plans for suicidal acts with all troubled adolescents. Once an assessment of the immediate risk of suicide is completed, a management scheme can be constructed. If the adolescent has a specific plan, immediate referral for acute intervention with a psychiatrist or other mental health professional is indicated. Chapter 21 addresses nursing issues related to the prevention and management of suicidal adolescents.

Sexuality (and Sex Education and Guidance)

Since the 1970s, sexual activity has increased among U.S. youth; at the same time, rates of sexually transmitted diseases (STDs), unintended pregnancy, and—beginning in the 1980s—human immunodeficiency virus (HIV) infection have increased among adolescents (Centers for Disease Control and Prevention, 1993). In the 1991 national Youth Risk Behavior Survey (YRBS), 69% of ninth through twelfth grade participants reported having had sexual intercourse in the 3 months prior to completing the survey. Many sexually active young people are engaging in behaviors that put them at risk for STDs and/or pregnancy, such as having sex with multiple partners and having sex without the use of condoms or other forms of contraception. In the YRBS 19% of students reported having four or more sexual partners during their lifetime. Although 82% of the sexually active students reported using some form of contraception during last intercourse, less than half (46%) reported condom use during last intercourse. The high prevalence of risky sexual behaviors among teens contributes to high rates of STDs and pregnancy in this age-group. In fact, *each year* 2.5 million U.S. adolescents—1 in 6—will acquire an STD (Yarber and Parrillo, 1992). About 1 million U.S. adolescents become pregnant each year; nearly 40% of these adolescents obtain abortions, slightly over 10% experience spontaneous abortion, and the remainder carry to term (U.S. Congress, 1991a).

Adolescence also appears to be a critical time in the development of sexual orientation. In a recent survey of seventh through twelfth graders in Minnesota, 88.2% of students described themselves as predominantly heterosexual; 10.7% were "unsure" of their sexual orientation; and 1.1% described themselves as bisexual or predominantly homosexual. Uncertainty about sexual orientation diminished in successively older age-groups, with corresponding increases in heterosexual and homosexual affiliation (Remafedi and others, 1992). Homophobia, the irrational fear of homosexuality in oneself or others, pervades our society at all levels (Taylor and Remafedi, 1993). In part because of the social stigma around homosexuality and the lack of socially sanctioned ways to explore their sexuality, gay, lesbian, and bisexual adolescents typically go through a period of identity confusion in their process of sexual identity development (Troiden, 1988). Sexual encounters with multiple same- and opposite-sex partners or engaging in other high-risk behaviors may be the means by which some young people deal with this confusion. In a 1986 survey, gay and bisexual adolescent males reported having sex with an average of 7 male partners in the previous year. One half of these teens had also had heterosexual experiences during the same year with an average of 5.6 female partners. Meetings in gay bars or public places accounted for the majority of encounters with male sexual partners. In nearly one third of the cases, the encounters were anonymous. Seventeen percent of the adolescents had been involved in prostitution, and over half were found to be abusing substances. Forty-five percent of boys had previously had an STD (Remafedi, 1987).

Obtaining a sexual history can be an important step in promoting sexual health and preventing sexually transmitted diseases and unintended pregnancies among young people. Given their sensitive nature, questions about sexuality should be prefaced by an explanation of their purpose and the limits of confidentiality. Initial questions can cover less sensitive topics such as milestones in pubertal development and, for girls, menstrual history (including age at menarche, timing of menstrual cycles, duration of menstrual flow, and symptoms of dysmenorrhea). Questions should also address dating behavior, same- and opposite-sex attractions, and same- and opposite-sex sexual behavior (e.g., "There are many ways people can be sexual with others, such as kissing, touching, and having oral, vaginal, and rectal intercourse. In what ways have you been sexual with others?"). Adolescents should be asked about a history of uninvited or nonconsensual sexual contact (e.g., "Has anyone ever touched you in a way that felt uncomfortable or wrong to you?"). Sexually active teens should be asked about their use of condoms, oral contraceptives, and other forms of contraception; the number of sexual partners they have had over the past 6 months; and the use of alcohol or other substances in connection with sexual activity. Sexually active adolescents should also be asked about any history of prior pregnancies or STDs. Sexually active teens who reveal a history of physical or sexual abuse, heavy use of alcohol or other drugs, or who have unstable social or economic support systems should be asked whether they have ever exchanged sex for money, shelter, or drugs.

Sexually active adolescents should be screened for STDs with laboratory tests for gonorrhea, chlamydia, and, for girls, a Pap test to detect human papilloma virus (HPV) infection or other cervical dysplasia. Males and females should be evaluated for HPV by visual inspection. Sexually active teens should have a serologic test for syphilis if they have lived in an area endemic for syphilis, have had other STDs, have had more than one sexual partner within the last 6 months, have exchanged sex for drugs or money, or are males who have engaged in sex with other males. Adolescents at risk for human immunodeficiency virus (HIV) infection should be offered confidential HIV-screening tests. HIV risk status includes a history of injecting drugs (including anabolic steroid injections), having had sexual intercourse in a geographic area with a high prevalence of HIV infection, having had other STD infections, having had more than one sexual partner in the last 6 months, having exchanged sex for drugs or money, being a male and having engaged in sex with other males, or having had a sexual partner who is at risk for HIV infection. The frequency of laboratory screening for STDs and HIV will depend on the sexual practices and STD history of the individual adolescent (American Medical Association, 1992).

All adolescents should receive health guidance regarding responsible sexual behaviors, including abstinence. Adolescents should receive information on how STDs, including HIV, are transmitted and on possible consequences of infection. Sexually active adolescents should be counseled about ways to reduce their risk of STDs and pregnancy, including limiting the number of sexual partners, using condoms consistently, using appropriate methods of birth control, and avoiding substance use in connection with sexual activity. Counseling should include instruction on how to use condoms effectively and methods of birth control. Adolescents should receive positive reinforcement for responsible sexual behaviors, including abstinence, consistent condom use, and appropriate use of birth control. Adolescents should also be counseled on ways to reduce their risk of sexual exploitation. Techniques for counseling adolescents to reduce risky sexual behaviors are discussed in detail in Chapter 20.

If an adolescent reports a history of sexual or physical abuse, further questions should be directed toward assessing for the occurrence of any ongoing abuse; the circumstances surrounding the abuse incident; and the presence of physical, emotional, or behavioral sequelae, including involvement in risk-taking behaviors. Nurses must be aware of local laws about reporting of abuse to authorities, and ethical and legal issues related to protecting the confidentiality of adolescent patients who report abuse.

Nurses need to acknowledge the possibilities of same-sex and bisexual attractions and relationships. Screening questions regarding sexual attractions and experiences should be phrased in ways that allow adolescents to discuss same- and opposite-sex preferences, such as using the term "partner" rather than "boyfriend" or "girlfriend." Health professionals who convey open and nonjudgmental attitudes about sexual orientation provide adolescents opportunities to talk about this sensitive topic and give parents who may be concerned about their adolescents' struggle with issues related to sexual orientation a source for discussing their questions or concerns.

Teenagers who question their sexual orientation should not be told that these feelings are only a passing phase. For the majority of young people, referral to an agency providing counseling and support services that might be needed is most appropriate. In addition to their special needs, gay, lesbian, and bisexual adolescents need the same sexuality education and information on STD/HIV transmission and prevention that is appropriate for all other adolescents.

In addition to being able to discuss issues related to sexual orientation, gay, lesbian, and bisexual teens often need a variety of support services. Because of long-standing biases against homosexuality in society, social support, including family support, positive adult role models, and healthy peer support networks, are critical for these young people. Health professionals who work with teens around sexual orientation issues are encouraged to seek out additional information and resources that address health needs and important health services for gay, lesbian, and bisexual adolescents (see Remafedi, 1990; Taylor and Remafedi, 1993).

HEALTH PROMOTION AMONG SPECIAL GROUPS OF ADOLESCENTS

Certain groups of adolescents—including adolescents of color and adolescents living in rural areas—experience health problems at disproportionate rates and face barriers to health care because of a lack of financial resources, limited availability of appropriate resources, or other factors.

Adolescents of Color

Children of color (i.e., children of African-American, Latino-Hispanic, Asian, American Indian, and Alaskan Native descent) are the fastest-growing population within the United States. In 1990, 30% of the U.S. population under the age of 19 was made up of children of color (Children's Defense Fund, 1991). By 2020, roughly 40% of the U.S. child population will be made up of minorities (Isaacs, 1993). Currently, half of African-American, Hispanic, and American Indian adolescents and 32% percent of Asian-American adolescents are poor or near-poor (below 150% of the federal poverty level). The disproportionate levels of health problems experienced by adolescents from these racial, ethnic, and tribal groups can be attributed, at least in part, to the effects of poverty and the lack of access to health care that is associated with being poor (U.S. Congress, 1991a).

It must be recognized that most of these children grow and develop normally and successfully meet the challenges of adolescence and young adulthood. Research has begun to identify factors that promote resiliency among minority adolescents from disadvantaged backgrounds, including those who grow up in poverty. Often these young people have come from families and communities that provide nurturing, supportive, and culturally rich environments (Isaacs, 1993). To be most effective, future health promotion interventions must include strategies that increase these protective factors in the lives of other adolescents growing up in high-risk environments.

However, too many minority adolescents experience predictable outcomes associated with living in environments where risk factors disproportionately outweigh protective factors. Higher percentages of minority children and adolescents have learning, emotional, and/or physical disabilities; have higher school drop-out rates and fewer opportunities for higher education; become parents at an early age; are incarcerated in youth detention facilities; and die as a result of homicide or unintentional injuries before reaching adulthood. The increase in health risk behaviors during adolescence, in combination with limited access to health care and effective preventive services, places these adolescents at significantly higher risk for adolescent pregnancy, STDs, HIV infection and acquired immunodeficiency syndrome (AIDS), chronic or other infectious diseases (such as hypertension, tuberculosis, and hepatitis), substance abuse, emotional problems, and violence. All of these health problems, which often lead to premature death or chronic disorders, are preventable (Isaacs, 1993).

Effective health promotion programs can make important contributions to the prevention of health problems among minority adolescents. There is a growing consensus that health promotion programs will be most effective if they are culturally competent. A ***culturally competent approach*** is one that both recognizes and incorporates—at all levels—the importance of culture, the assessment of relations across cultures, vigilance toward dynamics that result from cultural differences, the expansion of cultural knowledge, and the adaptation of programs to meet culturally specific needs (Dryfoos, 1991). Nurses, working with other health professionals and community leaders can be at the forefront of developing or adapting health promotion interventions that are culture specific. Several basic principles can be used to guide the development of culturally appropriate health promotion efforts (Isaacs, 1993):

- Health promotion messages can be most effective when they are conveyed through multiple community institutions. The content of these messages should be consistent across agencies, culturally appropriate, and couched in terms that deal with health destructive behaviors in a pragmatic rather than a judgmental manner (Nickens, 1990).
- Health promotion efforts should include involvement of peer groups, schools, communities, and families. In particular, families must be recognized as a positive source of cultural strength, as well as a primary source of information, education, and support for young people (Randall-David, 1989). Because "family" is defined differently by different cultures, a culture-specific definition of family must be the basis of developing interventions involving families. For example, prevention strategies that involve concerned relatives and friends have proved to be a highly successful approach to reaching Hispanic youth involved in high-risk behavior. Willingness of family and friends to be involved is rooted in Hispanic values of familialism and community (Marin, 1989).
- Those who develop strategies for minority adolescents and communities must draw on community-based values, traditions, and customs and work with knowledgeable persons from the community in developing focused interventions and communication channels (Office of Substance Abuse Prevention, 1992). The challenge for professionals, many of whom are from other cultures, is to develop collaborative relationships with community members that enable communities to identify health problems and their underlying causes and to design and evaluate programs that address identified needs.
- Health promotion interventions focused on minority adolescents may be most effective if they provide a generic framework and skills for developing relationships and problem solv-

ing that can be applied to any health-related decision. There is an emerging belief that this type of generic approach can be more effective than interventions focused on problem-specific entities (such as STDs, pregnancy, and substance use), since the behaviors that lead to many adolescent health problems are highly interrelated.

- Health promotion and prevention strategies must be developed and implemented in places where these adolescents are found. Adolescents who have left the school system are often at greater risk for health problems than those who remain in school. Health promotion messages must be incorporated into shelters for homeless and runaway youth, detention centers, residential programs, and community recreation centers to reach young people at highest risk.

To date, there has been little systematic evaluation of the effectiveness of health promotion interventions among minority adolescents (U.S. Congress, 1991a). Interventions that work must be documented so that these efforts can be disseminated and adapted for other communities of color.

Rural Adolescents

Outside of higher rates of accidental injuries (due in part to farm injuries) and lower rates of delinquency, there are few known differences in the health problems of rural and urban adolescents. Although research on the health status of rural adolescents is limited, it seems that rural adolescents experience many of the same health problems of adolescents in metropolitan areas (U.S. Congress, 1991a). However, rural adolescents face some unique barriers to health promotion, including more limited access to appropriate health services.

Rural adolescents' access to health care is limited by shortages of professionally staffed mental and physical health services, inadequately trained providers, transportation problems, and less access to Medicaid in rural states (U.S. Congress, 1990). Rural communities often lack adequately trained nurses, physicians, dentists, psychologists, social workers, and allied health professionals, in addition to modern equipment (Braden and Beauregard, 1994). Studies of a variety of health professionals have indicated that a substantial number feel inadequately prepared to address physical and psychosocial health issues of adolescents (Bearinger and others, 1992; Blum and Bearinger, 1990). In metropolitan areas providers who are unwilling or unable to address adolescents' concerns can refer to colleagues with expertise in adolescent health issues. The absence of adolescent health specialists combined with a limited network of agencies focused on adolescent health promotion exacerbates rural youths' problems with access to appropriate services. Finally, rural adolescents who live in poverty are less likely than their urban low-income counterparts to be covered by Medicaid (Rowland and Lyons, 1989) and thus to have financial coverage for health care services.

In addition to health promotion topics addressed with other populations of adolescents, prevention efforts focused on rural adolescents must include efforts to improve the safety of farm machinery and farming practices. Innovative efforts are needed to increase rural adolescents' access to health care services, including development and funding for school-linked health services, improvements in transportation, use of nonprofessionals and adult community members, better dissemination of information about availability of local health services, and access to further education in adolescent health for health care providers (U.S. Congress, 1991a).

NURSING CONSIDERATIONS

With continued increases in the numbers of adolescents in the United States—to a projected 24 million by the year 2000 (Millstein, Irwin, and Brindis, 1991)—and rising rates of many health-related problems of youth (Bearinger and Blum, 1994), there is an unprecedented need for adolescent health promotion. Nursing professionals can make significant contributions to health promotion among adolescents and their families. Grounded in an understanding of the biologic, cognitive, psychosocial, and social transitions of adolescence and their impact on health behavior, nursing interventions can address the developmental and health needs of adolescents. Working with colleagues from other disciplines, community members, parents, and adolescents

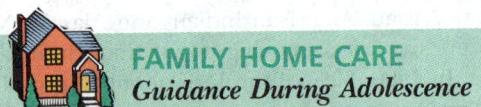

FAMILY HOME CARE

Guidance During Adolescence

Accept adolescent as a human being.
Respect adolescent's ideas, likes and dislikes, wishes.
Provide opportunity for choosing options and accept natural consequences of these choices.
Allow teenager to learn by doing, even when choices and methods differ from those of adults.
Provide adolescent with clear, reasonable limits.
Clarify house rules and consequences for breaking them.
Use family conferences to negotiate house rules.
Allow increasing independence within limitations of safety and well-being.
Be available but avoid pressing young person too far.
Respect adolescent's privacy.
Try to share adolescent's feelings of joy or sorrow.
Respond to feelings, as well as words.
Give space to a teenager who is in a bad mood.
Be available to answer questions, give information, and provide companionship.
Listen and try to be open to adolescent's views, even when they disagree with parental views.
Try to make communication clear.
Assist adolescent in selecting appropriate career goals and preparing for adult role.
Provide undemanding love.

Be aware that:

Adolescent is struggling for independence.
Adolescent is sensitive to feelings and behavior that affect him or her.
Message given to adolescent may not be message received.
Friends are extremely important to adolescent.
Adolescent has a strong need "to belong."
Adolescent sees things in black or white, good or bad.

themselves, nurses must become part of comprehensive approaches that deliver consistent messages across clinical, school, and community-based settings. Nurses can be at the forefront of developing and disseminating culturally appropriate health promotion interventions among special populations, including adolescents of color and rural teenagers. Nurses will also make significant contributions in areas not discussed in this chapter, such as in research and the formation of health policy (Bearinger and Gephart, 1987).

ANTICIPATORY GUIDANCE—CARE OF FAMILIES

The parents of the adolescent are usually as confused and perplexed as the youngster is about the changes and behavior of this stage of development. They also need support and guidance to help them through this trying time. They need to understand the changes taking place and to understand and accept the expected behaviors that accompany the process of detachment, to be prepared to "let go," and to promote the changed relationship from one of dependency to one of mutuality. Suggestions for anticipatory guidance of parents with an adolescent are listed in the Family Home Care box. Nurses interested in providing family-centered care are referred to the Bibliography for additional information on this expanding topic. (See also Communicating with Children, Chapter 6.)

KEY POINTS

- Adolescence is characterized by important biologic, cognitive, psychologic, and social change.
- The biologic events of puberty result in hormonal changes; changes in height, weight, strength, and endurance; and development of secondary sex characteristics.
- During adolescence, most individuals move from patterns of concrete thinking to abstract, hypothetical thinking.
- Major psychologic tasks of adolescence involve establishing a sense of identity along with behavioral, emotional, and value autonomy.
- According to Kohlberg's theory of moral development, adolescents begin to question existing moral values and learn to make choices; Gilligan observed differences in the way males and females make moral decisions.
- Spiritual development is characterized by the questioning of family values and ideals, a move to more philosophical thinking, and emphasis on personal religion.
- As adolescents establish identities separate from parents and families, relationships with peers often become more important.
- Biologic, cognitive, and psychosocial changes all affect sexual activity and sexual identity development of adolescents.
- Homosexual youth have unique issues to cope with in identity formation.
- The three primary causes of death during adolescence are injuries, homicide, and suicide.
- Major causes of adolescent morbidity include injury, sexually transmitted diseases, unintended pregnancy, and mental health problems, including depression, chronic illness, and eating disorders.
- To be most effective, adolescent health promotion efforts must actively involve teenagers at all stages.
- The availability of confidential health services is particularly important to adolescents.
- Certain groups of adolescents, including youth of color and rural youth, experience health problems at disproportionate rates and face barriers to health care because of limited access to appropriate, affordable resources.
- Motor vehicle injuries and drowning are the greatest causes of mortality from unintentional injuries in this age-group.

REFERENCES

American Academy of Pediatrics, Committee on Adolescence: Homosexuality and adolescence, *Pediatrics* 92(4):631-634, 1993.

American Medical Association: *Guidelines for adolescent preventive services,* Chicago, 1992, The Association.

American School Health Association, Association for the Advancement of Health, Education and Society for Public Health Education: *National adolescent student health survey: a report of the health of America's youth.* Reston, VA, 1989, Association for the Advancement of Health Education.

Annie E Casey Foundation and the Center for the Study of Social Policy: *KIDS COUNT data book: state profiles of child well-being,* Washington, DC, 1993, Center for the Study of Social Policy.

Attie I, Brooks-Gunn J, Petersen A: A developmental perspective on eating disorders and eating problems. In Lewis M, Miller S, editors: *Handbook of developmental psychopathology,* New York, 1990, Plenum Press.

Baumrind D: The influences of parenting style on adolescent competence and substance use, *J Early Adolesc* 11:56-95, 1991.

Bearinger L: Adolescent sexuality and media: health implications, *J Adolesc Health Care* 11(1):71-75, 1990.

Bearinger L, Blum R: Adolescent health care. In Wallace H, Nelson R, Sweeney P, editors: *Maternal and child health practices,* ed 4, Oakland, CA, 1994, Third Party.

Bearinger L, Gephart J: Priorities for adolescents' health, *MCN* 12(3):161-164, 1987.

Bearinger L, Gephart J: Interdisciplinary education in adolescent health, *J Pediatr Child Health* 29(suppl 1):S10-S15, 1993.

Bearinger L, McAnarney E: Integrated community health services: proceedings, *J Adolesc Health Care* 9(65):36S-40S, 1988.

Bearinger L and others: Nursing competence in adolescent health: anticipating the future needs of youth, *J Prof Nurs* 8(2):80-86, 1992.

Blum RW: Contemporary threats to adolescent health in the United States, *JAMA* 257:3390-3395, 1987.

Blum RW, Bearinger L: Knowledge and attitudes of health professionals toward adolescent health care, *J Adolesc Health Care* 11(4): 289-294, 1990.

Blum RW and others: *The state of adolescent health in Minnesota,* Minneapolis, 1989, University of Minnesota.

Blum RW and others: American Indian–Alaska Native youth health, *JAMA* 267(12):1637-1644, 1992.

Bracht N, Tsouros A: Principles and strategies of effective community participation, *Health Promot Int* 5(3):199-208, 1990.

Braden J, Beauregard K: *Health status and access to care of rural and urban populations,* AHCPR Pub No 94-0031, National Medical Expenditure Survey Research Findings 18, Agency for Health Care Policy and Research, Rockville, MD, 1994, Public Health Service.

Bronfenbrenner U: *The ecology of human development,* Cambridge, MA, 1979, Harvard University Press.

Brown B: Peer groups and peer cultures. In Feldman S, Elliot G, editors: *At the threshold: the developing adolescent,* Cambridge, MA, 1990, Harvard University Press.

Buhrmester D, Furman W: The development of companionship and intimacy, *Child Dev* 58:1101-1113, 1987.

Carnegie Council on Adolescent Development: *Turning points: preparing American youth for the 21st century,* Washington, DC, 1989, Carnegie.

Centers for Disease Control: Sexual behavior among high school students—United States, 1990, *MMWR* 40(51-52):885-888, 1992.

Centers for Disease Control and Prevention: Selected behaviors that increase risk for HIV infection, other sexually transmitted diseases, and unintended pregnancy among high school students—United States, 1991, *JAMA* 269(3):329-330, 1993.

Children's Defense Fund: *The state of America's children,* Washington DC, 1991, CDF.

Coleman E, Remafedi G: Gay, lesbian, and bisexual adolescents: a critical challenge to counselors, *J Counsel Dev* 68:36-40, 1989.

Comerci G: Normal pubescent growth and sexual maturation, *Semin Adolesc Med* 3:217-227, 1987.

Conger J: Current issues in adolescent development, *Master Lectures on Developmental Psychology,* Washington, DC, 1977, American Psychological Association.

Crockett L, Petersen A: Adolescent development: health risks and opportunities for health promotion. In Millstein, S, Petersen, A, Nightingale, E, editors: *Promoting the health of adolescents: new directions for the twenty-first century,* New York, 1993, Oxford University Press.

Dexheimer Pharris M, editor: *The community responds to youth violence: what works? What doesn't?* Monograph, 1994, Division of General, Pediatric, and Adolescent Health, University of Minnesota Medical School.

Dorn L, Crockett L, Petersen A: The relations of pubertal status to intrapersonal changes in young adolescents, *J Early Adolesc* 8:405-419, 1988.

Dryfoos J: Preventing high-risk behavior, *Am J Public Health* 81(2):157-158, 1991.

Elkind D: Understanding the young adolescent, *Adolescence* 13:128-134, 1978.

Elster A, Panzarine S, Holt K, editors: *American Medical Association State of the Art Conference on Adolescent Health Promotion: proceedings,* Arlington, VA, 1993, National Center for Education in Maternal and Child Health.

English A: Treating adolescents: legal and ethical considerations, *Med Clin North Am* 74(5): 1097-1112, 1990.

Entwisle D: Schools and adolescence. In Feldman S, Elliot G, editors: *At the threshold: the developing adolescent,* Cambridge, MA, 1990, Harvard University Press.

Epstein J: Parent involvement: what research says to administrators, *Educ Urban Soc* 19:119-136, 1987.

Erikson E: *Identity: youth in crisis,* New York, 1968, Norton.

Farel A: *Early adolescence and religion: a status study,* Carrboro, NC, 1982, Center for Early Adolescence.

Faust M: Alternative construction of adolescent growth. In Brooks-Gunn J, Petersen A, editors: *Girls at puberty: biological and psychosocial perspectives,* New York, 1983, Plenum Press.

Fell J, Nash C: The nature of the alcohol problem in U.S. fatal crashes, *Health Educ Q* 16:335-343, 1989.

Fingerhut L and others: *Firearm mortality among children, youth, and young adults, 1-34 years of age: trends and current status—United States, 1979-1990,* Washington, DC, 1991, US Government Printing Office.

Garmezy N: Resilience in children's adaptation to negative life events and stressed environments, *Pediatr Ann* 20(9):459-466, 1991.

Garn S, LaVelle M, Pilkington J: Comparisons of fatness in premenarcheal and postmenarcheal girls of the same age, *J Pediatr* 103:328-331, 1983.

Gilligan C: *In a different voice,* 1982, Cambridge, MA, 1982, Harvard University.

Gilligan C: *Adolescent development reconsidered,* Paper presented at the Invitational Conference on Health Futures of Adolescents, Daytona Beach, FL, 1986.

Gortmaker S, Dietz W, Sobal A: Increasing pediatric obesity in the United States, *Am J Dis Child* 141:535, 1987.

Graber J, Petersen A: Cognitive changes at adolescence: biological perspectives. In Gibson K, Petersen A, editors: *Brain maturation and cognitive development,* New York, 1991, Aldine de Gruyter.

Grant L, Demetriou E: Adolescent sexuality, *Pediatr Clin North Am* 35(6): 1271-1289, 1988.

Greenberger E, Steinberg L: *When teenagers work: the psychological and social costs of adolescent employment,* New York, 1986, Basic Books.

Greene A: Future time-perspective in adolescence: the present of things future revisited, *J Youth Adolesc* 15:99-113, 1986.

Greydanus D, Demarest D, Sears J: Sexual dysfunction in adolescents, *Semin Adolesc Med* 1(3):177-187, 1985.

Hamburg B: Subsets of adolescent mothers: developmental, biomedical, and psychosocial issues. In Lancaster J, Hamburg B, editors: *School-age pregnancy and parenthood: biosocial dimensions,* New York, 1986, Aldine de Gruyter.

Hamilton S: *Apprenticeship for adulthood: preparing youth for the future,* New York, 1990, Free Press.

Harter S: Self and identity development. In Feldman S, Elliott G, editors: *At the threshold: the developing adolescent,* Cambridge, MA, 1990, Harvard University Press.

Hayes C, editors: *Risking the future: adolescent sexuality, pregnancy, and childbearing,* vol 1, Washington, DC, 1987, National Academy Press.

Hill J: Research on adolescents and their families: past and present. In Irwin C Jr, editor: *Adolescent social behavior and health,* San Francisco, 1987, Jossey-Bass.

Hill J, Holmbeck G: Attachment and autonomy during adolescence. In Whitehurst G, editor: *Ann Child Dev,* Greenwich, CT, 1986, JAI Press.

Hoffman L: Effects of maternal employment in the two parent family, *Am Psychol* 44:283-292, 1989.

Ianni F: *The search for structure: a report on American youth today,* New York, 1989, Free Press.

Igoe J: Empowerment of children and youth for consumer self-care, *Am J Health Promot* 6:55-65, 1991.

Irwin C: *Toward a new health behavior model for adolescents,* Chicago, 1976, Society for Adolescent Medicine.

Irwin C, Vaughan E: Psychosocial context of adolescent development, *J Adolesc Health Care* 9:115-195, 1988.

Irwin C and others: *The health of America's youth: current trends in health status and utilization of health services,* San Francisco, 1991, University of California at San Francisco.

Isaacs M: Developing culturally competent strategies for adolescents of color. In Elster A, Panzarine S, Holt K, editors: *American Medical Association State of the Art Conference on Adolescent Health Promotion: proceedings,* Arlington, VA, 1993, National Center for Education in Maternal and Child Health.

Johnston L, O'Malley P, Bachman J: Press release of the 1990 national high school senior survey, Ann Arbor, 1991, University of Michigan, Institute for Social Research.

Kaluger G, Kaluger M: *Human development: the span of life,* ed 4, St Louis, 1988, Mosby.

Keating D, Clark L: Development of physical and social reasoning in adolescence, *Dev Psychol* 16:23-30, 1986.

Kirby D, and others: The effects of school-based health clinics in St. Paul upon school-wide birth rates, *Fam Plann Perspect* 25(1):12-16, 1993.

Klepp KI, Halper A, Perry C: The efficacy of peer leaders in drug abuse prevention, *J Sch Health* 56:407-411, 1986.

Kohlberg L, Gilligan C: The adolescent as philosopher: the discovery of the self in a post-conventional world. In Kagan J, Coles R, editors: *Twelve to sixteen: early adolescence,* New York, 1972, Norton.

Kreipe R: Principles of office counseling: the healthy adolescent, *Adolesc Med* 2(2):277-290, 1991.

Kuhn D, Amsel E, O'Loughlin M: *The development of scientific thinking skills,* San Diego, CA, 1988, Academic Press.

Lewis C: How adolescents approach decisions: changes over grades seven to twelve and policy implications, *Child Dev* 52:538-544, 1981.

Linn M: Content, context, and process in reasoning during adolescence: selecting model, *J Early Adolesc* 3:63-82, 1983.

Maccoby E, Martin J: Socialization in the context of the family: parent-child interaction. In Hetherington EM, editor: *Handbook of child psychology,* vol 4, *Socialization, personality and social development,* New York, 1983, John Wiley & Sons.

Marcia J: Development and validation of ego identity status, *J Pers Soc Psychol* 3:551-558, 1966.

Marin G: AIDS prevention among Hispanics: needs, risk behaviors, and cultural values, *Public Health Rep* 104(5):411-415, 1989.

McLanahan S, Bumpass L: Comment: a note of the effect of family structure on school enrollment. In Sandefun G, Tienda M, editors: *Divided opportunities,* New York, 1988, Plenum Press.

Millstein S: A view of health from the adolescent's perspective. In Millstein S, Petersen A, Nightingale E, editors: *Promoting the health of adolescents: new directions for the twenty-first century,* New York, 1993, Oxford University Press.

Millstein S, Irwin C: Concepts of health and illness: different constructs of variations on a theme? *Health Psychol* 6:515-524, 1987.

Millstein S, Irwin C, Brindis C: Sociodemographic trend and projections in the adolescent population. In Hendee W, editor: *The health of adolescents,* San Francisco, 1991, Jossey-Bass.

Millstein S, Petersen A, Nightingale E: Adolescent health promotion: rationale, goals, and objectives. In Millstein S, Petersen A, Nightingale E, editors: *Promoting the health of adolescents: new directions for the twenty-first century,* New York, 1993, Oxford University Press.

Mitchell J, Rothenberg M: Identifying psychiatric problems in an outpatient setting. *Consultant,* pp 267-281, 1984.

Murphey G: Testicular cancer, *Cancer* 33:100-104, 1983.

National Institute of Nursing Research: *Health promotion for older children and adolescents,* NIH Pub No 93-2420, Bethesda, MD, 1993, US Department of Health and Human Services, National Institutes of Health.

Neinstein L: *Adolescent health care: a practical guide,* ed 2, Baltimore, 1991, Williams & Wilkins.

Newacheck P, McManus M: Health insurance status of adolescents in the United States, *Pediatrics* 84:699-708, 1989.

Newcomb M, Bentler P: Substance use and abuse among children and teenagers, *Am Psychol* 44:242-248, 1989.

Nickens H: Health promotion and disease prevention among minorities, *Health Affairs,* 9(2):133-143, Summer 1990.

Office of Substance Abuse Prevention: *Technical assistance bulletin,* Rockville, MD, 1992, Department of Health and Human Services, Public Health Service.

O'Keefe G, Reid-Nash K: Socializing functions. In Berger C, Chafee S, editors: *Handbook of communication,* Newbury Park, CA, 1987, Sage.

Pallas A: School climate in American high schools, *Teachers College Record* 89:541-554, 1988.

Patterson G, Stouthamer-Loeber M: The correlation of family management practice and delinquency, *Child Dev* 55:1299-1307, 1984.

Pentz M: Benefits of integrating strategies in different settings. In Elster A, Panzarine S, Holt K, editors: *American Medical Association State of the Art Conference on Adolescent Health Promotion: proceedings,* Arlington, VA, 1993, National Center for Education in Maternal and Child Health.

Perry C, Jessor R: The concept of health promotion and the prevention of adolescent drug abuse, *Health Educ Q* 12:169-184, 1985.

Perry C, Kelder S: Prevention, *Ann Rev Addict Res Treat,* pp 453-472, 1992.

Perry C, Kelder S, Komro K: The social world of adolescents: family, peers, schools, and the community. In Millstein S, Petersen A, Nightingale E, editors: *Promoting the health of adolescents: new directions for the twenty-first century,* New York, 1993, Oxford University Press.

Perry C, Sieving R: *Peer involvement in global AIDS prevention among adolescents,* Paper prepared for World Health Organization Global Program on AIDS, 1991.

Piaget J: Intellectual evolution from adolescence to adulthood, *Hum Dev* 15:1-12, 1972.

Price J, and others: Differences in black and white adolescents' perceptions about cancer, *J Sch Health* 58:66-70, 1988.

Randall-David E: *Strategies for working with culturally diverse communities and clients,* Washington, DC, 1989, Association for the Care of Children's Health.

Regale G: *Proceedings: Surgeon General's workshop on drunk driving,* Rockville, MD, 1988, U.S. Department of Health and Human Services.

Remafedi G: Adolescent homosexuality: psychosocial and medical implications, *Pediatrics* 79:331, 1987.

Remafedi G: Fundamental issues in the care of homosexual youth, *Med Clin North Am* 74:1169-1179, 1990.

Remafedi G and others: Demography of sexual orientation in adolescents, *Pediatrics* 89(4):714-721, 1992.

Resnick M, Bearinger L: Physician attitudes and approaches to the problems of youth, *Pediatr Ann* 15(11):799-810, 1986.

Resnick M, Littman T, Blum R: Physicians' attitudes toward confidentiality of treatment for adolescents, *J Adolesc Health* 13:616-622, 1992.

Rest J, Davison M, Robbins S: Age trends in judging moral issues: a review of cross-sectional, longitudinal, and sequential studies of the Defining Issues Test, *Child Dev* 49:263-279, 1978.

Rosenberg M, Mercy J: Assaultive violence. In Rosenberg M, Fenley M, editors: *Violence in America: a public health approach,* New York, 1991, Oxford University Press.

Rowland D, Lyons B: Triple jeopardy: rural, poor and uninsured, *Health Serv Res* 23(6):975-1004, 1989.

Rutter M: Protective factors in children's responses to stress and disadvantage. In Kent M, Rolf J, editors: *Primary prevention of psychopathology,* vol 3, *Social competence in children,* Hanover, NH, 1979, University Press for New England.

Savin-Williams R, Berndt T: Friendship and peer relations. In Feldman S, Elliot G, editors: *At the threshold: the developing adolescent,* Cambridge, MA, 1989, Harvard University Press.

Schorr L, Schorr D: *Within our reach: breaking the cycle of disadvantage,* New York, 1988, Doubleday.

Schubiner H: Preventive health screening in adolescent patients, *Primary Care* 16:211-230, 1989.

Schultz J: Smoking-attributable mortality and years of potential life lost—United States, 1988, *MMWR* 40:62-71, 1991.

Seidman S, Rieder R: A review of sexual behavior in the United States, *Am J Psychiatry* 151(3):330-341, 1994.

Selman R: Toward a structural analysis of developing interpersonal relations concepts: research with normal and disturbed preadolescent boys. In Pick A, editor: *Minnesota symposia of child psychology,* vol 10, Minneapolis, 1976, University of Minnesota Press.

Simmons R: Social transition and adolescent development. In Irwin C Jr, editor: *Adolescent social behavior and health,* San Francisco, 1987, Jossey-Bass.

Simmons R, Blyth D: *Moving into adolescence,* New York, 1987, Aldine de Gruyter.

Simmons R and others: Entry into early adolescence: the impact of school structure, puberty, and early dating on self-esteem, 1979, *Am Sociol Rev* 44(6):948-967, 1979.

Spencer M, Markstrom-Adams C: Identity processes among racial and ethnic minority children in America, *Child Dev* 61:290-310, 1990.

Steinberg L: Latch-key children and susceptibility to peer pressure: an ecological analysis, *Dev Psychol* 22:433-439, 1986.

Steinberg L: *Adolescence,* ed 2, New York, 1989a, McGraw-Hill.

Steinberg L: Autonomy, conflict and harmony in the family relationship. In Feldman S, Elliot G, editors: *At the threshold: the developing adolescent,* Cambridge, MA, 1989b, Harvard University Press.

Steinberg L: Adolescent transitions and alcohol and other drug use prevention. In Goplerud E, editor: *Preventing adolescent drug use: from theory to practice* (OSAP Prevention Monograph 8), Rockville, MD, 1991, US Department of Health and Human Serivces.

Steinberg L, Elman J, Mounts N: Authoritative parenting, psychosocial maturity, and academic success among adolescents, *Child Dev* 60:1424-1436, 1989.

Steinberg L, Silverberg S: The vicissitudes of autonomy in early adolescence, *Child Dev* 57:841-851, 1986.

Steinberg L and others: Adolescents in the labor force: some costs and benefits to schooling and learning, *Educa Eval Pol Anal* 4:363-372, 1982.

Stipek D, McCroskey J: Investing in children: government and workplace policies for parents, *Am Psychol* 44:416-423, 1989.

Story M, Heald F, Dwyer J: Adolescent nutrition: trends and critical issues for the 1990s. In Sharbaugh C, editor: *Call to action: better nutrition for mothers, children, and families,* Washington, DC, National Center for Education in Maternal and Child Health.

Stringham P, Weitzman M: Violence counseling in the routine health care of adolescents, *J Adolesc Health Care* 9:389-393, 1988.

Sullivan H: *The interpersonal theory of psychiatry,* New York, 1953, Norton.

Taioli E, Wynder E: Effect of the age at which smoking begins on frequency of smoking in adulthood, *N Engl J Med* 325:968-969, 1991.

Taylor B, Remafedi G: Youth coping with sexual orientation issues, *J Sch Nurs* 9(2):26-39, 1993.

Tobin-Richards M: *Sex differences and similarities in heterosexual activity in early adolescence,* Paper presented at the biennial meeting of the Society for Research in Child Development, Toronto, 1985.

Troiden R: Homosexual identity development, *J Adolesc Health Care* 9:105-113, 1988.

Udry JR, Billy J: Initiation of coitus in early adolescence, *Am Sociol Rev* 52:841-855, 1987.

Udry JR and others: Serum androgenic hormones motivate sexual behavior in adolescent boys, *Fertil Steril* 43:90-94, 1985.

US Bureau of the Census: *School enrollment—social and economic characteristics of students: October 1986,* Current Population Report, Series P-20, No 429, Washington, DC, 1988, US Government Printing Office.

US Congress, Office of Technology Assessment: *Health care in rural America,* Pub No OTA-H-434, Washington, DC, 1990, US Government Printing Office.

US Congress Office of Technology Assessment: *Adolescent health, vol 1, Summary and policy options,* Pub No OTA-H-468, Washington DC, 1991a, US Government Printing Office.

US Congress, Office of Technology Assessment: *Adolescent health, vol 2, Background and the effectiveness of selected prevention and treatment services,* Pub No OTA-H-466, Washington, DC, 1991b, US Government Printing Office.

US Department of Health and Human Services, Public Health Service: *Healthy people 2000,* DHHS (PHS) Pub No 91-50212, Washington, DC, 1991, US Government Printing Office.

US Department of Health and Human Services, Public Health Service: *The Surgeon General's report on nutrition and health,* DHHS (PHS) Pub No 88-50210, Washington DC, 1988, US Government Printing Office.

US Preventive Services Task Force: The periodic health examination: age-specific charts, *Am Fam Physician* 41:189, 1990.

Walker L, de Vries B, Trevethan S: Moral stages and moral orientations in real-life and hypothetical dilemmas, *Child Dev* 58:842-858, 1987.

Werner E: High risk children in young adulthood: a longitudinal study from birth to 32 years, *Am J Orthopsychiatry* 52:72-81, 1989.

White K and others: Relationship maturity: a conceptual and empirical approach. In Meacham J, editor: *Contributions to human development,* vol 18, New York, 1987, S Karger.

Worthman C: Developmental dyssynchrony as normative experience: Kikuyu adolescents. In Lancaster J, Hamburg B, editors: *School-age pregnancy and parenthood: biosocial dimensions,* New York, 1986, Aldine de Gruyter.

Wuthnow R, Glock C: Religious loyalty, defection, and experimentation among college youth, *J Sci Study Relig* 12:157-180, 1973.

Yarber W, Parrillo A: Adolescents and sexually transmitted diseases, *J Sch Health* 62(7):331-338, 1992.

BIBLIOGRAPHY

General

American Academy of Pediatrics, Committee on Communications: Impact of rock lyrics and music videos on children and youth, *Pediatrics* 83:314-315, 1989.

Bane MJ, Ellwood DT: One fifth of the nation's children: why are they poor? *Science* 245: 1047-1053, 1989.

Boggs KU: Pubertal status and social support–seeking behavior in early adolescents, *J Pediatr Nurs* 3:229-236, 1988.

Brindis C, Lee P: Public policy issues affecting the health care delivery system of adolescents, *J Adolesc Health Care* 11:387-397, 1990.

Brown EF, Hendee WR: Adolescents and their music, *JAMA* 262:1659-1663, 1989.

Dornbusch SM and others: The relation of parenting style to adolescent school performance, *Child Dev* 58:1244-1257, 1987.

Duryea EJ, Hammes MJ: Cognitive development and the dynamics of decision-making among adolescents, *J Sch Health* 56:224-226, 1986.

Erikson EH: *Identity: youth and crisis,* New York, 1968, WW Norton.

Erikson EH: *Dimensions of a new identity,* New York, 1974, WW Norton.

Gilligan C, Ward JV, Taylor JM, editors: *Mapping the moral domain,* Cambridge, MA, 1988, Harvard University Press.

Gillis CL and others: *Toward a science of family nursing,* Menlo Park, CA, 1989, Addison-Wesley.

Goldenring JM, Cohen E: Getting into adolescent heads, *Contemp Pediatr* 5(7):75-90, 1988.

Groer MW and others: Adolescent stress and coping: a longitudinal study, *Res Nurs Health* 15(3):209-217, 1992.

Grubbs S and others: Self-efficacy in normal adolescents, *Issues Ment Health Nurs* 13:121-128, 1992.

Haggerty R: Care of the poor and underserved in America: older adolescents: a group at special risk, *Am J Dis Child* 145:569-571, 1991.

Hamburg D, Nightingale EO, Takanishi R: Facilitating the transitions of adolescence, *JAMA* 257:3405-3406, 1987.

Havens B, Swenson I: Menstrual perceptions and preparation among female adolescents, *JOGNN* 15:406-411, 1986.

Irwin CE, Shafer M: Adolescent medicine, *JAMA* 268(3):333-335, 1992.

Levine MD, McAnarney ER, editors: *Early adolescent transitions,* Lexington, MA, 1988, Lexington Books.

Moffit TE and others: Childhood experience and the onset of menarche: a test of a sociobiological model, *Child Dev* 63(1):59-67, 1992.

Morse IM, McKinnon D: Adolescents' response to menarche, *J Sch Health* 57:385-388, 1987.

Newman B, Newman P: The impact of high school on social development, *Adolescence* 22:525-533, 1987.

Offer D, Ostrov E, Howard KI: Adolescence: what is normal? *Am J Dis Child* 143:731-736, 1989.

Orr DP, Ingersoll GM: Adolescent development: a biopsychosocial review, *Curr Probl Pediatr* 18:443-499, 1988.

Piaget J: *The theory of stages in cognitive development,* New York, 1969, McGraw-Hill.

Pletsch PK and others: Self-image among early adolescents: revisited, *J Community Health Nurs* 8(4):215-231, 1991.

Puskar K, Lamb J: Life events, problems, stresses, and coping methods of adolescents, *Issues Ment Health Nurs* 12(3):267-281, 1991.

Rosella JD, Albrecht SA: Anticipatory guidance: alcohol, adolescents, and recognizing abuse and dependence, *Issues Compr Pediatr Nurs* 16(4):207-218, 1993.

Schmitt BD: Dealing with normal adolescent rebellion, *Contemp Pediatr* 7(7):55-60, 1990.

Schwartz ID, Root AW: Puberty in girls: normal or delayed? *Contemp Pediatr* 6(11):83-104, 1989.

Slap GB: Normal psychological and psychosocial growth in the adolescent, *J Adolesc Health Care* 7(suppl):13-23, 1986.

Slusher IL and others: State of the art of nursing research and theory development in adolescent health, *Issues Compr Pediatr Nurs* 16:1-11, 1993.

Steinberg L, Silberberg SS: The vicissitudes of autonomy in early adolescence, *Child Dev* 57:841-851, 1986.

Steinberg L and others: Impact of parenting practices on adolescent achievement: authorative parenting, school involvement, and encouragement to succeed, *Child Dev* 63(5):1266-1281, 1992.

Tanner JM: Issues and advances in adolescent growth and development, *J Adolesc Health Care* 8:470-478, 1987.

Thomas MA, Rebar RW: The endocrinology of normal and abnormal puberty, *Curr Opin Obstet Gynecol* 1:259-265, 1989.

Vaughn VC, Litt IF: *Child and adolescent development: clinical implications,* Philadelphia, 1990, WB Saunders.

Willits FK: Adolescent behavior and adult success and well-being: a 37-year panel study, *Youth Society* 20:68-87, 1988.

Health Promotion

Alderman EM, Fleischman AR: Should adolescents make their own health-care choices? *Contemp Pediatr* 10(1):65-82, 1993.

American Medical Association, Council on Scientific Affairs: Harmful effects of ultraviolet radiation, *JAMA* 262:380-384, 1989.

American Medical Association, Council on Scientific Affairs: Providing medical services through school-based health programs, *JAMA* 261:1939-1942, 1989.

Availability of comprehensive adolescent health services, *MMWR* 42(26):507-515, 1993.

Bearinger L, Gephardt J: Priorities for adolescent health: recommendations of a national conference, *MCN* 12:161-164, 1987.

Church JL, Baer KJ: Examination of the adolescent: a practical guide, *J Pediatr Health Care* 1:65-72, 1987.

Council on Scientific Affairs, American Medical Association: Confidential health services for adolescents, *JAMA* 269(11):1420-1424, 1993.

Craft MJ: Health care preferences of rural adolescents: types of service and companion choices, *J Pediatr Nurs* 2:3-12, 1987.

Cromer BA and others: Psychosocial determinants of compliance in adolescents with iron deficiency, *Am J Dis Child* 143:55-58, 1989.

Cromer BA and others: Compliance with breast self-examination instruction in high school students, *Clin Pediatr* 215-220, 1992.

Ell K, Northern H: *Families and health care: psychosocial practice,* New York, 1990, Adline de Gruyter.

Food and Nutrition Board, National Research Council: *Recommended dietary allowances,* ed 10, Washington, DC, 1989, National Academy of Sciences.

Greene J: Making adolescent space in a pediatric office, *Pediatr Nurs* 15:402-403, 1989.

Joffe A, Radius S, Gall M: Health counseling for adolescents: what they want, what they get, and who gives it, *Pediatrics* 82:481-485, 1988.

Kaufman KL and others: What, me worry? A survey of adolescents' concerns, *Clin Pediatr* 32(1):8-14, 1993.

Klerman LV: School absence—a health perspective, *Pediatr Clin North Am* 35:1253-1269, 1988.

Kulbok P, Earls FJ, Montgomery AC: Life-style and patterns of health and social behavior in high-risk adolescents, *Adv Nurs Sci* 11:22-35, 1988.

Lyons JAF: Adolescent health and school-based clinics, *Issues Compr Pediatr Nurs* 10:303-314, 1987.

Mahon NE, Yarcheski A, Yarcheski TJ: Health consequences of loneliness in adolescents, *Res in Nurs Health* 16(1):23-31, 1993.

Manning M: Health assessment of the early adolescent: challenges and clinical issues, *Nurs Clin North Am* 25(4):823-831, 1990.

Marks A, Fisher M: Health assessment and screening during adolescence, *Pediatrics* 80(suppl):135-158, 1987.

McAnarney ER: "Home alone": potential implications for adolescents, *Pediatrics* 92(1):146-147, 1993.

Mikhail BI: Reduction of risk factors for osteoporosis among adolescents and young adults, *Issues Compr Pediatr Nurs* 15:271-280, 1992.

Millstein SG: Adolescent health: challenges for behavioral scientists, *Am Psychol* 44:837-842, 1989.

Muscari ME: The "acting-out" adolescent: identification and management, *Pediatr Nurs* 18(4):362-366, 1992.

Newacheck PW: Adolescents with special health needs: prevalence, severity, and access to health services, *Pediatrics* 84:872-881, 1989.

Newacheck PW: Improving access to health services for adolescents from economically disadvantaged families, *Pediatrics* 84:1056-1063, 1989.

Olds RS: Promoting child health through comprehensive school health programs: an investment in America's future, *Fam Community Health* 11(4):32-40, 1989.

Panzarine S and others: Adolescent health care: a challenge for nursing educators, *J Nurs Ed* 27:278-280, 1988.

Richardson JL and others: Relationship between after-school care of adolescents and substance use, risk taking, depressed mood, and academic achievement, *Pediatrics* 92(1):32-38, 1993.

Sachs BP: Cognitive screening for adolescent health education, *J Pediatr Nurs* 2:113-119, 1987.

Smith KL, Turner JG, Jacobsen RB: Health concerns of adolescents, *Pediatr Nurs* 13:311-315, 1987.

Sobal J and others: Health concerns of high school students and teachers' beliefs about student health concerns, *Pediatrics* 81:218-223, 1988.

Wildey LS, Barton AP: Training in adolescent health for nurse practitioners, *J Pediatr Health Care* 2:195-199, 1988.

Sexuality and Sex Education

Adger H Jr, DeAngelis C: Sexuality education: our schools can do better, *Contemp Pediatr* 6(10):56-65, 1989.

Burke PJ: Adolescents' motivation for sexual activity and pregnancy prevention, *Issues Compr Pediatr Nurs* 10:161-171, 1987.

Crooks R, Baur K: *Our sexuality,* ed 4, Redwood City, CA, 1990, Benjamin/Cummings.

Hofferth SL, Hayes CD, editors: *Risking the future: adolescent sexuality, pregnancy and childbearing,* Washington, DC, 1987, National Academy Press.

Kenney RD: A guide to sexual abstinence counseling, *Contemp Pediatr* 6(12):83-95, 1989.

Lowry LW, McGinnis DG: Integenerational education in human sexuality, *MCN* 14:341-345, 1989.

Meeropool E: One of the gang: sexual development of adolescents with physical disabilities, *J Pediatr Nurs* 6(4):243-249, 1991.

Mellanby A, Phelps F, Tripp JH: Teenagers, sex, and risk taking, *Br Med J* 307(6895):25, 1993.

Remafedi G: Adolescent homosexuality: psychosocial and medical implications, *Pediatrics* 9:331-337, 1987.

Remafedi G: Homosexual youth: a challenge to contemporary society, *JAMA* 258:222-225, 1987.

Remafedi G: Male homosexuality: the adolescent's perspective, *Pediatrics* 79:326-330, 1987.

Roth B: Fertility awareness as a component of sexuality education: preliminary research findings with adolescents, *Nurse Pract* 18(3):40, 43, 47-48, 1993.

Sheehan MK, Ostwald SK, Rothenberger J: Perceptions of sexual responsibility: do young men and women agree? *Pediatr Nurs* 12:17-21, 1986.

Stout JW, Rivara FP: Schools and sex education: does it work? *Pediatrics* 83:375-379, 1989.

Taylor BA, Remafedi G: Youth coping with sexual orientation issues, *J Sch Nurs* 9(2):26-39, 1993.

Taylor MO: Teaching parents about their impaired adolescent's sexuality, *MCN* 14:109-112, 1989.

Wattleton F: American teens: sexually active, sexually illiterate, *J Sch Health* 57:379-380, 1987.

Woodcock A, Stenner K, Ingham R: "All these contraceptives, videos and that . . .": young people talking about school sex education, *Health Educ Res* 7(4):517-531, 1992.

Injury Prevention

American Academy of Pediatrics, Committee on Accident and Poison Prevention: Snowmobile statement, *Pediatrics* 82:798-799, 1988.

Carr M and others: Curling-iron cornea *N Engl J Med* 319:1672, 1988 (letter).

Christoffel KK, Christoffel T: Handguns: risks versus benefits, *Pediatrics* 77:781-782, 1986.

Epidemiologic Notes and Reports: Injuries associated with ultraviolet tanning devices—Wisconsin, *MMWR* 38:333-334, 1989.

Greensher J: Non-automotive vehicle injuries in adolescents, *Pediatr Ann* 17:114-121, 1988.

Jack MS: Personal fable: a potential explanation for risk-taking behavior in adolescents, *J Pediatr Nurs* 4:334-338, 1989.

Lawrence HS: Fatal nonpowder firearm wounds: case report and review of the literature, *Pediatrics* 85:177-181, 1990.

Lee EJ, Jacobson JM: Accident reports: survey of high school injuries, *Pediatr Nurs* 13:151-154, 1987.

Lee EJ, Jacobson JM, Levanas V: Stressful life events and accidents at school, *Pediatr Nurs* 15:140-142, 1989.

Meehan PJ, O'Carroll PW: Gangs, drugs, and homicide in Los Angeles, *Am J Dis Child* 146(6):683-687, 1992.

Myre LE, Black RE: Serious air gun injuries in children: update of injury statistics and presentation of five cases, *Pediatr Emerg Care* 3:168-170, 1987.

Orlowski J: Adolescent drownings: swimming, boating, diving, and scuba accidents, *Pediatr Ann* 17:125-132, 1987.

Paulson JA: The epidemiology of injuries in adolescents, *Pediatr Ann* 17:84-96, 1988.

Sadowski LS, Cairns RB, Earp JA: Firearm ownership among nonurban adolescents, *Am J Dis Child* 143:1410-1413, 1989.

Sheley JF, McGee ZT, Wright JD: Gun-related violence in and around inner-city schools, *Am J Dis Child* 146(6):677-682, 1992.

Spivak H, Prothrow-Stith D, Hausman AJ: Dying is no accident: adolescents, violence, and intentional injury, *Pediatr Clin North Am* 35:1339-1347, 1988.

Wintemute GJ, Teret SP, Kraus JF: Plastic handguns that resemble toy guns: new technology creates a uniquely hazardous product, *Pediatrics* 81:316-317, 1988.

CHAPTER 20

Physical Health Problems of Adolescence

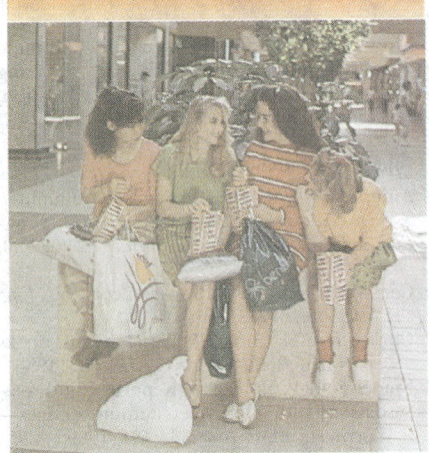

CHAPTER OUTLINE

RELATED TOPICS

Behavioral health problems of adolescence, Ch. 21
Disorders affecting the skin, Ch. 18
Genitalia (examination), Ch. 7
Health promotion of the adolescent and family, Ch. 19
Infection control, Ch. 27
Precocious puberty, Ch. 38

COMMON HEALTH CONCERNS OF ADOLESCENCE

ACNE

Adolescents are subject to the same skin conditions that affect the school-age child, such as bacterial, viral, and fungal infections; contact dermatitis; and drug reactions. However, there is one skin disorder that, although not limited to the adolescent age-group, appears predominantly at this time—acne vulgaris (common acne). Acne is the most common skin problem treated by physicians (Pochi, 1990). Acne involves anatomic, physiologic, biochemical, genetic, immunologic, and psychologic factors of significant importance.

It is estimated that about 85% of the population will have had acne by the end of the teenage years, and as many as 25% to 50% of children have evidence of the disorder before the age of 10. However, the peak incidence is in late adolescence, at age 16 to 17 in girls and 17 to 18 in males. The disorder is more common in males than in females (Rothman and Lucky, 1993). After this age period the disease usually decreases in severity, but it may persist well into adulthood. Early acne occurs in the midface region (mid-

■ Linda M. Kollar, RN, MSN, CPNP, revised this chapter.

forehead, nose, and chin) and later spreads to the lateral cheeks, lower jaw, back, and chest. The degree to which an individual is affected may range from nothing more than a few isolated comedones to a severe inflammatory reaction. Although the disease is self-limited and is not life-threatening, its significance to the affected adolescent is great, and it is a mistake to underestimate the impact that it can have on the person.

Etiology

The etiology of acne is still unclear, although a number of factors appear to be related to its development. Its distribution in families and a high degree of concordance in identical twins suggest a hereditary predisposition to acne. Androgens are implicated, since observations indicate a diminished effect on acne during pregnancy, virtual absence in castrated males and young children, and a higher incidence in adolescent males. The disease seems to be aggravated by emotional stress and a hot, humid environment. At least half of females with acne have a premenstrual flare-up of their acne. There is no positive evidence that any specific foods are factors, except perhaps on an individual basis. Medications with a direct androgenic effect will exacerbate acne. Systemic and topical steroids may induce acne lesions that slowly subside after the steroids have been discontinued.

Pathophysiology

Acne is a disease that involves the ***pilosebaceous follicles*** (the hair follicle and sebaceous gland complex) of the face, neck, shoulders, back, and upper chest—the so-called flush areas of the skin. However, there is no abnormality of the gland; it is the glandular secretion, sebum, initiated by androgenic hormones, that is involved in the pathogenesis of this disease. Increased sebum production begins at the time of adrenocortical maturation (adrenarche) and subtly continues to increase until the late teens. Acne severity is proportional to the sebum secretion rate, which is genetically determined (Rothman and Lucky, 1993).

There are two basic types of lesions seen in acne: (1) ***noninflamed lesions*** called comedones, consisting of compact masses of keratin, lipids, fatty acids, and bacteria that dilate the follicular duct, which may be plugged (***closed comedones,*** or whiteheads, with no visible opening) or open (***open comedones,*** or blackheads, with visible dilated openings that are discolored as fatty acids are oxidized by air); or (2) ***inflamed lesions*** that result when the follicular wall ruptures to produce papules, pustules, nodules, and cysts (Fig. 20-1). The inflammatory acne is responsible for the destructiveness and propensity for scarring. Individuals with acne usually have lesions of more than one morphology (Rothman and Lucky, 1993).

The maturation of the sebaceous glands begins as an early pubertal occurrence, and the development of acne as pubertal changes progress appears to be a result of hormones. Under the influence of the accelerated androgen secretion from the adrenal glands and gonads, the sebaceous gland increases in size with secretory productivity and resultant turnover of the follicular epithelium. These changes are accompanied by an alteration in the follicular lining that allows the accumulation and stagnation of sebum and keratinized material derived from the lining cells. Normally the growing hair shaft prevents this accumulation by functioning as a "pipe cleaner" and moving the material out of the follicle. In acne the small, fine, vellus hairs occupying sebaceous follicles are unable to move the fixed material and the acne lesion develops. The noninflammatory comedones may resolve or become infected pustules.

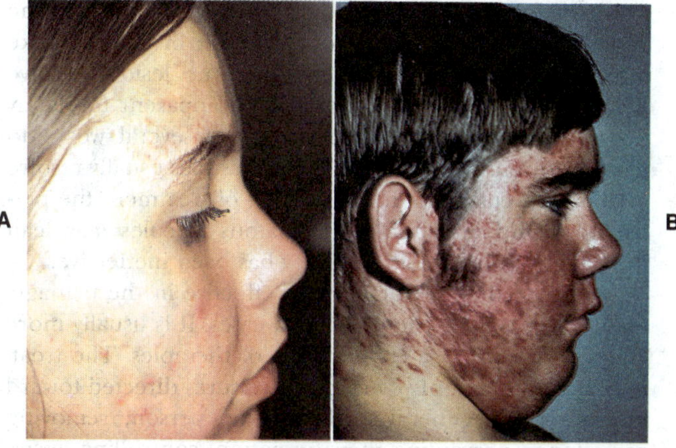

FIG. 20-1 Acne vulgaris. **A,** Comedones with a few inflammatory pustules. **B,** Papulopustular acne. (From Weston WL, Lane AT: *Color textbook of pediatric dermatology,* St Louis, 1991, Mosby.)

A normally harmless bacterium, *Propionibacterium acnes (P. acnes),* is present in larger amounts in persons with acne. Polymorphonuclear leukocytes enter the sebaceous follicle to ingest the bacteria. Hydrolytic enzymes and free fatty acids are released as a by-product of this ingestion. These fatty acids are the major tissue irritants in the sebum and initiate the inflammatory response. Inflammation is preceded by rupture of the distended follicles, which allows the follicular contents to leak into the dermis. The resultant damage causes a further wall-rupturing effect from leukocytes that invade the dermis. Those that become cystic are likely to form scars when they heal.

Adolescents' concern about their appearance tempts them to pick, finger, squeeze, and otherwise manipulate the lesions, which plays an important role in the perpetuation of acne. These mechanical factors may rupture the microcomedones, leading to inflammation and exacerbation of acne. Exposure to oily substances, chlorinated hydrocarbons, and coal tar distillates profoundly exaggerates acne, which may influence the choice of occupation among adolescents (e.g., to avoid working near fast-food grills).

Therapeutic Management

There is little evidence that treatment shortens the duration of the entire course of the disease. Acne can be psychologically difficult for adolescents who are especially sensitive about their appearance. Treatment can bolster self-esteem and prevent unnecessary scarring.

Successful management to a great extent depends on the

provider's understanding of the adolescent's goals and the adolescent's understanding of the cause of acne. Unlike many dermatologic conditions, the acne lesions resolve slowly, and improvement may not be apparent for many weeks. Individual comedones may take several weeks to months to resolve, and papules and pustules usually resolve in about 1 week. Also, in early stages of treatment the persistent postinflammatory erythematous macules may lead the patient to believe the therapy has been ineffective.

No single therapeutic agent is effective in the management of acne except in a few mild cases. It is usually more effective to employ a combination of therapies. The treatment most commonly consists of measures directed toward improving the general health of the person, removing comedones, preventing their formation, controlling excessive sebaceous gland activity, controlling infection, and preventing scar formation. The treatment consists of some general measures of care and specific treatments largely determined by the type of lesions involved and the preference of the practitioner. Although the combination of therapies and brands selected vary, the objectives are similar.

General Measures. A general explanation of the disease process and the plan of care is given to the adolescent, with emphasis on compliance to carry out the program faithfully for as long as the process persists. It is also important to obtain the cooperation, understanding, and support of the parents; therefore they should be present at the initial discussion. Adolescents should be reminded that acne occurs, to some degree, in almost all teenagers.

Improvement of the adolescent's overall health status is part of the general management. Adequate rest, moderate exercise, a well-balanced diet, reduction of emotional stress, and elimination of any foci of infection are all part of general health promotion. There is no convincing evidence to implicate any single dietary item or combination of foods in exacerbation of acne. Occasionally there is an aggravation of symptoms after each ingestion of a given food. In such instances the food is eliminated for a time to assess its influence on the disease.

Cleansing. Acne is not caused by dirt or oil on the surface of the skin. Gentle cleansing with a mild cleanser once or twice daily is usually sufficient. Antibacterial soaps are ineffective and may be too drying in combination with topical acne medications (Rothman and Lucky, 1993). For some adolescents hygiene of the hair and scalp appears to be related to the clinical activity of acne. In these persons acne of the forehead can be improved by brushing the hair away from the forehead and more frequent shampooing.

Medications. There is a wide range of types and combinations of topical agents for the treatment of acne, with selection depending on the type and severity of the lesions. ***Tretinoin (retinoic acid, Retin-A)*** is the only drug that effectively interrupts the abnormal follicular keratinization that produces microcomedones, the invisible precursors of the visible comedones. Tretinoin alone is usually sufficient for management of comedonal acne (Vershoore and others, 1993). Since tretinoin prevents the formation of new comedones, it takes at least 2 to 3 months for significant improvement to be apparent. Topical tretinoin is not associated with increased risk of birth defects (Jick and others, 1993) (see following discussion of isotretinoin).

Topical ***benzoyl peroxide*** kills *P. acnes* organisms and causes a reduction in free fatty acid concentrations on the skin surface (Rothman and Lucky, 1993). The most effective therapy involves the use of benzoyl peroxide, tretinoin, or a combination of these. Both agents can cause redness and peeling early in their use; therefore the treatment usually begins with graded increases in concentration and/or frequency of application according to the patient's tolerance. Both are available in cream or gel preparations. The usual regimen is to apply one medication in the morning and the other at night. They should not be applied together, since the benzoyl peroxide may oxidize the retinoic acid and render it impotent.

Since most patients also have some inflammatory lesions accompanying the comedones, a ***topical antibacterial agent*** is prescribed. Topical treatments are used to prevent new lesions, as well as to treat preexisting ones. The entire affected area must be treated, not just individual lesions. Clindamycin, tetracycline, erythromycin, and minocycline are the agents of choice. Combination treatment with topical retinoic acid and erythromycin gel has been shown to be more effective than either treatment alone. This advantage is due to the reduction of the initial flare-up of lesions; after 3 months of treatment retinoic acid is just as effective alone (Vershoore and others, 1993).

Systemic antibiotic therapy may be needed for some patients who do not respond to topical therapy for inflammatory acne. Oral antibiotics decrease bacteria colonization and free fatty acid concentration in the sebum. They also decrease inflammation by inhibiting neutrophil chemotaxis (Rothman and Lucky, 1993). Oral antibiotics are considered extremely safe even when given for years as part of acne treatment. The tetracycline group of antibiotics is the most successful oral antibiotic therapy for acne. They are relatively free of side effects with the exception of occasional gastrointestinal upset or vaginal candidiasis (Layton and Cunliffe, 1993).

The use of ***oral contraceptive pills (OCPs)*** has been found to produce good responses in adolescent females with acne. OCPs are unlikely to improve acne by their estrogenic effect alone. The clinician should choose OCPs with poorly androgenic progestins, such as norethisterone, when prescribing for young women with acne. An adolescent prescribed these agents should receive accurate information regarding use, risks, and side effects. See discussion of oral contraceptive agents later in this chapter.

Isotretinoin 13-cis-retinoic acid (Accutane), a very potent and effective oral agent, is reserved for severe, cystic acne. Isotretinoin decreases sebum production to nearly undetectable amounts, resulting in a decrease in *P. acnes* (Rothman and Lucky, 1993). Management of this regimen should be rendered only by a dermatologist. Patients with multiple, active, deep dermal, or subcutaneous cystic and nodular acne lesions are treated for 15 to 20 weeks, or until the total cyst count decreases by 70%. Prolonged remission often follows (American Academy of Pediatrics, 1992). The use of isotretinoin is limited as a universal treatment of inflammatory acne because of its side effects, which include dryness of skin and mucous membranes, musculoskeletal symptoms, and premature epiphyseal closure. The drug has also been found to be teratogenic and therefore unsuitable for pregnant women (Kochar and Penner, 1987). All sexually active teenagers should be identified before treatment, and the drug should be given only if they use an effective form of contraception during treatment and have received oral and written warning of the reproductive hazards of the drug (American Academy of Pediatrics, 1992).

Adolescents with scarring from acne need aggressive treatment to minimize new scar formation. The scars can be treated with collagen injections, chemical peeling, dermabrasion, and excision to improve the adolescent's appearance.

Teenagers with mild scarring may benefit from professional chemical peels using glycolic acid (70% to 80%) or home treatment with a glycolic acid cream or lotion (usually 8% to 12%). Glycolic acid is one of the chemicals known as alpha-hydroxy-acid (AHA) and is found in sugar cane. At low concentrations it causes exfoliation of the dead layer of skin (stratum corneum). The cream is applied once or twice a day. At higher concentrations the acid causes peeling of the epidermis (epidermolysis) (Van Scott and Yu, 1989).

Nursing Considerations

Assessment

The health screening interview should contain questions regarding the adolescent's concern about acne. Because acne is so common and its appearance may seem so mild, the health care provider may underestimate the relative importance of this phenomenon to the adolescent. The nurse should assess the individual adolescent's level of distress, current management, and perceived success of any regimen before initiating a referral. If adolescents do not perceive the acne to be a problem, they will not be motivated to follow the daily routine necessary to treat the acne. It is estimated that 80% to 90% of all cases of acne can be managed by the primary care provider without referral to a dermatologist (Atton and Tunnessen, 1988).

Nursing Diagnoses

Based on a thorough assessment, several nursing diagnoses are identified. The more common diagnoses for the adolescent with acne are included in the Nursing Care Plan on pp. 866-867. Others may apply in specific situations.

Planning

The goals for the adolescent with acne include the following:

1. Adolescent will demonstrate a reduction in the number and extent of lesions.
2. Adolescent will have a positive body image.
3. Adolescent will receive appropriate support and education about carrying out therapy properly.

Implementation

Once a treatment regimen has been prescribed, adolescents need ongoing support to comply effectively with management of the disorder and application of medications. Reinforcing and clarifying information is crucial, including causes of acne, rationale for treatment, correct use of medication, and expected side effects of therapy. Teenagers need supportive, caring individuals to help them maintain the persistence required to deal with this chronic condition.

Specific information regarding skin care helps enhance compliance. Teenagers are subject to the influence of commercial advertising from a variety of media. Information that dispels myths regarding use of abrasive cleansing products as a means of removing blackheads can prevent unnecessary costs. Washing with a mild, nonabrasive cleanser such as Dove (unscented) is adequate for cleansing.

Cosmetics do not cause acne, and contrary to once-popular belief, it does not make a difference if a cosmetic is oil-free or not (Bikowski, 1992). Cosmetic companies currently test the cosmetics on the male rabbit ear, which is more sensitive than human skin (Rothman and Lucky, 1993). Cosmetics that do not cause acne on the rabbit ear are labeled as ***noncomedogenic*** or ***nonacnegenic.*** Cosmetics should be removed at bedtime.

Certain acne preparations, such as retinoic acid and tetracycline, have been known to cause photosensitivity. Adolescents should be advised to apply the medication at night and use a sunscreen with a sun protective factor (SPF) of at least 15 in the daytime. Affected teenagers are also instructed to employ other measures that minimize sun exposure, such as wearing a hat or sun visor, to reduce exposure to potentially harmful ultraviolet rays (see Sunburn, Chapter 18).

Teenagers need to be educated about other factors that may aggravate acne and damage skin, such as too vigorous scrubbing. Picking, squeezing, and manual expression with fingernails break down ductal walls and cause acne to worsen. Other factors that exacerbate the lesions include wearing the hair over the face and application of oily hair preparations. Mechanical irritation, such as vinyl helmet straps that rub over areas predisposed to acne, can cause the development of lesions. Since acne lesions may not be limited to the face, adolescents need to be instructed to apply medication to other affected areas, such as the shoulders and back.

Medications. Because of the complexity of multiple medication regimens, an instruction sheet describing the etiology of acne and the therapy is helpful. Teenagers should be advised not to expect any visible improvement for 4 to 6 weeks after initiation of therapy. Initially the acne may appear worse as the microcomedones, not previously apparent, work their way to the surface of the skin. Also, medications often cause erythema, peeling, itching, burn-

NURSING CARE PLAN
The Adolescent with Acne

NURSING DIAGNOSIS: Impaired skin integrity related to presence of secretions, presence of infective organisms

PATIENT GOAL 1: Will exhibit signs of reduced inflammation and scarring

• **NURSING INTERVENTIONS/*RATIONALES***

Carefully cleanse skin with mild soap and water *to reduce risk of infection*

*Caution not to pick, squeeze, or otherwise manipulate lesions, *because this perpetuates acne and increases risk of infection*

Caution against too vigorous scrubbing *to prevent skin damage*

Impress the importance of following instructions, such as using only prescribed preparations

Instruct about shampooing, hairstyling, and the selection and use of cosmetics *because this can reduce number of lesions*

Apply peeling agent(s) as prescribed

*Administer antibiotics as prescribed *for inflammatory acne*

*Administer oral contraceptive pill (in selected female cases)

Stress to those on retinoic acid therapy and/or tetracycline the importance of avoiding exposure to sun; apply sunscreen for protection and wear hat or sun visor

• **EXPECTED OUTCOME**

Lesions heal with minimum scarring

PATIENT GOAL 2: Will exhibit signs of reduced number of lesions

• **NURSING INTERVENTIONS/*RATIONALES***

Avoid oily applications to the skin *because they aggravate acne by plugging pilosebaceous ducts*

Shampoo hair and scalp frequently (if prescribed)

Style hair off the forehead *because this is often beneficial in reducing forehead lesions*

Avoid use of cosmetic preparations, if possible; remove cosmetics at bedtime

Avoid face contact with other areas of the body (e.g., chin resting on hands, lying with face on arm)

• **EXPECTED OUTCOME**

Adolescent uses appropriate precautions

Adolescent exhibits signs of reduced number of lesions

PATIENT GOAL 3: Will comply with measures that promote general health

• **NURSING INTERVENTIONS/*RATIONALES***

Encourage adequate rest and moderate exercise, *since this is important for general health*

Help adolescent plan a well-balanced diet *to support body's natural defenses*

Help adolescent find mechanisms to reduce emotional stress, *since stress can contribute to acne*

Assess for any foci of infection and initiate measures to eliminate them

Eliminate any given food the adolescent has found that aggravates the symptoms *in order to assess its influence on acne*

• **EXPECTED OUTCOME**

Adolescent complies with measures that promote general health

NURSING DIAGNOSIS: Body image disturbance related to perception of facial lesions

PATIENT GOAL 1: Will demonstrate knowledge about acne and its treatment

• **NURSING INTERVENTIONS/*RATIONALES***

Dispel myths regarding the etiology of the condition *because myths associated with acne are common*

Reassure adolescent regarding unfounded fears

Provide accurate information about acne and the therapy to be implemented

• **EXPECTED OUTCOME**

Adolescent demonstrates an understanding of acne and its treatment

PATIENT GOAL 2: Will seek treatment for acne

• **NURSING INTERVENTIONS/*RATIONALES***

Be alert to cues that the adolescent wants to discuss the skin problem

Broach the subject of therapy for the adolescent with obvious skin lesions

Refer to health practitioner (e.g., dermatologist) who is sympathetic to the special needs of the adolescent

Discourage self-treatment with over-the-counter preparations *because these are usually not effective*

• **EXPECTED OUTCOMES**

Adolescent discusses feelings and concerns

Adolescent complies with suggestions

Adolescent seeks treatment

PATIENT GOAL 3: Will assume responsibility for care of skin

• **NURSING INTERVENTIONS/*RATIONALES***

Emphasize importance of gentle cleansing *because this is essential in treatment of acne*

Provide written instructions, including the cause of the lesions and the therapeutic regimen outlined, *to reinforce verbal instructions and provide for future referral*

Motivate the adolescent to assume responsibility for following through on instructions

Teach medication administration and other therapeutic and hygienic measures

Discourage "picking" at lesions *because this can increase number of lesions and risk of infection*

• **EXPECTED OUTCOME**

Adolescent assumes responsibility for care of skin lesions and complies with preventive measures

*Dependent nursing action.

NURSING CARE PLAN
The Adolescent with Acne—cont'd

PATIENT GOAL 4: Will receive adequate support

• **NURSING INTERVENTIONS/*RATIONALES***

Allow the adolescent to express feelings about the disorder, its effect on appearance, and the length of time required for therapy

Provide positive reinforcement for compliance *so that adolescent continues to comply with therapy*

Encourage maintenance of normal activities and interaction with peers *so that adolescent does not become isolated because of self-consciousness*

Explore job opportunities and after-school interests with the adolescent

Reinforce the efficacy of therapy and improvement in appearance

Assist adolescent with grooming *to enhance appearance and improve body image*

• **EXPECTED OUTCOME**

Adolescent discusses feelings and concerns regarding appearance and identifies positive aspects of appearance

NURSING DIAGNOSIS: Altered family processes related to the child with a troublesome skin problem

PATIENT (FAMILY) GOAL 1: Will demonstrate an understanding of adolescent's skin problem and therapy

• **NURSING INTERVENTIONS/*RATIONALES***

Explain acne and therapy prescribed *to increase family's understanding*

Assist family in helping adolescent assume greater responsibility for acne management

Explain the nature of adolescent development and the effect acne has on self-image and identity formation *so that family is more understanding and supportive*

• **EXPECTED OUTCOME**

Family demonstrates an understanding of the adolescent's skin problem and therapy

Family shows a supportive attitude

ing, and drying when first applied, tempting the adolescent to discontinue their use.

➤ **NURSING TIP** The adolescent can be advised that side effects may be minimized by delaying application of medicine until the skin is completely dry (20 to 30 minutes after cleansing).

Adolescents are instructed to apply the medication to the entire facial area, not just to the lesions. Furthermore, too heavy application, especially in skin crevices around the nose or chin, can result in redness and cracking of this skin. An innovative unit dose apparatus, which can be screwed to the top of the tube of retinoic acid, helps standardize the amount of medication that is applied daily. This minimizes the possibility of overapplication and increases the length of time between prescription refills, thereby decreasing expense (see Critical Thinking Exercise box).

The nurse needs to be aware of the potential side effects of therapy that may discourage compliance. Sexually active adolescent females taking OCPs and oral antibiotics should be instructed to use an additional form of contraception. Appropriate counseling before therapy is initiated and return visits to the nurse 2 weeks after initiation may decrease the dropout rate for treatment. Teenagers benefit greatly from the support received at this visit.

Expression of Comedones. In the past it was common to use comedone extractors to remove blackheads. This procedure has been shown to cause increased scarring. Topical tretinoin is the most effective medication for removing and preventing open and closed comedones (Bikowski, 1992).

CRITICAL THINKING EXERCISE
Acne

Kim, who is 16 years old, recently started "breaking out." During her visit to the dermatologist, she was diagnosed as having a mild form of acne and was told to cleanse her face twice a day and apply Retin-A and benzyl peroxide daily. Which instructions describe the correct skin care schedule?

1. Use a mild facial scrub in the morning and apply the Retin-A; at night use an astringent to remove makeup and apply benzyl peroxide.
2. Wash the face with soap in the morning and at night; wait 30 minutes after the night cleansing to apply Retin-A, followed by benzyl peroxide.
3. Wash the face with soap in the morning and apply benzyl peroxide; wash the face before bedtime and apply Retin-A.
4. Wash the face with soap in the morning and apply benzyl peroxide; wash the face in the evening and apply Retin-A about 30 minutes later.

The correct answer is 4. The most important aspects of the skin care regimen are to apply the topical preparation at different times of the day, because they are less effective when applied close together. Also, the face should be completely dry before applying Retin-A to reduce skin irritation. Although either preparation can be used first, it is preferable to suggest applying Retin-A at night, when the teenager has time to wait after cleansing the skin. Facial scrubs and astringents are not used, because they increase skin dryness.

❖ Evaluation

The effectiveness of nursing interventions is determined by continual reassessment and evaluation of care based on the following observational guidelines and expected outcomes:

1. Observe skin for evidence of exacerbation, reduction of lesions, and/or healing.
2. Interview adolescents regarding feelings and concerns.
3. Adolescent demonstrates the ability to carry out therapy.

Expected outcomes:
See Nursing Care Plan, pp. 866-867.

VISION CHANGES

Vision changes are common during the teenage years. The onset of refractory errors or worsening of previous errors peaks in adolescence as a result of the growth spurt. Other than myopia, new eye problems in this age-group are rare (Romano, 1990). Vision screening is usually performed within the school system by nurses. The main goal is to detect new refractive errors. Adolescents with vision changes are referred for contacts or glasses as appropriate.

HEALTH PROBLEMS OF THE MALE REPRODUCTIVE SYSTEM

PENILE PROBLEMS

Common congenital anomalies of the penis are almost always detected and corrected in infancy or early childhood, although some boys who need several operative procedures to repair a hypospadias (the most common congenital deformity of the penis) reach adolescence with a penis that looks different from those of their friends. A few who have received no medical care have uncorrected deformities that can cause serious psychologic problems during this sensitive period of development. These young boys need to be identified for surgical repair of the defect.

Uncircumcised males may encounter some problems during adolescence. Some young men have tight foreskins that cannot be retracted over the enlarging glans; some may not cleanse the area properly. These boys suffer more frequently from infection. Penile carcinoma was once thought to be related to circumcision. More recently it has been found that this carcinoma is associated with human papilloma virus types 16 and 18 (HPV 16, 18). Other factors such as phimosis and poor penile hygiene are critical cofactors in penile cancer development.

Trauma to the penis may occur in various ways, including burns and accidental injuries. The frenulum (the fold on the lower surface of the glans that connects it with the prepuce) can be torn after retraction of the foreskin, masturbation, or coitus. It can be frightening to the young boy but usually heals spontaneously with minimum care. However, any extensive bleeding may require suturing of the tissues.

Other problems include an adherent penis, a common condition in which the ventral surface of the penis adheres to the scrotum, producing a severe ventral curvature during erection and thus preventing satisfactory coitus. The adherent penis can be surgically corrected. Priapism is a rarer disorder consisting of painful, sustained penile erection without sexual desire. Treatment of priapism is directed toward treating conditions with which it is often associated, such as sickle cell disease, leukemia, the use of certain medications, and central nervous system lesions.

TESTICULAR TUMORS

Tumors of the testes are not a common condition, but when manifested in adolescence, they are generally malignant. Testicular cancer is the most common solid tumor in males 15 to 34 years of age. The usual presenting symptom is a heavy, hard, painless mass that is palpable on the anterior or lateral aspect of a testis. The tumor may be smooth or nodular and does not transilluminate unless accompanied by a hydrocele. The involved testicle hangs lower and is therefore more susceptible to trauma. Although not all scrotal masses are malignant, any firm swelling of the testes demands immediate evaluation. If a firm swelling is noted, the youth should be subjected to a minimum of preoperative palpation and referred immediately for surgical exploration. There is seldom delay in seeking medical advice if the mass is painful, but in the absence of pain the condition may go unattended for some time.

Treatment for testicular cancer consists of surgical removal of the affected testicle (orchiectomy) and the adjacent lymph nodes if affected. If metastases are evident in more distant nodes or organs, chemotherapy and radiation therapy are implemented (see Chapters 23 and 36).

Nursing Considerations

To supplement routine health assessment, every adolescent male should be taught to perform monthly ***testicular self-examination (TSE)***. This allows an opportunity for the adolescent to familiarize himself with his own anatomy and to ensure early detection of any abnormality. Each testicle is examined individually, preferably after a warm bath or shower, when scrotal skin is more relaxed, using the thumbs and fingers of both hands and applying a small amount of firm, gentle pressure. The normal testicle is a firm organ with a smooth, egg-shaped contour. The epididymis can be palpated as a raised swelling on the superior aspect of the testicle and should not be confused with an abnormality. The efficacy of teaching TSE to adolescent males has been tested and found to be successful (Klein, Berry, and Felice, 1990). The nurse can play an important role in providing this information to the adolescent male.

VARICOCELE

Varicocele usually presents as an asymptomatic scrotal mass or as scrotal aching after physical exercise (Nagar and Levran, 1993). A varicocele is characterized by elongation, dilation, and tortuosity of the veins of the spermatic cord superior to the testicle. The finding is rare in prepubertal children, but there is a dramatic increase in incidence at the onset of puberty. Varicoceles are found most often on the left side because of the greater length of the left spermatic vein and its entry into the left renal artery; the right spermatic vein enters the vena cava directly and at a lesser angle, which may be a source of future difficulty. A varicocele can be palpated as a wormlike mass situated above the testicle that decreases in size when the male is recumbent and becomes distended and tense when he is upright. There may be discomfort during sexual stimulation in some males.

In pubertal males the left testicle is usually larger than the right. However, when there is an associated varicocele, the left testicle is usually smaller than the right (Sawczuk and others, 1993). Testicular size and levels of dihydrotestosterone in seminal plasma decrease with increasing duration of the varicocele. Varicocelectomy is in general thought to be indicated when a man is found to have abnormal spermatogenesis, a normal partner, and a varicocele. Approximately 33% of infertile men have the condition as compared with 15% of fertile men. The adolescent with a varicocele is not likely to present for infertility evaluation; therefore the management is controversial (Sawczuk and others, 1993). The safety of the surgery, coupled with uncertainty regarding future fertility, presents an argument for surgical correction of a varicocele as soon as possible after diagnosis (Nagar and Levran, 1993).

EPIDIDYMITIS

Epididymitis is an inflammatory reaction of the epididymis of the testicle as a result of either infection or, occasionally, local trauma. The clinical presentation is an insidious onset of unilateral scrotal pain, redness, and swelling. Associated symptoms include urethral discharge, dysuria, fever, and pyuria. Epididymitis is not associated with gastrointestinal symptoms found in testicular torsion. The causative factors in the adolescent population are predominantly *Chlamydia trachomatis* and *Neisseria gonorrhoeae* (Paradise and Grant, 1992). Mild presentation of symptoms may mimic testicular torsion, which requires immediate surgical intervention. Therefore, immediate evaluation by a practitioner is indicated. Treatment consists of analgesics, scrotal support, bed rest, and initiation of appropriate antibiotic therapy.

TESTICULAR TORSION

Intravaginal torsion of the testicle is a condition in which the tunica vaginalis, which normally encases the testicle, fails to do so and the testis hangs free from its vascular structures. This condition can result in partial or complete venous occlusion with rotation around this vascular axis. In severe torsion the organ can become swollen and painful; the scrotum becomes red, warm, and edematous and appears to be immobile or fixed as a result of spasm of the cremasteric fibers. This type of torsion can occur at any time but is most common in prepubertal and postpubertal males (Hermann, 1989).

Typically, the adolescent will complain of pain that was either acute or insidious in onset and radiates to the groin. Nausea, vomiting, and abdominal pain may accompany the pain. Fever and urinary symptoms are generally not present. This is a surgical emergency for gonadal preservation.

Nursing Considerations

Nurses should be alert to the possibility of testicular torsion in adolescents who complain of scrotal pain. Since torsion often results from trauma to the scrotum, school nurses are the persons who are likely to encounter such injuries and should refer the adolescent for medical evaluation immediately.

GYNECOMASTIA

Some degree of bilateral or unilateral breast enlargement occurs frequently in young boys during puberty. It is estimated that approximately half of adolescent boys have transient gynecomastia, usually lasting less than 1 year (Biro and others, 1990). When the onset of gynecomastia is prepubertal or at Tanner stage 5 (see Fig. 19-8), the adolescent should be evaluated for rare adrenal or gonadal tumors, liver disease, or Kleinfelter syndrome. Gynecomastia has also been reported in males receiving oral ketoconazole for fungal infection.

If the condition persists or is extensive enough to cause embarrassment, plastic surgery is indicated for cosmetic and psychologic considerations. Administration of testosterone has no effect on breast development or regression and may even aggravate the condition.

Nursing Considerations

Treatment usually consists of assurance to the adolescent and his parents that this situation is benign and temporary. The adolescent may benefit from the knowledge that it occurs in more than 50% of his peers.

HEALTH PROBLEMS OF THE FEMALE REPRODUCTIVE SYSTEM

GYNECOLOGIC EXAMINATION

Whether it is her first experience or not, an adolescent is most likely apprehensive before a pelvic examination. Adolescents are extremely self-conscious about their bodies and the changes taking place. The girl will need continuing support in the form of anticipatory guidance regarding what she can expect and suggestions of what she can do to help herself relax during the procedure.

The ideal time to begin to prepare the young women for the pelvic examination is during childhood as she is maturing. External genitalia examination is always a part of a routine physical assessment; avoiding the genitals reinforces the attitude that sexuality is something to be avoided. During this time the child and her parents are informed that a pelvic examination should be performed during adolescence.

The timing of the initial pelvic examination is controversial, but examination and early assessment have several advantages. Criteria listing indications for a pelvic examination during adolescence are listed in the box on p. 870.

INDICATIONS FOR PELVIC EXAMINATION OF ADOLESCENT FEMALES

Menstrual disorders:
- Amenorrhea
- Irregular uterine/vaginal bleeding
- Dysmenorrhea unresponsive to therapy

Undiagnosed abdominal pain
Any sexually active adolescent
Request for a prescription contraceptive method
Suspected pelvic mass
Rape
Request by patient
Virginal 18-year-old

Ultrasound is becoming an important adjunct to the diagnosis of menstrual problems. The girl and her parents can be assured that her body is normal, which contributes to a positive body image. The pelvic examination provides an excellent opportunity for teaching about hygiene, body functions, and sexuality. The girl should be encouraged to ask questions about her changing body and its implications. The pelvic examination also allows opportunity for discussion about postponing sexual involvement and safer sex. Lack of knowledge is a large factor in risky sexual experimentation in adolescence. For those who object to examination in early adolescence, it can be delayed until middle adolescence or the onset of sexual activity. The pelvic examination should be made as nonstressful as possible.

The teenager is usually given the option of choosing a supportive person to be present during the pelvic examination. Suggested individuals might include a parent, best friend, boyfriend, or other health professional. The use of models and drawings and a display of equipment to be used facilitate understanding. Allowing the adolescent to handle the speculum may help to decrease some of the fear. The adolescent is given the choice of wearing a gown or her own clothing during the examination. Description of the examination, including information about the procedure and words that describe anticipated feelings and sensations experienced during the examination, has been demonstrated to reduce anxiety. Of major concern to the adolescent is fear of discovery of pelvic pathology. Reassurance regarding normal physical findings is extremely important (Millstein, Adler, and Irwin, 1988). The other major fear is that the examination will be very painful. The adolescent has often heard stories of gynecologic terror from other women. Ask the adolescent what she has heard about the examination to help dispel these myths and some of the fear.

Usually the stressful experience of being placed in stirrups in the traditional lithotomy position can be avoided. Most girls favor a semisitting position, which has the additional advantage of allowing eye contact during the procedure. Sometimes a pillow will help the patient feel more comfortable and less vulnerable. The provision of a mirror allows the girl to see what is taking place if she so desires and helps the examiner explain various aspects of anatomy. When possible, it is important to respect the adolescent's request for a female provider.

Numerous techniques have been described to teach women to relax during a pelvic examination, including breathing exercises, imagery, and other stress-reduction strategies (see Pain Management, Chapter 26). However, they are not effective with all individuals. When the examination is finished, the findings are discussed with the adolescent and necessary referrals are made if indicated. Written teaching materials are useful adjuncts to health education.

DELAYED MENARCHE/AMENORRHEA

It is not unusual for an adolescent to skip a menstrual period or two when establishing normal menstrual and ovulatory cycles. This is a result of an immature hypothalamic-pituitary-ovarian axis. In general, the later menarche occurs, the longer the period of anovulation. Two thirds of adolescent females will establish regular menstrual cycles by 2 years after menarche. This is of little concern unless it creates undue anxiety on the part of the girl or her parents, which can ordinarily be allayed by explanation and reassurance. Careful examination will reveal any congenital defects of the genital tract (a rare cause).

The average age of menarche is about 12.5 years, with a normal range of 9 to 16 years. In an evaluation for amenorrhea it is important to obtain an accurate history of secondary sexual characteristic development. ***Primary amenorrhea*** is defined as no menses by age 16 in the presence of normal secondary sexual characteristics, no menses 1 to 2 years after reaching Tanner stage V, or no menses 3 to 5 years after the onset of breast development.

Secondary amenorrhea is no menses for 3 to 6 months in a previously menstruating female when pregnancy has been excluded. Secondary amenorrhea is much more common than primary amenorrhea.

Primary Amenorrhea

Primary amenorrhea may be a result of absence or malformation of the female genital structures or the inability of normal structures to respond to hormonal stimulation. This can be of hypothalamic, pituitary, ovarian, or uterine origin and can include hypopituitarism, Turner syndrome, tumors, polycystic ovary disease, and infections. Primary amenorrhea in an adolescent who exhibits all the evidences of estrogen production and sexual maturation and complains of periodic (usually monthly) lower abdominal pain may have an imperforate hymen or transverse vaginal septum. The treatment is simple surgical perforation and drainage.

A group of systemic disorders that may affect the functions of the reproductive tract are thyroid hypofunction or hyperfunction, prolonged or severe infections, adrenal hyperplasia, diabetes mellitus, and other chronic diseases. Obesity or malnutrition (including protein, vitamin, or iron deficiencies) may also delay the onset of menstruation. Intensive physical exercise, such as gymnastics, can cause delayed puberty and growth (Theintz and others, 1993).

Secondary Amenorrhea

The most common cause of secondary amenorrhea in adolescence is pregnancy. Secondary amenorrhea is defined as absence of menses for at least three cycles or 6 months in females who have established cycles. Other factors, which disturb the hypothalamic-pituitary-gonadal axis and cause secondary amenorrhea, include physical or emotional stress, sudden environmental change, hyperthyroidism or hypothyroidism, chronic illness, sexually transmitted diseases (STDs), extreme weight loss or gain, anorexia nervosa, bulimia, ovarian disturbance, and extrinsic pharmacologic agents (Greydanus and Shearin, 1990).

Menstrual Irregularities in the Female Athlete

Over the past two decades more women of all ages have begun exercising earlier in life and with greater intensity. The most common clinical indications of potentially adverse effects of exercise on an adolescent's reproductive cycle include (1) delayed menarche, (2) anovulation associated with dysfunctional uterine bleeding (DUB), and (3) oligomenorrhea or amenorrhea with hypoestrogenic states (Shangold and others, 1990).

A higher incidence of delayed menarche has been observed in girls who start intense physical training before menarche. This is probably related to the postponing of critical body composition (17% body fat) associated with puberty. This delay can be associated with a hypoestrogenic state, which may lead to osteopenia and earlier osteoporosis. These adolescents are at increased risk for stress fractures (Greene, 1993).

Adolescents who exercise regularly and have menstrual bleeding more frequently than every 21 days or at intervals of 35 to 120 days are likely to have chronic anovulation. They usually produce estrogen but have inadequate progesterone. Unopposed estrogen can lead to endometrial hyperplasia and theoretic risk of endometrial adenocarcinoma (Greene, 1993).

Treatment of anovulation or hypoestrogen can be a 6-month trial of decreasing the intensity or duration of exercise and improving nutrition. If no improvement in symptoms is seen, low-dose oral contraceptive pills (OCPs) may be prescribed. OCPs will protect the endometrium and provide sufficient estrogen for bone density while providing contraception for the adolescent (Greene, 1993).

DYSMENORRHEA

A certain amount of discomfort during the first day or two of the menstrual flow is extremely common. Most women experience cramping, abdominal pain, backache, and leg ache, but in a few the pain is intolerable and incapacitating. Dysmenorrhea, or painful menses, is a source of morbidity in 1 in 6 adolescents (Rosenfield and Barnes, 1993). Primary dysmenorrhea is painful menses not related to any identifiable pathologic disorder. This is the most common cause of painful menses among adolescents. Primary dysmenorrhea occurs almost always in ovulatory cycles and commonly appears within 6 to 12 months of the onset of menarche, when ovulatory cycles are usually established. Painful menses is the leading cause of recurrent short-term school absenteeism (Sundell, Milson, and Andersch, 1990).

Dysmenorrhea beginning more than 2 years after menarche is more suggestive of secondary dysmenorrhea, painful menstruation secondary to pelvic pathology. Endometriosis and STDs are the most frequent causes of secondary dysmenorrhea in adolescents.

Etiology

The factor present in all instances of primary dysmenorrhea is occurrence of prior ovulation. Although it is not invariable, the symptoms do not occur during the first few postmenarchal months or during months of irregular anovulatory menses. Estrogen production alone does not appear to be related to uterine discomfort, and progesterone is associated with diminished uterine contractility.

There is a relationship between uterine contractility and the secretion of prostaglandins. Prostaglandins of the F classes cause uterine muscle contraction, vasoconstriction, and ischemia. The secretion of prostaglandins increases at about the twenty-fifth to the twenty-eighth day of the menstrual cycle and follows the decrease in progesterone secretion. Local discomfort may be related to vascular changes in the endometrial bed during menstruation caused by alternating vasoconstriction and vasodilation of endometrial vessels that induce local ischemia, edema, necrosis, and slough. Nerve terminals also become sensitive to prostaglandins by lowering the threshold of these nerve terminals to the action of chemical and physical stimuli. Most of the prostaglandin release occurs in the first 48 hours of menstruation; therefore pain is greater during the first 2 days. Nausea, vomiting, diarrhea, headache, and emotional changes that are associated with primary dysmenorrhea are also related to release of prostaglandins.

Research has demonstrated that the presence and severity of dysmenorrhea is increased in smokers as compared with nonsmokers. The severity increases significantly with the number of cigarettes per day. The exact mechanism remains unclear but may be related to decreased endometrial blood flow in girls who smoke (Sundell, Milson, and Andersch, 1990).

Psychogenic Dysmenorrhea. Adolescents who are found to have no demonstrable pelvic pathology and who do not respond to either prostaglandin inhibitors or oral contraceptives may have a psychogenic etiology for their menstrual cramps. Multiple causes of psychogenic pain have been identified. A prior episode of sexual assault or abuse may be a cause. The development of abstract thinking allows the adolescent to reflect on any previous episode of sexual abuse in a different perspective. Feelings of shame, guilt, blame, or anger may surface for the first time, and she may need to deal with these feelings within the context of a therapeutic counseling situation.

In the absence of abuse, other causes include familial conditioning, sex-role ambivalence, school avoidance, or a mechanism to avoid stressful situations. Clinical indexes of psychogenic pain have been described, including the onset of pain at menarche, pain that begins with the onset of menses and continues throughout the entire menstrual period, and a prior history of sexual abuse (Beach, 1988).

Clinical Manifestations

Typical complaints of the girl with dysmenorrhea are lower abdominal cramping and pain or discomfort. About 50% of females will also have systemic symptoms, including nausea and vomiting, fatigue, nervousness, diarrhea, and headache. The pain usually begins some hours before the appearance of visible vaginal bleeding, is most severe on the first day of menstruation, and may last from a few hours to a day but seldom exceeds 2 to 3 days. The symptoms and degree of discomfort vary considerably from one individual to another and from one period to another in the same woman. The pain may be only a mild fleeting discomfort or so severe as to be incapacitating, requiring absence from school. After adolescence the menstrual discomfort decreases with age and may resolve completely after childbirth.

Therapeutic Management

A careful history including menstrual and sexual history is necessary. In addition, a careful review of gastrointestinal and genitourinary systems to rule out problems in these organ systems is necessary. A thorough gynecologic examination is carried out to exclude any pelvic abnormalities. The pelvic examination may not be indicated in an adolescent who is not sexually active and responds to medical therapy.

The treatment of choice for adolescents is the administration of nonsteroidal antiinflammatory drugs (NSAIDs). These drugs block the formation of prostaglandins, leading to a reduction in uterine activity and the prevention of pain (Smith and Heltzel, 1991). Antiprostaglandins are taken for only 2 to 3 days of the menstrual cycle. Prophylactic use of NSAIDs has proved effective when begun a few days before the onset of the menses, approximately 11 days after ovulation. The relief appears to be the result of prostaglandin inhibition rather than analgesic effect.

A variety of drugs that are taken at the onset of the dysmenorrheic symptoms are available without prescription, such as ibuprofen and naproxen. The fenamates have the additional benefit of antagonizing the action of already-formed prostaglandins. Sometimes cyclic estrogen therapy to prevent ovulation provides dramatic and predictable relief from pain. Oral contraceptives are effective in approximately 90% of cases. Transcutaneous electrical nerve stimulation (TENS) hampers the perception of pain and has been found to be an effective nonpharmacologic source of relief from pain with dysmenorrhea.

Nursing Considerations

The nurse is most frequently the person to whom a young woman turns for advice regarding menstrual problems. Usually all that is needed is reassurance about this normal function. This also provides an opportunity to engage in health teaching concerning menstrual physiology and hygiene and the importance of a well-balanced diet, exercise, and general health maintenance. When assessment indicates a potential problem and need for evaluation, the girl should be referred to another health care provider.

Most of the prostaglandin inhibitors are available without prescription. Whatever drug the adolescent chooses to use, she needs to be told how the drug produces its effect, how to take the drug for maximum effect, and the side effects. The drug should be taken with food and a full glass of water. If no satisfactory relief is achieved, the adolescent is referred for further evaluation.

The nurse plays an important role in the identification of adolescents with dysmenorrhea. Research has demonstrated that adolescents need information regarding availability of effective treatment for dysmenorrhea. Only about 50% of women with dysmenorrhea take medication to relieve the symptoms, even though effective treatment is available.

PREMENSTRUAL TENSION SYNDROME (PMS)

Although PMS was first described in 1931, even with over 60 years of research it remains poorly defined. The natural history of PMS is not known. PMS includes a spectrum of normal to severe premenstrual changes, and there is no demarcated point in the spectrum at which it begins. A shortage of reliable scientific information has led to inconsistent and often ineffective medical intervention (Allen, McBride, and Pirie, 1991). There are more than 100 physical, psychologic, and behavioral symptoms that have been associated with the syndrome. The manifestations most frequently cited are headache, backache, increased fatigue, weight gain, irritability, crying spells, depression, bloating, and breast congestion. About 10% of women in the United States experience PMS severe enough to disrupt their lives (Helvacioglu and others, 1993). The initial evaluation consists of having the adolescent complete daily mood rating forms for two menstrual cycles.

A consistent association has been found between PMS and foods and beverages high in sugar or those that taste sweet; particularly chocolate, fruit juice, and beer. It is unknown whether this association is etiologic (Rossignol and Bonnlander, 1991).

Until the cause of PMS is determined, a specific cure will probably remain elusive. PMS clearly disappears from the onset of menopause or through the induction of a menopausal state from danazol (Rausch and Parry, 1993). Recent studies have shown a strong association of psychiatric disorders in patients complaining of PMS symptomatology (Helvacioglu and others, 1993). Depression and other symptoms related to depression are among the most common reported symptoms that occur in PMS. Antidepressant drugs, especially fluoxetine (Prozac), have been helpful in decreasing depression and mood changes.

Nursing Considerations

The nurse helps adolescents and their families experience the process of health. Nurses should empathize and support these young women. The nurse can provide information regarding direct-care measures, adequate rest, good nutrition, and regular exercise (Rausch and Parry, 1993). The nurse can also help the adolescent cope with the psychosocial aspect of the syndrome through counseling and support groups. Stress reduction techniques may also be helpful.

ENDOMETRIOSIS

Endometriosis is much more common in adolescents than has previously been thought. This painful disorder results in the formation of multiple small cysts on the ovaries, uterine surface, pelvic ligaments, or peritoneum that swell during the menstrual cycle, irritating nerve endings or creating adhesions between pelvic structures. The pain is localized in the lower abdomen, back, groin, thigh, and/or deep pelvis and may be cyclic or acyclic. It is aggravated by coitus but usually relieved by rest. The etiology is unknown but may be caused by the presence of endometrial tissue refluxed from the fallopian tubes during menstruation.

Laparoscopic examination is the gold standard for diagnosis. The goals of treatment are pain control and preservation of fertility. Oral contraceptive pills (OCPs) are used to induce a hypoestrogenated atrophic endometrium. Surgical interventions to remove the small cysts may be done. Recurrence is high, occurring in 6 months to a few years.

DYSFUNCTIONAL UTERINE BLEEDING (DUB)

DUB is abnormal vaginal bleeding that occurs in the absence of pregnancy, infection, neoplasms, or any other demonstrable pathologic condition or disease. DUB is usually associated with anovulation and presents commonly within 2 years of menarche, when more than 50% of cycles are anovulatory (Polaniczky and Slap, 1992). During adolescence, abnormalities in the timing (intervals of less than 20 days or greater than 40 days), length (greater than 8 days' duration), and amount (more than 80 ml) of menstrual flow can occur frequently. This irregularity is usually attributed to immaturity of the positive feedback mechanism between the hypothalamic-pituitary-gonadal axis and absence of the luteinizing hormone (LH) surge late in the menstrual cycle. The result is anovulatory cycles and tonic production of estrogen. The effect of the estrogen is an increase in the thickness of the endometrial lining without structural integrity. Without progesterone, menstrual flow is not limited. Not all anovulatory females have DUB. One contributing factor is the amount of endogenous estrogen. DUB is more common in overweight females, who are known to have increased endogenous estrogen from both fat storage and peripheral conversion of androgens to estrogens (Polaneczky and Slap, 1992).

A comprehensive health history and physical examination, including a pelvic examination, is indicated to ascertain the cause of bleeding. Initially it is important to assess the acuity and amount of blood loss and the possible need for hospitalization. Common causes of vaginal bleeding need to be ruled out before the diagnosis of DUB can be established. The most common reason for vaginal bleeding in adolescence is pregnancy. Other causes of vaginal bleeding can be related to anatomic anomalies, foreign bodies, endocrine disease, STDs, chronic illness, or previously undetected familial bleeding disorders (e.g., Von Willebrand disease).

Treatment of vaginal bleeding depends on determination of the underlying mechanism. The initial management is dependent on the amount of blood lost and the patient's symptoms. If the bleeding is infrequent and not associated with anemia, reassurance and a menstrual calendar for follow-up are often sufficient.

In persistent cases hormonal therapy, in the form of OCPs or cyclic medroxyprogesterone, has been beneficial. The adolescent needs to know that at the completion of the recommended regimen there will probably be a heavy flow with cramping for 3 to 4 days. If she is not given this information, she may believe that her condition is worse and assume that the treatment was ineffective. Untreated patients are at increased risk for endometrial hyperplasia and adenocarcinoma from the persistent unopposed estrogen stimulation of the endometrium. The OCPs are continued for several months, after which bleeding irregularities seldom recur. DUB may persist for up to 2 years in more than half of the cases.

Dilation and curettage may be necessary to control hemorrhage in severe cases or in those that do not respond to more conservative management. Supplemental iron is sometimes needed to correct anemia.

Nursing Considerations

Ordinarily only reassurance and attention to general health status are needed, with emphasis on a well-balanced diet, adequate rest, and moderate exercise. When OCPs are prescribed, the adolescent and her parents need careful explanation of the use of these medications. The high-dose estrogen OCPs can result in nausea and vomiting. Anticipatory supportive care includes preparation for procedures if these are a possibility.

VAGINITIS AND VULVITIS (VULVOVAGINITIS)

A small quantity of vaginal mucus is normal and in adolescent girls usually increases at the time of ovulation and before the onset of menstruation. It is characteristically clear and, except in rare instances when it appears in large amounts, causes no discomfort. In the normal state the vaginal pH is ≤4.5 because of the available lactic acid. However, some teenagers mistakenly believe it to be a sign of vaginal infection. After an examination the girl can generally be reassured. Since increased secretions may be associated with sexual excitement, this is an opportunity to discuss this process.

Leukorrhea is the term used to describe a glutinous, gray-white discharge, which can be caused by physical, chemical, or infectious agents. The symptoms of vaginitis are quite disruptive, and chronic symptoms can be an economic burden in office visits and treatment costs (Sparks, 1991). Physical causes include foreign bodies: a forgotten tampon or contraceptive sponge. It can also be caused by irritation from pinworms, bubble bath, douching, deodorant pads or tampons, or improper wiping after defecation. The resulting discharge may be purulent, blood tinged, or brown with an offensive odor. Removal of the offending material is usually all that is necessary.

Vulvovaginal candidiasis accounts for 20% to 30% of all causes of vaginitis (Sparks, 1991). It is well established that patients with diabetes or depressed cellular immunity and those taking oral antibiotics have an increased incidence of candidal infections. Pregnant adolescents also have an increased incidence of vaginal yeast infections.

The adolescent with vulvovaginal candidiasis will generally have vaginal pruritus and sometimes dysuria. The presence of the classic thick "cottage cheese–like" discharge is seen in a minority of patients. Most females have a minimal amount of a noncharacteristic discharge. The diagnosis is easily confirmed with microscopic evaluation. Treatment is generally with a vaginal cream containing a polyene or imidazole drug.

Trichomonas vaginalis is an anaerobic parasitic protozoan involved in 20% to 30% of all cases of vaginitis. Trichomonas is sexually transmitted and can be recovered from 60% to 100% of female partners of infected men and 30% to 85% of male partners of infected women (Sparks, 1991).

The infection is often asymptomatic and self-limiting in men. Women may be asymptomatic, but many will have a vaginal discharge and vulvovaginal soreness. Dysuria and an odor often accompany the symptoms. The diagnosis is confirmed with microscopic examination of a specimen from the vaginal flora.

Metronidazole is used for the treatment of trichomonas, in either a 2 g single dose or 500 mg b.i.d. for 7 days. Single-dose treatment is ideal in the adolescent population. Sexual partners should also be treated.

Bacterial vaginiosis is the most common etiology of vaginitis. The symptoms include a thin, homogeneous, malodorous vaginal discharge. The diagnosis can be confirmed by identification of clue cells with the microscope. The most effective treatment is metronidazole, 500 mg b.i.d.; the single-dose therapy is less effective for this infection.

Many of the infectious causes of vaginal discharge are sexually transmitted; these are discussed in relation to the specific organisms involved (see Sexually Transmitted Diseases, p. 885).

Nursing Considerations

Health teaching is important in the prevention and management of vaginitis. Girls should be taught at an early age to wipe from front to back after toileting. A careful history can often elicit other causes, such as use of irritating substances, foreign bodies, or sexual activity. The adolescent will need explanations of how the etiologic agent produced the irritation and the principles behind management. The discussion may also elicit questions and concerns the adolescent has regarding other aspects of her developing body and sexuality. With the availability of over-the-counter medications for the treatment of candidiasis, the nurse should stress the importance of an evaluation when an adolescent has a vaginal discharge to rule out other etiologies.

PELVIC INFLAMMATORY DISEASE (PID)

PID is an infection of the upper genital tract (endometrium, fallopian tubes, and ovaries), most commonly caused by sexually transmitted bacteria, such as *N. gonorrhoeae, C. trachomatis,* and a variety of other anaerobic bacteria. PID can have acute complications, such as perihepatitis and tubo-ovarian abscess. The long-term effects can include infertility due to tubal scarring, ectopic pregnancy, and chronic abdominal pain. It is estimated that each year 1 million females of reproductive age experience an episode of PID, with approximately 20% of cases occurring in teenagers.

Several risk factors associated with PID have been identified. Women under the age of 25 years have a 1 in 8 chance of experiencing PID compared with those over age 25 years, whose risk is 1 in 80. Nonwhite females are twice as likely to develop PID as white adolescents. Biologically the immature adolescent cervix is in the process of undergoing considerable change, and the area of transformation at the endocervical os is much larger. Adolescents have fewer protective antibodies, and cervical mucus is more easily penetrated by the bacteria (Cates, Rolfs, and Aral, 1990).

Presenting symptoms in the adolescent may be generalized, with fever, abdominal pain, urinary tract symptoms, and vague influenza-like manifestations, such as malaise, nausea, diarrhea, or constipation. A pelvic examination is indicated for every sexually active female who complains of lower abdominal pain to evaluate the possibility of PID.

PID is of major concern because of the devastating effects on the reproductive tract of affected adolescents. Outpatient management may be initiated, but hospitalization is preferred to ensure compliance, response to treatment, and preservation of future fertility (Shafer and Sweet, 1989; Paradise and Grant, 1992). Partner notification and treatment is essential.

HEALTH PROBLEMS RELATED TO SEXUALITY

The biologic maturation that forms the foundation of adolescent development and the transition to adulthood is accompanied by conflicting feelings, attitudes, and social practices related to the developing sexuality. During adolescence the sexual drive emerges, and adolescents begin to explore their ability to attract a partner. Frequently the physical urges precede emotional maturity. There is great social pressure to experiment with sex as well.

A number of environmental influences may be operating. Sexual enticements by the mass media to enhance physical attractiveness conflict with traditional religious and societal expectations for chastity. Easy access to cars, unsupervised time at home, and changing family composition have also contributed to the incidence of sexual experimentation among the adolescent population. Egocentrism and the concept of the personal fable (feelings of omnipotence, invulnerability, and immortality) lead to risk taking and experimentation. Several studies have found an association between cigarette smoking and early onset of sexual behaviors. Adolescents who use substances are more likely to become involved in risky sexual behavior (Gillmore and others, 1992). A number of studies have found that socioeconomic status, family structure and relationships, pubertal maturation, and various personality and behavioral characteristics are related to the timing and frequency of adolescent sexual activity (Fielding and Williams, 1991). More than 50% of adolescents have initiated sexual intercourse by 19 years of age. Although sexual activity among males in the United States is high, the majority of adolescent males have low numbers of sexual partners and low incidence of sexual intercourse. Less than 20% of adolescent males reported having more than one sexual relationship simultaneously (Sonenstein, Pleck, and Ku, 1991). The resulting social outcomes of adolescent sexual risk taking are teenage pregnancy and sexually transmitted diseases.

Prevention strategies must focus on educating and motivating sexually active teens to decrease the high-risk sexual behaviors. Delaying sexual intercourse, using condoms, choosing partners carefully, limiting sexual partners, and using reliable contraception will help to reduce the impact of sexual activity on the adolescent. Instruction in the skills needed to resist sexual intercourse has a stronger influence on reducing sexual activity than instructions on acquired immunodeficiency syndrome (AIDS) or birth control methods (Ku, Sonenstein, and Pleck, 1992).

ADOLESCENT PREGNANCY

Each year 1 in 10 adolescent girls in the United States becomes pregnant—approximately 1 million females under the age of 20 years. About 554,000 of these pregnancies result in a birth; more than 400,000 are terminated by abortion (McAnarney and Hendee, 1989). Sexually experienced white teens were less likely to become pregnant in 1988 than in 1980, but a higher proportion of teens were sexually experienced, so the overall pregnancy rate stayed about the same. The proportion of black teens who had premarital intercourse remained at about 58% from 1980 to 1988 with no overall change in the pregnancy rate. The decline in the pregnancy rate among sexually experienced white teenagers may be related to the sharp increase in condom use at first sexual intercourse. The proportion using a condom at first intercourse increased from 28% in 1980 to 1982 to 45% in 1983 to 1988 (Ventura, and others, 1992). Half of all premarital pregnancies occur in the first 6 months of sexual activity, and more than 20% occur in the first month (Fielding and Williams, 1991).

Today most teenage mothers choose to keep their babies; consequently, there are 1.3 million infants living with teenage mothers, about half of whom are married. In most cases teenage pregnancy is no longer considered to be biologically disadvantageous to the conceptus with early prenatal care. Teenage pregnancy is still regarded as socially, educationally, psychologically, and economically disadvantageous to the mother. The number one reason that females drop out of high school is because of pregnancy. More than 80% of single African-American mothers younger than 25 and more than 70% of single white mothers in the same age-group live in poverty (Children's Defense Fund, 1989).

Medical Aspects

With better facilities available for care, the mortality for teenage pregnancies is decreasing, but the morbidity remains high. Teenage girls and their unborn infants are at greater risk for complications of both pregnancy and delivery. The most frequent complications are premature labor and low-birth-weight infants, high neonatal mortality, iron deficiency anemia, fetopelvic disproportion, and prolonged labor. The pregnancies of adolescents less than 16 years old are more frequently complicated by obstetric problems and neonatal morbidity and mortality than those of adolescents ages 16 to 19. This may be related to incomplete growth and physiologic immaturity. Other research finds that since pregnancy can take place only after the girl has achieved an advanced state of growth and sexual maturity, the greater concerns are dietary habits, substance use (especially cigarettes), sexually transmitted diseases (STDs), the effects of poverty, and the onset of prenatal care (Stevens-Simon and McAnarney, 1993).

Although teenagers have special needs, the obstetric risk should be no greater than for any pregnant patient. When quality prenatal care is available early in the pregnancy, the progress and outcome of teenage pregnancies compare favorably with the obstetric performance of older women. (McAnarney and Hendee, 1989). However, adolescents often receive delayed or inadequate prenatal care. This delay in seeking care may be related to the adolescent not realizing she is pregnant or denying the pregnancy until the second or third trimester. Adolescents often lack the knowledge that early prenatal care is important (Kinsman and Slap, 1992).

The risk during a second pregnancy for the teen is much higher. An adolescent with a poor outcome in the first pregnancy has a threefold risk of repeating the poor outcome in the second pregnancy. The risk for preterm delivering recurring is double the rate in older women (Pope and others, 1993).

Developmental Factors. It does not necessarily follow that early biologic development is accompanied by early emotional and psychologic development. The physically mature young girl is still a teenager who must cope with the developmental tasks of adolescence. When the tasks of motherhood are superimposed on adolescent needs, the girl may be ill prepared to deal appropriately with either.

Complications of Pregnancy. The most serious complication of pregnancy is death. Girls under the age of 15 have a pregnancy death rate that is 60% higher than the rate for all women (Davis, 1989). This risk may be more of a socioeconomic factor than a biologic one.

Structural Factors. Labor may be prolonged in younger teenagers; this is directly related to fetopelvic incompatibility and is a reflection of teenagers' smaller stature and incomplete growth process. This is particularly true regarding girls 12 to 16 years of age. The incidence of prolonged labor is highest in girls younger than age 14. Girls who are 12 and 13 years old have the highest rate of cesarean births, primarily necessary because of cephalopelvic disproportion. However, older adolescents, 15 to 21 years of age, often have labors that are shorter than average, especially those girls who have previously delivered a baby. The critical point between pelvic disproportion and adequacy appears to occur around 15 years of age in the average adolescent.

Nutritional Needs. Caloric requirements during adolescence closely parallel the growth curve, and the need for protein, calcium, and iron is increased concomitantly. Young adolescents tolerate caloric restriction poorly, and the anabolic need for calories during pregnancy places an added burden on their bodies. The preconception weight is a major determinant of birth weight for infants born to adolescents (McAnarney, 1987). Weight gain recommendations for pregnant women should be based on their weight-for-height percentile or body mass index and not on their age (Stevens-Simon and McAnarney, 1992).

Since there is marked variation in the dietary needs of individual teenagers, no hard and fast rule can be laid down to describe an adequate diet for all pregnant girls. The diet must provide sufficient nutrients to meet growth needs of both the prospective mother and the unborn child without the threat of obesity or evidence of malnutrition. The best guide for determining nutritional needs is the Recommended Daily Allowance of the Food and Nutrition Board (1989) for adolescents and the additional 300 calories per day needed during the second and third trimesters of pregnancy. However, these do not take into consideration deviations and deficiencies. Pregnant teenagers exhibit food preferences, eating behaviors, and life-style habits that are similar to those of their nonpregnant peers. Frequent snacking on foods high in fat and sugar and low in essential nutrients results in below-recommended intakes of calcium, iron, zinc, folate, and vitamins B_6, A, and C—nutrients of special concern during pregnancy (Schneck and others, 1990).

Infants. There is a higher incidence of prematurity and low birth weight in infants born to teenagers. It is difficult to determine if this is a result of the developmental stage of the mother or a reflection of multiple factors associated with teenage pregnancies, including poor nutrition, lower socioeconomic status, concomitant disease, and late or no prenatal care. Adolescents with chlamydial infections during pregnancy are at increased risk for intrauterine growth retardation and preterm birth (Johns Hopkins, 1989). Several factors demonstrate a high degree of association with prematurity, such as first birth, immaturity, illegitimacy, and the young age of the mother, and can create an accumulative effect that places the pregnant teenager in a perilously high-risk situation.

Causal Factors

The causes of teenage pregnancy are complex, and attempts to disentangle the many facets have yet to be fully successful. Several factors have contributed to the rise in premarital births to teenagers. First, the trend toward earlier initiation of sexual activity, which started in the 1970s, continues. Second, only about 1 in 3 sexually active adolescents uses a reliable method of contraception consistently.

The majority of adolescents choose not to marry. When questioned, 92%, or 5 of 6 unmarried pregnant teens, report that their pregnancy was not intended (Trussell, 1988). Minority youth appear to be most at risk for unintended pregnancy. African-Americans and Hispanic adolescents experience the highest rates of pregnancy. Understanding the cultural meanings of childbearing and the impact of poverty on minority youth is essential before adequate intervention programs can be designed (Children's Defense Fund, 1989). Clearly, it is agreed that youth who delay childbearing until they have completed their own development and education are socially and economically better prepared to become parents.

Social and Economic Aspects

Poverty is often a result of teenage childbearing. Upchurch and McCarthy (1989) found that of women ages 21 to 29 who gave birth at age 17 or younger, only 55.5% had been able to complete high school. Since many of these young women are at considerable educational disadvantage, job opportunities are limited. Frequently they are employed in service-related positions (Children's Defense Fund, 1989). Adolescents with lower academic ability or those who drop out of school are more likely to have a repeat pregnancy.

Poor school performance usually precedes adolescent pregnancy. Unable to achieve academically, the youth views motherhood as a rite of passage into adult status (Davis, 1989). Adolescents with high educational expectations are significantly less likely than others to become pregnant (Plotnick, 1992). Another significant aspect of school dropout and accelerated maturity is the girl's alienation and isolation from her peers during a stage of development when identity formation is so closely allied with peer identification. She is deprived of the interrelationship with the adolescent social system that is so essential to the development of a sense of identity. The girl may believe that she no longer "belongs" to the peer group and does not qualify for membership in the older peer group of mothers. On the other hand, the pregnancy may provide the adolescent an entrance into a peer group.

Mother-Infant Relationship

Not only are infants of teenage mothers at risk medically, they are also at risk in other aspects of their existence. Although many adolescent mothers want their babies and are prepared to care for them in a mature manner, many others have unrealistic expectations for the child. The young mother often sees the infant as a plaything or a love object for herself. Children of adolescent mothers experience more developmental problems than children of adult mothers. The amount of cognitive stimulation in the child's early home environment is positively associated with the child's level of cognitive attainment (Moore and Snyder, 1991). Many children of adolescents are raised by a grandparent. Although some research has shown positive effects on child outcomes (Pope, and others, 1993), other studies have found that co-residence with the grandmother has potentially negative effects if the mother and grandmother are in conflict. When compared with adult mothers, adolescent mothers are found to be less sensitive, less verbal, and less responsive to their infant's cues (Panzarine and others, 1988).

A 17-year follow-up study of children born to adolescents in Baltimore revealed more emotional problems and drug use, and earlier sexual experience in children of teenage mothers (Furstenberg, Brooks-Gunn, and Morgan, 1987). These children read less well and are more likely to be retained in a grade than children of older women. Although all children of teenage mothers are at developmental risk, some children do well (Flanagan and others, 1994).

Researchers have also investigated the various factors that influence the mother-infant relationship. Maternal stresses, including changes in circumstances, influence her ability to cope and her sensitivity to the needs of the infant. Teenage mothers classify "stressful" as an argument with parent, boyfriend, or husband, whereas adult mothers tend to focus on problems directly involving the infant (Coll and Oh, 1987). Vocational and educational disadvantages to both teenage mothers and fathers further impinge on their coping abilities. It is important to recognize that not all adolescent mothers are alike. Some teenagers adjust well to the stresses and responsibilities of parenting, whereas others may lack the maturity or confidence to nurture optimally (East, Matthews, and Felice, 1994).

When socioeconomic status is controlled for, it has been found that younger adolescent mothers have lower acceptance of their children as compared with older adolescent mothers. The low acceptance continues when the child is preschool age, demonstrating that this is not a short-lived phenomenon (East, Matthews, and Felice, 1994). A review of 23 studies that assessed the relationship between maternal age and child maltreatment found conflicting results. Fourteen found that young maternal age was a risk factor, and nine found that young maternal age was not associated with increased risk of child maltreatment. None of the studies found a decreased risk of maltreatment with young maternal age (Stier and others, 1993).

There is also a positive correlation between the total amount of social support and the frequency of appropriate maternal behavior. It is important to assess who the adolescent feels she receives the most support from: it may be her family, her partner, a close friend, etc. Then the nurse can help her to access this support to her benefit.

The cognitive development of the adolescent influences the development of attitudes and realistic expectations regarding childbearing. To cope effectively and solve situational dilemmas, pregnant teenagers must be able to use the problem-solving approach to assess and evaluate consequences. The concrete thought and egocentrism of early adolescence can influence the mother's ability to evaluate the needs of the infant. Adolescent mothers lack knowledge of normal infant growth and development. This lack of knowledge may directly affect their perception, interpretation, and responsiveness to infant cues.

The characteristics of the infants also influence parental behavior. Teenage parents view their children as more temperamentally difficult than do adult parents (Fleming and others, 1993). Since temperamentally difficult infants have an adverse effect on sensitivity and responsiveness of parents, a parent-infant interaction that is not mutually satisfying can alter the parents' feelings of effectiveness and self-worth. This can alter their sensitivity and relationships with the infant.

Adolescent Fathers

Much of the research over the past decade has concentrated on how adolescent pregnancy affects young women. There is little research that has focused on teenage fatherhood because of the difficulty in sampling the fathers. Young men who have fathered a child have many decisions to make regarding marriage and living arrangements. These decisions can have consequences for the father, mother, and child. A young father may still play an active role in the life of his child whether he lives with the child or not. When male high school students were asked what they would do if they impregnated a girlfriend they had been dating for a year, blacks and whites were about equally likely to say they would be willing to live with their partner and child (Marsigilio, 1988). Socioeconomically disadvantaged adolescent males are likely to view paternity as a source of self-esteem and a rite of passage to adulthood (Marsigilio, 1993). Irrespective of their marital status or age at conception, a substantially higher proportion of teenage fathers are high school dropouts. Interestingly, teenage fathers whose first child was conceived within marriage have the poorest high school completion patterns (Marsigilio, 1987). Most teenage fathers are willing to accept their obligations and demonstrate strong paternal feelings for the newborn child. They also need to be made aware of their legal rights in relation to the child.

Nursing Considerations

It is evident from the preceding discussion that nurses play a central role in meeting the needs of pregnant teenagers. It is frequently the nurse to whom the young girl turns for help and guidance in her dilemma and on whom she relies for support and reassurance.

The first goal in nursing care of the pregnant teenager is to help her obtain prenatal care whether she elects to continue or terminate the pregnancy. Typically, adolescents are reluctant to seek medical help, in part because of anxiety but more often because of a tendency to deny the pregnancy. Early prenatal care is essential for the welfare of both mother and infant. For guidelines, teaching, and general support measures during pregnancy, the reader is directed to the excellent textbooks available on nursing care throughout the maternity cycle.

Basic to the implementation of any program of care is communication and the establishment of a trusting relationship. Initially the adolescent may appear apathetic and display little interest in discussing her pregnancy. It is important for the nurse to make every effort to put the adolescent at ease and avoid undue pressure. Conveying a nonjudgmental and genuine caring acceptance of the adolescent and her goals will assist the nurse in gaining the adolescent's confidence and trust. The girl may have encountered rejection and open criticism from authority figures and peers.

Communication takes time and patience. Asking open-ended questions and listening for cues will help identify physical, emotional, social, and cultural influences that might affect the adolescent's progress through the maternity cycle. Factors that might affect her physical status, such as smoking, drug use, and nutritional state and habits, need to be explored and confronted. Each teenager presents a unique situation in relation to background, life-style, support structure, and coping mechanisms. Listening to the teen is key to the development of the relationship. The nurse must listen for understanding, not truth. Understanding the situation from the adolescent's perspective is essential for a trusting relationship and effective communication.

Nutrition assessment should focus on the dietary adequacy of iron and calcium; multivitamins with folic acid are prescribed. The adolescent is referred for food supplement programs and other financial assistance (Women, Infants, and Children (WIC), Medicaid, Aid to Families with Dependent Children [AFDC], housing, and food stamps). Social work referral for thorough psychosocial assessment and planning is initiated. Programs that have been most successful are comprehensive in approach and use an interdisciplinary team concept.

The adolescent needs to know what is happening to her, what is expected of her, and how she can help in developing a plan of care. Adolescents have their own ideas about the type of help they need and support that would be beneficial. They should be consulted and provided with an opportunity to share their ideas. Social learning theory suggests that it is important to jointly choose goals that the adolescent believes are personally beneficial, attainable, and able to be maintained over time (Greenberg, 1989).

The adolescent will need help to improve her altered self-image, a crucial factor in adolescence. Giving her as much individual attention as possible; being a sympathetic listener; providing the opportunity for her to know, support, and be supported by other girls in the same situation; and helping her to experience success will facilitate progress toward achieving this goal.

The nurse also involves the family whenever possible. The parents of the girl and the father of the child need to express feelings and attitudes about the situation. The nurse should not make assumptions about whether or not the girl wishes to have these persons involved in her decisions and care. Rather, the nurse must determine the teenager's true feelings regarding these relationships.

Education regarding child care begins during pregnancy, and preparations should be made for continued education and assistance after the birth. Educational programs alone are probably not enough for high-risk youth. Research has shown home visiting programs to be helpful in the prevention of maltreatment of children with adolescent parents (Stier and others, 1993). Recognizing and referring high-risk teen parents for additional services is crucial. Referral should target adolescents with low self-esteem, teens less than 14 years of age, and those without a social support network in place. The adolescent and her labor partner should attend childbirth education classes designed to meet the developmental level of the adolescent.

Targeting teen parents for secondary pregnancy prevention is essential. The increased risk of recurrence and poor outcomes in subsequent pregnancies underscores the importance of these prevention programs.

ADOLESCENT ABORTION

In 1973 the landmark Supreme Court case of ***Roe v. Wade*** concluded that the right to an abortion rested within the rights of the individual. This right was not absolute but subject to certain state restrictions. Abortion is one of the most controversial moral issues in the United States. For example, 92% of Americans believe that a pregnant woman should be able to obtain an abortion if her own life is endangered, 83% believe she should be able to do so if there is a strong chance that the fetus has a serious defect, 86% believe an abortion should be available if the pregnancy is a result of a rape, and 43% said that a woman should be able to have an abortion for any reason (Klitsch, 1991). The right to an abortion is also determined by the stage of pregnancy. During the first trimester the woman and her care provider can arrive at a decision without government interference.

In recent years 26% of all abortions have been performed on women under age 20 (Henshaw, 1990). The rights of minors had a historical precedent when the Supreme Court ruled in 1967 that a juvenile had a right to a just trial before any sentencing could take place (otherwise known as the "mature minor" concept) (see Informed Consent, Chapter 27). This antecedent ruling allowed the reproductive rights of adults to be extended to minors. The requirement of parental notification in a minor's decision to have an abortion is being debated in state legislatures and in Congress. There is much debate as to whether the requirement of parental notification would be helpful or harmful to the adolescent. In a study of adolescents seeking abortion in states where parental notification is not required, only 39% of the minors had the abortion without the knowledge of either parent. More than half of those who did not involve a parent in the decision were over 16, and the majority of these involved an adult other than a parent (Henshaw and Kost, 1992). Supreme Court decisions have upheld state laws requiring parental consent or notification, but only if pregnant minors were allowed to go to court without involving their parents and if courts allowed mature minors to make their own decisions (Crosby and English, 1991).

In 1989 there were an estimated 233,000 unintended pregnancies, 161,000 births, and 162,000 abortions among adolescents ages 15 to 17. There were 9000 births and 14,000 abortions among girls age 14 and under (Ambriel and Lewis, 1992). Although abortion is a controversial and emotional issue, health care professionals involved in delivery of services to pregnant adolescents are confronted with this reality frequently. Since the law in this area is unsettled, changing rapidly, and varies by state, it is essential that nurses stay abreast of legal changes as they relate to reproductive rights of minors in the state in which they practice.

Other barriers to receiving an abortion include distance to the clinic, cost, and antiabortion harassment. Abortion services in the United States are offered primarily at free-standing abortion clinics, usually in major population centers. Abortions are not covered by insurance, and the cost may be prohibitive to many women, especially adolescents. More than half of the abortion providers report that picketing outside the agency occurs at least once a week (Henshaw, 1991).

The medical safety of a legal abortion has been well established. A higher mortality rate has been associated with a full-term pregnancy than with abortion. A variety of surgical procedures are available to the operator but are beyond the scope of this discussion. First-trimester abortions are performed as an outpatient procedure and require local anesthesia or mild sedation only. Complication rates have been reported to be 1% or less. Problems that arise after abortion are endometritis, hemorrhage, Rh sensitization, genital tract injury, retained fetal elements, and (in rare cases) pulmonary embolism or death (Greydanus and Shearin, 1990). Second-trimester abortions usually require hospital admission. The procedure is more complicated and is associated with greater risk from hemorrhage. Women who have an induced abortion are no more likely than other women to experience problems in bearing a healthy baby in subsequent pregnancies (Frank and others, 1991).

Abortion counseling criteria suggested in a policy statement by the American Academy of Pediatrics (1989) include three guiding principles: (1) the counselor should provide information in an unbiased format; (2) none of the options may be universally accepted by either the patient or the health care provider; and (3) the adolescent and other concerned individuals must be given adequate freedom to arrive at a working decision. The counselor must respect the moral decision and legal right of the adolescent to have an abortion; if unable to do so, the counselor should refer the adolescent to a care provider who can discuss all the options.

Although there is concern about the long-term emotional consequences for the female who has an abortion, there is no clear association between an adolescent's abortion history and her feelings of well-being and self-esteem. Women with greater numbers of births and those with at least one unwanted birth have been found to have generally lower levels of self-esteem than other women (Russo and Zierk, 1992).

Nursing Considerations

Early identification of pregnancy is essential, and nurses are in an optimum position to provide counseling on pregnancy options. Whatever option is chosen by the adolescent, referral should be initiated as quickly as possible to eliminate risk. Pelvic ultrasound may be indicated to assess gestational age correctly for those adolescents who cannot recall the date of their last menstrual period and when a bimanual examination is inconclusive.

Patient education regarding the medical aspects of the abortion before the procedure should be conducted verbally, and the patient should be provided with written instructions. Reviewing relaxation strategies to be used during the procedure is helpful. Parents or other significant adults are encouraged to be present during the medical procedure.

Finally, a discussion of future contraceptive needs is essential. The adolescent may be started on a hormonal method of contraception immediately after the abortion. Patients should be seen 2 weeks after an abortion to receive medical, contraceptive, and psychologic follow-up care.

CONTRACEPTION

Family planning services in general have developed and expanded during recent years, and with the increase in sexual activity among the teenage population, there is also an increased awareness of the need for contraceptive services as part of the health care of adolescents. Although all teenagers need sexuality education, not all of them are candidates for contraception. Among the large adolescent population, there are those who have made the decision to postpone sexual involvement, and there are also those who may wish to have a child.

Confidentiality is an important issue when discussing contraception with adolescents. Privacy is important to adolescents as they struggle to forge a personal identity and establish social relationships. Adolescents are particularly concerned about the judgements of others. The American Academy of Pediatrics Policy Statement "Confidentiality in Adolescent Health Care" states that "adolescents tend to underutilize existing health care resources," and that lack of confidentiality is "a significant access barrier to health care" (American Academy of Pediatrics, 1991). Health delivery systems must be structured to allow confidentiality, including methods for appointment scheduling, billing, record keeping, and follow-up that ensure privacy rights for adolescents (Cheng and others, 1993). Family-centered care and parental involvement in contraceptive choice is ideal for patient compliance. However, there are adolescents who need confidential care. The predominant feeling among health professionals is that parental notification is important but that the "parents' rights" view is not necessarily sensitive to the health needs and basic rights of youth. There is no evidence to substantiate the belief that providing contraceptive guidance contributes to sexual irresponsibility and promiscuity. Actually, a request for contraceptive information indicates a responsible effort on the part of the teenager to avoid an undesirable pregnancy.

Contraceptive Methods

A contraceptive method, to be safe and effective, must be suited to the individual. The choice is based on the adolescent's preference after being informed of all the benefits and disadvantages of the methods available. The adolescent must be motivated to use whatever method is cho-

TABLE 20-1 Advantages and Disadvantages of Contraceptive Methods in the Adolescent

METHOD	ADVANTAGES	DISADVANTAGES
Abstinence	100% effective in prevention of STDs and pregnancy No medical visit needed	Peer pressure for sex
Withdrawal Withdrawal of penis before ejaculation		High failure rate Some seminal fluid often released before ejaculation Ejaculate at vaginal orifice may enter vagina No STD protection
Rhythm Refrain from intercourse during fertile period	Encourages couple participation	Requires a predictable menstrual cycle, unusual in early and middle adolescence No STD protection High failure rates
Barrier methods Condom *Male:* Penile covering to trap sperm *Female:* Inserted into vagina with base covering part of perineum	No prescription needed Easy to use STD protection No medical complications	Interrupts sex May have decreased sensations Requires consistent use
Diaphragm Cervical covering to prevent sperm from reaching eggs Used with spermicidal jelly	May be inserted 4 to 6 hours before sex Effective when used correctly Few medical complications May be reused	Little STD protection Requires fitting by medical personnel Requires body awareness and comfort with touching oneself for insertion May increase incidence of urinary tract infection
Sponge Cervical covering Releases a spermicide	May be inserted up to 6 hours before sex Can be obtained without prescription	Minimal STD protection Requires body awareness and comfort with touching self May be difficult to remove Decreased effectiveness in parous woman
Spermicides Foam, jelly, cream, suppositories Inserted into vagina to kill sperm	Available without prescription Inexpensive Easy to use No major health concerns	High failure rate unless used with condom Interrupts sexual experience Messy
Oral contraceptives Estrogen and progesterone-like compounds that inhibit ovulation	Few medical complications in teens 99% effective if used correctly No interruption of sex Regulates menses, decreases dysmenorrhea and acne	Must use consistently Requires prescription Expensive No STD protection Small weight gain
Norplant Levonorgestrol slowly released into vascular system for 5 years Inhibits ovulation, thickens cervical mucosa; 6 small rods inserted into upper arm	No interruption of sex Long-term, highly effective protection against pregnancy Pregnancy prevention begins 24 hours after insertion Once removed, fertility returns immediately	No STD protection Significant weight gain Irregular menses Requires minor surgical procedure Expensive
Depo Provera Progestin that suppresses hormonal cycle and prevents ovulation Injection given every 3 months	No interruption of sex Invisible method	No STD protection Significant weight gain Irregular menses or amenorrhea Decreased libido Fertility may be delayed Must return to care provider every 3 months for injection
Postcoital Contraception Combined estrogen-progestin pill containing ethinyl estradiol; given within 72 hours of unprotected sex and repeated 12 hours later; prevents implantation	Useful in unplanned sexual intercourse	No STD protection May experience nausea Effectiveness dependent on phase of menstrual cycle Not intended for repeated use

sen. Factors associated with use of contraception include education, expectations, availability, cost of methods, parent education level, perception of high likelihood of pregnancy, perception of disadvantages of having a pregnancy, and low rate of disadvantages of birth control methods (Fielding and Williams, 1991). The provision of a birth control device is only part of a comprehensive sex education program. Partner involvement, when possible, has been shown to enhance user compliance. To make truly informed choices about contraception, adolescents need to know not only the efficacy of methods as they are actually used, but also their efficacy when used consistently. The advantages and disadvantages of various contraceptive methods recommended for use in adolescents are outlined in Table 20-1.

Nonprescription Methods. Sometimes, despite the effectiveness of prescription methods, teenagers use less effective methods to avoid the necessity for medical screening and supervision inherent in the use of prescription methods. Adolescents may report the use of withdrawal and reliance on "safe" periods in the menstrual cycle as their current method of contraception. Using the method of periodic abstinence, or the rhythm method, is very risky. When the rules are broken in this method, the couple is having unprotected sexual intercourse at times during the menstrual cycle when pregnancy is most likely to occur (Trussell and Grummer-Strawn, 1990). Factual knowledge about condoms and clarifying myths and misinformation about pregnancy prevention can help to reduce the incidence of unwanted pregnancy.

Because of the high incidence of STDs in the adolescent population, condom use should be discussed with all adolescents seeking contraceptive advice. The adolescent can then be assisted in choosing an additional method to prevent pregnancy.

The lack of female-controlled barrier methods known to protect against infection with STDs has led to the development of the female condom. The contraceptive efficacy of the female condom during typical use is similar to that of the diaphragm, sponge, or cervical cap. The female condom is nearly as effective in preventing pregnancy as the male condom without spermicidal lubricant. The female condom appears to have great potential for giving a woman control in reducing her risk of human immunodeficiency virus (HIV) infection (Trussell and others, 1994).

Prescription Methods. Pregnancy rates among teens using a prescription contraceptive method range from 7% to 13% per year (Winter and Breckenmaker, 1991). An adolescent choosing a prescription method of contraception requires a careful history and physical examination. Some medications or chronic illnesses may be a relative contraindication to some contraceptive methods.

Intrauterine devices (IUDs) and sterilization are common methods of birth control in the adult population but are not recommended for teenagers. IUDs increase the risk of pelvic inflammatory disease (PID) and its consequences, and nulliparous females are more likely to have difficulty during insertion of the device, to suffer cramping and bleeding, and to expel the IUD. Sterilization is contraindicated for adolescents, especially those who have not borne children (Hatcher and others, 1990; Tyrer, Rothbart, and Anderson, 1989).

REASONS FOR NOT SEEKING OR USING BIRTH CONTROL

Responses of teenagers at initial interview for contraception in order of frequency:

- Dangerous to use
- Waiting for closer relationship with partner
- Afraid family would find out
- Not having sex
- Afraid of examination
- Did not think had sex often enough for pregnancy
- Did not expect to have sex
- Thought wanted pregnancy
- Thought too young to get pregnant
- Partner objected
- Thought it cost too much
- Thought had to be older to get birth control

Modified from Zabin LS, Stark HA, Emerson MR: Reasons for delay in contraceptive clinic visit: adolescent clinic and nonclinic populations compared, *J Adolesc Health* 12:225-232, 1991.

Use of Contraception

In adolescents who are using contraception, the oral contraceptive pill (OCP) and the condom are the most popular methods. In fact, 80% of women in the United States have been on the pill at some time in their reproductive years. Condom use among adolescents has been on the rise over the past decade; however, consistent use of condoms remains infrequent (Shafer and Boyer, 1991; Sonenstein, Pleck, and Ku, 1989). When counseling adolescents regarding contraceptive use, the nurse needs to discuss effectiveness rates, being careful not to confuse theoretic effectiveness with typical user effectiveness. The unintended pregnancy rate for adolescents within the first year of use of a method is 26% (Mosher, 1990).

Delay in seeking contraceptive information is common. The median interval from onset of sexual intercourse until the first visit for contraception is 1 year. A pregnancy scare is usually the precipitating event for the contraception appointment. Reasons adolescents give for not making better use of contraception are listed in the box above.

Compliance in contraceptive use is related to many factors, including the following.

Lack of Information. Sometimes health professionals have a tendency to confuse a teenager's sophistication with knowledge. Although adolescents are acutely aware of their sexuality, their understanding of reproductive anatomy and physiology is incomplete. If they are using contraception, they often do so with little or no instruction and with only vague understanding. Misinformation is commonplace. Lacking a fundamental understanding of fertility, they often believe they are too young or have sex too infrequently to become pregnant. A majority of girls mistakenly believe that maximum fertility begins with menses and that the safe period occurs midway between menstrual periods.

Anxiety Regarding Contraception. Some adolescents are concerned that parents will be notified. Many have exaggerated ideas about the hazards of prescription methods, which correlates with misguided fears in the adult population. Other teens are fearful of the pelvic examination and delay seeking contraception to avoid the procedure.

Conflict About Sexual Activity. Many teenagers feel ambivalent regarding their sexual activity and avoid many contraceptives because their use seems too premeditated and implies that sex is planned rather than a spontaneous activity. Most of these girls believe that sex is all right if it was unplanned. This may often play a role in those adolescents who delay contraception, waiting for a relationship that is "close enough." A close relationship would allow the adolescents to accept and acknowledge their sexual activity.

Desire for Pregnancy. Some teens are seeking a pregnancy and will fail to use an effective method of contraception or use a prescribed method improperly. Some adolescents seek pregnancy as a legitimate rite of passage into adulthood or as a misdirected attempt to have someone to love them. Careful counseling and assistance with decision-making skills are essential when counseling the adolescent desiring pregnancy.

Nursing Considerations

Much of contraceptive education and service is assumed by nurses as part of sex education programs, family planning services, or postpartum health services. The introduction of contraceptive methods should ideally be associated with ongoing sex education. When they are included in this education process, the sexually active adolescent will consider contraceptives as a natural and logical part of intercourse. It is important that adolescents learn about sexuality, conception, and contraception from someone who can provide them with accurate information in a straightforward, nonjudgmental manner.

It is unrealistic to expect the adolescent to "just say no." Postponing sexual involvement requires effective communication and decision-making skills. Adolescents benefit from role-playing refusal skills in a safe environment. The nurse should also discuss with the adolescent how to introduce condoms into an existing relationship, as well as into new relationships. Young women who have ever requested a partner to use a condom are five times more likely to use a condom consistently over the next 6 months than women who have never made the request (Joffe and Radius, 1993). The nurse plays an important role in offering appropriate education, helping build confidence in adolescents' ability to make requests of their partners, and providing social support to the sexually active adolescent.

To make an informed decision, the adolescent needs a careful review of all methods available, including their advantages and disadvantages. When possible, this counseling should include the parent(s) and/or partner.

Compliance with a method will increase when the adolescent has a clear understanding of potential side effects. This is particularly important with methods, such as the hormonal implant, that require removal of the device by the care provider. For hormonal implant use to be fully voluntary, users must be able to have the implant removed whenever they want, for whatever reason, and without encountering perceived or actual barriers (Forrest and Kalser, 1993).

Adolescents need instructions in correct use of their contraceptive choice. Providing both verbal and written instructions is essential. The nurse should demonstrate the correct use of condoms to all sexually active adolescents.

An essential part of contraceptive services to teenagers is follow-up. Frequent follow-up to check effectiveness and general health will increase compliance. Close follow-up allows the care provider to monitor side effects, which may decrease compliance with the method.

An organization that provides education and services for adolescents, including both individual and group counseling, is the **Planned Parenthood Federation of America.*** It has branches in most cities in the United States.

RAPE

The adolescent girl is particularly vulnerable to sexual assault, and it is estimated that more than 50% of rape victims are between 15 and 19 years of age (Koss, Gidycz, and Wisniewski, 1987). Seven percent of 18- to 22-year-old Americans have experienced at least one episode of involuntary sexual intercourse. Females are more likely to report these experiences than males (Moore, Nord, and Peterson, 1989). In each instance the victim is potentially subjected to serious physical and/or emotional harm. There is no typical victim. Sexual assault victims are of all ages, ethnic groups, and economic groups, and are of either gender.

Legal definitions of rape vary from state to state but include the following categories: completed rape, attempted rape, and statutory rape. Most of the current definitions of rape have been expanded to include all forms of sexual victimization, including anal and oral, as well as genital, penetration. Sexual assault is not restricted to vaginal or anal penetration but includes every form of sexual activity, including voyeurism. To prove power over the victim, the assailant subjects the victim to sodomy and other types of demeaning sexual acts.

Statutory rape may be charged when the victim is unable to give consent legally by virtue of age (age varies from state to state but is usually less than 16 years), mental deficiency, psychosis, or an altered state of consciousness caused by sleep, drugs, or illness.

Assailants

Three relationships are identified for assault: stranger, nonstranger, and incest. Although all can have serious and long-lasting effects, they are presumed to be different in a number of important ways: in the nature of the dominant psychologic and cognitive behaviors they provoke, in the issues they raise for service providers and other potential helpers, and in the techniques that may be helpful for treating existing and new cases (Burgess, 1985).

Nonstranger Rapist. The majority of rapes are committed by a nonstranger, which is often referred to as ***acquaintance rape.*** The acquaintance may be a date, someone

*810 7th Ave., New York, NY 10019; (800) 230-PLAN.

who lives near the adolescent, someone who has contact with the victim through recreational activities, or someone in an official association with the teen. Some assailants wait for an opportunity when the victim is defenseless, such as the teenager at home alone with an uncle or cousin or the baby-sitter being driven home. In the United States 21% to 34% of women will be physically assaulted by an intimate partner. More than half of all women murdered in the 1980s were murdered by their partner (Browne, 1993).

The assailant may be another teenager known through social activity. The nature of sex-role learning in most cultures associates females with softness, nonassertiveness, and dependence on men. Young women are socialized to be alluring yet sexually unavailable and to assume the role of pacesetter in sexual situations. Males are conditioned to be strong, powerful, and aggressive (measures of masculinity) and to be aggressors in sexual situations. In a study questioning adolescents about attitudes toward violence, 32% of female teens believed forced sex was acceptable if the couple had dated a long time, 31% of girls and 54% of boys believed forced sex was acceptable if the woman had agreed to have sex but later changed her mind, and 27% of young women believed forced sex was acceptable if the woman had led the man on. In the same study 40% of the young men stated forced sex was acceptable if the man had spent a lot of money on the date (Parrot, 1989).

Acquaintance rape is frequently underreported because the victim may believe she contributed to the act in some way. The victim may not identify the experience as rape because it does not fit the standard concept of rape (ACOG Committee on Adolescent Health Care, 1993). Adolescents also report unwanted sexual activity that was not physically forced but was related to substance use, partner pressure, or peer pressure (Erickson and Rapkin, 1991).

Findings of studies also indicate that not only are teenagers at risk for rape by peers, but also they may face multiple assailants or "gang rapes." These variations on teenage rape include multiple assailants and a single victim, multiple assailants and multiple victims, and peer rape in tandem (e.g., offenders who group together specifically to rape).

Stranger Rapist. It is believed that stranger rapes probably account for nearly 50% of all rapes reported to police. Victims are frequently selected at random because they are apparently helpless.

Incest. The most commonly reported incestuous relationships are between a daughter and a male in a caretaking role (e.g., a father or stepfather). The average age of onset for an incestuous ongoing relationship is 8 to 9 years, and its duration is approximately 5 years (Kempe and Kempe, 1984). The victim's participation is gained through the application of authority, subtle pressure, persuasion, or misrepresentation of moral standards. For a further discussion of sexual abuse, see Child Maltreatment, Chapter 16.

Clinical Manifestations

Adolescents who have been raped arrive at the emergency room or practitioner's office under a variety of circumstances. They are usually brought in by parents, friends, or police, but some girls may seek medical help on their own. They may display a variety of manifestations, such as hysterical crying or giggling; agitation; feelings of degradation, anger or rage, helplessness; nervousness; and rapid mood swings. Adolescents may alternately appear calm and controlled, masking inner turmoil; they may be angry, confused, and filled with self-blame (American Academy of Pediatrics, 1989).

The rape victim may present with evidence of physical force, including roughness, nonbrutal beating (slapping), brutal beating (slugging, kicking), and choking or gagging. The predominant reaction of the victim is fear of the rape and of injury. Thus the victim is faced with the dilemma of submission or resistance. Resistance increases the victim's chance of escape but also increases the likelihood of violence against him or her.

Therapeutic Management

It is advisable to obtain parental consent for examination, but the examination may be performed without consent if the adolescent is legally mature or the parents are unavailable. A female observer should be present during the history taking and examination of female victims who are examined by a male practitioner. Whether a parent should be present during the examination is determined on an individual basis. The parent's presence is usually encouraged, but only if the parent is supportive. Often the presence of a parent or a police officer inhibits the person's ability to describe the incident.

Since rape is a legal matter to be determined by the courts, medical examination merely provides evidence of penetration, ejaculation, and, when possible, use of force. The last is difficult to determine, since many young women are left unmarked when forced to comply at the point of a weapon.

Initial Contact. The circumstances of the initial medical evaluation may be frightening and stressful. The initial contact with the rape victim must be supportive, and the fundamental goal is to do no further harm. The interrogating and associated activities have the potential to add to the trauma of the sexual assault. First, the victim needs to know that she is (1) all right and (2) not being blamed for the situation. The first approach is not one of repeated interrogation, but an attempt to reduce the victim's stress.

History. Although it is important to obtain a clear account of the circumstances of an alleged rape, it is equally essential to minimize any further psychologic trauma that might occur if the adolescent is forced to relive a very painful experience. The adolescent will in all likelihood have been questioned by family and the police. If the person is too upset, the detailed history may be delayed. The adolescent should not be further victimized by insensitive care and unnecessary trauma (American Academy of Pediatrics, 1989).

The history should be as complete as possible and must be taken and presented in the patient's own words, including any account of force or threats. Information includes the date, time, location, and an accurate description of all types of sexual contact. All related activities are included.

For example, evidence can be altered if the victim has bathed, urinated, defecated, douched, or changed clothing; therefore these activities are recorded. Use of a condom by the alleged assailant can alter evidence. For adequate care, other important data include the date of the last menstrual period, the date of last intercourse, use of contraception, and any possibility of a preexisting pregnancy or STD. The victim's behavior and emotional state are also recorded.

Examination. The physical examination is carried out as soon as possible, since physical evidence deteriorates rapidly. The adolescent is always told in advance in understandable terms exactly what to expect in the way of tests and procedures, and the explanation is accompanied by emotional support. The victim is examined thoroughly, including nongenital areas, for evidence of injury that might substantiate the use of force. Photographs are taken of bruises, lacerations, or scratches for evidence, and rips or tears in clothing and the presence of dirt or grass stains are noted and recorded. Perineal, vaginal, or rectal lacerations suggest rape.

Specimens are obtained from the vaginal cul-de-sac and are examined immediately to assess sperm mobility. A cervical smear is prepared and sent to the laboratory. Vaginal secretions are also tested for acid phosphatase, since this enzyme is not normally present in the female genital tract but is found in high concentrations in semen. This is especially important if the assailant has had a vasectomy or is infertile. Prostatic acid phosphatase has been found up to 22 hours after the alleged assault. The Pap smear is the most reliable test for documentation of sexual intercourse from 14 to 26 hours after the event. Forensic materials should be turned over to law enforcement officials promptly after collection (Paradise, 1990).

A baseline serology is drawn, and a gonococcal culture is obtained to prove that the victim did not have any preexisting infection. HIV testing should also be discussed with the victim. The adolescent is reexamined at appropriate intervals (4 to 6 weeks for syphilis; 2 to 3 days for gonorrhea) to determine if a disease was acquired from the assailant.

Treatment. Any injuries sustained by the victim that require surgical treatment are repaired. Most care providers prescribe prophylactic administration of antibiotics at the time of initial examination. Pregnancy prophylaxis with high-dose estrogen is offered to the victim who is not pregnant or using a contraceptive method.

Nursing Considerations

Many of the approaches described for the sexually abused child (see Chapter 16) apply to the adolescent. Sexual assault is a devastating experience with long-lasting effects. The primary goal of nursing care is not to inflict further stress on the victim, who is often angry, confused, frightened, embarrassed, and filled with self-blame. Young rape victims fear pregnancy, bodily injury, and the reactions of their parents and peers. Some believe that their bodies are permanently damaged and may even fear death as a consequence of the experience.

The nurse must do everything possible to reduce the stress of the interrogation and examination. Application of stress-reduction techniques during the process can help the adolescent manage the immediate experience. Although most health professionals and law enforcement officers are sensitive to the needs of the victim and attempt to make the process as nonstressful as possible, the nurse acts as the advocate for the adolescent and is alert for cues that the victim is being overstressed.

Follow-up care of the rape victim is essential and extends over a long period of time. Rape victims typically show very high levels of distress within the first week, which peaks in severity by 3 weeks following the assault, continues at high levels for the next month, and then begins to decrease by 2 to 3 months after the assault (Koss, 1993). Victims of sexual abuse have been noted to have an unusually high frequency of somatic complaints (Rapkin and others, 1990). Adolescents with a history of sexual abuse (rape, incest) have a significantly higher incidence of substance abuse. The nurse should include appropriate screening questions for substance use as well (Hernandez, 1992). Referral to a public health agency and/or mental health agency should be made as soon as possible with the victim's consent. Victims who live in areas with established rape crisis centers are referred to these facilities.

Aside from the universal need for emotional support, there are no firm guidelines for meeting the needs of rape victims. Their needs vary widely and depend on the nature of the incident, when it took place, the physical and emotional injuries sustained by the victim, the actions being considered as a result, the resources available for informal support, and the anticipated reactions of persons in the informal support network. Posttraumatic stress disorder (PTSD) occurs in many victims of rape (Goodman and others, 1993) (see Chapter 18). Acquaintance rape is as devastating to the victim as stranger rape (Koss, 1993). There are few reliable predictors of positive readjustment among rape survivors. In general, a young age at the time of assault is associated with increased distress. Women victimized in childhood are 2.4 times more likely than nonvictims to be assaulted as adults (Wyatt, Guthrie, and Notgrass, 1992).

Family Support. In addition to the needs of the adolescent rape victim, the nurse is also sensitive to the needs and reactions of the adolescent's parents. Some will be angry and blame the adolescent; others will feel guilty. Many reactions can be expected at the time of the incident, ranging from despair to extreme agitation. Frequently the parents require as much support and reassurance as the victim. Agitated, angry, or incapacitated parents are unable to provide support for their child. Meeting their needs can facilitate their ability to support the teenager during the crisis.

Prevention. With the increasing incidence of rape, many professionals are looking for additional means for preventing rape at all ages. Many schools and organizations arrange for classes on how to avoid an attack and how to behave in the event of an attempted rape. Rape trauma centers and most law enforcement agencies provide this service to groups. Every effort should be made to protect children and adolescents from injury and to teach them how to avoid situations that may promote an attack and how to behave in a threatening situation.

Nurses can be advocates for improving the community

environment and street lighting, providing safe housing and transportation, and improving the effectiveness of the criminal justice system. They can work toward educating adolescents about the relationship of risk-taking behaviors and sexual attack. These behaviors include drinking, taking drugs, and hitchhiking.

Nurses can also play an important role in educating individuals and groups about date rape. The course can help to challenge traditional sex role stereotypes. A date rape prevention program should include communication skills. A dating contract should be written by all adolescents to determine their own limits for physical contact before the situation arises. Ideally, this contract is written with their parents and shared with their date.

SEXUALLY TRANSMITTED DISEASES (STDS)

STDs represent one of the major causes of morbidity during adolescence and young adulthood and annually afflict approximately 10 million persons under the age of 25 years. Teenagers represent one of the groups at highest risk. The area of STD diagnosis and treatment has become exceedingly complex with the expansion from the five traditional venereal diseases (VDs) to the nomenclature of STD in the mid-1970s, which includes more than 20 different infections and associated syndromes.

Several unique characteristics—biologic, developmental, and environmental—place adolescents at risk for acquisition of STDs. Biologically the immature adolescent female undergoes major physiologic transformation in the area of the endocervix. The thin layer of columnar cells appears to favor attachment of infectious agents (e.g., *Chlamydia trachomatis,* human papilloma virus [HPV]), which accounts in part for the increased prevalence of these infections in adolescents. The unchallenged immune system does not provide localized antibody response at the cervical level when exposed repeatedly to infectious agents. During anovulatory cycles estrogen predominates, as demonstrated by the clear and watery cervical discharge. This may facilitate the transport of pathogens to the upper genital tract (Biro, 1992).

Developmentally teenagers experience biologic discontinuities wherein pubertal maturation precedes psychologic and cognitive maturity. For example, the average age of menarche has declined to 12.5 years, and the age of sexual debut has also declined; the majority of males and females are sexually active by age 19 years. The absence of future planning is often evident in their failure to see the implications of current behavior on future outcome, such as condom use to prevent STD or pregnancy, or the need to return for follow-up visits for contraceptive refill or STD treatment. During this time of evolving identity and emerging sexuality, the outcome is teenagers who have reproductive capabilities but insufficient maturity to make safe decisions and communicate effectively with their partner.

Recent data from a national sample of Canadian college students have shown that as young women have more sexual partners, their use of hormonal contraception increases. At the same time, the use of condoms declines. Nurses must continue to stress STD prevention and condom usage (Fisher, 1990).

Designing health care systems and providing in-service education for all health care personnel are essential to provision of services that meet the needs of adolescents. Environmental barriers to health care use by teenagers include high cost, lack of insurance, inconvenient timing of appointments, and inconvenient location of health facilities. Services need to be easily accessible and sensitive to the adolescent's developmental needs and desire for confidentiality. State statutes vary regarding the right to confidential testing and treatment for STDs. States without specific statutes outlining treatment can offer confidential care based on common law precedent. Nurses should review the guidelines in the state in which they are practicing.

GONORRHEA

Although gonorrhea as a clinical disease dates from the Old Testament, its differentiation from syphilis and its linkage to urethral discharge in men and serious pelvic complications in women (twentieth century) are more recent (Sparling, 1990).

Epidemiology

Several demographic factors have been described for persons who are at risk for acquiring gonorrhea. Adolescents 15 to 19 years of age have the highest overall incidence of gonococcal infection compared with any other age-group when rates are adjusted for sexual activity. Gonorrhea among nonwhites is 10 times more frequent than among whites. Part of this discrepancy can be explained by the fact that nonwhites are more likely to attend public health clinics, where reporting of the disease is better than in the private sector. Other known risk factors are low socioeconomic status, urban residence, early onset of sexual activity, single marital status, previous history of gonorrhea, and multiple sexual partners.

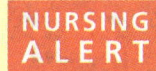

Prior infection is an important marker and should alert the clinician that the individual is at risk for reinfection.

Epidemiologic evidence suggests that there is a core group, or clustering of individuals, who are never treated or inadequately treated and thus serve as a reservoir for reinfection. This emphasizes the need for partner identification and appropriate treatment to interrupt this cycle of reinfection.

Gonorrhea is almost always sexually transmitted, except when it appears in the conjunctiva. Vertical transmission from the maternal cervix to the newborn's conjunctiva is the usual mode of infection. The incidence of gonococcal ophthalmia has decreased in developed countries by the routine application of prophylactic antibiotics to the eyes of newborn infants (see Chapter 8). Gonococcal infections do not confer lifelong immunity; therefore individuals are subject to reinfection.

Pathophysiology

The causative organism is *Neisseria gonorrhoeae,* a gram-negative diplococcus. The organisms have very specific survival requirements. They prefer a moist, alkaline environment (pH 7.2 to 7.6) and a temperature of 35° to 36° C (95° to 96.8° F). They quickly die on drying, on exposure to the weakest acids, and with an increase of 3° C in temperature. The gonococci survive only on the columnar and transitional epithelium; stratified epithelium is resistant to the onslaught. The organisms spread along the mucosa from the point of entry. They penetrate between the epithelial cells and, when they die, liberate an irritant that produces the inflammatory response, characterized by localized capillary dilation, edema, and leukocytosis. This process accounts for the purulent discharge and erosive balanitis and cervicitis sometimes observed in affected persons.

Clinical Manifestations

Symptoms can appear as early as 1 day or as late as 2 weeks after sexual contact. Gonococcal infection can occur in many diverse ways, with four basic presentations: asymptomatic, uncomplicated symptomatic, complicated symptomatic, and disseminated disease. The infection can involve a number of organs and a wide range of manifestations (Table 20-2). The pelvic inflammatory disease (PID) in females simulates the inflammatory process caused by other bacterial infections, and differential diagnosis is made for more definitive medical treatment. Since a large percentage of affected persons are asymptomatic, gonorrhea should be considered in the evaluation of all sexually active adolescents. Lack of clinical symptoms is especially characteristic of the rectal and pharyngeal infections.

There is a difference in the way the disease affects children. Whereas uncomplicated urogenital infection in postpubescent girls involves the cervix, in prepubescent girls it is seen as vulvovaginitis. Early complaints of vulvovaginitis include dysuria and perineal or vulvar discomfort, often associated with perianal soreness that is increased during defecation. Examination reveals edematous vaginal mucosa; a greenish yellow discharge may be present, and the perianal area often appears inflamed and edematous, with some discharge from anal crypts.

Diagnostic Evaluation

The diagnosis is established on identification of the organism from direct smear or culture techniques. In males the diagnosis is relatively easy. Since gram-negative diplococci are not normally present in the male genitourinary tract, their intracellular presence in smears is diagnostic. A false-negative result may be seen in the very early course of the disease, in old, untreated cases, in persons who have taken penicillin or a wide-spectrum antibiotic within a few hours of the examination, and in asymptomatic males (Biro, 1992). Asymptomatic males can be screened by detection of pyuria through leukocyte esterase activity in the urine (Shafer and others, 1989; Werner and Biro, 1991).

Homosexual males should receive pharyngeal, urethral, and rectal cultures. A routine pharyngeal culture for *N. gonorrhoeae* in heterosexual adolescents identifies an additional 1% of cases (Brown and others, 1989).

The diagnosis is more difficult in females, which has been a significant obstacle in effective control programs. Although cervical and urethral smears are fairly reliable in the acute phase of the disease, with less acute or asymptomatic cases there is a high yield of both false-positive and false-negative results by Gram stain. Specimens of pus from the urethra or cervix (not the vagina) should be cultured immediately on special media designed for detecting these organisms. Because of their adverse effects on organisms, surgical jelly or any fatty substance (including some types of

TABLE 20-2 Comparison Between Gonorrhea and Chlamydial Infection

CHARACTERISTICS	GONORRHEA	CHLAMYDIA
Incubation period	2-6 days; rare cases 10-16 days	8-21 days
Major site of infection	Urethritis (males) Cervicitis (females)	Urethritis (males) Cervicitis (females)
Local complications	Epididymitis, bartholinitis, salpingitis, prostatitis, PID, conjunctivitis, pharyngitis, proctitis	Epididymitis, bartholinitis, salpingitis, postpartum endometritis, PID, conjunctivitis (trachoma), proctitis
Systemic complications	Septicemia with resulting arthritis, dermatitis, endocarditis, meningitis, perihepatitis, peritonitis	Arthritis, perihepatitis, chronic conjunctivitis
Carrier state	Recognized, especially in women; can last for months; primary reservoir is the cervix; male urethra is a minor site	Recognized, especially in women; can last for months; primary reservoir is cervix; male urethra is a minor site
Effects of maternal infection on newborn	Less well established Ophthalmia neonatorum	Well-known; inclusion conjunctivitis and pneumonia
Treatment	Ceftriaxone or cefixime Single-dose treatment Treat for possible chlamydia infection as well Treat sexual contacts	Doxycycline b.i.d. for 7 days Azithromycin single-dose treatment Treatment of sexual contacts

swabs) should not be used in securing the specimen. The presence of menses is not a contraindication; the menstrual secretions provide an optimum environment for growth of the organism.

Therapeutic Management

The emergence of gonococcal strains resistant to penicillin has created new recommendations for treatment. Uncomplicated gonorrhea can be treated with a single intramuscular injection of ceftriaxone or a single oral dose of cefixime, ciproflaxin, or ciprofloxacin (U.S. Department of Health and Human Services, 1993). When treating pharyngeal infection, ceftriaxone or ciprofloxacin should be used. The antimicrobials known as quinolones should not be used in adolescents with less than Tanner stage 4 development because of the risk of myalgias. Another concern is the high incidence of coexistent chlamydial infection, which has been documented to occur in up to 45% of those individuals who have gonorrhea. Therefore coverage with antibiotics for chlamydia is also recommended to eradicate the coexistent infection. Treatment failure with this combination regimen is rare. Test of cure after completion of antibiotics is not indicated. A more cost-effective strategy is reexamination in 1 to 2 months after infection to detect either treatment failure or, more often, reinfection (U.S. Department of Health and Human Services, 1993). All sexual contacts should be traced and treated.

Complicated and disseminated infections may require longer antibiotic therapy, and complications are treated appropriately. In all cases of gonorrhea the long-term genitourinary problem in the male and possible occlusion of the fallopian tubes or tubo-ovarian abscesses in the female from untreated or repeated infections can lead to severe debilitation in later life, sterility, or even death. Therefore case finding and early treatment are imperative.

Prevention

Until a genuine prophylaxis against gonorrheal infections is available, preventive efforts must be directed toward finding and treating affected persons, locating and examining contacts of affected persons, and educating young people regarding the facts of the disease and its spread. The use of spermicide-coated latex condoms helps prevent transmission of the infection.

CHLAMYDIAL INFECTION

Chlamydial infection is a major type of STD in adolescents and young adults and is more common than gonorrhea in its incidence, transmission, range of infection sites, and carrier state. Over 4 million infections occur annually. An estimated $2.4 billion is spent annually on the direct and indirect cost of chlamydial illness (U.S. Department of Human Services, 1993). Like gonorrhea, the causative organism is responsible for a variety of disorders, including cervicitis, salpingitis, epididymitis, urethritis, peritonitis, conjunctivitis, pneumonia, and otitis media. However, the main infections are urethritis in males and cervicitis in females.

Pathophysiology

The disease is caused by *Chlamydia trachomatis,* an organism previously thought to be a virus but now know to be bacteria. Like viruses, chlamydiae are intracellular parasites during part of their life cycle. The organisms consist of alternating forms: the extracellular, or elementary, body and the intracellular, or initial, body. The elementary body attaches to the host cell, where it induces active phagocytosis and is ingested in a vesicle that serves as a setting for the next stage of the cycle.

Unlike other phagocytosed organisms, *C. trachomatis* is able to circumvent host cell defenses and become a part of the cell. Within the host cell the elementary body reorganizes into the larger initial body, which uses the cell's synthetic functions and energy sources for its own metabolic needs. It divides to produce microcolonies of chlamydiae. After 18 to 24 hours the initial bodies again reorganize into elementary bodies and exit from the disrupted host cell to infect new cells. The entire process takes about 40 hours, and the result is a slow, steady accumulation of intracellular inclusions that are diagnostic of the infection.

Clinical Manifestations

It is the minority of infected women that will have symptoms. When symptoms do occur, they are commonly vaginal discharge and dysuria (Biro, 1992). As the infection ascends to the endometrium and fallopian tubes, menstrual irregularities and lower abdominal pain may develop. Men also often have asymptomatic infections. Urethral discharge or dysuria are common symptoms for males. Rectal infections are generally asymptomatic; however, symptoms of proctitis may occur.

Diagnostic Evaluation

Diagnosis is cell culture or serologic evidence of infection. Because the staining techniques are insensitive, smears are not useful in the diagnosis of the disease. Development of rapid diagnostic tests for chlamydia allows for rapid, inexpensive diagnosis of this infection when expensive culture techniques are not available (Biro and others, 1994; Stamm and Mardh, 1990). As discussed with the diagnosis of gonorrhea, asymptomatic males can be effectively screened for chlamydial infection by using leukocyte esterase activity in uncentrifuged urine (Werner and Biro, 1991).

Therapeutic Management

The recommended treatment for uncomplicated chlamydial infections is doxycycline, 100 mg b.i.d. for 7 days, or azithromycin, 1 g orally in a single dose. If the adolescent is pregnant, erythromycin base, 500 mg q.i.d. for 7 days, or erythromycin ethylsuccinate, 800 mg q.i.d. for 7 days, is given (U.S. Department of Health and Human Services, 1993). When possible, single-dose therapy is ideal, but the cost may be prohibitive. Treatment of partners is imperative. A test of cure, 3 to 4 days after completion of treatment, is recommended in the adolescent population. Rates of chlamydial infection as high as 11% have been reported at test of cure in inner-city clinics serving adolescents (Smith and others, 1991).

HUMAN PAPILLOMAVIRUS (HPV)

Anogenital warts, caused by the human papillomavirus (HPV), are the most common STD in the United States. There is strong evidence linking HPV to the development of cervical dysplasia and carcinoma (Roye, 1992).

Individuals with HPV are more likely to develop carcinoma in situ; this risk more than doubles if the infection is diagnosed when the individual is less than 25 years old at the time of diagnosis (Mitchell, 1990). The behavioral risk factors for cervical malignancies include early age at first coitus, multiple sex partners, and cigarette smoking. Current smokers are more than two times as likely as other women to have cervical dysplasia (Parazzini and others, 1992).

HPV may present as condyloma acuminatum, subclinical papillomatosis, cervical dysplasia, or cervical cancer. The prevalence of abnormal cervical cytology in adolescence has increased over the last 20 years, from reports as low as 3% in 1977 to as high as 18.4% in 1991 (Roye, 1992). HPV can be found on any part of the male and female genitalia (U.S. Department of Health and Human Services, 1993).

The most visible type is ***condyloma acuminatum,*** a raised, polypoid mass with an irregular fingerlike surface and fissures, commonly described as having a "cauliflower" appearance. In females these warts are most commonly seen on the external genitalia or the vagina, cervix, or rectum. The shaft of the penis is the most common site in males, but warts may also appear on the meatus, anus, and scrotum. The presence of warts on the rectum or anus of males is frequently associated with anal intercourse; anal warts in females can be associated with autoinoculation.

Subclinical genital HPV infection is much more common than the warts that are exophytic (grows outward from surface). The previously common practice of treating areas that give a white appearance after application of acetic acid is no longer recommended. Acetowhitening is not a specific test for HPV. Subclinical infections in the absence of dysplasia are not treated. They will often regress spontaneously without treatment (U.S. Department of Health and Human Services, 1993).

Newer diagnostic techniques allow researchers to detect infection with HPV using DNA viral typing. Over 50 different viral types have been described. No easy method is currently available to predict those infections that will progress to cancer; therefore, all external lesions are treated.

Therapeutic Management

Treatment of external warts on females and males consists of topical applications of chemical agents, such as podophyllin (Podofilox) or trichloracetic acid (TCA). Cryotherapy may be used to treat low-level dysplastic lesions of the cervix. Other therapies include intravaginal and external applications of the antineoplastic drug, 5-fluorouracil; however, its use is limited to extensive and recurrent disease. Laser therapy, used to vaporize extensive lesions, is performed with the patient under general anesthesia and is associated with greater risk. Numerous clinical studies have shown that recurrence rates of at least 25% are present with all treatment modalities (U.S. Department of Health and Human Services, 1993). No studies have determined if the treatment of exophytic warts decreases transmission to partners.

Use of chemical agents requires special instructions. For example, the chemical agent podophyllin needs to be washed off 4 to 6 hours after application in order to prevent absorption of the chemical, which can be neurotoxic. Adolescents who may not follow through with this requirement may not be good candidates for this treatment modality. Teenagers have many questions regarding warts and their potential for causing cervical cancer; therefore education and reassurance are important. Adolescents need careful education regarding the risk for progression to cancer so that they will be compliant with follow-up care, which may be lengthy. The nurse plays an important role in educating the adolescent about the disease process, as well as in providing information regarding procedures and treatments.

HUMAN IMMUNODEFICIENCY VIRUS (HIV) INFECTION AND ACQUIRED IMMUNODEFICIENCY SYNDROME (AIDS)

Health professionals caring for teenagers express growing concern regarding the transmission of HIV and the development of AIDS among specific subgroups of adolescents. Presently, AIDS is considered to be universally fatal. Transmission of the virus takes place through sharing of body fluids infected with HIV. Major mechanisms of transmission for adolescents are through exchange of sexual fluids (semen, vaginal fluid, menstrual fluid, and blood) and receipt of blood or blood products infected with HIV (intravenous drug users [IVDUs] sharing unclean needles).

The reason for concern about HIV in teenagers is related to several factors. The trend toward younger age at first sexual intercourse and later age at first marriage provides a longer period when adolescents may be exposed to HIV and other STDs (Schwartz and Gillmore, 1990). Sexual partners of female adolescents are often several years older and may have already been infected. Since 1992 HIV infection has been the number one cause of death among men ages 25 to 44 (U.S. Department of Health and Human Services, 1993). The known high prevalence rates of other STDs and pregnancy among adolescents document that adolescents are sexually active without taking precautions to protect themselves against STDs. Although AIDS diagnoses among homosexual and bisexual men and among IV drug users are projected to reach a plateau during 1994, the number of AIDS diagnoses among persons whose HIV infection is attributed to heterosexual transmission of HIV is likely to increase through 1994 (Karon and others, 1992).

A long latency period between infection and the development of clinical AIDS has been demonstrated (average duration, 7 years). Since the greatest number of reported AIDS cases occur among young adults in their twenties, it can be inferred that many of these infections were acquired in adolescence. Adolescents infected with the virus can continue to spread the infection without knowing they have the disease (Hein, 1990).

DEGREES OF HIV RISK AND INTERVENTIONS AMONG ADOLESCENTS

CATEGORY 1

Teenagers who are currently not at risk for AIDS because of current life-style or absence of virus within their sphere of activities; very young, virginal; have received no transfusions; are not IV substance abusers

Issues:

- Worried but healthy; need to learn how to live in atmosphere of concern and maintain appropriate level of concern without undue anxiety; need help to differentiate between myths and facts
- Need for information on casual contacts; encourage to engage in activities that do not place them at risk
- Support decision making about sexual activities

CATEGORY 2

Sexually active teenagers who have not yet been exposed to HIV

Issues:

- Knowing (or not being able to "know") their partners
- Reconsider patterns of sexual behavior
- Use of contraceptives in general and condoms in particular

CATEGORY 3

Teenagers at risk for HIV acquisition because of exposure to infected individuals (IV drug users, sex partners of IV drug users, homosexuals or bisexuals, sex partners of homosexuals or bisexuals)

Issues:

- Decisions about HIV testing
- Knowledge of serostatus of partner(s)
- Need for barrier methods of contraception
- Reconsideration of patterns of sexual behavior
- Decision about continuing pregnancy
- Need for services geared to adolescent age-group for crisis intervention and follow-up of HIV-infected teenagers and partners

Modified from Hein K: Commentary on adolescent acquired immunodeficiency syndrome: the next wave of the human immunodeficiency virus epidemic? *J Pediatr* 114:144-149, 1989.

Degrees of risk have been identified for adolescents in relation to AIDS, with specific recommendations for education and intervention (see box at left; see also Acquired Immunodeficiency Syndrome, Chapter 35).

HEPATITIS B VIRUS (HBV)

Hepatitis B virus (HBV) is an infection of the liver that affects 300,000 persons annually, 10,000 of whom require hospitalization (see Chapter 33). Major concerns have been voiced because of the increased rate of infection, particularly among high-risk populations: IV drug users, sexual partners of HBV-infected individuals, homosexual males, and infants of HBV-infected pregnant women. It is estimated that infants whose mothers are positive for HBV will have a 70% to 90% chance of becoming infected, and nearly all of these infants will develop chronic HBV carrier status. Another area of concern is transmission of HBV through contaminated body fluids to health care workers.

Many potential negative outcomes can be avoided with primary prevention, adequately achieved through immunization. Currently immunization of all infants and adolescents is recommended. The immunization consists of a series of three injections. The goal is to target noninfected infants and adolescents before the onset of high-risk behaviors (see Immunizations, Chapter 12).

OTHER SEXUALLY TRANSMITTED GENITAL LESIONS

Many sores or lesions that appear on the genitals are the result of STDs. Experienced clinicians can correctly diagnose these lesions by visual examination only 60% of the time. A complete health history, physical examination, and appropriate diagnostic cultures are needed to determine the causative factors. Nurses who interact with adolescents

TABLE 20-3 Genital Lesions in Adolescents

DISEASE	MANIFESTATIONS	THERAPY	NURSING CONSIDERATIONS
Herpes simplex type 2	Prodrome: intense burning or itching at site of outbreak; often flulike symptoms Enlarged inguinal lymph nodes First lesions: clear, raised vesicles, very painful Recurrent lesions resolve more quickly and are less painful	Acyclovir (oral) Shortens clinical course in first episode Prophylaxis decreases recurrence rate	Immunocompromised patient at risk for overwhelming infection Sex partner only treated if lesion present Infection can be transmitted to infant during birth Adolescent needs education and support Increased risk for HIV with open lesion
Primary syphilis	Chancre: a hard, nontender, red, sharply defined lesion with indurated base, raised border, eroded surface, and scanty yellow discharge	Penicillin	Affected person more infectious during first year of disease May be transmitted to fetus Partner treatment necessary Increased risk for HIV with open lesion
Molluscum (viral)	Solitary clusters of raised, pearly white, firm, nontender papules Umbilicated dimpled lesions	Excision and expression of core material Cryotherapy	No known complications Sex partner only treated if lesions present

are in a primary position to obtain a health history and refer any sexually active adolescent for appropriate evaluation. Follow-up health education regarding any treatment regimen and prevention strategies is a major nursing role. Since many of the lesions are viral in nature, the nurse can assist the adolescent with communication techniques to inform future sexual partners about the potential for infection with the STD. A summary of the most common genital lesions seen in adolescents is outlined in Table 20-3.

NURSING CONSIDERATIONS

Nursing responsibilities encompass all aspects of STD education, prevention, and treatment. Primary prevention by avoiding exposure is the least expensive and most effective approach. The nurse can play a role in offering this education to children before they initiate sexual intercourse. The sexuality education of young people should include information about these diseases, such as their symptoms or lack of symptoms and treatment, as well as information dispelling the myths associated with their mode of transmission. These diseases are not contracted from toilet seats, drinking glasses, or bath towels. Most teens are uninformed or misinformed about these diseases. Helping to promote the inclusion of STD information and information on access to care in school sexuality education programs is an important function of the nurse. No matter what their area of practice, nurses are in a position to disseminate information, identify probable cases of STDs, and refer these cases for treatment.

The increasing incidence of STDs in young people is influenced to a great extent by the larger numbers of teens who engage in sexual activity at younger ages and with more partners. In addition, the changing pattern of contraceptive use is a contributing factor to more risky sexual activity. The hormonal contraceptive methods provide no protection against STDs. Unfortunately, many girls using these methods mistakenly believe they are also protected against STDs. To decrease the likelihood of infection, sexually active adolescents should be encouraged to always use a condom.

Essential measures for control of the disease include treating the disease, reporting it promptly, and tracking and treating contacts. When working with adolescents, nurses need highly developed interviewing skills and a nonjudgmental approach to elicit an accurate sexual history. Several characteristics of teenagers influence the way health professionals address specific issues related to STDs. Teenagers are often concrete thinkers, which affects the way they process information. Teenagers also have limited coping mechanisms to draw on to assist in dealing with such information. To gain the adolescent's cooperation, the nurse must convey acceptance, gain the adolescent's trust, and assure the adolescent of confidentiality.

KEY POINTS

- Adolescent health-seeking behaviors center on skin problems, abdominal discomfort, menstrual symptoms, and anxieties about physical development and sexual changes.
- Acne is prevalent in the adolescent years; medication and hygiene are the treatments of choice.
- The most frequent problems related to the male reproductive system are infections, scrotal conditions, and gynecomastia.
- The most frequent problems of the female reproductive system involve menstruation: delays, irregularities, discomfort, and infections.
- Adolescent pregnancy has profound social, educational, psychologic, and economic ramifications. The pregnancy necessitates special attention to nutrition, as well as psychologic and emotional support for the mother and father.
- Abortion as an alternative to birth is a highly controversial issue; there is evidence that it has no long-term psychologic sequelae for most women.
- Contraception is often not used because of lack of information, anxiety regarding use, conflict over sexual activity, and desire for pregnancy.
- Rape is a serious problem among adolescents; common forms are rape by a stranger, rape by a nonstranger, and incest.
- Sexually transmitted diseases are the most frequently occurring infectious diseases and a major cause of adolescent morbidity. Human immunodeficiency virus (HIV) infection is an increasingly important adolescent health problem.

REFERENCES

ACOG Committee on Adolescent Health Care: Adolescent acquaintance rape, *Int J Gynecol Obstet* 42:209-211, 1993.

Allen SS, McBride CM, Pirie PL: The shortened premenstrual assessment form, *J Reprod Med* 36:769-772, 1991.

Ambriel B, Lewis C: Social policy of adolescent abortion, *Child Youth Fam Serv Qu* 15:5-9, 1992.

American Academy of Pediatrics, Committee on Adolescents: Confidentiality in adolescent health care, *Pediatrics* 89:124-126, 1991.

American Academy of Pediatrics, Committee on Adolescents: Counseling the adolescent about pregnancy options, *Pediatrics* 83:135-137, 1989.

American Academy of Pediatrics, Committee on Drugs: Retinoid therapy for severe dermatological disorders, *Pediatrics* 90:119-120, 1992.

Atton AV, Tunnessen WW Jr: Acne update: help your patients help themselves, *Contemp Pediatr* 5(10):18-50, 1988.

Beach RK: Menstrual cramps need not be a curse, *Contemp Pediatr* 6(10):41-72, 1988.

Bikowski J: Effectively treating acne vulgaris, *Phys Sports Med* 20:100-107, 1992.

Biro FM: Adolescents and sexually transmitted diseases, *Matern Child Health Tech Bull,* Aug 1992.

Biro FM and others: Hormonal studies and physical maturation in adolescent gynecomastia, *J Pediatr* 116:450-455, 1990.

Biro FM and others: A comparison of diagnostic methods in adolescent girls with and without symptoms of chlamydia urogenital infection, *Pediatrics* 93:476-480, 1994.

Brown RT and others: Pharyngeal gonorrhea screening in adolescents: is it necessary? *Pediatrics* 84:623-625, 1989.

Browne A: Violence against women by male partners: prevalence and outcomes, and policy implications, *Am Psychol* 48:1077-1087, 1993.

Burgess AW: *The sexual victimization of adolescents,* DHHS Pub No (ADM) 858-1382, Washington, DC, 1985, US Government Printing Office.

Cates W, Rolfs RT, Aral SO: Sexually transmitted diseases, pelvic inflammatory disease and infertility: an epidemiological report, *Epidemiol Rev* 12:199-220, 1990.

Centers for Disease Control and Prevention: Update: mortality attributable to HIV infection among persons aged 25-44 years—United States, 1991 and 1992, *MMWR* 42(45)869-872, 1993.

Cheng TL and others: Confidentiality in health care: a survey of knowledge, perceptions, and attitudes among high school students, *JAMA* 269:1404-1407, 1993.

Children's Defense Fund: *Adolescent pregnancy: an anatomy of a social problem in search of comprehensive solutions,* Washington, DC, 1987, Adolescent Pregnancy Prevention Clearinghouse.

Coll CT, Oh W: The social ecology and early parenting of caucasian American mothers, *Child Dev* 58:955-963, 1987.

Crosby MC, English A: Mandatory parental involvement and judicial bypass laws: do they promote adolescent health? *J Adolesc Health* 12:143-147, 1991.

Davis S: Pregnancy in adolescents, *Pediatr Clin North Am* 36(89):665-680, 1989.

Davison DA: Trends in use of oral contraceptives, *Fam Plann Perspect* 22:169, 1990.

East PL, Matthews KL, Felice ME: Qualities of adolescent mothers' parenting, *J Adolesc Health* 15:163-168, 1994.

Erickson PI, Rapkin AJ: Unwanted sexual experiences among middle and high school youth, *J Adolesc Health* 12:319-325, 1991.

Fielding JE, Williams CA: Adolescent pregnancy in the United States: a review and recommendation for clinicians and research needs, *Am J Prev Med* 7:47-52, 1991.

Fisher WA: All together now, an integrated approach to preventing adolescent pregnancy and STD/HIV infection, *Siecus Rep* 18:23-35, 1990.

Flanagan PJ and others: Common behaviors of infants of teen mothers, *J Adolesc Health* 15:169-175, 1994.

Fleming BW and others: Assessing and promoting positive parenting in adolescent mothers, *Matern Child Nurs* 18:32-37, 1993.

Food and Nutrition Board: *Recommended dietary allowances,* Washington, DC, 1989, National Academy of Sciences—National Research Council.

Forrest JD, Kalser L: Question of balance: issues emerging from introduction of the hormonal implant, *Fam Plann Perspect* 25:127-132, 1993.

Frank PI and others: The effect of induced abortion on subsequent pregnancy outcomes, *Br J Obstet Gynecol* 98:1015-1024, 1991.

Furstenberg FF, Brooks-Gunn J, Morgan SP: Adolescent mothers and their children in later life, *Fam Plann Perspect* 19:142-151, 1987.

Gillmore MR and others: Substance use and other factors associated with risky sexual behavior among pregnant adolescents, *Fam Plann Perspect* 24:255-262, 1992.

Goodman LA and others: Male violence against women, *Am Psychol* 48:1054-1058, 1993.

Greenberg J: *Health education: learner centered instructional strategies,* Dubuque, Iowa, 1989, Wm C Brown.

Greene JW: Exercise induced menstrual irregularities, *Compr Ther* 19:116-120, 1993.

Greydanus DE, Shearin RB: *Adolescent sexuality and gynecology,* Philadelphia, 1990, Lea & Febiger.

Hatcher RA and others: *Contraceptive technology:* 1990-1992, New York, 1990, Irvington.

Hein K: Adolescent acquired immunodeficiency syndrome, *Am J Dis Child* 144:46-48, 1990.

Helvacioglu A and others: Premenstrual syndrome and related hormonal changes, *J Reprod Med* 38:864-870, 1993.

Henshaw SK: Induced abortion, a world review, *Fam Plann Perspect* 22:76-89, 1990.

Henshaw SK: The accessibility of abortion services in the United States, *Fam Plann Perspect* 23:246-252, 1991.

Henshaw SK, Kost K: Parental involvement in minors' abortion decisions, *Fam Plann Perspect* 24:196-207, 1992.

Hermann D: The pediatric acute scrotum, *Pediatr Ann* 18:198-204, 1989.

Hernandez JT: Substance abuse among sexually abused adolescents and their families, *J Adolesc Health* 13:658-662, 1992.

Jick SS and others: First trimester topical tretinoin and congenital disorders, *Lancet* 341:1181-1182, 1993.

Joffe A, Radius SM: Self-efficacy and intent to use condoms among entering college freshmen, *J Adolesc Health* 14(4):262-268, 1993.

Johns Hopkins Study of Cervicitis and Adverse Pregnancy Outcome: Association of *Chlamydia trachomatis* and *Mycoplasma hominis* with intrauterine growth retardation and preterm delivery, *Am J Epidemiol* 129:1247-1257, 1989.

Karon JM and others: Projections of the number of persons diagnosed with AIDS and the number of immunosuppressed HIV-infected persons—United States, 1992-1994, *MMWR* 41(RR-18):1-29, 1992.

Kempe RS, Kempe CH: *The common secret: sexual abuse of children and adolescents,* New York, 1984, WH Freeman & Co.

Kinsman SB, Slap GB: Barriers to adolescent prenatal care, *J Adolesc Health* 14:146-154, 1992.

Klein JF, Berry CC, Felice M: The development of a testicular self-examination instructional booklet, *J Adolesc Health Care* 11:235-239, 1990.

Klitsch M: Public abortion views unchanged, *Fam Plann Perspect* 23:148, 1991.

Kochar DM, Penner JD: Developmental effects of isotretinoin and 4 − 0 X 0 = isotretinoin: the role of metabolism in terato-genicity, *Teratology* 36:67-75, 1987.

Koss MP: Rape, *Am Psychol* 48:1062-1069, 1993.

Koss MP, Gidycz CA, Wisniewski N: The scope of rape: incidence and prevalence of sexual aggression and victimization in a national sample of higher education students, *J Consult Clin Psychol* 55:162-170, 1987.

Ku LC, Sonenstein FL, Pleck JH: The association of AIDS education and sex education with sexual behavior and condom use among teenage men, *Fam Plann Perspect* 24:100-196, 1992.

Layton AM, Cunliffe WJ: Phototoxic eruptions due to doxycycline—a dose related phenomenon, *Clin Exp Dermatol* 18:425-427, 1993.

Marsigilio W: Adolescent fathers in the United States: their initial living arrangements, marital experience and educational outcomes, *Fam Plann Perspect* 19:240-251, 1987.

Marsigilio W: Adolescent males' orientation toward paternity and contraception, *Fam Plann Perspect* 25:22-31, 1993.

Marsigilio W: Commitment to social fatherhood: prediction of adolescent males' intentions to live with their child and partner, *J Marriage Fam* 50:427-441, 1988.

McAnarney ER: Young maternal age and adverse neonatal outcome, *Am J Dis Child* 141:1053-1059, 1987.

McAnarney ER, Hendee R: The prevention of adolescent pregnancy, *JAMA* 262:74-77, 1989.

Millstein SG, Adler NE, Irwin CE: Sources of anxiety about pelvic examinations among adolescent females, *Sex Active Teenagers* 2(2):66-72, 1988.

Mitchell H: An update on human papillomavirus infection of the cervix, *Aust Fam Physician* 19(6):887, 890-894, 1990.

Moore KA, Snyder NO: Cognitive attainment among firstborn children of adolescent mothers, *Am Soc Rev* 56:612-618, 1991.

Moore KA, Nord CW, Peterson JL: Nonvoluntary sexual activity among adolescents, *Fam Plann Perspect* 21:110-114, 1989.

Mosher WD: Contraceptive practices in the United States: 1982-1988, *Fam Plann Perspect* 22:198-205, 1990.

Nagar H, Levran R: Impact of active case finding on the diagnosis and therapy of pediatric varicocele, *Gynecol Obstet* 177:3-40, 1993.

Panzarine S and others: Adolescent health care: a challenge for nursing education, *J Nurs Educ* 27:278-280, 1988.

Paradise JE: The medical evaluation of the sexually abused child, *Pediatr Clin North Am* 37:859-862, 1990.

Paradise JE, Grant L: Pelvic inflammatory disease in adolescents, *Pediatr Rev* 13:216-223, 1992.

Parazzini I and others: Risk factors for cervical intraepithelial neoplasia, *Cancer* 69:2276-2282, 1992.

Parrot A: Acquaintance rape among adolescents: identifying risk groups and intervention strategies, *J Soc Work Hum Sex* 8:47-61, 1989.

Plotnick RD: The effects of attitudes on teenage premarital pregnancy and its resolution, *Am Sociol Rev* 57:800-811, 1992.

Pochi PE: The pathogenesis and treatment of acne, *Ann Rev Med* 41:187-198, 1990.

Polaniczky MM, Slap GB: Menstrual disorders in the adolescent: dysmenorrhea and dysfunctional uterine bleeding, *Pediatr Rev* 13:83-87, 1992.

Pope SK and others: Low–birth weight infants born to adolescent mothers, *JAMA* 269:1396-1403, 1993.

Rapkin AJ and others: History of physical and sexual abuse in women with chronic pelvic pain, *Obstet Gynecol* 76:92-96, 1990.

Rausch JL, Parry BL: Treatment of premenstrual mood symptoms, *Psychiatr Clin North Am* 16:829-839, 1993.

Romano P: Vision and eye screening: test twice and refer once, *Pediatr Ann* 19:359-367, 1990.

Rosenfield RL, Barnes RB: Menstrual disorders in adolescence, *Adolesc Endocrinol* 22:491-505, 1993.

Rossignol AM, Bonnlander H: Prevalence and severity of the premenstrual syndrome, *J Reprod Med* 36:131-136, 1991.

Rothman KF, Lucky AW: Acne vulgaris, *Adv Dermatol* 8:347-374, 1993.

Roye CF: Abnormal cervical cytology in adolescents: a literature review, *J Adolesc Health* 13:643-650, 1992.

Russo NF, Zierk KL: Abortion, childbearing, and women's well-being, *Prof Psychol Res Pract* 23:256-261, 1992.

Sawczuk IS and others: Varicoceles' effect on testicular volume in prepubertal and pubertal males, *Urology* 41:466-468, 1993.

Schneck M and others: Low-income pregnant adolescents and their infants: dietary findings and health outcomes, *J Am Diet Assoc* 90:555-558, 1990.

Schwartz P, Gillmore MR: Sociological perspectives on human sexuality. In Holmes KK and others, editors: *STDs,* New York, 1990, McGraw-Hill.

Shafer M, Boyer CB: Psychosocial and behavioral factors associated with risk of STDs, including HIV infection, among urban high school students, *J Pediatr* 119:826-833, 1991.

Shafer MA, Sweet RL: Pelvic inflammatory disease in adolescent females, *Pediatr Clin North Am* 36:513-533, 1989.

Shafer MA and others,: Urinary leukocyte esterase screening test for asymptomatic chlamydial and gonococcal infections in males, *JAMA* 262:2562-2566, 1989.

Shangold M and others: Evaluation and management of menstrual dysfunction in athletes, *JAMA* 263:1665-1669, 1990.

Smith PB and others: Sexually transmitted disease treatment and return for test of cure of adolescents in a family planning clinic, *J Adolesc Health* 12:49-52, 1991.

Smith RP, Heltzel JA: Interrelation of analgesia and uterine activity in women with primary dysmenorrhea, *J Reprod Med* 36:260-264, 1991.

Sonenstein FL, Pleck JH, Ku LC: Sexual activity, condom use and AIDS awareness among adolescent males, *Fam Plann Perspect* 21:152-158, 1989.

Sonenstein FL, Pleck JH, Ku LC: Levels of sexual activity among adolescent males in the United States, *Fam Plann Perspect* 23:162-167, 1991.

Sparks JM: Vaginitis, *J Reprod Med* 36:745-752, 1991.

Sparling PF: Biology of *Neisseria gonorrhoeae.* In Holmes KK and others, editors: *Sexually transmitted diseases,* ed 2, New York, 1990, McGraw-Hill.

Stamm WE, Mardh PA: *Chlamydia trachomatis.* In Holmes KK and others, editors: *Sexually transmitted diseases,* ed 2, New York, 1990, McGraw-Hill.

Stevens-Simon C, McAnarney ER: Adolescent pregnancy: gestational weight gain and maternal and infant outcomes, *Am J Dis Child* 146:1359-1364, 1992.

Stevens-Simon C, McAnarney ER: Skeletal maturity and growth of adolescent mothers: relationship to pregnancy outcome, *J Adolesc Health* 13:428-432, 1993.

Stier DM and others: Are children born to young mothers at increased risk of maltreatment? *Pediatrics* 91:642-648, 1993.

Sundell G, Milson I, Andersch B: Factors influencing the prevalence and severity of dysmenorrhea in young women, *Br J Obstet Gynecol* 97:588-594, 1990.

Theintz GE and others: Evidence for a reduction of growth potential in adolescent female gymnasts, *J Pediatr* 122:306-313, 1993.

Trussell J: Teenage pregnancy in the United States, *Fam Plann Perspect* 20:262-272, 1988.

Trussell J, Grummer-Strawn L: Contraceptive failure of the ovulation method of periodic abstinence, *Fam Plann Perspect* 22:65-75, 1990.

Trussell J and others: Comparative contraceptive efficacy of the female condom and other barrier methods, *Fam Plann Perspect* 26:66-72, 1994.

Tyrer LB, Rothbart B, Anderson K: What every teen should know about contraceptives, *Contemp Pediatr* 6:68-94, 1989.

Upchurch DM, McCarthy J: Adolescent childbearing and high school completion in the 1980's: have things changed? *Fam Plann Perspect* 21:199-202, 1989.

US Department of Health and Human Services: 1993 sexually transmitted diseases treatment guidelines, *MMWR* 42(RR-14):1-102, 1993.

US Department of Health and Human Services: Recommendations for the prevention and management of *Chlamydia trachomatis* infections, *MMWR* 42(RR-12):1-39, 1993.

US Department of Health and Human Services: Update mortality attributable to HIV infection/AIDS among persons aged 25-44 years, United States, 1990 and 1991, *MMWR* 42(45):869-872, 1993.

Van Scott EJ, Yu RJ: Alpha hydroxy acids: procedures for use in clinical practice, *Cutis* 43:222-228, 1989.

Ventura SJ and others: Trends in pregnancies and pregnancy rates, United States, 1980-1988, *Month Vit Stat Rep* 41:1-11, 1992.

Verschoore M and others: Topical retinoids, their uses in dermatology, *Dermatol Clin* 11:107-116, 1993.

Werner MJ, Biro FM: Urinary leukocyte esterase screening for asymptomatic sexually transmitted diseases in adolescent males, *J Adolesc Health* 12:326-328, 1991.

Winter L, Breckenmaker LC: Tailoring family planning services to the special needs of adolescents, *Fam Plann Perspect* 23:24-35, 1991.

Wyatt GE, Guthrie D, Notgrass CM: Differential effects of women's child sexual abuse and subsequent sexual revictimization, *J Cons Clin Psychol* 60:167-173, 1992.

BIBLIOGRAPHY

Adolescent Health Care

Children's Safety Network: *Injury Prevention Professionals, A national directory,* Washington, DC, 1992, National Center for Education in Maternal and Child Health.

Elster A: *AMA guidelines for adolescent preventive services (GAPS): recommendations and rationale,* Baltimore, 1993, Williams & Wilkins.

English A: Treating adolescents: legal and ethical considerations, *Med Clin North Am,* 74:1097-1112, 1990.

Friedman SB, Fisher M, Schonberg SK, editors: *Comprehensive adolescent health care,* St Louis, 1992, Quality Medical.

McAnarney ER and others: *Textbook of adolescent medicine,* Philadelphia, 1992, WB Saunders.

Neinstein LS: *Adolescent health care: a practical guide,* ed 2, Baltimore, 1991, Urban & Schwarzenberg.

Strasburger VC, Brown RT: *Adolescent medicine: a practical guide,* Boston, 1991, Little, Brown.

Acne

Castiglia PT: Acne, *J Pediatr Health Care* 3:259-261, 1989.

Thomson EJ, Cordero JF: The new teratogens: accutane and other vitamin-A analogs, *MCN* 14:244-248, 1989.

Male Reproductive System

Fideleff H and others: Pubertal varicocele: correlation between clinical, Doppler, and hormonal findings, *Fertil Steril* 59:693-695, 1993.

Kursh ED, Resnick MI, editor: *Urology,* Oradell, NJ, 1987, Medical Economic Books.

Neinstein LS and others: Comfort of male adolescents during general and genital examination, *J Pediatr* 115:494-497.

Vaz RM, Best DL, Davis SW: Testicular cancer, *J Adolesc Health Care* 9:474-479, 1988.

Female Reproductive System

Cumming DC, Cumming CE, Kieren DK: Menstrual mythology and sources of information about menstruation, *Am J Obstet Gynecol* 164:472-476, 1991.

Doody KM, Carr BR: Amenorrhea, *Obstet Gynecol Clin North Am* 17:36-387, 1990.

Emans SJ, Goldstein DP: *Pediatric and adolescent gynecology,* Boston, 1990, Little, Brown.

Greydanus DE, Shearin RB: *Adolescent sexuality and gynecology,* Philadelphia, 1990, Lea & Febiger.

Lindow KB: Premenstrual syndrome: family impact and nursing implications, *JOGNN* 20:135-138, 1991.

Mortola JF and others: Diagnosis of premenstrual syndrome by a simple prospective, and reliable instrument: the calender of premenstrual experiences, *Obstet Gynecol* 76:302-307, 1990.

Shawky ZA, Refaie A: Dysfunctional uterine bleeding in adolescent and teenage girls, *Adolesc Pediatr Gynecol* 3:65-69, 1990.

Szydlo VL: Approaching an adolescent about a pelvic exam, *Am J Nurs* 16:1502-1506, 1988.

Sexuality

Cates W: Teenagers and sexual risk taking: the best of times and the worst of times, *J Adolesc Health* 12:84-94, 1991.

Ensminger ME: Sexual activity and problem behaviors among black, urban adolescents, *Child Dev* 61:2032-2046, 1990.

Howard M: *How to help your teenager postpone sexual involvement,* New York, 1989, Continuum.

Phinney VG and others: The relationship between early development and psychosexual behaviors in adolescent females, *Adolescence* 25:321-332, 1990.

Pregnancy

East PL, Matthews KL, Felice ME: Qualities of adolescent mothers' parenting, *J Adolesc Health* 15:163-168, 1994.

Fielding JE, Williams CA: Adolescent pregnancy in the United States: a review and recommendations for clinicians and research needs, *Am J Prev Med* 7:47-52, 1991.

Klerman LV: Adolescent pregnancy and parenting: controversies of the past and lessons for the future, *J Adolesc Health* 14:553-561, 1993.

School TO and others: Weight gain during pregnancy in adolescence: predictive ability of early weight gain, *Obstet Gynecol* 75:948-953, 1990.

Stevens KA, Pavlides C: Individualized prenatal nursing care of pregnant adolescents makes a difference, *JOGNN* 22:521-522, 1989.

Contraception

Berenson AB, Wiemann CM: Patient satisfaction and side effects with levonorgestrel implant use in adolescents 18 years of age or younger, *Pediatrics* 92:257-260, 1993.

Darney PD and others: Sustained-released contraceptives, *Curr Probl Obstet Gynecol Fertil* 13:90-125, 1990.

Dickey RP: *Managing contraceptive pill patients,* Durant, OK, 1993, Essential Medical Information Systems.

Hatcher RA and others: *Contraceptive technology,* rev ed 15, New York, 1990, Irvington.

Shoupe D and others: The significance of bleeding patterns in Norplant implant users, *Obstet Gynecol* 77:256-260, 1991.

Rape

Browne A: Violence against women by male partners, *Am Psychol* 48:1077-1087, 1993.

Corbett K, Gentry CS, Pearson W: Sexual harassment in high school, *Youth Soc* 25:93-103, 1993.

Eaton S: Sexual harassment at an early age: new cases are changing the rules for schools, *Harvard Educat Lett* 9:1-3, 1993.

Goodman LA and others: Male violence against women, *Am Psychol* 48:1054-1058, 1993.

Sexually Transmitted Diseases

Diclemente R: Predictors of HIV-preventive sexual behavior in a high-risk adolescent population: the influence of perceived peer norms and sexual communication on incarcerated adolescents' consistent use of condoms, *J Adolesc Health* 12:385-390, 1991.

Holmes KK and others: *Sexually transmitted diseases,* ed 2, New York, 1990, McGraw-Hill.

Rosenthal SL, Biro FM: A preliminary investigation of the psychological impact of sexually transmitted diseases in adolescent females, *Adolesc Pediatr Gynecol* 4:198-201, 1991.

Sugarman ST and others: Acquired immunodeficiency syndrome and adolescents, *Am J Dis Child* 145:431-436, 1991.

CHAPTER 21

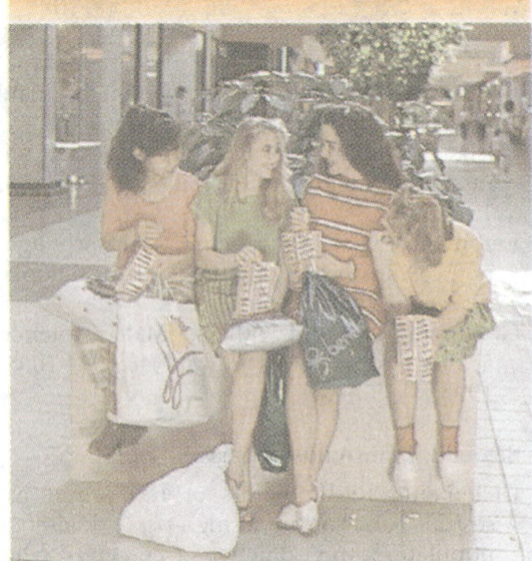

Behavioral Health Problems of Adolescence

CHAPTER OUTLINE

RELATED TOPICS

Childhood depression, Ch. 18
Cocaine exposure, Ch. 10
Communicating with children, Ch. 6
Fetal alcohol syndrome, Ch. 11
Health promotion of the adolescent and family, Ch. 19
Infants of mothers who smoke, Ch. 10
Narcotic-addicted infants, Ch. 10
Nutritional assessment, Ch. 6
Obesity, Ch. 13
Passive smoking, Ch. 32

EATING PROBLEMS/DISORDERS

ADIPOSE TISSUE

A multitude of factors create wide variations in fatness or thinness between individuals of all ages. Fat is contained in connective tissue cells that are usually referred to as adipose tissue; this tissue has a distinct lifetime pattern of development and distribution. Fat is characteristically found in subcutaneous tissues (except those of the eyelids, external ear, nose, scrotum, and backs of hands and feet, which contain very little), in the omentum, and in close relation to some viscera, such as the heart and kidneys. Although it contributes substantially to body weight, whether fat "grows" like other tissues is uncertain. The deposits of fat throughout the body function primarily as a means for storing energy. Therefore it is a labile tissue markedly affected by the nutrition of the individual. Another important role of adipose tissue is the production and regulation of hormones, most notably testosterone and estrogen. Abnormalities in body fat level can have profound effects on the regulation of these hormones, thus affecting menstrual regularity and reproductive capabilities.

Normal fat distribution during childhood follows a definite pattern. Fat first appears in the subcutaneous tissues of the fetus at approximately the sixth month of prenatal life. There is a rapid accumulation from the seventh month through the first 6 postnatal months, and the amount of subcutaneous fat present in the newborn correlates with the weight of the infant. However, by the end of the first year the infant who was lean at birth has approximately the same length and muscle mass as infants who were fatter initially. The significance of subcutaneous fat in relation to both the specialized "brown fat" and gestational age is discussed in relation to problems of prematurity and temperature regulation in the newborn (see Chapters 8 and 10).

■ Linda H. Bearinger, RN, MS, PhD, assisted in the revision of this chapter.
■ *Jamie Stang, RD, MPH, revised this section.

After 6 months of age the rate of fat accumulation declines rapidly and then decreases steadily in both sexes until 6 to 8 years of age. All children begin to slim down soon after the first birthday, but the decrease is somewhat less in girls than in boys; thus at any age girls have slightly more fat than boys. From the ages of 6 to 8 years fat again begins to accumulate slowly. It is during this period that obesity may begin in some children. Many children also put on excess fat just before the adolescent growth spurt.

Up until the onset of puberty there is little difference in fat accumulation and distribution in boys and girls. During the adolescent growth spurt the amount of fat in boys decreases sharply (especially in the limbs) and is not reestablished until early adulthood. Boys' increase in body weight and mass is primarily the result of accelerated bone and muscle growth. In many boys a preadolescent period of fat growth, often a source of social concern to both the child and his parents, precedes the general changes of adolescence. In girls the fat accumulation continues but assumes a typical distribution pattern that produces the feminine curves of the mature female.

The amount and distribution of fat also correlate with a genetically controlled body build that appears to be unrelated to caloric intake. In addition, culturally determined diets, amount of exercise, emotions, and numerous other factors that influence caloric consumption are reflected in increased fat deposits. It is now believed that the number of fat cells is established at an early age and that overfeeding during this time may have a significant influence on development of obesity at a later age.

OBESITY

Probably no problem related to adolescence is so apparent to others, is so difficult to treat, and has such long-term effects on psychologic and physical health status as obesity. It is the most common nutritional disturbance of children and one of the most challenging contemporary health problems at all ages. The prevalence of obesity is estimated at 25% to 30% of prepubertal children and from 18% to 25% of adolescents. Although the prevalence of obesity has increased 40% during the past 15 years in both children and adolescents, more rapid increases in prevalence have occurred among black children than among whites (Dietz, 1986). Also, in one study 26% of boys and 57% of girls were found to be at risk for compulsive overeating (Marston and others, 1988). Since adult obesity is associated with increased mortality and morbidity from a variety of complications, both physical and psychologic, the presence of adolescent obesity is a serious condition that deserves the interest and attention of health professionals.

The definition of obesity has always led to some confusion and, at best, is very imprecise. Because there is such variability in height and weight among normal healthy children, it is often difficult to determine the presence or extent of obesity by comparing a set of numbers with a standardized table of weights and heights. This is especially true in adolescence, when there is normally a period of rapid weight gain and linear growth together with varying rates of muscular development.

The greatest amount of confusion is related to the distinction between overweight and obesity. ***Obesity*** is an increase in body weight resulting from an excessive accumulation of fat or simply the state of being too fat. ***Overweight*** refers to the state of weighing more than average for height and body build, which may or may not include an increased amount of fat. It is possible for two children to have the same height and weight and for one to be obese whereas the other is not. This is particularly evident during early adolescence when there are considerable differences in the rates of muscular development. Obesity is easily recognized, although it is difficult to assess its severity, especially in children who are overweight to a lesser degree.

Etiology/Pathophysiology

Obesity results from a caloric intake that consistently exceeds caloric requirements and expenditure and may involve a variety of interrelated influences, including metabolic, hypothalamic, hereditary, social, cultural, and psychologic factors. Birth weight offers no clue in detection and prediction of childhood obesity; obese children do not have higher birth weights than nonobese children. However, there is a high correlation of childhood adiposity with both parental adiposity and children's daytime activity levels (Berkowitz and others, 1985). A brief description of some of the major theories regarding childhood obesity is presented here.

Genetic Factors. The incidence of obese children born to obese parents (80%) is significantly higher than the incidence of obese children born to parents who are thin or of normal weight (14%). Comparison of natural and adopted children shows a positive correlation for weight between children and their natural parents (Strunkard and others, 1986; Van Itallie, 1986). Moreover, studies of identical and fraternal twins reveal an extremely high correlation between identical twins—even identical twins who were reared in different environments—but not fraternal twins.

General body build seems to have some effect on obesity. Children who are inclined toward a rounded body build with soft body contours and larger amounts of subcutaneous fat are somewhat predisposed to the accumulation of fat. Some individuals may inherit a metabolic defect that interferes with the breakdown of fat once it has been stored in adipose tissue. This makes maintaining an ideal weight more difficult than it is for others.

It is almost impossible to distinguish between hereditary and environmental factors, since both may be operative in any situation, especially when other family members are also obese. Family and cultural eating patterns, as well as psychologic factors, play an important role; fat is still considered by many persons to be an indication of good health. The tendency toward obesity is manifested whenever environmental conditions are favorable toward excessive caloric intake, such as an abundance of food; limited access to low-fat foods, such as American Indians on reservations that are geographically isolated; and conditions creating reduced or minimal physical activity, such as excessive television viewing and the availability of automobiles.

Diseases. In less than 5% of cases childhood obesity can be attributed to an underlying disease. Such diseases include hypothyroidism, adrenal hypercorticoidism, hyperinsulinism, and dysfunction or damage to the central nervous system resulting from tumor, injury, infection, or vascular accident. Obesity is a frequent complication of muscular dystrophy, paraplegia, or other chronic illnesses that limit mobility.

Five recognized congenital syndromes have obesity as a feature (Laurence-Moon-Biedl, Prader-Willi, Vasquez, and Alstrom syndromes and pseudohypoparathyroidism). The most common of these is Prader-Willi syndrome, a disorder characterized by hypogonadism, slow intellectual development, short stature, and dysmorphic facial features, including a narrowed bifrontal diameter, almond-shaped eyes, and triangular-shaped mouth. These children are very hypotonic and will go to great lengths to obtain food.

Metabolic and Endocrine Factors. The complex interrelationships between hunger, satiety, the central nervous system, and the metabolism of carbohydrates, fats, and protein continue to be investigated in relation to their role in obesity. Theories advanced in an attempt to explain individual variability in energy requirements include increased metabolic efficiency in obese persons that facilitates fat storage; enhanced adipose tissue triglyceride synthesis; and retarded adipocyte lipolysis facilitating fat retention:

Brown fat theory—Obese people have less heat-producing brown fat than normal persons, and their brown fat works less efficiently. The body's heat production influences food intake. This may explain why some individuals are able to overeat and remain slim.

Adipose cell theory—Adipose tissue is hyperplastic, hypertrophic, or a combination of the two. ***Hyperplastic,*** or ***hypercellular, obesity*** occurs when the number of cells in adipose tissue is increased, producing lifelong and intractable obesity. Hyperplastic obesity is associated with earlier onset. ***Hypertrophic obesity*** is associated with an increase in cell size and therefore is more likely to be responsive to treatment. Obese children have larger cells that stay the same size once they reach a maximum, and their fat cells appear to increase in number during childhood.

Set point theory—Individuals have a programmed level, or set point, for body weight that remains relatively stable during adulthood. With increased caloric intake the metabolic rate increases to burn the excess; when intake is reduced, metabolism decreases to conserve energy.

Sodium (Na)/potassium (K) pump theory—Basal enzyme is used to keep potassium in and sodium out of body cells. Obese persons have less of the required substance and therefore use less energy to maintain equilibrium.

Lipoprotein lipase theory—This enzyme on fat cells is responsible for depositing globules in fat cells. When weight is lost, the body increases production of the enzyme to grasp and store fat. Obese persons are unable to inhibit this process during normal fat intake.

It has also been observed that on the whole, obese children tend to be taller than average with somewhat larger lean body mass. There is some evidence to indicate that growth is accelerated by overnutrition much the same as it is retarded by undernutrition. Consequently, children who are obese in infancy seem to attain relatively greater height than those with later-onset obesity.

Caloric Equilibrium. It is consistently observed that obese children are less active than lean children, but it is uncertain whether the inactivity creates the obesity or whether the obesity is responsible for the inactivity. Obesity in adolescents and children can be caused by overeating, low activity levels, or, in many cases, both factors. Interestingly, the rate of energy expenditure in obese children may be as high as or higher than that of children of average weight and the same stature (height). This is due in part to the increase in lean body tissue that accompanies the increase in body fat during weight gain. Caloric expenditure above and beyond that of children with average weight is required to mobilize excess energy stores and reduce body fat levels. It appears that in childhood, overeating is the dominant feature, whereas in adult life, reduced physical activity with normal intake is more likely to be the rule.

Although the intake of obese persons who are inactive may be lower than that of leaner persons, obese persons eat more at a given sitting and tend to eat more rapidly than nonobese persons. It appears characteristic that obese persons not only exhibit an overwhelming appetite, but also overeat when they are not hungry or have no appetite. They apparently respond to other cues, as well as to the hunger stimulus. It has also been shown that eating habits and frequency of food ingestion may produce alterations in enzyme activities in both adipose cells and muscle cells. Comparison of individuals who consume similar amounts of calories ingested either as one meal (gorging) or intermittently over a period of time (nibbling) shows an increase of body fat in the "gorgers." It appears that lipogenesis is accelerated following "gorging" patterns of food intake as compared with "nibbling" patterns. Obese adolescents are characteristically night eaters and often skip meals, particularly breakfast.

Sociocultural Factors. It is clear that patterns of eating are culturally and socially based. For some, the food preferences of the culture contribute to the development of obesity. Many cultures consider plumpness a sign of health, and some look on obesity as evidence of well-being. In other cultures obesity is a status symbol or an indication of affluence. It is not uncommon for obese children to be a product of families in which large meals are emphasized or children are admonished for leaving any food on their plates. Parents may have an exaggerated concept of the amount of food children should eat and expect them to eat more than they need.

In countries such as the United States and those in Western Europe, there is a marked difference in the prevalence of obesity between upper- and lower-class children, with differences frequently being apparent before 6 years of age. Lower socioeconomic groups have a greater prevalence of obesity, especially in girls. This obese state is established earlier and increases at a more rapid rate.

Psychologic Factors. Psychologic factors also affect

eating patterns, beginning in childhood. In infancy children first experience relief from discomfort through feeding and learn to associate eating with a sense of well-being, security, and the comforting presence of the nurturing person. Soon eating is deeply associated with the feeling of being loved. To the infant, to be fed is to be loved; satiety is security. In addition, the pleasurable oral sensation of sucking provides an additional connection between emotions and early eating behavior. Many parents use food, such as candy and other "treats," as a positive reinforcer for desired behavior, or as a way of compensating for their own feelings of guilt, especially if the child was unintended or, in contrast, is overvalued because of the loss of a previous child. This practice may soon acquire symbolic significance to the extent that the child continues to use food as a reward, a comfort, and a means by which to deal with feelings of depression or hostility.

Many individuals eat when they are not hungry, often as a response to psychologic cues such as boredom, loneliness, sadness, depression, or even tiredness. This is particularly characteristic of overweight individuals and may be an important factor in both the prevention and treatment of obesity. Difficulty in determining feelings of satiety can also lead to weight problems and may compound the factor of eating in response to emotional rather than physical hunger cues.

In some children overweight may be the normal state and may simply represent the upper end of the normal distribution curve. These children are most comfortable when they are well filled out, and they may or may not have emotional problems. Others may begin overeating in response to traumatic or upsetting events in their lives, such as the death of a parent or sibling; separation from a parent; parental divorce; physical, sexual, or emotional abuse; or school failure.

Obesity may be one manifestation of a disturbed way of life. Families of obese children may be socially introverted and may rely on family members for socialization. Television viewing may be the primary source of entertainment. Children may follow the family's social pattern of isolation and may tend to react to frustration with withdrawal or overeating. On school entrance the child may be unprepared for experiences outside the shelter of the family. Consequently, the child may turn to food for solace, which has become a means of coping with traumatic experiences, failure, and disappointment. Once obesity has developed, the family patterns of personal and social interaction tend to perpetuate it.

Obesity in Adolescence

Obesity in adolescence may appear simultaneously with the onset of adolescence, or it may have existed before puberty. Although there may be differences in the psychophysiologic dynamics in its development, the effect of the obesity on the teenager is the same. A great deal has been hypothesized about the psychogenic factors in obesity; however, the psychologic effects of being obese are undoubtedly underestimated. Obesity can be a serious deterrent to the social life of a child and, to an even greater extent, to the social life of a teenager. The common emotional sequelae of obesity in adolescence are poor body image, low self-esteem, social isolation, and feelings of rejection and depression.

Adolescent-onset obesity appears to be closely related to an inability to master the developmental tasks of adolescence; as a result young people regress to the self-satisfying tactic of overeating to compensate. Unfortunately, this mechanism only creates an additional obstacle to achieving developmental goals. The obesity, however, may ward off the pressures engendered by the internal changes of puberty and the outside world. In other words, the obesity becomes the safeguard. As long as they remain fat, adolescents have a vehicle for avoiding this repressed emotional material. They may come to view the obesity as the cause of all their disappointments. Consequently, they avoid taking the steps necessary for maturation. Eating is their means of coping with the normal drives of adolescence and more closely binds them to the family, who provides the food. Thus they become increasingly dependent on food as a means of gratification. This impedes the normal processes of separation and individuation, since they tend to shy away from their peers and become more closely bound to the family. Obesity during adolescence can also be a method of avoiding the issues of sexuality that normally occur during this developmental stage. The excess body fat can serve as a shield from unwanted sexual attention or advances by others. This can occur in childhood as well, usually in response to sexual abuse by others.

Vulnerable Personality. Obesity is most often a symptom in passive-dependent, compliant adolescents who are readily controlled by guilt and shame. They are easily influenced by outside forces (such as parents, peers, and school) that they consider to be more powerful than themselves. When faced with internal or external stress, these adolescents react with helplessness, ambivalence, and a tendency to seek support from someone they see as stronger than themselves, either adult or peer.

There are many psychologic implications in the development and perpetuation of obesity. It may represent aggression directed at the self, an attempt (in younger children) to grow bigger in order to physically deal with a hated person, or a means to bring shame and embarrassment to another (often the mother). Many overweight adolescents use obesity as a means of revenge. However, they easily become a scapegoat for the frustrations and anger of parents and others as a source of embarrassment and shame. A common problem is the ambivalence of parents who like to see their daughters eat but at the same time desire them to have slender figures.

Self-Concept and Obesity. Obese adolescents score higher on depression-measurement tests than thinner teenagers and significantly lower on body-image tests, indicating a less positive or a more impaired body concept. Unlike many disorders, an adolescent's obesity is a matter of general knowledge, continually on display for others to see. Some of the personality characteristics reflecting the psychologic effects of obesity have been likened to those of ethnic and racial minorities who have been subjected to ongoing discrimination. These include passivity, obsessive concern with the self-image, expectation of rejection, and progressive withdrawal. This sets into motion a cyclic pattern wherein adolescents expect rejection, feel awkward and out of place in social situations, isolate themselves from social contacts, and then experience actual rejection. Decreased opportunity for activity outside the home provides increased exposure to food, leading to an increase in obesity.

Obese adolescents, particularly obese girls, most often consider obesity undesirable and intensely dislike their figures and physical characteristics. They are concerned about their obesity, may be extremely self-deprecating, and judge other people in terms of their degree of weight. They may express contempt for fat persons and admiration for thin ones. Stylish, age-appropriate clothing is difficult to find and, when available, is restricted to special shops or departments. Sexual attractiveness is severely impaired or nonexistent; obese adolescents are much less likely to date than their nonobese peers.

There are three major factors that contribute to the development of a disturbed body image:

- Age of onset of the obesity. Body-image disturbances are primarily found in persons who were obese as children and adolescents or as adolescents alone.
- Presence of emotional disturbances or neuroses. A stable personality and a secure childhood appear to prevent body-image distortion, whereas emotional disturbances caused by the effects of a disturbed family will invite the development of a distorted body image.

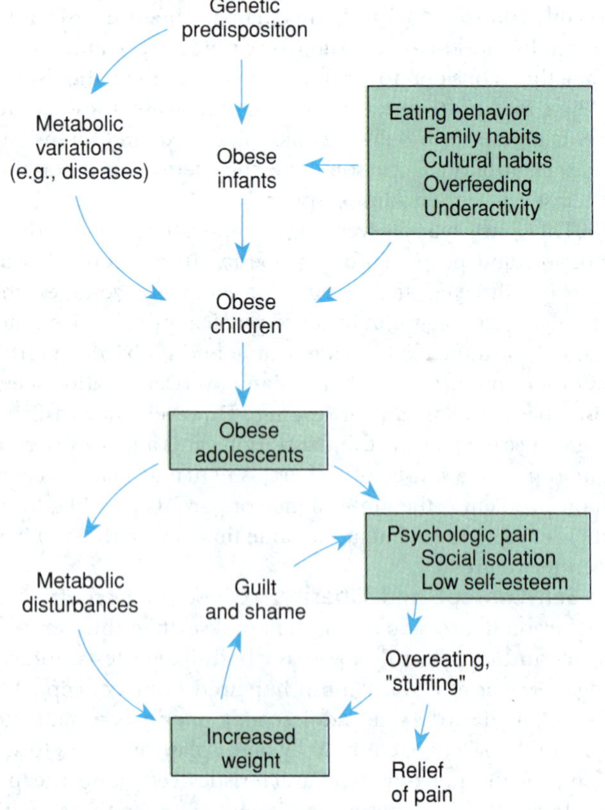

FIG. 21-1 Complex relationships in adolescent obesity.

- A negative evaluation of the obesity by others. The child internalizes the attitudes conveyed by significant others.

During adolescence, when the teen is establishing a sense of identity, derogatory views by peers and parents are incorporated into enduring views of the self. Fig. 21-1 shows interrelated factors that contribute to adolescent obesity. However, obesity does not necessarily imply low self-esteem. One study showed that although obese children had average self-esteem, lean children had higher self-esteem (Kaplan and Wadden, 1986).

Complications of Adolescent Obesity

The most prevalent complication of adolescent obesity is its persistence into adulthood, with remarkable resistance to treatment. The adult with long-standing obesity is subject to the development of associated medical complications that include hypertension, diabetes, coronary heart disease, stroke, and colorectal cancer. In males evidence suggests that obesity during adolescence (independent of current adult weight) significantly increases the risk of the last three conditions after 55 years of age (Must and others, 1992).

The most serious physical effect of severe obesity encountered in childhood is the pickwickian syndrome, named after the Charles Dickens character "Fat Boy Joe," who was continually falling asleep. Although the mechanism is unknown, narcolepsy associated with this obese state is thought to be caused by carbon dioxide narcosis from a decreased ventilatory capacity. There is an increased incidence of certain orthopaedic problems in obese children, especially Legg-Perthes disease and genu valgum (knock-knee). Probably the most destructive complications are the psychosocial problems that affect obese young people as a result of teasing, ridicule, and rejection by peers and family.

Diagnostic Evaluation

A careful history is taken regarding the development of obesity, and a physical examination is carried out to help differentiate simple obesity from increased fat resulting from organic causes. Psychologic assessment, accomplished via interviews with the teen and standardized personality tests, provides insight into personality and emotional problems that contribute to obesity and that might interfere with therapy. Appropriate diagnostic tests rule out suspected metabolic and endocrine disorders.

It is useful to have an estimation of the degree of obesity in order to have some idea of the component of body weight that can be modified. Several tests, both scientific and unscientific, can be employed to assess obesity. The most widely used means for determining obesity is measurement of skinfold thickness with special skinfold calipers. This device, calibrated in millimeters, allows the operator to control the pressure on the skinfold and provides a more precise measurement of its thickness. The Committee on Nutritional Anthropometry of the National Research Council recommends use of the triceps and subscapular areas for skinfold measurements (Chapter 7). The use of skinfold calipers to determine body fat measurements must be viewed with caution, however, since there is a great deal of variation in the estimation of fatness levels taken by health professionals who do not perform these measurements on a frequent basis.

A method of body composition measurement that is being recommended worldwide for use with adolescents is the ***body mass index (BMI),*** which expresses the relationship between height and weight (e.g., kilograms divided by meters squared [kg/m^2]). BMI is easily calculated, or the ratio can be found on BMI charts (Himes and Dietz, 1994). More sophisticated techniques have been developed for quantitating body fat and estimating its regional distribution. These include the ***bioelectric impedance*** method of determining body fat from measures of impedence of electrical current by way of electrodes attached to the arm and leg; ***computed tomography (CT),*** used to estimate subcutaneous and intra-abdominal fat deposition; ***magnetic resonance imaging (MRI),*** which provides clear images of fat deposits compared with tissues containing water and other components; and total-body ***neutron activation,*** which provides an estimation of water and fat, as well as calcium, protein, and other components.

Therapeutic Management

Because of the self-perpetuating nature of obesity, efforts to treat the condition have been universally disappointing. A high proportion of obese children become obese adults. Because most approaches to weight reduction and maintenance suffer from a lack of lasting success, a more effective and sustained approach is a preventive one—early recognition and establishment of control measures before the adolescent reaches an obese state. However, varying degrees of success have been achieved in some highly motivated individuals through weight-reduction techniques, including diet, exercise, behavior modification, and psychologic support.

Diet. Diet modification is essential to any weight-reduction program. The ideal diet regimen for children and adolescents should meet the criteria listed in the box below. Formal calorie-limited diets are difficult to maintain, and long-term maintenance is usually unsuccessful. The adoption of healthier eating habits—including those of increasing fiber and complex carbohydrates, modifying intake of fats (especially saturated fats), and eating only in response to physical hunger cues—can lead to gradual weight control and the development of desirable lifelong dietary habits. Significant caloric restriction, especially for children and adolescents who are still in the growth process, is never recommended (Table 21-1). Restriction of calories and nutrients can cause problems with physical growth and development, including delayed or stunted growth. Caloric restriction diets have been found to be effective for only short periods of time. Long-term weight reduction requires significant life-style changes, including the modification of eating habits and adoption of a more active life-style.

Physical Activity. Some type of regular physical activity is incorporated into a weight-reduction program. In the absence of exercise, both fat and lean body mass are generally lost and weight regained is primarily fat. Significant decreases in percentage of overweight have been observed in children who exercise in conjunction with diet when compared with those on a diet regimen alone (Epstein and others, 1985). For the self-conscious, reluctant teen it is often more effective to begin an exercise program at the time when some loss has been achieved from dieting and the loss has begun to level off somewhat. The teen is less likely to feel unwilling to engage in the activity. Parents should be reassured that tapering off in the rate of loss is not related to diet failure but to altered metabolism that must be balanced by maintaining or increasing activity. Activities should be those that emphasize self-improvement rather than competition.

Behavior Modification. Behavior modification approaches to weight loss are based on the observation that obese individuals have abnormal eating practices that can be altered. The attention is focused not on food but on the social and behavioral aspects surrounding food consumption. This approach has been used primarily with older children and adolescents.

Behavior weight modification programs appear to be more successful when the management includes a problem-solving component. Adolescents who are able to identify problems and determine possible solutions have significantly greater success with weight loss both immediately following the program and at follow-up evaluations (Graves, Meyers, and Clark, 1988).

Drugs. Prescribing appetite-suppressant drugs to children and adolescents is not favored by most practitioners.

ESSENTIALS OF GOOD WEIGHT MANAGEMENT FOR CHILDREN AND ADOLESCENTS

The diet should provide for:
- Weight maintenance or slow weight loss
- Meeting nutrient and energy needs
- Lack of hunger
- Preservation of lean body mass
- Increased physical activity
- Growth

TABLE 21-1 Average Calorie Requirements for Maintenance from Age 5 Years

AGE	BOYS	GIRLS
5	1350	1300
6	1400	1370
7	1600	1450
8	1650	1500
9	1750	1600
10	1800	1700
11	1900	1800
15	2400	2100
18	2500	2200

Data from Merritt RJ and others: Consequences of modified fasting in obese pediatric and adolescent patients. I. Protein-sparing modified fast, *J Pediatr* 96:13-19, 1980.

There is little, if any, convincing evidence that they are more effective than diet and exercise in maintaining long-term weight loss. Probably more important is a concern regarding habituation to amphetamines and similar drugs.

Surgical Techniques. Surgical techniques are available that bypass substantial portions of the intestine or occlude a large segment of the stomach to produce a marked diet restriction and hence weight loss. These shunting techniques are hazardous surgical procedures with many metabolic complications, including severe water and electrolyte depletion, persistent diarrhea, vitamin deficiency, internal herniation, and fatty infiltration and degeneration of the liver. Most nutrition and other health professionals find the use of surgical weight loss techniques to be unwarranted and ineffective in the long term. They should not be considered an easy or cosmetic approach to weight control in children or adolescents.

Nursing Considerations

Nurses are involved in many successful weight-loss programs. Few physicians are able or inclined to devote time to the long-term supportive care needed to maintain the motivation of obese adolescents. Although therapy involves a team approach that includes the nutritionist, nurse, physician, and adolescents and their families, nurses play a key role in the adherence to and maintenance of a promising program of weight reduction. Nurse practitioners are able to evaluate, treat, and follow overweight adolescents. They also assume an important position in recognizing potential weight problems and assisting parents and their adolescents in programs of prevention.

There are several factors related to the adolescent that health professionals must keep in mind when planning treatment for young people. First, weight gain and anabolism are normal and necessary to healthy development during adolescent years. Any weight-reduction program must protect the teenager from prolonged catabolism that may permanently impair growth. Second, energy-absorbing developmental tasks of adolescence are stressful enough in themselves that the psychologic stress of food deprivation may be more than an adolescent can handle.

❖ Assessment

The presence of obesity is obvious from appearance alone, and a gross determination can be made by a rough comparison of height and weight with standard growth charts. Adolescents who are 20% over the normal for their height and weight should be further evaluated. Evaluation includes a height and weight history of the young person, parents, and siblings, as well as eating habits, appetite and hunger patterns, and physical activities. It is useful to have an estimation of the degree of fatness in order to have some idea of the component of body weight that can be modified.

❖ Nursing Diagnoses

Based on a thorough assessment, several nursing diagnoses are identified. The more common diagnoses for the obese adolescent are included in the Nursing Care Plan on pp. 902-903. Others may apply in specific situations.

❖ Planning

The goals for the obese adolescent and the family include the following:

1. Adolescent will modify diet to provide loss of fat content without interfering with growth, normal activity, and psychologic well-being.
2. Adolescent will implement regular physical activity.
3. Adolescent will modify eating behavior.
4. Adolescent and family will receive psychologic support.

❖ Implementation

Reasons behind the desire to lose weight need to be explored with adolescents, but success is rarely achieved unless they are motivated to lose weight and take personal responsibility for dietary habits and physical activity. Teenagers who are forced by parents to seek help are seldom sufficiently motivated, become rebellious of parental nagging, and are unwilling to control dietary intake. A rigid approach or one based on parental enforcement of the regimen is doomed from the start. The strained relationships between parents and teenager are intensified by parental coercion. In addition, because adolescents get food outside the home, adults simply cannot control their food intake. The result may be an angry, sullen, and rebellious teen who gains, rather than loses, weight.

Nutrition Counseling. Adolescents are unusually sensitive to caloric restriction, both physically and psychologically. It is extremely difficult to achieve the ideal reduction in body fat without concurrent loss in lean body mass. Sharp restriction in calories may result in relatively large losses of lean body mass and is not recommended for children or adolescents.

Sometimes the most realistic approach, especially during growth, is simply to prevent an increase in body fat. By limiting calories, children who are still growing will eventually grow into their weight. This can be accomplished by adjusting three aspects of eating: (1) reducing the ***quantity*** eaten by purchasing, preparing, and serving smaller portions; (2) altering the ***quality*** consumed by substituting low-calorie foods for high-calorie foods (especially for snacks); and (3) altering ***situations*** by severing associations between eating and other stimuli, such as eating while watching television (Copeland and Baucom-Copeland, 1981).

The most successful diets are those that use ordinary foods in controlled portions rather than diets that require the avoidance of any specific food. The adolescent and parents are taught how to incorporate favorite foods into their diet and how to select substitutes that are also satisfying. The dieting teen should eat what the rest of the family eats, but less of it. When parents buy and prepare smaller amounts, tempting second helpings and leftovers are eliminated. To maintain a healthy diet, it is necessary to encourage the consumption of high-nutrient foods such as fruits, vegetables, whole grains, and low-fat dairy and protein products. Calories and fat should be kept to a healthy level without being significantly restricted. The family should avoid focusing on the fat or caloric content of foods or meals, since this can cause the child or adolescent to become "fat phobic" or "calorie conscious" to the point of believing that fat and calories are bad and thus trying to avoid all calories or fat.

For most teenagers snacking is an integral part of the daily routine, which makes dieting especially difficult for the obese adolescent. Consequently, adolescents who are serious about dieting should be helped in elimination or judicious selection of snack foods. For example, getting rid of high-calorie junk foods and placing snack foods out of sight help divert attention away from eating. Typically, snacking involves eating a quantity of one type of snack food; therefore substituting several items with lower caloric value for one item higher in calories can be more satisfying and not have the high caloric impact. Foods containing complex carbohydrates are more satisfying than those containing simple sugars.

No adolescent should be encouraged to initiate a reduction diet without a health assessment, evaluation, and counseling. It is also important to emphasize the undesirable nature of fad diets and crash programs that continually appear in various publications. Although some success has been achieved with low-carbohydrate, high-fat diets, their unpalatability and dietary boredom contribute to a high failure rate. Exotic diets have not been successful, and their unbalanced nature makes them potentially dangerous for growing children or adolescents. To be successful from all aspects, a dietary program should be nutritionally sound with sufficient satiety value, produce the desired weight loss, and be accompanied by nutrition education and continued support.

Behavior Modification. Altering eating behavior is essential to weight reduction, especially in maintaining long-term weight control. This approach emphasizes identification and elimination of inappropriate eating habits. Although the long-term effects of this method are still in need of evaluation, it appears to hold promise for the treatment of obesity in adolescents. The behavior modification programs are based on various concepts, primarily those that incorporate the following (Taitz, 1983):

- A description of the behavior to be controlled, such as eating habits
- Attempts to modify and control stimuli governing eating
- Development of eating techniques designed to control speed of eating
- Positive reinforcement for these modifications by a suitable reward system

Some of the techniques used in this approach are listed in the Nursing Care Plan on pp. 902-903.

Group Involvement. Some persons on weight-reduction programs find that the support and mutual reinforcement provided by a group of persons with a similar problem help them adjust to the changes needed for successful accomplishment of their goals, including weight loss. Commercial groups or diet workshops composed primarily of adults may be helpful to a few teenagers, but for most teenagers a group composed of other adolescents is more acceptable and usually more successful. Types of teenage groups include summer camps designed for obese young people and conducted by health professionals, school groups organized and led by a school nurse, and groups associated with special clinics.

Such groups not only are concerned with weight loss, but also emphasize the development of a positive self-image and encouragement of physical activity. Nutrition education and diet planning are essential elements of the group function, but equally important are discussions centered around better grooming and improvement of social skills. Improvement is measured by positive changes in all aspects of endeavor. For most, group support and reinforcement are basic to success.

Family Involvement. There is a definite connection between family environment and interaction and obesity (Huse and others, 1982a, 1982b). Involving the family facilitates weight loss, but the nature and extent of the involvement are related to the age of the child. With adolescents, parents need education in the purposes of the therapeutic measures and their role in management. The family is given nutrition education and is counseled regarding the reinforcement plan, altering the food environment, and maintaining proper attitudes. They can assist in monitoring the teen's eating behavior, food intake, and physical ac-

STAGES OF PROBLEM SOLVING RELATED TO WEIGHT CONTROL

Stage 0: Denial. Adolescents have not identified weight control as a personal problem and consider the obesity a result of causes outside themselves. They describe present and future goals that are incompatible with their present weight (e.g., becoming a model).

Objective of counseling: Help teens realize their responsibility in weight control.

Stage I: Awareness. Adolescents recognize that they have a weight-control problem; they feel guilty, helpless, and responsible and are able to identify inappropriate habits or behaviors causing the problem.

Objective of counseling: Direct energies into close self-examination of current energy-balance behaviors.

Stage II: Alterable causes. Adolescents recognize that weight control is a personal problem. They can identify inappropriate habits and behaviors but have not considered alternatives.

Objective of counseling: Help teens begin to formulate plans of action.

Stage III: Mechanisms. Adolescents understand the relationships of diet, activity, and weight control. They can identify factors in their lives that are responsible for weight gain and could be modified but have not made the behavioral changes needed for weight control.

Objective of counseling: Help adolescents select the most reasonable mechanisms of change in regard to obesity-producing factors identified in stage II and to make only those changes that seem reasonable to them.

Stage IV: Implementation. Adolescents have initiated habit and behavioral changes to control the weight problem. They are able to identify persons or situations that affect their ability to manage weight control. They are able to work through the problem-solving stages and handle new threats.

Objective of counseling: Encourage adolescents to exercise the plan whenever feasible and remind them that successful adoption will probably create new difficulties for which they must be alert.

NURSING CARE PLAN
The Adolescent Who Is Obese

NURSING DIAGNOSIS: Altered nutrition: more than body requirements related to dysfunctional eating patterns, hereditary factors

PATIENT/FAMILY GOAL 1: Will identify eating patterns and behaviors

• **NURSING INTERVENTIONS/*RATIONALES***

Guide adolescent and, at times, family to:
- Keep a record of everything eaten, including:
  - Time eaten
  - Amount eaten
  - Where food was consumed
  - Activity engaged in while eating
  - With whom the food was eaten or if it was eaten alone
  - Feelings at the time food was eaten (e.g., angry, depressed, lonely, elated)
- Identify food stimuli *because this often contributes to obesity*
  - Feelings of hunger
  - Television commercials
  - Smell or sight of food
- Assess eating environments *to determine possible effect on obesity*
  - Where food is eaten
  - With whom food is eaten, or eaten alone
  - Feelings at time of food consumption
  - Activity in which engaged while eating
- Analyze preceding data for patterns of eating and relationships of other factors as a basis for making adjustments

• **EXPECTED OUTCOME**

Adolescent's eating patterns and behaviors become apparent

PATIENT GOAL 2: Will demonstrate how to control food stimuli

• **NURSING INTERVENTIONS/*RATIONALES***

Encourage adolescent to do the following *in order to decrease temptation to overeat:*
- Separate eating from other activities
- Minimize food cues
- Get rid of "junk" food
- Prepare and serve only amounts to be eaten
- Put snacks out of sight
- Avoid purchase of problem foods such as "fast foods"
- Serve food from stove or other place out of reach of the established eating place

• **EXPECTED OUTCOME**

Adolescent demonstrates an understanding of eating patterns and endeavors to alter destructive patterns

PATIENT GOAL 3: Will change eating patterns

• **NURSING INTERVENTIONS/*RATIONALES***

Encourage adolescent to do the following *because changes in eating patterns can lessen risk of overeating:*
- Eat at a specific place reserved just for eating
- Eat orderly meals at regular hours
- Use smaller plates to make amounts of food appear larger
- Eat at slow pace
- Leave a small amount of food on plate
- Eliminate eating during television viewing
- Substitute healthy snacks such as raw vegetables for "junk" food snacks

• **EXPECTED OUTCOME**

Adolescent alters eating behaviors

PATIENT GOAL 4: Will alter activity patterns

• **NURSING INTERVENTIONS/*RATIONALES***

Encourage adolescent to:
- Use activities other than eating to deal with emotional stress, boredom, and fatigue, *since eating at these times often contributes to obesity*
- Engage in hobby activity, take a walk, straighten up room *in order to avoid overeating*
- Become involved in activities away from food

• **EXPECTED OUTCOME**

Adolescent engages in suitable activities according to age and interest

PATIENT GOAL 5: Will eat the prescribed diet

• **NURSING INTERVENTIONS/*RATIONALES***

Assist adolescent with meal planning

Employ strategies outlined above *so that child is more likely to adhere to prescribed diet*

• **EXPECTED OUTCOMES**

Adolescent conforms to prescribed diet plan

Adolescent evidences a steady weight loss (or weight maintenance in a growing child)

NURSING DIAGNOSIS: Activity intolerance related to sedentary life-style, physical bulk

PATIENT GOAL 1: Will increase physical activity

• **NURSING INTERVENTIONS/*RATIONALES***

Assess activity patterns and interests of adolescent

Arrange programmed activity such as running, swimming, cycling, aerobics, or after-school sports

Encourage routine activity such as walking, climbing stairs

Encourage activities that stress self-improvement rather than competition *in order to avoid sense of failure and feelings of rejection*

• **EXPECTED OUTCOME**

Adolescent engages in preferred exercise and activities regularly (specify)

NURSING CARE PLAN
The Adolescent Who Is Obese—cont'd

NURSING DIAGNOSIS: Ineffective individual coping related to little or no exercise, poor nutrition, personal vulnerability

PATIENT GOAL 1: Will receive adequate support

• **NURSING INTERVENTIONS/*RATIONALES***

Implement a school weight-loss program *to encourage attainment of goals*
- Employ a buddy system
- Use peers as sponsors and positive reinforcers
- Employ frequent weigh-ins conducted by involved adult, nurse, teacher, physical education instructor
- Provide reinforcement for weight change
  - Social—praise
  - Tangible—contract that earns simple rewards
- Graph positive weight changes and display graph where others in program can see it
- Provide nutrition education

Have a family member serve as a monitor at home *to help in progress toward goals and to encourage adolescent with positive statements daily*

• **EXPECTED OUTCOME**

Adolescent engages in school-based program (specify)

NURSING DIAGNOSIS: Self-esteem disturbance related to perception of physical appearance, internalization of negative feedback

PATIENT GOAL 1: Will have an opportunity to discuss feelings and concerns

• **NURSING INTERVENTIONS/*RATIONALES***

Encourage child to discuss his or her feelings and concerns *because this can facilitate coping*

Reinforce accomplishments *so that child is not discouraged in attainment of goals*

• **EXPECTED OUTCOMES**

Adolescent expresses feelings and concerns regarding problems

Adolescent maintains a positive attitude toward the weight-loss program

PATIENT GOAL 2: Will recognize ways to improve appearance

• **NURSING INTERVENTIONS/*RATIONALES***

Encourage good grooming, hygiene, and posture *to enhance appearance and promote self-esteem*

Assist with exploring positive aspects of appearance and ways to enhance these aspects

• **EXPECTED OUTCOME**

Adolescent shows measurable efforts to improve appearance (specify)

PATIENT GOAL 3: Will exhibit signs of improved self-esteem

• **NURSING INTERVENTIONS/*RATIONALES***

Relate to adolescent as an important, worthwhile individual *because this encourages development of self-esteem*

Encourage to set small, attainable goals for self

Encourage and support positive thinking (overweight persons are often negative thinkers) *to increase self-esteem*

Encourage in activities *to relieve boredom*

Encourage interaction with peers *because isolation and feelings of rejection may decrease self-esteem*

• **EXPECTED OUTCOMES**

Adolescent sets realistic short-term goals for self-improvement (specify)

Adolescent voices positive attitudes toward self

Adolescent engages in appropriate activities and interactions with peers (specify)

NURSING DIAGNOSIS: Altered family processes related to management of an obese adolescent

PATIENT/FAMILY GOAL 1: Will become involved in adolescent's weight-loss program

• **NURSING INTERVENTIONS/*RATIONALES***

Educate family regarding weight-loss program, including nutrition, relationship of food intake and exercise, psychologic support

Encourage family to:
- Use appropriate reinforcement
- Alter food and eating environment
- Maintain proper attitudes regarding program
- Assist in monitoring eating behavior, food intake, physical activity, weight change
- Eliminate food as a reward, *since this can contribute to obesity*
- Encourage adolescent with positive statements, *in order to increase self-esteem*

• **EXPECTED OUTCOMES**

Family becomes actively involved in adolescent's weight-loss program

Family supports adolescent in attainment of goals

tivity. More success has been achieved when counselors meet with adolescents and their parents separately (Brownell, Kelman, and Strunkard, 1983). Younger children and parents meet together, and parents are counseled alone when the children are very young.

Prognosis. Lifelong eating habits and psychologic problems make weight reduction extremely difficult and the failure rate very high. Some predictions can be made on the basis of experience. Weight reduction is more successful in older adolescents who have lean parents, who have a good academic performance, who have no affective disorder, and who have had no recent stressful life event (such as parents' divorce or a death).

Huse and others (1982a) determined that obese adolescents fit into various attitudinal stages indicating stages of problem solving. These stages of problem solving and their relation to weight control are outlined in the box on p. 901.

Prevention. Unfortunately, weight loss programs do not enjoy the successes of therapeutic interventions for most other disorders. The failure rate is dismally high. Consequently, the best approach is to identify the infant and child at risk and attempt to prevent obesity. Gradual accumulation of adipose tissue during childhood establishes a pattern of eating that is virtually irreversible by the time a child reaches adolescence (Taitz, 1983). Children who are at risk of obesity, or those considered likely to become fat, are worthy of attempts at prevention.

❖ EVALUATION

The effectiveness of nursing interventions is determined by continual reassessment and evaluation of care based on the following observational guidelines and expected outcomes:

1. Assess weight at regular intervals (usually weekly); discuss with adolescent his or her feelings, reactions, and concerns; analyze daily recordings (log) of activities (eating, behavior, exercise) and feelings.
2. Review physical activity program with teen.
3. Review log of eating behaviors; discuss observations with teen.
4. Interview adolescent about plan of care and progress toward short-term goals.

Expected outcomes:
See Nursing Care Plan, pp. 902-903.

ANOREXIA NERVOSA (AN)

AN is an eating disorder characterized by a refusal to maintain a minimally normal body weight (American Psychiatric Association, 1994). The term ***anorexia nervosa*** is an inaccurate description; the disorder is one in which individuals do not lack hunger but deny its existence. Emaciation is the result of self-inflicted starvation. AN occurs predominantly in middle- and upper-class white females between 12 and 35 years of age, and the incidence appears to be 0.5% to 1%. However, young school-age children (grades 3 through 9) admit preoccupation with diet and atypical eating habits (Maloney and others, 1989). Fewer than 10% of persons with AN are males.

Etiology/Pathophysiology

The onset of AN has two peaks: between 12 and 14 and between 16 and 17 years of age (Herzog and Copeland, 1985). Individuals who have this disorder are described as "good girls," perfectionists, academically high achievers, conforming, and conscientious. Typically, they have high energy levels, even when there is marked emaciation. There is a distinct psychologic component, and the diagnosis is based primarily on psychologic and behavioral criteria. Nevertheless, the physical manifestations of AN lend support to possible organic factors in the etiology. A strong extrinsic motive has, for some reason, suppressed the vital function of eating. Because the disorder predominantly involves females, the feminine pronoun is used in the ensuing discussions.

Psychologic Aspects. Dominating the psychologic aspects of AN are a relentless pursuit of thinness and a fear of fatness, which are usually preceded by a period of a year or two of mood disturbances and behavior changes. The weight loss is usually triggered by a traumatic interpersonal conflict, such as the onset of menstruation, that precipitates serious dieting, and this dieting continues out of control. Frequently there is an exaggerated misinterpretation of the normal fat deposition characteristic of the early adolescent period, or someone may comment that the adolescent is putting on weight. The weight loss may be a response to teasing, some change in her life (such as changing schools or going to college), or an incident that requires an independent decision that the teen is unprepared to make (such as a career choice). The association between previous childhood sexual abuse and AN is controversial. According to a review of several studies, the incidence of sexual abuse is no greater in individuals with AN than in the general population. However, sexual abuse should be considered a risk factor for the development of eating disorders (Connors and Morse, 1993).

The current emphasis on slimness is a significant factor contributing to the increasing incidence in this disorder among girls and young women. The standard for beauty is one exemplified by models in advertising. In most cultures, bigness is considered the ideal for men, and smallness is desired for women; and feminine success has long been tied with appearance. Consequently, the pressure to diet and be slim continues relentlessly. Young girls entering the growth phase of puberty when biologic fat accumulation is the normal course of development are particularly vulnerable. However, this standard is not universal. Women in countries where hunger and famine predominate do not consider extreme thinness a sign of beauty.

The syndrome of AN consists of three major areas of disordered psychologic functioning (see box on p. 905). Some current evidence suggests that AN is a symptom of family psychopathology that is not usually apparent until the child has improved. These girls are usually strongly dependent on their parents, and frequently an ambivalent mother-daughter relationship is present. There is often a history of family strife, with the AN being a symptom of the family's problems. Families are usually rigid, overly enmeshed, excessively controlling, and unable to display their feelings, and they have poor skills for resolving conflict (Joffe, 1990).

AREAS OF DISORDERED FUNCTIONING IN ANOREXIA NERVOSA

1. **Disturbed body image and delusional body concept.** The young girl identifies with her emaciation, defending the skeleton-like appearance as normal, actively maintains it, and denies that it is abnormal. She indicates that it is rewarding to achieve and maintain this emaciated state. She is increasingly fearful of weight gain and interprets the concern of others as attempts to make her fat.
2. **Inaccurate and confused perception and interpretation of inner stimuli.** Inaccurate hunger awareness is pronounced. The adolescent does not recognize signs of nutritional need in herself and is unable to assess the amounts of food taken. She may feel "full" after only a few bites and derives pleasure from the refusal of food. A preoccupation and tremendous involvement with food and related activities are associated with this eating behavior; the girl frequently assumes all meal planning and preparation for others. Girls with anorexia nervosa often increase their activity to help counteract the possibility of weight gain. This hyperactivity may continue until emaciation is far advanced.
3. **Paralyzing sense of ineffectiveness that pervades all aspects of daily life.** Teenagers with anorexia nervosa are overwhelmed by a deep sense of ineffectiveness. They are convinced that they only function in response to demands and wishes of others rather than doing as they want or choose. They have always been compliant children, but careful analysis reveals this to be mechanical obedience and overconformity that is not recognized as a reflection of a serious problem—a self-doubt regarding their ability to stand up for themselves or even the right for self-assertion.

Modified from Bruch H: Anorexia nervosa, *Nutr Today* 13(5):14-18, 1978.

Vulnerable girls are model daughters who are afraid to assume adult responsibilities. They usually find it difficult to formulate an identity and feel ineffective in their personal lives even if they appear successful and capable (Joffe, 1990). They usually feel out of control in all aspects of their lives and choose control of food intake to express their autonomy. Any interventions are viewed as an attempt to remove this control.

Organic Etiology. Evidence of organic etiology may implicate abnormalities of hypothalamic-pituitary and end-organ function in individuals with AN. This is based on the observation that secondary amenorrhea is a common finding and that appetite and satiety are hypothalamic functions. Associated symptoms manifested in AN that relate to hypothalamic dysfunction include abnormalities of thermoregulation, water conservation, and secretion of catecholamines.

Clinical Manifestations

The most obvious manifestation of this disorder is the severe and profound weight loss induced by self-imposed starvation. The adolescents identify with this skeleton-like appearance and do not regard it as abnormal or ugly. They attempt to hide their extreme thinness by wearing bulky sweaters and baggy pants, and they tend to overestimate the size of others. Adolescents with AN will often eat small amounts of food or play with food on their plates to give the impression that they are eating adequately and not experiencing disturbances in their eating habits. This can lead friends and family to disregard the possibility of AN. Surprisingly, they can display a marked preoccupation with food—preparing meals for others, talking about food, and hoarding food. Some become obsessed with fasting and engage in frequent strenuous exercise, self-induced vomiting, and/or taking laxatives in an attempt to speed up the weight-loss process.

TABLE 21-2 Some Characteristics of Eating Disorders

FACTORS	ANOREXIA NERVOSA	BULIMIA
Food	Turns away from food to cope	Turns to food to cope
Personality	Introverted Avoids intimacy Negates feminine role	Extroverted Seeks intimacy Aspires to feminine role
Behavior	"Model" child Compulsive/obsessive	Often "acts out" Impulsive
School	High achiever	Variable school performance
Control	Maintains rigid control	Loses control
Body image	Body distortion	Less frequent body distortion
Health	Denies illness	Recognizes illness Fluctuates
Weight	Body weight less than 85% of expected norm	Within 5 to 15 lb of normal body weight
Sexuality	Usually not sexually active	Often sexually active

These young people tend to withdraw from peer relationships and engage in self-imposed social isolation. They are continually striving for perfection, which may be demonstrated in other compulsive behaviors such as stinginess. They are usually overachievers, and their schoolwork is very important to them.

In the wake of the severe weight loss, these girls and young women exhibit physical signs of altered metabolic activity. They develop secondary amenorrhea, bradycardia, lowered body temperature, decreased blood pressure, and cold intolerance. They have dry skin and brittle nails and develop lanugo hair. The changes are usually reversible with adequate weight gain and improved nutritional status (see Table 21-1). Table 21-2 lists the differences between AN and bulimia.

Diagnostic Evaluation

Diagnosis is made on the basis of clinical manifestations and conformity to the criteria established by the American Psychiatric Association (1994) (see box on p. 906).

DIAGNOSTIC CRITERIA FOR ANOREXIA NERVOSA

1. Refusal to maintain body weight at or above a minimally normal weight for age and height (e.g., weight loss leading to maintenance of body weight less than 85% of that expected; or failure to make expected weight gain during period of growth, leading to body weight less than 85% of that expected)
2. Intense fear of gaining weight or becoming fat, even though underweight
3. Disturbance in the way in which one's body weight or shape is experienced, undue influence of body weight or shape on self-evaluation, or denial of the seriousness of the current low body weight
4. In postmenarcheal females, amenorrhea, i.e., the absence of at least three consecutive menstrual cycles. (A woman is considered to have amenorrhea if her periods occur only following hormone, e.g., estrogen administration.)

Specify type:

Restricting type: During the current episode of anorexia nervosa, the person has not regularly engaged in binge-eating or purging behavior (i.e., self-induced vomiting or the misuse of laxatives, diuretics, or enemas).

Binge-eating/purging type: During the current episode of anorexia nervosa, the person has regularly engaged in binge-eating or purging behavior (i.e., self-induced vomiting or the misuse of laxatives, diuretics, or enemas).

From American Psychiatric Association: *Diagnostic and statistical manual of mental disorders*, ed 4 (DSM-IV), Washington, DC, 1994, The Association.

Therapeutic Management

The treatment and management of AN involve three major thrusts: reinstitution of normal nutrition or reversal of the severe state of malnutrition, resolution of disturbed patterns of family interaction, and individual psychotherapy to correct deficits and distortions in psychologic functioning. Because of the psychogenic nature of the disorder, treatment is difficult and lengthy. Because most therapeutic interventions require a team approach, the bulk of management is discussed in relation to nursing considerations.

Nutrition. The initial goal is to treat the life-threatening malnutrition with strict adherence to dietary requirements. It sometimes necessitates intravenous and/or tube feedings, although such methods are usually reserved for severe situations. This is combined with psychotherapy with the family to improve the underlying psychologic misconceptions about the weight loss. Weight gain alone cannot be considered a cure for the disease and is an unreliable sign of progress. Relapses are frequent as the person reverts to previous eating patterns when removed from the therapeutic environment.

An adjunct to therapy is deconditioning by producing a mild euphoria incompatible with maintaining an anxiety about eating. There is a decided relationship between AN and depression. Decreasing the individual's consciousness of and vigilance about eating makes her less anxious and more amenable to other suggestions. Intervention includes the administration of antidepressant or antianxiety agents. However, these drugs must be carefully monitored because of their cardiovascular side effects.

Psychotherapy. Psychotherapy for anorexic adolescents is essential. The patient herself needs to be an active participant in the treatment process and to become aware of the impulses, feelings, and needs originating within herself. It is essential that the patient rely on her own thinking, become more realistic in her self-appraisal, and become capable of living as a self-directed, competent individual who can enjoy what life has to offer and no longer needs to manipulate the body and its functions in this bizarre way. Psychotherapy is aimed at helping the young person resolve the adolescent identity crisis, particularly as it relates to a distorted body image.

Adolescents whose illness can be clearly related to a dysfunctional family situation will need intensive family therapy. Many of those whose therapy plan is implemented in the hospital need a continued behavior modification program after discharge in order to maintain the desired weight.

Prognosis

Complete recovery rates for AN are less than ideal. Only 15% of affected individuals attain full recovery; 50% improve substantially, although they may relapse during times of stress. A few report a more favorable outcome with a small number of patients (Kreipe, Churchill, and Strauss, 1989). The mortality rate for this disorder is approximately 5% and is almost always associated with long-standing symptoms (Comerci, 1988) and such factors as depression, bulimia, and vomiting. Although the changes are often reversible, long-term effects of severe malnutrition may be evident. For many, AN will be a lifelong problem. The prognosis is best for teenagers in whom the disorder is diagnosed at a relatively early age, before abnormal eating patterns and other weight-loss techniques are established and emaciation has set in (Joffe, 1990).

Evidence indicates that patients restored to normal weight still demonstrate a very low self-esteem, are highly sensitive to social interactions, and remain "obsessoid" (Toner, 1986). There is a strong underlying suicidal tendency, and although patients may not be aware of it, the efforts to starve themselves may be a manifestation. This should be explored in psychotherapy.

Nursing Considerations

ASSESSMENT

Because AN is becoming increasingly prevalent in younger age-groups, pediatric nurses should be alert to the possibility of the disorder when weight loss becomes evident during a routine assessment. The health interview and nutritional assessment often provide clues and guidelines for further investigation.

❖ Nursing Diagnoses

Based on a thorough assessment, several nursing diagnoses are identified. The more common diagnoses for the adolescent with AN are included in the Nursing Care Plan on pp. 908-909. Others may apply in specific situations.

❖ Planning

The goals for the adolescent with AN and the family include the following:

1. Adolescent will normalize eating behaviors.
2. Adolescent will develop realistic perceptions of the body and food.
3. Adolescent will develop adaptive ways to cope with the distorted body image and interpersonal relationships.
4. Adolescent and family will receive support and guidance.

❖ Implementation

Nurses need to adopt and maintain a kind, supportive, yet firm manner in managing the care of a teen with AN without creating a passive-dependent attitude in the adolescent. The adolescent requires sustained support and reassurance as she copes with ambivalent feelings related to her own body concept and the desire to see herself as cooperative, reliable, and worthy of the kindness she receives. Encouraging the adolescent with education and activities that strengthen her self-esteem facilitates her resocialization process and social acceptance among her peers.

Diet. Rapid weight gain should be avoided. It can be medically unsafe, and it overwhelms the patient, who feels out of control immediately. Many of the deaths associated with AN occur during rehabilitation as a result of cardiovascular overload. A safe and reasonable target weight is calculated by the practitioner and dietitian—usually to attain 18% fat. Initially the adolescent resists the target weight as "too heavy," but without a target weight she feels out of control and believes people want her to gain weight indefinitely. Establishing a "maintenance weight range" of 1 kg over or under the target weight also helps the adolescent feel in control and teaches how weight is maintained through good dietary habits (e.g., uncontrollable weight gain is not inevitable when an individual consumes a normal diet).

It is also important for nurses to be aware of some of the physical side effects of AN. Patients with AN often limit their fluid intake, which can lead to urinary tract problems. Ketones and proteins are frequently detected in the urine as a result of fat and protein breakdown. Vital sign instability can be severe, including orthostatic hypotension; the heartbeat becomes irregular, and the pulse rate decreases markedly. The bradycardia and hypothermia can result in cardiac arrest.

Behavior Therapy. The behavior modification approach to therapy has both supporters and detractors. Providing privileges or activities for weight gain or positive eating behaviors has had some success, although this approach alone ignores the adolescent's individuality and does not address the conflict precipitating the disorder (Pipes and Trahms, 1993). A clearly defined behavior modification plan is communicated to the young person and maintained through a unified team approach by all persons involved in care.

The team responsible for the management of young people with AN arranges a carefully structured environment. A number of aspects are essential. First, there must be consistency. The team decides on an approach and adheres to it. The plan is structured with reality testing regarding caloric intake and body-image perception as an essential component. The team members provide a unified front to avoid any possibility of manipulation or inconsistency. Second, all members of the team must be involved. The responsibility of the program cannot be left to one person. The role and boundaries of each member are clearly spelled out and understood. Third, it is best to have continuity of team members. If possible, it is helpful to have the same staff persons all the time.

Fourth, communication among team members is essential, including clear communication with the patient regarding what is expected from her. Sometimes the limit-setting needed may seem unreasonable, and if the adolescent does not know the rationale for the limits, she may sabotage the entire program. It is also important to communicate with the family. Fifth, the plan must provide for support of patient, family, and staff. The patient needs positive feedback for accomplishments made in normalizing eating habits and behaviors. Meetings are held to discuss and process feelings and concerns. This includes group meetings of team members, immediate caregivers, and the patient.

All of those involved in therapy must keep in mind the adolescent's distorted sense of body image and self-awareness and her feelings of self-doubt, ineffectiveness,

TABLE 21-3 Behavior Modification Plan for Achieving Weight Gain in Anorexia Nervosa

WEIGHT (LB)*	PRIVILEGE LOST OR GAINED
70	Hospitalize In room; full bed rest No telephone, television, radio, phonograph, and so on No books, schoolwork, or craft materials No visitors
−3	Tube feeding
+¼	Bathroom privileges
+½	May have books, schoolwork, craft materials
+1	May have radio
+1½	May have television
+2	May have brief visit with parents
+2½	May have telephone
+3	May go out of room
+3½	May have friends visit
+5	May go home
−5	Rehospitalize with all restrictions
−8	Reinstitute tube feedings

From Hofmann AD, editor: *Adolescent medicine,* Menlo Park, CA, 1983, Addison-Wesley, p 324.

*Privileges should be accorded at ¼ lb gains in the beginning. Later they may be set at ½ lb intervals. This listing is only an example of one behavior modification approach.

NURSING CARE PLAN
The Adolescent with Anorexia Nervosa

NURSING DIAGNOSIS: Altered nutrition: less than body requirements related to self-starvation

PATIENT GOAL 1: Will consume nourishment adequate for weight gain

- **NURSING INTERVENTIONS/*RATIONALES***

Implement high-calorie diet as prescribed *to ensure nourishment adequate for gradual weight gain*
Explain nutritional plan to adolescent and family *to encourage compliance*
With dietitian and patient select balanced diet with the prescribed incremental increase in calories; *rapid weight gain is avoided because it can cause cardiovascular overload and give child an overwhelming sense of being out of control*
Help patient prepare an eating-habits diary *to assess adequacy of nutrition*

- **EXPECTED OUTCOME**

Adolescent evidences gradual weight gain

PATIENT GOAL 2: Will follow behavior modification plan (if implemented)

- **NURSING INTERVENTIONS/*RATIONALES***

Assure that all members of the health team determine an approach, understand the plan, and adhere to it consistently
Involve all team members, including the patient
Ensure continuity of caregivers (team members)
Provide for clear communication among team members and with the patient *so that patient understands precisely what is expected*
Consult with patient regarding progress
Avoid coercive techniques *because coercion is usually ineffective for long-term success*
Support patient in efforts (e.g., positive feedback for accomplishments)

- **EXPECTED OUTCOME**

Expectations are met consistently (specify)

PATIENT GOAL 3: Will reduce energy expenditure

- **NURSING INTERVENTIONS/*RATIONALES***

Monitor physical activity *to evaluate appropriateness for child's condition*
Supervise selection and performance of activity
Be alert to evidence of secretive exercising *because child may use exercising as a weight loss strategy*

- **EXPECTED OUTCOME**

Adolescent engages in quiet and specified activities

NURSING DIAGNOSIS: Body image disturbance related to altered perception

PATIENT GOAL 1: Will express self in acceptable ways

- **NURSING INTERVENTIONS/*RATIONALES***

Channel need for control and feeling of effectiveness in appropriate directions (rather than control of weight)
Obtain psychiatric referral as indicated *because psychotherapy is essential in treatment*
Encourage patient to monitor own care as appropriate *to provide a sense of control*

- **EXPECTED OUTCOME**

Adolescent expresses self in acceptable ways

PATIENT GOAL 2: Will receive adequate support

- **NURSING INTERVENTIONS/*RATIONALES***

Maintain open communications with adolescent *so that adolescent is able to express feelings and concerns*
Convey an attitude of caring and protection to adolescent
Avoid conveying an attitude of intrusion
Encourage participation in own care *so that adolescent has an appropriate sense of control*

- **EXPECTED OUTCOMES**

Adolescent expresses feelings and concerns
Adolescent becomes actively involved in own care and management

PATIENT GOAL 3: Will receive assistance in altering distorted self-image

- **NURSING INTERVENTIONS/*RATIONALES***

Support psychiatric plan of care *because this is essential in helping adolescent alter distorted self-image*

- **EXPECTED OUTCOMES**

Adolescent receives appropriate psychiatric care
Adolescent displays evidence of developing a positive self-image

NURSING DIAGNOSIS: Ineffective individual coping related to unrealistic perceptions

PATIENT/FAMILY GOAL 1: Will conform to therapeutic program

- **NURSING INTERVENTIONS/*RATIONALES***

Maintain consistency in therapeutic approach selected
Maintain vigilance to detect signs of sabotaging the therapeutic plan, such as self-induced vomiting, laxative or enema use, hoarding food, disposing of food, placing weighted material in clothing for weight-in, *because adolescent may use these methods to prevent weight gain*

NURSING CARE PLAN
The Adolescent with Anorexia Nervosa—cont'd

Provide positive reinforcement for progress
Be alert for signs of depression
Support psychotherapeutic measures
Help arrange for follow-up care *because treatment requires long-term care*

• **EXPECTED OUTCOME**
Adolescent and family conform to therapeutic program (specify behaviors)

NURSING DIAGNOSIS: Family coping: potential for growth related to ambivalent family relationships

PATIENT/FAMILY GOAL 1: Will recognize disturbed pattern of family interaction

• **NURSING INTERVENTIONS/*RATIONALES***
Observe family interaction *for assessment of coping patterns*
Explore feelings and attitudes of family members
Support psychotherapeutic measures for redirecting malfunctioning family processes
Help arrange for referral to individuals and groups that further therapeutic goals

• **EXPECTED OUTCOME**
Family patterns of interaction are recognized and evaluated

PATIENT/FAMILY GOAL 2: Will be prepared for home care

• **NURSING INTERVENTIONS/*RATIONALES***
Make certain both patient and family understand therapeutic plan
Arrange for follow-up care *because treatment needs to be long-term*
Refer to special agencies for additional information and support

• **EXPECTED OUTCOMES**
Family demonstrates an understanding of the etiology of the disorder and conforms to therapeutic program
Family uses resources available

and helplessness that prompt such self-damaging behavior in order to feel in control. The underlying principle in most behavior modification programs is to make conditions extremely uncomfortable and to grant privileges only as a reward for weight gain (Table 21-3). Patients who view the program as coercive and become depressed by this approach seldom maintain weight gain outside the hospital environment.

A ***behavioral contract***, an agreement that the patient makes with the others involved to change a maladaptive behavior, has proved to be effective in some cases. The written contract, constructed by the therapeutic team, is approved and signed by the patient. Unless the patient agrees to its terms, the contract can become the source of a power struggle. However, it can be an effective tool in that it places the responsibility for weight gain or other behavioral change on the patient (Carino and Chmelko, 1983).

Family Support. Family therapy seems to be effective when begun soon after the onset of illness, but it is less successful when the condition has existed for some time. Therapy is directed toward disengagement and redirection of malfunctioning processes in the family, but this usually requires individual psychotherapy for family members.

Nurses, patients, and families can find assistance and information from organizations that provide services for young persons suffering from this disorder. The **American Anorexia/Bulimia Association, Inc. (AABA),*** also provides information, referrals, counseling, programs, and activities aimed at combating eating disorders. The **National Association of Anorexia Nervosa and Associated Disorders, Inc. (ANAD),*** provides counseling, referral, and self-help programs for young people with AN. The **National Eating Disorders Organization**† provides information and support services for both patients and families. Another resource is **Anorexia Nervosa and Related Eating Disorders (ANRED).**‡

Prevention. There are no easy ways to prevent AN. However, public and professional awareness of signs and symptoms can help identify patients early so that treatment can be implemented in order to prevent or reduce the long-term adverse consequences. Some of the early signs of AN are outlined in the box on p. 910. Education about the disorder may help prevent some cases.

❖ EVALUATION

The effectiveness of nursing interventions is determined by continual reassessment and evaluation of care based on the following observational guidelines and expected outcomes:

1. Perform nutritional assessment, measure weight; review diet and nutritional intake (e.g., log); interview adolescent regarding food and eating behaviors; observe eating behaviors.
2. Interview adolescent regarding self-perceptions; observe behavior; confer with psychologist and other members of the health team regarding evidence of progress.

*Regents Hospital, 425 E. 61st St., New York, 10021; (212) 891-8686.

*P.O. Box 7, Highland Park, IL 60035; (708) 831-3438.
†445 E Grandville Rd., Worthington OH 43085; (614) 436-1112.
‡P.O. Box 5102, Eugene, OR 97405; (503) 344-1144.

EARLY SIGNS OF ANOREXIA NERVOSA

The adolescent:

Consumes an inappropriate diet (excessively strict) or may refuse to eat altogether

Develops peculiar eating habits such as toying with food, food "rituals," preparing and forcing food on family members without eating any herself

Engages in excessive exercise, such as compulsive jogging, running up and down stairs, rigorous calisthenics to burn off calories—often to the point of exhaustion

Withdraws from social interaction—starts to spend all her time in her room studying, exercising, or otherwise occupied

Ceases to have menstrual periods after sudden or excessive weight loss—sometimes almost as soon as dieting begins

Takes laxatives, diuretics, or enemas to speed intestinal transit time to lose added weight and empty intestines to flatten abdomen

Vomits deliberately—may go to bathroom after a meal and turn on faucets to avoid being heard

Denies hunger even after eating practically nothing for days or even weeks

Develops a distorted body image—states she "feels fat" as she becomes increasingly thinner

Loses weight—growing girls fail to achieve the 25th percentile on normal growth curves

3. Observe adolescent's behavior and interview young person regarding attitudes, concerns, and behaviors.
4. Interview family and confer with team members regarding progress; observe interpersonal interactions between adolescent and others, especially family members.

Expected outcomes:

See Nursing Care Plan, pp. 908-909.

BULIMIA

Bulimia (from the Greek meaning "ox hunger") refers to an eating disorder, similar to AN, that is characterized by repeated episodes of binge eating followed by inappropriate compensatory behaviors, such as self-induced vomiting; misuse of laxatives, diuretics, or other medications; fasting; or excessive exercise (American Psychiatric Association, 1994). The binge behavior consists of secretive, frenzied consumption of large amounts of high-calorie (or "forbidden") foods during a brief period of time (usually less than 2 hours). The binge is counteracted by a variety of weight control methods (purging), including self-induced vomiting, diuretic and laxative abuse, and rigorous exercise. These binge/purge cycles are followed by self-deprecating thoughts, a depressed mood, and an awareness that the eating pattern is abnormal.

Clinical Manifestations

Bulimia is observed more frequently in older adolescent girls and young women; male bulimics are uncommon. Persons with bulimia have many issues in common with other eating disorders—control being a major issue. Many begin with only occasional binges and purges "just for fun," enjoying the control over their weight while eating amounts of food that would normally produce obesity. As the disease progresses, the frequency of binges increases, the amount of food consumed increases, and the bulemic gradually loses control over the binge/purge cycle. The binge/purge cycle provides relief from feelings of guilt resulting from the enormous amounts of food consumed. The family becomes angry, and the individual with bulimia becomes frightened, frustrated, and increasingly guilt ridden, which only increases the symptoms in the self-destructive cycle.

The frequency of binging can be anywhere from once per week to seven or eight times per day. Because persons with bulimia usually binge on high-calorie foods, especially sweets, ice cream, and pastries, insulin production is stimulated to cope with the added carbohydrates. When the food is vomited, the unused insulin stimulates hunger and the desire to eat. An intake of 20,000 to 30,000 calories per day is not unusual. Bulimia was once thought to occur only in middle- or upper-income strata, but it now appears to occur across all socioeconomic levels.

Therapeutic Management

Therapy is similar to the management of AN. Hospitalization may be required, especially for complications, which are treated symptomatically. Intravenous fluids and potassium replacement are the essential elements of care, and cardiac monitoring is indicated. The integration of medical, psychologic, and nutritional approaches to eating disorders is essential in an effective treatment program. Each of the components provides a unique perspective to the individual, and therapy is often individualized to the person's needs.

Characteristically persons with bulimia are those who have been unsuccessful dieters, have low impulse control, and may have been self-conscious about being overweight in childhood. They may consciously or unconsciously suppress their feelings and have a strong desire to fit into the group.

Individuals with bulimia appear to fall into two categories: (1) those who consume vast quantities of food followed by purging but who, if unable to purge, still consume large amounts and (2) those who restrict their caloric intake, especially when unable to purge. Some bulimic women are of normal or (more often) slightly above normal weight; others become as underweight as individuals with AN. This latter type of bulimia, wherein individuals have a tendency to restrict intake, is also called ***bulimarexia.*** (See Table 21-2 for a comparison of AN and bulimia.)

Complications. Adolescents with bulimia suffer from several medical complications as a result of the frequent vomiting. Loss of fluids and electrolytes can occur very rapidly as in any other disorder characterized by gastrointestinal losses. Potassium depletion causes diminished reflexes, fatigue, and, if severe, possible cardiac arrhythmias. Potassium losses are more likely to occur with diuretic abuse. Laxative abuse can interfere with absorption of fat, protein, and calcium, as well as produce abdominal complaints, such as cramping, and sluggish bowel function.

DIAGNOSTIC CRITERIA FOR BULIMIA NERVOSA

1. Recurrent episodes of binge eating. An episode of binge eating is characterized by both of the following:
   a. Eating, in a discrete period of time (e.g., within any 2-hour period), an amount of food that is definitely larger than most people would eat during a similar period of time and under similar circumstances
   b. A sense of lack of control over eating during the episode (e.g., a feeling that one cannot stop eating or control what or how much one is eating)
2. Recurrent inappropriate compensatory behavior in order to prevent weight gain, such as self-induced vomiting; misuse of laxatives, diuretics, enemas, or other medications; fasting; or excessive exercise.
3. The binge eating and inappropriate compensatory behaviors both occur, on average, at least twice a week for 3 months.
4. Self-evaluation is unduly influenced by body shape and weight.
5. The disturbance does not occur exclusively during episodes of anorexia nervosa.

Specify type:

Purging type: During the current episode of bulimia nervosa, the person has regularly engaged in self-induced vomiting or the misuse of laxatives, diuretics, or enemas.

Nonpurging type: During the current episode of bulimia nervosa, the person has used other inappropriate compensatory behaviors, such as fasting or excessive exercise, but has not regularly engaged in self-induced vomiting or the misuse of laxatives, diuretics, or enemas.

From American Psychiatric Association: *Diagnostic and statistical manual of mental disorders,* ed 4 (DSM-IV), Washington, DC, 1994, The Association.

Vomiting produces a number of serious complications. Irritation from stomach acid causes erosion of tooth enamel and an increase in dental caries. Chronic esophagitis, chronic sore throat, difficulty swallowing, inflammation, and parotitis are frequent findings. Vomiting may be so severe that the patient suffers esophageal tears, hiatal hernia, and spontaneous bleeding in the eye. Anemia is common.

Diagnostic Evaluation

The diagnosis may be first suspected from the presence of complications. Final diagnosis is made on the basis of criteria established by the American Psychiatric Association (1994) (see box above). Distinctive hand lesions have also been observed in bulimic persons. The backs of the hands are often scarred and cut from repeated abrasion of the skin against the maxillary incisors during self-induced vomiting (Williams, Friedman, and Steiner, 1986).

Nursing Considerations

Nursing care is similar to care of the patient with AN. Acute care also involves careful monitoring of fluid and electrolyte alterations and observation for signs of cardiac complications.

"FEAR OF FAT" SYNDROME

Another phenomenon that affects some preteens and teenagers is the fear of becoming fat. In their enthusiasm to avoid becoming overweight, these young people restrict their caloric intake to the degree that they stop growing normally and pubertal changes do not take place. The disorder is distinct from AN in which the patients have a distorted body image. Adolescents who are afraid of obesity worry that overweight will make them physically unattractive, jeopardize their health, and shorten their life spans.

The desire for thinness in these adolescents is often triggered by the normal gain in weight and fat accumulation of adolescent growth and development (Attie and Brooks-Gunn, 1989). Dissatisfaction with their appearance often causes young people to resort to fad diets and severely reduce their intake far below the recommended daily allowances for nutrients. As many as 51% of underweight adolescents described themselves as extremely fearful of being overweight, and 36% were preoccupied with body fat (Moses, Banilivy, and Lifshitz, 1989). Unfortunately, to achieve low-calorie, low-fat diets, teenagers eliminate many basic foods such as milk, cheese, eggs, and meat without replacing them with other nutritious items such as cereal and bread. Their diets are lacking in essential minerals as well, especially zinc, a mineral closely tied to growth and onset of puberty (Lifshitz and Moses, 1988).

Many children worry about their weight long before adolescence, even when there is no reason for concern (Feldman, Feldman, and Goodman, 1988). In one study 45% of children (mean age 9.7 years) expressed a desire to be thinner, and 37% reported dieting in an attempt to lose weight; 10% reported binging, and 1% vomited in order to control weight (Maloney and others, 1989). The media emphasis on thinness and the nationwide emphasis on prevention of obesity may be detrimental to this vulnerable age-group.

Nurses encountering young people who self-impose unwarranted dieting need to focus their approach on education regarding normal body changes and the hazards of dieting. The risks of dieting are more serious than the risks associated with unwanted weight gain.

Although most authorities suggest a weight maintenance program for overweight children during the growth years, there are those who recommend that no child or adolescent in the growth-spurt period be encouraged or counseled to lose weight. Also, research on eating disorders might well focus on children in order to learn how preoccupation with weight begins and why thinness is thought to be so attractive (Feldman, Feldman, and Goodman, 1988).

SUBSTANCE ABUSE*

OVERVIEW

Although experimentation with drugs during adolescence is widespread, the majority of teens do not become high-risk users. National and state-wide surveys (Johnston, Bachman, and O'Malley, 1991, 1992; Blum, McKay, and Resnick,

*William W. Latimer, PhD, revised this section.

1989) indicate that although there is a steady increase in the incidence of adolescents using tobacco, alcohol, and marijuana between the ages of 12 and 18, experimentation with stimulants and inhalants is limited to 1 adolescent in 5, and to less than 1 in 10 with "hard" drugs such as hallucinogens, sedatives, and crack. Adolescents at greatest risk are not the estimated 80% to 90% of high school students who have tried alcohol or the 35% to 45% who have tried marijuana, but rather the estimated 5% who report daily use of alcohol during the past 30 days, and the 1% to 2% who use "hard" drugs regularly.

The etiology of substance abuse is poorly understood. Current research focuses on biopsychosocial risk and protective factors. For the majority of adolescents, experimentation with drugs occurs during a period in which a variety of behaviors are tried on for size and then discarded when the fit is not right. There are a number of theories about pathways leading to the abuse of substances. Although research has identified a variety of risk factors such as the presence of an enzyme (ALDH) that makes decomposition of ethanol in the body possible (Schuckit, 1987), the absence of family connectedness (Resnick, Harris, and Blum, 1993), and difficult temperament (Lerner and Vicary, 1984), no single factor or combination of factors is likely to explain the cause of adolescent substance abuse. The enormous impact of poverty, greater availability of substances, and neighborhood disorganization found in urban centers point to pervasive social-historical factors underlying adolescent substance abuse. Although there is much to learn about what leads an adolescent to abuse substances, most experts agree with a ***diathesis-stress model*** that presumes a biologic predisposition accompanied by psychosocial risk factors.

An adolescent abusing drugs has often adopted the use of substances as a means of coping with feelings of depression, anxiety, restlessness, or chronic feelings of boredom or emptiness. Since denial is often associated with substance abuse, nurses and other health professionals may not be aware of the abuse problem.

Definitions

The greatest area of misinformation and confusion is related to the terms applied to drug use. The most important differences among these terms is the distinction between voluntary and involuntary behavior and between culturally defined and physiologically identified events. ***Drug abuse, misuse,*** and ***addiction*** are culturally defined and are voluntary behaviors. ***Drug tolerance*** and ***physical dependence*** are involuntary behaviors based on physiologic changes. Consequently, an individual can be addicted to a narcotic with or without being physically dependent, whereas a person may be physically dependent on a narcotic without being addicted, such as patients who are experiencing pain.

The broad term "drug abuse," which is often applied to all forms of drug misuse, can be confusing and does not necessarily define the problem related to drug use. Many of the substances are controlled by law and involve severe penalties for their illegal use; others are sanctioned from a legal, social, and medical standpoint. Problems concerning drug use can therefore be defined as follows:

Legal—The drug being taken is strictly controlled by law and is accompanied by severe penalties for its use or possession.

Social—Use of a substance leads to disruptive or bizarre behavior that alienates the user from the rest of society; this results in a social problem.

Medical—Current or continued use of a substance may adversely affect the physical or mental health of an adolescent.

Individual—Focuses on the role that drug use plays in the individual's life and factors that contribute to the individual's need for the drug.

Patterns of Drug Use

Many factors influence the extent to which drugs are used by teenagers. The type of drug used, mode of administration, duration of use, frequency of use, and single or multiple drug use must be considered in determining the severity of the individual drug problem. Most drug use begins with experimentation. The individual may try a drug only once; it may be used occasionally; or it may become an integral part of a drug-centered life-style. Identification of the pattern of drug use in an individual facilitates the formulation of an approach to the problem. Patterns have been observed based on dose and frequency of use.

There are two broad categories of adolescents who use drugs: the ***experimenters*** and the ***compulsive users.*** There is a wide range of use between these groups that represents two ends of a continuum in terms of degree of use. Between the experimenters and compulsive users is a broad range of ***recreational users*** of drugs, principally drugs such as marijuana, cocaine, and alcohol. For many the goal is typically peer acceptance, and these users fit more closely with the experimenting, intermittent users. For others the goal is intoxication, and these users are more nearly like the compulsive users. The groups of greatest concern to health workers are those whose patterns of use involve high doses with the danger of overdose and those compulsive users with the threat of dependence, withdrawal syndromes, and altered life-style.

Types of Drugs Abused

Any drug can be abused, and most are potentially harmful to adolescents still going through formative life experiences. Although rarely considered drugs by society, the chemically active substances most frequently used are the xanthines and theobromines contained in chocolate and in common beverages such as tea, coffee, and colas. Common analgesics (e.g., Darvon Compound, Fiorinal), ethyl alcohol, and nicotine are others that, although recognized as drugs, are sanctioned by society. Any of these can produce mild to moderate euphoric and/or stimulant effects and can lead to physical and psychic dependence.

A great many factors determine personal preferences for gratification. Many drugs are not harmful for all teenagers, and some, used intermittently, will probably not produce ill effects or result in dependence. Reactions vary according to the drug used and its purity, the expectations of the user, and the context in which the drug is used. These factors determine to a great extent whether the experience is viewed as pleasant or unpleasant. The type of drugs used

TABLE 21-4 **Major Drugs Abused by Adolescents**			
CHEMICAL AGENT/ROUTE	**PHYSICAL SIGNS**	**BEHAVIOR**	**COMPLICATIONS**
OPIATES			
Heroin, morphine, methadone—injected subcutaneously or intravenously (IV), intranasal (sniffing), oral	Constricted pupils, respiratory depression, cyanosis Needle marks	Initial euphoria, tranquilization, lethargy, coma	Overdose: coma, respiratory arrest, death Injection site infection, hepatitis, abscesses, septicemia, tetanus, pulmonary complications, AIDS Withdrawal: muscle/stomach cramps, diarrhea, runny nose/eyes, restlessness, seizures, death Dental caries
DEPRESSANTS			
Barbiturates—secobarbital, amobarbital, pentobarbital, amobarbital/secobarbital—oral, IV	Slurred speech, ataxia, slowed reflexes, constricted pupils (barbiturates); dilated pupils (glutethimide)	Short attention span, impaired judgment, combativeness, violence	Overdose: respiratory depression, coma, death Injection site infection, hepatitis, septicemia, AIDS Withdrawal: hyperreflexia, irritability, seizures, death
Nonbarbiturates—methaqualone (Quaalude), ethchlorvynol (Placidyl)—oral	Poor coordination, tremors, ataxia, confusion, slurred speech, hyperreflexia, diplopia, general muscle weakness	Hyperexcitability; euphoria of methaqualone similar to opiate experience	Overdose: delirium and coma, convulsions, hepatic damage, respiratory arrest, death Withdrawal: similar to barbiturates and alcohol
Alcohol (ethanol)—oral	Poor coordination	Impaired judgment and perception, loss of inhibitions, emotional lability, quarrelsomeness, aggressiveness, hostility Lethargy	Hazards related to impaired judgment (e.g., automobile accidents, fights) Nutritional deficiencies Gastritis Overdose: coma, death, especially when used in combination with barbiturates Withdrawal: anxiety, tremors, hallucinations, hyperreflexia, seizures, death
MINOR TRANQUILIZERS			
Chlordiazepoxide (Librium), diazepam (Valium), meprobamate—oral	Nonspecific	Decreased anxiety and tension Occasional disinhibition	Similar to barbiturates but with reduced intensity
ORGANIC SOLVENTS			
Hydrocarbons and fluorocarbons—glue, cleaning fluid, lighter fluid, aerosol sprays, nail polish, gasoline—sniffed	Nonspecific	Euphoria, dysphoria, confusion, impaired perception and coordination Loss of consciousness	Asphyxia from plastic bags used to inhale fumes Lead poisoning Possible irreversible damage to central nervous system, kidneys, liver, and bone marrow
STIMULANTS			
Amphetamines—amphetamine sulfate, dextroamphetamine, methamphetamine—oral, subcutaneous, IV	Hypertension, weight loss, dilated pupils Sweating (when injected)	Psychologic and motor stimulation Hyperactivity, false bravado, euphoria, increased alertness, insomnia, anorexia, irritability, personality change	Injection site infection Paranoia, severe depression with suicidal tendency when drug stopped
Cocaine—intranasal, IV, smoke	Hypertension, tachycardia, hyperreflexia	Restlessness, hyperactivity, intense euphoria	Nausea/vomiting, inflammation/perforation of nasal septum
HALLUCINOGENS			
Cannabis—marijuana, hashish—smoke, oral	Occasionally tachycardia, delayed response time, poor coordination	Simple euphoria, mild intoxication, heightened sensory awareness, drowsiness	Occasionally depressive or anxiety reactions
LSD, PCP, DMT, STP, THC, mescaline—oral	Dilated pupils, reddened eyes, occasionally hypertension, hyperthermia, piloerection	Euphoria, heightened sensory awareness, increased appetite, hallucinations, confusion, paranoia	Primarily psychiatric: may intensify latent psychotic tendencies, panic, suicide possible, flashbacks

also varies according to geographic location, socioeconomic status, urban as opposed to suburban areas, and various historical periods.

A drug that is popular with one "generation" of adolescents may not be attractive to another, and changing trends are influenced by the adolescent's search for new and different experiences. The present concern is the rising use of alcohol, tobacco, cannibus, and hallucingens, as well as cocaine.

Drugs with mind-altering capacity that are available on the black market and that are of medical and legal concern are the hallucinogenic, narcotic, hypnotic, and stimulant drugs. In addition, health professionals are concerned about use of various volatile substances, such as gasoline, antifreeze, model airplane cement, organic solvents, and typewriter correction fluid, that are inhaled to achieve altered sensation in the user. Drugs available on the street are often mixed with other compounds and fillers so that the purity of the drug, its strength, and the nature of additives are highly variable. Many of the hazards associated with drug use are related to driving a car or operating equipment that may be harmful when carelessly used while under the influence of the drug. Some of the more commonly abused substances and their general manifestations are outlined in Table 21-4.

TOBACCO

Two trends have characterized the incidence of cigarette smoking among adolescents during the past 15 years (U.S. Department of Health and Human Services, 1994). Although an alarming number of teens smoke, fewer smoke today as compared with a peak in the mid-1970s. In 1989 the number of seniors who smoked cigarettes daily was one-third less than those smoking in 1976 (Johnston, 1985; Johnston, Bachman, and O'Malley, 1992). The second trend involves an increase in the proportion of girls smoking as compared with boys, leading to slightly higher smoking rates for girls than for boys.

Senior high school students who reported having smoked in the past 30 days ranged from 20% to 30% for boys and from 25% to 35% for girls (Johnston, Bachman, and O'Malley, 1992; Johnston, O'Malley, and Bachman, 1990). Also, approximately 11% of boys and girls reported smoking a half-pack or more daily. Although the number of smokers has declined in recent years, cigarette smoking is still considered to be the chief avoidable cause of death, with smoking leading to an excess mortality of approximately 400,000 people annually in the United States (U.S. Department of Health and Human Services, 1994).

The hazards of smoking at any age are undisputed; however, a preventive approach to teenage smoking is especially important for several reasons. There is a high probability that regular smoking in childhood leads to a lifetime habit with concomitant increases in morbidity and mortality.

Etiology

There are a variety of reasons why teenagers begin smoking in adolescence. The significant factors related to onset of smoking can be categorized as social, sociodemographic, psychosocial, and biologic. Once smoking behavior is established, smoking itself is thought to produce enough reinforcement to sustain the practice without the initial pressure.

Social Factors. Social pressures to smoke include imitation of the smoking behavior and attitudes of parents and other adults, the association of smoking with maturity or "mature" behavior, pressures from peers who view smoking as the popular thing to do, and the use of smoking as an outlet for real or imagined school, social, or home pressures. Other pressures come from advertisements aimed directly at teens.

Parental approval or disapproval of their children's smoking is an important force in predicting teenage smoking. In one study 34% of teenage smokers had smoked at least one cigarette in their homes, implying that smoking was accepted by the parents (Biglan and others, 1984). The social influence of same-sex family members or peers is an important factor, and the number of smokers in the immediate environment increases the probability of subsequent smoking by a youngster. When compared with families where neither parent smoked, twice as many boys and three times as many girls were smokers in families where both parents smoked (Evans, 1984). However, researchers have concluded that children are less likely to develop the smoking habit if someone in the family was a model for quitting. Having an ex-smoker model was influential enough to outweigh previous smoking effects on the child (Peterson and Peterson, 1986).

The social nature of smoking is also significant (Flay and others, 1983), as well as anticipation of enjoyment. However, the influence of friends on beliefs and behavior depends in part on the adolescent's tendencies toward rebelliousness and disobedience (McAlister, Krosnick, and Milburn, 1984).

The mass media have contributed to the incidence of smoking in adolescents. In advertisements smokers are engaged in activities and dressed in clothes suitable for adolescents, and the ads imply that smoking is associated with fun, risk taking, and sexual adventure, as well as a sign of maturity and autonomy (Davis, 1987). The ads also imply an association between smoking and youthful vigor, good health, good looks, and personal, social, and professional acceptance and success. Interest groups organized against smoking have recently attempted to ban the Joe Camel advertising campaign, accusing the cigarette company of deliberately targeting adolescents. To substantiate this argumant, they cite an extraordinary increase in smoking of Camel cigarettes among underage children and teens since the initiation of the Camel ad campaign (U.S. Department of Health and Human Services, 1994). Huang and others (1992) found that teens preferred cigarette advertisements using cartoons over those using human models or cigarette packages and words only. Perhaps even more disturbing is that by age 6 the faces of Mickey Mouse and Joe Camel were equally recognized (Fischer and others, 1991). The authors concluded that children's recognition of the cigarette logo and their positive associations with it may contribute to the onset of smoking during childhood and adolescence. Not surprisingly, DiFranza and others (1991) found that during the first 3 years of the Joe Camel campaign, the proportion of teen smokers preferring Camel cigarrettes over other brands rose from less than 1% to over 30%. Camel has denied the allegations and thus far has refused to modify its advertising. Countries such as the United Kingdom and Norway have banned all tobacco advertising (U.K. Department of Health, 1992; U.S. Department of Health and Human Services, 1994). The American Academy of Pediatrics (1994) recommends banning all forms of tobacco advertisement from print and electronic media.

Sociodemographic Factors. Sociodemographic factors that relate to levels of smoking include socioeconomic status, sex, and performance in school. A consistent, negative association has been observed between socioeconomic status and smoking (especially among boys), and there is a consistent correlation between low academic goals and performance and smoking (cited in Flay and others, 1983). At least 30% of persons who have not proceeded beyond a high school education are smokers, whereas less than 10% of college graduates smoke (Pierce and others, 1989). Rates of smoking are highest among adolescents who do not complete high school (Kandel, Raveis, and Kandel, 1984). Researchers report that students who focus on schoolwork and who have high educational goals for themselves are significantly less likely than their peers to develop a long-term smoking habit (Newcomb, McCarthy, and Bentler, 1989). Smokers have been found to be from families of lower socioeconomic levels and do not participate in school activities. Adolescents who participate in and dominate school activities tend to come from the upper end of the social continuum (Eckert, 1983).

Psychosocial Factors. Although theories explaining relationships between personality and smoking behavior may be suggested, research has been unable to document any significant differences between adolescents who do and those who do not smoke (Gerber and Newman, 1989). For example, although smokers may be anxious, there are enough nonsmoking adolescents experiencing anxiety to rule out this area of potential difference. Personality traits, such as anxiety, have been shown to predict how *much* an adolescent will smoke once having begun the habit, rather than discriminating between smokers and nonsmokers (Evans and others, 1979).

Biologic Factors. Biologic factors serve to both encourage and deter further experimentation of would-be smokers. Initial harshness, nausea, and irritation are sufficient to influence many youngsters not to try smoking again; to others it may represent a challenge to overcome. Smoking has been found to lower endurance by decreasing breathing capacity or ventilatory muscle endurance (Dessendorfer, Amsterdam, and Odland, 1983). Dependence is a result of nicotine, the primary alkaloid in tobacco. Nicotine exerts both stimulating and sedating effects on the central and peripheral nervous systems and on several organ systems. Attempts at stopping the smoking habit are accompanied by severe craving and withdrawal symptoms.

STAGES OF BECOMING A SMOKER

Preparation—Early learning experiences provided in the environment (e.g., parent or sibling smokers in the family)
Initiation—Trying the first cigarette; peer influences are more important than family influences in determining when cigarettes are first tried
Experimentation—Learning to smoke by repeated experimentation: decision to quit or continue
Regular smoking—Smoke sufficiently often to be considered a regular smoker

Data from Leventhal H, Cleary PD: The smoking problem: a review of the research and theory in behavioral risk modification, *J Personality Soc Psychol* 88:370-405, 1981.

Process of Becoming a Smoker

Researchers have identified three stages in the process of becoming a smoker: trying the first cigarette, experimental smoking (less than weekly), and regular smoking (at least weekly) (Flay and others, 1983). Some recognize a preparation or initiation stage in which psychosocial, environmental, and possibly biologic factors prepare certain youngsters to be smokers (see box above).

Smokeless Tobacco

The term ***smokeless tobacco*** refers to tobacco products that are placed in the mouth but not ignited (e.g., snuff and chewing tobacco). This increasingly popular substitute for cigarettes is now posing a serious hazard to children and adolescents, even school-age children, as well as young adults (U.S. Department of Health and Human Services, 1994). Significantly more boys (46%) than girls (4.7%) have tried smokeless tobacco by the twelfth grade. These products have also been proved to be carcinogenic, and regular use has been reported to cause other dental problems, including foul-smelling breath and tooth erosion or loss.

In a 1994 report of the Surgeon General (U.S. Department of Health and Human Services, 1994), two conclusions were drawn concerning the use of smokeless tobacco by adolescents: (1) smokeless tobacco use is associated with early indicators of periodontal degeneration and with lesions in the oral soft tissue, and (2) adolescent smokeless tobacco users are more likely than nonusers to become cigarette smokers.

Nursing Considerations

Prevention of regular smoking in teenagers appears to be the most effective way to reduce the overall incidence of smoking. Early education is one approach, but most school-based or large-scale public information campaigns have had no significant impact on smoking habits. A variety of methods have been employed to deal with the problem. Posters, charts, displays, statistics, and the use of examples of actual damaged lungs to communicate the hazards of smoking all have their supporters and doubters. Although some believe that these are a waste of time, others give evidence that many children are influenced by these "scare tactics." Presentation of films and demonstrations in science classes have proved to be of value in some schools.

For the most part, smoking-prevention programs that focus on negative long-term effects of smoking on health have been uniformly ineffective. Those emphasizing immediate effects and youth-to-youth programs have been somewhat more effective, but primarily in improving the teenagers' attitudes toward smoking (Silvis and Perry, 1987). Because smoking and smoking-related behavior function as key social symbols, antismoking campaigns must be addressed to the norms of the potential smokers, and anything that ridicules or threatens the social norms of the group can be unproductive or counterproductive. Also, investigators have found that teaching resistance to peer pressure to smoke may be effective in early adolescence but loses effectiveness as adolescents mature (Morgan and Grube, 1989). Emphasis on negative consequences of smoking is more likely to be effective with older adolescents.

Two areas of focus are gaining interest among health advocates: peer-led programming and use of media in smoking prevention (i.e., videotapes and films). Peer-led programs emphasizing social consequences of not smoking have proved most successful. If a significant number of influential peers can "sell" their classmates on the idea that the habit is not popular, the followers will imitate their behavior. Short-term rather than long-term consequences are emphasized (e.g., the effects of smoking on personal appearance, such as the unattractive stains on teeth and hands and the unpleasant odor that smoking gives to the breath and clothing).

Smoking bans in schools also accomplish several goals: (1) they discourage students from starting to smoke; (2) they reinforce knowledge of the health hazards of cigarette smoking and exposure to environmental tobacco smoke; and (3) they promote a smoke-free environment as the norm (School policies, 1989).

Nurses in schools and other agencies of the community are in a position to implement and reinforce teaching; to serve as consultants and counselors to student, teacher, and parent groups; and to be advocates in all areas in which antismoking campaigns might be effective. Several strategies are recommended (see box above, right). Information can also be obtained from **Stop Teenage Addiction to Tobacco (STAT),** a national organization devoted to educating the public and professionals.*

RECOMMENDED NONSMOKING STRATEGIES

Provide only a cursory mention of long-term health consequences (e.g., cardiovascular and cancer risks).

Discuss immediate physiologic consequences in some detail (e.g., changes in heart rate and blood pressure, minor respiratory symptoms, and blood carbon monoxide concentrations).

Mention alternatives to smoking for establishing a self-image that appears tough, independent, mature, or sophisticated (e.g., establishing a weight-lifting regimen, jogging and dancing, joining a Boys' Club or a Girls' Club, engaging in volunteer work for a hospital or political or religious group).

Mention the negative effects of smoking (e.g., earlier wrinkling of skin, yellow stains on teeth and fingers, tobacco odor on breath and clothing).

Mention the increasing ostracism of smokers by nonsmokers, both legal and informal, in places of work and public places.

Mention the increasing evidence that second-hand smoke is injurious to the health of nonsmokers who are regularly exposed, especially small children.

Acknowledge that many adults once believed that important social benefits were associated with smoking, but point out that the vast majority of adult smokers would now quit smoking if they could.

Arm the cooperative adolescent with arguments for dealing with peer pressure (e.g., by not smoking, a teenager demonstrates independence and nonconformity, traits normally prized by youth).

Request posters and pamphlets from local voluntary agencies (e.g., American Cancer Society, American Heart Association, and American Lung Association) to display prominently.

Modified from Wong-McCarthy WJ, Gritz ER: Preventing regular teenage cigarette smoking, *Pediatr Ann* 11:683-689, 1982.

ALCOHOL

Acute or chronic abuse of alcohol (ethanol), a socially accepted depressant, is responsible for many acts of violence, suicide, and accidental injury and death. Ethanol reduces inhibitions against aggressive and sexual acting out. Abrupt withdrawal is accompanied by severe physical and psychologic symptoms, and long-term use leads to slow tissue destruction, especially of the brain and liver cells.

Teenage drinking is not a new phenomenon, but because of its social acceptance, peer pressure, and easy accessibility, alcohol appears to have become the drug of choice. It is the most widely accepted drug, can be purchased legally by adults, is relatively inexpensive, is often used as part of a meal (wine, beer), and is approved by adults throughout the world when used in moderation. Young people may be afraid of hard drugs, but they feel comfortable with alcohol. Most have been exposed to alcohol all their lives.

Although there are racial, ethnic, and gender differences, the pattern of frequent, heavy drinking is likely to begin in the middle school years. Drinking increases with age and peaks between 18 and 22 years of age. Some surveys indicate that 11% of eighth graders consume the equivalent of 5.6 oz of absolute alcohol per week, and twelfth grade students have reported averaging two six-packs of beer per week, often consumed at one or two parties (Schwartz and others, 1986). The majority of teenagers in one study reported high self-esteem, good health, and few psychologic problems, and 63% reported having drunk alcohol at some time. The proportion of adolescents who report that they never drink alcohol becomes progressively smaller as teens get older (Schwartz and others, 1986).

Although the majority of adolescents who experiment with alcohol are not heavy users, social drinking remains a

*511 E. Columbus Ave., Springfield, MA 01105; (413) 732-STAT.

great concern primarily because of the disturbing rates of morbidity and mortality related to drunken driving. Alcohol is present in more than half of all fatal automobile crashes involving teens. In addition, approximately 10% of all fatal crashes involve adolescent drunken drivers.

The most noticeable effects of alcohol are on the central nervous system; these include changes in emotional and autonomic functions, such as judgment, memory, learning ability, and other intellectual capacities. Marked mood changes are characteristic of adolescent drinkers, who are described as hard to live with and unable to make up their minds. They can be identified by the way in which they use alcohol. Adolescent alcoholics often drink alone, cannot predictably control their use of alcohol, and protect their supply, afraid that they will be caught without anything to drink.

Teenage alcoholics often rely on alcohol as a defense against depression, anxiety, fear, and anger. They become increasingly tolerant to the drug, and there is an increased use of sedatives with alcohol. Some alcoholics have difficulty remembering things done while intoxicated and often intend to swear off the drug or cut down on its use. Not all of these characteristics are observed in the alcoholic, but if several of the signs are evident, individuals should be considered at risk and detoxification therapy should be initiated.

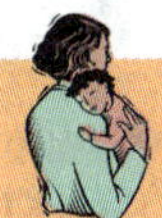

FAMILY FOCUS

Adolescent Alcohol Abuse

The two primary tasks of parenting an adolescent are to provide nurturing and to set appropriate limits (Nichols, 1987). Research on families with alcohol-abusing adolescents reveals serious deficiencies in one or both of these areas. A common health provider trap, however, given research findings and the sometimes implicit assumptions of practitioners, is to blame parents for their child's substance abuse problem. "Jane wouldn't be drinking so much if her mother weren't so critical and her father didn't ignore her." Further assessment often reveals the parents' own history of neglect and substance abuse. In short, parents' ability to set appropriate limits and provide nurturing are directly related to their own experiences as children. Equally harmful may be the practitioner who is overly eager to accept the axioms of popular literature about families with substance abuse problems. The greatest risk is to lose sight of the unique needs and circumstances of the individuals one is serving. One of the most difficult yet important challenges for health care providers is to establish a trusting relationship with families when attempting to help the adolescent who is struggling with a substance abuse problem.

Etiology

Social Factors. Parents, siblings, and peers all have a significant impact on adolescent alcohol use. Adolescents who develop drinking problems tend to come from families with negative communication patterns, inconsistent parental discipline, marital discord, and an absence of parent-child closeness. Substance abuse of an older brother has also been shown to have an effect on a younger brother's use independent of parental use (Brook and others, 1988). Several studies assessing family structure found a relationship between adolescent substance abuse and the overinvolvement of one parent, accompanied by distancing from the other (see Family Focus box).

While the family environment may provide the kindling for adolescent alcohol abuse, peers provide the spark. Knowing whether an adolescent associates with substance-using peers is the strongest predictor of an adolescent's use (Barnes and Welte, 1986). This is not to say that peer association causes adolescent substance abuse, but rather that in most cases adolescents who drink tend to have friends who also drink. The impact of peers on drug use has also been demonstrated among African-Americans, Asians, and Hispanics (Hartford, 1985; Newcomb and Bentler, 1986).

Sociodemographic Factors. Frequency of alcohol use is influenced by a variety of sociodemographic factors. Adolescents in urban areas drink more than their rural or suburban peers. More boys than girls experiment with alcohol initially, but by the twelfth grade these differences no longer exist. Good school performance and a commitment to education reduce risk; in contrast, school failure is associated with alcohol abuse (Friedman, 1983). School dropouts are at particularly high risk and have been shown to drink more than high school graduates (Mensch and Kandel, 1988).

Psychosocial Factors. Research on personality and alcohol abuse, particularly in the area of adolescence, is only beginning to investigate the interplay of complex factors that determine risk for alcohol abuse. Although aggressiveness early in life predicts subsequent alcohol use (Loeber, 1988), only one third of boys with aggressive behavior continue to be aggressive into adulthood (Loeber and Dishion, 1983). Children with attention problems, hyperactivity, and conduct problems are at risk for a variety of adverse outcomes in adolescence, including alcohol abuse. Personality traits associated with alcohol abuse include excessive and consistent rebelliousness and rejection of social norms (Jessor and Jessor, 1977). Children and adolescents with greater numbers and intensity of these traits (i.e., aggressive behavior and hyperactivity) which persist into adulthood, are at greatest risk for alcohol problems.

Biologic Factors. Research on the association between biochemical and genetic factors and adolescent alcohol abuse is mixed. Twin studies comparing concordance of alcoholism in monozygotic (identical) and dizygotic (nonidentical) twins indicate no genetic transmission for females, with variable results for males (Murray and Stabenau, 1982). One study found no relationship between genetic status and concordance of alcoholism between twin brothers, whereas another found that brothers with identical genotypes were twice as likely as nonidentical twins to be concordant for alcohol abuse.

Aldehyde dehydrogenase (ALDH) is an enzyme that assists with the breakdown of ethanol in the body. Absence of ALDH significantly reduces the likelihood that alcoholism will develop (Schuckit, 1987). Some researchers conclude that a tolerance to alcohol is what is inherited by people with the potential to develop alcoholism.

ADDITIONAL DRUGS

The majority of adolescents limit their experimentation with drugs to alcohol, tobacco, and marijuana. A much smaller proportion will try other drugs, some of which have serious consequences, including cocaine, barbiturates, narcotics, and hallucinogens. In 1989, however, a vast majority of high school seniors did not approve of even experimenting with "hard" drugs. Consistent with their self-report on use, most seniors also did not approve of regular use of alcohol, tobacco, and marijuana (Johnston, Bachman, and O'Malley, 1992).

Cocaine is the most potent antifatigue agent known, and although pharmacologically it is not a narcotic, it is legally categorized as such. Cocaine is available in two forms: water-soluble cocaine hydrocholoride administered by insufflation or "snorting" and a nonsoluble alkaloid (freebase) used primarily for smoking. "Crack" or "rock" is a purer and more menacing form of the drug; it can be produced cheaply and smoked in either water pipes or mentholated cigarettes. The increased use of cocaine is related to its availability and affordability, the false perception of safety in its use, its association with persons in glamorous occupations, its snob appeal, its reputation as a sexually enhancing drug, and peer pressure (Tarr and Macklin, 1987).

Cocaine creates a sense of euphoria, or an indefinable high. Withdrawal does not produce the dramatic symptoms observed in withdrawal from other substances. The effects are those more commonly seen in depression, including lack of energy and motivation, irritability, appetite changes, psychomotor retardation, and irregular sleep patterns. More serious symptoms include cardiovascular manifestations and seizures. Withdrawal is not to be confused with the so-called crash after a cocaine high, which consists of a long period of sleep. In 1989, 10% and 5% of high school seniors reported having tried cocaine and crack, respectively (Johnston, Bachman, and O'Malley, 1992). Answers to questions about health risks of cocaine can be obtained by calling the **National Cocaine Hotline.*** It also provides referrals to support groups and treatment centers.

Narcotics include opiates, such as heroin and morphine, and opioids (opiate-like drugs), such as hydromorphone (Dilaudid), fentanyl, meperidine (Demerol), and codeine. They produce a state of euphoria by removing painful feelings and creating a pleasurable experience of a specific quality and a sense of success accompanied by clouding of consciousness and a dreamlike state. Physical signs of narcotic abuse include constricted pupils, respiratory depression, and, often, cyanosis. Needle marks may be visible on arms or legs in chronic users. Withdrawal from opiates is extremely unpleasant unless it is controlled with supervised substitution of methadone.

Perhaps more important are the indirect consequences related to the illegal status of narcotic use and the problems associated with securing the drug—time-consuming searches and methods used to meet the high cost. Health problems result from self-neglect of physical needs (nutrition, cleanliness, dental care), overdose, contamination, and infection, including acquired immune deficiency syndrome (AIDS) and hepatitis B.

Central nervous system depressants include a variety of hypnotic drugs that produce physical dependence and withdrawal symptoms on abrupt discontinuation. They create a feeling of relaxation and sleepiness but impair general functioning. Drugs in this category include barbiturates and nonbarbiturates (e.g., methaqualone [Quaalude]), as well as alcohol. Barbiturates combined with alcohol produce a profound depressant effect. In 1989 slightly less than 10% of high school seniors reported having tried sedatives (Johnston, O'Malley, and Bachman, 1989).

The ***central nervous system stimulants,*** amphetamines and cocaine, do not produce strong physical dependence and can be withdrawn without much danger. However, psychologic dependence is strong, and acute intoxication can lead to violent, aggressive behavior or psychotic episodes manifested by paranoia, uncontrollable agitation, and restlessness. When combined with barbiturates, the euphoric effects are particularly addictive.

Methamphetamine can be snorted, injected, swallowed, or smoked and produces a burst of energy in its users, along with intense, alternating attacks of boldness and paranoia. It provokes excitement far more intense than that caused by crack and cocaine. The drug, with the street names "crank," "meth," and "crystal," is inexpensive and has a longer period of action than cocaine. Instead of a short (few minutes) high, as achieved with crack, a user can remain "up" for hours on a similar dose of crank.

About 11% of high school seniors reported using amphetamines within the previous year.

Hydrocarbon and fluorocarbon abuse includes glue "sniffing" and the inhalation of plastic cement, typewriter correction fluid, and other volatile substances (e.g., gasoline, gold and silver spray paint). Teens breathe these substances directly or place them in paper or plastic bags from which they rebreathe the fumes, which produce an immediate euphoria and altered consciousness. The substances are extremely hazardous, causing rapid loss of consciousness and respiratory arrest. Many persons taking these drugs do not have time to remove the bag from their heads and quickly become asphyxiated.

Mind-altering drugs or hallucinogens (psychedelic, psychotomimetic, psychotropic, or illusionogenic) are drugs that produce vivid hallucinations and euphoria. These drugs do not produce physical dependence, since they can be abruptly withdrawn without ill effect. However, acute and long-term effects are variable, and in some individuals the dissociative behavior may be unduly protracted. This category includes cannabis (marijuana, hashish) and lysergic acid diethylamide (LSD).

Marijuana is the third most widely used drug by teens after alcohol and tobacco. In 1989 more than 40% of high school seniors reported using marijuana in the past year, with about 18% reporting use in the past 30 days. Contrary to past stereotypes, marijuana use is not likely to be followed by use of "hard" drugs such as cocaine and heroin (Carroll, 1985).

Drug users have developed a specialized terminology for

*(800) COCAINE.

GLOSSARY OF DRUG JARGON

AMPHETAMINES

Bams
Beans
Benn
Bennies
Black beauties
Black cadillacs
Black dex
Bombido (injectable)
Browns
Cartwheels
Chalk
Co-pilots
Cranks
Cross
Crystal
Dexies
Dice
Doe
Drives
Eyeopeners
Fives (5 mg)
Footballs
Goofballs
Green hearts
Greenies
Greens
Heart(s)
Horse hearts
Jolly babies
Leapers
Lid rollers
Lightning
Meth
Orange hearts
Peaches
Pep pills
Rippers
Roses
Speed
Splash
Thrusters
Truck drivers
Wake-up
White crosses
White dexies
Whites
Yellow bams
Zeeters
Zip

BARBITURATES (GENERAL)

Barbs
Courage pills
Downers
Golf balls
Goofers
Idiot pills
Nimbie
Nimbles
Peanuts
Sleepers

BARBITURATES (SPECIFIC)

Blue birds (amobarbital)
Blue devils (amobarbital)
Blue heaven (amobarbital)
Canary (pentobarbital)
Christmas trees (mixtures)
Downers (amobarbital)
F-40s (secobarbital)
F-66s (amobarbital sodium and secobarbital sodium) (gorilla pills)
Mexican yellows (pentobarbital)
Nemmies (pentobarbital)
Pink ladies (secobarbital)
Pinks (secobarbital)
Rainbow (secobarbital; amobarbital)
Red birds (secobarbital)
Red devils (secobarbital)
Reds (secobarbital)
Seggy, seccy (secobarbital)
Tooies (tuinal)
Yellow jackets (pentobarbital)
Yellows (pentobarbital)

COCAINE

Bernies flake
C
Candy
Cecil
Charlie
Coca-cola
Coke
Cokomo (Kokomo)
Crack
Dust
Flake
Gift of the Sun God
Gold dust
Happy trails
Incentive
Lady snow
Leaf (the)
Movie star drug
Nose
Nose candy
Pimp
Pimp's drug
Rich man's drug
Rock
Schoolboy
Snow
Society high
Star-spangled powder
Stardust
White horse
White stuff

HEROIN

Big Harry
Blanco
Boy
Caballo
Chiva
Deuce (a $2 packet)
Doojee
Dust
H
Harry; hairy
Horse
Joy powder
Scag
Scat
Smack
Stuff
Sugar
Ticata
White lady
White stuff

MORPHINE

Dreamer
Dust
Emma (Miss)
Emsel
Hard stuff
Hocus
M
Monkey
Morf
Morpho
Unkie
White stuff

MARIJUANA

Acapulco gold (potent)
Bush
Butter
Flower
Grass
Griffo
Hemp
Hooch
Hooter
Indian hay
J
Jive
Joint
Kif
Mary Jane
Mohasky
Mooters
Mu
Mutah
Panama red
Pot
Reefer (cigarette)
Rockets
Smoke
Splimi
Stick (cigarette)
Straw
Superjoint
Texas tea
Tie stick (mixed with opium and tied to a popsicle stick)
Weed

LSD (LYSERGIC ACID DIETHYLAMIDE)

Acid
Blotter acid (on paper)
Blue microdot
Cube (the)
D (big)
Heavenly blue
Purple haze
Royal blue
Sugar
Wedding bells
Windowpane

PCP (PHENCYCLIDINE)

Angel dust
Busy bee
DOA
Elephant
Goon
Hog (also chloral hydrate)
Horse tranquilizer
Magic mist
Peace pills
Rocket fuel
Sherman's
White horizon
Wobble

OTHER HALLUCINOGENS

DMT (dimethyltryptamine): businessman's special
DMZ (Benactyzine)
DOM (4-methyl-2,5-dimethoxyamphetamine), STP
Hashish: black hash; black Russian (potent)
STP (dimethoxymethylamphetamine), DOM (syndicate acid, tranquility)
THC (tetrahydrocannabinol): hallucinogen in marijuana and hashish

MIXED SUBSTANCES

Chicago green (marijuana/opium)
Double trouble (amobarbital/secobarbital)
Fours (acetaminophen with 60 mg codeine)
Fuel (marijuana/insecticide)
Hog (phencyclidine/vegetable material [veterinary drug])
In-betweens (barbiturates/amphetamines)
Mickey Finn (chloral hydrate/alcohol)
Speedball (heroin/cocaine; Percodan/methedrine)
Star-spangled powder (heroin/cocaine)

MISCELLANEOUS

Alcohol: mountain dew, alley juice (methyl alcohol) moonshine (ethyl alcohol), sauce, hootch, booze, juice
Amyl nitrite: aimes, snappers
Chloral hydrate: joy juice
Ethchlorvynol (Placidyl): dyls, plastic red, K-H, K-N
Meperidine hydrochloride: Diane
Mescaline: chief, mesc, mescalito, mescal beans
Methadone: dolls, dollies fizzies (tablets)
Methaqualone (Quaalude): 714, ludes, sopors, westcoast, lemons
Opium for smoking: black stuff
Paregoric: licorice, bitter
Peyote: button, cactus, Hikori, Kikuli, Huatari, Wokouri, seni, tops
Tobacco: coffin, deck (pack), fag

the abused substances (see box on p. 919). The vocabulary varies in different localities, and new descriptive terms arise spontaneously wherever drugs are part of the environment.

Therapeutic Management

Adolescents experiencing toxic drug effects or withdrawal symptoms are frequently seen in emergency rooms. Experienced emergency room personnel are familiar with the management of acute drug toxicosis; the signs, symptoms, and behavioral characteristics of a variety of substances; and differences and similarities among them. When the drug is questionable or unknown, knowledge of these factors facilitates handling of the youngster and implementation of a treatment regimen.

The treatment for drug toxicity or withdrawal varies according to the drug and the method used. Every effort should be made to determine the type and amount of drug taken, the time it was taken, the mode of administration, and factors related to the onset of presenting symptoms.

It is helpful to know the patient's pattern of use. For example, if two types of drugs are involved, they may require different treatments. Gastric lavage may be employed when the drug has been ingested recently and the cough reflex is intact, but it would be of little value when the drug has been administered by the intravenous ("mainlined") or intranasal ("sniffed") route. Since the actual content of most street drugs is highly questionable, other pharmaceutical agents are administered with caution, except perhaps the narcotic antagonists in cases of suspected opiate overdose. It is necessary to assess for possible trauma sustained while the patient was under the influence of the drug.

Rehabilitation from hard drug use may require withdrawing the adolescent from the environment, as well as from the chemical agent. Programs must be suited to the individual and may involve foster home placement or a residential treatment setting, although many youngsters are handled in an ambulatory setting. Programs often include group sessions with other troubled adolescents. Information regarding help can be obtained from the **Center for Substance Abuse Treatment** hotline.*

CRITERIA FOR SUBSTANCE DEPENDENCE

A maladaptive pattern of substance use, leading to clinically significant impairment or distress, as manifested by three (or more) of the following, occurring at any time in the same 12-month period:

1. Tolerance, as defined by either of the following:
   a. A need for markedly increased amounts of the substance to achieve intoxication or desired effect
   b. Markedly diminished effect with continued use of the same amount of the substance
2. Withdrawal, as manifested by either of the following:
   a. The characteristic withdrawal syndrome for the substance
   b. The same (or a closely related) substance taken to relieve or avoid withdrawal symptoms
3. The substance is often taken in larger amounts or over a longer period than was intended.
4. There is a persistent desire or unsuccessful efforts to cut down or control substance use.
5. A great deal of time is spent in activities necessary to obtain the substance (e.g., visiting multiple doctors or driving long distances), use the substance (e.g., chain-smoking), or recover from its effects.
6. Important social, occupational, or recreational activities are given up or reduced because of substance use.
7. The substance use is continued despite knowledge of having a persistent or recurrent physical or psychological problem that is likely to have been caused or exacerbated by the substance (e.g., current cocaine use despite recognition of cocaine-induced depression, or continued drinking despite recognition that an ulcer was made worse by alcohol consumption).

Specify if:
With physiological dependence: Evidence of tolerance or withdrawal (i.e., either item 1 or 2 is present)
Without physiological dependence: No evidence of tolerance or withdrawal (i.e., neither item 1 nor 2 is present)

Course specifiers
Early full remission
Early partial remission
Sustained full remission
Sustained partial remission
On agonist therapy
In a controlled environment

From American Psychiatric Association: *Diagnostic and statistical manual of mental disorders,* ed 4 (DSM-IV), Washington, DC, 1994, The Association.

Nursing Considerations

Nurses in almost every setting are increasingly likely to have contact with adolescent drug abusers or to be in a position to serve as educator and patient advocate. The importance of nurses receiving training on substance abuse is also underscored by findings of a national survey that indicated that 40% of nurses working with adolescents reported insufficient skills in this area (Bearinger and others, 1992). Nurses are often in a position to serve as listener, confidant, and counselor to troubled teens. They are essential members of health teams whose efforts are directed toward short-term and long-term therapy for drug abusers.

Often observation or a description of the behavior is more valuable than a report by patients or their friends as to the chemical agent taken (see box above, right, for criteria). For example, aggressive behavior and disorientation are often seen in barbiturate, alcohol, stimulant, or hallucinogen intoxication but not in opiate intoxication. Overdose from either barbiturates or opiates can result in respiratory failure and coma. Pinpoint pupils are seen only in opiate toxicity. Nurses must be alert for life-threatening consequences of drug toxicity; therefore equipment and personnel should be available or the patient should be transferred to facilities that are prepared to provide supportive measures for physiologic depression and psychogenic phenomena.

Stimulation should be kept to a minimum for agitated, frightened youngsters. Treatment or tests that are not required immediately are best postponed. These teens primarily need psychologic support in a nonthreatening environment and close contact with a caring and understand-

*(800) 662-HELP.

ing person who can stay with them and help them maintain social contact.

Nurses in the schools also play an essential role, since they are likely to be the only health professionals with an opportunity to identify many adolescents with substance abuse problems who appear anxious, depressed, or angry. Assessment of potential substance abuse problems is an important part of evaluation. By assuring confidentiality, within appropriate limits and in a straightforward manner, nurses enable many adolescents to discuss problems openly, including problems involving substance abuse.

Obstetric and nursery personnel sometimes encounter the problem of drug dependence and withdrawal in newborn infants or in a compulsive drug-using mother. Affected infants are at risk and require special surveillance for complications of withdrawal; therefore the nursing staff should be aware of the drug dependence in those mothers who come to the hospital for delivery (see Chapter 10).

Long-Term Management. A major factor in the treatment and rehabilitation of young drug users is careful assessment, in the nonacute stage, to determine the function that the drug plays in these teens' lives. Administration of a standardized instrument such as the Personal Experience Inventory (Winters and Henly, 1989), a 33-scale inventory measuring drug use severity and associated psychosocial problems, helps to guide initial evaluation and subsequent treatment. Adolescents need help to identify the issues that motivated them to use drugs and to recognize their own role in self-destructive, inappropriate drug-abuse behavior before they can embark on a rehabilitation program.

The motivation phase of treatment is directed toward exploring the factors that influence drug use. It also involves establishing in the teen a feeling of self-worth and a commitment to self-help. It requires a trusting relationship between the adolescent and the health team and involves a thorough physical examination and assessment of psychologic, educational, and vocational status. A realistic appraisal of the adolescent's potential and efforts aimed at short-term goals, along with building self-esteem, lays the groundwork for a successful rehabilitation program.

Rehabilitation begins when teens decide that they can and are willing to change. Rehabilitation involves fostering healthy interdependent relationships with caring and supportive adults and exploring alternative mechanisms for problem solving while simultaneously reducing or eliminating drug use. Persons working with troubled young people must be prepared for recidivism, or the tendency to relapse, and maintain a plan for reentry into the treatment process.

The majority of treatment programs for adolescent substance abusers are based on adult 12-step models such as Alcoholics Anonymous. Research is very much needed to determine whether applying adult models to assist adolescents with change is warranted. **Toughlove*** is one such program. The Toughlove philosophy, first employed by Alcoholics Anonymous and Al-Anon, is based on the conviction that parents have the right and the responsibility to be the policymakers in the family, set limits on the behavior of their children, and take control of the household from out-of-control teenagers. The premise is that allowing teenagers to experience the negative consequences of their behavior will bring them closer to accepting help and/or changing their behavior (Newton, 1985). Parents no longer take responsibility for the teen's behavior and suffer the negative consequences. Adolescents are offered the choice of (1) getting treatment for mental health or their drug problem or (2) finding another place to live.

Pieper and Pieper (1992) criticize the Toughlove approach, contending that the uncompromising position adopted by parents is harmful to both the parents and their child. In contrast, treatment emphasizing self-caretaking is described as more useful as a long-term approach. The fact remains that knowledge of effective approaches to treatment of adolescent substance abuse is not clearly understood. Treatments sensitive to the developmental transitions of adolescence and the variety of biopsychosocial factors affecting substance use need to be developed and evaluated.

Other groups that provide support and counseling for families experiencing crises with their children include **Parents Anonymous*** and **Parental Stress, Inc.,**† both of which maintain crisis counseling on a 24-hour basis.

Prevention. Given the difficulty of treating substance abusers, prevention is the most effective policy. In recent years, a variety of programs have been applied with promising results. Successful programs reducing substance abuse risk have promoted parenting skills (Dishion, Kavanagh, and Reid, 1989), social skills among distractible children (Ketchel and Bieger, 1989), academic achievement (Latimer, 1991), and skills to resist peer influence (Botvin, 1986).

Nurses play an important role in each of these and other areas where prevention efforts are possible. Young people need to be educated regarding appropriate use of chemicals. More important, those associated with adolescents should listen to what they are saying, determine what is bothering them, and try to help them meet these needs before they resort to drugs.

Prevention programs all carry the implicit assumption that the variety of poor outcomes facing children at risk can be forestalled or at least reduced. Children need to feel they are loved, and to feel they are good at something that helps others. Parents need to provide love while setting appropriate limits. Substance abuse is only one of many outcomes facing children for whom these needs are consistently neglected. Nurses in a variety of settings are in a position to facilitate the healing of both adolescents and their families who have experienced the effects of substance abuse.

---

*P.O. Box 1069, Doylestown, PA 18901; (215) 348-7090.

*22330 Hawthorne Blvd., No. 208, Torrance, CA 90505; (800) 352-0386 (California) and (800) 421-0353 (elsewhere).

†(617) 742-7535 (Massachusetts) and (800) 632-8188 (elsewhere). Other sources of information include **National Clearinghouse for Alcohol and Drug Abuse Information,** P.O. Box 2345, Rockville, MD 20852, (800) 729-6686; **National Federation of Parents for Drug-Free Youth,** (800) 554-KIDS or (301) 585-5437 (Maryland); and **National Institute on Drug Abuse Prevention Branch,** (800) 638-2045 or (301) 443-2450 (Maryland).

SUICIDE*

Suicide is defined as the deliberate act of self-injury with the intent that the injury result in death. Most experts distinguish between suicidal ideation, suicide attempt, and suicide. ***Suicidal ideation*** involves preoccupation with thoughts about committing suicide and may be a precursor to suicide. Although it is not uncommon for adolescents to experience occasional suicidal thoughts, expressions of suicidal preoccupation should be taken seriously and an assessment should be conducted for appropriate referral. A ***suicide attempt*** is intended to cause injury or death but is unsuccessful. In anonymous student surveys, between 6% and 14% of junior and senior high school students reported having attempted suicide at least once (U.S. Congress, Office of Technology Assessment, 1991).

NURSING ALERT A history of a previous suicide attempt is a serious indicator for possible suicide completion in the future. Studies of adolescent suicides have found that as many as half had made previous attempts.

In the United States the suicide rate increases dramatically between the ages of 10 and 19. The sudden surge in the suicide rate between early and later adolescence reflects normal cognitive, physical, psychosocial, and spiritual changes that occur as a result of puberty and can best be understood in the social context in which they take place.

The major tasks of adolescence are (1) developing a coherent sense of personal identity, (2) establishing a clear gender identity, (3) establishing autonomy from parents, (4) beginning to master the ability to be in intimate relationships, (5) acquiring coping skills, (6) consolidating values, and (7) developing educational or vocational goals. It is quite likely that the rise in suicide and depression during the period of adolescence is due to cognitive development and the newly developed capacity for self-observation and future orientation (Rutter, 1987). Some young people experience a pervasive sense of despair when they look into the future and are faced with a discrepancy between what they have been led to anticipate and that which they are truly able to obtain. Self-hate and hopelessness may result. In part, the despair is a consequence of adolescents' newly developed cognitive ability to consider the abstract and hypothetical, which may paint a bleak futuristic picture for their lives. As adolescents struggle to establish their sense of self, they are constantly seeking external validation and confirmation of who they are. Introspection also becomes a prominent part of this process. Social experiences and peer relationships become more important during the adolescent years, and the increased need to belong and conform leads to an increased vulnerability to depression and suicidal thought. In the context of this intrapersonal and interpersonal searching, self-esteem becomes pivotal, moderating hopelessness and developing a strong sense of self.

Young people also focus on mastering empathy during the teen years. The ability to truly empathize with others creates a new awareness of the suffering of others. The capacity to passionately feel both joy and sorrow is exciting, yet frightening. For some, the pain seems overwhelming and endless. Because they most likely have not lived through intensely painful experiences, they have not developed the means to cope with deep emotions. They may feel alone in experiencing pain and sorrow and unable to recognize or express their need for support. Consequently, suicide becomes a means of escape. For adolescents who have not had guidance and experience in problem solving and coping with sorrow, suicide may seem the only option.

Today, the exposure of young people to both suicide and death is in stark contrast to the experiences of those who were adolescents before the onset of television and before the dramatic change in the nature of the extended family. Through electronic media, young people have been exposed to countless deaths, with suicide being romanticized and inaccurately portrayed. The frequency of ***contagion,*** or ***copycat, suicides*** among young people (i.e., increase in youth suicides after the suicide of one teenager is publicized) points to the perception of suicide as "glamorous." Young people have been desensitized to death by constant viewing of it on television; simultaneously, changes in families have insulated teens from death experiences. Because of improvements in health care and geographic mobility in the United States, which isolate family members from one another, young people are not as likely to participate in the painful emotional realities of sickness and death among older family members (Hoberman, 1989).

Over the past several decades the increasing youth suicide rate has paralleled increasing child poverty, increasing divorce rates, and decreasing parental involvement and support. As adolescents strive for a healthy autonomy from their parents and master skills required for interdependence with others, they begin to question and criticize their parents. They are attempting to discover their own identity and discern which qualities of their parents they want to take with them into their adult lives. This questioning and criticizing process can also generate a sense of guilt, insecurity, fear, and conflict. Even though they may be rebelling against their parents, during this stage young people desperately need to feel needed, wanted, and loved by their families; yet parent-child conflicts mask this need for feeling connected with their families. The relationship between expressions of hopelessness and despair, and family "connectedness" has been documented. In short, young people who feel that their families care about them are less likely to show suicidal behaviors (Resnick, Harris, and Blum, 1993).

The changing roles of young people in society have also had an impact on adolescent suicidality. With the period of adolescence being prolonged in the United States, roles for young people during this time can be unclear and difficult to formulate. The earlier onset of puberty and the growing need for higher educational attainment has increased the period of adolescence from 6 years to potentially 14 years. The extended time "in limbo" between childhood and adulthood has created greater role confusion for young people. At the turn of the century, young people had the opportunity to observe their parents' roles, but today

*Margaret Dexheimer Pharris, RN, MS, MPH, wrote this section.

the majority of parents are employed at jobs away from home, so that children do not have the opportunity to see their parents as vocational role models. The higher percentage of adolescents within the total population and the increased difficulties adolescents have obtaining jobs and being admitted to good colleges also contribute to a higher youth suicide rate (Offer and Schonert-Reichl, 1992). Role confusion, as well as prolonged adolescence, is associated with higher youth suicide and alcohol abuse rates.

Although most people emerge from adolescence with a healthy sense of who they are and where they are headed, the widespread belief that adolescence is a time of turmoil—of storm and stress—has created a sense that hopelessness and despair are a normal part of the second decade of life. *This is not so.* Four of every five young people do not experience adolescence as a time of despair (Offer and Schonert-Reichl, 1992). Thus, depressive symptoms, acting-out behaviors, and talk of suicide need to be taken seriously. They are *not* part of a common "phase" of adolescence; they are a call for help that needs the response of nurses and other professionals.

INCIDENCE

From 1979 to 1988 the suicide rate for children ages 10 to 14 years increased from 0.8 to 1.4 per 100,000 population, or 75%. For teenagers between 15 and 19 years of age, the rate increased from 8.4 to 11.3 per 100,000 population, or 34% (Mortality trends, 1993). Suicide is now the third leading cause of death among young people in the United States, with unintentional injuries ranking first and homicide second. In 1990 suicide was responsible for 4869 deaths, accounting for 13.3% of all deaths of persons 15 to 24 years of age (National Safety Council, 1993).

The incidence of youth suicide varies greatly by gender and by racial/ethnic background (Fig. 21-2). In 1990, for every 100,000 teens ages 15 to 19, suicide rates were 18.85 for all males and 3.71 for all females. Among black adolescents as compared with white adolescents, the rates were lower: 11.46 for black males and 1.93 for black females, as compared with 19.27 for white males and 4.00 for white females (National Center for Health Statistics, 1990). National ethnic data (i.e., other than black or white) are not available; however, regional data show that Latino teenagers have lower suicide rates than white teenagers but higher rates than black teenagers, and they have a higher male/female suicide ratio (Centers for Disease Control, 1991). Suicide rates for American Indian and Alaskan Native adolescents are between 2 and 3 times greater than the rates for all other adolescents; among American Indian adolescents ages 15 to 19, the rate is 26.3 per 100,000 (U.S. Congress, Office of Technology Assessment, 1989). Although American Indians have the highest suicide rates of any racial/ethnic group in the United States, there is great variation among tribes. Tribes with less social integration and less adherence to tribal traditions, but a high degree of individuality, generally have higher suicide rates than tribes that are tightly integrated and that adhere to traditional values and practices (Berlin, 1987; Long, 1986; May, 1987; Zimmerman, 1992). Asian-American and Jewish teenagers have a lower incidence of suicide than other ethnic groups (Maris, 1985). Internationally, youth suicide rates are higher in wealthy, industrialized countries and remarkably low in so-called developing countries (Zimmerman, 1992).

Also at higher risk for suicide are incarcerated youths in public correctional facilities, who have an estimated suicide rate 2.5 times higher than that of adolescents in the general population. Minors detained in adult jails are at especially high risk for suicide (U.S. Congress, Office of Technology Assessment, 1991).

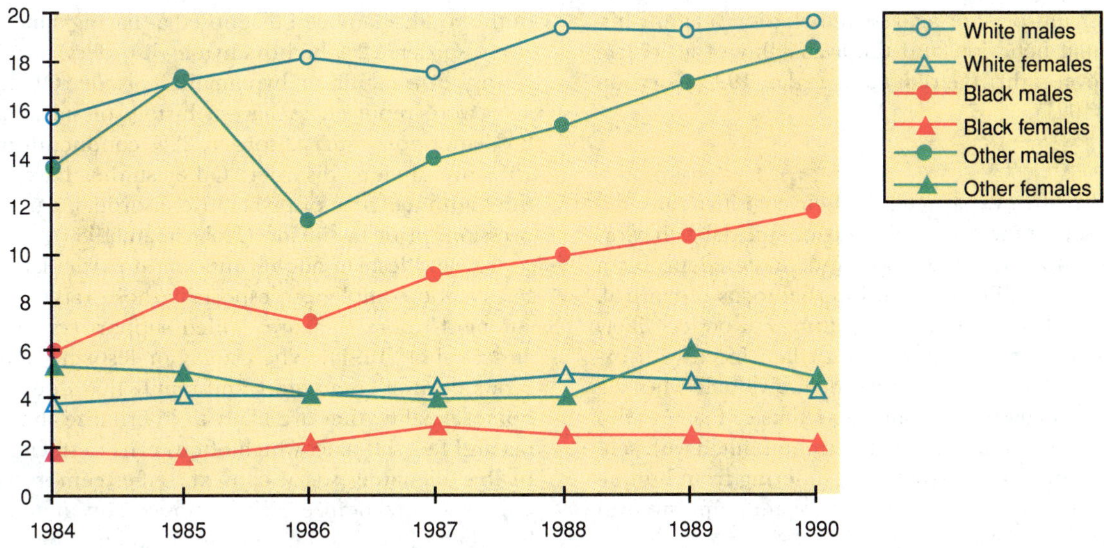

FIG. 21-2 U.S. suicide rates (per 100,000 population) among 15- to 19-year-olds. (From National Center for Health Statistics: *Mortality data tapes for number of deaths,* Washington, DC, 1990, US Bureau of Census Population Estimates.)

Even though the statistics reveal hopelessness and despair among young people, the true incidence of completed suicides in children and adolescents is not known because of general underreporting. Frequently deaths by suicide are reported as accidental because of pressures exerted by the family and society to avoid the cultural and religious stigma associated with self-destruction. There is also some degree of certainty that the high accident rate in persons in this age-group may reflect suicides masked by accidental death or homicide. Many theorists believe that the high youth homicide rate may have a strong suicidal component rooted in despair and hopelessness.

The true incidence of suicide attempts is even more difficult to measure. There exists no national reporting system for suicide attempts. Although there is a 5:1 male/female ratio for suicide completion, suicide attempts are far more common in females than in males (Hoberman, 1989). The major difference between suicide attempts and suicide completions is whether or not a lethal weapon is available. There is also a higher likelihood of successful suicide when the youth has consumed alcohol. Thus in societies where alcohol and lethal weapons are readily available to youths, there exists a higher incidence of youth suicide. A study showed that firearms were more likely to be present in the homes of suicide completers than in those of a control group of youths who had attempted suicide or who had suicidal ideation (Brent and others, 1988).

FACTORS ASSOCIATED WITH SUICIDE RISK

One of the most effective research methodologies used to study risk factors associated with suicide is that of psychologic autopsy, which involves data collection from the deceased person's family, friends, teachers, counselors, spiritual advisors, and educational and health care records. Psychologic autopsies show several factors associated with adolescent suicide. These include depression or other affective disorders, drug and alcohol abuse, family conflict, prior suicide attempt, antisocial or aggressive behavior, a family history of suicidal behavior, and the availability of a firearm (see box above, right) (Garland and Zigler, 1993; Garrison and others, 1991).

FACTORS ASSOCIATED WITH SUICIDE RISK

PAST HISTORY

- Family member, friend has made a suicide attempt
- Previous suicide attempt
- History of child abuse or neglect
- Past psychiatric hospitalization
- Death of a parent when child was young (3 to 5 years of age)

INDIVIDUAL FACTORS

- Marked, persistent depression
- Sees self as totally helpless—a victim of fate
- Impulsive
- Difficulty tolerating frustration
- Feelings of self-hatred or excessive guilt, feelings of humiliation
- Thinking disorder (wishes to join a deceased person, hears voices telling to kill self)
- Physical/body image problems (delayed puberty, chronic illness, disability, attention deficit hyperactivity disorder, learning disorders)
- Gay or lesbian in an unsupportive environment
- Alcohol or drug abuse
- A need to do things perfectly

FAMILY FACTORS

- Difficult home situation—long, bitter parent-child conflict
- Hostile parents
- Overt rejection by one or both parents
- Divorce or separation of parents
- Recent or impending move
- Family breakup or parental loss
- Exposure to unrealistically high parental expectations
- Parental indifference with very low expectations

SOCIAL/ENVIRONMENTAL FACTORS

- Incarcerated
- Lack of effective social support system
- Isolation
- Exposure to suicide of another
- Few social, vocational, educational opportunities
- Firearms in the home

Individual Factors

Adolescents' maturity, particularly their cognitive development, may determine the likelihood of suicidal behavior. Adolescents who have developed and mastered problem solving and social skills, have an internal locus of control, and have a positive sense of their future will be less likely to turn to suicide as an option even when faced with extreme stressors. On the other hand, individuals who see themselves as totally helpless and as victims of fate, or who are impulsive, unable to tolerate frustration, filled with self-hatred, experiencing excessive guilt, suffering from humiliation, withdrawn and aloof, or aggressive and impulsive will be more likely to take their own life.

In a study of young suicide completers, Brent and others (1988) found that 93% had at least one major psychiatric diagnosis. In interviewing parents, they found that 41% of the youths had been diagnosed as having a major depressive disorder, 22% had dysthymic disorders, and 7% had a history of a manic or hypomanic episode. Of this sample 41% were reported to have a history of substance abuse, 26% attention deficit disorder, 22% conduct disorder, and 15% overanxious disorder. Other studies have confirmed the high incidence of psychiatric disorders, particularly depression, prior to suicide (Hoberman, 1989).

Gay and lesbian adolescents are at particularly high risk for suicide completion, especially those raised in an environment where they are denied support systems (Bidwell and Deyher, 1991). When a gay or lesbian young person grows up in a community and family that does not accept homosexuality, they are likely to internalize the homophobia and feel self-hate, which often turns to suicidal feelings. In this alienating social context, self-esteem is challenged. Youths who recognize their homosexuality at an earlier age have been found to be more likely to attempt suicide than those who confront sexual orientation issues at a later age. Although similar data are not known for lesbian or bisexual young people, studies indicate that as many as 3 in 10 gay youths attempt suicide during adolescence (Remafedi, Farrow, and Deisher, 1991). In 1989 the Secretary of Health's Task Force on Youth Suicide (U.S. Department of Health and Human Services, 1989) reported that homosexual youths probably account for 30% of all teen suicides each year. In providing care that enhances support systems and nurtures opportunities for the healthy development of self-esteem in gay, lesbian, and bisexual adolescents and their families, nurses can play a significant role in reducing youth suicide rates in the United States.

Additional individual risk factors for suicidal behavior include poor academic progress, a history of being a victim of sexual abuse, learning disabilities, attention deficit disorder, chronic illness, disability, and antisocial behavior (especially assaultive behavior, which when experienced with suicidal feelings provides a strong risk indicator for suicide potential). Clearly, drug and alcohol use and abuse cannot be overlooked as strong contributing factors for suicide risk. More than 7 of 10 of all adolescent suicides are complicated by drug and alcohol use and abuse (Miller, Mahler, and Gold, 1991).

PROTECTIVE FACTORS FOR YOUTH SUICIDE

- Warm and caring family environment
- Self-esteem, locus of control, self-confidence
- Social skills
- Problem-solving skills
- Regular attendance at religious services
- Has an adult in their life who listens to them
- Perceives school personnel to be caring
- Parental support
- Parents have realistic, high expectations
- Family pays a lot of attention to them
- Cohesive family environment
- Supportive friendships
- Ability to manage negative affect, tolerate frustration and unfavorable events, think things through, actively problem solve, easily form close relationships, celebrate good things, and feel pleasure
- Family respects individuality

Family Factors

Families hold the greatest potential for protecting young people from suicidal behavior. Families who respect individuality; balance discipline with a supportive, understanding relationship; have good systems of communication; and have at least one attentive and caring parent available to the child protect adolescents from suicidal outcomes. In contrast, family risk factors for suicide include parental loss; family disruption; a family history of suicidality, substance abuse, or emotional disturbance; child abuse or neglect; unavailable parents; poor communication; isolation within an inflexible family system; family conflict; unrealistically high parental expectations; and parental indifference with low expectations.

A study comparing 473 suicidal and nonsuicidal youths found that youths in the nonsuicidal group were more likely to come from families where the parents were married; they reported better health and greater availability of someone to talk to; and they attended worship services more regularly than those in the suicidal group (Conrad, 1991). The author concluded that "a parent's show of affection is a very important way to make a difference in decreasing suicidal behaviors." Nursing interventions need to be designed in a manner that involves parents and enhances family cohesiveness (see box above, right). However, in working with families who have experienced the loss of a child through suicide, it is important to remember that while there is a higher risk of suicide in families who are under stress and who are less cohesive, youth suicide can and does happen in the context of a very caring and cohesive family environment.

Social/Environmental Factors

Important social/environmental influences that protect adolescents from suicidal behavior include good peer relationships, regular church attendance, strong social support within the community or school system, and available options for vocational and educational development. In contrast, factors associated with increased suicide risk include incarceration, isolation, acute loss of a boyfriend or girlfriend, lack of future options, increased size of the adolescent population, and availability of firearms in the home.

METHODS

Completed Suicide

Firearms are by far the most commonly used instruments in completed suicides among male and female adolescents, with the rate of suicide by firearms having increased 225% for 15- to 19-year-olds between 1968 and 1987 (U.S. Congress, Office of Technology Assessment, 1991). It is hypothesized that this increase is a result of the increased accessibility and availability of handguns. For adolescent males the second and third most common means of suicide, respectively, are hanging and carbon monoxide poisoning. For adolescent females they are overdose and carbon monoxide poisoning (Berman and Jobes, 1991).

Suicide Attempt

The most common method of suicide attempt is overdose or ingestion of a potentially toxic substance, such as drugs. A study of adolescent suicide attempters found that 83% overdosed as a means of attempting suicide (Spirito and others, 1992). The second most common method of suicide attempt is self-inflicted laceration.

PRECIPITATING FACTORS

Although suicide is often an impulsive act, it takes place against a backdrop of individual, family, and social risk factors and is often carried out in response to an exacerbation of long-standing stressors or in reaction to an acute precipitating factor. The most common factors precipitating adolescent suicide are a fight with a close friend; the breakup of an important relationship; failure in an important area, such as school activities; changing schools or moving; discovery of pregnancy plus family crisis and/or rejec-

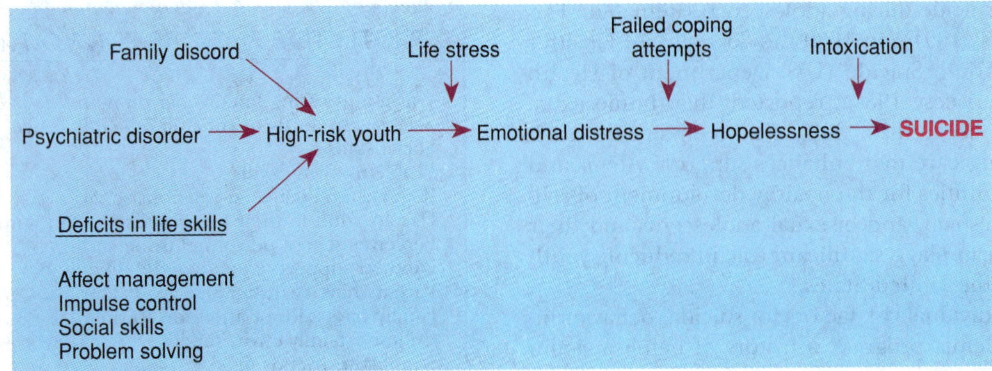

FIG. 21-3 The pathway from risk factors to completed suicide. (From Hoberman H: Completed suicide in children and adolescents: a review, *Resid Treat Child Youth* 7:61-88, 1989.)

PRECIPITATING FACTORS FOR SUICIDE

Increased depression and hopelessness
Fight with close friend
Failure to achieve specific goals in school, job, personal life
Breakup of important relationship
Friend moved away
Relocated to new community or school
Discovery of pregnancy combined with family stress and/or rejection by boyfriend
Death of close friend, relative, or pet
Argument within family
Shameful or humiliating experience
Trouble with police

tion by boyfriend; and death of a close friend, relative, or pet.

Fig. 21-3 presents a model for understanding the dynamics of the pathway from risk factors to completed suicide that incorporates multiple factors related to individual differences, as well as family and social contexts (see box above).

WARNING SIGNS OF SUICIDE

Preoccupation with themes of death—focuses on morbid thoughts
Wants to give away cherished possessions
Talks of own death, desire to die
Loss of energy—loss of interest, listlessness
Exhaustion without obvious cause
Changes in sleep patterns—too much or too little
Increased irritability, argumentativeness, or stubbornness
Physical complaints—recurrent stomachaches, headaches
Repeated visits to doctor, nurse practitioner, or emergency room for treatment of injuries
Reckless behavior
Antisocial behavior—engages in drinking, uses drugs, fights, commits acts of vandalism, runs away from home, becomes sexually promiscuous
Sudden change in school performance—lowered grades, cutting classes, dropping out of activities
Resists or refuses to go to school
Remains distant, sad, remote—flat affect, frozen facial expression
Describes self as worthless
Sudden cheerfulness following deep depression
Social withdrawal from friends, activities, interests that were previously enjoyed
Impaired concentration
Dramatic change in appetite

NURSING CONSIDERATIONS

Prevention

Nurses can play a pivotal role in reducing youth suicide rates in the general population. Nurses have the opportunity to provide anticipatory guidance to parents and adolescents in understanding normal adolescent development and normal feelings of young people as they move through the experiences of adolescence. They can teach parents how to be supportive and how to develop positive communication patterns in helping teens feel connected with and loved by their families. To foster healthy development, parents can be encouraged to provide teens with creative outlets and to assist young people in accepting strong emotions—pain, anger, frustration—as a normal part of the human experience.

NURSING ALERT Given what is known about youth suicide, nurses should ask parents, especially those of at-risk teenagers, if firearms are available in the house and, if so, recommend their removal. Parents must ensure that their children—especially children who are depressed, have poor problem-solving skills, or use drugs or alcohol—do not have access to firearms. Parents must be educated on the warning signs of suicide (see box above).

Nurses working in the community are in a strategic position to conduct educational programs in schools, places of worship, and community centers to help young people develop healthy, effective coping mechanisms and problem-solving skills. Nurses can teach parents, teachers, and youth workers about youth depression and stress. Informed parents are more likely to seek help for young people who report persistent, deep feelings of sadness, hopelessness, and suicidal feelings for psychologic evaluation and treatment. All who work with and nurture teenagers should keep in mind that depression in adolescents is manifested differently from that in adults. In teens it may be masked by impulsive, aggressive behaviors. Defiance, disobedience, and behavior problems can be indicative of underlying depression, suicidal ideation, and impending suicide attempts.

Prevention of youth suicide also involves advocating for social programs that reduce social isolation among young people, enhance opportunities for social support, and promote interaction with peers, as well as youth leaders and community workers. Young people need to be involved in a meaningful way in society. As adolescents gain meaningful roles in their schools and communities and experience a sense of competence and confidence in these roles, they become more able to cope with feelings of sadness and despair and are more able to be resilient when faced with stressful life events.

The clustering of suicides (i.e., "copycat" suicides) requires a change in the way both print and electronic media typically report youth suicide. Rather than romanticizing suicide, it needs to be portrayed as a poor means of coping with life's stressors and, at times, a response to underlying psychiatric disorders. In addition, to reduce "copycat" suicides, schools and communities must provide postvention programs when suicide has occurred. Information can be obtained from the **American Association of Suicidology.***

Health professionals must be alert to the warning signs of adolescent suicide. No threat of suicide should be ignored. Too often, suicidal threats or minor attempts are confused with bids for attention. It is also a mistake to be lulled into a false sense of security when the adolescent's depression is apparently relieved. The improvement in attitude may very well mean that the youngster has made the decision to carry out the threat.

Peers or other confidants are excellent sources of information and valuable observers. They are able to sense when a friend has undergone a marked personality change. It is important to emphasize that the peer who detects any change in a friend is a "potential rescuer" and should not remain quiet about the observations. A peer who believes that a friend may be suicidal should alert someone who is in a position to help—a parent, teacher, guidance counselor, or other person.

Care of the Suicidal Adolescent

In caring for young persons who express suicidal feelings, the nurse's first responsibility is to ensure their safety and protect them from harm. Any suicidal remarks must be taken seriously, and the young persons should not be left alone until the degree of their suicidality is assessed. An acronym for the assessment process is ***SLAP (specificity, lethality, accessibility,*** and ***proximity).*** The first step ***(specificity)*** is to ask adolescents if they feel suicidal, or feel as though they would like to take their own life. If so, what is their plan? Have they chosen a means of suicide, and do they have a specific plan? The second stage in assessment ***(lethality)*** involves determining the lethality of methods available to them. Do they plan to use a gun or knife? Have they chosen highly lethal medications, hanging, or carbon monoxide poisoning? The third stage ***(accessibility)*** involves determining the availability of the means of suicide, and the fourth stage ***(proximity)*** involves assessing whether they have determined a time to commit suicide and when.

Although confidentiality is the usual approach with adolescent counseling, in the case of self-destructive behaviors this cannot be honored. Suicidal behavior must be reported to the family and other professionals, and the adolescent is informed that this will be done. Such action conveys an important message to an attempter—that the nurse understands and cares.

NURSING ALERT Adolescents who express suicidal feelings and have a specific plan should be monitored at all times. They should not have access to belts, scarves, weapons, shoestrings, sharp objects, matches, or lighters. If they are intoxicated, they must be restrained or placed in a protective environment until they can be assessed by a psychiatrist or psychologist.

Understanding and caring demonstrated by the nurse to the adolescent are extremely therapeutic. Adolescents have a very deep need to be *normal* and will only feel more depressed and suicidal if they are stigmatized. Expressing a commitment to keeping them safe until they no longer feel so terribly sad and assuring them that they will indeed feel better with time are both helpful nursing actions. A person who feels extremely suicidal will welcome the security of being restrained if it is presented as an act of care, not punishment. Feeling actively suicidal is a very frightening experience, and the adolescent should not be left alone. By demonstrating care, open communication, and understanding, the nurse is modeling appropriate behavior for the young person's family. Time spent listening to family members and helping them understand will reduce the incidence of future suicidal actions.

The attempted, and especially the completed suicide of an adolescent is usually a major family crisis. In an attempted suicide the opportunity exists for the family and teenager to obtain help. Since these families are often already in conflict and at risk, nurses play an important role in referring them to appropriate mental health services. They should stress to parents the seriousness of the attempt and that this crisis offers the opportunity to avoid the tragedy of completed suicide. (See also Unexpected Childhood Death, Chapter 23.)

KEY POINTS

- The change, growth, and stress accompanying the transition to adulthood may predispose adolescents to faulty problem solving.
- Age of onset of obesity, presence of emotional disturbances or neuroses, and negative evaluation of obesity by others may all contribute to the development of a disturbed body image in the adolescent.

*2459 S. Ash, Denver, CO 80222; (303) 692-0985.

- Diet, exercise, and behavior modification are the hallmarks of treatment for obesity.
- The nurse's involvement in obesity control includes nutritional counseling, behavior modification, group programs, and family counseling.
- Anorexia nervosa, a disorder characterized by severe weight loss in the absence of obvious physical cause, consists of three areas of disordered psychologic functioning: disturbed body image and body concept of delusional proportions, inaccurate and confused perception and interpretation of inner stimuli, and paralyzing sense of ineffectiveness that pervades all aspects of daily life.
- Therapeutic management of anorexia involves reinstitution of normal nutrition, resolution of the disturbed patterns of family interaction, and individual psychotherapy to correct deficits and distortions in psychologic functioning.
- Individuals with bulimia can be classified into two categories: those who consume vast quantities of food followed by purging but who, if unable to purge, still consume large amounts and those who restrict their caloric intake, especially when unable to purge.
- Smoking is a widespread problem among teenagers; reasons for smoking include social pressure, mass media influence, and a need to develop a self-concept.
- Substance abuse is a severe problem in adolescence, and abusers include experimenters and compulsive users.
- Common types of drugs abused include alcohol, hydrocarbons and fluorocarbons, mind-altering drugs, narcotics, central nervous system depressants, and central nervous system stimulants.
- Suicide, the deliberate act of self-injury with the intent to kill, may occur in adolescents because of psychiatric disorders—primarily depression, family discord, and difficulties in coping with stress.
- Suicide is much more likely to occur if the adolescent has access to a firearm or has been drinking or using drugs.

REFERENCES

American Academy of Pediatrics, Committee on Substance Abuse: Tobacco-free environment: an imperative for the health of children and adolescents, *AAP News* 10(4):25, 27, 1994.

American Psychiatric Association: *Diagnostic and statistical manual of mental disorders,* ed 4 (DSM-IV), Washington, DC, 1994, The Association.

Attie I, Brooks-Gunn J: Development of eating problems in adolescent girls: a longitudinal study, *Dev Psychol* 25:70-77, 1989.

Barnes GM, Welte JW: Patterns and predictors of alcohol use among 7-12th grade students in New York State, *J Stud Alcohol* 47:53-62, 1986.

Bearinger LH and others: Nursing competence in adolescent health: anticipating the future needs of youth, *J Prof Nurs* 8(2):80-86, 1992.

Berkowitz RI and others: Physical activity and adiposity: a longitudinal study from birth to childhood, *J Pediatr* 105:734-738, 1985.

Berlin I: Suicide among American Indian adolescents: an overview, *Suicide Life Threat Behav* 17(3):218-232, 1987.

Berman AL, Jobes DA: *Adolescent suicide: assessment and intervention,* Washington, DC, 1991, American Psychological Association.

Bidwell R, Deyher R: Adolescent sexuality: current issues, *Pediatr Ann* 20(6):293-302, 1991.

Biglan A and others: A situational analysis of adolescent smoking, *J Behav Med* 1:109-114, 1984.

Blum RW, McKay C, Resnick MD: *The state of Minnesota adolescent health,* Monograph prepared by Adolescent Health Database Project, Minneapolis, Feb 1989, University of Minnesota.

Botvin GJ: Substance abuse prevention research: recent developments and future directions, *J Sch Health* 56:369-374, 1986.

Brent DA and others: Risk factors for adolescent suicide, *Arch Gen Psychiatry* 45:581-588, 1988.

Brook JS and others: The role of older brothers in younger brothers' drug use viewed in the context of parent and peer influences, *J Genet Psychol* 151:59-75, 1988.

Brownell KD, Kelman JH, Strunkard AJ: Treatment of obese children with and without their mothers: changes in weight and blood pressure, *Pediatrics* 71:515-523, 1983.

Carino CM, Chmelko P: Disorders of eating in adolescence: anorexia nervosa and bulimia, *Nurs Clin North Am* 18:343-352, 1983.

Carroll CR: *Drugs in modern society,* Dubuque, IA, 1985, Wm C Brown.

Centers for Disease Control: Attempted suicide among high school students—United States, 1990, *MMWR* 40(37):633-635, 1991.

Comerci GD: Eating disorders in adolescents, *Pediatr Rev* 10:1-6, 1988.

Connors ME, Morse W: Sexual abuse and eating disorders: a review, *Int Eat Dis* 13(1):1-11, 1993.

Conrad N: Where do they turn? Social support systems of suicidal high school adolescents, *J Psychosoc Nurs* 29(3):15-19, 1991.

Copeland ET, Baucom-Copeland S: Childhood obesity: a family systems view, *Am Fam Physician* 24(8):153-155, 1981.

Davis RM: Current trends in cigarette advertising and marketing, *N Engl J Med* 316:725-732, 1987.

Dessendorfer EA, Amsterdam EA, Odland TM: Adolescent smoking and its effect on aerobic exercise tolerance, *Phys Sports Med* 11:109-119, 1983.

Dietz WH: Prevention of childhood obesity, *Pediatr Clin North Am* 33:823-833, 1986.

Difranza JR and others: RJR Nabisco's cartoon camel promotes Camel cigarettes to children, *JAMA* 266(22):3149-3153, 1991.

Dishion TJ, Kavanagh K, Reid JB: *Child-rearing vs. peer interventions in the reduction of risk for adolescent substance use and adjustment problems: a secondary prevention strategy,* Paper presented at the Conference for the Advancement of Applied Behavior Therapy, Washington, DC, 1989.

Eckert P: Beyond the statistics of adolescent smoking, *Am J Public Health* 73:439-441, 1983.

Epstein LH and others: Effect of diet and controlled exercise on weight loss in obese children, *J Pediatr* 107:358-361, 1985.

Evans RI: Smoking prevention: overview, In Matarazzo J and others, editors: *Behavior health: a handbook of health enhancement and disease prevention,* New York, 1984, Wiley.

Evans RI and others: Smoking in children and adolescents: psychosocial determinants and prevention strategies. In *Smoking and health: a report of the Surgeon General,* DHEW Pub No (PHS) 79-50066, US Department of Health, Education, and Welfare, Washington, DC, 1979, US Government Printing Office.

Feldman W, Feldman E, Goodman JT: Culture versus biology: children's attitudes toward thinness and fatness, *Pediatrics* 81:190-194, 1988.

Fischer PM and others: Brand logo recognition by children aged 3 to 6 years: Mickey Mouse and Old Joe the camel, *JAMA* 266(22):3145-3148, 1991.

Flay BR and others: Cigarette smoking: why young people do it and ways of preventing it. In McGrath PJ, Firestone P: *Pediatric and adolescent behavioral medicine: issues in treatment,* New York, 1983, Springer.

Friedman AS: High school drug abuse clients. In *Clinical research notes,* Rockville, MD, 1983, Division of Clinical Research, National Institute on Drug Abuse.

Garland A, Zigler E: Adolescent suicide prevention: current research and social policy implications, *Am Psychol* 48(2):169-182, 1993.

Garrison C and others: The assessment of suicidal behavior in adolescents, *Suicide Life Threat Behav* 21(3):217-230, 1991.

Gerber RW, Newman IM: Predicting future smoking of adolescent experimental smokers, *J Youth Adolesc* 18:191-201, 1989.

Graves T, Meyers AW, Clark L: An evaluation of parental problem-solving training in the behavioral treatment of childhood obesity, *J Consult Clin Psychol* 56:245-250, 1988.

Hartford TC: Drinking patterns among black and non-black adolescents: results of a national survey. In Wright R, Watts TD, editors: *Prevention of black alcoholism: issues and strategies,* Springfield IL, 1985, Charles C Thomas.

Herzog DB, Copeland PM: Eating disorders, *N Engl J Med* 313:295-299, 1985.

Himes JH, Dietz WH: Guidelines for overweight in adolescent preventive services: recommendations from an expert committee, *Am J Clin Nutr* 59(2):307-316, 1994.

Hoberman HM: Completed suicide in children and adolescents: a review, *Resid Treat Child Youth* 7:61-88, 1989.

Huang PP and others: Black-white differences in appeal of cigarette advertisement among adolescents, *Tobacco Control* 1(4):249-55, 1992.

Huse DM and others: The challenge of obesity in childhood. I. Incidence, prevalence, and staging, *Mayo Clin Proc* 57:279-284, 1982a.

Huse DM and others: The challenge of obesity in childhood. II. Treatment guidelines by stage, *Mayo Clin Proc* 57:285-288, 1982b.

Jessor R, Jessor SL: *Problem behavior and psychosocial development: a longitudinal study of youth,* San Diego, 1977, Academic Press.

Joffe A: Too little, too much: eating disorders in adolescents, *Contemp Pediatr* 7(3):114-135, 1990.

Johnston LD: The etiology and prevention of substance use: what can we learn from recent historical changes? In Jones CL, Battjes RJ, editors: *Etiology of drug abuse: implications for prevention* (NIDA Research Monograph 56, DHHS Pub No ADM 86-1335, Washington, DC, 1985, US Government Printing Office.

Johnston LD, Bachman JG, O'Malley PM: *Monitoring the future: questionnaire responses from the nation's high school seniors 1987,* Ann Arbor, MI, 1991, Institute for Social Research, University of Michigan.

Johnston LD, Bachman JG, O'Malley PM: *Monitoring the future: questionnaire responses from the nation's high school seniors 1989,* Ann Arbor, MI, 1992, Institute for Social Research, University of Michigan.

Johnston LD, O'Malley PM, Bachman JG: *Drug use, drinking, and smoking: national survey results from high school, college, and young adult populations,* DHHS Pub No ADM 89-1638, Washington, DC, 1989, US Government Printing Office.

Johnston LD, O'Malley PM, Bachman JG: *National trends in drug use and related factors among American high school students and young adults, 1975-1989,* Washington DC, 1990, US Department of Health and Human Services, National Institute on Drug Abuse.

Kandel DB, Raveis VH, Kandel P: Continuity in discontinuities: adjustment in young adulthood of former school absentees, *Youth Soc* 15:325-353, 1984.

Kaplan KM, Wadden TA: *Childhood obesity and self-esteem, J Pediatr* 109:367-370, 1986.

Ketchel JA, Bieger G: *The efficacy of a psychosocially based drug prevention program for young adolescents,* Paper presented at the New England Educational Research Corporation Annual Meeting, Portsmouth, NH, April 1989.

Kreipe RE, Churchill BH, Strauss J: Long-term outcome of adolescents with anorexia nervosa, *Am J Dis Child* 143:1322-1327, 1989.

Latimer WW: *The University of Rhode Island Accommodation System for Students with Disabilities: a faculty handbook with special focus on learning disabilities,* Kingston, RI, 1991, University of Rhode Island Publications.

Lerner JV, Vicary JR: Difficult temperament and drug use: analyses from the New York longitudinal study, *J Drug Educ* 14:1-8, 1984.

Lifshitz F, Moses N: Nutritional dwarfing: growth, dieting, and fear of obesity, *J Am Coll Nutr* 7:367-370, 1988.

Loeber R: Natural histories of conduct problems, delinquency, and associated substance use: evidence for developmental progressions. In Lahey BB, Kazdin AE, editors: *Advances in clinical child psychology,* vol 2, New York, 1988, Plenum Press.

Loeber RT, Dishion T: Early predictors of male delinquency: a review, *Psychol Bull* 93:68-99, 1983.

Long KA: Suicide intervention and prevention with Indian adolescent populations, *Issues Ment Health Nurs* 8:247-253, 1986.

Maloney MJ and others: Dieting behavior and eating attitudes in children, *Pediatrics* 84:482-489, 1989.

Maris R: The adolescent suicide problem, *Suicide Life Threat Behav* 15:91-109, 1985.

Marston AR and others: Characteristics of adolescents at risk for compulsive overeating on a brief screening test, *Adolescence* 23:59-65, 1988.

May P: Suicide among American Indian youth: a look at the issue, *Child Today,* pp 22-25, July-Aug, 1987.

McAlister AL, Krosnick JA, Milburn MA: Causes of cigarette smoking: tests of a structural equation model, *Soc Psychol Q* 47:24-36, 1984.

Mensch BS, Kandel DB: Dropping out of high school and drug involvement, *Sociol Educ* 61:95-113, 1988.

Miller N, Mahler J, Gold M: Suicide risk associated with drug and alcohol dependence, *J Addict Dis* 10(3):49-61, 1991.

Morgan M, Grube JW: Adolescent cigarette smoking: a developmental analysis of influences, *Br J Dev Psychol* 7:179-189, 1989.

Mortality trends and leading causes of death among adolescents and young adults—United States, 1979-1988, *MMWR* 42(23): 459-462, 1993.

Moses N, Banilivy MM, Lifshitz F: Fear of obesity among adolescent girls, *Pediatrics* 83:393-398, 1989.

Murray RM, Stabenau JR: Genetic factors in alcoholism predisposition. In *Encyclopedia handbook of alcoholism,* New York, 1982, Gardner Press.

Must A and others: Long-term morbidity and mortality of overweight adolescents: a follow-up of the Harvard growth study of 1922 to 1935, *N Engl J Med* 327:1350-1355, 1992.

National Center for Health Statistics: *Mortality data tapes for number of deaths,* Washington, DC, 1990, US Bureau of Census Population Estimates.

National Safety Council: *Accident facts,* Itasca, IL, 1993, National Safety Council.

Newcomb MD, Bentler PM: Substance use and ethnicity: differential impact of peer and adult models, *J Psychol* 120:83-95, 1986.

Newcomb MD, McCarthy WJ, Bentler PM: Cigarette smoking, academic lifestyle, and social impact efficacy: an eight year study from adolescence to young adulthood, *J Appl Soc Psychol* 19:251-281, 1989.

Newton B: Tough love: help for parents with troubled teenagers—reorganizing the hierarchy in disorganized families, *Pediatrics* 76:691-694, 1985.

Nichols M: *The self in the system,* New York, 1987, Bruner/Mazel.

Offer D, Schonert-Reichl K: Debunking the myths of adolescence: findings from recent research, *J Am Acad Child Adolesc Psychiatry* 31(6):1003-1014, 1992.

Peterson CC, Peterson JL: Children and cigarettes: the effect of a model who quits, *J Appl Dev Psychol* 7:293-306, 1986.

Pieper MH, Pieper WJ: It's not tough, it's tender love: problem teens need compassion that the "tough-love" approach to childrearing doesn't offer them, *Child-Welfare* 71:369-377, 1992.

Pierce JP and others: Trends in cigarette smoking in the United States, *JAMA* 261:61-65, 1989.

Pipes PL, Trahms CM: *Nutrition in infancy and childhood,* ed 5, St Louis, 1993, Mosby.

Remafedi G, Farrow JA, Deisher RW: Risk factors for attempted suicide in gay and bisexual youth, *Pediatrics* 87:869-875, 1991.

Resnick MD, Harris L, Blum RW: The impact of caring and connectedness on adolescent health and well-being, *J Pediatr Child Health,* 295:15-95, 1993.

Rutter M: Psychosocial resilience and protective mechanisms, *Am J Orthopsychiatry* 57(3):316-331, 1987.

School policies and programs on smoking and health—United States, 1988, *MMWR* 38:202-203, 1989.

Schuckit MA: Biological vulnerability to alcoholism, *J Consult Clin Psychol* 55:301-309, 1987.

Schwartz RH and others: Drinking patterns and social consequences: a study of middle-class adolescents in two private pediatric practices, *Pediatrics* 77:139-143, 1986.

Silvis GL, Perry CL: Understanding and deterring tobacco use among adolescents, *Pediatr Clin North Am* 34:363-379, 1987.

Spirito A and others: Adolescent suicide attempts: outcomes at followup, *Am J Orthopsychiatry* 62:464-468, 1992.

Strunkard AJ and others: An adoption study of human obesity, *N Engl J Med* 314:193-198, 1986.

Taitz LS: *The obese child,* Boston, 1983, Blackwell Scientific Publications.

Tarr JE, Macklin M: Cocaine, *Pediatr Clin North Am* 34:319-331, 1987.

Toner BB: Long-term follow-up of anorexia nervosa, *Psychosom Med* 48:520-529, 1986.

US Congress, Office of Technology Assessment: *Indian adolescent mental health,* Washington, DC, 1989. US Government Printing Office.

US Congress, Office of Technology Assessment: *Adolescent health,* vol 2, *Background and the effectiveness of selected prevention and treatment services:* OTA-H-466, Washington, DC, 1991, US Government Printing Office.

US Department of Health and Human Services: *Preventing tobacco use among young people: a report of the surgeon general,* Atlanta, 1994, US Department of Health and Human Services, Public Health Service, Centers for Disease Control and Prevention, National Center for Chronic Disease Prevention and Health Promotion, Office on Smoking and Health.

US Department of Health and Human Services: Report of the Secretary's Task Force on Youth Suicide, vol 3, *Prevention and interventions in youth suicide,* Rockville, MD, 1989, US Department of Health and Human Services.

UK Department of Health: *Effect of tobacco advertising on tobacco consumption: a discussion document reviewing the evidence,* London, 1992, UK Department of Health, Economics and Operational Research Division.

Van Itallie TB: Bad news and good news about obesity, *N Engl J Med* 314:239-240, 1986.

Williams JF, Friedman IM, Steiner H: Hand lesions characteristic of bulimia, *Am J Dis Child* 140:28-29, 1986.

Winters KC, Henly GA: *The Personal Experience Inventory test and user's manual,* Los Angeles, 1989, Western Psychological Services.

Zimmerman J: Adolescent suicide: an analysis using Erikson's developmental framework, *Wis Med J,* 91(7):351-357, July 1992.

BIBLIOGRAPHY

General

Baumrind D: *Why adolescents take chances—and why they don't,* Paper presented at the National Institute for Child Health and Human Development, Bethesda, MD, Oct 1983.

Brophy J, Good TL: Teacher behavior and student achievement. In Wittrock MC, editor: Handbook of research on teaching, New York, 1986, MacMillan.

Jessor R, Jessor SL: *Problem behavior and psychosocial development: a longitudinal study of youth,* San Diego, CA, 1977, Academic Press.

Kandel DB, Andrews K: Processes of adolescent socialization by parents and peers, *Int J Addict* 22:319-342, 1987.

Obesity

Becque MD and others: Coronary risk incidence of obese adolescents: reduction by exercise plus diet intervention, *Pediatrics* 81:605-612, 1988.

Bray GA: Obesity: a blueprint for progress, *Contemp Nutr* 12(7), 1987.

Castiglia PT: Obesity in adolescence, *J Pediatr Health Care* 3:221-223, 1989.

Desmond S and others: Black and white adolescent's perceptions of their weight, *J Sch Health* 59(8):353-358, 1989.

Dietz WH Jr: Prevention of childhood obesity, *Pediatr Clin North Am* 33:823-833, 1986.

Dietz WH Jr: The overweight child: psychosocial effects and treatment, *Feelings* 31(1):1-4, 1989.

Dietz WH Jr, Gortmaker SL: Do we fatten our children at the television set? Obesity and television viewing in children and adolescents, *Pediatrics* 75:807-812, 1985.

Dwyer J: Child nutrition. In Sharbaugh C, editor: *Call to action: better nutrition for mothers, children and families,* Washington, DC, 1990, National Center for Education in Maternal and Child Health.

Garrow JS: Treatment of obesity, *Lancet* 340(8816):409-413, 1992.

Kaplan KM: Obesity in children, *Child Care Newslett* 5(2):1-3, 1986.

Klesges RC and others: Accuracy of self-reports of food intake in obese and normal-weight individuals: effects of parental obesity on reports of children's dietary intake, *Am J Clin Nutr* 48:1252-1256, 1988.

Mahan LK: Family-focused behavioral approach to weight control in children, *Pediatr Clin North Am* 34:983-996, 1987.

Mallory GB, Fiser DH, Jackson R: Sleep-associated breathing disorders in morbidly obese children and adolescents, *J Pediatr* 115:892-897.

Mellin LM: Adolescent obesity, *Contemp Nutr* 12(8), 1987.

Mendelson BK, White DR: Development of self-body-esteem in overweight youngsters, *Dev Psychol* 21:90-96, 1985.

Mogan J: Prevention of childhood obesity, *Issues Compr Pediatr Nurs* 9:33-38, 1986.

Moore DC: Body image and eating behavior in adolescent boys, *Am J Dis Child* 144:475-479, 1990.

Poissonnet CM, LaVelle M, Burdi AR: Growth and development of adipose tissue, *J Pediatr* 113:1-9, 1988.

Ravussin E, Swinburn BA: Pathophysiology of obesity, *Sci Pract* 340(8816):404-413, 1992.

Rocchini AP and others: Blood pressure in obese adolescents: effect of weight loss, *Pediatrics* 82:16-23, 1988.

Rosenbaum M, Leibel RL: Pathophysiology of childhood obesity, *Adv Pediatr* 35:73-138, 1988.

Serdula M and others: Do obese children become obese adults? A review of the literature, *Prev Med* 22:167-177, 1993.

Story M, Heald F, Dwyer J: Adolescent nutrition: trends and critical issues for the 1990s. In Sharbaugh C, editor: *Call to action: better nutrition for mothers, children and families,* Washington, DC, 1990, National Center for Education in Maternal and Child Health.

Story M and others: Demographic and risk factors associated with chronic dieting in adolescents, *Am J Dis Child* 145:994-998, 1991.

Stunkard AJ and others: The body-mass index of twins who have been reared apart, *N Engl J Med* 322:1483-1487, 1990.

Wadden TA and others: Obesity in black adolescent girls: a controlled clinical trial of treatment by diet, behavior modification, and parental support, *Pediatrics* 85:345-352, 1990.

Eating Disorders/Anorexia Nervosa and Bulimia

Abrams SA and others: Mineral balance and bone turnover in adolescents with anorexia nervosa, *J Pediatr* 123(2):326-331, 1993.

Arden MR and others: Alkaline urine is associated with eating disorders, *Am J Dis Child* 145:28-30, 1991.

Bachrach LK and others: Decreased bone density in adolescent girls with anorexia nervosa, *Pediatrics* 86:440-447, 1990.

Block PJ: Working with anorexic and bulimic adolescents, *Food Nutr News* 56:33-34, 1984.

Castiglia PT: Anorexia nervosa, *J Pediatr Health Care* 3:105-107, 1989.

Castiglia PT: Bulimia, *J Pediatr Health Care* 3:167-169, 1989.

Danziger Y and others: Parental involvement in treatment of patients with anorexia nervosa in a pediatric day-care unit, *Pediatrics* 81:159-162, 1988.

Drewnowski A, Hopkins S, Kessler R: The prevalence of bulimia nervosa in the U.S. college student population, *Am J Public Health* 78:1322-1325, 1988.

Epling WF, Pierce WD: Activity based anorexia, *Int J Eat Dis* 7:475-485, 1988.

Fallon A: Standards of attractiveness: their relationship toward body image perceptions and eating disorders, *Food Nutr News* 59(5):79-80, 1987.

Ferraro AR: Bulimia: a look from within, *Pediatr Nurs* 16:187-191, 1990.

Flood M: Addictive eating disorders, *Nurs Clin North Am* 24:65-69, 1989.

Garner D: Pathogenesis of anorexia nervosa, *Lancet* 431:1631-1634, 1993.

Garner DM, Garfinkel PE: *Handbook of psychotherapy for anorexia nervosa,* New York, 1985, Guilford Press.

Goodwin RA, Mickalide AD: Parent-to-parent support in anorexia nervosa and bulimia, *Child Health Care* 14:32-37, 1985.

Harding SE: Anorexia nervosa, *Pediatr Nurs* 11:275-277, 1985.

Hayes D, Ross CE: Concern with appearance, health beliefs, and eating habits, *J Health Soc Behav* 28:120-130, 1987.

Humphrey LL: Observed family interactions among subtypes of eating disorders using structural analysis of social behavior, *J Consult Clin Psychol* 57:206-214, 1989.

Inbody DR, Ellis JJ: Group therapy with anorexic and bulimic patients: implications for therapeutic intervention, *Am J Psychother* 39:411-420, 1985.

Kreipe RE, Forbes GB: Osteoporosis: a "new morbidity" for dieting female adolescents, *Pediatrics* 86:478-480, 1990.

Lakin JA, McClelland E: Binge eating and bulimic behaviors in a school-age population, *J Community Health Nurs* 4:143-164, 1987.

Litt IF, Glader L: Anorexia nervosa, athletics, and amenorrhea, *J Pediatr* 109:150-153, 1986.

Lowe MR, Caputo GD: Binge eating in obesity: toward the specification of predictors, *Int J Eat Dis* 10:49-55, 1991.

Lucas AR: Update and review of anorexia nervosa, *Contemp Nutr* 14(9), 1989.

Mansfield MJ, Emans SJ: Anorexia nervosa, athletics and amenorrhea, *Pediatr Clin North Am* 36:533-549, 1989.

Mitchell JE: Bulimia nervosa, *Contemp Nutr* 14(10), 1989.

Muscari ME: Identification and management of the early anorectic child, *J Pediatr Health Care* 1:196-203, 1987.

Muscari ME: Effective nursing strategies for adolescents with anorexia nervosa and bulimia nervosa, *Pediatr Nurs* 14:475-482, 1988.

Oppliger RA and others: Bulimic behaviors among interscholastic wrestlers: a statewide survey, *Pediatrics* 91(4):826-831, 1993.

Palla B, Litt IF: Medical complications of eating disorders in adolescents, *Pediatrics* 81:613-623, 1988.

Potts N: The secret pattern of binge/purge, *Am J Nurs* 84:32-35, 1984.

Rees JM: Eating disorders. In Mahan LK, Rees JM: *Nutrition in adolescence,* St Louis, 1984, Mosby.

Rigotti NA and others: The clinical course of osteoporosis in anorexia nervosa: a longitudinal study of cortical bone mass, *JAMA* 265:1133-1138, 1991.

Sanger E, Cassino T: Eating disorders—avoiding the power struggle, *Am J Nurs* 84:31-35, 1984.

Sciacca JP and others: Body mass index and perceived weight status in young adults, *Community Health* 16(3):159-168, 1991.

Shisslak C: Primary prevention of eating disorders, *J Consult Clin Psychol* 55:660-667, 1987.

Silber TJ and others: Prevalence of PCP use among adolescent marijuana users, *J Pediatr* 112:827-829, 1988.

Twiss JJ: The plight of a female adolescent—anorexia or bulimia: an overview, *Issues Compr Pediatr Nurs* 9:289-298, 1986.

Yates A: Current perspectives on the eating disorders. I. History, psychological and biological aspects, *J Am Acad Child Adolesc Psychiatry* 6:813-828, 1989.

Tobacco

Allen KF and others: Teenage tobacco use: data estimates from the Teenage Attitudes and Practices Survey, United States, 1989, Advance data from vital and health statistics, No 224, Hyattsville, MD, 1992, National Center for Health Statistics.

Altman DG and others: Reducing the illegal sale of cigarettes to minors, *JAMA* 261:80-83, 1989.

American Academy of Pediatrics, Committee on Adolescence: Tobacco use by children and adolescents, *Pediatrics* 79:479-481, 1987.

American Academy of Pediatrics, Committee on Substance Abuse: "Smokeless cigarettes" and other nicotine delivery devices, *Pediatrics* 87(3):410-411, 1991.

Goldstein AO and others: Relationship between high school student smoking and recognition of cigarette advertisements, *J Pediatr* 110:488-491, 1987.

Gottlieb A and others: Patterns of smokeless tobacco use by young adolescents, *Pediatrics* 91(1):75-78, 1993.

Haukkala A and others: Social inoculation against cigarette advertisements in a culture allowing cigarette advertising and in another banning it, *Fam Community Health* 17(1):13-18, 1994.

Jones R and others: The head start parent involvement program as a vehicle for smoking reduction intervention, *Fam Community Health* 17(1):1-12, 1994.

Karle H and others: Tobacco control for high-risk youth: tracking and evaluation issues, *Fam Community Health* 16(4):10-17, 1994.

Macdonald DI: Prevention of adolescent smoking and drug use, *Pediatr Clin North Am* 33:995-1005, 1986.

McMahon A, Maibusch RM: How to send quit-smoking signals, *Am J Nurs* 88:1498-1499, 1988.

Moss AJ: *Recent trends in adolescent smoking, smoking-uptake correlates, and expectations about the future,* Advance data from vital and health statistics, No 221, Hyattsville, MD, National Center for Health Statistics, 1992.

Myers MG, Brown SA: Smoking and health in substance-abusing adolescents: a two-year follow-up, *Pediatrics* 93(4):561-566, 1994.

Parkham DL and others: Adoption of health education-tobacco use prevention curricula in North Carolina school districts, *Fam Community Health* 16(3):56-57, 1993.

Pierce JP, Lee L, Gilpin EA: Smoking initiation by adolescent girls, 1944 through 1988: an association with targeted advertising, *JAMA* 271(8):569-636, 1994.

Selected tobacco-use behaviors and dietary patterns among high school students, *MMWR* 41(24):417-421, 1992.

Tonnesen P and others: Effect of nicotine chewing gum in combination with group counseling on the cessation of smoking, *N Engl J Med* 318:15-18, 1988.

Winklestein M: Adolescent smoking: influential factors, past preventive efforts, and future nursing implications, *Pediatr Nurs* 7(2):120-127, 1991.

Alcohol

American Academy of Pediatrics, Committee on Adolescence: Alcohol use and abuse: a pediatric concern, *Pediatrics* 79:450-453, 1987.

Barnes GM, Farrell MP, Cairns A: Parental socialization factors and adolescent drinking behaviors, *J Marriage Fam* 8:27-36, 1986.

Casswell S and others: What children know about alcohol and how they know it, *Br J Addict* 3:223-227, 1988.

Castiglia PT and others: Influences on children's attitudes toward alcohol consumption, *Pediatr Nurs* 15:263-266, 1989.

Felter R, Izsak E, Lawrence HS: Emergency department management of the intoxicated adolescent, *Pediatr Clin North Am* 34:399-421, 1987.

Killen JD: Evidence for an alcohol-stress link among normal weight adolescents reporting purging behavior, *Int J Eating Disorders* 6:349-356, 1987.

Kiltzner M and others: Screening for risk factors for adolescent alcohol and drug use, *Am J Dis Child* 141:45-49, 1987.

Lovato CY and others: Cigarette and alcohol use among migrant Hispanic adolescents, *Fam Community Health* 16(4):18-31, 1994.

Macdonald DI: How you can help prevent teenage alcoholism, *Contemp Pediatr* 3(11):50-72, 1986.

Macdonald DI: Patterns of alcohol and drug use among adolescents, *Pediatr Clin North Am* 34:275-288, 1987.

Petchers MK, Singer MI: Perceived-benefit-of-drinking scale: approach to screening for adolescent alcohol abuse, *J Pediatr* 110:977-981, 1987.

Rich J: Action stat! Acute alcohol intoxication, *Nursing 89* 19(9):33, 1989.

Rogers PD, Harris J, Jarmuskewicz J: Alcohol and adolescence, *Pediatr Clin North Am* 34:289-303, 1987.

Schuckit MA: Genetics and the risk of alcoholism, *JAMA* 254:2614-2617, 1985.

Shannon M and others: Cocaine exposure among children seen at a pediatric hospital, *Pediatrics* 83:337-342, 1989.

Smith DE, Schwartz RH, Martin DM: Heavy cocaine use by adolescents, *Pediatrics* 83:539-542, 1989.

Cocaine

Acee AM, Smith D: Crack, *Am J Nurs* 87:614-617, 1987.

Bateman DA, Heagarty MC: Passive freebase cocaine ("crack") inhalation by infants and toddlers, *Am J Dis Child* 143:25-27, 1989.

Brown BS and others: Kids and cocaine—a treatment dilemma, *J Subst Abuse Treat* 6:3-8, 1989.

Clouet D, Asghar K, Brown R, editors: *Mechanisms of cocaine abuse and toxicity,* NIDA Research Monograph 88, Washington, DC, 1988, US Government Printing Office.

Estroff TW, Schwartz RH, Hoffmann NG: Adolescent cocaine abuse, *Clin Pediatr* 28:550-555, 1989.

Farrar HC, Kearns GL: Cocaine: clinical pharmacology and toxicology, *J Pediatr* 115:665-675, 1989.

Heagarty MC: Crack cocaine: a new danger for children, *Am J Dis Child* 14:756-757, 1990.

Mofenson HC, Caraccio TR: Cocaine, *Pediatr Ann* 16:864-874, 1987.

Mofenson HC, Copeland P, Caraccio TR: Cocaine and crack: the latest menace, *Contemp Pediatr* 3(10):44-50, 1986.

Substance Abuse: Additional Drugs

Alderman EM, Schonberg SK, Cohen MI: The pediatrician's role in the diagnosis and treatment of substance abuse, *Pediatrics Rev* 13(8):314-318, 1992.

American Academy of Pediatrics, Committee on Adolescence, Committee on Bioethics, and Provisional Committee on Substance Abuse: Screening for drugs of abuse in children and adolescents, *Pediatrics* 84:396-398, 1989.

American Academy of Pediatrics, Committee on Substance Abuse: Role of the pediatrician in prevention and management of substance abuse, *Pediatrics* 91(5):1010-1013, 1993.

Anglin TM: Interviewing guidelines for the clinical evaluation of adolescent substance abuse, *Pediatr Clin North Am* 34:381-398, 1987.

Bertino JS, Reed MD: Barbiturate and nonbarbiturate sedative hypnotic intoxication in children, *Pediatr Clin North Am* 33:703-722, 1986.

Bloch J, Bloch JH, Keyes S: Longitudinally foretelling drug usage in adolescence: early childhood personality and environmental precursors, *Child Dev* 59:336-355, 1988.

Blum RW: Adolescent substance abuse: diagnostic and treatment issues, *Pediatr Clin North Am* 34:523-537, 1987.

Brown RT, Braden NJ: Hallucinogens, *Pediatr Clin North Am* 34:341-347, 1987.

Burpo RH: A step beyond "just say no," *MCN* 13:428-431, 1988.

Coulehan JL and others: Gasoline sniffing and lead toxicity in Navajo adolescents, *Pediatrics* 71:113-117, 1983.

DuPont RL: Teenage drug use: opportunities for the pediatrician, *J Pediatr* 102:1003-1007, 1983.

DuPont RL: Prevention of adolescent chemical dependency, *Pediatr Clin North Am* 34:495-505, 1987.

DuPont RL, Saylor KE: Depressant substance in adolescent medicine, *Pediatr Rev* 13(10):381-386, 1992.

DuRant RH and others: Use of multiple drugs among adolescents who use anabolic steroids, *N Engl J Med* 328(13):922-926, 1993.

Farrow JA, Rees JM, Worthington-Roberts BS: Health, developmental, and nutritional status of adolescent alcohol and marijuana abusers, *Pediatrics* 79:218-223, 1987.

Golb CS: Substance abuse: what turns casual use into chronic dependence? *Contemp Pediatr* 3(10):26-41, 1986.

Hahn E, Papazian K: Substance abuse prevention with preschool children, *J Community Health Nurs* 4:165-170, 1987.

Hoffmann NG, Sonis WA, Halikas JA: Issues in the evaluation of chemical dependency treatment programs for adolescents, *Pediatr Clin North Am* 34:449-459, 1987.

Huberty DJ and others: Family issues in working with chemically dependent adolescents, *Pediatr Clin North Am* 34:507-521, 1987.

Joshi NP, Scott M: Drug use, depression, and adolescents, *Pediatr Clin North Am* 34:1349-1364, 1987.

King NMP, Cross AW: Moral and legal issues in screening for drug use in adolescents, *J Pediatr* 111:249-250, 1987.

Klitzner M and others: *Substance abuse: early intervention for adolescents,* Princeton, NJ, 1993, The Robert Wood Johnson Foundation.

Kulberg A: Substance abuse: clinical identification and management, *Pediatr Clin North Am* 33:325-361, 1986.

Macdonald DI: Just say no, *J Pediatr* 114:673-675, 1989.

McHugh MJ: The abuse of volatile substances, *Pediatr Clin North Am* 34:333-340, 1987.

Morrison MA, Smith QT: Psychiatric issues of adolescent chemical dependence, *Pediatr Clin North Am* 34:461-480, 1987.

Murray S, Brewerton T: Abuse of over-the-counter dextromethorphan by teenagers, *South Med J* 86(10):1151-1153, 1993.

Muscari ME: The "acting-out" adolescent: identification and management, *Pediatr Nurs* 18(4):362-366, 1992.

Richardson JL: Relationship between after-school care of adolescents and substance use, risk taking, depressed mood, and academic achievement, *Pediatrics* 92(1):35-38, 1993.

Richardson JL and others: Substance use among eighth-grade students who take care of themselves after school, *Pediatrics* 84:556-566, 1989.

Robinson DP, Green JW: The adolescent alcohol and drug problem: a practical approach, *Pediatr Nurs* 14:305-310, 1988.

Schwartz RH: Are you ready to deal with the pot-smoking patient? *Contemp Pediatr* 4(4): 84-106, 1987.

Schwartz RH: Marijuana: an overview, *Pediatr Clin North Am* 34:305-317, 1987.

Schwartz RH, Comerci GD, Meeks JE: LSD: patterns of use by chemically dependent adolescents, *J Pediatr* 111:936-938, 1987.

Schwartz RH and others: Short-term memory impairment in cannabis-dependent adolescents, *Am J Dis Child* 143:1214-1219, 1989.

Strasburger VC: Prevention of adolescent drug abuse: why "just say no" just won't work, *J Pediatr* 114:676-681, 1989.

Swaim RC and others: Links from emotional distress to adolescent drug use: a path model, *J Consult Clin Psychol* 57:227-231, 1989.

Wheeler K, Malmquist J: Treatment approaches in adolescent chemical dependency, *Pediatr Clin North Am* 34:437-447, 1987.

Zarek D, Hawkins JD, Rogers PD: Risk factors for adolescent substance abuse, *Pediatr Clin North Am* 34:481-493, 1987.

Suicide

American Academy of Pediatrics, Committee on Adolescence: Suicide and suicide attempts in adolescents and young adults, *Pediatrics* 81:322-324, 1988.

Bakkala CF: The role of the school nurse in suicide prevention, *Sch Nurse* 6(1):13-15, 1990.

Baron P, Joly E: Sex differences in the expression of depression in adolescents, *Sex Roles* 18:1-7, 1988.

Berman AL, Schwartz RH: Suicide attempts among adolescent drug users, *Am J Dis Child* 144:310-314, 1990.

Brent DA and others: Firearms and adolescent suicide: a community case-control study, *Am J Dis Child* 147:1066-1071, 1993.

Christoffel KK and others: Adolescent suicide and suicide attempts: a population study, *Pediatr Emerg Care* 4:32-40, 1988.

Conrad N: Stress and knowledge of suicidal others as factors in suicidal behavior of high school adolescents, *Ment Health Nurs* 13:95-104, 1992.

Garrison CZ and others: Aggression, substance use, and suicidal behaviors in high school students, *Public Health* 83(2):179-184, 1993.

Gemma PB: Coping with suicidal behavior, *MCN* 14:101-103, 1989.

Gould MS, Shaffer D: The impact of suicide in television: evidence of imitation, *N Engl J Med* 315:690-694, 1986.

Gyulay JE: What suicide leaves behind, *Issues Compr Pediatr Nurs* 12:103-118, 1989.

Hergenroeder AC and others: The pediatrician's role in adolescent suicide, *Pediatr Ann* 15:787-798, 1986.

Hoffman Y: Surviving a child's suicide, *Am J Nurs* 87:955-956, 1987.

Kaminer Y, Robbins DR: Attempted suicide by insulin overdose in insulin-dependent diabetic adolescents, *Pediatrics* 81:526-528, 1988.

Kellermann AL: Suicide in the home in relation to gun ownership, *N Engl J Med* 327(7):467-472, 1992.

Mitchell K: Suicide: a preventable tragedy, *Pediatr Nurs* 11:165, 1985.

Muscari ME: Adolescent suicide attempts by acetaminophen ingestion, *MCN* 12:32-35, 1987.

Ostroff RB and others: Adolescent suicides modeled after television movies, *Am J Psychiatry* 142:989-1004, 1985.

Pfeffer CR: *The suicidal child,* New York, 1987, Atcom.

Pfeffer CR: Spotting the red flags for adolescent suicide, *Contemp Pediatr* 6(2):59-70, 1989.

Phillips DP, Carstensen LL: Clustering of teenage suicides after television news stories about suicide, *N Engl J Med* 315:685-689, 1986.

Rankin WW: Teenage suicide, *J Pediatr Nurs* 4:130-131, 1989.

Raskind SM: Suicide by burning: emotional needs of the suicidal adolescent on the burn unit, *Issues Compr Pediatr Nurs* 9:369-382, 1986.

Slap GB and others: Risk factors for attempted suicide during adolescence, *Pediatrics* 84: 762-772, 1989.

Smith JC, Mercy J, Rosenberg ML: Suicide and homicide among Hispanics in the Southwest, *Public Health Rep* 101(3):265-270, 1986.

Spotting the suicidal adolescent, *Emerg Med* 24(12):155-169, 1992.

Stivers C: Parent-adolescent communication and its relationship to adolescent depression and suicide proneness, *Adolescence* 23:291-295, 1988.

Valente SM: Assessing suicide risk in the school-age child, *J Pediatr Health Care* 1:14-20, 1987.

Velez CN, Cohen P: Suicidal behavior and ideation in a community sample of children: maternal and youth reports, *J Acad Child Adolesc Psychiatry* 27:349-356, 1988.

Winokur G, Black DW: Suicide—what can be done? *N Engl J Med* 327(7):490-491, 1992.

Young MJ: Two stories of adolescent suicide, *Clin Nurse Spec* 6(1):51-52, 1992.

UNIT VIII

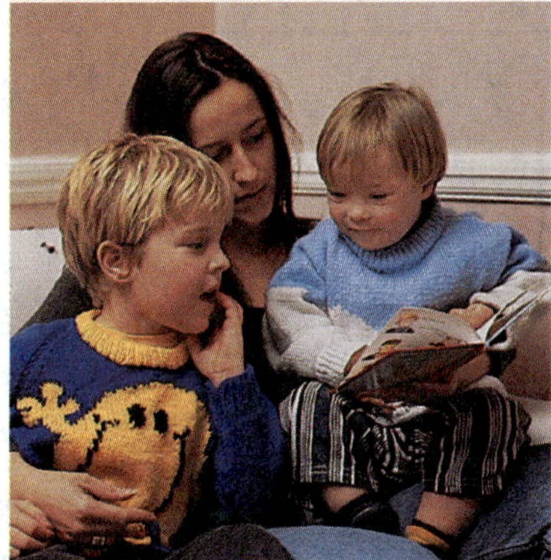

FAMILY-CENTERED CARE OF THE CHILD WITH SPECIAL NEEDS

CHAPTER 22 Family-Centered Care of the Child with Chronic Illness or Disability

CHAPTER OUTLINE

RELATED TOPICS

PERSPECTIVES IN THE CARE OF CHILDREN WITH SPECIAL NEEDS

SCOPE OF THE PROBLEM

Despite the interest and concern for children with special needs, exact definitions and incidence rates of chronic illness and disability do not exist. For the purposes of this chapter, see the definitions listed in the box at right. Statistics regarding chronic illness and disability are at best only estimates of the true prevalence of the problem and vary, depending on the definitions used, the methods of study, and the population investigated. In the United States an estimated 20% of children under 18 years of age experience mild chronic conditions, 9% experience chronic conditions of moderate severity, and 2% experience severe chronic conditions (Newacheck, Stoddard, and McManus, 1993; Newacheck and Taylor, 1992). Cancer and mental health problems without physical manifestations are not included in these figures. Two thirds of all cases of chronic illness are attributable to asthma and congenital heart defects; however, in terms of mortality, congenital heart defects and cancer are among the most lethal.

Survival rates affect the prevalence of chronic illness. While there has been little recent change in the survival patterns for certain chronic conditions, such as asthma or muscular dystrophy, other diseases have seen dramatic improvements in survival rates. Children with leukemia, Hodgkin disease, and other cancers have markedly improved survival rates. The median life expectancy for a child with cystic fibrosis has increased from 5 years of age in 1955 to 27 years today (Cystic Fibrosis Foundation, 1990). The most dramatic progress, however, has occurred in the treatment of spina bifida. In 1955, 90% of children born with spina bifida died in infancy; today, 90% to 95% survive infancy and have a normal life expectancy if they receive timely and appropriate medical intervention (Spina Bifida Association, 1990). In addition, technologic advances over the past several decades have resulted in increased survival rates of extremely premature infants and full-term low-birth-weight and very-low-birth-weight infants (≤1500 g) infants. The resulting progress for these children at risk contributes to the growing number of children with chronic and/or disabling conditions, many of whom remain dependent on technology.

Broadly expanding chronic conditions to include speech, learning, emotional, sensory, and cognitive disorders yields an even greater number of children who have a significant long-term condition. The vast majority of children with chronic illness or disability live at home with their families. Considering that the average American family has between three and four members, the number of individuals intimately affected by these children's illnesses and disabilities is staggering.

The impact of chronic illness and disability in children is wide-ranging. A child's activity level and developmental opportunities can be affected. Days can be lost from school.

■ Elizabeth Ahmann, RN, ScD, and Judy Holt Rollins, RN, MS, revised this chapter.

KEY TERMS REGARDING CHILDREN WITH SPECIAL HEALTH CARE NEEDS

Chronic illness—A condition that interferes with daily functioning for more than 3 months in a year, causes hospitalization of more than 1 month in a year, or (at time of diagnosis) is likely to do either of these

Congenital disability—A disability that has existed since birth but is not necessarily hereditary

Developmental delay—A maturational lag—an abnormal, slower rate of development in which a child demonstrates a functioning level below that observed in normal children of the same age

Developmental disability—Any mental and/or physical disability that is manifested before age 22 years and is likely to continue indefinitely

Disability—A functional limitation that interferes with a person's ability, for example, to walk, lift, hear, or learn

Handicap—A condition or barrier imposed by society, the environment, or one's own self; not a synonym for disability

Impairment—A loss or abnormality of structure or function

Technology-dependent child—A child between the ages of birth and 21 years with a chronic disability that requires the routine use of a medical device to compensate for the loss of a life-sustaining bodily function; daily ongoing care and/or monitoring is required by trained personnel

Modified from Research and Training Center on Independent Living (RTC/IL): *Guidelines for reporting and writing about people with disabilities,* ed 3, Lawrence, KS, 1990; Hobbs N, Perrin J, editors: *Issues in the care of children with chronic illness,* San Francisco, 1985, Jossey-Bass; and *Report to Congress and the Secretary by the Task Force on Technology Dependent Children: Fostering home and community-based care for technology-dependent children,* vol 2, US Department of Health and Human Services, Health Care Financing Administration, HCFA Pub No 88-02171, 1988.

Children with chronic illness or disability may be at an increased risk for behavior or emotional problems (Newacheck, McManus, and Fox, 1991; Patterson and Geber, 1991).

Parents may lose days from work, experience financial strain, and be challenged both emotionally and physically as they cope with care of the child. Siblings are affected, as can be extended family members.

The number of children and family members affected, as well as the range of effects, suggests that comprehensive nursing approaches are required to meet the needs of children, youth, and families. Clearly, nurses have a more crucial role than ever before in early screening, case finding, assessment, and diagnostic studies, as well as educational and supportive interventions that help families to cope adaptively and minimize the disruptive effects of the child's condition on both the child and the family. Another major responsibility is preventing disabling disorders by eliminating their known causes. Nurses are responsible for ensuring immunization programs, identifying infants and mothers who may be at risk prenatally or postnatally, identifying the disability early, promoting injury prevention policies and programs, and implementing innovative health education programs.

CHANGING TRENDS IN CARE

Several changes have occurred in providing services to children with special needs. Current emphasis is placed on a "noncategoric" approach, which avoids classifying needs and services by medical diagnoses, since most psychosocial and developmental needs of children with chronic conditions are not disease specific (Jones-Hessop and Stein, 1985). Influenced by technologic advances, economic considerations, and the need for more meaningful models of care, changes not only reflect the kinds of care and services children receive, but also indicate shifts in who provides that care and where services are provided.

Developmental Focus

Using a developmental approach rather than chronologic age emphasizes the child's abilities and strengths rather than disabilities. In the past, health professionals have viewed persons with a disability within a pathologic framework, probing for weaknesses and negative features. While much attention has been given to the technologic aspects of the child's care and health needs, less attention has been paid to the child's individuality, personality, or strengths; the family's needs; and the overall concerns of those who interact with these children. With use of the developmental model, attention is directed to the child's functional development, changes, and adaptation to the environment. Nurses often are in vital positions to redirect attention from the pathologic to the developmental model to meet the unique needs of the child and family.

Family Development

A developmental focus also considers family development. Duvall (1977) defined a model of family development based on the changing ages and developmental needs of both children and adults, as well as on the changing demands by external forces and crises as the family matures. Families are challenged to achieve specific developmental tasks at various stages in the family life cycle (e.g., leaving one's parents and forming a new relationship during the couple stage; accepting the influence of others on children's behavior during the school-age stage; refocusing on the marital role when children leave home) from the couple's courtship through their parenting years and into retirement (Carney, 1987). A family member's serious illness or disability can cause significant stress or crisis at any stage of the cycle. Just as with individual development, family development may be interrupted or even regress to an earlier level of functioning. Nurses can use the concept of family development to plan meaningful interventions and evaluate care (see Developmental Theory, Chapter 3).

Family-Centered Care

The importance of family-centered care—a philosophy that considers the family as the constant in the child's life—is especially evident in the care of children with special needs (see also Family-Centered Care, Chapter 1). As parents learn about the youngster's health care needs, they often become experts in delivering care. Health care providers, including nurses, are adjuncts to the child's care and need to form partnerships with parents. Collaboration is essential to forming trusting and effective partnerships. Collaborative relationships are characterized by communication, dialogue, active listening, awareness, and acceptance of differences (Bishop, Woll, and Arango, 1993).

Communicating with Families. Families whose child is ill react along what health care providers may view as a continuum from the "good" to the "difficult" family stereotype. Nurses readily form relationships with the "good" family, who perceives staff as having power or control and accepts this hierarchy (Satariano and Briggs, 1989). However, this is often not the case with the "difficult" family, who is characterized as being underinvolved or overinvolved in the child's care. Dixon (1993) describes four patterns of involvement in parents' relationships with nurses. ***Limited-contact*** parents choose to have limited involvement with the hospitalized child and nursing staff. These parents do not initiate relationships with nurses and are difficult to engage in decision making. ***Recipients of care*** believe nurses both know what is best for the child and should be in control. Their level of trust in professionals is very high, whereas their level of need for information is low. Parents who are ***monitors of care*** keep track of the performance of all hospital staff, seek care from nurses, and request detailed information. Finally, ***managers of care*** are in control of health-related decisions and use nurses for direct care and consultation. They are frequently involved in providing technologically complex care to their chronically ill child.

Nurses also exhibit patterns of behavior with respect to parents of ill children. First, facilitative nurses recognize the parent's roles with their child and try to remove barriers to their participation. Second, nurses who seek a high degree of control over their work may become "rule enforcers" with parents. Third, nurses may develop collegial relationships with parents over time, in which there is respect for the parents as experts concerning their child. Finally, nurses may avoid a parent whose values differ from their own or a parent who is overly demanding from the nurses' viewpoint.

The family and nurse come to share implicit and explicit expectations of one another, form views of one another, and negotiate roles regarding the child's care. Levels of control and trust are central to their interactions. The nurse who desires a high level of control will have very little difficulty with limited-contact or recipient-of-care parents but may experience conflict with monitor-of-care and manager-of-care parents, who also desire control. Parents who have a mistrust of professionals behave differently from those who have faith in the health care team. Nurses also trust parents differently, based on the judgment of the parenting they observe. Strategies for avoiding conflicts with families are described in Table 22-1. Care conferences, especially multidisciplinary meetings that include the family and key health professionals, provide an oppportunity for joint sharing of ideas and expression of feelings or concerns. Individual discussions, especially with the case manager, primary nurse, or clinical nurse specialist (advanced nurse practitioner), help establish a consistent and flexible plan of care that can prevent conflicts or deal with them before they become major issues. In family-centered care, the goal

TABLE 22-1 Strategies for Managing Parent-Nurse Interaction

PARENT CHARACTERISTICS	STRATEGIES
LIMITED CONTACT	
Have trust and mistrust	Do not force participation
May not accompany child; prefer to wait outside	Avoid authoritarian stance
Are very uncertain, quiet	Use simple terms and demystify surroundings
Use little verbal communication	Explain what will happen
Visit on limited or irregular basis	Point out how their presence helps child
RECIPIENT OF CARE	
Have total trust	Offer/provide information
Want nurse to make decisions	Allow unlimited contact with child
Offer numerous positive comments	Engage them in gaining child's cooperation
Are easily impressed with information	
Are prone to misunderstandings	
Comply with rules	
Focus on child while visiting	
MONITOR OF CARE	
Have high levels of mistrust	Believe that you can build trust
Have attitude that "mistakes can happen"	Negotiate, negotiate, negotiate!
Monitor everyone's performance	Be flexible regarding rules
Involved in all decisions	Avoid issues of control
Want high levels of information	Ask their opinion and use their suggestions
Know agency's hierarchy	
Seek care from nurses	
Ask for rule changes	
MANAGER OF CARE	
Are similar to Monitors, but less angry	Recognize them as experts about their child
Achieve complex coordination of child's chronic care	Recognize need for respite

Developed by Donna M. Dixon, Memorial Medical Center, Springfield, IL, 1993. Used with permission. Modified from Knafl KA, Cavallari KA, Dixon DM: *Pediatric hospitalization: family and nurse perspectives,* Glenview, IL, 1988, Scott, Foresman.

is to maintain the integrity of the family, empower family members to assume a leadership role, and support the family during stressful times (Baker, 1994).

Normalization

Normalization refers to establishing a normal pattern of living (see also Guidelines box on p. 957). It implies child and family access to services in as usual a fashion and environment as possible. Normalization permits the child and family to become or remain part of the community. Through application of the principles of normalization, the environment for the child is "normalized" and "humanized." The child and family live as normal a life as possible given the disability.

Home Care

Concurrent with the trend toward normalization has been the earlier discharge of children from acute or chronic care facilities to the family and community. ***Home care*** represents the return to a system and set of priorities in which family values are as important in the care of a child with a chronic health problem as they are in the care of other children. Home care seeks to achieve goals that are consistent with the developmental model (Stein, 1985):

1. Normalize the life of a child with special needs, including those with technologically complex care, in a family and community context and setting.
2. Minimize the disruptive impact of the child's condition on the family.
3. Foster the child's maximum growth and development.

With appropriate training and support, families today provide complex procedures and treatments in the home. Parents are challenged to retain a homelike setting among monitors, ventilators, and other sophisticated equipment. Throughout the text, home care is discussed as appropriate for specific conditions. Chapter 25 focuses on family-centered home care, and the process of transition from hospital to home is elaborated in Chapter 26.

Mainstreaming

Mainstreaming describes the process of integrating children with special needs into regular classrooms and child care centers. Just as the home is the natural environment for children, so school must also be included as an essential component of the child's overall physical, intellectual, and social development. Children who attend school have the advantages of learning and socializing with a wide group of peers. There is an increased focus on individualization as the academic needs of these children are planned along with those of the rest of the students. A variety of supplemental programs have been designed in the school system to accommodate special needs, thus providing these children with an equal educational opportunity. This change has largely resulted from the passage of Public Law 94-142, the Education for All Handicapped Children Act of 1975 (Downey, 1990). The 1990 amendments to the act (PL 101-476) changed its name to the Individuals with Disabilities Education Act (IDEA).

The 1975 law requires states to identify, diagnose, educate, and provide related services for children 5 to 18 years of age. The age range was extended in 1977 to include children between 3 and 21 years of age, with services for children between the ages of 3 and 5 remaining optional. Under the law, a multidisciplinary team designs an Individual Education Program (IEP), which contains specific educational and therapeutic strategies and goals for each eligible child. Parents may be involved in educational decisions and have the right to a hearing when the team's decision is viewed as inappropriate or harmful. Since many parents have little knowledge of this or other laws that establish rights for disabled children, nurses can provide an important service by informing them of the laws and where to obtain information.*

Early Intervention

Early intervention, or early childhood intervention, consists of any sustained and systematic effort to assist children from birth to age 3 years who are young, disabled, and developmentally vulnerable, as well as their families. Over the last 25 years much has been learned about service provision for very young at-risk children and children with disabilities and about how special services can support their development. Public Law 99-457, the Education of the Handicapped Act Amendments of 1986, made a giant step toward translating knowledge about early development into public policy. It directs states to develop and implement statewide comprehensive, coordinated, multidisciplinary interagency programs of early intervention services for infants and toddlers with disabilities, as well as their families.

A central component of the law's implementation is its focus on the family as a means of enhancing the child's development through the Individual Family Service Plan (IFSP). Developed jointly by families and professionals, the IFSP includes information about the infant/toddler's present level of development, family strengths and needs relating to enhancing development, major outcomes expected, services needed, identification of a case manager, and transition steps to preschool services.† All services and outcomes relate to the family's, as well as the child's, needs. The IFSP is a commitment to children and families that their strengths will be recognized and built on, that their needs will be met in a way that respects their beliefs and values, and that their hopes and aspirations will be encouraged and enabled.

Nurses have much to contribute to providing care for children covered by PL 99-457. Clinical skills and a traditional philosophy of family-focused care earn nurses a valuable place on interdisciplinary assessment and planning teams, often as case managers. Nurses can assess children in preschool settings, provide ongoing family and staff education, coordinate care with health care providers, develop health promotion programs for family and school staffs, and participate in community nursing networks (Hansen, Holaday, and Miles, 1990).

CULTURAL ISSUES

The United States does not have as clear a generalized culture as more homogeneous nations. For this reason, cultural competence is an important goal of nursing practice.

Issues of culture, ethnicity, and race affect health care services in a number of ways. Economic barriers are perhaps primary in access to care, but distribution of health care providers (particularly culturally competent providers), transportation difficulties, child care needs, and other factors also contribute (Newacheck, Stoddard, and McManus, 1993). Utilization may also be affected by the failure of health care providers to make the need for services understood in a context that is culturally relevant to the family. For example, Huber, Holditch-Davis, and Brandon (1993), in a study of a group of at-risk infants from low-income families, attribute a low rate of family follow-through on referrals for early intervention to parents simply not viewing their children as needing the services.

Groce and Zola (1993) point out that "many ethnic and minority populations, reflecting their own unique and longstanding cultural beliefs, practices, and support systems, do not define or address disability and chronic illness in the same manner as "mainstream" American culture (p. 1048)." As an example, Anderson (1986) has described problems faced by Chinese immigrants who did not share the dominant belief of Western health care providers in the "normalization" principles.

Communication can be a sensitive area. In some cultures families do not openly discuss certain topics. For this reason, some parents may simply feel uncomfortable participating in discussions about their child's condition (Munet-Vilaro and Vessey, 1990). Common health care terms may also be interpreted differently in different cultural groups. Patterson and Blum (1993) cite several examples, including the following:

- "Independent living" is espoused as a goal in the field of disabilities. The term may be interpreted as living alone, a goal that is culturally unacceptable to some groups.
- "Family support" may be interpreted by some families as implying that they are weak and in need of help.

While culture cannot completely explain how an individual will think and act, understanding cultural perspectives can help the nurse anticipate and understand why families may make certain decisions (Groce and Zola, 1993). Cultural attributes such as values and beliefs regarding illness or disability and its causation, social roles for the ill or disabled, family structure, the role of children, childrearing practices, self vs group orientation, spirituality, and time orientation also affect a family's response to illness or disability in a child.

Language issues aside, in working with people of other cultural backgrounds, nurses should place an emphasis on careful listening with an initial goal of understanding and articulating the family's perspective. The ability to interpret the mainstream medical culture to the family is also important (Stone and Hoffman, 1993). Furthermore, every effort should be made to incorporate traditional cultural beliefs of a family into treatment plans. Developing a plan of care in conjunction with the family, considering their preferences and priorities, is an important first step in formulating a plan of care that will best meet the family's needs, no matter what their cultural background (Ahmann, 1994).

*The *NICHCY New Digest,* vol 1, No 1, 1991, was entirely devoted to the topic "The Education of Children and Youth with Special Needs: What do the Laws Say?" (NICHCY, P.O. Box 1492, Washington, DC 20013.)

†The following resource is recommended for developing an IFSP: *Guidelines and Recommended Practices for the Individualized Family Service Plan* by B. Johnson, M. McGonigel, and R. Kaufmann, available from the Association for the Care of Children's Health, 7910 Woodmont Ave., Suite 300, Bethesda, MD 20814; (301) 654-6549.

THE CHILD AND FAMILY WITH SPECIAL NEEDS

REACTIONS OF FAMILIES TO A CHRONIC ILLNESS OR DISABILITY

When the diagnosis of a disability or chronic illness is made, the family progresses through a fairly predictable sequence of stages, regardless of the actual nature of the condition. Numerous investigators have studied families' responses and have postulated a number of "stages"; however, no one set of phases is universally accepted. The following discussion focuses on stages that are common to most families, with the exception of out-of-home placement. Not all families experience this process; persons may experience several "stages" simultaneously or may go back and forth between the stages; and each family member varies widely in the time needed to progress through any of the stages.

The nurse is cautioned to explore family reactions for all possible interpretations, not just negative ones. For example, too often a parent's angry reaction has been attributed to a stage of adjustment or a maladaptive reaction, rather than a rational response to, for instance, an insulting remark (Stone, 1989). Professionals are gradually replacing the past emphasis on the negative with a positive, more supportive stance in their interactions with families coping with the birth or diagnosis of a child with special needs.

Shock and Denial

The initial stage is a period of intense emotion and is characterized by shock, disbelief, and sometimes denial, especially if the disorder is not obvious, such as in chronic illness. Denial as a defense mechanism is a necessary cushion to prevent disintegration and is a normal response to grieving any type of loss. Probably all family members experience various degrees of adaptive denial as they learn of the impact that the diagnosis has on their lives. Denial becomes maladaptive when it prevents recognition of treatment or rehabilitative goals necessary for the child's optimum survival or development. For example, protracted denial may be seen in the response of a family to mental retardation; as long as the family can maintain a fiction of normality and handle the deviance within the present familial roles and values, there may exist no recognition of the diagnosis. Instead, the problem is explained as slow maturation or an easily remedied disorder. The denial may be enforced by the child's social development, which belies the degree of motor and speech retardation. Not infrequently, this ability to rationalize delayed development is successful until the child enters school and is compared with other children, making his or her differences blatantly evident. At this point the family may begin to recognize the diagnosis as a crisis and react with shock and disbelief.

Shock and denial can last from days to months, sometimes even longer. Examples of denial that may be exhibited at the time of diagnosis include (1) physician shopping, (2) attributing the symptoms of the actual illness to a minor condition, (3) refusal to believe the diagnostic tests, (4) delay in agreeing to treatment, (5) acting very happy and optimistic despite the revealed diagnosis, (6) refusing to tell or talk to anyone about the condition, (7) insisting that no one is telling the truth, regardless of others' attempts to do so, (8) denying the reason for admission, and (9) asking no questions about the diagnosis, treatment, or prognosis. Each of these mechanisms allows individuals to distance themselves from the onslaught of a tremendous emotional impact and to collect and mobilize their energies toward goal-directed, problem-solving behaviors.

In some instances, various indicators of denial can be viewed as adaptive. Searching for another professional opinion may mean that parents cannot obtain answers to their questions or that they are looking for a different approach to treatment that better meets the needs of their child and family. When parents discuss their strengths and the benefits they derive from caring for their child with special needs, it does not necessarily reflect refusal to accept their difficult circumstances. Sometimes delay in making decisions or failure to ask questions simply reflects a lack of information.

Partial denial, such as seeking additional professional consultations or occasionally acting as if nothing were wrong, is common for families with children who have life-threatening conditions. Without such a temporary protective mechanism, few people could survive the constant emotional drain of anticipating their own death or the death of a family member. Partial denial allows the child and family to absorb stressful information—or "dose" themselves—in amounts they can personally manage at the time.

Denial is probably the least understood and most poorly dealt with reaction. Health professionals typically label denial as "maladaptive" and actively attempt to strip it away by repeated and sometimes blunt explanations of prognosis.

Poor communication between parents and professionals can lead to misunderstandings. The term *hope,* for example, may translate as "hope for a cure" to one person and "hope for a pain-free death" to another. Nurses must avoid projecting personal interpretations of hope or other terms to parents when assessing parental reactions.

In children, the importance of denial has repeatedly been demonstrated as a factor in their positive coping with the diagnosis. Denial allows the child to maintain hope in the face of overwhelming odds and to function adaptively and productively. Like hope, denial may be an adaptive mechanism for dealing with loss that persists until a family or patient is ready or needs other responses. Relatives of critically ill patients also identify hope as a universal need (Hickey, 1990) (see Guidelines box on p. 958).

Adjustment

Adjustment gradually follows shock and is usually characterized by an open admission that the condition exists. This stage of partial acceptance (Fraley, 1990) may be accompanied by several responses, which are quite normal parts of the adaptation process. Probably the most universal of these feelings are ***guilt*** and ***self-accusation.*** Guilt is often greatest when the cause of the disorder is directly traceable to the parent, such as in genetic diseases or from accidental injury. However, it can occur even without any scientific or realistic basis for parental responsibility. Frequently the guilt stems from a false assumption that the disability is a result of personal failing or wrongdoing, such as not doing something correctly during pregnancy or the birth. Guilt may also be associated with cultural or religious beliefs. Some parents are convinced that they are being punished for some previous misdeed. Others may see the disorder as a sacrifice sent by God to test their religious strength and faith. With correct information, support, and time, most parents master guilt and self-accusation. The ability to master resentful and self-accusatory feelings of having "caused" the child's disorder is a crucial factor in determining the parents' acceptance of their child.

Children, too, may interpret their serious illness as retribution for past misbehavior. The nurse should be particularly sensitive to the child who passively accepts all painful procedures. This child may believe that such acts are inflicted as deserved punishment. It is always vital to assure children that what happens to them during diagnosis or treatment is to make them better.

Other common and normal reactions are ***bitterness*** or ***anger.*** Anger directed inward may be evident as self-reproaching or punitive behavior, such as neglecting one's health and verbally degrading oneself. Anger directed outward may be manifested in open arguments or withdrawal from communication and may be evident in the person's relationship with any number of individuals, such as the spouse, the child, and siblings. Passive anger toward the ill child may be evident in decreased visiting, refusal to believe how sick the child is, or inability to provide comfort. One of the most common targets for parental anger is members of the staff. Parents may complain about the nursing care, the insufficient time physicians spend with them, or the lack of skill of those who draw blood or start intravenous infusions.

Children are apt to respond with anger as well, and this includes the affected child, as well as the well siblings. Children are aware of the loss engendered by their illness or disability and may react angrily to the restrictions imposed or the feelings of being different. Siblings may also feel anger and resentment toward the ill child and parents for the loss of routine and parental attention. It is difficult for older children and almost impossible for younger children to comprehend the plight of the affected child. Their perception is of a brother or sister who has the undivided attention of their parents, is showered with cards and gifts, and is the focus of everyone's concern.

Children of various ages manifest anger differently. Young children may demonstrate their uncooperativeness by yelling, screaming, and physically fighting off the adversary. Older children may verbally express anger through abusive language. Passive anger, expressed in statements such as "I don't know" or "I don't care," usually evokes aggressive anger in others. Such passive anger may be misinterpreted as sullen, obnoxious, or hostile reactions. As a result, these statements are effective in keeping people at a distance, when the hidden message really is "I need to talk. Please help me understand what is happening."

CHARACTERISTICS OF PARENTAL OVERPROTECTION

- Sacrifices self and rest of family for the child
- Continually helps the child, even when the child is capable
- Is inconsistent with regard to discipline or employs no discipline; frequently different rules apply to the other siblings
- Is dictatorial and arbitrary, making decisions without considering the child's wishes, such as keeping the child from attending school
- Hovers and offers suggestions; calls attention to every activity, overdoing praise
- Protects the child from every possible discomfort
- Restricts play, often because of fear that the child will be injured
- Denies the child opportunities for growing up and assuming responsibility, such as learning to give own medications or perform treatments
- Does not understand the child's capabilities and sets goals too high or too low
- Monopolizes the child's time, such as sleeping with the child, permitting few friends, or refusing participation in social or educational activities

During the period of adjustment, four types of parental reactions to the child influence the child's eventual response to the disorder: ***overprotection,*** in which the parents fear letting the child achieve any new skill, avoid all discipline, and cater to every desire to prevent frustration; ***rejection,*** in which the parents detach themselves emotionally from the child but usually provide adequate physical care or constantly nag and scold the child; ***denial,*** in which parents act is if the disorder does not exist or attempt to have the child overcompensate for it; and ***gradual acceptance,*** in which parents place necessary and realistic restrictions on the child, encourage self-care activities, and promote reasonable physical and social abilities. Overprotection (see box above) is so common a parental reaction that it behooves the nurse to assess for its presence and to begin anticipatory guidance with the family when it may be appropriate. Many of these characteristics are also observed in the vulnerable child syndrome and could occur or continue should the child recover from illness or injury (see Chapter 10).

Reintegration and Acknowledgment

For many families the last stage is characterized by realistic expectations for the child and reintegration of family life with the illness or disability in proper perspective. Since a large portion of this phase is one of grief for a loss, total resolution is not possible until the child dies or leaves home as an independent adult. Therefore one can regard adjustment to chronic sorrow as "increased comfortableness" with everyday living.

This adjustment phase also involves social reintegration in which the family broadens its activities to include relationships outside of the home, with the child as an acceptable and participating member of the group. This last criterion often differentiates the reaction of gradual accep-

STRESSES OF FAMILIES WITH A CHILD WITH SPECIAL NEEDS

DAY-TO-DAY STRESSES

Constant attention
Reactions of other children and the larger community
Social relations
Effect on siblings
Marital relations

LIFE MAINTENANCE STRESSES

Financial stress, insurance
Housing
Transportation
Clothing and appliances
Need for support

WORRIES ABOUT THE FUTURE

Future children
Schooling and vocational training
Residential care

ANTICIPATED PARENTAL STRESS POINTS

Diagnosis of the condition—requires considerable learning, as well as dealing with emotional response
Developmental milestones—times children normally achieve walking, talking, self-care are delayed or impossible for the child
Start of schooling—particularly stressful are situations in which appropriate schooling will not be in a regular class placement
Reaching the ultimate attainment—situations, such as realizing that ambulation will be impossible or that the child will not learn to read, must be handled.
Adolescence—issues such as sexuality and independence become prominent
Future placement—decisions about placement must be made when the child becomes an adult or when the parents can no longer care for the child
Death of the child

ANTICIPATED SIBLING STRESS POINTS

Birth of another child—may be the affected sibling or the subsequent birth of an unaffected child
Diagnosis of condition—in certain illnesses, times of remission and exacerbations are difficult
Start of schooling—particularly stressful if friends reject the child with special needs
Adolescence—when dating begins, may be embarrassed to bring dates home
Future placement—may worry about responsibility for the affected sibling, especially if the parents are ill or die
Death of the child

tance during the adjustment period from total acceptance, or perhaps is more descriptive of the acknowledgment process.

Most parents of children with special needs tend to experience ***chronic sorrow***, an emotional response manifested through the life span of the parent-child interaction (Clubb, 1991). Acceptance is interspersed with periods of intensified sorrow for the loss. Grieving is most likely seen at each period of the child's development (e.g., entry into school, the onset of puberty), when the parent is again reminded of what could have been. Parental feelings of recurrent grief also surface when the child experiences a situational or developmental crisis (Fraley, 1990). Consequently, even families who have achieved a high level of adjustment and acceptance are at predictable times in need of support from professionals or other families who have coped successfully with similar experiences (see box at left).

Out-of-Home Placement

If strategies of coping cannot be employed to minimize the stress and disorganization of maintaining the child within the home to tolerable levels, the affected child may be permanently placed outside the home in a residential setting. Evolution of this phase is directly related to the degree of physical and mental disability.

This phase is not necessarily one of maladjustment. Placement may be the only option that will preserve the integrity of the family. Aging parents may be forced to accept this alternative as a result of progressive inability to meet the demands imposed by a severe disability. Relinquishing the role of primary caregiver is followed by an initial sense of loss, relief, guilt, and ambivalence, a pattern of reactions not unlike that seen following the death of a terminally ill child (see Chapter 23).

IMPACT OF THE CHILD'S CHRONIC ILLNESS OR DISABILITY ON FAMILY MEMBERS

Each family who has a child with special needs is affected by the experience. The effects on the parents and their responses are so critical that they directly influence the other members' reactions. In addition, the extended family is affected, and their response, as well as the community's acceptance of the child, can further assist or hinder the family's coping with the stresses imposed by caring for a child with special needs.

Parents

Besides grieving for the loss of a perfect child, parents may or may not receive positive feedback from transactions with their child. Many parents feel satisfaction and fulfillment from the parenting role. For others, parenting a child with a disability or chronic illness may be a series of unrewarding experiences that continually support the parents' feelings of inadequacy and failure. These responses may be most evident in parents who are responsible for the child's care. For example, they may become preoccupied with their ability to carry out certain procedures, perhaps overlooking the child's personal comfort and satisfaction or failing to offer praise for anything less than perfect cooperation or performance. They may pursue a frustrating activity until they achieve "success"—long after the child has become irritable and uncooperative. As a result, the parent can become caught in a pattern of interaction that is mutually unrewarding and minimally productive. For these parents several strategies may be helpful: education regarding what can reasonably be expected of their child, assistance in identifying the child's strengths, praise for a parental job well done, and finding respite care so that the parent can renew his or her own energies.

Parental Roles. Enormous demands may be placed on

parental time, energy, and financial resources to care for a child with chronic illness or disability. Depending on the roles assumed by each spouse, the wife often receives the brunt of the time and energy demands, and the husband shoulders the financial responsibilities. However, with changing sex roles, these responsibilities may be shared or shifted more heavily to one member. In a shared approach, parents often divide tasks in a very specific way, according to their skills or level of comfort. For example, the parent with patience for waiting may be the logical person to take the child for tests, examinations, and procedures. The parent who deals best with the sickness and side effects of treatment can ready the environment for the child's return home. It is important for nurses to realize that the absence of one parent from the hospital or clinic does not necessarily indicate that the shared parent pattern is not in effect (Clements, Copeland, and Loftus, 1990). On the other hand, making efforts to involve both parents in decision making and in learning how to care for the child's special needs can reduce some of the burden of care often placed inadvertently on mothers.

In some families changing sex roles mean added responsibilities for one parent. For example, the working mother may feel the need to continue employment to help defray the expenses, but she also incurs the added burden of additional child/home responsibilities. The result can eventually be marital conflicts as one partner views his or her share as unequal.

In addition, the partner who is not included in the caregiving activities may feel neglected, since much attention is directed toward the child, and resentful that he or she is not sufficiently informed to be competent in the care. Without active participation in the care of the child, the parent may have little appreciation of the time and energy involved in performing those activities. When the less competent partner does attempt to participate, the other parent frequently criticizes the less skillful efforts. As a result, communication may break down, and neither is able to support the other.

The nurse can assist the family in avoiding these patterns by providing anticipatory guidance early on. Guidance care addresses the stressors often cited as having an impact on the marriage: (1) the home care program with the burden of care assumed by primarily one parent, (2) the financial burden, (3) the fear of the child dying, (4) pressure from relatives, (5) the hereditary nature of the disease (if applicable), and (6) fear of pregnancy. Other causes of tension often center on the inconveniences associated with care, such as long waiting for appointments, lack of parking near care facilities, or lack of overnight accommodations (Kalnins, 1983). Certainly, these last stressors are within health professionals' domain to minimize, if not eliminate.

Mother/Father Differences. Mothers and fathers in the same family appear to experience distinct differences in adjusting and coping as parents of a child with special needs. Some mothers report a peaks-and-valleys, periodic crisis pattern, whereas fathers tend to experience their adjustment in terms of steady, gradual recovery. Some research suggests that mothers of children with certain conditions may be more susceptible to psychologic distress than fathers. Furthermore, mothers are more likely to have to deal with delaying or forfeiting personal goals (Fisman and Wolf, 1991).

The father of a child with special needs struggles with issues that may be quite distinct from those of the mother (Association for the Care of Children's Health, 1990). He may feel that his role of protector is challenged because he does not know how to help and cannot protect the family from the seemingly overwhelming recurring problems. Dreams of lineage, ego fulfillment, and athletic and vocational achievement are threatened and, in turn, may threaten the father's self-esteem. Because the traditional paternal role, particularly with sons, emphasizes joint recreation over caregiving, fathers seem to have more difficulty adjusting to a son with special needs than to a daughter with special needs. With today's increased emphasis on fathers' involvement in the lives of their children, this loss is felt more profoundly than in the past. The extensive stresses in the family can leave the father feeling depressed, weak, guilty, powerless, isolated, embarrassed, and very angry. Yet, fearful that he will lose control or be viewed as weak or ineffectual, the father will often hide his feelings and display an outward confidence that may lead others to believe that everything is fine. Feelings are further exacerbated by a health care system that frequently excludes and disregards men. Too often, the father feels like an afterthought in the care of his child (May, 1990).

Fathers worry about what the future holds for their children, as well as about the ability to manage the increasing financial burden. Some fathers escape in their work as a means for dulling the pain. Others view all of the difficulties of having a child with special needs as challenges to overcome and are not afraid to push limits and be assertive to acquire the needed services for their children (May, 1990).

Marital Relationship. Conflicts in parental role definition and differences in maternal and paternal coping patterns can place a strain on the marital relationship. Most families seem to manage this strain; research indicates that divorce rates are not substantially higher than those for the general population. A couple's marital functioning before the birth or diagnosis of a child with special needs may well be the best predictor of long-term marital adjustment (Kazak, 1989).

Single-Parent Families. Single-parent families are of special concern. The absence of a parent may be due to divorce or death, or the parents may never have married. As the only parent of a child who may require extensive, sophisticated, and lifelong care, the single parent may feel an enormous burden. Nurses must recognize that external sources of support and personal inner strength are particularly crucial for single parents to enable them to care for their child (Clements, Copeland, and Loftus, 1990). A special effort should be made to assist the single parent in finding financial and support services that can ease the burden of care. Nurses can also assist the single parent in identifying helping roles that may be acceptable to relatives and friends.

Siblings

Results of studies on how siblings are affected by having a brother or sister with special needs are inconsistent. Some confirm that brothers and sisters of children with chronic or disabling conditions are at high risk for maladjustment; others report no significant differences between siblings of children with special needs and siblings of children without chronic or disabling conditions; and still others note the absence of effects (Gallo and others, 1992). However, most investigators do agree that brothers and sisters of children with special needs are no more at risk for *severe* psychiatric problems than are siblings of children without chronic or disabling conditions.

Some difficulties for siblings arise from the demands of the child's condition. For example, at diagnosis the child with special needs by necessity becomes the focus of parental attention and concern. Frequent hospitalizations or trips to the physician or clinic disrupt the family routine. Siblings are pushed to the background, often staying at the homes of family and friends. The child's condition may interfere with holiday celebrations, vacations, and other special events. Siblings may resent these intrusions, which frequently demand self-sacrifice. Their parents may be unable to attend their school functions, ball games, or other activities, and, at times, may be physically and emotionally unavailable for them. The family's financial, as well as emotional, resources may be directed toward the child with special needs. When this occurs, there is often not only a decrease in normal family activities but a decrease in personal items for the other children as well.

Many of the difficulties siblings encounter are a result of the nature of the sibling relationship itself (see Chapter 14). It is within the sibling relationship that children learn to share, compete, and compromise with others close to them in status. The equality of this relationship is often lost when a brother or sister has special needs. The child with special needs is "out of tune," unable to contribute to the family or the sibling relationship in the usual way. Because identification is another characteristic of sibling relationships, some siblings believe that they, too, will "catch" the condition, a reasonable assumption considering experiences with contagious diseases, such as chickenpox. Identification, combined with a young child's egocentric thinking, may lead a sibling to feel responsible for a brother or sister's condition. For example, siblings may believe that playing rough with their brother or sister or even thinking bad thoughts about the sibling caused the condition.

Most brothers and sisters experience mixed and sometimes contradictory feelings. They may feel left out of new family developments and changing roles, guilty that they escaped getting the condition, or sad when their brother or sister is unable to participate in a particular activity or event. Some siblings feel embarrassed and ashamed; having a child in the family who is ill, disfigured, or disabled marks the family as "different." Siblings may actually experience a ***courtesy stigma***—a spoiled identity because of a close relationship with someone who is devalued and avoided because he or she is different. These painful feelings may lead to isolation and loneliness.

When parents give the child with special needs preferential treatment, siblings may feel resentful and jealous—feelings that are often distorted by their own sense of loss and concern. Older siblings in particular may resent stepping in as surrogate parents for their younger brothers and sisters. Siblings may be angry at parents for being unable to protect their brother or sister from getting the condition or angry at insensitive friends and classmates. Some siblings must also deal with anger from the child with special needs who resents them for escaping the experience.

Some siblings develop adjustment or behavior problems, especially younger male or older female siblings. Younger children having difficulty tend to become withdrawn and irritable, whereas older siblings tend to act out. Some typical problems include bed-wetting, headaches and other physical complaints, changes in school performance, school phobia, sleep problems, proneness to injury, depression, and severe separation anxiety. While characteristics of the illness or disability can affect the sibling's reaction (Lobato, 1990), sibling adjustment is not necessarily a function of the severity of the child's condition (Orsillo, McCaffrey, and Fisher, 1993).

Often overlooked is the positive caring between children with special needs and their brothers and sisters. Siblings can experience pride and satisfaction in their own contributions to the family, joy and excitement in their brother or sister's accomplishments, and genuine love. Some siblings say they sense more closeness in their families. Researchers have frequently noted more warmth, compassion, empathy, patience, and understanding in brothers and sisters of children with special needs. Ultimately, most brothers and sisters seem to adapt well, and many demonstrate high levels of self-confidence, independence, maturity, altruism, and tolerance.

Certain factors (e.g., family size, age between children) seem to influence sibling adjustment (Lobato, 1990; Rollins, 1990). However, the most important factors appear to be specific individual characteristics of the sibling and parental feelings, perceptions, and reactions. Siblings are more at risk for adjustment problems when parents are unaccepting of the child with special needs. Also, certain times seem to be more difficult for siblings (see box on p. 940).

How siblings react will have an important impact on the child's overall adjustment. When siblings act in a normal fashion, then a secure, stable training ground is provided for social relationships for the child with special needs.

Extended Family Members and Society

Two other groups of people may experience the effects of a child's chronic illness or disability: (1) the significant nonnuclear family members or friends and (2) society as a whole. Although extended family relationships are often helpful to parents in rearing a child with special needs, they may also be sources of stress. For example, grandparents or other well-meaning relatives may attempt to reassure the parents that the child "will grow out of" his or her slowness at a time when parents are struggling to accept reality.

Most grandparents experience some ambivalence: they love their grandchild and feel personal disappointment.

They often experience a double grief, both for their grandchild and for their child, the parent. The future is now unpredictable, not only for the grandchild, but for the child's parents as well (Burns and Madian, 1992). Grandparents do not often acknowledge these emotions, and they are left to adapt on their own. Support groups for grandparents, while uncommon, can be beneficial.

Although society's views of individuals with chronic illness or disability are changing toward a more accepting, nonjudgmental, and open attitude, parents, siblings, and the affected child frequently are victims of prejudice, ostracism, or criticism. A great deal of this stems from public ignorance and fear, and this remains a crucial area for intervention by health professionals. Another area in which society could better meet the needs of families of children with chronic illness or disability is in the development of support services such as respite care. Financing care and insurance practices that do not discriminate against individuals with chronic illness are other areas in which society could better support these children and their families.

CONCEPT OF FUNCTIONAL BURDEN

IMPACT OF CHILD WITH SPECIAL NEEDS

The child's need for medical and nursing care
The child's fixed deficits
The child's age-inappropriate dependency in activities of daily living
The disruptions caused by the care in the family routine
The psychologic burden of the prognosis on the family

FAMILY RESOURCES AND ABILITY TO COPE

The family's physical resources
The family's emotional resources
The family's educational resources
The family's social supports and available help
The competing demands for family members' time and energy

Data from Stein REK: Home care: a challenging opportunity, *Child Health Care* 14(2):90-95, 1985.

FACTORS AFFECTING THE FAMILY'S ADJUSTMENT

The diagnosis of a child with a serious health problem or disability is a major situational crisis that affects the entire family system. However, families can experience positive outcomes as they successfully deal with the many challenges that accompany a child with chronic illness or disability. One nursing goal is to assess which families are at greater or lesser risk for succumbing to the effects of the crisis. Several variables—available support system, perception of the event, coping mechanisms, reactions to the child, available resources, and concurrent stresses within the family—influence the resolution of a crisis. Although most families cope well, the needs of families at risk are great. If they receive emotional support and guidance early, there is an increased likelihood that they will also cope successfully.

Although it is easy to assume that families of children with the most severe illnesses or disabilities would have the poorest adjustment, the severity of the condition reflects only one part of the overall picture. The level of adjustment is significantly influenced by the ***functional burden*** on the individual family (Stein, 1985). This concept considers the issues related to caring for and living with the child in relation to the family's resources and ability to cope (see box above, right). The family of a child with multiple disabilities demanding complex care—yet having many resources and coping skills—may adjust more successfully to his or her situation than the family of a child with a less serious condition and a paucity of resources to counter the balance.

Available Support System

The significant others who are available to individuals for emotional strength during periods of crisis comprise their support system. Support systems may be available through a variety of relationships and may consist of one significant other, such as a spouse, or a group of significant others, such as the extended family or the health team.

Research indicates that the source of support is a determining factor in the effectiveness of certain forms of support. For example, expressive support is best provided by individuals with whom one has strong ties and who are like oneself. On the other hand, instrumental support can often be provided by those to whom the family has weaker ties and who can link the family to a broader, more diverse social network. Therefore, the most appropriate sources of informational support might include both professionals who have theoretic and practical knowledge and nonprofessionals—parents—whose experience equips them as experts. When professionals develop a strong therapeutic relationship with the family, they, too, can be appropriate sources of emotional support (see discussion on parent-professional partnerships in Chapter 1 and on p. 955).

Although a support system exists, it may not be effective unless the individual is able to use the system through mutual channels of communication.

Status of the Marital Relationship. The marital relationship is a prime source of potential support and overall is considered the best predictor of coping behavior and adjustment (Kazak, 1989; Trute, 1990). When the spouses can openly discuss their feelings, there tends to be much less guilt, anger, blame, and indecision. Each crisis during the long period of chronic illness is successfully resolved, lessening the accumulation and overlapping of multiple stresses.

Social Support Systems. Support systems may be available with significant others outside the marital relationship. For example, the single-parent family may have the support of extended family, such as that of the parent's own parents. Providing parents with written information they can share with extended family can often help them in reaching out to others during a difficult time. Occasionally, parents may be able to communicate with each other but are unable to talk with the child. This is particularly evident with very young children, who communicate least through verbalization, and with adolescents, who may be unwilling to discuss with or listen to adults. In this case the child is left without an available support system unless professionals share strategies with the family.

Ability to Communicate. Besides the availability of significant others, family members must have the ability to use the support system. Almost all methods of psychologic intervention, such as support through active listening, counseling, or crisis intervention, require verbal communication between two individuals. The ability to verbalize about feelings such as anger, fear, guilt, or anxiety helps individuals cope with the particular emotion. Verbalization allows for validation of feelings and thoughts.

Not all individuals are able to communicate well verbally. Some rely on religious faith and silent prayers for support. Others, such as children, communicate best through nonverbal methods, such as play, drawing, or writing. Some individuals may not be able to communicate with anyone because of their interpersonal withdrawal and social isolation. These individuals are most at risk because, even if a support system is available, they may be unable to share their problems with others.

Perception of the Illness/Disability

The meaning and significance of the child's condition are influenced by the individual's perception of the diagnosis. In particular, the association of guilt may complicate one's ability to realistically view the problem and ultimately resolve the associated grief. Guilt implies a feeling of control. The more guilt an individual has, the more control that person perceives was possible in the prevention or alteration of the diagnosis. Assessment of specific perceptions concerning the illness or disability aids in evaluating the individual's ability to cope with various aspects of the crisis and identifies possible areas for intervention.

Previous Knowledge. Although family members may be shocked to learn that their child has a serious illness or disability, they usually have some knowledge about the disorder from previous associations. It is important to explore the extent of that information, since there is a great tendency to compare the recently disclosed facts with the other knowledge. Because research indicates that people generally act in accordance with their beliefs, it is important to know what parents believe about their child's medical condition and if their beliefs are based on accurate information (Austin, 1990).

Influence of Religion. Religious beliefs and spirituality have various meanings for different people. For some, religion comprises the foundation of their support system—all of life revolves around their relationship with God. Healing and faith are synonymous, and any criticism of the family's spirituality can weaken their trust in the medical care. For others, it may intensify feelings of guilt, shame, bitterness, or punishment. For example, some individuals may interpret the illness as a punishment from God. They may exclaim, "What have I done to deserve this?" or "God, why are you punishing me in this way?" It is important to take such statements seriously and to explore reasons why the person believes that this is a punishment.

Imagined Cause. Although the cause of many disorders is unknown, parents and children usually supply their own answers. Sometimes this is associated with religious beliefs, but it may also be influenced by previous events. For example, children may interpret the reason for the illness as a punishment for not obeying others. Parents may be convinced that the disease was inherited. Sometimes there is a strong belief in curses, occult witchcraft, or devils as perpetrators of the disorder. Once the fantasied cause is revealed, the person can be helped to deal with the irrationalities of that thinking and, hopefully, will be relieved of feelings of guilt, blame, or anger.

Effects on the Family. How the child's illness or disability affects the family reveals how its members perceive the event. For example, the following statements could represent a particular reaction:

- **Denial**—"Everything is the same as it always was."
- **Inability to express feelings**—"We have more *things* to do."
- **Anger, blame, or bitterness**—"We never should have had children."
- **Resentment and hostility**—"My sister gets everything because she is sick."
- **Acceptance and ability to express feelings**—"The perspective of time has changed because we realize how precious and limited it is."

Coping Mechanisms

Coping mechanisms are those behaviors aimed at reducing the tension caused by a crisis. ***Approach behaviors*** are those coping mechanisms that result in movement toward adjustment and resolution of the crisis. ***Avoidance behaviors*** result in movement away from adjustment or maladaptation to the crisis. Several approach and avoidance behaviors used in coping with a chronic illness or disability are listed in the Guidelines box. None of the indexes can be used singly to assess the possible success or failure in resolving the crisis. Each behavior must be viewed in the context of all the variables affecting the family. For example, the observation of several avoidance behaviors in an emotionally healthy family may denote significantly less risk to the successful resolution of the crisis than an equal number of avoidance behaviors in an individual who has few available supports.

Two long-term coping strategies of familial adaptation to chronic and severe childhood illness have been significantly associated with a high level of family functioning (Venters, 1981). The first is the parents' ability to endow the illness with meaning within an existing spiritual or medical/scientific philosophy of life. There is an optimistic belief that all things work out for the good and a focus on the positive qualities of the situation. Statements such as "God has chosen our family to care for this special child" are reflective of the religious philosophy.

The second is an ability to share the burdens of the illness with individuals both inside and outside the family constellation. Intrafamilial relationships encourage togetherness of the family members and maintain a mutual acknowledgment that all members are important contributors to the family unit. Extrafamilial supports help preserve meaningful external contacts and provide needed help to the family.

Reactions to Previous Crises. Exploring the way in

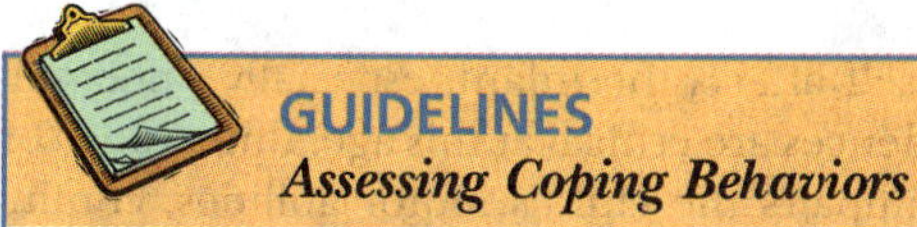

GUIDELINES
Assessing Coping Behaviors

APPROACH BEHAVIORS

Asks for information regarding diagnosis and child's present condition
Seeks help and support from others
Anticipates future problems; actively seeks guidance and answers
Endows the illness or disability with meaning
Shares burden of disorder with others
Plans realistically for the future
Acknowledges and accepts child's awareness of diagnosis and prognosis
Expresses feelings, such as sorrow, depression, and anger, and realizes reason for the emotional reaction
Realistically perceives child's condition; adjusts to changes
Recognizes own growth through passage of time, such as earlier denial and nonacceptance of diagnosis
Verbalizes possible loss of child

AVOIDANCE BEHAVIORS

Fails to recognize seriousness of child's condition despite physical evidence
Refuses to agree to treatment
Intellectualizes about the illness, but in areas unrelated to child's condition
Is angry and hostile to members of the staff, regardless of their attitude or behavior
Avoids staff, family members, or child
Entertains unrealistic future plans for child, with little emphasis on the present
Is unable to adjust to or accept a change in progression of disease
Continually looks for new cures with no perspective toward possible benefit
Refuses to acknowledge child's understanding of disease and prognosis
Uses magical thinking and fantasy, may seek "occult" help
Places complete faith in religion to point of relinquishing own responsibility
Withdraws from outside world; refuses help
Punishes self because of guilt and blame
Makes no change in life-style to meet needs of other family members
Resorts to excessive use of alcohol or drugs to avoid problems
Verbalizes suicidal intents
Is unable to discuss possible loss of child or previous experiences with death

which a family dealt with a previous crisis identifies their possible reactions to the present stressful event. The type of family structure frequently offers valuable clues to the general approach the family may use to solve the crisis.

In the authoritarian family one or both parents decide what is best for all its members. As a result, the type of coping behavior demonstrated is usually chosen by a specific individual, regardless of others' needs. In the laissez-faire family new coping mechanisms may be explored, but family members offer little direction, approval, or validation of the effectiveness of the behavior. Authoritative or democratic family members are flexible and have respect for each other's opinions, although the adults exercise direction and guidance for decision making. This last type of family usually demonstrates the most ability in exploring new coping mechanisms that are aimed at successful resolution of the crisis for the ultimate benefit of the entire family.

Reactions to the Child

An awareness of the family members' reactions to the child is important and can uncover the type of childrearing practices or attitudes that may support or hinder the child's optimum development and influence the family's adjustment (see Table 22-2 for assessment questions). Parental reactions are driven by feelings such as courage, love, fear, power, shame, pride, pity, guilt, caring, concern, and confusion. These reactions in turn affect attitudes and choice of childrearing practices, which can cause resounding effects throughout the family system.

Available Resources

Resources are the available means that exist or can be developed either within the family members, the family unit, or the community. For example, nurses can consider family members' age, intelligence, education, willingness and ability to learn the child's care, sense of humor, and sense of optimism as resources they can bring to a situation. Resources within the family unit, such as cohesion, adaptability, a sense of coherence, and hardiness, are aspects of the family system that can help considerably in the family's adjustment.

Community resources, such as health care resources, parent support groups, availability of respite care, alternatives for schooling, and educational facilities and recreational programs, are key elements in family adjustment. These kinds of resources are better developed in some areas than in others, meaning that what is available to a family depends largely on where they live. In an urban area, for example, families of children with special needs may find a greater number of programs and services for their children. Communities, like families, have different strengths.

How well the community meets the needs of families of children with special needs is influenced not only by the location of the community but by a balanced fit between family and community needs and resources. This fit is best achieved when the attitudes and beliefs shared by professionals in the community create a community climate or atmosphere that is supportive and empowering of families. Nurses who work with families of children with special needs are in unique positions to build professional understanding of family-centered care.

NURSING ALERT Be aware that many families may not have a telephone, a service most practitioners consider essential for families of children with special needs (Wissow and Warshow, 1990). Other families may have telephones but are reluctant to reveal the telephone number. To overcome these difficulties, use the following strategies:

1. Help family identify telephone access close to home (e.g., neighbor's home, nearby store).
2. Explore methods to obtain telephone service for family (e.g., social service agencies, charitable organizations).
3. Be sensitive to family's concern for privacy when asking for a telephone number; explain reason for needing number and to whom it will be given.

Concurrent Stresses Within the Family

The ability to deal with the already overwhelming stresses of a lifelong disability or illness is challenged when additional stresses are present. Ongoing stresses and strains in the family "pile up," increasing the family's vulnerability and reducing its ability to adapt and adjust to a child with special needs. For some family members, non-disease-related stressors are perceived as more stressful than those associated with a child's chronic condition. In a study of siblings of children with cancer, concurrent stressors—such as the pending remarriage of a parent—appeared to be causing some siblings more concern than having a brother or sister with cancer (Rollins, 1990).

Stressors may be situational or developmental. They may be related to marital difficulties, financial pressures, homelessness, or social isolation. With the alarming increase in drug abuse and wide spread alcohol abuse, it is reasonable to assume that a fair number of families may be struggling with a family member's alcohol or other drug problem. Even the more minor stresses such as arranging care for siblings, managing the home, and traveling to distant treatment centers can jeopardize the family's ability to cope successfully (see also box on p. 940).

Child or family developmental stressors predictably compound situational stress. For example, a common developmental stressor in the family life cycle is the birth of a first child, an event that requires adaptation by the spouse dyad. The birth of a child with a congenital health problem adds situational stress to the equation.

IMPACT OF CHRONIC ILLNESS OR DISABILITY ON THE CHILD

The child's reaction to chronic illness or disability depends to a great extent on his or her developmental level, temperament, and available coping mechanisms; on the reactions of significant others; and to a lesser extent on the condition itself. Knowledge of these variables is essential in providing the kind of support needed by these children to cope with a sometimes overwhelming situation.

Developmental Aspects

The impact of a chronic illness or disability is influenced by the age of onset. Chronic illness affects children of all ages, but the developmental aspects of each age-group dictate particular challenges, stresses, and risks for the child. The nurse must also recognize that children need to redefine their condition and its implications as they develop and grow. An understanding of these factors facilitates planning care to support the child and minimize the risks (see also Table 22-3).

Infancy. During infancy the child is engaged in the task of developing trust, which necessitates a reciprocal satisfying relationship between child and parent. When illness or disability occurs, this relationship is potentially affected. For example, a visible defect can retard parent attachment as the parent mourns the loss of the perfect child. In addition, prolonged illness may impose separations that prevent the child and parent from normal attachment and deprive the infant of the nurturing relationship.

The illness itself affects the infant, especially since sensorimotor experiences are critical at this age. Illness and/or disability often impairs the child's motor abilities, confining the child to a crib and lessening contact with the environment. Certainly, the messages transmitted to infants about their body are influenced by the amount of pain and discomfort they experience. Associating touch with pain can compromise the infant's ability to give and receive affection. Lack of pleasurable sensations can lead to an irritable and unhappy child. Consequently, parents may interpret the behaviors as evidence that they are inadequate in meeting the child's physical and emotional needs, which further affects the parent-child relationship and the acquisition of trust. Nursing intervention can be important in helping parents work with the irritable child in a way that encourages understanding and caring.

Nurses should advocate for policies and practices that will best meet the needs of the infant and family. Twenty-four-hour visitation in the NICU and other infant units is of primary importance. Showing parents how to touch and hold the infant will promote their confidence and competence. Kangaroo care has been shown to be both safe and beneficial to the infant. Mothers who choose to breast-feed can be encouraged, with a private space provided for them to nurse or pump and storage facilities made available for breast milk. Sibling visitation can be facilitated.

Toddler. The toddler is in the stage of autonomy; the need for mastery of locomotor and language skills is paramount. The child learning to walk and talk progresses toward becoming a separate person, both physically and psychologically. However, illness or disability can hinder mobility and deprive the child of mastery. In addition, overprotection can magnify the problem by setting limits on the child's exploration and experimentation for fear of injury or exertion. With limited opportunities for testing mastery, children may fear to venture on their own and thus develop little confidence in their abilities. Over time they may feel defeated and become apathetic, passive, and clinging. Nurse should help parents find ways to safely encourage toddler independence in both hospital and home settings.

Illness can impose separations that are detrimental to the toddler. Like the infant, separation is the most anxiety-producing event for toddlers. A chronic illness or disability can necessitate repeated hospitalizations and painful procedures. If the need to preserve the parent-child relationship is not appreciated in the hospital setting, the child may become depressed and eventually detach from the parent. Children seem to have a tremendous capacity to withstand stress, provided their attachment to the parent is preserved.

Preschooler. The preschooler is in the stage of initiative; numerous tasks are achieved during this age that can be severely hampered by chronic illness and disability. Impairment can limit the preschooler's learning about the environment, especially in terms of social development. Rather than being encouraged to play with peers and participate in nursery school activities, the chronically ill preschooler may be confined to the home, with socialization limited to the secure and tolerant family. Immature behavior may be tolerated because age-appropriate standards and discipline are not enforced. Consequently, when paired with children the same age or placed in school, the child is deficient in knowing how to act and can easily be criticized by peers who view him or her as a "baby." In fact, the child's illness or disability may provoke much less criticism than his or her inappropriate behavior. Faced with such reactions from others in contrast to the security of the home, the child may gradually choose a life of social isolation and loneliness, especially during the school-age years.

One of the major tasks of this period is establishing sexual identity, and one of the principal methods is through imitation of sex-related activities. However, the sick child may have fewer opportunities to engage in such activity and may view the parent predominantly in the caregiving role, since this may be the focus of their relationship.

In addition to sexual identity, the child's body image is forming. Children's knowledge of their body image is limited to what they see, feel, and use. If the child is chronically ill, body awareness is focused on the body's causing pain and anxiety. The child with a disability may have difficulty forming a mental image of impaired body parts, such as paralyzed extremities. This poorly developed sense of body integrity makes children especially fearful of intrusive or mutilating experiences, which can be frequent during prolonged illness.

One of the more critical influences of chronic illness or disability on preschoolers is the feeling of guilt that they "caused" the condition by a real or imagined misdeed. This is probably less of a factor if the child is born with the disorder than if it occurs during the preschool years. Such guilt can greatly affect the child's developing but fragile self-esteem. Unlike the child with a temporary physical impairment who has additional opportunities for achieving mastery and thus overcoming feelings of guilt and inferiority, the child with a chronic illness or disability experiences continual insults. Structuring situations to promote success can help a child develop a sense of competence and confidence.

School-Age Child. The child of school age is striving to achieve a sense of accomplishment while overcoming a sense of inferiority. Successful mastery of this task depends on the child's ability to cooperate and to compete with others. Consequently, physical impairments can greatly affect the ability to achieve and compete. For example, physical disability may hinder participation in sports and repeated absences from school caused by illness can place the child at an academic disadvantage. To repeat a grade can saddle the child with feelings of shame, inadequacy, and inferiority. However, the decision to remain in the same grade can also enhance feelings of success because the work requirements may be easier and new classmates provide a second chance for forming friendships.

During this age there is a transition from relationships with family members to strong identification with peers. Peers increasingly influence school-age children's view of themselves and their self-esteem. Anything that labels children as "different" can affect their sense of belonging to the group. Many children cope with their "differentness" by retreating from socialization. As they draw farther from the group, their sense of belonging diminishes, and intense loneliness and isolation dominate. Nurses can help families to promote social competence in their children (Breitmayer and others, 1992). For example, if children are helped to deal with their feelings of not being "normal and perfect" and to recognize their unique abilities, these children can cope very well. It is to be expected that not all children are able to master every task and that they will feel some degree of inferiority. If this is stressed to children with physical impairment, the burden to achieve is lessened.

As school-age children identify more with the peer group and authority figures outside the home, there is a concurrent striving for independence from the family. However, the ill child may be forced into an extended period of dependency either from the disorder or from parental overprotectiveness. Attempts to demonstrate independence may be manifested as resentment toward the parents, refusal to comply with treatment, or risk-taking behavior, such as cheating on the special diet. If parents can understand that these behaviors represent a normal phase of development, they may be more tolerant and able to find appropriate outlets for independence (e.g., increasing the child's responsibility for home care or increasing the child's control in non-disease-related activities).

Adolescence. The impact of illness or disability can be most detrimental during adolescence. A young child with impaired health reared in a home with loving parents who are sensitive to the child's needs generally copes well with the disorder. However, adolescence is different—even with all the benefits of parental love, the adolescent is striving for an independence from parents and in many ways must deal with the impact of impairment alone. As a result, coping may be more difficult and adolescents may be at greater risk for anxiety, depression, and adjustment problems (Grey, Cameron, and Thurber, 1991).

The major task of adolescents is to establish an identity of their own. Pubertal changes must be integrated into the self-image while the teenager is gaining control and mastery over increased physical capabilities and sexuality. During early adolescence this takes place primarily within the peer group. Illness or injury at this time interferes with teenagers' sense of mastery and control over a changing body. They are different at a stage of development when being different is unacceptable to the peer group, who may view a disability in one member as a threat to the established uniformity by which all are measured. At no time of life is an individual so vulnerable to the emotional stress of biologic impairment. Appearance, skills, and abilities are highly valued by peers; a teenager who is limited in any of these qualities is subject to rejection by this important group. This is especially marked when a physical disability interferes with sexual attractiveness.

These teenagers are faced with the task of incorporating their disability into the changing self-concept. The youngster who develops the illness or acquires the disability during the crucial adolescent years has more difficulty accomplishing this task than does the teenager who has been affected since childhood. It appears that the earlier the onset of a limiting condition, the better the individual is able to adapt to it. The youngster with a newly acquired disorder will have the additional task of grieving for a lost "perfection" while adjusting to the changes taking place as a natural course of events. The teenager places a great deal of emphasis on "fitting in" and is likely to feel rejected because of personal appearance or an inability to engage in activities expected of a healthy adolescent. The threat is greatest during middle adolescence, when the teenager has less available energy to cope with illness, since emotional resources are being used to meet the normal demands of this developmental phase.

The severity, type, and visibility of the illness also influence the adjustment process and appear to be sex related. Boys seem to be more concerned about diseases or therapies that interfere with their ability to function independently and to achieve vocational and academic goals and athletic prowess. Consequently, they may tolerate wearing a visible device or having a somewhat altered appearance as long as their physical and academic goals are not affected; for them confinement and restricted independence are less tolerable. While girls, too, are concerned about issues of independence and vocational and academic goals, they seem more upset by conditions that they perceive to interfere with their ability to attract important others and maintain relationships. Thus they may be more likely to tolerate restriction of movement and confinement, provided they continue to look attractive; disorders or treatments that affect their appearance may be devastating (Coupey and Cohen, 1984).

Adolescence is a time for achieving independence from the family and planning for future goals and responsibilities. Adolescents with long-term chronic illness tend to be less future directed and less independent than well peers (Orr and others, 1984). Enforced dependency from physical impairment can exacerbate the parent-child conflicts surrounding independence. Lack of understanding from both parties can result in bitter feelings and intrafamilial turmoil. The tendency toward rebellion may be directed at the disorder and reflected in decreased compliance with treatment, denying the disorder to preserve a sense of normalcy with peers, and risk-taking behavior that can place the teenager in jeopardy, such as driving a car despite a disorder that increases the chance of accident. Such behaviors can further strain an already tense parent-child relationship.

On the other hand, parents can promote independence by giving the adolescent a greater role in his/her own treatment regimen, encouraging the adolescent to develop a relationship with the physicians and nurses that is not mediated by parents, and promoting normalization principles.

Coping Mechanisms

Children's innate and learned coping mechanisms are very important in their ability to deal with their disorder. In a study of well children, their most common response to daily stressors was submission or endurance—quite possibly a fairly accurate view of the children's realization that they have little sense of control over daily life (Sorenson, 1990). Children with chronic conditions tend to use five distinct patterns of coping (see box above, right). Children with more positive and accepting attitudes about their chronic illness use a more adaptive coping style, characterized by optimism, competence, and compliance. They show fewer

COPING PATTERNS USED BY CHILDREN WITH SPECIAL HEALTH CARE NEEDS

Develops competence and optimism—Accentuates the positive aspects of the situation and concentrates more on what he or she has or can do rather than on what is missing and what he or she cannot do; is as independent as possible.

Feels different and withdraws—Sees self as being different from other children because of the chronic health condition, views being different as negative, sees self as less worthy than others, focuses on things he or she cannot do, and sometimes overrestricts activities needlessly.

Is irritable moody, and acts out—Uses proactive and self-initiated coping behaviors, although usually counterproductive in that the behaviors are not ego enhancing or socially responsible, nor do they result in desired outcomes; acts out irritability, which may or may not be associated with condition's symptoms.

Complies with treatment—Takes necessary medications/treatments, adheres to activity restrictions; also uses behaviors that indicate developing independence (e.g., assumes responsibility for taking medication).

Seeks support—Talks with adults, children, physicians, and nurses; develops plans to handle problems as they occur; uses downward comparison (i.e., realizes that others have it worse).

Modified from Austin J, Patterson J, Huberty T: Development of the coping health inventory for children, *J Pediatr Nurs* 6(3):166-174, 1991.

behavior problems at home and at school. The two maladaptive coping patterns, "feels different and withdraws" and "is irritable, moody, and acts out," are associated with poorer adaptation; children using these strategies have poorer self-concepts, more negative attitudes about their conditions, and more behavior problems at home and at school (Austin, Patterson, and Huberty, 1991). Individual characteristics that influence a child's ability to cope with stress are listed in the box on p. 949. In addition to these variables, the social support afforded these children is critically important. Therefore the better the family copes, the better the child is able to deal with the stressors imposed by the illness or disability.

Because it is often easier to recognize children who cope poorly with illness or disability, it is helpful to describe those behaviors typical of well-adjusted children. Well-adapted children gradually learn to accept their physical limitations but find achievement in a variety of compensatory motor and intellectual pursuits. They function well at home, at school, and with peers. They have an understanding of their disorder that allows them to accept their limitations, assume responsibility for care, and assist in treatment and rehabilitation regimens. Well-adjusted children express appropriate emotions, such as sadness, anxiety, and anger at times of exacerbations but confidence and guarded optimism during periods of clinical stability (Fig. 22-1). They are able to identify with other similarly affected individuals, promoting positive self-images and displaying pride and self-confidence in their ability to master a productive, successful life despite the disability.

INDIVIDUAL CHARACTERISTICS THAT AFFECT COPING IN CHILDREN

GENDER

Males are more vulnerable to stress than females.
Females are more likely to use emotional sensory and emotional expression responses than boys.
Males are more likely to use physical aggression in coping.

AGE

Children between ages 6 months and 4 years are considered most vulnerable.

TEMPERAMENT

The "difficult child" is considered more vulnerable than the easy child.
The more active, strong-willed child seems to cope better than the passive child.

PREEXISTING CONDITIONS

The child with preexisting anxiety is considered at greater risk for coping poorly.

SELF-CONCEPT

The child with low self-esteem and/or a low sense of self-direction is at greater risk for coping poorly.

SOCIAL SKILLS

The child with few social skills is at greater risk for coping poorly.

GENETIC FACTORS

Inborn traits influence the overall ability to adapt (e.g., vulnerability to alcoholism, sociopathy, mood disorders).

INTELLIGENCE

Children with above-average intelligence tend to have fewer psychiatric problems than children with lower intelligence.

HARDINESS/RESILIENCE

Positive behavioral patterns and favorable outcomes can be affected by a combination of temperament, familial traits, and support factors.

Data from Adams P, Fras I: *Beginning child psychiatry,* New York, 1988, Brunner/Mazel; Garmezy N: Resilience in children's adaptation to negative life events and stressed environments, *Pediatr Ann* 20(9):459-466, 1991; and Sorensen E: Children's coping responses, *J Pediatr Nurs* 5(4):259-267, 1990.

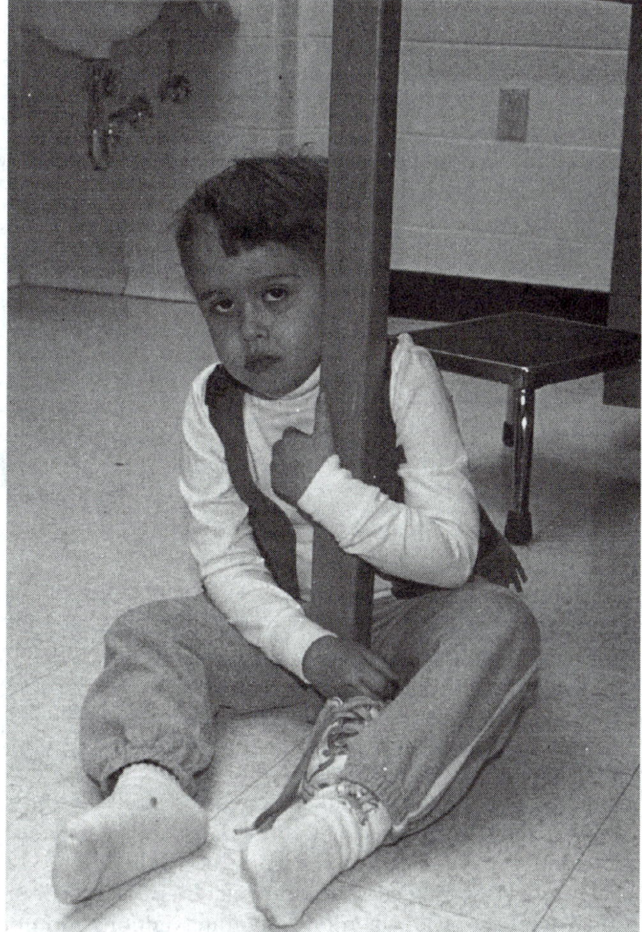

FIG. 22-1 Periods of sadness and anger are appropriate in the child's adjustment to a chronic illness or disability, especially during exacerbations of the disorder.

Responses to Parental Behavior

The parents' behavior toward the child, especially in terms of childrearing, is one of the most important influencing factors in the child's adjustment. For example, children who are reared by parents who establish reasonable limits tend to develop independence that is appropriate for their age and achievement commensurate with their limitations. They often display pride and confidence in their ability to cope successfully with the challenges imposed by their disorder. In contrast, children whose parents are overprotective tend to have marked dependency, fearfulness, inactivity, and lack of outside interests. Children who are raised by oversolicitous and guilt-ridden parents are often overly independent, defiant, and high-risk takers. Children who are reared by parents who emphasize their deficits and tend to "hide" or isolate them may appear as shy and lonely individuals. Anticipatory guidance by the nurse and encouragement of normalizing practices may assist parents in facilitating positive adjustment in their children.

Type of Illness or Disability

The type of illness or disability also influences the child's emotional response. Interestingly, some children with more severe disorders cope better than those with milder conditions. However, the presence of multiple conditions may place a child at risk for more behavioral problems (Newacheck, McManus, and Fox, 1991). Considering children's cognitive ability and their delay in achieving abstract thinking until adolescence, it is likely that an obvious condition is easier to accept because its limitations are concrete. For example, children who are blind or crippled are constantly reminded of their inability to run. However, children with hemophilia not only live by rules they do not understand but also only vaguely and occasionally sense their illness, such as when they run and accidentally initiate a bleeding episode. Therefore some chronic illnesses pose specific threats to children.

The onset of a crippling condition may generate a state of confusion for children, who may have trouble differentiating between actual body functions and their image of their bodies. They may also experience problems in identifying themselves and those extensions of self (e.g., wheelchairs, braces, crutches, or other mechanical or prosthetic devices) and may have tremendous difficulty in accepting functional aids.

NURSING CARE OF THE FAMILY AND CHILD WITH SPECIAL NEEDS

The major nursing goal is to help the family remain intact and functioning at maximum levels throughout the child's life. This involves not merely supporting the child and family during the critical period of the newborn phase when the infant is being diagnosed or when the parents encounter problems in the child of preschool or school age. It involves forming parent-professional partnerships that invite the parents' early input, encourage them to be accountable and responsible for the child's care, and do not reinforce the dangerous attitude that the professional will "fix" the child and give him or her back to the parents. It also reinforces the fact that it is not so much the condition itself that affects the child's progress and developmental outcomes but the family's ability to cope successfully with the child's problems. Thus long-term, comprehensive, systematic, family-centered approaches must be applied.

The nurse should strive to understand and accept individual response styles when planning interventions and not assume a common definition for what constitutes a need for help. Families that express no interest in psychosocial interventions are not necessarily resistant. A "cookbook" approach is ineffective; helpful programs must respond to individual needs.

A Nursing Care Plan for the child with special needs and the family is provided on pp. 967-971.

ASSESS THE FAMILY'S STRENGTHS AND LEVEL OF ADJUSTMENT

Since the nurse may meet a family during any phase of the adjustment process, it is essential to assess the family members' individual strengths, coping mechanisms, and reactions to the disorder. Ideally, assessment should begin as soon as the family learns the diagnosis. As part of a family-centered approach, the family should be an active participant in the process. Sample questions designed to elicit information for evaluating the family's adjustment are listed in Table 22-2. Families should always be informed of the purpose of the assessment process and, particularly, of the reasons for any personal questions. They should be given the opportunity to participate or not as they choose.

Several instruments can be used to assess the family's overall functioning and support system (see Chapter 6), and specific tools have been developed for families of children with chronic illness or disability. For example, the Coping Health Inventory for Parents (CHIPS) is an 80-item checklist providing self-report information about how parents perceive their overall response to the management of family life with a child with a chronic illness. Coping behaviors

TABLE 22-2 Assessment of Factors Affecting Family Adjustment

FACTORS AFFECTING ADJUSTMENT	ASSESSMENT QUESTIONS
Available support system	
Status of marital relationship	Whom do you talk to when you have something on your mind? (If answer is not the spouse, ask for the reason.)
Alternate support systems	When something is worrying you, what do you do? What helps you most when you are upset?
Ability to communicate	Does talking seem to help when you feel upset?
Perception of the illness/disability	
Previous knowledge of disorder	Have you ever heard the word (name of diagnosis) before? Tell me about it (if answer is yes).
Influence of religion	Has your religion or faith been of help to you? Tell me how (if answer is yes).
Imagined cause of disorder	What are your thoughts about the causes of the disorder?
Effects of illness or disability on family	How has your child's illness or disability affected you and your family? How has your life-style changed?
Coping mechanisms	
Reactions to previous crises	Tell me one time you've had another crisis (problem, bad time) in your family. How did you solve that problem?
Reactions to the child	Do you find yourself being a little more cautious with this child than with your other children?
Childrearing practices	Do you feel as comfortable disciplining this child as compared with your other children?
Attitudes	How is this child different from the siblings or other children of similar age? Describe your child's personality. Is it easy, difficult, or in-between? When you think of your child's future, what thoughts come to mind?
Available resources	What parts of your child's care are causing the most difficulty for you and/or your family? What services are available to help? What services do you need that presently are not available?
Concurrent stresses	What other problems are you facing now? (Be specific—ask about financial, marital, sibling, and extended family/friends concerns.)

(e.g., "believing that my child[ren] will get better" or "talking with the medical staff [nurses, social workers, etc.] when we visited the medical center") are listed, and parents are asked to record how "helpful" (0 to 3) the coping items are to them in managing the home illness situation (McCubbin and others, 1983). A number of other instruments can be used to assess various aspects of the family's needs and resources (Bailey and Simeonsson, 1988; Dunst, Trivette, and Deal, 1988; McCubbin and Thompson, 1987). Tools that a family may use to assess their resources and home environment are described in Chapter 25.

Regardless of the approach, assessment must be a continuous process because approach behaviors during one phase of the illness do not ensure reciprocal coping mechanisms in subsequent phases. Since support systems may change and perception of events may be altered at any point during the illness, nurses must continually evaluate the effectiveness of their interventions.

The nurse also assesses the parents' reaction to the child, using as a guideline the four categories of responses—overprotection, rejection, denial, and acceptance. Observing how parents interact with the child can provide valuable information (Bean, 1987):

- Do the parents cuddle the infant during feeding or maintain distance by positioning the baby on a bed or infant seat?
- Do they touch or stroke an older child who is fed in a high chair other than during actual feeding activities?
- During feeding, dressing, and play, do the parents periodically make direct eye contact with the child?
- Do the parents talk with the child and respond positively to vocalization?

The parents' and child's understanding of the condition is another significant assessment area. Parental knowledge fosters coping and is particularly important since most children seek information from the parents. One method of eliciting information is to ask how the person would explain the child's condition to a stranger. This approach frequently eliminates the use of medical jargon that the family has learned to conveniently cover up their true feelings. For example, if a parent explains that mental retardation means an IQ (intelligence quotient) of 75, the nurse can reinforce the accuracy of the information and add that often a stranger is unfamiliar with such numbers and needs to know what it means to have an IQ of 75.

While inquiring about the parents' level of understanding, the nurse also focuses on the child's and siblings' knowledge of the condition. It is not unusual for parents who appear well adjusted and knowledgeable to state that they have never told the children the truth. Although this is less of a problem when the condition is visible, it may occur when the disability can be cloaked in terms such as "a little behind" or "slow learner." Conflict arises when the child or siblings learn of the diagnosis from nonparental sources. (See also Informing Children of a Life-Threatening Diagnosis, Chapter 23.)

There are special challenges in assessing children's feelings about having a disability. The discussion on communication techniques in Chapter 6 focuses on several approaches to encourage children to discuss feelings about their diagnosis and future. For example, using drawing and play as a method of communication is appropriate in the child who may lack verbal skills or for any child dealing with difficult feelings.

Traditionally, the mother and child have been active participants and receivers of professional care, whereas fathers and siblings have been excluded. However, to achieve the goal of optimum development for the family unit, each member must be included. This involves scheduling office and/or home visits at times when other family members can be present. Although occasionally this necessitates appointments during evenings or early mornings, visits can also occur late in the afternoon or on weekends. Fathers often will change their work schedule to meet with a health professional once an invitation is extended.

The task of including other family members in a visit is approached positively. If they have not been included previously, they may interpret such an invitation as a portent of more bad news or an indication of their own difficulties. One way of welcoming others to join in a visit is to state that after hearing so often about the other siblings and the father, the nurse wishes to meet them. This casual approach is nonthreatening and implies friendly connotations.

Ideally a thorough assessment includes observing the child and family in a variety of settings, including the home and school. Tools that can be used to systematically assess the home environment are the Home Observation for Man-

GUIDELINES

Assessing Child's Home and School Environment

Observe the child's home and classroom behaviors, such as the ability to sit, follow directions, and comply with requests; determine appropriate responses to questions; and determine the child's independence in functioning.
Gather data on reported behavioral problems such as "hyperactivity," "noncompliance," or "stubbornness."
Observe the child's interactions with siblings and peers.
Observe the child's behaviors in structured and nonstructured activities.
Observe the parents' and teacher's appropriate and nonappropriate interactions with the child.
Observe the parents' and teacher's teaching strategies with the child. (Are school strategies consistent with home teaching?)
Observe the child's relationships with adults.
Determine the parents' and teacher's concerns and expectations of the child.
Administer standardized screening tools with the parent or teacher.
Observe the child's behavior before, during, and following a medication regimen.
Observe the child's eating patterns at home and at school.
Collaborate with the parents and teacher in future planning for the child.
Determine the effectiveness of programs of care for the child.
Coordinate parents, teachers, and others' plans for the child.
Assess the teacher's and/or school nurse's understanding of the child's disorder.

agement of the Environment (HOME) and the Home Screening Questionnaire (see Chapter 6).

The second most important environment for a child is school. Teachers exert a tremendous influence on the child's developmental progress, feelings of self-esteem, learning capacity, and formation of social relationships. Whenever feasible, the nurse should ask parents permission to visit the school to observe directly the child's behavior and interaction among teachers and classmates. A summary of objectives for home and school visits is presented in the Guidelines box on p. 951.

PROVIDE SUPPORT AT THE TIME OF DIAGNOSIS

The impact of the crisis usually occurs at the time of diagnosis, which may be at the time of birth, following a long period of physical and/or psychologic testing, or immediately after a tragic injury. It may begin before the diagnosis is made, when parents are aware that something is wrong with their child but before medical confirmation (Clements, Copeland, and Loftus, 1990).

The time of diagnosis is a critical time for parents. Although they may not hear or remember all that is said to them, they frequently sense a certain attitude of acceptance, rejection, hope, or despair that may influence their ability to absorb the shock and to begin adapting to the family's altered future. The affective tone of the communication is very important to parents (Krahn, Hallum, and Kime, 1993.)

Although it is usually the physician's responsibility to inform the family of the diagnosis, nurses are increasingly responsible for acting as a collaborator with the physician, giving follow-up information, and coordinating services with other agencies. Regardless of the exact role nurses assume, they must have guidelines to follow during the informing interview to provide the family with support during this critical time (see Guidelines box).

Parents are encouraged to be together when they are informed of their child's condition, thus avoiding the problem of one parent having to interpret complex findings and deal with the initial emotional reaction of the other. It also provides an opportunity to observe the interaction between the parents as they are confronted with the tragedy of discovering a serious problem in their child. Expressions on their faces, the times they look down, their ability to main-

GUIDELINES
Informing the Family of a Serious Condition

INITIAL DISCUSSION

- Discuss suspicions of a problem with parents when waiting for a definite diagnosis to help prepare them for a potentially serious diagnosis.
- Have both parents present or have a friend or family member accompany a single parent.
- Let the practitioner who knows the family best present the diagnosis with the primary nurse present.
- Share information about the child's diagnosis:
  - Use the correct terminology for the diagnosis.
  - Avoid names of symptoms to define the disorder that immediately have negative connotations. For example, instead of saying "Down syndrome is retardation," say, "Down syndrome is a chromosome abnormality." Once the dialogue has begun, tell parents other characteristics of the condition, (e.g., "A characteristic of Down syndrome is mental retardation").
  - Mention alternative names for the condition.
  - Discuss the possible range of functioning.
  - Explain other medical problems and how these are or are not related to the child's diagnosis.
- Be willing to repeat information if necessary.
- Convey kindness and understanding by sitting down near the parents, touching the parent's hand or shoulder, calling the child by name, and saying the parent's name during the conversation.
- Stress the personhood of the child by showing love, concern, and respect for the child as an individual.
- Allow parents to express emotion and to work through feelings naturally.
- Encourage parents to ask questions, and provide a telephone number for them to call with questions later or if they just want to talk more.
- Be patient if the parents continue to ask the same questions.
- Help parents feel competent and in control:
  - Assure parents that they will be kept informed to enable them to participate effectively in decision making regarding their child's treatment and care.
  - Provide parents with information about parent support groups or family resource centers, as well as knowledge about services and resources and financial assistance programs.
  - Ask for permission to call and give their name and phone number to a parent self-help organization, enabling the organization to reach out to them.
  - Discuss the siblings and assure parents that siblings tend to do well, especially if kept informed and included in the child's care.

ONGOING INFORMATION

- Share complete information with parents on an ongoing basis.
- Share information in manageable doses. Ask parents what information they want to receive at a given time to determine readiness and to avoid overload.
- Be sensitive to parents' reactions.
- Listen carefully when parents identify their needs, remembering that they may not always know the label of the service they require (e.g., that respite service is having someone else take over for a while so they can get some rest).
- Provide technical information in understandable terms, yet link these explanations with medical terminology.
- Explain why certain questions are being asked.
- Offer to share information with the child or with others involved in the child's care (e.g., brothers, sisters, grandparents, other extended family members, teachers, caregivers).
- Provide information on family support programs, referrals for specialty consultations and intervention programs, and opportunities to meet other parents whose child has a similar condition.

tain eye contact with the nurse, their behaviors that show they are avoiding what the nurse is saying, such as turning their heads, looking around, or looking away, or any other activity that shows that they are indeed dealing with a very difficult subject is observed.

The informing session should take place in a private, comfortable setting free of distractions and interruptions (Fig. 22-2). The atmosphere should be one in which parents feel free to express their emotions. If their feelings can be expressed and acknowledged, the parents can be helped to deal openly with them, and their need for further counseling can be determined. Their emotional needs are acknowledged by showing acceptance of such expressions as crying, sadness, anger, and disappointment. Emotional support is offered by having tissues available if a family member cries and demonstrating through facial and bodily language that indeed this is a difficult and painful period. Although touching is a powerful expression of empathy, it must be used wisely. For example, it can prematurely terminate free expression of feelings, especially when combined with statements such as "Everything will be all right." Nurses should also be aware of cultural issues regarding touching (see Chapter 2).

Parents should receive the kind of information they desire. Most parents report wanting a clear, simple explanation of the diagnosis, including what is and is not known about the diagnosis, a prediction of possible futures for the child, advice on what to do next, an opportunity to ask questions, a warm and sympathetic listener, and, most important, time. Clarification of explanations is elicited with such questions as, "Do you see what I mean?" or "Is this clear to you?" Technical terms are used with simple definitions. If the parents are unaware of the term, they are given written literature or at least a written summary of the diagnosis.

➤ **NURSING TIP** Develop a glossary of commonly used medical, technical, or disciplinary-specific terms; acronyms; and "initials" to distribute to parents. The list can stand alone or become a part of patient or parent handbooks.

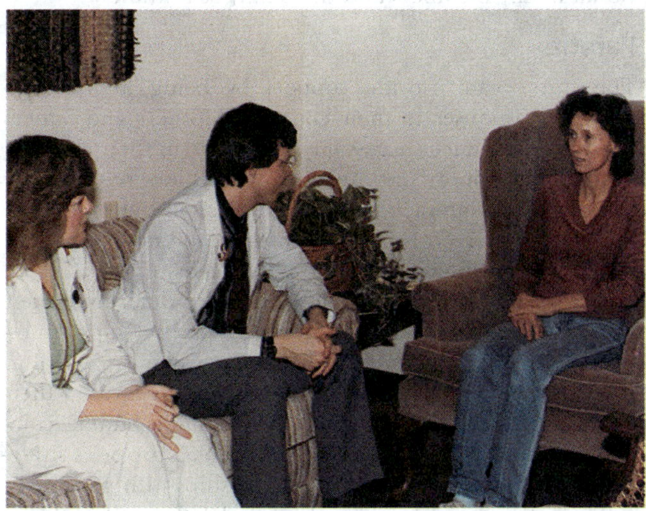

FIG. 22-2 Informing session should take place in a private, comfortable setting free of distractions and interruptions.

Finally, the informing conference should not end with the presentation of devastating news. Instead, the child's strengths, appealing behaviors, and potential for development are stressed, as well as available rehabilitation efforts or treatment. Parents are encouraged to view life with their child as very similar to life with other children. Their experiences should be thought of as a series of challenges that they are capable of handling, particularly with available professional feedback. The parents are assured that the nurse will be available to answer questions and to provide further assistance as it is needed in the future.

The preceding discussion relates primarily to the initial informing interview. However, because of the need for long-term follow-up, it is only one in a series of continuing discussions. In all interactions the family's input is solicited and incorporated into the plan of care (see also the Guidelines box on p. 955).

ACCEPT THE FAMILY'S EMOTIONAL REACTIONS

One of the most supportive interventions is to accept the family's emotional reactions to the diagnosis in as nonjudgmental a manner as possible. Although all families respond differently and in varying degrees of intensity, three responses are so common and often so poorly handled that they deserve special consideration.

Denial

Nurses' response to denial is a critical component of the individual's continuing need for this defense mechanism. The most effective method of support is active listening. Silence neither reinforces nor rejects denial (or any other emotional reaction) but implies a willingness and acceptance of the person's need for this behavior. However, silence alone can be misinterpreted. For example, if the person demonstrates denial, such as by saying, "I am sure the doctors made a mistake," and the nurse responds silently and leaves, the person may infer disapproval, agreement, avoidance, or rejection from this behavior.

To be effective, silence and listening must be accompanied by physical and mental concentration and use of body language to communicate interest and concern. Direct eye contact, touch, physical closeness, and body posture, such as sitting and leaning slightly forward, demonstrate silent but effective communication. Sometimes accepting people where they are, from their own perspective, is likely to give them the acknowledgment necessary to become more aware of their motives and to consider change.

Guilt

Since guilt is such a common response and can cause family members tremendous anxiety, they should be told directly that there is no known cause of the disorder when appropriate and that they are not to be blamed. Using the third-person technique (see Chapter 6) is valuable in eliciting thoughts of guilt. For example, with children an appropriate statement may be, "When people get sick, they often wonder if they did anything to

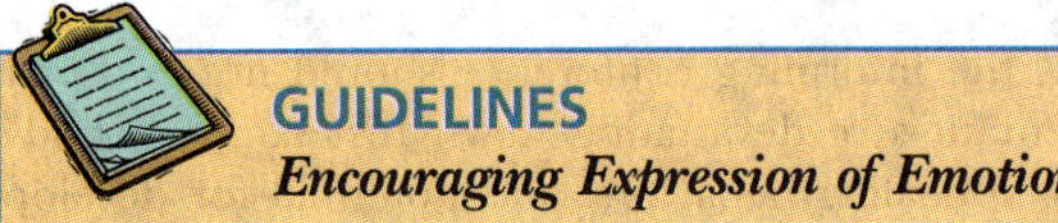

GUIDELINES
Encouraging Expression of Emotion

Describe the behavior: "You seem angry at everyone."
Give evidence of understanding: "Being angry is only natural."
Give evidence of caring: "It must be difficult to endure so many painful procedures."
Help focus on feelings: "Maybe you wonder why this happened to your child."

make themselves sick." This allows children an opportunity to explore any feelings of responsibility they harbor.

If family members are expressing feelings of guilt, it is important to allow them to talk about their feelings rather than quickly trying to dispel them with long "scientific" explanations. Statements such as "If you believe you are responsible for Johnny's condition, then no wonder you feel so bad," acknowledge the family member's feelings. This step is frequently appreciated and necessary before the facts can be presented and absorbed. An effective method in lessening guilt is to encourage the irrationality of thought. For example, one mother stated that her son probably developed cancer by sitting too close to the television, which she could have prevented by being more strict. By following her reasoning and talking about how *many* children sit close to the television and how *few* of them ever have cancer, the nurse was able to help the mother realize that this activity was not a cause.

Anger

Anger is one of the more difficult reactions to accept and deal with therapeutically. The responses to anger may be reciprocal anger, fear, acceptance, and/or encouragement. The first two reactions close off communication and express disapproval and rejection of the person. They most commonly occur when the listener views the anger as a personal assault. The last two responses allow the individual to ventilate his or her feelings in an atmosphere of nonjudgmental acceptance. Two basic rules for dealing with the angry person are to avoid losing one's temper and to encourage the person to talk. Guidelines for encouraging expression of emotions are provided in the Guidelines box above.

One essential element to the successful implementation of this process is to wait for the person to respond to a statement before proceeding to the next step. Since the objective of each statement is for the person to speak freely, the responses should avoid "yes" or "no" types of answers. For example, the behavior can be described, or the nurse can ask directly, "Are you angry?" The latter question, however, may hinder further expressive communication and places the burden of subsequent conversation on the nurse, who should be the listener.

HELP THE FAMILY COPE

In order for the family to meet the stresses of optimally adjusting to the child's condition, each member must be individually supported so that the family system is strong. Although the family unit can indefinitely support a member who is in need of assistance, its greatest strength lies in every member supporting each other. The nurse should bear in mind that the "member in need" is not necessarily the affected child but may be a parent or sibling who is dealing with stresses that require intervention.

Two recent theories offer some insight into family coping. The "chronic illness trajectory" model acknowledges that chronic conditions have a course that varies and changes over time (Corbin and Strauss, 1991). The course of the illness is affected by many medical and psychosocial factors, including technology, resources (instrumental, intrapersonal, and interpersonal), past experience, motivation, life-style, type and severity of illness, and the social climate. The majority of chronic illness management occurs in the home, not the hospital. This model suggests that the goal of nursing care in chronic illness is to help the family shape the course of the illness medically while maintaining quality of life for the child and family. This is done through assessment, teaching, monitoring, providing referrals, and so forth.

A second theory relates to family management styles. This theory, described by Knafl and Deatrick (1990), emphasizes the family's role in actively responding to a child's illness. Aspects of management style include:

- How the family defines the illness situation—what it means to them
- Management behaviors that the family applies, including alterations of family member roles, adapting life-style choices, and the like
- The sociocultural context, such as values and beliefs, as well as the political/economic climate

Knafl and Deatrick suggest that coping patterns and techniques can be learned. When nurses come to understand a family's management style, interventions can be targeted most appropriately to promote the growth of individual family members and the family as a whole.

Parents

The nurse can provide support by being attentive to families' responses to their children. Mothers and fathers need to experience success, joy, and pride in their children to give the support they need. Children, too, require support for their interactions, adjustments, and efforts. They must be reinforced for attempts to get to know their care providers and to communicate their needs to them.

Nurses must examine their attitudes to determine their ability to engage in parent-professional partnerships. An essential characteristic is the belief that parents are equal to professionals and that parents are experts regarding their child. The partnership is based on trust and is built by communication. The Guidelines box on p. 955 provides strategies for developing successful partnerships with parents.

Since the majority of mothers and fathers of children with special needs have little or no experience with children who have chronic or disabling conditions, the nurse can re-

GUIDELINES

Developing Successful Parent-Professional Partnerships

Promote primary nursing; in nonhospital settings designate a case manager.
Acknowledge the parents' overall competence and their unique expertise with their child.
Respect the parents' time as having equal value to that of other members of the child's health care team.
Explain or define any medical, technical, or disciplinary-specific terms.
Tell families, "I am not sure" or "I don't know" when appropriate.
Facilitate the family's effectiveness in team meetings:
- Provide families the opportunity to decide on the appropriate family members and professionals to include in assessment conferences and other meetings.
- Provide information to parents in a face-to-face meeting before convening any formal decision-making meeting about their child.
- Distribute meeting agendas to all participants, including the family, before the date of the meeting. Families, like all other team members, should always be made aware of why a meeting is being held, who will be there, and what to expect.
- Introduce other professionals who may be involved with the child to the parents before any group meeting.
- Provide parents with the same information as other participants so that they can contribute to any decision about their child (e.g., child development checklist, copies of assessment reports).
- Invite parents to speak first and often throughout any information-giving or decision-making meetings, to give their perspectives and describe their observations before professionals give theirs.
- Be open with families and with other professionals when there is disagreement about any aspect of assessment or programming.

Data from Bruder M: Parent and professional partnerships under PL 99-457, *Early Child Update* 5(2):1-2, 1989; Johnson B, McGonigel M, Kaufmann R, editors: *Guidelines and recommended practices for the Individualized Family Service Plan,* Washington, DC, 1989, Association for the Care of Children's Health; and Johnson BH, Jeppson ES, Redburn L: Caring for children and families: guidelines for hospitals, Bethesda, MD, 1992, Association for the Care of Children's Health.

mind them of their child's many strengths and normal traits and can role model appropriate interactions with the child. Above all, the nurse should ensure that the parents and siblings learn to perceive the child as a child first, with unique and individual characteristics and needs. The nurse needs to convey a humanistic, accepting approach of the child so that the parents can observe this acceptance. This attitude of liking, having concern for, and showing acceptance of the child should begin in early infancy and continue throughout the child's life.

Communication. Communication among all family members is encouraged. Parent group sessions are helpful in assisting parents in verbalizing thoughts and feelings to each other but often do not take into account siblings' or the child's viewpoint. Therefore the nurse may need to set up a family session, such as during a home or clinic visit. Although the ideal situation is to have all the members present at once, this is often not possible within the confines of traditional nursing practice. However, inviting members to participate at various visits is an appropriate alternative.

Parents are encouraged to discuss their feelings toward the child, the impact of this event on their marriage, and associated stresses, such as financial burdens. For most families, regardless of their income or insurance coverage, financial concerns exist. The costs of caring for a child with special needs can be overwhelming. Children with functional limitations account for one third of child hospital days; their hospital stays average twice as long; and they visit physicians twice as often as children without limitations (Horwitz and Stein, 1990). Direct medical expenses, in combination with out-of-pocket expenses for nonprescription medication, transportation, and so forth, can consume a high percentage of a family's income. In addition, the family wage earner may have to sacrifice job opportunities to remain close to a medical facility or to avoid losing insurance benefits.*

Fathers. While chronic illness often solidifies traditional male breadwinner and female caregiver roles in a family, families who open up these definitions and expand the boundaries of traditional roles can become stronger. Frequently the hospital and outpatient setting is less accepting and welcoming of direct involvement of fathers in decision making about or provision of the child's daily care. Furthermore, since many men have been socialized to bear burdens and not talk about feelings, men are often left without the emotional support so necessary to cope effectively. There are several ways nurses can encourage fathers to be involved in the life of their child with special needs (see Guidelines box on p. 956).

Coping Skills. Teaching the family how to cope with the child's chronic illness or disability can promote positive adaptation (Patterson and Geber, 1991). Cognitive, behavioral, and emotional tasks are part of the adaptive coping process:

- Cognitive tasks include learning about the disability, its prognosis, its management, and the like.
- Behavioral tasks include the actual management of the child's condition, doing daily therapies, monitoring the child, teaching self-care, and so forth.
- Emotional tasks include grieving the loss of normal functioning in the child, processing anger, and addressing limitations the condition places on all family members.

In addition, nurses can assist parents by identifying and building on family strengths, promoting child and family competence, and encouraging the development of a nurturing environment that addresses the needs of parents and siblings, as well as the child with special needs. Promoting normalization, teaching coping skills, and helping the family to use or further develop their social support networks are other nursing actions that can encourage and empower the parents and promote positive adaptation in the family

*Information regarding financial issues is available from the **Federation for Children with Special Needs,** 95 Berkeley St., Suite 104, Boston, MA 02116; (617) 482-2915.

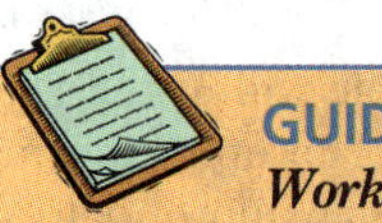

GUIDELINES
Working with Fathers

- Want and seek the involvement of fathers.
- Expect that fathers will be participants in decision making and involved in care provision.
- Regard fathers as able, effective parents, competent and capable of coping with the challenges they face.
- Invite the father to family meetings from the very beginning.
- Arrange appointments, meetings, or training sessions in the early morning, late afternoon, evening, or weekend to create minimal interference with the father's work schedule and give sufficient notice for fathers to accommodate their work schedule.
- Value the problem-solving, pragmatic approach and expertise that many men bring to the difficult challenges their families face (e.g., legislative advocacy, building adaptive devices, making videotapes).
- Show fathers a variety of ways to be involved in their child's care and support their involvement. Include them in training sessions on the child's care needs.
- Use social situations to introduce fathers to each other, such as family weekends, potluck dinners, and/or sporting events.
- Create and support father's support programs.
- Examine existing programs for families, from policy to implementation, for father's involvement.
- Involve fathers in program development and staff training.

Data from May J: *Fathers of children with special needs: new horizons,* Washington, DC, 1990, Association for the Care of Children's Health; May JE, Davis PB: Service delivery issues in working with fathers of children with special needs, *ACCH Network* 8(2):4, 1990; and Davis PB, May JE: Involving fathers in early intervention and family support programs, *Child Health Care* 20(2):87-91, 1991.

*Excellent resources on fathers' issues are presented in a training film, *Special Kids, Special Dads: Fathers of Children with Disabilities,* and a monograph, *Fathers of Children with Special Needs: New Horizons,* both of which are available from the Association for the Care of Children's Health, 7910 Woodmont Ave., Suite 300, Bethesda, MD 20814; (301) 654-6549.

and optimum mental health for the child (Patterson and Geber, 1991).

Community Resources. Community resources are often an important element in parent coping with chronic illness or disability. Numerous volunteer and community resources are available that provide assistance, rehabilitation, equipment, and funding for a variety of health problems.* National and local disease-oriented organizations may provide needed assistance and support to families that qualify. Many of these are discussed elsewhere in the text under the diagnosis. State and federal departments of health, mental health, social service, and labor may be able to help locate appropriate regional resources. For example, state **Programs for Children with Special Health Needs** (formerly Crippled Children's Services) provide financial assistance for children with many disabling conditions. Nurses should become acquainted with those in their communities and with vocational programs for special groups.

Although community resources may exist, it is often very difficult for parents to locate suitable services, and coordination among several agencies may be lacking. Fragmented care is one of the chief complaints from families, with specific problems of delayed referral and negative experiences with agency personnel cited as other concerns. Consequently, community networking for improved services is essential.*

Furthermore, case management can be a key service for families of children with special needs (Diehl, Moffitt, and Wade, 1991; Jackson, Finkler, and Robinson, 1992). Effective case management can result in both the use of more community services and better financial assistance for families. One study also documented better information, support, advocacy, and improved maternal satisfaction with a family-centered case management program (Marcenko and Smith, 1992).

Parent-to-Parent Support. The support a parent receives from another parent is unique and unobtainable from any other source. A growing number of hospitals and clinics now have a parent with a child who is chronically ill or disabled on staff. The services these parents provide are particularly valuable for parents of children with special needs who are likely to experience frequent and lengthy hospitalizations, as well as numerous routine clinic visits.

Just being with another parent who has shared similar experiences is helpful. A parent of a child with the same diagnosis is not always necessary, for parents in the process of adjusting to a child with special needs—or finding respite services, educational or rehabilitative services, special equipment vendors, or financial counseling—tread a common path. If the agency does not have a parent staff position, the nurse can contact parent groups, who will often send a representative. Another strategy is to ask another parent with a child who is chronically ill or disabled to talk to the parents.† The nurse should seek out a parent who is a good listener, has a nonjudgmental approach to differences in families, and possesses good advocacy and problem-solving skills.

The parent self-help group is another way to promote parent-to-parent support.‡ Group members feel less alone and have the opportunity to observe both coping and mastery role modeling from other members. Parents' groups

*A general source of information is the **National Information Center for Children and Youth with Disabilities,** P.O. Box 1492, Washington, DC 20013; (202) 884-8200 or (800) 695-0285. A comprehensive list of books and pamphlets for parents and teachers is available from the **National Easter Seal Society,** 23 W. Monroe St., Suite 1800, Chicago IL 60606; (312) 726-6200.

Guidelines for Developing Community Networks: Support for Families of Children with Chronic Illness or Handicapping Conditions,* available from the **Association for the Care of Children's Health, 7910 Woodmont Ave., Suite 300, Bethesda, MD 20814, (301) 654-6549; *Workbook Series for Providing Services to Children with Handicaps and Their Families,* available from **Georgetown University Child Development Center,** 3800 Reservoir Rd. N.W., Washington, DC 20007, (202) 687-8635.

†The *Parent Resource Directory* lists over 400 parents of children with chronic illness or disabilities in the United States and Canada, including addresses, phone numbers, the child's condition, and the health facility where the child receives care. It is available from the **Association for the Care of Children's Health,** 7910 Woodmont Ave., Suite 300, Bethesda, MD 20814; (301) 654-6549.

‡Information about self-help groups, as well as books and pamphlets, is available from the **National Self-Help Clearinghouse,** CUNY Graduate Center, 25 W. 43rd St., New York, NY 10036; (212) 642-2944.

are rich resources for information. Even if parents are unable to attend meetings, they can still benefit from group newsletters and other literature that often accompany membership. The nurse can foster parent participation in self-help groups by serving as a referral agent, a group advisory board member, a resource person, or an assistant in founding a group. Sometimes all that is required in starting a group is identifying one or two parents as leaders, sharing with them the names, telephone numbers, and addresses of other families, and guiding them in how to initiate a first meeting.*

➤ **NURSING TIP** Use cards and a file box to store information about parent self-help groups. The system facilitates adding new groups, updating old ones, and keeping cards in easy-to-retrieve alphabetic order.

Advocate for Empowerment. Nurses can advocate for methods that foster opportunities for parent empowerment. For example, nurses can suggest reimbursement for travel and child care, plus stipends to enable parents' voices to be heard at meetings and conferences. They can encourage parent membership on staff, committees, and boards. They can help keep parents informed of pending legislation on child health issues or take action when parents inform them.† Nurses can assess parental level of empowerment and provide the support and resources most needed at each level.

GUIDELINES
Promoting Normalization

Preparation. Prepare the child in advance for changes that may occur from the illness or disability; for example, the child is told in advance of the possible side effects of drug therapy.

Participation. Include the child in as many decisions as possible, especially those relating to his or her care regimen; for example, the child is responsible for taking medications or scheduling home treatments.

Sharing. Allow both family members and the child's peers to be a part of the care regimen whenever possible; for example, the child is given his or her medication when the other siblings receive their vitamins; the parent cooks the same menu for the whole family; and if the child is invited to another's home, the parent advises the family of the child's dietary restrictions.

Control. Identify areas where the child can be in control so that feelings of uncertainty, passivity, and helplessness are decreased; for example, the child identifies activities that are appropriate to his or her energy level and chooses to rest when fatigued.

Expectation. Apply the same family rules to the child with a chronic illness or disability as to the well siblings or peers; for example, the child is disciplined, expected to fulfill household responsibilities, and attends school in accordance with abilities.

The Child

Through ongoing contacts with the child, the nurse (1) observes the child's responses to the disorder, ability to function, and adaptive behaviors within the environment and with significant others; (2) explores the child's own understanding of the nature of his or her illness or condition; and (3) provides support while the child learns to cope with his or her feelings. Children are encouraged to express their concerns rather than allowing others to express them for them, since open discussions may reduce anxiety.

Parents sometimes convey concern because the child cannot express the anxieties he or she feels. If the child cannot or will not talk, the child may have to play out his or her feelings. He or she can be provided with toys to express threatening or stressful emotions. The nurse may find that the child responds best to drawing pictures or telling stories (see Chapter 6). Puppets can also be used. By demonstrating to parents how useful these techniques are, the nurse also helps them learn new ways of communicating with the child. For youngsters with extremely serious handicaps and/or persistent maladjustment, psychiatric evaluation and management may be needed.

One of the most important interventions is alleviating the child's feeling of being different and normalizing his or her life as much as possible. The principles in the Guidelines box are fundamental in implementing the normalizing process (Bossert and others, 1990; Krulik, 1980). Whenever possible, the nurse should help parents to assess the child's daily routine for indications of lack of normalizing practices. For example, the child who remains in a bedroom all day is in need of a restructured daily routine to provide activities in different parts of the house, such as eating in the kitchen with the family. Such children may also be aided by the inclusion of social, recreational, and academic activities that can be encouraged by applying normalization principles.

Children who are concerned that their condition detracts from their physical attractiveness need attention focused on the normal aspects of appearance and capabilities. Health professionals must help parents strengthen and consolidate the child's self-image by emphasizing the normal, while at the same time allowing children to express anger, isolation, fear of rejection, feelings of sadness, and loneliness. Anything that might improve attractiveness and contribute to a positive self-image is employed, such as makeup for a teenager with a scar, clothing that disguises a prosthesis, or a hairstyle or wig to cover a deformity or lost hair.

Children, particularly adolescents, are sensitive to the presence or absence of hope. Hopefulness is an internal quality that mobilizes humans into goal-directed action that may be satisfying and life-sustaining. A sense of hopefulness can produce increased participation in health-seeking be-

*The following resources are recommended: *Organizing and Maintaining Support Groups for Parents of Children with Chronic Illness and Handicapping Conditions* by Minna Newman Nathanson, available from the **Association for the Care of Children's Health,** 7910 Woodmont Ave., Suite 300, Bethesda, MD 20814, (301) 654-6549; and *The Self-Help Sourcebook: Finding and Forming Mutual Aid Self-Help Groups* by E.J. Madara and A. Meese, available from the **New Jersey Self-Help Clearinghouse,** Saint Clares–Riverside Medical Center, Denville, NJ 07834, (201) 625-9565.

†An excellent resource for becoming involved in political action is the *Public Affairs Public Issues Handbook,* available from the **American Cancer Society,** National Public Affairs Office, 316 Pennsylvania Ave., S.E., Suite 200, Washington, DC 20003; (202) 546-4011 or (800) ACS-2345.

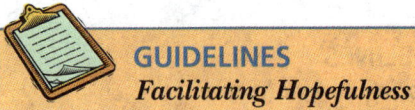

GUIDELINES
Facilitating Hopefulness

Give honest reports of conditions or events.
Encourage and participate with the child in physical activities (e.g., arrange activities, play games, or go for walks together).
Convey a fond, personal interest in the child (give hugs, ask follow-up questions from previous discussions).
Introduce conversations on neutral, non-disease-related or less sensitive topics (discuss child's favorite sports, tell stories).
Convey competence and gentleness when delivering care.
Provide information about other children in similar situations who are doing well.
Encourage the child to think ahead to more comfortable and preferred natural times.
Be lighthearted and initiate or respond to teasing or other playful interactions with the child.

Modified from Hinds P, Martin J, Vogel RJ: Nursing strategies to influence adolescent hopefulness during oncologic illness, *J Assoc Pediatr Oncol Nurs* 4(1/2):14-22, 1987.

haviors and an improved sense of well-being. Nurses can influence hopefulness through interpersonal and environmental means (see Guidelines box).

Siblings

As pointed out, the presence of a child with special needs in a family may result in parents paying less attention to the other children or expecting older siblings to take on greater responsibility for the care of the child. Siblings may respond by developing negative attitudes toward the child or by expressing anger in different forms. On the other hand, some research on siblings of chronically ill children suggests that siblings may demonstrate less hostility and anger toward the impaired sibling than that which exists between normal, comparison siblings (Faux, 1991).

Siblings may experience embarrassment associated with the stigma of a disorder such as mental retardation. Parents are then faced with the difficulty of responding to this embarrassment in an understanding and appropriate manner without punishing the siblings for feeling the way they do. Parents should talk with the siblings about how they view their affected sibling. For example, siblings of a child who is retarded may express fears about their ability to bear normal children. Adolescents in particular may not be able to discuss these vital issues with their parents and may prefer to consult with the nurse. Many siblings benefit from sharing their concerns with other young people who are experiencing a similar situation.* Support groups for siblings help decrease isolation, promote expression of negative feelings, and provide an opportunity to learn from each other (Heiney and others, 1990).

Many parents express concern about when and how to inform the other children in the family about the birth or the presence of a child who is disabled. The answer depends on each child's level of sophistication and understanding. However, it is usually best to inform the siblings before a neighbor or other nonfamily member does so. Nurses can show by their behavior that they see the parents as being capable in their own unique style of imparting information about the condition. However, they should make it clear that if the parents postpone informing the siblings, they assume the risk of hindering the siblings' ability to develop a realistic understanding of the problem. Uninformed siblings may fantasize or develop apprehensions that are out of proportion to the child's actual condition. Furthermore, if parents choose to be silent or deceptive about the issue, they are setting a negative precedent for the siblings to follow, rather than encouraging the siblings to cope with the experience in a healthy and nurturing way.

The nurse must be sensitive to the reactions of siblings and whenever possible intervene to promote positive adjustments. For example, siblings often mention that they are expected to take on additional responsibilities to help the parents care for the child. It is not unusual for them to express a positive reaction to assuming the extra duties but a negative response to feeling unappreciated for doing so. Such feelings can often be minimized by encouraging the siblings to discuss this with the parents and by suggesting to parents ways of showing gratitude, such as an increase in allowance, special privileges, and, most significantly, verbal praise (see Family Home Care box).

Extended Family Members and Society

The nurse must also be sensitive to family's cues regarding sources of stress from extended members, such as grandparents. For example, the nurse may encourage the parents to invite the grandparents to be present during one of the child's visits to a clinic, during the diagnostic workup, or to a parent conference or to provide appropriate literature. Including grandparents in a discussion in which they can share their concerns may help them deal with their feelings, thus reducing stress on the entire family. Grandparents' feelings of blame and anger, as well as any "cure fantasies" they harbor, can be brought out in the open and discussed if necessary. Grandparents can be helped to understand the effects of their behavior on the family with an appropriate statement, such as, "Your daughter is currently experiencing a great deal of pain and anguish. We realize that this is difficult for you as well as your daughter; however, you can be of tremendous help by being supportive toward her."

Considerable stress can also arise from nonfamilial sources, such as friends, neighbors, or strangers. Inability to cope with comments about the disorder or curious stares by others may foster the tendency to isolate and protect the child within the home. The family needs guidance in preparing for these inevitable experiences. One approach is encouraging parents to dress the child as much as possible like other children. Good grooming is very important in minimizing differences in appearance. Through role-playing parents can practice responses to comments such as "Is your child retarded?" or "Has he always been crippled?" Through parent groups family members can share experiences and learn from each other how they successfully deal with prob-

*For information on the **Sibling Information Network,** contact the Information Network, The A.J. Pappanikou Center: A-VAP, 62 Washington St., Middletown, CT 06457-2844; (203) 344-7500.

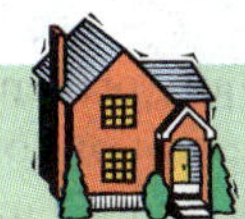

FAMILY HOME CARE
Supporting Siblings of Children with Special Needs

PROMOTE HEALTHY SIBLING RELATIONSHIPS

Value each child individually, and avoid comparisons. Remind each child of his or her positive qualities and contribution to other family members.

Help siblings see the differences and similarities between themselves and a child with special needs. Create a climate in which children can achieve successes without feeling guilty.

Teach siblings ways to interact with the child.

Seek to be fair in terms of discipline, attention, and resources; require the affected child to do as much for himself or herself as possible.

Let siblings settle their own differences; intervene only to prevent siblings from hurting one another.

Legitimize reasonable anger. Even children with special needs behave badly sometimes.

Respect a sibling's reluctance to be with or to include the child with special needs in activities.

HELP SIBLINGS COPE

Listen to siblings to let them know that their thoughts and suggestions are valued.

Praise siblings when they have been patient, have sacrificed, or have been particularly helpful. Do not expect siblings to always act in this manner.

Acknowledge the personal strengths siblings have and their ability to cope with stress successfully.

Provide age-appropriate information about the child's condition, and update when appropriate.

Let teachers know what is happening so they can be understanding and helpful.

Recognize special stress times for siblings and plan to minimize negative effects.

Schedule special time with siblings; have a friend or family member substitute when parent is unavailable.

Encourage siblings to join or help establish a sibling support group.

Use the services of professionals when needed. If parent feels that such a service is necessary, it should be provided in as vigorous a manner as a service for the child with special needs.

INVOLVE SIBLINGS

Seek out ways to realistically include siblings in the care and treatment of the child with special needs.

Limit caregiving responsibilities and give recognition when siblings perform them.

Develop a library of children's books on special needs.

Invite siblings to attend meetings to develop plans for the child with special needs (e.g., IEP, IFSP).

Discuss future plans with them.

Solicit their ideas on treatment and service needs.

Have them visit professionals who work with the child.

Help them develop competencies to teach the child new skills.

Provide opportunities for siblings to advocate for the child.

Allow siblings to set their own pace for learning and involvement.

Modified from Powell T, Ogle P: *Brothers and sisters—a special part of exceptional families,* Baltimore, 1985, Paul H Brooks; Spokane Washington Deaconess Medical Center Pediatric Oncology Unit: Tips for dealing with siblings, *The Candlelighters Childhood Cancer Foundation Quarterly Newsletter* 11(3, 4):7, 1987; and Carlson J, Leviton A, Mueller M: Services to siblings: an important component of family-centered practice, *The ACCH Advocate* 1(1):53-56, 1993.

ing questions or unkind remarks. Such interventions must include the siblings and the affected child, who also must face and deal with these events. Nurses can be instrumental in teaching young children about disabilities to familiarize them with the special needs and abilities of these individuals. For example, school nurses can simulate experiences such as having only one leg or being blind by using role-playing, they can use books or films, or they can invite community guests with physical limitations to visit the class.

FOSTER REALITY ADJUSTMENT

Fostering a reality adjustment primarily involves family education regarding the disorder, as well as general health care, developmental needs of the child, and realistic goal setting. Ideally, education should be aimed at preventing problems, rather than at relearning to change existing dilemmas. Like the interventions previously discussed, this goal requires an ongoing process that is part of assessment and emotional support of the family.

Educate About the Disorder and General Health Care

Educating the family about the disorder is actually an extension of revealing the diagnosis, especially those points listed in the Guidelines box on p. 952.* Education involves not only supplying technical information but also discussing how the condition will affect the child. For example, it is of little benefit to discuss mental retardation in terms of numbers. Rather, parents need to understand what the child can do in terms of self-help, academic learning, and independence. Similarly, the child who has lost a limb needs more than an explanation of the prosthetic leg. He or she must know the limitations it places on activity, as well as how to function with it and any special available opportunities.

Parents also need guidance on how the condition may interfere with or alter activities of daily living, such as eating, dressing, sleeping, and toileting. One area frequently affected is nutrition. Common problems are undernutrition as a result of food being inappropriately restricted, loss of appetite, vomiting, or motor deficits that interfere with feeding and overnutrition usually caused by a caloric intake in excess of energy expenditure or boredom and lack of stimulation in other areas. Although the child requires the same basic nutrients as other children, the daily require-

*Home care instruction sheets, which may be copied and given to families, are available in *Wong and Whaley's Clinical Manual of Pediatric Nursing* (Mosby).

ments may differ. Special nutritional considerations are discussed as appropriate throughout the text.

In addition to special nutritional needs, another very important area in which modifications may be needed is car safety. Children with conditions such as low birth weight or orthopaedic, neuromuscular, or respiratory problems often cannot safely use conventional care restraints. For example, children with hip spica casts cannot sit properly in child safety seats (see Developmental Dysplasia of the Hip, Chapter 11). Modifications can be made to some commercial models,* and for older children a special vest† is available that secures the child in a lying-down position to the back seat. Children in wheelchairs present special challenges because the wheelchair should be anchored with four points of attachment to the vehicle (two in front and two behind) and should always face forward (Richards, 1989). The family should consult the wheelchair manufacturer for specific instructions regarding safe car transportation.

Children with special needs require all the usual health care recommended for any child. Attention to injury prevention, immunizations, dental health, and regular physical examinations is essential. Nurses can play an important role in reminding parents of these aspects of care that are so often neglected when the concern is focused on the child's specific illness or disability. (See Recommendations for Health Supervision in Chapter 7 for assessing general aspects of health maintenance.) Specific discussions of nutrition, sleep and activity, dental health, and injury prevention are presented in the chapters on health promotion for specific age-groups. Immunizations are discussed in Chapter 12.

*Information on restraints for children with special needs is available from Automotive Safety for Children Program, Riley Hospital for Children, 534 N. Clinical Dr., Rm. 118, Indianapolis, IN 46202-5109; (317) 274-2977 or (800) KID-N-CAR (in Indiana).

†E-Z-On Vest is available from E-Z-On Products, 500 Commerce Way West, Suite 3, Jupiter, FL 33458; (407) 747-6920 or (800) 323-6598 (outside Florida).

Parents also need to be aware of the importance of communicating the child's condition in the event of a medical emergency. Young children are unable to give information about their disorder, and although older children may be reliable sources, after an accident they may be physically unable to speak. Therefore all children with any type of chronic condition that may affect medical care should wear some type of identification, such as a Medic-Alert bracelet,* which lists the medical condition and a collect phone number for emergency medical records and other personal information.

Children need information about their condition, the therapeutic plan, and how the disease or the therapy might affect their particular situation. Children nearing puberty also need to understand the maturation process and how their disability may alter this event. For example, the youngster with Crohn disease should understand that this disorder is associated with growth failure and delayed puberty; the child with diabetes needs to know that hormonal changes and increased growth needs will alter food and insulin requirements at this time; and the sexually active girl with sickle cell anemia or systemic lupus erythematosus needs to be aware of the hazards of pregnancy. The information should not be given all at once but timed appropriately to meet the changing needs of the youngsters, and it should be described and repeated as often as the situation demands (see Thinking Critically About . . . box).

*P.O. Box 1009, Turlock, CA 95381-1009; (800) ID-ALERT.

THINKING CRITICALLY ABOUT . . .

Approaches to Teaching Children About Their Illness or Disability

The traditional Piagetian approach to cognitive development has been the basis for most explanations of children's understanding of illness. Bibace and Walsh (1980, 1981) and Perrin and Gerrity (1981) have provided the most detailed systems of children's illness concepts using the Piagetian framework. This stage-based approach assumes that when a child is in a particular cognitive stage, the style of reasoning typical of that stage will apply to the child's understanding of illness.

Yet, the bulk of research examining children's illness concepts has been done on healthy children and fails to account for experience with illness as a factor in a child's understanding (Yoos, 1994). In fact, some research in child development and cognition suggests that domain-specific content knowledge (e.g., knowledge about a particular illness) may be more than an adjunct to cognition; it may be a critical element of the cognitive process. For example, Yoos (1991) found that school-age patients outperformed healthy adults in their total amount of knowledge about a disease, the cohesiveness of their knowledge structures, and the sophistication of their reasoning about aspects of the disease and its treatment. Children's awareness of concepts related to health and illness may thus reflect their access to relevant information as much or more than their cognitive maturity (Bird and Podmore, 1990).

Communication with children about their illness or disability is an integral part of nursing practice. Yoos (1994) suggests that the concept of cognitive stages may be useful to describe patterns in children but can be limiting if nurses assume that children are incapable of understanding certain medical information because of cognitive inabilities inherent in a specific stage. The child who is chronically ill or disabled has a need for a great deal of information about his or her condition to promote confidence, competence, and mastery. Over time, the child with a chronic condition may pick up bits of information, correct or incorrect, to meet that need. Rather than relying solely on the concept of cognitive stages, nurses should use individual assessments of both a child's knowledge base and knowledge deficits in the development of appropriate teaching strategies.

The subject of sexuality related to the effects of the disorder is a prominent concern of adolescents, but they rarely initiate a discussion of this sensitive topic. Any probable interference in sexual function because of the disability should be discussed openly and candidly with the teenager. Unfortunately, many nurses are reticent to discuss sexual issues with adolescents. Adults often underestimate the degree to which adolescents engage in unrealistic fantasies regarding sexual activities and related matters, or even sexual activity itself. In a study that compared parent and adolescent responses on perceived health care needs, parents were unaware of their teenagers' sexual activity (Dragone, 1990).

Throughout the long process of caring for a child with special needs, family members become expert in management of their child's care. Unfortunately, this expertise is often not recognized by health professionals who tend to be directive, rather than collaborative, in their approach to the family. This is particularly common during periods of hospitalization, when parents are placed in a "double-bind"—at home they are expected to care for their child yet in the hospital they are ignored as participants in care, especially treatment regimens. A supportive atmosphere must include coordination of care with family members, respect for their knowledge, and willingness to include their suggestions in the treatment plan.

Promote Normal Development

Aside from knowledge of the condition and its effect on the child's abilities, the family must be guided toward fostering appropriate development in their child. Although each stage may take longer to achieve, parents are guided toward helping the child fully realize potential in preparation for the next phase of development. See Table 22-3 for developmental aspects of chronic illness or disability and for supportive interventions. Several resources address promoting development specifically for the technology-dependent child (Ahmann and Bond, 1992; Ahmann and Lierman, 1992; Ahmann and Lipsi, 1992).

Early Childhood. During infancy the child is achieving basic trust through a satisfying, intimate, consistent relationship with his or her parents. However, the affected child's early existence may be stressful, chaotic, and unsatisfying. Consequently, he or she may need more parental support and expressions of affection to achieve trust. Likewise the parents require assistance in ways of meeting the infant's needs, such as how to hold a rigid or flaccid infant, how to feed a child with tongue thrust or episodes of dyspnea, and how to stimulate a child who seems incapable of achieving any skills. If hospitalizations are frequent or prolonged, every effort is made to preserve the parent-child relationship (see also Chapter 26).

During early childhood the goal is to achieve separation from mother, autonomy, and initiative. However, the natural parental response to having a sick child is overprotection. Parents need help in realizing the importance of brief separations from the child, including others in the child's care, and providing social experiences outside the home whenever possible. Respite care, which provides temporary relief for family members, is essential in allowing caregivers time away from the daily demands of caring for a child with special needs.

In spite of need, parents report extreme difficulty finding competent respite care. New respite programs have developed in response to this need. The **National Down Syndrome Society,** for example, designed a program to foster the skills of independence and socialization in children with Down syndrome, to provide a regular, planned respite for the children's parents, and to educate volunteer host families and communities about the potential of individuals with this genetic disorder.* The National Council on the Aging created **Family Friends,** a unique intergenerational program that uses older adult volunteers to assist and support families who have children with chronic illnesses living at home† (Kuehne, 1989). Still, many localities have no formal respite services available.

Young children also need the opportunity to develop independence. Frequently the child is able to learn self-help skills, such as holding the bottle, finger-feeding, and removing simple articles of clothing, but the parent continues to perform the act. Therefore the nurse must guide parents toward the usual milestones expected from the child. Initially this requires developmental assessment of functional age (see Developmental Assessment, Chapter 7). The self-contract is a useful tool for promoting independence and self-care. Although formalized self-contracts are most successful with school-age or older children, a simplified version can be effective with preschoolers (Wesolowski, 1988). For more on self-contracts see Chapter 27 under Compliance.

Periodically the child's developmental progress is evaluated. Since each child develops at his or her own rate, there are no rigid guidelines for expecting when particular skills will be achieved. However, lack of progress in any one area is investigated. For example, sometimes a delay in self-feeding is not caused by lack of motor skill but by the parents' impatience in waiting for the skill to develop. Cleaning up the spilled food may seem like one more unnecessary task unless the importance of using a cup or spoon is stressed. All that may be necessary to encourage parent participation are suggestions to avoid large accidents, such as pouring only a small amount of juice in a cup or having the child feed himself or herself mashed potatoes (a sticky food) rather than gelatin (a slippery food). Placing food on a tray or cookie sheet is also helpful in keeping the food within the child's reach.

Not all children with disabilities are capable of achieving all developmental milestones. For example, the child with mental impairment may never achieve cognitive skills above a preschool level. The child who is deaf may achieve only rudimentary verbal language. In these situations adjustments must be made to compensate for the lack of or se-

Down Syndrome Respite Manual, a "how-to" manual, contains step-by-step information for establishing this program and is available for $5.00 from the National Down Syndrome Society, 666 Broadway, Suite 810, New York, NY 10012; (212) 460-9330 or (800) 221-4602.

†Information is available from Family Friends, 1133 15th St., N.W., Suite 620, Washington, DC 20005; (202) 223-8215.

TABLE 22-3 Developmental Aspects of Chronic Illness or Disability in Children

DEVELOPMENTAL TASKS	POTENTIAL EFFECTS OF CHRONIC ILLNESS OR DISABILITY	SUPPORTIVE INTERVENTIONS
INFANCY		
Develop a sense of trust	Multiple caregivers and frequent separations, especially if hospitalized Deprived of consistent nurturing	Encourage consistent caregivers in hospital or other care settings Encourage parents to visit frequently or "room in" during hospitalization and to participate in care
Attach to parent	Delayed because of separation, parental grief for loss of "dream" child, parental inability to accept the condition, especially a visible defect	Emphasize healthy, perfect qualities of infant Help parents learn special care needs of infant for them to feel competent
Learn through sensorimotor experiences	Increased exposure to painful experiences over pleasurable ones Limited contact with environment from restricted movement or confinement	Expose infant to pleasurable experiences through all senses (touch, hearing, sight, taste, movement) Encourage age-appropriate developmental skills, e.g., holding bottle, finger feeding, crawling
Begin to develop a sense of separateness from parent	Increased dependency on parent for care Overinvolvement of parent in care	Encourage all family members to participate in care to prevent overinvolvement of one member Encourage periodic respite from demands of care responsibilities
TODDLERHOOD		
Develop autonomy	Increased dependency on parent	Encourage independence in as many areas as possible (e.g., toileting, dressing, feeding)
Master locomotor and language skills	Limited opportunity to test on own abilities and limits	Provide gross motor skill activity and modification of toys or equipment, such as modified swing or rocking horse Give choices to allow simple feeling of control (e.g., choice of what book to look at or what kind of sandwich to eat)
Learn though sensorimotor experience, beginning preoperational thought	Increased exposure to painful experiences	Institute age-appropriate discipline and limit-setting Recognize that negative and ritualistic behavior are normal Provide sensory experiences (e.g., water play, sandbox, finger paint)
PRESCHOOL		
Develop initiative and purpose Master self-care skills	Limited opportunities for success in accomplishing simple tasks or mastering self-care skills	Encourage mastery of self-help skills Provide devices that make task easier, e.g., self-dressing
Begin to develop peer relationships	Limited opportunities for socialization with peers; may appear "like a baby" to agemates Protection within tolerant and secure family may cause child to fear criticism and withdraw	Encourage socialization, such as inviting friends to play, daycare experience, trips to park Provide age-appropriate play, especially associative play opportunities Emphasize child's abilities; dress appropriately to enhance desirable appearance
Develop sense of body image and sexual identification	Awareness of body may center on pain, anxiety, and failure Sex role identification focused primarily on mothering skills	Encourage relationships with same-sex and opposite-sex peers and adults Help child deal with criticisms; realize that too much protection prevents child from realities of world
Learn through preoperational thought (magical thinking)	Guilt (thinking he or she caused the illness/disability or is being punished for wrongdoing)	Clarify that cause of child's illness or disability is not his or her fault or a punishment
SCHOOL AGE		
Develop a sense of accomplishment	Limited opportunities to achieve and compete, e.g., many school absences or inability to join regular athletic activities	Encourage school attendance; schedule medical visits at times other than school; encourage to make up missed work Educate teachers and classmates about child's condition, abilities, and special needs
Form peer relationship	Limited opportunities for socialization	Encourage sports activities, e.g., Special Olympics Encourage socialization, e.g., Girl Scouts, Campfire, Boy Scouts, 4-H Clubs, having a best friend or a club
Learn through concrete operations	Incomplete comprehension of the imposed physical limitations or treatment of the disorder	Provide child with knowledge about his or her condition Encourage creative activities, e.g., Very Special Arts

TABLE 22-3 Developmental Aspects of Chronic Illness or Disability in Children—cont'd

DEVELOPMENTAL TASKS	POTENTIAL EFFECTS OF CHRONIC ILLNESS OR DISABILITY	SUPPORTIVE INTERVENTIONS
ADOLESCENCE		
Develop personal and sexual identity	Increased sense of feeling different from peers and less able to compete with peers in appearance, abilities, special skills	Realize that many of the difficulties the teenager is experiencing are part of normal adolescence (rebelliousness, risk taking, lack of cooperation, hostility toward authority) Provide instruction on interpersonal and coping skills Encourage socialization with peers, including peers with special needs and those without special needs
Achieve independence from family	Increased dependency on family; limited job/career opportunities	Provide instruction on decision making, assertiveness, and other skills necessary to manage personal plans Encourage increased responsibility for care and management of the disease or condition, such as assuming responsibility for making and keeping appointment (ideally alone), sharing assessment and planning stages of health care delivery, contacting resources
Form heterosexual relationships	Limited opportunities for heterosexual friendships; less opportunity to discuss sexual concerns with peers	Encourage activities appropriate for age, such as attending mixed-sex parties, sports activities, driving a car
Learn through abstract thinking	Increased concern with issues such as why did he or she get the disorder, can he or she marry and have a family Decreased opportunity for earlier stages of cognition may impede achieving level of abstract thinking	Be alert to cues that signal readiness for information regarding implications of condition on sexuality and reproduction Emphasize good appearance and wearing stylish clothes, use of makeup Understand that adolescent has same sexual needs and concerns as any other teenager Discuss planning for future and how condition can affect choices

verely delayed achievement in one area. However, such adjustments must be based on an understanding of normal development. Since motor limitations are present in a majority of conditions, this disability is used as an example to illustrate psychologic implications in making developmental changes.

During early childhood the basic innate drive for movement is dominant. During toddlerhood there is rapid development of motor skills, which eventually becomes the basis for learning and coping with the complex world. Psychologically this period is critical for developing a desire for independence. Language development, bowel control, locomotion, and fine-motor control all converge to produce a feeling of competency. Gradually during the early school years this basic motor urge shifts to a more goal-directed, symbolic expression in which words and thoughts replace actions as a way of problem solving.

When the young child has a disability that interferes with motor development, there is the potential hazard of shifting to development of compensatory intellectual pursuits before the child is ready. If this occurs, achievement of autonomy and initiative may be compromised, setting the stage for emotional problems. Therefore intervention must be based on providing activities that allow maximum motor development. For example, if a child has paraplegia, it is not sufficient to strengthen the upper extremities to compensate for the lower ones. Rather the activity must take into account the child's need for social interaction, sense of control over the body, feeling of competence and achievement, and an outlet for aggression. Suitable activities may include ball throwing; swimming and water activities such as races, bubble blowing, and splashing; building blocks, or pounding with a hammer.*

With slight modifications, children with disabilities may be able to ride a tricycle by using self-adhering straps to secure the hands (Fig. 22-3).† Wheelchair races are always a popular activity. Programs such as the **Special Olympics**‡ offer children an opportunity to compete with their peers and to achieve athletic skill. Summer camps§ also provide chil-

*Information on a toy library system for children with sensory deficits, motor disabilities, and developmental delay is available from the **National Lekotek Center,** 2100 Ridge Ave., Evanston, IL 60201; (708) 328-0001 or (800) 366-7529.

†Allied Services Rehabilitation Hospital provides information about appropriate toys for disabled children and provides a toy adaptation service for its patients.

‡1350 New York Ave., N.W., Suite 500, Washington, DC 20005-1581; (202) 628-3630. Several pamphlets are available from the **National Easter Seal Society,** 230 W. Monroe St., Suite 1800, Chicago, IL 60606, (312) 726-6200; and the **American Alliance for Health, Physical Education, Recreation and Dance (AAHPERD),** 1900 Association Dr., Reston, VA 22091, (703) 476-3400, on sports and recreation for children with disabilities.

§A directory of camps for children with a variety of chronic illnesses or general physical disabilities is available for a fee from **American Camping Association,** Publications Service, 5000 State Rd., 67 N., Martinsville, IN 46151; (800) 428-CAMP. A camp list is also available for $0.50 from **Candlelighter's Childhood Cancer Foundation,** 7910 Woodmont Ave., Suite 460, Bethesda, MD 20814; (800) 366-2223.

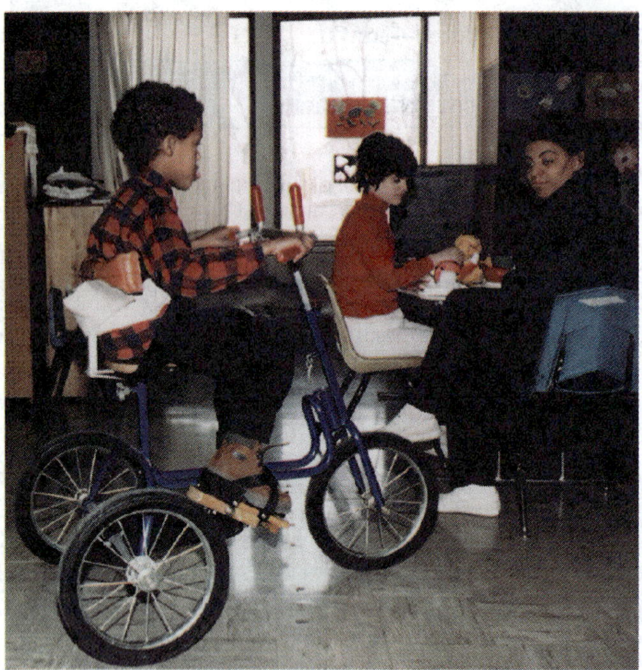

FIG. 22-3 A modified tricycle with block pedals, self-adhering straps for support, and modified seat and handlebars can help a child with disabilities gain mobility.

dren with unique opportunities to associate with similarly affected peers and develop a wide variety of skills, including increased independence in activities of daily living and special needs associated with their condition, such as administering medication. With innovation, many adaptations can be implemented in children's environments to increase their mobility and independence.* Technologic advances are mushrooming, especially in the application of computers, and parents should be directed to the latest developments that may help their child.

Children with special needs derive enormous benefits from expressive activities, such as art, music, poetry, dance, and drama. With adaptive equipment and imagination, children can participate in a variety of activities. Organizations such as **Very Special Arts** offer children an opportunity to celebrate and share their accomplishments.†

Another critical component for normal child development is discipline. Unfortunately this is one of the earliest childrearing practices eliminated when parents react with "over-benevolence." Not only does lack of discipline destroy the child's security because no boundaries exist on which to test behavior, it also fails to teach the child socially acceptable behavior and creates resentment and hostility among the siblings if different standards are applied to each child. The nurse's responsibility is to help parents learn successful methods of controlling behaviors before they become problems (see Chapter 14).

School Age. For school-age children, the major tasks are entry into school and achieving a sense of industry. While the importance of school in the life of all children is generally acknowledged, studies indicate that school absences are significantly higher among children with chronic illness, especially if psychosocial problems, such as behavior or family difficulties, coexist, than among their healthy peers. Some children, especially those with potentially terminal illnesses, may not return to school despite a long period of remission. The more school absences the child experiences, the greater the risk of poor academic achievement. For some children frequent absences may also lead to "school phobia." Psychosocial factors that contribute to the risk of school phobia include depression, change in appearance, fear of separation (child and parents), and resistance on the part of school personnel. To prevent school phobia, the child should resume school as quickly as possible following diagnosis. (See also School Phobia, Chapter 18.)

Preparation for entry or resumption of school is best accomplished through a team approach with the parents, child, school teacher, school nurse, and primary nurse in the hospital. Ideally, this planning should begin well before hospital discharge, provided the child is well enough to resume usual activities. A structured plan should be developed, with attention to those aspects of care that must be continued during school hours, such as administration of medication or other treatments (see Chapter 17). Special transportation needs should also be taken into consideration (School bus, 1993). Teachers need to be aware of the child's abilities in order to set realistic academic and athletic expectations (Larcombe and others, 1990). Parents' feelings regarding school resumption also need to be considered. Parents may have difficulty relinquishing the intensive parenting role, particularly if many of their other social attachments have weakened. A successful approach is to plan school attendance concurrently with the parents' recommencement of prediagnosis activities.

Children also need preparation before entering or resuming school. Having a tutor in the hospital or home as soon as children are physically able helps them realize that school will continue and gives them time to consider this prospect (Fig. 22-4). They need to investigate possible answers to the many questions others will ask. One method of anticipatory preparation is to role play, with the child as the "returned pupil" and the nurse as "other schoolmates." The nurse asks questions about the reason for the child's absence, the name of the disease, and so on. The child is thus provided with a safe opportunity to explore possible answers and to experience some of the possible reactions of others. If the child returns to school with some obvious physical change, such as hair loss, amputation, or visible scar, the nurse might also ask questions about these alterations to prompt preparatory responses from the child. The issue of ***sanctioned staring*** should be addressed with the child.

Initially the child may find it easier to attend half-day ses-

*An excellent publication is *The More We Do Together, Adapting the Environment for Children with Disabilities,* Monograph No. 31. Although it is out of print, a photocopy is available for $5.00 from the National Rehabilitation Information Center, (800) 227-0216.

†Very Special Arts has affiliate chapters in all 50 states and in selected sites internationally—yearly festivals are held throughout the world. Information is available from Very Special Arts, Education Office, John F. Kennedy Center for the Performing Arts, Washington, DC 20566; (202) 628-2800.

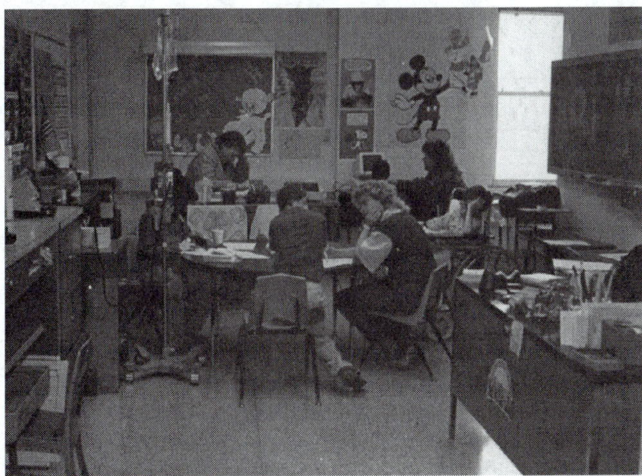

FIG. 22-4 Children with special needs should continue their schooling as soon as their condition permits.

sions or to participate in a limited number of activities. It is preferable to plan the school program with as much participation and leadership from the child as possible. Once children return, regular assessments of their progress are essential to assure a satisfactory adjustment. For example, some children appear to be doing well by investing all of their energies in academic endeavors to the detriment of social and/or physical activities. In essence the scholastic achievement may represent a retreat from other areas of school life that are equally important.

Classroom peers also need preparation, and a joint plan between the school teacher, nurse, and child is best. At a minimum the classmates should be given a description of the child's condition, prepared for any visible changes in the child, and allowed an opportunity to ask questions. The child should have the option of attending this session. As the child's condition changes, particularly if the illness is potentially fatal, school personnel, including the students, need periodic appraisal of the child's status and preparation for what to expect (see also Chapter 23).*

Children with special needs are encouraged to maintain or reestablish relationships with peers and to participate according to their capabilities in any age-appropriate activities. Alternative activities may be substituted for those that are impossible or that place a strain on their condition. It is important for these children to have the opportunity to interact with healthy peers, as well as to engage in activities with groups or clubs composed of similarly affected agemates. Such organizations as ostomy clubs, diabetic clubs, and cerebral palsy groups share information and provide support related to the special problems the members face.

Peer interaction is especially important in relation to cognitive development, social development, and maturation. Cognitive development is facilitated by interaction—by exploration of personal, social, and ethical values with peers, parents, and teachers. Youngsters whose isolation hampers their ability to interact with peers miss this opportunity to expand their thinking. Too many of these children withdraw to the passive companionship of television.

Adolescence. Adolescence can be a particularly difficult period for the teenager and family. All the needs discussed before apply to this age-group as well. Developing independence or autonomy, however, is a major task for the adolescent as planning for the future becomes a prominent concern. While the emphasis in the past has been on achieving independence from physical assistance, recent developments in the fields of special education, adolescent development, and family systems suggest redefining autonomy in terms of individuals' capacities to take responsibility for their own behavior, to make decisions regarding their own lives, and to maintain supportive social relationships (Crittenden, 1990). With this new definition, even individuals with severe impairment can be viewed as autonomous if they perceive their own needs and take responsibility for meeting them—either directly or by engaging the assistance of others. As adolescents become more autonomous, the nurse can help them discover and articulate how others can be of greatest assistance.

Physical symptoms are high on the teenager's list of health-related concerns (Dragone, 1990). Because adolescence is a time of enormous physical and emotional changes, it is important for the nurse to make a distinction between body changes that are related to disability and those that are a result of normal body development. It is a great comfort for these teenagers to know that many of the changes they experience are normal developmental outcomes.

A sense of feeling different from peers can lead to loneliness, isolation, and depression. Participation in groups of teenagers with chronic conditions or disabilities can alleviate feelings of isolation and smooth the transition to a meaningful relationship with one person in adulthood.*

Establish Realistic Future Goals

One of the most difficult adjustments is setting realistic future goals for the child and for those involved in the child's continued care. Sometimes the impact of this decision does not surface until the child finishes school or the parents near retirement, when a crisis can arise because all the family roles and relationships that maintained stability are now disrupted.

Planning for the future should be a gradual process. All along, the parents should cultivate realistic vocations for the child. For example, children with physical disabilities can be directed to intellectual, artistic, or musical pursuits. Children with developmental disabilities can be taught skills that can be performed in a special workshop. In this way the child's development proceeds in the direction of self-support through gainful employment.

*Several publications are available to help prepare school personnel, health professionals, and families for the child's return to school and are listed at the end of this chapter.

*Lasting Impressions, a well-developed psychosocial support program for adolescent cancer patients and their parents, provides an excellent model for supporting adolescents with cancer and other chronic conditions. For information about the program contact Beth Krietemeyer, BS, Center for Cancer Treatment and Research, 7 Richard Medical Park, Columbia, SC 29203.

THINKING CRITICALLY ABOUT . . .

Ethical Issues Young People and Families Face as a Result of Improved Survival from Chronic Illness

Chronically ill adolescents are faced with a number of serious ethical dilemmas as they enter adulthood. For example, should they share the truth of their condition with dating partners, prospective spouses, or potential employers? Should they seek a job with good health insurance rather than pursue a career with less employee benefits? Should they have the right to refuse further treatment, especially when the prospects for cure or even palliation are minimal? Whose wishes should be upheld when a conflict exists between the parents and young person? Should they transfer to adult care services? Will adult care practitioners be prepared to treat "childhood" diseases or conditions?

Such questions have no clear-cut answers. Rather, adolescents should be encouraged to weigh decisions, investigate alternatives, and choose their own solution (Silber, 1984). For example, in a study of adolescents with disabilities concerning their decision to have surgery, assessment of the teenager's view of surgery as "routine" or "nonroutine," the adolescent's and parents' goals, the alternatives to surgical intervention, how much power the teenager had in making the decision, and the young person's feelings regarding the decision-making process were important factors in arriving at an answer (Deatrick, 1984).

Consent and confidentiality are frequent dilemmas in providing care to any minor adolescent and are often made more complex by the teenager's health problem. For example, do these adolescents have the right to request health care without parents' knowledge or permission? If they are engaging in potentially hazardous activities, such as the teenager with cystic fibrosis who begins to smoke or the young man with hemophilia who engages in contact sports or tests HIV positive and becomes sexually active, should parents be informed? Two principles may be used in resolving such ethical questions: the principle of ***autonomy,*** which states that a person should have a say in any action that will affect him or her, and the principle of ***benevolence,*** which states that whenever something beneficial can be done, it should be done. Obviously, autonomy and benevolence support the adolescent's right to health care. However, in the best interests of the teenager, parents may need to be informed of activities that jeopardize their child's life (Silber, 1984).

With prolonged survival for many chronic illnesses, surviving young people must deal with new decisions and problems, such as marriage, employment, and insurance coverage (see Thinking Critically About . . . box). With appropriate guidance many of these individuals are capable of gainful employment* and may choose to marry and raise a family. For those whose conditions are genetic, there is the need for counseling regarding future offspring. Prospective spouses often benefit from an opportunity to discuss their feelings regarding marriage to an individual with continued health needs and possibly a limited life span. Health insurance coverage is a critical issue because some private carriers may no longer insure a young person who leaves home or may be unwilling to reinsure the person who is independent. Life insurance is another dilemma, especially when children have serious defects, such as congenital heart anomalies (Truesdell, Skorton, and Lauer, 1986). These issues are only beginning to receive attention but will become increasingly prominent as the number of survivors increases.

One solution that is gaining acceptance is transferring the older adolescent to adult care. The medical and psychosocial needs of adolescents approaching adulthood may be more easily managed by caregivers who are more familiar with adult issues.

Determining readiness for transfer is an important consideration. Arbitrary transfer to adult services based on age criterion alone can compromise both physical and psychosocial care for some young adults. Furthermore, age does not provide any information on how prepared the adolescent may be for transfer. Important considerations include knowledge of the condition and related treatments, medications, and precautions; child initiation and interest; and compliance with regimens.

Abrupt transfer to adult services can prove difficult for the young adult. Many adolescents have received care in the same medical setting since birth and have established trusting and meaningful relationships with practitioners and staff members. Increasingly, children with cystic fibrosis are identified as "in transition" at 16 years of age. To ease the transition, adult care practitioners work with the pediatric team in the pediatric clinic with 16- to 18-year-old adolescents and their families. At 18, most adolescents then move to the adult facility, where familiar faces await.

As more is learned about treating the adult phases of childhood conditions, more young adults will likely opt for adult services. In addition to assessing readiness, pediatric nurses can play a significant role in preparing adolescents and adult care providers for this important transition.

Unfortunately, vocational pursuits and independence are not realistic goals for all persons. Persons with multiple or severe disabilities may require lifelong care and assistance. In these situations parents must look to the time when they will no longer be able to care for their child. Residential placement may be very difficult unless the family mutually participates in the decision-making and planning process. Institutionalization should not be viewed as abandonment. Not infrequently, it is the only way to preserve the family unit. The nurse should help the family investigate suitable placements, discuss their feelings regarding

Text continued on p. 972.

*Information about employment is available from The President's Committee on Employment of People With Disabilities, 1331 F. St., N.W., Washington, DC 20004-1107; (202) 376-6200.

NURSING CARE PLAN
The Child with Chronic Illness or Disability

Nursing Diagnosis: Altered growth and development related to chronic illness or disability, parental reactions (overbenevolence), repeated hospitalization

PATIENT GOAL 1: Will attain maximum expected growth and developmental potential

• **NURSING INTERVENTIONS/*RATIONALES***
See Table 22-3

• **EXPECTED OUTCOME**
Child achieves appropriate physical, psychosocial, and cognitive development for age and abilities

Nursing Diagnosis: Altered family processes related to situational crisis (child with a chronic disease or disability)

PATIENT (FAMILY) GOAL 1: Will exhibit positive adjustment behaviors to the diagnosis

• **NURSING INTERVENTIONS/*RATIONALES***
Provide opportunity for family to adjust to discovery of diagnosis
Anticipate grief reaction to loss of the "perfect" child *because this usually occurs in the adjustment process*
Explore family's feelings regarding child and their ability to cope with the disorder
Encourage family to express their concerns
Repeat information as often as necessary *to reinforce family's understanding*
Serve as a role model regarding attitudes and behavior toward child

• **EXPECTED OUTCOMES**
Parents verbalize feelings and concerns regarding implications of the disease
Family demonstrates an attitude of acceptance and adjustment

PATIENT (FAMILY) GOAL 2: Will demonstrate understanding of disorder

• **NURSING INTERVENTIONS/*RATIONALES***
Help family to understand the disorder, its therapies, and implications
Reinforce information given by others *to promote better understanding*
Clarify misconceptions
Provide accurate information at a rate family can absorb *because information given too rapidly will not be learned*
Discuss advantages and limitations of therapeutic plan
Encourage family to ask questions and express concerns

• **EXPECTED OUTCOME**
Family demonstrates an understanding of the disease (specify)

PATIENT (FAMILY) GOAL 3: Will experience reduction of fear and anxiety

• **NURSING INTERVENTIONS/*RATIONALES***
Explore family's concerns and feelings of irritation, guilt, anger, disappointment, inadequacy and other feelings
Help family distinguish between realistic fears and unfounded fears; eliminate unfounded fears
Discuss with parents their fears regarding:
- Dealing with child's anxiety about condition
- Fear of dreadful developments
- Fear of death
- Fear of tests and procedures
- Child's ability to compete with peers

Explore their feelings regarding prescribed therapies

• **EXPECTED OUTCOME**
Family members discuss their fears and concerns

PATIENT (FAMILY) GOAL 4: Will exhibit positive adaptation behaviors to child

• **NURSING INTERVENTIONS/*RATIONALES***
Explore family's reaction to child and the disorder
Assess family's coping skills, abilities, and resources *so that these can be reinforced*
Help family to achieve a realistic view of child and capabilities and limitations
Foster positive family relationships *so that their ability to cope is maximized*
Assess interpersonal relationships within family, especially behaviors that reflect family's attitudes toward affected child
Intervene appropriately if there is evidence of maladaptation; refer for counseling if appropriate
Encourage parents in their attempts to promote child's development
Emphasize positive aspects of child's abilities or attributes
Help family gain confidence in their ability to cope with child, the disorder, and its impact on other family members

• **EXPECTED OUTCOMES**
Family verbalizes feelings and concerns regarding special needs of child and their effect on the family process
Family members demonstrate an attitude of confidence in their ability to cope

PATIENT (FAMILY) GOAL 5: Will exhibit ability to care for child

• **NURSING INTERVENTIONS/*RATIONALES***
Help family develop a thorough plan of care
Teach skills needed *to provide optimum care*
Interpret child's behavior to parents (e.g., anger, depression, regression, physical modifications as a result of disorder) *to prevent any unwarranted negative reaction (e.g., punishment) to child*
Help family plan for the future

• **EXPECTED OUTCOME**
Family sets realistic goals for selves, child, and others

Continued.

NURSING CARE PLAN
The Child with Chronic Illness or Disability—cont'd

PATIENT (FAMILY) GOAL 6: Will exhibit positive family relationship

- **NURSING INTERVENTIONS/*RATIONALES***

Identify family support systems (immediate family, extended family, friends, health service providers)
Assess systematically the number, affiliation, and interrelationships (if any) of persons the family sees as important
Help family to assign specific tasks to specific people *so that family receives support they need*
Reinforce positive coping mechanisms
Encourage family members to discuss their feelings about each other
Impress on parents the importance of providing as normal a life as possible for the affected child
Emphasize the growth and developmental progress of their child *to help family feel adequate in their maternal-paternal roles*
Help family foster child's development by stimulating child to age-appropriate goals consistent with activity tolerance

- **EXPECTED OUTCOMES**

Family demonstrates positive, growth-promoting behaviors
Family avails itself of support

PATIENT (FAMILY) GOAL 7: Will receive adequate support

- **NURSING INTERVENTIONS/*RATIONALES***

Be available to family *to provide support*
Listen to family members—singly or collectively
Allow for expression of feelings, including feelings of guilt, helplessness, and their perception of the impact that the condition may have (or does have) on the family
Refer to community agencies or special organizations providing assistance—financial, social, and support
Refer to genetic counseling if appropriate
Help family learn to expect feelings of frustration and anger toward child; reassure them that it is not a reflection on their parenting
Assist family in problem solving
Encourage interaction with other families who have a similarly affected child
  Introduce to families
  Provide information regarding support groups
Help families learn when to accept and when to "fight" for the care and services they feel are needed

- **EXPECTED OUTCOMES**

Family maintains contact with health providers
Family demonstrates an understanding of the needs of the child and the impact the condition will have on them
Problems are dealt with early
Family becomes involved with local agencies and support groups as needed

PATIENT (FAMILY) GOAL 8: Will be prepared for home care

- **NURSING INTERVENTIONS/*RATIONALES***

Teach skills needed *to ensure optimum home care*
Assess home situation, including family's strengths, weaknesses, and support systems
Help devise an individualized plan of care based on assessment of family's needs and resources
Encourage family involvement in care while still in the hospital *so that they are better prepared to assume child's care*
Encourage family to ask questions regarding posthospital care
Explore family's attitudes toward child's entry (or reentry) into the home
Help family acquire needed drugs, supplies, and equipment
Refer to special agencies, based on need assessment, *for on-going support and assistance*
Arrange for regular follow-up care *to assess effectiveness of home management*

- **EXPECTED OUTCOMES**

Family demonstrates an understanding of needed skills (specify skills and method of demonstration)
Family members avail themselves of resources within their community (specify)
Family complies with home care program

PATIENT (FAMILY) GOAL 9: Will participate in ongoing care

- **NURSING INTERVENTIONS/*RATIONALES***

Participate in follow-up care *to ensure continuity of care*
Coordinate team management of child and family
Be alert to comments by child or family members that indicate possible problems *so that problems are identified early*
Assess interpersonal relationships within family; especially behaviors that reflect family's attitudes toward child
Be alert for cues that signal undue anxiety and guilt: preoccupation with causative factors, constant analysis of effects of therapies, experimentation with diets and folk remedies, seeking magical cures
Be alert for overprotective behaviors such as assuming self-care activities for child, restricting child's activities or interaction with peers
Allow family to express discouragement at interference with activities and what appears to be slow progress

- **EXPECTED OUTCOMES**

Family participates in follow-up care
Family expresses both positive and negative reactions to child's progress
*Signs that may indicate family's difficulty in adjusting to child's condition are identified early

---
*Nursing outcome.

NURSING CARE PLAN

The Child with Chronic Illness or Disability—cont'd

PATIENT (SIBLINGS) GOAL 10: Will exhibit positive attachment behaviors with child

• **NURSING INTERVENTIONS/*RATIONALES***

Assess siblings *to identify areas of concern*
Communicate honestly with siblings about child's disease or disability
Provide opportunity for siblings to ask questions and express feelings, but avoid lengthy explanations before they ask *so that they are not overwhelmed*
Help parents talk to siblings about child's condition and interpret siblings' needs and questions
Encourage parents to spend special time with their children who are not ill or disabled
Help siblings and family understand that it is normal for them to sometimes have negative feelings about child
Prepare siblings in advance for any household changes, *since preparation encourages coping*
Allow sibling(s) to participate in child's care and therapy as appropriate
Help siblings learn how to explain child's condition to their peers and others
Acknowledge siblings' strengths and abilities to cope
Refer to sibling groups and networks composed of siblings of children with the same or similar conditions *for on-going support*
Assess siblings periodically *to determine their adjustment to the family situation*

• **EXPECTED OUTCOME**

Siblings verbalize or otherwise demonstrate their feelings and concerns
Parents include siblings in discussions about disabled child
Parents make an effort to spend time with other children
Siblings exhibit an understanding of household changes
Siblings assist with affected child's care (specify)
Siblings become involved in support groups (specify)

Nursing Diagnosis: Anxiety/fear related to tests, procedures, hospitalization, etc. (specify)

PATIENT GOAL 1: Will demonstrate understanding of hospitalization, procedures, etc. (specify)

• **INTERVENTIONS/*RATIONALES***

See Preparation for Procedures, Chapter 27
See Nursing Care Plan: The Child in the Hospital, Chapter 26

• **EXPECTED OUTCOME**

Child copes with stresses of procedures, tests, etc. (specify)

Nursing Diagnosis: High risk for injury (specify)

PATIENT GOAL 1: Will experience no injury

• **NURSING INTERVENTIONS/*RATIONALES***

Assess environment for hazards if indicated
Teach safety precautions *to decrease risk of injury*
Encourage activities that are compatible with the disease or disability

• **EXPECTED OUTCOME**

Child remains free of injury and complications

PATIENT GOAL 2: Will cope with limitations positively

• **NURSING INTERVENTIONS/*RATIONALES***

Help devise alternatives for restricted activities and help child cope with physical limitations *so that child's ability to cope is maximized*

• **EXPECTED OUTCOME**

Child demonstrates appropriate adaptation to limitations (specify)

PATIENT GOAL 3: Will experience no complications

• **NURSING INTERVENTIONS/*RATIONALES***

Stress importance of sound health practices and frequent health supervision *so that complications are less likely to develop*
Make certain child and family understand the therapeutic measures prescribed *to promote optimum health*
Encourage older child to choose activities but take responsibility for own safety
Plan with allied personnel (e.g., teachers, coaches, counselors) appropriate activities
Confer with school nurse (or other person) regarding any special needs of child
Discuss with parents any indicated limit-setting

• **EXPECTED OUTCOME**

Child maintains optimum health

Nursing Diagnosis: Diversional activity deficit related to environmental lack of diversion, physical limitations (specify), hospitalization

PATIENT GOAL 1: Will have opportunity to participate in diversionary activities

• **NURSING INTERVENTIONS/*RATIONALES***

Provide appropriate stimulation
Encourage activities appropriate to age, interest, and capabilities of child
Encourage physical exercise that does not overtax child (if indicated)
Incorporate therapeutic needs in play activities as appropriate
Supervise and encourage activities of daily living
Encourage child's natural tendency to be active
Encourage interaction with family and peers
Include child in planning and scheduling care *to ensure adequate time for diversionary activities*

Continued.

NURSING CARE PLAN
The Child with Chronic Illness or Disability—cont'd

• **EXPECTED OUTCOMES**
Child engages in age-appropriate activities within limits of capabilities
Child accepts efforts of family and caregivers

PATIENT GOAL 2: Will engage in appropriate exercise

• **NURSING INTERVENTIONS/*RATIONALES***
Encourage child to participate in normal childhood activities commensurate with interests and capabilities
Encourage and reinforce age-appropriate behaviors, experiences, and socialization with peers
Discourage physical inactivity *so that child receives needed exercise*

• **EXPECTED OUTCOME**
Child engages in nonsedentary activities within limits of disability

Nursing Diagnosis: Impaired social interaction related to hospitalization, confinement to home, frequent illness, activity intolerance, fatigue (specify)

PATIENT GOAL 1: Will experience positive interpersonal relationships

• **NURSING INTERVENTIONS/*RATIONALES***
Encourage child to maintain usual activities
Arrange for continued interpersonal contacts while hospitalized or otherwise confined
Provide opportunities for interaction with others, especially peers *for optimum growth and development*
Encourage regular school attendance (including daycare, beginning school, return to school)
Arrange for rest periods at school if needed so that child is better able to attend school
Promote peer contact whenever possible *so that relationships can develop and be maintained*
Encourage recreational outlets and after-school activities appropriate to child's interests and capabilities
Discourage activities that increase isolation from others

• **EXPECTED OUTCOMES**
Child engages in appropriate activities
Child associates with peers and family
Child attends school with reasonable regularity

Nursing Diagnosis: Self-care deficit (specify) related to specific impairment (specify)

PATIENT GOAL 1: Will engage in self-care activities

• **NURSING INTERVENTIONS/*RATIONALES***
Teach child about the disease and therapies *to ensure optimum safety and results*
Encourage child to assist in own care as age and capabilities permit
Provide and/or help devise methods to facilitate maximum functioning
Incorporate play that encourages desired behavior *to encourage cooperation and compliance*
Select toys and activities that allow maximum participation by child
Modify environment if needed (specify) *so that child can assume self-care activities*
Assist with self-care activities where needed (specify)
Avoid undue persistence to accomplish a goal
Provide incentives *to achieve desired behavior*
Instruct when to seek assistance from family or health care providers

• **EXPECTED OUTCOME**
Child engages in self-help activities commensurate with capabilities (specify activities and extent of involvement)

PATIENT GOAL 2: Will achieve sense of competence and mastery

• **NURSING INTERVENTIONS/*RATIONALES***
Capitalize on child's assets; help child compensate for liabilities
Praise child for accomplishments and "near" accomplishments, such as partial completion of a task, *to encourage sense of competency*
Ensure adequate rest before attempting energy-expending activities
Emphasize child's abilities and focus on realistic endeavors
Emphasize positive coping behaviors
Discourage activities that are beyond child's capabilities; promote and reinforce successful endeavors
Encourage participation in own care to the extent that child is able
Teach and encourage responsibility for use of equipment, appliances, testing, medication (specify)
Help child become adept at self-management to maximum capabilities

• **EXPECTED OUTCOMES**
Child takes responsibility for self-care according to age and capabilities (specify)
Child engages in appropriate activities without undue fatigue

Nursing Diagnosis: Body image disturbances related to perception of disability (self and others), feeling of differentness, inability to participate in specific activities (specify)

PATIENT GOAL 1: Will maintain positive attitude

• **NURSING INTERVENTIONS/*RATIONALES***
Convey an attitude of understanding, caring, and acceptance *to encourage positive body image*
Maintain open communications with child
Relate to child on appropriate cognitive level

NURSING CARE PLAN
The Child with Chronic Illness or Disability—cont'd

Serve as a role model for others *so that they are more accepting*

• EXPECTED OUTCOME
Child maintains a positive attitude (specify behaviors)

PATIENT GOAL 2: Will express feelings and concerns

• NURSING INTERVENTIONS/*RATIONALES*
Encourage verbalization of feelings and perceptions, especially feelings of "differentness"
Explore feelings concerning disease or disability and its implications: stress of being "different," physical limitations, difficulty competing, relationships with peers, self-image
Encourage child to discuss feelings about how he or she thinks others feel about the disorder

• EXPECTED OUTCOME
Child openly discusses feelings and concerns about the condition, therapies, and perceived reactions of others

PATIENT GOAL 3: Will cope with actual or perceived changes caused by illness

• NURSING INTERVENTIONS/*RATIONALES*
Acknowledge feelings and facilitate sharing feelings with family and other health professionals
Clarify misconceptions child may have acquired
Help child to identify positive aspects of situation *to facilitate coping*

• EXPECTED OUTCOME
Child discusses the disorder and feelings regarding limitations imposed by it

PATIENT GOAL 4: Will cope with disorder and its effects

• NURSING INTERVENTIONS/*RATIONALES*
Help child assess own strengths and assets; emphasize strengths
Identify coping behaviors *so that they can be reinforced*
Support positive coping mechanisms and extinguish negative ones
Help child set realistic goals *to facilitate coping*
Encourage as much independence as condition allows
Introduce child to other children who have adjusted well to this or a similar disorder
Suggest involvement with special groups and facilities for children with similar problems

• EXPECTED OUTCOMES
Child identifies own assets and strengths realistically
Child verbalizes positive suggestions for adjusting to the disability
Child becomes involved with special group activities

PATIENT GOAL 5: Will exhibit improved self-esteem and self-concept

• NURSING INTERVENTIONS/*RATIONALES*
Encourage an appealing physical appearance: good body hygiene, clean, straight teeth, good grooming, stylish hair and clothing, makeup for teenage girls
Assist with improving appearance and grooming
Point out positive aspects of own coping, appearance, and other capabilities
Promote constructive thinking in child; encourage child to maximize strengths
Reinforce positive behaviors
Help child to determine and engage in activities that foster self-esteem
Promote independence, *since this is an important part of self-esteem*

• EXPECTED OUTCOMES
Child demonstrates a positive appearance and attitude (specify)
Child appears clean, well-groomed, and attractively dressed
Child exhibits behaviors that indicate elevated self-esteem (specify)

PATIENT GOAL 6: Will exhibit appropriate sense of control

• NURSING INTERVENTIONS/*RATIONALES*
Channel need for control and feeling of effectiveness in appropriate directions
Encourage child to monitor own care as appropriate
Provide opportunities for child to make choices and participate in care when appropriate *to ensure sense of control*
Assess child with vocational planning when appropriate

• EXPECTED OUTCOME
Child becomes actively involved in own care and management

PATIENT GOAL 7: Will be prepared for discharge

• NURSING INTERVENTIONS/*RATIONALES*
Begin early in hospitalization to discuss "going home"
Help child develop independence and self-help capabilities
Encourage visits from friends *to help child assess the impact of any change in appearance or behavior that might interfere with returning to previous environments*

• EXPECTED OUTCOME
Child verbalizes and otherwise demonstrates interest in going home

See also:
Nursing Care Plan: The Child in the Hospital, Chapter 26
Nursing Care Plan: The Family of the Ill or Hospitalized Child, Chapter 26
Nursing Care Plan: The Child Who Is Terminally Ill or Dying, Chapter 23

this decision, and explore measures to maintain meaningful communication with the member who has a disability. The nurse can prepare and educate the public to smooth the transition and help normalize the experience for the child, the family, and the community.

KEY POINTS

- Trends in the treatment of children with chronic illness have focused on developmental stages, the child's strengths and uniqueness, family development, family-centered care, establishment of normalization, early discharge, home care, mainstreaming, and early intervention.
- Families' reactions to disability or chronic illness are manifested in the following stages: shock and denial, adjustment, reintegration and acknowledgment, and freezing out.
- In response to the child with chronic illness or disability, parents may be affected by feelings of inadequacy and failure; excessive demands on time, energy, and financial resources; and strain on spousal communication.
- Effects of chronic illness on siblings include changes in role status, irritability and physical complaints, jealousy, competition, anger, hostility, attention-seeking behavior, social withdrawal, and decline in school performance.
- Major factors affecting the family's adjustment to a child's chronic illness are the availability of a support system, their perception of the event, their coping mechanisms, reactions to the child, available resources, and concurrent stresses.
- The coping mechanisms parents use in dealing with the child with chronic illness are approach behaviors—movement toward adjustment and resolution of crisis—and avoidance behaviors—maladaptation or movement away from adjustment.
- The child's reaction to illness or disability depends on the child's developmental level and coping mechanisms, others' reactions, and the illness itself.
- A family-centered approach to care that enables and empowers parents offers the greatest opportunity for appropriate interventions that meet the unique needs of all family members.
- Mutual participation in care by child and parent facilitates better communication and alleviates feelings of parental inadequacy and child inferiority.
- Assessment of the family's coping mechanisms and reactions entails understanding the family's functioning and observing the child at home and at school.
- To help parents cope with their child's chronic illness, nurses must offer attentiveness, humanistic support, solicitation of suggestions for care, facilitation of communication, verbalization of feelings, and referral to volunteer and community agencies.
- Supporting the child involves encouraging self-expression, alleviating feelings of being different, and strengthening self-image.
- Fostering reality adjustment entails supplying information about the disorder, promoting normal development, andestablishing realistic future goals.

REFERENCES

Adams P, Fras I: *Beginning child psychiatry,* New York, 1988, Brunner/Mazel.

Ahmann E: "Chunky stew": appreciating cultural diversity while providing health care for children, *Pediatr Nurs* 20(3):320-324, 1994.

Ahmann E, Bond NJ: Promoting normal development in school age children and adolescents who are technology dependent: a family centered model, *Pediatr Nurs* 18(4):399-405, 1992.

Ahmann E, Lierman C: Promoting normal development in technology dependent children: an introduction to the issues, *Pediatr Nurs* 18(2):143-148, 1992.

Ahmann E, Lipsi K: Developmental assessment of the technology dependent infant and young child, *Pediatr Nurs* 18(3):299-305, 1992.

Anderson J: Ethnicity and illness experience: ideological structures and the health care delivery system, *Soc Sci Med* 22(11):1277-1283, 1986.

Association for the Care of Children's Health: Focusing on fathers of children with special needs, *ACCH Network* 8(2):1, 1990.

Austin J: Assessment of coping mechanisms used by parents and children with chronic illness, *MCN* 15(2):98-102, 1990.

Austin J, Patterson J, Huberty T: Development of the coping health inventory for children, *J Pediatr Nurs* 6(3):166-174, 1991.

Bailey D, Simeonsson R, editors: *Family assessment in early intervention,* Columbus, OH, 1988, Merrill.

Baker NA: Avoiding collisions with challenging families, *MCN* 19:97-101, 1994.

Bean M: Assessing families of children with developmental disabilities. In Wright L, Leahey M, editors: *Families and chronic illness,* Springhouse, PA, 1987, Springhouse.

Bibace R, Walsh M: Development of children's concepts of illness, *Pediatrics* 66:912-917, 1980.

Bibace R, Walsh M: *Children's conceptions of health, illness and body function: new directions for child development,* San Francisco, 1981, Jossey-Bass.

Bird JE, Podmore VN: Children's understanding of health and illness, *Psychol Health* 4:175-185, 1990.

Bishop KK, Woll J, Arango P: *Family/professional collaboration for children with special health care needs,* Burlington, 1993, Department of Social Work, University of Vermont.

Bossert E and others: Strategies of normalization used by parents of chronically ill school-age children, *Child Adolesc Psychiatr Ment Health Nurs* 3(2):57-61, 1990.

Breitmayer BJ and others: Social competence of school aged children with chronic illnesses, *J Pediatr Nurs* 7(3):181-188, 1992.

Burns CE, Madian N: Experiences with a support group for grandparents of children with disabilities, *Pediatr Nurs* 18(1):17, 1992.

Carney I: Working with families. In Orelove F, Sobsey D, editors: *Educating children with multiple disabilities: a transdisciplinary approach,* Baltimore, 1987, Paul H Brookes.

Clements D, Copeland L, Loftus M: Critical times for families with a chronically ill child, *Pediatr Nurs* 16(2):157-161, 224, 1990.

Clubb R: Chronic sorrow: adaptation patterns of parents with chronically ill children, *Pediatr Nurs* 17(5):461-466, 1991.

Corbin JM, Strauss A: A nursing model for chronic illness management based upon the trajectory framework, *Sch Inquiry Nurs Prac* 5(3):155-174, 1991.

Coupey S, Cohen M: Special considerations for the health care of adolescents with chronic illnesses, *Pediatr Clin North Am* 31(1):211-219, 1984.

Crittenden P: Toward a concept of autonomy in adolescents with a disability, *Child Health Care* 19(3):162-168, 1990.

Cystic Fibrosis Foundation: Personal communication Aug 13, 1990.

Deatrick JA: It's their decision now: perspectives of chronically disabled adolescents concerning surgery, *Issues Compr Pediatr Nurs* 7:17-31, 1984.

Diehl SF, Moffitt KA, Wade SM: Focus group interview with parents of children with medically complex needs: an intimate look at their perceptions and feelings, *Child Health Care* 20(3):170-178, 1991.

Dixon DM: *Parent participation during hospitalization: understanding differences,* Unpublished manuscript, Springfield, IL, 1993, Memorial Medical Center.

Downey W: Public Law 99-457 and the clinical pediatrician, *Clin Pediatr* 29(3):158-161, 1990.

Dragone M: Perspectives of chronically ill adolescents and parents on health care needs, *Pediatr Nurs* 16(1):45-50, 108, 1990.

Dunst C, Trivette C, Deal A: *Enabling and empowering families,* Cambridge, MA, 1988, Brookline Books.

Duvall E: *Marriage and family development,* ed 5, New York, 1977, JB Lippincott.

Faux SA: Sibling relationships in families with congenitally impaired children, *J Pediatr Nurs* 6(3):175-184, 1991.

Fisman S, Wolf L: The handicapped child: psychological effects of parental, marital, and sibling relationships, *Psychiatr Clin North Am* 14(1):199-217, 1991.

Fraley A: Chronic sorrow: a parental response, *J Pediatr Nurs* 5(4):268-273, 1990.

Gallo AM and others: Well siblings of children with chronic illness: parent's reports of their psychologic adjustment, *Pediatr Nurs* 18(1): 23-29, 1992.

Garmezy N: Resilence in children's adaptation to negative life events and stressed environments, *Pediatr Ann* 20(9):459-466, 1991.

Grey M, Cameron ME, Thurber FW: Coping and adaptation in children with diabetes, *Nurs Res* 40(3):144-149, 1991.

Groce NE, Zola IK: Multiculturalism, chronic illness, and disability, *Pediatrics* 91(5):1048-1055, 1993.

Hansen S, Holaday B, Miles M: The role of pediatric nurses in a federal program for infants and young children with handicaps, *J Pediatr Nurs* 5(4):246-251, 1990.

Heiney SP and others: The effects of group therapy on siblings of pediatric oncology patients, *J Assoc Pediatr Oncol Nurses* 7(3):95-100, 1990.

Hickey M: What are the needs of families of critically ill patients? A review of the literature since 1976, *Heart Lung* 19(4):401-415, 1990.

Horwitz S, Stein R: Health maintenance organizations vs indemnity insurance for children with chronic illness, *Am J Dis Child* 144:581-586, 1990.

Huber C, Holditch-Davis D, Brandon D: High risk preterm infants at 3 years of age: parental response to the presence of developmental problems, *Child Health Care* 22(2):107, 124, 1993.

Jackson B, Finkler D, Robinson C: A case management system for infants with chronic illnesses and developmental disabilities, *Child Health Care* 21(4):224-232, 1992.

Jones-Hessop D, Stein R: Uncertainty and its relation to the psychological and social correlates of chronic illness in children, *Soc Secur Med* 20(10):993-999, 1985.

Kalnins I: Cross-illness comparisons of separation and divorce among parents having a child with a life-threatening illness, *Child Health Care* 12(2):72-77, 1983.

Kazak A: Families of chronically ill children: a systems and social-ecological model of adaptation and challenge, *J Consult Clin Psychol* 57(1):25-30, 1989.

Knafl KA, Deatrick JA: Family management style: concept analysis and development, *J Pediatr Nurs* 5(1):4-14, 1990.

Krahn GL, Hallum A, Kime C: Are there good ways to give bad news? *Pediatrics* 91(3):578-582, 1993.

Krulik T: Successful "normalizing" tactics of parents of chronically ill children, *J Adv Nurs* 5(6):573-578, 1980.

Kuehne V: "Family friends": an innovative example of intergenerational family support services, *Child Health Care* 18(4):237-246, 1989.

Larcombe IJ and others: Impact of childhood cancer on return to normal schooling, *Br Med J* 301(6744):169-171, 1990.

Lobato D: *Brothers, sisters, and special needs,* Baltimore, 1990, Paul H. Brookes.

Marcenko MO, Smith LK: The impact of a family centered case management approach, *Soc Work Health Care* 17(1):87-100, 1992.

May J: *Fathers of children with special needs: new horizons,* Washington, DC, 1990, Association for the Care of Children's Health.

McCubbin H, Thompson A: *Family assessment inventories for research and practice,* Madison, 1987, The University of Wisconsin—Madison.

McCubbin H and others: CHIP—Coping Health Inventory for Parents: an assessment of parental coping patterns in the care of the chronically ill child, *J Marriage Fam* 45:359-370, 1983.

Munet-Vilaro F, Vessey J: Children's explanation of leukemia: a Hispanic perspective, *J Pediatr Nurs* 5(4):274-282, 1990.

Newacheck PW, McManus MA, Fox HB: Prevalence and impact of chronic illness among adolescents, *Am J Dis Child* 145(12):1367-1373, 1991.

Newacheck PW, Stoddard JJ, McManus M: Ethnocultural variations in the prevalence and impact of childhood chronic conditions, *Pediatrics* 91(5):1031-1039, 1993.

Newacheck PW, Taylor WR: Childhood chronic illness: prevalence, severity, and impact, *Am J Public Health* 82(3):364-371, 1992.

Orr DP and others: Psychosocial implications of chronic illness in adolescence, *J Pediatr* 104(1):152-157, 1984.

Patterson JM, Blum RW: A conference on culture and chronic illness in childhood: conference summary, *Pediatrics* 91(5):1025-1030, 1993.

Patterson JM, Geber G: Preventing mental health problems in children until chronic illness or disability, *Child Health Care* 20(3): 150-161, 1991.

Perrin EC, Gerrity PS: There's a devin (spell?) in your belly: children's understanding of illness, *Pediatrics* 67:841-849, 1981.

Richards DD: The challenge of transporting children with special needs, *AAP Safe Ride News,* pp 1-4, spring 1989.

Rollins J: Childhood cancer: siblings draw and tell, *Pediatr Nurs* 16(1):21-27, 1990.

Satariano HJ, Briggs NJ: The good family syndrome, *Pediatr Nurs* 15(3):285-286, 1989.

School bus transportation of children with special needs, *AAP News* 9(11), 1993.

Silber TJ: Ethical considerations in the care of the chronically ill adolescent. In Blum R, editor: *Chronic illness and disabilities in childhood and adolescence,* New York, 1984, Grune & Stratton.

Sorensen E: Children's coping responses, *J Pediatr Nurs* 5(4):259-267, 1990.

Spina Bifida Association: Personal communication, Aug 13, 1990.

Stein REK: Home care: a challenging opportunity, *Child Health Care* 14(2):90-95, 1985.

Stone D: Professional perceptions of parental adaptation to a child with special needs, *Child Health Care* 18(3):174-177, 1989.

Stone M, Hoffman R: *Cultural understanding: how far do you go?* Paper presented at ACCH conference on Caring for the Quilt: Incorporating Cultural Awareness into Pediatric Health Care, 1993.

Truesdell SC, Skorton DJ, Lauer RM: Life insurance for children with cardiovascular disease, *Pediatrics* 77(5):687-691, 1986.

Trute B: Child and parent predictors of family adjustment in households containing young developmentally disabled children, *Fam Relations* 39(3):292-297, 1990.

Venters M: Familial coping with chronic and severe childhood illness: the case of cystic fibrosis, *Soc Sci Med* 15A:289-297, 1981.

Wesolowski C: Self-contracts for chronically ill children, *MCN* 13(1):20-23, 1988.

Wissow L, Warshow M: Prevalence of home telephone service among families using an inner-city hospital's outpatient services, *Am J Dis Child* 144:426, 1990.

Yoos H: *Knowledge representation of a chronic illness: a study of kinds of expertise,* Unpublished doctoral dissertation, 1991, University of Rochester.

Yoos HL: Children's illness concepts: old and new paradigms, *Pediatr Nurs* 20(2):134-140, 1994.

BIBLIOGRAPHY

Adams EV: *Policy planning for culturally comprehensive special health services,* Bureau of Maternal and Child Health, US Department of Health and Human Services, 1990. Also available from CEDEN Family Resource Center, 1208 E. 7th St., Austin, TX 78702.

Ahmann E: An annotated bibliography on respite care for children and families, *Child Health Care* 14(3):183-186, 1986.

Ahmann E, Bond NJ: Promoting normal development in school age children and adolescents who are technology dependent: a family centered model, *Pediatr Nurs* 18(4): 399-405, 1992.

Ahmann E, Lierman C: Promoting normal development in technology dependent children: an introduction to the issues, *Pediatr Nurs* 18:143-148, 1992.

American Academy of Pediatrics: Health care financing for the child with catastrophic costs, *Pediatrics* 80(5):752-757, 1987.

American Academy of Pediatrics, Committee on Child Health Financing: Financing health care for the medically indigent child, *Pediatrics* 80(6):957-960, 1987.

American Academy of Pediatrics, Committee on Children With Disabilities: Screening for developmental disabilities, *Pediatrics* 78(3): 526-528, 1986.

American Academy of Pediatrics, Committee on Children With Disabilities: Transition of severely disabled children from hospital or chronic care facilities to the community, *Pediatrics* 78(3):531-534, 1986.

American Academy of Pediatrics, Committee on Children with Disabilities: Pediatric services for infants and children with special health care needs, *Pediatrics* 92(1):163-165, 1993.

American Nurses' Association: *HIV hepatitis B–hepatitis C blood borne diseases: nurses' risk, rights, and responsibilities,* Washington, DC, 1993, The Association.

ANA: AAN expert panel report: culturally competent health care, *Nurs Outlook* 40(6):277-283, 1992.

Anastaslow MJ, Harel S: *At risk infants: interventions, families, and research,* Baltimore, MD, 1992, Paul H Brooks.

Armstrong-Dailey A: Children's hospice care, *Pediatr Nurs* 16(4):337-339, 409, 1990.

Association for the Care of Children's Health: *Family support in the home,* Washington, DC, 1988, The Association.

Austin JK: Assessment of coping mechanisms used by parents and children with chronic illness, *MCN* 15(2):98-102, 1990.

Baldwin DS and others: Collaborative systems design for Part H of IDEA . . . Individuals with Disabilities Education Act, *Infants Young Child* 5(1):12-20, 1992.

Bartel NR, Thurman SK: Medical treatment and educational problems in children, *Phi Delta Kappan* 74(1):57-61, 1992.

Bluebond-Langner M and others: Children's knowledge of cancer and its treatment: impact of an oncology camp experience, *J Pediatr* 116(2):207-213, 1990.

Brewer EJ and others: Family-centered, community-based, coordinated care for children with special health care needs, *Pediatrics* 83(6):1055-1060, 1989.

Brookins GK: Culture, ethnicity, and bicultural competence: implications for children with chronic illness and disability, *Pediatrics* 91(5, Pt 2):1056-1062, 1993.

Brooks-Gunn J, Chase-Lansdale L: Children having children: effects on the family system, *Pediatr Ann* 20(9):467-481, 1991.

Brown J, Ritchie JA: Nurses' perceptions of their relationships with parents, *Matern Child Nurs J* 18:79-96, 1989.

Brown W, Thurman SK, Pearl LF: *Family centered early intervention with infants and toddlers: innovative cross disciplinary approaches,* Baltimore, MD, 1993, Paul H Brookes.

Burke SO and others: Hazardous secrets and reluctantly taking charge: parenting a child with repeated hospitalization, *Image: J Nurs Sch* 23(1):39-45, 1991.

Callery P, Smith L: A study of role negotiation between nurses and the parents of hospitalized children, *J Adv Nurs* 16:772-781, 1991.

Canning EH and others: Mental disorders in chronically ill children: parent-child discrepancy and physician identification, *Pediatrics* 90(5):692-696, 1992.

Cardoso P: A parent's perspective, *Child Health Care* 20(4):258-260, 1991.

Centers for Disease Control: Chronic disease reports in the Morbidity and Mortality Weekly Report, *MMWR* 38(suppl S-1):1-7, 1989.

Clark HB and others: Peer support group for adolescents with chronic illness, *Child Health Care* 21(4):233-238, 1992.

Clements DB, Copeland LG, Loftus M: Critical times for families with a chronically ill child, *Pediatr Nurs* 16(2):157-161, 224, 1990.

Cohen DS and others: Instruments to measure parent-child communication regarding pediatric cancer, *Child Health Care* 18(3):142-145, 1989.

Cohen MH, Martinson IM: Chronic uncertainty: its effect on parental appraisal of a child's health, *J Pediatr Nurs* 3(2):89-96, 1988.

Crowley A: Integrating handicapped and chronically ill children into day care centers, *Pediatr Nurs* 16(1):39-44, 1990.

Culley BS, Perrin EC, Chaberski MJ: Parental perceptions of vulnerability of formerly premature infants, *J Pediatr Health Care* 3(5):237-245, 1989.

Davis H: *Counselling parents of children with chronic illness or disability,* Baltimore, MD, 1993, Paul H Brookes.

Deatrick JA, Knafl KA: Management behaviors: day-to-day adjustments to childhood chronic conditions, *J Pediatr Nurs* 5(1):15-22, 1990.

Dunst CJ, Trivette CM, Deal A: *Supporting and strengthening families: methods, strategies and outcomes,* Cambridge, MA, 1993, Brookline Books.

Dunst CJ and others: Enabling and empowering families of children with health impairments, *Child Health Care* 17(2):71-81, 1988.

Ekvall SW: *Pediatric nutrition in chronic diseases and developmental disorders,* New York, 1993, Oxford University Press.

Fox HB, Newacheck PW: Private health insurance of chronically ill children, *Pediatrics* 85(1):50-57, 1990.

Freedman SA, Pierce PM, Reiss JG: REACH: a family-centered community-based case management model for children with special health care needs, *Child Health Care* 16(2):114-117, 1987.

Friedman MM: Transcultural family nursing: application to Latin and black families, *J Pediatr Nurs* 5(3):214-222, 1990.

Galbehouse B, Gitterman B: Maternal understanding of commonly used medical terms in a pediatric setting, *Am J Dis Child* 144:419, 1990.

Gallo AM and others: Stigma in childhood chronic illness: a well sibling perspective, *Pediatr Nurs* 17(1):21-27, 1991.

Gallo AM and others: Well siblings of children with chronic illness: parent's reports of their psychologic adjustment, *Pediatr Nurs* 18(1): 23, 1992.

Garmezy N: Resilience in children's adaptation to negative life events and stressed environments, *Pediatr Ann* 20(9):459-466, 1991.

Gergen PJ, Weiss KB: Changing patterns of asthma hospitalization among children: 1979 to 1987, *JAMA* 264(13):1688-1692, 1990.

Gill KM: Nurses' attitudes toward parent participation: personal and professional characteristics, *Child Health Care* 15(3):149-151, 1987.

Gortmaker SL and others: Chronic conditions, socioeconomic risks, and behavioral problems in children and adolescents, *Pediatrics* 85(3):267-276, 1990.

Grey M, Thurber FW: Adaptation to chronic illness in childhood: diabetes mellitus, *J Pediatr Nurs* 6(5):302-309, 1991.

Haas DL: Historical overview of the development of family centered community based, coordinated care in Michigan, *Issues Compr Pediatr Nurs* 15(1):1-15, 1992.

Harris JA, Newcomb AF, Gewanter HL: Psychosocial effects of juvenile rheumatic disease: the family and peer systems as a context for coping, *Arthritis Care Res* 4(3):123-130, 1991.

Hartman AF, Radin MB, McConnell B: Parent to parent support: a critical component of health care services for families, *Issues Compr Pediatr Nurs* 15(1):55, 1992.

Hass DL, Gray HB, McConnell B: Parent/professional partnerships in caring for children with special health care needs, *Issues Compr Pediatr Nurs* 15(1):39, 1992.

Healy A, Keesee P, Smith B: *Early services for children with special needs,* ed 2, Baltimore, 1989, Paul H Brookes.

Hewson M and others: Comprehensive team care, *MCN* 18(4):198-205, 1993.

Hinds PS, Martin J: Hopefulness and the self-sustaining process in adolescents with cancer, *Nurs Res* 37(6):336-340, 1988.

Ho HH, Miller A, Armstrong RW: Parent-professional agreement on diagnosis and recommendations for children with developmental disorders, *Child Health Care* 23(2):137-148, 1994.

Hochstadt NJ, Yost DM: The health care–child welfare partnership: transitioning medically complex children to the community, *Child Health Care* 18(1):4-11, 1989.

Hockenberry MJ, Coody DK, Bennett BS: Childhood cancers: incidence, etiology, diagnosis, and treatment, *Pediatr Nurs* 16(3):239-246, 256-257, 1990.

Horner MM, Rawlins P, Giles K: How parents of children with chronic conditions perceive their own needs, *MCN* 12(1):40-43, 1987.

How can one assess damage caused by treatment of childhood cancer? *Lancet* 34D(8822):758-759, 1992.

Immune Deficiency Foundation: Special editions insurance reimbursement issues, *IDF Newslett* 17, 1992.

Ireys HT, Nelson RP: New federal policy for children with special health care needs: implications for pediatricians, *Pediatrics* 90(3): 321-327, 1992.

Jackson PL: The primary care provider and children with chronic conditions. In Jackson PL, Vessey JA: *Primary care of the child with a chronic condition,* St Louis, 1992, Mosby.

Jellinek MS and others: Coping with the truly difficult parent, *Contemp Pediatr* 8(2):19-49, 1991.

Johnson B: The changing role of families in health care, *Child Health Care* 19(4):234-241, 1990.

Johnson B, McGonigel M, Kaufmann R, editors: *Guidelines and recommended practices for the Individualized Family Service Plan,* Washington, DC, 1989, Association for the Care of Children's Health.

Katcher AL, Haber JS: The pediatrician and early intervention for the developmentally disabled or handicapped child, *Pediatr Rev* 12(10):305-312, 1991.

Keeney SM: When children need rehabilitation, *Contin Care* 11(5):18-24, 1992.

Kelly M: Safe transport of technology dependent children, *MCN* 18(1):29-31, 1993.

Knafl KA and others: Parent's views of health care providers: an exploration of the components of a positive working relationship, *Child Health Care* 21(2):90-95, 1992.

Leff PT, Walizer EH: *Building the healing partnership: parents, professionals, and children with chronic illnesses and disabilities,* Cambridge, MA, 1992, Brookline Books.

Leonard BJ: Siblings of chronically ill children: a question of vulnerability versus resilience, *Pediatr Ann* 20(9):501-506, 1991.

Lewis C and others: Patient, parent, and physician perspectives on pediatric oncology rounds, *J Pediatr* 112(3):378-384, 1988.

Mahon MM: Chronic conditions and the family. In Jackson PL, Vessey JA: *Primary care of the child with a chronic condition,* St Louis, 1992, Mosby.

Malfair A: Supporting the child with special needs, *Can Nurse* 88(11):17-19, 1992.

Martinez NH, Schreiber ML, Hartman EW: Pediatric nurse practitioners: primary care providers and case managers for chronically ill children at home, *J Pediatr Health Care* 5(6):291-298, 1991.

Martinson IM and others: Impact of childhood cancer on healthy school age siblings, *Cancer Nurs* 13(3):183-190, 1990.

McAnear S: Parental reaction to a chronically ill child, *Home Health Care Nurse* 8(3):35-40, 1990.

McCarthy SM, Gallo AM: A case illustration of family management style, *J Pediatr Nurs* 7(6):395-402, 1992.

McClowry SG: Pediatric nursing psychosocial care: a vision beyond hospitalization, *Pediatr Nurs* 19(2):146-148, 1993.

McCubbin HI and others: Culture, ethnicity, and the family: critical factors in childhood chronic illness and disabilities, *Pediatrics* 91(5):1063-1070, 1993.

McLane JB: Lekotek: a unique play library for families with handicapped children, *Child Health Care* 14(3):178-182, 1986.

McManus MA, Newacheck PW: Health insurance differentials among minority children with chronic conditions and the role of federal agencies and private foundations in improving financial access, *Pediatrics* 91(5):1040-1047, 1993.

Mullis RL, Mullis AK, Kerchoff NF: The effect of leukemia and its treatment on self-esteem of school age children, *Matern Child Nurs J* 20(3-4):155-165, 1992.

Neff EJA, Dale JC: Assessment of quality of life in school aged children: a method—phase I, *Matern Child Nurs J* 19(4): Ninth Matern Child Nurs Conf Proc, Pt 3:313-320, 1990.

Nugent K and others: A practice model for a parent support group, *Pediatr Nurs* 18(1):11, 1992.

Numinen VJ and others: Building community based service systems for children with special needs: the Michigan locally based services program, *Issues Compr Pediatr Nurs* 15(1):17-37, 1992.

Office of Technology Assessment: *Technology-dependent children: hospital vs home care, a technical memorandum,* Washington, DC, 1987, US Government Printing Office.

O'Grady RS: Financing health care for children with chronic conditions. In Jackson PL, Vessey JA: *Primary care of the child with a chronic condition,* St Louis, 1992, Mosby.

Orsillo SM, McCaffrey RJ, Fisher JM: Siblings of head injured individuals: a population at risk, *J Head Trauma Rehabil* 8(1):102-115, 1993.

Palfrey J and others: Providing therapeutic services to children in special educational placements: an analysis of the related services provisions of Public Law 94-142 in five urban school districts, *Pediatrics* 85(4):518-526, 1990.

Patterson JM: Family resilience to the challenge of a child's disability, *Pedatr Ann* 20(9):491-499, 1991.

Patterson JM and others: Caring for medically fragile children at home: the parent-professional relationship, *J Pediatr Nurs* 9(2):98-106, 1994.

Perkins MT: Parent nurse collaboration: using the caregiver identity emergence phases to assist parents of hospitalized children with disabilities, *J Pediatr Nurs* 8(1):2-9, 1993.

Perrin EC, West PD, Culley BS: Is my child normal yet? Correlates of vulnerability, *Pediatrics* 83(3):355-363, 1989.

Perrin EC and others: Issues involved in the definition and classification of chronic health conditions, *Pediatrics* 91(4):787-793, 1993.

Pless IB, Power C, Peckham CS: Long-term psychosocial sequelae of chronic physical disorders in childhood, *Pediatrics* 91(6):1131-1136, 1993.

Podrasky DK, Sexton DL: Nurses' reactions to difficult patients, *Image: J Nurs Sch* 20(1):16-20, 1988.

Reed SB: Potential for alterations in family process: when a family has a child with cystic fibrosis, *Issues Compr Pediatr Nurs* 13(1):15-23, 1990.

Reflections on the rise in asthma morbidity and mortality, *JAMA* 264(13):1719-1720, 1990 (editorial).

Robinson CA: Roadblocks to family centered care when a chronically ill child is hospitalized, *Matern Child Nurs J* 16(3):181-193, 1987.

Rokusek C, Heinrichs E: Nutrition and feeding for persons with special needs: a practical guide and resource manual, ed 2, Pierre, SD, 1992, Department of Education and Cultural Affairs.

Savage TA, Culbert C: Early intervention: the unique role of nursing, *J Pediatr Nurs* 4(5):339-345, 1989.

Scharer K, Dixon DM: Managing chronic illness: parents with a ventilator-dependent child, *J Pediatr Nurs* 4:234-246, 1989.

Singer G, Powers LE: *Families, disability, and empowerment: active coping skills and strategies for family interventions,* Baltimore, MD, 1993, Paul H Brookes.

Sinnema G: Resilience among children with special health care needs and among their families, *Pediatr Ann* 20(9):483-486, 1991.

Spencer M, Markstrom-Adams C: Identity processes among racial and ethnic minority children in America, *Child Dev* 61:290-310, 1990.

Steele S: Nurse case management in a rural parent-infant enrichment program, *Issues Compr Pediatr Nurs* 14(4):259-266, 1991.

Strax TE: Psychological issues faced by adolescents and young adults with disabilities, *Pediatr Ann* 20(9):507-511, 1991.

Thome SE, Robinson CA: Health care relationships: the chronic illness perspective, *Res Nurs Health* 11:293-300, 1988.

Thorne S: *Negotiating health care: the social context of chronic illness,* Newbury Park, 1993, Sage.

Vessey JA, Caserza CL: Chronic conditions and child development. In Jackson PL, Vessey JA: *Primary care of the child with a chronic condition,* St Louis, 1992, Mosby.

Vincenti VB: Empowerment: its history and meaning, *Home Econ Forum* 6(2):7-14, 1993.

Walker DK and others: Perceived needs of families with children who have chronic health conditions, *Child Health Care* 18(4):196-201, 1989.

Wells PW and others: Growing up in the hospital. I. Let's focus on the child, *J Pediatr Nurs* 9(2):66-73, 1994.

Whyte DA: A family nursing approach to the care of a child with a chronic illness, *J Adv Nurs* 17(3):317-327, 1992.

Zagorsky ES: Caring for families who follow alternative health practices, *Pediatr Nurs* 19(1):71-75, 1993.

Zeltzer LK, LeBaron S: Fantasy in children and adolescents with chronic illness, *Dev Behav Pediatr* 7(3):195-198, 1986.

PUBLICATIONS FOR SCHOOL ATTENDANCE

Back to school: a handbook for teachers of children with cancer (also one for parents), Atlanta, 1989, American Cancer Society.

Lorn A, Martinez I: *When you have a visually handicapped child in your classroom: suggestions for teachers,* New York, 1985, American Federation for the Blind.

Morrow G: *Helping chronically ill children in school,* New York, 1985, Parker Publishing Co.

Students with cancer: a resource for the educator, U.S. Department of Health and Human Services, National Institutes of Health, NIH Pub. No. 87-2086, Washington, DC, 1987. (Order from Office of Cancer Communications, National Cancer Institute, Building 31, Room 10A24, Bethesda, MD 20892).

Suggestions for teachers and school counselors, Oak Brook, IL, 1983, The Compassionate Friends.

When your child is ready to return to school, Chicago, 1982, Association for Brain Tumor Research.

CHAPTER 23

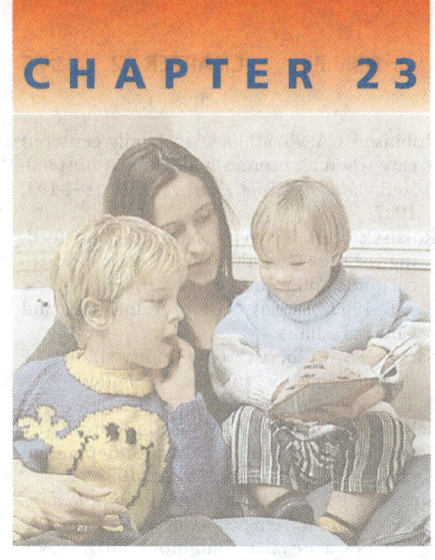

Family-Centered Care of the Child with Life-Threatening Illness

CHAPTER OUTLINE

RELATED TOPICS

The child with cancer, Ch. 36

Communicating with families, Ch. 6

Compliance, Ch. 27

Ethical decision making, Ch. 1

Family-centered care, Ch. 1

Family-centered care of the child with chronic illness or disability, Ch. 22

Family-centered home care, Ch. 25

Human immunodeficiency virus (HIV) infection and acquired immunodeficiency syndrome (AIDS), Ch. 35

Long-term sequelae of treatment, Ch. 36

Neonatal loss, Ch. 10

Pain assessment; pain management, Ch. 26

Sudden infant death syndrome, Ch. 13

FAMILY-CENTERED CARE

Although most childhood illnesses and many injuries and other trauma respond favorably to treatment, some do not. As a result, nurses may care for children and families facing sudden death or death after a prolonged illness. When a child and family face a prolonged and possibly terminal illness, health professionals are faced with the challenge of providing the best possible care to meet the physical, psychologic, and emotional needs of the child and family during the uncertain course of the illness and at the time of death. When death is sudden and unexpected, nurses are challenged to respond to grief and shock in families and provide comfort and support in the absence of a prior relationship.

Many factors affect the causes of death nurses are likely to encounter in children: developmental factors, medical advances and technology, and changing social patterns. Among infants, congenital anomalies, other complications of birth, and sudden infant death syndrome (SIDS) are leading causes of death (Statistical Abstract, 1993, Table 123). For some time, the leading cause of death among children over 1 year of age has been injuries (accidents). Among children 1 to 14 years of age, malignant neoplasms, congenital anomalies, homicide (and legal intervention), heart disease, and pneumonia and influenza follow in order as causes of death. From 1985 to 1990, human immunodeficiency virus (HIV) deaths more than tripled in the under 5 age-group and rose nearly sixfold among children ages 5 to 12 (Statistical Abstract, 1993, Table 131). Among youth 15 to 24 years of age, homicide (and legal intervention), suicide, malignant neoplasms, heart disease, and HIV infection follow accidents as the most prevalent causes of death (Statistical Abstract, 1993, Table 128).

A child diagnosed with a life-threatening illness or suffering serious, life-threatening trauma needs medical diagnosis and intervention, as well as nursing assessment and care—sometimes for a short time and sometimes over a lengthy period. The child also needs continuity with his or her family, and the family needs to continue in their central role of providing care, guidance, and nurturance for the child through the challenges they all face. The principles of family-centered care (see Chapters 1 and 22) provide a framework for nursing care of the child and family with a life-threatening diagnosis that respects the central role of the family.

Honest, unbiased, and complete communication is essential if families are to participate in caring for their child with a life-threatening condition. Parents need information about the diagnosis, prognosis, current treatment, treatment plans, treatment options, and pros and cons of the options. There may come a point when they will need information about how to communicate with their child about death, how to involve siblings, how to comfort their dying child, and how to recognize impending death. Information is best shared in a trusting relationship as part of an ongoing dialogue and presented in a sensitive, caring manner. Communication about the life-threatening illness

■ Elizabeth Ahmann, RN, ScD, revised this chapter.

COMMUNICATING WITH THE BEREAVED FAMILY

EXAMPLES OF NONTHERAPEUTIC STATEMENTS

Advice:	You should get out more. Stop feeling sorry for yourself. You need to be strong for your family.
Cheerfulness:	Now, now, don't cry; cheer up. Cheer up, you can always have another baby.
Interpretation:	It was God's will. It's better now because she is at peace.
Reassurance:	I know how you feel. God never gives us more than we can handle. Don't worry, everything will work out. At least, you still have the rest of your family.
Argument:	How can you say that? It's wrong to blame anyone. You should be glad his suffering is over.
Ignoring loss:	Remember, you're young and can still have another baby. It could be worse: he could have lived with severe brain damage.

EXAMPLES OF THERAPEUTIC STATEMENTS

Feeling-focused:	You seem confused and angry. You are still feeling the pain. Tell me more about how you are feeling.
Nonjudgmental questions:	Can I be of any help? Have you decided who the pallbearers will be?
Clarification:	Correct me if I'm wrong, but you intend to make all the arrangements. You feel the accident was your husband's fault? I'm not sure I understand. Tell me more about . . .
Explanations:	You can touch her and hold her if you wish.
Concern:	Your daughter's birthday is near. That must be painful to deal with.
Support, empathy:	It's OK to cry. It sounds like you have been doing some painful thinking.
Support, silence:	I'm here if you want to talk. (Silence) Hello. (Touch, silence)
Assessing coping and support:	Do you have friends and family who can help you now? You have been through a lot. How are you doing now? Is there someone who can drive you home?
Validating loss:	You have been through a very tough time. He was a special boy to all the staff. I will miss him.

Data from Davidowitz M, Myrick R: Responding to the bereaved: an analysis of "helping statements," *Death Educ* 8:1-10, 1984; Johnson L, Mattson S: Communication: the key to crisis prevention in pediatric death, *Crit Care Nurse,* pp 23-27, Dec 1992; and Segal S, Fletcher M, Meekison W: Survey of bereaved parents, *Can Med Assoc J* 134(1):38-42, 1986.

or injury, as well as communication at the time of death, requires tact and sensitivity. The box on p. 977 lists therapeutic and nontherapeutic approaches.

Collaboration should occur with parents regarding treatment goals and approaches to care at the time of death. A sense of participation in the outcome of the illness situation is not only the family's appropriate role, but is important in their coping with the child's condition and death (Price, 1992). In most instances there will be agreement between parents and professionals on how to approach the care of the child. When there is disagreement, respectful dialogue may clarify misunderstandings. An ethics consultant or committee may be called on in the unusual circumstance that differing points of view cannot be resolved easily (Rushton and Hogue, 1993). Generally, a family's wishes should be respected.

The nurse's role in working with the family should include empowering the family to care for their child in the ways they may choose. This is accomplished through information, support, encouragement, and training. A focus on the needs of the family also includes attention to emotional needs of parents and siblings and assistance with instrumental needs such as food, lodging, transportation, finances, and the like.

In working with families, nurses should be aware of the importance of culture. Culture influences how people view and make sense of the world. People often draw on their cultural heritage for strength, support, and meaning during challenging, stressful times. Nursing practice that is family centered will be respectful of culturally based needs and preferences in dealing both with life-threatening illness or injury and with death. Nurses can only come to know an individual family's needs by asking. In fact, in many circumstances, culturally based preferences may only be revealed in dialogue between the nurse and family members. Every effort should be made to respect a family's preferences once they are expressed (see Communicating with Families, Chapter 6).

REACTIONS OF THE FAMILY TO A LIFE-THREATENING ILLNESS

All families whose child has some type of physical or cognitive disability experience reactions to the loss of the "perfect" child that are similar, despite the diagnosis. The reader is urged to review the concepts in Chapter 22 and apply them to this discussion. The following section focuses on five phases in which there are significant differences in reactions to chronic disease vs life-threatening illness. In this section cancer is used as an example of life-threatening illness. A Nursing Care Plan for the child who is terminally ill or dying is presented on pp. 985-987.

Nurses should be aware that families' reactions to other life-threatening illnesses will be affected by the nature and course of the illness. For example, reactions to the diagnosis of AIDS/HIV may include guilt if parents were infected and passed the virus to the child, as well as realistic and serious stigma concerns. In facing the diagnosis and possible death of a child from AIDS/HIV, an infected parent must also face his or her own diagnosis and possible death (Lipson, 1993). Concerns about contagion affect the interactions between health care providers, the family, and the child as well. The complexity and sensitivity of issues such as these have implications for nursing care of the child and family (see Chapter 35).

Phase I—Revelation and Dawning Reality: Diagnosis and Treatment

When parents first learn of the diagnosis of cancer, their immediate reactions are similar to those of other families whose child has a chronic illness, except that the initial impact can be much more pessimistic and overwhelming because of the generally negative connotation regarding the disease. Principal concerns for children center around the diagnostic tests and treatments and their effects.

Almost immediately after the diagnosis is confirmed, induction therapy aimed at total remission of the disease begins. During this period families commonly react with quiet anger, depression, ambivalence, and bargaining. Much of the psychic energy is directed at waiting for the confirmation of a remission. If that does not occur, all the initial reactions may be repeated again, with increased anticipatory grieving.

Shock and Disbelief. Many parents relate that after they heard the diagnosis, they were deaf to everything else told to them. As one mother described, "All I heard the doctor say was the word 'leukemia.' I didn't hear anything else. All I could think of was that leukemia was fatal. I was certain my child was going to die. My husband heard the doctor say it was curable, but I didn't. I won't believe that until I see it. Even if my child is 50 years old, I will worry about it coming back." The pessimistic response of this mother is typical of many parents who are afraid to believe that their child will recover despite a favorable prognosis. Anticipatory grieving for the possible loss of the child is common, and if parents are not helped to understand the improved prognosis of these diseases, they may react by psychologically burying the child. This "alarm stage" of emotional chaos and belief in a terminal prognosis typically lasts a week to a month after the actual diagnosis but is highly influenced by the family's personal attitudes and sense of skepticism or faith (Brett and Davies, 1988).

Anger. Children often may feel angry, particularly because of all the traumatic procedures done to them as part of the diagnosis and treatment. Once they begin to feel better, they frequently express their anger through uncooperativeness. Parents receive the brunt of much of the child's anger and often find coping with it extremely difficult. A common reaction is to ignore it and try to pacify the child by giving in to requests whenever possible. Overprotectiveness and permissiveness are typical reactions during remission, and helping parents deal with the child's anger constructively during the hospitalization also prevents some of the potential future problems.

Reactions to Altered Body Image. One side effect of chemotherapy or cranial irradiation that has particular psychologic significance for children in different age-groups and for parents is hair loss.

Young children. For young children baldness has little significance. Preschoolers may attach superficial concern to the hair loss, particularly if it affects their sex role image. For example, one 4-year-old girl was disturbed about her baldness because she thought she looked like a boy. Once her parents emphasized her femaleness in dress, she was unconcerned about the temporary change.

Parents of young children may have a difficult adjustment. However, they may be unwilling to admit their concern and lack of acceptance. For example, the mother of a 3-year-old boy refused to openly discuss the hair loss in front of her son. She had decided to hide the change from him until new hair grew in. She had formulated a fantastic conspiracy to maintain the secret. For example, she planned to remove all mirrors in the house, to isolate him from children, to keep his head always covered with hats, and to buy a soft brush and groom the hair as if it were still present. She explained that this was necessary because he was very vain. When asked what she would do if he discovered the baldness, she calmly said, "I'll just tell him what happened." It was not possible for her to see the pitfalls of such a scheme until she verbalized her personal feelings about the hair loss.

School-age children. The reactions of school-age children depend on their preparation for the loss and the type of parental adjustment. Much of their anxiety relates to the anticipation of the loss rather than the actual baldness. Telling children about the change before it occurs, stressing that it is temporary, and suggesting ways of camouflaging it, such as with a wig, hat, or scarf, result in better adjustment to the altered body image.

➤ **NURSING TIP** If the hair is long enough, suggest that it be cut to save a swatch. The hair can be attached to a self-adhering fastener that is placed on the inside of a hat to make it appear as a full head of hair.

Adolescents. Adolescents have the most difficulty in accepting and adjusting to hair loss because it occurs at a time when peer acceptance and group conformity are essential. They need the opportunity to express their anger and fears of rejection without being judged or reproached. Sometimes parents try to reason with their adolescent child that the hair loss is a small sacrifice for a possible future recovery. Although true, it does little to comfort the adolescent in his or her present struggle.

Involving adolescents in selecting a wig or a hat that can be their trademark *before* the hair falls out provides them with a feeling of participation. Choosing a wig in advance allows them to secure a wig that is most similar to their own hair.

Nursing Considerations. The time of diagnosis is a critical period for the development of therapeutic relationships. Ideally, the primary nurse should be present with family members when the diagnosis is given. The same guidelines as discussed in Chapter 22 apply; parents want information that they consider critical—information related to the diagnosis and prognosis, disease process, need for additional diagnostic tests, immediate therapeutic plan, and availability of the practitioner. They value an open, sympathetic, direct, and uninterrupted discussion, with sufficient time to hear the information and ask questions. Information should be repeated and clarified as necessary.

In many instances the child's care is so complex that numerous specialists are involved. Consequently, the nurse becomes the only consistent person for the family. For example, in the case of a child with Wilms tumor, a pediatrician, urologist, surgeon, radiologist, and hematologist/oncologist participate in the medical/surgical care of the child. Even under the best of circumstances, parents can receive opposing messages from health team members and can become confused about who can answer their questions. The nurse is in an advantageous position to interpret those messages and to direct the parents to the most appropriate source of information.

In many instances care in the hospital is limited to a few days of diagnosis and initiation of treatment. However, in some cases an extended admission may be necessary. Many parents elect to stay with their child and to participate as much as possible in the care. Because the possibility of death in a child is a highly emotional experience, nurses may unknowingly usurp parents' roles or relinquish nursing responsibilities. They need to be aware of their approach toward parents and develop open dialogue with them in order to support the family in the way most comfortable for the parents. Planning the child's care *with* family members is a most effective way of communicating genuine concern and avoiding either hazard.

During the remission phase, parents, ill children, and siblings need reassurance that their reactions are normal and expected. The interventions discussed in Chapter 22 apply. Because of the shock usually experienced when a catastrophic illness is diagnosed, the needs of well family members, particularly siblings, may be neglected. Siblings can be helped to understand the reason for the abrupt change in family life by being kept informed of the child's condition and by continuing as much contact as possible with the hospitalized child (and absent parents if necessary) through visiting, telephone contact, letter writing, cards, or photographs.

Parents and children need thorough, detailed, and repeated explanations of the diagnostic tests and plan of therapy. They need reassurance that a change in the child's condition is most likely a result of therapy, not the disease. Decreasing the chance for the unexpected lessens the opportunities for increased anxiety. For example, forewarning the family about the side effects of therapy, such as alopecia, weight gain, constipation, stomatitis, and nausea and vomiting, as well as the necessary laboratory procedures, prepares them for these expected events and increases their sense of security and control.

Phase II—Reprieve: Remission and Maintenance Therapy

Once the child is in remission, there is a long period of hope for an eventual recovery and fear of a possible relapse. Parents commonly react with heightened vigilance by overprotecting the child, encouraging dependency, and liberalizing discipline. These reactions support the child's sick role and hinder optimum physical and emotional development. Family members may attempt to escape or avoid the problems of this period through social isolation.

Overprotectiveness. Although many children return home in relatively stable and much improved physical health, parents frequently treat them as invalids. One of the most common manifestations of overprotectiveness is parents' inability to set appropriate limits. It is understandable that, under the stress of potential loss, parents might respond by overindulging the child, giving in to every desire and wish. Although this is probably part of the grieving process during the initial phase of the illness, persistence of this reaction culminates in special problems during the often long period of remission.

For ill children, overprotection and "special" treatment increase their fears concerning serious illness and failure to recover. In addition, if they are given everything during periods of wellness, they will become very frustrated, unhappy, and demanding children during the terminal phase, when it will be impossible to meet all their requests.

Dependency. Closely associated with the overprotectiveness is increased dependency between parents and child. This is often evident in parents' unwillingness to send their child to school. If not helped toward reintegration of usual activities, they may use the hair loss or frequent visits for treatment as excuses for keeping the child home. The same needs and interventions regarding school that are discussed in Chapter 22 apply. However, school personnel may have special concerns.* A common, often unvoiced fear of school personnel is that the child will have some dramatic episode, such as massive hemorrhage, while in the classroom, and die (Klopovich and others, 1981). The nurse can assist parents in educating school personnel about the disease. During the discussion of the disease, the nurse should include the usual course of the illness and its specific implications (e.g., the child's increased susceptibility to common childhood diseases or unexpected epidemics such as chickenpox). The school nurse should be made aware of the need to report instances of contagious illness to the parents.

Several issues should also be approached with the schoolteacher and nurse, particularly other parents' questions about the disease, such as the chance of communicability, preparation of the class for expected physical changes, and possible future absences. During the terminal phase the parents should also discuss the likelihood of the child's death and the need for discussing this with the other students. Teachers of siblings who attend the same school should also be included in the discussions. For example, the siblings may be demonstrating in school their difficulties in adjusting to the child's illness. Such behavior may erroneously be interpreted as learning disabilities, behavioral or emotional problems, or delinquency, for example. Unless the teachers are aware of the extenuating circumstances, these children can be saddled with negative labels for the rest of their academic life.

Anxiety. In addition to the concerns discussed in the preceding paragraphs, there are many other anxiety-provoking stresses. The financial strain of a chronic illness is a constant worry. Job security is always a necessary consideration, because unemployment may jeopardize insurance coverage. There are also costs besides the actual medical care, such as transportation to the hospital, meals away from home, baby-sitting for other siblings, or temporary housing for distant medical care.* The nurse can provide assistance by referring the family to available organizations, such as the **Leukemia Society of America**† or the **American Cancer Society,**‡ who may be able to provide financial help, and to **The Candlelighters Childhood Cancer Foundation**§ for information and psychologic support.

Nutrition is also a continuing concern. Many drugs cause severe nausea and vomiting, thereby decreasing the child's appetite. The illness usually results in marked weight loss. Mealtime can become a battleground for family members. The nurse can assist families in preventing some of the problems by forewarning parents of the expected change in appetite and by suggesting ways of encouraging children to eat without causing a power struggle. For example, during the course of steroid therapy, appetite improves dramatically. Parents should be told that the increased hunger is a result of medication, not a change in the child's behavior or attitude. During periods of chemotherapy when the appetite is decreased, providing small, frequent meals of favorite foods often encourages some cooperation. Growth may also be slowed during the treatment phase from the various drugs and use of radiation. If parents are aware of some of these expected changes, they may be more accepting of the child's fluctuating appetite.

Nursing Considerations. Often remission and "going home" from the cancer center coincide, and a number of problems can be anticipated and often prevented by a thorough discussion at this time: maintenance of normal family patterns, school attendance, and relationships among family and friends. Because of the usual reaction by parents to overprotect the child, they should be advised to continue appropriate discipline of the child and siblings by resuming rules and limits in effect before the illness. The importance of resuming school and other daily activities as soon as possible is stressed, and other family members, particularly mothers, may benefit from resuming their previous functions, including employment. Parents are encouraged to schedule appointments for visits at times that least interfere with the child's daily routine, such as late on Friday, which leaves the weekend for recuperation from any unpleasant side effects (Fig. 23-1).

Ongoing compliance with medical treatment is a very im-

*See suggested readings on p. 975 for information concerning students with serious illness.

*Ronald McDonald Houses provide inexpensive homelike accommodations for families when distance to the hospital is a major factor. They are located in several large cities, and application for lodging is usually made through the social service department of the medical center.

†600 3rd Ave., New York, NY 10016; (212) 573-8484 or (800) 955-4572.

‡1599 Clifton Rd., NE, Atlanta, GA 30329-4251; (404) 329-7617. Also, Canadian Cancer Society, 10 Alcorn Ave., Suite 200, Toronto, Ontario M4V 3B1; (416) 961-7223.

§7910 Woodmont Ave., Suite 460, Bethesda, MD 20814; (301) 657-8401 or (800) 366-2223.

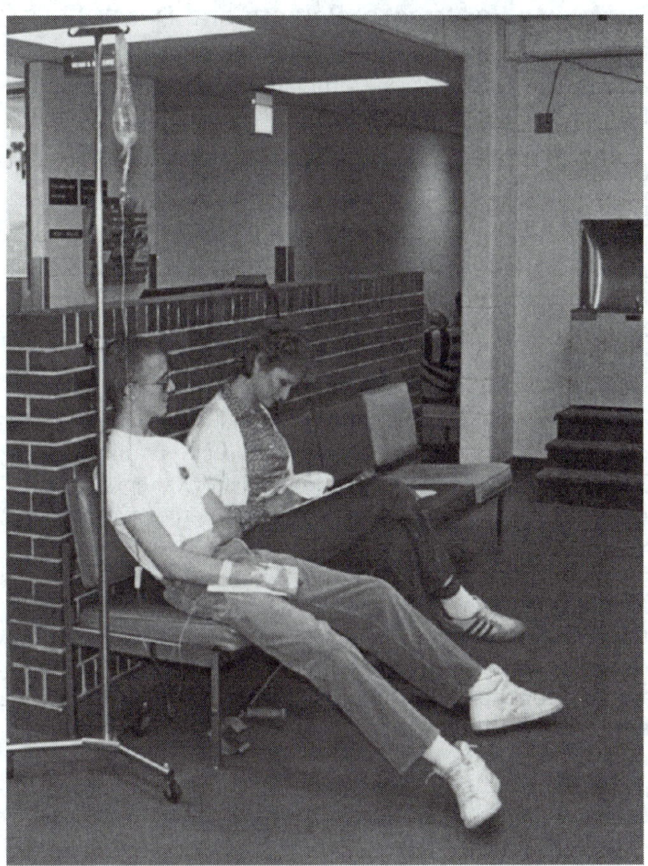

FIG. 23-1 Treatment often involves long periods of outpatient visits that should be scheduled at times that least interfere with the youngster's daily routine.

portant aspect of care, with the prognosis closely related to treatments. However, noncompliance is a serious problem among children with cancer, especially adolescents, who refuse to take the medication at home or keep treatment appointments. Not only can noncompliance affect the chance of survival, it can also cause unnecessary diagnostic tests and warranted change in treatment protocols. Strategies for enhancing compliance, especially in teenagers, are to include the youngster in treatment discussions, help the family set clear expectations and clarify roles (e.g., who is responsible for administering the drug or supervising the administration), and provide written instructions (Lansky, List, and Ritter-Sterr, 1988). (See also Compliance, Chapter 27.)

To avoid unnecessary social isolation, the parents need to be prepared for common responses of friends and relatives, such as staying away from the family, fearing the child's illness (especially concern for contagion), and giving unsolicited advice. Families can often avoid these problems by taking the initiative in informing others about the child's condition and asking directly that they remain in contact with each other. Being the first to express, "I know it's hard to know what to say and do in a situation like this," can put others at ease. A more difficult situation is the offering of unsolicited advice regarding treatment, particularly information about "new" but unproved methods. Parents can be encouraged to take a firm but tactful approach; they can comment that they will inquire about the method with their health professional but that they feel assured that their child is receiving the best care available. Many families benefit from associating with other similarly affected families. There is a special camaraderie between parents of children with cancer that seems to sustain them through the long ordeal (Lyman, 1987). Once such friendships develop, families often ask staff about other children's status. Staff may be concerned with sharing confidential information, but at least one study found families accepting of the practice (Patno, Young, and Dickerman, 1988). Staff could directly ask families for permission. Sources of information about self-help groups are discussed under Help the Family Cope, Chapter 22.

Because many children are treated in tertiary centers located at a distance from their home, there may not be one primary nurse who can act as liaison and coordinator among the nurses in the hospital, school, clinic, practitioner's office, and community. Often this results in a lack of preventive intervention. Nurses who are in a particularly advantageous position to become a primary link with the family are nurse practitioners (Hobbie and Hollen, 1993) and community nurses, and a nurse network should be established before discharge to ensure continuity of care.

Phase III—Recovery: Cessation of Therapy and Possible Cure

The maintenance period may be followed by cessation of therapy in the hope of a permanent recovery. Although this is a very happy time, it is mixed with feelings of grief, ambivalence, uncertainty, and concern for the future.

Denial and Ambivalence. At the time the decision is made to terminate therapy, many parents deny that treatment is no longer warranted. They may express ambivalence with such questions as "Are you sure that a longer period of drugs wouldn't guarantee a better chance for a cure?" There is difficulty in giving up the security of the rituals of medication, radiation therapy, and frequent examinations. Occasionally, health professionals erroneously label the ambivalence or denial as a psychologic need for the child's sick role.

In general, this reaction is characteristic of the grieving for the loss of security afforded by medical intervention and of the need for adjustment to the hazards of "waiting it out" again. Parents need almost as much support during this phase as they did when they were told of the diagnosis.

Overprotectiveness. Parents also relate a resurgence of the need to overprotect and isolate their child from any potential physical harm. As one mother stated, "I became fanatical about examining my child for signs of recurring illness when the drugs were stopped. If he had a runny nose or sore throat, I immediately took him to the doctor, requesting a blood count. I was so sure those leukemic cells had returned." She later compared this reaction to the ways in which she treated the child after his first remission. She added, "You would think that after 3 years of living with drugs, side effects, blood tests, and doctors, I would be thrilled to give it all up, but here I am, almost as shaky and nervous as if I had just found out he had the disease."

Uncertainty. The fear of cancer returning and the ever-present uncertainty of the child's survival are experienced by all family members. Mothers seem to bear the greatest burden of uncertainty, feeling concerned and often anxious about symptoms recurring. The fear of recurrence may worsen over time: even in situations of remission for as long as 12 years, family members have spoken of anxiety. This long-term anxiety can become disabling to some families (Clarke-Steffen, 1993; Cohen, 1993; Faulkner, Peace, and O'Keefe, 1993; Peace and others, 1992).

Concern for the Future. When cure is a realistic possibility, the family's concern for the *quantity* of life shifts to the *quality* of life. This is a legitimate concern, because chemotherapy and radiation are not without their immediate and long-term complications (Hollen and Hobbie, 1993). The need for continued medical supervision of these children cannot be overemphasized. (See Long-Term Sequelae of Treatment, Chapter 36.) Survivors worry most about their psychologic normalcy, schooling, and relationships with family and friends. They have concerns about having children, transmitting cancer to their offspring, and recurrence of their disease or another cancer. Some worry about employment discrimination, obtaining insurance, and access to future medical care.

For families who did not have the benefit of anticipatory guidance, the prospect of a cure may represent a rethinking of their childrearing practices. For example, these parents may have indulged the child and tolerated negative or regressive behaviors because of the thought of death. Now that the child's future is much more positive, there may be recognition that changes must occur to reestablish normal behavior. Such families benefit from professional guidance to gradually change behavioral patterns.

Nursing Considerations. Probably the most important component of care is acceptance of the family's mixed reactions to cessation of therapy. Parents need to feel comfortable in calling the nurse or clinic about any concern or problem. They also should be encouraged to verbalize their feelings and thoughts of cessation of therapy. It may be helpful for the nurse to acquaint them with another family who has progressed through this transition period.

Nurses working with these families must be aware of the long-term consequences of treatment and be vigilant of signs indicating problems, such as retarded growth or evidence of a second malignancy. Psychosocial problems may surface, and young people are particularly concerned about fertility and sexuality. Adolescents frequently equate the information about impaired fertility with impaired sexual performance, and even when such concerns are not voiced, they need clarification that sexual performance is not physiologically affected. Adolescent survivors should also receive information about the particular effects smoking tobacco and marijuana or consuming alcohol may have on their organs, which have already been compromised by radiation and chemotherapy (Hollen and Hobbie, 1993).

Phase IV—Recurrence: Relapse and Death

The most dreaded news other than the initial diagnosis is confirmation of a relapse. Although for many children the first relapse is followed by another remission, this and subsequent remissions are followed by subsequent relapses, with the final relapse being followed by death. The family's reactions during the terminal stage are influenced by their previous acceptance or denial of the child's illness. It is a period of intense anticipatory grieving, characterized by the relapse reactions of depression, loss of hope, and possibly acceptance. As the child's condition worsens, there is intensification of numerous fears.

Loss of Hope and Depression. One of the most difficult realizations for the family is the knowledge that with each relapse the chances for eventual recovery diminishes. The reality of possible death looms before them, particularly during the reinduction phase when a recurrent remission may or may not be feasible. Once another remission is attained, reason for hope is again present.

However, many families relate that after termination of the primary remission they never again feel as hopeful or optimistic. Some also discuss their silent preparation and grieving for the child's eventual death. Nurses need to be sensitive to such thoughts and aware of the possible beneficial aspects of this reaction, because repeated relapses are associated with poorer prognoses.

The usual reaction to loss of hope is depression. This may be the type of depression for past losses, but most often is anticipatory grieving for impending losses. Nurses need to carefully assess the reason for the depression and realistically plan intervention. For example, if another remission is likely, the nurse should plan to help the parents work through their depression. However, if this relapse is actually the commencement of the terminal stage, the nurse should plan to support the family in preparing for the death.

Fear of Death. The most prevalent fear is of death itself. Parents frequently ask about death through questions such as "What will he die from?" "How will we know she is dying?" and "What will happen when he dies?" It is important to listen sensitively to such questions because the real concern may be hidden behind the question. For example, when parents ask, "What will he die from?" they may not be so concerned with the medical cause of death, such as hemorrhage or infection, but may really be asking, "What is hemorrhage like?" Most people have a fantasy idea of how death will occur that is much more horrifying than the actual event. For example, parents will relate that their idea of hemorrhage is uncontrollable gushing of blood from every orifice. In reality it is usually internal bleeding and often oozing of blood from the nose. When the nurses are aware of the imagined events, they can clarify the misconceptions and supply the correct information.

Fear of Pain. The fear of uncontrollable pain is almost universal. Whatever bargaining occurs during the dying stage is for a peaceful, quiet, and quick death. Often parents will relate that the child has pain even when it appears that the child is comfortable. It is important for nurses to understand that pain is much more than physical. Watching one's child die is a pain that must certainly be immeasurable and that subjectively shadows one's perception of surrounding events. At the same time, pain control (discussed in Chapter 26) is an essential intervention in care of the dying child. Pain control measures should be administered on a preventive schedule, with adjustments made as needed to provide maximum comfort.

Fear of Loss of Control. A fear that is shared by the dying and the survivors is losing emotional and physical control as death approaches. Some parents attempt to cope with this fear by requesting that their child be heavily sedated during the terminal stage. However, the loss of control imposed by medication may make the child very distraught. Inasmuch as nurses usually regulate the administration of drugs, it is important for them to carefully assess the needs of both the child and the parents. Supporting parents at the time of impending death by being physically present, making the child as comfortable as possible, and talking to the awake child helps parents feel in control without the need for sedating the child.

Fear of Isolation and Loneliness. Parents fear that their child will die when they are not present. When the expectation is that death is near, nurses should know how to contact parents at any time they are not with the child. The hospital can supply pagers that can be used for this purpose. Dying children often request that their parents stay with them (Fig. 23-2), and this request should always be respected. No one need die in lonely isolation.

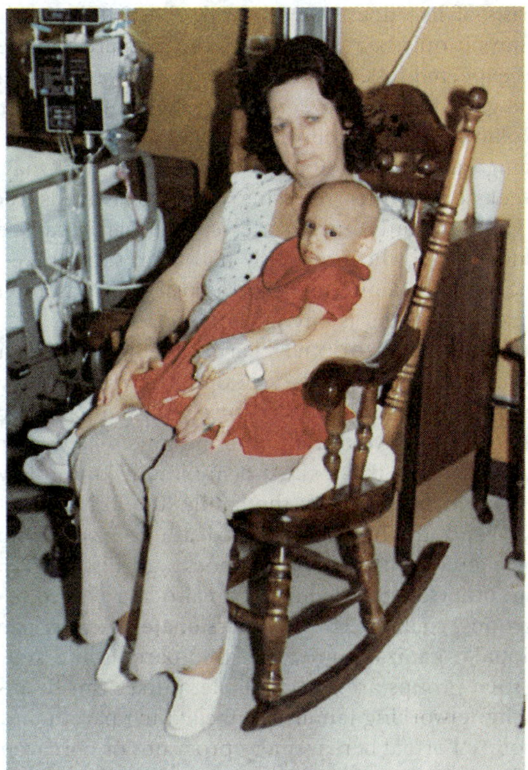

FIG. 23-2 For the dying child there is no greater comfort than the security and closeness of a parent.

Nursing Considerations. Relapse is a difficult phase for nurses because it often initiates a loss of hope and their own grieving process. One of the dangers during the phase of relapse is that nurses may transfer their feelings of pessimism or optimism to the parents. It is extremely important to assess one's own personal response to the relapse and then to plan the intervention according to the family's needs. This seems to be particularly critical during the final relapse. Nurses can help parents and children formulate realistic short-term goals and establish reasonable priorities of care. It is also the time to discuss with parents their wishes and expectations for the terminal phase. For some families the alternative of hospice or home care is a very significant and fulfilling means of sharing their child's last days (see p. 997).

During the terminal stage the fears of parents and children form the foundation for nursing care. These fears may be particularly worrisome for those parents who have chosen home care because they must assume primary responsibility for the child. The nurse's role includes preparing them to deal with each fear and providing assistance through home visits, telephone counseling, and the alternative of hospital admission at any time. As death approaches, nurses should recognize the physical signs (see box below) and summon parents who are not present to the child's bedside. Parents can also be informed of the physical signs of death so that they know what to expect. If death approaches sooner than expected, families should be prepared. Sometimes health professionals' need to deny death is so strong that parents are continually given messages of false hope that prevent them from preparing themselves for the worst news. Although others may think such false hope is helpful, in reality it may be extremely painful for family members to live in uncertainty.

The goal in caring for dying children is comfort, and no intervention is more important than control of pain. Anal-

PHYSICAL SIGNS OF APPROACHING DEATH

- Loss of sensation and movement in the lower extremities, progressing toward the upper body
- Sensation of heat, although body feels cool
- Loss of senses
  - Tactile sensation decreases
  - Sensitive to light
  - Hearing is last sense to fail
- Confusion, loss of consciousness, slurred speech
- Muscle weakness
- Loss of bowel and bladder control
- Decreased appetite/thirst
- Difficulty swallowing
- Change in respiratory pattern
  - Cheyne-Stokes respirations (waxing and waning of depth of breathing with regular periods of apnea)
  - "Death rattle" (noisy chest sounds from accumulation of pulmonary and pharyngeal secretions)
- Weak, slow pulse; decreased blood pressure

GUIDELINES
*Supporting Grieving Families**

GENERAL

Stay with the family; sit quietly if they prefer not to talk; cry with them if desired.
Accept the family's grief reactions; avoid judgmental statements (e.g., "You should be feeling better by now").
Avoid offering rationalizations for the child's death (e.g., "You should be glad your child isn't suffering anymore").
Avoid artificial consolation (e.g., "I know how you feel," or "You are still young enough to have another baby").
Deal openly with feelings such as guilt, anger, and loss of self-esteem.
Focus on feelings by using a feeling word in the statement (e.g., "You're still feeling all the pain of losing a child").
Refer the family to an appropriate self-help group or for professional help if needed.

AT THE TIME OF DEATH

Reassure the family that everything possible is being done for the child, if they wish lifesaving interventions.
Do everything possible to ensure the child's comfort, especially relieving pain.
Provide the child and family the opportunity to review special experiences or memories in their lives.
Express personal feelings of loss and/or frustrations (e.g., "We will miss him so much," or "We tried everything; we feel so sorry that we couldn't save him").
Provide information that the family requests and be honest.
Respect the emotional needs of family members, such as siblings, who may need brief respites from the dying child.
Make every effort to arrange for family members, especially parents, to be with the child at the moment of death, if they wish to be present.
Allow the family to stay with the dead child for as long as they wish and to rock, hold, or bathe the child.
Provide practical help when possible, such as collecting the child's belongings.
Arrange for spiritual support, such as clergy; pray with the family if no one else can stay with them.

AFTER THE DEATH

Attend the funeral or visitation if there was a special closeness with the family.
Initiate and maintain contact (e.g., sending cards, telephoning, inviting them back to the unit, or making a home visit).
Refer to the dead child by name; discuss shared memories with the family.
Discourage the use of drugs or alcohol as a method of escaping grief.
Encourage all family members to communicate their feelings rather than remaining silent to avoid upsetting another member.
Emphasize that grieving is a painful process that often takes years to resolve.

*"Family" refers to all significant persons involved in the child's life, such as the parents, siblings, grandparents, or other close relatives or friends.

gesics, especially opioids, are administered around the clock to prevent pain, with adjustments made in dosage and schedule as needed to maintain maximum comfort. This often requires increasing dosage of opioids beyond those normally recommended, decreasing the duration between doses, and changing routes of administration to comply with the child's needs and wishes. Whenever possible the oral route is preferred, but when no longer possible, continuous intravenous infusion administration may provide the greatest benefit. Parents and the child need to be reassured that the opioids are needed and that addiction is not a problem. If tolerance and/or physical dependence occur, these normal, involuntary responses to opioids are explained to prevent any misconception that they represent addiction. Parents may be particularly interested in helping their child by employing any nonpharmacologic measures that may augment pain relief and relaxation, such as cutaneous stimulation (e.g., rocking, stroking the skin) or diversion (e.g., reading to the child or playing music). (See also Chapter 26 for an extensive discussion of pain assessment and management.)

Both the family and the child may have heightened spiritual needs at the time of death. Spiritual support includes respect for the diverse beliefs of families, willingness to discuss matters of spirituality with them, and provision for the rituals and sacraments of organized religion or cultural preference. Many families desire a priest, minister, or rabbi, and the nurse can summon the clergy to be with the family. In those cases in which it may not be possible to reach a member of the clergy, the nurse may provide for the spiritual needs by praying with the family, reading from the Bible, or listening to the review of their life (see Guidelines box; see also Nursing Care Plan on pp. 985-987).

Phase V—The Beginning: Postdeath

The crisis of loss does not end with the child's death. In many ways it only begins. Families can prepare themselves for the expected loss, but when it occurs, there is a period of acute grief, followed by an extended phase of mourning (see p. 996). It is important for families to understand that mourning takes a long time. Whereas acute grief may last only weeks or months, resolving their loss is measured in years. Holidays and anniversaries can be particularly difficult, and people who previously had been supportive may now expect the family to have "adjusted." Consequently, prolonged mourning is often silent and lonely.

Nursing Considerations. Part of the difficulty in helping the bereaved family is lack of opportunity for follow-up in the traditional nursing structure. Consequently, many families never receive the support and guidance that could help them resolve the loss. At a minimum, one follow-up phone call or meeting with the family should be arranged, possibly 1 month after the child's death, to give the family time to overcome the phase of shock and disbelief (Jankovic and others, 1989). Families can also be referred to self-help groups, such as **The Compassionate Friends,*** an international organization for bereaved parents and siblings. When such groups are not available, nurses can be instrumental in networking families or facilitating parent and sibling groups. Formal bereavement programs or bereavement counseling can be helpful as well (see p. 996).

*P.O. Box 3696, Oak Brook, IL 60522-3696; (708) 990-0010.

NURSING CARE PLAN
The Child Who Is Terminally Ill or Dying

NURSING DIAGNOSIS: Altered growth and development related to terminal illness and/or impending death

PATIENT GOAL 1: Will receive adequate support during terminal phase

• **NURSING INTERVENTIONS/*RATIONALES***

Encourage family to remain near child as much as possible *to provide support through their presence*
Encourage child to talk about feelings; help family as they encourage child to express feelings
Provide safe, acceptable outlets for aggression
Answer questions as honestly as possible while maintaining a positive, hopeful approach
Explain all procedures and therapies, especially physical effect child will experience
Help child distinguish between consequences of therapies and manifestations of disease process
Structure hospital environment to allow for maximum self-control and independence within the limitations imposed by child's developmental level and physical condition
Respect child's need for privacy without neglecting child
Provide for presence of customary support systems

• **EXPECTED OUTCOMES**

Child expresses feelings freely
Child demonstrates an understanding of symptoms

PATIENT GOAL 2: Will exhibit minimal or no evidence of physical discomfort

• **NURSING INTERVENTIONS/*RATIONALES***

Appreciate that pain control is essential component of physical and emotional care during terminal stage
Provide pain relief around the clock *to prevent the recurrence of pain*
Encourage family to provide comfort measures child prefers (e.g., rocking, stroking)
Avoid excessive noise or light *that may irritate child*
Place all commodities within easy reach *to increase child's control and lessen need for excessive movement*
Use gentle, minimal physical manipulation
Avoid pressure (bedclothes, sheets) on painful areas
Experiment with using heat or cold on painful areas *(use cautiously because of easy skin breakdown)*
Whenever possible, make use of procedures (e.g., noninvasive temperature monitoring) *to minimize discomfort*
Change position frequently; if difficult for child, coordinate with pain relief from analgesics *to make moving easier and less distressing*
Avoid pressure on bony prominences or painful sites (water bed, flotation mattress); ensure good body alignment *to prevent skin breakdown*
Keep fresh air circulating in room (open window, use small fan)
Use pillows or other supports to prop child in comfortable position
Carry child (if possible) to other areas for diversion if desired
Place absorbent pads under hips *because child may be incontinent*
Help child to toilet if desired
Limit care to essentials
May need to forego usual hygienic measures such as bath or clothing change but provide comfort measures (e.g., mouth care, wiping forehead, gentle back rub)
*Administer anticholinergic drugs (atropine or scopolamine) *to reduce secretions (lessens "death rattle," which can be distressing to family)*

• **EXPECTED OUTCOME**

Child exhibits minimal or no evidence of physical discomfort

PATIENT GOAL 3: Will receive adequate emotional support at time of dying

• **NURSING INTERVENTIONS/*RATIONALES***

Preserve child's physical closeness with family members (e.g., parent may want to rock child in chair or lie next to child in bed)
Teach family about supportive interventions
Talk to child even though child may not appear to be awake
Position self and others where child can easily see face (e.g., sit at head of bed)
Speak to child in clear, distinct voice; avoid whispering
Avoid conversation about child in child's presence *to reduce anxiety/fear*
Offer calm reassurance and orient child to surroundings when awake
Phrase questions for "yes" or "no" answers *to conserve energy*
Avoid repeated measurements of vital signs, *which only disturb child*
Play favorite music *(may soothe child)*

• **EXPECTED OUTCOME**

Child appears calm and relaxed

NURSING DIAGNOSIS: Altered nutrition: less than body requirements related to loss of appetite, disinterest in food

PATIENT GOAL 1: Will receive optimum nutrition

• **NURSING INTERVENTIONS/*RATIONALES***

Offer any food and fluids child desires
Provide small meals and snacks several times a day
Avoid excessive encouragement to eat or drink
Avoid foods with strong odors *because they may cause nausea*
Provide pleasant environment for eating
Serve foods that require the least energy to eat (soups, shakes)
Feed slowly *to conserve energy*
*Administer antiemetic as prescribed if nausea/vomiting is a problem
Provide mouth care before and after eating; lubricate lips with petrolatum *to prevent cracking and promote comfort*

• **EXPECTED OUTCOME**

Child consumes some nutrients

---

*Dependent nursing action.

Continued.

NURSING CARE PLAN
The Child Who Is Terminally Ill or Dying—cont'd

NURSING DIAGNOSIS: Fear/anxiety related to diagnosis, tests, and therapies and prognosis

PATIENT GOAL 1: Will experience reduction of anxiety

- **NURSING INTERVENTIONS/*RATIONALES***

Limit interventions to palliation only; discuss need for nonpalliative treatment with family and physician
Explain all procedures and other aspects of care to child *to reduce anxiety and fear*
Remain with child or provide for constant attendance
Determine what child has been told about prognosis *so this information can be reinforced*
Determine what family wishes child to know about prognosis
Emphasize importance of honesty
Answer child's questions as openly and honestly as possible
Involve parents in child's care
Remain nonjudgmental regarding child's behavior

- **EXPECTED OUTCOME**

Child discusses fears without evidence of stress

NURSING DIAGNOSIS: Anticipatory grieving related to potential loss of a child

PATIENT (FAMILY) GOAL 1: Will receive adequate support

- **NURSING INTERVENTIONS/*RATIONALES***

Discuss the grieving process with family *so that family better understands normalcy of feelings*
Provide opportunities for family to express emotions
Help parents deal with their feelings, *allowing them more emotional reserve to meet the needs of their children*
Encourage parents to remain as near to child as possible, yet be sensitive to parents' needs
Provide information regarding child's status and anticipated reactions *to decrease anxiety/fear*
Help parents to understand behavioral reactions of their children, especially that concern for present crisis, such as loss of hair, may be much greater than for future ones, including possible death
Facilitate family's assistance with child's care
Provide comfort measures for child and family
Encourage family to maintain own health care needs
Provide as much privacy as possible
Assist family in assessing their need for referral services (e.g., hospice services, specific organizations for grieving families)
Encourage parents to honestly answer questions about dying rather than avoiding questions or using euphemisms
Encourage parents to share their moments of sorrow with their children
Discuss with parents appropriate involvement of siblings
Identify religious and cultural beliefs related to death (e.g., prayer, rites, rituals)
Provide preparation for postdeath services
Discuss with family their preferences for care if death is imminent
Arrange for appropriate spiritual care in accordance with family's beliefs and/or affiliations
Maintain contact with family
Provide support for families who choose home care for their child
See Guidelines box on p. 984.

- **EXPECTED OUTCOMES**

Family expresses fear, concerns, and any special desires for terminal child
Family demonstrates an understanding of child and his or her needs (specify)
Family members avail themselves of services as desired
See also:
Nursing Care Plan: The Child in the Hospital, Chapter 26
Nursing Care Plan: The Family of the Ill or Hospitalized Child, Chapter 26

PATIENT GOAL 2: Will exhibit no evidence of loneliness

- **NURSING INTERVENTIONS/*RATIONALES***

Offer calm reassurance to child
Reassure child of the love of others
Continue to set some limits for child *to provide a sense of security*
Spend time with child when not directly involved in care
Reinforce to child that what is happening is not child's fault *to decrease feelings of guilt*
Involve child in routine activities as tolerated
Maintain a "normal" atmosphere
Talk to child even though child may not appear to be awake
Situate self and others where easily visible to child
Speak to child in clear, distinct voice; avoid whispering
Avoid conversation about child's condition in presence of child *to decrease anxiety/fear*
Play favorite music and read stories to child
Orient child to surroundings when child is awake
Phrase questions for "yes" or "no" answers when possible *to conserve child's energy*

- **EXPECTED OUTCOME**

Child exhibits no evidence of loneliness

NURSING CARE PLAN
The Child Who Is Terminally Ill or Dying—cont'd

NURSING DIAGNOSIS: Anticipatory grieving related to imminent death of a child

PATIENT (FAMILY) GOAL 1: Will receive adequate support

- **NURSING INTERVENTIONS/*RATIONALES***

Be available to family
Inform family of what to expect at time of death
Convey an attitude of caring for both child and family
Encourage at least one family member to stay with child
Help family to provide care of child as they desire without forcing involvement
*Administer medications or other agents as prescribed *to reduce unpleasant manifestations*
Oxygen *for respiratory distress*
Anticonvulsants *for seizures*
Anticholinergic drugs *to reduce secretions ("death rattle")*
Analgesics *for pain*
Stool softeners/laxatives *for constipation*
Antiemetics *for nausea/vomiting*
Help and encourage family to express feelings appropriately
Encourage family to meet their own physical needs
Provide privacy
Provide for physical comfort of family
Provide emotional support and comfort to family
Encourage family to talk to child
Involve family and other children in decision making whenever possible, especially regarding alternatives for terminal care (hospital, home, hospice)
Support and assist family in giving explanations to other family members regarding child's status
Maintain nonjudgmental attitude toward behavior of family members

- **EXPECTED OUTCOMES**

Family members discuss their feelings
Family members are actively involved in child's care

PATIENT (FAMILY) GOAL 2: Will receive adequate support for home care

- **NURSING INTERVENTIONS/*RATIONALES***

Teach family physical care of child
Provide family with means for contacting health professionals at any time, (e.g., phone numbers)
Maintain daily contact with family (e.g., telephone call, home visit)
Refer to community agencies as appropriate *for ongoing support*
Reassure family that they can readmit child to the hospital at any time
Help plan with family what to do when the child dies and what to expect

- **EXPECTED OUTCOMES**

Family demonstrates ability to provide care for child
Family is in contact with appropriate support groups

*Dependent nursing action.

UNEXPECTED CHILDHOOD DEATH

Despite the fact that injuries are the leading cause of death among children, remarkably little research has been conducted of parental responses to sudden death. Similarly, little research has compared grief responses in survivors when the child's death was expected with those when the child's death was unexpected. One comparison of emotional and physical symptoms of parents whose child died after a chronic illness vs those whose child died after an accident found no difference between the two groups (Miles, 1985). However, parents of children who died suddenly did experience more guilt, a prolonged period of numbness and shock, intense loneliness and emptiness, anxious fear that someone else would die, and intense anger at those responsible for the injury (Miles and Perry, 1985). Another study found somewhat higher levels of depression among mothers experiencing the sudden loss of a child, as compared with mothers experiencing an anticipated loss (Leahy, 1991). Preliminary findings from a study done with Filipino children suggest that siblings of children who died suddenly may remain in the early stages of grief longer and may experience greater loneliness than siblings of children who died after an extended illness (Atuel, Williams, and Camar, 1988).

In long-term, potentially fatal illnesses, families may experience anticipatory grief. The parents mourn the loss of their child long before the death. Each time they see the pain the child must endure or experience the sudden loss of hope during a relapse, they are reminded of their child's uncertain future. This prolonged period of chronic anticipatory grief provides families with the precious opportunity to complete all "unfinished business," such as helping the child and siblings understand and cope with a fatal prognosis. Many families reflect on their changed perspective of time after learning of the diagnosis, particularly their heightened awareness of the value and worth of each day.

In sudden, unexpected death, however, the family is deprived of any of the advantages of anticipatory grief. There is no opportunity to prepare oneself or others for the death, and initial denial may be very strong. Because of this lack of time to prepare, many families feel great guilt and remorse for not having done something additional or different with the child. For example, they may berate themselves for depriving the child of some desired material object or privilege or, more painfully, for not having prevented the

STRATEGIES FOR INTERVENTION WITH SURVIVORS OF SUDDEN CHILDHOOD DEATH

ARRIVAL OF THE FAMILY

Meet the family immediately and escort to a private area.
A health care worker with bereavement training should remain with the family.
Provide information about the extent of illness or injury and treatment efforts.
If the health care worker must leave the family or the family requests privacy, return in 15 minutes so the family does not feel forgotten.
Provide tissues, telephone, coffee, and a Bible.

PRONOUNCEMENT OF DEATH

When available, the family's own physician should inform them of the child's death.
Alternatively, the physician or nurse should introduce themselves and establish calm, reassuring eye contact with the parents.
Honest clear communication that avoids misinterpretation is essential.
Nonverbal communication such as hugging, touching or remaining with the family in silence may be most emphathetic.
Acknowledge the family's guilt, attempt to alleviate it, and deal openly and nonjudgmentally with anger.
Provide information, answer questions, and offer reassurance that everything possible was done for the child.

VIEWING THE BODY

Offer the parents the opportunity to see the body; repeat the offer later if they decline.
Before viewing, inform the parents of bodily changes they should expect (tubes, injuries, cold skin).
A single staff member should accompany the family but remain inconspicuous.
Offer the opportunity to hold the child.
Allow the family as much time as they need.
Offer parents the opportunity for siblings to view the body.

FORMAL CONCLUDING PROCESS

Discuss and answer questions concerning autopsy and funeral arrangements; obtain signatures on the body release and autopsy forms.
Provide anticipatory guidance regarding symptoms of grief response and their normalcy.
Provide written materials about grief symptoms.
Escort the family to the exit or to their car if necessary.
Provide a follow-up phone call in 24 to 48 hours to answer questions and provide support.
Provide referrals to local support and resource groups (bereavement groups, bereavement counselors, SIDS groups, Parents of Murdered Children, and Mothers against Drunk Driving are examples).

Modified from Back K: Sudden, unexpected pediatric death: caring for the parents, *Pediatr Nurs* 17(6):571-574, 1991.

sudden death in some way. "If only I'd been a better parent" is a common feeling at this time.

Nursing intervention for families who experience the sudden death of a child must be sensitive to the special needs and concerns of these families. The box above outlines four major areas for intervention with survivors of sudden death. Arriving at the hospital and awaiting news of the child's condition is a vulnerable time. The communication of the child's death must be done with great sensitivity, and the physician or nurse should be prepared to handle feelings of denial, guilt, and anger without judgment. Offering an opportunity to view the body, even if it is disfigured, can be important, since a parent's imagined view of the child is often worse than the reality. Informing the family of what to expect when they view the child can lessen the shock. The need for autopsy and the fact that it will not influence an open viewing at a funeral should be explained. Finally, formal closure and follow-up with the family are important.

Families who experience a child's sudden death may experience recurrent memories of both the child and the death experience and may long grieve over missed opportunities (Kachoyeanos and Selder, 1993). Support and resource groups that may be useful to families include the **Sudden Infant Death Syndrome Alliance,* National Sudden Infant Death Syndrome Resource Center,† American Sudden Infant Death Syndrome Institute,* Mothers Against Drunk Driving,†** and **National Organization of Parents of Murdered Children, Inc.‡**

*10500 Little Patuxent Parkway, Suite 420, Columbia, MD 21044; (800) 221-7437 or (410) 964-8000.

†8201 Greensboro Dr., Suite 600, McLean, VA 22102; (703) 821-8955.

CHILDREN AND DEATH

CHILDREN'S UNDERSTANDING OF AND REACTIONS TO DYING AND DEATH

The concept of death is acquired through the sequential development of cognitive abilities and follows closely Piaget's stages. Although throughout childhood death is greatly influenced by the child's personal experiences with it and the explanations and attitudes offered by others, the abstract adult meaning of death as irreversible, inevitable, and universal is not understood by most children until preadolescence. Unless nurses understand how children perceive death, the fears associated with death in each age-group, and the personal meanings of death and bereavement during various stages of development, they cannot effectively counsel parents and children through the multiple crises associated with expected or unexpected death.

Knowledge about preschool and other children's concept of death is primarily based on the work of Maria Nagy (1948), who asked several hundred Hungarian children ranging in age from 3 to 10 years to draw pictures and write

*6065 Roswell Rd., Suite 876, Atlanta, GA 30328; (800) 232-SIDS (in Georgia: [800] 847-SIDS).

†P.O. Box 541688, Dallas, TX 75354-1688; (800) 438-6233.

‡100 E. 8th St., Rm. B41, Cincinnati, OH 45202; (513) 721-5683.

TABLE 23-1 Children's Concept of Death

COGNITIVE STAGE	CONCEPT
Sensorimotor (infancy, toddler)	No concept of death but reacts to loss
Preoperational thought (early childhood)	Death is temporary and reversible Death is seen as a departure or separation
Concrete operations (school age)	Death is irreversible but not necessarily inevitable Death may be personified and viewed as destructive Explanations for death are naturalistic and physiologic
Formal operations (later school age, adolescence)	Death is irreversible, universal, and inevitable Death is still seen as a personal but distant event Explanations for death are physiologic and theologic

down (if they were old enough) everything they could think of about death. From analyzing their responses, she concluded that there were three main stages of death interpretation. Although more recent studies have corroborated most of her findings, they have not found evidence of the personification seen in school-age children, but instead support for a concrete connotation of death, with naturalistic explanations about why people die, such as from old age or a gunshot wound (Table 23-1) (Wass, 1985). These findings may reflect differences in the religious and cultural orientation of the children studied by Nagy and those studied by current investigators.

The following discussion addresses reactions of children to their own impending death, as well as children's reactions to the death of others. Both areas contribute to understanding the perception of death among children. Furthermore, nurses may be called on to assist children and families in both types of situations.

Infants and Toddlers

Exactly how preverbal children view death is a mystery, because there is no way of reliably assessing their views of death. It is quite likely, on the basis of their cognitive abilities, that they have no concept of death. Toddler's egocentricity and vague separation of fact and fantasy make it impossible for them to comprehend absence of life. Although they may repeat what initially sounds like a correct definition of death, such as, "Grandpa is dead; he went to heaven," they may later refer to Grandpa as if he still exists. They can only perceive events in terms of their own frame of reference—living.

Reactions to Dying. Immobilization, regression to less independent levels of behavior, separation, intrusive or painful procedures, and alteration in ritualistic routine represent the greatest threats to seriously ill children in this age-group. However, they may perceive the seriousness of their condition from the parents' reactions of anxiety, sadness, depression, or anger. Although the children are unaware of the reason for such emotions, they are disturbed and upset by their parents' behavior. Helping parents deal with their feelings allows them more emotional reserve to meet the needs of their children. Encouraging them to stay in the hospital as much as possible and to participate in the child's care promotes the parents' and child's adjustment to a serious, potentially fatal illness or accident.

Reactions to Death. To the amazement and dismay of adults, toddlers may persist in wanting to visit the dead person, request that all that person's possessions and living quarters remain unchanged, and talk about the deceased as if nothing has happened. Dealing honestly and openly with such reactions is preferable to admonishing the child or trying to demonstrate what dead means. For example, the parent can restate that the person cannot visit because he or she is dead and in a special place (cemetery, heaven, or other explanation) and can offer to bring the child to visit the burial plot if possible.

Ritualism is extremely important to toddlers, so any change in the home following the death can produce anxiety. There is no harm in allowing the ritualism, such as setting an extra place at the table for the deceased person, because, for the child, imagining the person to be present is almost as real as life. What is important is to stress that, although the place is set at the table, the dead person will return only in thoughts and memories. As children grow older, form new attachments, and develop stronger ego defenses, they will be increasingly able and willing to let go of this fantasy person.

Preschool Children

Several characteristics of preschoolers' cognitive and psychologic development affect their conception of death. Because of their sense of precausality, they are unable to differentiate physical cause from logical or psychologic motivation. In addition, their egocentricity implies a tremendous sense of self-power and omnipotence. Therefore they believe that their thought is sufficient to cause events. The consequence of such magical thinking is the burden of guilt, shame, and punishment.

Concept of Death. Children between ages 3 and 5 have usually heard the word "death" and have some connotation of its meaning. They see death as a departure, possibly as a kind of sleep. They may recognize the fact of physical death but do not separate it from living abilities. The dead person in the coffin still breathes, eats, and sleeps. Death is temporary and gradual; life and death can change places with one another. Because of their immature concept of time, there is no real understanding of the universality and inevitability of death. Words such as "forever" and "everyone" have meaning only in the child's egocentric thinking. Waiting until Christmas may be "forever," and anybody the child denotes is "everyone."

Reactions to Dying. If preschoolers become seriously ill during this time, they may conceive of the illness as a punishment for their thoughts or actions. The usual diagnostic and treatment procedures, combined with enforced hospitalization, can confirm their belief that they are being punished. If the parents do not stay with them during hospitalization or prevent the traumatic procedures, they may be convinced that the parents are retaliating for the child's previous misdeeds or bad thoughts.

The same principles of magical thinking and omnipotence affect preschoolers when a sibling becomes critically ill or dies. One of the most significant types of death is sudden infant death syndrome (SIDS). Because it occurs unexpectedly to a healthy infant, who may have been rejected and unwanted by a jealous sibling, preschoolers find no evidence to support a physical cause of death. Indeed, the parents are frequently unaware of the reason for the fatality and may question any possible cause. If preschoolers are in any way accused or suspected of having harmed the infant, they may feel extremely guilty and responsible for the tragedy. On observing their parents' acute grief, they may interpret the anger or depression as a rejection of them.

When a child becomes ill, the well siblings experience the loss of routine and parental attention. It is natural for them to resent such disruptions and to blame the changes on the ill child. However, preschoolers have less ability than older children to understand the reasons for the parents' prolonged absence from the home. Even though parents may explain how ill the sibling is, what the hospital is like, and why they must be there, preschoolers only see the special attention and the material rewards that the ill sister or brother receives. Because they are also unable to differentiate causes for separation of the parents and ill child, they may fear that the parents may never return. If they should learn that the ill child may not get well or come home, they can interpret this to mean that the parents will also never return. Their greatest fear concerning death is separation from parents.

Reactions to Death. In relation to death, preschoolers may engage in activities that seem strange or abnormal to adults. For example, if a pet dies, preschoolers usually request a "funeral" or some ceremony to symbolize their loss. Perceptive parents realize that the function of such rites of passage is as important to the preschooler for the loss of a pet as to an adult for the loss of a significant person. After the "funeral" and "burial," preschoolers may dig up the remains. Many parents are confused by this behavior. However, children have no concept of the irreversible nature of death and must continually reassure themselves that the animal has not returned or gone somewhere else. If left alone to satisfy their curiosity, they will see that the dead animal is still in the ground.

Because young children accept the literal meaning of words, it is important for others to examine the implications of possible explanations for death. Those with a religious affiliation may equate death with an afterlife and explain that dead animals or people go to heaven. The act of digging up the dead pet may be a result of trying to ascertain whether the animal did go to heaven. Parents who are aware of the reason for this behavior can explain that the "soul" goes to heaven but the body remains in the earth. If parents dismiss this activity without some clarification, the child may interpret the religious message as a lie.

Another common euphemism for death is "gone to sleep." Again preschoolers attach the literal meaning of sleep to death and may fear going to sleep for fear of dying or never waking up. One 5-year-old child who had been told that her aunt died because she was very tired refused to engage in any strenuous activity and took naps frequently. Her parents became concerned about her sudden lassitude and finally asked her why she was always tired. The child exclaimed that she was *not* tired; she took naps to avoid fatigue because she did not want to die like her aunt. When the parents explained that her aunt was tired from old age and sickness, not from playing too much or sleeping too little, the child immediately resumed her usual behaviors.

Because of their limited defense mechanisms for dealing with loss, young children may react to a less significant loss with more outward grief than to the loss of a very significant person. This can be extremely disconcerting to parents who view their child's undisturbed behavior as evidence of lack of interest in or response to the tragedy. However, the reverse is most likely true. The loss is so deep, painful, and threatening that the child must deny it for the time being to survive its overwhelming impact. Behavioral reactions such as giggling, joking, attracting attention, or regressing to earlier developmental skills are signs indicating children's need to distance themselves from the tremendous loss. Understanding the function of such behaviors and supporting children through the reactions until such time as they feel enough self-control to grieve will help them gradually resolve the loss. Parents should expect grieving a significant loss to be a quite lengthy process in a young child.

School-Age Children

Although school-age children have a better understanding of causality, less egocentricity, and advanced perception of time, they still associate misdeeds or bad thoughts with causing death and feel intense guilt and responsibility for the event. However, because of their higher cognitive abilities, they respond well to logical explanations and comprehend the figurative meaning of words more than children in younger age-groups. Although they are less likely to interpret explanations in a purely literal sense, they are still prone to self-referenced definitions. For this reason, it is important for adults to clarify the meanings of statements and to repeatedly ask them what they think.

Concept of Death. Much of what pertains to the preschool period regarding the understanding of death also relates to school-age children, particularly those near 6 or 7 years of age. However, these children have a deeper understanding of death in the concrete sense. According to Nagy (1948), children of this age attempt to ascribe a more comprehensible meaning to the event by personifying death as a devil, God, ghost, or "bogeyman." Naturalistic-physiologic explanations of why death occurs and what happens to the dead body may be a preoccupation in this age-group. Factual explanations, such as "When you die, your body decays in the ground," are consistent with their concrete thinking.

By age 9 or 10 years most children have an adult concept of death. They realize that it is inevitable, universal, and irreversible. Their attitudes toward death are greatly influenced by the reactions and attitudes of others, particularly their parents.

Reactions to Dying. The increased ability of school-age children to comprehend and reason poses additional risks for them. They may fear the reason for the illness, communicability of the disease to themselves or others, consequences of the disease on their functioning and relationships with others, and the process of dying and death itself. They tend to fear the expectation of the event more than its realization. Their fear of the unknown is greater than that of the known; like preschoolers, their fantasy explanations for the unexpected or unknown are usually much more frightening and extreme than the actual situation. For this reason anticipatory preparation is very necessary and effective. These children respond well to explanations of the disease, names of drugs, and so on. Inasmuch as the developmental task of this age is industry, helping children who may be facing their own death to maintain control over their bodies by understanding what is happening to them and participating in what is done to them allows these youngsters to achieve independence, self-worth, and self-esteem and to avoid a sense of inferiority.

Because dying is loss of control over every aspect of living, the realization of impending death or failure to recover is a tremendous threat to their sense of security and ego strength. These children are likely to exhibit their fear more through verbal uncooperativeness than actual physical aggression. Health professionals may erroneously interpret this behavior as rude, impolite, insolent, or stubborn. In reality the words are conveying the same meaning as physical attempts to run away or to fight others off. This verbal "flight or fight" reaction to stress is a plea for some control and power. Encouraging children to talk about their feelings, allowing control where possible and appropriate, and providing outlets for aggression through play are means of dealing with this type of uncooperativeness.

Reactions to Death. School-age children are very interested in postdeath services, such as wakes, funerals, and burials. They may be inquisitive about what happens to the body—who dresses it, how the body feels, or what happens in an autopsy. Adults sometimes find these questions distressing, particularly when they concern the death of a significant person. However, such inquiries are a child's way of assimilating all the facts about death into a concrete, logical framework. Avoiding such questions or fabricating euphemistic stories only confuses and frustrates children's attempts at understanding what may happen *to them* if they should die.

Adolescents

By the time most children reach adolescence, they have a mature understanding of death, and as abstract thinking develops, there is more questioning of death and related topics, such as the religious meaning of afterlife. However, their other developmental needs, especially identity, make this an exceptionally difficult time for these young people to cope with the loss of a loved one or their own impending death.

Concept of Death. Although adolescents have a mature understanding of death, they are still very much influenced by "remnants" of magical thinking and are subject to the feelings of guilt and shame. Adolescents are exploring many new areas of interpersonal relationships and are likely to see deviations from accepted behavior as reasons for their illness. It is important to clarify that thoughts and activities, especially sexual experimentation, do not cause diseases such as cancer.

Reactions to Dying. Adolescents have the most difficulty in coping with death. Although they have reached the level of adult comprehension of the concept of death, they are least likely to accept cessation of life, particularly if it is their own. Developmentally, the rejection of death is understandable because the adolescents' tasks are to establish an identity by finding out who they are, what their purpose is, and where they belong. Any suggestion of being different or of nonbeing is a tremendous threat to the answers to such questions. Adolescents' concern is for the present much more than the past or future. Most recent research suggests that while adolescents with cancer are at an increased risk for psychological problems, most are generally well-adjusted and are meeting developmental tasks (Ritchie, 1992).

Adolescents strive for group acceptance and independence from parental constraints. As a result, they rely on peer rules and beliefs for personal direction and reject opposing parental demands. However, when they are faced with the crisis of serious illness, they may consider themselves alienated from peer associations and unable to communicate with their parents for emotional support. Therefore they may be virtually alone in their struggle for survival. Support groups or other means of networking adolescents facing death may be useful.

Healthy adolescents must deal with several maturational crises, such as acceptance of bodily changes and socialization of intensifying sexual impulses. Any threat to either task increases the vulnerability of adolescents to the stress of coping with such crises. The ravages of a terminal illness and the deleterious effects of chemotherapy may be greater concerns than the prospect of dying. Adolescents' orientation to the present compels them to worry about physical changes even more than the prognosis for future recovery. Parents and nurses benefit from understanding that denial and rationalization are the coping mechanisms most often used by adolescents with cancer (Ritchie, 1992).

Sometimes parents fail to understand the emotional impact on the adolescent of side effects from chemotherapy, such as hair loss, weight gain, fatigue, or skin eruptions. They wonder why the adolescent cannot accept the temporary altered body image for the possible benefit of the treatment. Intellectually adolescents can understand the necessity of treatment, but emotionally they have great difficulty in overcoming the feelings of being different, unable to equal others, and physically compromised because of the illness.

Nurses are in a most advantageous position in working with terminally ill adolescents; in the hospital setting they spend the greatest amount of time with them. They can structure the hospital admission to allow for maximum self-control and independence while allowing the adolescent the opportunity to learn to know the nurse. Answering adolescents' questions honestly, treating them as mature individuals, and respecting their needs for privacy, solitude, and personal expressions of emotions such as anger, sadness, or fear convey to adolescents the adult's true concern for their physical and emotional welfare. Nurses can help parents to communicate with their adolescent children by providing information on typical adolescent responses and coping patterns, acting as role models, avoiding alliances with either parent or child, and allowing parents the opportunity to ventilate their feelings of frustration, incompetence, or failure in an atmosphere of acceptance and nonjudgment.

Reactions to Death. The adolescent's reactions to death straddle the transition from childhood to adulthood. Although some teenagers are able to cope with death by expressing appropriate emotions, talking about the loss, and resolving the grief, others may appear undisturbed by the event, extremely angry, or unusually silent and withdrawn.

Because of their idealistic view of the world, they may criticize funeral rites as barbaric, money making, and unnecessary. Their fear of the unknown and inability to deal with these thoughts may prevent them from attending funeral services for others. They are sometimes horrified and angry over adults' concerns for practical matters such as immediate financial arrangements. Statements such as, "Daddy isn't even buried yet and you [mother] are worrying about his money," can cause great conflict and misunderstanding between child and parent. Helping adults understand why teenagers have such thoughts can avert an unnecessary and painful strain among family members.

Nursing Considerations

Nurses in almost any area of pediatrics have an opportunity to help families guide their children in developing positive attitudes toward death. First, they can counsel parents regarding children's age-specific understanding of death and appropriate ways to handle behaviors, such as digging up the dead pet.

Second, nurses can encourage parents to take advantage of "small deaths" to help children become familiar and more comfortable with loss. Observation and discussion of the seasons in nature, or the experience of the death of a pet, flowers, or a television character may present such an opportunity (Fig. 23-3). Certainly, such events should not be covered up, such as replacing a pet with a new one so the child thinks it is the same animal. Many children's books are available that present death in a sensitive and nonthreatening manner and, when read to children, offer opportunities for dialogue. (see also Communication Techniques, Chapter 6; sources of books are listed at the end of the chapter).

Third, nurses may take part in organized programs on death education, especially in the schools, or serve as resources for planning such programs (Wass and others, 1980). Through a formal curriculum devoted to this topic, youngsters are introduced to the many facets of death as a part of life. Such programs can also ease the reentry of children with life-threatening disorders back to school. When persons die who are known to children, such as classmates or teachers, special bereavement sessions can be instituted to help the students understand and deal with the loss.

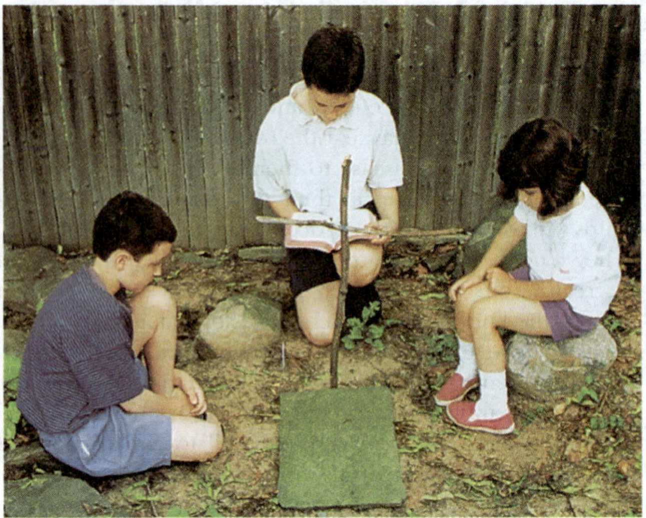

FIG. 23-3 Children learn about death and related rituals such as burial, through losses, such as death of a pet.

Finally, nurses can serve as resources to parents and others involved with children in answering questions about children and death. For example, many parents are concerned with how to handle "small deaths" constructively or whether young or school-age children should attend funeral or burial services of loved ones (see p. 999). Routine inquiry into such topics should be part of well-child care because it can promote healthy attitudes and prepare children to cope with loss when it occurs.

AWARENESS OF DYING IN CHILDREN WITH LIFE-THREATENING ILLNESS

One of the initial reactions of parents (and some health professionals) to the discovery of a life-threatening illness is to protect the child from the impact of the diagnosis. However, it is now widely understood that terminally ill children develop awareness of the seriousness of their diagnosis, even when protected from the truth. Anxiety may not always be attributable to fear of death but may be demonstrated in relationship to separation, pain, intrusive procedures, bodily change or mutilation, loneliness, immobilization, and punishment. Children as young as 2 or 3 years of age also perceive their parents' emotions and react accordingly.

Studies of children' experiences with life-threatening illness demonstrate that children learn about their situation through the acquisition of information, at which time they develop different conceptions of themselves. Five stages have been defined (Bluebond-Langner, 1978, 1989):

Stage I: Disease is a serious illness. New identity of "sick" child.

Stage II: Discovery of the relationship of medication and recovery. Learns the taboos of disease and death.

Stage III: Marked understanding of the purposes and implications of special procedures. Sense of well-being begins to fade and perceives self as different from other children.

Stage IV: Illness is viewed as a permanent condition. Sense of always being sick and never getting better.

Stage V: Realization that there is only a finite number of medications. Awareness (directly or indirectly) of the fatal prognosis.

Experience is considered the critical factor in the passage through these various stages. The experience of having a disease allows children to assimilate information by relating what they see and hear to what they feel and think. Experience also explains why age and intellectual ability are not related to the speed or completeness with which children pass through the various stages of awareness. Some 3- and 4-year-olds of average intelligence know more about their prognosis than very intelligent 9-year-olds who are still in their first remission, have had fewer clinical experiences, and are aware only that they have a serious illness (Greenham and Lohmann, 1982).

The time lapse between stages tends to be the same for all children regardless of age. Passage from the first stage to the second stage occurs rapidly on relapse. Passage through the second, third, and fourth stages takes somewhat longer, but passage to the fifth stage may take place as soon as the child learns of the death of another, and all knowledge from previous stages is quickly synthesized into a new self-awareness.

Informing Children of a Life-Threatening Diagnosis

Children need honest and accurate information about their illness, treatments, and prognosis. In most situations this best occurs as a gradual process over time, characterized by increasingly open dialogue between professionals, parents, and the child (Lipson, 1993). Providing an atmosphere of open communication early in the course of an illness facilitates answering difficult questions as the child's condition worsens (Lansky, List, and Ritter-Sterr, 1988). Providing appropriate literature about the disease, as well as the experience of illness and possible death, is also helpful.*

Exactly how and what to tell children about serious illness, dying, and death is a very individual matter. Families' wishes should generally be respected. However, parents may desire professional support and guidance in the process. Some principles and guidelines (see box above, right) can assist nurses and families in determining how to present facts and hope to a child in a way that fosters trust, enhances meaningful communication, and offers emotional support to the child.

THEMES THAT MAY ASSIST PARENTS IN DISCUSSING POSSIBLE DEATH WITH CHILDREN

The following themes may be useful to parents as they communicate with their children about their possible death. They should be used with cautious judgment, generally at the child's lead.

1. Death, like birth, is part of the natural order of things. It happens sooner for some, later for others.
2. Death has social significance. We have special feelings for the people we share our lives with.
3. Death is a separation. The child loses family and friends, and they lose the child.
4. The loss is never complete. The deceased lives on in some way. (The specific interpretation will be culturally or religiously based.)
5. The child will not be alone at death and after death. Parental presence and support are important to the child. (Cultural and religious beliefs will influence the interpretation of this point.)
6. Even a young child has touched others and influenced the world in some way. Children can be assured that they have contributed and have led full, happy lives.
7. The child should be reassured that all feelings are normal: sadness, tears, anger, and resentment are all OK.
8. The child should be reassured that it is all right not to want to discuss his or her illness. When the child wants to talk, adults will be ready to listen.
9. Silence is acceptable if the child prefers. So are confused or silly-sounding expressions of feelings.
10. While some of the experience leading to death may be painful, doctors will do what is necessary to minimize pain. Death itself will not hurt. After death the pain will never return.
11. When a loved one dies, people want a chance to say goodbye. Sometimes the person who is going to die will want to say goodbye to friends. Afterward, a funeral is a way many friends and relatives will say goodbye and gather to talk about how much they loved the child. People do not need to fear funerals.
12. Adults do not know much about death either and sometimes cry because they love the child and do not want to lose him or her. However, if a child has to die, parents, family, and friends will remember the happy times. The child's memory will live on in mind and spirit.

Modified from Deasy-Spinetta P, Spinetta J, Kung FH: *Emotional aspects of childhood leukemia: a handbook for parents,* New York (no date), Leukemia Society of America.

Developmental Age. A primary concern in any relationship with children is their age, because the level of comprehension is a function of children's cognitive development. As discussed earlier, children at various ages have different understandings and fears of death. The younger child fears separation, which can be imposed by any number of circumstances, only one of which is death or illness. The older child fears the results of illness, particularly pain or bodily injury, as well as death itself. Anyone working with children must be aware of such developmental variations and be sensitive to their verbal and nonverbal language.

*Excellent resources for children with cancer are *You and Leukemia: A Day at a Time* by L. Baker (1989, Saunders); *My Book for Kids with Cansur* by J. Gaes (1987, Melius & Peterson); and *What It Is I Have, Don't Want, Didn't Ask for, Can't Give Back, and How I Feel About It* (1983, Leukemia Society of America). More general resources for a child with serious or terminal illness include *Saying Goodbye* by J. Boulden and J. Boulden (1992, Boulden) and *When Someone Very Special Dies* and *When Someone Has a Very Serious Illness* by M. Heegard (1988, Woodland Press).

Sharing with parents any information and observations relevant to the child's experience is important. Communication techniques relevant to the child's developmental age should be used when communicating with the child (Chesterfield, 1992).

Previous Knowledge. Besides age, another essential principle is first to find out what the child is thinking and feeling. Before any explanations (true or false) are offered to children, they have invented their own. Answers to such questions as "What do you think is wrong with you?" or "What have you heard others say?" provide information on which to structure further explanations. Very often a child will respond with an answer of such detailed, accurate information that the only element lacking is the name of the disease. Other answers may reveal possible areas of misconception, which can then be clarified or refocused.

Sometimes health professionals, parents, and others hear the children's words but fail to comprehend their meaning. They erroneously assume that because children recite all the facts, they also understand their implications or have dealt with all their fears. This may not be so; intellectualizing about one's condition can be a powerful defense mechanism. For example, an adolescent who was undergoing serious open-heart surgery knew precisely every detail of the operation, preoperative and postoperative care, and involved risks. The medical and nursing staff considered her exceptionally well prepared. However, everyone had failed to ask her about how she felt. When the nurse asked her this before her surgery, the child answered, "I fear that I may die." Once this was verbalized, the child, her parents, and the nurse focused on her fears instead of on the facts of the illness.

Honesty. The last principle in explaining events such as death to children is honesty. Although the truth is usually the most difficult answer to give, in the long run it lessens many of the conflicts or problems that arise from lies, half-truths, or conspiracies. The truth provides answers for future questions. It also fosters trust. Children adeptly perceive the maxim: Do as I say, not as I do. It is very difficult to encourage children to be honest, to confide in others, and to openly discuss their fears if parents refuse to do the same.

Honesty is certainly not the easiest solution; the truth may prompt children to ask other distressing questions. The question many parents and health professionals dread the most is "Am I going to die?" When children have the answer to this question, the next question is "When?" Children need answers that are straightforward, yet caring. In telling children that a cure is no longer possible, one must also leave room for hope. The hope is redirected from care to comfort (Lansky, List, and Ritter-Sterr, 1988).

If given the opportunity, children will tell others how much they want to know. Asking questions such as, "If the disease came back, would you want to know?" "Do you want others to tell you everything, even if the news isn't good?" or "If someone were not getting better [or more directly, "were dying"], do you think they would want to know?" helps children set the limits of how much truth they can accept and cope with. Children need time to process many feelings and much information so that they can assimilate and hopefully accept the inevitable fact of mortality.

SIBLINGS' RESPONSES TO LIFE-THREATENING ILLNESS AND DEATH

The experience of a child with life-threatening illness and/or the child's death has profound effects on the family, including the siblings. Many of the siblings' responses to a prolonged life-threatening illness reflect those discussed in Chapter 22 regarding chronic illness or disability in a brother or sister. Predominant feelings of children when the sibling's diagnosis is potentially fatal, such as serious trauma or a disease such as cancer, include isolation and displacement—the parents devote the majority of their time to care for the ill or injured child, causing the siblings to feel left out of the parent/sick child partnership and regarded as unimportant family members.

Siblings may also express concern for their own health status, recognizing the possibility of death and at times manifesting physical symptoms similar to those of the child. Siblings' knowledge of the ill child's diagnosis is often inadequate, although many children perceive cancer to be the "scariest disease" (Martinson and others, 1990).

Sibling's responses to death arise in part from their cognitive understanding of death (see pp. 988-992). Two common feelings are guilt and shame. Guilt arises when children imagine their own responsibility for the illness or death. One 5-year-old child stated that her brother got sick when he caught her sore throat. Guilt may also be related to feeling both fortunate about not having the illness and jealous of the ill child's lavished attention. Shame at having a sibling in the family who is seriously ill, disfigured, or dying may be another source of guilt.

When a brother or sister dies, the sibling's reaction will depend on many factors, including the circumstances of the death, the quality of the prior sibling relationship, the age of the child, parental reactions, and family communication patterns (Bincer, 1989; Gibbons, 1992). Siblings grieve for the loss of the child, must deal with the stress of having grieving parents, and at times may feel like "the replaced child" or the "less special" child. For example, when a parent(s) memorializes the dead child, the surviving siblings are constantly reminded of this child's specialness and may feel that they can never "live up" to the memories or expectations (Davies, 1987).

Behavior problems such as acting out, poor school performance, and antisocial behavior may occur among children experiencing sibling death. Parents should inform the sibling's teachers of the death in the family. Despite these reactions, positive outcomes such as psychologic maturity and increased compassion can also result from the death of a sibling.

Siblings' adjustment may relate to the assistance and support they receive in their grieving process. Open communication within the family and the siblings' increased involvement with the ill child's care and death are likely to aid in positive adjustment. Nursing intervention should reflect these possibilities.

Nurses can suggest to parents that children need information about their sibling's illness and death, especially if the death was unexpected. Children need information about what is taking place both at the time of death and afterward (Dickinson, 1992). Parents should be encouraged to tell children directly that they did not cause the illness or death (except in rare instances of intentional killings) and that it is normal to feel guilty, jealous, or angry. Siblings' fears of becoming ill or dying should be addressed, and whenever possible the siblings should be involved in the child's care or other tasks helpful to the family, praised for their cooperation, and made to feel "special."

Siblings must grieve in their own ways and may occasionally need special attention from a parent. At times, siblings may need to talk about their memories of the child who died and express their longing, guilt, anger, and so forth. At other times, they will not dwell on the absent child, and parents should be assured that this is also quite normal (Bincer, 1989). Sometimes, however, siblings may protect their grieving parents by suppressing their own feelings or deciding not to discuss them (Faulkner, Peace, and O'Keefe, 1993). For this reason, sibling support groups can be beneficial (Opie and others, 1993; Raver, 1992).

GRIEF PROCESS IN EXPECTED AND UNEXPECTED DEATH

In response to any loss there is a grief reaction. ***Acute grief*** develops within hours to days and is characterized by somatic symptoms and intense subjective distress. ***Grief work,*** or ***mourning,*** refers to the lengthy process that begins with acute grief and extends into a period of reorganization of psychologic life, with attachment to new people and interests. ***Bereavement*** often refers to the period of mourning, although grief, mourning, and bereavement are used interchangeably.

Numerous investigators have contributed greatly to the present understanding of grief and bereavement, and those whose work is considered classic are presented in the following paragraphs. The "stages" of dying described by Kübler-Ross (1969) are not included here, because they were not based on work with children. The importance of the work of Kübler-Ross to the care of children and families lies in its emphasis on recognizing the dying person as being alive, and dying itself as a process in which the dying person is engaged. Care providers are most effective when actively engaging those coping with death and empowering them to address their remaining needs (Corr, 1993).

In expected death the child and family are generally involved in the plan for intervention both before and after the death. In unexpected death the survivors face the tremendous task of integrating the loss into their lives, with no opportunity for anticipatory grief. In either situation nurses can facilitate the grief process by being aware of expected psychologic and somatic reactions and by dialoguing with family members, ascertaining their needs, and supporting their efforts to cope, adapt, and grieve.

SYMPTOMATOLOGY OF NORMAL GRIEF

SENSATIONS OF SOMATIC DISTRESS

Feeling of tightness in the throat
Choking, with shortness of breath
Marked tendency to sighing
Empty feeling in the abdomen
Lack of muscular power
Intense subjective distress described as tension or mental pain

PREOCCUPATION WITH IMAGE OF THE DECEASED

Hears, sees, or imagines that the dead person is present
Slight sense of unreality
Feeling of emotional distance from others
May believe that he or she is approaching insanity

FEELINGS OF GUILT

Searches for evidence of failure in preventing the death
Accuses self of negligence or exaggerates minor omissions

FEELINGS OF HOSTILITY

Loss of warmth toward others
Tendency to irritability and anger
Wishes to not be bothered by friends or relatives

LOSS OF USUAL PATTERNS OF CONDUCT

Restlessness, inability to sit still, aimless moving about
Continual searching for something to do or what he or she thinks should be done
Lack of capacity to initiate and maintain organized patterns of activity

Modified from Lindemann E: Symptomatology and management of acute grief, *Am J Psychiatry* 101:141-143, 1944.

LINDEMANN: SYMPTOMATOLOGY OF GRIEF

Lindemann (1944) analyzed and described the reactions of adult survivors following the loss of significant others and found that acute grief has the following characteristics:

1. It is a definite syndrome with psychologic and somatic symptoms (see box above).
2. The syndrome may appear immediately after a crisis, be delayed, be exaggerated, or be apparently absent.
3. In place of the normal syndrome there may appear distorted reactions that represent one special aspect of the syndrome.
4. Through intervention, distorted reactions can be transformed into normal grief work with successful resolution.

The identification of "distorted" reactions is controversial. Lindemann described behaviors such as overactivity without a sense of loss, conspicuous change in social relationships, and acquiring symptoms of the deceased as maladaptive signs. More current research suggests that such behaviors may represent normal, but more variable, grief reactions. Psychosomatic symptoms such as compulsive-obsessive behavior and depression may be seen in parents years after the death of a child and do not reflect mental illness (Moore, Gilliss, and Martinson, 1988).

Anticipatory guidance may assist grieving family members. Health professionals should emphasize that grief reactions such as hearing the dead person's voice, feeling distant from others, or seeking reassurance that they did everything possible for the lost person are normal, necessary, and expected. They in no way signify poor coping, insanity, or an approaching mental breakdown. On the contrary, such behaviors signify that the survivor is working through the acute grief and are a necessary part of satisfactory resolution of the loss. These reactions do not mean it will be difficult to resume or restructure a meaningful role in the social environment.

PARKES: MOURNING

Whereas Lindemann's work focused on the symptoms of acute grief, several other researchers have attempted to analyze the behaviors and responses of the bereaved during the long and difficult process of mourning. Although there are numerous commonalities among the responses proposed by these authorities, the work of C. Murray Parkes with widows and widowers is considered classic (Glick, Weiss, and Parkes, 1974); according to Parkes' findings, the grief process consists of at least four phases (described below), which do not necessarily proceed in sequence but may occur simultaneously or disappear and recur at any time. Miles (1985a, 1985b) has described a similar model consisting of three stages of parental grieving. Contrary to the previous belief that mourning is completed in a year, data from clinical studies indicate that resolution of grief may take years. One study reported an *intensification* of grief during the third year (Rando, 1983). Another reported that the time since a child's death was not a factor in reducing the intensity of grief for families: some families manifest intense feelings of grief up to 20 years later (Neidig and Dalgas-Pelish, 1991).

Shock and Disbelief

Shock, numbness, and disbelief can be seen during the immediate phase of grief. As one parent described, "We were as prepared for our son's death as anyone could be, but it was a shock when in a moment his life was finished. I just can't get over the rapidity with which life ends." This temporary numbness protects the survivors from the overwhelming pain associated with grief. Often decisions are made automatically, and only certain details are remembered.

Expression of Grief

When the numbness fades, there begins a period of intense grief characterized by a yearning and loneliness for the deceased. During this stage many of the signs of acute grief are evident, and physical complaints such as inability to sleep and appetite changes are common. There is a tendency to review the events of the deceased's life and to evaluate the relationship with the loved one. At this time feelings of guilt and anger are common.

Disorganization and Despair

During this stage the pain of the loss is replaced primarily by emptiness, apathy, and deep depression. There is a feeling that life has no meaning and that the pain will never end. This is particularly relevant for parents. For example, mothers may feel a great emptiness from suffering a double loss—loss of their child and loss of the mothering role (Wong, 1980). Feelings of estrangement from other loved ones are common, and social isolation may foster the depression.

At times family members may need assistance in their grieving. Mothers, in particular, often feel a great sense of loneliness and emptiness, and part of their resolving the grief is finding a substitute role that is fulfilling and rewarding. Nurses can be instrumental in this process by (1) preparing the mother for anticipating the normal feelings of emptiness, loneliness, and sometimes even failure; (2) helping her reevaluate her role as parent and spouse, stressing that giving up the lost child must occur before she can reestablish emotional relationships; (3) encouraging her to explore fulfilling activities that use her special interests, talents, and qualifications; and (4) supporting her as her role changes, particularly assisting with communication between affected family members (Wong, 1980).

A child's death can challenge the marital relationship in several ways. Different grieving styles between the couple may hinder communication and support for each other. Differing needs and expectations can place a strain on the marriage (Schwab, 1992).

Nurses should also be aware of behaviors that indicate siblings' difficulty with resolving their grief, such as persistent blame and guilt, patterns of overactivity with aggressive and destructive outbursts, compulsive caregiving, persistent anxieties, excessive clinging to the parent, difficulty with forming new relationships, problems at school, or delinquency. In these situations professional assistance may be required, and the nurse can provide appropriate referral.

Reorganization

Reorganization refers to recovery from the loss. It is a very gradual process in which the survivors again find meaning in living, readjust to life without the deceased, develop new or renewed relationships, and learn to live with the memory of the deceased with much less pain. It never means that the loved one is forgotten and the pain is gone. There always remains a deep ache that is never totally replaced with happiness.

Resolution of grief may not always result in "letting go" of the loved one. Many survivors describe the pressure of an "empty space" in their lives years after the death of a child. Families attempt to fill the emptiness by keeping busy, often through altruistic involvements in self-help groups or by maintaining the connection with the lost child through recalling cherished memories. Feelings of emptiness intensity around holidays and anniversaries and with questions such as "How many children are in the family?" To exclude the dead child in the answer is to ignore his or her significance, but to include the child opens communication that makes many acquaintances uncomfortable.

BEREAVEMENT PROGRAMS

The ability of family members to work through their grief may be facilitated by a comprehensive bereavement program beginning at the time of the child's death and continuing for as long as is desired by the family (Johnson and others, 1993). The purpose of a bereavement program is to assist and support families in the process of coping with the devastating impact of the loss of a child and, hopefully, with grief resolution (Rose and Stewart, 1993). The components of such a program include initial contact and support by knowledgeable staff, information and reading materials relevant to the grief process, follow-up contacts by phone or mail, parent and sibling support groups, and referrals for counseling if indicated.* Parents should be given the option of participating in such a program, when available, but the desire not to participate should not be judged adversely by staff, since grief work is an individual process.

SPECIAL DECISIONS AT THE TIME OF DYING AND DEATH

Rarely are people prepared to cope with the numerous decisions that must be made when a loved one is dying or dies. When the death is expected, there is the opportunity to make plans in advance, such as where the child should spend the last days or what type of funeral arrangements are desired. When death is unexpected, the shock is sufficient to render the survivors incapable of making even simple decisions. Those in attendance at the death and those caring for the dying child can be instrumental in initiating decisions that may facilitate the grief process. The following is a brief review of selected instances when nurses can help parents make decisions related to the expected or unexpected death.

HOSPICE OR HOSPITAL CARE

When the child is dying of a terminal illness, parents should be given the choice of hospice† or hospital care for the terminal stage of illness. Hospital care refers to the traditional practices of caring for dying patients; hospice is a concept, not necessarily a facility. Hospice is holistic care for the patient and family that is intended to maximize the present quality of life whenever there is no reasonable expectation of cure. Hospice intends for the child to live life to the fullest without pain, with choices and dignity, and with family support (Armstrong-Dailey, 1990; Corr and Corr, 1992; Martinson, 1993; Sumner and Hurula, 1993). The three basic ways of providing hospice care are in a hospice, in a facility that employs the hospice concept, or in the child's home. If the home is chosen, the child may or may not die in the home. Reasons for final admission to a hospital vary but may be related to the parent's or sibling's wish to have the child die outside the home; exhaustion on the part of the caregivers; physical problems, such as sudden, acute pain or respiratory distress; and insufficient nursing services in the home (Martinson and others, 1986).

Hospice care is based on a number of important concepts that significantly set it apart from hospital care. First, the family are the principal caregivers, supported by a team of professional and volunteer staff. Second, the priority of care is comfort that considers the child's physical, psychologic, social, and spiritual needs. Pain and symptom control are primary concerns, and no extraordinary efforts are used to attempt a cure or prolong life. Third, the needs of the family are considered as important as those of the patient. Fourth, hospice is concerned with the family's post-death adjustment, and care may continue for a year or more.

With children, home care has been the more common environment for implementing the hospice concept and benefits the family in a variety of ways. Children who are dying are allowed the opportunity to remain with those they love and with whom they feel secure. Many children who were thought to be in imminent danger of death have gone home and lived longer than expected. Siblings feel more involved in the care and have more positive perceptions of the death. Parental adaptation has been more favorable, as shown by their perceptions of how the experience at home affected their marriage, social reorientation, religious beliefs, and views on the meaning of life and death. They also feel significantly less guilt after the child's death than families whose child died in the hospital (Lauer and others, 1983). There is also the economic advantage of home care, although private insurance may not cover the total cost of all outpatient and related services, and non–health care and indirect health care costs may be higher for families (Birenbaum and Clarke-Steffen, 1992).

Home care may engender stress for the family, particularly anxiety about what to expect at the time of death and how to provide the care. Questions frequently asked by parents are "How long will it be (before the child dies)?" and "How will he die?" Parents providing home care may experience more physical fatigue than if the child received hospital care. A potential stress is the lack of support from familiar hospital staff when a new agency provides home assistance.

Nurses working in hospice settings and with children dying at home are critical members of the health team. They often prepare the family for the home care experience, provide psychologic support for the family, and teach the physical care, especially comfort measures, such as pain control (see Chapter 26). They need to be available to the family and cognizant of times when the family may need relief from home care. If the child is at home, all families should have the option of admitting their child to the hospital if they feel they are unable to deal with the death. The child who dies at home must be pronounced dead, and hospice programs have provisions so this may proceed smoothly, or the police may be notified with an explanation of the circumstances to prevent unnecessary concern for abuse. Pro-

---

*A manual that can be useful in the development of a family-centered bereavement program is: *Whispers of Hope: A Hospital-Based Program for Bereaved Parents and Their Families* by T. Rose and E.S. Stewart (1993), available from Duke University Pediatric Brain Tumor Family Support Program, Durham, NC; (919) 684-5301.

†Information on hospice services for children is available from the National Hospice Organization, 1901 N. Moore St., Suite 901, Arlington, VA 22209; (800) 658-8898. A recommended resource is *Home Care: A Manual for Parents* by D. Moldow and I. Martinson, available from Children's Hospice International, 700 Princess St., Suite 3, Alexandria, VA 22314; (800) 24-CHILD.

viding the police with the number of the responsible practitioner is usually all that is necessary to confirm the cause of death. Some parents may wish to keep the body at home for the funeral service. Although state laws vary, usually the wake can be held at home, but if the body is not embalmed, it should not remain for any length of time (usually no longer than 24 to 48 hours). Unless the family can also dispose of the body or has special wishes (e.g., tissue donation or autopsy), arrangements need to be made for mortuary services.

RIGHT TO DIE

One of the benefits of hospice has been the recognition of patients' right to die as they wish, with emphasis on the *quality* of life. Unfortunately, this is not always the focus of care, especially in the traditional hospital setting. Many families are not given the option of terminating treatment when cure is unlikely, and staff may be reluctant to raise the question of "no code" or do not resuscitate (DNR) orders (withholding cardiopulmonary resuscitation in response to cardiac arrest). Some situations affecting quality of life, such as the dying child's right to refuse additional treatment, often pose difficult ethical questions (see Thinking Critically About. . . . box). The cessation of life-sustaining measures, such as artificial ventilation or tube feeding, in children who are in a persistent vegetative state remains a complex and controversial legal and ethical issue (McClung and Kamer, 1990).

As the group of health professionals who are most involved with families, nurses are in an excellent position to ensure that families are presented with the options available to them at the time of death. The nurse's first responsibility is to explore the family's wishes. This is best done in concert with the physician, but at times may need to be initiated by the nurse. Statements such as "Tell me about your thoughts for the kind of care you want your child to receive when he is dying" or "Have you considered the kinds of interventions you would like us to use when your child is near death?" can begin discussion of this sensitive but critical aspect of terminal care. Nurses can also assist the family in the decision-making process by minimizing environmental stressors, providing relevant essential information, discussing pain and suffering the child may experience, and encouraging the family to use formal and informal sources of support (relatives, pastors, professionals) as they face difficult decisions (Rushton and Glover 1990). If parents choose "DNR," they must be aware of exactly what will and will not be done for the child and assured that this does not mean "no care." For example, the family may wish that oxygen be given to the child for difficult breathing but not want active resuscitation. Once a decision is made, it must be communicated to all members of the health team and include a *written* medical order for the use or withholding of lifesaving measures. An order of "slow" or "delay" code is not legal (Saunders and Valente, 1986). Because the child's condition or the family's wishes may change, DNR orders are reviewed regularly.

VISUALIZATION OF THE BODY

Although most institutions recognize the need for parents to hold and spend time with the dead child, a dilemma may arise when the body is mutilated. Although the memory of the child's disfigurement can be extremely upsetting and generate concern for how much the child suffered, not seeing the body leaves the parents with imagined ideas of how their child looked, which can be worse than the reality and can delay the acceptance of the death (Miles and Perry, 1985). However, family members need preparation for this upsetting experience. They should be told what to expect and why certain parts of the body are covered or bandaged. It is desirable to place the body in a private room, without medical apparatus, and make it as presentable as the situation allows. Some people appreciate the presence of a nurse in the room with them; others desire privacy. Regardless of

THINKING CRITICALLY ABOUT . . .

The Dying Child's Right to Refuse Further Treatment

Traditionally, minor children (age of minority varies with state law) have not had the legal right to give informed consent for treatment or to refuse treatment. However, there is a growing concern for children in the end stage of fatal disease to have a voice in their care during the terminal phase. One of the major issues is the age at which children have the cognitive ability to understand the medical information, consider and comprehend the consequences of the decision—death, and choose freely among the options (Leikin, 1989). According to children's development of the death concept, a mature understanding of death does not occur until about 9 years of age. However, centers that have developed protocols for allowing informed choice by children document that youngsters as young as 6 years of age understand the implications of their disease as incurable and death as irreversible (Nitschke and others, 1982). These findings are consistent with those of Bluebond-Langner, who found that fatally ill children progress through a series of stages that shape their understanding of their disease and death (see pp. 992-993).

Other issues raised by opponents include the concern for dispelling hope in the child once death is pronounced imminent, parents' guilt if they later question the decision, and possible conflict between the child's and parents' wishes (Shumway, Grossman, and Sarles, 1983; Stanfill and Strong, 1985). Although there is insufficient research to answer these concerns, it seems unlikely that they will occur if the family is allowed to choose therapeutic alternatives in an atmosphere of professional support and with sufficient information. In addition, staff need to assess each child's capacity to understand the implications of refusing treatment, with documentation of the child's words and actions that support their conclusions (Foley, 1985).

how badly the body is harmed, parents may want to hold the child. Such options are offered and respected. Family members should be given as much time as they need to say good-bye; for many, viewing the body is a sign of closure to finish their good-byes and leave the hospital.

TISSUE DONATION/AUTOPSY

A topic that is rarely considered when a child dies is tissue donation. However, for some families this may be a meaningful act—one that benefits another human being despite the loss of their child. Unfortunately, initiating a discussion about tissue donation is often very stressful for staff, and there may be confusion regarding whose responsibility this is. In centers where transplants are performed, a full-time transplant coordinator is usually available to inform the family about organ donation and to take care of details. If such services are not available, the staff needs to discuss which members should discuss this topic with the family. Ideally, this should be the person who knows the family best, knows when the death is expected, or has the opportunity to spend time with the family when the death is unexpected. Often nurses are in an optimum position to suggest tissue donation after consultation with the attending physician. When possible; the topic should be raised before death occurs. The request should be made in a private and quiet area of the hospital and should be simple and direct, with questions such as "Are you a donor family?" or "Have you ever considered organ donation?" Most states have "required request" laws that mandate that the hospital make a request for tissue donation from the family of the deceased, especially if the patient is brain dead. A written consent from the family is required before donation can proceed (Giordano, 1989). When requests for organ donation are made, it should first be ascertained that families clearly understand the grave prognosis of their child. They should also be reassured that everything possible has been done or is being done to save or care for their child (Cerney, 1993). The option to donate organs should always be separate from the communication of impending or actual death (Meeting family needs, 1993).

Nurses need to be aware of common questions about organ donation to help families make an informed decision. Healthy children who die unexpectedly are excellent candidates for organ donation, although their age is a determinant of organ suitability. For example, very young donors present technical difficulties in organ removal (Williams, 1985). Children with cancer, chronic disease, or infection or who have suffered prolonged cardiac arrest may not be suitable candidates, although this is individually determined. The nurse should inquire if organ donation was discussed with the child or if the child ever expressed such a wish.* Any number of body tissues or organs can be donated (skin, eyes, bone, kidney, heart, liver, pancreas), and their removal does not mutilate or desecrate the body or cause any suffering. The family may have an open casket, and there is no delay in the funeral. There is no cost to the donor family, but organ donation does not eliminate funeral or cremation responsibilities. Most religions permit organ donation as long as the recipient benefits from the transplant, although Orthodox Judaism forbids it.

In cases of unexplained death, violent death, or suspected suicide, autopsy is required by law. In other instances it may be optional, and parents should be informed of this choice. The procedure, as well as forms that require signing, should be explained. The family should know that the child can be in an open casket following an autopsy.

SIBLINGS' ATTENDANCE AT BURIAL SERVICES

One of the most frequent concerns of parents is whether young or school-age children should attend funeral or burial services (see Thinking Critically About . . . box, p. 1000). Sharing moments of deep significance with parents helps children understand the experience and deal with their own feelings of shock, sorrow, and grief; depriving them of this opportunity may leave children with lifelong regrets (Fig. 23-4). However, children need preparation for postdeath services. They should be told what to expect, particularly how the deceased person will look if the coffin is open. Ideally the parent should explain the details to the child, but, if the parent's grief prevents this communication, a significant family member or friend should substitute.

It is often helpful to bring children to the funeral service before many visitors arrive. They are allowed private time to say good-bye but are spared some of the unpredictable emotional reactions of others, which can be very distressing to them. Allowing children to stay as long as they

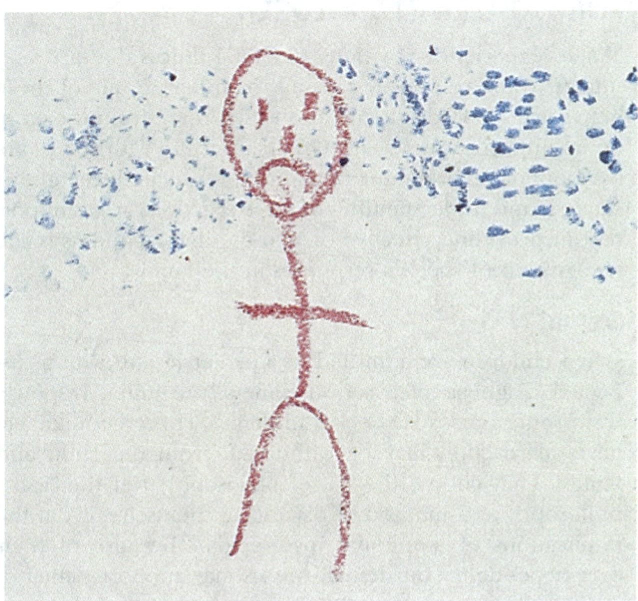

FIG 23-4 Drawing, made by 7-year-old child whose sister died in a car crash, shows the boy sad and crying (dots are tears) because he was not allowed to see his dead sibling.

*Information about being an organ donor is available from **The Living Bank,** P.O. Box 6725, Houston, TX 77265, (800) 528-2971; and from **The United Network for Organ Sharing (UNOS),** (800) 24-DONOR.

THINKING CRITICALLY ABOUT . . .

Children's Attending the Funeral or Burial Service of a Loved One

This question generates much controversy among the general public and professionals. Many lay people feel it is too frightening for children to be exposed to the dead and that it is better for them to remember the loved person as he or she was when alive. There is a general attitude of protecting children from unhappy or distressing events. However, among health professionals involved with children, there is a fairly general consensus that children should attend such services, and some authors suggest that no child is too young merely by virtue of age (Foley, 1986). Others recommend that the parents make the decision regarding attendance until children are 6 or 7 years of age, at which time children should choose (Zelauskas, 1981). Several retrospective studies indicate that attendance at funerals is both meaningful and useful to children (Dickinson, 1992; Silverman and Warden, 1992). Attendance at funerals helps children acknowledge the death, honor the deceased, and receive support and comfort. In addition, children, like adults, have "unfinished business," and visiting the dead person may represent an opportunity to complete those affairs. For example, the child may wish to say good-bye (verbally or written) or to leave a memento.

Unfortunately, little research has focused on the difference in adjustment between children who do or do not attend postdeath services. However, one study indicated substantial evidence of the benefit of involving children in the experience of their dying sibling. Lauer and others (1985) compared children's perceptions of their sibling's death at home vs in the hospital. The home care group (ages 5 to 23 years) reported they were prepared for the impending death, received consistent information and support from their parents, were involved in most activities, found the funeral experience comforting, and viewed their own involvement as the most important aspect of the experience. The non–home care group (ages 2 to 26 years) had opposite perceptions. Another study found that greater participation in the child's care and death, including funeral attendance, was associated with higher self-esteem in the siblings (Michael and Lansdown, 1986). Among adolescents, Kuntz (1991) found that seeing a parent who had died and being involved with the rituals surrounding the death promoted adaptive grieving. Thus it appears that increased involvement with the death, rather than isolation and "protection," benefits children.

wish, but respecting their need to leave, provides maximum control for them over their ability to grieve comfortably.

THE NURSE AND THE FATALLY ILL CHILD

NURSES' REACTIONS TO CARING FOR FATALLY ILL CHILDREN

Nurses experience reactions to a fatal illness that are very similar to the responses of family members. Some of these help nurses provide care by protecting them from the emotional impact of the event. Others interfere with the establishment of a therapeutic relationship with family members. Analysis and understanding of these reactions are as important in providing effective care to the dying child as is the recognition of specific responses in the family.

Denial

When children are admitted to a pediatric unit with a suspected diagnosis of a serious illness, the initial response from some nurses is shock and denial. However, their behavioral reaction may be withdrawal from the child and family. They choose the "cure" philosophy over the "care" philosophy as a method of distancing themselves from the implications of emotional involvement. Because of their own dependency on denial, nurses may support denial in parents. There are several methods of conveying this message, such as emphasizing only optimistic "survival statistics," negating the seriousness of the illness, focusing on "cheering up" the family, and engaging in casual conversation to avoid meaningful dialogue. Although this increases nurses' comfort in caring for the dying child. it does little to provide family members with an opportunity to progress beyond denial and begin anticipatory grieving.

Some denial is as important for nurses as it is for the child or parents; it protects nurses from the overwhelming reality of death. It would be extremely difficult to participate in the medical treatment plan without some expectation of a cure. Denial is also necessary to prevent feelings of failure. In general, the nursing and medical goal is curing illness and saving lives, not allowing patients to die. However, denial loses its beneficial functions when nurses refuse to admit the failure of treatment efforts and insist on adhering to the "curing" regimen, regardless of its effectiveness or value. Failure of treatment should not be equated with personal failure or failure to provide optimum nursing care.

Anger and Depression

Some nurses may be angry for having been assigned to the "leukemia case," because the very exposure to potential failure in a fatal illness is extremely threatening. Others may feel angry for having to subject the child to painful procedures or for being unable to relieve the child's physical and emotional suffering. Instead of anger, some nurses may feel depression for any of these reasons.

However, without an understanding of the reason for the emotion, nurses may project the anger onto others, particularly family members. They may be unable to tolerate the child's uncooperative behavior or the parents' continual requests for information. Anger fuels more anger, and parents react with hostility and think the members of the nursing staff are rejecting them. A vicious circle of resentment, mistrust, and frustration results.

Depression also has adverse effects on a therapeutic relationship, because nurses may withdraw from the child and parents as a method of controlling their sadness. Unaware of the reason for the avoidance, family members interpret it as evidence of inadequate care. This reaction also fosters a nonsupportive cycle of avoidance, withdrawal, resentment, and frustration. However, the messages are usually more covert than when the nurses' reaction is anger and may prevent a climax that could result in a solution to the problem.

Guilt

Nurses who feel unable to deal with fatal illness in a child often experience guilt. Nurses who become angry or depressed when caring for a dying child often reveal that they are very uncomfortable with this response but are unable to choose a more direct, constructive approach. They express guilt for having been intolerant of the child's or parents' behavior and, even more important, realize the missed opportunity to provide these individuals with professional support and guidance.

Nursing staff may experience guilt even when they can deal effectively with the family. There is often a feeling that the family's needs are never completely met. Such nurses tend to set expectations that are beyond anyone's ability to meet, such as the expectation that they are supposed to save lives, not let people die.

The one important difference between a dying child and an ill child is that there may be no second chance to meet the needs of the dying child. This finality is difficult to comprehend but can be a catalyst toward better understanding of one's own responses to dying. For example, when guilt makes one uncomfortable enough to seek alternate behavior patterns, there is an opportunity for change to occur, provided the individual is given some assistance and support.

Ambivalence

One of the most universal reactions of nurses is ambivalence in their feelings toward a dying child. There is the fluctuating adherence to hope for a cure and fear of a relapse. Sometimes the motivations for either are more for personal needs. For example, they may hope that the child recovers to avoid readmissions. Or they may wish for a remission so that discharge is assured. Such thoughts are certainly understandable in light of the emotional toll of nursing a dying child.

Ambivalence may be demonstrated in a particular type of bargaining. Rather than bargaining for extra time, nurses may hope that their colleagues are assigned the patient, or that a death may occur on a shift other than their own. Bargaining for a temporary absence from the dying child is a healthy response, because it denotes nurses' awareness of their own emotional limits. Nurses who are unable to recognize their personal emotional limits are in danger of seeking from the professional relationship their own needs for gratification, achievements, and fulfillment. This results in the loss of an objective evaluation of therapeutic interventions and the increased potential for subjective overinvolvement with the family.

Coping with Stress

Pediatric critical care and oncology nurses surveyed about stresses of their work rank the death of patients as most stressful (Benica, Longo, and Barnsteiner, 1992; Emery, 1993). The less experienced the nurse, the more likely death was rated as a stressor. Furthermore, nurses overestimated the percentage of deaths on their unit, suggesting that the experience overwhelms them.

One of the stress-related behaviors that can result from caring for dying children is ***burnout,*** a state of physical, emotional, and mental exhaustion. It occurs as a result of prolonged involvement with individuals in situations that are emotionally demanding. Nurses working in intensive care units are particularly prone to this occupational hazard, but staff nurses also can experience it when dealing with groups of children such as those who may die. To cope constructively, effectively, and therapeutically with children who are dying in spite of the stress generated, while avoiding burnout, requires deliberate and concerted effort on the part of the nurse.

Self-Awareness and Consciousness Raising. The initial step in effectively caring for a dying child is making a deliberate choice to become involved. Many nurses react negatively to the word "involvement" because they believe that professionals must remain uninvolved in order to maintain objectivity. Involvement does not displace objectivity. On the contrary, allowing oneself to feel with the other person expands one's ability to comprehend the meaning and depth of that emotion. According to Maslach (1979), the achievement of ***detached concern,*** in which the health care practitioner provides sensitive, understanding care by being sufficiently detached to make objective, rational decisions, is the ideal.

Involvement does have the potential risk of clouding objectivity, but awareness of one's reactions and investments in the care of a dying child minimizes this hazard. Developing awareness requires the willingness to investigate one's motivations for choosing to work in such an area and an understanding of the stresses inherent in the role, to review one's resolution of past losses, and to contemplate one's own fears of death. Often nurses realize that their cold, impersonal reaction to dying patients stems from previous unresolved conflicts or losses. Once they are able to talk about such experiences, they are usually able to gain insight into their behavior and begin to form alternative methods of reacting.

Knowledge and Practice. Intervening therapeutically with terminally ill children and their families requires more than self-awareness. It also necessitates basing nursing practice on sound theoretic formulations and empiric observations that serve as a general, concise analysis of the typical reactions of families. Although every individual is different and responds to events or crises in a way that is influenced by all of his or her previous life's experiences, there must be some beginning point for understanding the more typical responses of individuals and for making some decision as to their importance in the eventual resolution of the crisis. In this way nurses can plan care that meets the needs of each family member in terms of prevention as well as intervention of problems.

Nurses also must explore ethical issues surrounding the definition of death, the use of extraordinary, lifesaving measures vs passive or active euthanasia, and patient's rights to know and choose their own destiny. Once they have soundly formulated principles by which to practice, they need opportunities for decision making. When a team approach is used, nurses can be valuable members of the group, provided their own values are clarified and they have critically assessed the family's responses. (See Ethical Decision Making, Chapter 1.)

Support Systems. Support systems are essential to continued functioning in a high-stress environment. They allow for regeneration of energies by sharing feelings and concerns with others. Dealing with feelings about death in isolation can lead to repressed feelings such as denial, anger, depression, and grief. These feelings may be manifested in poor interactions between staff, inappropriate or unsupportive interactions with families, an inability to evaluate care plans or advocate for families, and a need to control (Hammer, Nichols, and Armstrong, 1992). Support is an important catalyst for processing feelings about death.

Social supports may be personal family members such as parents or spouses, extended relatives, and friends. Professional supports include colleagues, consultants, teachers, and supervisors. Peers may be sources of technical and practical advice. Since less experienced nurses rank death as more stressful, a mentoring relationship between a senior nurse and the less experienced nurse may provide support and role modeling, as well as assist in the development of effective coping strategies (Benica, Longo and Barnsteiner, 1992).

Other Strategies. Any number of other strategies may be used to reduce stress. These include maintaining good general health practices, especially regular exercise, and diversionary activities that are of personal interest beyond the workplace (Vachon and Pakes, 1985). Distancing techniques are also effective, such as leaving work at work, informing other staff not to contact them on their days off, periodically assuming less demanding assignments, and taking time off when needed. For caregivers who find the demands of this kind of nursing too emotionally draining, the ultimate distancing strategy is resignation (Munley, 1985).

A final technique is to focus on the positive aspects of the caregiving role. Despite the difficult times in caring for these children and families, there are many rewarding experiences that must be remembered. Dedicated efforts reap numerous rewards, and these must not be forgotten or minimized. Reflection on positive feedback from appreciative families can revitalize self-esteem and job satisfaction. Some hospice nurses succeed at their work by cognitive reframing that allows them to view success through a care rather than cure framework (Sumner and Hurula, 1993).

Some nurses find shared remembrance rituals to be useful in resolving grief (Hammer, Nichols and Armstrong, 1992; Zappa and Parks, 1993). Similarly, attending the funeral services can be a supportive act for both the family and the nurse and in no way detracts from the professionalism of care. For the family it conveys a sense of worth and caring by the nurse. For the nurse it can provide a sense of "closure" with the family and assist in the resolution of personal grief.

KEY POINTS

- A family-centered approach to care of the child and family facing life-threatening illness or death respects the central role of the family and emphasizes communication, collaboration, and cultural sensitivity.
- There are five phases of family reactions to a life-threatening illness such as cancer: Phase I—shock and disbelief, guilt, anger, anticipatory grieving, depression and ambivalence, bargaining; Phase II—overprotectiveness, dependency, social isolation, hope, fear, and anxiety; Phase III—denial and ambivalence, overprotectiveness, and concern for the future; Phase IV—heightened anticipatory grieving, loss of hope and despair, fear of death, fear of loss of control, and fear of isolation and loneliness; Phase V—acute grief and extended phase of mourning.
- Special needs of the family facing the unexpected death of a child include support while awaiting news of the child's status; a sensitive pronouncement of death; acknowledgement of feelings of denial, guilt and anger; an opportunity to view the body; closure; and referrals for support.
- To counsel families and children regarding death, nurses need to understand children's perceptions of death, the fears in each age-group, and personal meanings of death and bereavement during developmental stages.
- Toddlers' egocentricity and separation of fact from fantasy make death incomprehensible; they may still refer to a dead person as if the person exists.
- Because of their sense of precausality and self-power, preschoolers may believe that their thoughts actually cause another person's death.
- With their reasoning power and fear of the unknown, school-age children may feel intense guilt and responsibility about someone's death.
- Adolescents have difficulty accepting death because of their preoccupation with developing a sense of identity.
- Nurses may offer the following assistance in assessment and education about death: counseling parents about children's age-specific understanding of death, encouraging parents to help children become familiar and comfortable with loss, taking part in organized death education in schools, and serving as a resource to answer family's and children's questions.
- What children are told about their serious illness is the family's decision and can be based on several general principles regarding developmental age, previous knowledge, and honesty.
- Siblings have special needs, including the need for information, reassurance about their own health status, assurance that they are not responsible for the illness or death, and support for their own grieving process.
- According to Lindemann, acute grief is a syndrome with psychologic and somatic symptomatology that may appear after a crisis or be delayed, exaggerated, or apparently absent. Distorted reactions may represent one aspect of the syndrome and can be transformed into normal grief work.
- Parke's grief process consists of four phases that do not necessarily proceed in sequence and may recur at any time: shock and disbelief, expression of grief, disorganization and despair, and reorganization.

- Formal bereavement programs may assist families in coping with the loss of a child and in the process of grief resolution.
- Special decisions at the time of dying and death may involve hospital or hospice care, the child's right to die, visualization of the body, tissue donation/autopsy, and siblings' attendance at the funeral.
- In dealing with stress related to the dying patient, the nurse can cope successfully through self-awareness, consciousness raising, knowledge and practice, available support system, maintaining general good health, and focusing on the positive rewards of involvement with dying children and their families.

REFERENCES

Armstrong-Dailey A: Children's hospice care, *Pediatr Nurs* 16(4):337-339+, 1990.

Atuel TM, Williams PD, Camar MT: Determinants of Filipino children's responses to the death of a sibling, *Matern Child Nurs J* 17(2):115-134, 1988.

Benica SW, Longo CB, Barnsteiner JH: Perceptions and significance of patient deaths for pediatric critical care nurses, *Crit Care Nurs* 12(3):72-75, 1992.

Bincer W: *Siblings,* Cincinnati, 1989, Xerox/National Organization of Parents of Murdered Children.

Birenbaum LK, Clarke-Steffen L: Terminal care costs in childhood cancer, *Pediatr Nurs* 18(3):285-288, 1992.

Bluebond-Langner M: *The private worlds of dying children,* Princeton, NJ, 1978, Princeton University Press.

Bluebond-Langner M: Worlds of dying children and their well siblings, *Death Stud* 13:1-16, 1989.

Brett KM, Davies EMB: "What does it mean?" Sibling and parental appraisals of childhood leukemia, *Cancer Nurs* 11(6):329-338, 1988.

Cerney MS: Solving the organ donar shortage by meeting the bereaved family's needs, *Crit Care Nurse* 13(1):32-36, 1993.

Chesterfield P: Communicating with dying children, *Nurs Stand* 6(20):30-32, 1992.

Clarke-Steffen L: Waiting and not knowing: the diagnosis of cancer in a child, *J Pediatr Oncol Nurs* 10(4):146-153, 1993.

Cohen MH: The unknown and the unknowable—managing sustained uncertainty, *West J Nurs Res* 15(1):77-96, 1993.

Corr CA: Coping with dying: lessons that we should and should not learn from the work of Elisabeth Kübler-Ross, *Death Stud* 17(1):69-83, 1993.

Corr CA, Corr DM: Children's hospice care, *Death Stud* 16(5):431-449, 1992.

Davies B: Family responses to the death of a child: the meaning of memories, *J Palliative Care* 3(1):9-15, 1987.

Dickinson GE: First childhood death experiences, *Omega J Death Dying* 25(3):169-182, 1992.

Emery JE: Perceived sources of stress among pediatric oncology nurses, *J Pediatr Oncol Nurs* 10(3):87-92, 1993.

Faulkner A, Peace G, O'Keefe C: Future imperfect, *Nurs Times* 89(51):40-42, 1993.

Foley G: Conflicts in practice: the argument for, *J Assoc Pediatr Oncol Nurs* 2(3):22-24, 1985.

Foley GV: Facilitating death discussions with children. *Pediatrics: Nursing Update,* lesson 19, Princeton, NJ, 1986, Continuing Professional Educational Corp.

Gibbons MB: A child dies, a child survives: the impact of sibling loss, *J Pediatr Health Care* 6(2):65-72, 1992.

Giordano MS: What required-request laws mean to you, *Am J Nurs* 89(10):1296-1297, 1989.

Glick I, Weiss R, Parkes C: *The first year of bereavement,* New York, 1974, John Wiley & Sons.

Greenham DE, Lohmann RA: Children facing death: recurring patterns of adaptations, *Health Social Work* 7:89-94, 1982.

Hammer M, Nichols DJ, Armstrong L: A ritual of remembrance, *MCN* 17:310-313, Nov-Dec 1992.

Hobbie WL, Hollen PJ: Pediatric nurse practitioners specializing with survivors of childhood cancer, *J Pediatr Health Care* 7(1):24-30, 1993.

Hollen PJ, Hobbie WL: Risk-taking and decision making of adolescent long-term survivors of cancer, *Oncol Nurse Forum* 20(5):769-776, 1993.

Jankovic M and others: Meetings with parents after the death of their child from leukemia, *Pediatr Hematol Oncol* 6:155-160, 1989.

Johnson LC and others: The development of a comprehensive bereavement program to assist families experiencing pediatric loss, *J Pediatr Nurs* 8(3):142-146, 1993.

Kachoyeanos MK, Selder FE: Life transitions of parents at the unexpected death of a school-age and older child, *J Pediatr Nurs* 8(1):41-49, 1993.

Klopovich P and others: School phobia, *J Kans Med Soc* 82(3):125-127, 1981.

Kübler-Ross E: *On death and dying,* New York, 1969, Macmillan.

Kuntz B: Exploring the grief of adolescents after the death of a parent, *J Child Adolesc Psychiatr Ment Health Nurs* 4(3):105-109, 1991.

Lansky SB, List MA, Ritter-Sterr C: Psychiatric and psychological support of the child and adolescent with cancer. In Pizzo P, Poplack D, editors: *Principles and practice of pediatric oncology,* Philadelphia, 1988, JB Lippincott.

Lauer ME and others: A comparison study of parental adaptation following a child's death at home or in the hospital, *Pediatrics* 71(1):107-112, 1983.

Lauer ME and others: Children's perceptions of their sibling's death at home or hospital: the precursors of differential adjustment, *Cancer Nurs* 8(1):21-27, 1985.

Leahy JM: *The relationship of depression and type of bereavement, mode of death, and time since death in three groups of adult females,* doctoral dissertation, Garden City, NY, 1991, Adelphi University.

Leikin S: A proposal concerning decisions to forego life-sustaining treatment for young people, *J Pediatr* 115(1):17-22, 1989.

Lindemann E: Symptomatology and management of acute grief, *Am J Psychiatry* 101:141-148, Sept 1944.

Lipson M: What do you say to a child with AIDS? *Hastings Center Rep* 23(2):6-12, 1993.

Lyman MJ: The parent network in pediatric oncology: supportive or not? *Cancer Nurs* 10(4):207-216, 1987.

Martinson IM: Hospice care for children: past, present, and future, *J Pediatr Oncol Nurs* 10(3):93-98, 1993.

Martinson IM and others: Home care for children dying of cancer, *Res Nurs Health* 9(1):11-16, 1986.

Martinson IM and others: Impact of childhood cancer on healthy school-age siblings, *Cancer Nurs* 13(3):183-190, 1990.

Maslach C: The burn-out syndrome and patient care. In Garfield C, editor: *Stress and survival: the emotional realities of life-threatening illness,* St Louis, 1979, Mosby.

McClung JA, Kamer RS: Implications of New York's do-not-resuscitate law, *N Engl J Med* 323(4):270-272, 1990.

Meeting family needs in organ donation, *Progress Notes:* Newsletter of the Partnership for Organ Donation, p 7, winter 1993.

Michael S, Lansdown R: Adjustment to the death of a sibling, *Arch Dis Child* 61:278-283, 1986.

Miles MS: Emotional symptoms and physical health in bereaved parents, *Nurs Res* 34(2):76-81, 1985a.

Miles MS: Helping adults mourn the death of a child, Issues *Compr Pediatr Nurs* 8(1/6):219-241, 1985b.

Miles MS, Perry K: Parental responses to sudden accidental death of a child, *Crit Care Q* 8(1):73-84, 1985.

Moore IM, Gilliss DL, Martinson I: Psychosomatic symptoms in parents 2 years after the death of a child with cancer, *Nurs Res* 37(2):104-107, 1988.

Munley SA: Sources of hospice staff stress and how to cope with it, *Nurs Clin North Am* 20(2):343-355, 1985.

Nagy M: The child's view of death, *J Genet Psychol* 73:3-27, 1948.

Neidig JR, Dalgas-Pelish P: Parental grieving and perceptions regarding health care professionals' interventions, *Issues Compr Pediatr Nurs* 14(3):179-191, 1991.

Nitschke R and others: Therapeutic choices made by patients with end-stage cancer, *J Pediatr* 101(3):471-476, 1982.

Opie ND and others: The effect of a bereavement group experience on bereaved children's and adolescents' affective and somatic distress, *J Child Adolesc Psychiatry Ment Health Nurs* 5(11):20-26, 1992.

Patno KM, Young PC, Dickerman JD: Parental attitudes about confidentiality in a pediatric oncology clinic, *Pediatrics* 81(2):296-300, 1988.

Peace S and others: Childhood cancer: psychosocial needs: are they being met? *J Cancer Care* 1(1):3-13, 1992.

Price LJ: Metalogue on coping with illness: cases from Ecuador, *Qual Health Res* 2(2): 135-158, 1992.

Rando T: An investigation of grief and adaptation in parents whose children have died from cancer, *J Pediatr Psychiatry* 8(1):3-20, 1983.

Raver D: Siblings: "We will never forget," *Survivors* (Newsletter of Parents of Murdered Children), p 7, Nov 1992.

Ritchie MA: Psychosocial functioning of adolescents with cancer: a developmental perspective, *Oncol Nurs Forum* 19(10):1497-1501, 1992.

Rose TV, Stewart ES: *Whispers of hope: a hospital-based program for bereaved parents and their families,* Durham, NC: Duke University Medical Center Pediatric Brain Tumor Family Support Program, 1993.

Rushton CH, Glover JJ: Involving parents in decisions to forgo life-sustaining treatment for critically ill infants and children, *AACN Clin Issues Crit Care Nurs* 1(1):206-214, 1990.

Rushton CH, Hogue EE: When parents demand "everything," *Pediatr Nurs* 19(2):180-183, 1993.

Saunders JM, Valente SM: No code: the question that won't go away, *Nursing 86* 16(3):60-64, 1986.

Schwab R: Effects of a child's death on the marital relationship: a preliminary study, *Death Stud* 16(2):141-154, 1992.

Shumway CN, Grossman LS, Sarles RM: Therapeutic choices by children with cancer, *J Pediatr* 103(1):168, 1983 (letter).

Silverman PR, Warden JW: Children's understanding of funeral ritual, *J Death Dying* 25(4):319-331, 1992.

Stanfill P, Strong C: Conflicts in practice: the argument against, *J Assoc Pediatr Oncol Nurs* 2(3):25-26, 1985.

Statistical Abstracts of the United States 1993, ed 113, Lanham, MD, 1993, Bernian Press.

Sumner L, Hurula J: Pediatric hospice nursing: making the most of each moment, *Nursing 93* 50-55, Aug 1993.

Vachon MLS, Pakes E: Staff stress in the care of the critically ill and dying child, *Issues Compr Pediatr Nurs* 8(1-6):151-182, 1985.

Wass H: Concepts of death; a developmental perspective, *Issues Compr Pediatr Nurs* 8(1-6):3-24, 1985.

Wass H and others: *Death education: an annotated resource guide,* Washington, DC, 1980, Hemisphere.

Williams L: Organ procurement: what nurses need to know, *Crit Care Q* 8(1):27-30, 1985.

Wong D: Bereavement: the empty-mother syndrome, *MCN* 5(6):385-389, 1980.

Zappa S, Parks G: A remembrance ceremony to help families and staff work through the grieving process, *J Pediatr Oncol Nurs* 10(2):65-66, 1993 (abstract).

Zelauskas B: Siblings: the forgotten grievers, *Issues Compr Pediatr Nurs* 5:45-52, 1981.

BIBLIOGRAPHY

American Academy of Pediatrics, Committee on Pediatric Emergency Medicine: Death of a child in the emergency department, *Pediatrics* 93(5):861-862, 1994.

Antonacci M: Sudden death: helping bereaved parents in the PICU, *Crit Care Nurs* 10(4):65-66+, 1990.

Armstrong-Dailey A: Children's hospice care, *Pediatr Nurs* 16(4):337-339+, 1990.

Bachmann AT: Helping the survivors cope with sudden death, *Point of View* 26(2):6-7, 1989.

Back KJ: Sudden, unexpected pediatric death: caring for the parents, *Pediatr Nurs* 17(6): 571-575, 1991.

Baker JE, Sedeny MA, Gross E: Psychological tasks for children, *Am J Orthopsychiatry* 62(1):105-117, 1992.

Balk DE: Sibling death, adolescent bereavement and religion, *Death Stud* 15(1):1-20, 1991.

Bendor SJ: Anxiety and isolation in siblings of pediatric cancer patients: the need for prevention, *Soc Work Health Care* 14(3):17-35, 1990.

Black KJ: Sudden, unexpected pediatric death: caring for the parents, *Pediatr Nurs* 17(6): 571-575, 1991.

Bossert E, Martinson I: Kinetic family drawings—revised: a method of determining the impact of cancer on the family as perceived by the child with cancer, *J Pediatr Nurs* 5(3):204-213, 1990.

Bosworth T: Leukemia through a teenager's eyes, *MCN* 14(2):93-94, 1989.

Brahams D: Medicine and the law: a life-sustaining treatment for brain-damaged child, *Lancet* 339(8807):1472-1473, 1992.

Brett AS: Limitations of listing specific medical interventions in advance directives, *JAMA* 266(6):825-828, 1991.

Carlson JAS: The psychologic effects of sudden infant death syndrome on parents, *J Pediatr Health Care* 7(2):77-81, 1993.

Cassidy M: Supportive care and the dying child, *J Home Health Care Pract* 3(1):34-38, 1990.

Castiglia PT: Death of a parent, *J Pediatr Health Care* 2(3):157-159, 1988.

Castiglia PT: Death of a sibling, *J Pediatr Health Care* 2(4):211-213, 1988.

Chekryn J, Deegan M, Reid J: Impact on teachers when a child with cancer returns to school, *Child Health Care* 15(3):161-165, 1987.

Conrad NL: Spiritual support for the dying, *Nurs Clin North Am* 20(2):415-426, 1985.

Corr CA: Support for grieving children: the Doughy Center and the hospice philosophy, *Am J Hospice Palliative Care* 8(4):23-27, 1991.

Curnick S: Caring for a dying child at home, *Prof Care Mother Child* 1(2):55-57, 1991.

Czarniecki L, Dillman P: Pediatric HIV/AIDS, *Crit Care Nurs Clin North Am* 4(3):447-456, 1992.

Davies B: The family environment in bereaved families and its relationship to surviving sibling behavior, *Child Health Care* 17(1):22-31, 1988.

Davies B, Eng B: Factors influencing nursing care of children who are terminally ill, *Pediatr Nurs* 19(1):9-14, 1993.

Davis FD: Organ procurement and transplantation, *Nurs Clin North Am* 24(4):823-836, 1989.

Dufour DF: Home or hospital care for the child with end-stage cancer: effects on the family, *Issues Compr Pediatr Nurs* 12(5):371-383, 1989.

Dychkowski LB: Caring for the terminally ill child in the school setting, *Sch Nurse* 6(2):8-10, 12, 1990.

Erlen JA: The child's choice: an essential component in treatment decisions, *Child Health Care* 15(3):156-160, 1987.

Gaffney DA: Death in the classroom: a lesson in life, *Holistic Nurs Pract* 2(2):20-27, 1988.

Gary GA: Facing terminal illness in children with AIDS: developing a philosophy of care for patients, families, and caregivers, *Home Healthc Nurs* 10(2):40-43, 1992.

Gershan JA: Judaic ethical beliefs and customs regarding death and dying, *Crit Care Nurse* 5(1):32-34, 1985.

Gifford BJ, Cleary BB: Supporting the bereaved, *Am J Nurs* 90(2):48-53, 1990.

Gregory D, Longman A: Mothers' suffering: sons who died of AIDS, *Qual Health Res* 2(3):334-357, 1992.

Grogan LB: Grief of an adolescent when a sibling dies, *MCN* 15(1):21-24, 1990.

Hall MD: The way it is . . . caring for dying children, *Am J Nurs* 90(7):86, 1990.

Hammer M and others: A ritual of remembrance . . . grief suffered by nurses themselves, *MCN* 17(6):310-313, 1992.

Harr BD, Thistlethwaite JE: Creative intervention strategies in the management of perinatal loss, *Matern Child Nurs J* 19(2, Ninth Matern Child Nurs Conf Proc, pt 1):135-142, 1990.

Hazinski MF: Pediatric organ donation: responsibilities of the critical care nurse, *Pediatr Nurs* 13(5):354-357, 1987.

Henze SC: Crossed signals . . . DNR policies in home care, *Home Healthc Nurse* 8(2):13-14, 1990.

Hoekstra-Weebers JEH and others: A comparison of parental coping styles following the death of adolescent and preadolescent children, *Death Stud* 15(6):565-575, 1991.

Hogan NS, Balk DE: Adolescent reactions to sibling death: perceptions of mothers, fathers, and teenagers, *Nurs Res* 39(2):103-106, 1990.

Jefidoff A, Gasner R: Helping the parents of the dying child: an Israeli experience, *J Pediatr Nurs* 8(6):413-415, 1993.

Jezewski MA and others: Consenting to DNR: critical care nurses' interactions with patients and family members, *Am J Crit Care* 2(4):302-309, 1993.

Johnson SE: *After a child dies: counseling bereaved families,* New York, 1987, Springer.

Kachoyeanos MK, Selder FE: Life transitions of parents at the unexpected death of a school-age and older child, *J Pediatr Nurs* 8(1):41-49, 1993.

Kahn EC: A comparison of family needs based on the presence or absence of DNR orders, *Dimens Crit Care Nurs* 11(5):286-292, 1992.

Komp DM: Lessons from long-term survivors of childhood cancer, *Pediatrics* 84(5):910-911, 1989.

Krulik T, Holaday B, Martinson IM: *The child and family facing life-threatening illness,* Philadelphia, 1987, JB Lippincott.

Lantos JD, Berger AC, Zucker AR: Do-not-resuscitate orders in a children's hospital, *Crit Care Med* 21(1):52-55, 1993.

Leder SN: Life events, social support, and children's competence after parent and sibling death, *J Pediatr Nurs* 7(2):110-119, 1992.

Lewandowski W, Jones SL: The family with cancer: nursing interventions throughout the course of living with cancer, *Cancer Nurs* 11(6):313-321, 1988.

Markwell J: How children cope with death, *Health Visitor* 64(10):337-338, 1991.

Martinson IM: Impact of childhood cancer on family care in Taiwan, *Pediatr Nurs* 15(6):636-637, 1989.

Martinson IM, Nesbitt M, Kersey J: Children's adjustment to death of a sibling from cancer, *Adv Thanatol* 6:1-7, 1987.

Martinson IM and others: Home care for children dying of cancer. *Res Nurs Health* 9(1):11-16, 1986.

A matter of life and death . . . decision to designate a sick child as not for resuscitation, *Nurs Times* 88(27):55, 1992.

Miles A: Caring for families when a child dies, *Pediatr Nurs* 16(4):346-347, 1990.

Murphy SA: Preventive intervention following accidental death of a child, *Image J Nurs Sch* 22(3):174-179, 1990.

Norris MKG: How to manage tissue donation, *Am J Nurs* 89(10):1300-1302, 1989.

Nurses seek a voice in right-to-die cases, *Am J Nurs* 91(3):26, 1991.

Orlowski JP, Smith ML, Van Zwienen J: Pediatric euthanasia, *Am J Dis Child* 146(14):1440-1446, 1992.

Ott BB, Nieswiadomy RM: Support of patient autonomy in the do not resuscitate decision, *Heart Lung* 20(1):66-74, 1991.

Panchal JA: Beware a child suffers . . . loss of a brother or sister, *J Home Health Care Pract* 5(1):38-42, 1992.

Passarelli C: DNR orders in school? *J Sch Nurs* 8(4):4, 1992.

Pazola KJ, Gerberg AK: Privileged communication—talking with a dying adolescent, *MCN* 15(1):16-21, 1990.

Pengra H, Morgan D, Warren L: Nursing implementation of do not resuscitate policy into home healthcare, *Home Healthc Nurse* 10(2):32-39, 1992.

Perrone J: Adolescents with cancer: are they at risk for suicide? *Pediatr Nurs* 19(1):22-25, 1993.

Petix M: Explaining death to school-age children, *Pediatr Nurs* 13(6):394-396, 1987.

Pitel AU and others: Parent consultants in pediatric oncology, *Child Health Care* 14(1):46, 1985.

Rando TA, editor: *Parental loss of a child,* Champaign, IL, 1986, Research Press.

Saler L, Skolnick N: Childhood parental death and depression in adulthood: roles of surviving parent and family environment, *Am J Orthopsychiatry* 62(4):504-516, 1992.

Stewart G, Lie L: The emergency need for a SIDS support group for family child care, *J Pediatr Nurs* 8(3):185-189, 1993.

van Eys J: In my opinion . . . normalization while dying, *Child Health Care* 17(1):18-21, 1988.

Walker C: Siblings of children with cancer, *Oncol Nurs Forum* 17(3):355-360, 1990.

Worden JW: *Grief counseling and grief therapy,* New York, 1991, Springer.

RESOURCES FOR CHILDREN'S BOOKS ON DEATH*

Aradine C: Books for children about death, *Pediatrics* 57(3):372-378, 1976.

*Other sources of publications on life-threatening illness and death are **The Compassionate Friends,** P.O. Box 3696, Oak Brook, IL 60522-3696, (708) 990-0010; **Centering Corporation,** 1531 N. Saddle Creek Rd., Omaha, NE 68104, (402) 553-1200; **Pediatric Projects, Inc.,** P.O. Box 571555, Tarzana, CA 91357, (800) 947-0947; **Children's Hospice International,** 700 Princess St., Suite 3, Alexandria, VA 22314, (800) 24-CHILD; **National Cancer Institute,** Public Inquiries Office, Bldg. 31, Rm. 10A16, Bethesda, MD 20892, (301) 496-5583.

Bernstein J: Literature for young people: nonfiction books about death, *Death Educ* 3:111-119, 1979.

Bowden VR: Children's literature: the death experience, *Pediatr Nurs* 19(1):17-21, 32-33, 1993.

Delisle R, McNamee A: Children's perceptions of death: a look at the appropriateness of selected picture books, *Death Educ* 5:1-13, 1981.

Fassler J: *Helping children cope: mastering stress through books and stories,* New York, 1978, Free Press.

McBride M: Children's literature on death and dying, *Pediatr Nurs* 5(3):31-33, 1979.

Mills G: Books to help children understand death, *Am J Nurs* 79(2):291-295, 1979.

Seibert D, Drolet JO: Death themes in literature for children ages 3-8, *J Sch Health* 63(2):86-90, 1993.

Wass H: Books for children, *Issues Compr Pediatr Nurs* 8(1-6):373-376, 1985.

Wass H, Corr C, editors: *Helping children cope with death: guidelines and resources,* ed 2, Washington, DC, 1984, Hemisphere.

CHAPTER 24

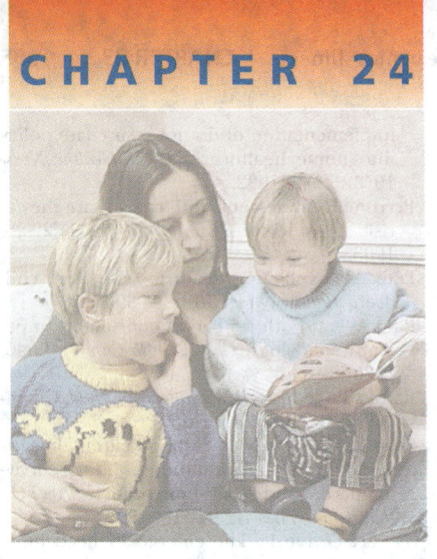

The Child with Cognitive, Sensory, or Communication Impairment

CHAPTER OUTLINE

RELATED TOPICS

Auditory testing, Ch. 7
Autism, Ch. 13
Defects caused by chemical agents, Ch. 11
Dental health: toddler, Ch. 14; school-age child, Ch. 17
Developmental assessment, Ch. 7
Family-centered care of the child with chronic illness or disability, Ch. 22
Fetal alcohol syndrome, Ch. 11
Hereditary influences on health promotion of the child and family, Ch. 5
Human immunodeficiency virus encephalopathy, Ch. 37
Language development, Ch. 4; infant, Ch. 12; toddler, Ch. 14; preschooler, Ch. 15
Limit-setting and discipline, Ch. 3
Optic, otic, and nasal administration (of medication), Ch. 27
Otitis media, Ch. 32
Play: infant, Ch. 12; toddler, Ch. 14; preschooler, Ch. 15; school-age child, Ch. 17
Preparation for hospitalization, Ch. 26
Toilet training, Ch. 14
Toy safety, Ch. 4
Vision testing, Ch. 7

COGNITIVE IMPAIRMENT

GENERAL CONCEPTS

Cognitive impairment is a general term that encompasses any type of mental difficulty or deficiency. In this chapter the term is used synonymously with ***mental retardation (MR)***. Although the needs and concerns of the family are a primary focus throughout the chapter, the reader is encouraged to review Chapter 22, which details the family's adjustment to disabilities in general.

The classic definition of MR has three components: subaverage intellectual functioning, deficits in adaptive behavior, and onset before 18 years of age (Batshaw, 1993). Recently the American Association on Mental Retardation (AAMR) significantly changed this definition by raising the upper limit of subaverage intellectual functioning from an intellectual quotient (IQ) of 70 to 75 and defining more clearly the deficit in adaptive behaviors. Adaptive limitations must occur in two or more of the following ten areas: communication, self-care, home living, social skills, leisure, health and safety, self-direction, functional academics, community use, and work (Luckasson, 1992).

It is critical to note that a low IQ alone is not the sole criterion for MR. For example, individuals with IQ scores near 75 may not be classified as retarded if they are able to adapt to the environment. Or, if cognitive impairment accompanied by adaptive limitations occurs from injury and disease after age 18, the person is not considered retarded.

The new definition also does not include a classification based on IQ scores as it did previously (Table 24-1). Rather, it emphasizes abilities, environments, supports, and empowerment. The intensity of needed support is classified as in-

■ Judith A. Vessey, RN,C, PhD, revised this chapter.

TABLE 24-1 Classification of Mental Retardation

LEVEL (IQ)*	PRESCHOOL (BIRTH-5 YEARS)—MATURATION AND DEVELOPMENT	SCHOOL AGE (6-21 YEARS)—TRAINING AND EDUCATION	ADULT (21 YEARS AND OLDER)—SOCIAL AND VOCATIONAL ADEQUACY
Mild—50-55 to approximately 70	Often not noticed as retarded by casual observer but is slower to walk, feed self, and talk than most children; follows same sequence in development as normal children	Can acquire practical skills and useful reading and arithmetic to a third to sixth grade level with special education; can be guided toward social conformity; achieves mental age of 8 to 12 years	Can usually achieve social and vocational skills adequate to self-maintenance; may need occasional guidance and support when under unusual social or economic stress; can adjust to marriage but not childrearing
Moderate—35-40 to 50-55	Noticeable delays in motor development, especially in speech; responds to training in various self-help activities	Can learn simple communication, elementary health and safety habits, and simple manual skills; does not progress in functional reading or arithmetic; achieves mental age of 3 to 7 years	Can perform simple tasks under sheltered conditions: participates in simple recreation; travels alone in familiar places; usually incapable of self-maintenance
Severe—20-25 to 35-40	Marked delay in motor development; little or no communication skills; may respond to training in elementary self-care (e.g., self-feeding)	Usually walks, barring specific disability; has some understanding of speech and some response; can profit from systematic habit training; achieves mental age of toddler	Can conform to daily routines and repetitive activities; needs continuing direction and supervision in protective environment
Profound—below 20-25	Gross retardation; minimum capacity for functioning in sensorimotor areas; needs total care	Obvious delays in all areas of development; shows basic emotional responses; may respond to skillful training in use of legs, hands, and jaws; needs close supervision; achieves mental age of young infant	May walk; needs complete custodial care; has primitive speech; usually benefits from regular physical activity

*Data from American Psychiatric Association: *Diagnostic and statistical manual of mental disorders (DSM-IV)*, ed 4, Washington, DC, 1994, The Association.

termittent, limited, extensive, or pervasive. The underlying assumption is that with appropriate supports over a prolonged period, the ability of the person with MR to function each day will generally improve. For educational purposes the terms ***educable mentally retarded,*** which corresponds to the mildly retarded group (about 85% of all people with MR), and ***trainable mentally retarded,*** which corresponds to children with moderate levels of MR (about 10% of the MR population), may be used (American Psychiatric Association, 1994).

Diagnosis

The diagnosis of MR is usually made after a period of suspicion by professionals and/or the family that the child's developmental progress is delayed. In some cases it is made at birth because of recognition of distinct syndromes, such as Down syndrome. At the other extreme, it is made after the child begins school and does poorly. In all cases a high index of suspicion for developmental delay is necessary for early diagnosis, and routine developmental screening (see Chapter 7) can assist in early identification. Delays are most commonly seen in speech development. Although gross motor skills such as walking may be delayed, poor motor progress is a poor predictor of MR (Montgomery, 1988). Other common misconceptions that delay early diagnosis include physical stereotyping ("all retarded children are dumb looking") and that children are too young to be tested. In fact, cute children may be retarded, and no child is too young to be evaluated.

Results of standardized tests are helpful in making the diagnosis of MR. The most commonly used tests for infants and preschoolers are the Bayley Mental and Motor Scales and the Wechsler Preschool and Primary Intelligence Scales (WPPIS). The most commonly used tests for older children are the Stanford-Binet Test and Wechsler Intelligence Scale for Children–Revised (WISC-R). These tests are administered only under favorable conditions and individually (never as a group test) by specially trained clinicians, such as psychometrists or child development specialists. Tests for assessing adaptive behaviors include the Vineland Social Maturity Scale and the AAMR Adaptive Behavior Scale. Informal appraisal of adaptive behavior may be made by those fully acquainted with the child (e.g., teachers, parents, or other care providers).

Etiology

The causes of severe MR are primarily genetic, biochemical, and infectious. In mild retardation, familial, social, and environmental causes predominate. Associated factors include maternal life-styles, such as poor nutrition, cigarette smoking, and chemical abuse, especially alcohol, all of which increase the risk of prematurity and intrauterine growth retardation (Task Force on Joint Assessment, 1985). Among individuals with severe retardation, chromosome

CAUSES OF MENTAL RETARDATION

Infection and intoxication—Any agent associated with abnormalities or malformations, such as rubella, syphilis, toxoplasmosis, maternal drug consumption (including alcohol), exposure to industrial chemicals, increased blood levels of lead, Rh incompatibility resulting in kernicterus, or maternal disorders, such as eclampsia
Trauma or physical agent—Injury to brain suffered during prenatal, perinatal, or postnatal period, including physical injury, lack of oxygen, or exposure to radiation
Metabolism or nutrition—Imbalances in fat, carbohydrates, and amino acids; inadequate nutrition; and metabolic or endocrine disorders, such as phenylketonuria or congenital hypothyroidism
Gross postnatal brain disease—Diseases characterized by skin eruptions, lesions, and tumors, such as neurofibromatosis and tuberous sclerosis
Unknown prenatal influence—Cerebral, spinal, and craniofacial malformations, such as microcephaly, hydrocephaly, meningomyelocele, and craniostenosis
Chromosome abnormalities—Chromosome aberrations resulting from radiation, viruses, chemicals, parental age, and genetic mutations, such as Down and fragile X syndromes
Other conditions originating in the perinatal period—Prematurity, low birth weight, and postmaturity
Psychiatric disorders with onset during child's developmental period—For example, autism
Environmental influences—Evidence of a deprived environment associated with a history of mental retardation among parents and siblings

disorders are common, with Down syndrome and fragile X syndrome making up the majority of these cases. Other identifiable disorders or syndromes, such as severe cerebral palsy, microcephaly, or infantile spasms, are also associated with MR. The prenatal, perinatal, and postnatal causes of MR are listed in the box above.

Prevention

Currently there is much concern with prevention of MR. ***Primary prevention strategies***—those designed to preclude the occurrence of the condition that causes retardation—include rubella immunization; genetic counseling, especially in terms of Down or fragile X syndrome; use of folic acid supplements during pregnancy to prevent neural tube defects; education regarding the dangers of ingesting alcohol during pregnancy and lead during childhood; adequate prenatal care and childhood nutrition; and reduction of nonintentional and intentional (abuse) head injuries. In the future, gene therapy for selected conditions will probably be a significant advance in preventing genetic disorders, such as phenylketonuria.

Secondary prevention activities—those designed to identify the condition early and institute treatment to avert cerebral damage—include prenatal diagnosis or carrier detection of disorders, such as Down syndrome, and newborn screening for treatable inborn errors of metabolism, such as congenital hypothyroidism, phenylketonuria, and galactosemia.

Tertiary prevention strategies—those concerned with treatment to minimize long-term consequences—include early identification of conditions and appropriate therapies and rehabilitation services. These include medical treatment of coexisting problems, such as hearing and visual impairment in Down syndrome, and programs for infant stimulation, parent training, preschool education, and counseling services to preserve the integration of the family unit.

NURSING CARE OF CHILDREN WITH COGNITIVE IMPAIRMENT

The goal of caring for children with MR is to promote their optimum social, physical, cognitive, and adaptive development as individuals within a family and community. General guidelines for coping with and adjusting to the child with special needs are discussed extensively in Chapter 22.

❖ ASSESSMENT

Nurses play a major role in identifying children with cognitive impairment. In the newborn and early infancy period few signs are present, with the exception of various syndromes that have distinctive features. However, after this age, delayed developmental milestones are the major clues to MR. In addition, nurses must have a high index of suspicion for early behavioral patterns that may suggest cognitive impairment (see box on p. 1009) and be aware of stereotypes that may delay diagnosis, such as "retarded children have to look dumb." Parental concerns, such as delayed development compared with siblings, need to be taken seriously. All children should receive regular developmental assessment, and the nurse is often the person responsible for performing such developmental screening tests (see Chapter 7). When delays are found, the nurse must use sensitivity and discretion in revealing this finding to parents and refer the child for diagnostic testing.

❖ NURSING DIAGNOSES

A number of nursing diagnoses are prominent in the nursing care of the child with cognitive impairment and the child's family; other diagnoses specific to individual cases become evident. The most common nursing diagnoses are outlined in the Nursing Care Plan on p. 1016.

❖ PLANNING

The goals for the child with MR and the family are as follows:

1. Child will be educated using effective teaching strategies.
2. Child's optimum development will be promoted.
3. Child will learn self-care skills.
4. Family will plan for future care.
5. Child will be cared for appropriately during hospitalization.

❖ IMPLEMENTATION

Educate Child and Family. To learn how to teach children with cognitive impairment, it is necessary to investigate their learning abilities and deficits. These children have a marked deficit in their ability to discriminate between two or more stimuli because of difficulty in recognizing the relevance of specific cues. Unfortunately, the ability to discriminate between symbols is essential in learning

EARLY BEHAVIORAL SIGNS SUGGESTIVE OF COGNITIVE IMPAIRMENT

Nonresponsiveness to contact
Poor eye contact during feeding
Diminished spontaneous activity
Decreased alertness to voice or movement
Irritability
Slow feeding

From Crocker A, Nelson R: Mental retardation. In Levine M and others: *Developmental-behavioral pediatrics*, Philadelphia, 1983, WB Saunders, p 760.

the alphabet for reading or numbers for arithmetic. However, these children can learn to discriminate if the cues are presented in an exaggerated, concrete form and all extraneous stimuli are eliminated. For example, the use of colors to exaggerate visual cues or music for auditory cues can help the child learn. The latter is particularly effective for teaching speech by singing a word in addition to saying it.

These children's deficits in discrimination also imply that concrete ideas are learned much more effectively than abstract concepts. Therefore, demonstration is preferable to verbal explanation, and learning is directed toward mastering a skill rather than understanding scientific principles underlying the procedure.

Another common deficit is in short-term memory. Whereas children with average intelligence can remember several words, numbers, or directions at one time, children with cognitive impairment are unable to do so. Thus they need simple, one-step directions. They respond to learning how to remember, such as by "clustering" pairs or triads together. This approach is helpful when trying to teach them their telephone number. Rather than having them memorize the entire seven-digit number, the teacher breaks it into pairs. After memorizing the pairs, the child puts them together.

Teaching through a step-by-step process requires a task analysis—each task is divided into its necessary components (see box on p. 1013). For example, if the child is learning to tie a shoe, the teacher must practice the skill, divide it into steps (task analysis), and teach each step completely before proceeding to the next activity.

One critical area of learning that has had a tremendous impact on education for cognitively impaired individuals is motivation. Programs based on the motivation principles of behavior modification, employing positive reinforcement for specific tasks or behaviors, have demonstrated marked improvement in children's ability to learn. Two techniques are especially important with this group of learners: ***fading*** (physically taking the child through each sequence of the desired activity and gradually fading out physical assistance so that the child becomes more independent) and ***shaping*** (waiting for the child to give a response that approximates the desired behavior, then reinforcing the child by social approval, such as touching or talking to him or her). Such principles can easily be implemented in the home in teaching self-help skills. Maintaining feelings of success in accomplishing specified goals also promotes a feeling of self-esteem in the child.

When behavior modification is employed, it is crucial not only to reinforce desirable behavior, but also to consistently ignore undesirable behavior. Ignoring the child is particularly difficult for many parents, because they may equate ignoring their child with being a "bad parent." Therefore the nurse must be especially supportive as the parent attempts negative reinforcement. The parent should realize that repetition plays an important part in the child's learning. As the child gains mastery, the parent is encouraged to decrease the social or physical reinforcement the child has been offered. The parent should understand that if a learning program does not move forward successfully, both parent and nurse will reevaluate the last sequence the child mastered to see if they are expecting too much too soon.

Advances in technology have greatly aided in providing active stimulation, especially in children who are severely retarded and may have physical disabilities that limit their range of capabilities. For example, with the use of specially designed switches, children are given control of some event in the environment, such as turning on the television. The television becomes reinforcement for activating the switch. Repetitive use of these switches provides an early, simplistic association with a technical device that may progress to the child using increasingly complex aids.

Early intervention programs have been widely promoted for children with developmental disabilities. Such children form an extensively diverse group, including those with MR, cerebral palsy, language and learning disabilities, sensory disorders, autism, and other conditions. Consequently, the types of programs vary widely in philosophy and interventions, and the issue of benefit from such programs is often confusing and conflicting.

One analysis of early intervention programs for infants with disabilities found that effectiveness was greatest in centers involving both parents and children in the interventions, in programs having a well-defined curriculum, and in centers that served a heterogenous group of children (possibly because these programs tended to enroll children at a younger age than programs targeted at a specific disability group) (Shonkoff and Hauser-Cram, 1987).

Nurses need to be aware of the types of programs in their community to direct families to groups whose philosophy is best suited to the family's needs. Early intervention programs are provided by a number of organizations. Under Public Law 101-476, The Individuals with Disabilities Education Act of 1990, states are encouraged to provide full early intervention services* and are required to provide educational opportunities for all children with disabilities from 0 to 21 years of age. Early intervention services are provided under public programs, such as Programs for Children with Special Health Needs or Head Start, or by pri-

*Information on early intervention programs in each state is available from the **National Down Syndrome Society,** 141 5th Ave., New York, NY 10011; (800) 221-4602.

vate organizations, such as the **National Easter Seal Society*** and the **Association for Retarded Citizens of the United States.†** Educational services that begin when the child reaches age 3 are provided by local school districts. Parents should inquire about these programs by contacting the appropriate agencies. The child's education should begin as soon as possible, not at 5 or 6 years of age. As children grow older, their education should be directed toward vocational training that prepares them for as independent a life-style as possible within their scope of abilities (American Academy of Pediatrics, 1986).

Promote Optimum Development. Optimum development requires appropriate guidance for establishing acceptable social behavior and personal feelings of self-esteem, worth, and security. These attributes are not simply learned, but also must arise from the genuine love and caring that exists among family members. However, families need guidance in providing an environment that fosters optimum development. Often it is the nurse who can provide continuing assistance in these areas of childrearing.

Communication. Verbal skills are often delayed more than other physical skills and are frequently the first clues of cognitive deficits. Since suggestions for promoting speech development are discussed on p. 1043, only brief comments are included here.

Language requires receptive skills (e.g., hearing), decoding skills (interpretation), and expressive skills (e.g., speech). Speech depends on basic receptive and encoding skills and also requires a structurally adequate oral vault and facial muscle coordination. Any of these may be impaired. For example, in children with Down syndrome the large protruding tongue often interferes with speech. These children may need tongue exercises to correct the tongue thrust or gentle reminders to keep the lips closed. Deficits in discrimination impede learning of different sounds. Often it helps to associate the sound with other stimuli, such as singing, which attracts and sustains the child's attention. Parents also must remember that since learning is slower, their teaching must continue longer. The nurse encourages them not to give up or believe that speech is hopeless.

Shaping techniques are useful in fostering meaningful vocalization. Every time the child vocalizes a sound that represents either a letter of the alphabet or an intelligible syllable, the parent responds with praise and social approval. Parents are instructed to record all meaningful vocalizations the child has learned in the past in order to continue reinforcing them. A written record also helps parents monitor evidence of progress in this area.

For some of these children, especially those with severe cognitive and physical impairments, speech acquisition is not possible and nonverbal methods of communication should be employed, such as sign language. Several nonverbal systems are available, but the clinician must be knowledgeable of the cognitive level required to learn and use the method. In order for these children to communicate, others in their environment need to learn the system as well.

Discipline. As discussed in Chapter 22, one of the first childrearing practices parents often neglect when they have a child with a disability is discipline. This not only can result in serious behavior problems, but also interferes with the child's developing a sense of security and self-control. It may also foster resentment from siblings who are forced to abide by a double standard.

Discipline must begin early. For children with cognitive impairment, limit-setting measures must be simple, consistent, and appropriate for their mental age. Control measures are based on teaching a specific behavior, not on having the child understand the reasons behind it. Stressing moral lessons is of little value to a child who cannot learn from self-criticism. Behavior modification, especially reinforcement of desired actions, and time-out are appropriate forms of behavior control (see Chapter 3).

Socialization. Acquiring social skills is complex; active rehearsal with role-playing and practice sessions, and positive reinforcement for desired behavior are successful approaches. Parents are encouraged early to teach their child socially acceptable behavior, such as waving good-bye, saying hello and thank you, responding to his or her name, greeting visitors but not being overly affectionate, and sitting modestly. The teaching of socially acceptable sexual behavior is especially important to minimize sexual exploitation (Williams, 1983). Parents also need to expose the child to strangers so he or she can practice manners, since there is not automatic transfer of learning from one situation to another.

Infant stimulation programs offer an opportunity for social experiences. As children grow older, they should have peer experiences similar to those of other children, including group outings, sports, and organized activity, such as Boy Scouts, Girl Scouts, or **Special Olympics.*** These children often experience greater success in individual and dual sports than in team sports and enjoy themselves with children of the same developmental age (American Academy of Pediatrics, 1987).

Adolescents with cognitive impairment also need social outlets for heterosexual experiences. Unfortunately, few schools or communities provide for this recreational need. The nurse can be instrumental in indirectly initiating such activities by encouraging parents to discuss these unmet social needs with educational staff. Clubs, sports, hobby projects, and dances can be organized for the teenagers to provide experience that teaches acceptable social behavior.

Sexuality. Adolescence may be a particularly difficult time for parents, especially in terms of the child's sexual behavior and needs, future plans to marry, and ability to be independent. Frequently, little anticipatory guidance has been offered parents to prepare the child for physical and sexual maturation, and the degree of the adolescent's interest in sex has been underestimated. Studies have found

*70 E. Lake St., Chicago, IL 60601; (312) 726-6200 or (800) 221-6827.
†2501 Avenue J, Arlington, TX 76006; (800) 433-5255.

*1350 New York Ave., N.W., Suite 500, Washington, DC 20005-4709; (202) 628-3630. In Canada: **Canadian Special Olympics, Inc.,** 40 St. Clair Ave. West, Suite 209, Toronto, Ontario M4V 1M6.

that as many as half of the youngsters with mild retardation (a proportion comparable to the general adolescent population), a third of the moderately retarded, and 9% of the severely retarded have had sexual intercourse, and less than one half of the total group used contraception (Chamberlain and others, 1984). These adolescents are especially vulnerable because of their lifelong dependence on caregivers, relatively powerless position in society, lack of sex education and personal safety, and inability to communicate sufficiently to describe the incident(s) (Tharinger, Horton, and Millea, 1990). In addition, these young people have increased rates of sexual abuse. To protect him or her from abusive sexual activities, parents must closely observe their teenager's activities and associates.

The question of contraceptive protection for female retarded adolescents is often a parental concern. Permanent contraception through sterilization is a special dilemma because of moral and ethical questions, as well as psychologic effects on the adolescent (see Thinking Critically About . . . box). Parents seem to be most interested in sterilization of daughters who are more severely retarded and for elimination of menses to avoid the problems of hygiene (Passer and others, 1984). Contraceptive choices that provide long-term protection, require little compliance, and often produce amenorrhea are subdermal levonorgestrel implants (Norplant) and intramuscular injections of medroxyprogesterone acetate (Depo-Provera) (Sharts-Hopko, 1993).

Parents of these adolescents are often very concerned about the advisability of marriage between two individuals with significant cognitive impairment. There is no conclusive answer; each situation must be judged individually. In many instances marriage would help the couple achieve a mutually satisfying and supportive relationship, meaningful companionship, and a more normal social/sexual adjustment. However, parenthood is usually not desirable because of the complexity of childrearing and the problem of perpetuating mental deficiency. The nurse should discuss this topic with parents and with the prospective couple, stressing suitable living accommodations and contraceptive methods to prevent pregnancy. If children are conceived, these parents require specialized assistance in learning to meet the needs of their offspring (Keltner and Tymchuk, 1992).

Many individuals who are retarded have normal and satisfying sexual relationships. Interest in sexuality is positively correlated with IQ level and gender; high-functioning males have significantly greater interest in sex than females (Ousley and Mesibov, 1991).

Nurses can help in this area by providing parents with information about sex education that is geared to the child's developmental level. For example, the adolescent female needs a *simple* explanation of menstruation and instructions on personal hygiene during the menstrual cycle.*

These adolescents also need practical sexual information regarding anatomy, physical development, and conception. Because of their easy persuasion and lack of judgment, they need a well-defined, concrete code of conduct with specific instructions for handling certain situations. Girls should know never to go alone anywhere with any person they do not know well. Boys should be warned of intimate advances from other males. Programs for teaching self-protection skills using instruction, modeling, rehearsal, feedback, and praise have been successful and have decreased sexual activity among these adolescents (Haseltine and Miltenberger, 1990; Warzak and Page, 1990).

Play. Children who are retarded have the same need for play as any other children. However, because of the child's slower development, parents may be less aware of

*Sources of information on sexuality and conception are the **Association for Retarded Citizens of the United States,** 2501 Ave. J, Arlington, TX 76006, (800) 433-5255; and **Planned Parenthood Federation of America,** 810 7th Ave., New York, NY 10019, (212) 541-7800.

THINKING CRITICALLY ABOUT . . .

Sterilization of Individuals Who Are Mentally Retarded

Although parents may ordinarily consent to any necessary medical or surgical treatment for their minor children, consent for sterilization is an exception (Williams, 1983). Currently the decision regarding sterilization of minors and incompetent adults, in particular those who are mentally retarded, is a moral and legal one. These individuals have the legal right to procreate and not be involuntarily sterilized, but generally are unable to exercise their rights (Krais, 1989). In addition, state laws vary; some allow no sterilization, and others permit review of sterilization requests.

Basically, two opposing viewpoints exist: those who believe that the *right to procreate* is fundamental and those who maintain that the *right not to procreate* is equally important and consider laws preventing sterilization to violate human rights (Passer and others, 1984). What are your views on this issue? What are the benefits or losses to society regarding these two viewpoints?

In allowing the young person who is mentally retarded to make an informed consent, a basic issue is the individual's level of competency. Assessing competency is a complex process. Silva (1984) presents a detailed review of elements and tests of competency and proposes that the main elements of decision-making competency are (1) internalization of a set of goals and values, (2) ability to comprehend and communicate information, and (3) ability to reason and make choices. Tests of competency must be employed on an individual basis, and nurses may be instrumental in presenting information in a simple and concrete manner that increases the person's understanding and level of competence. When a person is considered mentally incompetent, four areas need to be addressed: (1) identification of an appropriate decision maker, (2) alternatives to sterilization, (3) the person's best interests, and (4) current understanding of applicable laws (American Academy of Pediatrics, 1990).

the need to continue appropriate stimulation. They may also feel inadequate in playing with the child, since the usual reciprocal interaction and resulting satisfaction between child and parent may be slower in developing. Therefore the nurse guides parents toward selection of suitable toys and interactive activities. Since play has been discussed for children in each age-group in earlier chapters, only the exceptions for these children are discussed here.

The type of play is based on the child's developmental age, although the need for sensorimotor play may be prolonged. Parents should use every opportunity to expose the child to as many different sounds, sights, and sensations as possible. Appropriate play includes musical mobiles, stuffed toys, water play, floating toys, rocking chair or horse, swing, bells, and rattles. The child should be taken on outings, such as trips to the grocery store or shopping center; other people should be encouraged to visit in the home; and the child should be related to directly, through such means as cuddling, holding, talking to the child in the *en face* position, and giving "rides" on the parents' backs.

Toys are selected for their recreational and educational value. For example, a large inflatable beach ball is a good water toy, encourages interactive play, and can be used to learn motor skills, such as balance, rocking, kicking, and throwing. Attractive toys encourage a child to reach, thus assisting in the development of motor skills (Fig. 24-1). Musical toys that mimic animal sounds or respond with social phrases are excellent ways of encouraging speech. Toys should be simple in design so that the child can learn to manipulate them without help. For children with severe physical impairment, electronic switches can be used to allow them to operate toys (Fig. 24-2).

Safety is a major consideration in selection of toys. Toys that may be appropriate developmentally may present dangers to a child who is strong enough to break them. Even if more advanced toys are suitable for the child's physical skills, the parent must keep in mind the child's level of responsibility in using them properly. For example, the child may be physically able to use a bow and arrow but may lack the judgment in using it to shoot only at a target.

Supervision during play and other activities is stressed, since these children are slow to learn inherent dangers. Parents may need to place reminders around the house to prevent injuries, such as signs to keep the yard gate locked.

These children often lack the motivation to institute appropriate play activities on their own. As a result of boredom, they may resort to self-stimulatory behavior, such as rocking, twirling, masturbating, or finger-sucking, and self-injurious behaviors, such as head-banging or biting, hitting, or scratching themselves (Hyman and others, 1990). Such behaviors limit developmental progress and impede social acceptance. If such behaviors exist, appropriate play activities, especially as a method of distraction from self-stimulation, are discussed with the parents. Behavior techniques, such as ignoring children when they engage in such behavior and attending to them when they are behaving acceptably, should also be used.

Promote Independent Self-Help Skills. When a child with cognitive impairment is born, parents need assistance in promoting normal developmental skills that are almost automatically learned by other children. There is no way to predict when a child should be able to master self-help skills, and studies demonstrate that wide variability exists in the ages at which these children accomplish such functions (see Table 24-2). For the nurse to be successful in meeting this goal, the parents must be supported, included as the

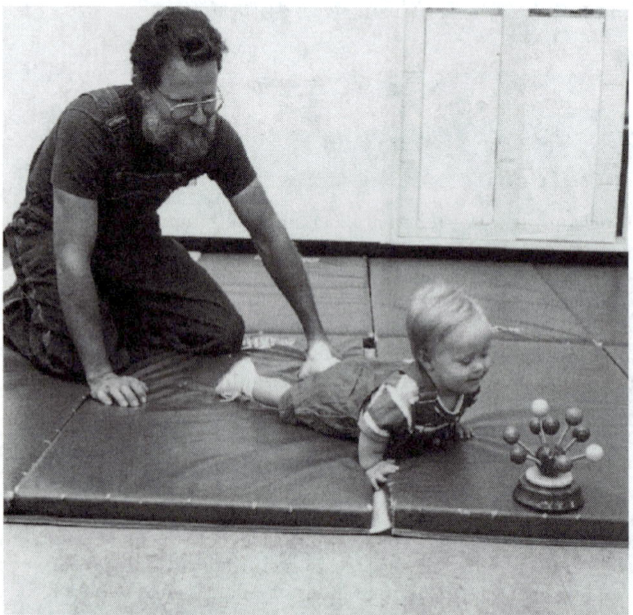

FIG. 24-1 Placing an attractive object out of child's reach encourages crawling movements.

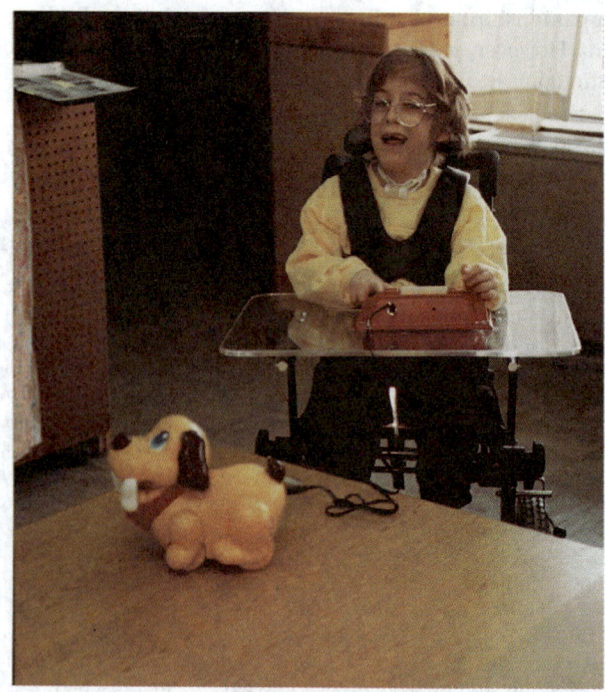

FIG. 24-2 A manual switch allows a child with cognitive impairment to play with a battery-operated toy.

primary rehabilitators with the child, and provided with detailed written descriptions of the stimulation program. Parents also need to be aware that numerous devices are commercially available that can aid in achievement of independence.*

Feeding. Self-feeding is recognized as the first major self-help skill that children learn. It involves the integration of fine and gross motor skills and visual perception. Most parents take for granted that they will be successful in teaching their children to feed themselves. Therefore the nurse must also be especially sensitive to the needs of the parent, as well as of the child, when assistance is offered.

Before beginning a self-feeding program, the nurse should do a task analysis, breaking the process of feeding into its smallest components (see box below). It is important to observe the child in an eating situation to determine whether any of these small steps that make up the entire task of self-feeding have been mastered. If so, the nurse should comment about them positively to the parent and child.

In addition to a task analysis, a number of other factors are assessed, such as the shape of the child's mouth and control of mouth, lip, and tongue movements (whether the tongue moves forward and backward or from side to side, whether there are rotary movements). The presence of teeth determines the textures and consistencies of food that may be offered to the child. The child's developmental readiness for self-feeding, such as the ability to maintain head and trunk support and to sit without support, eye-hand coordination, the firmness of the grasp, and ability to reach for an object, hold it, and release it, is examined. If the child has any physical impairments that interfere with holding or grasping the utensil, specially designed utensils can be substituted (Fig. 24-3) or homemade modifications can be used, such as building the handle up with a sponge or piece of wood or bending it to accommodate arm movement.

Further data are obtained from the parent by asking specifically about the family's approach to feeding. For example, who feeds the child regularly? Is the child fed when hungry or according to a prescribed schedule? What are the child's appetite patterns? Does the parent know when the child is full? What foods does the child like? How long does feeding take? A short feeding time, such as 10 or 20 minutes, might indicate that the child is being deprived of sensory experiences or appropriate interactions; a long time

*A resource for a wide variety of equipment, including self-help devices, is J.A. Preston, P.O. Box 89, Jackson, MI 49204; (517) 787-1600 or (800) 631-7277.

SAMPLE TASK ANALYSIS: SPOON FEEDING

1. Orients to the food by looking at it
2. Looks at the person
3. Reaches for it
4. Touches it
5. Grasps it
6. Lifts it
7. Delivers the spoon to the bowl
8. Lowers it into the food
9. Scoops food onto the spoon
10. Lifts it
11. Delivers the spoon to the mouth
12. Opens the mouth
13. Inserts the spoon into the mouth
14. Moves the tongue and mouth to receive the food
15. Closes the lips
16. Swallows the food
17. Returns the spoon to the bowl

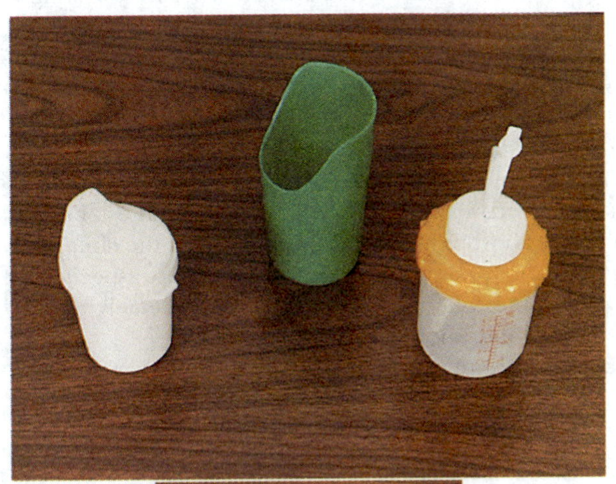

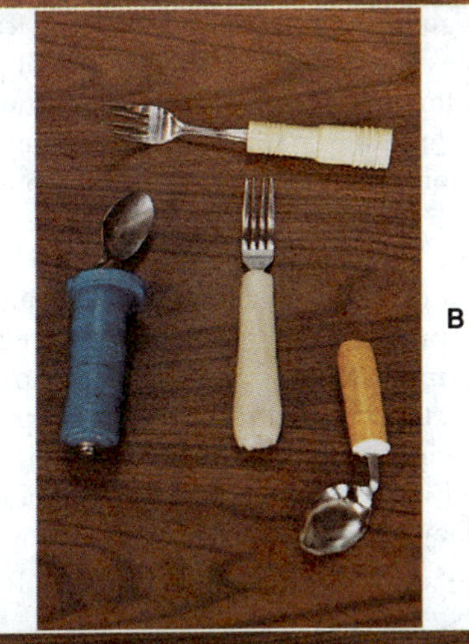

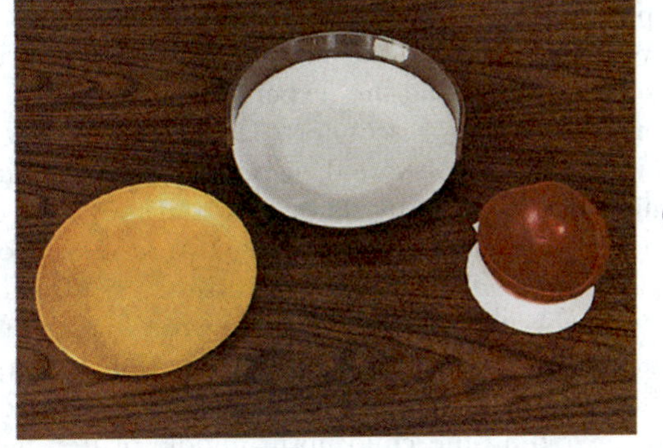

FIG. 24-3 Self-help aids for feeding. **A,** Modified drinking cups. **B,** Modified utensils. **C,** Modified dishes.

might indicate frustration and fatigue on the parent's part. Is the feeding environment described as quiet and nondistracting? What is the best time to begin teaching this new task? If the family is going on vacation, if someone is visiting, or if there has been a major stress in the family, this may not be the ideal time to begin a teaching program.

Preparation for the feeding activity is also discussed, such as proper placement of the child at the table and protection of the area against spills. The principle of normalization (see Chapter 22) is employed to make feeding a family activity. For example, the child is fed in the kitchen, at the table, or in a high chair in a sitting position, and with other family members whenever possible. Food should be served in attractive receptacles; offered in separate servings, not pureed or mixed together; served at the appropriate temperature, not routinely lukewarm; and be of sufficient variety and texture from each of the basic food groups.

Once the feeding program is begun, the nurse is in an important position to give parents supportive feedback. The parents' observational skills, their ability to share observations, keep records of the child's progress, and establish a goal that is appropriate and realistic for both the child and the parents are praised. By acknowledging these aspects, the nurse promotes mastery of a task that is extremely important to the child who is mentally retarded.

Toileting. Independent toileting is another major self-help skill that can be taught using behavior modification principles. It is usually started after self-feeding, since this is the normal sequence of development. Plans for a toileting program begin by assessing the child's physical and psychologic readiness (see Chapter 14). Because of physical or developmental limitations, certain signals may not be possible. For example, children who cannot walk can be trained once they are able to sit with good balance, and children with poor speech may need to rely on gesturing to signal their toileting needs.

Parents are interviewed regarding their readiness to pursue a toilet-training program that is characterized by a positive, consistent, individualized, nonpunitive, nonpressured style of teaching. It is important to explore the parents' willingness to participate, the time they have to invest in the program, the advantages they see, the inconveniences that toilet training may cause them, the reason they wish to start, and whether this is the best time for both the parents and the child to begin.

Any past attempts at toilet training the child are reviewed: When and why did the parents start training? What methods did they use? Did they experience feelings of frustration, indifference, or discomfort? How long did they attempt training, and what were their reasons for discontinuing training efforts? Looking back, how did they view the experience for themselves and the child? Were their efforts consistent? What did they do most consistently? Do they think it is important to try again? If the parents admit to using punishment in any form, including spanking, scolding, withholding privileges, using suppositories, withholding fluid, or getting the child up in middle of the night, the nurse must appeal to them to discontinue these unnecessary, ineffective methods.

As part of the procedure for determining the readiness of both parents and child to become involved in a successful toilet-training program, parents are asked to keep detailed records for 7 days. They should be cautioned to discontinue record keeping if the child becomes ill or if fluid intake is changed. Record keeping includes the following events:

1. The child ate or drank (indicate what), no matter how little was consumed.
2. The child's behavior was suddenly distinctly different (e.g., the child was noticeably quieter or louder, started fussing or tugging at clothes, pointed toward the bathroom, cried, or squirmed).
3. Parents gave the child positive attention related to toileting behaviors only, in the form of praise, concrete rewards, affection, or approval.
4. Parents gave attention in the form of scolding, threatening, or spanking if the child had wet or soiled the underclothes or did not tell them before eliminating.
5. The child indicated the need to go to the toilet by either gestures or words.
6. The child was noted to have dry underclothes.
7. The child was noted to have wet underclothes.

If possible, a toilet-training program should begin after such records are completed, because they show how parents are responding to the child's behaviors and at what times the child is most likely to eliminate.

The goal of any toilet-training program is to help the child achieve small goals and experience comfort and success and to help the parents simultaneously experience feelings of adequacy, minimum tension, and success. Parents should understand that they will be capitalizing on the times the child is most likely to eliminate and that they should respond immediately to any cues indicating this need.

A task analysis of toileting includes the same discrete steps as outlined for feeding (see box on p. 1013). A positive and relaxed attitude toward toilet training is important and differs little from the approach used with other children (see Chapter 14).

Dressing. Dressing skills develop without special training in most children, usually as a consequence of autonomy and imitation. For children who are retarded, special training is necessary to promote this skill. Factors that interfere with spontaneous learning include immature motor skills, lack of motivation, physical impairments, and lack of opportunity. The last variable should always be considered when assessing delayed development of independent dressing.

The level of independence in dressing varies according to the degree of retardation. Children with mild to moderate retardation and no accompanying physical limitations can become independent in all dressing skills, except for more complex tasks such as color coordination. Those who are severely retarded can achieve most dressing skills, except the ability to fasten complicated closures such as buttons or ties. Those who are profoundly retarded are usually able to assist in undressing and dressing but achieve no independent skills.

Children are considered mentally ready for dressing training if they can sit quietly for 3 to 5 minutes while working on a task, can watch what they are doing while working on a task, can follow physical gestures or cues, can follow verbal commands, and can relate clothing to the appropriate body part, such as socks with feet. As with other self-help skills, the child may not be able to master every task but should be evaluated for evidence of willingness to participate at his or her level of readiness. The use of teaching devices, such as dolls with mock closures, and reinforcement for success in managing the fasteners can increase the child's manipulative skills, which may be transferred to ready-to-wear clothing.

Choice of clothing is an important aspect of the training program. Clothes should be clean, up-to-date, and well fitted. They should be easy to put on and take off, easy to fasten, comfortable and nonrestricting, capable of disguising a physical disability, and easy to maintain. Suggested clothing includes undershirts with large neck openings; bras that have elastic straps and front fasteners; half-slips with flared design; underpants with elastic waists; boxer shorts for boys; slip-on polo shirts with large armholes and wide neck openings (not tight turtleneck sweaters); front-buttoning shirts or dresses; pants with elastic waistbands or large, side hook fasteners; wool or cotton ankle socks (not tight nylon knee socks); slip-on shoes; and apparel or shoes with self-adhering (Velcro) closures.

Grooming. Self-grooming is usually learned along with other independent skills, such as washing hands during toilet training. The same principles are followed in teaching grooming procedures as have already been discussed: assess the child's readiness and present level of competency, proceed with skills in the normal sequence of development, analyze the task into its component parts, and set up an individualized teaching program. As with self-dressing, a major factor in learning independent grooming is the opportunity to practice the skills.

Special mention must be made of dental hygiene. An odor-free mouth and clean teeth are essential in promoting a positive image. In addition, healthy teeth are necessary for proper chewing and speech. Diseased teeth and gums increase drooling and prevent proper preparation of food for subsequent digestion. Missing teeth interfere with proper tongue positioning for clear speech.

Many dental problems in these children are a result of neglected dental hygiene and excessive quantities of carbohydrates, including the use of candy to reward behavior. Some dental problems, such as periodontal disease, are associated with various genetic conditions, such as Down syndrome. Most dental problems are preventable with the dental hygiene practices discussed in Chapter 14.

If the child has physical impairments that limit the ability to brush, special devices may be necessary, such as a larger handle or a curved toothbrush, to reach all surfaces of the teeth. Electric toothbrushes or pressurized water devices may be a worthwhile investment for some children. Any strategies that help motivate the child to brush are used. For example, the parent can place a special "tooth calendar" on the wall and mark each date with stars to represent the number of brushings per day. At the end of a specified number of stars, the child can receive a special reward.

The child should be routinely taken to a dentist. It is important to prepare the child for such visits, since it is much more difficult to change an unsatisfactory experience than to prevent one. Once the child is traumatized by the experience, parents may be less inclined to take the child back for fear of temper tantrums or other resisting behavior. The nurse can assist families by locating dentists who are familiar with treating these children and discussing with parents preparatory procedures for the visit.

Help Families Adjust to Future Care. Not all families are able to cope with home care of these children, especially those who are severely or profoundly retarded and/or multiply disabled. Parents who do choose home care may not be able to continue with care responsibilities once they reach retirement or old age. The decision regarding residential placement is difficult for families. The nurse's role is to assist parents in exploring the reasons for desiring placement, especially of adolescents; investigating alternatives to home care before they become necessary; and establishing ways in which to maintain contact and communication with the family member. Guidelines for assessing out-of-home care facilities are listed in the Guidelines box.

A number of alternatives exist regarding out-of-home care, but the availability of these facilities varies widely, depending on the community's resources. Basically, care op

GUIDELINES
Assessing Out-of-Home Care Facilities

Clarify the facility's philosophy of care.
Assess the environment for adequacy of inanimate and animate stimuli for the residents.
Determine the appropriateness of amounts of stimuli in the environment.
Observe care provider–to–resident ratios.
Observe care personnel interacting with residents in a variety of teaching and learning experiences.
Determine the appropriateness of the setting for the person being considered for placement.
Observe the quality of physical care administered.
See if the residents are attended to regularly and consistently, instead of when inappropriate behaviors occur.
Determine if activities are age appropriate for the residents.
Determine the existence of structured and nonstructured activities.
Determine if individual plans of care are available and implemented.
Determine the functional levels of those who reside in settings (e.g., are they ambulatory and is speech encouraged)?
Determine if speech, physical, and occupational therapies are available.
Determine if each person is perceived as unique and distinct and if care is given to residents according to their needs.
Determine if and to what degree official standards of care are met.
Meet with parents of those who reside in special settings to hear their comments, both positive and negative.

NURSING CARE PLAN

The Child with Mental Retardation

NURSING DIAGNOSIS: Altered growth and development related to impaired cognitive functioning

PATIENT GOAL 1: Will achieve optimum growth and development potential

• **NURSING INTERVENTIONS/*RATIONALES***

Involve child and family in an early infant stimulation program *to help maximize child's development*

Assess child's developmental progress at regular intervals; keep detailed records to distinguish subtle changes in functioning *so that plan of care can be revised as needed*

Help family determine child's readiness to learn specific tasks *since readiness may not be easily recognized*

Help family set realistic goals for child *to encourage successful attainment of goals and self-esteem*

Employ positive reinforcement for specific tasks or behaviors *because this improves motivation and learning*

Encourage learning of self-care skills as soon as child achieves readiness

Reinforce self-care activities *to facilitate optimum development*

Encourage family to investigate special daycare programs and educational classes as soon as possible

Emphasize that child has same needs as other children (e.g., play, discipline, social interaction)

Before adolescence, counsel child and parents regarding physical maturation, sexual behavior, marriage, and family

Encourage optimum vocational training

• **EXPECTED OUTCOMES**

Child and family are actively involved in infant stimulation program

Family applies concepts and continues activities in home care of child

Child performs activities of daily living at optimum capacity

Family investigates educational programs

Appropriate limit-setting, recreation, and social opportunities are provided

Adolescent issues are explored as appropriate

PATIENT GOAL 2: Will achieve optimum socialization

• **NURSING INTERVENTIONS/*RATIONALES***

Emphasize that child has same need for socialization as other children

Encourage family to teach child socially acceptable behavior (e.g., saying "hello" and "thank you," manners, appropriate touch)

Encourage grooming and age-appropriate dress *to encourage acceptance by others and self-esteem*

Recommend programs that provide peer relationships and experiences (e.g., mainstreaming, Boy Scouts, Girl Scouts, Special Olympics) *to promote optimum socialization*

Provide adolescent practical sexual information and a well-defined, concrete code of conduct *because child's easy persuasion and lack of judgment may place child at risk*

• **EXPECTED OUTCOMES**

Child behaves in socially acceptable manner

Child has peer relationships and experiences

Child does not experience social isolation

NURSING DIAGNOSIS: Altered family processes related to having a child with MR

PATIENT (FAMILY) GOAL 1: Will receive adequate support

• **NURSING INTERVENTIONS/*RATIONALES***

Inform family as soon as possible at or after birth, *since family may suspect a problem and need immediate support*

Have both parents present at informing conference *to avoid problem of one parent having to relay complex information to the other parent and deal with the initial emotional reaction of the other*

Give family written information about the condition, when possible (e.g., a specific syndrome or disease), *for family to refer to later*

Discuss with family members benefits of home care; allow them opportunities to investigate all residential alternatives before making a decision

Encourage family to meet other families with a similarly affected child *so that they can receive additional support*

Refrain from giving definitive answers about the degree of retardation; stress the potential learning abilities of these children, especially with early intervention, *to encourage hope*

Demonstrate acceptance of child through own behavior *because parents are sensitive to the affective attitude of the professional*

Emphasize normal characteristics of child *to help family see child as an individual with strengths, as well as weaknesses*

Encourage family members to express their feelings and concerns *because this is part of the adaptation process*

• **EXPECTED OUTCOMES**

Family expresses feelings and concerns regarding the birth of a child with MR and its implications

Family members make realistic decisions based on their needs and capabilities

Family members demonstrate acceptance of child

PATIENT (FAMILY) GOAL 2: Will be prepared for long-term care of child

• **NURSING INTERVENTIONS/*RATIONALES***

As child grows older, discuss with parents alternatives to home care, especially as parents near retirement or old age, *so that appropriate long-term care can be provided*

Encourage family to consider respite care as needed *to facilitate family's ability to cope with child's long-term care*

Help family investigate residential settings, *since this may be needed for child's optimum care*

Encourage family to include affected member in planning and to continue meaningful relationships after placement

Refer to agencies that provide support and assistance

• **EXPECTED OUTCOMES**

Family identifies realistic goals for future care of child

Family avails themselves of supportive services

See also Nursing Care Plan: The Child with Chronic Illness or Disability, Chapter 22

tions range from the least to the most restrictive types of environments—foster homes, group residences, semi-independent living programs, and state and private institutions (Sirrocco, 1987). The current trend is toward noninstitutional care settings. Some communities have special vocational or day programs, which allow the individual an opportunity for some measure of gainful employment and the family temporary respite from care.

Care for the Child During Hospitalization. Caring for children with MR during hospitalization is a special challenge to nurses. Frequently nurses are unfamiliar with these children; nurses may cope with their feelings of insecurity and fear by ignoring or isolating the child. Not only is this approach nonsupportive, it may also be destructive for the child's sense of self-esteem and optimum development and may impair the parents' ability to cope with the stress of the experience. To prevent use of this nontherapeutic approach, nurses can use the mutual participation model in planning the child's care. Parents are encouraged to room with their child but should not be made to feel as if the responsibility is totally theirs.

Assessment of the child's abilities and special needs, as well as the family's or other caregiver's successful management techniques, is essential. Ideally the family should make a visit to the hospital before admission. A visit minimizes the unfamiliarity of the hospital setting and is an opportunity for staff members to allay any fears the parents or child may have. When the child is admitted, a detailed history (see Chapter 26) is taken, especially in terms of all self-help activity. During the interview the child's developmental age is assessed.

Questions about the child's abilities are approached positively. For example, rather than asking, "Is your child toilet trained yet?" the nurse may state, "Tell me about your child's toileting habits." The assessment should also focus on any special devices the child uses, effective measures of limit-setting, unusual or favorite routines, and any behaviors that may require intervention. For example, if the parent states that the child engages in self-stimulatory or self-injurious activities, the events that precipitate them and techniques the parents use to manage them are assessed. Once the functional level is known, the child is encouraged to be as independent as possible in the hospital setting.

Procedures are explained to the child using methods of communication that are at the appropriate cognitive level. Generally, explanations should be simple, short, and concrete, emphasizing what the child will *physically* experience. Demonstration either through actual practice or with visual aids is preferable to verbal explanation. The nurse repeats instructions often and evaluates the child's understanding by asking questions—"What did I say it will feel like?" "What will the doctor look like?" "Show me how you must lie," or "Where will the dressing be?" Parents are included in preprocedural teaching of their learning and to help the nurse learn effective methods of communicating with the child.

During hospitalization the nurse should also focus on growth-promoting experiences for the child. For example, hospitalization may be an excellent opportunity to emphasize to parents abilities the child does have but has not had the opportunity to practice, such as self-dressing. It may also be an opportunity for social experiences with peers, group play, or new educational/recreational activities. For example, one child who had had the habit of screaming and kicking demonstrated a definite decrease in these behaviors after learning to pound pegs and use a punching bag. Through social services the parents may become aware of specialized programs for the child. Nutritional counseling is available if the child is overweight or has evidence of specific deficiencies, such as iron deficiency. Hospitalization may also offer parents a respite from everyday care responsibilities and an opportunity to discuss their feelings with a concerned professional.

Assist in Measures to Prevent Retardation. Besides having a responsibility to families of a child with MR, nurses also need to be involved in programs aimed at preventing MR. Many of the familial, social, and environmental factors known to cause mild retardation are preventable. Counseling and education can reduce or eliminate such factors (e.g., poor nutrition, cigarette smoking, and chemical abuse), which also increase the risk of prematurity and intrauterine growth retardation. Consequently, the major interventions are directed at improving maternal health and educating women regarding the dangers of chemicals, including alcohol and nicotine, during pregnancy.

Other preventive strategies include taking part in immunization programs, especially for rubella; ensuring that neonatal screening is done on all newborns in the nurse's care; and helping identify families who may benefit from prenatal testing and genetic counseling.

❖ EVALUATION

The effectiveness of nursing interventions is determined by continual reassessment and evaluation of care based on the following observational guidelines and expected outcomes:

1. Observe techniques used to teach child and their success in accomplishing education; inquire if child is enrolled in early stimulation program.
2. Interview family regarding provision of appropriate socialization, discipline, and play for child; observe child's ability to communicate with others; if possible, interview child regarding feelings of self-worth.
3. Observe those activities of daily living that child can completely or partially perform.
4. Interview family regarding any plans for future care and their awareness of community services.
5. Check patient record for evidence of nursing admission history, especially for self-help activities; observe parent's involvement in child's care; observe social interaction of child and family with other patients.
6. Investigate community programs aimed at preventing retardation and inquire as to nursing involvement in these efforts.

Expected outcomes:
See Nursing Care Plan, p. 1016.

DOWN SYNDROME (DS)

Down syndrome, also known previously by the unacceptable name "mongolism" because of the particular facial charac-

TABLE 24-2 Relation Between Maternal Age and the Estimated Risk of Down Syndrome*

AGE	RISK OF DOWN SYNDROME
20	1/1667
25	1/1250
30	1/952
35	1/385
40	1/106
45	1/30
49	1/11

Modified from D'Alton ME, DeCherney AH: Prenatal diagnosis, *N Engl J Med* 328(2):114-120, 1993.
*Ages are at the expected time of delivery.

teristics that resemble those of the Mongol race, is the most common chromosome abnormality of a generalized syndrome, occurring in 1:800 to 1000 live births. It occurs slightly more often in whites than in blacks, although the incidence is unchanged in various socioeconomic classes (Pueschel, 1992).

Etiology

The cause of DS is not known. A number of theories, including genetic predisposition to nondisjunction, radiation prior to conception, and infection, have been proposed, but none of the hypotheses has been substantiated. Recent reports in cytogenetic and epidemiologic studies support the concept of multiple causality.

Although the etiology is unclear, the cytogenetics of the disorder are well established. Approximately 92% to 95% of all cases of DS are attributable to an extra chromosome 21 (group G), hence the name ***trisomy 21.*** Although children with trisomy 21 are born to parents of all ages, there is a statistically greater risk in older women, particularly those over 35 years of age (Table 24-2). For example, in women 30 years of age the incidence of Down syndrome is about 1 in 1500 live births, but in women age 40 it is about 1 in 100. However, the majority (about 80%) of infants with Down syndrome are born to women under age 35. In about 5% of cases the extra chromosome is from the father (Antonarakis, 1991). Paternal age is a factor.

About 4% to 6% of the cases may be caused by ***translocation of chromosome 21,*** where the third copy of this chromosome is attached to another chromosome. This type of genetic aberration is usually hereditary and is not associated with advanced parental age. From 2% to 3% of affected persons demonstrate ***mosaicism,*** which refers to cells with both normal and abnormal chromosomes. The degree of physical and cognitive impairment is related to the percentage of cells with the abnormal chromosome makeup. (For a discussion of the genetics involved in DS, see Chapter 5.)

Except for mosaicism, the mechanism by which the syndrome occurs has little effect on the characteristics displayed by the affected child and the management of the disorder. However, it is significant for purposes of genetic counseling. Whereas nondisjunction is usually a sporadic event associated with a low risk of recurrence (0.5% to 1%), a translocation is more often hereditary, with a recurrence risk of 10% to 15% if the mother is the carrier and 5% to 8% if the father is the carrier (Vessey, 1992). In DS caused by translocation, testing of the parents is necessary to identify the carrier and offer genetic counseling.

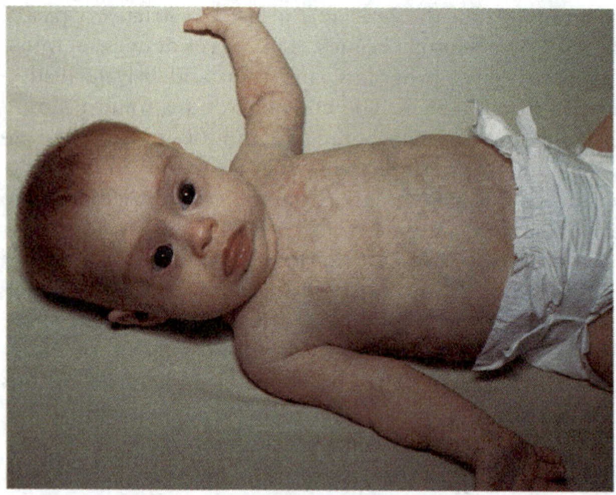

FIG. 24-4 Down syndrome in infant. Note small square head with upward slant to eyes, flat nasal bridge, protruding tongue, mottled skin, and hypotonia.

Clinical Manifestations

DS can usually be diagnosed by the clinical manifestations alone, although no one physical feature is diagnostic (see box on p. 1019 and Fig. 24-4), and there is considerable variation in phenotypic expression. In addition, some infants may have characteristics of DS, such as epicanthal folds, a narrow palate, short broad hands, and a transpalmar crease, but may be cytologically normal. A chromosome analysis is therefore done to confirm the genetic abnormality. The following are other outstanding features of the syndrome:

Intelligence—Varies from severely retarded to low-average intelligence but is generally within the mild to moderate range and may be related to parental intelligence (Pueschel, 1992). Initial development may appear near normal, although slow development, especially in speech, is characteristic and highly variable (see Table 24-3). Although some reports suggest a relative decline in IQ scores during early childhood, followed by a slight increase during adolescence (Carr, 1988), this needs further investigation, with the present emphasis being on early stimulation.

Social development—May be 2 to 3 years beyond the mental age, especially during early childhood. Temperamental characteristics show the same range as those found in unaffected peers, although there is a trend toward the easy-child pattern (Gunn and Perry, 1985).

Congenital anomalies—About 30% to 40% have congenital heart disease (CHD), especially septal defects. Other structural defects include renal agenesis, duodenal atresia, Hirschsprung disease, and tracheoesophageal fistula. Skeletal defects include patella dislocation, hip subluxation, and atlan-

CLINICAL MANIFESTATIONS OF DOWN SYNDROME

HEAD
*Separated sagittal suture
Brachycephaly
Skull rounded and small
Flat occiput
Enlarged anterior fontanel
Sparse hair (variable)

FACE
Flat profile

EYES
*Oblique palpebral fissures (upward, outward slant)
Inner epicanthal folds
Speckling of iris (Brushfield's spots)
Short, sparse eyelashes
Blepharitis

NOSE
*Small
*Depressed nasal bridge (saddle nose)

EARS
Small
Short pinna (vertical ear length)
Overlapping upper helices
Narrow canals

MOUTH
*High, arched, narrow palate
Small osseous orbit
Protruding tongue, may be fissured at lip and furrowed on the surface
Hypoplastic mandible
Downward curve (especially noted when crying)
Mouth kept open

TEETH
Delayed eruption
Alignment abnormalities common

CHEST
Shortened rib cage
12th rib anomalies
Pectus excavatum/carinatum
Microdontia
Periodontal disease

NECK
*Skin excess and lax
Short and broad

ABDOMEN
Protruding
Muscles lax and flabby
Diastasis recti
Umbilical hernia

GENITALIA
Small penis
Cryptorchidism
Bulbous vulva

HANDS
Broad, short
Stubby fingers
Incurved little finger (clinodactyly)
Transverse palmar crease
Characteristic dermal ridge patterns
Distally located axial triradius
Increased ulnar loops on fingers

FEET
*Wide space between big and second toes
*Plantar crease between big and second toes
Broad, stubby, short

MUSCULOSKELETON
*Hyperflexibility
*Muscle weakness
Hypotonia
Atlantoaxial instability

SKIN
Dry, cracked, and frequent fissuring
Cutis marmorata (mottling)

OTHER
Reduced birth weight

*Most common findings (Pueschel, 1992).

toaxial instability (instability of the first and second cervical vertebrae).

Sensory problems—Ocular problems include strabismus, nystagmus, astigmatism, myopia, hyperopia, head tilt, excessive tearing, and cataracts (Caputo and others, 1989). Hearing loss occurs in a large percentage of children with DS. Conductive, mixed, or sensorineural losses each account for approximately one third of the diagnoses (Roizen and others, 1993). Frequent otitis media, narrow canals, and impacted cerumen contribute to the problem.

Other physical disorders—These children have altered immune function, which contributes to numerous other conditions. Respiratory infections are very prevalent; when combined with cardiac anomalies, they are the chief cause of death, particularly during the first year (Declining mortality, 1990). The incidence of leukemia is several times more frequent than expected in the general population, and in about half of the cases the type is acute megakaryoblastic leukemia (Zipursky, Poon, and Doyle, 1992). Thyroid dysfunction, including Grave disease, goiter, chronic lymphocytic thyroiditis, and hypothyroidism, is common. The incidence of persistent primary congenital hypothyroidism has been reported as 30 times more frequent than in the general population (Fort and others, 1984). Acquired thyroid dysfunction also occurs frequently. Acquired cardiac disease, primarily valve dysfunction, has also been reported in adolescents (Geggel, O'Brien, and Feingold, 1993).

Growth—Growth in both height and weight is reduced, but weight gain is more rapid than growth in stature, often resulting in overweight by 36 months of age. Deficient growth rate is most marked during infancy and adolescence. Growth of children with moderate or severe CHD is more affected than those with mild or no CHD (Cronk and others, 1988).

Sexual development—May be delayed, incomplete, or both. Male genitalia may be underdeveloped, as well as secondary sex characteristics such as facial hair. The breast development of females is mild to moderate. Menstruation usually occurs at the average age, and postpubertal women can be fertile; a small number have had offspring, the majority of whom were born with some type of abnormality. Men with DS are infertile.

Therapeutic Management

Although there is no cure for DS, these children may require surgery to correct serious congenital anomalies, and they benefit from regular health care. Evaluation of sight and hearing is essential, and treatment of otitis media is required to prevent auditory loss, which can influence cognitive function (Libb and others, 1985). Neonatal and subsequent periodic testing of thyroid function is recommended. Special growth charts are available to monitor nutrition, height, weight, and general aspects of well-child care

(Cronk and others, 1988). Growth hormone therapy may be considered to increase height. Plastic surgery to alter phenotypic stigma is performed in some cases.

Fifteen percent to 20% of children with DS have atlantoaxial instability. Symptoms of the disorder include neck pain, weakness, and torticollis; however, most affected children are asymptomatic. Children with DS should be screened for atlantoaxial instability after their second birthday and before engaging in physically active exercise or sports or undergoing surgical or rehabilitative procedures (Pueschel, Scola, and Pezzullo, 1992). If children are diagnosed with atlantoaxial instability, surgery may be required, and they should refrain from participating in activities that may involve stress on the head and neck (American Academy of Pediatrics, 1984). If children become symptomatic, they should receive prompt attention, because they are at risk for spinal cord compression.

NURSING ALERT Report immediately any child with the following signs of spinal cord compression:
Persistent neck pain
Loss of established motor skills and bladder/bowel control
Changes in sensation

Prognosis. Life expectancy has improved in recent years but remains lower than that for the general population. Over 80% survive to age 30 years and beyond. Down syndrome is associated with earlier aging, and many individuals have neurologic changes associated with Alzheimer disease (Cooley and Graham, 1991).

Nursing Considerations

This discussion focuses on supporting parents at the time of diagnosis and preventing physical problems in the child. Long-term psychologic interventions for the child and family are discussed in Chapter 22, and decisions for the future are explored earlier in this chapter.

Support Family at Time of Diagnosis. Because of the characteristic facies and other physical characteristics, the infant with DS is usually diagnosed at birth. Generally, parents wish to know the diagnosis as soon as possible. Most parents prefer that both of them be present during the informing interview because it is a problem that both will have to face; they can emotionally support each other, and it eliminates the difficult task of revealing the diagnosis to the other partner.

The parents' responses to the child may greatly influence decisions regarding future care. Whereas some families willingly plan to take the child home, others consider foster care or adoption. The nurse must carefully answer questions regarding developmental potential, since the responses may influence the parents' decision. It is obvious from ranges such as those in Table 24-3 that these children's potential for developmental achievement varies greatly. Therefore it would be inaccurate and unfair to predict the child's intellectual capacity at birth. It is important to stress that a decision regarding placement will affect all of their lives and need not be made at the time of diagnosis. The nurse should emphasize every available source of assistance, such as parent groups, professional guidance, and literature, to help the family learn to live with the child and deal with childrearing problems.*

It may also be helpful for parents to know that studies of families who chose to rear the child at home report many favorable responses. Parental feelings toward the child usually are very positive; parents believe the experience of having this special child makes them stronger and more accepting of others. Behavioral problems among the siblings are similar to those found among families without children with DS, and divorce rates in the DS families are less than those in the general population (Carr, 1988; Cooper, 1989).

Assist Family in Preventing Physical Problems. Many of the physical characteristics of DS present nursing problems. The hypotonicity of muscles and hyperextensibility of joints complicate positioning. The limp, flaccid extremities resemble the posture of a rag doll; as a result, holding the infant is difficult and cumbersome. Sometimes parents perceive this lack of molding to their bodies as evidence of inadequate parenting. The extended body position promotes heat loss because more surface area is exposed to the environment. Parents are encouraged to swaddle or wrap the

TABLE 24-3 Developmental Milestones and Skills in Children with Down Syndrome

	AVERAGE (MONTHS)	RANGE (MONTHS)
MILESTONE		
Smiling	2	1½ to 3
Rolling over	6	2 to 12
Sitting	9	6 to 18
Crawling	11	7 to 21
Creeping	13	8 to 25
Standing	10	10 to 32
Walking	20	12 to 45
Talking, words	14	9 to 30
Talking, sentences	24	18 to 46
SKILL		
Eating		
Finger feeding	12	8 to 28
Using spoon/fork	20	12 to 40
Toilet training		
Bladder	48	20 to 95
Bowel	42	28 to 90
Dressing		
Undressing	40	29 to 72
Putting clothes on	58	38 to 98

From Pueschel SM: The child with Down syndrome. In Levine MD and others, editors: *Developmental behavioral pediatrics,* ed 2, Philadelphia, 1992, WB Saunders, p. 225.

*Sources of information include the **Association for Retarded Citizens of the United States,** 2501 Avenue J, Arlington, TX 76006, (800) 433-5255; **American Association on Mental Retardation,** 1719 Kalorama Rd., N.W., Washington, DC 20009, (202) 387-1968 or (800) 424-3688; the **National Down Syndrome Society,** 141 5th Ave., New York, NY 10011, (800) 221-4602; and the **National Down Syndrome Congress,** 1800 Dempster St., Park Ridge, IL 60068, (708) 823-7550 or (800) 232-6372.

infant tightly in a blanket before picking up the infant to provide security and warmth. The nurse also discusses with parents their feelings concerning attachment to the child, emphasizing that the child's lack of clinging or molding is a physical characteristic, not a sign of detachment or rejection.

Decreased muscle tone compromises respiratory expansion. In addition, the underdeveloped nasal bone causes a chronic problem of inadequate drainage of mucus. The constant stuffy nose forces the child to breathe by mouth, which dries the oropharyngeal membranes, increasing the susceptibility to upper respiratory tract and ear infections. Measures to lessen infection include clearing the nose with a bulb-type syringe,* rinsing the mouth with water after feedings, increasing fluid intake and using a cool-mist vaporizer to keep the mucous membranes moist and the nasal secretions liquefied, changing the child's position frequently, performing postural drainage and percussion if necessary, practicing good handwashing technique, and properly disposing of soiled articles, such as tissues (Steele and others, 1989). If antibiotics are ordered, the importance of completing the full course of therapy for successful eradication of the infection and prevention of growth of resistant organisms is stressed. Since hearing impairment is common and can interfere with development, the nurse should stress to parents the importance of auditory testing.

The large, protruding tongue and hypotonia also interfere with feeding, including breast-feeding, bottle-feeding, and introduction of solid foods. Parents need to know that the tongue thrust does not indicate refusal to feed but is a physiologic response. Parents are advised to use a small but long, straight-handled spoon to push the food toward the back and side of the mouth. If food is thrust out, it is refed. At times the family may require the assistance of a specially trained individual, such as a lactation expert or occupational therapist, to guide them in dealing with feeding problems.

Dietary intake needs supervision. Decreased muscle tone affects gastric motility, predisposing the child to constipation. Dietary measures such as increased fiber and fluid promote evacuation. The child's eating habits need careful monitoring to prevent obesity. Height and weight measurements should be obtained and plotted on specialized growth charts (Cronk and others, 1988) on a serial basis, especially during infancy, since excessive weight gain can impede motor development. The child receives calories in accordance with height and weight, not chronologic age.

During infancy the child's skin is pliable and soft. However, it gradually becomes rough and dry and is prone to cracking and infection. Skin care involves the use of minimum soap and application of lubricants. Lip balm is applied to the lips, especially when the child is outdoors, to prevent excessive chapping.

Promote Child's Developmental Progress. The hypotonicity affects muscular development. Supporting skills, such as rolling over, sitting up, standing, or pulling oneself to a sitting or standing position, may be delayed. These children should be involved in an early stimulation program that provides physical therapy to help them learn motor skills.

At regular intervals the child's developmental progress is assessed to ensure therapeutic adherence to a stimulation program. Developmental screening tests are inappropriate to evaluate indices of progress such as increased strength, balance, coordination, or muscle tone. Therefore, detailed written records of the child's motor abilities can be kept in order to distinguish subtle changes in functioning, as well as periodic formal testing.

The parents are encouraged to investigate special daycare programs for the child as soon as possible. They should also investigate the public school system for special education classes, including infant stimulation programs and preschools (see Critical Thinking Exercise box.) In essence, the same childrearing goals established for normal children are pursued for these children, with attention given to preventing the problems of overprotection and including family members, especially the father and siblings, in the caring role.

Assist in Prenatal Diagnosis and Genetic Counseling. Prenatal diagnosis of DS is possible through chorionic villus sampling and amniocentesis, since chromosome analysis of fetal cells can detect the presence of trisomy or translocation. However, sporadic cases in young women will not be identified when there is no indication for prenatal testing. However, testing for low maternal serum α–fetoprotein, high chorionic gonadotropin, and low unconjugated estriol levels may identify affected young women, who can then undergo amniocentesis (American Academy of Pediatrics, 1989; Haddow and others, 1992). There is also evidence that ultrasonography can detect anatomic peculiarities of DS (thickened nuchal fold and short femur

CRITICAL THINKING EXERCISE

Down Syndrome

Johanna, an 8-year-old with Down syndrome, has been mainstreamed into a regular second grade class. Johanna's teacher thinks Johanna is a behavior problem because she frequently leaves her seat in the back of the room, comes to the front, and then sits quietly on the floor. As the school nurse, you know that a likely explanation for this behavior is:

1. The class content is too advanced for Johanna, and she is bored.
2. Johanna is socially retarded, and she cannot be expected to behave like other children her age.
3. Johanna is having trouble hearing or seeing.
4. Johanna wants extra attention.

The correct answer is 3. Children with Down syndrome frequently have vision and hearing problems. Johanna's behavior suggests that she cannot see or hear what is happening in the class. The other answers are incorrect because Johanna's movement about the classroom is neither persistent nor disruptive. The nurse should do hearing and vision screening on Johanna as soon as possible.

*Home care instructions for using a bulb syringe are available in *Wong and Whaley's Clinical Manual of Pediatric Nursing* (Mosby).

length), with subsequent testing to confirm the diagnosis (Benzcerraf, Gelman, and Frigoletto, 1987).

The nurse's role in genetic counseling of women who are of advanced maternal age or who have a family history of DS includes discussing prenatal testing. If the fetus is affected, the nurse must allow the parents to express their feelings concerning elective abortion and support their decision to terminate or proceed with the pregnancy. (See also Nursing Care Plan: The Child with Down Syndrome.*)

FRAGILE X SYNDROME†

Fragile X syndrome is the most common inherited cause of MR and the second most common genetic cause of MR after DS. It has been described in all ethnic groups and races; the incidence of affected males is 1 in 1250; 1 in 2000 females are affected, and 1 in 700 females are carriers. Because its identification as a disorder is relatively new, many health professionals and educators lack the necessary familiarity with the manifestations for appropriate referral and management once it is diagnosed.

The syndrome is caused by an abnormal gene on the lower end of the long arm of the X chromosome. Chromosome analysis may demonstrate a fragile site (a region that fails to condense during mitosis and is characterized by a nonstaining gap or narrowing) in the cells of affected males and females and in carrier females. Since 1991, however, direct DNA analysis for the gene mutation causing fragile X syndrome has greatly increased the diagnostic accuracy of both affected and carrier individuals, as well as permitted prenatal diagnosis (Warren and Nelson, 1994). However, mentally impaired individuals without an established family history of fragile X are being evaluated; cytogenetic and DNA studies should be performed to rule out another chromosome abnormality as the cause of mental impairment (Cronister and Jacky, 1992).

This fragile site has been determined to be caused by a gene mutation that results in excessive repeats of nucleotide base pairs in a specific DNA segment of the X chromosome. The number of repeats in a normal individual is between 6 and 52. An individual with 50 to 200 base pair repeats is said to have a ***premutation*** and is therefore a carrier. When passed from a parent to a child, these base pair repeats can expand from 200 to 2000 or more, which is termed a ***full mutation.*** This expansion only occurs when a carrier mother passes the mutation to her offspring; it does not occur when a carrier father passes the mutation to his daughters. Male individuals with a full mutation are usually affected (80%) (i.e., have the physical and behavioral features and mental impairment); however, only 30% of females with a full mutation are affected. Interestingly, even females with a full mutation who do not appear to be affected, as well as carrier males and females with normal intelligence, may exhibit some learning disabilities and psychosocial disorders. These are only some of the features of this unusual disorder, which has been termed X-linked dominant with reduced penetrance. It is in distinct contrast to the classic X-linked recessive pattern where all carrier females are normal, all affected males have symptoms of the disorder, and no males are carriers. Consequently, genetic counseling of affected families is more complex than that for families with a classic X-linked disorder, such as hemophilia. Prenatal diagnosis of the fragile X gene mutation is not possible with direct DNA testing in a family with an established history, by amniocentesis or chorionic villus sampling (Brown and others, 1993).

CLINICAL MANIFESTATIONS OF FRAGILE X SYNDROME

PHYSICAL FEATURES

Long, wide, and/or protruding ears
Long, narrow face, with prominent jaw
In postpubertal males, enlarged testicles
Long palpebral fissures
High, arched palate
Strabismus
Increased head circumference
Mitral valve prolapse/aortic root dilation
Hypotonia
Hyperextensible finger joints
Transpalmar crease
Pes planus (flat feet)

BEHAVIORAL FEATURES

Mild to severe MR (occasional normal IQ with learning disabilities)
Speech delay; speech may be rapid, with stuttering and repetition of words
Short attention span, hyperactivity
Mouthing beyond expected age for behavior
Hypersensitivity to taste, sounds, touch
Intolerance to change in routine
Autistic-like behaviors
May exhibit aggressive behavior

Clinical Manifestations

The classic trend of physical findings in adult males with fragile X syndrome consists of a long face with a prominent jaw (prognathism); large, protruding ears, and large testes (macro-orchidism). However, in prepubertal children (Fig. 24-5) these features may be less obvious, and behavioral manifestations may initially suggest the diagnosis (see box above). In one study developmental delay was noted in all the children, with language delay seen in 95% of the subjects (Simko and others, 1989). The syndrome is strongly associated with autism; autistic-like behavior (e.g., rocking, talking to self, spinning, hand flapping, hand biting, poor eye contact, echolalia) is seen in many affected males, and males with autism may be positive for the fragile X chromosome (Chudley and Hagerman, 1987). Affected individuals tend to be strong in social skills and adaptive behavior, which means they may function or appear to function at a higher level than their IQ scores would predict.

In carrier females the clinical manifestations are extremely varied. Carrier and affected females may exhibit psychosocial deficits such as anxiety, withdrawal, and de-

*In *Wong and Whaley's Clinical Manual of Pediatric Nursing* (Mosby).
†Donna Phillips Smith, RN, MS, revised this section.

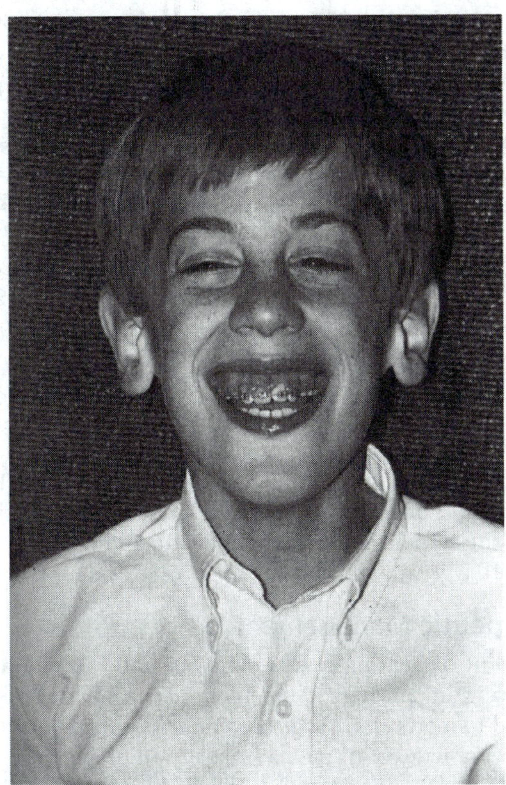

FIG. 24-5 Prepubertal fragile X male. (From Silverman AC, Hagerman RJ: Fragile X syndrome. In Jackson PL, Vessey JA: *Primary care of the child with a chronic condition,* St Louis, 1992, Mosby.)

pression (Freund, Reiss, and Abrams, 1993). Both affected sexes are fertile and therefore capable of transmitting the fragile X disorder.

Therapeutic Management

There is no cure for fragile X syndrome. Medical treatment may include the use of phenothiazines to control violent temper outbursts and central nervous system (CNS) stimulants to improve attention span and decrease hyperactivity. The use of folic acid, which affects the metabolism of CNS transmitters, is controversial.

All affected children require early speech and language therapy, occupational therapy to improve sensory integration, and special education assistance. Without appropriate intervention, progressive decline in IQ can occur (Chudley and Hagerman, 1987). Children with fragile X syndrome mimic the behavior of other children; therefore mainstreaming them with normal children may improve their behavior.

Prognosis. Individuals with fragile X syndrome are expected to live a normal life span. Their cognitive impairment may be ameliorated by behavioral and educational interventions.

Nursing Considerations

Since cognitive impairment is a fairly consistent finding in individuals with fragile X syndrome, the care afforded to these families is the same as for any child with MR. Because the disorder is hereditary, genetic counseling is necessary to inform parents and siblings of the risks of transmission. In addition, any male or female with unexplained or nonspecific mental impairment should be referred for chromosome analysis and DNA testing, as well as appropriate genetic counseling. Families with a member affected by the disorder should be referred to the **National Fragile X Foundation.***

SENSORY IMPAIRMENT

HEARING IMPAIRMENT

Hearing impairment is one of the most common disabilities in the United States. An estimated 1 in 1000 infants are born deaf. For infants admitted to the neonatal intensive care unit, the incidence rises sharply to approximately 1 to 3 per 100 neonates (National Institutes of Health, 1993). There are about 1 million hearing-impaired children ranging in age from birth to 21 years in the United States, and almost a third of these children have other disabilities, such as visual or cognitive deficits.

Definition and Classification

Hearing impairment is a general term indicating disability that may range in severity from mild to profound and includes the subsets of deaf and hard-of-hearing. ***Deaf*** refers to a person whose hearing disability precludes successful processing of linguistic information through audition, with or without a hearing aid. ***Hard-of-hearing*** refers to a person who, generally with the use of a hearing aid, has residual hearing sufficient to enable successful processing of linguistic information through audition. Other terms, such as "deaf and dumb," "mute," or "deaf-mute," are unacceptable. Hearing-impaired persons are not "dumb" and, if mute, have no physical speech defect other than that caused by the inability to hear.

Hearing defects may be classified according to etiology, pathology, or symptom severity. Each is important in terms of treatment, possible prevention, and rehabilitation.

Etiology. Hearing loss may be caused by a number of prenatal and postnatal conditions. These include a family history of childhood hearing impairment, anatomic malformations of the head or neck, low birth weight, severe perinatal asphyxia, perinatal infection (cytomegalovirus, rubella, herpes, syphilis, toxoplasmosis, and bacterial meningitis), chronic ear infection, cerebral palsy, Down syndrome, or administration of ototoxic drugs.

In addition, high-risk neonates who are surviving formerly fatal prenatal or perinatal conditions may be susceptible to hearing loss from the disorder or its treatment. For example, sensorineural hearing loss may be a result of continuous humming noises or high noise levels associated with incubators, oxygen hoods, or intensive care units, especially when combined with the use of potentially ototoxic antibiotics.

*1441 York St., Suite 215, Denver, CO 80206; (800) 688-8765 or (303) 333-6155.

Environmental noise is a special concern. Sounds loud enough to damage sensitive hair cells of the inner ear can produce irreversible hearing loss. Very loud, brief noise, such as gunfire, can cause immediate, severe, and permanent loss of hearing. Longer exposure to less intense but still hazardous sounds can also produce hearing loss (Consensus Conference, 1990). The exact sound level that produces hearing loss is unknown. As a general rule, sound appreciably louder than conversational speech is potentially harmful if the sound persists for a sufficient time.

Pathology. Disorders of hearing are divided according to location of the defect. ***Conductive*** or ***middle-ear hearing loss*** results from interference of transmission of sound to the middle ear. It is the most common of all types of hearing loss and most frequently is a result of recurrent serous otitis media. Conductive hearing impairment mainly involves interference with loudness of sound.

Sensorineural hearing loss, also called ***perceptive*** or ***nerve deafness,*** involves damage to the inner ear structures and/or the auditory nerve. The most common causes are congenital defects of inner ear structures or consequences of acquired conditions, such as bilirubin encephalopathy (kernicterus), infection, administration of ototoxic drugs, or exposure to excessive noise. Sensorineural hearing loss results in distortion of sound and problems in discrimination. Although the child hears some of everything going on around him or her, the sounds are distorted, severely affecting discrimination and comprehension. Ototoxic drugs cause hearing loss initially in high-frequency ranges that may not be detected by audiometry (Fausti and others, 1993).

Mixed conductive-sensorineural hearing loss results from interference with transmission of sound in the middle ear and along neural pathways. It frequently results from recurrent otitis media and its complications.

Central auditory imperception includes all hearing losses that do not demonstrate defects in the conductive or sensorineural structures. They are usually divided into organic or functional losses. In the ***organic type*** of central auditory imperception, the defect involves the reception of auditory stimuli along the central pathways and the expression of the message into meaningful communication. Examples are ***aphasia,*** an inability to express ideas in any form, either written or verbally; ***agnosia,*** the inability to interpret sound correctly; and ***dysacusis,*** difficulty in processing details or in discriminating among sounds.

In the ***functional type*** of hearing loss there is no organic lesion to explain a central auditory loss. Examples of functional hearing loss are conversion hysteria (an unconscious withdrawal from hearing to block remembrance of a traumatic event), infantile autism, and childhood schizophrenia.

Symptom Severity. Hearing impairment is expressed in terms of a ***decibel (dB),*** a unit of loudness (Table 24-4); it is measured at various frequencies, such as 500, 1000, and 2000 cycles per second, the critical listening speech range. Hearing impairment can be classified according to hearing-threshold level (the measurement of an individual's hearing threshold by means of an audiometer) and the degree of symptom severity as it affects speech (Table 24-5). These classifications offer only general guidelines regarding the effect of the impairment on any individual child, since children differ greatly in their ability to use residual hearing.

Therapeutic Management

Treatment of hearing loss depends on the cause and type of hearing impairment. Many conductive hearing defects respond to medical or surgical treatment, such as antibiotic therapy for acute otitis media or insertion of tympanostomy tubes for chronic otitis media. When the conductive loss is permanent, hearing can be improved with the use of a hearing aid to amplify sound.

Treatment for sensorineural hearing loss is much less satisfactory. Since the defect is not one of intensity of sound,

TABLE 24-4 Intensity of Sounds Expressed in Decibels

DECIBELS (DB)	REPRESENTATIVE SOUND
0	Softest sound normal ear can hear
10	Heartbeat, rustling of leaves
20	Whisper at 1.8 m (5 feet)
30-45	Normal conversation
60	Noise in average restaurant
70-80	Street noises
80	Loud radio in home
90-100	Train
120	Thunder, rock music
140	Jet airplane during departure
>140	Pain threshold

TABLE 24-5 Classification of Hearing Loss Based on Symptom Severity

HEARING LEVEL (DB)	EFFECT
Slight—<30 (hard of hearing)	Has difficulty hearing faint or distant speech Usually is unaware of hearing difficulty Likely to achieve in school but may have problems No speech defects
Mild—30-55 (hard of hearing)	Understands conversational speech at 3 to 5 feet but has difficulty if speech is faint or if not facing speaker May have speech difficulties
Moderate—55-70 (hard of hearing)	Unable to understand conversational speech unless loud Considerable difficulty with group or classroom discussion Requires special speech training
Profound—70-90 (deaf)	May hear a loud voice if nearby May be able to identify loud environmental noises Can distinguish vowels but not most consonants Requires speech training
Extreme—>90 (deaf)	May hear only loud sounds Requires extensive speech training

hearing aids are of less value in this type of defect. The use of cochlear implants (a surgically implanted prosthetic device) provides hope for some affected children. These implants use electrical stimulation to provide hearing and have proved to be effective in improving auditory discrimination and speech production skills in children who are profoundly deaf (Keveton and Balkany, 1991).

Disorders of central auditory imperception depend on the cause. Functional types, such as conversion hysteria, may require psychologic intervention, but others, such as autism, may not respond to any therapy.

Nursing Considerations

Tactile devices are another option for the profoundly deaf to improve their speech perception. A vibrotactile or electrotactile signal is used to transmit impulses to a point of stimulation, usually the fingers or hands. This information is then transmitted to the language-processing center in the brain (Sarant and others, 1993).

❖ Assessment

Assessment of children for hearing impairment is a critical nursing responsibility. Discovery of a hearing impairment within the first 6 to 12 months of life is essential to prevent social, physical, and psychologic damage to the child. Assessment involves (1) identifying those children who by virtue of their history are at risk (see box at right), (2) observing for behaviors that indicate a hearing loss, and (3) screening all children for auditory function. This discussion focuses on developmental/behavioral indices associated with hearing impairment. Auditory testing is presented in Chapter 7. There is controversy about who should be assessed and when they should be assessed. The National Institutes of Health (NIH) (1993) recommends that all infants who are admitted to the NICU be screened before discharge and that universal screening be implemented for all infants before age 3 months. Other specialists disagree, stating that universal screening can be complex, expensive, and not necessarily justified (Bess and Paradise, 1994). Wide variations in practice currently exist throughout the country.

Infancy. At birth the nurse can observe the neonate's response to auditory stimuli as evidenced by the startle reflex, head turning, eye blinking, and cessation of body movement. The infant may vary in the intensity of the response, depending on the state of alertness. However, a consistent absence of a reaction should lead to suspicion of hearing loss. Other clinical manifestations of hearing impairment in the infant are summarized in the box on p. 1026.

Childhood. The profoundly deaf child is much more likely to be diagnosed during infancy than the less severely affected one. If the defect is not detected during early childhood, the likelihood is that it will surface during entry into school, when the child has difficulty in learning. Unfortunately, some of these children are erroneously placed in special classes for students with learning disabilities or mental retardation. Therefore it is essential that the nurse suspect a hearing impairment in any child who demonstrates the behaviors listed in the box.

RISK CRITERIA FOR SENSORINEURAL HEARING IMPAIRMENT IN YOUNG CHILDREN

NEONATES (BIRTH TO 28 DAYS)

1. Family history of congenital or delayed-onset childhood sensorineural impairment
2. Congenital infection known or suspected to be associated with sensorineural hearing impairment such as toxoplasmosis, syphilis, rubella, cytomegalovirus, and herpes
3. Craniofacial anomalies including morphologic abnormalities of the pinna and ear canal, absent philtrum, low hairline, etc.
4. Birth weight less than 1500 g (<3.3 pounds)
5. Hyperbilirubinemia at a level exceeding indication for exchange transfusion
6. Ototoxic medications including but not limited to the aminoglycosides used for more than 5 days (e.g., gentamicin, tobramycin, kanamycin, streptomycin), and loop diuretics used in combination with aminoglycosides
7. Bacterial meningitis
8. Severe depression at birth, which may include infants with Apgar scores of 0 to 3 at 5 minutes and those who fail to initiate spontaneous respiration by 10 minutes or those with hypotonia persisting to 2 hours of age
9. Prolonged mechanical ventilation for a duration equal to or greater than 10 days (e.g., persistent pulmonary hypertension)
10. Stigmata or other findings associated with a syndrome known to include sensorineural hearing loss (e.g., Waardenburg or Usher syndrome)

RISK CRITERIA: INFANTS (29 DAYS TO 2 YEARS)

1. Parent/caregiver concern regarding hearing, speech, language, and/or developmental delay
2. Bacterial meningitis
3. Neonatal risk factors that may be associated with progressive sensorineural hearing loss (e.g., cytomegalovirus, prolonged mechanical ventilation, and inherited disorders)
4. Head trauma, especially with either longitudinal or transverse fracture of the temporal bone
5. Stigmata or other findings associated with syndromes known to include sensorineural hearing loss (e.g., Waardenburg or Usher syndrome)
6. Ototoxic medications including but not limited to the aminoglycosides used for more than 5 days (e.g., gentamicin, tobramycin, kanamycin, streptomycin) and loop diuretics used in combination with aminoglycosides
7. Children with neurodegenerative disorders such as neurofibromatosis, myoclonic epilepsy, Werdnig-Hoffmann disease, Tay-Sachs disease, Niemann-Pick disease, any metachromatic leukodystrophy, or any infantile demyelinating neuropathy
8. Childhood infectious diseases known to be associated with sensorineural hearing loss (e.g., mumps, measles)

From American Speech-Language Hearing Association: Joint Committee on Infant Hearing 1990 position statement, *ASHA* 33(suppl 5):3-6, 1991.

Of primary importance is the effect of hearing impairment on speech development. A child with a mild conductive hearing loss may speak fairly clearly but in a loud, monotone voice. A child with a sensorineural defect usually has difficulty in articulation. For example, inability to

CLINICAL MANIFESTATIONS OF HEARING IMPAIRMENT

INFANTS

Lack of startle or blink reflex to a loud sound
Failure to be awakened by loud environmental noises
Failure to localize a source of sound by 6 months of age
Absence of babble or inflections in voice by age 7 months
General indifference to sound
Lack of response to the spoken word; failure to follow verbal directions
Response to loud noises as opposed to the voice

CHILDREN

Use of gestures rather than verbalization to express desires, especially after age 15 months
Failure to develop intelligible speech by age 24 months
Monotone quality, unintelligible speech, lessened laughter
Vocal play, head banging, or foot stamping for vibratory sensation
Yelling or screeching to express pleasure, annoyance (tantrums), or need
Asking to have statements repeated or answering them incorrectly
Responding more to facial expression and gestures than verbal explanation
Avoidance of social interaction; often puzzled and unhappy in such situations; prefer to play alone
Inquiring, sometimes confused facial expression
Suspicious alertness, sometimes interpreted as paranoia, alternating with cooperation
Frequently stubborn because of lack of comprehension
Irritable at not making themselves understood
Shy, timid, and withdrawn
Often appear "dreamy," "in a world of their own," or markedly inattentive

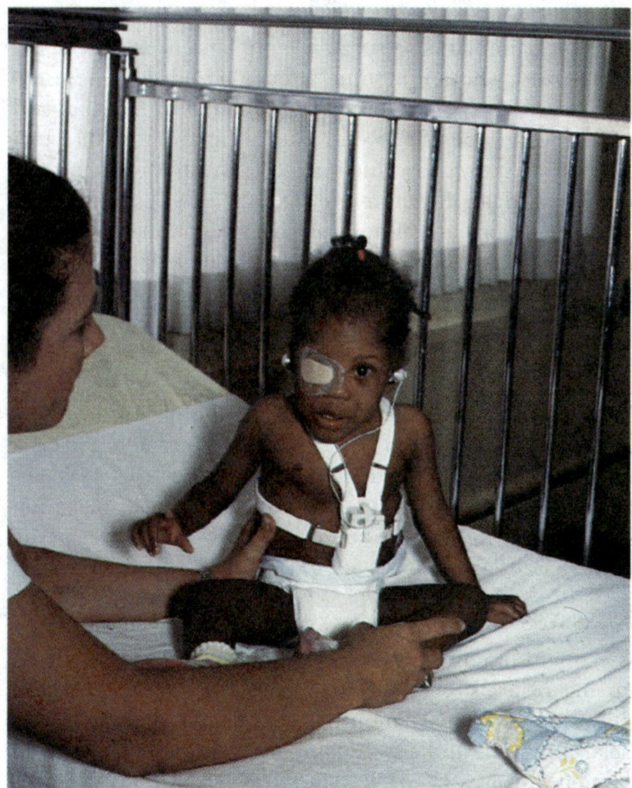

FIG. 24-6 On-the-body hearing aids are convenient for young children, such as this child with severe bilateral hearing loss. Note eye patching for strabismus.

hear higher frequencies may result in the word "spoon" being pronounced "poon." Children with articulation problems need to have their hearing tested.

NURSING ALERT When parents express concern about their child's hearing and speech development, refer the child for a hearing evaluation. Absence of well-formed syllables ("da," "na," "yaya") by 11 months of age should result in immediate referral (Eilers and Oller, 1994).

❖ NURSING DIAGNOSES

A number of nursing diagnoses are prominent in the nursing care of the child with hearing impairment and the child's family; other diagnoses specific to individual cases become evident. The most common nursing diagnoses are outlined in the Nursing Care Plan on pp. 1029-1030.

❖ PLANNING

The goals for the child with hearing impairment and the family are as follows:

1. Child will achieve optimum development through enhancement of the communication process and socialization.
2. Child and family will receive support.
3. Child will receive appropriate care during hospitalization.
4. An important nursing goal is to assist in measures to prevent hearing impairment.

❖ IMPLEMENTATION

Promote Communication Process. The nurse's initial role in rehabilitation is to encourage the family to participate in an auditory training program.* Rehabilitation training consists of using a hearing aid and learning lipreading (speech reading), sign language, and/or verbal communication.

Hearing aids. The nurse should be familiar with the types, basic care, and handling of hearing aids, especially when the child is hospitalized.† Types of aids include those worn in or behind the ear, models that are incorporated into an eyeglass frame, or types worn on the body with a wire connection to the ear (Fig. 24-6). One of the most common problems with a hearing aid is ***acoustic feedback,*** an an-

*Home training correspondence programs are sponsored by the **John T. Tracy Clinic,** 806 West Adams Blvd., Los Angeles, CA 90007; (213) 748-5481 or (800) 522-4582. Other sources of information on several aspects of hearing loss and on the International Parents' Organization are the **Alexander Graham Bell Association for the Deaf,** 3417 Volta Place, N.W., Washington, DC 20007, (202) 337-5220; and the **Canadian Hearing Society,** 271 Spadina Rd., Toronto, Ontario M5R 2V3, (416) 964-9595 or (800) 463-4327.

†Information about hearing aids is available from the **National Hearing Aid Society,** 20361 Middlebelt Rd., Livonia, MI 48152; (800) 521-5247 or (313) 478-2610 (in Michigan).

noying whistling sound usually caused by improper fit of the ear mold. Sometimes the whistling may be at a frequency that the child cannot hear but that is annoying to others. In this case, if children are old enough, they are told of the noise and asked to readjust the aid.

➤ **NURSING TIP** To reduce or eliminate whistling from a hearing aid, try reinserting the aid, making certain that no hair is caught between the ear mold and canal, cleaning the ear mold or ear, or lowering the volume of the aid.

As children grow older, they may be self-conscious about the device. Every effort is made to make the aid inconspicuous, such as an appropriate hairstyle to cover behind-the-ear or in-the-ear models, attractive frames for glasses, and placement of the on-the-body type where it is not seen, such as under a blouse or sweater. Children are given responsibility for the care of the device as soon as they are able, since fostering independence is a primary goal of rehabilitation.

NURSING ALERT Stress to parents the importance of storing batteries for hearing aids in a safe location out of reach of children and of teaching children (or supervising young children) not to remove the battery from the hearing aid. Batteries ingested are most often those from hearing aids, including the child's own aid (Litovitz and Schmitz, 1992).

Lipreading. Even though the child may become an expert at lipreading, only about 40% of the spoken word is understood, and less if the speaker has an accent, mustache, or beard. Exaggerating pronunciation or speaking in an altered rhythm further lessens comprehension. Parents can help the child understand the spoken word by using the suggestions in the Guidelines box. The child learns to supplement the spoken word with sensitivity to visual cues, primarily body language and facial expression (e.g., tightening the lips, muscle tension, and eye contact).

Sign language. Sign language, such as American Sign Language (ASL), Signed Exact English (SEE), or British Sign Language (BSL), is a visual-gestural language that uses hand signals that roughly correspond to specific words and concepts in the English language. Family members are encouraged to learn signing because using or watching hands requires much less concentration than lipreading or talking. Also, a symbol method enables some deaf children to learn more and to learn faster.

Cued speech. This method of communication is an adjunct to straight lipreading. It uses hand signals to help the hearing-impaired child distinguish between words that look alike when formed by the lips (e.g., "mat," "bat"). It is most commonly used by hearing-impaired children who are using speech rather than those who are nonverbal.

Speech therapy. The most formidable task in the education of a deaf child is learning to speak. Speech is learned through a multisensory approach, using visual, tactile, kinesthetic, and auditory stimulation. Since the usual mechanism for learning language (imitation and reinforcement) is not available to the deaf child, systematic formal education is required. Parents are encouraged to participate fully in the learning process.

Additional aids. Everyday activities present problems

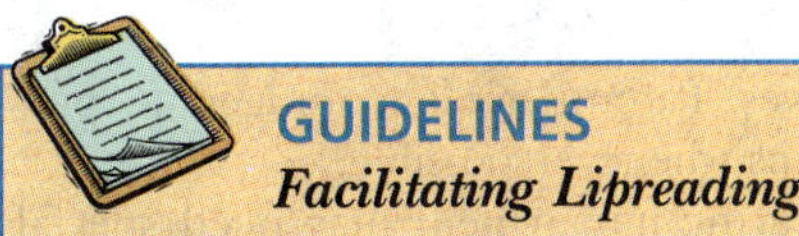

GUIDELINES
Facilitating Lipreading

Attract child's attention before speaking; use light touch to signal speaker's presence.
Stand close to child.
Face child directly or move to a 45-degree angle.
Stand still; do not walk back and forth or turn away to point or look elsewhere.
Establish eye contact and show interest.
Speak at eye level and with good lighting on speaker's face.
Be certain nothing interferes with speech patterns, such as chewing food or gum.
Speak clearly and at a slow and even rate.
Use facial expression to assist in conveying messages.
Keep sentences short.
Rephrase message if child does not understand the words.

for older children with hearing impairment. For example, they may not be able to hear the telephone, doorbell, or alarm clock. Several commercial devices are available to help them adjust to these dilemmas. Flashing lights can be attached to a telephone or doorbell to signal its ringing. Trained hearing ear dogs can provide great assistance to deaf individuals because they alert the person to sounds, such as someone approaching, a moving car, a signal to wake up, or a child's cry. Special teletypewriters or ***telecommunications devices for the deaf (TDD)*** help deaf people communicate with each other over the telephone; the typed message is conveyed via the telephone lines and displayed on a small screen.*

Any audiovisual medium presents dilemmas for these children, who can see the picture but cannot hear the message. However, with ***closed captioning,*** a special decoding device is attached to the television, and the audio portion of a program is translated into subtitles that appear on the screen.†

As deaf children learn to compensate for their lack of hearing, they become extremely perceptive to visual and vibratory changes. They often know when another person wishes to talk to them because the person will walk close by but not pass. They learn to be alert to other people approaching them by seeing their shadows or feeling the vibrations of their footsteps. They are acutely aware of facial expressions and may comprehend the unspoken word more quickly than the spoken word.

Socialization. Since socialization is extremely important to the child's development, the nurse discusses with the family methods of fostering social contact. If children attend a special school for the deaf, they are able to socialize with peers in that setting. Classmates become a potential source of close friendships because they communicate more

*Directory listings stating "TDD only" before a phone number indicate that regular telephone use is not possible; "TDD and voice" indicates that both TDD users and speaking/hearing people can use the telephone number.
†Additional information is available from the **National Captioning Institute, Inc.,** 5203 Leesburg Pike, Suite 1500, Falls Church, VA 22041; (703) 845-1992 or (703) 998-2400 (TDD Voice).

easily among themselves. Parents are encouraged to promote these relationships whenever possible.

Children with a hearing impairment may need special help in school or social activities. For those children wearing hearing aids, background noise should be kept to a minimum. Since many of these children are able to attend regular classes, the teacher may need assistance in adapting methods of teaching for the child's benefit. The school nurse is often in an optimum position to emphasize methods of facilitated communication, such as lipreading (see Guidelines box on p. 1027). Since group projects and audiovisual teaching aids may hinder the deaf child's learning, these educational methods should be carefully evaluated.

In a group setting, it is helpful for the other members to sit in a semicircle in front of the child. Since one of the difficulties in following a group discussion is that the deaf child is unaware of who will speak next, someone should point out each speaker. Speakers can also be given numbers, or their names can be written down as each person talks. If one person writes down the main topic of the discussion, the child is able to follow lipreading more closely. Such suggestions can increase the child's ability to participate in sports, clubs such as Boy Scouts or Girl Scouts, and group projects.

Support Child and Family. Once the diagnosis of hearing impairment is made, parents need extensive support to adjust to the shock of learning about their child's disability and an opportunity to realize the extent of the hearing loss. If the hearing loss occurs during childhood, the child also requires sensitive, supportive care during the long and often difficult adjustment to this sensory loss. Early rehabilitation is one of the best strategies for fostering adjustment. However, progress in learning communication may not always coincide with emotional adjustment. Depression or anger is common, and such feelings are a normal part of the grieving process. If possible, it may be helpful for the family to be involved in a parent support group. Such groups are often very helpful because other parents have dealt with the same issues and can offer practical advice and emotional support. (See also Chapter 22 for an extensive discussion of the emotional support of the child and family.)

Care for Child During Hospitalization. The needs of the hospitalized deaf child are the same as those of any other child, but the disability presents special challenges to the nurse (see Critical Thinking Exercise box). For example, verbal explanations must be supplemented with tactile and visual aids, such as books or actual demonstration and practice. Children's understanding of the explanation needs to be constantly reassessed. If their verbal skills are poorly developed, they can answer questions through drawing, writing, or gesturing. For example, if the nurse is attempting to clarify where a spinal tap is done, the child is asked to point to where the procedure will be done on the body. Since deaf children often need more time to grasp the full meaning of an explanation, the nurse needs to be patient, allowing ample time for understanding.

When communicating with the child, the nurse should use the same principles as those outlined for facilitating lipreading. Ideally nurses without foreign accents should be assigned to the child. The child's hearing aid is checked to ensure that it is working properly. If it is necessary to awaken the child at night, the nurse needs to remember that the child will not have the hearing aid on. To communicate, the child should place the device in the ear or use gestures. The nurse always makes sure that the child can see him or her before any procedures, even routine ones such as changing a diaper or regulating an infusion, are performed. It is important to remember that the child may not be aware of one's presence until alerted through visual or tactile cues.

Ideally parents are encouraged to room with the child. However, it must be conveyed to them that this is not to serve as a convenience to the nurse but as a benefit to the child. Although the parents' aid can be enlisted in familiarizing the child with the hospital and explaining procedures, the nurse also talks directly to the youngster, encouraging expression of feelings about the experience. If there is difficulty in understanding the child's speech, an effort is made to become familiar with his or her pronunciation of words. Parents often can be helpful by explaining the child's usual speech habits. Nonvocal communication devices that employ pictures or words that the child can point

CRITICAL THINKING EXERCISE

Hearing Impairment

Five-year-old Jason has a severe congenital hearing impairment. You have been assigned to care for him in the day surgery postanesthesia care unit (PACU), where he has just been admitted following a herniorrhaphy. As he emerges from anesthesia, he becomes more and more agitated. The most likely cause for his behavior is:

1. This is a normal reaction to anesthesia.
2. He is experiencing separation anxiety.
3. He is unable to communicate properly.
4. He is in pain.

The correct answer is 3. Because Jason became increasingly more agitated as he emerged from anesthesia, his behavior does not suggest the transitory confusion associated with the initial emergence from anesthesia. Rather, it suggests that as he became more aware of his surroundings and tried to communicate with the staff, Jason became increasingly frustrated. Reasons for this might include (a) not having his hearing aid in place; (b) having his arms restrained by IV's, pulse oximetry monitors, and a blood pressure cuff, thus restricting his use of sign language; (c) being unable to read the nurse's lips from a prone position; or (d) not having a nurse who could understand his speech or know/recognize his attempts to use sign language. While pain is a possibility and needs to be evaluated, it is common to give regional blocks during the surgery to keep children comfortable until after they are discharged home. It is unlikely that he is having separation anxiety, because this usually occurs in younger children.

NURSING CARE PLAN

The Child with Hearing Impairment

NURSING DIAGNOSIS: Sensory/perceptual alterations (auditory) related to hearing impairment

PATIENT GOAL 1: Will experience maximum hearing potential

• **NURSING INTERVENTIONS/*RATIONALES***

Help family investigate hearing aid dealers *to locate a reliable dealer*

Discuss types of hearing aids and their proper care *to ensure maximum benefit*

Stress to family importance of storing hearing aid batteries safely and of teaching children (or supervising young children) not to remove the battery *to prevent ingestion/aspiration of batteries*

Teach child how to regulate hearing aid *for maximum benefit*

Help child focus on all sounds in the environment and talk about them *to maximize hearing*

For older child, discuss methods of camouflaging the aid *to make it less conspicuous*

• **EXPECTED OUTCOMES**

Child acquires and uses hearing aid properly

Child does not ingest/aspirate hearing aid battery

NURSING DIAGNOSIS: Impaired verbal communication related to inability to hear auditory cues

PATIENT GOAL 1: Will engage in communication process within limits of impairment

• **NURSING INTERVENTIONS/*RATIONALES***

Encourage family to attend the rehabilitation program *in order to continue learning in the home;* encourage them to learn sign language *as a method of communication*

Teach language that serves a useful purpose *for communication*

Encourage use of language and books in the home *to stimulate verbal communication and promote normal development*

Encourage spontaneous language and correct speech *to promote speech development*

• **EXPECTED OUTCOMES**

Family continues communication practices in home environment

Family provides stimulation to child

PATIENT GOAL 2: Will demonstrate ability to lipread.

• **NURSING INTERVENTIONS/*RATIONALES***

Test child for visual problems *that may interfere with learning to lipread or use sign language*

Teach family and others involved with child (e.g., teacher) behaviors that facilitate lipreading (see box on p. 1027) *to promote communication process*

• **EXPECTED OUTCOMES**

Child communicates with others in manner taught (specify)

Persons communicating with child use good communication techniques

NURSING DIAGNOSIS: Altered growth and development related to impaired communication

PATIENT GOAL 1: Will achieve optimum independence level for age

• **NURSING INTERVENTIONS/*RATIONALES***

Help family transfer normal childrearing practices to this child *to promote optimum development*

Emphasize importance of attaining independence in self-care

Provide child with devices that foster independence (e.g., hearing ear dog, special signaling aids for telephone or doorbell)

Discuss with family importance of discipline and limit-setting, *since all children have these needs*

• **EXPECTED OUTCOMES**

Child performs activities of daily living appropriate to level of development

Appropriate discipline and limit-setting are provided

PATIENT GOAL 2: Will have opportunity to participate in activities for play and socialization

• **NURSING INTERVENTIONS/*RATIONALES***

Guide family in selection of toys *to maximize visual and tactile senses, as well as residual hearing*

Encourage child to participate in group activities (e.g., scouting, sports) *to promote socialization*

Help child follow group discussion by pointing out the speaker and arranging the group in a semicircle *to facilitate hearing and/or lipreading*

Help child develop friendships among hearing and deaf peers *to promote socialization*

Recommend closed-captioning television *for child's enjoyment*

• **EXPECTED OUTCOMES**

Child engages in activities appropriate to developmental level

Child has peer relationships and experiences

PATIENT GOAL 3: Will be provided educational opportunities within a regular classroom

• **NURSING INTERVENTIONS/*RATIONALES***

Discuss with teacher and children ways of communicating effectively with child (e.g., through facilitating lipreading) *to facilitate child's education*

Promote socialization with classmates *to encourage enjoyment of education*

Continued.

NURSING CARE PLAN
The Child with Hearing Impairment—cont'd

• **EXPECTED OUTCOMES**
Child attends school regularly
Child communicates with others in the classroom

NURSING DIAGNOSIS: Altered family processes related to diagnosis of deafness of a child

PATIENT (FAMILY) GOAL 1: Will adjust to child's hearing loss

• **NURSING INTERVENTIONS/*RATIONALES***
Anticipate grief reaction as part of adjustment to loss
Provide opportunities for family to express feelings and concerns *to promote adjustment*
Help family deal with feelings regarding previous responses to child when true nature of the problem was unknown *to minimize feelings of guilt*
Help family realize extent of child's disability and its tremendous influence on speech and language development
Discuss advantages and limitations of amplifying devices with different types of hearing loss *so that family can make informed decisions*
Encourage formal rehabilitation as soon as possible *to foster normal growth and development of child*

• **EXPECTED OUTCOMES**
Family expresses feelings and concerns regarding child's loss of hearing
Family demonstrates an understanding of the implications of hearing loss
Family becomes involved in appropriate programs

PATIENT (FAMILY) GOAL 2: Will receive emotional support

• **INTERVENTIONS/*RATIONALES***
Be available to family *for assistance and support*
Encourage family members to discuss their feelings regarding the disability *to enhance coping*
Stress child's abilities rather than disability *to promote child's optimum development*
Become familiar with techniques used for communication if following the family on a long-term basis
Refer family to appropriate community agencies for medical, psychiatric, educational, vocational, or financial assistance *to ensure that their overall needs are met*
Involve parents in local parent groups for deaf children *for continuing support*

• **EXPECTED OUTCOMES**
Family expresses feelings and concerns about the disability and its ramifications
Family members avail themselves of available resources

PATIENT (FAMILY) GOAL 3: Will demonstrate attachment to child

• **INTERVENTIONS/*RATIONALES***
Help family identify clues other than verbal ones that signify infant's communication with them, *because communication is an important part of attachment process*
Encourage family to stimulate child with visual and tactile cues, *since auditory cues are absent or diminished*
Stress importance of continuing to talk to child even though child may not hear their voices *to promote normalization*

• **EXPECTED OUTCOME**
Parents and child demonstrate a positive relationship

NURSING DIAGNOSIS: High risk for injury related to environmental hazards, infection

PATIENT (OTHERS) GOAL 1: Will not acquire or have greater hearing loss

• **INTERVENTIONS/*RATIONALES***
Infancy
Encourage immunization at appropriate age *to prevent acquired sensorineural hearing loss from childhood diseases*
Minimize noise levels in intensive care unit, *since this is associated with hearing loss*
Prevent ear infection; detect early *because this is the most common cause of impaired hearing*
Childhood
Assess hearing ability of infants and children receiving ototoxic antibiotics *for early detection*
Promote compliance with treatment regimens for otitis media, *since this is a common cause of impaired hearing*
Discuss with parents measures to prevent otitis media
Evaluate auditory ability of children prone to chronic ear or respiratory problems *for early detection of impaired hearing*
Assess sources of excessive noise in child's environment; institute appropriate measures to decrease sound levels (turn music lower, use ear protection) *because exposure to excessive noise is a cause of sensorineural hearing loss*
Participate in immunization programs for children *to prevent childhood diseases that may result in hearing loss*

• **EXPECTED OUTCOMES**
Infant or child does not develop hearing loss
Child is not exposed to excessive noise levels
Child is properly immunized

See also Nursing Care Plan: The Child with Chronic Illness or Disability, Chapter 22

to are also available (see Fig. 24-9). Such boards can also be made up by drawing pictures or writing the words of common needs on cardboard, such as *parent, food, water,* or *toilet.*

The nurse has a special role as child advocate with the deaf and is in a strategic position to alert other health team members and other patients to the child's special needs regarding communication. For example, the nurse should accompany other practitioners on visits to the child's room to ensure that they speak to the child and that the child understands what is said. Not infrequently caregivers forget that the child has the abilities to perceive and learn despite a hearing loss, and consequently they communicate only with the parents. As a result, the child's needs and feelings remain unrecognized and unmet.

Since deaf children often have difficulty in forming social relationships with other children, the child is introduced to roommates and encouraged to engage in play activities. The hospital setting can provide growth-promoting opportunities for social relationships. With the assistance of a child-life specialist, the child can learn new recreational activities, experiment with group games, and engage in therapeutic play. The use of puppets, doll-houses, role-playing with dress-up clothes, building with a hammer and nails, finger painting, playing with syringes, and water play can help the child express feelings that previously were suppressed.

Assist in Measures to Prevent Hearing Impairment. A primary nursing role is prevention of hearing loss. Since the most common cause of impaired hearing is chronic otitis media, it is essential that appropriate measures be instituted to treat existing infections and prevent recurrences (see Chapter 32). Children with histories of ear or respiratory infections or any other condition known to increase the risk of hearing impairment should receive periodic auditory testing.

To prevent the causes of hearing loss that begin prenatally and perinatally, pregnant women need counseling regarding the necessity of early prenatal care, including genetic counseling for known familial disorders; avoidance of all ototoxic drugs, especially during the first trimester; tests to rule out syphilis, rubella, or blood incompatibility; medical management of maternal diabetes; control of alcoholism; and adequate dietary intake. The necessity of routine immunization during childhood to eliminate the possibility of acquired sensorineural loss from rubella, mumps, or measles (encephalitis) is stressed.

Exposure to excessive noise pollution is a well-established cause of sensorineural hearing loss. The nurse should routinely assess the possibility of environmental noise pollution and advise children and parents of the potential danger. When individuals engage in activities associated with high-intensity noise, such as flying model airplanes, target shooting, or snowmobiling, they should wear ear protection such as earmuffs or earplugs (not ordinary dry cotton). However, any protection is better than none. Even common household equipment, such as lawn mowers and power vacuum cleaners, can be hazardous.

NURSING ALERT Suspect hazardous noise if the listener experiences (1) difficulty in communication while hearing the sound, (2) ringing in the ears (tinnitus) after exposure to the sound, or (3) muffled hearing after leaving the sound.

❖ EVALUATION

The effectiveness of nursing interventions is determined by continual reassessment and evaluation of care based on the following observational guidelines and expected outcomes:

1. Observe the techniques used to communicate with the child; inquire if child is enrolled in an auditory training program; inquire about socialization opportunities for the child (i.e., who are child's friends, what are his or her extracurricular activities).
2. Interview family regarding their adjustment to the sensory impairment; observe family members' relationship with the child; interview child regarding feelings about the sensory impairment and its effect on activities of daily living (especially important if impairment is recent).
3. Observe types of preparation/communication used to prepare child for hospitalization or procedures; observe parents' involvement in child's care; observe interaction of child and family with other patients.
4. Investigate community programs aimed at preventing or detecting hearing loss and inquire as to nursing involvement in these efforts.

Expected outcomes:
See Nursing Care Plan, pp. 1029-1030.

VISUAL IMPAIRMENT

Visual impairment is a common problem during childhood. In North America the prevalence of blindness and serious visual impairment in the pediatric population is estimated to be between 30 and 64 children per 100,000 population. Another 100 children per 100,000 have less serious impairment (Davidson, 1992). The nurse's role is one of assessment, prevention, referral, and, possibly, rehabilitation.

Definition and Classification

Legal blindness is defined as visual acuity of 20/200 or less and/or a visual field of 20 degrees or less in the better eye. ***Partially sighted*** is defined as visual acuity above 20/200 but worse than 20/70 in the better eye with correction. ***Visual impairment*** is a general term that includes both of these categories. Children who are visually impaired, including those who are legally blind, often have considerable useful vision and are able to use printed material, such as large-print books, as their major method of learning (Moller, 1993). Educational and governmental agencies in the United States use the legal definition of blindness to determine eligibility for services in regard to taxes, entrance into special schools, eligibility for aid, and other benefits.

Etiology

Visual impairment can be caused by a number of genetic and prenatal or postnatal conditions. These include peri-

TYPES OF VISUAL IMPAIRMENT

REFRACTIVE ERRORS

Myopia

Nearsightedness—Ability to see objects clearly at close range but not at a distance

Pathophysiology

Results from eyeball that is too long, causing image to fall in front of retina

Clinical manifestations

Rubs eyes excessively
Tilts head or thrusts head forward
Has difficulty in reading or other close work
Holds books close to eyes
Writes or colors with head close to table
Clumsy; walks into objects
Blinks more than usual or is irritable when doing close work
Is unable to see objects clearly
Does poorly in school, especially in subjects that require demonstration, such as arithmetic
Dizziness
Headache
Nausea following close work

Treatment

Corrected with biconcave lenses that focus rays on retina

Hyperopia

Farsightedness—Ability to see objects at a distance

Pathophysiology

Results from eyeball that is too short, causing image to focus beyond retina

Clinical manifestations

Because of accommodative ability, child can usually see objects at all ranges
Most children normally hyperopic until about 7 years of age

Treatment

If correction is required, use convex lenses to focus rays on retina

Astigmatism

Unequal curvatures in refractive apparatus

Pathophysiology

Results from unequal curvatures in cornea or lens that cause light rays to bend in different directions

Clinical manifestations

Depends on severity of refractive error in each eye
May have clinical manifestations of myopia

Treatment

Corrected with special lenses that compensate for refractive errors

Anisometropia

Different refractive strength in each eye

Pathophysiology

May develop amblyopia as weaker eye is used less

Clinical manifestations

Depends on severity of refractive error in each eye
May have clinical manifestations of myopia

Treatment

Treated with corrective lenses, preferably contact lenses, to improve vision in each eye so they work as a unit

AMBLYOPIA

Lazy eye—Reduced visual acuity in one eye

Pathophysiology

Results when one eye does not receive sufficient stimulation
Each retina receives different images, resulting in diplopia (double vision)
Brain accommodates by suppressing less intense image
Visual cortex eventually does not respond to visual stimulation, with loss of vision in that eye

Clinical manifestations

Poor vision in affected eye

Treatment

Preventable if treatment of primary visual defect, such as anisometropia or strabismus, begins before 6 years of age

STRABISMUS

"Squint" or cross-eye—Malalignment of eyes (Fig. 24-7)
Esotropia—Inward deviation of eye
Exotropia—Outward deviation of eye

Pathophysiology

May result from muscle imbalance or paralysis, poor vision, or congenital defect
Since visual axes are not parallel, brain receives two images, and amblyopia can result

Clinical manifestations

Squints eyelids together or frowns
Has difficulty in focusing from one distance to another
Inaccurate judgment in picking up objects
Unable to see print or moving objects clearly
Closes one eye to see
Tilts head to one side
If combined with refractive errors, may see any of the manifestations listed for refractive errors
Diplopia
Photophobia
Dizziness
Headache
Cross-eye

Treatment

Treatment depends on cause of strabismus
May involve occlusion therapy (patching stronger eye) or surgery to increase visual stimulation to weaker eye
Early diagnosis is essential to prevent vision loss

CATARACTS

Opacity of crystalline lens

Pathophysiology

Prevents light rays from entering eye and refracting them on retina

TYPES OF VISUAL IMPAIRMENT—cont'd

Clinical manifestations

Gradually less able to see objects clearly
May lose peripheral vision
Nystagmus (with complete blindness)
Gray opacities of lens
Strabismus
Absence of red reflex

Treatment

Requires surgery to remove cloudy lens and replace lens (intraocular lens implant, removable contact lens, prescription glasses)
Must be treated early to prevent blindness from amblyopia

GLAUCOMA

Increased intraocular pressure

Pathophysiology

Congenital type results from defective development of some component related to flow of aqueous humor
Increased pressure on optic nerve causes eventual atrophy and blindness

Clinical manifestations

Mostly seen in acquired types—loses peripheral vision
May bump into objects not directly in front
Sees halos around objects
May complain of mild pain or discomfort (severe pain, nausea, vomiting, if sudden rise in pressure)
Redness
Excessive tearing (epiphora)
Photophobia
Spasmodic winking (blepharospasm)
Corneal haziness
Enlargement of eyeball (buphthalmos)

Treatment

Requires surgical treatment (goniotomy) to open outflow tracts
May require more than one procedure

natal infections (herpes, chlamydia, gonococci, rubella, syphilis, or toxoplasmosis), retinopathy of prematurity, trauma, postnatal infections (meningitis), and disorders such as sickle cell disease, juvenile rheumatoid arthritis, Tay-Sachs disease, albinism, and retinoblastoma. In many instances, such as with refractive errors, the cause of the defect is unknown.

Refractive errors are the most common types of visual disorders in children. The term ***refraction*** means bending and refers to the bending of light rays as they pass through the lens of the eye. Normally, light rays enter the lens and fall directly on the retina. However, in refractive disorders the light rays either fall in front of the retina (myopia) or beyond it (hyperopia). Other eye problems, such as strabismus, may or may not include refractive errors, but they are very important because, if untreated, they result in blindness from amblyopia. These along with other, less frequent visual disorders are summarized in the box on pp. 1032-1033. In addition to these disorders, other visual problems can be a result of infection or trauma.

Trauma. Trauma is a common cause of blindness in children. Injuries to the eyeball and adnexa (supporting or accessory structures, such as eyelids, conjunctiva, and lacrimal glands) can be classified as penetrating or nonpenetrating. ***Penetrating wounds*** are most often a result of sharp instruments, such as sticks, knives, or scissors; propulsive objects, such as firecrackers, guns, bows and arrows, or slingshots; or a powerful contusion by a blunt object, which may occur during a fight or from a serious car accident. ***Nonpenetrating injuries*** may be a result of foreign objects in the eyes, lacerations, a blow from a blunt object such as a ball (baseball, softball, basketball, and racquet sports) or fist, or thermal or chemical burns.

Treatment is aimed at preventing further ocular damage and is primarily the responsibility of the ophthalmologist. It involves adequate examination of the injured eye (with the child sedated or anesthetized in cases of severe injury); appropriate immediate intervention, such as removal of the foreign body or suturing of the laceration; and prevention of complications, such as administration of antibiotics or steroids and complete bed rest to allow the eye to heal and blood to reabsorb (see Emergency Treatment box on p. 1035). The prognosis varies according to the type of injury. It is usually guarded in all cases of penetrating wounds because of the high risk of serious complications.

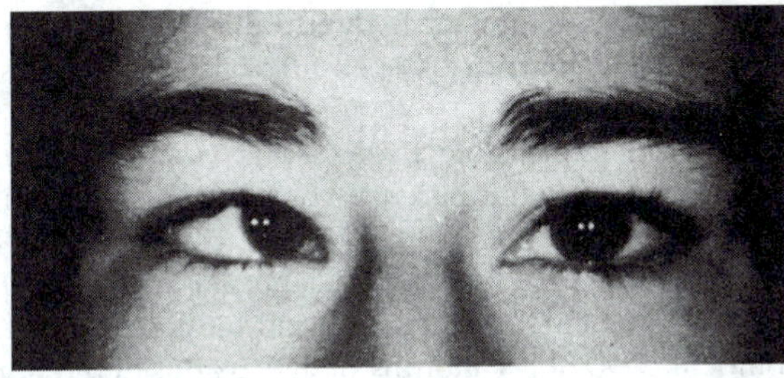

FIG. 24-7 Strabismus (esotropia). Note obvious malalignment of eyes. Light reflections are centered in the left cornea and to the side of the right cornea. (From Havener WH and others: *Nursing care in eye, ear, nose, and throat disorders,* ed 3, St Louis, 1974, Mosby.)

Infections. Infections of the adnexa and the structures of the eyeball or globe are not infrequent in children. The most common eye infection is conjunctivitis (see Chapter 16). Treatment is usually with ophthalmic antibiotics. Severe infections may require systemic antibiotic therapy. Steroids are used cautiously because they exacerbate viral infections such as herpes simplex, increasing the risk of damage to the involved structures.

Nursing Considerations

Nursing care of visually impaired children is a specialized area requiring additional training in vision testing and habilitation. However, general goals that focus on assessment, prevention, and rehabilitation of the child with visual impairment are every nurse's responsibility. In addition, nurses may have to care for a visually impaired child who is hospitalized and must know how to best meet the child's and family's special needs.

Assessment. Assessment of children for visual impairment is a critical nursing responsibility. Discovery of a visual impairment as early as possible is essential to prevent social, physical, and psychologic damage to the child. Assessment involves (1) identifying those children who by virtue of their history are at risk, (2) observing for behaviors that indicate a vision loss, and (3) screening all children for visual acuity and signs of other ocular disorders, such as strabismus. Clinical manifestations of various types of visual problems are given in the box on p. 1032. Vision testing is discussed in Chapter 7.

Infancy. At birth the nurse should observe the neonate's response to visual stimuli, such as following a light or object and cessation of body movement. The intensity of the response may vary, depending on the infant's state of alertness.

Of special importance in detecting visual impairment during infancy are the parents' concerns regarding visual responsiveness in their child. Their concerns, such as lack of eye contact from the infant, must be taken seriously. During infancy the child should be tested for strabismus. Lack of binocularity after 4 months of age is considered abnormal and must be treated to prevent amblyopia.

NURSING ALERT Suspect blindness if the infant does not react to light and in any-age child if parents express concern.

Childhood. Since the most common visual impairment during childhood is refractive errors, testing for visual acuity is essential. The school nurse usually assumes major responsibility for vision testing in schoolchildren. Besides refractive errors, the nurse should be aware of signs and symptoms that indicate other ocular problems. If a referral is made to the family requesting further eye testing, the school nurse is responsible for follow-up concerning the recommendation.

Support of Child and Family. The shock of learning that their child is blind or partially sighted is an immense crisis for families. Of all types of disabilities, many people fear loss of sight the most. Vision is involved in almost every activity of daily living. Parents need support during the initial phase of learning about the diagnosis and help to gain a realistic understanding of their child's abilities. The family is encouraged to investigate appropriate stimulation and educational programs for their child as soon as possible. Sources of information include state **Commissions for the Blind,** local schools for the blind, the **American Foundation for the Blind,*** **National Federation of the Blind,†** **National Association for Parents of the Visually Impaired, Inc.,‡** **National Association for Visually Handicapped,§** and **American Council of the Blind.‖**

When blindness is not congenital but acquired, newly blind children need a great deal of support to help them adjust to the disability. They are usually frightened and confused by the sudden or progressive loss of sight and benefit from an environment that provides security and familiarity.

Promotion of Parent-Child Attachment. A crucial time in the life of blind infants is when they and their parents are getting acquainted with each other. Pleasurable patterns of interaction between the infant and parents may be lacking if there is not enough reciprocity. For example, if the parent gazes fondly at the infant's face and seeks eye contact but the infant fails to respond because he or she cannot see the parent, a troubled cycle of responses may occur. The nurse can help parents learn to look for other cues that indicate the infant is responding to them, such as whether the eyelids blink; whether the activity level accelerates or slows; whether respiratory patterns change, such as faster or slower breathing when the parents come near; and whether the infant makes throaty sounds when they speak to the infant. In time parents learn that the infant has unique ways of relating to them. They are encouraged to show affection using nonvisual methods, such as talking or reading, cuddling, and walking the child.

Promotion of Child's Optimum Development. Promoting the child's optimum development requires rehabilitation in a number of important areas. These include learning self-help skills and appropriate communication techniques to become independent. Although nurses may not be directly involved in such programs, they can provide direction and guidance to families regarding the availability of programs and the need to promote these activities in their child.

Development and independence. Motor development depends on sight almost as much as verbal communication depends on hearing. From earliest infancy parents are encouraged to expose the infant to as many visual-motor experiences as possible, such as sitting supported in an infant seat or swing and being given opportunities for holding up the head, sitting unsupported, reaching for objects, and crawling.

Despite visual impairment, the child can become independent in all aspects of self-care. The same principles used for promoting independence in sighted children apply,

---

*15 W. 16th St., New York, NY 10011; (212) 620-2000.
†1800 Johnson St., Baltimore, MD 21230; (410) 659-9314.
‡2180 Linway Dr., Beloit, WI 53511; (800) 562-6265.
§22 W. 21st St., New York, NY 10010; (212) 889-3141.
‖1155 15th St., N.W., Suite 720, Washington, DC 20005; (202) 467-5081 or (800) 424-8666 (afternoons only).

Sources of information in Canada include the **Canadian National Institute for the Blind,** 1931 Bayview Ave., Toronto, Ontario M4G 4C8; **Low Vision Association of Canada,** 145 Adelaide St. West, Toronto, Ontario M5H 3H4; and **Blind Organization of Ontario,** 597 Parliament St., Suite B-3, Toronto, Ontario M4X 1W3.

with additional emphasis given to nonvisual cues. For example, the child may need help in dressing, such as special arrangement of clothing for style coordination and braille tags to distinguish colors and prints.

The blind child also must learn to become independent in navigational skills. The two main techniques are the ***tapping method*** (use of a cane to survey the environment for direction and to avoid obstacles) and ***guides,*** such as a human sighted guide or a dog guide, such as a Seeing Eye dog. Partially sighted children may benefit from ocular aids, such as a monocular telescope.

Play and socialization. Blind children do not learn to play automatically. Because they cannot imitate others or actively explore the environment as sighted children do, they depend much more on others to stimulate and teach them how to play. Parents need help in selecting appropriate play materials, especially those that encourage fine and gross motor development and stimulate the senses of hearing, touch, and smell. Toys with educational value are especially useful, such as dolls with various clothing closures.

Blind children have the same needs for socialization as sighted children. Since they have little difficulty in learning verbal skills, they are able to communicate with age-mates and participate in suitable activities. The nurse discusses with parents opportunities for socialization outside of the home, especially regular preschools. The trend is to include these children with sighted children to help them adjust to the outside world for eventual independence.

To compensate for inadequate stimulation, these children may develop ***blindisms*** (self-stimulatory activities, such as body rocking, finger flicking, or arm twirling). Such habits retard the child's social acceptance and are discouraged. Behavioral modification is often successful in reducing or eliminating blindisms.

Education. The main obstacle to learning is the child's total dependence on nonvisual cues. Although the child can learn via verbal lecturing, he or she is unable to read the written word or to write without special education. Therefore the child must rely on ***braille,*** a system that uses six raised dots to represent each letter and number. The child can then read the braille with the fingers and can write a message using a small typewriter-like device called a ***braille writer.*** However, unless others read braille, this type of communication is not useful for communicating with others. A more portable system for written communication is the use of a ***braille slate*** and ***stylus*** (Fig. 24-8) or a microcassette tape recorder. A recorder is especially helpful for leaving messages for others and for taking notes during classroom lectures. For mathematic calculations portable calculators with voice synthesizers are available.*

Records and tapes are significant sources of reading material other than braille books, which are large and cumbersome. The **Library of Congress**† has talking books, braille books, and a special records program, which are

*A catalog of numerous products for people with vision problems is available from the American Foundation for the Blind.

†Division for the Blind and Visually Handicapped, 1291 Taylor St., N.W., Washington, DC 20542; (202) 707-5100 or (800) 424-8567.

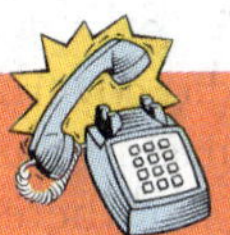

EMERGENCY TREATMENT
Eye Injuries

FOREIGN OBJECT

Examine eye for presence of a foreign body (evert upper lid to examine upper eye).
Remove a freely movable object with pointed corner of gauze pad lightly moistened with water.
Do not irrigate eye or attempt to remove a penetrating object (see below).
Caution child against rubbing eye.

CHEMICAL BURNS

Irrigate eye copiously with tap water for 20 minutes.
Evert upper lid to flush thoroughly.
Hold child's head with eye under tap of running lukewarm water.
Take to emergency room.
Have child rest with eyes closed.
Keep room darkened.

ULTRAVIOLET BURNS

If skin is burned, patch both eyes (make sure lids are completely closed); secure dressing with Kling bandages wrapped around head rather than tape.
Have child rest with eyes closed.
Refer to an ophthalmologist.

HEMATOMA ("BLACK EYE")

Use a flashlight to check for gross hyphema (hemorrhage into anterior chamber; visible fluid meniscus across iris; more easily seen in light-colored than in brown eyes).
Apply ice for first 24 hours to reduce swelling if no hyphema is present.
Refer to an ophthalmologist immediately if hyphema is present.
Have child rest with eyes closed.

PENETRATING INJURIES

Take child to emergency room.
Never remove an object that has penetrated eye.
Follow strict aseptic technique in examining eye.
Observe for:
- Aqueous or vitreous leaks (fluid leaking from point of penetration)
- Hyphema
- Shape and equality of pupils, reaction to light
- Prolapsed iris (not perfectly circular)

Apply a Fox shield if available (not a regular eye patch) and apply patch over unaffected eye to prevent bilateral movement.
Maintain bed rest with child in 30-degree Fowler position.
Caution child against rubbing eye.

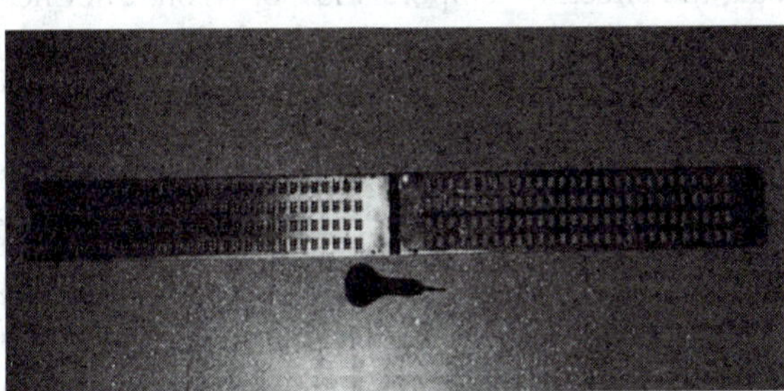

FIG. 24-8 Braille slate and stylus. The hinged slate consists of a series of open rectangles on one side and standard braille cells on the other. The paper is clamped or sandwiched between these two metal bars, and the appropriate dots are punched with the stylus.

EMERGENCY TREATMENT

available at many local and state libraries and directly from the Library of Congress. The talking book machine and tape player are provided at no cost to families, and there is no postage fee for returning the materials. **Recording for the Blind, Inc.,*** also provides texts and tapes of books, which are very helpful for secondary and college students who are blind.

Learning to use a regular typewriter is another form of writing but has the disadvantage of the blind person's being unable to check the accuracy of the typing. Computers eliminate this drawback; a home computer with a voice synthesizer can be adapted to speak each letter or word that has been typed.

The partially sighted child benefits from specialized visual aids, which produce a magnified retinal image. The basic devices are accommodation, such as bringing the object closer, special plus lenses, hand-held and stand magnifiers, telescopes, video projection systems, and large print. Special equipment is available to enlarge print. Information about services for the partially sighted is available from the **National Association for the Visually Handicapped** and **American Foundation for the Blind.** Children with diminished vision often prefer to do close work without their glasses and compensate by bringing the object very near to their eyes. This should be allowed. The exception is the child with vision in only one eye, who should always wear glasses for protection.

Care for child during hospitalization. Because nurses are more likely to care for children who are hospitalized for procedures that involve temporary loss of vision than for children who are blind, the following discussion concentrates primarily on the needs of such children. The nursing care objectives in either situation are to (1) reassure the child and family throughout every phase of treatment, (2) orient the child to the surroundings, (3) provide a safe environment, and (4) encourage independence. Whenever possible, the same nurse should care for the child to ensure consistency in the approach. These same principles also apply to a blind child who requires hospitalization.

When sighted children temporarily lose their vision, almost every aspect of the environment becomes bewildering and frightening. They are forced to rely on nonvisual senses for help in adjusting to the blindness without the benefit of any special training. Nurses have a major role in minimizing the effects of temporary loss of vision. They need to talk to the child about everything that is occurring, emphasizing aspects of procedures that are felt or heard. They should approach the child by always identifying themselves as soon as they enter the room. Since unfamiliar sounds are especially frightening, these are explained. Parents are encouraged to room with their child and participate in the care. Familiar objects, such as a teddy bear or doll, should be brought from home to help lessen the strangeness of the hospital. As soon as the child is able to be out of bed, he or she is oriented to the immediate surroundings. If the child is able to see on admission, this opportunity is taken to point out significant aspects of the room. The child is encouraged to practice ambulating with the eyes closed to become accustomed to this experience.

The room is arranged with safety in mind. For example, a stool or chair is placed next to the bed to help the child climb in and out of bed. The furniture is always placed in the same position to prevent collisions. Cleaning personnel are reminded of the need to keep the room in order. If the child has difficulty navigating by feeling the walls, a rope can be attached from the bed to the point of destination, such as the bathroom. Attention to details such as well-fitting slippers or robes that do not hang on the floor is important in preventing tripping. Unlike the child who is blind, these children are not familiar with navigating with a cane.

The child is encouraged to be independent in self-care activities, especially if the visual loss may be prolonged or potentially permanent. For example, during bathing the nurse sets up all the equipment and encourages the child to participate. At mealtime the nurse explains where each food item is on the tray, opens any special containers, prepares cereal or toast, but encourages the child in self-feeding. Favorite finger foods, such as sandwiches, hamburgers, hot dogs, or pizza, may be good selections. The child is praised for efforts at being cooperative and independent. Any improvements made in self-care, no matter how small, are stressed.

Appropriate recreational activities are provided, and if a child-life specialist is available, such planning is done jointly. Since children with temporary blindness have a wide variety of play experiences to draw on, they are encouraged to select activities. For example, if they like to read, they may enjoy being read to. If they prefer manual activity, they may appreciate playing with clay or building blocks or feeling different textures and naming them. If they need an outlet for aggression, activities such as pounding or banging on a drum can be helpful. Simple board and card games can be played with a "seeing partner" or if the opponent helps with the game. They should have familiar toys from home to play with, since familiar items are more easily manipulated than new ones. If parents wish to bring presents, they should be objects that stimulate hearing and touch, such as a radio, music box, or stuffed animal.

Occasionally children who are blind come to the hospital for procedures to restore their vision. Although this is an extremely happy time, it also requires intervention to help them adjust to sight. They need an opportunity to take in all that they see. They should not be bombarded with visual stimuli. They may need to concentrate on people's faces or their own to become accustomed to this experience. They often need to talk about what they see and to compare the visual images with their mental ones. The child may also go through a period of depression, which must be respected and supported. The nurse or parents should refrain from statements such as "How can you be so sad when you can see again?" Instead the child should be encouraged to discuss how it feels to see, especially in terms of seeing himself or herself.

Newly sighted children also need time to adjust to the ability to engage in activities that were impossible before.

*20 Roszel Rd., Princeton, NJ 08540; (609) 452-0606.

For example, they may prefer to use braille to read, rather than learning a new "visual approach," because of familiarity with the touch system. Eventually, as they learn to recognize letters and numbers, they will integrate these new skills into reading and writing. However, parents and teachers must be careful not to push them before they are ready. This applies to social relationships and physical activities, as well as learning situations.

Prevention. An essential nursing goal is to prevent visual impairment. This involves many of the same interventions discussed under hearing impairments, namely (1) prenatal screening for pregnant women at risk, such as those with rubella or syphilis infection and family histories of genetic disorders associated with visual loss; (2) adequate prenatal and perinatal care to prevent prematurity and iatrogenic damage from excessive administration of oxygen; (3) periodic screening of all children, especially newborns through preschoolers, for congenital blindness and visual impairments caused by refractive errors, strabismus, and so on; (4) rubella immunization of all children; and (5) safety counseling regarding the common causes of ocular trauma.

Safety counseling should include safe practices when working with, playing with, or carrying objects such as scissors, knives, and balls.

NURSING ALERT A face mask and helmet should be required gear for children playing baseball or softball (especially catcher, batter, umpire, and base runner), hockey, or football.

Following detection of eye problems, the nurse has a responsibility to prevent further ocular damage by ensuring that corrective treatment is employed. For the child with strabismus, this often necessitates occlusion patching of the stronger eye. Compliance with the procedure is greatest during the early preschool years. It is more difficult to encourage young school-age children to wear the occlusive patch because the poor visual acuity of the uncovered weaker eye interferes with schoolwork and the patch sets them apart from their peers. In school they benefit from being positioned favorably (closer to the chalkboard) and allowed extra time to read or complete an assignment. If treatment of the eye disorder requires instillation of ophthalmic medication, the family is taught the correct procedure (see Chapter 27).*

For the child with refractive errors, the nurse helps the child adjust to wearing glasses. Young children, who often pull glasses off, benefit from temporal pieces that wrap around the ears or an elastic strap attached to the frames and around the back of the head to hold the glasses on securely. Once children appreciate the value of clear vision, they are more likely to wear the corrective lenses.

Glasses should not interfere with any activity. Special protective guards are available to prevent accidental injury during contact sports, and all corrective lenses should be made from safety glass, which is shatterproof. Often corrective lenses improve visual acuity so dramatically that children are able to compete more effectively in sports. This in itself is a tremendous inducement to continue wearing glasses.

Contact lenses are a popular alternative. Several types are available, such as hard lenses, including gas-permeable ones, and soft lenses, which may be designed for daily or extended wear. Contact lenses offer several advantages over glasses, such as greater visual acuity, total corrected field of vision, convenience (especially with the extended wear type), and optimum cosmetic benefit. Unfortunately, they are usually more expensive and require much more care than glasses, including considerable practice to learn techniques for insertion and removal. If they are prescribed, the nurse can be very helpful in teaching parents or older children how to care for the lenses.

Since trauma is the leading cause of blindness, the nurse has the major responsibility of preventing further eye injury until the specific treatment is instituted. The major principles to follow when caring for an eye injury are outlined in the Emergency Treatment box on p. 1035. Since patients with a serious eye injury fear blindness, the nurse should stay with the child and family to provide support and reassurance. (See also Nursing Care Plan: The Child with Visual Impairment.*)

THE DEAF-BLIND CHILD

The most traumatic sensory impairment is loss of sight and hearing. One of the chief causes of deaf-blindness was congenital rubella syndrome, but immunization has decreased its incidence. Other causes are usually the result of one congenital sensory impairment combined with an acquired impairment, such as congenital blindness and acquired deafness from meningitis, or congenital deafness and acquired blindness from an eye injury. Most children with multisensory impairments have some residual hearing and vision to supplement the senses of touch, smell, and taste.

Auditory and visual impairments have profound effects on the child's development. They interfere with the normal sequence of physical, intellectual, and psychosocial growth. Although the child often achieves the usual motor milestones, they are delayed. Children only learn communication with specialized training. ***Finger spelling*** is one desirable method often taught to these children. The letters are spelled into the deaf-blind child's hand, and the child spells out ideas to the other person. Another type of tactile communication, the ***Tadoma method,*** involves the child placing the hand over the speaker's face and neck to monitor facial movements associated with speech production (Reed and others, 1989). Children with residual hearing can learn to speak. Whenever possible, speech is encouraged, since it allows communication with individuals not familiar with the preceding approaches.

Programs for these children vary. The John T. Tracy Clinic offers a home correspondence course for parents,

*Home care instructions for giving eye medications are available in *Wong and Whaley's Clinical Manual of Pediatric Nursing* (Mosby).

*In *Wong and Whaley's Clinical Manual of Pediatric Nursing* (Mosby).

and the **American Foundation for the Blind,** the **Helen Keller National Center,*** the **Perkins School for the Blind,†** and the **Foundation for the Junior Blind‡** provide special services; the last two organizations have residential educational programs.

Nursing Considerations

One of the major concerns of families with children who are deaf-blind is helping them establish communication. The nurse is in a vital position to help parents with this goal. Since infants may not coo, laugh, or make directed eye movements, they are limited in the cues they can send and receive. Therefore initiating and maintaining communication is the caregiver's responsibility. The nurse discusses with parents behaviors that signal the infant's recognition of them, such as quieting behavior, blinking, and change in respiration. The parents are encouraged to find ways of increasing stimulation for the child, especially cues that help the child identify each parent. For example, each person involved with the child should choose something that he or she, and only he or she, does, such as a kiss on the forehead or a stroke on the cheek. In this way the infant learns to discriminate among people in the environment.

As many sensory experiences as possible are provided, such as placing children in different positions during the day in relation to light and providing variation in stimuli so that they will be motivated to move toward, reach, touch, and explore the environment. Changing position also encourages muscle development and movement patterns. Sounds should be brought near and made interesting to these children. For example, they can participate in hearing by placing the hand on a radio or on a person's throat. Consistent tactile cues should be associated with a change of position and activities so that the movement is experienced as a positive, nonthreatening experience.

These children need secure, safe experiences while learning to walk and gaining confidence. Once ambulatory, they need help in exploring the environment on a gradual, *planned* basis. After they succeed in becoming well oriented to the environment, they are ready for a plan of locomotion. Sighted guide, trailing (movement directed by touching objects, such as the wall), and cane walking are three methods. An individually planned mobility program is based on the child's age, needs, and functional status and is shared with the child's therapist, teachers, parents, and siblings.

The future prospects for deaf-blind children are at best unpredictable. Sometimes congenital blindness and/or deafness is accompanied by other physical or neurologic handicaps, which further lessen the child's learning potential. The most favorable prognosis is often for children who have acquired deaf-blindness and have few, if any, associated disabilities. Their learning capacity is greatly potentiated by their developmental progress before the sensory impairments and the assistance of a trained companion. Although total independence, including gainful vocational training, is the goal, some deaf-blind children are unable to develop to this level. They may require life-long parental or residential care. The nurse working with such families helps them deal with future goals for the child, including possible alternatives to home care during the parents' advancing years. In this respect much of the nurse's role is similar to that discussed earlier for the child with cognitive impairment.

*Middle Neck Rd., Sands Point, NY 11050; (516) 944-8900 (voice/TDD).
†175 N. Beacon St., Watertown, MA 02172; (617) 924-3434.
‡5300 Angeles Vista Blvd., Los Angeles, CA 90043; (213) 295-4555.

COMMUNICATION IMPAIRMENT

GENERAL CONCEPTS

Communication impairment is a broad term that refers to the inability to (1) receive and/or process symbol systems for the spoken word, (2) represent concepts or symbol systems, and/or (3) transmit and use symbol systems. With severe communication impairment, other symbol systems, such as nonverbal methods (e.g., gestures, sign language, braille), may be needed to substitute for the spoken word.

Because of the complexity of communication, various classification systems are available and there is no universal agreement on one system. Basically, a communication impairment may occur in language, speech, or hearing or any combination of these. The problems encountered when hearing is affected are discussed earlier in this chapter. ***Language*** primarily refers to the symbol system used to convey thoughts or feelings to others. The two major types are ***receptive language,*** or understanding the spoken word, and ***expressive language,*** or speaking verbal symbols. ***Speech*** is the oral production of language, including articulation of sounds, rhythm, and tone.

Delayed development of language and speech is the most common symptom of developmental disability in children and affects from 5% to 10% of all children (Coplan, 1985). Speech problems are more prevalent than language disorders, and both impairments decline as children grow older. Males are affected three to four times more often than females (U.S. Department of Health and Human Services, 1988).

Etiology

The most common cause of communication impairment is mental retardation, followed by hearing impairment. Other causes include (1) central nervous system dysfunction, such as attention deficit disorders or learning disabilities; (2) severe emotional disturbance, such as autism and schizophrenia; (3) organic problems, such as cerebral palsy, cleft palate, vocal cord injury, and paralysis or foreshortening of the soft palate and uvula; and (4) some genetic disorders, such as cri-du-chat syndrome and Gilles de la Tourette syndrome. In some instances, such as in stuttering, the cause is unknown or speculative. Although the exact influence of environmental factors is controversial, the current thinking deemphasizes the importance of laziness, birth order, or bilingualism in relation to delayed language development (Coplan, 1985).

Language Impairment

Language disorders include an inability to:

1. Assign meaning to words (vocabulary)
2. Organize words into sentences
3. Alter word forms to indicate tense, possession, and plurality

Examples of language disorders are failure to develop vocabulary at the expected age, a reduced vocabulary for age, poor sentence structure, such as "Me see dog," or omitting words from the sentence, such as "Me fun." Such short or "telegraphic" phrases are normal during the first 2 years but should be replaced by more complete statements during the preschool years. Clinical manifestations of language disorders are presented in the box below.

Speech Impairment

Speech impairments include differences from normal in articulation, fluency, and voice production. ***Articulation*** errors refer to those sounds that a child makes incorrectly or inappropriately. For example, the child tends to distort or substitute a few consonants or blends, especially those that are learned last—*s, l, r,* and *th*—or the child omits many consonants, usually at the end of words, and substitutes the letters *t, d, k,* or *y* for them.

Dysfluencies, or ***rhythm disorders,*** usually consist of repetitions of sounds, words, or phrases. One of the most common and potentially serious dysfluencies is stuttering. ***Stuttering,*** or the less frequently used term ***stammering,*** describes dysfluent speech characterized by tense repetition of sounds or complete blockages of sounds or words. A stutter is sometimes referred to as a ***block*** when no sound comes out when the person tries to speak (Guitar, 1989).

Voice disorders are characterized by differences in pitch, loudness, and/or quality. Clinical manifestations of speech disorders are presented in the box at right.

CLINICAL MANIFESTATIONS OF LANGUAGE DISORDERS

ASSIGNING MEANING TO WORDS

First words not uttered before second birthday
Vocabulary size reduced for age or fails to show steady increase
Difficulty in describing characteristics of objects, although may be able to name them
Infrequent use of modifier words (adjectives or adverbs)
Excessive use of jargon past 18 months

ORGANIZING WORDS INTO SENTENCES

First sentences not uttered before third birthday
Short and incomplete sentences
Tendency to omit words (articles, prepositions)
Misuse of the "be," "do," and "can" verb forms
Difficulty understanding and producing questions
Plateaus at an early developmental level; uses easy speech patterns

ALTERING WORD FORMS

Omission of endings for plurals and tenses
Inappropriate use of plurals and tense endings
Inaccurate use of possession words

NONSPEECH COMMUNICATION

Many individuals who have severe disabilities, such as cerebral palsy, mental retardation, or multiple physical impairments, comprehend language but are unable to speak. Consequently, they benefit from communication methods that employ nonverbal symbols, such as sign language. Besides the use of hand or body gestures, numerous other communication systems exist. For example, ***Blissymbols*** are a highly stylized system of graphic symbols that represent words, ideas, and concepts (Murray, 1984). Although Blissymbols require education for their use, no reading skill is needed. These symbols or other self-explanatory graphics are usually arranged on a board, and the person points to the symbol(s) to convey a message; more sophisticated devices employ voice synthesizers that "speak" the symbol's meaning (Fig. 24-9). For children with physical limitations that prevent fine hand movements, numerous devices are available that facilitate isolating a symbol (Fig. 24-10). Nonverbal communication systems are allowing severely disabled indi-

CLINICAL MANIFESTATIONS OF SPEECH DISORDERS

DYSFLUENCY (STUTTERING)

Disturbance in the normal fluency and time patterning of speech (inappropriate for the individual's age), characterized by frequent occurrences of one or more of the following:
Sound and syllable repetitions
Sound prolongations
Interjections
Broken words (e.g., pauses within a word)
Audible or silent blocking (filled or unfilled pauses in speech)
Circumlocutions (word substitutions to avoid problematic words)
Words produced with an excess of physical tension
Monosyllabic whole-word repetitions (e.g., "I-I-I-I see him")
The disturbance in fluency interferes with academic or occupational achievement or with social communication.
If a speech-motor or sensory deficit is present, the speech difficulties are in excess of those usually associated with these problems.

ARTICULATION DEFICIENCY

Intelligibility of conversational speech absent by age 3 years
Omission of consonants at beginning of words by age 3 and at end of words by age 4
Persisting articulation faults after age 7
Omission of a sound where one should occur
Distortion of a sound
Substitution of an incorrect sound for a correct one

VOICE DISORDERS

Deviations in pitch (too high or too low, especially for age and sex); monotone
Deviations in loudness
Deviations in quality (hypernasality or hyponasality)

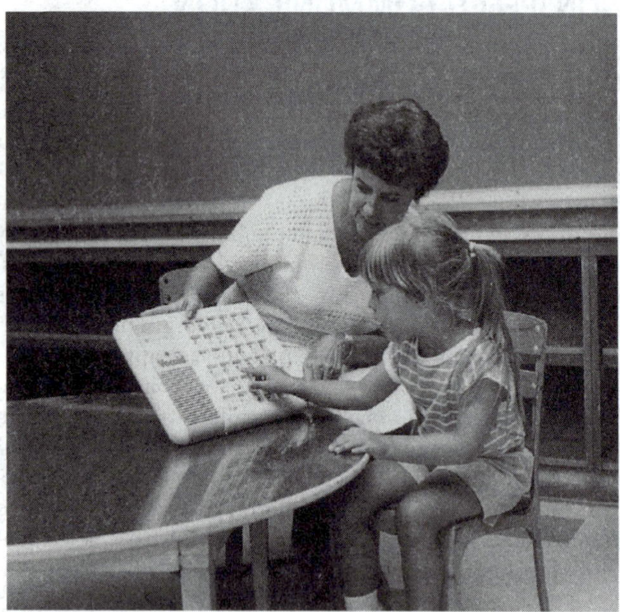

FIG. 24-9 The Vocaid is a communication board with a voice synthesizer. The child pushes the picture she wants, and that word or phrase is spoken. (Manufactured by Texas Instruments, Dallas, TX.)

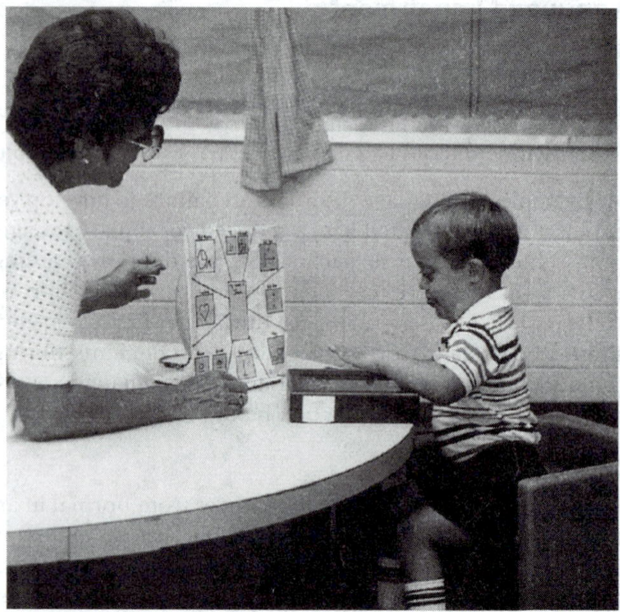

FIG. 24-10 Blissymbols can help a young child communicate nonverbally. This device uses a light behind each symbol; the light is rotated around the board by pressing the push panel.

viduals a much more meaningful life; many children are able to learn more and faster.*

NURSING CARE OF CHILDREN WITH COMMUNICATION IMPAIRMENT

Prevention

The primary intervention for communication disorders is prevention. Much of prevention directly relates to factors that predispose to causes of language/speech impairment, namely, mental retardation and hearing loss. Infants at risk for either condition (see boxes on pp. 1008 and 1025) should be referred for audiologic evaluation before 6 months of age so that audiologic and speech therapy can be initiated immediately, when required.

Prevention also involves early recognition of children at risk for language delays and involves timely intervention to promote adequate language development. Nurses are often able to provide education for families that fosters the child's communication skills. Specific interventions are presented in the Family Home Care box on p. 1043.

One area that is particularly important in terms of preventing communication impairment through appropriate parental guidance is stuttering. This hesitancy or dysfluency in speech pattern is a *normal* characteristic of language development during the preschool years. It occurs because children know what they want to say but hesitate or repeat words or sounds as they try to find the vocabulary to express themselves. Eventually their language skills parallel their other abilities, and speech becomes fluent.

However, when parents or other significant persons place undue emphasis or stress on this pattern of dysfluency, an abnormal speech pattern may result. Chances for reversal of stuttering are good until about 5 years of age. Therefore prevention must begin early. The nurse discusses with parents the normal dysfluencies in children's speech. When stuttering does occur, parents are advised to use the suggestions listed in the Family Home Care box to prevent inadvertently reinforcing the dysfluent pattern. If excessive concern of the parent or frustration and struggling behavior from the child are noted, the child is referred for language and speech evaluation.*

NURSING ALERT The critical point to remember is that the dysfluency must be arrested before the child develops an awareness or anticipation of the difficulty and begins to mistrust his or her speech skills.

❖ Assessment

Communication disorders can occur at any age but are most often found during childhood. The preschool period is considered critical to language development and therefore is a prime age for assessment and intervention. Failure to detect communication disorders during early childhood affects the development of social relationships and emotional

*Information about communication aids for children is available from the Crestwood Co., 6625 North Sidney Pl., Milwaukee, WI 53209; (414) 352-5678.

*Information about sources of assistance is available from the **Stuttering Resource Foundation,** 123 Oxford Rd., New Rochelle, NY 10804; (914) 632-3925 (Westchester) or (800) 232-4773 (outside local calling areas).

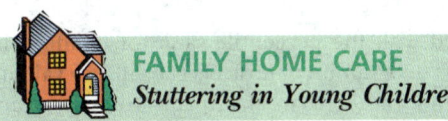

FAMILY HOME CARE
Stuttering in Young Children

TO BE ENCOURAGED

Viewing hesitancy and dysfluency as a normal part of speech development
Giving the child plenty of time and the impression that you are not rushed or in a hurry
Looking directly at the child while he or she is talking; being patient and never ridiculing or criticizing
Setting a good example by speaking clearly and articulating well
Identifying situations when stuttering increases, and avoiding them or ignoring the hesitancy
Minimizing stress, such as talking at the child's eye level; avoiding frequent questioning; and preventing interruptions while the child is speaking
Capitalizing on periods of fluent speech with positive reinforcement, such as singing songs or repeating nursery rhymes

TO BE AVOIDED

Practicing the natural tendency to "help" or finish the sentence for the child by supplying the word when the child has a block
Telling the child to stop and start over, to think before speaking, or to take it easy and go slowly
Showing great concern, embarrassment, or disapproval for hesitancy
Doing *anything* that emphasizes stuttering and calls the child's attention to speech skills
Promising a reward for proper speech

interactions, increases difficulty in developing academic skills, and lessens the chances for successful correction of deficit skills.

Assessment of abnormalities requires knowledge of normal language and speech development. Awareness of when children achieve such milestones enables nurses to distinguish when specific communication characteristics are expected and when they are considered deviations (Table 24-6). Nurses must also be aware of clinical manifestations of language and speech impairment (see boxes on p. 1039), as well as cognitive or hearing deficits (see boxes on pp. 1009 and 1026 and Cognitive Impairment, p. 1006).

Three methods are available for assessing speech and language development. ***Direct observation*** necessitates spontaneous language interaction between the child and the nurse. Suggestions for initiating conversation include showing children an object and asking them to describe it (asking children to name the object often results in one-word responses that are too limited for evaluation of speech, although appropriate for evaluation of language) or posing questions such as "If you could have three wishes, what would you want?" The word-imitative procedure may also be used by having children repeat sentences or words. This approach is valid because children are not able to reproduce statements using correct grammatical forms that they have not previously learned to use. Whenever possible, the child's conversation should be tape-recorded for serial documentation of progressive language/speech development and further evaluation by or consultation with a language or speech therapist.

Indirect assessment relies on parental information obtained through a history. Key questions that reflect problems in language or speech are listed in the Guidelines box on p. 1042. Information obtained from the history is criti-

TABLE 24-6 Normal Language/Speech Development During Early Childhood

AGE (YEARS)	DEVELOPMENT	INTELLIGIBILITY
1	Says two to three words with meaning Imitates sounds of animals Omits most final and some initial consonants	Usually no more than 25% intelligible to unfamiliar listener Height of unintelligible jargon at age 18 months
2	Uses two- to three-word phrases Has vocabulary of about 300 words Uses "I," "me," and "you" Articulation lags behind vocabulary	50% intelligible in context
3	Says four- to five-word sentences Has vocabulary of about 900 words Uses "who," "what," and "where" in asking questions Uses plurals, pronouns, and prepositions Often repeats and hesitates	75% intelligible
4-5	Has vocabulary of 1500 to 2100 words Able to use most grammatical forms correctly, such as past tense of verb with "yesterday" Uses complete sentences with nouns, verbs, prepositions, adjectives, adverbs, and conjunctions	At age 4 years, speech is 100% intelligible, although some sounds are still imperfect
5-6	Has vocabulary of 3000 words Comprehends "if," "because," and "why" Masters most sounds; still distorts *s, z, sh, ch,* and *j*	

GUIDELINES
Assessing Communication Impairment

KEY QUESTIONS FOR LANGUAGE DISORDERS

1. How old was your child when he (or she) began to speak his (or her) first words?
2. How old was your child when he (or she) began to put words into sentences?
3. Does your child have difficulty in learning new vocabulary words?
4. Does your child omit words from sentences (i.e., do sentences sound telegraphic?) or use short or incomplete sentences?
5. Does your child have trouble with grammar, such as the verbs "is," "am," "are," "was," and "were"?
6. Can your child follow two to three directions given at once?
7. Do you have to repeat directions or questions?
8. Does your child respond appropriately to questions?
9. Does your child ask questions beginning with "who," "what," "where," and "why"?
10. Does it seem that your child has made little or no progress in speech and language in the last 6 to 12 months?

KEY QUESTIONS FOR SPEECH IMPAIRMENT

1. Does your child ever stammer or repeat sounds or words?
2. Does your child seem anxious or frustrated when trying to express an idea?
3. Have you noticed certain behaviors, such as blinking the eyes, jerking the head, or attempting to rephrase thoughts with different words, when your child stammers?
4. What do you do when any of these occur?
5. Does your child omit sounds from words?
6. Does it seem like your child uses *t, d, k,* or *g* in place of most other consonants when speaking?
7. Does your child omit sounds from words or substitute the correct consonant with another one (such as "rabbit" with "wabbit")?
8. Do you have any difficulty in understanding your child's speech? How much of it is intelligible?
9. Has anyone else ever remarked about having difficulty in understanding your child?
10. Has there been any recent change in the sound of your child's voice?

cally important, and parental comments such as "He doesn't say much" or "Her use of words is so much slower than her older brother's was" must be taken seriously. However, caution must also be exercised in evaluating parental comments. Parents may be unaware of the child's difficulties because of lack of comparison with normal language development. Also, they may not realize the degree of unintelligible speech because of familiarity with the child's approximation of words. Conversely, parents may have unrealistic expectations regarding verbal development and may exaggerate the degree of dysfluency, misarticulation, or word usage.

Consequently, ***screening tests*** are a very important component of objective measurement of speech development. The ***Denver Articulation Screening Examination (DASE)*** (see Appendix B) employs the word-imitative procedure and is one of the most frequently used tests. The child repeats 22 words but pronounces 30 different sound elements. The raw score, or the number of correctly pronounced sounds, is then compared with the percentile rank for children in that age-group. The examiner must be careful to evaluate the specific sound rather than the quality of the entire word. For beginning examiners it is helpful to validate the final score by comparing the results with a different examiner, ideally a speech therapist. The child is also scored on intelligibility by selection of one of four possible categories: (1) easy to understand, (2) understandable half of the time, (3) not understandable, or (4) cannot evaluate. The DASE is a reliable, effective screening tool because it requires only 10 minutes for the examiner to perform and is designed to discriminate between significant speech delay and normal variations in the acquisition of speech sounds. It also detects common abnormal physical conditions such as hyponasality, hypernasality, tongue thrust, and lateral lisp.

The ***Early Language Milestone Scale (ELM)**** is a standardized screening instrument for assessing language development in children less than 3 years of age. The test focuses on expressive, receptive, and visual language, and the revised form includes intelligibility (Coplan and Gleason, 1988; Coplan and others, 1982). The ELM relies primarily on the parent's report, with occasional direct testing of the child, and takes 1 to 4 minutes to administer. The best age range for the ELM is 25 to 36 months (Walker and others, 1989).

A number of other tests are available to screen children for impaired language development. The ***Denver II,*** a revision of the Denver Developmental Screening Test, includes an expanded section on language items, and delays in that area provide an early indication for those children who require further evaluation (see Chapter 7). For children ages 2½ to 18 years the ***Peabody Picture Vocabulary Test–Revised*** is a useful screening instrument for word comprehension (Dunn and Dunn, 1981).

Referral. Following assessment and detection of language or speech problems, the nurse must make a decision regarding appropriate referral. The all-too-frequent advice of "let's wait and see what happens" or "your child will grow out of it" is often to the detriment of the child's future development. Since children normally vary greatly in their development of verbal skills, the nurse needs some guidelines for determining which child's development is abnormal. The Guidelines box on p. 1043 lists general recommendations for referring children for specialized audiologic and language evaluations. Information regarding available services for language, speech, and hearing can be obtained from the **American Speech-Language Hearing Association†** and the **Council for Exceptional Children‡** (see also p. 1026 for organizations devoted to hearing impairment).

Education

When a child is delayed in language development, it becomes very important to try to structure the parents' com-

*The complete testing kit can be purchased from Pro-Ed, Inc., (512) 451-3246 (call collect).

†10801 Rockville Pike, Rockville, MD 20852; (301) 897-5700 or (800) 638-8255.

‡Division for Children with Communication Disorders, 1920 Association Dr., Reston, VA 22091.

GUIDELINES
Referral Regarding Communication Impairment

AGE 2 YEARS

Failure to speak any meaningful words spontaneously
Consistent use of gestures rather than vocalizations
Difficulty in following verbal directions
Failure to respond consistently to sound

AGE 3 YEARS

Speech largely unintelligible
Failure to use sentences of three or more words
Omission of initial consonants
Frequent omission of final consonants
Use of vowels rather than consonants

AGE 5 YEARS

Stutters or has any other type of dysfluency
Sentence structure noticeably impaired
Substitutes easily produced sounds for more difficult ones
Omits word endings (plurals, tenses of verbs, etc.)

SCHOOL AGE

Poor voice quality (monotonous, loud, or barely audible)
Vocal pitch inappropriate for age
Any distortions, omissions, or substitutions of sounds after age 7 years
Connected speech characterized by use of unusual confusions or reversals

GENERAL

Any child with signs suggesting a hearing impairment (see p. 1025)
Any child who is embarrassed or disturbed by his or her speech
Parents who are excessively concerned or who pressure the child to speak at a level above that appropriate for the child's age

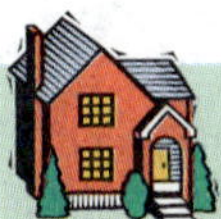

FAMILY HOME CARE
Helping a Child Learn Language

Provide listening opportunities:
- Select a small group of words connected to a specific activity (e.g., say "open" each time a door is opened).
- Repeat the word with the activity several times, then repeat the word but wait for the child to initiate the activity.

Choose vocabulary that is useful, easy to pronounce, and understandable to the child.

Encourage vocabulary development by having the child say the word rather than gesture before fulfilling a request (e.g., expect the child to say all or part of the word "drink" before giving a beverage).

Speak at a level slightly above the child's level (e.g., if the child speaks two words, use three- or four-word phrases).

Expand the statement, preserving the child's intent.*
- Expand the statement using the same noun.
  CHILD: Kitty jump
  ADULT: The kitty is on the chair.
- Replace the noun with a pronoun.
  CHILD: Kitty jump
  ADULT: She is jumping.
- Expand the statement adding new information.
  CHILD: Kitty jump
  ADULT: The dog is jumping, too.

Respond by indicating the meaning of the child's utterance, rather than its linguistic accuracy (or inaccuracy).*
  CHILD: Kitty jump
  ADULT: Yes, the kitty is jumping.

Substitute questions with statements about an observed activity (e.g., rather than asking, "What's that?" say, "Look at the kitten").

Reinforce the child's attempt to use language with verbal praise and affection.

---
*Data from US Department of Health and Human Services: Developmental speech and language disorders: hope through research, Pub No 188-2757, Bethesda, MD, 1988, Public Health Service, National Institutes of Health.

munication to expand the child's language, including new words, new sentence construction, and rules of grammar. The underlying principle is not to bombard children with words so that they learn more language, but to plan what will be said to them, what responses will be expected, and how they will be reinforced. Suggestions to help parents foster their child's attainment of language skills are presented in the Family Home Care box.

Parents should also be aware that children learn language through imitation. Therefore serving as role models by speaking clearly, fluently, and with proper grammar is essential to children's mastery of language and speech. Parents need guidance regarding normal language and speech development so that they expect neither too little nor too much from their child.

KEY POINTS

- The American Association on Mental Retardation (AAMR) defines mental retardation as significantly subaverage intellectual functioning, existing concurrently with related limitations in two or more adaptive skill areas (communication, self-care, home living, social skills, leisure, health and safety, self-direction, functional academics, community use, and work), and manifested before age 18 years.
- Diagnosis of cognitive impairment is based on standard developmental tests and an accurate history, and no child is too young to be assessed.
- Causes of severe mental retardation are primarily genetic, biochemical, and infectious. Mild retardation is associated primarily with familial, social, and environmental causes, whereas severe retardation is more likely to be associated with specific syndromes.
- Primary prevention efforts focus on support for the premature neonate and other high-risk newborns, rubella immunization, genetic counseling, education regarding alcohol, adequate prenatal nutrition, and reduction of nonintentional and intentional cerebral injuries.
- Secondary prevention activities include prenatal diagnosis or carrier detection.
- Tertiary prevention is aimed at minimizing long-term consequences through medical treatment.

- Education of children with cognitive impairment emphasizes sensory and verbal discrimination, improvement of short-term memory, motivation, and technologic support.
- Promoting optimum development may be achieved through family guidance regarding play, communication, discipline, socialization, and sexuality.
- Promotion of independent self-help skills is aimed at feeding, toileting, dressing, and grooming.
- For the hospitalized child with mental retardation, nurses must be aware of the child's abilities and needs, provide a familiar setting, and support families.
- Down syndrome, a chromosome abnormality, is characterized by subnormal intelligence, numerous physical stigmata, slowed social development, congenital anomalies, sensory problems, diminished growth and sexual development, and reduced life expectancy.
- Fragile X syndrome is characterized by mental retardation and phenotypic findings in affected males. It is considered the most common hereditary form of mental retardation and the second most common genetic cause after Down syndrome.
- Hearing defects may be categorized according to etiology, pathology, or symptom severity; prevention, treatment, and rehabilitation are based on these factors.
- Hearing disorders may be classified according to the location of the defect: conductive, sensorineural, mixed conductive-sensorineural, and auditory imperception.
- Some of the effects of hearing loss on growth and development are impaired knowledge of objects, emotional behavior, impaired academic learning, and decreased socialization.
- Prevention of hearing loss is the nurse's major responsibility. Efforts include treatment of infection, auditory testing, immunization, pregnancy and genetic counseling, and reduction of excessive noise.
- Rehabilitation for hearing loss involves parent education and support, hearing aids, lipreading, sign language, cued speech, speech therapy, and promotion of socialization.
- Visual impairments are often classified as legal blindness and partially sighted.
- Common visual impairments in childhood are refractive errors, amblyopia, strabismus, cataracts, glaucoma, trauma, and infections.
- Effects of visual impairment on development include impaired motor function, lack of stimulation, and diminished academic learning.
- Prevention of visual impairment focuses on prenatal screening, prenatal and perinatal care, periodic vision screening of all children, immunization, and safety counseling.
- Nursing goals in visual rehabilitation are helping the family and child adjust to the child's visual impairment, promoting parent-child attachment, fostering optimum development and independence, providing for play and socialization, and being aware of educational facilities.
- For the child undergoing ocular surgery, nursing care is aimed at reassuring the child and family throughout treatment, orienting the child to the surroundings, providing a safe environment, and encouraging independence.

REFERENCES

American Academy of Pediatrics, Committee on Bioethics: Sterilization of women who are mentally handicapped, *Pediatrics* 85(5):868-871, 1990.

American Academy of Pediatrics, Committee on Children with Disabilities: Role of the pediatrician in prevocational and vocational education of children and adolescents with developmental disabilities, *Pediatrics* 78(3):529-530, 1986.

American Academy of Pediatrics, Committee on Genetics: Prenatal diagnosis for pediatricians, *Pediatrics* 84(4):741-744, 1989.

American Academy of Pediatrics, Committee on Sports Medicine: Atlantoaxial instability in Down syndrome, *Pediatrics* 74(1):152-154, 1984.

American Academy of Pediatrics, Committee on Sports Medicine, Committee on Children with Disabilities: Exercise for children who are mentally retarded, *Pediatrics* 80(3):447-448, 1987.

American Psychiatric Association: *Diagnostic and statistical manual of mental disorders,* ed 4 (DSM-IV), Washington, DC, 1994, The Association.

Antonarakis SE and the Down Syndrome collaborative group: Parental origin of the extra chromosome in trisomy 21 as indicated by analysis of DNA polymorphisms, *N Engl J Med* 324:872, 1991.

Batshaw, ML: Mental retardation, *Pediatr Clin North Am* 40(3):465-692, 1993.

Benzcerraf B, Gelman R, Frigoletto F: Sonographic identification of second-trimester fetuses with Down's syndrome, *N Engl J Med* 317(22):1371-1376, 1987.

Bess FH, Paradise JL: Universal screening for infant impairment: not simple, not risk free, not necessarily beneficial, and not presently justified, *Pediatrics* 92:330-334, 1994.

Brown WT and others: Rapid fragile X carrier screening and prenatal diagnosis using a nonradioactive PCR test, *JAMA* 270(13):1569-1575, 1993.

Caputo AR and others: Down syndrome: clinical review of ocular features, *Clin Pediatr* 28(8):355-358, 1989.

Carr J: Six weeks to twenty-one years old: a longitudinal study of children with Down's syndrome and their families, *J Child Psychol Psychiatry* 29(4):407-431, 1988.

Chamberlain A and others: Issues in fertility control for mentally retarded female adolescents. I. Sexual activity, sexual abuse, and contraception, *Pediatrics* 73(4):445-450, 1984.

Chudley AE, Hagerman RJ: Fragile X syndrome, *J Pediatr* 110(6):821-831, 1987.

Consensus Conference: Noise and hearing loss, *JAMA* 263(23):3185-3190, 1990.

Cooley SC, Graham JM: Down syndrome—an update and review for the primary pediatrician, *Clin Pediatr* 30(4):233-253, 1991.

Cooper E: *Nurses' and parents' views of parents' adjustment to having a child with Down's syndrome,* unpublished master's thesis, Halifax, Nova Scotia, Canada, 1989, Dalhousie University.

Coplan J: Evaluation of the child with delayed speech or language, *Pediatr Ann* 14(3):202-208, 1985.

Coplan J, Gleason J: Unclear speech: recognition and significance of unintelligible speech in preschool children, *Pediatrics* 82(3, pt 2):447-452, 1988.

Coplan J and others: Validation of an early language milestone scale in a high-risk population, *Pediatrics* 70(5):677-683, 1982.

Cronister AE, Hagerman RJ: Fragile X syndrome, *J Pediatr Health Care* 3(1):9-19, 1989.

Cronister AE, Jacky P: Fragile X diagnostic testing update, *National Fragile X Foundation Newsletter,* pp 2-3, summer 1992.

Cronk C and others: Growth charts for children with Down syndrome: 1 month to 18 years of age, *Pediatrics* 81(1):102-110, 1988.

Davidson PW: Visual impairment and blindness. In Levine MD, Carey WB, Crocker AC, editors: *Developmental-behavioral pediatrics,* ed 2, Philadelphia, 1992, WB Saunders.

Declining mortality from Down syndrome—no cause for complacency, *Lancet* 335(8694): 888–889, 1990.

Dunn L, Dunn L: *The Peabody Picture Vocabulary Test—Revised,* Circle Pines, MN, 1981, American Guidance Service.

Eilers RE, Oller DK: Infant vocalizations and the early diagnosis of severe hearing impairment, *J Pediatr* 124:199-203, 1994.

Fausti SA and others: High-frequency testing techniques and instrumentation for early detection of ototoxicity, *J Rehabil Res* 30:333-341, 1993.

Fort P and others: Abnormalities of thyroid function in infants with Down syndrome, *J Pediatr* 104(4):545-549, 1984.

Freund LS, Reiss AL, Abrams MT: Psychiatric disorders associated with fragile X in the young female, *Pediatrics* 91(2):321-329, 1993.

Geggel, RL, O'Brien, JE, Feingold, M: Development of valve dysfunction in adolescents and young adults with Down syndrome and no known congenital heart disease, *J Pediatr* 122:821-823, 1993.

Grossman HJ, editor: *Manual on terminology and classification in mental retardation, American Association on Mental Deficiency,* ed 8, Baltimore 1983, Garamond Pridemark Press.

Guitar B: Stuttering, *Feelings Med Signif* 31(3): 9-12, 1989.

Gunn P, Perry P: The temperament of Down's syndrome toddlers and their siblings, *J Child Psychol Psychiatry* 26(6):973-979, 1985.

Haddow JE and others: Prenatal screening for Down's syndrome with use of maternal serum markers, *N Engl J Med* 327:588-593, 1992.

Haseltine B, Miltenberger RG: Teaching self-protection skills to persons with mental retardation, *Am J Ment Retard* 95(2):188-197, 1990.

Hyman SL and others: Children with self-injurious behavior, *Pediatrics* 85:437-441, 1990.

Keltner BR, Tymchuk AJ: Reaching out to mothers with mental retardation, *MCN* 17(3):136-140, 1992.

Keveton J, Balkany TJ: Status of cochlear implantation in children, *J Pediatr* 118:1-7, 1991.

Krais WA: The incompetent developmentally disabled person's right of self-determination, right to die, sterilization and institutionalization, *Am J Law Med* 15(2-3):333-361, 1989.

Libb JW and others: Hearing disorder and cognitive function of individuals with Down syndrome, *Am J Ment Defic* 90(3):353-356, 1985.

Litovitz T, Schmitz BF: Ingestion of cylindrical and button batteries: an analysis of 2382 cases, *Pediatrics* 89:747-757, 1992.

Luckasson R, editor: *Mental retardation: definition, classification and systems of support,* ed 9, Washington, DC, 1992, American Association on Mental Retardation.

Moller MA: Working with visually impaired children and their families, *Pediatr Clin North Am* 40(4):881-890, 1993.

Montgomery TR: Clinical aspects of mental retardation: the chief complaint, *Clin Pediatr* 27(11):529-531, 1988.

Murray F: Language for the handicapped, *Point of View* 21(3):8-9, 1984.

National Institutes of Health: *NIH consensus statement: early identification of hearing impairment in infants and young children,* vol 11, no 1, Washington, DC, 1993, NIH.

Ousley OY, Mesibov GB: Sexual attitudes and knowledge of high-functioning adolescents and adults with autism, *J Autism Dev Disord* 21(4):471-481, 1991.

Passer A and others: Issues in fertility control for mentally retarded female adolescents. II. Parental attitudes toward sterilization, *Pediatrics* 73(4):451-454, 1984.

Pueschel SM: The child with Down syndrome. In Levine MD and others, editors: *Developmental-behavioral pediatrics,* ed 2, Philadelphia, 1992, WB Saunders Co.

Pueschel, SM, Scola, FH, Pezzullo, JC: A longitudinal study of atlanto-dens relationships in asymptomatic individuals with Down syndrome, *Pediatrics,* 89:1194-1198, 1992.

Reed C and others: Analytic study of the Tadoma method: effects of hand position on segmental speech production, *J Speech Hear Res* 32:921-929, 1989.

Roizen NJ and others: Hearing loss in children with Down syndrome, *J Pediatr* 123:S9-12, 1993.

Sarant JZ and others: The effect of handedness in tactile speech perception, *J Rehabil Res* 30:423-435, 1993.

Sharts-Hopko NC: Depo-Provera, *MCN* 18(2): 128, 1993.

Shonkoff JP, Hauser-Cram P: Early intervention for disabled infants and their families: a quantitative analysis, *Pediatrics* 80(5):650-657, 1987.

Silva MC: Assessing competency for informed consent with mentally retarded minors, *Pediatr Nurs* 10(4):261-265, 306, 1984.

Simko A and others: Fragile X syndrome: recognition in young children, *Pediatrics* 83(4): 547-552, 1989.

Sirrocco A: *The 1986 inventory of long-term care places: an overview of facilities for the mentally retarded.* Advance data from Vital and Health Statistics, No 143, DHHS Pub No (PHS) 87-1250, Public Health Service, Hyattsville, MD, 1987.

Steele S and others: Home management of URI in children with Down syndrome, *Pediatr Nurs* 15(5):484-488, 1989.

Task Force on Joint Assessment of Prenatal and Perinatal Factors Associated with Brain Disorders: National Institutes of Health report on causes of mental retardation and cerebral palsy, *Pediatrics* 76(3):457-458, 1985.

Tharinger D, Horton CB, Millea S: Sexual abuse and exploitation of children and adults with mental retardation and other handicaps, *Child Abuse Negl* 14(3):301-312, 1990.

US Department of Health and Human Services: *Developmental speech and language disorders: hope through research,* Pub No 1 88-2757, Bethesda, MD, 1988, Public Health Service, National Institutes of Health.

Vessey JA: Down syndrome. In Jackson PL, Vessey JA: *Primary care of the child with a chronic condition,* St Louis, 1992, Mosby.

Walker D and others: Early Language Milestone Scale and language screening of young children, *Pediatrics* 83(2):284-288, 1989.

Warren ST, Nelson D: Advances in molecular analysis of fragile X syndrome, *JAMA* 271(7):536-542, 1994.

Warzak WJ, Page TJ: Teaching refusal skills to sexually active adolescents, *J Behav Ther Exp Psychiatry* 21(2):133-139, 1990.

Williams JK: Reproductive decisions: adolescents with Down syndrome, *Pediatr Nurs* 9(1):43-44+, 1983.

Zipursky A, Poon A, Doyle J: Leukemia in Down syndrome: a review, *Pediatr Hematol Oncol* 9(2):139-149, 1992.

BIBLIOGRAPHY

Mental Retardation

American Academy of Pediatrics, Committee on Children With Disabilities: Screening infants and young children for developmental disabilities, *Pediatrics* 93(5):863-865, 1994.

Batshaw ML, Perret YM: *Children with disabilities: a medical primer,* ed 3, Baltimore, MD, 1992, Paul H Brookes.

Brizee L, Sophos C, McLaughlin J: Nutrition issues in developmental disabilities, *Infants Young Child* 2(3):10-21, 1990.

Bromley B, Blacher J: Factors delaying out of home placement of children with severe handicaps, *Am J Ment Retard* 94(3):284-291, 1989.

Brown FR and others: Intellectual and adaptive functioning in individuals with Down syndrome in relation to age and environmental placement, *Pediatrics* 85:450-452, 1990.

Chomicki S, Wilgosh L: Health care concerns among parents of children with mental retardation, *Child Health Care* 21(4):206-212, 1992.

Crocker AC, Nelson RP: Mental retardation. In Levine MD and others, editors: *Developmental-behavioral pediatrics,* ed 2, Philadelphia, 1992, WB Saunders.

Cullen JC and others: Coping, satisfaction, and the life cycle in families with mentally retarded persons, *Issues Compr Pediatr Nurs* 14(3):193-207, 1991.

Davis BD, Steele S: Case management for young children with special health care needs, *Pediatr Nurs* 17(1):15-19, 1991.

Elkins TE and others: Reproductive health concerns in Down syndrome: a report of eight cases, *J Reprod Med* 35(7):745-750, 1990.

Elvik SL and others: Sexual abuse in the developmentally disabled: dilemmas of diagnosis, *Child Abuse Negl* 14(4):497-502, 1990.

Fagan JF and others: Selective screening device for the early detection of normal or delayed cognitive development in infants at risk for later mental retardation, *Pediatrics* 78(6): 1021-1026, 1986.

Forness SR, Hecht B: Special education for handicapped and disabled children: classification, programs, and trends, *J Pediatr Nurs* 3(2):75-88, 1988.

Friedrich WN, Cohen DS, Wilturner LT: Specific beliefs as moderator variables in maternal coping with mental retardation, *Child Health Care* 17(1):40-44, 1988.

Haefner HK, Elkins TE: Contraceptive management for female adolescents with mental retardation and handicapping disabilities, *Curr Opin Obstet Gynecol* 3(6):820-824, 1991.

Lynch EC, Staloch NH: Parental perception of physicians' communication in the informing process, *Ment Retard* 26(2):77-81, 1988.

Mahoney G, Finger I, Powell A: Relationship of maternal behavioral style to the development of organically impaired mentally retarded infants, *Am J Ment Defic* 90(3):296-302, 1985.

Morgan CD, Elias S: Prenatal diagnosis of genetic disorders, *J Perinat Neonat Nurs* 2(4):1-12, 1989.

Nehring WS: The nurse whose specialty is developmental disabilities, *Pediatr Nurs* 20(1): 78-81, 1994.

Oehler JM and others: How to target infants at highest risk for developmental delay, *MCN* 18(1):20-23, 1993.

Pipes PL, Glass R: Nutrition and feeding of children with developmental delays and related problems. In Pipes PL, Trahms CM, editors: *Nutrition in infancy and childhood,* ed 5, St Louis, 1993, Mosby.

Roth SP, Morse JS, editors: *A life-span approach to nursing care for individuals with developmental disabilities,* Baltimore, MD, 1994, Paul H Brooks.

Sameroff AJ and others: Intelligence quotient scores of 4-year-old children: social-environmental risk factors, *Pediatrics* 79(3):343-350, 1987.

Savage TA, Culbert C: Early intervention: the unique role of nursing, *J Pediatr Nurs* 4(5):339-345, 1989.

Steele S: Assessment of functional wellness behaviors in adolescents who are mentally retarded, *Issues Compr Pediatr Nurs* 9:331-340, 1986.

Steele S: Deinstitutionalization of persons with mental retardation/developmental disabilities, *Issues Compr Pediatr Nurs* 10:235-250, 1987.

Steele S: Assessing developmental delays in preschool children, *J Pediatr Health Care* 2(3):141-145, 1988.

Steele S: Fostering potentiality in persons with mental retardation, *Issues Compr Pediatr Nurs* 11:283-290, 1988.

Steele S: Preschool children with developmental delays: nursing intervention *J Pediatr Health Care* 2(5):245-252, 1988.

Stern F, Gorga D: Neurodevelopmental treatment (NDT): therapeutic intervention and its efficacy, *Infants Young Child* 1(1):22-32, 1988.

Sullivan-Volyai S: Practical aspects of toilet training the child with a physical disability, *Issues Compr Pediatr Nurs* 9(2):79-96, 1986.

Taylor MO: Teaching parents about their impaired adolescent's sexuality, *MCN* 14:109-112, 1989.

Varley CK, Fururkawa MJ: Psychopathology in young children with developmental disabilities, *Child Health Care* 19(2):86-92, 1990.

Vessey JA: Care of the hospitalized child with a cognitive developmental delay, *Holistic Nurs Pract* 2:48-54, 1988.

Williams DN: Becoming a woman: the girl who is mentally retarded, *Pediatr Nurs* 13(2):89-93, 1987.

Wolraich ML, Siperstein GN, O'Keefe P: Pediatricians' perceptions of mentally retarded individuals, *Pediatrics* 80(5):643-649, 1987.

Down Syndrome

Atlantoaxial instability in Down syndrome, *Lancet* 1(8628):24, 1989.

Brown FR and others: Intellectual and adaptive functioning in individuals with Down syndrome in relation to age and environmental placement, *Pediatrics* 85:450-452, 1990.

Churchill LR: Bone marrow transplantation, physician bias, and Down syndrome: ethical reflections, *J Pediatr* 114(1):87-88, 1989.

Cutler AT, Benezra-Obeiter R, Brink SJ: Thyroid function in young children with Down syndrome, *Am J Dis Child* 14:479-483, 1986.

Danner SC, Cerutti ER: *Nursing your baby with Down's syndrome,* Rochester, NY, 1984, Childbirth Graphics.

Davidson RG: Atlantoaxial instability in individuals with Down syndrome: a fresh look at the evidence, *Pediatrics* 81(6):857-865, 1988.

Goodwin BA, Huether CA: Revised estimates and projections of Down syndrome births in the United States and the effects of prenatal diagnosis utilization, 1970-2002, *Prenat Diagn* 7(4):261-271, 1987.

Hayes A, Batshaw ML: Down syndrome, *Pediatr Clin North Am* 40(3):523-535, 1993.

Lockitch G and others: Infection and immunity in Down syndrome: a trial of long-term low oral doses of zinc, *J Pediatr* 114:781-787, 1989.

Marino B and others: Ventricular septal defect in Down syndrome, *Am J Dis Child* 144:544-545, 1990.

May DC, Turnbull N: Plastic surgeons' opinions of facial surgery for individuals with Down syndrome, *Ment Retard* 30(1):29-33, 1992.

Msall ME, DiGaudio KM, Malone A: Health, developmental, and psychosocial aspects of Down syndrome, *Infants Young Child* 4(1): 35-45, 1991.

Pueschel SM, editor: *New perspectives on Down syndrome,* Baltimore, 1987, Paul H Brookes.

Pueschel SM, editor: *The young person with Down syndrome: transition from adolescence to adulthood,* Baltimore, 1988, Paul H Brookes.

Pueschel SM: Atlantoaxial instability, sport, and Down syndrome, *Lancet* 1(8635):438-439, 1989.

Quinn MM: Attachment between mothers and their Down syndrome infants, *West J Nurs Res* 13(3):382-396, 1991.

Rodgers PT, Coleman M, Buckley S: *Medical care in Down syndrome: a preventive medical approach,* New York, NY, 1992, Marcel Dekker.

Schneider DS and others: Patterns of cardiac care in infants with Down syndrome, *Am J Dis Child* 143:363-365, 1989.

Sharav T, Collins RM Jr, Baab PJ: Growth studies in infants and children with Down's syndrome and elevated level of thyrotropin, *Am J Dis Child* 142:1302-1306, 1988.

Spencer K, Carpenter P: Prospective study of prenatal screening for Down's syndrome with free β human chorionic gonadotrophin, *Br Med J* 307:764-769, 1993.

Steele S: Down syndrome: nursing interventions, newborn through preschool age years, *Issues Compr Pediatr Nurs* 13(2):111-126, 1990.

Walden BJ: The newborn infant with Down syndrome: realities and possibilities, *J Perinat Neonat Nurs* 2(4):72-82, 1989.

Van Riper M, Ryff C, Pridham K: Parental and family well-being in families of children with Down syndrome: a comparative study, *Res Nurs Health* 15:227-235, 1992.

Vessey JA, Swanson MN: Caring for the child with Down syndrome, *J School Nurs* 9(14):20-33, 1993.

Fragile-X Syndrome

Brown WT: The fragile X syndrome, *Neurol Clin* 7(1):107-121, 1989.

Crabbe LS and others: Cardiovascular abnormalities in children with fragile X syndrome, *Pediatrics* 41(4):714-715, 1993.

Cronister AE, Hagerman RJ: Fragile X syndrome, *J Pediatr Health Care* 3(1):9-19, 1989.

Fisch GS: What is associated with the fragile X syndrome? *Am J Genet* 48:112-121, 1993.

Hagerman RJ, Murphy MA, Wittenberger MD: A controlled trial of stimulant medication in children with the fragile X syndrome, *Am J Med Genet* 30(1-2):377-392, 1988.

Hagerman RJ, Sobesky WE: Psychopathology in fragile X syndrome, *Am J Orthopsychiatry* 59(1):142-152, 1989.

Hull C, Hagerman RJ: A study of the physical, behavioral, and medical phenotype, including anthropometric measures of females with fragile X syndrome, *Am J Dis Child* 147:1236-1241, 1993.

Nelson DL: Fragile X syndrome: review and current status, *Growth Genet Horm* 9(2):1-6, 1993.

Reiss AL, Freund L: Fragile X syndrome, *Biol Psychiatry* 27(2):223-240, 1990.

Schopmeyer BB, Lowe F, editors: *The fragile X child,* San Diego, 1992, Singular.

Silverman AC, Hagerman RJ: Fragile X syndrome. In Jackson PL, Vessey, JA: *Primary care of the child with a chronic condition,* St Louis, 1992, Mosby.

Simensen RJ, Rogers RC: Fragile-X syndrome, *Am Fam Physician* 39(5):185-193, 1989.

Simko A and others: Fragile X syndrome: recognition in young children, *Pediatrics* 83(4): 547-552, 1989.

Sutherland GR, Mulley JC: Diagnostic molecular genetics of the fragile X, *Clin Genet* 37(1):2-11, 1990.

Taylor AK and others: Molecular predictors of cognitive involvement in female carriers of fragile X syndrome, *JAMA* 271(7):507-514, 1994.

Webb T, Crawley P, Bundey S: Folate treatment of a boy with fragile X syndrome, *J Ment Defic Res* 34(pt 1):67-73, 1990.

Hearing Impairment

American Academy of Otolaryngology–Head and Neck Surgery Subcommittee on Cochlear Implants, Kveton J, Balkany TJ: Status of cochlear implantation in children, *J Pediatr* 118(25):1-7, 1991.

American Speech-Language Hearing Association: Guidelines for the audiologic assess ment of children from birth through 36 months of age, *ASHA* 33(suppl 5):37-43, 1991.

American Speech-Language Hearing Association: *How to buy a hearing aid*, Rockville, MD, The Association.

Badger T, Jones E: Deaf and hearing: children's conceptions of the body interior, *Pediatr Nurs* 16(2):201-205, 1990.

Balkany T: A brief perspective on cochlear implants, *N Engl J Med* 328:281-282, 1993 (editorial).

Beauchaine KL, Gorga MP: The identification and diagnosis of hearing loss in infants, *Clin Commun Dis* 1:21-29, 1991.

Boothroyd A, Geers AE, Moog JS: Practical implications of cochlear implants in children, *Ear Hear,* 12(4 suppl):81S-89S, 1991.

Cohen NL and others: A prospective, randomized study of cochlear implants, *N Engl J Med* 328:233-237, 1993.

Coplan J: Deafness: ever heard of it? Delayed recognition of permanent hearing loss, *Pediatrics* 79(2):206-213, 1987.

Cox RM: O the evaluation of a new generation of hearing aids, *J Rehabil Res* 30:297-304, 1993.

Epstein S, Reilly JS: Sensorineural hearing loss, *Pediatr Clin North Am* 36(6):1501-1520, 1989.

Grundfast KM, Lalwani AK: Practical approach to diagnosis and management of hereditary hearing impairment (HHI), *ENT J* 71:479-493, 1992.

Harrison LL: Minimizing barriers when teaching hearing-impaired clients, *MCN* 15(2): 113, 1990.

Jackson CB: Primary health care for deaf children, part I, *J Pediatr Health Care* 3(6):316-318, 1989.

Jackson CB: Primary health care for deaf children, part II, *J Pediatr Health Care* 4(1):39-41, 1990.

Kelly DP and others: Attention deficits in children and adolescents with hearing loss, *Am J Dis Child* 147:737-741, 1993.

Kravitz L, Selekman J: Understanding hearing loss in children, *Pediatr Nurs* 18:591-594, 1992.

McGarr N: Research on the use of sensory aids for hearing-impaired people, *Volta Rev* 91(5): 1-138, 1989.

Nadol JB: Hearing loss, *N Engl J Med* 329:1092-1102, 1993.

Oberklaid F, Harris C, Keir E: Auditory dysfunction in children with school problems, *Clin Pediatr* 28(9):397-403, 1989.

Paparella MM, Fox RY, Schachern PA: Diagnosis and treatment of sensorineural hearing loss in children, *Otolaryngol Clin North Am* 22:51-73, 1989.

Roizen NJ: Neurosensory hearing loss. In Capute AJ, Accardo PJ, editors: *Developmental disabilities in infancy and childhood*, Baltimore, 1991, Paul H Brookes.

Schilling LS, DeJesus E: Developmental issues in deaf children, *J Pediatr Health Care* 7:161-166, 1993.

Stewart JM, Downs MP: Congenital conductive hearing loss: the need for early identification and intervention, *Pediatrics* 91:355-359, 1993.

Thomas KA: How the NICU environment sounds to a preterm infant, *MCN* 14:249-251, 1989.

Thompson M, Thompson G: Early identification of hearing loss: listen to parents, *Clin Pediatr* 30(2):77-80, 1991.

Weibley T: Inside the incubator, *MCN* 14(2):96-100, 1989.

White KR, Behrens TR: The Rhode Island hearing assessment project: implications for universal newborn hearing screening, *Semin Hear* 14:1-86, 1993.

Zargi M, Boltezar IH: Effects of recurrent otitis media in infancy on auditory perception and speech, *Am J Otolaryngol* 13:366-372, 1992.

Vision Impairment

American Foundation for the Blind: *Directory of services for blind and visually impaired persons in the United States and Canada,* ed 24, New York, 1993, The Foundation.

Bailey C, Buckley R: Ocular prostheses and contact lenses. II. Contact lenses, *Br Med J* 302(6784):1066-1069, 1991.

Carr M and others: Curling-iron cornea, *N Engl J Med* 319:1672, 1988, (letter).

Catalano RA: Eye injuries and prevention, *Pediatr Clin North Am* 40:827-840, 1993.

DeRespinis PA: Cyanoacrylage nail glue mistaken for eye drops, *JAMA* 263(17):2301, 1990.

Dudley N: Aids for visual impairment, *Br Med J* 302(6761):1151-1153, 1990.

Friendly DS: Development of vision in infants and young children, *Pediatric Clin North Am* 40:693-704, 1993.

Garber N: Health promotion and disease prevention in ophthalmology, *J Ophthal Nurs Technol* 9(5):186-192, 1990.

King RA: Common ocular signs and symptoms in childhood, *Pediatric Clin North Am* 40:753-766, 1993.

Kodadek SM, Haylor MJ: Using interpretive methods to understand family caregiving when a child is blind, *J Pediatr Nurs* 5(1):42-49, 1990.

Kovalesky A: *Nurses guide to children's eyes,* New York, 1985, Grune & Stratton.

Lavrich JB, Nelson LB: Diagnosis and treatment of strabismus disorders, *Pediatr Clin North Am* 40:737-752, 1993.

Magramm I: Amblyopia: etiology, detection, and treatment, *Pediatr Rev* 13:7-14, 1992.

Menacker SJ: Visual function in children with developmental disabilities, *Pediatr Clin North Am* 40:659-673, 1993.

Moller AM: Working with visually impaired children and their families, *Pediatr Clin North Am* 40:881-890, 1993.

Nelson LB, Wilson TW, Jeffers JB: Eye injuries in childhood: demography, etiology, and prevention, *Pediatrics* 84(3):438-441, 1989.

Norris RM: Commonsense tips for working with blind patients, *Am J Nurs,* pp 360-361, March 1989.

Phillips S, Hartley JT: Developmental differences and interventions for blind children, *Pediatr Nurs* 14(3):201-204, 1988.

Repka MX: Common pediatric neuro-ophthalmologic conditions, *Pediatr Clin North Am,* 40:777-788, 1993.

Rollins JA: National Library Service for the Blind and Physically Handicapped, *Pediatr Nurs* 14(6):522, 1988.

Rubin SE, Nelson LB: Amblyopia: diagnosis and management, *Pediatr Clin North Am* 40:727-736, 1993.

Schraeder B, McEvoy-Shields K: Visual acuity, binocular vision, and ocular muscle balance in VLBW children, *Pediatr Nurs* 17(1):30-33, 1991.

Tongue AC: Refractive errors in children, *Pediatr Clin North Am* 34(6):1425-1437, 1987.

Multiple Impairments: Deaf-Blind

Luiselli JK: Training self-feeding skills in children who are deaf and blind, *Behav Mod* 17:457-473, 1993.

Programs for deaf-blind children and adults, *Am Ann Deaf* 138:205-209, 1993.

Communication Impairment

Accardo P, Whitman B: Toe walking: a marker of language disorders, *Clin Pediatr* 28(8):347-350, 1989.

Aram DM and others: Very low birthweight children and speech and language development, *J Speech Hear Res* 34:1169-1179, 1991.

Bashir AS, Stark RE, Graham JM: Communicative disorders. In Levine MD and others, editors: *Developmental-behavioral pediatrics,* ed 2 Philadelphia, 1992, WB Saunders.

Blamey P and others: Speech perception using combinations of auditory, visual, and tactile information, *Vet Admin J Rehabil Res Dev* 26(1):15-24, 1989.

Brady JP: The pharmacology of stuttering: a critical review, *Am J Psychiatry* 10:1309-1316, 1991.

Choi S, Cotton R: Surgical management of voice disorders, *Pediatr Clin North Am* 36(6): 1535-1549, 1989.

Fischel J and others: Language growth in children with expressive language delay, *Pediatrics* 82(2):218-227, 1989.

Hall D: Delayed speech in children, *Br Med J* 297(6659):1281-1282, 1988.

Kilmon CA, Barber N, Chapman K: Instruments for the screening of speech/language development in children, *J Pediatr Health Care* 5:61-70, 1991.

Klein SK: Evaluation for suspected language disorders in preschool children, *Pediatr Clin North Am* 38:1455-1467, 1991.

Lombardino L, Stapell J, Gerhardt K: Evaluating communicative behaviors in infancy, *J Pediatr Health Care* 1(5):240-246, 1987.

Menyuk P: Language development in a social context, *J Pediatr* 109(1):217-224, 1986.

Smith R and others: Effectiveness of a writing system using a computerized long-range optical pointer and 10-branch abbreviation expansion, *Vet Admin J Rehabil Res Dev* 26(1):51-62, 1989.

Speech dysfluency, *Lancet* 8637(1):530-532, 1989.

Weiss AL, Zebrowski PM: Disfluencies in the conversations of young children who suffer: some answers about questions, *J Speech Hear Res* 35:1230-1238, 1992.

CHAPTER 25

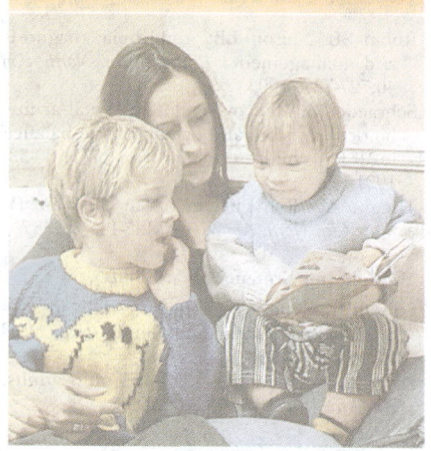

Family-Centered Home Care

CHAPTER OUTLINE

RELATED TOPICS

GENERAL CONCEPTS OF HOME CARE

Home care is not a new concept in pediatrics. Over time, the term has referred to parents caring for mildly ill children at home, to nursing home visits after children are discharged from the hospital, to hospice care, and, more recently, to care at home for children with more serious chronic illness and dependence on medical technology (Wong, 1991). As discussed in this chapter, ***home care*** refers to care provided for children with complex health care needs and their families in their places of residence for the purpose of promoting, maintaining, or restoring health or for maximizing the level of independence while minimizing the effects of disability and illness, including terminal illness. It differs from ***hospice care,*** which is a program of palliative and supportive care services providing physical, psychologic, social, and spiritual care for dying persons, their families, and other loved ones. Hospice services are available in both the home and inpatient settings (Strahan, 1993).

IMPETUS FOR HOME CARE

The initial impetus for home care for children with complex medical conditions came from parents' desire to have their child at home and from professionals' willingness to work with families to achieve this goal. Improving the quality of life for both the child and the family was the driving force in the efforts to move technology-dependent children from the hospital to the home setting.

Other factors eventually influenced the shift toward an emphasis on home care for this population. One factor, resulting from dramatic advances in medical care over the past two decades, is the substantial increase in the number of children requiring long-term complex medical care. Perhaps the greatest influence on the numbers of technology-dependent children results from advances in neonatal care.

■ Elizabeth Ahmann, RN, ScD, authored this chapter.

Portions of this text are modified from Ahmann E: An overview of issues in pediatric high tech home care. In Gorski L: *High tech home care manual,* Gaithersburg, MD, 1994, Aspen; and Ahmann E: Family-centered care: shifting our orientation, *Pediatr Nurs* 20(2):113-117, 1994.

Other factors that influence the numbers of technology-dependent children include improvements in trauma care and the survival of severe trauma victims; increased survival rates for children with leukemia and other cancers, chronic kidney disorders, sickle cell anemia, cystic fibrosis, spina bifida, and cardiac or intestinal malformations; more aggressive care for muscular dystrophy and degenerative neuromuscular disorders; and more children with acquired immunodeficiency syndrome (AIDS) (Office of Technology Assessment, 1987).

The cost of care is another critical factor. For third-party payers and the government, the cost of home care is generally less than the cost of hospital care for children dependent on medical technology and requiring substantial and complex care. Cost savings may be as high as 50% for premature infants with multiple problems (Richman, 1990). Similarly, cost savings to Medicaid in the range of 40% to 60% ($79,000 to $83,000) have been documented for home care of children with respiratory technology dependence (Fields and others, 1991). Costs to public and private insurers may be lower for home care because, at home, families absorb many of the costs of care, including medication, supplies, transportation, shelter, utilities, food, laundry, and housekeeping. Families generally provide at least some portion of the nursing care as well, and some may become unemployed or only partially employed to stay at home. The out-of-pocket expenses and loss of income can become a financial burden for the family (Birenbaum and Clarke-Steffen, 1992; Dowd and Vlastuin, 1990; Zanoa, 1992).

EFFECTIVENESS OF HOME CARE

The effectiveness of home care for many children has influenced the prevalence of the practice. However, home care may not be possible in all circumstances. A number of factors must be present to make it effective. First, the child's condition must be medically stable so that care can be managed in the home setting and supported by available home care equipment (Goldberg, 1990). Second, the family must want the child at home and must have the motivation and ability to learn the child's care. Families must also be able to live with the intrusion of the child's equipment, care schedule, and nurses and other providers in their daily life. Third, professionals and the community must be prepared to provide the necessary support to make home care successful. Services that support successful home care include those listed in the box below (left). Fourth, financial support, public and private, is essential.

Even if home care is initially successful for a child and family, changing factors may influence the plan. Alterations in the child's medical condition, the lack of adequate community resources, depletion of the family's financial resources, high levels of family stress and exhaustion, and disagreements between the family members and the health care team can all affect the success of home care (Harris, 1988). Changes in the home care plan or short- or long-term residential care may be alternatives if any of these occur.

DISCHARGE PLANNING AND SELECTION OF A HOME CARE AGENCY

Much of the success of home care for the child who is dependent on medical technology depends on careful planning and preparation. Despite the rapid growth of home care for technology-dependent children, negotiation with the insurance company may be required (Klug, 1991). General principles of discharge planning and transition to home care are addressed in Chapter 26. Discharge planning must begin early, be a multidisciplinary process, and involve the family. Early involvement of the home care agency promotes continuity of care and a smooth transition from hospital to home. The home care plan for a child with complex care requirements should address the many health and community services that may need to be mobilized (see box below, left). Comprehensive written home care instructions facilitate continuity of care across settings and providers (see box below).*

*Numerous home care instructions are available in *Wong and Whaley's Clinical Manual of Pediatric Nursing* (Mosby).

SERVICES THAT SUPPORT EFFECTIVE HOME CARE

- Adequate family training and preparation
- Professional caregivers trained in relevant nursing and communication skills
- Developmental intervention and support services
- Appropriately designed and well-maintained equipment
- Adequate social and psychologic support services
- High-quality respite care
- Appropriate home renovation
- Telephone service in the home
- Appropriate transportation
- Appropriate locally available emergency facilities
- Competent case management services

Modified from Office of Technology Assessment (OTA), Congress of the United States: *Technology dependent children: hospital v. home care—a technical memorandum* (OTA-TM-H-38), Washington, DC, 1987, US Government Printing Office.

MINIMUM CONTENTS OF WRITTEN HOME CARE INSTRUCTIONS

- A schedule of routine care needs
- Correct settings for any equipment required
- A list of signs, symptoms, and parameters (physical and behavioral) that are normal for the individual child
- A list of signs, symptoms, and parameters (physical and behavioral) that indicate a problem for the individual child
- Guidelines and a list for whom to contact about what problems
- An explanation of pertinent emergency procedures

From Ahmann E: An overview of issues in pediatric high tech home care. In Gorski L: *High tech home care manual,* Gaithersburg, MD, 1994, Aspen.

➤ **NURSING TIP** An excellent method of providing home care instructions is with video recordings. Once the family masters the procedures, consider video recording their performance on tape. Visual learning is most helpful for people who cannot read or are not fluent in English (Curry and Cullen, 1990).

The plans for transition from hospital to home should include family members (at least two persons) both learning and demonstrating all aspects of the child's care in the hospital. An in-hospital trial period during which parents provide total care for the child is generally beneficial as well. After a successful trial, the family may benefit from taking the child home on a brief pass before making final discharge plans. (This may need to be negotiated with the insurance company.) The home care nurse will play an important role in assessing this experience with the family. Whether or not the child is taken home on a pass, a predischarge home visit offers the home care nurse the opportunity to meet the family, help them assess their preparedness and the preparedness of the home environment, discuss plans for arranging the child's equipment at home (Fig. 25-1), reinforce prior discharge teaching, and implement any additional teaching that may be necessary.

CASE MANAGEMENT

Parents of children with complex care requirements often express frustration about the fragmentation of services and a desire for competent case management services (Diehl, Moffitt, and Wade, 1991). Traditional definitions of ***case management*** generally focus on cost control, attainment of desired clinical outcomes, and monitoring and evaluation of care provided. However, for optimum home care of the child who is technology dependent, case management—or care coordination—should be viewed more broadly.

Care coordination has several purposes. Its primary goal is ensuring continuity for the child and family across hospital, home, educational, therapeutic, and other settings. Care should be coordinated among multiple providers to reduce the complexity of care for the child, reduce fragmentation of care, and decrease the burden of care for the family. Care coordination should ensure that the medical, nursing, and health maintenance needs of the child are addressed, as well as the financial issues, psychosocial concerns, and educational issues of the child and family (Lobosco and others, 1991).

Care coordination is most effective if a single person works with the family to accomplish the many tasks and responsibilities involved (see box below). The nurse case manager should have a minimum of a baccalaureate degree in nursing and 3 years' experience (American Nurses Association, 1988). The nurse should also be knowledgeable about community resources, including the following: primary, secondary, and tertiary health care services; speech, language, hearing, and vision resources; respite care services; finan-

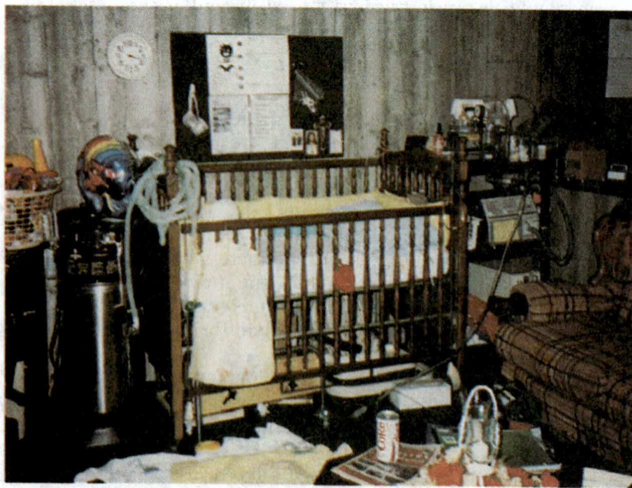

FIG. 25-1 An essential aspect of preparation for home is arranging equipment and supplies.

ASPECTS OF CARE COORDINATION

ASSESS NEEDS

Assess medical, nursing, and other needs of child.
Assess resources and needs of family.
Assess home environment.
Assess resources of community.

PLAN FOR COMPREHENSIVE CARE

Develop overall integrated plan of care.
Combine plans of various disciplines.
Highlight family goals.
Assure health maintenance needs are addressed.

LINK CLIENT(S) WITH SERVICE PROVIDER

Provide information about available services.
Initiate referrals to desired services.
Arrange appointments.
Assist with transportation arrangements.

COORDINATE SERVICES

Specify responsibilities of family and service providers.
Obtain agreements.
Help avoid service duplication.
Arrange conferences as necessary.
Assist in troubleshooting and problem solving between family and service providers.

MONITOR AND EVALUATE SERVICE PROVISION

Maintain regular contact with family and providers.
Review care plan on a regular basis.
Supervise quality of care.
Assess safety in provision of care.
Assess family satisfaction with care provided.

ADVOCATE FOR APPROPRIATE SERVICES

Address problem areas in home care services.
Encourage educational opportunities.
Negotiate insurance coverage.
Lobby for needed services and benefits.

PROVIDE ADMINISTRATIVE SUPPORT

Inventory equipment and supplies.
Assist in financial planning.
Complete paperwork for insurance, other agencies.
Oversee scheduling of provider visits and appointments.

From Ahmann E: An overview of issues in pediatric high tech home care. In Gorski L: *High tech home care manual,* Gaithersburg, MD, 1994, Aspen.

cial assistance programs; parent groups; advocacy groups; local, state, and federal public officials; transportation services; and private sector individuals with an interest in children with disabilities (Davis and Steele, 1991).

While professionals must always see part of their role as ensuring that integrated, coordinated care is provided, care coordination should promote the family's role as primary decision maker and enhance the family's capability to meet the special needs of the child and the family unit (Johnson, Jeppson, and Redburn, 1992; McGonigel, Kaufmann, and Johnson, 1991). Families may choose to be involved to varying degrees in the tasks involved in coordination of their child's care. Many parents will take on increasing responsibility for care coordination over time; they should be encouraged and supported in this role.

ROLE OF THE NURSE, TRAINING, AND STANDARDS OF CARE

The home care nurse must share a level of technical expertise with the critical care nurse while being able to adapt equipment, procedures, and the nursing process to the home setting. (See Chapters 27, 28, and 31 for specific technical skills that may be required in home care practice.) The need for technical expertise must be matched by a knowledge of child development and the ability to work creatively with the child challenged by chronic illness and technology dependence. When practicing in the home, the nurse must be comfortable making independent nursing judgments and problem solving with no immediate assistance. At the same time, the nurse must have excellent interpersonal skills, an ability to work with other professionals and the family, and, most important, an ability to respect family autonomy. (see box below.)

When working with a home care agency, nurses should expect to receive patient placements appropriate to their expertise. They should also expect orientation in the following areas: to the individual patient's care plan and equipment needs; to the agency's policies and procedures, including procedures for addressing any problems that may occur when care is provided in the home; to documentation procedures (reimbursement-driven documentation in home care differs from documentation practices in the hospital setting); and to legal liability issues. Supervision of practice, including occasional site visits by a nursing supervisor, should be provided.

ASPECTS OF THE ROLE OF THE HOME CARE NURSE

- Providing safe nursing care to the child
- Assisting families in assessing their strengths, resources, needs, and stressors
- Developing a comprehensive plan of care with the family
- Helping the family to promote optimum development in the child
- Providing information
- Referring families to sources of information and support
- Aiding families in case management tasks
- Supporting and empowering families in their efforts to problem solve, cope, and adapt to the challenges they face
- Providing appropriate documentation of care

Modified from Ahmann E: An overview of issues in pediatric high tech home care. In Gorski L: *High tech home care manual,* Gaithersburg, MD, 1994, Aspen.

Home care agencies, public or private, that participate in the Medicare or Medicaid programs must be certified by a federally designated state-certifying body and abide by federal and state regulations. Private agencies that do not participate in the federal programs are not mandated to meet the federal standards. The trend is for large, national, private agencies to develop a certifying process that will ensure greater credibility and acceptable standards of practice (Klug, 1992). The American Nurses Association (ANA) has developed standards of nursing practice for both community health and home care nurses that should guide practice in the home setting (ANA, 1986a, 1986b). Despite some important differences between pediatric and adult care in the home, as of this writing, no national standards specific to pediatric home care practice have been developed.

FAMILY-CENTERED HOME CARE

Technology dependence, chronic illness, and complex care requirements cross social, cultural, and economic boundaries. No matter what a family's background, family values must be respected in the provision of home care services. The home is the family's domain, and the child is at home because the family's central role is to nurture and raise their child. The ultimate responsibility for managing the child's health, developmental, and emotional needs lies with the family (Shelton, Jeppson, and Johnson, 1989). The nurse must respect the family's central role in the care of the child and must work in collaboration with the family in efforts to care for the child. Family-centered nursing practice is essential in the home setting.

The first of the nine key components of family-centered care (see Chapter 22) provides the philosophic basis for family-centered practice: recognition that the family is the constant in the child's life, whereas the service systems and personnel within those systems fluctuate (National Center for Family Centered Care, 1990). Professionals working with families of children with complex chronic problems must respect the family's central, caring role, their knowledge, and their particular and unique expertise (Cardoso, 1991; Diehl, Moffitt, and Wade, 1991). Families have the most intimate knowledge of the child's strengths and abilities, the challenges of providing care, and the abilities and needs of other family members (Bishop, Woll, and Arango, 1993). Believing that no one knows the child better than the family is critical to the success of any health care plan.

RESPECT FOR DIVERSITY

Respect for varied family structures and for racial, ethnic, cultural, and socioeconomic diversity among families is essential in home care (see also Chapter 2). Nurses work in close relationship with family members and in the family's own domain. The family's background and their life-style choices are respected. Particular attention is given to communication. The meaning of words used and the way they are said may affect various cultural groups in different ways. For example, the words "family support" may be interpreted by some families as an implication that they are weak and in need of help (Patterson and Blum, 1993). Families may also differ in their cultural view of children, in childrearing practices, and in their views of illness, its causes, and its meaning. The views of illness may influence the level of investment a family will make in the child's care. Families may have beliefs about health care and healing practices that are foreign to the nurse's background and experience (Groce and Zola, 1993; Hanson, Lynch, and Wayman, 1990; McCubbin and others, 1993; Patterson and Blum, 1993; Zagorsky, 1993). The home care nurse, aware that value systems drive behavior, needs to learn about the family's culture, ask questions without implying judgment, interpret the mainstream medical culture, and help families design interventions that meet their preferences (Stone and Hoffman, 1993).

Respect for family diversity and awareness of both family developmental stages (see Chapter 3) and the stages of a family's adjustment to illness in a child (see Chapter 22) will assist the home care nurse in recognizing and promoting family strengths and in respecting varied coping mechanisms. Labels such as "dysfunctional," "difficult," and "noncompliant" can reinforce negative expectations and shape behaviors of both parents and professionals (Johnson, Jeppson, and Redburn, 1992). On the other hand, emphasizing, identifying, and building on family strengths and coping mechanisms are strategies that promote a central goal in nursing care of the child and family: family empowerment (see Chapter 22). The nurse working with families should remain flexible and open-minded, since new family strengths may emerge over time and coping mechanisms may wax and wane with the stresses of caring for a child with serious or multiple problems (Quint and others, 1990).

PARENT-PROFESSIONAL COLLABORATION

Family-centered nursing practice is built on a foundation of parent-professional collaboration, which represents a shift from the traditional unidirectional relationships between health care providers and families. ***Collaborative relationships***, essential in the home care setting, are characterized by several features (Bishop, Woll, and Arango, 1993):

Communication—Including complete and unbiased sharing of information with parents about their child's care and prognosis

Dialogue—Exchanging of information and sharing of reactions and ideas

Active listening—Listening beyond the words to hear and understand concerns, including checking to be certain that interpretations are correct

Awareness and acceptance of difference—Willingness to examine one's own cultural biases and to accept that others may think and act out of different value systems

Negotiation—The process of examining different options, priorities, and preferences to best meet the needs of the child and family

The ***LEARN*** framework for communication with families can be useful in a collaborative practice approach (Berlin and Fowkes, 1983):

L **Listen** with sympathy and understanding to the family's perception of the problem.
E **Explain** your perception of the problem.
A **Acknowledge** and discuss the differences and similarities.
R **Recommend** treatment.
N **Negotiate** agreement.

Because of the attention it gives to both careful listening and acknowledging differences and similarities, the LEARN model is especially useful in cross-cultural communication.

Communication with the family should not be invasive. There is no need to collect information from the family that can be obtained from the child's records. The nurse should explain to the family the reason for questions, particularly those that the family may perceive as intrusive, and should inform families of who will have access to the information. The nurse must also assure families that they have a right to expect confidentiality in regard to the data collected. When working in the home, the nurse must respect the privacy of family members' communications with each other that may be overheard.

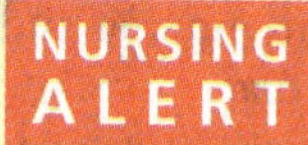

Home care nurses should restrict their communications with other professionals to clinically relevant information about the family.

Communication with family members should include sharing with the family, in a supportive manner, complete and unbiased information about all aspects of the child's condition and care (National Center for Family Centered Care, 1990). Parents often feel overwhelming frustration related to obtaining accurate information about their child's illness and its management. Parents want information given slowly and repeated as necessary over time; they want explanations in terms they can understand; and they want the opportunity to ask questions (Diehl, Moffitt, and Wade, 1991; Knafl and others, 1992), which should be answered in a straightforward manner. Stating "I don't know" is better than pretending to know or giving excuses. A plan can be made with the parents to gather relevant information when necessary. Information should be shared with families in a way that will have meaning in their cultural context (Huber, Holditch-Davis, and Brandon, 1993). Many parents report a preference for interactions with professionals that communicate empathy and concern. While they want accurate information, many parents prefer that providers moderate the amount of information on possible complications and unfavorable prognoses (Knafl and others, 1992). A resource guide for families in which they can record pertinent medical information can assist parents in managing their child's care (Lobosco and others, 1991).

Disagreements may arise between parents and nurses over proper procedures for care of the child (see Critical

Thinking Exercise box). In any situation that will not pose danger or risk for the child, nurses should respect parental preferences. If disagreements cannot be resolved, a home care supervisor or case manager should be contacted to assist with problem solving (Ahmann and Bond, 1992). If parents wish to alter a plan of treatment that is part of medical orders, the nurse should ask that they negotiate the change with the physician, since the nurse must follow the written medical orders (Klug, 1993).

Other options to help resolve conflicts include (Ahmann and Bond, 1992):

- Work with the family's priorities and reevaluate over time.
- Provide the family with additional information that may affect their perception of priorities.
- Share the nurse's perception of priorities and rationales without judgment.
- Suggest an additional priority goal if the family agrees.

THE NURSING PROCESS

In the home the family is a partner in each step of the nursing process. The use of formal self-report assessment tools can help families identify needs they may have for information, training, services, and support.* Assessment should also address family strengths and resources (see Family Assessment, Chapter 6). The principles of communication discussed previously guide data collection. The nurse's observations are shared neutrally, without value judgment, and in a way that preserves the family's own role in decision making (Bond, Phillips, and Rollins, 1994).

All of the information gathered as part of the assessment process is shared with the family. The nurse should recognize that the family's perception of their most important need will generally guide their behavior and consume their attention and energy (Dunst, Trivette, and Deal, 1988). Family priorities guide the planning process (Ahmann and Bond, 1992; Jackson, Finkler, and Robinson, 1992).

Both short- and long-term goals should be outlined and agreed on by the child, family, and professionals involved. The plan of care should integrate various disciplines that may be involved with the child in order to minimize duplication and consolidate care requirements. Cross-training of professionals and a transdisciplinary mode of treatment can also be useful when a child has multiple and complex care requirements (Ahmann and Lipsi, 1991, 1992). For example, certain physical or occupational therapy routines may be incorporated into the child's morning nursing pro-

*Self-report instruments to help families identify concerns, priorities, resources, and sources of support include *Family Needs Survey*, available from Frank Porter Graham Child Development Center, CB No. 180, University of North Carolina, Chapel Hill, NC 27599, (919) 966-2622; *How Can We Help?* available from Child Development Resources, P.O. Box 299, Lightfoot, VA 230980, (804) 220-1168; *Parent Needs Survey* (Seligman and Darling, 1989); and *Family Profile*, available from The Coordinating Center for Home and Community Care, 8258 Veterans Highway, Suite 13, Millersville, MD 21108, (410) 987-1048. Additional scales may be found in Appendix D of *Guidelines and Recommended Practices for the Individualized Family Service Plan*, edited by M. McGonigel, R. Kaufmann, and B. Johnson (1991); available from the Association for the Care of Children's Health, 7910 Woodmont Ave., Suite 300, Bethesda, MD 20814, (301) 654-6549; and in Dunst, Trivette, and Deal (1988).

CRITICAL THINKING EXERCISE
Family-Centered Home Care and Conflicts

A family wants to begin oral feeding of their 3-year-old daughter, Sarah, who is ventilator dependent and is being tube fed. They ask you, the nurse providing home care, to feed Sarah baby food. You recognize that Sarah has poor oral-motor skills, is at high risk of aspiration, and already has a compromised respiratory status. You:

1. Refuse to feed her baby food because the risk is too high.
2. Feed her baby food because the family has the right to make this decision for their child.
3. State your concerns to the family and leave the decision to them.
4. Acknowledge the family's desire, state your concerns, and explore options with the family and other providers before implementing a feeding plan with the family.

The correct answer is 4. While it may seem complicated to engage in communication, negotiation, and consultation over the seemingly simple issue of giving baby food to a 3-year-old, many issues must be considered.

The family may have legitimate reasons for wanting their daughter started on baby foods. The nurse should inquire about their reasons. They may feel that health care providers have overlooked this aspect of normal development. The family may be attempting to assist their daughter in achieving age-appropriate skills and may also want their daughter to participate in family mealtimes. These are legitimate, commendable goals, and the family should be supported in making such choices for their child. For this reason, option 1 is not the correct choice.

However, option 2 is not the correct choice, either. Before oral feeding begins, the nurse should be certain that the family understands possible risks of oral feeding (aspiration, pneumonia, possible difficulties treating pneumonia given the child's compromised respiratory status). Yet, option 3 is not the best choice the nurse could make. Professionals with expertise in the child's problems can provide invaluable guidance on approaching the desire for feeding in a way that may optimize success. (A child who is 3 years old and has not been fed orally will benefit from an oral-motor assessment by an occupational therapist with experience in this area. Speech therapists can also provide suggestions regarding oral-motor therapy. Specific plans with incremental steps to reduce oral-motor defensiveness and improve the ability to accept foods orally should precede feeding. Nutritional consultation may also be important as feeding plans shift, because of the risk of aspiration pneumonia.)

Option 4 encourages the nurse and the family to discuss the issue, plan for consultations and evaluation related to the child's oral-motor progress, and thereby arrange to meet the family's goals of oral feeding in safer incremental steps. Communication between the nurse and the family may also lead to other approaches to normalizing mealtimes for Sarah and her family. For example, Sarah's tube feeding could be scheduled to coincide with the family's mealtime. Sarah could also be taught to assist in the tube feeding with the eventual goal of taking over the feeding process herself.

Modified from Ahmann E, Bond NJ: Promoting normal development in school-age children and adolescents who are technology dependent: a family centered model, *Pediatr Nurs* 18:399-405, 1992.

SAMPLE FAMILY EVALUATION QUESTIONS

Please rate your home care nurse(s) in the following areas:

1. Knowledge of child growth and development
2. Understanding of your child's condition
3. Ability to evaluate and care for your child (vital signs, giving medications, IVs, tube feedings, tracheostomy care, etc.)
4. Knowledge of special equipment required in your child's care (monitor, ventilator, IV pump, oxygen, etc.)
5. Ability to provide suggestions and resources to improve your child's care
6. Communication skills with you and other family members
7. Communication with agencies and other health professionals
8. Respect for your family's priorities
9. Respect for your family's privacy

Please rate the agency on the following:

1. Provision of qualified nurses
2. Handling of the schedule
3. Frequency of case conferences
4. Problem solving

The following rating scale can be used: 1 = poor; 2 = fair; 3 = good; 4 = excellent

Name of nurse ______________

Modified from Grammatica G: Developing a quality home care program for children, *Pediatr Nurs* 15(1):33-35, 1989; and Klug R: Selecting a home care agency, *Pediatr Nurs* 18:504-507, 1992.

cedures, or speech therapy interventions may be conducted by the parent or nurse around eating times so that the entire day is not occupied by procedures. A written schedule of daily routines should be developed and followed by all caregivers.

Goals of care are supported by intervention strategies that reflect normalization (see Chapter 22) and the interests and abilities of the child and family. Nurses can help families explore a range of alternative strategies, services, and resources so that the family can choose the best match for their situation.

Family participation in evaluating a home care plan can occur on several levels. Families and care providers should regularly review the goals of care and then update the care plan as required. The nurse can also ask the family open-ended questions at regular intervals to assess their opinions on the effectiveness of care (Bond, Phillips, and Rollins, 1994). As part of the evaluation process, families should be acknowledged for their successes and accomplishments. Finally, families should be given an opportunity to evaluate the home care agency and other service providers on a periodic basis (see box above). The evaluations should be used by the agency to improve quality of care.

In addition to maintaining a sense of control over their child's care, families need to control their home and personal lives. For this reason, nurses should discuss "house rules" with the family, addressing issues such as the physical environment, private areas in the home, responsibility for maintaining the child's environment, and interactions with siblings (see Guidelines box).

GUIDELINES
Negotiating "House Rules" for Home Care

HOUSE RULES

Parking: Where to park and community regulations.
Access: Where to enter the home. Is knocking preferred or ringing the bell?
Personal belongings: Where does the nurse store own coat, boots, etc.? Does the family prefer slippers to shoes in the home?
Meals: Where may the nurse store own food? NOTE: This is very important given cultural diversity of clients.
Radio and television: Identify preferences regarding the usage. Remember this may help nurses to remain awake at night.
Patient room: The nurse is responsible for the child's immediate environment. Maintaining a clean working area and cleaning the room up at the end of the shift is the nurse's responsibility.
Telephone: Agency policy may dictate that all personal calls be limited to very brief time periods and be charged to the nurse making them. NOTE: Many nurses do need to check in with home at some interval during the evening.
Visitors: Identify who may enter the home when the parents are away (that is, child's friends or grandparents). A list of names should be available.
Privacy: Describe what parts of the home are off limits to the nurse and at what times.

CHILD

Routine: Specify times for playtime, bathtime, and bedtime. What does the parent want to participate in regarding these routines?
Mealtime: Specify where the family wants the child fed and if tube fed, specify a preference as to how and where it is done.
Clothing: Identify who picks out the child's clothes. Identify where the laundry is and who is responsible for washing the sick child's clothing.
Discipline: Discuss specific guidelines for discipline.
Homework: Discuss when it should be done and who is responsible for it being completed.

SIBLINGS

Discipline: Establish guidelines regarding how parents should be informed of siblings' conflicts and how discipline should be handled. NOTE: Parents or another caregiver must be in the home when siblings are home.
Patient care: Be specific regarding how children have helped with the child's care. Discuss any concerns regarding behavior that may compromise the child or siblings' safety.

NURSING

Parental notification: Specify what information the family wishes to be aware of immediately and what can wait until they are home.
Limits of responsibility: Specify duties the nurse may not perform, such as transportation of the child to care facilities.
Environment: Discuss the need to have adequate lighting and a comfortable working area.

Modified from Klug R: Clarifying roles and expectations in home care, *Pediatr Nurs* 19(4):375, 1993.

THINKING CRITICALLY ABOUT . . .

Family-Centered Home Care and Nurses' Roles and Responsibilities

While relevant in all settings, a family-centered approach to nursing practice seems most obviously fitting in the home care arena. The family's home is their domain, and their central role is all the more clear in the home setting. Working in the home makes the nurse all the more aware of the need for collaborative practice. At the same time, the challenges of defining the boundaries of what constitutes family-centered nursing practice may be most difficult for the nurse in the home setting. The traditional responsibilities of providers and parents cross over and must be blended in a new way (Lantos and Kohrman, 1992).

The following questions point to some of the more challenging areas when family-centered nursing practice is applied in the home care setting:

1. Where is the boundary between collaborating with families in home care nursing and becoming a part of the family system?

   Barnsteiner and Gillis-Donovan (1990) suggest that therapeutic relationships require the maintenance of well-defined boundaries between the nurse, the child, and the family that promote the family's control over the child's care. At the same time, Klug (1993) cautions that several factors challenge the maintenance of such clear boundaries: the informal home environment, the casual social conversations that occur with family members throughout the day, the participation by family members in care of the child, and the attempt by some families to reduce the stress of having a stranger in the home by incorporating the nurse as a member of the family.
2. Who determines the appropriate care of the child? Where are the boundaries between respecting parental decisions and choices that differ from those of the nurse?

   These questions can arise in the development of care plans (parents and nurse see different goals for the child), in carrying out procedures (parents and nurse have different methods for suctioning), and in styles of interacting with or disciplining a child. Ahmann and Bond (1992) outline a number of steps that the nurse can take in negotiating areas of disagreement with the family but suggest that in general the nurse should respect the family's choices even when the nurse has different priorities or approaches than the family. Klug (1993) suggests that a parent's authority should be respected unless either risk or harm is posed to the child or the written medical orders are not followed. Issues of legal liability cannot be overlooked (Hogue, 1992). Honest, respectful, communication and careful documentation are important when any disagreement arises. Agency policies will guide the nurse's practice (Hogue, 1992), and case managers or nursing supervisors may be called on to help negotiate areas of disagreement.
3. What is the responsibility of the nurse who may witness child neglect, abuse, or family violence?

   Some of what might be considered medical neglect may result from the family's feeling overwhelmed, not being fully educated about the proper care requirements, and/or denial. The nurse has a responsibility to address these issues with the family. At the same time, Hogue (1992) suggests that home care providers may have legal liability not only for their own actions, but even when it is parents who are "noncompliant" with medical orders. The frequency and severity of "noncompliance" will affect the nurse's responsibility. For example, one missed medication dose may be appropriately handled by documentation and counseling. On the other hand, regularly missed doses or one instance of turning off a ventilator alarm requires a more vigorous response. The point at which these instances cross the line into reportable medical neglect depend in part on the definitions of abuse or neglect in the state in which services are provided. Instances of child physical or sexual abuse that the nurse may observe generally require reporting. The nurse and the agency may have to determine whether the nurse should play any more direct role if such instances are observed.

These three questions have no clear, single answer. The answers emerge in thoughtful clinical practice with individual families and may differ from nurse to nurse and family to family. Awareness of the questions is important for thinking critically as challenging situations arise in practice.

Home care nursing encourages a close and rewarding relationship with the family. One of the most important aspects of this relationship is maintaining professional boundaries and a therapeutic role that is supportive but not intrusive. Some of these issues are discussed in the Thinking Critically About . . . box and under Therapeutic Relationship, Chapter 1.

PROMOTION OF OPTIMUM DEVELOPMENT, SELF-CARE, AND EDUCATION

There is little question that living at home offers most children with complex medical problems great social and emotional advantages over living in the hospital or other institutional setting. However, in infancy, and throughout the developmental stages, a child's medical condition(s) and the dependence on medical technology can place constraints on and pose challenges to ***normal development.*** For example, the child may have lengthy and repeated hospitalizations; developmental regression can occur in response to stress; fatigue may be due to underlying pathology, the flare of an illness, or medication side effects; and equipment requirements may impede mobility, exploration, and independence. The challenge of providing support for normal development in a child who is chronically ill and technology dependent is to optimize opportunities for develop-

INCORPORATING DEVELOPMENTAL SUPPORT INTO THE HOME CARE PLAN

The home care plan should:
- Provide for initial and periodic developmental assessments
- Involve the child and family in developmental assessment and planning
- Provide for complete information to the family regarding the child's developmental strengths, problems, needs, and prognosis
- Ensure referrals as necessary or appropriate for:
  - Early intervention services
  - Physical and/or occupational therapy
  - Speech, hearing, and/or vision assessments
  - Behavioral and/or emotional evaluation
  - Educational testing as appropriate
- Promote normalization practices, including:
  - Educational opportunities
  - Participation in recreational and community activities
  - Participating in household chores and responsibilities
  - Appropriate discipline and behavioral expectations
  - Family mealtimes
- Involve the child in age-appropriate self-care activities
- Ensure regular evaluation and revision of developmental plans

Modified from Ahmann E, Bond NJ: Promoting normal development in school-age children and adolescents who are technology dependent: a family centered model, *Pediatr Nurs* 18:399-405, 1992.

mentally appropriate experiences within the constraints posed by the medical condition and the equipment requirements (Ahmann and Lierman, 1992).

Home care plans are designed to promote optimum child development through assessment, planning, and referrals, and by interventions that address normalization issues and self-care (see box above). General principles for a family-centered assessment and planning process have been addressed earlier in this chapter and are applied in developmental assessment and planning as well.

Some parents may not pursue developmental intervention because they do not view their child as needing the services. In this case professionals need to explain the child's developmental needs to parents in ways that are meaningful from the parents' own cultural and socioeconomic perspectives (Huber, Holditch-Davis, and Brandon, 1993). Only then can parents make truly informed decisions. Once parents have been fully informed of the child's condition, likely developmental sequelae, and the expected benefits of intervention, developmental goals outlined by the child and family should guide planning and intervention (Ahmann and Bond, 1992).

Several principles underlie appropriate developmental intervention plans for children with complex medical problems (Ahmann and Lierman, 1992). First, understanding a child's medical condition ensures that the nurse and family can plan to maximize developmental opportunities at times when the child has the most energy and endurance and when stress signals that determine the child's tolerance for type, intensity, and duration of activity will be noted (Ahmann and Lipsi, 1991). Second, plans for developmental support must be flexible and tailored to the individual

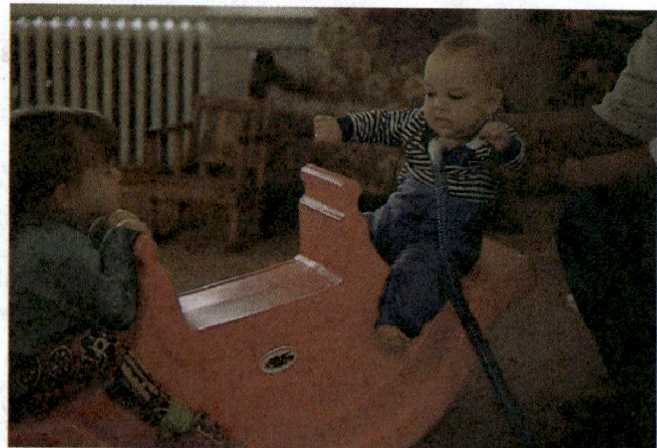

FIG. 25-2 Use of lengthy tubing facilitates freedom of movement.

child's abilities, interests, and needs. Third, familiarity with the child's medical equipment will facilitate the planning of creative ways to meet the child's developmental needs. For example, the use of lengthy oxygen tubing allows the active toddler freedom of movement during the day (Fig. 25-2); portable equipment of any type facilitates family outings; and mounting a ventilator to a wheelchair allows the adolescent greater independence.

Many developmental aspects of chronic illness or disability in children are discussed in Chapter 22 (see Promote Normal Development). Some additional factors apply when children are or have been dependent on medical technology and should be considered in developing plans to promote normal development (Ahmann and Lierman, 1992). These special needs may include:

- For infants, attention to promoting oral-motor development
- For toddlers, efforts to encourage mobility and exploration, and extra assistance with language development
- For preschoolers, assistance in self-care
- For school-age children, provision of games and tasks for mastery, and socialization opportunities
- For adolescents, increased independence in managing their own medical care

Promoting coping and capability can buffer stress and contribute to mental health and self-esteem in a child with chronic illness (Patterson and Geber, 1991). The extent to which a child is involved in his or her own care depends on many factors, including the child's developmental age, level of interest, and physical ability, as well as parental comfort and support. ***Self-care,*** both in activities of daily living and in regard to the medical condition, is important.

The frame of reference for self-care in activities of daily living should be the goal of attaining age-appropriate competence. Some modifications in the environment, in the medical equipment, and/or in the techniques for daily activities may be required to promote and support self-care (Ahmann and Bond, 1992). Aids for personal hygiene, selection of clothing, and dressing are discussed in Chapter 24, and several resources are also available (Jones, 1985).

Beyond infancy, every child can participate in the health care regimen. Toddlers can participate in simple ways such as holding equipment and discarding used supplies. School-age children may be able to clean medical equipment, restock supplies, and administer their own medications with supervision. Adolescents may be able to perform many of their own procedures, participate in decision making, and assume responsibility for scheduling caregivers' visits and out-of-home appointments (Ahmann and Bond, 1992). Most adolescents should not be left completely without supervision, since adolescent developmental issues, including denial and a sense of invulnerability and rebellion, may interfere with appropriate care. Effective teaching for self-care is focused at the child's own level of conceptual understanding and may be augmented by the use of dolls, other models and diagrams, simple explanations, and repetition (Vessey, Braithwaite, and Wiedmann, 1990; Yoos, 1988) (see Critical Thinking Exercise box).

For the school-age child or adolescent dependent on medical technology, ***educational planning*** is important. Despite laws that ensure a "free appropriate public education" to these children, conflict over payment for health care services in the school setting has often been an impediment to mainstreaming children with complex medical problems (Walker, 1991). When a child requiring special medical care is to be placed in an educational setting, the parents, child, school health coordinator, educational evaluation team, and education and administrative staff should meet to determine safe and appropriate placement, as well as necessary services and personnel to enable the child to attend school in the least restrictive environment. Planning for schooling of children with special medical needs should also take into account factors such as those listed in the box below. Training of educational staff and caregivers is essential to ensuring the child's safety in the educational setting* (Haynie, Porter, and Palfrey, 1989; Krier, 1993). Special assistance can also be beneficial in reintegrating previously schooled children, such as those with cancer, into the school setting (Katz and others, 1992). Parents may need assistance in developing the skills necessary to advocate effectively for their child in the educational system (DiGregorio-Hixson, Stoff and White, 1992).

CRITICAL THINKING EXERCISE

Home Care and the Adolescent

A 13-year-old girl has been diagnosed with Crohn disease following a period of 2 months' duration of bloody diarrhea, abdominal pain, and significant weight loss. Because of the chronic malabsorption and weight loss, continuous nasogastric tube feedings for 12 hours per night have been recommended as nutritional support therapy. In preparation for home care, which of the following nursing interventions should you question?

1. Provide education regarding symptoms or problems to be reported to the health care professionals.
2. Educate the girl regarding nasogastric tube insertion and administration of formula.
3. Provide emotional support regarding the new diagnosis and therapy.
4. Arrange for home care supplies and nursing visits at home as needed.

The correct answer is 2. Although an essential component of the nursing plan of care includes patient education and preparation for home care, there is no mention of including other family members in the teaching. While the adolescent should know how to insert the tube and administer the formula, she should not be expected to have sole responsibility for this procedure. Adolescents newly diagnosed with a chronic disease require emotional support regarding their prognosis, medical or nutritional care, and body image. Many children and adolescents with Crohn disease have gastrointestinal symptoms, extraintestinal symptoms, and growth delay, all of which can cause anxiety. Many adolescents will benefit from support from other patients their age with the same disease, as well as support and assistance from family members. Education should include the rationale for therapy, symptoms and problems to be monitored and reported, nasogastric tube insertion, administration of formula, and use of a feeding pump. Supplies for nasogastric tube feedings will need to be obtained, and a visiting nurse will likely be needed to monitor care and assist and educate the patient at home.

Contributed by Lynn Mattis, RN, MSN.

SAFETY ISSUES IN THE HOME

Safety is an important consideration in pediatric home care and should be addressed in the home care plan. First, before hospital discharge, emergency preparations must be made. The home should have a telephone.

*A thorough discussion of training issues, content, and guidelines for care in the school are provided in Haynie, Porter, and Palfrey, 1989.

SOME FACTORS TO CONSIDER WHEN PLACING A TECHNOLOGY-DEPENDENT CHILD IN THE SCHOOL SETTING

- The school health personnel must have pertinent medical and psychosocial information about the child.
- Persons familiar with the child's health care needs should attend an educational planning meeting with the family and school personnel.
- Appropriate placement and services should be identified and agreed on.
- A child-specific emergency plan must be developed in collaboration with the school administration, community emergency personnel, teacher, caregiver, and family.
- In-school health care needs must be specified in a written health care plan available to the administration, caregiver, and teacher.
- Safe transportation must be arranged.
- A series of educational meetings for school personnel should address roles, responsibilities, the child's condition, specialized needs, emergency procedures, and any specific skills that may be pertinent.
- The child and classmates should be prepared before school entry.

Modified from Haynie M, Porter SM, Palfrey JS: *Children assisted by medical technology in educational settings: guidelines for care,* Boston, 1989, The Children's Hospital (Project School Care).

➤ **NURSING TIP** If the family does not have a telephone, arrangements may be made with the telephone company to supply service. Alternatively, one or two nearby neighbors may agree to let the family use their services. In rural areas a local pharmacy, or police or ranger station may be willing to receive messages and relay them to the family.

The telephone and electric companies (if use of medical equipment requires electricity) are notified that the family needs to be placed on a priority service list so that the family will learn of any anticipated interruptions in service and receive priority in reinstatement of interrupted services. Prior contact with rescue squad and local emergency facility personnel can help ensure prompt and appropriate interventions if required (Ahmann, 1986).

Before hospital discharge, emergency protocols are developed and reviewed with both the parents and professional caregivers. Cardiopulmonary resuscitation (CPR) guidelines, if appropriate, should be posted near the child's bedside or in another accessible location. A list of emergency telephone numbers can be placed near each home phone and should include those of the rescue squad, emergency room, managing physician(s), nursing agency, and equipment vendor(s).

Another aspect of safety relates to the provision of care by appropriately trained individuals. Family members should receive thorough training in the child's care requirements and have the opportunity to demonstrate knowledge and confidence before hospital discharge. Professional staff caring for the child should have the appropriate background and training for the child's particular care needs. Because of the child's body size, special skill and caution are required in both the performance of procedures (e.g., gastrostomy feedings, suctioning) and in monitoring the use of equipment (e.g., ventilator settings, intravenous flow rates, and total fluid volumes) (see Chapters 27, 28, and 31).

The activity level and curiosity of young children raise additional safety considerations in the provision of home care. All medications, needles, syringes, and any contaminated materials are securely stored well out of the reach of curious hands. Special attention is paid to childproofing the control panels for ventilators, pumps, monitors, and other equipment. Use of clear plastic tape, covers, or panels to cover control knobs or buttons reduces the risk of accidental changes in settings. Electrical cords are kept short and out of reach, and safety covers are used on any open outlets. When not in use, equipment is unplugged, and any wires (e.g., lead wires for an apnea monitor) are stored out of reach.

Care at night poses other safety concerns. Care must be taken to prevent accidental strangulation on apnea, oximeter, or cardiac monitor wires or lengthy intravenous tubing during sleep. Parents or other caregivers need to be able to clearly hear monitor, ventilator, or pump alarms at night; an inexpensive intercom system or baby monitor can be used (Berry and Jorgenson, 1988).

➤ **NURSING TIP** Coiling extra tubing and taping it at the exit site, as well as running wires or tubes out the bottoms of pajamas, is a precaution against strangulation.

Safe transportation is a vitally important concern. Many of these children use wheelchairs and equipment that must be properly secured to the vehicle, including vans and buses. Additional information on car safety and general health supervision is in Chapter 22 (see Educate About the Disorder and General Health Care).

FAMILY-TO-FAMILY SUPPORT

Family-to-family support networks can be an important source of emotional and instrumental support, as well as empowerment for families of children with chronic health problems. Family-to-family support does not replace professional sources of support but, rather, is a unique resource promoting family strengths through shared experience (Johnson, Jeppson, and Redburn, 1992). Existing parent support groups may not necessarily meet an individual family's needs; when nurses refer a family to a particular group, they should inform the family of the group's purposes (Betz and others, 1990). The value of informal support networks should not be overlooked. Similarly, the support needs of fathers, grandparents, and siblings may be different from those of mothers (Gallo, 1991; Gallo and others, 1992; Graves and Ware, 1990) and should be acknowledged as part of the plan of care. (Some sources of information and support for families are listed at the end of this chapter.) Peer support for school-age children and adolescents with complex care themselves has also been shown to be beneficial (Clark and others, 1992).

KEY POINTS

- Effective home care depends on many factors, including the child's relative medical stability; the family's willingness, training, and ability to accommodate the child's care requirements; and professional, financial, and community support.
- Comprehensive, multidisciplinary discharge planning should begin early and should include the family and a home care representative in addition to hospital personnel.
- Thorough training of the family, including a trial of care, a predischarge pass to home, and a predischarge home visit, can ease the transition to home.
- Care coordination ensures continuity of care and reduces fragmentation of services. The family may assume varying degrees of care coordination over time.
- The home care nurse must share a level of technical expertise with the critical care nurse while being able to adapt equipment, procedures, and the nursing process to the home setting.
- Federal standards apply to agencies that participate in Medicare or Medicaid; standards of practice by The American Nurses Association can guide nurses in the home setting.
- Family-centered nursing practice is applied in the home setting; diversity in family structures, cultural backgrounds, strengths, and coping mechanisms is respected.
- Collaborative relationships are characterized by communication, dialogue, active listening, awareness and acceptance of difference, and negotiation.

- The nursing process is adapted to involve the family in each step and to preserve the family's central role in decision making.
- "House rules" agreed on by the nurse and family allow a family to maintain a feeling of control over their own environment when professionals are present.
- Home care plans are designed to promote optimum development of the child and focus on normalization, on the impact of the child's medical condition and technologic requirements on development, on self-care, and on educational needs.
- Safety in the provision of home care services involves emergency preparations and protocols, appropriate training of family and home care personnel, and safe use and childproofing of medical equipment.
- Family-to-family support networks can both provide emotional and instrumental support and encourage family empowerment.

REFERENCES

Ahmann E: *Home care for the high risk infant: a holistic guide to using technology,* Rockville, MD, 1986, Aspen.

Ahmann E, Bond NJ: Promoting normal development in school-age children and adolescents who are technology dependent: a family centered model, *Pediatr Nurs* 18:399-405, 1992.

Ahmann E, Lierman C: Promoting normal development in technology dependent children: an introduction to the issues, *Pediatr Nurs* 18:143-152, 1992.

Ahmann E, Lipsi KA: Early intervention for technology dependent infants and young children, *Infants Young Child* 3(4):67-77, 1991.

Ahmann E, Lipsi KA: Developmental assessment of the technology-dependent infant and young child, *Pediatr Nurs* 18:299-313, 1992.

American Nurses Association: *Standards of community health nursing practice,* Washington, DC, 1986a, The Association.

American Nurses Association: *Standards of home health nursing practice,* Washington, DC, 1986b, The Association.

American Nurses Association: *Nursing case management,* Washington, DC, 1988, The Association.

Barnsteiner J, Gillis-Donovan J: Being related and separate: a standard for therapeutic relationships, *MCN* 15:223-228, 1990.

Berry RK, Jorgenson S: Growing with home parenteral nutrition: maintaining a safe environment, *Pediatr Nurs* 14:155-157, 1988.

Berlin EA, Fowkes WC: A teaching framework for cross-cultural health care, *West J Med* 139(6):934-938, 1983.

Betz CL and others: A survey of self-help groups in California for parents of children with chronic conditions, *Pediatr Nurs* 16(3):293-296, 1990.

Birenbaum LK, Clarke-Steffen L: Terminal care costs in childhood cancer, *Pediatr Nurs* 18(3):285-288, 1992.

Bishop KK, Woll J, Arango P: *Family/professional collaboration,* Burlington, VT, 1993, Department of Social Work, University of Vermont.

Bond N, Phillips P, Rollin JA: Family-centered care at home for families with children who are technology-dependent, *Pediatr Nurs* 20(2):123-130, 1994.

Brooten D and others: A randomized clinical trial of early hospital discharge and home follow-up of very low birthweight infants, *N Engl J Med* 315:934-939, 1986.

Brooten D and others: Early discharge and specialist transitional care, *Image J Nurs Sch* 29(2):64-68, 1988.

Cardoso P: Family-centered care, *Child Health Care* 20(4):258-260, 1991.

Clark HB and others: Peer group support for adolescents with chronic illness, *Child Health Care* 21(4):233-238, 1992.

Curry R, Cullen J: Using videorecordings in pediatric nursing practice, *Pediatr Nurs* 16(5): 501-504, 1990.

Davis BD, Steele S: Case management for young children with special care needs, *Pediatr Nurs* 17:15-19, 1991.

DiGregorio-Hixson D, Stoff E, White PH: Parents of children with chronic health impairments: a new approach to advocacy training, *Child Health Care* 21(2):111-115, 1992.

Diehl SF, Moffitt KA, Wade SM: Focus group interview with parents of children with medically complex needs: an intimate look at their perceptions and feelings, *Child Health Care* 20(3):170-178, 1991.

Dowd E, Vlastuin L: Home care. In Craft M, Denehy J, editors: *Nursing interventions for infants and children,* Philadelphia, 1990, WB Saunders.

Dunst C, Trivette C, Deal A: *Enabling and empowering families,* Cambridge, MA, 1988, Brookline Books.

Fields A and others: Home care cost-effectiveness for respiratory technology-dependent children, *Am J Dis Child* 145(7): 729-733, 1991.

Gallo AM: Stigma in childhood chronic illness: a well sibling perspective, *Pediatr Nurs* 75:21-25, 1991.

Gallo AM and others: Well siblings of children with chronic illness: parents' reports of their psychological adjustment, *Pediatr Nurs* 18:23-27, 1992.

Goldberg AI: Children on ventilators: breathing easier at home, *Contemp Pediatr* 7:59-79, 1990.

Groce NE, Zola IK: Multiculturalism, chronic illness and disability, *Pediatrics* 91:1048-1055, 1993.

Graves JK, Ware ME: Parents' and health professionals' perceptions concerning parental stress during a child's hospitalization, *Child Health Care* 19(1):39-42, 1990.

Hanson M, Lynch E, Wayman K: Honoring the cultural diversity of families while gathering data, *Top Early Child Spec Educ* 10(1):112-131, 1990.

Harris PJ: Sometimes pediatric home care doesn't work, *Am J Nurs* 88:851-854, 1988.

Haynie M, Porter SM, Palfrey JS: *Children assisted by medical technology in educational settings: guidelines for care,* Boston, 1989, The Children's Hospital (Project School Care).

Hogue E: Parental noncompliance in home care, *Pediatr Nurs* 18(6):603-606, 1992.

Huber C, Holditch-Davis D, Brandon D: High-risk preterm infants at 3 years of age: parental response to the presence of developmental problems, *Child Health Care* 22(2):107-124, 1993.

Jackson B, Finkler DE, Robinson C: A case management system for infants with chronic illnesses and developmental disabilities, *Child Health Care* 21(4):224-232, 1992.

Johnson BH, Jeppson ES, Redburn L: *Caring for children and families: guidelines for hospitals,* Bethesda, MD, 1992, Association for the Care of Children's Health.

Jones ML: *Home care for the chronically ill or disabled child,* New York, 1985, Harper & Row.

Katz ER and others: Teacher, parent, and child evaluative ratings of a school reintegrative intervention for children with newly diagnosed cancer, *Child Health Care* 21(2):69-75, 1992.

Klug RM: Understanding private insurance for funding pediatric home care, *Pediatr Nurs* 17:197-198, 1991.

Klug RM: Selecting a home care agency, *Pediatr Nurs* 18:504-507, 1992.

Klug RM: Clarifying roles and expectations in home care, *Pediatr Nurs* 19:374-376, 1993.

Knafl K and others: Parents' view of health care providers: an exploration of the components of a positive working relationship, *Child Health Care* 21(2):90-95, 1992.

Krier JJ: Involvement of educational staff in the health care of medically fragile children, *Pediatr Nurs* 19(3):251-254, 1993.

Lantos JD, Kohrman AF: Ethical aspects of pediatric home care, *Pediatrics* 89(5):920-924, 1992.

Lobosco AF and others: Local coalitions for coordinating services to children dependent on technology and their families, *Child Health Care* 20(2):75-86, 1991.

McCubbin HI and others: Culture, ethnicity, and the family: critical factors in childhood chronic illness and disabilities, *Pediatrics* 91(5):1063-1070, 1993.

McGonigel M, Kaufmann R, Johnson B, editors: *Guidelines and recommended practices for the individualized family service plan,* ed 2, Bethesda, MD, 1991, Association for the Care of Children's Health.

National Center for Family Centered Care: *What is family-centered care?* Bethesda, MD, 1990, Association for the Care of Children's Health.

Office of Technology Assessment (OTA), Congress of the United States: *Technology dependent children: hospital v. home care—a technical memorandum* (OTA-TM-H-38), Washington, DC, 1987, US Government Printing Office.

Patterson JM, Blum RW: A conference on culture and chronic illness in childhood: conference summary, *Pediatrics* 91:1025-1030, 1993.

Patterson JM, Geber G: Preventing mental health problems in children with chronic illness or disability, *Child Health Care* 20(3): 150-161, 1991.

Quint R and others: Home care for ventilator-dependent children: psychosocial impact on the family, *Am J Dis Child* 144:1238-1241, 1990.

Richman R: Market memo: high-tech home care: what's in it for hospitals? *Strategic Manage* 8:1, 1990.

Seligman M, Darling D: *Ordinary families, special children: a systems approach to childhood disability,* New York, 1989, Guilford Press.

Shelton TL, Jeppson ES, Johnson BH: *Family-centered care for children with special care needs,* Washington, DC, 1989, Association for the Care of Children's Health.

Stone M, Hoffman R: *Cultural understanding: how far do you go?* Paper presented at the ACCH local conference on Incorporating Cultural Awareness into Pediatric Health-care, Washington, DC, April 30, 1993.

Strahan G: *Overview of home health and hospice care patients: preliminary data from the 1992 National Home and Hospice Care Survey;* advance data from vital and health statistics, No. 235, Hyattsville, MD, 1993, National Center for Health Statistics.

Vessey JA, Braithwaite KB, Weidmann M: Teaching children about their internal bodies, *Pediatr Nurs* 16:29-33, 1990.

Walker P: Where there is a way, there is not always a will: technology, public policy, and the school integration of children who are technology-assisted, *Child Health Care* 20(2): 68-74, 1991.

Wong DL: Transition from hospital to home for children with complex medical care, *J Pediatr Oncol Nurs* 8(1):3-9, 1991.

Yoos L: Cognitive development and the chronically ill child, *Pediatr Nurs* 14:375-378, 1988.

Zagorsky ES: Caring for families who follow alternative health care practices, *Pediatr Nurs* 19(1):71-75, 1993.

Zanoa JS: Beyond the stack of bills: what home care of cancer patients really costs, *Cancer Nurs News* 10(3):13, 1992.

BIBLIOGRAPHY

Aday LA, Aitken MJ, Wegener DH: *Pediatric home care: results of a national evaluation of programs for ventilator assisted children,* Chicago, 1988, Pluribus Press.

Ahmann E: An annotated bibliography on respite care for children and families, *Child Health Care* 14:183-186, 1986.

Ahmann E: Family-centered care: the time has come, *Pediatr Nurs* 20(1):52-53, 1994.

Aitken M: Matching models to environments: a planning guide to the selection of pediatric home care models, *Home Healthc Nurse* 7(2):12-21, 1989.

American Academy of Pediatrics, Ad Hoc Task Force on Home Care of Chronically Ill Infants and Children: Guidelines for home care of infants, children, and adolescents with chronic disease, *Pediatrics* 74(3):434-436, 1984.

American Academy of Pediatrics, Committee on Children with Disabilities: Pediatric services for infants and children with special health care needs, *Pediatrics* 92(1):163-165, 1993.

Brewer EJ and others: Family centered, community-based, coordinated care for children with special health care needs, *Pediatrics* 83:1055-1060, 1989.

Briggs NJ: Selecting a pediatric home care program, *Pediatr Nurs* 13:191, 1987.

Britton LJ, Johnston JD: Dependent on technology: a child grows up hospitalized, *Pediatr Nurs* 19(6):579-584, 1993.

Buehler JA, Lee HJ: Exploration of home care resources for rural families with cancer, *Cancer Nurs* 15(4):299-308, 1992.

Burns CE, Madian N: Experiences with a support group for grandparents of children with disabilities, *Pediatr Nurs* 18:17-22, 1992.

Cady C, Yoshioko RS: Using a learning contract to successfully discharge an infant on home total parenteral nutrition, *Pediatr Nurs* 17:67-74, 1991.

Corkery E: Discharge planning and home health care: what every staff nurse should know, *Orthop Nurs* 8(6):18-26, 1989.

Council of Scientific Affairs: Home care in the 1990s, *JAMA* 263(9):1241-1244, 1990.

Cress A: A quality safeguard-evaluation of medical stability at discharge, *Pediatr Nurs* 15(2):169-174, 1989.

Crummette B, Boatwright D: Case management in inpatient pediatric nursing, *Pediatr Nurs* 17(5):469-473, 1991.

Damato EG: Discharge planning from the neonatal intensive care unit, *J Perinat Neonat Nurs* 5(1):43-53, 1991.

Davis B, Steele S: Case management for young children with special health care needs, *Pediatr Nurs* 17(1):15-20, 1991.

Delaney N, Zolondick K: Day care for technology-dependent infants and children: a new alternative, *J Perinat Neonat Nurs* 5(1):80-85, 1991.

Doolittle RF: Biotechnology—the enormous cost of success, *N Engl J Med* 324(19):1360-1362, 1991.

Dowd E, Vlastuin L: Home care. In Craft M, Denehy J, editors: *Nursing interventions for infants and children,* Philadelphia, 1990, WB Saunders.

Dunst C and others: Enabling and empowering families of children with health impairments, *Child Health Care* 17(2):71-81, 1988.

Embon CM: Discharge planning for infants with bronchopulmonary dysplasia, *J Perinat Neonat Nurs* 5(1):54-63, 1991.

Gale C: Inadequacy of health care for the nation's chronically ill children, *J Pediatr Health Care* 3(1):20-27, 1989.

Gittler J: Case management for children with special health care needs. In Wallace HM, Ryan G, Oglesby AC, editors: *Maternal and child health practices,* ed 3, Oakland, CA, 1988, Third Party.

Goldberg AI, Monahan C: Home health care for children assisted by mechanical ventilation: physician's perspective, *J Pediatr* 114(3):378-83, 1989.

Haas DL: Family-centered, community-based, coordinated care for children with special health care needs, part II, *Issues Compr Pediatr Nurs* 15(2, entire issue), 1992.

Hamilton B, Vessey J: Pediatric discharge planning, *Pediatr Nurs* 18:475-480, 1992.

Hazlett E: A study of pediatric home ventilator management: medical, psychosocial, and financial aspects, *J Pediatr Nurs* 4(4):285-294, 1989.

Hewson M and others: Comprehensive team care, *MCN* 18(4):198-205, 1993.

Hochstadt N, Yost D: The health care–child welfare partnership: transitioning medically complex children to the community, *Child Health Care* 18(1):4-11, 1989.

Hochstadt NJ, Yost DM, editors: *The medically complex child: the transition to home care,* New York, 1991, Harwood Academic.

Hogue E: Liability for premature discharge, *Pediatr Nurs* 14(5):421-423, 1988.

Hogue E: Liability for premature discharge: an update, *Pediatr Nurs* 17(1):76-78, 1991.

Hogue E: Patient referrals: could nurses be violating federal and state antitrust laws? *Pediatr Nurs* 17(3):299-302, 1991.

Johnson B, McGonigel M, Kaufmann R, editors: *Guidelines and recommended practices for the Individualized Family Service Plan,* Washington, DC, 1989, Association for the Care of Children's Health.

Kasprisin C: Home care instructions. In Wong DL, Whaley LF: *Clinical manual of pediatric nursing,* ed 3, St Louis, 1990, Mosby.

Katz KS and others: Home-based care for children with chronic illness, *J Perinat Neonat Nurs* 5(1):71-79, 1991.

Kaufman J, Hardy-Ribakow D: Home care: a model of a comprehensive approach for technology-assisted chronically ill children, *J Pediatr Nurs* 2(4):244-249, 1987.

Kaufman J: An overview of public sector financing for pediatric home care, part I, *Pediatr Nurs* 17:280-281, 1991.

Kaufman J: An overview of public sector financing for pediatric home care, part II, *Pediatr Nurs* 17(4):380, 381, 422, 1991.

Kaufman J: Case management services for chil dren with special health care needs: a family-centered approach, *J Case Manage* 1(2):53-56, 1992.

Klein-Berndt S: Bronchopulmonary dysplasia in the family: a longitudinal case study, *Pediatr Nurs* 17:607-611, 1986.

Kruger SF, Rawlins P: Pediatric dismissal protocol to aid the transition from hospital care to home care, *Image* 16:120-125, 1984.

Ladden M: The impact of preterm birth on the family and society. II. Transition to home, *Pediatr Nurs* 16(6):620-626, 1990.

Larson L, Tollefson M, editors: *From hospital to home: an annotated bibliography,* Washington, DC, 1988, Association for the Care of Children's Health.

Leff P, Walizer E: *Building the healing partnership,* Cambridge, MA, 1992, Brookline Books.

Leighton EM, Davis RH, Anderson LJW: An orientation program for high-technology home care nursing, *Pediatr Nurs* 16:182-185, 1990.

Marrelli TM: *Handbook of home health standards and documentation: guidelines for reimbursement,* ed 2, St Louis, 1994, Mosby.

Martinson IM, Widmer A: *Home health care nursing,* Philadelphia, 1989, WB Saunders.

McClowry S: Pediatric nursing psychosocial care: a vision beyond hospitalization, *Pediatr Nurs* 19(2):146-148, 1993.

Monahan C, Manago R: Technology in pediatric home care: issues in monitoring for quality, *J Home Health Care Pract* 5(1):1-11, 1992.

Nissam LG, Sten MB: The ventilator assisted child: a case for empowerment, *Pediatr Nurs* 17:507-511, 1991.

Nugent K and others: A practice model for a parent support group, *Pediatr Nurs* 18:11-16, 1992.

Odle K: In my opinion . . . partnership for family-centered care: reality or fantasy? *Child Health Care* 17(2):85, 1988.

Patterson J: The role of the nurse manager in a case management delivery system, *Pediatr Nurs* 17(3):282, 1991.

Report to Congress and the Secretary by the Task Force on Technology-Dependent Children: *Fostering home and community-based care for technology-dependent children,* vol 2, 1988, US Department of Health and Human Services, Health Care Financing Administration, HCFA Pub No 88-02171.

Satariano H, Briggs N: The good family syndrome, *Pediatr Nurs* 15(3):285-286, 1989.

Scharer K, Dixon D: Managing chronic illness: parents with a ventilator-dependent child, *J Pediatr Nurs* 4(4):236-247, 1989.

Scharer K and others: Evaluating written discharge instructions in a pediatric setting, *J Nurs Qual Assur* 4(4):63-71, 1990.

Schuman A: Homeward bound: the explosion in pediatric home care, *Contemp Pediatr* 7:26-54, 1990.

Selekman J: Pediatric rehabilitation: from concepts to practice, *Pediatr Nurs* 17:11-14, 1991.

Sherman LP, Rosen CD: Development of a preschool program for tracheostomy dependent children, *Pediatr Nurs* 16:357-361, 1990.

Siarkowski-Amer K, Pigeon V: Documentation of discharge teaching before and after use of a discharge teaching tool, *J Pediatr Nurs* 6(5):296-301, 1991.

Smith SJ: Promoting family adaptation to the at-home care of the technology-dependent child, *Issues Compr Pediatr Nurs* 14(4):249-258, 1991.

Standiford DA and others: Extended day program: bringing preschool to the hospital, *Pediatr Nurs* 19(3):238-241, 1993.

Steele N, Harrison B: Technology-assisted children: assessing discharge preparation, *J Pediatr Nurs* 1(3):150-158, 1986.

Steele N, Morgan J: Emergency planning for technology-assisted children, *J Pediatr Nurs* 4(2):81-87, 1989.

Steele S: Nurse and parent collaborative case management in a rural setting, *Pediatr Nurs* 19(6):612-615, 1993.

Stein R: Home care: a challenging opportunity, *Child Health Care* 14(2):90-95, 1985.

Stein R: *Caring for children with chronic illness: issues and strategies,* New York, 1989, Springer.

Stein R, Jessop DJ: Does pediatric home care make a difference for children with chronic illness? Findings from the Pediatric Ambulatory Care Treatment Study, *Pediatrics* 73(6):845-853, 1984.

Sterling Y: Resource needs of mothers managing chronically ill infants at home, *Neonatal Network* 9(1):55-59, 1990.

Wegener DH, Aday LA: Home care for ventilator assisted children: predicting family stress, *Pediatr Nurs* 15:371-376, 1989.

Wheeler TW, Lewis CC: Home care for medically fragile children: urban versus rural settings, *Issues Compr Pediatr Nurs* 16:13-30, 1993.

SELECTED RESOURCES ON HOME CARE

Association for the Care of Children's Health
7910 Woodmont Ave., Suite 300
Bethesda, MD 20814
(301) 654-6549

National Association for Home Care
519 C Street, N.E.
Washington, DC 20002-5809
(202) 547-7424

National Father's Network
The Kindering Center
16120 Northeast 8th St.
Bellevue, WA 98008
(206) 747-4004

National Information Center for Children and Youth with Disabilities
PO Box 1492
Washington, DC 20013
(202) 884-8200 or (800) 695-0285

National Information Clearinghouse for Infants with Disabilities and Life Threatening Conditions

NIS
CDD/USC
Benson Building
Columbia, SC 29208
(800) 922-9234, ext. 201 (voice or TDD)
in South Carolina: (800) 922-1107.

Project Copernicus
(Family-Centered Care)
2911 E. Biddle St.
Baltimore, MD 21213
(410) 550-9700

Sibling Support Project
Children's Hospital and Medical Center
4800 Sand Point Way, N.E.
Seattle, WA 98105
(206) 368-4911

Skip (Sick Kids Need Involved People, Inc.)
545 Madison Ave., 13th Floor
New York, NY 10022
(212) 421-9160

PART II

Nursing Care of the Ill or Hospitalized Child

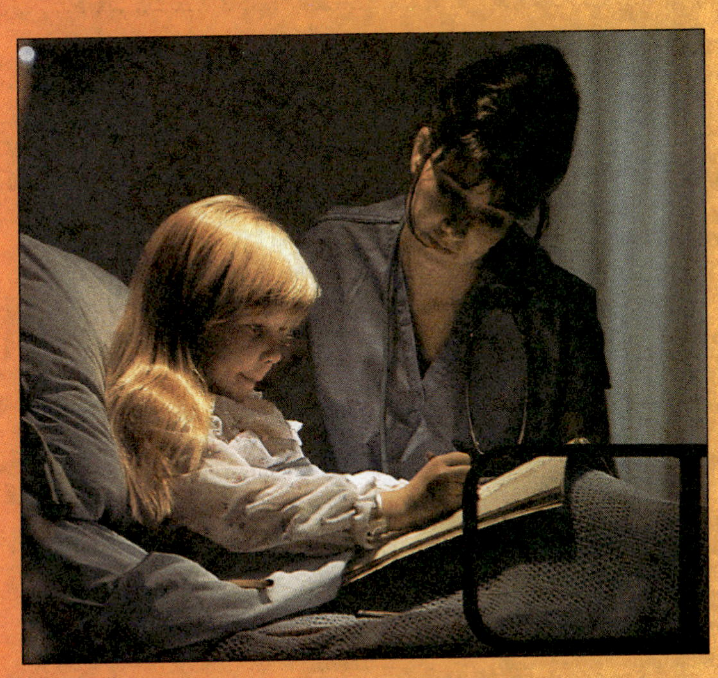

UNIT IX

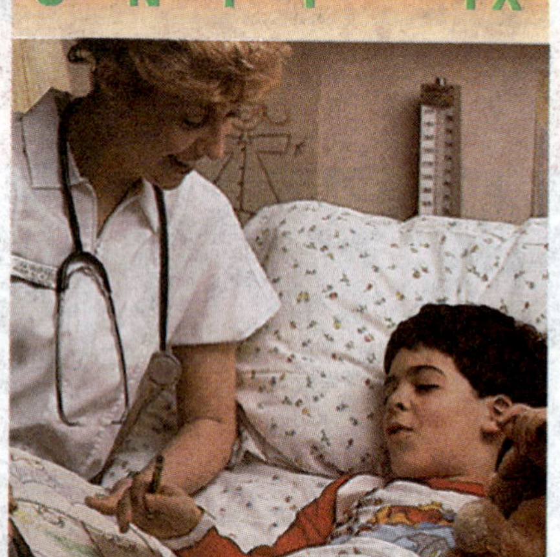

THE CHILD WHO IS HOSPITALIZED

CHAPTER 26

Family-Centered Care of the Child During Illness and Hospitalization

CHAPTER OUTLINE

RELATED TOPICS

Administration of medication, Ch. 27
Communication and health assessment of the child and family, Ch. 6
Compliance, Ch. 27
Family-centered care of the child with chronic illness or disability, Ch. 22
Family centered care of the child with life-threatening illness, Ch. 23
Family-centered home care, Ch. 25
Neonatal pain, Ch. 11
Nursing care of the surgical neonate, Ch. 11
Physical and developmental assessment of the child, Ch. 7
Preparation for procedures, Ch. 27
Social, cultural, and religious influences on child health promotion, Ch. 2
Surgical procedures, Ch. 27

For children and their families, illness and hospitalization constitute a stressful experience. It is often the first crisis children must confront. Children, especially during the early years, are particularly vulnerable to the crises of illness and hospitalization because (1) stress represents a change from the usual state of health and environmental routine, and (2) children have a limited number of coping mechanisms to resolve the stressful events. Children's reactions to these crises are influenced by their developmental age; previous experience with illness, separation, or hospitalization; available support system; their innate and acquired coping skills; and the seriousness of the diagnosis.

This chapter focuses on the various aspects of illness and hospitalization in children to assist nurses in providing the quality of care that promotes optimum resolution of the crisis and positive growth from the experience for the entire family unit.

STRESSORS AND REACTIONS RELATED TO DEVELOPMENTAL STAGE

Children's understanding of, reaction to, and method of coping with illness or hospitalization are influenced by the significance of individual ***stressors*** (those events that produce stress) during each developmental phase. The major stressors of separation, loss of control, bodily injury, and pain and children's behavioral reactions are discussed in this section. However, a review of the previous chapters on normal growth and development will facilitate a more thorough understanding of children's physical, psychosocial, and cognitive abilities and limitations. In addition, Chapters 22 and 23 present an in-depth discussion of children's and family members' reactions to a disability and chronic or life-threatening illness.

SEPARATION ANXIETY

The major stress from middle infancy throughout the preschool years, especially for children ages 15 to 30 months, is separation anxiety, also called ***anaclitic depression.*** The principal behavioral responses of these children to the three phases of separation anxiety are summarized in the box at right.

During the phase of ***protest,*** children cry loudly, scream for the parent, refuse the attention of anyone else, and are inconsolable in their grief (Fig. 26-1). They may continue this behavior for a few hours to several days. Some children may protest continuously, ceasing only from physical exhaustion. If a stranger approaches them, children will initially protest even louder.

During the phase of ***despair,*** the crying stops. The child is much less active, is disinterested in play or food, and with-

MANIFESTATIONS OF SEPARATION ANXIETY IN YOUNG CHILDREN

PHASE OF PROTEST

Observed behaviors during later infancy
- Cries
- Screams
- Searches for parent with eyes
- Clings to parent
- Avoids and rejects contact with strangers

Additional behaviors observed during toddlerhood
- Verbally attacks strangers (e.g., "Go away")
- Physically attacks strangers (e.g., kicks, bites, hits, pinches)
- Attempts to escape to find parent
- Attempts to physically force parent to stay

Behaviors may last from hours to days

Protest, such as crying, may be continuous, ceasing only with physical exhaustion

Approach of stranger may precipitate increased protest

PHASE OF DESPAIR

Observed behaviors
- Inactive
- Withdraws from others
- Depressed, sad
- Uninterested in environment
- Uncommunicative
- Regresses to earlier behavior (e.g., thumb-sucking, bed-wetting, use of pacifier, use of bottle)

Behaviors may last for variable length of time

Child's physical condition may deteriorate from refusal to eat, drink, or move

PHASE OF DETACHMENT

Observed behaviors
- Shows increased interest in surroundings
- Interacts with strangers or familiar caregivers
- Forms new but superficial relationships
- Appears happy

Detachment usually occurs after prolonged separation from parent; rarely seen in hospitalized children

Behaviors represent a superficial adjustment to loss

■ Judy Holt Rollins, RN, MS, revised this chapter.

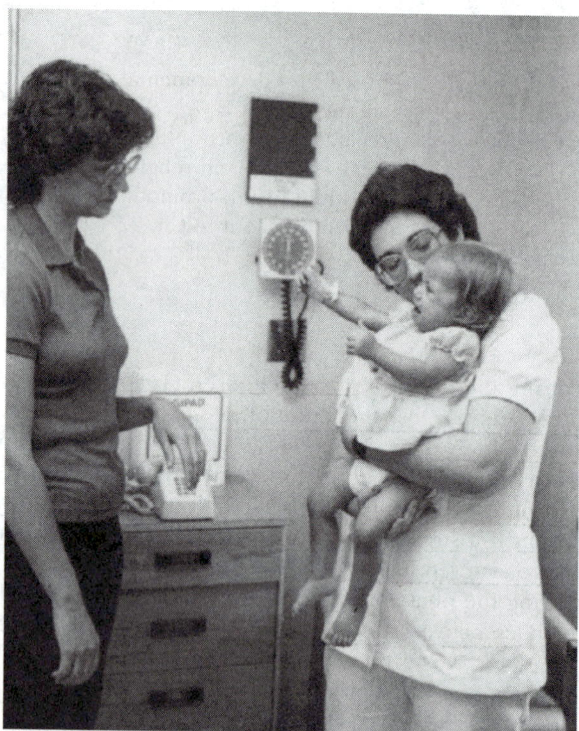

FIG. 26-1 In the protest phase of separation anxiety, children cry loudly and are inconsolable in their grief for the parent.

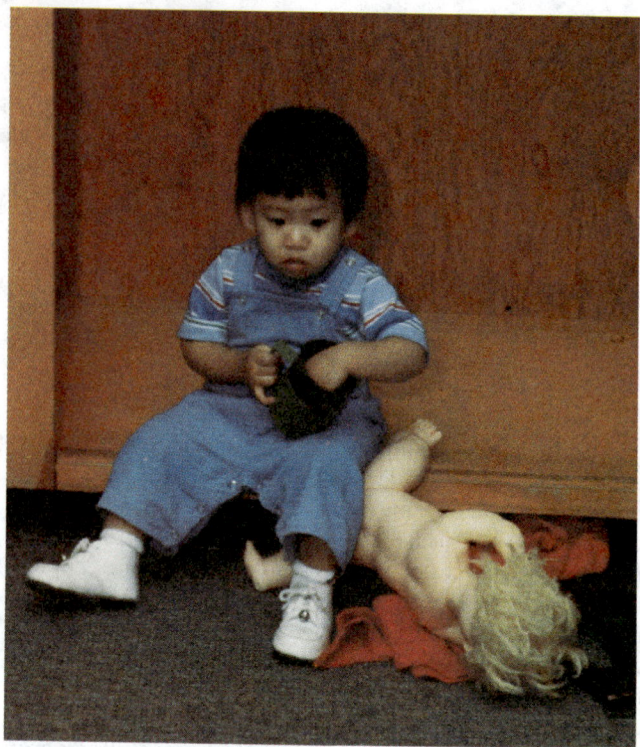

FIG. 26-2 During the despair phase of separation anxiety, children are sad, lonely, and disinterested in play or food.

draws from others. The child looks sad, lonely, isolated, and apathetic (Fig. 26-2). The major behavior characteristic is depression, a result of increasing hopelessness, grief, and mourning.

The third phase is ***detachment***, sometimes also called ***denial***. Superficially the child appears to have finally adjusted to the loss. The child becomes more interested in the surroundings, plays with others, and seems to form new relationships. However, this behavior is a result of resignation and is not a sign of contentment. The child detaches from the parent in an effort to escape the emotional pain of desiring the parent's presence. The child copes by forming shallow relationships with others, becoming increasingly self-centered, and attaching primary importance to material objects. This is the most serious phase, since reversal of the potential adverse effects is less likely to occur once detachment is established. However, in most situations the temporary separations imposed by hospitalization do not cause such prolonged parental absences that the child enters into detachment. In addition, considerable evidence suggests that, even with stresses such as separation, children are remarkably resilient, and permanent ill effects are rare.

While progression to detachment is uncommon, the initial phases are frequently observed even with very brief separations from either parent. Without an understanding of the meaning of each stage of behavior, health team members may erroneously label the behaviors as positive or negative. In the phase of protest, they may view the loud crying as "bad" behavior. Since the protesting increases if a stranger approaches, staff may interpret the reaction as evidence of their need to stay away. During the quiet, withdrawn phase of despair, they regard the child as finally "settling in" to the new surroundings and see the detachment behaviors as proof of a "good adjustment." The faster a child reaches this stage, the more likely the child will be regarded as the "ideal patient."

Since children seem to react "negatively" to visits by their parents, uninformed observers feel justified in restricting parental visiting privileges. For example, during the protest phase, children outwardly do not appear happy to see their parents. Instead, they may cry louder than before the parents' visit. If children are depressed, they may reject their parents or begin to protest once more. Often they cling to their parents in an effort to ensure their continued presence. Consequently, the parents' visits may be regarded as "disturbing" the child's adjustment to the surroundings. If the separation has progressed to the phase of detachment, children will respond no differently to their parents than to any other strange or familiar person.

Such reactions are distressing to parents, who may be unaware of their meaning. If they are regarded as intruders, parents will view their absence as "beneficial" to the child's adjustment and recovery. They may respond to the child's behavior by staying for short periods, decreasing the frequency of visits, or deceiving the child when it is time to leave. Consequently, a destructive cycle of misunderstanding and unmet needs results.

Early Childhood

Separation anxiety is most evident during the ages of 6 to 30 months and is the greatest stress imposed by hospitalization. If separation is avoided, young children have a tremendous capacity to withstand any other stress. During this time the typical reactions just described are seen. However, children in the toddler stage demonstrate more goal-directed behaviors. For example, they may verbally plead for their parents to stay and physically attempt to secure or find them. They may demonstrate displeasure on the parents' return or departure by having temper tantrums; refusing to comply to the usual routines of mealtime, bedtime, or toileting; or regressing to more primitive levels of development. However, temper tantrums, bed-wetting, or other behaviors may also be explained as expressions of anger or even a physiologic response to stress.

Since preschoolers are much more secure interpersonally than toddlers, they can tolerate brief periods of separation from their parents and are more inclined to develop substitute trust in other significant adults. However, the stress of illness usually renders them less able to cope with separation; as a result, they manifest many of the stage behaviors of separation anxiety. In general, the protest behaviors are more subtle and passive than those seen in younger children. Preschoolers may demonstrate separation anxiety through refusing to eat, difficulty in sleeping, crying quietly for their parents, continually asking when they will visit, or withdrawing from others. They may express anger indirectly by breaking their toys, hitting other children, or refusing to cooperate during usual self-care activities. Nurses need to be sensitive to these less obvious signs of separation anxiety to intervene appropriately.

Later Childhood

Previous research, usually based on adult recollections, indicated that the family does not play as important a role for school-age children as it does during the toddler and preschool years. However, in a recent study wherein children were asked about their fears when hospitalized, children ranked "being away from my family" higher than any other fear associated with hospitalization (Hart and Bossert, 1994). Although school-age children are better able to cope with separation in general, the stress and often accompanying regression imposed by illness or hospitalization may increase their need for parental security and guidance. This is particularly true for young school-age children who have only recently left the safety of the home and are struggling with the crisis of school adjustment. Middle and late school-age children may react more to the separation from their usual activities and peers than to absence of their parents. Their high level of physical and mental activity frequently finds no suitable outlets in the hospital environment. Even when they dislike school, they admit to missing its routine and associated activities and worry that they will not be able to compete or "fit in" with their classmates on returning to school. Feelings of loneliness, boredom, isolation, and depression are common. It is important to recognize that such reactions may occur more as a result of separation than from concern over the illness, treatment, or hospital setting.

School-age children may need and desire parental guidance or support from other adult figures but be unable or unwilling to ask for it. Because the goal of attaining independence is so important to them, they are reluctant to seek help directly for fear that they will appear weak, childish, or dependent. Cultural expectations to "act like a man" or to "be brave and strong" bear heavily on these children, especially males, who tend to react to stress with stoicism, withdrawal, or passive acceptance. Often the need to express hostile, angry, or other negative feelings finds alternate outlets, such as irritability and aggression toward parents, withdrawal from hospital personnel, inability to relate to peers, rejection of siblings, or subsequent problems in school.

For adolescents, separation from home and parents may be difficult. However, loss of peer-group contact may be a severe emotional threat because of loss of group status, inability to exert group control or leadership, and loss of group acceptance. Deviations within peer groups are poorly tolerated, and, although members may express concern for the adolescent's illness or need for hospitalization, they continue their group activities, quickly filling the gap of the absent member. During the temporary separation from their usual group, ill adolescents may benefit from group associations with other hospitalized age-mates.

LOSS OF CONTROL

One of the factors influencing the amount of stress imposed by hospitalization is the amount of control that persons perceive themselves as having. Lack of control increases the perception of threat and can affect children's coping skills. Many hospital situations decrease the amount of control a child feels. Although the usual sensory stimulations are lacking, the additional hospital stimuli of sight, sound, and smell may be overwhelming. Without an insight into the type of environment conducive to children's optimum growth, the hospital experience can at best temporarily slow development and at worst permanently retard it. Because the needs of children vary greatly depending on their age, the major areas of loss of control in terms of physical restriction, altered routine or rituals, and dependency are discussed for each age-group.

Infants

Infants are developing the most important attribute of a healthy personality—trust. Trust is established through consistent, loving care by a mothering person. Infants attempt to control their environment through emotional expressions, such as crying or smiling. In the hospital setting cues may be missed or misinterpreted, and routines may be established to meet the hospital staff's needs instead of the infant's needs. Inconsistent care and deviations from the infant's daily routine may lead to mistrust and a decreased sense of control (Wells and others, 1994).

Toddlers

Toddlers are striving for autonomy, and this goal is evident in most of their behaviors—motor skills, play, interpersonal relationships, activities of daily living, and communication.

When their egocentric pleasures meet with obstacles, toddlers react with negativism, especially temper tantrums. Any restriction or limitation of movement, such as the simple act of laying toddlers on their back, can cause forceful resistance and noncompliance.

Loss of control also results from altered routines and rituals. Toddlers rely on the consistency and familiarity of daily rituals to provide a measure of stability and control in their complex world of growing and developing. The hospitalization or illness severely limits their sense of expectation and predictability, since most details of the hospital environment differ from those of the home.

Toddlers' main areas for rituals include eating, sleeping, bathing, toileting, and play. When the routines are disrupted, difficulties can occur in any or all of these areas. The principal reaction to such change is regression. For example, when mealtime and food choices differ from those at home, toddlers often refuse to eat, demand a bottle, or request others to feed them. Although regression to earlier forms of behavior may seem to increase toddlers' security and comfort, in reality it is very threatening for them to relinquish their most recently acquired achievements.

Enforced dependency is a chief characteristic of the sick role and accounts for the numerous instances of toddler negativism. For example, rigid schedules, altered caregiving activities, unfamiliar surroundings, separation from parents, and medical procedures usurp toddlers' control over their world. Although most toddlers initially react negatively and aggressively to such dependency, prolonged loss of autonomy may result in passive withdrawal from interpersonal relationships and regression in all areas of development. Therefore the effects of the sick role are most severe in instances of chronic, long-term illnesses or in those families who foster the sick role despite the child's improved state of health.

Preschoolers

Preschoolers also suffer from loss of control caused by physical restriction, altered routines, and enforced dependency. However, their specific cognitive abilities, which make them feel omnipotent and all-powerful, also make them feel out of control. This loss of control in the context of their sense of self-power is a critical influencing factor in their perception of and reaction to separation, pain, illness, and hospitalization.

Preschoolers' egocentric and magical thinking limits their ability to understand events because they view all experiences from their own self-referenced perspective. Without adequate preparation for unfamiliar settings or experiences, preschoolers' fantasy explanations for such events are usually more exaggerated, bizarre, and frightening than the facts. One typical fantasy to explain the reason for illness or hospitalization is that it represents punishment for real or imagined misdeeds. The response to such thinking is usually feelings of shame, guilt, and fear.

Preschoolers' cognitive ability is also concrete. Explanations are understood only in terms of real events. Purely verbal instructions are often inadequate for them because of their inability to abstract and synthesize beyond what their senses tell them. When combined with their egocentric and magical powers, they can interpret any message according to their particular past experiences. Even with the best preparation for a procedure, they may misconstrue the details.

Transductive reasoning implies that preschoolers deduce from the particular to the particular, rather than from the specific to the general, or the general to the specific. For example, if preschoolers' concept of nurses is that they inflict pain, preschoolers will think that every nurse (or everyone wearing a similar uniform) will also inflict pain.

School-Age Children

Because of their striving for independence and productivity, school-age children are particularly vulnerable to events that may lessen their feeling of control and power. In particular, altered family roles; physical disability; fears of death, abandonment, or permanent injury; loss of peer acceptance; lack of productivity; and inability to cope with stress according to perceived cultural expectations may result in loss of control.

Because of the nature of the patient role, many routine hospital activities usurp individual power and identity. For these children, dependent activities such as enforced bed rest, use of a bedpan, inability to choose a menu, lack of privacy, help with a bed bath, or transport by a wheelchair or stretcher can be a direct threat to their security. Although all of these procedures seem routine and inconsequential, they allow no freedom of choice to children who want to "act grown-up." However, when children are allowed to exert a measure of control, regardless of how limited it may be, they generally respond very well to any procedure. For example, some of the most cooperative, satisfied, and contented patients are school-age children who help make their beds, choose their schedule of activities, assist in procedures, and help the nurses care for younger children. An increased sense of control usually results from a feeling of usefulness and productivity.

In addition to the hospital environment, illness may also cause a feeling of loss of control. One of the most significant problems of children in this age-group centers on boredom. When physical or enforced limitations curtail their usual abilities to care for themselves or to engage in favorite activities, school-age children generally respond with depression, hostility, or frustration. Keeping a normally active child on bed rest is no small challenge. However, emphasizing areas of control and capitalizing on quiet activities, particularly hobbies such as building models or collecting specific objects, promote their adjustment to physical restriction. Nursing judgment regarding selection of a roommate is one of the most important contributing factors to their overall adjustment to illness and hospitalization.

Adolescents

Adolescents' struggle for independence, self-assertion, and liberation centers on the quest for personal identity. Anything that interferes with this poses a threat to their sense of identity and results in a loss of control. Illness, which limits their physical abilities, and hospitalization, which separates them from usual support systems, constitute major situational crises.

The patient role fosters dependency and depersonalization. Adolescents may react to dependency with rejection, uncooperativeness, or withdrawal. They may respond to depersonalization with self-assertion, anger, or frustration. Regardless of which response they manifest, hospital personnel generally tend to regard them as difficult, unmanageable patients. Parents may not be a source of help because these behaviors serve to further isolate them from understanding the adolescent. Although peers may visit, they may not be able to offer the type of support and guidance needed. Sick adolescents often voluntarily isolate themselves from age-mates until they feel they can compete on an equal basis and meet group expectations. As a result, ill adolescents may be left with virtually no support systems.

Loss of control also occurs for many of the reasons discussed for school-age children. However, adolescents are more sensitive than younger children to potential instances of loss of control and dependency. For example, both groups seek information about their physical status and rely heavily on anticipatory preparation to decrease fear and anxiety. However, adolescents react not only to what information is supplied, but also to how it is conveyed. They may feel very threatened by others who relate facts in a derogatory manner. Adolescents want to know that others can relate to them on their own level. This necessitates a careful assessment of their intellectual abilities, previous knowledge, and present needs. It may also require the nurse's willingness to learn the adolescent's language.

BODILY INJURY AND PAIN

Fears of bodily injury and pain are prevalent among children. Recent research documents that young children, including newborns, react to painful stimuli. In caring for children, nurses must appreciate the concerns related to bodily harm and children's reactions to pain at different developmental periods. Developmental considerations related to children's understanding of illness and pain are summarized in Table 26-1. Developmental characteristics of children's reactions to pain are also important (see box on p. 1087).

Yoos (1994) cautions that these "stages" should be viewed rather as "patterns." Although the Piagetian structuralist perspective argues that changes in *cognitive structure* enable children to reach higher levels of reasoning, others argue that changes in *content* drive the system to higher levels. They assert that the ability to think at these higher levels is made possible by increasing knowledge and experience *within* a particular domain. Therefore illness experiences can produce child "experts" who may be better able to see underlying principles and connections about their particular illness or condition than a "novice" adult.

TABLE 26-1 Children's Developmental Concepts of Illness and Pain

COGNITIVE STAGE (AGE)	CONCEPT OF ILLNESS*	CONCEPT OF PAIN†
Preoperational thought (2 to 7 years)	*Phenomenism:* Perceives an external, unrelated, concrete phenomenon as the cause of illness (e.g., "being sick because you don't feel well") *Contagion:* Perceives cause of illness as proximity between two events that occurs by "magic" (e.g., "getting a cold because you are near someone who has a cold")	Conceives of pain primarily as physical, concrete experience Thinks in terms of magical disappearance of pain May view pain as punishment for wrongdoing Tends to hold someone accountable for own pain and may strike out at person
Concrete operational thought (7 to 10+ years)	*Contamination:* Perceives cause as a person, object, or action external to the child that is "bad" or "harmful" to the body (e.g., "getting a cold because you didn't wear a hat") *Internalization:* Perceives illness as having an external cause but as being located inside the body (e.g., "getting a cold by breathing in air and bacteria")	Conceives of pain physically (e.g., headache, stomachache) Able to perceive psychologic pain (e.g., someone dying) Fears bodily harm and annihilation (body destruction and death) May view pain as punishment for wrongdoing
Formal operational thought (13 years and older)	*Physiologic:* Perceives cause as malfunctioning or nonfunctioning organ or process; can explain illness in sequence of events *Psychophysiologic:* Realizes that psychologic actions and attitudes affect health and illness	Able to give reason for pain (e.g., fell and hit nerve) Perceives several types of psychologic pain Has limited life experiences to cope with pain as adult might cope despite mature understanding of pain Fears losing control during painful experience

*Data from Bibace R, Walsh ME: Development of children's concepts of illness, *Pediatrics* 66(6):912-917, 1980.
†Data from Hurley A, Whelan EG: Cognitive development and children's perception of pain, *Pediatr Nurs* 14(1):21-24, 1988.

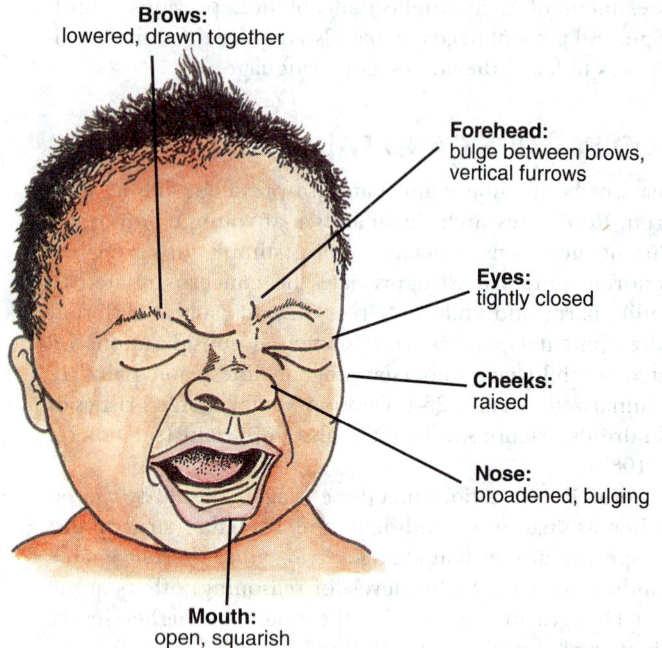

FIG. 26-3 Facial expression of physical distress is the most consistent behavioral indicator of pain in infants.

Infants

Of the research exploring children's development of illness concepts and how their understanding of illness relates to fears of bodily injury, no findings are available for preverbal children. Consequently, the following discussion is limited to infants' reactions to pain. Neonatal pain is discussed in Chapter 11.

Infants' response to pain after the neonatal period is quite similar to earlier reactions, although there is marked variability in measures of distress, especially initial cry and heart rate, which may decrease in some infants. The most consistent indicator of distress is a facial expression of discomfort (Izard, Hembree, and Huebner, 1987) (Fig. 26-3). Body movements include squirming, writhing, jerking, and flailing (Mills, 1989). The individual differences may be the result of temperamental characteristics, which require further research and study. Some infants may cry loudly following the procedure, whereas others are easily calmed by a gentle hug. It is important to recognize and respect such early signs of individuality and to realize that children who react less intensely may still be experiencing significant discomfort (Broome and others, 1990).

Infants less than 6 months of age seem to have no memory of previous painful experiences and react to a potentially stressful situation with less apprehension and fear than older children. However, after this time, children's response to pain is influenced by their recall of prior painful experiences and the emotional reaction of parents during the procedure. Older infants react intensely with physical resistance and uncooperativeness. They may refuse to lie still, attempt to push the person away, or try to escape with whatever motor activity they have achieved. Distraction does little to lessen their immediate reaction to pain, and anticipatory preparation, such as showing them the equipment, tends to increase their fear and resistance.

Toddlers

Toddlers' concept of body image, particularly the definition of body boundaries, is very poorly developed. Intrusive experiences, such as examining the ears or mouth or taking a rectal temperature, are very anxiety producing. Toddlers may react to such painless procedures as intensely as they do to painful ones.

Toddlers' reactions to pain are similar to those seen during infancy, except that the variables influencing the individual response are highly complex and varied. Memory, physical restraint, parent separation, emotional reactions of others, and lack of preparation partially determine the intensity of the behavioral response. In general, children in this age-group continue to react with intense emotional upset and physical resistance to any actual or perceived painful experience. Behaviors indicating pain include grimacing, clenching their teeth/lips, opening their eyes wide, rocking, rubbing, and aggressiveness, such as biting, kicking, hitting, or running away. Unlike adults, who usually decrease their activity when in pain, young children typically become restless and overly active; frequently this response is not recognized as a consequence of pain.

By the end of this age period, toddlers usually are able to communicate about their pain. Although they have not developed the ability to describe the type or intensity of the pain, they usually are able to localize it by pointing to a specific area.

Preschoolers

Concepts of illness begin during the preschool period and are influenced by the cognitive abilities of the preoperational stage. Preschoolers differentiate poorly between themselves and the external world. Their thinking is focused on externally perceived events, and causality is based on the proximity of two events. Consequently, children define illness according to what they are told or are given external evidence of, such as "You are sick because you have a fever." The cause of illness is seen as a concrete action the child does or fails to do, such as "Catching a cold because you go out into cold weather." Consequently, it implies a degree of responsibility and self-blame. Another explanation may be based on contagion, that the proximity of two objects or persons causes the illness (e.g., "A person gets a cold when someone else with a cold gets near him").

The psychosexual conflicts of children in this age-group make them very vulnerable to threats of bodily injury. Intrusive procedures, whether painful or painless, are threatening to preschoolers, whose concept of body integrity is still poorly developed. Preschoolers may react to an injection with as much concern for withdrawal of the needle as for the actual pain. They fear that the intrusion or puncture will not reclose and that their "insides" will leak out.

Concerns of mutilation are paramount during this age period. Loss of any body part is threatening, but preschool boys' fears of castration complicate their understanding of surgical or medical procedures associated with the genital area, such as circumcision, repair of hypospadias or epispadias, cystoscopy, or catheterization. Their limited comprehension of body functioning also increases their difficulty in understanding how or why body parts are "fixed." For example, telling preschoolers that their tonsils are to be removed may be interpreted as "taking out their voice," or having the penis "fixed" may be understood as cutting it off. Words such as "dye," "cut off," "take out," or "draw" (e.g., "draw some blood") are understood literally and can lead to confusion and fear (see Communicating with Children, Chapter 6).

Reactions to pain tend to be similar to those seen during toddlerhood, although some differences become apparent. For example, preschoolers respond more favorably to preparatory interventions, such as explanation and distraction, than younger children. Physical and verbal aggression are more specific and goal directed. Instead of showing total body resistance, preschoolers may push the offending person away, try to secure the equipment, or attempt to lock themselves in a safe place. Much more thought is evident in their plan of attack or escape.

Verbal expression in particular demonstrates their advanced development in response to stress. They may verbally abuse the attacker by stating, "Get out of here" or "I hate you." They may also use the more cunning approach of trying to persuade the person to give up the intended activity. A common plea is "Please don't give me a shot; I'll be good." Some statements are not only attempts to avoid the event but also evidence of children's perceptions about the experience.

Attempts to be comforted may also be evident through behaviors such as clinging to a parent, wanting to be held, or refusing to be left alone. A typical expression denoting the need for dependency is "Help me." It is important to recognize such requests as the need for support from others during a time of stress. Admonishing children to act grown-up or encouraging them to do things by stating, "I know you can do it yourself," deprives them of the support they are requesting and increases their own feelings of guilt and shame.

School-Age Children

Fears of the physical nature of the illness surface at this time. School-age children may be less concerned with pain than with disability, uncertain recovery, or possible death. Children with chronic illness are more likely to identify intrusive procedures as stressful, whereas children who are acutely ill are more likely to indicate physical symptoms (Bossert, 1994). Girls tend to express more and stronger fears than boys, and previous hospitalizations may have no effect on the frequency or intensity of these fears. Because of their developing cognitive abilities, school-age children are aware of the significance of different illnesses, the indispensability of certain body parts, potential hazards in treatment, lifelong consequences of permanent injury or loss of function, and the meaning of death. A major concern of hospitalized school-age children is their fear of being told that something is wrong with them (Hart and Bossert, 1994). They generally take a very active interest in their health or illness. Even those children who rarely ask questions usually reveal detailed knowledge of their condition by attentively listening to all that is said around them. They request factual information and quickly perceive lies or half-truths. Seeking information tends to be one way of their maintaining a sense of control despite the stress and uncertainty of illness.

The school-age child defines illness by a set of multiple concrete symptoms, such as signs of a cold, and views the cause as primarily germs or bacteria. The germs have a powerful, almost magical quality, so that in the child's mind, illness can be prevented by avoiding people with the germs. There is also the idea of contamination, which is similar to that seen in the younger age-group; for example, the illness occurs because of physical contact or because the child engaged in a harmful action and became contaminated. Consequently, feelings of self-blame and guilt may be associated with the reason for becoming ill.

School-age children begin to show concern for the potential beneficial and hazardous effects of procedures. Besides wanting to know if a procedure will hurt, they want to know what it is for, how it will make them better, and what injury or harm could result. For example, these children fear the actual procedure of anesthesia. Unlike preschoolers who fear the mask and the strange surroundings, school-age children fear what may happen while they are asleep, whether they will wake up, and if they may die. Preadolescents also worry about the procedure itself, particularly one that will result in visible changes in body appearance.

Intrusive procedures of a nonsexual nature, such as routine physical examination of the ears, nose, mouth, and throat, are generally well tolerated. However, concerns for privacy become evident and increasingly significant. Although school-age children may be cooperative during examination of, or procedures performed on, the genital area, it is usually very stressful for them, especially for preadolescents who are beginning pubertal changes. Nurses who respect children's need for privacy can provide them with much assurance and support.

By the age of 9 or 10, most school-age children show less fright or overt resistance to pain than younger children. They generally have learned passive methods of dealing with discomfort, such as holding rigidly still, clenching their fists or teeth, or trying to act brave by the "grin-and-bear-it" routine. If they do display signs of overt resistance, such as biting, kicking, pulling away, trying to escape, crying, or plea bargaining, they may deny such reactions later, especially to their peers for fear of embarrassment.

School-age children verbally communicate about their pain in respect to its location, intensity, and description. Unlike younger children, who may have difficulty choosing words to describe pain, children 8 years and older use a wide variety of words and phrases, such as hurting, sore, burning, stinging, aching, and "like a sharp knife" (Tesler and others, 1989).

School-age children also use words as a means of controlling their reactions to pain. For example, these children may ask the nurse to talk to them during a procedure. Some prefer to participate in a procedure, whereas others choose to distance themselves by not looking at what is happening. Most appreciate an explanation of the procedure and seem less fearful when they know what to expect. Others try to gain control by attempting to postpone the event. A typical request is "Give me the shot when I am finished with this." Although the ability to make decisions does increase their sense of control, unlimited procrastination results in heightened anxiety. When choices are allowed, such as selection of the injection site, it is best to structure the number of possible sites and to limit the number of "procrastination" techniques.

Similar to their more passive acceptance of pain is their nondirective request for support or help. School-age children will rarely initiate a conversation about their feelings or request someone to stay with them during a lonely or stressful period. Their visible composure, calmness, and acceptance often mask their inner longing for support. It is especially important to be aware of nonverbal clues, such as a serious facial expression, a halfhearted reply of "I am fine," silence, lack of activity, or social isolation, as signs of the need for help. Usually when someone identifies the unspoken messages and offers support, they readily accept it.

Adolescents

Although the development of body image begins at birth, its relevance is paramount during adolescence. Injury, pain, disability, and death are viewed primarily in terms of how each affects adolescents' views of themselves in the present. Any change that differentiates the adolescent from peers is regarded as a major tragedy. For example, diseases such as diabetes mellitus often present a more difficult adjustment period for children in this age-group than for younger children because of the necessary changes in the adolescent's life-style. Conversely, serious, even life-threatening illnesses that entail no visible body changes or physical restrictions may have less immediate significance for the adolescent. Therefore the nature of bodily injury may be more important in terms of adolescents' perception of the illness than its actual degree of severity.

Adolescents' rapidly changing body image during pubertal development often makes them feel insecure about their bodies. Illness, medical or surgical intervention, and hospitalization increase their existing concerns for normalcy. They may respond to such events by asking numerous questions, withdrawing, rejecting others, or questioning the adequacy of care. Frequently their fear for loss of control and body image change is demonstrated as overconfidence, conceit, or a "know-it-all" attitude.

Because of sexual changes, adolescents are very concerned about privacy. Lack of respect for this need can cause greater stress than physical pain. In addition, adolescents look for signs that indicate that they are developing normally and according to acceptable standards. When illness occurs, they fear that growth may be retarded, leaving them behind their peers. Although they may not voice this concern, they may demonstrate it by carefully observing others' reactions to them.

Adolescents typically react to pain with much self-control. Physical resistance and aggression are unusual at this age, unless the adolescents are totally unprepared for a procedure. As with older school-age children, they are very concerned with remaining composed and feel embarrassed and ashamed of losing control. They are able to describe their pain experience and to use any of the pain assessment tools developed for adults. However, they may be reluctant to disclose their pain unless the nurse is willing to listen closely and observe physical indications, such as limited movement, excessive quiet, or irritability. They may also believe that the nurse knows how they feel; thus they may see no need to ask for analgesia (Favaloro and Touzel, 1990).

EFFECTS OF HOSPITALIZATION ON THE CHILD

Children may react to the stresses of hospitalization before admission, during hospitalization, and after discharge. A child's conception of illness is even more important than age and intellectual maturity in predicting the level of adjustment before hospitalization (Carson, Gravley, and Council, 1992). Many children, especially those under 4 years of age, demonstrate temporary behavioral changes following discharge (see box below). These changes are a result of (1) separation from significant people, (2) a lack of opportunity to form new attachments, and (3) a strange environment.

Individual Risk Factors

A number of risk factors make certain children more vulnerable than others to the stresses of hospitalization (see box on p. 1073, left). It has also been noted that rural children exhibit significantly greater degrees of psychologic up-

POSTHOSPITAL BEHAVIORS IN CHILDREN

YOUNG CHILDREN

Some initial aloofness toward parents; may last from a few minutes (most common) to a few days

Frequently followed by dependency behaviors:
- Tendency to cling to parents
- Demand parents' attention
- Vigorously oppose any separation (e.g., staying at preschool or with a baby-sitter)

Other negative behaviors include:
- New fears (e.g., nightmares)
- Resistance to going to bed, night waking
- Withdrawal and shyness
- Hyperactivity
- Temper tantrums
- Food finickiness
- Attachment to blanket or toy
- Regression in newly learned skills (e.g., self-toileting)

OLDER CHILDREN

Negative behaviors include:
- Emotional coldness, followed by intense, demanding dependence on parents
- Anger toward parents
- Jealousy toward others (e.g., siblings)

set than urban children, possibly because urban children have opportunities to become familiar with a local hospital (Gillis, 1990). Perhaps because separation is such an important issue surrounding hospitalization for young children, children who are active and strong willed tend to fare better when hospitalized than youngsters who are passive. Consequently, nurses should be alert to children who passively accept all changes and requests; these children may need more support than the "oppositional" child.

The development of subsequent long-term emotional disturbance may be related to the length and number of hospital admissions and the type of hospital practices. A single hospitalization of 4 weeks or more and repeated hospital admissions have been associated with later disturbances. However, supportive practices, such as frequent family visiting, may lessen the detrimental effects of such admissions.

Changes in the Pediatric Population

The pediatric population in hospitals today has changed dramatically over the last two decades. A greater percentage of the children hospitalized today have more serious and complex problems than those hospitalized in the past. Many of these children are fragile newborns and children with severe injuries or disabilities who survived because of incredible technologic advances, yet were left with chronic or disabling conditions that require frequent and lengthy hospital stays. Research suggests that prior experience and familiarity with medical events related to hospitalization do not reduce fears in children (Hart and Bossert, 1994). Rather, prior experience may simply replace fear of the unknown with fear of the known. The nature of their conditions increases the likelihood that this group of children will experience more invasive and traumatic procedures while they are hospitalized. These factors make them more vulnerable to the emotional consequences of hospitalization and result in their needs being significantly different from those of the short-term patients of the past (see Chapter 22 for further discussion on children with special needs). The majority of these children are infants and toddlers, the age-group most vulnerable to the effects of hospitalization.

Concern in recent years has focused on the increasing numbers of these children "growing up in hospitals" (Britton and Johnston, 1993). Discharge is prolonged because of complex medical and nursing care, elusive diagnoses, complicated psychosocial issues, and inconsistent community resources (Wells and others, 1994). Without special attention devoted to meeting the child's psychosocial and developmental needs in the "artificial" hospital environment, the detrimental consequences of prolonged hospitalization may be severe.

Beneficial Effects of Hospitalization

While hospitalization can be and usually is stressful for children, it can also be beneficial. The most obvious benefit is the recovery from illness, but hospitalization also can present an opportunity for children to master stress and feel competent in their coping abilities. The hospital environment can provide children with new socialization experiences that can broaden their interpersonal relationships. The psychologic benefits need to be considered and maximized during hospitalization. Appropriate nursing strategies to achieve this goal are presented on p. 1102.

STRESSORS AND REACTIONS OF THE FAMILY OF THE CHILD WHO IS HOSPITALIZED

The crisis of childhood illness and hospitalization affects every member of the nuclear family and, to varying degrees, members of the extended family. The stressors and reactions of families have been discussed in detail in Chapter 22 in relation to chronic illness and in Chapter 23 in relation to life-threatening illness. In many respects they differ little regardless of the diagnosis except for their intensity and persistence, which are proportional to the degree of severity of the illness. Consequently, when a child is admitted to an intensive care facility, the family members' reactions and needs are typically greater than when a child is admitted with a less serious condition to the regular pediatric unit. The following discussion briefly reviews the common reactions of the family; specific reactions during intensive care admissions are discussed on p. 1121.

PARENTAL REACTIONS

Parents' reactions to illness in their child depend on a variety of influencing factors. Although one cannot predict which factors are most likely to influence their response, a number of variables have been identified (see box below).

RISK FACTORS THAT INCREASE CHILDREN'S VULNERABILITY TO THE STRESSES OF HOSPITALIZATION

"Difficult" temperament
Lack of fit between child and parent
Age (especially between 6 months and 4 years)
Male gender
Below-average intelligence
Multiple and continuing stresses (e.g., frequent hospitalizations)

FACTORS AFFECTING PARENTS' REACTIONS TO THEIR CHILD'S ILLNESS

Seriousness of the threat to the child
Previous experience with illness or hospitalization
Medical procedures involved in diagnosis and treatment
Available support systems
Personal ego strengths
Previous coping abilities
Additional stresses on the family system
Cultural and religious beliefs
Communication patterns among family members

Almost all parents respond to their child's illness and hospitalization with remarkably consistent reactions. Initially parents may react with ***disbelief,*** especially if the illness is sudden and serious. Following the realization of illness, parents react with ***anger, guilt,*** or both. They tend to search for self-blame regarding why the child became ill or to project anger at others for some wrongdoing. Even in the mildest of illnesses, parents question their adequacy as caregivers and review any actions or omissions that could have prevented or caused the illness. When hospitalization is indicated, parental guilt is intensified because they feel helpless in alleviating the child's physical and emotional pain.

Fear, anxiety, and ***frustration*** are common feelings expressed by parents. Fear and anxiety may be related to the seriousness of the illness and the type of medical procedures involved. Often a great deal of anxiety is related to the trauma and pain inflicted on the child because of the various procedures. Feelings of frustration are often related to lack of information about procedures and treatments, unfamiliarity with hospital rules and regulations, a sense of unwelcomeness from the staff, or fear of asking questions. Much frustration can be alleviated in a pediatric unit where parents are aware of what to expect and what is expected of them, are encouraged to participate in their child's care, and are regarded as the most significant contributors to the child's total health.

Parents eventually may react with some degree of ***depression.*** The depression usually occurs when the acute crisis is over, such as following hospital discharge or complete recovery. Mothers often comment on their feeling of physical and mental exhaustion after all the other family members have adapted to the crisis. Parents may also worry about and miss their other children, who may be left in the care of family, friends, or neighbors. Other reasons for anxiety and depression are related to concerns for the child's future well-being, including negative effects produced by the hospitalization and any subsequent financial burden incurred from the hospitalization.

SIBLING REACTIONS

Siblings' reactions to a sister's or brother's illness or hospitalization are discussed in Chapters 22 and 23 and differ little when a child becomes temporarily ill. They experience loneliness, fears, and worry. Their main reactions are anger, resentment, jealousy, and guilt. Various factors have been identified that influence the effects of the child's hospitalization on siblings. Although these factors are similar to those seen when a child has a chronic illness, Craft (1993) reported that the following are related specifically to the hospital experience and have been found to increase the effects on the sibling:

- Younger and experiencing many changes
- Cared for outside the home by care providers who are not relatives
- Received little information about their ill brother or sister
- Perceived their parents to be treating them differently as compared with before their sibling's hospitalization

Simon (1993) asked 45 siblings of children who were hospitalized their perceptions of the stress of the hospitalization of a brother or sister. The siblings' perceptions of the stress they experienced were equal to the level of stress of hospitalized children. No relationship between age or sex of the sibling was found. However, the perception of stress varied significantly in relation to the type of sibling relationship and frequency of sibling visitation, with those siblings who visited daily demonstrating a higher degree of perceived stress.

Parents are often unaware of the number of effects that siblings experience during the sick child's hospitalization and of the benefit of simple interventions to minimize such effects, such as explicit explanations about the illness and provisions for the siblings to remain at home. Although sibling visitation is advocated and is probably advantageous, effects on siblings who do visit the sick child are still evident but may be different. Those who do not visit may experience more difficulty concentrating in school, feelings of being less healthy, and nail biting, whereas those who visit are more likely to become angry (Craft and Wyatt, 1986).

Sibling visitation seems to increase the hospital-based parent's awareness of the changes older siblings are experiencing, but not those of younger siblings. This may be due to the tendency of parents and health professionals to include older sibling in discussions about the child, whereas younger sibling are sent to the playroom or given some toys to occupy their time (Craft and Craft, 1989).

ALTERED FAMILY ROLES

In addition to the effects of separation on family roles, loss of parenting, sibling, and offspring roles may affect each family member differently. One of the most common reactions of parents is specialized and intensified attention toward the sick child. The other siblings usually regard this as unfair and interpret the parents' attitude toward them as rejection. Although such responses are usually unconscious and unintended, they place unique burdens on ill children. For example, the ill child may feel obligated to play the sick role in order to meet parents' expectations, especially children who have had limited physical ability and regain normal health status, such as following corrective heart surgery. Parents, as well, may be unable to perceive the child's recovery and therefore need to continue the pattern of overprotection and indulgent attention.

Ill children may also feel jealousy and resentment from other siblings. Because of their singular position in the family, they may be denied the companionship of their brothers and sisters. Rivalry between siblings tends to be greatest in the sibling who is nearest the ill child's age. Without an understanding of the interpersonal dynamics between siblings, parents are likely to blame the well children for antisocial behavior. Illness may also result in children's loss of status within either their family or social group. For example, illness in the oldest child may temporarily terminate special privileges as "big" brother or sister.

NURSING CARE OF THE CHILD WHO IS HOSPITALIZED AND THE FAMILY

Children and their families require competent and sensitive care to minimize the potential negative effects of hospitalization and also to promote positive benefits from the experience. Interventions should focus on (1) eliminating or minimizing the stressors of separation, loss of control, and bodily injury and pain for children (see Nursing Care Plan: The Child in the Hospital, pp. 1104-1108); and (2) providing specific supportive strategies for family members, such as fostering family relationships and providing information (see Nursing Care Plan: The Family of the Ill or Hospitalized Child, pp. 1109-1112).

PREVENTING OR MINIMIZING SEPARATION

The primary nursing goal is to prevent separation, particularly in children under 5 years of age. Changes in hospitals' policies over recent years reflect a changed attitude toward parents; many hospitals no longer consider parents "visitors" and welcome their presence at all times throughout the child's hospitalization. However, this is not always possible, and measures to minimize the effects of separation must be implemented. The importance of a primary nurse for the child cannot be overemphasized. There is no substitute for the consistency provided by primary nursing and its advantages for the child and family.

Parent Participation and "Rooming-In"

Prevention of separation requires rooming-in facilities in pediatric hospital settings. Although some health facilities provide special accommodations for parents, the concept of "rooming-in" can be instituted anywhere. The first requirement is the staff's positive attitude toward parents. Unfortunately, although nurses often express explicit support for the concept of family-centered care (see Chapter 1), some of their practices and beliefs suggest otherwise (Berman, 1991). When hospital staff genuinely appreciate the importance of continued parent-child attachment, they foster an environment that encourages parents to stay. When parents are included in the care planning and are assured that they are a contributing factor to the child's recovery, they are more inclined to remain with their child and have more emotional reserves to support themselves and the child through the crisis. An empowerment model of helping allows the nurse to focus on parents' strengths and seek ways to promote growth and family functioning so that parents become empowered in caring for their child (Fig. 26-4).

Since the mother tends to be the usual family caregiver, she spends more time in the hospital than the father (Fig. 26-5). However, not all mothers feel equally comfortable in assuming responsibility for their child's care. Some may be under such great emotional stress that they need a temporary reprieve from total participation in caregiving activities. Others may feel insecure in participating in specialized ar-

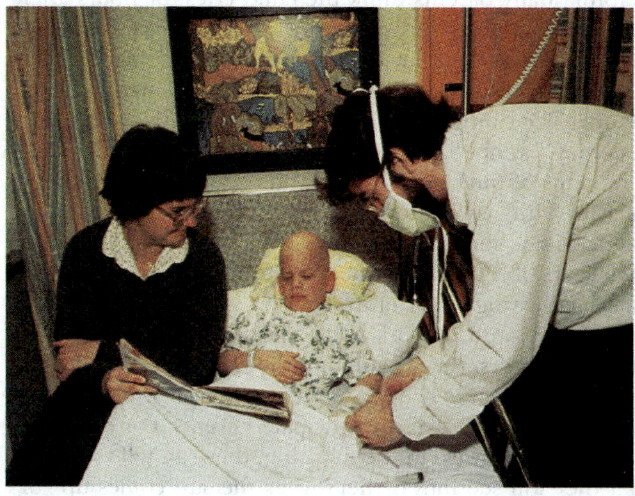

FIG. 26-4 Parental presence during hospitalization, including during procedures, provides emotional support for the child and empowers the parent in the caregiver role. (Courtesy St. Louis Children's Hospital.)

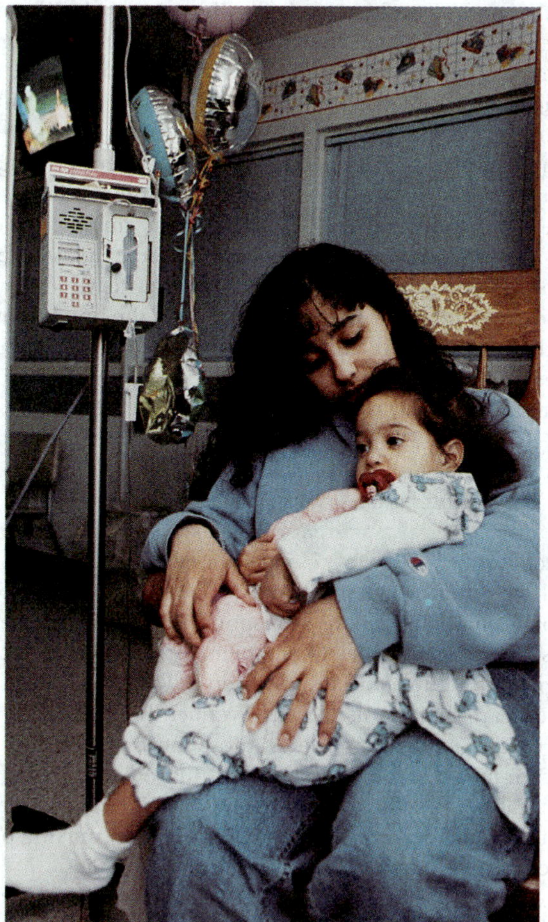

FIG. 26-5 Despite changing life-styles and sex roles, mothers tend to be the usual family caregiver and spend more time at the hospital than fathers.

eas of care, such as bathing the child after surgery. Individual assessment of each parent's preferred involvement is necessary to prevent the effects of separation while supporting parents in their needs as well. Parents and other family member should be both prepared and supported for the roles they choose (Johnson, Jeppson, and Redburn, 1992). Both underinvolvement and overinvolvement of parents in the child's care can be detrimental; therefore every effort is extended to help parents identify moderate amounts of visiting and participation. Reassuring parents of their essential role in the care of their child is often necessary, since parents may feel unimportant to the child when medical professionals "take over" (Ahmann, 1994).

With life-styles and sexual roles changing, some fathers may assume all or some of the usual mothering roles in the household. In this case it may be the father-child relationship that requires preservation. Fathers need to be included in the plan of care and respected for their parental role. For some fathers the child's hospitalization may represent an opportunity to alter their usual caregiving role and increase their involvement. Research indicates that fathers and mothers perceive different aspects of their child's hospitalization as stressful; therefore their support needs will vary (Graves and Ware, 1990). It is equally important to support the mother's role as family provider or parttime housekeeper in order to meet each parent's needs. In single-parent families the caregiver may not be a parent but an extended family member, such as a grandparent or aunt.

One of the potential problems with continuous parent visiting is neglect of the parent's need for sleep, nutrition, and relaxation. Often the sleeping accommodations are limited to a chair and sleep is disrupted by nursing procedures. After a few days parents can become exhausted but feel obligated to stay. Encouraging them to leave for brief periods, arranging for sleeping quarters on the unit but outside the child's room, and planning a schedule of alternating visiting with the other parent or with a family member can minimize the stresses for the parent.

➤ **NURSING TIP** If parents are reluctant to leave the hospital (usually for fear of not being there when the child awakens or the physician visits), try to arrange for them to have a remote "beeper" that can provide immediate communication regardless of their location.

All too often, nurses respond to parental participation by abandoning their patient responsibilities. Nurses need to restructure their roles to complement and augment the caregiving functions of parents. Even in units structured to provide care by parents, parents frequently feel anxiety in their caregiving responsibilities; those more involved in direct care may feel more anxiety than those less involved in direct care. Therefore, 24-hour responsibility may be too much for some parents. Assistance and relief by nursing personnel should always be available to these families.

Strategies to Minimize the Effects of Separation

When separation cannot be prevented, numerous strategies can be employed to minimize the effects of temporary separation on children. Ideally a primary nurse is assigned to meet the child's needs. Becoming a surrogate parent requires a thorough, detailed nursing history that specifically identifies the child's established daily routine. Usual daily activities such as food preparation and method of feeding help establish a complementary schedule of caregiving practices. It also helps the parent feel as if he or she is participating in the child's care but through another person. A nursing admission history for children is outlined in the box on pp. 1116-1117.

The nurse caring for the child must have an appreciation of the child's separation behaviors. As discussed earlier, the phases of protest and despair are normal. The child is allowed to cry. Even if the child rejects strangers, the nurse provides support through physical presence in the room. The nurse may say, "I know you are unhappy because you miss your mommy and daddy. It's all right to cry. I will sit here for awhile so you are not alone." This reinforces for children the nurse's awareness of their feelings without abandoning them. If detachment behaviors are evident, the nurse maintains the child's contact with the parents by frequently talking about them, encouraging the child to remember them, and stressing the significance of their visits, telephone calls, or letters.

The nurse can integrate stories related to separation themes and activities such as peek-a-boo and hiding-and-finding games into the child's routine care (Gaynard and others, 1990).

Separation may be equally as difficult for parents, especially when they do not understand the behaviors of separation anxiety. To avoid the immediate protest, parents may sneak out or lie to the child about leaving. As a result, the child does not learn that absence is associated with a guaranteed return but that absence means loss of parents. Helping parents recognize that separation behaviors are normal and expected can decrease their anxiety and may ease their fears about leaving without telling the child. Explaining to parents how the child reacts after they leave may also be helpful. Many parents think the child cries for hours after they leave, whereas in reality the child may cry for a few minutes but settle down when comforted by someone else.

Toddlers and preschoolers have a very limited concept of time. The young child's question, "Will my mommy come yesterday?" symbolizes a lack of understanding of usual measurements of time, such as days, hours, and weeks. Time is measured in associations, such as "Eating dinner when daddy comes home." Therefore, when helping parents with their fears of separation, nurses need to suggest ways of explaining leaving and returning. For example, if parents must leave to go to work or to make meals for the other family members, they should tell the hospitalized child the reason for leaving. They also need to convey the expected time of return in terms of anticipated events. For example, if the parents return in the morning, they can tell the child that they will see him or her "After the sun comes up" or "When [a favorite program] is on television."

The young child's ability to tolerate parental absence is very limited. Therefore parental visits should be frequent. For example, it is better for parents to visit three times a day for short periods than once a day for an extended time.

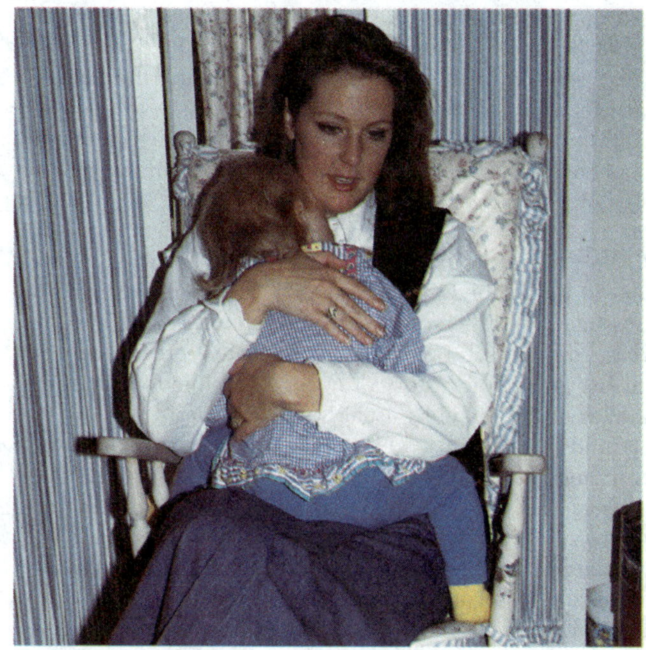

FIG. 26-6 When parents cannot visit, other significant persons can provide comfort to the child who is hospitalized.

This may necessitate that each parent visit at different times to lessen the length of separation. When parents cannot visit, the presence of other significant people can be comforting for the child (Fig. 26-6).

If parents leave after the child is asleep, they still need to communicate their absence. The parents of a 5-year-old boy solved this problem by devising a sign; on one side they drew a picture of a telephone and on the other a hamburger. Before they left, they turned the sign to the appropriate side to tell the child when he awoke that they were out using the telephone or eating.

For older children who know how to tell time, it is helpful to give them a clock or watch. However, these children have the same needs for honesty from their parents regarding visiting schedules. Because peer groups are also important, adolescents often appreciate planning visiting hours with their parents to provide them with some private time for friends.

Familiar surroundings also increase the child's adjustment to separation. If parents cannot room-in, they should leave favorite home articles with the child, such as a blanket, toy, bottle, feeding utensil, or article of clothing. Since young children associate such inanimate objects with significant people, they gain comfort and reassurance from such possessions. They make the association that if the parent left this, the parent will surely return. Placing an identification band on the toy lessens the chances of its being misplaced and provides a symbol that the toy is experiencing the same needs as the child. Other mementos of home include photographs and tape recordings of family members reading a story, singing a song, saying prayers before bedtime, relating events at home, or taking a "talking walk" through the home. The tapes can be played at lonely times, such as on awakening or before sleeping. Some units allow pets to visit, which can be a special event for a child and can have therapeutic benefits. Animals should be carefully screened for medical or behavioral problems, and patients should be screened for allergies.

Older children also appreciate familiar articles from home, particularly photographs, a radio, a favorite toy or game, and the usual pajamas. Often the importance of treasured objects for school-age children is overlooked or criticized. However, it is reported that about half of school-age children have a special object to which they formed an attachment in early childhood and that this is a normal and healthy phenomenon. Therefore such treasured or transitional objects can help even older children feel more comfortable in a strange environment.

The strange sights and sounds in the hospital that are commonplace for the nurse can be frightening and confusing for children. It is important for the nurse to try to evaluate stimuli in the environment from the child's point of view (considering also what the child may see or hear happening to other patients) and to make every effort to protect the child from frightening and unfamiliar sights, sounds, and equipment. The nurse should offer explanations or prepare the child for those experiences that are unavoidable. Combining familiar or comforting sights with the unfamiliar can relieve much of the harshness of medical equipment.

➤ **NURSING TIP** Soften medical equipment (e.g., clip a bear or other animal to a stethoscope; use paper, fabric, or stickers to transform an IV pump into a friendly animal) to create a pleasant and more familiar environment for children (Rollins, 1991).

Helping children maintain their usual nonhome contacts also minimizes the effects of separation imposed by hospitalization. This includes continuing school lessons during the illness and confinement, visiting with friends either directly or through letter writing or telephone calls, and participating in stimulating projects whenever possible (Fig. 26-7).

For extended hospitalizations, youngsters enjoy personalizing the hospital room to make it "home" by decorating the walls with posters and cards, rearranging the furniture (when possible), and displaying a collection or hobby. Growing plants can also be a constructive activity because it gives the child something to care for. Hardy and fast-growing plants are best, such as beans, sunflowers, and marigolds. A terrarium is useful for a child in an oxygen tent because it can be used to explain the oxygen cycle.

➤ **NURSING TIP** Recycle used IV bags and tubing as plant feeders/watering devices. This increases the child's understanding of medical equipment and makes the "unfamiliar" less threatening and fearful.

NURSING ALERT When considering plants, be aware that certain circumstances may preclude this activity, such as children with specific allergies or those who are susceptible to infections.

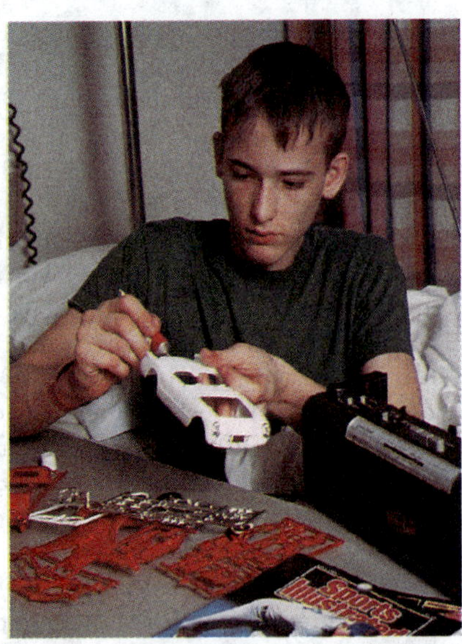

FIG. 26-7 For extended hospitalizations, children enjoy having projects to occupy their time. (Courtesy St. Louis Children's Hospital.)

MINIMIZING LOSS OF CONTROL

Feelings of loss of control result from separation, physical restriction, changed routines, enforced dependency, magical thinking, and altered roles within the family or peer group. Although some of these cannot be prevented, most of them can be minimized through individualized planning of nursing care.

Promoting Freedom of Movement

Younger children react most strenuously to any type of physical restriction or immobilization. Although some restraint, such as immobilizing an extremity for maintenance of an intravenous line, is frequently necessary, most physical restriction can be prevented if the nurse gains the child's cooperation.

For young children, particularly infants and toddlers, preserving parent-child contact is the best means of decreasing the need for or stress of restraint. For example, almost the entire physical examination can be done in a parent's lap, with the parent hugging the child for procedures such as otoscopy. For painful procedures the parents' preferences for assisting, observing, or waiting outside the room are assessed.

Environmental factors also influence the need for physical restraint. Keeping children in cribs or playpens may not represent immobilization in a concrete sense, but it certainly limits sensory stimulation. Increasing mobility by transporting children in carriages, wheelchairs, carts, wagons, or on stretchers or beds provides them with mechanical freedom.

In some cases physical restraint or isolation is necessary for recovery. Whenever possible, restraints should be removed to allow the child some period of supervised freedom, such as during the bath or when parents visit. When restraints or isolation cannot be discontinued, such as in severe burns, the environment can be manipulated to increase sensory freedom. For example, moving the bed toward the door or window; opening window shades; providing musical, visual, or tactile toys; and increasing interpersonal contact can substitute mental mobility for the limitations of physical movement.

Maintaining Child's Routine

Altered daily schedules and loss of rituals are particularly stressful for toddlers and early preschoolers and may increase the stress of separation. As stated previously, the nursing admission history provides a baseline for planning care around the child's usual home activities.

Children's response to loss of routine and ritualism is often demonstrated in problems with activities such as feeding, sleeping, dressing, bathing, toileting, and social interaction. Although some regression is to be expected in all these areas, sensitivity to the special needs of children can minimize the negative effects. For example, loss of appetite and marked food preferences are common in ill or hospitalized children. In addition, the food selections on hospital menus may differ greatly from preferred cultural or ethnic food preparation. Encouraging the child to eat while avoiding a battle is often a challenge, yet it is an essential nursing responsibility. Suggestions for feeding sick children are discussed in Chapter 27.

Although regression is expected and normal, nurses also have the responsibility of fostering children's optimum growth and development. Hospitalization can become a significant opportunity for learning and advancing. For example, extended hospitalization for long-term chronic illness or situations of failure to thrive, abuse, or neglect represent instances in which regression must be seen as an adjustment period, to be followed by plans for promoting appropriate developmental skills.

A frequently neglected aspect of altered routines is the change in the child's daily activities. A nonhospitalized child's day, especially during the school years, is structured with specific times for eating, dressing, going to school, playing, and sleeping. However, this time structure vanishes when the child is hospitalized. Although the nurses have a set schedule, the child is frequently unaware of it; new schedules are imposed that may be rigid or flexible. For example, some units have uniform nap and bedtimes for all children, whereas others allow children to stay up very late. Many children obtain significantly less sleep in the hospital than at home; the primary causes are delay in sleep onset and early termination of sleep because of hospital routines (Hagemann, 1981a, 1981b). Not only are hours of sleep disrupted, but waking hours are spent in passive activities. For example, few institutions impose any regulation on the amount of time the child spends watching television. Studies show that children spend an average of 8 hours a day watching television in the hospital, which is considerably more time than that spent at home (McCain and Bies, 1983).

One technique that can minimize the disruption in the child's routine is ***time structuring*** (Volz, 1981). This ap-

ERIC'S DAILY SCHEDULE:

7:00 AM – Breakfast, Watch TV, Brush Teeth, Wash up	3:00 PM – Tutor (M,W,F) Study Time (T,Th)
9:00 – Tub Room, Dressing Change	4:00 – Physical Therapy
10:00 – Rest, TV, Snack	5:00 – Dinner
11:00 – Physical Therapy	6:30 – Dressing Change
12:00 PM – Lunch	7:00 to 9:00 – TV, Reading, Snack, Friends Visit
1:00 – Playroom, Quiet Play, Rest, Friends Visit	9:00 – Brush Teeth, Wash up
	9:15 – Bedtime

FIG. 26-8 Time structuring is an effective strategy for normalizing the hospital environment and increasing the child's sense of control.

proach is most suitable for the noncritically ill school-age and adolescent child who has mastered the concept of time. It involves scheduling the child's day to include all those activities that are important to the child and nurse, such as treatment procedures, schoolwork, exercise, television, playroom, and hobbies. Together, the nurse, parent, and child then plan a daily schedule with time and activity written down (Fig. 26-8). This is left in the child's room, and a clock or watch is available for the child's use. Whenever possible, a calendar is also constructed with special events marked, such as favorite television programs, visits by friends or relatives, events in the playroom, and holidays or birthdays. If specific changes in treatment are expected (e.g., "beginning physical therapy in 2 days"), these are added.

➤ **NURSING TIP** Ask the young child to select or draw pictures or symbols to represent daily or weekly fun activities (e.g., favorite TV programs, family visits, playroom times). Draw a clock face with the hands of the clock depicting the time each event will occur next to the child's representation. Have the child compare the clock on the schedule with a clock or watch in the room. When the two match, the child knows that it is time for a favorite activity and exactly what that activity is.

Encouraging Independence

The dependent role of the hospitalized patient imposes tremendous feelings of loss on older children. Principal interventions should focus on respect for individuality and the opportunity for decision making. Although these sound simple, their efficacy lies with nurses who are flexible, tolerant, and personally secure. The last is particularly important because when decision making is geared toward the patient, nurses can feel threatened by a sense of lessened control.

Promoting children's control involves maintaining independence, and the concept of self-care can be most beneficial. ***Self-care*** refers to the practice of activities that individuals personally initiate and perform on their own behalf in maintaining life, health, and well-being (Orem, 1991). Although self-care is limited by the child's age and physical condition, most children beyond infancy can perform some activities with little or no help. Whenever possible, these activities are encouraged in the hospital. Other approaches include jointly planning care; time structuring; wearing street clothes; making choices in food selections, bedtime, and so on; continuing school activities; and rooming with an appropriate age-mate. For example, although school-age children may enjoy the responsibility of caring for a toddler or preschooler in their room, adolescents generally prefer quarters separate from the pediatric unit (see p. 1119).

BILL OF RIGHTS FOR CHILDREN AND TEENS

In this hospital you and your family have the right to:
- Respect and personal dignity
- Care that supports you and your family
- Information you can understand
- Quality health care
- Emotional support
- Care that respects your need to grow, play, and learn
- Make choices and decisions

From Association for the Care of Children's Health: *A pediatric bill of rights,* Bethesda, MD, 1991, The Association. A detailed explanation of each right plus a separate "Bill of Rights for Parents" is available for a fee from the Association for the Care of Children's Health, 7910 Woodmont Ave., Suite 300, Bethesda, MD 20814; (301) 654-6549.

Promoting Understanding

Loss of control can occur from feelings of having too little influence on one's destiny as well as from sensing overwhelming control or power over fate. Although preschoolers' cognitive abilities predispose them most to magical thinking and self-power, all children are vulnerable to misinterpreting causes for stresses such as illness and hospitalization.

Most children feel more in control when they know what to expect, because the element of fear is reduced. Anticipatory preparation and providing information help greatly to lessen stress and prevent lack of understanding (see Preparation for Procedures, Chapter 27).

Informing children of their rights while hospitalized fosters greater understanding and may relieve some of the feelings of powerlessness they typically experience. A recent addition to standards used to accredit hospitals recommends that hospitals providing services to children have a hospital-wide policy on the rights and responsibilities of these patients and of their parents and/or guardians (Joint Commission on Accreditation of Healthcare Organizations, 1992). An increasing number of hospitals and organizations have developed a "Bill of Rights" that is prominently displayed throughout the hospital or is presented to children and their families on admission (see box above for example).

PREVENTING OR MINIMIZING BODILY INJURY

Beyond early infancy all children fear bodily injury either from mutilation, bodily intrusion, body image change, disability, or death. In general, preparation of children for painful procedures decreases their fears. Manipulating procedural techniques for children in each age-group also minimizes fear of bodily injury. For example, since toddlers and young preschoolers are traumatized by insertion of a rectal thermometer, axillary temperatures or electronic temperature probes can effectively be substituted. Whenever procedures are performed on young children, the most supportive intervention is to do them as quickly as possible and maintain parent-child contact.

Because of young children's poorly defined body boundaries, the use of bandages may be particularly helpful. For example, telling children that the bleeding will stop after the needle is removed does little to relieve their fears, whereas applying a small Band-Aid usually provides much reassurance. The size of bandages is also significant to children in this age-group. The larger the bandage, the more importance is attached to the wound. Using successively smaller surgical dressings is one way of their measuring healing and improvement. Prematurely removing a dressing may cause them concern for their well-being.

In children who fear mutilation of body parts, repeatedly stressing the reason for a procedure and evaluating their understanding are essential to minimize fear. For example, explaining cast removal to preschoolers may seem simple enough, but the child's comprehension of the details may vary considerably from the explanation. Asking them to draw a picture of what they think will happen provides substantial evidence of how they perceive events.

Children may fear bodily injury from a great variety of sources. X-ray machines, use of strange equipment for examination, unfamiliar rooms, or awkward positions can be perceived as potentially hazardous. In addition, thoughts and actions can be imagined sources of bodily damage. For older children, masturbation or sex play may be perceived as powerful weapons of potential destruction. Therefore it is important to investigate imagined reasons, particularly of a sexual nature, for illness. Since children may fear revealing such thoughts, using protective techniques such as drawing or doll play may demonstrate previously undisclosed misconceptions.

Older children fear bodily injury of both internal and external origins. For example, school-age children are aware of the heart's significance and may fear the actual procedure as much as the pain, the stitches, and the possible scar. Adolescents may express concern for the surgery but be much more anxious over the resulting scar. An appreciation of each child's special concerns helps nurses focus on critical areas during preparation for procedures or when explaining the disease processes.

Children can grasp information only if it is presented according to their cognitive development. This necessitates an awareness of the words used to describe events or processes. The example of a 7-year-old who interpreted the physician's statement of "there's edema in your belly" as "there's a demon in your belly" is proof of the necessity of choosing words carefully and reevaluating the child's understanding of the message (Perrin and Gerrity, 1981).

When children are upset about their illness, their perception can be changed by (1) providing a somewhat different and less negative account of the disease or (2) offering an explanation that is characteristic of the next stage of cognitive development (Bibace and Walsh, 1980). An example of the first strategy is reassuring a preschool child who fears that after a tonsillectomy, another sore throat means a second operation. Explaining that once tonsils are "fixed," they do not need fixing again can help relieve the fear. An example of the second strategy is to explain that germs made the tonsils sick and even though germs can cause another sore throat, they cannot cause the tonsils to ever be sick again. This higher-level explanation is based on the school-age child's concept of germs as a cause of disease.

PAIN ASSESSMENT

Pain assessment is a critical component of the nursing process. Unfortunately, health professionals, including nurses, tend to underestimate the existence of pain in children. Several studies have documented the enormous disparity between medication practices with children and adults (see Thinking Critically About . . . box). One of the reasons for inadequate management of pain is a lack of understanding of what pain is—a personal phenomenon that *cannot* be experienced by any other individual. Therefore defining pain in terms of another's perceptions is inappropriate and inaccurate. An operational definition that is useful in clinical practice and is adopted by the World Health Organization (WHO) is: *pain is whatever the experiencing person says it is, existing whenever the person says it does* (McCaffery and Beebe, 1989). This definition implies a very important attitude toward patients—*that they are believed.* It includes both verbal and nonverbal expressions of pain.

Fallacies and Facts

Children are undertreated for pain for a number of complex and interrelated reasons, including professionals' misconceptions about pain; the complexities of pain assessment, particularly in nonverbal children; and the lack of information regarding currently available pain reduction techniques. A number of fallacies continue to flourish because of incorrect knowledge about pain in infants and children, despite these fallacies having been disproved by current research on pediatric pain (see box on p. 1082, bottom). Two fallacies that exist among nurses and probably promote undertreatment of pain the most are unrealistic fears about respiratory depression and addiction from opioids (Schmidt, Eland, and Weiler, 1994).*

*The term ***opioid*** refers to natural or synthetic analgesics with morphine-like actions. It is preferred to the term ***narcotic,*** which in a legal context refers to any substance that causes psychologic dependence, such as cocaine, which is not an opioid. The word "narcotic" also engenders fears of addiction in older children and parents that are unwarranted when opioids are used for pain control.

THINKING CRITICALLY ABOUT . . . *Undermedication of Pain in Children*

Several studies have examined the pattern of pain medication for children as compared with adults and have found remarkably consistent findings—that children have been undermedicated for pain. Eland and Anderson (1977) investigated the incidence of administration of analgesics to 25 hospitalized children for postoperative pain. Twelve of the children received a total of 24 doses of analgesics; the remaining 13 children were never given any medication for pain relief. In contrast, 18 adults with identical diagnoses received 372 opioid analgesic doses and 299 nonopioid analgesic doses for a total of 671 doses. One of the saddest findings was that more than twice as many children had pain medication ordered as received it. This lack of response to the need for pain medication directly relates to the nurses who failed to administer the analgesic.

Another study investigating analgesic prescriptions given to children and adults after open heart surgery found that all of the adults received medication, for a total of 564 doses, but only three fourths of the children were given medication, for a total of 237 doses during the first 3 postoperative days. This difference was even greater on the fifth postoperative day, when 83% of the adults continued to receive analgesics (a total of 136 doses) but only 12% of the children were medicated (a total of 10 doses) (Beyer and others, 1983). Another study on postoperative pain found that 75% of the children reported pain on the day of surgery and if orders for opioid or nonopioid analgesics were written, the nonopioid was given exclusively. In addition, the doses ordered were usually too small and/or too infrequent to be maximally effective. Most orders were written "PRN," which was often interpreted by nursing staff as "as little as possible" (Mather and Mackie, 1983). Younger children are less likely to have opioids offered, and "PRN" orders may place these children at a further disadvantage because of their inability to communicate their discomfort (Schechter, Allen, and Hanson, 1986). A review of analgesic use in the emergency department reported significantly low use in children with mild to moderate trauma, including children with painful fractures. Head injury was associated with especially low use of analgesics (Friedland and Kulick, 1994).

The situation is even more serious with infants. One analysis of anesthetic practices with newborns undergoing surgical ligation of patent ductus arteriosus found that 76% of the infants received only a muscle relaxant and nitrous oxide (Anand and Aynsley-Green, 1985). In a survey of nurses working in neonatal intensive care units, 79% believed that infants were undermedicated for pain. The same study found that more than half of the medications used for pain relief had no analgesic properties (Franck, 1987). A study comparing premedication for procedures found that infants in neonatal intensive care units received no premedication much more often than children in pediatric intensive care units (Bauchner, May, and Coates, 1992). Many of the procedures, such as arterial line or chest tube placement, are very painful and should be performed with at least a local anesthetic being given.

Fortunately, professionals' response to recognizing and treating pediatric pain has been improving. During the 1980s there was an impressive increase in the number of publications focusing on this topic (Guardiola and Banos, 1993). Studies, such as those described above, have prompted the American Academy of Pediatrics (1987) and the American Society of Anesthesiologists to publish jointly a statement on neonatal anesthesia that encourages the use of local or systemic pharmacologic agents "according to the usual guidelines for the administration of anesthesia to high-risk, potentially unstable patients." If medication is withheld, the decision should be based on the same medical criteria used for older patients, not on the infant's age or perceived degree of cortical maturity.

Guidelines are also available that help practitioners to assess and manage pain using methods based on the published scientific literature. In the United States the Agency for Health Care Policy and Research (AHCPR) has published guidelines developed by pain experts that focus on the issues of postoperative, procedure-related or trauma, and cancer pain. Other national and international organizations have also contributed research-based recommendations that nurses can use to improve pain control (see box on p. 1082, top).

In your agency, see if these references are readily available to staff. If not, order them, especially the free AHCPR publications, and distribute them, stressing that they provide state-of-the-art information. As you practice, carry your copy of the guidelines; mark sections, such as those discussing addiction and listing drug dosages, for quick reference. Compare your pain assessment and management interventions with those in the published guidelines, and make a commitment to increase your knowledge. *Remember: to effectively relieve pain, its management must be based on scientific research, not personal opinion or belief.* The questions in the Guidelines box on p. 1083 can help you identify prejudices that may interfere with pain relief practices.

Fear of Addiction. A major concern that prevents health professionals from adequately using opioids to relieve pain is an unwarranted fear of addiction. However, studies on addiction rates in patients treated with opioids have found an incidence of less than 1% (Friedman, 1990). The AHCPR Acute Pain Management Guideline Panel (1992) has made the following statement regarding addiction from opioid use in pain management for children: "There is no known aspect of childhood development or physiology that indicates any increased risk of physiologic or psychologic dependence from the brief use of opioids for acute pain management."

One of the reasons for the unfounded and prevalent fear regarding addiction is confusion between three terms: narcotic addiction, drug tolerance, and physical dependency. Health professionals and the public erroneously equate all three terms with addiction, when in reality these terms reflect completely different behavioral and physiologic actions:

Narcotic addiction—Behavioral, voluntary, pattern characterized by compulsive drug-seeking behavior leading to overwhelming involvement with use and procurement of drug for purposes other than medical reasons, such as pain relief

Drug tolerance—Physiologic, involuntary need for larger dose of opioid to maintain original analgesic effect

Physical dependence—Physiologic, involuntary effect mani-

SELECTED RESOURCES FOR GUIDELINES ON CHILDREN'S PAIN

Acute Pain Management: Operative or Medical Procedures and Trauma
Acute Pain Management in Infants, Children and Adolescents: Operative and Medical Procedures
Pain Control After Surgery: A Patient's Guide
Management of Cancer Pain
Management of Cancer Pain: Infants, Children, and Adolescents
Available at no charge from the Agency for Health Care Policy and Research Publications, P.O. Box 8527, Silver Spring, MD 20907; (800) 358-9295.

Principles of Analgesic Use in the Treatment of Acute Pain and Chronic Cancer Pain
Available from the American Pain Society, 5700 Old Orchard Rd., Skokie, IL 60077; (708) 966-0050.

Management of Acute Pain: A Practical Guide
Available from the International Association for the Study of Pain (IASP), 909 N.E. 43rd St., Suite 306, Seattle, WA 98105-6020; (206) 547-6409.

Handbook of Cancer Pain Management
Available from the Wisconsin Cancer Pain Initiative, 3675 Medical Sciences Center, University of Wisconsin Medical School, 1300 University Ave., Madison, WI 53706; (608) 262-0978.

Report of the Consensus Conference on the Management of Pain in Childhood Cancer
In *Pediatrics* 86(5, suppl):813-834, 1990; available from the American Academy of Pediatrics, P.O. Box 927, Elk Grove Village, IL 60009-0927; (800) 433-9016.

ANA Position Statements on Promotion of Comfort and Relief of Pain in Dying Patients and on the Role of the Registered Nurse in the Management of Patients Receiving IV Conscious Sedation for Short-Term Therapeutic, Diagnostic, or Surgical Procedures
Published in *The American Nurse,* pp 7-8, Feb 1992. May be available from American Nurses' Association Publications Distribution Center, P.O. Box 4100, Kearneysville, WV 25430; (800) 637-0323.

Oncology Nursing Society position paper on cancer pain
By Spross JA, McGuire DB: *Oncol Nurs Forum* 17(5):753, 1990.

ALSO AVAILABLE FOR FAMILIES:

Pain Control After Surgery: A Patient's Guide
Available at no charge from the Agency for Health Care Policy and Research Publications, P.O. Box 8527, Silver Spring, MD 20907; (800) 358-9295.

Children's Cancer Pain Can Be Relieved: A Guide for Parents and Families
Available from Wisconsin Cancer Pain Initiative, 3675 Medical Sciences Center, University of Wisconsin Medical School, 1300 University Ave., Madison, WI 53706; (608) 262-0978.

Pain Relief: How to Say No to Acute, Chronic, and Cancer Pain!
By Jane Cowles, 1993; available from MasterMedia Limited, 17 E. 89th St., New York, NY 10128; (212) 546-7650.

Questions and Answers About Pain Control: A Guide for People with Cancer and their Families
Available at no charge from the Office of Cancer Communications, Bldg. 31, Rm. 10A24, Bethesda, MD 20892, (800) 4-CANCER; and from local branches of the American Cancer Society, or call (800) ACS-2345.

FALLACIES AND FACTS ABOUT CHILDREN AND PAIN

Fallacy: Infants do not feel pain.
Fact: Infants demonstrate behavioral, especially facial, and physiologic, including hormonal, indicators of pain. Neonates have the neural mechanisms to transmit noxious stimuli by 20 weeks of gestation (Anand and Hickey, 1987, 1992; Marshall, 1989; Shapiro, 1989; Stevens, Johnston, and Horton, 1993). (See also Neonatal Pain, Chapter 11.)

Fallacy: Children tolerate pain better than adults.
Fact: Children's tolerance for pain actually *increases* with age (Haslam, 1969; Lander and Fowler-Kerry, 1991). Younger children tend to rate procedure-related pain higher than older children (Fradet and others, 1990; Humphrey and others, 1992; Wong and Baker, 1988).

Fallacy: Children cannot tell you where they hurt.
Fact: By 4 years of age, children can accurately point to the body area or mark the painful site on a drawing (Savedra and others, 1989, 1993; Van Cleve and Savedra, 1993); children as young as 3 years old can use pain scales, such as faces (Beyer, Denyes, and Villarruel, 1992; Wong and Baker, 1988).

Fallacy: Children always tell the truth about pain.
Fact: Children may not admit having pain to avoid an injection; because of constant pain, they may not realize how much they are hurting; children may believe that others know how they are feeling and not ask for analgesia (Favaloro and Touzel, 1990; Hester, 1989).

Fallacy: Children become accustomed to pain or painful procedures.
Fact: Children often demonstrate *increased* behavioral signs of discomfort with repeated painful procedures (Dolgin and others, 1989; Fitzgerald, Millard, and MacIntosh, 1988; Katz, Kellerman, and Siegel, 1980; Lander and Fowler-Kerry, 1991).

Fallacy: Behavioral manifestations reflect pain intensity.
Fact: Children's developmental level, coping abilities, and temperament, such as activity level and intensity of reaction to pain, influence pain behavior (Young and Fu, 1988; Wallace, 1989; Beyer, McGrath, and Berde, 1990). Children with more active, resisting behaviors may rate pain lower than children with passive, accepting behaviors (Broome and others, 1990).

Fallacy: Narcotics are more dangerous for children than they are for adults.
Fact: Narcotics (opioids) are no more dangerous for children than they are for adults. Addiction to opioids used to treat pain is extremely rare in children (Brozovic and others, 1986; Morrison, 1991; Rodgers and others, 1988; Rogers, 1990). Reports of respiratory depression in children are also uncommon (Berde and others, 1991; Billmire, Neale, and Gregory 1985; Dilworth and MacKellar, 1987). By 3 to 6 months of age healthy infants can metabolize opioids similarly to other children (Hertzka and others, 1989; Koren and others, 1985).

GUIDELINES

Exploring Attitudes, Beliefs, and Knowledge About Pain in Children

The following questions should help you understand what biases and misinformation may affect your ability and willingness to control pain:

Do you believe that infants feel pain similar to that felt by older children and adults?

Do you believe that it is ethical to inflict pain on children because they may not remember the painful event?*

Do you have a clear understanding of the difference between tolerance, physical dependence, and psychologic addiction?

Are you concerned that children, especially adolescents, receiving opioids (narcotics) for pain will become addicted?*

Does the fear of addiction or respiratory depression prevent you from giving an ordered opioid or choosing the higher dose when a dosage range is prescribed?*

Do you believe that larger doses of opioids can be given safely for increasing severity of pain?

When opioids or other analgesics are ordered PRN, do you tend to wait until the child is in severe pain before administering the next dose,* or do you give the next PRN dose to prevent severe pain from returning?

If children are old enough to rate pain, do you believe that your judgment based on the child's vital signs and behavior is more accurate in assessing the degree of pain than the child's pain rating?*

Do you believe that children who are easily distracted from pain have mild pain?*

Do you believe that sleep or sedation indicates pain relief* or that children may be exhausted from experiencing pain and therefore will sleep?

If a pain medication is ordered around the clock (ATC), would you wake the child for the next scheduled dose of an analgesic?

Is your goal in pain management to relieve pain to the level that the child can tolerate?*

Do you believe that drugs such as promethazine (Phenergan) or chlorpromazine (Thorazine) potentiate the effects of opioids?*

Are you more comfortable giving drugs such as diazepam (Valium) or midazolam (Versed) for sedation and amnesia rather than opioids for pain relief?*

Do you believe that parents can help in the assessment of pain?

Do you believe that meperidine (Demerol) is a safer drug than morphine?*

Do you believe that a specific procedure, illness, or operation is associated with a specific amount of pain and that children who experience more pain than typically expected are exaggerating their symptoms?*

Do you believe that nurses have the right to withhold pain medication because they believe the child is not suffering, despite a child's or parent's request for pain medication?

Do you believe that nurses have the responsibility to advocate better pain control for patients who have inadequate pain relief?

*If you have answered yes to these questions, your beliefs may adversely affect your pain management practices.

fested by withdrawal symptoms when chronic use of opioid is abruptly discontinued or opioid antagonist is administered

Fear of Respiratory Depression. Respiratory depression is the most serious side effect of opioids; however, it is a rare occurrence in children. Several studies document the safety of appropriately dosed opioids in infants and children (Beasley and Tibballs, 1987; Billmire, Neale, and Gregory, 1985; Dilworth and MacKellar, 1987). Evidence suggests that in children over 3 months of age (and possibly younger) opioids cause no greater respiratory depression than in adults (Hertzka and others, 1989; Olkkola and others, 1988). Respiratory depression is most likely to occur when the opioid is administered with other sedating drugs, such as promethazine (Phenergan), chlorpromazine (Thorazine), midazolam (Versed), or diazepam (Valium) (Yaster and others, 1990). Unlike many sedatives, opioids have the advantage of the antidote naloxone (Narcan), which rapidly reverses the respiratory depressant effect. Fortunately, the benzodiazepines, such as diazepam and midazolam, now have the drug flumazenil (Romazicon) to treat respiratory depression (see also p. 1098).

In addition, as tolerance to the analgesic effect of opioids occurs, tolerance to the respiratory depressant effect also occurs. Pain acts as a natural antagonist to the action of opioids. With increased pain, a patient can receive increased opioids and, except for constipation, will not experience increased side effects. Respiratory depression is rare in children receiving long-term opioid therapy (Paice, 1992).

Principles of Pain Assessment in Children

Since pain is both a sensory and an emotional experience, using several assessment strategies provides qualitative and quantitative information about pain. One approach to pain assessment in children is ***QUESTT*** (Baker and Wong, 1987):

Question the child.
Use pain rating scales.
Evaluate behavior and physiologic changes.
Secure parents' involvement.
Take cause of pain into account.
Take action and evaluate results.

Question the Child. Children's verbal statements and descriptions of pain are the *most* important factors in assessing pain. However, young children may not know what the word "pain" means and may need help in describing it using familiar language. Therefore using a variety of words to describe pain, such as "owie," boo-boo," "feel funny," "hurt," or the Spanish word "dolor," if appropriate, is necessary. Older children also benefit from using simple words to describe pain. Suggested questions for obtaining a history of the children's experiences with pain are presented in the box on p. 1084. Asking children to locate the pain is also helpful, and play can provide other means for helping children to reveal discomfort.

➤ **NURSING TIP** Ask child to point to where it hurts or to "where Mommy or Daddy would put a Band-Aid"; have child mark or color the painful area on a drawing of a hu-

PAIN EXPERIENCE HISTORY

CHILD FORM

Tell me what pain is.
Tell me about the hurt you have had before.
Do you tell others when you hurt? If yes, who?
What do you do for yourself when you are hurting?
What do you want others to do for you when you hurt?
What don't you want others to do for you when you hurt?
What helps the most to take your hurt away?

Is there anything special that you want me to know about you when you hurt? (If yes, have child describe.)

PARENT FORM

What word(s) does your child use in regard to pain?
Describe the pain experiences your child has had before.
Does your child tell you or others when he/she is hurting?
How do you know when your child is in pain?
How does your child usually react to pain?
What do you do for your child when he/she is hurting?
What does your child do for him/herself when he/she is hurting?
What works best to decrease or take away your child's pain?

Is there anything special that you would like me to know about your child and pain? (If yes, describe.)

Modified from Hester NO, Barcus CS: Assessment and management of pain in children, *Pediatr Nurs Update* 1:2-8, 1986.

man figure (Fig. 26-9); ask child to tell how a puppet, doll, or stuffed animal is feeling or to point out areas on these models that "hurt" or "don't feel good."

When asking children about pain, the nurse must remember that they may deny pain because they fear receiving an injectable analgesic or because they believe they deserve to suffer as punishment for some misdeed. They may also deny pain to a stranger but readily admit it to a parent. This behavior should not be interpreted as seeking attention from the parent, but as a valid indication of pain.

Use a Pain Rating Scale. Pain rating scales (tools) provide a subjective quantitative measure of pain. Although various pain scales exist (Table 26-2), not all of them are appropriate for young children. For the most valid and reliable pain intensity rating, a scale is selected that is suitable to the child's age, abilities, and preference. Scales using facial expressions are readily accepted by children and can be used by very young children. There is some evidence that children may prefer a faces scale to other tools (West and others, 1994; Wong and Baker, 1988).

Pain assessment scales for infants include the Postoperative Infant Pain Score (Barrier and others, 1989) and Neonatal Infant Pain Scale (NIPS) (Lawrence and others, 1993). More research is needed to establish the validity and clinical usefulness of these instruments. (See also Neonatal Pain, Chapter 11.)

It is best to use the same scale with children to avoid confusing them with different instructions and to use the pain assessment scale for pain only. Multiple uses of the scale (e.g., as a general measure of the child's feelings) can cause the child to lose interest in the scale. In introducing the pain scale, nurses should explain that this is one way for children to let nurses know how they are feeling. Ideally, children should be taught to use the scale before pain is expected, such as preoperatively. Familiarizing children with the scale facilitates its use when children are actually in pain.

Evaluate Behavioral and Physiologic Changes. Behavioral changes are common indicators of pain and are especially valuable in assessing pain in nonverbal children.

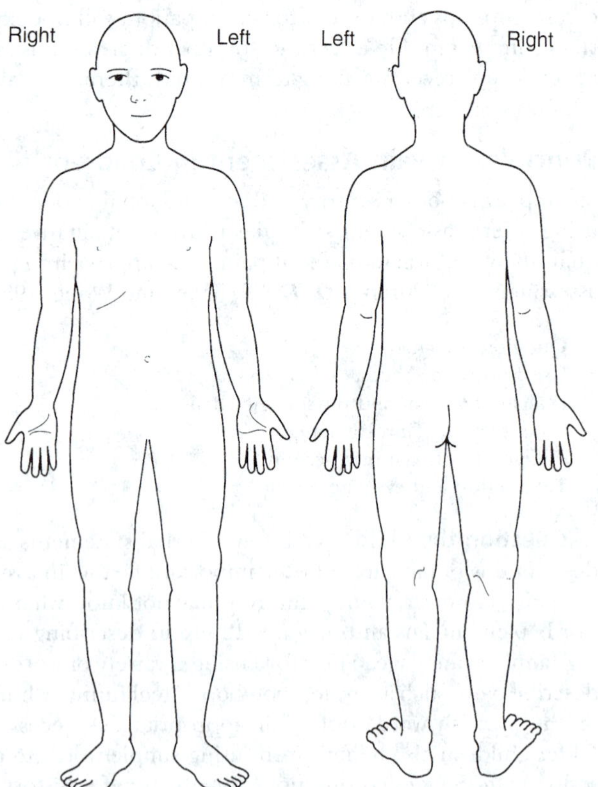

FIG. 26-9 Adolescent pediatric pain tool (APPT): body outlines for pain assessment. Instructions: "Color in the areas on these drawings to show where you have pain. Make the marks as big or as small as the place where the pain is." (From Savedra MC, Tesler MD, Holzemer WL, and Ward JA, School of Nursing, University of California–San Francisco, San Francisco, CA. Copyright © 1989, 1992.)

TABLE 26-2 Pain Rating Scales for Children

PAIN SCALE/DESCRIPTION	INSTRUCTIONS	RECOMMENDED AGE
FACES Pain Rating Scale* (Nix, Clutter, and Wong, 1994; Wong and Baker, 1988): Consists of six cartoon faces ranging from smiling face for "no pain" to tearful face for "worst pain"	Explain to child that each face is for a person who feels happy because there is no pain (hurt) or sad because there is some or a lot of pain. Face 0 is very happy because there is no hurt. Face 1 hurts just a little bit. Face 2 hurts a little more. Face 3 hurts even more. Face 4 hurts a whole lot, but Face 5 hurts as much as you can imagine, although you don't have to be crying to feel this bad. Ask child to choose face that best describes own pain. Record the number under chosen face on pain assessment record.	Children as young as 3 years
	 0  1 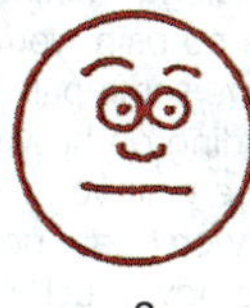 2  3  4 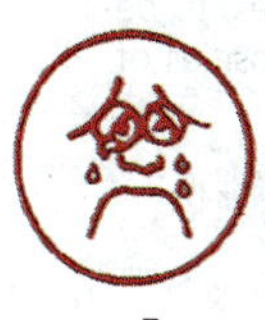 5	
Oucher† (Beyer, 1989): Consists of six photographs of child's face representing "no hurt" to "biggest hurt you could ever have"; also includes a vertical scale with numbers from 0 to 100; scales for African-American and Hispanic children have been developed (Villarruel and Denyes, 1991) and validated (Beyer, Denyes, and Villarruel, 1992)	***Photographs:*** Explain to child that face at bottom has "no hurt"; second picture, "just a little bit of hurt"; third picture, a "little bit more"; fourth picture, "even more hurt"; fifth picture, "*pretty* much hurt"; and last picture, "biggest hurt you could ever have." Ask child to choose face that best describes own pain. ***Numbers:*** Explain to child that 0 means you have "no hurt"; 0 to 29, "little hurts"; 30 to 69, "middle hurts"; 70 to 99, "big hurts"; and 100, "biggest hurt you could ever have." Ask child to choose any number between 0 and 100, not just numbers pictured on Oucher, that best describes own pain.	Children 3-13 years; use numeric scale if child can count to 100 by 1s and identify larger of any two numbers (as in original instructions), or by 10s (Jordan-Marsh and others, 1994); otherwise use photographic scale
Numeric Scale: Uses straight line with end points identified as "no pain" and "worst pain"; divisions along line are marked in units from 0 to 10 (high number may vary)	Explain to child that at one end of the line is a 0, which means that a person feels no pain (hurt). At the other end is a 10, which means the person feels the worst pain imaginable. The numbers 1 to 9 are for a very little pain to a whole lot of pain. Ask child to choose number that best describes own pain.	Children as young as 5 years, provided they can count and have some concept of numbers and their values of more or less
	No pain 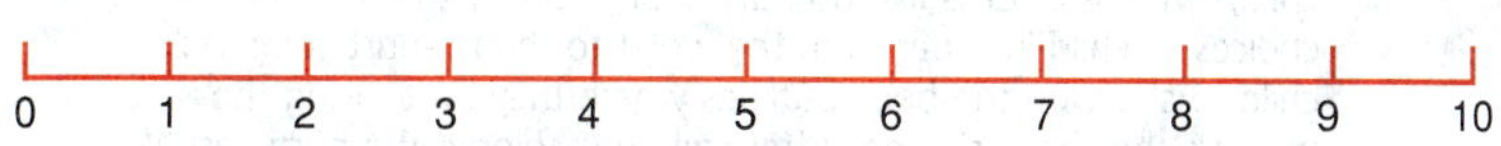 Worst pain; 0 1 2 3 4 5 6 7 8 9 10	
Poker chip tool‡: Uses four red poker chips placed horizontally in front of child	Tell child, "These are pieces of hurt." Beginning at the chip nearest child's left side and ending at the one nearest child's right side, point to chips and say, "This [the first chip] is a little bit of hurt and this [the fourth chip] is the most hurt you could ever have." For a young child or for any child who does not comprehend the instructions, clarify by saying, "That means this [the first chip] is just a little hurt; this [the second chip] is a little more hurt; this [the third chip] is more hurt; and this [the fourth chip] is the most hurt you could ever have." Ask child, "How many pieces of hurt do you have right now?" Children without pain will say they don't have any. Clarify child's answer by words such as "Oh, you have a little hurt? Tell me about the hurt." Elicit descriptors, location, and cause. Ask the child, "What would you like me to do for you?" Record number of chips selected.	Children as young as 4 to 4½ years, provided they can count and have some concept of numbers

*Several variations of faces scales exist. Complimentary copies of Wong/Baker FACES Scale are available from Purdue Frederick Co., 100 Connecticut Ave., Norwalk, CT 06856; (203) 853-0123, ext. 4010. For translations of FACES, see Appendix F.

†Oucher is available for a fee from Judith E. Beyer, PhD, RN, P.O. Box 47004, Aurora, CO 80047-0004.

‡Instructions for Poker Chip Tool and Word Graphic Rating Scale from Acute Pain Management Guideline Panel: *Acute pain management in infants, children, and adolescents: operative and medical procedures; quick reference guide for clinicians,* AHCPR Pub No 92-0020, Rockville, MD, 1992, Agency for Health Care Policy and Research, Public Health Service, US Department of Health and Human Services. Poker Chip Tool developed in 1975 by Nancy O. Hester, University of Colorado Health Sciences Center, Denver, CO. Spanish instructions from Jordan-Marsh M and others: *The Harbor-UCLA Medical Center Humor Project for Children,* Los Angeles, 1990, Harbor-UCLA Medical Center.

Continued.

TABLE 26-2 Pain Rating Scales for Children—cont'd

PAIN SCALE/DESCRIPTION	INSTRUCTIONS	RECOMMENDED AGE
	Spanish Instructions: Follow English instructions, substituting the following words. Tell parent, if present: "Estas fichas son una manera de medir dolor. Usamos cuatro fichas." Say to child: "Estas son pedazos de dolor: una es un poquito de dolor y cuatro son el dolor maximo que tu puedes sentir. Cuantos pedazos de dolor tienes?"	
Word Graphic Rating Scale[§] (Tesler and others, 1991): Uses descriptive words (may vary in other scales) to denote varying intensities of pain	Explain to child, "This is a line with words to describe how much pain you may have. This side of the line means no pain and over here the line means worst possible pain." (Point with your finger where "no pain" is, and run your finger along the line to "worst possible pain," as you say it.) "If you have no pain, you would mark like this." (Show example.) "If you have some pain, you would mark somewhere along the line, depending on how much pain you have." (Show example.) "The more pain you have, the closer to worst pain you would mark. The worst pain possible is marked like this." (Show example.) "Show me how much pain you have right now by marking with a straight, up-and-down line anywhere along the line to show how much pain you have right now." With a millimeter ruler, measure from the "no pain" end to the mark and record this measurement as the pain score.	Children as young as 5 years, although words may need explanation; words shown below were used with children ages 8 to 17 years
No pain	Little pain — Medium pain — Large pain	Worst possible pain
Visual Analogue Scale: Uses 10 cm horizontal line with end points marked "no pain" and "worst pain"	Ask child to place a mark on line that best describes amount of own pain. With a centimeter ruler, measure from the "no pain" end to the mark and record this measurement as the pain score.	Children as young as 4½ years; vertical or horizontal scale may be used (Walco and Ilowite, 1991)
Color Tool (Eland, 1993): Uses markers for child to construct own scale that is used with body outline	Present eight markers to child in a random order. Ask child, "Of these colors, which color is like . . .?" (the event identified by the child as having hurt the most). Place the marker away from the other markers. (Represents severe pain.) Ask child, "Which color is like a hurt, but not quite as much as . . .?" (the event identified by the child as having hurt the most). Place the marker with the marker chosen to represent severe pain. Ask child, "Which color is like something that hurts just a little?" Place the marker with the other colors. Ask child, "Which color is like no hurt at all?" Show the four marker choices to child in order from the worst to the no-hurt color. Ask child to show on the body outlines where they hurt, using the markers they have chosen. After child has colored the hurts, ask if they are current hurts or hurts from the past. Ask if child knows why the area hurts if it is not clear to you why it does.	Children as young as 4 years, provided they know their colors, are not color blind, and are able to construct the scale if in pain

§Word Graphic Rating Scale is part of the Adolescent Pediatric Pain Tool and is available for a fee from Pediatric Pain Study, University of California, School of Nursing, Department of Family Health Care Nursing, San Francisco, CA 94143-0606; (415) 476-4040.

Children's behavioral responses to pain change with age and follow a developmental trend (see box on p. 1087). However, children vary widely in their responses and may exhibit behaviors at one age that are more typically seen at a different age. In addition, temperament affects coping style, and children with more positive moods may appear to be in less pain than they actually are. Children who use passive coping behaviors (offering no resistance, cooperating) may rate pain as more intense than children who use active coping behaviors (resisting, attacking) (Broome and others, 1990). Cultural background may also play a role in children's pain responses, although the influence appears slight (Abu-Saad, 1984; Pfefferbaum, Adams, and Aceves, 1990). Cultural practices regarding pain are important (see Cultural Awareness box). Unfortunately, nurses often make judgments about pain based on behavior, which results in some children receiving inadequate pain medication (Wallace, 1989). (See also Critical Thinking Exercise box.)

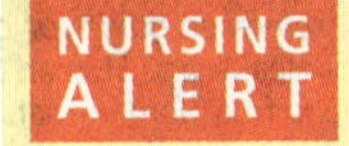

If children's behaviors appear to differ from their rating of pain, believe their pain rating.

DEVELOPMENTAL CHARACTERISTICS OF CHILDREN'S RESPONSES TO PAIN

YOUNG INFANTS

Generalized body response of rigidity or thrashing, possibly with local reflex withdrawal of stimulated area
Loud crying
Facial expression of pain (brows lowered and drawn together, eyes tightly closed, mouth open and squarish) (see Fig. 26-3)
Demonstrates no association between approaching stimulus and subsequent pain

OLDER INFANTS

Localized body response with deliberate withdrawal of stimulated area
Loud crying
Facial expression of pain and/or anger (same facial characteristics as pain but eyes may be open)
Physical resistance, especially pushing the stimulus away *after* it is applied

YOUNG CHILDREN

Loud crying, screaming
Verbal expressions of "Ow," "Ouch," or "It hurts"
Thrashing of arms and legs
Attempts to push stimulus away *before* it is applied
Uncooperative; needs physical restraint
Requests termination of procedure
Clings to parent, nurse, or other significant person
Requests emotional support, such as hugs or other forms of physical comfort
May become restless and irritable with continuing pain
All these behaviors may be seen in anticipation of actual painful procedure

SCHOOL-AGE CHILDREN

May see all behaviors of young child, especially *during* painful procedure but less in anticipatory period
Stalling behavior, such as "Wait a minute" or "I'm not ready"
Muscular rigidity, such as clenched fists, white knuckles, gritted teeth, contracted limbs, body stiffness, closed eyes, wrinkled forehead

ADOLESCENTS

Less vocal protest
Less motor activity
More verbal expressions, such as "It hurts" or "You're hurting me"
Increased muscle tension and body control

Data from Craig KD and others: Developmental changes in infant pain expression during immunization injections, *Soc Sci Med* 19(12):1331-1337, 1984; and Katz E, Kellerman J, Siegel S: Behavioral distress in children with cancer undergoing medical procedures: developmental considerations, *J Consult Clin Psychol* 48(3): 356-365, 1980.

Depending on the type and location of pain, children may display behaviors that indicate local body pain, such as pulling the ears for ear pain; rolling the head from side to side for head and ear pain; lying on the side with legs flexed for abdominal pain; limping for leg or foot pain; and refusing to move a body part. Children who experience chronic or repeated pain often develop effective behavioral coping strategies, such as squeezing a hand, talking, counting, relaxing, or thinking about pleasant events. Once these coping skills are identified, the child can be encouraged to use them in future experiences with pain.

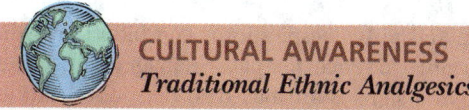

CULTURAL AWARENESS
Traditional Ethnic Analgesics

Many traditional ethnic remedies are used to relieve pain. Although they are widely available in the United States, they are not marketed as drugs and have not been subjected to standard tests for safety and effectiveness. One Chinese herbal product, Jin Bu Huan, has caused life-threatening poisoning in children (Jin Bu Huan, 1993). It is important to inquire about ethnic pain relievers and advise the family to store them out of children's reach to prevent unintentional ingestion.

CRITICAL THINKING EXERCISE
Pain Assessment

Stacy is 14 years old, and this is her second day following abdominal surgery. As you enter her room, she smiles at you and continues to talk and joke with her visitor. Stacy rates her pain a 4 on a scale of 0 to 5, no to worst pain, respectively. Her roommate, Jill, is 12 years old, and this is her third day following scoliosis surgery. She does not smile and is lying very still in bed. Jill rates her pain a 4 on the same scale. Based on your assessment, you write the following in their charts (choose two items):

1. Stacy: In no acute distress and appears comfortable, talking and joking with a visitor.
2. Jill: Rates her surgical pain a 4 on a 0 to 5 scale and is unable to move because of pain; she appears depressed.
3. Stacy: Rates her surgical pain a 4 on a 0 to 5 scale.
4. Jill: Rates her surgical pain a 4 on a 0 to 5 scale.

The correct answers are 3 and 4. The best estimate of pain is the person's self-report. Responses 1 and 2 are based on subjective impressions. In response 1 the adolescent's report of pain is totally disregarded. In response 2 there is no assessment data to support that Jill's behavior indicates inability to move or depression.

Physiologic responses indicating acute pain include flushing of the skin; increases in sweating, blood pressure, pulse, and respiration; decreases in oxygen saturation; restlessness; and dilation of the pupils. However, these signs vary considerably, and they may be produced by emotions such as fear, anger, or anxiety. They occur primarily in acute pain from stimulation of the sympathetic nervous system. If pain persists, the body begins to adapt, and these responses decrease or stabilize. Consequently, if nurses rely primarily on observing these physiologic indications before believing that pain exists, many instances of pain will go unrecognized.

One of the most valuable clues to pain is a change in behavior and vital signs after administration of an analgesic. Improved behavior (e.g., less irritability, cessation of crying) and decreased pulse, respirations, and blood pressure provide important evidence for pain management. Often the change in vital signs is attributed to the depressant effect of opioids, when in reality the return to more normal physiologic functioning is due to pain relief. However, no change in vital signs or behavior may mean that pain exists and that the analgesic was inadequate.

Secure Parents' Involvement. Parents know their child and are sensitive to changes in behavior. However, some parents may never have seen their child in severe pain and may equate certain responses, such as irritability or withdrawal, with discomfort. Others are aware that certain behaviors signal pain because the child has acted similarly during previous painful events. In addition, parents usually know what comforts their child, such as rocking, stroking, or talking (La Montagne, Johnson, and Hepworth, 1991). They are the most consistent persons caring for the child and want to be involved in pain relief (Watt-Watson, Everden, and Lawson, 1990). Encouraging their participation gives them control and a sense of helping.

To better assess the child's pain, the nurse can interview the parents about their child's previous pain experiences (see box on p. 1084). Ideally, this questioning should occur before the child is in pain, such as on admission to the hospital. Parents need to realize that their knowledge of their child is important in providing care. Parents sometimes leave the assessment of pain up to the nurse because "nurses are more experienced," and consequently parents do not report pain (Mills, 1989). Parents need to be taught nonverbal pain behaviors in children and encouraged to inform the staff when they occur.

Take Cause of Pain into Account. When children exhibit behaviors or other clues that suggest pain, reasons for discomfort should be investigated. Pathology may give clues to the expected intensity and type of pain. For example, pain associated with vaso-occlusive crises in sickle cell disease is severe. Pain caused by bone marrow puncture is typically greater than the discomfort associated with a venipuncture. However, it is a mistake to believe that certain conditions or procedures always produce a standard amount of pain. For example, sore throat pain may be mild or severe—only the child knows the intensity.

NURSING ALERT A golden rule to follow in pain assessment is: Whatever is painful to an adult is painful to an infant or child until proved otherwise.

Take Action and Evaluate Results. The reason for assessing pain is to relieve it. Total pain relief should be the goal, with the combined use of pharmacologic and nonpharmacologic interventions (see following discussion). However, complete relief may not be possible. When children are able, they can tell the nurse what level of pain is acceptable to them.

Regardless of the type of pain intervention, evaluation of the results is essential. No one pain reduction technique is effective for all children. Therefore a pain assessment record is used to monitor the effectiveness of the interven-

Pain Assessment Record

Directions for each column:

1. Record date and time of administering analgesic; assess analgesic effect ________ minutes later and then ________.
2. Use a pain rating scale if child understands its use. Name of scale ________. Ratings: No pain = ______. Worst pain = ______. Acceptable pain rating ______.
3. Record analgesic, dose, and route.
4. Record possible indications or effects of pain, such as shallow breathing due to incisional pain, parental request for pain relief; record indications or effects of pain relief, such as "moves easily, playing."
5. Record level of arousal, using sedation scale in box. Also, record any other side effects (e.g., nausea, itching).
6. R = respiratory function. Record breaths per minute and/or other observations of respiratory status (e.g., depth of respiration, change in color).
7. Signature or initials of person recording information.

SEDATION SCALE
0 = None
1 = Mild (occasionally drowsy; easy to arouse)
2 = Moderate (frequently drowsy; easy to arouse)
3 = Severe (somnolent; difficult to arouse)
S = Normal sleep (easy to arouse)

1 Date/ time	2 Pain rating	3 Analgesic	4 Possible effects/indications of pain or relief of pain	5 Arousal/ side effects	6 R	7 Signature

FIG. 26-10 Pain assessment record.

tions (Fig. 26-10). With nonverbal children, behavioral and physiologic signs are evaluated for evidence of pain relief. With verbal children, their statements about pain relief and pain ratings are also recorded. Changes in the medication regimen are made as needed to provide the maximum pain relief with the minimum side effects. Family members are often excellent allies for keeping a pain assessment record for the nurse.

NURSING ALERT Presenting practitioners with objective documentation of pain, rather than opinion, is more likely to lead to a favorable change in analgesic disorders (Walker and Wong, 1991).

PAIN MANAGEMENT

Relief of pain is a basic need and right of all children, yet physicians and nurses are often reluctant to order and administer analgesics and lack knowledge of well-documented approaches to pharmacologic pain control.

Effective pain management requires that health professionals be willing to try a number of interventions to achieve optimum results. Basically, pain-reducing methods can be grouped into two categories: nonpharmacologic and pharmacologic. Whenever possible, both should be used; however, nonpharmacologic measures should not be considered substitutes for analgesics.

Nonpharmacologic Management

A number of nonpharmacologic techniques exist for lessening the perception of pain and, when used with analgesics, can enhance these drugs' effectiveness. However, nonpharmacologic strategies can also produce a cooperative child who continues to suffer "in silence" (Zeltzer, Jay, and Fisher, 1989). Therefore nurses must carefully evaluate the effectiveness of the intervention in truly reducing pain and avoid setting an expectation of passive acceptance. Aside from this risk, nonpharmacologic methods are extremely safe and most are independent nursing functions. The methods either inhibit or modulate the transmission of noxious stimuli or increase descending control from the brain to the spinal cord.

Nonpharmacologic interventions include ***general strategies*** that are effective with most children, especially those who can benefit from explanations. However, ***specific nonpharmacologic strategies*** are more effective with certain children than with others (see Guidelines box on p. 1090). Experimentation with several strategies that are suitable to child's age, pain intensity, and abilities is often necessary to determine the most effective approach (Alexander and others, 1993).

NURSING ALERT Most specific nonpharmacologic strategies require children's understanding and cooperation. Therefore, try to match the strategy with the pain severity. Children in severe pain may not be able to expend the effort necessary to learn the technique, and those with very mild symptoms may not be motivated to learn. Therefore these strategies may be most useful with midrange pain (Cleeland, 1986).

In the selection of a pain reducer, it is best to use a strategy familiar to the child or to describe several strategies and let the child select the most appealing one. Parents should be involved in the selection process; they may be familiar with the child's usual coping skills and can help identify potentially successful strategies. Involving parents also encourages their participation in learning the skill with the child and acting as coach. If the parent cannot assist the child, other appropriate persons may include a grandparent, older sibling, nurse, or child-life specialist.

Children should learn a specific strategy *before* pain occurs or before it becomes severe. To reduce the child's effort, instructions for a strategy, such as distraction or relaxation, can be audiotaped and played during a period of discomfort. However, when learned, children often need help using the intervention during the procedure.

Pharmacologic Management

Using pharmacologic methods to control pain requires attention to four "rights": right drug, right dose, right route, and right time. Although nurses may not prescribe the medication, knowledge of these essential principles assists in optimally implementing analgesic orders and discussing with other practitioners possible strategies to improve pain control. In addition, observing for side effects of the drugs and using supportive approaches with children when administering the drug are important nursing interventions.

Right Drug. Nonopioids, including acetaminophen (Tylenol, paracetamol) and nonsteroidal antiinflammatory drugs (NSAIDs), are suitable for mild to moderate pain; opioids are needed for moderate to severe pain. A combination of the two analgesics attacks pain on two levels: nonopioids at the peripheral nervous system and opioids at the central nervous system. This approach provides increased analgesia without increased side effects. Several commercially available combinations, such as Tylenol with Codeine, may have increasing doses of the opioid but a constant dose of the nonopioid (see box on p. 1091). Therefore, before increasing the opioid, it may be preferable to increase the nonopioid component, for example, adding one plain Tylenol (300 mg) to Tylenol with Codeine No. 3 before advancing to Tylenol with Codeine No. 4. However, if this approach is not successful, the pain most likely requires a stronger opioid.

The action of various opioids differs. Morphine is considered the drug of choice. When morphine is not a suitable opioid, drugs such as hydromorphone (Dilaudid) and fentanyl (Sublimaze) are effective substitutes. Although fentanyl is used as an anesthetic in the operating room, it is classified as an analgesic. It can be safely administered by nurses (Willens, 1994).

Opioids are frequently combined with other drugs that are considered "potentiators." One common mixture is the "DPT," or "lytic" cocktail—Demerol, Phenergan, and Thorazine (see Thinking Critically About . . . box on use of DPT under Surgical Procedures, Chapter 27). However, there is little evidence that any drug potentiates the analgesic effect of opioids; rather, drugs such as promethazine (Phenergan) produce sedation, which is erroneously equated with analgesia.

GUIDELINES
Nonpharmacologic Pain Management

GENERAL STRATEGIES

Form a trusting relationship with child and family.
- Express concern regarding their reports of pain.
- Take an active role in seeking effective pain management strategies.

Use general strategies to prepare child for painful procedure (see Chapter 27).

Prepare child before potentially painful procedures but avoid "planting" the idea of pain. For example, instead of saying, "This is going to (or may) hurt," say, "Sometimes this feels like pushing, sticking, or pinching, and sometimes it doesn't bother people. You tell me what it feels like to you."
- Use "nonpain" descriptors when possible (e.g., "It feels like intense heat" rather than "It's a burning pain").
- This allows for variation in sensory perception, avoids suggesting pain, and gives child control in describing reactions.

Avoid evaluative statements or descriptions (e.g., "This is a terrible procedure" or "It really will hurt a lot").

Stay with child during a painful procedure.
- Encourage parents to stay with child if child and parent desire; encourage parent to talk softly to child and to remain near child's head.
- Involve parents in learning specific nonpharmacologic strategies and assisting child in their use.

Educate child about the pain, especially when explanation may lessen anxiety (e.g., that child's pain is expected after surgery and does not indicate something is wrong; reassure that child is not responsible for the pain).

For long-term pain control give child a doll, which becomes "the patient," and allow child to do everything to the doll that is done to the child; pain control can be emphasized through the doll by stating, "Dolly feels better after the medicine."

Teach procedures to child and family for later use.

SPECIFIC STRATEGIES

Distraction

Involve parent and child in identifying strong distractors.

Involve child in play; use radio, tape recorder, record player; have child sing or use rhythmic breathing.

Have child take a deep breath and blow it out until told to stop (French, Painter, and Coury, 1994).

Have child blow bubbles to "blow the hurt away."

Have child concentrate on yelling or saying "ouch" by focusing on "yelling loud or soft as you feel it hurt; that way I know what's happening."

Use humor, such as watching cartoons, telling jokes or funny stories, or acting silly with child.

Have child read, play games, or visit with friends.

Relaxation

With an infant or young child:
- Hold in a comfortable, well-supported position, such as vertically against the chest and shoulder.
- Rock in a wide, rhythmic arc in a rocking chair or sway back and forth, rather than bouncing child.
- Repeat one or two words softly, such as "Mommy's here."

With a slightly older child:
- Ask child to take a deep breath and "go limp as a rag doll" while exhaling slowly, then ask child to yawn (demonstrate if needed).
- Help child assume a comfortable position (e.g., pillow under neck and knees).
- Begin progressive relaxation: starting with the toes, systematically instruct child to let each body part "go limp" or "feel heavy"; if child has difficulty with relaxing, instruct child to tense or tighten each body part and then relax it.
- Allow child to keep eyes open, since children may respond better if eyes are open rather than closed during relaxation.

Guided Imagery

Have child identify some highly pleasurable real or pretend experience.

Have child describe details of the event, including as many senses as possible (e.g., "feel the cool breezes," "see the beautiful colors," "hear the pleasant music").

Have child write down or record script.

Encourage child to concentrate only on the pleasurable event during the painful time; enhance the image by recalling specific details, such as reading the script or playing the record.

Combine with relaxation.

Positive Self-Talk

Teach child positive statements to say when in pain (e.g., "I will be feeling better soon," "When I go home, I will feel better," "Relaxing will make me hurt less").

Thought Stopping

Identify positive facts about the painful event (e.g., "It does not last long").

Identify reassuring information (e.g., "If I think about something else, it does not hurt as much").

Condense positive and reassuring facts into a set of brief statements, and have child memorize them (e.g.: "Short procedure, good veins, little hurt, nice nurse, go home").

Have child repeat the memorized statements whenever thinking about or experiencing the painful event.

Cutaneous Stimulation

Includes simple rhythmic rubbing; use of pressure, electric vibrator; massage with hand lotion, powder, or menthol cream; application of heat or cold, such as an ice cube on the site before giving injection or application of ice to the site opposite the painful area (e.g., if right knee hurts, place ice on left knee).

A more sophisticated method is transcutaneous electrical nerve stimulation (TENS) (use of controlled low-voltage electricity to the body via electrodes placed on the skin).

Behavioral Contracting

Informal—May be used with children as young as 4 or 5 years of age:
- Use stars or tokens as rewards.
- Give uncooperative or procrastinating children (during a procedure) a limited time (measured by a visible timer) to complete the procedure.
- Proceed as needed if child is unable to comply.
- Reinforce cooperation with a reward if the procedure is accomplished within specified time.

Formal—Use written contract, which includes the following:
- Realistic (seems possible) goal or desired behavior
- Measurable behavior (e.g., agrees not to hit anyone during procedures)
- Contract written, dated, and signed by all persons involved in any of the agreements
- Identified rewards or consequences are reinforcing
- Goals can be evaluated

SELECTED COMBINATION OPIOID AND NONOPIOID ORAL ANALGESICS

NONASPIRIN PRODUCTS

Product	Contents
Darvocet-N 50	50 mg propoxyphene napsylate 325 mg actaminophen
Darvocet-N 100	100 mg propoxyphene napsylate 650 mg acetaminophen
Lortab	2.5, 5, or 7.5 mg hydrocodone bitartrate 500 mg acetaminophen
Lortab Liquid (each 5 ml)	2.5 mg hydrocodone bitartrate 120 mg acetaminophen
Percocet-5*	5 mg oxycodone HCl 325 mg acetaminophen
Tylenol with Codeine No. 1	7.5 mg codeine 300 mg acetaminophen
Tylenol with Codeine No. 2	15 mg codeine 300 mg acetaminophen
Tylenol with Codeine No. 3	30 mg codeine 300 mg acetaminophen
Tylenol with Codeine No. 4	60 mg codeine 300 mg acetaminophen
Tylenol and Codeine Elixir (each 5 ml)	12 mg codeine 120 mg acetaminophen 7% alcohol
Tylox*	5 mg oxycodone HCl 500 mg acetaminophen
Vicodin	5 mg hydrocodone 500 mg acetaminophen

ASPIRIN PRODUCTS†

Product	Contents
Darvon Compound	32 mg propoxyphene HCl 389 mg aspirin 32.4 mg caffeine
Darvon Compound-65	65 mg propoxyphene HCl 389 mg aspirin 32.4 mg caffeine
Darvon with A.S.A.	65 mg propoxyphene HCl 325 mg aspirin
Darvon-N with A.S.A.	100 mg propoxyphene napsylate 325 mg aspirin
Percodan*	4.5 mg oxycodone HCl 0.38 mg oxycodone terephthalate 325 mg aspirin
Percodan-Demi*	2.25 mg oxycodone HCl 0.19 mg oxycodone terephthalate 325 mg aspirin

*All medications require a prescription, but these are classified as schedule II drugs (like morphine), and each filling requires a written prescription that includes the patient's name and address, the practitioner's DEA (Drug Enforcement Agency) number, and the date. The prescription must be filled within 5 days.
†Aspirin is not recommended for children because of its possible association with Reye syndrome.

NURSING ALERT Meperidine (Demerol, pethidine) is not recommended for chronic use (or for more than 48 hours at a time), such as for postoperative pain control, because of the accumulation of its metabolite, ***normeperidine.*** Normeperidine is a central nervous system stimulant that can produce anxiety, tremors, myoclonus, and generalized seizures (Acute Pain, 1992; American Pain Society, 1992). Normeperidine's half-life is 15 to 20 hours, compared with 3 hours for meperidine, and the central nervous system excitation is not reversed with naloxone.

Assess the child at least every 8 hours for early signs of toxicity, such as tremors in the outstretched hand, episodes of twitching or jerking, or increased agitation or excitability (may be upset easily). If normeperidine toxicity is suspected, discontinue the meperidine immediately and notify the practitioner (Love, 1994). The pharmacist should complete an adverse drug reaction report to MedWatch*

Several drugs, known as ***adjuvant analgesics,*** may be used alone or with opioids to control pain symptoms, although they may or may not have analgesic properties.

Frequently used drugs to relieve anxiety, cause sedation, and provide amnesia are diazepam (Valium) and midazolam (Versed); however, they are not analgesics. Other adjuvants include tricyclic antidepressants (i.e., amitriptyline, imiprimine) and anticonvulsants for neuropathic pain (brief, lancinating pain); stool softeners, laxatives, and antiemetics for constipation and nausea/vomiting; steroids for inflammation and bone pain; and dextroamphetamine and caffeine for increased analgesia and decreased sedation.

At times health professionals question whether pain really exists and administer ***placebos*** to "see if the pain is real." This practice is unjustified and unethical; a positive response to a placebo, such as a saline injection, is common in patients who have a documented organic basis for pain. Therefore, the deceptive use of placebos does not provide useful information about the presence or severity of pain (Goodwin, Goodwin, and Vogel, 1979). In addition, the use of placebos can cause side effects similar to those of opioids, can destroy the client's trust in the health care staff, and raises serious ethical and legal questions (Perry and Heidrich, 1981). Therefore the use of placebos should be avoided (American Pain Society, 1992).

Right Dosage. The optimum dosage is one that controls pain without causing severe side effects. This usually requires ***titration,*** the gradual adjustment of drug dosage (usually by increasing the dose) until optimum pain relief without excessive sedation is achieved. Dosage recommendations, such as those in Tables 26-3 and 26-4, are only safe initial dosages, not optimum dosages. Children (except infants younger than about 3 months of age) metabolize drugs more rapidly than adults; younger children may require higher doses of opioids to achieve the same analgesic effect (Hertzka and others, 1989; Olkkola and others, 1988). Therefore, the therapeutic effect and duration of an-

*The FDA Medical Products Reporting Program, Food and Drug Administration, 5600 Fishers Lane, Rockville, MD 20852-9787; (800) FDA-1088.

TABLE 26-3 Nonsteroidal Antiinflammatory Drugs (NSAIDs) Approved for Children*

DRUG (TRADE NAME)	DOSE	COMMENTS
Acetaminophen (Tylenol and other brands)	10-20 mg/kg/dose every 4-6 hours not to exceed 5 doses in 24 hours	Available in drops (80 mg/0.8 ml), elixir (160 mg/5 ml), tablets (80 mg), swallowable caplets (160 mg), and rectal suppositories (several dosages) Nonprescription Higher dosage range may provide increased analgesia
Choline magnesium trisalicylate (Trilisate)	Children 37 kg or less: 50 mg/kg/day divided into 2 doses Children over 37 kg: 2250 mg/day divided into 2 doses	Available in elixir 500 mg/5 ml Prescription
Ibuprofen		
Children's Motrin	Children 6 months to 12 years: 5-10 mg/kg/dose every 6-8 hours not to exceed 40 mg/kg/day for fever Children over 12 years: 200-400 mg/dose every 6-8 hours	Available in suspension 100 mg/5 ml Prescription Recommended for fever reduction in children 6 months to 12 years, but also indicated for juvenile rheumatoid arthritis and mild to moderate pain in children over 12 years
Children's Advil	Children 6 months and older: 5-10 mg/kg/dose every 6-8 hours not to exceed 40 mg/kg/day for fever	Available in suspension 100 mg/5 ml Prescription Dosage recommendation is for juvenile rheumatoid arthritis and fever
Naproxen (Naprosyn)	Children over 2 years: 10 mg/kg/day divided into 2 doses	Available in elixir 125 mg/5 ml Prescription
Tolmetin (Tolectin)	Children over 2 years: 20 mg/kg/day divided into 3 or 4 doses	Available in scored 200 mg tablets Prescription

*All NSAIDs in the table except acetaminophen have significant antiinflammatory, antipyretic, and analgesic actions. Acetaminophen has a weak antiinflammatory action, and its classification as an NSAID is controversial. Patients respond differently to various NSAIDs; therefore, changing from one drug to another may be necessary for maximum benefit.

Acetylsalicylic acid (aspirin) is also an NSAID but is not recommended for children because of its possible association with Reye syndrome. The NSAIDs in the table have no known association with Reye syndrome. However, caution should be exercised in prescribing any salicylate-containing drug (e.g., Trilisate) for children with known or suspected viral infection.

Side effects of ibuprofen, naproxen, and tolmetin include nausea, vomiting, diarrhea, constipation, gastric ulceration, bleeding nephritis, and fluid retention. Acetaminophen and choline magnesium trisalicylate are well tolerated in the gastrointestinal tract and do not interfere with platelet function. NSAIDs except acetaminophen should not be given to patients with allergic reactions to salicylates. All the NSAIDs should be used cautiously in patients with renal impairment.

algesia vary. Children's dosages are usually calculated according to body weight, except in large children, where the weight formula may exceed the average adult dose. In this case the adult dose is used.

A reasonable starting dose of opioid for the neonate who is *not* mechanically ventilated is one fourth to one third of the recommended starting dose for older children. The infant is monitored very closely for signs of pain relief and respiratory depression. The dose is titrated to effect. Since tolerance can develop rapidly, very large opioid doses may be needed for continued severe pain (American Pain Society, 1992).

If pain relief is inadequate, the initial dosage is increased (usually by 50% if pain is moderate or by 100% if pain is severe) to provide greater analgesic effectiveness. Decreasing the interval between doses may also provide more continuous pain relief. A major difference between opioids and nonopioids is that nonopioids have a ***ceiling effect,*** which means that doses higher than the recommended dose will not produce greater pain relief. Opioids do not have a ceiling effect other than that imposed by side effects; therefore, larger dosages can be given safely for increasing severity of pain. (See Critical Thinking Exercise box on p. 1096.)

NURSING ALERT **A frequent error in attempts to improve pain control is to change to another analgesic. If an opioid, such as morphine, hydromorphone, or fentanyl, is used, rarely is the problem one of drug choice. Rather, the problem is usually one of inadequate dosage. If changing to another analgesic is warranted because of adverse side effects, the new drug should be at least equal in potency to the original analgesic.**

Parenteral and oral dosages of opioids are not the same. Because of the ***first-pass effect,*** an oral opioid is rapidly absorbed from the gastrointestinal tract and enters the portal circulation, where it is partially metabolized before reaching the central circulation. Therefore oral dosages must be larger to compensate for the partial loss of analgesic potency to achieve ***equianalgesia*** (equal analgesic effect). Conversion factors for selected opioids, when a change is made from intramuscular (IM) or intravenous (IV) to oral, are listed in Tables 26-4 and 26-5. Immediate conversion from

TABLE 26-4 Dosage of Selected Opioids for Children

DRUG	APPROXIMATE EQUIANALGESIC ORAL DOSE	APPROXIMATE EQUIANALGESIC PARENTERAL DOSE	RECOMMENDED STARTING DOSE (CHILDREN LESS THAN 50 KG BODY WEIGHT)[a]	
			ORAL	PARENTERAL[b]
Morphine[c]	30 mg q 3-4 hr (around-the-clock dosing) 60 mg q 3-4 hr (single dose or intermittent dosing)	10 mg q 3-4 hr	0.2-0.4 mg/kg oral q 3-4 hr 0.3-0.6 mg/kg oral time released q 12 hr	0.1-0.2 mg/kg IM q 3-4 hr 0.02-0.1 mg/kg IV bolus q 2 hr 0.015 mg/kg q 8 min PCA 0.01-0.02 mg/kg/hr IV infusion (neonates) 0.01-0.06 mg/kg/hr IV infusion (child)
Fentanyl (Sublimaze)	Not available	0.1 mg IV		0.5-1.5 µg/kg IV bolus q 0.5 hr 1-2 µg/hr IV infusion
Codeine[d]	130 mg q 3-4 hr	75 mg q 3-4 hr	1 mg/kg q 3-4 hr	Not recommended
Hydromorphone[c] (Dilaudid)	7.5 mg q 3-4 hr	1.5 mg q 3-4 hr	0.04-0.1 mg/kg oral q 4-6 hr	0.02-0.1 mg/kg IM q 3-4 hr 0.005-0.2 mg/kg IV bolus q 2 hr
Hydrocodone (in Lorcet, Lortab, Vicodin, others)	30 mg q 3-4 hr	Not available	0.2 mg/kg q 3-4 hr[f]	Not available
Levorphanol (Levo-Dromoran)	4 mg q 6-8 hr	2 mg q 6-8 hr	0.04 mg/kg q 6-8 hr	0.02 mg/kg q 6-8 hr
Meperidine (Demerol)[e]	300 mg q 2-3 hr	100 mg q 3 hr	Not recommended	0.75 mg/kg q 2-3 hr
Methadone (Dolophine, others)	20 mg q 6-8 hr	10 mg q 6-8 hr	0.2 mg/kg q 6-8 hr	0.1 mg/kg q 6-8 hr
Oxycodone (Roxicodone, also in Percocet, Percodan, Tylox, others)	30 mg q 3-4 hr	Not available	0.2 mg/kg q 3-4 hr[f]	Not available

Data from Acute Pain Management Guideline Panel: *Acute pain management: operative or medical procedures and trauma: clinical practice guideline,* AHCPR Pub No 92-0032, Rockville, MD, 1992, Agency for Health Care Policy and Research, Public Health Service, US Department of Health and Human Services; and Berde C and others: Report of the subcommittee on disease-related pain in childhood cancer, *Pediatrics* 86(5, pt 2):820, 1990.

IV, Intravenous; *IM,* intramuscular; *SC,* subcutaneous; *PO,* oral.

Note: Published tables vary in the suggested doses that are equianalgesic to morphine. Clinical response is the criterion that must be applied for each patient; titration to clinical response is necessary. Because there is not complete cross-tolerance among these drugs, it is usually necessary to use a lower than equianalgesic dose when changing drugs and to retitrate to response. **Caution:** Recommended doses do not apply to patients with renal or hepatic insufficiency or other conditions affecting drug metabolism and kinetics.

[a]**Caution:** Doses listed for patients with body weight less than 50 kg cannot be used as initial starting doses in infants less than 6 months of age. For nonventilated infants under 6 months of age, the initial opioid dose should be about one fourth to one third of the dose recommended for older infants and children. For example, morphine could be used at a dose of 0.03 mg/kg instead of the traditional 0.1 mg/kg.

[b]IM injections should not be used.

[c]For morphine, hydromorphone, and oxymorphone, rectal administration is an alternate route for patients unable to take oral medications, but equianalgesic doses may differ from oral and parenteral doses because of pharmacokinetic differences.

[d]**Caution:** Codeine doses above 65 mg often are not appropriate because of diminishing incremental analgesia with increasing doses but continually increasing constipation and other side effects.

[e]Should not be used chronically, particularly in patients with compromised renal function or for treatment of sickle cell crisis pain, because of accumulation of the metabolite, normeperidine, which causes central nervous system irritability (anxiety, tremors, myoclonus, and generalized seizures).

[f]**Caution:** Doses of aspirin and acetaminophen in combination with opioid/NSAID preparations must also be adjusted to the patient's body weight.

IM or IV to the suggested equianalgesic oral dose may result in a substantial error in the individual child. For example, the dose may be significantly more or less than what the child requires. Small changes ensure small errors.

Right Route. Several routes of administration exist (see box on pp. 1094-1095). Children should not have to endure pain, such as from IM injections, to achieve pain relief. Therefore the most effective and least traumatic route of administration should be selected.

A significant advance in the administration of IV or subcutaneous [SC] analgesics is the use of ***patient-controlled analgesia (PCA).*** As the name implies, the patient controls the amount and frequency of the analgesic, which is typically delivered through a special infusion device. Children who are physically able to "push a button" and who can understand the concept of "pushing a button" to obtain pain relief (usually during later preschool age) can use PCA (Gaukroger, Tomkins, and van der Walt, 1989; Gureno and Reisinger, 1991). Although it is controversial, parents and nurses have used the PCA system for the child (Riemondy

ROUTES AND METHODS OF ANALGESIC DRUG ADMINISTRATION

ORAL

Preferred because of convenience, cost, and relatively steady blood levels

Higher dosages of oral form of opioids required for equivalent parenteral analgesia

Peak drug effect occurs after 1½ to 2 hours for most analgesics

- Delay in onset of disadvantage when rapid control of severe pain or fluctuating pain is desired

SUBLINGUAL/BUCCAL/TRANSMUCOSAL

Tablet or liquid placed between cheek and gum (buccal) or under tongue (sublingual)

Highly desirable because more rapid onset than oral

- Avoids first-pass effect through liver, which normally reduces analgesia from oral opioids (unless sublingual/buccal form swallowed, which occurs often in children)

Few drugs commercially available in this form

- Many drugs can be compounded into a sublingual troche or lozenge (Pitorak, 1991; Wong and Redding, 1987)*

Fentanyl Oralet

- Fentanyl in hard confection base on a plastic holder used for preoperative sedation/analgesia

INTRAVENOUS (IV) (BOLUS)

Preferred for rapid control of severe pain

Provides most rapid onset of effect, usually in about 5 minutes

- Advantage for acute pain, procedural pain, and breakthrough pain

Initial bolus dose is controversial; one recommendation is one-half IM dose

Needs to be repeated hourly for continuous pain control

- Drugs with short half-life (morphine, fentanyl, hydromorphone) are preferred to avoid toxic accumulation of drug

INTRAVENOUS (CONTINUOUS)

Preferred over bolus and IM for maintaining control of pain

Provides steady blood levels

Easy to titrate dosage

Suggested initial dose is controversial; one approach to calculating hourly infusion rate is to divide IM dose by drug's expected duration for IM route

Full peak effect is delayed; best if combined with initial IV bolus dose

SUBCUTANEOUS (SC) (CONTINUOUS)

Used when oral and IV routes not available

Provides equivalent blood levels to continuous IV infusion

Suggested initial bolus dose to equal 2-hour IV dose; total 24-hour dose usually equal to total IV or IM 24-hour dose.

PATIENT-CONTROLLED ANALGESIA (PCA)

Generally refers to self-administration of drugs, regardless of route

Typically uses programmable infusion pump (IV or SC) that permits self-administration of boluses of medication at preset dose and time interval (***lockout interval*** is time between doses)

Best pain control may be achieved with initial bolus and continuous (basal or background) infusion of opioid

Optimum lockout interval not known, but must be at least as long as time needed for onset of drug

- Should effectively control pain during movement or procedures
- Longer lockout requires larger dose

May be used as a convenient analgesic delivery system for neonates; nurse pushes button for increased pain control

INTRAMUSCULAR (IM)

Available in many opioid preparations

Painful administration (hated by children)

Some drugs (e.g., meperidine) can cause tissue damage

Wide fluctuation in absorption of drug from muscle

Faster absorption from deltoid than gluteal sites

Shorter duration and more expensive than oral drugs

Time consuming for staff

INTRANASAL

Midazolam (Versed) has been used as nasal spray (Theroux and others, 1993)

- Although effective, may be traumatic route for children (Karl, Larach, and Ruffle, 1991; Lugo and others, 1993)
- Available commercially as Stadol NS (butorphanol); approved for those over 18 years of age (Schwesinger and others, 1992).

INTRADERMAL

Used primarily for skin anesthesia (e.g., for lumbar puncture, bone marrow aspiration, arterial puncture, skin biopsy)

Local anesthetics (lidocaine) cause stinging, burning sensation

- Duration of stinging may depend on type of "caine" used

To avoid stinging sensation associated with lidocaine:

- Buffer the solution by adding 1 part of sodium bicarbonate (1 mEq/ml) to 10 parts of 1% lidocaine (see Guidelines box on p. 1097)

TOPICAL/TRANSDERMAL

EMLA (eutectic mixture of local anesthetics [lidocaine/prilocaine]) cream (Juhlin and Evers, 1990)

- Eliminates or reduces pain from most procedures involving skin puncture
- Must be placed over puncture site under occlusive dressing for 1 hour or more before procedure
- Provides skin anesthesia for up to 4 hours

TAC (tetracaine/adrenalin/cocaine) or ***TC (without adrenalin)***

- Provides skin anesthesia about 15 minutes after application (Engebo, 1990)
- Gel (preferably) or liquid placed on wounds for suturing (nonintact skin) (Bonadio and Wagner, 1990, 1992)
- Must not be used on mucous membranes and denuded areas because of the risk of systemic absorption and toxicity
- Adrenalin must not be used on end arterioles (fingers, toes, tip of nose, penis, earlobes) because of vasoconstriction

---

Data primarily from American Pain Society: *Principles of analgesic use in the treatment of acute pain or chronic cancer pain*, ed 2, Skokie, IL, 1992, The Society; and McCaffery M, Beebe A: *Pain: clinical manual for nursing practice*, St Louis, 1989, Mosby.

*For further information about compounding drugs in troches or suppositories, contact Technical Staff, Professional Compounding Centers of America, P.O. Box 368, Sugarland, TX 77487; (800) 331-2498.

ROUTES AND METHODS OF ANALGESIC DRUG ADMINISTRATION—cont'd

TRANSDERMAL FENTANYL (DURAGESIC)

Available as "patch" for continuous cancer pain control (Miser and others, 1989)
Safety and efficacy not established in children under 12 years
Not appropriate for initial relief of acute pain because of long interval to peak effect (from 12 to 24 hours)
Orders for "rescue doses" of an opioid should be available for pain that "breaks through"
Has duration of up to 72 hours for prolonged pain relief
If respiratory depression occurs, several doses of naloxone may be needed

RECTAL

Alternative to oral or parenteral routes
Variable absorption rate
Generally disliked by children, but often preferred over IM injection
Acceptance may be culturally influenced
Many drugs can be compounded into rectal suppositories*

REGIONAL NERVE BLOCK

Use of long-acting anesthetic (bupivacaine) injected into site, usually at end of surgery
Provides prolonged analgesia postoperatively, such as following inguinal herniorrhaphy (Hinkle, 1987)
May be used to provide local anesthesia for surgery, such as dorsal penile nerve block for circumcision (Spencer and others, 1992).

INHALATION

Use of anesthetics, such as nitrous oxide or halothane, to produce partial or complete analgesia for painful procedures (Perin and Frase, 1985; Wattenmaker, Kasser, and McGravey, 1990)
Occupational exposure to high levels of nitrous oxide may cause side effects (Baird, 1992; Rowland and others, 1992)

EPIDURAL/INTRATHECAL

Involves catheter placed into epidural or intrathecal space for continuous drip or intermittent administration of opioid (with or without a long-acting anesthetic, e.g., bupivacaine)
Analgesia primarily from drug's direct effect on opiate receptors in spinal canal
Provides steady drug levels and long-lasting analgesia
Respiratory depression is very rare but may have slow and delayed onset; can be prevented by checking level of consciousness and respiratory rate and depth hourly for initial 24 hours
Nausea, itching, and urinary retention are common dose-related side effects

TABLE 26-5 Selected Analgesics (Equianalgesia)

TRADE (GENERIC) DRUG*	EQUAL TO ORAL MORPHINE (mg)	EQUAL TO IM/IV MORPHINE (mg)
Propoxyphene hydrochloride (Darvon) 65 mg	4.8	1.6
Propoxyphene napsylate + acetaminophen (Darvocet-N 50)	4.8	1.6
30 mg codeine + 300 mg acetaminophen (Tylenol No. 3)	7.2	2.4
Oxycodone 5 mg + 325 mg acetaminophen (Percocet)	7.2	2.4
Oxycodone 5 mg + 325 mg aspirin (Percodan)	7.2	2.4
Hydrocodone 5 mg + 500 mg acetaminophen (Vicodin)	9	3
Oxycodone 5 mg + 500 mg acetaminophen (Tylox)	9	3
Acetaminophen (Tylenol Extra Strength) 500 mg	4	1.3
Transdermal fentanyl patch (Duragesic) (based on 25 µg patch applied q 3 days = 50 mg oral morphine q 24 hr or divided into 6 doses = 8.3 mg)	8.3	2.77

Table by Betty R. Ferrell, PhD, FAAN, 1994
*Oral medication with exception of Fentanyl.

and others, 1991, Ruble and Billet, 1993; Webb, Paarlberg, and Sussman, 1991). Nurses can efficiently use the infusion device on any-age child to administer analgesics without the need for signing for and preparing opioid injections every time one is needed. When used as "nurse"- or "parent"-controlled analgesia, the concept of patient control is negated and may more often lead to excessive dosing.

PCA infusion devices typically allow for three methods or modes of drug administration to be used alone or in combination:

1. **Patient-administered boluses** that can only be infused according to the preset amount and lockout interval (time between doses); more frequent "pushing of the button" means no drug is delivered, but the patient may need the dose and time adjusted for better pain control
2. **Nurse-administered boluses** that are typically used to give an initial loading dose to increase blood levels rapidly and to relieve breakthrough pain (pain not relieved with the usual programmed dose)
3. **Continuous basal or background infusion** that delivers a constant amount of analgesic and prevents pain from returning during those times, such as sleep, when the patient cannot control the infusion; may decrease safety of PCA

At the present time the optimum use of these three modes is under investigation. However, as with any type of analgesic management plan, continued assessment of the child's pain relief is essential for the greatest benefit from PCA (see Critical Thinking Exercise box on p. 1096). Typi-

CRITICAL THINKING EXERCISE

Pain Management—Patient-Controlled Analgesia

Juan, 9 years old, is hospitalized for a fractured pelvis and multiple other trauma as a result of a motor vehicle injury. Since admission he has been receiving patient-controlled analgesia (PCA) ordered as "morphine, 1.0 to 1.5 mg/hr, lock-out 10 minutes; bolus dose 1.5 mg, not to exceed one dose per hour." In assessing his pain, you note that he rates the pain a 4 on a scale of 0 to 5, no to worst pain, respectively, and he has been pushing the PCA button an average of 15 times an hour. The first action you take is to:

1. Tell Juan that he is pushing the button too often; he should wait 10 minutes before using the PCA machine.
2. Administer the bolus dose of morphine and reassess pain in 10 minutes.
3. Increase the hourly dose of morphine from 1.0 to 1.5 mg and reassess pain in 1 hour.
4. Contact the surgeon about Juan's inadequate pain management.

The correct answer is 2. Juan's pain is inadequately treated, and your first intervention is to give the ordered bolus dose. If the bolus dose relieves the pain to an acceptable level for Juan, the next step is to increase the hourly dose of 1.5 mg. Since the PCA order allows titrating (adjusting) the dosage upward, this action precedes calling the surgeon. It is absolutely inappropriate to tell Juan to push the PCA button less often; this response disregards his need for improved pain control and eliminates a valuable assessment parameter, the number of PCA uses.

cal uses of PCA are for controlling pain from surgery, sickle cell crisis, trauma, and cancer.

Morphine is the drug of choice for PCA and is usually prepared in a concentration of 1 mg/ml. Other options are hydromorphone (0.2 mg/ml) and fentanyl (0.01 mg/ml). Because PCA is typically used for continuous and extended pain control, meperidine should not be administered (see Nursing Alert, p. 1091). In addition, morphine, as compared with meperidine (via PCA for an average of about 37 hours), produced significantly better pain relief and fewer side effects in children (Vetter, 1992). Another risk of using meperidine is confusion between its concentration (10 mg/ml) and that of morphine when the PCA pump is programmed, which can result in undermedication or overmedication.

Another advance is the use of the ***epidural*** or ***intrathecal route,*** primarily postoperatively or in selected cases of terminal care. A catheter is placed into the epidural or intrathecal space of the spinal column. An opioid (usually fentanyl or preservative-free morphine), often with a long-acting local anesthetic (usually bupivacaine) is instilled via continuous-drip or intermittent administration. Analgesia results primarily from the drug's direct effect on opiate receptors in the spinal cord, rather than in the brain, which is responsible for undesirable effects (e.g., sedation and respiratory depression [McIlvaine, 1990; Sabbe and Yaksh, 1990]). Respiratory depression is rare, but if it occurs, it develops slowly and is evident several hours after the infusion.

NURSING ALERT When the epidural or intrathecal route is used, check the child's level of consciousness and respiratory rate and depth hourly for the first 24 hours to detect delayed-onset respiratory depression (American Pain Society, 1992)

Other routes that have benefited from new products for pain control are the ***oral transmucosal*** and ***transdermal routes.*** Oral transmucosal ***fentanyl*** (Fentanyl Oralet) provides nontraumatic preoperative oral sedation (Feld and others, 1989; Streisand and others, 1989) (see Surgical Procedures, Chapter 27). Fentanyl is also available as a transdermal patch (Duragesic). It may be used for older children and adolescents who have chronic cancer pain.

One of the most significant improvements in the ability to provide atraumatic care to children is the anesthetic cream, ***ELMA,**** a eutectic mixture of local anesthetics (lidocaine 2.5% and prilocaine 2.5%). The eutectic mixture, whose melting point is lower than that of the two anesthestics alone, permits effective concentrations of the drug to penetrate *intact* skin. A thick layer of cream is applied under an occlusive transparent dressing for 1 hour or more before procedures, such lumbar, venous, arterial, finger, heel, or earlobe punctures; implanted port access; insertion of peripherally inserted central catheters (PICC lines); superficial biopsy; skin graft; laser treatment of port wine stains; removal of epicardial (pacing) wires, chest tubes, or hair (electrolysis); bone marrow examination; and IM or SC injections (Koren, 1993; Sherwood, 1993; Taddio and others, 1994; Uhari, 1993). For deeper pain, such as IM injections, the application time should be extended up to 2 hours. For venous cannulation, two sites should be anesthetized to provide an alternative area if needed. The duration of anesthesia is up to 4 hours. Studies have reported that the maximum penetration depth is 5 mm after a 2-hour application time (Bjerring and Arendt-Nielsen, 1990; Juhlin and Evers, 1990), but clinical experience suggests that the penetration of depth may be greater.

➤ **NURSING TIP** Transparent film, such as plastic wrap, can be placed over the cream, with the edges sealed to the skin with tape, to provide an occlusive dressing. Use only a small amount of tape on the skin to avoid the discomfort caused by its removal.

EMLA is approved for children over 1 month of age but has been safely used on newborns during circumcision (Weatherstone and others, 1993). It should be used cautiously on infants between the ages of 1 and 12 months who are receiving treatment with methemoglobin-inducing agents, such as sulfonamides, phenytoin (Dilantin), and acetaminophen (Tylenol). However, the use of these drugs is not a contraindication for applying EMLA, and there are no reports of methemoglobinemia due to EMLA when an infant received acetaminophen. Because of their dimin-

*For additional information about EMLA, contact Astra Pharmaceuticals, (800) 228-EMLA.

GUIDELINES
Using Buffered Lidocaine (BL)

Supplies: 8.4% sodium bicarbonate (1 mEq/ml), 1% to 2% lidocaine with or without epinephrine, syringe with removable needle, and a 30-gauge needle

Instructions:

- Use 1 part sodium bicarbonate to 10 parts lidocaine (i.e., draw up 1 ml of lidocaine and 0.1 ml of sodium bicarbonate).
- Change needle used to withdraw BL to 30-gauge needle for intradermal injection.
- For venipuncture or port access, inject 0.1 ml or less BL intradermally directly over intended puncture site; anesthesia occurs almost immediately.
- Suggested maximum dose of lidocaine for local anesthesia is 4.5 mg/kg.
- If buffering lidocaine vial (e.g., 20 ml lidocaine with 2 ml sodium bicarbonate), use solution for 7 days or less and preferably when freshly prepared.

ished levels of erythrocyte-methemoglobin reductase, infants less than 3 months old are more susceptible to prilocaine-induced methemoglobinemia (Lloyd, 1992), a very rare and reversible side effect. Methemoglobin is a dysfunctional form of hemoglobin that reduces the oxygen-carrying capacity of the blood, causing cyanosis and hypoxemia. The use of intravenous methylene blue promptly eliminates the methemoglobinemia (Farrington, 1993).

Other side effects are very mild and include pallor, erthema, or edema at the application site. The nurse should observe whether pallor or erythema has occurred, because skin changes indicate that EMLA has been absorbed. Since absorption appears to be diminished in some children with darkly pigmented skin and thick skin, the application time should be a minimum of 90 minutes. Because of the tendency of children to disturb the dressing, safety precautions during the application time are important to prevent other rare complications, such as eating the cream, rubbing the cream in the eye, or placing the dressing in the mouth, with its placement across the vocal cords or anesthetization of the pharynx (Norman and Jones, 1990).

NURSING ALERT To make the dressing less accessible, cover it with a self-adhering Ace-type bandage, such as Coban. Label the dressing with "EMLA applied," the date, and the time to distinguish it from other types of dressings (Powers, 1994). Instruct older children not to disturb the dressing. (Covering the dressing with an opaque material may reduce the attraction and discourage "fingering.") Supervise younger or cognitively compromised children throughout the application time.

The ***intradermal route*** is often used to inject a local anesthetic, typically lidocaine (Zylocaine), into the skin to reduce the pain from a lumbar puncture, bone marrow aspiration, or venous or arterial access. One problem with the use of lidocaine is the stinging and burning that initially occur. However, the used of ***buffered lidocaine*** reduces the stinging sensation (McKay, Morris, and Mushlin, 1987; Orlinsky and others, 1992) (see Guidelines box). Warming the lidocaine to 37° C (98.6° F) may also accomplish the same effect (Davidson and Boom, 1992).

SIDE EFFECTS OF OPIOIDS

GENERAL

- Constipation (possibly severe)
- Respiratory depression
- Sedation
- Nausea and vomiting
- Agitation, euphoria
- Mental clouding
- Hallucinations
- Orthostatic hypotension
- Pruritus
- Urticaria
- Sweating
- Miosis (may be sign of toxicity)
- Anaphylaxis (rare)

SIGNS OF TOLERANCE

- Decreasing pain relief
- Decreasing duration of pain relief

SIGNS OF PHYSICAL DEPENDENCE

- Initial signs of withdrawal:
  - Lacrimation
  - Rhinorrhea
  - Yawning
  - Sweating
- Later signs:
  - Restlessness
  - Irritability
  - Tremors
  - Anorexia
  - Dilated pupils
  - Gooseflesh

Right Time. The right timing for administering analgesics depends on the type of pain. For continuous pain control, such as for postoperative or cancer pain, a preventive schedule of medication ***around the clock (ATC)*** is effective. The ATC schedule avoids the low plasma concentrations that permit breakthrough pain. If analgesics are administered only when pain returns (a typical use of the PRN, or "as needed," order), pain relief may take several hours. This may require higher doses, leading to a cycle of undermedication of pain alternating with periods of overmedication and drug toxicity. This cycle of erratic pain control also promotes "clock watching," which may be erroneously equated with "addiction." Nurses can effectively use PRN orders by giving the drug at regular intervals, since "as needed" can be interpreted to mean "as needed to prevent pain."

Preventive pain control is best provided through continuous IV infusion rather than intermittent boluses. If intermittent boluses are given, the intervals between doses should not exceed the drug's expected duration of effectiveness. For extended pain control with fewer administration times, drugs that provide longer duration of action (e.g., some NSAIDs, time-released morphine, methadone, levorphanol) can be used.

NURSING ALERT Since "breakthrough" pain can occur even with optimum ATC scheduling, there should be an order for PRN "rescue" doses of an analgesic.

Continuous analgesia is not always appropriate, because not all pain is continuous. Frequently, temporary pain control is needed to provide analgesia before a scheduled procedure. When pain can be predicted, the drug's peak effect should be timed to coincide with the painful event. For example, with opioids the peak effect is approximately ½ to 1 hour for the IM or SC route (considerably less for the

GUIDELINES

Managing Opioid-Induced Respiratory Depression

If respirations are depressed:

Reduce infusion by 25% when possible.

Stimulate patient (shake gently, call by name, ask to breathe).

Administer oxygen (consider naloxone).

If patient cannot be aroused or is apneic (American Pain Society, 1992):

Administer naloxone (Narcan):

For children less than 40 kg: dilute 0.1 mg of naloxone in 10 ml of sterile saline to make 10 μg/ml solution and give 0.5 μg/kg.

For children over 40 kg: dilute 0.4 mg ampule in 10 ml of sterile saline and give 0.5 ml.

Administer bolus IV push every 2 minutes until effect is obtained.

Closely monitor patient. Naloxone's duration of antagonist action may be shorter than that of opioid, requiring repeated doses of naloxone

NOTE: Respiratory depression due to benzodiazepines (e.g., diazepam [Valium] or midazolam [Versed]) can be reversed with flumazenil (Romazicon). Pediatric dosing experience suggests 0.01 mg/kg (0.1 ml/kg) as loading dose followed by 0.005 mg/kg/min (0.05 ml/kg/min) until awake or to a maximum of 1 mg (10 ml) (Jones and others, 1991). The recommended initial dose for children 20 kg or more is 0.2 mg (2 ml) IV over 15 seconds; if no response after 45 seconds, administer same dose and repeat as needed at 60-second intervals for maximum dose of 1 mg (10 ml).

IV route); with nonopioids the peak effect occurs about 2 hours after oral administration. For rapid onset and peak of action, opioids that quickly penetrate the blood-brain barrier (e.g., IV fentanyl) provide excellent pain control. (See also Surgical Procedures, Chapter 27.)

Observe for Side Effects. Both NSAIDs and opioids have side effects, although the major concern is with those from opioids (see box on p. 1097). Respiratory depression is the most serious complication and is most likely to occur in sedated patients. The respiratory rate may decrease gradually or may cease abruptly; lower limits of normal are not established for children, but any significant change from a previous rate calls for increased vigilance. A slower respiratory rate does not necessarily reflect decreased arterial oxygenation; an increased depth of ventilation may compensate for the altered rate (Rowbotham and others, 1989). If respiratory depression or arrest occurs, the nurse must be prepared to intervene quickly (Pasero and McCaffery, 1994) (see Guidelines box).

Although respiratory depression is the most feared side effect, constipation is a common side, and sometimes serious, effect of opioids, which decrease peristaltic activity and increase anal sphincter tone. Prevention with stool softeners and laxatives is more effective than treatment once constipation occurs. Dietary treatment, such as increased fiber, is usually not sufficient to promote regular bowel evacuation. However, dietary measures, such as increased fluid, fruit, and bran intake, as well as activity, are encouraged.

Pruritus from epidural or intrathecal infusion can be treated with low doses of naloxone infused slowly or with IV nalbuphine. Pruritus from IV infusion usually responds to oral antihistamines. Nausea, vomiting, and sedation usually subside after 2 days of opioid administration, although oral or rectal antiemetics may be necessary.

Both tolerance and physical dependence can occur with prolonged use of opioids. Treatment of tolerance involves increasing the dose or decreasing the duration between doses. Treatment of physical dependence involves gradually reducing the dose over several days to prevent occurrence of withdrawal symptoms (similar to tapering of steroid dosages after chronic steroid therapy). The following are suggested guidelines for treating physical dependence (American Pain Society, 1992):

- Gradually reduce dose (similar to tapering of steroids):
  Give one half of previous daily dose in q 6 hr doses for first 2 days.
  Then reduce dose by 25% every 2 days.
- Continue this schedule until total daily dose of 0.6 mg/kg/day of morphine (or equivalent) is reached.
- After 2 days on this dose, discontinue opioid.
- May also switch to oral methadone, using one fourth of equianalgesic dose as initial weaning dose and proceeding as described above.

The use of methadone in tapering doses over 5 days is effective in reducing symptoms of withdrawal (Miser and others, 1986).

Use supportive statements when administering analgesics. The effectiveness of analgesics can be enhanced by a supportive attitude toward the child. By reinforcing the cause and effect of the medication and analgesia, the nurse can condition the child to expect pain relief, provided the regimen is likely to be effective. Although IM injections should *not* be given, when they are, children need to understand that the "little hurt from the needle will take away the bigger hurt for a long time."

Parents and older children may have concerns about the use of opioids because of fear of addiction. These concerns should be addressed with assurance that any such risk is extremely low. It may be helpful to ask the question, "If you did not have this pain, would you want to take this medicine?" The answer is invariably no, which reinforces the solely therapeutic nature of the drug. It is also important to avoid making statements to the family such as "We don't want you to get used to this medicine" or "By now you shouldn't need this medicine," which may reinforce the fear of becoming addicted.

PROVIDING DEVELOPMENTALLY APPROPRIATE ACTIVITIES

A primary goal of nursing care for the child who is hospitalized is to minimize threats to the child's development. Many strategies (e.g., minimizing separation) have been discussed and may be all that the short-term patient requires. However, children who experience prolonged or repeated hospitalization are at greater risk for developmental delays or regression. The nurse who provides opportunities for the child to participate in developmentally appropriate activities further normalizes the child's environment and helps reduce interference with the child's ongoing development (see Normalization, Chapter 22).

Play is the "work" of children of all ages and assumes a critical role in their development. Because of its other important purposes in the hospital setting, play is the focus of a separate discussion.

Perhaps at no other age is the concept of interference with normal development more crucial than when it is applied to the rapidly developing infant and toddler. The nurse plays a primary role in identifying children at risk and helping to plan, implement, and evaluate developmental intervention (see Chapters 12 and 14).

School is an integral part of the school-age child's and adolescent's development. Accreditation standards for hospitals serving children consider access to appropriate educational services a key factor in the accreditation decision process when a child's treatment requires a significant absence from school (Joint Commission on Accreditation for Healthcare Organizations, 1992). The nurse can encourage children to resume schoolwork as quickly as their condition permits, help them schedule and protect a selected time for studies, and help the family coordinate hospital educational services with their children's schools. Children should have the opportunity to "keep up" with art and music classes, as well as their academic subjects.

➤ **NURSING TIP** When adolescents must share a common activity room with younger patients, referring to the area as the "activity" room rather than the "playroom" may entice them to visit the room and participate in activities.

Although regression is expected and normal, nurses have the responsibility of fostering children's optimum growth and development. Hospitalization can become a significant opportunity for learning and advancing. Extended hospitalizations for long-term chronic illness or situations of failure to thrive, abuse, or neglect represent instances in which regression must be seen as an adjustment period, to be followed by plans for promoting appropriate developmental skills.

USING PLAY/EXPRESSIVE ACTIVITIES TO MINIMIZE STRESS

Play is one of the most important aspects of a child's life and one of the most effective tools for managing stress. Since illness and hospitalization constitute crises in the child's life and often involve overwhelming stresses, playing out fears and anxieties gives the child a means to cope with these stresses.

Play is essential to children's mental, emotional, and social well-being. As with their developmental needs, the need for play does not stop when children are ill or when they enter the hospital. On the contrary, play in the hospital serves many functions (see box above, right). Of all hospital facilities, no room probably does more to alleviate the stressors of hospitalization than the playroom. In this room children temporarily distance themselves from the fears of separation, loss of control, and bodily injury. They can work through their feelings in a nonthreatening, comfortable atmosphere and in the manner most natural for them. They also know that the boundaries of this room are safe from intrusive or painful procedures, strange faces, and probing questions. The playroom becomes a sanctuary of peace and safety in an otherwise frightening environment.

FUNCTIONS OF PLAY IN THE HOSPITAL

- Provides diversion and brings about relaxation
- Helps the child feel more secure in a strange environment
- Helps to lessen stress of separation and the feelings of homesickness
- Provides a means for release of tension and expression of feelings
- Encourages interaction and development of positive attitudes toward others
- Provides an expressive outlet for creative ideas and interests
- Provides a means for accomplishing therapeutic goals (see Use of Play in Procedures, Chapter 27)
- Places child in active role and provides opportunity to make choices and be in control

Engaging in such activities puts children in charge, removing them for a time from the usual passive role of recipients of a constant stream of "things" being done to them. In the hospital environment most decisions are made for the child; play and other expressive activities offer the child much-needed opportunities to make choices. Even if a child chooses not to participate in a particular activity, the nurse has offered the child a choice, perhaps one of but a few real choices the child has had that day (Rollins, 1993).

Children in various age-groups require different types of play facilities. Infants and toddlers need maximum safety, whereas school-age children and adolescents benefit most from group recreation. Providing space for special needs of children in each age-group can be difficult in overcrowded institutions, but innovative solutions can ensure practical answers. Playroom schedules can accommodate children in one age-group at one session and another group at a later time; for example, adolescents can use the facility in the evening when younger children are asleep. Older children can also congregate in one patient's room and listen to music, play games, or just talk about their experiences. If the location of the recreational session is rotated each evening, older children can look forward to arranging or setting up for the activities.

Diversional Activities

Almost any form of play can be used for diversion and recreation, but the activity should be selected on the basis of the child's age, interests, and limitations (Fig. 26-11). Children do not necessarily need special direction for using play materials. All they require is the raw materials with which to work and adult approval and supervision to help keep their natural enthusiasm or expression of feelings from getting out of control. Small children enjoy a variety of small, colorful toys they can play with in bed or in their room or

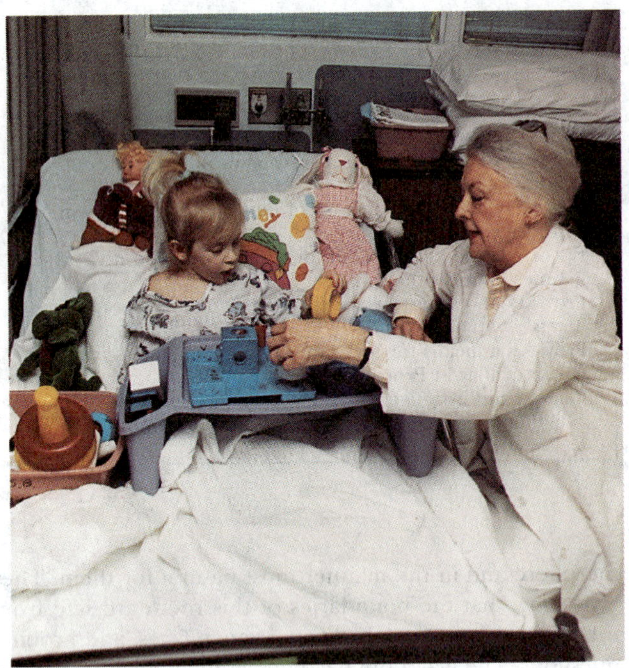

FIG. 26-11 Play materials for children in the hospital need to be appropriate for their age, interests, and limitations.

more elaborate play equipment, such as playhouses, sandboxes, rhythm instruments, and large boxes and blocks, that may be a part of the hospital playroom.

Games that can be played alone or with another child or an adult are popular with older children, as are puzzles; reading material; quiet individual activities such as sewing, stringing beads, and weaving; and Tinker-Toys, Lego blocks, and other building materials. Assembling models is an excellent pastime, but one should make certain that all pieces and necessary materials are included in the package so that the child is not disappointed.

Well-selected books are of infinite value to the child. Children never tire of stories. To have someone read aloud provides endless hours of pleasure and is of special value to the child who has limited energy to expend in play. A radio or television, part of most hospital room equipment, is a useful tool for entertaining a child, but parents and nurses should monitor program selection. Also, it should not be used as a substitute for social interaction or therapeutic play.

When supervising play for ill or convalescent children, it is best to select activities that are simpler than would normally be chosen according to the child's developmental level. These children usually do not have the energy to cope with more challenging activities. Other limitations also influence the type of activities. Special consideration must be given to the child who has limited movement, has a restricted extremity, or is isolated. Toys for isolated children must be capable of being disposed of or disinfected after use.

Toys. Parents of hospitalized children often ask nurses about the types of toys that would be best to bring for their child. Most want to bring new ones to cheer and comfort the child and assuage their own guilt feelings regarding the child's need for hospitalization. The nurse should tell the parents that, although wanting to provide these things for their child is natural, it is often better to wait awhile to bring new things, especially for younger children. Small children need the comfort and reassurance of familiar things, such as the stuffed animal the child hugs for comfort and takes to bed at night. These are a link with home and the world outside the hospital.

Large numbers of toys often confuse and frustrate a small child. A few small, well-chosen toys are usually preferred to one large, expensive one. Children who are hospitalized for an extended time benefit from changes. Rather than a confusing accumulation of toys, older toys should be replaced periodically as interest wanes.

➤ **NURSING TIP** Have parents provide the child with a shoe box, a child's small suitcase, or a knapsack to attach to the bed for an easy storage receptacle to prevent small items from becoming lost in the sheets or under the bed.

Children love putting things in and taking things out of a larger container. Many simple items, such as a small magnifying glass, a magnet, grooming aids, a small mirror, crayons and coloring books, colorful paper with scissors and paste, a magic slate, small dolls or toy soldiers, small cars, and beads to string, provide endless hours of amusement. The nurse is responsible for assessing the safety of the toys brought to the child.

A highly successful diversion for a child who is hospitalized for a length of time and whose parents are unable to visit frequently is for them to bring a box with seven small, inexpensive, and brightly wrapped items with a different day of the week printed on the outside. The child will eagerly anticipate the time for opening each one. When the parents know when their next visit will be, they can provide the number of packages that corresponds to the days between visits. In this way the child knows that the diminishing packages also represent the anticipated visit from the parent.

Expressive Activities

Play provides one of the best opportunities for encouraging emotional expression, including the safe release of anger and hostility. Nondirective play that allows children freedom for expression can be very therapeutic. Therapeutic play, however, should not be confused with the psychologic technique of play therapy. ***Play therapy*** is reserved for use by trained and qualified therapists who use the technique as an interpretative method with emotionally disturbed children. ***Therapeutic play***, on the other hand, is a very effective nondirective modality for helping children deal with their concerns and fears; at the same time, it often helps the nurse to gain insights into their needs and feelings.

Tension release can be facilitated through almost any activity. With younger ambulatory children, large-muscle activity such as use of tricycles and wagons is especially beneficial. Much aggression can be safely directed into games and activities that involve pounding and throwing. Bean-

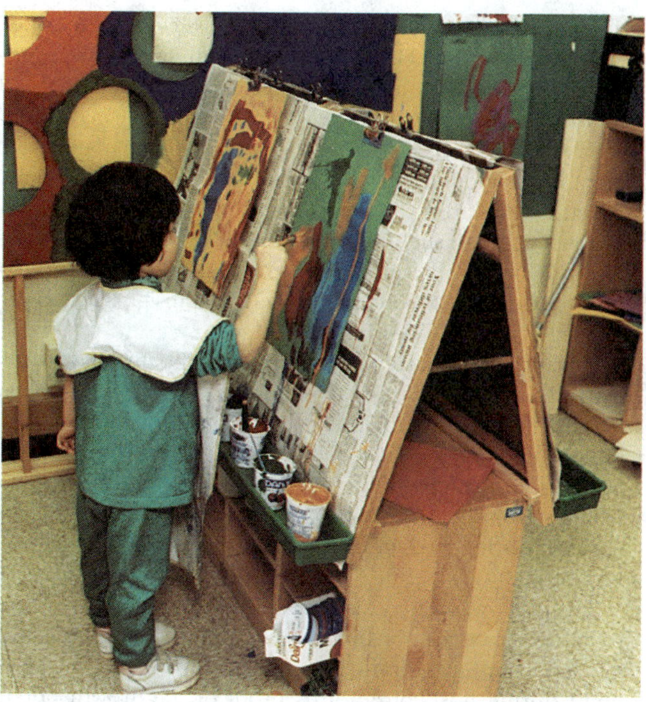

FIG. 26-12 Drawing and painting are excellent media for expression.

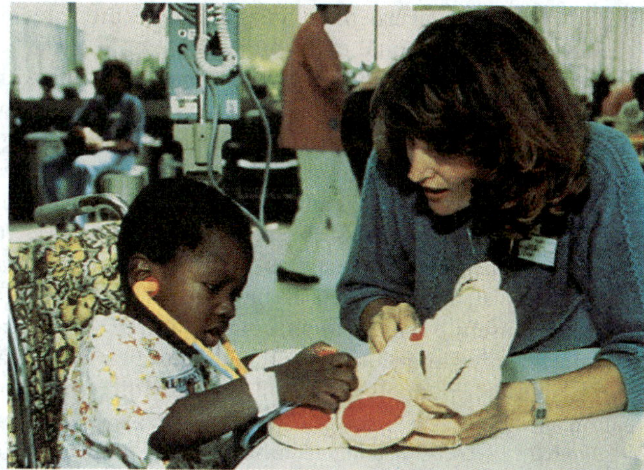

FIG. 26-13 Playing with miniature hospital equipment allows children to explore feelings and concerns and achieve mastery over hospital situations. (Courtesy St. Louis Children's Hospital.)

bags are often thrown at a target or open receptacle with surprising vigor and hostility. A pounding board is employed with enthusiasm by young children; clay and playdough are beneficial at any age. An angry child of 9 or 10 years of age may attack a mound of clay with the same intensity as a 3- or 4-year-old.

Creative Expression. The visual arts, music, dance/movement, and storytelling offer excellent opportunities for creative expression activities. A limited number of pediatric units have artist-in-residency programs to facilitate such activities. However, it can be relatively simple for nurses to support creative expression for children in hospital settings.

Drawing and painting are excellent media for expression (Fig. 26-12). Children are more at ease expressing their thoughts and feelings through art, because humans think first in images and later learn to translate these images into words. The child needs only to be supplied with the raw materials, such as crayons and paper; pots of bright poster color, large brushes, and an ample supply of newsprint supported on easels; or materials for finger painting. Children usually require little direction for self-expression; however, older children may be given some direction in what to paint or draw. For example, they may be asked to draw the hospital room or draw what they like or do not like about the hospital. Groups of children can enjoy this creative activity either working individually or, with older children, collaborating on a group project such as a mural painted on a long piece of paper. For children confined to bed, an old sheet (acquired from the laundry) spread over the bed and a large gown that extends down over the bedclothes to cover their own gown provide protection for clean linen.

While interpretation of children's drawing requires special training, observing changes in a series of the child's drawings over time can be helpful in assessing psychosocial adjustment and coping (Rae, 1991). The nurse can use children's drawings, stories, poetry, and other products of creative expression as a springboard for discussion of thoughts, fears, and understanding of concepts or events.

➤ **NURSING TIP** Have the child select a place he or she would like to visit. Help the child decorate the bed and equipment to suit the theme of the imaginary trip (e.g., truck, circus tent, spaceship, sky). At a set time each day, pretend to go with the child to the special place. Consider including props such as a suitcase or picnic basket (Hart and others, 1992).

Nurses can incorporate opportunities for musical expression into routine nursing care. For example, simple musical instruments, such as bracelets with bells, can be placed on infants' legs for them to shake to accompany mealtime music or dressing changes. Dance/movement suggestions may encourage a child to ambulate.

Holidays provide stimulus and direction for unlimited creative projects. The children can participate in decorating the pediatric unit, and making pictures and decorations for their rooms gives the children a sense of pride and accomplishment (see Nursing Tip above). This is especially beneficial for immobilized and isolated children. Making gifts for someone at home helps to maintain interpersonal ties.

Dramatic Play. Dramatic play is a well-recognized technique for emotional release, allowing children to reenact frightening or puzzling hospital experiences. Through use of puppets, replicas of hospital equipment, or some actual hospital equipment, children can play out the situations that are a part of their hospital experience (Fig. 26-13). Dramatic play enables children to learn about procedures and events that will concern them and to assume the roles of the adults in the hospital environment.

Puppets are universally effective for communicating with children. Most children view them as peers and readily communicate with them. Children will tell the puppet feelings that they hesitate to express to adults. Puppets can share children's own experiences and help them to find solutions to their problems. Puppets dressed to represent figures in the child's environment (e.g., a physician, nurse, child patient, therapist, and members of the child's own family) are especially useful. Small, appropriately attired dolls are equally effective in encouraging the child to play out situations, although puppets are usually best for direct conversation.

➤ **NURSING TIP** Make a simple puppet using a large handkerchief. Place some cotton balls in the center of the cloth and wrap a rubberband over the handkerchief and cotton balls to form a "head." Place the head over the index finger so that the rubberband secures it to the finger. Let the cloth drape over the front and back of the hand. The cloth forms four parts of the puppet: the index finger is the head, the thumb and other fingers are the arms, and the draped cloth is the body. Decorate the head by drawing features on it (Wong, 1993).

Play and other expressive activities must consider medical needs and any limitations imposed by the child's condition. For example, small children may eat paste and other creative media; therefore a child who is allergic to wheat should not be given finger paint made from wallpaper paste or playdough made with flour. A small child on a restricted salt intake should not play with modeling dough, since salt is one of its major constituents.* Treatment schedules and the institution's rules and policies must also be considered. At home play should be planned around the therapy regimen. However, play can be satisfactorily incorporated into the child's care if the nurse and others involved allow some flexibility and use creativity in planning for play.

MAXIMIZING POTENTIAL BENEFITS OF HOSPITALIZATION

While hospitalization generally represents a stressful time for children and families, it also presents an opportunity for facilitating positive change within the child and among family members. Therefore nursing interventions must also focus on maximizing the potential benefits of the experience.

Fostering Parent-Child Relationships

The crisis of illness or hospitalization can mobilize parents into more acute awareness of their children's needs. For example, one school-age child who was diagnosed with a serious physical condition commented to the nurse that he "enjoyed" the hospital because it was the first time that he had seen so much of his parents. He expressed concern over discharge because he anticipated the loss of the intensified love and attention. The nurse was able to discuss these feelings with the parents and to increase their awareness of their child's need for them.

Hospitalization provides opportunities for parents to learn more about their children's growth and development. When parents are helped to understand children's usual reactions to stress, such as regression or aggression, they are not only better able to support the child through the hospital experience but also may extend their insights into childrearing practices following discharge.

Difficulties in parent-child relationships that may result in feeding problems, negative behavior, and enuresis may decrease during hospitalization. The temporary cessation of such problems sometimes alerts parents to the role they may be playing in propagating the negative behavior. With assistance from health professionals, parents can restructure ways of relating to their children to foster more positive behavior.

Hospitalization may also represent a temporary reprieve or refuge from a disturbed home. Typically, abused or neglected children's dramatic physical and social improvement during hospitalization is proof of the growth potential of this experience. Hospitalized children temporarily are able to seek support, reassurance, and security from new relationships, particularly with nurses, hospitalized peers, and others.

Providing Educational Opportunities

Illness and hospitalization represent excellent opportunities for children and other family members to learn more about their bodies, each other, and the health professions. For example, during a child's admission for a diabetic crisis, the child may learn about the disease; the parents may learn about the child's needs for independence, normalcy, and appropriate limits; and each of them may find a new support system in the hospital staff.

The special tutoring that children may receive during extended hospitalization can help them advance their studies and concentrate on difficult subjects. The child's relationship with a tutor can foster a more positive attitude toward school and learning.

Illness or hospitalization can also help older children in choosing a vocational career. Frequently children have impressions of physicians or nurses that are disproportionately glorified or horrified. However, experience with different health professionals can influence their decision for or against a health career.

Promoting Self-Mastery

The experience of facing a crisis such as illness or hospitalization, coping successfully with it, and maturing as a result of it constitutes an opportunity for self-mastery. Younger children have the chance to test out fantasy vs reality fears. They realize that they were not abandoned, mutilated, castrated, or punished. In fact, they were loved, cared for, and treated with respect for their individual concerns. It is not unusual to hear children who have undergone hospitalization or surgery tell others of how "it was nothing" or proudly

*A national clearinghouse for research and education in visual and performing arts can be contacted at the **Center for Safety in the Arts,** 5 Beckman St., Suite 1030, New York, NY 10038; (212) 227-6220.

display their scars or bandages. For older children, hospitalization may represent an opportunity for decision making, independence, and self-reliance. They are proud of having survived the experience and may feel a genuine self-respect for their achievements. Nurses can facilitate such feelings of self-mastery by emphasizing aspects of personal competence in the child and not acknowledging uncooperative or negative behavior.

Providing Socialization

Hospitalization may offer children a special opportunity for social acceptance. Lonely, asocial, sometimes delinquent children find a sympathetic environment in the hospital. Children who are physically deformed or in some other way "different" from their age-mates may find an accepting social peer group. Although this does not always spontaneously occur, nurses can structure the environment to foster a supportive child group. For example, judicious selection of a roommate can help children gain a new friend and learn more about themselves. Forming relationships with significant members of the health care team, such as the physician, nurse, child-life specialist, or minister, can greatly enhance the child's adjustment in many areas of life.

Parents may also encounter a new social group in other parents who have similar problems. The waiting room or hallway "self-help" groups are part of every institution. Nurses can capitalize on this informal gathering by encouraging parents to discuss collectively their concerns and feelings. They can also refer parents to organized parent groups or can use the help and support of recovered hospitalized patients.

SUPPORTING FAMILY MEMBERS

The term ***family-centered care*** defines the focus of pediatric care because nursing of children cannot be optimally performed unless each family member is designated the "patient" or "client" (see Family-Centered Care, Chapter 1). Support involves the willingness to stay and listen to parents' verbal and nonverbal messages. Sometimes the support is not given directly by the nurse. For example, the nurse may offer to stay with the child to allow the parents time alone or may discuss with other family members the parents' need for extra relief. Often, extended relatives and friends want to help but do not know how. The nurse can suggest baby-sitting, preparing meals, tending the garden or home, doing laundry, or transporting the siblings to school as ways to lessen the parents' responsibilities. An ongoing parent support group held on the pediatric unit during the children's traditional "naptime" has also proved effective in helping parents share emotions and concerns related to hospitalization (Nugent and others, 1992).

Support may also be provided through the clergy. Parents with deep religious beliefs may appreciate the counsel of a clergy member, but because of their stress they may not have sufficient energy to initiate the contact. Nurses can be supportive by arranging for clergy to visit and by respecting and upholding parents' religious beliefs.

Support involves an acceptance of cultural, socioeconomic, and ethnic values. For example, health and illness are defined differently by various ethnic groups. For some, disorders that have few outward manifestations of illness, such as diabetes, hypertension, or cardiac problems, are not viewed as a sickness. Consequently, following a prescribed treatment may be seen as unnecessary. Nurses who appreciate the influences of culture are more likely to intervene therapeutically (see also Chapter 2 for an extensive discussion of cultural/religious influences on health care).

Parents need help in accepting their own feelings toward the ill child. If given the opportunity, parents often disclose their feelings of loss of control, anger, and guilt. They often resist admitting to such feelings because they expect others to disapprove of behavior that is less than perfect. Unfortunately, health personnel, including nurses, sometimes show little tolerance for deviation from the expected norm. This only increases the psychologic impact of a child's illness on family members. Helping parents identify the specific reason for such feelings and emphasizing that each is a normal, expected, and healthy response to stress provides them with an opportunity to lessen their emotional burden. Support may also include preparing siblings for hospital visits, assessing their adjustment, and providing appropriate interventions or referrals when needed.

Providing Information

One of the most important nursing interventions is to provide information regarding (1) the disease, its treatment, and prognosis; (2) the child's emotional, as well as physical, reaction to illness and hospitalization; and (3) the probable emotional reactions of family members to the crisis.

For many families the child's illness is their first contact with the hospital experience. Often parents are not prepared for the child's behavioral reactions to hospitalization, such as separation behaviors, regression, aggression, and hostility. Providing the parents with information about these normal and expected behavioral responses can lessen the parents' anxiety during the hospital admission (Vulcan

Text continued on p. 1108.

GUIDELINES

Helping Families Elicit Information

- Find out what the family wants to know.
- Teach them to avoid general questions, such as, "Why is my child sick?"
- Help them prepare specific questions, such as, "What is causing my child's pain?" or "What does this drug do?"
- Encourage the use of short and open-ended questions.
- Have the family write down the questions, preferably in a diary or journal that is kept in an accessible area, such as a pocket, to have available when needed.
- Encourage the family to speak up when they do not understand an answer and to have it explained in clearer or easier language.
- Have the family repeat the information to be certain they understand it and to record unfamiliar terms.

Modified from Norris L: Coaching the question, *Nursing 86* 16 (5):100, 1986.

NURSING CARE PLAN
The Child in the Hospital

NURSING DIAGNOSIS: Anxiety/fear related to separation from accustomed routine and support system; unfamiliar surroundings

PATIENT GOAL 1: Will experience minimized separation.

• **NURSING INTERVENTIONS/*RATIONALES***

Assign same nursing personnel as much as possible and a primary nurse *to provide the consistency that builds trust*
Arrange workload and schedule to allow personal contact with child
Encourage parents to room-in whenever possible *to prevent separation*
Provide an atmosphere of warmth and acceptance for both child and parents
Encourage parents and others to cuddle, hug, and otherwise demonstrate affection for child
Recognize child's separation behaviors as normal
- Allow child to cry, *since this is a normal response to separation*
- Provide support through physical presence

Maintain child's contact with parents and siblings
- Talk about child's parents frequently
- Encourage child to talk about and remember family members, pets
- Stress significance of parents' and siblings' visits, telephone calls, or letters

Help parents understand the behaviors of separation anxiety and suggest ways of supporting the child
- Explain to child when parents leave and when they will return
- Tell hospitalized child the reason for leaving
- Convey the expected time of return in terms of anticipated events. For example, if the parents will return in the morning, they can say they will see the child, "After the sun comes up," or, "When (a favorite program) is on television"
- Use a clock or calendar for an older child *so child can anticipate next family visit*
- Visit for short but frequent times rather than one long time; encourage parents and relatives to taken turns visiting
- Encourage siblings, grandparents, and other significant persons in child's life to visit
- Leave favorite articles from home, such as a blanket, toy, bottle, feeding utensil, or article of clothing, with child, *since this helps child tolerate separation*
- Respect treasured objects of older children, such as a stuffed animal
- Encourage family to provide photographs of family members and recordings of the parents' voices (e.g., reading a story, singing a song, saying prayers before bedtime, or relating events at home) *to familiarize the unfamiliar environment and to provide comfort during times of separation*

Play family recordings at lonely times, such as before sleep
Suggest that the family leave small gifts for the child to open each day: if the parents know when their next visit will be, have them leave the number of packages that correspond to the days between visits
Assign a "foster grandparent" or consistent volunteer to be with child if available

• **EXPECTED OUTCOMES**

Child has consistent caregivers
Parents visit as much as possible
Parents cooperate in care (specify)
Child accepts and responds positively to comforting measures
Child discusses the family, including pets
Parents demonstrate an understanding of separation behaviors
Siblings, grandparents, and other significant persons visit as much as possible
Family provides child with familiar and/or cherished articles from home
Assigned person spends time with child (specify amount)

PATIENT GOAL 2: Will express feelings

• **NURSING INTERVENTIONS/*RATIONALES***

Accept expression of feelings *so that child continues these expressions*
Provide an atmosphere that encourages free expression of feelings
Provide opportunities for the child to verbalize, "play out," or otherwise express feelings without fear of punishment
Encourage drawing and other expressive activities *because children often find it easier to express themselves in images instead of words*
Encourage keeping a journal or diary *to allow child to review progress and changes in feelings*

• **EXPECTED OUTCOME**

Child verbalizes or plays out feelings or concerns

PATIENT GOAL 3: Will remain calm

• **NURSING INTERVENTIONS/*RATIONALES***

Do nothing to make child more anxious, remembering that what may not provoke anxiety in an adult may make a child very anxious
Maintain calm, relaxed, and reassuring manner
Spend time with child and family *to establish rapport*
Give competent, consistent nursing care *to instill confidence in both parents and child*
Try to avoid intrusive procedures

• **EXPECTED OUTCOMES**

Child exhibits no signs of apprehension
Parents relate readily with personnel and calmly with child
Child rests quietly and calmly

NURSING CARE PLAN
The Child in the Hospital—cont'd

PATIENT GOAL 4: Will exhibit trusting behaviors

• **NURSING INTERVENTIONS/*RATIONALES***
Be positive in approach to child
Be honest with child *to encourage child to trust*
Convey to child the behaviors expected
Be consistent in expectations and relationships with child *because consistency is an important component of the development of trust*
Treat child fairly and help child to feel this
Encourage parents to maintain a truthful relationship with the child
Make certain child has call light or other signal device within reach

• **EXPECTED OUTCOMES**
Child develops rapport with primary nurse
Child maintains trust of family

PATIENT GOAL 5: Will experience feelings of security

• **NURSING INTERVENTIONS/*RATIONALES***
Maintain child's identity
Address child by name or usual nickname
Avoid assigning a nickname to child or converting a given name to its counterpart in another language (e.g., using Joe instead of José)
Avoid communicating any signals of rejection, distaste, or other negative feelings to child
Criticize or communicate disapproval of unacceptable *behavior,* not disapproval of the *child*
Communicate (verbally and nonverbally) that the child is a valued person
Discourage treatments or procedures in the child's room or playroom *to maintain these areas as "safe places"*

• **EXPECTED OUTCOMES**
Child interacts with staff
*Staff demonstrates respect for child

PATIENT GOAL 6: Will experience reduction of or no fear

• **NURSING INTERVENTIONS/*RATIONALES***
Explain routines, items, procedures, and events in a language and method appropriate to the child's developmental level; use simple language, drawings, and play *to facilitate understanding and mastery*
Reassure child and repeat reassurance as necessary
Ask child to explain reason for hospitalization and correct if necessary *to help absolve child from any guilt about being hospitalized*
Encourage parent(s) to participate in child's care
Encourage child to handle items that may seem strange or threatening *to reduce fear of the unknown*
Give encouragement and positive feedback for cooperation in care

• **EXPECTED OUTCOMES**
Child exhibits understanding of information presented (specify information and means of demonstration)
Child discusses procedures and activities without evidence of anxiety

PATIENT GOAL 7: Will be allowed to regress

• **NURSING INTERVENTIONS/*RATIONALES***
Recognize that regressive behavior is a feature of illness *so that it is not viewed as abnormal*
Accept regressive behavior and help child with dependency
Assist child in reconquering the negative counterpart of the psychosocial stage to which child has regressed (e.g., overcome mistrust; facilitate development of trust)

• **EXPECTED OUTCOME**
*Staff and parents exhibit an attitude of acceptance of regressive behaviors

PATIENT GOAL 8: Will experience adequate comfort level

• **NURSING INTERVENTIONS/*RATIONALES***
Provide pacifier, if appropriate, *to meet oral needs and to provide comfort*
Hold infant or young child when this does not interfere with therapy
Touch, talk, and otherwise comfort child who cannot be held
Provide sensory stimulation and diversion appropriate to child's level of development
Encourage family members to visit and allow them to comfort and care for child to the extent possible

• **EXPECTED OUTCOMES**
Child engages in nonnutritive sucking
Child exhibits no signs of distress
Family is involved in care

NURSING DIAGNOSIS: Anxiety/fear related to distressing procedures, events

PATIENT GOAL 1: Will be prepared for hospitalization

• **NURSING INTERVENTIONS/*RATIONALES***
Prepare child as needed *to reduce fear of the unknown and to promote cooperation*
Select appropriate preparatory materials
Involve parents *to enable them to serve as effective resources for their child*
Modify preparation in special situations (e.g., day hospital, emergency admission, ICU) (see box on p. 1115)

• **EXPECTED OUTCOME**
Child is prepared for hospital experience

*Nursing outcome.

Continued.

NURSING CARE PLAN
The Child in the Hospital—cont'd

PATIENT GOAL 2: Will exhibit decreased fear of bodily injury

• **NURSING INTERVENTIONS/*RATIONALES***
Recognize developmental fears associated with illness and procedures *to ensure appropriate intervention*
Provide age-appropriate explanations for procedures, especially those that are intrusive or involve the genitals, and include information about what body parts will not be affected, as well as those that will
Provide age-appropriate explanations for procedures the child may see or hear performed on other patients *to decrease child's fears*
Reassure child that certain body parts can be removed without producing harm (e.g., blood, tonsils, appendix)
Provide privacy for any procedure that exposes the body
Protect child from seeing unclothed patients
Use interventions that preserve child's concept of body integrity (e.g., bandages over puncture sites)

• **EXPECTED OUTCOME**
Child displays minimum fear of bodily injury

PATIENT GOAL 3: Will receive support during tests and procedures

• **NURSING INTERVENTIONS/*RATIONALES***
Prepare child for procedures according to age and level of understanding, including strategies for coping
Remain with child *to provide support by physical presence*
Prepare child and family for surgery if appropriate
Answer questions and explain purposes of activities
Keep child (and family) informed of progress

• **EXPECTED OUTCOME**
Child remains calm and cooperative during procedures

NURSING DIAGNOSIS: Powerlessness related to the health care environment

PATIENT GOAL 1: Will experience "homelike" atmosphere in the hospital environment

• **NURSING INTERVENTIONS/*RATIONALES***
Determine from parents or other caregiver the child's customary routine and the usual manner of handling the child (see box on pp. 1116-1117)
Maintain a routine similar to the one the child is accustomed to at home
Minimize a hospital-like environment as much as possible; allow child to sit at table to eat meals, wear own pajamas or street clothes
Use terms familiar to child, such as those for body functions
Encourage patients with extended hospitalizations to decorate room (e.g., pictures, bedspread from home) *to make it more "homelike"*
Encourage sibling visitation
Explore the possibility of pet visitation for children with extended hospitalizations

• **EXPECTED OUTCOME**
Child's routines and environment are similar to those at home (specify)

PATIENT GOAL 2: Will experience opportunities to exert control

• **NURSING INTERVENTIONS/*RATIONALES***
Allow child choices whenever possible, such as food selection, clothing, options for time of basic care (bath, play, bedtime), selection of television channels, choice of activities *to give child some measure of control*
Use time structuring with an older child (a jointly planned and written schedule of daily activities)
Permit freedom on the unit within defined and enforced limitations
Explain the reason for physically restraining a child to both child and parents
Encourage self-care according to child's abilities
Assign tasks to an older child, especially in extended hospitalization (e.g., making the bed, supervising younger children, distributing menus, collating charts)
Respect child's need for privacy

• **EXPECTED OUTCOMES**
Child participates in planning care (specify)
Child moves about the unit but respects limits
Child participates in care activities (specify activities)
Child assumes responsibility for tasks (specify)
*Child's need for privacy is maintained

NURSING DIAGNOSIS: Diversional activity deficit related to impaired mobility, musculoskeletal impairment, confinement to hospital or home, effects of illness

PATIENT GOAL 1: Will have opportunity to participate in activities

• **NURSING INTERVENTIONS/*RATIONALES***
Schedule therapies and periods of rest to allow for activities
Involve child in planning care to the extent of capabilities *to reduce feelings of passivity*
Arrange for and encourage interaction with others as feasible *to promote socialization*
Encourage visits from family and friends
Provide opportunity to socialize with noninfectious children

• **EXPECTED OUTCOMES**
Child helps plan care and schedule
Child interacts with family and other children

*Nursing outcome.

NURSING CARE PLAN
The Child in the Hospital—cont'd

PATIENT GOAL 2: Will have opportunity to participate in diversional activities

• **NURSING INTERVENTIONS/*RATIONALES***

Spend time with child

Query child and parents regarding child's favorite diversional activities

Change position of bed in room periodically *to alter sensory stimuli* if child is confined to bed

Provide activities appropriate to child's condition, physical limitations, and developmental level

Encourage family to caress and hold infant or child

Maintain accustomed routine at home and, when possible, if hospitalized

Consult with a child-life specialist *to provide diversional activities*

Encourage interaction with other children

Choose a roommate compatible in age, sex, and physical abilities

Monitor time spent watching television or playing electronic games vs interactive or creative activities

Allow ample time for play

Make play, art, music, and other expressive materials available to child

Encourage play activities and diversions appropriate to child's age, condition, and capabilities

Help facilitate an activity by acting under the child's instructions to perform tasks the child is unable to do

Use play as a teaching strategy and an anxiety-reducing technique

Promote the use of a separate activity room or area for adolescents

• **EXPECTED OUTCOMES**

Child engages in activities appropriate for age, interests, and physical limitations (specify activities)

Child receives attention and comfort

Child engages in age-appropriate play (specify)

NURSING DIAGNOSIS: Activity intolerance related to generalized weakness, fatigue, imbalance between oxygen supply and demand

PATIENT GOAL 1: Will maintain adequate energy levels

• **NURSING INTERVENTIONS/*RATIONALES***

Assess child's level of physical tolerance

Anticipate child's need for rest, as evidenced by irritability, short attention span, and fretfulness; assist child in those activities of daily living that may be beyond tolerance

Provide entertainment and quiet diversional activities appropriate to child's age and interest *to conserve energy*

Provide diversional play activities *that promote rest and quiet but prevent boredom and withdrawal*

Choose an appropriate roommate of similar age and interests and one who requires restricted activity *to decrease feelings of loneliness and sadness*

Instruct child to rest when feeling tired

Balance rest and activity when ambulatory

• **EXPECTED OUTCOMES**

Child plays and rests quietly and engages in activities appropriate to age and capabilities (specify)

Child exhibits no evidence of intolerance

Child tolerates increasingly more activity

PATIENT GOAL 2: Will receive optimum rest

• **NURSING INTERVENTIONS/*RATIONALES***

Provide quiet environment *to promote rest*

Organize activities for maximum sleep time

Schedule visiting to allow for sufficient rest

Keep visiting periods with friends and family short

Encourage parents to remain with child *to decrease separation and anxiety*

*Administer sedatives and analgesics as indicated if ordered for restlessness and pain

Encourage frequent rest periods

Enforce regular sleep times

Follow child's usual routine for bedtime, nap time

Implement measures to ensure sleep, such as quiet, darkened room

Be alert to signs that child is tired or overstimulated *to allow flexibility in scheduling or enforcing rest and sleep periods*

• **EXPECTED OUTCOMES**

Child remains calm, quiet, and relaxed

Child gets a sufficient amount of rest (specify)

NURSING DIAGNOSIS: High risk for injury/trauma related to unfamiliar environment, therapies, hazardous equipment

PATIENT GOAL 1: Will experience no injury

• **NURSING INTERVENTIONS/*RATIONALES***

Employ environmental safety measures *to prevent injuries*

Report any potential hazards (e.g., slippery floors, poor illumination, electrical hazards, damaged or malfunctioning furniture or equipment, unprotected windows, stairwells)

Dispose of small breakable items appropriately (thermometers, bottles)

Keep potentially hazardous articles out of child's reach

Check bathwater for temperature before bathing infant or child *to prevent burns*

Maintain surveillance of children in bathtub/shower

Keep crib sides up and securely fastened; use siderails for children who may fall out of bed

Use safety restraints only when absolutely necessary
- Remove as often as possible
- Discontinue as soon as possible

*Dependent nursing activity.

Continued.

NURSING CARE PLAN
The Child in the Hospital—cont'd

Check regularly for adequate circulation to the restrained area and any pressure points and that restraint is applied properly
Maintain hand contact while caring for a child in a crib with siderails down *to prevent falls*
Transport infants and children appropriately
Hold with proper support
Fasten safety belt on gurney, wheelchair
Alert parents and ancillary hospital personnel regarding child's physical tolerance and need for assistance during activity
Fasten safety belts in high chairs, swings

• EXPECTED OUTCOME
Child remains free of injury

NURSING DIAGNOSIS: Bathing/hygiene and dressing/grooming self-care deficit related to physical or cognitive disability, mechanical restrictions

PATIENT GOAL 1: Will engage in self-help activities

• NURSING INTERVENTIONS/*RATIONALES*
Allow child to help plan own daily routine and choose from alternatives when appropriate *to promote sense of control*
Encourage participation in self-care activities according to developmental level and capabilities *to promote mastery and decrease regression*
Provide devices, equipment, and methods to assist child in self-care
Advocate for child-sized features *that foster independence* (e.g., bathroom door handles low enough for children to reach)
Assist with dressing, grooming, bathing as indicated

• EXPECTED OUTCOME
Child engages in self-help activities to maximum capabilities

NURSING DIAGNOSIS: Toileting self-care deficit related to physical or cognitive disability, mechanical restrictions

PATIENT GOAL 1: Will exhibit normal elimination patterns

• NURSING INTERVENTIONS/*RATIONALES*
Solicit information from child and parents regarding child's normal patterns and procedures of elimination
Sit child in upright position when possible *to encourage elimination*
Employ special devices where appropriate (e.g., fracture pan, commode, elevated toilet seat)
Carry out bowel-training program with hydration, high-fiber diet, stool softeners, and mild laxatives if needed
Provide privacy *to promote relaxation needed for elimination*

• EXPECTED OUTCOME
Child has daily bowel movement

NURSING DIAGNOSIS: Altered patterns of urinary elimination related to discomfort, positioning

PATIENT GOAL 1: Will exhibit normal voiding

• NURSING INTERVENTIONS/*RATIONALES*
Solicit information from child and parents regarding child's normal patterns and procedures of elimination
Position child as upright as possible to void
Hydrate child *to ensure adequate urinary output for age*
Stimulate bladder emptying with warm water, running water, stroking suprapubic area
Catheterize as indicated

See also:
Nursing Care Plan: The Child with Chronic Illness or Disability, Chapter 22
Nursing Care Plan: The Child Undergoing Surgery, Chapter 27
Nursing Care Plan: The Child Who Is Terminally Ill or Dying, Chapter 23
Nursing Care Plan for specific health problem(s)

and Nikulich-Barrett, 1988). The family is equally unfamiliar with hospital rules, which often adds to feelings of confusion and anxiety. Therefore the family needs clear explanations about what to expect and what is expected of them. Nurses can also help family members become more adept at seeking information about their child's condition by asking questions that elicit meaningful information (see Guidelines box on p. 1103). In giving information, nurses need to be alert to information overload (see box on p. 191).

Parents also need to be aware of the effects of illness on the family and strategies that prevent negative changes. Specifically, parents should keep the family well informed and communicating as much as possible. They should treat all the children as equally and as normally as before the illness occurred. Discipline, which initially may be lessened for the ill child, should be continued to provide a measure of security and predictability. When ill children know that their parents expect certain standards of conduct from them, they feel certain that they will recover. When all limits are removed, they fear that something catastrophic will happen.

Helping parents understand and accept the meaning of posthospitalization behaviors in the sick child is necessary for them to tolerate and support such behaviors. Conse-

NURSING CARE PLAN
The Family of the Ill or Hospitalized Child

NURSING DIAGNOSIS: Anxiety/fear related to situational crisis, threat to role functioning, change in environment

FAMILY GOAL 1: Will adjust to hospital environment

• **NURSING INTERVENTIONS/*RATIONALES***

Introduce family to significant staff members
Describe hospital routine that affects child
Acclimate family to the new and strange surroundings (e.g., physical layout of unit, including playroom, unit kitchen, toilet, telephone, where they can stay, where they can store their belongings)
Direct family to areas they may need to use outside the unit (e.g., dining room, chapel)
Direct family to "destinations" (places within the hospital that are interesting to look at or talk about)
Provide an atmosphere that promotes questioning, expression of doubts and feelings
Be available to family *to facilitate their adjustment*
Be alert to signs of tension in family members
Provide for privacy

• **EXPECTED OUTCOMES**

Family demonstrates familiarity with hospital environment
Family members ask questions

FAMILY GOAL 2: Will feel a part of the health care team

• **NURSING INTERVENTIONS/*RATIONALES***

Employ a polite approach and demeanor
Greet family by name when they arrive on the unit
Encourage family's presence
Include family in planning patient care
Encourage family to select and assume specific roles in child's care
Offer encouragement for their efforts
Ask family to share with staff what they know about child's care and needs
Convey an attitude of collegiality with family, not competition

• **EXPECTED OUTCOME**

Family becomes involved in planning and carrying out care for the child

FAMILY GOAL 3: Will experience reduced apprehension

• **NURSING INTERVENTIONS/*RATIONALES***

Allow for expression of feelings about child's hospitalization and illness
Provide needed information *to alleviate fear of the unknown*
Prepare family for what to expect (e.g., procedures, behaviors)
Explore family's expectations
Explore family's concerns and feelings of irritation, guilt, anger, disappointment, inadequacy
Explore family's fears and anxieties regarding child's status and expectations of results of procedures or therapy
Introduce parents to other families who have a child in the hospital, especially a child who is similarly affected, *to facilitate family-to-family support*
Provide something constructive and meaningful for family to focus on (e.g., keeping record of intake and output, pain relief record, ensuring a specified amount of fluid intake, collecting a specimen)

• **EXPECTED OUTCOMES**

Family members verbalize feelings and concerns
Family demonstrates an understanding of procedures and behaviors (specify manner of demonstration and learning)
Family interacts with other families
Family complies with directions (specify)

FAMILY GOAL 4: Will be prepared for special procedures (e.g., radiology, diagnostic tests, surgery)

• **NURSING INTERVENTIONS/*RATIONALES***

Assess family's understanding of the procedure and its purpose
Provide needed information; clarify misconceptions
Explain special preparation needed (e.g., nothing by mouth [NPO], shaving, preprocedure medication or equipment)
Describe
- Where child will be during the procedure
- Whether family can be with child
- Where family can wait
- Approximate length of time procedure requires

Reassure family that they will be notified regarding progress of the procedure

• **EXPECTED OUTCOME**

Family demonstrates an understanding of procedures and tests (specify)

FAMILY GOAL 5: Will receive support during child's absence

• **NURSING INTERVENTIONS/*RATIONALES***

Provide a comfortable place for family to wait
Suggest activities to help reduce anxiety (e.g., go to the coffee shop or dining room, take a short walk [specify activity])
Be available to family *for support*
Make contact with family at frequent intervals *to relay information, provide comfort*

• **EXPECTED OUTCOME**

Family takes advantage of suggestions (specify)

Continued.

NURSING CARE PLAN
The Family of the Ill or Hospitalized Child—cont'd

FAMILY GOAL 6: Will adjust to child's appearance and behavior following procedure(s) or in special care unit

• **NURSING INTERVENTIONS/*RATIONALES***

Remain calm *to decrease family's anxiety*
Describe the environment, if appropriate (e.g., ICU)
Apply principles of learning to explanations
- Begin with small amounts of information
- Begin with very general information
- Allow ample time for family to absorb information and to ask questions
- Use age-appropriate explanations and techniques for siblings

Explain how child will look and the reasons for the child's appearance and equipment
Explain what child is experiencing
Prepare child and surroundings *to lessen the impact of the first impression*
- Tidy the bed
- Personalize the bed and bedside with a toy or other item(s)
- Provide chairs for family
- Be prepared for possible adverse reaction (e.g., fainting)

Convey an attitude of caring *about,* as well as *for,* the child
Accompany the family to the child's bedside
Allow time for follow-up discussion of questions and concerns

• **EXPECTED OUTCOME**

Family comes to child's bedside without evidence of distress

FAMILY GOAL 7: Will experience reduction of or no fear

• **NURSING INTERVENTIONS/*RATIONALES***

Help family distinguish between realistic and unfounded fears
Help eliminate unfounded fears
Discuss with family their fears regarding
- Child's signs and symptoms
- Child's anxiety
- Consequences of disease or therapy
- Deterioration of child's condition
- Tests and procedures
- Death

Answer questions honestly and compassionately

• **EXPECTED OUTCOME**

Family members verbalize fears and explore nature and ramifications of these fears

NURSING DIAGNOSIS: Powerlessness related to health care environment

FAMILY GOAL 1: Will experience a sense of control

• **NURSING INTERVENTIONS/*RATIONALES***

Encourage family's presence at times convenient for them; consider variations (e.g., cultural, occupational) in visiting
Encourage expression of concerns regarding child's care and progress
Explore family's feelings regarding prescribed therapies
Encourage family to assume as much control as possible in child's management
- Encourage participation in child's care
- Include family in setting goals for care
- Involve family in scheduling and other aspects of care
- Explain what family can do for child and how to handle child to maintain therapy (e.g., how to pick up the child who has an intravenous line)
- Employ family's suggestions regarding child's care whenever possible

• **EXPECTED OUTCOMES**

Family schedules time to be with child
Family readily discusses feelings and concerns
Family contributes to care and management of child
*Family's suggestions are incorporated into plan of care

NURSING DIAGNOSIS: Altered family processes related to situational crisis (threat to role functioning, hospitalization of a child)

FAMILY GOAL 1: Will demonstrate knowledge of child's illness

• **NURSING INTERVENTIONS/*RATIONALES***

Recognize family's concern and need for information, support
Assess family's understanding of diagnosis and plan of care
Reinforce and clarify health professional's explanation of child's condition, suggested procedures and therapies, and the prognosis
Use every opportunity to increase family's understanding of the disease and its therapies
Repeat information as often as necessary *to facilitate understanding*
Interpret technical information, *since family may not understand*
Help family interpret infant's or child's behaviors and responses
Do not appear rushed; if time is inappropriate, set a time for discussion as soon as feasible
- Keep appointment faithfully

• **EXPECTED OUTCOME**

Family demonstrates an understanding of the disease and its therapies (specify knowledge)

*Nursing outcome.

NURSING CARE PLAN
The Family of the Ill or Hospitalized Child—cont'd

FAMILY GOAL 2: Will experience reduction of or no guilt feelings

• **NURSING INTERVENTIONS/*RATIONALES***

Acknowledge feelings of guilt
Provide accurate and specific information regarding the cause of the illness
Clarify misconceptions and false assumptions

• **EXPECTED OUTCOME**

Family verbalizes their understanding of the cause of the illness (specify)

FAMILY GOAL 3: Will receive adequate support

• **NURSING INTERVENTIONS/*RATIONALES***

Respect parental rights
Convey an attitude of respectful caring for both child and family
Support and emphasize family's strengths and abilities
Provide feedback and praise
Refer to other professionals *for additional interpersonal and concrete support* (e.g., social service, clergy)

• **EXPECTED OUTCOMES**

Family exhibits behaviors that indicate a feeling of self-respect
Family uses supportive services

FAMILY GOAL 4: Will demonstrate positive coping behaviors toward child

• **NURSING INTERVENTIONS/*RATIONALES***

Determine family's understanding of the normal childhood responses to the stress of illness and hospitalization
Explain child's regression, magical thinking, egocentricity, separation anxiety, fears
Explain behavioral reactions generally expected of child (specify according to age and developmental level)
Explain what child is (family are) permitted to do in coping with child's behavior
Reinforce family's endeavors

• **EXPECTED OUTCOME**

Family demonstrates an understanding of child's unfamiliar behaviors (specify manner of demonstration—verbalization, physical attitude, behaviors with child)

FAMILY GOAL 5: Will assist child in coping effectively with hospitalization

• **NURSING INTERVENTIONS/*RATIONALES***

Help parents determine the best way to prepare child for hospitalization, procedures
Provide family with precise information about what will take place so they know what child is likely to experience
Encourage family to trust child's capacity to cope
Impress on family the need for honesty in relating to child
Encourage family to use play as a coping strategy
Suggest appropriate items to bring to child (e.g., pajamas, favorite toys)
See also Nursing Care Plan: The Child in the Hospital, p. 1104

• **EXPECTED OUTCOMES**

Family helps in planning strategies
Family is honest with child and staff
Family uses play as a tool for relating with child

FAMILY GOAL 6: Will experience positive relationships

• **NURSING INTERVENTIONS/*RATIONALES***

Recognize that family members know child best and are "cued in" to child's needs
Welcome unlimited family presence *to promote family relationships*
Encourage family to bring other significant family members to visit (e.g., siblings, grandparents, and [where permitted] pets)
Encourage family to provide child with significant, but manageable, items from home *to provide security*
Arrange for family members to have a meal together

• **EXPECTED OUTCOMES**

Child and family exhibit behaviors that indicate positive coping
Family is with child at appropriate times and in appropriate numbers
Child demonstrates an attitude of security with familiar persons and things

FAMILY GOAL 7: Will exhibit evidence of optimum health

• **NURSING INTERVENTIONS/*RATIONALES***

Stress importance of maintaining family members' health during child's illness and hospitalization
Encourage adequate rest *to promote health of family*
- Provide sleeping facilities where possible
- Encourage members to alternate visiting with child to allow some time at home
- Explore means for respite care of dependent family members

Assure family that child will receive optimum care in their absence
Provide relief for family from direct care of child as needed
Promote adequate nutrition
- Provide meals for parents if possible
- Direct family to nutritious resources for meals
- Encourage regular mealtimes away from unit
- Provide access to unit kitchen to store and prepare snacks

• **EXPECTED OUTCOMES**

Family shows no evidence of illness
Family members appear well rested
Family members eat regularly

Continued.

NURSING CARE PLAN
The Family of the Ill or Hospitalized Child—cont'd

FAMILY GOAL 8: Will experience smooth transition from hospital to home

• **NURSING INTERVENTIONS/*RATIONALES***
Assess family's learning needs
Outline and carry out a teaching plan
Determine services needed and make necessary referrals
Include family in planning and problem solving
Maintain open communication between family and health care providers

• **EXPECTED OUTCOME**
Child and family demonstrate the ability to provide needed care in the home

FAMILY GOAL 9: Will demonstrate knowledge of home care

• **NURSING INTERVENTIONS/*RATIONALES***
Assess family's knowledge to facilitate planning
Teach family the skills needed to carry out the therapeutic program (specify)
- Allow ample time for preparation
- Teach necessary techniques and observations
- Help family by demonstration
- Distribute appropriate home care instructions and/or other educational materials
- Encourage questions and expression of feelings and concerns
- Allow sufficient time for family to perform procedures under supervision

Inform parents of
- Signs of progress to observe for
- Any unfavorable signs to be alert for
- Problems that can be anticipated (e.g., care of equipment or devices)
- Behaviors that indicate special needs (e.g., pain medication, imminent seizures)
- A course of action to follow (e.g., seizure care)
- Make certain family knows how to contact appropriate persons if or when needed

Prepare family for possible posthospital behaviors of the child (see box on p. 1072)
Ensure family's comprehension of child's needs before discharge

• **EXPECTED OUTCOMES**
Family demonstrates procedures needed to care for child in the home (specify learning and method of demonstration)
Family is aware of how to seek help

FAMILY GOAL 10: Will demonstrate understanding of continuity of care

• **NURSING INTERVENTIONS/*RATIONALES***
Inform family of community resources available
Refer to agencies as appropriate (specify)
Help identify support group(s) for family
Be available to family by telephone or other means
Schedule follow-up appointments as needed

• **EXPECTED OUTCOMES**
Family seeks appropriate assistance
Family keeps appointments

See also:
- Nursing Care Plan: The Child in the Hospital, p. 1104
- Nursing Care Plan: The Child with Chronic Illness or Disability, Chapter 22
- Nursing Care Plan: The Child Who Is Terminally Ill or Dying, Chapter 23

quently, they should be forewarned of the usual continuance of such reactions following discharge. Parents who do not expect such reactions may misinterpret them as evidence of the child's "being spoiled" and demand perfect behavior at a time when the child is still reacting to the stress of illness and hospitalization. If the behaviors, especially the demand for attention, are dealt with in a supportive manner, most children are able to relinquish them and assume precrisis levels of functioning.

Nurses should also forewarn parents of the reactions of siblings to the ill child—particularly anger, jealousy, and resentment. Older siblings may deny such reactions because they provoke feelings of guilt. However, everyone needs outlets for emotions, and the repressed feelings may surface as problems in school, with age-mates, as psychosomatic illnesses, or in delinquent behavior.

Probably one of the most neglected areas involves giving information to siblings. Age frequently becomes the only factor that leads to an awareness of this problem, since older children may begin to ask questions or request explanations. However, even in this situation the information may be seriously inadequate. Children in every age-group deserve some explanation of the child's illness or hospitalization, preferably appropriate written information for older children. Although the exact wording may differ, the answer should focus on the following concerns: (1) "Will I get sick and have to go to the hospital?" (2) "Did I cause the illness?" (for actual or imagined reasons), and (3) "Will my parents abandon me if my brother or sister doesn't recover?" If parents or nurses address the explanations to these three questions, the siblings' own fears of illness, guilt, and abandonment are minimized.

Nursing approaches with siblings can be direct or indirect. Direct services might include (1) incorporating siblings into hospital admission programs; (2) liberalizing visiting regulations; (3) extending parent participation programs to include sibling involvement, such as through family dining or group play sessions; and (4) developing programs designed specifically for siblings, such as group sessions to discuss their concerns or posthospital discharge

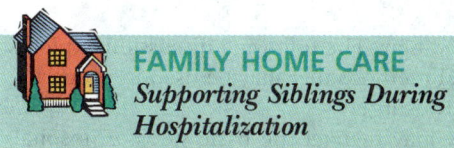

FAMILY HOME CARE
Supporting Siblings During Hospitalization

Trade off staying at the hospital with spouse or have a parent surrogate who knows the siblings well stay in the home.
Offer information about the child's condition to young siblings, as well as older siblings; respect the sibling who avoids information as a means of coping with the situation.
Arrange for children to visit their brother or sister in the hospital if possible.
Encourage phone visits and mail between brothers and sisters; provide children with phone numbers, writing supplies, and stamps.
Help each sibling identify an extended family member or friend to be their support person and provide extra attention during parental absence.
Make or buy inexpensive toys or trinkets for siblings, one gift for each day the child will be hospitalized.
- Wrap each gift separately and place in a basket, box, or other container at each child's bedside.
- Instruct siblings to open one gift each night at bedtime and to remember that he or she is in the parent's thoughts.

If the child's condition is stable and distance is not prohibitive, plan a special time at home with the siblings or have spouse or another relative or friend bring the children to meet parent(s) at a restaurant or other location near the hospital.
- Have extended family members or friends schedule a visit to the child in the hospital during parental absence.
- Arrange a pass for the child to leave the hospital to join the family if the child's condition permits.

Modified from Craft M, Craft J: Perceived changes in siblings of hospitalized children: a comparison of sibling and parent reports, *Child Health Care* 18(1):42-48, 1989; and Rollins J: *Brothers and sisters: a discussion guide for families,* Landover, MD, 1992, Epilepsy Foundation of America.

visits to evaluate the siblings' adjustment. Older siblings may not wish to attend a group; the nurse can be available for casual talks or for a tour, which may encourage the youngster to talk.

Indirect services, which can be influenced by any existing nursing role, involve helping parents understand, cope with, and support the siblings' reactions to the experience (see Family Home Care box). Measures such as ensuring siblings understand what is happening and providing for them to remain at home rather than with a neighbor or relative can help minimize some of the negative effects (Craft, Wyatt, and Sandell, 1985). Other interventions include helping the sick and well siblings maintain contact through telephone calls or sending tape recordings, letters, or postcards (see also Family Home Care box on p. 959).

PREPARATION FOR HOSPITALIZATION

The rationale for preparing children for the hospital experience and related procedures is based on the principle that fear of the unknown (fantasy) exceeds fear of the known. Therefore decreasing the elements of the unknown results in less fear. When children do not have paralyzing fear to cope with, they can direct their energies toward dealing with the other unavoidable stresses of hospitalization and benefit optimally from the growth potential of the experience.

For children past infancy and early toddlerhood, in-hospital and/or home preparation for hospitalization reduces their stress (Johnson, Jeppson, and Redburn, 1992). Even when children are too young to benefit from direct preparation, parents need prehospital counseling to lessen their fears and thus increase their ability to support the child psychologically. Prehospital counseling has two major goals:

1. To make the hospital less strange and frightening to parents and children
2. To establish a positive atmosphere and trusting relationship with hospital staff and family members

GUIDELINES IN PREPARING FOR HOSPITALIZATION

Although preparation for hospitalization is a common practice, there is no universal standard or program that is advocated in both general and children's hospitals. Some hospital admission programs focus on group preparation before actual admission, whereas others prepare each child either before or on the day of admission. There is also a trend to prepare well children for future hospitalizations, although the benefits and disadvantages are controversial (Azarnoff, 1985). The primary audience of most hospital preparation programs is children who are experiencing an initial hospitalization. However, readmission is also stressful; children's fear and fantasies may not subside with repeated hospital stays but may intensify. Also, concerns change as children develop and grow. These children need preparation as well, although the type of program needs to be individualized and may differ from the following guidelines for planning prehospital tours for groups or individual families who have not yet experienced hospital admission.

Ideally, preparatory procedures should be:

- Planned by the hospital staff before any child's admission to the hospital
- Appropriately designed for each child's developmental age
- Sufficiently individualized to account for different children's previous experience with hospitalization, present reason for admission, and available support system

In a growing number of hospitals ***child-life specialists,*** health care professionals with extensive knowledge of child growth and development and the special psychosocial needs of children who are hospitalized and their families, help prepare children for hospitalization, surgery, and procedures. A collaborative effort between the nurse, child-life specialist, and other members of the child's health care team will help ensure the best possible hospital experience for the child and family (American Academy of Pediatrics, Committee on Hospital Care, 1993).

In addition to the following discussion, the reader is also

encouraged to review Preparation for Procedures, Chapter 27.

Group Size and Timing of Preparation

Group size should be small (about 10 children to a group) to provide individualized attention and facilitate discussion. If tours are arranged for each child, the parents should be included and possibly the well siblings, although the actual benefit to these children has not been researched.

Prehospital admission programs should be scheduled for the time of day when staff members are most available and most treatment procedures are completed. They should occur before actual admission. However, no firm consensus exists on the timing of the event. Some authorities recommend preparing children 4 to 7 years of age about 1 week in advance so they can assimilate the information and ask questions. For older children the time may be longer. However, for young children, who may begin to fantasize about what they observed, 1 or 2 days before admission is sufficient time for anticipatory preparation (Petrillo and Sanger, 1980). Children ages 5 to 12 years prefer to know about impending hospitalization from several weeks to a few minutes before the event. Because standardized programs cannot adequately meet the needs of the full age range of pediatric patients, some hospitals have developed preparation programs that target a specific age-group, such as toddlers or adolescents (Johnson, Jeppson, and Redburn, 1992). The length of the session should be suited to the children's attention span—the younger the child, the shorter the program. The optimum approach is one that is individualized for each child and family.

Setting of the Tour

The setting of the tour should avoid any frightening aspects of the hospital environment and should typically include an inpatient room, the playroom (a highlight of the tour), the parents' waiting room, the nurses' station, and other special areas, such as the group dining room. Other areas that may be visited are the radiology department and laboratory area, the slumber or induction room, and the recovery room. Different hospitals may tailor this tour to include special rooms, such as the "OR playroom," where children and parents first go before any induction is administered. Children who are undergoing serious surgery requiring special postoperative care may be taken to visit the intensive care unit. Children scheduled for special tests, such as cardiac catheterization or cystoscopy, are sometimes shown these areas. Young children may respond better to shorter tours that concentrate on the areas of most concern, such as the pediatric unit, playroom, and recovery room. In any case, throughout the tour, the nurse (or other guide) must be alert to signs of concern or fear in the children. Strange noises, sights, sounds, and smells that are routine to hospital personnel can be frightening to children.

Preparatory Materials

The most suitable type of presentation for children includes a variety of preparatory materials, including films, lecture, demonstration, and play. The following discussion explores some of the typical methods that may be used in preparing children for elective surgery.

A puppet show may reenact the basic steps of hospitalization—admission procedures; preparation for surgery, the operating room, and the recovery room; and postsurgical treatment. The main focus of each scene is the use of concrete actions and models to familiarize the family members with what will occur. The puppets talk about children's common fears—pain, anesthesia, and parent separation. Although the sophistication of the materials varies, the basic characters should include a puppet family (mother, father, child) and hospital staff (physician, nurse) that are racially representative of the patient and hospital population. For example, both black and white dolls are required in many urban areas. Hospital equipment includes mask, cap, gloves, gown, intravenous bottle, stand, tubing, syringes, thermometer, blood pressure machine, stethoscope, scale, oxygen mask, suture removal set, bandages, bed, and sheets. If children are routinely admitted for diagnostic evaluations, miniature replicas of machinery (e.g., x-ray equipment) or slides as visual aids may be used. The use of scaled-down models is especially beneficial for young children, who may be frightened by the actual proportions of some equipment. However, the *intent* of what is conveyed greatly surpasses the sophistication of the materials used.

Opportunity for Discussion

Any type of preparatory program needs to provide ample opportunity for discussion both before and after the tour. During the tour family members are encouraged to ask questions and to familiarize themselves with the environment by sitting on a bed, using the electric bed controls, riding in a wheelchair, or handling the equipment in the special rooms. Ideally, the tour should also be an opportunity for meeting the child's primary nurse. Although this is not always possible because of staffing schedules, the nursing staff should be introduced to the children by name. Introducing them to one specific nurse, such as the head nurse or clinical specialist, helps them feel more comfortable in knowing who is available for questions or concerns during the hospital stay.

Following the tour there should be a question-and-answer period, monitored by a nurse. Sometimes the group is reticent about asking questions. In this case the nurse can stimulate discussion by posing a question to the audience or inviting the children to see and touch the puppets and equipment. Allowing children to play with the equipment and draw pictures about what they observed are excellent methods of evaluating the learning process and clarifying any misconceptions.

The tour may conclude with serving refreshments, which helps people relax, gather their thoughts, and ask a last-minute question. By informally visiting each table, the nurse has an excellent opportunity to discuss individual concerns. At this time the parents can also be invited to call the pediatric unit for any reason before admission, since questions may arise during this interval.

Prehospital Counseling by Parents

In many situations the preparation of children for hospitalization is left up to parents. Parents may abdicate this responsibility for a variety of reasons. For example, they sometimes think the child is too young to understand or is better off not knowing beforehand; often they are unable to prepare the child because of their own lack of knowledge and understanding.

Professionals can help parents prepare their children by adequately informing them of the specific details of hospitalization and related procedures, through both direct discussion and written material. Responsibility for such guidance often rests with office and clinic nurses. They can discuss with parents the appropriate timing of the preparation and the methods, such as picture books about going to the hospital (see p. 1131). Many hospitals develop their own books and photograph albums for this purpose. Nurses working with these parents should also assess their level of anxiety regarding the impending hospitalization to prevent emotional contagion to the child.

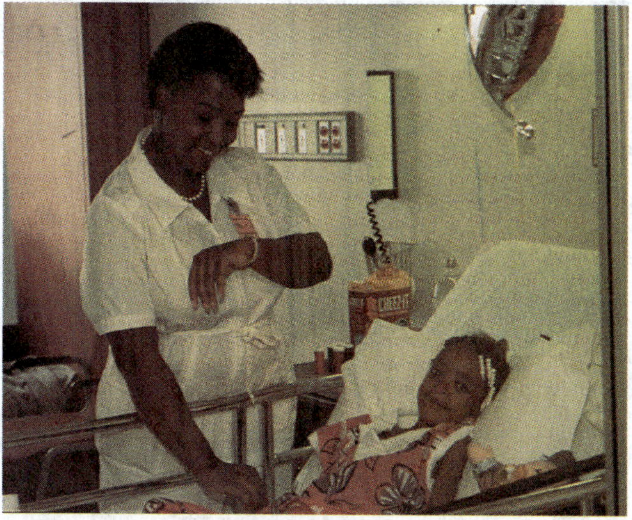

FIG. 26-14 The initial admission procedures allow the nurse to begin knowing the child and assessing his or her understanding of the hospital experience. (Courtesy St. Louis Children's Hospital.)

GUIDELINES
Hospital Admission

PREADMISSION

Assign a room based on developmental age, seriousness of diagnosis, communicability of illness, and projected length of stay.
Prepare roommate(s) for the arrival of a new patient; when children are too young to benefit from this consideration, prepare parents.
Prepare room for child and family, with admission forms and equipment nearby to eliminate need to leave child.

ADMISSION

Introduce primary nurse to child and family.
Orient child and family to inpatient facilities, especially to assigned room and unit; emphasize positive areas of pediatric unit.
- Room: Explain call light, bed controls, television, etc.; direct to bathroom, telephone, etc.
- Unit: Direct to playroom, desk, dining area, or other areas

Introduce family to roommate and his or her parents.
Apply identification band to child's wrist, ankle, or both (if not done).
Explain hospital regulations and schedules (e.g., visiting hours, mealtimes, bedtime, limitations [give written information if available]).
Perform nursing admission history (see box on pp. 1116-1117).
Take vital signs, blood pressure, height, and weight.
Obtain specimens as needed and order needed laboratory work.
Support child and perform or assist practitioner with physical examination (for purposes of nursing assessment).

GUIDELINES FOR EMERGENCY ADMISSION

Lengthy preparatory admission procedures are often impossible and inappropriate for emergency situations.
Unless an emergency is life-threatening, children need to participate in their care to maintain a sense of control.
Focus on essential components of admission counseling, including:
- Appropriate introduction to the family
- Use of child's name, not terms such as "honey" or "dear"
- Determination of child's age and some judgment about developmental age (if the child is of school age, asking about the grade level will offer some evidence for concurrent intellectual ability)
- Information about child's general state of health, any problems that may interfere with medical treatment (e.g., sensitivity to medication), and previous experience with hospital facilities
- Information about the chief complaint from both the parents and the child

GUIDELINES FOR ADMISSION TO INTENSIVE CARE UNIT

Prepare child and parents for elective ICU admission, such as for postoperative care after cardiac surgery.
Prepare child and parents for unanticipated ICU admission by focusing primarily on the sensory aspects of the experience and on usual family concerns (e.g., persons in charge of child's care, schedule for visiting, area where family can wait).
Prepare parents regarding child's appearance and behavior when they first visit child in ICU.
Accompany family to bedside to provide emotional support and answer questions.
Prepare siblings for their visit; plan length of time for sibling visitation; monitor siblings' reactions during visit to prevent them from becoming overwhelmed.

NURSING ADMISSION HISTORY ACCORDING TO FUNCTIONAL HEALTH PATTERNS*

HEALTH PERCEPTION–HEALTH MANAGEMENT PATTERN

Why has your child been admitted?
How has your child's general health been?
What does your child know about this hospitalization?
 Ask the child why he or she came to the hospital.
 If answer is "For an operation or for tests," ask the child to tell you about what will happen before, during, and after the operation or tests.
Has your child ever been in the hospital before?
 How was that hospital experience?
 What things were important to you and your child during that hospitalization? How can we be most helpful now?
What medications does your child take at home?
 Why are they given?
 When are they given?
 How are they given (if a liquid, with a spoon; if a tablet, swallowed with water; or other)?
 Does your child have any trouble taking medication? If so, what helps?
 Is your child allergic to any medications?
What, if any, forms of alternative medicine are being used?

NUTRITION-METABOLIC PATTERN

What are the family's usual mealtimes?
Do family members eat together or at separate times?
What are your child's favorite foods, beverages, and snacks?
 Average amounts consumed or usual size portions
 Special cultural practices, such as family eats only ethnic food
What foods and beverages does your child dislike?
What are your child's feeding habits (bottle, cup, spoon, eats by self, needs assistance, any special devices)?
How does your child like the food served (warmed, cold, one item at a time)?
How would you describe your child's usual appetite (hearty eater, picky eater)?
 Has being sick affected your child's appetite?
Are there any known or suspected food allergies? Is your child on a special diet?
Are there any feeding problems (excessive fussiness, spitting up, colic); any dental or gum problems that affect feeding?
What do you do for these problems?

ELIMINATION PATTERN

What are your child's toilet habits (diaper, toilet, trained–day only or day and night, use of word to communicate urination or defecation, potty chair, regular toilet, other routines)?
What is your child's usual pattern of elimination (bowel movements)?
Do you have any concerns about elimination (bed-wetting, constipation, diarrhea)?
What do you do for these problems?
Have you ever noticed that your child sweats a lot?

SLEEP-REST PATTERN

What is your child's usual hour of sleep and awakening?
What is your child's schedule for naps; length of naps?
Is there a special routine before sleeping (bottle, drink of water, bedtime story, nightlight, favorite blanket or toy, prayers)?
Is there a special routine during sleep time, such as waking to go to the bathroom?
What type of bed does your child sleep in?
Does your child have a separate room or share a room; if shares, with whom?
What are the home sleeping arrangements (alone or with others, e.g., sibling, parent, other person)?
What is your child's favorite sleeping position?
Are there any sleeping problems (falling asleep, waking during night, nightmares, sleep walking)?
Are there any problems awakening and getting ready in the morning?
What do you do for these problems?

ACTIVITY-EXERCISE PATTERN

What is your child's schedule during the day (nursery school, daycare center, regular school, extracurricular activities)?
What are your child's favorite activities or toys (both active and quiet interests)?
What is your child's usual television viewing schedule at home?
 What are your child's favorite programs?
 Are there any TV restrictions?
Does your child have any illness or disabilities that limit activity? If so, how?
What are your child's usual habits and schedule for bathing (bath in tub or shower, sponge bath, shampoo)?
What are your child's dental habits (brushing, flossing, fluoride supplements or rinses, favorite toothpaste); schedule of daily dental care?
Does your child need help with dressing or grooming, such as hair combing?
Are there any problems with the above (dislike of or refusal to bathe, shampoo hair, or brush teeth)?
What do you do for these problems?
Are there special devices that your child requires help in managing (eyeglasses, contact lenses, hearing aid, orthodontic appliances, artificial elimination appliances, orthopedic devices)?

NOTE: Use the following code to assess functional self-care level for feeding, bathing/hygiene, dressing/grooming, toileting:
 O: Full self-care
 I: Requires use of equipment or device
 II: Requires assistance or supervision from another person
 III: Requires assistance or supervision from another person and equipment or device
 IV: Is dependent and does not participate

COGNITIVE-PERCEPTUAL PATTERN

Does your child have any hearing difficulty?
 Does the child use a hearing aid?
 Have "tubes" been placed in your child's ears?
Does your child have any vision problems?
 Does the child wear glasses or contact lenses?
Does your child have any learning difficulties?
 What is the child's grade in school?
For information on pain, see box on p. 1084

SELF-PERCEPTION–SELF-CONCEPT PATTERN

How would you describe your child (e.g., takes time to adjust, settles in easily, shy, friendly, quiet, talkative, serious, playful, stubborn, easygoing)?
What makes your child angry, annoyed, anxious, or sad?
 What helps?

*The focus of the admission history is the child's psychosocial environment. Most of the questions are worded in terms of parental responses. Depending on the child's age, they should be addressed directly to the child when appropriate.

NURSING ADMISSION HISTORY ACCORDING TO FUNCTIONAL HEALTH PATTERNS—cont'd

How does your child act when annoyed or upset?
What have been your child's experiences with and reactions to temporary separation from you (parent)?
Does your child have any fears (places, objects, animals, people, situations)? How do you handle them?
Do you think your child's illness has changed the way he or she thinks about self (e.g., more shy, embarrassed about appearance, less competitive with friends, stays at home more)?

ROLE-RELATIONSHIP PATTERN

Does your child have a favorite nickname?
What are the names of other family members or others who live in the home (relatives, friends, pets)?
Who usually takes care of your child during the day/night (especially if other than parent, such as baby-sitter, relative)?
What are the parents' occupation and work schedules?
Are there any special family considerations (adoption, foster child, stepparent, divorce, single parent)?
Have any major changes in the family occurred lately (death, divorce, separation, birth of a sibling, loss of a job, financial strain, mother beginning a career, other)? Describe child's reaction.
Who are your child's play companions or social groups (peers, younger or older children, adults, prefers to be alone)?
Do things generally go well for your child in school or with friends?
Does your child use "security" objects at home (pacifier, thumb, bottle, blanket, stuffed animal or doll)? Did you bring any of these to the hospital?
How do you handle discipline problems at home? Are these methods always effective?
Does your child have any condition that interferes with communication? If so, what are your suggestions for communicating with your child?
Will your child's hospitalization affect the family's financial support or care of other family members, (e.g., other children)?
What concerns do you have about your child's illness and hospitalization?
Who will be staying with your child while hospitalized?
How can we contact you or another close family member outside of the hospital?

SEXUALITY-REPRODUCTIVE PATTERN

(Answer questions that apply to your child's age-group.)
Has your child begun puberty (developing physical sexual characteristics, menstruation)? Have you or your child had any concerns?
Does your daughter know how to do breast self-examination?
Does your son know how to do testicular self-examination?
How have you approached topics of sexuality with your child?
Do you feel you might need some help with some topics?
Has your child's illness affected the way he or she feels about being a boy or a girl? If so, how?
Do you have any concerns with behaviors in your child, such as masturbation, asking many questions or talking about sex, not respecting others' privacy, or wanting too much privacy?
Initiate a conversation about an adolescent's sexual concerns with open-ended to more direct questions and using the terms "friends" or "partners" rather than "girlfriend" or "boyfriend":
Tell me about your social life.
Who are your closest friends? (If one friend is identified, could ask more about that relationship, such as how much time they spend together, how serious they are about each other, if the relationship is going the way the teenager hoped.)
Might ask about dating and sexual issues, such as the teenager's views on sex education, "going steady," "living together," or premarital sex.
Which friends would you like to have visit in the hospital?

COPING-STRESS TOLERANCE PATTERN

(Answer questions that apply to your child's age-group.)
What does your child do when tired or upset?
If upset, does your child want a special person or object? If so, explain.
If your child has temper tantrums, what causes them and how do you handle them?
Whom does your child talk to when worried about something?
How does your child usually handle problems or disappointments?
Have there been any big changes or problems in your family recently?
How did you handle them?
Has your child ever had a problem with drugs or alcohol or tried suicide?
Do you think your child is "accident prone"? If so, explain.

VALUE-BELIEF PATTERN

What is your religion?
How is religion or faith important in your child's life?
What religious practices would you like continued in the hospital (e.g., prayers before meals/bedtime; visit by minister, priest, or rabbi; prayer group)?

HOSPITAL ADMISSION

The preparation that children require on the day of admission depends on their prehospital counseling. If they have been prepared in a formalized program, they will usually know what to expect in terms of initial medical procedures, inpatient facilities, and nursing staff. However, prehospital counseling does not preclude the need for support during procedures such as drawing blood, x-ray tests, or physical examination. For example, undressing young children before they feel comfortable in their new surroundings can be very upsetting. Causing needless anxiety and fear during admission may adversely affect the nurse's establishment of trust with these children. Therefore, nursing assistance during the admission procedure is vital, regardless of how well prepared any child is for the hospitalization. In addition, spending this time with the child gives the nurse an opportunity to evaluate understanding of subsequent procedures, such as surgery (Fig. 26-14). The usual admission procedures for children are outlined in the Guidelines box on p. 1115.

Nursing Admission History

The nursing admission history refers to a systematic collection of data about the child and family that allows the nurse to plan individualized care. The nursing admission history presented in the box on pp. 1116-1117 is organized according to the Functional Health Patterns outlined by Gordon (1994) (see Nursing Diagnosis, Chapter 1), which facilitates the formulation of nursing diagnoses. One of the main purposes of the history is to assess the child's usual health habits at home to promote a more normal environment in the hospital. Therefore questions related to activities of daily liv ing are a major part of the assessment. The questions found under the health perception–health management pattern are directed toward evaluation of the child's preparation for hospitalization and are key factors in determining if additional preparation is needed.

As with any history form, the questions are only guidelines; for maximum communication, nurses should ask these questions as a part of conversation, not as a direct questionnaire. Answers to questions that are broad and nonspecific, such as "What does your child know about this hospitalization?" need to be followed by more directive questions, such as "Tell me what you told him." Children may respond to questions regarding their knowledge of hospitalization with statements such as, "I don't know why I am here." Although this may be correct, frequently they have been given some explanation concerning the reason for hospitalization. Such an answer may mean that the explanation was inadequate, their anxiety blocked the recall, or they are testing out the explanation by prompting the nurse to supply additional information.

The nurse should also inquire about the use of any alternative medicine practices (see box below). In a national survey, over a third of adults had used at least one unconventional therapy within the previous year, yet 72% did not inform their medical doctor that they had done so (Eisenberg and others, 1993). It is reasonable to expect that many of these adults have children who also use alternative medicine practices. Use of the third-person technique may serve to give families permission to share this important information (e.g., "Many families tell me that their children benefit from megavitamins, acupuncture, relaxation, or music. I am wondering if this is true for your family").

Once the data are collected, they must be applied to the nursing process and communicated to other staff. It makes little sense to assess a child's home routine if none of this knowledge is integrated into the plan of care. Most nursing units have provisions for care plans in which specific information about the child's habits and needs are recorded.

ALTERNATIVE MEDICINE PRACTICES AND EXAMPLES

Nutrition, diet, and life-style/behavioral health changes—Macrobiotics, megavitamins, diets, life-style modification, health risk reduction/health education, wellness

Mind/body control therapies—Biofeedback, relaxation, prayer therapy, guided imagery, hypnotherapy, music/sound therapy, education therapy

Traditional and ethnomedicine therapies—Acupuncture, ayurvedic medicine, herbal medicine, homeopathic medicine, Native American medicine, natural products, traditional Oriental medicine

Structural manipulation and energetic therapies—Acupressure, chiropractic medicine, massage, reflexology, rolfing, therapeutic touch, Qi Gong

Pharmacologic and biologic therapies—Antioxidants, cell treatment, chelation therapy, metabolic therapy, oxidizing agents

Bioelectromagnetic therapies—Diagnostic and therapeutic application of electromagnetic fields (e.g., transcranial electrostimulation, neuromagnetic stimulation, electroacupuncture)

Physical Assessment

Although physical examinations by practitioners are a required part of the admission procedure, nurses should also use the valuable information gained from physical assessments in their planning of care (see Chapter 7). Subjecting children to two separate examinations is unnecessary if the nurse and other practitioners cooperate during the procedure. For example, when the nurse is present to support the child psychologically, the opportunity can also be used to observe the child's body for any bruises, rash, signs of neglect, deformities, or physical limitations.

The nurse should also listen to the heart and lungs to assess overall physical status. For example, it is impossible to evaluate improvement in respiratory function in a child admitted with pulmonary disease unless there are baseline data with which to compare subsequent findings. Collaboration also prevents the often frustrating and needless waste of the family's time in repeating histories and examinations, especially when the child has a chronic condition that requires many hospitalizations.

Placing the Child

Room assignments are usually made before the child is admitted to the pediatric unit. The minimum considerations for room assignment are age, sex, and nature of the illness. Ideally, however, room selection should be based on a variety of developmental and psychobiologic needs. Determining compatible roommates, both for the children and for rooming-in parents, greatly influences the growth potential from the hospital experience.

Although there are no absolute rules to govern room selection, in general, placing children of the same age-group and with similar types of illness in the same room is both psychologically and medically advantageous. However, there are many exceptions. For example, a school-age child may thrive on the responsibility of caring for a younger child. A child in traction may be very therapeutic for another child confined to bed because of a serious illness. A child who is very independent despite physical disabilities may help another child with similar or different limitations and the parents achieve deeper insight and acceptance of the disorder.

NURSING CARE DURING SPECIAL HOSPITAL SITUATIONS

In addition to a general pediatric unit, children may be admitted to special facilities, such as a day hospital, an adolescent unit, an isolation room, or an intensive care unit. Some admissions are unexpected and frequently constitute medical emergencies. Such situations require special preparation of the child and family and nursing care interventions based on an awareness of the child's needs and the unique stressors associated with these hospital facilities.

Day Hospital

The concept of a day hospital is to provide needed medical services for the child while eliminating the necessity of overnight admission. Among the benefits of a day hospital are (1) minimization of the stressors of hospitalization, especially separation from the family; (2) reduced chance of infection; and (3) economic saving. Admission to the day hospital usually is for surgical or diagnostic procedures, such as insertion of tympanostomy tubes, hernia repair, adenoidectomy, tonsillectomy, cystoscopy, or bronchoscopy.

Because of the limited contact with the child, nursing admission procedures are extremely important. Ideally, each child and family should receive preadmission counseling, including a tour of the facility and a review of the expected day's procedures. However, when this is not possible, surgery should be scheduled to allow some time for children to become acquainted with their surroundings and for nurses to assess, plan, and complement appropriate teaching.

Discharge instructions must also be explicit (see Discharge Planning and Home Care, p. 1122). Parents need guidelines on when to call their practitioner regarding a change in the child's condition. It is helpful for the nurse to make a follow-up telephone call or to specify a time for the family to report on the child's progress. Even hints for taking the child home in the car are appreciated.

➤ **NURSING TIP** Help the family prepare for the car ride with the discharged child by offering these suggestions:

Have a blanket and pillow in the car.

Take a basin or plastic bag in case of vomiting.

Use a cup with a cap and straw for the child to drink fluids.

Give any prescribed pain medication before leaving the facility.

Adolescent Unit

In recent years there has been increased awareness of children's needs based on developmental considerations. To meet the unique needs of adolescents, special units have been developed that provide privacy, increased socialization, and appropriate activities for these young people. Typically these units are set apart from the general pediatric facility so that the teenagers do not share space with younger children, who are often perceived as a threat to their maturity. These units also provide more flexible routines and activities, such as more group activity, wearing of street clothes, provisions to leave the adolescent unit temporarily, and access to the items so critical to teenagers—telephones, CD and tape players, video recorders, and televisions (Fig. 26-15). Because adolescents' food habits are rarely limited to the three traditional meals a day, a ready supply of snacks should be available. However, the most important benefit of these units is increased socialization with peers. In addition, staff members usually enjoy working with this age-group and are well suited to establishing the trust so essential for communication.

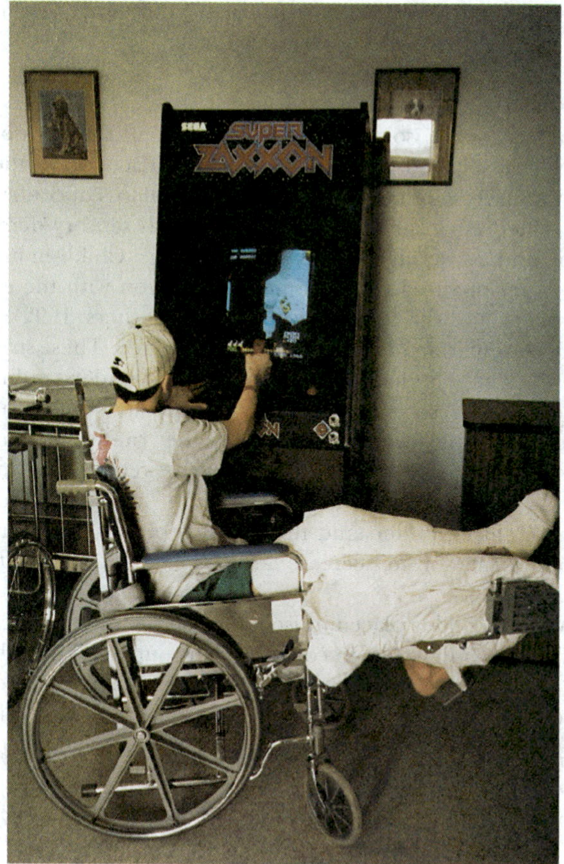

FIG. 26-15 Adolescent units include recreational activities that adolescents enjoy.

Despite the advantages of adolescent units, all young people require preparation for the experience. They need orientation to the unit, introduction to staff and other patients, and an atmosphere of warmth and welcome. Just as teenagers form "cliques" in normal social relationships, this same tendency occurs in the hospital. Staff must be aware of exclusiveness of group membership, especially when new patients are admitted. Scheduled and supervised group meetings are effective in preventing feelings of "nonbelonging" and in facilitating introductions and new friendships. They also provide an excellent opportunity for discussions about typical adolescent concerns (e.g., sexuality, drugs, drinking, parental relations) and special concerns of ill adolescents (e.g., peer rejection for being different) (Pazola and Gerberg, 1985).

Isolation

Admission to an isolation room increases all the stressors typically associated with hospitalization. There is further separation from familiar persons, additional loss of control, and added environmental changes, such as sensory deprivation and the strange appearance of visitors. Children may feel depersonalized from reduced interaction with the environment and the people in it (Hart and others, 1992). A child's orientation to time and place is affected. These stressors are compounded by children's limited understanding of isolation. Preschool children have difficulty understanding the rationale for isolation because they cannot comprehend the cause-and-effect relationship between germs and illness. They are likely to view isolation as punishment. Older children understand the causality better but still require information to decrease fantasizing or misinterpretation.

When a child is placed in isolation, preparation is essential for the child to feel in control. With young children the best approach is a simple explanation, such as "You need to be in this room to help you get better. This is a special place to make all the germs go away. The germs made you sick and you could not help that."

All children, but especially younger ones, need preparation in terms of what they will see, hear, or feel in isolation. Therefore they are shown the mask, gloves, and gown and are encouraged to "dress up" in them. Playing with the strange apparel lessens the fear of seeing "ghostlike" people walk into the room. Before entering the room, nurses and other health personnel should introduce themselves and let the child see their face before donning a mask. In this way the child associates them with significant experiences and gains a sense of familiarity in an otherwise strange and lonely environment.

When the child's condition improves, appropriate play activities are provided to minimize boredom, stimulate the senses, provide a real or perceived sense of movement, orient the child to time and place, provide social interaction, and reduce depersonalization.* Rather than dwelling on the negative aspects of isolation, the child can be encouraged to view this experience as challenging and positive. For example, the nurse can help the child look at isolation as a method of keeping others out and letting only special people in. Children often think of intriguing signs for their doors, such as "Enter at your own risk" or "Many have entered but few have left." These posterlike signs also encourage people "on the outside" to talk with the child about the ominous greetings.

Emergency Admission

One of the most traumatic hospital experiences for the child and parents is an emergency admission. The sudden onset of an illness or the occurrence of an injury leaves little time for preparation and explanation. Sometimes the emergency admission is compounded by admission to an intensive care unit or the need for immediate surgery. However, even in those instances requiring outpatient treatment, the child is exposed to a strange, frightening environment and to people who often inflict pain. Thus every medical emergency requires psychologic intervention to reduce the fear and anxiety frequently associated with the experience.

There is a wide discrepancy between what constitutes a medically defined emergency and a client-defined emergency. In pediatric populations most visits are for respiratory infections, with skin conditions, gastrointestinal disorders, and trauma such as poisoning accounting for the remainder of the cases. The most common reason parents give for bringing the child to the emergency room is concern about the illness worsening. However, practitioners generally do not consider the progressive symptoms as ne-

*An excellent resource for activities for children in isolation is *Therapeutic Play Activities for Hospitalized Children* by R.H. Hart and others (1992, Mosby).

CRITICAL THINKING EXERCISE

Postvention Counseling

David, 4 years old, is admitted to the hospital for an emergency appendectomy. The following day you ask him to describe his experiences. He describes the usual admission and preoperative procedures correctly but has no understanding of why they were done. His most prominent recollection focuses on all the needles he has received (blood tests, intravenous fluid, sedation).

When David tells you he thinks he got so many needles because he did not tell his mother about his stomachache soon enough, your most appropriate response is:

1. "Everyone who has an appendectomy needs to have blood tests, a tube in the hand because you can't drink right after surgery, and medicine to make you sleepy before surgery."
2. "You would still have had to have an appendectomy and those shots, even if you had told your mommy about your stomachache sooner."
3. "There were reasons for all of the needles. Your stomach probably didn't hurt badly in the beginning, so you didn't say anything until it hurt a lot. You didn't do anything wrong; that is not why you had to get shots."
4. "I wish you didn't have to get any shots, but you were a good boy."

The correct answer is 3. Although some of the other answers give the child good information, they do not fully answer his fear that he did something wrong and is being punished. Children who have little or no preparation before surgery often come to this conclusion. Without any other explanation, a young child will resort to magical thinking and provide his or her own explanation for the event. You should reassure the child that he did not cause bad things to happen.

Also refrain from labeling him a "good boy" or "big boy" for undergoing difficult procedures. If he is unable to do as well for another procedure, he may assume he is bad or is being a baby. Praise a child for doing well, trying hard to follow directions, or for any positive aspect of his behavior.

cessitating emergency care. Therefore the word "emergency" is perceived differently by various people. One of nursing's primary goals is to assess the parents' perception of the event and their reasons for considering it serious or life-threatening.

Lengthy preparatory admission procedures are often inappropriate for emergency situations. In such instances nurses must focus their nursing interventions on the essential components of admission counseling (see Guidelines box on p. 1115) and complete the process as soon as the child's condition is stabilized.

Unless an emergency is life-threatening, children need to participate in their care to maintain a sense of control. Because emergency rooms are frequently hectic, there is a tendency to rush through procedures in order to save time. However, the extra few minutes needed to allow children to participate may save many more minutes of useless resistance and uncooperativeness during subsequent procedures. Other supportive measures include ensuring privacy, accepting various emotional responses to fear or pain, preserving parent-child contact, explaining all events before or as they occur, and personally remaining calm.

At times, because of the child's physical condition, little or no preparatory counseling for emergency hospitalization can be done. In such situations the implementation of ***postvention,*** or counseling subsequent to the event, has therapeutic value. The process of postvention involves evaluating children's thoughts regarding admission and related procedures. It is similar to precounseling techniques; however, instead of supplying information, the nurse listens to the explanations offered by the child. Projective techniques such as drawing, doll play, or storytelling are especially effective. The nurse then bases additional information on what has already been revealed (see Critical Thinking Exercise box).

NEONATAL/PEDIATRIC ICU STRESSORS FOR THE CHILD AND FAMILY

PHYSICAL STRESSORS

Pain and discomfort (e.g., injections, intubation, suctioning, dressing changes, other invasive procedures)
Immobility (e.g., use of restraints, bed rest)
Sleep deprivation
Inability to eat or drink
Changes in elimination habits

ENVIRONMENTAL STRESSORS

Unfamiliar surroundings (e.g., crowding)
Unfamiliar sounds
- Equipment noise (e.g., monitors, telephone, suctioning, computer printout)
- Human sounds (e.g., talking, laughing, crying, coughing, moaning, retching, walking)

Unfamiliar people (e.g., health care professionals, patients, visitors)
Unfamiliar and unpleasant smells (e.g., alcohol, adhesive remover, body odors)
Constant lights (disturb diurnal rhythms)
Activity related to other patients
Sense of urgency among staff

PSYCHOLOGIC STRESSORS

Lack of privacy
Inability to communicate (if intubated)
Inadequate knowledge and understanding of situation
Severity of illness
Parental behavior (expression of concern)

SOCIAL STRESSORS

Disrupted relationships (especially with family and friends)
Concern with missing school/work
Play deprivation

Data primarily from Tichy AM and others: Stressors in pediatric intensive care units, *Pediatr Nurs* 14(1):40-42, 1988.

Intensive Care Unit (ICU)

Admission to an ICU can be a particularly traumatic event for both the child and the parents. The nature and severity of the illness and the circumstances surrounding the admission are major factors, especially for parents. Parents experience significantly more stress when the admission is unexpected rather than expected (Eberly and others, 1985). Stressors for the child and family are described in the box above, right. Parents report that their child's behavior and emotional responses, as well as alterations in their parental role, are the most stressful dimensions of the ICU experience (Miles and Mathes, 1991).

The family's emotional needs are important when a child is admitted to an ICU. While the same interventions that were discussed earlier for the stressors of separation, loss of control, and bodily injury and pain apply here, frequently they are not implemented or adjustments need to be made to accommodate the family's needs despite the often hectic and stressful atmosphere.

When an ICU admission is expected, such as for postoperative care after cardiac surgery, the child and parents should be prepared for the event. Some units advocate a tour, whereas others use picture books of the unit to familiarize the family with the environment and usual equipment. Dolls can be used to demonstrate the types of tubes that the child may have. Special care or effects of the tubes are discussed, such as the need to move despite the presence of chest tubes and inability to talk with an endotracheal tube. As much reassurance as possible should accompany the introduction of stressful information. For example, children should be reassured that they can talk when the tube is removed and that in the meantime they can use a communication board to convey their needs.

When parents first visit the child in the ICU, they need preparation for how the child will look and what the child is experiencing if awake. Ideally the nurse should accompany the family to the bedside to provide emotional support and answer any questions. If siblings visit, they need the same preparation as parents. Whether they should visit soon after the child is admitted or after the child's condition has stabilized is controversial. Early visiting minimizes the opportunity for siblings to fantasize about the experience and imagine fears that are probably greater than the actual situation (Shonkwiler, 1985). However, visiting early may be frightening, especially when the child is in pain or unresponsive and attached to numerous tubes and machinery. The length of time for sibling visitation should be planned ahead and monitored during the visit to prevent the well child from becoming overwhelmed.

Children admitted to the ICU need their parents' comfort and security, and parents are encouraged to stay with their child. If visiting hours are limited, the schedule should be flexible to accommodate parental needs. Family members should be given a schedule of the times permitted and assured that they can call the unit at any time. With liberalization of visiting hours, many parents think they must stay; nurses need to be sensitive to their needs, suggesting periodic respites from the stressful ICU environment.

Since altered parental roles are a major stress for parents, nurses need to implement interventions to minimize this concern, such as (1) educating and preparing parents for the expected role changes; (2) identifying ways in which parents can continue to fulfill parenting functions, such as helping with the bath or feeding and touching and talking to the child; and (3) determining new roles, such as helping with procedures. Use of the Nursing Mutual Participation Model of Care (NMPMC) has been found to lessen perceived stress of parents, especially stress related to alterations in the parental role in the ICU setting (Curley and Wallace, 1992). Information sharing can increase parents' sense of control and responsibility, but facts must be conveyed simply, repeated often, and monitored to prevent overwhelming family members. Since medical jargon abounds in a complex environment such as the ICU, unfamiliar terms need to be clarified and simpler terms substituted (see box under Preparation for Procedures: Psychologic Preparation, Chapter 27). Although several studies have described what parents perceive as most stressful, the most effective strategy may be to simply ask parents what is stressful and what they are doing to cope with the stressors they identify (Hughes and others, 1994). Assessment should be repeated periodically to account for changes in perceptions over time.

As in emergency admissions, there is a tendency in the ICU to perform procedures quickly and without attention to the child's preparational needs. Therefore nurses need to remember the special concerns of children in each age-group about bodily injury. Explaining each procedure, altering it whenever possible to decrease the child's fears, and supporting the child are essential. Giving children an object that symbolizes their courage, such as a "hero badge" or an "ICU diploma," helps them face their fears and anxiety. It is a positive memento of an otherwise stressful experience. Because of the numerous procedures performed on the child and the nature of the illness, pain management needs to receive a high priority.

Of particular importance in decreasing fear is ensuring that discussions that do not directly include the family are held where the child and family cannot overhear them. Casual conversation in the nursing station or in the halls can often be overheard and taken out of context. When discussions are held at the bedside, it is very easy to forget the patient and make remarks that are misunderstood. Usually a quiet reminder of how frightened the child can become from listening to these discussions is sufficient. If bedside conferences are necessary, the nurse interprets them for family members in language they can comprehend or, if appropriate, asks the family to leave the area during report.

Extensive monitoring makes a usual day-night cycle difficult in an ICU. However, some schedule should be established that maintains a similarity to daily events in the child's life. These include organizing care during normal waking hours, keeping regular bedtime schedules, including quiet times when televisions and radios are lowered or turned off, closing and opening drapes as appropriate, dimming lights, placing a curtain around the bed for privacy and decreased stimulation, and having clocks or calendars in easy view for older children. In particular, staff members must realize the need for quiet and refrain from loud talking or laughing. Equipment noise should be kept to a minimum by turning alarms as low as safely possible, performing treatments requiring equipment at one time, turning off bedside equipment not in use (e.g., suction, oxygen), and avoiding loud, abrupt noises (e.g., clattering bedpans, toilet flushing) (Snyder-Halpern, 1985). Such measures can reduce the sensory overload and the sleep deprivation commonly associated with ICU admissions.

Despite the stresses normally associated with ICU admission, a special security develops from being carefully monitored and receiving individualized care. Therefore planning for transition to the regular unit is essential and should include (1) assignment of a primary nurse on the regular unit who visits before the transfer; (2) continued visits by the ICU staff to assess the child's and parents' adjustment and to act as a temporary liaison with the nursing staff; (3) explanation of the differences between the two units and the rationale for the change to less intense monitoring of the child's physical condition; and (4) selection of an appropriate room, such as one close to the nursing station, and a compatible roommate.

DISCHARGE PLANNING AND HOME CARE

Most hospitalizations necessitate some type of discharge planning. Often this involves education of the family for continued care and follow-up in the home. Depending on the diagnosis, this may be relatively simple or considerably complex. With the current concern for cost containment and recognition of children's emotional needs, home care for children with technologically complex care, such as youngsters on ventilators, has become increasingly common. Preparing the family for home care demands a high degree of competence in planning and implementing discharge instruction. Although this is usually a team effort, nurses are often key individuals in initiating the process and collaborating with others in the planning and implementing stages. While it is not possible to discuss all the details needed for effective discharge planning and home care, this section presents a brief overview of the more critical aspects. More specific details are discussed throughout the text for conditions such as home apnea monitoring, tracheostomy care, or hyperalimentation, and numerous sources of information exist in the literature.

Assessment

Discharge planning for home care must begin with an assessment of the family's desire and capability in assuming care responsibilities. Ideally, at least two individuals should be committed to learning the skills needed for home care. A thorough assessment of the family and home environment should be done to ensure that the family's emotional and physical resources are sufficient to manage the tasks of home care (for a discussion of family and home assessment strategies, see Chapters 22 and 25). In addition to adequate family resources, an investigation of community services, including respite care, is needed to ensure that appropriate support agencies are available, such as emergency facilities, home health agencies, and equipment vendors. To coordinate the immense task of assessment and to plan implementation, a case coordinator should be appointed early in the discharge program (Stein, 1985).

Planning

Ideally, preparation for hospital discharge and home care begins during the admission assessment with the establishment of short- and long-term goals. These goals are concerned with the child's physical needs, as well as the psychologic needs of the child and family. For children who require complex care, discharge planning focuses on obtaining appropriate equipment and health care personnel for the home and on those skills that parents or children are expected to continue at home. In planning appropriate teaching, nurses need to assess (1) the actual and perceived complexity of the skill, (2) the parents' or child's ability to learn the skill, and (3) the parents' or child's previous or present experience with such procedures. (See Compliance, Chapter 27, for guidelines for effective teaching.)

The teaching plan should incorporate levels of learning, such as observing, participating with assistance, and finally acting without help or guidance. The skill should be divided into discrete steps, and each step taught to the family member until it is learned. Return demonstration of the skill should be requested before new skills are introduced. A record of teaching and performance provides an efficient checklist for evaluation. All families should receive detailed *written* instructions about home care before they leave the hospital, as well as telephone numbers for assistance (see Critical Thinking Exercise box).*

Transitional Care

Once the family is competent in performing the skill, they should be given responsibility for the care. Whenever possible, the family should have a transition or trial period to assume care with minimum supervision. This may be arranged on the unit, during a home pass, or in a facility (e.g., a motel) near the hospital. Some programs incorporate a hospital trial into their discharge criteria, necessitating that the family successfully manage this phase before discharge to home. Such transitions provide a safe practice period for the family, with assistance readily available when needed, and are especially valuable when the family lives at a distance to the treating center.

*Home care instructions for a wide variety of technical skills are available in *Wong and Whaley's Clinical Manual of Pediatric Nursing* (Mosby).

CRITICAL THINKING EXERCISE

Discharge Planning and Home Care

Two-year-old Rhonda comes from a rural home 150 miles from the medical center. Last month she suffered a severe case of meningitis that left her profoundly cognitively impaired. During her hospitalization her parents have called infrequently and have never visited, because they do not have a telephone or car as a result of their low income. Rhonda is now ready to be discharged from the tertiary care center. As the primary nurse who is responsible for Rhonda's discharge planning, you initiate which of the following activities:

1. Arrange for Rhonda to be institutionalized because her family will be unable to care for her.
2. Give a list of local services with an encouraging note about the importance of arranging follow-up care to the transport team to give to her parents.
3. Call and arrange for the public health nurse from Rhonda's district to make a home visit shortly after her return.
4. Arrange for a multidisciplinary case conference to discuss Rhonda's discharge.

The correct answer is 4. A multidisciplinary case conference including the parents can be arranged with some planning. The public health department can be asked to either escort Rhonda's parents to the medical center or arrange for them to participate over a speaker phone. The public health nurse from Rhonda's district also will be able to advise the team as to what services are available in Rhonda's community. Since Rhonda will need care from a variety of professionals, this conference will help ensure that there are no gaps or overlaps in services.

Providing Rhonda's parents with a list of agencies is inappropriate. First, they do not own their own phone. Second, the parents are not in the position of knowing what services they will need. Third, dealing with professional agencies is often an arduous task and one that parents should not be expected to do while adjusting to the child's disability. Although contacting the local public health nurse is a good idea, this should be done well in advance of discharge. This way the nurse could do a home assessment to help arrange for appropriate services. Institutionalization of children with mental retardation is considered a last resort. All other options should be explored first.

Evaluation and Continuing Support

Evaluation is a critical part of any discharge plan and assumes even more importance in home care of children with complex needs. Factors to consider in home care programs are need for subsequent hospitalization, child's developmental and physical progress, effects of home care on the family, actual vs expected use of resources by the family and home care team, financial costs and savings, and improved survival.

In most instances parents need only simple instructions

and understanding of follow-up care. However, the often overwhelming care assumed by some families necessitates continued professional support after discharge. Appropriate referrals and resources may include visiting nurse or home health agencies, private nurse services, the school system, physical therapist, mental health counselor, social worker, and various community agencies, including special organizations. Sharing the important issues surrounding the child's and family's needs is essential. Referral summaries should be concise, specific, and factual. When numerous support services are involved, periodic collaboration among the professionals involved and the family is an excellent strategy to ensure efficient implementation and comprehensive delivery of services.

KEY POINTS

- Children are particularly vulnerable to the stresses of illness and hospitalization because stress represents a change from the usual state of health and routine and because they possess limited coping mechanisms.
- The three phases of separation anxiety are protest, despair, and detachment.
- Feelings of loss of control are caused by unfamiliar environmental stimuli, physical restriction, altered routine, and dependency.
- Fear of bodily pain may be manifested in the following ways: infants—expressions, body movements; toddlers—intense emotional upset, physical resistance; preschoolers—aggression, verbal expression, dependency; school-age children—precise verbalization of pain, passive requests for support or help, procrastination technique; adolescents—self-control, irritability, limited movement.
- Because of their separation from significant people, children who are hospitalized may lack the opportunity to form new attachments in the strange environment and may exhibit negative behaviors after discharge.
- Family reactions are influenced by the seriousness of illness, experience with illness or hospitalization, diagnostic or therapeutic procedures, available support systems, personal ego strengths, coping abilities, additional stresses, cultural and religious beliefs, and family communication patterns.
- The following increase the negative effects of a brother's or sister's illness/hospitalization on siblings: fear of contracting illness, their younger age, a close relationship with the ill sibling, substitute child care, minimum explanation of the illness, and perceived changes in parenting.
- Nursing care of children who are hospitalized and their families is aimed at preventing or minimizing separation, decreasing loss of control, minimizing bodily injury and pain, using play and other expressive activities to lessen stress, maximizing potential benefits of hospitalization, and supporting family members.
- Pain assessment includes questioning the child, using pain rating scales, evaluating behavior and physiologic changes, securing parents' involvement, taking the cause of pain into account, and taking action.
- Pain management should incorporate both pharmacologic and nonpharmacologic methods. Pharmacologic methods focus on four rights: right drug, right dose, right route, and right time.
- Diversional or expressive play is an effective tool in minimizing stress.
- The nurse can maximize potential benefits of hospitalization by fostering parent-child relations, providing educational opportunities, promoting self-mastery, and encouraging socialization.
- Supporting family members involves listening to parents' verbal and nonverbal messages; providing clergy support; accepting cultural, socioeconomic, and ethnic values; and giving information to families and siblings.
- The major goals of prehospital counseling are to make the hospital less strange and frightening to parents and children and to establish a positive atmosphere and trusting relationships with staff and family members.
- In preparing families for hospitalization, the nurse should consider small group size and timing of the event, setting of the tour, inclusion of preparatory materials, time for discussion, and prehospital counseling for parents.
- Emergency admission or admission to a day hospital, isolation room, or intensive care unit requires additional intervention strategies to meet the child's and family's needs.

REFERENCES

Abu-Saad H: Cultural group indicators of pain in children, *Matern Child Nurs J* 13(3):187-196, 1984.

Acute Pain Management Guideline Panel: *Acute pain management in infants, children and adolescents,* AHCPR Pub No 92-0019, Rockville, MD, 1992, Agency for Health Care Policy and Research, Public Health Service, US Department of Health and Human Services.

Ahmann E: Family-centered care: shifting orientation, *Pediatr Nurs* 20(2):113-117, 1994.

Alexander M and others: A multidisciplinary approach to pediatric pain: an empirical analysis, *Child Health Care* 22(2):81-91, 1993.

American Academy of Pediatrics: Neonatal anesthesia, *Pediatrics* 80(3):446, 1987.

American Academy of Pediatrics, Committee on Hospital Care: Child life programs, *Pediatrics* 91(3):671-673, 1993.

American Pain Society: *Principles of analgesic use in the treatment of acute pain and chronic cancer pain,* ed. 3, Skokie, IL, 1992, The Society.

Anand K, Aynsley-Green A: Metabolic and endocrine effects of surgical ligation of patent ductus arteriosus in the human preterm neonate: are there implications for further improvement of postoperative outcome? *Mod Probl Paediatr* 23:143-157, 1985.

Anand KJS, Hickey P: Pain and its effects in the human neonate and fetus, *N Engl J Med* 317(21):1321-1329, 1987.

Azarnoff P: Preparing well children for possible hospitalization, *Pediatr Nurs* 11(1):53-56, 1985.

Baird P: Occupational exposure to nitrous oxide—not a laughing matter, *N Engl J Med* 327(14):1026-1027, 1992.

Baker C, Wong D: Q.U.E.S.T.: a process of pain assessment in children, *Orthop Nurs* 6(1):11-21, 1987.

Barrier G and others: Measurement of postoperative pain and narcotic administration in infants using a new clinical scoring system, *Intensive Care Med* 15:S37-S39, 1989.

Bauchner H, May A, Coates E: Use of analgesic agents for invasive medical procedures in pediatric and neonatal intensive care units, *J Pediatr* 121(4):647-649, 1992.

Beasley SW, Tibballs J: Efficacy and safety of continuous morphine infusion for postoperative analgesia in the paediatric surgical ward, *Aust NZ J Surg* 57:233-237, 1987.

Berde C and others: Patient-controlled analgesia in children and adolescents: a randomized, prospective comparison with intramuscular administration of morphine for postoperative analgesia, *J Pediatr* 118(3):460-466, 1991.

Berman H: Nurses' beliefs about family involvement in a children's hospital, *Issues Compr Pediatr Nurs* 14(3):141-153, 1991.

Beyer JE: *The Oucher: a user's manual and technical report,* Denver, CO, 1989, University of Colorado.

Beyer JE, Denyes MJ, Villarruel AM: The creation, validation and continuing development of the Oucher: a measure of pain intensity in children, *J Pediatr Nurs* 7(5):335-346, 1992.

Beyer JE, McGrath PJ, Berde CB: Discordance between self-report and behavioral pain measures in children aged 3-7 years after surgery, *J Pain Symptom Manage* 5(6):350-356, 1990.

Beyer J and others: Patterns of postoperative analgesic use with adults and children following cardiac surgery, *Pain* 17:71-81, 1983.

Bibace R, and Walsh ME: Development of children's concepts of illness, *Pediatrics* 66(6):912-918, 1980.

Billmire DA, Neale HW, Gregory RO: Use of IV fentanyl in the outpatient treatment of pediatric facial trauma, *J Trauma* 25(11): 1079-1080, 1985.

Bjerring P, Arendt-Nielsen L: Depth and duration of skin analgesia to needle insertion after topical application of EMLA cream, *Br J Anaesth* 64:173-177, 1990.

Bonadio WA, Wagner V: Efficacy of tetracaine-adrenaline-cocaine topical anesthetic without tetracaine for facial laceration repair in children, *Pediatrics* 86(6):856-857, 1990.

Bonadio W, Wagner V: Adrenaline—cocaine gel topical anesthetic for dermal laceration repair in children, *Ann Emerg Med* 21(12): 1435-1438, 1992.

Bossert E: Stress appraisals of hospitalized school-age children, *Child Health Care* 23(1):33-49, 1994.

Britton LJ, Johnston JD: Dependent on technology: a child grows up hospitalized, *Pediatr Nurs* 19(6):579, 1993.

Broome M and others: Children's medical fears, coping behaviors, and pain perceptions during a lumbar puncture, *Oncol Nurs Forum* 17(3):361-367, 1990.

Brozovic M and others: Pain relief in sickle cell crises, *Lancet* 2(8507):624-625, 1986.

Carson D, Gravley J, Council J: Children's prehospitalization conceptions of illness, cognitive development, and personal adjustment, *Child Health Care* 21(2):103-110, 1992.

Cleeland C: Behavioral control of symptoms, *J Pain Symptom Manage* 1(1):36-38, 1986.

Craft MJ: Siblings of hospitalized children: assessment and intervention, *J Pediatr Nurs* 8(5):289-297, 1993.

Craft M, Craft J: Perceived changes in siblings of hospitalized children: a comparison of sibling and parent reports, *Child Health Care* 18(1):42-48, 1989.

Craft MJ, Wyatt N: Effect of visitation upon siblings of hospitalized children, *Matern Child Nurs J* 15(1):47-59, 1986.

Craft MJ, Wyatt N, Sandell B: Behavior and feeling changes in siblings of hospitalized children, *Clin Pediatr* 24(7):374-378, 1985.

Curley MA, Wallace J: Effects of the nursing Mutual Participation Model of Care on parental stress in the pediatric intensive care unit: a replication, *J Pediatr Nurs* 7(6):377-385, 1992.

Davidson JA, Boom SJ: Warming lidocaine to *reduce pain associated with injection, Br Med J* 305(6854):617-618, 1992.

Dilworth NM, MacKellar A: Pain relief for the pediatric surgical patient, *J Pediatr Surg* 22:264-266, 1987.

Dolgin M and others: Behavioral distress in pediatric patients with cancer receiving chemotherapy, *Pediatrics* 84(1):103-110, 1989.

Eberly TW and others: Parental stress after the unexpected admission of a child to the intensive care unit, *Crit Care Q* 8(1):57-65, 1985.

Eisenberg DM and others: Unconventional medicine in the United States: prevalence, costs, and patterns of use, *N Engl J Med* 328(4):246-252, 1993.

Eland J: Children with pain. In Jackson OB, Saunders RB: *Child Health Nursing,* Philadelphia, 1993, JB Lippincott.

Eland JM, Anderson JE: The experience of pain in children. In Jacox A, editor: *Pain: a source book for nurses and other health professionals,* Boston, 1977, Little, Brown.

Engebo D: Safe and effective use of tetracaine, adrenaline, and cocaine (TAC) solution anesthetic for anesthetizing of lacerations, *J Emerg Nurs* 16(2):100-101, 1990.

Farrington E: Lidocaine 2.5%/prilocaine 2.5% EMLA Cream, *Pediatr Nurs* 19(5):484-486, 488, 1993.

Favaloro R, Touzel B: A comparison of adolescents' and nurses' postoperative pain ratings and perceptions, *Pediatr Nurs* 16(4): 414-417, 424, 1990.

Feld LH and others: Preanesthetic medication in children: a comparison of oral transmucosal fentanyl citrate versus placebo, *Anesthesiology* 71:374-377, 1989.

Fitzgerald M, Millard C, MacIntosh N: Hyperalgesia in premature infants, *Lancet* 6(8580): 292, 1988.

Fradet C and others: A prospective survey of reactions to blood tests by children and adolescents, *Pain* 40(1):53-60, 1990.

Franck L: A national survey of the assessment and treatment of pain and agitation in the neonatal intensive care unit, *JOGNN* 16:387-393, 1987.

French GM, Painter EC, Coury DL: Blowing away shot pain: a technique for pain management during immunization, *Pediatrics* 93(3):384-388, 1994.

Friedland LR, Kulick RM: Emergency department analgesic use in pediatric trauma victims with fractures, *Ann Emerg Med* 23(2): 203-207, 1994.

Friedman DP: Perspectives on the medical use of drugs of abuse, *J Pain Symptom Manage* 5(1):52-55, 1990.

Gaukroger P, Tomkins DP, van der Walt J: Patient-controlled analgesia in children, *Anaesth Intensive Care* 17(3):264-268, 1989.

Gaynard L and others: *Psychosocial care of children in hospitals,* Bethesda, MD, 1990, Association for the Care of Children's Health.

Gillis A: Hospital preparation: the children's story, *Child Health Care* 19(1):19-27, 1990.

Goodwin JS, Goodwin JM, and Vogel AV: Knowledge and use of placebos by house officers and nurses, *Ann Intern Med* 91:106-110, 1979.

Gordon M: *Nursing diagnosis: process and application,* ed 3, St. Louis, 1994, Mosby.

Graves JK, Ware ME: Parents' and health professionals' perceptions concerning parental stress during a child's hospitalization, *Child Health Care* 19(10):37-42, 1990.

Guardiola E, Banos J: Is there an increasing interest in pediatric pain? Analysis of the biomedical articles published in the 1980's, *J Pain Symptom Manage,* 8(7):449-450, 1993.

Gureno MA, Reisinger CL: Patient-controlled analgesia for the young pediatric patient, *Pediatr Nurs* 1991.

Hagemann V: Night sleep of children in a hospital. I. Sleep duration, *Matern Child Nurs J* 10:1-13, 1981a.

Hagemann V: Night sleep of children in a hospital. II. Sleep disruption, *Matern Child Nurs J* 10:127-142, 1981b.

Hart D, Bossert E: Self-reported fears of hospitalized school-age children, *J Pediatr Nurs* 9(2):83-90, 1994.

Hart R and others: *Therapeutic play activities for hospitalized children,* St Louis, 1992, Mosby.

Haslam DR: Age and the perception of pain, *Psychosom Sci* 15:86, 1969.

Hertzka R and others: Fentanyl-induced ventilatory depression: effects of age, *Anesthesiology* 70:213-218, 1989.

Hester NO: Comforting the child in pain. In Funk SG and others, editors: *Key aspects of comfort,* New York, 1989, Springer.

Hinkle AJ: Percutaneous inguinal block for the outpatient management of post-herniorrhaphy pain in children, *Anesthesiology* 67:411-413, 1987.

Hughes M and others: How parents cope with the experience of neonatal intensive care, *Child Health Care* 23(1):1-14, 1994.

Humphrey BG and others: The occurrence of high levels of acute behavioral distress in children and adolescents undergoing routine venipunctures, *Pediatrics* 90(1):87-91, 1992.

Hurley A, Whelan EG: Cognitive development and children's perception of pain, *Pediatr Nurs* 14(1):21-24, 1988.

Izard CE, Hembree EA, Huebner RR: Infants' emotion expressions to acute pain: developmental change and stability of individual differences, *Dev Pyschol* 23(1):105-113, 1987.

Jin Bu Huan toxicity in children—Colorado, 1983, *MMWR* 42(33):633-636, 1993.

Johnson BH, Jeppson ES, Redburn L: *Caring for children and families: guidelines for hospitals,* ed 1, Bethesda, MD, 1992, Association for the Care of Children's Health.

Joint Commission on Accreditation of Healthcare Organizations: *AMH92 accreditation manual for hospitals,* Chicago, 1992, The Commission.

Jones RDM and others: Antagonism of the hypnotic effect of midazolam in children: a randomized double-blind study of placebo and flumazenil administered after midazolam-induced anaesthesia, *Br J Anaesth* 66:660-666, 1991.

Jordan-Marsh M and others: Alternate Oucher form testing gender ethnicity and age variations, *Res Nurs Health* 17:111-118, 1994.

Juhlin L, Evers H: EMLA: a new topical anesthetic, *Adv Dermatol* 5:75-92, 1990.

Karl HW, Larach MG, Ruffle JM: Transmucosal midazolam for preinduction of anesthesia in pediatric patients: comparison of intranasal and sublingual routes, *J Pain Symptom Manage* 6(3):142, 1991.

Katz E, Kellerman J, Siegel S: Behavioral distress in children with cancer undergoing medical procedures: developmental considerations, *J Consult Clin Psychol* 48(3):356-365, 1980.

Koren G: Use of the eutectic mixture of local anesthetics in young children for procedure-related pain, *J Pediatr* 122:S30-S35, 1993.

Koren G and others: Postoperative morphine infusion in newborn infants: assessment of disposition characteristics and safety, *J Pediatr* 107(6):963-967, 1985.

LaMontagne LL, Johnson BD, Hepworth JT: Children's ratings of postoperative pain compared to ratings by nurses and physicians, *Issues Compr Pediatr Nurs* 14(4):241-247, 1991.

Lander J, Fowler-Kerry S: Assessment of sex differences in children's and adolescents' self-reported pain from venipuncture, *J Pediatr Psychol* 16(6):783-793, 1991.

Lawrence J and others: The development of a tool to assess neonatal pain, *Neonatal Network* 12(6):59-66, 1993.

Lloyd C: Chemically induced methaemoglobinemia in a neonate, *Br J Oral Maxillofac Surg* 30:63-5, 1992.

Love G: The dangers of normepederine toxicity, *Am J Nurs* 94(6):14, 1994.

Lugo RA and others: Complication of intranasal midazolum, *Pediatrics* 92(4):638, 1993 (letter).

Marshall RE: Neonatal pain associated with caregiving procedures, *Pediatr Clin North Am* 36(4):885-903, 1989.

Mather L, Mackie J: The incidence of postoperative pain in children, *Pain* 15:271-282, 1983.

McCaffery M, Beebe A: *Pain: clinical manual for nursing practice,* St Louis, 1989, Mosby.

McCain GC, Bies DC: Television viewing and the hospitalized child, *Pediatr Nurs* 9(1):33-35, 1983.

McIlvaine W: Spinal opioids for the pediatric patient, *J Pain Symptom Manage* 5(3):183-190, 1990.

McKay W, Morris R, Mushlin P: Sodium bicarbonate attenuates pain on skin infiltration with lidocaine, with or without epinephrine, *Anesth Analg* 66:572-574, 1987.

Miles MS and others: Maternal and paternal stress reactions when a child is hospitalized in a pediatric care unit, *Issues Compr Pediatr Nurs* 7:333-342, 1984.

Miles M, Mathes M: Preparation of parents for the ICU experience: what are we missing? *Child Health Care* 20(3):132-137, 1991.

Mills NM: Acute pain behavior in infants and toddlers. In Funk SG and others, editors: *Key aspects of comfort: management of pain, fatigue, and nausea,* New York, 1989, Springer.

Miser AW and others: Narcotic withdrawal syndrome in young adults after the therapeutic use of opiates, *Am J Dis Child* 140:603-604, 1986.

Miser A and others: Transdermal fentanyl for pain control in patients with cancer, *Pain* 37:15-21, 1989.

Morrison R: Update on sickle cell disease: incidence of addiction and choice of opioid in pain management, *Pediatr Nurs* 17(6):503, 1991.

Nix K, Clutter L, Wong DL: *The influence of the type of instructions in measuring pain intensity in young children using the FACES Pain Rating Scale,* Unpublished manuscript, 1994.

Norman J, Jones P: Complications of the use of EMLA, *Br J Anaesth* 64:403, 1990.

Nugent K and others: A practice model for a parent support group, *Pediatr Nurs* 18(1):11-16, 1992.

Olkkola K and others: Kinetics and dynamics of postoperative intravenous morphine in children, *Clin Pharmacol Ther* 44:128-136, 1988.

Orem D: *Nursing: concepts of practice,* ed 4, New York, 1991, Mosby.

Orlinsky M and others: Pain comparison of unbuffered versus buffered lidocaine in local wound infiltration, *J Emerg Med* 10:411-415, 1992.

Paice J: Pharmacologic management. In Watt-Watson JH, Donavon MK, editors: *Pain management: nursing perspectives,* St Louis, 1992, Mosby.

Pasero CL, McCaffery M: Avoiding opioid-induced respiratory depression, *Am J Nurs* 94(4):25-31, 1994.

Pazola KJ, and Gerberg AK: Teen group: a forum for the hospitalized adolescent, *MCN* 10(4):265-269, 1985.

Perin G, Frase D: Development of a program using general anesthesia for invasive procedures in a pediatric outpatient setting, *J Assoc Pediatr Oncol Nurses* 3(4):8-10, 1985.

Perrin EC, Gerrity PS: There's a demon in your belly: children's understanding of illness, *Pediatrics* 67(6):841-849, 1981.

Perry SW, Heidrich G: Placebo response: myth and matter, *Am J Nurs* 81(4):720-725, 1981.

Petrillo M, Sanger S: *Emotional care of hospitalized children,* ed 2, Philadelphia, 1980, JB Lippincott.

Pfefferbaum B, Adams J, Aceves, J: The influence of culture on pain in Anglo and Hispanic children with cancer, *J Am Acad Child Adolesc Psychiatry* 29(4):642-647, 1990.

Pitorak EF: Flavored morphine troches for cancer pain, *Oncol Nurs Forum* 18(3):601, 1991.

Porter J, Jick H: Addiction rare in patients treated with narcotics, *N Engl J Med* 302(2): 123, 1980.

Rae W: Analyzing drawings of children who are physically ill or hospitalized using the Ipsative method, *Child Health Care* 20(4):198-207, 1991.

Riemondy S and others: Nurse controlled analgesia: a new method of pediatric pain control, *J Pain Symptom Manage* 6(3):160, 1991 (abstract).

Rodgers BM and others: Patient-controlled analgesia in pediatric surgery, *J Pediatr Surg* 23(3):259-262, 1988.

Rogers A: The ABC of pediatric pain, *Prim Care Cancer* 10:7-8, 1990.

Rollins J: Supporting the child. In Smith DP and others, editors: *Comprehensive child and family nursing skills,* St Louis, 1991, Mosby.

Rollins J: Medical students as facilitators of the arts for children in hospitals, *Int J Arts Med* 2(1):7-13, 1993.

Rowbotham D and others: Transdermal fentanyl for the relief of pain after upper abdominal surgery, *Br J Anaesth* 63:56-59, 1989.

Rowland AS and others: Reduced fertility among women employed as dental assistants exposed to high levels of nitrous oxide, *N Engl J Med* 327(14):993-997, 1992.

Ruble K, Billett C: Innovative pain management for toddlers: parent-controlled analgesia, *Oncol Nurse Forum* 20(2):321, 1993.

Sabbe M, Yaksh T: Pharmacology of spinal opioids, *J Pain Symptom Manage* 5(3):191-203, 1990.

Savedra M, and others: Pain location: validity and reliability of body outline markings by hospitalized children and adolescents, *Res Nurs Health* 12:307-314, 1989.

Savedra MC and others: Assessment of postoperative pain in children and adolescents using the Adolescent pediatric pain tool, *Nurs Res* 42(1):5-9, 1993.

Schechter NL, Allen DA, Hanson K: Status of pediatric pain control: a comparison of hospital analgesic usage in children and adults, *Pediatrics* 77(1):11-15, 1986.

Schmidt K, Eland J, Weiler K: Pediatric cancer pain management: a survey of nurses' knowledge, *J Pediatr Oncol Nurs* 11(1):4-12, 1994.

Schwesinger WH and others: Transnasal butorphanol and intramuscular meperidine in the treatment of postoperative pain, *Adv Ther* 9(3):123-129, 1992.

Shapiro C: Pain in the neonate: assessment and intervention, *Neonatal Network* 8(1):7-21, 1989.

Sherwood KA: The use of topical anesthesia in removal of port-wine stains in children, *J Pediatr* 122:s36-s41, 1993.

Shonkwiler MA: Sibling visits in the pediatric intensive care unit, *Crit Care Q* 8(1):67-72, 1985.

Simon K: Perceived stress of nonhospitalized children during the hospitalization of a sibling, *J Pediatr Nurs* 8(5):298-304, 1993.

Snyder-Halpern R: The effect of critical care unit noise on patient sleep cycles, *Crit Care Q* 7(4):41-50, 1985.

Spencer DM and others: Dorsal penile nerve block in neonatal circumcision, *Am J Perinatol* 9(3):214-218, 1992.

Stein R: Home care: a challenging opportunity, *Child Health Care* 14(2):90-95, 1985.

Stevens BJ, Johnston CC, Horton L: Multidimensional pain assessment in premature neonates: a pilot study, *JOGNN* 26(5):531-541, 1993.

Streisand JB and others: Oral transmucosal fentanyl citrate premedication in children, *Anesth Analg* 69:28-34, 1989.

Taddio A and others: Use of lidocaine-prilocaine cream for vaccination pain in infants, *J Pediatr* 124(4):643-648, 1994.

Tesler MD and others: Children's words for pain. In Funk SG and others, editors: *Key aspects of comfort: management of pain, fatigue, and nausea,* New York, 1989, Springer Publishing.

Tesler M and others: The word-graphic rating scale as a measure of children's and adolescents' pain intensity, *Res Nurs Health* 14:361-371, 1991.

Theroux MC and others: Efficacy of intranasal midazolam in facilitating suturing of lacerations in preschool children in the emergency department, *Pediatrics* 91(3):624, 1993.

Tichy AM and others: Stressors in pediatric intensive care units, *Pediatr Nurs* 14(1):40-42, 1988.

Uhari M: A eutectic mixture of lidocaine and prilocaine for alleviating vaccination pain in infants, *Pediatrics* 92(5):719-721, 1993.

Van Cleve L, Savedra M: Pain location: validity and reliability of body outline markings for 4- to 7-year-old children who are hospitalized, *Pediatr Nurs* 19(3):217-220, 1993.

Vetter TR: Pediatric patient-controlled analgesia with morphine versus meperidine, *J Pain Symptom Manage* 7(4):204, 1992.

Villarruel AM, Denyes MJ: Pain assessment in children: theoretical and empirical validity, *Adv Nurs Sci* 14(2):32-41, 1991.

Volz DD: Time structuring for hospitalized, school-aged children, *Issues Compr Pediatr Nurs* 5:205-210, 1981.

Vulcan B, Nikulich-Barrett M: The effect of selected information on mothers' anxiety levels during their children's hospitalizations, *J Pediatr Nurs* 3(2):97-102, 1988.

Walco GA, Ilowite NT: Vertical vs horizontal visual analog scales of pain intensity in children, *J Pain Symptom Manage* 6(3):200, 1991.

Walker M, Wong DL: A battle plan for patients in pain, *Am J Nurs* 91(6):32-36, 1991.

Wallace M: Temperament: a variable in children's pain management, *Pediatr Nurs* 15(2):118-121, 1989.

Wattenmaker I, Kasser JR, McGravey A: Self-administered nitrous oxide for fracture reduction in children in an emergency room setting, *J Orthop Trauma* 4(1):35-38, 1990.

Watt-Watson JH, Evernden C, Lawson C: Parents' perceptions of their child's acute pain experience, *J Pediatr Nurs* 5(5):344-349, 1990.

Weatherstone KB and others: Safety and efficacy of a topical anesthetic for neonatal circumcision, *Pediatrics* 92(5):710-714, 1993.

Webb C, Paarlberg J, Sussman M: The use of a PCA device by parents or nurses for postoperative pain in children with cerebral palsy, *J Pain Symptom Manage* 6(3):160, 1991 (abstract).

Wells PW and others: Growing up in the hospital. I. Let's focus on the child, *J Pediatr Nurs* 9(2):66-73, 1994.

West N and others: Measuring pain in pediatric patients in the ICU, *J Pediatr Oncol Nurs* 11(2):64-68, 1994.

Willens JS: Giving fentanyl for pain outside the OR, *Am J Nurs* 94(2):24-28, 1994.

Wong D: Practice pointers, *School Healthwatch* 5(1):2, 1993.

Wong D, Baker C: Pain in children: comparison of assessment scales, *Pediatr Nurs* 14(1):9-17, 1988.

Wong D, Redding B: Lozenges can be "lifesavers," *Am J Nurs* 87(9):1129-1130, 1987.

Yaster M and others: Midazolam-fentanyl intravenous sedation in children: case report of respiratory arrest, *Pediatrics* 86(3):463-467, 1990.

Yoos HL: Children's illness concepts: old and new paradigms, *Pediatr Nurs* 20(2):134-140, 145, 1994.

Young M, Fu V: Influence of play and temperament on the young child's response to pain, *Child Health Care* 16(3):209-215, 1988.

Zeltzer LK, Jay SM, Fisher DM: The management of pain associated with pediatric procedures, *Pediatr Clin North Am* 36(4):941-964, 1989.

BIBLIOGRAPHY

Hospitalization: The Child and Family

Alexander D and others: Anxiety levels of rooming-in and non-rooming-in parents of young hospitalized children, *Matern Child Nurs J* 17(2):79-99, 1988.

American Academy of Pediatrics, Committee on Hospital Care: Staffing patterns for patient care and support personnel in a general pediatric unit, *Pediatrics* 93(5):850-854, 1994.

Balayewich C, Gasson A: Oh, Suzanna! A nursing challenge, *Axone* 15(1):9-12, 1993.

Banks E: Concepts of health and sickness of preschool- and school-aged children, *Child Health Care* 19(1):43-48, 1990.

Biehler B: Impact of role-sets on implementing self-care theory with children, *Pediatr Nurs* 18(1):30-34, 1992.

Bolig R, Weedle KD: Resiliency and hospitalization of children, *Child Health Care* 16(4):255-260, 1988.

Brown J, Ritchie JA: Nurses' perceptions of parent and nurse roles in caring for hospitalized children, *Child Health Care* 19(1):28-36, 1990.

Burke SO, Costello EA, Handley-Derry MH: Maternal stress and repeated hospitalizations of children who are physically disabled, *Child Health Care* 18(2):82-90, 1989.

Burke SO and others: Hazardous secrets and reluctantly taking charge: parenting a child with repeated hospitalizations, *Image J Nurs Sch* 23(1):39-45, 1991.

Caty S, Ritchie JA, Ellerton M: Helping hospitalized preschoolers manage stressful situations: the mother's role, *Child Health Care* 18(4):202-209, 1989.

Caty S, Ritchie JA, Ellerton ML: Mothers' perception of coping behaviors in hospitalized preschool children, *J Pediatr Nurs* 4(6):403-410, 1989.

Coffman S, Levitt MJ, Guacci-Franco N: Mothers' stress and close relationships: correlates with infant health status, *Pediatr Nurs* 19(2):135-140, 1993.

Cozad J: Children, hospitalization and stress, *Point View* 27(2):7-11, 1990.

Craft MJ, Craft JL: Perceived changes in siblings of hospitalized children: a comparison of sibling and parent reports, *Child Health Care* 18(1):42-48, 1989.

Curry NE: Enhancing dramatic play potential in hospitalized children, *Child Health Care* 16(3):142-149, 1988.

DelPo EG, Frick SB: Directed and nondirected play as therapeutic modalities, *Child Health Care* 16(4):261-267, 1988.

Denholm CJ: The adolescent patient at discharge and in the post-hospitalization environment: a review, *Matern Child Nurs J* 16(2):95-102, 1987.

Denholm CJ: Reactions of adolescents following hospitalization for acute conditions, *Child Health Care* 18(4):210-217, 1989.

Denholm CJ: Memories of adolescent hospitalization: results from a 4-year follow-up study, *Child Health Care* 19(2):101-105, 1990.

Denholm CJ, Ferguson RV: Strategies to promote the developmental needs of hospitalized adolescents, *Child Health Care* 15(3):183-187, 1987.

Elfert H, Anderson JM: More than just luck, *Can Nurse* 83(4):14-17, 1987.

Ellerton M, Ritchie JA, Caty S: Nurses' perceptions of coping behaviors in hospitalized preschool children, *J Pediatr Nurs* 4(3):197-205, 1989.

Faller HS: A child's perception of the hospital, *MCN* 13:38, 1988.

Flint NS, Walsh M: Visiting policies in pediatrics: parents' perceptions and preferences, *J Pediatr Nurs* 3(4):237-246, 1988.

Gaynard L, Goldberger J, Laidley L: The use of stuffed body-outline dolls with hospitalized children and adolescents, *Child Health Care* 20(4):216-224, 1991.

Goldberger J: Issue-specific play with infants and toddlers in hospitals: rationale and intervention, *Child Health Care* 16(3):134-141, 1988.

Greenberg LA: Teaching children who are learning disabled about illness and hospitalization, *MCN* 16(5):260-263, 1991.

Grey M: Stressors and children's health, *J Pediatr Nurs* 8(2):85-91, 1993.

Grimm DL, Pefley PT: Opening doors for the child "inside," *Pediatr Nurs* 16(4):368-369, 1990.

Hester NO: Health perceptions of school-age children, *Issues Compr Pediatr Nurs* 10:137-147, 1987.

Hudson C and others: Storytelling: a measure of anxiety in hospitalized children, *Child Health Care* 16(2):118-122, 1987.

Kennedy C, Gyr P, Garst K: A nursing tool to assess children upon hospital admission, *MCN* 16(2):78-82, 1991.

Kiely AB: *Volunteers in child health: management, selection, training, and supervision,* Bethesda, MD, 1992, Association for the Care of Children's Health.

Knafl KA, Cavallari KA, Dixon DM: *Pediatric hospitalization: family and nurse perspectives,* Boston, 1988, Scott, Foresman.

Kreger BE, Restuccia JD: Assessing the need to hospitalize children: pediatric appropriateness evaluation protocol, *Pediatrics* 84(2):242-247, 1989.

Kristjansdottir G: A study of the needs of parents of hospitalized 2- to 6-year-old children, *Issues Compr Pediatr Nurs* 14(1):49-64, 1991.

LaMontagne LL: Children's preoperative coping: replication and extension, *Nurs Res* 36(3):163-167, 1987.

Lipsi K, Clements-Shafer K, Rushton C: Developmental rounds: an intervention strategy for hospitalized infants, *Pediatr Nurs* 17(5):433-437, 468, 1991.

Logsdon DA: Conceptions of health and health behaviors of preschool children, *J Pediatr Nurs* 6(6):396-406, 1991.

Lynn MR: Siblings' responses in illness situations, *J Pediatr Nurs* 4(2):127-129, 1989.

Mabe P, Treiber F, Riley W: Examining emotional distress during pediatric hospitalization for school-aged children, *Child Health Care* 20(3):162-169, 1991.

Maheady DC: Health concepts of preschool children, *Pediatr Nurs* 12(3):195-197, 1986.

McBurney BH, Schultz C: Defining quality services in a general pediatric unit, *J Nurs Care Qual* 7(3):51-60, 1993.

McCain GC: Family functioning 2 to 4 years after preterm birth, *J Pediatr Nurs* 5(2):97-104, 1990.

McClowry SG: A review of the literature pertaining to the psychosocial responses of school-aged children to hospitalization, *J Pediatr Nurs* 3(5):296-311, 1988.

McClowry SG: The relationship of temperament to pre- and posthospitalization behavioral responses of school-age children, *Nurs Res* 39(1):30-35, 1990.

McClowry SG: Behavioral disturbances among medically hospitalized school-age children, *J Child Adolesc Psychiatr Ment Health Nurs* 4(2):62-67, 1991.

McClowry SG, McLeod SM: The psychosocial responses of school-age children to hospitalization, *Child Health Care* 19(3):155-161, 1990.

McCue K: Medical play: an expanded perspective, *Child Health Care* 16(3):157-161, 1988.

McLeod SM, McClowry SG: Using temperament theory to individualize the psychosocial care of hospitalized children, *Child Health Care* 19(2):79-85, 1990.

Merkens MJ: A pediatric chronic illness transition unit, *Child Health Care* 19(1):4-9, 1990.

Miller SA: Promoting self-esteem in the hospitalized adolescent: clinical interventions, *Issues Compr Pediatr Nurs* 10:187-194, 1987.

Miron J: What children think about hospitals, *Can Nurs* 86(3):23-25, 1990.

Nix KS: Children and the health care system. In Smith DP and others, editors: *Comprehensive child and family nursing skills,* St Louis, 1991, Mosby.

Nugent KE: Routine care: promoting development in hospitalized infants, *MCN* 14:318-321, 1989.

Nugent K and others: A practice model for a parent support group, *Pediatr Nurs* 18(1):11-16, 1992.

Oremland EK: Mastering developmental and critical experiences through play and other expressive behaviors in childhood, *Child Health Care* 16(3):150-156, 1988.

Pass MD, Pass CM: Anticipatory guidance for parents of hospitalized children, *J Pediatr Nurs* 2(4):250-258, 1987.

Porter CP, Villarruel AM: Socialization and caring for hospitalized African- and Mexican-American children, *Issues Compr Pediatr Nurs* 14(1):1-16, 1991.

Poster EC, Betz CL: Survey of sibling and peer visitation policies in Southern California hospitals, *Child Health Care* 15(3):166-171, 1987.

Powell GM and others: Maternal anxiety and the nature of sleep onset latency in hospitalized children, *Pediatr Nurs* 13(6):397-401, 1987.

Reynolds EA, Ramenofsky ML: The emotional impact of trauma on toddlers, *MCN* 13(2):106-109, 1988.

Robinson CA: Preschool children's conceptualizations of health and illness, *Child Health Care* 16(2):89-95, 1987.

Robinson CA: Roadblocks to family centered care when a chronically ill child is hospitalized, *Matern Child Nurs J* 16(3):181-193, 1987.

Ruddy-Wallace M: Temperament: assessing individual differences in hospitalized children, *J Pediatr Nurs* 2(1):30-36, 1987.

Saunders RB, Miller BB, Cates KM: Pediatric family care: an interdisciplinary team approach, *Child Health Care* 18(1):53-58, 1989.

Savedra M, Tesler M, Ritchie J: Parents' waiting: is it an inevitable part of the hospital experience? *J Pediatr Nurs* 2(5):328-332, 1987.

Schepp KG: Factors influencing the coping effort of mothers of hospitalized children, *Nurs Res* 40(1):42-46, 1991.

Schepp KG: Correlates of mothers who prefer control over their hospitalized child's care, *J Pediatr Nurs* 7(2):83-89, 1992.

Schum TT: Effects of hospitalization derived from a family diary: review of the literature, *Clin Pediatr* 28(8):366-370, 1989.

Slusher IL, McClure MJ: Infant stimulation during hospitalization, *J Pediatr Nurs* 7(4): 276-279, 1992.

Stevens MS: Which adolescents breeze through surgery? *Am J Nurs* 87(12):1564-1565, 1987.

Stevens MS: Application of a stress and coping framework to one adolescent's experience with hospitalization, *Matern Child Nurs J* 17(1):51-61, 1988.

Stevens MS: Benefits of hospitalization: the adolescent's perspective, *Issues Compr Pediatr Nurs* 11(4):197-212, 1988.

Stevens M: Coping strategies of hospitalized adolescents, *Child Health Care* 18(3):163-169, 1989.

Strickland MP: Children's adjustment to the hospital: a rural/urban comparison, *Matern Child Nurs J* 16(3):251-260, 1987.

Terry DG: The needs of parents of hospitalized children, *Child Health Care* 16(1):18-20, 1987.

Tedman M, Clatworthy S: Anxiety responses of 5- and 11-year-old children during and after hospitalization, *J Pediatr Nurs* 5(5):334-343, 1990.

Vessey JA, Braithwaite KB, Weidmann M: Teaching children about their internal bodies, *Pediatr Nurs* 16(1):29-33, 1990.

Vessey J, Mahon M: Therapeutic play and the hospitalized child, *J Pediatr Nurs* 5(5):328-333, 1990.

White MA and others: Distress and self-soothing bedtime behaviors in hospitalized children with non-rooming-in parents, *Matern Child Nurs J* 17(2):67-77, 1988.

White MA and others: Sleep onset latency and distress in hospitalized children, *Nurs Res* 39(3):134-139, 1990.

Wilson C: Use of children's artwork to evaluate the effectiveness of a hospital preparation program, *Child Health Care* 20(2):120-121, 1991.

Wilson CJ: Comparison of two methods of preparation for hospitalization, *Child Health Care* 16(1):24-27, 1987.

Winch AE, Christoph JM: Parent-to-parent links: Building networks for parents of hospitalized children, *Child Health Care* 17(2): 93-97, 1988.

Winkelstein ML, Carson VJ: Adolescents and rooming-in, *Matern Child Nurs J* 16(1):75-88, 1987.

Yap JN: The effects of hospitalization and surgery on children: a critical review, *J Appl Dev Psychol* 9:349-358, 1988.

Pain General Assessment

Aradine CR, Beyer JE, Tompkins JM: Children's pain perception before and after analgesia: a study of instrument construct validity and related issues, *J Pediatr Nurs* 3(1):11-23, 1988.

Beard J: Pain control: When your patient can't speak, *Am J Nurs* 94(4):22-23, 1994.

Beyer JE, Aradine CR: Content validity of an instrument to measure young children's perceptions of the intensity of their pain, *J Pediatr Nurs* 1(6):386-395, 1986.

Beyer JE, Knapp TR: Methodologic issues in the measurement of children's pain, *Child Health Care* 14(4):233-241, 1986.

Beyer JE, Levin CR: Issues and advances in pain control in children, *Nurs Clin North Am* 22(3):661-676, 1987.

Beyer JE, Wells N: The assessment of pain in children, *Pediatr Clin North Am* 36(4):837-854, 1989.

Bradshaw C, Zeanah PD: Pediatric nurses' assessments of pain in children, *J Pediatr Nurs* 1(5):314-322, 1986.

Carpenter PJ: New method for measuring young children's self-report of fear and pain, *J Pain Symptom Manage* 5(4):233-240, 1990.

Dale JC: A multidimensional study of infants' behaviors associated with assumed painful stimuli: phase II, *J Pediatr Health Care* 3(1):34-38, 1989.

Eland JM, Banner W: Assessment and management of pain in children. In Hazinski MF: *Nursing care of the critically ill child,* ed 2, St Louis, 1992, Mosby-Year Book.

Gujol MC: A survey of pain assessment and management practices among critical care nurses, *Am J Crit Care* 3(2):123-128, 1994.

Harbeck C, Peterson L: Elephants dancing in my head: a developmental approach to children's concepts of specific pains, *Child Dev* 63:138-149, 1992.

Hester NO: Pain in children. In Fitzpatrick JJ, Stevenson JS, editors: *Annual review of nursing research,* vol 11, New York, 1993, Springer.

Hurley A, Whelan EG: Cognitive development and children's perception of pain, *Pediatr Nurs* 14(1):21-24, 1988.

International Association for the Study of Pain: Pain terms: a current list with definitions and notes on usage, *Pain* 3:S216-S221, 1986.

Jacobsen PB and others: Analysis of child and parent behavior during painful medical procedures, *Health Psychol* 9(5):559-576, 1990.

Kuttner L, LePage T: Face scales for the assessment of pediatric pain: a critical review, *Can J Behav Sci* 21(2)198-209, 1989.

LaMontagne LL and others: Children's ratings of postoperative pain compared to ratings by nurses and physicians, *Issues Compr Pediatr Nurs* 14(4):241-247, 1991.

Lincoln LM: Children's response to acute pain: a developmental approach, *J Am Acad Nurse Practitioners* 4(4):139-141, 1992.

Mackey D, Jordan-Marsh M: Innovative assessment of children's pain, *J Emerg Nurs* 17(4):250-215, 1991.

McCaffery M: How reliable is your patient's pain assessment?, *Nursing 94* 24(1):19, 1994.

McCaffery M, Ferrel B: Opioid analgesics: nurses' knowledge of doses and psychological dependence, *J Nurs Staff Dev* 8(2):77-84, 1992.

McGrath PA: Evaluating a child's pain, *J Pain Symptom Manage* 4(4):198-214, 1989.

McGrath PJ, Craig KD: Developmental and psychological factors in children's pain, *Pediatr Clin North Am* 36(4):823-836, 1989.

McGrath PJ, Unruh A: *Pain in children and adolescents,* New York, 1988, Elsevier Science.

Miaskowski C and others: Assessment of patient satisfaction utilizing the American Pain Society's quality assurance standards on

acute and cancer-related pain, *J Pain Symptom Manage* 9(1):5-11, 1994.
Pasero CL: The right tool for the job, *Am J Nurs* 94(2)22, 1994.
Ross DM, Ross SA: *Childhood pain: current issues, research, and management,* Baltimore, 1988, Urban & Schwarzenberg.
Schechter NL: The undertreatment of pain in children: an overview, *Pediatr Clin North Am* 36(4):781-794, 1989.
Schechter NL and others: Individual difference in children's response to pain: role of temperament and parental characteristics, *Pediatrics* 87(2):171-177, 1991.
Stevens B: Development and testing of a pediatric pain management sheet, *Pediatr Nurs* 16(6):543-548, 1990.
Thorpe DM: Pain assessment. I. Matching the tool to patient needs, *Dimens Oncol Nurs* 3(2):19-25, 1989.
Walco GA, Ilowite NT: Vertical versus horizontal visual analogue scales of pain intensity in children, *J Pain Symptom Manage* 6(3):200, 1991.
Weissman DE and others: Educational role of cancer pain rounds, *J Cancer Educ* 4(2):113-116, 1989.
Wilkie DJ and others: Measuring pain quality: validity and reliability of children's and adolescents' pain language, *Pain* 41:151-159, 1990.
Wong D: Pediatric pain assessment scales: where do we go from here? *J Pediatr Oncol Nurs* 11(2):69-70, 1994.
Wong D, Baker C: The school nurse and the child in pain, *Sch Nurs* 5(2):14-28, 1989.

Pain Management

Beasley SW, Tibballs J: Efficacy and safety of continuous morphine infusion for postoperative analgesia in the paediatric surgical ward, *Aust NZ J Surg* 57:233-237, 1987.
Bell SG, Ellis LJ: Use of fentanyl for sedation of mechanically ventilated neonates, *Neonatal Network* 6:27-31, 1987.
Bhatt-Mehta V, Rosen DA: Management of acute pain in children, *Clin Pharm* 10:667-685, 1991.
Bonadio WA, Wagner V: Efficacy of TAC topical anesthetic for repair of pediatric lacerations, *Am J Dis Child* 142(2):203-205, 1988.
Broadman LM: Patient-controlled analgesia in children and adults. In Ferante FM, Ostheimer GW, Covino BG, editors: *Patient-controlled analgesia,* Boston, 1990, Blackwell Scientific Publications.
Broome M, Lillis P, Smith MC: Pain management with children: a meta-analysis of the research, *Nurs Res* 2:154-158, 1989.
Bostrom B, McCormick P, Hooke C: Painless procedures with propofol, *J Pediatr Oncol Nurs* 10(2):64-65, 1993.
Bucknell S, Sikorski K: Putting patient-controlled analgesia to the test, *MCN* 14(1):37-40, 1989.
Christoph R and others: Pain reduction in local anesthetic administration through pH buffering, *Ann Emerg Med* 17(2):117-120, 1988.
Crockett RK: Pain management in the pediatric emergency department, *Int Pediatr* 4(1):14-18, 1989.
Dalens B: Regional anesthesia in children, *Anesth Analg* 68:654-672, 1989.
Eland JM: The effectiveness of transcutaneous electrical nerve stimulation (TENS) with children experiencing cancer pain. In Funk SG and others, editors: *Key aspects of comfort,* New York, 1989, Springer.
Elander G, Hellstom G, Qvarnstrom B: Care of infants after major surgery: observation of behavior and analgesic administration, *Pediatr Nurs* 19(3):221-226, 1993.
Engebo D: Safe and effective use of tetracaine, adrenaline, and cocaine (TAC) solution anesthetic for anesthetizing of lacerations, *J Emerg Nurs* 16(2):100-101, 1990.
Frayling IM and others: Methaemoglobinaemia in children treated with prilocaine-lignocaine cream, *Br Med J* 301(6744):153-154, 1990.
French JP, Nocera M: Drug withdrawal symptoms in children after continuous infusions of fentanyl, *J Pediatr Nurs* 9(2):107-113, 1994.
Friedland LR, Kulick RM: Emergency department analgesic use in pediatric trauma victims with fractures, *Ann Emerg Med* 23(3):203-207, 1994.
Glare PG, Lickiss JN: Unrecognized constipation in patients with advanced cancer: a recipe for therapeutic disaster, *J Pain Symptom Manage* 7(6):369, 1992.
Gonzalez JC, Routh DK, Armstrong FD: Differential medication of child versus adult post-operative patients: the effect of nurses' assumptions, *Child Health Care* 22(1):47-59, 1993.
Goode IA, Betcher DL: EMLA, *J Pediatr Oncol Nurs* 11(1)38-41, 1994.
Gureno MA, Reisinger CL: Patient controlled analgesia for the young pediatric patient, *Pediatr Nurs* 17(3):251-254, 1991.
Halperin DL and others: Topical skin anesthesia for venous, subcutaneous drug reservoir and lumbar punctures in children, *Pediatrics* 84(2):281-284, 1989.
Harrison P: Lollipop successful in providing analgesia to children before painful procedures, *Can Med Assoc J* 145(5):521-524, 1991.
Hegenbath MA and others: Comparison of topical tetracaine, adrenaline, and cocaine anesthesia with lidocaine infiltration for repair of lacerations in children, *Ann Emerg Med* 19:63-67, 1990.
Heiney S: Helping children through painful procedures, *Am J Nurs* 1(11):20-24, 1991.
Hobbie C: Relaxation techniques for children and young people, *J Pediatr Health Care* 3(2):83-87, 1989.
Jay S and others: Cognitive, behavioral and pharmacologic interventions for children undergoing painful medical procedures, *J Consult Clin Psychol* 55:860-865, 1987.
Koren G, Maurice L: Pediatric uses of opioids, *Pediatr Clin North Am* 36(5):1141-1156, 1989.
Kuttner L: Favorite stories: a hypnotic pain reduction technique for children in acute pain, *Am J Clin Hyp* 30:44, 1988.
Leaby S, Hockenberry-Eaton M, Sigler-Price K: Clinical management of pain in children with cancer: selected approaches and innovative strategies, *Cancer Pract* 2(1):37-45, 1994.
Lindsley CB, Warady BA: Nonsteroidal antiinflammatory drugs: renal toxicity, a review of pediatric issues, *Clin Pediatr* 29(1):10-13, 1990.
Lipshitz M, Marino BL, Sanders ST: Choral hydrate side effects in young children: causes and management, *Heart Lung* 22(5):408-414, 1993.
McDonnell L, Bowden M: Breathing management: A simple stress and pain reduction strategy for use on a pediatric service, *Issues Compr Pediatr Nurs* 12:339-344, 1989.
Miser AW, Dothage JA, Miser JS: Continuous intravenous fentanyl for pain control in children and young adults with cancer, *Clin J Pain* 3:152-157, 1987.
Mofenson H, Caraccio T: Tack up a warning on TAC, *Am J Dis Child* 143(5):519, 1989.
Nelson PS and others: Comparison of oral transmucosal fentanyl citrate and an oral solution of meperidine, diazepam, and atropine for premedication in children, *Anesthesiology* 70:616-621, 1989.
Norton SJ: After effects of morphine and fentanyl analgesia: a retrospective study, *Neonatal Network* 7(3):25-28, 1988.
Pasero C, McCaffery M: Unconventional PCA: making it work for your patient, *Am J Nurs* 93(9):38-41, 1993.
Patterson D, Ware L: Coping skills for children undergoing painful procedures, *Issues Compr Pediatr Nurs* 11:113-143, 1988.
Roberts JR: Fentanyl patches, *Emerg Med* 25(6):17, 1993.
Roberts JR: Intranasal midazolam before suturing, *Emerg Med* 25(13):6, 1993.
Rodgers BM and others: Patient-controlled analgesia in pediatric surgery, *J Pediatr Surg* 23(3):259-262, 1988.
Rogers AG: The use and availability of rectal narcotics, *J Pain Symptom Manage* 1(4):292-230, 1986.
Ryan EA: The effect of musical distraction of pain in hospitalized school-aged children. In Funk SG and others: *Key aspects of comfort,* New York, 1989, Springer.
Sacchetti A and others: Pediatric analgesia and sedation, *Ann Emerg Med* 23:237-250, 1994.
Schechter NL, Altman A, Weisman S: Report of the Consensus Conference on the Management of Pain in Childhood Cancer, *Pediatrics* 86(5, suppl):813-834, 1990.
Selbst SM, Clark M: Analgesic use in the emergency department, *Ann Emerg Med* 19:1010-1013, 1990.
Shannon M, Berde CB: Pharmacologic management of pain in children and adolescents, *Pediatr Clin North Am* 36(4):855-871, 1989.
Steward DJ: Management of childhood pain: new approaches to procedure-related pain, *J Pediatr* 122(5, pt 2):entire issue, 1993.
Tipton G, DeWitt G, Eisenstein S: Topical TAC (tetracaine, adrenaline, cocaine) solution for local anesthesia in children: prescribing inconsistency and acute toxicity, *South Med J* 82(11):1344-1346, 1989.
Tobias JD: Indications and applications of epidural anesthesia in a pediatric population outside the perioperative period, *Clin Pediatr* 32(2):81-85, 1993.
Tobias JD and others: Oral ketamine premedication to alleviate the distress of invasive procedures in pediatric oncology patients, *Pediatrics* 90(4):537-541, 1992.
Tyler DC: Pharmacology of pain management, *Pediatr Clin North Am* 41(1):59, 1994.
Valente S: Using hypnosis with children for pain management, *Oncol Nurs Forum,* 18 (4), 699-704, 1991.
Weisman SJ, Schechter NL: The management of pain in children, *Pediatr Rev* 12(8):237-243, 1991.

Whitman HH: Sublingual morphine: a novel route of narcotic administration, *Am J Nurs* 84(7):939, 1984.

Wong DL: Managing pain. In Smith DP and others, editors: *Comprehensive child and family nursing skills,* St Louis, 1991, Mosby.

Wong DL: DPT pedi-cocktail: not a good mix, *Am J Nurs* 94(6):14-15, 1994.

Yaster M, Deshpande JK: Management of pediatric pain with opioid analgesics, *J Pediatr* 113(3):421-429, 1988.

Yaster M and others: Local anesthetics in the management of acute pain in children, *J Pediatr* 124(2)165-176, 1994.

Zajac J: Pediatric pain management, *Crit Care Nurse Q* 15(2):35-51, 1992.

Hospital Preparation and Special Admissions

Bernardo LM, Conway K, Bove M: The ABC method of emotional assessment and intervention: a new approach in pediatric emergency care, *J Emerg Nurs* 16(2):70-76, 1990.

Bolig R, Yolton KA, Nissen HL: Medical play and preparation: questions and issues, *Child Health Care* 20(4):225-229, 1991.

Brunnquell D, Kohen D: Emotions in pediatric emergencies: what we know, what we can do, *Child Health Care* 20(4):240-247, 1991.

Byers ML: Same day surgery: a preschooler's experience, *Matern Child Nurs J* 16(3):277-282, 1987.

Cagan J: Weaning parents from intensive care unit care, *MCN* 13:275-277, 1988.

Caine RM: Families in crisis: making the critical difference, *Focus Crit Care* 16(3):184-189, 1989.

Curley MA: Effects of the nursing mutual participation model of care on parental stress in the pediatric intensive care unit, *Heart Lung* 17(6, pt 1):682-688, 1988.

Curley MAQ: Caring for parents of critically ill children, *Crit Care Med* 21(9, suppl):S386-S387, 1993.

Deatrick JA, Knafl KA: Developing programs for hospitalized children: clinical significance of qualitative research, *J Pediatr Nurs* 3(2):123-126, 1988.

Doll-Speck L, Miller B, Rohrs K: Sibling education: implementing a program for the NICU, *Neonatal Network* 12(4)P:49-52, 1993.

Dracup K: Are critical care units hazardous to health? *Appl Nurs Res* 1(1):14-21, 1988.

Edwinson M, Arnbjornsson E, Ekman R: Psychologic preparation program for children undergoing acute appendectomy, *Pediatrics* 81(1):30-36, 1988.

Franck L, Epstein B, Adams S: Disaster preparedness for the ICN: Evolution and testing of one unit's plan, *Pediatr Nurs* 19(2):122-127, 1993.

Gillis AJ: Hospital preparation: the children's story, *Child Health Care* 19(1):19-27, 1990.

Glotzer D and others: Prior approval in the pediatric emergency room, *Pediatrics* 88(4):674-680, 1991.

Hazinski MF: Nursing care of the critically ill child: a seven-point check, *Pediatr Nurs* 11(6):453-461, 1985.

Heuer L: Parental stressors in a pediatric intensive care unit, *Pediatr Nurs* 19(2):128-131, 1993.

Jansen MT and others: Meeting psychosocial and developmental needs of children during prolonged intensive care unit hospitalization, *Child Health Care* 18(2):91-95, 1989.

Johnson PA, Nelson GL, Brunnquell DJ: Parent and nurse perceptions of parent stressors in the pediatric intensive care unit, *Child Health Care* 17(2):98-105, 1988.

Kasper JW, Nyamathi AM: Parents of children in the pediatric intensive care unit: what are their needs? *Heart Lung* 17(5):574-581, 1988.

Kidder C: Reestablishing health: factors influencing the child's recovery in pediatric intensive care, *J Pediatr Nurs* 4(2):96-103, 1989.

LaMontagne LL, Pawlak R: Stress and coping of parents of children in a pediatric intensive care unit, *Heart Lung* 19(4):416-421, 1990.

Lynch M: Preparing children for day surgery, *Child Health Care* 23(3):78-85, 1994.

Miles MS, Funk SG, Carelson J: Parental stressor scale: neonatal intensive care unit, *Nurs Res* 42(3):148-152, 1993.

Moore AC: Crisis intervention: a care plan for families of hospitalized children, *Pediatr Nurs* 15(3):234-236, 1989.

Munn VA, Tichy AM: Nurses' perceptions of stressors in pediatric intensive care, *J Pediatr Nurs* 2(6):405-411, 1987.

Ogilvie L: Hospitalization of children for surgery: the parents' view, *Child Health Care* 19(1):49-56, 1990.

Orsuto J, Sr, Corbo BH: Approaches of health caregivers to young children in a pediatric intensive care unit, *Matern Child Nurs J* 16(2):157-175, 1987.

Pawlak R, Chiafery M: Parental coping and activities during pediatric critical care, *Am J Crit Care* 1(2):76-80, 1992.

Philichi LM: Family adaptation during a pediatric intensive care hospitalization, *J Pediatr Nurs* 4(4):268-276, 1989.

Proctor DL: Relationship between visitation policy in a pediatric intensive care unit and parental anxiety, *Child Health Care* 16(1):13-17, 1987.

Rushton CH: Family-centered care in the critical care setting: myth or reality? *Child Health Care* 19(2):68-78, 1990.

Rushton CH: Strategies for family-centered care in the critical care setting, *Pediatr Nurs* 16(2):195-199, 1990.

Rushton CH: Child/family advocacy: ethical issues, practical strategies, *Crit Care Med* 21 (9, suppl):S387, 1993.

Small M, Engler A, Rushton C: Saying goodbye in the intensive care unit: helping caregivers grieve, *Pediatr Nurs* 17(1):103-105, 1991.

Stern HP and others: Communication, decision making, and perception of nursing roles in a pediatric intensive care unit, *Crit Care Nurs Q* 14(3):56-68, 1991.

Strobel SE, Keller CS: Metabolic screening in the NICU population: a proposal for change, *Pediatr Nurs* 19(2):113-117, 1993.

Terry DG: The needs of parents of hospitalized children, *Child Health Care* 16(1):18-20, 1987.

Thomas DO: How to deal with children in the emergency department, *J Emerg Nurs* 17(1):49-50, 1991.

Tichy AM and others: Stressors in pediatric intensive care units, *Pediatr Nurs* 14(1):40-42, 1988.

Titus S, Porter P: Orem's theory applied to pediatric residential treatment, *Pediatr Nurs* 15(5):465-468, 556, 1989.

Todres ID: Communication between physician, patient, and family in the pediatric intensive care unit, *Crit Care Med* 21(9, suppl):S383-S385, 1993.

Tompkins JM: Intrahospital transport of seriously ill or injured children, *Pediatr Nurs* 16(1):51-53, 1990.

Tse AM, Perez-Woods RC, Opie ND: Children's admissions to the intensive care unit: parents' attitudes and expectations of outcome, *Child Health Care* 16(2):68-75, 1987.

Tughan L: Visiting in the PICU: a study of the perceptions of patients, parents, and staff members, *Crit Care Nurs Q* 15(1):57-68, 1992.

Vessey J, Farley J, Risom L: Iatrogenic developmental effects of pediatric intensive care, *Pediatr Nurs* 17(3):229-232, 1991.

Voepel-Lewis T, Andrea CM, Magee SS: Parent perceptions of pediatric ambulatory surgery: using family feedback for program evaluation, *J Post Anesth Nurs* 7(2):106-114, 1992.

Welch TC: Ambulatory surgery centers: an aspect of surgical patient care, *Point View* 27(2):14-18, 1990.

Wilson CJ: Comparison of two methods of preparation for hospitalization, *Child Health Care* 16(1):24-27, 1987.

Wilson T, Broome ME: Promoting the young child's development in the intensive care unit, *Heart Lung* 18(3):274-281, 1989.

Wyckoff PM, Erickson MT: Mediating factors of stress on mothers of seriously ill, hospitalized children, *Child Health Care* 16(1):4-12, 1987.

Youngblut JM, Shiao SP: Child and family reactions during and after pediatric ICU hospitalization: a pilot study, *Heart Lung,* 22, 46-53, 1993.

Discharge Planning and Home Care

Cady C, Yoshioka R: Using a learning contract to successfully discharge an infant on home total parenteral nutrition, *Pediatr Nurs* 17(1):67-71, 74, 1991.

Crummette B, Boatwright D: Case management in inpatient pediatric nursing, *Pediatr Nurs* 17(5):469-473, 1991.

Curry R, Cullen J: Using videorecordings in pediatric nursing practice, *Pediatr Nurs* 16(5):501-504, 1990.

Davis B, Steele S: Case management for young children with special health care needs, *Pediatr Nurs* 17(1):15-20, 1991.

DeWitt PK and others: Obstacles to discharge of ventilator-assisted children from the hospital to home, *Chest* 103(5):1560-1565, 1993.

Foster SD: The role of education in discharge planning, *MCN* 13:403, 1988.

Giesy J: Teaching discharge management, *J Pediatr Nurs* 2(5):353-354, 1987.

Hogue E: Liability for premature discharge: an update, *Pediatr Nurs* 17(1):76, 78, 1991.

Isaacman DJ and others: Standardized instructions: do they improve communication of discharge information from the emergency department? *Pediatrics* 89(6):1204-1208, 1992.

Kasprisin C: Home care instructions. In Wong DL, Whaley LF: *Clinical manual of pediatric nursing,* ed 3, St Louis, 1990, Mosby.

Kelly JJ, Chu SY, Buehler JW: AIDS deaths shift from hospital to home: AIDS mortality project group, *Am J Public Health* 83(10):1433-1437, 1993.

McClowry SG: Pediatric nursing psychosocial care: a vision beyond hospitalization, *Pediatr Nurs* 19(2):146-148, 1993.

Miller MD and others: Ventilator-assisted youth: appraisal and nursing care, *J Neurosci Nurs* 25(5):287-295, 1993.

Nuttall P, Nicholes P: Cystic fibrosis: adolescent and maternal concerns about hospital and home care, *Issues Compr Pediatr Nurs* 15(3):199-213, 1992.

Scharer K and others: Evaluating written discharge instructions in a pediatric setting, *J Nurs Qual Assur* 4(4):63-71, 1990.

Sheikh L, O'Brien M, McCluskey-Fawcett K: Parent preparation for the NICU-to-home transition: staff and parent perceptions, *Child Health Care* 22(3):227-239, 1993.

Siarkowski-Amer K, Piegeon V: Documentation of discharge teaching before and after use of a discharge teaching tool, *J Pediatr Nurs* 6(5):296-301, 1991.

While AE: Consumer views of health care: a comparison of hospital and home care, *Child Care Health Dev* 18(2):107-116, 1992.

Wong DL: Transition from hospital to home for children with complex medical care, *J Pediatr Oncol Nurs* 8(1):3-9, 1991.

SELECTED BOOKS FOR CHILDREN

Banks A: *Hospital journal: a kid's guide to a strange place,* New York, 1989, Viking Penguin.

Chase F, Coleman L: *A visit to the hospital,* New York, 1974, Grosset & Dunlap.

Clark B: *Pop-up going to the hospital,* New York, 1970, Random House.

Collier J: *Danny goes to the hospital,* New York, 1970, WW Norton.

Howe J: *The hospital book,* New York, 1981, Crown.

Rey M, Rey H: *Curious George goes to the hospital,* New York, 1966, Houghton Mifflin.

Stein S: *A hospital story,* New York, 1974, Walker.

Weber A: *Elizabeth gets well,* New York, 1970, Thomas Y. Crowell.

OTHER RESOURCES

Association for Care of Children's Health, 7910 Woodmont Ave., Suite 300, Bethesda, MD 20814; (301) 654-6549.

Talks About the Hospital, a series written by Fred Rogers, is available from Family Communications, Inc., 4802 5th Ave., Pittsburgh, PA 15213; (412) 687-2990.

See also Bibliography in Chapter 6.

CHAPTER 27

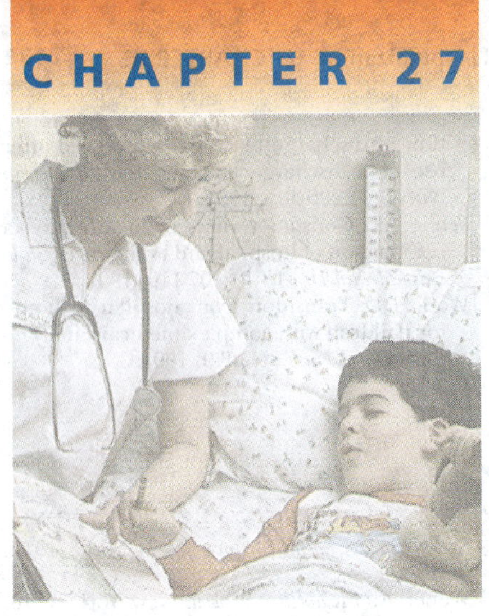

Pediatric Variations of Nursing Interventions

CHAPTER OUTLINE

RELATED TOPICS

Communicating with families, Ch. 6
Dental health: infant, Ch. 12; toddler, Ch. 14; preschooler, Ch. 15; school-age child, Ch. 17
Family-centered home care, Ch. 25
Febrile seizures, Ch. 37
Feeding resistance, Ch. 10
Injury prevention: infant, Ch. 12; toddler, Ch. 14; preschooler, Ch. 15; school-age child, Ch. 17; and adolescent, Ch. 19
Limit-setting and discipline, Ch. 3
Neonatal pain, Ch. 11
Nursing care of the surgical neonate, Ch. 11
Nutritional assessment, Ch. 6
Pain assessment; pain management, Ch. 26
Parenteral fluid therapy, Ch. 28
Preparation for hospitalization, Ch. 26
Skin care (neonatal), Ch. 10
Temperature (measurement), Ch. 7
Using play/expressive activities to minimize stress, Ch. 26
Venous access devices, Ch. 28
Wounds, Ch. 18

GENERAL CONCEPTS RELATED TO PEDIATRIC PROCEDURES

INFORMED CONSENT*

Informed consent refers to the legal and ethical requirement that patients must completely understand proposed treatments, including significant risks associated with treatment. Patients must also be informed of possible benefits of the proposed treatment, possible alternative treatments, and risks of nontreatment before giving informed consent. To obtain valid informed consent, three conditions must be met (Hogue, 1988):

1. The person must be capable of giving consent; he or she must be over the ***age of majority*** (age at which a child becomes an adult) and must be considered competent, that is, possess the mental capacity to make choices and understand their consequences.
2. The person must receive the information needed to make an intelligent decision.
3. The person must act voluntarily when exercising freedom of choice without force, fraud, deceit, duress, or other forms of constraint or coercion.

Many state legislatures have adopted laws (statutes) that address issues of informed consent. Nurses must understand what is required in their practices by reviewing applicable statutes in each jurisdiction in which they practice. There are, however, some general principles associated with informed consent that are generally applicable in all states. The following discussion of informed consent is presented in general terms and is not to be interpreted as legal advice. Although informing patients or parents of the risks, benefits, and alternatives of procedures is physicians' responsibility, nurses frequently are asked to secure patients' signatures on consent forms (see Thinking Critically About . . . box).

In caring for children, special dilemmas may arise regarding who may sign consent forms when a parent is unavailable. The age of majority is especially important when caring for adolescents, and competence is a key issue in decisions involving minors who are retarded or otherwise mentally incapacitated. Consequently, nurses need to be familiar with this highly significant and complex subject and must keep current on legal aspects of practice within their communities.

■ Kathryn A. Perry, APRN, RN,C, MSN, CNS, revised this chapter.
■ *Elizabeth E. Hogue, JD, revised this section.

PROCEDURES AND SITUATIONS REQUIRING INFORMED CONSENT

- Major surgery
- Minor surgery—cutdown, biopsy, dental extraction, suturing a laceration (especially one that may have a cosmetic effect), removal of a cyst, closed reduction of a fracture
- Diagnostic tests with an element of risk—bronchoscopy, needle biopsy, angiography, electroencephalogram, lumbar puncture, cardiac catheterization, ventriculography, bone marrow aspiration
- Medical treatments with an element of risk—blood transfusions, thoracentesis or paracentesis, radiation therapy, shock therapies
- Taking photographs for medical, educational, or other public use
- Removal of children from health care institutions against medical advice
- Postmortem examinations, except in unexplained deaths, such as sudden infant death, violent death, or suspected suicide
- Release of medical information

Requirements for Obtaining Informed Consent

Informed consent from a parent or legal guardian is usually required for medical or surgical treatment of children, including many diagnostic procedures. Informed consent must be obtained for each surgical or invasive diagnostic procedure and for certain situations that are not directly related to medical treatment (see box above).

Assent for proposed treatments should also be obtained from the child age 7 years or older who is at least in the concrete operations period. Assent requires that the child be informed about the proposed treatment or plan of care and agree or concur with the decisions made by the person(s) who can give informed consent. By including children in the decision-making process and gaining their acceptance, children are treated with respect (Erlen, 1987). Assent must also be obtained in research involving children. Considerable controversy surrounds the use of children as research subjects, and nurses involved in research must be aware of the legal and ethical guidelines and requirements

THINKING CRITICALLY ABOUT . . .

Informed Consent and Parental Right to the Child's Medical Chart

Does the right to certain types of information before giving valid informed consent include the right to review medical records? Since the process of consent continues throughout the patient's treatment, is there an ongoing right of parents to see their children's medical charts?

The answer to these questions varies depending on state law. Some state statutes give parents the unrestricted right to a copy of children's medical records. Other states have no statutes that address this point. In these states the best practice is to allow parents to review or have a copy of minors' charts under reasonable circumstances. That is, records should be available in a reasonable time. In addition, practitioners should avoid restrictive requirements such as review permitted only in the presence of a clinician. Rather, an appropriate practitioner should be available to answer any questions that parents may have during their review.

before initiating pediatric research (Rae and Fournier, 1986).

Eligibility for Giving Informed Consent

In most situations either a parent or legal guardian gives an informed consent. However, problems may arise when parents are not available to give consent, the child seeks certain treatments, the child is a so-called emancipated minor, or parents neglect or refuse treatment for their minor child. The judicial system may intervene in cases where the parents' views and the child's best interests conflict (Nix, 1991). However, laws significantly favor parental authority, and clear and convincing evidence must be presented before the court will intervene (Rhodes, 1988).

Problems may also occur when the child's parents are divorced. Generally speaking, both custodial and noncustodial parents may consent to treatment for their minor children. Consent from either divorced parent is sufficient; the consent of both parents is generally not required (Hogue, 1988).

Informed Consent of Parents or Legal Guardians. Parents have full responsibility for the care and rearing of their minor children, including legal control over them. Therefore, as long as children are minors, parents or persons designated as legal guardians for the child are required to give informed consent before medical treatment is rendered or any procedure is performed on the child. Parents also have a right to withdraw consent later.

Evidence of Consent. A signed consent form is only evidence that the process of informed consent has occurred; it is not legally required, although it may be an institutional policy. Verbal consent is also evidence of the process. For example, when parents are unavailable to sign consent forms, verbal consent may be obtained via telephone. Verbal consent may also be obtained from parents who are unable to sign, for example, because of injury. It is good risk management to have a witness to a parent's or guardian's verbal consent. Another nurse may be present or listening on a telephone extension. Both nurses record that informed consent was given and the name, address, and relationship of the person giving consent, together with their signatures indicating that they witnessed the consent.

Informed Consent of Mature and Emancipated Minors. State laws differ with regard to the so-called age of majority. Although some variation still exists, children become adults on their eighteenth birthdays in most states. Competent adults can give informed consent on their own behalf. Nonetheless, some courts have permitted minors to consent to their treatment based on the ***mature minors doctrine.*** This doctrine permits minors to give consent even though they are not technically adults as long as they understand the consequences of their decisions.

Statutes in many states permit minors to give consent on their own behalf to certain treatments, such as for:

- Sexually transmitted diseases
- Contraceptive services
- Pregnancy
- Drug or alcohol abuse

Pediatric nurses should carefully review laws in the states in which they practice to determine when minors may consent to treatment on their own behalf.

An ***emancipated minor*** is one who is legally under the age of majority but is recognized as having the legal capacity of an adult under circumstances prescribed by state law. Minors may become emancipated by the following:

- Pregnancy
- Marriage
- High school graduation
- Living independently
- Military service

GUIDELINES
Preparing Children for Procedures

Determine the details of the exact procedure to be performed.

Review the parents' and child's present level of understanding.

Plan the actual teaching based on the child's developmental age and existing level of knowledge.

Incorporate parents in the teaching if they desire, and especially if they plan to participate in the care.

Inform parents of their role during procedure, such as stand near child's head or in line of vision and talk softly to child.

While preparing the child and family, allow for ample discussion to prevent information overload and ensure adequate feedback.

Use concrete, not abstract, terms and visual aids to describe the procedure. For example, use a simple line drawing of a boy or girl (Fig. 27-1), and mark the body part that will be involved in the procedure.

Emphasize that no other body part will be involved.

If the body part is associated with a specific function, stress the change or noninvolvement of that ability (e.g., following tonsillectomy, the child can still speak).

Use words appropriate to the child's level of understanding (a rule of thumb for number of words is the age in years plus 1)

Avoid words/phrases with dual meanings (see Guidelines box on p. 1139) unless the child understands such words.

Clarify all unfamiliar words (e.g., "Anesthesia is a *special* sleep").

Emphasize the sensory aspects of the procedure—what the child will feel, see, smell, and touch and what the child can do during the procedure (e.g., lie still, count out loud, squeeze a hand, hug a doll).

Allow the child to practice those procedures that will require cooperation (e.g., turning, deep breathing, using an incentive spirometer or mask).

Introduce anxiety-laden information last (e.g., the preoperative injection).

Be honest with the child about the unpleasant aspects of a procedure but avoid creating undue concern. When discussing that a procedure may be uncomfortable, state that it feels different to different people and have the child describe how it felt.

Emphasize the end of the procedure and any pleasurable events afterward (e.g., going home, seeing the parent). Stress the benefits of the procedure to the child (e.g., "After your tonsils are fixed, you won't have as many sore throats").

Some states require emancipated minors to appear in court to prove their status. Such hearings usually result in court orders that are useful to nurses as proof of emancipation and the ability to consent to treatment. In other states one or more of the events just listed triggers emancipation without the need for any proof in court. Nurses who practice in such states are not necessarily required to seek proof of emancipation in order to accept consent from emancipated minors.

Consent to abortion is more complex. The U.S. Supreme Court has decided that parental consent is not required before performing abortions. The issue of parental notification before or after an abortion is still undecided.

Treatment Without Parental Consent. Exceptions to requiring parental consent before treating minor children occur when children need prompt medical or surgical treatment and a parent is not readily available to give consent or refuses to give consent. In the absence of parents or legal guardians, some providers permit persons in charge of the child to give informed consent for treatment. In emergencies, consent is not needed; it is implied according to the law (Hogue, 1988). Emergencies include danger to life or possibility of permanent injury.

Refusal to give consent can occur when the treatment, such as blood transfusions, conflicts with the parents' religious beliefs. All states recognize such exceptions and have statutory procedures to permit treatment if the life or health of such a minor is in jeopardy or if delayed treatment would create a risk to the health of the minor. The state is also able to intervene in situations that jeopardize the health and welfare of children, as in cases in which parents neglect or impose excessive or improper punishment on a child. In most communities there are procedures by which custody of the child can be transferred to a governmental or a private agency when parental neglect or abuse can be proved.

PREPARATION FOR PROCEDURES

Psychologic Preparation

Preparing children for procedures decreases their anxiety, promotes their cooperation, supports their coping skills and may teach them new ones, and facilitates a feeling of mastery in experiencing a potentially stressful event. Preparatory methods may be formal, such as group preparation for hospitalization (see Chapter 26). Most preparation strategies used by nurses are informal, focus on providing information about the experience, and are directed at stressful and/or painful procedures. Although research has been conducted on many types of preparation (e.g., using dolls, puppets, plays, books, videotapes, or slides), no one method is universally more effective than another. However, in general, young children respond better to play materials, and older youngsters benefit more from viewing peer-modeling films (Bates and Broome, 1986). Children often develop fantasies or distorted ideas in the absence of accurate information. Undefined threats or unexpected stress is more upsetting to the child than threats that are known, understood, and expected (Mansson, Fredrikzon, and Rosberg, 1992). Preparatory interventions are most effective in reducing behavioral distress (crying, resisting), followed by decreasing children's rating of pain, and last, by reducing

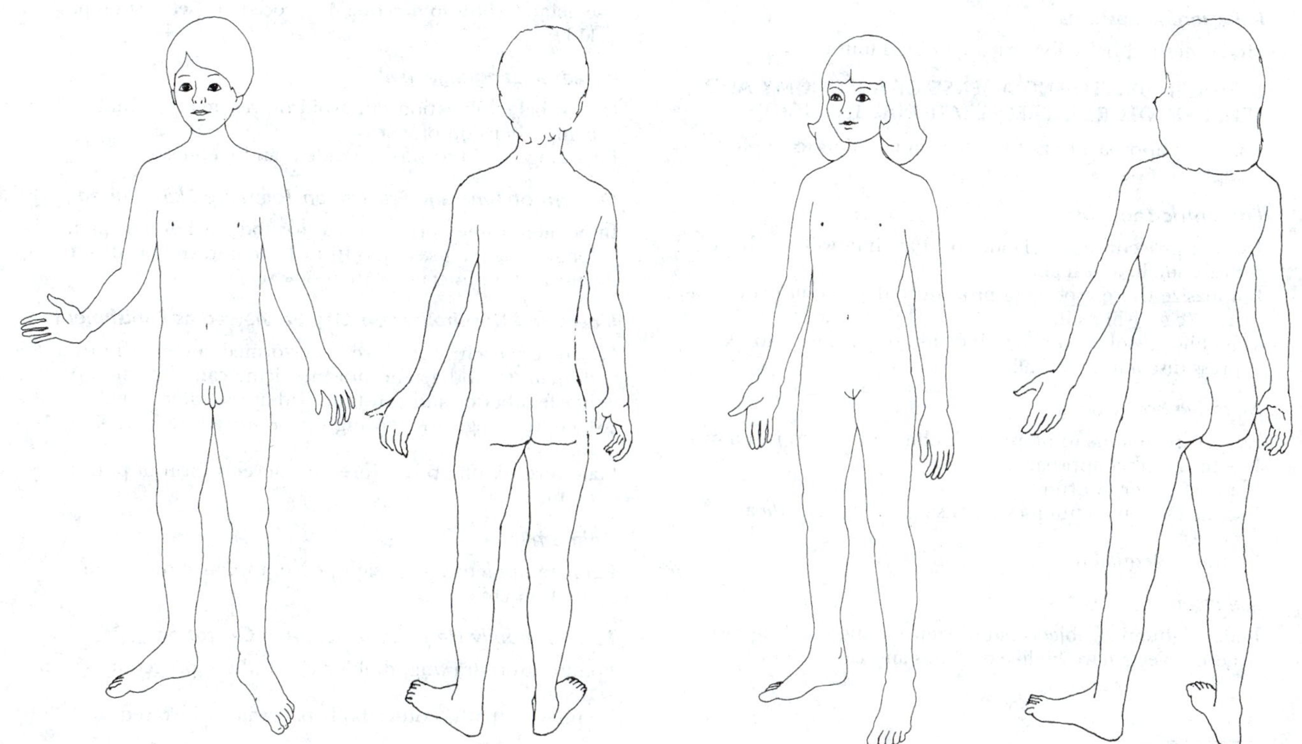

FIG. 27-1 Examples of line drawings to be used in preparing child for procedures.

GUIDELINES
Preparing Children for Procedures Based on Developmental Characteristics

INFANCY: DEVELOPING A SENSE OF TRUST AND SENSORIMOTOR THOUGHT

Attachment to Parent

*Involve parent in procedure if desired.
Keep parent in infant's line of vision.
If parent is unable to be with infant, place familiar object with infant (e.g., stuffed toy).

Stranger Anxiety

*Have usual caregivers perform or assist with procedure.
Make advances slowly and in nonthreatening manner.
*Limit number of strangers entering room during procedure.

Sensorimotor Phase of Learning

During procedure use sensory soothing measures (e.g., stroking skin, talking softly, giving pacifier).
*Use analgesics (e.g., local anesthetic, intravenous opioid) to control discomfort.
Cuddle and hug child after stressful procedure; encourage parent to comfort child.

Increased Muscle Control

Expect older infants to resist.
Restrain adequately.
Keep harmful objects out of reach.

Memory of Past Experiences

Realize that older infants may associate objects, places, or persons with prior painful experiences and will cry and resist at the sight of them.
*Keep frightening objects out of view.
*Perform painful procedures in a separate room, not in crib (or bed).
*Use nonintrusive procedures whenever possible (e.g., axillary or tympanic temperatures, oral medication).

Imitation of Gestures

Model desired behavior (e.g., opening mouth).

TODDLER: DEVELOPING A SENSE OF AUTONOMY AND SENSORIMOTOR TO PREOPERATIONAL THOUGHT

Use same approaches as for infant in addition to the following:

Egocentric Thought

Explain procedure in relation to what child will see, hear, taste, smell, and feel.
Emphasize those aspects of procedure that require cooperation (e.g., lying still).
Tell child it's okay to cry, yell, or use other means to express discomfort verbally.

Negative Behavior

Expect treatments to be resisted; child may try to run away.
Use firm, direct approach.
Ignore temper tantrums.
Use distraction techniques (e.g., singing a song *with* a child).
Restrain adequately.

Animism

Keep frightening objects out of view (young children believe objects have lifelike qualities and can harm them).

Limited Language Skills

Communicate using behaviors.
Use a few, simple terms familiar to child.
Give one direction at a time (e.g., "Lie down," then "Hold my hand").
Use small replicas of equipment; allow child to handle equipment.
Use play; demonstrate on doll but avoid child's favorite doll, since child may think doll is really "feeling" procedure.
Prepare parents separately to avoid child's misinterpreting words.

Limited Concept of Time

Prepare child shortly or immediately before procedure.
Keeping teaching sessions short (about 5 to 10 minutes).
Have preparations completed before involving child in procedure.
Have extra equipment nearby (e.g., alcohol swabs, new needle, Band-Aids) to avoid delays.
Tell child when procedure is completed.

Striving for Independence

Allow choices whenever possible but realize that child may still be resistant and negative.
Allow child to participate in care and to help whenever possible (e.g., drink medicine from a cup, hold a dressing).

PRESCHOOLER: DEVELOPING A SENSE OF INITIATIVE AND PREOPERATIONAL THOUGHT

Egocentric

Explain procedure in simple terms and in relation to how it affects child (as with toddler stress sensory aspects).
Demonstrate use of equipment.
Allow child to play with miniature or actual equipment.
Encourage "playing out" experience on a doll both before and after procedure to clarify misconceptions.
Use neutral words to describe the procedure (see box on p. 1139)

Increased Language Skills

Use verbal explanation but avoid overestimating child's comprehension of words.
Encourage child to verbalize ideas and feelings.

Concept of Time and Frustration Tolerance Skill Limited

Implement same approaches as for toddler but may plan longer teaching session (10 to 15 minutes); may divide information into more than one session.

Illness and Hospitalization May Be Viewed as Punishment

Clarify why each procedure is performed; a child will find it difficult to understand how medicine can make him or her feel better and can taste bad at the same time.
Ask child thoughts regarding why a procedure is performed.
State directly that procedures are never a form of punishment.

Animism

Keep equipment out of sight, except when shown to or used on child.

Fears of Bodily Harm, Intrusion, and Castration

Point out on drawing, doll, or child where procedure is performed.
Emphasize that no other body part will be involved.

*Applies to any age.

GUIDELINES

Preparing Children for Procedures Based on Developmental Characteristics—cont'd

Use nonintrusive procedures whenever possible (e.g., axillary temperatures, oral medication).
Apply a Band-Aid over puncture site.
Encourage parental presence.
Realize that procedures involving genitals provoke anxiety.
Allow child to wear underpants with gown.
Explain unfamiliar situations, especially noises or lights.

Striving for Initiative

Involve child in care whenever possible (e.g., hold equipment, remove dressing).
Give choices whenever possible but avoid excessive delays.
Praise child for helping and attempting to cooperate; never shame child for lack of cooperation.

SCHOOL-AGE CHILD: DEVELOPING A SENSE OF INDUSTRY AND CONCRETE THOUGHT

Increased Language Skills; Interest in Acquiring Knowledge

Explain procedures using correct scientific/medical terminology.
Explain reason for procedure using simple diagrams of anatomy and physiology.
Explain function and operation of equipment in concrete terms.
Allow child to manipulate equipment; use doll or another person as model to practice using equipment whenever possible (doll play may be considered "childish" by older school-age child).
Allow time before and after procedure for questions and discussion.

Improved Concept of Time

Plan for longer teaching sessions (about 20 minutes).
Prepare in advance of procedure.

Increased Self-Control

Gain child's cooperation.
Tell child what is expected.
Suggest ways of maintaining control (e.g., deep breathing, relaxation, counting).

Striving for Industry

Allow responsibility for simple tasks (e.g., collecting specimens).
Include in decision making (e.g., time of day to perform procedure, preferred site).
Encourage active participation (e.g., removing dressings, handling equipment, opening packages).

Developing Relationships with Peers

May prepare two or more children for same procedure or encourage one to help prepare another peer.
Provide privacy from peers during procedure to maintain self-esteem.

ADOLESCENT: DEVELOPING A SENSE OF IDENTITY AND ABSTRACT THOUGHT

Increasingly Capable of Abstract Thought and Reasoning

Supplement explanations with reasons why procedure is necessary or beneficial.
Explain long-term consequences of procedures.
Realize that adolescent may fear death, disability, or other potential risks.
Encourage questioning regarding fears, options, and alternatives.

Conscious of Appearance

Provide privacy.
Discuss how procedure may affect appearance (e.g., scar) and what can be done to minimize it.
Emphasize any physical benefits of procedure.

Concerned More with Present Than with Future

Realize that immediate effects of procedure are more significant than future benefits.

Striving for Independence

Involve in decision making and planning (e.g., choice of time; place; individuals present during procedure, such as parents; clothing to wear).
Impose as few restrictions as possible.
Suggest methods of maintaining control.
Accept regression to more childish methods of coping.
Realize that adolescent may have difficulty in accepting new authority figures and may resist complying with procedures.

Developing Peer Relationships and Group Identity

Same as for school-age child but assumes even greater significance.
Allow adolescents to talk with other adolescents who have had the same procedure.

signs of physiologic distress (heart rate, blood pressure, oxygen saturation) (Broome and Lillis, 1989; Broome, Lillis, and Smith, 1989).

General guidelines for preparing children for procedures are described in the Guidelines box on p. 1134, and age-specific guidelines that consider children's developmental needs and cognitive abilities are presented in the Guidelines box on pp. 1136-1137. In addition to these suggestions, nurses should consider the child's temperament, existing coping strategies, and previous experiences in individualizing the preparatory process. Children who are distractible and highly active, as well as those who are "slow to warm up," may need individualized sessions that are shorter for the active child but more slowly paced for the shy child (McLeod and McClowry, 1990). Youngsters who tend to cope well may need more emphasis on using their present skills, whereas those who appear to cope less adequately can benefit from more time devoted to simple coping strategies, such as relaxing, breathing, counting, squeezing a hand, or singing. Children with previous health-related experiences still need preparation for repeat or new procedures, but the nurse must assess what they know, correct misconceptions, supply new information, and introduce new coping skills as indicated by their previous reactions (Bates and Broome, 1986). Especially for painful procedures, the most effective preparation includes the provision of sensory-procedural information and helping the child develop coping skills, such as imagery or relaxation (Broome, 1990).

➤ **NURSING TIP** Prepare a basket (toy or treasure chest or cart) to keep near the treatment area. Items ideal for the basket include a Slinky; a sparkling "magic" wand (clear, acrylic tube sealed on both ends and partially filled with liquid in which is suspended metallic confetti); a soft foam ball; bubble solution; party blowers; pop-up books with foldout, three-dimensional scenes; real medical equipment, such as a syringe, adhesive bandages, and alcohol packets; toy medical supplies or a toy medical kit; marking pens; a note pad; and stickers. Have the child choose an item to use during a procedure, such as a party blower to help distract and relax the youngster. After the procedure, allow the child to choose a small gift, such as a sticker, or to play with items, such as medical equipment (Heiney, 1991).

Children also are different in their "information-seeking dimension"; some want to actively solicit information about the intended procedure, whereas others characteristically avoid information (Peterson and Toler, 1986). Parents can often guide nurses in deciding how much information is enough for the child, since parents know if the child is typically inquisitive or satisfied with short answers. Asking older children their preferences about the amount of explanation is also important. Questions such as "Do you like to know everything about new experiences or just the basic facts?" or "How much of an explanation do you want—just what you will experience or why things are done?" are also help-

THINKING CRITICALLY ABOUT . . .

Parental Presence During Their Child's Stressful Procedure

Health professionals have basically adopted two opposing philosophies in relation to parental presence during procedures. One view purports that parents should not be present, since the child may view the parent's presence and/or participation as complicity and then blame the parent for allowing such indignities to be inflicted on the child. Since children normally associate parents with a comforting, "make it better" role, these professionals believe that parents should be a source of comfort and security to the child, which is best served by reuniting the child and parents after the procedure. The opposite view holds that not allowing the parents to be present inflicts the additional stress of separation and deprives the child of the parents' support. No consensus exists on whether parents who are present with the child should participate in the procedure, such as assisting in restraint.

Many institutions routinely separate parents and children during painful or stressful situations. Although such policies are becoming more liberal, allowing parents to stay with the child during induction of anesthesia, recovery from anesthesia, and cardiopulmonary resuscitation during an arrest tends to remain restricted. However, when parents and children are asked their preference regarding visiting during these times, the results favor offering the family a choice.

Although relatively little research has focused on this important issue, most of the available research finds that parental presence is supportive. Vernon, Foley, and Schulman (1967) compared preschoolers' responses to stress during admission and anesthesia induction with the parent present or absent. They found no differences in the preschoolers' behavior during admission procedures but considerably more distress in children whose parent was not present during induction, especially at the final phase after the mask was placed on the face. Several more recent studies found similar results when parents were permitted to stay with unpremedicated children during induction anesthesia in an outpatient setting (Gauderer, Lorig, and Eastwood, 1989; Hannallah and Rosales, 1983; Schofield and White, 1989).

Shaw and Routh (1982) assessed the effect of parental presence on young children during an injection and found that the children separated from the parent cried less and for less time. They concluded that the increased negative behavior in the children when the parent was present did not necessarily indicate greater upset; rather, it showed the children's greater expression of emotion in a supportive atmosphere. Another study on parental presence during dental treatment did not find a statistically significant difference between children's stress levels and parental presence or absence. However, it did find that when the parents were with them, children were more relaxed (Venham, Bengston, and Cipes, 1978). While some health professionals maintain that parents are disruptive during a procedure, studies have found that most parents choose to participate, are cooperative, and even when they find the experience difficult and stressful, are able to support their children (Bauchner, Vinci, and Waring, 1989; Merritt, Sargent, and Osborn, 1990; Savedra, 1981). Parents can become stressed by the experience, and parents with high anxiety tend to cause more anxiety in the child, although the child may not behave any differently during the actual procedure (Broome and Endsley, 1989; Johnston and others, 1988).

Some of the most significant evidence in favor of parental presence during stressful procedures comes from children. When children are asked for their preference, the response is overwhelmingly in favor of having their parents stay with them. All children ages 4 to 18 years wanted their parents to accompany them during a bone marrow test (Hamner and Miles, 1988). More than 80% of children ages 5 to 11 years wanted parents at the time of anesthesia induction, and more than 90% wanted them to be in the postanesthesia care unit (Hanna and Sherlock, 1983). Seventy percent of adolescents ages 14 to 19 years preferred their parents to be present during cancer-related procedures (Weekes and Savedra, 1988). When school-age children were asked what would help most if they were in pain, 99.2% of them answered having their parents present, even though most realized that the parent could do nothing but be there (Ross and Ross, 1984). When parents were offered the choice of staying during an arrest, 100% stated they would choose this option again (Villarreal, 1992) (see also Cardiopulmonary Resuscitation, Chapter 31). When one hospital considered a policy of allowing parents in the operating room if the child was dying, the parent advisory committee simply asked, "What right has Children's Hospital to dictate to families how they should experience the death of a child or how they should grieve?" (Fina, 1994). Shouldn't this question apply to all "visiting" policies?

ful in tailoring information to avoid overpreparation or underpreparation. Drawings by the child may also be helpful in determining the level of understanding, misconceptions, and concerns about mutilation, body image, or loss of control that the child may not be able to put into words (Abbott, 1990; O'Malley and McNamara, 1993).

The exact timing of the preparation for a procedure varies with the child's age and the type of procedure. There are no exact guidelines to govern timing, but in general the younger the child, the closer the explanation should be to the actual procedure to prevent undue fantasizing and worrying. With complex procedures, more time may be needed for assimilation of information, especially with older children. For example, the explanation for an injection can immediately precede the procedure for all ages, but preparation for surgery may begin the day before for young children and a few days before for older children, although older children's preferences should be elicited (see Preparation for Hospitalization, Chapter 26).

Establish Trust and Provide Support. The nurse who has spent time with and who has established a positive relationship with a child will usually find it easier to gain cooperation. If the relationship is based on trust, the child will associate the nurse with caregiving activities that give comfort and pleasure most of the time and not as someone who brings discomfort and stress. If the nurse does not know the child, it is best if the nurse is introduced by another staff person whom the child trusts. The first visit with the child ideally focuses on the child first and then on explanation of the procedure only; performing the procedure should be avoided. When talking with the child, the nurse uses the same guidelines for communicating with children that are discussed in Chapter 6.

Consider Parental Presence. Children need support during procedures, and for young children the greatest source of support is the parents. However, controversy exists regarding the role parents should assume during the procedure, especially if discomfort is involved (see Thinking Critically About . . . box). Nurses need to consider the issues in deciding whether parental presence is beneficial. The parents' preferences for assisting, observing, or waiting outside the room should be assessed, as well as the child's preference for parental presence. The child's and parent's wishes are respected (Rollins and Brantly, 1991). Parents who wish to stay should be educated, since they do not automatically know what to do, where to be, and what to say to help the child through the procedure (Acute Pain Management Guideline Panel, 1992). Simple instructions such as clarifying where parents can stay in the room and positioning them where they have eye contact with the child provide support and lessen anxiety. Parents who do not want to be present are supported in their decision and encouraged to remain close by so that they can be available to console the child immediately following the procedure. Parents should also know that someone will be with their child to provide support. Ideally, this person should inform the parents after the procedure about how the child did.

Provide an Explanation. Children need an explanation for anything that involves them directly. Before performing a procedure, the nurse explains to children what is to be done and what is expected of them. The explanation should be short, simple, and appropriate to the child's level of comprehension. Long explanations are not necessary and may only increase anxiety in a small child. This is especially true regarding painful procedures. When explaining the procedure to parents with the child present, the nurse uses language appropriate to the child because unfamiliar words can be misunderstood (see Guidelines box). If the parents need additional preparation, this is done in an area away from the child. Teaching sessions are planned at times most conducive to the child's learning (e.g., after a rest period) and usual span of attention.

Special equipment is not necessary for preparing a child, but for young children who cannot yet think in concepts, using objects to supplement verbal explanation is important. Allowing children to handle actual items that will be used in their care, such as a stethoscope, sphygmomanometer, or oxygen mask, helps them to develop familiarity with these items and to reduce the threat often associated with their use. Miniature versions of hospital items such as gurneys and x-ray and intravenous equipment can be used to explain what the children can expect and permit them to safely experience situations that are unfamiliar and potentially frightening. Written and illustrated materials are also valuable aids to preparation.*

*Sources of preparatory materials are the *You're Gonna Do What?* series of diagnosis and treatment procedures, available from Arkansas Children's Hospital, Attn: Child Life Dept., 800 Marshall St., Little Rock, AR 72202, (501) 320-1199; *Talks About the Hospital Series* by Fred Rogers, available from Family Communications, Inc., 4802 5th Ave., Pittsburgh, PA 15213, (412) 687-2990; and *Hospital Friends,* available from the Centering Corp., 1531 N. Saddle Creek Rd., Omaha, NE 68104, (402) 553-1200.

GUIDELINES
Selecting Nonthreatening Words or Phrases

WORDS/PHRASES TO AVOID	SUGGESTED SUBSTITUTIONS
Shot, bee sting, stick	Medicine under the skin
Organ	Special place in body
Test	See how [specify body part] is working
Incision	Special opening
Edema	Puffiness
Stretcher, gurney	Rolling bed
Stool	Child's usual term
Dye	Special medicine
Pain	Hurt, discomfort, "owie," "boo-boo"
Deaden	Numb, make sleepy
Cut, fix	Make better
Take (as in "take your temperature or blood pressure")	See how warm you are Check your pressure; hug your arm
Put to sleep, anesthesia	Special sleep
Catheter	Tube
Monitor	TV screen
Electrodes	Stickers, ticklers
Specimen	Sample

➤ **NURSING TIP** Use photographs of children in different areas of the hospital (e.g., radiology department, operating room) to give children a more realistic idea of equipment they may encounter.

Physical Preparation

For most procedures, no special physical preparation is needed. However, some do require physical preparation, such as cleansing and shaving of the skin before surgery. One area of special concern is the administration of appropriate sedation and/or analgesia before stressful procedures. The drug is given before the procedure to allow time for the medication to reach its peak effect. Whenever possible, the intravenous (through an existing infusion), oral, transdermal, or rectal route is used rather than the intramuscular route because children dislike injections. Buffering lidocaine with sodium bicarbonate (10:1, 1% or 2% lidocaine:$NaCO_3$) will reduce pain caused by the injection of local anesthetic. EMLA, a eutectic mixture of local anesthetics, may be used to reduce the pain of venipunctures. It should be applied 1 to 2 hours before the procedure to intact skin. Some institutions are using short-acting anesthetics (e.g., ketamine), general anesthetics, or potent analgesics (e.g., fentanyl) to eliminate the pain and trauma associated with treatments, such as bone marrow tests, lumbar punctures, burn debridement, and suturing (Billmire, Neale, and Gregory, 1985; Forlini, Morin, and Treacy, 1987; Maunuksela, Rajantie, and Simes, 1986; Perin and Frase, 1985). (See also Preoperative Sedation, p. 1144, and Pain Management, Chapter 26.)

Performance of the Procedure

Supportive care continues during the procedure and can be a major factor in a child's ability to cooperate and achieve mastery. Ideally the same nurse who explains the procedure should perform it or assist. Before beginning, all equipment is assembled and the room is readied to prevent unnecessary delays and interruptions that only serve to increase the child's anxiety.

➤ **NURSING TIP** To avoid a delay during a procedure, have extra supplies handy. For example, have tape, bandages, alcohol swabs, and an extra needle in your pocket when giving an injection or performing a venipuncture.

If at all possible, procedures are performed in a special treatment room rather than the child's hospital room. Traumatic procedures should never be performed in "safe" areas, such as the playroom. If the procedure is lengthy, conversation that could be misinterpreted by the child is avoided. As the procedure is nearing completion, the nurse should inform the child that it is almost over in language the child understands.

Expect Success. Nurses who approach children with confidence and who convey the impression that they expect to be successful are less likely to encounter difficulty. It is best to approach a child as though cooperation is expected. Children sense anxiety in an adult and will respond to a perceived threat by striking out or actively resisting. Although it is not possible to eliminate such behavior in every child, a firm approach with a positive attitude from the nurse tends to convey a feeling of security to most children.

Involve the Child. As in any other aspect of care, involving children helps to gain their cooperation. Permitting them to make choices gives them some measure of control. However, a choice is given only in situations in which one is available. To ask children, "Do you want to take your medicine now?" or "I'm going to give you an injection now, okay?" leads them to believe that there is an option and provides them with the opportunity to legitimately refuse or delay the medication. This places the nurse in an awkward, if not impossible, position. It is much better to state firmly, "It's time to drink your medicine now." Children usually like to make choices, but the choice must be one that they do indeed have (e.g., "It's time for your medicine. Do you want to drink it plain or with a little water?").

Many children respond to tactics that appeal to their maturity or courage. This also gives them a sense of participation and achievement. For example, preschool children will be proud that they can hold the dressing during the procedure or remove the tape. The same is true for the school-age child, who often cooperates with minimum resistance.

Provide Distraction. A child who is occupied with an interesting activity is less likely to focus on the procedure. For example, when an injection is given, it is helpful to give the child something to do or something on which to focus attention. For example, asking the child to point the toes inward and wiggle them not only helps relax the gluteal muscles but provides a diversion. Other strategies for diverting attention are to have the child tightly squeeze the hands of a parent or an assistant, count aloud, sing a familiar song such as a nursery rhyme, or verbally express discomfort. (For other interventions that may lessen discomfort, see Nonpharmacologic [Pain] Management, Chapter 26.)

➤ **NURSING TIP** Help the child to select and practice a coping technique before the procedure. Consider having the parent or some other supportive person, such as a child-life specialist, "coach" the child in learning and using the coping skill.

Allow Expression of Feelings. The child should be allowed to express feelings of anger, anxiety, fear, frustration, or any other emotion. It is natural for children to strike out in frustration or to try to avoid stress-provoking situations. The child needs to know that it is all right to cry. Whatever the response, the nurse must accept the behavior for what it is. Telling a child with limited verbal skills, such as a toddler, to stop kicking, biting, or otherwise expressing frustration conveys to the child that he or she is not being understood. Behavior is children's primary means of communication and coping and should be permitted unless it inflicts harm on them or those caring for them.

Postprocedural Support

After the procedure the child continues to need reassurance that he or she performed well and is accepted and loved. If the parents did not participate, the child is united with them as soon as possible so that they can provide comfort.

Encourage Expression of Feelings. Planned activity after the procedure is helpful in encouraging constructive expression of feelings. For verbal children, reviewing the details of the procedure can clarify misconceptions and pro-

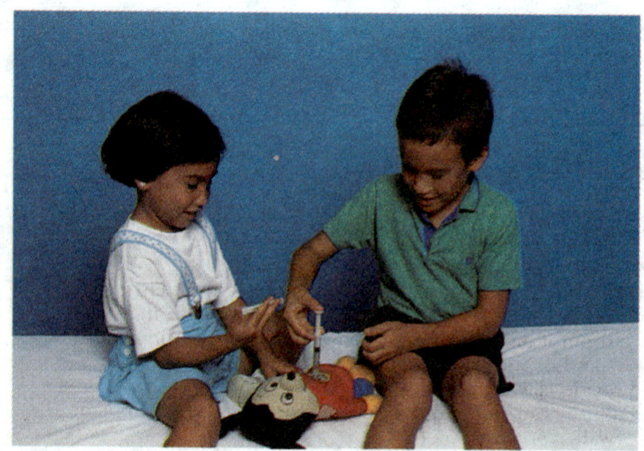

FIG. 27-2 Playing with syringes provides children with the opportunity to play out fears and concerns.

vide feedback for improving the nurse's preparatory strategies. Play is an excellent activity for all children. Infants and young children are given the opportunity for gross motor movement. Even older children are able to vent their anger and frustration in acceptable pounding or throwing activities. Playdough is a remarkably versatile medium for pounding and shaping. Dramatic play provides an outlet for anger and places the child in a position of control, in contrast to the position of helplessness in the real situation. Puppets may also be used to allow the child to communicate feelings in a nonthreatening way. One of the most effective interventions is therapeutic play, which includes well-supervised activities such as permitting the child to give an injection to a doll or stuffed toy to reduce the stress of injections (Fig. 27-2). (See next section and also Using Play/Expressive Activities to Minimize Stress, Chapter 26.)

Praise the Child. Children need to hear from adults that the youngsters did the best they could in the situation—no matter how they behaved. It is important for children to know that their worth is not being judged on the basis of behavior in a stressful situation. Reward systems, such as earning stars or tokens or saving the empty medicine cup as evidence of achievement, are often helpful. Children who require distasteful medications or injections over time can look with pride on a series of stars or stickers on a calendar, especially if an accumulated number represents a special privilege or reward.

Returning to the child a short while after the procedure helps the nurse to strengthen a supportive relationship. Relating with the child in a relaxed and nonstressful period allows him or her to see the nurse not only as someone associated with stressful situations but as someone with whom to share pleasurable experiences as well.

Use of Play in Procedures

The use of play is an integral part of relationships with children. As such, its value in specific situations is discussed throughout this book, such as in Chapter 26 in relation to hospitalization. Many institutions have very elaborate and well-organized play areas and programs under the direction of child-life specialists; other institutions have limited facilities. However, no matter what the institution provides for children, nurses can still include play activities as part of nursing care. Play can be used to teach, for expression of feelings, or as a method to achieve a therapeutic goal. Consequently, it should be included in preparing children for and encouraging their cooperation during procedures. Play sessions after procedures can be structured, such as directed toward needle play, or general, with a wide variety of equipment available for children to play with.

➤ **NURSING TIP** Play can also be spontaneous at the bedside and does not always require many supplies or much nursing time. Small items, such as finger puppets or a small bottle of bubbles, can be kept in the nurse's pocket for immediate use.

Even "routine" procedures such as temperature taking and oral administration of medication may be of concern to children (Ellerton, Caty, and Ritchie, 1985). Suggestions for incorporating play into nursing procedures and activities for the hospitalized child that facilitate learning and adjustment to a new situation are described in the box on p. 1142.

SURGICAL PROCEDURES

Preoperative Care

Children experiencing surgical procedures require both psychologic and physical preparation. In general, psychologic preparation is similar to that discussed earlier for any procedure and employs many of the same techniques used in preparing a child for hospitalization, such as films, books, play, and tours (see Chapter 26). However, some important differences exist. Even though children are asleep for the actual surgical intervention, they are subjected to numerous preoperative and postoperative procedures, which require a series of preparatory sessions to prevent overstressing the child with too much information. Six stress points before and after surgery have been identified as being significant in terms of causing anxiety (Visintainer and Wolfer, 1975):

1. Admission
2. The blood test
3. The afternoon of the day before surgery
4. Injection of preoperative medication
5. Before and during transport to the operating room
6. Return from the postanesthesia care unit (PACU)

Psychologic intervention consisting of systematic preparation, rehearsal of the forthcoming events, and supportive care at each of these points has been shown to be more effective than a single session preparation (which is a common method of preoperative preparation) or consistent supportive care without systematic preparation and rehearsal. Play is always an effective strategy in preparing children, and increased familiarity with medical procedures decreases anxiety (Siaw, Stephens, and Holmes, 1986).

Surprisingly little research has been conducted on children's perception of the surgical experience and their fears of the event. Although fear of anesthesia is thought

PLAY ACTIVITIES FOR SPECIFIC PROCEDURES

FLUID INTAKE

Make freezer pops using child's favorite juice.
Cut gelatin into fun shapes.
Make game of taking sip when turning page of book or in games such as "Simon Says."
Use small medicine cups; decorate the cups.
Color water with food coloring or powdered drink mix.
Have a tea party; pour at small table.
Let child fill a syringe and squirt it into mouth or use it to fill small, decorated cups.
Cut straws in half and place in small container (much easier for child to suck liquid).
Decorate straw: cut out small design with two holes and pass straw through; place small sticker on straw.
Use a "crazy" straw.
Make a "progress poster"; give rewards for drinking a predetermined quantity.

DEEP BREATHING

Blow bubbles with bubble blower.
Blow bubbles with straw (no soap).
Blow on pinwheel, feathers, whistle, harmonica, balloons, toy horns, party blowers.
Practice band instruments.
Have blowing contest using balloons, boats, cotton balls, feathers, marbles, Ping-Pong balls, pieces of paper; blow such objects on a table top over a goal line, over water, through an obstacle course, up in the air, against an opponent, or up and down a string.
Suck paper or cloth from one container to another using a straw.
Use blow bottles with colored water to transfer water from one side to the other.
Dramatize stories, such as "I'll huff and puff and blow your house down" from the Three Little Pigs.
Do straw-blowing painting.
Take a deep breath and "blow out the candles" on a birthday cake.
Use a little paint brush to "paint" nails with water and blow nails dry.

RANGE OF MOTION AND USE OF EXTREMITIES

Throw beanbags at fixed or movable target, wadded paper into wastebasket.
Touch or kick Mylar balloons held or hung in different positions (if child is in traction, hang balloon from trapeze).
Play "tickle toes"; wiggle them on request.
Play Twister game or "Simon Says."
Play pretend and guess games (e.g., imitate a bird, butterfly, horse).
Have tricycle or wheelchair races in safe area.
Play kick or throw ball with soft foam ball in safe area.
Position bed so that child must turn to view television or doorway.
Climb wall like a "spider."
Pretend to teach "aerobic" dancing or exercises; encourage parents to participate.
Encourage swimming if feasible.
Play video games or pinball (fine motor movement).
Play "hide and seek" game: hide toy somewhere in bed (or room if ambulatory) and have child find it using specified hand or foot.
Provide clay to mold with fingers.
Paint or draw on large sheets of paper placed on floor or wall.
Encourage combing own hair; play "beauty shop" with "customer" in different positions.

SOAKS

Play with small toys or objects (cups, syringes, soap dishes) in water.
Wash dolls or toys.
Bubbles may be added to bathwater if permissible; move bubbles to create shapes or "monsters."
Pick up marbles, pennies* from bottom of bath container.
Make designs with coins on bottom of container.
Pretend a boat is a submarine by keeping it immersed.
Read to child during soaks, sing with child, or play game, such as cards, checkers, or other board game (if both hands are immersed, move the board pieces for the child).
Sitz bath: give child something to listen to (music, stories) or look at (Viewmaster, book).
Punch holes in bottom of plastic cup, fill with water, and let it "rain" on child.

INJECTIONS

Let child handle syringe, vial, alcohol swab and give an injection to doll or stuffed animal.
Use syringes to decorate cookies with frosting, squirt paint, or target shoot into a container.
Draw a "magic circle" on area before injection; draw smiling face in circle after injection, but avoid drawing on puncture site.
Allow child to have a "collection" of syringes (without needles); make "wild" creative objects with syringes.
If multiple injections or venipunctures, make a "progress poster"; give rewards for predetermined number of injections.
Have child count to 10 or 15 during injection.

AMBULATION

Give child something to push.
- Toddler: push-pull toy
- School-age child: wagon or decorated IV stand
- Adolescent: a baby in a stroller or wheelchair

Have a parade; make hats, drums, etc.

EXTENDING ENVIRONMENT (PATIENTS IN TRACTION, ETC.)

Make bed into a private ship or airplane with decorations.
Put up mirrors so patient can see around room.
Move patient's bed frequently, especially to playroom, hallway, or outside.

*Small objects such as marbles or coins, as well as gloves or balloons, are unsafe for young children because of possible aspiration.

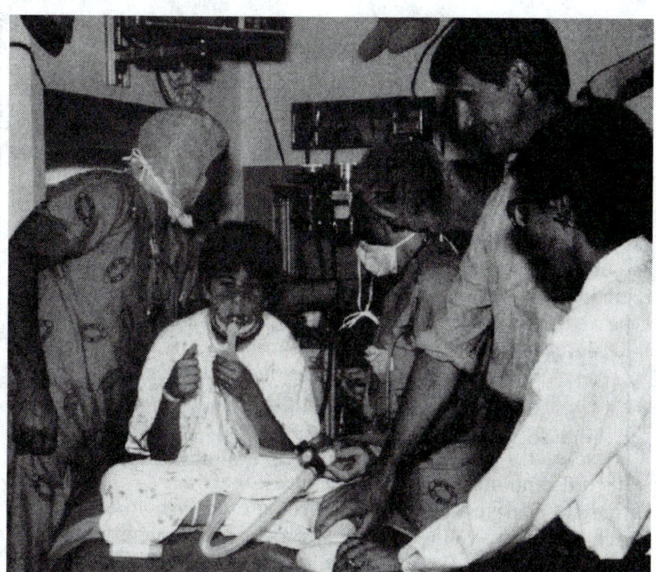

FIG. 27-3 Parental presence during induction of anesthesia can minimize the child's and parents' anxiety during the preoperative period.

to be a major concern among children, little evidence for this exists. One study of school-age children reported few remembered events and even fewer fears. Those events recalled more often were the ride to and arriving in the operating room, the preoperative or induction injection, waking up in pain, and not being allowed to eat or drink. The most feared events were the injection and the mask on the face. Although parents were not allowed to be with the children, more than 80% of the children wanted them during induction of anesthesia and in the PACU (Hanna and Sherlock, 1983).

Parental Presence. Parental presence during induction is becoming a more common practice, although few institutions endorse the policy (Fig. 27-3). Reports from parents who attend the induction are very favorable. Even though some may become anxious, most parents can control their anxiety, do not disrupt the induction, and support the child (Gauderer, Lorig, and Eastwood, 1989; Hanallah and Rosales; 1983; Schofield and White, 1989).

Some concern exists regarding the appropriateness of this practice for all parents. A few parents are visibly upset by the rapid succession of induction events, observing their child becoming limp, and leaving the child in the care of strangers (Vessey, Caserza, and Bogetz, 1990). Parents who are very anxious before surgery tend to become even more anxious after the induction, whereas the reverse is true of parents with little anxiety (Johnston and others, 1988).

However, based on the parents' favorable response to the practice and most children's desire to have parents with them during any stressful procedure (see Thinking Critically About . . . box on p. 1138), a policy of offering parents the option of attending the induction, combined with a program that prepares them for what to expect and what is expected of them, seems justified. When parents choose not to or are not allowed to attend the induction, leaving a

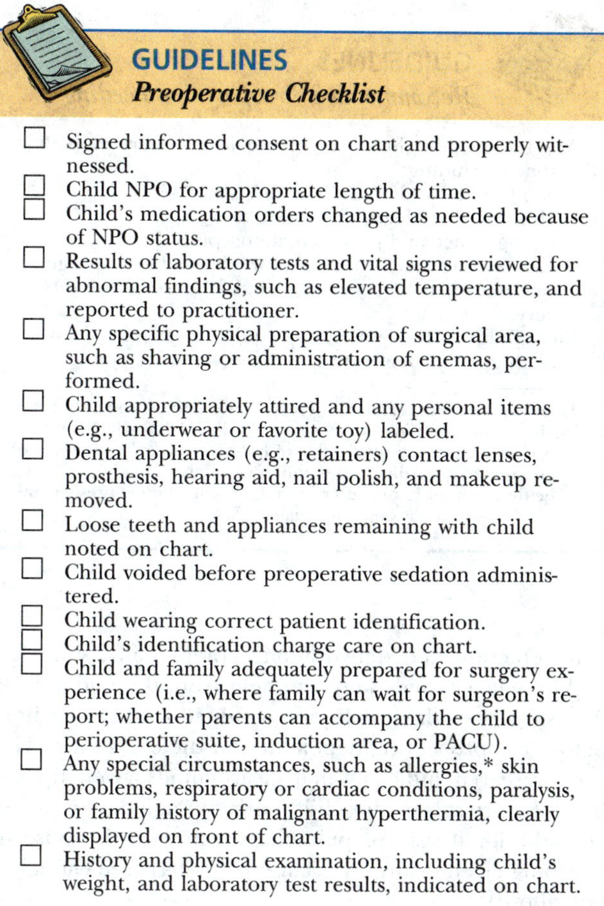

GUIDELINES
Preoperative Checklist

- ☐ Signed informed consent on chart and properly witnessed.
- ☐ Child NPO for appropriate length of time.
- ☐ Child's medication orders changed as needed because of NPO status.
- ☐ Results of laboratory tests and vital signs reviewed for abnormal findings, such as elevated temperature, and reported to practitioner.
- ☐ Any specific physical preparation of surgical area, such as shaving or administration of enemas, performed.
- ☐ Child appropriately attired and any personal items (e.g., underwear or favorite toy) labeled.
- ☐ Dental appliances (e.g., retainers) contact lenses, prosthesis, hearing aid, nail polish, and makeup removed.
- ☐ Loose teeth and appliances remaining with child noted on chart.
- ☐ Child voided before preoperative sedation administered.
- ☐ Child wearing correct patient identification.
- ☐ Child's identification charge care on chart.
- ☐ Child and family adequately prepared for surgery experience (i.e., where family can wait for surgeon's report; whether parents can accompany the child to perioperative suite, induction area, or PACU).
- ☐ Any special circumstances, such as allergies,* skin problems, respiratory or cardiac conditions, paralysis, or family history of malignant hyperthermia, clearly displayed on front of chart.
- ☐ History and physical examination, including child's weight, and laboratory test results, indicated on chart.

*For a discussion of latex allergy, see Spina Bifida/Myelodysplasia, Chapter 11.

favorite possession with the child and uniting the child and parents as soon as possible after surgery (preferably in the PACU) are important interventions. During surgery the family should have a designated place to wait and needs to be kept informed of the child's progress. They also should know where and when they can visit the child after surgery.

Aside from possibly being separated from the parents before and after surgery, children also may be cared for by a number of unfamiliar practitioners. Although the same supportive nurse should remain with the child through as many of the procedures as possible, the child may have other nurses, especially if the patient returns to a special care unit postoperatively. However, joint planning of care between the various nursing staffs, such as in pediatrics and the PACU, can overcome some of the disadvantages of unfamiliar nurses caring for the child. Many hospitals have surgical tours for children and parents to familiarize them with the strange environment and to introduce them to other individuals who will be involved in their care.

Besides psychologic preparation, children usually require various types of physical care before surgery, such as those listed in the Guidelines box above and in the Nursing Care Plan on pp. 1146-1149. Infants require special attention to fluid needs. They should not be without oral fluids for an extended period preoperatively to avoid glyco-

GUIDELINES
Recommended Preoperative Feeding

At 8 PM or midnight the evening before surgery, **stop all food,** including:
- Solid food, candy,* and chewing gum*
- Milk, milk products, and formulas†
- Orange juice and juice containing pulp

Breast-feeding may continue until **3 hours** before surgery.
Clear fluids may be continued until **2 hours** before surgery.
Clear fluids include water, apple juice, clear juice drinks, plain gelatin, clear broth, Pedialyte, and ice pops.

Modified from Schreiner MS: Preoperative and postoperative fasting in children, *Pediatr Clin North Am* 41(1):111-120, 1994.
*Hard sucking candy is probably of little concern, and a variety of opinions exist regarding the significance of gum chewing.
†The duration for fasting after formulas is uncertain at present, and shorter intervals may be appropriate.

EFFECTIVE PREMEDICATIONS FOR PROCEDURES

OPIOIDS*

Morphine sulfate, 0.05 to 0.10 mg/kg IV over 1 to 2 minutes given 5 minutes before procedure, or
Fentanyl, 1 to 2 μg/kg (0.001 to 0.002 mg/kg) IV 3 minutes before procedure, or
Meperidine (if morphine sulfate or fentanyl is not available), 0.5 to 1.0 mg/kg IV for 1 to 2 minutes given 2 to 5 minutes before procedure

SEDATIVES†

Diazepam (Valium), 0.2 to 0.3 mg/kg, maximum of 10 mg orally 45 to 60 minutes before procedure
Midazolam (Versed), 0.2 to 0.4 mg/kg, maximum to 15 mg (IV solution) orally 30 to 45 minutes or 0.05 mg/kg IV 3 minutes before procedure
Pentobarbital (Nembutal), 1 to 3 mg/kg IV boluses to a maximum of 100 mg until asleep
Chloral hydrate 20 to 75 mg/kg to a maximum dose of 100 mg/kg or 2.0 g given orally or rectally 60 minutes before procedure

Modified from Zeltzer LK and others: Report of the subcommittee on the management of pain associated with procedures in children with cancer, *Pediatrics* 86(suppl):826-831, 1990; and Coté CJ: Sedation for the pediatric patient, *Pediatr Clin North Am* 41(1):31-58, 1994.
*Provide analgesia and sedation.
†Provide sedation but no analgesia.

gen depletion and dehydration. Traditionally, solid food and nonclear liquids were withheld from the midnight before surgery, with clear liquids withheld from 4 to 8 hours before the procedure, depending on the child's age. However, research indicates that clear liquids given up to 2 hours before surgery for children of any age do not present any additional risk for pulmonary aspiration in those undergoing elective surgery (Schreiner, 1994) (see Guidelines box above).

Although most preoperative care procedures are routine, nurses should keep in mind that they can be anxiety provoking for children and parents. For example, for young children, having to wear a loose-fitting hospital gown without the security of underpants or pajama bottoms can be traumatic. Therefore these articles of clothing should be allowed.

Preoperative Sedation. The most upsetting event for children is generally the preoperative injection. Unfortunately, little research has been done on the necessity of this practice. If children have no preoperative pain, are well prepared psychologically for surgery, and have their parents nearby, preanesthetic medication may be unnecessary. Research on children who received no premedication, an oral sedative, or an opioid and an anticholinergic drug and whose parents accompanied them during induction found no difference in the ease of induction. The group receiving the opioid had better postoperative pain control but more nausea and vomiting (Schofield and White, 1989).

Numerous preanesthetic drug regimens are used with children, and no consensus exists on the optimum method. Drugs used should achieve five goals (American Academy of Pediatrics, 1992): (1) to guard the patient's safety and welfare; (2) to minimize physical discomfort or pain; (3) to minimize negative psychologic responses to treatment by providing analgesia, and to maximize the potential for amnesia; (4) to control behavior; and (5) to return the patient to a state in which safe discharge, as determined by recognized criteria, is possible. They should also be "atraumatic" by using oral, existing intravenous, or rectal routes. Several drug options exist, such as morphine, midazolam, diazepam, and fentanyl (see box above). The oral transmucosal preparation, Fentanyl Oralet, provides an effective and atraumatic form of preoperative sedation, especially in children without preexisting intravenous access. It consists of a lozenge on a plastic holder that is available in 200, 300, and 400 μg strengths. The recommended dose is 5 to 15 μg/kg; children over 40 kg may need the higher dosage. It is not recommended for children less than 15 kg. The peak effect occurs in 20 to 30 minutes from the start of administration, if the drug is sucked, not chewed and swallowed. If the lozenge is chewed, the drug is less effective because part of it is metabolized by the liver before entering the bloodstream. However, swallowing the drug rapidly does not increase the risk of respiratory depression during the first 15 to 30 minutes, the period of greatest risk for decreased respiration. A popular drug combination—meperidine (pethidine [Demerol]), promethazine (Phenergan), and chlorpromazine (Thorazine)—is no longer recommended (see Thinking Critically About . . . box).

The use of sedating drugs for procedures has serious associated risks, such as hypoventilation, apnea, airway obstruction, and cardiopulmonary impairment. They produce ***conscious sedation***—a medically controlled state of depressed consciousness that (1) allows protective reflexes to be maintained; (2) retains the patient's ability to maintain a patent airway independently and continuously; and (3) permits appropriate response by the patient to physical stimulation or verbal command (e.g., "Open your eyes").

The American Academy of Pediatrics (1992) has developed policies that provide guidelines for conscious seda-

THINKING CRITICALLY ABOUT . . . *The Drug Combination "DPT"*

The drug combination of meperidine (Demerol), promethazine (Phenergan), and chlorpromazine (Thorazine), also commonly known as "DPT," "pedi-cocktail," or "lytic cocktail," has been prescribed in pediatrics for many years. One premise behind the use of DPT was the belief that promethazine and chlorpromazine potentiated or increased the analgesic effect of meperidine. However, it is questionable whether any drug acts as an opioid potentiator. Rather, most add their primary effect, such as sedation or anxiolysis (reduction of anxiety), to the opioid's analgesic effect (McCaffery and Beebe, 1989). In fact, promethazine produces antianalgesia (Ros, 1987), and chlorpromazine produces initial antianalgesia followed by slight analgesia (Howland and Goldfrank, 1986). These effects alone make DPT an irrational choice for preprocedural or preoperative sedation.

Several recent reports argue strongly against DPT's continued use. Major criticisms of DPT include the following:

- It causes excessive central nervous system (CNS) depression; two thirds of 95 patients remained sedated (asleep) for 7 hours or more (Nahata, Clotz, and Krogg, 1985).
- It lowers the seizure threshold (Snodgrass and Dodge, 1989).
- Chlorpromazine may potentiate the actions and increase the toxicity of meperidine, leading to CNS depression, respiratory depression, and decreased blood pressure (Nahata, Clotz, and Krogg, 1985).
- Promethazine can cause extrapyramidal reactions (spasms of neck, face, tongue, and back; fixed eyeballs).
- It is usually administered intramuscularly, causing additional pain, especially from meperidine, which is irritating to the tissues. Because of the potential for respiratory depression, the intravenous route should not be used (Coté, 1994).

To emphasize its risks, the Acute Pain Management Guideline Panel (1992) of the Agency for Health Care Policy and Research (AHCPR) includes the following in its *Clinical Practice Guideline:* "Exercise caution when using the mixture of meperidine (Demerol), promethazine (Phenergan), and chlorpromazine (Thorazine), also known as DPT. DPT—given intramuscularly—has commonly been used for painful procedures. The efficacy of this mixture is poor when compared with alternative approaches, and it has been associated with a high frequency of adverse effects (Nahata, Clotz, and Krogg, 1985). It is not recommended for general use and should be used only in exceptional circumstances."

Although DPT is typically used before a single procedure, some clinicians prescribe DPT for pain relief from repeated treatments, such as burn care. Meperidine is not recommended for chronic dosing because of the accumulation of the metabolite normeperidine, a CNS stimulant that produces anxiety, tremors, myoclonus, and generalized seizures (American Pain Society, 1992).

In patients with normal renal function, normeperidine has a half-life of 15 to 20 hours; this time is extended greatly in patients with impaired renal function, especially those with sickle cell disease. The CNS effects have been observed in young, otherwise healthy patients given sufficiently high doses of meperidine. According to the Acute Pain Management Guideline Panel (1992), "meperidine should be reserved for very brief courses in otherwise healthy patients who have demonstrated an unusual reaction (e.g., local histamine release at the infusion site) or allergic response during treatment with other opioids such as morphine or hydromorphone."

Despite the well-documented risks of DPT and the AHCPR guidelines against its use, you may find some clinicians who are resistant or hard to convince. One reason is that prescribing DPT is an entrenched practice, and many may not be familiar with alternatives (see box on p. 1144). If so, you may refer them to another authority, the 1993 edition of *The Harriet Lane Handbook,* which no longer lists DPT among its suggested drugs for procedural sedation and/or analgesia (Johns Hopkins Hospital, 1993; Wong, 1994).

tion. These guidelines include provision of emergency equipment, such as a positive-pressure oxygen delivery system, airway management and breathing equipment, and an emergency cart. The patient's level of consciousness and responsiveness, heart rate, blood pressure, respiratory rate, and oxygen saturation (via pulse oximetry) must be monitored during the procedure by an individual present for this purpose.

The use of ***nitrous oxide*** for conscious sedation (defined as the administration of nitrous oxide—50% or less, with the balance as oxygen, without any other sedative, opioid, or other depressant drug before or concurrent with the nitrous oxide) does not require pulse oximetry monitoring, although it is strongly encouraged. The patient is able to maintain verbal communication throughout, and a second individual whose responsibility is to monitor the patient may also assist with the procedure. In all cases the patient's condition after the procedure is also documented.

Children may also fear induction of anesthesia by mask. Practices that can minimize anxiety related to inhalation anesthesia are (1) disguising the unpleasant odor of anesthetic gases by applying a pleasant-smelling substance on the mask; (2) using a transparent plastic mask rather than an opaque black mask and gradually bringing it toward the face; (3) directing a stream of gas toward the child's face from the bare tube until the child becomes drowsy, then using the mask; and (4) allowing the child to sit up rather than lie down for anesthesia induction (Jones, 1985).

Postoperative Care

After surgical procedures, various physical interventions and observations are required to prevent or minimize possible untoward effects (see Guidelines box, p. 1151, and Nursing Care Plan, pp. 1146-1149). Although most of these interventions are prescribed by physicians, it is the nurse's responsibility to exercise judgment in their implementation. For example, vital signs are taken as frequently as necessary until they are stable. Simply recording temperature, pulse, respiration, and blood pressure without comparing the present readings with previous ones is a useless techni-

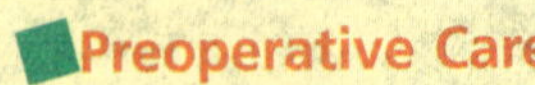

NURSING CARE PLAN
The Child Undergoing Surgery

Preoperative Care

NURSING DIAGNOSIS: High risk for injury related to surgical procedure, anesthesia

NURSE GOAL 1: Will receive fully informed consent and sign appropriate documents

• **NURSING INTERVENTIONS/*RATIONALES***

Inquire whether parents have any questions about procedure *to determine their level of understanding and to provide for additional information (from nurse or other professional)*

Check chart for signed informed consent form or obtain informed consent

Contact physician to determine if parents have been informed of procedure *because informed consent is physician's responsibility*

Obtain and/or witness signature if not obtained earlier

• **EXPECTED OUTCOMES**

Family receives fully informed consent

Family signs appropriate documents

PATIENT GOAL 2: Will receive proper hygiene measures

• **NURSING INTERVENTIONS/*RATIONALES***

Bathe child, groom hair

Provide mouth care *to promote comfort while NPO*

Cleanse operative site according to prescribed method, if ordered, *to minimize risk of infection*

• **EXPECTED OUTCOME**

Child is cleansed and prepared appropriately (specify)

PATIENT GOAL 3: Will receive proper preparation

• **NURSING INTERVENTIONS/*RATIONALES***

Carry out special procedure as prescribed (e.g., colonic enemas)

*Administer antibiotics as ordered, observing for known side effects

Order and/or assist with special tests such as radiographs

Consult with practitioner for appropriate change in schedule or route of administration of any medication child ordinarily receives

Attire child appropriately (e.g., special operating room gown)

Allow child to wear underwear or pajama bottoms, if possible, *to provide privacy*

Label personal articles and clothing

Remove any makeup and/or nail polish *to observe for cyanosis*

Remove jewelry and/or prosthetic devices (e.g., mouth retainers) *because they may be lost or interfere with anesthesia/surgery*

Check for loose teeth

Inform anesthesiologist, if detected, *to prevent aspiration of teeth during anesthesia*

• **EXPECTED OUTCOME**

Child is prepared appropriately (specify)

PATIENT GOAL 4: Will experience no complications

• **NURSING INTERVENTIONS/*RATIONALES***

Maintain child NPO (nothing by mouth) as ordered *to prevent aspiration during anesthesia* (clear liquids up to 2 hours before surgery for children at any age pose no additional risk for pulmonary aspiration during elective surgery)

Be sure child is well hydrated before NPO begins, especially infants *who are more at risk for dehydration*

Take and record vital signs

Report any deviations from admission readings, especially elevated temperature, *which may indicate infection*

Have child void before preoperative medication is administered *to prevent bladder distention or incontinence during anesthesia*

Record time of last voiding if unable to void

Be certain allergies are clearly indicated on chart *to decrease risk of adverse reaction*

Check laboratory values for any sign of systemic abnormality, such as infection (increased white blood cells), anemia (decreased hemoglobin and/or hematocrit), or bleeding tendencies (reduced platelets or prolonged bleeding or clotting time)

Keep small infants warm during transport and waiting time

• **EXPECTED OUTCOMES**

Child is NPO for designated time preoperatively

Child voids

Pertinent information about child is visible

PATIENT GOAL 5: Will experience no injury

• **NURSING INTERVENTIONS/*RATIONALES***

Check that identification band is securely fastened

Check identification band with surgical personnel *to ensure correct identification*

Fasten siderails of bed or crib *to prevent falls*

Use restraints during transport by stretcher (or other conveyance) *to prevent falls*

Do not leave child unattended

• **EXPECTED OUTCOMES**

Child is safe from immediate harm

Child is clearly and correctly identified

*Dependent nursing action.

NURSING CARE PLAN
The Child Undergoing Surgery—cont'd

NURSING DIAGNOSIS: Anxiety/fear related to separation from support system, unfamiliar environment, knowledge deficit

PATIENT GOAL 1: Will demonstrate optimum sense of security

- **NURSING INTERVENTIONS/*RATIONALES***

Institute preoperative teaching *to reduce anxiety/fear*
Orient child to strange surroundings
Explain where parents will be while child is in operating room
Have someone stay with child *to provide increased sense of security*

- **EXPECTED OUTCOME**

Child demonstrates minimum insecurity or anxiety

PATIENT/FAMILY GOAL 2: Will demonstrate understanding of surgery and postoperative care

- **NURSING INTERVENTIONS/*RATIONALES***

Prepare for postoperative procedures, as indicated (e.g., nasogastric tube, IV fluids, nothing by mouth, dressing changes, wound drains if necessary)
Explain reason for surgery; if special operative procedure is to be performed, explain basic principles and briefly outline care if needed *to reinforce information given by practitioner*
Explain all preoperative procedures (e.g., blood work, any other laboratory test)
In emergency situation, explain most essential components of surgery (e.g., where child will be before and after surgery, anesthesia, dressing)
Accept behavioral reactions of parents and child *because these can be highly variable*

- **EXPECTED OUTCOMES**

Child and family demonstrate an understanding of forthcoming events (specify methods of learning and evaluation)
*Family's behavioral reactions are accepted and supported

PATIENT GOAL 3: Will exhibit signs of optimum relaxation, sedation, and support before arriving in operating room

- **NURSING INTERVENTIONS/*RATIONALES***

*Administer preoperative sedation (preferably oral), if ordered, *to promote relaxation and sleep*
Place unfamiliar equipment out of child's view *to decrease anxiety/fear*
Place child in quiet room with minimum distraction *to promote relaxation and encourage sleep*
Do not leave child unattended
Explain what is happening, unless child is asleep
Encourage parents to stay with child as long as permitted and according to their wishes
Permit parent to hold child until child falls asleep, if desired
Encourage parents to accompany child as far as possible, preferably through induction of anesthesia
Allow significant objects to accompany child (e.g., a favorite toy) *to provide comfort and sense of security*

- **EXPECTED OUTCOMES**

Child falls asleep or lies quietly
Child is not left alone

NURSING DIAGNOSIS: Altered family processes related to a surgical procedure

PATIENT (FAMILY) GOAL : Will receive adequate support and reassurance

- **NURSING INTERVENTIONS/*RATIONALES***

Reinforce and clarify information given by practitioner
Explain associated diagnostic tests and procedures (e.g., x-ray examinations)
Explain child's schedule
  When child will receive premedication
  Time child will leave for surgery
  Where parents can wait for child to return
  Room to which child will return
  Postprocedural care and routines
Explore family's feelings regarding the procedure and its implications *to assess need for further intervention*
Include parents in preparation of child
Be available to family *to provide support and reassurance as needed*
See also Nursing Care Plan: The Family of the Ill or Hospitalized Child, Chapter 26

- **EXPECTED OUTCOMES**

Family demonstrates an understanding of procedure (specify demonstration) and related information (specify)
Family complies with directives (specify)

Postoperative Care

NURSING DIAGNOSIS: High risk for injury related to surgical procedure, anesthesia

NURSE GOAL 1: Receive child on return from surgery

- **NURSING INTERVENTIONS/*RATIONALES***

Place child in bed (unless transported in own bed or crib) using techniques appropriate to type of surgery *to prevent injury*
Hang IV apparatus and connect any needed equipment (e.g., suction apparatus, traction)
Place child in position of comfort and safety in accordance with surgeon's orders
Perform stat (immediate) activities

*Nursing outcome.

Continued.

NURSING CARE PLAN
The Child Undergoing Surgery—cont'd

• **EXPECTED OUTCOME**
Child is transferred to bed without injury and with minimum stress

PATIENT GOAL 2: Will exhibit signs of wound healing without evidence of wound infection

• **NURSING INTERVENTIONS/*RATIONALES***
Use proper handwashing techniques and other universal precautions, especially if wound drainage is present
Employ careful wound care *to minimize risk of infection*
Keep wound clean and dressings intact
Apply dressings *that promote moist wound healing* (i.e., hydrocolloid dressings [e.g., Duoderm])
Change dressings if indicated, whenever soiled; carefully dispose of soiled dressings
Carry out special wound care as prescribed (e.g., irrigation, drain care)
Cleanse with prescribed preparation (if ordered)
*Apply antibacterial solutions and/or ointments as ordered *to prevent infection*
Report any unusual appearance or drainage *for early detection of infection*
Place diapers below abdominal dressing *if appropriate to prevent contamination*
When child begins oral feedings, provide nutritious diet as ordered *to promote wound healing*

• **EXPECTED OUTCOME**
Child exhibits no evidence of wound infection

PATIENT GOAL 3: Will exhibit no evidence of complications

• **NURSING INTERVENTIONS/*RATIONALES***
Ambulate as prescribed *to decrease complications associated with immobility*
Maintain child NPO until fully awake *to prevent aspiration*
Encourage to void when awake
Offer bedpan
Boys may be allowed to stand at bedside
Notify practitioner if unable to void *to ensure appropriate intervention*
Maintain abdominal decompression, chest tubes, or other equipment, if prescribed
Provide diet as prescribed; advance as appropriate

• **EXPECTED OUTCOME**
Child exhibits no evidence of complications

NURSING DIAGNOSIS: Anxiety/fear related to surgery, unfamiliar environment, separation from support systems, discomfort

PATIENT GOAL 1: Will experience reduced anxiety

• **NURSING INTERVENTIONS/*RATIONALES***
Maintain calm, reassuring manner
Encourage expression of feelings *to facilitate coping*
Explain procedures and other activities before initiating
Answer questions and explain purposes of activities
Keep informed of progress
Remain with child as much as possible
Give encouragement and positive feedback for cooperation in care
Encourage parental presence as soon as permitted *to decrease stress of separation*
If emergency procedure, review child's memory of previous events *so that misconceptions can be clarified*

• **EXPECTED OUTCOMES**
Child rests quietly and calmly
Child discusses procedures and activities without evidence of anxiety

NURSING DIAGNOSIS: Pain related to surgical incision

PATIENT GOAL 1: Will experience no pain or reduction of pain to level acceptable to child

• **NURSING INTERVENTIONS/*RATIONALES***
Do not wait until child experiences severe pain to intervene *in order to prevent pain from occurring*
Avoid palpating operative area unless necessary
Insert rectal tube, if indicated, *to relieve gas*
Encourage to void, if appropriate, *to prevent bladder distention*
Administer mouth care *to provide comfort*
Lubricate nostril *to decrease irritation* from nasogastric tube if present
Allow child position of comfort if not contraindicated
Perform nursing activities and procedures (e.g., dressing change, deep breathing, ambulation) after analgesia
*Administer analgesics prescribed *for pain*
*Administer antiemetics as ordered *for nausea and vomiting*
Monitor effectiveness of analgesics

• **EXPECTED OUTCOME**
Child rests quietly and exhibits minimal or no evidence of pain (specify)

NURSING DIAGNOSIS: High risk for fluid volume deficit related to NPO status before and/or after surgery, loss of appetite, vomiting

PATIENT GOAL 1: Will receive adequate hydration

• **NURSING INTERVENTIONS/*RATIONALES***
Monitor IV infusion at prescribed rate *to ensure adequate hydration*
Attach pediatric IV apparatus if not done in operating room
Offer fluids as soon as ordered or child tolerates
Start with small sips of water and advance as tolerated

*Nursing outcome.

NURSING CARE PLAN
The Child Undergoing Surgery—cont'd

Encourage to drink
Tempt with favorite fluids, ice chips, or flavored ice pops

• **EXPECTED OUTCOMES**
Child exhibits no evidence of dehydration
Child takes and retains fluid when allowed (specify)

NURSING DIAGNOSIS: High risk for infection related to weakened condition, presence of infective organisms

PATIENT GOAL 1: Will maintain normal respiratory function

• **NURSING INTERVENTIONS/*RATIONALES***
Assess need for pain medication before respiratory therapy
Help to turn, deep breathe
Splint operative site with hand or pillow if possible before coughing (if coughing prescribed) *to minimize pain*
Assist with use of incentive spirometer or blow bottle
Perform percussion and vibration if indicated
Suction secretions if needed
Assess respirations, including breath sounds

• **EXPECTED OUTCOME**
Lungs remain clear

NURSING DIAGNOSIS: Altered family processes related to situational crisis (emergency hospitalization of child), knowledge deficit

PATIENT/FAMILY GOAL 1: Will receive adequate support and reassurance

• **NURSING INTERVENTIONS/*RATIONALES***
Explain all procedures *to reduce anxiety/fear*
Keep family informed of child's progress
Encourage expression of feelings *to facilitate coping*
Refer to public health nurse if indicated *for follow-up care*
Refer to appropriate agency or persons for specific help (e.g., social service, clergy)
See also Nursing Care Plan: The Child in the Hospital, Chapter 26
See also Nursing Care Plan: The Family of the Ill or Hospitalized Child, Chapter 26

• **EXPECTED OUTCOMES**
Family discusses child's condition and therapies comfortably
Family demonstrates an awareness of child's progress (specify method of evaluation)
Family members avail themselves of appropriate assistance

PATIENT (FAMILY) GOAL 2: Will demonstrate understanding of home care

• **NURSING INTERVENTIONS/*RATIONALES***
If dressing changes are required at home, teach parents sterile or aseptic procedures; provide written list of necessary equipment and instructions *for referral at home*
Instruct parents regarding administration of medications (if ordered), including possible side effects and untoward reactions, *to ensure adequate home care*
Instruct parents in care and management of special procedures (e.g., ostomy care, irrigations) *to ensure adequate home care*

• **EXPECTED OUTCOME**
Family demonstrates an understanding of instructions (specify methods of learning and evaluation)

cal function. Each vital sign is evaluated in terms of side effects from anesthesia and signs of impending shock or respiratory compromise (Table 27-1).

A change in vital signs that demands immediate attention is elevated temperature caused by ***malignant hyperthermia,*** a potentially lethal genetic myopathy. In susceptible children certain anesthetic agents trigger the disorder, producing elevated temperature, muscle rigidity, hypermetabolism, and muscle cell destruction. The symptoms may or may not occur during surgery; therefore, alert observation in the PACU and regular care unit is essential (Wlody, 1991). Treatment includes immediate discontinuation of triggering agents, hyperventilation with 100% oxygen, and intravenous dantrolene.

NURSING ALERT When taking the preoperative history, ask the family if any relatives have had anesthetic difficulties suggesting malignant hyperthermia; report findings immediately. Observe for early signs of the disorder:
Tachycardia
Rising blood pressure
Tachypnea
Mottled skin
Muscle rigidity

Providing comfort is a major responsibility after surgery. Pain is assessed and the child given analgesics as needed to provide comfort and facilitate cooperation in postoperative procedures, such as ambulating and deep breathing. Rou-

TABLE 27-1 Potential Causes of Postoperative Vital Sign Alterations in Children

ALTERATION	POTENTIAL CAUSE	COMMENTS
HEART RATE		
Increase	Decreased perfusion (shock) Elevated temperature Pain Respiratory distress (early) Medications (atropine, morphine, epinephrine)	Heart rate may increase to maintain cardiac output
Decrease	Hypoxia Vagal stimulation Increased intracranial pressure Respiratory distress (late) Medications (prostigmine)	Bradycardia is of more concern in the young child than tachycardia
RESPIRATORY RATE		
Increase	Respiratory distress Fluid volume excess Hypothermia Elevated temperature Pain	Body responds to respiratory distress primarily by increasing rate
Decrease	Anesthetics, opioids Pain	Decreased respiratory rate from opioids may be compensated by increased depth of respiration
BLOOD PRESSURE		
Increase	Excess intravascular volume Increased intracranial pressure Carbon dioxide retention Pain Medications (ketamine, epinephrine)	Serious in premature infants because it increases risk of intraventricular hemorrhage
Decrease	Vasodilating anesthetic agents (halothane, isoflurane, enflurane) Opioids (e.g., morphine) Shock (late sign)	Decreased blood pressure is late sign of shock because of elasticity and constriction of vessels to maintain cardiac output
TEMPERATURE		
Increase	Infection Environmental causes (warm room, excess coverings) Malignant hyperthermia	Fever associated with infection usually occurs later than fever of noninfectious origin Absence of fever does not rule out infection, especially in infants Malignant hyperthermia requires immediate treatment
Decrease	Vasodilating anesthetic agents (halothane, isoflurane, enflurane) Muscle relaxants Environmental causes (cool room) Infusion of cool fluids/blood	Neonates are especially susceptible to hypothermia with serious or fatal consequences

From Smith DP and others, editors: *Comprehensive child and family nursing skills,* St Louis, 1991, Mosby.

tinely scheduled intravenous analgesics and the use of patient-controlled anesthesia (PCA), rather than PRN (as necessary) orders, afford more satisfactory pain control (see Pain Management, Chapter 26).

Mouth care is another important aspect of care, because most children are allowed nothing orally until bowel sounds return (see p. 1159).

Since respiratory infections are a potential complication, every effort is taken to aerate the lungs and remove secretions. The lungs are auscultated regularly to identify abnormal sounds or any areas of diminished or absent breath sounds. To prevent hypostatic pneumonia, respiratory movement can be encouraged with incentive spirometers or other motivating activities (see p. 1142). If these measures are presented as games, the child is more likely to comply. The child's position is changed every 2 hours, and deep breathing is encouraged.

➤ **NURSING TIP** Because deep breathing is usually painful after surgery, have the child splint the operative site (depending on its location) by hugging a small pillow or a favorite stuffed animal.

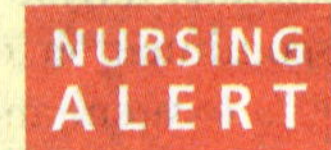

Early signs of respiratory involvement are abnormal rate, shallow depth, and cough. These findings are reported immediately.

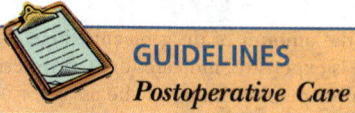

GUIDELINES
Postoperative Care

Ensure that preparations are made to receive child.
- Bed or crib is ready.
- Intravenous equipment, such as pumps, and any other relevant equipment, such as suction apparatus, oxygen flow meter, or Gomco suction, is at bedside.

Obtain baseline information:
- Take vital signs, including blood pressure (BP); keep BP cuff in place, deflated in order to lessen amount of disturbance to child.
- Take and record more frequently if any value fluctuates.
- Inspect operative area.
  - Check dressing if present.
  - Outline any bleeding area on dressing or cast with pen.
  - Reinforce, but do not remove, loose dressing.
  - Observe areas below surgical site for blood that may have drained toward bed.
  - Assess for bleeding and other symptoms in areas not covered with a dressing, such as throat following tonsillectomy.
- Assess skin color and characteristics.
- Assess level of consciousness, activity.

Notify physician of any irregularities in child's condition.

Assess for evidence of pain (see Pain Assessment, Chapter 26).

Review surgeon's orders after completing initial assessment, and check that any preoperative orders, such as seizure or cardiac medications, have been reordered and can be given by available routes (oral preparations may be contraindicated).

Monitor vital signs as ordered and more often if indicated.

Check dressings for bleeding or other abnormalities.

Check bowel sounds.

Observe for signs of shock, abdominal distention, bleeding.

Assess for bladder distention.

Observe for signs of dehydration.

Detect presence of infection:
- Take vital signs every 2-4 hours, as ordered.
- Collect or request needed specimens.
- Inspect wound for signs of infection—redness, swelling, heat, pain, purulent drainage.

During the recovery period, some time should be spent with children to assess their perception of surgery. Play, drawing, and storytelling are excellent methods of discovering their thoughts. With such information the nurse can support or correct their perceptions and assist children in achieving mastery for having endured a stressful procedure.

COMPLIANCE

One of the most significant nursing interventions concerning procedures that must be repeated in the hospital and/or continued at home is related to compliance. ***Compliance,*** also termed ***adherence,*** refers to the extent to which the patient's behavior in terms of taking medication, following diets, or executing other life-style changes coincides with the prescribed regimen. Reviews of compliance rates in children and adolescents with chronic diseases estimate that the rate of noncompliance ranges from 36% to more than 80% (Pidgeon, 1989). Since nurses are frequently responsible for teaching families about treatment protocols, they must have knowledge of factors that influence compliance, methods to measure compliance, and strategies to enhance adherence to prescribed treatment.

Assessment

In developing strategies to improve compliance, the nurse must first assess the patient's level of compliance. Since many children are too young to assume partial or total responsibility for their care, parents are usually the primary caregivers in terms of home management. Consequently, the nurse needs to assess their ability to carry out instructions. The first approach to assessment is knowledge of those factors that influence compliance. The second is to apply methods to assess more objectively the child's and parents' levels of compliance.

Factors That Influence Compliance. Research on compliance has identified several factors that influence compliance (see box below). The first area relates to factors about the patient. Contrary to what might be expected, no typical characteristics of noncompliers exist, and even education is not correlated with compliance (Rosenstock, 1988). Some evidence suggests that higher levels of self-esteem and increased autonomy favorably affect adolescent compliance (Pidgeon, 1989). However, family factors are important, and characteristics associated with good compli-

FACTORS THAT POSITIVELY INFLUENCE COMPLIANCE

INDIVIDUAL/FAMILY FACTORS
- High self-esteem
- Positive body image
- High degree of autonomy (increased locus of control)
- Supportive and well-adjusted family
- Effective family communication
- Family expectation for successful completion of therapy

CARE SETTING FACTORS
- Perceived satisfaction with care
- Positive interactions with practitioners
- Continuity of care
- Individualized care
- Minimum waiting time for appointments
- Convenient care setting

TREATMENT FACTORS
- Simple regimen
- Minimum disruption in usual life-style
- Short duration
- Inexpensive
- Visible benefits
- Tolerable side effects

ance include family support, family reminders, good communication, and expectations for successful completion of therapeutic regimen (Cromer and others, 1989; Meichenbaum, 1989; Pidgeon, 1989).

Factors relating to the care setting are very important in determining compliance and provide useful guidelines in planning strategies to improve compliance. Basically, any aspect of the health care setting that increases the family's satisfaction with the physical setting and the relationship with the practitioner positively influences adherence to the treatment regimen. In addition, the type of care required to manage the disorder is important. The more complex, expensive, inconvenient, longer, and disruptive the treatment protocol, the less likely the family is to comply. During long-term conditions that involve multiple treatments and considerable rearrangement of life-style, compliance is most severely affected.

Measurement of Compliance. While it is helpful to know those factors that influence compliance, especially in assessing the likelihood of compliance in a family, assessment must include more direct measurement techniques. A number of methods exist, each with its advantages and disadvantages. The most successful approach includes a combination of at least two of the following methods:

Clinical judgment. The nurse judges family compliance. This method is subject to bias and inaccuracy unless the nurse carefully evaluates the criteria used in evaluation.

Self-reporting. The family is asked about their ability to carry out the prescribed treatments. Although a simple method, most people overestimate their compliance by about 20%, even when they admit to lapses in treatment.

Direct observation. The nurse directly observes the patient or family perform the treatment. Although this approach is very effective in identifying errors related to the correct procedure, it is difficult to employ outside the health care setting. Also, the family's awareness of being observed frequently affects their performance.

Monitoring appointments. The family's attendance at scheduled appointments is recorded. Keeping appointments indicates general levels of compliance but only indirectly indicates compliance with the prescribed care.

Monitoring therapeutic response. The child's response in terms of benefit from treatment is monitored, preferably recorded on a graph or chart. Unfortunately, few treatments yield directly measurable results (e.g., decreased blood pressure, weight loss), making this a less satisfactory method for most types of therapies. Also, adherence does not ensure clinical improvement, and less than 100% may *achieve therapeutic results,* reinforcing partial compliance (Meichenbaum, 1989).

Pill counts. The nurse counts the number of pills remaining in the original container and compares the number missing with the number of days the medication should have been taken. Although this is a simple method, families may forget to bring the container or deliberately alter the number of pills to avoid detection. This method is also poorly suited to liquid medication, which is so often prescribed in pediatrics. A new technique is the use of pill container caps that record every opening as a presumptive dose (Cramer and others, 1989).

Chemical assay. For certain drugs, such as digoxin, theophylline, and phenytoin, measurement of plasma drug levels provides information on the amount of drug recently ingested. However, this method is expensive, indicates only short-term compliance, and requires precise timing of the assay for accurate results.

Compliance Strategies

Strategies to improve compliance are concerned with those interventions that encourage families to follow the prescribed treatment regimen. Ideally, such strategies should be implemented before or concurrent with the initiation of therapy to avoid compliance problems. When compliance problems are suspected, however, the nurse should assess why the child or family is having difficulty adhering to the treatment plan. A number of strategies have been identified as effective, but, as with measurement methods, no one approach is always successful, and the best results occur when at least two strategies are employed. The following is an overview of compliance strategies.

Organizational strategies refer to those interventions concerned with the care setting and the therapeutic plan. They include manipulating the factors listed in the box on p. 1151 that positively affect compliance. Depending on the individual situation, this may involve increasing the frequency of appointments, designating a primary practitioner, reducing the cost of medication by purchasing generic brands, reducing the disruption of the treatment on the family's life-style, and the use of "cues" to minimize forgetting. Numerous devices are available commercially or can be improvised for cueing, such as pill dispensers; watches with alarms; charts to record completed therapy; reminders such as messages on the refrigerator or morning coffeepot; and treatment schedules that incorporate the treatment plan into the daily routine, such as physical therapy after the evening bath.

Educational strategies are concerned with instructing the family about the treatment plan. Although education is an important component in enhancing compliance and patients who are more knowledgeable about their condition are more likely to comply, education alone does not ensure compliant behavior. Also, for education to be effective, it must incorporate teaching principles known to enhance understanding and retention of material (see Guidelines box). Written materials are essential, especially in any regimen requiring multiple or complex treatments, and need to be readable by the average individual, which appears to be at the fourth grade level (50% of health care clients have difficulty or are unable to read at a fifth grade level) (Streiff, 1986). One study found that 30% to 50% (depending on the educational level) of mothers failed to understand basic medical terms that residents presumed the mother would understand, such as *asthma, vitamin, fever, development,* and *virus* (Gablehouse and Gitterman, 1990). Including the culturally significant decision maker (e.g., maternal grandmother) in teaching sessions will help improve compliance (Faber, 1986).

Treatment strategies are related to the child's refusal or inability to take the prescribed medication. The family may also have difficulty following a prescribed treatment regimen. They may remember and understand the instructions

GUIDELINES
Effective Teaching of Family Members

- Establish rapport; reduce anxiety and fear.
- Assess what family knows and expects to learn, especially if they have concerns, and address their concerns before beginning teaching.
- Assess family's learning style; ask if they prefer having everything explained in detail or knowing only the major facts.
- Direct teaching to family decision maker and/or primary caregiver.
- Use a variety of teaching materials (lecture, demonstration, video or slide presentation, written material).
- Speak family's language, avoid jargon, and clarify all terms.
- Be specific when giving information; divide information into small steps.
- Keep information short, simple, and concrete.
- Introduce most important information first.
- Use "verbal" headings to organize information, such as, "There are two things you need to learn: how to give the medicine and what side effects to look for. First, how to give. . . . Second, what side effects. . . ."
- Stress importance of instructions and expected benefits; explain detrimental effects of inadequate treatment but avoid fear tactics.
- Evaluate teaching by eliciting feedback to ensure that family understands information.
- Repeat information as needed.
- Reward family for learning through verbal praise.
- Use "teachable" moments—times when family is most likely to accept new information (e.g., when symptoms are present).

but may not be able to give the medicine as prescribed. It is essential to assess the reason for refusal. For example, the child may not be able to swallow pills. In this case, perhaps they can be crushed or a liquid medication substituted. The opposite also may occur; the child is having difficulty drinking a liquid medication but is able to swallow pills. (See also Nursing Tip on p. 1182.)

Also assess the treatment/medication schedule to determine if it is reasonable for a home situation. While an every-6-hour or every-8-hour schedule is reasonable for hospitals, a parent would have difficulty getting up one or two times in the night when a medication could be given during the day at times that would be easy to remember (see Critical Thinking Exercise box).

Behavioral strategies encompass those interventions designed to modify behavior directly. Several strategies are effective in encouraging the desired behavior and are very useful with children. Ideally, positive reinforcement should be employed to strengthen the behavior and may consist of earning stars or tokens, which gains the child a special privilege or gift. A more formal method is the use of contracting (see following discussion). However, at times disciplinary techniques, such as time-out for young children (see p. 88) or withholding privileges for older children, may be needed to reduce noncompliance (Rapoff, 1986).

➤ **NURSING TIP** To encourage a child to perform a treatment for a certain time frame (e.g., soaking a foot), ask the child to soak during a favorite TV show, including commercials. This technique also helps evaluate compliance by asking the child what show was watched (Woolverton, 1991).

CRITICAL THINKING EXERCISE
Discharge Instructions

Ms. Jordan is getting ready to take 2-month-old Brittany home from the hospital after a 4-day admission for a severe ear infection and eye infection. Brittany will be going home taking an antibiotic that you have been giving every 8 hours and eye drops that you have been giving every 6 hours. The infant is fed about every 4 hours. Choose the appropriate home schedule.

1. 12 AM—Feed and give antibiotic and eye drops
   4 AM—Feed
   6 AM—Eye drops
   8 AM—Feed and give antibiotic
   12 PM—Feed and give eye drops
   4 PM—Feed and give antibiotic
   6 PM—Eye drops
   8 PM—Feed
2. 12 AM—Feed and give antibiotic
   4 AM—Feed
   8 AM—Feed and give eye antibiotic and eye drops
   12 PM—Feed and give eye drops
   4 PM—Feed and give antibiotic and eye drops
   8 PM—Feed and give eye drops
3. 12 AM—Feed and give antibiotic and eye drops
   6 AM—Feed and give antibiotic and eye drops
   10 AM—Feed and give eye drops
   2 PM—Feed and give antibiotic
   6 PM—Feed and give eye drops
   9 PM—Feed

The best answer is 2. Even though you followed the every-6-hour schedule for the eye drops in the hospital, it is unlikely that the parent could manage this at home. It is sometimes difficult getting eye drops into an infant's eyes, and giving the parent a schedule in which they must be given twice during the night would be difficult. Reducing the number of times the parent and infant must awaken during the night decreases the likelihood of a missed dose because the parent forgot to get up.

If this were an older child, the antibiotic schedule could also be altered to waking hours only so the child and parent would not have to awaken in the night for medication.

Although not every medication can be given on a more flexible schedule, most can. Ask the practitioner if the medication can be given three times a day instead of every 8 hours or four times a day instead of every 6 hours, etc. Medications or treatments given at unusual times are more likely to be missed. Discharge instructions should always be given keeping in mind the parent's ability to be compliant with them.

Contracting is a process in which the exact elements of desired behavior are explicitly outlined in the form of a written contract. Based on behavior modification, it is a very effective method of shaping behavior, especially with older children who are involved in the process of defining the rules of the agreement. Ideally, it should involve tangible rewards but may include negative consequences, such as demerits or "checks" for failing to comply. In deciding whether to use positive or negative reinforcers, the nurse should question parents about their opinion regarding powerful motivators for the child. Often the contract includes a commitment from the parent, such as agreeing to stop nagging about taking medication.

An effective contract includes the following:

- The goal or desired behavior is realistic and seems possible.
- The behavior is measurable (e.g., agreeing to take the drug before leaving for school without reminding).
- The contract is written and signed by all those involved in any of the agreements.
- The contract is dated, and if appropriate, a date is specified when a goal should be reached (e.g., number of pounds of weight loss in 2 weeks).
- The identified rewards or consequences are reinforcing.
- The goal can be evaluated (e.g., counting the number of tablets, using a scale for weight measurement).

More informal arrangements can be used with young children, such as rewarding desired behavior with stars, stickers, or other small novelties. Once the contract is implemented, it is evaluated at the end of the time specified in the agreement and revisions are made, such as extending the time or terminating the contract. If the contract has not been successful, every effort is made to ascertain if the goals were realistic, the time period was sufficient for accomplishing the goal, and the rewards or consequences were motivating. A successful contract may or may not work the next time.

GENERAL HYGIENE AND CARE

MAINTAINING HEALTHY SKIN

Skin, the largest organ of the body, is not merely a covering but also a complex structure that serves many functions, the most important of which is to protect the tissues that it encloses and to protect itself. Many routine nursing activities—maintaining an intravenous line, removing a dressing, positioning a child in bed, changing a diaper, using electrode patches, or maintaining restraints—have the potential to contribute to skin injury. Skin care must go beyond the daily bath and become a part of each nursing intervention. General guidelines for skin care are listed in the Guidelines box. Specific guidelines for skin care of neonates are provided in Chapter 10 under Skin Care.

Assessment of the skin is most easily accomplished during the bath, but often the nurse is not the one who bathes the child. In this case the nurse needs to plan a time to observe the child's skin and to request feedback from the caregiver. The skin is examined for any early signs of injury, especially in the child who is at risk. Risk factors include impaired mobility, protein malnutrition, edema, incontinence, sensory loss, anemia, and infection. Identification of risk factors helps to determine those children who need a more thorough skin assessment.

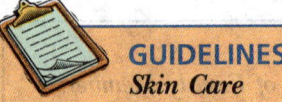

GUIDELINES
Skin Care

Cleanse skin with gentle soap (e.g., Dove) or cleanser (e.g., Cetaphil). Rinse well with plain warm water.

Provide daily cleansing of eyes, oral and diaper or perianal areas, and any areas of skin breakdown.

Apply moisturizing agents after cleansing to retain moisture and rehydrate skin; however, cleanse skin of any old cream before adding a new layer.

Use minimum tape/adhesive. On very sensitive skin, use a protective, pectin-based or hydrocolloid skin barrier between skin and tape/adhesives.

Use water or possibly adhesive remover (if skin is not fragile) when removing tape/adhesives.

Place pectin-based or hydrocolloid skin barriers directly over excoriated skin. Leave barrier undisturbed until it begins to peel off. With wet, oozing excoriations, place a small amount of stoma powder (as used in ostomy care) on site, remove excess powder, and apply skin barrier. Hold barrier in place for several minutes to allow barrier to soften and mold to skin surface.

Alternate electrode placement and thoroughly assess skin underneath electrodes at least every 24 hours.

Be certain fingers or toes are visible whenever extremity is used for IV or arterial line.

Reduce friction by keeping skin dry (may apply absorbent powder, such as cornstarch) and using soft, smooth bed linen and clothes.

Use a draw sheet to move a child in bed or onto a gurney to reduce friction and shearing injuries; do not drag the child from under the arms.

Identify children who are risk for skin breakdown before it occurs. Employ measures, such as pressure reducing or relieving devices, to prevent breakdown.

Do not massage reddened bony prominences because it can cause deep tissue damage; provide pressure relief to those areas instead.

Keep skin free of excess moisture (i.e., urine or fecal incontinence, wound drainage, excessive perspiration).

Routinely assess the child's nutritional status. A child who is NPO for several days and is only receiving IV fluid is nutritionally at risk, which can also affect the skin's ability to maintain its integrity. Hyperalimentation should be considered for these children before they are at risk.

When capillary blood flow is interrupted by pressure, the blood flows back into the tissue when the pressure is relieved. As the body attempts to reoxygenate the area, a bright-red flush appears. This ***reactive hyperemia,*** or flush, may be present for one half to three fourths as long as the time the pressure occluded the blood flow to the area.

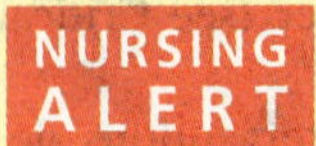

NURSING ALERT If the redness persists, this may be the first sign of skin breakdown, including the possibility of more extensive damage below the skin.

Staging of pressure ulcers is used to classify the amount of tissue damage that has occurred. The tissue in the wound must be visible in order to be staged; it is difficult to assess a wound that is covered with necrotic tissue or a scab (see box on p. 1155). Accurate documentation of redness or obvious skin breakdown is essential. Color, size (diameter and depth), location, presence of sinus tracts, odor, exudate, and response to treatment are observed and recorded at least daily. (For treatment of wounds, see Chapter 18; see also Critical Thinking Exercise box, p. 1156.)

The nurse must also have an understanding of the types

STAGING OF PRESSURE ULCERS

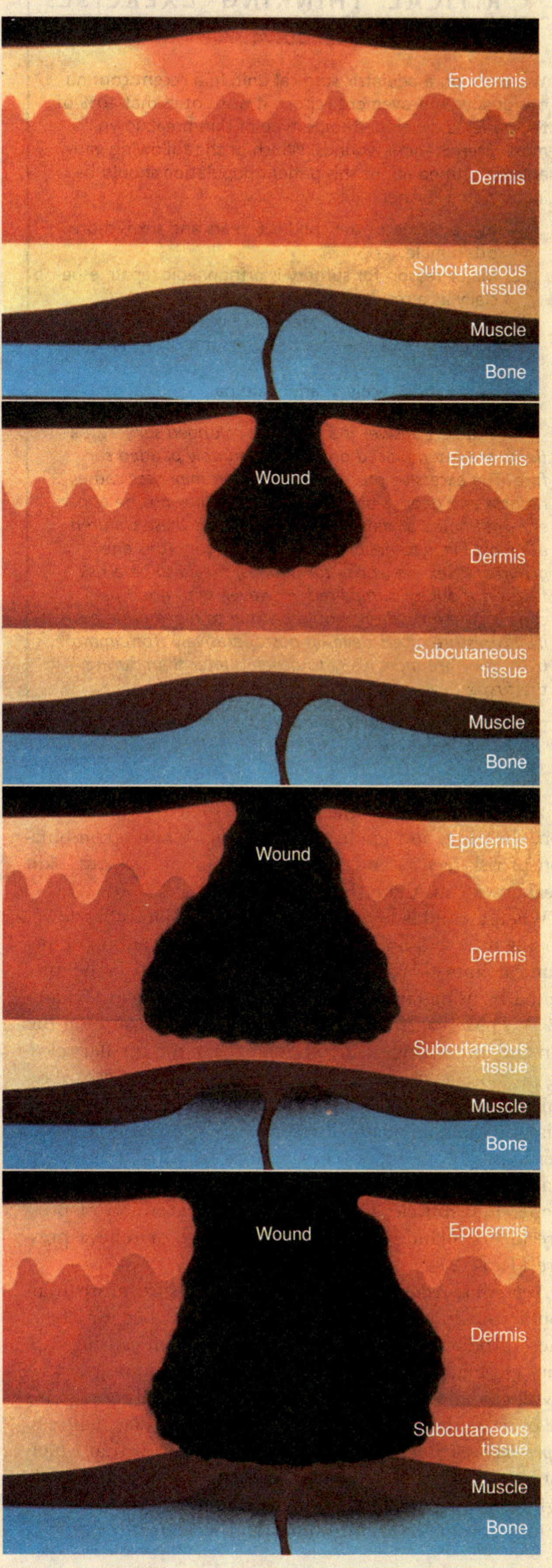

STAGE I

Nonblanchable erythema of intact skin; the heralding lesion of skin ulceration.* NOTE: Reactive hyperemia can normally be expected to be present for one half to three fourths as long as the pressure occluded blood flow to the area. This should not be confused with a Stage I pressure ulcer.

STAGE II

Partial-thickness skin loss involving epidermis and/or dermis. The ulcer is superficial and presents clinically as an abrasion, blister, or shallow crater.

STAGE III

Full-thickness skin loss involving damage or necrosis of subcutaneous tissue that may extend down to, but not through, underlying fascia. The ulcer presents clinically as a deep crater with or without undermining of adjacent tissue.†

STAGE IV

Full-thickness skin loss with extensive destruction, tissue necrosis or damage to muscle, bone, or supporting structures (e.g., tendon or joint capsule). NOTE: Undermining and sinus tracts may also be associated with Stage IV pressure ulcers.

From Panel for the Prediction and Prevention of Pressure Ulcers in Adults: *Pressure ulcers in adults: prediction and prevention,* Clinical Practice Guideline Number 3, AHCPR Pub No 92—0047, Rockville, MD, 1992, Agency for Health Care Policy and Research, Public Health Service, US Department of Health and Human Services. Illustrations courtesy ConvaTec, Princeton, NJ.

*Identification of Stage I pressure ulcers may be difficult in patients with darkly pigmented skin.

†When eschar is present, accurate staging of the pressure ulcer is not possible until the eschar has sloughed or the wound has been debrided.

CRITICAL THINKING EXERCISE

Risk of Skin Breakdown

You work on a pediatric surgical unit. In a recent continuous quality improvement report, it was noted that 10% of the patients developed some type of skin breakdown, most often Stage II wounds. Which of the following variables identified about this patient population should be investigated further?

1. Average age of the child is 6 years and sex is more often male.
2. Major reason for surgery is orthopaedic repair, especially as a result of trauma.
3. Average length of surgery is 4 hours, and average duration until appearance of wound is 24 to 48 hours.
4. All children received adequate pain medication.

The correct answer is 3. During prolonged surgery, patients are often placed on an inadequately padded surface. The excessive pressure on bony prominences causes redness and deeper tissue damage that may not be apparent until hours or days later. The fact that these children are most likely to need orthopaedic surgery (this age-group and sex are at risk for injuries) may also be a risk factor if mobility is impaired. However, with good pain control, these children should be able to move quite easily. If pressure ulcers develop postoperatively from immobility, they are most likely to develop later than during the first 2 days.

of mechanical damage that can occur, such as pressure, friction, shearing, and epidermal stripping. When a combination of risk factors and mechanical injury is present, skin breakdown can occur (Hagelgans, 1993).

When a child is identified as at risk for skin breakdown, nursing interventions are directed toward prevention of mechanical injury. Wounds caused by pressure can be prevented by using current technology and resources (Bryant, 1992). ***Pressure ulcers*** can develop when the pressure on the skin and underlying tissues is greater than the capillary closing pressure, causing capillary occlusion. If the pressure remains unrelieved, vessels can collapse, resulting in tissue anoxia and cellular death. Pressure ulcers most often occur over bony prominences. These lesions are usually very deep (stage IV), extending into subcutaneous tissue or even deeper into muscle, tendon, or bone. Prevention of pressure ulcers includes measures that reduce or relieve pressure (Table 27-2).

A ***pressure-reduction device*** reduces pressure more than would usually occur on a regular hospital bed or chair. These products do not prevent pressure from causing capillary closing; therefore, turning and repositioning are always included when using these devices. Most of these items are overlays that are placed on top of the regular mattress. A ***pressure-relief device*** maintains pressure below that which would cause capillary closing. These devices are usually high-technology beds that are used for patients who have multiple problems and cannot be turned effectively.

NURSING ALERT Convoluted foam mattress pads with a base of 2 inches (measured from where the convolutions begin, not the peak of the convolution) and soft padding, such as sheepskin, do not significantly reduce pressure when compared with a regular hospital mattress (Krouskop and others, 1985).

Friction and shear both contribute to pressure ulcers. ***Friction*** occurs when the surface of the skin rubs against another surface, such as the sheets on the bed. The skin may have the appearance of an abrasion. The skin damage is usually limited to the epidermal and upper layers. It most often occurs over the elbows or heels. Prevention of friction injury includes the use of protective sheepskin over the elbows or heels, moisturizing agents, transparent dressings over susceptible areas, and soft, smooth bed linen and clothing. By itself, friction does not cause tissue necrosis, but when it acts with gravity, it results in shear injury.

Shear is the result of the force of gravity pushing down on the body and friction of the body against a surface, such as the bed or chair. For example, when a patient is in the semi-Fowler position and begins to slide to the foot of the bed, the skin over the sacral area remains in the same place because of the resistance of the bed surface. The blood vessels in the area are stretched and may cause small vessel thrombosis and tissue death (Bryant, 1992). The same type of damage can occur when a patient is pulled up in the bed if the skin does not move with the patient. Prevention of shear injury includes using "lift sheets" when repositioning a patient, elevating the bed no more than 30 degrees for short periods, and using the knee gatch to interrupt the pull of gravity on the body toward the foot of the bed.

Epidermal stripping results when the epidermis is unintentionally removed with tape removal. These lesions are usually shallow and irregularly shaped. Prevention of epidermal stripping includes recognizing fragile skin, such as in neonates; using minimum tape; using solid-wafer skin barriers, transparent dressings, or laced binders to secure dressings (Montgomery straps) on areas in which tape must be changed frequently; using skin sealants under adhesives unless skin is fragile; and using porous tapes. Tape is placed so there is no tension, traction, or wrinkles on the skin. To remove tape, slowly peel the tape away while stabilizing the underlying skin. Adhesive remover may be used to break the adhesive bond but may be drying to the skin (Bryant, 1992). Wetting the tape with water may facilitate removal.

Chemical factors can also lead to skin damage. Fecal incontinence, especially when mixed with urine; wound drainage; or gastric drainage around gastrostomy tubes can erode epidermis. The skin can very quickly progress from redness to denudement if exposure continues. Moisture barriers, gentle cleansing as soon after exposure as possible, and skin barriers can be used to prevent damage caused by chemical factors (see also Diaper Dermatitis, Chapter 13).

BATHING

Unless contraindicated, most infants and children can be bathed in a tub at the bedside, on the bed, or in a stan-

TABLE 27-2 Pressure Reduction/Relief Devices

DESCRIPTION	ADVANTAGES	DISADVANTAGES	EXAMPLES*
OVERLAY†			
Foam: Varying density; 2-4 inch convoluted and nonconvoluted	Primarily pressure reduction, although in children may have pressure relief advantages; can be cut to fit cribs	Can soil with incontinent patient; inability to reduce skin moisture because of lack of airflow	Aerofoam, BioGard, Dura-Pedic, GeoMatt, Ultra Form Pediatric (does not include ordinary convoluted foam mattresses)
Gel/water filled: Pressure reduction; water or gel conforms to patient's contours	One-time charge; low cost for water; gels are expensive	Gravity displacement can lead to inadequate flotation; potential for leaks; heavy; question safety indications for CPR	Aqua-Pedics (water and gel), Tender Gel and Water, Theracare (water and gel)
Alternating-pressure mattress: An overlay with rows of air cells and pump; pump cycles air to provide inflation and deflation over pressure points	Constant low-volume airflow; managed excess skin moisture	Cost of pump rental; electric usage charge incurred by family; ongoing monitoring and maintenance of equipment; some complain pump is noisy	AeroPulse, AlphaBed, AlphaCare, BetaBed, Bio Flote, Dyna-CARE, Lapidus, PCA Systems, Pillo-Pump, Tenderair
Static air: Designed with interlocking air cells that provide dry flotation; inflated with a blower	May be more effective than foam; easy to clean; has been documented in adult studies to reduce pressure	Inflation level must be checked frequently by caregiver to maintain therapeutic levels; may cause increased perspiration because of plastic surface	DermaGard, K-Soft, Koala-Kair, Roho, Sof-Care, Tenderair
Low-air-loss specialty overlay: Multiple air-fluidized cushions that cover the entire bed; pressures can be set and controlled by a pump	Surface materials are constructed to reduce friction and shear and to eliminate moisture; pressure relief; can be used for prevention and/or treatment of ulcers	Surface mattress and pump are a rental item; cost of electricity used is incurred by family; not available for cribs	Acucair, Bio Therapy, CLINI-CARE, CRS 4000, RibCor Therapeutic Mattress Pad
SPECIALTY BEDS‡			
Low-air-loss beds: Bed surface consists of inflated air cushions; each section is adjusted for optimum pressure relief for patient's body size; some models have built-in scales	Provides pressure relief in any position; treatment for Stages III and IV pressure ulcers; available in pediatric crib sizes	Bed is more bulky than a hospital bed, and some homes may not be able to accommodate its size; reimbursement is questionable; family incurs electric bill	Air Plus, Flexicair, KinAir, Mediscus; Cribs: Pedcare, PediKair, PNEU-CARE/PEDI, Clinitron
Air-fluidized beds: Air is blown through glass beads to "float" patient	Treatment for deep pressure sores, burns, posterior flaps	Weighs 2400 pounds, which makes it unsuitable for home use; can be difficult to transfer patient; hard to position patient, especially for respiratory toileting	Clinitron, FluidAir Plus, Skytron
Kinetic therapy: Some bed surfaces consist of air cushions that are programmed to alternately inflate and deflate sections so the patient is rotated from side to side, or in some models, the bed frame rotates; some models are without air cushions	Indicated for patients with a high degree of immobility and severe respiratory distress, and who are hemodynamically unstable when moved	Used in acute care setting	***With air loss:*** BioDyne, Restcue, TheraPulse ***Without air loss:*** Keane Mobility RotoRest

Modified from Hagelgans NA: Pediatric skin care issues for the home care nurse, *Pediatr Nurs* 19(5):499-507, 1993.

*This list is a representative sampling of products that is not intended to be all inclusive. No endorsement of any product is intended. Within each category, products must be individually evaluated on their efficacy as comfort, pressure-reducing, or pressure-relieving devices. All products within a category do not necessarily perform equally.

†A device that is made to fit over a regular hospital mattress.

‡"High-tech" beds used in place of the standard hospital bed. These are usually used on a rental basis and are intended for short-term use. They usually provide pressure relief and eliminate shear, friction, and maceration.

dard bathtub located on the unit, which is often conveniently adapted for pediatric use. For infants and young children confined to bed, the towel method can be used. Two towels are immersed in a dilute soap solution and wrung damp. With the child lying supine on a dry towel, one damp towel is placed on top of the child and used to gently clean the body. This towel is discarded, then the child is dried and turned prone. The procedure is repeated using the second damp towel.

Infants and small children are *never* left unattended in a bathtub, and infants who are unable to sit alone are securely held with one hand during the bath. The infant's head is supported securely with one hand or the farther arm is firmly grasped in the nurse's hand while the head rests comfortably on the wrist. This provides secure control of the infant while the other hand is free to wash the infant's body (Fig. 27-4). Infants or children who are able to sit without assistance need only close supervision and a pad placed in the bottom of the tub to prevent slipping and loss of balance, which could result in a bumped head or submersion of the face.

Older children may enjoy a shower if it is available. School-age children may be reluctant to bathe, and many are not accustomed to a daily bath. However, most children who feel well require little encouragement to participate in their daily care. Nurses will need to use judgment regarding the amount of supervision the child requires. Some can be trusted to assume this responsibility unaided, whereas others will need someone in constant attendance. Children with cognitive impairments, physical limitations such as severe anemia or leg deformities, or suicidal or psychotic problems (who may commit bodily harm) require close supervision.

Areas that require special attention during bed baths and for children performing their own care are the ears, between skinfolds, the neck, the back, and the genital area. The genital area should be carefully cleansed and dried with particular care to skinfolds, and in uncircumcised boys, usually those over 3 years of age, the foreskin should be gently retracted and the exposed surfaces cleansed and then the foreskin replaced. If the condition of the glans indicates inadequate cleaning, such as accumulated smegma, inflammation, phimosis, or foreskin adhesions, teaching proper hygiene is indicated. In the Vietnamese and Cambodian cultures the foreskin is traditionally not retracted until adulthood (Krueger and Osborn, 1986). Older children have the tendency to avoid the genitalia; therefore they may need a gentle reminder.

Children who are ill or debilitated will need more extensive assistance with bathing and other aspects of hygienic care, but they should be encouraged to perform as much as they are able without overtaxing their energies. Increasing involvement can be expected with improved strength and endurance. Children with limited capacity for

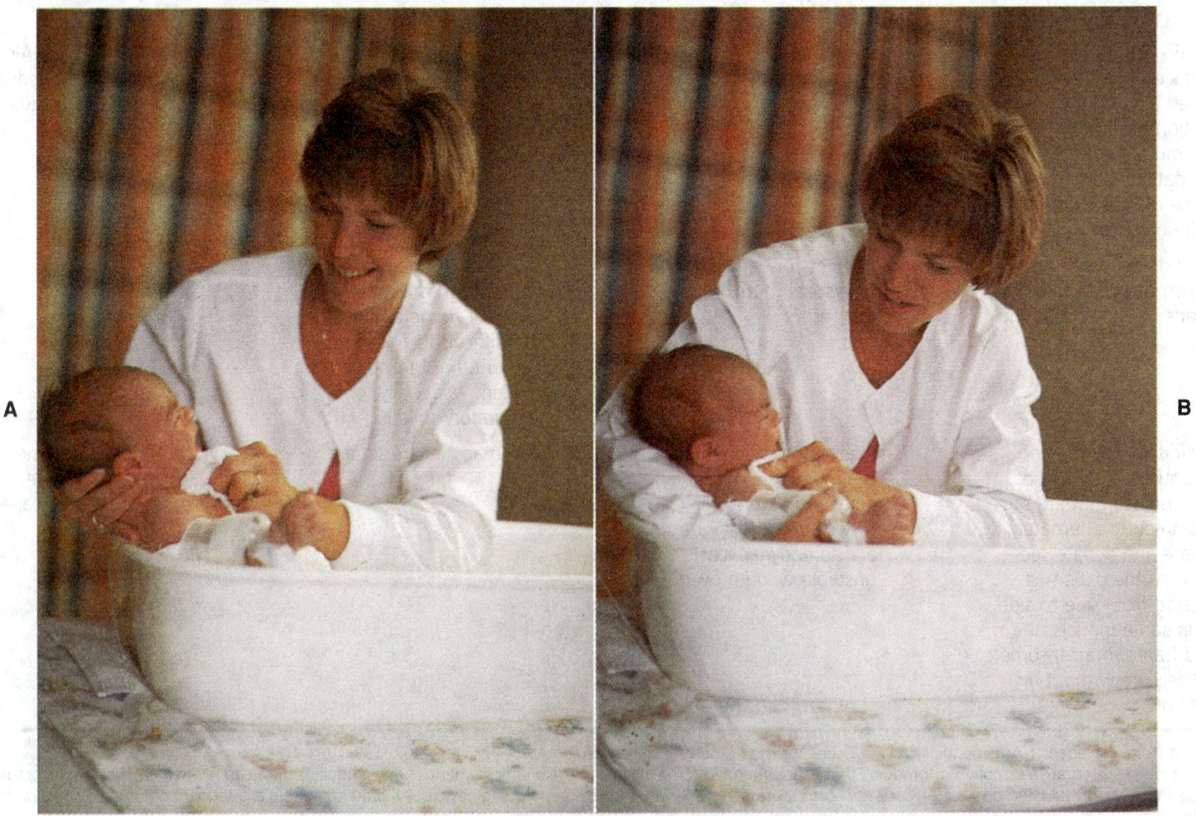

FIG. 27-4 Two methods of supporting infant during tub bath. **A,** Using hand to support neck and head. **B,** Using arm to support neck and head.

self-help but no other contraindications benefit greatly from tub baths. They can be transported to the tub and, with the aid of lifting devices and/or an appropriate number of persons to assist, gain the advantages of a tub bath.

ORAL HYGIENE

Mouth care is an integral part of daily hygiene and should be continued in the hospital. Infants and debilitated children will require the nurse or a family member to perform mouth care. Although young children can manage a toothbrush and are encouraged to use it, most will need assistance to perform a satisfactory job. Older children, although capable of brushing and flossing without assistance, sometimes need to be reminded that this is a part of their hygiene care. Most hospitals have equipment available for those children who do not have toothbrush or toothpaste of their own. (See Dental Health, Chapters 12, 14, 15, and 17; and Chapter 36 for mouth care of children with mucosal ulcers.)

HAIR CARE

Brushing and combing hair are a part of the daily care for all persons in the hospital, including infants and children. If the child does not have a brush or comb, many hospitals provide one as part of the usual admission kit. If not, the parents should be asked to bring hair care equipment for the child's use. Both boys and girls are helped to comb or brush their hair, or it is done for them, at least once daily. The hair is styled for comfort and in a manner pleasing to the child and parents. A satisfactory style for girls with longer hair is French braiding, which is created by starting with three equal portions of hair from the top of the scalp; as the hair is braided, segments of hair are added at successive intervals until all the hair has been incorporated into one or more neat, head-hugging braids. The ends are firmly anchored with an elastic hair band or barrette. The hair should not be cut without parental permission, although shaving hair to provide access to a scalp vein for intravenous needle insertion may be necessary.

If children are hospitalized for more than a few days, the hair may need shampooing. With infants, the hair may be washed during the daily bath or less frequently. For most children, washing the hair and scalp once or twice weekly is sufficient, unless there is an indication to wash it more frequently, such as following a high fever and profuse sweating. Some hospitals have shampoo basins, but almost any child can be conveniently transported by a gurney to an accessible sink or washbasin for shampooing. Those who are unable to be transported can receive a shampoo in their beds with adequate protection and/or specially adapted equipment or positioning. A convenient method involves positioning the child near the edge of the bed, placing towels under the shoulders, and draping a large plastic garbage bag at the edge of the bed with one open end under the shoulders and the hair placed inside the opening. The other end is opened and placed in a collection container. Water can be transported in a basin.

➤ **NURSING TIP** For a convenient source of water, fill an empty enema bag with warm water and hang the bag from an intravenous pole; use the clamp on the bag's tubing to adjust the flow of water (Bourgault, 1985).

Teenagers, with their normally increased oily sebaceous secretions, are particularly in need of frequent hair care and usually require more frequent shampoos. Commercial "dry shampoo" products may also prove useful on a short-term basis.

Black children require special hair care, and this need is frequently neglected or inadequately managed. For the black child with kinky hair, most standard combs are inadequate and may cause hair breakage and discomfort to the child. If a special comb with widely spaced teeth is not available on the unit, the parent can be reminded to bring a comb, if possible, for the child's use. It is also much easier to comb the hair after shampooing, when it is wet (Joyner, 1988). This type of hair requires a special hair dressing or pomade, which usually has a coconut oil base. The preparation is rubbed on the hands and then transferred to the hair to make it more pliable and manageable. The child's parents should be consulted regarding the preparation they wish to be used on their child's hair and asked if they can provide some for use during the child's hospitalization. Petroleum jelly should *not* be used. If braiding or plaiting the hair is desired, the hair should be damp and loosely woven. The hair tightens as it dries, which could result in tension folliculitis (Joyner, 1988).

FEEDING THE SICK CHILD

Loss of appetite is a symptom common to most childhood illnesses and is frequently the initial evidence of illness, preceding fever and other overt signs of infection. In most cases, children can be permitted to determine their own need for food. Since an acute illness is usually short, the nutritional state is seldom compromised. In fact, urging foods on the sick child may precipitate nausea and vomiting and in some cases even cause an aversion to the feeding situation that can extend into the convalescent period and beyond.

Refusing to eat may also be one way children can exert power and control in an otherwise helpless situation. For young children, loss of appetite may be related to the depression of separation from their parents and their natural tendency toward negativism. Parents' concern with eating can intensify the problem. Forcing a child to eat only meets with rebellion and reinforces the behavior as a control mechanism. Parents are encouraged to relax any pressure during an acute illness. Although it is best to encourage high-quality nutritious foods, the child may desire foods and liquids that contain mostly calories. Some well-tolerated foods include gelatin, diluted clear soups, carbonated drinks, flavored ice pops, dry toast, crackers, and hard candy. Even though these substances are not nutritious, they can provide necessary fluid and calories.

Dehydration is always a hazard when children are febrile or anorexic, especially when this is accompanied by vomiting or diarrhea. An adequate fluid intake is encouraged by

GUIDELINES
Feeding the Sick Child

Take a dietary history (see Chapter 6) and use information to make eating time as much like home as possible.
Encourage parents or other family members to feed child or to be present at mealtimes.
Have children eat at tables in groups; bring nonambulatory children to eating area in wheelchairs, beds, strollers, gurneys, or wagons.
Use familiar eating utensils, such as a favorite plate, cup, or bottle for small children.
Make mealtimes pleasant; avoid any procedures immediately before or after eating; make sure child is rested and pain free.
Have a nurse present at mealtimes to offer assistance, prevent disruptions, and praise children for their eating.
Serve small, frequent meals rather than three large meals or serve three meals and nutritious between-meal snacks.
Bring in foods from home, especially if food preparation is very different from hospital's; consider cultural differences.
Provide finger foods for young children.
Involve children in food selection and preparation whenever possible.
Serve small portions, and serve each course separately, such as soup first, followed by meat, potatoes, and vegetables, and ending with dessert; with young children camouflage size of food by cutting meat thicker so less appears on plate or by folding a cheese slice in half; offer second helpings; ensure a variety of foods, textures, and colors.
Provide food selections that are favorites of most children, such as peanut butter and jelly sandwiches, hot dogs, hamburgers, macaroni and cheese, pizza, spaghetti, tacos, fried chicken, corn on the cob, and fruit yogurt.
Avoid foods that are highly seasoned, have strong odors, are served hot, or are all mixed together, unless typical of cultural practices.
Provide fluid selections that are favorites of most children, such as fruit punch, cola, ginger ale, sweetened tea, ice pops, sherbet, ice cream, milk and milkshakes, eggnog, pudding, gelatin, clear broth, or creamed soups (see also box on p. 1142).
Offer nutritious snacks, such as frozen yogurt or pudding, ice cream, oatmeal or peanut butter cookies, hot cocoa, cheese slices or "kisses," pieces of raw vegetable or fruit, and dried fruit or cereal.
Make food attractive and different, for example:
- Serve a "picnic lunch" in a paper bag.
- Pack food in a Chinese-food container; decorate container.
- Put a "face" or a "flower" on a hamburger or sandwich with pieces of vegetable.
- Use a cookie-cutter to shape a sandwich.
- Serve pudding, yogurt, or juice frozen as a flavored ice pop.
- Make slurpies or snowcones by pouring flavored syrup on crushed ice.
- Add vegetable coloring to water or milk.
- Serve fluids through brightly colored or unusually shaped straws.
- Make "bowtie" sandwiches by cutting them in triangles and placing two points together.
- Slice sandwiches into "fingers."
- Grate mounds of cheese.
- Cut apples horizontally to make circles.
- Put a banana on a hot dog bun and spread with peanut butter.
- Break uncooked spaghetti into toothpick lengths and skewer cheese, cold meat, vegetables, or fruit chunks.

Praise children for what they do eat.
Do *not* punish children for not eating by removing their dessert or putting them to bed.

offering small amounts of favored fluids at frequent intervals and by providing salty foods if allowed. If diarrhea is present, high-carbohydrate liquids (e.g., carbonated beverages, gelatin, flavored ice pops) are avoided because they may aggravate the diarrhea by an osmotic effect (Ghishan, 1988). Also, replacing abnormal losses with plain water or undiluted broth, which may worsen the electrolyte imbalance, is not advocated. Fluids should not be forced, and the child is not wakened from rest to take fluids. Forcing fluids may create the same difficulties as urging unwanted food. Gentle persuasion with preferred beverages will usually meet with success. Using play techniques can also be very effective (see box on p. 1142).

In general, hot dogs, hamburgers, peanut butter and jelly sandwiches, fruit yogurt, milkshakes, spaghetti, tacos, macaroni and cheese, and pizza are favorite foods of most children. Although alone they may not typify well-balanced diets, they can be adjusted to include sufficient amounts from the basic four food groups. It is better to work with preferred food choices than with selections that children rarely eat. Approaches to food preparation that can increase the child's interest in eating are presented in the Guidelines box.

An understanding of children's feeding habits can also increase food consumption. For example, if children are given all their food at one time, they will generally eat the dessert first. Likewise, if they are presented with large portions, they often push the food away because the amount overwhelms them. If young children are not supervised during mealtime, they tend to play with the food rather than eat it. Therefore nurses should present food in the usual order, such as soup first, followed by small portions of meat, potatoes, and vegetables, and ending with dessert. The principles of conservation (see Cognitive Development, Chapter 15) can also be used to increase food consumption.

Once the child is feeling better, appetite usually begins to improve. It is also best to take advantage of any hungry period by serving high-quality foods and snacks. If the child still refuses to eat, nutritious fluids, such as prepared breakfast drinks, should be encouraged. Parents can be very helpful by bringing in these food items from home. This is especially important if the family's cultural eating habits differ from the hospital's food services.

When children are placed on special diets, such as clear liquids after surgery or during episodes of diarrhea, assessment of their intake and readiness to advance to more complex foods is essential.

NURSING ALERT Evidence of lack of readiness to advance the diet:
- Vomiting or diarrhea
- Decrease in appetite
- Abdominal cramping or distention
- Absence of bowel sounds
- Dehydration or weight loss

Regardless of the type of diet, charting the amount consumed is an important nursing responsibility. Descriptions need to be detailed and accurate, such as "4 ounces of orange juice, one pancake, no bacon, and 8 ounces of milk."

Comments such as "ate well" or "ate poorly" are inadequate. Charting the percentage of the meal eaten is also inadequate unless food is measured before serving.

NURSING ALERT Ask the parent if the child ate all of the food from the tray. Occasionally, a parent may eat something from the tray because the child did not eat or want it. The fact that a family member has eaten some of the food makes a marked difference in the report of how much the child ate.

If parents are involved in the child's care, they are encouraged to keep a list of everything eaten. Using a premeasured cup for fluids ensures a more accurate estimate of intake. A comparison of the intake at each meal can isolate food deficiencies, such as insufficient intake of meat or vegetables. Behaviors associated with mealtime also identify possible factors influencing appetite. For example, the observation, "Child eats well when with other children but plays with food if left alone in room," helps the nurse plan mealtime activities that stimulate the appetite.

CONTROLLING ELEVATED TEMPERATURES

An elevated temperature, most frequently from fever but occasionally caused by hyperthermia, is one of the most common symptoms of illness in children. This manifestation is frequently misunderstood and of great, but often unnecessary, concern to parents. To facilitate an understanding of fever, the following terms are defined:

Set point—The temperature around which body temperature is regulated by a thermostat-like mechanism in the hypothalamus

Fever (hyperpyrexis)—An elevation in set point such that body temperature is regulated at a higher level; may be arbitrarily defined as temperature above 38° C (100° F)

Hyperthermia—A situation in which body temperature exceeds the set point, which usually results from the body or external conditions creating more heat than the body can eliminate, such as in heat stroke, aspirin toxicity, or hyperthyroidism

Body temperature is regulated by a thermostat-like mechanism in the hypothalamus. This mechanism receives input from centrally and peripherally located receptors. When temperature changes occur, these receptors relay the information to the thermostat, which either increases or decreases heat production to maintain a constant set point temperature. However, during an infection, pyrogenic substances cause an increase in the body's normal set point, a process that is mediated by prostaglandins. Consequently the hypothalamus increases heat production until the core temperature reaches the new set point.

During the fever (febrile) state, shivering and vasoconstriction generate and conserve heat during the ***chill phase*** of fever, raising central temperatures to the level of the new set point. The temperature reaches a ***plateau*** when it stabilizes in the higher range. When the temperature is greater than the set point or when the pyrogen is no longer present, a crisis, or ***defervescence,*** of the temperature occurs (Holtzclaw, 1993).

Most fevers in children are of viral origin, are of relatively brief duration, and have limited consequences. In addition, fever probably plays a role in enhancing the developing of both specific and nonspecific immunity and aiding recovery and survival from infection (Reeves-Swift, 1990). Contrary to popular belief, neither the rise in temperature nor its response to antipyretics indicates the severity or etiology of infection, which casts doubt on the value of using fever as a diagnostic or prognostic indicator (Baker, Fosarelli, and Carpenter, 1987).

Therapeutic Management

Treatment of elevated temperature depends on whether it is due to a fever or hyperthermia. Because the set point is normal in hyperthermia, but increased in fever, different approaches must be used to lower body temperature successfully. An unusual presentation of elevated temperature is malignant hyperthermia; management of this emergency condition differs from the usual measures for fever or hyperthermia (see p. 1149).

Fever. The principal reason for treating fever is the relief of discomfort; no specific degree of fever requires treatment. Relief measures include pharmacologic and/or environmental intervention. The most effective intervention is the use of antipyretics to lower the set point.

Antipyretic drugs include acetaminophen, aspirin, and nonsteroidal antiinflammatory drugs (NSAIDs). Acetaminophen is the preferred drug; aspirin should not be given to children because of the possible association between aspirin use in children with influenza virus or chickenpox and Reye syndrome. A prescription NSAID, ibuprofen, is approved for fever reduction in children as young as 6 months of age (see Table 26-3). Dosage is based on the initial temperature level: 5 mg/kg of body weight for temperatures less than 39.1° C (102.5° F) or 10 mg/kg for temperatures greater than 39.1° C (102.5° F). The duration of fever reduction is generally 6 to 8 hours and is no longer with the higher dose (Watson and others, 1989). Nonprescription ibuprofen (Advil, Nuprin, Motrin IB, Medipren) is not approved for use in children under 12 years of age.

The recommended dosages of acetaminophen are listed in Table 27-3. It should be given every 4 hours, but no more than five times in 24 hours. Since body temperature normally decreases at night, three to four doses in 24 hours usually control most fevers. The temperature is usually retaken 30 minutes after the antipyretic is given to assess its effect but should not be repeatedly measured. The child's level of discomfort is the best indication for continued treatment.

Environmental measures to reduce fever may be used if tolerated by the child and if they do not induce shivering. Shivering is the body's way of maintaining the elevated set point by producing heat. Compensatory shivering greatly increases metabolic requirements above those already caused by the fever.

NURSING ALERT Treatment of shivering is directed at modifying or interfering with the rate of heat loss by warming the body with increased clothing (especially on the extremities), higher environmental temperature, and warm baths (Holtzclaw, 1990).

TABLE 27-3 Dosage Recommendations for Acetaminophen (Tylenol)*

AGE	WEIGHT (POUNDS)	DOSE (mg)	FORM†
Under 3 months	6-11	40	½ dropper
4-11 months	12-17	80	1 dropper or ½ tsp elixir
12-23 months	18-23	120	1½ droppers or ¾ tsp elixir or 1½ chewable tablets (80 mg)
2-3 years	24-35	160	2 droppers or 1 tsp elixir or 2 chewable tablets (80 mg)
4-5 years	36-47	240	1½ tsp elixir or 3 chewable tablets (80 mg)
6-8 years	48-59	320	2 tsp elixir or 4 chewable tablets (80 mg) or 2 swallowable tablets
9-10 years	60-71	400	2½ tsp elixir or 5 chewable tablets (80 mg) or 2½ swallowable tablets
11 years	72-95	480	3 tsp elixir or 6 chewable tablets (80 mg) or 3 swallowable tablets
12-14 years	96+	640	4 swallowable tablets

*Doses should be administered four or five times daily, but not to exceed five doses in 24 hours.
†1 dropper = 80 mg/0.8 ml; elixir = 160 mg/5 ml; chewable tablet = 80 mg each; junior-strength chewable tablets = 160 mg each; junior-strength swallowable tablets = 160 mg each.

Traditional cooling measures, such as minimum clothing, exposing the skin to the air, reducing room temperature, increasing air circulation, and cool moist compresses to the skin (e.g., the forehead), are effective if employed approximately 1 hour *after* antipyretic is given so that the set point is lowered. Cooling procedures such as sponging or tepid baths are ineffective in treating *febrile* children (these measures are used for hyperthermia) either when used alone or in combination with antipyretics, and they cause considerable discomfort (Newman, 1985).

Seizures associated with a fever occur in 3% to 4% of all children, usually in those between 3 months and 5 years of age. Although most children never have febrile seizures after the first occurrence, a younger age at onset and a family history of febrile seizures are associated with recurring episodes (Berg and others, 1990). For children who have febrile seizures, administration of antipyretics does not prevent recurrences (see Febrile Seizures, Chapter 37).

Hyperthermia. Unlike in fever, antipyretics are of no value in hyperthermia, because the set point is already normal. Consequently, cooling measures are used. Cool applications to the skin help to reduce the core temperature. Cooled blood from the skin surface is conducted to inner organs and tissues, and warm blood is circulated to the surface, where it is cooled and recirculated. The surface blood vessels dilate as the body attempts to dissipate heat to the environment and facilitate this cooling process.

Commercial cooling devices, such as cooling blankets or mattresses, are available to reduce body temperature. They are placed on the bed and covered with a sheet or lightweight blanket. Frequent temperature monitoring is essential to prevent excessive cooling of the body.

Traditionally, cool compresses have been used to decrease high temperature. However, no particular temperature of water is agreed on as optimum. For tepid tub baths, it is usually best to start with warm water and gradually add cool water until the desired water temperature of 37° C (98.6° F) is reached to accustom the child to the lower water temperature. Generally, the temperature of the water only has to be 1° to 2° (usually a warm temperature) less than the child's temperature to be effective (Kinmonth, Fulton, and Campbell, 1992). The child is placed directly in the tub of tepid water for 20 to 30 minutes while water is gently squeezed from a washcloth over the back and chest or gently sprayed over the body from a sprayer. In the bed or crib, cool washcloths or towels are used, exposing only one area of the body at a time. The sponging is continued for approximately 30 minutes.

NURSING ALERT Isopropyl alcohol should never be used for sponging; neurotoxic effects such as stupor, coma, and even death have been reported (Arditi and Killner, 1987).

After the tub or sponge bath, the child is dried and dressed in lightweight pajamas, nightgown, or diaper and placed in a dry bed. The temperature is retaken 30 minutes after the tub or sponge bath. The child is dried by gently rubbing the skin surface with a towel to stimulate circulation. The tub or sponge bath should not be continued or restarted until the skin surface is warm or if the child feels chilled. Chilling causes vasoconstriction, which defeats the purpose of the cool applications. In this condition little blood is carried to the skin surface; the blood remains primarily in the viscera to become heated.

Whether a temperature elevation in the critically ill child is caused by fever or hyperthermia, it should be treated more aggressively. The metabolic rate increases 10% for every 1° C increase in temperature and three to five times during shivering, increasing oxygen, fluid, and caloric requirements. If the child's cardiovascular or neurologic system is already compromised, these increased needs are especially hazardous (Bruce and Grove, 1992). In all children with elevated temperature, attention to adequate hydration is essential. Most children's needs can be met through additional oral fluids.

FAMILY TEACHING AND HOME CARE

Nurses have a unique opportunity for teaching the family about health care practices while the child is hospitalized. Although most children have learned self-care and hygiene in the home or at school, many have not. For some young children, this is their first introduction to the use of a toothbrush. Much health teaching can be accomplished even when the child is hospitalized for only a short time. The daily bath, handwashing before meals and after bowel and bladder evacuation, and conscientious dental hygiene are taught by example during routine care. Clean hair, nails, and clothing, as well as good grooming, are emphasized as essential to a pleasing appearance. Positive reinforcement of good hygiene practices helps to create a positive body image, promote the development of self-esteem, and prevent health problems (e.g., teaching girls to wipe the genital area from the front to back after toileting).

While sick children's appetites may be poor and not characteristic of their home eating habits, the hospital stay provides numerous opportunities for nurses to assess the family's knowledge of good nutrition and to implement teaching as needed to improve nutritional intake. Creative games can be employed that not only teach but provide diversion as well (Mandelbaum, 1983).

Parental education about elevated temperatures is essential, since many parents are unaware of what constitutes a fever, have unrealistic fears about the dangers of fever, and are apt to over- or undermedicate the febrile child (Gribetz and Cronley, 1987; Kilman, 1987). Parents also need to know that sponging is indicated for elevated temperatures from hyperthermia rather than fever and that ice water and alcohol are inappropriate, potentially dangerous, solutions. Parents should know how to take the child's temperature,* read the thermometer accurately, and have guidelines for seeking professional care (see Family Home Care box). Some of the newer temperature-measuring devices, such as plastic strip or digital thermometers, may be better suited for home use (see Temperature, Chapter 7). Many parents are unable to read a mercury thermometer or calculate the correct decimal point (Banco and Jayashekaramurthy, 1990). If the use of acetaminophen is indicated, the parents need instruction in administering the drug.* It is important to emphasize accuracy in both the amount of drug given and the time intervals at which the drug is administered.

Since many forms of acetaminophen are available, the nurse must be certain of the type being used in the home when discussing dosage. For example, the chewable tablets come in *two* strengths (80 mg and 160 mg), and the specially coated swallowable tablets for older children are 160 mg. Alert the parents to this because the tablets for older children may contain *twice* the amount of drug as the lower-dose chewable ones. If parents switch from the infant drops to the elixir, they are cautioned against using the dropper to measure the elixir, which is much less concentrated than the drops. Also, as children grow, the dosage needs to be recalculated. To ensure the correct dose, it is recommended that a dose for a small child be calculated on the basis of 15 mg/kg dose rather than 10 mg/kg/dose (Gribetz and Cronley, 1987).

*Home care instructions for measuring temperature and giving medications are available in *Wong and Whaley's Clinical Manual of Pediatric Nursing* (Mosby).

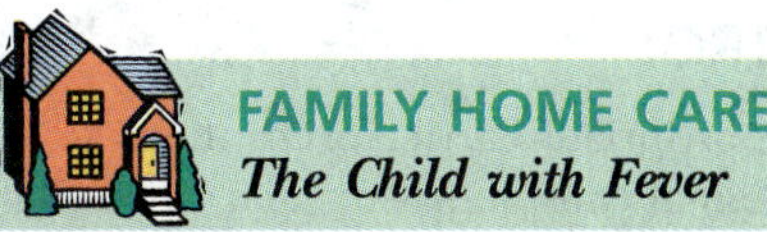

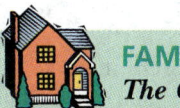

FAMILY HOME CARE
The Child with Fever

Call immediately if:
- Child is <2 months of age.
- Fever is >40.5° C (105° F).
- Child is crying inconsolably.
- Child is difficult to awaken.
- Child is confused or delirious.
- Child has had a seizure.
- Child has a stiff neck.
- Child has purple spots on the skin.
- Breathing is difficult, and child does not feel better after nose is cleared.
- Child is acting very sick.
- Child has an underlying risk factor for serious infection (e.g., sickle cell disease).

Call during office hours if:
- Child is 2 to 4 months old (unless fever is due to a diphtheria-pertussis-tetanus [DPT] vaccination).
- Fever is 40° to 40.5° C (104° to 105° F), especially if child is <2 years old.
- Burning or pain occurs with urination.
- Fever has been present for >72 hours.
- Fever has been present for >24 hours without an obvious cause or location of infection.
- Fever disappeared for >24 hours and then returned.
- Child has a history of febrile seizures.
- Parents have other questions.

Modified from Schmitt BD: Fever in childhood, *Pediatrics* 74(5, suppl):934, 1984.

SAFETY

Safety is an essential component of any patient's care, but children have special characteristics that require an even greater concern for safety. Since small children are separated from their usual environment and do not possess the capacity for abstract thinking and reasoning, it is the responsibility of everyone who comes in contact with them to maintain protective measures throughout their hospital stay. Nurses need a good understanding of the age level at which each child is operating and should plan for safety accordingly.

Name bands, a part of hospital safety practices, are particularly important for children in the pediatric age-group. Infants and unconscious patients are unable to tell or respond to their names. Toddlers may answer to any name or to a nickname only. Older children may exchange places, give an erroneous name, or choose not to respond to their own names as a form of joke, unaware of the hazards of such practices.

INFECTION CONTROL

Medical asepsis and appropriate barrier precautions to reduce the risk of nosocomial (hospital-associated) infections are essential in caring for children. Children are frequently infected with organisms, such as varicella (chickenpox), that are transmissible and may be dangerous to others, especially immunocompromised patients. In addition, children may not have developed good hygiene habits, such as handwashing after toileting. Young children are especially at risk for infection because of their high oral activity. Children in diapers present infection risks if caregivers do not practice meticulous cleaning techniques. Because of the importance of reducing the risk of nosocomial infection in children, a brief overview of the traditional and current trends in isolation practices is presented.

Although institutions can design their own system, most hospitals have adopted one of the following two basic systems for isolation precautions recommended by the Centers for Disease Control and Prevention (CDC) (1983)*:

Category-specific isolation precautions—Isolation categories group diseases for which similar isolation precautions are indicated. Instructions for each category include taking all the precautions necessary to prevent transmission of the most infectious disease in each category. Seven categories are used: strict isolation, contact isolation, respiratory isolation, tuberculosis isolation, enteric precautions, drainage/secretion precautions, and blood/body fluid precautions (replaced in 1987/1988 by Universal Blood and Body Fluid Precautions ["Universal Precautions"]).

Disease-specific isolation precautions—Each disease is listed with only the precautions needed to prevent transmission of that disease. Consequently, more variability exists in instructions with this system.

Both these systems are ***diagnosis driven;*** that is, the patient's diagnosis determines the type of precautions needed to interrupt the transmission of the infectious agent. However, these systems are not designed to provide protection when the infected person is undiagnosed. A problem with any diagnosis-driven approach to isolation precautions is that most communicable diseases are infectious before the diagnosis is made (Lynch and others, 1987).

Concern for possible transmission of infection such as hepatitis B and human immunodeficiency virus (HIV) from undiagnosed patients to other patients and health care workers prompted the CDC (1988) to issue guidelines for treating all patients as potentially infectious. This system developed by the CDC is known as ***universal precautions (UP).*** One type of UP is the ***body substance isolation (BSI)*** system. Important differences exist between these two systems (Table 27-4).

In 1991 the Occupational Safety and Health Administration (OSHA) changed federal legislation to reduce risks to health care workers from blood-borne pathogen exposures. The OSHA Bloodborne Pathogens Standard has now been implemented in all health care facilities in the United States. This standard requires facilities to use UP (U.S. Department of Labor, 1991).

NURSING ALERT Regardless of the system used, handwashing is the most critical infection control practice.

Nurses caring for young children are frequently in contact with body substances, especially urine, feces, and vomitus. In using BSI, nurses need to exercise judgment for those situations when gloves, gowns, or masks are necessary. For example, during feedings, gowns should be worn if the child is likely to vomit or spit up, which often occurs during burping. If aprons with minimum shoulder protection are worn, the child should be sitting on the nurse's lap, not upright against the shoulder, when the child is bubbled. The type of diaper may be an important aspect of infection control. Superabsorbent disposable diapers with elastic legs contain urine and feces better than cloth diapering systems, and their use can reduce fecal contamination in the environment (Van and others, 1991). Even when gloves are worn, the hands are washed thoroughly after removing the gloves, since studies have found both latex and vinyl gloves fail to provide consistent protection (Korniewicz, Laughton, and Butz, 1989; Larson, 1989) (see Thinking Critically About . . . box, p. 1167). An additional consideration regarding gloves is that some people are allergic to latex (see Spina Bifida/Myelodysplasia, Chapter 11).

Another essential practice of UP and BSI is that all needles (uncapped and unbroken) should be disposed of in a rigid, puncture-resistant container located near the site of use. Consequently, these containers are installed in patients' rooms. Since children are naturally curious, extra attention is needed in selecting a suitable container and a location that discourage access to the disposed needles. Needleless systems have been developed that allow secure syringe or intravenous tubing attachment to vascular access devices without the risk of needle stick injury to the child or nurse. These devices also help maintain intravenous line integrity. To encourage staff to practice BSI, reminders can be placed in strategic areas (Fig. 27-5).

ENVIRONMENTAL FACTORS

All the environmental safety measures for the protection of adults apply to children as well, such as good illumination, floors clear of fluid or other objects that might contribute to falls, and nonskid surfaces in showers and tubs. Electrical equipment is maintained in good working order, is used only by personnel familiar with its use, and is not in contact with moisture or near tubs, where it could prove to be a shock hazard. Beds of ambulatory patients are locked in place and at a height that allows easy access to the floor. Staff members practice proper care and disposal of small breakable items, such as thermometers and bottles, and know a well-organized fire plan. A special hazard for children is the danger of entrapment under an electronically controlled bed when it is activated to descend.

All windows should be securely screened and elevators and stairways made safe. Ideally, electrical outlets should be

*The CDC infection control guidelines are scheduled to be revised in late 1994 or in 1995.

TABLE 27-4 Comparison of Body Substance Isolation and Universal Precautions

BODY SUBSTANCE ISOLATION (BSI)*	CENTERS FOR DISEASE CONTROL AND PREVENTION (CDC) UNIVERSAL PRECAUTIONS (UP)†	COMMENTS
PURPOSE		
Reduces risk of cross-transmission of organisms, including human immunodeficiency virus (HIV), between patients and from patients to personnel Depends on the interaction between the caregiver and patient, regardless of diagnosis	Minimizes risk of blood-borne infection (HIV, hepatitis B virus [HBV]) Must also use category- or disease-specific isolation precautions for diagnosed infections Depends on type of patient contact and diagnosis	Major difference between BSI and UP: BSI system considers all patients potentially infectious for all pathogens (interaction driven); UP system considers all patients potentially infectious only for blood-borne infections and requires additional protections once diagnosis is made (diagnosis driven)
BODY SUBSTANCES CONSIDERED POTENTIALLY INFECTIOUS		
All, including: Blood Feces Urine Vomitus Wound and other drainage Oral secretions	Blood Semen Vaginal secretions Cerebrospinal fluid Synovial fluid Pleural fluid Peritoneal fluid Pericardial fluid Amniotic fluid Fluids *not* included unless they contain visible blood: Feces Nasal secretions Sputum Sweat Tears Urine and vomitus	UP do not apply to human breast milk or saliva except in special situations: Frequent exposure to breast milk (i.e., in breast milk banking) During dental procedures where saliva may be contaminated with blood
HANDWASHING		
Performed for 10 seconds with soap, running water, and friction any time the hands are visibly soiled and between most patient contacts even if gloves are worn Not necessary between sequential low-risk patient contacts involving intact skin, such as taking vital signs or administering medications	Immediately and thoroughly wash hands and other skin surfaces that are contaminated with body fluids to which UP apply	Handwashing is the single most important strategy for preventing infection transmission
GLOVES		
Must be used when contact with mucous membranes, nonintact skin, or moist body substances is likely to occur; changed between patient contacts	Must be worn when touching fluids to which UP apply The U.S. Occupational Safety and Health Administration (OSHA) Bloodborne Pathogen Standard requires gloves for all vascular access procedures‡	Washing or disinfecting gloves for reuse is not recommended Washing with surfactants may cause "wicking" (i.e., the enhanced penetration of liquids through undetected holes in the glove) Disinfecting agents can deteriorate the glove General CDC control practices for saliva include use of gloves for digital examination of mucous membranes and endotracheal suctioning
GOWNS OR PLASTIC APRONS		
Worn when it is likely that body substances will soil the clothing; changed between patient contacts	Same as BSI	With young children, use of a gown or plastic apron with adequate shoulder and chest protection may be needed during feeding and bubbling

*Data from Lynch P and others: Rethinking the role of isolation practices in the prevention of nosocomial infections, *Ann Intern Med* 107:243-246, 1987.
†Data from Centers for Disease Control: Update: Universal precautions for prevention of transmission of human immunodeficiency virus, hepatitis B virus, and other bloodborne pathogens in healthcare settings, *MMWR* 37(24):377-387, 1988.
‡Data from *Fed Register* 56(235):64175-64182, 1991.
NOTE: The American Academy of Pediatrics has published guidelines on infection control, but because they are limited only to HIV infection and depend on the prevalence of HIV infection in an area, which is rarely known, they are not included (Task Force on Pediatric AIDS, 1988).

Continued.

TABLE 27-4 Comparison of Body Substance Isolation and Universal Precautions—cont'd

BODY SUBSTANCE ISOLATION (BSI)*	CENTERS FOR DISEASE CONTROL AND PREVENTION (CDC) UNIVERSAL PRECAUTIONS (UP)†	COMMENTS
MASKS AND/OR EYE PROTECTION		
Worn when likely that the eyes and/or nose and mouth will be splashed with body substances or when personnel are working directly over large, open skin lesions	Same as BSI except only for substances considered infectious and as recommended by CDC guidelines (1983)	Benefit of masks in preventing transmission of airborne infection is questionable CDC guidelines (1983) recommend masks for protection from airborne infection UP system does not address masks except for protection from splashes, since HIV and HBV are not airborne. Eyeglasses generally adequate to provide eye protection, but need side shields. If splashing is likely, eye protection and masks or single-unit face shield should be used
NEEDLE/SYRINGE UNITS AND OTHER SHARP INSTRUMENTS		
Used needles not generally removed from disposable syringes, recapped or broken; all sharp instruments are disposed of in a rigid, puncture-resistant container located preferably near the site of use (e.g., patient's room, treatment rooms)	Same as BSI	Needle punctures are a leading cause of nosocomial (hospital-associated) transmission of blood-borne pathogens Gloves cannot prevent penetrating injuries caused by needles or other sharp instruments Adherence to proper handling of sharp instruments is essential If recapping is necessary, a one-handed scoop technique should be used
TRASH AND LINEN		
Bagged securely in leakproof containers and disposed of or cleaned according to institutional policy	Same as BSI	CDC recommendations include extensive discussions of environmental considerations for HIV transmission, although there is no evidence of casual or environmental transmission of HIV
PRIVATE ROOMS		
Desirable for children who soil the environment with body substances; required for children with airborne, communicable diseases unless they can share a room with roommate(s) known to be immune to the disease	Not addressed other than to use disease- or category-specific isolation precautions	According to CDC, diseases affecting children that require use of a private room for strict or respiratory isolation precautions are varicella (chickenpox), diphtheria, mumps, pertussis, measles, erythema infectiosum, epiglottitis, meningitis (*Haemophilus influenzae*, meningococcal), pneumonia (*H. influenzae*, meningococcal), and meningococcemia

provided with covers to prevent burns in small children, whose exploratory activities may extend to inserting objects into the small openings. Bath water is carefully checked before placing the child in it, and children must never be left alone in a bathtub. Infants are helpless in water, and small children (and some older ones) may turn on the hot water faucet and be severely burned.

Furniture is safest when it is scaled to the child's proportions, is sturdy, and is well balanced to prevent its being easily tipped over. Infants and small children must be securely strapped into infant seats, feeding chairs, and strollers. Baby walkers should be discouraged because they provide access to hazards, resulting in burns, falls, and poisonings. Infants, young children, and those who are weak, paralyzed, agitated, confused, sedated, or cognitively impaired are never left unattended on treatment tables, on scales, or in treatment areas. Even premature infants are capable of surprising mobility; therefore, portable incubators must be securely fastened when not in use. Beds of ambulatory patients should remain locked and at a height that allows easy access to the floor.

Crib sides are kept up and fastened securely unless an adult is at the bedside. It is safer to leave crib sides up, regardless of the child's ability to get out, even when the crib

THINKING CRITICALLY ABOUT . . .

The Effects of Fingernail Polish and Gloves on Hand Contamination

Clean hands, with a minimum presence of microorganisms, has always been the most important measure for controlling infection. Two recent studies looked at two different issues of concern: the use of fingernail polish and the use of gloves.

One controversy has been whether to allow surgical staff members to wear nail polish. The primary question has been that of the possibility of increased risk of surgical wound infections from the staff's hands. The argument against polish has been that microorganisms could be harbored in nail polish once it cracks, chips, or peels. As a result, in 1981 the Association of Operating Room Nurses (AORN), as well as a variety of nursing textbooks, recommended that nail polish should not be worn in the surgical environment. No studies have refuted or substantiated these recommendations.

However, a recent study compared microorganism counts on personnel's hands with and without nail polish. Twenty-six healthy volunteer subjects were compared over a period of time in groups randomly assigned to have polished or unpolished nails. Their results indicated that "nail polish did not pose a microbial risk under . . . test conditions . . . . In fact, the data are consistent with the hypothesis that polish, because of the hard, smooth surface, may actually seal crevices in which microorganisms could be harbored" (Baumgardner and others, 1993).

The study did raise two concerns about the use of polish: (1) the possibility that more seriously damaged nails could be adversely affected by nail polish and (2) the possibility that the presence of polish might have an effect on behavior in the surgical scrub; that is, the individual might be protective of the manicure and be "less inclined to perform a vigorous surgical scrub to protect the nails." Either of these cases, researchers asserted, could prove detrimental by fostering bacterial growth on the hands, although neither would reflect the direct effects of the polish itself. In conclusion, keeping nails short, clean, and healthy is probably more important than the effects of wearing nail polish.

In another study, researchers examined the efficacy of gloves as barriers to hand contamination during endotracheal tube care, digital rectal stimulation, and dental examination. Of the 135 gloves that were cultured, 86 were contaminated with gram-negative rods or enterococci on the outside of the gloves. In 11 of the 86 events, the health care worker's hands were contaminated, an event that occurred more frequently with vinyl (10 of 42) than with latex (1 of 44) gloves. Likewise, glove leaks occurred more frequently with vinyl (26 of 61) than with latex (6 of 70) gloves. However, there was not a strong correlation between glove leaks and contaminated hands; leaky gloves kept hands clean 77% of the time. Interestingly, health care workers were aware of the leaks in only 7 of the 32 instances. These results indicate that the absence of visible leaks cannot be used by personnel to assume that gloves are intact.

This study supported conclusions similar to those of the nail polish study. Although gloves provide "substantial protection," their use does not decrease the importance of routine handwashing after each patient contact (Olsen and others, 1993).

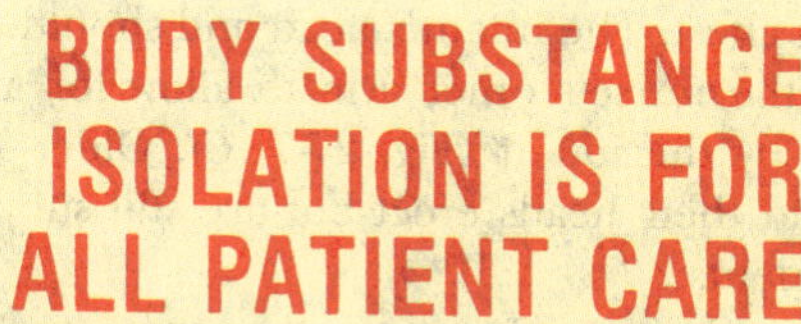

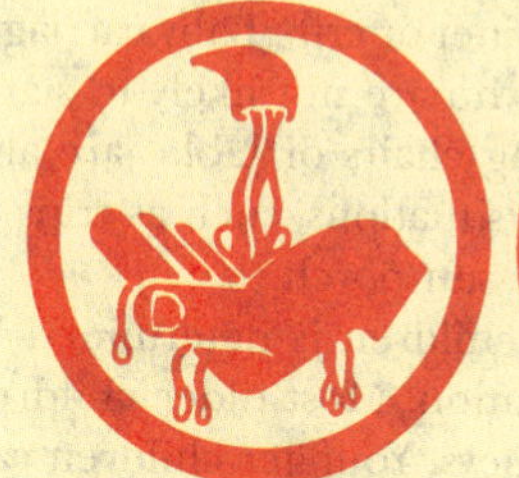
Wash hands.

Wear gloves when likely to touch body substances, mucous membranes or nonintact skin.

Wear plastic apron when clothing is likely to be soiled.

Wear mask/eye protection when likely to be splashed.

DO NOT RECAP.
Place intact needle/syringe units and sharps in designated disposal container. Do not break or bend needles.

FIG. 27-5 A decal can be displayed in a prominent location, such as on a towel dispenser, to remind personnel to use precautions with all body substances.

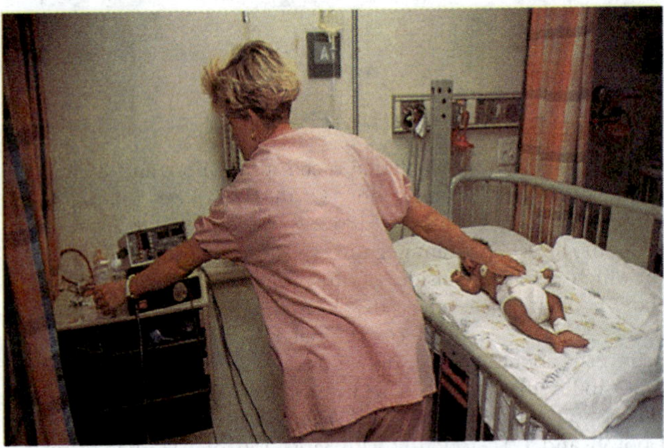

FIG. 27-6 Nurse maintains hand contact when back is turned.

is unoccupied, to remove the temptation to climb in. Anyone attending an infant or small child in a crib with the sides down should never turn away without maintaining hand contact with the child; that is, one hand is kept on the child's back or abdomen to prevent rolling, crawling, or jumping from the open crib (Fig. 27-6). Banco and Powers (1988) reported that falls from cribs by infants tended to occur when siderails had carelessly been left down. Children in beds, however, tended to fall despite raised siderails by climbing over them. A child who tends or seems inclined to climb over the sides of the crib is safest when placed in a specially constructed crib with a cover or a safety net over the top. If the net is used, it must be tied to the frame so that there is ready access to the child in case of emergency. Nets are never tied to the movable crib sides, and the knots are tied in a manner that permits quick release. (See also Injury Prevention, Chapter 12).

NURSING ALERT Do not place cribs within reach of heating units, appliances, dangling cords, outlets, or other objects that can be reached by curious hands.

Plants and flowers harbor gram-negative bacteria and molds that may be of risk to the immunocompromised child. These items may also pose the danger of poisoning to curious toddlers.

TOYS

Toys play a vital role in the everyday life of children, and they are no less important in the hospital setting. However, nurses are responsible for assessing the safety of toys brought to the hospital by well-meaning parents and friends. Toys should be appropriate to the child's age, condition, and treatment. For example, if the child is in an oxygen tent, electrical or friction toys or equipment cannot be placed in the tent, because sparks can cause oxygen to ignite. Toys are inspected to make certain that they are nonallergenic, washable, and unbreakable and that they have no small, removable parts that can be aspirated or swallowed or that can otherwise inflict injury on a child.

LIMIT-SETTING

Setting limits is essential to a child's safety. Children must understand where they are permitted to go and what they are permitted to do in the hospital. These limitations are made clear to them, consistently enforced, and repeated as frequently as necessary to make certain that they are understood. The nurse is responsible for where children are at all times. Children can easily wander off unnoticed, and their access to the tubs, laundry chutes, medication rooms/carts, and elevators must be prevented. Normally active older children often become restless when their activity is restricted and may resort to pillow fights, water fights, and other rough play that might endanger the safety of other children, staff, or visitors. Children in the hospital require surveillance, and appropriate tension-reducing activities can be planned and supervised by nurses and/or by the play therapist. A useful discipline technique is time-out (see Limit-Setting and Discipline, Chapter 3).

TRANSPORTING INFANTS AND CHILDREN

In the course of a hospital stay, infants and children usually need to be transported within the unit and to areas outside the pediatric unit. It is ordinarily safe to carry infants and small children for short distances within the unit, but for more extended trips the child should be securely transported in a suitable conveyance.

Small infants can be held or carried in the horizontal position with the back supported and the thigh grasped firmly by the carrying arm (Fig. 27-7, *A*). In the football hold the infant is carried on the nurse's arm with the head supported by the hand and the body held securely between the nurse's body and elbow (Fig. 27-7, *B*). Both these holds leave the nurse's other arm free for activity. The infant can be held in the upright position with the buttocks on the nurse's forearm and the front of the body resting against the nurse's chest. The infant's head and shoulders are supported by the nurse's other arm to allow for any sudden movement by the infant (Fig. 27-7, *C*). Older infants are able to hold their heads erect but are still subject to sudden movements.

Infants can be transported to other areas, such as the radiology department, in their bassinet or crib. Baby carriages are sometimes used for infants who are not likely to stand up. Strollers and wheeled feeding chairs or tables are also convenient transporters in some situations, such as trips to the playroom, nurse's station, or sun porch.

The method of transporting children is determined by their age, condition, and destination. Most older children are safe in wheelchairs or in gurneys. Younger children can be transported in their crib, on a gurney, in a wagon with raised sides, or in a wheelchair with a safety belt. Gurneys should be equipped with high sides and a safety belt, both of which are kept in place during transport.

RESTRAINTS

Some method of restraint frequently is needed to ensure a child's safety or comfort, to facilitate examination, or to

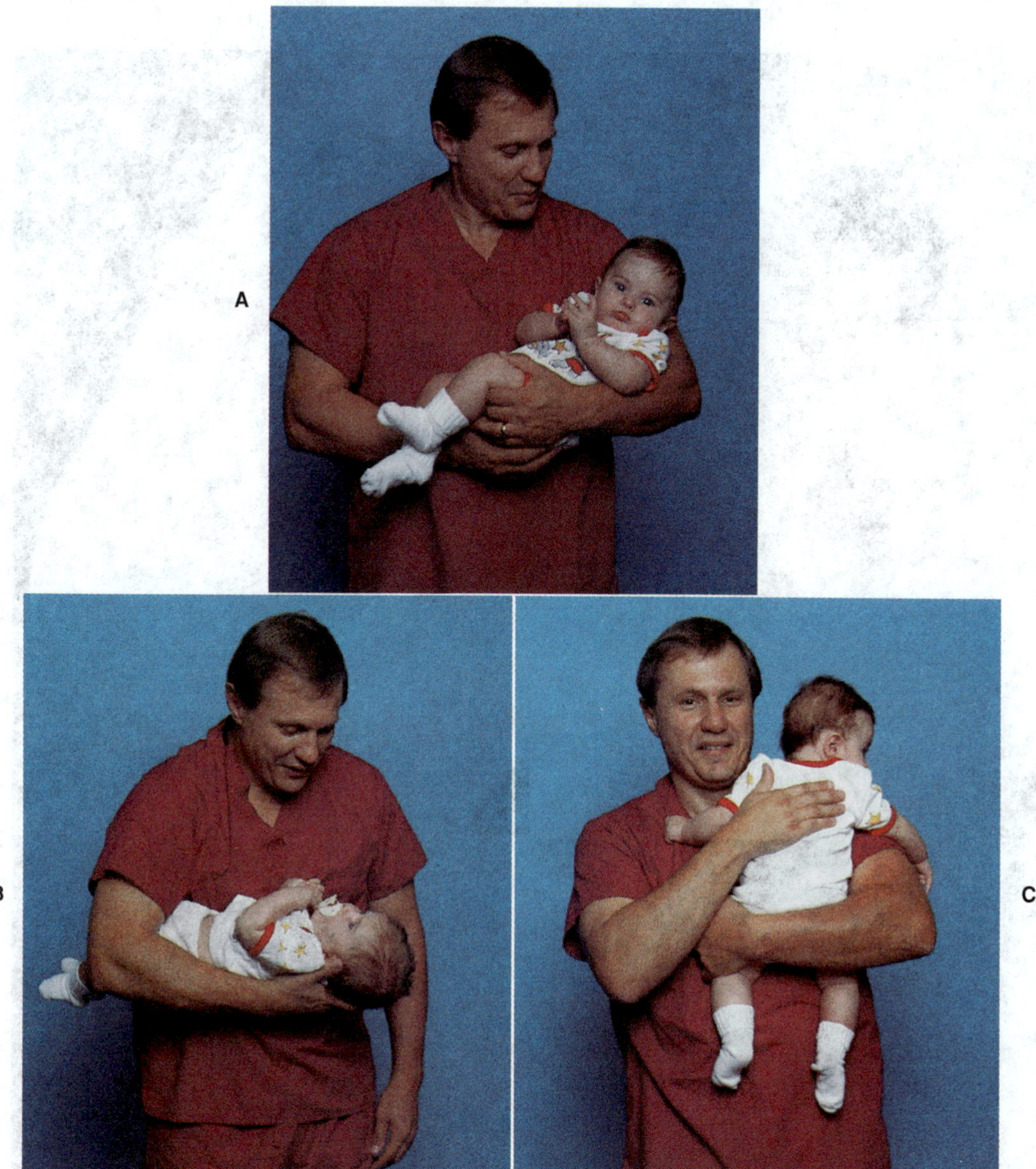

FIG. 27-7 Transporting infants. **A,** Infant's thigh firmly grasped in nurse's hand. **B,** Football hold. **C,** Back supported.

carry out procedures. Restraint can be accomplished with the hand or with physical devices. Restraining the child with the hand provides an element of human contact that is lacking in restraint by mechanical means. The use of physical devices may require a physician's order, although it is the nurse's responsibility to decide when mechanical restraints are needed. Restraints can often be avoided with adequate preparation of the child, parental or staff supervision of the child, and adequate protection of a vulnerable site, such as an infusion device.

Mechanical restraints are never used as a punishment or as a substitute for observation. When a child must be restrained, the child and parents need a simple explanation. If the restraint is applied for an extended time, the explanation must be repeated often to gain cooperation and to help the child understand that it is not a punishment. Restraining devices are not without risk and must be checked and documented every 1 to 2 hours. This ensures that restraints are accomplishing their purpose, that they are applied correctly, and that they do not impair circulation, sensation, or skin integrity.

Parents need to know the purpose of restraints, how to remove and reapply them, and the signs of complications from their use. Parents are sometimes upset when their child must be restrained and need to understand how they can help to ensure the maximum benefit and minimize the stress related to restraints. Children, too, should be prepared for the procedure or the circumstance for which the restraint is required.

Removing restraints whenever possible (at least every 2

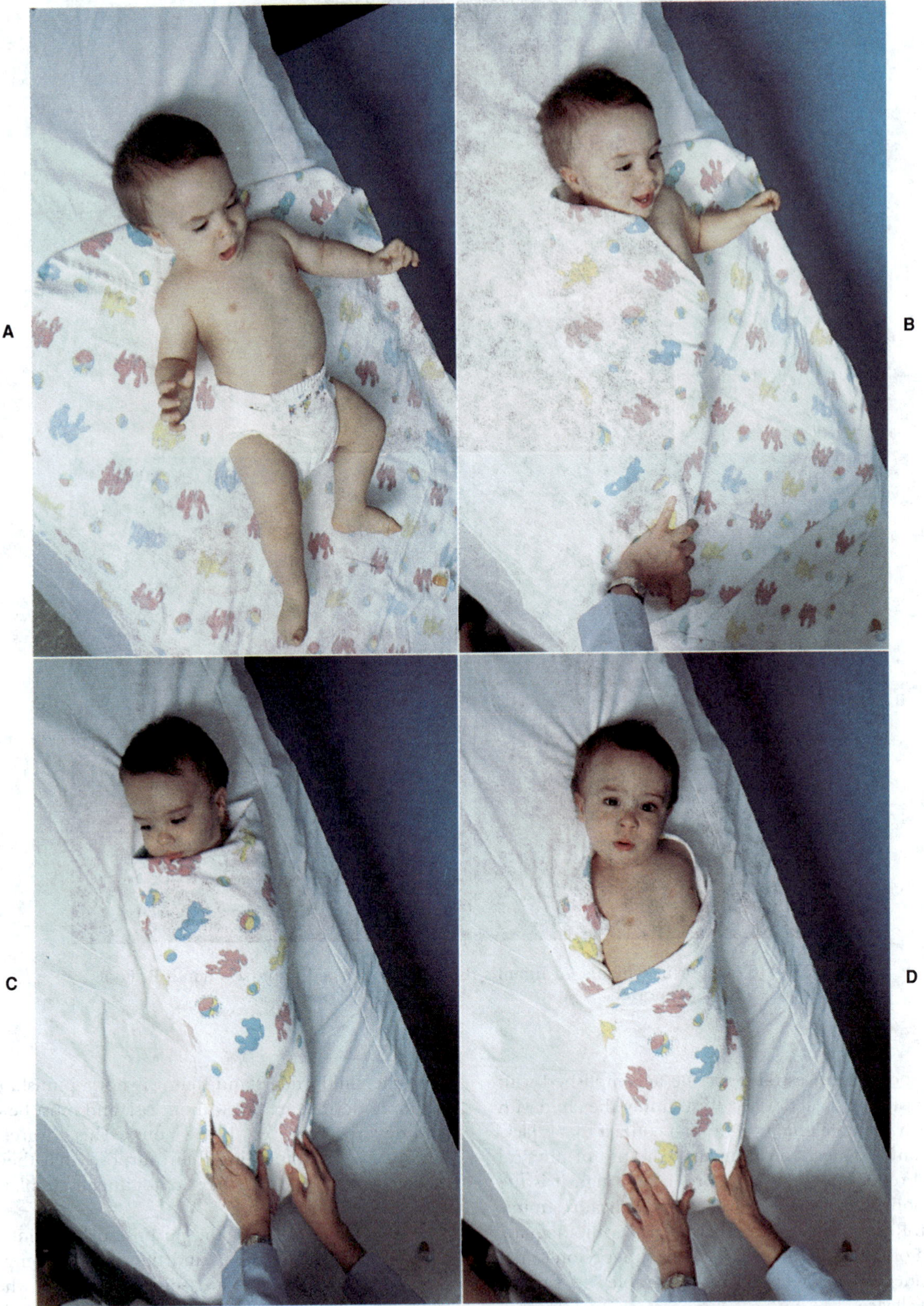

FIG. 27-8 Application of mummy restraint. **A,** Infant placed on folded corner of blanket. **B,** One corner of blanket brought across body and secured beneath the body. **C,** Second corner brought across body and secured, and lower corner folded and tucked or pinned in place. **D,** Modified mummy restraint with chest uncovered.

hours when children are awake) is an essential part of nursing care of children who are restrained for treatments or other purposes. Alternate methods may be devised to replace the need for passive restraints. Holding children for periods is a pleasant alternative, as is restraining them in a highchair, where they can observe nearby activities. If feasible, distraction techniques such as play and reading are employed to gain the child's cooperation without resorting to restraints. Parental participation is always encouraged.

A physician's order and parental consent are required for restraints used for reasons other than procedures. These requirements are controversial, and nurses should be aware of their agencies' policies. These requirements originated from some concerns in elderly persons.

Mummy Restraint

When an infant or small child requires short-term restraint for examination or treatment that involves the head and neck (e.g., venipuncture, throat examination, gavage feeding), the mummy device effectively controls the child's movements. A blanket or sheet is opened on the bed or crib with one corner folded to the center. The infant is placed on the blanket with shoulders at the fold and feet toward the opposite corner (Fig. 27-8, *A*). With the infant's right arm straight down against the body, the right side of the blanket is pulled firmly across the infant's right shoulder and chest and secured beneath the left side of the body (Fig. 27-8, *B*). The left arm is placed straight against the infant's side, and the left side of the blanket is brought across the shoulder and chest and locked beneath the infant's body on the right side (Fig. 27-8, *C*). The lower corner is folded and brought over the body and tucked or fastened securely with safety pins (Fig. 27-8, *D*). Safety pins can be used to fasten the blanket in place at any step in the process.

To modify the mummy restraint for chest examination, the folded edge of the blanket is brought over each arm and under the back, after which the loose edge is folded over and secured at a point below the chest to allow visualization and access to the chest.

Jacket Restraint

A jacket restraint is sometimes used as an alternative to the crib net to prevent the child from climbing out of the crib or to keep the child safe in various chairs. The jacket is put on the child with the ties in back so that the child is unable to manipulate them. The long tapes, secured to the understructure of the crib, keep the child inside the crib (Fig. 27-9). The jacket restraint is also useful as a means to maintain the child in a desired horizontal position. A Posey belt scaled to fit the child is an alternative device. The jacket-type restraint has been associated with accidental strangulation deaths in elderly persons (U.S. Department of Agriculture, 1992).

Arm and Leg Restraints

Occasionally, one or more extremities must be restrained or limited in motion. Several commercial restraining devices are available, including disposable wrist and ankle restraints, or a restraint can be fashioned from gauze tape, muslin strips, or a length of narrow stockinette. When this type of restraint is used, it must be appropriate to the child's size; it must be padded to prevent undue pressure, constriction, or tissue injury; and the extremity must be observed frequently for signs of irritation or impaired circulation. The ends of the restraints are never tied to the crib rails, since lowering of the rail will disturb the extremity, frequently with a jerk that may hurt or injure the child.

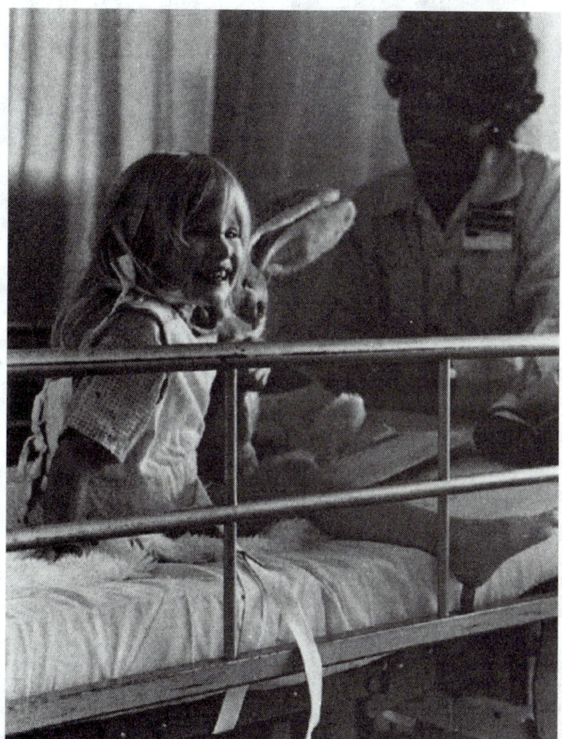

FIG. 27-9 Jacket restraint.

The ***clove hitch restraint*** is fashioned from a length of gauze or commercial ties. When properly applied, the restraint provides a snug fit with minimum danger of pulling too tightly. Fig. 27-10 illustrates the method of tying and applying a clove hitch restraint.

Elbow Restraint

Sometimes it is important to prevent the child from reaching the head or face, for example, after lip surgery, when a scalp vein infusion is in place, or to prevent scratching in skin disorders. For this purpose, elbow restraints fashioned from a variety of materials function very well. The most common form of elbow restraint consists of a piece of muslin long enough to reach comfortably from just below the axilla to the wrist, with a number of vertical pockets into which tongue depressors are inserted (Fig. 27-11). The restraint is wrapped around the arm and secured with tapes or pins. It may be necessary to pin the top of the restraint to the undershirt sleeve to prevent the restraint from slipping. Similar restraints can be made from readily available items.

➤ **NURSING TIP** Pad the ends of large-diameter towel rollers or appropriately sized plastic containers from which

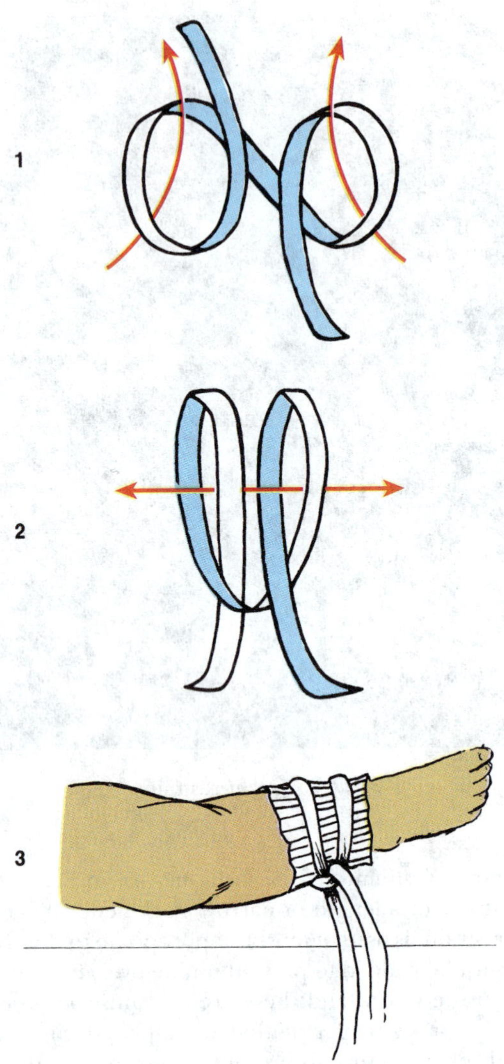

FIG. 27-10 Clove hitch restraint.

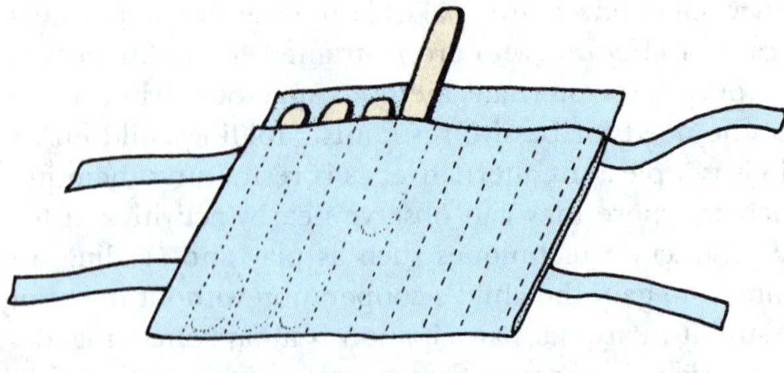

FIG. 27-11 Elbow restraint.

the tops and bottoms have been removed. Apply adhesive tabs to the top end, and pin the tabs to the child's sleeve to prevent the restraint from slipping from the extremity. Fashion adjustable restraints from tongue blades placed vertically against strips of adhesive and then covered with adhesive; secure with adhesive tabs as just described.

POSITIONING FOR PROCEDURES

Infants and small children are unable to cooperate for many procedures; therefore the nurse is responsible for minimizing their movement and discomfort with proper positioning. Older children usually need only minimum, if any, restraint. Careful explanation and preparation beforehand and support and simple guidance during the procedure are usually sufficient. For painful procedures the child should receive adequate analgesia and sedation to minimize pain and the need for excessive restraint. For local anesthesia use buffered lidocaine to reduce the stinging sensation or the topical anesthetic EMLA (see Pain Management, Chapter 26).

JUGULAR VENIPUNCTURE

The large, superficial external jugular vein is frequently used to obtain blood specimens from infants and young children. For easy access to the vein, the child is first placed in a mummy restraint in which the top edge of the restraint is low enough to permit access to the vein. The child is placed so that the head and shoulders extend over the edge of a table or a small pillow with the neck extended and the head turned sharply to the side (Fig. 27-12). One alternate method for restraining arms and legs is with the nurse holding the child's arms and legs at the same time that the child's head is restrained and positioned. It is important for the nurse holding the infant to maintain control of the infant's head without interfering with the operator's approach to the vein. The infant's crying during the procedure increases intravenous pressure, which facilitates visualization of the vein. Following venipuncture, digital pressure is applied to the site with a dry gauze square for 3 to 5 minutes or until bleeding stops. Care must be taken not to apply excessive pressure that might compromise circulation or breathing during or following the procedure.

FEMORAL VENIPUNCTURE

Other frequently used sites for venipuncture are the large femoral veins. The nurse restrains the infant by placing the child supine with the legs in a frog position to provide extensive exposure of the groin area. Both the arms and the legs of the infant can be effectively controlled by the nurse's forearms and hands (Fig. 27-13). Only the side used for the venipuncture is uncovered so that the operator is protected should the child urinate during the procedure. Pressure is applied to the site after the withdrawal of blood to prevent oozing from the site.

EXTREMITY VENIPUNCTURE

The most common sites of venipuncture are the veins of the extremities, especially the arm and hand. A convenient position for restraint is having one person on either side of the bed. The child's outstretched arm is partially stabilized by the technician drawing the blood. The other person

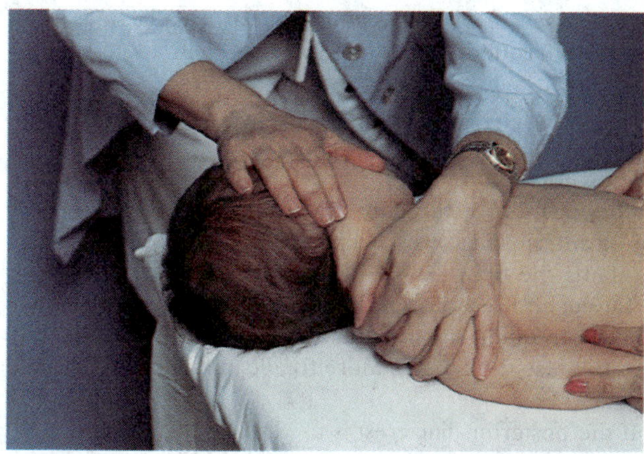

FIG. 27-12 Restraining child for jugular vein puncture.

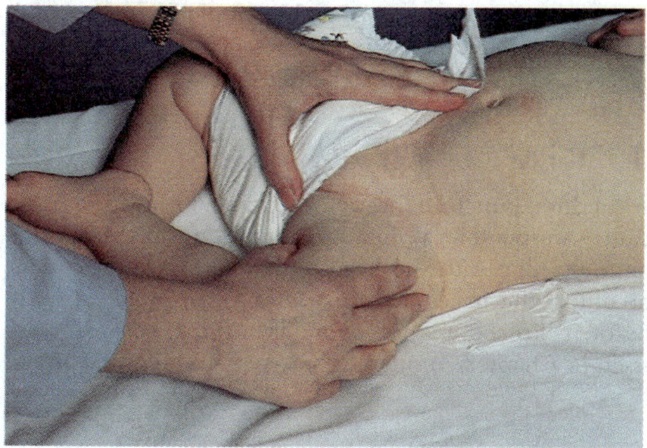

FIG. 27-13 Restraining infant for femoral vein puncture.

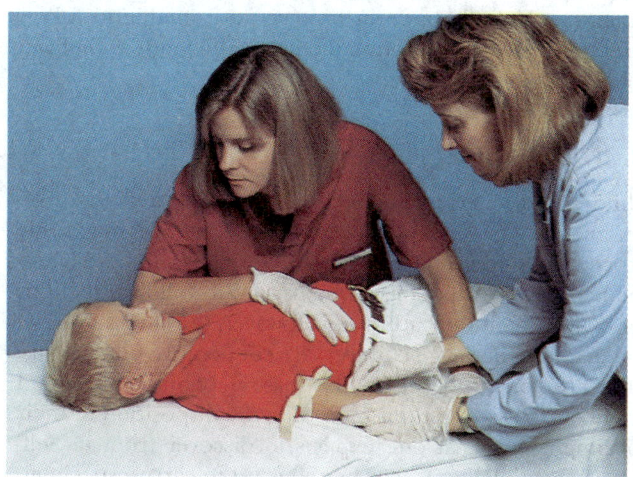

FIG. 27-14 Restraining child for extremity venipuncture. NOTE: Procedure is being performed in treatment room, not in child's hospital room.

leans across the child's upper body, preventing movement, and uses an arm to immobilize the venipuncture site. This type of restraint also comforts the child because of the close body contact and allows each person to maintain eye contact (Fig. 27-14).

LUMBAR PUNCTURE

The technique for lumbar puncture in infants and children is similar to that in the adult, although modifications are suggested in neonates, who have less distress in a side-lying position with modified neck extension than in flexion or a sitting position (Fig. 27-15, *A*). Neonates tend to have more cardiorespiratory changes during a lumbar puncture than do older infants regardless of positioning; therefore oximetry and heart rate monitoring are advisable (Lehmann and others, 1990). Pediatric lumbar puncture sets contain smaller spinal needles, but sometimes the practitioner will specify a particular size or type of needle that the nurse should make certain is placed on the tray.

Children are usually controlled best in the side-lying position, with the head flexed and the knees drawn up toward the chest. Even cooperative children need to be restrained to prevent possible trauma from unexpected, involuntary movement. They can be reassured that, although they are trusted, the restraint will serve as a reminder to maintain the desired position. It also provides a measure of support and reassurance to them.

The child is placed on the side with the back close to the edge of the examining table on the side from which the practitioner is working. The nurse maintains the child's spine in a flexed position by holding the child with one arm behind the neck and the other behind the thighs (Fig. 27-15, *B*). The flexed position enlarges the spaces between the lumbar vertebral spines, which facilitates access to the spinal fluid space. It is helpful to wrap the legs before positioning to decrease leg movement.

An alternate position used with small infants and some older children is the sitting position. The child is placed with the buttocks at the edge of the table and with the neck flexed so that the chin rests on the chest. The infant's arms and legs are immobilized by the nurse's hands (Fig. 27-15, *C*).

NURSING ALERT The sitting position may interfere with chest expansion and diaphragm excursion, and in infants the soft, pliable trachea may collapse. Therefore observe the child for difficulty with breathing.

Another position that employs close and comforting contact for the child involves holding the child upright against the nurse's (or parent's) chest with the child's legs wrapped around the adult's waist. The adult's arms are used to hug and restrain the child. For ease of the examiner, the adult should be standing. A small pillow is placed between the child's abdomen and the adult to help arch the child's back. If the pillow proves unsuccessful, a third person can place an arm in this space to achieve the desired position (Brown,

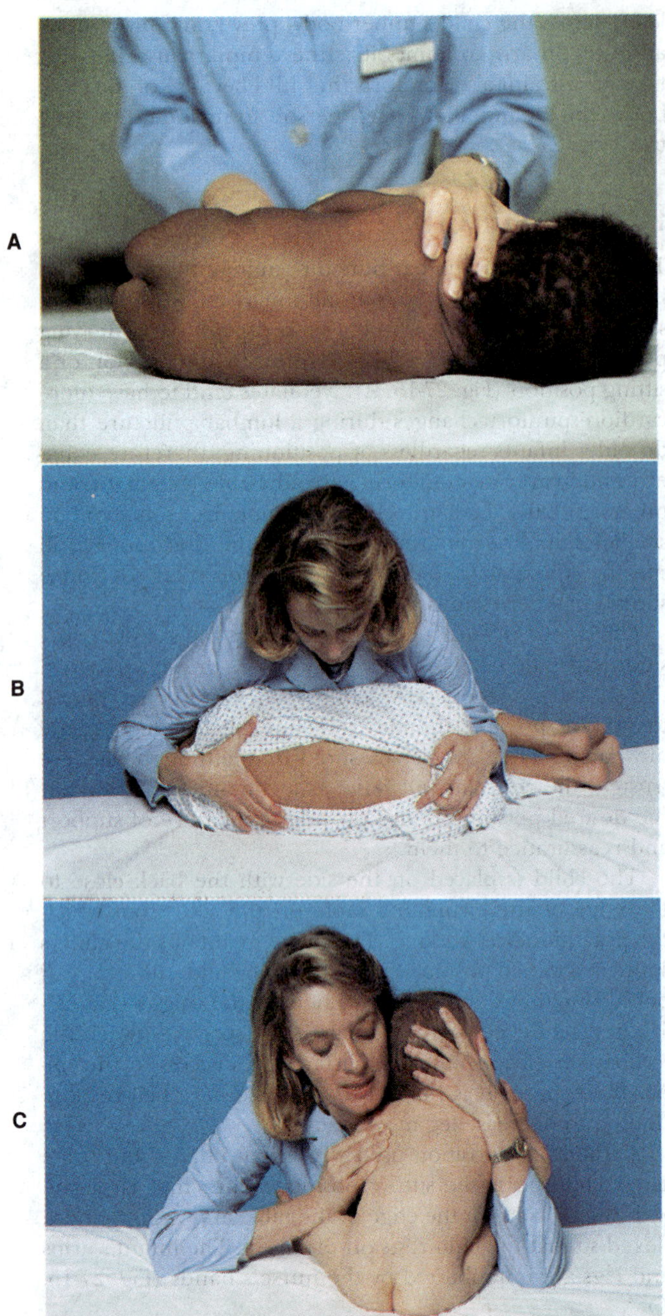

FIG. 27-15 **A,** Modified side-lying position for lumbar puncture. **B,** Older child in side-lying position. **C,** Infant sitting position allows for flexion of lumbar spine.

1984). Care should be taken that excessive pressure does not compromise circulation or breathing and that the nose and mouth are not covered by the restrainer's body.

Specimens and spinal fluid pressure are obtained, measured, and sent for analysis in the same manner as for the adult patient. Vital signs are taken as ordered, and the child is observed for any changes in level of consciousness, motor activity, or other neurologic signs. Post–lumbar puncture headache may occur and is related to postural changes; this is less severe when the child lies flat. Headache is seen much less frequently in young children than adolescents.

BONE MARROW ASPIRATION/BIOPSY

Position for a bone marrow aspiration or biopsy depends on the location of the chosen site. In children the posterior or anterior iliac crest is most frequently used, although in infants the tibia may be selected because of easy access to the site and restraint of the child. The sternum, which is the most frequent site in adults, is generally avoided in children because the bone is more fragile and adjacent to vital organs.

If the posterior iliac crest is used, the child is positioned prone. Sometimes a small pillow or folded blanket is placed under the hips to facilitate obtaining the bone marrow specimen. In children who have not received adequate analgesia or anesthesia, restraint is needed and is best applied with two people—one person to immobilize the upper body and a second person to immobilize the lower extremities. If the other sites are used, the child is placed supine and restraint is applied in a similar manner, with modifications for access to the tibia or anterior iliac crest.

OTHER PROCEDURES

For subdural puncture through a fontanel or burr hole, the infant is wrapped in a mummy restraint and placed in the supine position with the head accessible to the examiner. To control the head, the nurse uses a firm hold on each side of it. Procedures for immobilizing the head are discussed in Chapter 7 under Ears; Nose; Mouth and Throat.

COLLECTION OF SPECIMENS

Many of the specimens needed for diagnostic examination of children are collected in much the same way as they are for adults. Older children are able to cooperate if given proper instruction regarding what is expected from them. Infants and small children, however, are unable to follow directions or control body functions sufficiently to help in collecting some specimens.

URINE SPECIMENS

Children admitted to the hospital or seen in a clinic or office may require a urine specimen as a routine diagnostic procedure. Older children and adolescents will readily use the bedpan or urinal or can be trusted to follow directions for collection in the bathroom. However, they may have special needs. School-age children are cooperative but curious. They are concerned about the reasons behind things and are likely to ask questions regarding the disposition of their specimen and what one expects to discover from it. Self-conscious adolescents may be reluctant to carry a specimen bottle through a hallway or waiting room and appreciate a paper bag or other means for disguising the container. The presence of menses may be an embarrassment or a concern to teenage girls; therefore it is a good idea to ask them about this and make adjustments as necessary. The specimen can be delayed or a notation made on the laboratory slip to explain the presence of red blood cells.

Preschoolers and toddlers are less cooperative, primarily because they are usually unable to void on request. It is often best to offer them water or other liquids that they enjoy and wait about 30 minutes until they are ready to void voluntarily or set a timer to alert them to void shortly.

➤ **NURSING TIP** Wipe abdomen with alcohol pad and fan it dry; cooling effect often causes voiding within 2 minutes (Ellis, 1989). Apply pressure over suprapubic area or stroke paraspinal muscles (along spine) to elicit Perez reflex; in infants 4 to 6 months of age, reflex causes crying, extension of back, flexion of extremities, and urination.

Children will better understand what is expected if the nurse uses familiar terms for the function, such as "peepee," "wee-wee," or "tinkle." Some will have difficulty voiding in an unfamiliar receptacle. Potty chairs or a bedpan placed on the toilet are usually satisfactory. Toddlers who have recently acquired bladder control may be especially reluctant, since they undoubtedly have been admonished for "going" in places other than those approved by parents. A useful approach is to enlist the help of parents; they are likely to be successful, and this helps them to feel a part of the child's care.

For infants and toddlers who are not toilet trained, special urine collection devices are used. These devices are clear plastic, single-use bags with self-adhering material around the opening at the point of attachment. To prepare the infant, the genitalia, perineum, and surrounding skin are washed and dried thoroughly, since the adhesive will not stick to a moist, powdered, or oily skin surface. The collection bag is easiest to apply if attached first to the perineum, progressing to the symphysis (Fig. 27-16). With little girls the perineum is stretched taut during application to that area to ensure a leak-proof fit. With small boys the penis and sometimes the scrotum are placed inside the bag. The adhesive portion of the bag must be firmly applied to the skin all around the genital area to avoid possible leakage. The diaper is carefully replaced. For low-birth-weight infants, small bags with adhesive that is gentle to the skin are available.* Anatomically correct urine collection bags are also available.† The bag is checked frequently and removed as soon as the specimen is available, since the moist bag may become loosened on an active child. For some types of urine testing, such as checking specific gravity, ketones, sugar, and protein, urine can be aspirated directly from the diaper (Suri, 1988).

➤ **NURSING TIP** When using a urine collection bag, cut a small slit in the diaper and pull the bag through to allow room for urine to collect and to facilitate checking on the contents. To obtain small amounts of urine, use a syringe without a needle to aspirate urine directly from the diaper; if diapers with absorbent gelling material that trap urine are used, place a small gauze dressing, some cotton balls, or a

*Available from Hollister, Inc., 2000 Hollister Dr., Libertyville, IL 60048; (800) 323-4060.

†Available from ConvaTec, CN 5254, Princeton, NJ 08543-5254; (800) 422-8811.

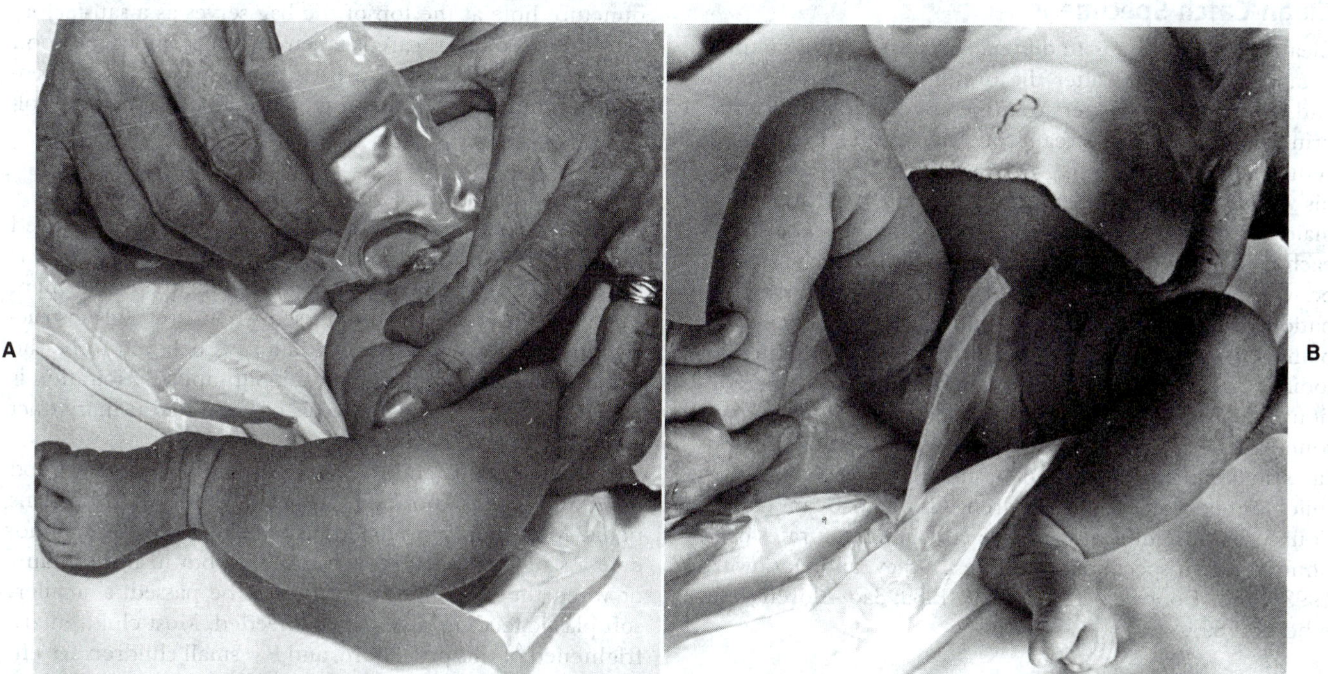

FIG. 27-16 Application of urine collection bag. **A,** For female infants, adhesive portion is applied to exposed and dried perineum first. **B,** Bag adheres firmly around perineal area to prevent urine leakage.

urine collection device* inside the diaper to collect urine and aspirate the urine with a syringe.

Immediate determination of urine specific gravity from a diaper sample is not essential. Studies report no significant change in specific gravities taken from diaper samples up to 4 hours after urination, provided that the diaper is folded closed and taped and is not exposed to air, heat, or light (Lybrand, Medoff-Cooper, and Monro, 1990; Stebor, 1989). Diapers exposed to the environment, especially when radiant heat is used, may lose moisture through evaporation, which may affect the accuracy of specific gravity measurement (Cooke, Werkman, and Watson, 1989).

Traditionally, specific gravity refractometers have been used on nursing units to measure specific gravity. However, current regulations have limited the refractometer's use to the laboratory. Urine dipsticks can be used on the nursing unit with reasonable accuracy.

When urine is collected for culture, the bag is removed immediately. If the urine is not tested within 30 minutes, the specimen is refrigerated or placed in a sterile container with a preservative (Goodman and others, 1985; Lewis and Alexander, 1980). Leaving the bag on the perineum for up to 30 minutes has been shown not to affect culture results (Schlager and others, 1990).

At times, parents may be requested to bring a urine sample to a health care facility for examination, especially when infants are unable to void during an outpatient visit. In this instance parents need instruction on applying the collection device and storage of the specimen.† Ideally the specimen should be brought to the designated place as soon as possible; if there is a delay, the sample should be refrigerated and the lapsed time reported to the examiner.

Clean-Catch Specimens

Clean-catch specimens traditionally refer to urine samples obtained for culture after the urethral meatus is cleaned and the first few milliliters of urine are avoided before the urine is collected (midstream specimen). In males the procedure consists of cleaning the perineum or tip of the penis with a soap- or antiseptic-soaked sterile pad, and in females it consists of wiping from front to back only once with each pad. This is repeated at least two times. The area may be wiped with sterile water to prevent accidental contamination of the urine with a solution that may destroy the pathogens, although minute amounts of antiseptic such as iodine do not alter bacterial counts. Although this traditional cleansing procedure is often practiced, studies have found that it does not significantly reduce contamination rates in infants, circumcised or uncircumcised males, or toilet-trained prepubertal children. Also, midstream collection does not significantly reduce contamination rates over nonmidstream specimens (Leisure, Dudley, and Donowitz, 1993; Lohr, Donowitz, and Dudley, 1989; Saez-Llorens and others, 1989).

*The Bard Sure Catch is available from Bard Urological Division, C.R. Bard, Inc., Covington, GA 30209; (800) 526-4467.

†Home care instructions for obtaining a urine sample are available in *Wong and Whaley's Clinical Manual of Pediatric Nursing* (Mosby).

Twenty-Four-Hour Collection

The need to collect urine voided over a 24-hour period creates a special challenge in infants and children. Collection bags and sometimes restraining methods are required in infants and small children. Older children require special instruction about notifying someone when they need to void or have a bowel movement so that urine can be collected separately and not discarded. Some older school-age children and adolescents can be trusted to take responsibility for collection of their own 24-hour specimens. These children can keep output records and transfer each voiding to the 24-hour collection container if this is permitted.

As in any 24-hour urine collection, the collection period always starts and ends with an empty bladder. At the time the collection begins, the child is instructed to void and the specimen is discarded. All urine voided in the subsequent 24 hours is saved in a container with a preservative or is placed on ice. Twenty-four hours from the time the precollection specimen was discarded, the child is again instructed to void, the specimen is added to the container, and the entire collection is taken to the laboratory for examination.

Infants and small children who are bagged for 24-hour urine collection require a special collection bag; frequent removal and replacement of adhesive collection devices can produce skin irritation. A thin coating of sealant, such as Skin-Prep, applied to the skin helps to protect it and aids adhesion unless its use is contraindicated, such as in a premature infant or a child with irritated skin. Plastic collection bags with collection tubes attached are ideal when the container must be left in place for a time. These can be connected to a collecting device or emptied periodically by aspiration with a syringe. When such devices are not available, a regular bag with a feeding tube inserted through a puncture hole at the top of the bag serves as a satisfactory substitute. However, care is taken to empty the bag as soon as the infant urinates to prevent leakage and loss of contents. An indwelling catheter may also be placed for the collection period.

Special Techniques

Bladder catheterization or ***suprapubic aspiration*** is employed when a specimen is urgently needed or when the child is unable to void or otherwise provide an adequate specimen. Catheterization is most often used when urethral obstruction or anuria caused by renal failure is believed to be the cause of the child's failure to void. Suprapubic aspiration is useful in clarifying the diagnosis of suspected urinary tract infection in acutely ill infants.

Catheterizing a child requires aseptic technique, good light, and gentle, thorough cleansing of the vulva or glans penis. Most children, including female infants, accommodate a size 6, 8, or 10 French catheter, but in male infants or when the larger catheters cannot be passed, a smaller, soft plastic feeding tube may be needed. Most children are frightened of this procedure, and few small children are entirely cooperative; therefore, even when the procedure is adequately explained, an assistant is needed to help restrain and reassure the child. Special care must be exercised when catheterizing young males to avoid trauma to the ductal and

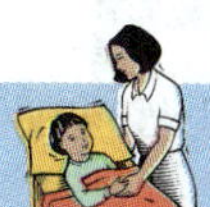

ATRAUMATIC CARE
Bladder Catheterization or Suprapubic Aspiration

Use distraction to help the child relax (blowing bubbles, deep breathing, singing a song, etc.).

Use a water-soluble jelly to lubricate the catheter. Lidocaine jelly can be used to anesthetize the area before insertion.

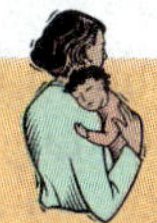

FAMILY FOCUS
Bladder Catheterization

Parents may be upset when their child is catheterized. Aside from the trauma the child experiences, some parents, especially those from different cultures, may fear that the procedure affects the daughter's virginity. To clarify this misconception, the family needs a detailed explanation of the genitourinary anatomy, preferably with a model that shows the separate vaginal and urethral openings.

glandular openings into the urethra, which might result in sterility.

Suprapubic aspiration, which is performed by a practitioner skilled in the procedure, involves aspirating bladder contents by inserting a 20- or 21-gauge needle in the midline approximately 1 cm above the symphysis and directed vertically downward. The skin is prepared as for any needle insertion, but the bladder should contain an adequate volume of urine. This can be assumed if the infant has not voided for at least 1 hour or the bladder can be palpated above the symphysis. This technique is especially useful for obtaining sterile specimens from young infants. The bladder is an abdominal organ at this time and is easily accessible.

Suprapubic aspiration is painful and has a higher failure rate than urethral catheterization; also, success depends more on the volume of urine in the bladder (Pollack, Pollack, and Andrew, 1994). (See Atraumatic Care and Family Focus boxes.)

STOOL SPECIMENS

Stool specimens are frequently collected in children to identify parasites and other organisms that cause diarrhea, to assess gastrointestinal function, and to check for occult (hidden) blood. Ideally, stool should be collected without contamination with urine, but in children wearing diapers, this is difficult unless a urine bag is applied. Children who are toilet trained should urinate first, flush the toilet, then defecate in the toilet or in a bedpan (preferably one that is placed on the toilet to avoid embarrassment) or a commercial potty hat.

➤ **NURSING TIP** To obtain a stool specimen, place plastic wrap over the toilet bowl to collect the stool. Use a tongue depressor or disposable spoon or knife to collect the stool.

An ample amount of stool is collected and placed in the appropriate container, which is covered and labeled. If several specimens are needed, the containers are marked with the date and time and kept in a specimen refrigerator. Special care is exercised in handling the specimen because of the risk of contamination.

BLOOD SPECIMENS

Although most blood specimens are obtained by the laboratory staff or physicians, nurses are increasingly responsible for specimen collection, especially if the child has an arterial or venous access device. However, whether the specimen is collected by the nurse or others, the nurse is responsible for making certain that specimens, such as serial examinations and fasting specimens, are collected on time and that the proper equipment is available, such as correct collection tubes and ice for blood gas samples.

Venous blood samples can be obtained by venipuncture or by aspiration from a peripheral or central access device. Withdrawing blood specimens through peripheral lock devices (also known as intermittent infusion devices, PRN adapters, and by the previous term, heparin locks) in small peripheral veins has met with varying degrees of success. Although it avoids an additional venipuncture for the child, attempting to aspirate blood from the peripheral lock may shorten the life of the device. When using an intravenous infusion site for specimen collection, it is important to consider the type of fluid being infused. For example, a specimen collected for glucose determination would be inaccurate if removed from a catheter through which glucose-containing solution is being administered.

➤ **NURSING TIP** To obtain a blood specimen from a central venous line or peripheral lock when the infusion solution may interfere with the test results, first aspirate a minimum quantity of blood equal to the volume of fluid in the catheter and discard; then aspirate the blood sample. For a blood culture, use the first sample of blood, since organisms are most likely to collect within the catheter itself (Schreiner, 1987).

NURSING ALERT On small or anemic children, keep track of the amount drawn and discarded over time. Frequent taking of blood specimens can rapidly decrease a child's blood count. Coordinate blood samples as much as possible to reduce the frequency.

Arterial blood samples are sometimes needed for blood gas measurement, although noninvasive techniques, such as transcutaneous oxygen monitoring and pulse oximetry, are being used more frequently. Arterial samples may be obtained by arteriopuncture using the radial, brachial, or femoral arteries; by deep heel puncture; or from indwelling arterial catheters. Adequate circulation should be assessed prior to arterial puncture by observing capillary refill or performing the Allen test, a procedure that assesses the circulation of the radial, ulnar, or brachial arteries (Millam, 1988; see also Blood Gas Determination, Chapter 31). Since unclotted blood is required, only heparinized collection tubes are used. In addition, no air bubbles should enter the tube, since they can alter blood gas concentration. Crying, fear, and agitation also affect blood gas values; therefore every effort is made to comfort the child. The blood samples are packed in ice to reduce blood cell metabolism and are taken to the laboratory for immediate analysis.

Capillary blood samples are taken from children by finger or earlobe stick methods, just as in the adult patient. The best method for taking peripheral blood samples from infants is by a heel stick. Before the blood sample is taken, the heel is warmed with warm, moist compresses for 5 to 10 minutes to dilate the vessels in the area. The area is cleansed with alcohol, and with the infant's foot firmly restrained with the free hand, the heel is punctured with a blade or an automatic lancet device. An automatic device, such as Tenderfoot* or Autolet, delivers a more precise puncture depth and is a less painful procedure than that achieved with a blade or lance (Paes and others, 1993). Although obtaining capillary blood gases is a common practice, these measures may not accurately reflect arterial values (Courtney and others, 1990).

The most serious complication of infant heel puncture is necrotizing osteochondritis from lancet penetration of the underlying calcaneus bone. To avoid this, the puncture should be no deeper than 2.4 mm and should be made at the outer aspect of the heel. The boundaries of the calcaneus can be marked by an imaginary line extending posteriorly from a point between the fourth and fifth toes and running parallel to the lateral aspect of the heel and another line extending posteriorly from the middle of the great toe and running parallel to the medial aspect of the heel (Fig. 27-17). In addition, repeated trauma to the walking surface of the heel can cause fibrosis and scarring that may interfere with locomotion. Frequent heel punctures have been associated with development of plantar warts at a later age.

*Available from International Technidyne Corp., 23 Nevsky St., Edison, NJ 08820; (800) 631-5945 or (908) 548-5700.

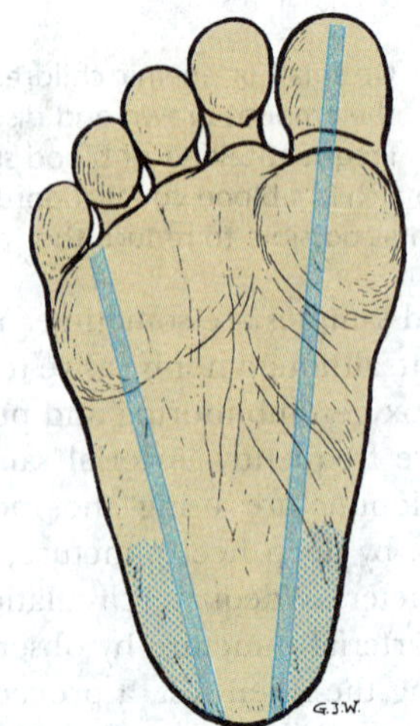

FIG. 27-17 Puncture site *(blue stippled area)* on sole of infant's foot.

The needed specimens are quickly collected, and pressure is applied to the puncture site with a dry gauze square until bleeding stops. The arm is kept extended, not flexed, while pressure is applied for a few minutes after venipuncture in the antecubital fossa to reduce bruising (Dyson and Bogod, 1987). The site is then covered with a Band-Aid. In young children, "spot" Band-Aids pose an aspiration hazard; their use should be avoided, or the Band-Aid should be removed as soon as the bleeding stops. Applying warm compresses to ecchymotic areas increases circulation, helps remove extravasated blood, and decreases pain.

No matter how or by whom the specimen is collected, children, even some older ones, fear the loss of their blood. This is particularly true for children whose condition requires frequent blood specimens. They mistakenly believe that blood removed from their bodies is a threat to their lives. Explaining to them that their blood is continually being produced by their bodies provides them with a measure of reassurance regarding this aspect of the stress-provoking

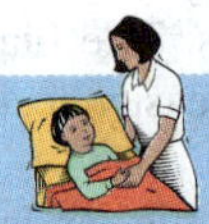

ATRAUMATIC CARE
Skin/Vessel Punctures and Multiple Blood Samples

To reduce the pain and distress associated with heel, finger, venous, or arterial punctures:

1. Apply EMLA topically over the site if time permits (at least 60 minutes) or use buffered lidocaine (injected intradermally near vein with 30-gauge needle) to numb the skin.
2. Use nonpharmacologic methods of pain and anxiety control (e.g., ask child to take a deep breath when the needle is inserted and again when the needle is withdrawn; ask child to count slowly and then faster and louder if pain is felt).
3. Emphasize that blood entering syringe or tube does not hurt.
4. Reassure young children that you did not "take their blood" away and that they have a lot more inside.
5. Place *small* bandage over puncture site to make removal easy and less painful and to reassure young children that their blood will not leak out.

For multiple blood samples:

1. Use an intermittent infusion device ("heparin lock") to collect additional samples from existing intravenous line; consider peripherally inserted central catheters (PICCs) early, not as a last resort.
2. Coordinate care to allow several tests to be performed on one blood sample using micromethods of testing.
3. Anticipate tests (i.e., type and cross-match for blood transfusion) and ask laboratory to save blood for additional testing.

Contrary to popular belief, a study of children ages 3 to 6 years found that asking them not to look at the "finger stick" to avoid the sight of blood or applying a decorated bandage did not lessen their rating of pain intensity (Johnston, Stevens, and Arbess, 1993).

procedure. When the blood is drawn, a simple comment such as, "Just look how red it is. You're really making a lot of nice red blood," confirms this information and affords them an opportunity to express their concern. A Band-Aid gives them added assurance that the vital fluids will not leak out through the puncture site.

Children also dislike the discomfort associated with venous, arterial, or capillary punctures. In fact, children have identified these procedures as the ones most frequently causing pain during hospitalization and arterial punctures as being one of the most painful of all procedures experienced (Wong and Baker, 1988). Toddlers are most distressed by venipunctures, followed by school-age children and then adolescents (Fradet and others, 1990; Humphrey and others, 1992). Consequently, nurses need to institute pain reduction techniques to lessen the discomfort of these procedures. (see Atraumatic Care box and Pain Management, Chapter 26).

RESPIRATORY SECRETION SPECIMENS

Collection of sputum or nasal discharge is sometimes required for diagnosis of respiratory infections, especially tuberculosis and respiratory syncytial virus (RSV). Older children and adolescents are able to cough as directed and supply sputum specimens when given proper directions. It must be made clear to them that a coughed specimen, not mucus cleared from the throat, is needed. It is helpful to demonstrate a deep cough so that communication is clear. Infants and small children are unable to follow directions to cough and will swallow any sputum produced when they do; therefore, gastric washings (lavage) may be used to collect a specimen. Sometimes a satisfactory specimen can be obtained by using a suction device such as a mucus trap if the catheter is inserted into the trachea and the cough reflex elicited. A catheter inserted into the back of the throat is not sufficient. For children with a tracheostomy, a specimen is easily aspirated from the trachea or major bronchi by attaching a collecting device to the suction apparatus.

Nasal washings are usually obtained to diagnose an infection of RSV. The child is placed supine, and 1 to 3 ml of sterile normal saline is instilled with a sterile syringe (without needle) into one nostril. The contents are aspirated using a small, sterile bulb syringe and are placed in a sterile container. Another method uses a syringe with 2 inches of 18- to 20-gauge tubing. The saline is quickly instilled and then aspirated to recover the nasal specimen. To prevent any additional discomfort to the child, all the equipment should be ready before beginning the procedure. Other respiratory secretion collection methods include nasopharyngeal swabs to diagnose *Bordetella pertussis* and throat cultures. Since obtaining throat and nasopharyngeal cultures may be traumatic to the child, using a gentle technique is important.

NURSING ALERT Do not attempt to obtain a throat culture if acute epiglottitis is suspected. The trauma from the swab may increase edema, possibly occluding the airway.

ADMINISTRATION OF MEDICATION

DETERMINATION OF DRUG DOSAGE

It is the physician's responsibility to prescribe drugs in the correct dosage to achieve the desired effect without endangering the child's health. However, nurses must have an understanding of the safe dosage of medications they administer to children as well as the expected action, possible side effects, and signs of toxicity. Unlike adult medications, there are few standardized dosage ranges for children in the pediatric age-groups, and with a few exceptions, drugs are prepared and packaged in average adult-dosage strengths.

Factors related to growth and maturation significantly alter an individual's capacity to metabolize and excrete drugs, and deficiencies associated with immaturity become more important with decreasing age. Immaturity or defects in any or all of the important processes of absorption, distribution, biotransformation, or excretion can significantly alter the effects of a drug. Newborn and premature infants with immature enzyme systems in the liver (where most drugs are broken down and detoxified), lower plasma concentrations of protein for binding with drugs, and immaturely functioning kidneys (where most drugs are excreted) are particularly vulnerable to the harmful effects of drugs. Beyond the newborn period, many drugs are metabolized more rapidly by the liver, necessitating larger doses or more frequent administration. This is particularly important in pain control, when the dosage may need to be increased or the interval between administering analgesics may need to be decreased (Singleton, Rosen, and Fisher, 1987).

Other factors that create problems in drug dosages in children include the difficulty in evaluating drug response. For example, how is a toxic manifestation such as ringing in the ears assessed in a preverbal child? In disease states, particularly in children, water losses and water requirements are both increased, whereas the fluid intake decreases. Since water is required to excrete the drug, dehydration poses the danger of toxic accumulation.

Various formulas involving age, weight, and body surface area (BSA) as the basis for calculations have been devised to determine children's drug dosage from a standard adult dose. Since the administration of medication is a nursing responsibility, nurses need not only a knowledge of drug action and patient responses, but also some resources for estimating safe dosages for children. The method most often used to determine children's dosage is based on BSA.

The most reliable method for determining children's dosage is to calculate the proportional amount of BSA to body weight. The ratio of BSA to weight varies inversely with length; therefore the infant who is shorter and weighs less than an older child or adult has relatively more BSA than would be expected from the weight.

The usual determination of BSA requires the use of the West nomogram (Fig. 27-18). BSA is estimated from the child's height and weight. Then this information is applied to a formula for dosage, such as either of the following formulas, which require different types of information:

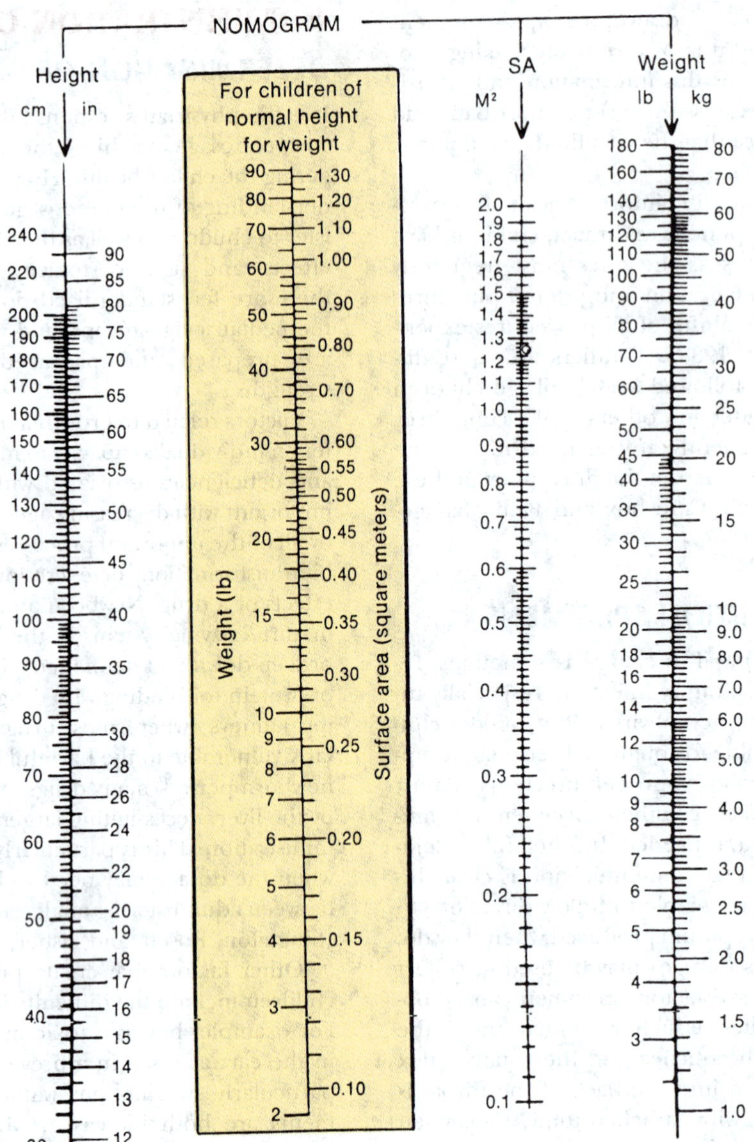

FIG. 27-18 West nomogram (for estimation of surface areas). Surface area is indicated where a straight line connecting height and weight intersects surface area (SA) column or, if patient is approximately of normal proportion, from weight alone (enclosed area). (From Behrman RE, Vaughan VC, editors: *Nelson textbook of pediatrics,* ed 14, Philadelphia, 1992, WB Saunders; modified from data of E Boyd by CD West.)

$$\frac{\text{BSA of child}}{\text{BSA of adult}} \times \text{Adult dose} = \begin{array}{c}\text{Estimated}\\ \text{child's dose}\end{array}$$

$$\text{BSA of child (m}^2\text{)} \times \text{Dose/m}^2 = \begin{array}{c}\text{Estimated}\\ \text{child's dose}\end{array}$$

PREPARATION FOR SAFE ADMINISTRATION

Checking Dosage

Administering the correct dosage of a drug is a shared responsibility between the physician who orders the drug and the nurse who carries out that order. Children react with unexpected severity to some drugs, and ill children may be especially sensitive to drugs. Therefore checking the dose if there is any doubt about its accuracy is a professional duty. When a dose is ordered that is outside the usual range or if there is some question regarding the preparation or the route of administration, the nurse should always check with the physician before proceeding with the administration, since the nurse is legally liable for any drug administered.

Administering some medications requires added safeguards. Even when it has been determined that the dosage is correct for a particular child, many drugs are potentially hazardous or lethal. Most hospital units or other facilities where medications are given to children have regulations requiring that specified drugs be double-checked by another nurse before they are given to the child. Among those drugs that require such safeguards are digoxin, heparin, chemotherapy, and insulin. Others that are frequently included are epinephrine, opioids, and sedatives. Even if this precaution is not mandatory, nurses would be wise to take such precautions for their own sense of security. Errors in decimal point placement may easily occur and may result in a tenfold or more dosage error (Koren, Barzilay, and Greenwald, 1986).

Identification

Before the administration of any medication, the child must be correctly identified, since children are not totally reliable in giving correct names on request. Infants are unable to give their name, toddlers or preschoolers may admit to any name, and school-age children may deny their identity in an attempt to avoid the medication. Children sometimes exchange beds during play. Parents may be present to identify their child, but the only safe method for identifying children is to check their hospital identification bands with the medication card.

Parents

Parents can be useful sources of information regarding the child and his or her capabilities. Nearly all parents have given some type of medication to their child and can describe the approaches that they have found to be successful. They can also provide information regarding the child's reaction to similar experiences if the child has been hospitalized before or has been given medication in a practitioner's office or clinic. In some cases it is less traumatic for the child if a parent gives the medication, provided the nurse prepares the medication and supervises its administration and the practice is consistent with hospital or ward policy. Children being given daily medications at home are accustomed to the parent's functioning in this capacity and are less apt to fuss than they would if the medication were administered by a stranger. Individual decisions need to be made regarding parental presence and participation, such as in helping with restraint during injections (see Thinking Critically About . . . box on p. 1138).

Child

Every child requires psychologic preparation for parenteral administration of medication and supportive care during the procedure (see pp. 1135-1139). Even if children have received several injections, they rarely become accustomed to the discomfort and have as much right to understanding and patience from those involved in giving the injection as any other child. Safe administration of any drug requires meticulous attention to the safeguards discussed here.

ORAL ADMINISTRATION

The oral route is preferred for administering medications to children whenever possible. Because of the ease of administration of oral medications, most are dissolved or suspended in liquid preparations. Although some children are able to swallow or chew solid medications at an early age, solid preparations are not recommended for young children. There is danger of aspiration in any oral preparation, but solid forms (pills, tablets, capsules) are especially hazardous if their administration causes extreme resistance or crying.

Most pediatric medications come in palatable and colorful preparations for added ease of administration. Some have a slightly unpleasant aftertaste, but most children will swallow these liquids with little if any resistance. The nurse should taste a minute amount of an oral preparation to ascertain if it is palatable or bitter. In this way, legitimate complaints of dislike from the child can be accepted and the taste camouflaged whenever possible. Most pediatric units have preparations available for this purpose.

➤ **NURSING TIP** To encourage the child's acceptance of oral medications:

- Give the child an ice pop or small ice cube to suck to numb the tongue before giving the drug.
- Mix the drug with a small amount (about 1 tsp) of sweet-tasting substance, such as honey (except in infants because of the risk of botulism), flavored syrups, jam, fruit purees, or ice cream; avoid essential food items, since the child may later refuse to eat them.
- Give a "chaser" of water, juice, a soft drink, or an ice pop or frozen juice bar after the drug.
- If nausea is a problem, give a carbonated beverage poured over finely crushed ice before or immediately after the medication.
- When medication has an unpleasant taste, have the child pinch the nose and drink the medicine through a straw. Much of what we taste is associated with smell.

Preparation

Selecting a vehicle to measure and administer a medication requires careful consideration. The devices available to measure medicines are not always sufficiently accurate for measuring the small amounts needed in pediatric nursing practice (Fig. 27-19). Although molded plastic cups offer reasonable accuracy in measuring moderate or large doses of liquids, paper cups are likely to have irregularly shaped or crumpled bottoms. Calibrations on the cups (especially the teaspoon mark) and the personal equation or interpretation of a given measure are highly variable. Measures less than a teaspoon are impossible to determine accurately with a medicine cup.

Many liquid preparations are prescribed in measurements of teaspoons. However, teaspoons and soup spoons are inaccurate measuring devices and are subject to error from a number of variables. For example, teaspoons vary greatly in capacity, and different persons using the same spoon will pour different amounts. This variability is also influenced by the adequacy of available light, the color of the liquid, and the size of the bottle from which it is poured. Therefore a drug ordered in teaspoons should be measured in milliliters—the established standard is 5 ml per teaspoon. A convenient hollow-handled medicine spoon is available to accurately measure and administer the drug* (see Fig. 27-19, *A*). Household *measuring* spoons can also be used when other devices are not available.

---

*Manufactured by Apex Medical Corp., P.O. Box 1235, Sioux Falls, SD 57101-1235; (800) 328-2935.

A

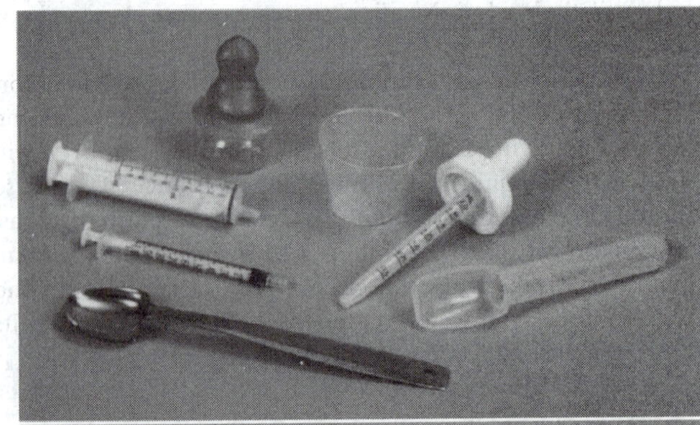

B

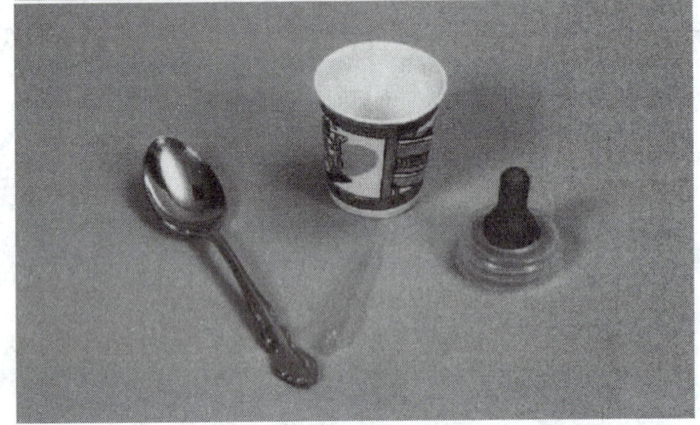

FIG. 27-19 **A,** Acceptable devices for measuring and administering oral medication to children *(clockwise):* measuring spoon, plastic syringes, calibrated nipple, plastic medicine cup, calibrated dropper, hollow-handled medicine spoon. **B,** Acceptable devices only for administering premeasured oral medication *(clockwise):* household teaspoon, paper cup, nipple, uncalibrated dropper.

Another unreliable device for measuring liquids is the drop, which varies to a greater extent than the teaspoon or measuring cup. Droppers are available in numerous sizes but, even with the standard USP dropper, the volume of a drop will vary according to the viscosity of the liquid measured. Viscid fluids produce much larger drops than thin liquids. Many medications are supplied with caps or droppers designed for measuring each specific preparation. These are accurate when used to measure that specific medication but are not reliable for measuring other liquids. Emptying dropper contents into a medicine cup invites additional error. Since some of the liquid clings to the sides of the cup, a significant amount of the drug can be lost.

NURSING ALERT Many pediatric medications are given by drops or dropper. A misunderstanding of these terms by parents can result in a potential overdose. In addition, many droppers that come with medications are marked in tenths of cubic centimeters. If a parent were to use a syringe instead of the dropper, 0.4 cc may be thought to be the same as 4 cc. Provide education to parents on correct methods for giving medication. Demonstrate the technique (Rudy, 1992).

The most accurate means for measuring small amounts of medication is the plastic disposable (never glass) syringe, especially the tuberculin syringe for volumes less than 1 ml. Not only does the syringe provide a reliable measure, but it also serves as a convenient means for transporting and administering the medication. The medication can be placed directly into the child's mouth from the syringe. For added safety, a short length of flexible tubing can be placed on the tip of the syringe to prevent mouth injury, although the tubing must be completely emptied of medication.

Young children and some older children have difficulty in swallowing tablets or pills. Since a number of drugs are not available in pediatric preparations, the tablet will need to be crushed before it can be given to these children. Commercial devices* are available, or simple methods can be employed for crushing tablets.

➤ **NURSING TIP** To minimize loss of the drug, crush the tablet between two spoons or place the tablet either in a medicine cup or between two small paper soufflé cups and use a pestle for crushing; collect the bits of pulverized medication that tend to cling to the sides of the cup or spoon and mix the crushed tablet with a palatable substance.

Another alternative is to have the pharmacist prepare the drug in a flavored, chewable troche or lozenge (Wong and Redding, 1987).

Not all drugs can be crushed (e.g., medication with an enteric or protective coating or formulated for slow release).* For some children, it may be possible to encourage swallowing the tablet or capsule by using a special glass designed with a shelf that holds the drug (manufactured by Apex Medical Corp.†). The child drinks normally, and the tablet is carried to the back of the throat. For children who must take solid oral medication for an extended period, training sessions using progressively larger candy to teach the child to swallow can be beneficial (Funk, Mullins, and Olson, 1984).

Since pediatric doses often require dividing adult preparations of medication, the nurse may be faced with the dilemma of accurate dosage. With tablets, only those that are scored can be halved or quartered accurately. If the medication is soluble, the tablet or contents of a capsule can be mixed in a small, premeasured amount of liquid and the appropriate portion given. If half a dose is required, the tablet is dissolved in 5 ml of water and 2.5 ml is given.

Administration

While administering liquids to infants is relatively easy, care must be observed to prevent aspiration. With the infant held in a semireclining position, the medication is placed in the mouth from a spoon, plastic cup, plastic dropper, or plastic syringe (without needle). The dropper or syringe is best placed along the side of the infant's tongue, and the liquid is administered slowly in small amounts, waiting for the child to swallow between deposits.

---

*Trademark Medical manufactures a pill crusher and has compiled a list of more than 190 medications that should not be crushed or chewed. Both are available from Trademark Medical, 1053 Headquarters Park, Fenton, MO 63026-2033; (314) 349-3265.

†See footnote on p. 1181.

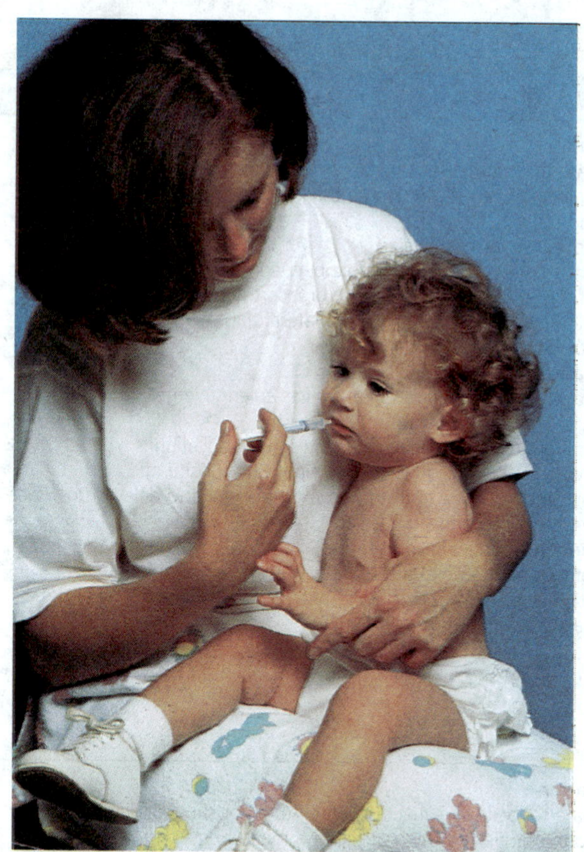

FIG. 27-20 Nurse partially restrains child for easy and comfortable administration of oral medication.

➤ **NURSING TIP** In infants up to 11 months of age and children with neurologic impairments, blowing a small puff of air in the face frequently elicits a swallow reflex (Orenstein and others, 1988).

Medicine cups can be used effectively for older infants who are able to drink from a cup. Because of the natural outward tongue thrust in infancy, medications may need to be retrieved from lips or chin and refed. Allowing the infant to suck the medication that has been placed in an empty nipple or inserting the syringe or dropper into the side of the mouth, parallel to the nipple, while the infant nurses are other convenient methods for giving liquid medications to infants. Medication is not added to the infant's formula feeding.

The young child who refuses to cooperate or resists consistently despite explanation and encouragement may require mild physical coercion. If so, it is carried out quickly and carefully. Every effort is made to determine why the child resists, and the reasons for this alternative are explained in such a way that the child will know that it is being carried out for his or her well-being and is not a form of punishment. There is always a risk in using even mild forceful techniques. A crying child can aspirate a medication, particularly when lying on the back. If the nurse holds the child in the lap with the child's right arm behind the nurse, the left hand firmly grasped by the nurse's left hand, and the head securely restrained between the nurse's arm and body, the medication can be slowly poured into the mouth (Fig. 27-20).

INTRAMUSCULAR (IM) ADMINISTRATION

Selecting the Syringe and Needle

The volume of medication prescribed for small children and the small amount of tissue for injection require that a syringe be selected that can measure very small amounts of solution. For volumes less than 1 ml, the tuberculin syringe, calibrated in one-hundredth increments, is appropriate. Very minute doses may require the use of a 0.5 ml, low-dose syringe. These syringes with specially constructed needles minimize the possibility of inadvertently administering incorrect amounts of a drug because of dead space, which allows fluid to remain in the syringe and needle after the plunger is pushed completely forward. A minimum of 0.2 ml of solution remains in a standard needle hub; therefore, when very small amounts of two drugs are combined in the syringe, such as mixtures of insulin, the ratio of the two drugs can be altered significantly. Measures that minimize the effect of dead space follow: (1) when two drugs are combined in the syringe, always draw them up in the same order to maintain a consistent ratio between the drugs; (2) use the same brand of syringe (dead space may vary); and (3) use one-piece syringe units (needle permanently attached to the syringe).

Dead space is also an important factor to consider when injecting medication, since flushing the syringe with an air bubble adds an additional amount of medication to the prescribed dose. This can be hazardous when very small amounts of a drug are given.

Consequently, flushing is not recommended, especially when less than 1 ml of medication is given. Syringes are calibrated to deliver a prescribed drug dose, and the amount of medication left in the hub and needle is not part of the syringe barrel calibrations. However, the air-bubble technique (drawing up about 0.2 ml or air into the syringe after withdrawing the medication) may be beneficial with certain drugs, such as iron dextran and diphtheria and tetanus toxoid, to avoid tracking the drug through the tissue (Chaplin, Shull, and Welk, 1985). Other techniques to minimize tracking include changing the needle after withdrawing the fluid from the vial and using the Z track method.

The needle length must be sufficient to penetrate the subcutaneous tissue and deposit the medication into the body of the muscle. Limited research is available on adequate needle length for children, although some traditional methods may be used. One study found that a 1-inch needle is necessary to adequately penetrate the vastus lateralis muscle in 4-month-old infants and probably is needed for 2-month-old infants (Hicks and others, 1989).

➤ **NURSING TIP** To estimate the needle length for IM injection, first grasp the lateralis or deltoid muscle and choose a needle length that is approximately half the distance between the thumb and the index finger. With the ventrogluteal or dorsogluteal site, only subcutaneous tissue is grasped, so choose a needle length that is slightly more

TABLE 27-5 Intramuscular Injection Sites in Children

SITE	DISCUSSION
VASTUS LATERALIS 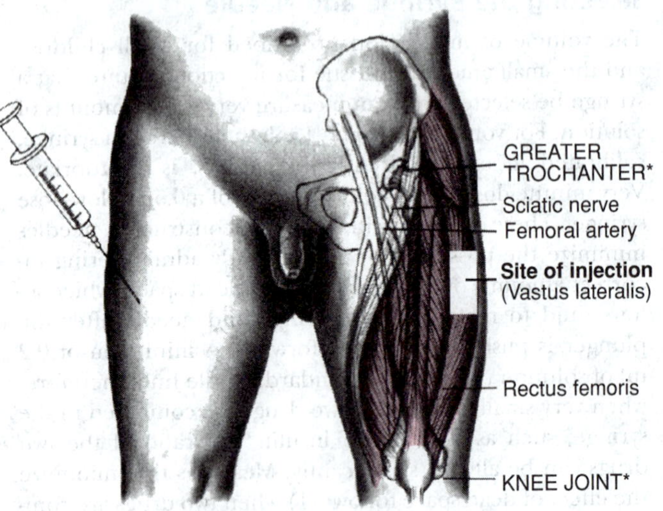 	**Location*** Palpate to find greater trochanter and knee joints; divide vertical distance between these two landmarks into thirds; inject into middle one third **Needle insertion and size** Insert needle at 45-degree angle between syringe and upper thigh in infants and in young children, or insert needle perpendicular to thigh or slightly angled toward lateral thigh 22 to 25 gauge, ⅝ to 1 inch† **Advantages** Large, well-developed muscle that can tolerate larger quantities of fluid (0.5 ml [infant] to 2.0 ml [child]) No important nerves or blood vessels in this location Easily accessible if child is supine, side lying, or sitting A tourniquet can be applied above injection site to delay drug hypersensitivity reaction if necessary **Disadvantages** Thrombosis of femoral artery from injection in midthigh area Sciatic nerve damage from long needle injected posteriorly and medially into small extremity
VENTROGLUTEAL 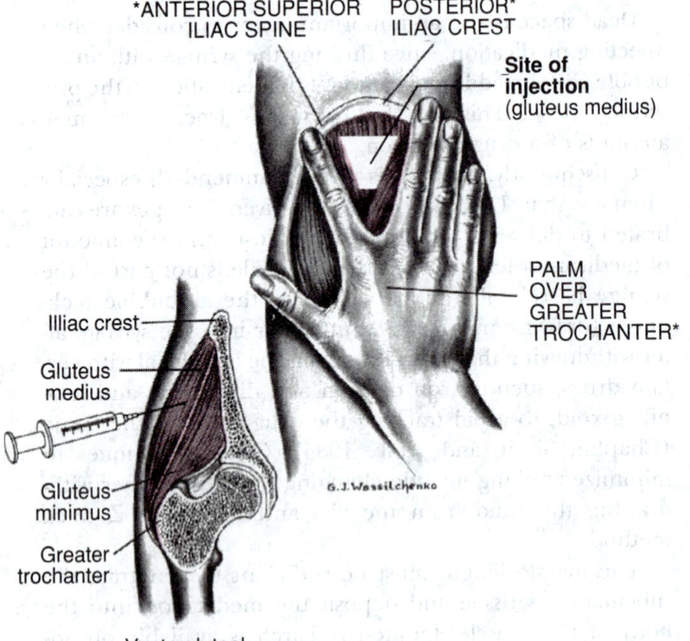 	**Location*** Palpate to locate greater trochanter, anterior superior iliac tubercle (found by flexing thigh at hip and measuring up to 1 to 2 cm above crease formed in groin), and posterior iliac crest; place palm of hand over greater trochanter, index finger over anterior superior iliac tubercle, and middle finger along crest of ilium posteriorly as far as possible; inject into center of V formed by fingers **Needle insertion and size** Insert needle perpendicular to site but angled slightly toward greater trochanter 22 to 25 gauge, ½ to 1 inch **Advantages** Free of important nerves and vascular structures Easily identified by prominent bony landmarks Thinner layer of subcutaneous tissue than in dorsogluteal site, thus less chance of depositing drug subcutaneously rather than intramuscularly Can accommodate larger quantities of fluid (0.5 ml [infant] to 2.0 ml [child]) Easily accessible if child is supine, prone, or side lying Less painful than vastus lateralis **Disadvantages** Health professionals' unfamiliarity with site Not suitable for use of a tourniquet

*Locations are indicated by asterisks on illustrations.
†Research has shown that a 1-inch needle is needed for adequate muscle penetration in infants 4 months old and possibly in infants as young as 2 months (Hicks and others, 1989). Other recommendations for needle size and volume of fluid are based on traditional practice and have not been verified by research.

TABLE 27-5 Intramuscular Injection Sites in Children—cont'd

SITE	DISCUSSION
DORSOGLUTEAL 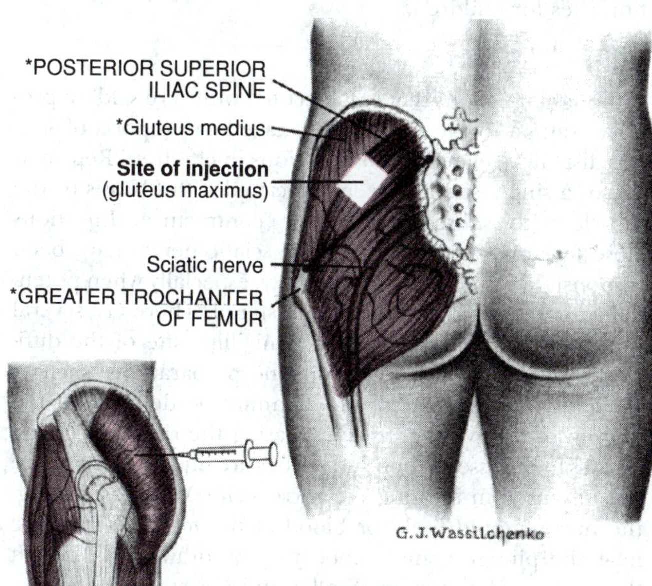 	**Location*** Locate greater trochanter and posterior superior iliac spine; draw imaginary line between these two points and inject lateral and superior to line into gluteus maximus or medius muscle **Needle insertion and size** Insert needle perpendicular to surface on which child is lying when prone 20 to 25 gauge, ½ to 1½ inches **Advantages** In older child, large muscle mass; well-developed muscle can tolerate greater volume of fluid (up to 2.0 ml) Child does not see needle and syringe Easily accessible if child is prone or side lying **Disadvantages** Contraindicated in children who have not been walking for at least 1 year Danger of injury to sciatic nerve Thick, subcutaneous fat, predisposing to deposition of drug subcutaneously rather than intramuscularly Not suitable for use of a tourniquet Inaccessible if child is supine Exposure of site may cause embarrassment in older child
DELTOID 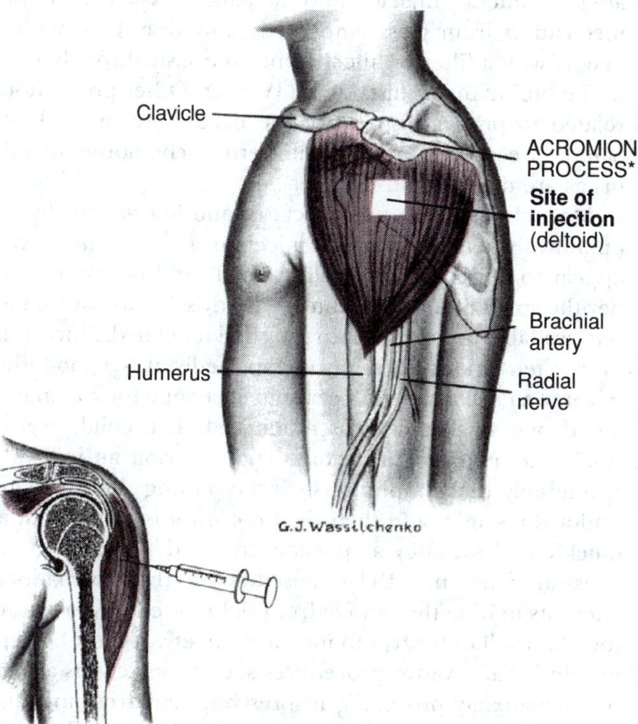 	**Location*** Locate acromion process; inject only into upper third of muscle that begins about two fingerbreadths below acromion **Needle insertion and size** Insert needle perpendicular to site with syringe angled slightly toward elbow 22 to 25 gauge, ½ to 1 inch **Advantages** Faster absorption rates than gluteal sites Tourniquet can be applied above injection site Easily accessible with minimum removal of clothing Less pain and fewer local side effects from vaccines as compared with vastus lateralis **Disadvantages** Small muscle mass; only limited amounts of drug can be injected (0.5 to 1.0 ml) Small margins of safety with possible damage to radial nerve and axillary nerve (not shown, lies under deltoid at head of humerus)

than half the distance. Choose a final needle length that allows for a small portion of the needle to be exposed at the skin surface as a precaution if the needle should break off from the hub.

The needle gauge should be as small as possible to deliver the fluid safely. Small gauges cause the least discomfort, but larger sizes are needed for viscous medication and when longer length needles are used (to prevent accidental bending).

Determining the Site

Factors that are considered when selecting a site for an IM injection on an infant or child include:

- The amount and character of the medication to be injected
- The amount and general condition of the muscle mass
- The frequency or number of injections to be given during the course of treatment
- The type of medication being given
- Factors that may impede access to or cause contamination of the site
- The ability of the child to assume the required position safely

Older children and adolescents usually pose few problems in selecting a suitable site for IM injections, but infants, with their small and underdeveloped muscles, have fewer available sites. It is sometimes difficult to assess the amount of fluid that can be safely injected into a single site. Usually 1 ml is the maximum volume that should be administered in a single site to small children and older infants. The muscles of small infants may not tolerate more than 0.5 ml. As the child approaches adult size, volumes approaching those given to adults may be used. However, the larger the amount of solution, the larger must be the muscle into which it is injected.

Injections must be placed in muscles large enough to accommodate the medication, but major nerves and blood vessels must be avoided. There is no universal agreement regarding the best IM injection site for children. The preferred site for infants is the vastus lateralis. General recommendations for using the gluteal sites are after children have been walking (length of suggested time varies but is usually a minimum of 1 year after walking), since the muscle develops with locomotion. Unfortunately, this recommendation is often applied to the ventrogluteal muscle site as well as the dorsogluteal site. However, significant differences exist between these two sites that warrant recognition. The ventrogluteal site is relatively free of major nerves and blood vessels, is a relatively large muscle with less subcutaneous tissue than the dorsal site, has well-defined landmarks for safe site location, and is easily accessible in several positions (Beecroft and Redick, 1990; Intramuscular injections, 1985). These advantages make it a preferred site over the dorsogluteal muscle and challenge the recommendation that the ventrogluteal site not be used until children have been walking. Although there are published recommendations regarding age, in clinical practice this site has been used in children as young as newborns. The deltoid muscle, a small muscle near the axillary and radial nerves, can be used for small volumes of fluid in children as young as 18 months of age. Its advantages are less pain and fewer side effects from the injectate (as observed with immunizations) as compared with the vastus lateralis (Ipp and others, 1989). Table 27-5 summarizes the four major injection sites and illustrates the location of the preferred IM injection sites for children.

Administration

Although injections that are executed with care seldom produce trauma to the child, there have been reports of serious disability related to IM injections in children. Repeated use of a single site has been associated with fibrosis of the muscle with subsequent muscle contracture. Injections close to large nerves, such as the sciatic nerve, have been responsible for permanent disability, especially when potentially neurotoxic drugs are administered. There are several reports of tissue damage from penicillin; one of the difficulties in administering the opaque preparations, such as Bicillin, is that aspirated blood cannot be detected at the bottom of the syringe, thus increasing the risk of injecting into a blood vessel. When such drugs are injected, great care must be used in locating the correct site. When aspirating, the nurse should look for blood at the *top* of the syringe near the plunger, since blood may be drawn up through the column of penicillin (Stoller and Losey, 1985).

A reported potential hazard with medication in glass ampules is the presence of glass particles in the ampule after the container is broken. When the medication is withdrawn into the syringe, the glass particles are also withdrawn and are subsequently injected into the patient. As a precaution, medication from glass ampules is only drawn through a needle with a filter or injected intravenously through a site in the tubing that is distal to an IV filter. Other precautions related to proper disposal of the needle are on p. 1166. Safety precautions for administering chemotherapeutic drugs are discussed in Chapter 36.

Most children are unpredictable and few are totally cooperative when receiving an injection. Even children who appear to be relaxed and constrained can lose control under the stress of the procedure. It is advisable to have someone available to help restrain the child if needed. Since children often jerk or pull away unexpectedly, it is a good idea to carry an extra capped needle to exchange for a contaminated one so that delay is minimized. The child, even a small one, is told that he or she is receiving an injection (preferably using a phrase such as "putting the medicine under the skin"), and then the procedure is carried out as quickly and skillfully as possible to avoid prolonging the stressful experience. Delay caused by lengthy explanations, attempts to hide the syringe from sight, or efforts to soothe the child will only serve to increase anxiety. It must be kept in mind that invasive procedures such as injections are especially anxiety provoking in preschool children and that small children usually associate any assault to the "behind" area with punishment. Since injections are painful, the nurse should employ excellent injection techniques and effective pain reduction measures to reduce discomfort (see Guidelines box).

Small infants offer little resistance to injections. Al-

GUIDELINES
Intramuscular Administration of Medication

Use safety precautions in administering medication (e.g., check child's identification).
Prepare medication.
- Select needle and syringe appropriate to the following:
  - Amount of fluid to be administered (syringe size)
  - Viscosity of fluid to be administered (needle gauge)
  - Amount of tissue to be penetrated (needle length)
- Maximum volume to be administered in a single site is 1 ml for older infants and small children.

Determine the site of injection (see Table 27-5); make certain muscle is large enough to accommodate volume and type of medication.
- Older children: select site as with adult patient; allow child some choice of site, if feasible.
- Following are acceptable sites for infants and small or debilitated children:
  - Vastus lateralis muscle
  - Ventrogluteal muscle
- Dorsogluteal muscle is insufficiently developed to be a safe site for infants and small children.

Administer medication.
- Provide for sufficient help in restraining child; children are often uncooperative, and their behavior is usually unpredictable.
- Explain briefly what is to be done and, if appropriate, what child can do to help.
- Expose injection area for unobstructed view of landmarks.
- Select a site where skin is free of irritation and danger of infection; palpate for and avoid sensitive or hardened areas. With multiple injections, rotate sites.
- Place child in a lying or sitting position; child is not allowed to stand because:
  - Landmarks are more difficult to assess.
  - Restraint is more difficult.
  - Child may faint and fall.
- Use a new, sharp needle with smallest diameter that permits free flow of the medication.
- Grasp muscle firmly between thumb and fingers to isolate and stabilize muscle for deposition of drug in its deepest part; in obese children, spread skin with thumb and index finger to displace subcutaneous tissue and grasp muscle deeply on each side.
- Allow skin preparation to dry completely before skin is penetrated.
- Have medication at room temperature.

Decrease perception of pain:
- Distract child with conversation.
- Give child something on which to concentrate (e.g., squeezing a hand or bed rail, pinching own nose, humming, counting, yelling "Ouch!").
- Place a cold compress or wrapped ice cube on site about a minute before injection, or apply cold to contralateral site.
- Say to child, "If you feel this, tell me to take it out, please."
- Have child hold a small Band-Aid and place it on puncture site after IM injection is given.

Insert needle quickly, using a dartlike motion.
Avoid tracking any medication through superficial tissues:
- Replace needle after withdrawing medication, or wipe medication from needle with sterile gauze.
- If withdrawing medication from an ampule, use a needle equipped with a filter that removes glass particles; then use a new, nonfilter needle for injection.
- Use the Z track and/or air-bubble technique as indicated.
- Avoid any depression of the plunger during insertion of the needle.

Aspirate for blood.
- If blood is found, remove syringe from site, change needle, and reinsert into new location.
- If no blood is found, inject into a relaxed muscle:
  - Dorsogluteal—place child on abdomen with legs and toes rotated inward.
  - Ventrogluteal—place child on side with upper leg flexed and placed in front of lower leg.

Inject medication slowly (over 20 seconds).
Remove needle quickly; hold gauze sponge firmly against skin near needle when removing it to avoid pulling on tissue.
Apply firm pressure to site after injection; massage site to hasten absorption unless contraindicated, as with irritating drugs.
Place a small Band-Aid on puncture site; with young children decorate Band-Aid by drawing a smiling face or other symbol of acceptance.
Hold and cuddle young child and encourage parents to comfort child; praise older child.
Allow expression of feelings.
Discard syringe and uncapped, uncut needle in puncture-resistant container located near site of use.
Record time of injection, drug, dose, and injection site.

though they squirm and may be difficult to hold in position, they can usually be restrained without assistance. The body of a larger infant can be securely restrained between the nurse's arm and body (Fig. 27-21). To inject into the body of a muscle, the muscle mass is firmly grasped between the thumb and fingers to isolate and stabilize the site. However, in obese children it is preferable to first spread the skin with the thumb and index finger to displace subcutaneous tissue and then grasp the muscle deeply on each side.

If medication is given around the clock, the nurse must be careful to wake the child before giving the injection. Although it may seem easier to surprise the sleeping child and do it as quickly as possible, performing the procedure in this way can cause the child to fear going back to sleep. If awakened first, children will know that nothing will be done to them unless forewarned. The Guidelines box summarizes

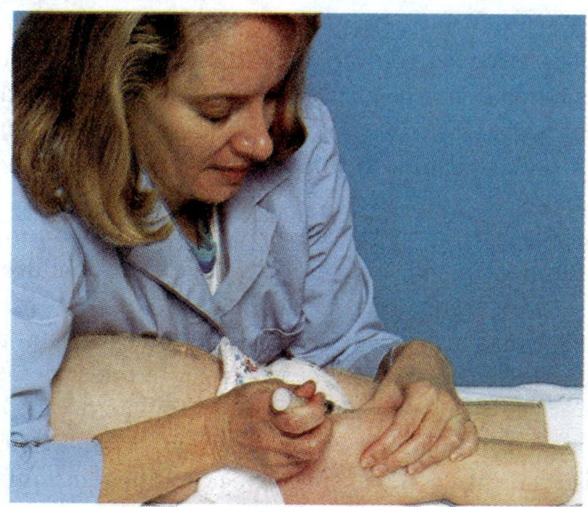

FIG. 27-21 Restraining small child for intramuscular injection. Note how nurse isolates and stabilizes muscle.

administration techniques that maximize safety and minimize the discomfort often associated with injections.

SUBCUTANEOUS AND INTRADERMAL ADMINISTRATION*

Subcutaneous and intradermal injections are frequently administered to children, but the technique differs little from the method used with adults. Examples of subcutaneous injections include insulin, hormone replacement, allergy desensitization, and some vaccines. Tuberculin (TB) testing, local anesthesia, and allergy testing are examples of frequently administered intradermal injections.

Techniques to minimize the pain associated with these injections include changing the needle if it pierced a rubber stopper on a vial, using 26- to 30-gauge needles (only to inject the solution), and injecting small volumes (up to 0.5 ml). The angle of the needle for the subcutaneous injection is typically 90 degrees. In children with little subcutaneous tissue, some practitioners insert the needle at a 45-degree angle. However, the benefit of using the 45-degree angle rather than the 90-degree angle remains controversial.

Although ***subcutaneous injections*** can be given anywhere there is subcutaneous tissue, common sites include the center third of the lateral aspect of the upper arm, the abdomen, and the center third of the anterior thigh. Some practitioners believe it is not necessary to aspirate before injecting subcutaneously; however, this is not universally accepted. Automatic injector devices do not aspirate before injecting.

When giving an ***intradermal injection*** into the volar surface of the forearm, the nurse should avoid the medial side of the arm, where the skin is more sensitive.

➤ **NURSING TIP** Families often need to learn injection techniques to administer medications, such as insulin, at home.* Begin teaching as early as possible to allow the family the maximum amount of practice time possible.

INTRAVENOUS (IV) ADMINISTRATION

The IV route for administering medications is frequently used in pediatric therapy. For some important drugs it is the only effective route of administration. This method is used for giving drugs to children who have poor absorption as a result of diarrhea, dehydration, or peripheral vascular collapse; children who need a high serum concentration of a drug; children who have resistant infections that require parenteral medication over an extended time; children who need continuous pain relief; and children who require emergency treatment.

Insertion sites and observation of the IV infusion are discussed in Chapter 28 under Parenteral Fluid Therapy and Venous Access Devices. However, several factors need to be considered in relation to IV medication. When a drug is administered intravenously, the effect is almost instantaneous and further control is limited. Most drugs for IV administration require a specified minimum dilution and/or rate of flow, and many are highly irritating or toxic to tissues outside the vascular system. In addition to the precautions and nursing observations related to IV therapy, factors to consider when preparing and administering drugs to infants and children by the IV route include:

- Amount of drug to be administered
- Minimum dilution of drug and if child is fluid restricted
- Type of solution in which drug can be diluted
- Length of time over which drug can be safely administered
- Rate of infusion that child and vessels can tolerate
- IV tubing volume capacity
- Time that this or another drug is to be administered
- Compatibility of all drugs that child is receiving intravenously and compatibility with infusion fluids

Before any IV infusion, the site of insertion is checked for patency. Medications are never administered with blood products. Only one antibiotic should be administered at a time.

IV infusion is suitable for children who can tolerate the necessary infusion rate and the extra fluid needed to administer the medication. For the very small infant or fluid-restricted child who is not able to tolerate the increased rate of fluids, other IV methods available are the direct technique and the retrograde technique. Although the medication must still be minimally diluted as recommended, the dose is administered closer to the child's vein, avoiding the need to also infuse the tubing volume.

For the ***direct technique,*** appropriately diluted medication is injected into the tubing at the site of the Y connection or through a stopcock in the direction of the child. A syringe pump may be used for a controlled rate. As syringe pumps become increasingly available, this method is being used more often for pediatric patients because of convenience, greater control over administration time, and the need to flush with less fluid when administering medication.

For the ***retrograde technique,*** appropriately diluted medication is injected into the IV tubing at the site of the Y connection or a stopcock, in the direction away from (retrograde) the child. The tubing is clamped, or the stopcock to the child is turned off. After the medication is injected, the tubing is unclamped or the stopcock opened, and the infusion resumes, with subsequent administration of the medication. This method does result in displacement of the fluid in the IV tubing, since the diluted medication is injected retrogradely. This fluid can be accommodated by an empty drip chamber (but not more than 3 ml) or by an empty syringe connected to an upper Y site or stopcock, which will accept the displaced fluid for discard. If the empty syringe method is used, the tubing volume between the two Y sites or stopcocks must be greater than the amount of diluted medication volume injected to avoid the medication reaching the discard syringe.

Regardless of the technique used, the nurse must know the minimum dilutions for safe administration of IV medications to infants and children.

---

*Home care instructions for giving subcutaneous injections are available in *Wong and Whaley's Clinical Manual of Pediatric Nursing* (Mosby).

NURSING ALERT An often unrecognized source of contamination for vascular access lines (peripheral and central) is stopcock ports. Unaccessed ports should be covered at all times with a sterile cap or syringe, which is changed if contaminated during access for medication administration or blood collection (Brosnan and others, 1988).

Several other methods of long-term venous access are available and include the peripheral lock device, central venous catheters, and implanted infusion ports (see Venous Access Devices, Chapter 28).

NASOGASTRIC, OROGASTRIC, OR GASTROSTOMY ADMINISTRATION

When a child has an indwelling feeding tube or a gastrostomy, oral medications are usually given via that route. An advantage of this method is the ability to administer oral medications around the clock without disturbing the child. A disadvantage is the risk of occluding or "clogging" the tube, especially when giving viscous solutions through small-bore feeding tubes. The most important preventive measure is adequate flushing after the medication is instilled (Leff and Roberts, 1988; Williams, 1989). See Guidelines box for guidelines for administration.

NURSING ALERT Sprinkle-type medication should be avoided. However, if there is no other option and the tube is large gauge (18 French or greater), but usually not a Foley catheter, it may be given by mixing the sprinkles with a small amount of pureed fruit and thinning with water. The fruit keeps the sprinkles suspended so they do not float to the top. Flush well. This procedure is not recommended for skin-level gastrostomy devices.

GUIDELINES
Nasogastric, Orogastric, or Gastrostomy Medication Administration in Children

- Use elixir or suspension (rather than tablets) preparations of medication whenever possible.
- Dilute viscous medication or syrup if possible with a small amount of water.
- If administering tablets, crush tablet to a very fine powder and dissolve drug in a small amount of warm water.
  - Never crush enteric-coated or sustained-release tablets or capsules.
- Avoid oily medications because they tend to cling to side of tube.
- Do not mix medication with enteral formula unless fluid is restricted. If adding a drug:
  - Check with pharmacist for compatibility.
  - Shake formula well and observe for any physical reaction (e.g., separation, precipitation).
  - Label formula container with name of medication, dosage, date, and time infusion started.
- Have medication at room temperature.
- Measure medication in calibrated cup or syringe.
- Check for correct placement of nasogastric or orogastric tube.
- Attach syringe (with adaptable tip but without plunger) to tube.
- Pour medication into syringe.
- Unclamp tube and allow medication to flow by gravity.
- Adjust height of container to achieve desired flow rate (e.g., increased height for faster flow).
- As soon as syringe is empty, pour in water to flush tubing.
  - Amount of water depends on length and gauge of tubing.
  - Determine amount before administering any medication by using a syringe to completely fill an unused nasogastric or orogastric tube with water. The amount of flush solution is usually 1½ times this volume.
  - With certain drug preparations (e.g., suspensions), more fluid may be needed.
- If administering more than one drug at the same time, flush the tube between each medication with clear water.
- Clamp tube after flushing, unless tube is left open.

RECTAL ADMINISTRATION

The rectal route for administration is less reliable but sometimes used when the oral route is difficult or contraindicated. Some of the drugs available in suppository form are aspirin, sedatives, analgesics (morphine), and antiemetics.* The difficulty in using the rectal route is that, unless the rectal ampulla is empty at the time of insertion, the absorption of the drug may be delayed, diminished, or prevented by the presence of feces. Sometimes the drug is later evacuated, securely surrounded by stool. However, the rectal route is used most frequently in children who are unable to take anything by mouth and are unlikely to have large amounts of stool. It is also used when oral preparations are unsuitable to control vomiting.

The wrapping on the suppository is removed, and the suppository is lubricated with water-soluble jelly or warm water. Using a glove or finger clot, the suppository is quickly but gently inserted into the rectum, making certain that it is placed beyond both the rectal sphincters. The buttocks are then held or taped together firmly to relieve pressure on the anal sphincter until the urge to expel the suppository has passed—5 to 10 minutes. Sometimes the amount of drug ordered is less than the dosage available. The irregular shape of most suppositories makes the process of dividing them into a desired dose difficult if not dangerous. If it must be halved, it should be cut lengthwise. However, there is no guarantee that the drug is evenly dispersed throughout the petrolatum base.

Rectal suppositories are usually inserted with the apex (pointed end) foremost. One study demonstrated easier insertion and a lower expulsion rate when the suppository was inserted with the base (blunt end) first. Reverse contractions or the pressure gradient of the anal canal may help the suppository to slip higher into the canal (Abd-El-Maeboud and others, 1991). This study, however, did not consider the issue of comfort on insertion.

If medication is administered via a retention enema, the same procedure is used. Drugs given by enema are diluted

*For information about compounding drugs in suppositories, contact **Technical Staff, Professional Compounding Centers of America (PCCA),** P.O. Box 368, Sugarland, TX 77487; (800) 331-2498.

in the smallest amount of solution possible to minimize the likelihood of being evacuated.

OPTIC, OTIC, AND NASAL ADMINISTRATION

There are few differences in administering eye, ear, and nose medication to children and to adults. The major difficulty is in gaining children's cooperation or employing restraining techniques. The infant's or young child's head is immobilized in the same manner as described in Fig. 7-31, *b*. Older children need only explanation and direction. Although the administration of optic, otic, and nasal medication is not painful, these drugs can cause unpleasant sensations, which can be eliminated with various techniques.

➤ **NURSING TIP** To reduce unpleasant sensations:

Eye—Apply finger pressure to the lacrimal punctum at the inner aspect of the lid for 1 minute to prevent drainage of medication to the nasopharynx and the unpleasant "tasting" of the drug.

Ear—Allow medications stored in the refrigerator to warm to room temperature before instillation.

Nose—Position the child with the head hyperextended to prevent strangling sensations caused by medication trickling into the throat rather than up into the nasal passages.

To instill eye medication, the child is placed supine or sitting with the head extended and is asked to look up. One hand is used to pull the lower lid downward; the hand that holds the dropper rests on the head so that it may move synchronously with the child's head, thus reducing the possibility of trauma to a struggling child or dropping medication on the face (Fig. 27-22). As the lower lid is pulled down, a small conjunctival sac is formed; the solution or ointment is applied to this area, never directly on the eyeball. Another effective technique is to pull the lower lid down and out to form a cup effect, into which the medication is dropped.

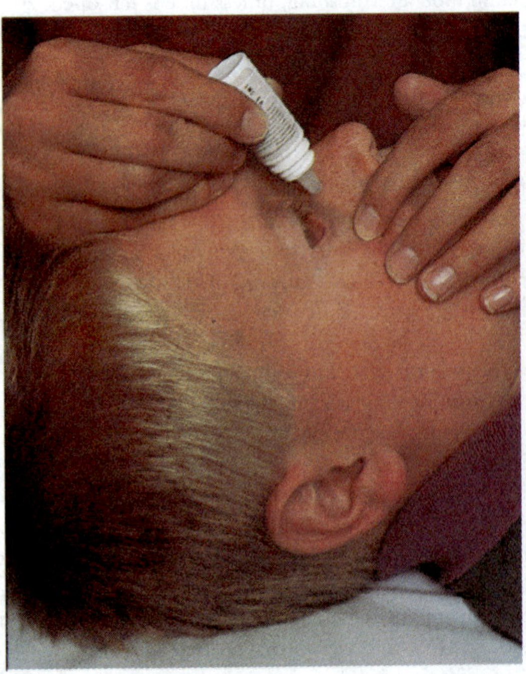

FIG. 27-22 Administering eye drops.

The lids are gently closed to prevent expression of the medication, and the child is asked to look in all directions to enhance even distribution of the preparation. Excess medication is wiped from the inner canthus outward to prevent contamination to the contralateral eye.

Instilling eye drops in infants can be difficult because they often clench the lids tightly closed. One approach is to place the drops in the nasal corner where the lids meet. The medication pools in this area, and when the child opens the lids, the medication flows onto the conjunctiva. For young children, playing a game can be helpful, such as instructing the child to keep the eyes closed until the count of 3, then to open them, at which time the drops are quickly instilled. Ointment can be applied when the child is sleeping by gently pulling down the lower lid and placing the ointment in the lower conjunctival sac.

NURSING ALERT If both eye ointment and drops are ordered, give drops first, wait 3 minutes, then apply the ointment to allow each drug to work. When possible, administer eye ointments before bedtime or naptime, since the child's vision will be blurred for a while.

Ear drops are instilled with the child restrained in the supine position and the head turned to the appropriate side. For children younger than 3 years of age, the external auditory canal is straightened by gently pulling the pinna downward and straight back. The pinna is pulled upward and back in children older than 3 years of age (see Fig. 7-25). To place the drops deep into the ear canal without contaminating the tip of the dropper, place a disposable ear speculum in the canal and administer the drops through the speculum. After instillation, the child should remain lying on the opposite side for a few minutes. Gentle massage of the area immediately anterior to the ear facilitates the entry of drops into the ear canal. The use of cotton pledgets prevents medication from flowing out of the external canal. However, they should be loose enough to allow any discharge to exit from the ear. Premoistening the cotton with a few drops of medication prevents the wicking action from absorbing the medication instilled in the ear.

Nose drops are instilled in the same manner as in the adult patient. Unpleasant sensations associated with medicated nose drops are minimized when care is taken to position the child with the head extended well over the edge of the bed or pillow (Fig. 27-23). Depending on their size, infants can be positioned in the football hold (see Fig. 27-7), in the nurse's arm with the head extended and stabilized between the nurse's body and elbow and the arms and hands immobilized with the nurse's hands, or with the head extended over the edge of the bed or a pillow. Following instillation of the drops, the child should remain in position for 1 minute to allow the drops to come in contact with the nasal surfaces.

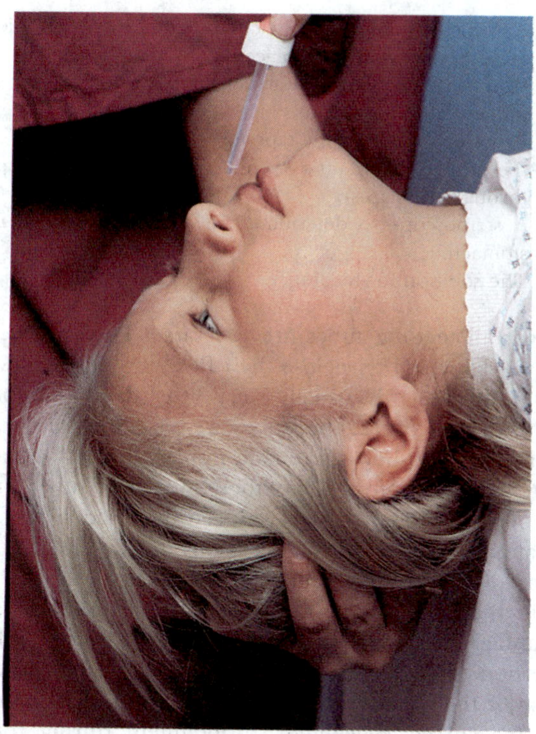

FIG. 27-23 Proper position for instilling nose drops.

FAMILY TEACHING AND HOME CARE

The nurse usually assumes the responsibility for preparing families to administer medications at home. The family should have an understanding of why the child is receiving the medication and the effects that might be expected, as well as the amount, frequency, and length of time the drug is to be administered. Instruction should be carried out in an unhurried, relaxed manner, preferably in an area away from busy ward or office routine, following the same guidelines for teaching outlined in the box on p. 1153.

The caregiver is carefully instructed regarding the correct dosage, and the nurse is responsible for preparing parents for the specifics of the task. Some persons have difficulty in understanding or interpreting terminology from the pharmacy, and just because they nod or otherwise indicate an understanding, it cannot be assumed that the message is clear. It is important to ascertain their interpretation of a teaspoon, for example, and to be certain they have acceptable devices for measuring the drug. If the drug is packaged with a dropper, syringe, or plastic cup, the nurse should show the point on the device that indicates the prescribed dose and demonstrate how the dose is drawn up into a dropper or syringe and measured and the bubbles eliminated. If the nurse has any doubts about the parent's ability to administer the correct dose, the parent should give a return demonstration. This is especially important when the drug has potentially serious consequences from incorrect dosage, such as insulin or digoxin, or when more complex administration is required, such as parenteral injections. When teaching a parent to give an injection, adequate time for instruction and practice must be allotted.

Home modifications are often necessary because the availability of equipment or assistance can differ from the hospital setting. For example, restraint is often required when giving medications to children, and the parent may need guidance in devising methods that allow for one person to restrain the child and safely give the drug. One successful method is described below.

➤ **NURSING TIP** To administer oral, nasal, or optic medication when only one person is available to restrain the child, use the following procedure:

- Place child supine on flat surface (bed, couch, floor).
- Sit facing child so that child's head is between operator's thighs and child's arms are under operator's legs.
- Place lower legs over child's legs to restrain lower body, if necessary.
- To administer oral medication, place small pillow under child's head to reduce risk of aspiration.
- To administer nasal medication, place small pillow under child's shoulders to aid flow of liquid through nasal passages.

The time that the drug is to be administered is clarified with the parent. For instance, when a drug is prescribed in association with meals, the number of meals that the family is accustomed to eat influences the amount of drug the child receives. Do they have meals twice a day or five times a day? When a drug is to be given several times during the day, together the nurse and parents can work out a schedule that accommodates the family routine. Occasionally a drug must be given at equal intervals throughout a 24-hour period. For example, telling them that the child needs 1 teaspoon of medicine four times a day is subject to misinterpretation, since parents may routinely schedule the doses at incorrect times. Instead, a preplanned schedule based on 6-hour intervals should be set up with the number of days required for therapeutic dosage listed. Written instructions should accompany all drug prescriptions.*

➤ **NURSING TIP** If parents have difficulty reading or understanding English, use colors to convey instructions. For example, mark each drug with a color and place the appropriate color on a calendar chart or on a drawing of a clock to identify when the drug needs to be given. If a liquid medication and syringe are used, also mark the syringe at the place the plunger needs to be with color-coded tape.

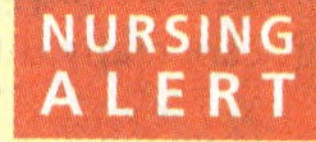

Dispose of any plastic covers that may be on the ends of syringes. These covers are small enough to be aspirated by young children (Botash, 1992).

GASTRIC FEEDING TECHNIQUES

Some children are unable to take nourishment by mouth because of conditions such as anomalies of the throat, esophagus, or bowel; impaired swallowing capacity; severe

---

*Home care instructions for giving medications are available in *Wong and Whaley's Clinical Manual of Pediatric Nursing* (Mosby).

debilitation; respiratory distress; or unconsciousness. These children are frequently fed by way of a tube inserted orally or nasally to the stomach ***(orogastric or nasogastric gavage)*** or duodenum/jejunum ***(enteral gavage)*** or by a tube inserted directly into the stomach (***gastrostomy***) or jejunum ***(jejunostomy)***. Such feedings may be intermittent or by continuous drip. Although the newer small-bore tubes may be used for enteral feedings, the following discussion is limited to gastric gavage and gastrostomy. Feeding resistance, a problem that may result from any long-term feeding method that bypasses the mouth, is discussed in Chapter 10. During normal feedings, infants are given a pacifier. Nonnutritive sucking has been shown to have several advantages, such as increased weight gain and decreased crying (Anderson, 1986). However, only pacifiers with a safe design must be used to prevent the possibility of aspiration. Using improvised pacifiers made from bottle nipples is not a safe practice.

When a child is concurrently receiving continuous-drip gastric or enteral feedings and parenteral (intravenous) therapy, the potential exists for inadvertent administration of the enteral formula through the circulatory system. The possibility for error increases when the parenteral solution is a fat emulsion, a milky appearing substance. Safeguards to prevent this potentially serious error include (Garvin and Franck, 1989):

- Use a separate, specifically designed enteral feeding pump mounted on a separate pole for continuous-feeding solutions.
- Label all tubing of continuous enteral feeding with brightly colored tape or labels.
- Use specifically designed continuous-feeding bags to contain the solutions instead of parenteral equipment, such as a burette.

GAVAGE FEEDING

Infants and children can be fed simply and safely by a tube passed into the stomach through either the nares or the mouth. The tube can be left in place or inserted and removed with each feeding. In older children it is usually less traumatic to tape the tube securely in place between feedings. When this alternative is used, the tube should be removed and replaced with a new tube according to hospital policy, specific orders, and the type of tube used. Meticulous handwashing is practiced during the procedure to prevent bacterial contamination of the feeding, especially during continuous-drip feedings.

Preparations

The equipment needed for gavage feeding includes:

- A suitable tube selected according to the size of the child and the viscosity of the solution being fed. Feeding tubes are available in silicone rubber, polyurethane, polyethylene, or polyvinylchloride. Polyurethane and silicone rubber tubes are smaller in diameter and more flexible than the others and are often referred to as small-bore tubes.
- A receptacle for the fluid; for small amounts a 10 to 30 ml syringe barrel or Asepto syringe is satisfactory; for larger amounts a 50 ml syringe with a catheter tip is more convenient.
- A syringe to aspirate stomach contents and/or to inject air after the tube has been placed.
- Water or water-soluble lubricant to lubricate the tube; sterile water is used for infants.
- Paper or nonallergenic tape to mark the tube and to attach the tube to the infant's or child's cheek (and nose, if placed through the nares).
- A stethoscope to determine the correct placement in the stomach.
- The solution for feeding.

Not all feeding tubes are the same. Polyethylene and polyvinylchloride types lose their flexibility and need to be replaced frequently, usually every 3 to 4 days. The polyurethane and silicone rubber tubes are indwelling and remain flexible so that they can remain in place longer and afford more patient comfort. Use of these small-bore tubes for continuous feeding has greatly reduced the incidence of complications, such as pharyngitis, otitis media, and incompetence of the lower esophageal sphincter (Wesley, 1988). While the increased softness and flexibility of the tubes are advantages, they also cause disadvantages, such as difficult insertion (may require a stylet, or metal guide wire), collapse of the tube during aspiration or gastric contents to test for correct placement, dislodgment during forceful coughing, and unsuitability for thick feedings (Moore and Green, 1985). Traditional methods for verifying placement are less reliable with the small-bore tubes (Metheny, 1988).

Procedure

Infants will be easier to control if they are first wrapped in a mummy restraint (see Fig. 27-9). Even tiny infants with random movements can grasp and dislodge the tube. Premature infants do not ordinarily require restraint, but if they do, a small towel folded across the chest and secured beneath the shoulders is usually sufficient. Care must be taken so that breathing is not compromised.

Whenever possible, the infant should be held during the procedure to associate the comfort of physical contact with the feeding. When this is not possible, gavage feeding is carried out with the infant or child on the back or toward the right side and the head and chest elevated. Feeding the child in a sitting position helps maintain the placement of the tube in the lowest position, thus increasing the likelihood of correct placement in the stomach.

The feeding tube can be passed through either the nose or the mouth. Since most young infants are obligatory nose breathers, insertion through the mouth causes less distress and helps to stimulate sucking. A tube passed through one of the nares in older infants and children is satisfactory once the tube is in place. An indwelling tube is almost always placed through the nose; the tube is alternated between nares with each insertion to minimize irritation, chance of infection, and possible breakdown of mucous membranes from pressure that occurs over time.

Two important issues remain unresolved regarding gavage feeding: measuring the insertion distance and checking the tube placement. Two standard methods of measuring tube length for insertion are (1) measuring from the nose to the bottom of the earlobe and then to the end of the xiphoid process or (2) measuring from the nose to the

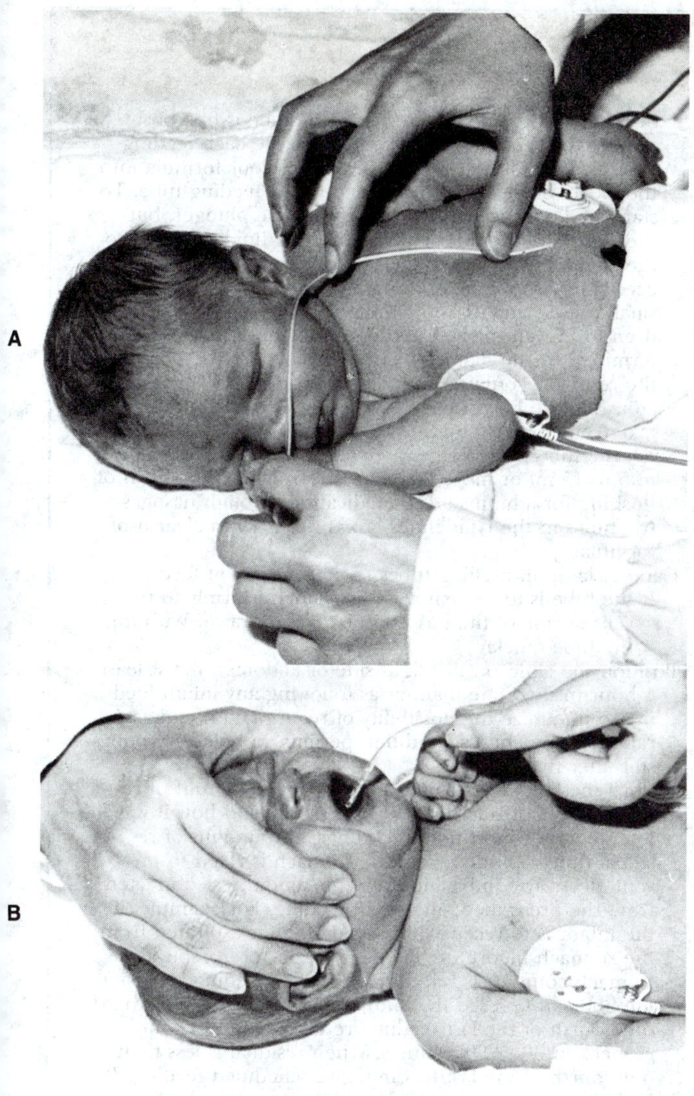

FIG. 27-24 Gavage feeding. **A,** Measuring tube for nasogastric feeding from tip of nose to earlobe and to midpoint between end of xiphoid process and umbilicus. **B,** Inserting the tube.

earlobe and then to a point midway between the xiphoid process and umbilicus (Fig. 27-24, *A*). However, research on using these methods in premature infants has found both placements to be too high (in the esophagus), although the second method provided better placement (Weibley and others, 1987). In a study on children 1 month to 18 years of age, the first method resulted in the *tip* of the tube, but not necessarily the side holes, being in the stomach 90% of the time. In the other 10% of the cases, the tip was above the esophageal sphincter (Welch and others, 1990). Studies have shown that height as a predictor of gastric tube insertion distance may provide a more valid measurement method (Ellett and others, 1992). For very-low-birth-weight infants, daily weight can be used to predict insertion length (Table 27-6). Until more definitive data are available, no method that results in a shorter distance than these methods should be used.

TABLE 27-6 Recommended Minimum Insertion Lengths for Orogastric Tubes in Very-Low-Birth-Weight Infants

	DAILY WEIGHT (G)			
	<750	750-999	1000-1249	1250-1499
Insertion length (cm)	13	15	16	17

From Gallaher KJ and others: Orogastric tube insertion length in very-low-birth-weight infants (<1500 grams), *J Perinatol* 13(2):128-131, 1993.

Unfortunately, "bedside" methods used to verify the placement of the tube have serious shortcomings (see Guidelines box). The only accurate method for testing tube placement is radiography, but this practice is not feasible before each feeding (Metheny, 1988). One method that appears promising is pH testing of aspirated fluid, since respiratory, gastric, and intestinal fluid have different pH (Metheny and others, 1989). Until pH is studied further, especially in children, nurses need to use the traditional methods with an awareness of their limitations. If doubt exists regarding correct placement, the physician should be consulted. The procedure for gavage feeding is described in the Guidelines box on p. 1194.

GASTROSTOMY FEEDING

Feeding by way of gastrostomy tube is a variation of tube feeding often used for children in whom passage of a tube through the mouth, pharynx, esophagus, and cardiac sphincter of the stomach is contraindicated or impossible. It is also used to avoid the constant irritation of a nasogastric tube in children who require tube feeding over an extended period. Placement of a gastrostomy tube may be performed with the child under general anesthesia or percutaneously using an endoscope and local anesthesia (Nelson and Hallgren, 1989). The tube is inserted through the abdominal wall into the stomach about midway along the greater curvature and secured by a purse-string suture. The stomach is anchored to the peritoneum at the operative site. The tube used can be a Foley, wing-tip, or mushroom catheter. Immediately after surgery the catheter may be left open and attached to gravity drainage for 24 hours or more.

Postoperative care of the wound site is directed toward prevention of infection and irritation. The area is cleansed at least daily or as often as needed to keep the area free of drainage. After healing occurs, meticulous care is needed to keep the area surrounding the tube clean and dry to prevent excoriation and infection. Daily applications of antibiotic ointment or other preparations may be prescribed to aid in healing and prevent irritation (see also p. 1196). Care is exercised to prevent excessive pull on the catheter that might cause widening of the opening and subsequent leakage of highly irritating gastric juices. Securely tape the tube to the abdomen, leaving a small loop of tubing at the exit site to prevent tension on the site.

For children on long-term gastrostomy feeding, a skin-level device (MIC-KEY, Bard Button, Gastroport) offers sev-

GUIDELINES
Nasogastric Tube Feedings in Children

Place the child supine with head slightly hyperflexed or in a sniffing position (nose pointed toward ceiling).

Measure the tube for approximate length of insertion, and mark the point with a small piece of tape.

Insert the tube that has been lubricated with sterile water or water-soluble lubricant through either the mouth or one of the nares to the predetermined mark. Since most young infants are obligatory nose breathers, insertion through the mouth causes less distress and helps to stimulate sucking. In older infants and children the tube is passed through the nose and alternated between nostrils. An indwelling tube is almost always placed through the nose.

- When using the nose, slip the tube along the base of the nose and direct it straight back toward the occiput.
- When entering through the mouth, direct the tube toward the back of the throat (Fig. 27-24, *B*).
- If the child is able to swallow on command, synchronize passing the tube with swallowing (see Nursing Tip on p. 1183).

Check the position of the tube by using *both* the following:

- Attach the syringe to the feeding tube and apply negative pressure. Aspiration of stomach contents indicates proper placement, but aspiration of respiratory secretions may be mistaken for stomach contents. However, absence of fluid is not necessarily evidence of improper placement. The stomach may be empty, the tube may not be in contact with stomach contents, or a small-bore flexible tube may collapse. Note the amount and character of any fluid aspirated and return the fluid to the stomach.
- With the syringe, inject a small amount of air (0.5 to 1 ml in premature or very small infants to 5 ml in larger children) into the tube while simultaneously listening with a stethoscope over the stomach area. Sounds of gurgling or growling will be heard if the tube is properly situated in the stomach, although it is possible to hear the air entering the stomach even when the tube is positioned above the gastroesophageal sphincter.
- Stabilize the tube by holding or taping it to the cheek, not to the forehead, because of possible damage to the nostril. To maintain correct placement, measure and record the amount of tubing extending from the nose or mouth to the distal port when the tube is first positioned. Recheck this measurement before each feeding.

Warm the formula to room temperature. Pour formula into the barrel of the syringe attached to the feeding tube. To start the flow, give a gentle push with the plunger, but then remove the plunger and allow the fluid to flow into the stomach by gravity. The rate of flow should not exceed 5 ml every 5 to 10 minutes in premature and very small infants and 10 ml/minute in older infants and children to prevent nausea and regurgitation. The rate is determined by the diameter of the tubing and the height of the reservoir containing the feeding and is regulated by adjusting the height of the syringe. A usual feeding may take from 15 to 30 minutes to complete.

Flush the tube with sterile water (1 or 2 ml for small tubes to 5 to 15 ml or more for large ones) or see discussion of flushing for administering medication through nasogastric tubes in the Guidelines box on p. 1189 to clear it of formula.

Cap or clamp indwelling tubes to prevent loss of feeding.

- If the tube is to be removed, first pinch it firmly to prevent escape of fluid as the tube is withdrawn. Withdraw the tube quickly.

Position the child on the right side or abdomen for at least 1 hour in the same manner as following any infant feeding to minimize the possibility of regurgitation and aspiration. If the child's condition permits, bubble the youngster after the feeding.

Record the feeding, including the type and amount of residual, the type and amount of formula, and how it was tolerated. For most infant feedings, any amount of residual fluid aspirated from the stomach is refed to prevent electrolyte imbalance, and the amount is subtracted from the prescribed amount of feeding. For example, if the infant is to receive 30 ml and 10 ml is aspirated from the stomach before the feeding, the 10 ml of aspirated stomach contents is refed plus 20 ml of feeding. Another method can be used in children. If residual is more than one fourth of the last feeding, return the aspirate and recheck in 30 to 60 minutes. When residual is less than one fourth of the last feeding, give scheduled feeding. If high aspirates persist and the child is due for another feeding, notify the practitioner.

eral advantages. The small, flexible silicone device protrudes slightly from the abdomen, is cosmetically pleasing in appearance, affords increased comfort and mobility to the child, is easy to care for, and is fully immersible in water. The one-way valve at the proximal end minimizes reflux and eliminates the need for clamping. However, the skin-level device requires a well-established gastrostomy site and is more expensive than the conventional tube. In addition, the valve may become clogged. When functioning, the valve prevents air from escaping; therefore the child may require frequent bubbling. With some devices, during feedings the child must remain fairly still, since the tubing easily disconnects from the opening if the child moves. With other devices, extension tubing can be securely attached to the opening (Fig. 27-25). The feeding is instilled at the other end of the tubing in a manner similar to that for a regular gastrostomy. The extension tubing may also have a separate medication port. Both the feeding and the medication ports have plugs attached. Some skin-level devices require a special tube to be able to decompress the stomach (check residual or decompress air), and some do not.

Positioning and feeding of water, formula, or pureed foods are done in the same manner and rate as for gavage feeding. After feedings the infant or child is positioned on the right side or in Fowler position, and the tube may be clamped or left open and suspended between feedings, depending on the child's condition. A clamped tube allows more mobility but is only appropriate if the child can tolerate intermittent feedings without vomiting or prolonged backup of feeding into the tube. Sometimes a Y tube is used to allow for simultaneous decompression during feeding. If a Foley catheter is used as the gastrostomy tube, very slight tension is applied and the tube is securely taped to maintain the balloon at the gastrostomy opening and prevent

GUIDELINES
Administration of Enemas to Children

AGE	AMOUNT (ml)	INSERTION DISTANCE (cm/inches)
Infant	120-240	2.5 (1)
2-4 years	240-360	5.0 (2)
4-10 years	360-480	7.5 (3)
11 years	480-720	10.0 (4)

leakage of gastric contents and the tube's progression toward the pyloric sphincter, where it may occlude the stomach outlet. As a precaution, the length of the tube is measured postoperatively and then remeasured each shift to be sure it has not slipped. A mark can be made above the skin level to further ensure its placement. When the gastrostomy tube is no longer needed, it is removed; the skin opening usually closes spontaneously by contracture.

PROCEDURES RELATED TO ELIMINATION

ENEMA

The procedure for giving an enema to an infant or child does not differ essentially from that for an adult, except for the type and amount of fluid administered and the distance for inserting the tube into the rectum (see Guidelines box). Depending on the volume, a syringe with rubber tubing, an enema bottle, or an enema bag should be used.

NURSING ALERT Proper insertion of the catheter tip, especially in infants, is essential to prevent rectal damage and perforation (see Fig. 7-7, *B*). If insertion of the enema tip causes discomfort, remove the tip and notify the physician.

An isotonic solution is used in children. Plain water is not used because, being hypotonic, it can cause rapid fluid shift and fluid overload. The Fleet enema (pediatric or adult sized) is not advised for children because of the harsh action of its ingredients (sodium biphosphate and sodium phosphate). Commercial enemas can be dangerous to patients with megacolon and to dehydrated or azotemic children. The osmotic effect of the Fleet enema may produce diarrhea, which can lead to metabolic acidosis. Other potential complications are extreme hyperphosphatemia, hypernatremia, and hypocalcemia, which may lead to neuromuscular irritability and coma (McCabe, Sibert, and Routledge, 1991).

➤ **NURSING TIP** If prepared saline is not available, it can be made by adding 1 teaspoon table salt to 500 ml (1 pint) tap water.

Since infants and young children are unable to retain the solution after it is administered, the buttocks must be held together for a short time to retain the fluid. The enema is administered and expelled while the child is lying with the buttocks over the bedpan and with the head and back supported by pillows. Older children are ordinarily able to hold the solution if they understand what to do and if they are not expected to hold it for too long. The nurse should have the bedpan handy or, for the ambulatory child, ensure that the bathroom is readily available before beginning the procedure. An enema is an intrusive procedure and thus threatening to the preschool child; therefore, a careful explanation is especially important to ease possible fear.

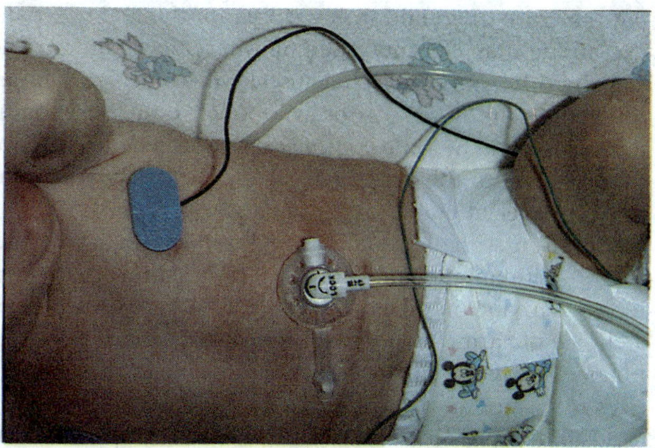

FIG. 27-25 Child with skin-level gastrostomy device (MIC-KEY), which provides for secure attachment of extension tubing to gastrostomy opening.

A preoperative bowel preparation solution given orally or through a nasogastric tube is increasingly being used instead of an enema. The polyethylene glycol–electrolyte lavage solution (Golytely) mechanically flushes the bowel without significant absorption, thereby avoiding potential fluid and electrolyte imbalances (Konings, 1989).*

OSTOMIES

Children may require stomas for various health problems. The most frequent causes are necrotizing enterocolitis and imperforate anus in the infant, less often Hirschsprung disease. In the older child the most frequent causes are inflammatory bowel disease, especially Crohn disease (regional enteritis), and ureterostomies for distal ureter or bladder defects.

Care and management of ostomies in the older child differ little from the care of ostomies in the adult patient. The major emphasis in pediatric care is the preparation of the child for the procedure and teaching care of the ostomy to the child and family. The basic principles of preparation are the same as for any procedure (see p. 1135). Simple, straightforward language is most effective, together with the use of illustrations and a replica model; for example, draw-

*Home care instructions for giving an enema are available in *Wong and Whaley's Clinical Manual of Pediatric Nursing* (Mosby).

ing a picture of a child with a stoma on the abdomen and explaining it as "another opening where bowel movements [or any other term the child uses] will come out." At another time the nurse can draw a pouch over the opening to demonstrate how the contents are collected. Using a doll to demonstrate the process is an excellent teaching strategy, and special books are available.*

Children with ileostomies are fitted immediately after surgery with an appliance to protect the skin from the proteolytic enzymes in the liquid stool. Parents are usually given a choice of caring for the colostomy with or without an appliance. Pediatric appliances are available in a variety of sizes to ensure an adequate fit.†

Ostomy equipment consists of a one- or two-piece system with a hypoallergenic skin barrier to maintain peristomal skin integrity. The pouch should be large enough to contain a moderate amount of stool and flatus but not so large as to overwhelm the infant or child. A backing helps minimize the risk of skin breakdown from moisture trapped between the skin and pouch. Small clips or rubber bands should be avoided to prevent choking in the young child.

Granulation tissue may grow around an ostomy site (Fig. 27-26). This moist, beefy red tissue is not a sign of infection. However, if it continues to grow, the excess moisture can cause irritation of the surrounding skin.

Protection of the peristomal skin is a major aspect of stoma care. Well-fitting appliances are important to prevent leakage of contents. Before the appliance is applied, the skin is prepared with a skin sealant that is allowed to dry. Then stoma paste is applied around the base of the stoma. The sealant and paste work together to prevent peristomal breakdown.

In infants with a colostomy left unpouched, skin care is similar to that of any diapered child. However, the peristomal skin is protected with a wafer barrier, such as a hydrocolloid dressing (e.g., Duoderm) or a barrier substance (e.g., zinc oxide ointment [Desitin], karaya products, or a mixture of zinc oxide ointment and karaya powder). If the skin becomes inflamed, denuded, or infected, the care is similar to the interventions used for diaper dermatitis (see Chapter 13). A product that helps protect healthy skin, heal excoriated skin, and minimize pain associated with skin breakdown is Ilex Dermalyte Protective Barrier Ointment.‡ The ointment adheres to denude weeping skin. It can be applied over topical antifungal and antibacterial agents if infection is present. If the infant is diapered, a coating of petrolatum is applied over the Ilex to prevent the gluteal creases and diaper from adhering to the ointment. When the area is cleaned, only the petrolatum is wiped off and reapplied. The Ilex is left intact to minimize trauma to the irritated skin. If Ilex is used under an appliance, an adhesive spray is applied over the ointment to help the appliance adhere.

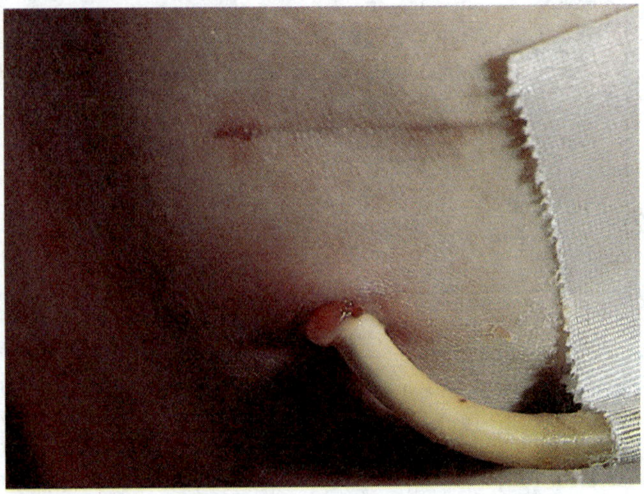

FIG. 27-26 Appearance of healthy granulation tissue around stoma.

With young children, protection of the pouch from being pulled off is also an important consideration. One-piece outfits keep exploring hands from reaching the pouch, and the loose waist prevents any pressure on the appliance. Keeping the child occupied with toys during the pouch change is also helpful. As children mature, their participation in ostomy care is encouraged. Even preschoolers can assist by holding supplies, pulling paper backings from the appliance, and helping clean the stoma area. Toilet training for bladder control needs to begin at the appropriate time as for any other child.

Older children and adolescents should eventually have total responsibility for ostomy care just as they would for usual bowel function. During adolescence, concerns for body image and the ostomy's impact on intimacy and sexuality emerge. The nurse should stress to teenagers that the presence of a stoma need not interfere with their activities. These youngsters can choose which ostomy equipment is best suited to their needs. Attractively designed and decorated pouch covers are well liked by teenagers (Erwin-Toth, 1988).

FAMILY TEACHING AND HOME CARE

Since these children are almost always discharged with a functioning colostomy, preparation of the family should begin as early as possible in the hospital. The family is instructed in the application of the device (if used), care of the skin, and instructions regarding appropriate action in case skin problems develop. Early evidence of skin breakdown or stomal complications, such as ribbonlike stools, excessive diarrhea, bleeding, prolapse, or failure to pass flatus or stool, is brought to the attention of the physician, the nurse, or the stoma specialist. The same principles are

Chris Has an Ostomy is available from the **United Ostomy Association, Inc.**, 36 Executive Park, Suite 120, Irvine, CA 92714-6744; (800) 826-0826.

†Little Ones Ostomy Products, ConvaTec, CN 5254, Princeton, NJ 08543-5254; (800) 422-8811.

‡Available from MEDCON Products, Inc., 50 Brigham Hill Rd., Grafton, MA 01519; (800) 443-6332.

applied as discussed earlier in this chapter for compliance, especially in terms of education (see p. 1153), and in Chapter 26 for discharge planning and home care.*

*Home care instructions on caring for a colostomy are available in *Wong and Whaley's Clinical Manual of Pediatric Nursing* (Mosby).

KEY POINTS

- Informed consent is valid when the person is capable of giving consent (is over the age of majority and is competent), the person is supplied with information needed to make an intelligent decision, and the person acts voluntarily when exercising freedom of choice.
- Informed consent is needed for major surgery, minor surgery, and diagnostic tests and medical treatments with an element of risk.
- The major principles in psychologic preparation of the child for surgery are to establish trust, provide support, and give an explanation in easy-to-understand terms.
- Most parents and children want to be together during stressful procedures and should be offered this opportunity, with guidance on how the parent can comfort the child.
- In the performance of a procedure the nurse should expect success, involve the child when possible in the procedure, provide distraction, and allow for expression of feelings.
- In giving postprocedural support, the nurse should encourage children to express their feelings and praise them for completion of the procedure.
- Six stressful times before and after surgery that produce anxiety in children are the day of admission, blood tests, the afternoon of the day before surgery, injection of preoperative medication, transportation to the operating room, and return from the postanesthesia care unit.
- Assessment of compliance entails measuring factors that affect compliance (through clinical judgment, self-reporting, and direct observation), monitoring therapeutic response, taking pill counts, and performing chemical assay.
- Compliance strategies may be classified as organizational, educational, and behavioral.
- Knowledge of the sick child's eating habits and favorite foods can help in maintaining adequate nutrition.
- Control of fever may be accomplished by pharmacologic means (administration of antipyretics); hyperthermia is controlled by environmental means (minimum clothing, increased air circulation, hypothermia mattress, and/or cool compresses).
- Infection control may be based on one of three basic systems: category-specific isolation precautions, disease-specific isolation precautions, or universal precautions. Only the system of universal precautions, especially body substance isolation, provides protection when the infected person is undiagnosed.
- Ensuring safety in the hospital setting is a major concern and can be achieved through environmental measures, infection control measures, limit-setting, and safe transportation.
- Restraints are used cautiously and typically require a medical order.
- Factors that affect drug dosage determination are growth and maturation, difficulty in evaluating drug response, and body surface area.
- Family teaching regarding medication administration includes telling parents why the child is receiving the drug, its possible effects, and the amount, frequency, and length of time the drug is to be administered.
- The major forms of gastric feeding for children are gavage feeding and gastrostomy feeding.
- In the care of children with ostomies, nurses play an important role in family support and instruction in care of the stoma site.

REFERENCES

Abbott K: Therapeutic use of play in the psychological preparation of preschool children undergoing cardiac surgery, *Issues Compr Pediatr Nurs* 13:265-277, 1990.

Abd-El-Maeboud K and others: Rectal suppository: common-sense and mode of insertion, *Lancet* 338(8770):798-800, 1991.

Acute Pain Management Guideline Panel: *Acute pain management: operative or medical procedures and trauma,* Clinical Practice Guideline, AHCPR Pub No 92-0032, Rockville, MD, 1992, Agency for Health Care Policy and Research, Public Health Service, US Department of Health and Human Services.

American Academy of Pediatrics, Committee on Drugs: Guidelines for monitoring and management of pediatric patients during and after sedation for diagnostic and therapeutic procedures, *Pediatrics* 86(6):1110-1115, 1992.

American Pain Society: *Principles of analgesic use in the treatment of acute pain and cancer pain,* ed 3, Skokie, IL, 1992, The American Society.

Anderson GC: Pacifiers: the positive side, *MCN* 11(2):122-124, 1986.

Arditi M, Killner M: Coma following use of rubbing alcohol for fever control, *Am J Dis Child* 141(3):237-238, 1987.

Baker M, Fosarelli P, Carpenter R: Childhood fever: correlation of diagnosis with temperature response to acetaminophen, *Pediatrics* 80(3):315-318, 1987.

Banco L, Jayashekaramurthy S: The ability of mothers to read a thermometer, *Clin Pediatr* 29(6):343-345, 1990.

Banco L, Powers A: Hospitals: unsafe environments for children, *Pediatrics* 82(5):794-797, 1988.

Bates T, Broome M: Preparation of children for hospitalization and surgery: a review of the literature, *J Pediatr Nurs* 1(4):230-234, 1986.

Bauchner H, Vinci R, Waring C: Pediatric procedures: do parents want to watch? *Pediatrics* 84(5):907-909, 1989.

Baumgardner CA and others: Effects of nail polish on microbial growth of fingernails, *AORN J* 58(1):85-88, 1993.

Beecroft P, Redick S: Intramuscular injection practices of pediatric nurses: site selection, *Nurs Educ* 15(4):23-28, 1990.

Berg AT and others: Predictors of recurrent febrile seizures: a metaanalytic review, *J Pediatr* 116(3):329-337, 1990.

Billmire D, Neale H, Gregory R: Use of IV fentanyl in the outpatient treatment of pediatric facial trauma, *J Trama* 25(11):1079-1080, 1985.

Botash SA: Syringe caps: an aspiration hazard, *Pediatrics* 90(1):92-93, 1992.

Bourgault A: A hair piece, *Nursing 85* 15(9):80, 1985.

Broome ME: Preparation of children for painful procedures, *Pediatr Nurs* 16(6):537-541, 1990.

Broome M, Endsley R: Maternal presence, childrearing practices, and children's response to an injection, *Res Nurs Health* 12:229-235, 1989.

Broome M, Lillis P: A descriptive analysis of pediatric pain management research, *J Appl Nurs Res* 2(2):74-81, 1989.

Broome M, Lillis P, Smith M: Pain interventions in children: a meta-analysis of the research, *Nurs Res* 38(3):154-158, 1989.

Brosnan KM and others: Contamination stopcock, *Am J Nurs* 88(3):320-323, 1988.

Brown SR: An anxiety reduction technique during lumbar punctures in infants and toddlers, *J Assoc Pediatr Oncol Nurs* 1(3):24-25, 1984.

Bruce JL, Grove SK: Fever: pathology and treatment, *Crit Care Nurse* 12(1):40-55, 1992.

Bryant RA, editor: Acute and chronic wounds: nursing management, St Louis, 1992, Mosby.

Chaplin G, Shull H, Welk PC III: How safe is the air-bubble technique for I.M. injections? *Nursing 85* 15(9):59, 1985.

Cooke R, Werkman S, Watson D: Urine output measurements in premature infants, *Pediatrics* 83(1):116-118, 1989.

Coté CJ: Sedation for the pediatric patient: a review, *Pediatr Clin North Am* 41(1):31-58, 1994.

Courtney SE and others: Capillary blood gases in the neonate: a reassessment and review of the literature, *Am J Dis Child* 144:168-172, 1990.

Cramer JA and others: How often is medication taken as prescribed? A novel assessment technique, *JAMA* 261(22):3273-3277, 1989.

Cromer BA and others: Psychosocial determinants of compliance in adolescents with iron deficiency, *Am J Dis Child* 143(1):55-58, 1989.

Dyson A, Bogod D: Minimizing bruising in the antecubital fossa after venipuncture, *Br Med J* 294(6588):1659, 1987.

Ellerton ML, Caty S, Ritchie JA: Helping young children master intrusive procedures through play, *Child Health Care* 13(4):167-173, 1985.

Ellett M and others: Predicting the distance for gavage tube placement in children using regression on height, *Pediatr Nurs* 18(2):119-121, 127, 1992.

Ellis R: Once more into the void, *Contemp Pediatr* 6(8):164, 1989.

Erlen JA: The child's choice: an essential component in treatment decisions, *Child Health Care* 15(3):156-160, 1987.

Erwin-Toth P: Teaching ostomy care to the pediatric client: a developmental approach, *J Enterostom Ther* 15:126-130, 1988.

Faber MM: A review of efforts to protect children from injury in crashes, *Fam Community Health* 4(3):25-41, 1986.

Fina DK: A chance to say goodbye, *Am J Nurs* 94(5):42-45, 1994.

Forlini J, Morin DM, Treacy S: Painless peds procedures, *Am J Nurs* 87(3):321-323, 1987.

Fradet C and others: A prospective survey of reactions to blood tests by children and adolescents, *Pain* 49(1):53-60, 1990.

Funk MJ, Mullins LL, Olson RA: Teaching children to swallow pills: a case study, *Child Health Care* 13(1):20-23, 1984.

Gablehouse BL, Gitterman BA: Maternal understanding of commonly used medical terms in a pediatric setting, *Am J Dis Child* 114:419, 1990.

Garvin G, Franck L: Preventing delivery of enteral formula via parenteral route, *Pediatr Nurs* 15(1):17-18, 1989.

Gauderer M, Lorig J, Eastwood D: Is there a place for parents in the operating room? *J Pediatr Surg* 24(7):705-707, 1989.

Ghishan FK: The transport of electrolytes in the gut and the use of oral rehydrating solutions, *Pediatr Clin North Am* 35(1):35-51, 1988.

Goodman LJ and others: A urine preservative system to maintain bacterial counts, *Clin Pediatr* 24(7):383-386, 1985.

Gribetz B, Cronley S: Underdosing of acetaminophen by parents, *Pediatrics* 80(5):630-633, 1987.

Hagelgans NA: Pediatric skin care issues for the home care nurse, *Pediatr Nurs* 19(5):499-507, 1993.

Hamner SB, Miles MS: Coping strategies in children with cancer undergoing bone marrow aspirations, *J Assoc Pediatr Oncol Nurs* 5(3):11-15, 1988.

Hanna WJ, Sherlock H: Recall and fears of anaesthesia and surgery in 50 Jamaican paediatric patients, *West Indian Med J* 32:75-82, 1983.

Hannallah R, Rosales J: Experience with parents' presence during anaesthesia induction in children, *Can Anaesth Soc J* 30(3):287-290, 1983.

Heiney SP: Helping children through painful procedures, *Am J Nurs* 20-24, 1991.

Hicks JF and others: Optimum needle length for diphtheria-tetanus-pertussis inoculation of infants, *Pediatrics* 84(1):136-137, 1989.

Hogue EE: Informed consent: implications for critical care nurses, *Pediatr Nurs* 14(4):315-316, 1988.

Holtzclaw BJ: Control of febrile shivering during amphotericin B therapy, *Oncol Nurs Forum* 17(4):521-524, 1990.

Holtzclaw BJ: Monitoring body temperature, *AACN Clin Issues Crit Care Nurs* 4(1):44-55, 1993.

Howland M, Goldfrank L: Meperidine usage in patients with sickle cell crisis, *Ann Emerg Med* 15(12):1506-1507, 1986.

Humphrey G and others: The occurrence of high levels of acute behavioral distress in children and adolescents undergoing routine venipunctures, *Pediatrics* 90(1):87-91, 1992.

Intramuscular injections: a guide to sites and techniques, Philadelphia, 1985, Wyeth Laboratories.

Ipp MM and others: Adverse reactions to diphtheria, tetanus, pertussis-polio vaccination at 18 months of age: effect of injection site and needle length, *Pediatrics* 83(5):679-682, 1989.

Johns Hopkins Hospital, *The Harriet Lane handbook,* ed 13, edited by Johnson KO, St Louis, 1993, Mosby.

Johnston CC, Stevens B, Arbess G: The effect of the sight of blood and use of decorative adhesive bandages on pain intensity ratings by preschool children, *J Pediatr Nurs* 8(3):147-151, 1993.

Johnston CC and others: Parental presence during anesthesia induction, *AAORN J* 47(1):187-194, 1988.

Jones ST: Reducing children's psychological stress in the operating suite, *Ophthalmic Plast Reconstr Surg* 1:199-203, 1985.

Joyner M: Hair care in the black patient, *J Pediatr Health Care* 2(6):281-287, 1988.

Kilman C: Parents' knowledge and practices related to fever management, *Pediatr Health Care* 1(4):173-179, 1987.

Kinmouth AL, Fulton Y, Campbell MJ: Management of feverish children at home, *Br Med J* 305(6862):1134-1136, 1992.

Konings K: Preop use of Golytely in pediatrics, *Pediatr Nurs* 15(5):473-474, 1989.

Koren G, Barzilay Z, Greenwald M: Tenfold errors in administration of drug doses: a neglected iatrogenic disease in pediatrics, *Pediatrics* 77(6):848-849, 1986.

Korniewicz D, Laughon B, Butz A: Integrity of vinyl and latex procedure gloves, *Nurs Res* 38:144-146, 1989.

Krouskop TA and others: Effectiveness of mattress overlays in reducing interface pressures during recumbency, *J Rehabil Res Dev* 22(3):7-10, 1985.

Krueger H, Osborn L: Effects of hygiene among the uncircumcised, *J Fam Pract* 22(4):353-355, 1986.

Larson E: Handwashing: it's essential—even when you use gloves, *Am J Nurs* 89(7):934-939, 1989.

Leff R, Roberts R: Enteral drug administration practices: report of a preliminary survey, *Pediatrics* 81(4):549-551, 1988.

Lehmann M and others: Upright or lying down: is one better for doing a lumbar puncture (LP)? *Am J Dis Child* 144:427, 1990.

Leisure MK, Dudley SM, Donowitz LG: Does a clean-catch urine sample reduce bacterial contamination? *N Engl J Med* 328(4):289-290, 1993.

Lewis JF, Alexander JJ: Overnight refrigeration of urine specimens for culture, *South Med J* 73(3):351-352, 1980.

Lohr J, Donowitz L, Dudley S: Bacterial contamination rates in voided urine collections in girls, *J Pediatr* 114(1):91-93, 1989.

Lybrand M, Medoff-Cooper B, Monro B: Periodic comparisons of specific gravity using urine from a diaper and collecting bag, *MCN* 15(4):238-239, 1990.

Lynch P and others: Rethinking the role of isolation practices in the prevention of nosocomial infections, *Ann Intern Med* 107:243-246, 1987.

Mandelbaum J: The food square: helping people of different cultures understand balanced diets, *Pediatr Nurs* 9(1):20-21, 1983.

Mansson ME, Fredrikzon B, Rosberg B: Comparison of preparation and narcotic-sedative premedication in children undergoing surgery, *Pediatr Nurs* 18(4):337-342, 1992.

Maunuksela E, Rajantie J, Simes M: Flunitrazepam-fentanyl-induced sedation and analgesia for bone marrow aspiration and needle biopsy in children, *Acta Anaesthesiol Scand* 30:409-411, 1986.

McCabe M, Sibert JR, Routledge PA: Phosphate enemas in childhood: cause for concern, *Br Med J* 302(6784):1074, 1991.

McCaffery M, Beebe A: *Pain: clinical manual for nursing practice,* St Louis, 1989, Mosby.

McLeod SM, McClowry SG: Using temperament theory to individualize the psychosocial care of hospitalized children, *Child Health Care* 19(2):79-85, 1990.

McMullen A and others: Heparinized saline or normal saline as a flush solution in intermittent intravenous lines in infants and children, *MCN* 18(2):78-85, 1993.

Meichenbaum D: Noncompliance, *Feelings Med Signif* 31(2):5-8, 1989.

Merritt K, Sargent J, Osborn L: Attitudes regarding parental presence during medical procedures, *Am J Dis Child* 144(3):270-271, 1990.

Metheny N: Measures to test placement of nasogastric and nasointestinal feeding tubes: a review, *Nurs Res* 37(6):324-329, 1988.

Metheny N and others: Effectiveness of pH measurements in predicting feeding tube placement, *Nurs Res* 38(5):280-285, 1989.

Millam DA: Getting into an artery, *Am J Nurs* 88(9):1214-1217, 1988.

Moore MC, Green HL: Tube feedings of infants and children, *Pediatr Clin North Am* 32(2):401-417, 1985.

Nahata MC, Clotz MA, Krogg EA: Adverse effects of meperidine, promethazine, and chlorpromazine for sedation in pediatric patients, *Clin Pediatr* 24:558-560, 1985.

Nelson C, Hallgren R: Gastrostomies: indications, management, and weaning, *Infants Young Child* 2(1):66-74, 1989.

Newman J: Evaluation of sponging to reduce body temperature in febrile children, *Can Med Assoc J* 132:641-642, 1985.

Nix KS: Obtaining informed consent. In Smith DP and others, editors: *Comprehensive child and family nursing skills,* St Louis, 1991, Mosby.

Olsen RJ and others: Examination gloves as barriers to hand contamination in clinical practice, *JAMA* 270(3):350-353, 1993.

O'Malley ME, McNamara ST: Children's drawings: a preoperative assessment tool, *AORN J* 57(5):1074-1089, 1993.

Orenstein S and others: The Santmyer swallow: a new and useful infant reflex, *Lancet* 1(8581):345-346, 1988.

Paes B and others: A comparative study of heelstick devices for infant blood collection, *Am J Dis Child* 147:346-348, 1993.

Perin G, Frase D: Development of a program using general anesthesia for invasive procedures in a pediatric outpatient setting, *J Pediatr Oncol Nurs* 3(4):8-10, 1985.

Peterson L, Toler S: An information seeking disposition in child surgery patients, *Health Psychol* 5(4):343-358, 1986.

Pidgeon V: Compliance with chronic illness regimens: school-aged children and adolescents, *J Pediatr Nurs* 4(1):36-47, 1989.

Pollack CV, Pollack ES, Andrew ME: Suprapubic bladder aspiration versus urethral catheterization in ill infants: success, efficiency, and complication rates, *Ann Emerg Med* 23(2):225-230, 1994.

Rae WA, Fournier CJ: Ethical issues in pediatric research: preserving psychosocial care in scientific inquiry, *Child Health Care* 14(4):242-248, 1986.

Rapoff MA: Helping parents to help their children comply with treatment regimens for chronic diseases, *Issues Compr Pediatr Nurs* 9(3):147-156, 1986.

Reeves-Swift R: Rational management of a child's acute fever, *MCN* 15(2):82-85, 1990.

Rhodes AM: Children and the law, *MCN* 13:171, 1988.

Rollins J, Brantly D: Preparing the child for procedures. In Smith DP and others, editors: *Comprehensive child and family nursing skills,* St Louis, 1991, Mosby.

Ros S: Outpatient pediatric analgesia—a tale of two regimens, *Pediatr Emerg Care* 3(4):228-230, 1987.

Rosenstock IM: Enhancing patient compliance with health recommendations, *J Pediatr Health Care* 2(2):67-72, 1988.

Ross DM, Ross SA: Childhood pain: the school-aged child's viewpoint, *Pain* 29(2):179-191, 1984.

Rudy C: A drop or a dropper: the risk of overdose, *J Pediatr Health Care* 6(1):40, 51-52, 1992.

Saez-Llorens X and others: Bacterial contamination rates for non-clean catch and clean catch midstream urine collections in uncircumcised boys, *J Pediatr* 114(1):93-95, 1989.

Savedra M: Parental responses to a painful procedure performed on their child. In Azarnoff P, Hardgrove C, editors: *The family in child health care,* New York, 1981, John Wiley & Sons.

Schlager TA and others: Bacterial contamination rate of urine collected in a urine bag from healthy non-toilet-trained male infants, *J Pediatr* 116(5):738-739, 1990.

Schofield NM and White JB: Interrelations among children, parents, premedication, and anaesthetists in paediatric day stay surgery, *Br Med J* 299(6712):1371-1375, 1989.

Schreiner MS: Preoperative and postoperative fasting in children, *Pediatr Clin North Am* 41(1):111-120, 1994.

Schreiner V: Don't discard this specimen, *Nursing '87* 17(10):5, 1987.

Shaw EG, Routh DK: Effect of mother presence on children's reaction to aversive procedures, *J Pediatr Psychol* 7(1):33-42, 1982.

Siaw SN, Stephens LR, Holmes SS: Knowledge about medical instruments and reported anxiety in pediatric surgery patients, *Child Health Care* 14(3):134-141, 1986.

Singleton MA, Rosen JI, Fisher DM: Plasma concentrations of fentanyl in infants, children and adults, *Can J Anaesth* 34(2):152-155, 1987.

Snodgrass WR, Dodge WF: Lytic/"DPT" cocktail: time for rationale and safe alternatives, *Pediatr Clin North Am* 36(5):1285-1291, 1989.

Stebor A: Posturination time and specific gravity in infant's diapers, *Nurs Res* 38(4):244-245, 1989.

Stoller KP, Losey R: Inadvertent intra-arterial injection of penicillin: an unseen danger, *Pediatrics* 75(4):785-786, 1985.

Streiff LD: Can clients understand our instructions? *Image* 18(2):48-52, 1986.

Suri S: Simplifying urine collection from infants and children without losing accuracy, *MCN* 13(12):438-441, 1988.

US Department of Agriculture: Potential hazards with protective restraint devices, *FDA Med Bull* 21(3), 1992.

US Department of Labor, Occupational Safety and Health Administration: *Occupational exposure to bloodborne pathogen,* final rule, 29 DFR part 1910.1030, Washington DC, 1991, US Government Printing Office.

Van R and others: The effect of diaper type and overclothing on fecal contamination in day-care centers, *JAMA* 265(14):1840-1844, 1991.

Venham LL, Bengston D, Cipes M: Parent's presence and the child's response to dental stress, *J Dent Child* 45(3):213-217, 1978.

Vernon DTA, Foley JM, Schulman JL: Effect of mother-child separation and birth order on young children's responses to two potentially stressful experiences, *J Pers Soc Psychol* 5(2):162-174, 1967.

Vessey J, Caserza L, Bogetz M: In my opinion . . . another Pandora's box? Parental participation in anesthetic induction, *Child Health Care* 19(2):116-118, 1990.

Villarreal P: *Personal communication,* San Antonio, 1992, University of Texas.

Visintainer MA, Wolfer JA: Psychological preparation for surgical pediatric patients: the effect of children's and parents' stress responses and adjustment, *Pediatrics* 56(2):187-202, 1975.

Watson PD and others: Ibuprofen, acetaminophen, and placebo treatment of febrile children, *Clin Pharmacol Ther* 46(1):9-17, 1989.

Weekes DP, Savedra MC: Adolescent cancer: coping with treatment-related pain, *J Pediatr Nurs* 3(5):318-328, 1988.

Weibley TT and others: Gavage tube insertion in the premature infant, *MCN* 12:24-27, 1987.

Welch JA and others: Staff nurses' experiences as co-investigators in a clinical research project, *Pediatr Nurs* 16(4):364-367, 396, 1990.

Wesley JR: Special access to the intestinal tract. In *Enteral feeding: scientific basis and clinical application,* Report of the 94th Ross Conference on Pediatric Research, Columbus, OH, 1988, Ross Laboratories.

Williams PJ: How do you keep medicines from clogging feeding tubes? *Am J Nurs* 89(2):181-182, 1989.

Wlody GS: Malignant hyperthermia, *Crit Care Nurs Clin North Am* 3(1):129-134, 1991.

Wong DL, Redding B: Lozenges can be "lifesavers," *Am J Nurs* 87(9):1129-1130, 1987.

Wong DL, Baker CM: Pain in children: comparison of assessment scales, *Pediatr Nurs* 14(1):9-17, 1988.

Wong DL: DPT or pedi-cocktail: not a good mix, *Am J Nurs* 94(6):15, 1994.

Woolverton E: Practice pointers, *School Health Watch* 2(4):2, 1991.

BIBLIOGRAPHY

Informed Consent

Appelbaum PS, Grisson T: Assessing patients' capacities to consent to treatment, *N Engl J Med* 319(25):1635-1638, 1988.

Davis AJ: Clinical nurses' ethical decision making in situations of informed consent, *Adv Nurs Sci* 11(3):63-69, 1989.

Erickson S and others: Gray areas: informed consent in pediatric and comatose adult patients, *Heart Lung* 16(3):323-325, 1987.

Erlen JA: The child's choice: an essential component in treatment decisions, *Child Health Care* 15(3):156-160, 1987.

Hogue EE: Consent for minors, *Pediatr Nurs* 15(4):404, 1989.

Leiken S: A proposal concerning decisions to forgo life-sustaining treatment for young people, *J Pediatr* 115(1):17-22, 1989.

Northrop CE, Kelly ME: *Legal issues in nursing,* St Louis, 1987, Mosby.

Rhodes AM: Consent for medical treatment, *MCN* 12(2):133, 1987.

Rhodes AM: Obtaining consent to treat minors, *MCN* 12(3):209, 1987.

Rhodes AM: When parents refuse to consent, *MCN* 12(4):289, 1987.

Rhodes AM, The rights of minors, *MCN* 13(4):281, 1988.

Rhodes AM: A minor's refusal of treatment, *MCN* 15(4):261, 1990.

Siantz MLD: Defining informed consent, *MCN* 13(2):94, 1988.

Silva M, Zeccolo R: Informed consent: the right to know and the right to choose, *Nurs Manage* 17(8):18-19, 1986.

Preparing for Procedures/Use of Play

Azarnoff P: Teaching materials for pediatric health professionals, *J Pediatr Health Care* 4(6):282-289, 1990.

Bates TA, Broome M: Preparation of children for hospitalization and surgery: a review of the literature, *J Pediatr Nurs* 1(4):230-239, 1986.

Broome ME: The relationship between children's fears and behavior during a painful event, *Child Health Care* 14(3):142-145, 1986.

Goldberger J, Wolfen J: Helping children cope with health-care procedures, *Contemp Pediatr* 7(3):141-162, 1990.

Hanson C, Strawser D: Family presence during cardiopulmonary resuscitation: Foote Hospital emergency department's nine-year perspective, *J Emerg Nurs* 18(2):104-106, 1992.

Mansson ME, Bjorkhem G, Wiebe T: The effect of preparation for lumbar puncture on children undergoing chemotherapy, *Oncol Nurs Forum* 20(1):39-45, 1993.

Perry SE: Teaching tools made by peers: a novel approach to medical preparation, *Child Health Care* 15(1):21-25, 1986.

Petrillo M, Sanger S: *Emotional care of hospitalized children,* ed 2, Philadelphia, 1980, JB Lippincott.

Pridham KF, Adelson F, Hansen MF: Helping children deal with procedures in a clinic setting: a developmental approach, *J Pediatr Nurs* 2(1):13-22, 1987.

Redman BK: *The process of patient education,* ed 7, St Louis, 1993, Mosby.

Rollins J, Brantly D: Preparing the child for procedures. In Smith DP and others, editors: *Comprehensive child and family nursing skills,* St Louis, 1991, Mosby.

Stanford G: Beyond honesty: choosing language for talking to children about pain and procedures, *Child Health Care* 20(4):261-262, 1991.

Streiff LD: Can clients understand our instructions? *Image* 18(2):48-52, 1986.

Waidley EK: Show and tell: preparing children for invasive procedures, *Am J Nurs* 85(7):811-812, 1985.

Zeltzer LK, Jay SM, Fisher DM: The management of pain associated with pediatric procedure, *Pediatr Clin North Am* 36(4):941-964, 1989.

Surgical Procedures

Addleman CD: What do you look for in the pediatric postanesthesia patient? *J Post Anesth Nurs* 3(1):3-10, 1988.

Atsberger DB, Shrewsbury P: Postoperative pain management: the PACU nurse's challenge, *J Post Anesth Nurs* 3(6):399-403, 1988.

Ashby D: Malignant hyperthermia: a potential crisis in the postanesthesia care unit, *J Pediatr Anesth Nurs* 5(4):279-281, 1990.

Avigne G, Phillips TL: Pediatric preoperative tours, *AORN J* 53(6):1458-1465, 1991.

Bender LH, Weaver K, Edwards K: Postoperative patient-controlled analgesia in children, *Pediatr Nurs* 16(6):549-554, 1990.

Berde CB: Pediatric postoperative pain management, *Pediatr Clin North Am* 36(4):921-940, 1989.

Carter JH, Hancock J: Caring for children: how to ease them through surgery, *Nursing 88* 18(10):46-50, 1988.

Coté CJ: NPO after midnight for children—a reappraisal, *Anesthesiology* 72(4):589-592, 1990.

Council on Scientific Affairs, American Medical Association: The use of pulse oximetry during conscious sedation, *JAMA* 270(12):1463-1468, 1993.

Gliniecki AM: Postanesthesia shaking: a review, *J Post Anesth Nurs* 7(2):89-93, 1992.

Heffline MS: A comparative study of pharmacological versus nursing interventions in the treatment of postanesthesia shivering, *J Post Anesth Nurs* 6(5):311-320, 1991.

Kaus SJ, Rockoff MA: Malignant hyperthermia, *Pediatr Clin North Am* 41(1):221-238, 1994.

Kennedy CM, Riddle II: The influence of the timing of preparation on the anxiety of preschool children experiencing surgery, *Matern Child Nurs J* 18(2):117-132, 1989.

Koren G: Use of the eutectic mixture of local anesthetics in young children for procedure-related pain, *J Pediatr* 122:S30-S35, 1993.

Krane EJ and others: Caudal morphine for postoperative analgesia in children: a comparison with caudal bupivacaine and intravenous morphine, *Anesth Analg* 66:647-653, 1987.

Litwack K: Practical points in the use of midazolam, *J Post Anesth Nurs* 3(6):408-410, 1988.

Maxwell LG, Deshpande JK, Wetzel RC: Preoperative evaluation of children, *Pediatr Clin North Am* 41(1):93-110, 1994.

McIlvaine WB: Perioperative pain management in children: a review, *J Pain Symptom Manage* 4(4):215-229, 1989.

Moushey R, Sinacore M, Diomede B: A perioperative teaching program: a collaborative process, *J Pediatr Nurs* 3(1):40-45, 1988.

Moyer S, Howe C: Pediatric pain intervention in the PACU, *Crit Care Nurs Clin North Am* 3(1):49-57, 1991.

Noonan AT and others: Family-centered nursing in the postanesthesia care unit: the evaluation of practice, *J Post Anesth Nurs* 6(1):13-16, 1991.

Ogilvie L: Hospitalization of children for surgery: the parents' view, *Child Health Care* 19(1):49-56, 1990.

Olkkola KT and others: Kinetics and dynamics of postoperative intravenous morphine in children, *Clin Pharmacol Ther* 44(2):128-136, 1988.

Puntillo KA: Dimensions of procedural pain and its analgesic management in critically ill surgical patients, *Am J Crit Care* 3(2):116-122, 1994.

Rivera WB: Practical points in the assessment and management of postoperative pediatric pain, *J Post Anesth Nurs* 6(1):40-42, 1991.

Rowland MA: Myths—and facts—about postop discomfort, *Am J Nurs* 90(5):60-64, 1990.

Rushton CH: The surgical neonate: principles of nursing management, *Pediatr Nurs* 14(2):141-151, 1988.

Schreiner M: The preopfast: not quite so fast, *Contemp Pediatr* 9(6):45-52, 1992.

Schreiner M and others: Ingestion of liquids compared with preoperative fasting in pediatric outpatients, *Anesthesiology* 72:593-597, 1990.

Steward DJ, editor: Management of childhood pain: new approaches to procedure-related pain, *J Pediatr* 122(5, pt 2):entire issue, 1993.

Strong NS: Assessing the postanesthesia patient, *Crit Care Nurs Q* 16(1):1-7, 1993.

Tobias JD and others: Postoperative analgesia: use of intrathecal morphine in children, *Clin Pediatr* 29:44-48, 1990.

van der Walt J and others: A study of preoperative fasting in infants aged less than three months, *Anaesth Intens Care* 18(4):527-531, 1990.

Vogelsang J, Hayes SR: Butorphanol tartrate (Stadol) relieves postanesthesia shaking more effectively than meperidine (Demerol) or morphine, *J Post Anesth Nurs* 7(2):94-100, 1992.

Wong DL: Pedicocktail not recommended, *Pediatr Nurs* 17(3):304, 1991.

Young MA and others: Latex allergy: a guideline for perioperative nurses, *AORN J* 56(3):488-502, 1992.

Zeltzer LK, Jay SM, Fisher DM: The management of pain associated with pediatric procedures, *Pediatr Clin North Am* 36(4):941-964, 1989.

Zuckerberg AL: Perioperative approach to children, *Pediatr Clin North Am* 41(1):15-30, 1994.

Compliance

Austin JK: Predicting parental anticonvulsant medication compliance using the theory of reasoned action, *J Pediatr Nurs* 4(2):88-95, 1989.

Baer CL: Compliance: the challenge for the future, *Top Clin Nurs* 7(4):77-85, 1986.

Burckhardt CS: Ethical issues in compliance, *Top Clin Nurs* 7(4):9-16, 1986.
Clark SR: Compliance and health behaviors, *Top Clin Nurs* 7(4):39-46, 1986.
Connaway N: My patient won't follow the medical plan treatment. What should I do to protect myself—legally? . . . home health care, *Home Healthc Nurs* 3(4):6-8, 1985.
DeFlorio IA, Duncan PA: Design for successful patient teaching, *MCN* 11:246-249, 1986.
Friedman IM, Litt IF: Promoting adolescents' compliance with therapeutic regimens, *Pediatr Clin North Am* 33(4):955-973, 1986.
Heyduk LJ: Medication education: increasing patient compliance, *J Psychosoc Nurs* 29(12): 32-35, 1991.
Hogue E: Parental noncompliance in home care, *Pediatr Nurs* 18(6):603-606, 1992.
Korsch BM: What do patients and parents want to know? What do they need to know? *Pediatrics* 74(5, suppl):917-920, 1984.
Littlefield LC: Therapeutic drug monitoring in ambulatory pediatrics, *J Pediatr Health Care* 1(2):113-116, 1987.
Lucas CM: Compliance and illness responses, *Top Clin Nurs* 7(4):47-56, 1986.
McCord MA: Compliance: self-care or compromise? *Top Clin Nurs* 7(4):1-8, 1986.
McHatton M: A theory for timely teaching, *Am J Nurs* 85(7):798-800, 1985.
Melnyk K: Barriers to care: operationalizing the variable, *Nurs Res* 39(2):108-112, 1990.
Miller A: When is the time ripe for teaching? *Am J Nurs* 85(7):801-804, 1985.
Morrison RA: Medication non-compliance, *Can Nurse* 89(4):15-18, 1993.
Padrick KP: Compliance: myths and motivators, *Top Clin Nurs* 7(4):17-22, 1986.
Russell FF, Mills BC, Zucconi T: Relationship of parental attitudes and knowledge to treatment adherence in children with PKU, *Pediatr Nurs* 14(6):514-516, 523, 1988.
Sallis JF: Improving adherence to pediatric therapeutic regimens, *Pediatr Nurs* 11(2): 118-120, 1985.
Spicher CM, Yund C: Effects of preadmission preparation on compliance with home care instructions, *J Pediatr Nurs* 4(4):255-262, 1989.
Stang H: Compliance: get parents in on the diagnosis, *Contemp Pediatr* 7(3):170, 1990.
Tyson RG: A prescription for compliance, *Contemp Pediatr* 10(4):5, 1993.
Williams RL and others: Educational strategies to improve compliance with an antibiotic regimen, *Am J Dis Child* 140(3):216-220, 1986.
Wysocki T and others: Behavior modification in pediatric hemodialysis, *ANNA J* 17(3):250-254, 1990.
Yoos L: Factors influencing maternal compliance to antibiotic regimens, *Pediatr Nurs* 10(2):141-147, 1984.

General Care and Hygiene/Fever

Baker RC and others: Severity of disease correlated with fever reduction in febrile infants, *Pediatrics* 83(6):1016-1019, 1989.
Burson JZ, Brannigan CN: The use of play in the nutritional support of hospitalized children, *Issues Compr Pediatr Nurs* 7(4-5):283-289, 1984.
Gildea JH: When fever becomes an enemy, *Pediatr Nurs* 18(2):165-167, 1992.
Goodrich C, March K: From ED to ICU: a focus on prevention of skin breakdown, *Crit Care Nurse* 15(1):1-13, 1992.
Hagelgans NA, Janusz HB: Pediatric skin care issues for the home care nurse, part 2, *Pediatr Nurs* 20(1):69-74, 76, 1994.
Herzog LW, Coyne LJ: What is fever? *Clin Pediatr* 32(4):142-146, 1993.
Hess CT: Patient support surface selection, *Contin Care* 11(6):35-50, 1992.
Hofman A and others: Pressure sores and pressure-decreasing mattresses: controlled clinical trial, *Lancet* 343(8897):568-571, 1994.
Ipp M, Jaffe D: Physicians' attitudes toward the diagnosis and management of fever in children 3 months to 2 years of age, *Clin Pediatr* 32(2):66-70, 1993.
Irwin M: Encourage oral intake—yes, but how? *Am J Nurs* 87(1):100-106, 1989.
Kauffman RE, Sawyer LA, Scheinbaum ML: Antipyretic efficacy of ibuprofen vs acetaminophen, *Am J Dis Child* 146(5):622-625, 1992.
Kilmon CA: Home management of children's fevers, *J Pediatr Nurs* 2(6):400-404, 1987.
Kleiman MB: Feverish children, frightened parents, *Contemp Pediatr* 6(3):161-167, 1989.
Kluger MJ: Fever revisited, *Pediatrics* 90(6):846-850, 1992.
Leung AK: Antipyretics in febrile children, *Lancet* 337(8748):1045, 1991.
McCarthy PL and others: Observation, history, and physical examination in diagnosis of serious illnesses in febrile children <24 months, *J Pediatr* 110(1):26-30, 1987.
Murphy KA: Acetaminophen and ibuprofen: fever control and overdose, *Pediatr Nurs* 18(4):428-432, 1992.
Reeves-Swift R: Rational management of a child's acute fever, *MCN* 15(2):82-85, 1990.
Singer L: When a sick child won't—or can't—eat, *Contemp Pediatr* 7(12):60-76, 1990.
Walson PD and others: Comparison of multidose ibuprofen and acetaminophen therapy in febrile children, *Am J Dis Child* 146(5):626-632, 1992.

Safety/Collection of Specimens

Amir J and others: The reliability of midstream urine culture from circumcised male infants, *Am J Dis Child* 147:969-970, 1993.
Blain-Lewis N: Comparative studies of bruising and healing after heelstick, *Neonatal Intensive Care* 5(5):18-21, 1992.
Brantly DK: Applying and maintaining restraints and restraining for procedures. In Smith DP and others, editors: *Comprehensive child and family nursing skills,* St Louis, 1991, Mosby.
DeGroot-Kosolcharoen J, Jones JJ: Permeability of latex and vinyl gloves to water and blood, *Am J Infect Control* 17:196-201, 1989.
Dennehy P: Heel blood sampling on older infants, *Neonatal Intensive Care* 5(5):21-23, 1992.
Fleischman AR: Clinical considerations for infant heel blood sampling, *Neonatal Intensive Care* 5(3):62-68, 1992.
Jackson MM: Implementing universal body substance precautions, *Occup Med* 4:39-44, 1989.
Jackson MM: Infection prevention and control for HIV and other infectious agents in obstetric, gynecologic and neonatal settings, *Clin Issues Perinat Women's Health Nurs* 1(1):115-121, 1990.
Jackson MM, Lynch P: The epidemiology of HIV infection, AIDS, and health-care worker risk issues, *Fam Community Health* 12(2):34-42, 1989.
Jackson MM and others: Why not treat all body substances as infectious? *Am J Nurs* 87(9):1137-1139, 1987.
Kelly PM: Are you ready to perform arterial punctures? *Nursing 87* 17(5):39-43, 1987.
Klein BS, Perloff WH, Maki DG: Reduction of nosocomial infection during pediatric intensive care by protective isolation, *N Engl J Med* 320:1714-1721, 1989.
Korniewicz D, Kirwin M, Larson E: Do your gloves fit the task? *Am J Nurs* 91(6):38-40, 1991.
Lander J, Fowler-Kerry S, Oberle S: Children's venipuncture pain: influence of technical factors, *J Pain Symptom Manage* 7(6):343-349, 1992.
Larson E: Handwashing: it's essential—even when you use gloves, *Am J Nurs* 89(7):934-939, 1989.
Lynch P and others: Implementing and evaluating a system of generic infection precautions: body substance isolation, *Am J Infect Control* 18(1):1-11, 1990.
Millam DA: Venous blood samples: sharpen your drawing skills, *Nursing 87* 17(12):56-61, 1987.
Pinheiro J, Furdon S, Ochoa LF: Role of local anesthesia during lumbar puncture in neonates, *Pediatrics* 91(2):379-382, 1993.
Preusser BA and others: Quantifying the minimum discard sample required for accurate arterial blood gases, *Nurs Res* 38:276-279, 1989.
Rutledge JC: Pediatric specimen collection for chemical analysis, *Pediatr Clin North Am* 36(1):37-47, 1989.
Suri S: Simplifying urine collection from infants and children without losing accuracy, *MCN* 13(12):438-441, 1988.
Weatherly KS, Young S, Andresky J: Needle stick injury in pediatric hospitals, *Pediatr Nurs* 17(1):95-99, 1991.

Administration of Medication

Beecroft PC, Redick S: Possible complications of intramuscular injections on the pediatric unit, *Pediatr Nurs* 15(4):333-376, 1989.
Bergeson PS: Immunizations to the deltoid region, *Pediatrics* 85(1):134, 1990 (letter).
Bergeson PS, Singer SA, Kaplan AM: Intramuscular injections in children, *Pediatrics* 70(6):944-948, 1982.
Birdsall C, Uretesky S: How do I administer medication by NG? *Am J Nurs* 84(10):1259-1260, 1984.
Dennis-Smithart R: Taking medication: the last straw, *Contemp Pediatr* 10(3):5, 1993.
Gahart BL: *Intravenous medications: a handbook for nurses and other allied health personnel,* ed 10, St Louis, 1994, Mosby.
Glassman SK, Measel CP: A makeshift minibottle: accurate small volume fluid or oral medication administration to infants, *Neonatal Network* 7(4):29-31, 1989.
Halperin D and others: Topical skin anesthesia for venous, subcutaneous drug reservoir and lumbar puncture in children, *Pediatrics* 84:281-284, 1989.

Knight MM and others: Medication education for children: is it worthwhile? *Child Adoles Psychiatr Men Health Nurs* 3(1):25-28, 1990.

Losek JD, Gyuro J: Pediatric intramuscular injections: do you know the procedure and complications? *Pediatr Emerg Care* 8(2):79-81, 1992.

Penatzer M and others: Common pediatric IV meds at a glance, *Pediatr Nurs* 14(1):56-58, 1988.

Raju TN and others: Medication errors in neonatal and paediatric intensive-care units, *Lancet* 2(8659):374-376, 1989.

Retting FM, Southby JR: Using different body positions to reduce discomfort during dorsogluteal injection, *Nurs Res* 31(4):219-221, 1982.

Smith SE: Eyedrop instillation for reluctant children, *Br J Ophthalmol* 75:480-481, 1991.

Taddio A and others: Effect of lidocaine-prilocaine cream on pain from subcutaneous injection, *Clin Pharm* 11:347-349, 1992.

Wink DM: Giving infants and children drugs: precision + caution = safety, *MCN* 16(6): 317-321, 1991.

Weir MR: Intravascular injuries from intramuscular penicillin, *Clin Pediatr* 27(2):85-90, 1988.

Wolf ZR: Medication errors and nursing responsibility, *Holistic Nurs Pract* 4(1):8-17, 1989.

Wooldridge JB, Jackson JG: Evaluation of bruises and areas of induration after two techniques of subcutaneous heparin injection, *Heart Lung* 17:476-482, 1988.

Wordell DC: Should you crush that tablet? *Nursing 88* 18(1):48-49, 1988.

Alternative Feeding Techniques/Elimination

Boarini JH: Principles of stoma care for infants, *J Enterostom Ther* 16(1):21-25, 1989.

Bockus S: Troubleshooting your tube feedings, *Am J Nurs* 91(5):24-28, 1991.

Embon CM: Ostomy care for the infant with necrotizing enterocolitis: nursing considerations, *J Perinat Neonat Nurs* 4(3):56-63, 1990.

Ferraro AR, Huddleston KC: Safe administration of small-volume enteral feedings: an alternative to intravenous pumps, *J Pediatr Nurs* 6(5):352-354, 1991.

Forgacs I, Macpherson A, Tibbs C: Percutaneous endoscopic gastrostomy, *Br Med J* 302(6839):1395-1396, 1992.

Garvin G: Discharge preparation of the pediatric patient with an ostomy, *Progression* 2(2):12-19, 1990.

Gauderer MWL: Gastrostomy techniques and devices, *Surg Clin North Am* 72(6):1285-1298, 1992.

Huddleston KC, Ferraro AR: Preparing families of children with gastrostomies, *Pediatr Nurs* 17(2):153-158, 1991.

Konigs K: Application of an ostomy pouch to a preterm infant, *Neonatal Network* 5(5):49-51, 1987.

Pulling R: The right place, *Can Nurse* 88(2):29-30, 1992.

Steele NF: The button: replacement gastrostomy device, *J Pediatr Nurs* 6(6):421-424, 1991.

Van Niel J: What's wrong with this peristomal skin? *Am J Nurs* 91(12):44-45, 1991.

Young RJ, Murray ND: Adapting intravenous pumps for enteral feeding, *MCN* 16:212-216, 1991.

U N I T X

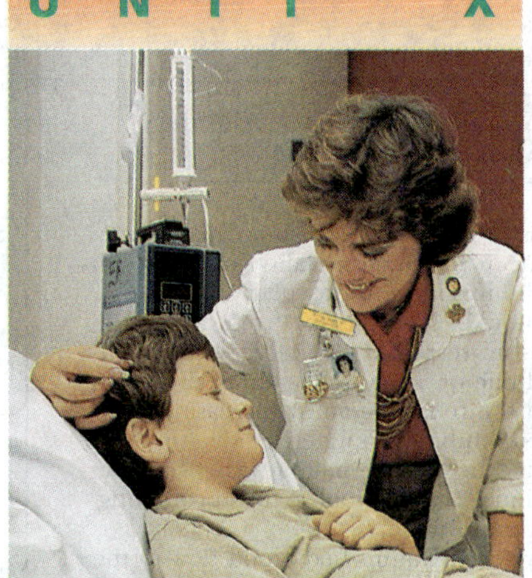

THE CHILD WITH DISTURBANCE OF FLUID AND ELECTROLYTES

CHAPTER 28 Balance and Imbalance of Body Fluids

CHAPTER OUTLINE

RELATED TOPICS

Burns, Ch. 29
The child with gastrointestinal dysfunction, Ch. 33
The child with renal dysfunction, Ch. 30
Collection of specimens, Ch. 27
Diarrhea, Ch. 29
Family-centered home care, Ch. 25
Gastric feeding techniques, Ch. 27
Intravenous administration (of medication), Ch. 27
Oral hygiene, Ch. 27
Pain management, Ch. 26
Preparation for procedures, Ch. 27
Shock states, Ch. 29
Vomiting, Ch. 29

DISTRIBUTION OF BODY FLUIDS

The distribution of body fluids, or ***total body water (TBW)***, involves the presence of ***intracellular (ICF)*** and ***extracellular (ECF)*** fluids. Water is the major constituent of body tissues, and the TBW in an individual ranges from 45% to 75% of total body weight.

The ICF refers to the fluid contained within the cells, whereas the ECF is the fluid outside the cells. The ECF is further broken down into several components: ***intravascular*** (contained within the blood vessels), ***interstitial*** (surrounding the cell and the location of most ECF), and ***transcellular*** (contained within specialized body cavities such as cerebrospinal, synovial, pleural, etc.). In the newborn about 50% of the body fluid is contained within the ECF, whereas a toddler's body fluid makes up about 30%.

■ Stephen Jones, RN,C, MS, PNP, revised this chapter.

PHYSICAL FORCES INFLUENCING FLUID BALANCE

Hydrostatic pressure—The pumping action of the heart increases fluid pressure in the arterial portion of the circulatory system, forcing fluid through the capillary walls into the interstitial spaces and from glomerular capillaries into the collecting tubules of the kidneys; it is the pressure created by the weight of fluid.

Osmotic pressure—The physical force, or "pull," created by a solution of higher concentration across a semipermeable membrane. Fluid in the solution of lesser concentration moves to the solution of greater concentration to equalize the concentration on each side of the membrane. Major osmotic forces in body fluids are sodium and intravascular proteins.

Diffusion—Random movement of molecules from a region of greater concentration to regions of lesser concentration. Rate of diffusion is influenced by the size and the distance across which the particle mass must diffuse (small particles move more rapidly than large ones), temperature (heat increases the rate of movement), and agitation (stirring hastens movement). **Facilitated diffusion** employs a carrier substance to assist solute movement across a membrane.

Active transport—A substance is transported by way of a carrier substance *against* a pressure gradient, from a region of lesser or equal concentration to a region of equal or higher concentration; examples include solutes such as sodium, potassium, and glucose.

Vesicular transport—A portion of a membrane engulfs a large molecule and releases it on the other side of the membrane. Substances move into cells by ***pinocytosis*** and out of cells by ***exocytosis***.

INTERNAL CONTROL MECHANISMS INFLUENCING FLUID BALANCE

Thirst—The impetus to ingest water is stimulated by increased solute concentration (osmolality) of extracellular fluid and/or diminished intravascular volume.

Antidiuretic hormone (ADH)—Released from the posterior pituitary gland in response to increased osmolality and decreased volume of intravascular fluid; promotes water retention in the renal system by increasing the permeability of renal tubules to water.

Aldosterone—Secreted by the adrenal cortex; enhances sodium reabsorption in renal tubules, thus promoting osmotic reabsorption of water.

Renin-angiotensin system—Diminished blood flow to the kidneys stimulates renin secretion, which reacts with plasma globulin to generate angiotensin, a powerful vasoconstrictor. Angiotensin also stimulates the release of aldosterone.

TABLE 28-1 Daily Maintenance Fluid Requirements

BODY WEIGHT (kg)	AMOUNT OF FLUID PER DAY
1-10	100 ml/kg
11-20	1000 ml plus 50 ml/kg for each kg >10 kg
>20	1500 ml plus 20 ml/kg for each kg >20 kg

The importance of body water to body function is related not only to its abundance but also to the fact that it is the medium in which body solutes are dissolved and all metabolic reactions take place. Since these metabolic processes are affected by even small alterations in fluid composition, precise regulation of the volume and composition of the fluid is essential. In healthy individuals, body water remains singularly constant, but marked alterations in either its volume or distribution that occur in many disease states can produce severely damaging physiologic consequences.

WATER BALANCE

Under normal conditions, the amount of water ingested closely approximates the amount of urine excreted in a 24-hour period, and the water in food and from oxidation balances that lost in feces and through evaporation. In this way, equilibrium is maintained.

Mechanisms of Fluid Movement

Water is retained in the body in a relatively constant amount and, with few exceptions, is freely exchangeable between all body fluid compartments. The proximity of the extravascular compartment to the cells allows for continual change in volume and distribution of fluids, largely determined by solutes (especially sodium) and physical forces (see box above, left). Transport mechanisms are the basis for all activity within the cells, and since they have limited ability to store materials, movement in and out of cells must be rapid. Internal control mechanisms are responsible for distribution and maintenance of fluid balance (see box above).

Maintaining Water Balance. Maintenance water requirement is the volume of water needed to replace obligatory fluid loss such as that from insensible water loss (through the skin and respiratory tract), evaporative water loss, and losses through urine and stool formation. The amount and type of these losses may be altered by disease states such as fever (with increased sweating), diarrhea, gastric suction, and sequestration of body fluids in a body space.

Basal maintenance calculations for required body water are based on the body's requirements for water in a normometabolic state, at rest; estimated fluid requirements are then increased or decreased from these parameters based on increased or decreased water losses, such as with elevated body temperature or congestive heart failure. Daily maintenance fluid requirements are outlined in Table 28-1.

Maintenance fluids contain both water and electrolytes and can be estimated from the child's age, body weight, degree of activity, and body temperature. ***Basal metabolic rate (BMR)*** is derived from standard tables and adjusted for the child's activity, temperature, and disease state. For example, for afebrile patients at rest the maintenance water require-

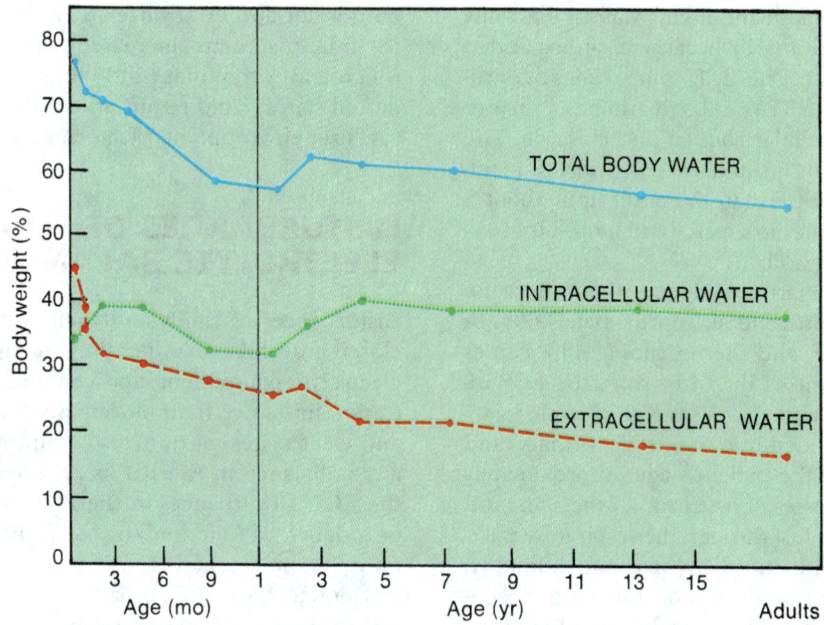

FIG. 28-1 Changes in total body water, extracellular water, and intracellular water in percentages of body weight. (Based on data from Fris-Hansen B: *Pediatrics* 28:169, 1961.)

ment is approximately 100 ml for each kilocalorie expended. Children with fluid losses or other alterations require adjustment of these basic needs to accommodate abnormal losses of both water and electrolytes as a result of a disease state. For example, insensible losses are increased when basal expenditure is increased by unusual activity in bed, fever, and hypermetabolic states. Hypometabolic states, such as hypothyroidism and hypothermia, decrease the BMR.

NURSING ALERT Nurses need to be alert for altered fluid requirements in various conditions:

Increased requirements:
- Fever (add 12% per rise of 1° C)
- Vomiting, diarrhea
- High-output renal failure
- Diabetes insipidus
- Burns
- Shock
- Tachypnea

Decreased requirements:
- Congestive heart failure
- Syndrome of inappropriate antidiuretic hormone (SIADH)
- Mechanical ventilation
- Postoperatively
- Oliguric renal failure
- Increased intracranial pressure

Changes in Fluid Volume Related to Growth

The percentage of TBW varies among individuals and in adults and older children is related primarily to the amount of body fat. Consequently, females, who have more body fat than males, and obese persons tend to have less water content in relation to weight.

The embryo is composed primarily of water with little tissue substance. As the organism grows and develops, a progressive decrease occurs in TBW, with the fastest rate of decline taking place during fetal life. The changes in water content and distribution that occur with age reflect the changes that take place in the relative amounts of bone, muscle, and fat comprising the body. At maturity the percentage of total body water is somewhat higher in the male than in the female and is probably a result of the differences in body composition, particularly fat and muscle content (Fig. 28-1).

Another important aspect of growth change as it corresponds to water distribution is related to the ICF and ECF compartments. In the fetus and prematurely born infant, the largest proportion of body water is contained in the ECF compartment. As growth and development proceed, the proportion within this fluid compartment decreases as the ICF and cell solids increase. The ECF diminishes rapidly from approximately 50% of body weight at birth to 30% at 2 years of age and 20% at maturity. The different effects on males and females become apparent at puberty.

Water Balance in Infants

Because of several characteristics, infants and young children have a greater need for water and are more vulnerable to alterations in fluid and electrolyte balance. Compared with older children and adults, they have a greater fluid intake and output relative to size. Water and electrolyte disturbances occur more frequently and more rapidly, and children adjust less promptly to these alterations.

The fluid compartments in the infant vary significantly from those in the adult, primarily because of an expanded extracellular compartment. The ECF compartment constitutes more than half of the TBW at birth and has a greater relative content of extracellular sodium and chloride. The infant loses a large amount of fluid at birth and still maintains a larger amount of ECF than the adult until about 2 years of age. This contributes to greater and more rapid water loss during this age period.

Fluid losses create compartment deficits that reflect the duration of dehydration. In general, approximately 60% of fluid is lost from the ECF, and the remaining 40% comes from the ICF. The amount of fluid lost from the ECF increases with acute illness and decreases with chronic loss.

Fluid losses may be divided into insensible, urinary, and fecal losses and vary with the patient's age. Approximately two thirds of insensible losses occur through the skin, and the remaining one third is lost through the respiratory tract. Insensible fluid loss is influenced by heat and humidity, body temperature, and respiratory rate. Infants and children have a much greater tendency to become highly febrile than do adults. Fever increases insensible water loss by approximately 7 ml/kg/24 hours for each degree rise in temperature above 99° F. Fever and increased surface area relative to volume are both factors that contribute to greater insensible fluid losses in young patients.

Surface Area. The infant's relatively greater body surface area (BSA) allows larger quantities of fluid to be lost through the skin. It is estimated that the BSA of the premature neonate is five times as great, and that of the newborn is two to three times as great, as that of the older child or adult. The proportionately longer gastrointestinal tract in infancy is also a source of relatively greater fluid loss, especially from diarrhea.

Metabolic Rate. The rate of metabolism in infancy is significantly higher than in adulthood because of the larger BSA in relation to the mass of active tissue. Consequently, there is a greater production of metabolic wastes that must be excreted by the kidneys. Any condition that increases metabolism causes greater heat production, with its concomitant insensible fluid loss and an increased need for water for excretion. The BMR in infants and children is higher to support growth.

Kidney Function. The kidneys of the infant are functionally immature at birth and are therefore inefficient in excreting waste products of metabolism. Of particular importance for fluid balance is the inability of the infant's kidneys to concentrate or dilute urine, to conserve or excrete sodium, and to acidify urine. Therefore the infant is less able to handle large quantities of solute-free water than is the older child and is more apt to become dehydrated when given concentrated formulas or overhydrated when given excessive water or dilute formula.

Fluid Requirements. As a result of these characteristics, infants ingest and excrete a greater amount of fluid per kilogram of body weight than do older children. Since electrolytes are excreted with water and the infant has limited ability for conservation, maintenance requirements include both water and electrolytes. The daily exchange of ECF in the infant is greatly increased over that of older children, which leaves the infant little fluid volume reserve in dehydrated states. Fluid requirements depend on hydration status, size, environmental factors, and underlying disease.

DISTURBANCES OF FLUID AND ELECTROLYTE BALANCE

Disturbances of fluids and their solute concentration are closely interrelated. Alterations in fluid volume affect the electrolyte component, and changes in electrolyte concentration influence fluid movement. Since intracellular water and electrolytes move to and from the ECF compartment, any imbalance in the ICF is reflected by an imbalance in the ECF. Disturbances in the ECF involve either an excess or a deficit of fluid and/or electrolytes; of these, fluid loss occurs more frequently.

Depletion of ECF, usually caused by gastroenteritis, is one of the most common problems encountered in infants and children (see Chapter 29). Until modern techniques for fluid replacement were perfected, it was one of the chief causes of infant mortality. Fluid and electrolyte problems related to specific diseases and their management are discussed throughout the book where appropriate. The major fluid disturbances, their usually causes, and clinical manifestations are outlined in Table 28-2; the most common disturbances, dehydration and edema, are elaborated further. Problems of fluid and electrolyte disturbance always involve both water and electrolytes; therefore, replacement includes administration of both, calculated on the basis of ongoing processes and laboratory serum electrolyte values.

In problems that involve alterations in the amount and composition of body fluid compartments, many areas are considered when planning management (see box below). The following discussion is concerned with the general concepts of two common fluid volume disturbances, dehydration and edema, that are features of a variety of conditions. Specific disorders are discussed in Chapters 29 and 30 and elsewhere in the book when appropriate.

AREAS OF CONCERN IN PLANNING MANAGEMENT OF FLUID PROBLEMS

- Volume of the body fluids (i.e., the water content of the patient)
- Osmolality of the body fluids, a factor that has an effect on the distribution of body water among the various compartments
- Hydrogen ion status (i.e., whether or not there has been a disturbance in the pH of body fluids or a disturbance in the homeostatic mechanisms that maintain the pH)
- Electrolyte deficits from cells as well as extracellular water
- Disturbances in the equilibrium between the mineral skeleton and body fluids
- Length of time alteration in fluid status has existed

TABLE 28-2 Disturbances of Fluid and Electrolyte Balance

MECHANISMS/SITUATIONS	MANIFESTATIONS	MANAGEMENT/NURSING CARE
WATER DEPLETION		
Failure to absorb or reabsorb water Complete sudden cessation of intake or prolonged diminished intake: Neglect of intake by self or caregiver—confused, psychotic, unconscious, or helpless Loss from gastrointestinal tract—vomiting, diarrhea, nasogastric suction, fistula Disturbed body fluid chemistry: inappropriate ADH secretion Excessive renal excretion: glycosuria (diabetes) Loss through skin or lungs: Excessive perspiration or evaporation—febrile states, hyperventilation, increased ambient temperature, increased activity (BMR) Impaired skin integrity—transudate from injuries Hemorrhage Iatrogenic: Overzealous use of diuretics Improper postoperative fluid replacement Use of radiant warmer or phototherapy	General symptoms: Thirst Variable temperature—increased (infection) Dry skin and mucous membranes Poor skin turgor Poor perfusion (decreased pulse, slowed capillary refill time) Weight loss Fatigue Diminished urinary output Irritability and lethargy Tachycardia Tachypnea Altered level of consciousness, disorientation Symptoms depend to some extent on proportion of electrolytes lost with water Laboratory findings: High urine specific gravity Increased hematocrit Variable serum electrolytes Variable urine volume Increased blood urea nitrogen (BUN) Increased serum osmolality	Provide replacement of fluid losses commensurate with volume depletion Provide maintenance fluids and electrolytes Determine and correct cause of water depletion Measure intake and output Monitor vital signs Monitor urine specific gravity
WATER EXCESS		
Water intake in excess of output: Excessive oral intake Hypertonic fluid overload Plain water enemas Failure to excrete water in presence of normal intake: Kidney disease Congestive heart failure Malnutrition	Edema: Generalized Pulmonary (moist rales or crackles) Intracutaneous (noted especially in loose areolar tissue) Elevated venous pressure Hepatomegaly Slow, bounding pulse Weight gain Lethargy Increased spinal fluid pressure Central nervous system manifestations (seizures, coma) Laboratory findings: Low urine specific gravity Decreased serum electrolytes Decreased hematocrit Variable urine volume	Limit fluid intake Administer diuretics Monitor vital signs Determine and treat cause of water excess Analyze laboratory electrolyte measurements frequently
SODIUM DEPLETION (HYPONATREMIA)		
Prolonged low-sodium diet Decreased sodium intake Fever Excess sweating Increased water intake without electrolytes Tachypnea (infants) Cystic fibrosis Burns and wounds Vomiting, diarrhea, nasogastric suction, fistulas Adrenal insufficiency Renal disease Diabetic ketoacidosis (DKA) Malnutrition	Associated with water loss: Same as with water loss—dehydration, weakness, dizziness, nausea, abdominal cramps, apprehension Mild—apathy, weakness, nausea, weak pulse Moderate—decreased blood pressure, lethargy Laboratory findings: Sodium concentration <130 mEq/L (may be normal if volume low) Urine specific gravity depends on water deficit or excess	Determine and treat cause Administer IV fluids with appropriate saline concentration

Continued.

TABLE 28-2 Disturbances of Fluid and Electrolyte Balance—cont'd

MECHANISMS/SITUATIONS	MANIFESTATIONS	MANAGEMENT/NURSING CARE
SODIUM EXCESS (HYPERNATREMIA)		
High salt intake—enteral or IV Renal disease Fever High insensible water loss: Increased temperature Increased humidity Hyperventilation Diabetes insipidus Hyperglycemia	Intense thirst Dry, sticky mucous membranes Flushed skin Temperature may be increased Hoarseness Oliguria Nausea and vomiting Possible progression to disorientation, convulsions, muscle twitching, nuchal rigidity, lethargy at rest, hyperirritable when aroused Lethargy findings: Serum sodium concentration ≥150 mEq/L High plasma volume Alkalosis	Determine and treat cause Administer fluids as prescribed Measure intake and output Monitor laboratory data Monitor neurologic status
POTASSIUM DEPLETION (HYPOKALEMIA)		
Starvation Clinical conditions associated with poor food intake Malabsorption IV fluid without added potassium Gastrointestinal losses—diarrhea, vomiting, fistulas, nasogastric suction Diuresis Administration of diuretics Administration of corticosteroids Diuretic phase of nephrotic syndrome Healing stage of burns Potassium-losing nephritis Hyperglycemic diuresis (e.g., diabetes mellitus) Familial periodic paralysis IV administration of insulin in ketoacidosis Alkalosis DKA	Muscle weakness, cramping, stiffness, paralysis, hyporeflexia Hypotension Cardiac arrhythmias, gallop rhythm Tachycardia or bradycardia Ileus Apathy, drowsiness Irritability Fatigue Laboratory findings: Decreased serum potassium concentration ≤3.5 mEq/L Abnormal ECG—notched or flattened T waves, decreased ST segment, premature ventricular contractions	Determine and treat cause Monitor vital signs, including electrocardiogram (ECG) Administer supplemental potassium Assess for adequate renal output before administration IV: administer K^+ slowly Oral: offer high-potassium fluids and foods Evaluate acid-base status
POTASSIUM EXCESS (HYPERKALEMIA)		
Renal disease Renal failure Adrenal insufficiency (Addison disease) Associated with metabolic acidosis Too rapid administration of IV potassium chloride Transfusion with old donor blood Severe dehydration Crushing injuries Burns Hemolysis Dehydration Potassium-sparing diuretics Increased intake of potassium (e.g., salt substitutes)	Muscle weakness, flaccid paralysis Twitching Hyperreflexia Bradycardia Ventricular fibrillation and cardiac arrest Oliguria Apnea—respiratory arrest Laboratory findings: High serum potassium concentration ≥5.5 mEq/L Variable urine volume Flat P wave on ECG, peaked T waves, widened QRS complex, increased PR interval	Determine and treat cause Monitor vital signs, including ECG Administer exchange resin, if prescribed Administer IV fluids as prescribed Administer IV insulin (if ordered) to facilitate movement of potassium into cells Monitor serum potassium levels Evaluate acid-base status
CALCIUM DEPLETION (HYPOCALCEMIA)		
Inadequate dietary calcium Vitamin D deficiency Rapid transit through gastrointestinal tract Advanced renal insufficiency Administration of diuretics Hypoparathyroidism Alkalosis Trapped in diseased tissues	Neuromuscular irritability Tingling of nose, ears, fingertips, toes Tetany Laryngospasm Generalized convulsions May be changes in clotting Positive Chvostek and Trousseau signs Hypotension	Determine and treat cause Administer calcium supplements as prescribed; administer slowly Monitor IV site; calcium may cause vascular irritation Monitor serum calcium levels Monitor serum protein levels

TABLE 28-2 Disturbances of Fluid and Electrolyte Balance—cont'd

MECHANISMS/SITUATIONS	MANIFESTATIONS	MANAGEMENT/NURSING CARE
Increased serum protein (albumin) Cow's milk formula—tetany of the newborn Exchange transfusion with citrated blood Inadequate parenteral administration in diseased states	Cardiac arrest Laboratory findings: Decreased serum calcium concentration (*N* = 8.8-10.8 mEq/L) or Increased serum protein Prolonged QT interval	
CALCIUM EXCESS (HYPERCALCEMIA)		
Acidosis Prolonged immobilization Conditions associated with increased bone catabolism Hypoproteinemia Kidney disease Hypervitaminosis D Hyperparathyroidism Hyperthyroidism Excessive IV or oral administration	Constipation Weakness, fatigue Nausea, vomiting Anorexia Dryness of mouth (thirst) Muscle hypotonicity Bradycardia/cardiac arrest Increased calcium concentration in urine may cause formation of kidney stones Laboratory findings: Increased serum calcium levels or Decreased serum protein levels Prolonged QRS complex or PR interval, shortened QT interval	Determine and treat cause Monitor serum calcium levels Monitor ECG

DEHYDRATION

Dehydration is a common body fluid disturbance encountered in the nursing of infants and children; it occurs whenever the total output of fluid exceeds the total intake, regardless of the underlying cause. Although dehydration can result from lack of oral intake (especially in elevated environmental temperatures), more often it is a result of abnormal losses, such as those that occur in vomiting or diarrhea, when oral intake only partially compensates for the abnormal losses. Other significant causes of dehydration are diabetic ketoacidosis and extensive burns.

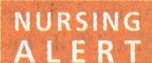

Whenever a child has a history of dehydration, nursing assessment should be geared toward the possibility of impending shock.

In early dehydration (during the first 2 days), fluid loss is derived from both the ECF and the ICF, since the increased osmolality of the diminished ECF volume causes fluid from the ICF compartment to move into the ECF compartment. As dehydration becomes chronic, the cellular losses become greater.

Types of Dehydration

Since sodium is the primary osmotic force that controls fluid movement between the major fluid compartments, dehydration is often described according to plasma sodium concentrations (i.e., isonatremic, hyponatremic, or hypernatremic). Other osmotic forces, however, such as glucose in diabetic dehydration and protein in nephrotic syndrome, may also play a dominant role. Consequently, dehydration is conventionally classified as (1) isotonic, (2) hypotonic, and (3) hypertonic.

Isotonic Dehydration. Isotonic (isosmotic or isonatremic) dehydration occurs in conditions in which electrolyte and water deficits are present in approximately balanced proportion. This is the primary form of dehydration occurring in children. The observable fluid losses are not necessarily isotonic, but losses from other avenues make adjustments so that the sum of all losses, or the net loss, is isotonic. Since no osmotic force is present to cause a redistribution of water between the ICF and ECF, the major loss is sustained from the ECF compartments. This significantly reduces the plasma volume and thus the circulating blood volume with its effect on skin, muscle, and kidneys. Shock is the greatest threat to life in isotonic dehydration, and the child with isotonic dehydration displays symptoms characteristic of hypovolemic shock. Plasma sodium remains within normal limits, between 130 and 150 mEq/L.

Hypotonic Dehydration. Hypotonic (hyposmotic or hyponatreic) dehydration occurs when the electrolyte deficit exceeds the water deficit. Since ICF is more concentrated than ECF in hypotonic dehydration, water transfers from the ECF to the ICF to establish osmotic equilibrium. This movement further increases the ECF volume loss, and shock is a frequent result. Because there is a greater proportional loss of ECF in hypotonic dehydration, the physical signs tend to be more severe with smaller fluid losses than in isotonic or hypertonic dehydration. Plasma sodium concentrations are typically less than 130 mEq/L.

Hypertonic Dehydration. Hypertonic (hyperosmotic or hypernatremic) dehydration results from water loss in ex-

TABLE 28-3 Intensity of Clinical Signs Associated with Varying Degrees of Isotonic Dehydration in Infants

	DEGREE OF DEHYDRATION		
	MILD	MODERATE	SEVERE
Fluid volume loss	<50 ml/kg	50-90 ml/kg	≥100 ml/kg
Skin color	Pale	Gray	Mottled
Skin elasticity	Decreased	Poor	Very poor
Mucous membranes	Dry	Very dry	Parched
Urinary output	Decreased	Oliguria	Marked oliguria and azotemia
Blood pressure	Normal	Normal or lowered	Lowered
Pulse	Normal or increased	Increased	Rapid and thready
Capillary filling time	<2 seconds	2-3 seconds	>3 seconds

cess of electrolyte loss and is usually caused by a proportionately larger loss of water and/or a larger intake of electrolytes. This type of dehydration is also the most dangerous and requires much more specific fluid therapy. This sometimes occurs in infants with diarrhea who are given fluids by mouth that contain large amounts of solute or in children receiving high-protein nasogastric tube feedings that place an excessive solute load on the kidneys. In hypertonic dehydration, fluid shifts from the lesser concentration of the ICF to the ECF. Plasma sodium concentration is greater than 150 mEq/L.

Since the ECF volume is proportionately larger, hypertonic dehydration consists of a greater degree of water loss for the same intensity of physical signs. Shock is less apparent in hypotonic dehydration. However, neurologic disturbances, such as seizures, are more likely to occur. Cerebral changes are serious and may result in permanent damage. These include disturbance of consciousness, poor ability to focus attention, lethargy, increased muscle tone with hyperreflexia, and hyperirritability to stimuli (tactile, auditory, bright light).

Degree of Dehydration

Traditionally, the magnitude of fluid loss has been described as a percentage (5%, 10%, 15%) and ascertained by a comparison of preillness weight and current weight, since any weight loss is substantially equivalent to the amount of water lost. However, water constitutes only 60% to 70% of infant weight, and adipose tissue, which contains little water, is highly variable in individual infants and children. Rather than percentage, a more accurate means of describing dehydration is to reflect acute loss (over 48 hours or less) in milliliters per kilogram of body weight (Finberg, 1990). For example, a 50 ml/kg loss is considered to be a mild fluid loss, whereas 100 ml/kg produces severe dehydration.

Clinical signs provide clues to the extent of dehydration (Table 28-3). The earliest detectable sign is usually tachycardia, followed by dry skin and mucous membranes, sunken fontanel, signs of circulatory failure (coolness and mottling of extremities), loss of skin elasticity, and delayed capillary filling time. (See also Table 28-4 for clinical manifestations of dehydration.)

Compensatory mechanisms attempt to maintain fluid volume by adjusting to these losses. Interstitial fluid moves into the vascular compartment to defend the blood volume in response to hemoconcentration and hypovolemia, and vasoconstriction of peripheral arterioles helps maintain pumping pressure. When fluid losses exceed the body's ability to sustain blood volume and blood pressure, circulation is seriously compromised and the blood pressure falls. This results in tissue hypoxia with accumulation of lactic acid, pyruvate, and other acid metabolites, which contributes to the development of metabolic acidosis.

Renal compensation is impaired by reduced blood flow through the kidneys, and little urine is formed. Increased serum osmolality stimulates the secretion of antidiuretic hormone (ADH) to conserve fluid and initiates the renin-angiotensin mechanisms in the kidney, causing further vasoconstriction. Aldosterone is released to promote sodium retention and conserve water in the kidneys. If dehydration increases in severity, urine formation is greatly diminished and metabolites and hydrogen ions that are normally excreted by this route are retained.

Shock, a common manifestation of severe depletion of ECF volume, is preceded by tachycardia and signs of poor perfusion and tissue oxygenation (by pulse oximeter readings). Peripheral circulation is poor as a result of reduced blood volume; therefore the skin is cool and mottled, with decreased capillary filling after blanching. Impaired kidney circulation often leads to oliguria and azotemia. While low blood pressure may accompany other symptoms of shock, in infants and young children it is usually a late sign and may herald the onset of cardiovascular collapse.

Diagnostic Evaluation

To initiate a therapeutic plan, several factors must be determined: the degree of dehydration based on physical assessment; the type of dehydration based on the pathophysiology of the specific illness responsible for the dehydrated state; specific physical signs other than general signs; initial plasma sodium concentrations; and associated electrolyte (especially serum potassium) and acid-base imbalances. Initial and regular ongoing evaluations are carried out to assess the patient's progress toward equilibrium and the effectiveness of therapy.

When examining an infant or younger child, one of the most important determinants is the weight, since this can

TABLE 28-4 Clinical Manifestations of Dehydration

	ISOTONIC (LOSS OF WATER AND SALT)	HYPOTONIC (LOSS OF SALT IN EXCESS OF WATER)	HYPERTONIC (LOSS OF WATER IN EXCESS OF SALT)
Skin			
Color	Gray	Gray	Gray
Temperature	Cold	Cold	Cold or hot
Turgor	Poor	Very poor	Fair
Feel	Dry	Clammy	Thickened, doughy
Mucous membranes	Dry	Slightly moist	Parched
Tearing and salivation	Absent	Absent	Absent
Eyeball	Sunken	Sunken	Sunken
Fontanel	Sunken	Sunken	Sunken
Body temperature	Subnormal or elevated	Subnormal or elevated	Subnormal or elevated
Pulse	Rapid	Very rapid	Moderately rapid
Respirations	Rapid	Rapid	Rapid
Behavior	Irritable to lethargic	Lethargic to comatose; convulsions	Marked lethargy with extreme hyperirritability on stimulation

assist in determining the percentage of total body fluid lost. Other important clinical manifestations include changing sensorium (irritability to lethargy), response to stimuli, integumentary (decreased elasticity and turgor), capillary refill (prolonged), heart rate (increased), sunken eyes, and in infants, sunken fontanels.

Therapeutic Management

Medical management is directed at correcting the fluid imbalance and treating the underlying cause. When the child is alert, awake, and not in shock, correction of dehydration may be attempted with oral fluid administration. Most dehydration is mild and can be managed at home by this method. Several commercial rehydration fluids are available for use (see Table 29-2). Oral rehydration management consists of rapid replacement of fluid loss over 4 to 6 hours, replacement of continuing losses, and providing for maintenance fluid requirements. Amounts and rates are determined from body weight and are increased if rehydration is incomplete or if excess losses continue. Full diet is usually withheld until the child is well hydrated and the basic problem in under control (see Diarrhea, Chapter 29).

Parenteral Fluid Therapy. Parenteral fluid therapy is initiated whenever the child is unable to ingest sufficient amounts of fluid and electrolytes to (1) meet ongoing daily physiologic losses, (2) replace previous deficits, and (3) replace ongoing abnormal losses. Patients who usually require IV fluids are those with severe dehydration, those with uncontrollable vomiting, those who are unable to drink for any reason (e.g., extreme fatigue, coma), and those with severe gastric distention.

Since dehydration constitutes a great threat to life, the first priority is the restoration of circulation by rapid expansion of the ECF volume in order to treat shock or prevent its occurrence. IV administration of fluid is begun immediately, even though the exact nature of the dehydration and the serum electrolyte values are not known. The solution selected is based on what is known regarding the probable type and cause of the dehydration. This usually involves an isotonic solution such as 0.9% sodium chloride or Lactated Ringer's, both of which are very close to the body's serum osmolality of 285 to 300 and do not contain dextrose (which is contraindicated in the early treatment stages of diabetic ketoacidosis).

A suggested formula is to replace one half the estimated deficit over the first 8 to 16 hours and one half over the next 16 to 24 hours, depending on the type of dehydration; thus the deficit is recovered within 24 to 48 hours. Maintenance fluid volumes are calculated and added to the infusion therapy during replacement therapy.

Sodium bicarbonate may be added, since acidosis is usually associated with severe dehydration, but potassium is not administered until kidney function is appropriate (or unless the child is known to be hypokalemic, such as in diabetic ketoacidosis). As the circulation improves, the glomerular filtration pressure increases to improve renal function, which is essential to electrolyte readjustments.

The goal of the next phase is the restoration of ECF volume. With improved circulation, water and electrolyte deficits can be evaluated and acid-base status corrected either directly through the administration of fluids or indirectly through improved renal function. Next, potassium lost in ICF must be replaced slowly by way of the ECF. Finally, the body fat and protein stores are replaced through diet. If the child is unable to eat or if feeding aggravates the condition (e.g., diarrhea), IV alimentation is provided to prevent serious malnourishment.

Although the initial phase of fluid replacement is rapid in both isotonic and hypotonic dehydration, it is contraindicated in hypertonic dehydration because of the risk of water intoxication, especially in the brain cells. There is an apparent lag time for sodium to reach a steady state when diffusing in and out of brain cells, whereas water diffuses almost instantaneously. Consequently, rapid administration of fluid will cause equally rapid diffusion of water into the dehydrated brain cells, causing marked cerebral edema. Since ECF volume is maintained relatively well in hypertonic as opposed to the other types of dehydration, shock is not a usual manifestation.

WATER INTOXICATION

Water intoxication, or water overload, is observed less often than dehydration. However, it is important that nurses and others who care for children are aware that this can occur and be alert to the possibility in certain situations. Patients who ingest excessive amounts of fluid develop a concurrent decrease in serum sodium and central nervous system symptoms. There is a large urinary output and, because water moves into the brain more rapidly than sodium moves out, the child may also exhibit irritability, somnolence, headache, vomiting, diarrhea, or generalized seizures. The affected child usually appears well hydrated but may be edematous or even dehydrated.

Fluid intoxication can occur during acute IV water overloading, too rapid dialysis, tap water enemas, or with too rapid reduction of glucose levels in diabetic ketoacidosis. Patients with central nervous system infections occasionally retain excessive amounts of water. Administration of inappropriate hypotonic solutions (e.g., 0.45% sodium chloride) may cause a rapid reduction in sodium and result in symptoms of water overload.

Infants are especially vulnerable to fluid overload. Their thirst mechanism is not well developed; therefore, they are unable to "turn off" fluid intake appropriately. A decreased glomerular filtration rate does not allow for repeated excretion of a water load, and ADH levels may not be maximally reduced. Consequently, infants are unable to excrete a water overload effectively.

Administration of inappropriately prepared formula is one of the more common causes of water intoxication. Families who cannot afford to buy enough expensive formula may dilute the formula to increase the volume or even substitute water for the formula. A family may run out of formula and dilute the remaining amount to make it last until they are able to purchase replacement formula. In addition, water is sometimes used for pacification. Water intoxication can also occur in infants who receive overly vigorous hydration during a febrile illness.

A number of clinicians have reported water intoxication in infants following swimming lessons (Bennett, Wagner, and Fields, 1983; Goldberg and others, 1982; Kropp and Schwartz, 1982). Although they hold their breath, some infants apparently swallow a large amount of water during repeated submersion. This is probably not a common occurrence, since parents who observe their infants swallowing water tend to keep the infant's head above water (Phillips, 1987). Anticipatory guidance to parents should include a discussion of swimming instruction and advice to stop a lesson if the child is observed to swallow unusual amounts of water or exhibit any symptoms of hyponatremia.

EDEMA

Edema represents an abnormal accumulation of fluid and subsequent tissue expansion within the interstitial tissue and develops when a defect in the normal circulation or a failure in the lymphatic drainage to remove the increased amounts occurs. The processes responsible for fluid removal include venous hydrostatic pressure, oncotic pressure of intravascular and interstitial spaces, an intact semipermeable capillary wall, tissue tension, and lymphatic flow.

Mechanisms of Edema Formation

A defect of any of the homeostatic mechanisms maintaining fluid balance can cause accumulation of interstitial fluid. Disequilibrium results from anything that (1) alters the retention of sodium, such as renal disease or hormonal influences; (2) affects the formation or destruction of plasma proteins, such as starvation or liver disease; or (3) alters membrane permeability, such as nephrotic syndrome or trauma.

Edema may be localized to a small or large area, such as that occurring in urticaria, infection, and pulmonary congestion, or it can be generalized, as in the hypoproteinemia of the nephrotic syndrome and starvation. A severe, generalized accumulation of great amounts of fluid in all body tissues is termed *anasarca.*

Increased Venous Pressure. The colloidal osmotic pressure (COP) of the plasma proteins draws fluid back into the vascular system as long as this force is greater than the venous hydrostatic pressure. However, when the venous pressure is increased, fluid tends to be retained in the interstitial spaces. This can occur when an individual remains in the same position for a long time, such as swollen ankles and feet after standing or sitting for long periods. Constrictive dressings or restraints applied too tightly to extremities will obstruct venous return, increase venous and capillary pressure, and cause edema. The most graphic pathologic illustrations are pulmonary edema caused by pulmonary circulation overload in cardiac defects with a left-to-right shunt and ascites caused by portal hypertension. Edema from any cause is increased in dependent areas because of this added factor of increased venous hydrostatic pressure and the gravitational effects in these areas.

Capillary Permeability. Damage to capillary walls or alteration in their permeability permits exudation of plasma protein into the interstitial space. Most often this occurs as local edema, such as manifested in inflammatory and hypersensitivity reactions. Capillary damage from burns allows extensive exudation of protein-rich fluid into the interstitial spaces to compound edema formation.

Diminished Plasma Proteins. A fall in plasma protein levels hampers the osmotic pull back into the vessels. Consequently, fluid remains in the interstitial spaces. Although other factors play a role, such as hydrostatic pressure of both the arterial vascular system and the tissues and Na^+ concentration, significantly low protein levels (below 4.5 mg/dl) are associated with edema. Examples of this are the massive albumin losses of the nephrotic syndrome, diminished serum protein from insufficient dietary protein, and (sometimes) hemodilution of plasma proteins from IV fluid administration in chronic dehydration.

Lymphatic Obstruction. Obstruction of lymph flow creates edema high in protein content. This occurs infrequently in childhood but can result from trauma to the lymphatic glands or removal of lymph nodes.

Tissue Tension. Tissue hydrostatic pressure is ordinarily of little consequence. However, it plays a significant role in determining distribution of edema fluid in certain pathologic conditions. Loose tissues allow a greater amount of fluid accumulation than tissues that are tightly bound by dense fibrous bands in which tissue pressure rapidly increases to limit further extravasation of fluid. Edema appears earlier and more readily in loose structures such as those in the periorbital and genital tissues. The alveolar structure of lung tissue is probably a contributing factor in pulmonary edema as well as in increased hydrostatic pressure in the pulmonary vessels.

Other Factors in Edema Formation. Any factor that causes Na^+ retention by the kidneys will produce or augment edema formation. This includes stimulation of the renin-angiotensin-aldosterone mechanisms for Na^+ reabsorption created by the diminished plasma volume in edema, which resulted from primary causes. The salt-retaining property of steroids is responsible for the edema associated with their administration.

Several types of edema exist, all of which can provide a palpable swelling of the interstitial space that is either localized or generalized. These include:

1. Peripheral edema, or localized or generalized palpable swelling of the interstitial space
2. Ascites, or the accumulation of fluid in the abdominal cavity (usually associated with renal or liver abnormalities)
3. Pulmonary edema, which occurs when there is an increase in the interstitial volume
4. Cerebral edema, which is a particularly threatening form of edema caused by trauma, infection, or other etiologic factors, including vascular overload or injudicious IV administration of hypotonic solutions
5. Overall fluid gain, especially seen in patients with kidney disease

Assessment

Generalized edema resulting from any of the above types can occur and is manifested by swelling in the extremities, face, perineum, and torso. A quick way to determine this severity is to measure the degree of pitting edema, as seen in Fig. 28-2.

Therapeutic Management

The primary goal in the management of edema is treatment of the underlying disease process, which is discussed in relation to the specific disorder. However, an essential aspect in the management of any fluid overload is early recognition, in which nurses play a vital role.

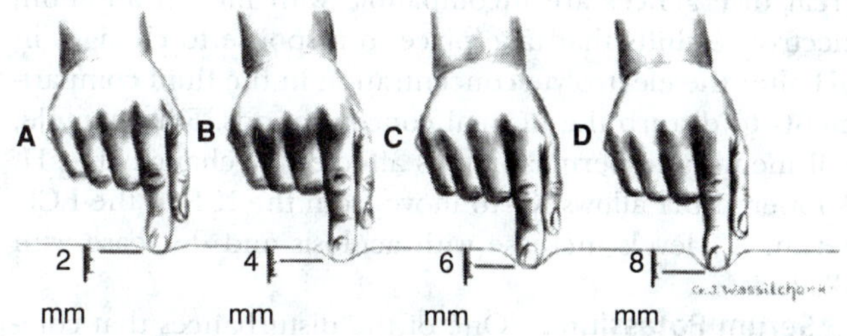

FIG. 28-2 Assessment of pitting edema. **A,** +1. **B,** +2. **C,** +3. **D,** +4. (From Bobak IM, Jensen MD: *Essentials of maternity nursing,* ed 2, St Louis, 1986, Mosby.)

DISTURBANCES OF ACID-BASE BALANCE

The ability of the body to regulate the acid-base status is one of the most crucial physiologic functions. Many disease states, such as diarrhea, vomiting, or febrile conditions, are complicated by disturbances in the acid-base balance, which are often more hazardous to the child's survival than the primary disease process. Sometimes simply providing adequate hydration, replacing electrolytes, and correcting acid-base disturbances are all that is needed to sustain an infant or child until the primary disorder has run its course.

ACID-BASE IMBALANCE

A disturbance of acid-base equilibrium in the direction of acidosis or alkalosis may come about in a variety of ways. However, very simply stated, ***acidosis (acidemia)*** results from either accumulation of acid or loss of base, and ***alkalosis (alkalemia)*** results from either accumulation of base or loss of acid.

Hydrogen Ion Concentration

The pH represents the concentration of H^+ in solution and only indicates whether the imbalance is more acidic or more alkaline. It does not reflect the nature of the imbalance, that is, whether it is of metabolic or respiratory origin. Body metabolism affects primarily the base bicarbonate (HCO_3); therefore alterations in the concentration of HCO_3 are termed ***metabolic*** disturbances of acid-base balance. Also, since the amount of carbon dioxide (CO_2) exhaled through the lungs affects the carbonic acid (H_2CO_3), changes in H_2CO_3 concentration are referred to as ***respiratory*** disturbances. Consequently, the simple disturbances (those with a single primary cause) are categorized as metabolic acidosis or alkalosis and respiratory acidosis or alkalosis.

It is also significant that the major signs and symptoms of hydrogen ion imbalances, acidosis and alkalosis, reflect central nervous system involvement. Depression of the CNS, manifested by lethargy, diminished mental capacity, delirium, stupor, and coma, is observed in acidosis of either metabolic or respiratory origin. On the other hand, alkalosis produces clinical manifestations of nervous system stimulation and excitement, including overexcitability, nervousness, tingling sensations, and tetany that may progress to convulsions. Persons with epilepsy are particularly susceptible to seizures, which can be precipitated by hyperventilation.

It is also important to note that eventually all body systems will become dysfunctional if the "normal" limits of pH are violated for very long. The extent and severity of signs and symptoms depend on the length of time the imbalance has existed and the magnitude or degree of the deviation from normal. A rapid, severe imbalance will seriously com-

TABLE 28-5 Laboratory Tests Employed in Assessment of Acid-Base Status

ABBREVIATION	TEST	NORMAL VALUES*	DESCRIPTION
pH	Partial pressure of hydrogen	Birth: 7.11-7.36 1 day: 7.29-7.45 Child: 7.35-7.45	Expression of hydrogen ion concentration
PCO_2	Partial pressure of carbon dioxide or carbon dioxide tension	Newborn: 27-40 Infant: 27-41 Girls: 32-45 Boys: 35-48	Measure of carbon dioxide tension; reflects carbonic acid (H_2CO_3) concentration of plasma
HCO_3 (serum) arterial	Carbon dioxide content or carbon dioxide combining power	Infant: 21-38 mEq/L Thereafter: 22-26 mEq/L	Concentration of base bicarbonate
BE	Base excess (whole blood)	Newborn: −2 to −10 Infant: −1 to −7 Child: +2 to −4 Thereafter: +2 to −2	Used to express extent of deviation from normal buffer base concentration; indicates quantity of blood buffers remaining after hydrogen ion is buffered

*Data from Behrman RE, Vaughan VC III, Editors: *Nelson textbook of pediatrics,* ed. 14, Philadelphia, 1992, Saunders.

promise the compensatory mechanisms to the point where it is incompatible with life, whereas the body will be able to compensate adequately for a mild, gradual distortion and produce few if any observable signs or symptoms.

TABLE 28-6 Summary of Simple Acid-Base Disturbances (Partially Compensated)

DISTURBANCE	PLASMA pH	PLASMA PCO_2	PLASMA HCO_3
Respiratory acidosis	↓	↑	↑
Respiratory alkalosis	↑	↓	↓
Metabolic acidosis	↓	↓	↓
Metabolic alkalosis	↑	↑	↑

Compensatory Mechanisms

Respiratory regulation in acid-base balance involves CO_2 regulation; that is, the rate and depth of alveolar ventilation will determine the concentration of CO_2 that is eliminated or retained. Renal processes, however, involve the regulation of HCO_3 via reabsorption, regeneration, and secretion of H^+ ion. When the fundamental acid-base ratio is altered for any reason, the body attempts to correct the deviation. In a simple disturbance, a single *primary* factor affects one component of the acid-base pair and is usually accompanied by a *compensatory* or *secondary* change in the component that is not primarily affected. For example, increased formation of metabolic acid rapidly reduces the HCO_3 in the formation of H_2CO_3. The respiratory mechanism immediately attempts to compensate for the imbalance by eliminating the H_2CO_3 through exhaled CO_2 and water. The imbalance is corrected when the kidneys excrete hydrogen and ammonium ions in exchange for reabsorbed sodium bicarbonate.

When the secondary changes (the hyperventilation and renal excretion of H^+ in the preceding example) succeed in preventing a distortion of the acid-base ratio and the pH is restored to normal, the disturbance is described as *compensated.* The *uncompensated* state exists when there is no compensatory effect and the pH remains uncorrected. The imbalance is said to be *corrected* when physiologic mechanisms fully correct the primary abnormality.

Laboratory Measurements

Several laboratory tests are employed to assess the nature and extent of acid-base disturbances. The importance of these data is readily apparent when a clinical observation such as hyperventilation can represent either the primary factor in respiratory alkalosis or a secondary or compensatory factor in metabolic acidosis. The laboratory tests of value in the assessment of acid-base status are outlined in Table 28-5. To determine the acid-base status, three variables—the respiratory component (PCO_2), the metabolic component (arterial HCO_3, or serum CO_2), and the serum pH—must be determined. Measurement of any two will allow computation of the third. A summary of relationships between these and other variables is outlined in Table 28-6.

Associated Disturbances in Acid-Base Balance

Physiologic functions of the body take place optimally when the pH is maintained within a normal range. The disequilibrium created by moderately altered pH can produce disordered function of physiologic and enzyme systems, but great divergences are incompatible with life. In addition, electrolyte shifts that take place in response to changes in pH alter the electrolyte concentration in the fluid compartments to disturb the normal concentrations. For example, cell membrane permeability is affected by changes in pH. A lowered pH allows K^+ to move from the ICF to the ECF. Serum K^+ levels increase with acidosis and decrease with alkalosis.

Serum Potassium. One of the disturbances that complicates both fluid losses and acid-base imbalance is an alteration of K^+ levels. During dehydration, fluid moves out of the ICF compartment into the ECF compartment in an attempt to balance the fluid losses. In doing so, K^+ also moves out, creating a total body K^+ depletion. Since renal function is drastically reduced in dehydration, normal excretion of K^+ does not take place. This causes elevated serum levels that can produce all the signs and symptoms of hyperkalemia. During rapid rehydration therapy for gastrointestinal losses and diabetic ketoacidosis, the ECF K^+ moves back into the ICF compartment, thereby posing the risk of hypokalemia unless there is an anticipated replacement. However, K^+ is not replaced until the ICF is sufficient to restore adequate renal function.

Serum Calcium. Disturbed ECF calcium (Ca^+) levels may occur in various types of dehydration. Usually the disturbance is in the form of reduced serum Ca^+ levels, especially where there is a concomitant potassium loss. Although hypocalcemia is a common finding, it rarely reaches a point of tetany in current practice, which includes adequate replacement of potassium losses. Immediate effects of Ca^+ imbalance associated with acidosis or alkalosis are tetany of metabolic alkalosis; long-term effects of chronic acidosis are related to bone resorption from renal disturbances.

Oxygen Combination. The capacity of oxygen (O_2) to combine with hemoglobin is also affected by changes in pH. The affinity of hemoglobin for O_2 decreases with a decrease in pH so that, in a state of acidosis, less O_2 will be picked up by the hemoglobin as blood travels through the lungs. However, O_2 is more easily released to the tissues when the pH is lowered. The opposite effects operate during an increase in pH.

Blood Flow. Blood flow in various areas is altered by changes in pH. Pulmonary circulation constricts in acidosis, whereas decreased pH (acidosis) causes vasodilation in systemic vessels.

RESPIRATORY ACIDOSIS

Respiratory acidosis results from diminished or inadequate pulmonary ventilation that causes an elevation in plasma P_{CO_2} and thus an increased concentration of dissolved H_2CO_2, which leads to elevated H_2CO_3 and H^+ concentration. Conditions that produce respiratory acidosis can originate at three levels in the respiratory system and result in inadequate gas exchange (see box below).

Compensation is mediated through the kidneys, which are stimulated to conserve and thus increase the plasma HCO_3 concentration and to excrete hydrogen ions. Laboratory findings in respiratory acidosis include elevated plasma HCO_3 concentration (greater than 29 mEq/L in older children, greater than 28 mEq/L in young children) and elevated P_{CO_2} (greater than 38 mm Hg, arterial).

The treatment of respiratory acidosis is aimed at correcting the primary defect and improving gas exchange at the alveolar level to provide more efficient removal of CO_2. Oxygen therapy is usually indicated, and if the condition warrants it, mechanical ventilation. Administration of buffers such as sodium bicarbonate to reduce H^+ concentration is usually not indicated, because it can result in fluid volume excess by causing an osmolar fluid shift from the blood to the intravascular space, which would only further compromise respiratory function and aggravate the acidosis. Sodium bicarbonate may be indicated with a $pH < 7.0$ if the cause is bronchial asthma or bronchospasm (Horne, Heitz, and Swearingen, 1991).

ORIGINS OF INADEQUATE GAS EXCHANGE

Factors that depress the respiratory center, such as head injury, depressant or narcotizing drugs, and infections of the central nervous system

Factors that affect the lung proper, such as obstructive pulmonary disease, pneumonia, cystic fibrosis, acute pulmonary edema, atelectasis, and occlusion of respiratory passages

Factors that interfere with the bellows action of the chest wall, including trauma to the chest wall, skeletal diseases or deformities, and diseases of the thoracic muscles or their innervation (e.g., muscular dystrophy or muscular atrophy)

RESPIRATORY ALKALOSIS

Conversely, respiratory alkalosis is caused by a primary increase in the rate and depth of pulmonary ventilation, resulting in unusually large amounts of CO_2 being exhaled or "blown off." This reduces the plasma P_{CO_2}, H_2CO_3, and H^+ concentration and leaves an excess of HCO_3. Conditions that cause stimulation of the respiratory center to produce hyperventilation are listed in the box below.

A frequent cause of hyperventilation in children is voluntary hyperventilation before underwater swimming. It is also a consideration in the care of persons having assisted ventilation. Incorrectly set mechanical ventilators can cause respiratory rates and tidal volumes in excess of physiologic needs.

Compensation of respiratory alkalosis takes place in the kidneys and consists of excretion of H_2CO_3 in association with Na^+ and K^+ to conserve H^+. Laboratory findings include elevated plasma pH (greater than 7.43), depressed plasma H_2CO_3 concentration (less than 23 mEq/L in older

CONDITIONS THAT PRODUCE HYPERVENTILATION

Primary central nervous system stimulation resulting from emotions, including hysteria, fear, apprehension, pain, anxiety; central nervous system infection (encephalitis); and certain drug reactions, such as early salicylate intoxication (a primary respiratory stimulant); mechanical ventilation

Reflex central nervous system stimulation from peripheral chemoreceptors as a result of hypoxia, which provides the stimulus for hyperventilation at high altitudes; fever or high environmental temperatures; congestive heart failure; and anemia

Reflex central nervous system stimulation from intrathoracic stretch receptors, which is believed to be the cause of hyperventilation in localized pulmonary disease

Pulmonary disorders: inhalation of irritants, asthma, pneumonia, and pulmonary edema children, less than 20 mEq/L in young children), and lowered P_{CO_2} (less than 35 mm Hg).

Treatment of respiratory alkalosis consists of correction of the primary defect and prevention of lost anions and the associated K^+ deficit. Rebreathing CO_2 slows respirations and provides rapid relief, as does O_2 therapy.

METABOLIC ACIDOSIS

Metabolic acidosis is a lowered plasma pH caused by any process that reduces the HCO_3 concentration. Metabolic acidosis can be produced by the gain of nonvolatile acids or the loss of HCO_3. Strong acid is gained, and HCO_3 is lost by several specific mechanisms and routes (see box below).

Compensation of metabolic acidosis is respiratory, with alveolar hyperventilation occurring immediately as the decrease in pH is sensed by the respiratory center. Strong acids are immediately buffered to generate the weaker H_2CO_3, which the respiratory system attempts to eliminate through increased alveolar ventilation. In this respiratory effort the breathing is deep and rapid—the Kussmaul or air-hunger type of respirations. HCO_3 conservation and excretion by the kidneys is a slower mechanism. Laboratory findings of uncompensated metabolic acidosis include lowered plasma pH (less than 7.33), diminished plasma HCO_3 concentration (less than 23 mEq/L in older children, less than 20 mEq/L in young children), and CO_2 combining power that is lowered and approximately equivalent to the plasma HCO_3 in concentration.

Treatment is directed at correcting the basic defect and replacing the excessive losses of HCO_3 with sodium or potassium bicarbonate or sodium lactate.

METABOLIC ACIDOSIS

Strong acid is gained by:
- Gain of exogenous acid (e.g., ammonium chloride) by ingestion or infusion (e.g., salicylates, methanol, ethylene glycol)
- Incomplete oxidation of fatty acids, which occurs in conditions such as diabetic ketoacidosis, starvation (including patients receiving nothing by mouth for therapeutic purposes)
- Incomplete oxidation of carbohydrate that produces large amounts of lactic acid as a result of primary lactic acidosis (rare) or secondary to tissue hypoxia from excessive exercise, serious trauma, and severe infection
- Inability of the renal system to excrete the normal, ongoing volume of inorganic acid metabolites, which results from the azotemic acidosis of advanced renal failure, renal tubular acidosis, and potassium-sparing diuretics

Base bicarbonate is lost by:
- Losses from the gastrointestinal tract—secretions distal to the pyloric sphincter contain large amounts of bicarbonate, which may be lost during conditions that produce diarrhea or vomiting, fistula drainage, and suction
- Losses as a result of inappropriate bicarbonate excretion in the kidneys because of renal tubular acidosis

METABOLIC ALKALOSIS

Metabolic alkalosis is represented by an elevated plasma pH that occurs when there is a reduction in H^+ concentration and an excess of HCO_3. This can be caused by a gain in base or a loss of acid (see box below).

Compensation in metabolic alkalosis theoretically should be respiratory; however, such compensation is irregular and unpredictable. In addition, renal correction is complicated by losses of Na^+, K^+, and Cl^-, which are lost in pyloric stenosis through vomiting. The kidneys will attempt to conserve the Na^+ and K^+ concentration at the expense of H^+ concentration and acid-base balance. Laboratory findings include elevated urine pH (often greater than 7; may be lowered if associated with K^+ depletion), elevated plasma pH (greater than 7.43), elevated plasma HCO_3 (greater than 29 mEq/L in older children, greater than 28 mEq/L in young children), and, if in conjunction with chloride deficit, reduced Cl^- concentration (less than 98 mEq/L).

Treatment of metabolic alkalosis is aimed at preventing further losses of acid and replacing lost electrolytes.

NURSING RESPONSIBILITIES IN FLUID AND ELECTROLYTE DISTURBANCES

Nursing observation and intervention are essential to the detection and therapeutic management of disturbances in fluid and electrolyte balance. Imbalances may be precipitated in a variety of circumstances, and the balance is so precarious, especially in infants, that changes can take place in a very short time. Therefore an important nursing responsibility is anticipation and perceptive observation for any signs of imbalance, particularly in those situations and conditions in which imbalance is likely to occur. Conditions in which changes can develop with surprising rapidity in young children include diarrhea; vomiting; sweating; fever; disorders such as diabetes, renal disease, and cardiac anomalies; administration of certain drugs such as diuretics and steroids; and trauma, such as major surgery, burns, and other extensive injury.

Nurses must be comfortable with equipment used to de-

METABOLIC ALKALOSIS

Loss of acid can result from the following:
- In children the most common cause of hydrogen ion depletion is loss of hydrochloric acid (HCl) incident to hypertrophic pyloric stenosis. The infant produces large amounts of HCl, which is vomited with repeated feedings. HCL is also lost in enteral tube drainage.
- Less often, hydrogen ions are lost through the kidneys in diuretic therapy, potassium depletion, or administration of adrenocortical hormones.

A gain in base is usually iatrogenic and relatively uncommon in children but can result from the following:
- Gain of exogeneous bicarbonate from ingestion or infusion
- Oxidation of salts or organic acid from infusion or ingestion of lactate, citrate, or acetate

liver fluids to infants and children and be familiar with the knowledge and techniques for assessment. An understanding of normal serum levels provides additional data on which to base assessments and interventions and to validate observations. Data that are helpful in assessment related to fluid and electrolyte balance are the medical diagnosis, the treatment that the child is receiving (especially medications and fluid therapies), laboratory reports, history, and records of intake and output. An important nursing role is teaching parents to recognize early signs of dehydration.

ASSESSMENT

Whether the child is at home, in the practitioner's office or clinic, or in the hospital, nursing assessment is an essential part of the nursing care plan. The assessment of suspected or potential fluid and electrolyte disturbance begins with the observation of general appearance. Ill children usually have drawn, flaccid expressions, and their eyes lack luster. Loss of appetite is one of the first behaviors observed in most childhood illnesses, and the infant's or child's activity level is diminished. The cry of an ill infant is less vigorous, often whining, and higher pitched than usual. The child is irritable, seeks the comfort and attention of the parent, and displays purposeless movements and inappropriate responses to people and familiar things. As the child's illness and level of dehydration become more severe, the irritability progresses to lethargy and even unconsciousness.

History

Much of the information regarding the child's behavior can be elicited from the parent. In addition to initial observations, a good history is extremely valuable to the assessment. The amount and type of intake and output (especially abnormal output) are important. An accurate estimate of fluid losses is beyond the capacity of history givers, but rough estimates of excessive fluid losses or diminished output can usually be obtained from information such as the number and consistency of stools the child has passed in the past 24 hours, the number of times the child voided, and the type and amount of food and fluid ingested or vomited. Parents frequently omit this information from their discussion with the health professional. They tell how much has been taken but not how much was excreted unless asked specifically for this information.

Both the type and the amount of intake provide valuable information. The quality and quantity can be determined: if intake is sustained, excessive, or curtailed. Loss early in diarrheal illness progresses rapidly, and the water losses can exceed sodium losses leading to hypernatremia. Hypernatremic dehydration indicates a significant interference with water intake. Also important is a history of normal or increased intake of an unusual fluid such as one containing sugar, tea, athletic hydration fluid (e.g., Gatorade), or other solute-containing fluids, which can contribute to hyponatremic dehydration in the face of abnormal losses (Finberg, 1990).

History of gradual weight gain and observations of any puffiness, especially in areas with less dense tissues (periorbital, scrotal), or "clothes fitting tighter" offer early clues to edema. History of excessive intake, especially when associated with diminished output, is important in assessing edema and water intoxication.

Clinical Observations

Tachycardia, the earliest manifestation of dehydration, can also be produced by fever and infection; therefore, these are considered in the assessment of dehydration. Dry skin and mucous membranes usually appear early. A sunken fontanel is a useful observation if the configuration of the fontanel is known when the infant is healthy. Signs of circulatory failure usually indicate severe dehydration, since compensatory mechanisms are able to sustain blood pressure in the low normal range for some time. Loss of skin elasticity, generally manifested in children less than 2 years of age, is measured by the time it takes for pinched abdominal skin to recoil. This sign is also observed in undernourished children. Also, in hypertonic dehydration the skin has a smooth, velvety feel before it develops disturbed elasticity.

Capillary filling time is assessed by pinching the abdominal skin, a toe, or a thumb and estimating the time that blood is observed to return. Capillary filling time in mild dehydration is less than 2 seconds, increasing to more than 3 seconds in severe dehydration. The technique is effective in children of all ages. However, it can be altered in the presence of heart failure, which affects circulation time, and hypertonic dehydration, in which fluid loss is primarily intracellular.

The observations outlined in Table 28-7 are also used to arrive at a meaningful assessment. When caring for the ill child, vital signs are assessed as often as every 15 to 30 minutes, and weight is recorded frequently during the initial phase of therapy. It is important to use the same scale each time the child is weighed and to predetermine the weight of any equipment or devices that must remain attached during the weighing process, including armboards and sandbags, as well as any clothing the child might be wearing. Routine weights should be taken at the same time each day.

Intake and Output Measurement

One of the most important roles of the nurse in fluid and electrolyte disturbance is related to intake and output (I & O). Accurate measurements are essential to the assessment of fluid balance. Measurements from all sources—including both gastrointestinal and parenteral intake and output from urine, stools, vomitus, fistulas, nasogastric suction, sweat, and drainage from wounds—must be taken and considered. Although the physician usually indicates when I & O are to be recorded, it is a nursing responsibility to keep an accurate I & O record on certain children:

- Receiving IV therapy
- After major surgery
- Severe thermal burns or injuries
- Renal disease or damage
- Congestive heart failure
- Dehydration
- Diabetes mellitus
- Oliguria

TABLE 28-7 Significance of Clinical Observations Related to Fluid and Electrolyte Effects

OBSERVATION	SIGNIFICANT VARIATION	POSSIBLE IMBALANCE	COMMENTS
Temperature	Elevated	Early water depletion Sodium excess	Elevated temperature will increase rate of water loss
	Lowered	Fluid volume deficit	Caused by reduced energy output Shock is outcome of severe fluid deficit
Pulse	Rapid, weak, thready, easily obliterated	Circulatory collapse may result from fluid deficit, hemorrhage, plasma-to-interstitial fluid shift	Pulse rate should include assessment of volume and quality as well as rate
	Bounding, easily obliterated	Impending circulatory collapse Sodium deficit	Pulse may be influenced by activity or emotions
	Bounding, not easily obliterated	Fluid volume excess Interstitial fluid-to-plasma shift	
	Weak, irregular, rapid	Severe potassium deficit	
	Weak, irregular, slowing	Severe potassium excess	
	Increased	Sodium excess Magnesium deficit	
	Decreased	Magnesium excess	
Respiration	Slow, shallow	Respiratory alkalosis	Rapid respirations increase water loss
	Rapid, deep	Metabolic acidosis	Not a reliable sign of respiratory alkalosis in infants
	Dyspnea	Fluid volume excess either general or pulmonary	
	Moist crackles	Fluid volume excess Pulmonary edema	
	Shallow	Potassium excess or deficit	
	Stridor	Severe calcium deficit	
Blood pressure	Increased	Fluid volume excess	Blood pressure not a reliable sign in young children
	Decreased	Sodium deficit Diminished vascular volume (loss of plasma-to-interstitial fluid shift) Severe potassium excess or deficit	Elasticity of blood vessels may keep blood pressure stable
Skin			
Color	Pallor	Protein deficit Fluid deficit Fluid compartment shifts	
	Flushed	Sodium excess	
Temperature	Cold, mottled extremities	Severe fluid volume deficit, even with fever Severe sodium depletion	Caused by decreased peripheral blood flow
Feel	Dry	Fluid depletion Sodium excess	
	Clammy, cold	Sodium deficit Plasma-to-interstitial fluid shift Hypotonic dehydration	
	Poor capillary filling	Fluid volume deficit	
Elasticity	Poor to very poor	Fluid depletion	Pinch of skin from abdomen or inner thigh is lifted and remains raised for several seconds
Pitting edema	Slight to severe	Fluid volume excess Plasma-to-interstitial fluid shift	Obese infants may appear normal
Mucous membranes	Dry Longitudinal wrinkles on tongue	Fluid volume depletion	
	Sticky; rough, red, dry tongue	Sodium excess Hypertonic dehydration	
Salivation and tearing	Absent	Fluid volume deficit	
Fontanel	Sunken	Fluid volume deficit	
	Bulging	Fluid volume excess	
Eyeballs	Sunken Soft	Fluid volume deficit	
Sensory alterations	Tingling in fingers and toes	Calcium deficit Alkalosis	Sensory alterations unreliable in infants and young children who are unable to communicate symptoms
	Abdominal cramps	Sodium deficit Potassium excess	

TABLE 28-7 Significance of Clinical Observations Related to Fluid and Electrolyte Effects—cont'd

OBSERVATION	SIGNIFICANT VARIATION	POSSIBLE IMBALANCE	COMMENTS
	Muscle cramps	Calcium deficit Potassium deficit	
	Lightheadedness	Respiratory alkalosis	
	Nausea	Calcium excess Potassium excess Potassium deficit	
	Thirst	Fluid deficit Sodium excess Calcium excess	May be difficult to assess in infants May be masked by nausea Any condition that reduces intravascular volume will stimulate thirst receptors
Neurologic signs	Hypotonia	Potassium deficit Calcium excess	
	Flaccid paralysis	Severe potassium deficit Severe potassium excess	
	Weakness	Metabolic acidosis	
	Hypertonia		
	Positive Chvostek sign	Calcium deficit	Children may develop calcium deficit easily, since growing bones do not readily relinquish calcium to circulation
	Tremors, cramps, tetany	Alkalosis with diminished calcium ionization Calcium deficit	
	Twitching	Magnesium deficit	
Behavior	Lethargy	Fluid volume deficit overload	Behavioral changes are among first indications of dehydration as reported by parents
	Irritability	Fluid volume deficit	
	Comatose condition	Hypotonic fluid deficit Profound acidosis of alkalosis	
	Lethargy with hyperirritability on stimulation	Hypertonic fluid deficit	
	Extreme restlessness	Potassium excess	
Weight	Loss	Fluid deficit	See Table 28-2
	Up to 5% (50 ml/kg)	Mild	
	5% to 9% (75 ml/kg)	Moderate	
	10% or higher (100 ml/kg)	Severe Protein or calorie deficiency	
	Gain	Edema—general or pulmonary Ascites	Check for hepatomegaly; children sequester excess fluid in liver
Urine	Increased (polyuria)	Interstitial fluid-to-plasma shift Increased renal solute load	Normal range Infant: 2-3 ml/kg/hr Toddler/preschooler: 2 ml/kg/hr School-age child: 1-2 ml/kg/hr Adolescent: 0.5-1 ml/kg/hr (varies with intake and other factors)
	Diminished	Mild fluid deficit Moderate to severe fluid deficit	
	Oliguria	Moderate to severe fluid deficit Plasma-to-interstitial fluid shift Sodium deficit Potassium excess Severe sodium excess Renal insufficiency	
	Specific gravity	Adequate hydration	Used to monitor hydration status in infants
	Low (≥1.010)	Fluid excess Renal disease Sodium deficit	Fixed low reading occurs in renal disease
	High (≥1.030)	Fluid deficit Sodium excess Glycosuria Proteinuria	
	pH		
	Acid	Acidosis—metabolic or respiratory Alkalosis accompanied by severe potassium deficit Fluid deficit	
	Alkaline	Alkalosis, metabolic or respiratory Hyperaldosteronism Acidosis accompanied by chronic renal infection and renal tubular dysfunction Diuretic therapy with carbonic anhydrase inhibitors	

- Receiving diuretic therapy
- Receiving corticosteroid therapy
- Respiratory distress

Infants or small children who are unable to use a bedpan or those who have bowel movements with every voiding will require the application of a collecting device (see Urine Specimens, Chapter 27). Collecting bags may not be suitable for all infants, for example, preterm and other infants whose fragile skin does not tolerate some types of self-adhesive appliances. If collecting bags are not used, wet diapers or pads are carefully weighed to ascertain the amount of fluid lost. This includes liquid stool, vomitus, and other losses. The volume of fluid in milliliters is approximately equivalent to the weight of the fluid measured in grams. The specific gravity as a measure of osmolality is determined with a refractometer or urine dipsticks and assists in assessing the degree of hydration.

➤ **NURSING TIP** 1 g wet diaper weight = 1 ml urine

Disadvantages of the weighed diaper method of fluid measurement include (1) inability to differentiate one type of loss from another because of admixture; (2) loss of urine or liquid stool from leakage or evaporation, especially if the infant is under a radiant warmer; and (3) additional fluid in diaper (superabsorbent disposable type) from absorption of atmospheric moisture (high-humidity incubators) (Hermansen and Buches, 1987 and 1988). Evaporative losses render measurements inaccurate unless the diaper is weighed and measured for specific gravity at least every 30 minutes when critical values are needed. Evaporative losses are greater in infants under radiant warmers or being treated with phototherapy. However, research indicates that accurate specific gravity measurements can be made for up to 2 hours on urine obtained from a diaper that has been removed from an infant, folded, and stored in a utility room (Lybrand, Medoff-Cooper, and Munro, 1990).

It is important to measure and record all intake, oral and parenteral, and output from all sources, including urine, stool, emesis, drainage tubes, fistulas, and wounds from which appreciable amounts of fluid are lost.

At home parents are advised to observe the number of times and how much the child voids. Infants younger than 1 year of age normally void every 1 to 2 hours; toddlers urinate approximately every 3 hours. As children get older, they void less frequently. The parents are instructed to notify the nurse or clinician if the child appears to be voiding an insufficient amount or persistently losing fluid through vomiting or diarrhea.

ORAL FLUID INTAKE

Under ordinary circumstances, an adequate oral intake is no problem in children who are able to respond to thirst cues. Hydration becomes a nursing problem when infants or children are unable to respond to the thirst mechanism and when fatigue or discomfort makes them reluctant to swallow. Children with elevated temperatures, those with continued gastrointestinal losses, those with labile diabetes, and children with cystic fibrosis are especially prone to dehydration. Occasionally, dehydration caused by inadequate intake has been observed in breast-fed infants.

A number of common fluids found in hospitals and in the home are acceptable for encouraging fluid intake and preventing dehydration, including diluted fruit juice, liquid or solid gelatin, sweetened tea, flavored ice pops, and sports electrolyte replacement drinks (e.g., Gatorade, Exceed) and infant solutions such as Infalyte and Pedialyte. Although traditional methods advocated the use of decarbonated cola or ginger ale, these are now not preferred because of their high glucose concentration and subsequent high osmolality (both are about 540), nor is straight apple juice (osmolality greater than 700) preferred. When teaching parents about fluid management, it is always wise to determine whether or not they understand the concept of clear liquids. It is important to emphasize that milk is not a liquid, since it forms curds when it comes in contact with stomach renin.

➤ **NURSING TIP** Any liquid through which newsprint can be read is considered to be clear.

When an electrolyte formula is prescribed, it is advisable to have the parents demonstrate their ability to prepare it, because a mistake or misunderstanding of measurements (e.g., substitution of a tablespoon for the teaspoon measure, using heaping rather than level measurements, or adding other ingredients, such as milk) can significantly alter the electrolyte concentration. Parents are cautioned about including broth as fluid intake. When prepared as directed on the labels, most commercial broths contain unusually high sodium concentrations. Parents should consult with a dietitian or the health practitioner for proper dilution of these fluids before offering them to a child who has large fluid losses. The caloric content and electrolyte composition of some common fluids are listed in Table 28-8.

Persuading a reluctant child to drink fluids can be a nurs-

TABLE 28-8 Sodium, Potassium, and Caloric Content of Selected Oral Fluids

FLUID	Na^+* (mEq/L)	K^+* (mEq/L)	CALORIES (kcal/L)
Water	0	0	0
Sugar water (5%)	0	0	200
Infalyte	50	25	126
Pedialyte	45	20	280
Coca-Cola	3.6	0	435
Pepsi-Cola	0	0	480
Ginger ale	4.5	0.1	300
7-Up	0.5	0	420
Sprite	7.6	0	400
Orange juice (unsweetened)	2	48.5	410
Apple juice	0.43	25	483
Gatorade	23.5	2.5	170
Grape juice	0.8	29.6	660
Jello (half strength)	5.5-16.5†	0.1-0.2	404

*Varies according to mineral content of water used for bottling.
†Varies according to flavor (Na^+ highest in wild cherry, lowest in grape and black raspberry).

ing challenge and is not uncommon in the care of infants and children. Older children will often respond to the challenge of meeting a specific goal for fluid intake (or deprivation) and can be active participants in planning an intake schedule. Contracts and rewards are effective strategies. However, young children require more creative tactics. Suggestions for encouraging children to drink fluids are discussed in Chapter 27. (See Chapter 27 also for a discussion of nasogastric alimentation.)

The Child Who Is NPO

Infants or children who are unable or not permitted to take fluids by mouth (NPO) have special needs. To ensure that they do not receive fluids, a sign can be placed in some obvious place, such as over their beds or pinned to their shirts, to alert others to the NPO status. Fluids are removed from the bedside to reduce the temptation. Drinking fountains and wash basins are monitored.

Oral hygiene, a part of routine hygienic care, is especially important when fluids are restricted or withheld (see Chapter 27). For young children who cannot brush their teeth or rinse their mouth without swallowing fluid, the mouth and teeth can be cleaned and kept moist by swabbing with a saline-moistened gauze. Judicious administration of ice chips provides moist, cool relief (if permitted by the practitioner). A thin layer of petrolatum (Vaseline) or other commercial lip aid helps to keep lips soft and prevents cracking and caking.

➤ **NURSING TIP** Water sprayed into the mouth from an atomizer is refreshing and relieves a dry mouth.

To meet the need to suck, infants should be provided with a pacifier, preferably an acceptable commercial variety. Aspiration of a nipple used to construct a pacifier has been reported (Millunchick and McArtor, 1986).

The child on restricted fluids provides an equal challenge. Limiting fluids is often more difficult for the child than NPO, especially when IV fluids are also eliminated. To make certain the child does not drink the entire amount allowed early in the day, the daily allotment is calculated to provide fluids at periodic intervals throughout the child's waking hours. Serving the fluids in small containers gives the illusion of larger servings. No extra liquid is left at the bedside if compliance is a problem.

PARENTERAL FLUID THERAPY*

Intravenous Infusion

Before an IV infusion is started, several preparatory activities must take place. All needed equipment is gathered so that the operator can proceed without interruption. More importantly, the child and the family must be prepared for this stressful procedure.

Solution. The composition of IV solution is selected on the basis of tonicity (osmolality) and electrolyte content. A solution that is ***isotonic*** has the same osmolality, or tonicity, as body fluids such as plasma. A ***hypertonic*** solution is one that has a greater concentration of solutes than plasma; a ***hypotonic*** solution has a lower concentration. Examples of isotonic solutions are 0.9% normal saline solutions, lactated Ringer's, and 5% dextrose in water; 10% glucose in water is a hypertonic solution; plain water and 0.2% sodium are hypotonic solutions. Although it is larger, one molecule of glucose has only half the osmolality of one molecule of NaCl because the NaCl ionizes in solution into two particles, the Na^+ and the Cl^- ions. Thus one molecule of NaCl exerts twice the osmotic pressure of one molecule of glucose.

Most common pediatric maintenance solutions include a combination of dextrose (usually 5% or 10%) and NaCl (usually 0.22% to 0.3%). The hypotonic solution is necessary for children, since their daily turnover of "free" water exceeds that of adults. Because infants and young children are subject to rapid fluid shifts, any IV solution given to them contains at least 0.2% NaCl to prevent brain edema, a disorder to which they are susceptible if given plain water. Glucose is rapidly metabolized; therefore the osmolality of 5% glucose is further diminished.

Equipment. For IV infusions in most children, a 22- to 24-gauge over-the-needle catheter is preferred. For small scalp veins a size 23 or 25 needle with flexible wings may be used. In situations in which fluids are urgently needed and there is difficulty in entering a vein, a polyethylene catheter inserted by the surgical cutdown procedure may be necessary. The vein of choice for this alternative is the internal saphenous vein located just anterior to the medial malleolus of the tibia or the external saphenous vein on the lateral side.

Other equipment needed includes alcohol and povidone-iodine swabs to clean the site, a tourniquet, an appropriate-sized padded armboard (when an extremity is used), rolled towels or small blankets for maintaining position of head or extremity, tape (or dressing and bacteriostatic ointment if hospital dictates), a T or J connector (an extension that makes changing tubing easier), transparent occlusive dressing (if needed), and an IV shield to protect the IV site after insertion. The prescribed solution, tubing, filter, and infusion pump are prepared in advance, ready to connect to the needle after insertion.

Infusion Pumps. There are several modifications in equipment used for IV infusion for children. A gravity drainage apparatus used for children is much the same as that for adults except that it is designed to deliver a reduced drop size (60 drops/ml) and contains a calibrated volume control chamber (e.g., a Buretrol or Solu-set) that regulates the amount of fluid that can be infused. A microdropper greatly facilitates calculation of flow rate because a prescribed number of milliliters per hour equals the number of drops per minute. For example, if the solution is to infuse at a rate of 30 ml per hour, the infusion is regulated to deliver 30 drops per minute.

A variety of infusion pumps are available, but all have a limited capacity, refillable from the bottle above or contained in syringe pumps, to minimize the possibility of overloading the circulation. Infusion devices are almost always used in pediatrics because they can accurately infuse very small amounts of fluid, as well as accurately provide the prescribed amount of IV solution. It is an important nursing

*Kathryn A. Perry, APRN, RN,C, MSN, CNS, revised this section.

responsibility to calculate the amount to be infused in a given length of time, set the infusion rate, and monitor the apparatus frequently (at least every 1 to 2 hours) to make certain that the desired rate is maintained, the integrity of the system remains intact, the site remains intact (free of infiltration or irritation), and the infusion does not stop.

Continuous infusion pumps, although convenient and efficient, are not without risks. Overreliance on the accuracy of the machine can cause either too much or too little fluid to be infused; therefore its use does not eliminate careful periodic assessment by the nurse. Excess pressure can build up if the machine is set at a rate faster than the vein is able to accommodate (or continues to pump when the needle is out of the lumen). This is especially true in very small infants. No matter what device is used, a thorough understanding of the apparatus is essential for safe fluid administration.

Preparing the Child and Parents

Children of any age are anxious and fearful of injections, and unless the IV infusion is implemented as an emergency procedure, there will be time to prepare them (see Preparation for Procedures, Chapter 27). Many children have never undergone the procedure, and those who have will remember the experience. It is useful to ask them what they think about the procedure and why it is needed for them specifically. Children's perceptions of the anticipated experience furnish information on misconceptions that need to be clarified and help the nurse prepare children for what they can expect. In addition, children's observations provide some insight into how to cope with a child's reactions during the insertion procedure and throughout the course of the IV therapy. For children who have repeated venipunctures, it is helpful to ask them or their parents where the vein has been successfully accessed.

Play, always an excellent stress-reducing technique, can be employed during the preparation process. Allowing children to handle the equipment and to "start" an IV infusion on a toy animal or doll helps familiarize them with the frightening aspects of the procedure. In some instances it may be helpful to introduce a child to another child who is coping well in the same situation.

It is best to arrange for a quiet, private setting for the child during the insertion. The assurance of privacy relieves the child of some anxieties concerning loss of control in front of others. It also avoids subjecting other children to the potentially stress-provoking scene. The child should be provided with some distracting activity, such as those described for injections, and perhaps be allowed to "help" by holding supplies such as a gauze square, helping to clean the site with alcohol, and assisting in taping the site after the procedure.

Children will usually cooperate better and feel more in command if they are allowed to sit up during the process, although this may not be possible even in some older, normally cooperative children. It is a mistake to assume that children will not lose control even after they promise to cooperate. It is wise to have ample assistance available in the event a child cannot control anxiety. The child need not be restrained until necessary, but the assistant should be prepared to grasp a child gently but firmly during the insertion. Explaining to children what is being done during each step of the procedure and how they can participate helps to obtain their cooperation and reduce their stress.

Application of EMLA, a topical anesthetic, or the intradermal use of buffered lidocaine to the injection site before needle insertion should be used to reduce the pain of injection. (See Chapter 26 for a discussion of pain management.) Parents are told about the procedure, including the reasons for the procedure, how long the needle must remain in place, and what they can expect during and after the insertion. They should be offered the option of remaining with their child or leaving (see Thinking Critically About . . . box on p. 1138).

The Procedure

The site selected for IV infusion depends on accessibility and convenience. Although it is possible to use any accessible vein in older children, attention must be directed toward the child's developmental, cognitive, and mobility needs when selecting a site. Whenever possible, it is best to avoid the child's favored hand in order to reduce the disability related to the procedure. A site is chosen that restricts the child's movements as little as possible—a site over a joint in an extremity is avoided, such as the antecubital fossa. An older child can help to select the site and thereby maintain some measure of control.

For veins in the extremities, it is best to start with the most distal sites, especially if irritating or sclerosing agents, such as chemotherapeutic drugs or hyperosmolar solutions (e.g., hyperalimentation), are to be used. If the vein is damaged, using distal sites initially preserves access to the vein in proximal sites. A scalp vein or a superficial vein of the wrist may also be used if larger veins are not accessible (Fig. 28-3). Arteries are avoided for peripheral IV therapy.

Most infants have one or two possible IV sites on each arm and foot and four to eight sites on the scalp. Since superficial veins of the scalp have no valves, they can be infused in either direction and are sometimes used for IV therapy in infants less than 9 months of age. The temporal and forehead areas are suitable and do not interfere with side-to-side head movements. Scalp veins have little subcutaneous tissue to obscure visualization of the vein, and there are no joints to interfere with movement. However, the use of a scalp vein site may require shaving the area around the site to better visualize the vein and provide a smoother surface on which to tape the tubing (Fig. 28-4). Shaving off a portion of the infant's hair is very upsetting to parents; therefore, they should *always* be told what to expect and reassured that the hair will grow in again rapidly (save the hair because parents often wish to keep it). As little as possible is removed directly over the insertion site. A rubber band slipped onto the head from brow to occiput will usually suffice as a tourniquet, although if the vessel is visible, a tourniquet may not be necessary in some infants.

➤ **NURSING TIP** A small adhesive tape tab slipped over the rubber band tourniquet provides a convenient way to grasp and remove the band.

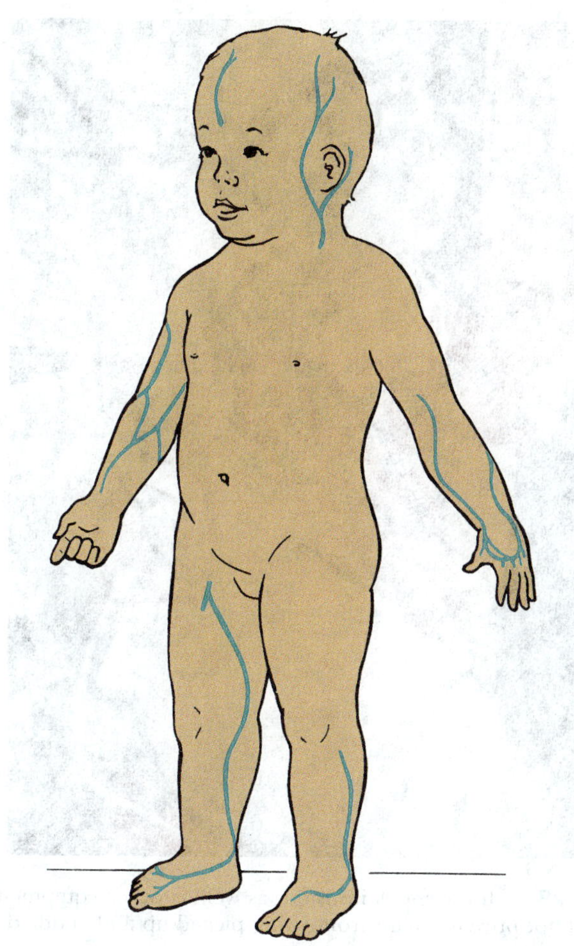

FIG. 28-3 Superficial veins used most often for intravenous infusion in infants and very young children. (From Kempe CH, Silver HK, O'Brien D: *Current pediatric diagnosis and treatment,* ed 9, Los Altos, CA, 1986, Lange Medical Publications.)

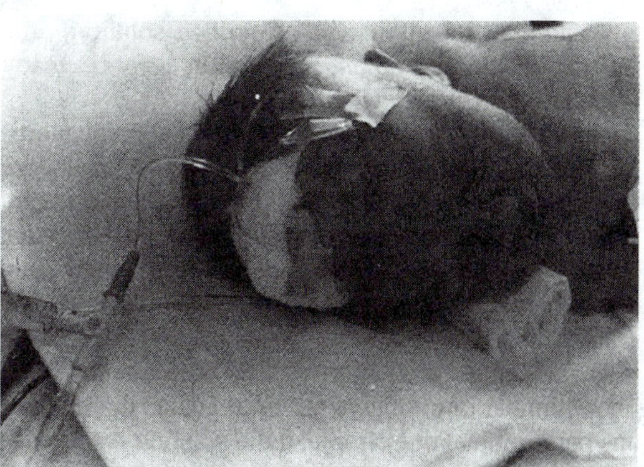

FIG. 28-4 Scalp vein infusion.

The extremity or head should be carefully restrained by an assistant for easier venipuncture and to minimize trauma resulting from the child's inadvertent movement. Extremities may be secured to the armboard when those sites are used, and head movements are restrained for scalp venipuncture. (See also Chapter 27 for additional restraining methods.) For a scalp site it is helpful to visualize the way in which the needle will be secured following insertion.

Locating a vein may be difficult because the veins are smaller and children have a significant amount of subcutaneous fat. When veins are not readily visible, applying a warm compress to the site or, when using an extremity, holding the limb in a dependent position below body level will help fill the veins for better visualization. Gentle tapping sometimes causes the veins to stand out. A flashlight held against the skin below the intended site sometimes assists in locating vessels; depth, however, may be hard to gauge. If these measures do not help, a tourniquet applied with light pressure medially to the site may be needed. Although the tourniquet makes the veins more visible and provides a more rapid blood return, the added venous pressure may cause fragile veins to "blow" when punctured, producing a hematoma.

➤ **NURSING TIP** A blood pressure cuff can also be used as a tourniquet and can give more control over the pressure needed to make the veins visible.

The needle or catheter must be placed in the direction of the blood flow, which creates no problem when an extremity is used. Scalp veins are more difficult to assess and may often actually be an artery; therefore palpation for a pulse on scalp sites is recommended. In general, the venous blood flows from the top of the head toward the neck. To test the direction before insertion, the forefinger is placed on the vein at the site chosen for venipuncture. While the finger gently presses the vein a second finger is used to "strip" the vein in the direction of the top of the head. The pressure from the second finger is released. If the vein fills distal to the compressing finger, the direction of flow is toward the stationary finger.

To maintain the integrity of the IV site, adequate protection of the site will be required for the child. An attempt is made to position the extremity in a natural anatomic position with the use of gauze pads or rolls as needed. A small board, well padded with plastic foam and a cloth or stockinette cover, provides a suitable means for immobilization (Fig. 28-5). When possible, the hand or arm is taped so that the fingers extend over the edge of the board. This allows more use of the fingers and reduces the chance of pulling the fingers out from under the tape. Some form of resilient padding is required to prevent areas of pressure necrosis over bony prominences such as the ankle or pressure on the peroneal nerve on the lateral aspect of the knees. To prevent trauma to the skin from removal of tape, gauze can be placed between the skin and the adhesive, or elastic self-adhering role bandages (e.g., Coban) can be applied around the extremity to secure the IV catheter or needle in older infants.

NURSING ALERT If any type of opaque covering is used to secure the IV line, the insertion site and extremity distal to the site should be visible to detect an infiltration. If these sites are not visible, they must be checked hourly to detect problems early.

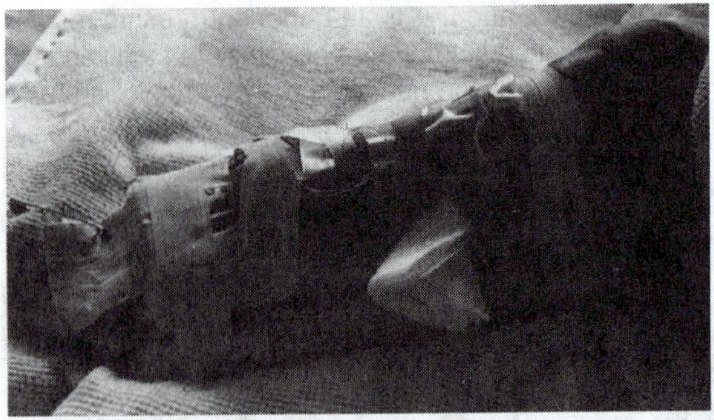

FIG. 28-5 Extremity immobilized with board and firmly secured to bedding with pins, if prescribed.

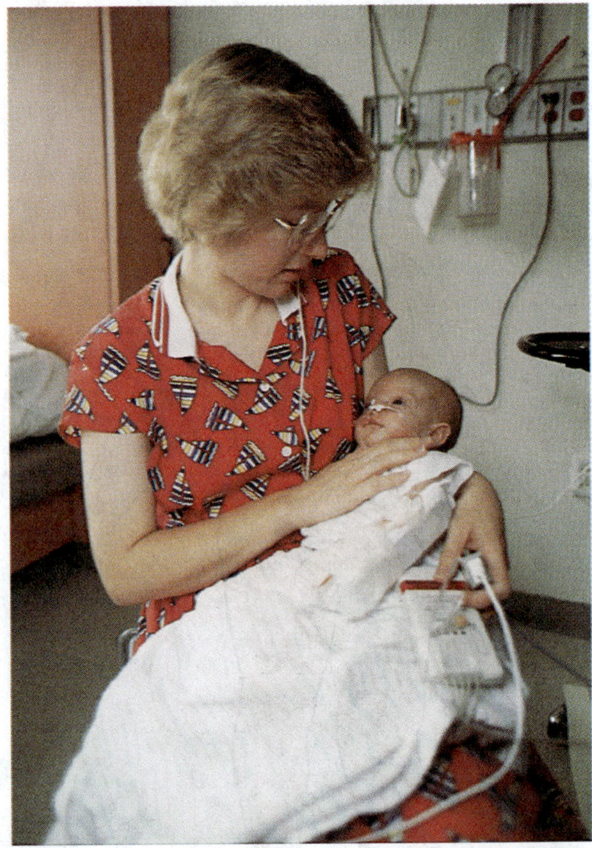

FIG. 28-6 Intravenous infusion, as well as other equipment, does not prevent infant from being picked up and cuddled.

Following insertion, the needle or catheter is firmly secured at the puncture site with nonallergenic tape and protected from becoming dislodged by immobilization of the extremity. The insertion site and about 1 to 2 inches of skin beyond the site are left uncovered for early detection of infiltration. Transparent dressings are ideal because they allow ready visualization of the insertion site. Some finger or toe areas are left unoccluded by dressings or tape to allow for assessment of circulation. The thumb is never immobilized because of the danger of contractures with limited movement later on. A plastic or wax paper cup that is cut in half (with the rigid edges covered with tape) and applied directly over the needle site will protect the infusion site. Some needle containers also make excellent protective covers, as do commercially available products such as IV shields. Whatever protection device is chosen, easy access to the IV site for assessment must be considered. A colorful and interesting sticker can be applied to the armboard or protecting device to add a positive note to the procedure.

Older children who are alert and cooperative can usually be trusted to protect the IV site. An IV infusion is not always a deterrent to mobility. When the child is feeling well and the insertion site is well secured, the child can be held or be walked, but precautions must be observed to preserve the integrity of the IV system.

Infants, small children, and uncooperative children require varying degrees of immobilization, and on rare occasions, complete restriction of movement may be needed to prevent removal of the IV infusion. The board is secured to the bed, and the remaining extremities that might be used to dislodge the needle or catheter are restrained. This includes feet as well as hands, since most infants will attempt to brush away the offending attachment by rubbing it against another extremity or body part.

Immobilization is intolerable to the naturally active child, and every effort should be extended to relieve the stress of immobilization (see Chapter 39). Frequent removal of the restraints provides the child with the opportunity to move the extremities. Whenever possible, the infant or child should be held and cuddled to help meet emotional needs during this trying time (Fig. 28-6). Range-of-motion exercises are employed on infants and children who are too ill or unable to move their extremities, but others should be encouraged to move their arms and legs. Most infants or small children will instinctively move their extremities when released. If not, a toy or other stimulus can provide incentive.

When it comes time to discontinue an IV infusion, many children are distressed by the thought of ***catheter removal.*** Therefore they need a careful explanation of the process and suggestions for helping. One way is to allow children to remove or help remove the tape from the site. It provides them with a measure of control and often encourages their cooperation. The procedure consists of turning off any pump apparatus, occluding the IV tubing, removing the tape, and pulling out the needle or catheter in the opposite direction of insertion, while exerting firm pressure at the site. A dry dressing (adhesive bandage strip) is placed over the puncture site. If a catheter was used for the IV infusion, the tip is inspected to make certain the catheter is intact and no portion remains in the vein.

Complications. The same precautions regarding maintenance of asepsis, prevention of infection, and observation for infiltration are carried out with patients of any age. When the fluid appears to be infusing too slowly or ceases, the usual assessment for obstruction within the apparatus, that is, kinks, screw clamps, shutoff valve, and positioning interference (e.g., a bent elbow), often locates the difficulty. When these actions fail to detect the problem, it may be necessary to carefully remove some of the tape and other material that obscure a clear view of the venipuncture site. Dependent areas, such as the palm and undersides of the extremity or the occiput and behind the ears, are examined.

Whenever possible, the IV infusion should be placed in an extremity to which the identification band (or bracelet) is not attached. Serious circulatory impairment can result from infiltrated solution distal to the band, which acts as a tourniquet preventing adequate venous return. To check for return blood flow through the catheter/needle, the solution bag is lowered below the level of the infusion site. A good blood return, or lack thereof, is not always an indicator of infiltration in small infants. Flushing the catheter/needle and observing for edema, redness, or streaking along the vein is an appropriate assessment of IV status (Wilson, 1992). If the tubing is connected to an infusion pump, it must be removed from the pump before lowering.

NURSING ALERT Different infusion pumps have preset pressures for infusion, delivery, and occlusion; therefore the pump's occlusion alarm is not entirely reliable to detect infiltrations.

Since IV therapy is often used in pediatrics and tends to be difficult to maintain, extravasation injuries are reported with relative frequency. A number of drugs are toxic to subcutaneous tissues and can result in varying degrees of tissue damage with extended hospitalization and treatment.

NURSING ALERT When an infiltration is observed (i.e., signs may include erythema, pain, edema, blanching, and streaking on the skin along the vein), immediately discontinue the infusion, elevate the extremity, notify the practitioner, and initiate the ordered treatment as soon as possible. Dry heat may be applied, except if the infused solution is sclerosing.

Drugs are available to diffuse extravasated fluid or neutralize the extravasated medication. One such drug is hyaluronidase, which is used in severe cases to diffuse extravasated fluids rapidly through the tissue and increase the absorption rate. When used, the IV infusion is discontinued, and with the needle still in place, the drug is injected into the site. If the catheter is removed, the drug is then injected (as prescribed) into the area surrounding the insertion site. Assessment and documentation of the site continues until the infiltration has completely resolved. Staging of IV infiltrates may be performed to evaluate treatment options (Flemmer and Chan, 1993).

Prevention of infection is a major nursing function during IV therapy. The infusion site is protected from trauma and entry of bacteria. When an IV infusion continues for several days or longer, the tubing and solution are changed at regular intervals according to hospital policy. Frequency ranges from every 24 to 72 hours—most often every 48 hours. To ensure that the equipment is changed regularly, it is labeled with the date and time that the new bag and tubing are attached. Any signs of inflammation such as redness or pain should be reported immediately. This usually requires removal of the infusion and restarting it at another site.

Intraosseous Infusion

Situations may occur in which rapid establishment of a systemic access is vital and venous access may be hampered by peripheral circulatory collapse, cardiopulmonary arrest, burns, or other conditions. Intraosseous infusion provides an alternate route for administration of fluids and medications until intravascular access can be attained. The technique has been used satisfactorily by paramedics, emergency department and critical care nurses, and physicians. A large-bore needle such as a bone marrow aspiration needle (e.g., Jamshadi) or an intraosseous needle is inserted into the medullary cavity of a long bone, most often the distal femur, proximal tibia, or distal tibia. Although a variety of needles can be used, the task has proved to be easier and faster with a bone marrow aspiration needle or an intraosseus needle. This procedure is usually reserved for children under 3 years of age who are unconscious or are receiving analgesics because the procedure is painful.

VENOUS ACCESS DEVICES (VADs)*

The ***peripheral lock,*** also known as an ***intermittent infusion device, saline well,*** or ***heparin lock,*** is used as an alternative for a keep-open infusion when extended access to a vein is required without the need for continuous fluid. It is most frequently employed for intermittent infusion of medication into a peripheral venous route. A short, flexible catheter (or occasionally a steel butterfly needle) is used as the lock device, and a site is selected where there will be minimum movement, such as the forearm. The needle/catheter is inserted and secured in the same manner as any IV infusion device, but the hub is occluded with a stopper.

The type of device used may vary among medical establishments, and the care and use of the peripheral lock are carried out according to the specific protocol of the institution or unit. However, the general concept is the same. The needle or catheter remains in place and is flushed with saline or heparin (1:10 units/ml) after infusion of the medication. The heparin solution prevents blood from clotting in the device between infusions.

Heparin is incompatible with many drugs, so the peripheral lock must be flushed with saline before and after administering medication. Controversy exists over saline vs heparin flush; many studies, however, show saline to be as effective in maintaining patency as heparin, with the only exception possibly being a 24-gauge catheter (McMullen and others, 1993). Children may be discharged with a peripheral lock in place in order to continue receiving medications without hospitalization; if so, this is usually reserved for children who require medications on a short-term basis and are referred to a home-based infusion company. Those with chronic illnesses who require repeated blood sampling or medications, long-term chemotherapy, or frequent hyperalimenation or antibiotic therapy are best managed with a central venous catheter.

➤ **NURSING TIP** Using a positive-pressure technique in which the flush syringe is slowly withdrawn from the periph-

■ *Janice Marie Wingo, RN, BSN, CPN, revised this section.

eral lock as the last 0.5 ml of flush is being injected may prevent backflow of blood into the infusion device, thus preventing clot formation in the catheter.

The children and parents are taught the procedure for care of the VAD before discharge from the hospital, including preparation and injection of the prescribed medication, the flush, and dressing changes. A protective device may be recommended for some active children to prevent their accidentally dislodging the needle. Many children take responsibility for preparing and administering medications. Both verbal and written step-by-step instructions* are provided for the learners.

*Home care instructions for caring for an intermittent infusion device are available in *Wong and Whaley's Clinical Manual of Pediatric Nursing* (Mosby).

Central Venous Access Devices

Central VADs have several different characteristics. The practitioner has to consider the best type of catheter for the individual patient's needs. Factors that can influence the decision include the reason for placement of the catheter (diagnosis), length of therapy, risk to the patient in placement of the catheter, and availability of resources to assist the family in maintaining the catheter (Camp-Sorrell, 1990; Masoorli and Angeles, 1990).

Central VADs can be categorized into three types:

1. Short-term or nontunneled catheters (subclavian, femoral, and jugular)
2. Short-term to moderate-term nontunneled catheters
3. Long-term, tunneled catheters and implanted ports (Table 28-9)

TABLE 28-9 Comparison of Long-Term Central Venous Access Devices

DESCRIPTION	BENEFITS	CARE CONSIDERATIONS
TUNNELED CATHETER (E.G. HICKMAN/BROVIAC CATHETER)		
Silicone, radiopaque, flexible catheter with open ends One or two Dacron Cuffs or Vitacuffs (biosynthetic material impregnated with silver ions) on catheter(s) enhances tissue ingrowth May have more than one lumen	Reduced risk of bacterial migration after tissue adheres to Dacron cuff or Vitacuff Easy to use for self-administered infusions	Requires daily heparin flushes Must be clamped or have clamp nearby at all times Must keep exit site dry Heavy activity restricted until tissue adheres to cuff Risk of infection still present Protrudes outside body; susceptible to damage from sharp instruments and may be pulled out; may affect body image More difficult to repair Patient/family must learn catheter care
GROSHONG CATHETER		
Clear, flexible, silicone, radiopaque catheter with closed tip and two-way valve at proximal end Dacron cuff or Vitacuff on catheter enhances tissue ingrowth May have more than one lumen	Reduced time and cost for maintenance care; no heparin flushes needed Reduced catheter damage—no clamping needed because of two-way valve Increased patient safety because of minimum potential for blood backflow or air embolism Reduced risk of bacterial migration after tissue adheres to Dacron cuff or Vitacuff Easily repaired Easy to use for self-administered IV infusions	Requires weekly irrigation with normal saline Must keep exit site dry Heavy activity restricted until tissue adheres to cuff Risk of infection still present Protrudes outside body; susceptible to damage from sharp instruments and may be pulled out; can affect body image Patient/family must learn catheter care
IMPLANTED PORTS (PORT-A-CATH, INFUS-A-PORT, MEDIPORT, NORPORT, GROSHONG PORT)		
Totally implantable metal or plastic device that consists of self-sealing injection port with top or side access with preconnected or attachable silicone catheter that is placed in large blood vessel	Reduced risk of infection Placed completely under the skin; therefore cannot be pulled out or damaged No maintenance care and reduced cost for family Heparinized monthly and after each infusion to maintain patency (Groshong port only requires saline) No limitations on regular physical activity, including swimming Dressing only needed when port accessed with Huber needle that is not removed No or only slight change in body appearance (slight bulge on chest)	Must pierce skin for access; pain with insertion of needle; can use local anesthetic (EMLA) or intradermal buffered lidocaine before accessing port Special noncoring needle (Huber) with straight or angled design must be used to inject into port Skin preparation needed before injection Hard to manipulate for self-administered infusions Catheter may dislodge from port, especially if child "plays" with port site (Twiddler syndrome) Vigorous contact sports generally not allowed

Short-term or ***nontunneled catheters*** are used in acute, emergency, and intensive care units. These catheters are made of polyurethane and are placed in large veins such as the subclavian, femoral, or jugular. A chest x-ray film should be taken to verify placement of the catheter tip before administration of fluids or medications.

Peripherally inserted central catheters (PICCs) can be used for short-term to moderate-length therapy. These catheters consist of silicone or polymer material and are placed by specially trained nurses (Brown, 1989). The most common insertion site is the antecubital area using the median, cephalic, or basilic vein. The catheter is threaded either with or without a guidewire into the superior vena cava. PICCs can be trimmed before insertion, and the decision can be made to insert the catheter "midline," which is considered between the insertion site and the head of the clavicle (Meares, 1992). If the catheter is threaded midline, total parenteral nutrition (TPN), should not be administered since the high concentration of glucose makes it irritating to the vessel and it should be infused through a central catheter.

The decision to insert a PICC needs to be made prior to several attempts at IV lines or blood sampling by phlebotomy. Once the antecubital veins have been punctured repeatedly, they are not considered to be a candidate for this type of catheter. Since this catheter is the least costly and has less chance of complications than other central VADs, it is an excellent choice for many pediatric patients. This catheter is also usually inserted either at the child's bedside or, more appropriately when available, the unit's treatment room.

NURSING ALERT Most PICC lines are not sutured into place, so care needs to be maintained when changing the dressing.

Long-term central VADs include tunneled and implanted infusion ports. They may have single, double, or triple lumens. Several lumens (multilumen catheters) allow more than one therapy to be administered at the same time. Reasons to use multilumen catheters include repeated blood sampling, TPN, administration of blood products or infusion of large quantities and/or concentrations of fluids, ability to administer incompatible drugs or fluids at the same time (through different lumens), and central venous pressure (CVP) monitoring.

With any of the central venous catheters, instilling medication through the injection cap is easily accomplished. With the implanted device, the port must be palpated for placement and stabilized, the overlying skin cleansed, and only special noncoring Huber needles used to pierce the port's diaphragm on the top or side, depending on the style. To avoid repeated skin punctures, a special infusion set with a Huber needle and extension tubing with Luer connection can be used (Fig. 28-7, *B*). With this attached, the injection procedure is the same as for the heparin device or venous catheters. To prevent infection, meticulous aseptic technique must be used anytime the devices are entered, including instillation of heparin or saline to prevent clotting.

With the patient under local or general anesthesia, the long-term catheter of choice is placed with aseptic technique. A vein, such as the jugular or subclavian, is entered through a small cutdown site, and the catheter is threaded to the junction of the superior vena cava and right atrium, confirmed by fluoroscopic dye injection, and then sutured in place. To stabilize the catheter and reduce the risk of infection, the remainder is tunneled beneath the skin to exit through a small incision at a convenient location on the anterior aspect of the chest or upper abdomen (Fig. 28-7, *A*). One or two Dacron cuffs or Vitacuff on the catheter remain in the subcutaneous tunnel; as tissue adheres to the cuff, the cuff provides a barrier to infection. The cutdown site is surgically closed, the catheter is sutured to the skin at the exit site, and a sterile dressing is applied.

Regardless of which catheter is used, the child and family are taught the care and management of the device with provision for practice under supervision (Fig. 28-8). It can be frightening to both child and parents to know that the catheter tip is situated near the heart. They need reassurance that with reasonable care they will do no harm to the apparatus. It is often useful to introduce the family to other

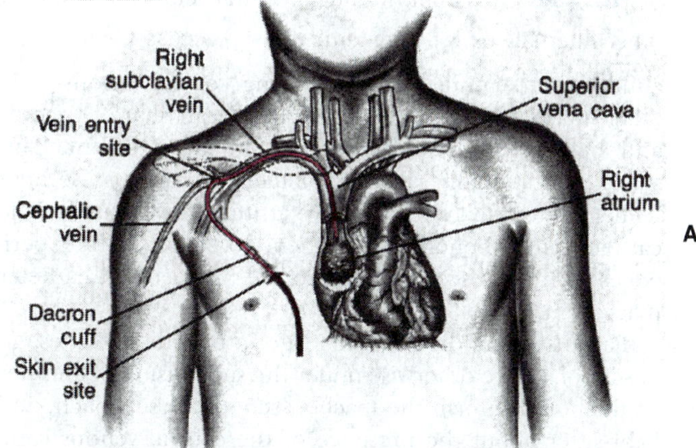

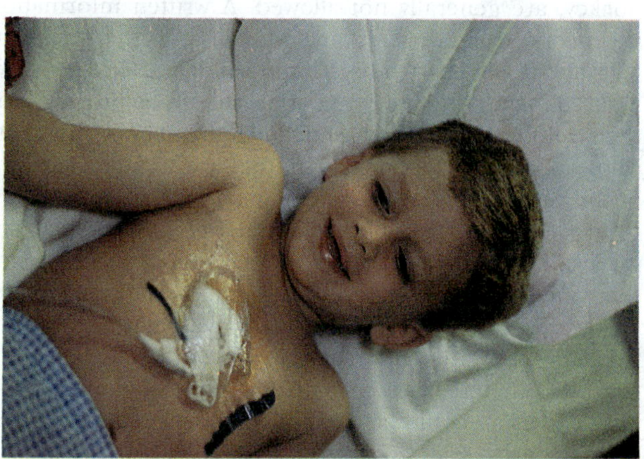

FIG. 28-7 Venous access devices. **A,** Central venous catheter insertion and exit site. **B,** Child receiving medication by way of an implantable port. Note needle and extension tubing inserted into port and secured with gauze dressings and a transparent dressing.

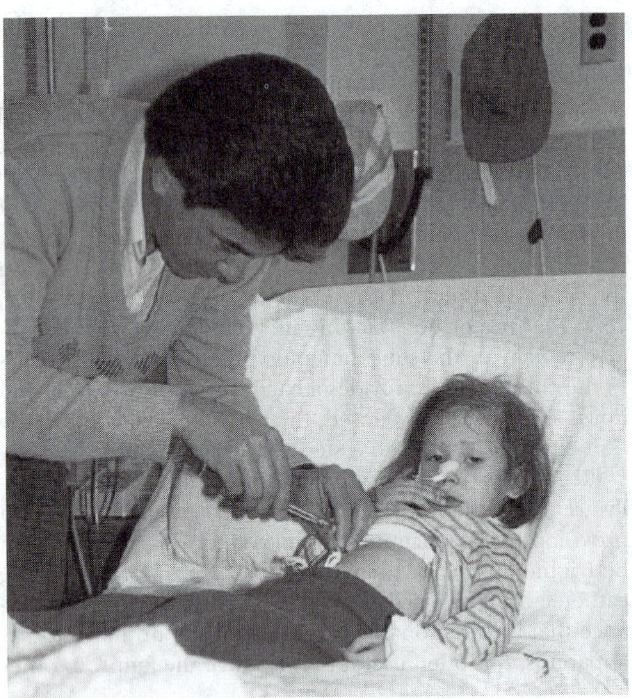

FIG. 28-8 A parent flushing a central venous catheter.

children and families who are using central venous catheters successfully and with whom they can share concerns and helpful tips regarding care and management. This sharing is especially valuable for teenage patients. Because teenagers usually have a positive attitude toward use of the catheter, it is beneficial for them to share their experiences with adolescents who face the prospects of catheter placement.

Parents of children who engage in outside activities, go to school, or are otherwise under the supervision of another adult should inform the teacher, school nurse, coach, and baby-sitter about the presence of the central venous catheter. Vigorous contact sports, such as football, soccer, and hockey, are generally not allowed. A written information sheet concerning the VAD, including its purpose, pertinent facts about any restrictions for the child, and directions related to management of the device, should be provided for their reference. Grandparents and other family members who care for the child are taught the care and management of the catheter by the nurse or the parents.

Procedures and published standards for catheter care vary widely among organizations, and there is no evidence that one method is superior over another. For example, some advocate covering the healed catheter site with a dressing; others do not. All companies that manufacture central catheters have patient and professional teaching kits. The user should become thoroughly familiar with the specific device selected for use.*

The catheter is not a deterrent to most activities, including showers or tub bathing. However, the practitioner is consulted before activities such as swimming or physical contact sports are attempted. Swimming is usually prohibited but may be allowed in certain situations. If the exit site is healed and the cuff adheres to the tissue, a transparent dressing can be placed over the catheter and exit site, and swimming may be permitted for a limited time, such as 1 hour or less, in a chlorinated pool. Most contact sports are prohibited because of the possibility of the catheter being hit or pulled.

➤ **NURSING TIP** A pocket sewn on the inside of a T-shirt provides a place in which to coil the catheter line while the child is at play if a dressing is not used.

Infection and an occluded catheter are two of the most common complications of central venous catheters. Although neither is an emergency, both require treatment: antibiotics for infection and a fibrinolytic agent, such as urokinase, for clots. Uncapping can be prevented by taping the cap securely to the catheter and the clamped line to the dressing. Leaks can be prevented by using a smooth-edged clamp only. Parents are cautioned to keep scissors away from the child to prevent accidental cutting of the catheter. If the catheter leaks, they are instructed to tape it above the leak and then clamp the catheter at the taped site. The child should be taken to the practitioner as soon as possible to prevent infection or clotting following a catheter leak.

NURSING ALERT If a central venous catheter is accidentally removed, apply pressure to the *entry* site to the vein, not the exit site on the skin (Marcoux, Fisher, and Wong, 1990).

Adolescents may benefit from the implanted ports, which consist of a small, circular "port of entry" that is placed under the skin (while the patient is under local or general anesthesia) over a bony prominence to provide a stable surface, usually under the distal third of the clavicle. A tunnel is created from the port to the point where the catheter enters a central vein leading to the entrance to the right atrium. Medication or other solution is injected with a special needle through the skin into the port. The device can remain situated indefinitely. Adolescents who are highly concerned about body image and may be troubled by the visible central venous catheter often prefer this method of venous access. One care consideration of an infusion port is that it requires repeated skin punctures, which may make it less acceptable to children. The use of a topical anesthetic, eutectic mixture of local anesthetics (EMLA), can make the puncture painless. (See also Pain Management, Chapter 26.)

INTRAVENOUS ALIMENTATION

Total parenteral nutrition (TPN), also known as intravenous alimentation or hyperalimentation, provides for the total nutritional needs of infants or children whose lives are threatened because feeding by way of the gastrointestinal tract is impossible, inadequate, or hazardous. Common conditions for which TPN is used therapeutically include chronic intestinal obstruction from peritoneal sepsis or adhesions, bowel fistulas, inadequate intestinal length, chronic nonremitting severe diarrhea, extensive body

*Home care instructions for caring for a central venous catheter are available in *Wong and Whaley's Clinical Manual of Pediatric Nursing* (Mosby).

burns, abdominal tumors treated by surgery, irradiation, and chemotherapy. TPN may also be initiated prophylactically when prolonged starvation is expected.

Hyperalimentation therapy involves IV infusion of highly concentrated solutions of protein, glucose, and other nutrients. The hyperalimentation solution is infused through conventional tubing with a special filter attached to remove particulate matter or microorganisms that may have contaminated the solution. A solution of glucose, lipids, and other nutrients can be mixed together in a bag and delivered through a volumetric pump (Bendorf, 1993). The highly concentrated solutions require infusion into a vessel with sufficient volume and turbulence to allow for rapid dilution. The wide-diameter vessels selected are the superior vena cava and innominate or intrathoracic subclavian veins approached by way of the external or internal jugular veins. In some situations the inferior vena cava from a femoral vein serves as an alternative route. Central VADs are ideal for long-term and home TPN.

The highly irritating nature of concentrated glucose precludes the use of the small peripheral veins in most instances. However, dilute glucose-protein hydrolysates that are appropriate for infusing into peripheral veins are being used with increasing frequency.

The major nursing responsibilities are the same as for any IV therapy: control of sepsis, monitoring of infusion rate, and assessment of the patient. The TPN solution must be prepared under rigid aseptic conditions best accomplished by specially trained technicians. In some institutions the solution and tubing are changed and the infusion site is redressed by specially trained nurses, using meticulous aseptic precautions.

General assessments such as vital signs, intake and output measurements, daily weights, and checking results of laboratory tests facilitate early detection of infection or fluid and electrolyte imbalance. Additional amounts of K^+ and Na^+ are often required in hyperalimentation; therefore, observation for signs of K^+ or Na^+ deficit or excess is part of nursing care. This is rarely a problem except in children with reduced renal function or metabolic defects.

The infusion is maintained at a constant rate by means of an infusion pump to ensure proper concentrations of glucose and amino acids. This requires accurate calculation of the rate required to deliver a measured amount in a given length of time. The hyperalimentation infusion rate should not be increased or decreased without the practitioner being made aware, since alterations can cause hyperglycemia or hypoglycemia.

Hyperglycemia may occur during the first day or two as the child adapts to the high-glucose load of the hyperalimentation solution. Although occurring infrequently, insulin may be required to assist the body's adjustment to the hyperglycemia. When this occurs, nursing responsibilities include blood glucose testing. To prevent hypoglycemia at the time hyperalimentation is discontinued, the rate of infusion is decreased gradually. The high concentration of glucose may produce an osmotic diuresis with the risk of hypertonic dehydration.

Because many children are treated with hyperalimentation regimens for long periods, it is especially important to be attuned to developmental needs. An infant stimulation program is initiated as early as feasible to prevent developmental delays (see Developmental Intervention and Care, Chapter 10). Delays in the areas of gross motor and language skills are observed most frequently in infants receiving long-term TPN (greater than 3 months), which may be caused by reduced mobility and social interaction (see Feeding Resistance, Chapter 10). The program is maintained throughout the hospital stay and extended into the home, where home hyperalimentation is implemented. In most instances, children achieve a satisfactory developmental level by 2 years of age.

Complications

Complications from TPN are numerous, and a major nursing responsibility is to prevent these when possible and to be alert to signs of their development. Complications either (1) are related to the infusate (metabolic complications) or (2) result from the presence of the indwelling catheter.

Metabolic complications are associated with the infant's or child's capacity for the various components of the hyperalimentation solution. Excessive intake of any of the components will create an imbalance, such as hyperglycemia, azotemia, acid-base disorders, anemia, bone demineralization, vitamin and mineral deficiencies, hyperosmotic dehydration and coma, fluid overload, and a variety of electrolyte imbalances.

Liver disease is the most important gastrointestinal complication in pediatric populations. The cause is obscure, but liver disease appears to be more prevalent in preterm infants who have minimum enteral feedings and who were begun on TPN at an early age. Affected children develop cholestasis, hepatocellular necrosis, and, in advanced disease, cirrhosis or hepatic failure. Manifestations include hepatomegaly, jaundice, and elevated serum transaminase, bilirubin, and alkaline phosphatase levels, which become evident approximately 2 weeks after initiation of TPN. Cholelithiasis is an uncommon but possible occurrence in pediatric patients. Therefore children receiving TPN should be assessed periodically for signs and symptoms of cholelithiasis and/or cholecystitis.

Catheter-related complications include those involving catheter placement, such as pneumothorax, hemothorax, perforation, and catheter dislodgment. However, the major complication associated with the catheter is infection: infection at catheter entrance site, catheter "seeding" sepsis, venous thrombosis with infection and embolization, and endocarditis.

Pediatric TPN generally has a higher concentration of calcium and phosphorus. This makes some TPN solutions more susceptible to precipitation. Fibrinolytic agents, such as urokinase, have no effect on precipitate. Hydrochloric acid has been used with success in clearing central VADs.

Home Total Parenteral Nutrition

Some children require total parenteral nutrition over an extended period, often weeks or months. For many children home total parenteral nutrition (HTPN) is an alternative for long-term hospitalization. The child must be one who is unable to maintain adequate enteral alimentation, has no medical problems requiring hospitalization, has a parent who is able to manage the home care (or is an older child who can participate in his or her own care), and has the potential to benefit from the treatment.

Before a home care program can be implemented, a thorough assessment is made of the family and the home situation. The parents must be capable of performing the technical aspects of the procedure and be able to adapt to the changes inherent in the home program. Psychosocial readiness of the family, family support systems, and practical considerations are investigated, including availability of a pharmacy to prepare the hyperalimentation solution, a physician to handle day-to-day emergency needs, and a cooperating insurance company or agency (because of the exorbitant cost of maintaining long-term parenteral feeding). In most areas home health care agencies are able to assume the major management of HTPN for families.

The needs of the particular child and the family situation are the basis for development and implementation of a care plan. The parents and child (when age and cognitively appropriate) learn to carry out the procedure under the supervision of a specially trained nurse; detailed, step-by-step instructions are written out. Before discharge the parents are prepared for taking over the child's total care. A room is provided at the hospital or the parent and child are housed at a nearby motel for 3 to 4 days. The parents assume full responsibility for the child's total care, with help readily available if needed. (At times, however, some teaching may begin at home because of policies of insurance companies and some health agencies.)

The emotional and economic benefits of this approach are readily apparent. The familiar environment and the atmosphere of normality are enormously therapeutic, and the stress of separation is avoided. With support from health professionals, a home care program can be the ideal alternative to hospitalization of a capable, motivated family of a child who requires TPN.

The family is encouraged to make the home life as normal as possible for the child within the limits imposed by the therapy. For example, having the infant or child at the table during mealtimes and including the child in family activities contribute to a normal family atmosphere. Quiet play should be encouraged during the HTPN, and it may be helpful to have a potty-chair available at the bedside. Toddlers who may crawl out of a crib may need to be protected from becoming tangled or catching IV tubing on the rail. It is also important to make certain the child's dental care is not neglected.

The family is referred to community agencies that provide support and practical assistance. The ***Oley Foundation,****
a nonprofit research and education organization, maintains a national registry of persons receiving HTPN and publishes a bimonthly newsletter for consumers, families, clinicians, and home care services.

*214 Hun Memorial, A23, Albany Medical Center, New Scotland Ave., Albany, NY 12208; (518) 262-5079.

KEY POINTS

- Water distribution and maintenance are determined by solutes, physical forces, internal control mechanisms, and boundary organs through which external exchanges occur.
- Infants are subject to fluid depletion because of their relatively greater surface area, their high rate of metabolism, and their immature kidney function.
- Management of fluid volume disturbances focuses on the following areas: volume of body fluids, osmolality, hydrogen ion status, electrolyte deficits, and disturbances in mineral skeleton and body fluid equilibrium.
- Fluid disturbances experienced by children are dehydration, water intoxication, and edema.
- Dehydration may be classified as isotonic, hypotonic, and hypertonic.
- Parental fluid therapy is initiated to meet ongoing daily physiologic losses, restore previous deficits, and replace ongoing abnormal losses.
- Fluid gains or losses from the interstitial spaces depend on the following factors: venous hydrostatic pressure, colloidal osmotic pressure, semipermeable capillary wall, tissue tension, and lymphatic flow.
- Edema formation is caused by increased venous pressure, capillary permeability, diminished plasma proteins, lymphatic obstruction, or decreased tissue tension.
- Disturbances in acid-base balance are respiratory acidosis, respiratory alkalosis, metabolic acidosis, and metabolic alkalosis.
- Respiratory acidosis may result from factors that depress the respiratory center, factors that affect the lung, and factors that interfere with the bellows action of the chest wall.
- Respiratory alkalosis results primarily from central nervous system stimulation.
- Metabolic acidosis is a lowered plasma pH caused by any process that reduces base bicarbonate concentration or increases metabolic acid formation.
- Metabolic alkalosis is an elevated plasma pH that occurs when there is a reduction of hydrogen ion concentration or an excess of base bicarbonate.
- Nursing assessment of fluid and electrolyte disturbances entails observation of general appearance, vital signs, daily weights, intake and output measurement, and review of relevant laboratory results.
- Long-term venous access is accomplished by intermittent intravenous devices; central venous catheters, including short-term (subclavian, femoral, and jugular), short-term to moderate-term (peripherally inserted central catheter), and long-term (tunneled) catheters and ports; or implanted ports.
- Intravenous alimentation provides total nutritional needs when feeding via the gastrointestinal tract is impossible, inadequate, or hazardous.
- Before initiating home total parenteral nutrition, the following factors are assessed: parents' ability to perform the procedure, existence of family support systems, availability of nearby pharmacies, and insurance coverage.

REFERENCES

Bendorf K: Transition from the hospital to the home for the infant requiring total parenteral nutrition, *J Perinat Neonat Nurs* 6(4):80-90, 1993.

Bennett HJ, Wagner T, Fields A: Acute hyponatremia and seizures in an infant after a swimming lesson, *Pediatrics* 72:125-127, 1983.

Brown JM: Peripherally inserted central catheters—use in home care, *J Intravenous Nurs* 12(3):144-150, 1989.

Camp-Sorrell D: Advanced central venous access: selection, catheters, devices, and nursing management, *J Intravenous Nurs* 13(6): 361-370, 1990.

Finberg L: Assessing the clinical clues to dehydration, *Contemp Pediatr* 7(4):45-57, 1990.

Flemmer L, Chan JSL: A pediatric protocol for management of extravasation injuries, *Pediatr Nurs* 19(4):355-368, 1993.

Goldberg GN and others: Infantile water intoxication after a swimming lesson, *Pediatrics* 70:599-600, 1982.

Hermansen MC, Buches M: Super diapers and premature infants, *Pediatrics* 79:1056-1057, 1987.

Hermansen MC, Buches M: Urine output determination from superabsorbent and regular diapers under radiant heat, *Pediatrics* 81:428-431, 1988.

Horne MH, Heitz UE, Swearingen PL: *Fluid, electrolyte, and acid-base balance,* St Louis, 1991, Mosby.

Horne MH, Swearingen PL: *Pocket guide; fluids, electrolytes, and acid-base balance,* St Louis, 1993, Mosby.

Kropp RM, Schwartz JF: Water intoxication from swimming, *J Pediatr* 101:947-948, 1982.

Lybrand M, Medoff-Cooper B, Munro BH: Periodic comparisons of specific gravity using urine from a diaper and collecting bag, *MCN* 15:238-239, 1990.

Marcoux C, Fisher S, Wong D: Central venous access devices in children, *Pediatr Nurs* 16:123-133, 1990.

Masoorli S, Angeles T: PICC lines: the latest home care challenge, *RN* 53(1):40-51, 1990.

McMullen A and others: Heparinized saline or normal saline as a flush solution in intermittent IV lines in infants and children, *MCN* 18(2):78-85, 1993.

Meares C: PICC and MLC lines: options worth exploring, *Nursing 92* 22(10):52-55, 1992.

Millunchick EW, McArtor RD: Fatal aspiration of a makeshift pacifier, *Pediatrics* 77:369-370, 1986.

Phillips KG: Swimming and water intoxication in infants, *Can Med J* 1136:1147, 1987 (letter).

Wilson D: Neonatal IVs: practical tips, *Neonatal Network* 11(2):49-53, 1992.

BIBLIOGRAPHY

General

Baliga R, Lewy JE: Pathogenesis and treatment of edema, *Pediatr Clin North Am* 34:639-648, 1987.

Balisteri W: Oral rehydration in acute infantile diarrhea, *Am J Med* 88(suppl 6A):305-335, 1990.

Barta MA: Correcting electrolyte imbalances, *RN* 50(2):30-33, 1987.

Carroll PF: Aspirated feeding solution, *Nursing 86* 16(1):33, 1986.

Chenevey B: Overview of fluid and electrolytes, *Nurs Clin North Am* 22:749-759, 1987.

Cusson R: Rice based oral rehydration fluid in the treatment of infant diarrhea, *J Pediatr Nurs* 7(6):414-415, 1992.

Figueroa D and others: A controlled trial of bismuth subsalicylate in infants with acute watery diarrheal disease, *N Engl J Med* 328(23):1653-1658, 1993.

Finberg L, Kravath R, Hellerstein S: *Water and electrolytes in pediatrics,* Philadelphia, 1993, WB Saunders.

Grisanti K, Jaffe D: Dehydration syndromes, *Emerg Med Clin North Am* 9(3):565-585, 1991.

Halpern J: Oral rehydration therapy: the best response to diarrheal dehydration, *J Emerg Nurs* 17(2):99-101, 1991.

Hazinski MF: Understanding fluid balance in the seriously ill child, *Pediatr Nurs* 14:231-236, 1988.

Lancaster LE: Renal and endocrine regulation of water and electrolyte balance, *Nurs Clin North Am* 22:761-772, 1987.

Lattanzi WE: Simplifying the approach to fluid therapy, *Contemp Pediatr* 6(2):72-88, 1989.

Lowrey SJ: Diminishing the risks of I.V. potassium chloride, *Nursing 88* 18(6):64, 1988.

O'Rourke ME: Reducing the risk of venous air embolism, *Am J Nurs* 88:886-890, 1988.

Pizarro D and others: Rice based oral electrolyte solutions, *N Engl J Med* 324:517-521, 1991.

Poyss AS: Assessment and nursing diagnosis in fluid and electrolyte disorders, *Nurs Clin North Am* 22:773-783, 1987.

Rahman ASM, Bari A, Molla AM: Rice ORT shortens the duration of watery diarrhea, *Trop Geogr Med* 43(1-2):23-27, 1991.

Reams PK, Deane DM: Bagged versus diaper urine specimens and laboratory values, *Neonatal Network* 6(6):17-20, 1988.

Romanski SO: Interpreting ABGs in four easy steps, *Nursing 86* 16(9):58-63, 1986.

Schwartz MW: Potassium imbalances, *Am J Nurs* 87:1292-1299, 1987.

Toto KH: When the patient has hyperkalemia, *RN* 50(4):34-37, 1987.

Toto KH: When the patient has hypokalemia, *RN* 50(3):38-41, 1987.

Young ME, Flynn KT: Third-spacing: when the body conceals fluid loss, *RN* 51(8):45-48, 1988.

Parenteral Therapy

Abrams L and others: Effect of peripheral IV infusion on neonatal axillary temperature measurement, *Pediatr Nurs* 15:630-632, 1989.

Axton SE, Fugate T: A protocol for pediatric IV meds, *Am J Nurs* 87:943-945, 1987.

Banta C: Hyaluronidase, *Neonatal Network* 11(6):103-105, 1992.

Barrus DH, Danek G: Should you irrigate an occluded I.V. line? *Nursing 87* 17(3):63-64, 1987.

Boykoff SL, Boxwell AO, Boxwell JJ: 6 ways to clear the air from an I.V. line, *Nursing 88* 18(2):46-48, 1988.

Brook J, Moss E: Air in the cavernous sinus following scalp vein cannulation, *Anaesthesia* 49:219-220, 1994.

Dick M and others: How to boost the odds of a painless IV start, *Am J Nurs* 92(6):49-50, 1992.

Dyson A, Bogod D: Minimizing bruising in the antecubital fossa after venipuncture, *Br Med J* 294:1659, 1987.

Everidge J: Achieving success in pediatric IV therapy, *J Emerg Med Serv* 14(7):94-96+, 1989.

Few BJ: Hyaluronidase for treating intravenous extravasations, *MCN,* 12:23, 1987.

Frederick V: Pediatric IV therapy: soothing the patient, *RN* 54(12):40-42+, 1991.

Hastings-Tolsma MT and others: Effect of warm and cold applications on the resolution of IV infiltrations, *Res Nurs Health* 16(3):171-178, 1993.

Hodler C, Alexander J: A new and improved guide to IV therapy: protocols for intravenous therapy, *Am J Nurs* 90(2):43-47, 1990.

Hutchinson D: Pediatric IV therapy: starting the line, *RN* 54(12):43-48, 1991.

Lenox AC: IV therapy: reducing the risk of infection, *Nursing 90* 20(3):60-61, 1990.

Maki DG and others: Prospective study of replacing administration sets for intravenous therapy at 48- vs 72-hour intervals, *JAMA* 258:1777-1781, 1987.

Millam DA: Managing complications of I.V. therapy, *Nursing 88* 18(3):34-42, 1988.

Moriarty-Sheehan M: Clearing up infusion pump problems, *RN* 49(7):40-41, 1986.

Neish SR and others: Intraosseous infusion of hypertonic glucose and dopamine, *Am J Dis Child* 142:878-880, 1988.

Nelson R, Miller H: Keeping air out of I.V. lines, *Nursing 86* 16(3):57-59, 1986.

Pettit J, Hughes K: Intravenous extravasation: mechanisms, management, and prevention, *J Perinat Neonat Nurs* 6(4):69-79, 1993.

Seigler RS, Tecklenberg, FW, Shealy R: Prehospital intraosseous infusion by emergency medical services personnel: a prospective study, *Pediatrics* 87:173-177, 1989.

Sherman JE, Sherman RH: I.V. therapy that clicks, *Nursing 89* 19(5):50-51, 1989.

Stanley M and others: Infiltration during intravenous therapy in neonates: comparison of Teflon and Vialon Catheters, *South Med J* 85(9):883-886, 1992.

Tietjen SD: Starting an infant's IV, *Am J Nurs* 90:44-47, 1990.

Viall CD: Your complete guide to central venous catheters, *Nursing 90* 20(2):34-41, 1990.

Yucha CB, Hastings-Tolsma M, Szeverenvi NM: Differences among intravenous extravasations using four common solutions, *J Intravenous Nurs* 16(5):277-281, 1993.

Long-Term Venous Access

Baranowski L: Central venous access devices: current technologies, uses, and management strategies, *J Intravenous Nurs* 16(3):167-194, 1993.

Birdsall C: What are dos and don'ts for Hickman/Broviac catheters? *Am J Nurs* 86:385, 1986.

Brosnan KM and others: Stopcock contamination, *Am J Nurs* 88:320-323, 1988.

Danek GD, Noris EM: Pediatric IV catheters: efficacy of saline flush, *Pediatr Nurs* 18(2): 111-113, 1992.

Dente-Cassidy AM: Myths and facts . . . about central venous catheters, *Nursing 91* 21(7): 30, 1991.

Favazza P, Brennan M, Carney K: The pediatric approach to home IV therapy: a case study, *Rx Home Care,* June 1987, pp 51-57.

Goode CJ and others: A meta-analysis of effects of heparin flush and saline flush: quality and cost implications, *Nurs Res* 40(6):324-330, 1991.

Harris LC, Rushton CH, Hale SJ: Implantable infusion devices in the pediatric patient: a viable alternative, *J Pediatr Nurs* 2:174-183, 1987.

Kelly C and others: A change in flushing protocols of central venous catheters, *Oncol Nurs Forum* 19(4):599-605, 1992.

Knox LS: Implantable venous access devices, *Crit Care Nurse* 7(1):70-73, 1987.

Marcoux C, Fisher S, Wong D: Central venous access devices in children, *Pediatr Nurs* 16(2):123-133, 1991.

Miller D: Tips on drawing blood through a heparin lock, *RN* 49(7):22-23, 1986.

Orr ME: Issues in the management of percutaneous central venous catheters: single and multiple lumens, *Nurs Clin North Am* 28(4): 911-919, 1993.

Ryder MA: Peripherally inserted central venous catheters, *Nurs Clin North Am* 28(4): 937-971, 1993.

Shearer J: Normal saline flush versus dilute heparin flush: a study of peripheral intermittent I.V. devices, *J Natl Intravenous Ther Assoc* 10(6):425-427, 1987.

Wachs T: Urokinase administration in pediatric patients with occluded central venous catheters, *J Intravenous Nurs* 13(2):100-102, 1990.

Whitney RG: Comparing long-term central venous catheters, *Nursing 91* 21(4):70-71, 1991.

Wildblood RA, Strezo PL: The how-to's of home IV therapy, *Pediatr Nurs* 13:42-46, 68, 1987.

Wurzel CL and others: Infection rates of Broviac-Hickman catheters and implantable venous devices, *Am J Dis Child* 142:536-540, 1988.

Intravenous Alimentation

Atkins JM, Oakley CW: A nurse's guide to TPN, *RN* 49(6):20-24, 1986.

Berry RK, Jorgensen S: Growing with home parenteral nutrition: adjusting to family life and child development, *Pediatr Nurs* 14:43-45, 1988.

Berry RK, Jorgensen S: Growing with home parenteral nutrition: maintaining a safe environment, *Pediatr Nurs* 14:155-157, 1988.

Birdsall C: When is TPN safe? *Am J Nurs* 85:73, 1985.

Committee on Nutrition: Commentary on parenteral nutriton, *Pediatrics* 71:547-552, 1983.

Dahlstrom KA and others: Nutritional status in children receiving home parenteral nutrition, *J Pediatr* 107:219-224, 1985.

Garvin G, Franck LS: Preventing delivery of enteral formula via parenteral route, *Pediatr Nurs* 15:17-18, 1989.

Geertsma MA and others: Feeding resistance after parenteral hyperalimentation, *Am J Dis Child* 139:255-256, 1985.

Greene HL and others: Guidelines for the use of vitamins, trace elements, calcium, magnesium, and phosphorus in infants and children receiving total parenteral nutriton: report of the Subcommittee on Pediatric Parenteral Nutrient Requirements from the Committee on Clinical Practice Issues of The American Society of Clinical Nutrition, *Am J Clin Nurs* 48:1324-1342, 1988.

O'Connor MJ, Ralston CW, Ament ME: Intellectual and perceptual-motor performance of children receiving prolonged home total parenteral nutrition, *Pediatrics* 81:231-236, 1988.

Orr MJ, Allen SS: Optimal oral experiences for infants on long-term total parenteral nutrition, *Nutr Clin Pract,* pp 288-295, 1986.

Wesley J: Home parenteral nutrition: indications, principles and cost-effectiveness, *Compr Ther* 9:29-36, 1983.

Zlotkin SH, Stallings VA, Pencharz PB: Total parenteral nutrition in children, *Pediatr Clin North Am* 32:381-400, 1985.

CHAPTER 29

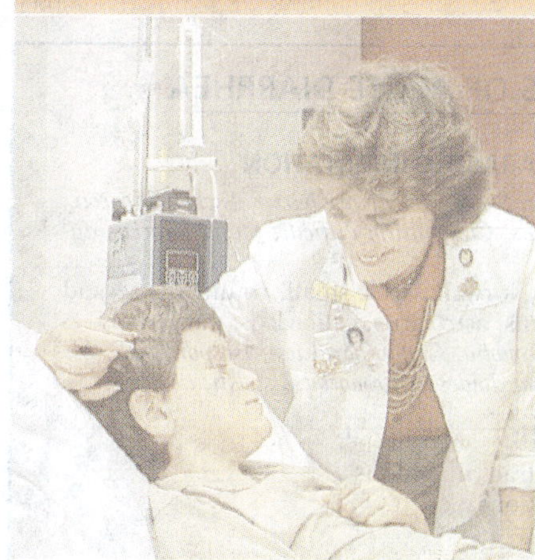

Conditions That Produce Fluid and Electrolyte Imbalance

CHAPTER OUTLINE

RELATED TOPICS

The child with cardiovascular dysfunction, Ch. 34
The child with gastrointestinal dysfunction, Ch. 33
Diaper dermatitis, Ch. 13
Disorders affecting the skin, Ch. 18
Family-centered care of the child with chronic illness or disability, Ch. 22
Family-centered home care, Ch. 25
Family-centered care of the child during illness and hospitalization, Ch. 26
Injury prevention: infant, Ch. 12; toddler, Ch. 14; school-age child, Ch. 17
Intestinal parasitic diseases, Ch. 16
Pain assessment; pain management, Ch. 26

GASTROINTESTINAL (GI) DISORDERS*

DIARRHEA

It is estimated that 500 million children worldwide suffer with diarrhea each year (Fitzgerald, 1989). For general practical purposes, diarrhea is usually classified as acute or chronic. ***Acute diarrhea*** is a leading cause of illness in children younger than 5 years of age; the dehydration that it causes is fatal for approximately 400 of these children a year in the United States (Kleinman, 1992). Most cases of acute diarrhea are caused by infectious agents, including viral, bacterial, and parasitic pathogens.

Chronic diarrhea is usually caused by chronic conditions such as malabsorption syndromes, inflammatory bowel disease, immune deficiency, food allergy, lactose intolerance, and chronic, nonspecific diarrhea. Chronic diarrhea may also be a result of inadequate management of acute infectious diarrhea.

Diarrhea is difficult to define, since stool frequency and consistency vary among individuals. Generally, diarrhea is present when there is an increase in stool frequency with an increased water content. Diarrhea varies in relation to

*Lynn E. Mattis, RN, MSN, revised this section.

CONSEQUENCES OF DIARRHEA

DEHYDRATION

Voluminous losses of fluid in frequent, watery stools
Losses when there is also vomiting
Reduced fluid intake resulting from nausea or anorexia
Increased insensible losses from fever, hyperpnea, and sometimes, high environmental temperature
Continued (although diminished) obligatory renal losses

ELECTROLYTE IMBALANCE

Losses of sodium, chloride, and potassium, and in some cases bicarbonate
Inadequate replacement of electrolytes when hypotonic or hypertonic solutions are used

METABOLIC ACIDOSIS

Increased absorption of short-chain fatty acids produced in the colon from bacterial fermentation of unabsorbed dietary carbohydrates
Accumulation of lactic acid from tissue hypoxia secondary to hypovolemia
Loss of bicarbonate in stools
Ketosis from fat metabolism when glycogen stores are depleted in untreated diarrheal dehydration or inadequate carbohydrate intake; may result in malnutrition

CAUSES OF ACUTE DIARRHEA

INFECTION AND PARASITIC INFESTATION

Bacteria: *Salmonella, Shigella, Campylobacter, Escherichia coli, Yersinia, Aeromonas, Clostridium difficile, Staphylococcus aureus*
Viruses: Rotavirus, Norwalk virus, small, round viruses, adenovirus, pestivirus, astrovirus, calicivirus, parvovirus
Parasites: *Giardia lamblia, Cryptosporidium, Isospora belli, Microsporidium, Strongyloides, Entamoeba histolytica*

ASSOCIATED WITH:

Upper respiratory tract infections
Urinary tract infections
Otitis media

DIETARY CAUSES

Overfeeding
Introduction of new foods
Reinstituting milk too soon after diarrheal episode
Osmotic diarrhea from excess sugar in formula
Excessive ingestion of sorbitol or fructose

MEDICATIONS

Antibiotics
Laxatives

TOXIC CAUSES

Ingestion of:
Heavy metals (arsenic, lead, mercury)
Organic phosphates

FUNCTIONAL CAUSES

Irritable bowel syndrome

OTHER CAUSES

Necrotizing enterocolitis
Hirschsprung enterocolitis

its severity, duration, associated symptoms, the age of the child, and the child's nutritional status.

Pathophysiology

Diarrhea is caused by abnormal intestinal water and electrolyte transport. The transport of fluid and electrolytes in the developing GI tract is related to the child's age. The intestinal mucosa of the young infant is more permeable to water than that of an older child. In young infants with increased intestinal luminal osmolality due to diarrhea, more fluid and electrolytes are lost than in older children (see box above). Diarrhea is due to several pathophysiologic processes.

Secretory diarrhea is generally due to bacterial enterotoxins that stimulate fluid and electrolyte secretion from the mucosal crypt cell, the principal secretory cells of the small intestine. ***Cytotoxic diarrhea*** is characterized by viral destruction of the mucosal cells of the villi of the small intestine. This results in a smaller intestinal surface area, with a decreased capacity for fluid and electrolyte absorption. ***Osmotic diarrhea*** is commonly seen in malabsorption syndromes, such as lactose intolerance, because the intestine cannot absorb nutrients or electrolytes. ***Dysenteric diarrhea*** is associated with an inflammation of the mucosa and submucosa in the ileum and colon caused by infectious agents such as *Campylobacter, Salmonella,* or *Shigella.* Edema, mucosal bleeding, and leukocyte infiltration occur.

ACUTE DIARRHEAL DISEASE

Acute diarrhea, a sudden increase in frequency and change in consistency of stools, is often caused by an infectious agent in the GI tract. It may also be associated with upper respiratory or urinary tract infections. Antibiotic therapy or laxative use can also lead to acute diarrhea in children (see box above). Acute diarrhea is usually self-limited (less than 14 days' duration) and will ultimately subside without specific treatment if dehydration does not create a serious complication.

Acute infectious diarrhea (infectious gastroenteritis) is caused by a wide variety of viral, bacterial, and parasitic pathogens. In the United States the incidence of acute infectious diarrhea is approximately 2½ episodes per person per year (Cohen, 1991). Infants and young children are at a high risk for the development of dehydration and malnutrition, the two major consequences of diarrhea.

Etiology

Most pathogens that cause diarrhea are spread by the fecal-oral route by contaminated food or water, or are spread from person to person, especially where there is close contact, such as in daycare centers. Living conditions play a role in infectious diarrhea. Lack of clean water, crowding, poor hygiene, nutritional deficiency, and poor sanitation are major risk factors, especially for bacterial or parasitic pathogens. The increased frequency and severity of diarrheal disease in infants is also related to age-specific alterations in susceptibility to pathogens. The immune system of infants

FACTORS THAT PREDISPOSE TO DIARRHEA

Age. As a general rule, the younger the child, the greater the susceptibility and the more severe the diarrhea. Diarrhea occurs more frequently in infancy, is a lesser threat in early childhood, and usually constitutes only a minor problem in older children.

Impaired health. Malnourished or debilitated children are more susceptible and tend to have more severe diarrhea.

Environment. Diarrhea occurs with greater frequency where there is crowding, substandard sanitation, poor facilities for preparation and refrigeration of food, and generally inadequate health care education. The frequency of diarrhea in infancy is closely related to the ingestion of contaminated milk; there is a lower incidence of diarrhea in breast-fed infants.

has not previously been exposed to many pathogens and has not acquired protective antibodies (see box above).

Rotavirus is the most common pathogen identified in young children in the United States who are hospitalized for diarrhea and dehydration, accounting for up to 50% of these admissions and causing up to 150 deaths annually (Cohen, 1991; Guarino and others, 1994). In addition, rotavirus is a significant nosocomial (hospital-acquired) pathogen. *Salmonella, Shigella,* and *Campylobacter* are the most frequently isolated bacterial pathogens, and *Giardia* and *Cryptosporidium* are the parasites that most commonly produce acute, infectious diarrhea (Table 29-1; see also Intestinal Parasitic Diseases, Chapter 16).

Other Causes of Acute Diarrhea. In addition to enteropathogens, acute diarrhea in children may be associated with respiratory and urinary tract infections. The mechanism for this is not clear. Ingestion of laxatives will also produce acute diarrhea, and excessive ingestion of sorbitol and fructose in common foods such as apple juice or in gum or candy can cause osmotic dietary diarrhea from the poorly absorbed carbohydrate.

Antibiotics such as ampicillin, amoxicillin, penicillin, cephalothin, and cefaclor are frequently associated with diarrhea. Antibiotics are thought to cause diarrhea because they alter the normal intestinal flora; the decreased colonic bacteria results in excessive malabsorbed carbohydrate and osmotic diarrhea (Treem, 1992). Antibiotics can also lead to colonization and toxin production by *Clostridium difficile,* which may cause diarrhea and pseudomembranous colitis.

Clinical Manifestations

The severity of the diarrhea, including the frequency and consistency of stools, is variable, depending on the individual and the etiologic agent. The most serious consequences of acute diarrheal disease are dehydration, electrolyte disturbances, and malnutrition. Dehydration may be mild, moderate, or severe (see Chapter 28 for clinical signs of dehydration). Metabolic acidosis may be present with severe diarrhea and dehydration. Malnutrition may contribute to the severity of the diarrhea and may be a consequence of diarrheal disease due to decreased dietary intake, malabsorption, and the catabolic response to infection. The infant's metabolic rate is higher than that of the adult, and this difference predisposes an infant to more rapid depletion of nutritional reserves during periods of malabsorption or diminished intake. Prolonged withholding of feeding or hypocaloric diets contribute to malnutrition in diarrheal disease.

Diagnostic Evaluation

The history provides valuable information regarding the duration, severity, associated symptoms, and potential cause of the diarrhea. The diagnostic assessment should include a physical examination and assessment of hydration status. Extensive laboratory evaluation is not indicated in a child with uncomplicated diarrhea and no evidence of dehydration (Bishop and Ulshen, 1988; Leung and Robson, 1989). Laboratory tests are indicated when a child is moderately to severely dehydrated.

Stool specimens should be examined in all children with diarrhea that persists for more than a few days. The presence of polymorphonuclear leukocytes suggests a bacterial infection. Cultures of the stool should be performed when blood or mucus is present in the stool, when symptoms are severe, when there is a history of travel to a developing country, and when polymorphonuclear leukocytes are found in the stool. An enzyme-linked immunosorbent assay (ELISA) may be used to confirm the presence of rotavirus, and the stool may be tested for the presence of *C. difficile* ("C. dif") toxin if there is a history of recent antibiotic use. The stool may need to be examined for ova and parasites when bacterial and viral cultures are negative and when diarrhea persists for more than a few days.

A stool pH of less than 6 and the presence of reducing substances may indicate the presence of carbohydrate malabsorption or secondary lactase deficiency. Measurement of stool electrolytes may help identify children with secretory diarrhea.

The urine specific gravity should be determined if dehydration is suspected. A complete blood count, serum electrolytes, creatinine, and blood urea nitrogen (BUN) may also be obtained in the child who appears dehydrated. The hemoglobin, hematocrit, creatinine, and BUN are often elevated in acute diarrhea and should normalize with rehydration.

Therapeutic Management

Therapeutic management is directed at correcting the fluid and electrolyte imbalances and preventing or treating malnutrition. The major goals in the management of acute diarrhea include (1) assessment of the fluid and electrolyte imbalance, (2) rehydration, (3) maintenance fluid therapy, and (4) reintroduction of adequate diet. Infants and children with acute diarrhea and dehydration should be treated first with ***oral rehydration therapy (ORT).*** In cases of severe dehydration and shock, parenteral fluids may be necessary. Early reintroduction of food is an important aspect of treatment of acute diarrhea in children. Antimicrobial agents are indicated for a few specific pathogens.

ORT is one of the major worldwide health care advances

TABLE 29-1 Infectious Causes of Acute Diarrhea

ORGANISM	PATHOLOGY	CHARACTERISTICS	COMMENTS
VIRAL AGENTS			
Rotavirus Incubation period: 1-3 days	Invade epithelium of small bowel mucosa Severely distorted mucosal architecture with atrophic mucosa and severe inflammatory changes Absorption of salt and water is decreased	Abrupt onset Fever (38° C or above) lasting approximately 48 hours Nausea/vomiting Abdominal pain Associated upper respiratory tract infection Diarrhea may persist for more than a week	Incidence higher in cool weather (80% in winter) Affects all age-groups; 6- to 24-month-old infants more vulnerable Usually mild and self-limited Important cause of nosocomial infections in hospitals and gastroenteritis in children attending daycare centers
Norwalk-like organisms Incubation period: 1-3 days	Mechanism of effect unknown Blunting of villi and inflammatory changes in lamina propria Reduced enzymes	Fever Loss of appetite Nausea/vomiting Abdominal pain Diarrhea Malaise	Source of infection: drinking water, recreation water, food (including shellfish) Affects all ages Self-limited (2-3 days)
BACTERIAL AGENTS			
Pathogenic *Escherichia coli* Incubation period: highly variable; depends on strain	Usually caused by enterotoxin production (small bowel) Reduces absorption and increases secretion of fluids and electrolytes	Onset gradual or abrupt Variable clinical manifestations Most—green, watery diarrhea with blood and mucus; becomes explosive Vomiting may be present from onset Abdominal distention Diarrhea Fever, appears toxic	Incidence higher in summer Usually interpersonal transmission but may transmit via inanimate objects A cause of nursery epidemics With symptomatic treatment only, may continue for weeks Full breast-feeding has a protective effect Symptoms generally subside in 3-7 days Relapse rate approximately 20%
Salmonella groups (nontyphoidal)—gram negative, nonencapsulated, nonsporulating Incubation period: 6-72 hours for gastroenteritis (usually less than 24); 3-60 days for enteric fever (usually 7-14)	Penetration of lamina propria (small bowel and colon) Local inflammation—no extensive destruction Stimulation of intestinal fluid excretion Systemic invasion of other sites	Rapid onset Variable symptoms—mild to severe Nausea, vomiting, and colicky abdominal pain followed by diarrhea, occasionally with blood and mucus Fever Hyperactive peristalsis and mild abdominal tenderness Symptoms usually subside within 5 days May have headache and cerebral manifestations (e.g., drowsiness, confusion, meningismus, or seizures) Infants may be afebrile and nontoxic May result in life-threatening septicemia and meningitis	Two thirds of patients are younger than 20 years of age; highest incidence in children younger than age 5 years, especially infants Highest incidence occurs from July through October, lowest from January through April Transmission primarily via contaminated food and drink—most from animal sources, including fowl, mammals, reptiles, and insects Most common sources are poultry and eggs In children—pets (e.g., dogs, cats, hamsters, and especially pet turtles) Communicable as long as organisms are excreted.
S. typhi	Rapid invasion of bloodstream from minor sites of inflammation Marked inflammation and necrosis of intestinal mucosa and lymphatics	Variable in infants Older children—irregular fever, headache, malaise, lethargy Diarrhea occurs in 50% at early stage Cough is common In a few days fever rises and is consistent; fatigue, cough, abdominal pain, anorexia, and weight loss develop; diarrhea begins	Decreased incidence in last decade Acute symptoms may persist for a week or more Transmitted by contaminated food or water (primary), infected animals (e.g., pet turtles)

TABLE 29-1 Infectious Causes of Acute Diarrhea—cont'd

ORGANISM	PATHOLOGY	CHARACTERISTICS	COMMENTS
Shigella groups—gram negative, nonmotile anaerobic bacilli Incubation period: 1-7 days, usually 2-4	Enterotoxin Stimulates loss of fluids and electrolytes Invasion of epithelium with superficial mucosal ulcerations *S. dysenteriae* forms exotoxin	Onset variable but usually abrupt Fever and cramping abdominal pain initially Fever—may reach 40.5° C Convulsions in about 10%—usually associated with fever Patient appears sick Headache, nuchal rigidity, delirium Watery diarrhea with mucus and pus starts about 12-48 hours after onset Stools preceded by abdominal cramps; tenesmus and straining follow Symptoms usually subside in 5-10 days	Approximately 60% of cases in children younger than age 9 years with more than one third between ages 1 and 4 years Peak incidence in late summer Transmitted directly or indirectly from infected persons Communicable for 1-4 weeks Self-limited disease Treat with antibiotics Severe dehydration and collapse can affect all patients Acute symptoms may persist for a week or more
Yersinia enterocolitica Incubation period: dose dependent; 1-3 weeks		Diarrhea—may be bloody Fever (>38.7° C) Abdominal pain in right lower quadrant (RLQ) Vomiting, diarrhea	Seen more frequently in winter Majority in first 3 years of life Transmitted by food and pets Can resemble appendicitis May be relapsing and last for weeks
Campylobacter jejuni Incubation period: 1-7 days or longer	Precise mechanism unclear Jejunum, ileum, and colon involvement Extensive ulceration with hemorrhagic ileitis Broadening and flattening of mucosa	Fever Abdominal pain—often severe, cramping, periumbilical Watery, profuse, foul-smelling diarrhea with blood Vomiting	Person-to-person transmission May be transmitted by pets (e.g., cat, dog, hamster) Food (especially chicken) and water-borne transmission Relapse possible Most patients recover spontaneously Antibiotics may speed recovery Peak incidence in summer
Vibrio cholerae (cholera) groups Incubation period: usually 2-3 days; range from few hours to 5 days	Enterotoxin causes increased secretion of chloride and possibly bicarbonate Intestinal mucosa congested with enlarged lymph follicles Intact mucosal surface	Sudden onset of profuse, watery diarrhea without cramping, tenesmus, or anal irritation, although children may complain of cramping Stools are intermittent at first, then almost continuous Stools are bloody with mucus	Rare in infants younger than 1 year old Mortality high in both treated and untreated infants and small children Transmitted via contaminated food and water Attack confers immunity
Clostridium difficile	Toxin stimulates colonic secretion by damaging epithelium	Diarrhea with blood in stools	May cause pseudomembranous colitis Follows antibiotic therapy
FOOD POISONING			
Staphylococcus Incubation period: 4-6 hours	Produce heat-stable enterotoxin	Nausea, vomiting Severe abdominal cramps Profuse diarrhea Shock may occur in severe cases May be a mild fever	Transferred via contaminated food—inadequately cooked or refrigerated (e.g., custards, mayonnaise, cream-filled or cream-topped desserts) Self-limited; improvement apparent within 24 hours Excellent prognosis
Clostridium perfringens Incubation period: 8-24 hours, usually 8-12	Produces heat-resistant and heat-sensitive toxins	Moderate to severe crampy, midepigastric pain	Self-limited illness Transmission by commercial food products, most often meat and poultry
Clostridium botulinum Incubation period: 12-26 hours (range, 6 hours to 8 days)	Highly potent neurotoxin	Nausea, vomiting Diarrhea Central nervous system (CNS) symptoms with curare-like effect Dry mouth, dysphagia	Transmitted by contaminated food products Variable severity—mild symptoms to rapidly fatal within a few hours Antitoxin administration

TABLE 29-2 Composition of Some Oral Rehydration Solutions

FORMULA	NA+ (mEq/L)	K+ (mEq/L)	CL− (mEq/L)	BASE (mEq/L)	GLUCOSE (g/L)
Pedialyte (Ross)*	45	20	35	30 (citrate)	25
Rehydralyte (Ross)	75	20	65	30 (citrate)	25
Infalyte (Mead Johnson)	50	25	45	34 (citrate)	30
WHO (World Health Organization)†	90	20	80	30 (bicarbonate)	20

*Note that there are many generic products available with compositions identical to Pedialyte.
†Must be reconstituted with water.

TABLE 29-3 Treatment of Acute Diarrhea

DEGREE OF DEHYDRATION	SIGNS/SYMPTOMS	REHYDRATION THERAPY*	REPLACEMENT OF STOOL LOSSES	MAINTENANCE THERAPY
Mild (5%-6%)	Increased thirst Slightly dry buccal mucous membranes	ORS 50 ml/kg within 4 hrs.	ORS 10 ml/kg (for infants) or 150-250 ml at a time (for older children) for each diarrheal stool	Breast-feeding, if established, should continue; regular infant formula if tolerated If lactose intolerance suspected, give undiluted lactose-free formula (or half-strength lactose-containing formula for brief period only); infants and children who receive solid food should continue their usual diet
Moderate (7%-9%)	Loss of skin turgor, dry buccal mucous membranes, sunken eyes, sunken fontanel	ORS 100 ml/kg within 4 hrs	Same as above	Same as above
Severe (>9%)	Signs of moderate dehydration plus one of following: rapid thready pulse, cyanosis, rapid breathing, lethargy, coma	Intravenous fluids (Ringer's lactate), 40 ml/kg/hr until pulse and state of consciousness return to normal; then 50 to 100 km/kg of ORS	Same as above	Same as above

*If no signs of dehydration are present, rehydration therapy is not necessary. Proceed with maintenance therapy and replacement of stool losses.

of the past decade. In developed countries, such as the United States, however, ORT has not been widely used because of the relative ease of access to intravenous fluids and entrenched patterns of care (Bezerra and others, 1992). ORT is effective, safer, less painful, and less costly than intravenous rehydration. As a result of studies conducted in the United States, The American Academy of Pediatrics (1985) and the Centers for Disease Control and Prevention (1992) recommend the use of ORT as the treatment of choice for most cases of dehydration caused by diarrhea.

Oral rehydration solutions (ORS) are successful in treating the great majority of infants with isotonic, hypotonic, or hypertonic dehydration. Table 29-2 shows the most commonly used solutions for oral rehydration. Glucose-mediated, enhanced sodium absorption forms the physiologic basis for the composition of these solutions. Recently, rice-based ORS has been developed as an alternative to the standard glucose ORS. These nutrient-based solutions may reduce vomiting, decrease diarrheal volume loss, and shorten the duration of disease (Santosham and Greenough, 1991).

Table 29-3 includes ORT guidelines for rehydration, replacement of stool losses, and maintenance therapy in dehydrated infants and children.

After rehydration in infants, ORS may be used during maintenance fluid therapy by alternating the solution with a low-sodium fluid such as water, breast milk, lactose-free formula, or half-strength lactose-containing formula. For older children, ORS can be given and a regular diet continued.

Ongoing stool losses should be replaced on a 1:1 basis with ORS. If the stool volume is not known, approximately 10 ml/kg or ½ to 1 cup of ORS should be given for each diarrheal stool.

Solutions for oral rehydration are useful in most cases of dehydration, and vomiting is not a contraindication. A child who is vomiting should be given ORS frequently in small amounts. For young children, the fluid can be given in a spoon or small syringe in 5 to 10 ml increments every 1 to 5 minutes by the child's caregiver. ORS may also be given by nasogastric or gastrostomy tube infusion in children who were feeding with this modality for other reasons.

Infants without clinical signs of dehydration do not need ORT. They should, however, receive the same fluids recommended for infants with signs of dehydration in the maintenance phase and for ongoing stool losses.

NURSING ALERT Diarrhea is not managed by encouraging intake of clear fluids by mouth, such as fruit juices, carbonated soft drinks, and gelatin. These fluids usually have a high carbohydrate content, a very low electrolyte content, and a high osmolality (Avery and Snyder, 1990). Caffeinated soda is avoided, because caffeine is a mild diuretic and may lead to increased loss of water and sodium. Chicken or beef broth is not given, because it contains excessive sodium and inadequate carbohydrate.

Early reintroduction of normal nutrients is desirable and is gaining more widespread acceptance. Recent studies indicate that continued feeding or early reintroduction of a normal diet is beneficial because of an improved nutritional outcome and because it may reduce the number of stools, reduce weight loss, and shorten the duration of illness (Brown, 1991; Brown, Gastanaduy, and Saavedra, 1988; Leung and Robson, 1989).

If an infant is breast-feeding, this method of feeding should be continued, and ORS should be used to replace ongoing losses. Available evidence indicates that continued human milk feeding during diarrheal illness results in reduced severity and duration of illness (Brown, 1991). Tolerance to human milk may be due to its low osmolality and its antimicrobial, enzymatic, and hormonal factors.

The use of nonhuman milk for infants and children with diarrhea remains controversial. Cow's milk and cow's milk formulas are of concern because maldigestion of lactose can occur in children with infectious diarrhea (Brown, 1991; Penny, Paredes, and Brown, 1989). Studies indicate that well-hydrated infants and children may resume full-strength nonhuman milk feeding immediately without adverse reactions (Brown, Peerson, and Fontaine, 1994; Chew and others, 1993). Many infants and children can be safely managed with a diet containing cow's milk. Some health care providers advocate the use of a lactose-free formula only in infants if milk or regular formula is not tolerated.

For older children, a regular diet can generally be offered once rehydration has been achieved. A BRAT diet (bananas, rice, apples, and toast or tea) is contraindicated for the child, and especially for the infant, with acute diarrhea because this diet has little nutritional value (low in energy and protein), is too high in carbohydrates, and is low in electrolytes. There is no contraindication to continue soft or pureed foods of all groups in the toddler. A diet of easily digestible foods such as cereals, cooked vegetables, and meats is adequate for the older child.

Intravenous fluids are required for severe dehydration and vomiting. Usually, saline solution containing 5% dextrose in water is administered. The initial volume should be 20 to 30 ml/kg and should be administered as a bolus. Therapy in the remainder of the first 24 hours should be aimed at completely correcting the remaining fluid and sodium deficits and replacing ongoing abnormal losses.

Enteric infections are generally self-limited conditions. Antimicrobial therapy is not indicated in the majority of children with acute diarrhea and is not available for enteric viruses. Specific antimicrobial therapy is indicated only for culture-proven bacterial or parasitic infections in which this therapy can reduce the duration of the illness, the severity of the symptoms, or the shedding and secondary spread of organisms. Antibiotics may be warranted before culture results are available in the febrile, ill-looking infant with dysenteric diarrhea (blood and polymorphonuclear cells in the stool). Indiscriminate use of antibiotics may lead to pseudomembranous colitis.

Antidiarrheal drug therapy with agents such as loperamide (Imodium A-D), diphenoxylate hydrochloride/atropine (Lomotil), Kaopectate, or Diasorb is not indicated in acute infectious diarrhea in infants and young children. Toxicity and adverse side effects may occur, such as worsening of the diarrhea because of slowing of motility and ileus or a decrease in diarrhea, with continuing fluid losses and dehydration.

The treatment of antibiotic-associated diarrhea is discontinuation of the antibiotic if possible and investigation for the presence of *C. difficile*. If laxatives or certain foods are the cause of diarrhea, their use should be discontinued (see Critical Thinking Exercise box, p. 1240).

Nursing Considerations

❖ Assessment

The nursing assessment of diarrhea begins with observation of the infant's or child's general appearance and behavior. The physical assessment includes all the parameters described for assessment of dehydration, such as decreased urinary output and weight, dry mucous membranes, poor skin turgor, sunken fontanel in the infant, and pale, cool, dry skin. With more severe dehydration, increased pulse and respiration, decreased blood pressure, and a prolonged capillary refill time (≥2 seconds) may indicate impending shock.

CRITICAL THINKING EXERCISE
Acute Diarrhea

A 6-month-old infant is brought to a primary care clinic because of diarrhea (three times as many stools as usual, which are watery in consistency), fever, and vomiting of 24 hours' duration. Following the initial examination of the infant, it is apparent that the baby has mild dehydration due to losses from the GI tract. The infant likely has acute infectious diarrhea. All of the following nursing considerations or interventions would be indicated in this situation except:

1. Ongoing assessment of the infant's fluid and electrolyte status
2. Education of the infant's caregivers regarding administration of oral rehydration solution (ORS)
3. Recommended delay of reintroduction of food for several days and administration of antidiarrheal medications
4. Education of the infant's caregivers regarding perineal skin care to prevent or diminish irritation

The correct answer is 3. Use of antidiarrheal medications is not recommended for acute infectious diarrhea. These drugs may be harmful, since adverse effects, such as slowed motility and ileus, may occur. The goals of management of acute diarrhea include assessment of hydration, provision of fluids for rehydration and maintenance, and reintroduction of an adequate diet. In this case, since the infant is mildly dehydrated, oral rehydration therapy (ORT) should be attempted. ORT is effective, safer, less painful, and less costly than intravenous rehydration. If ORS is administered in small quantities at frequent intervals, vomiting can be minimized.

Early reintroduction of normal nutrients is desirable, and delayed introduction of food may be harmful in terms of nutritional status and duration of illness. Breastfeeding should generally be continued, and most infants who receive cow's milk formulas may resume their usual feedings as soon as the infant is rehydrated. Occasionally, a soy formula will be recommended following an episode of acute infectious diarrhea if the infant demonstrates evidence of lactose malabsorption.

Perineal skin irritation is common with a diarrheal illness. Extra care is necessary in order to protect the skin or facilitate healing of excoriated skin. Gentle cleansing of the skin and use of protective ointments are often beneficial.

A history provides valuable information regarding probable etiologic agents, such as introduction of a new food, exposure to infectious agents, travel to an area of high susceptibility, contact with foods that might be contaminated, and contact with pets that are known to be sources of enteric infections. An allergic, drug, and dietary history may indicate food allergies, use of laxatives or antibiotics, and sources of excess sorbitol and fructose, such as apple juice.

❖ NURSING DIAGNOSES

Several nursing diagnoses become apparent on the basis of a thorough physical assessment. The major diagnoses appropriate for the infant or child are described in the Nursing Care Plan on pp. 1241-1242. Other diagnoses will be evident depending on the age and condition of the child and the etiology of the diarrhea.

❖ PLANNING

The goals for the dehydrated infant or child and for the family are as follows:

1. Infant or child will maintain adequate hydration.
2. Infant or child will maintain appropriate nutrition for age.
3. Infant or child will not spread infection (if etiologic agent) to others.
4. Family will receive appropriate support and education, especially regarding home care.

❖ IMPLEMENTATION

The management of most cases of acute diarrhea can take place in the home with proper education of the child's caregivers regarding the cause of diarrhea, potential complications, and appropriate therapy. Since most infections that cause acute diarrhea are spread by the fecal-oral route, personal hygiene, water supply, and food preparation are important considerations. Meticulous attention to perianal hygiene, disposal of soiled diapers, proper handwashing technique, hygienic food preparation, and isolation of infected persons will minimize transmission of infectious agents.

Caregivers are taught to monitor the child for signs of dehydration, especially the number of wet diapers or voidings, and to monitor fluids taken by mouth and the frequency and amount of stool losses. They need to be informed about ORT, including the administration of maintenance fluids and replacement of ongoing losses. ORT is time-consuming for the caregiver, but the benefits include safety, possibly cost, and less discomfort for the child as compared with intravenous therapy. ORS is administered in small quantities at frequent intervals. Vomiting is not a contraindication to ORT unless it is severe. Many parents and health care providers still follow earlier practices of either withholding feedings or providing clear fluids such as juices, broth, or gelatin or a BRAT diet. These practices are discouraged, and the parents are educated about the appropriate administration of fluids and a normal diet. A slightly higher stool output occurs with continuation of a normal diet initially and with ongoing replacement of stool losses. The stool pattern is outweighed by the benefits of a better nutritional outcome with fewer complications and a shorter duration of illness. The concerns and priorities of the parents should be explored in order to gain compliance with therapeutic management.

If the child with acute diarrhea and dehydration is hospitalized, nursing responsibilities include the same interventions that are often administered in the home. Appropriate precautions should be implemented to prevent possible spread of the infection. For example, everyone caring for the child must be aware of "clean" areas and "dirty" areas, especially in the hospital, where the sink in the child's room is used for many purposes. Food, eating and drinking utensils, toothbrushes, pacifiers, toys, and other personal items are stored away from the sink, diaper-changing surface, and

NURSING CARE PLAN
The Child with Acute Diarrhea (Gastroenteritis)

NURSING DIAGNOSIS: Fluid volume deficit related to excessive GI losses in stool or emesis

PATIENT GOAL 1: Will exhibit signs of rehydration and maintain adequate hydration

• **NURSING INTERVENTIONS/*RATIONALES***

*Administer oral rehydration solutions (ORS) *for both rehydration and replacement of stool losses* (see Table 29-2)
Give ORS frequently in small amounts, especially if child is vomiting, *because vomiting, unless severe, is not a contraindication to using ORS*
*Administer and monitor IV fluids as prescribed *for severe dehydration and vomiting*
*Administer antimicrobial agents as prescribed *to treat specific pathogens causing excessive GI losses*
After rehydration, offer child regular diet as tolerated *because studies show that early reintroduction of normal diet is beneficial in reducing number of stools and weight loss and shortening duration of illness*
Alternate ORS with a low-sodium fluid such as water, breast milk, lactose-free formula, or half-strength lactose-containing formula *for maintenance fluid therapy* (see Table 29-3)
Maintain strict record of intake and output (urine, stool, and emesis) *to evaluate effectiveness of interventions*
Monitor urine specific gravity every 8 hours or as indicated *to assess hydration*
Weigh child daily *to assess for dehydration*
Assess vital signs, skin turgor, mucous membranes, and mental status every 4 hours or as indicated *to assess hydration*
Discourage intake of clear fluids such as fruit juices, carbonated soft drinks, and gelatin *because these fluids usually are high in carbohydrates, low in electrolytes, and have a high osmolality*
Instruct family in providing appropriate therapy, monitoring intake and output, and assessing for signs of dehydration *to ensure optimum results and improve compliance with the therapeutic regimen*

• **EXPECTED OUTCOME**

Child exhibits signs of adequate hydration (specify)

NURSING DIAGNOSIS: Altered nutrition: less than body requirements related to diarrheal losses, inadequate intake

PATIENT GOAL 1: Will consume nourishment adequate to maintain appropriate weight for age

After rehydration, instruct breast-feeding mother to continue feeding breast milk *because this tends to reduce severity and duration of illness*
Avoid giving BRAT diet (bananas, rice, apples, and toast or tea) *because this diet is low in energy and protein, too high in carbohydrates, and low in electrolytes*
Observe and record response to feedings *to assess feeding tolerance*
Instruct family in providing appropriate diet *to gain compliance with therapeutic regimen*
Explore concerns and priorities of family members *to improve compliance with therapeutic regimen*

• **EXPECTED OUTCOME**

Child takes prescribed nourishment and exhibits a satisfactory weight gain

NURSING DIAGNOSIS: High risk for infection related to microorganisms invading GI tract

PATIENT (OTHERS) GOAL 1: Will not exhibit signs of gastrointestinal infection

• **NURSING INTERVENTIONS/*RATIONALES***

Implement body substance isolation or other hospital infection-control practices, including appropriate disposal of stool and laundry and appropriate handling of specimens *to reduce risk of spreading infection*
Maintain careful handwashing *to reduce risk of spreading infection*
Apply diaper snugly *to reduce likelihood of fecal spread*
Use superabsorbent disposable diapers *to contain feces and decrease chance of diaper dermatitis*
Attempt to keep infants and small children from placing hands and objects in contaminated areas
Teach children, when possible, protective measures *to prevent spread of infection,* such as handwashing after using toilet, etc.
Instruct family members and visitors in isolation practices, especially handwashing, *to reduce risk of spreading infection*

• **EXPECTED OUTCOME**

Infection does not spread to others

NURSING DIAGNOSIS: Impaired skin integrity related to irritation caused by frequent, loose stools

PATIENT GOAL 1: Skin will remain intact

• **NURSING INTERVENTIONS/*RATIONALES***

Change diaper frequently *to keep skin clean and dry*
Cleanse buttocks gently with bland, nonalkaline soap and water or immerse child in a bath for gentle cleansing *because diarrheal stools are highly irritating to skin*
Apply ointment such as zinc oxide *to protect skin from irritation* (type of ointment may vary for each child and may require a trial period)
Expose slightly reddened intact skin to air whenever possible *to promote healing;* apply protective ointment to very irritated or excoriated skin *to facilitate healing*
Avoid using commercial baby wipes containing alcohol on excoriated skin *because they will cause stinging*

*Dependent nursing action

Continued.

NURSING CARE PLAN
The Child with Acute Diarrhea (Gastroenteritis)—cont'd

Observe buttocks and perineum for infection, such as *Candida, so that appropriate therapy can be initiated*
*Apply appropriate antifungal medication *to treat fungal infection of skin*

• **EXPECTED OUTCOME**
Child has no evidence of skin breakdown

NURSING DIAGNOSIS: Anxiety/fear related to separation from parents, unfamiliar environment, distressing procedures

PATIENT GOAL 1: Will exhibit signs of comfort

• **NURSING INTERVENTIONS/*RATIONALES***
Provide mouth care and pacifier for infants *to provide comfort*
Encourage family visitation and participation in care as much as the family is able, *to prevent stress associated with separation*
Touch, hold, and talk to child as much as possible *to provide comfort and relieve stress*
Provide sensory stimulation and diversion appropriate for child's developmental level and condition *to promote optimum growth and development*

• **EXPECTED OUTCOMES**
Child exhibits minimal signs of physical or emotional distress
Family participates in child's care as much as possible

*Dependent nursing action

NURSING DIAGNOSIS: Altered family processes related to situational crisis, knowledge deficit

PATIENT (FAMILY) GOAL 1: Family will understand about child's illness and its treatment and will be able to provide care

• **NURSING INTERVENTIONS/*RATIONALES***
Provide information to family about child's illness and therapeutic measures *to encourage compliance with therapeutic regimen, especially at home*
Assist family in providing comfort and support to child
Permit family members to participate in child's care as much as they desire, *to meet needs of both child and family*
Instruct family regarding precautions *to prevent spread of infection*
Arrange for posthospitalization health care *for continued assessment and treatment*
Refer family to a community health care agency *for supervision of home care as needed*

• **EXPECTED OUTCOME**
Family demonstrates ability to care for child, especially at home

scale used to weigh diapers. The containment of feces is also a key factor in infection control. Research indicates that superabsorbent paper diapers with elastic legs permit less fecal leakage than cloth diapers with plastic coverings (Kubiak and others, 1993). Each hospital has a policy regarding necessary precautions. (See Infection Control, Chapter 27.)

➤ **NURSING TIP** To remind caregivers to keep diapers and other soiled articles away from clean areas, place signs identifying "clean" (e.g., the bed table) and "dirty" (e.g., the sink or bathroom) areas in the room. List on each sign what articles should be stored in each area.

Strict assessment of hydration status, daily weights, and measurement of intake and output and urine specific gravity are essential. The stools should be examined and tested for blood, pH, and reducing substances to determine carbohydrate malabsorption. Specimens may need to be collected for laboratory examination. Parenteral fluids may be required, and specialized nutritional support, such as semielemental formulas, continuous tube feedings, or parenteral nutrition, may be needed when oral nutrition is not tolerated.

Because diarrheal stools are highly irritating to the skin, extra care is needed to protect the skin in the perianal area from becoming excoriated. The skin is cleansed gently, and protective ointments such as zinc oxide may be applied. (See Diaper Dermatitis, Chapter 13.) Rectal temperatures are avoided because they can stimulate the bowel, increasing passage of stool.

Support for the child and family involves the same care and consideration as for all hospitalized children (see Chapter 26). Parents are kept informed of the child's progress and instructed in special care techniques, such as feeding, handwashing, and proper disposal of soiled diapers, clothes, and bed linen. Soiled diapers and linen should be discarded in receptacles close to the bedside.

❖ EVALUATION

The effectiveness of nursing interventions is determined by continued reassessment according to the following observational guidelines and expected outcomes:

1. Monitor fluid losses with careful intake and output measurements and daily weights.
2. Monitor food intake, especially calories.
3. Observe for evidence of complications from underlying disease (specify) and/or therapy.
4. Observe and interview family to determine extent and effectiveness of care.

CAUSES OF CHRONIC DIARRHEA*

MALABSORPTIVE CAUSES
Celiac disease
Pancreatic insufficiency (cystic fibrosis, chronic pancreatitis, Shwachman syndrome)
Short bowel syndrome
Lactose intolerance
Congenital enzyme deficiency (sucrase-isomaltase deficiency)

ALLERGIC CAUSES
Allergic gastroenteropathy
Eosinophilic gastroenteritis

IMMUNODEFICIENCY
Acquired hypoglobulinemia
Wiskott-Aldrich syndrome
Agammaglobulinemia
Severe combined immunodeficiency disease
Thymic hypoplasia
Selective IgA deficiency
Acquired immunodeficiency syndrome (AIDS)

INFLAMMATORY BOWEL DISEASE
Ulcerative colitis
Crohn disease

ENDOCRINE CAUSES
Hyperthyroidism
Congenital adrenal hyperplasia
Addison disease

MOTILITY DISORDERS
Hirschsprung disease
Intestinal pseudoobstruction

PARASITIC INFESTATIONS
Ascaris
Giardia

OTHER CAUSES
Radiation enteritis
Protein-losing enteropathy (Ménétrier disease, intestinal lymphangiectasia)
Secretory tumors (gastrinoma, carcinoma)

*See Chapter 33 for a discussion of chronic GI disorders.

Expected outcomes:
See Nursing Care Plan, pp. 1241-1242.

CHRONIC DIARRHEAL DISEASE

Chronic diarrhea is defined as an increase in stool frequency and increased water content with a duration of more than 14 days. It is often caused by chronic conditions such as malabsorption syndromes, inflammatory bowel disease, immune deficiency, food allergy, lactose intolerance, and chronic nonspecific diarrhea (see box above). Chronic diarrhea may also be a result of inadequate management of acute diarrhea. The etiology, pathophysiology, clinical manifestations, therapeutic management, and nursing considerations of many of these chronic conditions are discussed in Chapter 33.

INTRACTABLE DIARRHEA OF INFANCY

Intractable diarrhea of infancy is a syndrome defined as diarrhea occurring in the first few months of life that persists for longer than 2 weeks with no recognized pathogens and is refractory to treatment. The most common cause is acute infectious diarrhea that was not managed adequately from a nutritional point of view. This condition is sometimes referred to as postenteritis diarrhea or protracted diarrhea of infancy. The original etiologic agent will have disappeared, but the diarrhea persists.

Dehydration and electrolyte disturbances occur, as well as malnutrition. The diarrhea rapidly becomes self-perpetuating through a combination of secondary consequences: malnutrition deprives the infant of essential nutrients necessary for mucosal regeneration; the villi of the small intestine atrophy; and secondary digestive and absorptive disorders develop as a result of malnutrition, dysmotility, and overgrowth of bacteria. The significant mucosal injury leads to severe intolerance of most nutrients, perpetuating the cycle of malabsorption, diarrhea, and malnutrition, which may result in death.

Treatment consists primarily of nutritional support with oral feedings of a formula containing a protein hydrolysate, glucose polymers, and medium-chain triglycerides to maximize tolerance and nutrient absorption. Occasionally, continuous tube feedings or parenteral nutrition is necessary.

CHRONIC NONSPECIFIC DIARRHEA (CNSD)

CNSD, also known as irritable colon of childhood and toddlers' diarrhea, is a common cause of chronic diarrhea in children between 6 and 54 months of age. These children have loose stools, often with undigested food particles, with diarrhea greater than 2 weeks' duration. Children with CNSD are growing normally, have no evidence of malnutrition, no blood in the stool, and no enteric infection.

Often the history will reveal certain prior events, including a viral infection; the institution of dietary restrictions, such as avoidance of milk and dairy products; and previous antibiotic use. These events may be related to the origin of CNSD or influence the course of this disorder. The potential causes of CNSD include disordered small intestine motility, excessive fluid intake, dietary fat restriction, and carbohydrate malabsorption. Children with CNSD may have impaired intestinal motility, which causes rapid intestinal transit and impaired fluid absorption. Excessive fluid intake, in some children, may contribute to the initiation and perpetuation of CNSD.

It is apparent that specific dietary factors contribute to CNSD. Ingestion of a large quantity of osmotically active carbohydrates, which are poorly absorbed by the small intestine, contributes to diarrhea in many children with CNSD. Carbohydrates that are poorly absorbed include sorbitol and fructose. Sorbitol is found in significant concentration in common foods such as prunes, prune juice, pears, pear juice, peaches, apple juice, and sugar-free gum and candy. Fructose is found in significant quantities in many soft drinks, fruit juices, honey, figs, dried dates, prunes, and prune juice. Although fruit juice is considered a nutritious snack and is a fluid staple for children, fruit juice ingestion in excess may cause chronic diarrhea. A low-fat diet may contribute to diarrhea by causing an increase in the rate of gastric emptying and faster intestinal transit time, which contributes to malabsorption of fluid and nutrients. Many children with CNSD ingest low-fat diets with restricted milk and dairy products, for which large quantities of fruit and fruit juice are substituted. This pursuit of a healthful diet may contribute to CNSD.

The diagnosis of CNSD is one of exclusion. A history of prior illnesses and antibiotic use should be obtained. A dietary history, including fluid intake and quantities of fruit and fruit juice ingested, is important. The physical examination of the child with CNSD usually reveals normal growth, no blood in the stools, and no evidence of enteric infection. Chronic conditions such as pancreatic insufficiency, small bowel mucosal injury, and food allergy need to be excluded, often on the basis of the history and specific laboratory examinations. In a child less than 5 years of age, lactose intolerance suggests diffuse mucosal injury rather than CNSD (Treem, 1992).

The therapeutic management of CNSD may include the following measures: (1) avoidance of foods and liquids containing sorbitol and fructose, (2) increased fiber in the diet, (3) increased fat content in the diet, and (4) limitation of total fluid intake (Treem, 1992). CNSD often causes anxiety and frustration in the parents and affected child, but most cases resolve spontaneously or with simple treatment measures before the age of 4 or 5 years. The family needs reassurance that no significant morbidity is associated with CNSD.

VOMITING

Vomiting is the forceful ejection of gastric contents through the mouth. Vomiting is a well-defined, complex, coordinated process under central nervous system control that is usually accompanied by nausea and retching, whereas regurgitation is a simpler, more passive phenomenon that is effortless. There are many causes of vomiting, including acute infectious diseases, increased intracranial pressure (ICP), toxic ingestions, food intolerances and allergy, mechanical obstruction of the GI tract, metabolic disorders, and psychogenic problems. Vomiting is common in childhood, is usually self-limited, and requires no specific treatment, but complications can occur in children, including dehydration and electrolyte disturbances, malnutrition, aspiration, and Mallory-Weiss syndrome (small tears in the distal esophageal mucosa).

Etiology

The child's age, pattern of vomiting, and duration of symptoms help to determine the etiology. For example, chronic intermittent episodes of vomiting may indicate malrotation, whereas vomiting on a specific day at the same time before school is not likely to be a result of organic disease. The color and consistency of the emesis vary according to the etiology. Green, bilious vomiting suggests bowel obstruction. Curdled stomach contents, mucus, or fatty foods that are vomited several hours after ingestion suggest poor gastric emptying or high intestinal obstruction. Gastric irritation by certain medicines, foods, or toxic substances may cause vomiting.

Associated symptoms also help to identify the etiology. Fever and diarrhea accompanying vomiting suggest an infection. Constipation associated with vomiting suggests an anatomic or functional obstruction. Localized abdominal pain and vomiting often occur with appendicitis, pancreatitis, or peptic ulcer disease. A change in the level of consciousness or headache associated with vomiting indicates a central nervous system or metabolic disorder. Forceful vomiting is associated with pyloric stenosis.

Pathophysiology

The act of vomiting, including nausea and retching, is under central nervous system control. Two areas of the medulla are involved as the vomiting center. The medullary center is also activated by impulses from a second center, the chemoreceptive trigger zone, which is located in the floor of the fourth ventricle (see box below). Nausea is a sensation that may be induced by visceral, labyrinthine (inner ear), or emotional stimuli. It is characterized by the desire to vomit, with discomfort felt in the throat or abdomen. Nausea is often associated with autonomic symptoms, such as salivation, pallor, sweating, and tachycardia. Retching may occur with or without vomiting. Retching involves a series of spasmodic movements during inspiration, creating a negative intrathoracic pressure, and contraction of the abdominal muscles. Projectile vomiting is preceded and accompanied by vigorous peristaltic waves.

Vomiting is a well-recognized response to psychologic

SOURCES OF VOMITING STIMULI

Higher cortical centers—Either deep-seated or superficial psychologic disturbances. Stimuli include those associated with unpleasant sights, repugnant odors, and fright.

Chemosensitive trigger zone—Transmits impulses to cortical center; located on the floor of the fourth ventricle. Stimuli include chemical stimulation by drugs (e.g., apomorphine, morphine, ipecac, and some digitalis derivatives), toxins (e.g., from uremia, infections, or radiation), cerebral hypoxia, increased ICP, and disturbances of the semicircular canals of the inner ear.

Reflex excitement (vagal and sympathetic afferent nerves)—Results from disturbed GI and other viscera. Stimuli include irritation, inflammation, or mechanical disturbance in GI tract (e.g., distention or obstruction); irritation of other viscera (e.g., heart, renal pelvis, bladder); and pain.

stress. During stress, adrenaline levels rise, which may stimulate the chemoreceptor trigger zone. Nausea and vomiting is likely a protective mechanism to remove toxins from the system. Vomiting may follow ingestion of a contaminated feeding or GI infection, and it can be a learned behavioral response.

Diagnostic Evaluation

The diagnostic evaluation includes a thorough history and physical examination. The description of the vomitus; relationship to meals or specific foods; presence of pain, constipation, diarrhea, or jaundice; and behavior are important components of the history. Physical examination should include an assessment of the hydration status and an abdominal examination.

Further evaluation may include analysis of urine for protein or blood, serum electrolytes, and radiographic studies. A plain radiograph of the chest or abdomen or ultrasonography may reveal anatomic abnormalities. Brain scans are used to detect tumors. If esophagitis is suspected, endoscopy of the upper GI tract may be a valuable diagnostic procedure. A psychiatric evaluation may be indicated if cyclic vomiting, anorexia nervosa, bulimia, or self-poisoning is present. Self-induced vomiting and rumination may be a self-stimulation or gratification activity.

Therapeutic Management

The management of vomiting is directed toward detection and treatment of the cause of the vomiting and prevention of complications such as dehydration and malnutrition. Often vomiting is a symptom of a common infectious illness that is self-limited and will resolve with no specific treatment. Further investigation is indicated if there is dehydration, progressively severe vomiting, or persistent vomiting for more than 24 hours, or when the history and physical examination fail to suggest a diagnosis. If vomiting leads to dehydration, oral rehydration or parenteral fluids may be required.

Antiemetic drugs may be indicated when the vomiting can be anticipated, is of limited duration, and has a known cause. Antiemetic drugs may block the receptors in the chemoreceptor trigger zone (ondansetron [Zofran] or trimethobenzamide [Tigan]), enhance gastroduodenal peristalsis (metoclopramide [Reglan]), or compete for H_1-receptor sites (promethazine [Phenergan]). For children who are prone to motion sickness, it is often helpful to administer an appropriate dose of dimenhydrinate (Dramamine) before a trip.

Nursing Considerations

The major emphasis of nursing care of the vomiting infant or child is on observation and reporting of vomiting behavior and associated symptoms, and on the implementation of measures to reduce the vomiting. Accurate assessment of the type of vomiting, the appearance of the vomitus, and the child's behavior in association with the vomiting greatly aids in establishing a diagnosis of disorders that have vomiting as a clinical feature.

Nursing interventions are determined by the cause of the vomiting. When the vomiting is identified as a manifestation of improper feeding methods, establishing proper techniques through teaching and example will ordinarily correct the situation. If the vomiting is assessed as a probable sign of a GI obstruction, food is usually withheld or special feeding techniques are implemented. In situations in which vomiting is related to concurrent infection, dietary indiscretion, or emotional factors, efforts are directed toward maintaining hydration or preventing dehydration.

The thirst mechanism is the most sensitive guide to fluid needs, and ad libitum administration of a glucose-electrolyte solution to an alert child will restore water and electrolytes satisfactorily. It is important to include carbohydrates to spare body protein and to avoid ketosis resulting from exhaustion of glycogen stores. Small, frequent feedings of fluids or foods are preferable and more effective. Once vomiting has abated, more liberal amounts of fluids can be offered, followed by gradual resumption of the regular diet.

The vomiting infant or child is positioned to prevent aspiration and observed for evidence of dehydration. It is important to emphasize the need for the child to brush the teeth or rinse the mouth after vomiting to dilute hydrochloric acid that comes in contact with the teeth. A flavored mouthwash or brushing also helps freshen the mouth. Careful monitoring of fluid and electrolyte status must be exercised to avoid the possibility of hyperelectrolytemia.

SHOCK STATES*

SHOCK

Shock, or circulatory failure, is a complex clinical syndrome characterized by inadequate tissue perfusion to meet the metabolic demands of the body, resulting in cellular dysfunction and eventual organ failure. Although the causes are different, the physiologic consequences are the same: hypotension, tissue hypoxia, and metabolic acidosis.

Etiology

The most common type of circulatory failure in children is ***hypovolemic shock,*** which follows a reduction in circulating blood volume related to blood loss (e.g., trauma, major bleeding), plasma losses (e.g., burns, peritonitis), or extracellular fluid losses (e.g., diarrhea, dehydration) beyond the child's physiologic ability to compensate. ***Cardiogenic shock*** results from impaired cardiac muscle function resulting in decreased cardiac output. It is uncommon in children but may be seen following cardiac surgery and in children with acute arrhythmias, congestive heart failure, or cardiomyopathy. ***Distributive shock,*** or ***vasogenic shock,*** results from a vascular abnormality that produces maldistribution of blood supply throughout the body. This term includes (1) ***neurogenic shock,*** characterized by massive vasodilation due to the loss of sympathetic nervous system tone, which can occur with spinal cord injuries; (2) ***anaphylactic shock,*** characterized by a hypersensitivity reaction causing massive vasodilation and capillary leak, which may occur with drug or latex allergy, insect stings, or blood transfusion; and (3) ***septic***

*Patricia O'Brien, RN,C, MSN, PNP, revised this section.

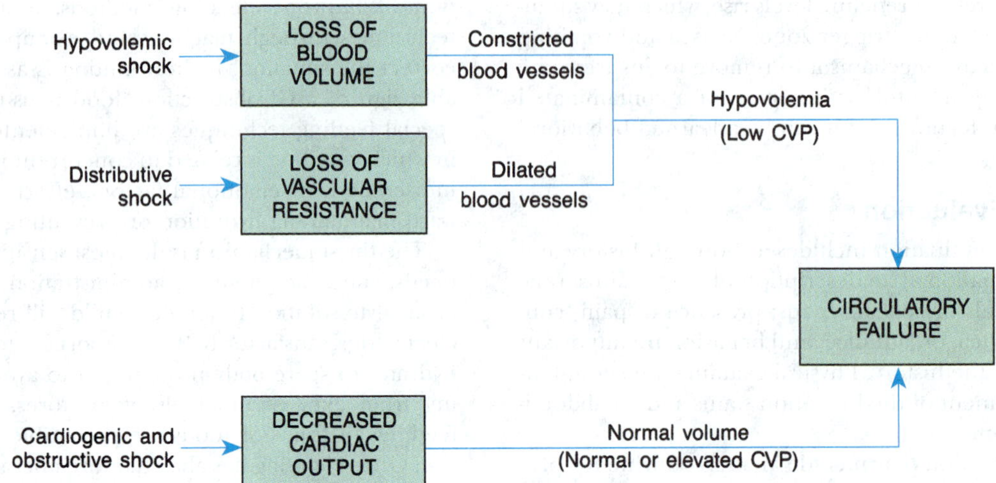

FIG. 29-1 Causes of circulatory failure in children. (Modified from Crone RK: *Pediatr Clin North Am* 27:525-538, 1980.)

shock, characterized by a decreased cardiac output and derangements in the peripheral circulation in response to a severe, overwhelming infection. Septic shock is the most common form of shock seen in newborns. The types of shock are listed in Fig. 29-1 and in the box on p. 1247.

Pathophysiology

The circulatory system of the healthy child is able to transport oxygen and nutrients to meet the essential needs of body tissues, which demand varying amounts of nutrients in relation to one another, to meet the demands of states such as exercise or illness, which increase the metabolic rate. The cardiac output and distribution to the various body tissues can change very rapidly in response to intrinsic (myocardial and intravascular) or extrinsic (neuronal) control mechanisms. In shock states these mechanisms are altered or challenged.

Reduced blood flow, as in hypovolemic shock, causes diminished venous return to the heart, low central venous pressure (CVP), low cardiac output, and hypotension. The reduced intravascular volume triggers a chain of compensatory mechanisms. Fluid is mobilized from the extracellular compartment. Vasomotor centers in the medulla are signaled, causing depressed vagal activity and increased sympathetic activity that increase the force and rate of cardiac contraction and constrict the arterioles and veins, thereby increasing peripheral vascular resistance.

Simultaneously, the lowered blood volume also leads to the release of large amounts of catecholamines, antidiuretic hormone, adrenocorticosteroids, and aldosterone in an effort to conserve body fluids. The catecholamines augment the vasomotor activity to produce vasoconstriction and reduce blood flow to the skin, kidneys, muscles, and splanchnic viscera in order to shunt the available blood to the brain and heart. Consequently, the skin feels cold and clammy, there is poor capillary filling, and glomerular filtration and urinary output are significantly reduced.

Impaired perfusion to peripheral tissues also produces metabolic alterations. Oxygen depletion causes the cells to revert to anaerobic glycolytic metabolism, forming pyruvic acid, which is then converted to lactic acid, thus producing lactic acidosis. The acidosis places an extra burden on the lungs as they attempt to compensate for the metabolic acidosis by increasing the respiratory rate. Impaired cellular uptake and metabolism of glucose create an early, transient hyperglycemia. When plasma fluid is lost, hemoconcentration and diminished blood flow increase the viscosity of the blood and further impair perfusion.

Prolonged vasoconstriction results in fatigue, and the release of vasodilator substances such as histamine leads to vasodilation. Venules, which are less sensitive to vasodilator substances, remain constricted for a time, causing massive pooling in the capillary and venular beds and transudation of plasma fluid into the tissues, which further depletes blood volume.

Complications of shock create further hazards. Central nervous system (CNS) hypoperfusion may eventually lead to cerebral edema, cortical infarction, or intraventricular hemorrhage. Renal hypoperfusion causes renal ischemia with possible tubular or glomerular necrosis and renal vein thrombosis. Reduced blood flow to the lungs can interfere with surfactant secretion and result in ***shock lung,*** or ***adult respiratory distress syndrome (ARDS),*** which is characterized by sudden pulmonary congestion and atelectasis with formation of a hyaline membrane. Gastrointestinal tract bleeding and perforation are always a possibility following splanchnic ischemia and necrosis of intestinal mucosa. Metabolic complications of shock may include hypoglycemia, hypocalcemia, and other electrolyte disturbances.

Shock syndromes characterized by vascular abnormalities (distributive shock) have a somewhat different pathophysiologic pattern of hemodynamic collapse. In neurogenic shock, sympathetic nervous system mechanisms that maintain vascular tone are interrupted, causing reduced

TYPES OF SHOCK

HYPOVOLEMIC SHOCK

Characteristics

Reduction in size of vascular compartment
Falling blood pressure
Poor capillary filling
Low central venous pressure (CVP)

Most Frequent Causes

Blood loss (hemorrhagic shock)—trauma, GI bleeding, intracranial hemorrhage
Plasma loss—increased capillary permeability associated with sepsis and acidosis, hypoproteinemia, burns, peritonitis
Extracellular fluid loss—vomiting, diarrhea, glycosuric diuresis, sunstroke

DISTRIBUTIVE SHOCK

Characteristics

Reduction in peripheral vascular resistance
Profound inadequacies in tissue perfusion
Increased venous capacity and pooling
Acute reduction in return blood flow to the heart
Diminished cardiac output

Most Frequent Causes

Anaphylaxis (anaphylactic shock)—extreme allergy or hypersensitivity to a foreign substance
Sepsis (septic shock, bacteremic shock, endotoxic shock)—overwhelming sepsis and circulating bacterial toxins
Loss of neuronal control (neurogenic shock)—interruption of neuronal transmission (spinal cord injury)
Myocardial depression and peripheral dilation—exposure to anesthesia or ingestion of barbiturates, tranquilizers, narcotics, antihypertensive agents, or ganglionic blocking agents

CARDIOGENIC SHOCK

Characteristic

Decreased cardiac output

Most Frequent Causes

Following surgery for congenital heart disease
Primary pump failure—myocarditis, myocardial trauma, biochemical derangements, congestive heart failure
Dysrhythmias—paroxysmal atrial tachycardia, atrioventricular block, and ventricular dysrhythmias; secondary to myocarditis or biochemical abnormalities (occasionally)

vascular resistance and peripheral pooling of blood; with this increased vascular capacity there is loss of effective circulating blood volume. Septic shock produces a hyperdynamic state in which there is often an elevated plasma volume and reduced peripheral resistance that leads to widespread vasodilation. In many cases there is a high cardiac output caused by the vasodilation in infected tissues and elsewhere plus a high metabolic rate resulting from the elevated body temperature. Degenerating tissues cause aggregation of red blood cells and sludging of the blood. Development of ***disseminated intravascular coagulation,*** triggered by either the degenerating tissue or bacterial toxins, consumes the clotting factors, which produces widespread hemorrhages. (See discussion in Chapter 35.)

Clinical Manifestations

Shock can be regarded as a form of compensation for circulatory failure and, because of its progressive nature, can be divided into three stages or phases: compensated, uncompensated, and irreversible. At all stages the principal differentiating signs are observed in the (1) degree of tachycardia and perfusion to extremities, (2) level of consciousness, and (3) blood pressure (BP). Additional signs or modifications of these more universal signs may be present depending on the type and cause of the shock.

Compensated Shock. When vital organ function is maintained by intrinsic mechanisms and the child's ability to compensate is effective, cardiac output and systemic arterial BP are usually normal or increased, but blood flow is generally uneven or maldistributed in the microcirculation. Early clinical signs are subtle, including apprehension, irritability, normal BP, narrowing pulse pressure, thirst, pallor, and diminished urinary output.

NURSING ALERT Unexplained mild tachycardia and a decrease in perfusion of the hands and feet are differentiating features of compensated shock.

Decompensated Shock. As shock progresses, perfusion in the microcirculation becomes marginal despite compensatory adjustments, and signs are more obvious and indicate early decompensation. These signs are tachypnea, moderate metabolic acidosis, oliguria, and cool, pale extremities with decreased skin turgor and poor capillary filling. The outcomes of circulatory failure that progress beyond the limits of compensation are tissue hypoxia, metabolic acidosis, and eventual dysfunction of all organ systems.

NURSING ALERT Tachycardia is pronounced; BP is maintained, but pulse pressure (difference between systolic and diastolic BP) becomes narrowed; there is poor capillary filling; and the child in decompensated shock exhibits decreased responsiveness, confusion, and sleepiness.

Irreversible Shock. Irreversible, or terminal, shock implies damage to vital organs such as the heart or brain of such magnitude that the entire organism will be disrupted regardless of therapeutic intervention. There is pronounced systemic vasoconstriction and hypoxia of visceral and cutaneous circulations with hypotension, acidosis, lethargy or coma, and oliguria or anuria. The child is totally obtunded. Thready, weak pulse; hypotension; periodic breathing or apnea; anuria; and stupor or coma are signs of impending cardiopulmonary arrest. Death occurs even if cardiovascular measurements return to normal levels with therapy.

Diagnostic Evaluation

The cause of shock can be discerned from the history and the physical examination. The extent of the shock is determined by measurement of vital signs, including CVP and capillary filling. Laboratory tests that assist in assessment are blood gas measurements, pH, and sometimes various liver function tests such as serum glutamic oxaloacetic transaminase (SGOT), bilirubin, and total serum protein (TSP). Coagulation status (prothrombin time [PT], partial thromboplastin time [PTT], platelet count, fibrinogen, fibrin) is evaluated when there is evidence of bleeding, such as oozing from a venipuncture site, bleeding from any orifice, or petechiae. Cultures of blood and other sites are indicated when there is a high suspicion of sepsis. Renal function tests are performed when impaired renal function is evident.

Therapeutic Management

Treatment of shock consists of three major thrusts: (1) ventilation, (2) fluid administration, and (3) improvement of the pumping action of the heart (vasopressor support). The first priority is to establish an airway and administer oxygen. Once the airway is assured, circulatory stabilization is the major concern. Placement of an intravenous catheter for rapid volume replacement is the most important action for reestablishment of circulation. Where individuals are familiar with and skilled in the technique, percutaneous cannulation of the internal jugular or subclavian veins is preferred. An alternative is rapid surgical cutdown cannulation of the saphenous vein. The vein is anatomically accessible, can accommodate the volumes of fluid needed, and is situated where it does not interfere with any resuscitation procedures that might be necessary. Another effective emergency method is intraosseous administration of fluids (see Chapter 28).

Ventilatory Support. The lung is the organ most sensitive to shock. The decrease in or redistribution of blood flow to respiratory muscles plus the increased work of breathing can rapidly lead to respiratory failure. Critically ill patients are unable to maintain an adequate airway. To place the lung at rest and improve ventilation, tracheal intubation is initiated early with positive-pressure ventilation and supplemental oxygen. Blood gases, oxygen saturation (using pulse oximetry), and pH are monitored frequently.

Increased extravascular lung water caused by edema—both hydrostatic and permeable—contributes to the development of respiratory complications. ***Hydrostatic edema*** occurs from elevation of pulmonary microvascular pressure as a result of left ventricular dysfunction; ***permeable edema*** occurs when damage to alveolar cell and pulmonary capillary epithelium causes fluid to leak into the interstitial space, resulting in ARDS (see Chapter 32). Therapy is directed toward maintaining normal arterial blood gas measurements, normal acid-base balance, and circulation. Efforts are made to remove fluid and prevent its accumulation by increasing oncotic pressure and decreasing microvascular hydrostatic pressure. Elevated oncotic pressure is promoted by diuresis with furosemide or mannitol, colloid administration, or both.

Cardiac Support. In many cases rapid restoration of blood volume is the main therapy needed in the resuscitation of the child in shock. An ***isotonic crystalloid solution*** (normal saline or lactated Ringer's solution) is usually the first choice for fluid replacement. Crystalloid is given in intravenous boluses of 10 to 20 ml/kg over 10 to 15 minutes and repeated as necessary. The child's response is assessed after each bolus. Successful resuscitation will be reflected by an increase in BP and a decrease in heart rate. An increased cardiac output will result in improved capillary circulation and skin color. ***Colloids,*** protein-containing fluids, are often administered to children in shock, albumin being the most common. Because albumin is a protein solution, it remains in the vascular space much longer than crystalloid fluids. A smaller volume of albumin can be given to increase the intravascular volume and support cardiac output as compared with a larger volume of crystalloid given to achieve the same effect. Blood administration is generally used only in situations of known blood loss, active bleeding, or markedly decreased hematocrit because of the infectious risks. Fresh-frozen plasma is used to correct coagulopathies, not as volume replacement.

For the critically ill child with shock and multisystem organ dysfunction, more aggressive monitoring is needed. Central venous measurements of right atrial pressure or pulmonary wedge pressure help guide fluid therapy. In children with persistent shock, a Swan-Ganz catheter should be placed for more accurate monitoring. Determination of arterial blood gases, hematocrit, serum electrolytes, glucose, and calcium concentrations provides additional information concerning composition of circulating blood. Correction of acidosis, hypoxemia, and any metabolic derangements is mandatory.

Vasopressor Support. Temporary pharmacologic support may be required to enhance myocardial contractility, to reverse metabolic or respiratory acidosis, and to maintain arterial pressure. The principal agents used to improve cardiac output and circulation are the ***sympathetic amines*** administered by constant infusion pump. Dopamine is the preferred drug in most situations because it also improves renal perfusion. Other agents used to improve cardiac output (e.g., dobutamine, isoproterenol, epinephrine) may also be used, depending on the situation.

Vasodilator medications are often used in combination with vasopressors. Common vasodilators are nitroprusside, Amrinone, and hydralazine. It is important that the patient has an adequate circulating blood volume before vasodilators are administered.

Metabolic acidosis is usually corrected with adequate tissue perfusion and improved renal function. This is accomplished with adequate ventilatory support, including oxygen, and restoration of blood volume and peripheral circulation. The administration of ***sodium bicarbonate*** may also be needed to correct acidosis resulting from shock. It should be given in small boluses that are diluted to avoid acute changes in osmolality. The major complications of bicarbonate administration are sodium overload and hyperosmolality.

Calcium chloride may be administered to improve cardiac function and to offset the reduced ionized calcium associated with large amounts of albumin, whole blood, or fresh-frozen plasma. ***Diuretics,*** such as furosemide (Lasix), cause a reduction in the ventricular filling pressures without changing cardiac output or heart rate and promote sodium and water excretion by the kidney in cases where pulmonary congestion is a problem.

Other Therapies. Peritoneal dialysis may be necessary if hyperkalemia, acidosis, hypervolemia, or altered mental status occurs. Nutritional support is provided by both enteral and parenteral routes. Prevention of infection is a primary concern because host resistance is depressed in patients in shock. Other complicating disorders, such as disseminated intravascular coagulation and gastrointestinal problems (e.g., paralytic ileus, stress ulceration), are managed appropriately. The ***intraaortic balloon pump (IABP)*** may be employed for the child with low cardiac output who is refractory to conventional medical management. ***Extracorporeal membrane oxygenation (ECMO)*** is used occasionally as a last resort where this therapy is available.

Nursing Considerations

The child in shock requires intensive observation and care, preferably in an intensive care environment.

NURSING ALERT When shock is a likely complication, the child is observed carefully for any early signs, such as irritability, unexplained increase in heart rate, thirst, pallor, or diminished urinary output. The appearance of any of these signs requires further evaluation and initiation of therapy.

The initial action in care of the child in shock is ensuring adequate tissue oxygenation (see Emergency Treatment box). The nurse should be prepared to administer oxygen by the appropriate route and to assist with any intubation and ventilatory procedures indicated. Other procedures and activities that require immediate attention are establishing an intravenous line, weighing the child (weight is needed to calculate drug dosages), obtaining baseline vital signs, placing an indwelling catheter, obtaining blood gas and other measurements, and administering medications as indicated.

The child is best positioned flat with legs elevated. Hypotensive patients show no benefit from the traditional Trendelenburg position. Head-down positioning tends to increase intracranial pressure, decrease diaphragmatic excursion and lung volume, and decrease venous return to the heart because of the altered thoracic pressure. Elevating the lower extremities decreases pooling in the extremities, thereby returning blood supply to the heart.

The nurse's responsibilities are to monitor vital signs, in particular BP, and intake and output, and to perform a general assessment of the level of consciousness, circulatory perfusion, and parenteral infusion sites. Intravenous medications are titrated according to patient responses, and vital signs are taken every 15 minutes during the critical periods and thereafter as needed. Urinary output is measured hourly, and blood gases, hematocrit, pH, and electrolytes are monitored frequently to assess the status of the child and the efficacy of therapy. Apnea and cardiac monitors are attached and monitored continuously. O_2 saturation monitors are an important addition to the child's care as a continuous measurement of oxygenation. In the initial stages of acute shock, the care of the child often requires the attendance of more than one nurse in order to manage all the necessary activities that must be carried out simultaneously.

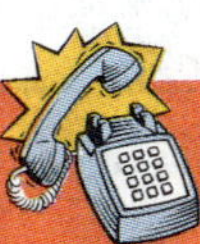

EMERGENCY TREATMENT
Shock

VENTILATION

Establish airway—be prepared for intubation.
Administer oxygen, usually 100% by mask.

FLUID ADMINISTRATION

Restore blood or fluid volume as ordered.

CARDIOVASCULAR SUPPORT

Administer vasopressors, especially epinephrine in dose of 0.01 mg/kg until maximum dose of 0.5 ml of 1:1000 dilution subcutaneously; may repeat if needed.

GENERAL SUPPORT

Keep child flat with legs raised above level of heart.
Keep child warm and calm.

IN ADDITION:

Septic shock—Administer broad-spectrum antibiotics intravenously.
Anaphylaxis—Remove allergen if possible; may place tourniquet above site of injection.

Family Support. Throughout the intense activity the parents must not be overlooked. Someone should contact them at frequent intervals to inform them about what is being done and if there is any improvement. Ideally, someone should remain with the parents to serve as a liaison between them and the intensive care team. However, this is not always feasible in such a critical situation. As soon as possible, they should be allowed to see the child. A member of the clergy may be called to help provide comfort and support.

SEPTIC SHOCK

Septic shock occurs when the host response to an infectious organism produces a systemic inflammatory response mediated by complex hormonal and chemical substances and results in compromised cardiac function, systemic perfusion, and tissue utilization of oxygen. Decreased cardiac output occurs, and alterations in the peripheral circulation, including massive vasodilation, decreased systemic vascular resistance, maldistribution of blood flow, and increased capillary permeability, are characteristic of septic shock. The incidence of septic shock is increasing in adults and children (Bone, 1991, Hazinski, 1990), possibly as a result of greater numbers of immunosuppressed patients and more widespread use of invasive devices in the seriously ill.

Three stages have been identified in septic shock (see box on p. 1250). In early septic shock there are chills, fever, and vasodilation with increased cardiac output that results in the warm, flushed skin reflecting vascular tone abnormalities and ***hyperdynamic, warm,*** or ***hyperdynamic-compensated responses.*** The patient has the best chance for survival from this stage. The ***normodynamic, cool,*** or ***hyperdynamic-uncompensated stage*** lasts for only a few hours. With advanc-

STAGES OF SEPTIC SHOCK

HYPERDYNAMIC STAGE (WARM SHOCK, PINK SHOCK)	NORMODYNAMIC STAGE (COOL SHOCK)	HYPODYNAMIC STAGE (COLD SHOCK)
Tachycardia	Tachycardia	Tachycardia
Tachypnea	Hyperventilation	Respiratory distress
Chills and fever	Normal temperature	Profound hypothermia
Skin flushed, warm	Skin cool	Skin cold, clammy
Warm extremities	Cool extremities	Cold, pale extremities
Bounding pulses	Normal pulses	Weak, thready pulses
Normal or elevated systemic blood pressure	Normal or slightly elevated systemic blood pressure	Severe hypotension
Wide pulse pressure	Normal to slightly narrow pulse pressure	Narrow pulse pressure
Normal urinary output or polyuria	Oliguria	Severe oliguria or anuria
Mental confusion	Depressed sensorium	Lethargy or coma
		Metabolic acidosis
		Multisystem organ failure

ing disease, signs progress through decompensatory manifestations, which deteriorate to signs of circulatory collapse indistinguishable from late shock of any cause. In the ***hypodynamic*** or ***cold stage*** of ***shock,*** cardiovascular function progressively deteriorates, even with aggressive therapy. This is the most dangerous stage of shock. A later and ominous development is disseminated intravascular coagulation (the major hematologic complication of septic shock), which is evidenced by petechiae or purpura fulminans, a severe form of subcutaneous hemorrhage (see Chapter 35).

Nursing Considerations

Nursing observations and care follow medical management as in all types of shock. Because many deaths from septic shock occur as a result of the pathophysiologic responses to the endotoxin and cardiac function is compromised early, the immediate concern is recognizing and treating the shock. Broad-spectrum antibiotics are administered, and the underlying source is identified as soon as possible to guide specific therapy.

As in any case of shock, pulmonary support is a major concern, but it is especially important in septic shock because the most common cause of death in septic shock is ARDS. In addition to multiple factors that increase vascular permeability in ARDS, endotoxin action causes direct damage to lung endothelium, resulting in noncompliant and atelectatic lungs. To optimize and maintain oxygen delivery, early institution of mechanical ventilation is often recommended.

NURSING ALERT To aid in early identification and management, nurses caring for children at risk for septic shock should be alert to early evidence of dysfunction—fever, tachycardia, and tachypnea.

ANAPHYLAXIS

Anaphylaxis is the acute clinical syndrome resulting from the interaction of an allergen and a patient who is hypersensitive. This antigen-antibody (IgE) reaction stimulates the release of chemical substances, primarily histamine, from mast cells. Histamine release causes vasodilation and increases capillary permeability, allowing fluid to leak into the interstitial space. Severe reactions are immediate in onset, are often life-threatening, and frequently involve multiple systems, primarily the cardiovascular, respiratory, gastrointestinal, and integumentary systems. Exposure to the antigen can be by ingestion, inhalation, skin contact, or injection. The most common allergens are listed in the left-hand box on p. 1251.

Prevention of a reaction is the primary goal. Preventing exposure is more easily accomplished in children known to be at risk, including those with (1) a history of previous allergic reaction to a specific antigen, (2) a history of allergy (atopy), (3) a history of severe reactions in immediate family members, and (4) a reaction to a skin test, although skin tests are not available for all allergens.

Pathophysiology

An anaphylactic reaction occurs as a result of interaction between an allergen and preexisting specific immunoglobulin E (IgE). When the antigen enters the circulatory system, a generalized reaction rapidly takes place. Vasoactive amines (principally histamine or histamine-like substances) are released from mast cells and cause vasodilation, bronchoconstriction, and increased capillary permeability. Consequently, there is increased venous capacity and pooling, reduced arterial pressure, and rapid loss of fluid into interstitial spaces, causing a marked decrease in venous return to the heart.

Clinical Manifestations

The onset of clinical symptoms usually occurs within seconds or minutes of exposure to the antigen, and the rapidity of the reaction is directly related to its intensity—the sooner the onset, the more severe the reaction. However, the onset may be delayed for as long as 2 hours. Typically, the reaction is preceded by one or more prodromal signs and symptoms, including vague complaints of uneasiness or impending doom, restlessness, irritability, severe anxiety, headache, dizziness, paresthesia, and disorientation. The

COMMON ALLERGENS ASSOCIATED WITH ANAPHYLAXIS

DRUGS/MEDICAL PRODUCTS

Antibiotics (penicillin, cephalosporins, tetracycline, aminoglycosides, streptomycin, amphotericin B)
Analgesics (aspirin, indomethacin, phenylbutazone)
Local anesthetics (lidocaine, procaine, bupivacaine, tetracaine)
Chemotherapeutic agents (adriamycin, bleomycin, cisplatin, cyclophosphamide, L-asparaginase, melphalan)
Antiepileptic drugs
Diagnostic contrast media (sulfobromophthalein sodium [BSP] dye, dehydrocholic acid [Decholin], iodinated contrast media, iopanoic acid [Telepaque])
Latex (gloves, catheters) (see also pp. 448-449; 450)

FOODS

Milk and milk products
Nuts and seeds
Legumes (peanuts, soybeans, beans, lentils)
Eggs
Seafood (fish, shellfish)
Wheat
Citrus fruits, strawberries
Chocolate

VENOMS

Hymenoptera (bee, yellow jacket, hornet, wasp, fire ant)
Snake
Jellyfish
Spider

BIOLOGIC AGENTS

Allergen extracts
Antisera (snake, tetanus, diphtheria)
Enzymes
Hormones
Immune globulin (gammaglobulin, blood, plasma)

POSSIBLE MANIFESTATIONS OF ANAPHYLACTIC REACTION

CARDIOVASCULAR

Tachycardia
Dysrhythmia
Hypotension
Relative hypovolemia

RESPIRATORY

Rhinitis—sneezing, nasal itching, rhinorrhea
Laryngeal edema—stridor
Bronchospasm—cough, wheezing

GASTROINTESTINAL

Nausea and vomiting
Abdominal pain
Diarrhea

CUTANEOUS (SKIN)*

Diffuse flushing, feeling of warmth
Urticaria (itching of skin and raised rash [hives])
Angioedema—periorbital, perioral

CENTRAL NERVOUS SYSTEM/OTHER

Sense of impending doom, sometimes loss of consciousness*
Headache*
Seizures

*Early signs

patient may lose consciousness. Cutaneous signs are the most common initial sign, and the child may complain of feeling warm. Angioedema is most noticeable in the eyelids, lips, tongue, hands, feet, and genitalia. Any or all of several reactions may affect one or more organ systems, as outlined in the box above, right.

Cutaneous manifestations are often followed by bronchiolar constriction. Bronchiolar constriction causes a narrowing of the airway, dilated pulmonary circulation produces pulmonary edema and hemorrhages, and there is often life-threatening laryngeal edema. Shock occurs as a result of mediator-induced vasodilation and sudden inadequacy of the circulation. The hypovolemia is further enhanced by increased capillary permeability and loss of intravascular fluid into the interstitial space. Laryngeal edema, with its acute upper airway obstruction and related hypovolemic shock, carries a more ominous prognosis.

Therapeutic Management

Successful outcome of anaphylactic reactions depends on rapid recognition of their severity and prompt institution of treatment (Sampson, Mendelson, and Rosen, 1992). The goals of treatment are to provide ventilation, restore adequate circulation, and prevent further exposure by identifying and removing the cause when possible.

A mild cutaneous reaction with no evidence of respiratory distress or cardiovascular compromise can be managed with antihistamines, such as diphenhydramine (Benadryl) and epinephrine. Moderate or severe distress presents a life-threatening emergency and requires immediate intervention. Severely unresponsive patients are transferred to hospital intensive care units when possible.

As in any shock state, the airway is the first concern. The most important drug is aqueous epinephrine 1:1000. The dose is 0.01 ml/kg to a maximum of 0.5 ml administered subcutaneously. With epinephrine 1:1000, the dose corresponds to 0.01 mg/kg. If the intravenous route is accessible, epinephrine 1:10,000 is used (0.1 ml/kg). Usually a single dose is effective, but additional doses are given if needed. The child should be observed for at least 6 hours, since late deterioration may occur. Other routes of administering epinephrine are intramuscular and via an airway, either nebulized or by injection through endotracheal tubes. In severe anaphylaxis, epinephrine by any route is better than none (Fisher, 1992).

Other drugs that may be used are aminophylline and diphenhydramine. Vasopressors may be required for severe shock from any cause. Corticosteroids are controversial, but some authorities advocate their use for control of persistent or recurrent symptoms. The time required for them to achieve their effect diminishes their value for emergency therapy.

The child is positioned and monitored the same as any

shock patient. If this is the initial anaphylactic reaction, it is especially important to identify the allergen and implement measures to prevent any future reaction. Medical identification should be carried by the patient at all times. Desensitization may be recommended in certain cases.

Nursing Considerations

The major nursing responsibility in anaphylaxis is anticipating which children are likely to develop a reaction, recognizing the early signs, and intervening appropriately. When an anaphylactic reaction is suspected, both immediate intervention and preparation for medical therapy are nursing responsibilities. Help will be needed and the practitioner should be notified, but the nurse must not leave the patient. The child is placed in a head-elevated position, unless contraindicated by hypotension, to facilitate breathing, and oxygen is administered. If the child is not breathing, cardiopulmonary resuscitation (CPR) is initiated.

If the cause can be determined, measures are implemented to slow the spread of the offending substance. For example, a tourniquet may be applied above the point of entry (e.g., sting, injection) or intravenous medication or dye infusion is discontinued. If an intravenous infusion line is not in place, one is established immediately and the flow rate is monitored carefully. Vital signs are monitored every 15 minutes, and urinary output is measured at regular intervals. Medications are administered as prescribed with regular assessment to monitor effectiveness and to detect signs of side effects of medication and fluid overload.

To prevent an anaphylactic reaction, parents are always asked about possible allergic responses to foods, medications, products such as latex, and environmental conditions (see Guidelines box [Taking a Drug Allergy History] on p. 201). These are displayed prominently on the patient's chart. The specific allergen is noted, as well as the type and severity of the reaction. Parents are excellent historians, especially when the child has displayed a dramatic reaction to a substance. Drugs, including related drugs (e.g., penicillin, nafcillin), that have produced a previous reaction are *never* given.

The child and the parents need as much reassurance as can be provided without giving false hope. They are kept informed of the child's progress, the reasons for the therapies, and what they can reasonably expect. It is a frightening experience and one that the family will remember and will make every effort to prevent recurring. The use of medical information in a convenient and visible form, such as a bracelet or necklace, is reinforced. For the child who is allergic to insect venom, the family is instructed to purchase an emergency kit to be kept with the child at all times (e.g., EpiPen Auto-Injector, or EpiPen Jr. Auto-Injector*). Both the family and the child, if the child is old enough and is likely to be away from the family (e.g., at school), are taught how to use the equipment (see also Chapter 27).

*Center Laboratories, 35 Channel Dr., Port Washington, NY 11050; (516) 767-1800.

NURSING ALERT Families should always inform other caregivers (e.g., daycare staff) and school personnel, especially the school nurse, of allergies in their children. These individuals should be prepared to respond immediately to a severe reaction.

TOXIC SHOCK SYNDROME (TSS)

TSS is a relatively rare disease that occurs predominantly (but not exclusively) in previously healthy young women during their menstrual periods. Studies have shown a striking relationship between the disease and the use of tampons (Centers for Disease Control, 1980), although other foci have been identified, including contraceptive sponges, nasal packing, and wounds. Some cases reported in children were unrelated to any identifiable foci. The number of reported cases peaked in 1980 at 1000 per year; it declined to less than 100 per year by 1987 (Broscious, 1991). However, a ***toxic shock–like syndrome*** also occurs from invasive group A streptococci; the incidence of this life-threatening disease appears to be increasing (Hoge and others, 1993; Working Group on Severe Streptococcal Infections, 1993).

CASE DEFINITION OF TOXIC SHOCK SYNDROME

1. Fever (temperature at or above 38.9° C [102° F])
2. Rash (diffuse macular erythroderma)
3. Desquamation 1 to 2 weeks after onset of illness, particularly of the palms and soles
4. Hypotension (systolic blood pressure at or below 90 mm Hg for adults or below the fifth percentile for age for children younger than 16 years of age, or orthostatic syncope)
5. Involvement of three or more of the following organ systems:
   a. Gastrointestinal (vomiting or diarrhea at onset of illness)
   b. Muscular (severe myalgia or creatine phosphokinase level above two times the upper limits of normal)
   c. Mucous membrane (vaginal, oropharyngeal, or conjunctival hyperemia)
   d. Renal (blood urea nitrogen or creatinine levels above two times the upper limits of normal or above five white blood cells per high-power field—in the absence of a urinary tract infection)
   e. Hepatic (total bilirubin, SGOT [serum glutamic oxaloacetic transaminase], or SGPT [serum glutamic pyruvic transaminase] above two times the upper limits of normal)
   f. Hematologic (platelets below 100,000/mm^3)
   g. Central nervous system (disorientation or alterations in consciousness without focal neurologic signs when fever and hypotension are absent)
6. Negative results on the following tests, if obtained:
   a. Blood, throat, or cerebrospinal fluid cultures
   b. Serologic tests for Rocky Mountain spotted fever, leptospirosis, or measles

From Centers for Disease Control: *MMWR* 29:442, 1980.

Pathophysiology

Evidence from several sources suggests that TSS occurs secondary to infection with phage group-1 *Staphylococcus aureus.* The organism is believed to produce an epidermal toxin, but the precise mode of transmission is not known. The disease has been observed primarily in women who use tampons during a menstrual period. The tampon may carry the organism from the fingers or the vulva into the vagina during insertion, the tampon might traumatize the vaginal wall and provide a focus of infection, or the tampon itself may provide a favorable environment for growth of the organism or elaboration of its toxin. Persistent use throughout the menstrual cycle also alters the vaginal mucosa by absorbing protective secretions and subjects it to greater mechanical trauma and microulcerations.

Clinical Manifestations

The sudden development of high fever, vomiting and diarrhea, profound hypotension, shock, oliguria, and an erythematous macular rash with subsequent desquamation are characteristic manifestations of TSS. Other manifestations might include headache, blurred vision, purulent conjunctivitis, abdominal guarding, and purulent vaginal discharge. Inasmuch as various signs and symptoms are associated with the disease and affected individuals seldom exhibit all of them, the Centers for Disease Control and Prevention has published a case definition of TSS (see box on p. 1252).

Complications include respiratory distress, cardiac dysfunction, hematologic changes (particularly disseminated intravascular coagulation), and abnormal liver function. Impaired perfusion to extremities may become severe, with eventual necrosis and loss of extremities.

Diagnostic Evaluation

The diagnosis is established on the basis of the criteria of the Centers for Disease Control and Prevention's TSS case definition. A history of tampon use contributes to the diagnosis. Additional laboratory tests include cultures from blood, vagina, cervix, and discharge from any suspected source of infection. Other laboratory tests are those that facilitate the management of shock.

Therapeutic Management

The management of TSS is the same as management of shock of any cause. Because the disease is highly varied in intensity, therapy is directed toward supportive care in mild cases to hospitalization and intensive care in severe cases. Appropriate parenteral antibiotics are usually administered after cultures are obtained. Preventing complications of impaired circulation demands constant observation and immediate therapeutic intervention for hypotension, pulmonary dysfunction, acidosis, hematologic changes, and renal impairment.

Nursing Considerations

Nursing care and observation of the acutely ill patient are the same as those described for shock of any cause. Because the disease is relatively rare, the major efforts of nursing are directed toward prevention. The association between the disease and the use of tampons provides some direction for education. Avoiding the use of tampons offers the most certain preventive measure, although this approach is probably unacceptable to most adolescent girls. Most young women prefer the freedom, comfort, and inconspicuousness that tampons afford and are unlikely to comply with this advice.

Adolescent girls who use tampons can be taught general hygiene measures, such as handwashing before insertion of the tampon and not to use a tampon that has been dropped or otherwise soiled. Tampons should be inserted carefully to avoid vaginal abrasion. Also, it is wise to modify their use. For example, tampons may be used intermittently during the menstrual cycle, alternating with sanitary napkins—perhaps using the napkins during the night, when at home during the day, and when flow is slight. Young girls are advised not to use superabsorbent tampons and not to leave any tampon in the body for more than 4 to 6 hours.

NURSING ALERT Patients who use tampons need to understand that they should remove the tampon and consult their health professional if they develop a sudden high fever, vomiting, diarrhea, muscle pain, dizziness, fainting or near fainting when standing up, or rash that resembles a sunburn.

BURNS*

OVERVIEW

Almost everyone has experienced a burn at some time. Burn injuries are usually attributed to extreme heat sources but may also result from exposure to cold, chemicals, or radiation. Most burns are relatively minor and do not require definitive medical treatment. However, burns involving a large body surface area, critical body parts, or the pediatric population frequently benefit from treatment in specialized burn centers. The American Burn Association has established criteria to guide decisions regarding the severity of injury and the need for transfer for specialized care.

Epidemiology and Etiology

Burn injuries represent one of the most severe traumas a body can sustain. Ongoing efforts toward education and burn prevention have failed to significantly reduce the incidence of thermal injury in the United States. Many of the victims are children, and approximately 75% of these burns are preventable. It is estimated that 35% of all burn injuries occur in the pediatric age-groups (East and others, 1988).

The American Burn Association estimates that 70,000 persons will require inpatient treatment for acute burn injuries annually. Studies of the National Burn Information Exchange indicate that 65% to 75% of all injuries occur in the home and that the group at highest risk is children under 2 years of age (Maley, 1986a). Scald injuries are the

*Marilyn E. Jenkins, RN, MBA, CNA, revised this section.

TABLE 29-4 Time/Temperature Relationship to Cause a Full-Thickness (Third-Degree) Burn

	TIME (SECONDS)	TEMPERATURE (°F)
Adult	30	130
	15	135
	5	140
	1.8	150
Young Children	10	130
	4	135
	1	140
	0.5	149

From Maley M: The final control: antiscald plumbing standards, *Information Exchange* 4:1-8, 1991.

single most common cause of burn injuries in children under age 3. Hot water is the most frequent burning agent, followed by grease. Two critical factors determine the risk of serious injury: the temperature of the material and the length of time the skin is exposed to the burning agent (Table 29-4).

Hot liquids in the kitchen account for 50% of the injuries in children under age 2 years. Pulling over containers of hot liquids or appliances is the greatest risk. An additional 21% of the injuries occur in the bathroom and are associated with hot tap water (Maley, 1993).

Burn injuries inflicted as a method of punishment account for 10% of all reported abuse and approximately 9% of all burns in the pediatric population (Silverstein and Wilson, 1988). Immersion in hot water is the most frequently seen injury, followed by contact burns with hot objects such as cigarettes. A high index of suspicion for abuse is raised by a burn distribution inconsistent with the reported incident, delay in seeking treatment, and a history of family instability and inability to deal with stress in crisis situations. Laws now exist in all states requiring the health care worker to report suspected child abuse.

The use of alternative heating devices such as kerosene heaters and wood-burning stoves has increased the risk of contact burns in all age-groups. Most contact burns result from the lack of shielding to prevent contact with hot surfaces. Flame burns involving flammable liquids such as gasoline account for approximately 30% of injuries seen in the pediatric population, especially over 8 years of age. Injuries are frequently made more severe by the ignition of clothing. The 3- to 8-year-old group is more frequently involved in accidents resulting from fire play.

Cigarettes are associated with the majority of fatal house fires and outnumber other causes by a factor of 2 to 1. The use of alternative heating sources is another common cause of house fires. The source of ignition is frequently a combustible material stored near the device, buildup of creosote in the chimney, spillage of fuel, or use of the wrong fuel. Many of these fires result in multiple deaths and injuries, especially in rural areas of the country. The majority of fatal house fires occur from October through March. The single most important element in the decrease in fire-related deaths seen since 1978 is the use of smoke detectors.

The majority of burns result from contact with thermal agents such as a flame, hot surfaces, or hot liquids. Electrical injuries occur most frequently during the spring and summer months and are associated with risk-taking behaviors in young males. Direct contact with high- or low-voltage current, as well as lightning strikes, is the most frequent mechanism of injury. The resistance of the tissue and the pathway of the electric current are responsible for the damage incurred. Electric current travels through the body on the path of least resistance—tissue, fluid, blood vessels, and nerves. A more localized burn is produced if the skin resistance is high at the area of contact, and a more systemic pattern of injury is produced if the skin resistance is low. Often compared with a crush injury, serious electrical trauma results from current passing through vital organs, muscle compartments, and nerve or vascular pathways. Loss of limbs, cardiac fibrillation, respiratory collapse, and burns are common sequelae following exposure to electrical energy. The very young child is particularly at risk for injury resulting from chewing on electrical cords.

Chemical burns are seen infrequently in the pediatric population but can cause extensive injury. The severity of injury is related to the chemical agent (acid, alkali, or organic compound) and the duration of contact. The mechanism of injury differs from other burns in that there is a chemical disruption and alteration of the physical properties of the body area exposed. Noxious agents exist in many cleaning products commonly found in the home. In addition to concern for localized damage, the potential for systemic toxicity must also be addressed. Of particular concern is the exposure of the eyes to chemical agents and the ingestion of caustic substances.

Although radiation injuries are rare, the most common sources in pediatrics are related to radiation exposure due to medical therapies and to ultraviolet light. The causative agent in all burns has important implications for the treatment and the prognosis of the pediatric patient. The nurse uses knowledge of the pathophysiologic processes of each type of injury in assessing the trauma, as well as in planning, implementing, and evaluating the care.

BURN WOUND CHARACTERISTICS

The physiologic responses, therapy, prognosis, and disposition of the injured child are all directly related to the amount of tissue destroyed; therefore the severity of the burn injury is assessed on the basis of the percentage of body surface area burned and the depth of the burn. Also important in determining the seriousness of injury are the location of the wounds, the age of the child, the causative agent, the presence of respiratory involvement, the general health of the child, and the presence of concomitant injuries. Psychosocial issues are also important considerations in planning for the optimum long-term outcome.

Extent of Injury

The extent of the burn is expressed as a percentage of the ***total body surface area (TBSA)*** injured. The child has differ-

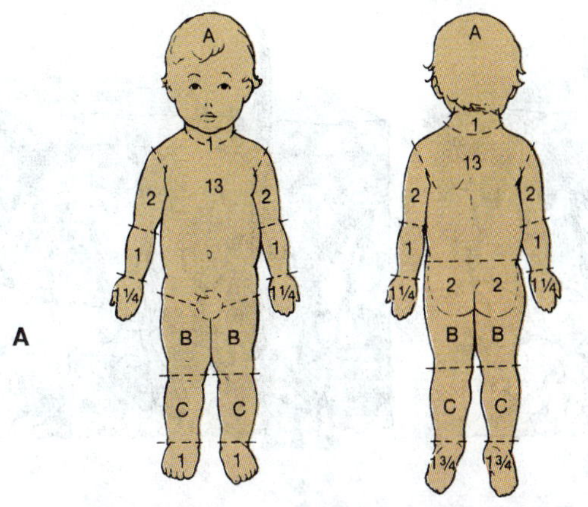

RELATIVE PERCENTAGES OF AREAS AFFECTED BY GROWTH

AREA	BIRTH	AGE 1 YR	AGE 5 YR
A = ½ of head	9½	8½	6½
B = ½ of one thigh	2¾	3¼	4
C = ½ of one leg	2½	2½	2¾

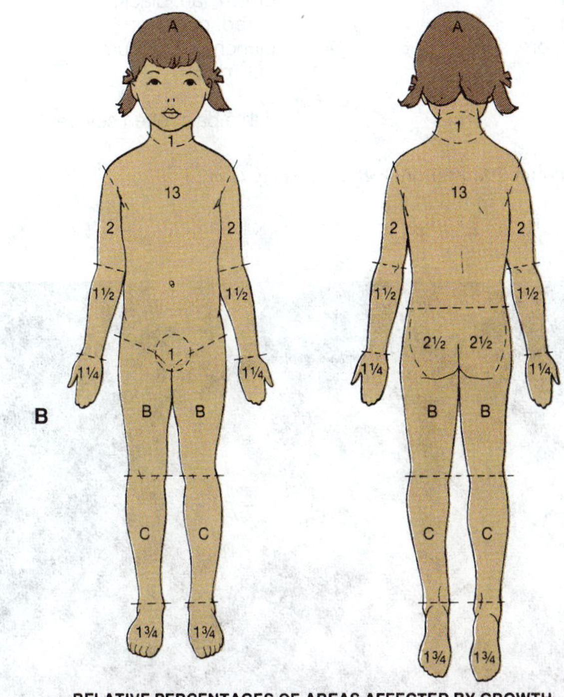

RELATIVE PERCENTAGES OF AREAS AFFECTED BY GROWTH

AREA	AGE 10 YR	AGE 15 YR	ADULT
A = ½ of head	5½	4½	3½
B = ½ of one thigh	4½	4½	4¾
C = ½ of one leg	3	3¼	3½

FIG. 29-2 Estimation of distribution of burns in children. **A,** Children from birth to age 5 years. **B,** Older children.

ent body proportions than the adult, resulting in inaccurate estimation of injury if the standard adult rule of nines is employed. The proportions of the child's trunk and arms are roughly the same as those of the adult. However, the infant's head and neck make up 18% of the TBSA, and each lower extremity accounts for 14% of the TBSA. As the child grows, percentages are deducted from the head and assigned to the legs. A ***modified rule of nines*** for the pediatric population proposes that for each year of life after age 2, 1% is deducted from the head and 0.5% is added to each leg (Helvig, 1993). It is generally more efficient to use any of a variety of charts designed to assign body proportions to children of different ages (Fig. 29-2).

Depth of Injury

A thermal injury is a three-dimensional wound and is also assessed in relation to the depth of injury. Traditionally the terms "first-," "second-," "third-," and "fourth-degree" have been used to describe the depth of tissue injury. However, with the current emphasis on wound healing, more descriptive terms related to the extent of destruction to the epithelializing elements of the skin are replacing the traditional terminology. First- and second-degree burns are classified as partial-thickness injuries, and third- and fourth-degree wounds are classified as full-thickness wounds. Partial-thickness wounds are further classified as superficial or deep in relation to the time required for healing to occur and the functional and cosmetic results anticipated. Since both terminologies are often used interchangeably, they are presented concomitantly in the chart describing the characteristics of burn wounds (Fig. 29-3).

Superficial (first-degree) burns are usually of minor significance. There is frequently a latent period followed by erythema. Tissue damage is minimal, protective functions of the skin remain intact, and systemic effects are rare. Pain is the predominant symptom, and the burn will heal in 5 to 10 days without scarring (Trofino and Braun, 1991). A mild sunburn is an example of a superficial first-degree burn.

Partial-thickness (second-degree) injuries involve the epidermis and varying degrees of the dermis. These wounds are painful, moist, red, and blistered. Superficial partial-thickness burns involve the epidermis and part of the dermis. Dermal elements are intact, and the wound should heal in approximately 14 days with variable amounts of scarring. The wound is extremely sensitive to temperature changes, exposure to air, and light touch. Deep dermal burns, although classified as second-degree or partial-thickness burns, in many respects resemble full-thickness injuries. Sweat glands and hair follicles remain intact. The burn may appear mottled with pink, red, or waxy white areas exhibiting blisters and edema formation (Fig. 29-4). Systemic effects are similar to those encountered with full-thickness burns. Although these wounds will heal spontaneously in approximately 30 days, they do so with extensive scarring.

Full-thickness (third-degree) burns are serious injuries that involve the entire epidermis and dermis and extend into subcutaneous tissue. Thrombosed vessels can be seen beneath the surface of the wound, and nerve endings, sweat glands, and hair follicles are destroyed. The burn varies in color from red to tan, waxy white, brown, or black and is distinguished by a dry, leathery appearance (Fig. 29-5). Normally, full-thickness burns lack sensation in the area of injury because of the destruction of nerve endings. However, most full-thickness burns occur with superficial and partial-thickness burns in which nerve endings are intact and exposed. Also, excised eschar and donor sites cause exposed

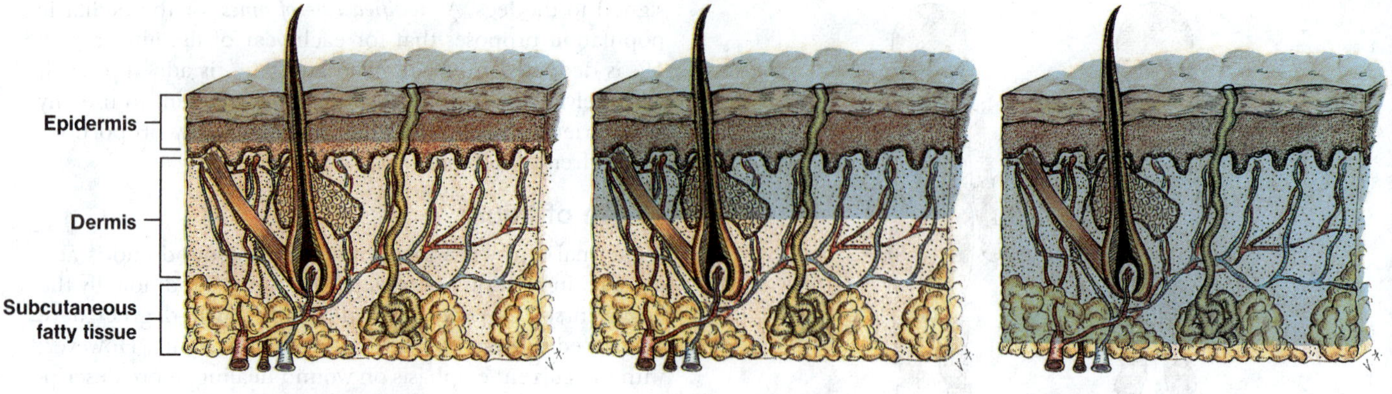

Epidermis
Dermis
Subcutaneous fatty tissue

	Superficial (first degree)	Partial-thickness (second degree)	Full-thickness (third degree)
Type of burn	Sunburn; low-intensity flash; brief scald	Scalds; flash flame	Fire; contact with hot objects
Appearance	Dry surface; red; blanches on pressure and refills	Blistered; moist; mottled pink or red, reddened; blanches on pressure and refills	Tough, leathery; brown, tan, black, or red; does not blanch on pressure; dull, dry
Sensation	Painful	Very painful	Variable pain, often severe

FIG. 29-3 Classification of burn depth. (Modified from Potter PA, Perry AG: *Basic nursing: theory and practice,* ed 2, St Louis, 1991, Mosby.)

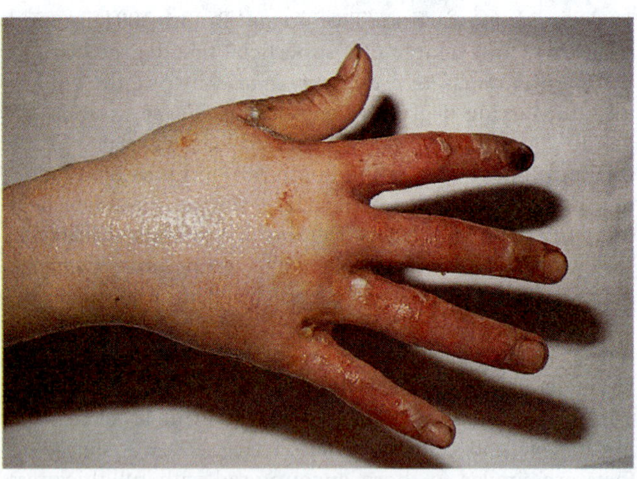

FIG. 29-4 Deep partial-thickness burn.

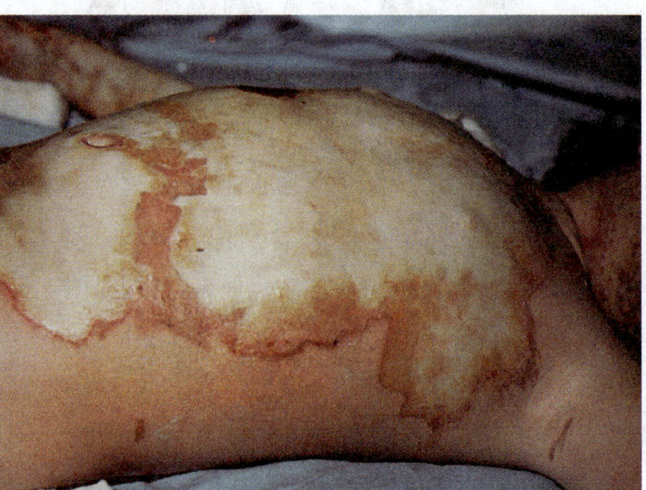

FIG. 29-5 Full-thickness thermal injury.

nerve fibers. Finally, as peripheral fibers regenerate, painful sensation returns. Consequently, children often experience severe pain that is related to the size and depth of the burn (Atchison and others, 1991). Full-thickness wounds are not capable of reepithelialization and require surgical excision and grafting to close the wound.

Fourth-degree burns are also full-thickness injuries and involve underlying structures such as muscle, fascia, and bone. The wound appears dull and dry, and ligaments, tendons, and bone may be exposed.

Severity of Injury

Burns are also appraised on the basis of their severity. This is useful in determining the disposition of the patient for treatment. Burn patients can usually be distinguished as (1) those with a major burn injury who require the services and facilities of a specialized burn center, (2) those with a moderate burn who may be treated in a hospital with expertise in burn care, and (3) those with minor injuries who are able to be treated on an outpatient basis (Table 29-5). The severity of the injury is determined by the extent and depth

TABLE 29-5 Severity Grading System Adopted by the American Burn Association

	MINOR*	MODERATE	MAJOR
Partial-thickness burns	<10% of TBSA	10%-20% of TBSA	>20% of TBSA
Full-thickness burns			All
Treatment	Usually outpatient; may require 1-2 day admission	Admission to hospital, preferably one with expertise in burn care	Admission to a burn center

From Vaccaro P, Trofino RB: Care of the patient with minor to moderate burns. In Trofino RB, editor: *Nursing care of the burn-injured patient,* Philadelphia, 1991, FA Davis.
*Minor burns exclude any burn involving the face, hands, feet, perineum, or crossing joints; electrical burns; any injury complicated by the presence of inhalation injury or concomitant trauma; children with psychosocial factors impacting the injury.

of the burn, the causative agent, the body area involved, the age, and concomitant injuries and illnesses.

Initial assessment to estimate the extent of skin damage is made by observation and simple diagnostic techniques. The extent of body surface area involvement is readily calculated, and the appearance of the wound provides clues to whether the injury involves the full thickness of the skin or only a portion of the skin layers. Touching injured surfaces to test for blanching and capillary refill indicates if circulation to the area is intact.

It is important to consider the cause of injury, as well as the duration of contact with the burning agent. In general, the more intense the heat source and the longer the contact, the deeper the resulting injury will be. Hot liquids may result in partial-thickness burns, whereas full-thickness injury is associated with flame burns. This may vary with the age of the child. Very young children are likely to sustain deeper injuries because of the thin nature of infant skin. This makes estimation of burn depth difficult in young children, especially following scald injuries. Inflicted injuries tend to be more severe than accidental burns because contact with the burning agent is prolonged. Electrical injuries may also be difficult to assess initially. Visible tissue destruction may appear minimal, and damage to underlying structures may be masked. The circumstances of the burn may also suggest the presence of associated injuries.

Certain areas of the body carry a higher risk of complications and require specialized care. Burns of the hands and feet and across joints may not necessarily involve a large body surface area, but injury and scar formation may interfere with normal growth and development. Specialized care is required to preserve maximum function. Burns to the face and neck, along with a history of the injury occurring in an enclosed space, raise a high index of suspicion of inhalation injury. In addition, airway compromise and hypoxia may result from edema formation, as well as pulmonary injury. Damage to the delicate cartilage of the nose and ears results in facial deformities. Facial burns may also involve the eyes and have long-term consequences for vision. Perineal burns are prone to infection and maceration in all patients, especially in young children who are not toilet trained. Scar bands and contractures in the perineal area may interfere with hygiene and mobility.

Children younger than 2 years of age have a significantly higher mortality than older children with burns of a similar magnitude. The infant has minimal protein stores, which are rapidly depleted during burn shock; an immature immune response, increasing the risk of infection and sepsis; and a greater amount of body water in proportion to size that is intolerant of rapid fluid shifts. In addition, the child has not achieved mature renal function. This negatively impacts the ability to retain sodium and water. These considerations, combined with the previously discussed fragility of the skin in the very young, increase the severity of injury.

Many patients sustaining thermal injuries may also suffer associated trauma. The circumstances of the accident may offer clues to related trauma. Children involved in house fires may have jumped from a window, sustaining fractures. Motor vehicle accidents and electrical injuries often result in concomitant injuries. Any suspicion of child abuse should alert the health care team to rule out other injuries.

PATHOPHYSIOLOGY

A burn injury represents a catastrophic insult that involves all organ systems. An understanding of the pathophysiology underlying thermal trauma is essential to provide appropriate nursing care to the pediatric burn victim.

Local Response

Damage to human skin by heat results in two types of injury: an immediate direct cellular response and a delayed response due to dermal ischemia. Irreversible cellular damage from protein denaturation occurs at temperatures exceeding 45° C (113° F). Three zones of injury demonstrate the evolution of local tissue damage (Fig. 29-6). The unstable area of injured cells, which may survive under ideal conditions, is designated as the zone of ***stasis.*** Progressive injury due to dermal ischemia may occur in this zone (see box on p. 1258).

Edema Formation. Thermal injury to the vessels in the two outer zones results in increased capillary permeability. At the same time, vasodilation causes an increase in hydrostatic pressure within the capillaries. The increased hydrostatic pressure, combined with the increased capillary permeability, causes loss of water, protein, and electrolytes from the circulating volume into the interstitial spaces. This shift is further enhanced by a diminishing intravascular on-

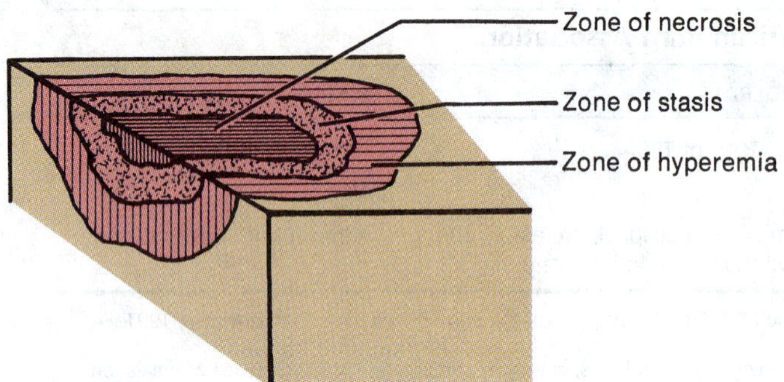

FIG. 29-6 Zones of injury in burn. (After Zawacki B: *Ann Surg* 180:98-102, 1974.)

ZONES OF BURN INJURY

Zone of coagulation (necrosis)—Area beneath obviously destroyed tissue; capillary flow has ceased and tissue destruction is irreversible; tissue is dead.
Zone of stasis—Area beneath and surrounding zone of coagulation; markedly reduced capillary flow; tissue severely damaged from heat but not coagulated. Tissue in this zone can be saved with prevention of further injury and adequate perfusion.
Zone of hyperemia—Area metabolically active; displays usual response to tissue injury.

cotic pressure, as protein and sodium are lost to the interstitial spaces. Although the edema involves both burned and unburned areas, at the site of injury the accumulation of edema fluid beneath and around the wound can reach extreme proportions until the extravasation of fluid is limited by tissue tension.

In addition, there are changes in the permeability of cells in and around the burned area that result in an abnormal exchange of electrolytes between cells and the interstitial fluid; specifically, sodium enters the cells in exchange for potassium, resulting in further depletion of intravascular sodium.

Fluid Loss. Without the protection of the skin, fluid loss at the air-wound interface can be extremely high. Fluid loss from burned skin is 5 to 10 times greater than from undamaged skin (Trofino and Braun, 1991). These losses are maximum at about the fourth day after injury but continue to pose problems until the denuded surfaces are grafted or healed.

Circulatory Status. Significant circulatory alterations take place in the zone of stasis located around the dead coagulated tissue. Heated red blood cells become spherical in shape. These heat-damaged cells, together with hemoconcentration from fluid shifts, depressed cardiac output, and tissue edema, reduce the blood flow in the burned area, resulting in capillary stasis. Thrombi develop that further impede circulation and produce tissue ischemia and necrosis. Hyperviscosity and impaired blood flow are also attributed to the release of substances, such as thromboplastin and clot-activating factors, from damaged cells that cause the production of microemboli, platelet adhesion and aggregation, and increased pain and edema. Circulation in the area around partial-thickness wounds ceases immediately after injury but is usually restored within 24 to 48 hours. In full-thickness burns, however, the vascular supply is completely occluded, and no appreciable circulation is reestablished until granulation takes place at the interface between burned and unburned skin.

Burn Wound. In superficial first-degree injuries, tissue damage is minimal. Protein loss is insignificant, and edema is barely perceptible. The burning sensation and pain resolve in 48 to 72 hours, and in 5 to 10 days the damaged epithelium peels off in small scales or sheets, leaving no scar.

Considerable edema and more severe capillary damage occur in partial-thickness burns. With reasonable care, superficial partial-thickness injuries heal spontaneously and uneventfully through the generative capacity of the stratum germinativum and epithelial cells of the lining of skin appendages. The wound should heal in approximately 14 days with minimal scarring.

Deep dermal burns heal more slowly by regeneration from the epithelial lining of skin appendages, sweat glands, and hair follicles. A thin epithelial covering develops in 25 to 35 days, but this type of burn may require several months to heal. Scarring is common, and infection or trauma can easily convert a partial-thickness wound to a full-thickness injury, especially in young children, with their normally thinner skin. Fluid loss and metabolic consequences may be considerable.

Cell destruction by coagulation necrosis takes place in full-thickness burns. Dead tissue and exudate convert to a thick, leathery eschar in 48 to 72 hours, which liquefies and begins to separate in 12 to 21 days if not surgically excised. This process is a result of autolysis, leukocyte digestion, and disintegration of collagen fibers. The dead avascular tissue provides an ideal environment for bacterial growth. If tissue is not grafted, new granulation tissue forms on the wound bed. The wound heals slowly by proliferation from the edges, with a high risk of infection and severe scarring. Full-thickness burns result in severe edema with fluid and electrolyte shifts and extensive metabolic changes.

Systemic Responses

Along with and subsequent to the pathophysiologic response at the site of injury, a number of systemic responses occur.

Cardiovascular System. The immediate postburn period is marked by dramatic alterations in circulation, known as ***burn shock.*** There is a precipitous drop in cardiac output that precedes any change in circulating blood or plasma volumes. The initial decrease in cardiac output (about 50% of normal resting values) is attributed to a circulating myocardial depressant factor, associated with severe burn injury, that affects the contractility of the heart muscle directly. As a result of fluid losses through denuded skin, increased capillary permeability, and vasodilation, the circulating volume decreases rapidly and cardiac output is reduced even further, usually leveling off at about 20% of normal resting values. Following adequate fluid resuscitation, cardiac output

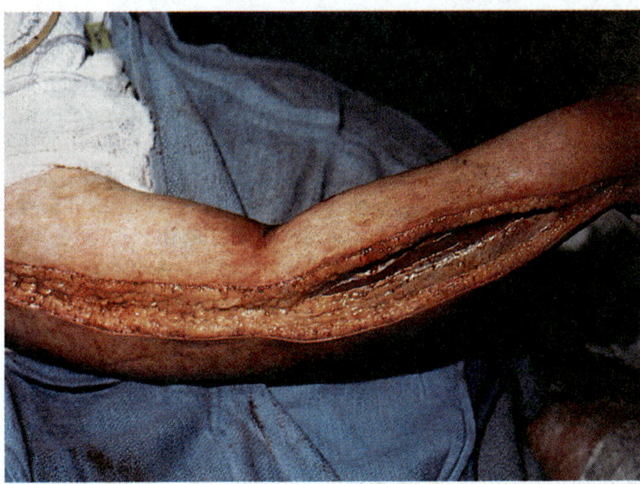

FIG. 29-7 Escharotomy/fasciotomy in a severely burned arm.

returns to normal spontaneously in 24 to 36 hours. If fluid is not replaced, cardiac output continues to decrease, resulting in inadequate perfusion, organ dysfunction, and ultimately death.

Capillary permeability with leakage of fluid takes place in uninjured areas, as well as in the burn wound. Severe edema due to the rapid fluid shift to the interstitial spaces and the shrinkage of drying eschar produces a tourniquet effect, resulting in a compartment syndrome. Compartments are composed of groups of muscles in the extremities that are surrounded by fibrous tissue. The inability of the fascia to expand in the presence of massive edema increases the pressure in the compartment, compromising circulation and entrapping nerves (Fig. 29-7).

Edema fluid accumulates rapidly in the first 18 hours after injury to reach a maximum in about 48 hours. Capillary permeability returns to normal, and fluid is reabsorbed, chiefly by way of the lymphatics. Reabsorption usually proceeds at the rate of fluid accumulation, although it may persist longer. Redistribution of fluid is often complex and unpredictable and is marked by diuresis.

In most children the cardiovascular system is able to withstand the demands placed on it, although shock is a prominent feature of large thermal injuries. Some children are prone to congestive heart failure and pulmonary edema. In addition, peripheral circulation in the infant is less efficient and more labile, which complicates burn response and therapy in this age-group.

Renal System. Loss of fluid from the intravascular compartment causes renal vasoconstriction that in turn leads to reduced renal plasma flow and depressed glomerular filtration. When adequate fluids are provided, the glomerular filtration rate returns to normal, and by the third or fourth postburn day, urinary output increases as edema fluid is mobilized and eliminated. In the first few days oliguria is more commonly the result of inadequate fluid replacement than of acute renal failure. If the child does not respond to treatment or if there is inadequate fluid resuscitation, acute renal failure may develop with significant kidney damage.

Blood urea nitrogen and creatinine levels are elevated as a result of tissue breakdown, decreased circulating volume, and oliguria. Hematuria may also be evident from the hemolysis of red blood cells, and oliguria may develop as a consequence of the increased pigment load. This is especially common following extensive electrical injury. Cell destruction releases large amounts of myoglobin, which occludes the kidney tubules and places the victim of electrical trauma at high risk for renal failure.

Gastrointestinal System. Perfusion of the GI tract and liver are decreased as a result of alterations in blood flow. Ischemia of the GI tract has been found to initiate and aggravate erosion and necrosis. Gastric acid production is initially suppressed for 48 to 72 hours after injury and then surpasses normal levels. Catecholamines may be a factor in the suppression. The accelerated acid production and autolysis of pepsin significantly increase the risk of erosion and ulceration.

Gastric dilation and paralytic ileus often occur following major burn injuries. Digestion virtually ceases in the stomach and the large intestine, but the small bowel maintains motility and absorptive capacity. Ileus is evident by absent or hypoactive bowel sounds on auscultation. Gastric decompression is necessary to empty the stomach and protect the child from acid aspiration until gastric motility is reestablished.

Metabolism. The metabolic rate in burn patients is greatly accelerated following initial resuscitation, and the nitrogen losses are far in excess of those seen in other types of injuries. The magnitude of energy requirements of the burned child frequently exceeds the usual needs of a normal, active child (Saffle and others, 1985). When the burn injury is extensive (>50% of TBSA), energy needs may approach twice the predicted basal requirements.

The stress of injury places high demands on the body. Stress-invoked glycogen breakdown depletes the energy stores in 12 to 24 hours, after which the body resorts to glyconeogenesis for high-energy needs. Blood glucose levels may be elevated as a result of insulin resistance. Rapid protein breakdown and muscle wasting occur in the burn patient if sufficient protein replacement is not provided.

Body temperature reflects the net balance between heat production and heat loss. Children with burn injuries typically exhibit an elevated body temperature, even in the absence of infection, as a result of the accelerated metabolism. Heat is lost as a result of the energy-consuming process of evaporation of water from the damaged skin surface. Infants and young children are especially vulnerable because of the large surface area relative to metabolically active tissue. Burning destroys a lipid layer and converts skin that is normally impermeable to water to a state that transmits water vapor at least four times as rapidly as unburned skin. In partial-thickness burns this loss is greatest on the day of injury; in full-thickness burns it rises slowly at first and then rapidly increases to reach a peak on about the fourth day after the burn. Evaporative losses continue until partial-thickness wounds are healed and full-thickness burns are grafted. Thus body stores of energy are rapidly depleted unless sufficient replacement is provided or losses are reduced.

Neuroendocrine System. As a response to stress of any origin, the hypothalamic-hypophyseal mechanism restores equilibrium by secreting trophic hormones, which stimulate various target organs of the neuroendocrine system. Adrenal activity is markedly increased. The medulla responds by secreting additional amounts of the catecholamines epinephrine and norepinephrine. Adrenocortical hormones reach a peak immediately after injury and remain elevated for some time. Aldosterone secretion, as well as a release of antidiuretic hormone, is sustained at a high level throughout hospitalization. Despite this increased adrenal activity, adrenal insufficiency is a rare complication.

Anemia and Metabolic Acidosis. The hematocrit is initially elevated because of hemoconcentration resulting from fluid shifts to the interstitial spaces and red blood cell destruction. In addition, a reduced red blood cell half-life results from increased cell fragility. A significant loss of circulating red blood cell mass is predominantly associated with deep burns.

Most burn patients exhibit some degree of metabolic acidosis as a result of the disruption of the buffering action of the body by the fluid shift to the extravascular spaces and the altered concentrations of potassium, sodium, chloride, and bicarbonate ions. Reduced blood volume and cardiac output result in diminished perfusion and tissue hypoxia with a shift to anaerobic metabolism. The resultant formation of metabolic acids is usually sufficiently compensated by respiratory mechanisms. Renal compensatory activities are impaired by the decreased blood flow.

Growth and Development. Alterations in growth patterns are frequently observed in children following extensive burn injuries; growth delays may persist during the convalescent period (Rutan and Herndon, 1990). Regression is universal in hospitalized children but is often extreme in burn patients. This response is related to separation anxiety, pain, restriction of behavior and activities, loss of control, and altered body image.

Complications

Thermally injured children are subject to a number of serious complications, both from the wound and from systemic alterations resulting from the injury. The immediate threat to life is related to airway compromise and profound shock. During healing, infection—both local and systemic sepsis—is the primary complication. Mortality associated with thermal trauma in children increases with the severity of injury and decreases as age advances. In children older than 3 years, the mortality rate is similar to that of adults. Below this age, survival of the burn and its associated complications is considerably lessened.

Pulmonary System. The impact of thermal injury on pulmonary function includes a full range of respiratory dysfunctions, including inhalation injury, aspiration of gastric contents, bacterial pneumonia, pulmonary edema and insufficiency, and emboli. Pulmonary complications remain the leading cause of death following thermal trauma. When inhalation injury accompanies surface burns, mortality approaches 56% as compared with 4.1% without inhalation injury in every age and burn size category (Thompson, Herndon, and Traber, 1986).

Inhalation injuries result from trauma to the tracheobronchial tree following inhalation of heated gases and toxic chemicals produced during combustion. Although direct thermal injury to the upper airway may occur, heat damage below the vocal cords is rare. Inspired heated air is cooled in the upper airway before reaching the trachea. Reflex closure of the cords and laryngeal spasm prevent full inhalation. Evidence of direct thermal injury to the upper airway includes burns of the face and lips, singed nasal hairs, and laryngeal edema. Clinical manifestation may be delayed as long as 24 to 48 hours. Wheezing, increasing secretions, hoarseness, wet rales, and carbonaceous secretions are signs of respiratory tract involvement. Upper airway obstruction is often an evolving phenomenon, occurring during vigorous fluid resuscitation and edema formation in the first 12 hours after injury. In such situations tracheal intubation may be necessary to preserve a patent airway.

Inhalation of carbon monoxide is suspected when the injury has occurred in an enclosed space (see Smoke Inhalation Injury, Chapter 32, for a discussion of carbon monoxide inhalation). Inhalation of other products of combustion, such as smoke and toxic chemicals, can produce varying degrees of pulmonary damage. Burning wood smoke is extremely irritating; smoke from burning plastic materials, especially polyvinyl chloride, release gases containing chlorine, sulfuric acid, and cyanide. Respiratory injury is manifested by mucosal erythema and edema followed by sloughing of the mucosa. A mucopurulent membrane replaces the mucosal lining and seriously compromises respiration and ventilation.

A common etiologic factor in respiratory failure in the pediatric population is bacterial pneumonia, which may be secondary to airway injury or contamination from intubation, or acquired through hematogenous spread of bacteria. Early in the postburn period, the largest percentage of pulmonary infections are the result of nosocomial exposure, immobility, and abdominal distention. The hematogenous variety occurs later and is related to the septic burn wound or other foci, such as phlebitis at the site of an invasive intravenous line. When inhalation injury and pneumonia are present concomitantly, a 60% increase in mortality has been observed (Carrougher, 1993).

A less common complication is pulmonary edema resulting from fluid overload or adult respiratory distress syndrome (ARDS) in association with gram-negative septicemia (see Chapter 32). This syndrome results from pulmonary capillary damage and the leakage of fluid into the interstitial spaces of the lung. A loss of compliance and interference with oxygenation are the consequences of pulmonary insufficiency in conjunction with systemic sepsis.

Deep burns, especially those circling the thorax, may cause restriction of chest excursion as a result of edema and inelastic eschar formation. Young children are particularly at risk because of the pliability of the skeletal structure. Hypoxia is relieved by longitudinal incisions along the anterior axillary lines combined with a transverse incision at the costal level. This procedure is referred to as an ***escharotomy*** and allows expansion of the chest wall to facilitate ventilation.

Wound Sepsis. Sepsis is a critical problem in the treatment of burns and is an ever-present threat following the shock phase. Initially, burn wounds are relatively pathogen-free, unless they are contaminated with potentially infectious material such as dirt or polluted water. However, dead tissue and exudate provide a fertile field for bacterial growth. Early colonization of the wound surface by a preponderance of gram-positive organisms (primarily staphylococcus) changes, on about the third postburn day, to predominantly gram-negative opportunistic organisms, particularly *Pseudomonas aeruginosa.* By the fifth postburn day bacterial invasion is well underway beneath the surface of the burn wound.

Characteristics of the burn wound contribute to the proliferation of pathogenic organisms. Vascular supply to full-thickness burns is occluded immediately, and no appreciable blood is supplied to the area for approximately 3 weeks after the injury. In partial-thickness wounds the circulation to the injured area is suspended for 24 to 48 hours. Circulation is then restored unless infection supervenes. Thrombosis from bacterial invasion will impair circulation sufficiently to convert partial-thickness wounds to full-thickness injuries. These large amounts of nonviable tissue also provide an excellent medium for the growth of microorganisms.

Occlusion of the local blood supply is believed to impair the delivery of both humoral and cellular defense mechanisms to the burned area. Initially there is a decrease in inflammatory and phagocytic cells to the wound, but the number of phagocytes gradually increases until they are present in abundance by the third postburn week, when granulation tissue is forming. Granulation tissue, with its rich blood supply, affords increasing resistance to infection. Inasmuch as organisms are normally a part of skin flora, cultures that reveal an organism concentration of 10^5/g of tissue have been arbitrarily chosen as the level of burn wound invasion.

The microflora present at any institution are influenced by the treatment modalities and the choice of antibiotics. A reduction in the percentage of specific bacteria and fungi recovered from burn wounds has occurred over the past 30 years. This reduction reflects improvements in patient management, aggressive excision and grafting of the wounds, and improved topical antimicrobial therapy. At the same time, the percentage of septicemias has remained relatively constant. Improved survival of patients with massive burn injuries and greater immunologic compromise would explain this apparent inconsistency (Holder, 1988).

NURSING ALERT Disorientation in the burned patient is one of the first signs of overwhelming sepsis. A spiking fever and diminished bowel sounds accompanied by paralytic ileus are noted and progressively increase over 48 to 72 hours, after which the temperature falls to subnormal limits. At this time the wound deteriorates, the white blood cell count is depressed, and septic shock becomes manifest.

Gastrointestinal System. Impaired gastric and large bowel motility is a common complication following burns

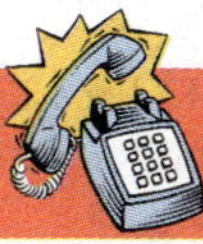

EMERGENCY TREATMENT
Burns

MINOR BURNS

Stop the burning process:
- Apply cool water to the burn or hold the burned area under cool running water.

Do not disturb any blisters that form.
Do not apply anything to the wound.
Cover with a clean cloth if risk of damage or contamination.
Remove burned clothing and jewelry.

MAJOR BURNS

Stop the burning process:
- Flame burns—smother the fire.
- Place victim in the horizontal position.
- Roll victim in a blanket or similar object; avoid covering the head.

Assess for an adequate airway and breathing.
If not breathing, begin mouth-to-mouth resuscitation.
Remove burned clothing and jewelry.
Cover wound with a clean cloth.
Transport to medical aid.
Begin IV and oxygen therapy.

greater than 20% of the TBSA. The small intestine, however, maintains its motility and absorptive capabilities. As long as gastric decompression is maintained, enteral nutrition can be safely supplied to the duodenum during periods of ileus (Gottschlich, Alexander, and Bower, 1990; Jenkins, Gottschlich and Alexander, 1989). GI motility is usually restored following adequate fluid resuscitation. Recurrence of an ileus later in the hospital course is suggestive of developing sepsis.

Superficial mucosal erosion, ***Curling ulcers,*** may be evident by 12 hours after injury and by 72 hours can be demonstrated in 67% of burn patients. The ulcers, however, are rare before 72 hours and are more commonly seen in the second or third postburn week (Fuchs and Gleason, 1988). The precise pathogenesis of gastroduodenal erosion remains undefined. However, certain factors are known to contribute to mucosal damage. There is an increasing incidence of Curling ulcers with increasing size of injury. Altered submucosal blood flow in the immediate postburn period and atrophy of the intestinal microvilli due to lack of enteral nutrition have also been implicated in the development of GI erosion. Impaired blood flow during septic episodes results in the progression of existing lesions. Prophylactic administration of antacids, histamine H_2-antagonists, or sucralfate, as well as the early initiation of enteral support, usually prevents the development of serious bleeding.

Central Nervous System. The reported incidence of burn-related encephalopathy has varied from 5% to 14% with the onset of symptoms following injury ranging from a few hours to several weeks (Kaye and Butler, 1988). The manifestations include hallucinations, personality changes, delirium, seizures, and coma. Postburn seizures appear to be unique to the pediatric burn patient. In most cases burn encephalopathy can be attributed to hypoxemia, hyponatremia, hypovolemia, septicemia, and drug administration. Although the cause is unidentified in one third of all cases, full neurologic recovery is usual, even with prolonged and serious manifestations.

THERAPEUTIC MANAGEMENT

The initial management of the burn patient begins at the scene of injury. Care rendered before arrival at the hospital can significantly impact morbidity and mortality. The clinical management of thermal trauma on admission to an emergency department differs depending on the severity of the injury.

Emergency Care

The first priority is to stop the burning process (see Emergency Treatment box on p. 1261). The child should then be transported immediately to the nearest medical facility for definitive treatment and evaluation for transfer to a burn center. The child and the family will be extremely frightened and anxious; sensitivity to their emotional state will provide reassurance during the transport process.

Stop the Burning Process. The chief aim of rescue in flame burns is to smother the fire, not fan it. Children tend to panic and run, which only serves to spread the flames and make assistance more difficult. The injured child should be placed in a horizontal position and rolled in a blanket, rug, or similar article, with care taken not to cover the head and face because of the danger of the inhalation of toxic fumes. If nothing is available, the victim should lie down and roll over slowly to extinguish the flames. Remaining in the vertical position may cause the hair to ignite or the inhalation of flames, heat, or smoke.

Major burns with large amounts of denuded skin should not be cooled. Heat is rapidly lost from burned areas, and additional cooling leads to a drop in core body temperature and potential circulatory collapse. Wet dressings also promote vasoconstriction because of cooling, resulting in impaired circulation to the burned area and increased tissue damage. Chemical burns present special circumstances and require flushing with copious amounts of water during transport to a medical facility. The use of neutralizing agents on the skin is contraindicated, since a chemical reaction is initiated and further injury may result. If the chemical is in powder form, the addition of water may spread the caustic agent. The powder should be brushed off if possible.

Burned clothing is removed to prevent further damage from smoldering fabric and hot beads of melted synthetic materials. Any jewelry is also removed to eliminate the transfer of heat from the metal and constriction due to edema formation. This also provides better access to the wound and precludes more painful removal later on.

Assess the Victim's Condition. As soon as the flames are extinguished, the condition of the victim is assessed. Airway, breathing, and circulation are the priority concerns. Cardiopulmonary and cerebral emergencies are always a consideration following trauma. Cardiopulmonary complications may result from exposure to electric current, inhalation of toxic fumes and smoke, hypovolemia, and shock. Emergency measures are instituted as appropriate.

Cover the Burn. The burn wound should be covered with a clean cloth to prevent contamination and alleviate pain by eliminating air contact. The child with extensive burns is covered to prevent hypothermia. No attempt should be made to treat the burn. Application of topical ointments, oils, or other home remedies is contraindicated.

Transport the Child to Medical Aid. The child with an extensive burn is not given anything by mouth to avoid aspiration in the presence of paralytic ileus and upper airway edema and to prevent water intoxication. The child is transported to the nearest medical facility. If this cannot be accomplished within a relatively short period of time, intravenous access should be established if possible with a large-bore catheter. Oxygen is administered if available at 100%. A report of the initial assessment and any interventions implemented is given to the medical facility assuming responsibility for the care of the child.

Provide Reassurance. Providing reassurance and psychologic support to both the family and the child helps immeasurably during postinjury crisis. Reducing anxiety helps to conserve energy needed to cope with the physiologic and emotional stress of a traumatic injury.

Management of Minor Burns

Treatment of burns classified as minor can usually be managed adequately on an outpatient basis when it is determined that the parent can be relied on to carry out instructions for care and observation. Patients with less than optimal circumstances may require close follow-up to ensure compliance with the treatment program.

The wound is cleansed with a mild soap and tepid water. Debridement of the wound includes removal of any embedded debris, chemicals, and devitalized tissue. Removal of intact blisters remains controversial. Some argue that blisters provide a barrier against infection; others maintain that blister fluid is an effective medium for the growth of microorganisms (Peate, 1992). Most practitioners favor covering the wound with an antimicrobial ointment to reduce the risk of infection and to provide some form of pain relief. The dressing consists of a fine-mesh gauze placed over the ointment and a light wrap of gauze dressing that avoids interference with movement. This helps to keep the wound clean and protect it from trauma. The caregiver is instructed to wash the wound twice a day, reapply the dressing, and return the child to the office or clinic as directed for wound observation.

Other practitioners prefer an occlusive dressing, such as a hydrocolloid, which is placed over the wound after cleansing. The dressing is changed once leakage occurs or at regular intervals, usually every 7 days (Hermans and Hermans, 1986). This method eliminates the discomfort associated with frequent dressing changes but impairs visualization of the wound surface.

If there is a high probability of infection or other complications or if there is doubt about the ability to carry out instructions, the parents may be directed to return daily for dressing changes and inspection, or a nurse may be assigned to make a home visit for that purpose. Frequent removal of the dressing is an effective mode of debridement. Soaking the dressing in tepid water before removal will help loosen the dressing and debris and reduce discomfort. Burns of the face are usually treated by exposure. The wound is washed and debrided in the same manner, and a thin film of antimicrobial ointment is applied twice a day.

A tetanus history is obtained on admission. When there is no history of immunization or more than 5 years have passed since the last immunization, tetanus prophylaxis is administered. Administration of antibiotics for minor burns is controversial. A mild analgesic, such as acetaminophen, is usually sufficient to relieve discomfort; the antipyretic effect of the drug also alleviates the sensation of heat.

Most minor burns heal without difficulty, but if the wound margin becomes erythematous, gross purulence is noted, or the child develops evidence of systemic reaction, such as fever or tachycardia, hospitalization is indicated. The child should also be evaluated for functional impairment, and the caregiver should be instructed in the exercise and ambulation program. Following wound healing, an evaluation of scar maturation and range of motion will indicate any need for further therapy.

Management of Major Burns

When a child with extensive burns is admitted to the hospital for treatment, a variety of assessments are conducted and therapies initiated. Of these, the priority concerns include the establishment and maintenance of an adequate airway, initiation of fluid administration, and evaluation and treatment of the wound. Although the order of implementation may vary from institution to institution, a number of procedures and activities are generally initiated on admission. Some are carried out simultaneously (see box above, right).

Other therapies, including nutritional support, positioning and splinting to prevent contractures, treatment of anemia and hypoproteinemia, psychosocial support, and rehabilitative aspects of burn management, are initiated as appropriate throughout the course of treatment.

Establishment of an Adequate Airway. The first priority of care is airway maintenance. Thermal injuries to the face, nares, and upper torso; a history of injury in an enclosed space; an examination of the oral and nasal membranes that reveals edema, hyperemia, and blisters; or evidence of trauma to the upper respiratory passages all suggest inhalation of noxious agents or respiratory burns. If there is evidence of respiratory involvement, 100% oxygen is administered and blood gas values, including carbon monoxide levels, are determined.

If the child exhibits changes in sensorium, air hunger, or other signs of respiratory distress, an endotracheal tube is inserted to maintain the airway. When severe edema of the face and neck is anticipated, intubation is performed before swelling makes tube placement difficult or impossible. A controlled intubation is preferred to an emergency procedure. Intubation allows for the delivery of humidified oxygen, the removal of secretions from respiratory passages, and the provision of ventilatory support.

Treatment may include bronchodilators to reduce bronchospasm. Bronchopulmonary hygiene to prevent atelectasis and pooling of secretions is employed to reduce the risk of pneumonia. Therapies include percussion and postural drainage, frequent position changes, and suctioning to remove secretions. Often placing the child in a semi-Fowler position with high-flow oxygen and maximum humidity is sufficient to relieve bronchospasm produced by trauma to the bronchial mucosa.

When full-thickness burns encircle the chest, constricting eschar may limit chest wall excursion. The child becomes increasingly difficult to ventilate. Escharotomy of the chest relieves this pressure and improves ventilation.

Fluid Replacement Therapy. The objectives of fluid therapy are compensation for water and sodium losses to the traumatized area and the interstitial spaces; replenishment of sodium deficits; restoration of circulating volume; provision of adequate perfusion; correction of acidosis; and improvement of renal function. Treatment for burn shock should be initiated in children with burns in excess of 15% to 20% of the TBSA.

Use of fluid and electrolyte therapy in the first 24 hours after injury remains controversial. The controversy is centered primarily around whether colloid solution should be a part of the resuscitation phase of fluid therapy. Those who favor crystalloid solutions believe that during this time the altered capillary membrane is unable to provide a structural barrier and that colloid solutions are of questionable value in restoring plasma oncotic pressure. In the young pediatric patient with a major burn injury, the replacement of serum proteins by colloid administration is appropriate, since hypoproteinemia may accentuate edema and serum concentrations have been shown to rapidly decrease during burn shock (Warden, 1992).

The composition of the fluid administered varies with

OUTLINE OF MAJOR BURN MANAGEMENT

- Ascertain the adequacy of the airway and provide oxygen, intubation, and ventilatory support as indicated.
- Insert a large-bore intravenous line, preferably through unburned skin, to deliver fluids at a sufficiently rapid rate to effect resuscitation.
- Remove clothing and jewelry and examine for secondary trauma.
- Obtain an admission weight.
- Insert a nasogastric tube to empty stomach content and maintain gastric decompression.
- Insert an indwelling Foley catheter to obtain specimens and monitor hourly output.
- Evaluate the burn wound and determine the extent and depth of injury.
- Calculate fluid requirements and establish the appropriate regimen.
- Provide intravenous medication for control of pain and anxiety only after adequate oxygenation is ensured and fluid resuscitation is initiated.
- Obtain baseline laboratory studies.
- Perform escharotomy and/or fasciotomy to the chest and extremities for constricting circumferential eschar or elevated compartment pressures, and impaired circulation.
- Apply topical antimicrobials and dressings to the burn wounds.
- Obtain a history regarding the injury and other pertinent data.
- Administer appropriate tetanus prophylaxis.

the philosophy of the individual practitioner and may consist of an isotonic saline solution, a near-isotonic solution, or even a hypertonic saline solution. A decreased tolerance of children to hypertonic solutions may result in hypernatremia, hyperosmolality, and intracellular dehydration. Many formulas have been proposed as guidelines for fluid administration following burn injury. Perhaps the most commonly employed regimen is the Parkland formula. It is important to remember that whatever formula is used during resuscitation, it serves only as a guideline and that individual adjustments must be made based on the patient's response to therapy. Fluid replacement is maintained at a rate that will provide an hourly urinary output of 30 ml in older children and 1 to 2 ml/kg in children weighing less than 30 kg. Other parameters monitored during fluid resuscitation include vital signs, capillary refill, and sensorium.

Some common reasons for patients to require fluids well in excess of the calculated volume include underestimation of burn size (particularly in pediatric patients), pulmonary injury that sequesters resuscitation fluid in the lung, electrical injury with greater tissue destruction than is visible, and delay in the initiation of fluid resuscitation (Faldmo and Kravitz, 1993). Irreversible burn shock that persists despite aggressive fluid resuscitation remains a significant cause of death in the immediate postburn period. Exchange transfusion consisting of the replacement of circulating volume by banked whole blood provides a therapeutic modality that may benefit the patient who fails to responds to conventional resuscitation. Inflammatory response factors, thought to be important in burn shock, are removed, thus lowering the concentration present in the body and restoring capillary integrity and substantially reducing fluid requirements (Heink, 1992).

NURSING ALERT Capillary refill and alterations in sensorium and urinary output are the most reliable indicators for assessing the adequacy of fluid resuscitation in burned children. Blood pressure can remain normotensive even in a state of hypovolemia.

After the initial 24 to 48 hours, the capillary seal is restored. Fluid requirements decrease to a constant that persists until wound coverage is achieved. Colloid solutions such as albumin or plasma are useful to maintain plasma volume. Fluid balance may continue to be a problem throughout the course of treatment, especially during periods of increased evaporative loss from the burn wound. Approximately 48 to 72 hours after injury, interstitial fluid returns to the vascular compartment and diuresis occurs to eliminate excess fluids. Increasing intake to match urinary output during this phase can result in circulatory overload.

Nutrition. The enhanced metabolic requirements and the accompanying catabolism of severe burns make nutritional needs of paramount importance and often difficult to provide. The metabolic rate of children with burn injuries increases linearly with increasing burn size to a maximum of 150% to 200% of normal (Harmel, Vane, and King, 1986; Ireton and others, 1986). The diet must provide sufficient calories to meet augmented needs, as well as increased quantities of protein to diminish nitrogen deficits. Studies have shown that high-protein dietary supplementation can accelerate wound healing and improve host defense. The burn patient should derive 20% to 25% of energy needs from protein (Alexander and others, 1980).

Many burn patients are able to eat; a high-protein, high-calorie diet is encouraged as soon as possible after resolution of paralytic ileus. However, many of these children have poor appetites and are unable to meet energy requirements solely by oral feeding. Most children with burns in excess of 25% of the TBSA require supplementation with tube feeding. Absence of bowel sounds does not preclude enteral nutrition. Since the small bowel maintains motility and absorptive capabilities, the placement of a small-bore feeding tube into the duodenum allows for the safe delivery of enteral nutrition during periods of paralytic ileus associated with trauma, sepsis, and anesthesia (Jenkins, Gottschlich, and Warden, 1994). Protection from aspiration is achieved by means of a nasogastric tube to decompress the stomach.

If nutritional requirements cannot be met entirely by the enteral route, parenteral hyperalimentation can be used to supplement intake. However, enteral nutrition is preferred because it eliminates the risk of catheter-related sepsis, maintains intestinal integrity and function, and allows more efficient utilization of nutrients, especially protein (Herndon and others, 1987). Early initiation of enteral support, along with aggressive management of complications, allows successful enteral alimentation in most burned children (Dominioni and others, 1984; Gottschlich and others, 1988).

To facilitate growth and proliferation of epithelial cells, administration of vitamins A and C is begun early in the postburn period. Zinc is also supplemented by some practitioners because zinc stores are depleted during catabolism. Zinc appears to play a role in wound healing and epithelialization (Gottschlich and Warden, 1990).

Medication. Controversy exists regarding the use of antibiotics during the first few days after injury. Antibiotics are usually not administered prophylactically in the absence of identified pathogens. The administration of systemic antibiotics to control wound colonization is not indicated, since decreased circulation to the injured area prevents delivery of the medication to areas of deepest injury. Surveillance cultures and monitoring of the clinical course provide the most reliable indicators of developing infection. Appropriate antibiotics can then be instituted to treat the identified organism. Beta-streptococcus cultured from the throat or wounds is particularly destructive to grafted tissue. Otitis media should not be overlooked as a source of fever in the pediatric population.

Some form of sedation and analgesia is required in the care of burned children. Morphine sulfate is the drug of choice for severe burn injuries. Morphine has extensive distribution, although it is eliminated rapidly; continuous infusion or frequent administration is needed for pain management in burns. Morphine is administered intravenously and titrated to individual need. The unstable circulatory status and edema formation preclude intramuscular or subcutaneous administration. The addition of scheduled methadone to intermittent morphine administration for painful procedures has proved effective in managing burn pain in some children (Schmidt and others, 1989). Nonopioid/opioid combinations, such as acetaminophen with codeine, are often effective for less severe injuries.

The use of short-acting anesthetic agents, such as ketamine and nitrous oxide, has proved beneficial in eliminating procedural pain. Ketamine is a dissociative anesthetic agent that can be administered either orally, intravenously, or intramuscularly. Unconsciousness following intravenous administration occurs within 30 seconds and lasts approximately 10 minutes (Groeneveld and Inkson, 1992). Pharyngeal reflexes remain intact, thus ensuring a patent airway. The use of ketamine has proved to be a safe and effective method of pain control with minimal risk to the patient (Hendricks and others, 1991) (Fig. 29-8).

Nitronox is a useful short-term analgesic mixture of gases on a fixed ratio of 50% nitrous oxide and 50% oxygen. Initiation of action is approximately 1 minute with peak effect reached in 3 to 5 minutes. It is eliminated from the body, mostly via the lungs, within 2 to 5 minutes. Nitronox is useful to alleviate anxiety and raise the threshold of pain during procedures. The child must be able to follow instructions and may self-administer the Nitronox with assistance. No treatment should last longer than 30 minutes, and the child should be monitored continuously during the procedure. Side effects of nitrous oxide administration may include excitability, shortness of breath, nausea, and/or vomiting. It is not recommended for children who are sedated, hypotensive, unconscious, pregnant, or intoxicated or for those with abdominal distension or chest injuries (Selbst, 1993).

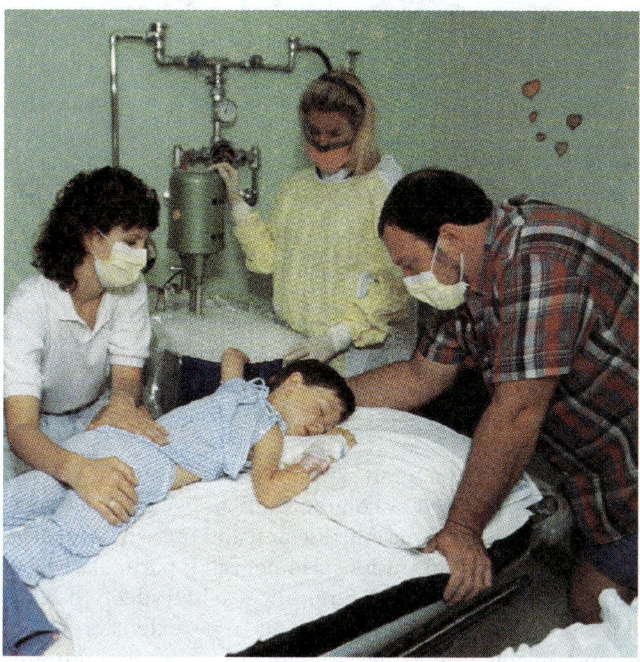

FIG. 29-8 Pain control during burn care. Child is well sedated with oral ketamine and midazolam.

Management of the Burn Wound

After the initial period of shock and the restoration of fluid balance, the primary concern is the burn wound. The objectives of wound management include the prevention of infection, removal of devitalized tissue, and closure of the wound. The application of dressings and topical antimicrobial therapy reduce pain by minimizing the exposure to air.

Primary Excision. In children with large, full-thickness burn wounds, excision is performed as soon as the patient is hemodynamically stable after initial resuscitation. Since the burn wound is precipitating the exaggerated physiologic response, many associated complications do not resolve until the eschar is excised and the wound is closed (Finkelstein and others, 1992). Early excision of deep partial-thickness and full-thickness burns has reduced the incidence of infection and the threat of sepsis (Petersen, Umphred, and Warden, 1982).

Debridement. Hydrotherapy is employed to cleanse the wound and involves soaking in a tub or showering once or twice a day for no more than 20 minutes. Hydrotherapy helps to cleanse not only the wound but the entire body and also aids in maintenance of range of motion.

Partial-thickness wounds require debridement of devitalized tissue to promote healing. Debridement is very painful and requires some type of analgesia before the procedure. The water acts to loosen and remove sloughing tissue, exudate, and topical medications. Mesh gauze serves to entrap the exudative slough and is readily removed during hydrotherapy (Fig. 29-9). Any loose tissue is carefully trimmed away before the wound is redressed (Fig. 29-10).

Topical Antimicrobial Agents. Several methods are used for covering the burn wound (see box on p. 1266). All meet the objective of preparation for permanent wound coverage and all employ some type of topical agent. Before the development of effective topical agents for reducing the incidence of invasive organisms, wound sepsis was the major cause of mortality from burn injury. Topical agents do not eliminate organisms from the wound but can effectively inhibit bacterial growth. To be effective, a topical application must be nontoxic, capable of diffusing through eschar,

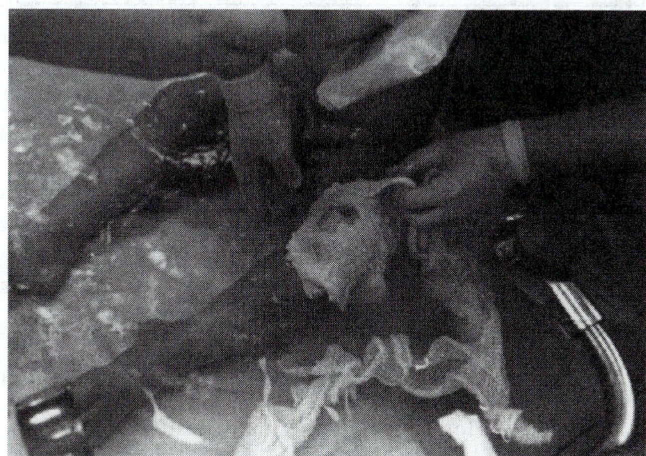

FIG. 29-9 Removal of dressing during hydrotherapy.

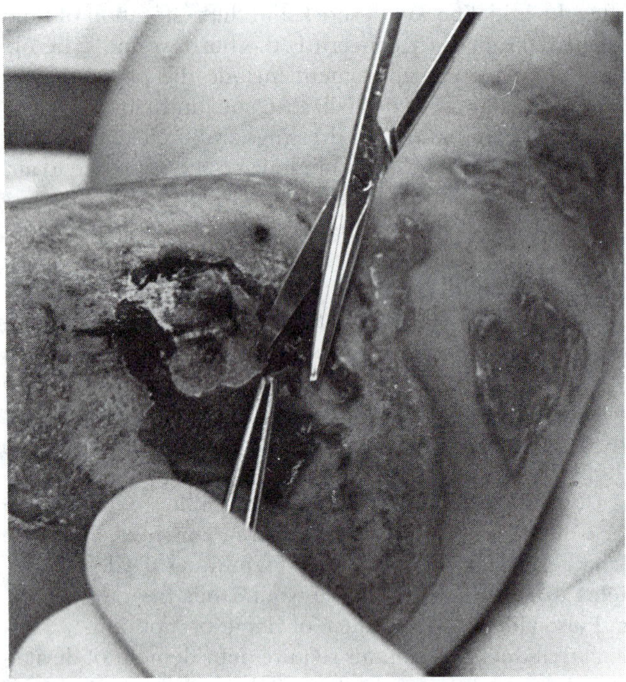

FIG. 29-10 Dead skin and debris are carefully trimmed away before dressing is applied.

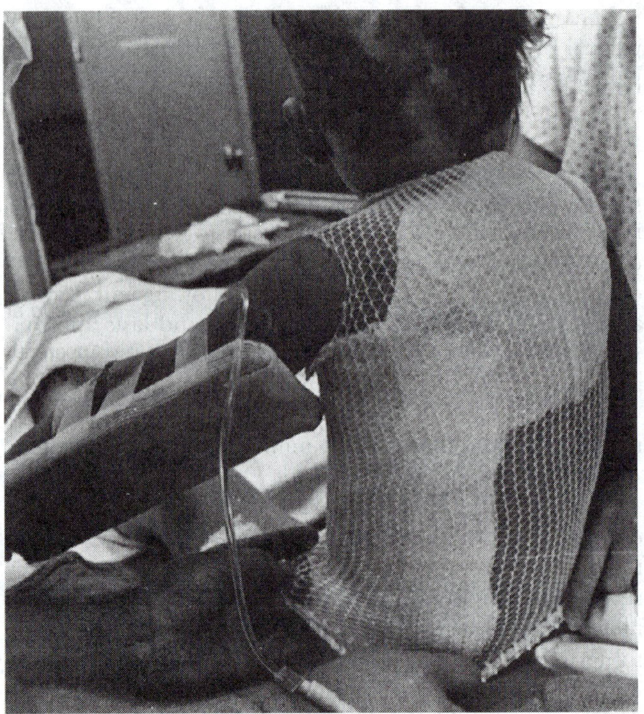

FIG. 29-11 Burn wound covered with gauze dressings and secured with tabular elastic netting.

METHODS OF BURN WOUND MANAGEMENT

Exposure—Wounds are left open to air; crust forms on partial-thickness wounds, and eschar forms on full-thickness burns.

Open—Topical antimicrobial agent is applied directly to the wound surface, and the wound is left uncovered.

Modified—Antimicrobial is applied directly or impregnated into thin gauze and applied to the wound; gauze or net secures the area (Fig. 29-11).

Occlusive—Antimicrobial is impregnated in gauze or applied directly to the wound; multiple layers of bulky gauze are placed over the primary layer and secured with gauze or net.

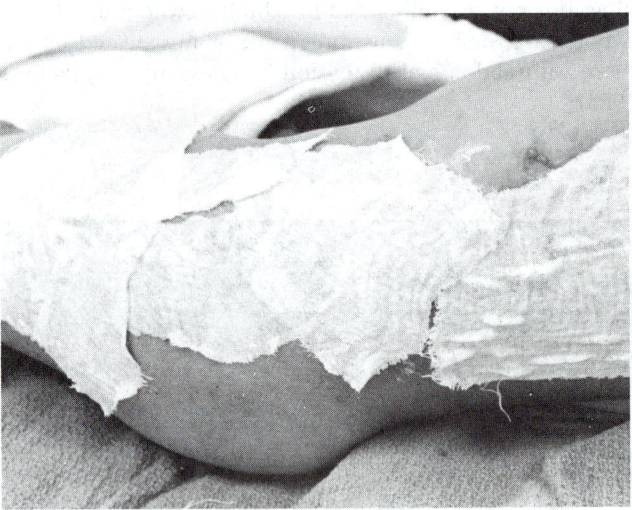

FIG. 29-12 Gauze impregnated with ointment applied to burn wound.

harmless to viable tissue, inexpensive, and easy to apply. It should not encourage the development of resistent strains of bacteria and should produce minimum electrolyte derangement (Fig. 29-12). The significant properties of commonly used agents are summarized in Table 29-6.

Biologic Skin Coverings. Temporary closure of the burn wound by the use of material other than the patient's own skin has become commonplace. Biologic dressings are used during the acute phase of therapy to cover the wound surface, protect the wound from bacterial contamination, reduce fluid and protein loss, and increase the rate of epithelialization (Herndon and others, 1985). In addition, biologic dressings markedly reduce pain and facilitate movement of joints to retain range of motion.

Allograft or homograft skin is obtained from human cadavers and processed by commercial skin banks. Donors are screened for communicable diseases, and the skin is tracked much like blood transfusions. Homograft is particularly useful in the coverage of surgically excised deep partial-thickness and full-thickness wounds in extensive burns when available donor sites are limited. Severe immunosuppression occurs in massively burned children, and the allograft becomes adherent (Fig. 29-13). The homograft can

TABLE 29-6 Comparison of Common Topical Preparations

AGENT	DRESSINGS	ADVANTAGES	DISADVANTAGES
Silver nitrate 0.5% ($AgNO_3$)	Exposure, modified or occlusive; impedes joint movement; dressings changed twice daily; keep dressing moist, rewet at least every 2 hours	Greatly reduces evaporative losses; does not interfere with wound healing; bacteriostatic action against major burn flora, including *Pseudomonas* and *Staphylococcus;* inexpensive	Does not penetrate eschar; ineffective on established burn wound infections; little effect on *Klebsiella* and *Aerobacter* groups; stains skin, clothing, linens; makes assessment of the wound difficult because of staining; hypotonicity pulls electrolytes from the wound, depleting sodium, potassium, chloride, and magnesium; stings on application
Silver sulfadiazine 1% (AgSD)	Occlusive; motion of joints maintained; applied twice daily; do not use with a history of allergy to sulfa	Little pain on application; bactericidal by altering DNA and cell metabolism; effective against gram-positive and gram-negative bacteria; easy to apply; nontoxic	Transient neutropenia; does not penetrate eschar; forms proteinaceous gel on wound surface that is painful to remove; occasional rashes and pruritus; decreases granulocyte formation
Mafenide acetate 10% (Sulfamylon)	*Cream:* Usually exposure; do not apply to face; apply twice daily *Solution:* Occlusive; keep dressing moist (rewet at least every 2 hours); protect solution from light	Penetrates eschar and diffuses rapidly into burn wound and underlying tissues; effective in deep flame, electrical, and infected wounds; biostatic against many gram-positive and gram-negative organisms, including *Pseudomonas* and *Clostridium*	Difficult and painful to remove cream; pain on application; metabolic acidosis, hypercapnia, and carbonic anhydrase inhibition; inhibits wound healing; hypersensitivity in some patients
Povidone-iodine (Betadine ointment)	Exposure, modified or occlusive Change dressing 2-3 times daily	Microbicidal against gram-positive, gram-negative organisms, yeast, fungi, and viruses; ease of application	Painful on application; elevation of protein-bound iodine may result in metabolic acidosis; stains clothes, linens, and the wound, making evaluation difficult; allergic reaction to iodine
Bacitracin	Exposure, modified; motion of joints maintained; change dressing twice daily	Bactericidal and bacteriostatic against gram-positive organisms; low toxicity; painless application; ease of application	Limited activity against gram-negative organisms; allergic reaction in sensitive individuals

remain in place until suitable donor sites become available (Frank and others, 1983). Typically, rejection is seen approximately 14 days after application. The use of homograft is limited by the availability of tissue banks and a supply of suitable donors.

Xenograft from a variety of species, most notably pigs, is commercially available. Split-thickness pigskin adheres less than allografts because of a progressive, degenerative necrosis (Pruitt and Levine, 1984). Pigskin dressings are replaced daily or every 2 to 3 days. They are particularly effective in children with partial-thickness scald burns of the hands and face, since they allow relatively pain-free movement, which reduces contracture formation and has the added benefit of improving appetite and morale (Fig. 29-14).

When applied early to a superficial partial-thickness injury, biologic dressings appear to accelerate wound healing. They create an environment at the wound surface that is conducive to epithelial growth, in contrast to topical antimicrobial agents, which may slow epithelialization. Biologic dressings must be applied to clean wounds. If the dressing covers areas of heavy microbial contamination, infection occurs beneath the dressing. In the case of partial-thickness burns, such infection may convert the wound to a full-thickness injury. It is important to observe the wound daily for any sign of an infectious process.

Synthetic Skin Coverings. A number of satisfactory skin substitutes are available for the management of partial-thickness burn wounds. Ideally, the dressing should provide many of the properties of human skin: adherence, elasticity, durability, and hemostasis. Synthetic skin substitutes are readily available, have an indefinite shelf life, and are relatively inexpensive.

Synthetic dressings, composed of a variety of materials, can be used very successfully in the management of superficial partial-thickness burns and donor sites. Examples in-

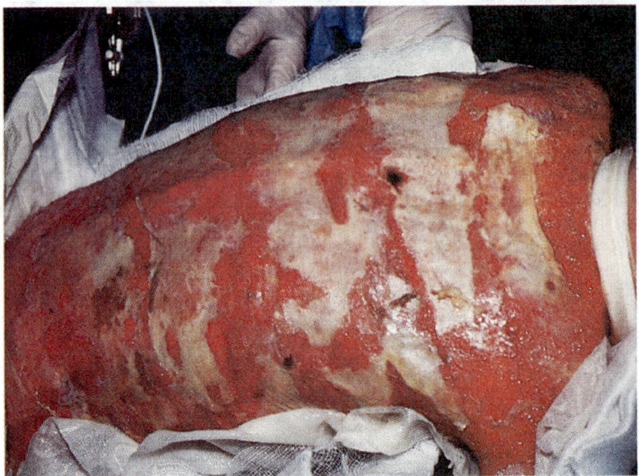

FIG. 29-13 Adherent homograft applied to excised full-thickness wound.

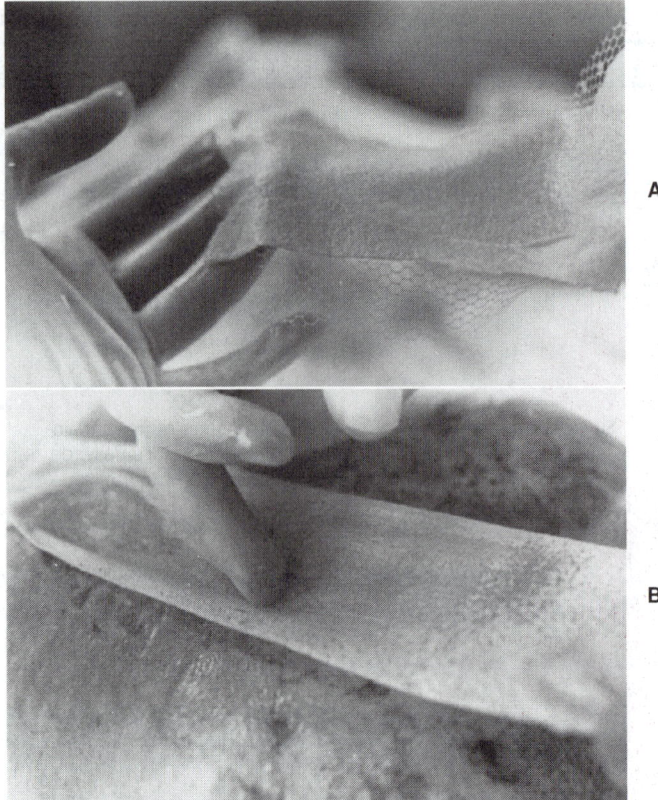

FIG. 29-14 Porcine dressing, **A,** removed from net backing and, **B,** applied to wound.

clude adherent elastic films, hydroactive materials, or colloidal suspensions that are usually permeable to air, vapor, and fluids. Another product that consists of a nylon fabric bonded to a silicone rubber membrane is used by many burn centers. Calcium alginate is gaining popularity for the treatment of donor sites with both patients and staff because of its significant reduction in discomfort.

As with biologic dressings, it is important that the wound be free of debris before the dressing is applied. Evidence of purulence, erythema, or cellulitis around the wound edges or temperature elevation may indicate that the wound has become infected beneath the dressing. Prompt discontinuance of the synthetic dressing is indicated. All synthetic dressings are reputed to hasten wound healing and to reduce discomfort.

Permanent Skin Coverings. Permanent coverage of deep partial-thickness and full-thickness burns is usually accomplished with a split-thickness skin graft. This graft consists of the epidermis and a portion of the dermis removed from an intact area of skin by a special instrument, the dermatome (Fig. 29-15). If all of the wounds cannot be grafted at once, there are priority areas for coverage: the face, hands, joint surfaces, and neck. These preferential sites are chosen to hasten healing, establish function, and improve the patient's sense of well-being.

With extensive burns it is often difficult to find enough viable skin to cover the wounds; therefore, available donor sites are used to the best advantage by special techniques. The various types of split-thickness skin grafts are described in the first box on p. 1269. Sheet grafts are used in areas where cosmetic results are most visible; mesh grafts result in a less desirable cosmetic and functional outcome. Requirements for the successful vascularization of any graft are listed in the second box on p. 1269.

Until the blood supply to the grafted skin is established, it is nourished by osmotic interchange with the recipient bed. Wound healing takes place as the area releases fibrin that attaches the graft to the bed. The fibrin is infiltrated

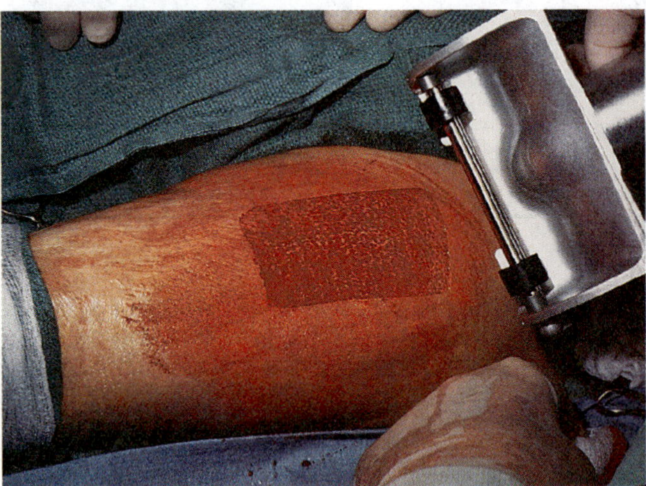

FIG. 29-15 Removal of split-thickness skin graft with a dermatome.

by leukocytes, fibroblasts, and the capillary buds of the granulation tissue. This process begins within hours of grafting, and vascularization is established after 3 days. Within 2 weeks the graft is attached to the recipient bed by connective tissue.

The donor site is dressed with synthetic wound coverings or fine-mesh gauze until the dressing separates at 10 to 14

TYPES OF SKIN GRAFTS

TEMPORARY GRAFTS

Allografts (homografts)—Skin that is obtained from genetically different members of the same species who are free of disease.

Xenografts (heterografts)—Skin that is obtained from members of a different species, primarily pigskin.

PERMANENT GRAFTS

Autografts—Tissue obtained from undamaged areas of the patient's own body.

Isografts—Histocompatible tissue obtained from genetically identical individuals.

METHODS OF APPLYING SPLIT-THICKNESS GRAFTS

Sheet graft—A sheet of skin, removed from the donor site, is placed intact over the recipient site and sutured in place (Fig. 29-16).

Mesh graft—A sheet of skin is removed from the donor site and passed through a mesher, which produces tiny slits in the skin. The meshing allows the expansion of the skin to cover 1½ to 9 times the area of the sheet graft (Fig. 29-17).

REQUIREMENTS FOR A SUCCESSFUL GRAFT

Sufficient nourishment until the new blood supply is established from the base of the recipient bed

Primary tissue contact (i.e., actual contact between the surface of the graft and a recipient bed that is free of bacteria and necrotic skin)

Avoidance of bleeding, hematoma formation, and fluid accumulation beneath the graft

Prevention of infection

Prevention of mechanical trauma

days when the wound is healed (Housinger, Wondrely, and Warden, 1993). Dressings are not changed on donor sites to avoid damage to newly healed, delicate epithelium. Healed donor sites are available for reharvesting in patients with extensive burns and limited undamaged skin. The quality of skin from donor sites is decreased when multiple grafts are taken (Fig. 29-18).

Cultured Epithelium. When burns are extensive and donor sites for split-thickness skin grafting are limited, it is possible to culture cells from a full-thickness skin biopsy and produce coherent sheets that can be applied to clean, excised full-thickness wounds. Some children have been successfully treated with this autologous cultured epithelium (Boyce and others, 1993). Long-term followup studies are currently being conducted to determine pathologic changes and functional properties. Epithelial cell culture grafts offer the possibility of an unlimited source of autografts in patients with extensive burns.

NURSING CONSIDERATIONS

Nursing care of the pediatric burn patient represents a challenge to the nurse's knowledge of anatomy and physiology,

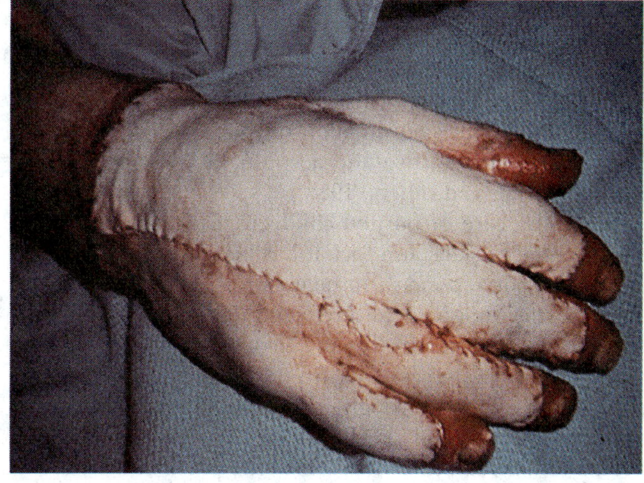

FIG. 29-16 Sheet graft.

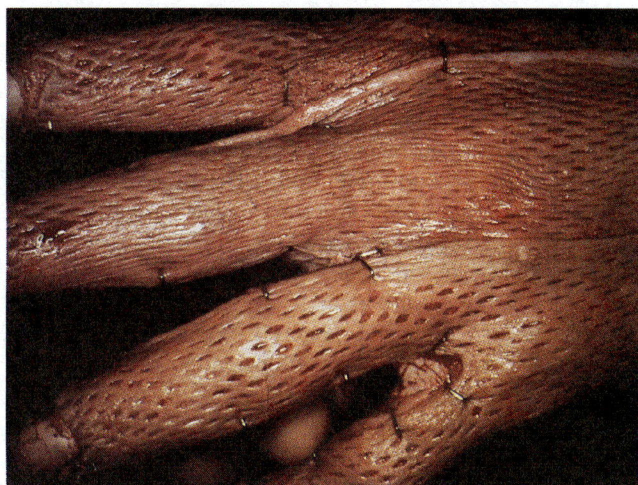

FIG. 29-17 Mesh graft.

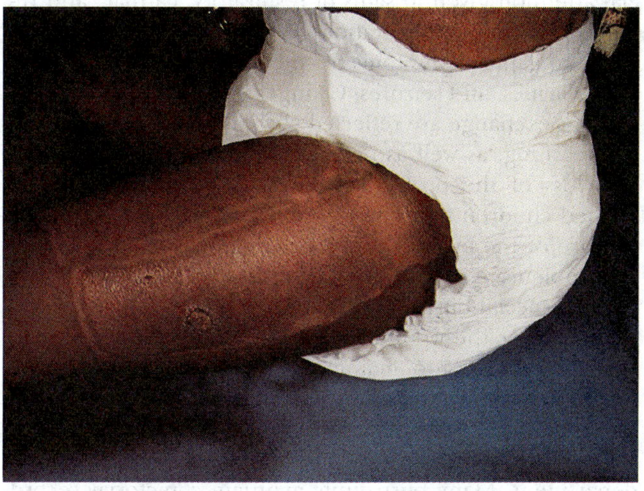

FIG. 29-18 Healed donor site.

the behavioral sciences, and pathophysiology. Patient outcome following thermal injury is the result of the collaboration of a professional multidisciplinary team using a family-centered care approach. The nurse is given much responsibility for the coordination of the team activities and functions as an assertive and accountable member of the team (Warden and others, 1988).

Since the care of burned children encompasses such a broad range of skills and foci, it has been divided into segments that correspond with the major phases of burn treatment. The acute phase, also referred to as the emergent or resuscitative phase, involves the first 24 to 48 hours. The management phase extends from the completion of adequate resuscitation through wound coverage. The rehabilitative phase begins once the majority of the wounds are healed and rehabilitation becomes the predominant focus of the plan of care. This phase continues until all reconstructive procedures and corrective measures have been accomplished and often extends over a period of months or years.

Acute Phase

The primary emphasis during the emergent phase is the treatment of burn shock and management of the pulmonary status. Monitoring vital signs, output, fluid infusion, and respiratory parameters are ongoing activities in the hours immediately following injury. The intravenous infusion is begun immediately and is regulated to maintain urinary output of at least 1 to 2 ml/kg in children weighing less than 30 kg; an output of 30 to 50 ml/hr is expected in children weighing more than 30 kg. Urinary output and specific gravity, vital signs, laboratory data, and objective signs of adequate hydration guide the rate of fluid administration.

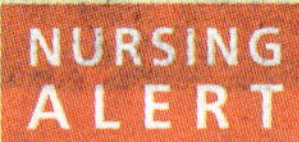

Assessment of sensorium is another important indicator of the adequacy of hydration.

Children are observed for changes in all parameters. They require constant observation and assessment with special attention given to signs of respiratory, cardiac, and renal complications. Alterations in electrolyte balance can produce clinical symptoms of confusion, weakness, cardiac irregularities, and seizures. Changes in respiratory function and gas exchange are reflected clinically by increased work of breathing, as well as by alterations in blood gas values. The loss of the protective function of the skin exposes burned children to an increased risk of hypothermia.

Care of the burn wound is secondary to the more critical problems of respiratory and cardiac failure. When transfer to a special burn care facility is anticipated, it is important to cover the wounds with sterile sheets and wrap the child in blankets to maintain body temperature during transfer. The burn wound can be evaluated and dressed following arrival at the burn center. If no burn unit is available, the wound is cleansed and dressed in the emergency department. Many burn units maintain a pictorial record of the wound to record progress and for legal purposes, especially in cases of suspected child abuse. The burn wound is treated according to the protocol of the specific burn facility. Baseline cultures are obtained on admission. It is the nurse's responsibility to monitor infection control procedures and ensure that staff and visitors comply with established protocols to prevent cross-contamination in the burn unit.

Throughout the acute phase of care the psychosocial needs of the children and their families should not be overlooked. The child is frightened, uncomfortable, and often confused. Children may be isolated from familiar persons and surroundings; the often overwhelming physical needs at this time are the primary focus of the staff and parents. In addition to concern for their child, the family experiences guilt, which has nothing to do with the burn injury. This guilt is instead related to the fact that the parents did not or could not protect their child. Consistency in the information presented and the attitude of the staff creates a sense of familiarity and stability during the emergent phase.

Management and Rehabilitative Phases

After the patient's condition is stabilized, the management phase begins. The multidisciplinary team concentrates on preventing wound infections, closing the wound as quickly as possible, and managing the numerous complications that may occur. The rehabilitative phase begins when permanent wound closure has been achieved, although rehabilitation issues are identified on admission and are included in the plan of care throughout the hospital course.

❖ Assessment

Wound assessment is of major importance, as is comprehensive assessment of the child's general condition and behaviors. Observation for signs of complications, especially infection, and the assessment of the need for and effectiveness of pain management are important nursing functions.

❖ Nursing Diagnoses

Based on a thorough assessment, several nursing diagnoses are identified. The more common diagnoses for the child with burns are included in the Nursing Care Plan on pp. 1276-1278. Others may apply in specific situations.

❖ Planning

The goals for the child with a burn injury and the family are as follows:

1. Child will experience reduction of pain.
2. Child will exhibit evidence of wound healing.
3. Child will receive adequate nutrition and will achieve reduction in metabolic losses.
4. Child will not experience acute complications during management phase.
5. Child will not experience long-term complications during rehabilitative phase.
6. Child and family will receive emotional support.

❖ Implementation

The management phase of burn care involves intensive nursing care, which can be difficult for the patient, the family, and the nursing staff. Except for minor burn injuries, care usually takes place in a burn unit and involves members of a variety of disciplines, such as physical therapy, nutrition, social services, and respiratory care.

Comfort Management. The severe pain of the wound and resultant therapies, the anxiety generated by these experiences, sleep deprivation, itching related to wound healing, and the conscious and unconscious interpretations of traumatic events contribute to psychologic reactions and behaviors frequently observed in burned children. It is always difficult to deal with a child in pain, and to inflict pain on helpless children is contrary to the empathetic nature of nursing. Interventions may include medications (including intravenous morphine and short-term anesthetics), relaxation techniques, distraction therapy, cutaneous stimulation by touching, and family participation.

It is important to offer thorough age-appropriate explanations to the child before procedures to reduce anxiety associated with an unfamiliar environment and frightening treatments. Compounding the pain is the child's interpretation of it and of the procedure; this is closely related to the developmental level of the child. There are often feelings of anger, guilt, and depression, and, as in all illnesses, regressive behavior. When children appear to accept pain with little or no response, psychologic consultation is in order. Consistency in caregivers is important. When this is not possible, a carefully developed, multidisciplinary plan of care will provide consistency in approach, explanation, and intervention that will reduce fear (Rieg and Jenkins, 1991).

Care of the Burn Wound. The nurse has a major responsibility for cleansing, debriding, and applying topical medications and dressings to the burn wound. Because dressing removal is a painful procedure, children should receive adequate analgesia before the scheduled dressing change. Medication should be administered so that the peak effect of the drug coincides with the procedure. Children who have an understanding of the procedure to be performed and some perceived control demonstrate less maladaptive behavior. Children respond well to participation in decisions and the actual procedure as their condition allows (see Guidelines box).

GUIDELINES

Reducing the Stress of Burn Care Procedures

Have all materials ready before beginning.
Administer appropriate analgesics.
Remind the child of the impending procedure to allow sufficient time to prepare.
Allow the child to test and approve the temperature of the water.
Allow the child to select the area of the body on which to begin.
Allow the child to request a short rest period during the procedure.
Allow the child to remove the dressings if desired.
Provide something constructive for the child to do during the procedure (e.g., holding a package of dressings or a roll of gauze).
Inform the child when the procedure is near completion.
Praise the child for cooperation.

Nonpharmacologic interventions are effective means of coping with pain for some children. By the age of 7, a child can begin to understand that pain is necessary for healing. Distraction therapy, deep breathing, and relaxation techniques may facilitate the procedure. Some children benefit from parental participation as well. Medical play is a technique that is often effective in helping the younger child to gain some mastery over the procedure. Techniques that work best for the individual patient are incorporated into the plan of care and consistently implemented during the dressing change procedure (Helvig, 1993).

Outer dressings are removed; any dressings that have adhered to the wound can be more easily removed by the application of tepid water. Loose or easily detached tissue is also debrided during the cleansing process. Children can be encouraged to participate in dressing removal. Providing something constructive for the child to do helps them to focus on something other than the procedure. In dressing the wound, it is important that all areas be clean, that medication be amply applied, and that no two burned surfaces touch each other, such as fingers or toes, or the ears touching the side of the head. If touching, the burned surfaces will heal together, causing deformity and/or dysfunction.

Topical medications may be applied directly to the wound with a clean gloved hand or impregnated into fine-mesh gauze before application. Dressings are then applied to assist in absorption of exudate, debridement of the wound, and increased patient comfort. All dressings applied circumferentially should be wrapped in a distal to proximal manner. The dressing is applied with sufficient tension to remain in place but not so tightly as to impair circulation or limit motion. Elastic bandages are applied over dressings to prevent epithelial breakdown, decrease edema formation, stimulate circulation, and improve mobility. The bandage is applied in a figure-eight to promote optimum circulation. A stable dressing is especially important when the child is ambulatory.

Burns that involve the eyelids require special care to prevent corneal ulceration. No solution other than water or saline should come in contact with the eyes during the cleansing process. Vigorous debridement is avoided in this area of thin, delicate tissue. The patient is assessed throughout the healing process for the ability to close the eyes. Inability to close the eyes because of contracture formation, administration of paralytic agents, or corneal burns requires the instillation of ophthalmic ointment and the covering of the eyes with a patch to prevent further corneal damage (Walter, 1993).

Universal precautions, including the use of protective garb and barrier techniques, should be followed when caring for all patients with thermal injuries. Frequent hand and forearm washing is the single most important element of the infection control program. Strict policies for the cleaning of the environment and patient care equipment should be implemented to minimize the risk of cross-contamination. All visitors and members of other departments should be oriented to the infection control policies, including the importance of hand and forearm washing and donning of protective garb. All visitors should be screened for infection and contagious diseases before patient contact (Weber and Tompkins, 1993).

Nutrition. Oral feedings are usually encouraged unless the child is intubated or paralytic ileus persists. Because children frequently lack an appetite, a great deal of encouragement, help, and patience is required on the part of the nursing staff. Consultation between the parent and dietitian helps to determine food preferences. Children who are old enough to participate should be included in meal planning.

Nourishing snacks are provided between scheduled meals. Painful procedures should not be scheduled around meals; most children are too physically exhausted and emotionally upset to eat at this time. Many children eat better in an atmosphere more nearly like what they are accustomed to at home. When their condition allows, children enjoy sitting at a table for meals and interacting with other children.

Children who require enteral supplementation by tube feeding must be monitored on an ongoing basis for intolerance and tube malposition. The nurse should monitor and record any indications of abdominal distention, diarrhea, or electrolyte and metabolic derangement. Accurate documentation of oral, parenteral, and enteral nutritional intake is essential to evaluate the adequacy of nutritional support.

Prevention of Complications: Acute Care. The maintenance of body temperature is important to the burned child. The environment should be maintained between 28° and 33° C (82.4° and 91.4° F) to minimize metabolic expenditure and maximize comfort (Herndon and others, 1985). Large areas of the body should not be exposed simultaneously during dressing changes. Using warmed solutions, linens, occlusive dressings, heat shields, and warming blankets assists in the prevention of hypothermia. The optimum environment for the burned child can be very uncomfortable for persons attending the child.

The chief danger in this phase of care is infection: wound infection, generalized sepsis, or bacterial pneumonia. It is important to conduct accurate and ongoing assessments of all parameters that provide clues to the early diagnosis and treatment of infectious complications. In addition to signs of a developing wound infection, systemic symptoms of sepsis include a change in the level of consciousness, a rising or falling white blood cell count, hypothermia or hyperthermia, loss of the progression of wound healing, increasing fluid requirements, hypoactive or absent bowel sounds, tachycardia, tachypnea, and thrombocytopenia.

Children are reluctant to move when doing so causes pain and are likely to assume a position of comfort. Unfortunately, the most comfortable position is frequently one that encourages the formation of contractures and loss of function. Ongoing efforts to prevent contractures include the positioning and splinting of involved extremities in extension, active and passive physical therapy, and the encouragement of spontaneous movement when feasible. In addition to the maintenance of proper body alignment, frequent position changes are important to improve capillary perfusion to common pressure areas and bronchopulmonary hygiene. Low–air loss beds are beneficial for the child with posterior grafts or the morbidly obese. Areas of par-

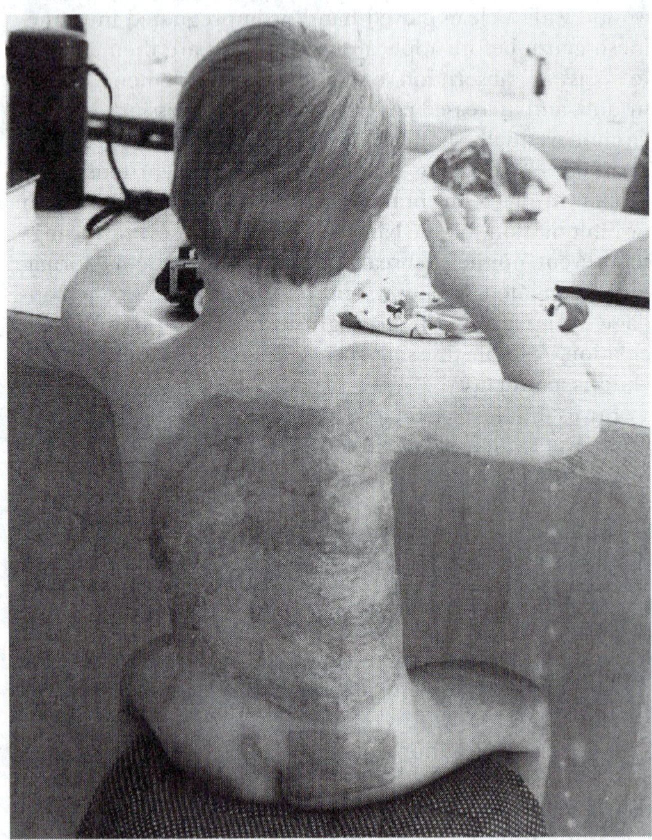

FIG. 29-19 Extensive scars from flame burn. Note donor graft site on right buttock.

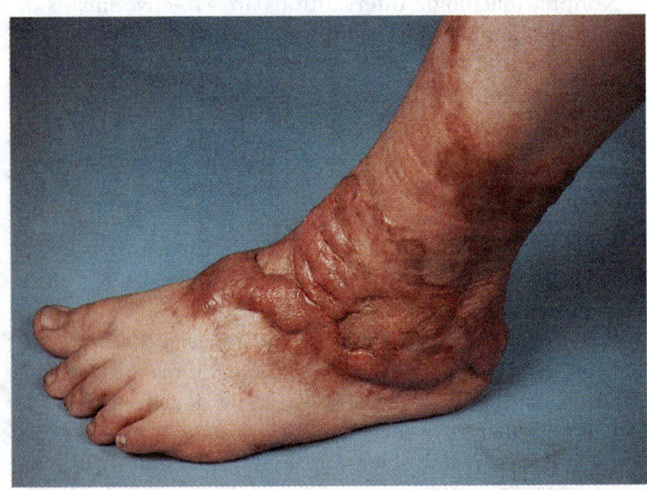

FIG. 29-20 Hypertrophic immature scar.

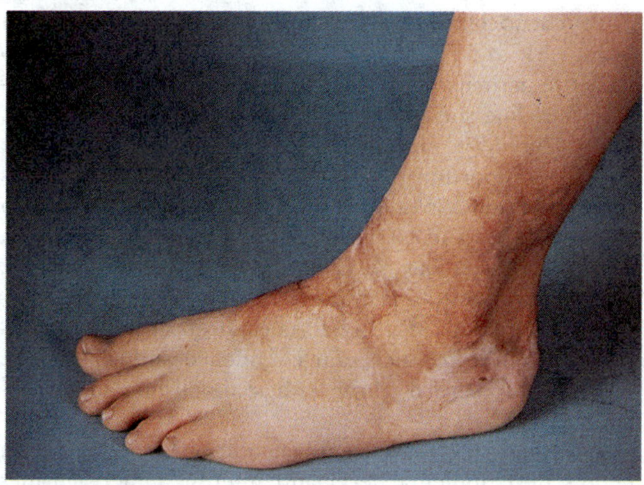

FIG. 29-21 Flat, mature scar after pressure.

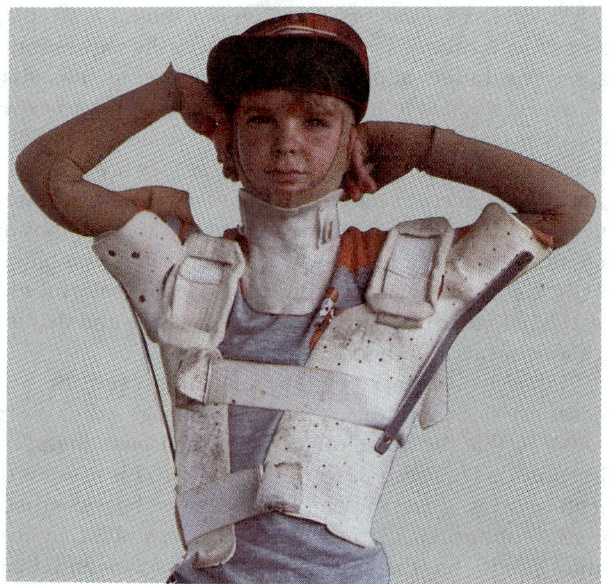

FIG. 29-22 Child in elasticized (Jobst) garment and "airplane" splints.

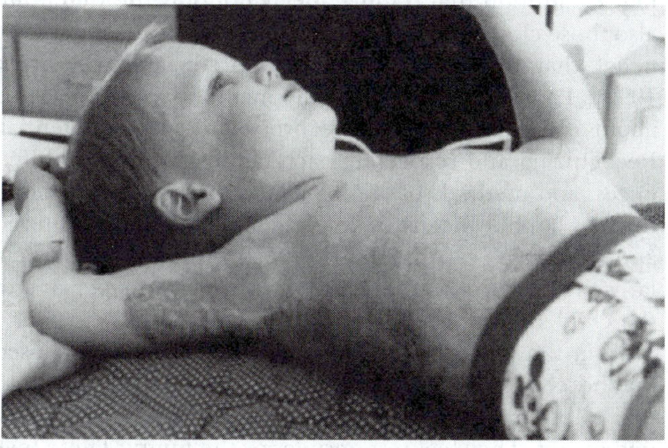

FIG. 29-23 Daily physical therapy to prevent contracture deformity is continued at home.

ticular concern for pressure area development in the pediatric population are the posterior scalp, heels, and areas exposed to mechanical irritation from splints and dressings.

Prevention of Complications: Long-Term Care. The rehabilitative phase of care begins once wound coverage has been achieved. Scar formation becomes a major problem as burn wounds heal (Fig. 29-19). The scar tissue is metabolically active and highly vascular; collagen is deposited in an undefined pattern. Contractile properties of the scar tissue can result in disabling contractures, deformity, and disfigurement. As long as the scar is raised, red, and firm, it is considered to be active (Fig. 29-20). Hypertrophic scarring typically reaches a peak approximately 4 to 6 months after wound healing, and most scars mature or become inactive in 1 to 2 years. The mature scar is characterized by pigmented color, flattening, and an increase in the suppleness of the tissue (Fig. 29-21).

Uniform pressure applied to the scar decreases the blood supply and forces the collagen into a more normal alignment. When the pressure is removed, the blood supply to the scar is immediately increased, so periods without pressure should be brief to avoid nourishment of the hypertrophic tissue. Continuous pressure to areas of scarring can be achieved by elastic bandages or commercially available pressure garments. Since these custom-made garments are often worn for months, revision may be required as the child grows. It is much easier to prevent scarring and contracture of the wound than to resolve an existing problem. Splints and appliances may also be needed until wound maturation is achieved (Fig. 29-22). Part of home care frequently includes the continuation of regular physical therapy (Fig. 29-23).

Scar tissue has some properties that are significant, particularly for growing children. Intense itching occurs in healing burn wounds and scar tissue until the scar is no longer active. It is usually treated with hydroxyzine (Atarax) or diphenhydramine (Benadryl) and frequent applications of a moisturizer, such as Eucerin, cocoa butter, or Nivea. Massage therapy during the application of moisturizers is also beneficial to stretch scar tissue and aid in contracture prevention. Scar tissue has no sweat glands, and children with extensive scarring may experience difficulty during hot weather. Caregivers should be alerted to this possibility and be prepared to institute alternate methods of cooling when necessary.

Scar tissue does not grow and expand as does normal tissue, which may create difficulties, especially in functional areas such as the hands and over joints. Additional surgery is sometimes required to allow independent functioning in daily activities, to improve cosmetic appearance, or to restore anatomic integrity. Reconstructive surgery employs various techniques, including local or distant flaps, full- or partial-thickness grafts, tissue expanders, or pedicle flaps.

The nursing activities in the rehabilitative phase of treatment focus on the child and family's adaptation to the burn injury and their ability to reintegrate into the community. The multidisciplinary team approach remains the model for support of the patient and family (Fig. 29-24). In 1989, burn nurses identified rehabilitation, discharge planning, and

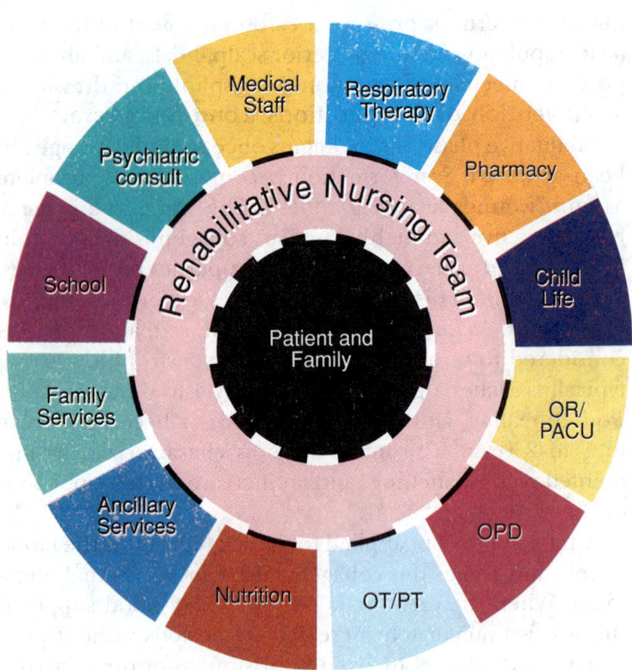

FIG. 29-24 Multidisciplinary approach to rehabilitation of the pediatric burn patient.

follow-up care as three areas of priority for nursing research. Given the long tradition of a team approach to burn care, it is not surprising that the participants identified a collaboration with other disciplines as the means to best address rehabilitation issues (Bayley and others, 1992).

The psychologic pain and sequelae of severe burn injury are as intense as the physical trauma. The impact of severe burns taxes the capabilities at all ages, but very young children, who suffer acutely from separation anxiety, and adolescents, who are developing an identity, are probably the most affected psychologically. Toddlers cannot understand why the parents they love and who have protected them can leave them in such a frightening and unfamiliar place. Adolescents, in the process of achieving independence from the family, find themselves in a dependent role with a damaged body. Being different from others at a time when conformity with their peers is so important is difficult to accept.

Anticipation of the return to school can be an overwhelming and frightening prospect. It is essential for health care professionals to recognize the importance of preparing teachers and classmates for the child's return. Teachers need to be provided with information to assist the child and family and to promote the child's optimum adjustment. Hospital-sponsored school reentry programs use a variety of methods to provide education and information about the implications of the injury, garments and appliances, and the need for support and acceptance. Telephone calls, videotapes, packets of information, and visits by members of the health care team offer opportunities to aid reintegration into the school environment—a focal point of the child's life.

Psychosocial Support of the Child. Children should begin early to do as much for themselves as possible and to be active participants in their care. Loss of control and perceived helplessness may result in acting-out behaviors. Nurses should be sensitive to these feelings and allow the child the opportunity for choices and decision making as their condition allows. At the same time, it is important to set boundaries and establish a daily schedule to provide a sense of predictability, security, and control. During illness, children regress to a previous developmental level that allows them to deal with stress. As children begin to participate in their care, they gain confidence and self-esteem. Fears and anxieties diminish with accomplishment and self-confidence.

Activities are selected and encouraged based on each child's developmental level and interest. Quiet activities such as reading, coloring, and games are always appropriate. Critically ill children enjoy tapes and stories, even though they may not be able to actively participate in play. Television is a satisfactory diversion but should not replace contact with others. Play that encourages the expression of anger, frustration, and guilt is especially therapeutic. Medical play is a valuable tool to teach children what to expect and their role in the treatment process. School-age children benefit by continuing study activities as they are able.

Children need to feel they look nice. The burns, dressings, and medical equipment do little to foster a positive self-image. Small things, such as careful hair combing, a bright ribbon or pajamas, a pretty blanket, or colorful stickers will help them feel better about themselves and that they are worthwhile to others.

Children need to know that their injury and the treatments are not punishment for real or imagined transgressions and that the nurse understands their fear, anger, and discomfort. They also need body contact. This is often difficult to arrange for the child with massive burns; stroking areas of unburned skin is comforting. Even older children enjoy sitting on the nurse's or parent's lap and being cuddled and hugged. This can be a comfort in times of stress or a reward, but most of all it should be kept in mind that it is a natural part of childhood.

Psychosocial Support of the Family. There is a growing recognition that trauma affects not only the victim but also those closest to the child. Severe trauma challenges the belief that the world is safe and predictable (Munster, 1993). Parents and other family members are concerned about the child's survival, recovery and future potential. Recognizing and respecting each family's strengths, differences, and methods of coping allows the nurse to respond to their unique needs by implementing a family-centered approach to care (Ahmann, 1994). It is the family, particularly the parents, who are the most significant persons in the child's life.

As in any emergency situation, all attention is focused on the child, and the parents feel powerless and ineffectual. Most parents feel overwhelming guilt, whether justified or not. They feel responsible for the injury. These feelings may impede the child's rehabilitation. Parents may indulge the child and allow noncompliant behaviors that affect physical and emotional recovery.

Nurses are in an opportune position to assist parents in coping with the stresses of the child's illness and their own feelings of guilt and helplessness. The parents need to be informed of the child's progress and helped in their efforts to cope with their feelings while providing support to their child. The nurse is the person who can help them understand that it is not selfish to look after themselves and their own needs in order to better meet the needs of their child. For parents whose response to the injury is severe or whose response to stress is manifested in destructive behavior, definitive professional help may be needed.

The parents are members of the multidisciplinary team and participate in the development of the plan of care. It is important to address their input in order to consider all aspects of the physical, emotional, social, and cultural factors impacting the child and family and to establish a realistic home therapy program. The family's willingness to assume responsibility for care and their ability to implement the therapeutic regimen are assessed. Home, school, and other environmental factors are explored; financial concerns and available community resources are discussed; and a specific plan of care for the child, with an anticipated follow-up program, is developed.

Caring for the Caregiver. Burn care is a very complex and demanding specialty. Nurses who choose this field of nursing reap many rewards and endure many stresses. Ongoing support from peers, the multidisciplinary team, and nursing management is important to assist burn nurses in caring for themselves and to continue to render quality care to their patients.

❖ Evaluation

The effectiveness of nursing interventions is determined by the continual reassessment and evaluation of care based on the following observational guidelines and expected outcomes:

1. Observe child's behavior during all aspects of care; listen for verbal cues; use a pain assessment tool to evaluate the effectiveness of analgesia.
2. Observe the burn wound and patient's general condition.
3. Observe child's eating behavior and the amount of food consumed; weigh weekly or as indicated.
4. Inspect the burn wound for signs of infection; take vital signs; observe for evidence of respiratory complications, gastric bleeding, altered hemoglobin, and neurologic signs.
5. Observe for evidence of healing, scar formation, and contracture; assess the effectiveness of physical therapy and appliances (splints, pressure garments).
6. Observe child's and family's behaviors; interview child and family regarding concerns.

Expected outcomes:

See Nursing Care Plan, pp. 1276-1278.

Prevention of Burn Injury

Burn prevention is the responsibility of all members of the community. Nurses have an obligation to participate in educational efforts directed at parents, children, and others on the prevention of burn injuries and fire-related deaths. The best cure is prevention of the problem.

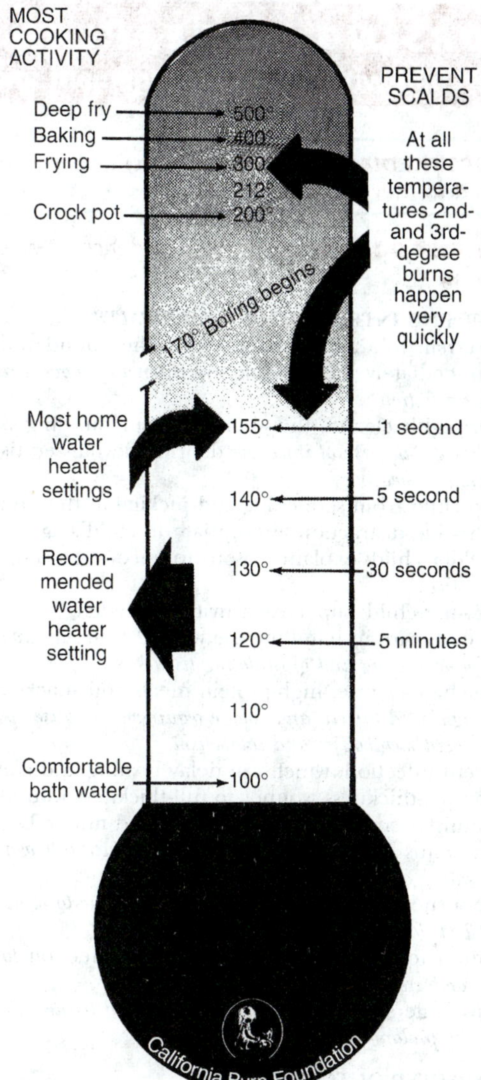

FIG. 29-25 Temperatures associated with common burn injuries in the home. NOTE: Most authorities recommend that water heaters be kept at the lowest safe setting of 120° F. (Courtesy California Burn Foundation, Canoga Park, CA.)

Infants and toddlers are most frequently injured by hot liquids in the kitchen and bathroom. These injuries often occur as a result of inadequate supervision of this curious and energetic age-group. Prevention efforts are targeted at parents and other caregivers; education includes the importance of adequate supervision and the establishment of safe play areas in the home. Hot liquids should be kept out of reach; tablecloths and dangling appliance cords are often pulled by toddlers, spilling hot grease and liquids on the small child. Electrical cords and outlets represent a poten-

NURSING CARE PLAN
The Child with Burns: Management and Rehabilitative Stages

NURSING DIAGNOSIS: Impaired skin integrity related to thermal injury

PATIENT GOAL 1: Will exhibit evidence of wound healing

• **NURSING INTERVENTIONS/*RATIONALES***

Shave hair to a 2-inch margin from the wound and area immediately surrounding the burn *to remove a reservoir for infection*

Thoroughly cleanse the wound and surrounding skin *to decrease the risk of infection;* debride devitalized tissue *to promote healing*

Keep child from scratching and picking at the wound

Provide distraction appropriate to child's age

Older child: explain reasons to encourage cooperation

Young child: supervise activity as needed

Maintain care in handling the wound *to avoid damaging epithelializing and granulating tissues*

Offer high-calorie, high-protein meals and snacks *to meet augmented protein and calorie requirements caused by increased metabolism and catabolism*

Prevent infection, which can delay healing and convert partial-thickness wounds to full-thickness wounds

Administer supplementary vitamins and minerals—vitamins A, B, C, iron, and zinc—*to facilitate wound healing and epithelialization*

Pad burned ears *to prevent tissue necrosis due to minimal blood flow to cartilage*

Monitor for signs/symptoms of wound infection *to ensure prompt recognition and treatment*

Wrap fingers and toes separately *to avoid tissue adherence from prolonged contact*

• **EXPECTED OUTCOME**

Wounds heal without evidence of damage or inflammation

PATIENT GOAL 2: Will maintain integrity of skin graft

• **NURSING INTERVENTIONS/*RATIONALES***

Position for minimal mechanical disturbance of graft site

Restrain if necessary *to prevent graft from being dislodged*

Maintain splints or dressings *if needed for protection of the graft*

Observe grafts for evidence of hematoma/fluid accumulation; aspirate or express fluids *to ensure contact of the graft with the base*

• **EXPECTED OUTCOME**

Skin graft remains intact

NURSING DIAGNOSIS: Pain related to skin trauma, therapies

PATIENT GOAL 1: Will experience reduction of pain to a level acceptable to the child

• **NURSING INTERVENTIONS/*RATIONALES***

Assess need for medication (see Pain Assessment, Chapter 26)

Recognize that burn pain is often overwhelming, engulfing, and irrepressible

Position in extension to minimize pain resulting from exercising to regain extension

Implement passive and active exercising *to minimize contracture formation*

Reduce irritation to prevent increased pain

Touch/stroke unburned areas *to provide physical contact and comfort*

Employ appropriate nonpharmacologic pain-reduction techniques (see Pain Management, Chapter 26)

Promote control and predictability during painful procedures (see box on p. 1271)

Anticipate the need for pain medication and administer before the onset of severe pain and at regular intervals *to prevent recurrence* (see Pain Management, Chapter 26)

• **EXPECTED OUTCOME**

Child exhibits reduction of pain to level acceptable to child

NURSING DIAGNOSIS: High risk for infection related to denuded skin, presence of pathogenic organisms, and altered immune response

PATIENT GOAL 1: Will exhibit no evidence of wound infection

• **NURSING INTERVENTIONS/*RATIONALES***

Implement and maintain infection control precautions according to unit policy

Maintain careful handwashing by members of staff and visitors *to minimize exposure to infectious agents*

Wear clean or sterile gown, cap, mask, and gloves when handling wound area *to minimize exposure to infectious agents*

Debride eschar, crust, and blisters *to eliminate the reservoir for organisms*

Avoid patient contact with persons who have upper respiratory or skin infection

Cover the wound and/or patient according to the protocol of the unit *to provide a barrier to organisms*

Administer good oral hygiene

*Apply prescribed topical antimicrobial preparation and dressings to the wound *to control bacterial proliferation*

Obtain baseline and serial wound cultures *to ascertain any increase or changes in wound flora*

Monitor closely for signs of sepsis and infection (disorientation, tachypnea, temperature above 39.5° C [103° F], hypothermia, distention of the abdomen or intestinal ileus, change in wound appearance)

*Dependent nursing action.

NURSING CARE PLAN

The Child with Burns: Management and Rehabilitative Stages—cont'd

• **EXPECTED OUTCOMES**
Possible sources of infection are eliminated
Wound displays minimal or no evidence of infection

NURSING DIAGNOSIS: Altered nutrition: less than body requirements related to increased catabolism and metabolism, loss of appetite

PATIENT GOAL 1: Will receive optimum nourishment

• **NURSING INTERVENTIONS/*RATIONALES***
Encourage oral feeding (see Feeding the Sick Child, Chapter 27)
Provide high-calorie, high-protein meals and snacks *to avoid protein breakdown and meet augmented caloric requirements*
Provide foods child likes, *to stimulate appetite*
Allow self-help *to encourage cooperation*
Provide meals when child is most likely to eat well
Provide attractive meals and surroundings *to encourage eating*
Provide companionship at meals *to create a more homelike environment*
Use "contract" with older children *to encourage compliance*
Administer supplemental enteral feedings as prescribed *to meet calculated needs*
Obtain weekly weight *to monitor nutritional status*
Record accurate intake and output *to evaluate sufficiency of intake*
Monitor for diarrhea/constipation and institute prompt treatment *to avoid feeding intolerance*

• **EXPECTED OUTCOME**
Child consumes a sufficient amount of nutrients (specify) and maintains preburn weight

NURSING DIAGNOSIS: Impaired physical mobility (specify level) related to pain, impaired joint movement, scar formation

PATIENT GOAL 1: Will achieve optimum physical functioning

• **NURSING INTERVENTIONS/*RATIONALES***
Carry out range-of-motion exercises *to maintain optimum joint and muscle function*
Encourage mobility if child is able to move extremities
Ambulate as soon as feasible
Splint involved joints in extension at night and during rest periods *to minimize contracture formation*
Encourage and promote self-help activities *to increase mobility*
Administer analgesia before painful activity (e.g., physical therapy) *so that child is more likely to cooperate and be mobile*
Encourage participation in activities of daily living and play activities *to incorporate exercise into enjoyable events*
Use lotion and massage on healed areas before exercise *to soften tissues and promote relaxation*

PATIENT GOAL 2: Will exhibit minimal scarring

• **NURSING INTERVENTIONS/*RATIONALES***
Position in a functional attitude for minimal deformity and optimum functioning
Apply splints as ordered and designed *to minimize contracture*
Wrap healing tissue with elastic bandage or dress in elastic garments as ordered *to help reduce scar hypertrophy by compressing collagen and decreasing vascularity*
Carry out physical therapy *to minimize deformity related to scar contracture formation*
Provide treatment for pruritus *to minimize scratching and irritation of newly healed tissue*

• **EXPECTED OUTCOME**
Wound heals with minimal scar formation; joints remain flexible and functional

NURSING DIAGNOSIS: Body image disturbance related to perception of appearance and mobility

PATIENT GOAL 1: Will receive adequate emotional support

• **NURSING INTERVENTIONS/*RATIONALES***
Convey positive attitude toward child *to demonstrate acceptance and so that child expects to get better*
Encourage parents to participate in care *to prevent the stress of separation and prepare for reintegration into the community*
Encourage as much independence as condition allows *to give child a sense of control*
Arrange for continued schooling *to encourage optimum development and sense of normalcy*
Promote peer contact where possible *to decrease isolation*
Be honest with child and family *to create a trusting nurse-client relationship*
Encourage activities appropriate to age and capabilities *to promote normalcy and increase self-esteem*
Prepare peers for child's appearance *to encourage acceptance and support*
Provide opportunities for child and family to discuss the impact of the change in appearance and life-style *to increase coping*
Support behaviors suggesting adaptation *to build on strengths*

• **EXPECTED OUTCOMES**
Child accepts efforts of family and caregivers
Child engages in activities with others according to age and capabilities

Continued.

NURSING CARE PLAN

The Child with Burns: Management and Rehabilitative Stages—cont'd

PATIENT GOAL 2: Will demonstrate improved body image

• **NURSING INTERVENTIONS/*RATIONALES***

Explore feelings concerning physical appearance *to facilitate coping with body image changes*

Discuss feelings about returning to home, family, school, and friends *to build coping mechanisms*

Provide reinforcement of positive aspects of appearance and capabilities *to recognize and build on strengths*

Point out evidence of healing *to encourage a sense of hope*

Discuss aids that camouflage disfigurement *to facilitate coping*

- Wigs
- Clothing (e.g., turtleneck sweaters)
- Makeup

Provide recreational and diversional activities *to promote a sense of normalcy*

Promote constructive thinking in child *to encourage positive coping*

Help child devise a plan to address and cope with the reactions of others *to increase the sense of control*

• **EXPECTED OUTCOMES**

Child discusses feelings and concerns regarding appearance and the perceived reactions of others

Child verbalizes positive suggestions for adjusting to appearance and community/peer response

PATIENT GOAL 3: Will engage in self-care activities

• **NURSING INTERVENTIONS/*RATIONALES***

Assist with self-care activities as needed

Encourage self-care according to capabilities

Begin early in hospitalization to discuss "going home" *so that child expects to get better*

Accept regressive behavior where appropriate *because this is how child is coping with stress*

Help child develop independence and self-help capabilities *to increase self-esteem*

• **EXPECTED OUTCOMES**

Child verbalizes and otherwise demonstrates interest in going home

Child engages in self-help activities

NURSING DIAGNOSIS: Altered family processes related to situational crisis (child with a serious injury)

PATIENT GOAL 1: Will be prepared for discharge and home care

• **NURSING INTERVENTIONS/*RATIONALES***

Teach wound care to caregiver *to achieve proficiency and increase confidence*

Discuss diet, rest, and activity *to assist in planning for a home care regimen*

Explore attitudes toward child's reentry into the family *to facilitate coping and identify a possible need for intervention*

Explore family's concept regarding child's capabilities and the possible restrictions and freedom they will allow *to assist them in planning realistically for an altered life-style*

Help family set realistic goals for themselves, the child, and other family members *to clarify and validate the plan of home care*

Help family acquire needed equipment and supplies *to reduce anxiety*

• **EXPECTED OUTCOMES**

Family demonstrates an understanding of child's needs and the impact child's condition will have on them

Family sets realistic goals for selves, child, and others

PATIENT/FAMILY GOAL 2: Will participate in follow-up care

• **NURSING INTERVENTIONS/*RATIONALES***

Coordinate team management of child and family for ongoing care *to provide continuity*

Arrange for return visits

Assess the needs of the family *to determine appropriate plan of care*

Arrange for referral agencies based on needs assessment

Collaborate with school nurse *to help with child's reintegration into school and the world of peers*

Visit the school, if possible, to prepare teacher and peers *to encourage acceptance of child*

• **EXPECTED OUTCOMES**

Family maintains contact with health providers

Child attends school regularly and interacts with agemates

See also:
Nursing Care Plan: The Child in the Hospital, Chapter 26
Nursing Care Plan: The Family of the Ill or Hospitalized Child, Chapter 26

tial risk to small children, who may chew on accessible cords and insert objects into outlets.

In 1974 the Consumer Product Safety Commission recommended a reduction of hot water heater thermostats to a maximum of 120° F. The "dial-down" recommendation has been suggested by utility companies, burn treatment centers, medical personnel, and others interested in public safety. However, many hot water heaters remain set well above the safe level (Maley, 1991). Small children are especially at risk for scald injuries from hot tap water because of their decreased reaction time and agility, their curiosity, and the thermal sensitivity of their skin (Fig. 29-25).

The increased use of microwave ovens has resulted in burn injuries associated with the appliance because of the extremely hot internal temperatures generated in heated items. Baby formula, jelly-filled pastries, and hot liquids and dishes may result in cutaneous scalds or ingestion of overheated liquids (Maley, 1986b; Maley, 1990). Parents should use caution when removing items from the microwave oven and always test the food before giving it to the child.

As children mature, risk-taking behaviors increase. Matches and lighters are very dangerous in the hands of the young; over a 2-year period 5800 structure fires resulting in 170 deaths and 1200 injuries were caused by children playing with lighters (U.S. Consumer Product Safety Commission, 1992). The Consumer Product Safety Commission has developed standards for child-resistant lighters (Maley, 1992), but such legislation will not eliminate all lighter-related accidents. Adults must remember to keep potentially hazardous items out of the reach of children; a lighter, like a match, is a tool for the use of adults.

Education related to fire safety and survival should begin with the very young. "Stop, drop, and roll" to extinguish a fire can be practiced, as well as the safe exit from the home in case of fire. Materials, such as coloring books, are available from many fire departments and burn foundations. Community burn prevention programs also provide opportunities to educate children and parents about fire, burn hazards, and prevention behaviors (Harrell, Hoelker, and Maley, 1994).

Additional information on burn care and prevention can be obtained from the **American Burn Association*** and the **National Safety Council.*** The **Alisa Ann Ruch Burn Foundation**† provides assistance to burn victims and burn centers. The **Shriners Burn Institutes** are staffed to treat pediatric patients following acute burn injuries and those requiring rehabilitative and reconstructive services as a result of scarring and functional impairment. Information can be obtained from local Shrine Temples and Clubs, from Shriners Hospitals, or by contacting the **International Shrine Headquarters.**‡ The Alisa Ann Ruch Foundation and Shriners Hospitals for Crippled Children support research to improve burn care and treatment and promote public education in burn prevention.

*New York–Cornell Medical Center, 525 E. 68th St., Room L-706, New York, NY 10021; (800) 548-BURN.

*444 N. Michigan Ave., Chicago, IL 60611; (800) 621-7615.

†20944 Sherman Way, Suite 115, Canoga Park, CA 91303; (818) 883-7700.

‡2900 Rocky Point Dr., Tampa, FL 33607; (800) 237-5055; in Florida: (800) 282-9161.

KEY POINTS

- Gastrointestinal disorders of childhood that frequently cause fluid depletion and electrolyte disturbance are diarrhea and vomiting.
- The four general types or mechanisms of diarrhea are secretory, cytotoxic, osmotic, and dysenteric diarrhea.
- The treatment for acute diarrhea consists primarily of oral rehydration and provision of an adequate diet.
- Burns are caused by thermal, electrical, chemical, or radioactive agents.
- The severity of burn injury is assessed on the basis of the percentage of body surface area burned, depth, location, age, etiologic agent, concomitant injuries, and general health.
- Emergency measures for severe burns include stopping the burning process; assessing for airway, breathing, and circulation; covering the burn; transporting the child to the hospital; and providing reassurance to the child and family.
- Management of minor burns consists of facilitating wound healing, relieving discomfort, and preventing complications.
- Management of major burn injuries involves facilitating wound healing, relieving discomfort, replacing destroyed skin, preventing and/or treating complications, and providing rehabilitation.
- Active participation by the child and family is important in the care of the child with thermal trauma.

REFERENCES

Ahmann E: Family-centered care: the time has come, *Pediatr Nurs* 20:52-53, 1994.

Alexander JW and others: Beneficial effects of aggressive protein feeding in severely burned children, *Ann Surg* 192:505-517, 1980.

American Academy of Pediatrics, Committee on Nutrition: Use of oral fluid therapy and posttreatment feeding following enteritis in children in a developed country, *Pediatrics* 75:358-361, 1985.

Atchison NE and others: Pain during burn dressing change in children: relationship to burn area, depth and analgesic regimens, *Pain* 47:41-45, 1991.

Avery M, Snyder J: Oral therapy for acute diarrhea: the underused simple solution, *N Engl J Med* 323(13):891-894, 1990.

Bayley EW and others: Research priorities for burn nursing: rehabilitation, discharge planning, and follow-up care, *J Burn Care Rehabil* 13:471-476, 1992.

Bezerra JA and others: Treatment of infants with acute diarrhea: what's recommended and what's practiced, *Pediatrics* 90(1):1-4, 1992.

Bishop W, Ulshen M: Bacterial gastroenteritis, *Pediatr Clin North Am* 35(1):69-87, 1988.

Bone RC: Gram-negative sepsis, *Chest* 100:802-807, 1991.

Boyce ST and others: Skin anatomy and antigen expression after burn wound closure with composite grafts of cultures, skin cells and biopolymers, *Plast Reconstr Surg* 91:632-641, 1993.

Broscious S: Toxic shock syndrome and its potential complications, *Crit Care Nurse* 11(4):28-35, 1991.

Brown K: Dietary management of acute childhood diarrhea: optimal timing of feeding and appropriate use of milks and mixed diets, *J Pediatr* 118(4):S92-S98, 1991.

Brown K, Gastanaduy A, Saavedra J: Effect of continued oral feeding on clinical and nutritional outcomes of acute diarrhea in children, *J Pediatr* 12(19):191-200, 1988.

Brown KH, Peerson JM, Fontaine O: Use of nonhuman milks in the dietary management of young children with acute diarrhea: a meta-analysis of clinical trials, *Pediatrics* 93(1):17-27, 1994.

Carrougher GJ: Inhalation injury, *AACN Clin Issues* 4:367-377, 1993.

Centers for Disease Control: Follow-up on toxic-shock syndrome, *MMWR* 29:441-445, 1980.

Centers for Disease Control and Prevention: The management of acute diarrhea in children: oral rehydration, maintenance, and nutritional therapy, *MMWR* 41(RR-16): entire issue, 1992.

Chew F and others: Is dilution of cows' milk formula necessary for dietary management of acute diarrhoea in infants aged less than 6 months? *Lancet* 341:194-197, 1993.

Cohen M: Etiology and mechanisms of acute infectious diarrhea in infants in the United States, *J Pediatr* 118(4):S34-S39, 1991.

Dominioni L and others: Prevention of severe, postburn hypermetabolism and catabolism by immediate intragastric feeding, *J Burn Care Rehabil* 5:106-112, 1984.

East MK and others: Epidemiology of burns in children. In Carvajal HF, Parks DH, editors: *Burns in children: pediatric burn management,* St Louis, 1988, Mosby.

Faldmo L, Kravits M: Management of acute burns and burn shock resuscitation, *AACN Clin Issues* 4:351-366, 1993.

Finkelstein JL and others: Pediatric burns: an overview, *Pediatr Clin North Am* 39:1145-1163, 1992.

Fisher M: Treating anaphylaxis with sympathomimetic drugs, *Br Med J* 305:1107-1108, 1992.

Fitzgerald J: Management of acute diarrhea, *Pediatr Infect Dis J* 8(8):564-569, 1989.

Frank DH and others: Comparison of Biobrane, porcine, and human allograft as biologic dressings for burn wounds, *J Burn Care Rehabil* 4:186-190, 1983.

Fuchs GJ, Gleason WA: Gastrointestinal complications in burned children. In Carvajal HF, Parks DH, editors: *Burns in children: pediatric burn management,* St Louis, 1988, Mosby.

Gottschlich MM, Alexander JW, Bower RH: Enteral nutrition in patients with burns or trauma. In Rombeau JL, Caldwell MD, editors: *Enteral and tube feeding,* Philadelphia, 1990, WB Saunders.

Gottschlich MM, Warden GD: Vitamin supplementation in the burn patient, *J Burn Care Rehabil* 11:275-279, 1990.

Gottschlich MM and others: Diarrhea in tube-fed burn patients: incidence, etiology, nutritional impact and prevention, *JPEN J Parenter Enteral Nutr* 12:338-345, 1988.

Groeneveld A, Inkson T: Ketamine: a solution to procedural pain in burned children, *Can Nurse* 88(8):28-31, 1992.

Guarino A and others: Oral immunoglobulins for treatment of acute rotaviral gastroenteritis, *Pediatrics* 93(1):12-16, 1994.

Harmel RP, Vane DW, King DR: Burn care in children: special considerations, *Clin Plast Surg* 13:95-105, 1986.

Harrell D, Hoelker L, Maley MS: Community burn prevention, *Proc Am Burn Assoc* 26:66, 1994.

Hazinski MF: Shock in the pediatric patient, *Crit Care Nurs Clin North Am* 2:309-323, 1990.

Heink NR: Fluid resuscitation and the role of exchange transfusion in pediatric burn shock, *Crit Care Nurse* 12(7): 50-56, 1992.

Helvig E: Pediatric burn injuries, *AACN Clin Issues* 4:433-442, 1993.

Hendricks L and others: Subanesthetic ketamine for painful nonoperative procedures in pediatric burn patients, *Proc Am Burn Assoc* 23:52, 1991.

Hermans M, Hermans R: Burns: Duoderm, an alternative dressing for smaller burns, *Burns* 12:214-219, 1986.

Herndon DN and others: Treatment of burns in children, *Pediatr Clin North Am* 32:1311-1332, 1985.

Herndon DN and others: Failure of TPN supplementation to improve liver function, immunity, and mortality in thermally injured patients, *J Trauma* 27:195-204, 1987.

Hoge CW and others: The changing epidemiology of invasive group A streptococcal infections and the emergence of streptococcal toxic shock–like syndrome, *JAMA* 269:384-389, 1993.

Holder IA: The burn wound: microbiological aspects. In Carvajal HF, Parks DH, editors: *Burns in children: pediatric burn management,* St Louis, 1988, Mosby.

Housinger TA, Wondrely L, Warden GD: The use of Biobrane for pediatric donor sites, *J Burn Care Rehabil* 14:26-28, 1993.

Ireton CS and others: Evaluation of energy expenditures in burn patients, *J Am Diet Assoc* 86:333-339, 1986.

Jenkins M, Gottschlich MM, Alexander JW: Enteral alimentation in the early postburn phase. In Blackburn GL, Bell SJ, Mullen JL, editors: *Nutritional medicine: a case management approach,* Philadelphia, 1989, WB Saunders.

Jenkins M, Gottschlich M, Warden G: Enteral support during operative procedures, J Burn Care Rehabil 15:199-205, 1994.

Kaye EM, Butler IJ: Neurologic complications of burns in childhood. In Carvajal HF, Parks DH, editors: *Burns in children: pediatric burn management,* St Louis, 1988, Mosby.

Kleinman RE: We have the solution: now what's the problem? *Pediatrics* 90(1):113-115, 1992.

Kubiak M and others: Comparison of stool containment in cloth and single-use diapers using a simulated infant feces, *Pediatrics* 91(3):632-636, 1993.

Leung A, Robson W: Acute diarrhea in children, *Postgrad Med* 86(8):161-173, 1989.

Maley M: How many people do get burned? *Rekindle/ISFSI* 4:17-18, 1986a.

Maley M: Microwave oven-associated burns, *Rekindle/ISFSI* 12:10-12, 1986b.

Maley MP: Microwave oven–related burn injuries: summary focus on the risk to children, *The Voice/ISFSI* 12:19, 1990.

Maley M: The final control: anti-scald plumbing standards, *Information Exchange* 4:1-8, 1991.

Maley M: The child resistant lighter—an update, *Information Exchange* 8:1-3, 1992.

Maley M: Scald in the kitchen, *Information Exchange* 9:1-5, 1993.

Munster AM: *Severe burns: a family guide to medical and emotional recovery,* Baltimore, 1993, Johns Hopkins University Press.

Peate WF: Outpatient management of burns, *Am Fam Physician* 45:1321-1330, 1992.

Penny ME, Paredes P, Brown KH: Clinical and nutritional consequences of lactose feeding during persistent postenteritis diarrhea, *Pediatrics* 84:835-844, 1989.

Petersen SR, Umphred E, Warden GD: The incidence of bacteremia following burn wound excision, *J Trauma* 22:274-279, 1982.

Pruitt BA, Levine NS: Characteristics and uses of biologic dressings and skin substitutes, *Arch Surg* 119:312-322, 1984.

Rieg LS, Jenkins M: Burn injuries in children, *Crit Care Clin North Am* 3:457-470, 1991.

Rutan RL, Herndon DN: Growth delay in post-burn pediatric patients, *Arch Surg* 125:392-395, 1990.

Saffle JR and others: Use of indirect calorimetry in the nutritional management of burned patients, *J Trauma* 25:32-39, 1985.

Sampson HA, Mendelson MD, Rosen JP: Fatal and near-fatal anaphylactic reactions to food in children and adolescents, *N Engl J Med* 327:380-384, 1992.

Santosham M, Greenough W: Oral rehydration therapy: a global perspective, *J Pediatr* 118(4):S44-S51, 1991.

Schmidt L and others: The use of scheduled methadone and morphine sulfate to control postoperative pain in the adolescent burn patient, *Proc Am Burn Assoc* 21:47, 1989.

Selbst SM: Pain management in the emergency department. In Schechter N, Berde C, Yaster M: *Pain in infants, children, and adolescents,* Baltimore, 1993, Williams & Wilkins.

Silverstein P, Wilson R: Prevention of pediatric burn injuries. In Carvajal HF, Parks DH, editors: *Burns in children: pediatric burn management* St Louis, 1988, Mosby.

Thompson PB, Herndon D, Traber D: Effects on morbidity of inhalation injury, *J Trauma* 26:163-165, 1986.

Treem W: Chronic nonspecific diarrhea of childhood, *Clin Pediatr* pp 413-420, July, 1992.

Trofino RB, Braun AE: Pathophysiology of burns. In Trofino RB, editor: *Nursing care of the burn-injured patient,* Philadelphia, 1991, FA Davis.

U.S. Consumer Product Safety Commision: Child-resistant lighter standard moves forward, *News from CPSS,* Release no. 92-123, July 29, 1992.

Vaccaro P, Trofino RB: Care of the patient with minor to moderate burns. In Trofino RB, editor: *Nursing care of the burn-injured patient,* Philadelphia, 1991, FA Davis.

Walter P: Burn wound management, *AACN Clin Issues* 4:378-387, 1993.

Warden GD: Burn shock resuscitation, *World J Surg* 16:16-23, 1992.

Warden GD and others: Multidisciplinary team approach to the pediatric burn patient, *QRB* 14:219-226, 1988.

Weber JM, Tompkins DM: Improving survival: infection control and burns, *AACN Clin Issues* 4:414-423, 1993.

Working Group on Severe Streptococcal Infections: Defining the group A streptococcal toxic shock syndrome, *JAMA* 269:390-391, 1993.

BIBLIOGRAPHY

Diarrhea

Bhan M and others: Efficacy of mung bean (lentil) and pop rice based rehydration solutions in comparison with the standard glucose electrolyte solution, *J Pediatr Gastroenterol Nutr* 6:392-399, 1987.

Booth IW: Dietary management of acute diarrhoea in childhood, *Lancet* 341(8851):996, 1993.

Buzby M: Chronic diarrhea: management in pediatrics, *J Pediatr Health Care* 3(3):163-165, 1989.

Conway S, Ireson A: Acute gastroenteritis in well-nourished infants: comparison of four feeding regimens, *Arch Dis Child* 64:87-91, 1989.

Ford-Jones E and others: The incidence of viral-associated diarrhea after admission to a pediatric hospital, *Am J Epidemiol* 131(4):711-718, 1990.

Galaeno N and others: Comparison of two special infant formulas designed for their treatment of protracted diarrhea, *J Pediatr Gastroenterol Nutr* 7:76-83, 1988.

Ghishan FK: The transport of electrolytes in the gut and the use of oral rehydration solutions, *Pediatr Clin North Am* 35(1):35-51, 1988.

Grill B: Oral rehydration, food allergy, and specialized nutrition, *Curr Opin Pediatr* 1:384-393, 1989.

Hamilton J: Viral enteritis, *Pediatr Clin North Am* 35(1):89-101, 1988.

Khuffash F, Sethi S, Shaltout A: Acute gastroenteritis: clinical features according to etiologic agents, *Clin Pediatr* 27(8):365-368, 1988.

Kleinman R: Milk protein enteropathy after acute infectious gastroenteritis: experimental and clinical observations, *J Pediatr* 118(4):S111-S115, 1991.

Lebenthal E, Lu R: Glucose polymers as an alternative to glucose in oral rehydration solutions, *J Pediatr* 118(4):S62-S69, 1991.

Lifshitz F, Ament M: Role of juice carbohydrate malabsorption in chronic nonspecific diarrhea in children, *J Pediatr* 120(5):825-829, 1992.

Margolis P and others: Effects of unrestricted diet on mild infantile diarrhea, *Am J Dis Child* 144:162-164, 1990.

Pickering L: Therapy of acute infectious diarrhea in children, *J Pediatr* 118(4):S18-S128, 1991.

Pizarro D and others: Comparison of efficacy of a glucose/glycine/glycylglycine electrolyte solution versus the standard WHO/ORS in diarrheic dehydrated children, *J Pediatr Gastroenterol Nutr* 7:882-222, 1988.

Smith G: Home treatment of mild, acute diarrhea and secondary dehydration of infants and small children: an educational program for parents in a shelter for the homeless, *J Prof Nurs* 4:60-63, 1988.

Infectious Gastroenteritis

Cohen M, Balistreri WF: Diagnosing and treating diarrhea, *Contemp Pediatr* 6(3):89-114, 1989.

Hoffman RE, Shillam PJ: The use of hygiene, cohorting, and antimicrobial therapy to control an outbreak of shigellosis, *Am J Dis Child* 144:219-221, 1990.

Shock

Barry W and others: Intravenous immunoglobulin therapy for toxic shock syndrome, *JAMA* 267(24):3315-3316, 1992.

Berro EA, Bechler-Karsch A: A closer look at septic shock, *Pediatr Nurs* 19:289-297, 1993.

Morriss FC: Analphylaxis. In Levin DL, Morriss FC, editors: *Essentials of pediatric intensive care*, St Louis, 1990, Quality Medical.

Pamillo JE: Pathogenetic mechanisms of septic shock, *N Engl J Med* 328:1471-1477, 1993.

Resnick SD: Toxic shock syndrome: recent developments in pathogenesis, *J Pediatr* 116:321-328, 1990.

Rice V: Shock, a clinical syndrome: an update, part 1, *Crit Care Nurse* 11:20-27, 1991.

Rice V: Shock, a clinical syndrome: an update, part 2, *Crit Care Nurse* 11:74-82, 1991.

Rice V: Shock, a clinical syndrome, an update, part 3, *Crit Care Nurse* 11:34-39, 1991.

Rice V: Shock, a clinical syndrome, an update, part 4, *Crit Care Nurse* 11:28-32, 35-43, 1991.

Strodtbeck F, Joyce B: Shock in newborns and children, *Crit Care Nurs Q* 11:75-83, 1988.

Wahl SC: Shock: how to detect it early, *Nursing 89* 19(1):53-59, 1989.

Wynn SR: Anaphylaxis at school, *J School Nurs* 9:5-11, 1993.

Toxic Shock Syndrome

Resnick SD: Toxic shock syndrome: recent developments in pathogenesis, *J Pediatr* 116:321-328, 1990.

Burns

Baker MD, Chiaviello C: Household electrical injuries in children, *Am J Dis Child* 143:59-62, 1989.

Bessey PQ, Wilmore DW: The burned patient. In Kinney JM and others, editors: *Nutrition and metabolism in patient care,* Philadelphia, 1988, WB Saunders.

Blakeney P and others: Social competence and behavioral problems of pediatric survivors of burns, *J Burn Care Rehabil* 14:65-72, 1993.

Blumenfield M, Schoeps MM: *Psychological care of the burn and trauma patient,* Baltimore, 1992, Williams & Wilkins.

Cockington RA: Ambulatory management of burns in children, *Burns* 15:271-273, 1989.

Desai MH and others: *Candida* infection with and without nystatin prophylaxis, *Arch Surg* 127:159-162, 1992.

Herndon DN, Rutan RL, Rutan TC: Management of the pediatric patient with burns, *J Burn Care Rehabil* 14:3-8, 1993.

Kinner MA, Daly WL: Skin transplantation, *Crit Care Nurs Clin North Am* 4:173-178, 1992.

Kravitz M and others: Sleep disorders in children after burn injury, *J Burn Care Rehabil* 14:83-90, 1993.

Martinez S: Ambulatory management of burns in children, *J Pediatr Health Care* 6:32-37, 1992.

Marvin JA, Carrougher G, Bayley E: Burn nursing Delphi study: pain management, *J Burn Care Rehabil* 13:685-694, 1992.

Matsuda T and others: High-dose vitamin C therapy for extensive deep dermal burns, *Burns* 18:127-131, 1992.

Meyer WJ and others: Parental well-being and behavioral adjustment of pediatric survivors of burns, *J Burn Care Rehabil* 15:62-68, 1994.

Miller AC, Hickman LC, Lemasters GK: A distraction technique for control of burn pain, *J Burn Care Rehabil* 13:576-580, 1992.

O'Neill JA: Inhalation injury in children. In Haponik EF, Munster AM, editors: *Respiratory injury: smoke inhalation and burns,* New York, 1990, McGraw-Hill.

Osgood PF, Szyfelbein SK: Management of burn pain in children, *Pediatr Clin North Am* 36:1001-1013, 1989.

Reeves SU, Warden G, Staley MJ: Management of the pediatric burn patient. In Richard RL, Staley MJ, editors: *Burn care and rehabilitation: principles and practice,* Philadelphia, 1994, FA Davis.

Rosenstein DLW: A school reentry program for burned children. I: Development and implementation of a school reentry program, *J Burn Care Rehabil* 8:319-322, 1987.

Schwanholt C, Daugherty MB, Gaboury T: Splinting the pediatric palmar burn, *J Burn Care Rehabil* 13:460-464, 1992.

Smith GA, Savinski-Bozinko G: Giving emergency care for burns: *Nursing 89* 19(9):55-62, 1989.

Stoddard FJ, Stroud L, Murphy JM: Depression in children after recovery from severe burns, *J Burn Care Rehabil* 13:340-347, 1992.

Tredget EE and others: Epidemiology of infections with *Pseudomonas aeruginosa* in burn patients: the role of hydrotherapy, *Clin Infect Dis* 15:941-949, 1992.

Warden GD: Burn patients: coming of age? The 1993 presidential address to the American Burn Association, *J Burn Care Rehabil* 14:581-588, 1993.

Wright TF and others: Hardiness, stress, and burnout among intensive care nurses, *J Burn Care Rehabil* 14:376-381, 1993.

Zingg BM: Managing burns in children: an intraoperative nursing care plan, *AORN J* 54:568-575, 1991.

CHAPTER 30

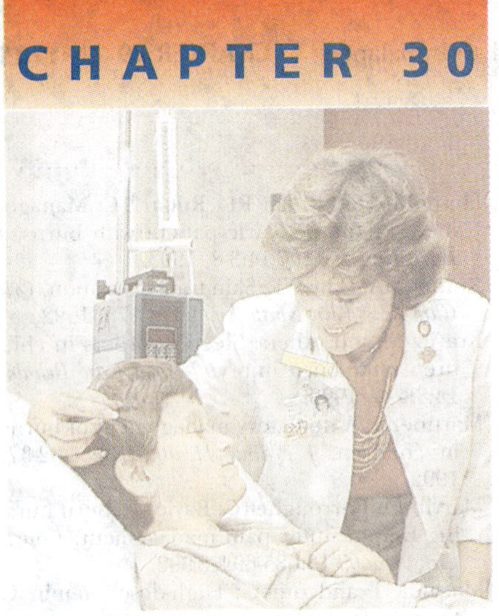

The Child with Renal Dysfunction

CHAPTER OUTLINE

RELATED TOPICS

Administration of medication, Ch. 27
Collection of specimens, Ch. 27
Defects of the genitourinary tract, Ch. 11
Family-centered care of the child with chronic illness or disability, Ch. 22
Family-centered home care, Ch. 25
Physical examination: genitalia, Ch. 7

RENAL STRUCTURE AND FUNCTION

The primary responsibility of the kidney is to maintain the composition and volume of the body fluids in equilibrium. To maintain this constant internal environment, the kidney must respond appropriately to alterations in the internal environment caused by variations in dietary intake and extrarenal losses of water and solutes. This is accomplished by the formation of urine (the product of glomerular filtration), tubular reabsorption, and tubular secretion. ***Reabsorption*** is the transport of a substance from the tubular lumen to the blood in surrounding vessels. ***Secretion*** is transport in the opposite direction (i.e., from the blood to the lumen). These processes can be active or passive. ***Excretion*** is the elimination of a substance from the body, in this case urine.

A secondary function of the kidney is the production of

■ Teresa L. Hall, RN, MS, and Mikel Gray, RN, PhD, PNP, CURN, revised this chapter.

certain humoral substances. One such substance is an enzyme, ***erythropoietin stimulating factor (ESF,*** or ***erythrogenin),*** which acts on a plasma globulin to form erythropoietin, which in turn stimulates erythropoiesis in the bone marrow. Its production is increased in the presence of hypoxia and androgens. Few red blood cells are formed in the absence of erythropoietin, which accounts in some measure for the anemia associated with advanced renal disease. Another enzyme, ***renin,*** is also secreted by the kidney in response to reduced blood volume, decreased blood pressure, or increased secretion of catecholamines. Renin stimulates the production of the angiotensins, which produce arteriolar constriction and an elevation in blood pressure and stimulate the production of aldosterone by the adrenal cortex.

RENAL PHYSIOLOGY

The structural and functional unit of the kidney is the nephron, which is composed of a complex system of tubules, arterioles, venules, and capillaries (Fig. 30-1). The nephron consists of the ***Bowman capsule,*** enclosing a tuft of capillaries, which is joined successively to the ***proximal convoluted tubule,*** the ***loop of Henle,*** the ***distal convoluted tubule,*** and the ***straight*** or ***collecting duct.*** Collecting tubules join larger ducts, and all of the larger collecting ducts of one renal pyramid join to form a single duct that opens into a ***minor calyx.*** A number of calyces empty into one of several ***major calyces*** that converge into the ***renal pelvis.*** The renal pelvis narrows after it leaves the kidney and forms what then becomes a ***ureter,*** through which urine drains into the ***urinary bladder.***

The blood supply to the kidneys constitutes about one fifth of the total cardiac output; therefore profuse bleeding can accompany renal trauma. Because interstitial tissue is sparse, individual nephrons with their blood vessel component are closely packed together. Each nephron is supplied by a sizable ***afferent arteriole,*** which separates into capillary loops that comprise the glomerular tuft. Blood leaves by a smaller ***efferent arteriole.*** From there the efferent arterioles branch into a ***peritubular capillary*** network and hairpin loops called the ***vasa recta,*** which parallel the Henle loops and the collecting ducts. The total surface area of the renal capillaries is approximately equal to the total surface of the tubules.

The ***Bowman capsule*** is composed of two cellular layers that separate the blood from the glomerular filtrate—the capillary endothelium and a layer of tubular epithelial lining cells. Situated between these layers is the basal lamina, or basement membrane. The permeability of this glomerular membrane is a result of its structure; the capillary endothelium is fenestrated with pores or ***fenestrae,*** and the outer surface of the glomerular epithelium consists of fingerlike projections ***(pseudopodia,*** or ***podocytes),*** which cover the entire surface to form slits called ***slit pores.*** The basement membrane has no visible openings but behaves as if it con-

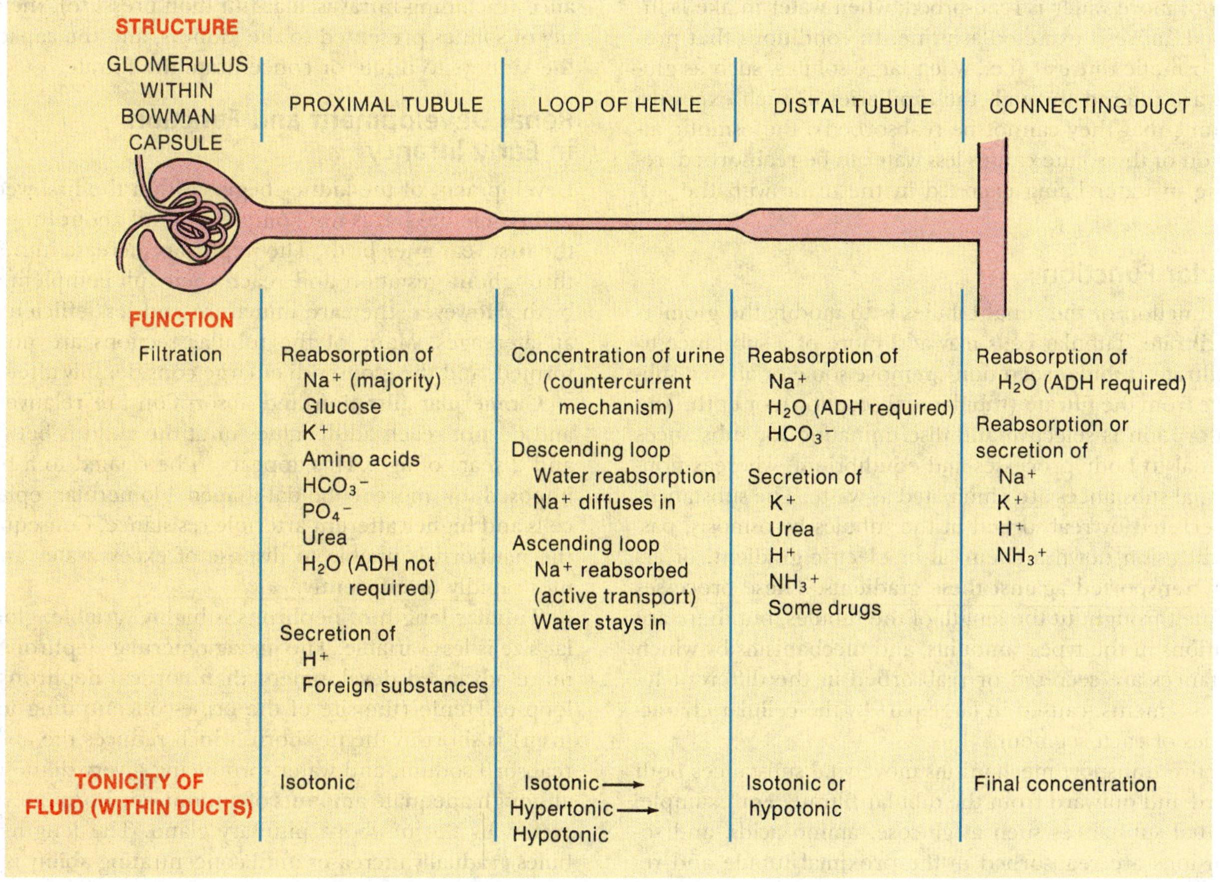

STRUCTURE
GLOMERULUS WITHIN BOWMAN CAPSULE
PROXIMAL TUBULE
LOOP OF HENLE
DISTAL TUBULE
CONNECTING DUCT
FUNCTION
Filtration
Reabsorption of
Na+ (majority)
Glucose
K+
Amino acids
HCO_3^-
PO_4^-
Urea
H_2O (ADH not required)
Secretion of
H+
Foreign substances
Concentration of urine (countercurrent mechanism)
Descending loop
Water reabsorption
Na+ diffuses in
Ascending loop
Na+ reabsorbed (active transport)
Water stays in
Reabsorption of
Na+
H_2O (ADH required)
HCO_3^-
Secretion of
K+
Urea
H+
NH_3^+
Some drugs
Reabsorption of
H_2O (ADH required)
Reabsorption or secretion of
Na+
K+
H+
NH_3^+
TONICITY OF FLUID (WITHIN DUCTS)
Isotonic
Isotonic
Hypertonic
Hypotonic
Isotonic or hypotonic
Final concentration

FIG. 30-1 Major functions of nephron components.

tains pores or channels. Consequently, the glomerular filtrate, which has essentially the same composition as plasma except for the large protein molecules and cellular elements, passes through these three layers and does so at a very rapid rate. The structure of these layers becomes altered in kidney disease.

Glomerular Filtration

Filtration through the glomerular capillaries is governed by the same mechanism as filtration across other capillaries in the body (i.e., the size of the capillary bed, the permeability of the capillaries, and the hydrostatic and osmotic pressure gradients across the capillaries). The filtration capacity of the glomerulus is the product of three pressure forces—glomerular hydrostatic pressure, colloidal osmotic (oncotic) pressure (COP), and intracapsular pressure—and permeability of the glomerular capillaries.

Blood enters the nephron at a substantial pressure. This hydrostatic pressure forces plasma fluid and solutes through the capillary membrane into the collecting apparatus of the unit. As this filtrate travels through the renal tubules, water and solutes are selectively reabsorbed back into the vascular compartment. That which is not reabsorbed is excreted as urine. Filtration takes place as long as hydrostatic pressure within the glomerular capillaries exceeds the opposing COP of the plasma proteins. If the pressure becomes equal through decreased hydrostatic pressure or decreased COP, no further filtration takes place. In a state of dehydration, more water is reabsorbed; when water intake is increased, more is excreted as urine. In conditions that produce osmotic diuresis (i.e., when large solutes, such as glucose, are filtered through the capillaries in such excessive amounts that they cannot be reabsorbed), the osmotic attraction of the solute causes less water to be reabsorbed, resulting in water being excreted in the urine with the solute.

Tubular Function

The function of the renal tubules is to modify the glomerular filtrate. Tubular cells may add more of a substance to the filtrate (tubular secretion), remove some or all of a substance from the filtrate (tubular reabsorption), or both. The reabsorption is selective and discriminating for substances essential to body processes and equilibrium, whereas nonessential substances are eliminated as waste. The substances are secreted or reabsorbed in the tubules by osmosis, passive diffusion down a chemical or electric gradient, or actively transported against these gradients. These processes operate throughout the length of the tubules, but there are variations in the types, amounts, and mechanisms by which substances are secreted or reabsorbed in the different tubular segments, caused in large part by the cellular characteristics of each segment.

Active transport mechanisms move vital substances both inward and outward from the tubular filtrate. For example, essential substances such as glucose, amino acids, and sodium ions are reabsorbed in the proximal tubule and returned directly to the blood. Active transport mechanisms, as elsewhere, have a limited capacity, or threshold, for moving the solute. When the maximum of the transport mechanism is reached, no more of the substance is reabsorbed, and the remainder is excreted in the urine. For example, when blood glucose concentrations exceed their transport capacity, the surplus remains in the filtrate to be excreted in the urine (glycosuria). When two substances share a common transport mechanism, the first substance may be blocked by the addition of a second substance (selective inhibition). The effect of many therapeutic agents (e.g., diuretics) depends on this process.

Electrolytes are moved by both active transport and diffusion, and the transport of some, particularly sodium, has important effects on other substances. For example, sodium is actively transported from all parts of the nephron. The movement of sodium ions produces both an electric and an osmotic gradient, which causes chloride ions and water to diffuse from the tubules in an effort to establish equilibrium. This is the obligatory water reabsorption in the kidneys. There is a limit to the concentration gradient against which sodium can be transported out; therefore when larger than normal amounts of sodium ions remain in the tubules, water is obliged to remain with the sodium.

Under normal conditions the kidneys are able to adjust the urine and solute excretion in response to the requirements for body water and electrolyte balance. They are able to excrete or conserve both water and most electrolytes in addition to excreting end products of protein metabolism, principally urea. The volume of urine excreted by the kidneys in a given period of time depends on the water balance (including intravascular filtration pressure), the quantity of solutes presented to the kidneys, and the capacity of the kidneys to dilute or concentrate the filtrate.

Renal Development and Function in Early Infancy

Development of the kidney begins within the first weeks of embryonic life but is not completed until about the end of the first year after birth. The nephrons increase in number throughout gestation and reach their full complement by birth. However, they are immature and less efficient than at later ages. Many of the tubular sections are not fully formed, and the glomeruli enlarge considerably after birth.

Glomerular filtration and absorption are relatively low and do not reach adult values until the child is between 1 and 2 years of age. This appears to be related to a barrier imposed by more cuboidal-shaped glomerular epithelial cells and higher afferent arteriole resistance. Consequently, the newborn is unable to dispose of excess water and solutes rapidly or efficiently.

Tubular length of nephrons is highly variable; glomerular size is less variable. The juxtaglomerular nephrons show more advanced development than cortical nephrons. The loop of Henle (the site of the urine-concentrating mechanism) is short in the newborn, which reduces the ability to reabsorb sodium and water, producing a very dilute urine, although adequate amounts of antidiuretic hormone are secreted by the newborn pituitary gland. The length of tubules gradually increases until concentrating ability reaches adult levels about the third month of life. Urea synthesis and excretion are slower during this time, and the newborn retains large quantities of nitrogen and essential electrolytes in order to meet needs for growth in the first weeks of life. Consequently, the excretory burden is minimized. The lower concentration of urea, the principal end product of nitrogen metabolism, also reduces concentrating capacity, since it also contributes to the concentration mechanism.

Other characteristics of the newborn's kidneys create differences in renal function from that of older children and adults. Because of some as yet undetermined cause, newborn infants are unable to excrete a water load at rates similar to those of older persons. Hydrogen ion excretion is reduced, acid secretion is lower for the first year of life, and plasma bicarbonate levels are low. As a result of these inadequacies of the kidney, along with less efficient blood buffers, the newborn is more liable to develop severe metabolic acidosis. Sodium excretion is reduced in the immediate newborn period, and the kidneys are less able to adapt to deficiencies and excesses of sodium. For example, an isotonic saline infusion may produce edema because of impaired ability to eliminate excess. Conversely, inadequate reabsorption of sodium from tubules may increase sodium losses in disorders such as vomiting or diarrhea. Moreover, infants have a diminished capacity to reabsorb glucose and, during the first few days, to produce ammonium ions.

The kidney functions during fetal life and produces urine that contributes to the amniotic fluid volume. The 24-hour urine volume is low at birth, rapidly increases in the neonatal period, and steadily increases with normal growth (see Appendix D).

RENAL PELVIS AND URETERS: STRUCTURE AND FUNCTION*

The ***renal pelvis*** is a funnel-shaped structure that originates at the major calyces and terminates in the funnel-shaped ureteropelvic junction. The ***ureter*** is a thin mucomuscular tube that extends from the ureteropelvic to the ureterovesical junction in the base of the bladder. Three areas—the ureteropelvic junction, the ureterovesical junction, and the segment nearest the sacroiliac junction—are particularly narrow and prone to obstruction when a solid body (such as a urinary calculus ["stone"]) passes.

The principal function of the renal pelvis and ureter is the transport of urine from the kidney to the bladder. Urine is moved via a process called ***peristalsis,*** whereby muscular movements originating in the renal pelvis propel a bolus of urine toward the urinary bladder for storage and eventual evacuation when the child urinates. The renal pelvis stores only a relatively small volume of urine (approximately 15 ml in adults) before a contraction is triggered that pushes the urine toward the bladder. The forward movement of urine from the kidney to the bladder is called ***efflux,*** whereas abnormal or backward urine movement is termed ***reflux.*** Aside from mechanical stretching, ureteral peristalsis is modulated by neurogenic and hormonal factors (Gray, 1992).

The ***ureterovesical junction*** joins the ureters and bladder. It comprises three principal components: the lowest segment of the ureter, the trigone muscle, and the adjacent bladder wall. The ureters allow the passage of urine from the upper urinary tracts while preventing regurgitation of urine from the bladder to the ureters. During bladder filling, intravesical pressure remains relatively low and the detrusor muscle remains in a relaxed state. A peristaltic contraction of the ureter propels urine into the bladder. During micturition, the intravesical pressure rises as the detrusor muscle contracts; that raises the potential for harmful reflux into the upper urinary tracts. Several mechanisms in the normal ureterovesical junction act together to prevent reflux. The terminal (intravesical) ureteral segment tunnels through the bladder wall at an oblique angle. During bladder contraction, tension in the detrusor muscle squeezes the intravesical ureter closed. This process is enhanced by the trigone muscle that surrounds the ureteral orifice of the terminal ureter. In addition, the longitudinally arranged muscle of the intravesical ureter contracts, providing further resistance from reflux. Anatomic defects of the ureterovesical junction, such as lateral displacement of the ureter or reduced length of the intravesical ureter, predispose the child to primary reflux. Voiding dysfunction associated with infections and high bladder pressures predispose the child to secondary reflux (Kramer, 1992).

*Mikel Gray, RN, PhD, PNP, CURN, wrote this section and the following section on the urethrovesical unit.

URETHROVESICAL UNIT: STRUCTURE AND FUNCTION

The ***urethrovesical unit*** consists of the bladder, urethra, and pelvic muscles; it is also called the ***lower urinary tract*** (Gray, 1992). The ***urinary bladder*** is a muscle-lined sac that stores and empties itself of urine. In the infant the bladder lies entirely in the abdomen. The bladder assumes its place in the true pelvis shortly before puberty. This change in position is caused by maturation of the pelvic bone rather than migration of the bladder and urethra.

The bladder is characterized by two inlets, the ***ureteral orifices,*** and a single outlet, the ***urethral orifice.*** The base of the bladder is a relatively fixed, triangular area consisting of the bladder neck and trigone. The body of the bladder, in contrast, is distensible, changing from a tetrahedron (four-sided) shape when the bladder is relatively empty to a nearly spherical shape as the bladder fills.

One of the four layers of the bladder wall consists of smooth muscle bundles that promote bladder evacuation via micturition. Collectively, this muscular tunic is called the ***detrusor.*** The muscular tunic of the bladder wall also contains ***collagen,*** a tough, nonelastic substance that maintains the integrity of the bladder wall while preventing overdistention. Certain pathologic factors, including denervation of the bladder and obstruction of the outlet, may cause an overabundance of collagen in the detrusor muscle. This causes a loss of bladder compliance (distensibility), abnormally high filling pressures, and trabeculation of the bladder wall.

The ***urethra*** is a mucomuscular tube that connects the external meatus and the bladder. The ***male urethra*** originates at the bladder neck, piercing the prostate and pelvic floor before tunneling through the posterior portion of the penis and terminating at the glans penis. The proximal portion of the urethra comprises the sphincter mechanism, whereas the distal portion serves as a conduit for the passage of urine or semen. The urethral meatus is a vertical slit located at the summit of the glans penis.

The ***female urethra*** follows a relatively short, straight course compared with the male. It originates at the bladder base and terminates at an external meatus located immediately superior to (in front of) the vaginal orifice. The distal two thirds of the female urethra is fused with the vaginal wall.

The primary responsibilities of the bladder are to store urine manufactured by the kidneys and evacuate this urine at regular intervals via the process of micturition. During infancy, the bladder is expected to empty spontaneously; by the fourth year of life (or earlier), the child is expected to gain control of detrusor and urethral sphincter function. Control of the urethrovesical unit is referred to as ***urinary continence.*** Continent individuals are expected to hold their urine for a period of at least 2 hours while awake. During sleeping hours, they may arise once to urinate, although many children and young adults sleep for 8 hours or more without interruption. Three factors—anatomic integrity of the lower urinary tract, detrusor control, and competence of the urethral sphincter mechanism—must function normally for continence to be achieved and maintained (Gray, 1992).

Detrusor control requires successful integration of neurologic structures in the brain, spinal cord, and peripheral nervous systems. The ***brain*** influences bladder function via its inhibitory role on detrusor contractions. The ***stable detrusor*** contracts only when its owner gives permission. Several areas of the brain act together to control detrusor stability. Pathology of one of these areas is known to produce ***detrusor instability,*** or the loss of control over detrusor contractions.

The ***spinal cord*** influences lower urinary tract function because it transmits messages between the brain and the target organ. Two areas in the spinal cord are particularly significant. The ***thoracolumbar cord*** (spinal levels T10 to L2) influences bladder and urethral sphincter function. Sympathetic impulses from the brain travel to the bladder body and smooth muscle of the urethra, causing relaxation of the detrusor muscle and contraction of urethral smooth muscle. This combination of actions promotes bladder filling and storage of urine. The ***sacral spinal cord*** (spinal segments S2 to S4) influences the bladder muscle, promoting micturition. Parasympathetic impulses travel from these nuclei, causing contraction of the detrusor muscle and, indirectly, promoting relaxation of smooth muscle in the urethra.

Two ***peripheral nerve plexuses*** directly influence the control of the detrusor muscle. The pelvic plexus provides parasympathetic innervation to the bladder and urethra, and the inferior hypogastric plexus provides sympathetic innervation (Bradley, 1986).

The final mechanism responsible for the attainment and maintenance of continence is the ***urethral sphincter mechanism.*** Traditionally, two sphincters are described. The ***internal sphincter*** consists of the smooth muscle of the bladder and proximal urethra, and the ***external sphincter*** consists of the periurethral striated muscle. However, more recent explanations of the components of the sphincter mechanism have challenged this conception, and it is better to describe a single mechanism consisting of elements of compression and elements of tension.

Elements of compression are necessary for the urethra to form a watertight seal between episodes of urination. The softness (collapsibility) of the urethral wall is important for continence, particularly when the urethral integrity is altered by placement of a catheter. The watertight seal of the urethra is further enhanced by the mucus produced by the epithelium. The mucus reduces surface tension, promoting collapse of the walls and sealing the microscopic fissures against urinary leakage.

The vascular cushion also acts as an element of compression in addition to producing tension, contributing to urethral closure during physical stress. The vascular cushion or network of the arterioles, venules, and arteriovenous communications in the urethra promotes urethral compression by transmitting pressure from the muscles surrounding the urethra and those intrinsic to its walls. The vascular cushion contributes to urethral closure pressure because it is filled with an incompressible fluid with its own intrinsic pressure.

The ***elements of tension*** in the urethral sphincter mechanism consist of the vascular cushion, intrinsic smooth and skeletal muscles, and periurethral striated muscle. These muscles are specially innervated to maintain tension needed for urethral closure between episodes of micturition and to provide an extra measure of urethral tension needed when significant physical exertion stresses sphincter closure. The pelvic muscles receive somatic innervation, allowing voluntary interruption of the urinary stream, as well as added protection against precipitous rises in abdominal pressure (Staskin and others, 1985).

Clinical Manifestations

As in most disorders of childhood, the incidence and type of kidney or urinary tract dysfunction change with the age and maturation of the child. In addition, the presenting complaints and the significance of these complaints vary with maturation. For example, a complaint of enuresis has greater significance at age 8 years than at age 4. In the newborn, urinary tract disorders are associated with a number of obvious malformations of other body systems, including the curious and unexplained but frequent association between malformed or low-set ears and urinary tract anomalies. Important signs and symptoms that suggest possible renal or genitourinary tract disease in children at different ages are outlined in the box on p. 1287.

Many of the clinical manifestations are common to a variety of childhood disorders, but their presence is an indication to obtain further information from the past history, family history, and laboratory studies as part of a complete physical examination. Suspected renal disease can be further evaluated by means of radiographic studies and renal biopsy.

SIGNS AND SYMPTOMS OF URINARY TRACT DISORDERS OR DISEASE AT DIFFERENT AGES

NEONATAL PERIOD (BIRTH TO 1 MONTH)

Poor feeding
Vomiting
Failure to gain weight
Rapid respiration (acidosis)
Respiratory distress
Spontaneous pneumothorax or pneumomediastinum
Frequent urination
Screaming on urination
Poor urinary stream
Jaundice
Seizures
Dehydration
Other anomalies or stigmata
Enlarged kidneys or bladder

INFANCY (1 TO 24 MONTHS)

Poor feeding
Vomiting
Failure to gain weight
Excessive thirst
Frequent urination
Straining or screaming on urination
Foul-smelling urine
Pallor
Fever
Persistent diaper rash
Seizures (with or without fever)
Dehydration
Enlarged kidneys or bladder

CHILDHOOD (2 TO 14 YEARS)

Poor appetite
Vomiting
Growth failure
Excessive thirst
Enuresis, incontinence, frequent urination
Painful urination
Swelling of face
Seizures
Pallor
Fatigue
Blood in urine
Abdominal or back pain
Edema
Hypertension
Tetany

Laboratory Tests

Both urine and blood studies contribute vital information for detection of renal problems. The single most important test is probably routine urinalysis. Specific urine and blood tests provide additional information.

Glomerular filtration rate is a measure of the amount of plasma from which a given substance is totally cleared in 1 minute. Clearance is calculated from the ratio of substance excreted to the concentration of that substance in the plasma. A number of substances can be used, but the most useful clinical estimation of glomerular filtration is the clearance of ***creatinine,*** an end product of protein metabolism in muscle and a substance that is freely filtered by the glomerulus and secreted by renal tubular cells. The production and secretion of creatinine remain relatively constant from day to day, and its appearance in the urine is determined by the serum level. When the collection is complete and accurately timed, the results are fairly reliable and compare favorably with clearance of other substances, such as inulin, that require special equipment to evaluate and long immobilization of the child.

Any significant degree of renal disease can diminish the glomerular filtration rate, but diseases of the glomerulus and renal vascular disease have the most immediate effect. The nurse's responsibility in this test is collection of urine, usually a 12- or 24-hour specimen.

The major urine and blood tests are outlined in Tables 30-1 and 30-2. Special tests and nursing responsibilities are briefly described in Table 30-3.

Nursing Considerations

Nursing responsibilities in assessment of renal disorders and/or diseases begins with observation of the child for any manifestations that might indicate dysfunction. The most significant ongoing assessments in children with renal conditions are accurate measurement and recording of ***weight; intake*** and ***output;*** and ***blood pressure*** (see Chapter 7) These assessments are necessary not only for children with known renal dysfunction, but also for those children at risk for developing renal complications (e.g., children in shock, postoperative patients).

In addition to the general manifestations of renal conditions (see box at left), many conditions have specific characteristics that distinguish them from other disorders. These are discussed as appropriate throughout the chapter.

The nurse is generally the one who is responsible for preparing infants, children, and parents for tests and collection of urine and (sometimes) blood specimens (see Preparation for Procedures, Chapter 27, and Collection of Specimens, Chapter 27, for observation and laboratory analysis). Nurses observe the characteristics of urine collected, often perform any of a number of tests on urine specimens (e.g., urine specific gravity, protein, blood, glucose, ketones), and assist with more complex diagnostic tests (e.g., radiography, cystoscopy). Nurses must be familiar with significant laboratory tests, their implications, and preprocedural care.

NURSING ALERT Use of Fleet enemas in children with acute or chronic renal failure is potentially lethal because of hyperphosphatemia. Requests for Fleet enemas in this situation should not be implemented without careful investigation.

GENITOURINARY TRACT DISORDERS

URINARY TRACT INFECTION (UTI)

UTI is a clinical condition that may involve the urethra, bladder (lower urinary tract), and/or the ureters, renal pelvis, calyces, and renal parenchyma (upper urinary tract). Because it is often impossible to localize the infection, the

TABLE 30-1 Urine Tests of Renal Function

TEST	NORMAL RANGE	DEVIATIONS	SIGNIFICANCE OF DEVIATIONS
PHYSICAL TESTS			
Volume	Age related	Polyuria	Osmotic factors (urinary glucose level in diabetes mellitus)
		Oliguria	Retention caused by obstructive disease Inadequate bladder emptying caused by neurogenic bladder or obstructive disorder
		Anuria	Obstruction of urinary tract; acute renal failure
Specific gravity	With normal fluid intake: 1.016-1.022 Newborn: 1.001-1.020	High	Dehydration Presence of protein or glucose Presence of radiopaque contrast medium after radiologic examinations
	Others: 1.001-1.030	Low	Excessive fluid intake Distal tubular dysfunction Insufficient antidiuretic hormone Diuresis
		Fixed at 1.010	Chronic glomerular disease
Osmolality	Newborn: 50-600 mOsm/L Thereafter: 50-1400 mOsm/L	High or low	Same as for specific gravity More sensitive index than specific gravity
Appearance	Clear pale yellow to deep gold	Cloudy Cloudy reddish pink to reddish brown Light Dark Red	Contains sediment Blood from trauma or disease Myoglobin following severe muscle destruction Dilute Concentrated Trauma
CHEMICAL TESTS			
pH	Newborn: 5-7 Thereafter: 4.8-7.8 Average: 6	Weak acid or neutral	If associated with metabolic acidosis, suggests tubular acidosis If associated with metabolic alkalosis, suggests potassium deficiency Urinary infection Metabolic alkalosis
		Alkaline	Metabolic alkalosis
Protein level	Absent	Present	Abnormal glomerular permeability (e.g., glomerular disease, changes in blood pressure) Most kidney disease Orthostatic in some individuals
Glucose level	Absent	Present	Diabetes mellitus Infusion of concentrated glucose-containing fluids Glomerulonephritis Impaired tubular reabsorption
Ketone levels	Absent	Present	Conditions of acute metabolic demand (stress) Diabetic ketoacidosis
Leukocyte esterase	Absent	Present	Can identify both lysed and intact white blood cells via enzyme detection
Nitrites	Absent	Present	Most species of bacteria convert nitrates to nitrites in the urine
MICROSCOPIC TESTS			
White blood cell count	Less than 1 or 2	More than 5 polymorphonuclear leukocytes/field	Urinary tract inflammatory process
		Lymphocytes	Allograft rejection Malignancy
Red blood cell count	Less than 1 or 2	4-6/field in centrifuged specimen	Trauma Stones Glomerular injury Infection Neoplasms

TABLE 30-1 Urine Tests of Renal Function—cont'd

TEST	NORMAL RANGE	DEVIATIONS	SIGNIFICANCE OF DEVIATIONS
Presence of bacteria	Absent to a few	More than 100,000 organisms/ml in centrifuged specimen	Urinary tract infection
Presence of casts	Occasional	Granular casts	Tubular or glomerular disorders Degenerative process in advanced renal disease
		Cellular casts White blood cell Red blood cell Hyaline casts	Pyelonephritis Glomerulonephritis Proteinuria; usually transient

TABLE 30-2 Blood Tests of Renal Function

TEST	NORMAL RANGE (mg/dl)	DEVIATIONS	SIGNIFICANCE OF DEVIATIONS
Blood urea nitrogen (BUN)	Newborn: 4-18 Infant, child: 5-18	Elevated	Renal disease—acute or chronic (the higher the BUN, the more severe the disease) Increased protein catabolism Dehydration Hemorrhage High protein intake Corticosteroid therapy
Uric acid	Child: 2.0-5.5	Increased	Severe renal disease
Creatinine	Infant: 0.2-0.4 Child: 0.3-0.7 Adolescent: 0.5-1.0	Increased	Severe renal impairment

broad designation UTI is applied to the presence of significant numbers of microorganisms anywhere within the urinary tract (except the distal one third of the urethra, which is usually colonized with bacteria).

Infection of the urinary tract may be present with or without clinical symptoms. As a result, the site of infection is often difficult to pinpoint with accuracy. Various terms used to describe urinary tract disorders are listed in the box at right.

The peak incidence of UTI not caused by structural anomalies occurs between 2 and 6 years of age. Except for the neonatal period, females have a 10 to 30 times greater risk for developing UTI than males. Approximately 3% to 5% of girls will have one or more episodes of UTI before puberty (Jodal and Winberg, 1987). The likelihood of recurrence is 50% or greater in girls; the recurrence rate is lower in boys (Edelmann, 1988).

UTI in newborns differs in some respects from infections occurring in older children. In this group males outnumber females. The rate of recurrence of UTI in neonates is estimated at 25% (Cepero-Akselrad, Ramirez-Seijas, and

CLASSIFICATIONS OF URINARY TRACT INFECTIONS OR INFLAMMATIONS

Bacteriuria—Presence of bacteria in the urine
Asymptomatic bacteriuria—Significant bacteriuria with no evidence of clinical infection (usually defined as greater than 100,000 colony-forming units [CFU])
Symptomatic bacteriuria—Bacteriuria accompanied by physical signs of urinary infection (dysuria, suprapubic discomfort, hematuria, fever)
Recurrent UTI—Repeated episode of bacteriuria or symptomatic UTI
Persistent UTI—Persistence of bacteriuria despite antibiotic treatment
Febrile UTI—Bacteriuria accompanied by fever and other physical signs of urinary infection; presence of a fever typically implies a pyelonephritis
Cystitis—Inflammation of the bladder
Urethritis—Inflammation of the urethra
Pyelonephritis—Inflammation of the upper urinary tract and kidneys
Urosepsis—Febrile urinary tract infection coexisting with systemic signs of bacterial illness; blood culture reveals presence of urinary pathogen

TABLE 30-3 Radiologic and Other Tests of Urinary System Function

TEST	PROCEDURE	PURPOSE	COMMENTS AND NURSING RESPONSIBILITIES
Intravenous pyelography (IVP) (intravenous urogram; excretory urogram)	Intravenous injection of a contrast medium Medium secreted and concentrated by tubules X-ray films made 5, 10, and 15 minutes after injection; delayed films (30, 60 minutes, etc.) are obtained if obstruction suspected	Defines urinary tract Provides information about integrity of kidneys, ureters, and bladder Retroperitoneal masses visualized when they shift position of ureters	Preparation for test: Infants less than 2 years of age—no solid food, omit one bottle on morning of examination; studies should be done early to avoid withholding of fluids Children aged 2-14 years—give cathartic evening before examination, nothing orally after midnight,* enema (Fleet [See Nursing Alert, p. 1287] or soapsuds) morning of examination
Retrograde pyelography	Contrast medium injected through ureteral catheter	Visualizes pelvic calyces, ureters, and bladder	Prepare the child for cystoscopy
Renal angiography	Contrast medium injected directly into renal artery via catheter placed in femoral artery (or umbilical artery in newborn) and advanced to renal artery	Visualizes renal vascular system, especially for renal arterial stenosis	Give cathartic if ordered Give preoperative medication if ordered Observe for reaction to contrast medium Monitor vital signs following procedure
Radioisotope imaging studies	Contrast medium injected intravenously; computer analysis to measure uptake or washout (excretion) for analysis of organ function	*DTPA* radioisotope used to measure glomerular filtration rate; estimate of differential renal function and renal washout to determine presence and location of upper urinary tract obstruction *DMSA* radioisotope allows visualization of renal scars and differential renal function; ureters and bladder are not visualized *MAG 3* radioisotope combines features of DTPA (evaluation of upper urinary tract obstruction) with features of DMSA radioisotope (differential renal function)	Insert or assist with insertion of intravenous infusion Monitor intravenous infusion Urethral catheterization may accompany DTPA radioisotope scan; prepare child for catheterization when indicated
Voiding cystourethrography	Contrast medium injected into bladder through urethral catheter until bladder is full; films taken before, during, and after voiding	Visualizes bladder outline and urethra, reveals reflux of urine into ureters, and shows complications of bladder emptying	Prepare child for catheterization
Radionuclide (nuclear) cystogram	Radionuclide-containing fluid injected through urethral catheter until bladder is full; images generated before, during, and after voiding	Alternative to voiding cystourethrography in children with allergy to intravesical contrast material Allows evaluation of reflux, although visualization of anatomic details is relatively poor	Prepare child for catheterization Reassure patient and parents that allergic response to contrast materials is avoided by use of radionuclide
Scout film	Flat plate roentgenogram of abdomen and pelvis for kidney, ureters, bladder (KUB)	Detects and establishes renal outlines, presence of calculi, or opaque foreign bodies in bladder	Prepare as for routine x-ray film
Cystoscopy	Direct visualization of bladder and lower urinary tract through small scope inserted via urethra	Investigation of bladder and lower tract lesions; visualizes urethral openings, bladder wall, trigone, and urethra	Give nothing orally after midnight* Carry out preoperative preparations

*Current research supports oral intake of clear fluids up to 2 hours before test (see Surgical Procedures, Chapter 27).

TABLE 30-3 Radiologic and Other Tests of Urinary System Function—cont'd

TEST	PROCEDURE	PURPOSE	COMMENTS AND NURSING RESPONSIBILITIES
Renal biopsy	Removal of kidney tissue by open or percutaneous technique for study by light, electron, or immunofluorescent microscopy	Yields histologic and microscopic information about glomeruli and tubules; helps to distinguish between types of nephrotic syndromes Distinguishes other renal disorders	Give nothing orally 4-6 hours before test* Premedicate as ordered Prepare setup for procedure Assist with procedure Take vital signs Apply pressure to area with pressure dressing and, if feasible, a sandbag Bed rest for 24 hours Observe for abdominal pain, tenderness Monitor input and output; surgical incision may be required in infants
Renal/bladder ultrasound	Transmission of ultrasonic waves through renal parenchyma, along ureteral course, and over bladder	Allows visualization of renal parenchyma, renal pelvis without exposure to external beam radiation or radioactive isotopes Visualization of dilated ureters and bladder wall also possible	Noninvasive procedure
Testicular (scrotal) ultrasound	Transmission of ultrasonic waves through scrotal contents and testis	Allows visualization of scrotal contents, including testis Testicular ultrasound is used to identify masses, and Doppler-enhanced ultrasound is used to differentiate hyperemia of epididymo-orchitis from ischemia of torsion	Noninvasive procedure
Computed tomography (CT)	Narrow-beam x-rays and computer analysis provide precise reconstruction of area	Visualizes vertical or horizontal cross section of kidney Especially valuable to distinguish tumors and cysts	Noncontrast scan is noninvasive Contrast enhanced CT scan preparation is similar to IVP
Urine culture and sensitivity	Collection of sterile specimen	Determines presence of pathogens and the drugs to which they are sensitive	Does not require specific parental permission Send specimen to laboratory immediately after collection Catherization, clean-catch, or suprapubic specimen
Urodynamics	Set of tests designed to measure bladder filling, storage, and evacuation functions Uroflowmetry is a test to determine efficiency of urination Cystometrogram is a graphic comparison of bladder pressure as a function of volume Sphincter electromyogram is a test of pelvic muscle function during bladder filling and evacuation Voiding pressure study is a comparison of detrusor contraction pressure, sphincter EMG, and urinary flow	Determine characteristics of voiding dysfunction Used to identify type (cause) of incontinence or urinary retention Especially valuable for voiding dysfunction complicated by urinary infection, urinary retention, or neurogenic bladder dysfunction	Prepare child for catheterization Insertion of a rectal tube will produce feelings of rectal fullness or pressure Insertion of needles may be required for sphincter electromyography
Whitaker perfusion test	Injection of contrast material through renal pelvis and ureters Pressures are measured in renal pelvis and urinary bladder	Determine presence of obstruction causing upper urinary tract dilation	Prepare child for insertion of a spinal needle or perfusion catheter in renal pelvis (anesthesia often required)

Castaneda, 1993). At all ages asymptomatic bacteriuria is more common than symptomatic disease, and recurrence is not uncommon, especially in girls. The overall recurrence rate in older children is estimated at 30% (Cepero-Akselrad, Ramirez-Seijas, and Castaneda, 1993). An increased incidence of UTI is observed in adolescents, especially those with evidence of sexual activity.

Etiology

A variety of organisms can be responsible for UTI. *Escherichia coli* (80% of cases) and other gram-negative enteric organisms are most frequently implicated; all are common to the anal, perineal, and perianal region. Other organisms associated with UTI include *Proteus, Pseudomonas, Klebsiella, Staphylococcus aureus, Haemophilus,* and coagulase-negative *Staphylococcus.* A number of factors contribute to the development of UTI. These include anatomic, physical, and chemical conditions or properties of the host urinary tract.

Anatomic and Physical Factors. The structure of the lower urinary tract is believed to account for the increased incidence of bacteriuria in females. The short urethra, which measures about 2 cm (¾ inch) in young females and 4 cm (1½ inches) in mature women, provides a ready pathway for invasion of organisms. In addition, the closure of the urethra at the end of micturition may return contaminated bacteria to the bladder.

The longer male urethra (as long as 20 cm [8 inches] in an adult) and the antibacterial properties of prostatic secretions inhibit the entry and growth of pathogens. Reports indicate an increased incidence of UTI in infants less than 1 year of age who are not circumcised as compared with infants who are circumcised (Herzog, 1989; Roberts, 1988; Wiswell and Geschke, 1989). The presence of a foreskin is associated with a greater quantity of periurethral bacteria that can ascend the urethra easily (Wiswell and others, 1988; Fussell and others, 1988). The incidence of renal scarring is greatest in patients whose first infection occurs during infancy.

The single most important host factor influencing the occurrence of UTI is urinary stasis. Ordinarily urine is sterile, but at 37° C (98.6° F) it provides an excellent culture medium. Under normal conditions the act of completely and repeatedly emptying the bladder flushes away any organisms before they have an opportunity to multiply and invade surrounding tissue. However, urine that remains in the bladder allows bacteria from the urethra to rapidly become established in the rich medium.

Incomplete bladder emptying (stasis) may result from reflux (see p. 1295 for a discussion of reflux), anatomic abnormalities (especially those involving the ureters), dysfunction of the voiding mechanism, or extrinsic ureteral or bladder compression. The pressure of overdistention within the bladder may increase the risk of infection by decreasing host resistance, probably as a result of lessened blood flow to the mucosa. This frequently occurs in neurogenic bladder or as a consequence of voluntarily holding back urine despite the urge to void.

Extrinsic factors that may be responsible for functional bladder neck obstruction are chronic and intermittent constipation and pregnancy. In both conditions, the full rectum or uterus displaces the bladder and posterior urethra in the fixed and limited space of the bony pelvis, causing obstruction, incomplete micturition, and urinary stasis. Treating constipation along with antibiotic therapy for UTI reduces the recurrence of infection, whereas failure to relieve the fecal retention in spite of adequate treatment of the UTI may result in recurrence.

Other extrinsic factors that can contribute to UTI include catheters, especially short-term indwelling catheters, and administration of antimicrobial agents. Antimicrobials alter the host's normal perineal flora, allowing easier colonization with uropathogens. Tight clothing or diapers, poor hygiene, and local inflammation, such as from vaginitis, masturbation, or pinworm infestation, may also increase the risk of ascending infection. The essential oils in bubble baths and shampoos can irritate the urethra of both boys and girls, causing painful and frequent urination. Consequently, bubble baths are discouraged. There is no evidence that plain tub baths increase the risk of UTI, but infections have been related to the use of hot tub or whirlpool baths. Sexual intercourse may produce transient bacteriuria in females and is associated with an increased risk of UTI.

Altered Urine and Bladder Chemistry. Several mechanical and chemical characteristics of the urinary tract promote urine sterility. Adequate fluid intake promotes urinary transport and lowers the concentration of pathogens (and nutrients) in the urine. Diuresis also enhances the antibacterial properties of the renal medulla, probably as a result of increased blood flow hastening leukocytosis and promoting mechanical removal of pathogens.

While many common urinary pathogens favor an alkaline medium, the urine is slightly acidic. Intake of specific beverages, including cranberry or apple juice and ascorbic acid, has been recommended to lower the urinary pH, increasing its antiinfective potential. The intake of cranberry juice (300 ml/day) reduced the frequency of bacteriuria with pyuria in older women (Avorn and others, 1994). Similar research is needed in children, especially with juices, such as cranberry-apple, that may appeal more to children.

Pathophysiology

Following invasion by bacteria, the lower urinary tract's first line of defense is complete evacuation by voiding. Inflammation in the bladder and urethral walls will be apparent within 30 minutes of invasion by a bacterial pathogen. Polymorphoneucleocytes rapidly migrate to the bladder wall, which will become completely injected within 2 hours. Complete evacuation of the bladder is particularly important for the eradication of bacteria from the urine. Urination not only removes bacteria and associated toxins contained in the urine, it also allows more efficient destruction of remaining bacteria left on the thin film of urine that is closely adherent to the vesical wall.

Recurrent infection of the urinary bladder predisposes the individual to transient episodes of vesicoureteric reflux. Following resolution of the infection, the reflux is not detectable on voiding cystourethrography. While it is known that certain adherent bacteria promote urinary system dilation, the relationship between bladder wall inflammation and utereovesical junction competence remains unclear (Kramer, 1992).

Clinical Manifestations

The clinical manifestations of UTIs depend on the age of the child. In newborn infants and children less than 2 years of age the signs are characteristically nonspecific. They more nearly resemble gastrointestinal tract disorders: failure to thrive, feeding problems, vomiting, diarrhea, abdominal distention, and jaundice. Newborns may have fever or hypothermia and/or sepsis. Other evidence that may be observed includes frequent or infrequent voiding, constant squirming and irritability, strong-smelling urine, and abnormal stream. A persistent diaper rash may also be a helpful clue.

The classic symptoms of UTI are often observed in children over 2 years of age. These include enuresis or daytime incontinence in the child who has been been toilet trained, fever, strong- or foul-smelling urine, increased frequency of urination, dysuria, or urgency. They may also complain of abdominal pain or costovertebral angle tenderness (flank pain). Some will present with hematuria; preschoolers may vomit. There is a high frequency of obstructive uropathy in young infants and boys that is characterized by dribbling of urine, straining with urination, or a decrease in the force and size of the urinary stream. High fever and chills accompanied by flank pain, severe abdominal pain, and leukocytosis suggest pyelonephritis. However, flank pain and tenderness may be the only indication of pyelonephritis on physical examination.

Manifestations in adolescents are more specific. Symptoms of lower tract infections include frequency and painful urination of a small amount of turbulent urine that may be grossly bloody. Fever is usually absent. Upper tract infection is characterized by fever, chills, flank pain, and lower tract symptoms, which may appear 1 or 2 days after the upper tract symptoms.

Many UTIs in children are asymptomatic or atypical in clinical presentation, and many complaints may be unrelated to the urinary tract. Many are treated as respiratory or gastrointestinal infections. It is important that these children be identified so that treatment can be initiated. Significant scarring can take place, especially in infants and very young children.

Diagnostic Evaluation

The diagnosis of UTI depends on a high degree of suspicion, evaluation of the history and physical examination, and urinalysis and culture. Urine characteristic of possible infection appears cloudy, hazy, or thick with noticeable strands of mucus and pus; it also smells fishy and unpleasant even when fresh. A presumptive UTI diagnosis can be made on the basis of microscopic examination of the urine, which often reveals pyuria (5 to 8 white blood cells/ml of uncentrifuged urine) and the presence of at least one bacterium in a Gram stain. However, a normal urinalysis may also be present in conditions of asymptomatic bacteriuria.

The diagnosis of UTI is confirmed by the detection of bacteria in a urine culture, but urine collection is often difficult, especially in infants and very small children (see Collection of Specimens, Chapter 27). Several factors may alter a urine specimen. Contamination of a specimen by organisms from sources other than the urine is the most frequent cause of false-positive results. Bag urine specimens are frequently contaminated by perineal and perianal flora and are usually considered inadequate for a definitive diagnosis. Clean-catch urine specimens have been determined to be no better than a regular midstream specimen. Unless the specimen is a first morning sample, a recent high fluid intake may indicate a falsely low organism count. Therefore children should not be encouraged to drink large volumes of water in an attempt to obtain a specimen quickly.

The most accurate tests of bacterial content are suprapubic aspiration (children less than 2 years of age) and properly performed bladder catheterization (as long as the first few milliliters are excluded from collection). Care of a urine specimen obtained for culture is an important nursing aspect related to diagnosis. The specimen should be taken to the laboratory for culture immediately. If culture is delayed, the sample can be placed in a refrigerator for up to 24 hours, but storage can result in loss of formed elements such as blood cells and casts (Bailie, 1986).

Tests to detect bacteriuria are being used with increased frequency in screening for UTI. The plastic dipstick, Chemstrip, and agar-coated slide tests are quick and inexpensive methods for detecting infection before obtaining final culture results. The presence of nitrites on dipstick analysis of urine has been shown to have a predictive value of as much as 100% (Lohr and others, 1993). The absence of nitrites and leukocyte esterase in combination has been shown to have 100% negative predictive value (Woodward and Griffiths, 1993) (see Table 30-1). These test results are being used to initiate treatment of UTI while culture results are pending. It is important to remember that some organisms that cause urinary tract infections are non–nitrite producing (e.g., pseudomonas).

Localization of the infection site may involve more specific tests, including ureteral catheterization, bladder washout procedures, and radioisotope renography. Other tests, such as ultrasonography, voiding cystourethrogram (VCUG), intravenous pyelogram (IVP), and DSMA (dimercaptosuccinic acid) scan may be performed after the infection subsides to identify anatomic abnormalities contributing to the development of infection and existing kidney changes from recurrent infection.

Therapeutic Management

The objectives of treatment of children with UTI are to (1) eliminate current infection, (2) identify contributing factors to reduce the risk of recurrence, (3) prevent systemic spread of the infection, and (4) preserve renal function (Rushton, 1992). Antibiotic therapy is guided by laboratory culture and sensitivity tests. Nonetheless, empiric therapy, based on the child's past history and presenting symptoms, may be necessary when fever or systemic illness complicates UTI. Common antiinfective agents used for UTI include the penicillins, sulfonamide (including trimethoprim and sul-

TABLE 30-4 Common Side Effects of Urinary Antiinfective Drugs

DRUG	SIDE EFFECTS	NURSING MANAGEMENT
Trimethoprim/sulfamethoxazole (Bactrim, Septra)	Renal toxicity	Administer with water, maintain adequate fluid intake
Nitrofurantoin (Macrodantin)	Nausea/gastrointestinal upset	Administer with meals or snack
Carbenicillin (Geocillin, Geopen)	Diarrhea	Administer with Lactinex, 2 tablets, given with antibiotic
	Nausea related to medication odor, foul taste	Administer with ice water; advise patient to swallow rapidly and avoid smelling drug; drug may need to be discontinued if intolerance is marked
Cephalexin (Keflex)	Nausea, mild diarrhea	Administer with meals or snack

Modified from Gray M: *Genitourinary disorders,* St Louis, 1992, Mosby.

fisoxazole in combination), the cephalosporins, nitrofurantoin, and the tetracyclines. All antibiotics may cause side effects or may prove ineffective because of bacterial resistance (Table 30-4).

Children with suspected pyelonephritis and fever are admitted to the hospital and given appropriate antibiotics intravenously for a minimum of 48 hours. Blood and urine cultures are obtained on admission and following therapy. Urine cultures are usually repeated at monthly intervals for 3 months and at 3-month intervals for 6 months. Children under age 5 years with a documented UTI, regardless of gender, should have radiographic evaluation (Andrich and Majd, 1992; Cepero-Akselrad, Ramirez-Seijas, and Castaneda, 1992). If anatomic defects such as primary reflux or bladder neck obstruction are present, surgical correction of these abnormalities may be necessary to prevent recurrent infection or may indicate the need for prophylactic antibiotics and careful follow-up. Follow-up study is an important component of medical management, since the relapse rate is high and recurrent infection tends to occur 1 to 2 months after termination of treatment. The aim of therapy and careful follow-up in such cases is to prevent morbidity and reduce the chance of renal scarring.

Prognosis. With prompt and adequate treatment at the time of diagnosis, the long-term prognosis for UTIs is usually excellent. However, the hazard of progressive renal injury is greatest when infection occurs in young children (especially under 2 years of age) and is associated with congenital renal malformations and reflux. Therefore early diagnosis of children at risk is particularly important during infancy and toddlerhood.

Nursing Considerations

Objectives of nursing care include identification of children with UTI and education of parents and child regarding prevention and treatment of infection. Aside from the influence of renal abnormalities, females between the ages of 2 and 6 years are in general a high-risk group. Since they are not a captive population, mass screening is difficult. However, the annual health examination should include a routine urinalysis. In addition, nurses should instruct parents to observe regularly for clues suggesting UTI. Unfortunately, the signs of UTI are not as evident as those of upper respiratory tract infection. Therefore many cases go undetected because no one thought to investigate this very common problem.

NURSING ALERT A child who exhibits the following should be evaluated for urinary tract infection:
Incontinence in a toilet-trained child
Strong-smelling urine
Frequency and/or urgency

Since infants and young children are unable to express their feelings and sensations verbally, it is difficult to detect discomfort they may be experiencing from dysuria. A careful history regarding voiding habits, stooling pattern, and episodes of unexplained irritability may assist in detecting less obvious cases of UTI. Consequently, parents should be encouraged to observe for specific clues of UTI in suspected cases (see Critical Thinking Exercise box).

When infection is suspected, collecting an appropriate specimen is essential. It is the nurse's responsibility to take every precaution to obtain acceptable, clean-voided specimens in order to avoid the use of other collecting procedures except when absolutely indicated.

➤ **NURSING TIP** To detect UTI in infants and toddlers, check the diaper every ½ hour (increases the opportunity for observing the stream for such findings as straining or fretting before voiding begins, signs of discomfort before and during urinating, intermittent starting and stopping of the stream, and frequent dripping of small amounts of urine).

Frequently other tests are performed to detect anatomic defects. Children are prepared for these tests as appropriate for their age. Children who are old enough to understand need an explanation of the procedure, its purpose, and what they will experience (see Preparation for Procedures, Chapter 27). Sometimes a simple description of the urinary system is helpful. Especially for preschool children, the nurse must clarify that the urinary tract is separate from any sexual function and that the test is for a problem that

CRITICAL THINKING EXERCISE

Urinary Tract Infection and Constipation

During your assessment of Ginger, a 4-year-old admitted to the hospital for severe urinary tract infection, her mother tells you that Ginger has bowel movements every third to fourth day. They are usually large, hard-formed stools, and Ginger sometimes has trouble evacuating the stool. You should:

1. Explain to the mother that this may be normal for Ginger, because her mother has the same pattern and Ginger will have less trouble as she gets older.
2. Explain to the mother the relationship of diet to constipation as you develop a line of inquiry to elicit the fat content of Ginger's diet.
3. Explain to the mother that the diarrhea associated with the antibiotics Ginger is now receiving should correct the constipation.
4. Explain to the mother the relationship between chronic constipation and urinary tract infections as you move into a complete elimination history.

The correct response is 4. While Ginger may have an elimination pattern similar to her mother's, 3 to 4 days is a long interval between stools, even for an adult. In this instance the presence of a large stool mass within the colon is likely to cause pressure on the bladder and urethra and not allow the bladder to empty completely. Stasis of urine within the bladder can then lead to infection. While a diet and fluid intake history is part of the assessment of children with urinary tract infections and constipation, the fat content of Ginger's diet is not the most critical information at this time. Finally, Ginger may or may not develop diarrhea secondary to her antibiotic regimen. However, one bout of diarrhea will not eliminate the constipation, which has been present over a long period of time.

they did not cause. It is not uncommon for children to associate blame for perceived wrongdoing (e.g., masturbation) or unacceptable thoughts with the reason for the illness or the tests. For young children under 3 to 4 years of age, the procedure can be explained on a doll. For those who are older, a simple drawing of the bladder, urethra, ureters, and kidneys makes the explanation more understandable.

Children may be treated as outpatients to avoid overnight separation from home for such procedures. In such cases nurses must be careful not to overlook the need for adequate preparation so that if surgery is subsequently indicated, the child will be able to encounter the impending operation with facts and understanding from these procedures, which will help to decrease fear and anxiety of more extensive medical-surgical intervention.

Since antiinfective drugs are indicated in treatment of UTI, the nurse teaches the patient and parents the appropriate dosage and scheduling and provides suggestions for administration of the agent.* Certain drugs are available in liquid form; others are available in a capsule or pill form only. Generally, capsules can be separated or pills crushed, and their contents may be mixed with a small volume of food or chilled liquid to mask a disagreeable taste. A simple suggestion is to introduce a medicine in divided doses mixed with a flavored gelatin in an ice cube tray. Other medications are best tolerated with a small portion of partly frozen grape or apple juice.

*Home care instructions for giving medications to children are available in *Wong and Whaley's Clinical Manual of Pediatric Nursing* (Mosby).

Adequate fluid intake is always indicated during an acute UTI. It is recommended that a person drink 30 ml/kg, or approximately 15 ml/lb of body weight (Pearson and Larson, 1992). In certain instances forcing fluids (drinking greater than 15 ml/lb of body weight) may be feasible. The patient should primarily drink clear liquids. Caffeinic beverages or carbonated beverages are avoided, since they have a potentially irritative effect on the bladder mucosa. The child who is febrile and unable to drink liquids is given intravenous hydration until the fever resolves and oral liquids are tolerated.

Prevention. Prevention is the most important goal in both primary and recurrent infection, and most preventive measures are simple, ordinary hygienic habits that should be a routine part of daily care. Any signs of intestinal parasites (e.g., scratching between the legs and around anal area) should be investigated and treated appropriately. Sexually active adolescent females are advised to urinate as soon as possible after intercourse to flush out bacteria introduced during sex play. Parents and older children are taught health practices that prevent UTI (see Guidelines box, p. 1296).

Children who experience recurrent febrile UTIs or those with recurrent infections complicated by vesicoureteric reflux may be given a suppressive or prophylactic antibiotic for a period of months or several years. The medication is commonly administered once a day; the patient and parents are advised to give the antibiotic before sleep, since this represents the longest period without voiding. A sulfonamide/trimethoprim, nitrofurantoin, or cephalosporin is often used for antibiotic prophylaxis.

VESICOURETERAL REFLUX (VUR)

VUR refers to the retrograde flow of bladder urine into the ureters. Reflux increases the chance for and perpetuates infection, since with each void urine is swept up the ureters and then allowed to empty after voiding. Therefore the residual urine from the ureters remains in the bladder until the next void. The International Classification System describes the degree of reflux from the bladder into upper genitourinary tract structures (see box on p. 1296).

Primary reflux results from a congenital anomaly affecting the ureterovesical junction. Ectopic or orthotopic implantation of the ureter, abnormal tunneling of the intramural ureteral segment, and defects in the configuration of the ureteral orifice are associated with primary reflux. Primary reflux has shown a familial pattern; the incidence of reflux in siblings of affected children is as high as 45%. ***Secondary reflux*** occurs as a result of an acquired condition. UTI can produce transient reflux, and children with reflux

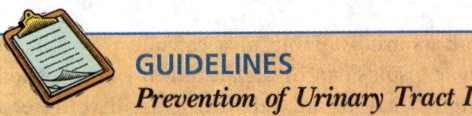

GUIDELINES
Prevention of Urinary Tract Infection

FACTORS PREDISPOSING TO DEVELOPMENT	MEASURES OF PREVENTION
Short female urethra close to vagina and anus	Perineal hygiene—wipe from front to back Avoid tight clothing or diapers; wear cotton panties rather than nylon Check for vaginitis or pinworms, especially if child scratches between legs
Incomplete emptying (reflux) and overdistention of bladder	Avoid "holding" urine; encourage child to void frequently, especially before a long trip or other circumstances where toilet facilities are not available Empty bladder completely with each void Avoid straining at stool
Concentrated and alkaline urine	Encourage generous fluid intake Acidify urine with juices such as cranberry and a diet high in animal protein

are at greater risk for recurrent (and febrile) urinary infections. Neuropathic bladder dysfunction, particularly when poor bladder compliance coexists with bladder outlet obstruction, may produce reflux as urine seeks to escape the high pressures of the lower urinary tract. VUR has also been associated with ureteropelvic junction (UPJ) obstruction. Whether this reflux is primary or secondary to the UPJ obstruction is unknown (Kramer, 1992).

Reflux with infection can lead to kidney damage, since refluxed urine ascending into the collecting tubules of the nephrons allows the microorganisms to gain access to the renal parenchyma, initiating renal scarring. The shape of renal papillae and the angle of entry of collecting ducts change with advancing age, making intrarenal reflux difficult. Therefore most renal scars associated with reflux occur at a very young age and are present at the time of diagnosis; few develop after 5 years of age. However, between 30% and 60% of children with VUR have evidence of renal scarring, and scarring is almost always found in association with reflux. Therefore VUR is an important cause of renal damage, and careful examination for its presence is indicated. Careful routine follow-up is a critical part of management of children with UTIs, and children with reflux, documented by voiding cystoureterography, are assessed repeatedly during ensuing years.

Therapeutic Management

Conservative, nonoperative therapy is effective in controlling infection in most cases of VUR. There is a high incidence of spontaneous resolution over time—approximately 20% to 30% for each 2-year period throughout childhood. An 80% probability of remission may occur in grades I and II reflux when managed medically (Hensle and Burbige, 1986). Therapy consists of continuous low-dose antibacterial therapy with frequent urine cultures, which can usually be done at home by the dip slide or Chemstrip methods. This long-term therapy requires medical supervision and reliable, cooperative parents. Surgical correction of reflux may be required for grades IV and V reflux. Grade III is managed conservatively unless there are complications.

VESICOURETERAL REFLUX GRADING SYSTEM

Grade I:	VUR into the lower ureter only
Grade II:	Ureteral and pelvic filling without calyceal dilation
Grade III:	Ureteral and pelvic filling with mild calyceal blunting
Grade IV:	Marked distention of pelvis, calyces, and ureter
Grade V:	Massive VUR associated with severe hydronephrosis

The major indications for surgical intervention include significant anatomic abnormality at the ureterovesical junction, recurrent UTIs, high grades of VUR, noncompliance with medical therapy, intolerance to antibiotics, and VUR after puberty in females. Antireflux surgery consists of reimplantation of the ureters. Postsurgical antibiotic therapy is continued until a voiding cystourethrogram demonstrates no further VUR. Postoperative excretory urograms are performed before discharge, at 3 months, and at 1 year and 3 years after surgery to assess renal growth. Accelerated renal growth is observed in some children after surgery.

Nursing Considerations

The primary nursing goal in children receiving medical therapy is encouraging compliance. The importance of maintaining the medical regimen should be emphasized to parents and older children. The medications prescribed are usually well tolerated by children, but parents may need help in encouraging children to take the medication. The methods described in Chapter 27 provide some guidelines for administration and encouraging compliance. The importance of hygiene and a frequent voiding schedule are also discussed.

GLOMERULAR DISEASE

ACUTE GLOMERULONEPHRITIS (AGN)

AGN as a classification includes a number of distinct entities. It may be a primary event or a manifestation of a systemic disorder (Table 30-5), and the disease can range from minimal to severe. The common features include oliguria, edema, hypertension and circulatory congestion, hematuria, and proteinuria. Most are postinfectious and have been associated with pneumococcal, streptococcal, and viral in-

TABLE 30-5 Renal Involvement Associated with a Systemic Disease Process

DISEASE	MECHANISM	RENAL MANIFESTATION	COMMENTS
Systemic lupus erythematosus (SLE)	Deposition of autoantibody-antigen complexes in kidney	Variable degrees of hematuria and proteinuria More severe—nephrotic syndrome, hypertension, renal insufficiency	Responsive to corticosteroid and antimetabolite therapy Renal failure most common cause of death from SLE Rare before adolescence but may occur in school-age children
Anaphylactoid (Henoch-Schönlein) purpura	Unknown	Hematuria (gross or microscopic) Less common—edema, hypertension Nephrotic syndrome with oliguria and hypertension indicates severe involvement Rarely—acute renal failure	Incidence from 20% to 70% of cases Renal involvement most serious manifestation of the disease More common in children over age 6 years Responsive to corticosteroid therapy Management similar to that for persistent glomerulonephritis
Sickle cell disease	Infarction of renal vessels by sickled cells (especially medullary) Results in decreased circulation in vasa recta and impaired sodium and chloride ion reabsorption in collecting ducts	Hematuria Nephrotic syndrome Defective urine collection Progressive glomerulonephritis	Irreversible with increasing age Severe urinary tract infections with bacteremia not uncommon
Polyarteritis nodosa	Fibroid necrosis of arterial walls Large vessels—patchy renal infarction Microscopic vessels—necrotizing glomerulitis	Proteinuria Hematuria Severe hypertension	Kidney involvement of secondary importance in infancy Variable course Long-term prognosis guarded
Bacterial endocarditis	Focal or diffuse, immune-complex deposition related to chronic bacteremia Some embolization of glomeruli by bacteria and fibrin from endocardial vegetations	Proteinuria Hematuria	Seen in about 50% of cases Renal involvement seldom of major significance
Prolonged bacteremia (infected atrioventricular shunts)	Immune-complex deposition with exudation and cellular proliferation	Variable degrees of persistent nephrotic syndrome	Vigorous antibiotic therapy and/or removal of infected shunt required

fections. All postinfectious diseases are presumed to result from immune complex formation and glomerular deposition, and the clinical presentations may be indistinguishable.

Acute poststreptococcal glomerulonephritis (APSGN) is the most common of the noninfectious renal diseases in childhood and the one for which a cause can be established in the majority of cases. APSGN can occur at any age but affects primarily early school-age children, with a peak age of onset of 6 to 7 years. It is uncommon in children younger than 2 years of age, and males outnumber females 2:1 (Jordan and Lemire, 1982).

Etiology

It is now generally accepted that APSGN is an immune-complex disease (i.e., a reaction that occurs as a by-product of an antecedent streptococcal infection with certain strains of the group A β-hemolytic streptococcus). Most streptococcal infections do not cause APSGN. A latent period of 10 to 14 days occurs between the streptococcal infection and the onset of clinical manifestations. The peak incidence of disease corresponds to the incidence of streptococcal infections. Disease secondary to streptococcal pharyngitis is more common in the winter or spring, but when associated with pyoderma (principally impetigo), it may be more prevalent in later summer or early fall, especially in warmer climates. Multiple cases tend to occur in families. Second attacks are rare.

Pathophysiology

The mechanism by which the reaction takes place is still speculative. The most popular proposal to explain the pathologic process is that the streptococcal infection is followed by the release of a membranelike material from the specific organism into the circulation. Because it is antigenic, antibody is formed, and after the appropriate period of time, an immune-complex reaction occurs. These immune complexes become trapped in the glomerular capillary loop.

The kidney itself appears normal or moderately enlarged, but microscopic examination reveals a diffuse proliferative and exudative process. Glomerular capillary loops are almost obliterated by swelling, and infiltration with polymorphonuclear leukocytes adds to the appearance of increased cellularity. Consequently, the glomeruli appear dense and bloodless. Further examination reveals discrete nodules or "humps" on the basement membrane, which are identified as deposits of immune complexes. These deposits are not evident after about 6 weeks.

Endothelial cell proliferation and edema occlude the capillary lumen of affected glomeruli, and the afferent arteriole is probably constricted by vasospasm, both of which significantly reduce the glomerular filtration rate. This occurs without a proportional decrease in renal blood flow and results in a reduced capacity to form filtrate from the glomerular plasma flow. Vascular and tubular changes are mild and nonspecific; therefore, tubular function is less severely impaired.

The decreased filtration of plasma results in an excessive accumulation of water and an avid retention of sodium. These cause expanded plasma and interstitial fluid volumes that lead to circulatory congestion and edema. It is unclear whether the decreased glomerular filtration rate, increased capillary permeability, or vascular spasm is responsible for these various manifestations. The cause of the hypertension associated with acute glomerulonephritis is also unexplained. Plasma renin activity is low during the acute phase, but the hypervolemia may be a factor.

Clinical Manifestations

Typically, affected children are in good health until they experience the antecedent infection. In some instances there is no history of an infection, or it is described only as a mild cold. The onset of nephritis appears after an average latent period of about 10 days. Since the child appears well during this time, the association is not recognized by parents.

Initial signs of nephrotic reaction include puffiness of the face, especially around the eyes (periorbital edema), anorexia, and passage of dark-colored urine. The edema is more prominent in the face in the morning but spreads during the day to involve the extremities and abdomen. The edema is only moderate and may not be appreciated by someone unfamiliar with the child's normal appearance. The urine is cloudy, smoky brown, or what parents describe as resembling tea or cola, and severely reduced in volume.

NURSING ALERT A child who exhibits the following should be evaluated for possible acute glomerulonephritis:

Orbital edema, which parents report is worse in the morning
Loss of appetite
Decreased output
Dark-colored urine revealed by examination
Antecedent streptococcal infection

The child is pale, irritable, and lethargic, and appears unwell but seldom expresses specific complaints. Older children may complain of headaches, abdominal discomfort, and dysuria. Vomiting is not uncommon. On examination there is usually a mild-to-moderate elevation in blood pressure (diastolic, 80 to 120 mm Hg; systolic, 120 to 180 mm Hg). Occasionally a child will have an atypical mode of onset with severe symptoms such as convulsions (secondary to cerebral ischemia and/or hypertension), pulmonary and circulatory congestion, minimal urine findings, or hematu-

TABLE 30-6 Comparison of Poststreptococcal Glomerulonephritis and Nephrotic Syndrome

MANIFESTATIONS	ACUTE POSTSTREPTOCOCCAL GLOMERULONEPHRITIS	MINIMAL-CHANGE NEPHROTIC SYNDROME
Streptococcal antibody titers	Present	Absent
Blood pressure	Elevated	Normal or decreased
Edema	Primarily periorbital and peripheral	Generalized severe
Circulatory congestion	Common	Absent
Proteinuria	Moderate	Massive
Hematuria	Gross or microscopic	Microscopic or none
Casts	Present	Present
Azotemia	Present	Absent
Serum potassium levels	Increased	Normal
Serum protein levels	Minimal reduction	Markedly decreased
Serum lipid levels	Normal	Elevated
Fatigue	Present	Present
Age at onset (years)	5-7	2-3

ria in the absence of hypertension and edema. For a comparison between APSGN and minimal-change nephrotic syndrome, see Table 30-6.

Clinical Course. The acute edematous phase of glomerulonephritis usually persists from 4 to 10 days but may persist for 2 or 3 weeks, during which time the child remains listless, anorexic, and apathetic. The weight fluctuates, the urine remains thick and smoky brown in color, and the blood pressure may suddenly reach dangerously high levels at any time during this phase.

The first sign of improvement is a small increase in urinary output with a corresponding decrease in body weight, followed in 1 or 2 days by copious diuresis. With diuresis the child begins to feel better, the appetite improves, and the blood pressure decreases to normal with the reduction of edema. Gross hematuria diminishes, in part because of dilution of the red blood cells in the more dilute urine, but microscopic hematuria may persist for weeks or months. The blood urea nitrogen level decreases during diuresis, but it, along with a slight to moderate proteinuria, may persist for several weeks.

Prognosis. Almost all children correctly diagnosed as having APSGN recover completely, and specific immunity is conferred so that subsequent recurrences are uncommon. Deaths from complications still occur but are, fortunately, rare. A few of these children may develop chronic disease, but many of these cases are believed to be (probably) different glomerular diseases misdiagnosed as poststreptococcal disease.

Complications. The major complications that may develop during the acute phase of glomerulonephritis are hypertensive encephalopathy, acute cardiac decompensation, and acute renal failure. Normally, cerebral blood flow responds to acute arterial hypertension by vasoconstriction. However, acute and severe hypertension may cause this protective autoregulation of cerebral blood flow to fail, leading to hyperperfusion of the brain and cerebral edema. The premonitory signs of encephalopathy are headache, dizziness, abdominal discomfort, and vomiting. If the condition progresses there may be transient loss of vision and/or hemiparesis, disorientation, and generalized convulsions of the tonic/clonic type.

Cardiac decompensation during the acute edematous phase of nephritis is caused by hypervolemia and not by cardiac failure. Signs of circulatory congestion are evident, however. The heart is enlarged, and increased pulmonary vascular markings are evident on roentgenographic examination. Increased pulmonary capillary permeability is also believed to be an important factor in the development of pulmonary edema.

Acute renal failure with persistent oliguria or anuria is an uncommon complication but one that requires an appropriate treatment regimen.

Diagnostic Evaluation

Urinalysis during the acute phase characteristically shows hematuria, proteinuria, and increased specific gravity. The specific gravity is moderately elevated and seldom exceeds 1.020. Proteinuria generally parallels the hematuria, and the content usually shows 3+ or 4+ but is not the massive proteinuria seen in nephrotic syndrome. Gross discoloration of urine reflects its red blood cell and hemoglobin content. Microscopic examination of the sediment shows many red blood cells, leukocytes, epithelial cells, and granular and red blood cell casts. Bacteria are not seen, and urine cultures are negative.

Blood examination reveals normal electrolytes (sodium, potassium, and chloride ions) and carbon dioxide levels, unless the disease has progressed to renal failure. Azotemia resulting from impaired glomerular filtration is reflected in elevated blood urea nitrogen and creatinine levels in at least 50% of cases. When proteinuria is heavy, there may be changes associated with nephrotic syndrome (i.e., transient hypoproteinemia and hyperlipidemia).

Cultures of the pharynx are positive for streptococci in only a few cases, and the numbers are not significantly greater than the normal carrier incidence in many communities. Positive cultures help to establish a diagnosis. Cultures should be obtained from other household members, and persons positive for group A streptococci should receive a course of antistreptococcal therapy.

Some serologic tests may help in diagnosis. Antibody responses to the extracellular products of the streptococci provide indirect evidence of previous streptococcal infection. These include antistreptolysin O (ASO), antistreptokinase (ASKase), antihyaluronidase (AHase), antideoxyribonuclease-B (ADNase-B), and antinicotyladenine dinucleotidase (ANADase). The ASO titer is the most familiar and readily available test for streptococcal antibodies. ASO appears in the serum about 10 days after the initial infection and persists for 4 to 6 weeks; however, there is no correlation between the degree of elevation and its duration and the severity or prognosis of the glomerulonephritis. It is a useful diagnostic tool when nephritis follows a pharyngeal infection but is of less value after pyoderma. An ASO titer of 250 Todd units or higher is of diagnostic significance, as is a rising titer in two samples taken a week apart. More consistent and reliable antibody tests following streptococcal skin infections are elevated AHase and ADNase-B titers.

Nonspecific acute-phase reactants that reflect acute inflammatory processes, such as the erythrocyte sedimentation rate (ESR), C-reactive protein (CRP), and serum mucoprotein tests, are elevated during the early stages of acute disease and then gradually return to normal as healing takes place. The ESR is sometimes used as a guide to the progress of the nephritis.

Since glomerulonephritis is an immune-complex disease, there is reduced total serum complement activity in the early stages of acute disease. The simpler measurements of the C3 complement component (beta$_1$ C globulin) are used as an index of total complement activity. The test is most useful in children with no edema or minimal urine findings.

Other studies that are employed include a chest x-ray examination, which shows characteristic generalized cardiac enlargement, pulmonary congestion, and pleural effusion during the edematous phase of acute disease. Electrocardiography reveals elevation or depression of the ST segment, prolonged QRS and ST segments, lengthening of the P-R interval, and flattened or inverted T waves. Renal biopsy for diagnostic purposes is seldom required but may be useful in the diagnosis of atypical cases.

Correlations between laboratory and morphologic findings indicate a significant relationship between creatinine clearance and severity of glomerular damage. Greater damage is reflected in a reduced creatinine clearance and is also associated with a higher blood urea nitrogen level. An increased excretion of cellular protein is associated with increasing glomerular capillary obliteration. There appears to be no correlation between the extent of glomerular damage and ASO titer, oliguria, or blood pressure.

Therapeutic Management

No specific treatment is available for acute glomerulonephritis, but recovery is spontaneous and uneventful in most cases. Management consists of general supportive measures and early recognition and treatment of complications. Children who have normal blood pressure and a satisfactory urinary output can generally be treated at home. Those with substantial edema, hypertension, gross hematuria, and/or significant oliguria should be hospitalized because of the unpredictability of complications. Short hospitalization is the rule in uncomplicated cases; prolonged hospitalization is required only for children with severely impaired renal function.

General Measures. Bed rest may be recommended during the acute phase, but ambulation does not seem to have an adverse effect on the course of the disease once the gross hematuria, edema, hypertension, and azotemia have abated. Since they are generally listless and experience fatigue and malaise, most children voluntarily restrict their activities during the most active phase of the disease.

Fluid Balance. Regular measurement of vital signs, body weight, and intake and output is essential in order to monitor the progress of the disease and to detect complications that may appear at any time during the course of the disease. A record of daily weight is the most useful means to assess fluid balance and should be kept for children treated at home, as well as for those who are hospitalized. Water restriction is seldom necessary unless the output is significantly reduced (less than 2 to 3 dl/24 hr). In these children the water allowed is equivalent to the calculated insensible loss plus the volume of urine excreted. Children on a regimen of restricted fluids, especially those who are severely edematous or those who have lost weight, should be observed for signs of dehydration.

Diuretics are usually of limited value, since very little sodium reaches the distal tubules as a result of the reduced filtration rate. However, diuretic therapy, usually furosemide, is helpful if significant edema and fluid overload are present. Digitalis may be employed sometimes, although there is question regarding its effectiveness in acute nephritis. Rarely, children with acute glomerulonephritis develop acute renal failure with oliguria that significantly alters the fluid and electrolyte balance. These children require careful management that may include peritoneal dialysis or hemodialysis.

Loss of glomerular filtration may produce electrolyte imbalances in children with severe forms of APSGN, especially hyperkalemia, acidosis, hypocalcemia, and hyperphosphatemia. Management of these electrolyte disturbances is described under acute renal failure.

Hypertension. Acute hypertension must be anticipated and identified early. Blood pressure measurements are taken every 4 to 6 hours. Significant but not severe hypertension is controlled with hydralazine (Apresoline), usually in conjunction with a diuretic. Oral hydrochlorothiazide is used to control mild hypertension. Seizure activity associated with hypertensive encephalopathy requires anticonvulsant therapy as well as antihypertensive agents (see Renal Failure, p. 1312, for management of severe hypertension).

Nutrition. Dietary restrictions depend on the stage and severity of the disease, especially the extent of edema. Regular diet is permitted in uncomplicated cases, but the intake of sodium is usually limited (no salt is added to foods). Moderate sodium restriction is usually instituted for children with hypertension or edema. Foods with substantial amounts of potassium are generally restricted during the period of oliguria. Protein restriction is reserved only for children with severe azotemia resulting from prolonged oliguria. The loss of appetite associated with the disease usually limits the protein intake sufficiently. During the acute stage calories may be restricted to carbohydrates and fats.

Antibiotics. Antibiotic therapy is indicated only for those children with evidence of persistent streptococcal infections. The antibiotics do not alter the course of the disease but are often recommended to prevent transmission of nephritogenic streptococci to other family members (Fish and Fouser, 1986). Authorities are divided in their use of prophylactic antimicrobials for other family members.

Nursing Considerations

Nursing care of the child with glomerulonephritis involves careful assessment of the disease status, with regular monitoring of vital signs (including frequent measurement of blood pressure), fluid balance, and behavior. Vital signs provide clues to the severity of the disease and early signs of complications. They are carefully measured, and any abnormalities are reported and recorded. The volume and character of urine are noted, and the child is weighed daily. Assessment of the child's appearance for signs of cerebral complications is an important nursing function, since the severity of the acute phase is variable and unpredictable. The child with edema, hypertension, and gross hematuria may be subject to complications, and anticipatory preparations such as seizure precautions and intravenous equipment are included in the nursing care plan.

For most children a regular diet is allowed, but it should contain no added salt. Foods high in sodium and salted treats are eliminated, and parents and friends should be advised not to bring items such as potato chips or pretzels. However, the total amount of salt ingested is usually less than prescribed because of poor appetite. Fluid restriction, if prescribed, is more difficult, and the amount permitted should be evenly divided throughout the waking hours and served in small cups to give the illusion of larger servings. Meal preparation and service require special attention, since the child has a poor appetite and is indifferent to meals during the acute phase. Again, collaboration with parents and the dietitian and special consideration for food preferences facilitate meal planning.

During the acute phase children are generally quite content to lie in bed, and activities should be those that require little expenditure of energy. As they begin to feel better and their symptoms subside, activities should be planned to allow for frequent rest periods and avoidance of fatigue.

Children with mild edema and no hypertension, as well as convalescent children being treated at home, need follow-up care. Parents are instructed regarding general measures, including activity, diet, and prevention of infection. Strenuous activity is usually restricted until there is no evidence of proteinuria or macroscopic hematuria.

Health supervision is continued with weekly, followed by monthly, visits for evaluation and urinalysis. Parent education and support in preparation for discharge and home care include education in home management and the need for follow-up care and health supervision.

CHRONIC OR PROGRESSIVE GLOMERULONEPHRITIS

The majority of cases of renal glomerular disease are acute glomerulonephritis, minimal-change nephrotic syndrome, and glomerulonephritis associated with systemic diseases. These pose relatively few problems of diagnosis, and their natural course is fairly predictable. A few cases present a prolonged course and a poor ultimate prognosis. They are a rather heterogeneous group, defined by correlating the clinical manifestations, pathologic conditions, and natural course of the individual diseases.

Persistent glomerulonephritis is used to describe those cases of glomerulonephritis that have no specific histologic picture but that fail to show the rapid recovery expected in acute nephritis. ***Chronic glomerulonephritis (CGN)*** describes advanced glomerular disease, which includes a variety of different disease processes. ***Rapidly progressive glomerulonephritis*** is used to describe an acute illness with severe, acute onset resembling acute poststreptococcal glomerulonephritis but that causes rapidly progressive deterioration of renal function in weeks to months.

Pathophysiology

In most cases of CGN, immunologic mechanisms can be implicated either through direct attack on the kidney or secondary to the accumulation of immune complexes in the glomerular filter or fibrin deposition from previously damaged glomeruli. Either can contribute to further glomerular damage and can initiate chronic changes in the glomerular structure. In many cases there is no history of an attack of acute glomerular disease. In other cases it may represent one of a succession of exacerbations of a preexisting disease. CGN that is not associated with other diseases may go undetected for years and be relatively asymptomatic until kidney destruction produces marked reduction in renal function. Consequently, the disease is more common in adolescents than in younger children. Renal insufficiency with all its manifestations occurs as the ultimate event.

Clinical Manifestations

The clinical manifestations and laboratory findings reflect deteriorating renal function. Nephrotic syndrome frequently develops. Hypertension, edema, proteinuria, cardiac failure, dyspnea, osteodystrophy, and anemia are common manifestations of progressive disease.

Diagnostic Evaluation

Laboratory findings may include proteinuria, with casts and red and white blood cells. Failing renal function is evidenced by elevated blood urea nitrogen, creatinine, and uric acid levels. Electrolyte alterations include metabolic acidosis, decreased sodium from the chronic salt-losing state, elevated potassium, elevated phosphorus, and decreased calcium levels. As the disease progresses, urine specific gravity eventually stabilizes at an isotonic state (about 1.012) as a result of the inability of the kidney to reabsorb solutes or respond to antidiuretic hormone. The renal insufficiency may extend from 5 to 15 years and even longer, or rapid deterioration may progress to end-stage renal disease (ESRD).

Therapeutic Management

Early in the course of the disease, treatment is appropriate to the underlying disease and is largely symptomatic in most cases. Efforts are directed toward providing optimal conditions for the child's physical, psychologic, and social development. As few restrictions as feasible are imposed, and the child is allowed to live as normal a life as possible for as long as possible. Drug treatment offers little lasting benefit, although diuretic therapy may be helpful occasionally for edema or hypertension. Marked hypertension is controlled with antihypertensive agents, and anemia may require periodic transfusion with fresh packed cells. Salt is only moderately restricted. Ultimately, dialysis and transplantation may restore relatively good health; however, these alternatives are usually not available until renal failure is far advanced. (See Chronic Renal Failure, p. 1318, for more detailed management of specific problems.) Children with rapidly progressive glomerulonephritis are usually referred to a center specializing in renal disease.

Nursing Considerations

The problems of CGN and those encountered in chronic renal insufficiency from any cause are discussed in association with chronic renal failure.

NEPHROTIC SYNDROME

Nephrotic syndrome is the most common presentation of glomerular injury in children. It is defined as massive proteinuria, hypoalbuminemia, hyperlipemia, and edema, but the disorder is a clinical manifestation of a large number of distinct glomerular disorders in which increased glomerular permeability to plasma protein results in massive urinary protein loss. Following a description of the three major forms of nephrotic syndrome, the remainder of the discussion is devoted to minimal-change disease.

Types of Nephrotic Syndrome

Nephrotic syndrome can be classified as primary, when the syndrome is restricted to glomerular injury, or secondary, when it develops as part of a systemic illness. Although it may have several different histologic variations, the most common form of the primary disease is minimal change nephrotic syndrome. A congenital form is also recognized.

Minimal-Change Nephrotic Syndrome (MCNS). Approximately 80% of cases of nephrotic syndrome in children occur in the absence of recognizable systemic disease or preexisting renal disease and are categorized as idiopathic. MCNS can present at any age but is predominantly a disease of the preschool child. The disease is rare in children younger than 6 months of age, uncommon in infants younger than 1 year of age, and unusual after the age of 8. The incidence of the disease in North America is approximately 2:100,000 children per year, and males outnumber females 2:1. In adolescence the ratio is 1:1.

The cause of MCNS (also known as idiopathic nephrosis, "minimal-lesion" nephrosis, childhood nephrosis, lipoid nephrosis, or uncomplicated nephrosis) remains obscure. Often a nonspecific illness, usually a viral upper respiratory tract infection, precedes the manifestations by 4 to 8 days but is considered to be a precipitating factor rather than a cause.

Secondary Nephrotic Syndrome. Nephrotic syndrome may occur after or in association with glomerular damage of known or presumed etiology. Prominent among causes of glomerular damage is acute or chronic glomerulonephritis. Less commonly, secondary nephrotic syndrome occurs during the course of collagen diseases (such as disseminated lupus erythematosus and anaphylactoid purpura) or as a result of toxicity to drugs (such as trimethadione and heavy metals), stings, or venom. Nephrotic syndrome is the major presenting symptom of renal disease in pediatric patients with acquired immunodeficiency syndrome (AIDS). Diverse, rare causes are sickle cell disease, hepatitis, malaria, cyanotic heart disease, diabetes mellitus, amyloidosis, tuberculosis, infected ventriculojugular shunts, renal vein thrombosis, or malignancies.

Congenital Nephrotic Syndrome. The hereditary form of nephrotic syndrome is caused by a recessive gene on an autosome. Infants who have nephrotic syndrome are

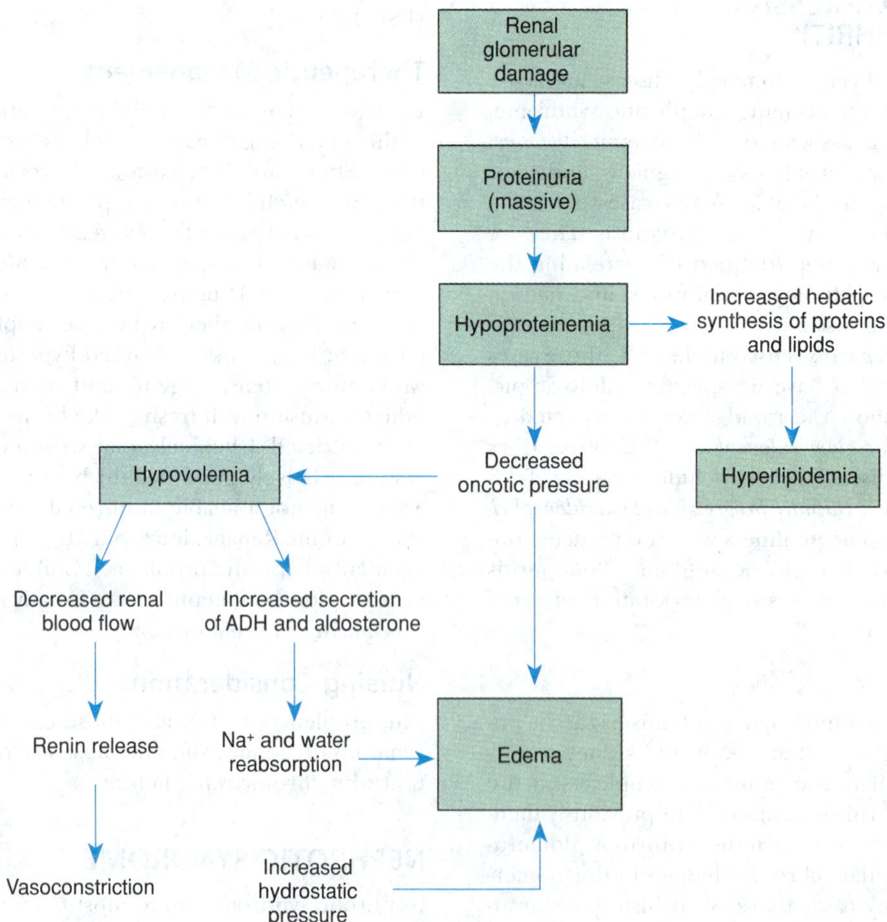

FIG. 30-2 Sequence of events in nephrotic syndrome.

small for gestational age, and proteinuria and edema are manifested early. The disease does not respond to the usual therapy, and death in the first year or two of life is the rule if the infant does not receive a successful renal transplant.

Pathophysiology

The pathogenesis of MCNS is not understood. There may be a metabolic, biochemical, or physiochemical disturbance in the basement membrane of the glomeruli that leads to increased permeability to protein, but the causes and mechanisms are only speculative.

The glomerular membrane, which is normally impermeable to albumin and other large proteins, becomes permeable to proteins, especially albumin, which leak through the membrane and are lost in urine (hyperalbuminuria). This reduces the serum albumin level (hypoalbuminemia), which decreases the colloidal osmotic pressure in the capillaries. As a result, the hydrostatic pressure exceeds the pull of the colloidal osmotic pressure, and fluid accumulates in the interstitial spaces and body cavities, particularly the abdominal cavity (ascites). The shift of fluid from the plasma to the interstitial spaces reduces the vascular fluid volume (hypovolemia), which in turn stimulates the renin-angiotensin system and the secretion of antidiuretic hormone and aldosterone. Tubular reabsorption of sodium and water is increased in an attempt to increase intravascular volume. The elevation of serum cholesterol, phospholipids, and triglycerides is unexplained. The sequence of events in nephrotic syndrome is diagrammed in Fig. 30-2.

Clinical Manifestations

A previously well child begins to gain weight, which progresses insidiously over a period of days or weeks. Puffiness of the face, especially around the eyes, is apparent on arising in the morning but subsides during the day, when swelling of the abdomen and lower extremities is more prominent. The generalized edema develops so slowly that parents may consider it to be a sign of healthy growth. Although an acute infection may precipitate severe generalized edema ***(anasarca)***, the usual course is one of progressive weight gain until either a rapid or a gradual increase in edema prompts the family to seek medical evaluation. Usually present are periorbital edema, abdominal swelling from ascites, and labial or scrotal swelling (Fig. 30-3). Edema of the intestinal mucosa may cause diarrhea, loss of appetite, and poor intestinal absorption. The volume of urine is decreased, and it appears darkly opalescent and frothy.

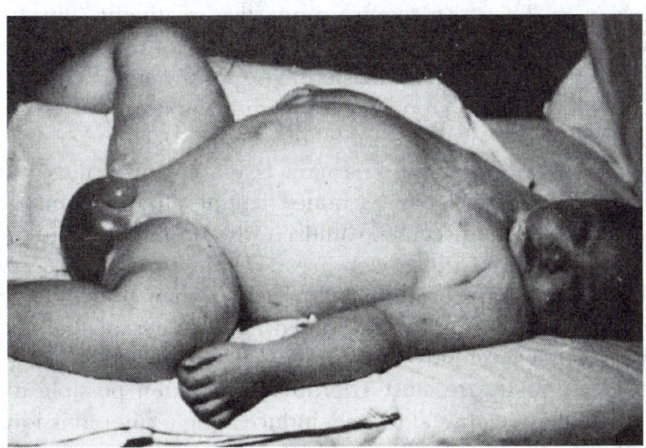

FIG. 30-3 Two-year-old child with nephrosis. (From Shirkey HC, editor: *Pediatric therapy*, ed 6, St Louis, 1980, Mosby.)

Extreme skin pallor is often present, and the child has a tendency toward skin breakdown during periods of edema. The child is irritable and may be easily fatigued or lethargic but does not appear seriously ill. Weight loss from poor appetite and loss of protein is not uncommon, although it is frequently obscured by edema. Changes in the nails appear as white (Muercke) lines parallel to the lanula, which are caused by prolonged hypoalbuminemia. The blood pressure is usually normal or slightly decreased. The child is more susceptible to infection, especially cellulitis, pneumonia, peritonitis, or septicemia.

NURSING ALERT A child who exhibits the following should be evaluated for the possibility of nephrotic syndrome:

Weight gain over that expected based on previous pattern
Parent observation that the child's clothes fit tightly
Decreased urinary output
Pallor, fatigue

In children with MCNS, in rare instances there is significant or persistent hypertension, gross or persistent hematuria, significant or persistent azotemia (presence of increased nitrogenous products in the blood), or depression of serum $\beta 1_c$ globulin.

Diagnostic Evaluation

The diagnosis of MCNS is made on the basis of the history and clinical manifestations (edema, proteinuria, hypoalbuminemia, and hypercholesterolemia in the absence of hematuria and hypertension) in children between the ages of 2 and 4 years. Massive proteinuria is reflected in urinary excretion of protein that frequently reaches levels in excess of 2 $g/m^2/day$ of body surface, with relatively greater clearance of low-molecular-weight proteins. Hyaline casts from high protein and sluggish flow and oval fat bodies, as well as a few red blood cells, can be found in the urine of most affected children, although there is seldom gross hematuria. Specific gravity is high and proportionate to the amount of protein concentration. If hypovolemia is not significant and the child is well hydrated, the glomerular filtration rate is usually normal.

Total serum protein concentrations are reduced, with the albumin fractions significantly reduced (less than 2 g/dl) and plasma lipids elevated. Serum cholesterol may be as high as 450 to 1500 mg/dl. Hemoglobin and hematocrit are usually normal or elevated, and the platelet count is high (500,000 to 1,000,000) as a result of hemoconcentration. Serum sodium concentration is usually low, about 130 to 135 mEq/L.

If renal biopsy is performed, it provides information regarding the glomerular status and type of nephrotic syndrome, response to drugs and probable course of the disease. Under the microscope the foot processes of the basement membrane appear fused. The major focuses in differential diagnosis are to establish the edema as renal in origin and to distinguish minimum-change nephrotic syndrome from other glomerulopathies with nephrotic syndrome as a manifestation.

Therapeutic Management

The medical management consists of both general and specific measures. The primary objective is to reduce the excretion of urinary protein and maintain a protein-free urine. Additional objectives include prevention or treatment of acute infection, control of edema, establishment of good nutrition, and readjustment of any disturbed metabolic processes. Children with severe symptoms or whose disease is newly recognized are hospitalized for assessment and observation for evidence of infection, response to therapy, and parental education.

General Measures. General treatment is principally supportive. During the edema phase the child is often placed on bed rest, but activity is not restricted during remission. Children can be remarkably active with no evidence that restriction affects the ultimate outcome. Acute and intercurrent infections are treated with appropriate antibiotics, and efforts are made to eliminate possible infection.

Diet. The child who is in remission is allowed a regular diet; however, during periods of massive edema, salt is restricted in the form of no added salt at the table and excluding foods with very high salt content. This is usually tolerated by the child for a time, but it should be adjusted to the child's appetite and must not interfere with nutrient intake. Although edema cannot be removed by a low-sodium diet, its rate of increase may be reduced. Water is seldom restricted. A diet generous in protein is logical, but there is no evidence that it is beneficial or alters the outcome of the disease. The presence of azotemia and renal failure is a contraindication for high-protein intake.

Corticosteroid Therapy. The response of most affected children to corticosteroids has established these drugs as prime therapeutic agents in management of nephrotic syndrome. Corticosteroid therapy is begun as soon as the diagnosis has been determined and is administered orally in a dosage of 2 mg/kg of body weight or 60 mg/m^2/day in evenly divided doses. Prednisone, the safest and least expensive drug, is the steroid of choice. The drug is continued until the urine is free from protein and remains normal for 10 days to 2 weeks.

The course of the disease is fairly predictable. There is little change during the first few days of therapy. In most patients diuresis occurs as the urinary protein excretion diminishes within 7 to 21 days after the initiation of steroid therapy. Other clinical manifestations stabilize or return to normal shortly thereafter. Almost 95% of patients between 1 and 10 years of age with no hypertension, hematuria, or renal insufficiency and who have satisfactory laboratory measurements of C3 complement and a renal clearance of IgG will have complete resolution of proteinuria with therapy.

CLASSIFICATION OF NEPHROTIC SYNDROME ACCORDING TO STEROID RESPONSE

1. **Steroid-sensitive** (20% to 40%)—Response to a single short course of steroids without evidence of relapse after cessation of therapy.
2. **Frequent relapsers** or **steroid-dependent** (60% to 80%)—Respond to steroids and can be tapered off completely; have three or more relapses in a 6- to 12-month period; remit when placed on steroids but tend to relapse on lowered dosage.
3. **Steroid-unresponsive** or **steroid-resistant**—Never respond to steroids or become resistant to steroids at some point during the course of disease.

Modified from McEnery PT, Strife CF: Nephrotic syndrome in childhood, *Pediatr Clin North Am* 89:875-894, 1982.

If the child has not responded to therapy within 28 days of daily steroid administration, the likelihood of subsequent response diminishes rapidly. When the child is free of proteinuria and edema, the total daily dose of prednisone is usually given for a time as a single dose every 48 hours. The dose is gradually tapered to discontinuation over a variable period, from several weeks to months, depending on the medical philosophy. Once a satisfactory response is achieved, steroid therapy is reduced to every other day (q.o.d.). This dosage is less likely to depress pituitary-adrenal function and produces fewer side effects during prolonged therapy. If a tendency to relapse is demonstrated, the number of relapses can be reduced with administration of a low-dose, q.o.d. schedule of prednisone therapy that continues for 6 months to 1 year (provided remission is achieved and successful tapering to low-dose q.o.d. therapy occurs).

Children with MCNS are often described according to their response to corticosteroid therapy (see box above). Children with MCNS typically relapse one to three times per year. Steroid-dependent children tend to have frequent relapses over many years and receive large amounts of steroids, which results in cushingoid features and growth retardation. They also require supportive treatment (diuretics, diet). The prognosis for steroid-unresponsive children is less predictable than for steroid-responsive children.

Children who require frequent courses of steroid therapy are highly susceptible to complications of steroids, such as growth retardation, cataracts, obesity, hypertension, gastrointestinal bleeding, bone demineralization, infections, and hyperglycemia. Children who do not respond to steroid therapy, those who have frequent relapses, and those in whom the side effects threaten their growth and general health may be considered for a course of therapy using other immunosuppressant medications.

Immunosuppressant Therapy. It is often possible to reduce the relapse rate and induce long-term remission with administration of an oral alkylating agent, usually cyclophosphamide (Cytoxan), alternating with prednisone. Both drugs are administered for up to 2 to 3 months, after which cyclophosphamide is discontinued abruptly and the prednisone is decreased by decrements. Chlorambucil has also proved to be effective when given with corticosteroids. The two drugs share many characteristics, and response to both appears to depend on dose, duration of therapy, age, and duration of the disease.

Significant side effects of cyclophosphamide must be considered and discussed with parents of children for whom this drug is contemplated. Leukopenia must be anticipated, and evidence suggests that cyclophosphamide may cause azoospermia with potential sterility in males treated for more than 2 to 3 months and variable effects on gonadal function in females.

Diuretics. One characteristic of the edema of nephrotic syndrome is its usual lack of responsiveness to diuretic agents. However, in cases in which edema interferes with respiration or there is hypotension, hyponatremia, or evidence of skin breakdown, loop diuretics are sometimes useful, usually furosemide in combination with metolazone. In addition, plasma expanders such as salt-poor human albumin may be administered to severely edematous children requiring prompt control; however, they must be administered frequently, since the glomeruli are readily permeable to albumin in the acute stage (Haws and Baum, 1993).

Prognosis. The prognosis for ultimate recovery in most cases is good. It is a self-limiting disease, and in children who respond to steroid therapy the tendency to relapse decreases with time. With early detection and prompt implementation of therapy to eradicate proteinuria, progressive basement membrane damage is minimized, so that when the tendency to exacerbations is past, renal function is usually normal or near normal. It is estimated that approximately 80% of affected children have this favorable prognosis, although half the children have relapses even after 5 years, and 20% after 10 years (Kim and Grupe, 1986).

Nursing Considerations

❖ Assessment

Continuous monitoring of fluid retention or excretion is an important nursing function. Strict and accurate records of intake and output are essential but may be difficult in very young children. Application of collection bags is highly irritating to edematous, sensitive skin that is already subject to breakdown. Other methods of monitoring progress include examination of the urine for specific gravity and albumin, daily weight, and measurement of abdominal girth. Assessment of edema such as increased or decreased swelling around the eyes and dependent areas, the degree of pitting (if noted), and the color and texture of the skin are part of nursing care. Vital signs are monitored to detect any early signs of complications such as shock or an infective process.

❖ Nursing Diagnoses

Constant reassessment and evaluation reveal a number of nursing diagnoses that are relevant to the care of these children and their families (see Nursing Care Plan, pp. 1306-1307). Others will be apparent in specific situations.

❖ Planning

The goals for the child with nephrotic syndrome and the family are as follows:

1. Child will exhibit no evidence of fluid accumulation.
2. Child will receive appropriate volume of fluid.
3. Child will exhibit no evidence of skin breakdown or infection.
4. Child will receive optimum nutrition.
5. Child and family will express feelings and concerns.
6. Child will receive adequate rest.

❖ Implementation

Children hospitalized with MCNS may be placed on bed rest during the edema phase of the disease. They seldom offer resistance, since they are usually lethargic and easily fatigued, and their cumbersome edematous bulk is not conducive to movement. Most are content to lie in the prone position. These children must be encouraged and helped to turn regularly to prevent tissue breakdown. Areas that are particularly edematous, such as the scrotum, abdomen, and legs, may require support, and skin surfaces should be cleaned and separated with clothing, cotton, or antiseptic powder to prevent intertrigo.

Infection is a constant source of danger to edematous children and those receiving corticosteroid therapy. These children are particularly vulnerable to upper respiratory tract infection; therefore, they must be kept warm and dry, turned frequently, and protected from contact with infected roommates, visitors, or personnel. Spontaneous peritonitis can occur secondary to migration of intestinal bacteria across the bowel wall and into the peritoneum. Vital signs are monitored to detect any early signs of an infective process.

Loss of appetite that accompanies active nephrosis creates a perplexing problem for nurses. During this time the combined efforts of nurse, dietitian, parents, and the child are needed to formulate a nutritionally adequate and attractive diet. Salt is usually restricted, but not eliminated, during the edema phase. Every effort should be made to serve attractive meals with a minimum of fuss, but it usually requires a considerable amount of ingenuity and enticement to get the child to eat. Games, rewards, and special treats often help, but each child is unique, and it may require considerable trial and error to arrive at a successful strategy. Also, the same strategy may not work consistently (see Feeding the Sick Child, Chapter 27).

As the edema subsides, children are allowed increased activity. Although they are easily fatigued, they are usually able to adjust activities according to their individual tolerance but may require guidance in selection of play activities. Suitable recreational and diversional activities are an important part of their care. Once edema fluid has been lost, children are allowed to resume their usual activities with discretion. Irritability and mood swings accompanying the inactivity, disease process, and steroid therapy are not unusual manifestations in these children, which create an additional challenge to the nurse and the family.

Family Support and Home Care. Many children are treated at home during exacerbations. Parents are taught

NURSING CARE PLAN
The Child with Nephrotic Syndrome

NURSING DIAGNOSIS: Fluid volume excess (total body) related to fluid accumulation in tissues and third spaces

PATIENT GOAL 1: Will exhibit no or minimal evidence of fluid accumulation

• **NURSING INTERVENTIONS/*RATIONALES***

Assess intake relative to output
- Measure and record intake and output accurately
- Weigh daily (or more often, if indicated) *to assess fluid retention*

Assess changes in edema
- Measure abdominal girth at umbilicus *to assess ascites*
- Monitor edema around eyes and dependent areas *because these are common sites of edema*
- Note degree of pitting, if present
- Note color and texture of skin

Test urine for specific gravity, albumin *because hyperalbuminuria is manifestation of nephrotic syndrome*

Collect specimens for laboratory examination

*Administer corticosteroids as prescribed *to reduce excretion of urinary protein*

*Administer diuretics if ordered *to provide temporary relief from edema*

Limit fluids as indicated *during massive edema*

• **EXPECTED OUTCOME**

Child exhibits no or minimal evidence of fluid accumulation (specify parameters)

PATIENT GOAL 2: Will receive appropriate volume of fluid

• **NURSING INTERVENTIONS/*RATIONALES***

Regulate fluid intake carefully *so that child does not receive more than prescribed amount*

Monitor intravenous infusion *to maintain prescribed intake*

Employ strategies to prevent undesired intake
- Use small containers for fluid intake *so that volume does not appear so restricted*
- Divide allowed intake into small volumes spread over entire day
- Spray mouth with atomizer (mist) *to prevent feeling of dryness*
- Offer chewing gum and sugarless hard candies

Keep lips lubricated *for comfort and to prevent cracking*

• **EXPECTED OUTCOME**

Child receives no more fluid than prescribed

NURSING DIAGNOSIS: High risk for (intravascular) fluid volume deficit related to protein and fluid loss, edema

PATIENT GOAL 1: Will exhibit no or minimal evidence of intravascular fluid loss or hypovolemic shock

• **NURSING INTERVENTION/*RATIONALE***

Monitor vital signs *to detect physical evidence of fluid depletion*

Assess pulse quality and rate *for signs of hypovolemic shock*

Measure blood pressure *to detect hypovolemic shock*

Report any deviations from normal *so that prompt treatment is instituted*

**Administer salt-poor albumin if prescribed as a plasma expander*

• **EXPECTED OUTCOME**

Child exhibits no or minimal evidence of intravascular fluid loss or hypovolemic shock

NURSING DIAGNOSIS: High risk for infection related to lowered body defenses, fluid overload

PATIENT GOAL 1: Will exhibit no evidence of infection

• **NURSING INTERVENTIONS/*RATIONALES***

Protect child from contact with infected persons *to minimize exposure to infective organisms*
- Place in room with noninfectious children
- Restrict contact with persons who have infections, including family, other children, friends, and staff members
- Teach visitors appropriate preventive behaviors (e.g., handwashing)

Observe medical asepsis

Use good handwashing

Keep child warm and dry *because of vulnerability to upper respiratory infection*

Monitor temperature *for early evidence of infection*

Teach parents signs and symptoms of infections

• **EXPECTED OUTCOMES**

Child and family apply good health practices

Child exhibits no evidence of infection

*Dependent nursing action.

NURSING CARE PLAN
The Child with Nephrotic Syndrome—cont'd

NURSING DIAGNOSIS: High risk for impaired skin integrity related to edema, lowered body defenses

PATIENT GOAL 1: Will maintain skin integrity

• **NURSING INTERVENTIONS/*RATIONALES***
Provide meticulous skin care
Avoid tight clothing *that may cause pressure areas*
Cleanse and powder opposing skin surfaces several times per day *to prevent skin breakdown*
Separate opposing skin surfaces with soft cotton *to prevent skin breakdown*
Support edematous organs, such as scrotum, *to relieve pressure areas*
Cleanse edematous eyelids with warm saline wipes
Change position frequently; maintain good body alignment *because child with massive edema is usually lethargic, easily fatigued, and content to lie still*
Use pressure-relieving or pressure-reducing mattresses or beds as needed *to prevent ulcers* (see Maintaining Healthy Skin, Chapter 27)

• **EXPECTED OUTCOME**
Child's skin displays no evidence of redness or irritation

NURSING DIAGNOSIS: Altered nutrition: less than body requirements related to loss of appetite

PATIENT GOAL 1: Will receive optimum nutrition

• **NURSING INTERVENTIONS/*RATIONALES***
Offer nutritious diet
Restrict sodium during edema and steroid therapy
†Administer supplementary vitamins and iron as ordered
Enlist aid of child, parents, and dietitian in formulation of diet *to encourage optimum nutrition despite loss of appetite*
Provide cheerful, clean, relaxed atmosphere during meals *so that child is more likely to eat*
Serve small quantities initially *to stimulate appetite;* encourage seconds
Provide special and preferred foods *to encourage child to eat*
Serve foods in an attractive manner *to stimulate appetite*
See also Feeding the Sick Child, Chapter 27

• **EXPECTED OUTCOME**
Child consumes an adequate amount of nutritious food

NURSING DIAGNOSIS: Body image disturbance related to change in appearance

PATIENT GOAL 1: Will express feelings and concerns

• **NURSING INTERVENTIONS/*RATIONALES***
Explore feelings and concerns regarding appearance *to facilitate coping*
Point out positive aspects of appearance and evidence of diminished edema *so that child feels encouraged*
Explain to child and family that symptoms associated with steroid therapy will subside when medication is discontinued
Encourage activity within limits of tolerance
Encourage socialization with persons without active infection *so that child is not lonely and isolated*
Provide positive feedback *so that child feels accepted*
Explore areas of interest and encourage their pursuit

• **EXPECTED OUTCOMES**
Child discusses feelings and concerns
Child engages in activities appropriate to interests and abilities

NURSING DIAGNOSIS: Activity intolerance related to fatigue

PATIENT GOAL 1: Will receive adequate rest

• **NURSING INTERVENTIONS/*RATIONALES***
Maintain bed rest initially if severely edematous
Balance rest and activity when ambulatory
Plan and provide quiet activities
Instruct child to rest when he or she begins to feel tired
Allow for periods of uninterrupted sleep

• **EXPECTED OUTCOMES**
Child engages in activities appropriate to capabilities
Child receives adequate rest and sleep

NURSING DIAGNOSIS: Altered family processes related to a child with a serious disease

PATIENT (FAMILY) GOAL 1: Will receive adequate support

• **NURSING INTERVENTIONS/*RATIONALES* AND EXPECTED OUTCOMES**
See Nursing Care Plan: The Family of the Ill or Hospitalized Child, Chapter 26

See also Nursing Care Plan: The Child in the Hospital, Chapter 26

*Dependent nursing action.

to detect signs of relapse and to bring the child for treatment at the earliest indications. Unless the edema and proteinuria are severe or the parents, for some reason, are unable to care for the ill child, home care is preferred. Parents are instructed in urine testing for albumin, administration of medications, and general care. Salt is restricted to no additional salt during relapse and steroid therapy, but a regular diet is suitable for the child in remission. Parents are instructed regarding avoiding contact with infected playmates, but the child is permitted to attend school. It is important for parents of children on corticosteroid therapy to be aware of the common side effects of steroid therapy, such as rounding of the face, increased appetite, abdominal distention, and hirsutism, and to distinguish some of these from the edema formation of the disease. They should be reassured that the symptoms will disappear gradually after discontinuation of the drug. The child should receive close medical and/or nursing observation to detect unusual but more serious side effects (see Critical Thinking Exercise box).

CRITICAL THINKING EXERCISE
Nephrotic Syndrome

Jerome is an 8-year-old boy with relapsing nephrotic syndrome who has become steroid dependent. He is being seen in the outpatient clinic for follow-up assessment. During your initial assessment you identify the following: (1) weight has increased 2 kg in the last 2 weeks; (2) blood pressure is 100/70; (3) mother reports that Jerome is not urinating very much and she does not know how much he has been drinking; (4) while you are measuring Jerome's abdominal girth, he guards his abdomen and complains of stomachache; (5) his temperature is 38° C (100.4° F) orally. Of the following correct actions, you should first:

1. Examine Jerome's abdomen more thoroughly while eliciting a 24-hour recall of illness symptoms from his mother.
2. Elicit a 24-hour recall of food and fluid intake from Jerome and his mother together.
3. Obtain a clean-catch urine specimen. Divide the specimen so that you can perform a dipstick analysis immediately and retain the other specimen for possible urinalysis and culture after consultation with the primary health practitioner.
4. Explore the mother's understanding of Jerome's illness and its relationship to his current condition to begin outlining your teaching plan for this family.

The correct response is 1. One of the complications of severe nephrotic syndrome is peritonitis, which can occur secondary to migration of intestinal bacteria across the bowel wall and into the protein-rich acidic fluid. Jerome's mother has already said that she does not know what he has been drinking. Therefore your only possibility of assessing his intake is to elicit the recall while they are together. While his weight gain and reduced urinary output are major concerns, they are secondary to peritonitis. (It should be recognized that children on strict fluid restrictions are prone to obtain fluids from unauthorized sources.) Obtaining a urine specimen for dipstick analysis is part of the initial assessment for Jerome. In this instance the fever and abdominal pain are the first priority. As with option 3, the fourth choice must be addressed, along with evaluation of the current stress level in the home, after the fever and pain have been addressed.

The prolonged course of the relapsing form of nephrotic syndrome is taxing to both the child and the family. The up-and-down course of remissions and exacerbations with periodic disruption of family life by hospitalization places a severe strain on the child and the family, both psychologically and financially. Parents and children over 5 or 6 years of age need reassurance regarding this characteristic of the course of the disease so that they will not become discouraged with the frequent relapses. At the same time, it is important to impress on them the importance of long-term care to gain their cooperation. A satisfactory response is more likely when relapses are detected and therapy is instituted early, and remissions are prolonged when instructions are carried out faithfully. For example, one child had an exacerbation when his mother reduced the dosage of his drug because it was so expensive.

Social isolation is a concomitant problem for these children. Isolation is related to frequent hospitalization or confinement during relapse, the risk of infection that may precipitate an exacerbation, lack of energy, and the child's reluctance to face friends at home or school because of the changes in appearance resulting from the disease or the medication. Both parents and child need someone to listen to their complaints, to assist them in coping with both short-term and long-term problems associated with the disease, and to find solutions to their problems. Continuous support of the child and family is one of the major nursing considerations.

❖ EVALUATION

The effectiveness of nursing interventions is determined by continual reassessment and evaluation of care based on the following observational guidelines and expected outcomes:

1. Measure intake and output and examine urine for albumin.
2. Monitor vital signs and assess skin for evidence of breakdown or infection.
3. Assess appetite and eating behaviors.
4. Observe and interview child and family regarding their understanding of the disease, therapies, and compliance with prescribed regimen.

Expected outcomes:

See Nursing Care Plan, pp. 1306-1307.

RENAL TUBULAR DISORDERS

Disorders of renal tubular function include a variety of conditions in which there are one or more abnormalities in specific mechanisms of tubular transport or reabsorption, whereas initially glomerular function is normal or comparatively less impaired. Eventually there may be more widespread kidney destruction with renal failure. In some cases the dysfunction has little, if any, effect on renal function. These disorders may be permanent or transient and may originate as primary defects or arise as a secondary effect of metabolic disease or exogenous toxins. Renal tubular disorders may be congenital (usually displaying characteristic patterns of genetic transmission), appear without evidence of hereditary transmission, or be acquired as a result of known or unknown causes.

Unlike the classic manifestations of glomerular diseases, edema and hypertension are absent and the blood urea nitrogen level and routine urinalysis are usually normal. Proteinuria may be demonstrated but only by elaborate tests. Manifestations of tubular disorders are primarily metabolic disturbances or deficiencies, such as failure to thrive, metabolic bone disease, or persistent acidosis. The variety of these disorders is extensive and the incidence rare.

TUBULAR FUNCTION

The function of the proximal tubules is the reabsorption of substances from the glomerular filtrate, including sodium, potassium, chloride, bicarbonate, glucose, phosphate, and amino acids. A number of disorders feature impairment of reabsorption of one or more filtrate constituents, and most involve defects in the transport mechanisms for these substances. Impaired tubular reabsorption of any specific substance will cause that substance to appear in the urine, usually with reduced levels in the blood.

The primary functions of the distal renal tubules are acidification of urine, potassium secretion, and the selective and differential reabsorption of sodium, chloride, and water, which determines the final urinary concentration. Since the contribution of the distal tubule to urine composition depends in part on the volume and composition of the filtrate from the proximal tubule, the net contribution of the distal tubule is related to proximal tubular function and glomerular filtration.

RENAL TUBULAR ACIDOSIS

Renal tubular acidosis is a syndrome of sustained metabolic acidosis in which there is impaired reabsorption of bicarbonate and/or excretion of net hydrogen ion, but in which glomerular function is normal or comparatively less impaired. On the basis of underlying pathophysiology, renal tubular acidosis is divided into ***proximal renal tubular acidosis,*** which results from a defect in bicarbonate absorption, and ***distal renal tubular acidosis,*** which results from inability to establish an adequate gradient of pH between blood and tubular fluid.

Proximal Tubular Acidosis (Type II)

Proximal tubular acidosis is caused by impaired bicarbonate reabsorption in the proximal tubule. It may occur as an isolated defect (primary); however, more often it appears in association with other proximal tubular disorders (secondary). As a result of a depressed renal threshold, bicarbonate reabsorption in the proximal tubule is incomplete, causing the plasma concentration of bicarbonate to stabilize at a lower level than normal. This results in a hyperchloremic metabolic acidosis. There is no impairment of distal tubular integrity or, in most cases, of the distal acidifying mechanism. A more complex abnormality in the proximal tubules is the ***Fanconi syndrome*** in which transport mechanisms are damaged by the accumulation of toxic metabolites or the tubular epithelium is damaged by heavy metals such as lead or arsenic.

The cause of the primary disorder is unknown, but it appears to be almost entirely restricted to male infants. The major clinical manifestation and presenting symptom is growth failure. Tachypnea from hyperchloremic metabolic acidosis is also evident. Dehydration, vomiting, episodic fever, nephrolithiasis secondary to hypercalciuria, muscle weakness or paralysis as a result of hypokalemia, and episodes of severe, life-threatening acidemia (sometimes triggered by a concurrent infection) may be seen also.

Complications are rare. The disorder appears to be transient and resolves spontaneously in time.

Distal Tubular Acidosis (Type I)

Distal tubular acidosis is caused by the inability of the kidney to establish a normal pH gradient between tubular cells and tubular contents. Its most characteristic feature is the inability to produce a urinary pH below 6.0 despite the presence of severe metabolic acidosis.

Distal renal tubular acidosis may occur as a primary, isolated defect or in association with other diseases or disorders. Most secondary causes are rare. The primary disorder is usually considered to be a hereditary defect with a variable degree of expression and a greater penetrance in females. After the age of 2 years the child usually has growth failure, although there is often a history of vomiting, polyuria, dehydration, anorexia, and failure to thrive. Evidence of bone demineralization (see hypophosphatemic rickets) may be present, along with, occasionally, the formation of urinary calculi (urolithiasis) in older children.

The inability to secrete hydrogen ion causes an accumulation of the ion in the body, which soon depletes the available hydrogen buffer, producing a sustained acidosis. Acidosis retards normal somatic growth, and demineralization of bone occurs as bone salts are mobilized to buffer the excessive hydrogen ions. Increased serum levels of both calcium and phosphorus contribute to the development of stones within the renal system. Both sodium and potassium are secreted in larger amounts. Serum potassium levels are depleted as the distal tubules excrete large amounts of potassium ions in an attempt to conserve sodium, since hydrogen ions are unable to participate in the exchange. Hyponatremia stimulates increased aldosterone secretion, which further aggravates the hypokalemia. With the depletion of bicarbonate ions, more chloride is reabsorbed in the proximal tubule to create a hyperchloremia.

Prognosis. The primary disorder is usually permanent, but with early diagnosis and therapy secondary effects on growth and stone formation can be avoided. When it occurs as a secondary complication and renal damage is prevented, the prognosis is good.

Therapeutic Management

Treatment of both proximal and distal disorders consists of administration of sufficient bicarbonate or citrate to balance metabolically produced hydrogen ions and maintain the plasma bicarbonate level within normal range and to correct associated electrolyte disorders, especially hypokalemia. Proximal disorders require large volumes of bicarbonate to compensate for urinary losses; in distal disorders the alkali required to maintain a normal plasma concentration is low. Most authorities favor a mixture of sodium and potassium bicarbonate (or citrate) in order to prevent deficiencies of either cation. The citrate solutions (Bicitra, Polycitra, or Shohl solution) are usually more easily tolerated than bicarbonate solutions. Shohl solution is very effective but has the disadvantage of requiring preparation by a pharmacist.

Nursing Considerations

Nursing goals include recognizing the possibility of renal tubular acidosis in children who fail to thrive or display other symptoms suggestive of the disorders and referring these children for medical evaluation. Helping parents understand the importance of compliance in administration of medications on a long-term basis is a primary goal of nursing management (see Compliance, Chapter 27, and Administration of Medication, Chapter 27). Children who must continue the medication indefinitely are taught the importance of taking the medications as soon as they are old enough to assume responsibility for their own care.

NEPHROGENIC DIABETES INSIPIDUS (NDI)

NDI is the major disorder associated with a defect in the ability to concentrate urine. In this disorder the distal tubules and collecting ducts are insensitive to the action of antidiuretic hormone or its exogenous counterpart, vasopressin. The nature of the defect is unknown but it occurs primarily in males, which supports X-linked recessive inheritance. The disease is more variable in female carriers of the defective gene who may exhibit only a mild defect in urine-concentrating ability. The differential diagnosis for NDI should include chronic obstructive renal disorders, sickle cell disease, renal tuberculosis, and other renal disorders, which may cause high urinary output with failure of the kidney to respond to vasopressin.

Clinical Manifestations

The disease is manifested in the newborn period by vomiting, unexplained fever, failure to thrive, and severe recurrent dehydration with hypernatremia. The passage of copious amounts of dilute urine, which produces severe dehydration and hypoelectrolytemia, is a serious threat to life during this period and may be responsible for the high incidence of mental and motor retardation found in affected persons. Growth retardation is probably related to diminished food intake and poor general health because of uncontrolled polydipsia. Diagnosis is suspected on the basis of the patient and family history and confirmed by a urine osmolality value consistently below that of plasma. Lack of response to vasopressin administration rules out other causes.

Therapeutic Management

Therapy involves provision of adequate volumes of water to compensate for urinary losses. As a result of an insatiable thirst, most of the child's time is spent drinking and voiding, with little time for activity and stimulation. These children may go to great lengths to satisfy their thirst. A low-sodium/low-solute diet and the use of chlorothiazide or ethacrynic acid diuretics to increase the reabsorption of sodium and water in the proximal tubule help to reduce the amount of tubular fluid delivered to the distal tubules and diminish the volume of water excreted. Urinary output has been reported to be reduced when prostaglandin inhibitors such as tolmetin sodium, indomethacin, ibuprofen, and aspirin are administered in conjunction with chlorothiazide (Libber, Harrison, and Spector, 1986). Supplemental potassium may be required to prevent hypokalemia as a result of thiazide therapy. If the disease is recognized early and treatment instituted and maintained, normal growth can be expected, and a normal life span anticipated.

Nursing Considerations

Nursing goals for children and families with NDI are to recognize signs of the disorder early and assist them in coping with the long-term inconvenience of the continual thirst and elimination problems. Families need to be taught to administer medications and help with diet planning for those on sodium restriction and who need supplemental potassium. The problem of ensuring adequate hydration is lifelong, and families need to adapt to away-from-home fluid needs and to avoid activities that contribute to dehydration when fluids may not be available. Genetic counseling is recommended.

MISCELLANEOUS RENAL DISORDERS

HEMOLYTIC-UREMIC SYNDROME (HUS)

HUS is an uncommon acute renal disease that is characterized by a triad of manifestations: acute renal failure, hemolytic anemia, and thrombocytopenia. HUS occurs primarily in infants and small children between the ages of 6 months and 3 years. It has been recognized predominantly in whites and, although it occurs worldwide, is more prevalent in South Africa, Argentina, and the West coasts of North and South America. HUS represents one of the main causes of acute renal failure in early childhood (Rizzoni and others, 1988).

Etiology

In the majority of cases no causative agents have been identified, although recent theories implicate genetic factors, prostacyclin deficiency, neuraminidase and agglutination, endotoxins (especially *Shigella* endotoxin), antithrombin-III deficiency, deficiency of antioxidants, and reduced platelet aggregation. The appearance of the disease has been associated with *Rickettsia,* viruses (especially Coxsackie, ECHO, and adenovirus), *Escherichia coli,* pneumococci, *Shigella,* and *Salmonella* and may represent an unusual response to these infections. Multiple cases of HUS caused by enteric infection of the *E. coli* 0157:H7 serotype have been traced to undercooked meat.

The disease usually follows an acute gastrointestinal or upper respiratory tract infection and tends to occur in scattered outbreaks in small geographic areas. HUS is clinically and pathologically similar to thrombocytopenic purpura, except for the hypertension that is associated with HUS. Some have speculated that thrombocytopenic purpura may be the adult version of the hemolytic-uremic syndrome of infancy and early childhood.

Pathophysiology

The primary site of injury appears to be the endothelial lining of the small glomerular arterioles, although other organs and tissues may be involved (e.g., the liver, brain, heart, pancreatic islet cells, and muscles). The endothelium becomes swollen and occluded with deposition of platelets and fibrin clots (intravascular coagulation). Red blood cells are damaged as they move through the partially occluded blood vessels. These fragmented red blood cells are removed by the spleen, causing acute hemolytic anemia. Fibrinolytic action on the precipitated fibrin causes these fibrin-split products to appear in the serum and urine. The platelet aggregation within damaged blood vessels or the damage and removal of platelets produce the characteristic thrombocytopenia.

Clinical Manifestations

The disease is preceded by a prodromal period during which there is an episode of diarrhea and vomiting. Less often the illness is an upper respiratory tract infection or, occasionally, varicella, measles, or a urinary tract infection.

The hemolytic process persists for several days to 2 weeks. During this time the child is anorectic, irritable, and lethargic. There is marked and rapid onset of pallor, accompanied by hemorrhagic manifestations such as bruising, purpura, or rectal bleeding. Severely affected patients are anuric and are frequently hypertensive. Convulsions and stupor suggest central nervous system involvement, and there may be signs of acute heart failure. Mild cases demonstrate anemia, thrombocytopenia, and azotemia; urinary output may be reduced or increased.

Diagnostic Evaluation

The triad of anemia, thrombocytopenia, and renal failure is sufficient for diagnosis. Renal involvement is evidenced by proteinuria, hematuria, and the presence of urinary casts; blood urea nitrogen and serum creatinine levels are elevated. A low hemoglobin and hematocrit and a high reticulocyte count confirm the hemolytic nature of the anemia.

Therapeutic Management

In general, treatment is directed toward control of the complications and hematologic manifestations of renal failure. The initial supportive measures for most children are those used in managing renal failure—fluid replacement (calculated with great care), treatment of hypertension, and correction of acidosis and electrolyte disorders. The most consistently effective treatment is early and repeated hemodialysis or peritoneal dialysis, which is instituted in any child who has been anuric for 24 hours or who demonstrates oliguria with uremia or hypertension and seizures. Blood transfusions with fresh, washed packed cells are administered for severe anemia but are used with caution to prevent circulatory overload from added volume.

Once vomiting and diarrhea have resolved, the child is restarted on enteral nutrition. Sometimes parenteral nutrition is required for children with severe, persistent colitis and in those in whom tissue catabolism is marked. There is no substantial evidence that heparin, corticosteroids, or fibrinolytic agents are beneficial, and in some instances they may aggravate the condition. The usefulness of plasma infusion for treatment of HUS is currently being studied.

Prognosis. With prompt treatment the recovery rate is about 95%, but residual renal impairment ranges from 10% to 50% in various areas. Death is usually caused by residual renal impairment or central nervous system injury.

Nursing Considerations

Nursing care is the same as that provided in acute renal failure and, for children with continued impairment, includes management of chronic disease. Because of the sudden and life-threatening nature of the disorder in a previously well child, parents are often ill-prepared for the impact of hospitalization and treatment. Therefore support and understanding are especially important aspects of care.

FAMILIAL GLOMERULOPATHY (ALPORT SYNDROME)

The syndrome of chronic hereditary nephritis consists of hematuria, high-frequency sensorineural deafness, ocular disorders, and chronic renal failure. The disease appears to be inherited as an autosomal-dominant trait, which suggests a possible X-linked dominant trait, although rare male-to-male transmission occurs. It is uncommon but not rare and accounts for a significant percentage of persistent glomerular disease in childhood.

The clinical manifestations are indistinguishable from mild acute nephritis. Initial symptoms include hematuria, proteinuria, malaise, and mild edema. Onset of gross hematuria may be associated with an acute respiratory infection. The average age of onset is 6 years, but the condition may be noted in infancy. It begins slowly and progresses until uncontrollable renal failure develops in adolescence or early adulthood. There is usually a positive family history. Most untreated boys develop severe symptoms, whereas affected girls generally have a milder disease and a normal life expectancy.

Treatment is symptomatic and supportive. Dialysis and renal transplantation are ultimate therapeutic measures for renal involvement. Hearing loss and ocular disorders should receive appropriate attention, and families should be counseled regarding the genetic implications of the disease.

UNEXPLAINED PROTEINURIA

Often apparently healthy children with no suggestion of renal disease will demonstrate proteinuria on routine urinalysis. The percentage of children with unexplained proteinuria ranges from 1% at 6 years of age to 11% at puberty, reaching a maximum prevalence at age 13 in girls and age 16 in boys.

Unexplained proteinuria can be categorized as (1) transient (inconstant), (2) persistent, or (3) orthostatic, or postural. ***Transient proteinuria*** is a common finding with no known cause, but it sometimes increases with febrile illness, exercise, cold, or emotions.

Persistent proteinuria usually signifies renal disease. ***Orthostatic proteinuria*** is seen in 3% to 5% of adolescents and young adults, and, although proteinuria is evident in the recumbent as well as the erect position, it is readily detected by qualitative tests. Reactions of 2+ or 3+ are frequently encountered. The cause is unknown, but minor glomerular changes occur in many instances. The condition is benign and generally resolves over a period of time.

In cases of unexplained proteinuria, it is important to confirm or exclude renal disease with appropriate diagnostic tests. Repeated examination for proteinuria, an orthostatic test, urine culture, and (if proteinuria is persistent) more definitive tests, including 24-hour protein excretion, renal ultrasound, and renal scan, are indicated.

RENAL TRAUMA

Serious injuries of the genitourinary tract are not uncommon in the pediatric age-group, the peak incidence occurring between the ages of 10 and 20 years. The kidneys are among the organs most often injured in children, despite their relatively protected location. However, the kidneys in children are more mobile than they are in the adult, and the outer borders are less well protected. They are separated from the skin surface by only 2 to 3 cm (¾ to 1¼ inches) in young children. Most injuries are of the nonpenetrating or "blunt" type, usually involving falls, athletic injuries, and motor vehicle accidents. Penetrating trauma (e.g., gunshot or stab wound) occurs much less frequently in children. In many children preexisting renal abnormalities, particularly congenital anomalies associated with mild to moderate hydronephrosis, are found that were unrecognized before the accident.

Renal injury can be suspected in children who complain of flank pain, and frequently there are abrasions or contusions on the overlying skin. Hematuria is consistently present, but the amount of blood in the urine is not a reliable indicator of the seriousness of the injury. Many relatively insignificant injuries are associated with grossly bloody urine, whereas some of the most severe injuries are found in children with only microscopic hematuria (see box above, right).

Renal rupture involves the actual splitting open of the kidney capsule, causing extravasation of blood or a mixture of blood and urine into the surrounding retroperitoneal space. Renal vascular injury, although unusual, requires immediate recognition and surgical intervention. Since the volume per minute blood flow through the kidney is greater (25% of cardiac output) than to any other abdominal organ, injury to the kidney may result in a rapid loss of blood.

In active children there may or may not be a history of unusual trauma. Abdominal or flank pain and tenderness are caused by bleeding around the kidney and may or may not be associated with fever. Clots passing down the ureter may cause pain similar to that of renal colic, and dysuria is common. Patients with more severe injuries may complain of nausea or abdominal pain. There may be a palpable abdominal mass caused by loss of blood and/or urine into the retroperitoneum. The fibrous capsule enclosing the kidney prevents expansion of a hematoma; therefore exsanguination and shock are seldom observed, even in severe renal trauma.

The diagnosis is made on the basis of intravenous pyelography, angiography, and/or retrograde pyelography. Unsuspected hydronephrosis often is first detected as a result of traumatic injury.

CLASSIFICATION ACCORDING TO EXTENT OF RENAL INJURY

Type I: A relatively mild renal contusion in which the capsule, parenchyma, and collecting system are usually intact but subcapsular bleeding frequently occurs into the parenchyma and appears in the urine. Renal contusion is an important cause of gross hematuria in active children.

Type II: Laceration of the kidney, injury to a major renal vessel, or injury to the collecting system with intracapsular extravasation of urine.

Type III: Multiple renal lacerations or injury to the main renal artery.

Therapeutic Management

Severe injury requires close observation in the hospital intensive care unit, as well as blood replacement if there is severe internal or external bleeding. In most cases bleeding subsides spontaneously. Surgical exploration is indicated in multiple injuries, extravasation of blood around the kidneys, or disruption of the major vessels or the collecting system. Children with less severe injuries, such as contusions only, are placed on bed rest. They should remain on bed rest for 3 days after cessation of gross bleeding, since the substance released from injured renal tissue (urinary urokinase) has strongly fibrinolytic properties that may precipitate serious bleeding. The prognosis depends on the nature and extent of the injury.

Nursing Considerations

Nursing management is directed toward recognizing and assisting in the diagnosis of renal injury. Care of both the child and the family is primarily supportive. All the concepts related to emergency hospitalization and care are implemented (see Chapter 26). Postsurgical care, if indicated, is the same as for any other surgical patient.

RENAL FAILURE

Renal failure is the inability of the kidneys to excrete waste material, concentrate urine, and conserve electrolytes. The disorder can be acute or chronic and affects most of the systems in the body. Two terms that are often used in relation to renal failure need some clarification: ***azotemia*** is the accumulation of nitrogenous waste within the blood; ***uremia*** is a more advanced condition in which retention of nitrogenous products produces toxic symptoms. Azotemia is not life-threatening, whereas uremia is a serious condition that often involves other body systems.

ACUTE RENAL FAILURE (ARF)

ARF is said to exist when the kidneys suddenly are unable to regulate the volume and composition of urine appropriately in response to food and fluid intake and the needs of the organism. The principal feature is oligoanuria* associated with azotemia, acidosis, and diverse electrolyte disturbances. ARF is not common in childhood, but the outcome depends on the cause, associated findings, and prompt recognition and treatment.

Etiology

ARF can develop as a result of a large number of related or unrelated clinical conditions—poor renal perfusion, acute renal injury, or the final expression of chronic, irreversible renal disease. The most common cause in children is transient renal failure resulting from dehydration or other causes of poor perfusion that respond to restoration of fluid volume. Causes of ARF are usually classified as prerenal, intrinsic renal, and postrenal causes. This implies that only renal causes are characterized by damage to the renal parenchyma, whereas prerenal and postrenal causes can be more easily remedied. However, severe or long-standing prerenal or postrenal etiologies can produce severe secondary renal damage.

Prerenal Causes. Prerenal causes of ARF are most common in children and are always related to reduction of renal perfusion in an anatomically and physiologically normal kidney and collecting system. Dehydration secondary to diarrheal disease or persistent vomiting is the most frequent cause of prerenal failure in infants and children. Surgical shock and trauma (including burns) are also common causes. Hypovolemia and decreased renal perfusion cause a decreased glomerular filtration rate and stimulate the secretion of renin, aldosterone, and antidiuretic hormone, which further diminish urine flow. Extended and severe hypoperfusion (secondary to such procedures as cardiac surgery) can produce cortical or tubular necrosis; however, when medical care is available, this is seldom allowed to occur. The azotemia that accompanies this type of renal failure generally is rapidly reversible with prompt attention to expansion of the extracellular fluid volume. Prerenal failure is often difficult to distinguish from tubular or cortical necrosis.

Intrinsic Renal Causes. Intrinsic renal causes of ARF comprise the largest group that requires extended management. These include diseases and nephrotoxic agents that damage the glomeruli, tubules, or renal vasculature. Glomerular disease is the most common cause of glomerular damage, whereas tubular destruction is more often caused by ischemia or nephrotoxins. Vascular damage is an uncommon cause of renal failure in childhood. The type and extent of damage determine the degree and duration of renal insufficiency, and it is difficult to predict in any given case whether or not acute necrosis will develop.

Postrenal Causes. ARF resulting from obstructive uropathy is uncommon in children except during the first year of life. However, renal function can be restored by relief of the obstruction. The degree of recovery depends on the duration of the renal failure.

Pathophysiology

ARF is usually reversible, but the deviations of physiologic function can be extreme, and mortality in the pediatric age-group is still high. There is severe reduction in the glomerular filtration rate, an elevated blood urea nitrogen level, and decreased tubular reabsorption of sodium from the proximal tubule. Consequently, there is increased concentration of sodium in the distal tubule, which causes stimulation of the renin mechanism. The local action of angiotensin causes vasoconstriction of the afferent arteriole, which further reduces glomerular filtration and prevents urinary losses of sodium. There is a significant reduction in renal blood flow.

The pathologic conditions that produce acute renal failure caused by glomerulonephritis, hemolytic-uremic syndrome, and other renal disorders have been discussed in relation to those disease processes. The necrotic processes within the nephron can be cortical, tubular, or both.

Cortical Necrosis. Complete cortical necrosis usually results from severe ischemia, infection, or intravascular coagulation and represents a severe, irreversible cause of acute renal failure. In the pediatric age-group this occurs as a fatal event most frequently during the neonatal period as a result of hypoxia and shock. When cortical destruction is incomplete, some recovery of renal function may occur. Intravascular coagulation is believed to play a significant role as an intermediate factor in the development of ARF, especially in cases related to sepsis.

Tubular Necrosis. Damage to the renal tubules can be broadly classified as (1) secondary to renal ischemia and (2) associated with the ingestion or inhalation of substances toxic to the kidneys. Renal tubules are particularly vulnerable to a wide variety of toxic agents that produce vasoconstriction and to focal patches of ischemia that cause a uniform necrosis of the tubular epithelium down to, but not including, the basement membrane. A lesion produced by sustained reduction in renal blood flow involves the basement membrane as well, which may become fragmented and ruptured to the extent that the continuity of tubular structure is disrupted. The lesions may affect any segment of the tubules, appearing at irregular intervals along with normal segments throughout the kidney.

Healing of tubular lesions is accomplished by reepithelialization in the areas with intact basement membrane. In those areas in which the basement membrane has been disrupted, such healing is unable to take place, and connective tissue grows through the ruptured membrane, thus pre-

*The definition of oligoanuria varies extensively, from 1.8 to 4 dl/m^2/24 hours, in the literature.

venting reestablishment of tubular integrity. Individual cells within the nephron are capable of regeneration, but the entire nephron is not capable of this.

Clinical Course. The clinical course of the child with ARF is variable and depends on the cause. In reversible ARF there is a period of severe oliguria, or the low-output phase, followed by an abrupt onset of diuresis, or a high-output phase, followed by a gradual return to, or toward, normal urine volumes. The length of the oliguric phase in older children and adolescents is 10 to 14 days, although it is highly variable at all ages. It tends to be shorter (3 to 5 days) in infants, children, and milder cases. The onset of the diuretic phase appears unexpectedly and over several days proceeds in stepwise fashion from very low to above-normal urine volumes. During the oliguric phase manifestations of uremia are present but may also be accompanied by other clinical disorders that make assessment difficult, such as infection, anoxia, and shock.

Clinical Manifestations

In many instances of ARF the infant or child is already critically ill with the precipitating disorder, and the explanation for development of oliguria may or may not be readily apparent. Often the underlying illness overshadows the renal failure and frequently assumes the priority of care (e.g., the patient who is in shock from endotoxemia, the infant who is severely dehydrated from gastroenteritis, or a child who is subject to seizures as a result of hypertensive encephalopathy associated with acute glomerulonephritis).

The prime manifestation of ARF is oliguria, generally a urinary output of less than 50 ml/24 hr. Anuria is uncommon except in obstructive disorders. Other symptoms related to ARF include edema, drowsiness, circulatory congestion, and cardiac arrhythmia from hyperkalemia. Seizures may be caused by hyponatremia or hypocalcemia and tachypnea from metabolic acidosis. With continued oliguria, biochemical abnormalities can develop rapidly, and circulatory and central nervous system manifestations appear.

Diagnostic Evaluation

When a previously well child develops ARF without obvious cause, a careful history is taken to reveal symptoms that may be related to glomerulonephritis, to obstructive uropathy, or regarding exposure to nephrotoxic chemicals, such as ingestion of heavy metals or inhalation of carbon tetrachloride or other organic solvents or drugs, such as methicillin, sulfonamides, neomycin, polymyxin, and kanamycin. Laboratory data reflect the kidney dysfunction—hyperkalemia, hyponatremia, metabolic acidosis, hypocalcemia, anemia, or azotemia (Table 30-7).

Therapeutic Management

The most effective management of ARF is prevention. The development of ARF is a known risk in certain situations. This should be anticipated and recognized, and adequate therapy should be implemented (e.g., fluid therapy for children with hypovolemia in such conditions as dehydration, burns, and hemorrhage). Nephrotoxic drugs should be used with caution or avoided in children with renal disease, and all personnel should be knowledgeable about precautions related to their administration. For example, a generous fluid intake is needed for children receiving antimetabolite drugs and after radiotherapy.

The treatment of ARF is directed toward (1) treatment of the underlying cause, (2) management of the complications of renal failure, and (3) provision of supportive therapy within the constraints imposed by the renal failure. Treatment of poor perfusion resulting from dehydration consists of volume restoration, as described in the treatment of dehydration (see Chapter 28). If oliguria persists after restoration of fluid volume or if the renal failure is caused by intrinsic renal damage, the physiologic and biochemical

TABLE 30-7 Laboratory Findings Associated with Acute Renal Failure

CLINICAL PROBLEM	MECHANISM	CLINICAL CONSIDERATIONS
Azotemia Elevated BUN levels	Ongoing protein catabolism Significantly decreased excretion	Lower rate of production in neonates and persons with depleted protein stores Increased in situations involving large amounts of necrotic tissue or extravasated blood
Elevated plasma creatinine levels	Continued production Significantly decreased excretion	Production less affected by other factors More sensitive measure of intensity of azotemia Low in neonate because of small muscle mass relative to size
Metabolic acidosis	Continued endogenous acid production Significantly decreased excretion Depletion of extracellular and intracellular fluid buffers	Compensatory hyperventilation Opisthotonos Major threat to life
Hyponatremia	Dilution of extracellular fluid Decreased excretion of water	May develop cerebral signs
Hyperkalemia	Ongoing protein catabolism Decreased excretion compounded by metabolic acidosis	Most important electrolyte to be considered in acute renal failure May contribute to cardiac arrhythmia With ECG changes, major threat to life May be lost from gastrointestinal tract
Hypocalcemia	Associated with metabolic acidosis and hyperphosphatemia	During alkali therapy, may cause tetany

abnormalities that have resulted from kidney dysfunction must be corrected or controlled. Central venous pressure monitoring is usually implemented.

Initially a Foley catheter is inserted to rule out urine retention, to collect available urine for electrolytes and analysis, and to monitor results of diuretic administration. The catheter may or may not be removed. Many authorities who believe that it serves little purpose during the oliguric phase and predisposes to bladder infection prefer collection bags for measuring urine output. Others maintain a catheter for hourly urine measurements.

Oliguria. When there is persistent oliguria in the presence of adequate hydration and no lower tract obstruction, mannitol, furosemide, or both may be administered rapidly as a test to provoke a flow of urine. When glomerular function is intact, the administration of these substances will behave as nonreabsorbable solute in the tubular fluid to evoke an osmotic diuresis. The presence of mannitol in tubular fluid and the obligatory water that follows it also serve to dilute the concentration of any nephrotoxin that may be present in the tubules below toxic levels. The furosemide blocks reabsorption of tubular filtrate. If urine flow is generated to the extent of 6 to 10 ml/kg of body weight in 1 to 3 hours, the initial dosage is reduced and continued, if needed, to sustain the flow. If no urine is produced within 2 hours after the single dose, the drugs are not repeated, and an oliguric regimen is instituted to control water balance and other abnormalities.

Fluid and Calories. The amount of exogenous water provided should not exceed the amount needed to maintain zero water balance. It is calculated on the basis of estimated endogenous water formation and losses from sensible (primarily gastrointestinal) and insensible sources. No allotment is calculated for urine as long as oliguria persists.

The child with ARF has a tendency to develop water intoxication and hyponatremia, which make it difficult to provide calories in sufficient amounts to meet the needs of the child and reduce the tissue catabolism, metabolic acidosis, hyperkalemia, and uremia. If the child is able to tolerate oral foods, concentrated food sources high in carbohydrate and fat but low in protein, potassium, and sodium may be provided. However, many children have functional disturbances of the gastrointestinal tract, such as nausea and vomiting; therefore the intravenous route is generally preferred, and nourishment usually consists of essential amino acids or a combination of essential and nonessential amino acids administered by the central venous route.

Control of water balance in these patients requires careful monitoring of feedback information, such as accurate intake and output, body weight, and electrolyte measurements. In general, during the oliguric phase no sodium, chloride, or potassium is given unless there are other large, ongoing losses. Regular measurement of plasma electrolyte, pH, blood urea nitrogen, and creatinine levels is required to assess the adequacy of fluid therapy and to anticipate complications that require specific treatment.

Hyperkalemia. An elevated serum potassium level is the most immediate threat to the life of the child with ARF. Potassium ions are not being excreted, whereas at the same time release of potassium from cells is accelerated by acidosis, stress, and tissue breakdown in cases associated with internal bleeding or trauma. Since cardiac arrhythmia and cardiac arrest may result, electrocardiograms as well as serum potassium ion levels are monitored regularly. Hyperkalemia can be minimized and sometimes avoided by eliminating potassium from all food and fluid, by reducing tissue catabolism, and by correcting acidosis.

NURSING ALERT Any of the following signs of hyperkalemia constitute an emergency situation and should be reported immediately:

Serum potassium concentrations in excess of 7 mEq/L

Presence of ECG abnormalities, such as prolonged QRS complex, depressed ST segment, high peaked T waves, bradycardia, or heart block

Several measures are available to reduce the serum potassium concentration, and the priority of implementation is usually based on the rapidity with which the measures are effective. Temporary measures that produce a rapid but transient effect are:

1. Calcium gluconate, 0.5 ml/kg, administered intravenously over 2 to 4 minutes, with continuous ECG monitoring, exerts a protective effect on cardiac conduction.
2. Sodium bicarbonate, 2 to 3 mEq/kg, administered intravenously over 30 to 60 minutes, elevates the serum pH to cause a transient shift of extracellular fluid potassium into the intracellular fluid. However, there is risk of hypocalcemia, tetany, and fluid overload.
3. Glucose, 50%, and insulin, 1 U/kg, administered intravenously, accelerate glycogen synthesis, causing glucose and potassium to move into the cells. Insulin facilitates the entry of glucose into cells.

These effects produce only transient protection by redistributing existing potassium stores; they do not remove potassium from the body. However, they provide relief while more definitive but slower-acting measures are being implemented. Potassium can be removed by:

1. Administration of an ion-exchange resin such as polystyrene sodium sulfonate (Kayexalate), 1 g/kg, administered orally or rectally, to bind potassium and remove it from the body. This requires time to be effective, and a sodium ion is exchanged for each potassium ion. This increased sodium concentration adds to the body fluids, which may contribute to fluid overload, hypertension, and cardiac failure.
2. Dialysis (discussed on p. 1325). Hemodialysis is efficient but requires specialized facilities. Peritoneal dialysis is simpler and can be carried out in almost any hospital setting. Indications for dialysis in ARF are continued oliguria associated with any of the following:
   - Severe, persistent acidosis
   - Inability to reduce serum potassium levels to a safe range with other methods
   - Clinical uremic syndrome, consisting of nausea and vomiting, drowsiness, and progression to coma
   - Circulatory overload, hypertension, and evidence of cardiac failure

A popular philosophy is to institute dialysis after 24 to 48 hours of oliguria, regardless of other symptoms. Supporters of this approach believe that early and frequent dialysis is associated with reduced morbidity and mortality and that it permits improved nutrition with relaxed diet restrictions. The combination of dialysis and nutrition tends to reduce the complications of ARF.

Hypertension. Hypertension is a frequent and serious complication of ARF, and, to detect it early, blood pressure determinations are taken every 4 to 6 hours. The most common cause of hypertension in ARF is overexpansion of the extracellular fluid and plasma volume together with activation of the renin-angiotensin system. The goal of therapy is to prevent hypertensive encephalopathy and avoid overtaxing the cardiovascular system.

When there is a threat of encephalopathy, labetalol (a beta and alpha blocker) may be administered intravenously as bolus infusions or a continuous drip. Sodium nitroprusside may be given but requires close monitoring. For less urgent situations, hydralazine, clonidine, or verapamil may be given intravenously. Oral drugs used for acute hypertension include nifedipine, captopril, minoxidil, hydralazine, propranolol, or furosemide (Lasix).

Other Complications. Other complications that may occur with ARF are anemia, convulsions and coma, cardiac failure, and pulmonary edema. ***Anemia*** is frequently associated with ARF, but transfusion is not recommended unless the hemoglobin level drops below 6 g/dl. Transfusions consist of fresh, packed red blood cells given slowly to reduce the likelihood of increasing blood volume, hypertension, and hyperkalemia.

Seizures occur rather often when renal failure progresses to uremia and are also related to hypertension, hyponatremia, and hypocalcemia. Treatment is directed to the specific cause when known. More obscure etiologies are managed with antiepileptic drugs.

Cardiac failure with pulmonary edema is almost always associated with hypervolemia. Treatment is directed toward reduction of fluid volume, with water and sodium restriction and administration of diuretics. Digitalis is ineffective and can be hazardous.

Diuretic, or High-Output, Phase. When the output begins to increase, either spontaneously or in response to diuretic therapy, the intake of fluid, potassium, and sodium must be monitored, and adequate replacement must be provided to prevent depletion and its consequences. In some cases the high-output phase is mild and lasts only a few days; in others enormous amounts of electrolyte-rich urine are passed.

Prognosis. The prognosis of ARF depends largely on the nature and severity of the causative factor or precipitating event and the promptness and competence of management. The mortality rate is less than 20%. The outcome is least favorable in children with rapidly progressive nephritis and cortical necrosis. Children in whom ARF is a result of hemolytic-uremic syndrome or acute glomerulitis may recover completely, but residual renal impairment or hypertension is more often the rule. Complete recovery is usually expected in children whose renal failure is a result of dehydration, nephrotoxins, or ischemia. ARF following cardiac surgery is less favorable. It is often impossible to assess the extent of recovery for several months.

Nursing Considerations

Nursing care of the infant or child with ARF involves care of the underlying cause plus careful observation and management of the renal status. The major goal is reestablishment of renal function, with emphasis on providing an adequate caloric intake to minimize reduction of protein stores, prevention of complications, and monitoring of fluid balance, laboratory data, and physical manifestations. The probability of dialysis must be considered, and the necessary equipment made available in anticipation of such an eventuality. Because the child requires intensive observation and often specialized equipment, admission to an intensive care unit where equipment and personnel trained in its use are available is the usual disposition.

❖ Assessment

Meticulous attention to the fluid intake and output is mandatory, including all the physical measurements discussed previously in relation to problems of fluid balance. Monitoring of fluid balance and vital signs is continuous, and observers are constantly on the alert for signs of complications so that appropriate interventions can be implemented.

NURSING ALERT Diminished urinary output and lethargy in a child who is dehydrated, in shock, or recently postoperative should be evaluated for possible acute kidney failure.

❖ Nursing Diagnoses

A number of diagnoses are evident following a thorough assessment of the child with ARF (see Nursing Care Plan, p. 1317). Others will be noted, depending on the age of the child, the cause of the renal failure, and any concomitant complications.

❖ Planning

The major goals for the child with ARF and the family are as follows:

1. Child will maintain appropriate fluid volume.
2. Child will maintain normal electrolyte levels.
3. Child will maintain blood pressure within acceptable limits.
4. Child will experience minimized risk of infection.
5. Child and family will receive adequate support.

❖ Implementation

The major nursing task in the care of the infant or child with ARF is monitoring and assessing fluid and electrolyte balance. Limiting fluid intake requires ingenuity on the part of caregivers to cope with the child who is thirsty. Rationing the daily intake in small amounts of fluid served in containers that give the impression of larger volumes is one strategy. Older children who understand the rationale of fluid limits can help determine how their daily ration should be distributed.

Meeting nutritional needs is sometimes a problem, since the child may be nauseated and getting the child to eat concentrated foods without fluids may be difficult. When nourishment is provided by the intravenous (IV) route, careful

NURSING CARE PLAN
The Child with Acute Renal Failure

NURSING DIAGNOSIS: Fluid volume excess related to failure or compromised renal regulatory mechanisms

PATIENT GOAL 1: Will maintain appropriate fluid volume

• NURSING INTERVENTIONS/*RATIONALES*

Assist with dialysis *to maintain excretory function*

Monitor progress *to assess adequacy of therapy and detect possible complications*

• EXPECTED OUTCOME

Child exhibits no evidence or complications of accumulated fluid and waste products between dialysis sessions

PATIENT GOAL 2: Will maintain appropriate fluid volume through regulation of fluid intake

• NURSING INTERVENTIONS/*RATIONALES*

*Administer intravenous or oral fluids as prescribed

Closely monitor intravenous infusion *to maintain prescribed intake and prevent fluid overload*

Measure and record intake and output accurately

Weigh daily (or more often if indicated)

Employ strategies to prevent undesired intake

- Remove fluids from access by child
- Use small containers for fluid intake *so that volume does not appear so restricted*
- Divide allowed intake into volumes spread over 24 hours to avoid period of no fluid allowance
- Spray mouth with atomizer (avoid excess use, which would increase intake) *to prevent feeling of dryness*
- Keep lips lubricated *for comfort and to prevent cracking*

• EXPECTED OUTCOME

Child exhibits no evidence of fluid gain

NURSING DIAGNOSIS: High risk for injury related to accumulated electrolytes and waste products

PATIENT GOAL 1: Will maintain normal electrolyte levels

• NURSING INTERVENTIONS/*RATIONALES*

*Assist with dialysis *to maintain excretory function*

*Administer Kayexalate as prescribed *to reduce serum potassium levels*

*Provide diet low in protein, potassium, and sodium, if prescribed, *to reduce excretory demand on kidneys*

Observe for evidence of accumulated waste products (hyperkalemia, hypernatremia, uremia) *to ensure prompt treatment*

• EXPECTED OUTCOME

Child exhibits no evidence of waste product accumulation

*Dependent nursing action.

PATIENT GOAL 2: Will maintain blood pressure within acceptable limits

• NURSING INTERVENTIONS/*RATIONALES*

*Administer antihypertensives as prescribed *to reduce blood pressure*

Avoid situations that increase child's anxiety and apprehension, *since these factors can raise blood pressure*

Provide quiet, calm environment

• EXPECTED OUTCOME

Child's blood pressure remains within acceptable limits (specify)

NURSING DIAGNOSIS: Potential for infection related to lowered body defenses, fluid overload

PATIENT GOAL 1: Will experience minimized risk of infection

• NURSING INTERVENTIONS/*RATIONALES*

Protect child from contact with infected persons *to minimize exposure to infective organisms*

- Place in room with noninfectious children
- Restrict contact with persons who have infections, including family, other children, friends, and staff members
- Teach visitors appropriate preventive behaviors (e.g., handwashing)

Observe medical asepsis

- Practice good handwashing

Keep child warm and dry *because of vulnerability to upper respiratory infection*

Monitor temperature *for early evidence of infection*

• EXPECTED OUTCOMES

Child and family apply good health practices

Child exhibits no evidence of infection

NURSING DIAGNOSIS: Altered family processes related to a child with a serious disease

PATIENT (FAMILY) GOAL 1: Will receive adequate support

• NURSING INTERVENTIONS/*RATIONALES* AND EXPECTED OUTCOMES

See Nursing Care Plan: The Family of the Ill or Hospitalized Child, Chapter 26

See also Nursing Care Plan: The Child in the Hospital, Chapter 26

monitoring is essential to prevent fluid overload. IV fluid management related to fluid overload can become a major challenge in the face of nutritional requirements and administration of IV medications. The IV drugs being used may be nephrotoxic, which can require a specified volume of solution for delivery. In some instances blood products must also be delivered. Collaborating to prevent fluid overload while delivering medications and calories requires a concerted effort. In addition, nursing measures, such as maintaining an optimum thermal environment, reducing any elevation of body temperature, and reducing restlessness and anxiety, are employed to decrease the rate of tissue catabolism.

The nurse must be continually alert for changes in behavior that indicate the onset of complications. Infection from reduced resistance, anemia, and general morbidity is a constant threat. Fluid overload and electrolyte disturbances can precipitate cardiovascular complications such as hypertension and cardiac failure. Fluid and electrolyte imbalances, acidosis, and accumulation of nitrogenous waste products can produce neurologic involvement manifested by coma, seizures, or alterations in sensorium.

Although children with ARF are usually quite ill and voluntarily diminish their activity, infants may become restless and irritable, and children are often anxious and frightened. Frequent, painful, and stress-producing treatments and tests must be performed. The presence of a supportive, empathetic nurse can provide comfort and stability in a threatening and unnatural environment.

Family Support. Providing support and reassurance to parents is among the major nursing responsibilities. The seriousness and emergency nature of ARF are stressful to parents, and most feel some degree of guilt regarding the child's condition, especially when the illness is the result of ingestion of a toxic substance, dehydration, or a genetic disease. They need reassurance and a sympathetic listener. They also need to be kept informed of the child's progress and provided explanations regarding the therapeutic regimen. The equipment and the child's behavior are sometimes frightening and anxiety provoking. Nurses can do much to help parents comprehend and deal with the stresses of the situation.

❖ Evaluation

The effectiveness of nursing interventions is determined by continual reassessment and evaluation of care based on the following observational guidelines and expected outcomes:

1. Carry out frequent assessment of vital signs and behaviors.
2. Observe eating behaviors and energy expenditure; monitor intake of protein and calories; carefully monitor intake and output, weigh daily or more often as prescribed.
3. Monitor vital signs, sensorium and other neurologic signs; evaluate laboratory results and observe for signs of electrolyte imbalance.
4. Observe and interview child and family regarding their understanding of the disease and therapies; encourage child and family to express their feelings and concerns.

Expected outcomes:
See Nursing Care Plan, p. 1317.

CHRONIC RENAL FAILURE (CRF)

The kidneys are able to maintain the chemical composition of fluids within normal limits until more than 50% of functional renal capacity is destroyed by disease or injury. CRF or insufficiency begins when the diseased kidneys can no longer maintain the normal chemical structure of body fluids under normal conditions. Progressive deterioration over months or years produces a variety of clinical and biochemical disturbances that eventually culminate in the clinical syndrome known as ***uremia.*** When the kidneys can no longer function, even with medical intervention, and the patient must resort to dialysis for clearing wastes, the term ***end-stage renal disease (ESRD)*** is applied. The pattern of renal dysfunction is remarkably uniform no matter what disease process initiates the advanced disease.

Etiology

A variety of diseases and disorders can result in CRF. The most frequent causes of CRF before age 5 years are congenital renal and urinary tract malformations (particularly renal hypoplasia and dysplasia and obstructive uropathy) and vesicoureteral reflux. Glomerular and hereditary renal disease predominate in children 5 to 15 years of age. Glomerular diseases that most frequently lead to CRF are chronic pyelonephritis, chronic glomerulonephritis, and glomerulonephropathy associated with systemic diseases such as anaphylactoid purpura and lupus erythematosus. Hereditary nephritis, congenital nephrotic syndrome, Alport syndrome, polycystic kidney, and several other hereditary disorders result in renal failure in childhood. Renal vascular disorders such as hemolytic-uremic syndrome, vascular thrombosis, or cortical necrosis are less frequent causes.

Pathophysiology

Early in the course of progressive nephron destruction, the child remains asymptomatic with only minimal biochemical abnormalities. Unless its presence is detected in the process of routine assessment, signs and symptoms that indicate advanced renal damage frequently emerge only late in the course of the disease. Midway in the disease process, as increasing numbers of nephrons are totally destroyed and most others are damaged in varying degree, the few that remain intact are hypertrophied but functional. These few normal nephrons are able to make sufficient adjustments to stresses to maintain reasonable degrees of fluid and electrolyte balance. Definitive biochemical examination at this time will reveal restricted tolerance to excesses or restrictions. As the disease progresses to the end stage, because of severe reduction in the number of functioning nephrons, the kidneys are no longer able to maintain fluid and electrolyte balance, and the features of the uremic syndrome appear.

The pathophysiology of specific biochemical abnormalities is briefly summarized in the following sections.

Retention of Waste Products. A moderate decrease in renal function is not associated with a rise in fasting blood urea nitrogen concentration. With progressive nephron destruction and diminished function, the serum level of these end products of protein metabolism increases.

However, the blood urea nitrogen level is affected by protein intake, whereas the creatinine concentration depends on muscle mass; therefore creatinine is a more reliable index of renal failure.

Water and Sodium Retention. The damaged kidneys are able to maintain sodium and water balance under normal circumstances, although the few remaining functional nephrons are required to increase their rate of filtration and reabsorption in proportion to their numbers. The limitations of this capacity become apparent under stress. The nature of abnormalities in adjustment depends on the underlying renal disease: infants and small children with kidney dysplasia or urinary obstructive disease tend to excrete large volumes of dilute urine low in sodium content; children with glomerular disease tend to retain both sodium and water as a result of a greater reduction in glomerular filtration than of tubular reabsorption; and children with defective sodium reabsorption from tubular disease tend to lose sodium with a corresponding osmotic water loss. Consequently, sodium excesses may cause edema and hypertension, whereas sodium deprivation can result in hypovolemia and circulatory failure. Only in ESRD is markedly reduced glomerular filtration inadequate to handle normal amounts of sodium and water. Retention of these substances leads to edema and vascular congestion.

Hyperkalemia. Dangerous hyperkalemia is an infrequent occurrence in CRF until the end stage. However, the kidneys are unable to adjust readily to increased ingestion of potassium, and they require a longer period of time to rid the body of this excess.

Acidosis. A sustained metabolic acidosis is characteristic of CRF; it results from the inability of the damaged kidney to excrete a normal load of metabolic acids generated by normal metabolic processes. There is reduced capacity of the distal tubules to produce ammonia and impaired reabsorption of bicarbonate. Although there is continual hydrogen ion retention and bicarbonate loss, the plasma pH is maintained at a level compatible with life by other buffering mechanisms, particularly the bone salt (see following sections).

Calcium and Phosphorus Disturbances. One of the distressing features of CRF is its effect on calcium and phosphorus homeostasis. Profound and complex disturbances in the metabolism of these substances result in significant bone demineralization and impaired growth. This appears to be related to several factors (see top box at right). The result of these complex disturbances in calcium, phosphorus, and bone metabolism produces growth arrest or retardation, bone pain, and deformities known as ***renal osteodystrophy,*** sometimes called ***renal rickets,*** since the disorganization of bone growth and demineralization are similar to that caused by vitamin D–resistant rickets.

Anemia. A consistent feature of chronic renal insufficiency is anemia that appears to result from several factors (see middle box at right).

Growth Disturbance. One of the most striking effects of CRF in childhood, and one that can have profound psychologic and social consequences for the developing child, is retarded growth. The cause is poorly understood but may be related to nutritional and biochemical factors (see box above).

Sexual maturation may be delayed or may not occur in children with CRF, and secondary amenorrhea frequently develops in girls past puberty. CRF can also cause sexual dysfunction by creating imbalances in gonadal hormone levels. Decreased testosterone levels impair spermatogenesis in males; decreased estrogen, luteinizing hormone, and progesterone cause anovulation and menstrual irregularities (usually amenorrhea) in females. Autonomic neuropa-

FACTORS RELATED TO BONE DEMINERALIZATION IN CHRONIC RENAL FAILURE

1. In a state of acidosis there is dissolution of the alkaline salts of bone, which serve as buffers, and the release of phosphorus and calcium into the bloodstream.
2. Reduced glomerular filtration and excretion of inorganic phosphate lead to an elevation of plasma phosphate with a concomitant decrease in serum calcium.
3. Decreased serum calcium concentration stimulates the secretion of parathyroid hormone (PTH), which results in resorption of calcium from bones. Under normal circumstances parathyroid hormone inhibits the tubular reabsorption of phosphates.
4. Diseased kidneys are unable to complete the synthesis of vitamin D to its most active form, 1,25-dihydroxycholecalciferol, which is necessary for the absorption of calcium from the gastrointestinal tract and deposition of calcium in bone. This acquired resistance to vitamin D decreases calcium absorption, permits retention of phosphorus, and contributes to secondary hyperparathyroidism.

CAUSES OF ANEMIA IN CHRONIC RENAL FAILURE

1. Shortened life span of red blood cells caused by some extracorpuscular factor associated with the uremic state
2. Impaired red blood cell production resulting from decreased production of erythropoietin
3. Increased tendency to bleed, associated with a prolonged bleeding time, probably related to impaired platelet function
4. Superimposed nutritional anemia

PROBABLE CAUSES OF GROWTH FAILURE IN CHRONIC RENAL FAILURE

1. Renal osteodystrophy
2. Poor nutrition associated with dietary restrictions (especially protein) and loss of appetite
3. Biochemical abnormalities associated with renal failure, such as sustained acidosis, hyperkalemia, chronic hyposmolarity secondary to hyposthenuria (secretion of urine with low specific gravity), and phosphorus depletion

thy and anemia are also factors that can alter sexual function.

Other Disturbances. Children with CRF are more susceptible to infection, especially pneumonia, urinary tract infection, and septicemia, although the reason for this is not entirely clear. Hyperventilation, a manifestation of the respiratory compensatory mechanism for metabolic acidosis, and pulmonary edema may contribute to upper respiratory tract infection. These children become extraordinarily sensitive to changes in vascular volume that may cause, in addition to pulmonary overload, cerebral symptoms and circulatory manifestations such as hypertension and cardiac failure.

Numerous neurologic manifestations appear with advanced renal failure, although no specific toxin or biochemical defect has been identified. However, disturbances in enzyme function, disturbances in water and electrolyte balance, altered calcium ion concentration, hypertension, and accumulation of various "uremic toxins" have been implicated.

Clinical Manifestations

The first evidence of difficulty is usually loss of normal energy and increased fatigue on exertion. For example, the child may prefer quiet, passive activities rather than participation in more active games and outdoor play. The child is usually somewhat pale, but the change is often so inconspicuous that it may not be evident to parents or others. Sometimes the blood pressure is elevated. Growth is affected early in the development of chronic renal failure, and falling behind on the growth chart is often the first measurable sign.

As the disease progresses, other manifestations may appear. The child eats less well (especially breakfast); shows less interest in normal activities, such as schoolwork or play; and has a decreased or increased urinary output and a compensatory intake of fluid. For example, a child who has achieved bladder control may wet the bed at night. Pallor becomes more evident as the skin develops a characteristic sallow, muddy appearance as a result of anemia and deposition of urochrome pigment in the skin. The child may complain of headache, muscle cramps, and nausea. Other signs and symptoms include weight loss, facial puffiness, malaise, bone or joint pain, growth retardation, dryness or itching of the skin, bruised skin, and sometimes sensory or motor loss. Amenorrhea is common in adolescent girls.

Therapy is generally instigated before the appearance of the ***uremic syndrome***, although there are occasions in which the symptoms may be observed. Manifestations of untreated uremia reflect the progressive nature of the homeostatic disturbances and general toxicity. Gastrointestinal symptoms include loss of appetite, and nausea and vomiting. Bleeding tendencies are apparent in bruises, bloody diarrheal stools, stomatitis, and bleeding from the lips and mouth. There is intractable itching, probably related to hyperparathyroidism, and deposits of urea crystals appear on the skin as "uremic frost" (Greaves, 1992). There may be an unpleasant "uremic" odor to the breath. Respirations become deeper as a result of metabolic acidosis, and circulatory overload is manifested by hypertension, congestive heart failure, and pulmonary edema. Neurologic involvement is reflected by progressive confusion, dulling of the sensorium, and, ultimately, coma. Other signs may include tremors, muscular twitching, and seizures.

Diagnostic Evaluation

The diagnosis of CRF is usually suspected on the basis of any of a number of clinical manifestations, a history of prior renal disease, and/or biochemical findings. The onset is usually gradual, and the initial signs and symptoms are vague and nonspecific. Laboratory and other diagnostic tools and tests are of value in assessing the extent of renal damage, biochemical disturbances, and related physical dysfunction. Often they can help establish the nature of the underlying disease and differentiate between other disease processes and the pathologic consequences of renal dysfunction.

Therapeutic Management

In irreversible renal failure the goals of medical management are to promote effective renal function, to maintain body fluid and electrolyte balance within acceptable limits, to treat systemic complications, and to promote as active and normal a life as possible for the child for as long as possible. This becomes increasingly difficult as the disease progresses toward its inevitable end. Even therapeutic measures designed to relieve one manifestation may prove detrimental to another. For example, antihypertensive agents may further impair renal function.

Activity. Children are allowed unrestricted activity and to set their own limits regarding rest and extent of exertion. They are encouraged to attend school. When the effort is too great, home tutoring is arranged.

Diet. Regulation of diet has been seen as the most effective means, short of dialysis, for reducing the quantity of materials that require renal excretion. The goal of the diet in renal failure is to provide sufficient calories and protein for growth while minimizing the excretory demands made on the kidney, to limit metabolic bone disease (osteodystrophy), and to minimize fluid and electrolyte disturbances. Dietary protein intake is limited only to the recommended daily allowance (RDA) for the child's age. Restriction of protein intake below the RDA is believed to negatively impact growth and neurodevelopment (Raymond and others 1990). Dietary phosphorus may need to be restricted. It should be remembered that any attempt to restrict dietary intake in children potentially restricts caloric intake and can impact growth.

Protein in the diet should include foods of high biologic value. When given with meals, substances that bind phosphorus in the intestines prevent its absorption and allow a more liberal intake of phosphorus-containing protein. Sodium and water are not usually limited, unless there is evidence of edema or hypertension.

Potassium is not restricted as long as creatinine clearance remains at acceptable limits (greater than or equal to 30 to 35 ml/min). Restrictions are instituted for patients with oliguria or anuria, however. Restrictions of any or all these minerals may be imposed in later stages or at any time in which factors cause abnormal serum concentrations.

Because of modified dietary intake, altered metabolism, and poor appetite, some dietary supplementation is usually needed. Because fat-soluble vitamins can accumulate in patients with CRF, vitamins A, E, and K are not supplemented beyond normal dietary intake. Vitamin D is prescribed, and water-soluble vitamin supplementation may be required if the diet is inadequate. Other dietary needs are discussed in relation to osteodystrophy and anemia. Dietary management of the child with renal failure is a difficult and complex problem that necessitates collaboration with a registered dietician who is knowledgeable of pediatric nutrition and the impact of renal failure.

Osteodystrophy. Measures directed at prevention or correction of the calcium/phosphorus imbalance are reduction of dietary phosphorus, administration of a phosphorus-binding agent, provision of supplemental calcium, control of acidosis, and administration of vitamin D.

Dietary phosphorus can be controlled by the reduction of protein and milk intake. Phosphorus levels can be further reduced by the oral administration of phosphorus-binding agents that combine with the phosphorus to decrease gastrointestinal absorption and thus the serum levels of phosphate.

Calcium carbonate preparations can be used as phosphorus binders. These medications act as (1) phosphate binders, (2) calcium supplements, and (3) alkalizing agents. Calcium carbonate preparations can be given with meals to bind phosphorus if the child is hyperphosphatemic or mildly hypocalcemic. If given 1 to 2 hours after meals, they act as calcium supplements for children with stable phosphorus but low calcium levels. Calcium acetate can also be used.

Aluminum hydroxide gels are also effective phosphorus binders. However, aluminum phosphate binders have been shown to cause aluminum loading when used on a continuous basis in children; therefore these substances are used only for very short periods to treat severe or unresponsive hyperphosphatemia (Sedman, 1986). These children should be monitored for aluminum accumulation and evidence of aluminum intoxication, such as altered sensorium, inability to talk, ataxia, or seizures.

When serum phosphate levels are within a normal range, appropriate vitamin D therapy is instituted. The drugs that are administered to increase the absorption of calcium through the gastrointestinal tract include dehydrotachysterol (Hytakerol) or 1,25-dihydroxyvitamin D_3 (Rocaltrol). The serum calcium level is monitored weekly during periods when the drugs are being changed or regulated. Parathyroid hormone levels are measured every 2 to 3 months.

Osseous deformities that result from renal osteodystrophy, especially those related to ambulation, are troublesome and require correction if they occur. Careful attention to the management of osteodystrophy and bone growth can prevent deformities from occurring in some children.

Acidosis. Pharmacologic treatment of acidosis is initiated early in children who have chronic renal insufficiency. In addition to reducing the formation of metabolic acids by decreasing the dietary intake of protein, acidosis is alleviated by alkalizing agents such as sodium bicarbonate or a combination of sodium and potassium citrate (Bicitra, Polycitra, or Shohl solution*). Correction of acidosis is best attempted after calcium levels are elevated, since rapid correction may precipitate tetany in a hypocalcemic child.

Anemia. Because the anemia associated with renal failure is related to decreased production of erythropoietin, it usually cannot be successfully managed with hematinic agents. However, sufficient sources of folic acid and iron should be provided in the diet, although this is difficult when protein sources are restricted. Inadequate intake and iron losses that may occur are managed by supplemental iron, usually ferrous sulfate. Providing adequate sources of ascorbic acid at the same time that iron-rich foods or supplement are given enhances the absorption.

The medication, recombinant human erythropoietin (rHuEPO), corrects anemia (improving energy level and general well-being) and eliminates the need for frequent blood transfusions in patients with CRF (Eschbach and Adamson, 1989). Injectable iron supplements may be required in conjunction with rHuEPO.

Hypertension. Hypertension of advanced renal disease may be managed initially by cautious use of a low-sodium diet, fluid restriction, and perhaps diuretics such as thiazides or furosemide. Strict restriction of sodium intake may be necessary in oliguric patients. Severe hypertension may require the use of a combination of a beta blocker and a vasodilator (propranolol and hydralazine). Other drugs that may be used include nifedipine, atenolol, minoxidil, prazosin, captopril, or labetalol singly or in combinations.

Growth Retardation. One major consequence of CRF is growth retardation, especially in the preadolescent. These children grow poorly both before and after initiation of hemodialysis. Depletion of body protein is characteristic of children with CRF, in addition to a number of metabolic abnormalities. The use of recombinant human growth hormone to accelerate growth in children with growth retardation secondary to CRF has been approved by the FDA. Studies are now being conducted in various pediatric centers to evaluate the use of recombinant human growth hormone following renal transplant. Evidence indicates marked acceleration in growth velocity in children treated with growth hormone (Koch and others, 1989).

Miscellaneous Complications. Intercurrent infections are treated with appropriate antimicrobials at the first sign of infection. Most of these drugs are excreted through the kidneys; therefore, the dosage is usually reduced in proportion to the decrease in renal function, and the interval between doses is extended in these children to avoid possible toxic effects from accumulation. Any drug eliminated through the kidneys is administered with caution. Serum levels of ototoxic and/or nephrotoxic drugs (e.g., gentamycin or kanamycin) are assessed regularly to ensure a safe nontoxic level.

*Each milliliter of Shohl solution contains 1 mEq of citrate ion, which metabolizes to yield 1 mEq of bicarbonate. Citric acid exerts no effect on acid-base balance but enhances the palatability of the mixture.

Dental defects are common in children with chronic kidney disease, and the earlier the onset of the disease the more severe are the dental manifestations. These include hypoplasia, hypomineralization, tooth discoloration, alteration in size and shape of teeth, malocclusion (secondary to deficient skeletal growth), ulcerative stomatitis, occasional oral hematomas, and an increase in calcific deposits around the teeth. Regular dental care is especially important in these children. Other nondental complications are treated symptomatically (e.g., chlorpromazine [Thorazine] or prochlorperazine [Compazine] is given for nausea, antiepileptics are given for seizures, and diphenhydramine [Benadryl] is given for pruritus). Once evidence of ESRD appears in a child, the disease runs its relentless course and terminates in death in a few weeks, unless waste products and toxins are removed from body fluids by dialysis and/or kidney transplantation. Since these techniques have been adapted for infants and small children, the outlook for these patients has improved remarkably. These alternatives are implemented in most cases of renal failure once palliative management is no longer effective.

Nursing Considerations

The child with CRF is a prime example of an individual whose life is maintained by drugs and artificial means, and the multiple stresses placed on these children and their families are often overwhelming. The unrelenting course of the disease process is one of progressive deterioration. There is no means to prevent the irreversible progress of renal insufficiency, nor is there any known cure. As the affected child progresses from renal insufficiency to uremia and then to dialysis and transplantation with a need for intensity of therapy, the need for supportive nursing care is also intensified. Team effort is more important than ever and involves coordination of personnel from medicine, nursing, social services, physical/occupational therapy, dietetics, and psychologic or psychiatric specialties.

Progressive disease places a number of stresses on the child and the family. There is a continuing need for repeated examinations that often entail painful procedures, side effects, and frequent hospitalizations. Diet therapy can become progressively more restrictive and intense, and parents may need help in learning to select appropriate foods, in reading labels carefully for sodium and potassium content, and in modifying meals to accommodate the special needs of the child. The child is required to take a variety of medications. Compliance is difficult when long-term therapies are involved. Ever present in all aspects of the treatment regimen is the agonizing realization that without treatment death is the inevitable outcome.

ESRD presents the same nonspecific stresses on child and family as any other chronic (Chapter 22) or life-threatening (Chapter 23) illness. The reactions and adaptation of the child and family depend on the age and developmental stage of the child, the cultural and socioeconomic background of the family, the quality of the interpersonal relationships of family members, and the communication patterns within the family. In general the problems observed and emotional responses to the stress of the illness are influenced less by the nature of the illness than by the family relationships and the personalities of its members.

One of the first and most noticeable changes is the alteration in physical appearance—fluctuations in weight, anemia, and failure to grow. Children must adjust to the fact that they will always be different from their peers in some ways. They will be shorter, often more tired, and unable to participate in all the activities that are attractive to young people. Children who have had diversion procedures, dialysis shunts, and other surgeries or who urinate into a bag need to learn positive coping strategies for the alterations in their body image and for the questions and potential teasing of peers. It is not difficult or unusual for children with chronic conditions to exhibit behavioral regression. This is particularly so for children with renal failure, since their appearance is often of a child much younger than their chronologic age.

School is often difficult for these children. Frequent absences for illnesses, evaluations, or treatments disrupt the educational process and socialization. Teachers and school systems are not always sympathetic to the rights and needs of a child with a chronic illness (e.g., the right to equal education and the need for flexibility and special help at times), which places an additional burden on the parents. Sometimes a teacher will pass a failing child because of pity.

In some families illness and stressful experiences act as a unifying force; in others stress aggravates preexisting problems and contributes to family disharmony. The relentless nature of the disease and its therapies not only place physical and emotional stresses on the family but are also a chronic drain on the family finances. Insurance rarely covers the full cost of the multiple hospitalizations and outpatient expenses. ESRD care is funded by the federal Medicare program, for which most children qualify. However, hidden costs abound, such as transportation to special treatment centers, meals, and sometimes lodging away from home. Some temporary assistance may be provided by private foundations, churches, and community groups, and nurses should become familiar with those in the area of their practice that can be of financial and educational service to these families. For example, the **National Kidney Foundation*** and numerous other agencies provide services and information for families, including pamphlets and descriptive literature. Particularly useful are booklets written for children with renal disease.†

Some specific stresses related to ESRD and its treatment are predictable. When it first becomes apparent that kidney failure is inevitable, both parents and child experience great depression and anxiety. Acceptance is particularly difficult if renal failure progresses rapidly after the diagnosis.

*National Kidney Foundation, 30 E. 33rd St., New York, NY 10016; (212) 889-2210 or (800) 622-9010.

†Recommended resources for children and parents are *Sidney Kidney* by H.H. Pamplin, J.A. Light, and L.R. Hyman (1974, Walter Reed Army Medical Center); and *Understanding Kidney Failure: A Handbook for Parents* by F. Orrbine and N.N. Wolfish, available for $2.00 from Children's Hospital of Eastern Ontario Foundation, 385 Smyth Rd., Ottawa, Ontario, Canada K1H 8L2.

Denial and disbelief are usually pronounced, especially among parents. Denial can also develop when progression to ESRD has been prolonged and both the parents and the child develop a denial pattern of believing it will never occur.

Once the kidney failure is established and symptoms become progressively more distressing, the initiation of hemodialysis is usually perceived as a positive experience; and after the initial concerns of implementing the treatment, the child begins to feel better, and parental anxiety is relieved for a time. (See Nursing Care Plan: The Child with Chronic Renal Failure.*)

TECHNOLOGIC MANAGEMENT OF RENAL FAILURE

Technologic advances in the care of children with acute and chronic renal failure have provided a means for maintaining excretory function in acute disease and for prolonging life in those with ESRD. The primary modalities are hemodialysis, peritoneal dialysis, hemofiltration, and transplantation.

Dialysis is the process of separating colloids and crystalline substances in solution by the difference in their rate of diffusion through a semipermeable membrane. This movement across the membrane is accomplished by three processes: osmosis, diffusion, and ultrafiltration (see box below).

Methods of dialysis currently available for clinical management of renal failure are:

1. **Hemodialysis,** in which blood is circulated outside the body through artificial cellophane membranes that permit a similar passage of water and solutes
2. **Peritoneal dialysis,** wherein the abdominal cavity acts as a semipermeable membrane through which water and solutes of small molecular size move by osmosis and diffusion according to their respective concentrations on either side of the membrane
3. **Hemofiltration,** in which blood filtrate is circulated outside the body by hydrostatic pressure exerted across a semipermeable membrane and replaced (simultaneously) by electrolyte solution

*In *Wong and Whaley's Clinical Manual of Pediatric Nursing* (Mosby).

PROCESSES OF FLUID AND ELECTROLYTE MOVEMENT

Osmosis—Passive movement of water from a solution of lower concentration to a solution of higher concentration of particles

Diffusion—Random movement of particles from an area of greater concentration to an area of lower concentration

Ultrafiltration—Movement of fluid, under pressure, through filtering material with minute pores

The choice of whether to use hemodialysis, peritoneal dialysis, or hemofiltration is determined by the nature of the renal failure (acute vs chronic), the cause of the renal failure, and patient/parent preference. Hemodialysis is more efficient than peritoneal dialysis, but is technically more difficult in infants and very young children. Hemofiltration may be a viable substitute for dialysis in these children. As a rule, dialysis is reserved for children who are in end-stage renal failure, since it requires creation of an access and special equipment. It may be used acutely for such conditions as severe metabolic acidosis, accidental poisoning, intractable heart failure, hypernatremia, hyperkalemia, hepatic coma, and acute renal failure.

The absolute indications for dialysis are life-threatening electrolyte abnormalities, severe volume overload, and children with bilateral neoplastic disease or bilateral nephrectomies performed for various reasons, including intractable hypertension. Although each child is assessed on an individual basis, indications for instituting dialysis in CRF are biochemical abnormalities including elevated BUN, acidosis, severe hyperphosphatemia, elevated potassium, and anemia requiring transfusion (placing child at risk for fluid overload). Other indications include deteriorating CNS function or congestive heart failure that is unresponsive to other therapy. Growth failure, severe osteodystrophy, insufficient caloric intake, and inability to carry out normal activities are sometimes criteria for dialysis.

Most children show rapid clinical improvement with the implementation of dialysis, although it is directly related to the duration of uremia before dialysis and the extent to which dietary regulations are followed. Growth rate and skeletal maturation improve, but recovery of normal growth is uncommon. In many cases sexual development, although delayed, has progressed to completion. Females generally remain amenorrheic while on hemodialysis. Those on peritoneal dialysis may have menses.

HEMODIALYSIS

Hemodialysis is the preferred dialytic method for children with acute conditions such as life-threatening hyperkalemia or poisoning with dialyzable compounds. Protein loss is less extensive than with peritoneal dialysis. However, it is not recommended for small children, whose delicately balanced cardiovascular dynamics may be upset by the rapid changes in blood volume and systemic blood pressure that may occur with hemodialysis. In addition, it may be difficult to place vascular access for hemodialysis in small children.

Hemodialysis is the preferred form of dialysis for certain family situations in which any one person is unable to take the time and responsibility to perform the procedures at home. It is best suited to children who live close to the dialysis center, since they must come to the center as often as three or more times a week for treatments. Children who are not good candidates for peritoneal dialysis because of family noncompliance, recurrent peritoneal infections, or unstable living conditions must elect to have hemodialysis.

Procedure

Hemodialysis requires the use of special dialysis equipment—the hemodialyzer, or so-called artificial kidney. Hemodialyzers are available in three forms—coil, parallel flow (plate), and hollow fiber—but not all are suited to pediatric patients. Hollow fiber dialyzers are preferable for children because their blood compartment is relatively small and rigid (Novello, 1986a). Pediatric dialysis can be safely carried out when the fluid volume required to fill both the hemodialyzer and blood tubing does not exceed 10% of the child's calculated blood volume.

Hemodialysis also requires blood access by three types of means: grafts, fistulas, or external access devices. An arteriovenous fistula is an access in which a vein and artery are connected surgically. The preferred site is the radial artery and a forearm vein. Sometimes alternate vessels are used, including the tibial artery and the long saphenous vein, especially for home dialysis. An alternative to the external Teflon shunt is the creation of a subcutaneous (internal) arteriovenous fistula by anastomosing a segment of a saphenous vein autograft or a bovine arterial xenograft to the brachial artery and brachiocephalic vein, which produces dilation and thickening of the superficial vessels of the forearm to provide easy access for repeated venipuncture. Fewer complications and less restriction of activity are observed with this approach. Both the graft and the fistula require needle insertion at each dialysis. For short-term external vascular access, percutaneous catheters are inserted in the femoral, subclavian, or internal jugular veins, even in very small children. For long-term external vascular access, cuffed, dual-lumen catheters can be surgically placed similarly to other central venous access devices. They are ready to be used immediately, and no needles are required.

Various hemodialysis schedules are employed, but most centers recommend dialysis three times a week for 4 to 6 hours, depending on the size of the child. For a complete description of the highly specialized process of hemodialysis, the reader is directed to the numerous references available on this topic.

Dietary limitations are necessary in chronic dialysis to avoid biochemical complications and to facilitate adequate dialysis. Fluid and sodium are restricted to prevent fluid overload, with its associated symptoms of hypertension, cerebral manifestations, and congestive heart failure. Potassium is restricted to prevent complications related to hyperkalemia; phosphorus restriction helps to prevent parathyroid hyperactivity and its attendant risk of abnormal calcification in soft tissues. Limited protein intake reduces high levels of blood urea nitrogen. Fluid is usually limited to 5 dl/m^2/day plus an amount equal to daily urinary output.

Seizures during or after hemodialysis are not uncommon. The cause is uncertain, but they probably result from cerebral edema caused by alterations in osmolality in the brain when the blood urea nitrogen level is lowered rapidly. Hyponatremia may be a factor as well. Seizures are most likely to occur at the time dialysis is first initiated, when large changes in serum osmolality may occur.

Home Hemodialysis

With appropriate cannulization and proper training and education of both the child and the parents, hemodialysis can be performed at home. Time spent in transportation is eliminated, the environment is more pleasant and secure, and the child is able to assume a more active role in the treatment program. Home dialysis is especially advantageous for children waiting for a transplant who live a great distance from the dialysis center or for children who have had one or more kidney transplant failures.

Home hemodialysis units are available to some children, and the preparation and management are similar to that required for hemodialysis in the hospital. The patient is equipped with a dialysis unit that is used with the vascular access established for outpatient dialysis. Parents of children on home hemodialysis must know how to operate the equipment, connect the unit to the vascular access, and assess the status of the child.

Nursing Considerations

Initiating a hemodialysis regimen is a traumatic and anxiety-provoking experience for most children. After surgery for implantation of the graft, fistula, or long-term external access device, the initial experience with the hemodialysis machine and its implication is frightening to most children. They need reassurance about the nature of the preparations for dialysis and the conduct of the treatment. They are anxious concerning repeated venipunctures (with implanted shunts and for blood chemistries) and the sight of their blood leaving their body and entering the machine. Pain management (see Chapter 26) should include the use of EMLA, a topical anesthetic, to reduce or eliminate the discomfort of needle punctures. Anxiety can also be caused by the child's physiologic response to the treatment (e.g., nausea and vomiting, cramps, or seizures). These are usually individual responses related to the child's overall well-being and degree of compliance with the total medical regimen. Once the initial fear of the machine has been resolved, children can be helped to develop strategies for dealing with restricted activity and movement for the duration of each treatment (Fig. 30-4).

Adolescents, with their increased need for independence and their urge for rebellion, may adapt less well. They resent the control and enforced dependence imposed by the rigorous and unrelenting therapy program. They resent dependency on a machine, parents, and professional staff. Depression, hostility, or both are common in adolescents undergoing hemodialysis. The adverse consequences of the disease include the need for diet restrictions, limitations in physical activity (resulting from lack of energy, frequent illnesses, and specific restrictions related to access), and the sense of being different from other children. Withdrawal from peers and social isolation are the rule, and noncompliance with the therapeutic regimen is not uncommon.

Body changes related to the disease process, such as growth retardation, skin color, and lack of sexual maturation, are stress provoking. Dietary restrictions are particularly burdensome for both children and parents. Children

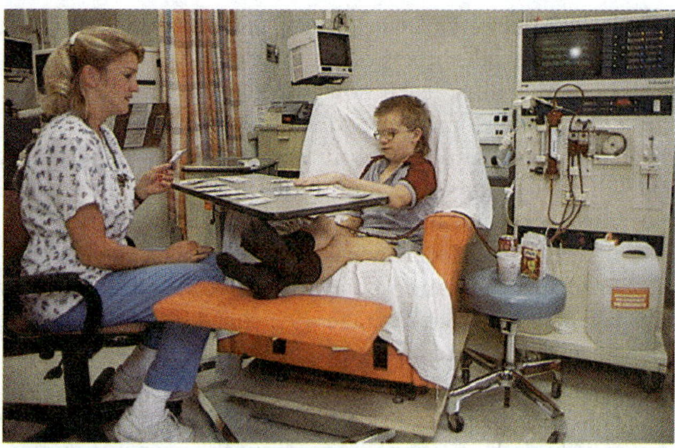

FIG. 30-4 Diversional activities help lessen the boredom children can experience during hemodialysis.

feel deprived when unable to eat foods previously enjoyed and unrestricted for other family members. Consequently, failure to cooperate is not uncommon. Diet restrictions are interpreted as punishment and, since they may not be able to fully understand the purpose of the restrictions, some will sneak forbidden food items at every opportunity. Allowing children, especially adolescents, maximum participation in and responsibility for their own treatment program is helpful. The extent of compliance and adjustment depends on the personalities of the involved persons, the quality of their relationships, and their coping mechanisms.

After weeks, months, or years of hemodialysis, the parents and the child feel anxiety associated with the prognosis and continued pressures of the treatment. The relentless need for treatment interferes with family plans and activities, including school. Graft and fistula problems are not uncommon and present a common source of aggravation. The occurrence of seizures during dialysis is highly stressful to both the child and the family. Most families and children on hemodialysis look to renal transplantation as a desirable alternative to long-term treatment.

PERITONEAL DIALYSIS (PD)

For ***acute conditions*** PD is quick, relatively easy to learn, safe to perform, and requires a minimal amount of equipment and specially trained nurses. PD is a slow, gentle process, which decreases the stress on body organs that can occur with the rapid chemical and volume changes of hemodialysis. The procedure is indicated for neonates, children with severe cardiovascular disease, or those with bleeding abnormalities who are poor risks for vascular access and heparinization.

Chronic PD is the preferred form of dialysis for children/parents who are independent, families who live a long distance from the medical center, infants, school-age children, and adolescents, who prefer fewer dietary restrictions and a gentler form of dialysis. Chronic peritoneal dialysis is most often performed at home.

Contraindications for use of PD include recent abdominal surgery, peritoneal adhesions and scarring, or paralytic ileus. A higher rate of infection (peritonitis and pneumonia) is observed with this modality, as well as a lower rate of efficiency in children with hypotension and reduced visceral blood flow as compared with hemodialysis.

Procedure

In acute situations PD catheter insertion may be accomplished at the bedside; catheters for long-term use are placed surgically in the operating room with the patient under anesthesia. A catheter is inserted through the anterior abdominal wall, and the catheter cuff is sutured into place. Chronic PD catheters are tunneled through a subcutaneous tract before exiting the skin in a manner similar to implantation of central venous access devices. At the time of dialysis, a commercially prepared dialysis solution (dialysate) is allowed to flow by gravity through the catheter into the peritoneal cavity, where it remains while equilibrium between plasma and dialysis fluid takes place. Approximately 30 to 50 ml/kg of dialysate is instilled at each cycle. The fluid is then allowed to flow by gravity drainage into a receptacle, and fresh dialysate is again instilled.

In PD, each pass or cycle is characterized by inflow time, dwell time, and drain time. The length of each portion of the cycle is part of the dialysis prescription. The times vary according to the goals of the treatment (i.e., removal of water, solute, electrolyte, or all of these). The procedure is usually continued until renal function is restored, poisons are reduced, or (in prolonged need) the patient is switched to a form of chronic PD—***continuous ambulatory peritoneal dialysis (CAPD)*** or ***continuous cycling peritoneal dialysis (CCPD)***. An acute PD catheter may remain in place for several weeks provided that aseptic technique is adhered to by all who enter the system.

Home Dialysis

The development of satisfactory methods for CAPD and its alternative, CCPD, has provided additional means for managing ESRD at home. In both methods commercially available sterile dialysate solution is instilled into the peritoneal cavity through the surgically implanted indwelling catheter. The warmed solution is allowed to enter the peritoneal cavity by gravity and remains a variable length of time according to the procedure used.

In CAPD the dialysate is instilled, the line is clamped off, and the empty solution bag is rolled up and worn attached to the abdomen or thigh or even placed in a pocket. The solution is allowed to remain in the peritoneum for 4 to 6 hours. The bag is then unrolled and placed on the floor, the line is unclamped, and the fluid is drained into the bag by gravity. Another heated bag is hung, and the process is repeated so that there is fluid in the abdomen continuously. The procedure is performed three times during the day and once at night. For an active child CAPD has proved to be a satisfactory alternative to hemodialysis that can be continued for an indefinite time.

CCPD is a modification of CAPD and intermittent peritoneal dialysis. The dialysis exchange is performed only at night using an automatic dialysis machine, which controls the timed cycles of inflow and outflow of dialysate. The catheter is opened only at night rather than four times a day, although an additional exchange may be prescribed during the day. The nighttime dialysis allows the child more freedom during the day and relieves parents from having to perform multiple exchanges (Alliapoulos and others, 1984).

The care and management of the procedure are the responsibility of the parents of young children. School nurses can perform the procedure for younger school-age children. Older children and adolescents are able to carry out the procedure themselves, thus providing them with some control and less dependency. This is especially important for adolescents.

Complications. CAPD and CCPD are presently considered to be the methods of choice for most children who require dialysis because they are easier to initiate and maintain than hemodialysis. Peritonitis is the major complication of home peritoneal dialysis. The patients are treated intraperitoneally with antibiotics, and some may require catheter replacement. Although the risk of infection is continuously present, most practitioners believe that it is not great enough to discourage the use of these methods.

However, other complications have been noted in patients on home peritoneal dialysis. Tunnel infections are evidenced by swelling, warmth, and tenderness along the subcutaneous catheter tract; however, they can be managed with administration of antibiotics or catheter replacement. Peritoneal leaks and ventral hernias caused by the sustained intraabdominal pressure that develops within the peritoneum have also been found in a significant number of children. Most of these patients respond to reduction in dialysate volume.

Nursing Considerations

The availability of home dialysis has offered a greater degree of freedom for persons undergoing long-term dialysis. The need for a residence convenient to a dialysis unit and the necessity for frequent trips to the unit are eliminated except for monthly evaluations. The nurse is responsible for teaching the family. Education focuses on (1) the disease, its implications, and the therapeutic plan; (2) the possible psychologic effects of the disease and the treatment; and (3) the technical aspects of the procedure.

The family must learn how to take vital signs before and after the dialysis and how to interpret the significance of blood pressure and temperature variations. They need to know how to vary the composition of the dialysate to compensate for variations in the vital signs and to maintain an accurate record of all aspects of the treatment.

Parents of the young child using CAPD are taught how to exchange bags and manage the procedure at home. Even newborn infants are able to benefit from peritoneal dialysis. Older children can be taught to take responsibility for their own treatments as much as possible. The family is encouraged to ask questions throughout the preparation time, including those that clarify anatomy and physiology, mechanical functioning, and side effects of the disease and the treatment. The peritoneal dialysis schedule is outlined to meet the individual needs of the patient and the family. Most schedules are arranged for uninterrupted sleep at night and to coordinate the dialysis with school and other activities. The diet, medication, and activity are discussed, and feelings about the entire therapeutic program are explored with the child and the family.

Infection is the greatest hazard of peritoneal dialysis; therefore the family is instructed to contact the appropriate persons at the earliest evidence of peritonitis. In most instances of peritonitis the infection can be controlled with administration of antibiotics. Unfortunately, there is a high incidence of peritonitis, and repeated infections may necessitate replacement of the catheter or its removal and abandonment of the peritoneum as an access route.

The importance of emotional, as well as material, support cannot be overemphasized. The National Kidney Foundation, mentioned previously, provides a number of services and information for families of children with renal disease. A relatively new organization, the **American Association of Kidney Patients (AAKP),*** has been organized to promote the interest and welfare of kidney patients. It provides education and support for patients and public education regarding all areas of kidney disease (see Critical Thinking Exercise box).

*Suite LL1, 1 Davis Blvd., Tampa, FL 33606; (813) 254-2558.

THINKING CRITICALLY ABOUT . . . *Medical Care Rationing*

The criteria for selection of renal transplant recipients sometimes create dilemmas for professionals. In most cases the decision is simply a matter for the transplant team and the family to resolve for the benefit of the child involved. However, in some situations, especially in view of the scarcity of donor kidneys and the expense of the procedure, the solution is less clear. The matter creates more questions than answers.

For example, should a child without a severe mental or physical disability take priority over one with these disabilities? Should financial responsibility be a consideration? Some youngsters with renal transplants have discontinued taking their medications, thereby either causing damage to their kidney or losing the graft. Should these youngsters receive a second transplant? Should very young children whose families have proved to be too unreliable in complying with a therapeutic regimen be given a transplant when the success of the graft depends on following a prescribed therapeutic plan? Are very young, unwed adolescent mothers likely to be less compliant in following the prescribed medical regimen? Can persons on limited incomes manage to acquire the costly medications? If not, should the government subsidize payment?

What solutions to these dilemmas are available and how are decisions justified? Who should make the decisions?

CONTINUOUS ARTERIOVENOUS HEMOFILTRATION (CAVH)

A third type of dialysis used primarily in acute care settings is CAVH, a gentle form of dialysis that employs specialized equipment (filter, pump, tubing connected to a vascular access) to ultrafiltrate blood continuously at a very slow rate. With this procedure, fluid balance may be achieved within 24 to 48 hours after initiation. CAVH is a procedure used to remove excess fluid from patients with severe oliguric fluid overload.

CAVH is an ideal form of dialysis for children with fluid overload from surgical procedures (such as cardiovascular surgery) who do not have severe biochemical abnormalities. It is frequently used for critically ill children who require volume-expanding fluids such as hyperalimentation solution, albumin, or packed red cells. It creates space for the infusion of these replacement solutions in fluid-sensitive patients. CAVH has proved to be a highly successful alternative form of dialysis for critically ill children who might not survive the rapid volume changes that occur with hemodialysis and peritoneal dialysis. In the event that an artery cannot be accessed for CAVH, an alternative hemofiltration method is ***continuous veno-venous hemofiltration (CVVH).*** The process is similar to CAVH. Whereas CAVH can sometimes be performed entirely by gravity, CVVH requires a blood pump to maintain flow through the filter.

TRANSPLANTATION

Renal transplantation is now an acceptable and effective means of therapy in the pediatric age-group. Although peritoneal dialysis and hemodialysis are life-preserving and are able to be carried out in the home in a large number of cases, neither method is compatible with a normal life-style. Transplantation, on the other hand, offers the opportunity for a relatively normal life. It is presently regarded as the preferred form of treatment for children with chronic renal failure.

Kidneys for transplant are available from either of two sources: a living related donor (LRD), usually a parent or sibling, or a cadaver donor (CD), wherein the family of a dead or brain-dead patient consents to donation of a healthy kidney. The criteria for selection of kidney recipients are quite liberal, but uniform criteria have not been established among the various centers that specialize in the procedure. In general, there is no limit to age. In some cases a person's mental status (e.g., mental retardation, emotional instability, or noncompliant behavior) may be reason to defer transplantation until the recipient's psychoemotional status improves and it is reasonable to assume that the posttransplant regimen will be carried out (Novello, 1986b) (see Thinking Critically About . . . box).

Children who have ESRD secondary to malignancies must be cancer-free for a specified period of time prior to transplantation (usually 1 year). Generalized infection must be eradicated before attempted transplantation, and the recipient should have adequate bladder capacity. Some children may have bladder augmentation or other genitourinary surgery as preparation for transplantation. Children with abnormal urinary tracts may be subject to more posttransplant urologic complications and infection than they would otherwise be.

There is a high incidence of disease recurrence in the transplanted kidneys of children who have had focal segmental glomerulosclerosis, mesangiocapillary glomerulonephritis, hemolytic uremic syndrome, primary hyperoxaluria, or sickle cell nephritis (Iglesias and Richard, 1993). It should be recognized that many children with these systemic illnesses, as well as those with previous cancers of the renal system and those with anomalous urinary tracts, have had successful renal transplants.

Procedure

The kidney graft is placed in the extraperitoneal space, usually the anterior iliac fossa; the renal artery is anastomosed to the internal iliac or hypogastric artery; the renal vein is anastomosed to the hypogastric vein; and the ureter is implanted into the bladder or anastomosed to the recipient's ureter. Small children receiving a large donor kidney may require placement within the abdomen with vessel anastomoses to the aorta and inferior vena cava. Unless there is

CRITICAL THINKING EXERCISE

End-Stage Renal Disease

Jamie is a 20-month-old boy with end-stage renal disease secondary to obstructive uropathy. He is currently in the hospital for replacement of his peritoneal dialysis catheter. In reviewing his admission data base, you identify that his initial oral polio vaccine series does not appear to be complete and that he has not had an MMR vaccine. Of the following actions, which is the most critical given that you would interview his primary caretaker to verify that the immunization status is correct?

1. Include instructions on the need for completing Jamie's infant immunizations and the locations of local immunization clinics in your discharge teaching with Jamie's parents.
2. Bring the immunization status to the attention of Jamie's primary health care practitioner as soon as possible.
3. Recognize that Jamie's chronic condition has contributed to his incomplete immunization status and that his immunizations will be completed before he receives a renal transplant.
4. Recommend that Jamie receive the oral polio vaccine and MMR in 4 to 6 weeks when he has recovered from his surgery.

The most appropriate action at this time is 2. The primary health care practitioner can potentially order the immunizations to be given before discharge from this hospitalization. Jamie's immunization status is most likely related to his chronic illness. However, he must receive the immunizations before becoming eligible for renal transplantation because both vaccines contain live viruses that the immunosuppressive medications required after renal transplantation would preclude. Jamie's recent surgery is not a contraindication to vaccination at this time, and waiting simply delays his transplant eligibility. Educating his parents is also appropriate; however, the objective at this time is immediate immunization.

medical contraindication, the recipient's failed kidneys are left in place. Severe hypertension, neoplasm, large, continuous protein losses, and obstructive uropathy are the usual causes of nephrectomy.

The primary goal in transplantation is the long-term survival of the grafted tissue. The means by which this is attempted is (1) securing tissues that are antigenically similar to that of the recipient and (2) suppressing the recipient's immune mechanism.

Selection of Donor Tissue

The source of a donor kidney is either a live person or a cadaver soon after death. The closer the genetic relationship between the donor and recipient, the better the possibility of long-term survival. The only truly compatible tissue match is that between identical twin siblings. The next best possible match is a sibling, then a parent, and finally an uncle or aunt. In some states use of siblings is impossible until the possible donor is of age to give consent for removal of a kidney. Unrelated donors are least likely to be compatible. Careful immunologic studies are carried out to determine the donor whose kidney is least likely to be rejected by the recipient.

Suppression of the Immune Response

After the best possible tissue match is obtained for a transplant, the survival time can be significantly lengthened by suppressing the immune response of the recipient. The immunosuppressant therapy of choice in kidney transplantation is corticosteroids (prednisone) in conjunction with cyclosporine and azathioprine. Other therapies include antilymphoblast globulin or monoclonal antibodies, administered intravenously for 14 days after transplant.

The administration of these drugs is not without hazard. The major problem encountered with nonspecific immunosuppression is that it not only suppresses the immune response to the grafted tissue but also suppresses the body's capacity to respond to other antigenic stimuli. Consequently, the child is vulnerable to overwhelming infections.

Prednisone is a powerful immunosuppressant and anti-inflammatory agent that acts to stabilize cell walls, reduce migration of white blood cells into the inflamed area, and inhibit deposition of fibrin and collagen. It also depresses T-cells, B-cells, and phagocytes. A number of complications that are directly attributable to corticosteroid therapy are cause for concern in children receiving steroid therapy. Interference with calcium absorption retards linear growth, and in most centers alternate-day administration is being used in an effort to improve growth rates and to decrease other long-term side effects. Other corticosteroid-induced side effects may include the characteristic cushingoid facies, cataracts, fluid and sodium retention, gastric ulcer, and obesity.

Cyclosporine is a powerful immunosuppressant that acts to decrease production of T-cells. Side effects of this drug are arterial hypertension, which may appear within 3 weeks of transplant; hirsutism; and nephrotoxicity, a major concern in renal transplantation. Maintenance doses of cyclosporine are determined by serum blood levels. Low therapeutic cyclosporine levels usually prevent untoward side effects, as well as rejection. After the initial intravenous therapy immediately following the transplant, the drug is administered orally. When the liquid form is used, each center has specific instructions for administering cyclosporine. The concerns are that the complete dose will be taken and absorption of the medication will be maximized.

Azathioprine is a powerful immunosuppressant that interferes with cellular protein synthesis. The problem related to the toxic effect of azathioprine is mainly neutropenia, which is usually managed by reduced dosage. (See Chapter 36 for a discussion of immunosuppressant therapy and related nursing care.)

Rejection

Rejection of a transplanted kidney is the most frequent cause of transplant failure. Rejection can be one of three types—hyperacute, acute, or chronic. Hyperacute rejection is irreversible, develops immediately or within a few hours after revascularization, and is related to circulating antibodies preformed in the recipient against the donor tissue antigens. These are seen in second transplants or in persons sensitized from blood transfusions.

Acute rejection usually occurs between the first few days and 6 months after transplantation but may occur as late as 1 or 2 years later. Rejection is evidenced by both biochemical and clinical abnormalities. The most frequent finding is fever, which is usually accompanied by swelling and tenderness over the graft, hypertension, and diminished urinary output. A severe reaction may cause oliguria. Increases in serum blood urea nitrogen and creatinine levels are laboratory evidence of decreased transplant function. Most acute rejection episodes respond to intravenous administration of methylprednisolone sodium succinate (Solu-Medrol), antilymphoblast globulin, or monoclonal antibodies.

NURSING ALERT The child with a recent kidney transplant (a few days) or one who was grafted approximately 6 months previously who exhibits any of the following should be evaluated immediately for possible rejection:

- Fever
- Swelling and tenderness over graft area
- Diminished urinary output
- Elevated blood pressure

Chronic rejection is characterized by slow, gradual deterioration of renal function that typically begins 6 months or more after transplantation. Evidence of rejection may be heralded by proteinuria and/or hematuria, and the rejection may have symptomatology indistinguishable from the original kidney disease. No present therapy can halt the progressive process, which inevitably leads to loss of the implanted kidney.

Prognosis

The overall graft survival rate for kidneys from living related donors is 89% at 1 year and 80% at 3 years. For cadaver kidneys the graft survival rate is 74% at 1 year and 62% at 3 years (McEnery and others, 1992). Posttransplant complications include infection, hypertension, steroid toxicity, hyperlipidemia, aseptic necrosis, malignancy, and growth retardation (Ettenger and Fine, 1987). Long-term graft survival is not guaranteed, and many children require a second or third transplant. Successful renal transplantation does improve rehabilitation of children with CRF, both educationally and psychologically.

Nursing Considerations

The possibility of renal transplantation often comes as a hope for relief from the rigors of dialysis or the restriction of a conservative management regimen. Most children and families respond well to a kidney transplant. Children with successful renal transplants are usually able to resume life activities similar to those of their unaffected age-mates by 1 year following the transplant. The rehabilitation of children with renal transplants is influenced primarily by their pattern of functioning before becoming ill. It is important to remember that transplantation is a treatment that makes a much less negative impact on the normal life activities of a child. However, stresses remain for the child and family in relation to the uncertainty of the future, the child's health and well-being, social isolation, and financial burdens (Uzark, 1992).

A variety of serious emotional and psychologic conflicts may arise as a consequence of donor selection, including ambivalence of donors faced with surgery and relinquishing a kidney, feelings of guilt if one should prove to be unacceptable as a donor, and the emotional impact of having a live relative–donated kidney rejected by the recipient. This especially can result in guilt feelings when a parent is the donor.

The child recipient responds in various ways to a kidney transplant. The concept of having a foreign body, especially a cadaver kidney, inside their own body is sometimes disturbing to children. They often speculate about the age, sex, personality, and physical characteristics of the donor. They may fear that the kidney will wear out if it came from an older person. Some children are distressed to find that their donor kidney came from a person of the opposite sex. Corticosteroid therapy, necessary in kidney transplants, creates undesirable side effects (e.g., growth failure, obesity, characteristics of Cushing syndrome [see Fig. 38-3], acne, and hirsutism) that are frequently a source of emotional and social problems for older children. Characteristic facial changes (coarseness, thickened nares, puffy cheeks, prominent supraorbital ridges, and mandibular prognathism) have also been reported in children receiving cyclosporine (Reznik and others, 1987).

The most frequent reason for noncompliance in childhood renal transplant recipients is dislike of undesirable side effects. The cosmetic implications of the side effects can be overwhelming, especially to adolescent girls. Deliberate discontinuation of the drugs is most commonly observed in teenage girls. Noncompliance is also seen frequently in children from poorly communicating families who are not very supportive (see Compliance, Chapter 27).

Working with children and their families during the various stages of renal failure, dialysis, and transplantation is a difficult and challenging experience. Nurses must become familiar with the family; assess family strengths, weaknesses, and coping mechanisms; and be prepared to provide intensive support and guidance during the prolonged experience. The child and family need help in accepting what is happening to them, learning anticipatory guidance regarding predictable stresses, and dealing constructively with the physical, emotional, and financial burdens that are an ongoing part of this prolonged disability.

KEY POINTS

- The main function of the kidney is to maintain the composition and volume of body fluids in equilibrium.
- Common inflammatory disorders of the genitourinary tract include urinary tract infection, nephrotic syndrome, and acute glomerulonephritis.
- Management of UTIs is directed at eliminating infection, detecting and correcting functional or anatomic abnormalities, preventing recurrences, and preserving renal function.
- Vesicoureteral reflux is the retrograde flow of bladder urine into the ureters.
- Common features of acute glomerulonephritis are oliguria, edema, hypertension, circulatory congestion, hematuria, and proteinuria.
- Therapeutic management of acute glomerulonephritis is maintenance of fluid balance, treatment of hypertension, and antibiotic therapy.
- Nephrotic syndrome is characterized by increased glomerular permeability to protein.
- Management of nephrotic syndrome is aimed at reducing excretion of protein, reducing or preventing fluid retention by tissues, and preventing infection and other complications; dietary control; corticosteroid therapy; immunosuppressant therapy; use of diuretics; and use of antimicrobials.
- Primary functions of the distal renal tubules are acidification of urine, potassium secretion, and selective and differential reabsorption of sodium, chloride, and water.
- The most common renal tubular disorders are renal tubular acidosis and nephrogenic diabetes insipidus.
- Management of hemolytic-uremic syndrome is aimed at control of hematologic manifestations and complications of renal failure.
- In acute renal failure, management is directed at determining treatment of the underlying cause, management of complications of renal failure, and supportive therapy.
- Abnormalities in chronic renal failure are waste product retention, water and sodium retention, hyperkalemia, acidosis, calcium and phosphorus disturbance, anemia, hypertension, and growth disturbances.
- When the child will need home dialysis, the nurse educates the family about the disease, its implications, the therapeutic plan, possible psychologic effects of the disease, and the treatment and technical aspects of the procedure.
- The major concerns in renal transplantation are tissue matching and prevention of rejection, as well as psychologic concerns involve self-image as related to possible body changes as a result of the effects of corticosteroid therapy.

REFERENCES

Alliapoulos JC and others: Comparison of continuous cycling peritoneal dialysis with continuous ambulatory peritoneal dialysis in children, *J Pediatr* 105:721-725, 1984.

Andrich MP, Majd M: Diagnostic imaging in the evaluation of the first urinary tract infection in infants and young children, *Pediatrics* 90(3):436-441, 1992.

Avorn J and others: Reduction of bacteriuria and pyuria after ingestion of cranberry juice, *JAMA* 271(10):751-754, 1994.

Bailie MD: Rapid screening and diagnosis of UTI, *Contemp Pediatr* 3:33-41, 1986.

Bradley WE: Physiology of the urinary bladder. In Walsh PC and others, editors: *Campbell's urology,* Philadelphia, 1986, WB Saunders.

Cepero-Akselrad A, Ramirez-Seijas F, Castaneda A: Urinary tract infection in children, *Int Pediatr* 8(3):314-325, 1993.

Edelmann CM Jr: Urinary tract infection and vesicoureteral reflux, *Pediatr Ann* 17:568-582, 1988.

Eschbach JW, Adamson JW: Guidelines for recombinant human erythropoietin therapy, *J Kidney Dis* 14:2-8, 1989.

Ettenger RB, Fine RN: Renal transplantation. In Holiday MA, Barratt TM, Vernmier RL, editors: *Pediatric nephrology,* Baltimore, 1987, Williams & Wilkins.

Fish AJ, Fouser LS: Glomerulonephritis. In Gellis SS, Kagan BM, editors: *Current pediatric therapy 12,* Philadelphia, 1986, WB Saunders.

Fussell EN and others: Adherence of bacteria to human foreskins, *J Urol* 140:997-1001, 1988.

Gray ML: *Genitourinary disorders,* St Louis, 1992, Mosby.

Greaves MW: Itching—research has barely scratched the surface, *N Engl J Med* 326(15):1016-1017, 1992.

Haws RM, Baum M: Efficacy of albumin and diuretic therapy in children with nephrotic syndrome, *Pediatrics* 91(6):1142-1146, 1993.

Hensle TW, Burbige KA: Vesicoureteral reflux. In Gellis SS, Kagan BM, editors: *Current pediatric therapy 12,* Philadelphia, 1986, WB Saunders.

Herzog LW: Urinary tract infections and circumcision: a case-control study, *Am J Dis Child* 143:348-350, 1989.

Iglesias JH, Richard GA: Pediatric renal transplantation, *Int Pediatr* 8(3):373-386, 1993.

Jodal IU, Winberg J: Management of children with unobstructed urinary tract infection, *Pediatr Nephrol* 1:647-650, 1987.

Jordan SC, Lemire JM: Acute glomerulonephritis, *Pediatr Clin North Am* 29:857-873, 1982.

Kim MS, Grupe WE: The nephrotic syndrome. In Gellis SS, Kagan BM, editors: *Current pediatric therapy 12,* Philadelphia, 1986, WB Saunders.

Koch VH and others: Accelerated growth after recombinant human growth hormone treatment of children with chronic renal failure, *J Pediatr* 115:365-371, 1989.

Kramer SA: Vesicouteteral reflux. In Kelalis PP, King LR, Belman AB, editors: *Clinical pediatric urology,* Philadelphia, 1992, WB Saunders.

Libber S, Harrison H, Spector D: Treatment of nephrogenic diabetes insipidus with prostaglandin synthesis inhibitors, *J Pediatr* 108:305-311, 1986.

Lohr JA and others: Making a presumptive diagnosis of urinary tract infection by using a urinalysis performed in an on-site laboratory, *J Pediatr* 122(1):22-25, 1993.

McEnery PT and others: Renal transplantation in children, *N Engl J Med* 326(26):1727-1732, 1992.

Novello AC: Hemodialysis. In Gellis SS, Kagan BM, editors: *Current pediatric therapy 12,* Philadelphia, 1986a, WB Saunders.

Novello AC: Renal transplantation. In Gellis SS, Kagan BM, editors: *Current pediatric therapy 12,* Philadelphia, 1986b, WB Saunders.

Pearson BD, Larson JM: Urine control by elders: Noninvasive strategies. In Funk SG and others, editors: *Key aspects of elder care,* New York, 1992, Springer.

Raymond NG and others: An approach to protein restriction in children with renal insufficiency, *Pediatr Nephrol* 4:145-148, 1990.

Reznik VM and others: Changes in facial appearance during cyclosporin treatment, *Lancet* 1:1405-1406, 1987.

Rizzoni G and others: Plasma infusion for hemolytic-uremic syndrome in children: results of a multicenter controlled trial, *J Pediatr* 112:284-290, 1988.

Roberts JA: URI: an argument for circumcision, *Contemp Pediatr* 5(8):42-54, 1988.

Rushton HG: Nonspecific infections. In Kelalis PP, King LR, Belman AB, editors: *Clinical pediatric urology,* Philadelphia, 1992, WB Saunders.

Sedman AB: Chronic renal failure. In Gellis SS, Kagan BM, editors: *Current pediatric therapy 12,* Philadelphia, 1986, WB Saunders.

Staskin DR and others: Pathophysiology of stress incontinence, *Clin Obstet Gynecol* 12:357, 1985.

Uzark K: Caring for families of pediatric transplant recipients: psychosocial implications, *Crit Care Nurs Clin North Am* 4(2):255-261, 1992.

Wiswell TE, Geschke DW: Risks from circumcision during the first month of life compared with those for uncircumcised boys, *Pediatrics* 83:1011-1015, 1989.

Wiswell TE and others: Effect of circumcision status on periurethral bacterial flora during the first year of life, *J Pediatr* 113:442-446, 1988.

Woodward MN, Griffiths DM: The use of dipsticks for routine analysis of urine from children with acute abdominal pain, *Br Med J* 306:1512, 1993.

BIBLIOGRAPHY

General

Perelstein EM: Renal tubular acidosis, *Int Pediatr* 8(3):326-333, 1993.

Urinary Tract Infection/Reflux

Alon U and others: Ultrasonography in the radiologic evaluation of children with urinary tract infection, *Pediatrics* 78:58-64, 1986.

Brogna L, Lakaszawski ML: The continent urostomy, *Am J Nurs* 86:160-163, 1986.

Burns MW: Pediatric urinary tract infection: diagnosis, classification and significance, *Pediatr Clin North Am* 34:1111-1120, 1987.

Conti MT, Euthropius L: Preventing UTI's: What works? *Am J Nurs* 87:307-309, 1987.

Conway JJ, Cohn RA: Evolving role of nuclear medicine for the diagnosis and management of urinary tract infection, *J Pediatr* 124(1):87-90, 1994.

Edelmann CM Jr: Urinary tract infection and vesicoureteral reflux, *Pediatr Ann* 17:568-582, 1988.

Heldrich FJ: Pinning down the diagnosis of UTI, *Contemp Pediatr* 5:52-78, 1988.

Jodal U and others: Infection pattern in children with vesicoureteral reflux randomly allocated to operation or long-term antibacterial prophylaxis, *J Urol* 148:1650-1652, 1992.

Johnson CE and others: Renal ultrasound evaluation of urinary tract infections in children, *Pediatrics* 78:871-878, 1986.

Lerner GR, Fleischmann LE, Perlmutter AD: Reflux nephropathy, *Pediatr Clin North Am* 34:747-770, 1987.

Steele BT, De Maria J: A new perspective on the natural history of vesicoureteric reflux, *Pediatrics* 90(1):30-32, 1992.

Van Gool JD and others: Historial clues to the complex of dysfunctional voiding, urinary tract infection and vesicoureteral reflux, *J Urol* 148:1699-1702, 1992.

Woodward JR, Rushton HG: Reflux uropathy, *Pediatr Clin North Am* 34:1349-1364, 1987.

Glomerular Diseases

Berns JS and others: Steroid responsive nephrotic syndrome of childhood: a long-term study of clinical course, histopathology, efficacy of cyclophosphamide therapy, and effects of growth, *Am J Kidney Dis* 9:108-114, 1987.

Brodehl J, Ehrich JHH: Short versus standard prednisone therapy for initial treatment of idiopathic nephrotic syndrome in children, *Lancet* 1:380-383, 1988.

Schnaper HW: The immune system in minimal change nephrotic syndrome, *Pediatr Nephrol* 3:101-110, 1989.

Tejani A and others: Cyclosporin A–induced remission in relapsing nephrotic syndrome in children, *Kidney Int* 33:729-734, 1988.

Ueda N and others: Intermittent versus long-term tapering prednisolone for initial therapy in children with idiopathic nephrotic syndrome, *J Pediatr* 112:122-126, 1988.

Vernier RL, Chavers B: Glomerular permeability: new concepts, *Pediatr Ann* 17:590-600, 1988.

Warshaw BL, Hymes LC: Daily single-dose and daily reduced-dose prednisone therapy for children with the nephrotic syndrome, *Pediatrics* 83:694-699, 1989.

Wynn SR and others: Long-term prognosis for children with nephrotic syndrome, *Clin Pediatr* 27:63-68, 1988.

Hemolytic-Uremic Syndrome

Cleary TG: Cytotoxin-producing *Escherichia coli* and the hemolytic uremic syndrome, *Pediatr Clin North Am* 35:485-501, 1988.

Havens PL and others: Laboratory and clinical variables to predict outcome in hemolytic-uremic syndrome, *Am J Dis Child* 142:961-964, 1988.

Kavi J, Wise R: Causes of the haemolytic uraemic syndrome, *Br Med J* 298:65-67, 1989.

Novillo AA and others: Haemolytic uremic syndrome associated with faecal cytotoxin and verotoxin neutralizing antibodies, *Pediatr Nephrol* 2:288-290, 1988.

Siegler RL: Management of hemolytic-uremic syndrome, *J Pediatr* 112:1014-1020, 1988.

Renal Failure

Bock GH and others: Disturbances of brain maturation and neurodevelopment during chronic renal failure in infancy, *J Pediatr* 114:231-238, 1989.

Crittenden MR, Holaday B: Physical growth and behavioral adaptations of children with renal insufficiency, *ANNA J* 16:87-92+, 1989.

Doolittle RF: Biotechnology—the enormous cost of success, *N Engl J Med* 324(19):1360-1362, 1991.

Fine RN, Salusky IB, Ettenger RB: The therapeutic approach to the infant, child, and adolescent with end-stage renal disease, *Pediatr Clin North Am* 34:789-801, 1987.

Foreman JW, Chan JCM: Chronic renal failure in infants and children, *J Pediatr* 113:793-800, 1988.

Gaudio KM, Siegel NJ: Pathogenesis and treatment of acute renal failure, *Pediatr Clin North Am* 34:771-787, 1987.

Gertner JM: Phosphorus metabolism and its disorders in childhood, *Pediatr Ann* 16:957-965, 1987.

Kling PJ and others: Pharmacoginetics and pharmacodynamics of erythtopoietin during therapy in an infant with renal failure, *J Pediatr* 121(5):822-825, 1992.

Langman C: Childhood uremic bone disease, *Pediatr Ann* 16:974-978, 1987.

McCrory WW and others: Effects of dietary phosphate restriction in children with chronic renal failure, *J Pediatr* 111:410-412, 1987.

Obrecht JA, Gallo AM, Knafl KA: A case of illustration of family management style in childhood end stage renal disease, *ANNA J* 19(3):255-260, 1992.

Quinlan M: Nursing assessment and management of malnutrition in uremic infants, *ANNA J* 15:19-22, 1988.

Trachtman H, Gauthier B: Parenteral calcitriol for treatment of severe renal osteodystrophy in children with chronic renal insufficiency, *J Pediatr* 110:966-970, 1987.

Weiss R: Management of chronic renal failure, *Pediatr Ann* 17:584-589, 1988.

Dialysis/Transplantation

Bell S: CAVH in pediatrics: Meeting the challenge, *ANNA J* 15:25-26, 1988.

Dirkes SM: Making a critical difference with CAVH, *Nursing 89* 19(11):57-60, 1989.

Doyle CL, Flanigan MJ, Mabe C: Tidal peritoneal dialysis vs. continuous cyclic peritoneal dialysis: children's preference, *ANNA J* 19(3):249-254, 1992.

Gharbieh PA: Renal transplant: surgical and psychologic hazards, *Crit Care Nurse* 8(6):58-70, 1988.

Gold LM and others: Psychosocial issues in pediatric organ transplantation: the parents' perspective, *Pediatrics* 77:738-743, 1986.

Gorynski L, Knight F: A peer group for adolescent dialysis patients, *ANNA J* 19(3):262-264, 1992.

House RM, Thompson TL II: Psychiatric aspects of organ transplantation, *JAMA* 260:535-539, 1988.

Kelley JE and others: Surgical aspects of pediatric dialysis, *Int Pediatr* 8(3):367-372, 1993.

Malti J, Wellons D: CAPD: a dialysis breakthrough with its own burdens, *RN* 51:46-52, 1988.

McFarland K: Pediatric peritoneal dialysis, *Pediatr Nurs* 14:426-429, 1988.

Moskop JC: Organ transplantation in children: ethical issues, *J Pediatr* 110:175-179, 1987.

Neff EJ: Nursing the child undergoing dialysis, *Issues Compr Pediatr Nurs* 10:173-185, 1987.

Pascual JF, Lopez JD, Molina M: Hemofiltration in children with renal failure, *Pediatr Clin North Am* 34:803-818, 1987.

Sander V, Murray C, Robertson P: School and the in-center pediatric hemodialysis patient, *ANNA J* 16:72-74, 1989.

Sheldon CA, McLorie GA, Churchill BM: Renal transplantation in children, *Pediatr Clin North Am* 34:1209-1232, 1987.

Sheldon CA and others: Surgical considerations in childhood end-stage renal disease, *Pediatr Clin North Am* 34:1187-1208, 1987.

Sinai-Trieman L, Salusky IB, Fine RN: Use of subcutaneous recombinant human erythropoietin in children undergoing continuous cycling peritoneal dialysis, *J Pediatr* 114:550-554, 1989.

Suddaby EC, Bell SB, Murphy KJ: Continuous hemofiltration in infants and children, *Pediatr Nurs* 16:79-82, 1990.

Tejani A, Fine RN: Cadaver renal transplantation in children, *Clin Pediatr* 32(4):194-202, 1993.

Tejani A and others: Factors predictive of sustained growth in children after renal transplantation, *J Pediatr* 122(3):397-402, 1993.

Weichler NK: Caretakers' informational needs after their children's renal or liver transplant, *ANNA J* 20(2):135-139, 1993.

UNIT XI

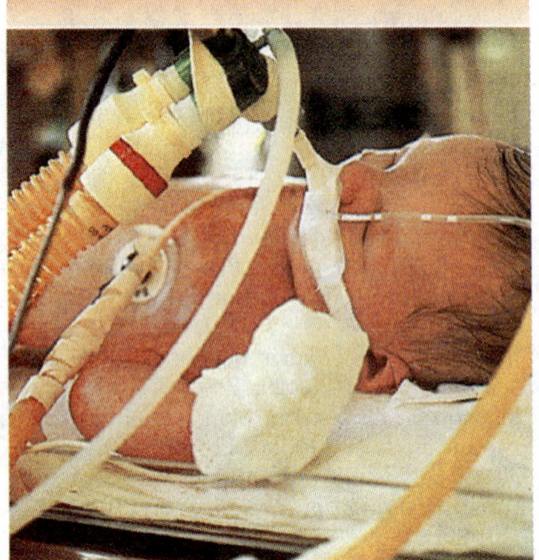

THE CHILD WITH PROBLEMS RELATED TO TRANSFER OF OXYGEN AND NUTRIENTS

CHAPTER 31 The Child with Disturbance of Oxygen and Carbon Dioxide Exchange

CHAPTER OUTLINE

RELATED TOPICS

The child with respiratory dysfunction, Ch. 32
Family-centered home care, Ch. 25
High risk related to disturbed respiratory function, Ch. 10
Discharge planning and home care, Ch. 26
Physical examination: chest, lungs, Ch. 7
Preparation for procedures, Ch. 27
Shock, Ch. 29

RESPIRATORY TRACT STRUCTURE AND FUNCTION

Disorders involving the respiratory tract, many of which can be life-threatening, occur frequently in infancy and childhood. Anatomically, a number of differences influence the manner in which children, particularly infants, respond to respiratory disturbances.

The ***respiratory tract*** consists of many complex structures that function under neural and hormonal control. The primary responsibility of these structures is to distribute air and exchange gases so that cells are supplied with oxygen (O_2) for body metabolism while carbon dioxide (CO_2), the volatile product of metabolism, is removed. The organs of the respiratory system—nose, pharynx, larynx, trachea, bronchi, and lungs—provide the means whereby gases enter the body. The circulatory system then distributes gases to and from the millions of cells throughout the body. All the structures of the respiratory system except the minute air sacs (alveoli) of the lung tissue function in air distribution. It is within the alveoli that the gas exchange takes place.

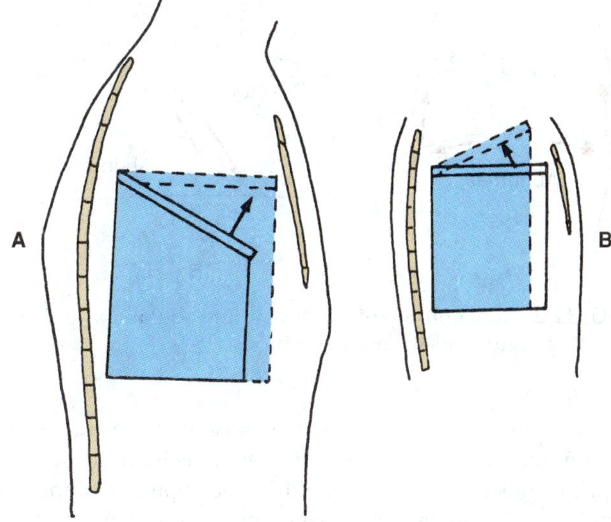

FIG. 31-1 Mechanisms of respiratory excursion. **A,** Downward and lateral position of rib in adult and expansion of lung capacity on thoracic inspiration. **B,** More horizontal position of rib in infant and decreased expansion of lung capacity of thoracic inspiration.

STRUCTURE

The ***thoracic cavity,*** which is encased in the bony framework provided by the ribs, vertebrae, and sternum, consists of three major partitions: the ***three-lobed lung*** on the right, the ***two-lobed lung*** on the left, and the space between them—the ***mediastinum***—which contains the esophagus, trachea, large blood vessels, and heart. The entire thoracic cavity is lined by the smooth ***parietal pleura,*** which adheres to the ribs and superior surface of the diaphragm. Each lung is encased in a separate ***visceral pleural sac*** that, when inflated, lies against the parietal pleura. Normally the two pleural membranes are separated by only enough fluid to lubricate the surface for painless movement during filling and emptying of the lungs. In disease states this space may contain air ***(pneumothorax)*** or fluid ***(pleural effusion)***—more specifically serum ***(hydrothorax),*** blood ***(hemothorax),*** or pus (***pyothorax,*** also known as ***empyema***). Inflammation of the pleura causes the painful friction of pleurisy during respiratory movements.

Chest

The chest has a relatively round configuration at birth but changes gradually to one that is more or less flattened in the anteroposterior (front-to-back) diameter in adulthood. In certain lung diseases chronic overinflation causes changes in these measurements. For example, in severe obstructive lung disease (e.g., asthma, cystic fibrosis) the anteroposterior measurement approaches the transverse (side-to-side) measurement to produce the so-called ***barrel chest.*** Periodic measurements provide clues to the course of the lung disease or the efficacy of therapy. For example, increased size indicates progressive obstructive lung disease.

The elliptic shape of the ribs and the angle at which they are attached to the spine allow the thorax to change size during respiration. Contraction of the intercostal muscles lifts the ribs from a downward angle to a more horizontal angle, which increases both the anteroposterior and the lateral dimensions of the chest (Fig. 31-1, *A*). This also changes the diameter of the bronchi; the diameter increases during inspiration and decreases during expiration, an important factor when the bronchi are narrowed as a result of obstruction or inflammation. Contraction and relaxation of the diaphragm cause the chest cavity to lengthen and shorten, which also increases the volume of the chest cavity during inspiration. Normal expiration is passive, although contraction of the internal intercostal muscles pulls the rib cage downward, and contraction of the abdominal muscles forces the diaphragm upward to decrease the chest size actively (see Fig. 7-34).

An adult's ribs articulate with the vertebrae and sternum from a downward and lateral angle, also causing the chest cavity to enlarge. In the newborn infant, however, the ribs articulate with the spine at a horizontal rather than a downward slope and, if raised further, decrease the diameter of the chest (Fig. 31-1, *B*). Therefore the infant relies almost entirely on diaphragmatic-abdominal breathing. During inspiration the diaphragm is forced downward, increasing the available space for lung expansion; the intercostal muscles serve primarily as stabilizing forces. Also facilitating respiration are the processes of compliance—or the elastic properties of lung tissue, which allow them to expand and recoil—and resistance, which affects the quantity of flow through the airways (see p. 1336).

Variations also occur in lung volume relative to posture. In the upright position the evenly distributed weight of the abdominal contents contributes to uniform application of negative intrathoracic pressure. However, in the supine position the abdominal contents apply weight caudally to cre-

■ Stephen Jones, RN,C, MS, PNP, revised this chapter.

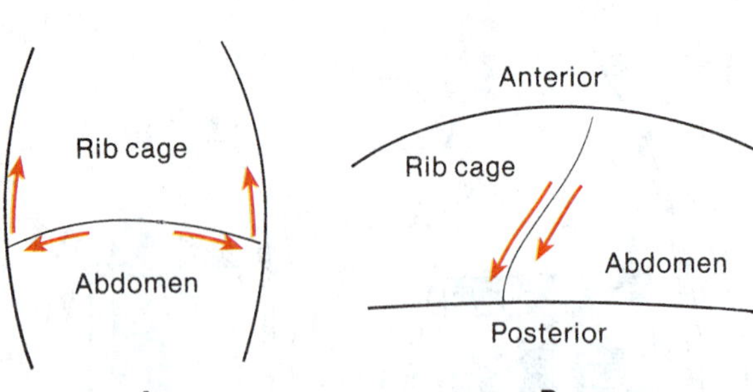

FIG. 31-2 Relationship of diaphragm and abdominal contents in, **A,** upright, and **B,** supine positions.

ate a nonuniform distribution of positive pressure to the diaphragm. Consequently, lung volume is increased in the upright position and decreased in the supine position. In addition, the mechanical attachment of the diaphragm to the rib cage is such that contraction will elevate the rib cage in the upright position but in the supine position tends to pull in the rib cage (Fig. 31-2).

In the newborn the diaphragm is attached higher in front and consequently is longer. Therefore this already stretched diaphragm is unable to contract as far or as forcefully as that of the older infant or child. Young infants are also less able to withstand diaphragmatic fatigue because of fewer energy-producing components. Abdominal distention from gas or fluid can impede diaphragmatic excursion significantly.

Airways

The rigid ***nasal structures,*** which are lined with ciliated mucous membranes, serve as passageways for air, warming and moistening air, filtering it of impurities, and destroying microorganisms that come in contact with immune defenses in the mucosa. In infancy the nasal passages are narrow, and infants are primarily nose-breathers, which substantially increases airway resistance. Any factor that decreases the size of the passages and further increases airway resistance, such as nasal mucosal swelling and mucous accumulation, hampers infants' breathing and feeding.

The ***upper airway*** (oronasopharynx, pharynx, larynx, and upper part of the trachea) is shared by both the respiratory and the alimentary tracts, and many of the muscles in this area participate in several complex acts. However, the sequence of airway muscle activation is different in breathing and swallowing. The upper airway dilates during inspiration and constricts during exhalation. During certain activities these dimensions are modified; for example, inspiration is short during crying, coughing, and sneezing, but with crying the larynx and pharynx dilate. The net result of swallowing is closure of the upper airway with interruption of airflow. Consequently the timing and magnitude of muscle activation have important implications for airway size and patency.

The ***pharynx*** is also a passageway for the entry and exit of air, and it plays a role in phonation by helping produce vowel sounds. The pharynx contains the palatine and lingual tonsils, which are involved in infection control.

The ***larynx,*** situated at the upper end of the trachea, is constructed of a rigid circular framework of cartilage and contains the epiglottis and the glottis (vocal cords). These structures prevent solids or liquids from entering the airway during swallowing, and the vibrations of the vocal cords produce voice sounds. In infancy the ***glottis*** is located more cephalad (toward the head) than in later childhood, and the laryngeal reflexes are very active. The ***epiglottis*** is longer and projects further posteriorly in infants. The narrowest portion of the larynx is at the level of the ***cricoid cartilage.*** In the infant and young child the ciliated columnar epithelium below the vocal cords is loosely bound with areolar tissue and is therefore more susceptible to edema formation. Swelling of the glottis and epiglottis produces hoarseness and often life-threatening obstruction of this narrow portion of the airway.

The ***lower airway*** is made up of the lower trachea, mainstem bronchi, segmental bronchi, subsegmental bronchioles, terminal bronchioles, and alveoli. The ***trachea,*** which is composed of smooth muscle supported by C-shaped rings of cartilage, ensures an open airway to the bronchi and lungs. The trachea divides at the ***carina*** into two primary ***bronchi.*** The right one is situated slightly more vertical than the left, which causes aspirated objects to lodge more frequently in the right bronchus. Each bronchus enters the lung on its respective side, where it divides into secondary bronchi that continue to branch and divide into progressively smaller ***bronchioles.*** The entire bronchial tree is lined with mucous membrane and is composed of spiral smooth muscle supported by rings of cartilage. As the bronchioles become smaller, the cartilaginous rings become increasingly irregular and then disappear completely in the smallest bronchioles, the walls of which consist of only a single layer of cells (Fig. 31-3). There is a range of 23 to 26 levels of branches divided into two categories: the ***conducting airways*** and the ***terminal respiratory units.*** These branch levels, called ***generations,*** are divided into five types (Thompson and others, 1993).

All the structures are subject to obstruction from edema or foreign objects, but the degree of obstruction from constriction of smooth muscle differs. The diameter of the relatively rigid upper airway is less subject to constriction than the lower airways, which contain very little cartilaginous support. The highly reactive bronchiolar smooth muscle of the lower airways can cause life-threatening obstruction during bronchoconstriction. The airway cartilage in young infants is very soft and compressible; therefore the intrathoracic airways are highly reactive to stimuli, such as vagal nerve stimulation.

The airways of the newborn have very little smooth muscle, but in children 4 to 5 months of age they contain sufficient muscle to cause narrowing in response to irritating stimuli. By 1 year of age, smooth muscle development and reactivity are comparable to those in the adult. Growth of the respiratory system follows the general growth curve during the early weeks of life, but the airways grow faster than the thoracic and cervical portions of the vertebral column. Consequently, the larynx and trachea descend in relation to the upper spine. For example, the bifurcation of

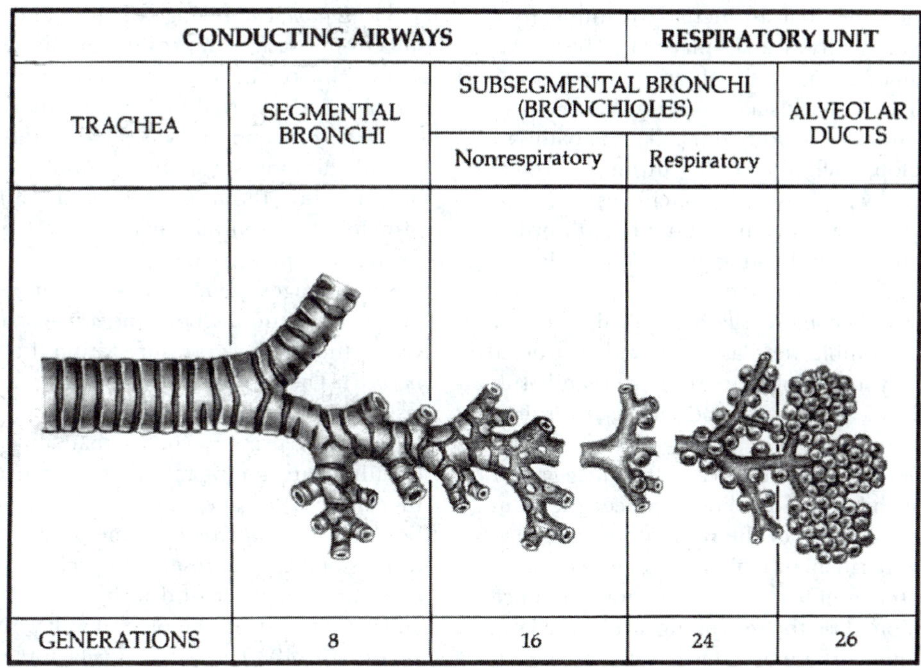

FIG. 31-3 Structures of the lower airway. (From Thompson JM and others: *Mosby's clinical nursing,* ed 3, St Louis, 1993, Mosby.)

the trachea that lies opposite the third thoracic vertebra in the infant descends to a position opposite the fourth in adulthood (Fig. 31-4). Likewise, the cricoid cartilage descends from a position opposite the fourth cervical vertebra in the infant to opposite the sixth cervical vertebra in the adult. These anatomic changes produce differences in the angle of access to the trachea at various ages and must be considered when the infant or child is to be positioned for resuscitation and airway clearance.

The function of the tracheobronchial tree is to distribute air to the alveoli of the lung. A variety of diseases and conditions, such as mucosal swelling, muscular contraction, and mechanical obstruction by mucus or a foreign body, can cause localized or generalized airway occlusion.

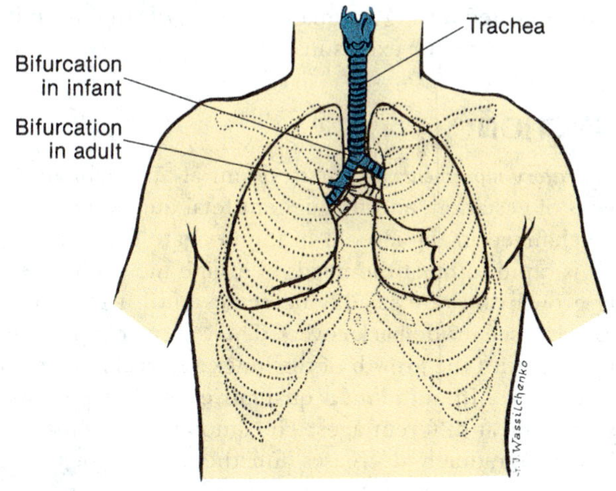

FIG. 31-4 Difference in level of bifurcation of trachea in infant and adult.

Respiratory Units

The two cone-shaped lungs consist of the bronchi, bronchioles, and innumerable small ***air sacs,*** or ***alveoli.*** Through these thin-walled sacs, gas exchange occurs by simple diffusion between the inspired air and the bloodstream. The amount of gas exchanged depends on many factors, including the amount and composition of air inhaled, thickness of the alveolar wall, adequacy of circulation to the alveoli, and substances within the alveoli that either prevent their inflation (e.g., surface-active substance surfactant) or prevent gas exchange (e.g., fluids).

With age, changes take place in the air passages that increase respiratory surface area. The major changes are in the number and size of alveoli and in the increased branching of terminal bronchioles. Whereas the number of conducting airways is complete early in fetal life, the air sacs are shallow with wide necks but have few shared walls, or ***septa,*** at birth. This promotes patency but limits surface area for gas exchange. The alveoli are large with thick septa that have little elastic recoil (not unlike the emphysemic lung). During the first year bronchioles continue to branch, and the globular alveoli formed earlier in the terminal units rapidly increase in number with each generation. These alveoli partition and divide existing alveoli to form smaller lobular units separated by thinner septa, thus enlarging the area available for gas exchange.

Alveoli increase steadily in number, but it is unclear when septal division ceases and an increase in size begins. It appears to occur sometime during middle childhood, although evidence indicates that an increase in number of alveoli for each terminal airway takes place at puberty. Approximately nine times as many alveoli are present at age 12 years than at birth. In later stages of growth, the structures lengthen and enlarge. In addition, collateral pathways of ventilation develop, including pores through alveolar walls and possibly pathways between bronchioles.

All of these factors are significant to respiratory disorders in young children. Infants and young children have less alveolar surface area for gas exchange, the narrowly branching peripheral airways become easily obstructed, and lack of collateral pathways inhibits ventilation beyond obstructed units. Consequently, young children are more readily subject to obstruction and atelectasis, especially as a result of repeated infection.

A variety of pathologic conditions can affect ***lung growth.*** A postural defect such as kyphoscoliosis reduces the number of alveoli. Rare infections of the respiratory tract (e.g., coxsackievirus) can permanently alter lung development, resulting in decreased numbers of small airways. Replication of alveoli is inhibited, so the remaining alveoli are large but decreased in number. Lung growth can also be enhanced by changes in hormone levels. Glucocorticosteroids, thyroxine, and prolactin enhance lung development, and lack of thyroid hormone results in immature lungs. Biochemical substances that enhance lung growth are theophylline, estrogen, isoxsuprine, epidermal growth factor, and heroin injected during pregnancy. Lung growth is inhibited by phenobarbital or excess insulin.

FUNCTION

Respiratory movements are first evident at approximately 20 weeks of gestation, and throughout fetal life amniotic fluid is exchanged in the alveoli. In the neonate the respiratory rate is rapid to meet the needs of a high metabolism. During growth the rate steadily decreases until it levels off at maturity (see inside back cover). The volume of air inhaled increases with the growth of the lungs and is closely related to body size. In addition, a qualitative difference exists in expired air at different ages. The amount of O_2 in the expired air gradually decreases and the amount of CO_2 increases during growth.

Ventilation, the passage of air in and out of the lungs, results from changes in pressure gradients created by changes in the size of the thoracic cavity. Contraction of the diaphragm and external intercostal muscles increases the size of the thorax and decreases the intrathoracic pressure. As a result, air moves from the atmosphere, which has a higher pressure, into the lungs, which have a lower pressure. The principles of ***artificial ventilation*** are based on this concept. Artificial respiratory devices increase the pressure entering the air passages ***(positive-pressure breathing devices),*** lower the pressure around the body ***(negative-pressure ventilator),*** or increase the negative pressure within the thoracic cavity ***(rocking bed).*** The shorter abdominal length of infants makes this last method ineffectual.

The two primary forces that affect the mechanics of breathing are compliance and resistance; conditions that either increase or decrease these two forces are listed in the box below. ***Compliance*** is a measure of chest wall and lung distensibility. It represents the relative ease with which the chest and lungs expand with increasing volume and then collapse away from the pleural wall with decreasing volume (elastic recoil). The two major factors determining compliance are (1) ***alveolar surface tension surfactant,*** which is maintained by a lipoprotein at the air-fluid interface that allows alveolar expansion and prevents alveolar collapse, and (2) ***elastic recoil,*** the tendency of the lungs to return to the resting state after inspiration (a passive process that requires no muscular effort). Other factors influencing compliance include the degree of tissue hydration, lung blood volume, surface forces at the air-fluid interface, and chest and/or lung tissue pathology (i.e., fibers of elastin or collagen). Factors that interfere with compliance and recoil increase the work of breathing.

Compliance is normally very high in the newborn and infant because of a more pliant (flexible) rib cage. This greater compliance causes the rib cage to be easily distorted with increased negative pressure in the pleural cavity or when factors inhibit the stabilizing action of the intercostal muscles. As the child grows, chest wall compliance decreases and elastic recoil increases; therefore ventilation becomes progressively more efficient. In pathologic states an increase in compliance indicates that the lungs or chest wall is abnormally easy to inflate and has lost some elastic re-

CONDITIONS AND DISEASES AFFECTING LUNG COMPLIANCE AND RESISTANCE

COMPLIANCE		RESISTANCE	
DECREASED	**INCREASED**	**INCREASED**	**DECREASED**
Pulmonary edema	Lobar emphysema	Asthma	Normal lung fields
Pneumothorax	Asthma	Cystic fibrosis	
Atelectasis		Bronchopulmonary dysplasia (BPD)	
Pulmonary fibrosis		Bronchiolitis	
Absence of muscles of breathing		Tracheostenosis	
Neuromuscular conditions		Conditions with high amount of secretions	
Surfactant deficiency			
Distended fluid spaces			
Engorged blood vessels			

coil, such as in asthma. A decrease in compliance indicates that the lungs or chest wall is abnormally stiff or difficult to inflate, such as in respiratory distress syndrome (McCance and Huether, 1994).

Resistance is determined primarily by airway size. Three sources of resistance must be overcome during breathing: tissue resistance in the chest wall (about 20% resistance), tissue resistance in the lungs (about 15% resistance), and, most important, flow resistance in the airways (this is most likely to increase with any kind of respiratory disease). The four factors determining resistance are flow rate velocity, gas viscosity, length of airway, and airway diameter. If any of the first three variables increases, then resistance to air flow will also increase. If airway diameter decreases, then resistance increases exponentially.

The small diameter of children's airways increases the potential risk of any condition that reduces airway size. The example in Fig. 31-5 illustrates the difference that airway size plays in older children's and infants' responses to airway compromise.

NURSING ALERT Any condition that decreases or increases compliance and/or increases airway resistance results in increased work of breathing (increased respiratory rate, retractions, nasal flaring). If respiratory muscle fatigue develops, respiratory failure can occur.

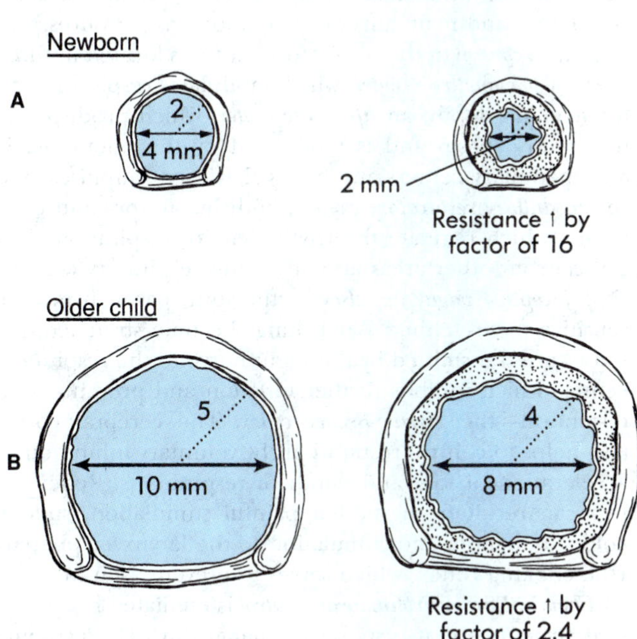

FIG. 31-5 Effects of 1 mm of circumferential edema in a small neonate and an older child. **A,** The neonate possesses a larynx of approximately 4 mm diameter and 2 mm radius. If 1 mm of circumferential edema develops, it will halve the airway radius and increase resistance to air flow by a factor of 16. **B,** The older child possesses a larynx approximately 10 mm in diameter and 5 mm in radius. The 1 mm of circumferential edema will reduce the radius by 20% (from 5 mm to 4 mm) and increase resistance to air flow by a factor of 2.4. (From Hazinski MF, editor: *Nursing care of the critically ill child,* ed 2, St Louis, 1992, Mosby.)

The diameter of the airways and thus the airflow are determined by the balance of forces that tend to widen or narrow the airways. One of these is neural regulation of bronchial smooth muscles mediated through autonomic nerves. Sympathetic impulses relax the airways; parasympathetic impulses constrict them. Reflex constriction occurs in response to irritating inhalants such as dust, smoke, or sulfur dioxide; arterial hypoxemia and hypercapnia; cold air; and some drugs, such as acetylcholine and histamine. Other factors that alter airway size are peribronchial pressure, which tends to narrow the airways, and intraluminal pressure, which tends to keep airways open. For example, forced expiration causes increased peribronchial pressure and hence narrowing of the airways; a positive-pressure breathing apparatus increases intraluminal pressure, keeping the airways open.

Gas Exchange*

Gases in the blood are measured by the ***partial pressures (tensions)*** of the individual gases and are expressed in millimeters of mercury, also called ***torr.*** With O_2 therapy it is important to understand the relationship between the concentration of the inspired gas and the partial pressure of that gas in the arteries (PaO_2). Inspired O_2 is expressed as the ***fraction of inspired O_2 (FIO_2),*** with 1.0 meaning 100% O_2, 0.5 meaning 50% O_2, and so on. Patients breathing room air would have an FIO_2 of 0.21, since ambient air contains 21% O_2. Understanding the relationship between inspired gases and their partial pressures in the blood begins with a knowledge of gases in ambient air and how the pressure they exert creates a gradient between the alveoli and capillary blood.

Ambient air is composed of 21% O_2, trace amounts of CO_2, and 79% nitrogen (N). Water vapor (H_2O) also exerts a pressure. The water vapor does not change with the barometric pressure (PB) but exerts a constant pressure of 47 mm Hg when the gas is fully saturated at body temperature. Each contributes to the total PB as follows:

$$P_B = PO_2 + PCO_2 + PN_2 + PH_2O$$

The significance of inspired gases lies in the FIO_2 and the pressure it exerts (PIO_2). At sea level this can be calculated as follows:

$$PIO_2 = FIO_2 \times (P_B - PH_2O)$$
$$PIO_2 = 0.21 \times (760 - 47)$$
$$PIO_2 = 0.21 \times 713$$
$$PIO_2 = 150 \text{ mm Hg}$$

When the FIO_2 is increased, the pressure exerted also increases:

$$PIO_2 = 0.50 \times (760 - 47)$$
$$PIO_2 = 0.50 \times 713$$
$$PIO_2 = 356.5 \text{ mm Hg}$$

As the inspired gas travels down the airway and reaches the alveoli, the pressure drops as CO_2 is added to the mixture.

*Kathleen Rossman, RRT, wrote this section.

Ambient air contains only traces of CO_2. As the gas diffuses from the capillary blood to the alveoli, however, the amount and pressure of CO_2 in the alveoli increase to the CO_2 levels in the venous blood. By subtracting the PCO_2 from the PIO_2, the alveolar O_2 pressure (PAO_2) can be determined. The $PACO_2$ is first divided by 0.8. This correlation factor, or respiratory quotient (RQ), is used to calculate the ratio of O_2 absorbed to CO_2 eliminated. The alveolar pressure can then be expressed as:

$$PAO_2 = PIO_2 - (PACO_2 \div 0.8)$$
$$PAO_2 = 150 - (40 \div 0.8)$$
$$PAO_2 = 150 - 50$$
$$PAO_2 = 100 \text{ mm Hg}$$

Since normal venous PO_2 is approximately 40 mm Hg, a gradient is created when the PAO_2 is 100 mm Hg and diffusion occurs between the alveoli and capillary blood. When the patient's PaO_2 decreases, the FIO_2 can be raised to increase the PAO_2, thereby increasing the gradient for diffusion.

Because CO_2 is more soluble than O_2, it diffuses 21 times faster; therefore diffusion of CO_2 from the blood to the alveoli is not impaired. The amount of O_2 that diffuses into the blood and the amount of CO_2 removed by the lungs depend on several factors (see box below).

Oxygen/Carbon Dioxide Transport. Once O_2 has diffused from the alveolus to the pulmonary capillary, it is transported throughout the body in two ways. A small amount (PaO_2) is transported as a solute dissolved in the plasma and the water of red blood cells. A larger portion (40 to 70 times as much) is carried by hemoglobin as ***oxyhemoglobin.*** Since each gram of hemoglobin can combine with 1.34 ml of O_2, the transport capacity is largely determined by the amount of hemoglobin present. For example, children with severe anemia tend to be fatigued, be somewhat cyanotic, and breathe more rapidly. In addition, increasing the amount of O_2 delivered to the alveoli can increase the amount carried by the blood only in relation to the amount of hemoglobin present. For example, at a PaO_2 of 100 mm Hg, hemoglobin is 97.5% saturated. Hemoglobin saturation is commonly termed ***arterial oxygen saturation (SaO_2)*** or ***oxyhemoglobin saturation.*** The nonlinear relationship between the PaO_2 and the SaO_2 is described by the oxyhemoglobin dissociation curve (Fig. 31-10).

CO_2 is carried in the blood in a number of ways. A small amount ($PaCO_2$) is transported dissolved in the plasma and the water of red blood cells. A large amount (more than half) hydrates to form carbonic acid, which dissociates and is carried as bicarbonate and hydrogen ions. The remaining CO_2 combines with certain plasma proteins and hemoglobin. The association of CO_2 with hemoglobin is accelerated by an increasing $PaCO_2$ and a decreasing PaO_2 and is decreased by the opposite conditions. The diffusion of CO_2 into the alveoli is very rapid. Thus the equilibrium between the $PaCO_2$ of the pulmonary capillaries and the alveoli is achieved promptly.

Transport between blood and tissue cells is accomplished down a diffusion gradient, just as it is between the blood and the alveoli.

Regulation of Respiration. The mechanisms that control respiration can be divided into two large categories: (1) a ***neural system*** that maintains a coordinated, rhythmic respiratory cycle and regulates the depth of respiration and (2) a ***chemical (neurohumoral)*** system that regulates alveolar ventilation and maintains normal blood gas pressures.

Neural control in the respiratory center is located in three areas: a ***pneumotaxic center,*** which modulates respiratory frequency and depth; an ***apneustic center,*** which produces an inspiratory spasm and is modulated by the pneumotaxic and medullary centers and by vagal afferent impulses; and the ***medullary respiratory centers,*** both inspiratory and expiratory, which regulate the rhythmicity of respirations. Impulses from other areas also affect the respiratory centers. ***Proprioceptive vagal impulses*** in the lung parenchyma are sensitive to stretching. When lungs become stretched, impulses are transmitted by the vagus nerve to the respiratory center, which inhibits further inflation and prevents overdistention—the ***Hering-Breuer reflex.*** The cerebral cortex also helps to control respirations by voluntary inhibition or acceleration of rate and depth of respirations. Reflex apnea can result from sudden painful stimulation, sudden cold stimulation, and stimulation to the larynx or pharynx (the choking reflex, which serves to prevent aspiration).

Chemical, or ***neurohumoral, control*** is mediated by specialized structures that respond to changes in pH, PCO_2, and PO_2—***central chemoreceptors,*** probably located in the medulla, and ***peripheral chemoreceptors,*** located in the great vessels. Peripheral chemoreceptors of greatest physiologic importance are the carotid bodies, located at the division of the common carotid artery into its external and internal branches, and the aortic bodies that lie between the ascending aorta and the pulmonary artery. CO_2 and hydrogen ions control respiration by acting directly on the respiratory center; the peripheral chemoreceptors respond to changes in PO_2. Thus an increase in ventilation can result from either

FACTORS AFFECTING GAS DIFFUSION IN ALVEOLI

Pressure gradient between alveolar air and capillary blood—In order for gases to diffuse across this gradient, the gas molecules must pass through the barrier of liquid surfactant lining the alveolus. Disease can greatly increase this barrier, thus interfering with the diffusion process.

Alveolar ventilation, or **amount of air that reaches the alveoli**—Any obstruction to air passing from the upper airways through the bronchi to the alveoli decreases the volume of air available for diffusion. ***Minute ventilation (MV)*** is the amount of air inhaled in a normal breath ***(tidal volume [TV])*** multiplied by the respiratory rate. Factors affecting the respiratory rate or TV may decrease the amount of air available for diffusion.

Relationship between amount of alveolar air and alveolar perfusion—Factors that decrease the amount of alveolar perfusion increase the ventilation/perfusion ratio. Factors or disease states that increase or decrease the amount of alveolar air also create a ventilation/perfusion mismatch and abnormal levels of PO_2 or PCO_2 in the blood.

(1) stimulation of the respiratory center by an increased $Paco_2$ or pH or (2) a decreased Pao_2, which stimulates the carotid and aortic bodies. These bodies then transmit signals to the brain to excite the respiratory center.

The lungs also have an important role in ***acid-base balance.*** Less rapid than the chemical buffers, the respiratory mechanism begins to act within 1 to 3 minutes to make adjustments in pH by eliminating or retaining CO_2. When the levels of CO_2 are altered sufficiently, the respiratory centers in the brain respond by either increasing or decreasing the rate and depth of respirations. For example, when the pH of the blood drops, as from increased exercise, a compensatory increase in respirations rids the body of the CO_2 derived from carbonic acid, which is formed from buffered acid metabolites. CO_2 buildup from breath-holding produces the same response, again increasing the carbonic acid and reducing the serum pH. Therefore the lungs are the compensatory organs in metabolic disturbances and respond quite rapidly.

Defenses of the Respiratory Tract

The respiratory tract has several anatomic and biochemical characteristics that provide natural defenses against the many biologic and inanimate agents that can damage respiratory tissues. Intact defenses help to repel and resist the impact of injurious agents; factors that reduce the integrity of these mechanisms increase the vulnerability of these tissues to invasion and disease. Respiratory tract defenses include:

Lymphoid tissues—Faucial, lingual, and pharyngeal tonsils (adenoids) and other pharyngeal lymphoid tissues form a protective circle around the entrance to the respiratory tract. These help to localize and contain invading organisms so that they can be destroyed by the body's humoral defense mechanisms.

Mucous blanket—The epithelium of the respiratory tract secretes a sticky mucus to which airborne organisms adhere.

Ciliary action—The mucus secreted by the columnar epithelium of the respiratory tract is kept flowing, carrying microorganisms and other foreign agents away from the lungs to be coughed or swallowed.

Epiglottis—The epiglottis and the epiglottis reflex protect the respiratory tract from invading material, including infectious exudate from the upper tract, and prevent such material from being aspirated into the lower tract.

Cough—The expulsive force of the cough reflex propels foreign material out of the lower tract.

Tracheobronchial dynamics—The tracheobronchial tree elongates and dilates on inspiration and shortens and narrows on expiration.

Position changes—Changes in body position encourage drainage of tracheobronchial passages.

Lymphatics—Lymphatics draining the terminal bronchi and bronchioles remove invading organisms, which are filtered and destroyed in the regional lymph nodes.

Humoral defenses—Organisms and other foreign material are removed and/or destroyed by phagocytes, enzymes, and immunoglobulins, especially immunoglobulin A (IgA), secreted by the bronchial epithelium.

Although effective, these natural barriers are frequently breached. For example, some children have conditions that predispose them to infection as a result of interference with the efficiency of these mechanisms (e.g., chronic asthma, cystic fibrosis, and the various immunodeficiency disorders). Frequent, intense exposure to organisms that accompanies conditions of crowding or continual exposure to irritating substances in the air results in breakdown of healthy defenses. Concurrent illness, malnutrition, or fatigue reduces the efficiency of natural defenses. Also, drying of the mucous membranes inhibits the activity of humoral defenses, such as immunoglobulins.

ASSESSMENT OF RESPIRATORY FUNCTION

PHYSICAL ASSESSMENT

The nurse can obtain much information about the child's respiratory status from simple observations of physical signs and behavior. However, to make a useful assessment, the nurse needs to know what to look for and what it means (see Physical Examination: Chest, Chapter 7). ***Auscultation*** of the lung fields is helpful in identifying specific pathologies and in assessing the child's responses to treatment. Also, auscultation is essential when determining airway patency. ***Palpation*** and ***percussion*** provide information regarding areas of pain and tissue density. Breath sounds and their terminology are also described in Chapter 7.

Respiration

Much can be determined from the configuration of the chest and the pattern of respiratory movement, including rate, regularity, symmetry of movements, depth, effort expended in respiration, and use of accessory muscles of respiration. To assess deviations from the usual, the observer must know the normal type and rate of respiration in relation to the child's size and age (see inside back cover). Respirations (ventilations) are best determined when the child is sleeping or quietly awake.

Tachypnea (rapid ventilations) is observed with anxiety, elevated temperature, severe anemia, and as a result of metabolic acidosis. It may also be associated with respiratory alkalosis caused by psychoneurosis and with central nervous system disturbances. The progress of disorders that contribute to low compliance, such as the pneumonias, pulmonary edema, and pleural effusion, can be followed and evaluated by observing changes in respiratory rate.

Alterations in the depth of respirations—too deep ***(hyperpnea)*** or too shallow ***(hypopnea)***—are recognized as abnormal only in the extremes. Hyperpnea is noted with fever, severe anemia, respiratory alkalosis associated with psychosis, central nervous system disturbances, and respiratory acidosis that accompanies disorders such as diabetes mellitus or diarrhea. Hypoventilation is less easily detected and occurs with metabolic alkalosis in conditions such as pyloric stenosis and respiratory acidosis that accompanies diaphragmatic paralysis or central nervous system depression.

Associated Observations

Associated observations also contribute to assessment. ***Retractions,*** or a sinking in of soft tissues relative to the carti-

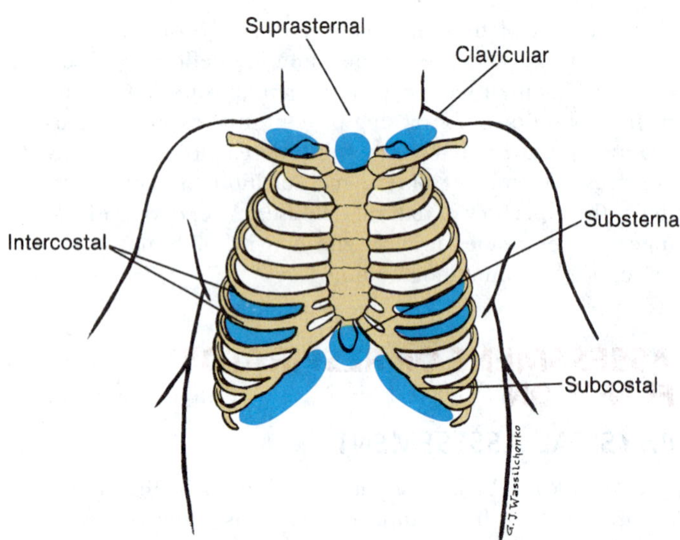

FIG. 31-6 Location of retractions.

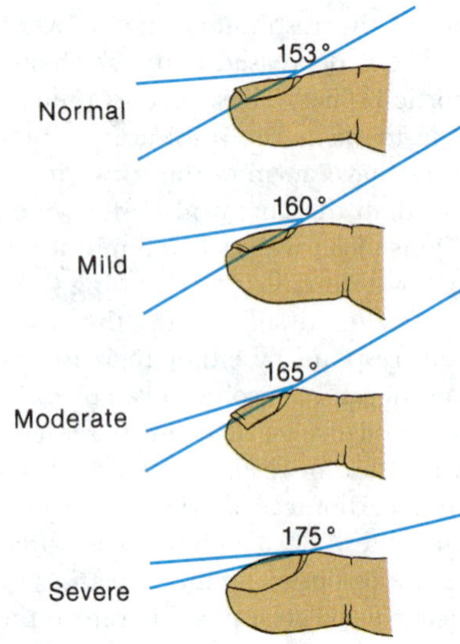

FIG. 31-7 Stages of clubbing. Degree of angle formed above finger at skin-nail junction indicates extent of clubbing. Angle greater than 160 degrees and decided curvature of nail are good criteria for presence of clubbing. (Modified from Waring WW: The history and physical examination. In Chernick V, editor: *Kendig's disorders of the respiratory tract in children,* ed 5, Philadelphia, 1990, WB Saunders.)

laginous and bony thorax, may be noted in some pulmonary disorders. Although slight intercostal retractions are normal, in disease states (particularly in severe airway obstruction) retraction becomes extreme. Subcostal retraction, observed anteriorly at the lower costal margins, indicates a flattened diaphragm, since it not only lowers the floor of the thorax but also pulls on the rib cage in response to a greater than normal decrease in intrathoracic pressure. In severe obstruction, retractions extend to the supraclavicular areas and the suprasternal notch. (See Fig. 31-6 for location of retractions.)

Nasal flaring can be a sign of increased work of breathing and may be a very significant finding in an infant. The enlargement of the nostrils helps reduce nasal resistance and maintain airway patency. Nasal flaring may be intermittent or continuous and should be described as minimal or marked.

Head bobbing in a sleeping or exhausted infant is a sign of dyspnea. The head, supported on the caregiver's arm only at the suboccipital area, will bob forward with each inspiration. This is caused by neck flexion resulting from contraction of the scalene and sternocleidomastoid muscles. ***Noisy breathing*** such as "snoring" is frequently associated with hypertrophied adenoidal tissue, choanal obstruction, polyps, or a foreign body in the nasal passages.

Grunting is frequently a sign of chest pain, suggesting acute pneumonia or pleural involvement. It is also observed in pulmonary edema and is a characteristic of respiratory distress syndrome. It serves to increase end-expiratory pressure and thus prolong the period of O_2 and CO_2 exchange across the alveolocapillary membrane.

Color changes of the skin, especially mottling, pallor, and cyanosis, are noted. Except for the peripheral bluish discoloration resulting from circulatory stasis in the newborn or the mottling or peripheral cyanosis resulting from a cool environment, mottling and cyanosis are significant and usually indicate cardiopulmonary disease.

Chest pain may be a complaint of older children and may have a variety of causes, both pulmonary and nonpulmonary. It may be caused by disease of any of the chest structures—esophagus, pericardium, diaphragm, pleura, or chest wall. ***Parietal pleural pain*** is usually localized over the affected area and is aggravated by respiratory movements. The pain of ***diaphragmatic pleural irritation*** may be referred to the base of the neck posteriorly and anteriorly or to the abdomen. Most pleural pain is related to respiration; therefore respiratory movements are shallow and rapid.

Clubbing, or proliferation of tissue about the terminal phalanges, accompanies a variety of conditions, frequently those associated with chronic hypoxia, primarily cardiac defects and chronic pulmonary disease. Although clubbing often worsens with lung disease, it does not reflect disease progression accurately (Orenstein, 1989). The degree of clubbing is determined by the extent to which the nail base is lifted on the dorsal surface of the phalanx by the tissue proliferation. The greater the angle formed above the finger or toe at the skin-nail junction, the more pronounced the clubbing, especially when there is a decided curvature to the nail (Fig. 31-7).

Cough is often associated with respiratory disease, although it may suggest some other disorder (see left-hand box on p. 1341). It serves as a protective mechanism, as well as an indicator of some form of irritant. A cough can be initiated voluntarily but is usually a result of a complex reflex consisting of three components: afferent nerve fibers, the cough center, and efferent nerve fibers. Much of the respiratory epithelium contains afferent receptors that are sensitive to mechanical or chemical stimuli. These receptors are concentrated in the areas of the larynx, the carina,

CAUSES OF COUGH

Inflammatory disorders
- Asthma, infections

Lung disease
- Cystic fibrosis, bronchiolitis, retained foreign body, congenital malformations

Focal or anatomic lesions
Psychogenic or habit cough
Postnasal drip and/or sinusitis

COUGH ASSESSMENT

Onset and duration
Type—Dry, hacking, moist, barking, brassy, paroxysmal (a sudden attack, outburst, or intensification of symptoms)
Progress—Better, worse, unchanged, persistent
Pattern—Daytime, nighttime, both, different intensity with time or activity
Associated symptoms—Sore throat, dyspnea, pain and its location
Secretions—Sputum presence, consistency, color, frequency, evidence of swallowing sputum, postnasal drip

and the bifurcations of the large and medium-sized bronchi. When a stimulus is applied to these areas, impulses are transmitted via the vagus nerve to the cough center in the brainstem. Efferent impulses travel via the vagus, phrenic, and spinal motor nerves to the larynx, intercostal muscles, diaphragm, abdominal muscles, and pelvic floor. An inspiratory gasp and closure of the glottis are followed by contraction of muscles in the chest wall, diaphragm, abdomen, and pelvic floor. The resulting compression and increase in pleural, alveolar, and subglottic pressure cause a sudden opening of the glottis and immediate release of trapped air at extremely rapid expiratory flow rates, which forces undesirable material from the respiratory tract.

Inflammation or infection almost anywhere in the upper or lower respiratory tract may produce coughing. Some types of cough are characteristic of specific diseases. For example, a severe cough is associated with measles and cystic fibrosis, and the paroxysmal cough accompanied by an inspiratory "whoop" is pathognomonic of pertussis. A brassy cough is part of the symptomatology of croup and foreign body aspiration. Because there are no cough receptors in the alveoli, a cough may be absent in a child with pneumonia in the early stages of the disease, but is a common feature during active pneumonia and recovery. Cough is assessed according to the features listed in the box above, right.

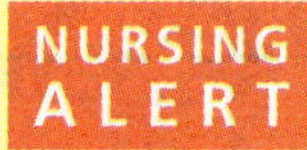

Coughing is not normal and should be investigated further.

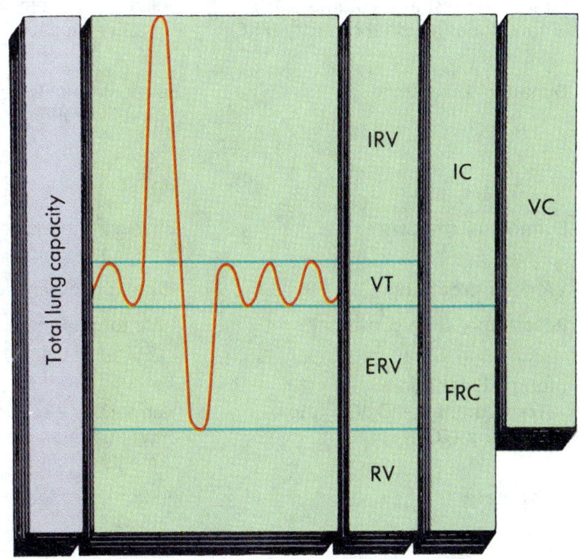

FIG. 31-8 Divisions of total lung capacity. Total lung capacity *(TLC)* is the maximum amount of air contained in the lungs. The total lung capacity is divided into four primary volumes: *IRV,* inspiratory reserve volume; *VT,* tidal volume, *ERV,* expiratory reserve volume; and *RV,* residual volume. ***Capacities*** are combinations of two or more lung volumes. These include inspiratory capacity *(IC)*, functional residual capacity *(FRC)*, and vital capacity *(VC)*. (From Shapiro BA, Harrison RA, Walton R: *Clinical application of blood gases,* ed 3, St Louis, 1982, Mosby.)

DIAGNOSTIC PROCEDURES

Various procedures are available for assessing respiratory function and diagnosing respiratory disease. Understanding how the tests are carried out helps nurses caring for children with respiratory disorders to devise the best strategies for preparing the children for the tests, gaining their cooperation, and supporting them during the procedure. Moreover, this knowledge provides nurses with information on which to base nursing interventions, such as positioning, use of supplemental O_2, and assistance with coughing or deep breathing.

Pulmonary Function Tests

Noninvasive pulmonary mechanics can easily be measured at the bedside of infants and children with the use of pneumotachography or spirometry. This information is sometimes limited in diagnosis, since the same functional abnormality may occur in different diseases. These tests are useful to evaluate the severity and course of a disease and to study the effects of treatment. A listing of the measured parameters is provided in Table 31-1 and Fig. 31-8.

Radiology and Other Diagnostic Procedures

Radiography is used frequently in diagnostic evaluation of children. Although no definitive information exists on the effects of low-dose radiation, measures are carried out to protect vulnerable areas from possible damage. When possible, technicians and others try to prevent unnecessary exposure of the child (and personnel), and the more radiosensitive areas are protected. Careful protection of the im-

TABLE 31-1 Pulmonary Function and Blood Gas Tests Used in Children

TEST	MEASUREMENT	SIGNIFICANCE
Forced vital capacity (FVC) (peak flow)	Maximum amount of air that can be expired after maximum inspiration	Reduced in obesity Reduced in obstructive airway disease Normal in restrictive disease
Forced expiratory volume in 1 (FEV_1) or 3 (FEV_3) seconds	Amount of air that can be forced from the lungs after maximum inspiration in 1 and 3 seconds	Normally 80% of FVC in 1 second Reduced in obstructive disease
Tidal volume (TV or V_T)	Amount of air inhaled and exhaled during any respiratory cycle	Multiplied by respiratory rate to provide minute volume Information needed to determine rate and depth of artificial ventilation
Functional residual volume (FRV); functional residual capacity (FRC)	Volume of air remaining in the lungs after passive expiration	Allows for aeration of alveoli Increased in hyperinflated lungs of obstructive lung disease
Dynamic compliance	Relationship between change in volume and pressure difference	Reflects elastic recoil of lung Normal volume but decreased airflow in obstructive disease (e.g., asthma) Normal flow but decreased volume in restrictive disease (e.g., pulmonary fibrosis)
Pulmonary resistance	Changes in pressure with changes in flow on inspiration and expiration	
Work of breathing	Total work expended moving lung and chest	
Respiratory time constancy	Time for proximal and alveolar airway pressure to equilibrate	
Blood oxygenation		
Transcutaneous O_2/CO_2 monitoring (TCM)	Skin surface electrodes heated and applied to well-perfused areas of the trunk; measurements in mm Hg	Provides continuous and reliable trends of arterial O_2 and CO_2 Noninvasive
Oximetry	Photometric measurement of O_2 saturation (SaO_2) Measurements in percentages	Provides continuous noninvasive measurements of hemoglobin saturation
Capnography	Measures CO_2 during inhalation and exhalation cycle and produces a graph of CO_2 concentration over time	Provides end-tidal CO_2 levels to determine trends and identify shunts
Arterial puncture	Arterial blood obtained from temporal (neonates), brachial, radial, posterior tibial, and femoral arteries	Obtains blood for gas analysis (Po_2, Pco_2, pH)
FEV_1 or FEV_3/FVC	Percentage of maximum inspiration that is expired in 1 or 3 seconds	Normally 95% of FVC in 3 seconds Reduced in obstructive disease

mature gonads of the infant or child with lead shields is essential. Other sensitive areas are the thyroid gland, ocular lens, and bone marrow.

Although nurses have limited control over the length, frequency, and correct application of the x-ray beam, they can make certain that the infant or child receives proper protection from possible hazards. Lead shields, correctly placed and consistently applied to areas not needed for diagnostic purposes, are essential. Play and modification of methodology can be used effectively to reduce the trauma sometimes associated with the procedure and to gain the child's cooperation. Special radiologic examinations used in respiratory diagnosis are outlined in Table 31-2.

Several other procedures are employed in diagnosing lung disorders (Table 31-3). Most require specialized equipment and skills. All require some type of preparation of the child.

Blood Gas Determination

Blood gas measurements are sensitive indicators of change in respiratory status in acutely ill patients (see Table 31-4). They provide valuable information regarding lung function, lung adequacy, and tissue perfusion and are essential for monitoring conditions involving hypoxemia, CO_2 retention, and pH. For the nurse who cares for the acutely ill respiratory patient, this information provides cues for decision making regarding therapeutic interventions, such as adjusting the ventilator, increasing chest physiotherapy, administering O_2, or positioning the child for maximum ventilation. Both invasive and noninvasive (see Atraumatic Care box, p. 1344) methods are available.

Pulse oximetry provides a continuous or intermittent noninvasive method of determining oxygen saturation (SaO_2) to guide oxygen therapy. A sensor comprising a light-emitting diode (LED) and a photodetector is placed in op-

TABLE 31-2 Radiologic Examinations

TEST	DESCRIPTION	PURPOSE	COMMENT
Radiography	Pictures obtained by passing x-rays through body and recording them on sensitized film	Produces images of internal structures of chest, including air-filled lungs, airways, vascular markings, heart, and great vessels	Requires preparation, cooperation, and immobilization of child
Fluoroscopy	Electronically intensified image to allow its projection on viewing screen	Used primarily to study diaphragmatic excursion and respiratory motion of the lungs Examination of barium-filled esophagus to outline mediastinal abnormalities	Requires preparation and immobilization of child
Bronchography	Contrast medium is instilled directly into bronchial tree through opaque catheter inserted via orotracheal tube	Most valuable to demonstrate and inspect bronchiectasis Detects distal bronchial obstruction Detects malformations	Carried out with child under general anesthesia or sedation Used less frequently than other examinations Prepare child for anesthesia
Barium swallow	Esophagus is outlined when barium solution or colloid is swallowed	Esophageal displacement defines mediastinal masses Detects swallowing disorders and malformations (e.g., tracheoesophageal fistula)	Valuable adjunct for diagnosis Performed under fluoroscope Prepare child for procedure
Angiography	Injection of dye to produce image of pulmonary vasculature	Investigation of pulmonary vascular anomalies and pulmonary hypertension	Performed with child under general anesthesia Prepare child for anesthesia
Computed tomography (CT)	Sequence of x-rays, each representing a cross section or "cut" through lung tissue at different depth	Useful in identifying presence of calcium or a cavity within a lesion, hilar adenopathy, mediastinal masses, or abnormalities	Usually reserved for children old enough to be able to suspend respiration voluntarily Prepare child for procedure
Magnetic resonance imaging (MRI)	Use of large magnet and radio waves to produce two- or three-dimensional image	Clearly identifies soft tissues	Requires cooperation and usually sedation of child Prepare child for procedure or anesthesia
Radioisotope scanning	Intravenous injection of albumin labeled with radioisotopes or inhalation of radioactive aerosols or xenon gas followed by radiation scanning	Delineates defects in pulmonary arterial perfusion and diseased areas of lung Detects location of aspirated foreign body	Requires cooperation of child or sedation Prepare child for procedure
Ultrasonography	Transmission of sound waves through chest	Identifies opacification	Limited use in diagnosis of respiratory disorders Prepare child for procedure

TABLE 31-3 Diagnostic Procedures Used in Respiratory Disorders

PROCEDURE	DESCRIPTION	PURPOSE
Tracheal aspiration	Sputum obtained by direct aspiration from trachea	Obtains secretions for examination, culture
Bronchoscopy	Direct observation of tracheobronchial tree via bronchoscope	Localizes abnormalities in major airways Provides access to (1) remove aspirated foreign bodies from major airways, (2) remove obstructive mucous plugs, and (3) perform bronchial lavage
Lung puncture	Needle aspiration of lung fluid via syringe and needle through intercostal space	Obtains lung aspirate for histologic study or culture
Lung biopsy	Removal of lung tissue via open thoracotomy or closed-needle procedures	Diagnosis of protracted pulmonary disease unexplained by other means
Brush biopsy	Material for biopsy obtained with nylon brush on end of wire passed through tube placed via nose, pharynx, trachea, and airways (via fluoroscope) to involved lung segment	Obtains material for culture and histologic examination
Percutaneous transtracheal aspiration	Needle and catheter aspiration of tracheal secretions through thyroid cartilage	Obtains secretions for laboratory examination and culture

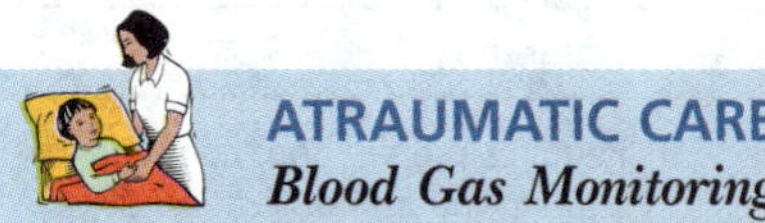

ATRAUMATIC CARE
Blood Gas Monitoring

For continuous monitoring of blood gases, noninvasive measurements are used whenever possible. Also, oximetry should be used before arterial punctures are performed when information about O_2 saturation is sufficient to evaluate the child's condition.

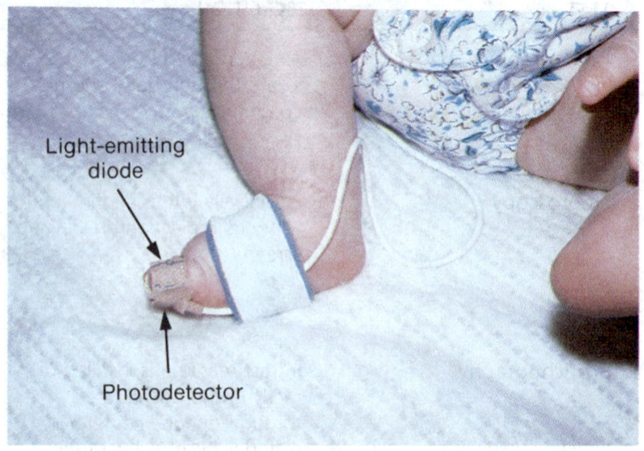

FIG. 31-9 Oximeter sensor on great toe. Note that sensor is positioned with light-emitting diode opposite photodetector. Cord is secured to foot to minimize movement of sensor.

position around a foot, hand, finger, toe, or earlobe, with the LED placed on top of the nail when digits are used (Fig. 31-9). The diode emits red and infrared lights that pass through the skin to the photodetector. The photodetector measures the amount of each type of light absorbed by ***functional hemoglobins*** (those capable of carrying O_2). Hemoglobin saturated with oxygen ***(oxyhemoglobin)*** absorbs more infrared light than does hemoglobin not saturated with oxygen ***(deoxyhemoglobin)***. A microprocessor determines the difference between absorption of the red and infrared light, and the percentage of the total normal hemoglobin that is oxygenated is displayed. Pulsatile blood flow is the primary physiologic factor that influences accuracy of the pulse oximeter.

Another noninvasive method is ***transcutaneous monitoring (TCM)***, which provides continual monitoring of transcutaneous partial pressure of O_2 in arterial blood ($tcPaO_2$) and, with some devices, of CO_2 in arterial blood ($tcPaCO_2$). An electrode is attached to the warmed skin to facilitate arterialization of cutaneous capillaries. The site of the electrode must be changed every 3 to 4 hours to prevent burning the skin, and the machine must be calibrated with every site change. This monitoring is used frequently in neonatal intensive care units, but it may not reflect PaO_2 in infants with impaired local circulation or in older infants whose skin is thicker.

The PaO_2 can be correlated with the SaO_2 by means of the ***oxyhemoglobin dissociation curve*** (Fig. 31-10), although changes in PaO_2 do not cause identical (linear) changes in SaO_2. Rather, the S-shaped curve has two important segments. Once PaO_2 is >80 to 100 mm Hg, the curve is almost horizontal, and the hemoglobin is virtually saturated (95% and above). At this point, further increases in the PaO_2 will only increase the dissolved oxygen in the blood and will not, under normal conditions, contribute significantly to the arterial O_2 content. At a PaO_2 of <60 to <50 mm Hg, the curve is nearly vertical. At this point, even small reductions in the PaO_2 will produce a significant reduction in the hemoglobin saturation (below 90%) and thus in the arterial O_2 content.

➤ **NURSING TIP** A quick formula for calculating correlation of PaO_2 with SaO_2 is the 30-60, 60-90 rule. Assuming a normal pH, $PaCO_2$, and body temperature, this rule can apply: when $PaO_2 = 30$, $SaO_2 = 60$; when $PaO_2 = 60$, $SaO_2 = 90$.

Oximetry is insensitive to hyperoxia because hemoglobin approaches 100% saturation for all PaO_2 readings above approximately 100 mm Hg, which is a dangerous situation for the premature infant at risk for developing retinopathy of prematurity (see Chapter 10). Therefore, the premature infant being monitored with oximetry should have upper limits identified, such as 90% to 95%, and a protocol should be established for decreasing O_2 when saturations are high (Harbold, 1989).

The degree to which O_2 combines with hemoglobin is affected by several factors. A shift of the curve to the left causes an increased affinity of hemoglobin for O_2, but the O_2 is not easily released to the tissues. This represents an increase in the SaO_2 if it is measured against the same PaO_2 of the normal oxyhemoglobin dissociation curve. This left shift can be caused by an increase in blood pH or a decrease in arterial CO_2 pressure ($PaCO_2$), body temperature, or 2,3-diphosphoglycerate (2,3-DPG), a substance in the red blood cells.

A shift of the curve to the right causes a decreased affinity of hemoglobin for O_2, but improved O_2 release to the tissues. This represents a lower SaO_2 if measured against the same PaO_2 of the normal oxyhemoglobin dissociation curve. This rightward shift can be caused by a decrease in blood pH or an increase in $PaCO_2$, body temperature, or 2,3-DPG.

Oximetry offers several advantages over TCM. Oximetry (1) does not require heating the skin, thus reducing the risk of burns; (2) eliminates a delay period for transducer equilibration; and (3) maintains an accurate measurement regardless of the patient's age or skin characteristics or the presence of lung disease.

NURSING ALERT It is important to make certain that sensory connectors and oximeters are compatible. Wiring that is incompatible can generate considerable heat at the tip of the sensor, causing second- and third-degree burns under the sensors (Murphy, 1990). Pressure necrosis can also occur from sensors attached too tightly. Therefore inspect the skin under the sensor frequently.

Applying the sensor correctly is essential for accurate SaO_2 measurements. Since the sensor must identify every pulse beat to calculate the SaO_2, movement can interfere with sensing. Some devices synchronize the oxygen satura-

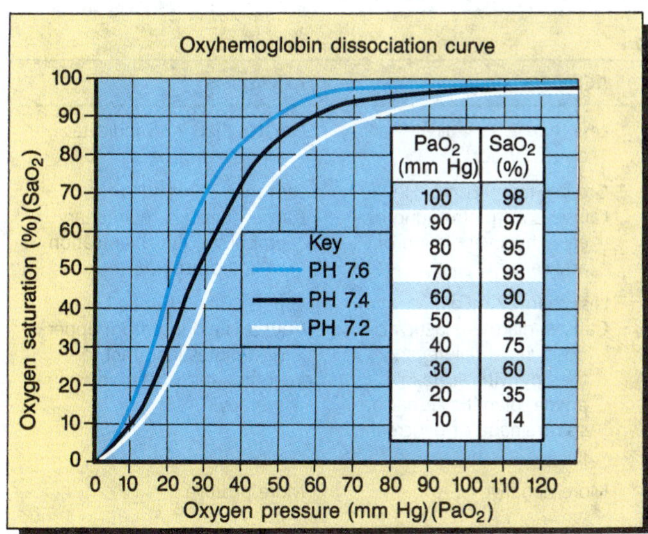

FIG. 31-10 Oxyhemoglobin dissociation curve. Changes in the affinity of hemoglobin for oxygen shift the position of the oxyhemoglobin dissociation curve. ***Standard curve*** (black): Assumes normal pH (7.4), temperature, PCO_2, and 2,3-DPG levels. ***Shift to left*** (blue): Increases O_2 affinity of Hb: increased pH; decreased temperature, PCO_2, and 2,3-DPG. ***Shift to right*** (white): Decreases O_2 affinity of Hb: decreased pH; increased temperature, PCO_2, and 2,3-DPG

tion reading with the heartbeat, thereby reducing the interference caused by motion. Sensors are not placed on extremities used for blood pressure monitoring or with indwelling arterial catheters, since pulsatile blood flow can be affected. It is recommended that the probe site be changed at least every 4 to 8 hours in preterm infants.

➤ **NURSING TIP** ***For the infant:*** Tape the sensor securely to the great toe and tape the wire to the sole of the foot (or use a commercial holder that fastens with a self-adhering closure). Place a snugly fitting sock over the foot. ***For the child:*** Tape the sensor securely to the index finger and tape the wire to the back of the hand. Use self-adhering Ace-type wrap (e.g., Coban) around the finger and/or hand to further secure the sensor and wire.

Ambient light from ceiling lights and phototherapy, as well as high-intensity heat and light from radiant warmers, can interfere with readings. Therefore the sensor should be covered to block these light sources. Intravenous dyes; green, purple, or black nail polish; nonopaque synthetic nails; and possibly ink used for footprinting can also cause inaccurate SaO_2 measurements. The dyes should be removed or, in the case of porcelain nails, a different area used for the sensor. Skin color, thickness, and edema do not affect the readings. Elevated levels of dyshemoglobins (carboxyhemoglobin, methemoglobin, and fetal hemoglobin) affect the accuracy of the device because it is able to distinguish only between two types of functional hemoglobins (Blumer, 1991).

Arterial blood gas (ABG) sampling may be performed on blood from an artery or a capillary. Some controversy surrounds the collection of "arterialized" capillary blood for blood gas measurements; however, many believe it to be a safe, convenient, and relatively accurate method. The blood samples are obtained by taking a deep heel stick after dilation of the vascular bed by warming (see Fig. 27-17). The first drop of blood is discarded, and subsequent blood is collected directly into heparinized capillary tubes held in a horizontal position. The tube is delivered to the laboratory as soon as possible.

ABG samples may also be obtained through an indwelling catheter (e.g., arterial line, multilumen catheter, or Swan-Ganz catheter), or by arteriopuncture. The artery most frequently used is the radial artery, since there are no nearby veins. The temporal, posterior tibial, and umbilical arteries can be used effectively in the newborn. The femoral and brachial arteries may also be used. The radial and posterior tibial arteries are the first choice for intermittent arterial blood sampling because of the collateral circulation present. Adequacy of collateral circulation is determined by the ***Allen test,*** which should be performed before arterial puncture is attempted. To perform the test, the extremity distal to the puncture site is elevated and blanched by squeezing gently (such as making a fist). The two arteries supplying blood flow to the extremity (such as the radial and ulnar arteries in the wrist) are then occluded. The extremity is lowered, and pressure is removed from *one* artery (such as the ulnar). Color return to the blanched extremity in less than 5 seconds indicates collateral circulation.

NURSING ALERT Nurses should perform the Allen test as a precautionary measure regardless of whether or not they perform the arterial puncture.

Normal ABG values are much the same for all ages and depend on the concentration of O_2 the child is breathing. The arterial PO_2 should rise in proportion to the O_2 concentration being inhaled. Therefore when ABG values are evaluated, the following are considered: the percentage of O_2 administered (if any); the child's body temperature (as little as 1° F can alter the blood gas values 5% to 8%); and the presence of anxiety (if children hyperventilate, CO_2 is exhaled) or crying (can cause breath-holding and apnea, resulting in decreased PaO_2).

Unclotted whole or capillary blood is required; therefore a heparinized syringe or capillary tube is used to draw blood samples. No air bubbles should enter either vessel to alter the blood gas concentration. Many institutions use prepackaged ABG sampling kits. These kits allow air-free samples to be drawn without the need for heparin dilutions. The amount collected depends on the child's size. Depending on the laboratory facilities, as little as 0.1 ml may be sufficient in small infants. Table 31-4 lists normal ABG and pH measurements on room air at sea level.

The significance of ABG determination is related primarily to the relationships among these three parameters: pH, PO_2, and PCO_2. Much of this is discussed in relation to acid-base imbalance in Chapter 28. Sometimes a specified schedule of testing is ordered; at other times the sample is to be drawn as indicated by clinical observations. Any change in a blood gas value must be compared with the other values and with previous readings, as well as with the child's clinical appearance and behavior, medical history, and associ-

TABLE 31-4 Blood Gas Analysis

COMPONENT	DEFINITION	NORMAL VALUE	ACIDOSIS	ALKALOSIS
pH	Indicates acid-base status of body	7.35-7.45	Less than 7.35 indicates an excess of acid	Greater than 7.45 indicates an excess of base
Pco_2	Pressure exerted by dissolved CO_2 in blood Under control of lungs Respiratory component	35-45 mm Hg	Greater than 45 mm Hg Causes: obstructive lung disease, hypoventilation of any cause	Less than 35 mm Hg Causes: hypoxia, pulmonary embolism, hyperventilation of any cause
HCO_3	Buffers effect of acid in blood Under control of kidneys Metabolic component	22-26 mEq/L	Less than 22 mEq/L Causes: diarrhea, lactic acidosis, renal failure, shock, therapy with acetazolamide, diabetic ketoacidosis, drainage of pancreatic juice	Greater than 26 mEq/L Causes: fluid loss from upper gastrointestinal tract, diuretics, corticosteroid therapy
Base excess (BE)	Reflects status of all bases in blood	± 2	More negative	More positive
Po_2	Pressure exerted by dissolved O_2 in blood Indicates effectiveness of oxygenation by lungs	80-100 mm Hg	Less than 80 mm Hg: hypoxia Causes: obstructive lung disease, high CO_2 levels, low Fio_2, hypoventilation	Greater than 100 mm Hg: hyperoxygenation Causes: high Fio_2, hyperventilation

Modified from Johns Hopkins Hospital: *The Harriet Lane handbook,* edited by Johnson KB, ed 13, St Louis, 1993, Mosby.
NOTE: The Sao_2 printed with blood gas reports cannot be used as a standard to confirm oximetry readings. Blood gas analyzers provide only approximate blood O_2 saturations based on calculations using measured blood gases, pH, and Pao_2.

ated physiologic factors. Other factors that influence blood gas levels include the amount and method of O_2 administration, the assessment of the child, and the nature of the respiratory disorder.

Signs that indicate the need for blood examination include a change in color (e.g., mottling, pallor, cyanosis, or duskiness), depth or rate of respirations (e.g., shallow and rapid), behavior or sensorium, and sometimes other vital signs. The nurse may or may not be able to obtain the blood sample by arteriopuncture, depending on the institution's policies. Nurses are usually able to withdraw the sample from an arterial catheter, and they should become skilled in the techniques of drawing blood and flushing the line. No matter who obtains the sample, the nurse is responsible for its speedy transport for analysis.

The results of the gas analysis provide the nurse with information on which to base further nursing action. Nurses must be able to understand the report's significance to implement nursing interventions (e.g., changing the position, performing suction, administering prescribed drugs, or notifying the attending physician) according to the interpretation of the gas analysis. Because of the increased use of continuous noninvasive monitoring, painful arterial punctures can be minimized.

RESPIRATORY THERAPY

OXYGEN THERAPY

The indication for administration of O_2 is ***hypoxemia*** (reduced blood oxygenation). O_2 is administered by mask, hood, nasal cannula, face tent, O_2 tent, or ventilator (Table 31-5). The mode of delivery is selected on the basis of the concentration needed and the child's ability to cooperate in its use. The concentration of O_2 delivered should be regulated according to the individual child's needs. There are hazards related to its use; therefore O_2 should not be continued after the indication for its use is no longer present. Since medical-grade O_2 from piped systems or tanks is anhydrous, humidification of the gas before administration to the patient is usually indicated.

O_2 therapy is primarily carried out in the hospital, although increasing numbers of children are receiving O_2 in the home. It is the responsibility of the nurse or respiratory care practitioner to ensure uninterrupted delivery of the appropriate O_2 concentration and monitoring of the child's response to the therapy.

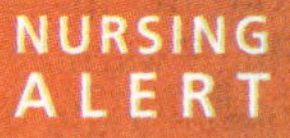

Oxygen is a drug and is prescribed by dose.

Oxygen Administration

O_2 delivered to infants is best tolerated by ***plastic hood*** (Fig. 31-11). Low and high concentrations of O_2 can be easily maintained in this head hood, and most nursing procedures can be continued without interrupting the O_2 delivery. This is not possible when delivering O_2 directly into the incubator. At least 4 to 5 L/min of flow is needed to maintain O_2 concentrations and remove the exhaled CO_2.

The humidified O_2 is not allowed to blow directly into the face of an infant in a hood. Cold fluid or air applied to the face stimulates receptors that trigger the diving reflex, which causes bradycardia and shunting of blood from peripheral to central circulation. The O_2 hood should not rub

TABLE 31-5 Advantages and Disadvantages of Various Oxygen-Delivery Systems

SYSTEM	ADVANTAGES	DISADVANTAGES
Oxygen masks	Various sizes available Ability to provide a predictable concentration of oxygen (with Venturi mask) whether child breathes through nose or mouth.	Skin irritation Fear of suffocation Accumulation of moisture on face Possibility of aspiration of vomitus Difficulty in controlling O_2 concentrations
Nasal cannula	Provision of constant oxygen flow even while child eats and talks Possibility of more complete observation of child because nose and mouth remain unobstructed	Discomfort for the child Possibility of causing abdominal distention and discomfort or vomiting Difficulty of controlling O_2 concentrations if child breathes through mouth Inability to provide mist if desired
Oxygen tent	Achievement of lower O_2 concentrations (FiO_2 of 0.3-0.5) Child receives increased inspired O_2 concentration even while eating.	Necessity for right fit around bed to prevent leakage of gas Cool and wet tent environment Poor access to patient—inspired O_2 levels will fall whenever tent is entered
Oxygen hood, face tent	Achievement of high O_2 concentrations (FiO_2 up to 1.00) Free access to patient's chest for assessment	High humidity environment Need to remove patient for feeding and care

Modified from Hazinski MF, editor: *Nursing care of the critically ill child,* ed 2, St Louis, 1992, Mosby.

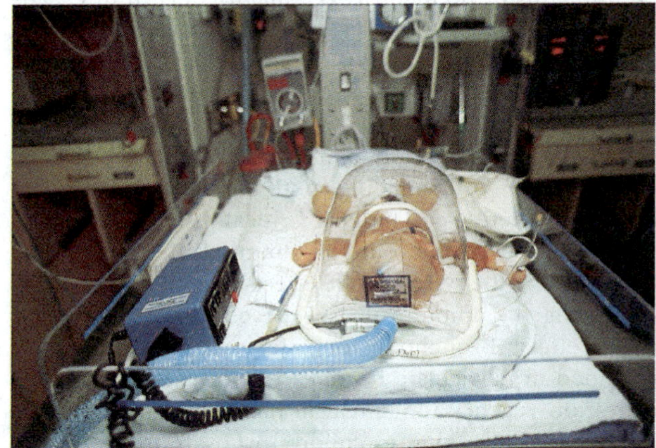

FIG. 31-11 Oxygen administered to infant by means of a plastic hood. Note oxygen analyzer (blue machine).

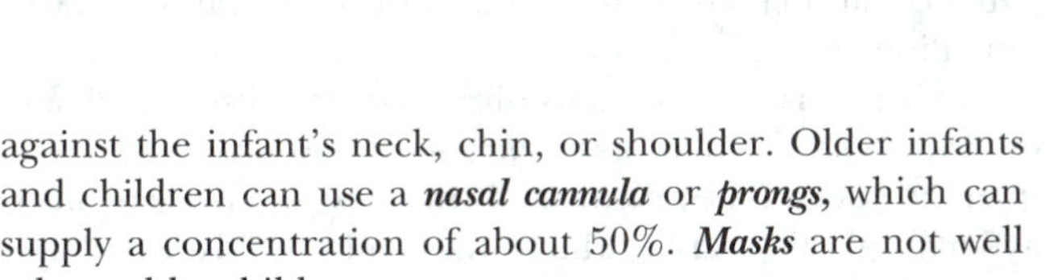

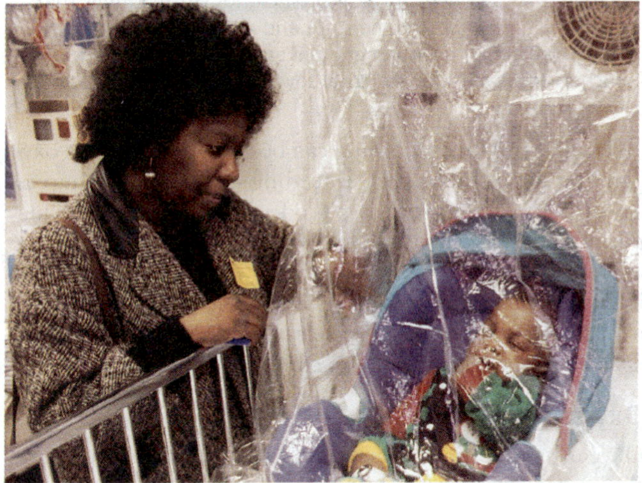

FIG. 31-12 The tent provides a comfortable method for oxygen administration.

against the infant's neck, chin, or shoulder. Older infants and children can use a ***nasal cannula*** or ***prongs,*** which can supply a concentration of about 50%. ***Masks*** are not well tolerated by children.

For most children beyond early infancy, the ***oxygen tent*** is the most satisfactory means for O_2 administration (Fig. 31-12). A tent does not require any device to come into direct contact with the face, but the concentration of O_2 within the tent is difficult to control and to maintain above 30% to 50%. The comfort to the child makes it the method of choice except in cases of marked respiratory distress. A major difficulty with the use of the tent is keeping the tent closed so that O_2 concentration is maintained.

To reduce O_2 loss, nursing care is planned carefully so that the tent is opened as little as possible. Since O_2 is heavier than air, loss will be greater at the bottom of the tent; therefore the tent is tucked in snugly without open edges. The bottom of the tent should be examined more often when the child is restless and fussy and liable to pull the covers loose. Some tents are even open at the top. Because of the rapid diffusing qualities of CO_2, the levels of the gas do not build up within these enclosures.

After the tent has been opened for an extended period of time, it is flushed with O_2 by increasing the flow meter for a few minutes to quickly raise the O_2 and mist concentration. The flow meter is then reset to the prescribed number of liters.

The enclosed tent becomes very warm; therefore some

type of cooling mechanism is provided. Although the cool environment can reduce fever and airway inflammation, it can also produce hypothermia and cold stress. Since O_2 is drying to the tissues, the gas is humidified, which causes moisture to condense on the tent walls.

NURSING ALERT Keep the child warm and dry by checking the temperature inside the tent and the child's bedding and clothing frequently. Adjust the temperature and change clothing as often as needed.

The reactions of children to the oxygen tent are variable. Some, especially older children, feel comfortable in the tent and like the cozy, close privacy it affords. Others, more often younger children, may be frightened by the forced enclosure. The plastic walls distort their view of the world and constitute a barrier between them and their source of comfort, their parent. Their distress can be minimized if they are able to see someone nearby and are reassured that they will not be left alone. A favorite toy or object can accompany the child inside the tent. Other familiar items can be placed at the foot of the bed or otherwise in view.

NURSING ALERT Inspect all toys for safety and suitability (e.g., vinyl or plastic—not stuffed items that absorb moisture and are difficult to keep dry). The high O_2 environment makes any source of sparks (such as mechanical or electrical toys) a potential fire hazard.

In most instances the child can be removed from the oxygen tent for activities such as feeding and bathing, whereas in other cases the child is placed in the tent only during periods of rest. Still other children may require O_2 continuously and can be removed from the tent or incubator only if an oxygen source is held close to the child's face. Any change in color, increased respiratory effort, or restlessness is an indication to return the child to the oxygen tent.

Oxygen Toxicity

Oxygen is essential to life and a valuable therapeutic aid. Prolonged exposure to high O_2 tensions, however, can be damaging to lung tissue. Although the exact pathogenesis of the pulmonary changes is unclear, evidence indicates damage to lung capillaries, which causes diffuse microhemorrhagic changes, diminished mucus flow, inactivation of surfactant, and altered ciliary function. The total effect appears to be the direct result of "lung burn" and is therefore a result of the PAO_2 and not the PaO_2. The result of these changes is a gradual impairment of alveolar ventilation.

Atelectasis may occur as a result of the "washing out" of nitrogen from the alveoli by the high concentrations of O_2. This is more likely to occur in persons with low tidal volume and retention of mucus or other secretions.

Oxygen-induced CO_2 narcosis is a physiologic hazard of O_2 therapy that may occur in persons with chronic pulmonary disease. It is seldom encountered in children except those with cystic fibrosis. These children have chronic alveolar hypoventilation with a concomitant chronic CO_2 retention and hypoxemia. In these patients the respiratory center has adapted to the continuously higher $PaCO_2$ levels, and therefore hypoxia becomes the more powerful stimulus to respiration. When the PaO_2 is elevated during O_2 administration, the hypoxic drive is removed, causing progressive hypoventilation and increased $PaCO_2$ levels, and the child rapidly becomes unconscious. CO_2 narcosis can also be induced by the administration of sedation in these patients.

Other suspected toxic effects of O_2 include changes in the renal tubules, sympathoadrenal medullary stimulation precipitating neurogenic seizures, and an increased rate of destruction of red blood cells. In preterm infants the risk of retinopathy of prematurity is a major concern in O_2 administration (see Chapter 10).

AEROSOL THERAPY

Continuous administration of mist, or aerosolized water, for the treatment of inflammatory conditions of the airways has no proven benefit (see Thinking Critically About . . . box). Using the airway as the route of administration can be useful in avoiding the systemic side effects of certain drugs and in reducing the amount of drug necessary to achieve the desired effect. Bronchodilators, steroids, and antibiotics, suspended in particulate form, can be inhaled so that the medication reaches the small airways. Aerosol therapy is particularly challenging in children who are too young to cooperate in controlling the rate and depth of breathing. Administration of medications by this route requires skill, patience, and creativity on the part of the respiratory care practitioner.

Medications can be aerosolized or nebulized with air or with O_2-enriched gas. ***Hand-held nebulizers*** are frequently used. The medicated mist is discharged into a small plastic mask, which the child holds over the

THINKING CRITICALLY ABOUT . . . *Mist Therapy*

Continuous administration of mist, or aerosolized water, for the treatment of inflammatory conditions of the airways is a common practice that has no proven benefit (Alderson and Warren, 1984), although clinical improvement has been noted in some cases (e.g., the use of a mist tent or a very humid environment, such as a steamy bathroom, for the treatment of croup). For other pathologic conditions, however, mist therapy can be detrimental. For example, bronchoconstriction in children with asthma can be exacerbated by mist therapy.

The notion that inhaled mist can influence the viscosity of mucus in dehydrated children is erroneous; inhaled mist does not affect the water content of expectorated mucus. If dehydration is evident, oral or parenteral rehydration will normalize the water content of respiratory mucus.

nose and mouth. To avoid particle deposition in the nose and pharynx, the child is instructed to take slow, deep breaths through an open mouth during treatment. For home use, an air compressor is necessary to force air through the liquid medication to form the aerosol. Relatively compact, portable units can be rented from health equipment companies.

The ***metered dose inhaler (MDI)*** is a self-contained, hand-held device that allows for intermittent delivery of a specified amount of medication. Many bronchodilators are available in this form and are used successfully by children with asthma (see Chapter 32). For children less than 5 or 6 years of age, a ***spacer device*** attached to the MDI can help coordinate breathing and aerosol delivery and allows the aerosolized particles to remain in suspension for a longer time.

A major nursing responsibility during aerosol therapy is to assess the effectiveness of the treatment and the patient's tolerance of the procedure. Assessment of breath sounds and work of breathing should be performed before and after treatments. Young children who become upset with a mask held close to the face may become fatigued from fighting the procedure and may appear worse during and immediately after the therapy. Careful assessment is needed by the nurse and practitioner to determine if the treatment is of value. It may be necessary to spend a few minutes calming the child after the therapy, allowing vital signs to return to baseline levels, in order to accurately assess changes in breath sound and work of breathing.

BRONCHIAL (POSTURAL) DRAINAGE

Bronchial drainage is indicated whenever excessive fluid or mucus in the bronchi is not being removed by normal ciliary activity and cough. Positioning the child to take maximum advantage of gravity facilitates removal of secretions. The effect is sometimes dramatic in children with chronic lung disease characterized by thick mucus secretions, such as asthma and cystic fibrosis.

Postural drainage is carried out three to four times daily and is more effective when it follows other respiratory therapy, such as bronchodilator and/or nebulization medication. Bronchial drainage is generally performed before meals (or 1 to 1½ hours after meals) to minimize the chance of vomiting and is repeated at bedtime. The length and duration of treatment depend on the child's condition and tolerance level—usually 20 to 30 minutes. There are positions to facilitate drainage from all major lung segments (Fig. 31-13), but all positions are not used at each session. Children will usually cooperate for four to six positions, but more than six tend to exceed their limits of tolerance. Older children can be expected to tolerate longer periods.

In the hospital an older child can be positioned over an elevated knee rest. Small children and infants can be positioned with pillows or on the therapist's lap and legs (Fig. 31-14). Infants should not be placed in the Trendelenburg position, because they do not have an autonomic regulation of blood flow to the head. Special modifications of the techniques are required in children whose conditions contraindicate the standard positioning, such as head injuries, some types of surgical incisions or burns, and casts or traction. At home small children can be positioned on a padded ironing board.* Children who require postural drainage over months or years may benefit from specially constructed tables padded and adjusted to their individual needs. The position used and the frequency and duration of treatment are individualized.

CHEST PHYSIOTHERAPY (CPT)

CPT usually refers to the use of postural drainage in combination with adjunctive techniques that are thought to enhance the clearance of mucus from the airway. These techniques include manual percussion, vibration, and squeezing of the chest; cough; forceful expiration; and breathing exercises. However, the efficacies of techniques, both individually and combined, are controversial (Kyff, 1987). Postural drainage in combination with forced expiration has been shown to be beneficial, but the benefit of other techniques has yet to be demonstrated.

The most common technique used in association with postural drainage is manual ***percussion*** of the chest wall. Nurses are often responsible for this maneuver if respiratory care coverage is not available; therefore they should become skilled in the technique. The patient is dressed in a light shirt and placed in a postural drainage position. The practitioner then gently but firmly strikes the chest wall with a cupped hand (Fig. 31-15, *A*). A "popping," hollow sound should be the result, not a slapping sound. Percussion should be done over the rib cage only and should be painless. Percussion can be performed with a soft circular mask (adapted to maintain air trapping) or a percussion cup marketed especially for the purpose of aiding the loosening of secretions (Fig. 31-15, *B*).

Vibration can be used to help move secretions cephalad during exhalations. Hand-held vibrators should be approved for use in an O_2-enriched environment (tent, head hood). Larger children may benefit from a more powerful vibrator. This therapy is subject to patient tolerance, and oximetry is an excellent monitoring tool for therapy tolerance.

Chest physiotherapy is contraindicated when patients have pulmonary hemorrhage, pulmonary embolism, end-stage renal disease, increased intracranial pressure, osteogenesis imperfecta, or minimum cardiac reserves. Chest physiotherapy is a time-consuming procedure and is effective for only certain patients. After an exhaustive review of the literature, Sutton (1988) has offered guidelines for performing chest physiotherapy (see Guidelines box, p. 1352).

Squeezing is sometimes a useful maneuver while the child is in the drainage position. The child is directed to take a deep breath and then exhale through the mouth rapidly and as completely as possible. The depth of the expiratory effort is increased by brief, firm pressure from the practitioner's hands compressing the sides of the chest. This decreases the volume of the tracheobronchial tree and fa-

*Home care instructions are available in *Wong and Whaley's Clinical Manual of Pediatric Nursing* (Mosby).

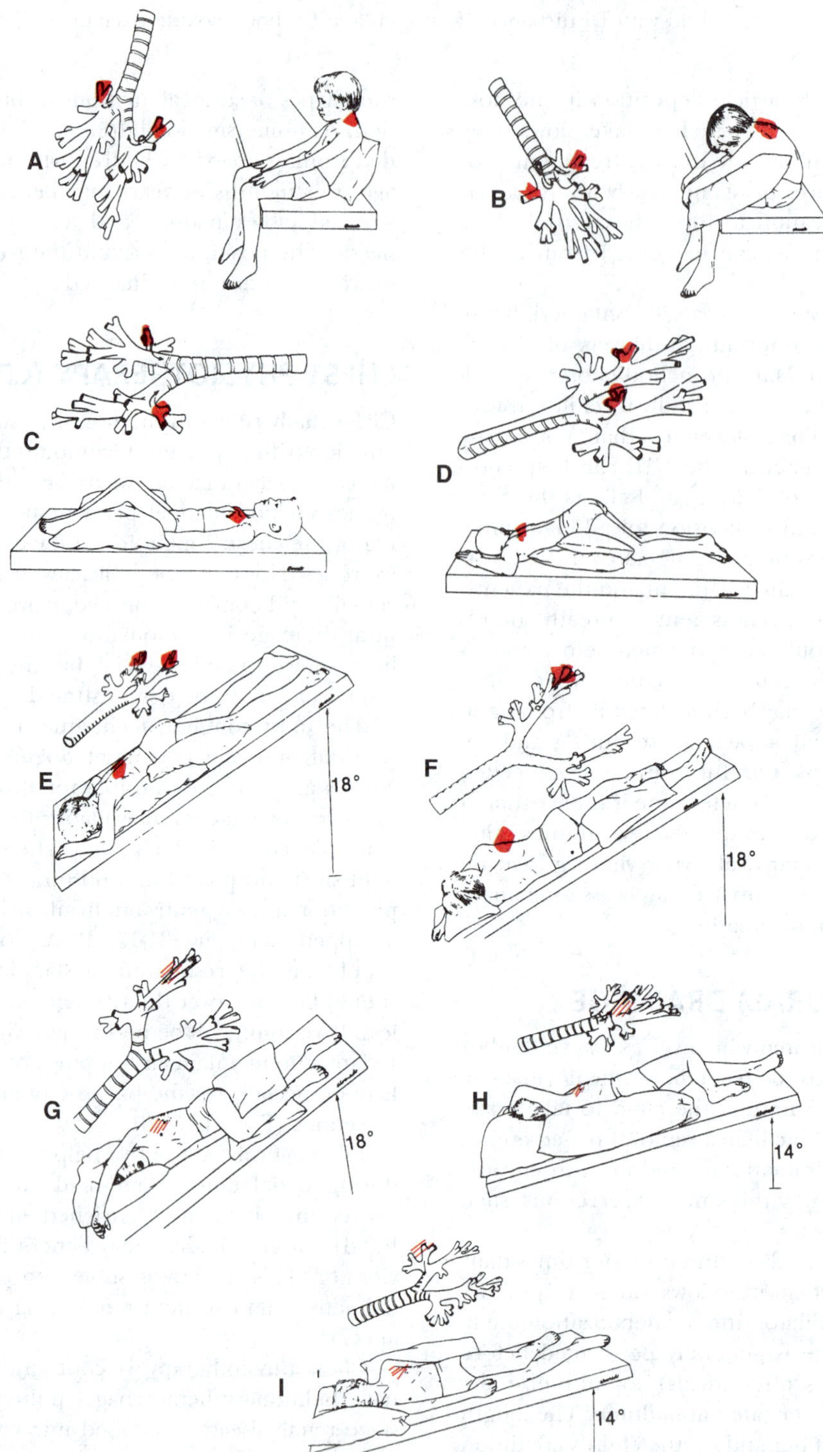

FIG. 31-13 Bronchial drainage positions for all major lung segments of child. For each position, model of tracheobronchial tree is projected beside child to show segmental bronchus *(striped)* being drained and pathway *(arrow)* of secretions out of bronchus. Drainage platform is horizontal unless otherwise noted. Striped area on child's chest indicates area to be cupped or vibrated by therapist. **A,** Apical segment of right upper lobe and apical subsegment of apical-posterior segment of left upper lobe. **B,** Posterior segment of right upper lobe and posterior subsegment of apical-posterior segment of left upper lobe. **C,** Anterior segments of both upper lobes; child should be rotated slightly away from side being drained. **D,** Superior segments of both lower lobes. **E,** Posterior basal segments of both lower lobes. **F,** Lateral basal segments of right lower lobe; left lateral basal segment would be drained by mirror image of this position (right side down). **G,** Anterior basal segment of left lower lobe; right anterior basal segment would be drained by mirror image of this position (left side down). **H,** Medial and lateral segments of right middle lobe. **I,** Lingular segments (superior and inferior) of left upper lobe (homologue of right middle lobe).
(From Chernick V, editor: *Kendig's disorders of the respiratory tract of children,* ed 5, Philadelphia, 1990, WB Saunders.)

cilitates the expression of secretions. The inspiration after the activity often stimulates a deep, productive cough (reinforced by the operator).

Deep breathing is often encouraged when the child is relaxed and in the desired position for drainage. The child is directed to take several deep breaths using diaphragmatic breathing. The use of deep breathing enlarges the tracheobronchial tree, enabling air to circulate around and through secretions that are not affected by usual tidal volumes. Expirations after these deep breaths often carry secretions and may stimulate a cough. Other methods that can be employed to stimulate deep breathing are use of blow bottles of various types and incentive spirometers, and incorporation of play that extends the expiratory time and increases expiratory pressure. For example, such play may include using items such as pinwheel toys, moving small items by blowing through a straw, blowing cotton balls or a Ping-Pong ball on a table, preventing a tissue from falling by blowing it against a wall, blowing up balloons (under supervision), singing loudly (especially songs with a lot of words between breaths), or blowing soap bubbles.

With or without stimulation, children are encouraged to

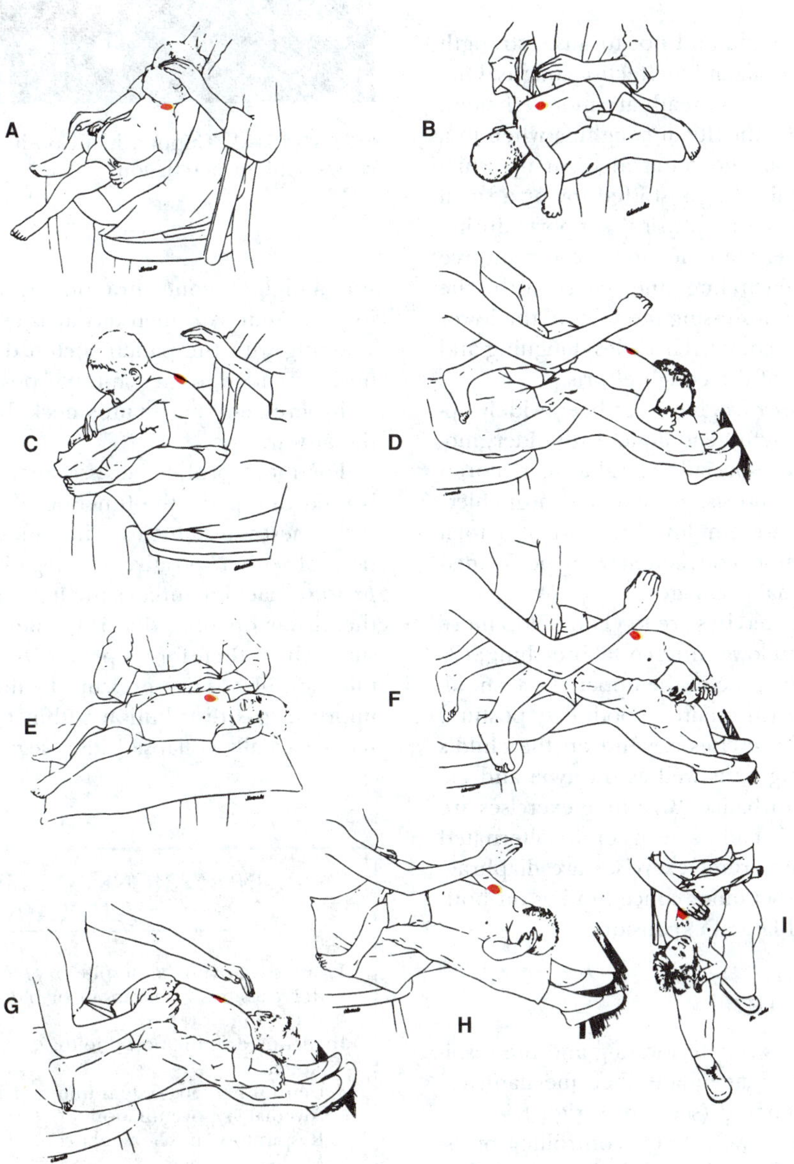

FIG. 31-14 Bronchial drainage positions for major segments of all lobes in infant. Procedure is most easily carried out in therapist's lap. Therapist's hand on chest indicates area to be cupped or vibrated. **A,** Apical segment of left upper lobe. **B,** Posterior segment of left upper lobe. **C,** Anterior segment of left upper lobe. **D,** Superior segment of right lower lobe. **E,** Posterior basal segment of right lower lobe. **F,** Lateral basal segment of right lower lobe. **G,** Anterior basal segment of right lower lobe. **H,** Medial and lateral segments of right middle lobe. **I,** Lingular segments (superior and inferior) of left upper lobe. (Modified from Cystic Fibrosis Foundation: *Infant segmental bronchial drainage,* Rockville, MD, The Foundation.)

GUIDELINES
Performing Chest Physiotherapy

Chest physiotherapy should be used for patients who have increased sputum production. It is probably of no value to the uncomplicated postoperative patient or the patient with pneumonia.
Forced expiration combined with postural drainage is more effective than cough alone.
Percussion and vibration have no proven value.
Appropriate use of bronchodilators before chest physiotherapy will enhance mucus clearance.

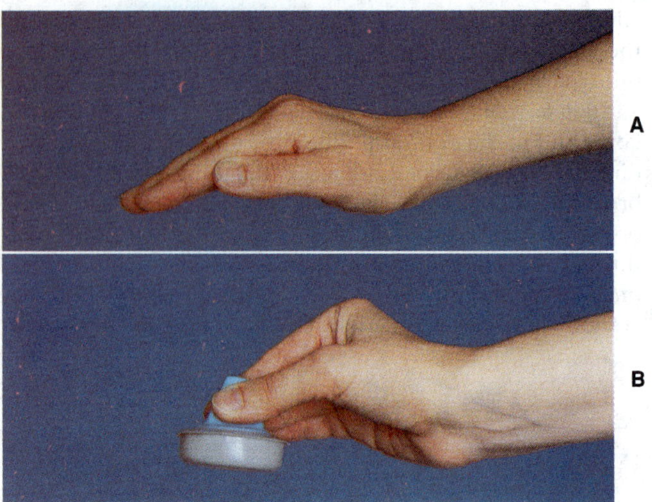

FIG. 31-15 **A,** Cupped hand position for percussion. **B,** Device for infant percussion.

cough, not to suppress a cough, and not to waste strength and energy with repeated weak and ineffective coughs. One or two hard coughs after a deep breath are more efficient. Since many children have difficulty in coughing when in a dependent position, they are encouraged to sit up while they cough. Having the child hug a stuffed toy or a small pillow offers comfort, as well as physical support, during coughing. As an alternative, the practitioner can reinforce the child's efforts by encircling the chest with the practitioner's hands and compressing the sides of the lower chest in synchrony with the cough. This is less fatiguing and increases the effectiveness of the cough efforts.

Breathing and ***postural exercises*** have not been widely applied to children but are useful techniques with older, motivated children. They are especially of value to children with kyphoscoliosis, cystic fibrosis, asthma, and bronchiectasis. Breathing exercises are employed as part of a total therapy program and are more convenient when performed in association with bronchial drainage.

The goals of breathing exercises are to (1) develop more effective diaphragmatic and lower intercostal breathing; (2) relax all muscles, especially those of the upper chest, shoulder girdle, and neck; and (3) attain a good, easy posture. The number and type of exercises depend on the child's age, motivation, and strength, as well as the type and extent of the physiologic disturbance. Breathing exercises are selected to meet the specific child's needs or are alternated in their use. The most important exercises are diaphragmatic breathing and side bending, concentrating on both abdominal expansion and lateral expansion.

ARTIFICIAL VENTILATION

If a child's respiratory status is deteriorating and the respiratory effort is excessive or inadequate, then mechanically assisted ventilation is considered (see box at right).

A variety of methods are available for controlling or assisting ventilation. Temporary assistance can be provided by a hand-operated self-inflating ventilation bag with a mask and a nonreturnable valve to prevent rebreathing, commonly referred to as a ***bag-valve-mask.*** With the mask placed on the nose and mouth, the bag is rhythmically compressed, forcing gas from the bag into the patient's airways. The self-inflating bag should also be the type with a reservoir so that a much greater percentage of O_2 can be delivered. To ensure a high O_2 concentration, O_2 should be delivered at 10 to 15 L/min. An open airway is established by correct positioning with the patient's chin directed forward and the neck extended to the "sniffing" position. It is important not to hyperextend an infant's neck, because this can occlude the airway.

For more prolonged assistance, mechanical ventilation is used to replace the function of the diaphragm and thoracic chest wall muscles. The lungs are inflated by application of either positive or negative pressure. A ***positive-pressure*** machine inflates the lungs by creating a pressure at the airway opening that is greater than intraalveolar pressure, which then forces pressurized gas into the lungs. Application of positive pressure by mechanical means usually improves gas distribution within the lung and often reinflates partially collapsed lung segments. The overall effect

INDICATIONS FOR MECHANICAL VENTILATION

Progressive hypoxia, despite oxygen therapy, measured by decreasing O_2 saturations or blood gas analysis (high $Pa{CO_2}$ and low pH)
Inadequate ventilation due to:
- Apnea
- Central nervous system injury or infection
- Alveolar hypoventilation
- Respiratory muscle weakness
- Medication toxicity
- Infectious pathology
- Foreign body obstruction

Excessive work of breathing, manifested by retractions, tachypnea, decreasing O_2 saturation, abnormal respiratory patterns
Inadequate respiratory effort
Hyperventilation due to increased intracranial pressure (ICP)

is improvement of gas exchange. ***Negative-pressure ventilators*** create a subatmospheric pressure around the chest wall and inside the chest, thus allowing air to move into the chest. This form of ventilation is occasionally used for patients with neuromuscular disease, such as Werdnig-Hoffmann.

Ventilators are usually classified according to the factors that regulate cycling. The method by which inspiration is terminated can be categorized as pressure cycled, volume cycled, or time cycled (see box below). Newer modes of ventilatory support include ***high-frequency ventilation,*** or ***"jet" ventilation,*** where O_2 is delivered under high pressure at a rapid cycling rate. Another type is ***extracorporeal membrane oxygenation (ECMO),*** which provides both pulmonary and cardiac support using external oxygenation technology. Ventilators are attached to the patient by endotracheal tube or tracheostomy.

NURSING ALERT Patients requiring mechanical ventilation should always have a self-inflating ventilation bag with a reservoir at the bedside. When the patient's condition or the ventilator's operation is in doubt, the ventilation bag is used.

Care of the Patient

The regulation and maintenance of mechanical ventilators are the responsibility of respiratory care practitioners. However, nurses should understand the function of the ventilator being used and be able to detect signs of malfunction and deviations from the desired settings. The nurse also promotes the effectiveness of ventilation by suctioning, positioning, ensuring that adequate humidification is in use, and providing support and reassurance to the child receiving mechanical ventilation and to the family. (See Chapter 10 for assisted and controlled ventilation in the neonate.)

NURSING ALERT The use of a mechanical ventilator does not guarantee that the child is actually being ventilated. Nursing assessment of ventilatory status, therefore, is essential.

TYPES OF VENTILATORS

Pressure-cycled ventilator—Terminates the respiratory cycle when a preset inspiratory pressure is reached. Volume will differ greatly, depending on the flow rate of the delivery of gas. The compliance of the lung will affect the tidal volume even though the pressure will remain constant.

Volume-cycled ventilator—Terminates respiration when a preset volume (tidal volume) is delivered. The compliance and resistance of the lung will change the pressure needed to deliver the preset volume.

Time-cycled ventilator—Terminates inspiration when a preset time is reached. Tidal volume is greatly affected by the compliance of the ventilator tubing, compliance and resistance of the lung, and flow rate of the delivered gas. The duration of the inspiratory pressure will be affected by the preset inspiratory time and the flow rate of the delivered gas.

Nursing assessment of the child requiring mechanical ventilation focuses on physical examination, vital signs, pulmonary status, oxygenation, and airway patency (e.g., obstruction or dislodgment), as well as laboratory analysis and pulse oximetry. Other important criteria to assess include nutritional status, intake and output (urinary output should be at least 2 ml/kg/hr for the younger child and 1 ml/kg/hr for the older child), and skin integrity (especially around the face and lips for the child with an endotracheal tube, and around the neck and stoma for the child with a tracheostomy).

Weaning the patient from a ventilator involves gradual physical and psychologic withdrawal from dependence on the mechanical device. Criteria for beginning the weaning process vary with the primary disease and the practitioner's preference.

The child who is to be extubated is allowed nothing by mouth to avoid the risk of aspiration. Steroids may be administered before the extubation to control laryngeal edema. Sedation or other respiratory depressants are contraindicated so that the child can be observed for respiratory activity. The child is placed on a cardiac and apnea monitor if one is not already attached. Resuscitation and reintubation equipment is available at the bedside. Chest physiotherapy and suctioning are ordinarily performed just before tube removal, and cool mist is begun immediately after extubation. The child is monitored for respiratory distress, and ABG measurements are observed. The most common complications are airway edema, fatigue, and atelectasis. Airway edema often responds to nebulized racemic epinephrine, which can be given several times to prevent reintubation.

Endotracheal Airways

An artificial airway is usually used in association with artificial ventilation and in children with upper airway obstruction (see box on p. 1354). Endotracheal (ET) intubation can be accomplished by the ***nasal (nasotracheal), oral (orotracheal),*** or ***direct tracheal (tracheostomy)*** routes. Oral intubation is usually the method of choice for emergency situations, but for prolonged intubation a nasotracheal tube is used. Nasotracheal intubation facilitates oral hygiene and provides more stable fixation, which reduces the complication of tracheal erosion and the danger of accidental extubation.

➤ **NURSING TIP** The size of an ET tube can be determined in three ways:

Using patient length and the Broselow resuscitation tape*

$$\text{ET tube size} = \frac{\text{Age (years)}}{4} + 4$$

"Pinky" rule: the diameter of a child's pinky is approximately the size of the trachea.

Although newborn infants have been successfully maintained on ET tubes for longer periods, in older children who require intubation for an extended period of time, tracheostomy is usually considered. The decision to change

*Vital Signs, 20 Campus Rd., Totowa, NJ 07512; (800) 932-0760.

INDICATIONS FOR POSSIBLE INTUBATION

Airway obstruction
Respiratory arrest
Neuromuscular compromise or paralysis
Inadequate ventilation
Hypoxemia despite supplemental O_2
Pulmonary toilet
Respiratory acidosis

from an ET tube to a tracheostomy is made on an individual basis. The tracheostomy allows the child to speak (by temporarily occluding the opening with a clean fingertip or with a special device) and eat and also facilitates clearing of secretions. Suctioning an ET tube is carried out with the same care as suctioning a tracheostomy.

Complications. The most severe complication related to immediate intubation is hypoxia with accompanying bradycardia. Patients must be closely monitored during intubation attempts, and if hypoxia occurs, the procedure is discontinued until vital signs are stable. Ventilation with bag-valve-mask and O_2 is reinstituted. Other complications include trauma to the mouth and teeth, epistaxis, creation of air leaks, and vagal-mediated changes in vital signs. The most common sequela of intubation is a sore throat, which disappears within 48 to 72 hours without therapy, although a humidified atmosphere is beneficial. Other complications include traumatic laryngitis, infection, glottic edema, and mucosal lesions of the larynx secondary to pressure exerted by the rigid ET tube. The most severe sequela of intubation is laryngeal stenosis secondary to fibrosis.

TRACHEOSTOMY

Tracheostomy consists of a surgical opening in the trachea between the second and fourth tracheal rings (Fig. 31-16). The procedure is performed in infants and children for a variety of reasons. Congenital or acquired structural defects, such as subglottic stenosis, tracheomalacia, and vocal cord paralysis, account for most tracheostomies in this age-group and require a long-term tracheostomy. A tracheostomy may be performed in an emergency situation for epiglottitis, croup, or foreign body aspiration. These tracheostomies are placed for a short term until the infection is clear. An infant or child requiring long-term ventilatory support may also have a tracheostomy.

Pediatric tracheostomy tubes are usually made of plastic or Silastic (Fig. 31-17), the most common being Hollinger, Jackson, Aberdeen, and Shiley tubes. These tubes are constructed with a more acute angle than adult tubes, and they soften at body temperature, conforming to the contours of the trachea. Since these materials resist the formation of crusted respiratory secretions, they are made without an inner cannula. Some children require a metal tracheostomy tube (usually made of sterling silver or stainless steel), which contains an inner cannula. The principal advantage of metal tubes is their nonreactivity and decreased chance for an allergic reaction.

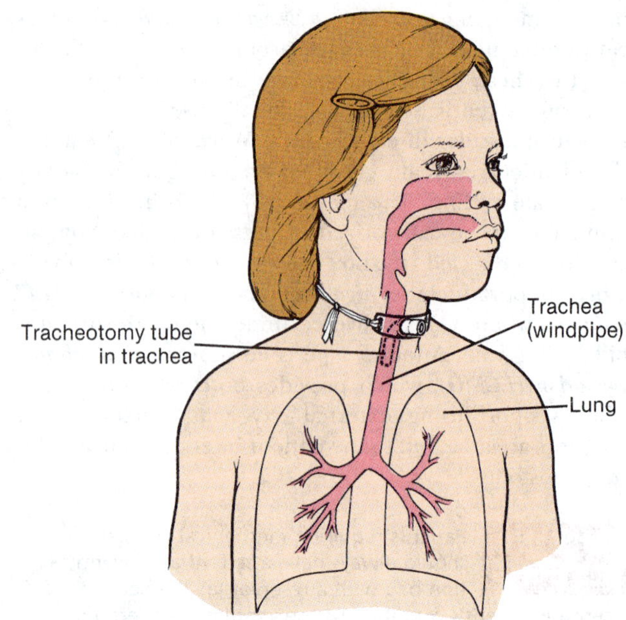

FIG. 31-16 Tracheostomy tube in trachea and securely tied with cloth tape.

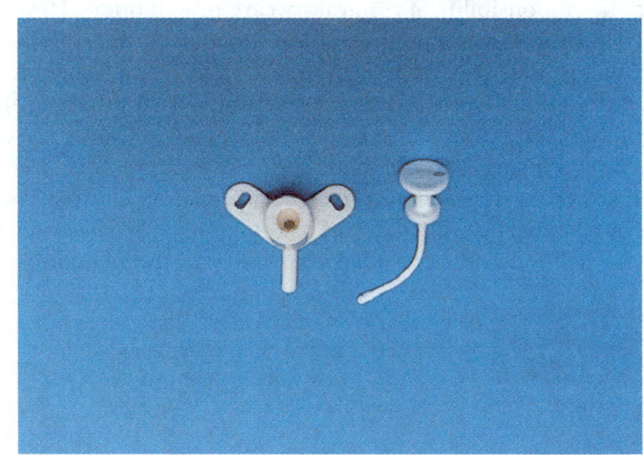

FIG. 31-17 Silastic pediatric tracheostomy tube and obturator.

Tracheostomy Care

Before the tracheostomy is performed, it is important to prepare the child and family. Preoperative teaching should include the child (if age appropriate), family, and other primary caregivers and should address the child's appearance with a tracheostomy in place, the communication method to be used following the procedure, and postoperative procedures. Medical play, allowing a hands-on experience with tracheostomy supplies, should be encouraged, as well as a tour of the pediatric intensive care unit to assist in decreasing anxiety.

The child returns from the operating room with the tracheostomy tube in place and long sutures (stay sutures) taped to the chest. These sutures are attached to the tra-

THINKING CRITICALLY ABOUT . . . *Suctioning and Catheter Length*

Traditional technique for suctioning endotracheal (ET) or tracheostomy tubes recommends advancing a suction catheter into the tube until it meets resistance, then withdrawing it slightly and applying suction. However, studies indicate that this approach causes trauma to the tracheobronchial wall. This trauma can be avoided by inserting the catheter and advancing it to the premeasured depth of just to the tip (especially in infants) or no more than 0.5 cm beyond the tube (Kleiber, Krutzfield, and Rose, 1988).

Calibrated catheters are easier to use for premeasured suctioning technique, but unmarked catheters can also be used. To measure the length for catheter insertion, place the catheter near a sample ET or tracheostomy tube (same size as child's tube) with the end of the catheter at the correct position. Grasp the catheter with a sterile-gloved hand to mark the length and insert the catheter until the hand reaches the stoma.

cheal rings and can be used to hold the tracheostomy stoma open in the event of accidental decannulation. In approximately 5 days a tract is formed in the trachea, subcutaneous tissue, and skin, at which time the stay sutures are no longer required. The nurse should tell the child that removal of the stay sutures is not painful.

Children who have undergone a tracheostomy require a 7- to 10-day hospital stay. During this time the child is closely monitored for the development of complications such as hemorrhage, edema, aspiration, and the entrance of free air into the pleural cavity. The focus of postoperative nursing care is maintaining a patent airway, facilitating the removal of pulmonary secretions, providing humidified air or O_2, cleansing the stoma, monitoring the child's ability to swallow, and teaching while simultaneously preventing complications (the most dangerous being related to accidental decannulation and tube obstruction).

Since the child may be unable to signal for help, direct observation and use of respiratory and cardiac monitors is essential. Respiratory assessments (including breath sounds and work of breathing, vital signs, tightness of the tracheostomy ties, and the type and amount of secretions) are performed every 15 minutes until the patient is stable and then every 1 to 2 hours for the first 24 hours. Assessments thereafter are every 2 to 4 hours or more frequently if needed. Some bleeding from the surgical site can be expected, but profuse bleeding is unusual and the practitioner should be notified immediately if this occurs. Copious amounts of bloody secretions are also uncommon and should be considered a sign of hemorrhage.

The child is positioned with the head of the bed raised, or in the position most comfortable to the child, with the call light easily available. Suction catheters, suction source, gloves, sterile saline, sterile gauze for wiping away secretions, scissors, an extra tracheostomy tube of the same size with ties already attached, another tracheostomy tube one size smaller, and the obturator are kept at the bedside. A source of humidification is provided, since the normal humidification and filtering functions of the airway have been bypassed. Intravenous fluids ensure adequate hydration until the child is able to swallow sufficient amounts of fluids.

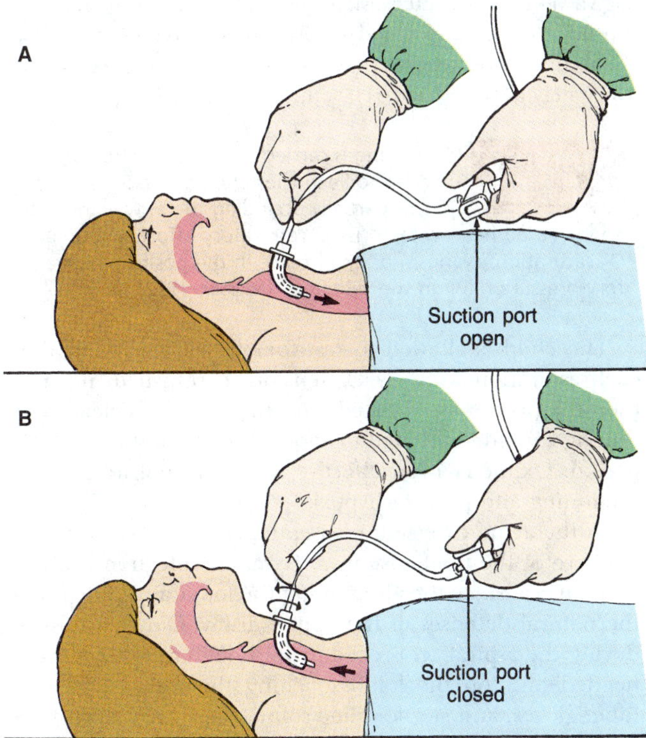

FIG. 31-18 Tracheostomy suctioning. **A,** Insertion, port open. **B,** Withdrawal, port occluded. Note that catheter is inserted just slightly beyond end of tracheostomy tube.

Suctioning. The airway must remain patent and requires frequent suctioning during the first few hours after a tracheostomy to remove mucous plugs and excessive secretions. Proper vacuum pressure and suction catheter size are important to prevent atelectasis and decrease hypoxia from the suctioning procedure. Vacuum pressure should range from 80 to 100 mm Hg. Unless secretions are thick and tenacious, the lower range of negative pressure is recommended. Tracheal suction catheters are available in a variety of sizes. The catheter selected should have a diameter one half the diameter of the tracheostomy tube. If the catheter is too large, it can block the airway. The catheter is constructed with a side port so that the catheter is introduced without suction and removed while simultaneous intermittent suction is applied by covering the port with the thumb (Fig. 31-18). The catheter is inserted to 0.5 cm beyond or just to the end of the tracheostomy tube (see Thinking Critically About . . . box).

A small amount of sterile isotonic saline (a few drops to 0.5 to 2 ml, depending on the child's size) injected into the tube may help loosen secretions and crusts for easier aspiration, although the value of this practice is unproved. Only sterile saline without preservatives can be used.

NURSING ALERT Suctioning should require no more than 5 seconds (American Heart Association, 1994).

Counting 1—one thousand, 2—one thousand, 3—one thousand, and so on while suctioning is a simple means for monitoring the time. Without a safeguard the airway may be obstructed for too long a period. Hyperventilating the child with 100% O_2 before and after suctioning (using a bag-valve-mask or increasing the FiO_2 ventilator setting) should also be performed to prevent hypoxia. Closed tracheal suctioning systems that allow for uninterrupted O_2 delivery may also be used (Hart and Mahutte, 1992).

NURSING ALERT Suctioning is carried out *only as often as needed* to keep the tube patent. Signs of mucus partially occluding the airway include an increased heart rate, a rise in respiratory effort, a drop in O_2 saturation, cyanosis, or an increase in the positive inspiratory pressure (PIP) on the ventilator (Musser, 1992).

The child is allowed to rest for 30 to 60 seconds after each aspiration to allow O_2 tension to return to normal; then the process is repeated until the trachea is clear. Suctioning should be limited to about three aspirations in one period. Oximetry is an effective feedback tool to monitor suctioning and prevent hypoxia.

In the acute care setting, aseptic technique is used during care of the tracheostomy. Secondary infection is a major concern, since the air entering the lower airway bypasses the natural defenses of the upper airway. Gloves are worn during the aspiration procedure, although a sterile glove is needed only on the hand touching the catheter. A new tube, gloves, and sterile saline solution are used each time (see Critical Thinking Exercise box).

Routine Care. The tracheostomy stoma requires daily care. Assessments of the stoma area include observations for signs of infection and breakdown of the skin. The skin is kept clean and dry, and secretions around the stoma may be gently removed with half-strength hydrogen peroxide. Hydrogen peroxide should not be used with sterling silver tracheostomy tubes, because it tends to pit and stain the silver surface. The nurse should be aware of wet tracheostomy dressings, which can predispose the peristomal area to skin breakdown. Several products are available to prevent or treat excoriation. The Allevyn tracheostomy dressing is a hydrophilic sponge with a polyurethane back that is highly absorptive. Other possible barriers to help maintain skin integrity include the use of hydrocolloid wafers (such as Duoderm CGF and Hollister Restore) under the tracheostomy flanges, as well as use of extra-thin hydrocolloid wafers under the chin.

The tracheostomy tube is held in place with tracheostomy ties made of a durable, nonfraying material. The ties are changed daily and when soiled. New ties are looped through the flanges (Fig. 31-19) and tied snugly in a triple knot at the side of the neck *before* the soiled ties are cut and removed. Some nurses have found that threading the ties through a piece of ¼-inch surgical tubing cushions the ties; others have found the tubing to be irritating to the skin. The ties should be tight enough to allow just a fingertip to be inserted between the ties and the neck (Fig. 31-20). It is easier to ensure a snug fit if the child's head is flexed rather than extended while ties are being secured. Ties fastened with self-adhering closures are also available. These devices, such as the Dale tracheostomy tube holder, are made of a soft, cushioning, and slightly stretchy material that is very comfortable. They are becoming increasingly popular because of their ease of use and ability to maintain better skin integrity. One should still be aware, however, of the safety factor and use them on children who are unlikely to pull and undo the fastener.

Routine tracheostomy tube changes are usually carried

CRITICAL THINKING EXERCISE

Planning for Home Tracheostomy Care

Jose Munoz, 18 months old, has been ventilator dependent since birth. He is presently hospitalized with pneumonia that has responded well to antibiotic therapy. You are discussing plans for discharge and home care with the family. Jose lives with his mother and her parents. Home nursing support is available only during the day. The family does not want to take Jose home, because he is frequently suctioned at night. Your initial intervention is to:

1. Talk with the night nurses about their suctioning program.
2. Design a plan for the family that allows them to each assume responsibility for night care with scheduled suctioning times.
3. Arrange with social service to request additional financial support for the family.
4. Suggest that Jose stay in the hospital until he needs less frequent suctioning.

The correct answer is 1. If the family managed with daytime nursing assistance before this hospitalization and the pneumonia has resolved, the child should not require intensive suctioning. In talking with the night staff, you find that the nurses suction anytime they walk past the room and hear Jose "gurgling." They also do not use premeasured suctioning technique. You discuss with them a program of premeasured suctioning only as needed to reduce the production of secretion that may be from tracheal irritation.

The other three responses assume that the frequent suctioning is needed and are not appropriate initial interventions. Suctioning should not be performed on a set schedule, but only as needed. Seeking additional financial support for nighttime nurses will not help the family return to the prehospital home care arrangements. Jose should be discharged as soon as possible to avoid nosocomial infection, promote normalization for a toddler, and contain health care costs. In this case changing the suctioning regimen decreased the frequency to a minimum of once or twice a night—a level of care the family was able to manage.

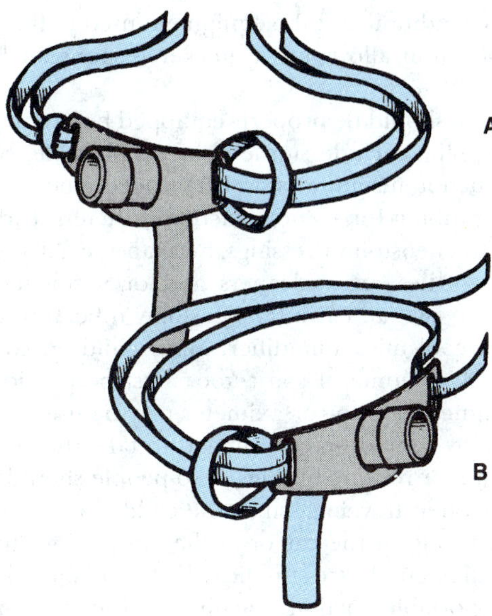

FIG. 31-19 Pediatric tracheostomy tube. **A,** Cloth tape secured at both sides to be tied in back. **B,** Cloth tape secured on one side and looped through other side to be tied at side.

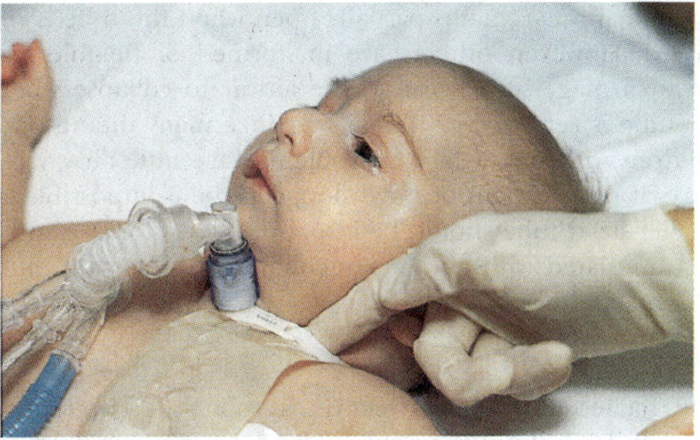

FIG. 31-20 Tracheostomy ties are snug but allow one finger to be inserted.

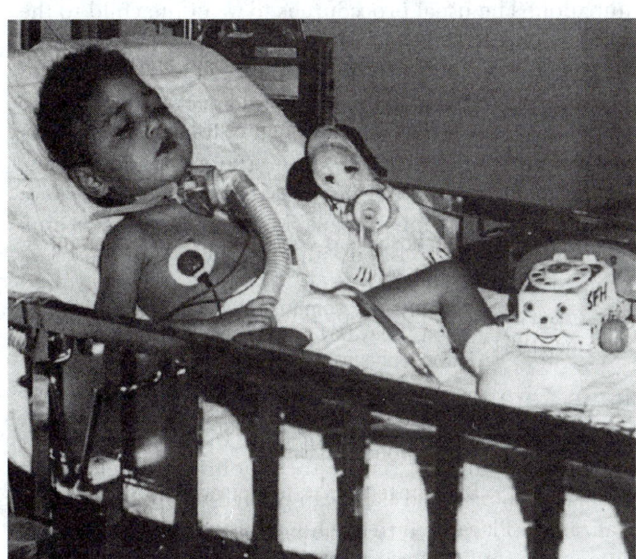

FIG. 31-21 Child with a tracheostomy and a mist collar.

out weekly after a tract has been formed to minimize formation of granulation tissue. The first change is usually performed by the surgeon; subsequent changes are performed by the nurse and, if the child is discharged home with the tracheostomy, by either a parent or a visiting nurse. Ideally two caregivers participate in the procedure to assist with positioning the child.

Changing the tracheostomy tube is accomplished using sterile technique. The new, sterile tube is prepared by inserting the obturator and attaching new ties. The child is suctioned before the procedure to minimize secretions, then restrained and positioned with the neck slightly extended. One caregiver cuts the old ties and removes the tube from the stoma. The new tube is inserted gently into the stoma (using a downward and forward motion that follows the curve of the trachea), the obturator is removed, and the ties are secured. The adequacy of ventilation must be assessed after a tube change because the tube can be inserted into the soft tissue surrounding the trachea; therefore breath sounds and respiratory effort are carefully monitored.

Supplemental O_2 is always delivered with a humidification system to prevent drying of the respiratory mucosa (Fig. 31-21). Humidification of room air for an established tracheostomy can be intermittent if secretions remain thin enough to be coughed or suctioned from the tracheostomy. Direct humidification via tracheostomy mask can be provided during naps and at night so that the child is able to be up and around unencumbered during much of the day. Room humidifiers are also used successfully (Lichtenstein, 1986). The system chosen depends on the viscosity (thickness) of the secretions and the practitioner's preference.

The inner cannula, if used, should be removed with each suctioning, cleaned with sterile saline and pipe cleaners to remove crusted material, dried thoroughly, and reinserted.

Emergency Care: Tube Occlusion and Accidental Decannulation. Occlusion of the tracheostomy tube is life-threatening, and infants and children are at greater risk than adults because of the smaller diameter of the tube. Maintaining patency of the tube is accomplished with suctioning and routine tube changes to prevent formation of crusts that can occlude the tube.

NURSING ALERT Life-threatening occlusion is apparent when the child displays signs of respiratory distress and a suction catheter cannot be passed to the end of the tube despite several attempts and instillation of saline. This situation requires an immediate tube change.

Accidental decannulation also requires immediate tube replacement. Some children have a fairly rigid trachea, so that the airway remains partially open when the tube is removed. However, others have malformed or flexible tracheal cartilage, which causes the airway to collapse when the tube is removed or dislodged. Since many infants and children with upper airway problems have little airway reserve, if replacement of the dislodged tube is impossible, a smaller-sized tube should be inserted. If the stoma cannot be cannulated with another tracheostomy tube, oral intubation should be performed.

Decannulation

The tracheostomy tube is removed as soon as it is no longer needed. Diseases of short duration (e.g., croup) usually allow early removal, but some conditions (e.g., tracheomalacia, tracheostenosis, paralysis) may require that the tube remain in place indefinitely. Opinions differ regarding the best means for removing the tube, especially after lengthy intubation. The usual procedure is to wean the child to the smallest possible tracheostomy tube. Once this has been accomplished and the child's respiratory status is unimpaired for 24 hours, the tube is occluded, with removal within the next 24 hours. A small bandage is usually placed over the open stoma, which will close within a short period of time. The procedure is carried out in a hospital setting where continuous observation is available and emergency reintubation can be accomplished without delay, if necessary. Following successful decannulation, the child remains under close observation in the hospital for an additional 48 hours (Blumer, 1991).

Home Care of the Child with a Tracheostomy*

The early return of the infant or child with a tracheostomy to a home setting can reduce the amount of developmental delay and/or social handicap related to prolonged hospitalization. Placement in the home also allows for reestablishment of routines and a regular schedule of normal activities. Physical and/or occupational therapy, as well as speech therapy, is continued in the home setting. Nursing care may also be continued in the home through private-duty care or by routine, frequent nursing visits.

Preparing the family to care for the child with a tracheostomy at home is multifaceted. Teaching sessions should be short, and written material must accompany instructions to reenforce what is being taught.† The family must be able to demonstrate tracheostomy care before the child is discharged from the hospital. This home-based care of a tracheostomy includes suctioning the tracheostomy, cleaning the stoma, changing the tracheostomy ties, changing the tracheostomy tube, adjusting or adapting the home environment, and recognizing warning signs of obstruction, infection, or a worsening condition.

To prepare for any emergency, the family must be taught infant or child cardiopulmonary resuscitation (CPR). The local utilities company and local EMS should be notified of the child's condition and the equipment used in the home. Prior notification allows for a quicker response if help is needed.

The home should be properly equipped before the child arrives. Supplies include sterile saline, a portable, battery-operated suction machine (as well as a DeLee suction trap), connecting tubing for suction, suction catheters, hydrogen peroxide, tracheostomy dressings, twill tape or self-adhering tracheostomy ties, pipe cleaners and/or a tracheostomy brush, sterile jars, an extra tracheostomy tube, a ventilator bag, and a cool mist humidifier. Many children continue receiving O_2 at home; if so, it, too, must be provided. Finally, an apnea monitor or oximeter may be used.

The family should be encouraged to take the child out of the home for routine outings. Two people should always be present when traveling, since the child may need attention while riding in the car or at the destination. In addition to routine child care supplies, the family should always bring the portable suction machine, sterile suction catheters, an extra tracheostomy tube, and a complete sterile tracheostomy care kit.

Management of the Tracheostomy. Clean technique and thorough, strict handwashing is taught for suctioning, cleaning the tracheostomy site, and changing the tracheostomy tube. One sterile suction catheter per day is usually sufficient. After initial use, the catheter is rinsed with sterile water and then stored between uses in a sterile cup or jar.

Skin at the tracheostomy site is assessed for areas of breakdown and/or drainage. The area can be cleansed with an antibacterial soap and water.

The family is encouraged not to oversuction the child, since this causes increased mucus production and irritation to the mucosal lining. The care provider should be alert to changes in the child's secretions regarding the amount, color, and/or viscosity. Awareness of these changes can prompt early medical interventions if necessary.

When dealing with the child's secretions, the family must be able to take care of a plugged, clogged, and/or obstructed tracheostomy tube. This situation can result in life-threatening circumstances. The family must be able to remove the plugged tube and replace it with a clean one.

Older children and adolescents should be taught to care for their tracheostomies. The child should be encouraged to assume as much of his or her care as is developmentally appropriate. Independence is enhanced as the child takes responsibility for tracheostomy care.

Home Environment. Changes in the home environment may be necessary before bringing the child home. Toys, blankets, clothing, and pets that shed fine hair or lint, as well as aerosols, powders, dust, and smoke, should be avoided. Fine particles from any of these items can accumulate in the tracheostomy tube and obstruct the airway. Toys that have small removable parts (that could become foreign bodies if placed in the tracheostomy tube) should also be eliminated.

Clothing should have a loose-fitting collar that does not cover the tracheostomy tube opening. When the child is outside, the artificial nose or a thin cloth such as a ban-

*Amy Verst, RN, MSN, PNP, ATC, revised this section.

†Home care instructions for tracheostomy care, postural drainage, and cardiopulmonary resuscitation are available in *Wong and Whaley's Clinical Manual of Pediatric Nursing* (Mosby).

danna can be placed loosely over the tracheostomy tube to prevent cold air, dust, dirt, or sand from entering the tube. The latter also camouflages the tracheostomy and allows a sense of normalcy to occur.

Bathing can be performed in a tub filled with shallow water, although it is important to ensure that no water or soap enters the tracheostomy tube. If this does occur, the tracheostomy should be suctioned immediately. Older children may shower if they are able to tolerate plugging the tube while under the shower spray.

Vocalization. The life of a child with a tracheostomy should be normalized. After the child returns home, routines should be established that allow the child to renew skills and enhance childhood development. Verbalization and speaking are major tasks that are often overlooked. Vocalization for the child with a tracheostomy has recently become a reality. Several tracheostomy speaking valves have been created to aid in the development of uninterrupted speech without the necessity of finger occlusion. When the speaking valve is used, air enters through the tracheostomy but is expelled over the vocal cords and through the mouth and nose. This creates a more normal passage of air through the upper airway.

Many benefits are afforded to the child with a speaking valve. An improved self-image is developed, since the tracheostomy can be disguised and finger occlusion for speech is not needed. The ability to swallow improves, since pressure can now accumulate because of the decreased amount of air released from the tracheostomy. This also allows for the creation of back pressure into the lungs. The lungs then remain open for improved gas exchange. Other advantages of this redirection of air by a speaking valve into the upper airway include improved senses of smell and taste. Secretion production is decreased because of normal evaporation, and secretions can now be coughed into the mouth, decreasing the amount of suctioning required.

Several speaking valves are available. The ***Passy Muir*** valve* is a one-way valve that attaches to the hub of all types and sizes of tracheostomies. It can be used in infants and in children who are ventilator assisted.

The Pilling Company† makes two types of speaking valves for adolescents and adults. The first, the ***Kistner valve***—a part of all Kistner tracheostomy tubes—is made of thin, soft plastic and does not protrude into the trachea. (Jackson metal tracheostomy tubes can also be used with a Kistner valve.) The second type is the ***Tucker valve,*** which is built into the inner cannula as a one-way leaflet. The leaflet opens on inspiration to allow air in and closes on expiration to force air into the upper airway. The Tucker valve inner cannula can be used with Tucker tracheostomy tubes sizes 4 to 9 and with Jackson tracheostomy tubes sizes 4 to 8. Tucker valves can only be used with sterling silver tracheostomy tubes.

*Further information can be obtained from Passy & Passy, Inc., 451 Campus Dr., Suite 273, Irvine, CA 92715; (714) 856-2634 or (800) 634-5397 (outside California).

†Further information can be obtained from The Pilling Co., 420 Delaware Dr., Fort Washington, PA, 19034; (800) 523-6507.

Tracheostomy speaking valves are inappropriate for use in children with an inflated cuff tracheostomy, laryngectomy, severe tracheostenosis, and copious or excessive secretions, and in unconscious or seriously ill children.

Socialization. School-age children can be placed in a regular classroom environment and participate in school activities as their physical abilities will allow. They should be encouraged to interact with their peers to facilitate socialization. Participation in ability-appropriate extracurricular activities should also be advocated.

Many children with tracheostomies benefit from attending summer camps for children with tracheostomies who may or may not be ventilator dependent.* Camping environments provide the child with independent living and a normal camping experience. Some camping sites allow the family to vacation together yet provide special care and assistance for the child with a tracheostomy.

RESPIRATORY EMERGENCY

RESPIRATORY FAILURE

Inadequacy of the O_2-supplying role results in blood ***hypoxemia*** and tissue ***hypoxia;*** inadequate CO_2 removal causes ***hypercapnia.*** Often both gases may be insufficiently exchanged. In general, the term ***respiratory insufficiency*** is applied to two conditions: (1) children with increased work of breathing in whom gas exchange function remains near normal and (2) children who are unable to maintain normal blood gas tensions and develop hypoxemia and acidosis secondary to CO_2 retention.

Respiratory failure is defined as the inability of the respiratory apparatus to maintain adequate oxygenation of the blood, with or without CO_2 retention. This process denotes pulmonary dysfunction that generally results in impaired alveolar gas exchange, which can lead to hypoxemia and/or hypercarbia.

Respiratory arrest is the cessation of respiration.

Apnea is absence of airflow (breathing) for more than 15 seconds. Apnea can be (1) ***central,*** in which respiratory efforts are absent; (2) ***obstructive,*** in which respiratory efforts are present; and (3) ***mixed,*** in which both central and obstructive components are present.

Effective pulmonary gas exchange requires clear airways, normal lungs and chest wall, and adequate pulmonary circulation. This functional pulmonary unit plus normal respiratory control mechanisms ensures adequate total alveolar ventilation and perfusion, which are reflected in O_2 and CO_2 tensions in arterial blood leaving the lung. Anything that affects these functions or their relationships can compromise respiration.

Respiratory dysfunction may have an abrupt or an insidious onset. Respiratory failure therefore can occur as an emergency situation or may be preceded by gradual and progressive deterioration of respiratory function. Most clini-

*Information about camps is available from Aequitron Medical Ventilator Users Network. Contact Jan Nelson, Aequitron Medical, 14800 28th Ave., N., Minneapolis, MN 55447; (800) 497-4979 or (612) 557-8256, ext. 256.

cal manifestations are nonspecific and are affected by variations among individual patients and differences in the severity and duration of inadequate gas exchange.

The diagnosis of respiratory failure is determined by the combined application of three sources of information:

1. Presence or history of a condition that might predispose to respiratory failure
2. Observation of respiratory failure
3. Measurement of ABGs and pH

Conditions That Predispose to Respiratory Failure

Respiratory disorders are more conveniently classified according to three dominant functional abnormalities, although all three types may be present in the disease. In ***obstructive lung disease*** there is increased resistance to airflow in either the upper or the lower respiratory tract. Obstruction can result from anomalies (e.g., tracheomalacia, choanal atresia, vocal paralysis), aspiration (e.g., meconium, mucus, vomitus, foreign body), infection (e.g., epiglottitis, pneumonia, pertussis, severe tonsillitis), tumors (e.g., hemangioma), anaphylaxis, and laryngospasm from local irritation (e.g., intubation, drowning, aspiration).

In ***restrictive lung disease*** there is impaired lung expansion resulting from loss of lung volume, decreased distensibility, or chest wall disturbance. Causes of pulmonary restriction include respiratory distress syndrome, pneumonia, cystic fibrosis, pneumothorax, pulmonary edema, plural effusion, near-drowning, diaphragmatic hernia, abdominal distention, muscular dystrophy, and paralytic conditions (e.g., polio, botulism).

In ***primary inefficient gas transfer*** there is insufficient alveolar ventilation for CO_2 removal or impaired oxygenation of pulmonary capillary blood as a result of dysfunction of the respiratory control mechanism or a diffusion defect. Causes of ***respiratory center depression*** include cerebral trauma (birth injuries); intracranial tumors; central nervous system infection (meningitis, encephalitis, sepsis); overdose with barbiturates, opioids, benzodiazepines (diazepam [Valium], or midazolam [Versed]); severe asphyxia (hypercapnia, hypoxemia); and tetanus. ***Pulmonary diffusion defects*** include pulmonary edema, fibrosis, embolism, or hypertension; collagen disorders; *Pneumocystis carinii* infection; anemia; and hemorrhage.

Recognition of Respiratory Failure

Respiratory failure that occurs as a result of acute obstruction of a major airway or cardiac arrest is sudden and readily apparent. Gradual and more covert development of signs and symptoms is less easily recognized. Insufficient alveolar ventilation from any cause ultimately leads to hypoxemia and hypercapnia. However, situations occur in which severe respiratory distress may be present without significant CO_2 retention, and hypoxemia may occur without clinically detectable cyanosis. Therefore evaluation of respiratory adequacy is based on both clinical assessment and laboratory studies. Nursing observation and judgment are vital to successful management of respiratory failure. Nurses must be able to assess a situation and initiate appropriate action within moments.

SIGNS OF RESPIRATORY FAILURE

CARDINAL SIGNS

Restlessness
Increase in respiratory effort
Tachypnea
Tachycardia
Diaphoresis

EARLY BUT LESS OBVIOUS SIGNS

Mood changes, such as euphoria or depression
Headache
Altered depth and pattern of respirations
Hypertension
Exertional dyspnea
Anorexia
Increased cardiac output and renal output
Central nervous system symptoms (decreased efficiency, impaired judgment, anxiety, confusion, restlessness, irritability, depressed level of consciousness)
Flaring nares
Chest wall retractions
Expiratory grunt
Wheezing and/or prolonged expiration
Absent or decreased breath sounds

SIGNS OF MORE SEVERE HYPOXIA

Hypotension or hypertension
Dimness of vision
Somnolence
Stupor
Coma
Dyspnea
Depressed respirations/agonal respirations
Bradycardia
Cyanosis, peripheral or central
Apnea

Unless respiratory arrest occurs suddenly, signs of hypoxemia and hypercapnia are usually subtle in their development and become more obvious as respiratory failure progresses. The unknowing observer may attribute early signs such as mood changes and restlessness to other causes, and some signs can be altered by other factors. The signs of respiratory failure are outlined in the box above.

In clinical situations in which impaired ventilation can be anticipated or clinical manifestations indicate impending hypoxemia, serial measurements of blood gases should be obtained and monitored to detect impending respiratory failure, and therapy should be implemented before respiratory acidosis becomes extreme.

MANAGEMENT AND RELATED NURSING CONSIDERATIONS

The interventions used in the management of respiratory failure are often dramatic, requiring special skills, and are frequently emergency procedures. If respiratory arrest occurs, the primary objectives are to recognize the situation and immediately initiate resuscitative measures, such as suctioning, CPR, and/or intubation. When the situation is not an arrest, the suspicion of respiratory failure is confirmed by assessment and the severity is defined by ABG analysis.

NURSING OBSERVATIONS FOR THE CHILD WITH RESPIRATORY FAILURE

Visual inspection of skin color to estimate level of arterial O_2 saturation
Observation of respiratory effort or distress—nasal flaring, grunting, gasping, retraction, agonal
Observation of diaphragmatic movement, lung expansion, and use of accessory muscles—depth, symmetry, inspiration/expiration ratio
Auscultation of thorax to assess:
- Breath sounds—presence, intensity, quality, symmetry
- Abnormal sounds—stridor, wheezes, crackles, rubs, crepitation, increase or decrease in sounds
- Tube placement and need for endotracheal suction when child is intubated

Interventions such as supplemental oxygen, positioning, stimulation, suctioning, and early intubation may avert an arrest. When severity is established, an attempt is made to determine the underlying cause by thorough evaluation.

Treatment of respiratory dysfunction involves both specific and nonspecific therapy. Specific therapies are directed toward reversal of the causative factors. However, sometimes nonspecific measures are needed to maintain oxygenation and enhance CO_2 removal until specific methods take effect. The major reasons for implementing nonspecific treatments are (1) unknown etiology, (2) lack of specific treatment for a known cause, (3) lack of time for a specific treatment to take effect, and (4) need for specialized personnel or equipment for specific treatment.

The principles of management are to (1) treat the underlying cause, (2) correct hypoxemia/hypercapnia, (3) maintain ventilation and maximize oxygen delivery, (4) minimize extrapulmonary organ failure, (5) apply specific and nonspecific therapy to control oxygen demands, and (6) anticipate complications. Monitoring the patient's condition is critical, and some of the techniques employed to maintain oxygenation and assist ventilation are described in the previous section.

Observation and Monitoring

The child is monitored to evaluate the cause of the failure, help determine a course of action, and assess the patient's response to treatment. If close continuous monitoring is required, the child is transferred to an intensive care unit. The child is kept as comfortable as possible, and observation is geared toward general appearance, responsiveness, pulse oximetry, and vital signs. The child is positioned to allow maximum lung expansion and comfort, such as sitting upright and/or leaning forward. Appropriate treatment modalities are applied according to the specific functional disturbance and the underlying etiology.

The child's cardiac and respiratory status are monitored by observation and by electronic means. However, no monitoring equipment can replace conscientious nursing observations (see box above), which should focus primarily on the child's airway, oxygenation, ventilation, and skin perfusion.

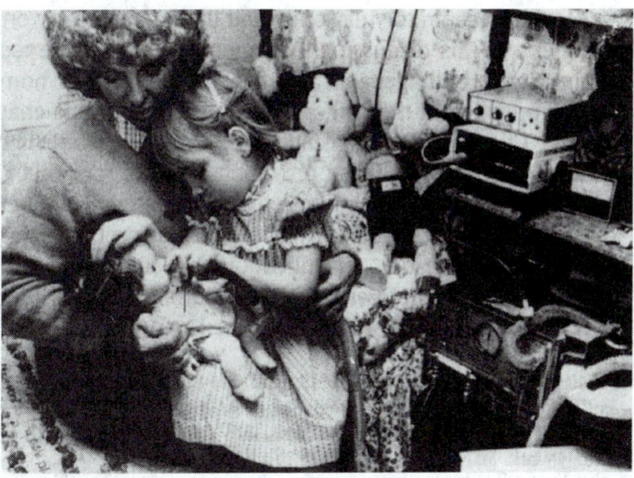

FIG. 31-22 Child with a tracheostomy being managed at home.

Since a goal of therapy is to control the O_2 demands of the body, assessments of fever and pain should be frequent. Both conditions (as well as cold stress) can dramatically increase O_2 requirements, especially in younger children, and therefore increase respiratory effort. Oxygenation can be measured by the use of pulse oximetry or blood gases.

Family Support

Children who are fatigued and in distress before a procedure, such as a tracheostomy, will probably fall into a restful sleep after establishment of an airway. However, unless they remain unconscious or semiconscious, they will probably be anxious and frightened when they are unable to communicate. Children who are old enough to write and not too fatigued can use a pad of paper and a pencil or spelling board to express their needs and concerns. Other alternative means for communication are pictures illustrating various items and activities. Simple sign language has proved to be an effective and easily learned communication medium (Hall and Weatherly, 1989).

It is often a terrifying experience for young children to discover that they are unable to make vocal sounds, including crying. It is also stressful to parents to watch their children plead with frightened eyes and cry noiselessly. It is important to talk to children and reassure them that their voices will return when the tube is removed. Children can also be taught to occlude the opening with a clean finger so that they can use the vocal cords to communicate.

Parents have numerous concerns relative to tracheostomies, ET tubes, and ventilators. If time allows before intubation or a tracheostomy, the reasons for the decision to implement the therapy, the expected results, and the approximate length of time it will remain in place should be discussed with them. Parental concern is centered around the (often) life-threatening implications generated by the need for the procedure and the possible long-term effects on the child, both physiologic and psychologic, regarding a tracheostomy. Parents are concerned about the visible

THINKING CRITICALLY ABOUT . . . *Parental Presence During CPR*

Although parents are increasingly welcome to stay during procedures (see Chapter 27), few acute care facilities allow parents to stay during CPR or a "code." Health professionals' reasons for this decision include believing the experience is too upsetting for the family, fearing the family will need care that will interfere with the staff's resuscitation efforts, experiencing discomfort being "watched" by the family, and fearing increased legal liability if the family knows what has been done or not done.

In reality, when parents do observe their child's CPR, these reasons are not supported. One study found that parents who were given the choice of staying during the code unanimously stated that they would choose this option again. Parents did not interfere with the resuscitation, they were assured that everything was done for their child, and they considered being present one of the most important memories of this difficult experience (Villarreal, 1992).

Of family members who stayed during CPR of an adult patient, 76% said their adjustment to death was easier and 64% felt their presence was beneficial to the dying person; 71% of staff members endorsed the policy (Hanson and Strawser, 1992).

Based on these findings, we need to question the wisdom of excluding parents during CPR. All may not choose to be present, but shouldn't they be given the opportunity? Whose benefit is served by family exclusion? If the main reason is the staff's own fears and anxieties about being observed and possibly judged on their performance, is depriving the family of their wishes justified? Consider out-of-hospital arrests; EMS personnel routinely perform CPR with family and strangers watching. Why is this public rescue attempt considered acceptable but an inhospital code considered a private event?

wound and the scar. Parents who must face the possibility of caring for the child with a tracheostomy at home have additional worries regarding their ability to assume this responsibility (see p. 1358 and Fig. 31-22).

For those families whose child has a respiratory arrest, support focuses on keeping the family informed of the child's status and helping them cope with a near-death experience or an actual death (see Chapter 23). Knowing that their child requires CPR is a frightening and often overwhelming experience for parents. Uncertainty regarding outcome—both mortality and morbidity—is a primary concern. Traditionally, family members are not allowed to be present during resuscitation efforts (see Thinking Critically About . . . box). Nurses can serve as the family's advocate by either being present with them or making sure a support person, such as the clergy, is present. Following the child's recovery or death, the family needs continued support and thorough medical information regarding lifesaving measures, the prognosis if the child survives, and the cause of death if the child dies.

CARDIOPULMONARY RESUSCITATION (CPR)*†

Cardiac arrest in the pediatric population is less often of cardiac origin than from prolonged hypoxemia secondary to inadequate oxygenation, ventilation, and circulation (shock). Some causes include injuries, suffocation (e.g., foreign body aspiration), smoke inhalation, sudden infant death syndrome (SIDS), and infection. Respiratory arrest is associated with a better survival than cardiac arrest. Once cardiac arrest occurs, the outcome of resuscitative efforts is poor. Most children either die or survive with significant neurologic morbidity, especially if the cardiac arrest occurred outside of a hospital (Zaritsky, 1993).

*Kathryn A. Perry, APRN, RN,C, MSN, CNS, revised this section.

†Home care instructions for CPR are available in *Wong and Whaley's Clinical Manual of Pediatric Nursing* (Mosby).

Complete apnea signals the need for rapid and vigorous action to prevent cardiac arrest. In such situations nurses must be prepared to initiate action immediately. In the hospital, emergency equipment should be readily available in areas in which respiratory arrest might take place, and the status of this resuscitation equipment should be checked at least once daily. Regardless of the cause of the arrest, some very basic procedures are carried out, modified somewhat according to the child's size.

NURSING ALERT Rescuers who have infections (regardless of type) that may be transmitted by blood or saliva or who believe they have been exposed to such an infection should not perform mouth-to-mouth resuscitation if the circumstances allow other immediate or effective methods of ventilation (e.g., use of a bag-valve-mask) (Special Communications, 1989).

Outside the hospital situation, the first action in an emergency is to quickly assess the extent of any injury and determine whether the child is unconscious. A child who is struggling to breathe but is conscious should be transported immediately to an advanced life support (ALS) facility, allowing the child to maintain whatever position affords the most comfort. However, attempting to transport a child by automobile wastes valuable time in obtaining help. Transport by an emergency medical service (EMS) is recommended or preferable. Services in larger communities can institute ALS immediately or en route to a medical facility.

An unconscious child is managed with care to prevent additional trauma if a head or spinal cord injury has been sustained. The circumstances in which the child is found offer some clues to a possible injury. For example, a child who has been thrown from a bicycle or fallen from a tree is more likely to have sustained trauma than a child who is discovered in bed. The child should be turned as a unit with firm support to the head and neck to prevent rolling, twisting, or tilting backward or forward.

One-rescuer CPR

		ACTIONS		
	Objectives	**Adult (over 8 yr)**	**Child (1 to 8 yr)**	**Infant (under 1 yr)**
A. AIRWAY	1. Assessment: Determine unresponsiveness.	Tap or gently shake shoulder.		
		Say, "Are you okay?"		Speak loudly.
	2. Get help.	Activate EMS.	Shout for help. If second rescuer available, have person activate EMS.	
	3. Position the victim.	Turn on back as a unit, supporting head and neck if necessary (4-10 seconds).		
	4. Open the airway.	Head-tilt/chin-lift.		
B. BREATHING	5. Assessment: Determine breathlessness.	Maintain open airway. Place ear over mouth, observing chest. Look, listen, feel for breathing (3-5 seconds).*		
	6. Give 2 rescue breaths.	Maintain open airway.		
		Seal mouth to mouth.		Mouth to nose/mouth.
		Give 2 slow breaths. Observe chest rise. Allow lung deflation between breaths.		
		1½ to 2 seconds each	1 to 1½ seconds each	
	7. Option for obstructed airway.	a. Reposition victim's head. Try again to give rescue breaths.		
			b. Activate EMS.	
		c. Give 5 subdiaphragmatic abdominal thrusts (the Heimlich maneuver).		c. Give 5 back blows. c. Give 5 chest thrusts.
		d. Tongue-jaw lift and finger sweep.	d. Tongue-jaw lift, but finger sweep only if you see a foreign object.	
		If unsuccessful, repeat a, c, and d until successful.		
C. CIRCULATION	8. Assessment: Determine pulselessness.	Feel for carotid pulse with one hand; maintain head-tilt with the other (5-10 seconds).		Feel for brachial pulse: keep head-tilt.
CPR	Pulse absent: Begin chest compressions: 9. Landmark check.	Run middle finger along bottom edge of rib cage to notch at center (top of sternum).		Imagine a line drawn between the nipples.
	10. Hand position.	Place index finger next to finger on notch:		Place 2-3 fingers on sternum. 1 finger's width below line. Depress ½-1 in.
		Two hands next to index finger. Depress 1½-2 in.	Heel of one hand next to index finger. Depress 1-1½ in.	
	11. Compression rate.	80-100 per minute	100 per minute	At least 100 per minute
	12. Compressions to breaths.	2 breaths to every 15 compressions	1 breath to every 5 compressions	
	13. Number of cycles.	4	20 (approximately 1 minute)	
	14. Reassessment.	Feel for carotid pulse.		Feel for brachial pulse.
		If no pulse, resume CPR, starting with compressions.	If alone, activate EMS. If no pulse, resume CPR, starting with compressions.	
	Pulse present; not breathing: Begin rescue breathing.	1 breath every 5 seconds (12 per minute)	1 breath every 3 seconds (20 per minute)	

FIG. 31-23 One-rescuer CPR. (Modified from Chandra NC, Hazinski MF, editors: *Textbook of basic life support for healthcare providers,* Dallas, 1994, American Heart Association.)

*If victim is breathing or resumes effective breathing, place in recovery position: (1) move head, shoulders, and torso simultaneously; (2) turn onto side; (3) leg not in contact with ground may be bent and knee moved forward to stabilize victim; (4) victim should not be moved in any way if trauma is suspected and should not be placed in recovery position if rescue breathing or CPR is required.

Two-rescuer CPR for children over 8 years of age

Step	Objective	Actions
1. AIRWAY	**One rescuer (ventilator):** Assessment: Determine unresponsiveness.	Tap or gently shake shoulder.
		Shout, "Are you okay?"
	Call for help.	Activate EMS.
	Position the victim.	Turn on back if necessary (4-10 sec).
	Open the airway.	Use a proper technique to open airway.
2. BREATHING	Assessment: Determine breathlessness.	Look, listen, and feel (3-5 sec).
	Ventilate twice.	Observe chest rise: 1-1.5 sec/inspiration.
3. CIRCULATION	Assessment: Determine pulselessness.	Feel for carotid pulse (5-10 sec).
	State assessment results.	Say "No pulse."
	Other rescuer (compressor): Get into position for compressions.	Hand, shoulders in correct position.
	Locate landmark notch.	Landmark check.
4. COMPRESSION/ VENTILATION CYCLES	**Compressor:** Begin chest compressions.	Correct ratio compressions/ventilations: 5/1
		Compression rate: 80-100/min (5 compressions/3-4 sec).
		Say any helpful mnemonic.
		Stop compressing for each ventilation.
	Ventilator: Ventilate after every 5th compression and check compression effectiveness.	Ventilate 1 time (1.5-2 sec/inspiration).
	(Minimum of 10 cycles.)	Check pulse occasionally to assess compressions.
5. CALL FOR SWITCH	**Compressor:** Call for switch when fatigued.	Give clear signal to change.
		Compressor completes 5th compression.
		Ventilator completes ventilation after 5th compression.
6. SWITCH	Simultaneously switch:	
	Ventilator: Move to chest.	Move to chest.
		Become compressor.
		Get into position for compressions.
		Locate landmark notch.
	Compressor: Move to head.	Move to head.
		Become ventilator.
		Check carotid pulse (5 sec).
		Say "No pulse."
		Ventilate once (1.5-2 sec/inspiration).
7. CONTINUE CPR	Resume compression/ventilation cycles.	Resume Step 4.

FIG. 31-24 Two-rescuer CPR. NOTE: Two-rescuer CPR for children ages 1 to 8 years can be performed similarly to that for adults with appropriate changes in chest compressions and ventilations. (Modified from Chandra NC, Hazinski MF, editors: *Textbook of basic life support for healthcare providers,* Dallas, 1994, American Heart Association.)

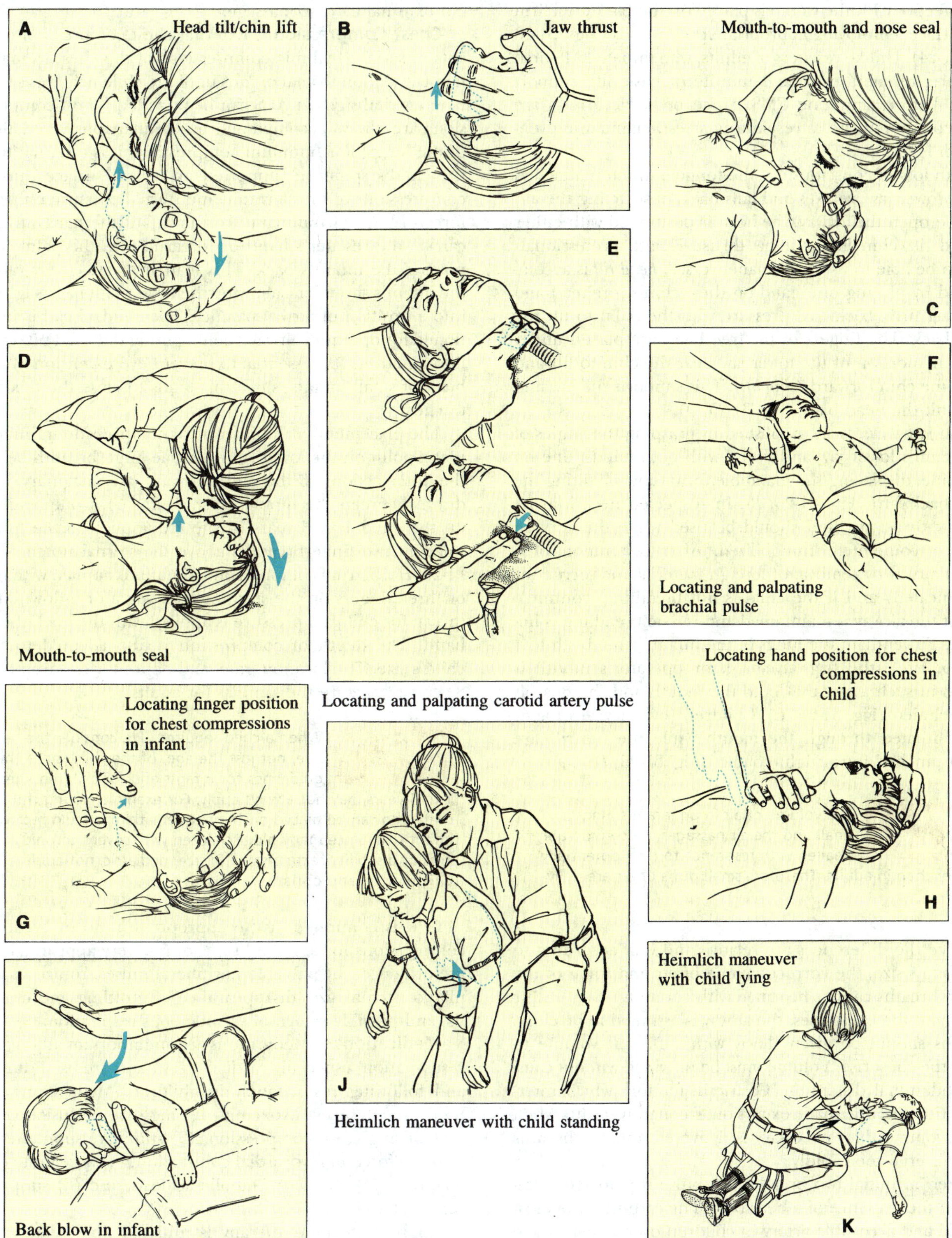

FIG. 31-25 Procedures for cardiopulmonary resuscitation, **A** to **H,** and airway obstruction, **I** to **K.** (From Chandra NC, Hazinski MF, editors: *Textbook of basic life support for healthcare providers,* Dallas, 1994, American Heart Association.)

Resuscitation Procedure

For effective CPR the victim is placed on the back on a firm flat surface, employing appropriate precautions (Figs. 31-23 and 31-24). Unlike rescuers of adults, who initiate EMS first, pediatric rescuers provide 1 minute of basic life support (BLS) before activating EMS. Since pediatric arrests are most commonly due to respiratory arrest, maintaining ventilation is primary.

With loss of consciousness the tongue, which is attached to the lower jaw, relaxes and falls back, obstructing the airway. To open the airway, the head is positioned with either a head tilt/chin lift or a jaw thrust. Health professionals should be able to use both maneuvers. A ***head tilt*** is accomplished by placing one hand on the victim's forehead and applying firm, backward pressure with the palm to tilt the head back. The fingers of the free hand are placed under the bony portion of the lower jaw near the chin to lift and bring the chin forward ***(chin lift)***. This supports the jaw and helps tilt the head back (Fig. 31-25, *A*).

The ***jaw thrust*** is accomplished by grasping the angles of the victim's lower jaw and lifting with both hands, one on each side, displacing the mandible forward while tilting the head backward (Fig. 31-25, *B*). In suspected neck injuries the jaw thrust method should be used while the cervical spine is completely immobilized. After restoration of a patent airway by removal of foreign material and secretions (if indicated) and if the child is not breathing, continuation of the airway is maintained and rescue breathing is initiated. To ventilate the lungs in the infant (from birth to 1 year of age), the bag-valve-mask or operator's mouth is placed in such a way that both the mouth and the nostrils are included (Fig. 31-25, *C*). Children (over 1 year of age) are ventilated through the mouth while the nostrils are firmly pinched for airtight contact (Fig. 31-25, *D*).

NURSING ALERT The volume of air in an infant's lungs is small and the air passages are considerably smaller, with resistance to flow potentially higher than in adults. Therefore small puffs of air are delivered.

Since the differences are relative and vary according to the child's size, the correct volume of air and force of the rescue breaths cannot be stated with certainty. If air enters freely and the chest rises, the airway is assumed to be clear. Breaths should be given slowly with sufficient volume to make the chest rise. Volume must be provided without causing abdominal distention. Gastric distention, which interferes with diaphragmatic excursion, frequently occurs when more volume than necessary is delivered and the breaths are delivered too rapidly.

After an initial two breaths, the pulse is palpated to ascertain the presence of a heartbeat. The carotid is the most central and accessible artery in children over 1 year of age (Fig. 31-25, *E*). However, the very short and often fat neck of the infant renders the carotid pulse difficult to palpate. Therefore it is preferable to use the brachial pulse, located on the inner side of the upper arm midway between the elbow and the shoulder (Fig. 31-25, *F*). Absence of a carotid or brachial pulse is considered sufficient indication to begin external cardiac massage.

Chest Compression. External chest compression consists of serial, rhythmic compressions of the chest to maintain circulation to vital organs until the child achieves spontaneous vital signs or ALS can be provided. Chest compressions are always accompanied by simultaneous ventilation of the lungs. For optimum compressions it is essential that the child's spine be supported on a firm surface during compressions of the sternum, and sternal pressure must be forceful but not traumatic. For an infant the hard surface can be the rescuer's hand or forearm, with the palm supporting the infant's back. This maneuver effectively raises the infant's shoulders, allowing the head to tilt back slightly, into a position of airway patency. The child's head is positioned for optimum airway opening using the head tilt/chin lift maneuver. It is essential to prevent overextension of the head of small infants, since this tends to close the flexible trachea.

The placement of the fingers for compression in infants is at a point on the lower sternum one fingerbreadth below the intersection of the sternum and an imaginary line drawn between the nipples (Fig. 31-25, *G*). Compressions on the child 1 to 8 years of age are applied to the lower sternum two fingerbreadths above the sternal notch (Fig. 31-25, *H*). Sternal compression to infants is applied with two or three fingers on the sternum exerting a firm downward thrust; for children pressure is applied with the heel of one hand. The depth of compression is also adapted to the child's size. The location, rate, and depth for children over 8 years of age are the same as for adults.

NURSING ALERT When a child requires CPR, consider the size, not just the age, of the child, since the guidelines for infants and for children ages 1 to 8 years may not always apply. For example, young children who can be placed on the rescuer's thigh should receive infant CPR. Since many older children with severe chronic illness or disability remain small in size, pediatric, not adult CPR, may be appropriate.

CPR is continued at the appropriate ratio of breaths/compressions for age until signs of recovery appear. These are evidenced by palpable peripheral pulses, return of pupils to normal size, disappearance of mottling and cyanosis, and possibly return of spontaneous respiration.

Medications. Medications are an important adjunct to resuscitation, especially cardiac arrest, and are used during and following resuscitation in children. Medications are used to (1) correct hyoxemia, (2) increase perfusion pressure during chest compression, (3) stimulate spontaneous or more forceful myocardial contraction, (4) accelerate cardiac rate, (5) correct metabolic acidosis, and (6) suppress ventricular ectopy.

Appropriate fluid therapy is initiated immediately for children in the hospital or by EMS personnel during transport (see Parenteral Fluid Therapy, Chapter 28, and Shock, Chapter 29). A complete supply of emergency medications is kept and maintained in all EMS vehicles and on all hospital units. The supply is checked on a regular basis (usu-

TABLE 31-6 Drugs for Pediatric Cardiopulmonary Resuscitation

DRUG/DOSE	ACTION	IMPLICATIONS
Epinephrine HCl IV/IO: 0.01 mg/kg (1:10,000)* ET: 0.1 mg/kg (1:1000)*	Adrenergic Acts on both alpha- and beta-receptor sites, especially heart and vascular and other smooth muscle	Most useful drug in cardiac arrest Disappears rapidly from bloodstream after injection May produce renal vessel constriction and decreased urine formation
Sodium bicarbonate 1 mEq/kg	Alkalinizer Buffers pH	Infuse slowly and only when ventilation is adequate
Atropine sulfate 0.02 mg/kg/dose Minimum dose: 0.1 mg Maximum single dose: infants and children, 0.5 mg; adolescents, 1.0 mg	Anticholinergic-parasympatholytic Increases cardiac output, heart rate by blocking vagal stimulation in heart	Used to treat bradycardia after ventilatory assessment
Calcium chloride 10% 20 mg/kg	Electrolyte replacement Needed for maintenance of normal cardiac contractility	Used only for hypocalcemia, calcium blocker overdose, hyperkalemia, or hypermagnesemia Administer slowly
Lidocaine HCl 1 mg/kg	Antidysrhythmic Inhibits nerve impulses from sensory nerves	Used for ventricular dysrhythmias only
Bretylium 5 mg/kg; may be increased to 10 mg/kg	Antidysrhythmic Inhibits release of norepinephrine in postganglionic nerve endings that control ventricular tachycardia	Used if lidocaine is not effective Administer rapidly
Adenosine 0.1 to 0.2 mg/kg Maximum single dose: 12 mg	Antidysrhythmic Causes a temporary block through the atrioventricular (AV) node and interrupts the reentry circuits	Administer rapidly Very effective Minimal side effects
INFUSIONS		
Epinephrine HCl infusion 0.1-1.0 μg/kg/min	Adrenergic See above	Titrated to desired hemodynamic effect
Dopamine HCl infusion 2-20 μg/kg/min	Agonist Acts on alpha receptors, causing vasoconstriction Increases cardiac output	Titrated to desired hemodynamic response
Dobutamine HCl infusion 2-20 μg/kg/min	Adrenergic direct-acting beta$_1$-agonist Increases contractility and heart rate	Titrated to desired hemodynamic response Little vasoconstriction, even at high rates
Lidocaine HCl infusion 20-50 μg/kg/min	Antidysrhythmic Increases electrical stimulation threshold of ventricle	See above Lower infusion dose used in shock Used for ventricular tachycardia

**IV,* Intravenous route; *IO,* intraosseous route; *ET,* endotracheal route.

ally once on each 8-hour shift). Resuscitation medications are listed in Table 31-6.

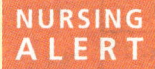

When administering drugs during CPR (or a "code"), use a saline flush between medications to prevent drug interactions.

AIRWAY OBSTRUCTION

Attempts at clearing the airway should be considered for (1) children in whom aspiration is witnessed or strongly suspected and (2) unconscious, nonbreathing children whose airways remain obstructed despite the usual maneuvers to open them. When aspiration is strongly suspected, the child is encouraged to continue coughing as long as the cough remains forceful. If the cough becomes ineffective, mechanical maneuvers should be used in an attempt to dislodge the object.

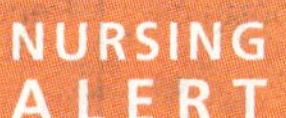

In a conscious choking child attempt to relieve the obstruction only if:
The child is unable to make any sounds.
The cough becomes ineffective.
There is increasing respiratory difficulty with stridor.

Although there is controversy concerning the optimum method for relieving foreign body obstruction in children, there is agreement that no blind finger sweeps should be used. The methods currently recommended are a combination of ***back blows*** and ***chest thrusts*** in infants and the ***Heimlich maneuver*** in children. Because of the risk of injury to

Foreign body airway obstruction management
Signs of life-threatening obstruction

The truly choking child *cannot speak, becomes cyanotic,* and *collapses*				
		Actions		
	Objectives	**Adult (over 8 yr)**	**Child (1 to 8 yr)**	**Infant (under 1 yr)**
CONSCIOUS VICTIM	1. Assessment: Determine airway obstruction.	Ask, "Are you choking?" Determine if victim can cough or speak.		Observe breathing difficulty, ineffective cough, no strong cry.
	2. Act to relieve obstruction.	Perform up to 5 subdiaphragmatic abdominal thrusts (Heimlich maneuver).		Give 5 back blows.
				Give 5 chest thrusts.
	Be persistent.	Repeat Step 2 until obstruction is relieved or victim becomes unconscious.		
VICTIM WHO BECOMES UNCONSCIOUS	3. Position the victim: call for help.	Turn on back as a unit, supporting head and neck, face up, arms by sides. Call out, "Help!" Activate EMS. If second rescuer available, have person activate EMS.		
	4. Check for foreign body.	Perform tongue-jaw lift and finger sweep.	Perform tongue-jaw lift. Remove foreign object only if you actually see it.	
	5. Give rescue breaths.	Open the airway with head-tilt/chin-lift. Try to give rescue breaths. If airway is obstructed, reposition head and try to ventilate again.		
	6. Act to relieve obstruction.	Perform up to 5 subdiaphragmatic abdominal thrusts (Heimlich maneuver).		Give 5 back blows.
				Give 5 chest thrusts.
	7. Be persistent.	Repeat steps 4-6 until obstruction is relieved.		
UNCONSCIOUS VICTIM	1. Assessment: Determine unresponsiveness.	Tap or gently shake shoulder. Shout, "Are you okay?"	Tap or gently shake shoulder.	
		If unresponsive, activate EMS.		
	2. Call for help: position the victim.	Turn on back as a unit, supporting head and neck, face up, arms by sides.		
			Call out for help.	
	3. Open the airway.	Head-tilt/chin-lift.		Head-tilt/chin-lift, but do not tilt too far.
	4. Assessment: Determine breathlessness.	Maintain an open airway. Ear over mouth; observe chest. Look, listen, feel for breathing. (3-5 seconds)		
	5. Give rescue breaths.	Make mouth-to-mouth seal.		Make mouth-to-nose-and-mouth seal.
		Try to give rescue breaths.		
	6. If chest is not rising, try again to give rescue breaths.	Reposition head. Try rescue breaths again.		
	7. Activate the EMS system.		If airway obstruction not relieved after about 1 minute, activate EMS as rapidly as possible.	
	8. Act to relieve obstruction.	Perform up to 5 subdiaphragmatic abdominal thrusts (Heimlich maneuver).		Give 5 back blows.
				Give 5 chest thrusts.
	9. Check for foreign body.	Perform tongue-jaw lift and finger sweep.	Perform tongue-jaw lift. Remove foreign object only if you actually see it.	
	10. Rescue breaths.	Open the airway with head-tilt/chin-lift. Try again to give rescue breaths. If airway is obstructed, reposition head and try to ventilate again.		
	11. Be persistent.	Repeat steps 8-10 until obstruction is relieved.		

FIG. 31-26 Foreign body airway obstruction management. (Modified from Chandra NC, Hazinski MF, editors: *Textbook of basic life support for healthcare providers,* Dallas, 1994, American Heart Association.)

abdominal organs, abdominal thrusts are not recommended for infants.

Infants

A choking infant is placed face down over the rescuer's arm with the head lower than the trunk and the head supported (Figs. 31-25, *I;* 31-26). For additional support the rescuer should support the arm firmly against the thigh. Up to five quick, sharp, back blows are delivered between the infant's shoulder blades with the heel of the rescuer's hand. Less force is required than would be applied to an adult. After delivery of the back blows, the rescuer's free hand is placed flat on the infant's back so that the infant is "sandwiched" between the two arms, making certain the neck and chin are well supported. While the rescuer maintains support with the infant's head lower than the trunk, the infant is turned and placed supine, supported on the rescuer's thigh, where up to five quick downward chest thrusts are applied in rapid succession in the same location as external chest compressions described for CPR. Back blows and chest thrusts are continued until the object is removed or the infant becomes unconscious.

Children

The Heimlich maneuver, a series of subdiaphragmatic abdominal thrusts, is recommended for children over 1 year of age. The maneuver creates an artificial cough that forces air, and with it the foreign body, out of the airway. The procedure is carried out with the child in a standing, sitting, or lying position (Fig. 31-25, *J* and *K*). In the conscious choking child, upward thrusts are delivered to the upper abdomen with the fisted hand at a point just below the rib cage (Figs. 31-25, *J;* 31-26). To prevent damage to the internal organs, the rescuer's hands should not touch the xiphoid process of the sternum or the lower margins of the ribs. Up to five thrusts are repeated in rapid succession until the foreign body is expelled.

It is neither necessary nor desirable to squeeze or compress the arms during the procedure. It is not a punch or a bear hug. The child may vomit after relief of the obstruction and should be positioned to prevent aspiration. After breathing is restored, the child should receive medical attention and be assessed for complications.

The success of the technique is primarily a result of the obstruction occurring at the end of a maximum respiration. The victim is most likely to choke on food during inspiration; therefore the tidal volume plus expiratory reserve volume is present in the lungs. When pressure is exerted on the diaphragm by the maneuver, the food bolus is ejected with considerable force by this trapped air.

KEY POINTS

- The major functions of the respiratory tract are to distribute air and exchange gases to supply cells with oxygen (O_2) and to remove carbon dioxide (CO_2).
- Several anatomic features predispose infants and young children to airway obstruction and atelectasis: there is less alveolar surface for gas exchange; narrowly branching peripheral airways become easily obstructed; and lack of collateral pathways inhibits ventilation beyond obstructed units.
- Gas exchange depends on the amount and composition of gases inhaled, thickness of the alveolar wall, adequacy of circulation to the alveoli, and substances within the alveoli that prevent their inflation or gas exchange.
- The amount of O_2 that diffuses into the blood depends on a pressure gradient between alveolar air and capillary blood, the total functional surface area of the alveolocapillary membrane, minute volume, and alveolar ventilation.
- Defense mechanisms of the respiratory tract include the lymphatic system, mucus secretions, ciliary action, epiglottis, cough reflex, tracheobronchial dynamics, body position changes, and humoral defenses.
- Complete assessment of respiratory function involves a detailed history, physical examination, pulmonary function tests, radiography, and blood gas determination.
- Pulse oximetry is a noninvasive method of determining the O_2 saturation in the blood. One limitation of the technology is that it does not identify dangerously high O_2 levels.
- Improvement in respiratory function may be accomplished with measures such as O_2 therapy, positioning, humidification, aerosol therapy, and artificial ventilation.
- O_2 for administration must always be humidified.
- Chest physiotherapy is useful for patients with increased sputum production but is contraindicated for some.
- Implications for possible intubation include airway obstruction, respiratory arrest, pulmonary toilet, neuromuscular compromise and/or paralysis, and hypoxemia.
- Respiratory failure is defined as the inability of the respiratory system to maintain adequate oxygenation of the blood, with or without CO_2 retention.
- Management of respiratory failure is to provide O_2, maintain ventilation, apply appropriate therapy, and anticipate complications.
- Endotracheal and tracheostomy suctioning involves premeasured insertion of the catheter, application of suction for 3 to 4 seconds when withdrawing the catheter, and supplemental O_2 before and after suctioning.
- Occlusion of the endotracheal and tracheostomy tube is life-threatening; therefore equipment for replacing a tube must always be at hand.
- Pediatric cardiopulmonary resuscitation (CPR) includes 1 minute of ventilations and compressions before summoning emergency help.
- Two essentials of CPR are to support the patient's spine and to apply forceful, but not traumatic, sternal pressure.
- The Heimlich maneuver is reserved for children for whom aspiration is witnessed or strongly suspected. A combination of back blows and chest thrusts is used for infants with obstructed airways.

REFERENCES

Alderson SH, Warren RH: Pediatric aerosol therapy guidelines, *Clin Pediatr* 23:553-557, 1984.

Blumer JL: *A practical guide to pediatric intensive care,* ed 3, St Louis, 1991, Mosby.

Hall SS, Weatherly KS: Using sign language with tracheostomized infants and children, *Pediatr Nurs* 15:362-267, 1989.

Hanson C, Strawser D: Family presence during cardiopulmonary resuscitation: Foote Hospital emergency department's nine-year perspective, *J Emerg Nurs* 18(2):104-106, 1992.

Harbold LA: A protocol for neonatal use of pulse oximetry, *Neonatal Network* 8(1):41-42, 55-57, 1989.

Hart TP, Mahutte CK: Evaluation of a closed-system, directional-tip suction catheter, *Respir Care* 37(11):1260-1265, 1992.

Kleiber C, Krutzfield N, Rose EF: Acute histologic changes in tracheobronchial tree associated with different suction catheter insertion techniques, *Heart Lung* 17:10-14, 1988.

Kyff JV: Current thoughts on chest physical therapy, *Respir Manage* 17(6):70-73, 1987.

Lichtenstein MA: Pediatric home tracheostomy care: a parent's guide, *Pediatr Nurs* 12:41-48, 69, 1986.

McCance KL, Huether SE: *Pathophysiology: The biological basis for disease in adults and children,* ed 2, St Louis, 1994, Mosby.

Murphy KG and others: Severe burns from a pulse oximeter, *Anesthesiology* 73:350, 1990.

Musser V: How do you use shallow-suction technique in children? *Am J Nurs* 92(5):79-83, 1992.

Orenstein DM: *Cystic fibrosis: a guide for patient and family,* New York, 1989, Raven Press.

Special Communications: Risk of infection during CPR training and rescue: supplemental guidelines, *JAMA* 262:2714-2715, 1989.

Sutton PP: Chest physiotherapy: time for reappraisal, *Br J Dis Chest* 82:127-137, 1988.

Thompson JM and others: *Mosby's clinical nursing,* ed 3, St Louis, 1993, Mosby.

Villarreal P: Personal communication, University of Texas, San Antonio, 1992.

Zaritsky A: Outcome of pediatric cardiopulmonary resuscitation, *Crit Care Med* 21(9, suppl):S325-S327, 1993.

BIBLIOGRAPHY

General

Ahmann E, Lipsi KA: Early intervention for technology-dependent infants and young children, *Infants Young Child* 3(4):67-77, 1991.

Brown MA, Swanson C: Understanding children with chronic lung disease: respiratory supports and treatments, part 2, *Infants Young Child* 5(3):57-66, 1993.

Dudell G, Cornish JD, Bartlett RH: What constitutes adequate oxygenation? *Pediatrics* 85:39-41, 1990.

Lareau S, Larson JL: Ineffective breathing pattern related to airflow limitation, *Nurs Clin North Am* 22:179-191, 1987.

Soud T: Airway breathing, circulation, and disability: what is different about kids? *J Emerg Nurs* 81(2):107-119, 1992.

Wilmott RW: Pursuing the cause of persistent cough, *Contemp Pediatr* 4(10):26-43, 1987.

Wolff, PS: An ingenious way to treat psychogenic cough, *MCN* 13:118-120, 1988.

Pulmonary Assessment

Ahrens T: Respiratory monitoring in critical care, *AACN Clin Issues Crit Care Nurs* 4(1):56-65, 1993.

Birdsell C: How do you measure transcutaneous oxygen? *Am J Nurs* 87:1273-1274, 1987.

Birdsell C: How and when do you use pulse oximetry? *Am J Nurs* 87:158-165, 1989.

Carroll P: Clinical application of pulse oximetry, *Pediatr Nurs* 19(2):150-151, 1993.

Chatburn RL: Evaluation of pediatric pulmonary function: theory and application, *Respir Care* 34:597-608, 1989.

Comer DM: Pulse oximetry: implications for practice, *JOGNN* 21(1):35-41, 1992.

Durren M: Getting the most from pulse oximetry, *J Emerg Nurs* 18(4):340-342, 1992.

Ehrhardt BS, Graham M: Pulse oximetry: an easy way to check oxygen saturation, *Nursing 90* 20:50-54, 1990.

Fruthaler GJ: Snurgles and gurgles: respiratory sounds that worry parents, *Contemp Pediatr* 5(7):42-46, 1988.

Gramlich T: Pulse oximetry, *Emergency* 24(8):25-27, 1992.

Hader CF, Sorensen ER: The effects of body position on transcutaneous oxygen tension, *Pediatr Nurs* 14:469-473, 1988.

Hess D, Kacmarek RM: Techniques and devices for monitoring oxygenation, *Respir Care* 38(6):646-671, 1993.

Hickenlooper GB, Sowan NA: Comparison of cardiorespiratory fitness tests for children, *Pediatr Nurs* 14:485-487, 491, 1988.

Miller P: Using pulse oximetry to make clinical nursing decisions, *Orthop Nurs* 11(4):39-42, 1992.

Reimer JM, Schreiber MD, Dimand RJ: Portable transcutaneous O_2 and CO_2 monitors and pulse oximeters during transport of critically ill newborn infants, *J Air Med Transport* 11(8):9-13, 1992.

Rooth G, Huch A, Huch R: Transcutaneous oxygen monitors are reliable indicators of arterial oxygen tension (if used correctly), *Pediatrics* 9:283-286, 1987.

Rotello LC and others: A nurse-directed protocol using pulse oximetry to wean mechanically ventilated patients from toxic oxygen concentrations, *Chest* 102(6):1833-1835, 1992.

Russell R, Helms P: Comparative accuracy of pulse oximetry and transcutaneous oxygen in assessing arterial saturation in pediatric intensive care, *Neonatal Intensive Care* 5(1):38-40, 1992.

Salyer JW, Chatburn RL, Dolcini DM: Measured vs calculated oxygen saturation in a population of pediatric intensive care patients, *Respir Care* 34:342-348, 1989.

Salyer JW, Lewis D: Pulse oximetry: application in the pediatric and neonatal critical care unit, *AACN Clin Issues Crit Care Nurs* 1(2):339-347, 1990.

Sherman JM: New options for examining children's airways, *Contemp Pediatr* 6(1):30-44, 1989.

Sobel DB: Burning of a neonate due to a pulse oximeter: arterial saturation monitoring, *Pediatrics* 89(1):154-155, 1992.

Webster H, Chellis MJ: Physiologic monitoring of infants and children, *AACN Clin Issues Crit Care Nurs* 4(1):180-196, 1993.

Respiratory Therapy/Suctioning

AARC Clinical Practice Guideline: Endotracheal suctioning of mechanically ventilated adults and children with artificial airways, *Respir Care* 38(5):500-504, 1993.

Bailey C and others: Shallow versus deep endotracheal suctioning in young rabbits: pathologic effects on the tracheobronchial wall, *Pediatrics* 82:746-751, 1988.

Czarnik RE and others: Differential effects of continuous versus intermittent suction on tracheal tissue, *Heart Lung* 20(2):144-151, 1991.

Fiorentini A: Potential hazards of tracheobronchial suctioning, *Intens Crit Care Nurs* 8(4):217-226, 1992.

Glass C and others: Nurses' ability to achieve hyperinflation and hyperoxygenation with a manual resuscitation bag during endotracheal suctioning, *Heart Lung* 22(2):158-165, 1993.

Hartsell MB: Chest physiotherapy and mechanical vibration, *J Pediatr Nurs* 2:135-137, 1987.

Hoffman LA, Mazzocco MC, Roth JE: Fine tuning your chest PT, *Am J Nurs* 87:1566-1572, 1987.

Hodge D: Endotracheal suctioning and the infant: a nursing care protocol to decrease complications, *Neonatal Network* 9(5):7-15, 1991.

Kerr M, Menzel L, Rudy E: Suctioning practices in the pediatric intensive care unit, *Heart Lung* 20(3):300, 1991.

Knox AM: Performing endotracheal suction on children: a literature review and implications for nursing practice, *Intensive Crit Care Nurs* 9(1):48-54, 1993.

Mancinelli-Van-Atta J, Beck SL: Preventing hypoxemia and hemodynamic compromise related to endotracheal suctioning, *Am J Crit Care* 1(3):62-79, 1992.

Noll ML, Hix C, Scott G: Closed tracheal suction systems: effectiveness and nursing complications, *AACN Clin Issues Crit Care Nurs* 1(2):327-328, 1990.

Runton N: Suctioning artificial airways in children: appropriate technique, *Pediatr Nurs* 18(2):115-118, 1992.

Shorten DR, Byrne PJ, Jones RL: Infant responses to saline instillations and endotracheal suctioning, *JOGNN* 20(6):464-469, 1991.

Smith SJ: Suctioning the airway, *Emergency* 25(3):41-45, 1993.

Tolles CL, Stone KS: National survey of neonatal endotracheal suctioning practices, *Neonatal Network* 9(2):7-14, 1990.

Wilson G and others: Evaluation of two endotracheal suction regimes in babies ventilated for respiratory distress syndrome, *Neonatal Network* 11(7):43-45, 1992.

Witmer MT, Hess D, Simmons M: An evaluation of the effectiveness of secretion removal with the Ballard closed-circuit suction catheter, *Respir Care* 36(8):844-848, 1991.

Artificial Mechanical Ventilation

Ahmann E, Lipsi KA: Early intervention for technology-dependent infants and young children, *Infants Young Child* 3(4):67-77, 1991.

Boegner E: Modes of ventilatory support and weaning parameters in children, *AACN Clin Issues Crit Care Nurs* 1(2):378-386, 1990.

Dixon M, Holmes RB: The care of a ventilator-dependent child on a general pediatric unit, *J Pediatr Nurs* 2:184-192, 1987.

Dougherty JM: Negative pressure devices in pediatric practice, *Pediatr Nurs* 16:135-138, 1990.

Gordin P: High-frequency jet ventilation for severe respiratory failure, *Pediatr Nurs* 15(6):625-629, 1989.

Mallory GB Jr, Stillwell PC: The ventilator-dependent child: issues in diagnosis and management, *Arch Phys Med Rehabil* 72(1):43-55, 1991.

Turner BS: Maintaining the artificial airway: current concepts, *Pediatr Nurs* 16(5):487-493, 1990.

Warner J, Norwood S: Psychosocial concerns of the ventilator-dependent child in the pediatric intensive care unit, *AACN Clin Issues Crit Care Nurs* 2(3):432-445, 1991.

Whitford KM: Health care needs of ventilator-dependent children, *Pediatr Nurs* 14:216-219, 1988.

Withiam-Wilson MJ: Accidental breathing circuit disconnections in the neonatal or pediatric critical care setting, *Pediatr Nurs* 17(3):283-286, 293, 1991.

Endotracheal Airways/Tracheostomy

Beard B, Monaco FJ: Tracheostomy discontinuation: impact of tube selection on resistance during tube occlusion, *Respir Care* 38(3):267-270, 1993.

Corbo BH: Endotracheal intubation: adolescent ICU experiences, *Crit Care Q* 8(1):35-46, 1985.

Hummel PA, Kleiber C: Spontaneous endotracheal tube extubation in infants and children, *Focus Crit Care* 16(4):311-318, 1989.

McGee L: Case study: maintaining skin integrity during the use of tracheostomy ties, *Ostomy Wound Manage,* 30(5):37-40, 1990.

Runton N, Zazal GH: The decannulation process in children, *J Pediatr Nurs* 4:370-373, 1989.

Sherman LP, Rosen CD: Development of a preschool program for tracheostomy dependent children, *Pediatr Nurs* 16(4):357-361, 1990.

Simon BM, McGowan JS: Tracheostomy in young children: implications for assessment and treatment of communication and feeding disorders, *Infants Young Child* 1(3):1-9, 1989.

Turner BS: Maintaining the artificial airway: current concepts, *Pediatr Nurs* 16(5):487-493, 1990.

Home Care

Anderson KL: Long-term oxygen therapy: indications and guidelines for use, *Home Healthc Nurse* 7(3):40-48, 1989.

Andrews MM, Nielson DW: Technology dependent children in the home, *Pediatr Nurs* 14:111-114, 151, 1988.

Burnes L: Tracheostomy care: preparing parents for discharge, *MCN* 17(6):293, 1992.

Harrison LL: Teaching parents to provide home-care for ventilator-dependent children, *MCN* 14:281, 1989.

Hazinski MF: Pediatric home tracheostomy care: a parent's guide, *Pediatr Nurs* 12:41-48, 69, 1986.

Kaufman J, Hardy-Ribakow D: What parents need to know about trach care, *RN* 51:99-104, 1988.

Kennelly C: Tracheostomy care: parents as learners, *MCN* 12:264-267, 1987.

Kenney MM: Hospital to home: care of the child with a tracheostomy, *Neonatal Network* 6(1):21-24, 1987.

Leighton EM, Davis RH, Anderson LJW: An orientation program for high-technology home care nursing, *Pediatr Nurs* 16:182-185, 1990.

O'Pray M: Working with families with infants with respiratory equipment in the home, *Issues Compr Pediatr Nurs* 10:113-121, 1987.

Paulson PR: Nursing considerations for discharging children home on low-flow oxygen, *Issues Compr Pediatr Nurs* 10(4):209-214, 1987.

Quint RD and others: Home care for ventilator-dependent children: psychosocial impact on the family, *Am J Dis Child* 144(11):1238-1241, 1990.

Scharer K, Dixon DM: Managing chronic illness: parents with a ventilator-dependent child, *J Pediatr Nurs* 4:236-247, 1989.

Ronczy NM, Beddome M: Preparing the family for home tracheotomy care, *AACN Clin Issues Crit Care Nurs* 1(2):367-377, 1990.

Wegener DH, Aday LA: Home care for ventilator-assisted children: predicting family stress, *Pediatr Nurs* 15(4):371-376, 1989.

Wessel GL, Prumo MO, Harrison P: School placement and the oxygen-dependent child, *J Pediatr Nurs* 6:435-436, 1989.

Respiratory Emergencies/CPR

Brown R, Ioli JG: A pediatric resuscitation poster: development and multiple uses, *Pediatr Nurs* 19(1):56-58, 1993.

Buzz-Kelly L, Gordin P: Teaching CPR to parents of children with tracheostomies, *MCN* 18(3):158-163, 1993.

Chandra NC, Hazinski MF, editors: *Textbook of basic life support for healthcare providers,* Dallas, 1994, American Heart Association.

Hazinski MF: Advances and controversies in cardiopulmonary resuscitation in the young, *J Cardiovasc Nurs* 6(3):74-85, 1992.

Raphaely RC: Acute respiratory failure in infants and children, *Pediatr Ann* 15:315-321, 1986.

Singhal N and others: Attitudinal and resource changes after a neonatal resuscitation training program, *Neonatal Network* 11(4):37-40, 1992.

Stroud T: Airway, breathing, circulation, and disability: what is different about kids? *J Emerg Nurs* 18(2):107-116, 1992.

Wright S, Norton C, Kesten K: Retention of infant CPR instruction by parents, *Pediatr Nurs* 15:37-41, 1989.

CHAPTER 32

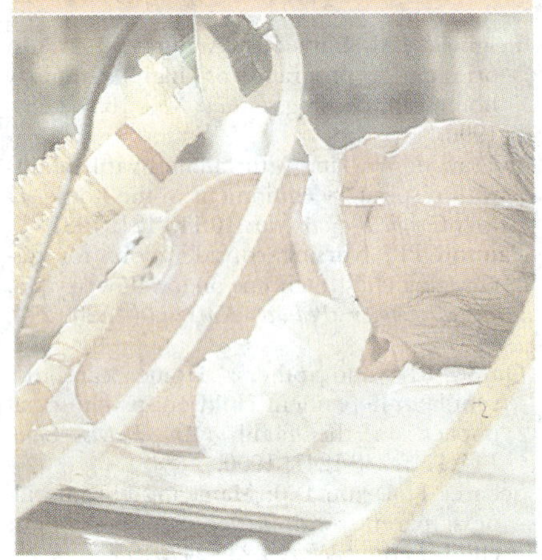

The Child with Respiratory Dysfunction

CHAPTER OUTLINE

RELATED TOPICS

Administration of medication, Ch. 27
The child with disturbance of oxygen and carbon dioxide exchange, Ch. 31
Compliance, Ch. 27
Controlling elevated temperatures, Ch. 27
Family-centered care of the child with chronic illness or disability, Ch. 22
Family-centered home care, Ch. 25
High risk related to disturbed respiratory function, Ch. 10
Immunizations, Ch. 12
Infection control, Ch. 27
Ingestion of injurious agents, Ch. 16
Maintaining healthy skin, Ch. 27
Pain assessment; pain management, Ch. 26
Physical examination: ears, nose, mouth and throat, chest, lungs, Ch. 7
Surgical procedures, Ch. 27
Tobacco (use), Ch. 21

RESPIRATORY INFECTION

GENERAL ASPECTS OF RESPIRATORY INFECTIONS

Infections of the respiratory tract are described in a number of different ways according to the general areas of involvement in the more common infections. The *upper respiratory tract,* or *upper airway,* consists primarily of the nose and pharynx. The *lower respiratory tract* consists of the bronchi and bronchioles (which constitute the reactive portion of the airway because of their smooth muscle content and ability to constrict) and the alveoli. Authorities disagree about the designation for the structurally stable portion of the airway (including the epiglottis, larynx, and trachea). Some consider these structures to be part of the lower airway, whereas others categorize them as upper airway struc-

■ Stephen Jones, RN,C, MS, PNP, revised this chapter.

tures. For this discussion, the trachea is considered with lower tract disorders, and infections of the epiglottis and larynx are categorized as croup syndromes.

Respiratory infections seldom fall neatly into discrete anatomic areas. Infections tend to spread from one structure to another because of the contiguous nature of the mucous membrane lining the entire tract. Consequently, infections of the respiratory tract involve several areas rather than a single structure, although the effect on one may predominate in any given illness.

Etiology and Characteristics

Respiratory infections account for a large majority of acute illnesses in children. The etiology and course of these infections are influenced by a number of factors, including the age of the child, season, living conditions, and preexisting medical problems.

Infectious Agents. The respiratory tract is subject to a wide variety of infective organisms, but the largest percentage of infections are caused by viruses, particularly in the upper respiratory passages. These infections account for a large majority of acute illnesses in children. Other agents that may be involved in primary or secondary invasion include group A β-hemolytic streptococci, staphylococci, *Haemophilus influenzae, Chlamydia trachomatis, Mycoplasma,* and pneumococci.

Age. The pattern of respiratory infection varies considerably with the age of the child. Infants under age 3 months have a lower infection rate, presumably because of the protective function of maternal antibodies. The infection rate soars from age 3 to 6 months, the time between the disappearance of maternal antibodies and the infant's own antibody production. The viral infection rate continues to be high during the toddler and preschool years but drops steadily. By the time the child reaches 5 years of age, viral respiratory infections are much less frequent, but the incidence of *Mycoplasma pneumoniae* and group A β-streptococcal infections increases.

Some of the viral agents produce a mild illness in older children but cause severe lower respiratory tract illness or croup in infants. The amount of lymphoid tissue increases throughout middle childhood, and repeated exposure to organisms confers increasing immunity as the child grows older; thus older children have a greater resistance to most organisms. Whooping cough is a relatively harmless tracheobronchitis in childhood but a serious disease in infancy.

Size. Anatomic differences influence the degree to which children respond to respiratory tract infections. The diameter of the airways is smaller in young children than in older children and is therefore subject to considerable narrowing from edematous mucous membranes and increased production of secretions. In addition, the distance between structures within the tract is shorter anatomically in the young child; therefore organisms move more rapidly down the respiratory tract for more extensive involvement. Also, the relatively short and open eustachian tube in infants and young children allows pathogens easy access to the middle ear.

Resistance. The ability to resist invading organisms depends on several factors. Deficiencies of the immune system place the child at risk for any infectious process. The general conditions that appear to decrease resistance to infection are malnutrition, anemia, fatigue, and chilling of the body. Conditions affecting the respiratory tract that weaken its defenses and predispose to infection include allergies (e.g., allergic rhinitis), asthma, cardiac anomalies that have a tendency to cause pulmonary congestion, and cystic fibrosis of the pancreas. Daycare attendance, especially if the caregivers smoke, also increases the likelihood of infection (Holberg, Wright, and Martinez, 1993; Hurwitz and others, 1991).

Seasonal Variations. The most common respiratory tract pathogens appear in epidemics during the winter and spring months, but mycoplasma infections occur more often in autumn and early winter. Infection-related asthma (e.g., asthmatic bronchitis) occurs more frequently during cold weather.

Clinical Manifestations

Infants and young children, especially those between 6 months and 3 years of age, react more severely to acute respiratory tract infection than older children, and they are often more ill than their local manifestations would indicate. Young children display a number of generalized signs and symptoms, as well as local manifestations, that differ from those seen in older children and adults. An infant or child may display any or all of the signs and symptoms listed in the box on p. 1374.

Nursing Considerations

Because respiratory infections are common in children, they are the illnesses most frequently observed by nurses.

❖ Assessment

The general assessment of the respiratory system follows the guidelines described in Chapter 7 (for nose, mouth and throat, chest, and lungs), and normal vital signs can be found on the inside back cover. In addition, special attention is given to the specific observations outlined in the box on p. 1374 using the components in the box on p. 1375.

❖ Nursing Diagnoses

After a thorough assessment, a number of nursing diagnoses may be identified. The most likely diagnoses are outlined and discussed in the Nursing Care Plan on pp. 1377-1379. Others may be apparent in individual cases.

❖ Planning

The goals for the child with an acute respiratory infection and the family are as follows:

1. Child will exhibit normal respiratory efforts.
2. Child will receive adequate rest.
3. Child will remain comfortable.
4. Child will not spread primary infection to others.
5. Child's temperature will remain within normal limits.
6. Child will maintain normal hydration and adequate nutrition.

SIGNS AND SYMPTOMS ASSOCIATED WITH RESPIRATORY INFECTIONS IN INFANTS AND SMALL CHILDREN

FEVER
May be absent in newborn infants
Greatest at ages 6 months to 3 years
  Temperature may reach 39.5° to 40.5° C (103° to 105° F) even with mild infections
Often appears as first sign of infection
May be listless and irritable or somewhat euphoric and more active than normal, temporarily; some children talk with unaccustomed rapidity
Tendency to develop high temperatures with infection in certain families
  May precipitate febrile seizures (see Chapter 37)
  Febrile seizures uncommon after 3 or 4 years of age

MENINGISMUS
Meningeal signs without infection of the meninges
Occurs with abrupt onset of fever
Accompanied by:
  Headache
  Pain and stiffness in the back and neck
  Presence of Kernig and Brudzinski signs
Subsides as the temperature drops

ANOREXIA
Common with most childhood illnesses
Frequently the initial evidence of illness
Almost invariably accompanies acute infections in small children
Persists to a greater or lesser degree throughout febrile stage of illness; often extends into convalescence

VOMITING
Small children vomit readily with illness
A clue to the onset of infection
May precede other signs by several hours
Usually short lived, but may persist during the illness

DIARRHEA
Usually mild, transient diarrhea but may become severe
Often accompanies respiratory infections, especially viral infections
Is frequent cause of dehydration

ABDOMINAL PAIN
Common complaint
Sometimes indistinguishable from pain of appendicitis
Mesenteric lymphadenitis may be cause
Muscle spasms from vomiting may be a factor, especially in nervous, tense children

NASAL BLOCKAGE
Small nasal passages of infants easily blocked by mucosal swelling and exudation
Can interfere with respiration and feeding in infants
May contribute to the development of otitis media and sinusitis

NASAL DISCHARGE
Frequently accompanies respiratory infections
May be thin and watery (rhinorrhea) or thick and purulent
  Depends on the type and/or stage of infection
Associated with itching
May irritate upper lip and skin surrounding the nose

COUGH
Common feature of respiratory disease
May be evident only during the acute phase
May persist several months after a disease

RESPIRATORY SOUNDS
Sounds associated with respiratory disease:
  Cough
  Hoarseness
  Grunting
  Stridor
  Wheezing
Auscultation:
  Wheezing
  Crackles
  Absence of sound

SORE THROAT
Frequent complaint of older children
Young children (unable to describe symptoms) may not complain even when highly inflamed
  Often, child will refuse to take oral fluids or solids
  Elastic nature of the tissues in young children may cause less pressure on nerve endings

7. Child will experience no complications.
8. Child and family will receive information, especially for home care, and support.

❖ IMPLEMENTATION

Ease Respiratory Efforts. Most acute respiratory infections are mild and cause few distressing symptoms. Although children may feel uncomfortable and have a "stuffy" nose and some mucosal swelling, respiratory distress is uncommon. The interventions described in the remainder of the discussion are usually sufficient to relieve most minor discomfort and ease respiratory efforts. However, children with croup or epiglottitis may develop sufficient swelling to obstruct the airway. These children are hospitalized for observation and therapy (see discussions of specific disorders). Positioning for optimum respiration and observation for signs of respiratory distress are primary nursing interventions.

The atmosphere in homes heated during the winter months is often very dry. Warm or cool mist has been a common therapeutic measure for symptomatic relief of respiratory discomfort. The moisture soothes inflamed membranes and seems to be especially beneficial when there is hoarseness or any laryngeal involvement. Mist tents are frequently used in the hospital for humidifying the air and relieving discomfort. However, use of steam vaporizers in the home should be discouraged because of the hazards related to their use and the little evidence to support their efficacy. Alternate measures are available, such as humidification systems. Shallow pans with wide surface areas for evaporation increase humidity but should be placed where they do not pose a safety hazard.

COMPONENTS FOR ASSESSING RESPIRATORY FUNCTION

RESPIRATIONS

The pattern of respirations is observed for rate, depth, ease, and rhythm of breathing:

Rate—Rapid (tachypnea), normal, or slow for the particular child

Depth—Normal depth, too shallow (hypopnea), too deep (hyperpnea); usually estimated from the amplitude of thoracic and abdominal excursion

Ease—Effortless, labored (dyspnea), orthopnea, associated with intercostal and/or substernal retractions (inspiratory "sinking in" of soft tissues in relation to the cartilaginous and bony thorax), pulsus paradoxus (blood pressure falls with inspiration and rises with expiration), flaring nares, head bobbing (head of sleeping child with suboccipital area supported on caregiver's forearm bobs forward in synchrony with each inspiration), grunting, or wheezing

Labored breathing—Continuous, intermittent, becoming steadily worse, sudden onset, at rest or on exertion, associated with wheezing, grunting, associated with pain

Rhythm—Variation in rate and depth of respirations

OTHER OBSERVATIONS

In addition to respirations, particular attention is addressed to the following:

Evidence of infection—Check for elevated temperature, enlarged cervical lymph nodes, inflamed mucous membranes, and purulent discharges from the nose, ears, or lungs (sputum)

Cough—Observe the characteristics of the cough (if present); for example, under what circumstances the cough is heard (e.g., night only, on arising), the nature of the cough (paroxysmal with or without wheeze, "croupy" or "brassy"), frequency of cough, associated with swallowing or other activity, character of the cough (moist and dry), productivity

Wheeze—Expiratory or inspiratory, high-pitched or musical, prolonged, slowly progressive or sudden, associated with labored breathing

Cyanosis—Note distribution (peripheral, perioral, facial, trunk as well as face), degree, duration, associated with activity

Chest pain—May be a complaint of older children. Note location and circumstances: localized or generalized, referred to base of neck or abdomen, dull or sharp, deep or superficial, associated with rapid, shallow respirations or grunting

Sputum—Older children may provide sputum sample by coughing, whereas young children may need use of bulb suction to provide a sample. Note volume, color, viscosity, and odor

Bad breath—May be associated with some lung infections

A time-honored method of producing steam is the shower. Running a shower of hot water into the empty bathtub or open shower stall with the bathroom door closed produces a quick source of steam. Keeping a child in this environment for 10 to 15 minutes offers the same advantages as the mist tent without the fear and restraint often associated with the confines of a tent. A small child can be held on the lap of a parent or other adult. Older children can sit in the bathroom under the supervision of an adult.

➤ **NURSING TIP** A large, wet beach towel hung with one end in shallow water in the bathtub will increase humidity if the bathroom door remains open.

Promote Rest. Children who have an acute febrile illness should be placed on bed rest. This is usually not difficult while the temperature is elevated but may be difficult when children, particularly young children, feel fairly well. When parents take the advice seriously and consistently keep them in bed, most children learn to cooperate during illness. Often children are more apt to comply if they are allowed to lie quietly on a couch where they can watch television or participate in an alternate quiet activity. If children are unreasoning and expend an inordinate amount of energy in protest, allowing them to play quietly on the floor serves the purpose of rest better than allowing them to cry excessively in bed. A number of entertainment devices, based on individual interests, can be used to keep children quiet.

Promote Comfort. Older children are usually able to manage nasal secretions with little difficulty. Parents are instructed about the correct administration of nose drops and throat irrigations, if ordered. For very young infants, who normally breathe through their noses, an infant nasal aspirator or a rubber ear syringe is helpful in removing nasal secretions before feeding. This practice, followed by instillation of saline nose drops, may be all that is necessary to clear nasal passages and promote feeding. Saline nose drops can be prepared at home by dissolving 1 teaspoon of salt in 1 pint of warm water.*

For older infants and children who can better tolerate decongestants, vasoconstrictive nose drops may be administered 15 to 20 minutes before feeding and at bedtime. Two drops are instilled, and since this shrinks only the anterior mucous membranes, 2 more drops are instilled 5 to 10 minutes later. Phenylephrine (Neo-Synephrine) 0.25% is the usual choice of decongestant nose drops, although others, such as ephedrine 1%, may be prescribed. Older cooperative children often prefer nasal sprays. They are taught to compress the plastic container at the moment of inspiration to gain relief. Spray bottles and bottles of nose drops should be used for one child only and only for one illness, since they become easily contaminated with bacteria. Nose drops or sprays should not be administered for more than 3 days to avoid rebound congestion.

Hot or cold applications sometimes provide relief for other children with painful cervical adenitis. An ice bag or heating pad applied to the neck may decrease the discomfort, but safety precautions must be observed to prevent burns. The ice bag or heating device must be covered, and the heating pad should not be set at high ranges.

Prevent Spread of Infection. Careful handwashing should be carried out when caring for children with respiratory infections. Children and families are taught the correct disposal of respiratory secretions and proper behavior related to airborne droplets (coughing and sneezing). They

*Home care instructions for administration of nose drops and nasal aspiration are available in *Wong and Whaley's Clinical Manual of Pediatric Nursing* (Mosby).

are taught to use a tissue or their hand to cover their nose and mouth when they cough or sneeze and to dispose of the tissues properly, as well as wash their hands.

Every endeavor should be made to remove affected children from contact with other children. Ideally, ill children should be isolated in a separate bedroom at the first sign of illness. This is seldom a problem with an only child but is often difficult when living arrangements are crowded and there are several children in the family. If no separate bedroom is available, the other children perhaps could sleep on a couch or cot, or with relatives or friends. An effort should be made to teach well children to stay away from ill children if the living conditions allow for segregation, although this may be difficult or impossible to enforce.

Reduce Temperature. If the child has a significantly elevated temperature, controlling the fever becomes a major nursing task. The parent should know how to take a child's temperature and read the thermometer accurately. Most parents are able to do this, but nurses cannot make this assumption. Those who cannot will require instruction in use of the thermometer.*

If the practitioner has prescribed acetaminophen, parents may need help administering the drug. Most parents can read the label and calculate the desired dose, but some have difficulty and will require careful instruction or precise direction.* It is important to emphasize accuracy in both the amount of drug given and the time intervals at which the drug is administered in order to avoid accumulation effects. Cool liquids are encouraged to help reduce the temperature and to minimize the chances of dehydration. (See Controlling Elevated Temperatures, Chapter 27.)

Promote Hydration. Dehydration is always a hazard when children are febrile or anorexic, especially when vomiting or diarrhea is also present. Adequate fluid intake should be encouraged by offering small amounts of favorite fluids at frequent intervals. High-calorie liquids, such as colas, fruit juices, water flavored and sweetened with corn syrup, or similar drinks, help prevent catabolism and dehydration but should be avoided if diarrhea is present. Oral rehydration solutions, such as Infalyte or Pedialyte, should then be considered for infants, and sports drinks, such as Gatorade or Exceed, should be considered for older children. Fluids should not be forced, and children should not be awakened to take fluids. Forcing fluids may create the same difficulties as urging unwanted food. Gentle persuasion with preferred beverages will usually be successful.

Parents should know how to assess their child's level of hydration (see Chapter 28). They are advised to observe the frequency of voiding and notify the nurse or practitioner if there appears to be insufficient voiding.

➤ **NURSING TIP** Counting the number of wet diapers in a 24-hour period is a satisfactory method of assessing output in infants and toddlers.

Provide Nutrition. Loss of appetite is characteristic of children with acute infections, and in most cases, children can be permitted to determine their own need for food. Many children show no decrease in appetite, and others respond well to certain foods, such as gelatin, soup, and puddings (see also Feeding the Sick Child, Chapter 27). Since the illness is relatively short, the nutritional state is seldom compromised. In fact, urging foods on anorexic children may precipitate nausea and vomiting and in some cases even cause an aversion to the feeding situation that can extend into the convalescent period and beyond.

Family Support and Home Care. Small children with respiratory infections are irritable and often difficult to comfort. Therefore the family needs support, encouragement, and practical suggestions for care. Since most care involves comfort measures and administration of medication, a primary goal of education is related to these activities.

In addition to antipyretics and nose drops, the child may require antibiotic therapy. It is usually the nurse who instructs the parents about continuing medication begun in the hospital or initiating medications at home, especially antibiotics. Parents of children who are sent home with oral antibiotics need to understand the importance of regular administration and continuing the drug for the prescribed length of time, regardless of whether the child appears to be ill.

Parents are also cautioned against giving the child any medications that are not approved by the health practitioner. Adverse effects have been noted in children who have received some preparations intended for adults (e.g., some long-acting nose drops [Neo-Synephrine II] and dextromethorphan cough squares [mistaken for candy]). They are also cautioned about giving the child unprescribed antibiotics left over from a previous illness. Self-medication with unprescribed antibiotics is a significant problem. It should be emphasized that some drugs interact with others to produce serious side effects, and such a likelihood is increased when medications are administered to children without consultation with the practitioner. The nurse is in an excellent position to provide drug information to families. (See Chapter 27 for administration of medications and teaching parents.)

❖ EVALUATION

The effectiveness of nursing interventions is determined by continual reassessment and evaluation of care based on the following observational guidelines and expected outcomes:

1. Observe child's respiratory effort and movement.
2. Observe signs and symptoms for progress toward status before illness.
3. Observe child's behavior and activity.
4. Observe other family members and contacts for evidence of infection.
5. Take temperature.
6. Observe for signs of adequate hydration.
7. Observe eating behavior.
8. Assess child for evidence of complications, such as dehydration, weight loss, or spread of infection to other areas of the body.
9. Observe family's behavior and interview members regarding their feelings and concerns.

*Home care instructions for measuring temperature and administration of medication are available in *Wong and Whaley's Clinical Manual of Pediatric Nursing* (Mosby).

NURSING CARE PLAN
The Child with Acute Respiratory Infection

NURSING DIAGNOSIS: Ineffective breathing pattern related to inflammatory process

PATIENT GOAL 1: Will exhibit normal respiratory function

• **NURSING INTERVENTIONS/*RATIONALES***

Position for maximum ventilation (i.e., open airway and permit maximum lung expansion)

Allow position of comfort (e.g., tripod position of child with epiglottitis or maintain head elevation of at least 30 degrees)

Check child's position frequently to ensure child does not slide down *to avoid compressing the diaphragm*

Avoid constricting clothing or bedding

Use pillows and padding to maintain open airway (e.g., in infant or child with hypotonia)

*Provide increased humidity and supplemental oxygen by placing child in small tent or hood (infant) or administer via nasal cannula or mask (prefered methods for children older than infancy because of safety issues)

Promote rest and sleep by scheduling appropriate activity and rest periods

Encourage relaxation techniques

Teach child and family measures to ease respiratory efforts (i.e., appropriate positioning)

For most respiratory illnesses use cool-mist humidifier in child's room

For spasmodic croup create warm mist by running hot water in a closed bathroom (warm mist, often used for children with spasmodic croup, may be helpful because of its relaxing effect, but mostly because child is being held upright in the shower)

• **EXPECTED OUTCOMES**

Respirations remain within normal limits (see inside back cover for normal variations)

Respirations are unlabored

Child rests and sleeps quietly

PATIENT GOAL 2: Will receive optimum oxygen supply

• **NURSING INTERVENTIONS/*RATIONALES***

Position for maximum ventilatory efficiency (see Goal 1, above)

Use pulse oximetry to monitor oxygen saturations

Place in a cool, humidified environment, using appropriate oxygen delivery system

*Provide oxygen as prescribed and/or needed

• **EXPECTED OUTCOMES**

Child breathes easily

Respirations remain within normal limits (see inside back cover for normal variations)

Oxygen saturation is ≥95%

NURSING DIAGNOSIS: Fear/anxiety related to difficulty breathing, unfamiliar procedures, and possibly environment (hospital)

PATIENT GOAL 1: Will experience reduction of fear/anxiety

• **NURSING INTERVENTIONS/*RATIONALES***

Explain unfamiliar procedures and equipment to child in developmentally appropriate terms

Establish rapport with child and parents

Remain with child during procedures

Use calm, reassuring manner

Provide frequent attendance during acute phase of illness

Provide comfort measures child prefers (e.g., rocking, stroking, music)

Provide attachment objects (e.g., familiar toy, blanket)

Encourage family-centered care with increased parental attendance and, when possible, involvement

Do nothing to make child more anxious or fearful

Instill confidence in both parents and child

Try to avoid any intrusive or painful procedures

Be aware of child's rest/sleep cycle or pattern in planning nursing activities

Assess and implement appropriate pain management therapy (i.e., sedatives and/or analgesics) (see Pain Assessment; Pain Management, Chapter 26).

Provide diversional activities appropriate to child's cognitive ability and condition

*Administer medications that promote improved ventilation (e.g., bronchodilators, expectorants) as prescribed

• **EXPECTED OUTCOMES**

Child exhibits no signs of respiratory distress or physical discomfort

Parents remain with child and provide comfort

Child engages in quiet activities appropriate for age, interest, condition, and cognitive level

NURSING DIAGNOSIS: Ineffective airway clearance related to mechanical obstruction, inflammation, increased secretions, pain

PATIENT GOAL 1: Will maintain patent airway

• **NURSING INTERVENTIONS/*RATIONALES***

Position child in proper body alignment *to allow better lung expansion and improved gas exchange, as well as to prevent aspiration of secretions (prone, semiprone, side lying)*

Suction secretions from airway as needed

Limit each suction attempt to 5 seconds with sufficient time between attempts to allow reoxygenation

Position supine with head in "sniffing" position with neck slightly extended and nose pointed to ceiling

Avoid neck hyperextension

*Dependent nursing action.

Continued.

NURSING CARE PLAN
The Child with Acute Respiratory Infection—cont'd

Assist child in expectorating sputum
Administer expectorants if prescribed
Perform chest physiotherapy
Give nothing by mouth *to prevent aspiration of fluids* (e.g., child with severe tachypnea)
*Administer appropriate pain management
Have emergency equipment available *to avoid delay in treatment if needed*
Avoid throat examination and culture with suspected epiglottitis, *because it could cause airway obstruction*
Assist child in splinting any incisional/injured area *to maximize effects of coughing and chest physiotherapy*

• **EXPECTED OUTCOMES**
Airways remain clear
Child breathes easily; respirations are within normal limits (see inside back cover)

PATIENT GOAL 2: Will expectorate secretions adequately

• **NURSING INTERVENTIONS/*RATIONALES***
Ensure adequate fluid intake *to liquefy secretions*
Provide humidified atmosphere *to prevent crusting of nasal secretions and drying of mucous membranes*
Explain importance of expectoration to child and family
Assist child in coughing effectively; provide tissues
Remove accumulated mucus; suction if needed
*Administer pain medications as indicated before attempt to clear airway
Provide nebulization with appropriate solution and equipment as prescribed
Assist with splinting *so child will experience minimal discomfort*
*Perform percussion, vibration, and postural drainage *to facilitate drainage of secretions*

• **EXPECTED OUTCOME**
Older child expectorates secretions without undue stress and fatigue; younger child will be able to have a productive cough

NURSING DIAGNOSIS: High risk for infection related to presence of infective organisms

PATIENT GOAL 1: Will exhibit no signs of secondary infection

• **NURSING INTERVENTIONS/*RATIONALES***
Maintain aseptic environment, using sterile suction catheters and good handwashing
Isolate child as indicated *to prevent nosocomial spread of infection*
Administer antibiotics as prescribed *to prevent or treat infection*
Provide nutritious diet according to child's preferences and ability to consume nourishment *to support body's natural defenses*
Encourage good chest physiotherapy
Teach child and/or family manifestations of illness

• **EXPECTED OUTCOME**
Child exhibits evidence of diminishing symptoms of infection

PATIENT GOAL 2: Will not spread infection to others

• **NURSING INTERVENTIONS/*RATIONALES***
Use universal precautions (see Infection Control, Chapter 27)
Instruct others (parents, members of staff) in appropriate precautions
Teach affected children protective methods to prevent spread of infection (e.g., handwashing, disposal of soiled tissues)
Limit the number of visitors/family members/siblings and screen for any recent illness
Try to keep infants and small children from placing hands and objects in contaminated areas
Assess home situation and implement protective measures as feasible in individual circumstances
*Administer antimicrobial medications if prescribed

• **EXPECTED OUTCOME**
Others remain free from infection

NURSING DIAGNOSIS: Activity intolerance related to inflammatory process, imbalance between oxygen supply and demand

PATIENT GOAL 1: Will maintain adequate energy levels

• **NURSING INTERVENTIONS/*RATIONALES***
Assess child's level of physical tolerance
Assist child in those activities of daily living that may be beyond tolerance
Provide diversional activities appropriate to child's age, condition, capabilities, and interest
Provide diversional play activities that promote rest and quiet but prevent boredom and withdrawal
Provide rest and sleep periods appropriate to age and condition
Instruct child to rest when feeling tired
Balance rest and activity when ambulatory

• **EXPECTED OUTCOMES**
Child plays and rests quietly and engages in activities appropriate to age and capabilities (specify)
Child exhibits no evidence of increased respiratory distress
Child tolerates increasingly more activity

PATIENT GOAL 2: Will receive optimum rest

• **NURSING INTERVENTIONS/*RATIONALES***
Provide quiet environment
Organize activities for maximum sleep time
Do not perform nonessential treatments or procedures *to maximize rest*

*Dependent nursing action.

NURSING CARE PLAN
The Child with Acute Respiratory Infection—cont'd

Schedule visiting to allow for sufficient rest
Encourage parents to remain with child
Schedule treatments or other activities around the needs of the child *so that fatigue will be minimized.*
*Administer sedatives and analgesics as indicated if ordered for restlessness and pain
Encourage frequent rest periods and regular sleep times
Follow child's usual routine for bedtime and nap time
Implement measures to ensure sleep, such as quiet, darkened room

• **EXPECTED OUTCOMES**
Child remains calm, quiet, and relaxed
Child rests a sufficient amount (specify)

NURSING DIAGNOSIS: Pain related to inflammatory process, surgical incision

PATIENT GOAL 1: Will experience no pain or reduction of pain/discomfort to level acceptable to child

• **NURSING INTERVENTIONS/*RATIONALES***
Use local measures (gargles, troches, warmth or cold) to reduce throat pain
Apply heat or cold as appropriate to affected area
Administer analgesic as prescribed (see Pain Management, Chapter 26)
Assess response to pain control measures (see Pain Assessment, Chapter 26)
Encourage diversional activities appropriate to age, condition, capabilities

*Dependent nursing action.

• **EXPECTED OUTCOME**
Child has no pain or acceptable level of pain

NURSING DIAGNOSIS: Altered family process related to illness and/or hospitalization of a child

PATIENT (FAMILY) GOAL 1: Will experience reduction of anxiety and increased ability to cope

• **NURSING INTERVENTIONS/*RATIONALES***
Recognize parental concern and need for information and support
Explore family's feelings and "problems" surrounding hospitalization and child's illness
Explain therapy and child's behavior
Provide support as needed
Encourage family-centered care and encourage family to become involved in their child's care

• **EXPECTED OUTCOME**
Parents ask appropriate questions, discuss child's condition and care calmly, and become involved positively in child's care

See also
Nursing Care Plan: The Family of the Ill or Hospitalized Child, Chapter 26
Nursing Care Plan: The Child in the Hospital, Chapter 26

Expected outcomes:
See Nursing Care Plan, pp. 1377-1379.

UPPER RESPIRATORY TRACT INFECTIONS (URIs)

ACUTE VIRAL NASOPHARYNGITIS

Acute nasopharyngitis (the equivalent of the "common cold") is caused by any of a number of different viruses, usually rhinoviruses, respiratory syncytial virus (RSV), adenovirus, influenza virus, or parainfluenza virus.

Clinical Manifestations

Symptoms of nasopharyngitis are more severe in infants and children than in adults. Fever is common, especially in young children. Older children have low-grade fevers, which appear early in the process. In children 3 months to 3 years, fevers occur suddenly and are associated with irritability, restlessness, and decreased appetite and activity. Nasal inflammation may lead to obstruction of passages, producing open-mouth breathing. Other symptoms (e.g., vomiting, diarrhea) may also be evident in some children.

The initial symptoms in older children are dryness and irritation of nasal passages and sometimes the pharynx, followed in a few hours by sneezing, chilly sensations, muscular aches, an irritating nasal discharge, and sometimes cough. Nasal inflammation may lead to obstruction, and continual wiping away of secretions causes skin irritation to nares.

The disease is self-limited and usually resolves within 4 to 10 days without complications. Occasionally, and especially if a fever recurs, a child might experience otitis media (particularly infants); this usually occurs early or after the initial phase of nasopharyngitis is past. Pneumonia is a less frequent complication; when it does occur, it is usually observed more often in infants.

Therapeutic Management

Children with nasopharyngitis are managed at home. There is no specific treatment, and effective vaccines are not available. Antipyretics are usually prescribed for mild fever and discomfort (see Chapter 27 for management of fever). Decongestants may be prescribed for children and infants over 6 months of age in an effort to shrink swollen nasal passages. The decongestants that exert their effect by vasoconstriction are usually less effective when taken orally than when applied topically as nose drops. Since these drugs affect *all* vascular beds, they should be given with caution to children with diabetes.

Cough suppressants containing dextromethorphan may be prescribed for a dry, hacking cough. Some preparations contain up to 22% alcohol; they should not be administered to young children continuously and must be stored securely away from children.

Antihistamines are largely ineffective in treatment of nasopharyngitis. The drugs have a weak atropine-like effect that tends to dry secretions, but they can cause drowsiness and, paradoxically, have a stimulatory effect on children. There is no support for the usefulness of expectorants, and antibiotics are usually contraindicated because they can sensitize a child who may need the drugs in a severe illness.

Prevention. Nasopharyngitis is so widespread in the general population that it is impossible to prevent. In addition, children are more susceptible to colds because they have not yet developed resistance to many types of viruses. Very young infants are subject to relatively serious complications; therefore some attempt should be made to protect them from exposure. Rest is recommended until the child is free of fever for at least 1 day.

Nursing Considerations

A cold is often the parents' first introduction to an illness in their infants. Parents are assisted in managing the infant or child as described for general care. Most of the distress of nasopharyngitis is related to the nasal obstruction, especially in small infants. Placing the child in a prone position (unless respirations are compromised) and elevating the head of bed (assists with drainage of secretions), suctioning, and vaporization may help provide relief. Saline nose drops and gentle suction with a bulb syringe, particularly before feeding, are sometimes useful.

Maintaining adequate fluid intake is essential during any infectious process. Although a child's appetite for solid foods is usually diminished for several days, it is important to offer favorite fluids to prevent dehydration. Fluids can be cool or warm, depending on individual preference. See Nursing Considerations, p. 1381, for other interventions.

Because nasopharyngitis is spread from secretions, the best means for prevention is avoiding contact with affected persons. This goal is difficult in places where large numbers of people are confined in a small area for a long time, such as classrooms. Family members with a cold should try to "keep it to themselves" by carefully disposing of tissues; not sharing towels, glasses, or eating utensils; covering the mouth and nose with tissues when coughing or sneezing; and washing the hands thoroughly after nose blowing or sneezing. The most frequent carriers of infection are the human hands, which deposit viruses on doorknobs, faucets, and other everyday objects. Therefore children should be taught to wash their hands thoroughly before putting them near their nose, mouth, or eyes.

Family Support. Support and reassurance are important elements of care for families of young children with recurrent URIs. Because URIs are so frequent in children less than 3 years of age, families may feel they are on an endless roller coaster of illness. They can be reassured that frequent colds are a normal part of childhood and that by 5 years of age, their children will have developed immunity to many viruses. Parents who work outside the home should expect to have to take time off to care for ill children during the fall and winter months. If the children are cared for routinely in daycare centers, the infection rate will be higher than if they were being cared for in the home. Parents should know the signs of respiratory complications and be counseled to notify a health professional if any signs of complications appear or if the child does not improve within 2 or 3 days (see box above).

EARLY EVIDENCE OF RESPIRATORY COMPLICATIONS

Parents are instructed to notify the health professional if any of the following are noted:
- Evidence of earache (see p. 1387)
- Respirations faster than 50 to 60 per minute
- Fever over 101° F
- Listlessness
- Increasing irritability with or without fever
- Persistent cough 2 days or more
- Wheezing
- Crying
- Refusal to eat
- Restlessness and poor sleep patterns

Modified from National Association of Pediatric Nurse Associates and Practitioners (NAPNAP): *Baby's first cold,* New York, 1989, Winthrop Consumer Products. Copies available from NAPNAP, 1101 Kings Hwy., N., No. 206, Cherry Hill, NJ 08034; (609) 667-1773.

ACUTE STREPTOCOCCAL PHARYNGITIS

Group A β-hemolytic streptococci (GABHS) infection of the upper airway (strep throat) is not in itself a serious disease, but affected children are at risk for serious sequelae: acute rheumatic fever (ARF), an inflammatory disease of heart, joints, and central nervous system (see Chapter 34), and acute glomerulonephritis, an acute kidney infection (see Chapter 30). Permanent damage can result from these sequelae, especially ARF, which has demonstrated a recent resurgence in the United States. However, only 21% to 50% of children with streptococcal infections have a history of pharyngitis, and by 15 years of age the likelihood that group A is responsible is only about 15% (McMillan, 1988).

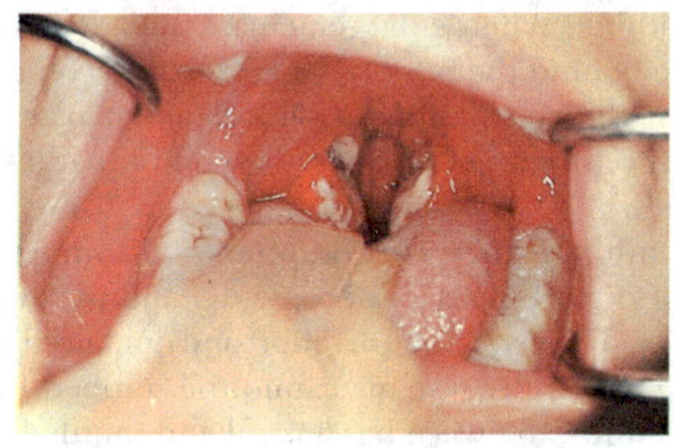

FIG. 32-1 Tonsillitis and pharyngitis. (From Thompson JM and others: *Clinical nursing*, St Louis, 1986, Mosby.)

Clinical Manifestations

GABHS is generally a relatively brief illness that varies greatly in severity from subclinical (no symptoms) to comparatively severe toxicity. The onset is generally abrupt and characterized by pharyngitis, headache, fever, and (especially in small children) abdominal pain. The tonsils and pharynx may be inflamed and covered with exudate (50% to 80% of cases) (Fig. 32-1), which usually appears by the second day of illness. Anterior cervical lymphadenopathy (30% to 50% of cases) usually occurs early, and the nodes are often tender. Pain can be relatively mild to severe enough to make swallowing difficult. Clinical manifestations usually subside in 3 to 5 days unless complicated by sinusitis or parapharyngeal, peritonsillar, or retropharyngeal abscess. Nonsuppurative complications may appear after the onset of GABHS—acute nephritis in about 10 days and rheumatic fever in an average of 18 days (Feigin, 1990).

Diagnostic Evaluation

Clinical diagnosis of GABHS infection can present difficulties. Although 80% to 90% of all cases of acute pharyngitis are viral, a throat culture should be performed to rule out GABHS and (in some cases) *Corynebacterium diphtheriae.* Because some children normally harbor streptococci in their throats, a positive culture is not always conclusive evidence of active disease. Since most streptococcal infections are short-term illnesses, antibody (antistreptolysin O) responses do not appear until relatively late and are useful only for retrospective diagnosis.

Rapid identification of GABHS is possible with diagnostic test kits that can be used in the office or clinic setting. However, because of their questionable sensitivity, they are not yet considered to be a substitute for culture, especially if the organism is endemic in the community.

Therapeutic Management

If streptococcal sore throat infection is present, oral penicillin is prescribed in a dose sufficient to control the acute local manifestations and to maintain an adequate level for at least 10 days to eliminate any organisms that might remain to initiate rheumatic fever symptoms. Penicillin does not appear to prevent the development of acute glomerulonephritis in susceptible children; however, it may prevent the spread of a nephrogenic strain of GABHS to others in the family. Penicillin usually produces a prompt response within 24 hours. Occasionally patients require retreatment if the organism is not eradicated.

A combination of penicillin and rifampin is more effective in eradicating GABHS than penicillin alone and is recommended for carriers and persons resistant to penicillin. Erythromycin or a cephalosporin may be used for children who are sensitive to penicillin. Manifestations are treated symptomatically.

Nursing Considerations

The nurse is often the person who performs a throat smear for culture and instructs the parents about administering penicillin and analgesics as prescribed. Most children prefer to remain in bed during the acute phase of the illness. Cold or warm compresses to the neck may provide relief. In children old enough to cooperate, warm saline gargles offer some relief of throat discomfort. Pain may interfere with oral intake, and the child should not be forced to eat. Cool liquids or ice chips are usually more acceptable than solids and are encouraged.

Special emphasis is placed on correct administration of oral medication and completing the course of antibiotic (see Administration of Medication, Chapter 27, and Compliance, Chapter 27). If injections are required, they must be administered deep into a large muscle mass (e.g., the vastus lateralis or gluteus muscle). Parents need to be aware of the residual tenderness, which may cause the child to limp for a day or two. Local applications of heat are helpful in relieving some of the discomfort.

Prevention. No satisfactory method of immunization is available for prevention of streptococcal disease. The organism is spread by close contact with affected persons—direct projection of large droplets or physical transfer of respiratory secretions containing the organism. As a result, spread of infection is common in families, classrooms, and daycare centers. Children with streptococcal infection are noninfectious to others within a few hours after initiation of antibiotic therapy. The streptococcus is not virulent when dried but is acquired from close droplet transmission; therefore, fomites are not usually a hazard.

It is important to know when the organism is epidemic in the community so that families can be on the alert for symptoms. Directors of daycare centers and school officials should share infectious disease information with parents. Obtaining throat cultures from children who are close family contacts of patients with streptococcal infection is advised. The administration of antibiotics before the onset of symptoms prevents most cases of streptococcal disease.

TONSILLITIS

The tonsils are masses of lymphoid tissue located in the pharyngeal cavity. Their function is to filter and protect the respiratory and alimentary tracts from invasion by pathogenic organisms. They also may have a role in antibody formation. Although the size of tonsils varies, children generally

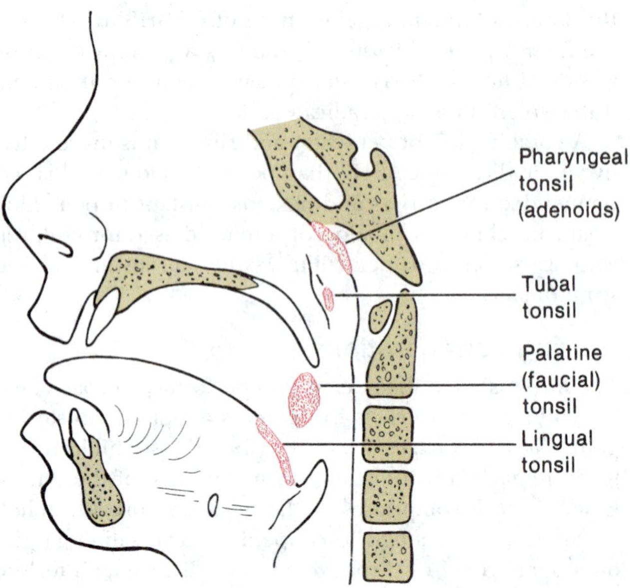

FIG. 32-2 Location of various tonsillar masses.

have much larger tonsils than adolescents or adults. This difference is thought to be a protective mechanism at a time when young children are especially susceptible to URI.

Pathophysiology

Several pairs of tonsils are part of a mass of lymphoid tissue encircling the nasal and oral pharynx, known as ***Waldeyer tonsillar ring*** (Fig. 32-2). The ***palatine,*** or ***faucial, tonsils*** are located on either side of the oropharynx, behind and below the pillars of the fauces (opening from the mouth). A free surface of the palatine tonsils is usually visible during oral examination. The palatine tonsils are those removed during tonsillectomy. The ***pharyngeal tonsils,*** also known as the ***adenoids,*** are located above the palatine tonsils on the posterior wall of the nasopharynx. Their proximity to the nares and eustachian tubes causes difficulties in instances of inflammation. The ***lingual tonsils*** are located at the base of the tongue and only rarely are removed. The ***tubal tonsils,*** found near the posterior nasopharyngeal opening of the eustachian tubes, are not part of the Waldeyer tonsillar ring.

Etiology

Tonsillitis usually occurs in association with pharyngitis. Because of the abundant lymphoid tissue and the frequency of URIs, tonsillitis is a very common cause of morbidity in young children. The causative agent may be viral or bacterial.

Clinical Manifestations

The manifestations of tonsillitis are chiefly caused by inflammation. As the palatine tonsils enlarge from edema, they may meet in the midline (kissing tonsils), obstructing the passage of air or food. The child has difficulty swallowing and breathing. When enlargement of the adenoids occurs, the space behind the posterior nares may become blocked, making it difficult or impossible for air to pass from the nose to the throat. As a result, the child breathes through the mouth.

If mouth breathing is continuous, the mucous membranes of the oropharynx become dry and irritated. There may be an offensive mouth odor and impaired senses of taste and smell. Because air cannot be trapped for proper speech sounds, the voice has a nasal and muffled quality. A persistent, harassing cough is also common. Because of the proximity of the adenoids to the eustachian tubes, this passageway is frequently blocked by swollen adenoids, interfering with normal drainage and frequently resulting in otitis media and/or difficulty hearing.

Therapeutic Management

The diagnosis is established from visual examination of the throat. Most children with tonsillitis respond to medical treatment. However, a significant number undergo surgical intervention, although the exact criteria for this common procedure are controversial.

Medical. Since the illness is self-limiting, treatment of viral pharyngitis is symptomatic. Throat cultures positive for GABHS infection warrant antibiotic treatment. It is important to differentiate between viral and streptococcal infection in febrile exudative tonsillitis. Since the majority of infections are of viral origin, early rapid tests can eliminate unnecessary antibiotic administration. In general, viral tonsillitis has been found to be more common in children younger than 3 years of age and GABHS more common in children 6 years or older (Putto, 1987).

Surgical. Surgical treatment of chronic tonsillitis is a very controversial subject. Many authorities believe that most of these surgeries are unwarranted. Others, who have seen children improve measurably after tonsillectomy and adenoidectomy, continue to recommend it for selected patients. There is a small number of severely affected children for whom surgery is clearly indicated, a larger number for whom it is not indicated, and a considerable number who fall between these two extremes. These are the children over whom most of the controversy occurs.

Tonsillectomy (removal of the palatine tonsils) is indicated for massive hypertrophy that results in difficulty breathing or eating. Absolute indications are malignancy and obstruction of the airway that result in cor pulmonale. ***Adenoidectomy*** (removal of the adenoids) is recommended for those children in whom hypertrophied adenoids obstruct nasal breathing. Their removal may be warranted in the child under 3 years of age and should be performed without a tonsillectomy. Follow-up after adenoidectomy should include assessment of hearing, smell, and taste for expected improvement. Contraindications to either tonsillectomy or adenoidectomy are (1) cleft palate, since both tonsils help minimize escape of air during speech; (2) acute infections at the time of surgery, since the locally inflamed tissues increase the risk of bleeding; and (3) uncontrolled systemic diseases or blood dyscrasias.

Generally, removal of the tonsils should occur after 3 or

4 years of age because of the problem of excessive blood loss in small children and the possibility of regrowth or hypertrophy of lymphoid tissue. The tubal and lingual tonsils often enlarge to compensate for the lost lymphoid tissue, resulting in continued pharyngeal and eustachian tube obstruction.

Nursing Considerations

Nursing care of the child with tonsillitis mainly involves providing comfort and minimizing activities or interventions that might precipitate bleeding. A soft to liquid diet is generally preferred. A cool-mist vaporizer helps keep the mucous membranes moist during periods of mouth breathing. Warm salt-water gargles, throat lozenges, and analgesic/antipyretic drugs such as acetaminophen (Tylenol) are useful to promote comfort.

If surgery is needed, the child requires the same psychologic preparation and physical care as for any other procedure (see Chapters 26 and 27). The following discussion focuses on specific nursing care for tonsillectomy and adenoidectomy (T & A), although both procedures may not be performed.

A complete history is taken, with special notation of any bleeding tendencies, since the operative site is highly vascular. Baseline vital signs are important for postoperative monitoring and observation. Signs of any URI are noted and reported, and bleeding and clotting times are included in the usual laboratory work requests. During physical assessment the presence of any loose teeth is noted. (See also Surgical Procedures, Chapter 27.)

Until they are fully awake, children are placed on the abdomen or side to facilitate drainage of secretions, and any needed suctioning is performed carefully to avoid trauma to the oropharynx. When alert, children may prefer sitting up, although they should remain in bed for the remainder of the day. They are discouraged from coughing frequently, clearing their throat, and blowing their nose, any of which may aggravate the operative site.

Some secretions are common, particularly dried blood from surgery. All secretions and vomitus are inspected for evidence of fresh bleeding (some blood-tinged mucus is expected). Dark-brown (old) blood is usually present in the emesis, as well as in the nose and between the teeth. If parents do not expect this, they may be frightened at a time when they need to be calm and reassuring for their children.

The throat is very sore after surgery. An ice collar may provide relief, but many children find it bothersome and prefer not to have it. Most children experience moderate pain after a T &/or A and should receive pain medication for at least the first 24 hours (Rauen and Holman, 1989). Analgesics are ordered but may need to be given rectally or intravenously to avoid the oral route. Since pain is continuous, pain control should be continuous or administered at regular intervals (see Pain Management, Chapter 26). Irritable children may require mild sedation to lessen crying, which irritates the operative site, increasing the chance of bleeding.

Food and fluid are restricted until children are fully alert and there are no signs of hemorrhage. Cool water, crushed ice, flavored ice pops, or dilute fruit juice is given first, although fluids with a red or brown color are avoided to distinguish fresh or old blood in emesis from the ingested liquid. Citrus juice may cause discomfort and is usually poorly tolerated. Milk, ice cream, or pudding is not offered until clear fluids are retained, because milk products coat the mouth and throat, causing the child to clear the throat more often, which may initiate bleeding. Soft foods, particularly gelatin, cooked fruits, sherbet, soup, and mashed potatoes, are started on the first or second postoperative day or as the child tolerates feeding. The pain from surgery often inhibits intake, reinforcing the need for adequate pain control.

Postoperative hemorrhage is unusual but can occur. Therefore the nurse observes the throat directly for evidence of bleeding, using a good source of light and, if necessary, carefully inserting a tongue depressor. Other signs of hemorrhage are increased pulse (greater than 120 beats/min), pallor, frequent clearing of the throat or swallowing by a younger child, and vomiting of bright-red blood. Restlessness, an indication of hemorrhage, may be difficult to differentiate from general discomfort after surgery. Decreasing blood pressure is a much later sign of shock and usually indicates at least 8% to 10% fluid volume loss.

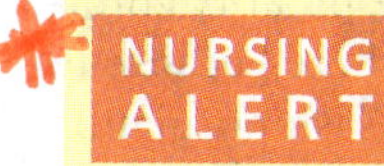

The most obvious early sign of bleeding is the child's continuous swallowing of the trickling blood. While the child is sleeping, the frequency of swallowing is noted.

If continuous bleeding is suspected, the physician is notified immediately, since a child can lose a considerable amount of blood before overt signs of blood loss are observed. Surgery may be required to ligate a bleeding vessel. Airway obstruction may occur as a result of edema or accumulated secretions and is indicated by signs of respiratory distress, such as stridor, drooling, restlessness or agitation, increasing respiratory rate, and, if severe, progressive cyanosis. Suction equipment and oxygen should be available after tonsillectomy.

Family Support and Home Care. Discharge instructions include (1) avoiding foods that are irritating or highly seasoned, (2) avoiding the use of gargles or vigorous toothbrushing, (3) discouraging the child from coughing or clearing the throat or putting objects in the mouth, (4) using mild analgesics or an ice collar for pain, and (5) limiting activity to decrease the potential for bleeding. Hemorrhage may occur up to 10 days after surgery as a result of tissue sloughing from the healing process. Any sign of bleeding warrants immediate medical attention. Objectionable mouth odor and slight ear pain with a low-grade fever are common for a few days postoperatively. However, persistent severe earache, fever, or cough requires medical evaluation. Most children are ready to resume normal activity within 1 to 2 weeks after the operation.

A T &/or A often represents the first hospitalization experience for the child and family. Since the surgery is usually an elective procedure, there is ample opportunity to prepare both children and parents for this event. Both need reassurance about what to expect at the time of admission, before and after surgery, and at discharge. Some children (usually older children) will be admitted as a "same-day surgery" and be discharged home after a recovery period. Others will remain in the hospital; for those, parents are encouraged to visit often or room-in if possible and participate in their child's care. Children are honestly apprised of postoperative discomfort and reassured that they will be able to talk. Sometimes children believe that the procedure will immediately "make the throat all better" and are dismayed to find that it still hurts after the surgery. Ideally, children should have an opportunity to discuss the experiences to gain a feeling of mastery and to overcome any fears or misconceptions. (See also Nursing Care Plan: The Child with a Tonsillectomy.*)

INFECTIOUS MONONUCLEOSIS

Infectious mononucleosis is an acute, self-limiting infectious disease that is common among young persons up to 25 years of age. The disease is characterized by an increase in the mononuclear elements of the blood and by general symptoms of an infectious process. The course is usually mild but occasionally can be severe or, rarely, accompanied by serious complications. Although not a respiratory condition, infectious mononucleosis is discussed here because its principal areas of involvement include the lymph glands, such as the tonsils, in the neck.

Etiology/Pathophysiology

The herpeslike ***Epstein-Barr (EB) virus*** is the principal cause of infectious mononucleosis. It appears in both sporadic and epidemic forms, the sporadic cases being more common. The mechanism of spread has not been proved, although it is believed to be transmitted by direct intimate contact with oral secretions. It also appears to be only mildly contagious, and the period of communicability is unknown. The incubation period following exposure is 4 to 6 weeks. There is enlargement of lymph nodes from mononuclear infiltration and variable infiltration of most body tissues.

Clinical Manifestations

The onset of symptoms of infectious mononucleosis appears anywhere from 10 days to 6 weeks after exposure and may be acute or insidious. The common presenting symptoms vary greatly in type, severity, and duration. The characteristics of the disease are malaise, sore throat, and fever with generalized lymphadenopathy and splenomegaly that may persist for several months. Most often the symptoms appear insidiously with fatigue, lack of energy, and sore throat that may not become prominent. The youngster's chief complaint is difficulty in maintaining the usual level of activity. This is often attributed to lack of sleep, a URI, or both. In many instances the manifestations never arouse enough concern to bring the affected individual to medical attention. Many cases of infectious mononucleosis are no doubt never recognized as such. The clinical manifestations of infectious mononucleosis are usually less severe (often subclinical or unapparent) and the convalescent phase is shorter in younger children than in older children and young adults. Many young children do not develop all the expected clinical and laboratory findings; often a complication is the only or presenting symptom.

A skin rash is present in a few cases, most often a discrete macular eruption most prominent over the trunk. More young children have rashes, and older children have abdominal pain. Other symptoms may include headache and epistaxis. The tonsils may be enlarged, reddened, and sometimes covered with a diphtheria-like membrane. The youngster may have a severe sore throat. Failure to thrive, otitis media, and episodes of recurrent tonsillopharyngitis are more closely associated with childhood disease. In about half of the cases, the spleen is enlarged, sometimes to the point of a risk of possible rupture. Hepatic involvement to some degree is almost always present, often associated with jaundice, which may cause the disease to be confused with infectious hepatitis. The extensive mononuclear infiltration produces symptoms related to any body tissue so that the clinical picture can resemble that of many conditions, including neurologic manifestations and cardiac involvement.

Diagnostic Evaluation

The diagnosis is established on the basis of clinical manifestations, absolute increase in atypical leukocytes in a peripheral blood smear, and a positive heterophil agglutination test. Differential diagnosis depends on the clinical symptoms present. For example, the pharyngitis may simulate symptoms of other diseases such as diphtheria and streptococcal pharyngitis. Lymphadenopathy, fever, and malaise are all characteristic of numerous disorders. Jaundice, nervous system manifestations, and skin eruptions each similarly indicate a variety of conditions. The leukocyte count may be normal or low, but usually lymphocyte leukocytosis develops.

The ***heterophil antibody test*** determines the extent to which the patient's serum will agglutinate sheep red blood cells. In infectious mononucleosis a titer of 1:160 is considered diagnostic, although a rising titer during the earlier stages is the best indicator. Because young children have a lower rate of heterophil antibody responses, the diagnosis may be overlooked in this group.

The ***spot test (Monospot),*** a slide test of high specificity, has been developed for the diagnosis of infectious mononucleosis. It is rapid, sensitive, inexpensive, and easy to perform, and it has the advantage that it can detect significant agglutinins at lower levels, thus permitting earlier diagnosis. Blood is usually obtained for the test by finger puncture and is placed on special paper. If the blood agglutinates, forming fragments or clumps, the test is positive for the infection.

Therapeutic Management

No specific treatment exists for infectious mononucleosis. Common symptoms are ordinarily relieved by simple rem-

---

*In *Wong and Whaley's Clinical Manual of Pediatric Nursing* (Mosby).

edies. A mild analgesic is usually sufficient to relieve the bothersome symptoms of headache, fever, and malaise. Bed rest is encouraged for fatigue but is not imposed for any specified time. Affected youngsters are instructed to regulate activities according to their own tolerance unless complicating factors are present. If the spleen is enlarged, for example, activities in which they might receive a blow to the abdomen or chest are avoided.

A short course of oral penicillin is sometimes prescribed for sore throat, especially if β-hemolytic streptococci are present. Administration of ampicillin frequently precipitates a maculopapular rash in affected persons; therefore its use is contraindicated. Sore throat, which can be severe, can be relieved by gargles, hot drinks, analgesic troches, or analgesics, including opioids. The use of corticosteroids has demonstrated effectiveness in reducing respiratory distress from tonsillar hypertrophy, hemolytic anemia, thrombocytopenia, and neurologic complications. Although steroids can shorten the course of the illness, their use is reserved for complicated cases.

Prognosis. The course of infectious mononucleosis is self-limiting and usually uncomplicated. Contrary to popular belief, mononucleosis is not necessarily a difficult, prolonged, disabling disease, and the prognosis is generally good. Acute symptoms usually disappear within 7 to 10 days, and the persistent fatigue subsides within 2 to 4 weeks. A number of affected youngsters may need to restrict activities for 2 to 3 months; the disease rarely extends for longer periods.

Complications are uncommon but can be serious and require appropriate management. Liver involvement is present to some degree in almost all cases and may become chronic. Neurologic complications are seen in some outbreaks and vary in severity and outcome. Other complications include pneumonitis, myocarditis, hemolytic anemia, thrombocytopenia, and ruptured spleen. Some evidence also indicates a depressed cellular immune reactivity during the course of the disease and for some time afterward; thus, live vaccines are best avoided until several months after recovery.

NURSING ALERT Advise family to seek medical evaluation of the youngster if:

Breathing becomes difficult.
Abdominal pain develops.
Sore throat pain is so severe that the child is unable to eat or drink.

Nursing Considerations

Nursing responsibilities are directed toward providing comfort measures to relieve the symptoms and helping affected youngsters and their families determine appropriate activities according to the stage of the disease and their interests. They may need diet counseling to select foods that contain sufficient calories to meet growth and energy needs but are easy to swallow. Every effort should be made to prevent a secondary infection; therefore, the adolescent is counseled to limit exposure to persons outside the family, especially during the acute phase of illness.

The protracted nature of the illness and its associated weakness and fatigue frequently cause depression and resentment on the part of usually vigorous, active teenagers. It is important to spend time with youngsters to listen to their concerns and to allow them to express their feelings and vent their anger. Adolescents need reassurance that the limitations are only temporary, that social activities—so essential at this stage of development—can be resumed after the acute phase, and that they will have sufficient autonomy to determine the extent of their capabilities and the rate of resumption of activities.

INFLUENZA

Influenza, or "flu," one of the most common disorders, has been overused in diagnosis of relatively nondescript respiratory infections. Influenza is caused by three of the orthomyxoviruses, which are antigenically distinct: types A and B, which cause epidemic disease, and type C, which is unimportant epidemiologically. The viruses may undergo significant changes from time to time. Major changes that occur at intervals of years (usually 5 to 10) are called ***antigenic shift;*** minor variations within the same subtypes, ***antigenic drift,*** occur almost annually. Consequently, antigenic drift that takes place over several years can alter the virus sufficiently to result in susceptibility of individuals to a type for which they were previously immunized or infected.

The disease is spread from one individual to another by direct contact (large-droplet infection) or by articles recently contaminated by nasopharyngeal secretions. There is no predilection for a specific age-group, but attack rates are highest in young children who have not had previous contact with a strain. It is frequently most severe in infants. During epidemics, infection among school-age children is believed to be a major source of transmission in a community. Influenza is more common during the winter months.

The disease has a 1- to 3-day incubation period, and affected persons are most infectious for 24 hours before and after onset of symptoms. The virus has a peculiar affinity for epithelial cells of the respiratory tract mucosa, where it destroys ciliated epithelium with metaplastic hyperplasia of the tracheal and bronchial epithelium with associated edema. The alveoli may also become distended with a hyaline-like material. The viruses can be isolated from nasopharyngeal secretions early after onset of the infection, and serologic tests identify the type by complement fixation or the subgroups by hemagglutination inhibition.

Clinical Manifestations

The manifestations of influenza may be subclinical, mild, moderate, or severe. In most cases of overt illness, the throat and nasal mucosa are dry, and there is a dry cough and a tendency toward hoarseness. A sudden onset of fever and chills is accompanied by flushed face, photophobia, myalgia, hyperesthesia, and sometimes prostration. Subglottal croup is common, especially in infants. The symptoms last for 4 to 5 days. Complications include severe viral pneumonia (often hemorrhagic), encephalitis, and secondary bacterial infections, such as otitis media, sinusitis, or pneumonia.

Therapeutic Management

Uncomplicated influenza in children usually requires only symptomatic treatment: acetaminophen for fever, dextromethorphan for cough (if needed), and sufficient fluids to maintain hydration. Amantadine hydrochloride (Symmetrel) has been effective in reducing symptoms associated with type A disease if administered within 24 to 48 hours after onset. It is ineffective against type B or C influenza or other viral diseases. It should not be given to children under 1 year of age but is recommended for unvaccinated high-risk children, as is late immunization. Children with influenza (or other similar viruses) should not receive aspirin because of its possible link with Reye syndrome.

Prevention. Inactivated influenza viral vaccines are safe and effective for prevention of influenza provided the antigens in the vaccine correlate with circulating influenza viruses. For information on immunization, see Chapter 12.

Nursing Considerations

Nursing care is the same as for any child with a URI, including helping the family to implement measures to relieve symptoms. The greatest danger to affected children is development of a secondary infection.

NURSING ALERT Prolonged fever or appearance of fever during early convalescence is a sign of secondary bacterial infection and should be reported to the practitioner for antibiotic therapy.

OTITIS MEDIA (OM)

OM is one of the most prevalent diseases of early childhood. It has been determined that approximately 70% of children have had at least one episode and 33% have had three or more episodes by 3 years of age, accounting for more than 30 million visits per year at a cost of over $3 billion (Williams and others, 1993). The incidence is highest in children ages 6 months to 2 years; it then gradually decreases with age, except for a small increase at age 5 or 6 years, the time of school entry. OM occurs infrequently in children over 7 years of age. Boys are affected more frequently than girls in children less than school age; later the sexes are affected equally. The incidence of acute otitis media (AOM) is highest in the winter months. Children living in households with many members (especially smokers) are more likely to have OM than those living with fewer persons, and children with siblings or parents who had a history of chronic OM have a higher incidence than those who do not. In fact, it is estimated that 8% of cases of OM with effusion (OME) and 17% of the days the child has OME may be attributed to exposure to tobacco smoke (Etzel and others, 1992).

OM has been defined in a variety of ways. The acute, more severe disease has been known as "suppurative," "purulent," or "bacterial" OM, and OME is known as "serous," "secretory," "nonsuppurative," and "glue ear." The standard terminology that has been established to describe OM is outlined in the box above.

STANDARD TERMINOLOGY FOR OTITIS MEDIA

Otitis media—An inflammation of the middle ear without reference to etiology or pathogenesis
Acute otitis media (AOM)—A rapid and short onset of signs and symptoms lasting approximately 3 weeks
Otitis media with effusion (OME)—An inflammation of the middle ear in which a collection of fluid is present in the middle ear space
Subacute otitis media—Middle ear effusion lasting from 3 weeks to 3 months
Chronic otitis media with effusion—Middle ear effusion that persists beyond 3 months

Etiology

AOM is most frequently caused by *Streptococcus pneumoniae* and *Haemophilus influenzae.* The etiology of the noninfectious type is unknown, although it is frequently the result of blocked eustachian tubes from the edema of URIs, allergic rhinitis, or hypertrophic adenoids. Chronic OM is frequently an extension of an acute episode. Passive smoking has been established as a significant factor in the development of OM. It has been suggested that smoke inhalation increases the risk of a blocked eustachian tube by impairing mucociliary function, causing congestion of soft nasopharyngeal tissues, or predisposing patients to URI (Strachan, Jarvis, and Feyerabend, 1989). Daycare attendance is also a risk factor for OM (Alho and others, 1993).

A relationship has been observed between the incidence of OM and the feeding methods in early infancy. Infants fed breast milk have a lower incidence of OM compared with formula-fed infants (Teele and others, 1989). Other studies, however, indicate that the mean number of episodes decreases significantly with an increased duration and exclusivity of breast-feeding (Duncan and others, 1993). Breast-feeding may protect infants against respiratory viruses and allergy by the presence of increased secretory immunoglobulin A (IgA) and limits the exposure of the eustachian tube and middle ear mucosa to microbial pathogens and foreign proteins. Also, reflux of milk up the eustachian tubes is less likely in breast-fed infants because of the semivertical positioning during breast-feeding compared with bottle-feeding. The admonition is to "prop the baby, not the bottle."

Pathophysiology

OM is primarily the result of a dysfunctioning eustachian tube. The eustachian tube is part of a contiguous system composed of the nares, nasopharynx, eustachian tube, middle ear, and mastoid antrum and air cells (see Fig. 7-26). Eustachian tubes have three important functions relative to the middle ear: (1) protection of the middle ear from nasopharyngeal secretions, (2) drainage of secretions pro-

> **FACTORS PREDISPOSING TO DEVELOPMENT OF OTITIS MEDIA**
>
> The eustachian tubes are short, wide, and straight and lie in a relatively horizontal plane (Fig. 32-3).
> The cartilage lining is undeveloped, making the tubes more distensible and therefore more likely to open inappropriately.
> The normally abundant pharyngeal lymphoid tissue readily obstructs the eustachian tube openings in the nasopharynx.
> Immature humoral defense mechanisms increase the risk of infection.
> The usual lying-down position of infants favors the pooling of fluid, such as formula, in the pharyngeal cavity.

duced in the middle ear into the nasopharynx, and (3) ventilation of the middle ear to equalize air pressure within the middle ear with atmospheric pressure in the external ear canal and replenishment of oxygen that has been absorbed.

Mechanical or functional obstruction of the eustachian tube causes accumulation of secretions in the middle ear. Intrinsic obstruction can be caused by infection or allergy, whereas extrinsic obstruction is usually the result of enlarged adenoids or nasopharyngeal tumors. Persistent collapse of the tube during swallowing can cause functional obstruction associated with decreased stiffness or an inefficient opening mechanism. Eustachian tube obstruction results in negative middle ear pressure and, if persistent, produces a transudative middle ear effusion. Drainage is inhibited by sustained negative pressure and impaired ciliary transport within the tube. When the passage is not totally obstructed, contamination of the middle ear can take place by reflux, aspiration, or insufflation during crying, sneezing, nose blowing, and swallowing when the nose is obstructed.

Several factors predispose infants and young children to development of otitis media (see box above).

Complications. The consequences of prolonged middle ear disorders can be either functional or structural. The principal functional consequence is ***hearing loss,*** although loss in most children is conductive in nature and mild in severity. The causes of hearing loss are negative middle ear pressure, the presence of effusion in the middle ear, or structural damage to the tympanic membrane. However, the most feared consequence of hearing loss is its adverse effect on development of speech, language, and cognition. Children who have prolonged periods of middle ear effusion perform less well on speech and language tests than those who have few if any middle ear diseases.

Structural complications or sequelae involve primarily the tympanic membrane. ***Tympanic membrane retraction*** or ***retraction pocket*** occurs when continued negative middle ear pressure draws the tympanic membrane inward, and in areas of low-tensile strength or atrophic segments of the drum head, retraction pockets appear. This retraction may result in impaired sound transmission, perforation of the thinned-out areas, or infection in the pockets and, later, cholesteatoma.

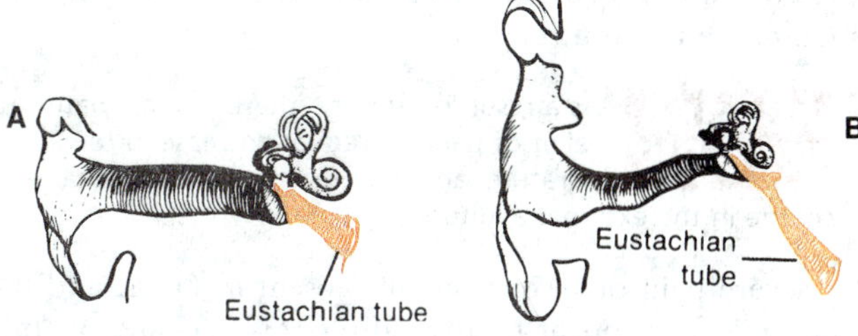

FIG. 32-3 Comparison of anatomic position of eustachian tube in, **A,** child and, **B,** adult.

Tympanosclerosis (eardrum scarring) is the deposition of hyaline material into the fibrous layer of tympanic membrane. It is often seen in children with inflammatory middle ear disease or those with repeated tympanoplasty tube placement. Eardrum ***perforation*** is a common complication in AOM and often accompanies chronic disease. Persistent perforation is a complication of tympanostomy tube placement. Surgery is required to close some perforations.

Adhesive otitis media (glue ear) is a thickening of the mucous membrane by proliferation of fibrous tissue that can cause fixation of the ossicles with a resultant hearing loss. ***Chronic suppurative otitis media,*** an inflammation of the middle ear and mastoid, is evidenced by perforation and discharge (otorrhea) for up to 6 weeks' duration. ***Labyrinthitis,*** infection of the inner ear, and ***mastoiditis,*** infection of the mastoid sinus, are rare since the advent of antibiotic therapy. ***Meningitis*** and other suppurative intracranial complications are possible complications of extension of infection from the middle ear or mastoid. However, these complications occur infrequently when adequate antibiotic therapy is implemented.

Cholesteatoma is one of the least common but most potentially dangerous sequelae of OME. A cholesteatoma is formed when the keratinizing, stratified, squamous epithelial cell lining desquamates to form scales that accumulate within the middle ear space. As it enlarges, the cholesteatoma erodes all the structures it encounters, especially bone, destroying the ossicles and gaining entry to the inner ear and meninges. Clinical signs are a foul-smelling, grayish yellow discharge, sometimes pain, and permanent progressive hearing loss. Treatment is surgical excision of the entire cholesteatoma.

Clinical Manifestations

As purulent fluid accumulates in the small space of the middle ear chamber, pain results from the pressure on surrounding structures. Infants become irritable and indicate their discomfort by holding or pulling at their ears and rolling their head from side to side. Young children usually verbally complain of the pain. A temperature as high as 40° C (104° F) is common, and postauricular and cervical lymph glands may be enlarged. Rhinorrhea, vomiting, and diarrhea, as well as signs of concurrent respiratory or pharyngeal infection, may also be present. Loss of appetite typically occurs, and sucking or chewing tends to aggravate the pain. In children with OME, exudate will accumulate and pressure will increase, with the potential for the tympanic membrane to rupture.

NURSING ALERT As a result of rupture, there is immediate relief of pain, a gradual decrease in temperature, and the presence of purulent discharge in the external auditory canal.

Severe pain or fever is usually absent in OME, and the child may not appear ill. Instead there is a feeling of "fullness" in the ear, a popping sensation during swallowing, and a feeling of "motion" in the ear if air is present above the level of fluid. Since chronic serous OM is the most frequent cause of conductive hearing loss in young children, audiometry may reveal deficient hearing.

Diagnostic Evaluation

In AOM, otoscopy reveals an intact membrane that appears bright red and bulging, with no visible landmarks or light reflex. The usual landmarks of the bony prominence from the long and the short process of the malleus are obscured by the outwardly bulging membrane. In OME, otoscopic findings may include a slightly injected, dull-gray membrane, obscured landmarks, and a visible fluid level or meniscus behind the eardrum if air is present above the fluid.

Several tests provide an assessment of mobility of the tympanic membrane. Pneumatic otoscopy and tympanometry are discussed under Auditory Testing (Chapter 7). Acoustic reflectometry measures the level of sound transmitted and reflected from the middle ear to a microphone located in a probe tip placed against the ear canal opening and directed toward the tympanic membrane. The information provides a measure of canal length and presence of effusion. The greater the cancellation of transmitted sound by reflected sound, the greater the probability of middle ear effusion.

Diagnosis is usually based on clinical manifestations, but if purulent discharge is present, it should be cultured and a specific antibiotic chosen for that organism.

Therapeutic Management: Acute Otitis Media (AOM)

In treating AOM, administration of antibiotics is the mainstay of therapy. A variety of antibiotics may be prescribed individually or in combination, with amoxicillin the antibiotic of choice because of its ease of use, relatively inexpensive cost, and availability. Many studies, however, have examined the use of other antibiotics for their efficacy and ease of administration. An important consideration for deciding which drug to prescribe is compliance by the parent in giving the antibiotic; therefore, several studies have examined the use of single-dose medication. Another consideration for the use of an antibiotic involves whether the organism causing the OM is a β-lactamase-producing organism, with *S. pneumoniae, H. influenzae,* and *Moraxella catarrhalis* being the most commonly identified pathogens. The number of β-lactamase-producing organisms has risen to include 10% to 40% of *H. influenzae* and 70% to 100% of *M. catarrhalis* strains in the past 2 decades (Owen and others, 1993).

In addition to amoxicillin, other oral antibiotics frequently prescribed include sulfonamides, trimethoprim-sulfamethoxazole (Bactrim, Septra), erythromycin-sulfisoxazole (Pediazole), and the cephalosporins, which, in many settings, are becoming the first-line drugs because of their broad-spectrum activity, dosage schedule, decreased side effects, and bactericidal activity against β-lactamase-producing pathogens. Many of these antibiotics may be effective in treating symptoms (e.g., pain) and in returning fluid to a sterile state but may not be effective in eliminating the eustachian tube blockage. As indicated, with the continual rise of β-lactamase-producing strains, the cephalosporins are proving to be beneficial, with third-generation drugs such as cefixime (Suprax) or second-generation cefaclor (Ceclor) showing good results (Williams and others, 1993).

There has also been research on the use of intramuscular (IM) single-dose drugs, with the cephalosporin ceftriaxone (Rocephin) being studied the most. Outcomes have been positive based on elimination of symptoms, with researchers indicating that a single IM injection is as effective as 10 days of oral amoxicillin for treating uncomplicated AOM in children (Green and Rothrock, 1993). There are several issues to consider with this therapy: (1) the cost; (2) broadening the indications and use of this cephalosporin for outpatient management of a common disease and possibly hastening the emergence of resistant bacteria; and (3) the use of painful IM treatments for controlling a common, frequently self-limited disease (see Atraumatic Care box).

Other measures may be considered in treating the child with OM. For fever or discomfort, analgesic/antipyretic drugs such as acetaminophen or ibuprofen may be given. The use and efficacy of antihistamines and decongestants in treating AOM is questionable; their main role may be in prevention. Although they may promote comfort, ear drops are usually not recommended, because they tend to obscure a clear view of the tympanic membrane.

Children with AOM should be seen after antibiotic therapy to evaluate the effectiveness of the treatment and to identify potential complications, such as effusion or hearing impairment. It is often difficult for parents to determine hearing loss; therefore, audiometric testing should be done. (Screening tests for hearing are discussed in Chapter 7.)

Therapeutic Management: Recurrent Otitis Media

Trying to manage children with recurrent AOM is often frustrating; therefore, other therapies have been examined, including chemoprophylaxis with long-term antibiotic therapy, steroid use, immunotherapy, and surgery. The use of antibiotics has been already discussed. For children re-

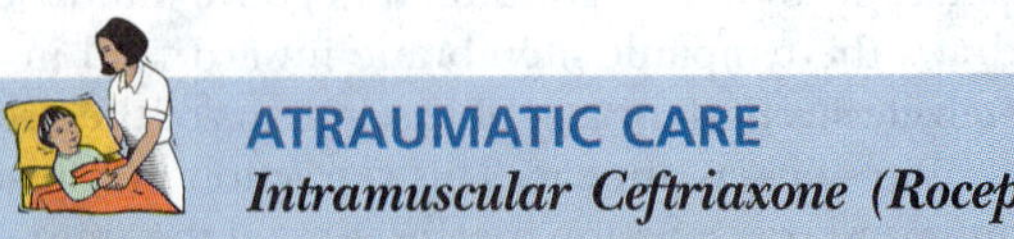

ATRAUMATIC CARE
Intramuscular Ceftriaxone (Rocephin)

To reduce the pain from IM administration of ceftriaxone, use lidocaine 1% as the diluent (Schichor and others, 1994).

ceiving long-term therapy, an evaluation once a month is usually done to detect any evidence of effusion, and any acute infection during prophylaxis is treated with an alternate antibiotic regimen. According to recently published guidelines by AHCPR, steroids are not recommended for treatment of OME in children of any age.* It is important to note, however, that the suggestion was that antibiotics (e.g., amoxicillin, ampicillin, sulfisoxazole, or trimethoprim-sulfamethoxazole) should be the first therapy to be tried and that the routine use of steroid therapy in unselected children with OME is not warranted. Furthermore, although a short course of antibiotics appears to be effective in short-term clearance, the effect tends to be limited and is of relatively short duration (Williams and others, 1993).

There is an increasing indication for the use of immunotherapy, with the new pneumococcus vaccine showing a better response than the previous polysaccharide one. A newer concept is a vaccine "cocktail" that would protect against pneumococcus, *Haemophilus*, and other contributing bacteria. The *H. influenzae* type b conjugate vaccine provides high protective efficacy for meningitis and epiglottitis but has not yet been proved effective against OM (Black and others, 1991). A new immune globulin being studied is the bacterial polysaccharide immune globulin (BPIG), with initial results being positive, as well as showing a significant time spent free of AOM (Gray, 1993; Shurin and others, 1993).

From a surgical standpoint, myringotomy with tubes is very effective in eliminating fluid, pain, and hearing loss secondary to the presence of recurrent and chronic OM where there is not spontaneous perforation of the tympanic membrane. Tubes are usually placed in the anteroinferior quadrant of the membrane. If, however, a eustachian tube remains blocked, fluid will return after a fairly rapid spontaneous healing of the myringotomy. Adenoidectomy may be successful in treating OM if a blocked eustachian tube secondary to hypertrophy of adenoids is the cause, whereas tonsillectomy is not generally considered a beneficial treatment (Maw and Bawden, 1993). Mastoidectomy may be performed when antibiotic therapy has failed and the child's life is threatened by infection, with tympanoplasty (middle ear reconstructive surgery) possibly being done after surgery.

Therapeutic Management: Otitis Media with Effusion (OME)*

Many children may have fluid that persists in the middle ear for weeks or months; these children usually have some impairment of hearing. The major goal of therapy, therefore, is to establish and maintain an aerated middle ear that is free of fluid with a normal mucosa and ultimately to achieve normal hearing. The medical management of recurrent OM, as well as OME, is often open ended and seemingly uncertain (Williams and others, 1993) in regard to antimicrobial and surgical management. As already indicated, with OM and recurrent OM, many preventive, prophylactic, and active treatment modalities are available.

When medical interventions are unsuccessful in achieving the goals of therapy, surgical management is often considered. Many children will benefit from myringotomy and tympanostomy tube placement. This therapy allows for mechanical drainage of the fluid, which will promote better healing of the membrane and prevent scar formation and loss of elasticity. The tubes (or ventilatory pressure-equalizer [PE] tubes, grommets, or dottles) facilitate continued drainage of fluid and also allow ventilation of the middle ear. The primary objective is to allow the eustachian tube a period of recovery while the tubes perform their functions. The surgery is relatively benign, but it is important to remember that tubes may tend to become plugged and often require reinsertion. Complications of repeated or long-term tube placement are tympanosclerosis, localized or diffuse atrophy of the membrane, persistent perforation, or, rarely, cholesteatoma. It has also been shown that adenoidectomy and tube insertion for children with OME and hearing loss are beneficial, and that children in households where there was no smoking also did considerably better and were free of symptoms longer (Maw and Bawden, 1993).

Prognosis. Most cases of OM resolve eventually. However, hearing loss, typically conductive, is considered the most common complication of OM. The degree of hearing loss can vary from none to severe. Although conductive hearing loss is most associated with OM, sensorineural hearing loss may also be present, especially in severe forms of chronic or recurrent OM, because of the toxic products from fluids into the cochlea through the tympanic membrane. The longer the fluid is present, the greater the sensorineural hearing loss. Children who are prone to OM should be referred to a pediatric otolaryngologist and possibly a pediatric allergist for identification and treatment of the etiology of their eustachian tube dysfunction. They also should be referred to a speech/language pathologist for primary prevention counseling. In addition, the child should ideally be followed by an audiologist to evaluate the adequacy of hearing.

Nursing Considerations

Nursing objectives for the child with AOM include the following: (1) relieve pain, (2) facilitate drainage when possible, (3) prevent complications or recurrence, (4) educate family in care of the child, and (5) provide emotional support to the child and family.

Analgesics are often very helpful to reduce severe earache. High fever, particularly in infants, should be reduced with antipyretic drugs to avoid febrile convulsions. The application of heat may reduce pain in some children but may aggravate discomfort in others. Local heat should be placed over the ear while the child lies on the affected side. This position also facilitates drainage of the exudate if the eardrum has ruptured or if myringotomy was performed. An ice compress placed over the affected ear may also provide comfort, since it reduces edema. If the child is cooperative,

*Near publication, the "Otitis Media with Effusion in Young Children" guidelines were published. The reader is encouraged to review this document: AHCPR Pub. No. 94-0620 (overview), 94-0623 (quick reference guide), and 94-0624 (parent guide); available in English and Spanish from AHCPR Publications Clearinghouse, OME/AAP, P.O. Box 8547, Silver Spring, MD 20907; (800) 358-9295.

either procedure can be tried to determine which offers maximum relief.

If the ear is draining, the external canal may be cleansed with sterile cotton swabs or pledgets soaked in hydrogen peroxide. If ear wicks or lightly rolled sterile gauze packs are placed in the ear after surgical treatment, they should be loose enough to allow accumulated drainage to flow out of the ear; otherwise the infection may be transferred to the mastoid process. Parents should be told to keep these wicks dry during shampoos or baths. Occasionally drainage is so profuse that the pinna and surrounding skin become excoriated from exudate. This is prevented by frequent cleansing and application of various moisture barriers (e.g., Aloe Vesta, Proshield Plus) or petrolatum jelly (e.g., Vaseline).

Parents require some anticipatory guidance regarding temporary hearing loss that accompanies OM. For example, they may need to speak louder, at closer proximity, and while facing the child. They are reminded that the child is not ignoring them but is unaware of being spoken to. Persistent difficulty in hearing beyond the acute stage should be evaluated.

The child may not be able to localize where a sound is coming from, since awareness and understanding of speech are reduced either unilaterally or bilaterally, depending on the degree of hearing deficit. The family should also be aware of possible behavioral changes with hearing loss, including inattentiveness to or lack of awareness of environmental sounds; requests for repetition in conversation or mishearing of content; softer or louder voice than usual; poor attention span and fidgety behavior when in a group (e.g., classroom) listening situation; aggressiveness and low frustration tolerance because of the frustration of frequent communication breakdown; and impaired speech and language skills.

Preventing recurrence requires adequate parent education regarding antibiotic therapy. Antibiotics are frequently considered "miracle" drugs or a "one-dose" cure for everything. Since the symptoms of pain and fever usually subside within 24 to 48 hours, the rapid outward signs of recovery support such thinking. Nurses must emphasize that although the child looks well in a couple of days, the infection is not completely eradicated until all the prescribed medication is taken. At the risk of alarming parents, it is important to stress the potential complications of OM, especially hearing loss, which can be prevented with adequate treatment and follow-up care (see Administration of Medication, Chapter 27, and Compliance, Chapter 27).*

A concern presented by the use of tympanostomy tubes is the possibility of water entering the middle ear. Several studies indicate that small amounts of water pose little hazard and that even swimming without earplugs or occlusive bathing caps carries no higher risk for an increased incidence of OM. However, diving, jumping, and submerging may be forbidden by some practitioners. Bath and shampoo water should be kept out of the ear, if possible, since soap reduces the surface tension of water, facilitating entry through the tube. Lake water, as well as bath water, is contaminated; therefore wearing earplugs, although not watertight, prevents total flooding of the external canal and provides sufficient protection. Parents should be aware of the appearance of a grommet (usually a tiny, white plastic, spool-shaped tube) so that they can observe if it falls out. They are reassured that this is normal and requires no immediate intervention (Isaacson and Rosenfeld, 1994).

Parents sometimes ask about preventing ear discomfort in their infants during ascent or descent of an airplane. During ascent, air in the middle ear expands, but decompression takes place through a normal eustachian tube. If the tissues are congested with a URI, the passage of air may be blocked. A nasal-mucosa shrinking spray or oral decongestant before the trip may be helpful. During descent, the air within the middle ear decreases as atmospheric pressure increases. Swallowing is the simplest and most effective method for inflating the middle ear on descent; therefore feeding or offering a pacifier to infants during descent is beneficial.

Reducing the chances of OM is possible with some simple measures, such as sitting or holding an infant upright for feedings. Forceful nose blowing during a URI is discouraged to avoid forcing organisms to ascend through the eustachian tube. Early detection of possible middle ear effusion is a primary nursing goal in prevention of complications. Infants and preschool children should be screened for effusion, and all schoolchildren, especially those with learning disabilities, should be tested for middle ear effusion. Frequent audiologic evaluations, medical consultation, and education of parents and children are advised when middle ear effusion is detected. (See also Nursing Care Plan: The Child with Acute Otitis Media.*)

OTITIS EXTERNA

Infections of the external ear may result from normal ear flora (*Staphylococcus epidermidis* and *Corynebacterium,* primarily) that assume pathogenic characteristics under conditions of excessive wetness or dryness. Ordinarily the external ear canal is protected by a waxy, water-repellent coating composed of highly viscid secretions of the sebaceous glands and the watery, pigmented secretions of apocrine glands in combination with exfoliated surface cells. Inflammation occurs when this environment is altered by swimming, bathing, or increased environmental humidity ***(swimmer's ear);*** by infection, dermatoses, or insufficient cerumen; or by trauma from a foreign body or a finger.

Secondary invasion of foreign pathogens also occurs. In addition to the resident flora, the offending agents can be *Pseudomonas aeruginosa* (most common), *Enterobacter aerogenes, Proteus mirabilis, Klebsiella pneumoniae,* streptococci, and fungi such as *Candida* and *Aspergillus.* The ear canal becomes irritated, and maceration takes place.

The predominant symptom of external ear infection is ear pain accentuated by manipulation of the pinna, especially pressure on the tragus. The pain often appears to be

*Home care instructions for administration of medications are available in *Wong and Whaley's Clinical Manual of Pediatric Nursing* (Mosby).

*In *Wong and Whaley's Clinical Manual of Pediatric Nursing* (Mosby).

out of proportion to the degree of inflammation. Conductive hearing loss may be present as a result of the edema, secretions, and accumulation of debris within the canal. Edema, erythema, and a cheesy green-blue-gray discharge and tenderness appear as the infection progresses. The external canal may be so tender and swollen that visualization is difficult. There may be fever. In advanced cases the pain is intense, constant, and aggravated by jaw motion or ear manipulation.

Therapeutic objectives include relief of pain, edema, and itching and restoration of normal flora, cerumen, and canal epithelium. Analgesics are prescribed for pain. Debris is removed with gentle suction and wisps of cotton on metal cotton carriers. Otic preparations containing neomycin with either colistin or polymyxin and corticosteroids are instilled in the canal. A gauze wick is usually inserted to facilitate the medication reaching the site of inflammation. The wick is removed after swelling and pain have subsided, but the drops are continued for at least 3 days after relief of pain. The best management for external ear inflammation is prevention.

Nursing Considerations

Nurses can teach parents or patients to apply simple measures to prevent recurrent infections. Children are advised to limit their stay in the water to less than an hour, if possible, and ears should dry completely (1 to 2 hours) before children enter the water again. Shaking the head and judicious use of the corner of a towel can remove most excess water. The ear canal can also be dried with a small tuft of cotton (not a swab). Placing a combination of white vinegar and rubbing alcohol (50/50) in both ear canals on arising, at bedtime, and at the end of each swim (the most common cause of otitis externa) is effective in preventing recurrence. The solution must remain in the canal for 5 minutes (Marcy, 1989). Youngsters are cautioned not to pick at the ears with a pencil, cotton swab, bobby pin, or other object, which can injure or infect the ear canal.

➤ **NURSING TIP** To keep the ear dry, pull the auricle up and out to straighten the canal, then use a conventional hair dryer, set on low or no heat, held at a distance of 18 to 24 inches for 30 seconds, three times a day (Hands, 1987).

CROUP SYNDROMES

Croup is a general term applied to a symptom complex characterized by hoarseness, a resonant cough described as "barking" or "brassy" (croupy), varying degrees of inspiratory stridor, and varying degrees of respiratory distress resulting from swelling or obstruction in the region of the larynx. Acute infections of the larynx are of greater importance in infants and small children than they are in older children, in part because of the increased incidence in children in this age-group and the smaller diameter of the airway, which renders it subject to significantly greater narrowing with the same degree of inflammation (Fig. 32-4).

Croup is a common respiratory disease of childhood and occurs more often in boys than in girls (Quan, 1992). The number of croup cases increases in the late autumn through early winter months and occurs primarily in children 6 months to 3 years of age, especially those 2 years of age (Cressman and Myer, 1994; Solar and Eldadah, 1990). Hospitalization is necessary for 1% to 15% of children with croup, and intubation is required in 1% to 5% of hospitalized children (Quan, 1992; Skolnik, 1989).

Acute respiratory infections of the nonreactive airway involve all areas to some extent and are seldom restricted to one area. ***Croup syndromes*** affect to varying degrees the larynx, trachea, and bronchi. However, laryngeal involvement often dominates the clinical picture because of the severe effects on the voice and breathing. Croup syndromes are usually described according to the primary anatomic area affected, that is, epiglottitis (or supraglottitis), laryngitis, laryngotracheobronchitis (LTB), and tracheitis. In general, LTB tends to occur in very young children, whereas epiglottitis is more characteristic of older children (see Table 32-1 for a comparison of croup syndromes).

Since croup is one of the most benign conditions causing upper airway obstruction, it is vitally important to identify correctly and distinguish what type of croup syndrome is actually occurring (i.e., spasmodic croup or LTB) as opposed to a potentially life-threatening condition such as epiglottitis, bacterial tracheitis, foreign-body aspiration, or a peritonsillar abscess. The key differences between LTB and epiglottitis are the absence of cough, the presence of

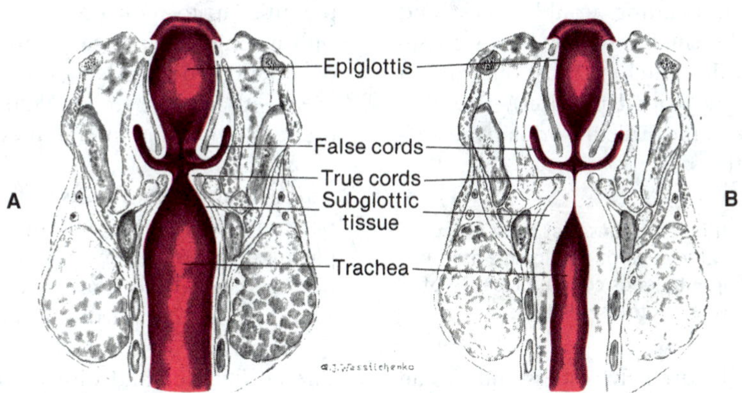

FIG. 32-4 **A,** Normal larynx. **B,** Obstruction and narrowing resulting from edema of croup.

TABLE 32-1 Comparison of Croup Syndromes

	ACUTE EPIGLOTTITIS (SUPRAGLOTTITIS)	ACUTE LARYNGO-TRACHEOBRONCHITIS	ACUTE SPASMODIC LARYNGITIS (SPASMODIC CROUP)	ACUTE TRACHEITIS
Age-group affected	1-8 years	3 months–8 years	3 months–3 years	1 month–6 years
Etiologic agent	Bacterial, usually *H. influenzae*	Viral	Viral with allergic component	Bacterial, usually *S. aureus*
Onset	Rapidly progressive	Slowly progressive	Sudden; at night	Moderately progressive
Major symptoms	Dysphagia Stridor aggravated when supine Drooling High fever Toxic Rapid pulse and respirations	URI Stridor Brassy cough Hoarseness Dyspnea Restlessness Irritability Low-grade fever Nontoxic	URI Croupy cough Stridor Hoarseness Dyspnea Restlessness Symptoms waken child Symptoms disappear during day Tends to recur	URI Croupy cough Stridor Purulent secretions High fever No response to laryngotracheobronchitis (LTB) therapy
Treatment	Antibiotics Airway protection	Humidity Racemic epinephrine	Humidity	Antibiotics

dysphagia, and the high degree of toxicity in children with epiglottitis. *These children usually look worse than they sound, in contrast to children with croup, who sound worse than they look.*

ACUTE EPIGLOTTITIS

Acute epiglottitis, or acute supraglottitis, is a serious obstructive inflammatory process that occurs principally in children between 2 and 5 years of age, but can occur from infancy to adulthood. The disorder requires immediate attention. The obstruction is supraglottic, as opposed to the subglottic obstruction of laryngitis. The responsible organism is usually *Haemophilus influenzae;* LTB and epiglottitis do not occur together.

Clinical Manifestations

The onset of epiglottitis is abrupt, less often preceded by cold symptoms and more often by a sore throat, and can rapidly progress to severe respiratory distress. The child usually goes to bed asymptomatic to awaken later complaining of sore throat and pain on swallowing. The child has a fever, appears sicker than clinical findings would suggest, and presents a classic picture: the child generally insists on sitting upright, leaning forward, with chin thrust out, mouth open, and tongue protruding (tripod position). Drooling of saliva is common because of the difficulty or pain on swallowing and excessive secretions.

NURSING ALERT Three clinical observations that have been found to be predictive of epiglottitis are absence of spontaneous cough, presence of drooling, and agitation (Mauro and others, 1988).

The child is irritable and extremely restless and has an anxious, apprehensive, and frightened expression. The voice is thick and muffled, with a froglike croaking sound on inspiration. The child is not hoarse. Suprasternal and substernal retractions may be visible. The child seldom struggles to breathe, and slow, quiet breathing provides better air exchange. The sallow color of mild hypoxia may progress to frank cyanosis. The throat is red and inflamed, and a distinctive, large, cherry-red, edematous epiglottis is visible on careful throat inspection. *Throat inspection should be attempted only when immediate intubation can be performed if needed.*

Therapeutic Management

The course of epiglottitis may be fulminant, with respiratory obstruction appearing suddenly. Progressive obstruction leads to hypoxia, hypercapnia, and acidosis followed by decreased muscular tone, reduced level of consciousness, and, when obstruction becomes more or less complete, a rather sudden death. A presumptive diagnosis of epiglottitis constitutes an emergency.

The child suspected of epiglottitis should be examined where facilities are available for coping with this type of emergency. The child is best transported while sitting in a parent's lap to reduce distress. Examination of the throat with a tongue depressor is contraindicated until properly experienced personnel and equipment are at hand to proceed with immediate intubation or tracheostomy in the event that the examination precipitates further or complete obstruction.

If a lateral neck film is indicated, the same experienced personnel should accompany the child to the radiology department. However, most practitioners prefer that the child not be transported but remain on the parent's lap in the examination area during portable radiology.

Endotracheal intubation or tracheostomy is usually considered for the child with *H. influenzae* epiglottitis with severe respiratory distress. It is recommended that the intubation or tracheostomy and any invasive procedure, such

CRITICAL THINKING EXERCISE

Croup Syndrome

Kim Lee, 4 years old, is admitted to the emergency department with a sore throat, pain on swallowing, drooling, and a fever of 39° C (102.2° F). She looks ill, is agitated, and prefers to sit up and lean over. Which of the following medical orders should you question?

1. Obtain a complete blood count (CBC) and throat culture STAT.
2. Place child on oxygen saturation monitor.
3. Start an IV of 5% dextrose in normal saline to run at 30 ml/hr.
4. Have pediatric-size tracheostomy tray available.

The correct answer is 1. This child's symptoms suggest epiglottitis. The nurse should question the order for a throat culture because the procedure can precipitate obstruction of the airway. The CBC and other interventions are appropriate.

as starting an intravenous infusion, be performed in the operating room. Whether or not there is an artificial airway, the child requires intensive observation by experienced personnel. The epiglottal swelling usually decreases after 24 hours of antibiotic therapy, and the epiglottis is near normal by the third day. Intubated children are generally extubated at this time.

Children with suspected bacterial epiglottitis are given antibiotics intravenously, followed by oral administration to complete a 7- to 10-day course. The use of corticosteroids for reducing edema may be beneficial during the early hours of treatment; most intubated children will have had a course of corticosteroids for 24 hours before extubation.

Prevention. The American Academy of Pediatrics (1994) recommended that all children beginning at 2 months of age receive one of the *H. influenzae* type B conjugate vaccines. Since administration of the vaccine has become a routine part of the regular immunization schedule, a decline in the incidence of epiglottitis has occurred. Patients now tend to be older and have disease caused by other organisms (Gorelick and Baker, 1994). (See also Immunizations, Chapter 12.)

Nursing Considerations

Epiglottitis is a serious and frightening disease for the child, family, and health professionals. It is important to act quickly but calmly and provide support without unduly increasing anxiety. The child is allowed to remain in the position that provides the most comfort and security, and parents are reassured that everything possible is being done to obtain relief for their child.

NURSING ALERT Nurses who suspect epiglottitis should not attempt to visualize the epiglottis directly with a tongue depressor or take a throat culture but should refer the child to a physician immediately (see Critical Thinking Exercise box).

Acute care of the child is that described for the child with acute respiratory distress and artificial airways in Chapter 31. Continuous monitoring of respiratory status, including blood gases, is part of nursing observations, and the intravenous infusion is maintained as described in Chapter 28.

ACUTE LARYNGITIS

Acute infectious laryngitis is a common illness in older children and adolescents. Infants and smaller children experience more generalized involvement (see following section on laryngotracheobronchitis). Viruses are the usual causative agents and the principal complaint is hoarseness, which may be accompanied by other upper respiratory symptoms (e.g., coryza, sore throat, nasal congestion) and systemic manifestations (e.g., fever, headache, myalgia, malaise). Associated complaints vary with the infecting virus. For example, adenoviruses and influenza viruses are responsible for more systemic involvement; parainfluenza viruses, rhinoviruses, and respiratory syncytial virus (RSV) cause more mild illness (Wald, 1990).

Therapeutic Management and Nursing Considerations

The disease is almost always self-limited without long-term sequelae. Treatment is symptomatic with fluids and humidified air (see Nursing Care Plan on p. 1377).

ACUTE LARYNGOTRACHEOBRONCHITIS (LTB)

LTB is the most common type of croup experienced by children admitted for hospitalization and primarily affects children less than 5 years of age. Organisms usually responsible for LTB are the parainfluenza virus type 1, followed by virus types 3 and 2, RSV, influenza A and B, and *Mycoplasma* pneumoniae (Quan, 1992). The disease is usually preceded by a URI, which gradually descends to adjacent structures. It is characterized by gradual onset of low-grade fever.

Inflammation of the mucosa lining the larynx and trachea causes a narrowing of the airway. When the airway is significantly narrowed, the child struggles to inhale air past the obstruction and into the lungs, producing the characteristic inspiratory stridor and suprasternal retractions; other classic manifestations include cough and hoarseness. The typical child with LTB is a toddler who develops the classic barking or seallike cough and acute stridor after several days of coryza. The child may be in slight to moderate respiratory distress, with some mild wheezing and a low-grade fever. When the child is unable to inhale a sufficient volume of air, symptoms of hypoxia become evident. As the work of forcing air past the obstruction increases, negative pressure generated in the thoracic cavity also increases, leading to leakage of pulmonary vascular fluid into interstitial spaces and causing uneven ventilation and hypoxia. Obstruction severe enough to prevent adequate exhalation of carbon dioxide causes respiratory acidosis, and, eventually, the child experiences respiratory failure. (See progression of symptoms outlined in the box on p. 1394.)

PROGRESSION OF SYMPTOMS IN LARYNGOTRACHEOBRONCHITIS

STAGE I

Fear
Hoarseness
Croupy cough
Inspiratory stridor when disturbed

STAGE II

Continuous respiratory stridor
Lower rib retraction
Retraction of soft tissue of neck
Use of accessory muscles of respiration
Labored respiration

STAGE III

Signs of anoxia and carbon dioxide retention
Restlessness
Anxiety
Pallor
Sweating
Rapid respiration

STAGE IV

Intermittent cyanosis
Permanent cyanosis
Cessation of breathing

As described by Forbes. From Krugman S and others: *Infectious diseases of children,* ed 9, St Louis, 1992, Mosby.

Therapeutic Management

The major objective in medical management of infectious LTB is maintaining an airway and providing for adequate respiratory exchange. Children with mild croup (no stridor at rest) are managed at home. Parents are taught the signs of respiratory distress so that professional help can be summoned early if needed. Children who progress to stage II respiratory symptoms should receive medical attention, usually with hospitalization.

High humidity with cool mist provides relief for most children (Quan, 1992; Ruddy, 1993). A cool-air vaporizer can be used at home. In the hospital setting, huts for infants or mist tents for toddlers are sometimes used to provide increased humidity and supplemental oxygen.

The cool-temperature therapy modalities assist by constricting edematous blood vessels. Cool droplets are heavier than warm vapor and can therefore penetrate lung fields better. In the home environment some suggestions to provide cool air are: taking the child outside to breathe in cool night air; use of a cold-water vaporizer or humidifier; standing in front of the freezer; and taking the child to a cool basement or garage.

Controversy has surrounded the use of mist therapy to treat croup. Studies have failed to demonstrate any improvement in subglottic edema with mist therapy, and it has been suggested that the apparent effectiveness of mist therapy is probably due to the calming effect of the caregiver's or parent's presence (Quan, 1992; Ruddy, 1993). Despite this, mist therapy remains the first-line home and emergency department therapy for mildly distressed children (Quan, 1992).

It is also essential to allow children with mild croup to continue to drink beverages they like and to encourage parents to try whatever comforting measures work best with their child (e.g., being held, rocked, walked, sung to). If the child is unable to take oral fluids, intravenous fluid therapy might be indicated. Children with severe respiratory distress (traditionally, for infants with a respiratory rate >60 breaths/min) should not be given anything by mouth to prevent aspiration and decrease the work of breathing.

Nebulized epinephrine (racemic epinephrine) is often used in children with more severe disease, stridor at rest, retractions, or difficulty breathing (Quan, 1992; Ruddy, 1993). The α-adrenergic effects cause mucosal vasoconstriction and subsequent decreased subglottic edema. The onset of action is rapid, with detectable clinical improvement within 10 to 15 minutes, although symptoms frequently reappear—typically called "relapse" as opposed to "rebound"—within 2 hours (Ruddy, 1993; Skolnick, 1989). In a significant number of children, however, improvement persists and additional treatments are not necessary. Despite its adrenergic effects, racemic epinephrine is generally well tolerated, and tachycardia only rarely occurs (Quan, 1992).

The use of corticosteroids is beneficial because the antiinflammatory effects decrease subglottic edema. The onset of action is clinically detectable as early as 6 hours after administration, with continued improvement over 12 to 24 hours (Kairys, Olmstead, and O'Connor, 1989).

Combination therapy, with racemic epinephrine and corticosteroids, has also recently undergone trials with good success, even by administering in the emergency department and then discharging the child home (Kelley and Simon, 1992; Ledwith and Shea, 1993). In implementing this protocol, recommendations to follow include the following (Kelley and Simon, 1992): (1) choose patients who have access to additional care in case they need it; (2) observe the child in the emergency department for a minimum of 2 to 3 hours after the treatment; and (3) discharge only if the child is free of significant stridor or retractions at rest. For inpatients, similar results have been reported, with children showing improvement of symptoms 12 and 24 hours from initiation of therapy (Kairys, Olmstead, and O'Connor, 1989; Kunkel and Baker, 1992; Wusson, Krug, and Yamashita, 1992). There was also a significantly lower intubation rate in the corticosteroid group (Kairys, Olmstead, and O'Connor, 1989); for children who were intubated, the duration of intubation was shorter and the need for reintubation less (Tibballs, Shawn, and Landau, 1992). Children receiving corticosteroids also demonstrated improvement in both pulse oximetry and respiratory rate (Stoney and Chakrabarti, 1991; Super and others, 1989).

Nursing Considerations

The most important nursing function in the care of children with croup is continuous, vigilant observation and accurate assessment of respiratory status. Cardiac, respiratory, and noninvasive blood gas monitoring equipment supplement visual observations. Changes in therapy are frequently based on nurses' observations and assessment of a child's status, response to therapy, and tolerance of procedures. The trend away from early intubation of children with LTB emphasizes the importance of nursing observation and the ability to recognize impending respiratory failure so that intubation can be implemented without delay. Intubation equipment should be readily accessible and taken with the child during transport to other areas (e.g., radiology, operating room).

NURSING ALERT Early signs of impending airway obstruction include increased pulse and respiratory rate; substernal, suprasternal, and intercostal retractions; flaring nares; and increased restlessness.

To conserve energy, children are given every opportunity to rest. Infants or small children find that being enclosed within a mist tent, coughing, having laryngeal spasms, and needing intravenous therapy are additional sources of distress. Infants and small children prefer sitting upright, and most want to be held. Children need the security of the parent's presence. Since crying increases respiratory distress and hypoxia, a child's individual tolerance for these therapies must be assessed. An extremely fussy child may do better when held in the parent's lap with cool mist directed toward the child's face.

The rapid progression of croup, the alarming sound of the cough and stridor, and the child's apprehensive behavior and ill appearance combine to create a very frightening experience for the parents. They need reassurance regarding the child's progress and an explanation of treatments. They may feel guilty for not having suspected the seriousness of the condition sooner. The family should be allowed to remain with their child as much as possible, especially when this decreases the child's distress.

The nurse can provide them with an opportunity to express their feelings, thus minimizing any blame or guilt. They need frequent reassurance provided in a calm, quiet manner and education regarding what they can do to make their child more comfortable. Fortunately, as the crisis subsides and the child responds to therapy, breathing becomes easier and recovery is generally prompt. Home care after discharge includes continued humidity, adequate hydration, and nourishment. Parents are encouraged to ask questions about home care and preparation for discharge. Referral to a public health agency for follow-up care may be advisable.

ACUTE SPASMODIC LARYNGITIS

Acute spasmodic laryngitis (spasmodic croup, "midnight croup," or "twilight croup") is distinct from laryngitis and LTB and characterized by paroxysmal attacks of laryngeal obstruction that occur chiefly at night. Signs of inflammation are absent or mild, and there is frequently a history of previous attacks lasting for 2 to 5 days followed by uneventful recovery. It usually affects children ages 1 to 3 years. Some children appear to be predisposed to the condition; allergy and psychogenic factors are implicated in some cases.

The child goes to bed well or with some very mild respiratory symptoms but awakes suddenly with characteristic barking, metallic cough, hoarseness, noisy inspirations, and restlessness. The child appears anxious, frightened, and prostrated. Dyspnea is aggravated by excitement; however, there is no fever, the attack subsides in a few hours, and the child appears well the next day.

Therapeutic Management and Nursing Considerations

Children with spasmodic croup are managed at home, with cool mist being recommended for the child's room. Warm mist provided by steam from hot running water in a closed bathroom may be helpful. The two primary reasons these techniques are effective are the upright positioning of the child and the comfort of having a parent hold the child. Humidification helps to a certain degree, but warm temperatures will not help to relieve the constriction. Sometimes the spasm is relieved by sudden exposure to cold air (as when the child is taken out into the night air to see the practitioner). Parents are usually advised to have the child sleep in humidified air until the cough has subsided so that subsequent episodes may be prevented. Children with moderately severe symptoms may be hospitalized for observation and therapy with cool mist and racemic epinephrine, as for LTB. Patients may respond to corticosteroid therapy. The disease is usually self-limited.

BACTERIAL TRACHEITIS

Bacterial tracheitis, an infection of the mucosa of the upper trachea, is a distinct entity with features of both croup and epiglottitis. The disease is seen in children ages 1 month to 6 years and may be a serious cause of airway obstruction—severe enough to cause respiratory arrest. It is believed to be a complication of LTB, and although *Staphylococcus aureus* is the most frequent organism responsible, group A β-hemolytic streptococci and *H. influenzae* have also been implicated.

Many of the manifestations of bacterial tracheitis are similar to those of LTB but are unresponsive to LTB therapy. There is a history of previous URI with croupy cough, stridor unaffected by position, toxicity, and high fever. A prominent manifestation is the production of thick, purulent tracheal secretions. Respiratory difficulties are secondary to these copious secretions.

Therapeutic Management and Nursing Considerations

Bacterial tracheitis requires vigorous management. Humidified oxygen, antipyretics, and antibiotics are prescribed. Most children require endotracheal intubation and frequent tracheal suctioning to prevent airway obstruction. The emphasis in this disorder is early recognition in order to prevent catastrophic airway obstruction.

INFECTIONS OF THE LOWER AIRWAYS

The *reactive portion* of the lower respiratory tract includes the bronchi and bronchioles in children. Cartilaginous support of the large airway is not fully developed until adolescence. Consequently, the smooth muscle in these structures represents a major factor in the constriction of the airway, particularly in the bronchioles, that portion that extends from the bronchi to the alveoli.

Table 32-2 compares some of the major features of bronchial and bronchiolar infections.

BRONCHITIS

Bronchitis (sometimes referred to as *tracheobronchitis*) describes inflammation of large airways (trachea and bronchi), which is almost invariably associated with a URI. Viral agents are the primary cause of the disease, although *Mycoplasma pneumoniae* is a common cause in children older than 6 years of age. The condition is characterized by a dry, hacking, and nonproductive cough that is worse at night and becomes productive in 2 to 3 days.

Bronchitis is a mild self-limiting disease that requires only symptomatic treatment, including analgesics, antipyretics, and humidity. Cough suppressants may be useful to allow rest but can interfere with cough clearance of secretions (Neddenriep, Taussig, and Mietens, 1989). Most patients recover uneventfully in 5 to 10 days.

RESPIRATORY SYNCYTIAL VIRUS (RSV)/BRONCHIOLITIS

Bronchiolitis is an acute viral infection with maximum effect at the bronchiolar level. The infection occurs primarily in winter and spring and is rare in children over 2 years of age. Although few children with bronchiolitis require hospitalization, it can be a serious disease.

Although adenoviruses and parainfluenza viruses can cause acute bronciolitis, ***respiratory syncytial virus (RSV)*** is responsible for at least 50% of children admitted for bronchiolitis (Hall, 1993; Jury, 1993; Kuzel and Clutter, 1993) and is recognized as the single most important respiratory pathogen in infancy and early childhood. It is estimated that more than 95,000 children are hospitalized each year at a cost of over $300 million (LaVia and others, 1993; Marks, 1992). The numbers are high, but it is important to realize that this represents only about 5% of the total number of children who contract RSV. It is also important to note that almost all children have contracted RSV infection by age 4 years (Hall, 1993; Kuzel and Clutter, 1993).

Etiology

RSV is a paramyxovirus containing a single strand of ribonucleic acid (RNA) and is related to parainfluenza virus. There are two major subgroups of RSV strains: A (the more virulent) and B. More children develop bronchiolitis and pneumonia from RSV subgroup A infections than from subgroup B infections during years of major outbreaks.

The disease usually begins in the fall, reaches a peak during the winter, and then decreases during the spring. In tropical regions, peaks of activity are less pronounced and outbreaks tend to occur in rainy seasons (Hall, 1993).

Pathophysiology

RSV affects the epithelial cells of the respiratory tract. The ciliated cells swell, protrude into the lumen, and lose their cilia. RSV produces a fusion of the infected cell membrane with cell membranes of adjacent epithelial cells, thus forming a giant cell with multiple nuclei. At the cellular level this fusion results in multinucleated masses of protoplasm, or "syncytia," being created.

TABLE 32-2 Comparison of Conditions Affecting the Bronchi

	VIRAL-INDUCED ASTHMA*	BRONCHITIS	BRONCHIOLITIS
Description	Exaggerated response of bronchi to infection Bronchospasm, exudation, and edema of bronchi	Usually occurs in association with URI Seldom an isolated entity	More common infectious disease of lower airways Maximum obstructive impact at bronchiolar level
Age-group affected	Late infancy and early childhood	Affects children in first 4 years of life	Usually children 2-12 months; rare after age 2 Peak incidence approximately age 6 months
Etiologic agents	Most often viruses but may be any of a variety of URI pathogens	Usually viral Other agents (e.g., bacteria, fungi, allergic disorders, airborne irritants) can trigger symptoms	Viruses, predominantly respiratory syncytial viruses; also adenoviruses, parainfluenza viruses, and *M. pneumoniae*
Predominant characteristics	Wheezing, productive cough	Persistent dry, hacking cough (worse at night) becoming productive in 2-3 days	Dyspnea, paroxysmal nonproductive cough, tachypnea with retractions and flaring nares, emphysema, may be wheezing
Treatment	Bronchodilators	Cough suppressants if needed	Oxygen mist Ribavirin if severe

*See Asthma, p. 1416.

These processes cause the bronchiole mucosa to swell, and lumina are subsequently filled with mucus and exudate; the walls of the bronchi and bronchioles are infiltrated with inflammatory cells, and peribronchiolar infections may occur. As luminal epithelial cells are shed into the bronchioles when they die, the lumina are frequently obstructed; this occurs most on expiration. In time, this could result in hyperinflation of the infant's lung and air trapping. The variable degrees of obstruction produced in small air passages by these changes lead to hyperinflation, obstructive emphysema resulting from partial obstruction, and patchy areas of atelectasis. Dilation of bronchial passages on inspiration allows sufficient space for intake of air, but narrowing of the passages on expiration prevents air from leaving the lungs. Thus air is trapped distal to the obstruction and causes progressive overinflation ***(emphysema)***.

Transmission

The transmission of RSV is predominantly through direct contact with respiratory secretions, mainly as a result of inoculation from hand to eye, nose, or other mucous membranes; by direct inoculation by large-particle aerosols; or by self-inoculation from contaminated fomites (Hall, 1993; Kuzel and Clutter, 1993; Marks, 1992).

RSV in secretions has been found to survive for hours on countertops, gloves, paper tissues, and cloth and for half an hour on skin; it remains infectious when transferred from hands or objects. Distant spread of RSV by small-particle aerosols (airborne transmission) has not been documented (Hall, 1993).

Clinical Manifestations

The younger the infant, the greater the likelihood that severe lower respiratory tract disease requiring hospitalization will occur. The peak incidence for RSV is 2 to 5 months of age (Hall, 1993; Jury, 1993), but reinfection with RSV is extraordinarily common at all ages, with the highest rates being reported from daycare centers. The severity of RSV tends to diminish with age and repeated infections.

The illness usually begins with a URI because of its portal of entry after an incubation of about 5 to 8 days, with symptoms such as rhinorrhea and fever often appearing first. OM and conjunctivitis may also be present. In time, a cough may develop. If the disease progresses, it becomes a lower respiratory tract infection and manifests typical symptoms (see box below, left). With infants there may be several days of URI symptoms or no characteristics except slight lethargy, poor feeding, or irritability; fever is usually present during this initial phase but is usually low grade. If the illness progresses to involve the lower tract, fever might actually disappear; the presence or degree of fever, therefore, does not reflect the severity of illness.

Once the lower airway is involved, classic manifestations include signs of altered air exchange, such as wheezing, retractions, crackles, dyspnea, tachypnea, and diminished breath sounds.

SIGNS AND SYMPTOMS OF RESPIRATORY SYNCYTIAL VIRUS

INITIAL

Rhinorrhea
Pharyngitis
Coughing/sneezing
Wheezing
Diffuse rhonchi, rales, and wheezing
Intermittent fever

WITH PROGRESSION OF ILLNESS

Increased coughing and wheezing
Air hunger
Tachypnea and retractions
Cyanosis

SEVERE ILLNESS

Tachypnea >70 breaths/min
Listlessness
Apneic spells
Poor air exchange; poor breath sounds

Diagnostic Evaluation

Because RSV infection may be manifested as a URI, it is often difficult to identify this specific etiologic agent by clinical criteria alone. The most difficult distinction to make in infants is between RSV and intrinsic reactive airway disease or asthma, because these conditions also involve the lower airway and have similar symptoms of airway resistance.

With RSV the identification has been simplified by the development of various tests done on nasal or nasopharyngeal secretions, using either rapid immunofluorescent antibody (IFA) or enzyme-linked immunosorbent assay (ELISA) techniques for RSV antigen detection. Both rapid tests have sensitivities and specificities of about 90%. The other, more traditional test still being done is the viral culture; this is becoming obsolete, however, because it may take several days to get a result.

Therapeutic Management

Treatment of bronchiolitis is based on the severity of symptoms and includes high humidity, adequate fluid intake, rest, and medications. Most children with bronchiolitis can be managed at home; however, hospitalization is usually recommended for children with complicating conditions, such as underlying lung or heart disease, associated debilitated states, or questionable adequacy of caregiver. The child who is tachypneic, has marked retractions, seems listless, or has a history of poor fluid intake should also be admitted (Guerra, Kemp, and Shearer, 1990). Mist therapy is generally combined with oxygen by hood or tent in concentrations sufficient to alleviate dyspnea and hypoxia, after which mist alone is continued for mild dyspnea. Fluids by mouth may be contraindicated because of tachypnea, weakness, and fatigue; therefore, intravenous fluids are preferred until the crisis of the disease has passed.

Clinical assessments, noninvasive oxygen monitoring, and blood gas values guide therapy. Medical therapy for bronchiolitis is controversial. Bronchodilators, corticosteroids, cough suppressants, and antibiotics have not proved to be effective in uncomplicated disease and are not recommended for routine use. Corticosteroids, theophylline, and furosemide have all been used for intubated and ventilated infants and children. ***Ribavirin,*** an antiviral agent (synthetic nucleoside analog) is the only specific therapy available for RSV infection (it also has therapeutic activity against influenza and parainfluenza), and improvement has been demonstrated in children with lower respiratory tract involvement (Hall, 1993; Jury, 1993). Some investigators question the unclear evidence of benefit from the drug (Ray, 1988; Wald, Dashefsky, and Green, 1988), and others cite potential toxic effects to health care workers from its use (Guglielmo, Jacobs, and Locksley, 1989). The Academy of Pediatrics (1993) recommends the criteria for use of ribavirin that are in the box at right. Several studies are examining the use of high-dose, short-duration therapy in which ribavirin is administered for 2 hours, three times a day, for 3 days; to date, the results have proved to be as effective as the traditional time frames (Englund and others, 1990).

Controversy has also surrounded the possible toxicity of ribavirin, since it produced teratogenic effects on laboratory rodents from studies done in the late 1970s and early 1980s. To date, all the studies done have indicated not only ribavirin's efficacy but also its safety in both patients and health care personnel taking care of children receiving the drug (Englund and others, 1990). Both the Academy of Pediatrics (1993) and the Canadian Pediatric Society (1991) have issued statements in support of the use and safety of ribavirin.

Attempts to produce a safe and effective vaccine have been going on since RSV was first discovered. At present, the greatest success has been with the newly developed genetic engineering techniques of vaccine production (Hall, 1993). In an attempt to combat the infection, especially in high-risk situations, research is also being done into the use of prophylactic administration of RSV immune globulin (Groothius and others, 1993; McIntosh, 1993). The initial conclusion is that monthly administration of high doses of RSV intravenous immune globulin (IVIG) was safe and effective in significantly decreasing both the incidence and the severity of RSV infection in high-risk children.

Nursing Considerations

Children admitted to the hospital with suspect RSV infection may be assigned separate rooms or grouped with other RSV-infection children over age 2 years. A variety of infection control procedures have been employed over the years, the most important of which is consistent handwashing and not touching the nasal mucosa or conjunctiva. The routine use of gowns and masks has not been shown to be of additional benefit, although gowns may help diminish the potential for fomite spread during close contact when infectious secretions may contaminate clothing (Hall, 1993). Other isolation procedures of potential benefit are those aimed at diminishing the number of hospital personnel, visitors, and uninfected patients in contact with the child. Another measure includes making patient assignments so that nurses assigned to children with RSV are not taking care of other patients who may be considered high risk.

Nurses taking care of children receiving ribavirin are advised to follow the suggestions in the box at right. Patient care sometimes warrants opening the tent while the small-particle aerosol generator (SPAG) is still running; in these cases it is recommended that one first shut the machine off and wait a few moments before opening the tent. Gloves and gowns are not essential, since dermal absorption appears to be negligible (Academy of Pediatrics, 1993). Scavenger devices are commercially available to help decrease the escape of aerosolized ribavirin.

RECOMMENDATIONS FOR THE USE OF RIBAVIRIN

1. Ribavirin should be used with children at high risk for complications caused by other conditions:
   - Infants at high risk for severe or complicated RSV infection, including those with bronchopulmonary dysplasia, cystic fibrosis, and other chronic lung conditions
   - Premature infants
   - Children with immunodeficiency (especially those with AIDS or severe combined immunodeficiency disease)
   - Recent transplant recipients
   - Patients undergoing chemotherapy for malignancy
   - Infants who are severely ill (values for arterial oxygen tension of less than 65 mm Hg and increasing concentration of carbon dioxide arterial pressure are useful indicators)
   - All patients mechanically ventilated for RSV infection
2. Ribavirin treatment should also be considered for hospitalized infants who may be at increased risk of progressing from a mild to a more complicated course:
   - Young age (less than 6 weeks)
   - Underlying condition such as multiple congenital anomalies, certain neurologic or metabolic diseases (e.g., severe cerebral palsy)
3. Rapid diagnostic techniques to identify RSV antigen in respiratory secretions should be performed when the child is admitted to the hospital; if rapid tests are not available, ribavirin treatment should begin on patients in recommended categories who:
   - Have bronchiolitis or pneumonia clinically compatible with RSV infection,
   - Are admitted during the RSV season (November through April)

   Treatment is discontinued if an agent other than RSV is found; treatment is continued if no agent is identified but:
   - The most likely clinical diagnosis remains RSV infection
   - The infant is severely ill
4. Ribavirin is:
   - Nebulized by a small-particle aerosol generator (SPAG) into an oxygen hood, tent, or mask from a solution containing 20 mg of ribavirin per milliliter of water
   - Administered for 12 to 20 hours per day
   - Usually given for 3 to 5 days
5. Contact isolation of patients with RSV remains in effect.
6. Precautions for health care personnel and visitors include the following:
   - Informing about the potential but unknown risks of environmental exposure to ribavirin
   - Advising pregnant women not to care directly for patients who are receiving ribavirin
   - Lowering environmental exposure to ribavirin by
     —Temporarily stopping aerosol administration when the hood or tent is open
     —Administering drug in well-ventilated rooms (at least six air changes per hour)

Modified from American Academy of Pediatrics, Committee on Infectious Diseases: Use of ribavirin in the treatment of respiratory syncytial virus infection, *Pediatrics* 92(3):501-504, 1993.

PNEUMONIA

Pneumonia refers to various disorders that differ in terms of the causative agent, course of the disease, pathology, and prognosis. The one common identifying feature of all pneumonias is that each involves a degree of inflammation, most frequently from infection. The common site for inflammation is the pulmonary parenchyma, with the causative agent usually introduced into the lungs through inhalation or the bloodstream. Pneumonia is common in childhood but occurs more frequently in infancy and early childhood. Clinically, pneumonia may occur either as a primary disease or as a complication of some other illness.

Pneumonia can be classified according to morphology, etiologic agent, and clinical form. Although morphologic classification is typically used (see box below), the most useful classification is generally considered to be based on the etiology, with the possibility of viral, bacterial, mycoplasma, and aspiration of foreign substances. Less often, pneumonia may be caused by histomycosis, coccidioidomycosis, and other fungi. Other terms that describe pneumonias are hemorrhagic, fibrinous, and necrotizing.

The clinical manifestations of pneumonia vary greatly, depending on the etiologic agent, the age of the child, the child's systemic reaction to the infection, the extent of the lesions, and the degree of bronchial and bronchiolar obstruction. The etiologic agent is identified largely from the clinical history, the child's age, the general health history, the physical examination, radiography, and the laboratory examination.

VIRAL PNEUMONIA

Viral pneumonias occur more frequently than bacterial pneumonias and are seen in children of all age-groups. They are often associated with viral URIs, and the pathologic changes involve interstitial pneumonitis with inflammation of the mucosa and the walls of bronchi and bronchioles. Virtually every type of microorganism is capable of producing pneumonia, with viruses representing the single most frequent cause: RSV in infants and parainfluenza, influenza, and adenovirus in older children. There are few clinical symptoms to distinguish between the responsible organisms, and differentiations between viruses can be made only by laboratory examination.

Clinical Manifestations

The onset may be acute or insidious, and symptoms are variable, ranging from mild fever, slight cough, and malaise to high fever, severe cough, and prostration. Early in the course of the illness, the cough is likely to be unproductive or productive of small amounts of whitish sputum. Breath sounds may include a few wheezes or fine crackles. Radiography reveals diffuse or patchy infiltration with a peribronchial distribution.

Therapeutic Management and Nursing Considerations

The prognosis is generally good, although viral infections of the respiratory tract render the affected child more susceptible to secondary bacterial invasion. Treatment is usually symptomatic and includes measures to promote oxygenation and comfort, such as oxygen administration with cool mist, chest physiotherapy and postural drainage, antipyretics for fever management, fluid intake, and family support. Although some authorities recommend antimicrobial therapy in hope of reducing or preventing secondary bacterial infection, it is usually reserved for children in whom the presence of such infection is demonstrated by appropriate cultures.

> **TYPES OF PNEUMONIA**
>
> **Lobar pneumonia**—All or a large segment of one or more pulmonary lobes is involved. When both lungs are affected, it is known as bilateral or "double" pneumonia.
>
> **Bronchopneumonia**—Begins in the terminal bronchioles, which become clogged with mucopurulent exudate to form consolidated patches in nearby lobules; also called lobular pneumonia.
>
> **Interstitial pneumonia**—The inflammatory process is more or less confined within the alveolar walls (interstitium) and the peribronchial and interlobular tissues.

PRIMARY ATYPICAL PNEUMONIA

Mycoplasma pneumoniae is the most common cause of pneumonia in children between ages 5 and 12 years (Moffet, 1989). It occurs principally in fall and winter months and is more prevalent in crowded living conditions.

Clinical Manifestations

The onset may be sudden or insidious and is usually accompanied by general systemic symptoms, including fever, chills (in older children), headache, malaise, anorexia, and muscle pain (myalgia). These symptoms are followed by rhinitis, sore throat, and a dry, hacking cough. The cough, initially nonproductive, produces seromucoid sputum that later becomes mucopurulent or blood streaked. The duration and degree of fever vary widely and may last from several days to 2 weeks. Dyspnea occurs infrequently.

Radiographic examination reveals evidence of pneumonia before physical signs are apparent. There may be fine crepitant crackles over various areas of the lung fields, but consolidation is usually not demonstrated. The pathologic process consists of interstitial round cell infiltration and edema of alveolar septa and varying distribution of areas of inflammation, necrosis, and ulceration of the mucosal lining of bronchi and bronchioles. Areas of consolidation and emphysema are present.

Therapeutic Management and Nursing Considerations

Most affected persons recover from acute illness in 7 to 10 days with symptomatic treatment, followed by a week of convalescence. Hospitalization is rarely necessary.

BACTERIAL PNEUMONIA

Bacterial pneumonia is often a serious infection. The pathogenetic mechanisms involved are often aspiration or hematogenous dissemination. The cause varies depending on the age and underlying illness of the child and the degree of immunosuppression or competency. The child presents with an underlying lower airway condition, which then requires further examination.

Etiology and Epidemiology

Etiology of bacterial pneumonia varies with the age of the child. *Streptococcus pneumoniae* (pneumococcus), group A streptococcus, staphylococcus, or enteric bacilli are the most likely agents in infants under 3 months of age. Chlamydial infection is also a cause of pneumonia in this age-group. In the 3-month to 5-year age-group, pneumococcal infection and *Haemophilus influenzae* type b (Hib) are common causes, although *H. influenzae* is causing fewer infections because of the Hib vaccine. Mycoplasma pneumonia is found more frequently in children over 5 years of age, with streptococcus and staphylococcus being the most common causes in otherwise healthy children.

Clinical Manifestions

Clinical manifestations of bacterial pneumonia in normal children (see box below) usually appear acutely with fever and toxic appearance; infants and younger children develop more severe symptoms than older children. The older child may complain of headache, chills, abdominal pain, or chest pain. Respiratory distress may or may not be present. Initially, cough is usually hacking and nonproductive, and breath sounds are diminished or heard as scattered crackles. When consolidation is present, breath sounds may be tubular in quality with no adventitious noises. As the infection resolves, coarse crackles and wheezing are heard and the cough becomes productive with purulent sputum.

Lack of specific signs indicating infection makes diagnosis in infancy particularly difficult. First evidence of infection is often irritability or lethargy and poor feeding. Abrupt fever may be accompanied by seizures. Respiratory distress is evident with air hunger, tachypnea, and circumoral cyanosis. Because pneumonia in newborns carries a high morbidity and mortality, bacterial infection should be suspected in those with respiratory symptoms and therapy initiated.

Staphylococcal pneumonia is rare but particularly progressive and must be treated aggressively. The onset is rapid, with rapid deterioration. Conjunctivitis and furuncles are signs of a probable staphylococcal infection.

GENERAL SIGNS OF PNEUMONIA

- Fever: usually quite high
- Respiratory
  - Cough: unproductive to productive with whitish sputum
  - Tachypnea
  - Breath sounds: rhonchi or fine crackles
  - Dullness with percussion
  - Chest pain
  - Retractions
  - Nasal flaring
  - Pallor to cyanosis (depends on severity)
- Chest x-ray film: diffuse or patchy infiltration, with peribronchial distribution
- Behavior: irritable, restless, lethargic
- Gastrointestinal: anorexia, vomiting, diarrhea, abdominal pain

Diagnostic Evaluation

The key to a preliminary diagnosis is finding pulmonary infiltrates on radiographic examination, usually revealing lobar consolidation and, in some severe cases, pleural effusion. Laboratory studies performed, including Gram stain and culture of sputum, nasopharyngeal specimens, blood cultures, and lung aspiration and biopsy, may indicate many different positive results. The white blood cell count may be elevated, but it may be normal for infants with staphylcoccal disease. In addition, children with staphylcoccal disease usually have an elevated antistreptolysin O titer.

Therapeutic Management

Antimicrobial therapy has significantly reduced the morbidity and mortality from bacterial pneumonia. Therapy with penicillin G, intramuscularly or intravenously, or for penicillin-allergic children, erythromycin, trimethoprim-sulfamethoxazole, clindamycin, chloramphenicol, or cephalosporins, is effective in the treatment of pneumococcal pneumonia and is implemented as soon as the diagnosis is suspected. Because staphylococcal infections are caused by penicillinase-producing (penicillin G–resistant) staphylococci, semisynthetic penicillins are administered. In the hospital, medications are given parenterally for rapid action and maximum effect. Sometimes a single daily dose of procaine penicillin G or oral penicillin every 6 to 8 hours for 7 to 10 days may be given for pneumococcal pneumonia.

Most older children with pneumococcal pneumonia can be treated at home, especially if the condition is recognized and treatment initiated early. Antibiotic therapy, bed rest, liberal oral intake of fluid, and administration of antipyretics for fever constitute the principal therapeutic measures. Hospitalization is indicated when pleural effusion or empyema accompanies the disease and is mandatory for children with staphylococcal pneumonia. Pneumonia in the infant or young child is best treated in the hospital, since the course of illness is more variable and complications are more common in very young patients. In addition, intravenous fluid administration is frequently necessary, and oxygen may be required if the child is in respiratory distress.

Prognosis. The prognosis for pneumococcal infections is generally good, with rapid recovery when they are recognized and treated early. The course of staphylococcal pneumonia is generally prolonged. The prognosis varies with the length of the illness before treatment, although early recognition and treatment are usually beneficial.

Use of pneumococcal polysaccharide vaccine is recommended for use in selected individuals such as children over age 2 years who are at risk of acquiring pneumococcal infection or are at risk of serious disease. (See Immunizations, Chapter 12.)

Complications. At present, the classic features and clinical course of pneumonia are rarely seen because of early and vigorous antibiotic and supportive therapy. However, many children, especially infants, with staphylococcal pneumonia develop empyema, pyopneumothorax, or tension pneumothorax. Pneumococci are the most common cause of acute otitis media and a frequent complication of pneumococcal infection. Pleural effusion is not uncommon in children with lobar (pneumococcal) pneumonia. A diagnostic thoracentesis is performed if fluid is suspected to be in the pleural cavity. Nonpurulent effusions, such as occur in pneumococcal pneumonia, do not require surgical drainage.

Continuous closed chest drainage is instituted when purulent fluid is aspirated, a frequent finding in staphylococcal infections. If a large amount of purulent drainage is obtained, an appropriate antibiotic is instilled into the cavity and the suction is discontinued for approximately 1 hour after the instillation. Closed drainage is continued until drainage fluid is free of pathogens—rarely more than 5 to 7 days. Sometimes repeated pleural taps are sufficient to remove fluid; however, the purulent drainage accumulates so rapidly and is so highly viscous that continuous drainage is preferred. In addition, continuous drainage is less traumatic to the child than repeated thoracentesis.

Thoracentesis. Dyspnea resulting from pressure from fluid accumulation in the pleural cavity requires removal by thoracentesis. Thoracentesis is also performed to obtain fluid for culture or to instill antibiotics directly into the pleural cavity. Equipment and preparation for the procedure are the same as for an adult. Nursing responsibilities include obtaining and setting up equipment, preparing the child physically and psychologically, and assisting the practitioner with the procedure. If continuous closed chest drainage is anticipated, this equipment should also be available. Thoracentesis is performed with the child in a sitting position, preferably with arms and trunk bent forward over pillows or over an overbed table with a pillow. Infants are positioned in a semirecumbent position on the unaffected side. The child will need to be physically restrained in the desired position by the nurse. The nurse provides explanation, offers emotional support during the procedure, and observes the child for any changes in color, respiration, and pulse and any alterations in behavior (e.g., coughing) and sensorium.

After the procedure the child is made comfortable, and observations and recording of physical and emotional responses are continued. The amount and description of the fluid obtained and any medication instilled are recorded, and specimens are sent to the laboratory for culture. Continuous closed chest drainage is managed according to the same protocol as for the child with a thoracotomy.

Nursing Considerations

Nursing care of the child with pneumonia is primarily supportive and symptomatic but necessitates thorough respiratory assessment and administration of oxygen and antibiotics. The child's respiratory rate and status, as well as general disposition and level of activity, are frequently assessed. Isolation procedures are instituted according to hospital policy; rest and conservation of energy are encouraged by relief of physical and psychologic stress. The child is disturbed as little as possible by clustering care to encourage the child's regular sleep cycle. If the cough is disturbing, judicious use of antitussives, especially before rest times and meals, is often helpful. To prevent dehydration, fluids are frequently administered intravenously during the acute phase. Oral fluids, if allowed, are given cautiously to avoid aspiration and to decrease the possibility of aggravating a fatiguing cough.

Children may be placed in a mist tent, with cool humidification moistening the airways and providing an atmosphere that assists in temperature reduction. Children often require frequent clothing and linen changes to prevent chilling in the damp atmosphere. They are usually more comfortable in a semierect position but should be allowed to determine the position of comfort. Lying on the affected side (if pneumonia is unilateral) splints the chest on that side and reduces the pleural rubbing that often causes discomfort. If needed, oxygen can be delivered into the mist tent or be administered via nasal cannula. Fever is usually controlled by the cool environment and administration of antipyretic drugs as prescribed. Temperature is monitored regularly to detect a rise that might trigger a febrile seizure.

Vital signs and chest sounds are monitored to assess the progress of the disease and to detect early signs of complications. Children with ineffectual cough or those with difficulty handling secretions, especially infants, require suctioning to maintain a patent airway. A simple bulb suction syringe is usually sufficient for clearing the nares and nasopharynx of infants, but mechanical suction should be readily available if needed. Older children can usually handle secretions without assistance. Postural drainage and chest physiotherapy are generally prescribed every 4 hours or more often, depending on the child's condition.

The hospitalized child is apprehensive, and many of the treatments and tests are frightening and stress producing. It is important to involve the entire family in as much of the care as appropriate and to encourage questions and facilitate effective communication regarding provision of care. Reducing anxiety and apprehension reduces psychologic distress in the child, and when the child is more relaxed, the respiratory efforts are lessened. Easing respiratory efforts makes the child less apprehensive, and encouraging the presence of the caregiver provides the child with a customary source of comfort and support.

CHLAMYDIAL PNEUMONIA

Chlamydia trachomatis is an intracellular microorganism that has a number of properties similar to gram-negative bacteria. It is currently classified as a specialized bacterium. The organism is responsible for one of the most common sexually transmitted diseases, and newborn infants acquire pulmonary infection from their mothers via ascending infection just before or in the process of birth.

Chlamydial pneumonia is a severe, diffuse disease; its onset is in children between 1 and 3 months, and it is characterized by a persistent cough and tachypnea, but minimum or absent fever. Radiographs show nonspecific abnormalities. Treatment with erythromycin and sulfa drugs shortens the course of the illness. Nursing care is the same as for any infant with pneumonia.

OTHER INFECTIONS OF THE RESPIRATORY TRACT

PERTUSSIS (WHOOPING COUGH)

Pertussis, or whooping cough, is an acute respiratory infection caused by *Bordetella pertussis* that occurs chiefly in children younger than 4 years of age who have not been immunized. It is highly contagious and is particularly threatening in young infants, who have a higher morbidity and mortality rate. (See Table 16-1 for signs, symptoms, and management of pertussis.) The incidence is highest in the spring and summer months, and a single attack confers lifetime immunity. Pertussis vaccine is effective, but the immunity diminishes with time after the initial infection or immunization. A small number of immunized adolescents develop an asymptomatic case of pertussis (Cromer, Goydos, and Hackell, 1993).

TUBERCULOSIS (TB)

TB is an ancient disease that, although controlled in most developed countries, remains a health hazard and the leading cause of death throughout many parts of the world (Jackson, 1993; Starke and Jacobs, 1992). In the United States the incidence of TB is increasing; the age-group affected most is 25 to 44 years old (54.5% increase from 1985 to 1992). The disease has also increased significantly in children, with a 36.1% increase in those up to 4 years old and a 34.1% increase in children ages 5 to 14 years (Jackson, 1993). The increases are attributed in part to the many foreign-born persons emigrating to the United States, since statistics show that more than two thirds of the reported TB cases now occur in nonwhite and ethnic groups (Gaffney, Dennis, and Carneiro, 1994; Jackson, 1993), as well as in persons with other risk factors, especially HIV infection (see box at right) (American Academy of Pediatrics, 1994b).

Etiology

TB is caused by *Mycobacterium tuberculosis,* an acid-fast bacillus (i.e., the organism is not readily decolorized by acids after staining). The main types of tubercle bacilli that cause disease in humans are the human *(M. tuberculosis)* and the bovine *(M. bovis)*. Children are susceptible to both varieties, and in parts of the world where TB in cattle is not controlled or pasteurization of milk is not practiced, the bovine type is a common source of infection in children.

Although the causative agent is the tubercle bacillus, other factors influence the degree to which the organism is able to produce an altered state in the host. Also emerging are multidrug-resistant strains of *M. tuberculosis,* which have caused a number of outbreaks in hospitals (Beck-Sague and others, 1992; Centers for Disease Control, 1993; Pearson and others, 1992). This resistance occurs probably because of patient/family noncompliance with the long therapeutic regimen (Jackson, 1993). Resistance to the bacillus can be modified by many factors (see box below).

Pathophysiology

The source of infection in children is usually an infected member of the household, either adult or teenager, but any frequent visitor to the household, such as a baby-sitter, could expose the child. Transmission of *M. tuberculosis* usually occurs when the child inhales microdroplets (usually 1 to 5 μ in size) into the respiratory tract after someone has coughed or sneezed, when they disperse the organisms into the air. Although the lung is the most frequent portal of entry in humans, the organism *M. bovis* can gain entrance to the body by ingestion of infected milk. When the *M. tuberculosis* droplet is inhaled, it passes down the bronchial tree, implanting in either a bronchiole or alveolus, and then starts to multiply every 18 to 24 hours (Jackson, 1993).

FACTORS AFFECTING RESISTANCE TO TUBERCULOSIS

HEREDITY

No positive evidence to indicate hereditary tendency
Evidence that resistance to infection may be genetically transmitted

SEX

Early years: no sex differences in incidence
Later childhood and adolescence: morbidity and mortality higher in girls than in boys

AGE

Diminished resistance to infection in infancy
- Delay in development of acquired immunity
- Diminished capacity to resist extension of infective process

Increased tendency to develop disease during puberty and adolescence
- New infection superimposed on a previous one
- Increased contacts
- Indigenous reinfection stimulated by metabolic changes or suboptimum diets during a period of rapid growth

STRESS STATES

Temporary stressful circumstances (e.g., injury or illness, undernutrition, emotional distress, chronic fatigue) may increase susceptibility to infection
Increased secretion of adrenal steroids suppresses protective inflammatory response and permits infection to spread
Therapeutic administration of corticosteroids (similar effect)

NUTRITION

Active disease inversely proportional to state of nutrition
Excellent nutrition is essential to young children's recovery from disease

INTERCURRENT INFECTION

Infectious diseases (especially human immunodeficiency virus [HIV], measles, pertussis) may activate latent tuberculosis
Noncompliance with therapy

There is a proliferation of epithelial cells that surround and encapsulate the multiplying bacilli in an attempt to wall off the invading organisms, thus forming the typical ***tubercle.*** During the inflammatory process, some of the bacilli leave the focal area and are carried to the regional lymph nodes that drain the anatomic area of the organism; as a result, the child develops a fever. Radiographic examinations may be positive if such tests are made, as in cases when the child is known to have been exposed. The tuberculin test is positive. Outcomes of pulmonary TB can vary.

Extension of the primary lesion at the original site causes progressive tissue destruction as it spreads within the lung, discharges material from foci to other areas of the lungs (e.g., bronchi or pleura), or produces pneumonia. Erosion of blood vessels by the primary lesion can cause widespread dissemination of the tubercle bacillus to near and distant sites ***(miliary TB).*** Organisms deposited in the upper lung zones, bones, kidneys, and brain may find favorable environments for growth, but certain organs and tissue, such as bone marrow, liver, and spleen, appear to inhibit multiplication of the bacilli.

For children not immunosuppressed or compromised, a strong cell-mediated immune response provides specific immunity that usually limits further multiplication of the bacilli. These children will remain asymptomatic, and the lesions will usually heal. ***TB infection*** is manifested by a positive skin test only. In a small percentage of persons with newly acquired TB, replication of the organism continues, and ***TB disease*** will ensue, as evidenced by a positive chest radiograph, positive sputum culture, and signs of disease.

Clinical Manifestations

Clinical manifestations of TB in children are extremely variable. The disease may be asymptomatic or produce a broad range of symptoms, including general responses such as fever, malaise, anorexia, and weight loss or more specific symptoms related to the site of infection (e.g., lungs, bone, brain, kidneys). Lung disease may or may not include cough (which progresses slowly over weeks to months), aching pain and tightness in the chest, and (rarely) hemoptysis.

As increasing amounts of lung tissue become involved, the respiratory rate increases, the lung on the affected side does not expand as well as the other, auscultation reveals diminished breath sounds and crackles, and there is dullness to percussion. In children (usually infants) who are unable to contain the spread of infection, the fever persists; the generalized symptoms are manifest; and they develop pallor, anemia, weakness, and weight loss.

Diagnostic Evaluation

Several tests and procedures are used to establish a diagnosis. Diagnosis is based on information derived from physical examination, history, reaction to tuberculin tests, radiographic examinations, and organism cultures. In addition, it must be determined whether or not the lesion is in the active, quiescent, or healed stage.

History. Symptoms generally do not contribute significantly to a diagnosis. History of possible contact with a person known to be infected or subsequently found to be infected is helpful. All contacts of an affected child are examined for the disease.

Tuberculin Test. The tuberculin test is still the single most important test to determine whether a child has been infected with the tubercle bacillus. A primary infection initiates a hypersensitivity reaction to the protein fraction of the tubercle bacillus, which can be detected 2 to 10 weeks after the infection.

Two types of tuberculin preparations are used for skin tests: ***old tuberculin (OT)*** and ***purified protein derivative (PPD)*** of tuberculin. The PPD is used most widely, and the standard dose is 5 tuberculin units (TU) in 0.1 ml of solution, injected intradermally ***(Mantoux test).*** Also sometimes used are the ***multiple-puncture tests (MPTs),*** such as the Tine, which may contain OT or PPD. The MPTs have several problems that may severely limit their usefulness (American Academy of Pediatrics, 1994b):

1. The exact dose of tuberculin antigen introduced into the skin cannot be standardized and therefore is not appropriate for diagnostic testing.
2. The booster phenomenon occurs, which represents an increase in reaction to a skin test caused by repetitive testing. This incidence increases with age and is greater in geographic areas where exposure to nontuberculous mycobacteria is common in children previously vaccinated with bacillus Calmette-Guérin (BCG).
3. The MPTs have been associated with high rates of false-positive and false-negative results as compared with the Mantoux test.
4. The use of MPTs has led to the practice of allowing nonprofessionals, such as parents, to interpret the skin tests and report findings by telephone or mail.

Recommendations for skin testing follow (American Academy of Pediatrics, 1994b):

1. Routine annual skin testing for tuberculosis (Mantoux) in children with no risk factors in low-prevalence communities is not indicated. In such settings, positive skin reactions are most likely to be falsely positive.
2. Children at high risk should be tested annually, using Mantoux tests. These groups include:
   - Contacts of adults with infectious tuberculosis
   - Those who are from, or have parents who are from, regions of the world with high prevalence of tuberculosis
   - Those with abnormalities on chest roentgenogram suggestive of tuberculosis
   - Those with clinical evidence of tuberculosis
   - HIV-seropositive persons
   - Those with immunosuppressive conditions
   - Those with other medical risk factors: Hodgkin disease, lymphoma, diabetes mellitus, chronic renal failure, malnutrition
   - Incarcerated adolescents
   - Children frequently exposed to the following adults: HIV-infected individuals, homeless persons, users of intravenous and other street drugs, poor and medically indigent city dwellers, residents of nursing homes, migrant farm workers
3. Children who have no risk factors but who reside in high-prevalence regions and children whose history for risk factors is incomplete or unreliable may receive periodic Mantoux tests, such as at 1, 4 to 6, and 11 to 16 years of age. Such a decision should be based on the local epidemiology of tuberculosis.
4. Tuberculin skin testing can be done at the same time that

DEFINITION OF POSITIVE MANTOUX SKIN TEST (5 TU-PPD) IN CHILDREN*

REACTION ≥5 mm

Children in close contact with persons who have known or suspected infectious cases of tuberculosis:
- Households with active or previously active cases if (1) treatment cannot be verified as adequate before exposure, (2) treatment was initiated after period of child's contact, or (3) reactivation is suspected

Children suspected to have tuberculous disease:
- Chest roentgenogram consistent with active or previously active tuberculosis
- Clinical evidence of tuberculosis

Children with immunosuppressive conditions† or HIV infection

REACTION ≥10 mm

Children at increased risk of dissemination from:
- Young age: less than 4 years of age
- Other medical risk factors, including Hodgkin disease, lymphoma, diabetes mellitus, chronic renal failure, and malnutrition

Children with increased environmental exposure:
- Born, or whose parents were born, in regions of the world where tuberculosis is highly prevalent
- Frequently exposed to adults who are HIV infected, homeless, users of intravenous and other street drugs, poor and medically indigent city dwellers, residents of nursing homes, incarcerated or institutionalized persons, and migrant farm workers

REACTION ≥15 mm

Children 4 years of age or older without any risk factors

From American Academy of Pediatrics, Committee on Infectious Diseases: *1994 Red Book: Report of the Committee on Infectious Diseases,* ed 23, Elk Grove Village, IL, 1994, The Academy, p 485.
*These recommendations should apply regardless of whether BCG has been previously administered.
†Including immunosuppressive doses of corticosteroids.

CIRCUMSTANCES PRODUCING FALSE-NEGATIVE REACTIONS TO TUBERCULIN TESTS

Tuberculin reaction suppressed by:
- Intercurrent diseases (e.g., viral diseases such as measles, rubella, influenza, mumps, varicella, and probably others [about 4 weeks])
- Viral vaccines (e.g., measles, mumps, and rubella vaccines [about 4 weeks])
- Corticosteroids and other immunosuppressive agents

Cellular immunodeficiency disease

Severe malnutrition

Too early testing before the body develops a sensitivity to the protein fraction of the tubercle bacillus

Use of impotent, outdated testing material—Mixture that has been prepared for too long or has been exposed to sunlight

Faulty technique (e.g., deep injection, no wheal formed, improper measurement of solution, or leaking of solution from a defective or loosely fitting syringe)

Overwhelming tuberculosis infections—End-stage and terminal miliary disease; may cause allergy to disappear

measles vaccine (usually MMR) is given. If testing is indicated in a child who does not have clinical or roentgenographic manifestations suggestive of tuberculosis, and cannot be done concurrently, testing should be postponed for 4 to 6 weeks.

5. All results (positive or negative) should be read routinely by qualified medical personnel.

Test results are determined according to instructions provided by the manufacturer. A ***positive reaction*** indicates that the person has been infected and has developed a sensitivity to the protein of the tubercle bacillus; it does not confirm the presence of active disease. Once individuals react positively, they will continue to do so. A positive reaction in a previously negative reactor indicates the person has been infected since the last test. Guidelines for interpreting the Mantoux skin test are listed in the box above.

In theory, tuberculin testing should not be carried out before or at the same time as measles immunization. Exacerbation of TB is known to occur with natural measles infection and could result from the live attenuated measles virus vaccine. Furthermore, viral interference from the vaccine may cause a false-negative reaction. However, in actual practice, neither of these possibilities is considered a contraindication to measles immunization, especially in the event of an epidemic.

Various factors can affect the response to the test and produce false reactions. A negative reaction usually means that the child has never been infected with the organism. However, circumstances may produce a false-negative reaction (see box above).

Bacteriologic Examination. A definitive diagnosis is made by demonstrating the presence of mycobacteria in culture. The organism is identified from microscopic examination of properly prepared and stained smears from early-morning gastric washings or from sputum, pleural fluid, urine, spinal fluid, draining lymph nodes, and other body fluids.

Radiographic Studies. Radiographic examinations are usually carried out, but numerous chronic intrathoracic diseases may simulate tuberculous lesions; therefore the use of x-ray examinations is chiefly supplementary to other diagnostic methods.

Classification. Based on the results of skin testing and other tests, the following classification may be used for individuals exposed to and/or infected with TB (American Thoracic Society, 1990):

- Class 0: No TB exposure
- Class 1: TB exposure, no evidence of infection
- Class 2: TB infection, no disease
- Class 3: TB, clinically active
- Class 4: TB, not clinically active
- Class 5: TB suspect (diagnosis pending)

Therapeutic Management

Medical management of tuberculous lesions in children consists of adequate nutrition, chemotherapy, general supportive measures, prevention of unnecessary exposure to other infections that further compromise the body's defenses, prevention of reinfection, and sometimes surgical procedures.

Chemotherapy is the single most important therapeutic modality available for management of TB. A variety of chemical agents can be used, and a regimen involving two or more drugs simultaneously has been found to be effective and is usually the mode of choice.

Preventive therapy is intended to keep latent infection from progressing to clinically active tuberculosis, as well as being used for primary prevention to prevent initial infection in persons in high-risk situations. The most common drug used for this is isoniazid (INH) for 9 months and up to 12 months for the HIV-infected child. This is given daily in a single dose, usually 10 mg/kg orally, with a maximum dose of 300 mg. The drug has no effect on the child's reaction to tuberculin; therefore the test continues to be useful in detecting acquired infection.

For the child with clinically active tuberculosis, the goal is to achieve sterilization of the tuberculous lesion. A 6-month regimen consisting of INH, rifampin, and pyrazinamide (PZA) given daily for the first 2 months is recommended. After this 2-month period, a regimen of INH and rifampin given twice weekly is acceptable if administration of the drugs is observed directly. Additional medications used less frequently include streptomycin (intramuscular injection only) and ethambutol (American Academy of Pediatrics, 1994a).

NURSING ALERT Direct observation means that a health care worker or other responsible, mutually agreed on individual is present when medications are administered to the patient. If the reliability of self-administration of medications is in doubt, directly observed, twice-weekly therapy administered by a health care professional must be provided.

The rationale for multiple drug therapy is based on three characteristics of the bacillus. Metabolic rates of bacilli vary in different lesions. For example, bacilli in well-oxygenated lesions (e.g., open cavities) replicate rapidly; the organism in a low-oxygen environment can remain dormant for extended periods (Starke, 1988). Also, *M. tuberculosis* is particularly prone to mutation to drug-resistant strains, and drugs vary in their ability to penetrate the blood-brain barrier (Engel, 1989). Sometimes a short course of corticosteroids may be used (in conjunction with antituberculosis drugs) to diminish the inflammatory response, especially in meningitis.

Surgical procedures may be required to remove the source of infection in tissues that are inaccessible to chemotherapy or that are destroyed by the disease. Orthopaedic procedures for correction of bone deformities, bronchoscopy for removal of a tuberculous granulomatous polyp, or resection of a portion of a diseased lung may also be performed.

Prognosis. Most children recover from primary TB infection and may be unaware of its presence. However, very young children have a higher incidence of disseminated disease. It is a serious disease during the first 2 years of life, during adolescence, and in children infected with HIV. Except in cases of tuberculous meningitis, death seldom occurs in treated children. Antibiotic therapy has decreased mortality and hematogenous spread from primary lesions.

Prevention. The only certain means to prevent TB is to avoid contact with the tubercle bacillus. Maintaining an optimum state of health with adequate nutrition and avoiding fatigue and debilitating infections promote natural resistance but do not prevent infection.

Pasteurization of milk and routine testing and elimination of diseased cattle have helped reduce the incidence of bovine tuberculosis. Infants and children should be given only pasteurized milk from TB-free cattle.

Of concern to hospital personnel is that the infected child and/or family members may spread the disease when visiting in the hospital. Most children with TB need not be isolated and can be hospitalized on an open ward if they are receiving chemotherapy. Children and adolescents with infectious pulmonary TB, that is, those whose sputum smears show acid-fast bacillus, should be on isolation precautions until effective chemotherapy has been initiated, their sputum smears show a diminishing number of organisms, and their cough is improving. Masks are indicated only when the child is coughing and does not reliably cover the mouth. Gowns are indicated only if needed to prevent gross contamination of clothing. Family members should be managed with these precautions when visiting until they are demonstrated not to have infectious TB.*

Limited immunity can be produced by administration of ***BCG (bacillus Calmette-Guérin)*** vaccine containing bovine bacilli with reduced virulence. The freshly prepared vaccine, injected intradermally, produces definite although incomplete protection (about 50%) against TB (Colditz and others, 1994). In most instances, positive tuberculin reactions develop after inoculation. The distribution of BCG vaccine is controlled by local or state health departments, but the vaccine is not used extensively, even in areas with a high prevalence of disease. BCG vaccination is not generally recommended for use in the United States. However, it may be recommended for long-term protection of infants and children with negative tuberculin skin tests who are at high risk for continuing exposure to persons with infectious TB and who cannot be placed on long-term preventive therapy or when an issue of noncompliance exists (American Thoracic Society, 1992).

Nursing Considerations

Hospitalization is seldom necessary except for needed diagnostic tests. Only those children with the more serious forms are placed in the hospital for therapy; others are managed satisfactorily at home. Therefore the major nursing care of children with TB involves nurses in ambulatory settings: outpatient departments, schools, and especially public health agencies.

---

*As of this writing, the Centers for Disease Control and Prevention (CDC) are revising their 1990 *Guidelines for Preventing the Transmission of Tuberculosis in Health-Care Facilities,* which may be published in late 1994 or in 1995.

Asymptomatic children are able to lead an essentially unrestricted life. They can and should attend school (or daycare), but older children are restricted from vigorous activities such as competitive games and contact sports during the active stage of primary TB. They should be protected from stresses, including parental anxieties, overprotection, and pressures regarding nutritional intake. The regular immunization schedule should be continued. Care should be exerted to maintain an optimum health status with proper diet, adequate rest, and avoidance of infection.

Diagnosis. Nurses assume several important roles in management of the disease, including assisting with radiographic examinations, performing skin tests, and obtaining specimens for laboratory examination. Skin tests, whether used as screening tools or diagnostic aids, must be carried out correctly in order for the results to be accurate. A wheal 6 to 10 mm in diameter is formed in the skin when the solution is injected. If a wheal is not formed, the procedure is repeated.

Sputum specimens are difficult or impossible to obtain in an infant or young child, since they swallow any mucus coughed from the lower respiratory tract. Therefore the best means for obtaining material for smears or culture is by gastric washing, that is, aspiration of lavaged contents from the fasting stomach. The procedure is carried out and the specimen obtained early in the morning before the customary breakfast time.

Ambulatory Care. Nursing supervision of the child at home involves teaching parents and child about the disease and its ramifications. Since children usually acquire the disease from an adult in the home, parents often feel guilty. Historically the disease has been regarded with fear, and numerous misconceptions need to be clarified. Reducing parental anxieties helps them to deal with the illness more constructively and to collaborate more effectively in planning for the child's continued care. The success of therapy depends on the acceptance and cooperation of the family. Therefore promoting compliance with drug therapy is essential (see Compliance, Chapter 27). The nurse can help the family to understand the rationale of diagnostic procedures and therapy and the importance of maintaining the therapeutic plan over the extended period needed for recovery. Promoting optimum general health and preventing intercurrent infections and reinfections with the tubercle bacillus are also of primary importance. Excellent patient education materials can be obtained from the **American Lung Association.***

Case Finding. Case finding and follow-up of known contacts are important nursing responsibilities. Every case of tuberculosis identified in the community involves nurses in follow-up of known contacts—contacts from whom the affected person may have acquired the disease and persons who may have been exposed to the diseased individual. Early diagnosis affords a means for early protection or treatment and prevents further spread of the disease.

*1740 Broadway, New York, NY 10019-4374; (212) 315-8700.

PULMONARY DISTURBANCE CAUSED BY NONINFECTIOUS IRRITANTS

FOREIGN BODY ASPIRATION

Small children characteristically explore matter with their mouths and are therefore particularly prone to aspirate foreign bodies into the air passages. Aspiration of foreign bodies can occur at any age but is most commonly seen in older infants and children ages 1 to 3 years. Children under 4 years of age account for 20% of all deaths caused by inhaled foreign material (Blumer, 1991). Aspiration of a foreign body presents a serious and sometimes fatal condition. Severity is determined by the location, type of object aspirated, and extent of obstruction. For example, dry vegetable matter, such as a seed, nut, or piece of carrot or popcorn, that does not dissolve and that may swell when wet creates a particularly difficult problem. The high fat content of potato chips and peanuts may cause the added risk of lipoid pneumonia. "Fun foods" of any kind are among the worst offenders.

More than 90% of deaths from food-related asphyxiation occur in children less than 5 years of age and 65% occur in infants. Offending foods in the order of frequency of aspiration are hot dog, round candy, peanut or other nut, grape, cookie or biscuit, other meat, carrot, apple, and peanut butter. Round foods are the most frequent offenders. The first four items together make up more than 40% of all aspirated food items.

A sharp or irritating object produces irritation and edema. A round, pliable object that does not readily break apart is more likely to occlude an airway than an object with a different shape. Latex balloons (uninflated, inflated, or in broken pieces) are especially hazardous. It takes only a small piece of the pliable, impermeable latex to totally occlude the airway. A small object may cause little if any pathologic change, whereas an object of sufficient size to obstruct a passage can produce various changes, including atelectasis, emphysema, inflammation, and abscess.

Pathophysiology

A foreign body may be arrested in any portion of the air passages from the larynx to the bronchi. Three fourths of inhaled foreign bodies lodge in a mainstem or lobar bronchus, with less than 5% finding their way into more distal portions of the lung field and the remaining 20% lodging in the trachea (Blumer, 1991). The site is usually determined by the size, weight, and configuration of the object. For example, heavy objects such as bullets, coins, and nails are more likely to drop into the most dependent portions of the tracheobronchial tree. The object may remain in the same location or change its situation in the airway. It can be coughed from a smaller to a larger airway and reaspirated in a different passage—or it might be ejected forcefully into the mouth and subsequently swallowed.

Signs characteristic of obstruction caused by a foreign body in a bronchus can be explained by the same mechanisms that control the flow of fluids in pipes (Fig. 32-5). During normal respiration the caliber of bronchi and bron-

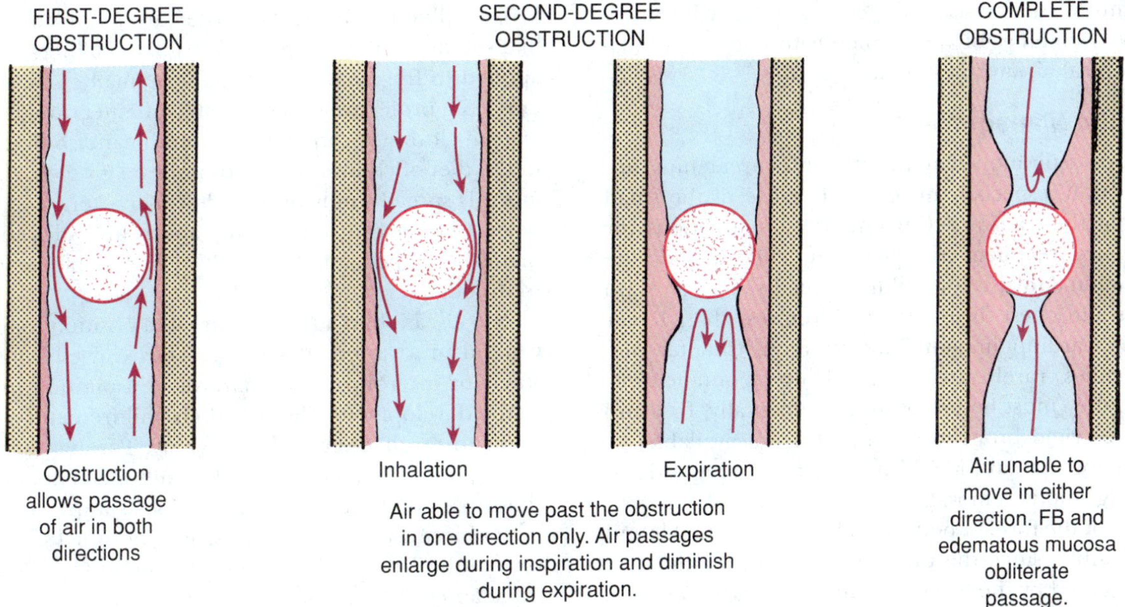
FIRST-DEGREE OBSTRUCTION
SECOND-DEGREE OBSTRUCTION
COMPLETE OBSTRUCTION
Obstruction allows passage of air in both directions
Inhalation
Expiration
Air able to move past the obstruction in one direction only. Air passages enlarge during inspiration and diminish during expiration.
Air unable to move in either direction. FB and edematous mucosa obliterate passage.

FIG. 32-5 Mechanisms of airway obstruction by foreign body *(FB)*.

chioles becomes larger during inspiration and smaller during expiration. When a small object partially obstructs a passage, air passes around the obstruction during both inspiration and expiration (bypass valve). In this type of obstruction a wheeze is heard. A somewhat larger obstruction will allow air to enter the distal portion when bronchioles enlarge during inspiration, but when they diminish in caliber during expiration, the lumen becomes occluded and air becomes trapped distal to the obstruction (check valve). This type of obstruction produces obstructive emphysema. When there is complete blockage of the bronchus by a foreign body or by the foreign body and swollen mucosa, air is unable to move in either direction (stop valve), and the air distal to the obstruction is soon absorbed, leaving an area of obstruction atelectasis. The right bronchus, with its shorter length and straighter angle, is the usual site of bronchial obstruction.

Clinical Manifestations

Initially, a foreign body in the air passages produces choking, gagging, or coughing, but symptoms usually depend on the site of obstruction and on the interval between aspiration and presentation. Laryngotracheal obstruction most commonly causes dysnpea, cough, stridor, and hoarseness because of a decreased air entry. Cyanosis may also occur if the obstruction becomes worse. Bronchial obstruction, on the other hand, usually produces cough (frequently paroxysmal), wheezing, and asymmetric breath sounds, with diminished air entry into the lower airways.

If the obstruction progresses, the child's face may become livid, and sometimes the child falls unconscious and dies of asphyxiation if the object is not removed. If obstruction is partial, hours, days, or even weeks often pass without symptoms after the initial period. Secondary symptoms are related to the anatomic area in which the foreign body is lodged and are usually caused by a persistent respiratory infection focused distally to the obstruction. A history of recurrent intractable pneumonia is reason to consider a foreign body in an airway. Often, by the time secondary symptoms appear, the parents have forgotten the initial episode of coughing and gagging. The most common symptoms observed in children brought to medical attention are stridor, wheezing, sternal retraction, and cough (Esclamado and Richardson, 1987).

Diagnostic Evaluation

The diagnosis of a foreign body is usually suspected on the basis of the history and physical signs. Initial diagnostic testing usually includes anteroposterior and lateral chest x-ray films. Radiographic examination reveals opaque foreign bodies but may be of limited use in localizing vegetable matter. Therefore the presence of airway foreign bodies cannot be excluded based on normal radiographic studies. Rigid bronchoscopy is usually required for a definitive diagnosis of foreign bodies in the larynx and trachea. Fluoroscopic examination is a valuable aid in detecting and localizing foreign bodies in the bronchi.

On fluoroscopy, a check-valve–obstructed lung will remain expanded, the diaphragm will remain low and fixed on the obstructed side, and the heart and mediastinum will shift to the unobstructed side during expiration. In a stop-valve obstruction the heart and mediastinum are drawn to the obstructed side and remain there during both inspiration and expiration. The diaphragm on the obstructed side remains high, whereas that on the unobstructed side moves normally.

In children with equivocal clinical manifestations and diagnostic results, flexible bronchoscopy may be used to provide a definitive diagnosis. This technology can be safely and relatively comfortably performed with conscious sedation and topical airway anesthesia.

Therapeutic Management

Foreign body aspiration may result in life-threatening airway obstruction, especially in infants because of the small diameters of their airways. Current recommendations for the emergency treatment of the choking child include the use of abdominal thrusts for children over 1 year of age and back blows and chest thrusts for children less than 1 year of age (see Cardiopulmonary Resuscitation, Chapter 31). Foreign bodies rarely are coughed up spontaneously. Therefore, they must be removed instrumentally, first and preferably by rigid bronchoscopy, and if not available, by direct laryngoscopy and Magill forceps for supraglottic or glottic foreign body removal.

Removal of the foreign body must be done as quickly and soon as possible, since the progressive local inflammatory process triggered by the foreign material hampers removal, a chemical pneumonia soon develops, and vegetable matter begins to macerate within a few days, causing it to be even more difficult to remove. After removal of the foreign body, the child is placed in a high-humidity atmosphere, and any secondary infection is treated with appropriate antibiotics.

Nursing Considerations

A major role of nurses caring for a child who has aspirated a foreign body is to keep the child as quiet as possible and monitor respiratory status while waiting for surgical removal of the object. The child and the family are naturally upset and frightened, but an agitated child can cause a foreign body to descend and lodge farther down in the respiratory tree (e.g., from the larynx or trachea into the right stem bronchus).

All persons working with children should be prepared to deal effectively with aspiration of a foreign body. Choking on food or other material should not be fatal. Two very simple procedures, back blows and the Heimlich maneuver, which can be used by both health professionals and lay persons, can save lives. It is the obligation of nurses to learn the techniques and teach them to parents and other groups. (See Figs. 31-25 and 31-26.)

To aid a child who is choking, nurses need to recognize the signs of distress. Not every child who gags or coughs while eating is truly choking.

NURSING ALERT The child in distress (1) *cannot speak,* (2) *becomes cyanotic,* and (3) *collapses.* These three signs indicate that the child is truly choking and requires immediate and quick action. The child can die within 4 minutes. Follow-up care after the foreign body is removed includes chest physiotherapy as indicated, monitoring for respiratory distress, and education of the parents.

Prevention. Small children should not be allowed access to enticing small objects that they might place in their mouth. Rubber balloons are high-risk items for children; Mylar balloons are the only safe variety for children. Unlikely items (foil tabs from soft drink containers, Band-Aids applied to fingers of infants or very small children, plastic tabs from protective coverings on containers and from price tags on clothing) can be hazardous. Peanut butter, a staple in the diet of children, should never be given to a child unless it is spread thinly on bread or a cracker. A spoonful of peanut butter can obstruct the airway and stick to mucous membranes, becoming difficult or impossible for the child to dislodge.

Nurses, as child advocates, are in a position to teach prevention in a variety of settings. They can educate parents singly or in groups about hazards of aspiration in relation to the developmental level of their children and encourage them to teach their children safety. Parents teach by example; therefore, they should be cautioned about behaviors that their children might imitate, for example, holding foreign objects, such as pins, nails, and toothpicks, in their lips or mouth. Prevention based on the child's age is discussed in Chapters 12 and 14.

FOREIGN BODY IN THE NOSE

Children will sometimes introduce a foreign object into the nose. This includes such items as food, crayons, small toys, pieces of plastic, beans, beads, erasers, wads of paper, and small stones. A foreign body can be suspected when there is evidence of local obstruction with sneezing, mild discomfort, and (rarely) pain. The irritation produces local mucosal swelling and, with items that increase in size as they absorb moisture (hygroscopic), the signs of obstruction and discomfort increase with time. Infection usually follows, as evidenced by foul breath and a purulent or bloody discharge from one nostril.

Although the object is usually situated anteriorly, unskilled attempts at removal may move it further posteriorly. Removal is carried out as soon as possible to prevent the risk of aspiration and to prevent local tissue necrosis. Removal can usually be accomplished with topical anesthesia and either forceps or suction. Sometimes phenylephrine added to the topical anesthesia will help shrink swollen membranes. Infection and irritation usually disappear promptly after removal.

ASPIRATION PNEUMONIA

The general term ***aspiration pneumonia*** refers to the type of pneumonia occurring when food, secretions, inert materials, or volatile compounds or liquids enter the lung. When this occurs, inflammation and degradation of the airway passages occur. Many conditions increase the risk of aspiration (see box on p. 1409). Aspiration of fluid or food substances is a particular hazard in the child who has difficulty with swallowing or is unable to swallow because of paralysis, weakness, debility, congenital anomalies such as cleft palate or tracheoesophageal fistula, or absent cough reflex (unconscious) or who is force fed, especially while crying or breathing rapidly.

Clinical signs of the aspiration of oral secretions may not

> **CONDITIONS THAT INCREASE RISK OF ASPIRATION**
>
> **ALTERED LEVEL OF CONSCIOUSNESS**
>
> Central nervous system injury or disease (e.g., meningitis, seizures, paralysis, trauma, poisoning, toxic ingestion)
> Sedation
> General anesthesia
> Cardiopulmonary resuscitation
>
> **DYSPHAGIA**
>
> Esophageal dysmotility
> Neurologic deficit
> Gastroesophageal reflux
>
> **MECHANICAL DISRUPTION OF DEFENSIVE BARRIERS**
>
> Endotracheal tube
> Tracheostomy
> Cleft lip/palate
>
> **PERSISTENT VOMITING**
>
> Gastrointestinal infection
> Chemotherapy
> Emetic (e.g., ipecac)
> Postanesthesia
>
> Modified from Hazinski MF, editor: *Nursing care of the critically ill child*, ed 2, St Louis, 1992, Mosby.

be distinguishable from other forms of acute bacterial pneumonia; for example, if vegetable matter has been aspirated, manifestations may not appear for several weeks after the event. Classic symptoms include an increasing cough or fever with foul-smelling sputum, deteriorating chest radiographs, and other signs of lower airway involvement. These deviations may persist for weeks, however, while the child starts to feel better.

The newborn may develop a severe pneumonia from aspirating amniotic fluid and debris during the process of birth. Rarely, aspiration causes immediate death from asphyxia; more often the irritated mucous membrane becomes a site for secondary bacterial infection. In addition to fluids, food, vomitus, and nasopharyngeal secretions, other substances that cause pneumonia are hydrocarbons, lipids, powder, and barium.

Hydrocarbon Pneumonia

Children frequently develop pneumonia secondary to the ingestion of various forms of hydrocarbons, such as kerosene, gasoline, solvents, and lighter fluid (butane, may be inhaled also). Petroleum distillates are generally impure substances and contaminated with heavy metals or other toxic chemicals that can cause systemic as well as local effects. Many, but not all, hydrocarbons are made from petroleum (e.g., turpentine is made from pine oil), and many are found in the home or garage.

Hydrocarbons are usually packaged in attractive containers, and many have a pleasant aroma. Therefore they are frequently ingested accidentally by young children. They are not often swallowed with the intent of committing suicide, however. On the average, children will swallow less than 30 ml (often about 3 to 4 ml). They begin coughing severely and swallow no more. Although central nervous system abnormalities, gastrointestinal irritation, myocardiopathy, and renal toxicity can all occur, the most serious complication is pneumonitis.

Distillates that have high volatility (evaporate quickly), decreased viscosity (thinner solution), and low surface tension are more likely to be aspirated and produce respiratory complications. Lower viscosity enhances penetration into more distal airways; lower surface tension facilitates spread over a larger area of lung surface. Consequently, ingestion of lighter fluid, kerosene, or gasoline frequently causes a pathologic condition, whereas ingestion of petroleum jelly, tar, or lubricating oil rarely does.

Pathogenesis. The severity of the lung injury depends on the pH of the aspirated material, the presence of bacteria, and the volatility/viscosity of the substance. The pathogenesis of the pulmonary involvement is the subject of conflicting interpretations, but the most generally accepted explanation is irritation from aspiration during swallowing, vomiting, or gastric lavage. Reactions include bronchospasm, atelectasis, and emphysema. Pathologic changes consist of signs of inflammation (edema, hyperemia, infiltration of polymorphonuclear cells), vascular thrombosis and hemorrhage, and necrosis of bronchial, bronchiolar, and alveolar tissues. Further resulting conditions include pulmonary hemorrhage, necrosis, surfactant impairment, and pulmonary edema. Even in small amounts, the hydrocarbon spreads over the surface of tissues and the lungs and interferes with gas exchange. Inert fluids aspirated may fail to produce a chemical or bacterial pneumonia, but they still can decrease lung compliance and cause hypoxemia.

Clinical Manifestations. Acid aspiration may produce immediate pulmonary symptoms that worsen over the first 24 hours. Coughing and vomiting occur almost immediately after ingestion, which probably contributes to the aspiration. Central nervous system symptoms may consist of agitation and restlessness, confusion, drowsiness, or coma. The temperature is elevated (37.8° C to 40° C or [100° F to 104° F]). (See also Ingestion of Injurious Agents, Chapter 16.)

After swallowing, coughing, and choking, the child becomes short of breath, and older children complain of dyspnea. There are varying degrees of cyanosis, tachycardia, tachypnea, nasal flaring, and retractions. Intercostal retractions, grunting, cough, and fever may appear within 30 minutes or be delayed for a few hours. Localized areas of dullness are felt on percussion and moderately intense wheezes and crackles are usually heard. Severe injury causes hemoptysis and pulmonary edema that develop rapidly, more severe cyanosis, and death within 24 hours of aspiration.

Therapeutic Management. Inducing the child to vomit is contraindicated because of the renewed danger of aspiration. Hydrocarbons are readily absorbed by the gastrointestinal tract and excreted by the lungs. Bronchitis or pneumonia usually develops early (within the first 24 hours) but may be delayed. Recovery from pulmonary involvement occurs in most instances despite a severe clinical course.

Death, if it occurs, is generally the result of hepatic failure complicated by pulmonary factors. Treatment is the same as for any lower respiratory tract inflammation and consists of high humidity, oxygen, hydration, and treatment of any secondary infection. Further treatment modalities include support of the respiratory system using supplemental oxygen to maintain oxygen saturations >95%, as well as preparing for possible endotracheal intubation.

Lipoid Pneumonia

Oily substances aspirated into the respiratory passages cause progressive changes in lung tissues. First, an interstitial proliferative inflammation occurs that may include an exudative pneumonia. The next stage involves a diffuse, chronic, proliferative fibrosis that is often complicated by acute bronchopneumonia. The final stage features multiple localized nodules or tumorlike paraffinomas. There are no characteristic manifestations. Cough is usually present, and dyspnea is seen in severe cases. Secondary bronchopneumonia infections are common. The outcome depends on the extent of pulmonary damage, the general condition of the infant, and discontinuing the oily inhalation. No specific treatment exists.

Powder

The use of powder has been discouraged for infants; however, although the incidence has decreased, a significant number of infants suffer talcum powder aspiration. Commercial talcum powder is predominantly a mixture of talc (hydrous magnesium silicate) and other silicates. Severe respiratory distress occurs immediately as a result of an inflammatory reaction in small bronchioles initiated by deep inhalation of the extremely light powder. (See Chapter 12 for further discussion of powder inhalation.)

Nursing Considerations

Care of the child with aspiration is the same as that described for the child with pneumonia from other causes. However, the major thrust of nursing care is aimed at prevention of aspiration. Proper feeding techniques should be carried out for weak, debilitated, and uncooperative children, and preventive measures are used to prevent aspiration of any material that might enter the nasopharynx.

Oily nose drops and oil-based vitamin preparations are not appropriate for infants and small children. Solvents, lighter fluid, and other hydrocarbon substances should be kept away from older infants and small children who are apt to put anything in their mouths and who may be attracted by the slightly sweet smell.

Infants and debilitated children should be positioned on the right side after feedings to minimize the possibility of aspirating vomitus or regurgitated feeding. Nurses play a major role in education for injury prevention (see Injury Prevention, Chapters 12 and 14).

For children who have aspirated, therapy is primarily supportive, including interventions to decrease bronchospasm, monitoring of oxygen saturations, fluid and electrolyte management, and administering of antibiotics.

ADULT RESPIRATORY DISTRESS SYNDROME (ARDS)

ARDS was first described in adults and is now recognized as occurring in children. It has been associated with many clinical conditions and injuries, such as sepsis, aspiration, near-drowning, pulmonary contusion and long bone fractures, immunodeficiency, metabolic derangements, infections, drug overdose, and multisystem trauma (Sarnaik and Lieh-Lai, 1994). It is characterized by respiratory distress and hypoxemia that occur within 72 hours after any of the above conditions and may be described as shock lung, wet lung, stiff lung, congestive atelectasis, and posttraumatic lung. The diagnosis of ARDS is likely when the child with a known precipitating factor develops tachypnea, hypoxia, and diffuse pulmonary infiltrates on chest radiographs.

The hallmark of ARDS is increased permeability of the alveolocapillary membrane that results in pulmonary edema. There are essentially three stages of injury: acute phase developing into a latent period, followed by the development of acute respiratory failure, with the final stage involving a recuperative period usually characterized by severe pulmonary abnormalities. During the acute phase the alveolocapillary membrane is damaged, with an increasing pulmonary capillary permeability and resulting interstitial edema. The later stages are characterized by pneumocyte and fibrin infiltration of the alveoli, with the start of either the healing process or fibrosis. When fibrosis occurs, the child may demonstrate respiratory distress and the need for mechanical ventilation.

With ARDS, the lungs become stiff, gas diffusion is impaired, and eventually there is bronchiolar mucosal swelling and congestive atelectasis. The net effect is decreased functional residual capacity and increased intrapulmonary right-to-left shunting of pulmonary circulation. Surfactant secretion is reduced, and the atelectasis and fluid-filled alveoli provide an excellent medium for bacterial growth.

The child entering into ARDS may first demonstrate only symptoms caused by the injury or infection but, as the condition deteriorates, will manifest hyperventilation, tachypnea, increasing respiratory effort, cyanosis, and a decreasing oxygen saturation. At times, the developing hypoxemia is not responsive to oxygen administration.

Therapeutic Management

Based on these symptoms, it is vitally important to begin and continue with careful monitoring and provision of oxygenation and ventilatory function: pulse oximetry is an important tool to use in determining effectiveness of therapy. Most treatment modalities, however, are supportive and involve the approaches listed in the Guidelines box.

When delivering oxygen, it is extremely important to monitor saturations and amount being delivered, since increased levels can promote atelectasis by reabsorption. The use of endotracheal intubation and positive end-expiratory pressure (PEEP) may be required to ensure maximum oxygen delivery by increasing functional residual capacity, reducing intrapulmonary shunting, and shifting pulmonary fluids to secondary areas of the lungs.

GUIDELINES
Management of the Child with Adult Respiratory Distress Syndrome (ARDS)

1. Prevent infection; treat the precipitating disease.
2. Maintain intravascular volume and hydration status.
3. Monitor urinary output.
4. Treat fever.
5. Establish and maintain neutral thermal environment.
6. Maintain tissue oxygenation:
   a. Oxygen administration
   b. Correct and appropriate position to improve functional residual capacity
   c. Mechanical ventilation when needed, with PEEP therapy
   d. Suctioning
7. Employ comfort measures and treat pain.
8. Provide psychologic and emotional support.
9. Provide nutritional support, with appropriate calories given via tube feeding for child unable to tolerate oral intake.
10. Initiate pharmacologic therapy:
    a. Surfactant
    b. Nonsteroidal antiinflammatory drugs (NSAIDs)
    c. Immunotherapy with monoclonal antibodies

Recent developments in the treatment of ARDS include (1) medications to interrupt the formation or activation of mediators contributing to progression of intrapulmonary shunting and lung injury, such as nonsteroidal antiinflammatory drugs (NSAIDs); (2) immunotherapy with monocolonal antibodies that work against the specific toxins causing the lung injury; and (3) human and artificial surfactant to reduce the severity of and sequelae from RDS and that may be useful in treating lung disease associated with ARDS and near-drowning (Hazinski, 1992).

Prognosis. In spite of advances in understanding and treating ARDS, mortality remains high and in children may range from 35% to 90%. The precipitating disorder influences the outcome; the worst prognosis is associated with uncontrolled sepsis, bone marrow transplantation, cancer, and multisystem involvement with hepatic failure. In children who recover, persistent cough and exertional dyspnea may remain. However, minimal data exist on long-term complications (Sarnaik and Lieh-Lai, 1994).

Nursing Considerations

Nursing care involves careful monitoring of pulse, heart rate, perfusion, capillary filling, and urinary output, as well as assessment of respiratory status. Blood gas analysis and pulse oximetry are important evaluation tools. Respiratory distress is a frightening situation for both the child and the parents, and attention to their psychologic needs is a major element in the care of these children. Since the mortality rate of ARDS is high, the family is kept informed of the child's progress and made aware of the possibility of death. (See also Family-Centered Care of the Child with Life-threatening Illness, Chapter 23.)

SMOKE INHALATION INJURY

A number of noxious substances that may be inhaled are toxic to humans. They are primarily products of incomplete combustion and cause more deaths from fires than flame injuries. The severity of the injury depends on the nature of the substances generated by the material being burned, whether the victim is confined in a closed space, and the duration of contact with the smoke.

General Aspects

Possible inhalation injury is suspected when there is a history of flames in a closed space whether or not burns are present. Sooty material around the nose or in the sputum, singed nasal hairs, or mucosal burns of the nose, lips, mouth, or throat are all signs that the affected person demands observation for possible pulmonary injury from inhalants. A hoarse voice and cough are further evidence of airway involvement, and increased inspiratory and expiratory stridor indicates severe damage to the upper passages. Signs of respiratory distress are also indicated by tachypnea, tachycardia, and diminished or abnormal breath sounds, including crackles, and wheezes.

Three distinct stages occur with the above manifestations in the child suffering from inhalation injury: (1) pulmonary insufficiency, usually during the initial 12 hours; (2) pulmonary edema, usually after 6 to 72 hours, with an increase in the lung fluid and interstitial edema; and (3) bronchopneumonia, usually after 72 hours with a resulting airway obstruction or atelectasis. Strangulation may also occur from the cervical eschar secondary to a severe burn (Ruddy, 1994).

Smoke inhalation causes three different types of injury: heat, local chemical, and systemic.

Heat Injury. Heat causes thermal injury to the upper airways, but since air has low specific heat, the injury goes no further than the upper airway. Reflex closure of the glottis prevents injury to lower airways. Heat may reach the middle airway occasionally but it rarely penetrates to the lungs.

Chemical Injury. A wide variety of gases may be generated during the combustion of materials such as clothing, furniture, and floor coverings. Acids, alkalis, and their precursors in smoke can produce chemical burns. These substances can be carried deep into the respiratory tract, including the lower respiratory tract, in the form of insoluble gases. Soluble gases tend to dissolve in the upper respiratory tract.

Synthetic materials are especially toxic, producing gases such as oxides of sulfur and nitrogen, acetaldehyde, formaldehyde, hydrocyanic acid, and chlorine. Heated plastics are the source of extremely toxic vapors, including chlorine and hydrochloric acid from polyvinylchloride and hydrocarbons, aldehydes, ketones, and acids from polyethylene. Irritant gases such as nitrous oxide or carbon dioxide combine with water in the lungs to form corrosive acids; aldehydes cause denaturation of proteins, cellular damage, and edema of pulmonary tissues. Chemical burns to the airways are similar to burns on the skin, except they are painless because the tracheobronchial tree is relatively insensitive to pain.

Inhalation of small amounts of noxious irritants produces alveolar and bronchiolar damage that can lead to obstructive bronchiolitis. Severe exposure causes further injury, including alveolocapillary damage with hemorrhage, necrotizing bronchiolitis, inhibited secretion of surfactant, and formation of hyaline membranes—manifestations of ARDS described in the previous section.

Systemic Injury. Gases that are nontoxic to the airways (e.g., carbon monoxide, hydrogen cyanide) can cause injury and death by interfering with or inhibiting cellular respiration. Carbon monoxide (CO) is a colorless, odorless gas with an affinity for hemoglobin 200 to 250 times greater than that of oxygen. CO combines at the same point on the hemoglobin molecule as does oxygen; therefore, when it enters the bloodstream, CO readily binds reversibly with hemoglobin to form ***carboxyhemoglobin (COHb)***. Normal COHb blood levels are <1%. COHb levels should be measured by arterial blood gas analysis. Because CO combines more readily and is released less readily, very low levels of tissue oxygen levels must be reached before appreciable amounts of oxygen are released from the hemoglobin. Therefore, tissue hypoxia reaches dangerous levels before oxygen is available to meet tissue needs.

NURSING ALERT The oxygen saturation (Sao_2) obtained by pulse oximetry will be normal because the device measures only oxygenated and deoxygenated hemoglobin; it does not measure dysfunctional hemoglobin, such as COHb.

Accidental poisoning is most often the result of exposure to fumes from heaters or smoke from structural fires, although poorly ventilated recreational vehicles with improperly operated or maintained gas lamps or stoves and cooking in underventilated areas with charcoal grills or hibachis are also frequent causes. CO is produced by incomplete combustion of carbon or carbonaceous material such as wood or charcoal.

The signs and symptoms of CO poisoning are secondary to tissue hypoxia and vary with the level of COHb. Mild manifestations include headache, visual disturbances, irritability, and nausea, whereas more severe intoxication causes confusion, hallucinations, ataxia, and coma (see box above, right). CO may increase cerebral blood flow, increase cerebral capillary permeability, and increase cerebrospinal fluid pressure, all of which contribute to the central nervous system (CNS) signs observed. The bright, cherry-red lips and skin often described are less often observed; more frequently, pallor and cyanosis are seen.

INHALATION INJURY RELATED TO CARBOXYHEMOGLOBIN CONCENTRATION

SIGNS AND SYMPTOMS	PERCENT OF COHb CONCENTRATION
Usually none (often questioned)	0-5
Tightness across forehead, may or may not be headache, cutaneous blood vessel dilation	5-15
Throbbing headache plus above	15-30
Severe headache, weakness, dizziness, dimmed vision, nausea, vomiting, cardiovascular collapse (especially infants, anemic children, and those with pulmonary disease)	30-40
Same as above but worse, with greater possibility of cardiovascular collapse, syncope, coma, and lactic acidemia	40-50
Syncope, tachycardia, poor cardiac output, seizures, Cheyne-Stokes respirations, death*	50-60
Coma, seizures, decreased cardiac output, respiratory depression and failure, death if not treated*	60-80

*Death can occur with lower concentrations in infants and in children with pulmonary disease or anemia.

Therapeutic Management

The treatment of children with smoke toxicity is largely symptomatic, but the most widely accepted treatment is placing the child on humidified 100% oxygen as quickly as possible and closely monitoring for signs of respiratory distress and impending failure. Blood gases are drawn to determine baseline arterial blood gases and COHb levels. Surprisingly, arterial oxygen partial pressure may be within normal limits unless there is marked respiratory depression. If CO poisoning is confirmed, 100% oxygen is continued until COHb levels fall to the nontoxic range of about 10%.

Early endotracheal intubation is recommended in many cases because upper airway edema frequently occurs and makes later intubation very difficult. Indications for intubation include full-thickness burns of the face or neck; children with altered sensorium with inability to protect the airway, such as a gag reflex; visible edema on bronchoscopy; and clinical signs indicating obstruction such as stridor, wheezing, or grunting.

When a hyperbaric oxygen chamber is available, its use is greatly advocated for COHb levels >25% or when coma is present (Ruddy, 1994). This therapy should be employed at the time of presentation even if the level has fallen because of significant CO remaining in the tissue. The usual therapy involves 30- to 90-minute intervals in the chamber, which will approximately double the amount of dissolved oxygen present in the blood; therefore oxygen delivery should improve.

Other therapies that may be used but that remain controversial include transfusion with washed red blood cells to increase the oxygen carried to tissues, and hypothermia to reduce the tissue demand for oxygen and to prevent CNS complications.

Respiratory distress may occur early in the course of smoke inhalation as a result of hypoxia, or patients who are breathing well on admission may later develop sudden respiratory distress. Therefore intubation and/or tracheostomy equipment should be available at the bedside. More often, distress is related to transient edema of the airways, which can occur at any level in the tracheobronchial tree. Controversy exists regarding tracheostomy, but many prefer this procedure when the obstruction is proximal to the larynx and reserve nasotracheal intubation for lower tract involvement.

The use of corticosteroids, although controversial, may be of value in reducing edema, and bronchodilators are often given intravenously or by nebulizer. Broad-spectrum antibiotics are also sometimes administered prophylactically.

Nursing Considerations

Nursing care of the child with inhalation injury is the same as that for any child with respiratory distress. Vital signs and other respiratory assessments are performed frequently, and the pulmonary status is carefully observed and maintained. Pulmonary physiotherapy is usually part of the therapeutic program, as well as mechanical ventilation if needed. Fluid requirements for children experiencing inhalation injury are greater than those with surface burns alone. As mentioned, one concern is the development of pulmonary edema; therefore, accurate monitoring of intake and output is essential.

In addition to the observation and management of the physical aspects of inhalation injury, the nurse also deals with the psychologic needs of a frightened child and distraught parents. As with any accidental injury, the parents feel overwhelming guilt, even when the injury occurred through no fault of their own. More often, however, the injury could have been prevented, which compounds their guilt feelings. They need much support and reassurance, as well as information about the child's condition, treatment, and progress.

The increased use of wood-burning stoves as a primary or supplementary source of heat has produced additional air-pollutant particles in residential air. Investigators have noted an increase in respiratory illness in infants and children from households heating with wood-burning stoves (Honicky, Osborne, and Akpom, 1985). A family assessment that reveals frequent respiratory infections in children during the cold winter months should alert the nurse to this possibility.

PASSIVE SMOKING

Numerous researchers have investigated the effects of environmental pollution on children's health and have determined that the worst pollutant is parental smoking, especially maternal smoking. Children exposed to environmental tobacco smoke have an increased number of respiratory illnesses, such as bronchitis, pneumonia, asthma, and otitis media, as compared with children of nonsmoking parents. Also, the number of illnesses is positively correlated with the number of cigarettes smoked. The incidence of respiratory disease related to passive smoking also correlates with the number of smoking members of the family. Maternal cigarette smoking may be associated with increases of 20% to 35% in the rates of respiratory illnesses and respiratory symptoms. Paternal smoking is associated with smaller increases. Children of smoking parents have reduced performance on pulmonary function tests, especially forced expiratory volume (FEV). Maternal smoking may have a deleterious effect on fetal growth and increases the risk of spontaneous abortion, premature rupture of the membranes, and delivery of a stillborn infant. Living in a household with smoking residents also increases the risk of becoming a smoker. Based on these findings, the U.S. Environmental Protection Agency (EPA) (*Respiratory health effects,* 1992) concluded that there is a *causal* relationship between environmental tobacco smoke exposure and reductions in pulmonary function.*

The American Academy of Pediatrics has renewed its statement on hazards of passive smoking (American Academy of Pediatrics, 1994c). The report states: "The dangers to children of both active and passive tobacco exposure, including smokeless forms, are so well established that pediatricians should make the elimination of this threat a major issue as they pursue the goal of a tobacco-free generation by the year 2000."

Nursing Considerations

Passive smoking during childhood may well be the most important precursor of chronic lung disease in the adult. Nurses and other health care professionals need to be aware of this problem and include this information in all health assessments of children, especially those with respiratory illnesses. In families where smokers refuse to quit, house rules should be established for reducing smoke in the child's environment (see Family Home Care box). Nurses should also inform caregivers of the health hazards of children's exposure to environments of tobacco smoke, set an example for children and families, and become advocates for "no smoking" ordinances in public places, prohibition of advertising

*For a copy of the EPA report *Respiratory Health Effects of Passive Smoking,* write to CERI, US EPA, 26 W. Martin Luther King Dr., Cincinnati, OH 45268; (513) 569-7562.

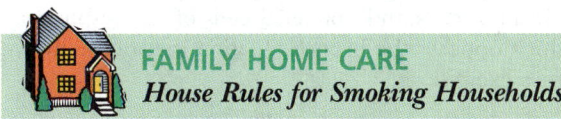

Do not smoke in same room with children.
Restrict smoking to an isolated, preferably outdoor, area.
Do not smoke in motor vehicles with children.
Do not smoke in rooms children use.

tobacco products in the media, and inclusion of health warnings of sidestream smoke on tobacco products.

LONG-TERM RESPIRATORY DYSFUNCTION

ALLERGIC RHINITIS

Allergic rhinitis is the most common of all allergic disorders and, although not life-threatening, is a significant cause of morbidity in all age-groups. The manifestations may be episodic or perennial. ***Seasonal allergic rhinitis,*** also known as "hay fever" or "summer cold," occurs during certain months of the year and does not develop until the individual has been sensitized by two or more pollen seasons. Although the peak incidence is in the postadolescent teenage group, younger children are also affected. It is estimated that 8% to 10% of children within the United States will experience allergic rhinitis each year (Virant, 1992).

Pathophysiology

The development of allergic rhinitis requires two conditions: a familial predisposition to develop allergy and exposure of a sensitized person to the allergen. Inhalants in the form of microscopic airborne particles, including pollens, mold, animal danders, and environmental dusts, are the principal allergens. It is thought that water-soluble allergens diffuse into the respiratory epithelium from airborne foreign particles that enter the upper respiratory tract with each inhalation.

In the allergic child, symptoms are mediated by the production of antigen-specific immunoglobulin E (IgE) by the child's B lymphocytes, with the primary defect probably being excessive production of interleukin 4 (IL-4) or a deficient level of gamma interferon (Virant, 1992). Clinical disease occurs when an allergen reacts with antigen-specific IgE on the child's nasal mast cells. Several mediators are released at this time, but the most significant is ***histamine,*** which is a potent vasodilator acting directly on local receptors to include vasodilation and edema. This, in turn, triggers neural reflexes, inducing mucus hypersecretion and sneezing. In this context, allergic rhinitis should be viewed as an inflammatory disease. After diffusion, IgE antibody production is stimulated in the genetically susceptible child, and subsequent sensitization of respiratory tissues takes place. Repeated exposure of these sensitized membranes to specific aeroallergens results in antigen-antibody interactions with the release of mast cell mediators, inflammation, and clinical allergic disease. In exercise-induced bronchospasm, cold, dry air triggers a release of bronchoactive substances in mast cells and epithelial cells of the respiratory tract, which opposes the bronchodilation that normally accompanies exercise.

Clinical Manifestations

Children who have allergic rhinitis may have a history of watery rhinorrhea, nasal obstruction, sneezing, or nasal pruritus. Symptoms may be seasonal (e.g., during the spring or summer pollen periods) or perennial and also include

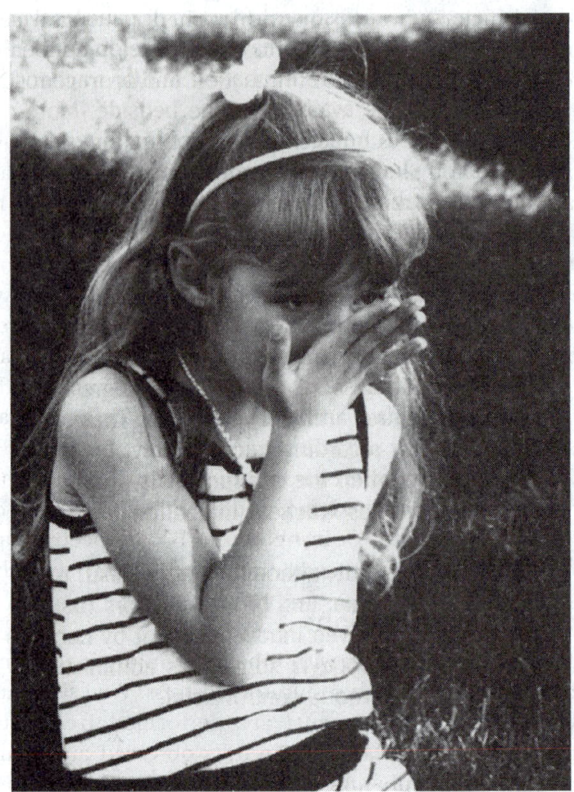

FIG. 32-6 "Allergic salute."

itching of the nose, eyes, palate, pharynx, and conjunctiva. The nasal stuffiness sometimes progresses to partial or total obstruction of airflow, and mucus secretion with postnasal drainage can occur. Nasal itching is troublesome, and the affected child attempts to alleviate the symptoms by rubbing the nose—the "allergic salute" (Fig. 32-6).

On physical examination, these children may display dark circles or "allergic shiners" beneath their eyes; these are secondary to obstruction of normal outflow from regional lymphatics and veins. If the nasal obstruction is severe, the child will probably be an obligate mouth-breather. Another common, more specific facial finding is a horizontal nasal crease across the lower third of the nose due to frequent rubbing induced by the nasal pruritus. The child may develop facial tics and mannerisms in an attempt to avoid scratching the nose (Simons, 1988). Other classic facial features include an open mouth caused by chronic nasal obstruction ("allergic gape") and radiating lines in the lower orbitopalpebral grooves ***(Dennies lines)***.

Other symptoms may appear during peak symptom periods, including tearing and soreness of the eyes and gelatinous conjunctival discharge in the morning, irritability, fatigue, depression, and loss of appetite.

When allergic rhinitis is suspected, it is important to obtain information regarding clinical signs of related disorders, including middle ear disease, complaints of ear pain, delayed speech or language development, chronic cough or wheezing, exercise intolerance, eczema, or urticaria. Finally, it is important to obtain a history of potential allergen triggers or environmental changes that could have precipitated this episode. Chronic rhinitis leading to significant nasal obstruction can lead to various abnormalities in growth and development and in psychosocial and intellectual development (Pearlman, 1988).

Diagnostic Evaluation

Diagnosis of allergic rhinitis is based on a thorough history and physical examination. Since allergic rhinitis is often associated with atopic dermatitis or asthma, examination of the skin and chest is indicated (Simons, 1988). Other tests that may be used include mucus examination for eosinophils, superficial biopsy of nasal mucosa, fiberoptic rhinoscopy, blood examination for elevated eosinophils, and various challenge tests. Nasal blood flow and nasal airflow measurements are sometimes used.

Sensitization Testing. Tests for sensitization to specific allergens include skin tests and the radioallergosorbent and related tests. ***Skin testing*** involves injection of specific allergens and remains the most commonly used diagnostic test for allergy. The allergenic extract is introduced into the epidermis by (1) scratch, prick, or puncture; (2) a single intradermal injection of a dilute concentration of specific allergen; or (3) serial dilution (threefold or tenfold) injections to determine the end point of reactivity. After a suitable time period (10 to 30 seconds), the size of the resultant wheal and flare reaction is measured to assess the patient's sensitivity. The magnitude of the wheal and flare response correlates roughly with the severity of symptoms produced by natural exposure to the same allergen; however, a positive skin test does not always indicate the presence of clinical reactivity (Wood and Sampson, 1987).

Skin testing and immunotherapy are generally safe procedures, but they are not without risk. Severe and even fatal reactions can occur within a short time, depending on the type of extract used and sensitivity of the individual. To minimize the risk of severe reactions the American Academy of Allergy and Immunology (1990) recommends the patient remain under observation for at least 20 minutes after injection and longer for high-risk patients. In other countries (e.g., United Kingdom), in which extracts unapproved in the United States are used, the recommended waiting period is 2 hours.

NURSING ALERT Onset of a reaction is often insidious. Mild initial symptoms may include local pruritus, pallor, flushing, cyanosis, shortness of breath, dyspnea, cough, malaise, or abdominal pain. Later developments include hypotension, airway obstruction, chest pain, ventricular fibrillation, and loss of consciousness (Lockey and others, 1987).

If the history, physical examination, and results of nasal cytology all suggest allergic rhinitis, skin testing should be performed for relevant inhalant allergens such as dust mites, animal danders, molds, and pollens. Positive skin tests verify the presence of specific IgE.

Radioallergosorbent (RAST) testing should be reserved for the child who has significant dermatographism or eczema and in whom skin testing is likely to be unreliable or difficult to interpret. There is general agreement that this test should be used as a supplemental test rather than a screening tool. The RAST test, which measures only IgE, requires one serum sample; in the case of an extremely allergic child who already has an elevated serum IgE level, this test can produce significant false-positive results for allergic rhinitis (Virant, 1992).

Therapeutic Management

Therapy is directed toward avoidance of offending allergens, and use of medication and immunotherapy (hyposensitization or desensitization). Avoidance measures involve removing allergens from the environment and are usually effective for allergy to foods, drugs, and animals (see Family Home Care box on p. 1427).

If a patient is unable to avoid the allergens, symptoms can be controlled with drugs in many cases. However, treatment should be highly individualized. Four main classes of drugs are used: H_1-receptor antagonists (antihistamines), adrenergic and anticholinergic drugs, disodium cromoglycate (cromolyn), and topical corticosteroids.

Antihistamines are the preferred medications because of their ability to counteract the effects of histamine. Dosage and efficacy of antihistamine are frequently limited by the appearance of undesirable side effects such as sedation, restlessness, dry mouth, urinary retention, and constipation. Any of the many types of drugs should be taken on a regular basis rather than "as needed" for the relief of preexisting symptoms (Virant, 1992). If nasal obstruction is a prominent feature, relief can often be obtained from an α-adrenergic decongestant given singly or in combination with an antihistamine. Nasal or oral administration often provides symptomatic relief; caution should be taken, however, with long-term use because of "rebound effects" (return of symptoms) and habituation. Cromolyn sodium is used prophylactically on a regular basis and is effective in preventing both the early and the late responses to antigen. Generally, however, cromolyn should be considered an adjunct to antihistamine therapy during allergic symptoms and as a primary treatment only if the antihistamines are ineffective or intolerable. Finally, topical nasal corticosteroids (e.g., fluticasone propionate) are a safe, effective alternative to the use of cromolyn sodium and can be used effectively on a short-term basis during periods of exacerbation (Grossman and others, 1993; Lumry and others, 1991).

Immunotherapy may be necessary if drug therapy and avoidance of allergens are ineffective in controlling symptoms or if drugs evoke undesirable side effects. The process of immunotherapy typically involves a series of injections with extracts of the specific allergens that cause symptoms for the child. Initially, treatment is given weekly with dilute exposures, and the tolerated dosage is then gradually increased. This process takes about 4 to 8 months to complete, and once this level is reached, maintenance treatment is continued every 3 to 4 weeks for 3 to 5 years (Virant, 1992). Immunotherapy appears to be most effective in reducing symptoms caused by seasonal pollen-related allergy.

Nursing Considerations

Nurses can help by recognizing the existence of rhinitis and referring children for diagnosis and therapy.

➤ **NURSING TIP** To distinguish allergies from colds, be aware that:

Allergies are seldom accompanied by fever; colds are.

Allergies tend to cause itching in the child's eyes and nose; colds do not.

Allergies usually trigger constant and consistent bouts of sneezing; colds are characterized by sporadic sneezing.

The major nursing goal in care of the child with allergic rhinitis is preparation for skin tests and desensitization injections, which are the source of greatest stress to children. It is difficult to make them understand how inflicting discomfort regularly over a long time is going to make them better. Adolescents can intellectualize the rationale behind the procedures and tolerate the discomfort but still need the support that is provided by sympathetic nursing.

To help allay children's fears of skin tests, they need a careful and thorough explanation of what is to be done and how many "pricks" are involved (usually series of eight on each site, for a total of 30 tests). Very young, anxious patients may benefit from one prick on the arm to demonstrate how it feels. The skin is pierced with a stylet rather than a regular needle and syringe; then a drop of allergen is placed on the site. A helpful strategy is to have the child count off the number of pricks with the nurse as a distraction. For intradermal skin injection, EMLA, a topical anesthetic, reduces or eliminates pain without altering test results (Wolf and others, 1994).

ASTHMA

Asthma is defined as "airway obstruction or a narrowing that is characterized by bronchial irritability after exposure to various stimuli" and that is reversible either spontaneously or with treatment. When the symptoms (shortness of breath, wheezing, and/or chest tightness) become worse, either abruptly or progressively, the child is experiencing an exacerbation (American Academy of Pediatrics, 1994d).

The incidence, severity, and mortality associated with asthma have risen steadily throughout the world (Bloomberg and Strunk, 1992; Weitzman and others, 1992). The increasing numbers may result from increasing air pollution, poor access to medical care, and/or underdiagnosis and undertreatment. Asthma is the most common chronic disease of childhood (Murphy and Kelly, 1993), as well as the primary cause of school absences, and is responsible for a major proportion of pediatric admissions to emergency rooms and hospitals (Larter and Kieckhefer, 1992). The cost of treating asthma in children is more than $1 billion yearly (Cloutier, 1993). Although the onset of asthma may be at any age, 80% to 90% of children have their first symptoms before 4 or 5 years of age, and it is estimated that 5% to 10% of children in the United States have manifestations of asthma at some time during childhood (Ellis, 1987). Boys are affected more frequently than girls until adolescence, when the trend reverses. The severity of the disease varies greatly among children and is not influenced by sex.

Asthma can be classified as ***intermittent,*** in which the child is symptom-free for extended periods without medication, and ***chronic,*** which describes the child who requires frequent or continuous medical therapy. Both intermittent and chronic disease are variable in intensity, and the choice of therapy depends on both the classification and the severity.

Etiology

Although the exact etiology of asthma remains equivocal, evidence suggests that the disease occurs from hypersensitivity to environmental substances that trigger an allergic reaction (Larter and Kieckhefer, 1992). A strong relationship exists between viral infections and asthma induction in infants, with allergens playing a less important role in this age-group because it takes time for allergic sensitivity to develop. Although allergic reactions to food may occur in infants, foods are not common triggers of asthma (National Heart, 1991). Studies in children with asthma suggest, however, that allergy influences the persistence and severity of the disease (Groth and Hurewitz, 1992). Important triggers that tend to induce exacerbations are listed in the box below. There tends to be a family predisposition toward hyperactivity of the airways, but this relationship remains just one variable as a potential cause of asthma.

The allergic reaction in the airways is significant for two reasons: (1) it can cause an immediate reaction, with obstruction occurring, and (2) it can precipitate a late bronchial obstructive reaction several hours after the initial exposure. This delayed bronchial response is associated with an increase in the airway hyperresponsiveness to nonimmunologic stimuli and can persist for several weeks or more after a single allergen exposure (National Heart, 1991).

While allergy does provide an explanation for triggering asthma, there are instances where no allergic process can

TRIGGERS TENDING TO PRECIPITATE AND/OR AGGRAVATE ASTHMATIC EXACERBATIONS

Allergens
- **Outdoor:** Trees, shrubs, weeds, grasses, molds, pollens, air pollution, spores
- **Indoor:** Dust and/or dust mites, mold, cockroach antigen

Irritants: tobacco smoke, wood smoke, odors, sprays
Exposure to occupational chemicals
Exercise
Cold air
Changes in weather or temperature
Environmental change: moving to new home, starting new school, etc.
Colds and infections
Animals: cats, dogs, rodents, horses
Medications: aspirin, nonsteroidal antiinflammatory drugs (NSAIDs), antibiotics, beta blockers
Strong emotions: fear, anger, laughing, crying
Conditions: gastroesophageal reflux, tracheoesophageal fistula
Food additives: sulfite preservatives
Foods: nuts, milk/dairy products
Endocrine factors: menses, pregnancy, thyroid disease

be detected. Theories that attempt to explain the airway reaction include (1) a basic defect in the β-adrenergic receptors on leukocytes and (2) increased cholinergic activity in the airways (Duffs and Platts-Mills, 1992). Asthma is an extremely complex disorder involving biochemical, immunologic, infectious, endocrine, and psychologic factors.

NURSING ALERT Risk factors for asthma include:
Age
Heredity
Gender
Children of young mothers under age 20
Smoking
Ethnicity: African-Americans at greatest risk
Previous life-threatening attacks
Lack of access to medical care
Psychologic and psychosocial problems

Pathophysiology

There is general agreement that heightened airway reactivity is characteristic of children with asthma, with the single most important component of this hyperreactivity being bronchospasm and obstruction (Fig. 32-7). The reasons for this are less clear, and most theories do not explain all types and causes of asthma. Some theories attribute the hyperreactivity to (1) an exaggeration of the normal defenses of the respiratory tract, (2) abnormal tissue reactions in the bronchioles, possibly immunologically induced, or (3) an imbalance of normally balanced responses. However, the mechanisms responsible for the obstructive symptoms are many and involve multiple factors (Fig. 32-8). These factors can then lead to and cause the classic characteristics of inflammation and hyperresponsiveness, which can then lead to airway obstruction. Once this cycle is started, further mechanisms include accumulation of tenacious secretions from mucous glands and spasm of the smooth muscle of the bronchi and bronchioles, which, in time, may only further decrease the diameter of airways and enhance the obstructive process.

The mechanisms contributing to airway inflammation are multiple and involve a number of different pathways. It is unlikely that asthma is caused by either a single cell or a single inflammatory mediator; rather, it appears that asthma results from complex interactions among inflammatory cells, mediators, and the cells and tissues present in the airways (National Heart, 1991). The sequence for the initial trigger in an asthmatic episode may occur as follows:

1. An initial release of inflammatory mediators from bronchial mast cells, macrophages, and epithelial cells
2. Migration and activation of other inflammatory cells
3. Alterations in epithelial integrity and autonomic neural control of airway tone
4. Increase in the airway smooth muscle responsiveness, which then results in several physiologic manifestations, such as wheezing and dyspnea with eventual obstruction

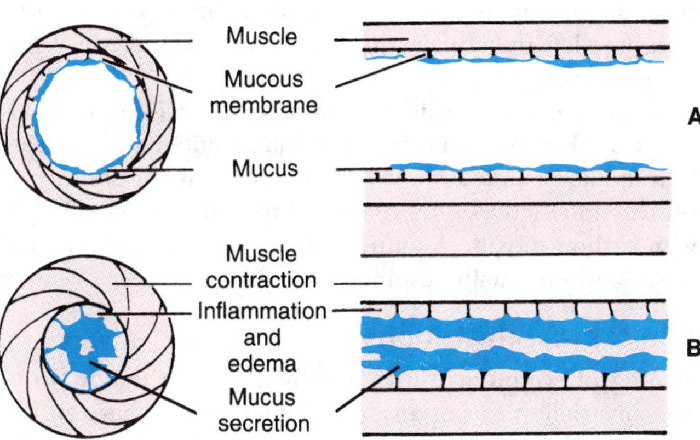

FIG. 32-7 Mechanisms of obstruction in asthma.

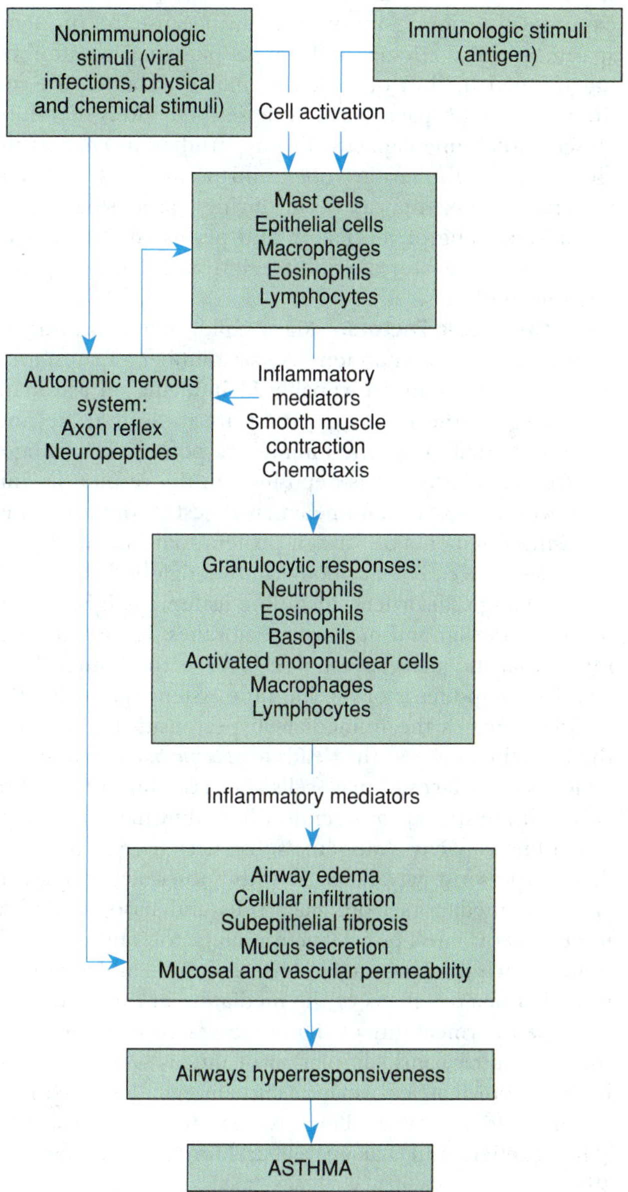

FIG. 32-8 Proposed pathways in pathogenesis of bronchial inflammation and airway hyperresponsiveness. (From National Heart, Lung, and Blood Institute, National Institutes of Health: *Guidelines for the diagnosis and management of asthma,* Pub No 91-3042, Bethesda, MD, Aug 1991.)

The role that each of these mechanisms plays varies from child to child, as well as during the course of the disease. In some children, smooth muscle contraction is the major factor early in the episode, followed by mucosal edema and increased mucus secretion, which are predominant in contributing to the obstruction. In others, the sequence of the responses is reversed.

NURSING ALERT Airflow is determined by the size of the airway lumen, degree of bronchial wall edema, mucus production, smooth muscle contraction, and muscle hypertrophy.

Exacerbations. Exacerbations are acute or subacute episodes of progressively worsening shortness of breath, cough, wheezing, chest tightness, or some combination of these changes. They also are characterized by decreases in expiratory airflow. Airways narrow because of bronchospasm, mucosal edema, and mucus plugging, with air being trapped behind occluded or narrowed airways. Functional residual capacity rises because the child is breathing close to total lung capacity; this hyperinflation enables the child to keep the airways open and permits gas exchange to occur. Hypoxemia can occur during episodes because of the mismatching of ventilation and perfusion. This is seen as increasing carbon dioxide tension and decreasing oxygen tension levels.

Immunologic Factors. Many children with asthma exhibit an allergic component. A vast number of substances in the environment are capable of inducing an asthmatic response, but the most significant are those that are antigenic (i.e., that evoke the immune response). The antigen (or foreign substance) is deposited on the respiratory mucosa, where lysozymes immediately digest its outer coating, releasing fragments of foreign protein that initiate the immune sequence. The antibody (immunoglobulin) most active in allergic disorders, including asthma, is IgE, located primarily in skin and mucous membranes. It has also been found that the allergic response involves the humoral and cellular components of the immune system (Finn, 1992).

IgE mediates the immediate hypersensitive reaction in the bronchial mucosa that leads to ***specific tissue binding.*** IgE attaches to surfaces of mast cells and basophils, where it reacts with the specific antigen to which they have developed a bonding capacity. Antigenic substances trigger an immediate hypersensitivity reaction with subsequent release of chemical mediators from mast cells and basophils: histamine, leukotrienes, platelet-activating factor, and other substances, including prostaglandins, serotonin, and various kinins. The major effects of the mediators in the airways are increased permeability of the blood vessels, contraction of smooth muscle, and stimulation of mucus secretion. Studies have shown a clear relationship among allergic skin test reactivity to airborne allergens, serum IgE, and asthma (Hill, Szefler, and Larsen, 1992; Morgan and Martinez, 1992).

Vagal Stimulation. Normally the balance of vagal and sympathetic nerve influences maintains the tone of bronchial smooth muscle. Irritant receptors on the bronchial mucosa stimulated by various antigenic (pollens, dust) or nonantigenic (smoke, fumes, cold) stimuli trigger a reflex bronchospasm that narrows the airway. This normal reflex mechanism is designed to protect the alveoli from harmful stimuli in the bronchi; however, in the person with asthma the bronchial constriction is abnormally severe. Acetylcholine, a neurotransmitter, mediates the vagal response.

Ventilation. The rigid cartilaginous rings of the upper airways act to modify the constrictive forces, but in the smaller bronchi and the bronchioles the cartilage has been replaced by membranous tissue. The smooth muscle, arranged in spiral bundles around the airway, causes narrowing and shortening of the airway, which significantly increases airway resistance to airflow. Since the bronchi normally dilate and elongate during inspiration and contract and shorten on expiration, the respiratory difficulty is more pronounced during the expiratory phase of respiration.

Increased resistance in the airway causes forced expiration through the narrowed lumen. The volume of air trapped in the lungs increases as airways are functionally closed at a point between the alveoli and the lobar bronchi by the combined mechanisms just described. As the severity of the asthma increases, the airways close at higher residual volume. This gas trapping is the central physiologic feature in the clinical manifestations of asthma, since it forces the individual to breathe at a higher and higher lung volume. This in turn increases the elastic work of breathing and decreases the mechanical efficiency of respiratory muscles. Consequently, the person with asthma fights to inspire sufficient air, and hyperinflation of alveoli increases the diameter of the airways by exerting lateral traction on bronchiolar walls. Gas exchange is facilitated, but more energy is required during inspiration to overcome the tension of already stretched elastic lung tissues. The expenditure of effort for breathing causes fatigue, decreased respiratory effectiveness, and increased oxygen consumption and cardiac output at a time when gas exchange and cardiac output are already compromised. In addition, the inspiration occurring at higher lung volumes reduces the effectiveness of the cough. The child becomes progressively dyspneic, cyanotic, and tachypneic.

Gas Exchange. The degree to which impaired respiration interferes with gas exchange depends to a large measure on the ratio of poorly ventilated and hyperextended alveoli to well-ventilated alveoli. When the number of poorly ventilated alveoli increases, the degree of arterial hypoxemia also increases; with complete airway obstruction, a right-to-left pulmonary shunt with total absence of ventilation occurs.

While there are a sufficient number of well-ventilated alveolocapillary units, perfusion remains adequate and carbon dioxide elimination is not impaired. As the severity of obstruction increases, there is a reduced alveolar ventilation with carbon dioxide retention, hypoxemia, respiratory acidosis, and eventually respiratory failure.

Clinical Manifestations

Timing of symptoms varies greatly among patients. Bronchoconstriction in response to an allergen can have an immediate, histamine-type pattern or a late response with airway hypersensitivity lasting for days, weeks, or months. Since a second wave of symptoms sometimes appears 6 to 8 hours after the initial antigen exposure, patients should have sufficient medicine to control late-response symptoms if they occur. Once again, the classic manifestations are dyspnea, wheezing, and coughing.

Children may experience a prodromal itching localized at the front of the neck or over the upper part of the back. An asthmatic episode usually begins with children feeling uncomfortable or irritable and increasingly restless. They may also complain of a headache, feeling tired, or their chest feeling tight. After this, respiratory symptoms include a hacking, paroxysmal, irritative, and nonproductive cough caused by bronchial edema. Accumulated secretions, acting as a foreign body, stimulate the cough. As the secretions become more profuse, the cough becomes rattling and productive of frothy, clear, gelatinous sputum. Bronchial spasm and mucosal edema reduce the size of the bronchial lumen, which is, as a result, more easily occluded by mucous plugs.

A common symptom of asthma is coughing in the absence of respiratory infection, especially at night. This may disrupt sleep, leading to excessive fatigue during the day and poor school performance. Wheezing may be mild or discernible only on auscultation at the end of expiration, or severe enough to be audible. The child is frequently short of breath.

The child with a more severe episode is short of breath and tries to breathe more deeply; the expiratory phase becomes prolonged and is accompanied by an audible wheezing. The child often appears pale but may have a malar flush and red ears. The lips assume a deep, dark-red color that may progress to cyanosis observed in the nail beds and skin, especially around the mouth. The child is restless and apprehensive with an anxious facial expression. Sweating may be prominent as the exacerbation progresses. Younger children have a tendency to assume the tripod sitting position, whereas older children have a tendency to sit upright with shoulders in a hunched-over position, hands on the bed or chair, and arms braced to facilitate the use of accessory muscles of respiration. The child speaks with short, panting, broken phrases. Infants and small children are restless, irritable, and difficult to make comfortable. The severity of the episode can be evaluated on the basis of sweating and the child's refusal to lie down. A nonsweating child who remains upright is moderately ill; one who remains recumbent is the least ill.

The prolonged expiratory phase is less apparent in infants and young children because of a more pliable chest and the normal rapid respiratory rate. Therefore, expiratory and inspiratory dyspnea are more difficult to differentiate. Infants may display intercostal, suprasternal, subcostal, and sternal retractions.

Examination of the chest reveals hyperresonance on percussion. Breath sounds are coarse and loud, with sonorous crackles throughout the lung fields. Expiration is prolonged. Coarse rhonchi can be heard, as well as generalized inspiratory and expiratory wheezing that becomes more high pitched as obstruction progresses. With minimal obstruction, wheezing may be only mild (discernible only on auscultation at the end of expiration) or even absent but can be accentuated by rapid, deep breathing.

With severe spasm or obstruction, breath sounds and crackles may become inaudible. Cough is ineffective despite repeated, hacking maneuvers. This represents lack of air movement and may be misinterpreted as improvement by unknowing examiners.

NURSING ALERT Shortness of breath with air movement in the chest restricted to the point of absent breath sounds accompanied by a sudden rise in respiratory rate is an ominous sign indicating ventilatory failure and imminent asphyxia.

Children with chronic asthma develop generalized vascularization, mucosal thickening, and hypertrophy of the mucous glands and fibers of the bronchial musculature. With repeated episodes the thoracic cavity becomes fixed in a hyperaerated state (barrel chest), with depressed diaphragm, elevated shoulders, and increased use of accessory muscles of respiration.

Diagnostic Evaluation

Asthma is underdiagnosed in childhood and is often mislabeled as "wheezy bronchitis." This can result in the misuse of cough suppressants, antihistamines, and antibiotics (not indicated in the treatment of asthma) and ineffective use of bronchodilators (Neddenriep, Schumacher, and Lemen, 1989). The diagnosis of asthma is based on the child's medical history, physical examination, and laboratory test results.

Generally, chronic cough in the absence of infection or diffuse wheezing during the expiratory phase of respiration is sufficient to establish a diagnosis. Several observations provide assistance in differential diagnosis of other conditions (see box below). Localized, monophonic wheezing may indicate the obstruction of a single bronchus, caused by foreign body aspiration, bronchial stenosis, or intrathoracic tumor. Stridor, heard primarily on inspiration, usually indicates an extrathoracic obstruction such as laryngotra-

CONDITIONS THAT MAY MIMIC ASTHMA

OBSTRUCTION INVOLVING LARGE AIRWAYS

Foreign body in trachea, bronchus, or esophagus
Vascular rings
Laryngotracheomalacia
Enlarged lymph nodes
Tumor laryngeal webs
Tracheostenosis or bronchostenosis
Vocal cord paralysis

OBSTRUCTION INVOLVING BOTH LARGE AND SMALL AIRWAYS

Bronchiolitis: viral or obliterative
Cystic fibrosis
Bronchopulmonary dysplasia
Aspiration from swallowing dysfunction; gastroesophageal reflux; tracheoesophageal fistula
Pulmonary edema
Acute inflammation of the airways

cheomalacia, croup, or epiglottitis. Coarse crackles due to increased mucus secretion are often heard in conjunction with reactive airways, but fine crackles, characteristic of congestive heart failure or pneumonia, are absent. Most children with asthma are well nourished and do not display signs of chronic hypoxia. Poor growth, digital clubbing, or chronic bacterial infection is more likely to be caused by cystic fibrosis, heart disease, or cancer.

Pulmonary function tests (PFTs) provide an objective and reproducible method of evaluating the presence and degree of lung disease, as well as the response to therapy (Mueller and Eigen, 1992). In assessing respiratory function, the parameters most often measured include lung volumes, flows, timed volumes, and airway reactivity, while revealing air trapping and decreased expiratory flow. Spirometry can generally be performed reliably on children by the age of 5 or 6 years and includes either the traditional and simple mechanical spirometer often used in clinics, offices, and the home or the new computerized versions. One of the key measurements is the ***peak expiratory flow rate (PEFR)***, or the greatest flow velocity that can be obtained during a forced expiration. It is important to note that PFTs do not confirm the diagnosis; rather, they place the disease into physiologic categories. Three zones of measurement are typically used to interpret PEFR. The zone system is adapted to a traffic light so that the categories are easier to use and remember (see Guidelines box). Applications of PEFR measurements are described in Table 32-3.

Each individual child's PEFR varies according to age, height, sex, and race. The child's value may be consistently higher or lower than average predicted norms. Each child needs to establish his or her ***personal best value.*** A personal best value can be established during a 2- to 3-week period during which the child records PEFR at least twice a day. The present PEFR is then compared with the personal best (National Heart, 1991).

Because allergic rhinitis and eczema often accompany symptoms of allergic asthma, bronchial challenges using the cholinergic agent methacholine or histamine are performed occasionally to assess airway responsiveness to an allergen. Although the test is highly specific and sensitive, it puts the child at risk for a serious asthma episode and should be done under close observation in a qualified laboratory or clinic.

Skin testing is useful in identifying specific allergens, and those obtained by the puncture technique correlate better than intracutaneous tests with symptoms and measurements of specific IgE antibody. Provocative testing, direct exposure of the mucous membranes to a suspected antigen in increasing concentrations, helps to identify inhaled allergens. The RAST test helps identify antigens against various foods and is often useful in determining appropriate therapy.

In addition to these tests, other important tests include laboratory (complete blood count [CBC] with differential)

GUIDELINES
*Interpreting Peak Expiratory Flow Rates**

- ***Green (80% to 100% of personal best)*** signals all clear. Asthma is under reasonably good control. No symptoms are present, and the routine treatment plan for maintaining control can be followed.
- ***Yellow (50% to 80% of personal best)*** signals caution. Asthma is not well controlled. An acute exacerbation may be present. Maintenance therapy may need to be increased. Call the practitioner if the child stays in this zone.
- ***Red (below 50% of personal best)*** signals a medical alert. Severe airway narrowing may be occurring. An immediate bronchodilator should be taken. Notify the practitioner if the PEFR measure does not return immediately and stay in yellow or green zones.

*These zones are guidelines only. Specific zones and management may be individualized for each child by the practitioner.

TABLE 32-3 Applications of Peak Expiratory Flow Rate

OFFICE AND EMERGENCY ROOM	HOSPITAL	HOME	SCHOOL
Rapid, objective identification of severity Follow response to therapy	Bedside assessment of prebronchodilator and postbronchodilator function Follow response to therapy	Monitor asthma to increase or decrease therapy as necessary Early detection of decreases in PEFR that may indicate onset of an exacerbation of asthma Follow trends for diurnal variation in PEFR that predict instability of asthma and need for increased therapy Report changes over the phone to assist practitioner with recommendations when called Identify "triggers" of asthma (e.g., seasons, environmental exposures, viral infections, exercise)	Guide decisions by school personnel when student has acute episodes of asthma at school Identify exercise-induced asthma Increase sports participation by using PEFR to determine need to increase treatment Detect asthma that is not under control

Modified from National Heart, Lung, and Blood Institute: Guidelines for the diagnosis and management of asthma. In National Asthma Education Program: *Expert Panel Report,* Bethesda, MD, 1991, US Department of Health and Human Services, 1991, p 20.

and chest x-ray films. The CBC may show a slight elevation in the white blood cell (WBC) count during acute asthma, but elevations to more than 12,000/mm^3 or an increased percentage of band cells may indicate respiratory infection. The presence of eosinophilia of greater than 500/mm^3, however, tends to suggest an allergic or inflammatory disorder. Frontal and lateral x-ray films show infiltrates and hyperexpansion of the airways, with the anteroposterior (AP) diameter on physical examination indicating an increased diameter (suggestive of barrel chest).

Therapeutic Management: General

The overall goal of asthma management is to prevent disability and to minimize physical and psychologic morbidity—to assist the child in living as normal and happy a life as possible. This includes facilitating the child's social adjustments in the family, school, and community and normal participation in recreational activities and sports. To accomplish these goals, several treatment principles need to be followed (National Heart, 1991):

1. Since asthma is a chronic condition with acute exacerbations, treatment requires a continuous-care approach to prevent an episode and control symptoms.
2. Prevention of exacerbations is an extremely important principle of therapy. This includes avoidance of triggers, avoidance of allergens, and the use of medications as needed.
3. Therapy should include efforts to reduce underlying inflammatory components and relieve or prevent symptomatic airway narrowing.
4. Asthma therapy has several integral components: patient education, environmental control, and pharmacologic therapy, as well as the use of objective measures to monitor the severity of disease and course of therapy.

Allergen Control. The goal of nonpharmacologic therapy is prevention and reduction of the child's exposure to airborne allergens and irritants. Basic to any therapeutic plan is an evaluation of the child's general health and an assessment of the specific allergenic factors and the nonspecific factors that precipitate symptoms. ***House dust mites*** and other components of house dust are the agents identified most often in children allergic to inhalants. The most important method to eliminate dust mites is to keep the humidity in the house under 50%, the level below which dust mites do not survive (Cloutier, 1993; Duffs and Platt-Mills, 1992). Other recommendations for controlling allergens are in the Family Home Care box, p. 1427.

Specific allergens are identified by skin testing, and steps are taken to eliminate or avoid the offending allergens. Often, simply removing the offending environmental factors will decrease the frequency of asthma episodes, for example, removal of a dog or cat from the home of a child sensitive to animal dander. Nonspecific factors that may trigger an episode, such as extremes of temperature, are sometimes controlled by dehumidifiers or air conditioners.

Drug Therapy. Most children do not require continuous medication. The goal is to control the acute exacerbation; therefore, early recognition and treatment at the onset are most important. Preventing rapid relief of the bronchospasm reduces the need for drastic measures and increases the likelihood that relief will be complete. Medical management of asthma varies considerably among practitioners. Several drugs are prescribed, often in combination, to reverse or prevent bronchospasm.

Pharmacologic therapy is used to treat reversible airflow obstruction and airway hyperresponsiveness. Consensus reports have indicated the need to use antiinflammatory drugs as the primary agents to control chronic childhood asthma, as well as to consider the use of cromolyn sodium as a first-line agent (Larsen, 1992; Murphy and Kelly, 1992, 1993). Medications available include the following categories:

1. Antiinflammatory agents, such as corticosteroids, cromolyn sodium or cromolyn-like compounds, and other agents
2. Bronchodilators, such as β-adrenergic agonists and methylxanthines
3. Anticholinergic agents.

Corticosteroids. Corticosteroids are the most effective antiinflammatory drugs for the treatment of reversible airflow obstruction and are highly effective in controlling symptoms and reducing bronchial hyperreactivity in chronic asthma (Djukanovic and others, 1992; Ernst and others, 1992; Murphy and Kelly, 1993; National Heart, 1991; Van Essen-Zandvliet and others, 1992). Most trials have shown a significant improvement of all asthma parameters, including decreasing symptoms, emergency visits, and medication requirements.

Corticosteroids may be administered parenterally, orally, or by aerosol. Oral medications are metabolized slowly, with an onset of action up to 3 hours after administration and peak effectiveness occurring within 6 to 12 hours. Acute short-term therapy is typically begun with high dosages, which can be maintained for 5 to 10 days; this therapy should be maintained until PEFRs are stable and near normal levels. Oral steroids should be continued only if shown to reduce chronic symptoms substantially or reduce the frequency of severe episodes and should not be used alone without maximizing other forms of therapy. Long-term use is limited by the risk of significant adverse effects, such as osteoporosis, hypertension, Cushing syndrome, impaired immune mechanisms, and hypothalamic-pituitary-adrenal suppression (National Heart, 1991).

Inhaled corticosteroids are safe and effective and should be attempted to determine whether oral corticosteroid treatment can be reduced or eliminated. Their use appears to result in few or no side effects; at the same time, it has been demonstrated that the use of high doses of inhaled corticosteroids reduces the need for the long-term use of oral steroids (Peter and others, 1993).

Cromolyn and nedocromil sodium. Cromolyn sodium is currently the best nonsteroidal antiinflammatory drug for asthma (National Heart, 1991). Although the exact mechanism of how it works is not known, it appears to act superficially to inhibit mast cell degranulation in both early-phase and late-phase allergen-induced airway narrowing and acute airway narrowing after exposure to exercise, cold dry air, and sulfur dioxide. There is no way to reliably predict whether a child will respond to the drug. Cromolyn sodium produces only minimal side effects, such as occasional coughing on inhalation of the powder formulation, and may be given via nebulizer or MDI.

A new drug, approved and released in the United States in 1994, is nedocromil sodium, a topical medication that has both antiallergic and antiinflammatory properties (Murphy and Kelly, 1993; Sedgwick and others, 1992; Warner and others, 1992). One study showed that nedocromil was of significant benefit when added to sustained-release theophylline and could be substituted for theophylline in theophylline-dependent adults (Callaghan, Teo, and Clancy, 1992). Several studies are currently examining the drug in use with children, but the prospects for nedocromil are very positive.

β-Adrenergic agents. β-Adrenergic agonists (primarily albuterol, metaproterenol, and terbutaline) are the medications of choice for treatment of acute exacerbations of asthma and for the prevention of exercise-induced asthma. These drugs bind with the beta receptors on the smooth muscle of airways, where they activate adenylate cyclase and convert adenosine monophosphate (AMP) to cyclic AMP (cAMP). It is believed that the increased cAMP enhances binding of intracellular calcium (Ca) to the cell membrane, reducing the availability of Ca and thus allowing smooth muscle to relax. Other effects of the drug help stabilization of mast cells to prevent release of mediators. Most β-adrenergics used in asthma therapy affect only beta-2 receptors, which help eliminate bronchospasm. Beta-1 effects, which are reflected in increased heart rate and gastrointestinal disturbances, have been minimized.

β-Adrenergic agonists can be given via inhalation or as oral or parenteral preparations. The inhaled drug, administered by ***metered-dose inhaler (MDI)*** or nebulizer, has a more rapid onset of action than the oral form but is more costly. The MDI may have a spacing unit or reservoir attached, which makes it easier for small children to use. Inhalation also reduces troublesome systemic side effects: irritability, tremor, nervousness, and insomnia.

Inhaled β-adrenergics can be taken two to four times daily for acute symptoms. Children with exercise-induced bronchospasm are advised to use the drug prophylactically 10 to 15 minutes before exercise. Small children who have difficulty using the MDI can obtain effective relief with nebulization. The medication is mixed with saline or cromolyn and then nebulized with compressed air. Children are instructed to breathe normally with the mouth open to provide a direct route to the trachea.

Aerosol or inhaled therapy is comparable to or better than oral therapy in producing bronchodilation and causes fewer systemic adverse effects. Because asthma is an airway disease, inhaled therapy with the beta-2 agonist delivered directly to the airways is usually preferable to systemic therapy. Most literature indicates that MDIs are as effective as nebulizers in delivering the medication (Handling, 1993; Kerem and others, 1993). There has been some research into the efficacy of regular use (as opposed to as-needed use) of potent inhaled beta-2 agonists and diminished control of asthma, but additional work needs to be done regarding the issue of tolerance.

Methylxanthines. The methylxanthines, principally theophylline, have been used for decades to relieve symptoms and prevent asthma attacks. Theophylline, however, is now considered as a third-line agent and perhaps even unnecessary for treating asthma exacerbations (Hill; Szefler, and Larsen, 1992; Murphy and Kelly, 1993; Weinberger, 1993). It is a relatively weak bronchodilator as compared with the β-adrenergics, and since asthma is now believed to be an inflammatory condition, other drugs are of increased benefit (Stempel and Szefler, 1992). It was shown that theophylline, even at therapeutic concentrations, did not additionally benefit children hospitalized with severe asthma who were being treated frequently with nebulized albuterol and methylprednisolone intravenously (Carter and others, 1993: Meltzer and others, 1992).

Questions surrounding theophylline have largely focused on safety issues rather than efficacy (Murphy and Kelly, 1993). The most recent review of 125 pediatric intoxications over 5 years suggests a more severe outcome at lower concentrations for chronic toxicity (Shannon and Lovejoy, 1992). When theophylline is used, it may be taken intravenously, intramuscularly, orally, or rectally (seldom used). The drug is also available in sustained-release form for oral ingestion. In addition to its bronchodilator effect, theophylline is also a central respiratory stimulant and increases respiratory muscle contractility. One also needs to consider factors that may affect metabolization of the drug (see box at left). It is generally agreed that theophylline should be used when the child is not responsive to other inhaled medications and for treating chronic asthma (Stempel and Szefler, 1992; Weinberger, 1993).

Monitoring serum concentrations is an important component of both acute care and long-term management. Monitoring is required for children who fail to exhibit the expected bronchodilator effect, as well as for those who develop an adverse effect on the usual dose. Although theophylline has been accepted to have a therapeutic level of 10 to 20 μg/ml, a more conservative approach would be to aim for levels of 5 to 15 μg/ml (National Heart, 1991). The signs and symptoms of theophylline intoxication involve

FACTORS AFFECTING THEOPHYLLINE CLEARANCE

SUBSTANCES THAT ACCELERATE CLEARANCE

Phenytoin
Rifampin
Phenobarbital
Valproic acid
Cigarette and marijuana smoking

FACTORS THAT DELAY CLEARANCE

Age: Neonates, infants
Medication: Antibiotics (especially erythromycin), cimetidine (Tagamet), carbamazepine (Tegretol), quinoline, oral contraceptives, propranolol (Inderal), furosemide, allopurinol
Illnesses: Liver or heart dysfunction, congestive heart failure, fever for more than 24 hours, acute viral illness
Other: Obesity

many different organ systems, with gastrointestinal symptoms—nausea and vomiting—being the most common early events. Cardiopulmonary effects include tachycardia, arrhythmias, and stimulation of the respiratory center (tachypnea), with diuresis, irritability, and even seizures possible.

There have been reports that theophylline may cause behavior problems and poor school performance (Gutstadt and others, 1989; Rachelefsky and others, 1986). Because theophylline causes central nervous system stimulation, it may produce behavioral disturbances in children, with impairment of learning. One study (not specifically examining the theophylline issue) suggested a modestly increased risk of academic problems among children with asthma compared with well children, with fair-poor health twice as likely to have a reported learning disability as those in good-excellent health (Fowler, Davenport, and Garg, 1992). In general, however, most research, as well as a review conducted by the Food and Drug Administration, tends to refute the hypothesis that theophylline adversely affects school performance (Fitzpatrick and others, 1992; Fowler, Davenport and Garg, 1992; Lindgren and others, 1992; Murphy and Kelly, 1993; National Heart, 1991) and causes behavioral changes (Bender and others, 1991, 1992).

The dose of theophylline varies with age. Children under 12 months of age metabolize the drug faster than adults, so the dose per kilogram must be higher. Because absorption also varies among individuals, it is important to follow serum levels of the drug until a therapeutic dose is achieved.

Anticholinergics. Anticholinergic therapy, the oldest form of bronchodilator therapy for asthma, works by reducing the intrinsic vagal tone to the airways and blocking reflex bronchoconstriction caused by inhaled irritants. The principal reasons these agents are not favored is because of the length of time for onset of action and adverse side effects such as drying of respiratory secretions, blurred vision, and cardiac and CNS stimulation. The primary drugs used are atropine or its derivative ipratropium, which does not cross the blood-brain barrier and therefore elicits no CNS effects. Ipratropium has been shown to be effective during status asthmaticus when used in nebulized form in combination with β-adrenergic agents (National Heart, 1991).

Heliox. For children manifesting bronchospasm or difficulty in ventilation, heliox (helium/oxygen mixture) has been used. Helium is nonreactive with biologic membranes and is virtually insoluble in lung tissue. Carbon dioxide diffuses more readily through a mixture of helium/oxygen than through air because of the decreased density, resulting in less turbulent airflow.

Steroids, β-agonists, and cromolyn sodium attempt to reduce the work of breathing by dilating the airways and reducing airway edema, thus recreating laminar flow. Unfortunately, although bronchodilation may start rapidly with these drugs, complete reversal of the hypoventilation and respiratory acidosis may not occur for prolonged periods, making heliox a useful adjunct therapy. Each therapy works by completely different mechanisms, but the goal accomplished is the same: decreased work of breathing. The helium effect lasts only as long as the gas is used and does not have any inherent bronchodilating effect; definitive therapy with bronchodilators must be started at the same time.

Helium can be delivered from premixed tanks, which may be blended in a stand-alone unit or within a ventilator. An oxygen analyzer must be place in-line after mixing the gases to measure the concentration of oxygen the patient is actually receiving. No significant untoward effects from helium have been reported, even for individuals using the gas for weeks at a time at different altitudes (Gluck, 1993). The usual ratio of helium to oxygen is either 60%:40% or 70%:30%. One study showed significant improvement in aeration (Shiue and Gluck, 1989). Another study indicated a significant decrease in airway resistance for patients on ventilators within 5 minutes of the start of heliox, as well as significant acid-base correction within 20 minutes of therapy initiation (Gluck, Onorato, and Castriotta, 1990).

Chest Physiotherapy. Chest physiotherapy (CPT) is a standard adjunct to treatment of chronic asthma. This includes breathing exercises, physical training, and inhalation therapy. These therapies help produce physical and mental relaxation, improve posture, strengthen respiratory musculature, and develop more efficient patterns of breathing. For the motivated child, breathing exercises and controlled breathing are of value in preventing overinflation and improving the strength of respiratory muscles and the efficiency of the cough. Stretch exercises sometimes help increase the flexibility of the ribs. Sit-ups and leg exercises strengthen abdominal muscles and aid expiration.

Hyposensitization. The role of hyposensitization in childhood asthma has not been clarified. In many cases the child demonstrates multiple sensitivities, which makes such therapy impractical. Moreover, the injections can be expensive and uncomfortable. When the allergen can be defined and cannot be avoided or controlled satisfactorily by drugs, specific hyposensitization is seriously considered. Immune therapy is not recommended for allergens that can be eliminated effectively, for example, food sensitivities, drugs, and animal dander. Inhalant allergens such as house dust, pollens, and molds are most often the allergens considered for immune therapy.

Injection therapy is usually limited to clinically significant allergens. The initial dose of the offending allergen(s), based on the size of the skin reaction, is injected subcutaneously. The amount is increased at weekly intervals until a maximum tolerance is reached, after which a maintenance dose is given at 4-week intervals. This may be extended to 5- or 6-week intervals during the off-season for seasonal allergens. Successful treatment is continued for a minimum of 3 years and then stopped. If no symptoms appear, acquired immunity is said to be retained; if symptoms recur, treatment is reinstituted.

Exercise. Airway obstruction often develops in children with asthma. ***Exercise-induced bronchospasm,*** or ***exercise-induced asthma (EIA),*** does not represent a unique syndrome but rather an example of the airway hyperactivity common to all persons with asthma. This bronchoconstriction is not limited to children with asthma but also occurs in children with allergic rhinitis. EIA is defined as an acute, reversible, usually self-terminating airway obstruction that develops 5 to 15 minutes after strenuous exercise and lasts 15 to 60 minutes after the onset (Pierson, 1988). Usually, the episode subsides spontaneously in ½ to 1 hour. The severity of an attack increases as the exercise becomes increasingly strenuous. Patients with a history of EIA often have normal pulmonary function tests and are only symptomatic with exercise (American Academy of Pediatrics, 1989).

The problem is rare in activities that require only short bursts of energy (e.g., baseball, sprints, gymnastics, skiing) compared with those that involve endurance exercise (e.g., soccer, basketball, distance running). Swimming, even long-distance swimming, is well tolerated by children with EIA, partly because they are breathing air fully saturated with moisture, but the type of breathing required may also play a role. Exhaling underwater prolongs each expiration and increases the end-expiratory pressure within the respiratory tree (essentially pursed-lip breathing).

Children with asthma are often excluded from exercise by parents, teachers, and physicians, as well as by the children themselves because they are reluctant to provoke an episode. This can seriously hamper peer interaction and physical health. It has been found that moderate or even strenuous exercise is advantageous for children with asthma. The majority of these children can participate in activities at school and in sports with minimum difficulty, provided the asthma is under control. Participation is encouraged but should be evaluated on an individual basis in terms of tolerance for duration and intensity of effort. Appropriate prophylactic treatment with β-adrenergic agents or cromolyn sodium before exercise will usually permit full participation in strenuous exercise. Restrictions are invoked only when the child's condition makes it necessary.

Therapeutic Management: Specific

Children are subject to asthmatic exacerbations at varying intervals, with severity ranging from wheezing to life-threatening status asthmaticus. The modes of management vary according to the frequency and severity of the disease, as described in Table 32-4.

Several protocols have been developed for treating the child experiencing an asthmatic episode at home, in the emergency department, or in the hospital (National Heart, 1991). Successful home management of acute asthma begins before symptoms develop, and subtle signs, such as coughing or changes in activity level, are noticed. An example of an initial assessment and emergency treatment protocol is described in Table 32-5.

Status Asthmaticus. Children who continue to display respiratory distress despite vigorous therapeutic measures, especially injections of epinephrine, are considered to be in ***status asthmaticus.*** The severity of an attack can be categorized as outlined in Table 32-4. The condition may develop gradually or rapidly, often coincident with complicating conditions such as pneumonia that can influence the duration and treatment of the exacerbation. Status asthmaticus is a medical emergency that can result in respiratory failure and death if untreated.

Persistent hypoventilation leads to accumulation of carbon dioxide, with a decrease in arterial pH and respiratory acidosis. As a result, compensatory buffering mechanisms become overtaxed and the pH may drop to dangerous levels. Vomiting and dehydration cause further reduction of arterial pH by promoting retention of acids. Therapy for status asthmaticus is directed toward correction of dehydration and acidosis, improvement of ventilation, and treatment of any concurrent infection.

Several scoring systems have been devised for assessing the severity of bronchial obstruction, and most involve blood gas and pH measurements, presence of cyanosis, use of accessory muscles, breath sounds, and mental alertness. A child suspected of status asthmaticus is usually admitted to a pediatric intensive care unit for close observation and

TABLE 32-4 Estimation of Severity of Acute Exacerbation in Children with Asthma

SIGN/SYMPTOM	MILD	MODERATE	SEVERE
Peak expiratory flow rate	70%-90% predicted or baseline	50%-70% predicted or baseline	<50% predicted or baseline
Respiratory rate	Normal to 30% above mean	30%-50% increase above mean	>50% increase above mean
Alertness	Normal	Normal	May be decreased
Dyspnea	Absent or mild, speaks in complete sentences	Moderate, speaks in phrases or partial sentences	Severe, speaks only in single words or short phrases
Accessory muscle use	No intercostal to mild retractions	Moderate intercostal retractions with tracheosternal retractions, use of sternocleidomastoid muscles, chest hyperinflation	Moderate intercostal retractions, tracheosternal retractions with nasal flaring during inspiration, chest hyperinflation
Color	Good	Pale	Possibly cyanotic
Auscultation	End-expiratory wheeze only	Inspiratory and expiratory wheezing	Breath sounds inaudible
Oxygen saturation*	>95%	90%-95%	<90%
$Pco_{2(opt)}$	<35	<40	>40

From American Academy of Pediatrics, Provisional Committee on Quality Improvement: Practice parameter: the office management of acute exacerbations of asthma in children, *Pediatrics* 93(1):119-126, 1994.

*Oxygen saturation values are optional and will have to be adjusted for altitude. These values assume that the patient is at sea level.

TABLE 32-5 Initial Assessment and Emergency Treatment of Acute Exacerbations of Asthma in a Child Who Is Capable of Using a Peak Flow Meter*

ASSESSMENT	RECOMMENDED ACTIONS
Does the patient have: Altered level of consciousness Marked dyspnea, speaks only in single words or short phrases Severe intercostal or sternocleidomastoid retractions Cyanosis, pallor, or diaphoresis Inaudible breath sounds Subcutaneous or other extrapulmonary air Oxygen saturation <90% if oximeter available Peak expiratory flow rate <50% of predicted norm or baseline Pco_2 >40 mm Hg if arterial blood gases are available	If any of these conditions exist: Give oxygen by ventimask or nasal cannula. If unable to generate PEFR, give epinephrine subcutaneously (SC), 0.01 mL/kg/dose of 1:1000 epinephrine with a maximum dose of 0.3 mL or SC terbutaline 0.005-0.010 mg/kg/dose with a maximum dose of 0.25 mg. If able to generate PEFR, give nebulized albuterol 0.15 mg/kg/dose or 0.03 mL/kg/dose up to a maximum of 5 mg with 6 L/min of O_2 flow. Give systemic steroids at a prednisone equivalent of 2 mg/kg. Consider transfer to an appropriate emergency setting at an Fio_2 of 0.40 or greater and intermittent albuterol treatments every 20 min or continuous albuterol treatments at 0.5 mg/kg/hr if initial response is inadequate. If patient responds well to initial albuterol treatment, repeat twice every 20 minutes and provide *follow-up treatment.*
Does the patient have a history of: Steroid-dependent asthma Panic attacks with acute exacerbations Duration of asthma >12 hours History of respiratory failure Premonitions of death ≥2 visits to office or ED in 24 hours >3 visits in 48 hours Paroxysmal attacks especially at night	THIS IS A HIGH-RISK PATIENT. Begin therapy immediately as outlined above for moderate or severe exacerbation, regardless of the severity of the current episode. These are high-risk factors that should be considered in the decision to urgently transfer the patient to an appropriate emergency setting. If there is not a prompt clinical response to therapy, consider transfer and give systemic steroids (oral or parenteral) at a prednisone equivalent of 2 mg/kg before transfer.

From American Academy of Pediatrics, Provisional Committee on Quality Improvement: Practice parameter: the office management of acute exacerbations of asthma in children, *Pediatrics* 93(1):119-126, 1994.
*NOTE: This table presents only *one part* of the treatment of acute asthmatic episodes.

continuous cardiorespiratory monitoring.

The child is given intravenous fluids and nothing by mouth except liquids if the condition permits. Intravenous infusion provides a means for hydration and administering medications. Correction of dehydration, acidosis, hypoxia, and electrolyte derangements is guided by frequent determination of arterial pH, blood gases, and serum electrolytes. Bronchospasm is relieved by giving nebulized albuterol (either intermittent or continuous) along with corticosteroids (either oral or intravenous). For the child not responding to either of these therapies, oral theophylline or aminophylline may be considered.

Humidified oxygen is administered by nasal prongs, hood, or face mask to maintain an arterial oxygen tension greater than 65 mm Hg but less than 100 mm Hg to avoid the danger of oxygen narcosis. Mist tents do not allow for the close observation needed for the severely affected child. Since oxygen is a stimulus for respiration, high levels may significantly depress respirations. Controlled ventilation with endotracheal intubation may be needed if the condition progresses to respiratory failure, but it is rarely needed for more than 12 hours.

With a pH lower than 7.25, sodium bicarbonate is usually administered to correct acidosis, since values this low tend to impair systemic, pulmonary, and coronary blood flow; normal pH enhances the response of bronchial smooth muscle to bronchodilator therapy. Antibiotics are frequently prescribed, since infection may be masked or may not always be evident and is always a threatening complication. As the attack subsides, fluids and medication are given orally (adrenergic agonists may be administered by MDI), and discharge plans are begun, especially for follow-up care.

Prognosis. The outlook for children with asthma varies widely. An impressive number of children become asymptomatic at puberty, but no factor can predict which children will "outgrow" their asthma. Some develop other forms of allergy in adulthood. It has been postulated that just as the skin manifestations of infancy (eczema) shift to the bronchi in childhood, there may be another shift in the susceptible tissues (shock organ) at adulthood—most frequently to the nose.

The prognosis for control or disappearance of symptoms will differ from children who have rare and infrequent episodes to those who are constantly wheezing or are subject to status asthmaticus. In general, severe and numerous symptoms, that have been present for a long time, combined with a family history of allergy, increase the likelihood of a poor prognosis. Many who outgrow their exacerbations are subject to exercise-induced asthma as adults, and the associated disorders of growth impairment, chest deformity, and airway obstruction are maintained throughout life.

The relationship between childhood asthma and the development of chronic obstructive pulmonary disease (COPD) in adulthood has not been determined satisfactorily. Parental smoking has been clearly associated with increased risk of wheezing, respiratory symptoms, and lower respiratory tract illness, all components of asthma (Morgan and Martinez, 1992). Smoking is the major risk factor for development of COPD, although numerous persons who had asthma have developed COPD without smoking.

Deaths from asthma have been relatively uncommon, especially in young age-groups, but the increases have been reported within the United States as well as worldwide (McFadden and Gilbert, 1992). The death rate from asthma increased 46% in the period 1980-1989 despite advances in therapy (American Academy of Pediatrics, 1994d). The adolescent age-group appears to be the most vulnerable, with the greatest increase occurring in ages 10 to 14 years. No reliable data exist to explain this increase. Factors that have been postulated include exposure of atopic persons to more allergens, change in severity of the disease, abuse of drug therapy (toxicity), failure of families and practitioners to recognize severity of asthma, and psychologic factors, such as denial or refusal to accept the disease (Friday and Fireman, 1988). Risk factors for asthma deaths appear to be onset at an early age, frequent attacks, difficult-to-manage disease, adolescence, history of respiratory failure, psychologic problems (refusal to take medications), dependency on or misuse of drugs (high use), presence of physical stigmata (barrel chest, intercostal retractions), and abnormal pulmonary function tests (see Family Focus box).

The regular use of β-adrenergic drugs, especially fenoterol (not used in the United States), administered by MDI has been associated with increased risk of death or near-death. Whether their heavy use is directly responsible for the increased risk or indirectly indicates the severity of the asthma is unknown (Burrows and Lebowitz, 1992; Spitzer and others, 1992).

Traditional viewpoints and research have held that asthma is not a curable disease. Exciting new data, however, are challenging this, and science is beginning to better understand the pathophysiology and subsequent goals of therapy (Sullivan, 1992). This is based on research that examined spontaneous remissions, remissions induced by antigen removal or use of specific antigen immunotherapy, and the use of corticosteroids and other medications (e.g., gold, cancer chemotherapy). Much of the future research will involve examining the pathophysiologic mechanisms that may be vulnerable to eradication by combination therapy, along with aggressive antiinflammatory drugs.

Nursing Considerations: Acute Care

Children who are admitted to the hospital with acute asthma are ill, anxious, and uncomfortable. In most instances, children are admitted as an emergency with status asthmaticus and are in acute distress. The importance of continual observation and assessment cannot be overemphasized.

NURSING ALERT The child who sweats profusely and remains sitting upright and refuses to lie down is in severe distress. Also, the child who suddenly becomes agitated, or the agitated child who suddenly becomes quiet, may be seriously hypoxic and requires immediate intervention.

An intravenous infusion is begun immediately, and medication, usually corticosteroids and theophylline, is administered to relieve bronchospasm. The child is monitored closely and continuously during theophylline or terbutaline administration for relief of respiratory distress and signs of side effects or toxicity. Pulse, respiration, and blood pressure are taken and recorded every 5 minutes during rapid infusion and every 15 minutes for at least an hour after the drug has been initiated. Theophylline levels should be checked at 1, 8, and 24 hours into infusion, since toxicity can occur with serum levels greater than 20 μg/ml.

NURSING ALERT Side effects from theophylline include nausea, vomiting, headache, irritability, and insomnia. Early signs of toxicity are nausea, tachycardia, and irritability; seizures and dysrhythmias occur at blood theophylline levels greater than 30 μg/ml.

Some practitioners prefer to administer aerosol β_2-adrenergics and corticosteroids. If aerosol medications are administered, the β-adrenergics are administered first to open the airways before administration of antiinflammatory agents.

It is especially important that the child receive sufficient fluid either orally or intravenously to replace losses through diaphoresis and hyperventilation. Liquids are best tolerated if they are warm or at room temperature. Cold liquids can trigger reflex bronchospasm and should be avoided. Nourishment is provided in small, frequent feedings to avoid abdominal distention that might interfere with diaphragm excursion.

NURSING ALERT Dehydration should be corrected slowly; overhydration can increase the accumulation of interstitial pulmonary fluid to exacerbate small airway obstruction.

Older children usually prefer the high-Fowler position, although they may be more comfortable sitting upright or leaning slightly forward. When possible, the nurse communicates in such a way that a child need only reply in a few words to avoid fatigue. Shortness of breath makes talking difficult. Oxygen is indicated for relief of dyspnea and cyanosis; however, it is not administered indiscriminately but regulated according to the blood gas analysis, pulse oximetry, and objective observation of color, respiratory effort, and sensorium. Associated treatments such as intermittent positive-pressure breathing or postural drainage and tests (e.g., blood gases, PFTs) may be performed by specialized personnel or may be the nurse's responsibility.

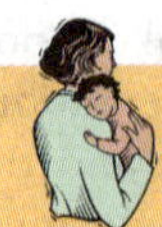

FAMILY FOCUS
Asthma: Factors Affecting Prognosis

Psychologic factors play an important role in children who die during an asthmatic episode. Those who die tend to have significant psychologic problems, such as extreme reactions to separation or loss, a history of family turmoil, and expressed hopelessness or despair that leads to depression. Their families are less likely to recognize the severity of the asthma and the need to comply with therapy. In this situation appropriate family education concerning the risks of the child's disease if treatment is inconsistent can be lifesaving (Klinnert, Miller, and Mrazek, 1990).

Children in status asthmaticus are apprehensive and anxious. Moreover, they are usually tired from respiratory efforts and loss of sleep. The calm, efficient presence of a nurse helps to reassure them that they are safe and will be cared for during this stressful period. It is important to assure children that they will not be left alone and that their parents are allowed to be near and available when needed.

Parents need reassurance, too. They want to be informed of their child's condition and therapies. They are upset, apprehensive about the child's condition, and feeling guilty. Often they feel that they may have in some way contributed to the child's condition or could have prevented the episode. They may even feel, consciously or unconsciously, anger toward the child for continuing to display symptoms despite their efforts to prevent or control the exacerbation. Reassurance about their efforts expended on the child's behalf and their parenting capabilities can help alleviate their stress. All efforts to reduce parental apprehension will, in turn, help reduce the child's distress. Anxiety is easily communicated to the child from parents and members of the staff.

Nursing Considerations: General Care

Nursing care of children with asthma involves both acute and long-term care and includes therapies and observations described in previous discussions of respiratory disturbances. Nurses who are involved with children in the home, clinic, or practitioner's office play an important role in helping the children and their families learn to live with the condition. The disease can be tolerated if it does not interfere with family life, physical activity, or school attendance or if it does not require hospitalization.

❖ Assessment

Nurses are involved in the initial assessment and workup to determine the cause and extent of the asthma. Physical assessment of asthma involves the same observations and techniques described in Chapters 7 and 31. In addition, some physical characteristics of chronic respiratory involvement are noted and evaluated, including chest configuration (e.g., barrel chest), posturing, and type of breathing. A history of the current and previous episodes and likely precipitating factors or events provides important information.

Nurses assist with various diagnostic tests, pulmonary function tests, and skin testing as well as a general health assessment. Also, the child and family are assessed as to the degree to which the disorder (if previously diagnosed) interferes with everyday activities, the disorder alters the child's self-concept, and the child and family comply with the prescribed therapy.

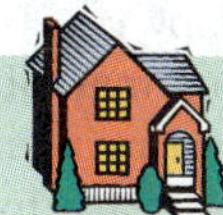

FAMILY HOME CARE
"Allergy-Proofing" the Home

Keep humidity between 40% and 50%; use dehumidifier if available.
Have carpets cleaned professionally frequently or remove them, including carpeting on concrete.
- Avoid vacuuming carpets, which sends allergens into the air, although it does remove waste particles of dust mite.
- If available, use central vacuum cleaner with collecting bag outside of home or use cleaner filters (e.g., high-efficiency particulate air [HEPA] filters).

Use chemical agents to kill mites or alter antigens in house.
- Treating carpet with 3% tannic acid solution or benzylbenzoate (available in foam for mattresses and furniture and in powder for carpets) kills dust mites; keep child away from treated areas during and several hours after chemical application.*

If possible, use an air-cleaning device, such as electrostatic precipitator; approximate-size units can be used in child's room.
Have air and heat ducts professionally cleaned annually; change or clean filters monthly.
Place airtight plastic, vinyl, or hypoallergenic covers on mattress, box spring, and pillows.*
Use foam rubber mattress and pillows or Dacron pillows and synthetic blankets.
Launder blankets and sheets in hot water (over 48.8° C [120° F]).
Store nothing under bed; keep closets and storage areas uncluttered.
Use washable shades rather than blinds or curtains.
Use child's bedroom for sleeping, not playing.
Remove from room unnecessary furniture, rugs, stuffed or real animals, toys, books, upholstered furniture, plants, aquariums, wall hangings, etc.
Cover or replace upholstered furniture; avoid rattan or wicker furniture.
Cover walls with washable paint or wallpaper.
Limit child's exposure to animals.
Change child's clothes after playing outdoors; wash hair nightly if outside and pollen count is high.
Keep child indoors while lawn is being mowed, bushes/trees are being trimmed, or pollen count is high.
Keep windows and doors closed during pollen season; use air conditioner if available.
Cover heating vents with filter material (e.g., cheesecloth) to prevent circulation of dust, especially when heat is turned on after summer.
Use smooth cotton or synthetic fabric for bedcovers, curtains, and scatter rugs and launder weekly.
Wet mop bare floors weekly.
Wet dust (or use Endust) and clean room weekly; child should not be present during housecleaning activities.
Encase wool or feather items in nonallergenic coverings.*
Limit or avoid child's exposure to tobacco and wood smoke.
Avoid odors or sprays (e.g., perfumes, talcum powder, room deodorizers, fresh paint).
Avoid cellar (basement) as play area and use dehumidifier in damp cellar.
Clean showers and tile areas; spray with antimold agent (e.g., Lysol).
Keep vaporizers and air conditioners (including automobile air conditioner) clean and free of mold.

*A source of information is Allergy Control Products, Inc., 96 Danbury Rd, Ridgefield, CT 06877; (800) 422-DUST.

❖ NURSING DIAGNOSES

Based on a thorough assessment, several nursing diagnoses are identified. The more common diagnoses for the child with asthma are included in the Nursing Care Plan on pp. 1431-1433. Others may apply in specific situations.

❖ PLANNING

The goals for a child with asthma and the family include the following:

1. Child will not experience an asthmatic episode.
2. Child will exhibit improved ventilatory capacity.
3. Child will maintain optimum health.
4. Child will not develop complications.
5. Child will engage in normal activities for age.
6. Child and family will receive appropriate support and education regarding the disease and its management.

❖ IMPLEMENTATION

The major emphasis of nursing care is directed toward outpatient management by the family. Parents are even able to manage acute exacerbations if they maintain contact with the practitioner and know how to observe for the expected response and signs of probable toxicity.

Avoid Allergens. As indicated on p. 1421, the primary goal of asthma management is avoidance of an exacerbation. Parents need to know the nature of the disease and, when the allergens are determined, how they can avoid and/or relieve asthmatic episodes. The nurse assists the parent in modifying the environment to reduce contact with the offending allergen(s) (see Family Home Care box, p. 1427). The parents are cautioned to avoid exposing a sensitive child to excessive cold, wind, or other extremes of weather, smoke, sprays, or other irritants. Passive smoking has been associated with exacerbation of symptoms in children with hyperresponsive airways, especially in boys and older children (Morgan and Martinez, 1992; Murray and Morrison, 1989; National Heart, 1991).

Although foods are an unusual cause of asthma, foods known to provoke symptoms should be eliminated from the diet. Food additives, especially monosodium glutamate (MSG); sulfites, such as sulfur dioxide; sodium and potassium salts of sulfite, bisulfite, and metabisulfite; and dyes have been reported to produce allergic responses in sensitive persons. Families are taught to read labels carefully for the presence of these substances.

Since approximately 2% to 6% of children with asthma are sensitive to aspirin, nurses caution the parents to use other analgesic/antipyretic drugs for discomfort or fever. Acetaminophen appears to be a safe drug for these children and is recommended as the analgesic of choice (National Heart, 1991). Those children with aspirin-induced asthma may also be sensitive to nonsteroidal antiinflammatory drugs and tartrazine (yellow dye number 5, a common food coloring). Other drugs that should be avoided by children with asthma are antihistamines (dry airway secretions, making expectoration difficult), cough suppressants (impair clearance of secretions), and sedatives (depress respirations and aggravate hypoventilation).

Relieve Bronchospasm. Parents and older children need to learn how to use the medications prescribed to relieve bronchospasm. They are taught to recognize early signs and symptoms of an impending attack so that it can be controlled before symptoms become distressing. Most children can recognize prodromal symptoms well before an attack (about 6 hours) so that preventive therapy can be implemented. Some objective signs that parents may observe include rhinorrhea, cough, low-grade fever, irritability, itching (especially in front of neck and chest), apathy, anxiety, sleep disturbance, abdominal discomfort, and loss of appetite. A variety of easy-to-use, inexpensive peak expiratory flow meters (PEFMs) are available for use in the home to help assess the extent of the child's symptoms (see Family Home Care box above).

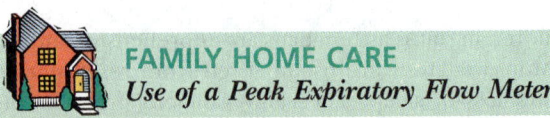

FAMILY HOME CARE
Use of a Peak Expiratory Flow Meter

1. Before each use, make sure the sliding marker or arrow on the PEFM is at the bottom of the numbered scale.
2. Stand up straight.
3. Remove gum or any food from the mouth.
4. Close your lips tightly around the mouthpiece. Be sure to keep your tongue away from the mouthpiece.
5. Blow out as hard and as quickly as you can, a "fast hard puff."
6. Note the number by the marker on the numbered scale.
7. Repeat entire routine three times.
8. Record the *highest* of the three readings, not the average.
9. Measure your peak expiratory flow rate (PEFR) close to the same time and same way each day (i.e., morning and evening; before and/or 15 minutes after taking medication).
10. Keep a chart of your PEFRs.

Older children who use a nebulizer or aerosol device to deliver adrenergic drugs need to learn how to use the device correctly (Rachelefsky, 1992). The MDI (Fig. 32-9) combines portability with a rapid and reliable dose for patients managed at home. The objective of the device is to distribute the prescribed medication directly to the narrowed airways. It is important that the child learns to breathe slowly and deeply for better distribution to narrowed airways (see Family Home Care box, p. 1429). Rapid inspiration causes the drugs to move through unobstructed bronchioles to patent airways, where they are less needed. The length of time between puffs varies according to the acuity of the episode and the location of the child—home, emergency department/clinic, or hospital.

Young children and those who are otherwise unable to manipulate the device or coordinate breathing with activation of the MDI are able to use special chambers called ***spacers.*** These permit an operator to deliver the medication from the MDI into the spacer from which the child inhales (see Critical Thinking Exercise box).

The child and parents also need to be cautioned about the adverse effects of prescribed drugs and the dangers of overuse. They should know that it is important to use them when needed but not indiscriminately or as a substitute for avoiding the symptom-provoking allergen. Parents and

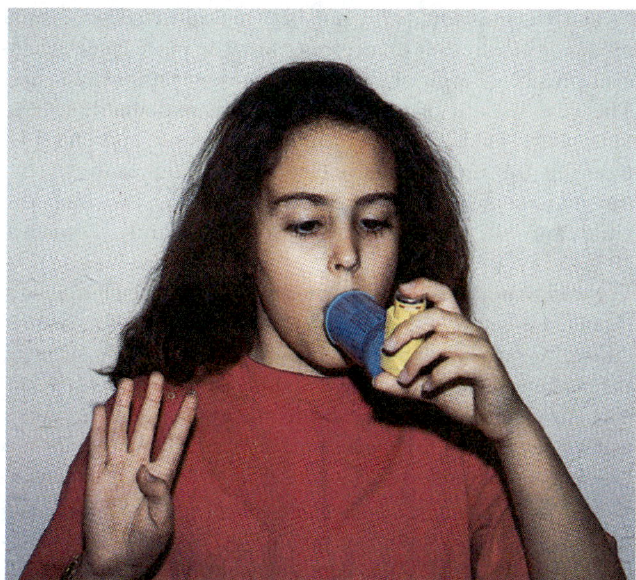

FIG. 32-9 Child using metered-dose inhaler with spacer. Fingers are used for counting to 10 seconds.

child are taught to report any changing reaction to a drug or if the drug appears to be losing its effectiveness, as evidenced by more frequent need for the drug. Parents are also cautioned against purchasing generic substitutions for prescribed theophylline, since dosage varies considerably. Also, over-the-counter preparations may contain duplicate medications that increase the dosage of a prescribed drug (e.g., Bronkaid R, which contains theophylline). Toxicity has been reported from this practice (Keyes, 1987).

Maintain Health and Prevent Complications. The child should be protected from a respiratory infection that can trigger an attack or aggravate the asthmatic state, especially in young children, whose airways are mechanically smaller and more reactive. Also, the equipment used for the child, such as nebulizers, must be kept absolutely clean to decrease the chances of contamination with bacteria and fungi. Oral candidiasis is a major complication of aerosolized steroids; therefore children with severe asthma who are taking steroids by this route are taught to rinse the mouth thoroughly with water after each treatment to minimize the risk of infection.

Breathing exercises and controlled breathing are taught and encouraged for the motivated youngster, and the nurse can help to select activities suitable to the child's capacity. Anything that promotes proper diaphragmatic breathing, side expansion, and generally improved mobility of the chest wall is encouraged by many practitioners.

➤ **NURSING TIP** Play techniques that can be used as breathing exercises for younger children to extend their expiratory time and increase expiratory pressure include blowing cotton balls or a Ping-Pong ball on a table, blowing a pinwheel, or preventing a tissue from falling by blowing it against the wall.

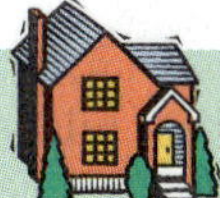

FAMILY HOME CARE
*Use of a Metered-Dose Inhaler**

STEPS FOR CHECKING HOW MUCH MEDICINE IS IN THE CANISTER

1. If the canister is new, it is full.
2. If the canister has been used repeatedly, it might be empty. (Check product label to see how many inhalations should be in each canister.)
3. To check how much medicine is left in the canister, put the canister (not the mouthpiece) in a cup of water.
   a. If the canister sinks to the bottom, it is full.
   b. If the canister floats sideways on the surface, it is empty.

STEPS FOR USING THE INHALER

1. Remove the cap and hold inhaler upright.
2. Shake the inhaler.
3. Tilt the head back slightly and breathe out.
4. With the inhaler in an upright position, insert the mouthpiece:
   a. About 3 to 4 cm from the mouth *or*
   b. Into an aerochamber *or*
   c. Into the mouth, forming an airtight seal between the lips and the mouthpiece
5. At the end of a normal expiration, depress the top of the inhaler canister firmly to release the medication (into either the aerochamber or the mouth), and breathe in slowly (about 3-5 seconds). Relax the pressure on the top of the canister.
6. Hold the breath for at least 5 to 10 seconds to allow the aerosol medication to reach deeply into the lungs.
7. Remove the inhaler and breathe out slowly through the nose.
8. Wait 1 minute between puffs (if additional one is needed).
9. To determine if child is using an inhaler properly, have child use the device in front of a mirror. If vapor does not appear on the mirror, the inhaler is being used correctly.

Adapted from National Heart, Lung, and Blood Institute, National Institutes of Health: *Guidelines for the diagnosis and management of asthma,* Pub No 91-3042, Bethesda, MD, Aug 1991.

*NOTE: Inhaled dry powder capsules require a different inhalation technique. To use a dry powder inhaler, it is important to close the mouth tightly around the mouthpiece of the inhaler and inhale rapidly.

CRITICAL THINKING EXERCISE
Asthma

Traditional thinking about the pathophysiology of asthma has changed in recent years. Which one of the following treatments reflects this better understanding of the mechanisms involved in an asthmatic episode?

1. Peak expiratory flow meter (PEFM)
2. Metered-dose inhaler (MDI)
3. Allergy hyposensitization
4. Chest physiotherapy

The correct answer is 2. Inflammation of the bronchial airways is now recognized as a critical component in the pathophysiology of asthma. MDIs are used to deliver corticosteroids to decrease the inflammation. The PEFM is an assessment device; the other two choices have been used traditionally.

➤ **NURSING TIP** To reduce the probability of an asthmatic episode triggered by cold air, teach the child to breathe through the nose (not the mouth). Also, a reservoir of warm air can be created by having the child wear a mask or swaddling the nose and mouth in a scarf when in cold air.

Asthma camps have become popular in recent years as a means of encouraging physical activity in a more homogeneous, controlled, and less competitive environment. Although not all persons subscribe to this practice, some support the benefits, which are primarily that the denominator of asthma is removed as a factor. Everyone at the camp has asthma; therefore, no child is different from the others.

Promote Normal Activities. Self-care is the hallmark of effective asthma management, and self-management programs are important in helping the child and family to learn as much as possible about the factors that precipitate an asthma episode and the most effective means of bringing the disease under control.

It is important to realize that self-care does not mean self-treatment. Therefore, especially for younger children, comanagement concepts are important: the child, family, and health care provider are all working together as a team. Among the essential features of effective programs, as indicated by the National Heart, Lung, and Blood Institute (1991), are the four Rs:

1. Reaching agreement on goals and what is expected of an asthma treatment program
2. Rehearsal of important techniques such as how to use the MDI, nebulizer, and PEFM, as well as what to do should an asthmatic episode occur
3. Repetition both within formal self-management courses and at office visits
4. Reinforcement in the form of praise of mastery of skills and compliance with therapy

Most self-management programs convey four principles to the child and family regarding the disease and its management. First, asthma is a very common disease, and to have asthma is annoying but not disgraceful. Even though emotions have been implicated in asthma, psychologic aspects are primarily a response to it rather than a cause. Emotions and stress can be major triggers, but the disease, not the individual, is responsible for the symptoms. Absolution of the individual from the responsibility for the etiology makes the concept of a therapeutic plan more sensible and acceptable.

Second, persons with asthma are able to live full and active lives. Learning about others who have accomplished their goals (e.g., Theodore Roosevelt) and meeting children of the same age who are dealing effectively with their disease, including engaging in age-related activities (e.g., sports), provide positive examples of what is possible.

Third, it is much easier to prevent than to treat an asthmatic episode. The importance of compliance with a therapeutic program and learning the activities or factors that trigger an episode are emphasized. Sustained-release medications and appropriate drug administration before exercise or with a respiratory infection have made it possible for children with asthma to avoid an exacerbation.

Fourth, individuals do not become addicted to asthma medication, but they do prefer to breathe more freely whenever possible. Emphasis is on management rather than cure. The cost/benefit of each medication is explained, and attempts are made to assess the "wheezogenic" potential by tapering the medication periodically to demonstrate that the management process is a dynamic one in which the child and the parent are active participants (Lewiston, 1986).

Several approaches are used to facilitate self-management. Self-contained programs and brochures for patient education are available throughout the national office of the **Asthma and Allergy Foundation of America (AAFA).*** The **American Lung Association†** also has brochures about asthma available through the local offices. One that is highly recommended is *Superstuff,* a workbook for elementary and junior high school children that includes self-management techniques using a variety of educational aids. An excellent and highly recommended publication is *Children with Asthma: A Manual for Parents.*‡ Self-management instruction in group settings (e.g., camps for children with asthma) is a very popular means for education and training. Three such packaged programs are available that have proved successful. Many are funded by organizations with support from local health professionals, institutions, and interested families. One, *ACT (Asthma Care Training),* a five-session program with the theme "You're in the Driver's Seat," using driving and traffic analogies, is available without charge through the AAFA. *WOW (Winning Over Wheezing)* is a cassette-workbook developed for group instruction.§

Asthma education and awareness are an important aspect of asthma management. Although the principles of self-management are very general and the programs designed for general use, each child and family have their own special needs that require individualized care and attention.

Child and Family Support. The nurse working with children with asthma can provide them with support in a number of ways. Many asthmatic children voice frustration about the ways their episodes interfere with their goal achievements and social lives. They need education about their disease, and they need to realize that it is not as bad as they might think. Children, their families, and their peers need to know what to do to prevent an exacerbation and what to do during one. These children need reassurance from the health team and reinforcement of their coping mechanisms. Last of all, they need "grit"—the courage to help them live and cope with their condition one day at a time.

Both short- and long-term adaptation of affected children to the disease depends to a great extent on the family's acceptance of the disorder. The task of living day-to-day with affected children involves the family continually. There are

---

*1125 15th St., Washington, DC, 20005; (202) 466-7643.

†National office: 1740 Broadway, New York; NY 10019; (212) 315-8700.

‡Available from Pedipress, Inc., 125 Red Gate Lane, Amherst, MA 01002; (413) 549-7798.

§*Winning Over Wheezing,* Rhone-Poulenc-Rorer, Inc., 500 Virginia Dr., Fort Washington, PA 19304.

NURSING CARE PLAN
The Child with Asthma

NURSING DIAGNOSIS: High risk for suffocation related to interaction between individual and allergen(s)

PATIENT GOAL 1: Will experience no asthmatic episode

• **NURSING INTERVENTIONS/*RATIONALES***

Teach child and family how to avoid conditions or circumstances that precipitate asthmatic episode

Assist parents in eliminating allergens or other stimuli that trigger exacerbation (see p. 1416 for complete listing), such as:

- Meal planning to eliminate allergenic foods
- Removal of pets
- Modification of environment: "allergy-proof" home, especially no smoking in home

Avoid extremes of environmental temperature

- When child is exposed to cold air, recommend breathing through nose (not mouth) and wearing a mask or scarf, or cupping hand over nose and mouth *to create a reservoir of warm air to breathe*

Assist parents in obtaining and/or installing device to control environment (dehumidifier, air conditioner, electronic air filter)

Teach child and family to recognize early signs and symptoms *so that an impending episode can be controlled before it becomes distressful*

Teach child and family correct use of bronchodilators and antiinflammatory drugs (e.g., corticosteroids, cromolyn sodium), adverse effects, and dangers of overuse or underuse of drugs

Teach child to understand how equipment works

Teach child correct use of inhalers, nebulizers, and peak expiratory flow meters

Teach child and family prophylactic treatment when appropriate (e.g., prevent exercise-induced bronchospasm by using medication before exercise)

Explain to child and family possible benefits of hyposensitization therapy when allergen(s) can be defined and cannot be avoided (e.g., pollen, mold) or controlled satisfactorily by drugs

*Administer hyposensitization therapy if prescribed

• **EXPECTED OUTCOMES**

Family makes every effort to remove or avoid possible allergens or precipitating events

Child/family are able to detect signs of an impending episode early and implement appropriate actions

Child/family are able to administer medications and use inhalers and other equipment

PATIENT GOAL 2: Will experience optimum health

• **NURSING INTERVENTIONS/*RATIONALES***

Encourage sound health practices *to support body's natural defenses:*

- Balanced, nutritious diet
- Adequate rest
- Good hygiene
- Appropriate exercise
- Follow-up care

Prevent respiratory infection *since it can trigger an attack or aggravate the asthmatic state*

- Avoid exposure to infection
- Take meticulous care of equipment *to avoid bacterial and/or fungal growth*
- Use good handwashing

• **EXPECTED OUTCOMES**

Child and parents practice sound health practices

Child exhibits no evidence of infection

NURSING DIAGNOSIS: Ineffective airway clearance related to allergenic response and inflammation in the bronchial tree

PATIENT GOAL 1: Will exhibit evidence of improved ventilatory capacity

• **NURSING INTERVENTIONS/*RATIONALES***

Instruct and/or supervise breathing exercises and controlled breathing *to promote proper diaphragmatic breathing, side expansion, and improved chest wall mobility*

Use play techniques for breathing exercises with young children (e.g., blow a pinwheel or blow cotton balls on table *to extend expiratory time and increase expiratory pressure)*

Teach correct use of prescribed medications

Teach correct use of peak expiratory flow meter, nebulizer, and metered-dose inhaler if indicated

Teach family to perform percussion and postural drainage and to encourage coughing if indicated

Encourage physical exercise

- Recommend activities requiring short bursts of energy (e.g., baseball, sprints, skiing), *since they may be better tolerated than those requiring endurance exercise* (e.g., soccer, distance running)
- Recommend swimming *because child breathes air saturated with moisture, and exhaling underwater prolongs expiration and increases end-expiratory pressure*
- Restrict physical activity only when child's condition makes it necessary

Encourage good posture *for maximum lung expansion*

Assist child and family in selecting activities appropriate to child's capabilities and preferences

• **EXPECTED OUTCOMES**

Child breathes easily and without dyspnea

Child exhibits improved ventilatory capacity (specify)

Child engages in activities according to abilities and interest (specify)

*Dependent nursing action.

Continued.

NURSING DIAGNOSIS: Activity intolerance related to imbalance between oxygen supply and demand

PATIENT GOAL 1: Will receive optimum rest

• **NURSING INTERVENTIONS/*RATIONALES***

Encourage activities appropriate to child's condition and capabilities (specify)
Provide ample opportunities for sleep, rest, and quiet activities

• **EXPECTED OUTCOMES**

Child engages in appropriate activities (specify)
Child appears rested

NURSING DIAGNOSIS: Altered family processes related to having a child with a chronic illness

PATIENT/FAMILY GOAL 1: Will exhibit positive adaptation to the condition

• **NURSING INTERVENTIONS/*RATIONALES***

Foster positive family relationships
Reinforce positive coping mechanisms of child and family
Use every opportunity to increase parents' and child's understanding of the disease and its therapies, *since adequate knowledge is related to family's timely use of preventive and emergency intervention*
Reinforce the need for responding to early signs of impending asthma episode using prescribed medications as needed *to decrease potential for a severe exacerbation*
Intervene appropriately if there is evidence of maladaptation
Be alert to signs of parental rejection or overprotection
Be alert to signs that child is depressed and make appropriate referral for psychologic support, *since depressed children, especially adolescents, may not comply with therapies as a means of passive suicide*
Teach child and family how to give respiratory treatments *to eliminate any confusion* regarding medication or inhalers/nebulizers
Encourage family to contact school personnel (e.g., nurse, teachers, coaches, principal) to develop a consistent plan of care for school setting
Refer family to appropriate support groups and community agencies

• **EXPECTED OUTCOMES**

Family copes with symptoms and effects of the disease and provides a normal environment for the child
See Nursing Care Plan: The Child with Chronic Illness or Disability, Chapter 22

Status Asthmaticus (Special Needs)

NURSING DIAGNOSIS: High risk for suffocation related to bronchospasm, mucus secretions, edema

PATIENT GOAL 1: Will experience cessation of bronchospasm

• **NURSING INTERVENTIONS/*RATIONALES***

Establish intravenous infusion *for administration of medication and hydration*
*Administer aerolized bronchodilators and either oral or IV corticosteroids as prescribed *to relieve bronchospasm*
Carefully monitor IV aminophylline infusion or oral theophylline *for maximum efficacy and minimum side effects*
- Closely monitor vital signs before, during, and after administration
- Monitor serum aminophylline or theophylline levels
- Observe for side effects of theophylline: nausea, headache, irritability, insomnia, hyperactivity
- Observe for signs of theophylline toxicity: nausea, tachycardia, irritability (when levels exceed 20 mg/ml), and seizures and dysrhythmias (at levels greater than 30 mg/ml)
- Interview parents to determine medications given before admission to avoid possible overdose

Have emergency equipment and medications readily available *to prevent delay in treatment*

• **EXPECTED OUTCOMES**

Child breathes more easily
Child does not suffocate
Child demonstrates no evidence of theophylline toxicity

PATIENT GOAL 2: Will exhibit normal respiratory function

• **NURSING INTERVENTIONS/*RATIONALES***

Administer humidified oxygen by tent, face mask, or cannula *to maintain satisfactory oxygenation*
Closely monitor oxygen saturations and blood gases via pulse oximetry *to detect early or impending hypoxia*
Closely monitor percentage of oxygen delivered, *since high levels may depress respirations*
Position *for optimum lung expansion*
- High-Fowler position
- Provide overbed table with pillows on which to lean if more comfortable for child

Implement measures to reduce fear/anxiety *to decrease respiratory efforts and oxygen consumption*
Encourage relaxation techniques (see p. 1423) *to decrease anxiety and promote lung expansion*
Administer sedatives and tranquilizing agents, if prescribed, with extreme caution and when agitation is not caused by anoxia, *since these drugs can depress respirations and mask signs of anoxia*
Organize activities to allow for rest, sleep, and minimum expenditure of energy

*Dependent nursing action.

• **EXPECTED OUTCOMES**
Child's respirations are unlabored and within normal limits (see inside back cover)
Child rests and sleeps comfortably
Child does not experience decreased oxygen saturations

PATIENT GOAL 3: Will successfully expel bronchial secretions

• **NURSING INTERVENTIONS/*RATIONALES***
Provide adequate hydration, oral or intravenous, *to liquefy secretions for easier removal*
Maintain NPO, if necessary, *to prevent aspiration of fluids and food*
Provide humidified atmosphere *to prevent drying of mucous membranes*
Encourage child to cough effectively
  Provide tissues
  Explain need to remove secretions
Suction, using correct technique, only when necessary
Do not use chest physiotherapy (CPT) during an acute episode since will only agitate an already anxious, dyspneic child and aggravate the episode; CPT may be started as soon as signs of airway obstruction significantly subside
Position, if necessary, *to prevent aspiration of secretions*
  Semiprone
  Side-lying

• **EXPECTED OUTCOMES**
Secretions are adequately and easily expelled
Child coughs effectively
Child does not aspirate secretions, food, or fluids

NURSING DIAGNOSIS: High risk for fluid volume deficit related to difficulty taking fluids, insensible fluid losses from hyperventilation and diaphoresis

PATIENT GOAL: Will exhibit adequate hydration

• **NURSING INTERVENTIONS/*RATIONALES***
Maintain intravenous infusion at appropriate rate, *since fluid therapy will enhance liquifaction of secretions* (IV usually run two-thirds to three-quarters maintenance [unless dehydration present] in order to minimize the risk of pulmonary edema because of high inspiratory pressures)
Encourage oral fluids
  Offer fluids when acute respiratory distress subsides *to decrease risk of aspiration*
  Avoid cold liquids *since they can trigger reflex bronchospasm*
  Give fluids (and food) in small, frequent feedings *to avoid abdominal distention that might interfere with diaphragmatic excursion*
  Use play techniques appropriate to child's age *to encourage fluid intake*
Measure intake and output
Correct dehydration slowly, *since overhydration can increase the accumulation of interstitial pulmonary fluid, leading to increased airway obstruction*

• **EXPECTED OUTCOME**
Child exhibits adequate hydration

NURSING DIAGNOSIS: High risk for injury (respiratory acidosis, electrolyte imbalance) related to hypoventilation, dehydration

PATIENT GOAL 1: Will not experience acidosis

• **NURSING INTERVENTIONS/*RATIONALES***
Closely monitor blood pH, *since pH less than 7.25 impairs systemic, pulmonary, and coronary blood flow, and normal pH enhances effect of bronchodilators*
*Administer sodium bicarbonate as ordered *to prevent or correct acidosis*
Maintain intravenous infusion *for administration of emergency medications and to prevent dehydration*
Prevent vomiting and subsequent dehydration; initially, child will experience alkalosis, but if vomiting becomes severe or uncontrolled, can lead to acidosis
Implement measures to improve ventilation; hypoventilation may cause an *accumulation of carbon dioxide, which will decrease pH*

• **EXPECTED OUTCOME**
Child exhibits no evidence of respiratory acidosis

PATIENT GOAL 2: Will exhibit normal serum electrolytes

• **NURSING INTERVENTIONS/*RATIONALES***
Closely monitor serum electrolytes since dehydration, as well as medications, can alter normal serum electrolytes
Maintain intravenous infusion at appropriate rate
Prevent dehydration and vomiting *since they cause electrolyte imbalances*

• **EXPECTED OUTCOME**
Child exhibits normal serum electrolytes

NURSING DIAGNOSIS: Altered family processes related to emergency hospitalization of child

PATIENT/FAMILY GOAL: Will experience reduction of anxiety

• **NURSING INTERVENTIONS/*RATIONALES***
Keep parents informed of child's condition
Encourage expression of feelings, especially severity of condition and prognosis
Allow parents to be with child as much as possible by encouraging family-centered care concepts
Point out any evidence of improvement *to encourage positive coping behaviors*
If/when possible, schedule treatments and care to child's routines
Reduce sensory stimuli by maintaining quiet, relaxed environment

• **EXPECTED OUTCOMES**
Family verbalizes concerns and spends time with child
Family exhibits no signs of distress

See also:
  Nursing Care Plan: The Family of the Ill or Hospitalized Child, Chapter 26
  Nursing Care Plan: The Child in the Hospital, Chapter 26

periodic crises and the ever-present threat of a crisis, requiring parental vigilance, sleepless nights, frequent emergency trips to the hospital, and often overwhelming medical expenses. Throughout these stresses, parents are expected and encouraged to promote as normal a life as possible for their children without neglecting the needs of siblings.

❖ EVALUATION

The effectiveness of nursing interventions is determined by continual reassessment and evaluation of care based on the following observational guidelines and expected outcomes:

1. Interview family about removal or avoidance of known allergens.
2. Observe child for evidence of respiratory symptoms.
3. Assess child's general health.
4. Observe child and interview family about any infections or other complications.
5. Interview child about daily activities.
6. Determine the degree to which the family and child understand the child's condition and the extent to which the therapies are carried out.

Expected outcomes:
See Nursing Care Plan, pp. 1431-1433.

CYSTIC FIBROSIS (CF)

CF, a condition characterized by exocrine (or mucus-producing) gland dysfunction that produces multisystem involvement, is the most common lethal genetic illness among white children, adolescents, and young adults. In the early 1950s the life expectancy was extremely short; by 1966 the median age was 7.5 years; and by 1990 it had increased to 27.6 years (Fitzsimmons, 1993; McMullen, 1992; Patterson and others, 1993). It is estimated that 3.3% of white persons in the United States are symptom-free carriers. Although it is estimated that more than 95% of documented cases affect white persons (1 in 3500 births), the disease is also present in Hispanics (1 in 11,500 births), African-Americans (1 in 14,000 births), and Asians (1 in 25,000 births) (Fitzsimmons, 1993). Canada (32 years) and the United States (27+ years) have the highest median age, whereas Latin America has the lowest (6 years); the major difference is access to health care facilities and antibiotics (Canada Cystic Fibrosis Foundation, 1990). It is estimated that individuals born with CF in the 1990s can be expected to survive into their 40s; the outlook looks even better when one considers the advances in new therapies, impact of protein and gene therapy, continued aggressive chest physiotherapy, aerosolized antibiotic therapy, and nutritional education (Collins, 1992; Elborn, Shale, and Britton, 1991).

Etiology

CF is inherited as an autosomal recessive trait; the affected child inherits the defective gene from both parents, with an overall incidence of 1:4 (see Chapter 5). In 1989 researchers discovered that the mutated gene responsible for CF was located on the long arm of chromosome 7, along with its protein product, ***cystic fibrosis transmembrane regulator (CFTR)*** (Kerem and others, 1989). Since that time, almost 300 alterations that diverge from the original sequence of the gene have been reported; at least 230 of these are associated with disease. Among them, the ΔF508 is the most common alteration, found in about 70% of all known CF chromosomes (Tizzano and Buchwald, 1993). Variance in the mutation does result in some phenotypic variation, but concordance for ΔF508 leads to both pancreatic deficiency and pulmonary disease (Fulginiti and Lewy, 1993).

Pathophysiology

With the discovery of the CFTR gene, research is continuing to determine its multisystem effects on the body. CF is characterized by several apparently unrelated clinical features: increased viscosity of mucous gland secretions, a striking elevation of sweat electrolytes, an increase in several organic and enzymatic constituents of saliva, and abnormalities in autonomic nervous system function. Although both sodium and chloride are affected, the defect appears to be primarily a result of abnormal chloride movement (Quinton, 1989); the CFTR appears to function as a chloride channel (Bear and others, 1992). Further evidence indicates that ΔF508 is closely related to pancreatic insufficiency. The role of CFTR, however, is not definitive. While it has been found lining the membrane of epithelial cells in the reabsorptive part of sweat glands, its effects on bronchopulmonary disease are not clear (Koch and Hoiby, 1993).

Some evidence indicates overactivity of the autonomic nervous system, which stimulates the cholinergic glands. This theory is plausible, since this system innervates all exocrine glands, but findings are not conclusive. Patients with CF demonstrate decreased pancreatic secretion of bicarbonate and chloride (Kopelman and others, 1988), and the primary transport abnormality in CF involves an electrogenic chloride channel or its regulation (Orlando and others, 1989). An increase in sodium and chloride in both saliva and sweat is characteristic of children with CF and forms the basis for one of the most reliable diagnostic procedures, the sweat chloride test.

The sweat electrolyte abnormality is present from birth throughout life and is unrelated to the severity of the disease or the extent to which other organs are involved. The sodium and chloride content of sweat in children with CF is two to five times greater than that of the controls in 98% to 99% of affected children.

The primary factor, and the one responsible for the multiple clinical manifestations of the disease, is mechanical obstruction caused by the increased viscosity of mucous gland secretions (Fig. 32-10). Instead of forming a thin, freely flowing secretion, the mucous glands produce a thick, inspissated mucoprotein that accumulates and dilates them. Small passages in organs such as the pancreas and bronchioles become obstructed as secretions precipitate or coagulate to form concretions in glands and ducts.

Respiratory Tract. Because of the increased viscosity of bronchial mucus, there is greater resistance to ciliary action (probably secondary to infection and ciliary destruction), a slower flow rate of mucus, and incomplete expectoration, which also contributes to the mucous obstruction. This re-

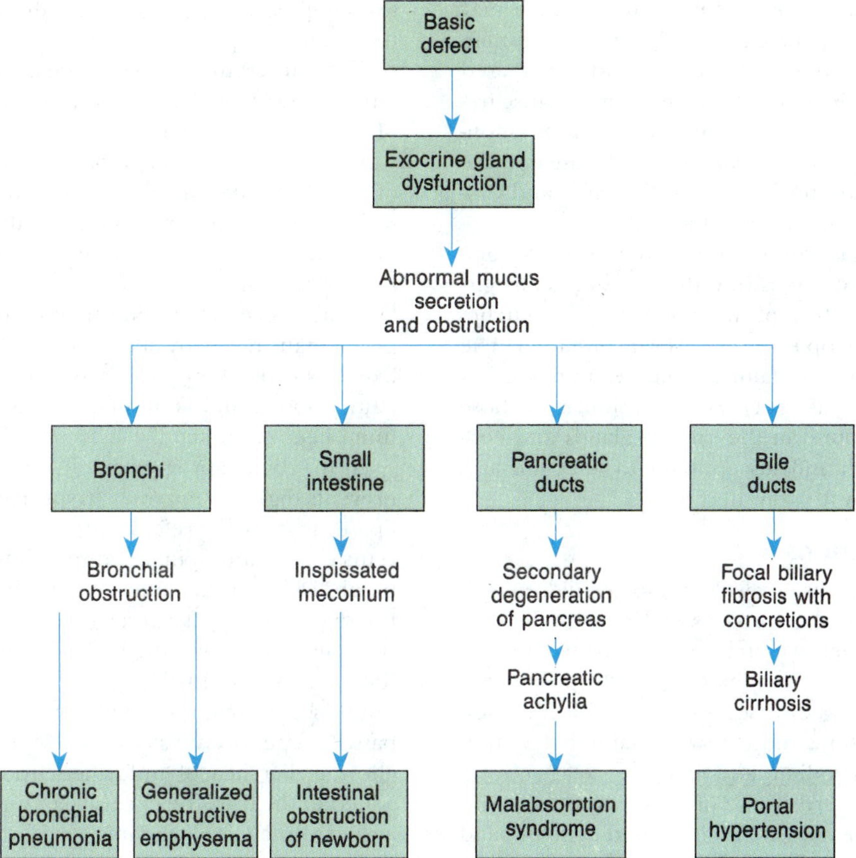

FIG. 32-10 Various effects of exocrine gland dysfunction in cystic fibrosis.

tained mucus serves as an excellent medium for any bacterial growth. Reduced O_2–CO_2 exchange causes variable degrees of hypoxia, hypercapnia, and acidosis. In severe, progressive lung involvement, compression of pulmonary blood vessels and progressive lung dysfunction frequently lead to pulmonary hypertension, cor pulmonale, respiratory failure, and death.

Pulmonary complications are present in almost all children with CF, but the onset and extent of involvement are variable. Symptoms are produced by stagnation of mucus in the airways with eventual bacterial colonization leading to destruction of lung tissue. The abnormally viscous and tenacious secretions are difficult to expectorate and gradually obstruct the bronchi and bronchioles, causing scattered areas of atelectasis and emphysema. The stagnant mucus offers a favorable environment for bacterial growth. Infection usually begins in the early years with *Staphylococcus aureus, Haemophilus influenzae,* and *Streptococcus pneumoniae; Pseudomonas aeruginosa* predominates in later years. *P. aeruginosa* infection is not specific for CF but occurs much more frequently in CF than in other diseases characterized by chronic airways obstruction (Koch and Hoiby, 1993). The bacteria develop resistance to multiple drugs and are almost impossible to eradicate. Multiple antibodies developed by the patient to the bacteria are ineffective in controlling infection, and the host is able to tolerate large concentrations of bacteria without overt evidence of worsening.

Gradual progression of pulmonary disease follows chronic infection, bronchial epithelium is destroyed, and infection spreads to peribronchial tissues, resulting in weakening of bronchial walls and peribronchial fibrosis. The pattern is chronic, progressive fibrosis with decreased O_2–CO_2 exchange and a concurrent alteration in pulmonary vasculature. Chronic hypoxemia causes contraction and hypertrophy of medial muscle fibers in pulmonary arteries and arterioles, leading to pulmonary hypertension and eventual cor pulmonale. Pneumothorax may occur when peripheral bullae rupture; hemoptysis can occur when the bronchial wall is eroded through to an artery.

Gastrointestinal Tract. The extent of gastrointestinal involvement varies. In the pancreas of many patients, the thick secretions block the ducts, leading to cystic dilations of the acini (small lobes of the gland), which then undergo degeneration and progressive diffuse fibrosis. This event prevents essential pancreatic enzymes from reaching the duodenum, which causes marked impairment in the digestion and absorption of nutrients, particularly fats, proteins, and, to a lesser degree, carbohydrates. Disturbed absorption is reflected in excessive stool fat ***(steatorrhea)*** and protein ***(azotorrhea)***.

The endocrine function of the pancreas often remains unchanged, since the islets of Langerhans are normal but may decrease in number as pancreatic fibrosis progresses. However, the incidence of diabetes mellitus is greater in these children than in the general population, which may be caused by changes in pancreatic architecture and diminished blood supply over time. Consequently, with increased survival, insulin-dependent diabetes is becoming a more frequent finding in the CF population. There is no relationship between the progression of pulmonary disease and the development of diabetes mellitus in CF (Wheeler and Colten, 1988). Diabetic ketoacidosis is rare.

In the liver, focal biliary obstruction and fibrosis are common and become more extensive with time, eventually giving rise to a distinctive type of multilobular biliary cirrhosis. A few children develop extensive liver involvement. The gallbladder is small and contains a firm, gelatinous material that also fills the cystic duct. Findings similar to those in the pancreas are found in the salivary glands and contribute to a dry mouth and susceptibility to infection as a result of interference with salivation.

Clinical Manifestations

The clinical manifestations vary widely among children with CF and change as the disease progresses. However, the hallmark processes that elicit symptoms are (1) pancreatic enzyme deficiency due to duct blockage; (2) progressive chronic obstructive lung disease associated with infection and intestinal destruction; and (3) sweat gland dysfunction resulting in increased sodium and chloride sweat concentrations. The usual pattern is one of failure to thrive, with an increased weight loss despite an increased appetite, and gradual deterioration of the respiratory system. The diagnosis is not readily apparent in many cases, especially when there is no familial evidence of disease. Some children display symptoms at birth; others may not develop symptoms for weeks, months, or years. Some show only mild forms of the disease with limited impairment of digestion and respiratory problems, whereas others have severe malabsorption and life-threatening pulmonary complications. Although most affected children display both pulmonary and GI symptoms, a few have only enzyme deficiency without pulmonary disease; a few have only pulmonary disease without pancreatic insufficiency.

Respiratory Tract. Initial pulmonary manifestations are often wheezing respirations and a dry, nonproductive cough. Eventually diffuse bronchial and bronchiolar obstruction leads to irregular aeration with progressive pulmonary disturbance and secondary infection. Dyspnea increases, the cough often becomes paroxysmal, and the mucoid impactions within the small air passages cause a generalized obstructive emphysema and patchy areas of atelectasis.

Progressive pulmonary involvement with hyperaeration of functioning alveoli produces the overinflated, barrel-shaped chest in which the anteroposterior diameter approaches the lateral diameter. When ventilation and subsequent diffusion and gas exchange are significantly impaired, cyanosis and clubbing of fingers and toes may occur. The child has repeated episodes of bronchitis and bronchopneumonia and is subject to chronic sinusitis and nasal polyps. The incidence of ear, nose, and throat surgeries is higher in this group of children when compared with the general population.

Gastrointestinal Tract. The earliest postnatal manifestation of CF is ***meconium ileus,*** which occurs in 7% to 10% of newborns with the disease (McMullen, 1992). Thick, puttylike, tenacious, mucilaginous meconium blocks the lumen of the small intestine usually at or near the ileocecal valve, which gives rise to signs of intestinal obstruction, including abdominal distention, vomiting, failure to pass stools, and rapid development of dehydration with associated electrolyte imbalance. Thick intestinal secretions continue to be problematic for many people with CF throughout life. Gumlike masses in the cecum can obstruct the bowel, causing pain, nausea, and vomiting. This is referred to as "meconium ileus equivalent."

As the disease progresses, obstruction of pancreatic ducts prevents digestive enzymes (trypsin, chymotrypsin, amylase, lipase) from being released into the duodenum, which prevents conversion of ingested food into compounds that can be absorbed by the intestinal mucosa. Consequently, the nondigested food is excreted (chiefly unabsorbed fats and proteins), increasing the bulk of feces to two or three times the normal amount. The bulky nature of the stools may go unnoticed at first, but usually by 6 months of age the child passes large, loose stools with normal frequency or a chronic diarrhea of unformed stools. As solid foods are added to the diet, the excessively large stools become frothy and extremely foul smelling.

Because so little is absorbed from the intestine, affected children have difficulty maintaining weight despite a healthy appetite and diet. Unable to compensate for the fecal losses, children lose weight and exhibit marked wasting of tissues and failure to grow. The abdomen is distended, the extremities are thin, and the sallow skin droops from wasted buttocks. The impaired ability to absorb fats results in a deficiency of the fat-soluble vitamins A, D, E, and K, which causes easy bruising. Anemia is a common complication. These GI symptoms are similar to those seen in children with celiac disease, and failure to thrive is a frequent initial diagnosis in young children with CF.

The most common GI complication associated with CF in poorly treated children is ***prolapse of the rectum,*** which occurs most often in infancy and early childhood and is related to large, bulky stools and lack of supportive fat pads around the rectum. Children of all ages are subject to peptic ulcers, pancreatic insufficiency, and intestinal obstruction from inspissated or impacted feces. Abdominal distention is common, abdominal cramps may be excessive, and foul-smelling flatus is a common complaint. Malabsorption and malnutrition are other commonly associated problems.

Reproductive System. Reproductive systems of both males and females with CF are affected. Females with CF have normal fallopian tubes and ovaries. Fertility can be inhibited by highly viscous cervical secretions, which act as a plug, blocking sperm entry, but many more women are becoming pregnant and delivering viable infants (Fitzsimmons, 1993). With few exceptions males are sterile, which may be caused by blockage of the vas deferens with abnormal secretions or by failure of normal development of the wolffian duct structures (vas deferens, epididymis, and seminal vesicles), resulting in decreased or absent sperm production.

Integumentary System. The consistent finding of abnormally high sodium and chloride concentrations in the sweat is a unique characteristic of CF. Parents frequently observe that their infants taste "salty" when they kiss them. The chloride channel defect in sweat glands prevents reabsorption of sodium and chloride, which leaves the affected person at risk for abnormal salt loss, dehydration, and hypochloremic and hyponatremic alkalosis during hyperthermic conditions. This is especially important to the infant because of limited fluid stores and the potential for inadequate sodium intake with most commercially prepared infant formulas.

The disease is sometimes expressed in other ways, for example, hypoelectrolytemia caused by massive losses through sweat, especially in high environmental temperatures or febrile episodes. Infants with CF who fail to thrive frequently demonstrate hypoalbuminemia resulting from diminished absorption of protein, which in severe cases causes generalized edema.

Diagnostic Evaluation

An initial evaluation is conducted with overall appraisal in the areas of general activity, physical findings, nutritional status, and findings on chest radiographs. The diagnosis of CF is suspected in the child who fails to thrive and/or has frequent upper respiratory infections and is established on the basis of duplicate sweat chloride tests. Diagnosis of CF requires a positive sweat test result in the presence of either clinical symptoms consistent with CF or a family history of CF.

The ***quantitative sweat chloride test (pilocarpine iontophoresis)*** involves stimulating the production of sweat, collecting the sweat, and measuring the sweat electrolytes. The quantitative analysis requires a minimum of 50 mg of sweat; 75 to 100 mg is preferable. Two separate samples are collected to ensure the reliability of the test for any individual. Because newborns do not have active sweat glands, it is often difficult to obtain an adequate sample for analysis. Therefore, if results are questionable, the test is repeated at a later date. The test should be performed only by personnel skilled in the procedure.

Normally, sweat chloride content is less than 40 mEq/L, with a mean of 18 mEq/L. A chloride concentration greater than 60 mEq/L is diagnostic of CF; levels of 40 to 60 mEq/L are highly suggestive of the disease. Children with questionable results are followed carefully for any evidence of pulmonary system symptoms so that treatment can be implemented immediately.

Chest radiography reveals characteristic patchy atelectasis and obstructive emphysema. Pulmonary function tests are sensitive indexes of lung function, providing evidence of abnormal small airway function in CF. Other diagnostic tools that may aid in diagnosis include stool fat and/or enzyme analysis. Stool analysis requires a 72-hour sample with accurate recording of food intake during that time. Radiographs, including barium enema, are used for diagnosis of meconium ileus.

Screening

The impact of genetic discoveries on understanding the etiology and treatment of CF is only beginning to unfold at the same time that approaches to detection are changing to reflect new technologies. The standard methods of diagnosis rely either on detection of abnormal chloride secretion in sweat or, in newborns, on elevated immunoreactive trypsinogen (Fulginiti and Lewy, 1993). Carrier screening is available and reliable for siblings and family members of a child with CF (Beaudet and others, 1989). Development of deoxyribonucleic acid (DNA) probes, however, has enabled the identification of the disease in families who have an individual affected with CF. The tests detect the major gene defect (ΔF508) for CF, which is located in about 70% of white patients and 30% of black patients. Heterozygote screening and prenatal testing will continue to be studied and researched during the 1990s. In the meantime, there is an increased demand to implement screening processes for detection of CF in the general population (McMullen, 1992; Mennie, Gilfillan and Compton, 1992). While technologically possible, a number of mass population screening issues remain unstudied and unanswered: public and professional education, human resource needs, and the effects of information on legislative and health insurance systems. Before mass screening can be a feasible endeavor, pilot screening programs are needed to determine the impact of these issues, and a larger percentage of the gene mutations must be identified (Wilford and Fost, 1990).

Therapeutic Management

The improved survival rate of patients with CF during the past two decades is attributable largely to antibiotic therapy and improved nutritional management. Goals of therapy, therefore, include the following: (1) to prevent or minimize pulmonary complications; (2) to ensure adequate nutrition for growth; and (3) to assist the child and family in adapting to a chronic disorder. In attempting to attain these, there is a multisystem approach to treatment modalities. Current and future technologies are examining the methods of lessening the effects of the CFTR and are preparing for direct attacks on the defect rather than relying on management of the end results (i.e., traditional treatment for pulmonary and GI complications). Some of these new modalities include (Fulginiti and Lewy, 1993; McMullen, 1992; Tizzano and Buchwald, 1993):

1. Blockade of the "sodium pump" by the aerosolized drug amiloride hydrochloride (changes transmembrane chloride transport in respiratory epithelia and inhibits sodium and thus water reabsorption)
2. Use of various substances intended to alter the characteristically abnormal mucus in the airways (e.g., DNase I)
3. Aerosolized agents such as α_1-antitrypsin to inhibit neutrophil elastase (a powerful enzyme that causes inflammation)
4. Drugs that promote chloride secretion
5. Replacement gene therapy

Management of Pulmonary Problems. Management of pulmonary problems is directed toward prevention and treatment of pulmonary infection by improving aeration, removing mucopurulent secretions, and administering antimicrobial agents. Most children will develop respiratory symptoms by 3 years of age. Young children normally have small airways and are predisposed to frequent viral infections. The large amounts and viscosity of respiratory secretions in children with CF contribute to the likelihood of infection. Once infection becomes established in relatively defenseless lungs, it is difficult to eradicate.

Prevention of infection involves a daily routine of ***chest physiotherapy (CPT)*** to maintain pulmonary hygiene (see Chapter 31). In theory, postural drainage and percussion of the lungs loosen and move secretions toward the glottis to facilitate expectoration. Numerous studies have been conducted to evaluate the efficacy of the procedure. Several researchers have pursued the concept that exercise, deep breathing, and directed coughing are just as effective in preventing pulmonary deterioration. However, patients have been found to regress when conventional CPT is discontinued (Reisman and others, 1988). Therefore, although it is time-consuming for the child and family, CPT remains the cornerstone of pulmonary therapy.

CPT is usually performed twice daily (on rising and in the evening) and more frequently if needed, especially during pulmonary infection. Bronchodilator medication delivered in an aerosol helps open bronchi for easier expectoration and is administered before CPT when the patient exhibits evidence of reactive airway disease and/or wheezing. Mist therapy is of little proven value.

Another form of aerosolized medication is ***recombinant human deoxyribonuclease (DNase)***, a drug developed from the original DNA medications that were found to decrease the viscosity of mucus. The dosing schedule may involve inhalation three times a day, 5 days a week, for 2 weeks. It is well tolerated and has no major adverse effects (minor reactions are typical of the patient's underlying disease before treatment). In addition, improvements in spirometry, PFTs, and dyspnea scores have been seen, as well as a reduction in the viscosity of sputum (Aitken and others, 1992).

Forced expiration, or "huffing," with the glottis partially closed helps move secretions from small airways so that subsequent coughing can move secretions forcefully from large airways. Several studies indicate this maneuver enhances the pulmonary function of patients with CF (Bain, Bishop, and Olinsky, 1988).

Physical exercise is an important adjunct to daily CPT. Exercise not only stimulates mucus secretion, it also provides a sense of well-being and increased self-esteem. In some instances, exercise can be substituted for CPT. Any aerobic exercise that is enjoyed by the patient should be encouraged. The ultimate aim of exercise is to establish a good habitual breathing pattern.

Pulmonary infections are treated as soon as they are recognized. Some practitioners prefer to prescribe oral antibiotics prophylactically at the time of diagnosis; others begin therapy when pulmonary symptoms arise. Sputum culture and sensitivity guide the choice of antibiotic. The trend is toward aggressive therapy even for milder disease.

Colonization with *P. aeruginosa* signals progressive involvement. Although the bacteria are impossible to eradicate, they can be successfully controlled for many years. Inhaled antibiotics are administered as a prophylactic measure in some centers, but once the organism has become established, antibiotic therapy is most effective given intravenously. Patients with CF metabolize antibiotics more rapidly than normal; therefore drug dosage is often higher than would be expected. The antibiotic selected (usually aminoglycosides, cephalosporins, or semisynthetic penicillins) depends on sensitivity of the organism. Duration of therapy depends on the patient's response, measured with clinical indicators including cough, fatigue, and exercise intolerance in addition to tests such as pulmonary function tests PFTs, chest radiography, and O_2 and CO_2 measurements.

Intravenous antibiotics are often administered at home as an alternative to hospitalization as long as the family agrees and regular monitoring for toxicity can be accomplished. Home care is widely accepted as both medically safe and less costly. Most children have central venous access devices for home administration of intravenous medications. When pulmonary function does not improve with outpatient management, hospitalization may be recommended for continued antibiotic therapy and vigorous CPT.

Oxygen administration is usually recommended for children with acute episodes, but since many of these children have chronic CO_2 retention, the unsupervised use of O_2 can be harmful (see Oxygen Toxicity, Chapter 31).

Pneumothorax is most often caused by rupture of subpleural blebs through the visceral pleura and usually occurs in patients with more advanced disease; it is estimated that 5% to 8% of all patients will eventually have a pneumothorax (Fiel, 1993). Common signs and symptoms are usually nonspecific and include tachypnea, tachycardia, dyspnea, pallor, and cyanosis. Some pneumothoraces resolve spontaneously, whereas others require more aggressive therapy, such as chest tube insertion. For those patients unresponsive to such therapy, other options include partial pleurectomy, limited surgical pleurodesis, chemical pleurodesis, and oversewing or stapling of the subpleural blebs (Fiel, 1993). For most patients the benefits of surgery far outweigh the risks.

Blood streaking of the sputum is common in children over 10 years of age, is usually associated with exacerbation of bacterial infection of the airway, and most often requires no specific treatment. Hemoptysis greater than 300 ml in 24 hours for the older child (less for a younger child) indicates a potentially life-threatening event and needs to be treated immediately. Sometimes bleeding can be controlled with bed rest, cough suppressants, and antibiotics. If hemoptysis persists, the site of bleeding should be localized via bronchoscopy and cauterized or embolized (Fiel, 1993). Adjunct therapy includes administration of vitamin K and intravenous antibiotics.

Nasal polyps occur in about 10% of children with CF, and this finding should increase the suspicion of CF. Treatment includes extended use of antibiotics, nasal cromolyn sodium, corticosteroids, intermittent use of nasal decongestants, and warm mist and saline nasal rinses for comfort. If these measures are ineffective, surgical interventions are considered (McMullen, 1992).

Lung transplantation is a final therapeutic option for a few end-stage patients. Heart-lung and double-lung procedures have been successfully performed in children with advanced pulmonary vascular disease and hypoxia. The obstacles surrounding this technique are availability of donated organs and complications from surgery (Fiel, 1993).

Management of Gastrointestinal Problems. The principal treatment for pancreatic insufficiency is replacement pancreatic enzymes, which are administered with meals and snacks to ensure that digestive enzymes are mixed with food in the duodenum. Enteric-coated products prevent the neutralization of enzymes by gastric acids, thus allowing activation to occur in the alkaline environment of the small bowel. The amount of enzymes depends on the severity of the insufficiency, the response of the child to enzyme replacement, and the philosophy of the practitioner. Usually 1 to 5 capsules are administered with a meal, and a smaller amount is taken with snacks. Capsules can be swallowed whole or taken apart and the contents sprinkled on a small amount of food to be taken at the beginning of the meal. The amount of enzyme is adjusted to achieve normal growth and a decrease in the number of stools to two or three per day.

Children with CF require a well-balanced, high-protein, high-calorie diet (high calorie because of the impaired intestinal absorption). In fact, they often require up to 150% of the recommended daily allowances to meet their needs for growth. Breast-feeding with enzyme supplementation should be continued whenever possible for parents who prefer this method and, when necessary, supplemented with a higher-calorie-per-ounce formula. For formula-fed infants, commercial cow's milk formulas are usually adequate, although frequently a hydrolysate formula with medium-chain triglycerides (e.g., Pregestimil or Alimentum) may be recommended. Enzymes are mixed into cereal or fruit, such as applesauce. Since the uptake of fat-soluble vitamins is decreased, water-miscible forms of these vitamins (A, D, E, K) are given, along with multivitamins and the enzymes. While fat restriction is not necessary (Luder and others, 1989), one concern is that other nutrients might not be provided from a diet with increased fats. When high-fat foods are eaten, the child is encouraged to add extra enzymes. Pancreatic enzymes should be taken within 30 minutes of eating, and the beads should not be chewed or crushed: by destroying the enteric coating, inactivation of the enzymes and excoriation of oral mucosa can occur.

Children with CF should thrive with adequate replacement therapy and calorie intake. Failure to thrive despite adequate nutritional support usually indicates deterioration of pulmonary status. Occasionally, patients will be placed on supplemental tube feedings or parenteral alimentation in an effort to build up nutritional reserves if there has been a history of inability to maintain weight.

Meconium ileus and meconium ileus equivalent, or total or partial intestinal obstruction, can occur at any age. Constipation is often the result of a combination of malabsorption (either from inadequate pancreatic enzyme dosage or a failure to take the enzymes), decreased intestinal motility, and abnormally viscous intestinal secretions. These problems usually do not require surgical interventions and may be treated with Go-LYTELY or Colyte (osmotic solutions given orally or by nasogastric tubes), other laxatives, stool softeners, or rectal administration of meglumine diatrizoate (Gastrografin) or acetylcysteine (Mucomyst). Once the obstruction has been relieved, a low-fat diet and long-term use of some combination of stool softener, mild stimulant, bulk laxative, and added bulk to the diet may be recommended (McMullen, 1992).

Rectal prolapse occurs in about 25% of children, usually in the first 3 years of life (McMullen, 1992). The first episode of rectal prolapse is frightening to both parents and child. Its reduction usually requires immediate guidance and intervention, which is managed by simply guiding the rectum back into place with a gloved, lubricated finger. Further management usually involves attempting to decrease the bulk of daily stools through enzyme replacement.

Salt depletion through sweating can be a problem during hot weather or physical exertion. Most children are able to adjust salt to their needs, and older children often exhibit a preference for salty foods. Salt supplementation is often needed during hot weather or febrile periods and should include use of fluids such as Gatorade or Exceed, which provide an adequate supply of electrolytes.

Some experimentation is being conducted to evaluate the use of recombinant human growth hormone, much the same as in children with growth hormone deficiency (see Chapter 38). The objective of growth stimulation is to improve physical strength and endurance, thereby promoting activity (e.g., exercise) and, ultimately, respiratory function.

Prognosis. Despite more than 40 years of progress and a recent surge in new treatment modalities, CF remains a progressive and incurable disease. The pulmonary involvement ultimately determines the patient's outcome, since pancreatic enzyme deficiency is less of a problem if adequate nutrition is ensured. With advances in technology, parents and adolescents are now being challenged to set future goals that may include college, careers, social relationships, and marriage. Concurrently, they are faced with increasing morbidity and higher rates of CF complications as they grow older.

Nursing Considerations

Assessment of the child with CF involves both pulmonary and GI observations. Pulmonary assessment is the same as that described for asthma (see p. 1427), with special attention to lung sounds, observation of cough, and evidence or degree of finger clubbing. GI assessment primarily involves observing the frequency and nature of the stools and abdominal distention. The observer is also alert to evidence of failure to thrive (e.g., weight loss, wasting, pallor, fatigue). Family members are interviewed to determine the child's eating and eliminating habits, to observe salty perspiration, and to confirm a history of frequent respiratory infections or bowel obstruction in infancy.

On initial contact, frequently in the hospital setting, nurses are involved in performing or assisting with diagnostic tests, primarily sweat for laboratory analysis of chloride content and, less often, stool specimens for trypsin and fat.

The child, usually an infant, needs comfort during the procedures; young children need distraction while they are confined during iontophoresis. Even short periods of inactivity seem long to an active child. Children beyond very early childhood need an explanation of the strange, and sometimes painful, procedures and the equipment used for tests and treatments.

At first the respiratory equipment is frightening, especially in infants and very young children. The child needs support and guidance in using the equipment. Accepting uncharacteristic behavior and explaining this normal stress response to parents are important nursing functions.

Parents are anxious and puzzled. Few of them have any understanding of the disease process and the long-term implications it has for their family. They need careful explanations of the disease, how it might affect their family, and what they can do to provide the best possible care for their child.

The shock associated with the diagnosis is overwhelming to parents. They must face the impact of the chronic, life-threatening nature of the disease and the prospect of intensive treatment, for which they must assume a major part of the responsibility and for which they are ill prepared. They often fear that they will be unable to provide the care the child needs. One of the most difficult aspects of the diagnosis is the implications inherent in its etiology, that is, the recognition that each parent contributed the gene responsible for the defect in their child.

Hospital Care. When the child is hospitalized for confirmation of the diagnosis or for pulmonary complications, aerosol therapy is instituted or continued. Respiratory therapy is usually initiated and supervised by a trained respiratory therapist or physiotherapist. In institutions with large support staffs, they may provide all treatments. Otherwise, it becomes the responsibility of the nurse to perform the prescribed aerosol therapy and CPT and to teach supervised breathing exercises. CPT should not be performed before or immediately after meals. Planning the activity so that it does not coincide with meals is difficult in the hospital situation. However, it is very important and is often overlooked by nursing personnel.

Oxygen is cautiously administered to children in respiratory distress, and the child requires frequent assessment. The hazard of oxygen narcosis is a constant threat in children with long-standing disease who receive oxygen (see Chapter 31). The child requires close observation to assist with cough and expectoration.

The diet is implemented for the newly diagnosed child or continued for the child who is hospitalized for pulmonary disease. Children in the early stages of the disease maintain a good appetite, and some will eat excessively. With infection and increased lung involvement, however, the appetite diminishes. Eventually it becomes a challenge to tempt failing appetites (see Feeding the Sick Child, Chapter 27). Some younger children may object to the extra fluids that are encouraged to prevent dehydration. Food is considered therapy for these patients. The caloric intake should be increased significantly. Pancreatic enzymes are supplied for each meal or snack, and adequate salt is provided, especially for febrile children.

Frequent skin care is carried out to prevent irritation and skin breakdown over bony prominences. Particular attention is necessary after use of the bedpan or when the diaper is changed. Careful cleansing helps to reduce irritation and odor from offensive stools, and the use of moisture barriers will protect the skin. (See also Diaper Dermatitis, Chapter 13, and Maintaining Healthy Skin, Chapter 27.)

The child will need support for the many treatments and tests that are a necessary part of the hospital therapy. Intravenous fluids and blood tests are almost always a part of the treatment, and the child soon associates hospitalization with these stress-provoking procedures. Because these children are usually quite thin with little muscle mass, careful selection of injection sites is required.

Support to both child and family is a vital part of nursing care. The progressive nature of the disease makes each illness requiring hospitalization a potentially life-threatening event. Skilled nursing care and sympathetic attention to the emotional needs of the child and family help them cope with the stresses associated with repeated respiratory infections and hospitalization.

When discussing the nature of the illness and the genetic etiology, families should be informed of services in the community that provide genetic counseling. The inheritance of CF is straightforward and offers little confusion if explained in the context of flipping two coins. It is important that the family fully understands the 1:4 likelihood of an affected child with each pregnancy (see Chapter 5).

Home Care. After the diagnosis is confirmed and a treatment program determined, preparation for home care is implemented. The plan of care should be flexible enough so that family activities are disrupted as infrequently as possible. Parents will need help in finding inhalation equipment available for home use that best meets their needs. They will need opportunities to learn about the practice the use of the equipment, as well as some of the problems they may encounter.

They need to learn about the preferred diet of nutritious meals with tolerated fat and ample protein and carbohydrate and the administration of pancreatic enzymes. Children usually adjust well to taking pancreatic enzymes. For infants and young children, the enzymes can be mixed with pureed fruit, such as applesauce, and fed with a spoon. Capsules are suitable for older children. It is important to stress to parents that the enzymes, in the amount regulated to the child's needs, should be administered about 30 minutes before all meals and snacks. They are cautioned about not restricting salt, especially during hot weather, and ensuring an adequate fluid intake, since dehydration aggravates the thick mucus secretions. Oral hygiene is important because of interference with salivation and the increased susceptibility to oral infections.

One of the most important aspects of educating parents for home care is teaching chest physiotherapy and breathing exercises. The success of a therapy program depends on conscientious performance of these treatments regularly as prescribed. The number of times these therapies are performed each day is determined on an individual basis, and often parents readily learn to adjust the number and intensity of the treatments to the child's needs. Although it is usually the physiotherapist who instructs the parents, nurses frequently follow up the care in the home and assist the family with innovative approaches to therapy. For example, using games and normal childhood activities to achieve the desired end reduces the likelihood that treatment will meet with resistance from the child. When additional respiratory exercises are introduced to established routines, the family will need to be reeducated in new techniques, such as "huffing."

Postural drainage can be achieved with simple activities that are fun, such as hanging by the knees from a bar or low-hanging trapeze that can be easily built in the backyard (or indoors), turning somersaults, or playing "wheelbarrow" with the child suspended head down and propelling with the hands while the adult holds on to the feet. Most children respond to a challenge, such as, "How long can you stand on your head?" Small children can "stand on their heads" with their heads on the cushion of a large chair with or without an adult holding on to their feet. Parents soon learn to respond to cues from their children and incorporate spontaneous activities into the treatment regimen.

For pulmonary infection, home intravenous antibiotics are typically prescribed. Home intravenous care is preferred for willing and competent families, since it reduces tension and usually brings a sense of belonging to the family members. With the use of the venous access devices, such as peripherally inserted central catheters (or PICC lines), the parents and child are taught the technique of direct administration into the intravenous line.* (See also Venous Access Devices, Chapter 28.) Unfortunately, around-the-clock administration may be difficult for families because it may require waking at least once during the night to give the drug.

The nurse can assist the family in contacting resources that provide help to families with affected children. The various special child health services, many local clinics, private agencies, service clubs, and other community groups often offer equipment and medications either free or at reduced rates. The **Cystic Fibrosis Foundation**† has chapters throughout the United States to provide education and services to families and professionals.

Family Support. One of the most important and difficult aspects of providing care for the family of a child with CF is coping with the emotional needs of the child and family. The diagnosis, treatment, and prognosis are fraught with many problems, frustrations, and feelings. The diagnosis with all its implications evokes feelings of guilt and self-recrimination in parents. These feelings may be particularly marked if the newly diagnosed child is the second affected child in the family, and the parents had been counseled about the 1:4 risk of such an event occurring.

The long-range problems are those encountered in the care of a child with a chronic illness (see Chapter 22). Both the child and the family must make many adjustments, the success of which depends on their ability to cope and also on the quality and quantity of support they receive from outside sources. Combined efforts of a variety of health professionals offer the most comprehensive services to families. It is often the responsibility of the nurse to organize and coordinate these services, to assess the home situation, and to collect the data needed to evaluate the effectiveness of the services in meeting the family's needs.

For the family, the illness means modification of numerous family activities. Meals require planning in order not to place too many restrictions on the affected child or deprive the other members of the family. Limits on mobility restrict family recreational activities, especially when the child's therapy includes respiratory equipment that is not transportable. CPT must be continued wherever the child may be. In addition, members of the family hesitate to take the child too far from familiar and trusted medical care. The illness even determines the family's place of residence and employment, since the child's condition dictates that the family live near medical care facilities that offer the specialized care the child needs.

The persistent need for treatment several times daily also places a strain on the family. Someone must perform the procedures, such as percussion and vibration, even on older children who are able to assume responsibility for their own exercises and respiratory therapy. Children often balk at the treatments, and the parents are placed in the position of insisting on compliance. Sometimes the stress and anxiety related to this continual routine generate feelings of resentment, which are frequently focused on one aspect of the regimen, such as the diet or equipment. When possible, occasional trusted respite care should be made available to the parent or parents to allow them the opportunity to leave the situation for short periods without undue anxiety about the child's welfare.

The affected child also may become resentful about the disease, its relentless routine of therapy, and the necessary curtailment it places on activities and relationships. The child's activities are interrupted or built around treatment, medications, and diet that impose hardships (such as carrying medication to school and other places where the child may eat away from home), and the growth retardation associated with most chronic illnesses may be trying. Any of these aspects of the disease may be the cause of ridicule from other children. However, the child should be encouraged to attend school and join age-appropriate groups, such as scouting, to foster a life that is as normal and productive as possible.

Families afflicted with CF have psychologic hurdles similar to those of all families coping with a child with a chronic illness (see Chapter 22), and a constant source of anxiety for both parents and child is the ever-present fear of death. However, despite the prognosis of a shortened life span, numerous hospitalizations, and unpleasant complications, children with CF have been found to be well adjusted (Co-

*Home care instructions for giving medications to children are available in *Wong and Whaley's Clinical Manual of Pediatric Nursing* (Mosby).

†6931 Arlington Rd., Bethesda, MD 20814-3205; (800) FIGHT CF or (301) 951-4422. In Canada: **Canadian Cystic Fibrosis Foundation,** 586 Eglinton Ave., E., Suite 204, Toronto, Ontario M4P 1P2. Two excellent publications available from the Cystic Fibrosis Foundation are *What Everyone Should Know About Cystic Fibrosis* and *Cystic Fibrosis: A Summary of Symptoms, Diagnosis, and Treatment.* For information about specialized medications, especially Pulmozyne, and equipment for CF and other pulmonary diseases, contact **Cystic Fibrosis Pharmacy, Inc.,** H.H.C.S. Pharmacy Services, 633 E. Colonial Drive, Orlando, FL 32803; (800) 741-4427.

wen and others, 1986). Patients and their siblings show generally healthy self-esteem, and family functioning is normal.

As the disease progresses, however, family stress should be expected, and the patient may become angry and noncompliant. It is important for the nurse to recognize the changing needs of the family. Families should be made aware of sources for counseling as stressful setbacks occur. Patients need to be guided into activities that enable them to express anger, sorrow, and fear without guilt.

As life expectancy continues to rise for children with CF, issues related to marriage, childbearing, and career choice become more pressing. Men must be informed at some point that they will be unable to produce offspring. It is important that the distinction be made between sterility and impotence. Normal sexual relationships can be expected. Female patients may be able to bear children but must be made aware of the possible deleterious effects on the respiratory system created by the burden of pregnancy. They need to know that their children will be carriers of the CF gene.

Life as an independent adult, the goal that most families have for their children, should be encouraged for children with CF. From the time that children can take partial responsibility for their own care (e.g., CPT and taking enzymes), independence and accountability should be fostered. Although the prognosis for these children has improved, many do not survive through the second decade of life. Anticipatory grieving and other aspects related to care of a child with a terminal illness are part of nursing care (see Chapter 23). (See also Nursing Care Plan: The Child with Cystic Fibrosis.*

*In *Wong and Whaley's Clinical Manual of Pediatric Nursing* (Mosby).

KEY POINTS

- Acute infection of the respiratory tract is the most common cause of illness in infancy and childhood.
- The incidence and severity of respiratory tract infections are influenced by the infectious agent involved, the child's age, and the child's natural defenses.
- Symptoms of respiratory tract infections include fever, febrile convulsions, anorexia, vomiting, diarrhea, abdominal pain, nasal blockage and discharge, wheezing, cough, respiratory sounds, and presence or absence of sore throat.
- Common respiratory tract infections of childhood include acute nasopharyngitis, acute pharyngitis, influenza, tonsillitis, and otitis media.
- Severe bleeding from the tonsil site can occur within 6 hours after surgery or 5 to 10 days after tonsillectomy.
- Factors that predispose children to otitis media are the shape and position of eustachian tubes, undeveloped cartilage lining, abundant pharyngeal lymphoid tissue, immature humoral defense mechanisms, and the recumbent position (in infants).
- The most common upper respiratory infections are categorized as croup syndromes, which include acute laryngotracheobronchitis, acute spasmodic laryngitis, and acute epiglottitis.
- Epiglottitis is a medical emergency and is characterized by high fever, toxic appearance, and difficulty swallowing.
- The primary nursing function in the care of children with croup is observation for signs of respiratory embarrassment and relief of laryngeal obstruction.
- Lower airway conditions constitute the majority of respiratory problems in children and are usually viral in nature (excluding foreign body aspiration).
- Common infections of the lower airway include bacterial tracheitis, asthmatic bronchitis, bronchitis, bronchiolitis, and pneumonia.
- Pneumonias are generally classified either by site (lobar, bronchial, or interstitial) or by etiologic agent (viruses, bacteria, mycoplasmas, or associated with foreign bodies).
- Management of uncomplicated bronchiolitis and viral pneumonia is symptomatic in otherwise healthy infants.
- In tuberculosis, resistance to the bacillus can be altered by heredity, sex, age, stress states, poor nutrition, intercurrent infection, and noncompliance with therapy.
- Signs of choking include inability to speak, color change, and decreased level of activity.
- Inhaled objects are rarely coughed up spontaneously; therefore they must be removed by direct laryngoscopy or bronchoscopy.
- Inducing a child to vomit is contraindicated in the event of hydrocarbon ingestion because of the danger of hydrocarbon aspiration.
- Asthma is now thought to occur mostly because of hypersensitivity to environmental substances that trigger a complex allergic response; therefore an important component of therapy is elimination of environmental allergens, or triggers.
- Asthma can be triggered by a variety of agents and is characterized by bronchospasm, edema of the bronchial mucosa, and increased bronchial mucus secretion, which can result in the classic manifestations of cough, dyspnea, and wheeze.
- The mainstays of treating asthma include use of bronchodilators, antiinflammatory agents, oxygen, and rest.
- Cystic fibrosis is the most frequently occurring inherited disease of white children and is transmitted by the autosomal recessive gene, CFTR, located on chromosome 7.
- Diagnosis of cystic fibrosis is based on family history, absence of pancreatic enzymes, chronic pulmonary involvement, and an abnormally high sweat chloride concentration, with the pilocarpine (or sweat test) being the most commonly used diagnostic test.

REFERENCES

Aitken M and others: Recombinant human DNase inhalation in normal and cystic fibrosis subjects: a phase 1 study, *JAMA* 267(14):1947-1951, 1992.

Alho OP and others: Control of the temporal aspect when considering risk factors for acute otitis media, *Arch Otolaryngol Head Neck Surg* 119:444-449, 1993.

American Academy of Allergy and Immunology, Executive Committee: The waiting period after allergen skin testing and immunotherapy, *Pediatrics* 85:526-527, 1990.

American Academy of Pediatrics, Committee on Infectious Diseases: *Haemophilus influenzae* type b conjugate vaccine: immunization of children 2 to 15 months of age, *AAP News* 6(11):19 and 23, 1990.

American Academy of Pediatrics, Committee on Infectious Diseases: Use of ribavirin in the treatment of RSV, *Pediatrics* 92(3):501-504, 1993.

American Academy of Pediatrics, Committee on Infectious Diseases: *1994 Red Book: Report of the Committee on Infectious Diseases,* ed 23, Elk Grove Village, IL, 1994a, The Academy.

American Academy of Pediatrics, Committee on Infectious Diseases: Screening for tuberculosis in infants and children, *Pediatrics* 93(1):131-134, 1994b.

American Academy of Pediatrics, Committee on Substance Abuse: Tobacco-free environment: an imperative for the health of children and adolescents, *Pediatrics* 93(5):866-868, 1994c.

American Academy of Pediatrics, Provisional Committee on Quality Improvement: Practice parameter: The office management of acute exacerbations of asthma in children, *Pediatrics* 93(1):119-126, 1994d.

American Academy of Pediatrics, Section on Allergy and Immunology and Section on Diseases of the Chest: Exercise and the asthmatic child, *Pediatrics* 84:392-393, 1989.

American Thoracic Society: Diagnostic standards and classification of tuberculosis, *Am Rev Respir Dis* 142:725-735, 1990.

American Thoracic Society: Control of tuberculosis in the United States, *Am Rev Respir Dis* 146(6):1623-1633, 1992.

Bain J, Bishop J, Olinsky A: Evaluation of directed coughing in cystic fibrosis, *Br J Dis Chest* 82:138-148, 1988.

Bear C and others: Purification and functional reconstruction of the cystic fibrosis transmembrane conductance regulator (CFTR), *Cell* 68:809-818, 1992.

Beaudet A and others: Linkage disequilibrum, cystic fibrosis, and genetic counseling, *Am J Hum Genet* 44:319-326, 1989.

Beck-Sague C and others: Hospital outbreak of multidrug-resistant *Mycobacterium tuberculosis* infections: factors in transmission to staff and HIV-infected patients, *JAMA* 268:1280-1286, 1992.

Bender B, Milgron H: Theophylline-induced behavior change in children, *JAMA* 267(19):2621-2624, 1992.

Bender B and others: Psychological change associated with theophylline treatment of asthmatic children: a 6 month study. *Pediatr Pulmonol* 11:233-242, 1991.

Bloomberg G, Strunk R: Crisis in asthma care, *Pediatr Clin North Am* 39(6):1225-1241, 1992.

Blumer JL: *A practical guide to pediatric intensive care,* ed 3, St Louis, 1991, Mosby.

Burrows B, Lebowitz M: The β-agonist dilemma, *N Engl J Med* 326(8):560-561, 1992.

Callaghan B, Teo N, Clancy L: Effects of the addition of nedocromil sodium to maintenance bronchodilator therapy in the management of chronic asthma, *Chest* 101:787-792, 1992.

Canada Cystic Fibrosis Foundation: *Report of the Canadian Patient Data Registry 1989,* Toronto, 1990, The Foundation.

Canadian Pediatric Society Committee on Infectious Disease and Immunization: Position statement: Ribavirin: is there a risk to hospital personnel? 144(3):285-286, 1991.

Carter E and others: Efficacy of intravenously administered theophylline in children hospitalized with severe asthma, *J Pediatr* 122(3):470-76, 1993.

Centers for Disease Control: Outbreak of multidrug-resistant tuberculosis at a hospital, *MMWR* 42:427-434, 1993.

Cloutier M: Quick: what's the first-line therapy for acute asthma? *Contemp Pediatr* 10(3):76-94, 1993.

Colditz GA and others: Efficacy of BCG vaccine in the prevention of tuberculosis, *JAMA* 271(9):698-702+, 1994.

Collins F: Cystic fibrosis: molecular biology and therapeutic implications, *Science* 256: 774-779, 1992.

Cowen L and others: Psychologic adjustment of the family with a member who has cystic fibrosis, *Pediatrics* 77:745-752, 1986.

Cressman WR, Myer CM: Diagnosis and management of croup and epiglottitis, *Pediatr Clin North Am* 41(2):265-276, 1994.

Cromer BA, Goydos J, Hackell J: Unrecognized pertussis infection in adolescents, *Am J Dis Child* 147:575-577, 1993.

Djukanovic R and others: Effect of an inhaled corticosteroid on airway inflammation and symptoms in asthma, *Am Rev Respir Dis* 145:669-674, 1992.

Duff A, Platts-Mills T: Allergens and asthma, *Pediatr Clin North Am* 39(6):1277-1291, 1992.

Duncan B and others: Exclusive breast-feeding for at least 4 months protects against otitis media, *Pediatrics* 91(5):867-872, 1993.

Elborn J, Shale D, Britton J: Cystic fibrosis: current survival and population estimates to the year 2000, *Thorax* 46:881-885, 1991.

Ellis EF: Allergic disorders. In Behrman RE, Vaughan VC III: *Nelson textbook of pediatrics,* ed 13, Philadelphia, 1987, WB Saunders.

Engel NS: Multiple drug therapy for pediatric tuberculosis, *MCN* 14:169, 1989.

Englund J and others: High-dose, short-duration ribavirin aerosol therapy in children with suspected RSV infection, *J Pediatr* 117:313-320, 1990.

Ernst P and others: Risk of fatal and near-fatal asthma in relation to inhaled corticosteroid use, *JAMA* 268(24):3462-3464, 1992.

Esclamado RM, Richardson MA: Laryngotracheal foreign bodies in children, *Am J Dis Child* 141:259-262, 1987.

Etzel R and others: Passive smoking and middle ear effusion among children in day care, *Pediatrics* 90(2):228-232, 1992.

Feigin RD: Group A streptococcal infections. In Oski FA and others, editors: *Principles and practice of pediatrics,* Philadelphia, 1990, JB Lippincott.

Fiel S: Clinical management of pulmonary disease in cystic fibrosis, *Lancet* 341(8852):1070-1074, 1993.

Finn A: Allergy and inflammation, *Emerg Med* 24(12):47-58, 1992.

Fitzpatrick MF and others: Effect of therapeutic theophylline levels on the sleep quality and daytime cognitive performance of normal subjects, *Am Rev Respir Dis* 145:1355-1358, 1992.

Fitzsimmons S: The changing epidemiology of cystic fibrosis, *J Pediatr* 122(1):1-9, 1993.

Fowler M, Davenport M, Garg R: School functioning of children with asthma, *Pediatrics* 90(6):939-944, 1992.

Friday GA, Fireman P: Morbidity and mortality of asthma, *Pediatr Clin North Am* 35:1149-1162, 1988.

Fulginiti V, Lewy J: Pediatrics: update on cystic fibrosis, *JAMA* 270(2):246-248, 1993.

Gaffney K, Dennis J, Carneiro C: Think TB: new focus for family assessment, *Pediatr Nurs* 20(1):37-38, 1994.

Gluck E, Onorato D, Castriotta R: Helium-oxygen mixture in intubated patients with status asthmaticus and respiratory acidosis, *Chest* 98(3):693-698, 1990.

Gorelick MH, Baker MD: Epiglottitis in children, 1979 through 1992: effects of *Haemophilus influenzae* type b immunization, *Arch Pediatr Adolesc Med* 148(1):47-50, 1994.

Gray BM: Immune globulin administration as an approach to prevention of acute otitis media, *J Pediatr* 123:739-741, 1993.

Green S, Rothrock S: Single-dose intramuscular ceftriaxone for acute otitis media in children, *Pediatrics* 91(1):23-29, 1993.

Groothius JR and others: Prophylactic administration of respiratory syncytial virus immune globulin to high-risk infants and young children, *N Engl J Med* 329:1524-1530, 1993.

Grossman J and others: Fluticasone propionate aqueous nasal spray is safe and effective for children with seasonal allergic rhinitis, *Pediatrics* 92(4):594-599, 1993.

Groth H, Hurewitz A: The diagnosis: bronchial asthma, *Emerg Med* 24(12):31-40, 1992.

Guerra IC, Kemp JS, Shearer WT: Bronchiolitis. In Oski FA and others, editors: *Principles and practice of pediatrics,* Philadelphia, 1990, JB Lippincott.

Guglielmo BJ, Jacobs RA, Locksley RM: The exposure of health care workers to ribavirin aerosol, *JAMA* 261:1880-1881, 1989 (letter).

Gutstadt LB and others: Determinants of school performance in children with chronic asthma, *Am J Dis Child* 143:471-475, 1989.

Hall C: Respiratory syncytial virus: what we know now, *Contemp Pediatr* 10(1):92-110, 1993.

Handling the severe asthma attack: inhalers versus nebulizers, *Emerg Med* 25(13):49-51, 1993.

Hands B: Blow-drying for otitis externa, Can Med Assoc J 137:1077, 1987.

Hazinski MF: *Nursing care of the critically ill child,* ed 2, St Louis, 1992, Mosby.

Hill M, Szefler S, Larsen G: Asthma pathogenesis and the implication for therapy in children, *Pediatr Clin North Am* 39(6):1205-1223, 1992.

Holberg CJ, Wright AL, Martinez FD: Child day care, smoking by caregivers, and lower respiratory tract illness in the first 3 years of life, *Pediatrics* 91:885-892, 1993.

Honicky RE, Osborne JS III, Akpom CA: Symptoms of respiratory illness in young children and the use of wood-burning stoves for indoor heating, *Pediatrics* 75:587-593, 1985.

Hurwitz ES and others: Risk of respiratory illness associated with day-care attendance: a nationwide study, *Pediatrics* 87:62-69, 1991.

Isaacson G, Rosenfeld RM: Care of the child with tympanostomy tubes: a visual guide for the pediatrician, *Pediatrics* 93(6):924-929, 1994.

Jackson M: Tuberculosis in infants, children and adolescents: new dilemmas with an old disease, *Pediatr Nurs* 19(5):437-442, 1993.

Jury D: More on RSV and ribavirin, *Pediatr Nurs* 19(1):89-92, 1993.

Kairys S, Olmstead E, O'Connor G: Steroid treatment of laryngotracheitis: a meta-analysis of the evidence from randomized trials, *Pediatrics* 83:683-693, 1989.

Kelley P, Simon J: Racemic epinephrine use in croup and disposition, *Am J Emerg Med* 10:181-184, 1992.

Kerem B and others: Identification of the cystic fibrosis gene: genetic analysis, *Science* 245:1073-1080, 1989.

Kerem E and others: Efficacy of albuterol administered by nebulizer versus spacer device in children with acute asthma, *J Pediatr* 123(2):313-317, 1993.

Keyes WG: Theophylline toxicity caused by an over-the-counter antiasthmatic preparation, Clin Pediatr 26:630-633, 1987.

Klinnert M, Miller B, Mrazek D: Asthma fatalities: who's at risk? *Contemp Pediatr* 7(11):81-98, 1990.

Koch C, Hoiby N: Pathogenesis of cystic fibrosis, *Lancet* 341(8852):1065-1069, 1993.

Kopelman H and others: Impaired chloride secretion, as well as bicarbonate secretion, underlies the fluid secretory defect in the cystic fibrosis pancreas, *Gastroenterology* 95:349-355, 1988.

Kunkel N, Baker M: Aerosolized epinephrine use in treatment of croup, *Am J Dis Child* 146:470, 1992.

Kuzel R, Clutter D: Current perspectives on respiratory syncytial virus infection, *Postgrad Med* 93(1):129-132, 1993.

Larsen GL: Asthma in children, *N Engl J Med* 326:1540-1545, 1992.

Larter N, Kieckhefer G: Asthma. In Jackson P, Vessey J: *Primary care of the child with a chronic condition,* St Louis, 1992, Mosby.

LaVia W and others: Clinical profile of pediatric patients hospitalized with respiratory syncytial virus infection, *Clin Pediatr* 32(8):450-454, 1993.

Ledwith C, Shea L: The use of nebulized racemic epinephrine in the outpatient treatment of croup, Paper presented at the AAP section on Emergency Medicine, Washington, DC, 1993.

Lewiston NJ: Asthma self-management programs and education, *Pediatr Ann* 15:127-136, 1986.

Lindgren S and others: Does asthma or treatment with theophylline limit children's academic performance? *N Engl J Med* 327:926-930, 1992.

Lockey R and others: Fatalities from immunotherapy (IT) and skin testing (ST), *J Allergy Clin Immunol* 79:660-677, 1987.

Luder E and others: Efficacy of a nonrestricted fat diet in patients with cystic fibrosis, *Am J Dis Child* 143:458-464, 1989.

Lumry W and others: Fluticasone propionate is safe and effective for children with seasonal allergic rhinitis, *J Allergy Clin Immunol* 87:152, 1991.

Marcy SM: A summer refresher: swimmer's ear, *Contemp Pediatr* 6(5):90-91, 1989.

Marks M: Respiratory syncytial virus infections, *Clin Pediatr* 31(11):688-691, 1992.

Mauro RD and others: Differentiation of epiglottitis and laryngotracheobronchitis in the child with stridor, *Am J Dis Child* 142:679-682, 1988.

Maw R, Bawden R: Spontaneous resolution of severe chronic glue ear in children and the effect of adenoidectomy, tonsillectomy, and insertion of ventilation tubes (grommets), *Br Med J* 306:756-760, 1993.

McFadden E, Gilbert I: Asthma, *N Engl J Med* 327(27):1928-1937, 1992.

McIntosh K: Respiratory syncytial virus: successful immunoprophylaxis at last, *N Engl J Med* 329(21):1572-1573, 1993.

McMillan JA: Sore throats in teens: strep and beyond, *Contemp Pediatr* 5(3):20-30, 1988.

McMullen A: Cystic fibrosis. In Jackson PL, Vessey JA: *Primary care of the child with a chronic condition,* St Louis, 1992, Mosby.

Meltzer E and others: Long term comparison of three combinations of albuterol, theophylline, and beclomethasone in children with chronic asthma, *J Allergy Clin Immunol* 90:2-11, 1992.

Mennie M, Gilfillan A, Compton M: Prenatal screening for cystic fibrosis, *Lancet* 340(8813):214-216, 1992.

Moffet H: *Pediatric infectious disease,* ed 3, Philadelphia, 1989, JB Lippincott.

Morgan W, Martinez F: Risk factors for developing wheezing and asthma in childhood, *Pediatr Clin North Am* 39(6):1185-1203, 1992.

Mueller G, Eigen H: Pediatric pulmonary function testing in asthma, *Pediatr Clin North Am* 39(6):1243-1257, 1992.

Murphy S, Kelly H: Evolution of therapy for childhood asthma, *Am Rev Respir Dis* 146:544-546, 1992 (editorial).

Murphy S, Kelly W: Asthma, inflammation, and airway hyperresponsiveness in children, *Curr Opin Pediatr* 5:255-265, 1993.

Murray AB, Morrison BJ: Passive smoking by asthmatics: its greater effect on boys than on girls and on older than on younger children, *Pediatrics* 84:451-459, 1989.

National Heart, Lung, and Blood Institute, National Institutes of Health: *Guidelines for the diagnosis and Management of Asthma,* Pub No 91-3042, Bethesda, MD, Aug 1991.

Neddenriep D, Schumacher MJ, Lemen RJ: Asthma in childhood, *Curr Probl Pediatr* 19:331-385, 1989.

Neddenriep D, Taussig LM, Mietens C: Infections of the lower respiratory tract. In Eichenwald HF, Ströder J, editors: *Current therapy in pediatrics—2,* Philadelphia, 1989, BC Decker.

Orlando RC, others: Colonic and esophageal transepithelial potential difference in cystic fibrosis, *Gastroenterology* 96:1041-1048, 1989.

Owen M and others: Efficacy of cefixime in the treatment of acute otitis media in children, *Am J Dis Child* 147:81-86, 1993.

Patterson J and others: Family correlates of a 10-year pulmonary health trend in cystic fibrosis, *Pediatrics* 91(2):383-389, 1993.

Pearlman D: Chronic rhinitis in children, *J Allergy Clin Immunol* 81:962-966, 1988.

Pearson M and others: Nosocomial transmission of multidrug-resistant *Mycobacterium tuberculosis:* a risk to patients and health care workers, *Ann Intern Med* 117:191-196, 1992.

Peter JFM and others: Long-term effect of inhaled corticosteroids on growth rate in adolescents with asthma, *Pediatrics* 91(3):1121-1126, 1993.

Pierson WE: Exercise-induced bronchospasm in children and adolescents, *Pediatr Clin North Am* 35:1031-1040, 1988.

Putto A: Febrile exudative tonsillitis: viral or streptococcal? *Pediatrics* 80:6-11, 1987.

Quan L: Diagnosis and treatment of croup, *Am Fam Physician* 46(3):747-755, 1992.

Quinton P: Defective epithelial ion transport in cystic fibrosis, *Clin Chem* 35:726-730, 1989.

Rachelefsky GS and others: Behavior abnormalities and poor school performance due to oral theophylline use, *Pediatrics* 78:1133-1138, 1986.

Rachelefsy G and others: An update on the diagnosis and management of pediatric asthma: based on the National Heart, Lung, and Blood Institute Expert Panel report, *Nurse Practitioner* 18(2):51-52+, 1993.

Rauen KK, Holman JB: Pain control in children following tonsillectomies: a retrospective study, *J Nurs Qual Assur* 3(3):45-53, 1989.

Ray CG: Ribavirin: ambivalence about an antiviral agent, *Am J Dis Child* 142:488-489, 1988 (editorial).

Reisman J and others: Role of conventional physiotherapy in cystic fibrosis, *J Pediatr* 113:632-636, 1988.

Respiratory health effects of passive smoking: lung cancer and other disorders, Washington, DC, Dec 1992, Office of Health and Environmental Assessment, Office of Research and Development, US Environmental Protection Agency.

Rosenfeld R: New concepts for steroid use in otitis media with effusion, *Clin Pediatr* 31:615-621, 1992.

Ruddy R: Croup—has management changed? *Contemp Pediatr* 10(12):21-32, 1993.

Ruddy RM: Smoke inhalation injury, *Pediatr Clin North Am* 41(2):317-336, 1994.

Sarnaik AP, Lieh-Lai M: Adult respiratory distress syndrome in children, *Pediatr Clin North Am* 41(2):337-363, 1994.

Schichor A and others: Lidocaine as a diluent for ceftriaxone in the treatment of gonorrhea: does it reduce the pain of the infection? *Arch Pediatr Adolesc Med* 148(1):72-75, 1994.

Sedgwick J and others: Inhibition of eosinophil density change and leukotriene C4 generation by nedocromil sodium, *J Allergy Clin Immunol* 90:202-209, 1992.

Shannon M, Lovejoy F: Effect of acute versus chronic intoxication on clinical features of theophylline poisoning in children, *J Pediatr* 121:125-130, 1992.

Shiue S, Gluck E: The use of helium-oxygen mixture in support of patients with status asthmaticus and respiratory acidosis, *J Asthma* 26(3):177-180, 1989.

Shurin P and others: Bacterial polysaccharide immune globulin for prophylaxis of acute otitis media in high-risk children, *J Pediatr* 123:801-810, 1993.

Simons FER: Allergic rhinitis: recent advances, *Pediatr Clin North Am* 35:1053-1074, 1988.

Skolnick N: Treatment of croup: a critical review, *Am J Dis Child* 143:1945-1949, 1989.

Solar M, Eldadah M: Croup in older children: case report of two school-age children with croup, *Clin Pediatr* 29:581-582, 1990.

Spitzer WO and others: The use of β-agonists and the risk of death and near death from asthma, *N Engl J Med* 326(8):501-506, 1992.

Starke JR: Modern approach to the diagnosis and treatment of tuberculosis in children, *Pediatr Clin North Am* 35:441-464, 1988.

Starke J, Jacobs R: Resurgence of tuberculosis, *J Pediatr* 120(6):839-853, 1992.

Stempel D, Szefler S: Management of chronic

asthma, *Pediatr Clin North Am* 39(6):1293-1309, 1992.
Stoney P, Chakrabarti M: Experience of pulse oximetry in children with croup, *J Laryngol Otol* 105:295-298, 1991.
Strachan DP, Jarvis MJ, Feyerabend BT: Passive smoking, salivary cotinine concentrations and middle ear effusion in 7 year old children, *Br Med J* 298:1549-1552, 1989.
Sullivan T: Is asthma curable? *Pediatr Clin North Am* 39(6):1363-1381, 1992.
Super DM and others: A prospective randomized double-blind study to evaluate the effect of dexamethasone in acute laryngotracheitis, *J Pediatr* 115:323-329, 1989.
Teele DW and others: Epidemiology of otitis media during the first seven years of life in children in Greater Boston: a prospective cohort study, *J Infect Dis* 160:83-94, 1989.
Tibballs J, Shawn F, Landau L: Placebo controlled trial of prednisolone in children intubated for croup, *Lancet* 340:745-750, 1992.
Tizzano E, Buchwald M: Recent advances in cystic fibrosis research, *J Pediatr* 122(6):985-988, 1993.
Van Essen-Zandvliet E and others: Effects of 22 months of treatment with inhaled corticosteroids and/or B_2 agonists on lung function, airway responsiveness, and symptoms in children with asthma, *Am Rev Respir Dis,* 1992.
Virant F: Allergic rhinitis, *Pediatr Rev* 13(9):323-328, 1992.
Wald ER: Croup. In Oski FA and others, editors: *Principles and practice of pediatrics,* Philadelphia, 1990, JB Lippincott.
Wald ER, Dashefsky B, Green M: In re Ribavirin: a case of premature adjudication? *J Pediatr* 112:154, 1988.
Warner JO and others: Asthma: a followup statement from an international paediatric asthma consensus group, *Arch Dis Child* 67:240-248, 1992.
Weinberger M: Theophylline: when should it be used? *J Pediatr* 122(3):403-405, 1993.
Weitzman M and others: Recent trends in the prevalence and severity of childhood asthma, *JAMA* 268(19):2673-2677, 1992.
Wheeler WB, Colten HR: Cystic fibrosis: current approach to diagnosis and management, *Pediatr Rev* 9:241-248, 1988.
Wilfond B, Fost N: The cystic fibrosis gene: medical and social implications for heterozygote detection, *JAMA* 263:2777-2783, 1990.
Williams R and others: Use of antibiotics in preventing recurrent acute otitis media and in treating otitis media with effusion, *JAMA* 270(11):1344-1351, 1993.
Wolf SI and others: EMLA cream for painless skin testing: a preliminary report, *Ann Allergy* 73(1):40-42, 1994.
Wood RA, Sampson HA: A practical guide to allergy testing, *Contemp Pediatr* 4(special issue):8-20, 1987.
Wusson K, Krug S, Yamashita T: Duration of clinical response to racemic epinephrine in children with croup, *Am J Dis Child* 146:506-510, 1992.

BIBLIOGRAPHY

Respiratory Infection

Brook I, Leyva FD: Microbiology of tonsillar surfaces in infectious mononucleosis, *Arch Pediatr Adolesc Med* 148(2):171-173, 1994.
Carabott JA and others: Oral fluid intake in children following tonsillectomy, *Pediatr Nurs* 18(2):124-126, 1992.
Cefaratt J, Steinberg E: An alternative method for delivery of ribavirin to nonventilated pediatric patients, *Respir Care* 37(8):877-881, 1992.
Clark G: Childhood tuberculosis cases escalate: disease makes comeback; new strains develop, *AAP News* 10(5):1, 8-9, 11, 1994.
Cohen B, Brady M: Practices surrounding ribavirin administration, *Pediatr Nurs* 18(3):253-257, 1992.
Dahl K and others: A nursing procedure for the safe administration of ribavirin in a PICU, *Heart Lung* 21(3):287, 1992.
Dooley S and others: Nosocomial transmission of tuberculosis in a hospital unit for HIV infected patients, *JAMA* 267:2632-2635, 1992.
Everett D: For a child with pneumonia, there's no place like home, *RN* 53(3):85-88, 1990.
Filippell M, Rearick T: Respiratory syncytial virus, *Nurs Clin North Am* 28(3):651-671, 1993.
Gladu JM, Ecobichon DJ: Evaluation of exposure of health care personnel to ribavirin, *J Toxicol Environ Health* 28:1-12, 1989.
Groothuis J and others: Early ribavirin treatment of RSV infection in high risk children, *J Pediatr* 117:792-798, 1990.
Harris J and others: Respiratory syncytial virus: a pediatric nursing plan of care, *J Pediatr Nurs* 7(2):128-132, 1992.
Mauro RD, Poole SR: Is it croup? A guide to diagnosis and treatment, *Contemp Pediatr* 5(10):51-70, 1988.
Miller H: Respiratory syncytial virus and the use of ribavirin, *MCN* 17(5):238-241, 1992.
Nederhand K and others: Respiratory syncytial virus: A nursing perspective, *Pediatr Nurs* 15(4):342-345, 1989.
Ophir D, Elad Y: Effects of steam inhalation on nasal patency and nasal symptoms in patients with common cold, *Am J Otolaryngol* 3:149-153, 1987.
Piontek-Lentz T: Ribavirin: ready for RSV season, *Neonatal Network* 7(2):29-35, 1989.
Rhodes A: A reemerging public health issue, *MCN* 18:175, 1993.
Rodriquez W and others: Environmental exposure of primary care personnel to ribavirin aerosol when supervising treatment of infants with RSV, *Antimicrob Agents Chemother* 31:1143-1146, 1987.
Sanchez J and others: Treatment of NICU survivors requiring mechanical ventilation due to RSV, *Pediatr Res* 31(4, pt 2):35A, 1992.
Sheahan SL, Seabolt JP: *Chlamydia trachomatis* infections: a health problem of infants, *J Pediatr Health Care* 3:144-149, 1989.
Skoner D, Caliguiri L: The wheezing infant, *Pediatr Clin North Am* 35:1011-1030, 1988.
Smith D and others: A controlled trial of aerosolized ribavirin in infants receiving mechanical ventilation for severe RSV infection, *N Engl J Med* 325:24-29, 1991.
Smith TD, Wilkinson V, Kaplan EL: Group A *Streptococcus*-associated upper respiratory tract infections in a day-care center, *Pediatrics* 83:380-384, 1989.
Snell J: Economic and long term benefits of ribavirin therapy on RSV infection, *Lung* 168:S422-S429, 1990.
Spicer CM, Yund C: Effects of preadmission preparation on compliance with home care instructions, *J Pediatr Nurs* 4:255-262, 1989.
Szilagyi PG: What can we do about the common cold? *Contemp Pediatr* 7(2):23-49, 1990.
Todisco T, de Benedictis FM, Dottorini M: Viral and *Mycoplasma pneumoniae* pneumonias in school-age children: three-year follow-up of respiratory function, *Pediatr Pulmonol* 6:232-236, 1989.
Vallejo J, Starke J: Tuberculosis and pregnancy, *Clin Chest Med* 13(4):693-707, 1992.
Waisman Y and others: Prospective randomized double-blind study comparing L-epinephrine and racemic epinephrine aerosols in the treatment of laryngotracheitis, *Pediatrics* 89:302, 1992.

Otitis Media

Bluestone CD: Modern management of otitis media, *Pediatr Clin North Am* 36:1371-1387, 1989.
Casselbrant M and others: Efficacy of antimicrobial prophylaxis and of tympanostomy tube insertion for prevention of recurrent acute otitis media, *Pediatr Infect Dis J* 11:278-286, 1992.
Dyson AT, Holmes AE, Duffitt DV: Speech characteristics of children after otitis media, *J Pediatr Health Care* 1:261-265, 1987.
Fireman P: Otitis media and nasal disease: a role for allergy, *J Allergy Clin Immunol* 82:917-926, 1988.
Fireman P: Otitis media and its relationship to allergy, *Pediatr Clin North Am* 35:1075, 1090, 1988.
Kleinman LC and others: The medical appropriateness of tympanostomy tubes proposed for children younger than 16 years in the United States, *JAMA* 271:1250-1255, 1994.
Le C: Otitis revisited: are ear tubes the answer? *Contemp Pediatr* 9(9):24-45, 1988.
Mandel E and others: Antibiotic therapy for otitis media with effusion, *JAMA* 269(4):516-517, 1993.
Roberts JE and others: Otitis media in early childhood and cognitive, academic, and classroom performance of the school-age child, *Pediatrics* 83:477-485, 1989.
Stool S, Field J: The impact of otitis media, *Pediatr Infect Dis J* 8(suppl 1):S11-S14, 1989.

Noninfectious Irritants

Crawford WA: On the health effects of environmental tobacco smoke, *Arch Environ Health* 43:34-37, 1988.
Eliopoulos C and others: Hair concentrations of nicotine and cotinine in women and their newborn infants, *JAMA* 271:621-623, 1994.
Evans D and others: The impact of passive smoking and effects on emergency room visits of urban children with asthma, *Am Rev Respir Dis* 135:567-572, 1987.
Frankowski BL, Secker-Walker RH: Advising

parents to stop smoking, *Am J Dis Child* 143:1091-1094, 1989.

Friedman EM: Foreign bodies in the pediatric aerodigestive tract, *Pediatr Ann* 17:640-647, 1988.

Greenberg RA and others: Ecology of passive smoking by young infants, *J Pediatr* 114:774-780, 1989.

Holroyd HJ: Foreign body aspiration: potential cause of coughing and wheezing, *Pediatr Rev* 10:59-63, 1988.

Irons TG, Kenney RD: Let's get parents to stop smoking, *Contemp Pediatr* 5(3):107-118, 1988.

Kenna MA: Foreign bodies in the air and food passages, *Pediatr Rev* 10:25-31, 1988.

Laks Y, Barzilay Z: Foreign body aspiration in childhood, *Pediatr Emerg Care* 4:102-106, 1988.

Lavengood TDW: Involuntary smoking—children in crisis, *Pediatr Nurs* 14:93-95, 1988.

Lybarger PM: Inhalation injury in children: nursing care, *Issues Compr Pediatr Nurs* 10:33-50, 1987.

Mohler SE: Passive smoking: a danger to children's health, *J Pediatr Nurs* 1:298-304, 1987.

Pierson WE, Koenig JQ, Bardana EJ Jr: Potential adverse health effects of wood smoke, *West J Med* 151:339-342, 1989.

Miscellaneous Respiratory Conditions

McConnell EA: Giving intradermal injections, *Nursing 90* 20(3):70, 1990.

Reed JL, Keegan MJ: Fat embolism syndrome: a complication of trauma, *Crit Care Nurse* 13(3):33-37, 1993.

Rooklin AR, Gawchik SM: Allergic rhinitis—it's that time again! *Contemp Pediatr* 11(4):19-41, 1994.

Royall JA, Levin DL: Adult respiratory distress syndrome in pediatric patients. I. Clinical aspects, pathophysiology, pathology, and mechanisms of lung injury, *J Pediatr* 112:169-180, 1988.

Royall J, Levin DL: Adult respiratory distress syndrome in pediatric patients. II. Management, *J Pediatr* 112:335-347, 1988.

Asthma

Blue CL: Exercise-induced asthma: the "silent asthma," *J Pediatr Nurs* 2:167-174, 1988.

Capen CL and others: The team approach to pediatric asthma education, *Pediatr Nurs* 20(3):231-237, 1994.

Clark NK, Gotsch A, Rosenstock I: Patient, professional and public education on behavioral aspects of asthma: a review of strategies for change and needed research, *J Asthma* 39(4):241-255, 1993.

Davis J, Wasserman E: Behavioral aspects of asthma in children, *Clin Pediatr* 31(11):678-681, 1992.

DiGiullo G and others: Hospital treatment of asthma: lack of benefit from theophylline given in addition to nebulized albuterol and intravenously administered corticosteroid, *J Pediatr* 122(3):464-466, 1993.

Dworkin G, Kattan M: Mechanical ventilation for status asthmaticus in children, *J Pediatr Nurs* 114:545-549, 1989.

Fitzpatrick M and others: Therapeutic theophylline levels on the sleep quality and daytime cognitive performance of normal subjects, *Am Rev Respir Dis* 145:1355-1358, 1992.

Frost L, Kieckhefer GM, Rubino C: Incorporating research into a community asthma program, *Pediatr Nurs* 14:197-200, 1988.

Furukawa C: Stepping up the treatment of children with asthma, *Pediatrics* 92(1):144-146, 1993.

Gurwitz D: Family education: effective treatment for asthma, *Contemp Pediatr* 4(3):55-64, 1987.

Isles A, Robertson C: Treatment of asthma in children and adolescents: the need for a different approach, *Med J Aust* 158(11):761-763, 1993.

Karsch AB: Assessment and management of status asthmaticus, *Pediatr Nurs* 20(3):217-223, 1994.

Kieckhefer GM: Testing self-perception of health theory to predict health promotion and illness management, *J Pediatr Nurs* 2:381-391, 1987.

Lyttle B, Hollestelle A: Asthma: assessment and management in a pediatric hospital, *Can Fam Physician* 39:7933-7938, 1993.

Mendlowitz DR and others: Understanding respiration and digestion: a developmental comparison of healthy and asthmatic children, *Child Health Care* 17:45-49, 1988.

National Institutes of Health: *Teach your patients about asthma,* Bethesda, MD, 1992, National Asthma Education Program.

Plaut TF: Helping asthma patients breathe easier, *Contemp Pediatr* 6(special issue):59-76, 1989.

Plaut TF: What a peak flow meter can do for children with asthma, *Contemp Pediatr* 6(special issue):33-52, 1989.

Ramsey AM, Siroky AS: The use of puppets to teach school-age children with asthma, *Pediatr Nurs* 14:187-190, 1988.

Reid M: Complicating features of asthma, *Pediatr Clin North Am* 39(6):1327-1341, 1992.

Rolnick SJ: Self-management of pediatric asthma: four programs being studied, *J Pediatr Nurs* 2:264-266, 1988.

Salerno M, Hoss K, Hoss R: Allergen avoidance in the treatment of dust-mite allergy and asthma, *Nurse Practitioner* 17(10):53-56, 61, 65, 1992.

Sharts-Engel N: Inhaled steroids for children with asthma, *MCN* 17(2):112, 1992.

Stillwell P: Keeping ahead of childhood asthma, *Clin Pediatr* 32(2):97-99, 1993.

Strauss RE and others: Aminophylline therapy does not improve outcome and increases adverse effects in children hospitalized with acute asthmatic exacerbations, *Pediatrics* 93(2):205-206, 1994.

Taylor W: Impact of childhood asthma on health, *Pediatrics* 90(5):657-662, 1992.

Theophylline precautions, *Emerg Med* 25(3):51-52, 1993.

Tozcinski K: Update on common allergic diseases, *Pediatr Nurs* 19(4):410-414, 1993.

Traver GA, Martinez M: Asthma update. I. Mechanisms, pathophysiology, and diagnosis, *J Pediatr Health Care* 2:221-226, 1988.

Traver GA, Martinez M: Asthma update. II. Treatment, *J Pediatr Health Care* 2:227-233, 1988.

Treatment of chronic asthma in children, *Can Med Assoc J* 145(6):637-638, 1991.

Wenger NMR, Walsh M: Children's perspectives on coping with asthma, *Pediatr Nurs* 20(3):224, 1994.

Zimo DA, Gaspar M, Akhter J: The efficacy and safety of home nebulizer therapy for children with asthma, *Am J Dis Child* 143:208-211, 1989.

Cystic Fibrosis

Brissette S and others: Nursing care plan for adolescents and young adults with advanced cystic fibrosis, *Issues Compr Pediatr Nurs* 10:87-97, 1987.

Cassey J and others: Totally implantable system for venous access in children with cystic fibrosis, *Clin Pediatr* 27:91-95, 1988.

Dibble SL, Savedra MC: Cystic fibrosis in adolescence: a new challenge, *Pediatr Nurs* 14:299-303, 1988.

Gibson C: Perspective in parental coping with a chronically ill child: the case of cystic fibrosis, *Issues Compr Pediatr Nurs* 11:33-41, 1988.

Gutteridge C, Kuhn RJ: Pulmozyme-Dornase Alfa, *Pediatr Nurs* 20(3):278-279, 1994.

Handyside A, Lesko J, Tarin J: Birth of a normal girl after in vitro fertilization and preimplantation diagnostic testing for cystic fibrosis, *N Engl J Med* 327:905-909, 1992.

Hanning R, Blimkie C, Bar-Or O: Relationships among nutritional status and skeletal and respiratory muscle function in cystic fibrosis: does early dietary supplementation make a difference? *Am J Clin Nutr* 57(4):580-587, 1993.

Kerem E and others: Wheezing in infants with cystic fibrosis: clinical course, pulmonary function, and survival analysis, *Pediatrics* 90(5):703-706, 1992.

Loftus T: Helping cystic fibrosis patients with high-tech home care, *Caring* 6(6):22-27, 1988.

Madden B and others: Intermediate-term results of heart-lung transplantation for cystic fibrosis, *Lancet* 339(8809):1583-1587, 1992.

Myer PA: Parental adaptation to cystic fibrosis, *J Pediatr Health Care* 2:20-28, 1988.

Nuttall P, Nicholes P: Cystic fibrosis: adolescent and maternal concerns about hospital and home care, *Issues Compr Pediatr Nurs* 15:199-213, 1992.

Reed SB: Potential for alterations in family process: when a family had a child with cystic fibrosis, *Issues Compr Pediatr Nurs* 13:15-23, 1990.

Screening for cystic fibrosis, *Lancet* 340 (8813):209-210, 1992 (editorial).

Walker LS, Ford MB, Donald WD: Cystic fibrosis and family stress: effects of age and severity of illness, *Pediatrics* 79:239-246, 1987.

CHAPTER 33

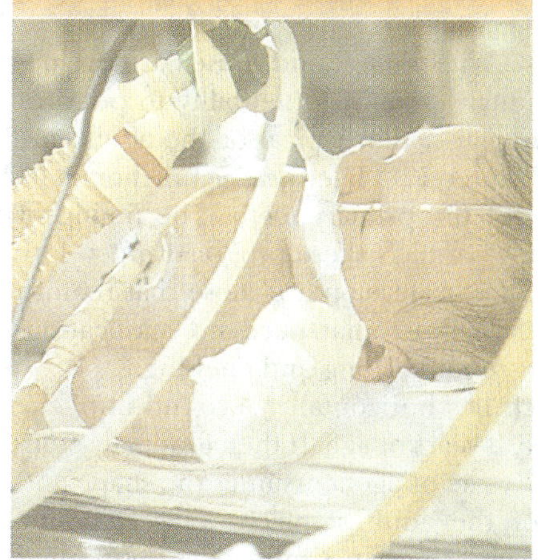

The Child with Gastrointestinal Dysfunction

CHAPTER OUTLINE

RELATED TOPICS

Central venous access devices, Ch. 28
Cystic fibrosis, Ch. 32
Disorders of the gastrointestinal tract, Ch. 11
Encopresis, Ch. 18
Feeding resistance, Ch. 10
Gastric feeding techniques, Ch. 27
Gastrointestinal disorders, Ch. 29
Intestinal parasitic diseases, Ch. 16
Nursing care of high-risk newborns, Ch. 10
Ostomies, Ch. 27
Pain assessment: pain management, Ch. 26
Preparation for procedures, Ch. 27
Procedures related to elimination, Ch. 27
Sudden infant death syndrome, Ch. 13
Surgical procedures, Ch. 27

GASTROINTESTINAL (GI) STRUCTURE AND FUNCTION

The primary function of the GI tract is the digestion and absorption of nutrients. The GI tract also has secretory, barrier, endocrine, and immunologic functions (see box below). The extensive surface area of the GI tract and its digestive function represent the major means of exchange between the human organism and the environment. Thus any dysfunction of the GI tract can cause significant problems with the exchange of fluids, electrolytes, and nutrients. This section provides an overview of the development and

■ Lynn E. Mattis, RN, MSN, revised this chapter.

FUNCTIONS OF THE GASTROINTESTINAL TRACT

Process and absorb nutrients necessary to maintain metabolic processes and to support growth and development
Perform an excretory function for both digestive residue and other waste products that pour into the intestine from the blood or are excreted in the bile
Provide detoxification while other routes of elimination (kidneys, liver, skin) are still immature
Participate in maintaining fluid and electrolyte balance in infancy

anatomy of the GI tract and the functions of digestion and absorption.

DEVELOPMENT OF THE GASTROINTESTINAL TRACT

The development of the GI tract (from mouth to anus) occurs in several stages from conception through birth. The GI tract may be divided into three parts in intrauterine life: ***foregut*** (esophagus, stomach, and proximal duodenum), ***midgut*** (distal duodenum, jejunum, ileum, cecum, and proximal colon), and ***hindgut*** (distal colon and rectum). The ***salivary glands, liver, gallbladder,*** and ***pancreas*** are outgrowths of the foregut and midgut.

The ***esophagus*** develops from the foregut and can be identified by 4 weeks of gestation. It elongates rapidly after the fourth week to a length of approximately 10 cm at term. The ***stomach*** is identifiable by 4 weeks of gestation and continues to develop during the second trimester. From the fifth week of gestation until term, the intestine lengthens a thousandfold.

The third trimester is the period of most extensive and rapid growth of the gut. The ***small intestine*** is approximately 250 to 300 cm long at term, and the ***large intestine*** is approximately 30 to 50 cm at term. The small intestine grows in length a small amount in childhood to approximately 4 m by adulthood.

During pregnancy the fetus receives nutrients via the placenta. At birth the full-term infant is capable of adaptation to extrauterine nutrition. This adaptation process includes coordinated sucking and swallowing, efficient gastric emptying and intestinal motility, regulation of digestive secretions and enzymes, efficient digestion and absorption, and excretion of waste products. The capacity of the infant to adapt to enteral nutrition depends on the gestational age at birth and the type of nutrients to which the GI tract is exposed. Many processes necessary for this adaptation are not fully developed until 33 to 34 weeks of gestation.

Many preterm infants less than 34 weeks of gestation require gavage feeding regardless of their birth weight (Weaver, 1991). The rate of gastric emptying may also be affected by prematurity. The motility of the small intestine is disorganized in infants less than 30 weeks of gestation. Intestinal motility increases as the gestational age increases, but it is not known if the introduction of enteral feeding initiates coordinated motor activity. ***Meconium,*** a thick greenish black material consisting of epithelial cells, digestive tract secretions, and residue of swallowed amniotic fluid, is normally expelled from the intestine shortly after birth and provides evidence of patency of the GI tract.

At term, the mechanical functions of digestion are relatively immature. ***Swallowing*** is an automatic reflex action for the first 3 months, and the infant has no voluntary control of swallowing until the striated muscles in the throat establish their cerebral connections. This begins at approximately 6 weeks of age. By 6 months the infant is capable of swallowing, holding food in the mouth, or spitting it out at will. The mechanism of ***sucking*** is also a reflexive activity in the newborn, and the muscular action of the tongue has a typical forward thrust. With neural and muscular development, the infant gradually acquires the ability to perform the coordinated muscular action typical of the adult type of swallowing (see Chapter 12). The ***chewing*** function is facilitated by eruption of the primary teeth. The timing of dietary changes closely parallels these progressive developmental capabilities. First to develop are those that require merely swallowing, then those that need no mastication, and finally those that require biting and chewing.

The ***stomach,*** which lies horizontally, is round until the child is approximately 2 years of age. It then gradually elongates until at about 7 years of age it assumes the shape and anatomic position of the adult stomach. This anatomic placement of the stomach in infancy influences positioning practices during and after feeding (see Chapter 8). At birth the stomach capacity is small, but it increases rapidly with age.

The frequency and character of stools are affected by the rate of peristalsis and the nature of ingested food. The frequent, yellow stools of the neonate gradually assume a more adult regularity and character in the infant. The emptying time of the stomach is slower in the newborn and decreases in older infants and children. The stomach capacity has implications for determining the amount and frequency of feedings during this period of growth.

The ***secretory cells*** of the GI tract are believed to be functional at birth. However, since most of the digestive enzymes depend on a specific pH relationship that is gradually acquired with age, their efficiency may be impaired. The newborn produces only small amounts of saliva, which contains some of the starch-splitting enzyme amylase; therefore its primary purpose at this time is to moisten the mouth and throat. By the end of the second year, the salivary glands have increased in size about 5 times to reach their full size and function.

DIGESTION

Three processes—digestion, absorption, and metabolism—are necessary in order for the body to convert nutrients into forms it can use and are actually a continuum of events. ***Nutrients*** are composed of seven major substances: carbohydrates, proteins, fats, vitamins, minerals, water, and electrolytes. ***Digestion*** is the initial preparation of food for use by the body. Two basic activities are involved: mechanical or muscular activity producing GI motility (movement) and chemical or enzymatic activity resulting from GI secretions.

Mechanical digestion occurs through a series of neuromuscular actions that move and mix food along the GI tract at a rate suitable for digestion and absorption. Three types of muscles in the stomach and intestines contribute to this motility: (1) ***circular muscles*** churn and mix food particles; (2) ***longitudinal muscles*** propel the food mass; and (3) ***sphincter muscles*** (the lower esophageal, pyloric, ileocecal and anal sphincters) control passage of the food mass to the next segment. The nervous system regulates these muscular actions. The ***intramural plexus*** forms the complex network of nerves within the GI wall that control smooth muscle contractions.

Chemical digestion involves five general types of GI secretions: (1) ***enzymes*** (specific actions on degradation of nutrients), (2) ***hormones*** (stimulate or inhibit GI secretions), (3) ***hydrochloric acid*** (produce the pH necessary for the activity of specific enzymes), (4) ***mucus*** (lubricates and protects the GI tract), and (5) ***water and electrolytes*** (transport nutrients for digestion and absorption). Numerous cells and glands produce these secretions. The cells that secrete mucus and GI hormones are found primarily in the ***mucosa*** of the stomach and small intestine. The ***salivary glands*** secrete enzymes, and the ***gastric glands*** secrete enzymes and hydrochloric acid. The ***pancreas*** also secretes enzymes, and the liver secretes bile.

Mechanical and chemical digestion begins in the mouth. ***Biting*** and ***chewing*** mix food with saliva and reduce the food into a ***bolus.*** The saliva moistens the food to aid in swallowing. Salivary ***amylase*** begins the process of digestion of complex carbohydrates or starches.

The next phase of digestion is ***swallowing,*** or ***deglutition.*** Safe swallowing requires coordination of the oral and pharyngeal phases of swallowing to prevent food material from entering the airway. The coordination of swallowing is controlled by the interaction of the cranial nerves and the muscles of the mouth, pharynx, and esophagus. The ***oral phase*** of swallowing is voluntary. The ***pharyngeal phase*** is involuntary and consists of elevation of the palate, uvula, and larynx, followed by a peristaltic wave. The ***upper esophageal sphincter (UES)*** then relaxes to allow passage of the bolus into the esophagus. ***Peristalsis*** (wavelike movements that squeeze food along the entire length of the alimentary tract) moves the food through the esophagus, and the ***lower esophageal sphincter (LES)*** relaxes to allow the food to enter the stomach.

Once a bolus of food has entered the stomach, the LES contracts to prevent food from refluxing (returning) into the esophagus. The ***stomach*** stores, mixes, and empties the food during digestion. The ***gastric glands*** secrete enzymes, hydrochloric acid, and mucus, which mix with the food to continue the process of digestion. The enzyme ***pepsin,*** formed from pepsinogen, begins the breakdown of whole proteins into polypeptides. ***Hydrochloric acid,*** secreted by the parietal cells, aids in the digestion of proteins. The hormone ***gastrin*** is released in the stomach in response to food. Gastrin stimulates the parietal cells to produce more hydrochloric acid. When the pH is very low, a feedback mechanism stops secretion of gastrin to prevent excessive acid formation. The ***mucus*** serves primarily to form a protective barrier between the acid and the gastric mucosa.

Partially digested food and watery secretions ***(chyme)*** are delivered to the small intestine. Up to this time, most of the digestion has been mechanical. The major part of chemical digestion, as well as several types of movement that aid in mechanical digestion, occurs in the small intestine. The small intestine secretes a large number of enzymes, each of which is specific for one of the fundamental types of nutrients. The mucosa of the small intestine secretes ***disaccharidases (maltase, lactase,*** and ***sucrase)*** that convert maltose, lactose, and sucrose to monosaccharides (glucose, fructose, and galactose). ***Amino peptidase*** and ***dipeptidase*** convert polypeptides to smaller peptides and amino acids.

Secretions from the liver and pancreas complete the process of chemical digestion. The ***pancreas*** produces several enzymes that digest nutrients. ***Amylase*** converts starch to disaccharides. ***Trypsin*** and ***chymotrypsin*** convert proteins and polypeptides to smaller polypeptides. ***Lipase*** converts fats to glycerides and fatty acids. These pancreatic enzymes become active only after the inactive forms are secreted into the small intestine. For example, the enzyme ***enterokinase,*** secreted by the intestinal mucosal glands, is necessary for trypsinogen to be converted into trypsin. Otherwise, activated enzymes would digest the pancreas and pancreatic duct.

Another important aid in digestion and absorption in the small intestine is ***bile.*** Bile is produced in the liver and stored by the gallbladder. When fat enters the small intestine, the hormone ***cholecystokinin,*** which stimulates the gallbladder to release bile, is secreted by the intestinal mucosal glands. Bile, an emulsifying agent for fats that facilitates the digestion of fats by lipase, is necessary for the absorption of the fat-soluble vitamins A, D, E, and K. Absence of bile causes increased amounts of ingested fat to appear in the feces ***(steatorrhea),*** as well as a deficiency of these vitamins.

ABSORPTION

After digestion of the food is complete, the simplified nutrient end products—monosaccharides (glucose, fructose, and galactose) from carbohydrates, fatty acids and glycerides from fats, and small peptides and amino acids from proteins—are ready for absorption. Vitamins and minerals are also released as a result of digestion. Water and electrolytes contribute to the fluid food mass that is finally absorbed.

The principal site for absorption of nutrients in the GI tract is the ***small intestine.*** The inner mucosa of the small intestine consists of folds and projections that are progressively smaller in size. These mucosal folds, villi, and microvilli, increase the inner surface area approximately 600 times over the outer serosa, yielding an extremely large surface for absorption.

The ***mucosal folds*** are elevated folds along the mucosa. The ***villi*** can be seen by light microscope and are small fingerlike projections covering the mucosal folds. The villi increase the surface area further. Each villus has a vascular supply, including ***venous*** and ***arterial capillaries*** and ***lacteals*** (lymphatic vessels in the small intestine that contain the substance chyle). The ***microvilli,*** numerous minute projections on the surface of each villus (visible by electron microscope), form the ***brush border*** (Fig. 33-1).

There are several mechanisms of absorption by the small intestine, including passive diffusion, carrier-mediated diffusion, active energy-driven transport, and engulfment. ***Passive diffusion (osmosis)*** occurs across the epithelial membrane in the direction from higher concentration to lower concentration. ***Carrier-mediated diffusion*** occurs as molecules are carried across the epithelial cells of microvilli by a molecule that serves as a vehicle. Large molecules must be combined with a smaller molecule to pass from a greater pressure gradient to a lesser one. For example, vitamin B_{12} re-

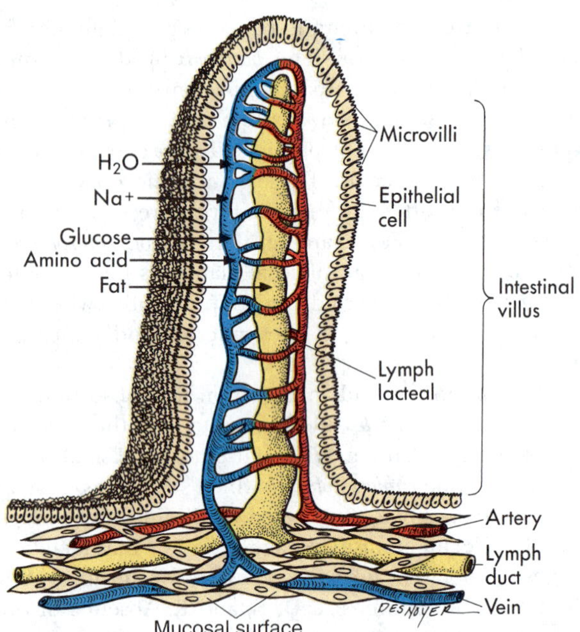

FIG. 33-1 Intestinal villus. Presence of intestinal villi and microvilli increases absorptive surface area of the intestinal mucosa. Most absorbed substances enter the blood in intestinal capillaries, with the exception of fat, which enters lymph by way of the intestinal lacteals. (From Thibodeau GA, Patton KT: *Anatomy and physiology,* ed 2, St Louis, 1993, Mosby.)

CLINICAL MANIFESTATIONS OF GASTROINTESTINAL DYSFUNCTION IN CHILDREN

Failure to thrive—Deceleration from established growth pattern or consistently below the 5th percentile for height and weight on standard growth charts; sometimes accompanied by developmental delays

Spitting up or regurgitation—Passive transfer of gastric contents into the esophagus or mouth

Vomiting—Forceful ejection of gastric contents; involves a complex process under central nervous system control that causes salivation, pallor, sweating, and tachycardia; usually accompanied by nausea

- ***Projectile vomiting***—Vomiting accompanied by vigorous peristaltic waves and typically associated with pyloric stenosis or pylorospasm

Nausea—Unpleasant sensation vaguely referred to the throat or abdomen with an inclination to vomit

Constipation—Passage of firm or hard stools or infrequent passage of stool with associated symptoms such as difficulty expelling the stools, blood-streaked stools, and abdominal discomfort

Encopresis—Overflow of incontinent stool causing soiling; often due to fecal retention or impaction

Diarrhea—Increase in the number of stools with an increased water content as a result of alterations of water and electrolyte transport by the GI tract; may be acute or chronic

Hypoactive, hyperactive, or absent bowel sounds—Evidence of intestinal motility problems that may be caused by inflammation or obstruction

Abdominal distention—protuberant contour of the abdomen that may be caused by delayed gastric emptying, accumulation of gas or stool, inflammation, or obstruction

Abdominal pain—Pain associated with the abdomen that may be localized or diffuse, acute or chronic; often caused by inflammation, obstruction, or hemorrhage

Gastrointestinal bleeding—May be from an upper or lower GI source and may be acute or chronic

- ***Hematemesis***—Vomiting of bright red blood or denatured blood that results from bleeding in the upper GI tract or from swallowed blood from the nose or oropharynx
- ***Hematochezia***—Passage of bright red blood per rectum, usually indicating lower GI tract bleeding
- ***Melena***——Passage of dark-colored, "tarry" stools due to denatured blood, suggesting upper GI tract bleeding or bleeding from the right colon

Jaundice—Yellow coloration of the skin and sclerae associated with liver dysfunction

Dysphagia—Difficulty swallowing caused by abnormalities in the neuromuscular function of the pharynx or upper esophageal sphincter or by disorders of the esophagus

Dysfunctional swallowing—Impaired swallowing due to central nervous system defects or structural defects of the oral cavity, pharynx, or esophagus; can cause feeding problems or aspiration

Fever—Common manifestation of illness in children with GI disorders; usually associated with dehydration, infection, or inflammation

quires intrinsic factor to be carried into the intestinal circulation.

In ***active energy-driven transport,*** nutrients require energy to be absorbed and to cross the intestinal epithelial membrane. This mechanism is referred to as a ***pump.*** The pump transports molecules across the membrane by means of energy supplied by the cell's metabolism. The sodium pump, which transports glucose, is an example of this mechanism.

Engulfment, or ***pinocytosis,*** is the process that allows large macromolecules to be absorbed by the epithelial cells of the villi. The epithelial cell engulfs the macromolecule and opens to allow the particle to enter the interior of the cell. The particle then enters the capillary blood. Some whole proteins and fat droplets are transported by this mechanism.

Following absorption by these mechanisms, the end products of carbohydrates and proteins are absorbed into the intestinal capillaries and enter the portal blood circulation of the liver, to be carried to the body tissues. The transfer of end products of fat digestion is unique in that the fat molecules pass between the cells of the intestinal mucosa and into the lacteals of the villi. From there, they enter the larger lymph vessels and then the portal blood flow at the thoracic duct. Exceptions include the medium- and short-chain fatty acids, which can be absorbed directly into the blood circulation of the villi. Most of the fats commonly consumed are long-chain fatty acids, however, which are transported by way of the lacteals.

Fat-soluble vitamins are absorbed with digested fats in the presence of bile. Water-soluble vitamins, vitamin B complex, and vitamin C are absorbed readily in the small intestine. Absorption of vitamin B_{12} takes place only in the ileum. The majority of water and electrolyte absorption also takes place in the small intestine.

The ***large intestine*** completes the process of absorption and functions primarily to absorb sodium and additional

TABLE 33-1 Gastrointestinal Diagnostic Procedures

TEST	DESCRIPTION	PURPOSE	COMMENTS
Stool examination	Gross, microscopic, and chemical examination of stool specimen	To detect presence of normal and abnormal constituents	Most tests demand a fresh specimen Provide samples from several areas of the stool
Ova and parasites (O & P)	Microscopic examination of stool contents for presence of parasites or their eggs	To aid in diagnosis of parasitic infections	Requires several fresh specimens placed in a special preservative
Bacterial culture	Sample contents are grown on culture medium	To confirm diagnosis of bacterial pathogens	Avoid external contamination of stool Deliver a fresh specimen to laboratory promptly in a clean cup Serologic tests will determine the presence of bacterial toxins
Stool assay for viral pathogens	ELISA (enzyme-linked immunosorbent assay)	To detect presence of viral pathogens	Standard ELISA test available for detection of rotavirus and adenovirus
Quantitative fat	Determination of presence of abnormal quantities of fat	To aid in diagnosis of pancreatic insufficiency or malabsorption syndrome	Requires a 72-hour cumulative specimen and a simultaneous food intake record to determine a coefficient of absorption
Reducing substances (sugars)	One Clinitest tablet is added to a small amount of liquid stool suspended in 10 drops of water; resulting color is compared with urine testing chart to determine amount of reducing sugars	To detect carbohydrate malabsorption by measuring stool-reducing substances	Easily and quickly administered screening test Test should be carried out as soon as possible after collection Test modified for detection of sucrose, which is not a reducing sugar Test can be performed on unit Positive results suggest carbohydrate malabsorption
pH	Nitrazine pH paper is dipped into liquid stool, and color is compared with chart provided	To screen for carbohydrate malabsorption	A pH of <5.5 indicates carbohydrate malabsorption
Occult blood guaiac test (Hemoccult, SmithKline Diagnostics)	Stool is smeared on guaiac paper, and 2 drops of developing solution are added to reverse side, which reveals blue color in presence of blood	To detect presence of blood in stool	Easily and quickly administered screening test Small amounts of blood (e.g., from bleeding mouth, gums, and nose) may give positive results
Orthotolidine test (Hematest, Ames Co.)	Hematest tablet and water are added to stool smeared on filter paper, which turns blue in presence of blood	To detect presence of blood in stool	False-positive results can be caused by red meats and iron
Gastric acidity	Stomach secretions are removed by suction via nasogastric tube (NG) tube; serial specimens are needed; samples are tested for pH	To measure gastric acidity	Requires fast before test Children: nothing after midnight Infant less than 1 year of age: nothing 4 to 6 hours before test NG tube placed so that tip lies in most dependent area of stomach Child needs preparation for tube insertion

Continued.

TABLE 33-1 Gastrointestinal Diagnostic Procedures—cont'd

TEST	DESCRIPTION	PURPOSE	COMMENTS
Pancreatic function	Pancreatic secretions are collected via duodenal tube under stimulated conditions and analyzed for water, ions, and enzymes Serial samples are collected	To determine functional secretory capacity of pancreas	Requires preprocedure fast Drawbacks include expense and invasiveness Pancreatic enzyme supplements interfere with test Child needs preparation for tube insertion
Radiography			
Plain films	Anteroposterior and lateral radiographs of abdomen and pelvis	To detect foreign body or mass, reveal bowel gas patterns, and detect obstruction or perforation in GI tract	Requires no special physical preparation Child needs preparation for procedure
Contrast studies—upper GI series, lower GI series	Radiopaque media (barium or water-soluble contrast) or air is swallowed or administered as an enema	To assess structure and function of GI tract and to detect luminal abnormalities, mucosal defects, or masses	Barium enema sometimes requires cleansing enemas and oral cathartics before procedure Contrast material may be given by nasogastric (NG) or gastrostomy tube Contrast enemas may reduce intussusception Children need preprocedure preparation for swallowing contrast media, NG tube insertion, or enema Encourage fluids following procedure
Ultrasonography (sonography)	Measures and records reflection of pulsed or continuous high-frequency sound waves	To locate, measure, and delineate abdominal organs	Noninvasive techniques No radiation involved Doppler studies demonstrate presence and direction of blood flow often requiring IV contrast material Child needs preparation for procedure
Computed tomography (CT)	Pinpoint x-ray beam is directed on horizontal or vertical plane to provide series of "cuts" or "slices" that are fed into computer and assembled in image displays on video screen and transferred to permanent record	To visualize horizontal and vertical cross section of abdomen at any axis To distinguish density of various tissue structure of organs To detect blunt trauma and masses	Usually noninvasive, but may require oral or IV contrast material May require sedation Child needs preparation for procedure
Magnetic resonance imaging (MRI)	Images are formed by reemission of radio signals by atomic nuclei stimulated in a magnetic field	Permits visualization of internal body structures in any plane Permits soft tissue discrimination unavailable with many techniques	Usually noninvasive, but may require oral or IV contrast material May require sedation for lengthy immobilization; time of test is long Child requires preparation for procedure No exposure to ionizing radiation No magnetic material can be present in scanner
Manometry			
Esophagus	A multilumen catheter is inserted into esophagus, and pressure of water in catheter is sensed by a transducer and recorded	Useful for evaluation of dysphagia, esophageal spasm, achalasia, dysmotility	May require sedation Child needs preparation for procedure

TABLE 33-1 Gastrointestinal Diagnostic Procedures—cont'd

TEST	DESCRIPTION	PURPOSE	COMMENTS
Rectal	Records reflex responses of anal sphincter to transient rectal balloon distention	To measure anal sphincter function, especially for screening for constipation, Hirschsprung disease	Child needs preparation for procedure
Biopsy			
Liver	Removal of small piece of living tissue for microscopic examination by needle with child under sedation and local anesthesia, or surgically with an open-wedge sample	To detect biliary obstruction, hepatitis, cirrhosis, and metabolic abnormalities	Requires sedation and analgesia Child needs preparation for procedure
Esophagus, stomach, intestine	A small sample of mucosal tissue is taken by forceps for microscopic examination	To detect mucosal abnormalities	Requires sedation or general anesthesia Child needs preparation for procedure
Endoscopy			
Upper GI endoscopy, colonoscopy, flexible sigmoidoscopy, anoscopy	Fiberoptic endoscope is introduced into areas to be examined Endoscope has flexible-tip light source and aspiration and instrument channel	Direct visualization of lumen of GI tract to evaluate appearance and integrity of mucosa, detect lesions, and provide access for biopsy Allows for instrumental removal of foreign objects or sclerotherapy	Lower GI endoscopy requires bowel cleansing with magnesium citrate or Golytely (colonic lavage solution) before procedure and clear liquid diet 48 hours before procedure Child must be NPO for 4-8 hours before upper GI endoscopies Requires sedation or general anesthesia Child needs preparation for procedure
Esophageal pH monitoring	A small probe that measures pH is placed through nose into distal one third of esophagus and is connected to a recording device that monitors pH over time	To determine frequency and time of clearance of gastric acid refluxed into esophagus (GER) Usually done over 24 hours of monitoring	Effects of feeding, positioning, sleep, and other events on GER can be determined Child needs preparation for procedure
Breath hydrogen test	Hydrogen is generated in colon by bacterial fermentation of undigested carbohydrates and is then absorbed into blood, where it diffuses into expired air via lungs A 10%-12% solution of a particular carbohydrate is administered orally, and hydrogen breath is measured at fixed intervals and analyzed by gas chromatography	A rise in expired hydrogen after oral loading with a specific carbohydrate indicates its malabsorption or bacterial overgrowth	Noninvasive Hydrogen is not a product of any known metabolic reaction in humans Amount of hydrogen expired in each breath is related to amount of carbohydrate presented to colonic bacteria Child needs preparation for collecting breath sample
D-Xylose absorption test	10% D-xylose solution is administered orally; serum D-xylose is measured fasting and 30, 60, 90, and 120 minutes after D-xylose dose, or urine is collected for 5 hours and D-xylose excretion in urine is measured	To evaluate absorptive capacity of duodenojejunal mucosa Diagnosis of small bowel malabsorption caused by celiac disease	Requires 4-8 hour fast before administration of D-xylose May require multiple venipunctures if serum D-xylose is measured Long, time-consuming test Child requires preparation for all aspects of procedure (see Blood Specimens, Chapter 27)

water. The remainder of the products of digestion pass into the large intestine through the ileocecal valve. The muscular activity of the large intestine propels the mass forward. Most of the water and sodium is absorbed into the bloodstream in the proximal half of the colon. The colonic bacteria synthesize vitamin K, vitamin B_{12}, and some of the vitamin B complex. Bacteria also affect the color and odor of the stool and gas formation. The odor is primarily caused by products of bacterial action and depends on the type of colonic flora and ingested food. (Defects in digestion or absorption notably alter the odor, as well as the appearance, of feces.) Color is the result of bilirubin end products converted by bacteria to urobilinogen and then oxidized to urobilin (stercobilin). The ***feces*** that are excreted consist of undigested residue, water, bacteria, and mucus. Defecation occurs when the internal and external anal sphincters relax following distention of the rectum by feces.

ASSESSMENT OF GASTROINTESTINAL FUNCTION

The most common consequences of GI disease in children include malabsorption, fluid and electrolyte disturbances, malnutrition, and poor growth (see Dehydration, Chapter 28, and Acute Diarrheal Disease, Chapter 29). A thorough GI assessment includes history questions, general observations, clinical examination, and specific tests and procedures. The most important basic nursing assessments include measurement of intake and output, heights and weights, abdominal examination, and simple stool and urine tests.

Numerous clinical manifestations provide clues to specific GI problems (see box on p. 1450). In some cases only one manifestation may be observed; others may involve several signs and symptoms as part of the disease complex or syndrome.

A number of tests may be employed to assess GI function (see Table 33-1), and nurses are often responsible for collecting specimens (see Collection of Specimens, Chapter 27). Since children may refuse to drink contrast media, generally dislike enemas, and are frightened of unfamiliar equipment, they need preparation for procedures and collection of specimens (see Preparation for Procedures, Chapter 27).

INGESTION OF FOREIGN SUBSTANCES

Children are prone to ingesting foreign substances, since they may put their hands or any attractive object or substance in their mouth. Infants and small children in particular explore items with the mouth instinctively. Older children often place items in their mouth and accidentally swallow them. Rarely, a child deliberately swallows unusual objects or substances. Hands come into contact with dirt and contaminated objects that may contain lead, bacteria, or parasites (see Chapter 16).

PICA

Pica is an eating disorder characterized by the compulsive and excessive ingestion of both food and nonfood substances. ***Food picas*** include the excessive eating of ordinary foods or unprepared food substances, such as coffee grounds or uncooked cereals. ***Nonfood picas*** include the ingestion of substances such as clay, soil, stones, laundry starch, paint chips, ice, hair, paper, rubber, and feces. Pica is more common in children, women (especially during pregnancy), individuals who are autistic or mentally retarded, and those with anemia or chronic renal failure (Anderson, Akmal, and Kittur, 1991). In some cultures pica is an accepted practice based on the presumed nutritional or therapeutic properties or on religious or superstitious beliefs (Korman, 1990).

There are several theories regarding the cause of pica, including psychologic theories (compulsive neurosis) and nutritional theories (craving caused by a nutrient deficiency). Pica has been found to be clearly associated with both iron and zinc deficiencies, although controversy exists regarding whether pica is the cause or the result of the deficiency. Pica has also been reported to be the presenting symptom in children with celiac disease thought to be caused by iron deficiency.

In some instances pica is relatively harmless. However, when the ingested substance contains a toxic ingredient (e.g., lead in paint), the consequences can cause serious complications. Surgical complications, such as intestinal obstruction, perforation, inflammation or hemorrhage, can result.

Pica may be detected by the history, physical examination, and radiologic studies. However, it is often unrecognized, and children may deny any unusual eating behaviors. Pica should be considered when children known to be at risk for this condition develop abdominal pain, other GI symptoms, or anemia. Children exhibiting signs of this disorder should be evaluated, and if a potentially harmful substance is involved, it should be removed from the environment of the child. Nursing education regarding the dangers of pica, especially lead (see Chapter 16), and assistance in helping families remove the substance are important aspects of care.

FOREIGN BODIES

Ingestion of a variety of foreign bodies is common in infants and children. Most foreign bodies, such as marbles, small coins, beads, and small closed safety pins, pass through the GI tract without difficulty. Larger items and long or sharp objects, such as hairpins, pull tabs from beverage cans, needles, nails, tacks, and large or open safety pins, may become impacted in the GI tract. Foreign bodies tend to become impacted at normally narrow sites of the GI tract or at areas of pathologic narrowing. The proximal third of the esophagus is the most common site of foreign body impaction in children (Brady, 1991). Foreign bodies, including food boluses, are more likely to become impacted in the esophagus of children with motility disorders or other esophageal abnormalities. Pathologic narrowing of the intestine or intestinal stomas can also be the cause of foreign body obstruction.

Foreign bodies are generally classified as sharp, dull, pointed, blunt, toxic, or nontoxic. Small button batteries found in watches, cameras, calculators, and toys are the most common toxic foreign bodies ingested. Impaction by toxic foreign bodies can lead to local damage from pressure necrosis and corrosive action or burns from the battery's alkaline contents (Brady, 1991).

The infant or child who has ingested a foreign body may or may not be symptomatic. Older children may give a history of foreign body ingestion, but young or cognitively impaired children may not be able to give this kind of history. Occasionally the circumstances may indicate foreign body ingestion, such as the onset of symptoms following eating or following play with small objects. The most common symptoms include difficulty swallowing (dysphagia) or a foreign body sensation. Respiratory symptoms, including stridor, coughing, and choking, may occur from compression of the trachea by an esophageal foreign body. Sharp objects or blunt objects, after prolonged impaction, may cause perforation in the GI tract. Symptoms of perforation include chest or abdominal pain and GI bleeding.

In addition to the history, physical examination occasionally may contribute to the evaluation. Pulmonary findings may be present, and some gastric or intestinal foreign bodies may be palpable. Radiographs are indicated when foreign body ingestion is suspected. Some objects are not radiopaque, however, and a contrast study may be necessary.

The length, width, and character of foreign bodies determines whether the foreign body should be removed or left to pass spontaneously. The majority of foreign bodies pass spontaneously. The progress may be followed radiographically, and all stools should be examined to detect passage of the object. The child should be fed the usual diet. Sharp, pointed, long, toxic, and impacted foreign bodies often need to be removed, usually by endoscopy. Surgical removal is rarely indicated except in instances of perforation or vascular injury. Traditional interventions, such as magnetic or Foley catheter removal, are used less frequently, because they can increase the risk that the foreign body will be dropped, potentially causing pulmonary aspiration (Brady, 1991). An alternative to removal involves advancing the foreign body carefully into the stomach for continued travel through the GI tract (Bonadio and others, 1988).

Nursing Considerations

The primary nursing intervention is prevention of foreign body ingestion through family teaching. All children who are old enough to understand are taught not to put anything in their mouth except food. Infants and young children who cannot follow such advice must have their environment protected for them.

Prevention includes supervision, as well as ongoing education as the child matures. Any small items, diaper pins, or sharp objects are placed out of the area where an infant is usually cared for, plays, or sleeps. As the infant becomes more mobile and exploration increases, the environment is inspected carefully for any hazardous objects. The caregivers should search the floor carefully on hands and knees and remove small objects that are accessible to inquisitive young children. Any potentially dangerous items are placed out of reach of a young child or discarded where they cannot be retrieved easily. Toys are carefully examined for any small or removable parts that could be accidentally ingested. Infants or young children should not be allowed to play with marbles, coins, or objects with small batteries.

Once an object is swallowed, parents need guidelines on seeking treatment (see Emergency Treatment box). When no treatment is advised and the object is left to pass spontaneously, parents should examine all stool for verification that the object has passed safely through the GI tract, usually in 3 to 4 days. For children in diapers, this is easily accomplished by squeezing the stool between the diaper to locate the object, but in toilet-trained children it requires more effort. A piece of plastic wrap placed across the toilet bowl to collect the stool makes it easier to examine the feces. A tongue blade or similar disposable object may be needed to break up the stool for inspection.

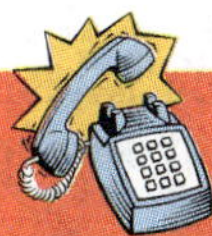

EMERGENCY TREATMENT
Foreign Body Ingestion

1. Seek medical treatment immediately if:
   a. Any sharp or large object or a battery was ingested.
   b. There are signs that the object may have been aspirated (i.e., coughing, choking, inability to speak, or difficulty breathing) (see Chapter 31 for emergency treatment of acute airway obstruction).
   c. There are signs of GI perforation (i.e., chest or abdominal pain, evidence of bleeding in vomitus, stool, hematocrit, or vital signs).
   d. There are signs that the object may be lodged in the esophagus (i.e., increased salivation, drooling, gagging, or difficulty swallowing).
   e. There are signs that the object may be lodged in the pharynx (i.e., discomfort in the throat or chest—more likely with a fish or chicken bone or large piece of meat).
2. Seek medical advice even if the object is smooth and small (usually less than the size of a nickel).
3. If no treatment is advised, check the stool for passage of the object; do not give laxatives.

DISORDERS OF MOTILITY

CONSTIPATION

Constipation is the infrequent passage of firm or hard stools or of small, hard masses associated with symptoms such as difficulty in expulsion of stool, blood-streaked bowel movements, and abdominal discomfort. The frequency of bowel movements alone is not considered a strict diagnostic criteria, because it varies widely among children. Having extremely long intervals between defecation is termed ***obstipation.*** Constipation with fecal soiling is referred to as ***enco-***

presis (see Chapter 18). The following discussion is concerned primarily with causes and treatment of simple constipation during childhood.

Constipation may arise secondary to a variety of organic disorders of the GI tract or in association with a wide range of systemic disorders. Structural disorders of the intestine, such as strictures, ectopic anus, and Hirschsprung disease, may be associated with constipation. Systemic disorders associated with constipation include hypothyroidism; hypercalcemia due to hyperparathyroidism, or vitamin D excess; and chronic lead poisoning. Constipation may also be a side effect of drugs, such as antacids, diuretics, phenytoin (Dilantin), antihistamines, and opioids (narcotics), and iron supplementation. Spinal cord lesions may be associated with loss of rectal tone and sensation; affected children are prone to chronic fecal retention and overflow incontinence.

The majority of children have ***idiopathic*** or ***functional constipation,*** because no underlying cause can be clearly identified. Chronic constipation may be initiated by environmental or psychosocial factors. Transient illness, overzealous toilet training attempts, personality, and emotional factors may play a role in the etiology of constipation. The suppression of the urge to defecate may be one cause of constipation. Stool-withholding behavior may lead to significant fecal retention. The more distended the rectum becomes with stool, the more feces are required to produce the necessary mass to stimulate defecation. Eventually, the sensation or urge to defecate may be lost. Some children with chronic constipation and encopresis have abnormal defecation dynamics; the external anal sphincter contracts rather than relaxes during attempts to defecate (Loening-Baucke, 1989).

Normally the ***newborn*** passes a first meconium stool within 24 to 36 hours of birth. Any infant who does not do so should be assessed for evidence of intestinal atresia or stenosis, Hirschsprung disease (congenital aganglionic megacolon), hypothyroidism, meconium plugs, or meconium ileus. ***Meconium plugs*** are caused by meconium that has reduced water content and are usually evacuated following digital examination, but they may require enemas with normal saline or contrast medium.

Meconium ileus, often the initial manifestation of cystic fibrosis, is the luminal obstruction of the distal small intestine by abnormal meconium. Treatment is the same as for a meconium plug. Early surgical intervention may be necessary to evacuate the small intestine.

The age of onset of constipation is frequently during ***infancy,*** or under 1 year of age (Hatch, 1988). Medical causes such as Hirschsprung disease, hypothyroidism, and strictures must be ruled out in chronic cases of constipation. The history should always include frequency of bowel movements, the composition of the diet, and whether the constipation is recent or has been present since birth.

One cause of constipation in infancy is related to dietary practices. It is almost unknown in breast-fed infants, who typically have softer stools than bottle-fed infants, although frequency can occasionally be decreased. Constipation may accompany the change from human milk or modified cow's milk formula to whole cow's milk. Some bottle-fed infants pass hard stools and develop anal fissures. Stool-withholding behavior may begin at this age in response to pain on defecation.

Most constipation in ***early childhood*** is due to environmental changes or is related to normal development when a child begins to attain control over bodily functions. A child who has experienced discomfort during bowel movements may deliberately try to withhold stool. The rectum accommodates the stool accumulation, and the urge to defecate passes. When bowel contents are ultimately evacuated, the accumulated feces are passed with even greater pain, reinforcing the desire to withhold stool.

Constipation in ***school-age children*** may represent an ongoing chronic problem or may develop for the first time. The onset of constipation at this age is often due to environmental changes, stresses, and changes in toileting patterns. A common cause of new-onset constipation at school entry is fear of using school bathrooms, which are noted for their lack of privacy. Also, early and hurried departure for school immediately after breakfast may impede bathroom use. Most schools will liberalize bathroom rules for individual children who have been identified and have a parent or health professional intervene on their behalf. Encopresis often causes additional emotional stress for the school-age child (see Chapter 18).

Therapeutic Management

Treatment of constipation depends on the cause. Meconium plugs are usually evacuated following digital examination. To facilitate their removal, as well as passage of meconium ileus, irrigations of normal saline or the iodinated contrast medium diatrizoate meglumine (Gastrografin) may be needed.

Management of the infant should include education of the parents concerning normal bowel habits. Short, transient periods of constipation usually require no intervention. Mild constipation usually resolves as solid food is introduced in the diet. Occasionally the use of glycerin suppositories, malt extract, or lactulose may be required if passage of hard stools or anal fissures persist.

The management of simple constipation consists of a plan to keep the bowel relatively empty of stool and dietary management to prevent further constipation. Management of chronic constipation should shrink the distended rectum back to normal size by keeping it evacuated of stool. This is best accomplished by using a combination of therapies. The program should incorporate bowel cleansing, maintenance therapy to prevent stool retention, modification of diet, bowel habit training, and behavioral modification.

There is not total agreement as to the most effective means to clean the bowel, but saline or mineral oil enemas are often recommended initially to remove impacted stool. The enemas may be accompanied by bisacodyl (Dulcolax) suppositories. Sometimes, manual removal of the impaction may be required. These procedures need to be repeated until all stool is evacuated. Occasionally a polyethylene glycol electrolyte solution (Golytely) by oral or nasogastric (NG) tube administration is necessary for severe fecal impaction. Rarely, surgical disimpaction is required.

Maintenance therapy should allow easy passage of stool and prevent stool retention. Maintenance therapy includes mineral oil, a stool softener, and/or an oral laxative such as senna (Fletcher's Castoria, Senokot). Cisapride, a prokinetic drug that increases GI motility and has few side effects, may also be used (Staino and others, 1991). A high-fiber diet is provided; fiber adds bulk to the stool by retaining water and facilitating intestinal propulsion of stool. Increasing fluid intake may be beneficial for some children and is recommended for those receiving a diet high in fiber or fiber supplements (Metamucil, Fiberall). Prunes are a high-fiber food that appears to directly stimulate contraction of the intestinal wall, but the substance responsible for these actions has not been clearly identified (Goldfinger, 1991).

The role foods play in causing constipation has not been well researched. Calcium-rich products may reduce stooling from a local action on intestinal mucosa (Frithz, Wictorin, and Ronquist, 1991).

Effective counseling is an essential element of the treatment plan for children with chronic constipation. Bowel function, the purpose of interventions, and the need for persistence should be explained to the child and family. Erroneous concepts concerning this condition should be corrected.

Retraining therapy involves habit training, reinforcement for sitting on the toilet and defecation, and emotional support. A regular toilet time should be established once or twice a day, preferably after a meal. A reasonable amount of time (5 to 10 minutes) should be spent attempting to defecate completely. Biofeedback may be indicated as a form of behavioral modification and a means to teach children to relax the anal sphincter during defecation (Benninga, Buller, and Taminiau, 1993).

Nursing Considerations

Unfortunately, constipation tends to be self-perpetuating. A child who has difficulty or discomfort when attempting to evacuate the bowels has a tendency to retain the bowel contents, and thus constipation becomes a chronic problem. Nursing assessment begins with a history of bowel habits, diet, events that may be associated with the onset of constipation, drugs or other substances that the child may be taking, and the consistency, color, frequency, and other characteristics of the stool. If there is no evidence of a pathologic condition that requires further investigation, the major task of the nurse is to educate the parents regarding normal stool patterns and to participate in the education and treatment of the child.

Dietary modifications are usually essential in preventing constipation. The diet should be high in fiber. Parents will benefit from guidance in dietary planning, especially regarding foods that have a high fiber content (see box above, right). If bran is added to the diet, creative ways to disguise the consistency, such as adding it to cereal, peanut butter, mashed potatoes, fruit shakes, and baked goods, is helpful. Beans are often found in Mexican dishes children enjoy and can be added to soups, salads, and stews. A good source of fiber is corn and popcorn beyond the age when foreign body aspiration is a hazard.

Children and parents also need reassurance concerning the mild nature of the condition. Many mothers are unduly concerned about constipation in their infants and consider the condition dangerous (Potts and Sesney, 1992). If the child needs enemas or medication, the family is given appropriate instructions.* It is important to discuss with them their attitudes and expectations regarding toilet habits and the treatment plan.

HIGH-FIBER FOODS

BREAD, GRAINS

Whole-grain bread or rolls
Whole-grain cereals
Bran
Pancakes, waffles, and muffins with fruit or bran
Unrefined (brown) rice

VEGETABLES

Raw vegetables, especially broccoli, cabbage, carrots, cauliflower, celery, lettuce, and spinach
Cooked vegetables, such as those listed above, and asparagus, beans, brussels sprouts, corn, potatoes, rhubarb, squash, string beans, and turnips

FRUITS

Prunes, raisins, or other dried fruits
Raw fruits, especially those with skins or seeds, other than ripe banana or avocado

MISCELLANEOUS

Legumes (beans), popcorn, nuts, seeds
High-fiber snack bars

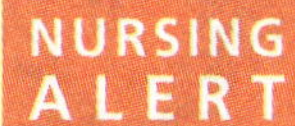

Mineral oil must be given carefully to avoid the risk of aspiration.

HIRSCHSPRUNG DISEASE (CONGENITAL AGANGLIONIC MEGACOLON)

Hirschsprung disease is a congenital anomaly that results in mechanical obstruction from inadequate motility of part of the intestine. It accounts for about one fourth of all cases of neonatal intestinal obstruction. It may not be diagnosed until later in infancy or childhood. The incidence is 1 in 5000 live births. It is four times more common in males than in females and follows a familial pattern in a small number of cases. Hirschsprung disease is associated with other anomalies, such as Down syndrome. Depending on its pre-

*Home care instructions for administering oral medications and enemas are available in *Wong and Whaley's Clinical Manual of Pediatric Nursing* (Mosby). See also the following patient education aid: Understanding constipation in your child, *Patient Care* 21(5):126-127, 1987.

sentation, it may be an acute, life-threatening condition or a chronic disorder.

Pathophysiology

The term ***congenital aganglionic megacolon*** describes the primary defect, which is the absence of autonomic parasympathetic ganglion cells in the submucosal (Meissner) and myenteric (Auerbach) plexuses in one or more segments of the colon. Lack of innervation produces the functional defect (i.e., absence of propulsive movements [peristalsis]), which causes accumulation of intestinal contents and bowel distention proximal to the defect (megacolon) (Fig. 33-2). In addition, failure of the internal anal sphincter to relax contributes to clinical manifestations of obstruction, because it prevents evacuation of solids, liquids, and gas.

Hirschsprung disease results from failure of craniocaudal migration of ganglion cell precursors along the GI tract between the fifth and twelfth weeks of gestation. The aganglionic segment almost always includes the rectum and some portion of the distal colon, but the entire colon or part of the small intestine may be involved. Rarely, skip segments or total intestinal aganglionosis may occur.

Intestinal distention and ischemia may occur as a result of distention of the bowel wall, which contributes to the development of ***enterocolitis*** (inflammation of the small bowel and colon), the leading cause of death in children with Hirschsprung disease (Kirschner, 1991).

Clinical Manifestations

Clinical manifestations vary according to the age when symptoms are recognized, the length of the affected bowel, and the occurrence of complications, such as enterocolitis. In the newborn the primary signs and symptoms are failure to pass meconium within 24 to 48 hours after birth, food refusal, vomiting, and abdominal distention.

During infancy inadequate weight gain, constipation, abdominal distention, and episodes of diarrhea and vomiting are likely to occur. Bloody diarrhea, fever, and severe lethargy are ominous signs because they often signify the presence of enterocolitis, which greatly increases the risk of fatality. Enterocolitis may also be present without diarrhea and is first evidenced by unexplained fever and poor feeding.

During childhood the symptoms become chronic and include constipation, passage of ribbonlike, foul-smelling stools, and abdominal distention. Fecal masses may be palpable. Fecal soiling is uncommon, but fecal impactions recur frequently. The child usually has a poor appetite and poor growth.

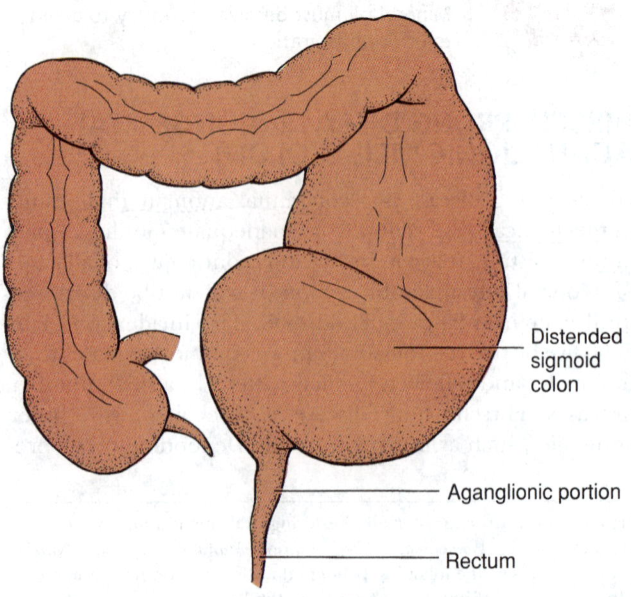

FIG. 33-2 Hirschsprung disease.

Diagnostic Evaluation

In the neonate diagnosis is suspected on the basis of clinical signs of intestinal obstruction or failure to pass meconium. In infants and children the history is an important part of diagnosis and typically details a chronic pattern of constipation. On examination the rectum is empty of feces, the internal sphincter is tight, and leakage of liquid stool and accumulated gas may occur if the aganglionic segment is short. A barium enema often demonstrates the transition zone between the dilated proximal colon (megacolon) and the aganglionic distal segment. However, this typical megacolon and narrow distal segment may not develop until the age of 2 months or later in some affected children.

To confirm the diagnosis, rectal biopsy is performed either surgically to obtain a full-thickness biopsy or by suction biopsy for histologic evidence of the absence of ganglion cells. A noninvasive procedure that may be used is ***anorectal manometry,*** in which a catheter with a balloon attached is inserted into the rectum. The test records the reflex pressure response of the internal anal sphincter to distention of the balloon. A normal response is relaxation of the internal sphincter followed by a contraction of the external sphincter. In Hirschsprung disease the external sphincter contracts normally but the internal sphincter fails to relax.

Therapeutic Management

The vast majority of children with Hirschsprung disease require surgery rather than medical therapy with frequent enemas. Once the child is stabilized with fluid and electrolyte replacement, if needed, surgery is performed with a high rate of success. The surgical management consists primarily of the removal of the aganglionic portion of the bowel in order to relieve obstruction, restore normal motility, and preserve the function of the external anal sphincter. In most cases this is accomplished in two stages. First, a temporary ostomy is created proximal to the aganglionic segment, which relieves obstruction and allows the normally innervated dilated bowel to return to its normal size.

Following this initial surgery a second complete, corrective surgery is performed, usually when the child weighs approximately 20 pounds (Kirschner, 1991). There are several definitive operations that can be performed, including the Swenson, Duhamel, Boley, and Soave procedures. The ***Soave procedure*** is often performed and consists of pulling the end of the normal bowel through the muscular sleeve of the rectum, from which the aganglionic mucosa has been removed. The ostomy is usually closed at the time of the final, definitive surgery. Simpler operations, such as an anorectal myomectomy, may be indicated in very-short-segment disease.

Prognosis. Most children with Hirschsprung disease require surgery rather than medical therapy. Once the child is stabilized with fluid and electrolyte replacement, if needed, the temporary colostomy is performed with a high rate of success. Following the later pull-through procedure, anal stricture and incontinence are potential complications that may occur and require further therapy, including dilations or bowel-retraining therapy.

Nursing Considerations

Many of the nursing concerns depend on the child's age and the type of treatment. Nursing observation of passage of meconium and bowel patterns in the neonatal period is an important factor in early diagnosis. If the disorder is diagnosed during the neonatal period, the main objectives are helping the parents adjust to the congenital disorder in their child, fostering infant-parent bonding, preparing them for the medical/surgical intervention, and assisting them in caring for the colostomy after discharge.

When the disorder is not discovered during this period, the nurse can facilitate establishing a diagnosis by carefully listening to the history, with a special emphasis on bowel habits. In Hirschsprung disease, several areas must be investigated: (1) frequency of bowel movements; (2) character of stools, particularly ribbonlike and foul-smelling stools; and (3) onset of constipation, especially if present since birth. Other clues in the history and physical examination include poor feeding habits, fussiness and irritability, distended abdomen, and signs of undernutrition, such as thin extremities, pallor, muscle weakness, and fatigue.

In unusual cases when the child is managed with occasional enemas, the nurse needs to teach the parents the correct procedure, as well as inform them of the dangers associated with using tap water, concentrated salt solutions, soap solutions, or phosphate preparations. Normal saline solution can be purchased without a prescription from a pharmacy or can be prepared at home by adding 1 level measuring teaspoon of noniodized salt to 1 pint of tap water. Since the instructions for preparing the solution and administering the enema require several steps, all of the directions should be written down, as well as verbally explained. See Chapter 27 for suggested amounts of solution according to the child's age. The following discussion is limited to care of the child undergoing surgical correction.

Preoperative Care. Much of the child's preoperative care depends on the age, clinical condition, and type of surgical procedure. Preoperative preparation entails many of the same procedures that are common to any surgery (see Chapter 27). In the newborn, whose bowel is sterile, no additional preparation is required. However, children beyond the newborn period need bowel emptying with repeated saline enemas and reduction of bacterial flora with oral antibiotics and colonic irrigations, using antibiotic solution before the second definitive surgical procedure.

In children with enterocolitis, emergency preoperative care includes frequent monitoring of vital signs and blood pressure for signs of shock; monitoring fluid and electrolyte replacements, plasma, or other blood derivatives; and observing for symptoms of bowel perforation, such as fever, increasing abdominal distention, vomiting, increased tenderness, irritability, dyspnea, and cyanosis.

Since progressive distention of the abdomen is a serious sign, abdominal circumference is measured at the largest diameter, usually at the level of the umbilicus. The point of measurement is marked with a pen to ensure reliability. It is best to record the measurement in serial order so that a change will be readily apparent (see Atraumatic Care box).

Older children need to be emotionally prepared and educated for an ostomy (see Ostomies, Chapter 27). The infant's or child's caregivers also need preparation before surgery. Since a colostomy represents a change in body function, the nurse should investigate the caregiver's previous knowledge of this procedure. Family members may have misconceptions regarding an ostomy or may have concerns regarding the appearance or care of the stoma. Education and emotional support are the most helpful nursing interventions at this time.

Teaching children and family members about an ostomy is best done by a verbal explanation, as well as through the use of a drawing and/or a teaching doll. It is important to stress to parents and older children that the colostomy for Hirschsprung disease is temporary. The nurse should also keep in mind that although a temporary colostomy is favorable in terms of future help and adjustment, it also necessitates additional surgery, which may be very stressful to parents and children.

Since poor feeding and poor growth are frequently associated with Hirschsprung disease, the caregivers should be informed that these problems generally improve following surgical intervention. Education and support should alleviate some of the child's and family members' anxiety and stress, and they should be reassured that the outcome for health and adjustment is often good.

Postoperative Care. Postoperative care following a colostomy or pull-through procedure is similar to that following any abdominal surgery. The infant or child should have nothing by mouth and will often have an NG tube to suction. Intake and output, including NG tube losses and stool from the ostomy, are measured. Intravenous fluids are monitored to maintain adequate hydration and electrolyte balance. An abdominal assessment, including monitoring of

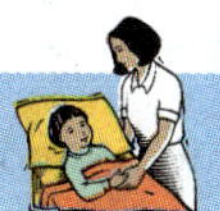

ATRAUMATIC CARE
Abdominal Circumference Measurements

To reduce any stress to the acutely ill child when frequent measurements of abdominal circumference are needed, leave the tape measure in place beneath the child. Measure the abdomen at the same time that vital signs are taken to avoid frequently disturbing the child.

return of bowel sounds and passage of stool, will indicate when oral feeding can be initiated. Following a colostomy procedure, ostomy care is an important nursing responsibility. Ongoing education of the older child and caregivers regarding ostomy care will begin with preparation for their discharge home.

When family members initially visit their child postoperatively, they are often anxious about the numerous tubes and intravenous lines attached to various body parts. The nurse should explain the function of each piece of equipment, stressing features that permit the child to be safely moved and handled, such as length of tubing, use of armboards and intravenous sites, and tape to secure the NG tube to the nose. Parents are encouraged and assisted in holding and comforting their child.

Home Care. Postoperatively, parents need instruction concerning colostomy care at home, including skin care, emptying and changing the ostomy appliance, and monitoring for problems* (see Ostomies, Chapter 27). During the early postoperative period, including parents and the older child in dressing changes can enhance teaching of colostomy care when an appliance is fitted and promote gradual acceptance of the body change. Even a preschooler can be included in the care by handing articles to the parent, rolling up the colostomy bag after it had been emptied, or applying cream to the surrounding skin. Since these children may have had difficulties with bowel training before surgery because of constipation and erratic stool patterns, the period during the temporary ostomy can relieve the pressures previously associated with bowel control. Older children should be involved in colostomy care to the point of total responsibility.

In some institutions an enterostomal therapist is available to provide additional expert assistance in planning for home care, such as preparation of the skin, application of the collecting appliance, care of the appliance, control of odor, and signs of complications, such as ribbonlike stools, excessive diarrhea, bleeding, prolapse, or failure to pass flatus or stool.

Sometimes families require financial assistance and additional psychologic support, and referral to a social worker or other service agency may be necessary. Additional supervision of care, reinforcement of child and family education, and support is often required in the home setting to maintain continuity of care. A referral to a home health care agency for home nursing visits can meet this need. (See also Nursing Care Plan: the Child with Hirschsprung Disease [Megacolon].†)

GASTROESOPHAGEAL REFLUX (GER)

Best defined as the passive transfer of gastric contents into the esophagus, GER occurs occasionally in everyone; the frequency, persistence, and complications are what may make it abnormal. Approximately 1 in 300 to 1 in 1000 children have a significant or pathologic problem. In the past much emphasis was placed on the resting or baseline pressure of the lower esophageal sphincter (LES). Studies have been unable to show a relationship between baseline LES pressure and abnormal reflux. GER most likely occurs during transient and inappropriate relaxations of the LES. The exact cause is not known, but potential causes of this inappropriate relaxation of the LES may be related to the central nervous system or to a developmentally exaggerated enteric reflex (Hillemeier, 1991). Several factors appear to favor GER, including gastric distention, increased abdominal pressure caused by coughing, central nervous system disease, delayed gastric emptying, hiatal hernia, and gastrostomy placement. Some children are especially prone to develop GER; these include children who have undergone tracheoesophageal or esophageal atresia repair, or who have neurologic disorders, scoliosis, asthma, or cystic fibrosis.

Clinical Manifestations

The most common clinical manifestation of GER is passive regurgitation or emesis. Many other less common symptoms that may appear in children with a significant problem include poor weight gain, heme-positive emesis or stools, anemia, irritability or heartburn, gagging or choking after a feeding, apnea, or recurrent pneumonias.

Recurrent reflux of acidic gastric contents can lead to ***esophagitis,*** which can cause bleeding from the esophageal mucosa. If the blood loss is significant, anemia can develop. Esophagitis can also cause discomfort in the chest area, which may be manifested as unusual irritability or poor intake of nutrients. Poor weight gain and poor growth may occur in a child with an insufficient intake of nutrients or with a very large amount of regurgitation.

Multiple respiratory abnormalities have been linked to GER, but it is often difficult to distinguish whether respiratory problems are the result or a contributing cause of reflux. In newborns, particularly premature infants, a few symptoms, such as apnea and bradycardia, have been attributed to GER. In addition, microaspiration may occur in some infants and children with GER. The cause may include a swallowing disorder leading to aspiration of refluxed gastric contents or an esophagovagal reflex rather than GER.

Diagnostic Evaluation

The history and physical examination is an important part of the diagnostic evaluation for GER. The history should include questions regarding feeding habits, frequency and characteristics of emesis, behavior, and respiratory symptoms, including the time at which they occur and any associated events. The physical examination should include a stool guaiac test and assessment of growth and nutritional status.

Several diagnostic studies are available to further evaluate GER. Generally, the initial study is the upper GI series. This study does not provide much useful information for the purpose of diagnosing GER, but it is important to exclude anatomic obstructions, such as an esophageal, gastric, or duodenal web; pyloric mass; or malrotation.

One frequently used study to aid in the evaluation of

*Home care instructions for caring for the child with a colostomy are available in *Wong and Whaley's Clinical Manual of Pediatric Nursing* (Mosby).
†In *Wong and Whaley's Clinical Manual of Pediatric Nursing* (Mosby).

GER is ***esophageal pH monitoring.*** This consists of a probe placed through the nose down to the distal esophagus and connected to a pH monitoring device. A 24-hour pH probe study provides information regarding the frequency of acid reflux, the amount of time there is acid in the distal esophagus, and the time it takes for the acid to be cleared from the esophagus. The effects of feeding, positioning, sleep, and other events on GER can be determined. Occasionally a pH probe study can be done simultaneously with a cardiorespiratory recording monitor to address the relationship of GER and respiratory symptoms.

Fiberoptic endoscopy may be performed when GER is suspected in order to assess whether esophagitis is present. The esophagus is examined visually for evidence of inflammation or ulceration. Mucosal biopsies are obtained to assess for microscopic changes consistent with GER and to determine the severity of reflux.

Scintigraphy and manometry are also used in the diagnosis of GER. During ***scintigraphic studies*** a radionuclide is added to the infant's formula, and a gamma counter detects the presence of formula refluxed to the esophagus or lungs. Scintigraphy is a useful tool for assessing delayed gastric emptying, which may contribute to GER. Esophageal manometry has limited value as a diagnostic tool for GER in terms of providing useful clinical information.

Therapeutic Management

Therapeutic management of GER depends on its severity and on whether complications such as poor growth, esophagitis, or respiratory problems are present. For the majority of infants with reflux, only conservative management is indicated to minimize the symptoms until the problem resolves. Small, frequent feedings are often beneficial to decrease the amount of regurgitation. Occasionally, continuous NG tube feedings are indicated if severe regurgitation and poor growth are present.

There are controversies regarding both thickened feedings and positioning therapy as a treatment for GER. Thickened feedings have been shown to increase formula caloric density, decrease regurgitation, decrease crying time, and increase sleep time (Orenstein, Magill, and Brooks, 1987). The percent of time with reflux with thickened versus unthickened feedings, however, was not found to be significant except in infants maintained in the 30-degree prone position (Bailey and others, 1986). Coughing has also been shown to be more frequent after thickened feedings than after unthickened feedings (Orenstein, Shalaby, and Putnam, 1992). Thickened feedings may benefit some infants with reflux and emesis.

Positioning therapy has been a topic of much controversy and research (see Thinking Critically About . . . box). At this time, the available information suggests that either the flat prone or head-elevated prone position following feeding and at night is a reasonable measure to treat infants with GER.

Pharmacologic therapy is sometimes used as an adjunct therapy to treat infants and children with GER. Antacids or histamine-receptor antagonists (H_2 blockers), such as cimetidine (Tagamet), ranitidine (Zantac), or famotidine (Pepcid), reduce the amount of acid present in gastric contents and may prevent esophagitis. Omeprazole (Prilosec) more completely suppresses gastric acid secretion than do H_2 blockers. This drug is generally reserved for infants and children who do not respond adequately to H_2 blockers, since the long-term effects of omeprazole are not known. Antacids can be used in addition to antisecretory medications to treat symptoms.

Prokinetic medications are often prescribed as a treatment for GER. Both metoclopramide (Reglan) and bethanechol (Urecholine) may decrease reflux. Metoclopramide has been found to mildly increase resting LES pressure and to increase the rate of gastric emptying. Studies provide mixed reviews regarding the effectiveness of metoclopramide for GER; in some cases it may increase the number of reflux episodes (Machida and others, 1988). Metoclopramide may be most useful in the treatment of children with GER accompanied by delayed gastric emptying. The side effects of metoclopramide include restlessness, drowsi-

THINKING CRITICALLY ABOUT . . . *Positioning in Gastroesophageal Reflux*

Positioning therapy for infants with GER has changed in the past decade. Earlier, the upright position in an infant seat was recommended for infants with reflux. Meyers and Herbst (1982) found the 30-degree upright prone position to be superior to the supine or upright position. Orenstein and Whitington (1983) found the elevated prone position in a harness to be superior to positioning in an infant seat. The prone position was also associated with more sleep time and decreased crying time, with potential beneficial behavioral effects (Orenstein, 1990a). The latest of this series of studies examined whether the head-elevated prone position was better than the flat prone position for infants with GER. No significant differences between flat prone and head-elevated prone position were found (Orenstein, 1990b). The author concluded that the head-elevated prone position is probably not worth the extra effort required to maintain this position. The American Academy of Pediatrics Task Force on Infant Positioning and SIDS (1992) recommended that healthy infants, when being put down to sleep, be positioned on their side or back; however, prone may be the position of choice for infants with symptoms of GER or other conditions.

These recommendations have led to considerable discussion and controversy regarding the best sleeping position for healthy infants and those with GER, in relation to prevention of sudden infant death syndrome (SIDS) (see Chapter 13).

What recommendations do you see being given to families? Consider the challenges in maintaining a 30-degree upright prone position, especially in an older infant, and issues related to skin care on pressure points, especially the knees and elbows.

ness, and extrapyramidal reaction, which are associated with prolonged or high doses of the drug.

Cisapride, a recently approved prokinetic drug, increases LES pressure, promotes gastric emptying, and has fewer central nervous system side effects than metoclopramide. It could supersede other agents as the preferred medication for GER (Orenstein, 1992).

Bethanechol has also been shown to greatly increase LES pressure, but it has not been proved to decrease reflux by pH probe studies (Hillemeier, 1991). Bethanechol also has side effects, including respiratory symptoms such as wheezing.

Surgical management as a treatment for GER is selected for those children with severe complications, such as recurrent aspiration pneumonia, apnea, acute life-threatening events (ALTEs), and severe esophagitis, who generally have failed medical therapy. The ***Nissen fundoplication,*** which involves a 360-degree wrap of the fundus of the stomach around the distal esophagus, is the most common surgical procedure for reflux. A gastrostomy is usually performed at the same time for decompression of the stomach postoperatively. Fundoplication combined with pyloroplasty may be performed in children with GER who also have delayed gastric emptying. Unfortunately, complications can occur following fundoplication; therefore the decision to perform this procedure should be carefully considered. Postoperative problems include small bowel obstruction, failure with continued GER, wrap hernia, retching, gas-bloat syndrome, and dumping syndrome. For children with neurologic impairment who are continuously tube fed, an alternative to fundoplication with gastrostomy tube placement is a nonsurgical percutaneous gastrojejunostomy and placement of a jejunostomy tube (Albanese and others, 1993).

Prognosis. The majority of infants with GER have a mild problem that generally improves by about 1 year of age and requires only observation or medical therapy. Over 60% of children with reflux will be symptom-free by 18 months of age (Herbst, 1989). If GER is severe and remains unsuccessfully treated, multiple complications can occur. Esophageal strictures caused by persistent esophagitis with scarring are one of the most significant complications. Recurrent respiratory distress or aspiration pneumonia is another serious complication that is an indication for surgery. Failure to thrive caused by GER can often be managed with medical therapy and nutritional support.

Nursing Considerations

Nursing care is directed at (1) identifying children with symptoms suggestive of GER; (2) educating parents regarding home care, including feeding, positioning, and medications when indicated; and (3) if appropriate, caring for the child undergoing surgical intervention. For the majority of infants, parental reassurance of the benign nature of the condition and its relationship to physiologic maturity is the most important intervention. To help parents cope with the inconvenience of regurgitation, simple measures such as using bibs and protective clothes during feeding and prone positioning after feeding are beneficial.

It may be a challenge to maintain the desired position for the infant who does benefit from upright prone positioning. The 30-degree elevation of the head of the bed can be created by using a wedge or extra bedding under the mattress. A commercially available harness may be helpful in maintaining the infant in the head-elevated prone position (Fig. 33-3).

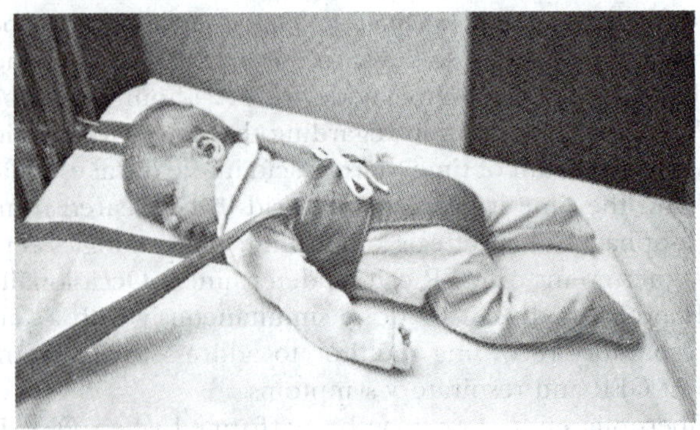

FIG. 33-3 Five-week-old infant positioned in harness. (From Orenstein SR, Whitington PF: Positioning for prevention of infant gastroesophageal reflux, *J Pediatr* 103:534-537, 1983.)

➤ **NURSING TIP** An improvised harness using a baby blanket can be made for the infant with GER. Place the infant prone on the blanket, bring the ends of the blanket up between the infant's legs, and secure all corners of the blanket to the mattress with safety pins on either side of the infant's trunk.

When the infant is older and more mobile, maintaining correct positioning becomes increasingly difficult. An alternative frame has been described that consists of a cradle bed, bassinet, or board with a firm wooden base and a wooden spindle or large dowel that protrudes through the center of the mattress. To protect areas such as the infant's knees and elbows, the mattress is covered with a sheepskin or soft blanket, and pressure areas are inspected for signs of redness.

Feeding modification may require some rescheduling of the family's routine to accommodate more frequent feeding times. If formula is thickened with cereal (generally, 1 teaspoon to 1 tablespoon of rice cereal per ounce of formula is recommended), the nipple opening may need to be enlarged for easier sucking. Usually breast-feeding may continue, and the mother may provide more frequent feeding times or express the milk for thickening with rice cereal. When regurgitation is severe and growth is a problem, continuous nasogastric feedings may decrease the amount of emesis and provide constant buffering of gastric acid. Special preparation of caregivers is required when this type of nutritional therapy is indicated.

Nonnutritive sucking tends to hasten clearance of refluxed material from the esophagus. In infants with GER, nonnutritive sucking was found to affect the frequency of reflux episodes—increasing reflux in prone infants and decreasing it in seated infants (Orenstein, 1988). Nonnutritive sucking also reduces crying behavior.

Other practical measures include avoiding rough play following feedings and avoiding feeding just before bedtime. The success or failure of management often is directly related to the nurse's role in providing thorough education regarding all aspects of the prescribed treatment plan.

Postoperative nursing care is similar to that for other types of abdominal surgery (see Chapter 27). Gastric decompression by an NG tube or gastrostomy must be maintained to avoid distention in the immediate postoperative period. Usually the NG tube should not be replaced by the nurse if it is accidentally removed, because of the risk of injury to the operative site. When postoperative ileus resolves, the NG tube is removed or the gastrostomy tube is elevated in preparation for feeding. If bolus feedings are initiated through the gastrostomy, the tube may need to remain vented for several days or longer to avoid gastric distention from swallowed air. Edema surrounding the surgical site and a tight gastric wrap may prohibit the infant from expelling air through the esophagus. Some infants benefit from clamping of the tube for increasingly longer intervals until they are able to tolerate continuous clamping between feedings. During this time, if the infant displays increasing irritability and evidence of cramping, some relief may be provided by venting the tube.

Preparation for Home Care. If medical management is prescribed or surgery performed, nursing responsibilities include educating caregivers about administering drugs at home,* special feeding regimens or formula preparation, gastrostomy care, and postoperative care (see Chapter 27). After surgery, reflux is completely controlled in most cases, with these children attaining normal health and growth. If a gastrostomy tube is inserted during surgery, it may be removed after several months unless nutritional supplementation is needed. In severe cases of gas-bloat or dumping syndrome, continuous tube feedings may be better tolerated. Caregivers should be aware of potential postoperative problems, such as difficulty vomiting, gas-bloat symptoms, or discomfort with large solid-food meals, and seek guidance from their health care provider as needed.

IRRITABLE BOWEL SYNDROME (IBS)

In IBS the small and large intestine experience abnormal motility. IBS and recurrent abdominal pain are conditions that may appear in childhood or adolescence (see Recurrent Abdominal Pain, Chapter 18). Children with IBS often have alternating diarrhea and constipation, flatulence, and lower abdominal pain. Many children are evaluated for inflammatory bowel disease, lactose intolerance, parasitic infection, or laxative abuse. Most of these children appear active and healthy, and experience normal growth. Affected children are more likely to have a history of colic with feeding difficulties and a family history of bowel problems.

Therapeutic Management

The long-range goal of treatment is development of regular bowel habits and relief of symptoms. As with other variants of functional abdominal pain, environmental modifications or psychosocial intervention may relieve stress and GI symptoms. A high-fiber diet with psyllium supplements (i.e., Metamucil, Fiberall) is often beneficial for the treatment of IBS. Antispasmodics, antidiarrheal drugs, and simethicone may benefit some children.

Nursing Considerations

The primary nursing goal is family support and education. The disorder is very stressful to children and parents. Support and reassurance that although the symptoms of the disorder are difficult to deal with, the disorder is not generally a threat to the child's health are helpful. Nurses can help the child and family to identify and implement strategies that decrease symptoms, including eating slowly, avoiding carbonated beverages, adding fiber to the diet, and relieving environmental stressors.

INFLAMMATORY CONDITIONS

ACUTE APPENDICITIS

Appendicitis, inflammation of the ***vermiform appendix*** (blind sac at the end of the cecum), is the most common reason for abdominal surgery during childhood. Although uncommon in children younger than 2 years of age, it is associated with increased complications and mortality in this agegroup. Primarily an acute disorder, appendicitis rapidly progresses to perforation and peritonitis if it remains undiagnosed. It is a significant pediatric problem, because early diagnosis is frequently delayed as a result of children's inability to verbalize symptoms, and the common signs may be mistaken for other illnesses.

Etiology

Appendicitis occurs when there is stasis or obstruction within the lumen of the appendix, but the mechanism that may lead to obstruction varies. Obstruction can occur with hardened fecal material ***(fecalith)***, foreign bodies, microorganisms, or parasites. The proximal portion of the appendix may be kinked by a congenital peritoneal fold. Appendiceal obstruction has also been attributed to hyperplasia of the submucosal lymphoid tissue, presumably as a result of intercurrent infection, and to fibrous stenosis resulting from an earlier inflammation or a tumor. Dietary habits also play a role. Children with high-fiber diets have a lower incidence of appendicitis than those whose fiber intake is low (Shandling, 1991). Fiber increases the bulk and softness of the stool—a factor that minimizes the chance of obstruction and promotes evacuation.

Pathophysiology

With acute obstruction the outflow of mucous secretions is blocked, and pressure builds within the lumen, resulting in compression of blood vessels and ischemia. Subsequent necrosis causes perforation or rupture with fecal and bacterial contamination of the peritoneal cavity. The resulting inflammation spreads rapidly throughout the abdomen ***(peritonitis)***—especially in young children, who are unable

*Home care instructions for administration of medications and nasogastric and gastrostomy feedings are available in *Wong and Whaley's Clinical Manual of Pediatric Nursing* (Mosby).

to localize infection and who have a thinner appendiceal wall. The omentum, which is not fully developed, is less efficient in walling off the inflammation, sealing perforated viscera, and confining an intraperitoneal disease process. The proximity of all abdominal and pelvic organs favors the spread of peritonitis to accessory digestive and reproductive organs. Progressive peritoneal inflammation results in functional intestinal obstruction of the small bowel ***(ileus)***, since intense GI reflexes severely inhibit bowel motility. Since the peritoneum represents a major portion of total body surface, the loss of extracellular fluid to the peritoneal cavity leads to electrolyte imbalance and hypovolemic shock.

Clinical Manifestations

The most common symptom of appendicitis is colicky abdominal pain and tenderness with guarding of the abdomen. Initially the pain is generalized or periumbilical; however, it usually descends to the lower right quadrant. The most intense site of pain may be at the ***McBurney point***, located midway between the right anterosuperior iliac crest and the umbilicus. This pain is severe, localized (may become diffuse), and constant. Movement, such as an automobile or gurney ride or movement of the examination table, usually aggravates the pain. Nausea, vomiting, and anorexia typically occur *after* the pain starts. Diarrhea, as well as other common signs of childhood illness, such as upper respiratory tract congestion, poor feeding, lethargy, or irritability, may accompany appendicitis. The child may not be able to walk well, complaining of pain in the right hip due to inflammation in the psoas or iliopsoas muscles. There is usually a low-grade fever in appendicitis without perforation; a temperature greater than 39° C (102.2° F) indicates perforation or a viral illness. Absent bowel sounds indicate a perforated appendix with peritonitis.

NURSING ALERT Signs of peritonitis in addition to fever usually include sudden relief from pain after perforation; subsequent increase in pain, which is usually diffuse and accompanied by rigid guarding of the abdomen; progressive abdominal distention; tachycardia; rapid, shallow breathing as the child refrains from using abdominal muscles; pallor; chills; irritability; and restlessness.

Diagnostic Evaluation

The diagnosis is based primarily on the history and physical examination. The cardinal sign of appendicitis is an abrupt onset of constant, localized, and severe pain on abdominal examination. Laboratory evaluation includes a white blood cell count with a differential that is usually elevated but is seldom higher than 15,000 to 20,000 mm^3 with an elevated percentage of bands (often called "shift to the left"), indicating an inflammatory process.

A barium enema or upper GI series with small bowel follow-through may aid in the diagnosis of appendicitis. Ultrasonography should be used to aid in the differentiation of pediatric abdominal pain from other causes (Siegel, Carel, and Surratt, 1991).

Diagnosis is not always straightforward. Numerous infectious and inflammatory processes have features in common. For example, fever, vomiting, abdominal pain, and an elevated blood count are associated with inflammatory bowel disease, acute infectious diarrhea, pelvic inflammatory disease, urinary tract infection, right lower lobe pneumonia, mesenteric adenitis, Meckel diverticulum, and intussusception. In adolescent females the symptoms may be caused by an ectopic pregnancy. Also, diagnosis may be delayed in infants and small children because of the young child's difficulty in verbalizing symptoms, resulting in prolonged symptoms before diagnosis and the presence of associated illness. Consequently, the risk of perforation is greater. One study found that about half of affected adolescents did not "look sick," as judged by the examiner (Reynolds and Jaffe, 1990). Therefore health care providers must have a high degree of suspicion for appendicitis in the differential diagnosis of sudden-onset severe abdominal pain.

Therapeutic Management

The treatment for appendicitis before perforation is surgical removal of the appendix (appendectomy). Usually antibiotics are administered preoperatively. Intravenous fluids and electrolytes are often required before surgery. The operation is usually performed through a right lower quadrant incision. Often the child is discharged from the hospital in 2 to 3 days.

Ruptured Appendix. Management of the child diagnosed with peritonitis caused by a ruptured appendix begins with intravenous administration of fluid and electrolytes, systemic antibiotics, and decompression of the GI tract with a nasogastric (NG) tube preoperatively. Postoperative management includes intravenous fluids and electrolytes, continued administration of antibiotics (gentamicin, ampicillin, and metronidazole or clindamycin), and NG tube suction for abdominal decompression until intestinal motility returns.

In some instances the wound is closed following irrigation of the peritoneal cavity. Many surgeons, however, leave the wound open (delayed closure) to prevent wound infection and abscess formation. A drain may be used to permit transperitoneal drainage.

The treatment of a localized perforation with an appendiceal abscess is controversial. Some surgeons prefer to treat these children with antibiotics and intravenous fluids and allow the abscess to drain spontaneously. An elective appendectomy is then performed 2 to 3 months later.

Prognosis. Complications are uncommon following a simple appendectomy, and recovery is usually rapid and complete. The mortality rate from perforating appendicitis has improved from nearly certain death a century ago to 1% or less at the present time (Samelson and Reyes, 1987). Complications, however, including wound infection and intraabdominal abscess, are not uncommon. Early recognition of the illness is important to prevent complications.

Nursing Considerations

❖ Assessment

Because successful treatment of appendicitis is based on prompt recognition of the disorder, a primary nursing objective is to assist in establishing a diagnosis. Since abdominal pain is a common childhood complaint, the nurse needs to make some preliminary assessment of the severity of the pain (see Chapter 26). One of the most reliable estimates is the degree of change in behavior. A child who stays home from school and voluntarily lies down or refuses to play is much more likely to have considerable pain than a child who is absent from school but plays contentedly at home. The younger nonverbal child may assume a rigid, side-lying position with the knees flexed and have decreased range of motion of the right hip. For those nurses involved in primary ambulatory care, the responsibility of recognizing a possible case of appendicitis and prompt medical and/or surgical referral is particularly important. A detailed history and thorough abdominal examination cannot be overemphasized. Palpating the abdomen should be delayed until all other assessments have been made. The child is instructed to point with one finger to the site of the abdominal pain. Rebound tenderness may be present but is not always a sufficiently reliable test in children. Light palpation will satisfactorily elicit pain without causing excessive trauma (see Atraumatic Care box). Other techniques for assessment of the abdomen are discussed in Chapter 7.

NURSING ALERT In any instance in which severe abdominal pain is expected, the nurse must be aware of the danger of administering laxatives or enemas. Such measures stimulate bowel motility and increase the risk of perforation.

❖ Nursing Diagnoses

Based on a thorough assessment, several nursing diagnoses are identified. The more common diagnoses for the child with acute appendicitis are included in the Nursing Care Plan on p. 1466. Others may apply in specific situations.

❖ Planning

The goals for the child with acute appendicitis and the family include the following:

1. Child and family will be prepared for surgical intervention.
2. Child will receive postoperative care as described for the child undergoing surgery in Chapter 27.
3. Child with peritonitis will not experience postoperative complications, such as spread of infection.
4. Child and family will receive support and education.

❖ Implementation

Physical preparation of the child with appendicitis is similar to that for any child undergoing surgery (see Chapter 27). In situations in which medical treatment is required to correct problems associated with peritonitis, the nurse must anticipate expected procedures and set up equipment as quickly as possible to prevent any delay in preparing the child for surgery. Psychologic preparation of the child and parents is similar to that used in other emergency situations (see Chapter 27).

Postoperative Care. Postoperative care for the nonperforated appendix is the same as for most abdominal operations. Care of the child with a ruptured appendix and peritonitis involves more complex care. The course of recovery is considerably longer and may require up to 2 weeks of hospitalization.

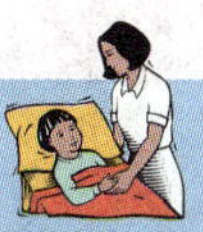

ATRAUMATIC CARE
Palpating the Abdomen for Abdominal Pain

Because children associate the stethoscope with "listening," use the bell piece for initial palpation of the abdomen for tenderness. Children usually endure pressure from the stethoscope that they would not tolerate from a probing hand. Follow with manual palpation, using a gentle touch without lifting the hand from the abdomen while observing the child's face for signs of discomfort.

Ask the child to lift the heels and drop them to the floor two or three times, to hop on one foot, or to "puff out" or "pull in" the abdomen to check for tenderness without more painful probing.

The child is maintained on intravenous fluids and antibiotics; is allowed nothing by mouth; and remains on low, intermittent gastric decompression until there is evidence of return of intestinal motility. Listening for bowel sounds and observing for other signs of bowel activity (such as passage of stool) are part of the routine assessment.

A drain is often placed in the wound during surgery, and frequent dressing changes with meticulous skin care are essential to prevent excoriation of the surgery area. If the wound is left open, moist dressings (usually saline-soaked gauze), as well as wound irrigations with antibacterial solution, are used to provide an optimum healing environment.

Pain management is an essential part of the child's care. Not only is the incision painful, but also the repeated dressing changes and irrigations can cause considerable distress. Since pain is continuous during the first few postoperative days, analgesics, especially opioids, are given around the clock. Procedures are performed when the analgesics have exerted their peak effect. (See also Pain Assessment; Pain Management, Chapter 26).

Psychosocial care after surgery is also important. Sudden, acute illnesses cause unique stress, since there is little time for preparation or planning. Parents and older children need an opportunity to express their feelings and concerns regarding the events surrounding the illness and hospitalization. The nurse can provide important education and psychosocial support to promote adequate coping, with alleviation of anxiety for both the child and the family.

❖ Evaluation

The effectiveness of nursing interventions is determined by continual reassessment and evaluation of care based on the following observational guidelines:

1. Observe child preoperatively for reaction to the situation and compliance with care.
2. Observe for documentation regarding child's emotional and physical needs, especially assessment of pain and administration of analgesics.
3. Monitor child for evidence of infection.
4. Interview and observe child and family for evidence of their understanding of the condition, especially its sudden onset and the need for surgery.

NURSING CARE PLAN

The Child with Appendicitis

Preoperative Care

NURSING DIAGNOSIS: Pain related to inflamed appendix

PATIENT GOAL 1: Will experience no pain or reduction of pain to level acceptable to child

• **NURSING INTERVENTIONS/*RATIONALES***

See Pain Assessment; Pain Management, Chapter 26
Allow position of comfort (usually with legs flexed) *because it may vary among children*
Provide small pillow *for splinting of abdomen*
*Administer analgesia *to provide pain relief*

• **EXPECTED OUTCOME**

Child rests quietly, reports and/or exhibits no evidence of discomfort

NURSING DIAGNOSIS: High risk for fluid volume deficit related to decreased intake and losses secondary to loss of appetite, vomiting

PATIENT GOAL 1: Will receive fluids for adequate hydration

• **NURSING INTERVENTIONS/*RATIONALES***

Maintain NPO *to minimize losses through vomiting and minimize abdominal distention*
Maintain integrity of infusion site *for intravenous fluids and electrolytes*
*Administer intravenous fluids and electrolytes as prescribed
Monitor intake and output *to assess hydration*

• **EXPECTED OUTCOMES**

Child receives sufficient fluids to replace losses
Child exhibits signs of adequate hydration (specify)

NURSING DIAGNOSIS: High risk for infection related to possibility of rupture

PATIENT GOAL 1: Will experience minimized risk of infection

• **NURSING INTERVENTIONS/*RATIONALES***

Closely monitor vital signs, especially for increased heart rate and temperature and rapid, shallow breathing, *to detect ruptured appendix*
Observe for other signs of peritonitis (e.g., sudden relief of pain [sometimes] at time of perforation, followed by increased, diffuse pain and rigid guarding of the abdomen, abdominal distention, bloating, belching [from accumulation of air], pallor, chills, and irritability) *for appropriate treatment to be initiated*
Avoid administering laxatives or enemas, *because these measures stimulate bowel motility and increase risk of perforation*
Monitor WBC count *as indicator of infection*

• **EXPECTED OUTCOMES**

Child remains free of symptoms of peritonitis
Signs of peritonitis are recognized early (specify)

*Dependent nursing action.

Postoperative Care

See Postoperative Care in Nursing Care Plan: The Child Undergoing Surgery, Chapter 27

Ruptured Appendix

NURSING DIAGNOSIS: High risk for spread of infection related to presence of infective organisms in abdomen

PATIENT GOAL 1: Will experience minimized risk of spread of infection

• **NURSING INTERVENTIONS/*RATIONALES***

Provide wound care and dressing changes as prescribed *to prevent infection*
Monitor vital signs and WBC count *to assess presence of infection*
*Administer antibiotics as prescribed

• **EXPECTED OUTCOME**

Child demonstrates resolution of peritonitis as evidenced by lack of fever, clean wound, normal WBC

NURSING DIAGNOSIS: High risk for injury related to absence of bowel motility

PATIENT GOAL 1: Will not experience abdominal distention, vomiting

• **NURSING INTERVENTIONS/*RATIONALES***

Maintain NPO in early postoperative period *to prevent abdominal distention and vomiting*
Maintain NG tube decompression *until bowel motility returns*
Assess abdomen for distention, tenderness, presence of bowel sounds *to assess presence of peristalsis*
Monitor passage of flatus and stool *as indicator of bowel motility*

• **EXPECTED OUTCOME**

Child does not exhibit signs of discomfort; abdomen remains soft and nondistended; child does not vomit

NURSING DIAGNOSIS: Altered family processes related to illness and hospitalization of child

PATIENT (FAMILY) GOAL 1: Will receive adequate support

• **NURSING INTERVENTIONS/*RATIONALES***

Encourage expression of feelings and concerns *to enhance coping*
Encourage child to discuss hospital admission and treatments *in order to clarify misconceptions*
See Nursing Care Plan: The Child in the Hospital, Chapter 26
See Nursing Care Plan: The Family of the Ill or Hospitalized Child, Chapter 26

• **EXPECTED OUTCOMES**

Child and family express feelings and concerns
Child and family demonstrate understanding of hospitalization and treatments

Expected outcomes:
See Nursing Care Plan, p. 1466.

MECKEL DIVERTICULUM

Meckel diverticulum is a remnant of the fetal omphalomesenteric duct that connects the yolk sac with the primitive midgut during fetal life. Normally the structure is obliterated by the seventh to eighth week of gestation, when the placenta replaces the yolk sac as the source of nutrition for the fetus. Failure of obliteration may result in an ***omphalomesenteric fistula*** (a fibrous band connecting the small intestine to the umbilicus), known as Meckel diverticulum.

Meckel diverticulum is a true diverticulum because it arises from the antimesenteric border of the small intestine and includes all layers of the intestinal wall. The position of the diverticulum is variable, although it is usually found within 100 cm of the ileocecal valve (Brown and Olshaker, 1988). Most diverticula are 1 to 10 cm long (Turgeon and Barnett, 1990).

Meckel diverticulum is the most common congenital malformation of the GI tract and is present in 1% to 3% of the population. It is more common in males than in females, and complications are several times more frequent in males. Often it exists without ever causing symptoms. Most symptomatic cases are seen in childhood.

Pathophysiology

The symptomatic complications of Meckel diverticulum are caused by bleeding, obstruction, or inflammation. Gastric mucosa is the most common ectopic tissue found in a Meckel diverticulum. Bleeding, which is the most common problem in children, is caused by peptic ulceration or perforation because of the unbuffered acidic secretion. Several mechanisms may cause obstruction. Intussusception may be led by the Meckel diverticulum. Obstruction may also be caused by entanglement of the small intestine around a fibrous cord, by trapping of a loop of intestine under the band, by incarceration within a hernia sac, or by volvulus of the intestinal segment containing the diverticulum. Diverticulitis occurs when peptic ulceration or obstruction leads to inflammation.

Clinical Manifestations

Signs and symptoms are based on the specific pathologic process, such as inflammation, bleeding, or intestinal obstruction. The most common clinical manifestations include painless rectal bleeding, abdominal pain, or signs of intestinal obstruction. Hematochezia or currant jelly–like stool is the most common symptom in young children, and bleeding may be mild or profuse. The bleeding may be significant enough to cause hypotension. Obstruction occurs more often in adults, but volvulus and intussusception are common presentations in children with Meckel diverticulum.

Diagnostic Evaluation

Diagnosis is usually based on the history, physical examination, and radiographic studies. Radionucleotide scintigraphy (Meckel scan) confirms the diagnosis in 90% of the cases (Turgeon and Barnett, 1990). It consists of intravenous injection of a contrast agent, which accumulates in functional gastric mucosa, including ectopic locations. Laboratory studies are usually part of the general workup to rule out any bleeding disorder and to evaluate the severity of the anemia. Abdominal radiographs, barium enema, and arteriography have generally been unsuccessful as aids in diagnosis.

Therapeutic Management

The standard treatment for symptomatic Meckel diverticulum is surgical removal. In instances in which severe hemorrhage increases the surgical risk, medical intervention to correct hypovolemic shock (e.g., blood replacement, intravenous fluids, and oxygen) may be necessary. In diverticulitis antibiotics may be used preoperatively to control infection. If intestinal obstruction has occurred, appropriate preoperative measures are used to correct fluid and electrolyte imbalances and prevent abdominal distention.

Prognosis. If Meckel diverticulum is diagnosed and treated early, full recovery is likely. The mortality rate of untreated Meckel diverticulum has been reported to range from 2.5% to 15% (Brown and Olshaker, 1988). The serious complications of untreated Meckel diverticulum include GI hemorrhage and bowel obstruction.

Nursing Considerations

Nursing objectives are the same as for any child undergoing surgery (see Chapter 27). When intestinal bleeding is present, specific preoperative considerations include (1) frequent monitoring of vital signs and blood pressure, (2) keeping the child on bed rest, and (3) recording the approximate amount of blood lost in stools.

Postoperatively the child will require intravenous fluids and an NG tube for decompression and evacuation of gastric secretions. Since the onset of illness is usually rapid, psychologic support is important, as in other acute conditions, such as appendicitis. It is important to remember that massive rectal bleeding is most often traumatic to both the child and the parents and may significantly affect their emotional reaction to hospitalization and surgery.

INFLAMMATORY BOWEL DISEASE (IBD)

IBD is a general designation for two chronic intestinal disorders—ulcerative colitis (UC) and Crohn disease (CD). The term should not be confused with irritable bowel syndrome, which refers to a functional disorder (see p. 1463). Although UC and CD are grouped under the classification of IBD because they have similar epidemiologic, immunologic, and clinical features, they are two distinct conditions with very significant differences.

In addition to GI symptoms, each of these diseases is characterized by extraintestinal and systemic inflammatory responses. Exacerbations and remissions without complete resolution are another feature of IBD. In the pediatric population, growth failure is a unique and important problem associated with IBD, especially in CD. CD is often the more disabling condition with more serious complications, and medical and surgical treatment is often less effective than in UC.

CD is now more common than UC in the pediatric population, although the incidence of both UC and CD has increased significantly in the past few decades. The onset of both diseases often occurs in late childhood or adolescence. The incidence in males and females is similar, with a slightly higher incidence of CD in females.

Etiology

The exact cause of IBD is unknown, although there is evidence for a multifactorial etiology. It is proposed that IBD is the result of one or more environmental influences, such as infectious organisms, dietary habits, and environmental toxins, that promote disease in genetically susceptible individuals. For example, there is a familial tendency in about 20% to 25% of cases; individuals from higher socioeconomic levels and more whites than nonwhites are affected; the incidence is several times greater in Jews living in Europe and North America than in the general population; and there is a higher occurrence of disease in urban settings than in rural areas.

The inflammatory response is probably immunologically mediated. A primary role for psychologic factors in the pathogenesis of IBD has not been supported by evidence, although psychologic problems may occur secondary to IBD, and may intensify symptoms and influence the course of the disease.

Ulcerative Colitis (UC)

Pathophysiology and Clinical Manifestations. The inflammation is limited to the colon and rectum, with the distal colon and rectum often the most severely affected. Inflammation usually is limited to the mucosa and submucosa and involves continuous segments along the length of the bowel with varying degrees of ulceration, bleeding, and edema. Water and electrolytes are poorly absorbed by the inflamed mucosa of the colon, resulting in loose stools. Thickening of the bowel wall and fibrosis are unusual, but long-standing disease can result in shortening of the colon and strictures.

The presentation of ulcerative colitis may be mild, moderate, or severe, based on the extent of mucosal inflammation and systemic symptoms. Most include bloody diarrhea or occult fecal blood, abdominal pain, and varying degrees of systemic manifestations and growth abnormalities (Jackson and Grand, 1991).

One of the earliest signs of UC may be growth failure with decreased linear growth velocity (Jackson and Grand, 1991). Growth failure is most likely due to chronic poor dietary intake caused by anorexia due to GI symptoms. UC often presents with the insidious onset of diarrhea, possibly with hematochezia, and usually without fever or weight loss. The course of the disease may remain mild with intermittent exacerbations. Some children and adolescents present with grossly bloody diarrhea, cramps, urgency with defecation, mild anemia, fever, anorexia, weight loss, and moderate signs of systemic illness. Severe UC is characterized by very frequent bloody stools, abdominal pain, significant anemia, fever, and weight loss. ***Extraintestinal manifestations*** are less common in UC than in CD and may precede colitis. The erythrocyte sedimentation rate may be elevated, indicating the presence of a systemic response to an inflammatory process. Enlarged lymph nodes (lymphadenopathy), arthritis, and the skin lesions of erythema nodosum may be present.

Crohn Disease (CD)

Pathophysiology and Clinical Manifestations. The chronic inflammatory process of CD may involve any part of the GI tract from mouth to anus but most commonly affects the terminal ileum. CD usually does not involve a continuous segment of the intestine, and frequently there are areas of inflammation with intact mucosa in between. As with UC, the extent of the disease involvement correlates with the clinical manifestations. The inflammation may result in ulcerations, fibrosis, adhesions, stiffening of the bowel wall, stricture formation, and fistulas to other loops of bowel, bladder, vagina, or skin. The characteristics of UC and CD are listed in Fig. 33-4.

Common presenting manifestations of CD include diarrhea, abdominal pain with cramps, fever, and weight loss. Mild GI symptoms, poor growth, and extraintestinal manifestations may be present for several years before overt GI symptoms are present.

Nonspecific GI symptoms such as satiety, nausea, and burning epigastric pain may be present. Gastroduodenal abnormalities and symptoms are usually due to the Crohn disease rather than peptic ulcer disease, although the symptoms of each are similar. With small intestinal involvement, diarrhea with malabsorption is present as a result of mucosal inflammation, partial bowel obstruction with stasis and bacterial overgrowth, or fistulas. Both malabsorption and anorexia are factors that contribute to the growth problems that are so prevalent in CD.

The disease process can also involve the colon, causing diarrhea, cramps, and urgency with defecation. Signs of colitis, such as gross rectal bleeding or stool with occult blood, are similar to those seen in UC. Perianal disease, including skin tags, abscesses, fissures, and fistulas, is a feature of CD.

Extraintestinal manifestations, including erythema nodosum, large joint arthritis, uveitis, mouth ulcers, liver disease, and renal calculi, are common in CD. Children with CD often have anemia and an elevated white blood cell count and erythrocyte sedimentation rate during exacerbations of the disease. The arthritis associated with CD is a nondestructive synovitis of the large joints that does not cause joint deformity. Skin lesions of erythema nodosum or erythema multiforme usually resolve when the intestinal inflammation is well controlled. Liver disease, usually mild, occurs in a small number of children, but sclerosing cholangitis can cause significant liver dysfunction. Uveitis (inflammation of the uveal tract of the eye, including the iris, ciliary body, and choroid) occurs in only a small number of children. Approximately one third of children and adolescents with

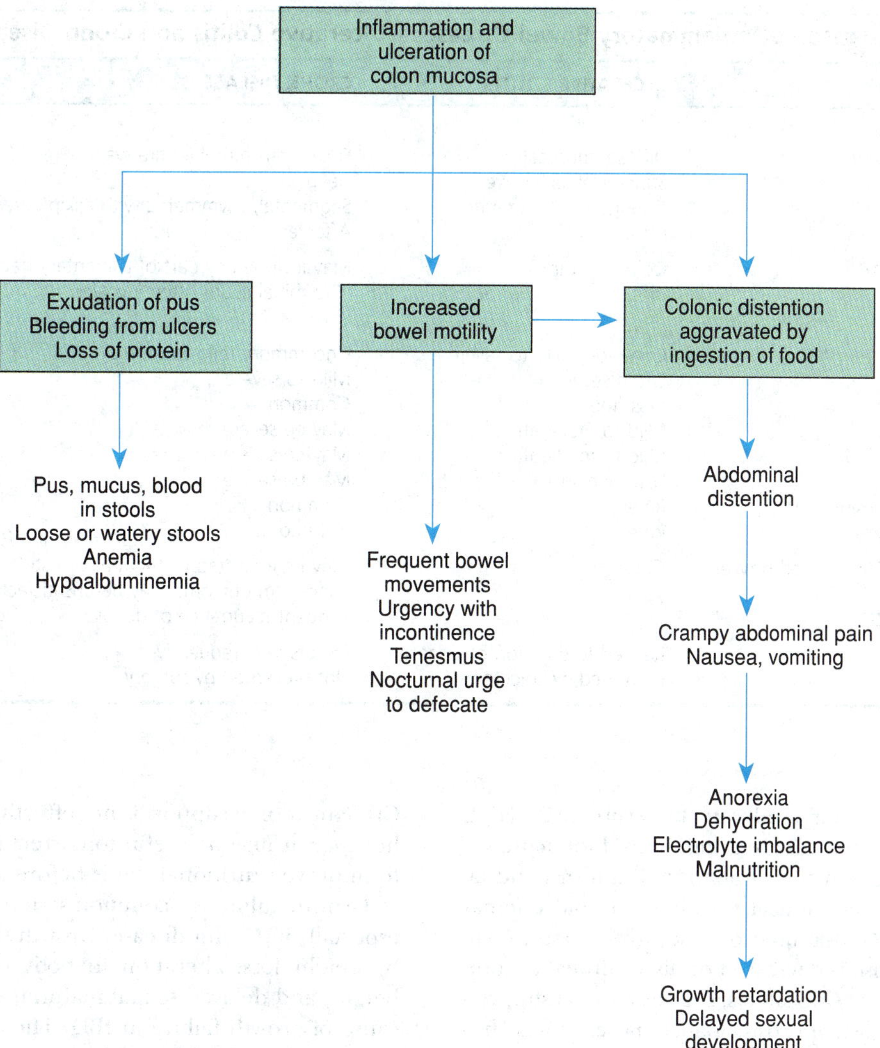

FIG. 33-4 Effects of ulcerative colitis or Crohn disease.

IBD have growth failure and delay in sexual maturation (Seidman, 1989). (See Table 33-2 for characteristics of UC and CD.)

Diagnostic Evaluation

The diagnosis of UC and CD is based on a combination of findings from the history, physical examination, laboratory evaluation, and other diagnostic tests. Laboratory tests include a complete blood count to evaluate anemia and an erythrocyte sedimentation rate to assess the systemic reaction to the inflammatory process. Levels of total protein, albumin, iron, zinc, magnesium, vitamin B_{12}, and fat-soluble vitamins are measured, because they may be low in children with CD. Stool is examined for the presence of blood, leukocytes, and infectious organisms.

An upper GI series with small bowel follow-through is necessary to evaluate small bowel disease in children suspected of having CD; the terminal ileum may be rigid and narrowed with partial obstruction. A CT scan may be indicated to evaluate abscesses or bowel wall thickening. A barium or air contrast enema is usually performed in children with suspected colitis unless the colitis is severe.

Diagnosis of IBD is usually confirmed following endoscopy of the lower and upper GI tracts. The bowel is examined grossly for ulcerations or strictures. Multiple mucosal biopsies are obtained during endoscopy, and the tissue is examined for microscopic changes consistent with inflammation caused by IBD.

Therapeutic Management

The goals of therapy for IBD are (1) to control the inflammatory process in order to reduce or eliminate the symptoms, (2) to obtain long-term remission, (3) to promote normal growth and development, and (4) to allow as normal a life-style as possible. Treatment must be individualized and managed according to the type and severity of the disease and the response to therapy.

Medical Treatment. Corticosteroids are the most ef-

TABLE 33-2 Comparison of Inflammatory Bowel Diseases—Ulcerative Colitis and Crohn Disease

CHARACTERISTICS	ULCERATIVE COLITIS	CROHN DISEASE
Pathologic changes		
Extent of involvement	Diffuse, mucosal	Focal, transmural (entire wall)
Ulceration	Superficial, extensive	Deep
Distribution of lesions	Contiguous, symmetric	Segmental, asymmetric with "skip" areas
Lymph nodes	Normal	Affected
Areas of involvement	Colon, rectum	May include any part of alimentary tract from mouth to anus; terminal ileum often involved
Clinical features		
Intestinal bleeding	Common, mild to severe	Uncommon, mild to severe
Diarrhea	Often severe	Mild to severe
Abdominal pain	Less frequent	Common
Anorexia	Mild to moderate	May be severe
Weight loss	Mild to moderate	May be severe
Growth retardation	Usually mild	May be severe
Anal and perianal lesions	Rare	Common
Fistulas and strictures	Rare	Common
Surgical resection of affected bowel	Curative	May be indicated if strictures or fistulas are present Long-term outcome may be unsatisfactory because of frequent recurrence of disease
Risk of carcinoma	Related to duration of disease Prevented by colectomy	Occurs less frequently Not prevented by surgery

fective drugs for treating moderate to severe IBD. High doses of intravenous steroids are administered for acute exacerbations and are then transitioned to oral forms and tapered according to the clinical response. Steroid enemas may be used with rectosigmoid disease involvement. Generally, the steroid dose is decreased or discontinued as soon as possible to minimize side effects, such as adrenal suppression, hypertension, osteoporosis, glaucoma, cataracts, hirsutism, diabetes, altered body composition, and growth retardation.

Sulfasalazine is useful in the treatment of UC and CD. Since this drug interferes with the absorption of folic acid, daily supplements of folic acid are often prescribed. Side effects of sulfasalazine include allergic responses, headache, nausea, vomiting, neutropenia, and oligospermia. Sulfasalazine is a combination of 5-aminosalicylate and sulfapyridine. Since many of the side effects are due primarily to the sulfapyridine, alternative nonabsorbable salicylate drugs without sulfapyridine, including olsalazine and mesalamine, may be prescribed.

Metronidazole may be useful as an adjunctive therapy in children with CD or with complications such as perianal disease or small bowel bacterial overgrowth. Other immunosuppressive drugs, including 6-mercaptopurine, azathioprine, and cyclosporine A, have been used with success in selected children with IBD. The major risk of these drugs is bone marrow suppression, which can cause leukopenia and opportunistic infections.

Nutritional Support. Nutritional support is a very important component of therapeutic management of IBD. There is some evidence to support the importance of nutritional support as an adjunctive therapy, and possibly as a primary therapy in lieu of corticosteroids, in children with CD. Nutritional support is not effective as a therapy for UC; however, it may be useful to correct growth retardation or to improve nutritional status before surgery.

Growth failure is a common serious complication of IBD, especially in Crohn disease. Growth failure is characterized by weight loss, alteration in body composition, retarded height, and delayed sexual maturation. Malnutrition is the cause of growth failure in IBD. The cause of the malnutrition is multifactorial and includes inadequate dietary intake, excessive GI losses, malabsorption, drug-nutrient interactions, and increased nutritional requirements (Seidman, 1989). Inadequate dietary intake occurs as a result of anorexia associated with chronic disease and episodes of increased disease activity. Excessive losses of nutrients occur secondary to intestinal mucosal inflammation and diarrhea. Stool losses include protein, blood, electrolytes, and minerals. Malabsorption due to mucosal injury and bacterial overgrowth is common in CD. Carbohydrate, lactose, fat, vitamin, and mineral malabsorption can occur in small bowel disease. Vitamin B_{12} and folic acid deficiencies are common in children with disease or resection of the terminal ileum. Increased nutritional requirements are present with increased inflammatory activity, fever, fistulas, and periods of rapid growth, such as adolescence.

The goals of nutritional support include (1) correction of specific nutrient deficits and replacement of ongoing losses, (2) provision of adequate energy and protein for healing, and (3) provision of adequate nutrients to promote normal growth. Nutritional support may include both enteral and parenteral nutrition. A well-balanced, high-protein, high-calorie diet is recommended for children whose symptoms do not prohibit an adequate oral intake. There is little evidence that avoiding specific foods influences the severity of the disease. Foods containing fiber (which is mechanically difficult to digest), such as seeds, popcorn, and corn, may produce symptoms and obstruction in children with intestinal strictures. Supplementation with multivitamins, iron, and folic acid is generally recommended.

Enteral formulas, given by mouth or by continuous NG tube infusion (often at night), may be required to correct nutritional deficiencies and growth retardation. Both polymeric and elemental formulas may correct malnutrition and promote catch-up growth. Elemental formulas have been used successfully to improve nutritional status, as well as to induce remission, in children and adolescents with CD. Several studies have demonstrated that a diet consisting of elemental formula induced remission of the disease either without steroids or with diminished dosage of steroids (Belli and others, 1988).

Total parenteral nutrition (TPN) has been shown to improve nutritional status in children with IBD. Short-term remission of symptoms has been achieved following TPN, although complete "bowel rest" has not been proved to reduce inflammation or to add to the benefits of improved nutrition achieved by TPN (Jackson and Grand, 1991). TPN is primarily indicated as therapy for children with feeding intolerance produced by GI symptoms or in instances where obstruction or fistulas are present. TPN may be useful in nutritional rehabilitation before surgery.

Surgical Treatment. Surgery is indicated for UC when medical and nutritional therapies fail to prevent significant complications. Surgical options include a ***subtotal colectomy*** and ***ileostomy*** with a rectal stump left as a blind pouch. A ***J-pouch*** or ***Kock pouch,*** consisting of terminal ileum, may be created to aid in continence. An ***ileoanal pull-through*** preserves the normal pathway for defecation. Removing the colon ***(total colectomy)*** is curative.

Surgery may be required in children with CD when complications cannot be controlled by medical and nutritional therapy. Segmental intestinal resections are performed for small bowel obstructions or fistulas. Partial colonic resection is not curative, however, since the disease often recurs.

Prognosis. IBD is a chronic disease, often with exacerbations followed by relatively long periods of remission. The outcome of the disease process is influenced by the severity and the region of bowel affected and by compliance with therapy. Malnutrition, growth failure, intestinal strictures and fistulas, and GI bleeding are serious complications of IBD. The overall prognosis for UC is good; surgery to remove the diseased colon often provides a cure. There is no cure for CD.

Carcinoma of the colon is a long-term complication of UC and, less often, of CD. In UC (not CD), removal of the diseased bowel prevents development of carcinoma.

Nursing Considerations

Many of the nursing considerations relate directly to the therapeutic management of IBD. However, the scope of nursing responsibilities includes (1) continued guidance of families in terms of dietary management and drug compliance; (2) adjusting to a disease of remissions and exacerbations, or to one of chronic illness; and (3) when indicated, preparing the child and parents for the possibility of diversionary bowel surgery.

Since nutritional support is a very important component of therapy, encouraging the anorectic child to consume sufficient quantities of food is often a challenge. An approach that is more likely to meet with success involves including the child in meal planning; encouraging small, frequent meals or snacks rather than three large meals a day; and encouraging high-protein, high-calorie foods, such as milk shakes, cream soups, puddings, and custard (if lactose is tolerated). (See also Feeding the Sick Child, Chapter 27.)

A nutritionist should be consulted to provide dietary counseling for the child and family members. Nurses have an important role in preparing children and families to administer NG tube feedings or TPN, if either is indicated, as short- or long-term therapy. The purpose and the expected outcomes of these therapies should be carefully explained. The child and family members' anxieties should be acknowledged, and they should be given adequate time to demonstrate the skills necessary to continue the therapy at home if needed. A referral to a home health agency to ensure continuity of care is beneficial for the child receiving home nutritional support (see Family-Centered Home Care, Chapter 25).

Mouth ulcers may occur in children with CD. These ulcers generally resolve with good control of the disease process, but they may contribute to poor oral intake. Gentle mouth care and the avoidance of hot liquids or foods usually will minimize discomfort (see Stomatitis, Chapter 16).

The importance of continued drug therapy despite remission of symptoms must be stressed to the child and caregivers. Failure to adhere to the pharmacologic regimen can result in exacerbation of the disease process (see Compliance, Chapter 27).

Attending to the emotional aspects of a chronic condition requires a thorough assessment of those stress factors that are disease related. Frequently the nurse can be instrumental in helping these children adjust to the problems of growth retardation, delayed sexual maturation, dietary restrictions, feelings of being different or sickly, inability to compete with peers, and necessary absence from school during the exacerbations of the illness (see Chapter 22). Complications of IBD, especially growth failure, can negatively affect self-esteem, school performance, and social interactions. Nurses can promote positive coping skills by educating the child regarding the disease and the rationale for all therapies. Many children benefit from peer support provided by other children with IBD (see Chapter 22).

In the event that a permanent ileostomy is required, the nurse can assist the child and family in accepting and adjusting to the change by teaching them how to care for the ileostomy, emphasizing the positive aspects of surgery (particularly, accelerated growth and sexual development, permanent recovery, and eliminated risk of colonic cancer) and stressing the normality of life despite bowel diversion. Introducing the child and parents to other ostomy patients, especially those of the child's age, can be the greatest therapeutic measure in fostering eventual acceptance. The family should discuss the option of a continent ostomy with the child's surgeon.

Because of the chronic and often lifelong nature of the disease, families benefit from many of the services provided by organizations such as the **Crohn's and Colitis Foundation of America, Inc. (CCFA),*** which has branches in many major communities and provides education regarding the management of IBD. If diversionary bowel surgery is indicated, the **United Ostomy Association**† and the **International Association for Enterostomal Therapy**‡ are available to assist with ileostomy care and provide important psychologic support through their self-help group. (See also Nursing Care Plan: The Child with Inflammatory Bowel Disease.§)

PEPTIC ULCER DISEASE (PUD)

PUD is a chronic condition causing a circumscribed loss of tissue of the mucosal, submucosal, and sometimes muscular layer in parts of the GI tract exposed to acid-pepsin gastric secretions. Ulcers are described as gastric or duodenal and as primary or secondary. A ***gastric ulcer*** involves the mucosa of the stomach, and a ***duodenal ulcer*** involves the pylorus or duodenum. ***Primary ulcers*** occur in the absence of a predisposing factor. ***Secondary ulcers,*** or ***stress ulcers,*** occur as a result of the stress of a severe underlying disease or injury (e.g., severe burns, sepsis, multisystem organ failure), or ingestion of an ulcerogenic drug (e.g., salicylates, nonsteroidal antiinflammatory agents, ferrous sulfate).

Stress ulcers occur more frequently in infancy and early childhood. In older children and adolescents the majority of ulcers are primary. The incidence of ulcers in boys is two to three times greater than the incidence in girls, although this difference is less in very young children.

Etiology

The etiology of PUD in children is unknown, although both genetic and environmental factors appear to be important. There is an increased familial incidence and an increased incidence in persons with blood group O.

There is a significant relationship between the bacterium *Helicobacter pylori* (previously called *Campylobacter pylori*) and ulcers. *H. pylori,* known to colonize the gastric mucosa, has been identified in 90% to 100% of adult patients with PUD (Nord, 1988). It may cause ulcers by weakening the gastric mucosal barrier and allowing acid to damage the mucosa.

In addition to ulcerogenic drugs, both alcohol and smoking are known to contribute to ulcer formation. There is no conclusive evidence to implicate particular foods, such as caffeine-containing beverages or spicy foods, as a cause of PUD. Polyunsaturated fats and fiber may play a role in ulcer prevention.

Psychologic factors may play a role in the development of PUD. Stressful life events and dependency, passiveness, and hostility have all been implicated as contributing factors in PUD. Many psychologic studies, however, are uncontrolled, which makes it difficult to determine the pathogenesis of emotional factors in PUD.

Pathophysiology

Most likely, the pathogenesis of PUD is due to an imbalance between destructive factors that promote the formation of peptic ulcers and protective factors that guard against ulcer formation (Ziller and Netchvolodoff, 1993). The gastroduodenal epithelium secretes a layer of water-insoluble mucus gel that serves as a protective barrier against hydrogen ions, which are neutralized by the bicarbonate within the mucus. Prostaglandins appear to play a role in mucosal defense, because they stimulate both mucus and alkali secretions. Abnormalities of the mucus-bicarbonate barrier, such as infection, are likely to contribute to ulcer formation.

The most important endogenous destructive factors include gastric acid and pepsin production. When abnormalities in the protective barrier exist, the mucosa is vulnerable to damage by acid and pepsin. Exogenous factors, such as aspirin and nonsteroidal antiinflammatory drugs, have been shown to cause gastric ulcer by inhibition of prostaglandin synthesis. The pathogenesis, manifestations, and complications of PUD are outlined in Fig. 33-5.

Clinical Manifestations

The clinical manifestations of PUD vary according to the age of the child and the location of the ulcer (Table 33-3). Common clinical manifestations include chronic abdominal pain, especially when the stomach is empty, such as during the night or early morning; recurrent vomiting; hematemesis; melena; chronic anemia; and abdominal tenderness.

Diagnostic Evaluation

Diagnosis is based on the history (pattern of pain), physical examination (pain in the epigastric area), and diagnostic testing, such as radiographs, barium studies, and endoscopy. Endoscopy of the upper GI tract is the most reliable test to diagnose PUD. Laboratory tests include a complete blood count and stool analysis for occult blood.

Therapeutic Management

The major goals of therapy for children with PUD are to relieve discomfort, promote healing, and prevent complications and recurrence. The management is primarily medical and consists of administration of medications to treat the infection or reduce or neutralize gastric acid secretion. Whenever possible, known stressors are reduced.

Antacids are widely prescribed in the initial treatment of peptic ulcers. Antacids have mucosal protective properties and neutralize acid. Aluminum or magnesium antacids are administered 1 and 3 hours after each meal and at bedtime. The frequency may be reduced as healing occurs, but ant-

*444 Park Ave., South, New York, NY 10016; (212) 679-1570.

†36 Executive Park, Suite 120, Irvine, CA 92714-6744; (714) 660-8624.

‡2081 Business Center Dr., Suite 290, Irvine, CA 92715; (714) 476-0268. In Canada: **Canadian Foundation for Ileitis and Colitis,** 21 St. Clair Ave., East, Suite 301, Toronto, Ontario M4TL 1L9, (416) 920-5035; **United Ostomy Association, Canada,** 5 Hamilton Ave., Hamilton, Ontario L8V 2L3, (416) 389-8822.

§In *Wong and Whaley's Clinical Manual of Pediatric Nursing* (Mosby).

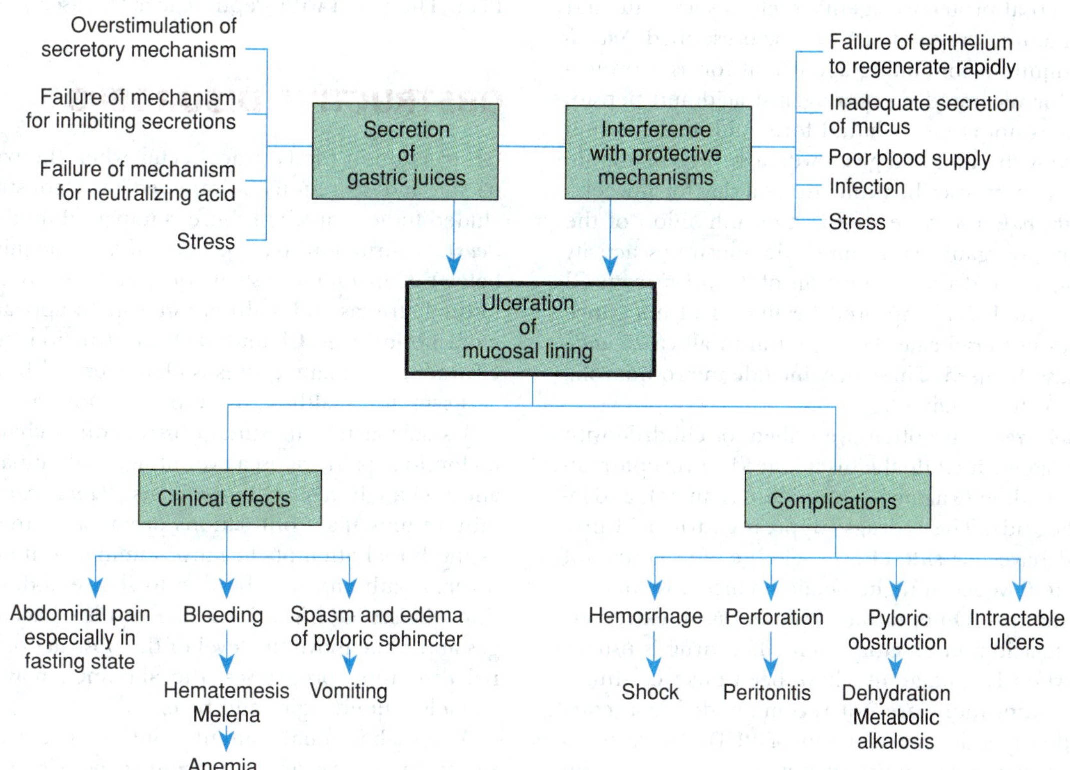

FIG. 33-5 Possible causes and effects of peptic ulcer.

TABLE 33-3 Clinical Manifestations of Peptic Ulcers

TYPE OF ULCER	MANIFESTATIONS	COMMENTS
NEONATES		
Usually gastric and secondary	Perforation may occur Often massive hemorrhage Same as seen in stress ulcers	May be catastrophic More likely in infants with hypoxia, sepsis, difficult labor/delivery, or nasogastric feeding
INFANTS TO 2-YEAR-OLD CHILDREN		
Gastric or duodenal, primary or secondary	Poor eating, vomiting, irritability, melena, hematemesis Vague discomfort	Primary ulcers more likely to be gastric with slow onset Usually bleed rather than perforate
2- TO 6-YEAR-OLD CHILDREN		
Gastric or duodenal	Vomiting, generalized or epigastric pain, melena, hematemesis Wake at night crying with pain	Diagnosis often made on basis of history Duodenal ulcers 5:1 over gastric Perforation more likely in secondary ulcers
6- TO 9-YEAR-OLD CHILDREN		
Usually duodenal and primary	Pain—burning or tenderness in epigastrium related to fasting state, melena, hematemesis, vomiting	May be related to emotional stress
CHILDREN OVER 9 YEARS		
Usually duodenal	Vomiting, epigastric pain, melena, hematemesis	More typical of adult type Chances of recurrence greater than 50%

acids are often prescribed for several weeks. Diarrhea is a common side effect of magnesium-containing antacids, and compliance with the frequent dosing schedule may be a problem.

Other mucosal protective agents, such as sucralfate and bismuth-containing preparations, may be prescribed. ***Sucralfate*** is an aluminum-containing agent that forms a protective barrier for ulcerated mucosa against acid and pepsin. Sucralfate does not come in liquid form, although the pill can be mixed with water and given with a syringe or spoon. This drug may be prescribed four times a day for 6 weeks. ***Bismuth compounds*** also have an effect on inhibition of the growth of microorganisms. Bismuth demonstrates activity against *H. pylori,* and the eradication of *H. pylori* from GI tissue is associated with improved healing of ulcers. Since bismuth does not eradicate the organism in all cases, ***antibiotics*** may also be used. These may include metronidazole, amoxicillin, or tetracycline.

Antisecretory agents are often prescribed for children with PUD. These agents include the histamine (H_2) receptor antagonists cimetidine (Tagamet), ranitidine (Zantac), and famotidine (Pepcid). These drugs suppress gastric acid production and have few side effects. The general course of therapy is 4 to 6 weeks. A nightly maintenance dose may be given for 6 months. Omeprazole (Prilosec) is an extremely potent gastric acid antisecretory agent. This drug is usually prescribed when H_2 antagonists have been unsuccessful.

Dietary modifications are not recommended as a component of therapeutic management of PUD. There is no evidence that dietary factors contribute to ulcer formation or that special diets are effective in the treatment of PUD.

Surgical intervention may be required in the management of complications of PUD, such as hemorrhage, perforation, or gastric outlet obstruction. Ligation of the source of bleeding or closure of a perforation may be performed. A vagotomy and pyloroplasty may be indicated in children with recurring ulcers despite aggressive medical treatment.

Prognosis. The long-term prognosis for PUD is variable. Many ulcers can be successfully treated with medical therapy; however, primary duodenal peptic ulcers frequently recur. Complications, such as GI bleeding, can occur that extend into adulthood. The effect of maintenance drug therapy on long-term morbidity remains to be established with further studies.

Nursing Considerations

The main nursing objective is to promote healing of the inflamed mucosa through compliance with the medication regimen. If an analgesic/antipyretic is needed for other reasons during the course of therapy, acetaminophen, not aspirin, is used. Drug compliance is essential and can be a problem with frequent administration of antacids. Therefore strategies to improve compliance are instituted early in the course of therapy (see Chapter 27). The child and caregiver should be educated about the disease process and the rationale for drug therapy.

Although the exact role stress plays in the pathogenesis of PUD in children is unclear, the nurse should be aware of those family and environmental conditions that may have precipitated or may aggravate the condition. Children may benefit from psychologic counseling and from learning how to cope more constructively with stresses in their lives, such as from school, family, and friends. (See also Nursing Care Plan: The Child with Peptic Ulcer Disease.*)

OBSTRUCTIVE DISORDERS

Obstruction in the GI tract occurs when the passage of nutrients and secretions is impeded by a constricted or occluded lumen, or when there is impaired motility ***(paralytic ileus)***. Obstructions may be congenital or acquired (see box below). Congenital obstructions, such as esophageal or intestinal atresias and malrotation, usually appear in the neonatal period (see Chapter 11). Obstruction in part of the GI tract from many causes is characterized by similar signs and symptoms, although the progression may vary greatly.

Usually, acute intestinal obstruction is characterized by abdominal pain, nausea, vomiting, abdominal distention, and a change in stooling patterns. ***Pain*** is caused by intermittent muscular contractions proximal to the obstruction as the bowel attempts to move luminal contents along the normal path and may be due to severe abdominal distention. ***Abdominal distention*** is the result of accumulation of gas and fluid above the level of the obstruction. As abdominal distention progresses, the abdomen may become extremely tender, rigid, and firm.

When abdominal contents continue to accumulate, nausea and vomiting occur. ***Vomiting of gastric contents*** is often the first sign of a high obstruction, such as obstruction of the pylorus, and ***vomiting of bile-stained material*** is a sign of obstruction of the small intestine. Persistent vomiting can lead to dehydration and electrolyte disturbances. ***Constipation*** and ***obstipation*** (prolonged absence of defecation) are early signs of low obstructions and later signs of higher obstructions. In acute conditions such as intussusception, the clinical manifestations are apparent within a few hours of the onset of the disorder. In other conditions such as pyloric stenosis, the signs and symptoms may have a more gradual onset. ***Bowel sounds*** may initially be hyperactive,

*In *Wong and Whaley's Clinical Manual of Pediatric Nursing* (Mosby).

CAUSES OF INTESTINAL OBSTRUCTION IN CHILDREN

CONGENITAL	ACQUIRED
Atresia	Pyloric stenosis
Incarcerated hernia	Intussusception
Imperforate anus	Postoperative adhesions or strictures
Meckel diverticulum	Tumor
Hirschsprung disease	Foreign body
Stricture	
Malrotation	
Volvulus	
Meconium plug	
Meconium ileus	
Annular pancreas	

then diminish or cease. ***Respiratory distress*** may occur when the diaphragm is pushed up into the pleural cavity as a result of severe abdominal distention.

HYPERTROPHIC PYLORIC STENOSIS (HPS)

HPS occurs when the circular muscle of the pylorus becomes thickened, causing constriction of the pylorus and obstruction of the gastric outlet. This condition usually develops in the first few weeks of life, causing projectile vomiting, dehydration, metabolic alkalosis, and failure to thrive. HPS is more common in firstborn children, and males are affected five times more frequently than females. Inheritance is polygenic, with an increased risk in siblings and offspring of affected persons. HPS is seen less frequently in black and Oriental infants than in white infants. It is more likely to affect a full-term infant than a premature one. The precise etiology of pyloric stenosis is not known.

Pathophysiology

The circular muscle of the pylorus is grossly enlarged as a result of both hypertrophy (increased size) and hyperplasia (increased mass). This produces severe narrowing of the pyloric canal between the stomach and the duodenum. Consequently, the lumen at this point is partially obstructed. Over a period of time, inflammation and edema further reduce the size of the opening until the partial obstruction may progress to complete obstruction. The muscle is thickened to as much as twice its usual size (2 to 3 cm). The hypertrophied pylorus may be palpable as an olivelike mass in the upper abdomen.

Pyloric stenosis is not a congenital disorder. Evidence suggests that local innervation may be involved in the pathogenesis. In most cases this is an isolated lesion; however, it may be associated with intestinal malrotation, esophageal and duodenal atresia, and anorectal anomalies (Fig. 33-6).

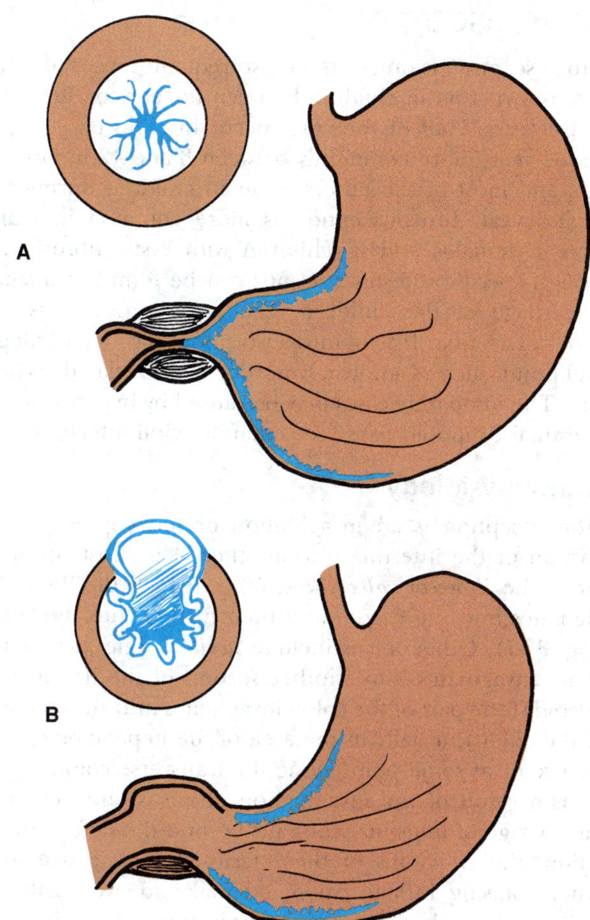

FIG. 33-6 Hypertrophic pyloric stenosis. **A,** Enlarged muscular tumor nearly obliterates pyloric channel. **B,** Longitudinal surgical division of muscle down to submucosa establishes adequate passageway.

Clinical Manifestations

Infants with HPS present with vomiting; the emesis contains milk or formula and is not bile stained. The vomiting usually starts in the second or third week of life, but it may not appear until several months of age. The vomiting usually becomes forceful and projectile. Initially the infant may be hungry and irritable, and later becomes lethargic, dehydrated, and malnourished. Gastric peristalsis may be visible on examination, and the olive-shaped mass in the epigastrium just to the right of the umbilicus may be palpated.

Diagnostic Evaluation

The diagnosis of HPS is often made following the history and physical examination. The olivelike mass is most easily palpated when the stomach is empty, the infant is quiet, and the abdominal muscles are relaxed. When there is doubt about the diagnosis, radiographic or ultrasound studies should be obtained. A plain film may show a dilated stomach, and ultrasound studies confirm the presence of a pyloric mass. Barium studies show the elongated and narrowed pyloric canal.

Laboratory findings reflect the metabolic alterations created by severe depletion of both water and electrolytes from extensive and prolonged vomiting. There are decreased serum levels of both sodium and potassium, although these may be masked by the hemoconcentration from extracellular fluid depletion. Of greater diagnostic value are a decrease in serum chloride levels and increases in pH and bicarbonate (carbon dioxide content), indicative of metabolic alkalosis. The blood urea nitrogen will be elevated as evidence of dehydration.

Therapeutic Management

Surgical relief of the pyloric obstruction by pyloromyotomy is the standard therapy for this disorder. Preoperatively, the infant must be rehydrated, and metabolic alkalosis is corrected with parenteral fluid and electrolyte administration. Replacement fluid therapy usually delays surgery for 24 to 48 hours. The stomach is decompressed with a nasogastric (NG) tube. In infants with no evidence of fluid and electrolyte imbalance, surgery is performed without delay.

The surgical procedure is performed through a right upper quadrant incision and consists of a longitudinal incision through the circular muscle fibers of the pylorus down to but not including the submucosa (***pyloromyotomy,*** sometimes called ***Fredet-Ramstedt procedure***) (Fig. 33-6, *B*). The procedure has a very high success rate.

Feedings are usually begun 4 to 6 hours postoperatively, beginning with small, frequent feedings of glucose, water, or electrolyte solution. If clear fluids are retained, about 24 hours after surgery formula is started in the same small increments. The amount and the interval between feedings are gradually increased until a full feeding schedule is reinstated, which usually takes about 48 hours. The infant is often discharged from the hospital by the second or third postoperative day.

Prognosis. The prognosis is excellent, and the mortality is low. Postoperative complications include persistent pyloric obstruction and wound dehiscence. Approximately 15% of infants with HPS also have gastroesophageal reflux (Milla, 1991).

Nursing Considerations

Nursing care involves primarily observation for clinical features that help establish the diagnosis, careful regulation of fluid therapy, and reestablishment of normal feeding patterns. Nurses are in a position to recognize signs of HPS in infants and to refer them for medical evaluation. The possibility of HPS should be considered in the very young infant who fails to gain weight and has a history of vomiting after meals. Assessment is based on observation of eating behaviors, evidence of characteristic clinical manifestations, and hydration and nutritional status.

Preoperatively the emphasis is placed on restoring hydration and electrolyte balance. The infant is allowed nothing by mouth and is given intravenous fluids of glucose and electrolytes based on serum electrolyte values, usually sodium chloride solution with added potassium (when there is adequate urinary output). Careful monitoring of the intravenous infusion and strict monitoring of intake, output, and urine specific gravity measurements are important nursing responsibilities. Accurate description of any vomiting, as well as the number and character of stools, is recorded.

Observations include assessment of vital signs, particularly those that indicate fluid or electrolyte imbalances. The infant is especially prone to metabolic alkalosis from loss of hydrogen ions, and depletion of potassium, sodium, and chloride, all of which are contained in gastric secretions. The skin and mucous membranes are assessed for alterations in hydration status, and daily weights should be obtained (see Chapter 28 for manifestations of fluid and electrolyte disturbances). It is the responsibility of the nurse to ensure that the NG tube is patent and functioning properly and to measure and record the type and amount of drainage.

As with any child in the hospital, parents are encouraged to visit and become involved in the child's care. Most parents need support and reassurance that the condition is caused by a structural problem and is not a reflection of their parenting skills and capacities.

Postoperative Care. Postoperative vomiting is not uncommon, and most infants, even with successful surgery, exhibit some vomiting during the first 24 to 48 hours. Intravenous fluids are administered until the infant is taking and retaining adequate amounts by mouth. Therefore much of the same care that was instituted before surgery is continued postoperatively, including observation of vital signs, monitoring of intravenous fluids, and careful monitoring of intake and output. In addition, the infant is observed for responses to the stress of surgery and for evidence of pain. Appropriate analgesics are given.

The NG tube may be maintained after surgery for a short time. Feedings are usually instituted within 24 hours postoperatively, beginning with clear liquids containing glucose and electrolytes. They are offered in small quantities at frequent intervals as ordered by the physician. If the infant has been breast-fed, breast milk, expressed by the mother, may be given by bottle when the infant is able to tolerate feedings, or the mother is instructed to limit nursing time and gradually increase the time to previous patterns. Supervision of feedings is an important part of postoperative care. Care of the operative site consists of observation for any drainage or signs of inflammation and care of the incision as directed by the surgeon. Poorly nourished infants may have problems with wound healing. (See also Nursing Care Plan: The Child with Hypertrophic Pyloric Stenosis.*)

INTUSSUSCEPTION

Intussusception is one of the most frequent causes of intestinal obstruction in children between the ages of 3 months and 5 years. Half of the cases occur in children younger than 1 year, more commonly between 3 and 12 months of age, and most of the others occur in children during the second year. Intussusception is more common in males than in females and in children with cystic fibrosis. Although specific intestinal lesions can be found in a small percentage of the children, generally the cause is not known. Less than 10% of intussusceptions have a pathologic lead point, such as a polyp, lymphoma, or Meckel diverticulum. The idiopathic cases may be caused by hypertrophy of intestinal lymphoid tissue secondary to viral infection.

Pathophysiology

Intussusception is an invagination or telescoping of one portion of the intestine into another. The most common site is the ***ileocecal valve (ileocolic),*** in which the ileum invaginates into the cecum and then further into the colon (Fig. 33-7). Other forms include ***ileoileal*** (one part of the ileum invaginates into another section of the ileum) and ***colocolic*** (one part of the colon invaginates into another area of the colon), usually in the area of the hepatic or splenic flexure or at some point along the transverse colon.

As a result of the invagination, there is obstruction to the passage of intestinal contents beyond the defect. In addition, the two walls of the intestine press against each other, causing inflammation, edema, and eventually decreased blood flow. Ischemia, perforation, peritonitis, and shock are serious complications of intussusception.

---

*In *Wong and Whaley's Clinical Manual of Pediatric Nursing* (Mosby).

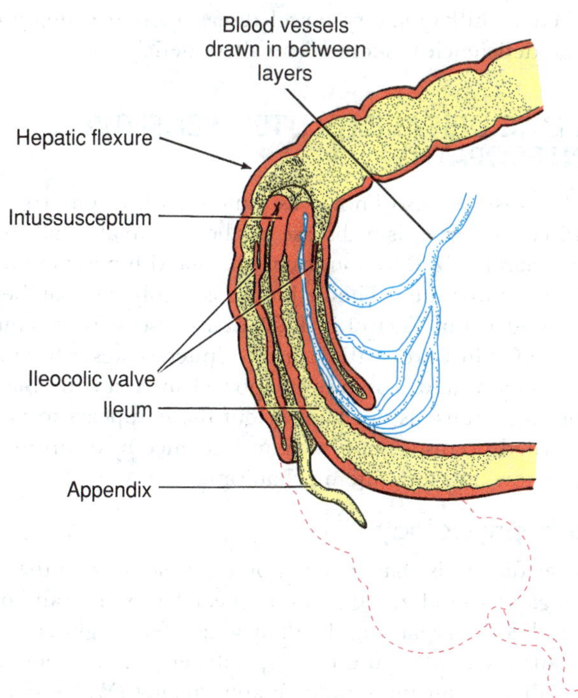

FIG. 33-7 Ileocolic intussusception.

Clinical Manifestations

The classic presentation of intussusception is a healthy, thriving child, usually between 3 and 12 months of age, who suddenly has an episode of acute colicky abdominal pain. Typical behavior includes screaming and drawing the knees up to the chest. These episodes of severe pain are characterized by intervals in which the child appears normal and comfortable.

During this initial period, vomiting usually occurs, the abdomen is soft, and the child may pass a normal stool. A sausage-shaped mass may be felt in the upper right quadrant. The classic currant jelly–like stool (stool mixed with blood and mucus) occurs later in the disease, and the abdomen becomes tender and distended. With atypical cases, lethargy may be the primary presenting symptom (Hickey, Sodhi, and Johnson, 1990; Knudson, 1988). If treatment is not sought, the child may become acutely ill, with fever and prostration, and exhibit signs of peritonitis (see p. 1464).

NURSING ALERT The classic signs and symptoms of intussusception may not be present; a more chronic picture may occur, characterized by diarrhea, anorexia, weight loss, occasional vomiting, and periodic pain. The older child may have pain without other signs or symptoms. Since this condition is potentially life-threatening, be aware of such signs and closely observe and refer these children for further medical investigation.

Diagnostic Evaluation

Frequently the diagnosis can be made on subjective findings alone. However, definitive diagnosis is based on a barium enema, which clearly demonstrates the obstruction to the flow of barium. Initially an abdominal radiograph is obtained to detect intraperitoneal air, which would contraindicate a barium enema. A rectal examination reveals mucus, blood, and occasionally a low intussusception itself.

Therapeutic Management

In many cases the initial treatment of choice is nonsurgical hydrostatic reduction, traditionally by barium enema. In this procedure correction of the invagination is carried out at the same time as the diagnostic testing. The force exerted by the flowing barium is usually sufficient to push the invaginated portion of the bowel into its original position, similar to pushing an inverted "finger" out of a glove.

The use of barium as the contrast agent is becoming less routine. Presently a high percentage of radiologists use water-soluble contrast and air pressure to reduce intussusceptions (Meyer, 1992). The increased use of water-soluble contrast reflects concern regarding the risk of barium peritonitis. The administration of air pressure to reduce intussusception is as successful as and more rapid than barium, without the risk of peritonitis (Tamanaha and others, 1987). Intravenous fluids, nasogastric decompression, and antibiotic therapy may be given before attempts at hydrostatic reduction are made.

Since this procedure is not always successful and is not recommended if there are clinical signs of shock or perforation, the child may require surgical intervention. Surgery involves manually reducing the invagination and, where indicated, resecting any nonviable intestine.

Prognosis. Nonoperative reduction is successful in more than 75% of cases. The risk of recurrence is about 10%. Surgery is required for those patients in whom the contrast enema was unsuccessful. If untreated, approximately 10% of children will have spontaneous reduction or chronic intussusception. The other 90% of untreated children will suffer from complications such as perforation, peritonitis, and sepsis (Knudson, 1988). With early diagnosis and treatment, serious complications and death are very uncommon.

Nursing Considerations

The nurse can assist in establishing a diagnosis by obtaining the history of the child's physical and behavioral symptoms. Although parents may not know the medical problem, they are astute in detecting a change in the child's behavior.

NURSING ALERT A report of severe colicky abdominal pain in a child with vomiting and currant jelly–like stools is a significant clue to intussusception.

As soon as intussusception is suspected, the nurse begins to prepare the parents for the immediate need for hospitalization, the usual nonsurgical techniques, and the possibility of surgery. It is important at this time to explain the basic defect of intussusception and how an intussusception is corrected with contrast enemas.

➤ **NURSING TIP** Intussception is easily demonstrated by pushing the end of a "finger" on a rubber glove back into itself or using the example of a telescoping rod. The principle of reduction by hydrostatic pressure can be simulated by filling the glove with water, which pushes the finger into a fully extended position.

Even though nonsurgical intervention is often successful, preoperative procedures may be performed. For the child with signs of electrolyte imbalance, hemorrhage, or peritonitis, additional medical preparations such as replacement fluids, antibiotics, and nasogastric suctioning may be indicated. All stools are examined before hydrostatic reduction or surgery.

NURSING ALERT Passage of a normal brown stool usually indicates that the intussusception has reduced itself. This is immediately reported to the physician, who may choose to alter the diagnostic/therapeutic plan of care.

Following hydrostatic reduction, the nurse observes for passage of barium or water-soluble contrast material with stools. The child should be admitted to the hospital for 12 to 24 hours for observation. The parents should be educated about the risk of recurrence. If intussusception recurs, hydrostatic reduction is usually attempted. A laparotomy is considered for multiple recurrences. If surgical reduction or bowel resection is performed, postoperative care is similar to that following any abdominal surgery (see Chapter 27).

Family Support. Since this hospitalization may be the child's first separation from the parents, it is especially important to preserve the parent-child relationship by encouraging rooming-in. It may also be the parents' first experience with hospital care for their child, necessitating their preparation for procedures such as intravenous therapy, frequent vital sign and blood pressure monitoring, and special orders, such as nothing by mouth. Because of the rapidity of the onset, diagnosis, and treatment, parents may be left with the feeling of stunned numbness. They may ask few questions, or they may constantly make inquiries, sometimes the same ones several times. If the nurse realizes the circumstances surrounding this condition, the parents' reactions are more likely to be understood and accepted. (See also Nursing Care Plan: The Child with Intussusception.*)

MALABSORPTION SYNDROMES

Malabsorption syndromes are characterized by chronic diarrhea and malabsorption of fluid and nutrients. An important complication of malabsorption syndromes in children is failure to thrive. Malabsorption may be caused by a ***decreased intestinal surface area*** (short bowel syndrome), ***pancreatic insufficiency*** resulting in decreased pancreatic enzymes for digestion (cystic fibrosis, chronic pancreatitis, Schwachman syndrome), and ***inadequate macronutrient digestion*** at the brush border level with decreased brush border enzymes due to villous injury (celiac disease, food allergy, infection, inflammatory bowel disease) or to primary enzyme deficiencies (sucrase-isomaltase deficiency).

*In *Wong and Whaley's Clinical Manual of Pediatric Nursing* (Mosby).

CELIAC DISEASE (GLUTEN-SENSITIVE ENTEROPATHY)

Celiac disease, also known as gluten-sensitive enteropathy and celiac sprue, is a disease of the proximal small intestine characterized by abnormal mucosa with permanent intolerance to gluten. The incidence is highly variable, being reported as 1 in 300 to 1 in 4000. Celiac disease is seen more frequently in Europe than in the United States, where it is uncommon, and it is rarely reported in Asians or Blacks. The exact cause is not known, but there appears to be an inherited predisposition with an influence by environmental factors and immune mechanisms.

Pathophysiology

Celiac disease is characterized by an intolerance to the protein ***gluten*** found in the grain of wheat, barley, rye, and oats. Two theories regarding the damaging effect of gluten in celiac disease are that there is a specific enzyme deficiency or that there is an immunologic abnormality (Walker-Smith, 1991). The mucosa of the small intestine becomes damaged, and villous atrophy, hyperplasia of the crypts, and infiltration of the epithelial cells with lymphocytes occur. Villous atrophy leads to malabsorption due to the reduced absorptive surface area (see Fig. 33-1 and the discussion of absorption on p. 1449).

Clinical Manifestations

Symptoms of celiac disease most often appear between the ages of 1 and 5 years. There is usually an interval of several months between the introduction of gluten into the diet and the onset of symptoms. The clinical manifestations are variable. Diarrhea may be acute or insidious, and the stools are often described as watery and pale, with an offensive odor. Anorexia is often present, as well as abdominal pain. Some children have severe abdominal distention and muscle wasting, particularly in the buttocks and extremities. Vomiting, anemia, and constipation can also be manifestations of celiac disease. Behavioral changes such as extreme irritability and fretfulness may be present.

Diagnostic Evaluation

The definitive diagnosis of celiac disease is based on a jejunal biopsy that demonstrates the appearance of small, flat intestinal mucosa with hyperplastic villous atrophy while the child is eating adequate amounts of gluten. Second, the diagnosis is confirmed following a full clinical remission and resolution of the jejunal mucosal abnormalities after withdrawal of gluten from the diet. The presence of antigliadin, antireticulin, and antiendomysial IgG and IgA antibodies, and their disappearance when gluten is removed from the diet, aids in the diagnosis (Walker-Smith and others, 1990). A new method for the rapid detection of serum IgG and IgA antigliadin antibodies permits screening for the disease and monitoring the response to therapy (Not and others, 1993).

Therapeutic Management

Treatment of celiac disease consists primarily of dietary management. Although a gluten-free diet is prescribed, it is difficult to remove every source of this protein. Also, some patients are able to tolerate restricted amounts of gluten. Since gluten is found mainly in the grains of wheat and rye, but also in smaller quantities in barley and oats, these four foods are eliminated. Corn, rice, and millet are substitute grain foods.

Children with untreated celiac disease may have lactose intolerance, especially if their mucosal lesions are extensive. Lactose intolerance usually improves as the mucosa heals with gluten withdrawal. Specific nutritional deficiencies, such as iron, folic acid, and fat-soluble vitamin deficiencies, are treated with appropriate supplements.

Prognosis. Celiac disease is generally regarded as a chronic disease; its severity varies greatly among children. The most severe symptoms usually occur in early childhood and again in adult life. Most children who comply with dietary management are healthy and remain free of symptoms and complications. Strict dietary avoidance of gluten may minimize the risk of developing lymphoma, especially of the small intestine, one of the most serious complications of the disease.

Nursing Considerations

The main nursing consideration is helping the child adhere to dietary management. This involves considerable time in explaining the disease process to the child and the parents, the specific role of gluten in aggravating the disorder, and those foods that must be restricted. It is especially difficult to maintain a diet indefinitely when the child has no symptoms and temporary transgressions result in no difficulties. Although the chief source of gluten is cereal and baked goods, grains are frequently added to processed foods as thickeners or fillers. To compound the difficulty, gluten is added to many foods as hydrolyzed vegetable protein, which is derived from cereal grains. The nurse must advise parents of the necessity of reading all label ingredients carefully to avoid hidden sources of gluten.

Many of children's favorite foods contain gluten, including bread, cake, cookies, crackers, donuts, pies, spaghetti, pizza, prepared soups, some processed ice cream, many types of chocolate candy, milk preparations such as malts, hot dogs, luncheon meats, meat gravy, and some prepared hamburgers. Many of these products can be eliminated from the infant's or young child's diet fairly easily, but monitoring the diet of the school-age child or adolescent is much more difficult. Luncheon preparation away from home is particularly difficult, since bread, luncheon meats, and instant soups are not allowed. For families on restricted food budgets, adherence to the diet adds an additional financial burden, since many inexpensive or convenient foods cannot be used.

It is important to stress long-range complications, as well as to remind parents of the child's physical status before dietary treatment—and dramatic improvement following treatment. The nurse can be instrumental in allowing the child to express concerns and frustration while focusing on ways in which the child can still feel normal. The child and parents can be encouraged to find new recipes using suitable ingredients, such as Mexican or Chinese dishes that use corn or rice. A nutritionist should be consulted to provide children and their families with detailed dietary instructions and education.

Several resources are available to assist children and parents in all aspects of coping with celiac disease. The **American Celiac Society*** and the **Celiac Sprue Association/United States of America†** are organizations that provide support and guidance to families and supply educational materials concerning gluten-free diet, food sources, recipes, and travel information.‡

SHORT BOWEL SYNDROME (SBS)

SBS is a malabsorptive disorder that occurs as a result of decreased mucosal surface area, usually due to extensive resection of the small intestine. Malabsorption may be exacerbated by other factors, such as bacterial overgrowth and dysmotility. The most common causes of SBS in children include congenital anomalies (jejunal and ileal atresia, gastroschisis), ischemia (necrotizing enterocolitis), and trauma or vascular injury (volvulus [twisting of bowel on itself]). Other causes of SBS in infants and children include bowel resection due to long-segment Hirschsprung disease and omphalocele. Radiation enteritis can also lead to SBS. The prognosis for infants with SBS has dramatically improved in the past 20 to 30 years, primarily from advances in parenteral nutrition and enteral feeding.

Therapeutic Management

The goals of therapy for infants and children with SBS include the following: (1) preserve as much length of bowel as possible during surgery; (2) maintain optimum nutritional status, growth, and development while intestinal adaptation occurs; (3) stimulate intestinal adaptation with enteral feeding; and (4) minimize complications related to the disease process and therapy.

Nutritional Support. Nutritional support becomes the long-term focus of care for children with SBS. The ***initial phase*** of therapy includes ***total parenteral nutrition (TPN)*** as the primary source of nutrients for the child. Occasionally, additional parenteral fluids are required to manage fluid and electrolyte losses.

Numerous complications are associated with SBS and long-term TPN. ***Central venous catheter infections*** can occur from contamination of the parenteral nutrition solutions, administration sets, or the catheter itself. The GI tract can also be a source of microbial seeding of the catheter in children with SBS. Small intestine bacterial overgrowth and

---

*Dept. N83, 45 Gifford Ave., Jersey City, NJ 07304; (201) 432-2107.

†3213 Rocklyn Dr., Des Moines, IA 50322; (515) 270-9689. In Canada: **Canadian Celiac Association, Inc.,** 1087 Meyerside Dr., Suite 5, Mississauga, Ontario L5T 1M5; (416) 673-8200.

‡A booklet, *Pointers for Parents: Coping with Celiac Sprue,* which provides information on shopping, cooking, and living with an affected child, is available from Clinical Dietetics Dept., Children's Memorial Hospital, 2300 Children's Plaza, Chicago, IL 60614; (312) 880-4000.

bowel atrophy, which may foster increased intestinal permeability of bacteria, may contribute to bacterial translocation and increase the risk of central line infections.

Metabolic complications of parenteral nutrition may occur secondary to the composition of the parenteral nutrition solution or to impaired metabolic function. Potential metabolic complications include electrolyte disturbances, hyperglycemia, hypoglycemia, and hyperlipidemia.

Technical complications include catheter occlusion, catheter migration, venous thrombosis, and pulmonary embolus. The catheter may also become damaged or perforated, resulting in leakage of the TPN solution and increasing the risk of microbial contamination. When the major blood vessels become thrombosed following multiple central venous catheterizations, a lack of adequate central venous access may become a significant problem for the child in need of long-term parenteral nutrition.

Cholestasis and ***liver dysfunction*** may occur as a complication of parenteral nutrition in a small number of children with SBS. In some cases cholestasis may be severe enough to progress to cirrhosis and liver failure. The incidence and severity of the cholestasis is multifactorial; however, prolonged TPN, as well as lack of enteral feeding, play independent and significant roles.

The introduction of ***enteral feeding*** constitutes the ***second phase*** of nutritional support and is instituted as soon as possible following surgery. Generally, a continuous infusion of a partially elemental formula via nasogastric (NG) or gastrostomy tube is recommended. These special formulas contain glucose, sucrose and glucose polymers, hydrolyzed proteins, and medium-chain triglycerides, which are more readily absorbed. Continuous feedings are advantageous over bolus feedings because of enhanced absorption and tolerance. Enteral feedings are gradually advanced as tolerated. Dehydration and severe metabolic acidosis are contraindications to increasing the enteral feeding concentration or rate. Oral feedings of partially elemental formula, electrolyte solutions, water, and small amounts of solids may be offered in addition to tube feedings so that the child can learn to suck and swallow. Oral feedings help to minimize problems with oral hypersensitivity and food aversion when the bowel can tolerate more complex foods.

As enteral feedings are gradually advanced, TPN can be decreased in terms of calories, fluid, and total hours of infusion per day. The total caloric intake must be adjusted to maintain normal growth.

A ***final phase*** of nutritional support occurs when exclusively enteral feedings can sustain adequate growth and development. During this phase the continuous feedings of partially elemental formula may be decreased as tolerance and acceptance of oral foods increases. The risk of development of specific nutritional deficiencies increases once TPN is discontinued. Malabsorption of fat-soluble vitamins (A, D, E, and K) and trace minerals (iron, selenium, zinc) is common in children with SBS. Vitamin B_{12} deficiency often occurs following resection of the ileum. Serum vitamin and mineral levels should be obtained, and enteral supplementation of vitamins and minerals may be required.

Adaptation Process. Long-term survival without TPN depends on the ability of the small intestine to increase its absorptive capacity so that nutritional needs may be provided through the enteral route. Many children develop the ability to live without TPN because of the adaptation response of the small intestine following massive resection. The compensatory increase in the mucosal surface area occurs primarily by villus hyperplasia. The small intestine length and diameter increase a small amount in children as well. This ***adaptation response*** is characterized by an increase in cell number and cell mass per villus column. The increased villus length and increased number of enterocytes available for absorption per centimeter of bowel allows for a gradual increase in absorption of nutrients. The capacity for adaptation is greater after proximal small bowel resection than after distal resection.

Stimulation of the adaptation process is an important goal of therapy; the primary stimulus is enteral feeding. Atrophy of the mucosa of the intestine occurs when no intraluminal nutrition is provided, even though nutrients are given parenterally. Intraluminal nutrients stimulate the mucosal adaptation through several mechanisms: (1) direct contact of nutrients with the mucosal surface appears to stimulate intestinal hyperplasia; (2) trophic hormones are secreted in response to intraluminal nutrients, which stimulate production of enterocytes; and (3) trophic upper GI secretions are released by stimulation from the presence of intraluminal nutrients (Vanderhoof and others, 1992).

Medical and Surgical Therapy. Common problems associated with SBS are treated medically. ***Bacterial overgrowth*** is likely to occur when the ileocecal valve is absent or when stasis due to a partial obstruction or a dilated segment of bowel with poor motility exists. Alternating cycles of broad-spectrum antibiotics may be used to reduce bacterial overgrowth; treatment may decrease the risk of bacterial translocation and subsequent central venous catheter infections.

Another complication of bacterial overgrowth and carbohydrate malabsorption is ***metabolic acidosis.*** Malabsorbed carbohydrates are fermented by bacteria in the intestine, and short-chain fatty acids are produced that accumulate in the bloodstream, causing acidosis. The treatment for metabolic acidosis may include antibiotic therapy, low-carbohydrate formulas, and supplemental administration of citrate or bicarbonate.

Gastric acid hypersecretion is caused by a disruption of normal feedback mechanisms from the small intestine to the stomach following bowel resection. Histamine receptor antagonist drugs are administered to treat this problem.

Although nutritional and medical therapy are the primary forms of treatment for SBS, additional surgery may be indicated. If severe dilation of the small bowel occurs with subsequent complications, an ***intestinal tapering procedure*** may be beneficial. Many other surgical interventions, including intestinal valves, antiperistaltic segments, recirculating loops, and intestinal lengthening procedures, have been attempted in order to delay intestinal transit time or increase absorptive surface area. None of these surgical procedures is sufficiently safe and successful to be used routinely (Thompson, 1993). ***Intestinal transplantation*** has been

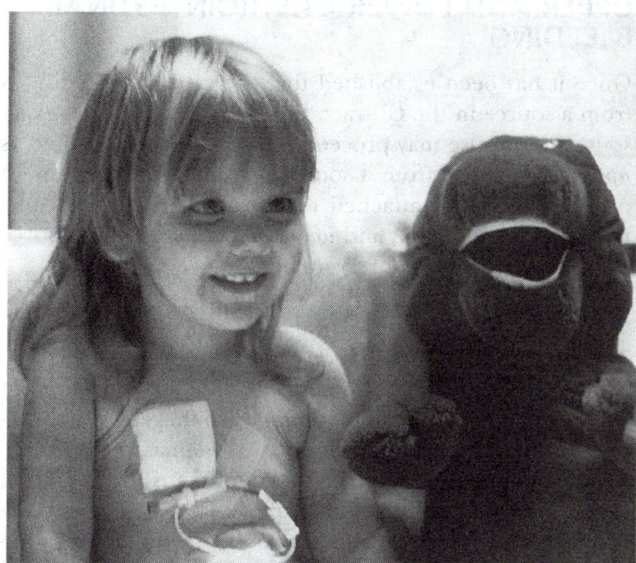

FIG. 33-8 Two-year-old child with a central venous catheter for long-term parenteral nutrition.

performed successfully in children; however, the experience is limited, and the long-term results are unknown. Only those children with a permanent dependence on TPN or severe complications of long-term parenteral nutrition are considered candidates for transplantation.

Prognosis. The prognosis for infants with SBS has improved with advances in parenteral nutrition and the understanding of the importance of enteral nutrition. The prognosis depends in part on the length of the residual small intestine and on whether the ileocecal valve was preserved. Ultimate survival may be possible with as little as 11 cm of jejunoileum with an ileocecal valve and as little as 25 cm of jejunoileum without an ileocecal valve (Dorney and others, 1985). However, more recently the prognosis for children with even less residual small bowel without an ileocecal valve has improved. Small bowel transplantation or liver and small bowel transplantation may further improve the prognosis in the near future.

Nursing Considerations

The most important components of nursing care for children with SBS include administration and monitoring of nutritional therapy. During TPN therapy care must be taken to minimize the risk of complications related to the central venous access device, such as catheter infections, occlusions, dislodgment, or accidental removal. For example, the catheter is secured away from the diaper area to prevent contamination of the line from stool or gastrostomy tube drainage. All connections are taped, and the tubing is secured to (Fig. 33-8) and covered by the child's clothing. (See also Chapter 28 regarding care of central venous access devices.)

Care of enteral feeding tubes and monitoring enteral feeding tolerance are other important ongoing nursing responsibilities. The NG tube will need to be changed periodically, and proper tube placement will need to be checked at least once a day. The gastrostomy tube will require daily site care and monitoring for signs of tube migration or local infection. Assessing enteral feeding tolerance includes daily measuring of intake and output, and urine-specific gravity; frequent weights; daily stool testing for occult blood, reducing substances, and pH; and monitoring for vomiting, abdominal distention, and increased frequency and volume of stools (see Critical Thinking Exercise box).

CRITICAL THINKING EXERCISE
Short Bowel Syndrome

The parents of a 2-year-old boy with short bowel syndrome call their health care professional to report that their child has passed many more stools than usual with an increased watery consistency in the past 24 hours. He also has a fever of 39° C (102.2° F) and has vomited several times. The boy is admitted to the hospital. During the initial period of nursing assessment, you would monitor:

1. Stool pH, urine pH, vital signs
2. Vital signs, weight, urine specific gravity, measurement of intake and output
3. Vital signs, stool-reducing substances, stool culture
4. Urine specific gravity, stool for blood, electrolytes

The correct answer is 2. Since dehydration and electrolyte disturbances are common with diarrhea, important initial nursing interventions include assessment of the child's hydration status, including vital signs, weight, urine specific gravity, and measurement of intake and output. Children with chronic malabsorption may have severe diarrhea and are particularly susceptible to dehydration and electrolyte imbalance with an acute episode of illness such as infectious gastroenteritis. Additional factors contributing to dehydration include vomiting and fever.

Laboratory analyses, including serum electrolytes, blood urea nitrogen, and creatinine, will also be necessary in order to guide the fluid and electrolyte therapy. Stool samples may need to be obtained to detect bacterial or viral pathogens. However, obtaining these tests is not an independent nursing function. Ongoing assessment may include testing of stool-reducing substances and pH (to detect carbohydrate malabsorption) and stool Hematest (to detect bleeding from intestinal mucosal inflammation or ischemia).

Home Care. When long-term TPN is required, preparation of the family for home care of the child is a major nursing responsibility. Preparation for home nutritional support is initiated as early as possible to prevent lengthy hospitalizations with subsequent problems such as developmental delays and family stresses.

Many infants and children can be successfully cared for at home with enteral and parenteral nutrition if the family is thoroughly prepared and provided with adequate support services. Most of these children and families will benefit from home nursing care to assist with and supervise therapy. Nurses can advocate, on behalf of patients and families, for necessary services and supplies for home care. Careful follow-up care by a multidisciplinary nutritional support service is essential. Most home health agencies now provide portable enteral and parenteral equipment, which enables the child and family to maintain a more normal and active life-style.

In addition to TPN, central venous catheter care, and tube feedings,* nursing care of infants with SBS should include nonnutritive sucking, oral stimulation, and provision of small amounts of oral feeding as prescribed in order to prevent later food aversion. Inadequate oral stimulation during a critical period in infancy may result in difficulty establishing successful oral feeding at a later date (Tuchman, 1991). Food aversion may require treatment by a multidisciplinary feeding team using behavioral therapy (see Feeding Resistance, Chapter 10).

Many infants with SBS have an intestinal ostomy performed at the time of the initial bowel resection. Routine ostomy care is another important nursing responsibility.* Since infants and children with SBS have chronic diarrhea, perineal skin irritation is often a problem following ostomy closure. Frequent diaper changes, gentle perineal cleansing, and protective skin ointments help prevent skin breakdown (see also Diaper Dermatitis, Chapter 13).

When hospitalization is prolonged, the child's developmental and emotional needs must be part of the nursing plan of care. This often requires special efforts to promote normal family adjustment and adaptation to hospital routines. It may be months to years before the child will no longer require specialized nutritional support. The family members require psychosocial support in addition to thorough education in order to cope successfully with a chronic condition such as SBS.

GASTROINTESTINAL BLEEDING

GI bleeding in infants and children is common and may range from a mild problem to a life-threatening situation. Most actual or apparent instances of GI bleeding in children cause great anxiety in the parents or caregivers. Ingestion of certain substances such as red food coloring in gelatin, soft drinks, amoxicillin, and certain foods such as tomatoes, cranberries, and beets may look like blood when vomited or passed per rectum. Bismuth, spinach, dark chocolate, and iron supplements may lead to dark stools that may be mistaken for melena. Blood may also be vomited or passed per rectum, but the origin of the blood may not be the GI tract. In the newborn, swallowed maternal blood at the time of delivery may account for some episodes of apparent GI bleeding. A bleeding site on the nipple of a nursing mother may lead to heme-positive stools in the breast-fed infant. Finally, blood can be swallowed during epistaxis and then be passed as hematemesis or melena.

*See Chapters 27 and 28 for additional nursing care related to these procedures. Home care instructions for caring for a central venous catheter, giving nasogastric tube feedings, giving gastrostomy feedings, and caring for the child with a colostomy are available in *Wong and Whaley's Clinical Manual of Pediatric Nursing* (Mosby).

UPPER AND LOWER GASTROINTESTINAL BLEEDING

Once it has been established that the cause of bleeding is from a source in the GI tract, the investigation of the exact source and cause may proceed. The causes are classified as ***upper GI bleeding,*** from a source proximal to the ligament of Treitz, which is attached to the duodenum at its junction with the jejunum, and ***lower GI bleeding,*** from a source distal to the ligament of Treitz.

Etiology

The esophagus is a common site of upper GI bleeding. Esophagitis due to gastroesophageal reflux may lead to chronic and often occult blood loss. Esophageal varices secondary to portal hypertension may cause massive bleeding. Peptic inflammation (gastritis and duodenitis) or ulceration is the most common cause of upper GI bleeding in children. Hemorrhagic gastritis may occur in the newborn infant following a difficult delivery or asphyxia. In this circumstance gastric perforation is a serious complication that requires emergent treatment. Less common causes of upper GI bleeding include bleeding disorders, vascular malformations, GI duplications, Mallory-Weiss syndrome (an esophageal tear caused by protracted vomiting), and hematobilia (bleeding into biliary passages).

In lower GI bleeding, small amounts of bright red blood in the stool of a healthy child most commonly is from an anal fissure. Colonic polyps are another common cause of passage of bright red blood per rectum in toddlers and older children. Bleeding associated with diarrhea may indicate a serious problem. Enteric infections remain the leading cause, but necrotizing enterocolitis, hemolytic-uremic syndrome, inflammatory bowel disease, and food allergy should be considered. Other causes are intussusception with the passage of blood per rectum (see p. 1476) or Meckel diverticulum with the painless passage of currant jelly–like stools (see p. 1467).

Pathophysiology

The GI tract has an extensive surface area and a rich vascular supply. Bleeding can occur from anywhere along the GI tract from a vein, artery, or vascular malformation. Children with coagulopathies, including hemophilia A or B, have an incidence of GI bleeding of 10% to 25% (Berry and Perrault, 1991). Many of these children have peptic ulcer disease. Children with liver disease may also have deficiency of many coagulation factors because of poor synthetic function and malabsorption of vitamin K, which also predisposes the child to GI bleeding.

Portal hypertension may lead to GI bleeding, because the formation of portosystemic shunts can result in dilated venous channels in vulnerable locations such as the esophagus and stomach. These dilated venous channels ***(varices)*** may bleed briskly, causing severe GI hemorrhage.

Diagnostic Evaluation

The diagnosis of GI bleeding is often made on the basis of the history and physical examination. ***Hematemesis*** is the vomiting of bright red blood or denatured blood that looks like "coffee grounds," usually representing an upper GI source of bleeding. ***Hematochezia*** is the passage of bright red blood per rectum, indicating a lower GI source of bleeding. This blood may precede or follow a bowel movement or be mixed with or coat the stool. Bright red blood that coats the stool may be due to a hard bowel movement, hemorrhoids, or anal fissures. Blood mixed with stool indicates a bleeding source proximal to the rectum. Blood passed alone following a bowel movement is most likely due to bleeding in the perianal or rectal area, possibly caused by a polyp. Blood with mucus in the stool indicates an inflammatory or infectious condition, and currant jelly–like stools indicate vascular compromise, such as intussusception. ***Melena*** is the passage of black, tarry stools that contain denatured (digested) blood and suggests an upper GI source of bleeding. Occasionally, bright red blood may be passed per rectum from an upper GI source of bleeding when the bleeding is massive. It is important to test emesis or stool for the presence of occult blood to differentiate true bleeding from the ingestion of food containing food coloring.

Laboratory tests, including a hemoglobin and hematocrit, blood urea nitrogen, and creatinine, and coagulation studies are often necessary in order to evaluate the extent of blood loss and to determine if a coagulopathy is present. Gastric lavage and aspiration through a nasogastric (NG) tube should be performed in the presence of hematemesis or severe rectal bleeding, or whenever the site of bleeding is in doubt.

Additional diagnostic procedures depend on whether the bleeding source is in the upper or lower GI tract. If an upper GI source of bleeding is likely, endoscopy of the upper GI tract is the most accurate method of identifying a bleeding site. Angiography or barium studies may also be performed. The diagnostic approach to lower GI bleeding depends on the nature and severity of bleeding. Stools should be tested, and a rectal examination is performed. Plain radiographs, ultrasonography, or barium studies may provide information regarding the cause of bleeding. A sigmoidoscopy or colonoscopy may be performed depending on the child's history and physical examination. If bleeding is brisk, a radionuclide-tagged red blood cell scan may locate the site of bleeding.

Therapeutic Management

Treatment of GI bleeding in children depends on its severity and cause. The first step in management of acute GI bleeding is to assess the magnitude of blood loss and restore the child's hemodynamic stability. Severe bleeding necessitates hospitalization. Intravenous fluids (normal saline or lactated Ringer's solution) are administered rapidly. Oxygen therapy is indicated if the bleeding is severe. Transfusion of blood products may be required if the blood loss is significant, and any existing coagulopathy should be corrected.

Upper GI mucosal lesions are usually treated with histamine (H_2) receptor antagonists (cimetidine [Tagamet], ranitidine [Zantac], or famotidine [Pepcid]) and antacids to reduce acidity and promote mucosal healing. Variceal hemorrhage can be treated with peripheral vasopressin infusion and endoscopic sclerotherapy to hasten tissue fibrosis. Balloon tamponade to place pressure on the bleeding area may be performed as a temporary measure until endoscopic sclerotherapy can be done.

Therapy for lower GI bleeding is directed toward the primary underlying condition. The treatment may include medical or surgical management. Surgery may be required if the bleeding is severe despite aggressive medical intervention.

Nursing Considerations

The infant or child with acute and severe GI bleeding requires emergency care. Initial management includes assessment of the magnitude of bleeding and hemodynamic status and assistance with resuscitation efforts (see Critical Thinking Exercise box).

CRITICAL THINKING EXERCISE

Hematemesis

A 6-month-old infant is seen in the emergency room. The parents brought the infant to the hospital because he spit up formula with blood streaks. In the emergency room the infant is tachypneic, tachycardia, and febrile with a temperature of 39° C (102.2° F). A chest x-ray film shows pneumonia. The infant is admitted to the hospital to receive antibiotics and for observation. Several hours after admission to the inpatient unit, the mother calls the nurse when the infant vomits a large amount of bright red blood. The infant is pale and lethargic. All of the following should be included in the initial nursing actions except:

1. Call for assistance and estimate amount of blood loss.
2. Obtain vital signs and monitor capillary refill, skin color, and behavior.
3. Prepare to pass a nasogastric tube, obtain blood for laboratory analyses, and start an intravenous line.
4. Test stool for blood (Hematest or Hemoccult).

The correct answer is 4. Since this infant has acute severe gastrointestinal bleeding, initial nursing actions include an assessment of hemodynamic status for possible shock (option 2). The infant should not be left unattended, and the nurse should call for assistance, since further vomiting and potential aspiration may occur. The nurse should also anticipate that a nasogastric tube will need to be inserted to lavage the stomach and monitor for further bleeding. Blood will need to be drawn, including a hemoglobin, hematocrit, platelet count, white blood cell count, and a type and crossmatch for potential transfusion. An intravenous line will need to be inserted to administer fluids and possibly blood products.

Once the patient is stabilized, additional information and evaluation will be necessary in order to identify the cause of the bleeding. In this case a potential cause of bleeding is stress-induced gastritis or peptic ulceration due to infection. Hematest of the stool will add no useful information at this point.

NURSING ALERT Monitor closely for signs of shock: restlessness; increased respiratory and heart rate; poor capillary refill; pallor; cool, clammy extremities; and decreased blood pressure (a late sign). Call for assistance immediately if these signs are observed.

Oxygen should be administered, and suction equipment should be available. An intravenous catheter should be inserted, and preparation should be made for the administration of intravenous fluids, usually normal saline or lactated Ringer's solution. Blood should be drawn for laboratory analysis, including a hemoglobin, hematocrit, blood urea nitrogen, creatinine, coagulation studies, and type and crossmatch. The nurse should be prepared to insert an NG tube to help locate the site of bleeding and to lavage the stomach with normal saline at room temperature if upper GI bleeding is suspected. After the child is stabilized, ongoing monitoring in an intensive care setting may be indicated.

In cases of mild or chronic bleeding, there is more time for a thorough history and diagnostic evaluation. This type of evaluation often takes place on an outpatient basis. Important nursing responsibilities include assisting with the history and physical examination, diagnostic procedures, and education regarding the therapeutic plan.

The parent or caregiver of a child with GI bleeding may be extremely anxious and panic stricken. They need reassurance that most instances of bleeding are self-limited and can be treated successfully. In life-threatening situations, special emotional support is required by the health care team, including physicians, nurses, and social workers. The family is kept informed about the source, cause, and treatment of the bleeding.

HEPATIC DISORDERS

The liver is an active vital organ whose functions can be divided into several groups: (1) vascular functions of storing and filtering blood; (2) secretory function of producing bile; (3) metabolism of carbohydrate, protein, and fat; (4) synthesis of blood-clotting components and storage of iron and vitamins (A, D, B_{12}, and K); and (5) detoxification and excretion of certain drugs and metabolic substances. Many disorders can cause liver dysfunction in children, including biliary atresia (see Chapter 11), hepatitis, and cirrhosis.

ACUTE HEPATITIS

Hepatitis, an acute or chronic inflammation of the liver, is a significant health threat to children, especially when it is caused by hepatitis B virus (see Chapter 12). Thousands of cases of hepatitis in children are reported each year to the Centers for Disease Control and Prevention, and it is likely that many other cases occur that are not reported. Many recent advances in the prevention, detection, and management of children with viral hepatitis have occurred that should change the epidemiology of this disease.

Etiology

Hepatitis in children may be caused by a virus, a chemical or drug reaction, or some other disease process. The majority (90%) of cases of viral hepatitis are caused by five viruses, including:

- Hepatitis A virus (HAV, previously designated infectious hepatitis)
- Hepatitis B virus (HBV, previously designated serum hepatitis)
- Hepatitis C virus (HCV, previously designated parenterally transmitted non-A, non-B hepatitis virus [PT-NANB])
- Hepatitis D virus (HDV, delta agent)
- Hepatitis E virus (enterically transmitted non-A, non-B hepatitis virus [ET-NANB])

In addition, cytomegalovirus (CMV), Epstein-Barr virus (EBV), and herpes simplex virus (HSV) may occasionally cause hepatitis. The clinical symptoms of these viruses are similar. Epidemiologic features and serologic testing are used to differentiate the causes. Table 33-4 compares the features of HAV, HBV, and HCV.

Hepatitis A is usually an acute condition causing mild illness. HAV is the most common form of acute viral hepatitis. There is no chronic or carrier state. HAV is a contagious disease that is spread directly or indirectly by the fecal-oral route, through ingestion of raw shellfish from polluted waters, direct exposure to infected fecal material, or close contact with an infected person. HAV can affect individuals at any age, but the highest incidence occurs among preschool or school-age children. Many outbreaks of HAV occur in daycare centers (especially those with children in diapers) and in custodial care facilities. The incubation period is approximately 4 weeks. Many affected children are asymptomatic, but mild nausea, vomiting, and diarrhea may occur.

Hepatitis B (previously called serum hepatitis) can be an acute and/or chronic infection, ranging from an asymptomatic limited infection to fatal fulminant (rapid and severe) hepatitis. HBV transmission is usually via the parenteral route through the exchange of blood, or any bodily secretion or fluid, either directly or from contaminated objects, such as used "sharps" (e.g., needles). Intimate physical contact and spread from mother to infant is a potential source of infection. Contaminated fluids splashed into the mouth or eyes can also cause infection. Hepatitis B has been acquired following blood transfusion, but this likelihood has been reduced as a result of blood product screening procedures. Transplanted organs can also serve as a source of HBV. Adults whose occupations are associated with considerable exposure to blood or blood products, such as health care workers, are at an increased risk of contracting HBV.

Most HBV in children is acquired perinatally. Newborn infants are at risk for hepatitis if the mother is infected with HBV or was a carrier of HBV during pregnancy. Possible routes of maternal-fetal (infant) transmission include (1) leakage of virus across the placenta late in pregnancy or during labor, (2) ingestion of amniotic fluid or maternal blood, and (3) breast-feeding, especially if the mother has cracked nipples. The infectivity of colostrum and breast

TABLE 33-4 Comparison of Types A, B, and C Hepatitis

CHARACTERISTICS	TYPE A	TYPE B	TYPE C
Incubation period	15-40 days, average 30 days	50-180 days, average 50 days	14-180 days, average 50 days
Period of communicability	Unknown	Variable	Begins before onset of symptoms
	Virus in blood and feces 2 to 3 weeks before onset of jaundice and for about 1 week after onset of jaundice	Virus in blood or other body fluids during late incubation period and acute stage of disease; may persist in carrier state for years	May persist in carrier state for years
Mode of transmission	Principal route—fecal-oral Rarely—parenteral	Principal route—parenteral Less frequent route—oral, sexual, any body fluid Perinatal transfer—transplacental blood (last trimester), at delivery, or during breast-feeding, especially if mother has cracked nipples	Principal route—parenteral Nonparenteral spread possible
Clinical features			
Onset	Usually rapid, acute	More insidious	Variable
Fever	Common and early	Less frequent	Less frequent
Anorexia	Common	Less frequent	Less frequent
Nausea and vomiting	Common	Sometimes present	Sometimes present
Rash	Rare	Sometimes present	Rare
Arthralgia	Rare	Common	Rare
Pruritus	Rare	Sometimes present	Rare
Jaundice	Present (many cases anicteric)	Present	Present
Immunity	Present after one attack; no crossover to type B or C	Present after one attack; no crossover to type A or C	Present after one attack; no crossover to type A or B
Carrier state	No	Yes	Yes
Chronic infection	No	Yes	Yes
Prophylaxis			
Immune globulin (IgG)	Passive immunity Successful, especially in early incubation period and preexposure prophylaxis	Passive immunity Inconsistent benefits; probably of no use	Passive immunity May be successful if given immediately after exposure
HAV vaccine	Under development		
HBV immune globulin (HBIG)	No benefit	Postexposure protection possible if given immediately after definite exposure	No benefit
HBV vaccine (see Table 12-10)		Provides active immunity Universal vaccination recommended for all newborns	
Mortality	0.1% to 0.2%	0.5% to 2.0% in uncomplicated cases; may be higher in complicated cases	1% to 2% in uncomplicated cases; may be higher in complicated cases

milk is controversial. The severity of hepatitis in the infant varies from no liver disease to a fulminant or chronic, active type.

HBV infection occurs in children in other high-risk situations: (1) individuals with hemophilia or other disorders who have received multiple transfusions, (2) children and adolescents involved in intravenous drug abuse, (3) institutionalized children, and (4) preschool children in endemic areas (Balistreri, 1988). The incubation period for HBV infection ranges from 50 to 180 days. HBV can cause a carrier state and lead to chronic hepatitis with eventual cirrhosis or hepatocellular carcinoma in adulthood.

Hepatitis C has been called "non-A, non-B hepatitis" because of the absence of HAV and HBV serologic markers of infection. HCV transmission appears to be largely parenteral, although other routes may occasionally be responsible (Carey and Patel, 1992). HCV is the primary cause of posttransfusion hepatitis, and before heat treatment of clotting factor concentrates, patients with hemophilia who needed replacement therapy were at risk for acquiring hepatitis C (Kanesaki and others, 1993). The clinical course is variable. The incubation period ranges from 14 days to 6 months. Some children may be asymptomatic, but hepatitis C often becomes a chronic condition and can cause cirrhosis and hepatocellular carcinoma. About 50% of individuals infected with HCV develop chronic disease (Carey and Patel, 1992). Although aplastic anemia is a rare complication of all forms of viral hepatitis, it is more common with hepatitis C.

Hepatitis D occurs in children already infected with HBV. Hepatitis D virus is a defective RNA virus that requires the helper function of HBV. The incubation period is from 21 to 90 days. Both acute and chronic forms of hepatitis D tend to be more severe than hepatitis B and can lead to cirrhosis. HDV occurs mostly in drug addicts and individuals with hemophilia.

Hepatitis E is enterically transmitted non-A, non-B hepatitis. Transmission may occur through the fecal-oral route or from contaminated water. The incubation period is 2 to 9 weeks. This illness is uncommon in children, does not cause chronic liver disease, is not a chronic condition, and has no carrier state. However, it can be a devastating disease among pregnant women, with a mortality rate of 10% to 20% (Krugman, 1992).

Pathophysiology

The pathologic changes occur primarily in the parenchymal cells of the liver and result in variable degrees of swelling, infiltration of liver cells by mononuclear cells, and subsequent degeneration, necrosis, and fibrosis. Structural changes within the hepatocyte are thought to account for altered liver functions, such as impaired bile excretion, elevated transaminase levels, and decreased albumin synthesis. The disorder may be self-limiting, with regeneration of liver cells without scarring, leading to a complete recovery. There are, however, forms of hepatitis that do not result in complete return of liver function. These include ***fulminant hepatitis,*** which is characterized by a severe acute course with massive destruction of the liver tissue causing liver failure and a high mortality, and ***subacute*** or ***chronic active hepatitis,*** characterized by progressive liver destruction and the potential for development of cirrhosis.

Clinical Manifestations

The clinical manifestations and course of uncomplicated acute viral hepatitis are similar for most of the hepatitis viruses. Usually the prodromal or ***anicteric phase*** (absence of jaundice) lasts 5 to 7 days. Anorexia, malaise, lethargy, and easy fatigability are the most common symptoms. Fever may be present, especially in adolescents. Nausea, vomiting, and epigastric or right upper quadrant abdominal pain or tenderness may occur. Arthralgia and skin rashes may occur and are more likely in children with hepatitis B than in those with hepatitis A. The transaminases, rather than the bilirubin, will often be elevated in acute hepatitis, and hepatomegaly may be present. Some mild cases of acute viral hepatitis will not cause symptoms or will be mistaken for influenza.

In young children most of the prodromal symptoms disappear with the onset of jaundice, or the ***icteric phase.*** Many children with acute viral hepatitis, however, never develop jaundice. If jaundice occurs, it is often accompanied by dark urine and pale stools.

Children with chronic active hepatitis may be asymptomatic, but more commonly have nonspecific symptoms of malaise, fatigue, lethargy, weight loss, or vague abdominal pain. Hepatomegaly may be present, and the transaminases are often very high, with mild to severe hyperbilirubinemia.

Fulminant hepatitis is due primarily to hepatitis B or hepatitis C. Many children with fulminant hepatitis develop symptoms characteristic of viral hepatitis and then rapidly develop manifestations of liver failure, including encephalopathy, coagulation defects, ascites, deepening jaundice, and increasing white blood cell count. Changes in mental status or personality indicate impending liver failure. Although children with acute hepatitis may have hepatomegaly, a rapid decrease in the size of the liver (indicating loss of tissue due to necrosis) is a serious sign of fulminant hepatitis. Complications of fulminant hepatitis may be present, including GI bleeding, sepsis, renal failure, and disseminated coagulopathy.

Diagnostic Evaluation

Diagnosis is based on the history, physical examination, and serologic markers for hepatitis A, B, and C. No liver function test is specific for hepatitis, but serum aminotransferase (ALT) levels are markedly elevated. Serum bilirubin levels peak 5 to 10 days after clinical jaundice appears. Histologic evidence from liver biopsy may be required to aid in establishment of the diagnosis and to assess the severity of the liver disease. Diagnosis of hepatitis B is confirmed by the detection of various antibodies that are produced in response to the infection or antigens that are part of HBV. HAV is diagnosed by the presence of hepatitis A antibody (anti-HAV). During the initial infective period anti-HAV of the IgM class is present, but after about 3 to 6 months this antibody declines and anti-HAV of the IgG class increases. Therefore detection of anti-HAV IgM indicates active infection, and anti-HAV IgG indicates past infection and immunity (Krugman, 1992). Antibodies to different HCV antigens can also be detected (Kanesaki and others, 1993).

Several antibodies and antigens are important in the diagnosis of HBV and include:

HBsAg—Hepatitis B surface antigen (found on the surface of the virus)
anti-HBs—Antibody to HBsAg
HBcAg—Hepatitis B core antigen (found on the inner core of the virus)
anti-HBc—Antibody to HBcAg
HBeAg—Hepatitis Be antigen (another component of the HBV core)
anti-HBe—Antibody to HBeAg

Tests are available for detection of all the HBV antigens and antibodies except HBcAg. A test has been developed to detect HBV DNA in serum; most HBeAg-positive sera have detectable HBV DNA. The presence of HBsAg and HBeAg indicates active infection. Neonatal infection is most likely to occur in infants born to mothers who are HBeAg-positive. In contrast, hepatitis B is much less likely to occur in infants whose mothers are HBsAg-positive but HBeAg-negative and have antibodies to HBeAg (Krugman, 1992).

Clinical improvement is usually associated with a decrease in or disappearance of these antigens, followed by the appearance of their antibodies. Anti-HBc of the IgM class is seen early in the disease, followed by a rise in anti-HBc of the IgG class. Since the antibodies persist indefinitely, they are used to identify the ***carrier state*** (individuals with HBV who have no clinical disease but are able to transmit the organism).

An assay for anti-HCV antibodies is now available. Tests have shown that the antibody is not detectable until 5 to 20 weeks following the onset of symptoms. Therefore the assay will not detect most cases of acute HCV infection (Ergun and Miskovitz, 1990).

The history should include questions to seek evidence of (1) contact with a person known to have hepatitis, especially a family member; (2) unsafe sanitation practices, such as contaminated drinking water; (3) eating certain foods, such as clams or oysters (especially from polluted water); (4) multiple blood transfusions; (5) ingestion of hepatotoxic drugs, such as salicylates, sulfonamides, antineoplastic agents, acetaminophen, anticonvulsants, and many other medications; and (6) parenteral administration of illicit drugs or sexual contact with a person who uses these drugs.

Therapeutic Management

Treatment options for viral hepatitis are limited. The goals of management include early detection, support and monitoring of the disease, recognition of chronic liver disease, and prevention of spread of the disease. No specific effective therapy for either acute or chronic hepatitis B or hepatitis C exists. Special high-protein, high-carbohydrate, low-fat diets are generally not of value. The use of corticosteroids alone or with immunosuppressive drugs is generally not advocated at this time. Hospitalization is required in the event of coagulopathy or fulminant hepatitis. Human interferon-α has shown promise as a therapeutic agent in chronic hepatitis B and chronic hepatitis C infections (Bacon, 1991). Antiviral therapy with acyclovir may be considered for active hepatitis B infection (Bruckstein, 1989). The selection of therapy for hepatitis depends on the severity of inflammation and the cause of the disorder.

Prevention. Proper handwashing and universal precautions can prevent the spread of viral hepatitis. Prophylactic use of standard immune globulin (IG) is effective in preventing hepatitis A in situations of preexposure (such as anticipated travel to areas where HAV is prevalent) or within 2 weeks of exposure.

Hepatitis B immune globulin (HBIG) is effective in preventing HBV infection following one-time exposures such as accidental needle punctures or other contact of contaminated material with mucous membranes and should be given to newborns whose mothers are HBsAg-positive. HBIG is prepared from plasma that contains high titers of antibodies against HBV. HBIG should be given within 72 hours of exposure.

Vaccines have been developed to prevent HBV infection, and immunization is recommended for all newborns and for high-risk groups (see Immunizations, Chapter 12). It is possible to prevent hepatitis D by preventing hepatitis B (Lisanti and Talotta, 1992). A vaccine for HAV is being developed.

Prognosis. The prognosis for children with hepatitis is variable and depends on the type of virus and the child's age and immunocompetency. Hepatitis A and E are usually mild and brief illnesses with no carrier state. Hepatitis B can cause a wide spectrum of acute and chronic illness. Infants are more likely than older children to develop chronic hepatitis. Chronic HBV infection leads to cirrhosis in 25% to 30% of cases (Ergun and Miskovitz, 1990). Hepatocellular carcinoma during adulthood is a potentially fatal complication of chronic HBV infection. Hepatitis C frequently becomes chronic, and cirrhosis may develop in these children. The highest mortality occurs in hepatitis D. Fulminant hepatic failure occurs in approximately 1% to 2% of cases of viral hepatitis, regardless of the etiology (Balistreri, 1988) and is associated with a mortality rate of 60% to 90%, with higher mortality in older children (Krugman, 1992).

Nursing Considerations

Nursing objectives depend largely on the severity of the hepatitis, the medical treatment, and factors influencing the control and transmission of the disease. Since children with mild viral hepatitis are frequently cared for at home, explaining any medical therapies and infection control measures is frequently the clinic or office nurse's responsibility. In instances in which further assistance is needed for parents to comply with such instructions, a public health nursing referral may be necessary.

A regular diet and a realistic schedule of rest and activity adjusted to the child's condition are encouraged. Since school-age children rarely transmit hepatitis virus to their peers, they can often return to school as soon as they feel well.

Handwashing is the single most effective measure in prevention and control of hepatitis in any setting (for a discussion of preventive measures in the daycare center, see Chapter 15; see also Infection Control in Chapter 27). Parents and children need an explanation of the usual ways in which hepatitis A (fecal-oral route) and hepatitis B (parenteral route) are spread.* Parents should also be aware of the recommendation for universal vaccination against HBV for newborns (see Chapter 12).

In young people with HBV infection who have a known or suspected history of illicit drug use, the nurse has the additional responsibility of helping them realize the associated dangers of drug abuse, stressing the parenteral mode of transmission of hepatitis and encouraging them to seek counseling through a drug program. (See also Nursing Care Plan: The Child with Acute Hepatitis.†)

CIRRHOSIS

Cirrhosis occurs as an end stage of many chronic liver diseases, including biliary atresia and chronic hepatitis. Severe

*Home care instructions for preventing AIDS and hepatitis infection are available in *Wong and Whaley's Clinical Manual of Pediatric Nursing* (Mosby).
†In *Wong and Whaley's Clinical Manual of Pediatric Nursing* (Mosby).

liver damage can be caused by infectious, autoimmune, or toxic factors and by chronic diseases, such as hemophilia and cystic fibrosis, in long-term survivors. A cirrhotic liver is irreversibly damaged.

Pathophysiology

Cirrhosis occurs as a result of hepatocyte injury with necrosis, fibrosis, regeneration, and eventual degeneration. Diminished parenchymal cell mass causes regeneration of tissue with nodular areas of proliferating hepatocytes that stretch the surrounding connective tissue. Hepatocytes respond to injury with deposition of collagen that forms fibrous connective tissue. This scar tissue and nodular areas of regeneration impair the intrahepatic blood flow. Ongoing necrosis and self-perpetuation of this pathologic process are the result of cirrhosis.

Failure of hepatocellular function and portal hypertension occur with cirrhosis. Cirrhosis often leads to complications, including ascites, severe cholestasis, encephalopathy (hepatic coma), and GI bleeding.

Clinical Manifestations

Clinical manifestations of cirrhosis develop from the features commonly seen with all chronic liver disorders. Children with cirrhosis often exhibit jaundice, poor growth, anorexia, muscle weakness, and lethargy. Ascites, edema, GI bleeding, anemia, and abdominal pain may be present in children with impaired intrahepatic blood flow. Pulmonary function may be impaired in children with cirrhosis because of pressure against the diaphragm due to hepatosplenomegaly and ascites. Dyspnea and cyanosis may occur, especially on exertion. Intrapulmonary arteriovenous shunts may develop, which can also cause hypoxemia. Spider angiomas and prominent blood vessels on the upper torso are often present.

Diagnostic Evaluation

The diagnosis of cirrhosis is based on (1) the history, especially in regard to prior liver disease, such as hepatitis; (2) physical examination, particularly hepatosplenomegaly or a sudden decrease in liver size; (3) laboratory evaluation, especially liver function tests, such as bilirubin and aminotransferases, ammonia, albumin, cholesterol, and prothrombin time; and (4) liver biopsy for characteristic changes. Doppler ultrasonography of the liver and spleen is useful to confirm ascites, to evaluate the blood flow through the liver and spleen, and to determine the patency and size of the portal vein if liver transplantation is being considered.

NURSING ALERT The most common complication from percutaneous liver biopsy is internal bleeding (Cohen and others, 1992). Monitor vital signs and laboratory values, especially hematocrit, for evidence of hemorrhage and shock.

Therapeutic Management

Unfortunately, there is no successful treatment to arrest the progression of cirrhosis. The goals of management include monitoring liver function and managing specific complications such as esophageal varices and malnutrition. Assessment of the child's degree of liver dysfunction is important so that the child may be evaluated for transplantation at the appropriate time.

Liver transplantation has improved the prognosis substantially for many children with cirrhosis. Average 4-year survival rates are about 64% following orthotopic liver transplantation (Lloyd-Still, 1991). Unfortunately, many children die while waiting for a suitable donor. (See also Biliary Atresia, Chapter 11.)

Nutritional support is an important therapy for children with cirrhosis and malnutrition. Supplements of fat-soluble vitamins are often required, and mineral supplements may also be indicated. In some instances aggressive nutritional support in the form of continuous tube feedings or parenteral nutrition may be necessary.

Esophageal and gastric varices are a life-threatening complication of portal hypertension. Acute hemorrhage is managed with intravenous fluids, blood products, vasopressin, and gastric lavage. Balloon tamponade with a Sengstaken-Blakemore tube may be indicated. Endoscopic sclerotherapy is often used to treat varices.

Ascites may be managed by sodium restriction and diuretics. Severe ascites with respiratory compromise may be managed with administration of albumin or by paracentesis.

Although the full mechanism of hepatic encephalopathy is unknown, failure of the damaged liver to remove endogenous toxins, such as ammonia, plays a role. Treatment is directed at limiting the ammonia formation and absorption that occur in the bowel, especially with the drugs neomycin and lactulose. Since ammonia is formed in the bowel by the action of bacteria on ingested protein, neomycin reduces the number of intestinal bacteria so that less ammonia is produced. The fermentation of lactulose by colonic bacteria produces short-chain fatty acids, which lowers the colonic pH, thereby inhibiting bacterial metabolism. This decreases the formation of ammonia from bacterial metabolism of protein.

Prognosis. The success of liver transplantation has revolutionized the approach to liver cirrhosis. Liver failure

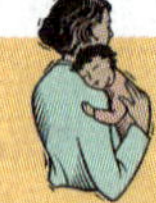

FAMILY FOCUS

End-Stage Liver Disease

In many cases the child and family must cope with an uncertain progression of the disease. The only hope for long-term survival may be liver transplantation. Transplantation can be very successful, but the waiting period may be long, since there are many more children in need of organs than there are donors. The procedure is very expensive and is only performed at designated medical centers, which are often far from the family's home. The nurse should recognize the unique stresses of coping with end-stage liver disease and waiting for transplantation, and should assist the family in coping with these stressors. The assistance of social workers and support from other parents can be very beneficial.

and cirrhosis are currently indications for transplantation. Liver transplantation reflects the failure of other medical and surgical measures to prevent or treat cirrhosis. Careful monitoring of the child's condition and quality of life are necessary in order to evaluate the need for and timing of transplantation.

Nursing Considerations

Nursing care of the child with cirrhosis is influenced by several factors, including the cause of the cirrhosis, the severity of complications, and the prognosis. The prognosis is often poor unless successful liver transplantation occurs. Therefore nursing care of this child is similar to that for any child with a life-threatening illness (Chapter 23). Hospitalization is required when complications such as hemorrhage, severe malnutrition, or hepatic failure occur. Nursing care is directed at monitoring of the child's condition and interventions aimed at treatment of specific complications. If liver transplantation is an option, the family needs support during this time (see Family Focus box).

KEY POINTS

- The essential functions of the GI system are to process and absorb nutrients necessary to maintain metabolic processes and support growth and development, to perform excretory functions, to provide detoxification, and to maintain fluid and electrolyte balance.
- Digestion is the catabolism of foodstuffs (water, vitamins, minerals, carbohydrates, proteins, and fats) from their original complex form to simple, assimilable nutrients.
- The small intestine is the principal absorptive site in the GI system.
- Most ingested foreign bodies pass through the alimentary tract without difficulty. Those lodged in the esophagus or objects with sharp edges require further evaluation.
- Constipation is usually managed by diet therapy and measures to keep the bowel relatively empty of stool.
- Hirschsprung disease requires surgical removal of aganglionic segments of bowel.
- Nursing care of gastroesophageal reflux is aimed primarily at instructing caregivers regarding home care feeding and positioning, and caring for the child undergoing surgical intervention.
- Although the cause of appendicitis is poorly understood, it is commonly a result of obstruction of the lumen, often by a fecalith. Common signs and symptoms are colicky abdominal pain, guarding of the abdomen, and fever.
- Meckel diverticulum is a congenital malformation of the GI tract characterized by rectal bleeding.
- Inflammatory bowel disease refers to ulcerative colitis and Crohn disease. Chronic diarrhea and growth abnormalities are common features.
- Management of inflammatory bowel disease includes nutritional support, sufasalazine, corticosteroids or other immunosuppressive drugs, antibiotics, and general supportive therapy. Surgical removal of inflamed bowel may be necessary.
- Peptic ulcers are poorly understood, but a likely cause is interference with the normal protective mechanisms of the mucosal lining.
- General signs of GI obstruction include abdominal pain, nausea and vomiting, abdominal distention, and a decline in the amount of stool excreted.
- Hypertrophic pyloric stenosis is characterized by projectile vomiting without loss of appetite, dehydration, and metabolic alkalosis. Therapy is surgical pyloromyotomy.
- Intussusception is a cause of intestinal obstruction during infancy. Treatment is either nonsurgical hydrostatic reduction or surgical reduction.
- Malabsorption syndromes are disorders associated with some degree of impaired digestion and/or absorption. They include digestive defects, absorptive defects, and anatomic defects.
- The prognosis for children with short bowel syndrome improved dramatically as a result of advances in parenteral and enteral nutritional support, which is the primary therapy for this condition. Home care is an important component of these children's quality of life.
- Celiac disease is characterized by an intolerance for gluten. The major role of the nurse in the management of celiac disease is helping the parents and child adhere to diet therapy.
- GI bleeding may be upper or lower GI tract bleeding, and initial management should include assessment of the magnitude of bleeding and restoration of hemodynamic stability.
- Viral hepatitis is caused by at least five types of virus—hepatitis A virus, hepatitis B virus, hepatitis C virus, hepatitis D virus, and hepatitis E virus.
- Hepatitis A virus is spread by the fecal-oral route, whereas hepatitis B and C viruses are transmitted primarily by the parenteral route. The single most effective measure in prevention and control of hepatitis in any setting is handwashing.
- Universal immunization against hepatitis B virus is recommended for all newborns.
- Liver transplantation offers hope to children with end-stage liver disease.

REFERENCES

Albanese CT and others: Percutaneous gastrojejunostomy versus Nissen fundoplication for enteral feeding of the neurologically impaired child with gastroesophageal reflux, *J Pediatr* 123:371-375, 1993.

American Academy of Pediatrics Task Force on Infant Positioning and SIDS: Positioning and SIDS, *Pediatrics* 89(6):1120-1126, 1992.

Anderson J, Akmal M, Kittur D: Surgical complications of pica, *Am Surgeon* 57(1):663-667, 1991.

Bacon B: Managing chronic hepatitis, *Postgrad Med* 90(5):103-112, 1991.

Bailey D and others: Lack of efficacy of thickened feeding as treatment for gastroesophageal reflux, *J Pediatr* 110(2):187-189, 1986.

Balistreri W: Viral hepatitis, *Pediatr Clin North Am* 35(2):375-407, 1988.

Belli D and others: Chronic intermittent element diet improves growth failure in children with Crohn's disease, *Gastroenterology* 94(3):603-610, 1988.

Benninga MA, Buller HA, Taminiau JA: Biofeedback training in chronic constipation, *Arch Dis Child* 68(1):126-129, 1993.

Berry R, Perrault J: Gastrointestinal bleeding. In Walker A and others, editors: *Pediatric gastrointestinal disease,* Philadelphia, 1991, BC Decker.

Bonadio WA and others: Esophageal bougienage technique for coin ingestion in children, *J Pediatr Surg* 23:917-918, 1988.

Brady P: Esophageal foreign bodies, *Gastroenterol Clin North Am* 20(4):691-701, 1991.

Brown C, Olshaker J: Meckel's diverticulum, *Am J Emerg Med* 6(2):157-163, 1988.

Bruckstein A: Chronic hepatitis: the challenge of diagnosis and treatment, *Postgrad Med* 85(7):67-74, 1989.

Carey W, Patel G: Viral hepatitis in the 1990's. III. Hepatitis C, hepatitis E, and other viruses, *Cleve Clin J Med* 59(6):595-601, 1992.

Cohen MB and others: Complications of percutaneous liver biopsy in children, *Gastroenterology* 102:629-632, 1992.

Dorney S and others: Improved survival in very short small bowel of infancy with use of long-term parenteral nutrition, *J Pediatr* 107:521-525, 1985.

Ergun G, Miskovitz P: Viral hepatitis, *Postgrad Med* 88(5):69-76, 1990.

Friede A and others: Transmission of hepatitis b virus from adopted Asian children to their American families, *Am J Public Health* 78:26-29, 1988.

Frithz G, Wictorin B, Ronquist G: Calcium-induced constipation in a prepubescent boy, *Acta Paediatr Scand* 80(10):964-965, 1991.

Goldfinger SE: Prunes and constipation, *Harvard Health Lett* 16:8, 1991.

Hatch T: Encopresis and constipation in children, *Pediatr Clin North Am* 35(2):257-277, 1988.

Herbst J: Gastroesophageal reflux. In Lebenthal E, editor: *Textbook of gastroenterology and nutrition in infancy,* New York, 1989, Raven Press.

Hickey R, Sodhi S, Johnson W: Two children with lethargy and intussusception, *Ann Emerg Med* 19(4):390-392, 1990.

Hillemeier A: Reflux and esophagitis. In Walker W and others, editors: *Pediatric gastrointestinal disease,* Philadelphia, 1991, BC Decker.

Jackson W, Grand R: Crohn's disease. In Walker W and others, editors: *Pediatric gastrointestinal disease,* Philadelphia, 1991, BC Decker.

Kanesaki T and others: Hepatitis C virus infection in children with hemophilia: characterization of antibody response to four different antigens and relationship of antibody response, viremia, and hepatic dysfunction, *J Pediatr* 123:381-387, 1993.

Kirschner B: Hirschsprung's disease. In Walker W and others, editors: *Pediatric gastrointestinal disease,* Philadelphia, 1991, BC Decker.

Knudson M: Intussusception, *Postgrad Med* 83(8):201-212, 1988.

Korman S: Pica as a presenting symptom in childhood celiac disease, *Am J Clin Nutr* 51:139-141, 1990.

Krugman S: Viral hepatitis: A, B, C, D and E—infection, *Pediatr Rev* 13(6):203-212, 1992.

Lisanti P, Talotta D: Hepatitis update: the delta virus, *AORN J* 55(3):790-800, 1992.

Lloyd-Still JD: Impact of orthotopic liver transplantation on mortality from pediatric liver disease, *J Pediatr Gastroenterol Nutr* 12:305-309, 1991.

Loening-Baucke V: Factors determining outcome in children with chronic constipation and faecal soiling, *Gut* 30:999-1006, 1989.

Machida H and others: Metoclopramide in gastroesophageal reflux of infancy, *J Pediatr* 112(3):483-487, 1988.

Meyer J: The current radiologic management of intussusception: a survey and review, *Pediatr Radiol* 22:323-325, 1992.

Meyers W, Herbst J: Effectiveness of positioning therapy for gastroesophageal reflux, *Pediatrics* 69(6):768-772, 1982.

Milla P: Motor disorders including pyloric stenosis. In Walker W and others, editors: *Pediatric gastrointestinal disease,* Philadelphia, 1991, BC Decker.

Nord K: Peptic ulcer disease in the pediatric population, *Pediatr Clin North Am* 35(1):117-137, 1988.

Not T and others: A new, rapid, noninvasive screening test for celiac disease, *J Pediatr* 123(3):425-427, 1993.

Orenstein SR: Effect of nonnutritive sucking on infant gastroesophageal reflux, *Pediatr Res* 24:38-40, 1988.

Orenstein SR: Effects on behavior state of prone versus seated positioning for infants with gastroesophageal reflux, *Pediatrics* 85(5):765-767, 1990a.

Orenstein SR: Prone positioning in infant gastroesophageal reflux: is elevation of the head worth the trouble? *J Pediatr* 117(2):184-187, 1990b.

Orenstein SR: Gastroesophageal reflux, *Pediatr Rev* 13(5):174-182, 1992.

Orenstein SR, Magill H, Brooks P: Thickening of infant feedings for therapy of gastroesophageal reflux, *J Pediatr* 110(2):181-186, 1987.

Orenstein SR, Shalaby T, Putnam P: Thickened feedings as a cause of increased coughing when used as therapy for gastroesophageal reflux in infants, *J Pediatr* 121(6):913-915, 1992.

Orenstein SR, Whitington P: Positioning for prevention of infant gastroesophageal reflux, *pediatrics* 103(4):534-537, 1983.

Potts MJ, Sesney J: Infant constipation: maternal knowledge and beliefs, *Clin Pediatr* 31(3):143-148, 1992.

Reynolds SL, Jaffe DM: Quick triage of children with abdominal pain, *Emerg Med* 22(14):39-42, 1990.

Samelson S, Reyes H: Management of perforated appendicitis in children—revisited, *Arch Surg* 122:691-695, 1987.

Seidman E: Nutritional management of inflammatory bowel disease, *Gastroenterol Clin North Am* 17(1):129-155, 1989.

Shandling B: Appendicitis. In Walker W and others, editors: *Pediatric gastrointestinal disease,* Philadelphia, 1991, BC Decker.

Siegel MJ, Carel C, Surratt S: Ultrasonography of acute abdominal pain in children, *JAMA* 266:1987-1989, 1991.

Staiano A and others: Effect of cisapride on chronic idiopathic constipation in children, *Dig Dis Sci* 36(6):733-736, 1991.

Tamanaha K and others: Air reduction of intussusception in infants and children, *J Pediatr* 111(5):733-735, 1987.

Thompson J: Surgical considerations in the short bowel syndrome, *Surg Gynecol Obstet* 176:89-101, 1993.

Tuchman D: Disorders of deglutition. In Walker W and others, editors: *Pediatric gastrointestinal disease,* Philadelphia, 1991, BC Decker.

Turgeon D, Barnett J: Meckel's diverticulum, *Am J Gastroenterol* 85(7):777-781, 1990.

Vanderhoof J and others: Short bowel syndrome, *J Pediatr Gastroenterol Nutr* 14(4):359-370, 1992.

Walker-Smith J: Celiac disease. In Walker W and others, editors: *Pediatric gastrointestinal disease,* Philadelphia, 1991, BC Decker.

Walker-Smith J and others: Revised criteria for diagnosis of coeliac disease, *Arch Dis Child* 65:909-911, 1990.

Weaver L: Anatomy and embryology. In Walker W and others, editors: *Pediatric gastrointestinal disease,* Philadelphia, 1991, BC Decker.

Ziller S, Netchvolodoff C: Uncomplicated peptic ulcer disease, *Postgrad Med* 93(4):126-138, 1993.

BIBLIOGRAPHY

Disorders of Motility

Andze G and others: Diagnosis and treatment of gastroesophageal reflux in 500 children with respiratory symptoms: the value of pH-monitoring, *J Pediatr Surg* 26(3):295-300, 1991.

Boyle J: Gastroesophageal reflux in the pediatric patient, *Gastroenterol Clin North Am* 18(2):315-337, 1989.

Clayden G: Management of chronic constipation, *Arch Dis Child* 67:340-344, 1992.

Di Lorenzo C and others: Gastric emptying with gastro-oesophageal reflux, *Arch Dis Child* 62:449-454, 1987.

Dipalma J: Metoclopramide: a dopamine receptor antagonist, *Am Fam Physician* 41(3):919-921, 1990.

Ellett ML: Constipation/encopresis: a nursing perspective, *J Pediatr Health Care* 4(3):141-146, 1990.

Evans K: Pediatric management problems . . . chronic constipation, *Pediatr Nurs* 16(6):590-591, 1990.

Fonkalsrud E and others: Surgical treatment of the gastroesophageal reflux syndrome in infants and children, *J Pediatr Surg* 154:11-17, 1987.

Fonkalsrud E and others: Operative treatment for the gastroesophageal reflux syndrome in children, *J Pediatr Surg* 24(6):525-529, 1989.

Foster P, Cowan G, Wrenn E: Twenty-five years' experience with Hirschsprung's disease, *J Pediatr Surg* 25(5):531-534, 1990.

Galmiche J and others: Double-blind comparison of cisapride and cimetidine in treatment of reflux esophagitis, *Dig Dis Sci* 35(5):649-655, 1990.

Grunow J, Al-Hafidh A, Tunell W: Gastroesophageal reflux following percutaneous endoscopic gastrostomy in children, *J Pediatr Surg* 24(1):42-45, 1989.

Hinder R and others: Relationship of a satisfactory outcome to normalization of delayed gastric emptying after Nissen fundoplication, *Ann Surg* 210(4):458-465, 1989.

Hlusko D, McMurray J: Gastroesophageal reflux: treatment and nursing care, *Neonatal Network* 9(5):33-36, 1991.

Hyman P, Abrams C, Dubois A: Gastric emptying in infants: response to metoclopramide depends on the underlying condition, *J Pediatr Gastroenterol Nutr* 7:181-184, 1988.

Jolley S and others: Gastric emptying in children with gastroesophageal reflux. II. The relationship to retching symptoms following antireflux surgery, *J Pediatr Surg* 22(10):927-930, 1987.

Keren S and others: Studies of manometric abnormalities of the rectoanal region during defecation in constipated and soiling children: modification through feedback therapy, *Am J Gastroenterol* 83(8):827-831, 1988.

Kaluser A and others: Behavioral modification of colonic function: can constipation be learned? *Dig Dis Sci* 35(10):1271-1275, 1990.

Konings K: Preop use of Golytely in pediatrics, *Pediatr Nurs* 15:473-474, 1989.

Marshall J: Gastroesophageal reflux disease, *Postgrad Med* 85(7):92-125, 1990.

Orenstein SR, Lofton S, Orenstein D: Bethanechol for pediatric gastroesophageal reflux: a prospective, blind, controlled study, *J Pediatr Gastroenterol Nutr* 5:549-555, 1986.

Orenstein SR, Orenstein D: Gastroesophageal reflux and respiratory disease in children, *J Pediatr* 112(6):847-858, 1988.

Orenstein SR and others: Reliability and validity of an infant gastroesophageal reflux questionnaire, *Clin Pediatr* 32(8):472-484, 1993.

Silk D: Fibre and enteral nutrition, *Gut* 30:246-264, 1989.

Sondheimer J: Resolving chronic constipation in children, *Patient Care* 21(5):108-112, 114, 116-118, 1987.

Sondheimer J: Gastroesophageal reflux: update on pathogenesis and diagnosis, *Pediatr Clin North Am* 35(1):103-116, 1988.

Sterling C, Schaffer S, Jolley S: Home management related to medical treatment for childhood gastroesophageal reflux, *Pediatr Nurs* 19(2):167-173, 1993.

Sterling C and others: Nursing responsibility in the diagnosis, care, and treatment of the child with gastroesophageal reflux, *J Pediatr Nurs* 6(6):435-440, 1991.

Tolia V and others: Randomized, prospective double-blind trial of metoclopramide and placebo for gastroesophageal reflux in infants, *J Pediatr* 115(1):141-145, 1989.

Turnage R and others: Late results of fundoplication for gastroesophageal reflux in infants and children, *Surgery* 105(4):457-464, 1989.

Understanding chronic constipation in your child, *Patient Care* 21(5):126-127, 1987.

Wheatley M and others: Long-term follow-up of brain-damaged children requiring feeding gastrostomy: should an antireflux procedure always be performed? *J Pediatr Surg* 26(3):301-305, 1991.

Zahr LK, Trentini P: Gastroesophageal reflux, fundoplication, and dumping: literature review and case study, *Issues Compr Pediatr Nurs* 12:385-393, 1989.

Inflammatory Conditions

Aiges H and others: Home nocturnal supplemental nasogastric feedings in growth-retarded adolescents with Crohn's disease, *Gastroenterology* 97(4):905-910, 1989.

Christie P, Hill G: Effect of intravenous nutrition on nutrition and function in acute attacks of inflammatory bowel disease, *Gastroenterology* 99:730-736, 1990.

Cooke D: Inflammatory bowel disease: primary health care management of ulcerative colitis and Crohn's disease, *Nurse Pract* 16(8):27-39, 1991.

De Giacomo C and others: Omeprazole treatment of severe peptic disease associated with antral G cell hyperfunction and hyperpepsinogenemia I in an infant, *J Pediatr* 117(6):989-993, 1990.

Drumm B and others: Peptic ulcer disease in children: etiology, clinical findings, and clinical course, *Pediatrics* 82(3):410-414, 1988.

Ellett ML, Schibler K: Adolescent psychosocial adaptation to inflammatory bowel disease, *J Pediatr Health Care* 2:57-66, 1988.

Elmore J, Dibbind A, Curci M: The treatment of complicated appendicitis in children, *Arch Surg* 122:424-427, 1987.

Gamal R, Moore T: Appendicitis in children aged 13 years and younger, *Am J Surg* 159:589-592, 1990.

Garretson D, Frederich D, Frederich M: Meckel's diverticulum, *Am Fam Physician* 42(1):115-119, 1990.

Gazzard B: The quality of life in Crohn's disease, *Gut* 28:378-381, 1987.

Giaffer M, North G, Holdsworth C: Controlled trial of polymeric versus elemental diet in treatment of active Crohn's disease, *Lancet* 335:816-819, 1990.

Gilbert G, Chan C, Thomas E: Peptic ulcer disease, how to treat it now, *Postgrad Med* 89(4):91-98, 1991.

Kirschner B: Inflammatory bowel disease in children, *Pediatr Clin North Am* 3(1):189-208, 1988.

Kisumoto and others: Complications and diagnosis of Meckel's diverticulum in 776 patients, *Am J Surg* 164:382-383, 1992.

Mezoff A, Balistreri WF: New GI therapies: any better than antiacids? *Contemp Pediatr* 7(4):101-123, 1990.

Mollitt A, Mitchum D, Tepas J: Pediatric appendicitis: efficacy of laboratory and radiologic evaluation, *South Med J* 81(12):1477-1479.

Peppercorn M: Advances in drug therapy for inflammatory bowel disease, *Ann Intern Med* 112(1):50-60, 1990.

Perkal M, Seashore J: Nutrition and inflammatory bowel disease, *Gastroenterol Clin North Am* 18(3):567-577, 1989.

Perrone VE: Inflammatory bowel disease. In Jackson PL, Vessey JA: *Primary care of the child with a chronic condition,* St Louis, 1992, Mosby.

Putnam T, Gagliano N, Emmens R: Appendicitis in children, *Surg Gynecol Obstet* 170:527-532, 1990.

Rappaport W, Peterson M, Stanton C: Factors responsible for the high perforation rate seen in early childhood appendicitis, *Am Surg* 55(10):602-605, 1989.

Rogers A: Medical treatment and prevention of peptic ulcer disease, *Postgrad Med* 88(5):57-60, 1990.

Rosen S, Rogers A: Peptic ulcer disease, a problem-oriented symposium, *Postgrad Med* 88(5):41-55, 1990.

Rothrock and others: Clinical features of misdiagnosed appendicitis in children, *Ann Emerg Med* 20(1):45-50, 1991.

Soll A and others: Nonsteroidal antiinflammatory drugs and peptic ulcer disease, *Ann Intern Med* 14(4):307-319.

Stange E and others: Cyclosporin-A treatment in inflammatory bowel disease, *Dig Dis Sci* 34(9):1387-1392, 1989.

Obstructive Disorders

Bisset G, Kirks D: Intussusception in infants and children: diagnosis and therapy, *Radiology* 168:141-145, 1988.

Bonadio W: Intussusception reduced by barium enema, *Clin Pediatr* 27(12):601-604, 1988.

Deluca S: Hypertrophic pyloric stenosis, *Am Fam Physician* 47(8):1771-1773, 1993.

Golladay E, Broadwater J, Molitt D: Pyloric stenosis—a timed perspective, *Arch Surg* 122:825-826, 1987.

Rollins M and others: Pyloric stenosis: congenital or acquired? *Arch Dis Child* 64:138-147, 1989.

Sapala S: Pediatric management problems, *Pediatr Nurs* 14(6):520-521, 1988.

Skipper R, Boeckman C, Klein R: Childhood intussusception, *Surg Gynecol Obstet* 171:151-153, 1990.

West K and others: Intussusception: current management in infants and children, *Surgery* 102(4):704-709, 1987.

Malabsorption Syndromes

Caniano D, Starr J, Ginn-Pease M: Extensive short-bowel syndrome in neonates: outcome in the 1980s, *Surgery* 105(2):119-124, 1989.

Colaco J and others: Compliance with gluten free diet in coeliac disease, *Arch Dis Child* 62:706-708, 1987.

Edes T: Clinical management of short-bowel syndrome, *Postgrad Med* 88(4):91-95, 1990.

Edes T and others: Essential fatty acid sufficiency does not preclude fat-soluble-vitamin deficiency in short-bowel syndrome, *Am J Clin Nutr* 53:499-502, 1991.

Galea M and others: Short-bowel syndrome: a collective review, *J Pediatr Surg* 27(5):592-596, 1992.

Guandalini S and others: Diagnosis of coeliac disease: time for a change? *Arch Dis Child* 64:1320-1325, 1989.

Hansmann M and others: Small bowel transplantation in a child, *AJCP* 42(5):686-692, 1989.

Iacono G and others: Extreme short bowel syndrome: a case for reviewing the guidelines for predicting survival, *J Gastroenterol Nutr* 16(2):216-219, 1993.

Kelly D and others: Rise and fall of coeliac disease 1960-85, *Arch Dis Child* 64:1157-1160, 1989.

Kurkchubasche A, Smith S, Rowe M: Catheter sepsis in short-bowel syndrome, *Arch Surg* 127:21-25, 1992.

Lin C and others: Nutritional assessment of children with short-bowel syndrome receiving home parenteral nutrition, *Am J Dis Child* 141:1093-1098, 1987.

Murray N, Vanderhoof J: Short bowel syndrome in children and adults, *J Enterostom Ther* 14(4):168-173, 1987.

Pokorny W, Fowler C: Isoperistaltic intestinal lengthening for short bowel syndrome, *Surg Gynecol Obstet* 172:39-43, 1991.

Todo S and others: Intestinal transplantation in composite visceral grafts or alone, *Ann Surg* 216(3):223-234, 1992.

Todo S and others: Intestinal transplantation in humans under FK 506, *Transplant Proc* 25(1):1198-1199, 1993.

Trier J: Diagnosis and treatment of celiac sprue, *Hosp Pract* 30:41-54, 1993.

Vanderhoof J: Short bowel syndrome. In Lebenthal E, editor: *Textbook of gastroenterology and nutrition,* New York, 1989, Raven Press.

Wise B: Neonatal short bowel syndrome, *Neonatal Network* 11(7):9-15, 1992.

Zahr LK and others: The short bowel syndrome: an update and a case study, *J Pediatr Nurs* 7(3):189-195, 1992.

Gastrointestinal Bleeding

Ament ME: Diagnosis and management of upper gastrointestinal tract bleeding in the pediatric patient, *Pediatr Rev* 12(4):107-116, 1990.

Cochran EB and others: Prevalence of, and risk factors for, upper gastrointestinal tract bleeding in critically ill pediatric patients, *Crit Care Med* 20(11):1519-1523, 1992.

Hill ID, Bowie MD: Endoscopic sclerotherapy for control of bleeding varices in children, *Am J Gastroenterol* 86(4):472-476, 1991.

Jonides L: Rectal bleeding, *J Pediatr Health Care* 6(6):377, 390, 1992.

Marshall J: Acute gastrointestinal bleeding, *Postgrad Med* 87(4):63-69, 1990.

Mertes J: Action stat! G.I. bleeding, *Nursing 89* 19(8):37, 1989.

Raine PA: Investigation of rectal bleeding, *Arch Dis Child* 66(3):279-280, 1991.

Silber G: Lower gastrointestinal bleeding, *Pediatr Rev* 12(3):85-93, 1990.

Hepatic Disorders

Bodenhorn K: Hepatitis B: the challenge for nurses, *J Pediatr Health Care* 6(1):41-42, 1992.

Bruckstein A: Chronic hepatitis: the challenge of diagnosis and treatment, *Postgrad Med* 85(7):67-74, 1989.

Buisuttil RW and others: Liver transplantation in children, *Ann Surg* 213(1):48-57, 1991.

Carey W, Patel G: Viral hepatitis in the 1990's. I. Current principles of management, *Cleve Clin J Med* 59(4):317-325, 1992.

Carey W, Patel G: Viral hepatitis in the 1990's. II. Hepatitis B and delta virus, *Cleve Clin J Med* 59(4):393-401, 1992.

Ergun G, Miskovitz P: Viral hepatitis, *Postgrad Med* 88(5):69-76, 1990.

Garland J, Werlin S, Rice T: Ischemic hepatitis in children: diagnosis and clinical course, *Crit Care Med* 16(12):1209-1212, 1988.

Marx J: Viral hepatitis, *Nursing 93* 23(1):34-42, 1993.

Nowicki M, Balistreri W: Hepatitis A to E: building up the alphabet, *Contemp Pediatr* 9(11):118-128, 1992.

Pasquale M, Cerra F: Sengstaken-Blakemore tube placement, *Crit Care Clin* 8(4):743-753, 1992.

Peck SN, Griffith DJ: Reducing portal hypertension and variceal bleeding, *Dimens Crit Care Nurs* 7(5):269-279, 1988.

Smith J: Hepatitis C: a major public health problem, *J Adv Nurs* 18:503-506, 1993.

Utili R and others: Prolonged treatment of children with chronic hepatitis B with recombinant α_{2a}-interferon: a controlled, randomized study, *Am J Gastroenterol* 86(3):327-330, 1991.

Whitington PF, Balistreri WF: Liver transplantation in pediatrics: indications, contraindications, and pretransplant management, *J Pediatr* 118(2):169-177, 1991.

UNIT XII

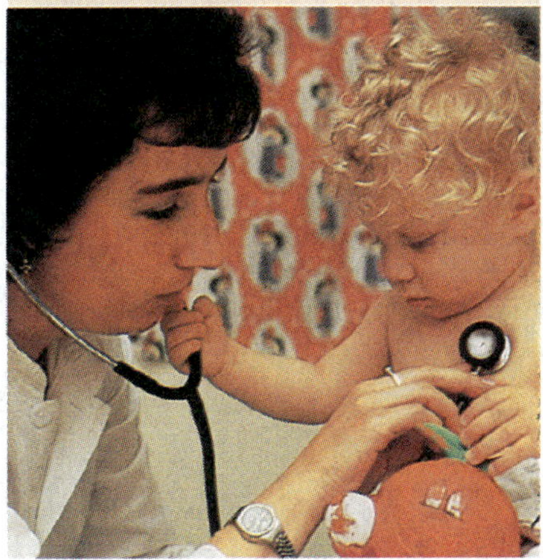

THE CHILD WITH PROBLEMS RELATED TO PRODUCTION AND CIRCULATION OF BLOOD

CHAPTER 34 The Child with Cardiovascular Dysfunction

CHAPTER OUTLINE

RELATED TOPICS

Birth of a child with a physical defect, Ch. 11
Compliance, Ch. 27
Controlling elevated temperatures, Ch. 27
Heart (physical assessment), Ch. 7
High risk related to cardiovascular/hematologic complications, Ch. 10
Family-centered care of the child with chronic illness or disability, Ch. 22
Family-centered care of the child with life-threatening illness, Ch. 23
Neonatal loss, Ch. 10
Neonatal pain, Ch. 11
Nursing care of the surgical neonate, Ch. 11
Pain assessment; pain management, Ch. 26
Physiologic measurements, Ch. 7
Preparation for procedures, Ch. 27
Skin (physical assessment), Ch. 7
Surgical procedures, Ch. 27
Tissue donation/autopsy, Ch. 23
Transplantation, Ch. 30
Vulnerable child syndrome, p. 388

CARDIAC STRUCTURE AND FUNCTION

Cardiovascular disorders in children are divided into two major groups: congenital cardiac defects and acquired heart disorders. ***Congenital heart defects*** are anatomic abnormalities present at birth that result in abnormal cardiac function. The clinical consequences of congenital heart defects fall into two broad categories, congestive heart failure and hypoxemia. ***Acquired cardiac disorders*** refer to disease processes or abnormalities that occur after birth and can be seen in the normal heart or in the presence of congenital heart defects. They result from various factors, including infection, autoimmune responses, environmental factors, and familial tendencies.

Understanding the effects of congenital and acquired heart defects requires knowledge of the normal heart's structure and function, including embryologic development, fetal circulation, and the changes that occur with postnatal growth. Basic cardiac physiology is presented in this section; altered hemodynamics are discussed on p. 1504.

CARDIAC DEVELOPMENT AND FUNCTION

The heart is a muscular four-chambered organ whose primary purpose is to pump blood throughout the body. It is located slightly to the left of the sternum in the space between the two pleural cavities, called the ***mediastinum.*** The main mass of the heart is formed by the muscular tissue, the ***myocardium.*** Lining the inner surface of the myocardium is the ***endocardium,*** a thin layer of endothelial tissue. The heart also has its own special covering, a double-walled membrane called the ***pericardium.*** Between the two layers is a slight space ***(pericardial space),*** which is filled with a few drops of serous fluid ***(pericardial fluid).*** These layers provide for frictionless movement of the heart muscle.

The interior of the heart is divided into four chambers. The two upper chambers are called ***atria;*** the two bottom chambers are ***ventricles.*** The atria are divided into the right atrium (RA) and the left atrium (LA) by the atrial septum. The ventricles are divided into the right ventricle (RV) and the left ventricle (LV) by the ventricular septum. Located within the heart are four ***valves,*** whose main function is to prevent the backflow of blood. The ***tricuspid valve,*** so named because it has three leaflets, or cusps, of endocardial tissue projecting into the ventricles, is located between the RA and the RV. The ***mitral valve*** has two leaflets and is located between the LA and the LV. Together these two valves are often termed ***atrioventricular (AV) valves.*** The valve leaflets are attached to the heart muscle by several cordlike structures called ***chordae tendineae.*** The ***semilunar valves*** are located in the pulmonary artery (PA) ***(pulmonic valve)*** and the aorta ***(aortic valve).*** Heart sounds (S_1 and S_2) are related to the vibrations that result during closing of these valves (see Chapter 7).

Embryologic Development

The heart and other components of the circulatory system (blood, blood vessels, lymph) begin to develop from the mesoderm during the fourth week of gestation and are completed by the eighth week. Cardiac development parallels the embryo's increasing nutritional needs.

During the third week, two endocardial tubes fuse to become the heart tube. As the tube elongates, it begins to coil to the right (dextra or D-looping). This looping occurs by approximately the twenty-eighth day, when the heart begins to beat. Concentrations of mesenchymal cells enlarge and cause their lining (endocardium) to bulge into the heart lumen. These internal bulges are called ***endocardial cushions*** and eventually merge to divide the heart chambers.

The developing heart tube bulges until it finally lies in the pericardial cavity. The tube remains attached to the pericardium at its cephalic and caudal ends but is free at the midsection. During the fifth week the midcardiac tube grows rapidly and assumes a characteristic convoluted shape with identifiable structures. These structures ultimately give rise to the heart chambers and vessels and include (1) a ***common atrium;*** (2) a ***common ventricle;*** (3) the ***bulbus cordis,*** which eventually helps form the outflow tracts of the ventricles; (4) the ***sinus venosus,*** which develops into the ***inferior*** and ***superior vena cava*** and ***coronary sinus;*** and (5) the ***truncus arteriosus,*** which divides into the PA and aorta and also gives rise to the aortic arch.

The formation of the heart's internal structures, particularly the cardiac septa (partitions), takes place almost simul-

■ Patricia O'Brien, RN,C, MSN, PNP; Annette L. Baker, RN, MSN; and Jeanne T. Boisvert, RN, BSN, revised this chapter.

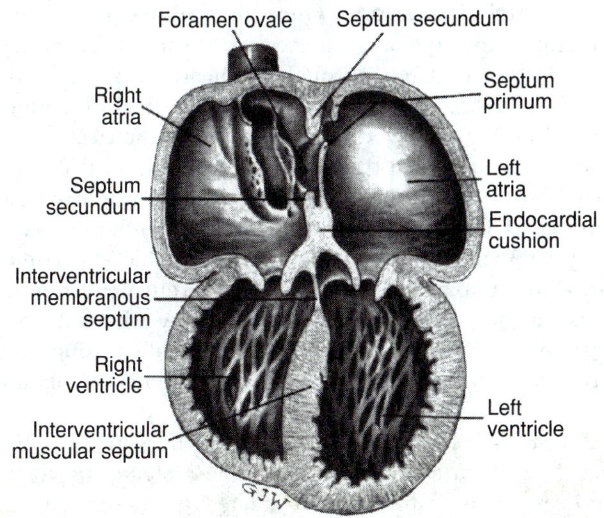

FIG. 34-1 Septal development of the heart.

taneously. The ***atrial septum*** is formed by the growth of both the ***septum primum*** and the ***septum secundum*** at about the fourth week of fetal growth. Overlapping of the septum primum and septum secundum before fusion results in a temporary flap opening known as the ***foramen ovale.***

The ***ventricular septum*** develops from the joining of the muscular and membranous ventricular septa during the fourth to eighth weeks of growth. The ***muscular septum*** develops when the right and left ventricular chambers fuse, whereas the ***membranous septum*** develops out of an intricate growth of the endocardial cushions, conal cushions, and conotruncal septum (Fig. 34-1). During this partitioning process, congenital defects may result if the formation of various structures is disturbed.

Fetal Circulation. The structure of the fetal heart provides for a pattern of circulation that is very different from that required during postnatal life. During fetal life the lungs are essentially nonfunctional and the liver is only partially functional; therefore less blood is needed in these organs than is required after birth. The fetal brain requires the highest oxygen concentration. The characteristics of fetal circulation ensure that the most vital organs and tissues receive the maximum concentration of vital materials.

Blood carrying oxygen and nutritive materials from the placenta enters the fetal system through the umbilicus via the large umbilical vein (Fig. 34-2, *A*). The blood then travels to the liver, where it divides; part of the blood enters the portal and hepatic circulation of the liver, and the remainder travels directly to the inferior vena cava (IVC) by way of the ***ductus venosus.*** Because of the higher pressure of blood entering the RA from the IVC, it is directed posteriorly in a straight pathway across the RA and through the foramen ovale to the LA. In this way the better-oxygenated blood enters the LA and LV to be pumped through the aorta to the head and upper extremities. Blood from the head and upper extremities entering the RA from the superior vena cava (SVC) is directed downward through the tricuspid valve into the RV. From here it is pumped through the PA, where the major portion is shunted to the descending aorta via the ***ductus arteriosus.*** A small amount flows to and from the nonfunctioning fetal lungs. Blood is returned to the placenta from the descending aorta through the two umbilical arteries.

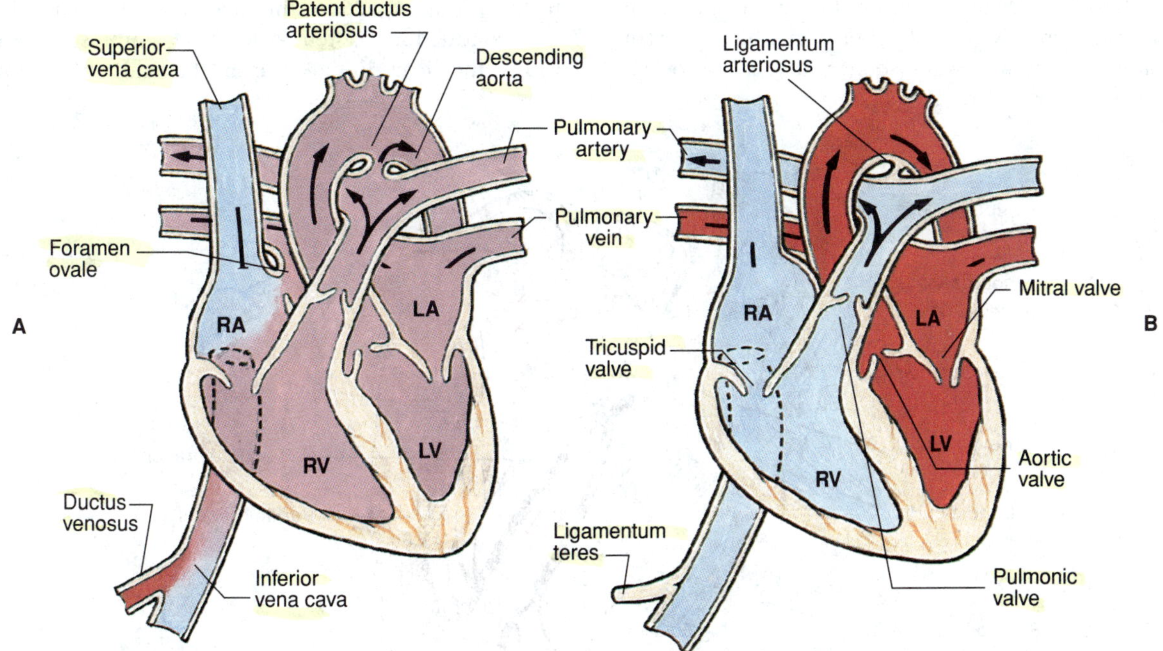

FIG. 34-2 Changes in circulation at birth. **A,** Prenatal circulation. **B,** Postnatal circulation. Arrows indicate direction of blood flow. Although four pulmonary veins enter the LA, for simplicity this diagram shows only two. *RA,* Right atrium; *LA,* left atrium; *RV,* right ventricle; *LV,* left ventricle.

Before birth, the high pulmonary vascular resistance created by the collapsed fetal lung causes greater pressures in the right side of the heart and the PAs. At the same time, the free-flowing placental circulation and the ductus arteriosus produce a low systemic vascular resistance in the remainder of the fetal vascular system. With the clamping of the umbilical cord and the expansion of the lungs at birth, the hemodynamics of the fetal vascular system undergo pronounced and abrupt changes. These changes are the direct result of cessation of the placental blood flow and the beginning of lung respiration. The changes occurring at birth are discussed in Chapter 8, and the circulatory changes in the heart are shown in Fig. 34-2, *B*.

Postnatal Development

In infancy the size of the heart in relation to total body size is larger, and the heart occupies a larger space within the mediastinum. The ventricle walls are more or less equal in thickness at birth. With the increased demand of the postnatal peripheral circulation, the left side becomes thicker than the right and pressures on the left side of the heart rise. Right-sided pressures decrease because the right ventricle is pumping blood to the low-pressure pulmonary bed. An increase in heart size accompanies the adolescent growth spurt, with a resulting increase in blood pressure and decrease in heart rate. The heart rate at any age shows an inverse relationship to body size (see inside back cover).

The arteries and veins elongate to keep pace with expanding body dimensions, and the vessel walls thicken to cope with the increased pressure. The systolic blood pressure after birth is low, reflecting the weaker LV of the neonate. With the developing strength and power of the left side of the heart, the systolic pressure rises rather sharply during the first 6 weeks and continues to rise but at a much slower rate until shortly before puberty, at which point it rises rapidly to adult levels (see inside back cover).

Postnatal Circulation. Once the cardiorespiratory system adjusts to the changes necessary to support extrauterine life, the circulation through the heart assumes a pathway that allows for oxygenation of venous blood by the lungs and delivery of saturated blood to the systemic circulation. Blood returning from the body via the SVC and IVC is received in the RA. It flows to the RV through the tricuspid valve. The RV pumps the blood through the pulmonic valve into the PA and then to the lungs, where the blood becomes saturated with oxygen. The blood is then returned from the lungs via the pulmonary veins into the LA, where it flows through the mitral valve to the LV, and finally through the aortic valve to the aorta and into the systemic circulation (see Fig. 34-2, *B*).

Arteries are thicker-walled blood vessels with thin muscular layers that carry highly oxygenated blood away from the heart to the capillary bed, which supplies oxygen and nutrients to the tissues. Veins are thin-walled blood vessels that return desaturated blood to the heart. The arterial system provides resistance to blood flow to maintain blood pressure and circulation. The venous system acts as a collecting system and a reservoir to accommodate changes in circulating blood volume. Both work together to provide equilibrium and maintain blood pressure.

The heart muscle receives its blood supply through the coronary circulation. The right and left ***coronary arteries***, which arise above the aortic valve, supply all the myocardium. The heart is the first organ to receive blood with each heartbeat; the brain is next. These two organs depend most on adequate oxygen levels for normal function. ***Coronary veins*** collect the blood and return it directly to the RA or through the coronary sinus, which drains into the RA.

Conduction System. To maintain an orderly and effective pumping action, the heart has a specialized electrical conduction system—electrical impulses generated within the heart initiate the mechanical contraction lead-

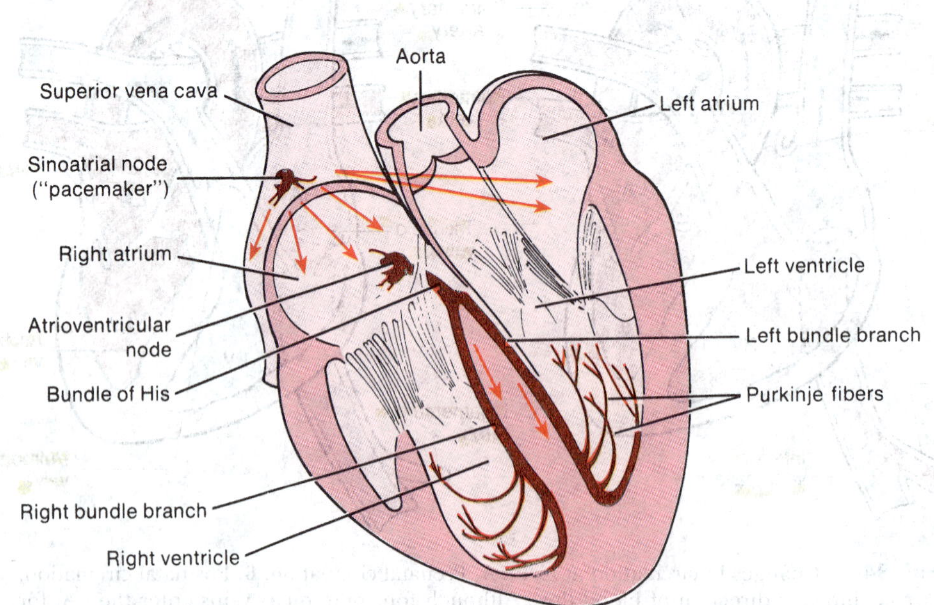

FIG. 34-3 Conduction system of the heart.

ing to the circulation of blood. Although all myocardial cells are capable of developing an action potential and depolarizing without external stimulation, certain specialized cells make up the heart's normal conduction system. These structures include the (Fig. 34-3):

1. **Sinoatrial (SA)** node, located within the RA wall near the opening of the SVC
2. **Atrioventricular (AV) node,** also located within the RA but near the lower end of the septum
3. **Atrioventricular bundle (bundle of His),** which extends from the AV node along each side of the interventricular septum and then divides into right and left bundle branches
4. **Purkinje fibers,** which extend from the AV bundle into the walls of the ventricles

The SA node is normally the heart's pacemaker and initiates an impulse. The impulse spreads from the SA node throughout the atria to cause depolarization. As the atria depolarize, impulses spread to the AV node to conduct to the ventricles. The AV node is the major pathway by which the impulses from the atria can be transmitted to the ventricles. The impulses then spread to the AV bundle and Purkinje fibers to cause simultaneous depolarization of the ventricles.

A ***cardiac cycle*** is composed of sequential contraction ***(systole)*** and relaxation ***(diastole)*** of both the atria and the ventricles. First, the atria contract, ejecting blood into the relaxed ventricles. Then, as the atria relax, the ventricles contract to eject blood into the PA and aorta. During diastole, blood enters the atria from the systemic and pulmonary veins, thus completing one cardiac cycle.

Basic Cardiac Physiology

The heart is basically a complex pump, ejecting blood throughout the body. The heart and lungs function together to deliver oxygen to the tissues and remove waste products such as carbon dioxide. The primary function of the cardiopulmonary system is to provide effective oxygen transport to meet the body's metabolic needs. To perform this function, the heart must maintain an adequate cardiac output. By definition, ***cardiac output*** is the volume of blood ejected by the heart in 1 minute. It is derived by multiplying the heart rate (HR) (number of beats per minute) by the stroke volume. ***Stroke volume*** is the amount of blood ejected by the heart in any one contraction. Stroke volume is influenced by three factors: preload, afterload, and contractility.

Cardiac output = HR × Stroke volume
↑
Preload
Afterload
Contractility

HR is influenced by the autonomic nervous system. The sympathetic fibers increase HR, and the parasympathetic fibers, acting through the vagus nerve, decrease HR. Levels of circulating catecholamines and other hormones also influence HR. Generally, an increase in HR will increase cardiac output, and a decrease or irregularity in HR (bradycardia, dysrhythmia) will impair cardiac output. However, a very fast HR shortens diastole and impairs coronary artery perfusion, causing eventual impairment of cardiac muscle function.

In simple terms, ***preload*** is the volume of blood returning to the heart, or the circulating blood volume. In physiologic terms, preload refers to myocardial fiber length. If the amount of blood delivered to the heart increases, then the myocardial fibers lengthen, and a greater amount of blood is pumped out of the heart. The circulating blood volume is most easily assessed clinically using the central venous pressure (CVP).

Afterload refers to the resistance against which the ventricles must pump when ejecting blood (ventricular ejection). Conditions that make it more difficult for the heart to pump blood forward into the circulation (e.g., severe hypertension) increase the afterload. It is determined by several complex factors, primarily the relative resistances of the systemic circulation ***(systemic vascular resistance)*** and the pulmonary circulation ***(pulmonary vascular resistance)***. Clinically, without the aid of hemodynamic monitoring, measurement of arterial blood pressure gives some indication of afterload—higher blood pressure, greater afterload.

Contractility refers to the efficiency of myocardial fiber shortening, or the ability of the cardiac muscle to act as an efficient pump. There is no simple bedside technique to assess contractility, although an echocardiogram may be useful. Contractility is often inferred in clinical practice. Assessments of peripheral tissue perfusion (pulses, warmth of extremities, and capillary refill) and urinary output can be helpful. Decreased contractility is suspected if the extremities are cool with thready pulses and urinary output is diminished. Certain states are known to depress contractility (e.g., hypoxia, acidosis). It is often decreased following cardiac surgery in the early postoperative period.

Adequate systemic perfusion depends on an appropriate HR, adequate circulating blood volume, efficient pump function, appropriate systemic and pulmonary vascular resistances, capillary permeability, and tissue utilization of oxygen. The body makes frequent adjustments in the various determinants of cardiac output to maintain a steady state.

Several clinical examples are useful to illustrate these principles. The ***Starling law (Frank-Starling curve)*** demonstrates that an increase in ventricular end-diastolic volume (caused by an increased preload) somewhat increases stroke volume. Since the myocardial fibers can stretch only to a certain point and still function effectively, any increase in volume beyond this point impairs cardiac output. When decreased cardiac output results from decreased preload (e.g., in hypovolemia due to blood loss), treatment involves providing volume, either with intravenous fluids or blood products. If decreased cardiac output results from a dramatic increase in afterload (e.g., severe hypertension) that increases the myocardial workload, treatment involves reducing afterload with vasodilating drugs. Contractility can be enhanced by medications such as digoxin or intravenous inotropic medications such as dopamine or dobutamine. Adjustments in HR are the most common response to changes in cardiac output; HR is slowest during sleep and can more than double with strenuous physical exercise.

ASSESSMENT OF CARDIAC FUNCTION

History

Assessment of all functional health patterns helps to establish a thorough history from the family. In taking a history, the nurse should elicit the parents' concerns. Often they have vague, nonspecific complaints, such as "Baby doesn't feed well" or "Baby is too quiet," that offer clues to a less obvious cardiac defect. Parents of children with congenital or acquired heart disease will often report one or more of the following:

- Poor weight gain, poor feeding habits, fatigue during feeding, sweating with feeding
- Frequent respiratory infections and difficulties (tachypnea, dyspnea, shortness of breath, persistent cough)
- Cyanosis
- Evidence of exercise intolerance

A history of previous cardiac defects in a sibling, maternal rubella infection during pregnancy, the use of medications or chemicals during pregnancy, or chronic illness in the mother can be important clues to the diagnosis of congenital heart disease. Children with chromosome abnormalities, such as Turner, Down, or Holt-Oram syndromes, are likely to have associated congenital heart defects, and the history is essential in evaluating their overall health.

In evaluating acquired heart disease, a history of a viral infection or toxic exposure is important if myocarditis is suspected. A history of a previous streptococcal infection is essential in rheumatic fever.

Physical Examination

Assessment of vital signs is helpful in screening patients for diseases of the cardiovascular system. An abnormally fast heart rate ***(tachycardia)*** or slow heart rate ***(bradycardia)*** may indicate cardiac disease. A fast respiratory rate ***(tachypnea)*** may indicate congestive heart failure. Hypertension is diagnosed by serial blood pressure measurements. Differences in blood pressure between upper and lower extremities may indicate coarctation of the aorta (see p. 1522).

NURSING ALERT A systolic blood pressure value 8 to 10 mm Hg higher in the arm than in the leg should be considered a significant finding in terms of coarctation of the aorta (Park, Lee, and Johnson, 1993).

Several aspects of physical examination may yield evidence of heart disease. (See Chapter 7 for a general discussion of physical assessment of the heart.) During inspection, a general examination of skin color (particularly the presence of cyanosis), position of comfort, and overall nutritional status is performed. During palpation, the point of maximum intensity and the apical impulse should be established, since they may offer clues to the position of the heart. The presence of a thrill, a soft vibration over the heart that reflects the transmitted sound of a heart murmur, should be noted. The quality of chest activity ("active precordium"), quality and symmetry of all pulses, warmth of extremities, and presence or absence of edema are assessed. Locating the hepatic and splenic borders for evidence of organ enlargement is also important.

Auscultation of heart sounds begins with assessment of heart rate and rhythm. The normal heart sounds S_1 and S_2 are auscultated, and the normal physiologic splitting of S_2 is noted. The presence of additional heart sounds, such as a gallop or a murmur, is noted. Auscultation of lung sounds, in particular noting the presence of crackles, wheezing, grunting, or decreased or absent breath sounds in some areas, is also important in the assessment of cardiovascular disease.

Murmurs are heart sounds that reflect the flow of blood within the heart. They may occur in systole or diastole or occur in both (a continuous murmur). They may reflect blood flow through a normal heart (particularly in periods of increased cardiac output such as fever, anemia, or rapid growth) or reflect abnormalities within the heart or the great arteries. (See Chapter 7 for a more detailed discussion of heart murmurs.) About 50% of children have an innocent murmur at some point (Newburger, 1992b). Innocent murmurs are present in infants and children with normal cardiac anatomy and heart function.

TESTS OF CARDIAC FUNCTION

A variety of invasive and noninvasive tests may be employed in the diagnosis of heart disease. Table 34-1 briefly outlines cardiac diagnostic procedures. The more frequently conducted tests are described here. Cardiac catheterization, which generates more anxiety than any other cardiac test, is discussed in detail; it may be used for diagnostic and interventional purposes.

Radiography

A chest x-ray examination is the most frequently ordered radiographic test for children with suspected cardiac problems. A chest film provides a permanent record of (1) the heart's size and configuration, its chambers, and the great vessels; and (2) the pattern of blood flow, especially in the pulmonary vessels. Fluoroscopy is used mainly in conjunction with cardiac catheterization.

Electrocardiography

An electrocardiogram (ECG) measures the electrical activity of the heart and records it on graph paper. This allows the evaluation of the sequence and magnitude of the electrical impulses generated by the heart (Fig. 34-4). The normal ECG consists of the P wave, P-R interval, QRS complex, T wave, Q-T interval, and ST segment:

P-wave—Represents the spread of the impulse over the atria (atrial depolarization). The sinus node's electrical activity is not represented in the ECG.

P-R interval—Represents the time that elapses from the beginning of atrial depolarization to the beginning of ventricular depolarization. It is termed P-R instead of P-Q because the Q wave is frequently absent.

QRS complex—Represents ventricular depolarization. It is ac-

TABLE 34-1 Procedures for Cardiac Diagnosis

PROCEDURE	DESCRIPTION
Chest radiograph (x-ray)	Provides information on heart size and pulmonary blood flow patterns
Electrocardiography (ECG or EKG)	Graphic measure of the electrical activity of the heart
Holter monitor	24-hour continuous ECG recording used to assess dysrhythmias
Echocardiography	Use of high-frequency sound waves obtained by a transducer to produce an image of cardiac structures
Transthoracic	Done with transducer on chest
M-Mode	One-dimensional graphic view used to estimate ventricular size and function
Two-dimensional (2-D)	Real-time, cross-sectional views of heart used to identify cardiac structures and cardiac anatomy
Doppler	Identifies blood flow patterns and pressure gradients across structures
Fetal	Imaging fetal heart in utero
Transesophageal (TEE)	Transducer placed in esophagus behind the heart to obtain images of posterior heart structures or in patients with poor images from chest approach
Cardiac catheterization	Imaging study using radiopaque catheters placed in a peripheral blood vessel and advanced into heart to measure pressures and oxygen levels in heart chambers and visualize heart structures and blood flow patterns
Hemodynamics	Measures pressures and oxygen saturations in heart chambers
Angiography	Use of contrast material to illuminate heart structures and blood flow patterns
Biopsy	Use of special catheter to remove tiny samples of heart muscle for microscopic evaluation; used in assessing infection, inflammation, or muscle dysfunction disorders; also to evaluate for rejection following heart transplant
Electrophysiology (EPS)	Employ special catheters with electrodes to record electrical activity from within heart; used to diagnose rhythm disturbances
Exercise stress test	Monitoring of heart rate, blood pressure, ECG, and oxygen consumption at rest and during progressive exercise on a treadmill or bicycle

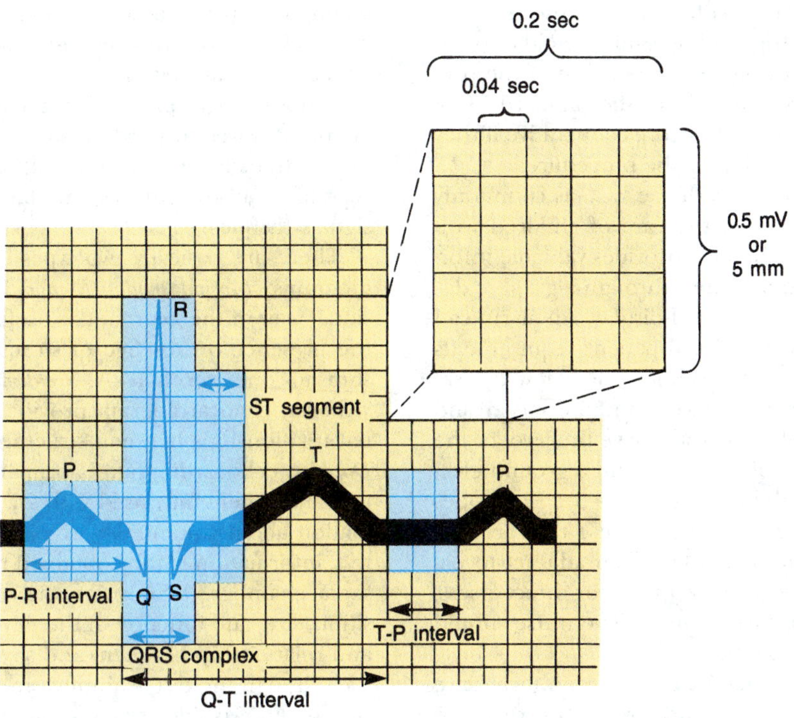

FIG. 34-4 Normal electrocardiogram pattern. Inset *(upper right)* shows conventional time and voltage or amplitude (height) calibrations.

tually composed of three separate waves—the Q, the R, and the S—that result from the currents generated when the ventricles depolarize before their contraction.

T wave—Represents ventricular repolarization.

Q-T interval—Represents ventricular depolarization and repolarization. This interval varies with heart rate—the faster the rate, the shorter the Q-T interval. Therefore in children this interval is normally shorter than in adults.

ST segment—Represents the time that the ventricles are in absolute refractory period, the period between ventricular depolarization and repolarization.

Information supplied by an ECG includes heart rate and rhythm, abnormalities of conduction, muscular damage (ischemia), hypertrophy, effects of electrolyte imbalance, the influence of various drugs, and pericardial disease. The ECG gives no direct information about the mechanical performance of the heart as a pump.

Special uses of the ECG include (1) continuous ambulatory monitoring, which employs a Holter monitor, a transistorized tape recorder attached to chest leads, and (2) exercise stress assessment, in which the ECG is monitored during controlled exercise, usually on a treadmill.

An ECG is taken by placing leads or electrodes on the skin to transmit electrical impulses back to a recording machine. Usually the electrodes are attached to the extremities and chest with adhesive, such as hydrogel, or with a suction bulb. An electrolyte lubricant is placed between the skin and the lead to increase conductivity. Chest leads must be positioned correctly because even minor misplacement can cause considerable inaccuracy in the recording. The standard adult ECG has 12 leads (6 limb leads and 6 chest leads). The standard pediatric ECG has actually 15 leads with the addition of leads on the right side of the chest and on the left lateral chest area. Although all these tests are painless, the leads can be frightening. Children old enough to understand can benefit from an explanation of the procedure. The child must remain still for the standard ECG; infants and young children may be more cooperative if they are held in the parent's lap during the procedure.

Bedside cardiac monitoring with the ECG is commonly used in pediatrics, especially in the care of children with heart disease. The bedside monitor provides valuable information about heart rate and rhythm through a graphic display of the ECG tracing and a digital display. An alarm can be set with parameters for individual patient requirements and will sound if the heart rate is above or below the set parameters. Gelfoam electrodes are commonly used and placed on the right side of the chest (above the level of the heart) and on the left side of the chest, and a ground electrode is placed on the abdomen (Fig. 34-5). Electrodes should be changed every 1 to 2 days because they are irritating to the skin. Bedside monitors are an adjunct to patient care and should never be substituted for direct assessments and auscultation of heart sounds. The nurse should assess the patient, not the monitor.

➤ **NURSING TIP** Electrodes for cardiac monitoring are often color coded: white for right, green (or red) for ground, and black for left. Always check to ensure that these colors are placed correctly.

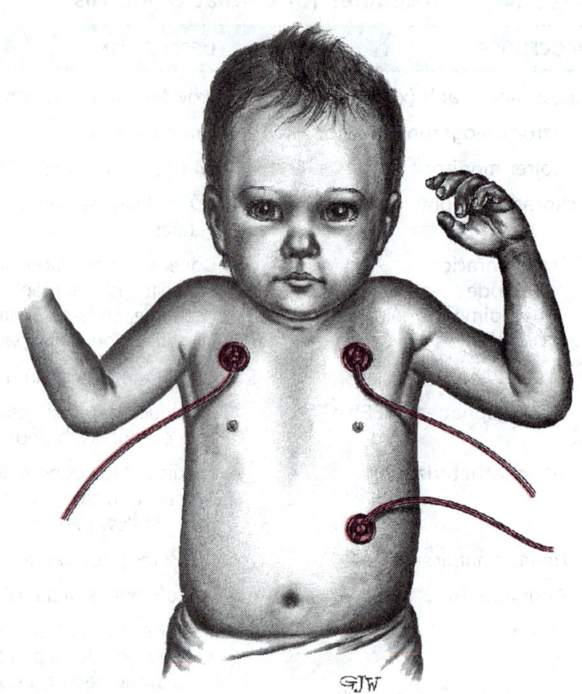

FIG. 34-5 Electrode placement for standard chest lead II in cardiac monitoring.

Echocardiography

Echocardiography is one of the most frequently used tests for detecting cardiac dysfunction in children. Recent improvements in echocardiographic techniques have made it increasingly possible to confirm the diagnosis without resorting to cardiac catheterization. In increasing instances a prenatal diagnosis of congenital heart disease can be made by fetal echocardiography.

Echocardiography involves the use of ultra-high-frequency sound waves to produce an image of the heart's structure. A transducer placed directly on the chest wall delivers repetitive pulses of ultrasound and processes the returned signals (echoes).

There are basically two types of transthoracic echocardiograms. ***Motion mode (M-mode)*** provides a one-dimensional view of the heart and is useful in determining its size, the presence or absence of structures, and their relationship to one another. A ***two-dimensional (2-D)***, or ***cross-sectional***, echocardiogram provides information about spatial relationships between structures. A ***pulse***, or ***continuous Doppler***, echocardiogram is primarily a velocity-sensing system and is generally used with 2-D "echo" to provide information about volume flow rate. Depending on the type of test, information can be obtained regarding the integrity of septa; chamber size; position and contractility; presence, position, size, and function of the valves; velocity of blood flow; and relationship between, and size of, the great vessels.

Although the test is noninvasive, painless, and associated with no known side effects, it can be traumatic for children. The child must lie quietly in the standard echocardiographic positions; crying, nursing, or sitting up often leads to diagnostic errors or omissions. Therefore infants and young children may need a mild sedative; older children benefit from psychologic preparation for the test. The distraction of a videotape is often helpful.

Transesophageal echocardiograms (TEEs) can provide information in cases where it is difficult to obtain information using the transthoracic approach. A transducer is passed into the esophagus to an area behind the atria. This procedure is more complicated and may require intubation to protect the airway of smaller children. Patients require IV sedation before this test.

Cardiac Catheterization

The most diagnostic invasive procedure is cardiac catheterization, in which a radiopaque catheter is inserted through a peripheral blood vessel into the heart. It is usually combined with angiography (angiocardiography), in which a radiopaque contrast material is injected through the catheter and into the circulation. Cardiac catheterization provides information regarding:

- ***Oxygen saturation*** of blood within the chambers and great vessels
- ***Pressure changes*** within these structures
- Changes in ***cardiac output*** or ***stroke volume*** (the amount of blood pumped out of the LV into the aorta with each contraction)
- ***Anatomic abnormalities,*** such as septal defects or obstruction to flow

Cardiac catheterization may be diagnostic, interventional, or electrophysiologic. Until recently, diagnostic catheterization was the only option. The two main types of ***diagnostic cardiac catheterizations*** are (1) ***right-sided,*** or ***venous, catheterization,*** in which the catheter is introduced from a vein into the RA; and (2) ***left-sided,*** or ***arterial, catheterization,*** in which the catheter is threaded by way of a systemic artery retrograde into the aorta and LV, or from a right-sided approach to the LA by means of a septal puncture or through an existing abnormal septal opening. In children the most common method is a right-sided catheterization, since septal defects permit entry into the left side of the heart.

The catheter is usually introduced through a percutaneous puncture into the femoral vein (the catheter is threaded over a guidewire inserted through a large-bore needle). Rarely, a cutdown procedure is needed to gain access to the vein, but this approach is associated with an increased risk of infection, hemorrhage, and obstruction. Once the vessel is entered, the catheter is guided through the heart with the aid of fluoroscopy. As the tubing is advanced, the child may feel pressure at the insertion site and vasospasm (fluttering) of the small vessels. Once the catheter is within the heart, blood samples and pressure readings are taken for analysis. Then the contrast material may be injected, and films are taken of the dilution and circulation of the material. As the contrast medium is administered, the child may experience warmth, nausea, vomiting, restlessness, or headache.

Interventional cardiac catheterization has become an alternative to surgery in some congenital heart defects, such as isolated valvular pulmonic stenosis and patent ductus arteriosus (Table 34-2).

TABLE 34-2 Current Interventional Cardiac Catheterization Procedures in Children

DIAGNOSIS	INTERVENTION
Transposition of the great arteries	Balloon atrioseptostomy Well established May also be done under echocardiography
Valvular pulmonary stenosis Distal pulmonary artery stenosis Recurrent coarctation of the aorta Rheumatic mitral valve	Balloon dilation Accepted alternative to surgery
Native coarctation of the aorta Valvular aortic stenosis	Balloon dilation Requires further follow-up
Patent ductus arteriosus Atrial septal defect Ventricular septal defect	Transcatheter device closure Clinical trials Devices under investigation
Some tachydysrhythmias	Radiofrequency ablation to destroy accessory pathway

Electrophysiologic studies are increasingly being used to evaluate and treat dysrhythmias. ***Diagnostic electrophysiologic catheterizations*** employ catheters with tiny electrodes that record the heart's electrical impulses directly from the conduction system. ***Interventional electrophysiologic catheterizations*** use radiofrequency ablation to destroy accessory pathways, which cause some tachydysrhythmias.

Nursing Considerations. Cardiac catheterization has become a routine diagnostic procedure and may be done on an outpatient basis. Catheterization is not, however, without risks, especially in neonates and seriously ill infants and children. Typical reactions include acute hemorrhage from the entry site (more likely with interventional procedures because larger catheters are used), low-grade fever, nausea, vomiting, loss of a pulse in the catheterized extremity (usually transient, resulting from a clot, hematoma, or intimal tear), and transient dysrhythmias (generally catheter induced). Rare risks include stroke, seizures, tamponade from myocardial perforation, and death (Roberts, 1989). Therefore, good nursing judgment and physical assessment before and after the procedure are essential.

Preprocedural care. A complete nursing assessment is necessary to ensure a safe procedure with a minimum of complications. This assessment should include an accurate height (essential to correct catheter selection) and weight. Obtaining a history of allergic reactions is important, since some of the contrast agents used are iodine based. Specific attention to signs and symptoms of infection is crucial. Severe diaper rash may be a reason to cancel the procedure if femoral access is required. Since assessment of pedal pulses is important after catheterization, the nurse should assess and mark pulses (dorsalis pedis, posterior tibial) be-

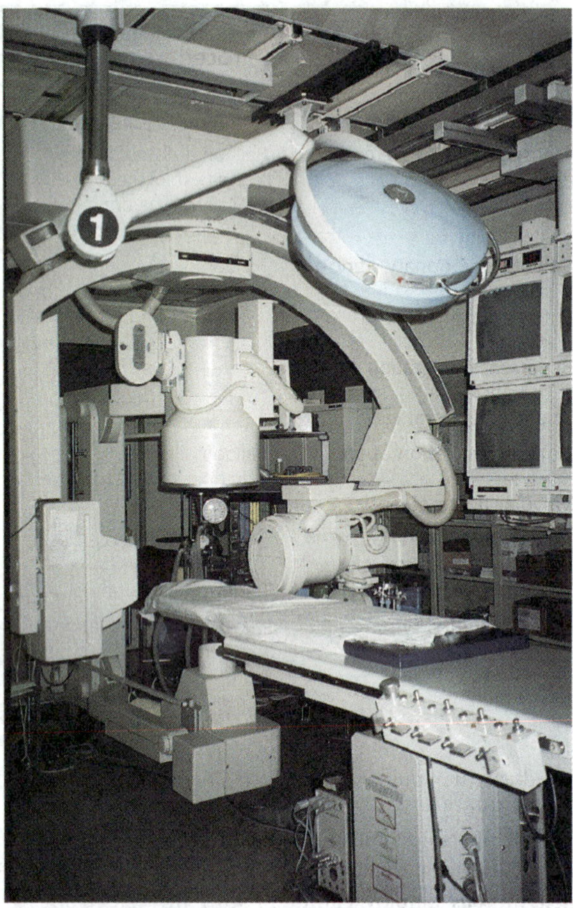

FIG. 34-6 Cardiac catheterization laboratory.

fore the child goes to the catheterization room. The presence and quality of pulses in both feet are clearly documented. Baseline oxygen saturation in children with cyanosis is also recorded.

Preparing the child and family for the procedure is the joint responsibility of physician, nurse, and parents. School-age children and adolescents benefit from a description of the catheterization laboratory (Fig. 34-6) and a chronologic explanation of the procedure emphasizing what they will see, feel, and hear. Preparation materials such as picture books, videotapes, or tours of the catheterization laboratory may be helpful. Preparation should be geared to the child's developmental level (see Chapter 27). The child's caregivers often benefit from the same explanations. Additional information, such as the expected length of the catheterization, description of the child's appearance after catheterization, and usual postprocedure care, should be outlined.

Before the test the child is usually given an analgesic and a sedative/anxiolytic drug combination, such as meperidine (pethidine [Demerol]) and midazolam (Versed). Chloral hydrate is often used in infants, and morphine sulfate is used in children with unrepaired tetralogy of Fallot. General anesthesia is usually unnecessary except in selected interventional procedures. Typically, the child is allowed nothing by mouth before catheterization, although polycythemic infants and children may require intravenous fluids to prevent dehydration, and neonates may need dextrose solution for up to 2 hours before the procedure to prevent hypoglycemia. Usually the morning dose of all oral medications is withheld, although this is clarified beforehand with the practitioner.

CRITICAL THINKING EXERCISE
Cardiac Catheterization

Tommy, a 4-year-old with tetralogy of Fallot, has just returned from the catheterization laboratory. He has vomited, and his mother calls you to the bedside to tell you that he is bleeding. You arrive to find Tommy crying and sitting up in a puddle of blood. The first thing you do is:

1. Increase the rate of his intravenous fluids.
2. Give an antiemetic and keep Tommy NPO (nothing by mouth).
3. Call the cardiologist.
4. Lie Tommy down, remove the dressing, and apply direct pressure above the catheterization site.

The correct answer is 4. This may be an arterial bleed, and Tommy is at risk for losing a large amount of blood in a short time. Your first priority should be to control the bleeding. Pressure is applied above the visible catheterization site where the vessel was entered. Placing the child flat decreases the effect of gravity on the rate of bleeding and is the appropriate position in case of shock. When this is done, you can notify the practitioner and replace fluids and control emesis as ordered.

Postprocedural care. Essentially, the care following cardiac catheterization is the same as general postoperative care. However, since children are not anesthetized during the procedure, they usually return directly to their room. Patients are often placed on a cardiac monitor and a pulse oximeter for the first few hours following catheterization.

The most important nursing responsibility is observation of the following for signs of complications (see Critical Thinking Exercise box):

- Pulses, especially below the catheterization site, for equality and symmetry (pulse distal to the site may be weaker for the first few hours after catheterization but should gradually increase in strength)
- Temperature and color of the affected extremity, since coolness or blanching may indicate arterial obstruction
- Vital signs, which are taken as frequently as every 15 minutes, with special emphasis on heart rate, which is counted for 1 full minute for evidence of dysrhythmias or bradycardia
- Blood pressure, especially for hypotension, which may indicate hemorrhage from cardiac perforation or bleeding at the site of initial catheterization
- Dressing, for evidence of bleeding or hematoma formation in the femoral or antecubital area
- Fluid intake, both intravenous and oral, to ensure adequate hydration. (Blood loss in the catheterization laboratory, the child's NPO status, and diuretic actions of dyes used during the procedure put children at risk for hypovolemia and dehydration.)

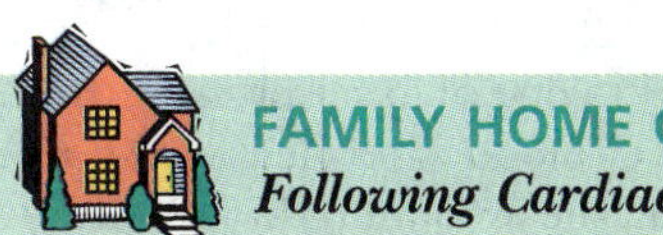

FAMILY HOME CARE
Following Cardiac Catheterization

Remove pressure dressing the day after catheterization. Cover site with an adhesive bandage strip for several days.
Keep site clean and dry. Avoid tube baths for several days; may shower.
Observe site for redness, swelling, drainage, and bleeding. Monitor for fever, Notify practitioner if these occur.
Avoid strenuous exercise for several days. May attend school.
Resume regular diet without restrictions.
Use acetaminophen or ibuprofen for pain.
Keep follow-up appointments per practitioner's instruction.

Modified from Children's Hospital (Boston) Cardiovascular Program, 1994.

- Infants are particularly at risk for hypoglycemia. They should receive dextrose containing IV fluids, and blood glucose levels should be checked.

NURSING ALERT If bleeding occurs, direct continuous pressure is applied 2.5 cm (1 inch) *above* the percutaneous skin site to localize pressure over the vessel puncture.

If venous vasospasm occurs, apply warmth to the opposite extremity, not the affected extremity, to improve circulation to the affected leg or arm.

Depending on hospital policy, the child may be kept in bed with the affected extremity maintained straight for 4 to 6 hours after venous catheterization and 6 to 8 hours after arterial catheterization to facilitate healing of the cannulated vessel. If younger children have difficulty complying, they can be held in the parent's lap with the leg maintained in the correct position. The child's usual diet can be resumed as soon as tolerated, beginning with sips of clear liquids and advancing as the condition allows. The child is encouraged to void to clear the contrast material from the blood. Generally, there is only slight discomfort at the percutaneous site. Acetaminophen can be given for pain. The catheterization site is covered with an occlusive waterproof pressure dressing (usually a foam tape dressing tightly applied) to prevent bleeding and contamination that could cause infection. The dressing is left on until the next day. Home care instructions are outlined in the Family Home Care box.

CONGENITAL HEART DISEASE (CHD)

The incidence of CHD in children is generally reported to be 4 to 10:1000 live births (Hoffman, 1990). CHD is the major cause of death (other than prematurity) in the first year of life. Although there are more than 35 well-recognized defects, the most common heart anomaly is ventricular septal defect (VSD) (Table 34-3). Reports on its incidence indicate that the diagnosis of VSD is increasing in frequency in the United States. Although the reason for this is not known, at least part of it probably results from improved detection of small, isolated VSDs, primarily with echocardiography (Martin, Perry, and Ferencz, 1989).

TABLE 34-3 Percentage Distribution of Selected Congenital Heart Defects and Association with Other Conditions

DEFECT	PERCENTAGE OF SPECIFIC DEFECTS*	DISORDERS ASSOCIATED WITH INCREASED INCIDENCE OF DEFECT†
Ventricular septal defect	32.1	Down syndrome Holt-Oram syndrome Fetal alcohol syndrome
Transposition of great arteries	2.6	Diabetes or prediabetes in mother
Tetralogy of Fallot	3.8	Down syndrome Fetal alcohol syndrome
Coarctation of aorta	6.7	Turner syndrome Apert syndrome
Patent ductus arteriosus	8.3	Rubella syndrome Down syndrome
Hypoplastic left heart syndrome	3.1	—
Atrioventricular valve defect	3.6	Down syndrome
Pulmonic stenosis	8.6	Rubella syndrome Noonan syndrome
Atrial septal defect	7.4	Noonan syndrome Holt-Oram syndrome Down syndrome Fetal alcohol syndrome
Aortic stenosis	3.8	Turner syndrome
Truncus arteriosus	1.7	—

*U.S. multicenter data. From Hoffman JJ: Congenital heart disease: incidence and inheritance, *Pediatr Clin North Am* 37(1):31, 1990.
†Data from Noonan JA: Association of congenital heart disease with syndromes or other defects, *Pediatr Clin North Am* 25(4):797-816, 1978.

The etiologic factor in CHD is not known in more than 90% of cases. However, several factors are associated with a higher-than-expected incidence of the defect. These include prenatal factors such as (1) maternal rubella during pregnancy, (2) maternal alcoholism, (3) maternal age over 40 years, and (4) maternal insulin-dependent diabetes. Heart defects are found in a much higher percentage of stillbirths, spontaneous abortions, and low-birth-weight infants, especially those small for age (Hoffman, 1990). Children with CHD are also more likely to have extracardiac defects, such as tracheoesophageal fistula, renal agenesis, and diaphragmatic hernias.

Several genetic factors are also implicated in CHD, although the influence is multifactorial. The risk of recurrence in families with an affected parent is variable: 1% to

3% if the father is affected and 2% to 10% if the mother is affected; the risk is possibly higher for left-sided obstructive lesions (Nora and Nora, 1988). The risk of recurrence in siblings is 1% to 3% overall. Certain chromosome aberrations, such as Down and Holt-Oram syndromes, are associated with increased risk of cardiac defects.

ALTERED HEMODYNAMICS

To understand the physiology of heart defects, it is necessary to review the role of pressure gradients, flow, and resistance within the circulation. Blood flows because of pressure gradients in different parts of the body and because of the heart's pumping action. As with any fluid, blood flows from an area of high pressure to one of low pressure and takes the path of least resistance. The rate of flow is directly proportional to the pressure gradient (i.e., the higher the pressure gradient, the greater the rate of flow) and inversely proportional to the resistance (i.e., the higher the resistance, the less the rate of flow). However, increased resistance does not always decrease flow. If the proximal cardiac chamber can increase the driving pressure proportionately, flow can remain unchanged.

Normally the pressure on the right side of the heart is lower than that on the left side, and the resistance in the pulmonary circulation is less than that in the systemic circulation. Likewise, vessels entering or exiting from these chambers have corresponding pressures (e.g., lower pressure in the PA and higher pressure in the aorta). Therefore, if an abnormal connection exists between the heart chambers, such as a septal defect, blood flows from an area of higher pressure (left side) to one of lower pressure (right side). This directional flow of blood is termed a ***left-to-right shunt.*** If the opening is small, the amount of blood shunted to the atrium or ventricle may be minimal.

An understanding of saturations within the heart is also helpful in understanding CHD. The blood returning to the heart via the great veins, the SVC and the IVC, should have the lowest oxygen saturation because the tissues should have extracted oxygen, leaving the venous blood desaturated. Saturations in the RA, RV, and PA should be equal. Blood returning from the lungs to the heart through the pulmonary veins should be fully saturated, the most oxygen-rich blood in the body. Saturations on the left side of the heart should all be equal, with fully saturated blood entering the aorta and first supplying the heart muscle through the coronary arteries and then supplying the brain (Fig. 34-7). Normally, saturated blood circulates separately from desaturated blood. Depending on the type of defect, mixing of saturated and desaturated blood may occur. The amount of mixed blood that reaches the systemic circulation is a significant feature of several cardiac anomalies and results in varying degrees of hypoxemia and cyanosis.

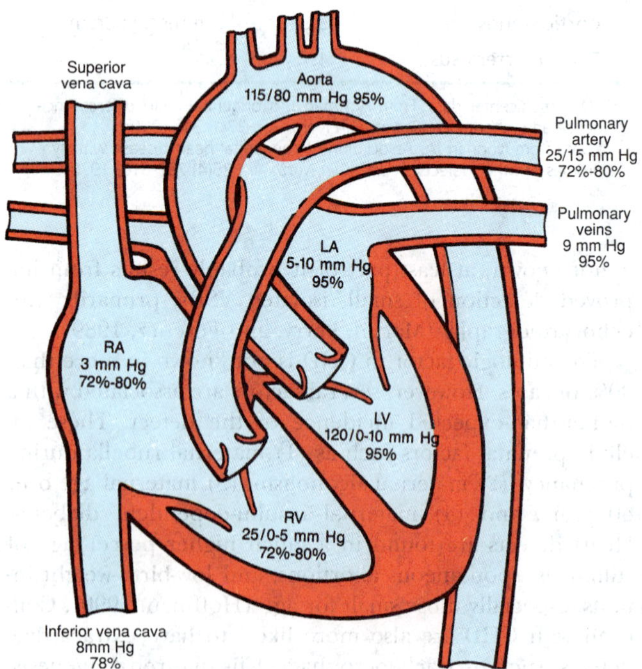

FIG. 34-7 Normal chamber pressures (mm Hg) and oxygen saturations (SaO_2) in cardiac chambers and great arteries. For simplicity, only two of the four pulmonary veins are shown. See Fig. 34-2 for abbreviations.

CLASSIFICATION AND CLINICAL CONSEQUENCES

Congenital heart defects have been divided into two categories. Traditionally, a physical characteristic, cyanosis, has been used as the distinguishing feature, dividing the anomalies into ***acyanotic*** and ***cyanotic defects.*** In clinical practice this system is problematic because children with acyanotic defects may develop cyanosis. Also, more often, those with cyanotic defects may be pink and have more clinical signs of congestive heart failure (CHF). Because of the complexity of many defects and the variability of their clinical manifestations, the cyanotic-acyanotic classification system has proved inadequate and misleading.

Another classification system, based on ***hemodynamic characteristics,*** or movements involved in circulation of blood, is more frequently used. The defining characteristic is blood flow patterns: (1) increased pulmonary blood flow, (2) decreased pulmonary blood flow, (3) obstruction to blood flow out of the heart, and (4) mixed blood flow, in which saturated and desaturated blood mix within the heart or great arteries. Both classification systems are outlined in Fig. 34-8.

With the hemodynamic classification system, the clinical manifestations of each group are more uniform and predictable. Defects that allow blood flow from the high-pressure left side of the heart to the lower-pressure right side (left-to-right shunt) result in increased pulmonary blood flow and cause CHF. Obstructive defects impede blood flow out of the ventricles; obstruction on the left side of the heart results in CHF, whereas severe obstruction on the right side causes cyanosis. Defects that cause decreased pulmonary blood flow result in cyanosis. Mixed lesions present a variable clinical picture based on degree of mixing and amount of pulmonary blood flow; hypoxemia (with or without cyanosis) and CHF usually occur together. (For

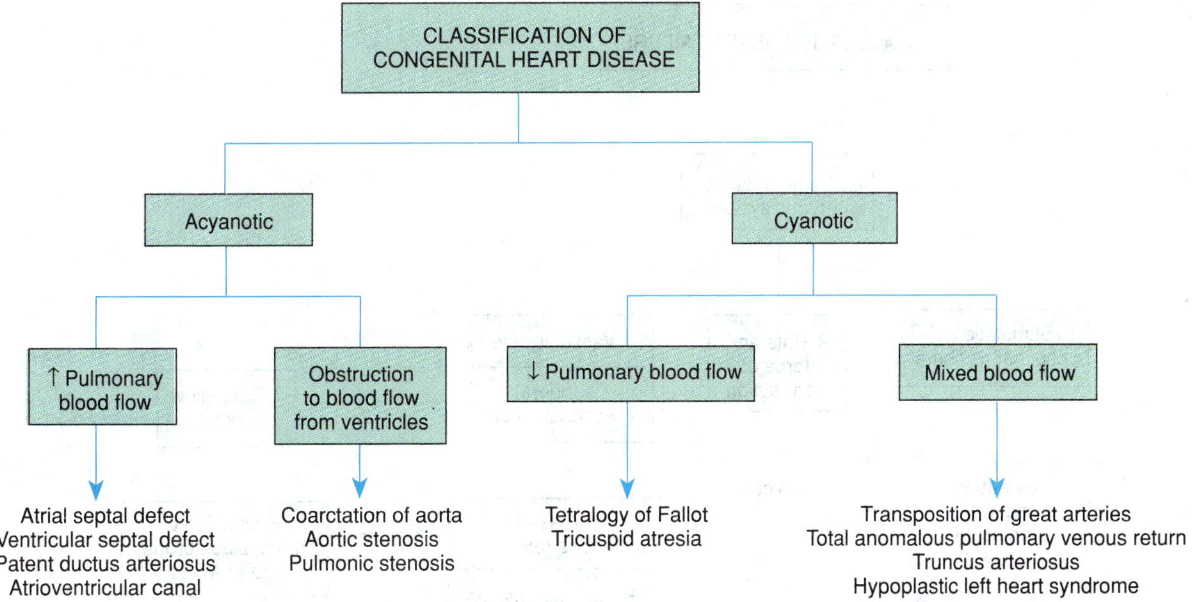

FIG. 34-8 Comparison of acyanotic-cyanotic and hemodynamic classification systems of congenital heart disease.

more detailed explanations, see specific defects later in this chapter.)

Depending on the severity of the cardiac defect and the altered hemodynamics, two principal clinical consequences can occur: CHF and hypoxemia. The conditions can occur alone or together. Nursing care plays a critical role in the early identification and supportive management of these conditions.

CONGESTIVE HEART FAILURE (CHF)

Congestive heart failure is inability of the heart to pump an adequate amount of blood to the systemic circulation to meet the body's metabolic demands. Causes of CHF can be classified according to the following changes:

Volume overload, especially with left-to-right shunts that may cause the RV to hypertrophy in order to compensate for the additional blood volume

Pressure overload, primarily resulting from obstructive lesions, such as valvular stenosis or coarctation of the aorta

Decreased contractility, primarily factors that affect the contractility of the myocardium, such as cardiomyopathy or myocardial ischemia from severe anemia or asphyxia, heart block, acidemia, and low levels of potassium, glucose, calcium, or magnesium

High cardiac output demands, in which the body's need for oxygenated blood exceeds the heart's cardiac output (even though the volume may be normal), such as in sepsis, hyperthyroidism, and severe anemia

In children CHF occurs most frequently secondary to congenital heart defects in which structural abnormalities result in an increased volume load or increased pressure load on the ventricles. For example, septal defects can cause large left-to-right shunts, resulting in a volume load on the RV. Obstruction to flow out of the LV, such as narrowing of the aorta (coarctation of the aorta), can cause increased pressure inside the ventricle. CHF can also be a result of an excessive workload on a normal myocardium. Myocardial failure, in which the contractility of the heart muscle is impaired, can result from cardiomyopathy, drugs, electrolyte imbalances, dysrhythmias, and other causes. Diseases in other organ systems, particularly the lungs, also can cause CHF. Obstructive changes in the lungs result in increased pulmonary vascular resistance, which increases the right ventricular workload. In time the right side of the heart has difficulty pumping blood forward to the lungs, becomes dilated, and hypertrophies; then signs and symptoms of right-sided heart failure are seen. ***Cor pulmonale*** is the term for CHF resulting from obstructive lung diseases such as cystic fibrosis or bronchopulmonary dysplasia.

Pathophysiology

Theoretically, heart failure may be divided into two classifications: right-sided failure and left-sided failure. In ***right-sided failure*** right ventricular function is suboptimal. RV end-diastolic pressure rises, causing increased central venous pressure and systemic venous engorgement. Systemic venous hypertension causes hepatomegaly and may cause edema in the extremities. In ***left-sided failure*** left ventricular dysfunction occurs and LV end-diastolic pressure rises, resulting in increased pressure in the LA and also in the pulmonary veins. The lungs become congested with blood, causing elevated pulmonary pressures and pulmonary edema.

Although each type of heart failure produces different signs and symptoms, clinically it is unusual to observe solely right- or left-sided failure in children. Since both sides of the heart depend on adequate function of the other side,

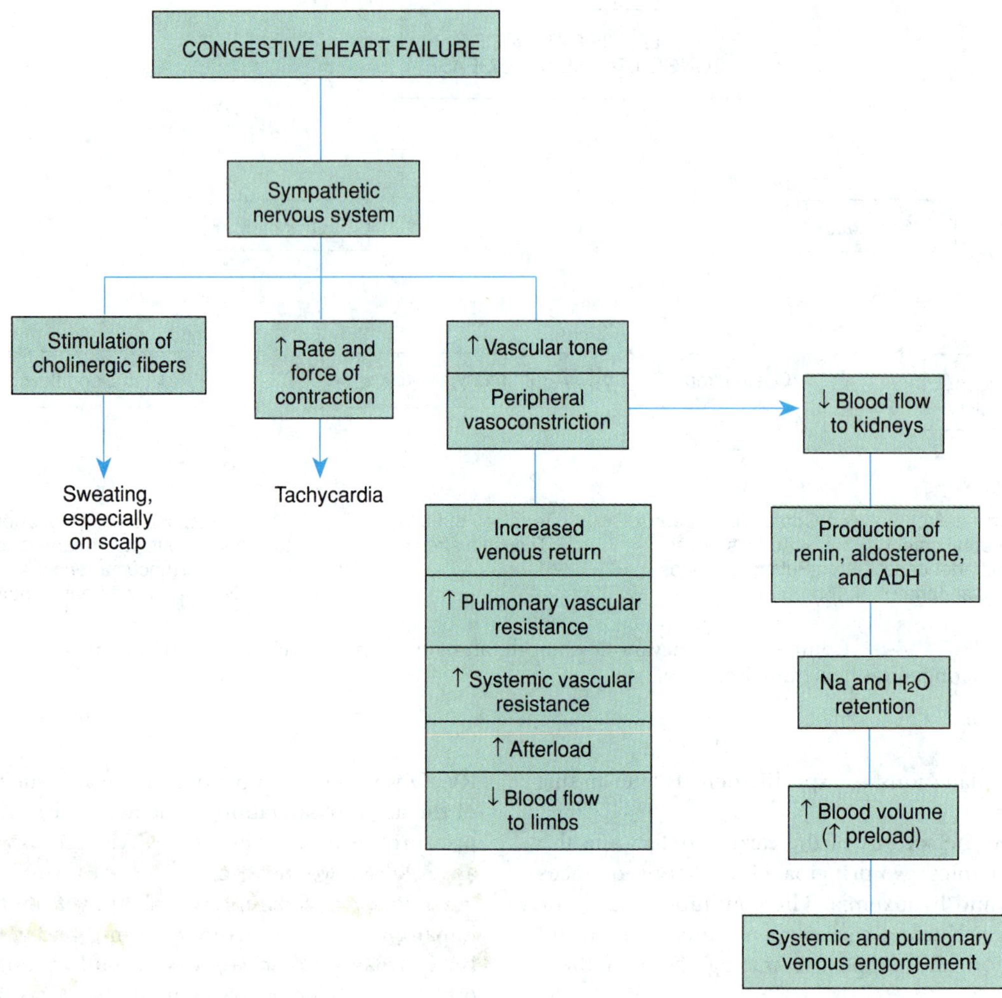

FIG. 34-9 Pathophysiology of congestive heart failure.

failure of one chamber causes a reciprocal change in the opposite chamber.

Compensatory Mechanisms. The heart initially tries to meet the body's demand for increased cardiac output through several compensatory mechanisms called the ***cardiac reserve.*** These include hypertrophy and dilation of the cardiac muscle and stimulation of the sympathetic nervous system (Fig. 34-9).

Hypertrophy and dilation of the cardiac muscle. In response to the need to increase cardiac output, the cardiac muscle hypertrophies, developing greater tension. It is able to generate increased pressure within the ventricle, pumping blood out of the heart at a higher pressure. Also, the cardiac muscle can dilate and increase the stretch of its fibers, which increases the force of contraction. However, both hypertrophy and dilation have potentially negative effects. Hypertrophy may result in decreased ventricular compliance over time. Decreased compliance requires a higher filling pressure to produce the same stroke volume. The increased muscle mass impairs oxygenation to the heart muscle. Beyond a certain amount of dilation, the force of contraction decreases and the heart fails. (See discussion of Starling law, p. 1497.)

Stimulation of the sympathetic nervous system. When the cardiac output begins to fall, stretch receptors and baroreceptors in the blood vessels stimulate the sympathetic nervous system, releasing catecholamines. Catecholamines increase the force and rate of myocardial contraction, as manifested by tachycardia. They cause peripheral vasoconstriction, resulting in increased systemic vascular resistance, increased venous return, and reduced blood flow to the limbs, viscera, and kidneys. Sympathetic cholinergic fibers cause sweating.

While initially successful in increasing cardiac output, prolonged sympathetic stimulation also has negative effects. By shortening the diastolic period, tachycardia increases oxygen consumption by the heart muscle, eliminates the heart's resting phase, and impairs coronary artery perfusion. A continued increase in systemic vascular resistance increases the afterload on the heart muscle, which requires extra work by the heart muscle and reduces systemic blood flow.

The renal system is particularly sensitive to reductions in blood flow and renal perfusion, activating the renin-angiotensin-aldosterone mechanism. Renin-angiotensin secretion causes vasoconstriction and leads to an increase in

CLINICAL MANIFESTATIONS OF CONGESTIVE HEART FAILURE

IMPAIRED MYOCARDIAL FUNCTION

Tachycardia
Sweating (inappropriate)
Decreased urinary output
Fatigue
Weakness
Restlessness
Anorexia
Pale, cool extremities
Weak peripheral pulses
Decreased blood pressure
Gallop rhythm
Cardiomegaly

PULMONARY CONGESTION

Tachypnea
Dyspnea
Retractions (infants)
Flaring nares
Exercise intolerance
Orthopnea
Cough, hoarseness
Cyanosis
Wheezing
Grunting

SYSTEMIC VENOUS CONGESTION

Weight gain
Hepatomegaly
Peripheral edema, especially periorbital
Ascites
Neck vein distention (children)

aldosterone secretion, which causes retention of salt and water. Retention of salt and water causes an increase in preload. Although at first helpful to the failing heart, the sodium and water retention becomes excessive, resulting in signs of systemic venous congestion and fluid overload.

Clinical Manifestations

As the compensatory mechanisms are exceeded, the child will exhibit signs of CHF because of decreased myocardial contraction, increased preload, and increased afterload. The signs and symptoms of CHF can be divided into three groups: (1) impaired myocardial function, (2) pulmonary congestion, and (3) systemic venous congestion (see box above). Because these hemodynamic changes occur from different causes and at differing times, the clinical presentation may vary among children.

Impaired Myocardial Function. One of the earliest signs of CHF is ***tachycardia*** (sleeping heart rate greater than 160 beats/min in infants) as a direct result of sympathetic stimulation. It is elevated even during rest but becomes extremely rapid with the slightest exertion. Ventricular dilation and excess preload result in extra heart sounds S_3 and S_4, referred to as ***gallop rhythm. Diaphoresis*** is often seen, especially on the head during exertion. Children are easily fatigued, have poor exercise tolerance, and are often irritable. Decreased cardiac output results in ***poor perfusion,*** manifested by cold extremities, weak pulses, slow capillary refill, low blood pressure, and mottled skin. Extreme pallor or duskiness are ominous signs.

Pulmonary Congestion. ***Tachypnea*** (respiratory rate greater than 60 breaths/min in infants) occurs in response to decreased lung compliance. Tachypnea can lead to hypoxemia because oxygen does not reach the alveoli for gas exchange in adequate amounts with fast breathing rates. ***Mild cyanosis*** results from impaired gas exchange and is relieved with oxygen administration. ***Dyspnea*** is caused by a decrease in the distensibility of the lungs. Inability to feed with resultant poor weight gain is primarily a result of tachypnea and dyspnea on exertion. ***Costal retractions*** occur as the pliable chest wall in the infant is drawn inward during attempts to ventilate the noncompliant lungs. Initially dyspnea may only be evident on exertion, but it may progress to the point that even slight activity results in labored breathing. In infants dyspnea at rest is a prominent sign and may be accompanied by flaring nares.

As the LV fails, blood volume and pressure increase in the LA, pulmonary veins, and lungs. Eventually the pulmonary capillary pressure exceeds the plasma osmotic pressure, forcing fluid into the interstitial space and finally causing ***pulmonary edema.*** Increased interstitial lung water also decreases compliance (ability to expand) of the lungs and increases the work of breathing.

Orthopnea (dyspnea in the recumbent position) is caused by increased blood flow to the heart and lungs from the extremities. It is relieved by sitting up because blood pools in the lower extremities, decreasing venous return. In addition, this position decreases pressure from the abdominal organs on the diaphragm. In infants orthopnea may be evident in their inability to lie supine and their desire to be held upright.

Edema of the bronchial mucosa may produce ***wheezing*** from obstruction to airflow. Mucosal swelling and irritation result in a persistent, dry, hacking ***cough.*** As pulmonary edema increases, the cough may be productive from increased secretions. Pressure on the laryngeal nerve results in ***hoarseness.*** A late sign of heart failure is ***gasping*** and ***grunting respirations.***

Infants with CHF have an increased metabolic rate and require additional caloric intake to grow. The work of the heart and breathing demands all the infant's energy, leaving little for normal activity. As a result of poor weight gain and activity intolerance, infants with CHF demonstrate ***developmental delays.*** Because of the physical energy and strength needed to sit up, pull to stand, and walk, these infants are delayed most in gross motor activities. The fine motor, social, and cognitive aspects of development seem less impaired. Following surgical correction, most children will catch up to their peers with time. Older children with severe CHF will have decreased exercise tolerance and persistent developmental delays.

Systemic Venous Congestion. Systemic venous congestion from right-sided failure results in increased pressure and pooling of blood in the venous circulation. ***Hepatomegaly*** occurs from pooling of blood in the portal circulation and transudation of fluid into the hepatic tissues. The liver may be tender on palpation, and its size is an indication of the course of heart failure.

Edema forms as the sodium and water retention causes systemic vascular pressure to rise. The earliest sign is ***weight gain.*** However, as additional fluid accumulates, it leads to swelling of soft tissue that is dependent and favors the flow of gravity, such as the sacrum and scrotum (when recumbent) and loose periorbital tissues. In infants edema is usually generalized and difficult to detect. Gross fluid accumulation may produce ***ascites*** and ***pleural effusions.***

Distended neck and ***peripheral veins*** result from a consistently elevated central venous pressure. Normally neck and hand veins collapse when the head or hands are raised above the level of the heart, since the blood drains by gravity back to the heart. However, when the venous pressure is high, it slows venous return, causing the veins to remain distended. Distended neck veins are difficult to detect in the short, fat neck of infants and are usually observed only in older children.

Diagnostic Evaluation

Diagnosis is made on the basis of clinical symptoms such as tachypnea and tachycardia at rest, dyspnea, retractions, activity intolerance (especially during feeding in infants), weight gain caused by fluid retention, and hepatomegaly. A chest x-ray film demonstrates cardiomegaly and increased pulmonary vascular markings due to increased pulmonary blood flow. Ventricular hypertrophy appears on the ECG.

Therapeutic Management

The goals of treatment are to (1) improve cardiac function (increase contractility and decrease afterload), (2) remove accumulated fluid and sodium (decrease preload), (3) decrease cardiac demands, and (4) improve tissue oxygenation and decrease oxygen consumption.

Improve Cardiac Function. Two groups of drugs are used to enhance myocardial performance in CHF: (1) digitalis glycosides, which improve contractility, and (2) angiotensin-converting enzyme inhibitors, which reduce the afterload on the heart, making it easier for the heart to pump.

Digitalis has three major actions. It (1) increases the force of contraction (positive inotropic), (2) decreases the heart rate (negative chronotropic) and slows the conduction of impulses through the AV node (negative dromotropic), and (3) indirectly enhances diuresis by increased renal perfusion. The beneficial effects are increased cardiac output, decreased heart size, decreased venous pressure, and relief of edema.

In pediatrics, ***digoxin (Lanoxin)*** is used because of its rapid onset and decreased risk of toxicity as a result of a relatively short half-life (1½ days) compared with other digitalis preparations. It is available as an elixir (50 μg/ml) for oral administration or in a parenteral preparation (0.1 mg/ml). For infants the dose is often calculated in micrograms (1000 μg = 1 mg). Because digoxin has a very narrow margin of safety, the dosage must be calculated exactly; premature infants are more sensitive to digoxin and require smaller doses because the drug accumulates in the blood faster than in full-term infants and children (Friedman, 1992).

Treatment is based on a digitalizing dose, given intravenously or orally, in divided doses over 24 hours to bring the child's serum digoxin level into the therapeutic range. A maintenance dose, usually one eighth of the digitalizing dose, is given orally twice a day to maintain blood levels (Table 34-4). During digitalization the child is monitored with an ECG to observe for the desired effects (prolonged P-R interval and reduced ventricular rate) and detect side effects, especially dysrhythmias.

TABLE 34-4 Oral Digoxin Dosage in Infants and Children*

AGE	TOTAL DIGITALIZING DOSE†	DAILY MAINTENANCE DOSE‡
Premature infant	20	5
Full-term infant	30	8-10
<2 years	40-50	10-12
2-10 years	30	8-10

*Dosage in μg/kg of body weight except as indicated.
†Total dose given in several divided doses over 12 to 24 hours.
‡Maintenance dose given in two divided doses.

Digoxin is the only oral inotropic agent generally available for infants and children, although other oral inotropic agents are being used in clinical trials in adults. For patients in severe CHF, intravenous inotropic agents such as dopamine, dobutamine, or amrinone are used to improve contractility. They are generally given in intensive care unit (ICU) settings.

A newer group of drugs that has proved beneficial in the treatment of CHF are the ***angiotensin-converting enzyme (ACE) inhibitors.*** As their name implies, these drugs inhibit the normal function of the renin-angiotensin system in the kidney. The production of renin triggers the production of angiotensin I and angiotensin II, which cause vasoconstriction and aldosterone secretion. The ACE inhibitors block the conversion of angiotensin I to angiotensin II so that instead of vasoconstriction, vasodilation occurs. Vasodilation results in decreased pulmonary and systemic vascular resistance, decreased blood pressure, a reduction in afterload, and decreased right and left atrial pressures. It also reduces the secretion of aldosterone, which reduces preload by preventing volume expansion from fluid retention and decreases the risk of hypokalemia. Renal blood flow is improved, which enhances diuresis.

Two ACE inhibitors are currently used in pediatrics: ***captopril (Capoten),*** given three times a day, and ***enalapril (Vasotec),*** given twice a day. Captopril is used in infants and young children because it can be given in smaller doses; its principal side effects are hypotension, renal dysfunction, and cough. Captopril may also have some immune-based side effects, including fever and allergic reactions. Since enalapril has the same principal side effects but fewer immune-based side effects, patients may be switched from one preparation to the other (see box on p. 1548) (Opie, 1991). Additional drugs in this class are now available for adults; they may be seen in pediatric use in the future.

NURSING ALERT Because ACE inhibitors also block the action of aldosterone, the addition of potassium supplements or spironolactone (Aldactone) to the drug regimen of patients taking diuretics is usually not needed and may cause hyperkalemia.

Remove Accumulated Fluid and Sodium. Treatment consists of diuretics, possible fluid restriction, and possible sodium restriction. Diuretics are the mainstay of therapy to eliminate excess water and salt to prevent reaccumulation.

TABLE 34-5 Diuretics Used in Congestive Heart Failure

DRUG	ACTION	COMMENTS	NURSING CONSIDERATIONS
Furosemide (Lasix)	Blocks reabsorption of sodium and water in proximal renal tubule and interferes with reabsorption of sodium in loop of Henle and in most proximal portion of distal tubule	Drug of choice in severe CHF Causes excretion of chloride and potassium (hypokalemia may precipitate digitalis toxicity)	Begin to record output as soon as drug is given Observe for dehydration caused by profound diuresis Observe for side effects (nausea and vomiting, diarrhea, ototoxicity, hypokalemia, dermatitis, postural hypotension) Encourage foods high in potassium and/or give potassium supplements Monitor chloride and acid-base balance with long-term therapy
Chlorothiazide (Diuril)	Acts directly on distal tubules and possibly proximal tubules to decrease sodium, water, potassium, chloride, and bicarbonate absorption Decreases urinary diluting capacity	Less frequently used drug Causes hypokalemia, acidosis from large doses May be given on alternate days or for 4 or 5 days and stopped for 2 days to allow for reabsorption of potassium	Observe for side effects (nausea, weakness, dizziness, paresthesia, muscle cramps, skin eruptions, hypokalemia, acidosis) Encourage foods high in potassium and/or give potassium supplements
Spironolactone (Aldactone)	Blocks action of aldosterone, allows retention of potassium	Weak diuretic Has potassium-sparing effect; frequently used with thiazides, furosemide Poorly absorbed from gastrointestinal tract Takes several days to achieve maximum actions	Observe for side effects (skin rash, drowsiness, ataxia, hyperkalemia) Do not administer potassium supplements
Bumetanide (Bumex)	Loop diuretic similar to furosemide Much more potent than furosemide (1 mg = 40 mg furosemide)	May be used for severe CHF when furosemide is less effective Use cautiously because of profound diuresis and electrolyte imbalances	Monitor for dehydration and electrolyte imbalances Observe for side effects (similar to those for furosemide) Observe for renal toxicity and electrolyte disturbances
Metolazone (Zaroxolyn)	Unique thiazide diuretic Appears effective in patients with reduced renal function	Chronic diuretic; useful in long-term therapy, not for acute diuresis Duration of action: 24 hours Use cautiously (once a day or several times weekly) because of profound diuresis and electrolyte imbalances	Observe for side effects, especially dehydration, nausea, vomiting, electrolyte imbalances Provide foods high in potassium and/or administer potassium supplements

The most commonly used agents are listed in Table 34-5. Since furosemide and the thiazides cause loss of potassium, potassium supplements and rich dietary sources of the electrolyte are given.

NURSING ALERT A fall in the serum potassium level enhances the effects of digoxin, increasing the risk of digoxin toxicity. Increased serum potassium diminishes digoxin's effect. Therefore serum potassium levels (normal range 3.5 to 5.5 mmol/L) must be carefully monitored.

Fluid restriction may be required in the acute states of CHF and must be carefully calculated to avoid dehydrating the child, especially if cyanotic CHD and significant polycythemia are present. Infants rarely need fluid restrictions because CHF makes feeding so difficult that they struggle to take maintenance fluids.

Sodium-restricted diets are used less often in children than in adults to control CHF because of their potential negative effects on the child's appetite and ultimate growth. If salt intake is restricted, the diet usually consists of avoiding additional table salt and highly salted foods. Low-salt formulas are available but used infrequently because infants need a normal sodium source to offset the sodium depletion of chronic diuretic therapy. Most infant formulas have slightly more sodium than breast milk.

Decrease Cardiac Demands. To lessen the workload on the heart, metabolic needs are minimized by (1) providing a neutral thermal environment to prevent cold stress in infants, (2) treating any existing infections, (3) reducing the effort of breathing (semi-Fowler position), (4) using medication to sedate an irritable child, and (5) providing rest and decreasing environmental stimuli.

Improve Tissue Oxygenation. All the preceding measures serve to increase tissue oxygenation either by improving myocardial function or by lessening tissue oxygen demands. In addition, supplemental cool humidified oxygen may also be administered to increase the amount of available oxygen during inspiration. Oxygen administration is especially helpful in patients with pulmonary edema, intercurrent respiratory infections, and increased pulmonary vascular resistance (oxygen is a vasodilator that decreases pulmonary vascular resistance).

> **NURSING ALERT** Oxygen is a drug and is only administered with an appropriate order. There are some uncommon circumstances in patients with complex hemodynamics in which oxygen can be detrimental.

An oxygen hood is preferred with young infants to provide increased concentration of the gas. A nasal cannula or face tent may be useful with older infants and children. Nasal cannulas are ideal for long-term oxygen administration because the child can be ambulatory and can easily eat and drink. Cool humidification is necessary to counteract the drying effect of oxygen. The amount of cool humidity is carefully regulated to prevent chilling.

Nursing Considerations

The infant or child with CHF is usually quite ill and may be admitted to an intensive care unit. Expert nursing care is essential to reduce the cardiac demands that strain the failing heart muscle. During this time the child and family require emotional support; for some children severe CHF represents end-stage cardiac disease.

❖ Assessment

Nurses need to be alert to signs of CHF in children with CHD and in infants with suspected CHD (see box on p. 1507). Signs of CHF indicate a worsening clinical condition; the earlier they are detected, the sooner treatment can be begun.

> **NURSING ALERT** The early signs of CHF are:
> Tachycardia, especially during rest and slight exertion
> Tachypnea
> Profuse scalp sweating, especially in infants
> Fatigue and irritablility
> Sudden weight gain
> Respiratory distress

❖ Nursing Diagnoses

Following a thorough assessment, several nursing diagnoses are evident (see Nursing Care Plan, pp. 1513-1514). Others may become apparent in special circumstances and with children in different age-groups.

❖ Planning

The goals for the infant or child with CHF and the family are as follows:

1. Child will exhibit improved cardiac output.
2. Child will experience decreased cardiac demands.
3. Child will exhibit improved respiratory function.
4. Child will maintain adequate nutritional status.
5. Child will exhibit no evidence of fluid excess.
6. Child and family will receive adequate support and education.

❖ Implementation

Although the objectives of nursing care are the same, the interventions differ depending on the child's age. Interventions for infants are quite different from those for older children.

Assist in Measures to Improve Cardiac Function. The nurse's responsibility in administering digoxin includes observing for signs of toxicity, calculating and administering the correct dosage, and instituting parental teaching regarding drug administration at home. The child's apical pulse is always checked before administering digoxin. As a general rule the drug is not given if the pulse is below 90 to 110 beats/min in infants and young children or below 70 beats/min in older children (the cutoff point for adults is 60). However, since the pulse rate varies in children in different age-groups, the written drug order should specify at what heart rate the drug is withheld. The nurse should also use judgment in evaluating the pulse rate. If it is significantly lower than the previous recording, the dose should be withheld until the practitioner is notified.

The apical rate is taken because a pulse deficit (radial pulse rate lower than apical) may be present with decreased cardiac output. It is auscultated for 1 full minute to evaluate alterations in rhythm. If the child is monitored by means of an ECG, a rhythm strip is obtained and attached to the chart for rate and rhythm analysis, such as abnormal lengthening of the P-R interval (more than a 50% increase over predigitalization interval) and dysrhythmias.

Digoxin is a potentially dangerous drug because the margin of safety of therapeutic, toxic, and lethal doses is very narrow. Many toxic responses are extensions of its therapeutic effects. Therefore the nurse must maintain a high index of suspicion for signs of toxicity when administering digoxin. The most common signs of digoxin toxicity in infants and children are bradycardia (though other dysrhythmias may occur), anorexia, nausea, and vomiting. Although vomiting should alert the nurse to observe for other evidence of cardiac toxicity, one episode of vomiting does not warrant cessation of the drug, because vomiting from other causes frequently occurs, especially in infants. Vomiting associated with digoxin toxicity is often unrelated to feedings, and infants are usually less interested in feeding with a recent decrease in oral intake. When in doubt regarding the cause of the vomiting and if another dose of digoxin should be given, the nurse should seek the practitioner's advice before administering the next dose. When there is concern about possible digoxin toxicity, the digoxin drug level is checked.

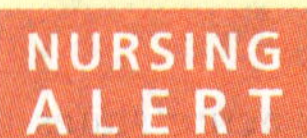

> Therapeutic serum digoxin levels range from 0.8 to 2 μg/L. Observe for signs of toxicity, especially bradycardia and vomiting.

Other extracardiac signs of toxicity are neurologic or visual disturbances, which are extremely difficult to identify in children and consequently are of little value in assessing toxicity in infants.

Since digoxin toxicity can occur from accidental overdose, great care must be taken in properly calculating and measuring the dosage. When converting milligrams to micrograms to milliliters, the nurse carefully checks the placement of the decimal point, since an error causes a significant change in dosage. For example, 0.1 mg is 10 times the dosage of 0.01 mg.

NURSING ALERT Infants rarely receive more than 1 ml (50 µg, or 0.05 mg) in one dose; a higher dose is an immediate warning of a dosage error. To ensure safety, compare the calculation with another staff member before giving digoxin.

If digoxin toxicity occurs, especially as a result of a drug overdose, all subsequent doses are withheld. The child is closely monitored for dysrhythmias, which are treated appropriately if they occur. Digoxin-specific Fab fragments are used as an antidote to digoxin in cases of severe digitalis toxicity (Woolf, 1992). Because of the long half-life of digoxin (1.5 days), it may be several days before the blood level returns to normal (Opie, 1991).

These same principles are taught to parents in preparation for discharge, although the correct dose in milliliters is usually specified on the container, thus reducing potential errors in calculation. The nurse observes the parent measuring the elixir in the dropper and stresses the level mark as the meniscus of the fluid that is observed at eye level. Other instructions for administering digoxin are listed in the Family Home Care box.

Parents are also advised of the signs of toxicity. According to the practitioner's preference, they may be taught to take the pulse before giving the drug. A return demonstration of the procedure from both parents or principal caregivers is included as part of the teaching plan. Their level of anxiety in counting the pulse is assessed, since overconcern about the heart rate may result in excessive withholding of the drug.

Afterload reduction. For patients receiving ACE inhibitors for afterload reduction, the nurse should carefully monitor blood pressure before and after dose administration, observe for symptoms of hypotension, and notify the practitioner if blood pressure is low. Serum electrolytes should be monitored. Because ACE inhibitors also block the action of aldosterone, they act as potassium-sparing agents. Most patients do not need potassium supplements or spironolactone (Aldactone) while receiving these medications. Numerous medications affecting the kidney can potentiate renal dysfunction, so children taking multiple diuretics along with an ACE inhibitor require careful assessment.

Decrease Cardiac Demands. The infant requires rest and conservation of energy for feeding. Every effort is made to organize nursing activities to allow for uninterrupted periods of sleep. Whenever possible, parents are encouraged to stay with their infant to provide the holding, rocking, and cuddling that help children sleep more soundly. To minimize disturbing the infant, changing bed linen and complete bathing are done only when necessary. Feeding is planned to accommodate the infant's sleep and wake patterns. The child is fed when hungry, such as when sucking

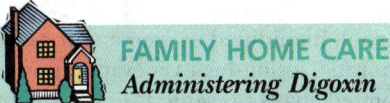

FAMILY HOME CARE
Administering Digoxin

- Give digoxin at regular intervals, usually every 12 hours, such as 8 AM and 8 PM.
- Plan the times so that the drug is given *1 hour before* or *2 hours after* feedings.
- Use a calendar to mark off each dose that is given or post a reminder, such as a sign on the refrigerator.
- Have the prescription refilled *before* the medication is completely used.
- Administer the drug carefully by slowly directing it on the side and back of the mouth.
- Do not mix it with other foods or fluids, since refusal to consume these results in inaccurate intake of the drug.
- If the child has teeth, give water after administering the drug; whenever possible, brush the teeth to prevent tooth decay from the sweetened liquid.
- If a dose is missed and more than 4 hours has elapsed, withhold the dose and give the next dose at the regular time; if less than 4 hours has elapsed, give the missed dose.
- If the child vomits, do not give a second dose.
- If more than two consecutive doses have been missed, notify the physician or other designated practitioner.
- Do not increase or double the dose for missed doses.
- If the child becomes ill, notify the physician or other designated practitioner immediately.
- Keep digoxin in a safe place, preferably a locked cabinet.
- In case of accidental overdose of digoxin, call the nearest poison control center immediately; the number is usually listed in the front of the telephone directory.

Modified from Jackson PL: Digoxin therapy at home: keeping the child safe, *MCN* 4(2):105-109, 1979.

on fists rather than when crying for a bottle, since the stress of crying exhausts the limited energy supply. Since infants with CHF tire easily and may sleep through feedings, smaller feedings every 3 hours may be helpful. Gavage feedings may be instituted to provide adequate nutrition and allow the infant to rest.

Every effort is made to minimize unnecessary stress. With infants, this primarily involves preserving the parent-child relationship and meeting their needs to reduce frustration. Older children need an explanation of what is happening to them to decrease anxiety about their illness and necessary treatments such as cardiac monitoring, oxygen administration, and medications. Outlining a plan for the day, preparation for tests and procedures, providing quiet activities, and providing adequate rest periods are all helpful interventions with older children. Some infants and children require sedation during the acute phase of illness to allow them to rest.

Temperature is carefully monitored for hyperthermia (a sign of infection) or hypothermia (loss of heat to ambient air). Fever is reported, since infection must be promptly treated. Fever increases oxygen demands and is poorly tolerated. If body temperature is low, the child is kept warm with additional blankets or the use of a radiant heater. Maintaining body temperature is very important for the child who is receiving cool, humidified oxygen and for one who tends to be diaphoretic, losing heat via evaporation.

Skin breakdown from edema is prevented with frequent change of position and use of pressure-relieving or pressure-reducing mattresses or beds. The skin, especially over the sacrum, is checked for evidence of redness from pressure. Respiratory infections can exacerbate CHF and should be appropriately treated and prevented if possible. The child is protected from persons with respiratory infections and has a noninfectious roommate. With an older child, it is advantageous to choose a roommate who is also confined to bed and relatively quiet in order to promote a restful environment. Good handwashing technique is practiced before and after caring for any hospitalized child. Antibiotics may be given to combat respiratory infection. The nurse ensures that the drug is given at equally divided times over a 24-hour schedule to maintain high blood levels of the antibiotic.

Reduce Respiratory Distress. Careful assessment, positioning, and oxygen administration can reduce respiratory distress. Respirations are counted for 1 full minute during a resting state. Any evidence of increased respiratory distress is reported, since this may indicate worsening heart failure.

Infants should be positioned to encourage maximum chest expansion, with the head of the bed elevated; they should sit up in an infant seat or be held at a 45-degree angle. Children prefer to sleep on several pillows and remain in a semi-Fowler or high Fowler position during waking hours. Shirts and diapers are pinned loosely to allow maximum chest expansion. Safety restraints, such as those used with the infant seats, are applied low on the abdomen and loosely enough to provide safety and maximum expansion.

The infant or child is often given humidified supplemental oxygen via oxygen hood or tent, nasal cannula, or mask. The child's response to oxygen therapy is carefully evaluated by noting respiratory rate, ease of respiration, color, and especially oxygen saturations, as measured by oximetry.

Maintain Nutritional Status. Meeting the nutritional needs of infants with CHF or serious cardiac defects is a nursing challenge. The metabolic rate of these infants is greater because of poor cardiac function and increased heart and respiratory rates. Their caloric needs are greater than those of the average infant because of their increased metabolic rate, yet their ability to take in adequate calories is hampered by their fatigue. Feeding for a fragile infant with serious CHD is similar to exercise in an adult, and they often do not have the energy or cardiac reserve to do extra work. The nurse seeks measures to enable the infant to feed easily without excess fatigue and to increase the caloric density of the formula.

The infant should be well rested before feeding and fed soon after awakening so as not to expend energy on crying. A 3-hour feeding schedule works well for many infants. (Feeding every 2 hours does not provide enough rest in between feedings, and a 4-hour schedule requires an increased volume of feeding, which many infants are unable to take.) The feeding schedule should be individualized to the infant's needs. A soft preemie nipple or a slit in a regular nipple to enlarge the opening decrease the energy expenditure of the infant while sucking. Infants should be well supported and fed in a semi-upright position. The infant may need to rest frequently and may need to have the jaw and cheeks stroked to encourage sucking. Generally, giving an infant about a half hour to complete a feeding is reasonable. Prolonging the feeding time can exhaust the infant and decrease the rest period between feedings.

Infants with feeding difficulties are often gavage fed using a nasogastric tube to supplement their oral intake and ensure adequate calories. If they are very stressed and fatigued, in respiratory distress, or tachypneic to 80 to 100 breaths/min, oral feedings may be withheld and all nutrition given by gavage feedings. Gavage feedings are usually a temporary measure until the infant's medical status improves and nutritional needs can be met through oral feedings. Some infants with severe CHF, neurologic deficits, or significant gastroesophageal reflux may need placement of a gastrostomy tube to allow adequate nutrition (see Critical Thinking Exercise box).

Increasing the caloric density of formulas by concentration and then adding corn or MCT oil or polycose is frequently done. Infant formulas provide 20 calories per ounce, and the use of additives can increase the calories to 30 calories or more per ounce. This allows the infant to obtain more calories despite a smaller volume intake of formula. The caloric density of the formula needs to be increased slowly (by 2 calories per ounce per day) to prevent

Critical Thinking Exercise

Congestive Heart Failure

A 6-week-old infant is admitted from the clinic in congestive heart failure following diagnosis of a ventricular septal defect. On admission, HR is 170, RR is 84, BP is 76/40, and O_2 saturation is 96%. He is very tired and irritable and has mild retractions but no edema. He has been feeding poorly for several days. He is started on digoxin and lasix. In planning fluid and nutrition for the next 12 hours, you would expect the following interventions to be ordered:

1. Push bottle feedings every 3 hours.
2. Make him NPO and run IV fluids at one-half maintenance.
3. Place a nasogastric feeding tube and institute gavage feedings to meet maintenance fluid requirements.
4. Begin infant on high-calorie formula and bottle-feed every 4 to 5 hours.

The correct answer is 3, begin gavage feedings. The infant is in mild respiratory distress with tachypnea and is very tired. Bottle-feedings would be too tiring, and he would not receive adequate fluids or nutrition. Gavage feedings will allow the infant to rest and supply needed nutrition. Enteral feedings are always preferred over IV hydration because more calories can be given. Fluid restriction is not needed, because the infant is behind on fluid intake, and lasix therapy has begun, so further fluid restriction would risk dehydration.

NURSING CARE PLAN
The Child with Congestive Heart Failure

NURSING DIAGNOSIS: Decreased cardiac output related to structural defect, myocardial dysfunction

PATIENT GOAL 1: Will exhibit improved cardiac output

• **NURSING INTERVENTIONS/*RATIONALES***

*Administer digoxin (Lanoxin) as ordered, using established precautions *to prevent toxicity*
- Make certain dosage is within safe limits
- Infants rarely receive more than 1 ml (50 μg or 0.05 mg) in one dose; *a higher dose is an immediate warning of a dosage error*
- Ascertain correct preparation for route
- Check dosage with another nurse *to ensure safety*
- Count apical pulse for 1 full minute before giving drug
  - Withhold medication and notify practitioner if pulse rate is less than 90 to 110 beats/min (infants) or 70 to 85 beats/min (older children), depending on previous pulse readings
- Recognize signs of digoxin toxicity (nausea, vomiting, anorexia, bradycardia, dysrhythmias)
- Often an ECG rhythm strip is taken *to assess cardiac status before administration*
- Ensure adequate intake of potassium
- Observe for signs of hypokalemia (muscle weakness, hypotension, dysrhythmias, tachycardia or bradycardia, irritability, drowsiness) or hyperkalemia (muscle weakness, twitching, bradycardia, ventricular fibrillation, oliguria, apnea)
- Monitor serum potassium levels *because decrease enhances digoxin toxicity*

*Administer medications to decrease afterload, as ordered
- Check blood pressure
  - Observe for signs of hypotension
- Monitor electrolyte levels

Attach cardiac monitor if ordered

• **EXPECTED OUTCOMES**

Heartbeat is strong, regular, and within normal limits for age (see inside back cover)

Peripheral perfusion is adequate

NURSING DIAGNOSIS: Ineffective breathing pattern related to pulmonary congestion

PATIENT GOAL 1: Will exhibit improved respiratory function

• **NURSING INTERVENTIONS/*RATIONALES***

Place in inclined posture of 30 to 45 degrees *to encourage maximum chest expansion;* tilt mattress support of incubator: place older infant in infant seat

Avoid any constricting clothing or restraints around abdomen and chest

*Administer humidified oxygen as prescribed

Assess respiratory rate, ease of respiration, color, and oxygen saturations as measured by oximetry

• **EXPECTED OUTCOME**

Respirations remain within normal limits, color is good, and child rests quietly (see inside back cover for normal variations in respirations)

PATIENT GOAL 2: Will experience reduction of anxiety

• **NURSING INTERVENTIONS/*RATIONALES***

Employ flexible feeding schedule *that reduces fretfulness associated with hunger*

Handle child gently

Hold and comfort infant

Employ comfort measures found effective for individual child

Encourage family to provide comfort and solace

Explain equipment and procedures to child *to decrease anxiety*

• **EXPECTED OUTCOME**

Child rests quietly and breathes easily

NURSING DIAGNOSIS: Fluid volume excess related to fluid accumulation (edema)

PATIENT GOAL 1: Will exhibit no evidence of fluid excess

• **NURSING INTERVENTIONS/*RATIONALES***

*Administer diuretics as prescribed

Maintain accurate intake and output

Weigh daily at same time and on same scale *to assess fluid gain or loss*

Assess for evidence of increased or decreased edema

Maintain fluid restriction, if ordered

Provide skin care for children with edema

Change position frequently *to prevent skin breakdown associated with edema*
- Use alternating-pressure mattress

• **EXPECTED OUTCOME**

Infant exhibits evidence of fluid loss (frequent urination, weight loss)

NURSING DIAGNOSIS: Activity intolerance related to imbalance between oxygen supply and demand

PATIENT GOAL 1: Will exhibit no additional respiratory or cardiac stress

• **NURSING INTERVENTIONS/*RATIONALES***

Maintain neutral thermal environment *because hypothermia or hyperthermia increases need for oxygen*
- Place newborn in incubator or under warmer
- Keep infant warm
- Treat fever promptly

*Dependent nursing action.

Continued.

NURSING CARE PLAN
The Child with Congestive Heart Failure—cont'd

Feed small volumes at frequent intervals (every 2 to 3 hours) using soft nipple with moderately large opening, *since infants with CHF tire easily*
Implement gavage feeding if infant becomes fatigued before taking an adequate amount
Time nursing activities to disturb child as little as possible
Implement measures to reduce anxiety
Respond promptly to crying or other expressions of distress

• EXPECTED OUTCOME
Child rests quietly

NURSING DIAGNOSIS: High risk for infection related to reduced body defenses, pulmonary congestion

See Infection Control, Chapter 27
See Nursing Care Plan: The Child with Congenital Heart Disease. p. 1538

NURSING DIAGNOSIS: Altered family processes related to a child with a life-threatening illness

PATIENT (FAMILY) GOAL 1: Will receive adequate support

• NURSING INTERVENTIONS/*RATIONALES* AND EXPECTED OUTCOMES
See Nursing Care Plan: The Family of the Ill or Hospitalized Child, Chapter 26

PATIENT (FAMILY) GOAL 2: Will be prepared for home care

• NURSING INTERVENTIONS/*RATIONALES*
Teach family:
- Medication administration and side/toxic effects
- Signs and symptoms of CHF and to report them to designated practitioner
- Feeding techniques and nutritional requirements
- Positioning
- Need for rest
- Growth and developmental considerations
  - Growth is slowed
  - Gross motor skills may be delayed more than fine motor skills

Refer to outpatient services and community resources as needed *for ongoing support*

• EXPECTED OUTCOMES
Family demonstrates an understanding of the condition and required care at home
Family uses appropriate community resources

diarrhea or formula intolerance. Breast-feeding mothers may be encouraged to provide the infant with alternating feedings of breast milk and high-calorie formulas. Some lactating mothers will prefer to feed the child expressed breast-milk that has been fortified with Similac or Enfamil powder, polycose, or corn oil to increase caloric intake. A supplemental nurser may also be helpful. A diet plan specific to the individual infant's needs is calculated and prescribed by the nutritionist in collaboration with the other health personnel. The nurse needs to reinforce this information with the parents as necessary.

Assist in Measures to Promote Fluid Loss. When diuretics are given, the nurse records fluid intake and output and monitors body weight at the same time each day to evaluate benefit from the drug. Since profound diuresis may cause dehydration and electrolyte imbalance (loss of sodium, potassium, chloride, bicarbonate), the nurse observes for signs indicating either complication, as well as signs and symptoms suggesting reactions to the drugs. Diuretics should be given early in the day to children who are toilet trained to avoid the need to urinate at night. If potassium-losing diuretics are given, the nurse encourages foods high in potassium, such as bananas, oranges, whole grains, legumes, and leafy vegetables, and administers prescribed supplements.

➤ **NURSING TIP** Mix the potassium supplement elixir with fruit juice (red punch or grape juice works well) to disguise the bitter taste and to prevent intestinal irritation from a concentrated solution.

NURSING ALERT Observe for signs of hypokalemia (muscle weakness, hypotension, dysrhythmias, tachycardia or bradycardia, irritability, drowsiness) or hyperkalemia (muscle weakness, twitching, bradycardia, ventricular fibrillation, oliguria, apnea) from supplement overdose.

Fluid restriction is rarely necessary in infants because of their difficulty in feeding. However, if fluids are restricted, the nurse plans fluid intake schedules for a 24-hour period, allowing for most fluids during waking hours. With toddlers and preschoolers it is psychologically advantageous to give small amounts of liquid in small cups so that the containers appear full. Suitable utensils are decorated medicine cups, paper Dixie cups, doll-sized teacups, or measuring cups. It is also important to avoid leaving extra fluids at the bedside, since older children may help themselves to additional servings. Older children's cooperation is gained by placing them in charge of recording fluid intake.

If salt is limited, the nurse discusses food sources of sodium with the family and discourages their bringing salt-containing treats to the child. At mealtime the child's tray is checked to make sure the appropriate diet is given.

Support Child and Family. CHF is a serious complication of heart disease. Parents and older children are usually acutely aware of the critical nature of the condition. Since stress places additional demands on cardiac function, the nurse should focus on reducing anxiety through anticipatory preparation, frequent communication with the parent regarding the child's progress, and constant reassurance that everything possible is being done.

Home care involves many of the same interventions discussed under Plan for Discharge and Home Care (see p. 1537). The nurse teaches the family about the medications that need to be administered and alerts them to the signs of worsening CHF that require medical attention, such as increased sweating, decreased urinary output (noted in fewer wet diapers or infrequent use of the toilet), or poor feeding. Compliance is a major issue, and every effort is extended to improve the family's adherence to the medication schedule (see Chapter 27). Written instructions regarding correct administration of digitalis (digoxin) are essential (see Family Home Care box on p. 1511), including an explanation regarding signs of toxicity.

If CHF is the end stage of a severe heart defect, the nurse cares for this child the same as for any child who is terminally ill, using the principles discussed in Chapter 23.

❖ EVALUATION

The effectiveness of nursing interventions for the family and the child with CHF is determined by continual reassessment and evaluation of care based on the following observational guidelines and expected outcomes:

1. Monitor heart rate and quality, respiratory rate and efforts, and color, and observe behaviors that provide clues to expended effort.
2. Observe nutritional intake, feeding behaviors, and weight.
3. Monitor intake, output, and weight.
4. Interview and observe behaviors of family.

Expected outcomes:

See Nursing Care Plan, pp. 1513-1514.

HYPOXEMIA

Hypoxemia refers to an arterial oxygen tension (or pressure, PaO_2) that is less than normal and can be identified by a decreased arterial oxygen saturation (SaO_2) or a decreased PaO_2. ***Hypoxia*** is a reduction in tissue oxygenation that results from low SaO_2 and PaO_2 and results in impaired cellular processes. ***Cyanosis*** is a blue discoloration in the mucous membranes, skin, and nail beds of the child with reduced oxygen saturation. It results from the presence of deoxygenated hemoglobin (hemoglobin not bound to oxygen) in a concentration of 5 g/dl of blood or more. Cyanosis is usually apparent when SaO_2 is 80% to 85% (Nadas, 1992). Determination of cyanosis is subjective. It can vary depending on skin pigment, quality of light, color of the room, or clothing worn by the child. The presence of cyanosis may not accurately reflect arterial hypoxemia, because both SaO_2 and the amount of circulating hemoglobin are involved. Children with severe anemia may not be cyanotic despite severe hypoxemia, because the hemoglobin level may be too low to produce the characteristic blue color. Conversely, patients with polycythemia may appear cyanotic despite a near-normal PaO_2.

Altered Hemodynamics

Heart defects that cause hypoxemia and cyanosis result from desaturated venous blood (blue blood) entering the systemic circulation without passing through the lungs. Three types of defects cause cyanosis in the infant. The first results from severe obstruction to pulmonary blood flow and blood shunting from the right side to the left side of the heart, or ***right-to-left shunting.*** Tetralogy of Fallot is the most common example. The second is mixing of arterial and venous blood within the chambers of the heart itself; a single ventricle is an example. The third defect, transposition of the great arteries, presents a unique situation in which the pulmonary and systemic circulations are parallel rather than in sequence. Fully oxygenated blood returns to the lungs, and desaturated blood returns to the body. Newborns with transposition of the great arteries depend on intracardiac mixing from a patent foramen ovale, septal defect, or ductus arteriosus to allow oxygenation.

Infants and children with some complex cardiac anomalies can be both hypoxemic and cyanotic and have symptoms of CHF. Defects resulting in one functional ventricle, hypoplastic left heart syndrome, and transposition of the great arteries with a ventricular septal defect are examples.

Adolescents and young adults may become cyanotic because of unrepaired septal defects in which the increased pulmonary blood flow over many years results in pulmonary vascular changes. ***Eisenmenger complex (syndrome)*** refers to the clinical situation in which a left-to-right shunt becomes a right-to-left shunt because of a progressive increase in pulmonary vascular resistance. With increasing pulmonary vascular thickening, the resistance in the pulmonary circulation can exceed or equal that in the systemic circulation, causing a reversal of blood flow from the right to the left ventricle.

Clinical Manifestations

Over time, two physiologic changes occur in the body in response to chronic hypoxemia: polycythemia and clubbing. Persistent hypoxemia stimulates erythropoiesis, resulting in ***polycythemia,*** an increased number of red blood cells. Theoretically, a greater number of red blood cells increases the oxygen-carrying capacity of the blood. However, this increased red blood cell formation may result in anemia if iron is not readily available for the formation of hemoglo-

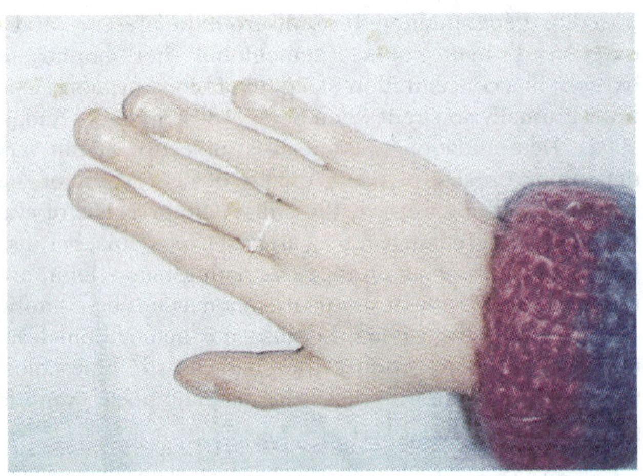

FIG. 34-10 Clubbing of the fingers.

bin. In addition, polycythemia increases the viscosity of the blood and tends to crowd out platelets and other coagulation factors. ***Clubbing,*** a thickening and flattening of the tips of the fingers and toes, is thought to occur because of chronic tissue hypoxemia and polycythemia (Fig. 34-10).

Infants with mild hypoxemia may be asymptomatic except for cyanosis and exhibit near-normal growth and development. Those with more severe hypoxemia may exhibit fatigue with feeding, poor weight gain, tachypnea, and dyspnea. The position of comfort for these infants is either flaccid with extremities extended (in contrast to the normal flexed position) or side-lying with the knees toward the chest. Both positions are thought to be a response to tissue hypoxia and an attempt to reduce oxygen demands. Flaccidity is usually a sign of severe cardiovascular compromise.

Squatting, most characteristic of children with unrepaired tetralogy of Fallot, is seen in toddlers and older children as an unconscious attempt to relieve chronic hypoxia, especially during exercise. The squatting position is helpful because flexing the legs (1) reduces the return of venous blood from the lower extremities, which is very desaturated, and (2) increases systemic vascular resistance, which diverts more blood flow into the pulmonary artery. Placing an infant in the knee-chest position (recommended during hypercyanotic spells) has the same beneficial hemodynamic effects as squatting. Because of early surgical intervention before walking, squatting is rarely seen.

Severe hypoxemia resulting in tissue hypoxia is manifested by clinical deterioration and signs of poor perfusion. The infant is pale and dusky with increased cyanosis, cool to touch with diminished pulses, and lethargic with signs of respiratory distress, including hyperpnea and gasping respirations. Tissue hypoxia causes metabolic acidosis, leading to hyperventilation and a rapidly worsening clinical course unless prompt treatment is instituted.

Hypercyanotic spells, also referred to as blue spells or "tet" spells because they are often seen in infants with tetralogy of Fallot, may occur in any child whose heart defect includes obstruction to pulmonary blood flow and communication between the ventricles (see Fig. 34-8). The infant becomes acutely cyanotic and hyperpneic because sudden infundibular spasm decreases pulmonary blood flow and increases right-to-left shunting (the proposed mechanism in tetralogy of Fallot). With other anomalies an increase in oxygen requirements, which the infant is unable to meet, may cause a spell. Hypoxia causes acidosis, which further increases pulmonary vascular resistance, which further decreases pulmonary blood flow; thus a vicious cycle ensues. Spells, rarely seen before 2 months of age, occur most frequently in the first year of life and more often in the morning, and they may be preceded by feeding, crying, or defecation. Because profound hypoxemia causes cerebral hypoxia, hypercyanotic spells require prompt assessment and treatment to prevent brain damage or possibly death.

Persistent cyanosis as a result of cyanotic cardiac defects places the child at risk for significant neurologic complications. Polycythemia and the resultant increased viscosity of the blood increase the risk of thromboembolic events. ***Cerebrovascular accidents*** (CVAs, strokes) may occur in about 2% of patients; infants with severe cyanosis and iron deficiency anemia are at greatest risk (Rosenthal, 1989). They may occur spontaneously but often follow an acute febrile illness, a hypoxic spell, or cardiac catheterization. Signs and symptoms of CVA include sudden paralysis, altered speech, extreme irritability or fatigue, and seizures. There is a 2% incidence of brain abscess in this patient population (Newburger, 1992b). Right-to-left shunting of blood in cyanotic heart defects allows bacteria to colonize the brain, which is vulnerable because of hypoxemia and poor perfusion of the cerebral microcirculation. Rarely seen in children under age 2 years, it should be suspected in older children with fever, headaches, focal neurologic signs, or seizures. Prompt treatment with antibiotics and surgical drainage is critical because death or significant neurologic impairment may result. Also, children who are cyanotic, especially those with systemic-to-pulmonary shunts, are at increased risk of ***bacterial endocarditis*** (see p. 1540).

Negative developmental consequences, particularly in the area of motor and cognitive development, may result from chronic hypoxemia (Newburger and others, 1984). Fifty percent of postnatal brain growth occurs in the first year of life, so chronic hypoxemia, poor growth, and nutrition during this period can have significant adverse effects. If the risks of CVA, brain abscess, periods of profound cyanosis and hypoxia during hypercyanotic spells, and multiple surgeries, hospitalizations, and cardiac catheterizations are added, the possibility of neurologic insult resulting in developmental delays becomes significant and increases with each year of life. Minimizing these risks is an important factor in the trend toward early corrective surgical repair of cyanotic defects in infancy.

Children who are cyanotic from birth are generally smaller than their peers, exhibit poor weight gain, have dyspnea on exertion, fatigue easily, and have poor exercise tolerance. Hematologic abnormalities are also seen, such as thrombocytopenia, abnormal platelet function, fewer coagulation factors, and prolonged clotting time. These hematologic changes increase the likelihood of postoperative bleeding.

Diagnostic Evaluation

Cyanosis in the newborn can be the result of cardiac, pulmonary, metabolic, or hematologic disease, although cardiac and pulmonary causes occur most often. To distinguish between the two, a hyperoxia test may be helpful. The infant is placed in a 100% oxygen environment, and blood gases are monitored. A PaO_2 of 150 mm Hg or more suggests lung disease, and a PaO_2 of less than 100 mm Hg suggests cardiac disease (problem is related to inadequate perfusion of the pulmonary bed) (Driscoll, 1990). An accurate history, chest radiograph (demonstrating reduced pulmonary blood flow), and especially an echocardiogram contribute to the diagnosis of cyanotic heart disease.

Therapeutic Management

Newborns generally exhibit cyanosis within the first few days of life as the ductus arteriosus, which provided pulmonary blood flow, begins to close. Prostaglandin E_1, which causes vasodilation and smooth muscle relaxation, thus increasing dilation and patency of the ductus arteriosus, is administered intravenously to reestablish pulmonary blood flow. The use of prostaglandins has been lifesaving for infants with ductus-dependent cardiac defects. The increase in oxygenation allows the infant to be stabilized and for a complete diagnostic evaluation to be performed before further treatment is needed.

Hypercyanotic spells occur suddenly, and prompt recognition and treatment are essential. In the hospital setting, spells are often seen during blood drawing or intravenous insertion, when the child is highly agitated, or following cardiac catheterization. Treatment of a hypercyanotic spell is outlined in the Guidelines box. Morphine, administered subcutaneously or through an existing intravenous line, is helpful in reducing infundibular spasm. Generally, a spell indicates the need for prompt surgical treatment (Driscoll, 1990). In some instances propranolol (Inderal) may be given in the interim to prevent infundibular spasm.

The cyanotic infant and child are well hydrated to keep the hematocrit and blood viscosity within acceptable limits to reduce the risk of CVA. Fevers are carefully evaluated because bacteremia can result in bacterial endocarditis. The infant is monitored closely for anemia because of the risk of CVAs and the reduced arterial oxygen-carrying capacity that occurs. Iron supplementation and possibly blood transfusion are used as needed. Older children and adolescents may require serial phlebotomy to reduce blood viscosity and minimize the risk of CVA. The goal is to reduce the hematocrit to approximately 60% by removing small aliquots of blood and replacing blood with normal saline or other intravenous solutions to maintain intravascular volume. This procedure is a temporary measure but may relieve symptoms of dyspnea, headache, and malaise for short periods and can be repeated every 1 or 2 months if polycythemia is severe.

Respiratory infections or reduced pulmonary function from any cause can worsen hypoxemia in the cyanotic child. Aggressive pulmonary hygiene, chest physiotherapy, administration of antibiotics, and use of oxygen to improve arterial saturations are important interventions.

Palliative Surgery. Severely hypoxemic newborns with cardiac defects not amenable to corrective repair may have a palliative surgical procedure called a ***shunt.*** The shunt serves the same purpose as the ductus arteriosus: to increase blood flow to the lungs through a systemic artery–to–pulmonary artery connection. Currently a ***modified Blalock-Taussig shunt*** using a Gore-Tex or Impra tube graft to create a communication between the right or left subclavian artery and the pulmonary artery on the same side is the preferred procedure. Because of the higher resistance in the systemic circulation, blood flows from the subclavian artery to the pulmonary artery and to the lungs for oxygenation. The small diameter of the subclavian artery (as opposed to the aorta) automatically restricts the volume of blood flow to the pulmonary artery. This procedure sacrifices the brachial and radial pulse on the affected side, and the hand initially may be slightly cooler and paler until collateral circulation develops. Table 34-6 outlines the different shunt procedures, including past ones rarely performed today and those used in specific clinical situations. Corrective surgical

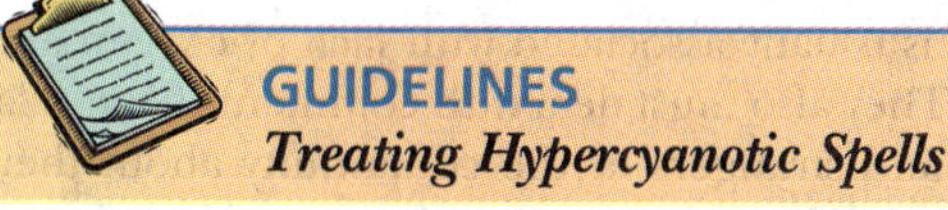

GUIDELINES
Treating Hypercyanotic Spells

Place infant in knee-chest position (Fig. 34-11).
Employ calm, comforting approach.
Administer 100% oxygen by face mask.
Give morphine subcutaneously or through existing intravenous line.
Begin intravenous fluid replacement and volume expansion, if needed.
Repeat morphine administration.

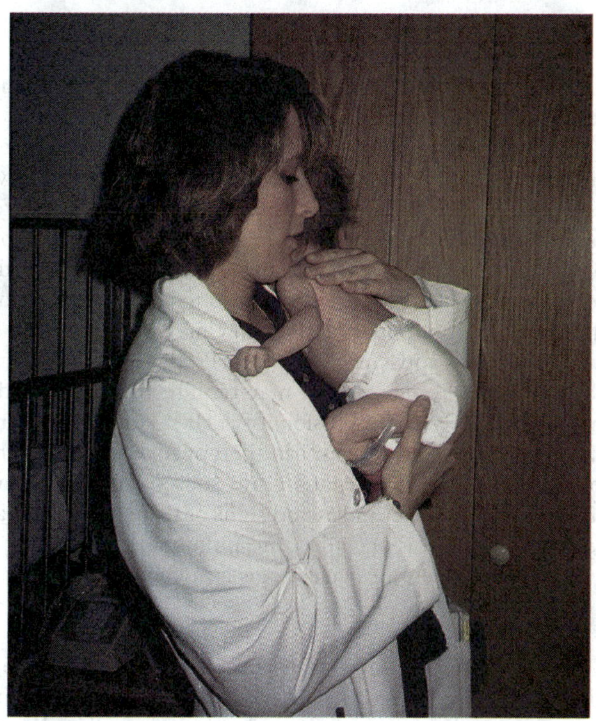

FIG. 34-11 Infant held in knee-chest position.

TABLE 34-6 Shunt Procedures for Children with Cardiac Defects

TYPE OF SHUNT/LOCATION	COMMENTS
Potts Descending aorta to left pulmonary artery	Rarely performed Shunt often excessive, causing CHF May be difficult to take down at time of definitive repair
Waterston Ascending aorta to right pulmonary artery	Rarely performed Shunt often excessive, causing CHF Kinking at anastomosis can cause obstruction of right pulmonary artery, requiring reconstruction at time of definitive repair
Blalock-Taussig (BT) Subclavian artery to pulmonary artery	Replaced by modified version More difficult to perform in small infants because of small subclavian artery Ligation of subclavian artery may cause growth retardation in affected arm
Modified Blalock-Taussig Subclavian artery or pulmonary artery using Gore-Tex or Impra tube graft	Shunt flow sometimes excessive, requiring use of diuretics Possibility of thrombosis; antiplatelet therapy may be used postoperatively Easy to ligate at time of definitive correction Shunt size fixed and may become too small as child grows
Central Ascending aorta to main pulmonary aorta using Gore-Tex graft	Length of shunt acts to restrict blood flow, limiting symptoms of CHF; may require diuretics Uncommon; used when BT shunt or modified BT shunt cannot be done Easy to perform and remove at time of repair
Glenn Superior vena cava to side of right pulmonary artery, which is ligated from main pulmonary artery Blood flow to right lung only	Used as a second shunt procedure if complete repair not possible High mortality in infants under age 6 months Superior vena cava syndrome may occur Pulmonary arteriovenous fistulas may occur many years later Difficult to take down at time of definitive repair
Bidirectional Glenn (cardiopulmonary anastomosis) Superior vena cava to side of right pulmonary artery Blood flow to both lungs	Done as a second shunt; often as a staging step to a Fontan procedure Can be incorporated into eventual modified Fontan procedure Relieves cyanosis and decreases volume overload on ventricle

Modified from O'Brien P: Surgical repair of cyanotic cardiac defects in young adults, *Nurs Clin North Am* 19(3):524, 1984.

repair is always preferred to a palliative shunt procedure if it can be performed at low risk. Corrective techniques are described with the cardiac defect.

Following a shunt procedure, the infant must be assessed for signs of increased or decreased pulmonary blood flow. If the shunt is too small or narrowed, the newborn may remain severely hypoxemic, with oxygen saturations below 70%. Surgically revising the shunt or placement of an additional shunt may be needed. More often the shunt is too large and the pulmonary blood flow may be excessive, resulting in signs and symptoms of CHF and oxygen saturations above 85%. The infant may require digoxin and diuretic therapy (see discussion of CHF). Some surgeons place infants on low-dose aspirin therapy for several months to prevent platelet aggregation and subsequent narrowing of the shunt. Acute cyanosis and signs of tissue hypoxia may occur if the shunt is occluded and pulmonary blood flow is severely limited; shunt occlusion is a medical emergency.

Nursing Considerations

The general appearance of infants and children with significant cyanosis poses unique concerns. Blue lips and fingernails are obvious signs of their hidden cardiac defect. Clubbing and small, thin stature in older children further indicate severe heart disease. Body image concerns are important; these children are often teased about their appearance and singled out as different. Adolescents are especially concerned about their body image, and cyanosis can become a particular issue for them. Many children, when asked what surgery will do, reply, "Make me pink." Their joy and excitement following surgery are evident when they see their pink fingers. Accentuating the normal and positive and being careful not to call attention to their cyanosis are helpful interventions. Meeting other children who are cyanotic in the clinic or hospital reassures them that they are not the only ones who are blue.

Parents are often fearful of their child's bluish color, since cyanosis is usually associated with lack of oxygen and severe illness. They also must deal with comments from relatives, friends, and strangers in the community about their child's abnormal color. They need a simple explanation of hypoxemia and cyanosis and reassurance that cyanosis does not imply a lack of oxygen to the brain. Their questions and fears need to be addressed in a calm, supportive manner, and positive aspects of their child's growth and development are emphasized. They are taught the treatment for hypercyanotic spells (see box on p. 1517).

Dehydration must be prevented in hypoxemic children

because it potentiates the risk of CVAs. Fluid status is carefully monitored, with accurate intake and output and daily weight measurements. Maintenance fluid therapy is the minimum requirement, supplemental fluids should be readily available, and gavage feeding or intravenous hydration is given to children unable to take adequate oral fluids. Fever, vomiting, and diarrhea can cause dehydration and require prompt treatment. Parents are instructed in the importance of adequate fluid intake and measures to prevent dehydration. An oral electrolyte solution such as Pedialyte should be available at home in the event the infant is unable to tolerate the usual formula. The practitioner should be notified of fever, vomiting, diarrhea, or other problems.

Preventive measures and accurate assessment of respiratory infection are important nursing considerations. Any compromise in pulmonary function will increase the infant's hypoxemia. Good handwashing and protection from individuals with an obvious respiratory infection are important. Aggressive pulmonary hygiene, treatment with antibiotics or antiviral agents as indicated, and supplemental oxygen to decrease hypoxemia are necessary measures. Infants may need to be gavage-fed or given parenteral hydration if respiratory distress prevents oral feeding.

NURSING ALERT Intracardiac shunting of blood from the right side (desaturated) to the left side of the heart allows air in the venous system to go directly to the brain, resulting in an air embolism. Therefore all intravenous lines should have filters in place to prevent air from entering the system, and the entire tubing and any syringes used for flushing or administering medication are checked for air. Any air is removed, and all connections are taped securely.

DEFECTS WITH INCREASED PULMONARY BLOOD FLOW

In this group of cardiac defects, intracardiac communications along the septum or an abnormal connection between the great arteries allows blood to flow from the high-pressure left side of the heart to the lower-pressure right side of the heart (Fig. 34-12). Increased blood volume on the right side of the heart increases pulmonary blood flow at the expense of systemic blood flow. Clinically patients demonstrate signs and symptoms of CHF. Atrial and ventricular septal defects and patent ductus arteriosus are typical anomalies in this group (see box on pp. 1519-1521).

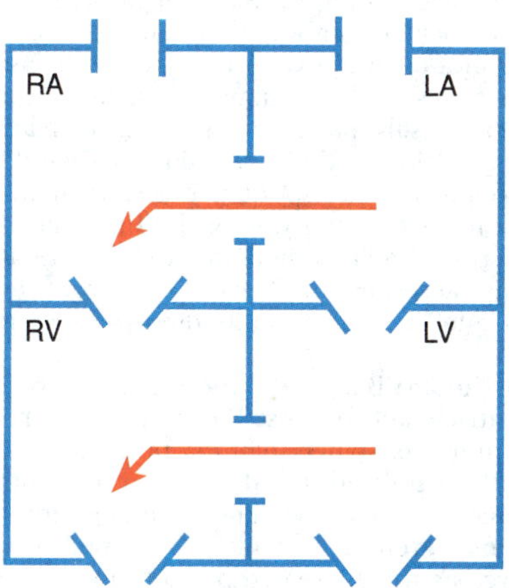

FIG. 34-12 Hemodynamics in defects with increased pulmonary blood flow.

DEFECTS WITH INCREASED PULMONARY BLOOD FLOW

ATRIAL SEPTAL DEFECT (ASD)

Description: Abnormal opening between the atria, allowing blood from the higher-pressure left atrium to flow into the lower-pressure right atrium. There are three types:

- ***Ostium primum (ASD 1)***—Opening at lower end of septum; may be associated with mitral valve abnormalities
- ***Ostium secundum (ASD 2)***—Opening near center of septum
- ***Sinus venosus defect***—Opening near junction of superior vena cava and right atrium; may be associated with partial anomalous pulmonary venous connection

Pathophysiology: Because left atrial pressure slightly exceeds right atrial pressure, blood flows from the left to the right atrium, causing an increased flow of oxygenated blood into the right side of the heart. Despite the low pressure difference, a high rate of flow can still occur because of low pulmonary vascular resistance and the greater distensibility of the right atrium, which further reduces flow resistance. This volume is well tolerated by the right ventricle because it is delivered under much lower pressure than in a ventricular septal defect. Although there is right atrial and ventricular enlargement, cardiac failure is unusual in an uncomplicated atrial septal defect. Pulmonary vascular changes usually occur only after several decades if the defect is unrepaired.

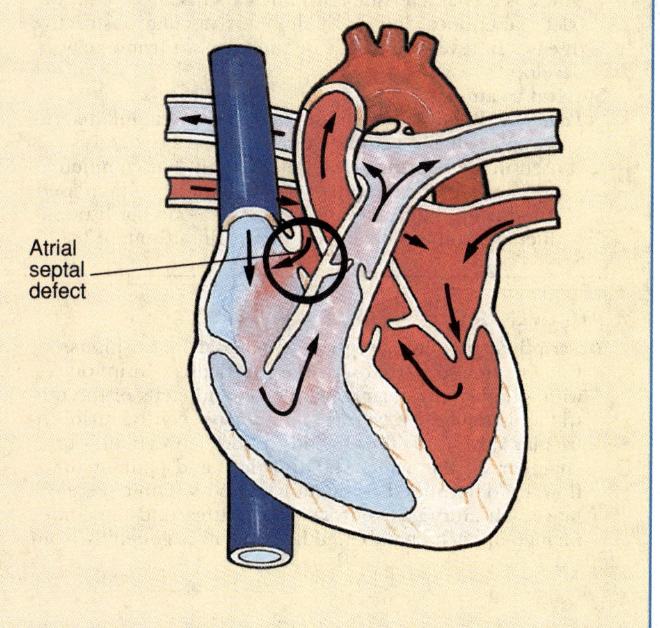

Continued.

DEFECTS WITH INCREASED PULMONARY BLOOD FLOW—cont'd

ATRIAL SEPTAL DEFECT (ASD)—cont'd

Clinical manifestations: Patients may be asymptomatic. They may develop congestive heart failure. There is a characteristic murmur. Patients are at risk for atrial dysrhythmias (probably caused by atrial enlargement and stretching of conduction fibers) and pulmonary vascular obstructive disease and emboli formation later in life from chronic increased pulmonary blood flow.

Surgical treatment: Surgical Dacron patch closure of moderate to large defects similar to closure of ventricular septal defects. Open repair with cardiopulmonary bypass is usually performed before school age. In addition, the sinus venosus defect requires patch placement, so the anomalous right pulmonary venous return is directed to the left atrium with a baffle. The ASD 1 may require repair or, rarely, replacement of the mitral valve.

Nonsurgical treatment: ASD 2 may also be closed using devices during cardiac catheterization. This technique is in clinical trials in some centers.

Prognosis: Very low operative mortality, less than 1%.

VENTRICULAR SEPTAL DEFECT (VSD)

Description: Abnormal opening between the right and left ventricles. May be classified according to location: membranous (accounting for 80%) or muscular. May vary in size from a small pinhole to absence of the septum, resulting in a common ventricle. Frequently associated with other defects, such as pulmonary stenosis, transposition of the great vessels, patent ductus arteriosus, atrial defects, and coarctation of the aorta. Many VSDs (20% to 60%) are thought to close spontaneously. Spontaneous closure is most likely to occur during the first year of life in children having small or moderate defects. A left-to-right shunt is caused by the flow of blood from the higher-pressure left ventricle to the lower-pressure right ventricle.

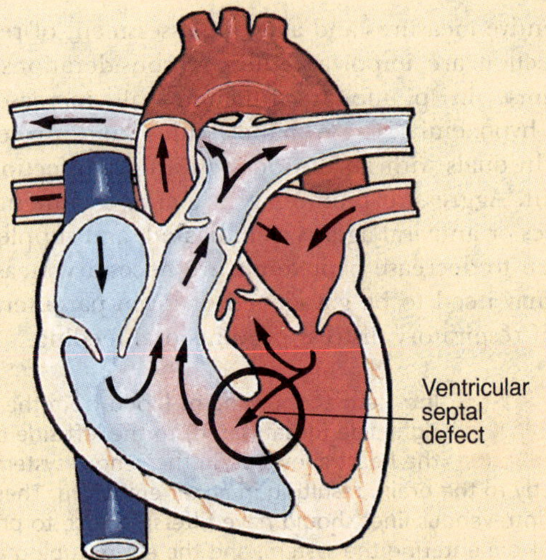

Pathophysiology: Because of the higher pressure within the left ventricle and because the systemic arterial circulation offers more resistance than the pulmonary circulation, blood flows through the defect into the pulmonary artery. The increased blood volume is pumped into the lungs, which may eventually result in increased pulmonary vascular resistance. Increased pressure in the right ventricle as a result of left-to-right shunting and pulmonary resistance causes the muscle to hypertrophy. If the right ventricle is unable to accommodate the increased workload, the right atrium may also enlarge as it attempts to overcome the resistance offered by incomplete right ventricular emptying. In severe defects Eisenmenger syndrome may develop (see p. 1515).

Clinical manifestations: Congestive heart failure is common. There is a characteristic murmur. Patients are at risk for bacterial endocarditis and pulmonary vascular obstructive disease. In severe defects, Eisenmenger syndrome may develop.

Surgical treatment:

Palliative: Pulmonary banding in symptomatic infants. Although palliation using a pulmonary artery band is used in some institutions, data suggest that complete primary repair can be performed without an increased risk during the first year of life. Age alone has little influence on the outcome of the repair, although younger infants are frequently sicker in the postoperative period.

Complete repair: Small defects are repaired with a purse-string approach. Large defects usually require a knitted Dacron patch sewn over the opening. Both procedures are performed via cardiopulmonary bypass. The repair is generally approached through the right atrium and the tricuspid valve. Postoperative complications include residual VSD and conduction disturbances.

Nonsurgical treatment: Device closure during cardiac catheterization is under clinical trials in some centers for closure of muscular defects that carry a high operative risk.

Prognosis: Risks depend on the location of the defect, number of defects, and other associated cardiac defects. Single membranous defects have a low mortality (less than 5%); multiple muscular defects can have a risk of more than 20%.

ATRIOVENTRICULAR CANAL (AVC) DEFECT

Description: Incomplete fusion of endocardial cushions. Consists of a low atrial septal defect that is continuous with a high ventricular septal defect and clefts of the mitral and tricuspid valves, creating a large central atrioventricular valve that allows blood to flow between all four chambers of the heart. The directions and pathways of flow are determined by pulmonary and systemic resistance, left and right ventricular pressures, and the compliance of each chamber, although flow is generally from left to right. It is the most common cardiac defect in children with Down syndrome.

Pathophysiology: The alterations in the hemodynamics depend on the defect's severity and the child's pulmonary vascular resistance. Immediately after birth, while the newborn's pulmonary vascular resistance is high, there is minimum shunting of blood through the defect. Once this resistance falls, left-to-right shunting occurs and pulmonary blood flow increases. The resultant pulmonary

DEFECTS WITH INCREASED PULMONARY BLOOD FLOW—cont'd

vascular engorgement predisposes to development of CHF.

Clinical manifestations: Patients usually have moderate to severe congestive heart failure. There is a characteristic murmur. There may be mild cyanosis that increases with crying. Patients are at high risk for developing pulmonary vascular obstructive disease.

Surgical treatment:

Palliative: Pulmonary artery banding for infants with severe symptoms that are caused by increased pulmonary blood flow in some centers. Other centers believe complete repair can be performed in infants.

Complete repair: Surgical repair consists of patch closure of the septal defects and reconstruction of the AV valve tissue (either repair of the mitral valve cleft or fashioning two AV valves). If the mitral valve defect is severe, a valve replacement may be needed. Postoperative complications include heart block, CHF, mitral regurgitation, dysrhythmias, and pulmonary hypertension.

Prognosis: Operative mortality is about 10%. Potential later problem is mitral regurgitation, which may require valve replacement.

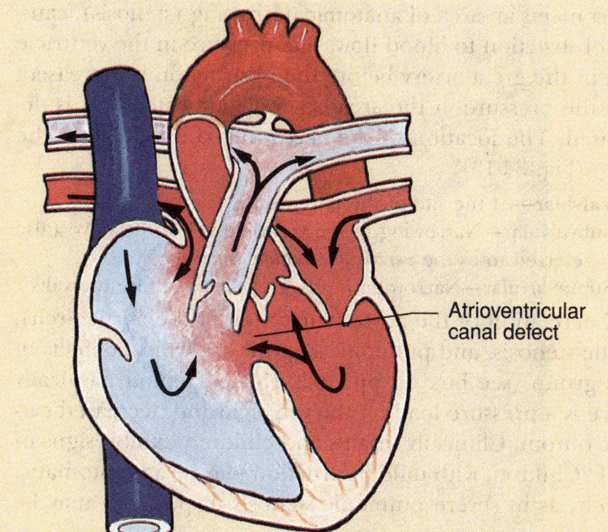

PATENT DUCTUS ARTERIOSUS (PDA)

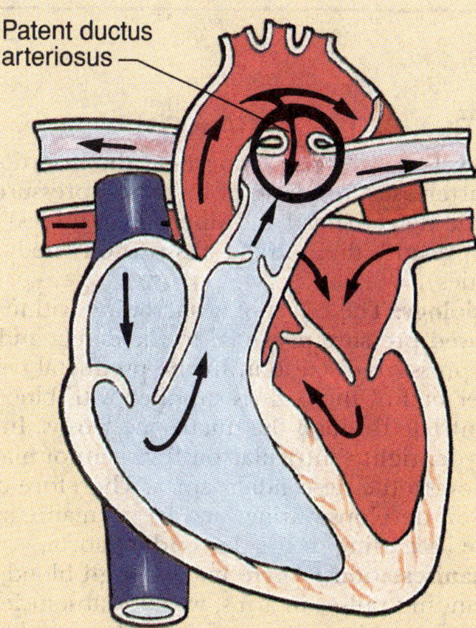

Description: Failure of the fetal ductus arteriosus (artery connecting the aorta and pulmonary artery) to close within the first weeks of life. The continued patency of this vessel allows blood to flow from the higher-pressure aorta to the lower-pressure pulmonary artery, causing a left-to-right shunt.

Pathophysiology: The hemodynamic consequences of PDA depend on the size of the ductus and the pulmonary vascular resistance. At birth the resistance in the pulmonary and systemic circulations is almost identical, thus equalizing the resistance in the aorta and pulmonary artery. As the systemic pressure exceeds the pulmonary pressure, blood begins to shunt from the aorta, across the duct, to the pulmonary artery (left-to-right shunt).

The additional blood is recirculated through the lungs and returned to the left atrium and left ventricle. The effect of this altered circulation is increased workload on the left side of the heart, increased pulmonary vascular congestion and possibly resistance, and potentially increased right ventricular pressure and hypertrophy.

Clinical manifestations: Patients may be asymptomatic or show signs of congestive heart failure. There is a characteristic machinery-like murmur. A widened pulse pressure and bounding pulses result from runoff of blood from the aorta to the pulmonary artery. Patients are at risk for bacterial endocarditis and pulmonary vascular obstructive disease in later life from chronic excessive pulmonary blood flow.

Medical management: Administration of indomethacin (prostaglandin inhibitor) has proved successful in closing a patent ductus in premature infants and some newborns.

Surgical treatment: Surgical division or ligation of the patent vessel via a left thoracotomy. A newer technique, visual assisted thoracoscopic surgery (VATS), uses a thoracoscope and instruments placed through three small incisions on the left side of the chest to place a clip on the ductus. It is used in some centers and eliminates the need for a thoracotomy, thereby speeding postoperative recovery.

Nonsurgical treatment: Closure with placement of an occluder device during cardiac catheterization is done in some institutions.

Prognosis: Both procedures can be done at low risk with less than 1% mortality.

OBSTRUCTIVE DEFECTS

Obstructive defects are those in which blood exiting the heart meets an area of anatomic narrowing (stenosis), causing obstruction to blood flow. The pressure in the ventricle and in the great artery before the obstruction is increased, and the pressure in the area beyond the obstruction is decreased. The location of the narrowing is usually near the valve (Fig. 34-13):

Valvular—At the site of the valve itself

Subvalvular—Narrowing in the ventricle below the valve (also referred to as the ***ventricular outflow tract***)

Supravalvular—Narrowing in the great artery above the valve

Coarctation of the aorta (narrowing of the aortic arch), aortic stenosis, and pulmonic stenosis are typical defects in this group (see box on pp. 1522-1524). Hemodynamically there is a pressure load on the ventricle and decreased cardiac output. Clinically infants and children exhibit signs of CHF. Children with mild obstruction may be asymptomatic. Rarely, as in severe pulmonic stenosis, hypoxemia may be seen.

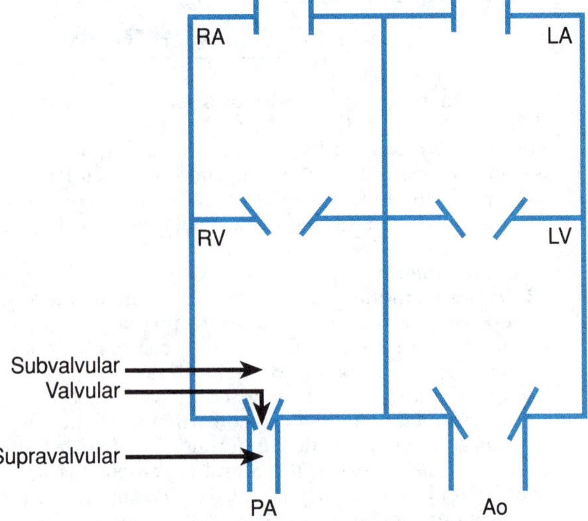

FIG. 34-13 Obstruction to ventricular ejection can occur at the valvular level (shown), below the valve (subvalvular), or above the valve (supravalvular). Pulmonary stenosis is shown here.

OBSTRUCTIVE DEFECTS

COARCTATION OF THE AORTA (COA)

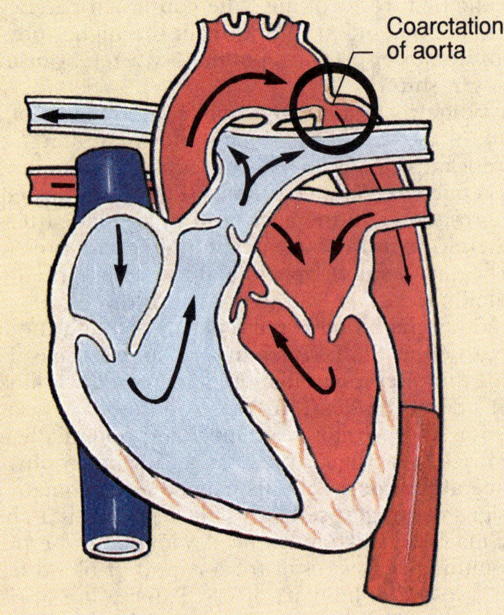

Description: Localized narrowing near the insertion of the ductus arteriosus, resulting in increased pressure proximal to the defect (head and upper extremities) and decreased pressure distal to the obstruction (body and lower extremities).

Pathophysiology: The effect of a narrowing within the aorta is increased pressure proximal to the defect and decreased pressure distal to it. In the preductal type of COA the lower half of the body is supplied with blood by the right ventricle through the ductus arteriosus. In the postductal type, right ventricular outflow cannot maintain blood flow to the descending aorta. Therefore collateral circulation develops during fetal life to maintain flow from the ascending to the descending aorta.

Clinical manifestations: There may be high blood pressure and bounding pulses in arms, weak or absent femoral pulses, and cool lower extremities with lower blood pressure. There are signs of congestive heart failure in infants. Often these patients' hemodynamic condition deteriorates rapidly, and they are admitted to the intensive care unit near death, usually severely acidotic and hypotensive. Mechanical ventilation and inotropic support are often necessary before surgery. Older children may experience dizziness, headaches, fainting, and epistaxis resulting from hypertension. Patients are at risk for hypertension, ruptured aorta, aortic aneurysm, or stroke.

Surgical treatment: Either resection of the coarcted portion with an end-to-end anastomosis of the aorta or enlargement of the constricted section using a graft of prosthetic material or a portion of the left subclavian artery. Because this defect is outside the heart and pericardium, cardiopulmonary bypass is not required and a thoracotomy incision is used. Postoperative hypertension (greater than 160 mm Hg) is treated with intravenous sodium nitroprusside or amrinone, followed by oral medications, such as captopril, hydralazine, and/or propranolol. Residual permanent hypertension after repair of COA seems to be related to age and time of repair. To prevent both hypertension at rest and exercise-provoked systemic hypertension after repair, elective surgery for COA is advised within the first 2 years of life. There is a 5% to 10% risk of recurrent narrowing in patients who underwent surgical repair as infants. (Hellenbrand, 1990) Percutaneous balloon angioplasty techniques have proved very effective in relieving residual postoperative coarctation gradients.

Nonsurgical treatment: Balloon angioplasty as a primary intervention for COA is being performed in some centers, but concerns about inadequate relief of gradients, risk of aneurysm formation, and restenosis have limited its widespread use. More clinical experience and longer follow-up are needed (Friedman, 1992).

Prognosis: Less than 5% mortality in patients with isolated coarctation; increased risk in infants with other complex cardiac defects.

OBSTRUCTIVE DEFECTS—cont'd

AORTIC STENOSIS (AS)

Description: Narrowing or stricture of the aortic valve, causing resistance to blood flow in the left ventricle, decreased cardiac output, left ventricular hypertrophy, and pulmonary vascular congestion. The prominent anatomic consequence of AS is the hypertrophy of the left ventricular wall, which eventually will lead to increased end-diastolic pressure, resulting in pulmonary venous and pulmonary arterial hypertension. Left ventricular hypertrophy also interferes with coronary artery perfusion and may result in myocardial infarction or scarring of the papillary muscles of the left ventricle, causing mitral insufficiency. ***Valvular stenosis,*** the most common type, is usually caused by malformed cusps resulting in a bicuspid rather than tricuspid valve or fusion of the cusps. ***Subvalvular stenosis*** is a stricture caused by a fibrous ring below a normal valve; ***supravalvular stenosis*** occurs infrequently. Valvular AS is a serious defect for the following reasons: (1) the obstruction tends to be progressive; (2) sudden episodes of myocardial ischemia, or low cardiac output, can result in sudden death; and (3) surgical repair rarely results in a normal valve. This is one of the rare instances in which strenuous physical activity may be curtailed because of the cardiac condition.

Pathophysiology: A stricture in the aortic outflow tract causes resistance to ejection of blood from the left ventricle. The extra workload on the left ventricle causes hypertrophy. If left ventricular failure develops, left atrial pressure will increase; this causes increased pressure in the pulmonary veins, resulting in pulmonary vascular congestion (pulmonary edema).

Clinical manifestations: Infants with severe defects demonstrate signs of decreased cardiac output with faint pulses, hypotension, tachycardia, and poor feeding. Children show signs of exercise intolerance, chest pain, and dizziness when standing for long periods. There is a characteristic murmur. Patients are at risk for bacterial endocarditis, coronary insufficiency, and ventricular dysfunction.

Valvular Aortic Stenosis

Surgical treatment: Aortic valvotomy under inflow occlusion.

Prognosis: Aortic valvotomy in critically ill neonates and infants still carries a mortality of 10% to 20% in major medical centers (Park, 1988). Results of aortic valvotomy in older children are very good, with mortality close to 0%. However, aortic valvotomy remains a palliative procedure, and approximately 25% of patients require additional surgery within 10 years for recurrent stenosis. A valve replacement may be required at the second procedure.

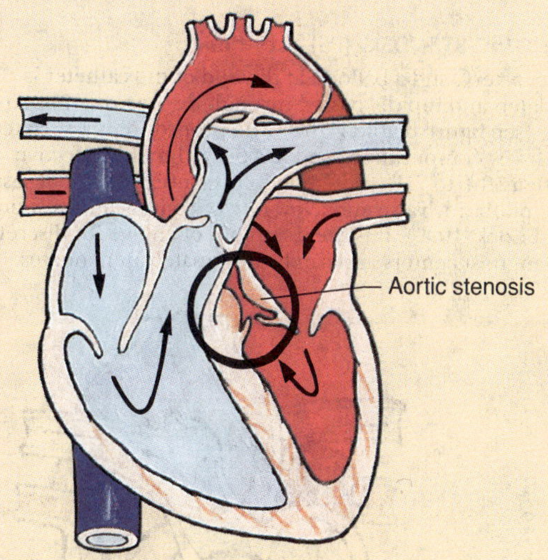

Nonsurgical treatment: Dilating narrowed valve with balloon angioplasty in the catheterization laboratory.

Prognosis: The incidence of side effects and complications, including aortic insufficiency or valvular regurgitation, tearing of the valve leaflets, loss of pulse in the catheterized limb, or serious dysrhythmias, is about 40%. In critically ill neonates the mortality rate is similar to that of surgery, approximately 15% to 30% (Perry and others, 1989).

Subvalvular Aortic Stenosis

Surgical treatment: May involve incising a membrane if one exists or cutting the fibromuscular ring. If the obstruction results from narrowing of the left ventricular outflow tract and a small aortic valve annulus, a patch may be required to enlarge the entire left ventricular outflow tract and annulus and replace the aortic valve, an approach known as the ***Konno*** procedure. An aortic homograft with a valve may also be used (***extended aortic root replacement***), or the pulmonary valve may be moved to the aortic position and replaced with a homograft valve (***Ross*** procedure).

Prognosis: Mortality from surgical repairs of subvalvular AS is less than 2% in major centers; however, about 10% of these patients develop recurrent subaortic stenosis and require additional surgery (Friedman, 1992). All operations to replace the aortic root and enlarge the left ventricular outflow tract require further evaluation.

PULMONIC STENOSIS (PS)

Description: Narrowing at the entrance to the pulmonary artery. Resistance to blood flow causes right ventricular hypertrophy and decreased pulmonary blood flow. ***Pulmonary atresia*** is the extreme form of PS in that there is total fusion of the commissures and no blood flows to the lungs. The right ventricle may be hypoplastic.

Pathophysiology: When PS is present, resistance to blood flow causes right ventricular hypertrophy. If right ventricular failure develops, right atrial pressure will increase and this may result in reopening of the foramen ovale, shunting of unoxygenated blood into the left atrium, and systemic cyanosis. If PS is severe, CHF occus, and systemic venous engorgement will be noted. An associated defect such as a PDA partially compensates for the obstruction by shunting blood from the aorta to the pulmonary artery and into the lungs.

Clinical manifestations: Patients may be asymptomatic; some have mild cyanosis or congestive heart failure. Newborns with severe narrowing will be cyanotic. There is a characteristic murmur. Cardiomegaly is evident on chest x-ray film. Patients are at risk for bacterial endocarditis, with progressive narrowing causing increased symptoms.

Surgical treatment: In infants, transventricular (closed) valvotomy ***(Brock)*** procedure. In children, pulmonary valvotomy with cardiopulmonary bypass.

Nonsurgical treatment: Balloon angioplasty in the cardiac catheterization laboratory to dilate valve. A catheter is inserted across the stenotic pulmonic valve into the pulmo-

Continued.

OBSTRUCTIVE DEFECTS—cont'd

PULMONIC STENOSIS (PS)—cont'd

nary artery, and a balloon at the end of the catheter is inflated and rapidly passed through the narrowed opening (see figure below, right). The procedure is associated with few complications and has proved highly effective, with a 50% to 75% reduction in pressure gradient across the pulmonic valve and a low rate of complications (Radtke and Lock, 1990). It is the treatment of choice for discrete PS in most centers and can be done safely in neonates.

Prognosis: Low risk for both procedures; less than 2% mortality. Both balloon dilation and surgical valvotomy leave the pulmonic valve incompetent because they involve opening the fused valve leaflets; however, these patients are clinically asymptomatic. Long-term problems with restenosis or valve incompetence may occur.

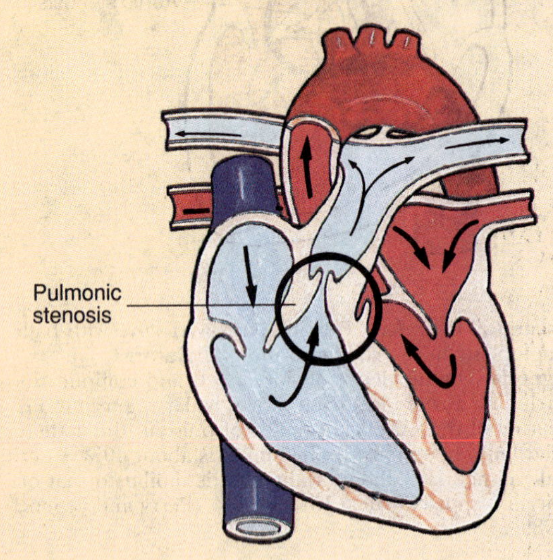

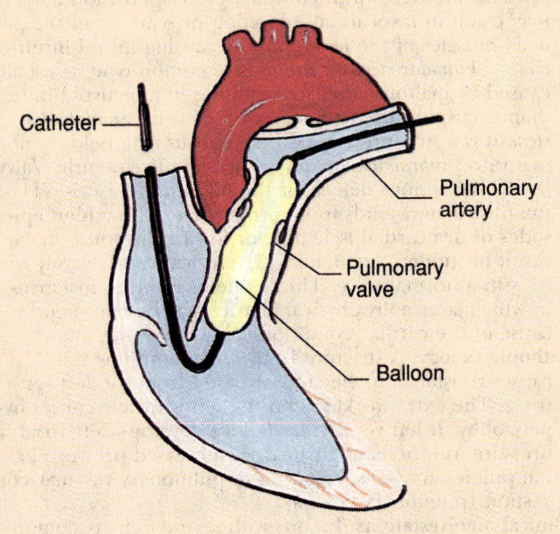

DEFECTS WITH DECREASED PULMONARY BLOOD FLOW

In this group of defects, there is obstruction of pulmonary blood flow and an anatomic defect (ASD or VSD) between the right and left sides of the heart (Fig. 34-14). Because blood has difficulty exiting the right side of the heart via the pulmonary artery, pressure on the right side increases, exceeding left-sided pressure. This allows desaturated blood to shunt right to left, causing desaturation in the left side of the heart and in the systemic circulation. Clinically these patients are hypoxemic and usually appear cyanotic. Tetralogy of Fallot and tricuspid atresia are the more common defects in this group (see box on pp. 1525-1526).

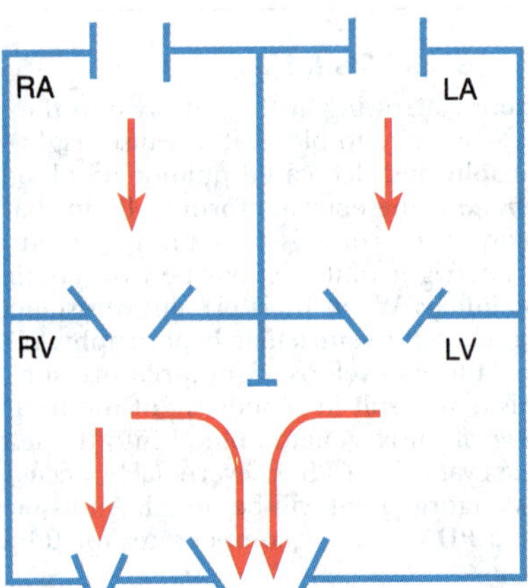

FIG. 34-14 Hemodynamic defects with decreased pulmonary blood flow. For abbreviations, see Fig. 34-2.

DEFECTS WITH DECREASED PULMONARY BLOOD FLOW

TETRALOGY OF FALLOT (TOF)

Description: The classic form includes four defects: (1) ventricular septal defect, (2) pulmonic stenosis, (3) overriding aorta, and (4) right ventricular hypertrophy.

Pathophysiology: The altered hemodynamics vary widely, depending primarily on the degree of pulmonary stenosis, but also on the size of the VSD and the pulmonary and systemic resistance to flow. Because the VSD is usually large, pressures may be equal in the right and left ventricles. Therefore the shunt direction depends on the difference between pulmonary and systemic vascular resistance. If pulmonary vascular resistance is higher than systemic resistance, the shunt is from right to left. If systemic resistance is higher than pulmonary resistance, the shunt is from left to right. Pulmonic stenosis decreases blood flow to the lungs and, consequently, the amount of oxygenated blood that returns to the left heart. Depending on the position of the aorta, blood from both ventricles may be distributed systemically.

Clinical manifestations:

Infants: Some infants may be acutely cyanotic at birth; others have mild cyanosis that progresses over the first year of life as the pulmonic stenosis worsens. There is a characteristic murmur. There are acute episodes of cyanosis and hypoxia, called blue spells or tet spells (see p. 1516). Anoxic spells occur when the infant's oxygen requirements exceed the blood supply, usually during crying or after feeding.

Children: With increasing cyanosis, there may be clubbing of the fingers, squatting, and poor growth.

Patients are at risk for emboli, cerebrovascular disease, brain abscess, seizures, and loss of consciousness or sudden death following an anoxic spell.

Surgical treatment:

Palliative shunt: In infants who cannot undergo primary repair, a palliative procedure to increase pulmonary blood flow and increase oxygen saturation may be performed. The preferred procedure is the ***Blalock-Taussig*** or ***modified Blalock-Taussig shunt,*** which provides blood flow to the pulmonary arteries from the left or right subclavian artery (see Table 34-6). In general, however, shunts are avoided because they may result in pulmonary artery distortion.

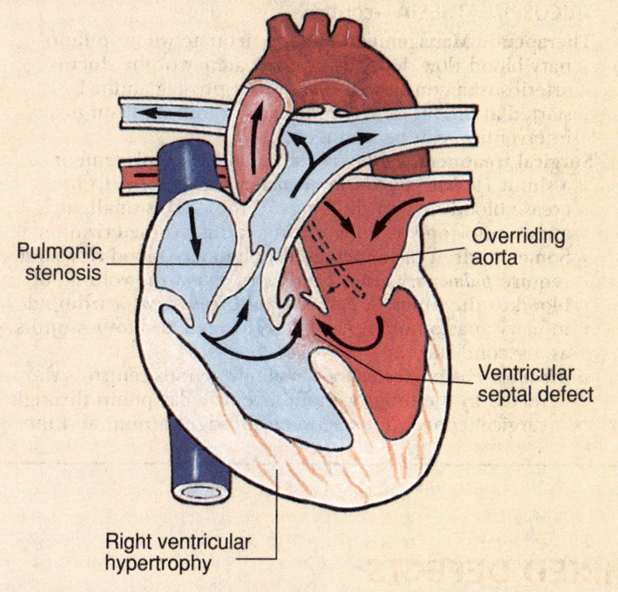

Complete repair: Elective repair is usually performed in the first year of life. Indications for repair include increasing cyanosis and the development of hypercyanotic spells. Complete repair involves closure of the VSD and resection of the infundibular stenosis, with a pericardial patch to enlarge the right ventricular outflow tract. The procedure requires a median sternotomy and the use of cardiopulmonary bypass.

Prognosis: The operative mortality for total correction of TOF is less than 5%. With improved surgical techniques there is a lower incidence of dysrhythmias and sudden death; surgical heart block is rare. CHF may occur postoperatively.

TRICUSPID ATRESIA

Description: Failure of the tricuspid valve to develop, consequently no communication from right atrium to right ventricle. Blood flows through an atrial septal defect or a patent foramen ovale to the left side of the heart and through a ventricular septal defect to the right ventricle and out to the lungs. It is often associated with pulmonic stenosis and transposition of the great arteries. There is complete mixing of unoxygenated and oxygenated blood in the left side of the heart, resulting in systemic desaturation and varying amounts of pulmonary obstruction, causing decreased pulmonary blood flow.

Pathophysiology: At birth the presence of a patent foramen ovale (or other atrial septal opening) is required to permit blood flow across the septum into the left atrium; the PDA allows blood flow to the pulmonary artery into the lungs for oxygenation. A VSD allows a modest amount of blood to enter the right ventricle and pulmonary artery for oxygenation. Pulmonary blood flow usually is diminished.

Clinical manifestations: Cyanosis is usually seen in the newborn period. There may be tachycardia and dyspnea. Older children have signs of chronic hypoxemia with clubbing. Patients are at risk for bacterial endocarditis, brain abscess, and stroke.

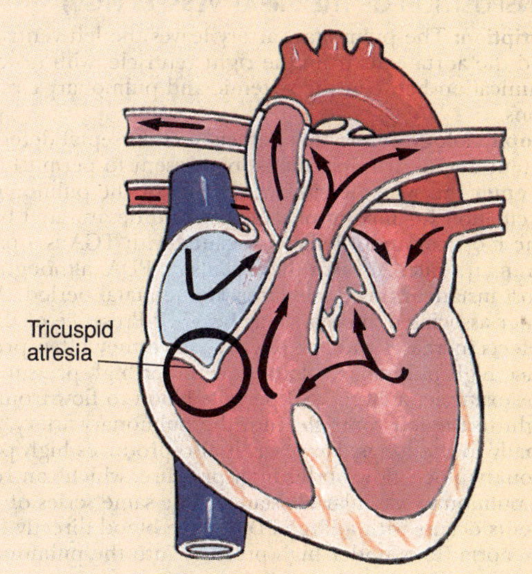

Continued.

DEFECTS WITH DECREASED PULMONARY BLOOD FLOW—cont'd

TRICUSPID ATRESIA—cont'd

Therapeutic Management: For the neonate whose pulmonary blood flow depends on the patency of the ductus arteriosus, a continuous infusion of prostaglandin E_1 is started at 0.1 mg/kg of body weight/min until surgical intervention can be arranged.

Surgical treatment: ***Palliative*** treatment is the placement of a shunt (***pulmonary-to-systemic artery anastomosis***) to increase blood flow to the lungs. If the ASD is small, an atrial septostomy is done during cardiac catheterization. Some children have increased pulmonary blood flow and require ***pulmonary artery banding*** to lessen the volume of blood to the lungs. A ***bidirectional Glenn shunt*** (cardiopulmonary anastomosis) may be performed at 6 to 9 months as a second stage.

Modified Fontan procedure—Systemic venous return is directed to the lungs without a ventricular pump through surgical connections between the right atrium and the pulmonary artery. A fenestration (opening) in the right atrial baffle is sometimes done to relieve pressure. Patient must have normal ventricular function and a low pulmonary vascular resistance for the procedure to be successful. The modified Fontan procedure separates oxygenated and unoxygenated blood inside the heart and eliminates the excess volume load on the ventricle but does not restore normal anatomy or hemodynamics.

Prognosis: Surgical mortality is greater than 10%. Postoperative complications include dysrhythmias, systemic venous hypertension, pleural and pericardial effusions, elevated pulmonary vascular resistance, and ventricular dysfunction. While initial results have been encouraging, long-term survival and morbidity must await future studies.

MIXED DEFECTS

Many complex cardiac anomalies are classified together in the *mixed* category (see box on pp. 1526-1529) because survival in the postnatal period depends on mixing of blood from the pulmonary and systemic circulations within the heart chambers. Hemodynamically, fully saturated systemic blood flow mixes with the desaturated pulmonary blood flow, causing a relative desaturation of the systemic blood flow. Pulmonary congestion occurs because the differences in pulmonary artery pressure and aortic pressure favor pulmonary blood flow. Cardiac output decreases because of a volume load on the ventricle. Clinically, these patients have a variable picture that combines some degree of desaturation (although cyanosis is not always visible) and signs of CHF. Some defects, such as transposition of the great arteries, cause severe cyanosis in the first days of life and later cause CHF. Others, such as truncus arteriosus, cause severe CHF in the first weeks of life and mild desaturation.

MIXED DEFECTS

TRANSPOSITION OF THE GREAT ARTERIES (TGA) OR TRANSPOSITION OF THE GREAT VESSELS (TGV)

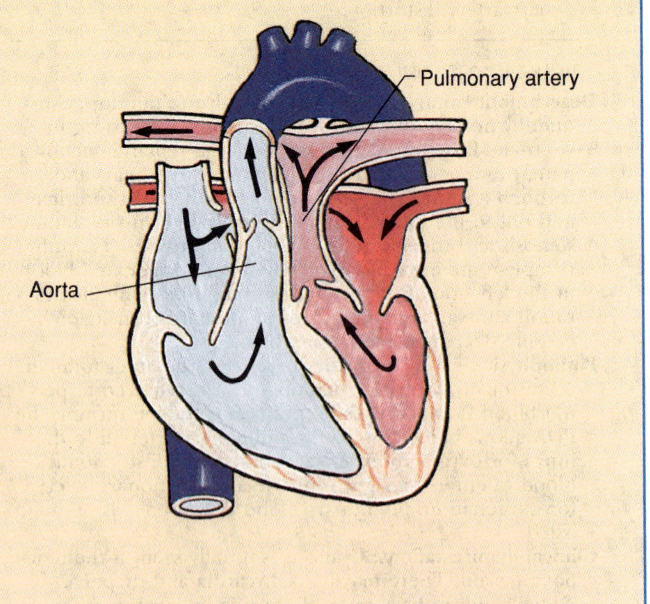

Description: The pulmonary artery leaves the left ventricle, and the aorta exits from the right ventricle, with no communication between the systemic and pulmonary circulations.

Pathophysiology: Associated defects such as septal defects or patent ductus arteriosus must be present to permit blood to enter the systemic circulation and/or the pulmonary circulation for mixing of saturated and desaturated blood. The most common defect associated with TGA is a patent foramen ovale. At birth there is also a PDA, although in most instances this closes after the neonatal period. Another associated anomaly may be VSD. Presence of these defects increases the risk of CHF, since they often produce high pulmonary blood flow under high pressure. For example, a large VSD permits blood to flow from the right to the left ventricle, into the pulmonary artery, and finally to the lungs. However, it also produces high pulmonary blood flow under high pressure, which can result in pulmonary vascular resistance. The same series of events occurs with a large PDA, since blood directly from the aorta flows under high pressure into the pulmonary artery and lungs.

Clinical manifestations: Depend on the type and size of the associated defects. Children with minimum communication are severely cyanotic and depressed at birth. Those

MIXED DEFECTS

with large septal defects or a patent ductus arteriosus may be less severely cyanotic but may have symptoms of congestive heart failure. Heart sounds vary according to the type of defect present. Cardiomegaly is usually evident a few weeks after birth.

Therapeutic Management:

To provide intracardiac mixing: The administration of intravenous prostaglandin E_1 may be initiated to temporarily increase blood mixing if systemic and pulmonary mixing is inadequate to provide an oxygen saturation of 75% or to maintain cardiac output. During cardiac catheterization a balloon atrial septostomy ***(Rashkind procedure)*** may also be performed to increase mixing and maintain cardiac output over a longer period.

Surgical treatment:

Arterial switch procedure: Procedure of choice performed in first weeks of life. Involves transecting the great arteries and anastomosing the main pulmonary artery to the proximal aorta (just above the aortic valve) and anastomosing the ascending aorta to the proximal pulmonary artery. The coronary arteries are switched from the proximal aorta to the proximal pulmonary artery, creating a new aorta. Reimplantation of the coronary arteries is critical to the infant's survival, and they must be reattached without torsion or kinking to provide the heart with its supply of oxygen. The advantage of the arterial switch procedure is the reestablishment of normal circulation, with the left ventricle acting as the systemic pump. Potential complications of the arterial switch include narrowing at the great artery anastomoses or coronary artery insufficiency.

Creation of an intraatrial baffle to divert venous blood to the mitral valve and pulmonary venous blood to the tricuspid valve using the patient's atrial septum ***(Senning procedure)*** or a prosthetic material ***(Mustard procedure)***. Performed in first year of life. A disadvantage is the continuing role of the right ventricle as the systemic pump and the late development of right ventricular failure and rhythm disturbances. Other potential postoperative complications include loss of normal sinus rhythm, baffle leaks, and ventricular dysfunction.

Rastelli procedure: Operative choice in infants with TGA, VSD, and severe PS. It involves closure of the VSD with a baffle, directing left ventricular blood through the VSD into the aorta. The pulmonic valve is then closed, and a conduit is placed from the right ventricle to the pulmonary artery, creating a physiologically normal circulation. Unfortunately, this procedure requires multiple conduit replacements as the child grows.

Prognosis: Operative mortality is about 5% to 10% with all procedures; with atrial level repairs there is a later risk of dysrhythmias and ventricular dysfunction.

TOTAL ANOMALOUS PULMONARY VENOUS CONNECTION (TAPVC)

Description: Rare defect characterized by failure of the pulmonary veins to join the left atrium. Instead, the pulmonary veins are abnormally connected to the systemic venous circuit via the right atrium or various veins draining toward the right atrium, such as the superior vena cava. The abnormal attachment results in mixed blood being returned to the right atrium and shunted from the right to the left through an ASD. The type of TAPVC is classified according to the pulmonary venous point of attachment as:

Supracardiac—Attachment above the diaphragm, such as to the superior vena cava (most common form) (Fig. 34-26)

Cardiac—Direct attachment to the heart, such as to the right atrium or coronary sinus

Infracardiac—Attachment below the diaphragm, such as to the inferior vena cava (most severe form)

TAPVC is also called total anomalous pulmonary venous return (TAPVR) or total anomalous pulmonary venous drainage (TAPVD).

Pathophysiology: The right atrium receives all the blood that normally would flow into the left atrium. As a result, the right side of the heart hypertrophies, whereas the left side, especially the left atrium, may remain small. An associated ASD or patent foramen ovale allows systemic venous blood to shunt from the higher-pressure right atrium to the left atrium and into the left side of the heart. As a result, the oxygen saturation of the blood in both sides of the heart (and ultimately, in the systemic arterial circulation) is the same. If the pulmonary blood flow is large, pulmonary venous return is also large and the amount of saturated blood is relatively high. However, if there is obstruction to pulmonary venous drainage, pulmonary venous return is impeded, pulmonary venous pressure rises, and pulmonary interstitial edema develops and eventually contributes to CHF. Infracardiac TAPVC is often associated with obstruction to pulmonary venous drainage and is a surgical emergency.

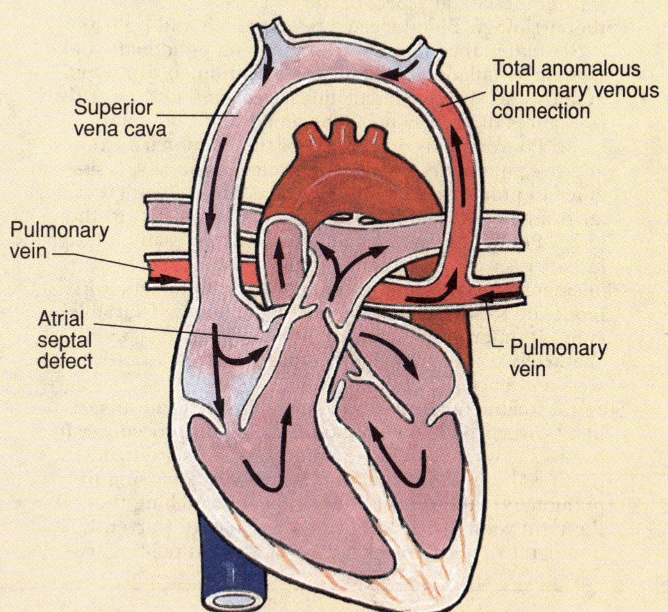

Clinical manifestations: Most infants develop cyanosis early in life. The degree of cyanosis is inversely related to the amount of pulmonary blood flow—the more pulmonary blood, the less cyanosis. Children with unobstructed TAPVC may be asymptomatic until pulmonary vascular resistance decreases during infancy, increasing pulmonary blood flow, with resulting signs of CHF. Cyanosis becomes worse with pulmonary vein obstruction; once obstruction occurs, the infant's condition usually deteriorates rapidly. Without intervention, cardiac failure will progress to death.

Surgical treatment: Corrective repair in early infancy. The surgical approach varies with the anatomic defect. In gen-

Continued.

MIXED DEFECTS—cont'd

TOTAL ANOMALOUS PULMONARY VENOUS CONNECTION (TAPVC)—cont'd

eral, however, the common pulmonary vein is anastomosed to the left atrium, the ASD is closed, and the anomalous pulmonary venous connection is ligated. The cardiac type is most easily repaired; the infracardiac type has the highest morbidity and mortality because of the higher incidence of pulmonary vein obstruction. Potential postoperative complications include reobstruction; bleeding; dysrhythmias, particularly heart block; pulmonary artery hypertension; and persistent heart failure.

Prognosis: The cardiac type has a surgical mortality of less than 5%; the incidence of morbidity is greater with the other types and increases with the presence of pulmonary vein obstruction.

TRUNCUS ARTERIOSUS (TA)

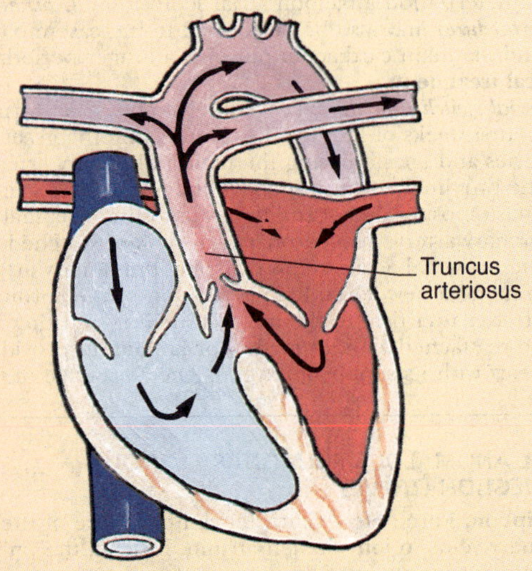

Description: Failure of normal septation and division of the embryonic bulbar trunk into the pulmonary artery and the aorta, resulting in a single vessel that overrides both ventricles. Blood from both ventricles mixes in the common great artery, causing desaturation and hypoxemia. Blood ejected from the heart flows preferentially to the lower-pressure pulmonary arteries, causing increased pulmonary blood flow and reduced systemic blood flow. There are 3 types:

Type I—A single pulmonary trunk arises near the base of the truncus and divides into the left and right pulmonary arteries.

Type II—The left and right pulmonary arteries arise separately from the posterior aspect of the truncus.

Type III—The pulmonary arteries arise independently from the lateral aspect of the truncus.

Pathophysiology: Blood ejected from the left and right ventricles enters the common trunk, mixing pulmonary and systemic circulations. Blood flow is distributed to the pulmonary and systemic circulations according to the relative resistances of each system. The amount of pulmonary blood flow depends on the size of the pulmonary arteries and the pulmonary vascular resistance. Generally, resistance to pulmonary blood flow is less than systemic vascular resistance, resulting in preferential blood flow to the lungs. Pulmonary vascular disease develops at an early age in patients with truncus arteriosus.

Clinical manifestations: Most infants are symptomatic with moderate to severe congestive heart failure and variable cyanosis, poor growth, and activity intolerance. There is a characteristic murmur. Patients are at risk for brain abscess and bacterial endocarditis.

Surgical treatment: Early repair in the first few months of life. Corrective repair is a modified Rastelli procedure. It involves closing the VSD so that the truncus arteriosus receives the outflow from the left ventricle, excising the pulmonary arteries from the aorta, and attaching them to the right ventricle by means of a homograft. Currently, homografts (segments of cadaver aorta and pulmonary artery that are treated with antibiotics and cryopreserved) are preferred over synthetic conduits to establish continuity between the right ventricle and pulmonary artery. Homografts are more flexible and easier to use during the procedure and appear less prone to obstruction. Postoperative complications include persistent heart failure, bleeding, pulmonary artery hypertension, dysrhythmias, and residual VSD. These children require additional procedures to replace the conduit as its size becomes inadequate in relation to the children's growth.

Prognosis: Mortality is greater than 10%; future operations are required to replace the conduits.

HYPOPLASTIC LEFT HEART SYNDROME (HLHS)

Description: Underdevelopment of the left side of the heart, resulting in a hypoplastic left ventricle and aortic atresia. Most blood from the left atrium flows across the patent foramen ovale to the right atrium, to the right ventricle, and out the pulmonary artery. The descending aorta receives blood from the patent ductus arteriosus supplying systemic blood flow.

Pathophysiology: An ASD or patent foramen ovale allows saturated blood from the left atrium to mix with desaturated blood from the right atrium and to flow through the right ventricle and out into the pulmonary artery. From the pulmonary artery the blood flows to the lungs, then through the ductus arteriosus into the aorta and out to the body. The amount of blood flow to the pulmonary and systemic circulations depends on the relationship between the pulmonary and systemic vascular resistances. The coronary and cerebral vessels receive blood by retrograde flow through the hypoplastic ascending aorta.

Clinical manifestations: There is mild cyanosis and signs of congestive failure until the patent ductus arteriosus closes, then progressive deterioration with cyanosis and decreased cardiac output, leading to cardiovascular collapse. It is usually fatal in the first months of life without intervention.

Therapeutic management: Neonates require stabilization with mechanical ventilation and inotropic support preoperatively. A prostaglandin E_1 infusion is needed to main-

MIXED DEFECTS—cont'd

tain ductal patency, ensuring adequate systemic blood flow.

Surgical treatment: Several-staged approach: First stage is ***Norwood procedure***—anastomosis of the main pulmonary artery to the aorta to create a new aorta, shunting to provide pulmonary blood flow, and creation of a large atrial septal defect. Postoperative complications include imbalance of systemic and pulmonary blood flow, bleeding, low cardiac output, and persistent heart failure. Second stage is often a ***bidirectional Glenn shunt*** done at 6 to 9 months of age to relieve cyanosis and reduce the volume load on the right ventricle. The final repair is a ***modified Fontan procedure*** (see Tricuspid Atresia in box on p. 1526).

Transplantation: Some programs believe that heart transplantation in the newborn period is the best option for these infants. Problems include the shortage of newborn organ donors, risk of rejection, long-term problems with chronic immunosuppression, and infection (see Heart Transplantation, p. 1556).

Prognosis: Mortality risks of more than 25% with both surgery and transplantation. Currently, only about half the patients survive to complete the last stage, the modified Fontan procedure. This may improve in the future. Because of the high-risk nature of both surgical palliation and neonatal heart transplantation, some cardiologists continue to recommend no treatment for this defect.

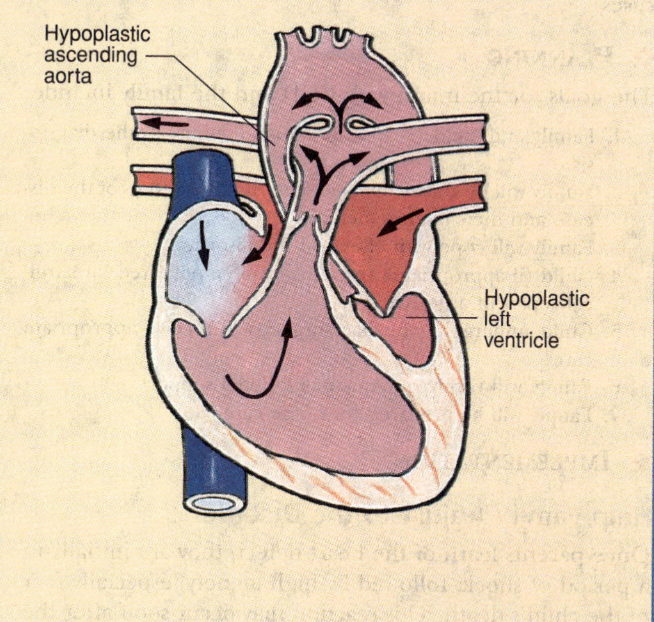

NURSING CARE OF THE FAMILY AND CHILD WITH CONGENITAL HEART DISEASE

When a child is born with a severe cardiac anomaly, the parents are faced with the immense psychologic and physical tasks of adjusting to the birth of a child with special needs. The reactions and nursing interventions required to support the family differ little from those discussed in Chapters 11 and 22. The following discussion is primarily directed (1) toward the family of an infant who has a serious heart defect and requires home care before definitive repair and (2) toward preparation and care of the child and family when heart surgery is performed. For nursing care related to the child with hypoxemia and CHF, the reader should refer to earlier discussions of these topics.

❖ Assessment

Nursing care of the child with a congenital heart defect begins as soon as the diagnosis is suspected. Prenatal diagnosis of congenital heart defects is becoming increasingly frequent. New demands are being placed on nurses to counsel and support families, as well as assess the fetus with known heart defects as families prepare for the birth of these infants.

Many children do not display symptoms of heart disease until the child's growth and/or energy expenditure exceeds the heart's ability to supply oxygenated blood to the tissues. Since the onset of symptoms may be gradual, the child may curtail activity, so that the signs of exercise intolerance are less obvious. However, a careful history yields important clues to this change. For example, infants are normally extremely mobile, and their energies are directed toward learning gross motor skills. Most infants suck vigorously and fall asleep after finishing a feeding. It is very unusual to hear of a child who prefers to sit rather than crawl or walk or who falls asleep shortly after beginning a feeding. Likewise, a child who needs frequent rests or naps after limited play periods may also be exhibiting exercise intolerance. Such histories should alert the nurse to assess cardiac function.

Other clues are a history of poor weight gain; poor feeding habits, especially the need to pause during feeding; poor suck; difficulty in coordinating sucking, swallowing, and breathing; frequent respiratory infections; cyanosis; and squatting. Since parents may not view any of these findings as abnormal, the nurse must specifically ask about them during a health assessment.

Another indication of heart defects is murmurs. Chapter 7 discusses the usual distinguishing characteristics between innocent and organic murmurs. Nurses who perform primary health assessments must be knowledgeable of the differences in order to correctly refer children with heart murmurs of possible organic origin to a cardiologist. There has been controversy over informing parents of innocent murmurs, since some practitioners believe that the parent may be unduly worried and transfer that concern to overprotectiveness of the child. However, this problem can be avoided by stressing to parents that although a murmur was heard, no heart disease is present, no further cardiac study is needed, and the heart is normal.

❖ Nursing Diagnoses

Many nursing diagnoses are apparent following a thorough assessment of the child and family. Some of these are developed in the Nursing Care Plan on pp. 1538-1539. Others will become evident based on assessment of individual cases.

❖ Planning

The goals for the infant with CHD and the family include:

1. Family and child (if appropriate) will adjust to the diagnosis.
2. Family will be knowledgeable regarding symptoms of the disease and their management.
3. Family will cope with effects of the disorder.
4. Child (if appropriate) and family will be prepared for surgical repair of a defect.
5. Child undergoing cardiac surgery will receive appropriate care.
6. Family will receive adequate emotional support.
7. Family will be prepared for home care.

❖ Implementation

Help Family Adjust to the Disorder

Once parents learn of the heart defect, they are initially in a period of shock, followed by high anxiety, especially fear of the child's death. This reaction may occur soon after the child's birth or at a later period in life. Whatever its timing, the family needs a period of grief before assimilating the meaning of the defect. Unfortunately, the demands for medical treatment may not allow this, necessitating that the parents be informed of the condition in order to give informed consent for diagnostic/therapeutic procedures. The nurse can be instrumental in supporting parents in their loss, assessing their level of understanding, supplying information as needed, and helping other members of the health team to understand the parents' reactions.

Severely distressed newborns usually remain in the hospital. This can seriously affect parent-infant attachment unless parents are encouraged to hold, touch, and look at their child. Every effort must be made by health personnel to foster attachment. (See Chapter 10 for suggestions for promoting attachment between parents and their hospitalized newborn.)

The effect of a child with a serious heart defect on the family is complex. No member, regardless of the degree of positive adjustment, is unaffected. Mothers frequently feel inadequate in their mothering ability because they gave birth to a child with a defect and are unable to keep their child well. Mothers often feel constantly exhausted from the pressures of caring for these children and the other family members. Likewise, fathers and siblings may feel neglected and resentful, a reaction similar to the feelings of family members toward other chronic conditions (see Chapter 22). Often parents do not feel confident leaving the child in another's care because they believe that the child will be upset by a change in routine and that the baby-sitter will be unable to cope with the child's symptoms. This often sets up a trap for parents, especially mothers, who become locked into the child's care with no relief. Although the parents' fears are justified, they can be minimized by gradually teaching someone (a reliable relative or neighbor) how to care for the child.

The need to maintain discipline and set consistent limits cannot be overemphasized. Using behavior modification techniques, either concrete awards (e.g., a favorite food) or social reinforcement (e.g., approval), can be effective. However, it is most beneficial if employed *before* the child learns to control the family. Therefore guiding parents toward the need for discipline while the child is in infancy is necessary to prevent later problems. It also teaches these children how to tolerate frustration and delayed gratification, which often are lacking because of immediate satisfaction of all their needs.

Another problem that may develop within family relationships is the child's overdependency. This is often the result of parental fear that the child may die and overcompensation through what has been termed the benevolent overreaction (see Chapter 22). The best approach to dealing with this dilemma is prevention. Parents need guidance to recognize the eventual hazards of continuing dependency and protectiveness as the child grows older, and the nurse can assist parents in learning ways to foster optimum development. Unless parents are helped to see what activities the child can do, they may focus on physical limitations and encourage dependency.

The child also needs opportunities for social development. These children do not need to be isolated from known sources of infection or prevented from playing with other children because of concern regarding overexertion. Such practices only add to the dangers of increased dependency in the home environment. Parents need to be encouraged to seek appropriate social activity, especially before kindergarten.

Frequently the continuing unremitting stresses of care—physical exhaustion, financial costs, emotional upset, fear of death, and concern for the child's future—are not fully appreciated by those caring for the family. Even when the child's condition is stabilized or corrected, the family may need to make new adjustments in their life-style. Introducing them to other families with similarly affected children can help them adjust to the daily stresses.*

Educate Family About the Disorder

Once parents are ready to hear about the heart condition, it is essential that they be given a clear explanation based on their level of understanding. Lack of familiarity with the cardiovascular system may be a major reason for lack of parental understanding, and it is usually helpful to review the basic structure and function of the heart before describing the defect (Kaden and others, 1985). A simple diagram, pictures, or a model of the heart can be most helpful in visualizing the heart and the congenital defect. Parents appreciate receiving written information about the specific condition.† Health care professionals should take advantage of

*Some local American Heart Associations have organized parent groups.

†Books for parents include *If Your Child Has a Congenital Heart Defect: A Guide for Parents,* available from the American Heart Association, 7320 Greenville Ave., Dallas, TX 75231, (214) 373-6300; and *The Heart of a Child: What Families Need to Know About Heart Disorders in Children,* by C.A. Neill, E.B. Clark, and C. Clark, available from Johns Hopkins University Press, 701 W. 40th St., Baltimore, MD 21211-2190; (410) 516-6900.

subsequent encounters with the family to assess parental understanding of the condition and clarify information as needed.

Another fact to remember is that different health personnel may convey the same information using different diagrams and medical terms. To prevent this from becoming a problem, which often happens when several health team members work with a family, the same type of diagram should be used, and the parents should write down any unclear terms or ask for clarification. Sometimes it is helpful to provide the family with a glossary of frequently used words for reference.

Parents are primarily interested in two types of information—prognosis and surgery. They are frequently upset about indefinite answers to either. The family should be assured that the health care team will be honest in keeping them informed of the child's condition and of decisions regarding future procedures and treatments. The nurse needs to be aware of alterations in the plan of therapy in order to convey similar messages to the family.

Children of various ages have different ideas about their heart. Children between ages 4 and 6 years have heard about the heart, know its approximate anatomic location in the chest or back, illustrate it as valentine shaped, characterize it by the sounds *tick-tock* or *thump,* and visualize blood as free-flowing (not in vessels). Children ages 7 to 10 have a clearer concept of the heart, realizing that it is not shaped like a valentine and that it has vital functions, such as, "It makes you live." However, their knowledge of its integrated functions to pump blood through a system of vessels to all parts of the body is still hazy. By age 10 or 11, children have a much more involved concept of the heart, with knowledge of veins, valves, pumping action, and circulation. They are beginning to appreciate why death occurs when the heart stops.

Information given to the child must be tailored to the child's developmental age. As the child matures, the level of information is revised to meet the child's new cognitive level. Preschoolers need basic information about what they will experience more than what is actually occurring physiologically. School-age children benefit from a concrete explanation of the defect. Preadolescents and adolescents often appreciate a more detailed description of how the defect affects their heart. Children of all ages need to express their feelings concerning the diagnosis.

Help Family Cope with Effects of the Disorder

Parents also need an explanation regarding the symptoms of the disease. Many children have few symptoms but may develop CHF. Therefore parents should be aware of early signs of worsening physical status, such as sweating, sudden weight gain, decreased exercise tolerance, poor feeding, and increased breathing effort. These symptoms need medical evaluation, but the family is assured the symptoms usually respond quickly to therapeutic intervention.

Another area of parental concern is the child's level of physical activity. Children do not need to restrict activity, and the best approach is to treat the child normally and allow self-limited activity. Deliberately attempting to prevent crying should be avoided because it can establish a maladaptive parental pattern of relating to the infant. Exceptions to self-determined activity primarily involve strenuous recreational and competitive sports.

NURSING ALERT Although decisions regarding activity restrictions are made on an individual basis on the cardiologist's advice, children with aortic stenosis or insufficiency are usually not permitted to engage in strenuous activity (Fyler, 1992).

Infants and children with CHD require good nutrition. Providing infants with adequate nutrition is especially difficult because of their high caloric requirements and inability to suck effectively because of fatigue and tachypnea. Instructing parents in feeding methods that decrease the work of the infant and giving high-calorie formula are important interventions. (See p. 1512 for a discussion on feeding the infant with CHF.)

Children with severe cardiac defects are often anorexic. Encouraging them to eat can be a tremendous challenge. Because of the parents' concern over eating, children learn early to manipulate parents through eating, such as making unrealistic demands for foods that are not available. The nurse advises parents of this potential problem, since prevention yields greater success than intervention. For example, the child should be given a choice of available high-nutrient foods. Suggestions for encouraging sick children to eat are discussed in Chapter 27.

The family also needs to be knowledgeable regarding the therapeutic management of the disorder, especially in terms of the medications that the child is receiving. Parents are taught the correct procedure for giving drugs* and cautioned to keep them in a safe area to prevent accidental ingestion (see Family Home Care box on p. 1511).

Prepare Child and Family for Surgery

Few surgical procedures demand as much planning for preoperative preparation and postoperative care as does heart surgery. The general principles for preparing children for procedures, such as surgery, are discussed in Chapter 27, and the reader is urged to review them. This discussion focuses on those measures specific to the cardiovascular procedure. Technical differences exist between closed- and open-heart surgery, since the latter involves the use of cardiopulmonary bypass (extracorporeal circulation). Consequently, there are some additions to physical care postoperatively in open-heart surgery. However, in general the term *heart surgery* is used regardless of the actual procedures, and the same nursing interventions apply.

The child is usually admitted to the hospital 1 day before surgery for diagnostic tests. This interval allows time to prepare the child and parents for surgery, although with the present concern on health care costs, less time may be appropriated for admission procedures. With infants the focus of preoperative teaching is directed to the parents.

*Home care instructions on giving medications to children are available in *Wong and Whaley's Clinical Manual of Pediatric Nursing* (Mosby).

Since much information is conveyed, it is important to schedule teaching to prevent information overload and to be alert to signs of overload (see box on p. 191). No well-documented research exists on how extensive preoperative preparation should be, and the nurse must use considerable judgment in planning the aspects of teaching. Preparation can be divided into three categories: equipment, environment, and procedures. The following discussion assumes that the child and/or parents have an understanding of the defect.

Introduce Child and Family to the Environment. Ideally, when the child is admitted, a plan should be made to provide consistent caregivers. In some institutions the nurse who will care for the child postoperatively in the intensive care unit is also assigned to the child at admission to facilitate forming a relationship with the family and to share preoperative teaching, such as introduction to the recovery room and intensive care unit. To increase familiarity, all nurses should call the child and parents by name and refer to themselves by name. Wearing a name tag reinforces this point. Postoperatively the family will feel more at ease if they recognize familiar names, faces, and voices.

If a visit to the recovery room and/or intensive care unit is planned, it should take place when there is minimum activity in the area, the parents can accompany the child, and the child is well rested. Usually the day before surgery is ample time to allow the child to ask questions and to prevent undue fantasizing about the experience. If a visit is not included in the teaching plan, the nurse can use a book, preferably with pictures or photographs of the actual rooms, to explain the environment to the child.

During the visit to the intensive care unit, the child and parents should experience everything that directly affects the child's care, such as the sounds of ECG monitors, oxygen tents, and placement of the bed. All positive, nonfrightening aspects of the environment are emphasized, such as the play area, visitors' section, pictures or mobiles in the room, or television. If it is a pediatric intensive care unit, the nurse can introduce the family to other children who may be recovering from surgery. The child should be protected from the frightening sights in the unit, and equipment not in view postoperatively, such as equipment located behind or below the bed, needs less attention. The child and parents are encouraged to ask questions or to explore further any equipment in the room, but they should not be pushed to assimilate more information than they appear to be tolerating.

Familiarize Child and Family with Equipment. Some of the equipment, such as the stethoscope, sphygmomanometer, and thermometer, will already be familiar to the child and parents. However, the nurse emphasizes that procedures involving such equipment will be done more frequently. The child is told about the placement of the oximeter sensor on the skin, usually the finger.

Types of equipment new to many families are the oxygen mask, suction, chest tubes, endotracheal tubes, incentive spirometers, nasogastric tube, and intravenous tubing. Each of these is shown and demonstrated either on a doll or on the child, if he or she appears ready. With a younger child, miniaturized equipment suitable for use with a doll or puppet is often less anxiety producing than the actual samples. If other children in the unit have an intravenous infusion or are in oxygen tents, the older child may benefit from seeing them, but this must be planned carefully to avoid frightening the child.

Several intravenous lines are inserted perioperatively: (1) a peripheral line for infusion of fluids; (2) a venous pressure line, inserted into the right subclavian or jugular vein; and (3) an arterial line for direct measurement of arterial pressure. Younger children need only know the location of each tubing and that both arms may be restrained to prevent dislodging the tubing. Older children may appreciate knowing the reason for each infusion, especially when venous and arterial measurements are taken. Since the lines are inserted during surgery, they are not painful, only uncomfortable because of the restricted movement.

The type and size of dressing the child will have after surgery are discussed and can be shown on a doll. Usually one of two types of incisions is made: a ***median sternotomy,*** which splits the sternum, or a ***lateral thoracotomy,*** which extends from the midaxillary line to the scapula. Frequently no sutures are visible because subcuticular, absorbable sutures may be used. If this is done, it should be pointed out to the child and parents, who may fear the incision will open. Sometimes a butterfly incision is used for cosmetic reasons in girls instead of the regular median sternotomy.

The child may be told about chest tubes and their purpose in draining fluid from around the heart and lungs. A picture of the equipment used for drainage can be shown to the child, or the setup can be simulated by attaching one end of the tubes to a doll with a chest dressing and the other end to small bottles (e.g., empty medicine vials). The nurse stresses that the child must move even though the tubes are in place. It can be demonstrated on the doll that the tubing is long enough to permit turning. Since this information may be anxiety producing, it is best left to the end of teaching or eliminated if the child appears too anxious.

An endotracheal (ET) tube is inserted during surgery and may be left in place for ventilatory assistance and tracheobronchial suctioning. However, it may be best to prepare older children for the ET tube only if *prolonged* ventilatory support is planned. The ET tube can be presented as a "breathing tube" that is placed in the nose or mouth. The nurse explains that while the tube is in, the child will feel it in the throat and will not be able to talk, but nothing is wrong. The child can express desires by pointing or using a picture communication board. The nurse stresses that the tube will be removed as soon as possible, often during the first postoperative day.

Preoperative physical care differs little, if any, from that for any other surgery and is discussed in Chapter 27. The child should be assured that the parents will be there when the child wakes up; they should be allowed to accompany their child as far as possible to the operating suite (see Thinking Critically About . . . box on p. 1138). After all the equipment and procedures have been explained, it is important to talk about "getting well" and going home. If a doll was used during the preparatory session, the tubes can be removed and the doll can be dressed in regular clothes in anticipation of discharge.

Provide Postoperative Care

Immediate postoperative care is usually provided by specially trained nurses in intensive care units. Many of the procedures, such as arterial pressure and central venous pressure (CVP) monitoring and the observations related to vital functions, require advanced educational training (the reader should refer to critical care texts for further information). However, nurses caring for the child before surgery and during the convalescent period need to be familiar with the major principles of care.

Observe Vital Signs and Arterial/Venous Pressures. Vital signs and blood pressure (BP) are recorded frequently until stable. Heart rate and respirations are counted for 1 full minute, compared with the ECG monitor, and recorded with activity. The heart rate is normally increased after surgery. The nurse observes cardiac rhythm and notifies the practitioner of any changes in regularity. Dysrhythmias may occur postoperatively secondary to administration of anesthetics, acid-base and electrolyte imbalance, hypoxia, surgical intervention, or trauma to conduction pathways.

At least hourly the lungs are auscultated for breath sounds. Diminished or absent sounds most likely indicate an area of atelectasis, which necessitates further medical assessment. Auscultation guides the nurse's selective use of postural drainage and percussion to those pulmonary lobes most in need. It also allows a more objective evaluation of effective ventilation.

Temperature changes are typical during the early postoperative period. Hypothermia is expected immediately after surgery from hypothermia procedures, effects of anesthesia, and loss of body heat to the cool environment. During this period the child is kept warm to prevent additional heat loss. Infants may be placed under radiant heat warmers. During the next 24 to 48 hours the body temperature may rise to 37.7° C (100° F) or slightly higher as part of the inflammatory response to tissue trauma. After this period an elevated temperature is most likely a sign of infection and warrants immediate investigation for probable cause.

Intraarterial monitoring of BP is almost always done following open-heart surgery. Residual vasoconstriction after cardiopulmonary bypass makes indirect blood pressure readings less reliable, and intraarterial monitoring permits continuous rather than intermittent observation. A catheter is passed into the radial artery or the dorsalis pedis or posterior tibial artery, and the other end is attached to an electronic monitoring system, which provides a continuous recording of the BP. Continuous BP readings are compared with those taken indirectly with a sphygmomanometer or oscillometry (Dinamap). A discrepancy between the two may indicate a change in peripheral vascular resistance, a malfunction in the electronic device, or human error in using the wrong-size blood pressure cuff. The nurse also observes for potential complications of intraarterial monitoring, such as arterial thrombosis, infection, air emboli, or blood loss through the catheter. Prevention of each of these hazards is similar to care for any other type of infusion.

The intraarterial line is maintained with a low-rate constant infusion of heparinized saline to prevent clotting. The amount of irrigant is recorded as intake fluid. The dressing at the site is changed daily.

Intracardiac monitoring lines provide data on cardiac function and output. They are placed intraoperatively and may be present in the left atrium, pulmonary artery, or right atrium. Placement of a catheter in the right atrium allows for measurement of the pressure in the right side of the heart. Therefore it indicates right atrial filling pressure, right ventricular function, the relationship between blood volume (venous return) and cardiac output, and early signs of right-sided CHF. The CVP catheter is inserted into the superior vena cava or inferior vena cava, and the other end is attached to a monitor.

CVP continually changes according to blood volume, heart rate, and myocardial function. If the blood volume decreases, such as in shock, the CVP falls. If the efficiency of the left side of the heart decreases, the resistance to right ventricular ejection will ultimately result in an elevated CVP but decreased intraarterial pressure. CHF and/or hypervolemia raise the CVP.

The complications of CVP lines are similar to those of other infusions, with the addition of atrial dysrhythmias from irritation of the atrial wall; hemothorax, pneumothorax, or hydrothorax from accidental puncture as the catheter enters the thorax; and fluid overload, since the intravenous line is kept patent by a continuous drip. The nurse observes for signs and symptoms indicative of each of these risks.

Maintain Respiratory Status. The child is generally maintained on mechanical ventilation in the immediate postoperative period. When weaning and extubation are completed, humidified oxygen is delivered by mask or hood to prevent drying of mucosa. The child is kept warm and dry, since excessive chilling from wet linens causes an increased metabolic need and consequent increased cardiac demand. The child is encouraged to turn and deep breathe at least hourly. Every measure is employed to enhance ventilation and decrease pain, such as splinting of the operative site and use of analgesics.

Suctioning is performed only as needed. Deep suctioning is performed carefully to avoid vagal stimulation (cardiac dysrhythmias) and laryngospasm, especially in infants. Suctioning is intermittent and maintained for no more than 5 seconds to prevent depleting the oxygen supply. Supplemental oxygen is administered with a manual resuscitation bag before and after the procedure to prevent hypoxia. Heart rate is monitored after suctioning to detect changes in rhythm or rate, especially bradycardia. The child should always be positioned facing the nurse to permit assessment of the child's color and tolerance to the procedure.

NURSING ALERT During suctioning, observe for signs and symptoms of respiratory distress, such as tachypnea, use of accessory muscles for breathing, and restlessness.

Chest tubes are inserted into the pleural and/or mediastinal space during surgery or in the immediate postoperative period to remove secretions and air in order to allow reexpansion of the lung. The chest tube is attached to a water-seal drainage system, usually a disposable type such as Pleur-Evac. The purpose of the underwater drainage is to prevent air from traveling up the tube into the pleural space, causing a pneumothorax. The nursing considerations include the following: (1) do not interrupt water-seal drainage unless the chest tube is clamped, (2) check for tube patency (fluctuation in the water-seal chamber), and (3) maintain sterility.

Drainage is checked hourly for color and quantity. Immediately postoperatively the drainage may be bright red, but afterward it should be serous. The largest volume of drainage occurs in the first 12 to 24 hours, and drainage is greater in extensive heart surgery.

NURSING ALERT Chest tube drainage greater than 3 ml/kg/hr for more than 3 consecutive hours is excessive and may indicate postoperative hemorrhage (Hazinski, 1992). The surgeon is notified immediately, since cardiac tamponade can develop rapidly and is life-threatening.

Chest radiographs are taken when the tubes are inserted to check their location and after they are removed to evaluate the inflation of the lungs. Chest tubes are usually removed on the second to third postoperative day. Lung expansion is evidenced by decreased fluctuation in the tube and absence of drainage.

Removal of chest tubes is a painful, frightening experience (see Atraumatic Care box). Children are forewarned that they will feel a sharp, momentary pain. After the suture is cut, the tubes are quickly pulled out at the end of full inspiration to prevent intake of air into the pleural cavity. A purse-string suture (placed when the tubes were inserted) is pulled tight to close the opening. A petrolatum-covered gauze dressing is immediately applied over the wound and securely taped on all four sides to the skin so that an airtight seal is formed. The dressing is checked for signs of drainage and any evidence of infection.

Provide Maximum Rest. After heart surgery, maximum rest should be provided to decrease the workload of the heart and promote healing. Nursing care is planned according to the child's usual activity and sleep patterns. The simplest way to ensure individualized, efficient, high-quality care is to plan at the beginning of the shift the nursing procedures to be done. Periods of rest are identified. The schedule should be shared with parents to allow them to visit at the most advantageous times, such as after a rest period when no special treatments are anticipated.

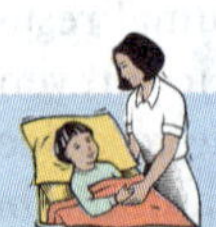

ATRAUMATIC CARE
Chest Tube Removal

Analgesics such as intravenous fentanyl (2 to 3 μg/kg) or morphine sulfate (0.1 mg/kg), often in combination with midazolam (Versed), should be given before the procedure. Some practitioners use EMLA, a topical anesthetic placed on the site, for at least 1 hour under an occlusive dressing to decrease discomfort, especially when the sutures are pulled, although the "pulling pain" through the chest is typically felt.

Provide Comfort. Heart surgery is both painful and frightening for children, and providing comfort is a primary nursing concern. Unfortunately, children are often poorly medicated for pain after surgery, especially children who are unable to verbally communicate discomfort (see Pain Assessment, Chapter 26). However, studies show that adequate analgesia and anesthesia decrease the body's stress response to surgery and improve postoperative morbidity and mortality (Anand and Hickey, 1992; Wessel, 1993) (see also Neonatal Pain, Ch. 11).

Continuous intravenous opioid infusions, particularly morphine and fentanyl, are safe and effective methods of pain control (Maguire and Maloney, 1988). Patient-controlled analgesia may be used with children old enough to understand the concept, and epidural morphine is another option (Rosen and Rosen, 1989). Paralyzing agents such as pancuronium (Pavulon) or metocurine (Metubine) may also be used with the analgesics for children who are very agitated or hemodynamically unstable. Children receiving opioid infusions for a prolonged period are weaned slowly from the medication to prevent withdrawal symptoms.

Most patients need intravenous analgesics for pain control during the immediate postoperative period. Following removal of lines and tubes, pain may be controlled with oral medications such as codeine with acetaminophen (Tylenol) or oxycodone and acetaminophen (Tylox). Nonsteroidal antiinflammatory agents such as intravenous ketorolac (Toradol) or oral ibuprofen may be used to provide relief of moderate postoperative pain.

Acetaminophen alone provides adequate pain relief for most children at discharge. Sternotomy incisions are usually well tolerated, with some discomfort when walking and coughing. Thoracotomy incisions are usually more painful because the incision is through muscle; a more aggressive pain management plan with round-the-clock medications for several days is often necessary to allow for adequate rest, ambulation, and pulmonary hygiene.

In addition to pharmacologic pain control, every effort is made to minimize the discomfort of procedures, such as using a firm pillow or favorite stuffed animal placed against the chest incision during coughing, and performing treatments *after* pain medication is given, preferably at a time that coincides with the drug's peak effect. Nonpharmacologic measures are employed to lessen the perception of pain, and parents are encouraged to comfort their child as much as possible. (See also Pain Management, Chapter 26.)

Monitor Fluids. Intake and output of all fluids must be accurately calculated. Intake is primarily intravenous fluids; however, a record of fluid used to flush the arterial and CVP lines or to dilute medications is also kept. Output includes hourly recordings of urine (usually a Foley catheter is inserted and attached to a closed collecting device), drainage from chest and nasogastric tubes, and blood drawn for analysis. Urine is analyzed for specific gravity to assess the kidneys' concentrating ability and to assess approximately the body's degree of hydration. Renal failure is a potential risk from a transient period of low cardiac output.

NURSING ALERT The signs of renal failure are decreased urinary output (less than 1 ml/kg/hr) and elevated levels of blood urea nitrogen and serum creatinine (Hazinski, 1992).

Fluids are restricted during the immediate postoperative period to prevent hypervolemia, which places additional demands on the myocardium, predisposing the child to cardiac failure. Two factors influence increased blood volume. In open-heart surgery the cardiopulmonary pump is primed with a large volume of fluid (usually electrolyte solution), which may greatly dilute the patient's blood. The large fluid volume also diffuses into the interstitial spaces, causing total-body edema and pulmonary edema. Postoperatively the increased interstitial fluid diffuses back into the systemic circulation, where it can be excreted by the kidney. Diuretics help accelerate this process.

In addition, the physiologic changes of open- or closed-heart surgery stimulate the adrenal cortex to secrete aldosterone, which increases renal reabsorption of sodium. This results in water retention but increased excretion of potassium. Concurrently the hypothalamus secretes additional antidiuretic hormone (ADH), which causes the distal and collecting tubules to reabsorb more water. Not only can this process result in hypervolemia, but it also may cause electrolyte imbalances, principally hypokalemia. Decreased potassium affects myocardial function and may increase the risk of dysrhythmias. The nurse assesses electrolyte imbalances by observing for signs of hypokalemia (see Table 34-5) and checking all blood electrolyte reports.

Fluid requirements are based on the child's weight and body surface area. The child is weighed daily, and the same scale is used at approximately the same time each day to avoid errors in measurement. The child is usually given nothing by mouth for the first 24 hours. If an ET tube is inserted, oral fluids are usually withheld until the child is extubated. Fluid restriction may be imposed even when oral fluids are given. The nurse calculates the distribution over a 24-hour period based on the child's preoperative weight and drinking habits. The distribution should allow for the majority of fluid to be given during the child's most wakeful and active periods.

Plan for Progressive Activity. Fatigue and weakness are common after heart surgery, as a result of both the surgical trauma to the heart and sleep deprivation during the immediate postoperative period. However, moderate activity is essential to prevent pulmonary and vascular complications. Initially, turning, coughing, and deep breathing are sufficient to promote respiratory expansion. However, passive range-of-motion exercises, especially to the lower extremities, are instituted to prevent venous stasis. All infusion sites are inspected for evidence of thrombophlebitis and emboli. The areas are passively exercised to promote circulation.

A progressive schedule of ambulation and activity is planned, based on the child's preoperative activity patterns and postoperative cardiovascular and pulmonary function. Toys that were enjoyed before surgery are provided to encourage movement. It is important to plan the activity at times when the child is well rested, is comfortable (usually has had analgesic medication), and is not scheduled for any strenuous procedure or treatment immediately afterward.

Ambulation is initiated early, usually by the second postoperative day, when chest tubes, arterial lines, and assisted ventilatory equipment may be removed. The nurse begins ambulation for this child the same as for a child who had undergone any other postsurgical procedure, progressing from sitting on the edge of the bed and dangling the legs to standing up and to sitting in a chair. Heart rate and respirations are carefully monitored to assess the degree of cardiac demand imposed by each activity. Tachycardia, dyspnea, cyanosis, desaturation, progressive fatigue, or dysrhythmias indicate the need to limit further energy expenditure. Even if the child is able to ambulate to a chair with a moderate increase in heart rate, the effort required to return to bed must be considered. After ambulation a rest period is scheduled.

Observe for Complications of Heart Surgery. Several complications can occur after heart surgery, most of which are related to open-heart surgery and use of cardiopulmonary bypass. Many of the procedures discussed in the preceding paragraphs are aimed at preventing these problems. Only those that have not already been discussed are included here. A serious complication, bacterial endocarditis, is discussed on p. 1540.

Hematologic changes. While passing through the heart-lung machine, blood is exposed to substantial trauma by direct contact with oxygen, mechanical action, foreign substances, and massive doses of anticoagulants. The result of mechanical trauma is red blood cell hemolysis and potential renal tubular necrosis. Heparinization of the blood during extracorporeal circulation can result in clotting abnormalities from decreased thrombin and prothrombin, decreased platelets, and altered platelet aggregation.

Hemolysis of red blood cells results in blood loss and anemia, which may require packed red blood cell transfusion. The nurse monitors results of complete blood counts to identify the severity of the hemolysis. All urine is tested for the presence of blood. If transfusions are required, the child is closely observed for signs of reaction (see Table 35-2) and fluid overload. The necessity of measuring urinary output hourly has already been discussed.

Since blood clotting mechanisms are affected, signs of hemorrhage, especially bleeding from the chest tubes and a fall in arterial/venous pressures, are important observations. Hemorrhage is more likely to occur in patients who have repair of cyanotic heart defects because of the associated physiologic thrombocytopenia.

Normally the filter and bubble trap on the heart-lung machine remove air emboli, tiny clots, fat debris, and organisms from the arterialized (oxygenated) blood before its return to the body. However, impure blood entering the systemic circulation can cause fat emboli, thromboemboli, and infection anywhere in the body, but most importantly in the brain.

Cardiac changes. Cardiac failure may result from increased workload on ventricles that have been hypertrophied before surgery. Consequently, signs of heart failure are watched for, including elevation of the CVP.

Low cardiac output syndrome and ***decreased peripheral perfusion*** can occur from hypothermia or inability of the left ventricle to maintain systemic circulation. The most important signs of adequate peripheral perfusion are rapid capillary refill, good skin color, warm extremities, and strong pulses. Evidence of low cardiac output is similar to signs of shock (i.e., decreased BP, decreased pulse pressure, cool extremities, metabolic acidosis, and oliguria). Low cardiac output states are aggressively treated with intravenous inotropic medications such as dopamine, dobutamine, and amninone. If maximum medical therapy is failing, cardiac assist devices such as the intraaortic balloon pump, ECMO, or a ventricular assist device may be used in some centers in certain circumstances. These are new therapies with many complications and mixed results, and further study is needed before they are widely used in infants and children (Suddaby and O'Brien, 1993).

Dysrhythmias can result from electrolyte imbalance, especially hypokalemia, and surgical intervention to the septum or myocardium. The heart rate and rhythm are carefully monitored by observing the ECG pattern and by counting the apical pulse for 1 full minute. Dysrhythmias that impair cardiac performance are bradycardia, tachycardia, extrasystole, or heart block. When assessing dysrhythmias, nurses need to be aware of normal rates for age to determine abnormally fast and slow rhythms. The child is assessed for signs of decreased cardiac output, since in some children a faster than normal rate may be required to maintain an adequate cardiac output in the postoperative period. Epicardial pacing wires may be inserted during surgery for managing cardiac dysrhythmias postoperatively.

Cardiac tamponade is compression of the heart by blood and other effusion (clots) in the pericardial sac, which severely restricts the normal heart movement. A characteristic sign is ***paradoxic pulse pressure,*** in which the systolic pressure drops during inspiration because accumulated blood compresses the heart, resulting in a drop in cardiac output. Other signs include a rising venous pressure, falling arterial pressure, narrowing pulse pressure, tachycardia, dyspnea, cyanosis, apprehension, and a compensatory posture of sitting and leaning forward. Any evidence of this potentially fatal complication is immediately reported. Treatment consists of prompt pericardiocentesis to remove the blood or fluid. If active hemorrhage and coagulopathy are present, steps are taken to enhance blood clotting.

Pulmonary changes. Areas of atelectasis are common immediately after surgery as a result of deflation of the lung during cardiopulmonary bypass. Other pulmonary complications include pneumothorax, especially caused by faulty chest tubes; pulmonary edema from increased pulmonary blood flow or heart failure; and pleural effusion caused by persistent venous congestion. Signs of pneumothorax are persistent decreased breath sounds, sudden dyspnea, tachycardia, rapid shallow respirations, cyanosis, and sometimes sharp chest pain. Signs of pulmonary edema are tachypnea, rales, wheezing, moist dyspneic respirations, tachycardia, cyanosis, and restlessness. Signs and symptoms of pleural effusions include increased respiratory rate, vomiting, decreased breath sounds, fatigue, irritability, and decreased oxygen saturation (see Critical Thinking Exercise box).

Neurologic changes. ***Cerebral edema*** and ***brain damage*** may occur during open-heart surgery. Although the exact cause is unknown, it is thought to be a result of tissue ischemia or emboli. The nurse checks the equality of strength and reflexes in both extremities for evidence of paralysis; assesses the pupil size, equality, and reaction to light and accommodation; and assesses the child's orientation to the environment. Any evidence of cerebral damage is immedi-

CRITICAL THINKING EXERCISE

Postoperative Cardiac Care

Four-year-old Amy is 3 days postoperative following repair of coarctation of the aorta. She has a left thoracotomy and a chest tube in place. During your assessment you note an absence of breath sounds in the left upper lobe, a mildly elevated respiratory rate of 32, and a decreased O_2 saturation of 90%. She is not in any respiratory distress but is complaining of left shoulder pain. The chest tube has drained 30 ml of serous fluid in the past 12 hours. Which of the following is the best course of action?

1. You should consider a possible pneumothorax, carefully check the chest tube placement and connections, and notify the practitioner.
2. You should reassure her that decreased or absent breath sounds on the affected side are typical of patients with thoracotomy incisions.
3. You should administer codeine and acetaminophen as ordered, since her respiratory findings are likely due to pain.
4. You should consider a pleural effusion, check the amount of chest tube drainage, and change her position frequently to promote drainage of the pleural space.

The correct answer is 1. A pneumothorax is a common complication in patients with chest tubes, and Amy is experiencing typical symptoms of absent breath sounds, increased respiratory rate, decreased O_2 saturation, and pain. The chest tube is carefully assessed to make sure it is properly in place, all connections are tight and there is no air leak, and the Pleurevac is functioning correctly. The practitioner is notified and will likely request a chest x-ray film, which will distinguish between a pneumothorax, a pleural effusion, or atelectasis. A pneumothorax due to a leak in the chest drainage system will continue to worsen and may lead to significant respiratory distress. Therefore it needs to be promptly assessed and treated. If her symptoms are related to atelectasis, then chest physical therapy, pain management to decrease splinting, frequent position changes and ambulation are all indicated.

ately reported. The nurse also observes for focal or generalized ***seizure*** activity, which may be secondary to electrolyte imbalance.

Postpericardiotomy syndrome. This syndrome of fever, leukocytosis, pericardial friction rub, and/or pericardial and pleural effusion can occur anytime the pericardium is opened, either in the immediate postoperative period or after surgery, typically around day 7 to 21. The cause is unknown, although etiologic theories include a viral infection, autoimmune response to myocardial tissue, or a reaction to blood in the pericardium. It is self-limited and is treated with rest, salicylates, and sometimes steroids. Pericardiocentesis and/or pleurocentesis may be needed to treat large effusions.

Provide Emotional Support

Children may become depressed after surgery. This is thought to be caused by preoperative anxiety, postoperative psychologic and physiologic stress, and sensory overstimulation. Typically, the child's disposition improves on leaving the intensive care unit (see Chapter 26).

Children may also be angry and uncooperative after surgery as a response to the physical pain and to the loss of control imposed by the surgery and treatments. They need an opportunity to express feelings, either orally or through activity. The nurse can be supportive by reassuring children that the procedures that require cooperation, such as coughing and deep breathing, are difficult to perform; by praising them for efforts to cooperate; and by refraining from expecting too much "courage" or "bravery." This approach allows children to express feelings with the nurse's acceptance, regardless of their emotional response. Children also may express feelings of anger or rejection toward parents. The nurse must reassure parents that this is normal and that with continued support the anger will subside.

The nurse can support the parents by being available for information and explaining all the procedures to them. The first few postoperative days are particularly difficult because parents see their child in pain and realize the potential risks from surgery. They often are overwhelmed by the physical environment of the intensive care unit and feel useless because they can do so little for their child. The nurse can minimize such feelings by including parents in caregiving activities if they wish, such as a partial bath, turning, or positioning for postural drainage; by providing information about the child's condition; and by being sensitive to their emotional and physical needs. The importance of their presence in making the child feel more secure is stressed, even if they do not provide physical care.

Plan for Discharge and Home Care

Ideally, discharge planning begins on admission for cardiac surgery and includes an assessment of the parents' adjustment to the child's altered state of health. As mentioned earlier, one of the most common parental reactions is overprotection, and the nurse needs to be aware of times when the family may need help in recognizing the child's improved health status. With surgical correction of heart anomalies occurring during infancy, there is less likelihood

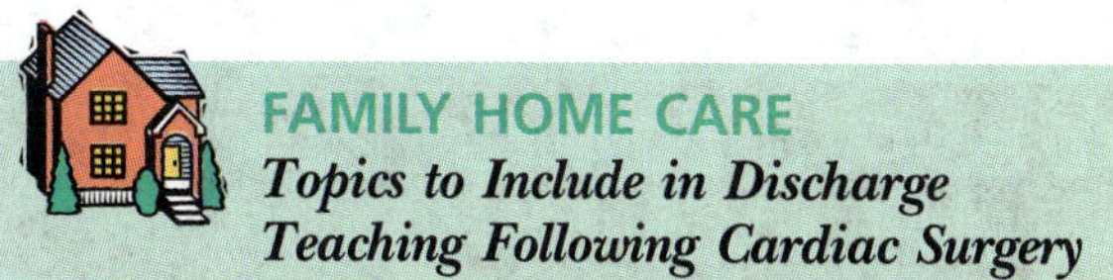

FAMILY HOME CARE
Topics to Include in Discharge Teaching Following Cardiac Surgery

- Medication teaching (for digoxin, see p. 1511)
- Activity restrictions
- Diet and nutrition
- Wound care (include dressings if any, suture removal, bathing)
- Bacterial endocarditis prophylaxis (see p. 1540)
- Follow-up appointments (cardiologist, primary care provider)
  - Community agencies as needed (visiting nurse service, early developmental intervention)
- When to call practitioner; signs and symptoms of postoperative problems
- Review of cardiac defect and surgical repair

of this pattern of overdependency developing. Many of these children are at risk for the vulnerable child syndrome (see p. 388).

The family will need verbal as well as written instructions on medication, nutrition, activity restrictions, subacute bacterial endocarditis, return to school, wound care, and signs and symptoms of infection or complications. Referrals to community agencies may be warranted to assist parents in the transition from hospital to home and to reinforce the teaching (see Family Home Care box).

The parents will also need clear instructions on when to seek medical care, such as for a change in the child's behavior or an unexplained fever. Follow-up with the cardiologist is also arranged before discharge. Appropriate medical identification, such as a bracelet, is indicated for children with a pacemaker or a heart transplant and for those receiving anticoagulation therapy or antidysrhythmic medication.

The nurse also discusses common behavior disturbances that may occur after discharge, such as nightmares, sleep disturbances, separation anxiety, and overdependence. A supportive, consistent response is essential to allow the child to overcome the surgical experience. The child may work out feelings and fears through therapeutic play, and this should be encouraged.

Although surgical correction of heart defects has improved dramatically, it is still not possible to totally reverse many of the complex anomalies. For many children repeat procedures are required to replace conduits or grafts or to manage complications, such as restenosis. Consequently, the long-term prognosis is uncertain, and full recovery is not always possible. For these families medical follow-up and continued emotional support are essential. The nurse can often serve as an important primary health professional and as a resource for referrals when needed.

❖ EVALUATION

The effectiveness of nursing interventions for the family and the child with CHD is determined by continual reassessment and evaluation of care based on the following observational guidelines and expected outcomes:

NURSING CARE PLAN
The Child with Congenital Heart Disease

NURSING DIAGNOSIS: High risk for cardiac output related to structural defect

PATIENT GOAL 1: Will exhibit improved cardiac output

• **NURSING INTERVENTIONS/*RATIONALES***

*Administer digoxin as ordered, using established precautions *to prevent toxicity* (see p. 1510 and Family Home Care box, p. 1511)

*Administer afterload reduction medications as ordered (see p. 1511)

*Administer diuretics as ordered (see p. 1514)

• **EXPECTED OUTCOME**

Heart rate, blood pressure, and peripheral perfusion are normal for age (see inside back cover)

Urinary output is adequate (between 0.5 to 2 ml/kg, depending on age)

NURSING DIAGNOSIS: Activity intolerance related to imbalance between oxygen supply and demand

PATIENT GOAL 1: Will maintain adequate energy levels without additional stresses

• **NURSING INTERVENTIONS/*RATIONALES***

Allow for frequent rest periods and uninterrupted periods of sleep

Encourage quiet games and activities

Help child select activities appropriate to age, condition, and capabilities

Avoid extremes of environmental temperature *because hyperthermia or hypothermia increases the need for oxygen*

Implement measures to reduce anxiety

Respond promptly to crying or other expressions of distress

• **EXPECTED OUTCOMES**

Child determines and engages in activities commensurate with capabilities

Child receives appropriate amount of rest/sleep (specify)

NURSING DIAGNOSIS: Altered growth and development related to inadequate oxygen and nutrients to tissues; social isolation

PATIENT GOAL 1: Will follow growth curve for weight and height

• **NURSING INTERVENTIONS/*RATIONALES***

Provide well-balanced, highly nutritious diet *to achieve adequate growth*

Monitor height and weight; plot on growth charts *to determine growth trend*

May administer iron supplements *to correct anemia*, if ordered

• **EXPECTED OUTCOME**

Child achieves adequate growth (specify)

PATIENT GOAL 3: Will have opportunity to participate in age-appropriate activities

• **NURSING INTERVENTIONS/*RATIONALES***

Encourage age-appropriate activities

Emphasize that child has same need for socialization as other children

Allow child to set own pace and activity limits *because child will rest when tired*

• **EXPECTED OUTCOMES**

Child engages in age-appropriate activities

Child does not experience social isolation

NURSING DIAGNOSIS: High risk for infection related to debilitated physical status

PATIENT GOAL 1: Will exhibit no evidence of infection

• **NURSING INTERVENTIONS/*RATIONALES***

Avoid contact with infected persons

Provide for adequate rest

Provide optimum nutrition *to support body's natural defenses*

• **EXPECTED OUTCOME**

Child remains free of infection

NURSING DIAGNOSIS: Altered family processes related to having a child with a heart condition

See Nursing Care Plan: The Child with Chronic Illness or Disability, Chapter 22

PATIENT/FAMILY GOAL 1: Will experience reduction of fear and anxiety

• **NURSING INTERVENTION/*RATIONALE***

Discuss with parents and child (if appropriate) their fears and concerns regarding child's cardiac defects and physical symptoms, *since these frequently cause anxiety/fear*

• **EXPECTED OUTCOME**

Family discusses their fears and anxieties

PATIENT GOAL 2: Will exhibit positive coping behaviors

• **INTERVENTIONS/*RATIONALES***

Encourage family to participate in care of child while hospitalized *to facilitate better coping at home*

*Dependent nursing action.

NURSING CARE PLAN
The Child with Congenital Heart Disease—cont'd

Encourage family to include others in child's care *to prevent their own exhaustion*
Assist family in determining appropriate physical activity and disciplining methods for child

• **EXPECTED OUTCOME**
Family copes with child's symptoms in a positive way

PATIENT (FAMILY) GOAL 3: Will demonstrate knowledge of home care

• **INTERVENTIONS/*RATIONALES***
Teach skills needed for home care
- Administration of medications
- Feeding techniques
- Interventions for conserving energy and those directed toward relief of frightening symptoms
- Signs that indicate complications
- Where and whom to contact for help and guidance

Anticipate need for further information and support
Refer family to local chapter of the American Red Cross *for instruction in cardiopulmonary resuscitation*

• **EXPECTED OUTCOMES**
Family demonstrates ability and motivation for home care
Family members learn cardiopulmonary resuscitation technique

NURSING DIAGNOSIS: High risk for injury (complications) related to cardiac condition and therapies

PATIENT (FAMILY) GOAL 1: Will recognize signs of complications early

• **INTERVENTIONS/*RATIONALES***
Teach family to recognize signs of complications
- Congestive heart failure (CHF) (for complete list see box on p. 1507)
  - Early signs:
    - Tachycardia, especially during rest and slight exertion
    - Tachypnea
    - Profuse scalp sweating, especially in infants
    - Fatigue and irritation
    - Sudden weight gain
    - Respiratory distress
- Digoxin toxicity
  - Vomiting (earliest sign)
  - Nausea
  - Anorexia
  - Bradycardia
  - Dysrhythmias
- Increased respiratory effort—retraction, grunting, cough, cyanosis
- Hypoxemia—cyanosis, restlessness
- Cardiovascular collapse—pallor, cyanosis, hypotonia

Teach family to intervene during hypercyanotic spells
- Place child in knee-chest position with head and chest elevated
- Remain calm
- Administer 100% oxygen by face mask if available
- Call practitioner

• **EXPECTED OUTCOME**
Family recognizes signs of complications and institutes appropriate action

PATIENT/FAMILY GOAL 2: Will demonstrate understanding of diagnostic tests and surgery

• **INTERVENTIONS/*RATIONALES***
Explain or clarify information presented to family by the practitioner and surgeon
Prepare child and parents for the procedure
Assist with family's decision regarding surgery
Explore feelings regarding surgical options

• **EXPECTED OUTCOME**
Family demonstrates an understanding of procedures (e.g., tests, surgery) (specify learning and manner of demonstration)

See also:
- Nursing Care Plan: The Child in the Hospital, Chapter 26
- Nursing Care Plan: The Family of the Ill or Hospitalized Child, Chapter 26
- Nursing Care Plan: The Child Undergoing Surgery, Chapter 27

1. Interview family and observe their behavior with the infant or child.
2. Encourage family to discuss their feelings and concerns; observe their understanding of the diagnosis and treatment.
3. Interview child and observe his or her behavior and concerns; encourage the verbal child to express feelings; interview family and observe family interactions and relationships.
4. Interview family regarding their understanding of the condition and the proposed surgery.
5. Monitor and observe infant or child and family preoperatively and postoperatively.
6. Interview child and family regarding response to cardiac surgery.
7. Observe and interview child and family regarding their understanding of home care needs, ability to carry out care, and compliance with the plan of care.

Expected outcomes:
See Nursing Care Plan, pp. 1538-1539.

ACQUIRED CARDIOVASCULAR DISORDERS

Acquired cardiac disorders refer to disease processes or abnormalities that occur after birth and can be seen in the normal heart or in the presence of congenital heart defects. They occur for a variety of reasons, including infection, autoimmune responses, environmental factors, and familial tendencies. Nursing care often plays a critical role in the identification and supportive management of these cardiovascular disorders.

BACTERIAL (INFECTIVE) ENDOCARDITIS (BE)

BE or infective endocarditis (IE), or subacute bacterial endocarditis (SBE), is an infection of the valves and inner lining of the heart. Although it can occur without underlying heart disease, it most often is a sequela of bacteremia in the child with acquired or congenital anomalies of the heart or great vessels. It especially affects children with valvular abnormalities, prosthetic valves, recent cardiac surgery with invasive lines, and rheumatic heart disease with valve involvement. In addition, a growing problem is endocarditis associated with drug abuse (Kaplan and Shulman, 1989). The most common causative agent is *Streptococcus viridans;* other causative agents are *Staphylococcus aureus,* gram-negative bacteria, and fungi, such as *Candida albicans.* Endocarditis associated with open-heart surgery is most often caused by *S. aureus,* coagulase-negative staphylococci, or diphtheroids (Kaplan, 1990).

Pathophysiology

The microorganisms usually grow on a section of the endocardium that has been subjected to abnormal blood streaming and turbulence, such as occurs when the flow of blood is restricted by an anatomic narrowing or forced through an abnormal opening. Growth may also begin where the abnormal jet of blood strikes the opposing endocardium, causing a thickening of the lining. Changes in the endocardium predispose it to the growth of invading organisms.

Organisms may enter the bloodstream from any site of localized infection. The most common portals of entry are oral from dental work *(S. viridans);* urinary tract, such as from urinary tract infection after catheterization (gram-negative bacilli); heart, from cardiac surgery, especially if synthetic material is used (valves, patches, conduits); and the bloodstream from long-term indwelling catheters. The microorganisms grow on the endocardium, forming vegetations (verrucae), deposits of fibrin, and platelet thrombi. The lesion may grow to invade adjacent tissues, such as aortic and mitral valves and myocardium, and may break off and embolize elsewhere, especially in the spleen, kidney, central nervous system, lung, skin, and mucous membranes.

Clinical Manifestations

The onset of symptoms is usually insidious, with unexplained low-grade, intermittent fever. Other common nonspecific symptoms are anorexia, malaise, myalgias, arthralgias, headache, and weight loss. A new murmur or a change in a previously existing one is frequently found as a result of damage to valves or perforation of the myocardium. Another finding, especially in those with prolonged illness, is splenomegaly. Other signs that result from emboli formation elsewhere in the body include splinter hemorrhages (thin black lines) under the nails, Osler nodes (red, painful intradermal nodes with white centers found on the pads of the phalanges), Janeway spots (painless hemorrhagic areas on the palms and soles), and petechiae on the oral mucous membranes.

Diagnostic Evaluation

Several laboratory findings may indicate BE, such as ECG changes (prolonged P-R interval), radiographic evidence of cardiomegaly, anemia, elevated erythrocyte sedimentation rate, leukocytosis, and microscopic hematuria. Definitive diagnosis can be made after growth of the organism and identification of the causative agent in the blood. Usually several blood specimens are drawn for culturing to rule out contamination during venipuncture and dilution technique. Strict sterile technique is practiced in obtaining cultures to avoid contamination. As soon as an organism is isolated, sensitivity studies are done to determine appropriate antibiotic therapy. Vegetation formation and myocardial abscess may be visualized on 2-D echocardiography.

Therapeutic Management

Treatment is administration of high-dose antibiotics (usually penicillin, ampicillin, methicillin, cloxacillin, streptomycin, and/or gentamicin for specific bacteria or amphotericin B and/or flucytosine for fungi) given intravenously for at least 4 to 6 weeks. Blood cultures are taken periodically to evaluate the response to antibiotic therapy. In instances when antibiotic therapy is unsuccessful, CHF develops, or recurrent systemic emboli are present, surgical intervention is warranted. This may include replacing damaged valves with prostheses, debriding and draining myocardial abscesses, excising areas of infection, and removing vegetations (Kaplan and Shulman, 1989).

Successful early medical treatment, especially with BE, occurs in approximately 80% of affected patients. However, cases diagnosed late, those cause by antibiotic-resistant organisms or fungi, or those occurring in infants or patients without preexisting heart disease carry a higher mortality and may necessitate surgical intervention. Death is most often caused by CHF, myocardial infarction from coronary emboli, or cardiac perforation. Nonfatal complications result from embolism to other organs, especially to the central nervous system (causing hemiplegia, aphasia, meningitis, convulsions), kidney (resulting in hematuria, proteinuria), spleen, and bowel.

Prevention of BE in susceptible children is of utmost importance and includes all children with CHD except those with (1) isolated ASD secundum and (2) surgical repair of ASD secundum, VSD, and PDA without residual effects after 6 months. In addition, patients with mitral valve prolapse without valvular regurgitation do not require prophylaxis (Dajani and others, 1990). Prevention involves administration of prophylactic antibiotic therapy shortly before

PROCEDURES REQUIRING PROPHYLAXIS FOR BACTERIAL ENDOCARDITIS

All dental procedures likely to induce gingival or mucosal bleeding, including professional teeth cleaning (not simple adjustment of orthodontic appliances or shedding of deciduous teeth)
Tonsillectomy and/or adenoidectomy
Surgical procedures or biopsy involving respiratory or intestinal mucosa
Bronchoscopy with a rigid bronchoscope
Incision and drainage of infected tissue
Genitourinary and gastrointestinal procedures, including most diagnostic and therapeutic procedures that are invasive (sclerotherapy for esophageal varices, esophageal dilation, cystoscopy, urethral dilation, urethral catheterization or surgery if urinary tract infection is present, prostatic surgery, vaginal hysterectomy and vaginal delivery in presence of infection)

Data from Dajani AS and others: Prevention of bacterial endocarditis: recommendations by the American Heart Association, *JAMA* 264(22):2919-2922, 1990.

and briefly after procedures known to increase the risk of entry of organisms (see box above). Drugs of choice include amoxicillin, ampicillin, clindamycin, gentamicin, and vancomycin. The drugs may be given orally or parenterally, depending on the procedure to be performed. Published recommendations provide guidelines for antibiotic prophylaxis, but they are complex and must be individualized for the child (Dajani and others, 1990).

Nursing Considerations

Ideally the objective of nursing care is counseling parents of high-risk children concerning the need for prophylactic antibiotic therapy before procedures such as dental work. The family's regular dentist should be advised of existing cardiac problems in the child as an added precaution to ensuring preventive treatment. These children should also maintain the highest level of oral health to reduce the chance of bacteremia from oral infections. (See also discussion on dental care in Chapter 14.)

Parents should also have a high index of suspicion regarding potential infections. Without unduly alarming them, the nurse stresses that any unexplained fever, weight loss, and change in behavior (lethargy, malaise, anorexia) must be brought to the practitioner's attention. Such symptoms should not be self-diagnosed as a cold or flu. Early treatment is important in preventing further cardiac damage, embolic complications, and growth of resistant organisms.

Treatment of endocarditis requires long-term hospitalization for the duration of parenteral drug therapy. In some cases intravenous antibiotics may be administered at home with nursing supervision for part of the treatment course. Nursing goals during this period are (1) preparation of the child for intravenous infusion, usually with an intermittent-infusion device, and several venipunctures for blood cultures; (2) observation for side effects of antibiotics, especially inflammation along venipuncture sites; (3) observation for complications, including embolism and CHF; and (4) prevention of boredom and depression, especially from restricted mobility caused by hospitalization and need for partial bed rest (if required). Follow-up after treatment is also important, and the nurse can be instrumental in arranging for convenient appointments.

RHEUMATIC FEVER (RF)

RF is a poorly understood autoimmune reaction to group A, beta-hemolytic, streptococcal pharyngitis. It is a self-limited disease that involves the joints, skin, brain, serous surfaces, and heart. If not for cardiac valve damage (referred to as ***rheumatic heart disease***), RF would be of little consequence (Fyler, 1990). In the 1920s, however, rheumatic heart disease was the leading cause of death in individuals between 5 and 20 years of age (Bland, 1987).

Recently, in developed countries, RF and rheumatic heart disease have become uncommon, probably as a result of antibacterial control of streptococcal infection, successful treatment of rheumatic heart disease, and a change in the organism itself. However, RF remains a devastating problem in developing (third world) countries and has reappeared in some parts of the United States (Veasy, Tani, and Hill, 1994).

Etiology

Strong evidence supports a relationship between upper respiratory infection with group A streptococci and subsequent development of RF (usually within 2 to 6 weeks). In almost all cases of RF a previous infection with group A streptococci can be documented by laboratory evidence of rising antibody titers. Prevention or treatment of group A streptococcal infection prevents RF.

Pathophysiology/Clinical Manifestations

The principal manifestations of RF are observed in the heart, joints, skin, and central nervous system. Inflammatory hemorrhagic bullous lesions, called ***Aschoff bodies,*** are formed, which cause swelling, fragmentation, and alterations in the connective tissue. Aschoff bodies are found in virtually all patients with clinical rheumatic activity. These lesions are found in the heart, blood vessels, brain, and serous surfaces of the joints and pleura (Fyler, 1992).

The major cardiac manifestation of rheumatic fever is ***carditis*** involving the endocardium, pericardium, and myocardium. In the acute illness, clinical signs and symptoms reflect valvulitis, myocarditis, and pericarditis. Clinically rheumatic carditis is almost always associated with a murmur of valvulitis (Special Writing Group, 1992). The presence of an apical systolic murmur reflecting mitral regurgitation is a common clinical finding in acute rheumatic carditis. This murmur is a long, high-pitched, blowing murmur that begins with the first heart sound (S_1) and continues throughout systole. Other murmurs in the acute phase may reflect aortic regurgitation. In addition, myocarditis produces tachycardia that is out of proportion to the degree of fever, especially during rest or sleep. Signs and symptoms of congestive heart failure may result, and cardiomegaly may be demonstrated by chest x-ray examination. Signs and symptoms of pericarditis include muffled heart sounds due to pericardial effusion. In addition, the patient may demonstrate a pericardial friction rub and complain of chest pain. Pericardial effusions can be documented by echocardiography. Patients with mitral or aortic valve involvement may experience progressive valvar damage as time goes on. The development of stenosis (primarily mitral stenosis) may eventually require surgical intervention.

The second major manifestation is ***polyarthritis*** caused by edema, inflammation, and effusions in joint tissue. The arthritis is reversible and migratory, favoring large joints such as the knees, elbows, hips, shoulders, and wrists. The affected joint is swollen, hot, red, and exquisitely painful for 1 to 2 days, after which a different joint is affected. Joint manifestations usually accompany the acute febrile period, most often in the first 1 to 2 weeks; however, they can persist for 4 weeks in untreated patients.

The third major manifestation is ***erythema marginatum.*** This is a distinct, erythematous macule with a clear center and wavy, well-demarcated border. This transitory, nonpruritic rash is most often found on the trunk and proximal portion of extremities.

The fourth major manifestation is the development of ***subcutaneous nodules,*** which are small (0.5 to 1 cm), nontender swellings that persist indefinitely after onset of the disease and gradually resolve with no resulting damage. They are rare but may be found in crops over bony prominences, such as feet, hands, elbows, scalp, scapulae, and vertebrae.

The last major manifestation reflects central nervous system involvement characterized by ***chorea,*** which is referred to as ***St. Vitus dance*** or ***Sydenham chorea.*** Chorea is characterized by sudden, aimless, irregular movements of the extremities, involuntary facial grimaces, speech disturbances, emotional lability, and muscle weakness that can be profound. It is usually exaggerated by anxiety and attempts at deliberate fine motor activity and is relieved by rest, especially sleep.

In addition to these major manifestations, minor manifestations that may support the diagnosis include arthralgia and fever, which may be low grade and which often spikes in the late afternoon. Laboratory findings reflect an inflammatory process. Other vague signs and symptoms include unexplained epistaxis, abdominal pain that may be severe enough to simulate appendicitis, weakness, fatigue, pallor, anorexia, and weight loss.

Diagnostic Evaluation

There is no single symptom or laboratory test that can definitively diagnose RF. Rather, the diagnosis is based on a set of guidelines recommended by the American Heart Association. These guidelines were recently revised so that they are designed to aid only in the diagnosis of the initial episode of rheumatic fever (see box above, right). Clinical and laboratory findings are divided into major and minor manifestations and must be accompanied by evidence of recent streptococcal infection in the majority of instances.

GUIDELINES FOR THE DIAGNOSIS OF INITIAL ATTACK OF RHEUMATIC FEVER (JONES CRITERIA, 1992 UPDATE)*

MAJOR MANIFESTATIONS	MINOR MANIFESTATIONS
Carditis	Clinical findings
Polyarthritis	Arthralgia
Chorea	Fever
Erythema marginatum	Laboratory findings
Subcutaneous nodules	Elevated acute-phase reactants
	Erythrocyte sedimentation rate
	C-reactive protein

SUPPORTING EVIDENCE OF ANTECEDENT GROUP A STREPTOCOCCAL INFECTION

Positive throat culture or rapid streptococcal antigen test
Elevated or rising streptococcal antibody titer

From *JAMA* 268(15):2070, 1992.
*If supported by evidence of preceding group A streptococcal infection, the presence of two major manifestations or of one major and two minor manifestations indicates a high probability of acute rheumatic fever.

Although the majority of patients with RF meet criteria, there are three circumstances where exceptions are allowed. In patients who have chorea as the only symptom and in patients who present late with continued carditis, the late diagnosis may preclude supporting manifestations and laboratory findings. Finally, a recurrence of RF in a patient with a previous history may not fulfill the standard Jones criteria. However, if there is a single major or several minor manifestations in a patient with a history of prior disease along with evidence of recent group A streptococcal infection, the diagnosis may be made without classic adherence to the criteria.

Streptolysin-O (O because it is oxygen labile) is a streptococcal extracellular product that produces lysis of the red blood cell. ***Antistreptolysin-O titers (ASLO)*** measure the concentration of antibodies formed in the blood against this product. Normally the titers begin to rise about 7 days after onset of the infection and reach maximum levels in 4 to 6 weeks. Therefore a rising titer demonstrated by at least two antistreptolysin-O tests is the most reliable evidence of recent streptococcal infection. Normal values are between 0 and 120 Todd units. Elevations over 333 Todd units indicate recent streptococcal infection in children.

Therapeutic Management

The goals of medical management are (1) eradication of hemolytic streptococci, (2) prevention of permanent cardiac damage, (3) palliation of the other symptoms, and (4) prevention of recurrences of RF. Penicillin is the drug of choice, with erythromycin as a substitute in penicillin-sensitive children. Salicylates are used to control the inflammatory process, especially in the joints, and reduce the fever and discomfort. Salicylates should not be instituted before diagnosis, since it may mask the polyarthritis. Prednisone may be indicated in patients with pancarditis and valvar involvement (Fyler, 1992). Bed rest is recommended during the acute febrile phase but need not be strict.

Prophylactic treatment against recurrence of RF is started after the acute therapy and involves monthly intramuscular injections of benzathine penicillin G (1.2 million U), two daily oral doses of penicillin (200,000 U), or one daily dose of sulfadiazine (1 g). The duration of long-term prophylaxis is uncertain. Because of the risk of BE in rheumatic heart disease, the same prophylaxis discussed earlier is implemented. The antibiotic regimens used to prevent recurrences of RF are inadequate for the prevention of BE.

Children who have had acute RF are susceptible to recurrent RF for the rest of their lives and should be followed medically for at least 5 years. Children and families must be aware of the need for continuing antibiotic prophylaxis for dental work, infection, and invasive procedures.

Nursing Considerations

The objectives of nursing care for the child with RF are to (1) encourage compliance with drug regimens, (2) facilitate recovery from the illness, (3) provide emotional support, and (4) prevent recurrence of the disease. Since compliance is a major concern in long-term drug therapy, every effort is made to encourage adherence to the therapeutic plan (see Compliance, Chapter 27). When compliance is poor, monthly injections may be substituted for daily oral administration of antibiotics, and children need preparation for this often dreaded procedure.

Interventions during home care are primarily concerned with providing rest and adequate nutrition. Usually, once the febrile stage is over, children can resume moderate activity and their appetite improves. If carditis is present, the family must be aware of any activity restrictions and may need help in choosing less strenuous activities for the child.

One of the most disturbing and frustrating manifestations of the disease is chorea. The onset is gradual and may occur weeks to months after the illness, sometimes even occurring in children who have not been diagnosed with RF. It may be mistaken for nervousness, clumsiness, behavioral changes, inattentiveness, and learning disability. It is usually a source of great frustration to the child because the movements, incoordination, and weakness severely limit physical ability. The child needs an opportunity to verbalize feelings. Of utmost importance is stressing to parents and schoolteachers the involuntary, sudden nature of the movements, that the chorea is transitory, and that all manifestations eventually disappear.

Nurses also have a role in prevention, primarily in screening school-age children for sore throats that may be caused by group A streptococci. This may involve actively participating in throat culture screening programs or referring children with a possible streptococcal infection for testing. (See also Nursing Care Plan: The Child with Rheumatic Fever.*)

*In *Wong and Whaley's Clinical Manual of Pediatric Nursing* (Mosby).

KAWASAKI DISEASE (KD) (MUCOCUTANEOUS LYMPH NODE SYNDROME)

KD is an acute systemic vasculitis of unknown cause. Approximately 80% of cases occur in children under the age of 5 years, with peak incidence in the toddler age-group. The acute disease is self-limited. Without treatment, however, approximately 20% to 25% of children develop cardiac sequelae. Damage to the blood vessels that supply the heart muscle (the coronary arteries) and damage to the heart muscle itself can occur. The most common sequela is dilation of the coronary arteries, resulting in ***ectasia*** (dilation) or aneurysm formation. Infants less than 1 year of age are at the greatest risk for heart involvement. KD has become a leading cause of acquired heart disease in children in the United States (Leung and others, 1993).

KD is seen in every racial group. However, it occurs most frequently in Japan and in children of Japanese heritage regardless of where they live. Blacks are affected slightly more than whites, and males are affected more than females, with approximately a 1.6:1 ratio (Rauch, 1987). The reported incidence is greater in children of higher socioeconomic backgrounds for unknown reasons.

The etiology of KD remains unconfirmed. Although KD is not spread by person-to-person contact, several factors support infectious etiologic factors. It is often seen in geographical and seasonal outbreaks, with most cases reported in the late winter and early spring. Recent but controversial evidence suggests that superantigens that include toxins from group A streptococci and *Staphylococcus aureus* may be responsible for KD (Leung and others, 1993).

Pathophysiology

Although KD is best known for damage to the cardiovascular system, it involves all the small and medium-sized blood vessels (Newburger and Burns, 1989). During the acute stage of the illness there is progressive inflammation of the small vessels (capillaries, venules, arterioles) along with pancarditis. This vasculitis progresses to the medium-sized muscular arteries (12 to 25 days), potentially damaging the walls of the vessels and leading to the formation of coronary artery aneurysms in some children. In addition, aneurysms of the peripheral cervical, axillary, brachial, iliac, and renal arteries can occur, although this is rare. Inflammation gradually subsides and eventually ceases in 6 to 8 weeks. Over time, damaged, ectatic vessels respond by myointimal proliferation. The walls of the vessel heal inward, and the internal diameter may eventually return to normal in one half to two thirds of patients (Takahashi and others, 1987). The smaller the aneurysm, the more likely it is to heal. Even if the lumen size is restored, the vessel is never completely normal again. The affected vessel walls thicken and are subject to scarring, calcification, and stenosis, especially at the distal ends of the aneurysm.

Almost all of the morbidity and mortality resulting from KD is due to cardiac complications. Coronary thrombosis may result from sluggish and turbulent blood flow in a dilated vessel. In the long term, stenosis and scarring may also lead to impeded blood flow, predisposing the patient to myocardial ischemia and infarction. At greatest risk for development of cardiac sequelae are infants and those children with prolonged fever.

Clinical Manifestations

KD manifests in three phases: acute, subacute, and convalescent. The ***acute phase*** begins with an abrupt onset of high fever that is unresponsive to antibiotics and antipyretics. Over the next week or so, the diagnostic symptoms become evident. The bulbar conjunctiva of the eyes become reddened, with clearing around the iris (limbal sparing). The eyes are generally dry, without drainage. Inflammation of the pharynx and the oral mucosa develops, with red, cracked lips and the characteristic "strawberry tongue" (the normal coating of the tongue sloughs off, leaving the large papillae exposed, resembling a strawberry). The rash of KD differs from child to child but is never vesicular. It is most often accentuated in the perineum. Often the area affected by the rash may desquamate. In addition, the child's hands and feet become edematous, and the palms and soles become erythematous. The child may have cervical lymphadenopathy (at least a single node 1.5 cm or larger). During this stage the child is typically *very* irritable and inconsolable. Complications during this period include myocarditis with resultant ECG changes, decreased left ventricular function, and occasional symptoms of CHF. Approximately one third of patients will develop a temporary arthritis beginning in the small joints.

The ***subacute phase*** begins with resolution of the fever and lasts until all outward clinical signs of KD have disappeared. During this phase the child is at greatest risk for the development of coronary artery aneurysms. If changes in the arteries occur, they generally become evident by echocardiography during the second week of illness. Damaged vessels continue to stretch and will reach their maximum diameter approximately 4 weeks from the onset of illness. Thrombocytosis and hypercoagulability place the child at risk for coronary thrombosis. During this period the child often has the characteristic periungual desquamation (peeling that begins under the fingertips and toes) of the hands and feet. Arthritis may be evident during this phase and usually affects the larger weight-bearing joints. Irritability persists during this phase.

In the ***convalescent phase*** all the clinical signs of KD have resolved. The laboratory values, however, have not yet returned to normal. The erythrocyte sedimentation rate may remain elevated, reflecting lingering inflammation. Thrombocytosis may still be present. Arthritis may continue into this stage, and coronary complications may remain a concern. This phase is complete when all blood values return to normal (6 to 8 weeks after onset). At the end of this stage parents report that the child appears to have returned to normal in terms of temperament, energy, and appetite.

Cardiac Involvement. The most serious complication of KD is the potential for myocardial infarction, which generally results from thrombotic occlusion of a coronary aneurysm. The group at highest risk for thrombus formation are children with "giant" aneurysms (greater than 8 mm in diameter). The main symptoms of acute myocardial infarction in children are abdominal pain, vomiting, restlessness, unconsolable crying, pallor, and shock. Complaints of chest pain are more typical in older children (Kato, Ichinose, and Kawasaki, 1986).

Diagnostic Evaluation

Currently no specific diagnostic test exists for KD. Therefore the diagnosis is established on the basis of clinical findings and associated laboratory results (see box below).

These criteria should be used as guidelines. Many children with KD do not fulfill standard diagnostic criteria, and infants often have an atypical presentation. It is therefore important to consider KD as a possible diagnosis in any infant or child with prolonged elevated temperature that is unresponsive to antibiotics and is not attributable to another cause.

Several associated laboratory findings, when combined with clinical data, can be helpful in making the diagnosis. The typical child with KD is anemic and has a leukocytosis with a "shift to the left" (increased immature white blood cells) during the acute phase. An elevated erythrocyte sedimentation rate reflects ongoing inflammation and generally persists for 6 to 8 weeks. Microscopic urinalysis reveals a sterile pyuria with mononuclear cells. This will not be evident with a regular dipstick, because the white blood cells are not polymorphonuclear neutrophils. A transient elevation of liver enzymes typically occurs. Thrombocytosis with hypercoagulability becomes evident in the subacute phase and peaks 3 to 4 weeks after the onset of fever.

Echocardiograms are used to monitor myocardial and coronary artery status. A baseline echocardiogram should be obtained at the time of diagnosis for comparison with future studies. In addition, follow-up echocardiograms should be performed at approximately 2 weeks after onset and again at 4 to 6 weeks from the onset of fever to determine the diameter of the coronary arteries, as well as left ventricular contractility and valvular function. If cardiac involvement is evident, more frequent studies may be necessary.

DIAGNOSTIC CRITERIA FOR KAWASAKI DISEASE

The child must exhibit five of the following six criteria, including fever:

1. Fever for 5 or more days (often diagnosed with shorter duration of fever if other symptoms are present)
2. Bilateral conjunctival injection (inflammation) without exudation
3. Changes in the oral mucous membranes, such as erythema, dryness, and fissuring of the lips; oropharyngeal reddening; or "strawberry tongue" (large papillae are exposed)
4. Changes in the extremities, such as peripheral edema, erythema of the palms and soles, and periungual desquamation (peeling) of the hands and feet
5. Polymorphous rash
6. Cervical lymphadenopathy (one lymph node >1.5 cm)

Therapeutic Management

The current treatment of KD includes high-dose intravenous gamma globulin along with salicylate therapy. Gamma globulin reduces the duration of fever and the incidence of coronary artery abnormalities when given within the first 10 days of the illness. A single large infusion of 2 g/kg over 8 to 12 hours is the standard treatment (Newburger and others, 1991).

Aspirin is given initially in an antiinflammatory dose (80 to 100 mg/kg/day in divided doses every 6 hours) to control fever and symptoms of inflammation. Once fever has subsided, aspirin is continued at an antiplatelet dose (3 to 5 mg/kg/day). Low-dose aspirin is continued in patients without echocardiographic evidence of coronary abnormalities until the platelet count has returned to normal (6 to 8 weeks). If the child develops coronary abnormalities, salicylate therapy is continued indefinitely. Additional anticoagulatory therapy, such as coumadin, may be indicated in those children with giant aneurysms (>8 mm), who are at the greatest risk for morbidity and mortality (American Heart Association, 1994).

Prognosis. Most children with KD recover fully following treatment. However, when cardiovascular complications occur, serious morbidity may result. Death occurs rarely and almost always results from ischemia due to coronary thrombosis or stenosis.

Nursing Considerations

The nursing care of children with KD is challenging. Inpatient care focuses on symptomatic relief, emotional support, medication administration, diagnostic assistance, and education of the child and family.

In the initial phase the nurse must monitor the child's cardiac status carefully. Intake and output and daily weight measurements are recorded. Although the child may be reluctant to eat and therefore may be partially dehydrated, fluids need to be administered with care because of the usual finding of myocarditis. The child should be assessed frequently for signs of CHF, including decreased urinary output, gallop rhythm, tachycardia, and respiratory distress. Cardiac monitoring is suggested in the following cases: before the initial ECG and echocardiogram are completed and shown to be normal, during the infusion of intravenous gamma globulin (because of the large fluid load), for children less than 1 year of age, and for any child with cardiac symptoms. Sedation is generally required before echocardiography in children under 3 years of age, since the child needs to remain completely still for up to an hour.

Most nursing care focuses on symptomatic relief. To minimize skin discomfort, cool cloths, nonscented lotions, and soft, loose clothing are helpful. During the acute phase, mouth care, including lubricating ointment to the lips, is important for the mucosal inflammation. Clear liquids and soft foods can be offered. Elevated temperatures need to be carefully monitored. Acetaminophen can be given for fever (see Controlling Elevated Temperatures, Chapter 27). If arthritis develops, passive range of motion may be indicated and can be done most easily during the child's bath.

The administration of gamma globulin should follow the same guidelines as for any blood product, with frequent monitoring of vital signs. Patients must be watched for allergic reactions (see Table 35-2). Cardiac status needs monitoring because of the large volume being administered to patients who may have myocarditis and/or diminished left ventricular function. Intravenous patency is checked because extravasation can result in tissue damage. Hypercoagulability and venous fragility often make it difficult to maintain intravenous access in children with KD (McEnhill and Vitale, 1989).

Patient irritability is perhaps the most challenging problem. These children need to be placed in a quiet environment that promotes adequate rest. Their parents need to be supported in their efforts to comfort an often inconsolable child. They may need time away from their child, and nurses can often provide respite care for the family. Parents need to understand that irritability is a hallmark of KD and that they need not feel guilty or embarrassed about their child's behavior.

Discharge Teaching. Parents need accurate information about the progression of KD, including the importance of follow-up monitoring and when they should contact their practitioner. Irritability is likely to persist for up to 2 months after the onset of symptoms. Peeling of the hands and feet is painless and occurs primarily in the second and third weeks. Arthritis, especially of the larger weight-bearing joints, may persist for several weeks. Children are typically most stiff in the mornings, during cold weather, and after naps. Passive range of motion in the bathtub is often helpful in increasing flexibility. Any live immunizations (e.g., measles-mumps-rubella) should be deferred for 3 months after the administration of gamma globulin, since the body might not produce the appropriate amount of antibodies.

Some children develop recurrent fever and symptoms. Temperature should be recorded after discharge until the child has been afebrile for several days. Parents should be educated about the signs and symptoms of KD; if any occur together with a temperature of 38.4° C (101° F) or above, they are instructed to notify their practitioner.

Parents also need to be instructed about the administration of salicylates and, if the child is receiving high doses, made aware of the signs of aspirin toxicity—ringing in the ears (tinnitus), headache, dizziness, and confusion. The only side effect of low-dose aspirin is easy bruising. In addition, the aspirin should be stopped and the practitioner notified if the child is exposed to chickenpox or influenza because of the drug's possible association with Reye syndrome.

All parents should understand the unlikely but real possibility of myocardial infarction, as well as the signs and symptoms of cardiac ischemia in a child. At discharge the ultimate cardiac sequela is generally not known, since changes occur up to a month after the onset of KD. In addition, the parents of children with known severe coronary artery sequelae may be taught cardiopulmonary resuscitation.* Finally, children with coronary abnormalities may require indefinite antiplatelet therapy with low-dose aspirin.

---

*Home care instructions for measuring a child's temperature for administering oral medication, and for infant and child cardiopulmonary resuscitation are available in *Wong and Whaley's Clinical Manual of Pediatric Nursing* (Mosby).

In this situation contact sports should be avoided, and yearly administration of influenza vaccine is indicated.

SYSTEMIC HYPERTENSION

Hypertension is the consistent elevation of BP beyond values considered the upper limits of normal. The two major categories of hypertension are ***essential,*** or ***primary*** (no identifiable cause), and ***secondary*** (subsequent to an identifiable cause) hypertension. Traditionally, primary hypertension has been considered a disease of older adults and is a major health problem. Hypertension is the most common cause of cerebrovascular accident and is a major risk factor in myocardial infarction. However, in recent years there has been increasing interest in this disorder in children and in whether early detection may decrease later morbidity and mortality. Some evidence suggests that primary hypertension of adulthood may begin in childhood. However, findings reveal that many adults with high BP had normal BP as children and that children with high BP have normal BP as adults (Gillman and others, 1993). These findings emphasize the importance of BP evaluation for all individuals at each health visit.

Etiology

Most instances of hypertension observed in young children occur secondary to a structural abnormality or an underlying pathologic process, although this is being challenged by screening programs of relatively healthy children. The most common cause of secondary hypertension is renal disease (90%), followed by cardiovascular, endocrine, and some neurologic disorders. Miscellaneous conditions such as lead poisoning and ingestion of excessive amounts of licorice are causes unique to children. As a rule, the younger the child and the more severe the hypertension, the more likely it is to be secondary. The conditions associated with secondary hypertension in children and adolescents are listed in the box at right.

The causes of primary hypertension are undetermined. There is evidence that both genetic and environmental factors play a role. In younger children hypertension is most commonly due to secondary causes; however, in adolescents primary hypertension is seen more often than the secondary forms. The incidence of hypertension is greater in children with a family history of hypertension. American blacks have a higher incidence of hypertension than whites. In the black population hypertension develops earlier and is frequently more severe, resulting in mortality at an earlier age. Environmental factors that contribute to the risk of developing hypertension include obesity, salt ingestion, smoking, and stress.

CONDITIONS ASSOCIATED WITH SECONDARY HYPERTENSION IN CHILDREN

RENAL DISORDERS

Congenital defects
- Polycystic kidney, ectopic kidney, horseshoe kidney, etc.
- Obstructive anomalies
- Hydronephrosis

Renal tumor
- Wilms tumor
- Renovascular

Abnormalities of renal arteries

Renal vein thrombosis

Acquired disorders
- Glomerulonephritis—acute or chronic
- Pyelonephritis
- Nephritis associated with collagen disease

CARDIOVASCULAR DISEASE

Coarctation of aorta
Arteriovenous fistulas
Patent ductus arteriosus
Aortic or mitral insufficiency

METABOLIC AND ENDOCRINE DISEASES

Adrenal tumors
- Adenoma
- Phenochromocytoma
- Neuroblastoma
- Cushing syndrome
- Adrenogenital syndrome
- Hyperthyroidism
- Aldosteronism
- Hypercalcemia
- Diabetes mellitus

NEUROLOGIC DISORDERS

Space-occupying lesions of cranium (increased intracranial pressure)
- Tumors, cysts, hematoma
- Cerebral edema
- Encephalitis (including Guillain-Barré and Reye syndromes)

MISCELLANEOUS CAUSES

Drugs (corticosteroids, oral contraceptives, pressor agents, amphetamines)
Burns
Genitourinary surgery
Trauma (e.g., stretching of femoral nerve with leg traction)
Insect bites (e.g., scorpion)
Intravascular overload (blood, fluid)
Hypernatremia
Toxemia of pregnancy
Heavy metal poisoning

Clinical Manifestations

Although clinical manifestations associated with hypertension depend largely on the underlying cause, some observations can provide clues to the practitioner that an elevated blood pressure may be a factor. Adolescents and older children with hypertension complain of frequent headaches, dizziness, and/or changes in vision. In infants or young children who cannot communicate symptoms, observation of behavior provides clues, although gross behavioral changes may not be apparent until complications are present. Parents of infants and small children who have been treated for hypertension report that their child had previously been irritable, often indulged in an abnormal degree of head banging or rubbing, and may have wakened screaming in the night (when blood pressure tends to be highest).

TABLE 34-7 Classification of Hypertension by Age-Group

AGE-GROUP	SIGNIFICANT HYPERTENSION (mm Hg)	SEVERE HYPERTENSION (mm Hg)
Newborn		
(7 days)	Systolic BP ≥ 96	Systolic BP ≥ 106
(8-30 days)	Systolic BP ≥ 104	Systolic BP ≥ 110
Infant (<2 years)	Systolic BP ≥ 112 Diastolic BP ≥ 74	Systolic BP ≥ 118 Diastolic BP ≥ 82
Children (3-5 years)	Systolic BP ≥ 116 Diastolic BP ≥ 76	Systolic BP ≥ 124 Diastolic BP ≥ 84
Children (6-9 years)	Systolic BP ≥ 122 Diastolic BP ≥ 78	Systolic BP ≥ 130 Diastolic BP ≥ 86
Children (10-12 years)	Systolic BP ≥ 126 Diastolic BP ≥ 82	Systolic BP ≥ 134 Diastolic BP ≥ 90
Adolescents (13-15 years)	Systolic BP ≥ 136 Diastolic BP ≥ 86	Systolic BP ≥ 144 Diastolic BP ≥ 92
Adolescents (16-18 years)	Systolic BP ≥ 142 Diastolic BP ≥ 92	Systolic BP ≥ 150 Diastolic BP ≥ 98

From American Academy of Pediatrics: Report of the Second Task Force on Blood Pressure Control in Children—1987, *Pediatrics* 79(1):1-25, 1987.

Diagnostic Evaluation

It is clear from the increasing numbers of hypertensive or potentially hypertensive children and adolescents being identified that a BP determination should be a routine part of annual assessment in children. In addition, any child who is ill should have BP measurements taken, since the signs and symptoms of hypertension in children are often vague. The BP of children at any age should be measured if they are diagnosed as having or suspected of having coarctation of the aorta, unexplained heart failure, unexplained heart murmurs, unexplained seizures or other neurologic signs, an abdominal mass or masses, edema, ascites, and/or evidence of renal failure, hypernatremia, failure to thrive, respiratory distress, and hyperlipidemia.

No definitive cutoff values are used in the diagnosis of hypertension in the pediatric patient. The American Academy of Pediatrics (1987) has suggested the classification in Table 34-7. ***Significant hypertension*** is considered a BP persistently between the 95th and 99th percentiles for age and sex. ***Severe hypertension*** is a blood pressure persistently at or above the 99th percentile for age and sex. It is important to note that a child who is large for age may normally have a higher BP than a child who is of average size.

Before a diagnosis is made, BP should be measured on at least three separate occasions. To obtain an accurate reading, care is taken to quiet the child or relax the adolescent while the measurement is recorded to avoid false readings caused by excitement. The chief cause of falsely elevated BP readings is the use of improperly fitting, narrow cuffs. Therefore attention to correct measurement technique is essential (see Blood Pressure, Chapter 7). Twenty-four-hour BP monitoring devices detect changes in pressure throughout the day, thus giving a more realistic picture. These devices are best used with older children who are able to tolerate being attached to an ambulatory monitor.

In children with suspected primary hypertension, initial laboratory data are also obtained. This generally includes a urinalysis, renal function studies such as a creatinine and blood urea nitrogen, a lipid profile, complete blood count, and electrolytes. More intensive tests may be indicated for those with probable secondary hypertension.

Therapeutic Management

Therapy for secondary hypertension involves diagnosis and treatment of the underlying cause. In those cases amenable to surgical repair, the nature of the condition, the type of surgery, and the age of the child are all important considerations. Children or adolescents with consistently elevated BP readings from no known cause or those with secondary hypertension not amenable to surgical correction may be treated with a combination of nonpharmacologic and pharmacologic interventions. Dietary practices and life-style changes are important in the control of hypertension both for children and for adults. Nonpharmacologic measures, such as limitation of dietary salt, weight control, increased exercise, and avoidance of stress and smoking, carry no risk and should be instituted first, except in severe cases. Since the long-term effects of antihypertensive agents on children are not known, drug treatment of asymptomatic children with mild or borderline hypertension is not recommended.

Since obesity and hypertension are closely related, a weight reduction program is recommended for overweight youngsters. In salt-sensitive children, high salt intake increases the risk of hypertension for those genetically predisposed and aggravates existing hypertension unless salt intake is limited. Modifying salt intake in children is difficult and takes time and support. Regular exercise augments weight reduction and alone has been shown to normalize blood pressure. The exercise regimen is tailored to the child's interest. Aerobic exercise, such as swimming, running, or cycling, is highly recommended. Stress reduction strategies may be beneficial and include biofeedback and relaxation. Smoking is discouraged. If the adolescent is taking oral contraceptives, these may need to be discontinued and other contraceptive options provided.

Drug therapy in children is instituted with caution. Indications for antihypertensive drug therapy include significant elevations of BP resistant to nonpharmacologic intervention. The American Academy of Pediatrics Second Task Force on Blood Pressure Control in Children (1987) recommends beginning with one drug and adding other agents only if control is not obtained. Compliance with antihypertensive drug regimens is often difficult.

The oral antihypertensive drugs used most often in children include the beta blockers (propranolol), ACE inhibitors, diuretics, and occasionally a vasodilator (hydralazine). Calcium channel blockers remain controversial for the pediatric population. Pharmacologic intervention is tailored to meet the needs of individual children and is determined by the hypotensive effect produced and the appearance of any side effects. The goal is to achieve a normotensive state throughout the day without accompanying side effects. With many antihypertensive drugs, minimal data are available regarding their side effects in children. Therefore any behavioral or physical changes that occur after institution of therapy should be considered a possible effect, and therapy may need to be revised.

Nursing Considerations

The nurse is a valuable link in the health care delivery system in relation to hypertension in the pediatric age-group. Active in detection, diagnosis, and therapy in any setting—hospital, school, clinic, private office, public health services, and private practice—nurses are frequently the persons who operate well-child care and follow-up units and are usually the primary contact between health services and the child and family.

A BP measurement should always be a part of the routine assessment of infants and children. In carrying out the procedure, it is important to use the correct cuff size. Any questionable reading is repeated. When an elevated pressure is detected, the procedure should be carried out in the supine, sitting, and standing positions as feasible. In addition, initial comparisons should be made between the upper and lower extremities.

Nursing counseling and guidance of affected children is a challenge. Education aimed at the understanding of hypertension and its implication over the life span is essential in promoting patient and family compliance with both nonpharmacologic and pharmacologic therapies (see Compliance, Chapter 27).

Home BP measurements can facilitate surveillance in youngsters with chronic hypertension and can document effectiveness of therapy. A family member can be instructed in how to take and record accurate BP measurements, thus decreasing the number of trips to a health care facility. This individual needs to understand when to contact the practitioner regarding elevated values. When this option is not feasible, the school nurse can often be a valuable resource in monitoring BP.

The nurse plays an important role in assessing individual families and providing targeted information regarding nonpharmacologic modes of intervention, such as diet, weight loss, smoking, and exercise programs. If extensive dietary counseling is required, the child should be referred to a registered nutritionist with expertise in working with children and adolescents. Exercise regimens should be individualized. Schoolchildren and young adolescents generally prefer team sports rather than individual training, which they may view as a burden rather than an enjoyable activity. If peers and family members can be encouraged to participate in any of the management strategies, the child's compliance is likely to be greater.

Young hypertensive women should avoid oral contraceptives because of their pressor effects. Other options need to be presented before this form of birth control is discontinued (see Contraception, Chapter 20).

If drug therapy is prescribed, the nurse needs to provide information to the family regarding the reasons for drug therapy, how the drug works, and possible side effects (see box below). It is important to explain that the drug needs to be taken consistently to achieve any prolonged control of BP. The need for follow-up is stressed, especially since antihypertensive therapy can sometimes be safely discontinued if BP remains under control over time.

ANTIHYPERTENSIVE DRUGS COMMONLY USED IN THE TREATMENT OF PEDIATRIC HYPERTENSION, WITH NURSING INTERVENTIONS*

BETA BLOCKERS

Actions: Blocks response to beta stimulation
Depresses renin output

Propranolol (Inderal)
- Monitor pulse and blood pressures (can cause bradycardia and hypotension).
- Instruct to take with meals.
- Advise that drug may cause fatigue, a decrease in exercise tolerance, weakness, and cold extremities.
- Warn males of possible impotence.

Atenolol (Tenormin)
- Monitor pulse and blood pressures (can cause bradycardia and hypotension).
- Advise that drug can be given once a day.
- Instruct patients not to discontinue abruptly (needs to be withdrawn over a 2-week period).

ACE INHIBITORS

Action: Acts primarily by interfering with the production of angiotensin II, a potent vasoconstrictor

Captopril (Capoten)
- Monitor blood pressure and pulse.
- Instruct to take 1 hour before meals to increase absorption.
- Instruct patient to report any evidence of infection.
- Advise to avoid rapid position changes (can initially cause dizziness).

Enalapril (Vasotec)
- Monitor blood pressure and pulse (may cause hypotension).
- Instruct to report any swelling of face or lips and difficulty breathing (may rarely cause laryngeal edema).
- Instruct to report any evidence of infection.
- Advise not to use potassium supplements (can increase serum levels).

VASODILATOR

Actions: Acts on vascular smooth muscle
Thought to produce its effect by direct action on blood vessels to cause arterial vasodilation

Hydralazine (Apresoline)
- Instruct to take with meals.
- Advise that drug may cause drowsiness and to use caution operating machinery or doing other hazardous activity.
- Instruct to report if sore throat, fever, muscle and joint aches, or skin rash develops.

DIURETICS

(See Table 34-5)

*For the use of all drugs, instruct child or adolescent (and family) to:
- Rise slowly from a horizontal position and avoid sudden position changes.
- Take drug as prescribed.
- Notify practitioner if unpleasant side effects occur, but do not discontinue drug.
- Avoid alcohol and stay on prescribed diet.

Learning needs vary greatly depending on developmental levels and individual differences. Some children and families require a great deal of support, education, and guidance, whereas others need only education and periodic follow-up. A positive approach is essential; negative feedback will serve only to alienate the family. Exploring the reasons for difficulty in compliance can often provide realistic alternatives. Continued education, support, and reinforcement for positive behavior is a major nursing responsibility.

HYPERLIPIDEMIA (HYPERCHOLESTEROLEMIA)

Hyperlipidemia is a general term for excessive lipids (fat and fatlike substances); ***hypercholesterolemia*** refers to excessive cholesterol in the blood. High lipid or cholesterol levels are believed to play an important role in producing ***atherosclerosis*** (fatty plaques on the arteries), which eventually can lead to coronary artery disease (CAD), a primary cause of morbidity and mortality in the adult population. The risk of premature CAD has been shown to increase directly with plasma concentrations of total cholesterol and certain types of lipids. Interventions that decrease low-density lipoproteins (LDLs) and increase high-density lipoproteins (HDLs) have been shown to lower the risk for CAD (LaRosa and others, 1990). Current research indicates that a presymptomatic phase of atherosclerosis begins in childhood. As a result, preventive cardiology is focusing on the screening and management of lipid levels in childhood. The goal is to identify those children at high risk and intervene early.

The rationale for lipid screening and management in children is evolving, as lipid levels have been followed from childhood into adulthood. Children who demonstrate cholesterol levels in the upper percentiles seem to have an increased risk of remaining in the upper percentiles into adulthood. The more severely affected children are generally the ones targeted for dietary and possibly pharmacologic intervention. On the other hand, children in the lower percentiles are unlikely to have high cholesterol levels as adults. Cholesterol in childhood appears to be a major population predictor for adult cholesterol levels (Newburger, 1990). From known data on lipid levels and their relationship to cardiovascular disease in adults, some experts believe that children with hypercholesterolemia may suffer an increased risk of cardiovascular disease in adulthood.

To date, no definitive studies can predict the long-term risk of heart disease for children with hyperlipidemia. Research in this area is logistically difficult to complete because of the long period of clinical follow-up extending over 40 to 60 years. As a result, pediatric guidelines are inferred from adult data. Life-style habits, including diet, exercise patterns, and smoking, all known to be potential risk factors for cardiovascular disease, are normally established at a young age.

Cholesterol, a fatlike steroid alcohol, is part of the lipoprotein complex in plasma that is essential for cellular metabolism. ***Triglycerides,*** natural fats synthesized from carbohydrates, are used for energy. Both are major lipids transported on lipoproteins, a combination of lipids and proteins, which include:

Chylomicrons—Produced in the intestine in response to the intake of dietary fat. These are the principal transporters of dietary fat (triglycerides) from the intestine to the blood and ultimately to the fatty tissue. Chylomicrons are usually not present in the blood after a 12- to 14-hour fast.

Very-low-density lipoproteins (VLDLs)—Contain high concentrations of triglycerides, moderate concentrations of cholesterol, and little protein.

Low-density lipoproteins (LDLs)—Contain low concentrations of triglycerides, high levels of cholesterol, and moderate levels of protein. The end-product of VLDL synthesis, LDLs are the major carriers of cholesterol to the cells. Cells used cholesterol for synthesis of membranes and steroid production. Elevated levels of circulating LDL is a strong risk factor in cardiovascular disease.

High-density lipoproteins (HDLs)—Contain very low concentrations of triglycerides, relatively little cholesterol, and high levels of protein. HDLs transport free cholesterol to the liver for secretion in the bile. High levels of HDL are thought to protect against cardiovascular disease.

The formula used for a standard fasting lipid profile that reflects total cholesterol (TC) is:

$$\text{TC} = \text{LDL} + \text{HDL} + \frac{\text{Triglycerides}}{5}$$

LDL concentration can be calculated from this formula. It is considered accurate as long as the fasting triglyceride level is <450 mg/dl.

$$\text{LDL} = \text{TC} - \left(\text{HDL} + \frac{\text{Triglycerides}}{5}\right)$$

Diagnostic Evaluation

Diagnosis of hyperlipidemia is based on analysis of blood for a full lipid profile. Two samples drawn in the fasting state (12 hours) should be analyzed, and the average of the values used for diagnosis. Blood samples should be collected after having the child sit for 5 minutes, and the tourniquet should be applied immediately before the needle puncture, since posture and vascular stasis may affect results. Diagnostic values for acceptable, borderline, and high

TABLE 34-8 Classification of Total and Low-Density Lipoprotein (LDL) Cholesterol Levels in Children and Adolescents from Families with Hypercholesterolemia or Premature Cardiovascular Disease

CATEGORY	TOTAL CHOLESTEROL, mg/dl	LDL-CHOLESTEROL, mg/dl
Acceptable	<170	<110
Borderline	170-199	110-129
High	≥200	≥130

From National Cholesterol Education Program: Report of the Expert Panel on Blood Cholesterol Levels in children and adolescents, *Pediatrics* 89(3, pt 2):527, 1992.

THINKING CRITICALLY ABOUT . . . *Cholesterol Screening for Children*

Practitioners' opinions differ regarding lipid screening in childhood. In 1992 the National Cholesterol Education Program (NCEP) issued a concensus statement that provides guidelines for cholesterol screening in the pediatric population. Currently, selective screening is recommended for children who have a family history of premature cardiovascular disease (<55 years old) or children who have at least one parent with high blood cholesterol (>240 mg/dl). In addition, if a child's complete family history is not available, practitioners may consider screening. Finally, cholesterol values should be obtained in children who have any individual risk factors, such as a history of diabetes, Kawasaki disease, hypertension, or obesity.

Selective screening is favored by many experts because high blood cholesterol aggregates in families as a result of shared genetic and environmental factors (NCEP Guidelines, 1992). In addition, the most severely affected children generally come from families where there is a high incidence of early heart disease.

Advocates of selective screening oppose universal screening for various reasons. Screening is costly, and the laboratory data may vary significantly from center to center, resulting in inappropriate diagnosis. Since a prudent diet is now recommended for children over 2 years of age, universal screening will not alter management for most, and no valid evidence indicates that cholesterol-lowering diets prevent death from heart disease in adults (Feldman, 1990; Finberg, 1990).

Those favoring universal screening believe that selective screening is too limited and overlooks many children with hyperlipidemia. With varying family constellations a common situation today, family history may be incomplete. In addition, a negative history from a parent may be inaccurate, since approximately half of well-educated adults do not know their own cholesterol levels (Strong and Dennison, 1988).

In your practice, how many adult family members know their "numbers"? Also, observe how often pediatric practitioners ask about parents' cholesterol levels and heart disease as part of the child's health assessment. From your observations do you believe that selective screening is being implemented?

total cholesterol and LDL cholesterol levels are listed in Table 34-8.

Screening children for hypercholesterolemia is a controversial issue, with some authorities advocating universal screening and others proposing selective screening. Current guidelines recommended by the National Cholesterol Education Program (NCEP) (1992) recommend a strategy that combines two complementary approaches: (1) a ***population approach*** that aims to lower the average levels of blood cholesterol among all American children through population-wide changes in nutrient intake and eating patterns, and (2) an ***individualized approach*** based on selective screening (see Thinking Critically About . . . box).

Therapeutic Management

Treatment of high cholesterol is primarily dietary. The NCEP guidelines recommend a two-step dietary approach that restricts the intake of cholesterol and fat. Children with borderline LDL cholesterol are advised to follow the ***step one diet.*** It recommends the same nutrient intake as for the general population (i.e., less than 10% of total calories from saturated fatty acids, no more than 30% of calories from total fat, less than 300 mg/day of cholesterol, and adequate calories to support growth and development and to reach or maintain desirable body weight). Children with high LDL cholesterol levels initially are also placed on this diet. If these dietary modifications fail to achieve satisfactory levels of LDL after 3 months of therapy, the ***step two diet*** is initiated. The dietary restrictions include a further reduction of saturated fatty acid intake to 7% of calories and of cholesterol intake to less than 200 mg/day.

For children with severe hypercholesterolemia who fail to respond to dietary modifications, drug therapy may be necessary. Two drugs recommended for treatment are the bile acid–binding resins or sequestrants ***cholestyramine*** and ***colestipol.*** These two drugs act by binding bile acids in the intestinal lumen. Because they are not absorbed by the intestine, they do not produce systemic toxicity and are safe for children. Cholestyramine (Questran) and colestipol (Colestid) are both powders that are mixed with water or juice just before ingestion. Some patients cannot tolerate the medication because of the taste and the side effects, the most significant being constipation, abdominal pain, gastrointestinal bloating, flatulence, and nausea. Patients often complain of the "gritty" consistency of the medication. The average dose for a child is 4 g three times daily or 6 g twice daily.

NURSING ALERT The Report of the Expert Panel on Blood Cholesterol Levels in Children and Adolescents regarding recommendations for fat intake are not intended for infants from birth to 2 years of age, whose fast growth requires a higher percentage of calories from fat. Toddlers 2 to 3 years of age may safely make the transition to the recommended eating pattern as they begin to eat with the family. No treatment recommendations are made for any child younger than 2 years of age.

Patients should be instructed to take one multivitamin supplement with iron daily, since cholestyramine may interfere with the absorption of fat-soluble vitamins. It may also interfere with the absorption of other medications, which should be given earlier than 1 hour before or 6 hours after the resin-binding agent is ingested. The results of a complete blood count, chloride and folate levels, and serum concentrations of vitamins A, D, and E should be evaluated yearly.

Niacin (nicotinic acid) decreases TC and LDL levels and increases HDL cholesterol. It is generally administered to older children who do not tolerate resin-binding agents well. Some patients require niacin as adjunct therapy along with bile acid–binding resins.

NURSING ALERT Although available without a prescription, niacin is treated as a prescription medicine in children, and its use is monitored closely by a health care professional with clinical and laboratory monitoring, especially liver function tests (Colletti and others, 1993).

Patients taking niacin often complain of itching, gastrointestinal distress, and flushing episodes, especially when initially taking the drug. Flushing can be avoided if the patient is premedicated with aspirin (160 mg/day) approximately ½ hour before the dose. The initial dose of niacin for children, using a time-release or long-acting preparation, is 125 to 250 mg twice daily. This can be increased to a maximum dose of 30 mg/kg/day. Side effects are uncommon in patients taking less than 1000 g/day. Liver function tests should be monitored routinely in patients taking niacin, since it can cause elevated liver enzymes and bilirubin.

Nursing Considerations

Nurses play an important role in the screening, education, and support of children with hyperlipidemia and their families. When a child is referred to a lipid clinic, it is essential that the family be adequately prepared for the first visit. Generally, the parents will be asked to keep a dietary history of the child before this visit. Sometimes they will need to complete a questionnaire regarding the child's normal dietary habits over the preceding year. Families are instructed to keep their child fasting for at least 12 hours before screening. Therefore it is important to schedule the blood test early in the morning and to arrange for nourishment immediately thereafter. At the visit a complete family history is taken, including the health of both parents and all first-degree relatives, including questions about early heart disease, hypertension, strokes (CVAs), sudden death, hyperlipidemia, diabetes, and endocrine abnormalities. Nurses may also uncover risk factors when obtaining a health history for other purposes. It is therefore important that nurses be familiar with current screening practices and the availability of resources for children with positive family histories.

Parents and extended families are informed about cholesterol and hyperlipidemia. This education should include a brief introduction to the different lipoprotein categories, including cholesterol, HDL, LDL, and triglycerides. Also, behavioral risk factors for heart disease, such as smoking and exercise, are reviewed. For management to be effective, parents need to understand the rationale for dietary and/or pharmacologic intervention. The key is prevention of future cardiovascular disease.

Stringent dietary guidelines may become an issue of control and a source of great stress for many families. Children are not viewed as having a disease. Rather, the positive aspects of healthy eating, regular exercise, and avoiding smoking are emphasized. Basic dietary changes are encouraged for the whole family so that the affected sibling is not singled out. The focus is positive, with emphasis on what can be eaten, such as substituting chicken and fish for hot dogs and hamburgers and frozen yogurt for ice cream (Table 34-9). Cultural differences must be considered and recommendations individualized. For example, it is more realistic to suggest frying food in a monounsaturated oil such as canola than to forbid fried food altogether in families where this is common practice. Substitution rather than elimination needs to be emphasized. Visual aids are often helpful, especially for children (e.g., test tubes depicting the amount of fat in a hot dog). Diets should be flexible and individually tailored by a nutritionist experienced in combining recommendations that meet both the nutritional demands of the growing child and lipid modifications. Parents are encouraged to participate in dietary and educational sessions, ask questions, and share ideas and experiences.

Parents often feel guilty about the hereditary component of hyperlipidemia. Many of these same parents believe they

TABLE 34-9 Low-Cholesterol Substitutes for Common Foods

FOODS HIGH IN CHOLESTEROL AND SATURATED FATS	SUBSTITUTIONS LOW IN CHOLESTEROL AND SATURATED FATS
Red meat	Skinless chicken, broiled or baked Turkey Tofu Meatless main dishes (e.g., vegetarian chili or lasagna) Fish
Hot dogs	Low-fat hot dogs
Processed luncheon meats and fast foods	Turkey Low-fat ham Tuna fish Grilled, skinless chicken or salads
Regular milk (4% fat)	Skim milk
Ice cream	Nonfat frozen yogurt Sherbert without cream Frozen fruit juice bars
Butter, shortening, lard	Olive oil, canola oil, Fat-free margarine Fat-free mayonnaise
Cheddar/American cheese	Part-skim mozzarella sticks Fat-free yogurt Fat-free cottage cheese Fat-free American cheese
Egg noodles	Yolkless noodles Other grains (rice and pasta)
Potato chips	Pretzels Plain popcorn Vegetable sticks
Chocolate	Cocoa-containing foods
Cookies/crackers	Low-fat cookies/crackers (graham, animal, saltines)

Adapted from National Cholesterol Education Program, *Pediatrics* 89(suppl):525-584, 1992.

have failed if the diet alone is not making a significant difference in their child's lipid profile. They are reassured that a dietary approach alone is often not sufficient, especially for children with values greater than the 95th percentile.

Parents of children who require pharmacologic therapy need to understand the purpose, dosage, and possible side effects of the various drugs. Medication schedules should remain flexible and should not interfere with the child's daily activities. As an example, children of elementary school age may have better compliance if they take a resin-binding agent (e.g., cholestyramine, colestipol) twice a day (i.e., before school and at night) rather than the standard three times a day. Follow-up phone calls by the nurse between visits allow parents to discuss their concerns and ask any questions that have arisen.

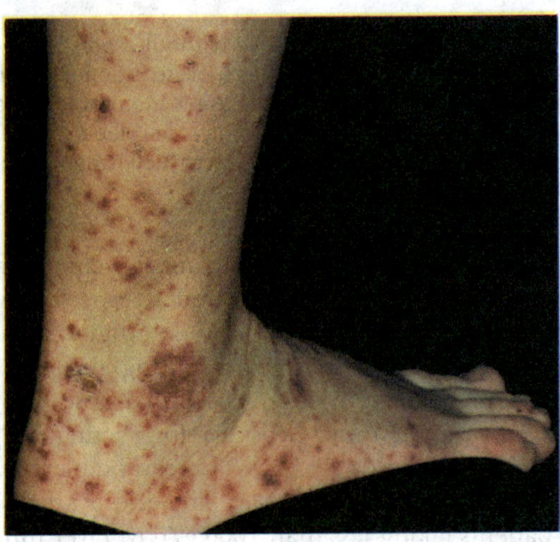

FIG. 34-15 Henoch-Schönlein purpura. (From Habif TP: *Clinical dermatology: a color guide to diagnosis and therapy,* ed 2, St Louis, 1990, Mosby.)

HENOCH-SCHÖNLEIN PURPURA (HSP)

HSP, also referred to as allergic vasculitis, allergic purpura, or anaphylactoid purpura, is a relatively common acquired disorder in children characterized by a nonthrombocytopenic purpura, arthritis, nephritis, and abdominal pain.

The etiology is unknown, but the disease often follows an upper respiratory tract infection, and allergy or drug sensitivity plays a role in some instances. The disease occurs in children ages 6 months to 16 years but more frequently in children ages 2 to 11 years. It is observed more often in white children than in other races and in boys almost twice as often as in girls.

Pathophysiology

The disease is characterized by inflammation of small blood vessels, and the manifestations observed are influenced by the size and distribution of the affected vessels. A generalized vasculitis of dermal capillaries (and to a lesser extent small arterioles and veins) causing extravasation of red blood cells produces the petechial skin lesions. Inflammation and hemorrhage may also occur in the gastrointestinal tract, synovium, glomeruli, and central nervous system.

Clinical Manifestations

The onset of the disease may be abrupt with the simultaneous appearance of several manifestations or gradual with the sequential appearance of different manifestations. The primary feature, however, is a symmetric purpura that involves the buttocks and lower extremities but may extend to include the extensor surfaces of the upper extremities and, less commonly, the upper trunk and face (Fig. 34-15). The rash may be associated with maculopapular lesions, urticaria, and erythema. There is often marked edema of the scalp, eyelids, lips, ears, and dorsal surfaces of the hands and feet—especially in infants and younger children.

Arthritic effects are evident in two thirds of affected children and range from asymptomatic swelling around a single joint to painful tender swelling of several joints, most often the knees and ankles. The involvement is periarticular and resolves in a few days without permanent damage or deformity.

Two thirds of the children have gastrointestinal involvement manifested by recurrent colicky midabdominal pain, often associated with nausea and vomiting. The stools contain gross or occult blood and mucus.

Renal involvement occurs in up to 50% of affected children and is potentially the most serious long-term complication. Initially the nephritis is manifested as hematuria, casts, and proteinuria. Although the majority of children with renal involvement recover completely, some develop chronic renal disease with eventual renal failure.

Diagnostic Evaluation

Diagnosis is usually established on the basis of the history and clinical manifestations. Laboratory tests are used to assess gastrointestinal and renal involvement and to determine adequacy of hemostatic function. Tests for occult blood in the stool are performed. Increased levels of immunoglobin A are a frequent finding.

Therapeutic Management

Management is primarily supportive, with close observation for signs of renal or gastrointestinal manifestations. Edema, rash, malaise, and arthralgia are usually managed with appropriate analgesics, such as nonsteroidal antiinflammatory drugs, and mild sedation is necessary. Corticosteroids may be prescribed for relief of more severe edema, arthralgia, and colicky abdominal pain. The nephropathy requires careful monitoring of fluid and electrolyte balance, salt intake, and blood pressure. Antihypertensive agents may be needed (Lanzkowsky, Lanzkowsky and Lanzkowsky, 1992).

The majority of children recover without the need for hospitalization, and in most instances a single acute episode clears spontaneously within a month. Others may have periodic recurrences for as long as 2 to 3 years before attaining permanent remission from symptoms. Rarely, death occurs from severe gastrointestinal complications, acute renal failure, or central nervous system involvement. Children with HS nephritis should receive long-term follow-up (Goldstein and others, 1992).

Nursing Considerations

Nursing care of the child hospitalized with HSP is primarily supportive, with vigilant observation for signs of complications. Vital signs are taken and recorded at regular intervals, specimens are obtained for laboratory examination, and medication is administered as prescribed. Urine and stools are carefully observed for fresh and occult blood.

If the child suffers from joint pain, positioning, careful movement, and administration of analgesics help reduce discomfort. Nonnarcotic analgesics also relieve the discomfort of fever and malaise. More severe involvement such as gastrointestinal symptoms and nephritis is managed as for any such disorder (see appropriate nursing care).

Concern about the unsightly appearance of the rash is common. The child and parents can be reassured that it is only a temporary phenomenon, and the child can be encouraged to wear clothing that helps hide the rash, such as long sleeves, pants, and a robe. Emphasizing good grooming and attractive apparel helps promote a more positive self-image.

CARDIOMYOPATHY

Cardiomyopathy refers to abnormalities of the myocardium in which the cardiac muscles' ability to contract is impaired. Although the incidence of cardiomyopathy in infants and children is small, it accounts for about 5% of all cardiac deaths in childhood, and about one half of the survivors have chronic cardiac disability. Possible etiologic factors include familial or genetic causes, infection, deficiency states, metabolic abnormalities, and collagen vascular diseases (Hohn and Stanton, 1987). Most cardiomyopathies in children are considered ***primary*** or ***idiopathic,*** in which the cause is unknown and the cardiac dysfunction is not associated with systemic disease. Some of the known causes of ***secondary*** cardiomyopathy are anthracycline toxicity (the antineoplastic agents doxorubicin [Adriamycin] and daunomycin), hemochromatosis (from excessive iron storage), Duchenne muscular dystrophy, Kawasaki disease, collagen diseases, and thyroid dysfunction.

Cardiomyopathies can be divided into three broad clinical categories according to the type of abnormal structure and dysfunction present: dilated cardiomyopathy, hypertrophic cardiomyopathy, and restrictive cardiomyopathy. ***Dilated cardiomyopathy*** is characterized by ventricular dilation and greatly decreased contractility resulting in symptoms of CHF. This is the most common type of cardiomyopathy in children. Its cause is often unknown, although carnitine and selenium deficiency, metabolic diseases, drug toxicities, dysrhythmias, and infection causing myocarditis should be considered. The clinical findings are of CHF with tachycardia, dyspnea, hepatosplenomegaly, fatigue, and poor growth. Dysrhythmias may be present and may be more difficult to control with worsening heart failure. Chest radiography demonstrates cardiomegaly and congested lung fields. The echocardiogram demonstrates poor ventricular contractility, a dilated left ventricle, and reduced shortening and ejection fraction. Cardiac catheterization with endomyocardial biopsy is usually done to assist with diagnosis and identify a possible infectious cause.

Hypertrophic cardiomyopathy is characterized by an increase in heart muscle mass without an increase in cavity size, usually occurring in the left ventricle and associated with abnormal diastolic filling. A large subgroup of this category is idiopathic hypertrophic subaortic stenosis, or obstructive cardiomyopathy, which has a familial association. Infants of diabetic mothers may have a hypertrophic cardiomyopathy that resolves with time (Lees and King, 1989). Clinical findings may include signs of CHF, especially in infants, and anginal chest pain. Dysrhythmias and syncope are also seen, and sudden death is a possibility. Chest radiography shows a mildly enlarged heart; the ECG demonstrates left ventricular hypertrophy, often with ST-T changes. The echocardiogram is most helpful and demonstrates asymmetric septal hypertrophy and an increase in left ventricular wall thickness, with a small left ventricular cavity.

Restrictive cardiomyopathy, rare in children, describes a restriction to ventricular filling caused by endocardial or myocardial disease or both. It is characterized by diastolic dysfunction and absence of ventricular dilation or hypertrophy (Hohn and Stanton, 1987). Symptoms are of CHF (see p. 1507).

Therapeutic Management

Treatment is directed toward correcting the underlying cause whenever feasible. However, in most affected children this is not possible, and treatment is aimed at managing CHF (see p. 1508) and dysrhythmias. Digoxin, diuretics, and aggressive use of afterload reduction agents have been found helpful in managing symptoms in those with dilated cardiomyopathy. Digoxin and inotropic agents are usually not helpful in the other forms of cardiomyopathy, since increasing the force of contraction may exacerbate the muscular obstruction and actually impair ventricular ejection. Beta blockers such as propranolol (Inderal) or calcium channel blockers such as verapamil (Calan) have been used to reduce left ventricular outflow obstruction and improve diastolic filling in those with hypertrophic cardiomyopathy.

Careful monitoring and treatment of dysrhythmias are essential. Anticoagulants may be given to reduce the risk of thromboemboli, a complication of the sluggish circulation through the heart. For worsening heart failure and signs of poor perfusion, intravenous inotropic support with dobutamine for several days has been successfully used in children, with symptomatic improvement lasting beyond the infusion. Severely ill children may benefit from mechanical ventilation, oxygen administration, and intravenous afterload reduction agents such as nitroprusside or amrinone. Heart transplantation may be a treatment option for patients who have worsening symptoms despite maximum medical therapy (see p. 1556).

Nursing Considerations

Because of the poor prognosis in most children with cardiomyopathy, nursing care is consistent with that for any child with a life-threatening disorder (see Chapter 23). One of the most difficult adjustments for the child may be the realization of failing health and the need for restricted activity, especially the normally active youngster with idiopathic hypertrophic subaortic stenosis. The child should be included in decisions regarding activity and allowed to discuss feelings, particularly if the disease follows a progressively fatal course. Once symptoms of CHF or dysrhythmias develop, the same nursing interventions are implemented as discussed on pp. 1510-1515. If cardiac transplantation is considered, the needs of the child and family are great in terms of psychologic preparation and postoperative care. The nurse plays an important role in assessing the family's understanding of the procedure and long-term consequences. Children of school age and older should be fully informed to give their assent to the procedure (see Informed Consent, Chapter 27).

CARDIAC DYSRHYTHMIAS

Classification

Dysrhythmias, or abnormal heart rhythms, can be classified according to various criteria, such as the effect on heart rate and rhythm:

Bradydysrhythmias—Abnormally slow rate
Tachydysrhythmias—Abnormally rapid rate
Conduction disturbances—Irregular heart rate

Before classifying an infant or child with an abnormal rate, nurses must be familiar with the standards of normal heart rate for the particular age-group (see inside back cover). Heart rate variations considered normal for a particular child can vary tremendously.

Bradydysrhythmias. The most common bradydysrhythmia in children is ***complete atrioventricular block (AV block),*** also referred to as complete heart block (Fig. 34-16). This can be either congenital or acquired, as seen in postoperative patients following surgery in the area of the AV valves and ventricular septum.

Sinus bradycardia in children can be due to the influence of the autonomic nervous system, as with hypervagal tone, or in response to hypoxia and hypotension. Once the infant receives adequate oxygenation and any acidosis is eliminated, the heart rate will often return to baseline. Sinus bradycardias are also known to develop after atrial inversion (baffle) procedures (Mustard or Senning).

Not all bradycardias originate in the sinus node. ***Junctional*** or ***nodal rhythms*** are common in the postoperative patient. The impulse for these rhythms originates further down the conduction system, in the AV node. Identification is marked by a normal QRS complex, which may be preceded by an inverted P wave or followed by an inverted P wave, or there may be completed absence of the P wave on the ECG. Often little change occurs in the heart rate or cardiac output. If there is no significant compromise to the patient's cardiac status, no treatment is necessary.

Tachydysrhythmias. ***Sinus tachycardia*** secondary to fever, anxiety, pain, anemia, dehydration, or any other etiologic factor requiring increased cardiac output should be ruled out first before diagnosing an increased heart rate as pathologic. ***Supraventricular tachycardia (SVT)*** one of the most common dysrhythmias found in children, refers to a rapid regular heart rate of 200 to 300 beats/min (Fig. 34-17). The onset of SVT is often sudden, and the duration is variable. Infants and young children with SVT may be unable to communicate the rapid heart rate, and the clinical course can progress to CHF. Important signs in the infant and young child are poor feeding, extreme irritability, and pallor.

Conduction Disturbances. Most rhythm disturbances are seen postoperatively in the child undergoing cardiac surgery and are of little significance. ***AV blocks*** are most often related to edema around the conduction system and resolve without treatment. Temporary epicardial wires are placed in most patients at surgery; if a rhythm disturbance occurs, temporary pacing can be employed. Just before discharge, the health practitioner removes the wires by pulling slowly and deliberately down on them from the site of insertion. In some cases, permanent pacemaker implantation may be necessary to treat complete AV blocks that do not resolve in the initial postoperative period.

Premature contractions can occur from an atrial, ventricular, or junctional focus. Their significance depends on the degree of compromise and the presence or absence of underlying CHD.

Diagnostic Evaluation

Several advances in the diagnosis of cardiac dysrhythmias have greatly improved the understanding and treatment of these conditions in children. The basic diagnostic procedure is the ECG, including 24-hour Holter monitoring. However, more definitive procedures include both noninvasive and invasive techniques.

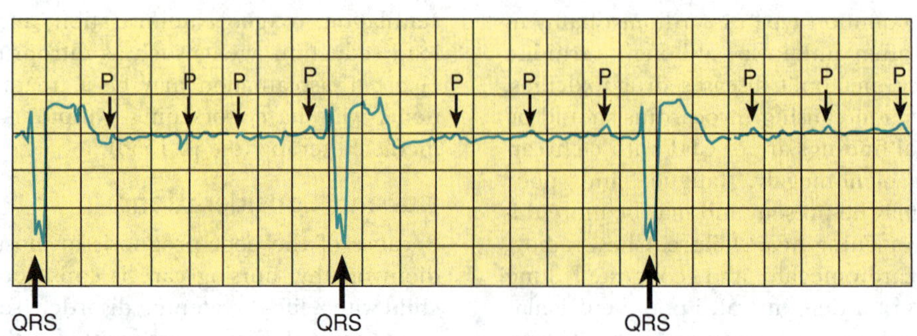

FIG. 34-16 Complete heart block. Note slow rhythm and several P waves not followed by a QRS complex.

Electrophysiologic cardiac catheterization allows for identification of the conduction disturbance and immediate investigation of drugs that may control the dysrhythmia. Electrode catheters are introduced transvenously and directed toward the right side of the heart. The heart is then selectively stimulated to induce dysrhythmias. Once a dysrhythmia occurs, different antidysrhythmic drugs are administered intravenously to monitor which pharmacologic agent is most successful in terminating the dysrhythmia. Patients and families undergoing this procedure are prepared in the same manner as any patient undergoing cardiac catheterization (see p. 1501).

Another procedure that may be employed is ***transesophageal recording.*** An electrode catheter is passed to the lower esophagus and, when in position at a point proximal to the heart, is used to stimulate and record dysrhythmias.

Therapeutic Management. Treatment of dysrhythmias depends on the cause and severity. Whenever possible, the underlying cause is treated. However, in some cases it is necessary to use antidysrhythmic drugs, with the goal being control, not cure. A permanent pacemaker may be needed in some children, such as those with postsurgical AV block or, less frequently, congenital AV block. The pacemaker takes over or assists in the conduction function of the heart. The surgical implantation of a pacemaker is usually a low-risk procedure. Once the wire has been introduced, a small incision is made and a pocket formed under the muscle to house and protect the generator. Continuous ECG monitoring is necessary during the recovery phase to assess pacemaker function. The nurse should be aware of the programmed rate and expected individual generator variations. A baseline ECG strip is obtained for future comparison.

Pacemaker functions have become dramatically more sophisticated; they can control heart rate according to activity, cardiac output, and respirations. In addition, some models can be programmed for overdrive pacing or cardioversion when the generator detects accelerated rates beyond established normal values.

The treatment of SVT depends on the degree of compromise imposed by the dysrhythmia. In some instances vagal maneuvers, such as applying ice to the face, massaging the carotid artery (on *one* side of the neck only), or having an older child perform a Valsalva maneuver (e.g., exhaling against a closed glottis, blowing on the thumb as if it were a trumpet for 30 to 60 seconds), have reversed the SVT.

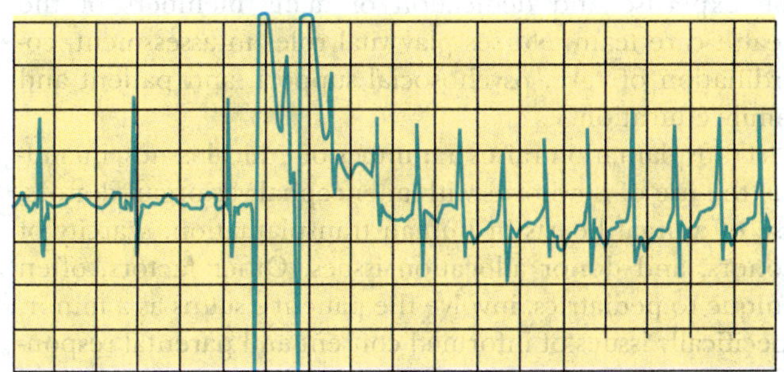

FIG. 34-17 Supraventricular tachycardia (SVT). Note normal sinus rhythm (three PQRST complexes) on the left and abrupt onset of a very fast rhythm (SVT) on the right.

When vagal maneuvers fail, adenosine may be used to end the episode of SVT. When given as a rapid intravenous bolus, adenosine impairs AV node conduction and allows normal conduction to resume. The desired effect usually occurs in 10 to 20 seconds. Its very short half-life (less than 10 seconds) minimizes side effects, such as flushing, headache, chest discomfort, dyspnea, and dizziness (Zempsky and Dick, 1993).

If cardiac output is significantly compromised or signs of CHF exist, electrical cardioversion can be employed in the intensive care setting. ***Transesophageal atrial overdrive pacing*** is accomplished through placement of a protected lead into the esophagus, behind the left atrium of the heart. The lead is then attached to a stimulator capable of pacing at very rapid rates to interrupt the tachydysrhythmia. ***Synchronized cardioversion*** is the timed delivery of a preset amount of energy through the chest wall in an attempt to reestablish an organized rhythm.

Nursing Considerations

An initial nursing responsibility is recognition of an abnormal heartbeat, either in rate or rhythm. When a dysrhythmia is suspected, the apical rate is counted for 1 full minute and compared with the radial rate, which may be lower because all the apical beats are not felt. Consistently high or low heart rates should be regarded as suspicious. Accurate nursing assessment is essential.

The onset and diagnosis of a cardiac dysrhythmia are frightening experiences for parents and the older child. Sometimes the dysrhythmia rapidly leads to heart failure and an emergency medical crisis. In this situation parents need much support to express their feelings, understand the diagnosis, and comply with home therapy, such as daily drug administration. In working with the family, the nurse must not forget the impact of the diagnosis of a heart problem. As one mother stated, "The heart is the body"; there is acute awareness of the necessity of the heart as a vital organ. Often an unspoken fear of potential death exists even if the dysrhythmia is benign, and repeated explanations are needed to allay the anxiety. In dealing with parents of an infant diagnosed with a dysrhythmia, the nurse must be sensitive to the care needed by parents facing the birth of a child with a congenital anomaly (see Chapter 11).

A primary focus of nursing care is education of the family regarding the specific treatment of the dysrhythmia. Following the first episode of SVT, parents should be taught to take a radial pulse for 1 full minute. If medication is prescribed, instructions regarding accurate dosage and the importance of administering the correct dose at specified intervals are stressed.

When a ***pacemaker*** is implanted, the education of the parents and child includes an explanation of the device, a description of the component parts, the surgical procedure, and discharge teaching. The pacemaker is made up of two basic parts, the pulse generator and the lead. The ***pulse generator*** is composed of the battery and the electronic circuitry. The function is to produce the electrical impulse sent to the heart and to receive and respond to signals produced by the heart. The *lead* is an insulated, flexible wire that conducts the electrical impulse from the pulse generator to the heart. Two types of leads are available, transvenous and epicardial. The child's size and the heart's structure determine which lead is more appropriate. ***Transvenous leads*** are inserted into a large vein, often the subclavian, and advanced into the right side of the heart. Placement is secured by engaging a small corkscrew or fish-hook attachment at the end of the lead into the endocardium. ***Epicardial leads*** are directly attached to the epicardial layer of the heart. Parents should be aware of which type of lead their child has in place.

Discharge teaching includes information about the signs and symptoms of infection, general wound care, and any specific limitations to activity. Instructions for telephone transmission of ECG readings are also given. Telephone transmission can be used to transmit ECG strips and also to monitor battery life and pacemaker function. Children with pacemakers should wear a medical alert device, and their parents should have a pacer identification card with specific pacer data in case of an emergency.

In life-threatening dysrhythmias, the family needs support and concise information regarding the medical interventions. Most important, families need to be assured that effective pain management will be employed during cardioversion. Following the child's conversion to normal rhythm, the family may need to learn cardiopulmonary resuscitation.*

HEART TRANSPLANTATION

Heart transplantation has become a treatment option for infants and children with worsening heart failure and a limited life expectancy despite maximum medical and surgical management. Indications for cardiac transplantation in children are cardiomyopathy and end-stage congenital heart disease. An important and controversial group of patients with congenital heart disease are infants with hypoplastic left heart syndrome who undergo heart transplantation as their initial treatment.

According to Kriett and Kaye (1992), nearly 1000 heart transplants have been performed in infants and children less than 10 years of age, the majority being done in infants. In their study the 1-year actuarial survival (predicted life expectancy) for children ages 1 to 18 was 76%; for infants it was 71%. The 5-year actuarial survival rates were 67% and 61%, respectively. In another study of infants from 3 hours to 12 months of age, the overall survival was 83%, with the best results in very young infants (Bailey and others, 1993).

The heart transplant procedure may be orthotopic or heterotopic. ***Orthotopic heart transplantation*** refers to removing the recipient's own heart and implanting a new heart from a donor who has had brain death but a healthy heart. The donor and recipient are matched by weight and blood type. ***Heterotopic heart transplantation*** refers to leaving the recipient's own heart in place and implanting a new heart to act as an additional pump or "piggyback" heart; this type of transplant is rarely done in children.

Before transplantation, potential recipients are carefully evaluated to identify problems in other organ systems that might preclude or increase the risk of transplantation. A psychosocial evaluation of the patient and family is done to identify possible problems in complying with the complex medical regimen following transplantation and in providing needed support systems. Patients are listed on a national computer network organized by the **United Network for Organ Sharing (UNOS)** to match donors and recipients. Because of the limited donor supply, from 10% to 25% of infants waiting for heart transplants will die before receiving a donor heart (see also Tissue Donation/Autopsy, Chapter 23).

The posttransplant course is complex. Although heart function is greatly improved or normal following transplantation, the risk of rejection is serious. Rejection of the heart is diagnosed primarily by endomyocardial biopsy and several noninvasive tests. Immunosuppressants must be taken for life and have many systemic side effects. Infection is always a risk. Potential long-term problems that may limit survival include chronic rejection, causing coronary artery disease; renal dysfunction and hypertension resulting from cyclosporine administration; lymphoma; and infection (Zuberbuhler, Fricker, and Griffith, 1989). In the short term, following successful transplantation, children are able to return to full participation in age-appropriate activities and appear to adapt well to their new life-style (Bailey and others, 1993; Baum and others, 1991). The long-term prognosis is unknown.

Nursing Considerations. Nursing care following transplantation is demanding and complex, with careful attention to both the physical needs of the child and the emotional needs of the child and family. Immunosuppressants and nursing implications are discussed in Chapter 30 in relation to renal transplantation. Care of the immunosuppressed child is reviewed in Chapter 36. Psychosocial concerns and appropriate interventions for the child with a life-threatening disorder are presented in Chapter 23. Successfully caring for a child following a heart transplant requires the expertise and dedication of many members of the health care team. Nurses play vital roles in assessment, coordination of care, psychosocial support, and patient and family education.

Transplantation raises a number of ethical issues, including the use of newborns with anencephaly as organ donors, use of animal hearts in human transplantation, scarcity of donors, and donor allocation issues. Other factors, often unique to pediatrics, involve the patient's status as a minor, specifically issues of informed consent and parental responsibility and authority.

*Home care instructions are available in *Wong and Whaley's Clinical Manual of Pediatric Nursing* (Mosby).

KEY POINTS

- Congenital heart disease is the most common form of cardiac disease in children.
- Major categories to investigate in the cardiac history are poor weight gain, poor feeding habits, and fatigue during feeding; frequent respiratory infections and difficulties; and evidence of exercise intolerance.
- The most common tests used in assessing cardiac function are radiography, electrocardiography, echocardiography, and cardiac catheterization.
- Cardiac catheterization procedures can be divided into three groups: (1) diagnostic procedures, including angiography, that measure pressures and saturations to establish cardiac diagnosis; (2) interventional procedures, in which catheters or balloon devices are used to correct cardiac defects; and (3) electrophysiologic procedures for diagnosis and treatment of dysrhythmias.
- Cardiac catheterization provides important information about oxygen saturation of blood within the chambers and great vessels, pressure changes, changes in cardiac output or stroke volume, and anatomic abnormalities.
- Several prenatal factors may predispose children to congenital heart disease: maternal rubella during pregnancy, maternal alcoholism, maternal age above 40 years, and maternal insulin-dependent diabetes.
- Congenital heart defects can be divided into four main groups, as determined by hemodynamic patterns: (1) defects that result in increased pulmonary blood flow, (2) obstructive defects, (3) defects that result in decreased pulmonary blood flow, and (4) mixed defects.
- Cardiac output is determined by the interaction of several factors: preload, afterload, contractility, and heart rate.
- Clinical consequences of congenital heart defects include congestive heart failure (CHF) and hypoxemia. A child can have both hypoxemia and CHF, although usually they occur independently.
- Clinical manifestations of CHF are impaired myocardial function (tachycardia, cardiomegaly), pulmonary congestion (dyspnea, tachypnea, orthopnea, cyanosis), and systemic congestion (hepatosplenomegaly, edema, distended veins).
- Nursing measures in the care of a child with CHF are to assist in improving cardiac function, decrease cardiac demands, reduce respiratory distress, maintain nutritional status, promote fluid loss, and provide family support.
- Clinical manifestations of hypoxemia are cyanosis, polycythemia, clubbing, and delayed growth and development. The child is at increased risk for hypercyanotic spells, cerebrovascular accidents, brain abscess, and bacterial endocarditis.
- Caring for the child with congenital heart disease (CHD) and the family requires helping them adjust to the disorder and cope with the effects of the defect and fostering growth-promoting family relationships.
- Preoperative care of the child with a congenital defect involves introducing the child and family to the hospital and preparing them for preoperative and postoperative procedures.
- Providing postoperative care includes observing vital signs and arterial/venous pressures, maintaining respiratory status, allowing maximum rest, providing comfort, monitoring fluids, planning for progressive activities, giving emotional support, observing for complications of surgery, and planning for discharge and home care.
- Acquired cardiovascular disorders include bacterial endocarditis, rheumatic fever, systemic hypertension, cardiac dysrhythmias, Kawasaki disease, cardiomyopathy, and hyperlipidemia.
- Prevention of bacterial endocarditis in certain children with CHD involves administration of prophylactic antibiotics when specific procedures are performed.
- Acute rheumatic fever is a systemic inflammatory disease that can damage the cardiac valves and is associated with previous group A streptococcal infection. Its incidence has increased in some areas of the United States.
- Kawasaki disease is an extensive inflammation of small vessels and capillaries that may progress to involve the coronary arteries, causing aneurysm formation. The administration of gamma globulin is an important aspect of treatment.
- Education of the child and family with hypertension focuses on drug therapy, diet control, and appropriate exercise.
- Cholesterol screening in children is controversial; currently children with known risk factors for hyperlipidemia are screened and treated as needed. The influence of childhood cholesterol levels on later development of coronary artery disease is under investigation.
- Henoch-Schönlein purpura is characterized by a nonthrombocytic purpura and variable joint and visceral abnormalities. Nursing care is primarily supportive, with observation for complications and provision of comfort being key nursing goals.
- Cardiomyopathy, or abnormality of the myocardium, is a serious, often fatal, disorder. Heart transplantation may offer more favorable options for some children than drug or other regimens.
- Common dysrhythmias in children include slow rhythms (bradycardias, heart block) and fast rhythms (sinus tachycardia, supraventricular tachycardia).
- Heart transplantation has been extended to infants and children with cardiomyopathy and complex congenital heart defects involving ventricular dysfunction, such as hypoplastic left heart syndrome.

REFERENCES

American Academy of Pediatrics: Report of the Second Task Force on Blood Pressure Control in Children–1987, *Pediatrics* 79(1):1-25, 1987.

American Academy of Pediatrics, Committee on Nutrition: Indications for cholesterol testing in children, *Pediatrics* 83(1):141-142, 1989.

American Heart Association, Committee on Rheumatic Fever, Endocarditis, and Kawasaki Disease: Guidelines for long-term management of patients with Kawasaki disease, *Circulation* 89(2):916-922, 1994.

Anand KJS, Hickey PR: Halothane-morphine compared with high-dose sufentanil for anesthesia and postoperative analgesia in neonatal cardiac surgery, *N Engl J Med* 326:1-9, 1992.

Bailey LL and others: Bless the babies: one hundred fifteen late survivors of heart transplantation during the first year of life, *J Thorac Cardiovasc Surg* 105(5):805-815, 1993.

Baum D and others: Pediatric heart transplantation at Stanford: results of a 15 year experience, *Pediatrics* 88(2):203-214, 1991.

Bland EF: The way it was, *Circulation* 76:1190-1195, 1987.

Colletti RB and others: Niacin treatment of hypercholesterolemia in children, *Pediatrics* 92(1):78-82, 1993.

Dajani AS and others: Prevention of bacterial endocarditis: recommendations by the American Heart Association, *JAMA* 264(22): 2919-2922, 1990.

Driscoll DJ: Evaluation of the cyanotic newborn, *Pediatr Clin North Am* 37(1):1-23, 1990.

Feldman W: Routine cholesterol surveillance in childhood, *Pediatrics* 86(1):150-151, 1990 (letter).

Finberg L: Pediatrics, *JAMA* 263(19):2672-2673, 1990.

Friedman WF: Congenital heart disease in infancy and childhood. In Braunwald E, editor: *Heart disease: a textbook of cardiovascular medicine,* ed 4, Philadelphia, 1992, WB Saunders.

Fyler DF, editor: Rheumatic fever. In *Nadas' pediatric cardiology,* Philadelphia, 1992, Hanley & Belfus.

Gillman MW and others: Identifying children at high risk for the development of essential hypertension, *J Pediatr* 122:837-846, 1993.

Goldstein AR and others: Long-term follow-up of childhood Henoch-Schonlein nephritis, *Lancet* 339:280-282, 1992.

Hazinski MF: *Nursing care of the critically ill child,* ed 2, St Louis, 1992, Mosby.

Hellenbrand WE and others: Balloon angioplasty for aortic recoarctation: results of valvuloplasty and angioplasty, *Am J Cardiol* 65:793, 1990.

Hoffman JI: Congenital heart disease: incidence and inheritance, *Pediatr Clin North Am* 37(1):31, 1990.

Hohn AR, Stanton RE: Myocarditis in children, *Pediatr Rev* 9(3):83-88, 1987.

Kaden GG and others: Physician-patient communication: understanding congenital heart disease, *Am J Dis Child* 139(10):995-999, 1985.

Kaplan EL: Myocarditis, pericarditis, and infective endocarditis. In Moeller JH, Neal WA, editors: *Fetal, neonatal, and infant cardiac disease,* Norwalk, CT, 1990, Appleton & Lange.

Kaplan EL, Shulman ST: Infective endocarditis. In Adams FH, Emmanouilides GC, Riemenschneider TA, editors: *Moss' heart disease in infants, children, and adolescents,* ed 4, Baltimore, 1989, Williams & Wilkins.

Kato H, Ichinose E, Kawasaki T: Myocardial infarction in Kawasaki disease: clinical analyses in 195 cases, *J Pediatr* 108(6):923-927, 1986.

Kriett JM, Kaye MP: The Registry of the International Society of Heart Transplantation ninth official report–1992, *J Heart Lung Transplant* 11(4):599-606, 1992.

Lanzkowsky S, Lanzkowsky L, Lanzkowsky P: Henoch-Schoenlein purpura, *Pediatr Rev* 13(4):130-137, 1992.

LaRosa JC and others: The cholesterol facts: a joint statement by the American Heart Association and the National Heart, Lung, and Blood Institute, *Circulation* 81(5):1721-1733, 1990.

Lees MH, King DH: Heart disease in the newborn. In Adams FH, Emmanouilides GC, Riemenschneider TA, editors: *Moss' heart disease in infants, children, and adolescents,* ed 4, Baltimore, 1989, Williams & Wilkins.

Leung DYM and others: Toxic shock syndrome toxin–secreting *Staphylococcus aureus* in Kawasaki syndrome, *Lancet* 342:1385-1388, 1993.

Maguire DP, Maloney P: A comparison of fentanyl and morphine use in neonates, *Neonatal Network* 7(1):27-35, 1988.

Martin GR, Perry LW, Ferencz C: Increased prevalence of ventricular septal defect: epidemic or improved diagnosis, *Pediatrics* 83(2):200-203, 1989.

McEnhill M, Vitale K: Kawasaki disease: new challenges in care, *MCN* 14:406-410, 1989.

Nadas AS: Hypoxemia. In Fyler DC, editor: *Nadas' pediatric cardiology,* Philadelphia, 1992, Hanley & Belfus.

National Cholesterol Education Program: Report of the expert panel on blood cholesterol levels in children and adolescents, *Pediatrics* 89:525-584, 1992.

Newburger JW: Management of dyslipidemia in childhood and adolescence. In Fyler DF, editor: *Nadas' pediatric cardiology,* Philadelphia, 1992a, Hanley & Belfus.

Newburger JW: Central nervous system sequelae of congenital heart disease. In Fyler DC, editor: *Nadas' pediatric cardiology,* Philadelphia, 1992b, Hanley & Belfus.

Newburger JW: Innocent heart murmurs. In Fyler DC, editor: *Nadas' pediatric cardiology,* Philadelphia, 1992c, Hanley & Belfus.

Newburger JW, Burns JC: Kawasaki syndrome, *Cardiol Clin* 7(2):453-465, 1989.

Newburger JW and others: Cognitive function and age at repair of transposition of great arteries in children, *N Engl J Med* 310:1495-1499, 1984.

Newburger JW and others: A single intravenous infusion of gammaglobulin as compared with four infusions in the treatment of acute Kawasaki syndrome, *N Engl J Med* 324(23):1623-1639, 1991.

Nora JJ, Nora AH: Update on counseling the family with a first degree relative with a congenital heart defect, *Am J Med Genet* 29:137-142, 1988.

Opie LH, editor: *Drugs for the heart,* ed 3, Philadelphia, 1991, WB Saunders.

Park MK: *Pediatric cardiology for the practitioner,* ed 2, St Louis, 1988, Mosby.

Park MK, Lee D, Johnson GA: Oscillometric blood pressures in the arm, thigh, and calf in healthy children and those with aortic coarctation, *Pediatrics* 91(4):761-765, 1993.

Perry SB and others: Interventional catheterization of left heart lesions, including aortic and mitral valve stenosis and coarctation of the aorta, *Cardiol Clin* 7(2):341-349, 1989.

Radtke W, Lock JE: Balloon dilation, *Pediatr Clin North Am* 37(1):193-214, 1990.

Rauch AM: Kawaski syndrome: critical review of U.S. epidemiology, *Prog Clin Biol Res* 250:33-44, 1987.

Roberts PJ: Caring for patients undergoing therapeutic cardiac catheterization, *Crit Care Nurs Clin North Am* 1(2):275-288, 1989.

Rosen KR, Rosen DA: Caudal epidural morphine for control of pain following open heart surgery in children, *Anesthesiology* 70(3):418-421, 1989.

Rosenthal A, Dick M: Tricuspid atresia. In Adams FH, Emmanouilides GC, Riemenschneider TA, editors: *Moss' heart disease in infants, children, and adolescents,* ed 4, Baltimore, 1989, Williams & Wilkins.

Special Writing Group of the Committee on Rheumatic Fever, Endocarditis, and Kawasaki Disease of the Council on the Cardiovascular Disease in the Young of the American Heart Association: Guidelines for the diagnosis of rheumatic fever: Jones Criteria, 1992 (update), *JAMA* 268:2069-2073, 1992.

Strong WB, Dennison BA: Pediatric preventive cardiology: atherosclerosis and coronary heart disease, *Pediatr Rev* 9(10):303-314, 1988.

Suddaby EC, O'Brien AM: ECMO for cardiac support in children, *Heart Lung* 22:401-407, 1993.

Takahashi M and others: Regression of coronary aneurysms in patients with Kawasaki syndrome, *Circulation* 75:387-394, 1987.

Veasy LG, Tani LY, Hill HR: Persistence of acute rheumatic fever in the intermountain area of the United States, *J Pediatr* 124:9-16, 1994.

Wessel DL: Hemodynamic responses to perioperative pain and stress in infants, *Crit Care Med* 21(9, suppl):S361-S362, 1993.

Woolf AD and others: The use of digoxin-specific fab fragments for severe digitalis intoxication in children, *N Engl J Med* 326(26):1739, 1992.

Zempsky WT, Dick M: Acute SVT: the case for adenosine, *Contemp Pediatr* 10(9):87-97, 1993.

Zuberbuhler JR, Fricker FJ, Griffith BP: Cardiac transplantation in children, *Cardiol Clin* 7(2):411-418, 1989.

BIBLIOGRAPHY

Diagnostic Procedures

Apple S, Thurkauf GE: Preparing for and understanding transesophageal echocardiography, *Crit Care Nurse* 12:29-34, 1992.

Barber G: Pediatric exercise testing, *Curr Opin Cardiol* 6(11):107-109, 1991.

Benson LN, Freedom RM: Interventional cardiac catheterization, *Curr Opin Pediatr* 1(1): 106-109, 1989.

Caire JB, Erickson S: Reducing distress in pediatric patients undergoing cardiac catheterization, *Child Health Care* 14(3):146-152, 1986.

DiLucente L, Goresan J: Transesophageal echocardiography: application to the postoperative cardiac surgery patient, *DCCN* 10:74-80, 1991.

Gardner RM, Hujes M: Fundamentals of physiologic monitoring, *AACN Clin Issues Crit Care Nurs* 4(1):11-24, 1993.

Glasier CM and others: Extracardiac chest ultrasonography in infants and children: radiographic and clinical implications, *J Pediatr* 114(4, pt 1):540-544, 1989.

Hellenbrand WH: Interventional cardiac catheterization, *Curr Opin Cardiol* 6(1):110-118, 1991.

Hochrein MA: Heart smart: a guide to cardiac tests, *Am J Nurs* 92(12):22-25, 1992.
McConnell JR and others: Magnetic resonance imaging of the brain in infants and children before and after cardiac surgery, *Am J Dis Child* 144(3):374-378, 1990.
Reidy SJ, O'Hara PA, O'Brien P: Streptokinase use in children undergoing cardiac catheterization, *J Cardiovasc Nurs* 4(1):46-56, 1989.
Sondheimer HM: Cardiac catheterization—a new role in the 90s, *Contemp Pediatr* 7(3):91-106, 1990.
Vargo L: Evaluation of cardiac size on the neonatal chest x-ray, *Neonatal Network* 12(3):65-67, 1993.
Webster H, Chellis MJ: Physiologic monitoring of infants and children, *AACN Clin Issues Crit Care Nurs* 4(1)180-197, 1993.

Congestive Heart Failure

Aronson JK, Hardman M: Digoxin, *Br Med J* 305(6862):1149-1152, 1992.
Brown KK: Boosting the failing heart with inotropic drugs, *Nursing 93* 23(6):34-44, 1993.
Dahlmann AR: Captopril, *Neonatal Network* 7(5):41-43, 1989.
Delgizzi LJ, Ueda JN: Using inotropic and vasodilating agents in pediatric patients with cardiac disease, *AACN Clin Issues Crit Care Nurs* 1(1):131-147, 1990.
Hagedorn MI, Gardner SL: Physiologic sequelae of prematurity: the nurse practitioner's role, part III, *J Pediatr Health* 4(5): 229-236, 1990.
Kaplan S: New drug approaches to the treatment of heart failure in infants and children, *Drugs* 39(3):388-393, 1990.
Linday L and others: Digoxin inactivation by the gut flora in infancy and childhood, *Pediatrics* 79(4):544-548, 1987.
Malinowski P, Yablonski C: Congenital heart disease in infants: nursing assessment, *Crit Care Q* 9(2):6-23, 1986.
Noerr B: Captopril, *Neonatal Network* 9(5):69-71, 1991.
Park JK, Hsu DT, Gersony WM: Intraaortic balloon pump management of refractory congestive heart failure in children, *Pediatr Cardiol* 14(1):19-22, 1993.
Shaddy RE, Teitel DF, Brett C: Short-term hemodynamic effects of captopril in infants with congestive heart failure, *Am J Dis Child* 142:100-105, 1988.
Werner NP: Congestive heart failure: pathophysiology and management throughout infancy, *J Perinat Neonat Nurs* 7(3):59-76, 1993.
Zalzstein E and others: Once-daily versus twice-daily dosing of digoxin in the pediatric age group, *J Pediatr* 116(1):137-139, 1990.

Congenital Heart/Cardiovascular Disease

Allen H and others: Insurability, *Circulation* 86(2):703-710, 1992.
Arfken CL and others: Mitral valve prolapse: associations with symptoms and anxiety, *Pediatrics* 85(3):311-315, 1990.
Beekman RH, Rocchini AP, Rosenthal A: Therapeutic cardiac catheterization for pulmonary valve and pulmonary artery stenosis, *Cardiol Clin* 7(2):331-340, 1989.
Benson DW: Changing profile of congenital heart disease, *Pediatrics* 83(4):790-791, 1989.
Callow LB: Postoperative nursing management of the infant with TAPVC, *DCCN* 10(3):140-149, 1991.
Callow LB: Current strategies in the nursing care of infants with HLHS undergoing 1st stage palliation with the Norwood procedure, *Heart Lung* 21(5):463-470, 1992.
Cardiovascular health and disease in children: current status, *Circulation* 89(2):923-930, 1994.
Castaneda AR and others: Transposition of the great arteries: the arterial switch operation, *Cardiol Clin* 7(2):369-376, 1989.
Clark EB: Cardiac embryology: its relevance to congenital heart disease, *Am J Dis Child* 140(1):41-44, 1986.
Clery JD: Two inotropic agents: dopamine and dobutamine, *Pediatr Nurs* 14(5):414, 1988.
Cohen DM: Surgical management of congenital heart disease in the 1990's, *Am J Dis Child* 146:1447-1452, 1992.
Cullen S, Celermajer DS, Dean field JE: Exercise in congenital heart disease, *Cardiol Young* 1(2):129-135, 1991.
De La Cruz MV, Gomez CS, Cayre R: The developmental components of the ventricles: their significance in congenital heart malformations, *Cardiol Young* 1(2):123-128, 1991.
Ferencz C and others: Congenital cardiovascular malformations associated with chromosome abnormalities: an epidemiologic study, *J Pediatr* 114(1):79-85, 1989.
Ferry PC: Neurologic sequelae of open-heart surgery in children, *Am J Dis Child* 144(3):369-373, 1990.
Freedom RM: The hypoplastic left heart syndrome: evolving trends in therapy and present concerns, *Curr Opin Pediatr* 1(1):90-93, 1989.
Hellenbrand WE, Mullins CE: Catheter closure of congenital cardiac defects, *Cardiol Clin* 7(2):351-368, 1989.
Ilbawi M: Current status of surgery for congenital heart diseases, *Clin Perinatol* 16(1): 157, 1989.
Jensen CA: Nursing care of a child following an arterial switch procedure for transposition of the great arteries, *Crit Care Nurs* 12(8):51-57, 1992.
Johnson AB, Davis JS: Treatment options for the neonate with HLHS, *J Perinat Neonat Nurs* 5(2):84-92, 1991.
Kirklin J, Barret-Boyes B: *Cardiac surgery*, New York, 1992, John Wiley & Sons.
Latson LA and others: Transcatheter closure of patent ductus arteriosus in pediatric patients, *J Pediatr* 115(4):549-553, 1989.
Lin A, Garver K: Genetic counseling for congenital heart defects, *J Pediatr* 113(6):1105-1108, 1988.
Morris CD, Menashe VD: 25 year mortality after surgical repair of congenital heart defects in childhood: a population based cohort study, *JAMA* 266:3447-3452, 1991.
Nora, JJ: Chance and ventricular septal defect (letter), Pediatrics 77(6):930-931, 1986.
Norris MKG, editor: Pediatric and neonatal cardiology, *Crit Care Nurs Clin North Am* 6:111-236, 1994.
Norwood WI: Hypoplastic left heart syndrome, *Ann Thorac Surg* 52:688-695, 1991.
O'Brien P, Elixson, M: The child following the Fontan procedure: nursing strategies, *AACN Clin Issues Crit Care Nursing* 1(1):46–58, 1990.
O'Fallon WM, Weidman WH, editors: Long term follow-up of congenital aortic stenosis, pulmonary stenosis, and ventricular septal defect, Report from the Second Joint Study on the natural history of congenital heart defects (NHS-2), *Circulation* (suppl) 87(2): I1-I126, 1993.
Rao PS: Balloon valvuloplasty and angioplasty in infants and children, *J Pediatr* 114(6):907-914, 1989.
Salzer HR and others: Growth and nutritional intake of infants with congenital heart disease, *Pediatr Cardiol* 10(1):17-23, 1989.
Siebert JR and others: Ebstein's anomaly and extracardiac defects, *Am J Dis Child* 143:570-572, 1989.
Smith JB, Vernon-Levett P: Hypoplastic left heart syndrome: treatment options, *MCN* 14:180-183, 1989.
Smith JB, Vernon-Levett P: Care of infants with HLHS, *AACN Clin Issues Crit Care Nurs* 4(2):329-339, 1993.
Smith MS and others: Symptomatic mitral valve prolapse in children and adolescents: catecholamines, anxiety, and biofeedback, *Pediatrics* 84(2):290-295, 1989.
Swetnam SM, Yabek SM, Alverson DC: Hemodynamic consequences of neonatal polycythemia, *J Pediatr* 110(3):443-447, 1987.
Talner NS, Lister G: Perioperative care of the infant with congenital heart disease, *Cardiol Clin* 7(2):419-438, 1989.
Tong E: An overview of artificial heart valve replacement in infants and children, *J Cardiovasc Nurs* 6(3):30-43, 1992.
Vet TW, Ottenkamp J: Correction of atrioventricular septal defect, *Am J Dis Child,* 143: 1361-1365, 1989.

Heart Transplantation

Addonizio L: Cardiac transplantation in the pediatric patient, *Prog Cardiovasc Dis* 33(1): 19-34, 1990.
Bernstein D: Update on cardiac transplantation in infants and children, *Crit Care Med* 21(9, suppl):S354-S355, 1993.
Johnston J: Role of the pediatric nurse in selection and support of potential donors for heart transplantation, *Focus Crit Care* 18(2):167-171, 1991.
Johnston J: Cardiac transplant in early infancy, *Crit Care Nurs Clin North Am* 4(3):521-535, 1992.
Lake KD, Kilkenny JM: The pharmacokinetics and pharmacodynamics of immunosuppressive agents, *Crit Care Nurs Clin North Am* 4:205-221, 1992.
Lyons M: Immunosuppressive therapy after cardiac transplantation: teaching pediatric patients and their families, *Crit Care Nurse* 13(1):39-45, 1993.
Mahon PM: OKT3 and heart transplantation: an overview, *Crit Care Nurs* 11(8):42-47, 1991.
Moodie DS, Stillwell PC: Thoracic organ transplantation in children, *Clin Pediatr* 32(6):322-328, 1993.
Muirhead J: Heart transplantation in children: indications, complications, and management, *J Cardiovasc Nurs* 6(3)44-55, 1992.
Noonan DM and others: Nursing considerations for neonates awaiting heart transplant for HLHS, *J Pediatr Nurs* 6(5):327-330, 1991.
O'Brien P, Hanley FH: New directions in pediatric heart transplantation, *Crit Care Nurs Clin North Am* 4:193-203, 1992.
Pezze JL, Whiteman K: Transplantation's newest weapon: FK506, *Am J Nurs* 91(10):40-42, 1991.

Porter R and others: Perceived stress and coping strategies among cardiac transplant patients during the organ waiting period, *Heart Lung* 21(3):292, 1992.

Smith S, editor: *Tissue and organ transplantation: indications for professional nursing practice,* St Louis, 1990, Mosby.

Uzark K: Caring for families of pediatric transplant recipients: psychosocial implications, *Crit Care Nurs Clin North Am* 4:255-263, 1992.

Nursing Care

Abbott K: Therapeutic use of play in the psychological preparation of preschool children undergoing cardiac surgery, *Issues Compr Pediatr Nurs* 13(4):265-277, 1990.

Combs VL, Marino BL: A comparison of growth patterns in breast and bottle fed infants with congenital heart disease, *Pediatr Nurs* 19(2)175-179, 1993.

Craig J: The postoperative cardiac infant: physiologic basis for neonatal nursing interventions, *J Perinat Neonat Nurs* 5(2):60-70, 1991.

Fisk R: Management of the pediatric cardiovascular patient after surgery, *Crit Care Q* 9(2):75-82, 1986.

Foldy SM, Gorman JB: Perioperative nursing care for congenital cardiac defects, *Crit Care Nurs Clin North Am* 1(2):289-296, 1989.

Hardingham K: The pediatric cardiovascular surgery patient: a case study, *J Cardiovasc Nurs* 7(2):80-85, 1993.

Kashani IA, Higgins SS: Counseling strategies for families of children with congenital heart disease, *Pediatr Nurs* 12(1):38-40, 1986.

Kulik L and others: Pharmacologic interventions for the neonate with compromised cardiac function, *J Perinat Neonat Nurs* 5(2):71-84, 1991.

Lobo ML: Parent infant interactions during feeding with infants with congenital heart defects, *J Pediatr Nurs* 7(2):97-105, 1992.

Malinowski P, Yablonski C: Congenital heart disease in infants: nursing assessment, *Crit Care Q* 9(2):6-23, 1986.

Monett Z, Moynihan P: Cardiovascular assessment of neonatal heart, *J Perinat Neonat Nurs* 5(2):50-59, 1991.

O'Brien P, Boisvert JT: Discharge planning for children with heart disease, *Crit Care Nurs Clin North Am* 1(2):297-305, 1989.

Polacek TL and others: Effect of positioning on arterial oxygenation in children with atelectasis following heart surgery, *Heart Lung* 21(5):457-462, 1992.

Rotondi P: Intensive care unit management of the postoperative cardiac surgery patient, *Crit Care Q* 9(2):49-63, 1986.

Uzark K: Counseling adolescents with congenital heart disease, *J Cardiovasc Nurs* 6(3):65-73, 1992.

Uzark K, Messiter E, Rosenthal A: Promoting dental health care in children with congenital heart disease, *Pediatr Nurs* 12(2):96-99, 1986.

Bacterial Endocarditis

Hansen D and others: Bacterial endocarditis in children: trends in its diagnosis, course, and prognosis, *Pediatr Cardiol* 13(4):198-203, 1992.

Kaplan EL: Bacterial endocarditis prophylaxis, *Pediatr Ann* 21(4):249-255, 1992.

Saiman L, Prince A, Gersony W: Pediatric infective endocarditis in the modern era, *J Pediatr* 122(6):847-853, 1993.

Scrima DA: Infective endocarditis: nursing considerations, *Crit Care Nurse* 7:47-56, 1987.

Snelson C, Cline BA, Luby C: Infective endocarditis: a challenging diagnosis, *Dimens Crit Care Nurs* 12(1):4-16, 1993.

Rheumatic Fever

Bisno AL: Group A streptococcal infections and acute rheumatic fever, *N Engl J Med* 325(11):783-793, 1991.

Forster J, editor: Rheumatic fever: keeping up with the Jones criteria, *Contemp Pediatr* 10:51-60, 1993.

Freund B and others: Acute rheumatic fever revisited, *J Pediatr Nurs* 8:167-176, 1993.

Griffiths SP: Rheumatic fever. In Hoekelman RA and others, editors: *Primary pediatric care,* ed 2, St Louis, 1992, Mosby.

Griffiths SP, Gersony WM: Acute rheumatic fever in New York City (1969 to 1988): a comparative study of two decades, *J Pediatr* 116(6):882-887, 1990.

Grimes DE, Woolbert LF: Facts and fallacies about streptococcal infection and rheumatic fever, *J Pediatr Health Care* 4(4):186-192, 1990.

Kaplan EL: Pharmacokinetics on benzathine penicillin G: serum levels during the 28 days after intramuscular injection of 1,200,000 units, *J Pediatr* 115(1):146-150, 1989.

Swedo S and others: Sydenham's chorea: physical and psychological symptoms of St. Vitus dance, *Pediatrics* 91:706-713, 1993.

Kawasaki Disease

Akagi T and others: Outcome of coronary artery aneurysms after Kawasaki disease, *J Pediatr* 121(5):689-694, 1992.

American Academy of Pediatrics, Committee on Infectious Diseases: Intravenous γ-globulin use in children with Kawasaki disease, *Pediatrics* 82(1):122, 1988.

Burns JC: Kawasaki disease, *Curr Opin Pediatr* 1:13-15, 1989.

Fatica NS and others: Rug shampoo and Kawasaki disease, *Pediatrics* 84(2):231-234, 1989.

Fujita Y and others: Kawasaki disease in families, *Pediatrics* 84(4):666-669, 1989.

Gersony WM: Long-term issues in Kawasaki disease, *J Pediatr* 121(5):731-733, 1992.

Glode MP and others: Effect of intravenous immune globulin on the coagulopathy of Kawasaki syndrome, *J Pediatr* 115(3):469-473, 1989.

Koike K, Freedom RM: Kawasaki disease, with a focus on cardiovascular manifestations, *Curr Opin Pediatr* 1(1):135-141, 1989.

Nash DJ: Kawasaki disease: application of the Roy adaptation model to determine interventions, *J Pediatr Nurs* 2(5):308-315, 1987.

Rowley AH, Shulman ST: Current therapy for acute Kawasaki syndrome, *J Pediatrics* 118(96):987-991, 1991.

Shreve B: Kawasaki disease: early treatment/positive results, *Pediatr Nurs* 19(6):607-610, 1993.

Sundel R, Newburger JW: Kawasaki disease. In Cooke JR, Frohlich ED: *Current management of hypertensive and vascular diseases,* St Louis, 1992, Mosby.

Suzuki A and others: Aortocoronary bypass surgery for coronary arterial lesions resulting from Kawasaki disease, *J Pediatr* 116(4):567-573, 1990.

Systemic Hypertension

Carmon M and others: Cardiovascular screening programs: implications for school nurses, *Pediatr Nurs* 16(5):509-511, 1990.

Daniels SR: Primary hypertension in childhood and adolescence, *Pediatr Ann* 21(4):224-234, 1992.

De Swiet M, Dillon MJ: Hypertension in children, *Br Med J* 299(6697):469–470, 1989.

Falkner B: Essential hypertension in children, *Curr Opin Pediatr* 1(1):131-134, 1989.

Gillman MW and others: Identifying children at high risk for the development of essential hypertension, *J Pediatr* 122:837-846, 1993.

Jung FF, Ingelfinger JR: Hypertension in childhood and adolescence, *Pediatr Rev* 14(5):169-179, 1993.

Rocchini A, editor: Childhood hypertension, *Pediatr Clin North Am* 40(1):entire issue, 1993.

Rocchini AP and others: Blood pressure in obese adolescents: effect of weight loss, *Pediatrics* 82(1):16-23, 1988.

Sinaiko AR, Gomez-Marin O, Prineas RJ: Prevalence of "significant" hypertension in junior high school-aged children: the children and adolescent blood pressure program, *J Pediatr* 114(4, pt 1):664-669, 1989.

Hyperlipidemia (Hypercholesterolemia)

American Academy of Pediatrics, Committee on Nutrition: Statement on cholesterol, *Pediatrics* 90(3):469-673, 1992.

Cardiovascular risk factors from birth to 7 years of age: the Bogalusa heart study, *Pediatrics* 80(5):entire issue, 1987.

Cortner JA, Coates PM, Gallagher PR: Prevalence and expression of familial combined hyperlipidemia in childhood, *J Pediatr* 16(4):514-519, 1990.

Davidson DM, Smith RM, Qaqundah PY: Cholesterol screening in children during office visits. *J Pediatr Health Care* 4(1):11-17, 1990.

Davidson DM and others: School-based blood cholesterol screening, *J Pediatr Health Care* 3(1):3-8, 1989.

Dennison BA and others: Parental history of cardiovascular disease as an indication for screening for lipoprotein abnormalities in children, *J Pediatr* 115(2):186-194, 1989.

Einhorn PT, Rifkind BM: Cholesterol measurement in children, *Am J Dis Child* 147(4):373-377, 1993.

Freedman DS and others: Tracking of serum cholesterol levels in a multiracial sample of preschool children, *Pediatrics* 90:80-86, 1992.

Gidding SS: Rationale for lowering serum cholesterol levels in American children, *Am J Dis Child* 147(4):386-392, 1993.

Gillman MW: Screening for familial hypercholesterolemia in childhood, *Am J Dis Child* 147(4):393-396, 1993.

Granot E, Deckelbaum RJ: Hypocholesterolemia in childhood, *J Pediatr* 115(2):171-185, 1989.

Hayman LL and others: Reducing risk for heart disease in children, *MCN* 13:442-448, 1988.

Hayman LL and others: Which child is at risk for heart disease? *MCN* 13:328-333, 1988.

Jacobson MS, Lillienfeld DE: The pediatrician's role in atherosclerosis prevention, *J Pediatr* 112(5):836-841, 1988.

Lannon CM, Earp J: Parent's behavior and attitudes toward screening children for high serum cholesterol levels, *Pediatrics* 89:1159-1163, 1992.

Lauer RM, Lee J, Clarke WR: Factors affecting the relationship between childhood and adult cholesterol levels: the Muscatine study, *Pediatrics* 82(3):309-318, 1988.

Lifshitz F, Moses N: A complication of dietary treatment of hypercholesterolemia, *Am J Dis Child* 143:537-542, 1989.

Mietus-Snyder M and others: Effects of nutritional counseling on lipoprotein levels in a pediatric lipid clinic, *Am J Dis Child* 147(4):378-381, 1993.

Mistretta EF, Stroudy S: Hypercholesterolemia in children: risk and management, Pediat Nurs 16(2):152–154, 1990.

Neufeld EJ, Newburger JW: How should children with hypercholesterolemia be managed? *Choices Cardiol* 7:233-236, 1993.

Nolan R: Child hypercholesterolemia: implications for nurse practitioners, *Pediatr Nurs* 20(11):46-50, 1994.

Polansky SM, Bellet PS, Sprecher DL: Primary hyperlipidemia in a pediatric population: classification and effect of dietary treatment, *Pediatrics* 91:92-96, 1993.

Sanchez-Bayle M and others: Diet therapy for hypercholesterolemia in children and adolescents: a follow-up. *Arch Pediatr Adolesc Med* 148(1):28-32, 1994.

Schifman V, Hannaman KN: Cholesterol: a practical teaching plan for children and adolescents, *Issues Compr Pediatr Nurs* 12(5): 359-369, 1989.

Cardiomyopathy

Colan SD and others: Cardiomyopathies. In Fyler DC, editor: *Nadas' pediatric cardiology,* Philadelphia, 1992, Hanley & Belfus.

Friedman RA, Moadk JP, Garson A. Clinical course of idiopathic dilated cardiomyopathy in children, *J Am Coll Cardiol* 18:152-156, 1991.

Maron BJ: Cardiomyopathies. In Adams FH, Emmanouilides GC, Riemenschneider TA, editors: *Moss' heart disease in infants, children, and adolescents,* ed 4, Baltimore, 1989, Williams & Wilkins.

Purcell JA: Cardiomyopathy, *Am J Nurs* 89(1): 57-75, 1989.

Richardson PJ, Why HJ: Myocarditis and dilated cardiomyopathy: a pathogenetic link? *Heart Failure* 8:27-31, 1992.

Cardiac Dysrhythmias

Alpern D, Uzark K, Dick M: Psychosocial responses of children to cardiac pacemakers, *J Pediatr* 114(3):494-501, 1989.

Cox DM: Complete heart block in the pediatric patient, *J Emerg Nurs* 18(6):497-500, 1992.

Farrington E: Adenosine, *Pediatr Nurs* 17(6): 590, 1991.

Gillette PC and others: Dysrhythmias. In Adams FH, Emmanouilides GC, Riemenschneider TA, editors: *Moss' heart disease in infants, children, and adolescents,* ed 4, Baltimore, 1989, Williams & Wilkins.

Hanisch DG and others: Complex dysrhythmias in infants and children, *AACN Clin Issues Crit Care Nurs* 3(1):255-269, 1992.

Higgins SS, Hardy CE, Higashino SM: Should parents of children with congenital heart disease and life-threatening dysrhythmias be taught cardiopulmonary resuscitation? *Pediatrics* 84(6):1102-1104, 1989 (letter).

Klitzner TS: Arrhythmias in the general pediatric population: an overview, *Pediatr Ann* 20(7):347-349, 1991.

Lerman B, Belardinelli L: Cardiac electrophysiology of adenosine, *Circulation* 83(5): 1499-1506, 1991.

Moulton L and others: Radiofrequency catheter ablation for supraventricular tachycardia, *Heart Lung* 22:3-14, 1993.

Ralston MA and others: Use of adenosine for diagnosis and treatment of tachyarrhythmias in pediatric patients, *J Pediatr* 124(1):139-143, 1994.

Suddaby E, Riker S: Defibrillation and cardioversion in children, *Pediatr Nurs* 17(5):477-481, 1991.

Till J and others: Efficacy and safety of adenosine in treatment of SVT in infants and children, *Br Heart J* 62:204-211, 1989.

Van Hare GF and others: Percutaneous radiofrequency catheter ablation for supraventricular arrhythmias in children, *J Am Coll Cardiol* 17:1613-1620, 1991.

Walsh EP, Saul JP: Transcatheter ablation for pediatric tachyarrhythmias using radiofrequency electrical energy, *Pediatr Ann* 20(7): 386-392, 1991.

Zeigler V: Adenosine in the pediatric population: nursing implications, *Pediatr Nurs* 17(6):600-602, 1991.

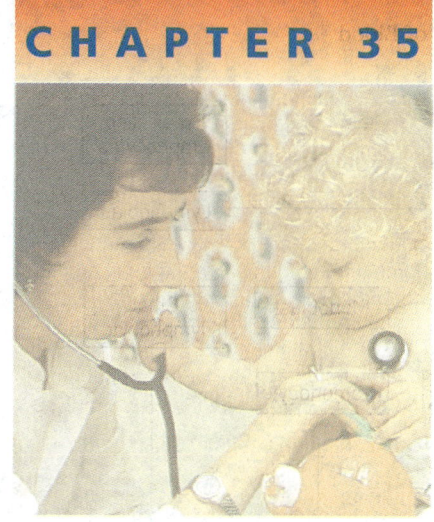

CHAPTER 35

The Child with Hematologic or Immunologic Dysfunction

CHAPTER OUTLINE

RELATED TOPICS

Administration of medication, Ch. 27
Bone marrow aspiration/biopsy, Ch. 27
Bone marrow transplantation, Ch. 36
Collection of specimens, Ch. 27
Compliance, Ch. 27
Family-centered care of the child with chronic illness or disability, Ch. 22
Family-centered care of the child during illness and hospitalization, Ch. 26
Family-centered care of the child with life-threatening illness, Ch. 23
Hemolytic disease of the newborn, Ch. 9
Human immunodeficiency virus encephalopathy, Ch. 37
Human immunodeficiency virus infection and acquired immunodeficiency syndrome, Ch. 20
Immunizations, Ch. 12
Infection control, Ch. 27
Leukemias, Ch. 36
Lymphomas, Ch. 36
Pain assessment; pain management, Ch. 26
Physical examination: skin, Ch. 7
Preparation for procedures, Ch. 27

THE HEMATOLOGIC SYSTEM AND ITS FUNCTION

ORIGIN OF FORMED ELEMENTS

Blood has two major components: a fluid portion called plasma and a cellular portion known as the formed elements of the blood. The two components are approximately equal in volume. ***Plasma*** is about 90% water and 10% solutes. The principal solutes are albumin, electrolytes, and proteins. Among the proteins are clotting factors, globulins, circulating antibodies, and fibrinogen. The ***cellular elements*** are red blood cells (RBCs, erythrocytes), white blood cells (WBCs, leukocytes), and platelets (thrombocytes).

The major ***hemopoietic organs*** (blood-forming organs) of the body are the ***red bone marrow (myeloid tissue)*** and the ***lymphatic system,*** which consists of lymph (fluid), lymphatic vessels, and lymphoid structures—the lymph nodes, spleen, thymus, and tonsils. Although the lymphatic system plays an important role in regulating blood cells, the lymph vessels

■ Christina Algiere Kasprisin, RN, MS, revised this chapter.

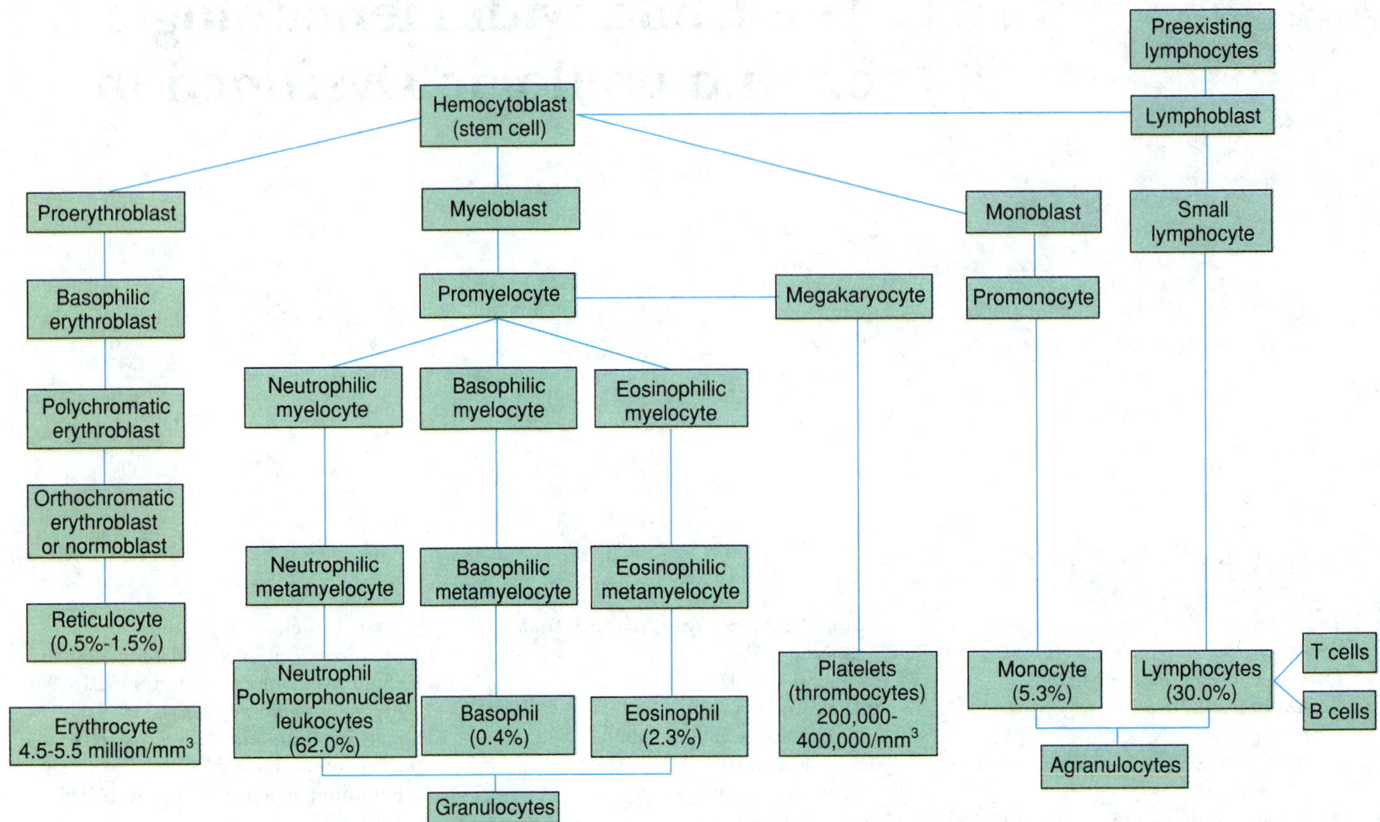

FIG. 35-1 Formation of blood cells. Erythrocyte values are averages for older children. (For blood values at each age, see Appendix D.)

and fluids do not produce cells. The ***lymph nodes*** regulate the manufacture of WBCs. The ***spleen*** and ***liver*** are prime organs for hematopoiesis in the young fetus and cell removal in postnatal life. ***Macrophages*** (formerly called reticular cells) are cells of mesodermal origin that are widely dispersed in the lining of the vascular and lymph channels. Macrophages form a network and are capable of phagocytosis (ingestion and digestion of foreign substances), formation of immune bodies, and differentiation into other cells, such as hemocytoblasts, myeloblasts, or lymphoblasts.

All of the formed elements of the blood, except to some extent the agranulocytes, are believed to be formed in myeloid tissue during postnatal life. During embryonic development the mesenchyme, spleen, liver, thymus, and yolk sac serve as additional sites of blood cell formation. In certain blood disorders these sites, particularly the spleen, can be stimulated to produce blood cells, and constitute ***extramedullary hemopoiesis.*** In infants and young children all of the bone contains red marrow (so called because of its color from the formation of erythrocytes), but as bone growth ceases near the end of adolescence, only the ribs, sternum, vertebrae, and pelvis continue to produce blood cells. The remainder of the bone marrow becomes yellow from deposition of fat. However, in conditions of increased demand for blood cells, the yellow marrow can revert to red marrow as another hemopoietic source.

Although the progressive development of each blood cell is fairly well delineated, there is considerable controversy regarding the origin of the blood cell. One of the most widely held theories (monophyletic) is that each blood cell originates from a primordial (primitive) cell called a ***blast,*** or ***stem, cell.*** This ***hemocytoblast*** in turn gives rise to the erythroblast, myeloblast, monoblast, lymphoblast, and megakaryoblast (Fig. 35-1).

Red Blood Cells (RBCs, Erythrocytes)

The erythrocyte is formed from the hemocytoblast in the red bone marrow. As illustrated in Fig. 35-1, the hemocytoblast forms the proerythroblast. The initial cell of this series has a deep blue (basophilic)–staining cytoplasm and therefore is called a ***basophilic erythroblast.*** The chief change in the erythroblast is accumulation of hemoglobin in the cytoplasm. As the basophilic material decreases and the amount of hemoglobin increases, the cell is called a ***polychromatic erythroblast,*** which describes its mixture of staining properties. At the same time as the nucleus is decreasing in size, the basophilic material disappears, so that the cell is uniformly stained by eosin dye, hence the name ***orthochromatic erythroblast,*** or ***normoblast.*** Finally, the normoblast completely loses its nucleus by a process of extrusion as it squeezes through the pores of the membrane into the capillary. As a result of losing its nucleus, the cell caves in on both sides, giving the mature erythrocyte its characteristic appearance as a biconcave disk. During each of these stages the different cells continue to undergo mitosis so that increasingly greater numbers of cells are produced. Since the mature RBC does not have a nucleus, it is unable to multiply.

The ***reticulocyte*** is the last stage of development before the mature erythrocyte. Reticulocytes are slightly larger than erythrocytes and indicate active RBC production ***(erythropoiesis)***. Ordinarily the total proportion of circulating reticulocytes is between 0.5% and 1.5%. The ***reticulocyte,*** or ***retic, count*** is a simple laboratory test frequently used to indirectly analyze hemopoiesis.

Regulation of Erythrocyte Production. The usual life span of the mature erythrocyte is 120 days. Apparently, as RBCs grow old, their membranes become fragile and eventually rupture. The contents of the cell fragment as they circulate through the blood vessels and are phagocytized by the macrophages in the spleen, liver, and bone marrow. The hemoglobin is broken down into the iron-containing pigment hemosiderin and the bile pigments biliverdin and bilirubin. Most of the iron is reused by the bone marrow for production of new RBCs or stored in the liver and other tissues for future use. The bile pigments are excreted by the liver in bile.

Normally there is a homeostatic balance between the regulation of RBC production and destruction. This balance ensures adequate tissue oxygenation and a blood viscosity that allows the blood to flow freely through the vessels. The basic regulator of erythrocyte production is believed to be tissue oxygenation and renal production of ***erythropoietin*** (also called ***erythropoietic stimulating factor***). In states of tissue hypoxia, erythropoietin is released by the kidneys into the bloodstream. As a result, the bone marrow is stimulated to produce new RBCs. The major activity seems to be an increase in both the maturation rate and mitosis of all stages of erythrocyte production, but primarily at the stem cell level.

During this rapid increase of RBC production, the circulating erythrocytes may not be totally mature. Consequently, the number of reticulocytes may increase dramatically (as high as 30% or more of the total RBC count). Even normoblasts may appear in the blood. If this rise in erythrocyte and reticulocyte count does not occur, it may indicate bone marrow failure.

Once tissue oxygenation is adequate, the production of erythropoietin ceases. Thus tissue oxygen requirements control both the stimulation and termination of erythrocyte production. It is important to note that it is the ability of RBCs to transport oxygen to the tissues in response to their needs, not the circulating numbers of erythrocytes, that is the basic regulatory mechanism. Oxygen transport depends on both the number of circulating RBCs and the amount of normal hemoglobin in the cell. This explains why ***polycythemia*** (increase in the number of erythrocytes) occurs in conditions of prolonged tissue hypoxia, such as cyanotic heart defects (see Chapter 34). If the circulating numbers of erythrocytes controlled erythropoietin release, this feedback mechanism would control erythrocyte production at a constant level (4.5 to 5.5 million/mm^3 of blood) regardless of existing tissue hypoxia.

Colony-stimulating factors (CSFs) are a naturally occurring group of glycoproteins. They were first discovered and characterized from their effect on growth and differentiation of marrow cells. Recombinant DNA technology has enabled the production of large quantities of highly purified CSFs that are nearly identical to the naturally occurring substances. Three CSFs—***granulocyte CSF (G-CSF), granulocyte-macrophage CSF (GM-CSF),*** and ***erythropoietin***—are available commercially.

The use of G-CSF and GM-CSF has been beneficial as adjunct therapy in hematologic and oncologic disorders. Patients receiving the growth factors use less antibiotics and have shorter hospitalizations than patients who are not given the drugs (Furman and Crist, 1992).

Erythropoietin is currently being used for several clinical indications. The most dramatic results have been achieved with children who are anemic secondary to chronic renal failure. Erythropoietin is able to induce an increase in hematocrit sufficient to eliminate the need for RBC transfusions. Current research is investigating the use of erythropoietin in the anemia of prematurity, in hemoglobinopathies, and with G-CSF.

Functions of Erythrocytes. The major function of RBCs is to transport hemoglobin, which in turn carries oxygen to all cells of the body. However, erythrocytes have other significant functions: (1) they contain quantities of carbonic anhydrase, an enzyme that catalyzes the reaction between carbon dioxide (CO_2) and water, allowing large quantities of CO_2 to react with blood for transportation to the lungs, and (2) the hemoglobin, a protein, serves as an acid-base buffer, which, in combination with CO_2, maintains the blood pH at a constant level.

Hemoglobin (Hgb)

Hgb is a complex molecule composed of four globin chains. The type of Hgb in the cells depends on both the stage of life and any abnormalities in the genes that regulate the production of hemoglobin. ***Fetal Hgb,*** composed of two alpha and two gamma chains, has a greater affinity for oxygen and is best suited to the fetal environment. During the latter part of pregnancy, the fetus begins developing ***adult Hgb*** (two alpha and two beta chains). When a defect in Hgb synthesis is present (e.g., sickle cell disease or thalassemia), fetal Hgb may be produced into adulthood. Research is currently underway to develop cell-free hemoglobin that can be used for oxygen and CO_2 transport.

White Blood Cells (WBCs, leukocytes)

The leukocytes refer to a number of cells with similar yet distinct functions. They are divided into two major classifications—granulocytes and agranulocytes—based on the presence or absence, respectively, of granules within the cytoplasm of the cells.

Granulocytes. There are three types of granulocytes: ***neutrophils, basophils,*** and ***eosinophils.*** The name of each of these refers to the characteristic staining property of the granule during laboratory analysis. Neutrophils stain neutral to the dyes, whereas basophils stain a purple color to the basic methylene blue dye, and eosinophils take on a red color to the acidic eosin dye. Because the nuclei of neutrophils have two or more lobules that are connected by fine chromatin strands, the terms ***polymorphonuclear*** (meaning "many-formed nuclei") ***leukocytes,*** or simply ***polys*** or ***segs*** (segmented or mature neutrophils), and ***bands*** (immature neutrophils with the nuclei connected), may be used collectively to refer to the neutrophils.

The granulocytes, like erythrocytes, are produced in the bone marrow. For this reason these cells are sometimes referred to as ***myelogenous leukocytes.*** It is believed that these cells originate from primitive stem cells, which develop into myeloblasts. As Fig. 35-1 illustrates, the genesis of neutrophils, basophils, and eosinophils is similar to the stages observed during erythrocyte production. The differentiation of myeloblasts into various mature WBCs is primarily the result of specialization within the cytoplasm and degeneration of the nucleus. Unlike the erythrocyte, however, all of the WBCs are nucleated.

Increased numbers of bands in the peripheral circulation (referred to as a ***shift to the left*** on the complete blood count) indicate an accelerated production of granulocytes to meet the body's needs, such as in bacterial infection. The ***absolute neutrophil count (ANC)*** reflects the body's ability to handle bacterial infections. If the ANC is less than 1000, there is a serious risk of infection; if it is less than 500, a severe risk of infection is present.

Agranulocytes. The agranulocytes comprise two cell types, the ***monocytes*** and ***lymphocytes.*** Characteristically, these cells do not develop granules, and the nuclei are not lobulated. They are believed to have their origin in various lymphogenous organs and for this reason are sometimes referred to as ***lymphogenous leukocytes.*** However, since stem cells and reticular cells are capable of differentiating into monocytes or lymphocytes, the origin of these cells is frequently designated as the ***lymphomyeloid complex,*** which includes the bone marrow, lymph nodes, spleen, liver, thymus, subepithelial lymphoid tissue (tonsils, vermiform appendix, and intestinal lymphoid tissues), and connective tissues (mesenchymal cells of the reticuloendothelial system).

The monocytes follow the same sequence of development from the stem cell as the granulocytes (see Fig. 35-1). The monocytes in turn have the ability to exit the vessels and develop into ***macrophages,*** large cells that are highly effective phagocytes. ***Kupfer cells*** are macrophages located in the liver. ***Histiocytes*** are macrophages in the connective tissue. These names are remnants of the old reticular endothelial system.

Lymphocytopoiesis (lymphocyte formation) is believed to take place anywhere in the lymphomyeloid complex. Lymphocytes develop from blast (stem) cells (see Fig. 35-1). The lymphocyte has the potential to develop into other cells. For example, lymphocytes may become T-cells or B-cells (see p. 1600).

Regulation of Leukocyte Production. The exact life span of the leukocytes is not as clearly defined as that of the erythrocytes, because their existence in the circulation is primarily for transportation to extravascular areas, where they reside in reservoirs or where they are needed to resist infection. Therefore their survival rate has been divided into three phases: (1) the ***hemopoietic phase,*** extending from the development of the blast cell to the delivery of the mature leukocyte into the circulation; (2) the ***intravascular phase,*** the period within the circulation; and (3) the ***extravascular phase,*** the time spent in the viscera or tissues.

Granulocytes have a half-life of 6 to 8 hours in the blood and, after entering the tissues, die over 4 to 5 days. Agranulocytes live for an extended period because they remain in inflamed tissue areas longer than the granulocytes. Because monocytes wander back and forth between the blood and tissues and are capable of becoming macrophages, their half-life in the blood is 8 to 10 hours, but their half-life in the tissue is 60 to 90 days.

The regulation of leukocytes is based on the body's need for them. Tissue damage from bacterial or viral agents promotes leukocyte circulation and production. However, ***leukocytosis*** (increase in leukocytes) results from tissue destruction from almost any factor, such as hemorrhage, neoplastic disease, toxicity, operative procedures, chemical and thermal injury, or tissue ischemia.

The leukocytes probably die as a result of their activity at the site of injury and are phagocytized by other newly formed WBCs. Effective control of the inflammatory process with subsequent tissue recovery most likely results in a feedback mechanism to the bone marrow and causes lymphogenous organs to cease increased production of WBCs.

Functions of Leukocytes. Although all of the leukocytes play some role in the immune process, each of the WBCs plays a specific role. Neutrophils and monocytes are effective phagocytes and as a result are primarily involved in inflammatory reactions. ***Neutrophilia*** (increased numbers of neutrophils) is most evident in an acute inflammation, whereas ***monocytosis*** (increased number of monocytes) is more evident in chronic conditions. The reason for this is that as the affected area becomes acidic from tissue necrosis, neutrophils, which prefer a neutral environment, become less efficient, and the monocytes, which become macrophages, become more powerful. These cells also increase during chronic inflammation. The other functions of lymphocytes in terms of the immune process are discussed on p. 1600.

The function of eosinophils is still not completely known. They seem to have parasiticidal properties because they can selectively destroy parasites. They may also function in the immediate type of allergic or anaphylactic hypersensitivity reactions, since ***eosinophilia*** (increased numbers of eosinophils) is well documented in such conditions. Eosinophils also are thought to release a substance called ***profibrinolysin,*** which, when activated to form fibrinolysin, digests ***fibrin,*** thereby helping dissolve a clot.

The function of basophils is also not completely understood, although ***basophilia*** (increased numbers of basophils) occurs during the healing phase of inflammation and during prolonged inflammation. Basophils in the blood exit the vessels and become mast cells in the tissue. They are responsible for histamine release, resulting in increased permeability of the vessels to allow WBCs to exit the vessels at the site of injury.

Platelets

Platelets are actually small fragments of cells. They are smaller than blood cells, do not possess a cellular structure, and consist of a clear substance containing granules. The origin of platelets is the megakaryocyte, which is part of the myelogenous group of WBCs (see Fig. 35-1). Platelets are formed when the megakaryocytic membrane invaginates, fuses within the cell to separate the cytoplasm, and then fragments.

Regulation of Platelet Production. The life span of platelets has been estimated as 8 to 10 days. Apparently, the body regulates platelets to maintain a fairly constant level (between 200,000 and 400,000/mm^3). Platelet production is probably regulated by a hormone, thrombopoietin, but the source and mode of action of this substance are unknown. Old platelets are most likely removed by the liver and spleen.

Function of Platelets. The term ***thrombocyte*** means "clot" (thrombo) and "cell" (cyte) and accurately describes the main function of platelets. When there is a break in the continuity of a blood vessel, the platelets, which are normally round or oval disks, come in contact with the wet vessel surface and dramatically change their shape to become swollen spheres with long, irregular projections called ***pseudopodia*** (false feet). As a result, the platelets begin to adhere to the wet endothelium and to each other. The initial platelets at the site of injury release substances that attract other thrombocytes to the area. This causes a layering of platelets, which eventually forms a ***plug.*** This plug is large enough to partially or totally occlude the opening in the vessel wall but small enough to allow blood flow to continue unimpaired through the vessel.

In small vessel tears, the platelet plug is sufficient to produce hemostasis, and additional blood coagulation is not necessary. However, when platelet counts are low, these numerous small ruptures, which occur continually in the body as a result of general functioning, are not repaired. Consequently, small hemorrhagic areas called ***petechiae*** form under the skin. Their appearance is similar to reddish freckles or tiny spiderwebs.

Platelets also influence hemostasis by releasing a substance called ***serotonin*** at the site of injury. This substance is a vasoconstrictor that produces vascular spasm to decrease the amount of blood flow to the injured area.

ASSESSMENT OF HEMATOLOGIC FUNCTION

Several tests can be performed to assess hematologic function, including additional procedures to identify the cause of the dysfunction. The following discussion is limited to a description of the most common and one of the most valuable tests, the ***complete blood count (CBC).*** Other procedures, such as those related to iron, coagulation, and immune status, are discussed throughout the chapter as appropriate.

The CBC consists of the following determinations: RBC count, WBC count, hematocrit (Hct), hemoglobin (Hb or Hgb), differential WBC, RBC indices (mean corpuscular volume [MCV], mean corpuscular hemoglobin [MCH], mean corpuscular hemoglobin concentration [MCHC]), and peripheral smear. Additional tests may be included, such as the reticulocyte count, RBC volume distribution width (RDW), and platelet count. Each of these is summarized in Table 35-1. Most of the determinations can be performed on a small quantity of blood (micromethod) and are automatically computed. The nurse should be familiar with the significance of the findings from the CBC and aware of normal values for age, which are listed in Appendix D.

The history and physical examination are essential to identification of hematologic dysfunction, and the nurse is often the first person to suspect a problem based on information from these sources. Comments by the parent regarding the child's lack of energy, food diary of poor sources of iron, frequent infections, and bleeding that is difficult to control offer clues to the more common disorders affecting the blood. A careful physical appraisal, especially of the skin, can reveal findings such as pallor, petechiae, or bruising that may indicate minor or serious hematologic conditions. Nurses need to be aware of the clinical manifestations of blood diseases in order to assist in recognizing symptoms and establishing a diagnosis.

RED BLOOD CELL DISORDERS

ANEMIA

Anemia is defined as reduction of RBC volume or hemoglobin (Hgb) concentration to levels below normal. It is not a disease itself but a manifestation of an underlying pathologic process. The anemias are the most common hematologic disorders of infancy and childhood.

Classification

Anemias can be classified using two basic approaches: (1) ***etiology*** or ***pathophysiology,*** the causes of erythrocyte and hemoglobin depletion, or (2) ***morphology,*** the characteristic changes in RBC size, shape, and color as described below:

Size—Cell size; for example, ***normocytes*** (normal), ***microcytes*** (smaller than normal), or ***macrocytes*** (larger than normal)

Shape—Irregularly shaped RBCs; for example, ***poikilocytes*** (irregularly shaped cells), ***spherocytes*** (globular cells), and ***drepanocytes*** (sickle cells)

Staining characteristics or color—Reflects the hemoglobin concentration; for example, ***normochromic*** (sufficient or normal amount) or ***hypochromic*** (reduced amount)

The morphologic classification provides an orderly method for ruling out certain diagnoses when establishing a cause for a particular anemia. However, the etiologic approach provides direction for planning nursing care. For example, anemia with reduced hemoglobin concentration may be caused by a dietary depletion of iron, and the principal intervention is replenishing iron stores.

The basic causes of anemia are (1) excessive blood loss, (2) increased destruction of RBCs, or (3) impaired or decreased rate of production. Each of these causes affects the amount of hemoglobin that is available to carry oxygen to

TABLE 35-1 Tests Performed as Part of the Complete Blood Count

TEST (AVERAGE VALUE)*	DESCRIPTION	COMMENTS
Red blood cell (RBC) count (4.5-5.5 million/mm)^3	Number of RBCs/mm^3 of blood	Indirectly estimates Hgb content of blood Reflects function of bone marrow
Hemoglobin (Hgb) determination (11.5-15.5 g/dl)	Amount of Hgb/dl of whole blood	Total blood Hgb primarily depends on number of circulating RBCs, but also on amount of Hgb in each cell
Hematocrit (Hct) (35%-45%)	Percentage or volume of packed RBCs to whole blood	Indirectly measures Hgb content Is approximately three times Hgb content
RBC indices		
Mean corpuscular volume (MCV) (77-95 μm^3)	Average of mean volume (size) of a single RBC $MCV = \frac{Hct\ (\%) \times 10}{RBC\ count\ (millions/mm^3)}$	MCV and MCH depend on accurate counts of RBCs, whereas MCHC does not; therefore MCHC is often more reliable All indices depend on *average* cell measurements and do not show individual RBC (anisocytosis) variations MCV values expressed as cubic microns (μm^3) or femtoliters (fl)
Mean corpuscular hemoglobin (MCH) (25-33 pg/cell)	Average or mean quantity (weight) of Hgb of a single RBC $MCH = \frac{Hgb\ (g)/dl \times 10}{RBC\ count\ (millions/mm^3)}$	MCH values expressed as picograms (pg) or micromicrograms (μμg)
Mean corpuscular hemoglobin concentration (MCHC) (31%-37% Hgb [g]/dl RBC)	Average concentration of Hgb in a single RBC $MCHC = \frac{Hgb\ (g)/dl \times 100}{Hct\ (\%)}$	MCHC values expressed as % Hgb (g)/cell or Hgb (g)/dl RBC
RBC volume distribution width 13.4% ± 1.2%		Average size of RBCs
Reticulocyte count (0.5%-1.5% erythrocytes)	% Reticulocytes to RBCs	Index of production of mature RBCs by red bone marrow Decreased count indicates depressed bone marrow function Increased count indicates erythrogenesis in response to some stimulus When reticulocyte count is extremely high, other forms of immature RBCs (normoblasts, even erythroblasts) may be present Indirectly estimates hypochromic anemia
White blood cell (WBC) count (4.5-13.5 × 10^3 cells/mm^3)	Number of WBCs/mm^3 of blood	Total number of WBCs is less important than differential count
Differential WBC count	Inspection and quantification of WBC types present in peripheral blood	Values are expressed as percentages; to obtain absolute number of any type of WBCs, multiply its respective percentage by total number of WBCs
Neutrophils (polys) (54%-62%) (3.0-5.8 × 10^3 cells/mm^3)		Primary defense in bacterial infection; capable of phagocytizing and killing bacteria
Bands (3%-5%) (0.15-0.4 × 10^3 cells/mm^3)		Immature neutrophil Increased numbers in bacterial infection Also capable of phagocytosis and killing
Eosinophils (1%-3%) (0.05-0.25 × 10^3 cells/mm^3)		Named for their staining characteristics with eosin dye Increased in allergic disorders, parasitic diseases, certain neoplasms, and other diseases
Basophils (0.075%) (0.015-0.030 cells/mm^3)		Named for their characteristic basophilic stippling Contain histamine, but their function is unknown
Lymphocytes (25%-33%; 1.5-3.0 × 10^3 cells/mm^3)		Involved in development of antibody and delayed hypersensitivity

*See Appendix D for normal values according to ages.

TABLE 35-1 Tests Performed as Part of the Complete Blood Count—cont'd

TEST (AVERAGE VALUE)*	DESCRIPTION	COMMENTS
Monocytes (3%-7%)		Large phagocytic cells that are involved in early stage of inflammatory reaction
Absolute neutrophil count (ANC) (>1000)	% Neutrophils and bands × WBC count	Indicates body's capability to handle bacterial infections
Platelet count (150-400 × $10^3/mm^3$)		Cellular fragments that are necessary for clotting to occur
Stained peripheral blood smear	Visual estimation of amount of Hgb in RBCs and overall size, shape, and structure of RBCs	Various staining properties of RBC structures may be evidence of immature forms of erythrocyte Shows variation in size and shape of RBCs—microcytic, macrocytic, poikilocytic (variable sizes)

the cells. An ***etiologic classification*** is based on the various conditions that can result from any of these physiologic changes.

Acute or chronic hemorrhage results in loss of plasma and all formed elements of the blood. After acute hemorrhage the body replaces plasma within 1 to 3 days, maintaining blood volume. However, this results in a low concentration of RBCs, which are gradually replaced within 3 to 4 weeks. During this period there is usually a normocytic, normochromic anemia, provided there are sufficient iron stores for hemoglobin synthesis.

In chronic blood loss the actual number of RBCs may be normal because of continual replacement. However, insufficient iron is available to form hemoglobin as quickly as it is lost. As a result, erythrocytes are usually microcytic and hypochromic.

Excessive destruction or ***hemolysis*** of erythrocytes can occur from a defect within the RBC (intracorpuscular) that shortens the life span of the cell, preventing production from keeping pace with destruction. The two examples, sickle cell anemia and thalassemia, have decreased erythrocyte life spans because of a hemoglobin defect.

Extracorpuscular factors are those conditions that cause hemolysis in otherwise normal RBCs. A classic example is blood group incompatibility, such as hemolytic disease of the newborn or incompatibility secondary to mismatched blood transfusion. Other causes can be toxic drugs, burns, poisonings (such as from lead), infections such as malaria, and splenic sequestration (hypersplenism).

Impaired or decreased production can occur as a result of either bone marrow failure or deficiency of essential nutrients. ***Bone marrow failure*** may be caused by (1) replacement of bone marrow by fibrosis or by neoplastic cells, such as in leukemia; (2) depression of marrow activity from irradiation, chemicals, or drugs; or (3) interference with bone marrow activity from other systemic diseases, such as severe infection, chronic renal disease, widespread malignancy (without marrow infiltration), collagen diseases, or hypothyroidism. When depression of the hematologic system is extensive, aplastic anemia develops.

The reason for various systemic disorders affecting erythrocyte production varies according to the condition. For example, in ***severe chronic infection*** there is evidence that depression of erythropoiesis is caused by a defect in the conversion of protoporphyrin into hemoglobin. In addition, there is some degree of hemolysis, although the exact mechanism is not known.

The most common childhood anemia is a result of ***iron deficiency.*** Besides iron as an essential component of hemoglobin synthesis, RBC production depends on amino acids; vitamins B_6, B_{12}, and C; folic acid; copper; and possibly cobalt. Chronic malnutrition causes anemia as a result of generalized protein, mineral, and vitamin deficiencies.

Pernicious anemia develops when the gastric mucosa fails to secrete sufficient amounts of intrinsic factor, which is essential for absorption of vitamin B_{12}. Deprived of vitamin B_{12}, the bone marrow produces fewer but larger (macrocytic) RBCs. The erythrocytes are usually immature and, because of their extremely fragile cell membranes, are rapidly destroyed during circulation.

Pathophysiology and Clinical Manifestations

The basic physiologic defect caused by anemia is a decrease in the oxygen-carrying capacity of blood and consequently a reduction in the amount of oxygen available to the cells. When the anemia has developed slowly, the child usually adapts to the declining hemoglobin level, and most children seem to have a remarkable ability to function quite well despite low levels of hemoglobin. Also, compensatory mechanisms such as a shift in the oxyhemoglobin dissociation curve may delay the development of any obvious signs (see p. 1345).

When the Hgb falls sufficiently to produce clinical manifestations, the signs and symptoms are due to tissue ***hypoxia.*** Muscle weakness and easy fatigability are common. The skin is usually pale, and it may take on a waxy pallor in severe anemia. Cyanosis is typically not evident, because it is the result of the quantity of deoxygenated Hgb in arterial blood. Hgb levels generally must *exceed* 5 g/dl before cyanosis is evident. Anemia is caused by decreased Hgb and/or RBCs, not inadequate oxygen saturation of existing Hgb.

Central nervous system manifestations include headache, dizziness, light-headedness, irritability, slowed thought processes, decreased attention span, apathy, and depression.

Growth retardation resulting from decreased cellular metabolism and coexisting anorexia is a common finding in chronic severe anemia. It is frequently accompanied by delayed sexual maturation in the older child.

The effects of anemia on the circulatory system can be profound. A reduction in Hgb concentration that results in decreased oxygen-carrying capacity of the blood is associated with a compensatory increase in heart rate and cardiac output. Initially this greater cardiac output compensates for the lower oxygen-carrying capacity of the blood, since blood replenished with oxygen returns to the tissues at a faster than normal rate. As the blood flows faster and more turbulently, a heart murmur may be heard. However, if the body's demand on the pumping action of the heart increases, such as during exercise, infection, or emotional stress, cardiac failure may ensue.

Diagnostic Evaluation

In general, anemia may be suspected from findings on the history and physical examination, such as lack of energy, easy fatigability, and pallor, but unless the anemia is severe, the first clue to the disorder may be alterations in the CBC, such as decreased RBCs, and decreased Hgb and Hct levels. Although anemia is sometimes defined as an Hgb below 10 or 11 g/dl, this arbitrary cutoff is inappropriate for all children, because Hgb levels normally vary with age (see Appendix D).

Various findings on the CBC are also significant, such as increased reticulocytes, which indicate the body's response to an increased demand for RBCs. A peripheral smear may demonstrate significant changes in the shape of RBCs, such as sickled cells. Tests to measure the amount of Hgb in a single cell are helpful in determining the cause of the anemia (see Table 35-1). Sometimes a bone marrow aspiration may be necessary to evaluate the body's ability to produce normal cells. For example, in leukemia the bone marrow is ***hyperplastic*** (producing increased numbers of cells), whereas in aplastic anemia the bone marrow is ***hypoplastic*** (producing decreased numbers of cells) or ***aplastic*** (producing no cells).

Tests for hematologic function do not always reflect the *immediate* changes occurring in the blood. For example, in acute massive hemorrhage the Hgb and Hct may not be reliable, since the plasma volume may not reequilibrate for several hours. Without the hemodilution caused by the reexpansion of the vascular space, the Hgb and Hct may be close to normal and the RBC loss may not be apparent. Consequently, assessing the quantity of blood loss in a seriously ill child may be difficult. The estimated volume of blood loss must be analyzed in conjunction with the total blood volume of the child to determine the percent of blood loss. Blood specimens obtained from central lines may more accurately reflect the patient's status than specimens obtained from an extremity, because of the vasoconstriction of the peripheral vasculature. Decreased blood pressure changes are a late sign because of the compensatory mechanisms.

Therapeutic Management

The objective of medical management is to reverse the anemia by treating the underlying cause. In nutritional anemias the specific deficiency is replaced. In blood loss from acute hemorrhage, RBC transfusion may be given. In severe anemia, supportive medical care may include oxygen therapy, restoration of adequate blood volume, intravenous fluids, and bed rest. In addition to these general measures, more specific interventions may be implemented depending on the cause, and these are discussed in the next sections.

Nursing Considerations

❖ Assessment

The physical examination yields valuable evidence regarding the severity of the anemia and some indication of its possible etiology. In interviewing the family, the nurse stresses the following areas: (1) nutrition, especially dietary intake of iron; (2) past history of chronic, recurrent infection; (3) eating habits, particularly pica and ingestion of lead-based paint or other toxic agents; (4) bowel habits and presence of frank blood in stools or black, tarry stools as a result of chronic blood loss; and (5) familial history of hereditary diseases, such as sickle cell disease or thalassemia.

The nurse should also be aware of the significance of blood tests. For example, if the blood studies show a microcytic, hypochromic anemia suggestive of iron deficiency but the parent reports an iron-rich diet, the nurse needs to pursue the nutritional history for possible discrepancies.

❖ Nursing Diagnoses

A variety of nursing diagnoses may be evident following assessment of anemia. Some of the general aspects of nursing management are included in the Nursing Care Plan on pp. 1575-1576. Others become apparent in specific situations.

❖ Planning

The goals for the infant or child with anemia and the family include the following:

1. Child and family will receive adequate support and education.
2. Child will exhibit minimal physical or emotional exertion.
3. Child will experience no complications from anemia or its treatment.

Prepare Child for Laboratory Tests. Since several blood tests may be ordered, the child may experience multiple finger sticks and/or venipunctures. However, these invasive procedures need not be painful (see Blood Specimens, Chapter 27). The nurse also has the responsibility of preparing the child for the tests by (1) explaining the significance of each test, particularly why the tests are not done at one time; (2) physically being with the child during the procedure whenever possible; and (3) allowing the child to play with the equipment on a doll and/or participate in the actual procedure (e.g., by cleansing the finger with an alcohol swab).

Older children may appreciate the opportunity to observe the blood cells under a microscope or in photographs. This is especially important if a serious blood disorder, such as leukemia, is suspected, since it serves as a foundation for explaining the pathophysiology of the disorder.

➤ **NURSING TIP** Suggested explanations for teaching children about blood components are:

Red blood cells—Carry the oxygen you breathe from your lungs to all parts of your body.

White blood cells—Help keep germs from causing infection.

Platelets—Small parts of cells that help make bleeding stop; platelets help your body stop bleeding by forming a clot (scab) over the hurt area.

Plasma—The liquid portion of blood; has clotting factors that help make bleeding stop.

Bone marrow is not a routine hematologic test but is essential for definitive diagnosis of the leukemias, lymphomas, and certain anemias. Information for preparing the child is in Chapter 27.

Decrease Tissue Oxygen Needs. Since the basic pathology in anemia is a decrease of oxygen-carrying capacity in the RBCs, a nursing responsibility is to minimize tissue oxygen needs when anemia is severe enough to affect the child's energy level. In most instances of anemia this is not necessary, but when it is, several important interventions are implemented. These same interventions apply to any child with a nursing diagnosis of fatigue or activity intolerance.

The child's level of tolerance for activities of daily living and play is assessed, and adjustments are made to allow as much self-care as possible without undue exertion. During periods of rest the nurse takes vital signs and observes behavior to establish a baseline of nonexertion energy expenditure. During periods of activity the nurse repeats these measurements and observations to compare them with resting values.

NURSING ALERT Signs of exertion include tachycardia, palpitations, tachypnea, dyspnea, shortness of breath, hyperpnea, breathlessness, dizziness, light-headedness, diaphoresis, and change in skin color. The child looks fatigued (sagging, limp posture; slow, strained movements; inability to tolerate additional activity).

Once a baseline of physical tolerance has been established, the nurse anticipates those activities that are physically taxing, such as dressing, feeding, or getting out of bed, and allows for conservation of energy by assisting the child as needed. However, since dependency can be threatening, the child is allowed as much control in the environment as possible. For example, a child with severe anemia may be unable to walk to the bathroom but may be able to use a bedside commode or be transported in a wheelchair to the lavatory rather than having to use a bedpan. Scheduling activities throughout the day with planned rest periods in between maximizes the child's energy potential without causing undue exertion. Safety measures are anticipated and implemented, (e.g., staying with the child when out of bed and raising siderails when in the bed to prevent falls).

Diversional activities are planned that promote rest but prevent boredom and withdrawal. Since short attention span, irritability, and restlessness are common in anemia and increase stress demands on the body, appropriate activities are planned, such as listening to music; using a tape recorder; watching television; playing video games; reading or listening to stories or comics; continuing a favorite hobby, such as stamp collecting; coloring or drawing; playing board and card games; or being wheeled in a carriage or chair. Choosing the appropriate roommate, such as a child of similar age with a diagnosis that also requires restricted activity, is another helpful intervention.

If infants or young children are hospitalized, the importance of preventing separation from parents must be considered. Crying and fretfulness place increased stress demands on the body, which increases oxygen needs. Parents may need help in understanding the importance of their presence.

Children with anemia are prone to infection because tissue hypoxia causes cellular dysfunction and the disturbed metabolic processes weaken the host's defenses against foreign agents. Infection also worsens the anemia by increasing metabolic needs and in instances of chronic infection also interferes with erythropoiesis and shortens the survival time of RBCs. All the usual precautions are taken to prevent infection, such as practicing thorough handwashing, appropriate room selection in a noninfectious area, restricting visitors or hospital personnel with active infection, and maintaining adequate nutrition. The nurse also observes for signs of infection, particularly temperature elevation and leukocytosis. However, an elevated WBC count sometimes occurs in anemia without the presence of systemic or local infection.

Observe for Complications. Multiple blood samples may present a problem with cumulative blood loss, necessitating blood replacement. This situation occurs most often in infants with severe anemia. To prevent this, blood may be withdrawn through a continuous intravenous line and replaced after the exact amount needed has been tested and discarded. As a precaution, a record is kept of the volume of blood being withdrawn. Using micromethods of testing whenever possible minimizes the amount of blood required for the test. The nurse needs to observe for cumulative effects of blood loss, particularly signs of shock and increased hypoxia, and to explain to parents the necessity of multiple blood samples and the reason for blood replacement (see Cultural Awareness box and Critical Thinking Exercise box, p. 1572).

The main complication of anemia is cardiac decompensation, which can result from excessive demands on the heart as a result of increased metabolic needs or of cardiac overload during rapid blood transfusion. Signs and symptoms of heart failure are tachycardia, dyspnea, rales, moist respirations, cough, shortness of breath, and sweating. Obviously, preventing heart failure through minimizing hypoxia and transfusing blood slowly is of first priority. Packed RBCs are usually administered to prevent circulatory hypervolemia. When blood transfusions are required in severe anemia to increase the Hgb level, all the usual precautions for administering blood and observing for signs of transfusion reactions are instituted (Table 35-2). Technologic advances in blood banking and transfusion medicine enable the administration of only the blood component needed by the child (Table 35-3).

Although hemolytic reactions are rare, ABO incompatibility remains the most common cause of death from blood transfusion, and human error is usually responsible (admin-

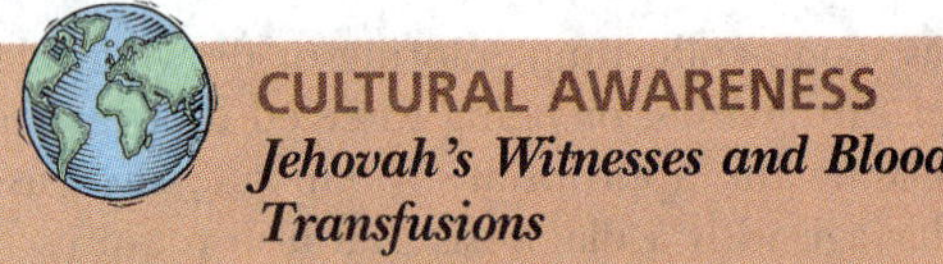

CULTURAL AWARENESS
Jehovah's Witnesses and Blood Transfusions

Jehovah's Witnesses are members of a worldwide religious group that strongly opposes the use of blood products, especially blood transfusions, for themselves and their children. They believe that the Bible forbids eating the blood of any flesh, and they consider blood transfusions to be equivalent to oral ingestion of blood. Among the members there are differing interpretations of the prohibition of blood, from loss of salvation to a forgivable sin.

Transfusions of whole blood, packed RBCs, WBCs, platelets, and plasma (fresh or frozen) are forbidden. Banking of the person's own blood or salvage from suction during surgery is also forbidden, because Witnesses believe that blood that has left the body should be discarded.

The use of albumin, immune globulin, and factor concentrates, as in hemophilia, is an individual decision. Nonblood plasma expanders, such as saline solution, Ringer's lactate, and hetastarch, are acceptable, and Witnesses may give blood for a sample.

The nurse's role is to be an advocate for the family and a consultant to other members of the health team regarding the family's beliefs. The nurse should ensure that the family is aware of all alternatives to transfusions and the consequences of each option (Quintero, 1993). With advances in health care, more products are being developed, such as recombinant factor VIII concentrate, that are considered nonblood products. When the child's life is in danger, a court order may be obtained to give temporary custody to the state, which then removes the parent's right to refuse treatment.

CRITICAL THINKING EXERCISE
Blood Transfusion

Five-year-old Courtney Hale has been admitted to the hospital for tests to rule out aplastic anemia. Your initial assessment of Courtney reveals a very pale girl with extreme fatigue and slightly labored breathing. In obtaining data from Mrs. Hale, you learn that the family members are Jehovah's Witnesses. They are allowed to receive medical care with the exception of blood products.

The laboratory results reveal that Courtney has a hemoglobin of 6.5 g/dl. The practitioner has decided that a blood transfusion is necessary. The father tells you that if Courtney receives blood, she will be "damned" and she will not be with them on Judgment Day. The practitioner refuses to treat the child without transfusions. What should you do?

1. Prepare to obtain a court order to transfuse packed red blood cells.
2. Make arrangements to transfer the patient to another institution.
3. Try to convince the father that his daughter's life is in danger.
4. Respect the family's religious beliefs.

The correct answer is 4. You need to act as an advocate for the family. Attempting to persuade them to change their religious beliefs is probably futile and will only alienate them. A court order to grant temporary custody to the state is usually granted only if the child's life is in danger. In this case the immediate life-threatening nature of the child's condition is doubtful. Both the decision for a court order and a transfer to another agency are complex processes that nurses may participate in, but not decide.

istration of wrong type to patient or mislabeling of blood product) (Linden, Paul, and Dressler, 1992). Blood is usually matched between the donor and recipient for blood groups (A, B, AB, or O) and Rh factors (positive or negative). However, AB-type RBCs can be transfused to individuals with blood types A, B, and AB, and Rh-negative RBCs can be used for Rh-positive individuals. (See Chapter 9 for a discussion of blood groups and ABO and Rh incompatibility.)

When blood is mismatched, the A or B antiagglutinin is mixed with RBCs containing A or B agglutinogens, respectively, and agglutination (clumping) of the RBCs occurs. The agglutinins, which are bivalent, attach themselves to two different erythrocytes at the same time, causing the cells to clump together and clog small blood vessels. Over a few hours to days, the entrapped cells degenerate and hemolyze, liberating excessive quantities of Hgb into the circulation. The eventual hemolysis of large numbers of RBCs decreases the blood volume, causing circulatory failure and ***shock.*** Treatment is aimed at replacing lost blood and using plasma volume expanders.

Acute kidney shutdown and eventual ***renal failure*** are the result of renal vasoconstriction from antigen-antibody complexes derived from the RBC surface. The greatly reduced blood flow causes complete renal failure and death within 7 to 12 days. Treatment involves promoting diuresis with rapid dilute intravenous fluids and diuretics, such as furosemide and mannitol, and alkalinizing body fluids, which render Hgb more soluble.

Another consequence of hemolysis is the release of large quantities of phospholipids, which are capable of stimulating ***disseminated intravascular coagulation (DIC)*** (p. 1598). As a result, the plasma is depleted of the necessary coagulation factors needed to prevent hemorrhage. Without treatment with heparin to prevent the coagulation and blood components to initiate clotting, death from generalized hemorrhage can occur.

Besides the nursing precautions and responsibilities outlined in Table 35-2, some general guidelines that apply to all transfusions include:

- Take vital signs, including blood pressure, *before* administering blood to establish baseline data for intratransfusion and posttransfusion comparison, then every 15 minutes for 1 hour while blood is infusing.
- Check the identification of the recipient with the donor's blood group and type, regardless of the blood product used.
- Administer the first 50 ml of blood or ⅕ volume (whichever is smaller) *slowly* and stay with the child.
- Administer with normal saline on a piggyback setup.
- Administer blood through an appropriate filter to eliminate

TABLE 35-2 Nursing Care of the Child Receiving Blood Transfusions

COMPLICATION	SIGNS/SYMPTOMS	PRECAUTIONS/NURSING RESPONSIBILITIES
IMMEDIATE REACTIONS		
Hemolytic Reactions		
Most severe type, but rare Incompatible blood Incompatibility in multiple transfusions	Chills Shaking Fever Pain at needle site and along venous tract Nausea/vomiting Sensation of tightness in chest Red or black urine Headache Flank pain Progressive signs of shock and/or renal failure	Verify patient identification Identify donor and recipient blood types and groups before transfusion is begun; verify with another nurse or other practitioner Transfuse blood slowly for first 15 to 20 minutes and/or initial ⅕ volume of blood; remain with patient Stop transfusion immediately in event of signs or symptoms, maintain patient intravenous line, and notify practitioner Save donor blood to re-crossmatch with patient's blood Monitor for evidence of shock Insert urinary catheter and monitor hourly outputs Send samples of patient's blood and urine to laboratory for presence of hemoglobin (indicates intravascular hemolysis) Observe for signs of hemorrhage resulting from disseminated intravascular coagulation (DIC) Support medical therapies to reverse shock
Febrile Reactions		
Leukocyte or platelet antibodies Plasma protein antibodies	Fever Chills	May give acetaminophen for prophylaxis Leukocyte-poor RBCs are less likely to cause reaction Stop transfusion immediately; report to practitioner for evaluation
Allergic Reactions		
Recipient reacts to allergens in donor's blood	Urticaria Flushing Asthmatic wheezing Laryngeal edema	Give antihistamines for prophylaxis to children with tendency toward allergic reactions Stop transfusion immediately Administer epinephrine for wheezing or anaphylactic reaction
Circulatory Overload		
Too rapid transfusion (even a small quantity) Excessive quantity of blood transfused (even slowly)	Precordial pain Dyspnea Rales Cyanosis Dry cough Distended neck veins	Transfuse blood slowly Prevent overload by using packed RBCs or administering divided amounts of blood Use infusion pump to regulate and maintain flow rate Stop transfusion immediately if signs of overload Place child upright with feet in dependent position to increase venous resistance
Air Emboli		
May occur when blood is transfused under pressure	Sudden difficulty in breathing Sharp pain in chest Apprehension	Normalize pressure before container is empty when infusing blood under pressure Clear tubing of air by aspirating air with syringe at nearest Y connector if air is observed in tubing; disconnect tubing and allow blood to flow until air has escaped only if a Y connector is not available
Hypothermia	Chills Low temperature Irregular heart rate Possible cardiac arrest	Allow blood to warm at room temperatures (less than 1 hour) Use approved mechanical blood warmer or electric warming coil to rapidly warm blood; never use microwave oven Take temperature if patient complains of chills; if subnormal, stop transfusion

Continued.

TABLE 35-2	**Nursing Care of the Child Receiving Blood Transfusions—cont'd**	
COMPLICATION	**SIGNS/SYMPTOMS**	**PRECAUTIONS/NURSING RESPONSIBILITIES**
Electrolyte Disturbances		
Hyperkalemia (in massive transfusions or in patients with renal problems)	Nausea, diarrhea Muscular weakness Flaccid paralysis Paresthesia of extremities Bradycardia Apprehension Cardiac arrest	Use washed RBCs or fresh blood if patient is at risk
DELAYED REACTIONS		
Transmission of Infection		
Hepatitis Human immunodeficiency virus (HIV) Malaria Syphilis Bacteria or viruses Other	Signs of infection (e.g., jaundice) Toxic reaction: high fever, severe headache or substernal pain, hypotension, intense flushing, vomiting/diarrhea	Blood is tested for antibodies to HIV, hepatitis C virus, and hepatitis B core antigen; in addition, blood is tested for hepatitis B surface antigen (HBsAg) and alanine aminotransferase (ALT), and a serology test is performed for syphilis; positive units are destroyed; individuals at risk for carrying certain viruses are deferred from donation Report any sign of infection and, if occurring during transfusion, stop transfusion immediately, send sample for culture and sensitivity tests, and notify physician
Alloimmunization		
(Antibody formation) Occurs in patients receiving multiple transfusions	Increased risk of hemolytic, febrile, and allergic reactions	Use limited number of donors Observe carefully for signs of reactions
Delayed Hemolytic Reaction	Destruction of RBCs and fever 5 to 10 days after transfusion	Observe for posttransfusion anemia and decreasing benefit from successive transfusions

TABLE 35-3 Description of Blood Components

COMPONENT	APPROXIMATE VOLUME (ml/U)	INDICATIONS	DOSE
Whole blood	500	Symptomatic anemia with large-volume deficit	Volume of whole blood = weight (kg) × change in Hct desired × 2
Packed RBCs	300	Symptomatic anemia	Volume PRBC = weight (kg) × change in Hct desired
RBCs, leukocytes removed	275-300	Symptomatic anemia, febrile reactions from leukocyte antibodies	Same as for RBCs
Fresh frozen plasma	220	Deficit of labile and stable plasma coagulation factors and thrombotic thrombocytopenic purpura (TTP)	Varies
Cryoprecipitate with antihemophilic factor (AHF)	15—containing 80 or more units of factor VIII (FVIII-c) and at least 150 mg of fibrinogen	Hemophilia A von Willebrand disease Hypofibrinogenemia Factor XIII deficiency	Varies
Platelets—random donor	50	Bleeding from thrombocytopenia or platelet function abnormality	0.1 U/kg will raise the count by 40,000/mm^3 at 1 hour
Platelets produced by pheresis	300	Same as random donor	
Granulocytes (pheresis)	220	Neutropenia with infection	
Factor VIII concentrate	Varies	Hemophilia A	1 U/kg body weight for each 0.02 U/ml (2%) increase
Prothrombin complex (factors II, VII, IX, and X)	Varies	Hereditary II, VII, IX, X deficiency Hemophilia B (IX deficiency)	

NURSING CARE PLAN
The Child with Anemia

NURSING DIAGNOSIS: Anxiety/fear related to diagnostic procedures/transfusion

PATIENT/FAMILY GOAL 1: Will become knowledgeable about the disorder, diagnostic tests, and treatment

• **NURSING INTERVENTIONS/*RATIONALES***

Prepare child for tests *to relieve anxiety/fear*

Remain with child during tests and initiation of transfusion *to provide support and observe for possible complications*

Explain purpose of blood components *to increase understanding of disorder, diagnostic tests, and treatment*

• **EXPECTED OUTCOMES**

Child and family display minimal anxiety

Child and family demonstrate an understanding of the disorder, diagnostic tests, and treatment

NURSING DIAGNOSIS: Activity intolerance related to generalized weakness, diminished oxygen delivery to tissues

PATIENT GOAL 1: Will receive adequate rest

• **NURSING INTERVENTIONS/*RATIONALES***

Observe for signs of physical exertion (tachycardia, palpitations, tachypnea, dyspnea, shortness of breath, hyperpnea, breathlessness, dizziness, light-headedness, sweating, and change in skin color) and fatigue (sagging, limp posture, slow, strained movements, inability to tolerate additional activity) *to plan appropriately for rest*

Anticipate and assist in those activities of daily living that may be beyond child's tolerance *to prevent exertion*

Provide diversional play activities *that promote rest and quiet but prevent boredom and withdrawal*

Choose appropriate roommate of similar age and interests who requires restricted activity *to encourage compliance with need for rest*

Plan nursing activities *to provide sufficient rest*

Assist with activities requiring exertion

• **EXPECTED OUTCOMES**

Child plays and rests quietly and engages in activities appropriate to capabilities

Child does not exhibit signs of physical exertion or fatigue

PATIENT GOAL 2: Will exhibit normal respirations

• **NURSING INTERVENTIONS/*RATIONALES***

Maintain high-Fowler position for *optimum air exchange*

Administer supplemental oxygen if needed *to increase oxygen to tissues*

Take vital signs during periods of rest *to establish baseline for comparison during periods of activity*

• **EXPECTED OUTCOME**

Patient breathes easily; respiratory rate and depth are normal (see inside back cover)

PATIENT GOAL 3: Will experience minimal emotional stress

• **NURSING INTERVENTIONS/*RATIONALES***

Anticipate child's irritability, short attention span, and fretfulness by offering to assist child in activities rather than waiting for request for help

Encourage parents to remain with child *to minimize stress of separation*

Provide comfort measures (e.g., pacifier, rocking, music) *to minimize stress*

Encourage child to express feelings *to minimize anxiety/fear*

See also Nursing Care Plan: The Child in the Hospital, Chapter 26

• **EXPECTED OUTCOME**

Child remains calm and quiet

PATIENT GOAL 4: Will receive appropriate blood elements

• **NURSING INTERVENTIONS/*RATIONALES***

*Administer blood, packed cells, platelets as prescribed (see Table 35-2)

*Administer hematopoetic growth factors as prescribed, *to stimulate blood cell formation*

• **EXPECTED OUTCOME**

Child receives appropriate blood elements without incident

NURSING DIAGNOSIS: Altered nutrition: less than body requirements related to reported inadequate iron intake (less than RDA); knowledge deficit regarding iron-rich foods

PATIENT GOAL 1: Will receive adequate supply of iron

• **NURSING INTERVENTIONS/*RATIONALES***

Provide diet counseling to caregiver, especially in regard to:

Food sources of iron (e.g., meat, liver, fish, egg yolks, green leafy vegetables, legumes, nuts, whole grains, iron-fortified infant cereal and dry cereal) (see also Chapter 11) *to ensure that child receives adequate supply of iron*

Feed milk as supplemental food in infant's diet after solids are begun *because overingestion of milk decreases child's intake of iron-rich solid foods*

Teach older child about importance of adequate iron in the diet *to encourage compliance*

• **EXPECTED OUTCOME**

Child receives at least minimum daily requirement of iron

*Dependent nursing action.

Continued.

NURSING CARE PLAN
The Child with Anemia—cont'd

PATIENT GOAL 2: Will consume iron supplements

- **NURSING INTERVENTIONS/*RATIONALES***

*Administer iron preparations as prescribed

Instruct family regarding correct administration of oral iron preparation

Give in divided doses (specify) *for maximum absorption*

Give between meals *to increase absorption in upper gastrointestinal tract*

Administer with fruit juice or multivitamin preparation *because vitamin C appears to facilitate absorption of iron*

Do not give with milk or antacids, *since they decrease absorption*

*Administer liquid preparation with dropper, syringe, or straw *to avoid contact with teeth and possible staining*

Assess characteristics of stools *because adequate dosage of oral iron turns stool a tarry green color*

- **EXPECTED OUTCOMES**

Family relates a diet history that verifies child's compliance with these suggestions

Child is given iron supplement as evidenced by green, tarry stools

Child takes medication appropriately

See also Nursing Care Plan: The Family of the Ill or Hospitalized Child, Chapter 26

*Dependent nursing action.

particles in the blood and prevent the precipitation of formed elements—gently shake the container frequently.

- Use blood within 30 minutes of its arrival from the blood bank; if it is not used, return to the blood bank—do not store in a regular unit refrigerator.
- Infuse a unit of blood (or the specified amount) within 4 hours. If the infusion will exceed this time, the blood should be divided into appropriate-size quantities by the blood bank, with the unused portion refrigerated under controlled conditions.
- If a reaction of any type is suspected, take vital signs, stop the transfusion, maintain a patent intravenous line with normal saline and new tubing, notify the practitioner, and do not restart the transfusion until the child's condition has been medically evaluated.

Blood is usually administered to children by infusion pump; therefore the usual precautions and management related to pumps apply. When the blood is started with a standard transfusion set, the filter chamber is filled to allow the total filter to be used. The drip chamber is partially filled with blood to permit counting of the drops. In adjusting the flow rate, it is important to remember that blood administration sets do not use microdrops (60 drops/ml) but regular drops (usually 10 or 15 drops/ml). Therefore this must be considered when calculating the flow rate.

Oxygen may be administered to provide optimum environmental conditions for hemoglobin saturation. However, oxygen is of limited value because each gram of hemoglobin is able to carry a limited amount of the gas. In addition, prolonged supplemental oxygen can decrease erythropoiesis. Therefore the child is monitored closely for evidence of decreasing benefit from oxygen. One of the first signs of hypoxia is restlessness.

❖ EVALUATION

The effectiveness of nursing interventions is determined by continual reassessment and evaluation of care based on the following observational guidelines and expected outcomes:

1. Interview child and family regarding their understanding of diagnostic procedures and the blood disorder, as well as regarding their feelings and concerns.
2. Monitor therapeutic interventions and child's tolerance for activity.
3. Assess child for evidence of infection and/or complications of therapies.

Expected outcomes:

See Nursing Care Plan, pp. 1575-1576.

IRON DEFICIENCY ANEMIA

Anemia caused by an inadequate supply of dietary iron is the most prevalent nutritional disorder in the United States and the most common mineral disturbance. Almost 16% of lower-income children 6 to 24 months of age are anemic (Wimberly and Parks, 1991). Adolescents are also at risk because of their rapid growth rate combined with poor eating habits (Raunikar and Sabio, 1992). Premature infants are especially at risk because of their reduced fetal iron supply.

There has been a decrease in the prevalence of iron deficiency anemia during the past 15 years. This in part can be linked to families' participation in the Women, Infants, and Children (WIC) program, which provides iron-fortified formula for the first year of life (Oski, 1993). However, iron deficiency is still a significant health problem for children from low-income families (Francis, Williams, and Yarandi, 1993).

Etiology

Iron deficiency anemia can be caused by any number of factors that decrease the supply of iron, impair its absorption, increase the body's need for iron, or affect the synthesis of Hgb (see box on p. 1577). Although the clinical manifestations and diagnostic evaluation are quite similar regardless of the cause, the therapeutic and nursing considerations depend on the specific reason for the iron deficiency. The fol-

CAUSES OF IRON DEFICIENCY ANEMIA

1. **Inadequate supply of iron**
   a. Deficient dietary intake
      (1) Rapid growth rate
      (2) Excessive milk intake, delayed addition of solid foods
      (3) Poor general eating habits
   b. Inadequate iron stores at birth
      (1) Low birth weight, premature, multiple births
      (2) Severe iron deficiency in mother (hemoglobin level below 9 g/dl)
      (3) Fetal blood loss at or before delivery
2. **Impaired absorption**
   a. Presence of iron inhibitors
      (1) Phytates, phosphates, or oxalates
      (2) Gastric alkalinity
   b. Malabsorptive disorders
   c. Chronic diarrhea
3. **Blood loss**
   a. Acute or chronic hemorrhage
   b. Parasitic infestation
4. **Excessive demands for iron required for growth**
   a. Prematurity
   b. Adolescence
   c. Pregnancy
5. **Inability to form hemoglobin**
   a. Lack of vitamin B_{12} (pernicious anemia)
   b. Folic acid deficiency

lowing discussion is limited to iron deficiency anemia resulting from inadequate iron in the diet.

At birth the full-term infant's supply of iron is approximately 300 mg, or 75 mg/kg of body weight. The majority of iron has been transferred from the mother at the rate of 4 mg per day during the last trimester. The bulk of the iron is stored in the circulating hemoglobin of the erythrocytes; the rest is deposited in the liver, spleen, and bone marrow. Maternal iron stores are adequate for the first 5 to 6 months of age in the full-term infant but only for about 2 to 3 months in premature infants or infants of multiple births. When exogenous sources of iron are not supplied to meet the infant's growth demands following depletion of fetal iron stores, iron deficiency anemia results. Physiologic anemia should not be confused with iron deficiency anemia resulting from nutritional causes (see Chapter 12).

Pathophysiology

Iron is required for the production of Hgb. One molecule consists of ***protein (globin)*** combined with four molecules of a ***pigmented compound (heme)***. Each molecule of heme contains one atom of iron. When iron stores are deficient, the production of Hgb is reduced. Consequently, the main effect of iron deficiency is decreased Hgb and reduced oxygen-carrying capacity of the blood.

Clinical Manifestations

The clinical manifestations are directly attributed to the reduction in the amount of oxygen available to tissues and resemble those seen in any type of anemia. Usually the signs are insidious and obscure, and the severity is directly related to the duration of the dietary deficiency.

Although the majority of infants with iron deficiency anemia are underweight, many are overweight because of excessive milk ingestion (known as ***milk baby***). These children become anemic for two reasons. Milk, a poor source of iron, is given almost to the exclusion of solid foods, and some infants fed cow's milk have an increased fecal loss of blood. This asymptomatic loss of hemoglobin has been thought to cause iron deficiency (Ziegler and others, 1990), but not all studies support this relationship (Fuchs and others, 1993). Although chubby, these infants are pale, usually demonstrate poor muscle development, and are prone to infection. The skin color may be described as porcelain-like.

Although the mechanism is unknown, iron deficiency anemia enhances the leakage of plasma proteins in infants, causing edema, retarded growth, and decreased serum concentration of the proteins albumin, gamma globulin, and transferrin, a protein that binds iron and transports it through the plasma. Other, less common manifestations of iron deficiency include glossitis, angular stomatitis, and koilonychia (concave or "spoon" fingernails). The precise relationship of iron deficiency anemia to behavioral and intellectual functioning is not clear, but increasing evidence suggests that iron deficiency, alone or with anemia, results in impaired cognitive skills that may or may not reverse after correction of the iron-deficient state (Idjradinata and Pollitt, 1993; Lozoff, Jimenez, and Wolf, 1991; Walter and others, 1989).

Diagnostic Evaluation

Laboratory tests that measure or describe Hgb, the morphologic changes in the RBC, and iron concentration are usually performed. The RBC count may be normal, borderline, or moderately reduced. Typically, the nearly normal number of erythrocytes is strikingly out of proportion to the low Hgb concentration. RBCs are typically small in size in a lowered Hct (usually below 33%), since the microcytic RBCs pack together into a smaller volume, regardless of their actual number. The small RBCs also decrease the mean corpuscular volume (MCV). For infants near 1 year of age, an MCV below 70 μm^3 is considered diagnostic, whereas in the preschool and older child an MCV of 75 μm^3 is usually the lower limit of normal.

The reticulocyte count is usually normal or slightly reduced because of decreased stores of iron. However, in severe anemia when tissue hypoxia exerts an erythropoietic response, the reticulocyte count may be elevated to 3% or 4%. The level of erythrocyte protoporphyrin (EP), the immediate precursor of heme, becomes elevated in RBCs whenever heme synthesis is disturbed.

In terms of differential diagnosis, a stool analysis for occult blood (guaiac test) is commonly performed to confirm or rule out the possibility of chronic fecal blood loss, especially from milk intolerance or structural anomalies such as diverticulitis.

Iron Studies. In addition to those tests that indirectly indicate the level of iron by the effects of iron deficiency on the RBC, several other tests are usually performed that more directly measure the amount of circulating iron. The ***serum-iron concentration (SIC)*** measures the amount of circulating iron and normally is about 70 μg/dl in infants and slightly higher in older children. Lower limits of serum iron vary not only with age but also with time of day; they are highest in the morning, when the test should be performed.

The ***total iron-binding capacity (TIBC)*** measures the amount of ***transferrin,*** or iron-binding globulin, which is necessary for the transport of iron in the bloodstream. When combined with transferrin, the iron is loosely bound to the globulin molecule so that it can be released easily to tissue cells anywhere in the body. In iron deficiency anemia the TIBC is elevated above the normal range of 350 μg/dl (6 months to 2 years) or 450 μg/dl (children older than 2 years and adults). The elevated TIBC represents the body's compensatory mechanisms to absorb more exogenous sources of iron during states of deficiency than normally. The combination of a reduced SIC and an elevated TIBC is of significant diagnostic value because it is not found in any other condition, except hypochromic, microcytic anemia caused by inadequate intake or absorption of iron. The ***transferrin saturation*** is calculated by dividing the SIC by the TIBC and multiplying the result by 100 to express the value as a percentage. A transferrin saturation of 10% suggests anemia.

Therapeutic Management

Prevention is the primary goal and is achieved through optimum nutrition and appropriate iron supplementation. In infants the American Academy of Pediatrics (1992) recommends the following guidelines to prevent iron deficiency:

- Use only breast milk or commercial infant formula for the first 12 months.
- Begin iron supplementation (preferably iron-fortified commercial formula or in breast-fed infants, iron-fortified infant cereal) to provide 1 mg/kg/day of iron by 4 to 6 months of age in full-term infants and by 2 months in preterm infants.
- Administer iron (ferrous sulfate) drops at a dose of 2 to 3 mg/kg/day to a maximum of 15 mg/day to breast-fed preterm infants after 2 months of age and iron-fortified infant cereal when solid foods are introduced.
- Limit the amount of formula to no more than 1 L/day to encourage intake of iron-rich solid foods.

Once the diagnosis of iron deficiency anemia is made, therapeutic management focuses on increasing the amount of supplemental iron the child receives. This is usually done through dietary counseling and the administration of oral iron supplements. In formula-fed infants the most convenient and best sources of supplemental iron are iron-fortified commercial formula and iron-fortified infant cereal (Walter and others, 1993). Iron-fortified formula provides a relatively constant and predictable amount of iron and is not associated with an increased incidence of gastrointestinal symptoms, such as colic, diarrhea, or constipation. Infants under 12 months of age should not be given fresh cow's milk to decrease the possibility of iron deficiency from gastrointestinal blood loss occurring from allergy to the milk protein.

Dietary addition of iron-rich foods may not provide sufficient supplemental quantities of the mineral. Oral supplements of ferrous iron are given because this form is more readily absorbed than ferric iron, resulting in higher Hgb levels. Ingested iron is absorbed largely from the duodenum, and absorption is facilitated by an acid environment. Children absorb an average of 10% to 20% of oral iron supplements, but during periods of iron deficiency they absorb an additional 5% to 10%. Oral iron supplements are prescribed in daily doses of 10 to 15 mg for approximately 4 months to replace body stores. Ideally the daily dose of iron should be given in two or three divided doses between meals. Side effects of oral iron therapy include nausea, gastric irritation, diarrhea or constipation, and anorexia, but they occur infrequently, especially in infants. If the iron produces vomiting and diarrhea, it should be administered with meals and in gradually increasing doses.

Response to oral iron therapy is reflected in a peak increase in reticulocyte count by the fifth to the tenth day of administration. Following the reticulocyte rise, the Hgb and Hct levels and RBC count increase. The hemoglobin level rises an average of 0.17 to 0.25 g/dl/day; therefore a substantial increase should occur by the end of 1 month.

If the Hgb is very low or if levels fail to rise after 1 month of oral therapy, intramuscular or intravenous iron is administered. Transfusions are indicated for the most severe anemia and in cases of serious infection, cardiac dysfunction, or surgical emergency where anesthesia is required. Packed RBCs, not whole blood, are used to minimize the chance of circulatory overload. Supplemental oxygen is administered when tissue hypoxia is severe.

Prognosis. The prognosis for a child with this condition is very good. However, there is evidence that if the iron deficiency anemia is long-standing, mild cognitive impairment may result (Idjradinata and Pollitt, 1993).

Nursing Considerations

The main nursing objective is prevention of nutritional anemia through parent education. Nurses need to be aware of recommendations regarding iron supplementation during infancy and appropriate sources of dietary iron. One of the difficulties in terms of infant feeding is encouraging parents to limit the quantity of milk, use iron-fortified infant formulas, and introduce solid foods when they believe milk is best for the infant and equate the resultant weight gain with a "healthy child." Although milk is an excellent food, it is deficient in iron, vitamin C, zinc, and fluoride. Sources of each of these nutrients and the role they play in preventing deficiencies need to be discussed with the family, especially the person who is responsible for feeding the infant. For example, the mother may have less decision-making power regarding feeding than the grandmother who cares for the child.

It is also stressed that overweight is not synonymous with good health. If the infant has obvious signs of anemia such as pallor, listlessness, frequent infections, and muscular weakness, they are pointed out as evidence of suboptimum health. In some instances it is helpful to chart the hemoglobin or hematocrit values to visually impress on parents the change in iron levels. Often increased blood values correspond to improved physical status and reinforce the benefit of dietary or oral iron supplementation.

Instructing parents regarding proper administration of oral iron supplements is an essential nursing responsibility. Several factors affect the absorption of iron, such as stomach acidity (see Table 13-2). Ideally iron supplements are administered in two divided doses between meals when the presence of free hydrochloric acid is greatest and are accompanied by a citrus fruit or juice, which helps reduce iron to its most soluble state. An inadequate dietary intake of calcium helps bind and remove agents such as phosphates and phytates that react with iron to render it insoluble. In cultures in which tea is drunk as a common beverage, iron should be administered with some other liquid, because the tannins in tea form an insoluble complex with iron from foods other than meat (Merhav and others, 1985). When adequate dosage is reached, the stools usually turn a tarry green color. The nurse advises parents of this normally expected change and inquires about its occurrence on follow-up visits. Absence of the greenish-black stool may be a clue to poor compliance. If compliance is an issue, every effort should be made to institute strategies to improve adherence to the medication regimen, such as administering the drug once a day at the most convenient time (see Compliance, Chapter 27).

Oral iron supplements are available in liquid or tablet form. Since liquid preparations may temporarily stain the teeth, the medication is taken through a straw or given through a syringe or medicine dropper placed toward the back of the mouth. Brushing the teeth after administration of the drug lessens the discoloration.

NURSING ALERT Because iron ingested in excessive quantities is toxic, even fatal, parents should keep no more than a 1-month supply in the home and store it safely away from the reach of children.

Iron dextran, if ordered, must be injected deeply into a large muscle mass using the Z-tract method, and the injection site is *not* massaged after injection to minimize skin staining and irritation. Since no more than 1 ml should be given in one site, multiple injections are sometimes required. Careful observation is required because of the risk of adverse reactions, such as anaphylaxis with intravenous administration. A test dose is recommended before routine use.

Counseling families whose children are anemic is often a difficult and challenging task. Meal planning must be based on their budget, cultural pattern, and food preferences. Often this requires more than a brief discussion with the mother or usual caregiver about foods high in iron (see Table 13-2). For teaching to be effective, the nurse may need to offer recipes, assist in planning a shopping list, and investigate food prices for economy. Since the physical effects of anemia are insidious, parents may not consider their child ill and consequently may view the medication and diet changes as unnecessary. Stressing what the physical and behavioral improvements will be and what effect the improved diet will have on all family members may encourage parents to adhere to the treatment plan.

Diet education of teenagers is especially difficult, especially since teenage girls are particularly prone to following weight-reduction diets. Emphasizing the effect of anemia on appearance (pallor) and energy level (difficulty maintaining popular activities) may be useful. (See Chapter 13—Mineral Disturbances and Table 13-2—for sources of iron-rich foods.)

SICKLE CELL ANEMIA (SCA)

SCA is one of a group of diseases collectively termed ***hemoglobinopathies,*** in which normal adult hemoglobin ***(hemoglobin A [HbA])*** is partly or completely replaced by abnormal ***sickle hemoglobin (HbS). Sickle cell disease (SCD)*** includes all those hereditary disorders, the clinical, hematologic, and pathologic features of which are related to the presence of HbS. Even though SCD is sometimes used to refer to SCA, this use is incorrect. Other correct terms for SCA are ***SS*** and ***homozygous sickle cell disease.***

In the United States the most common forms of SCD are:

1. **Sickle cell trait,** the heterozygous form of the disease (HbA and HbS or HbAS)
2. **Sickle cell anemia,** the homozygous form of the disease (HbSS)
3. **Sickle cell–C disease,** a heterozygous variant of SCD, including both HbS and HbC
4. **Sickle cell–hemoglobin E disease,** a variant of SCD in which glutamic acid has been substituted for lysine in the number 26 position of the beta chain
5. **Sickle thalassemia disease,** a combination of sickle cell trait and β-thalassemia trait

Of the SCDs, SCA is the most common form in black Americans in the United States, followed by sickle cell–C disease and sickle β-thalassemia. Another beta chain variant, hemoglobin E, is found primarily in people of Southeast Asian origin. People who carry the trait for hemoglobin E are completely asymptomatic, but those who are homozygous exhibit a disease clinically similar to hemoglobin C disease.

SCA is found primarily in the black race, although infrequently it affects whites, especially those of Mediterranean descent. The incidence of the disease varies in different geographic locations. Among American blacks, the incidence of sickle cell trait is about 8%. In West Africa the incidence is reported to be as high as 40% among native blacks. The high incidence of sickle cell trait in these individuals is believed by some to be the result of selective protection of trait carriers against malaria caused by *Plasmodium falciparum.*

Mode of Transmission

The gene that determines the production of HbS is situated on an autosome. The expected pattern of transmission from two parents who carry the heterozygous gene HbAS is illustrated in Fig. 5-6. Therefore, when both parents have sickle cell trait, there is a 25% chance of their producing an offspring with SCA. In the United States it is estimated that one in 12 black persons carries the trait; therefore the risk of two black parents having a child with the disease is 0.7%. The occurrence of other forms of SCD is the result of union between two individuals who carry the heterozygous form of hemoglobin variants.

Basic Defect

The basic defect responsible for the sickling effect of erythrocytes is in the globin fraction of hemoglobin, which is composed of 574 amino acids. HbS differs from HbA in the substitution of only one amino acid (valine) for another (glutamine) at the sixth position of the β-polypeptide chain. Under conditions of dehydration, acidosis, hypoxia, and temperature elevations, the relatively insoluble HbS changes its molecular structure to form long, slender crystals. These filamentous crystals cause distortion of the cell membrane from a pliable disk to a crescent- or sickle-shaped RBC. The filamentous forms are associated with much greater viscosity than the normal holly leaf structure of HbA.

In most instances the sickling response is reversible under conditions of adequate oxygenation and hydration. During this time the RBCs are indistinguishable from normal erythrocytes on peripheral examination. RBCs with HbS can sickle and unsickle under adverse conditions. After repeated cycles of sickling and unsickling, the RBC becomes irreversibly sickled.

Although the defect is inherited, the sickling phenomenon is usually not apparent until later in infancy because of the presence of fetal hemoglobin (HbF). HbF is composed of two alpha and two gamma polypeptide chains. At 32 weeks' gestation, the production of beta and delta chains begins. These combine with alpha chains to form the major adult hemoglobins, HbA (two alpha and two beta chains) and HbA_2 (two alpha and two delta chains). As long as HbF persists, sickling does not occur, because there are no beta chains carrying the defect. The newborn has from 60% to 80% fetal hemoglobin, but this rapidly decreases during the first year, so that the child is at risk for sickle cell–related complications (Sickle Cell Disease Guideline Panel, 1993).

Sickle Cell Trait. Persons with sickle cell trait have the same basic defect, but only about 35% to 45% of the total hemoglobin is HbS. The remainder is HbA. Normally these individuals are asymptomatic. Although rare, complications have been described in individuals with sickle cell trait. Nonpainful, gross hematuria is the major complication seen primarily in the teenage and adult years. Under conditions of extreme or prolonged deoxygenation, such as riding in an unpressurized aircraft or military training, splenic sequestration with profound anemia can occur, resulting in death.

Pathophysiology and Clinical Manifestations

The clinical features of SCA are primarily the result of (1) ***obstruction*** caused by the sickled RBCs and (2) increased RBC ***destruction*** (Fig. 35-2). The entanglement and enmeshing of rigid sickle-shaped cells with one another intermittently block the microcirculation, causing vaso-occlusion. The resultant absence of blood flow to adjacent tissues causes local hypoxia, leading to tissue ischemia and infarction (cellular death). Most of the complications seen in SCA can be traced to this process and its impact on various organs of the body.

Initially the ***spleen*** may become enlarged from congestion and engorgement with sickled cells. This repeated insult to the splenic sinuses results in infarction. The functioning cells are gradually replaced with fibrotic tissue, until by the age of 5 years the spleen is decreased in size and totally replaced by a fibrous mass ***(functional asplenia).*** Without the spleen to filter bacteria and to promote the release of large numbers of phagocytic cells, these individuals are highly susceptible to infection.

The ***liver*** is also altered in form and function. Liver failure and necrosis are the result of severe impairment of hepatic blood flow from anemia and capillary obstruction. The liver is usually enlarged as a result of blood stasis and is occasionally tender. With progressive focal necrosis and subsequent scarring, cirrhosis eventually occurs.

Kidney abnormalities are probably the result of the same cycle of congestion of glomerular capillaries and tubular arterioles with sickle cells and hemosiderin, tissue necrosis, and eventual scarring. The principal results of kidney ischemia are hematuria, inability to concentrate urine, enuresis, and occasionally nephrotic syndrome.

Bone changes include hyperplasia and congestion of the bone marrow, resulting in osteoporosis, widening of the medullary spaces, and thinning of the cortices. As a result of the weakening of bone, especially in the lumbar and thoracic regions, skeletal deformities, particularly lordosis and kyphosis, may occur. From chronic hypoxia, the bone becomes susceptible to osteomylitis, frequently from *Salmonella.* Aseptic necrosis of the femoral head from chronic ischemia is an occasional problem.

Changes in the ***central nervous system*** are primarily vascular from the same cyclic reaction of occlusion, ischemia, and infarction. Stroke or cerebrovascular accident is a major complication and can result in permanent paralysis or death (Balkaran and others, 1992). Any number of neurologic symptoms can herald a minor cerebral insult, such as headache, aphasia, weakness, convulsions, visual disturbances, or unilateral hemiplegia. Loss of vision is usually the result of progressive retinopathy and retinal detachment. One study suggests cognitive impairment from sickle cell anemia. Affected children scored 1 standard deviation (SD) below siblings on most cognitive measures (Swift and others, 1989).

Heart problems are mainly attributable to the stress of chronic anemia, which can eventually result in decompensation and failure. Cardiomyopathy is visualized on chest x-ray examination, and a systolic flow murmur is frequently present as a consequence of the anemia.

With the formation of sickled erythrocytes, mechanical fragility is increased, thereby decreasing the life span of the RBC. Hemolysis occurs both during intravascular circulation and as a result of stagnation of sickled cells in the congested spleen. Although the body attempts to compensate through stimulated erythropoietic activity, as evidenced by

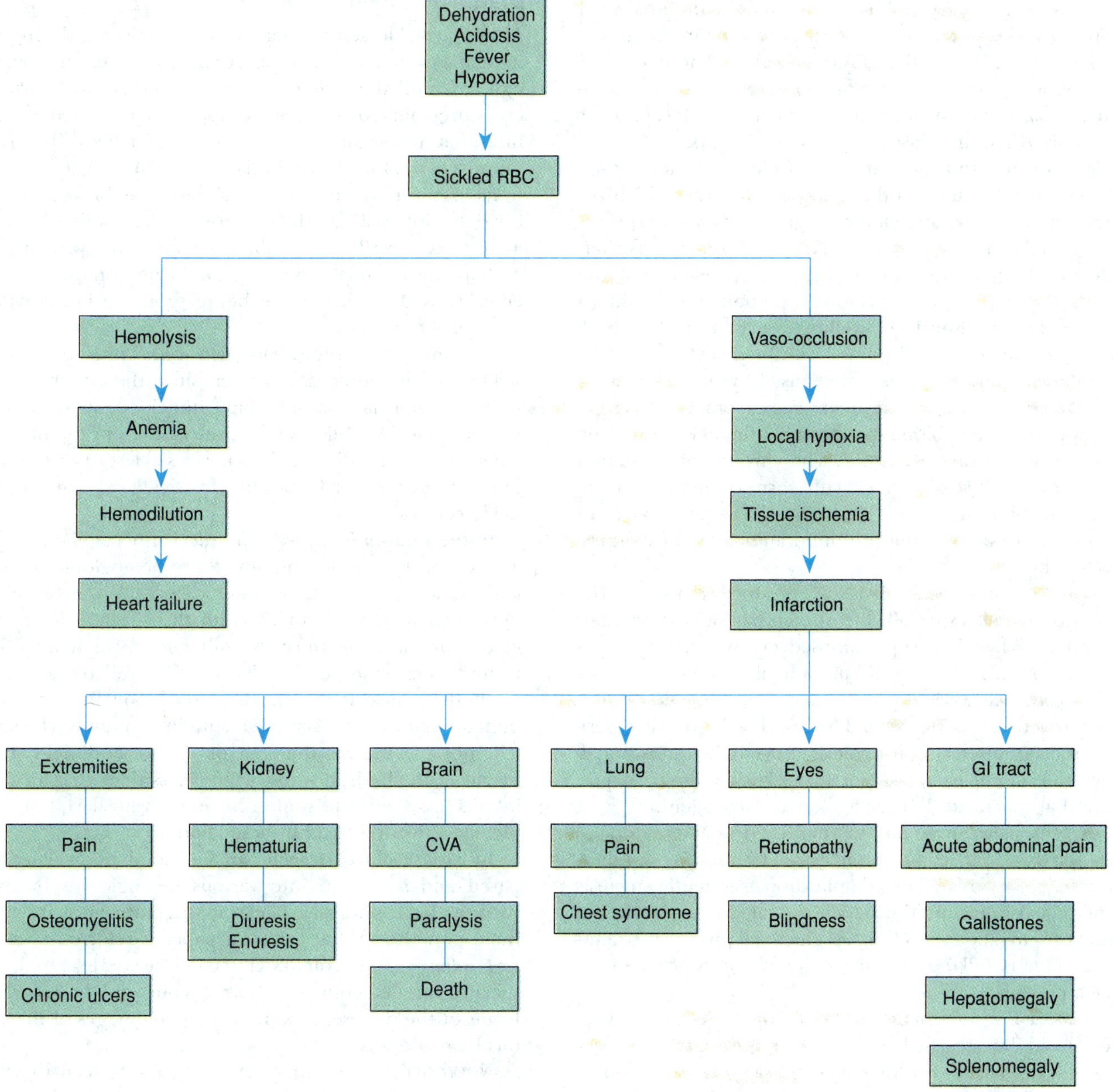

FIG. 35-2 Tissue effects of sickle cell anemia.

a hyperplastic bone marrow, the rate of destruction exceeds the rate of production. A normocytic, normochromic anemia results. With increased hemolysis, hemosiderosis (increased storage of iron) is present in the liver, spleen, bone marrow, kidneys, and lymph nodes (see p. 1589).

Other Signs and Symptoms. In addition to the effects of sickling on various organ structures, the child with SCA may have a variety of complaints, such as exercise intolerance, anorexia, jaundiced sclera, and gallstones. Chronic leg ulcers are common in adolescents and adults and are thought to be a result of decreased circulation due to vaso-occlusion and tissue ischemia. Other generalized effects include growth retardation in both height and weight, delayed sexual maturation, and decreased fertility. If the child reaches adulthood, sexual development and adult height are usually achieved.

Sickle Cell Crises. The clinical manifestations of SCA vary markedly in severity and frequency. The most acute symptoms of the disease occur during periods of exacerbation called ***crises.*** There are several types of episodic crises—vaso-occlusive, acute splenic sequestration, aplastic, hyperhemolytic, stroke, chest syndrome, and infection. The crises may occur individually or concomitantly with one or more other crises.

Vaso-occlusive crises (VOCs) are the most common and non-life-threatening crises. They are the result of sickled cells obstructing the blood vessels, causing occlusion, ischemia, and potentially necrosis. A child with a VOC alone may have mild to severe bone pain, acute abdominal pain from visceral hypoxia or gallstones, priapism (an unwanted, prolonged penile erection), and arthralgia. The pain is often migratory, with presence of a low-grade fever, but without an exacerbation of anemia. Pain may be localized or generalized and may last from minutes to days.

VOCs can result in a variety of skeletal problems. One of the more frequent is the ***hand-foot syndrome,*** which occurs primarily in young children ages 6 months to 2 years. It is caused by infarction of short tubular bones and is characterized by pain and swelling of the soft tissue over the hands and feet. It usually resolves spontaneously within a couple of weeks. Localized swelling over joints with arthralgia can occur from erythrostasis with sickle cells.

Splenic sequestration crises are caused by the spleen's sequestering (pooling) large quantities of blood, causing a precipitous drop in blood volume and ultimately shock. The crisis may be acute or chronic. The chronic manifestation is termed ***hypersplenism.*** The acute form occurs most commonly in children between 2 months and 5 years of age and may result in death from profound anemia and cardiovascular collapse.

Aplastic crisis is diminished RBC production, usually triggered by a viral (especially the human parvovirus) or other infection. When it is superimposed on the existing rapid destruction of RBCs, a profound anemia results.

Megaloblastic anemia is attributed to an excessive nutritional need for folic acid and/or vitamin B_{12} during periods of pronounced erythropoiesis. Since infection is not always antecedent to aplastic or hypoplastic crises, it is possible that folic acid deficiency is a causative agent.

Hyperhemolytic crisis occurs when there is an accelerated rate of RBC destruction characterized by anemia, jaundice, and reticulocytosis. This complication frequently suggests other coexisting conditions, such as viral illness, transfusion reactions to alloantibodies, or glucose-6-phosphate dehydrogenase (G6PD) deficiency, which is also common in black persons.

A ***stroke*** is a sudden and severe complication, often with no related illnesses. Sickled cells block the major blood vessels in the brain, resulting in cerebral infarction, which causes variable degrees of neurologic impairment. Repeat strokes causing progressively greater brain damage occur in 60% of children who have already experienced one stroke.

Chest syndrome, which is clinically similar to pneumonia, is associated with chest pain, fever, pneumonia-like cough, and associated anemia. It is believed that a VOC or infection results in sickling in the small blood vessels of the lungs, with ensuing occlusion, stasis, and anemia. Repeated episodes of chest syndrome may cause restrictive lung disease and pulmonary hypertension.

Overwhelming infection, especially due to *Streptococcus pneumonia* and *Haemophilus influenzae type b* as a result of defective splenic function, is the major cause of death in children under the age of 5 with SCD. Repeated insults on the splenic sinuses by sickled cells result in impaired filtration and function, allowing the development of septicemia and possibly subsequent death.

Diagnostic Evaluation

Although sickle cell anemia has been reported during the neonatal period and early part of infancy, it may not be recognized until the toddler and preschool period, during a crisis precipitated by an acute upper respiratory or gastrointestinal infection. However, early diagnosis (before 3 months of age) facilitates initiation of appropriate interventions to minimize complications. Several tests are available for detecting SCD. Although most of the routine hematologic tests described in Table 35-1 are done primarily to evaluate the anemia, this discussion focuses on the tests specifically used to detect the homozygous or heterozygous form of the disease.

Examination of the ***stained blood smear*** may reveal a few sickled red blood cells. However, since the erythrocyte assumes its normal discoid shape under adequate oxygenation, no sickled cells may be present even in the homozygous form of the disease. Whenever sickle cells are found, the diagnosis is usually positive for sickle cell anemia, not sickle cell trait.

In the ***sickle-turbidity test (Sickledex)*** anticoagulated blood is mixed with a special solution. Since hemoglobin S is normally much less soluble than hemoglobin A or F (as well as other variants), when mixed with this solution it forms a cloudy or turbid mixture. All other forms of hemoglobin result in a clear suspension. This test is a reliable screening method because it can be done on blood from a finger puncture and yields accurate results in 3 minutes. However, it is not specific for the trait or disease and yields false-negatives in children whose Hgb is less than 10 g/dl or in infants less than 4 to 6 months of age who have not completely converted to adult hemoglobin.

In ***hemoglobin electrophoresis*** the blood is specially prepared and separated into various hemoglobins by high-voltage electrophoresis. The resulting pattern of the separated peptides as it appears on paper is referred to as ***fingerprinting*** of the protein. This test is accurate, rapid, and specific for detecting the homozygous and heterozygous forms of the disease, as well as the percentages of the various hemoglobins.

Newborn Screening. Screening for SCA in the newborn period can identify children with hemoglobinopathies. Early diagnosis can facilitate parent education and medical intervention. There has been a decrease in the death rate from splenic sequestration. Parents are taught to palpate the child's abdomen and seek medical attention at the first sign of complications (Sickle Cell Disease Guideline Panel, 1993).

Therapeutic Management. The aims of therapy are (1) to prevent the sickling phenomenon, which is responsible for the pathologic sequelae, and (2) to treat the medical emergency of sickle cell crisis. Three general forms of treatment are available: supportive/symptomatic, specific, and curative. Research is investigating hydroxyurea and erythropoietin, which may increase the concentration of fetal hemoglobin and ultimately reduce complications (Charache, 1994; Rodgers and others, 1993). A promising area of research is bone marrow transplant as a possible cure for SCD (Johnson and others, 1994; Vermylen and Cornu, 1994) (see Chapter 36). Limiting factors include proper patient selection (Bray and others, 1994), as well as the availability of suitable donors (Mentzer and others, 1994). This technology raises many ethical issues regarding patient access and availability of therapy (Secundy, 1994).

Medical management is directed at supportive and symptomatic treatment of crises, especially in children with chest syndrome or cardiac failure. Although specific treatments are warranted in different types of crises, the main general objectives include (1) bed rest to minimize energy expenditure and oxygen utilization at the child's discretion; (2) hydration for hemodilution through oral and intravenous therapy; (3) electrolyte replacement, since hypoxia results in metabolic acidosis, which also promotes sickling; (4) analgesics for the severe abdominal and joint pain (see Nursing Considerations); (5) blood replacement to treat anemia and to reduce the viscosity of the sickled blood; and (6) antibiotics to treat any existing infection. The administration of pneumococcal, *Haemophilus influenzae* type b, and meningococcal vaccines is recommended for these children because of their susceptibility to infection from functional asplenia (see Immunizations, Chapter 12). In addition, it is recommended that they receive prophylaxis with oral penicillin by 4 months of age. The nurse assumes an important role in helping the family to comply with a medication regimen (Day, Brunson, and Wang, 1992).

Short-term oxygen therapy may be helpful in severe crises, especially in children with cardiac failure. Although oxygen may prevent more sickling, it usually is not effective in reversing sickling or in pain reduction, because with the vessels clogged with cells, the oxygen is not able to reach the enmeshed sickled RBCs (Zipursky and others, 1992). In addition, prolonged administration of oxygen can depress bone marrow activity, further aggravating the anemia.

The use of blood transfusions is another important component of care. An RBC transfusion is used in aplastic, hyperhemolytic, and splenic sequestration crises. Exchange transfusions have been successful in reducing the number of circulating sickle cells and therefore slowing down the vicious cycle of hypoxia, tissue ischemia, and injury. They are used in chest syndrome and after a stroke to prevent recurrence and further cerebral damage. Routine transfusions to maintain the Hgb above 10 g/dl in children with central nervous system disease can minimize the chances of further neurologic problems. In the event of surgery, exchange or partial exchange transfusions are given preoperatively to prevent anoxia and suppress the formation of new sickle cells and postoperatively to replace lost blood. However, multiple transfusions carry the risk of hepatitis, transfusion reactions, and hemosiderosis (Charache, Lubin, and Reid, 1989). To reduce iron overload and hemosiderosis, home subcutaneous chelation therapy may be started (see p. 1590). Although the appropriate time for beginning treatment is controversial, chelation is often initiated after 4 years of regular transfusions (Day and others, 1993).

In children with recurrent life-threatening splenic sequestration, splenectomy may be a lifesaving measure. However, because the spleen usually atrophies on its own through progressive fibrotic changes, routine splenectomy is not recommended because of the risk of overwhelming infection. However, surgical or autosplenectomy has several advantages, since the spleen is the major site of sickling, sequestration, and destruction of RBCs.

Prognosis. The prognosis varies. The greatest risk is usually in children under 5 years of age, and the majority of deaths in these children are caused by overwhelming infection. However, as the child grows older, the crises usually become less severe and less frequent, although death in early adulthood is not uncommon. Consequently, SCA is a chronic illness with a potentially terminal outcome. Physical and sexual maturation are delayed in adolescents with SCA. Although adults achieve normal height, weight, and sexual function, the delay may present problems to the teenager (Mankad, 1992). Bone marrow transplantation offers the hope of a cure for some children, although the mortality related to the procedure is significant (Kodish and others, 1991).

Nursing Considerations

❖ Assessment

Many nurses are involved in screening programs for SCA to identify persons with the abnormal Hgb in order to implement therapy for homozygotes and provide genetic counseling for heterozygotes. Young children from families of at-risk racial or geographic origin who exhibit any of the signs previously described are advised to seek medical attention immediately.

Assessment of the child in sickle cell crisis involves all areas and systems that can be affected by circulatory obstruction, including vital signs, neurologic signs, vision, and hearing, as well as the respiratory, gastrointestinal, renal, and musculoskeletal systems. It is also important to assess the location and intensity of pain.

❖ Nursing Diagnoses

Nursing diagnoses are derived from observation and assessment of children at risk or who demonstrate evidence of SCD. Some of the general aspects of nursing management are included in the Nursing Care Plan on pp. 1586-1587. Others will become apparent, depending on the state of the child's health, the organs involved, and the individual needs of the child and family.

❖ Planning

The primary goals for the child with SCD and the family are as follows:

1. Child will experience minimal effects of sickling.
2. Family and child (when appropriate) will receive adequate education regarding the sickling phenomenon, possible consequences, and genetic counseling.
3. Child and family will adjust to a lifelong, potentially fatal hereditary disease.

❖ Implementation

Minimize Tissue Deoxygenation. Anything that increases cellular metabolism also results in tissue hypoxia. For the child this includes (1) frequent rest periods during physical activities; (2) avoiding contact sports if the spleen is enlarged, since rupture will cause massive internal hemorrhage; (3) avoiding environments of low oxygen concentration, such as high altitudes or nonpressurized airplane flights; and (4) avoiding known sources of infection. If the child has even a mild infection, the parents must seek medical attention at once.

Promote Hydration. The importance of hemodilution in preventing sickling and later in delaying the vaso-occlusion–hypoxia–ischemia cycle has already been discussed. The nurse calculates the child's fluid requirements (approximately 150 ml/kg/day), which is the minimum daily fluid intake (Charache, Lubin, and Reid, 1989). The nurse also assesses the child's usual fluid consumption to evaluate its adequacy and makes adjustments based on this knowledge. It is not sufficient to advise parents to "force fluids" or "encourage drinking." They need specific instructions on how many glasses or bottles of fluid are required. Many foods are also a source of fluid, particularly soups, gelatin, and puddings.

Children can be encouraged to drink by giving them a "special" cup or glass, using a straw, taking advantage of thirsty times, such as on awakening or after playing, serving frequent, small portions, and leaving the cup in easy reach for self-service. Flavored ice pops and crushed ice "slurpies" are sources of fluid commonly accepted by children (see also p. 1142).

Since the kidneys' ability to concentrate urine is impaired, the child is especially prone to dehydration. Dilute urine or low specific gravity is no longer a valid sign of adequate hydration. Parents are taught to observe for other indications of fluid loss, such as dry mucous membranes, dry diapers, weight loss, and a sunken fontanel in infants. In addition, without the ability to conserve water by concentrating urine, the child is prone to dehydration from environmental factors, particularly overheating. The nurse alerts parents to the need for wearing proper indoor and outdoor clothing and avoiding excess exposure to the sun.

Increased fluids combined with renal diuresis result in the problem of enuresis. Parents who are unaware of this fact frequently employ the usual measures to discourage bed-wetting, such as limiting fluids at night, and many revert to punishment and shame to force bladder control. The nurse discusses this problem with parents, stressing the child's inability to master prolonged control. Reminding the child to urinate frequently is helpful during the day, and waking him or her once during the night may prove beneficial if the child's sleep patterns are not disturbed. Parents who are toilet training their toddlers should be aware of the more frequent pattern of urination and increased difficulty in learning control. Enuresis should be regarded as a complication of the disease, such as joint pain or some other symptom, to alleviate parental pressure on the child and to prevent any fluid restriction.

Minimize Crises. Since infection is the major cause of death due to the body's inability to resist infection, the nurse stresses to parents the importance of adequate nutrition, frequent medical supervision, proper handwashing, and isolation from known sources of infection. The last measure must be tempered with an awareness of the child's need for living a normal life. Overprotection can be as devastating emotionally as an infection is physically. Parents need to be aware of the necessity of seeking prompt medical care at the first sign of any infection.

The family should be taught the signs and symptoms of crises and advised to seek medical attention immediately. Teaching parents spleen palpation for earlier detection of splenic sequestration can reduce mortality from this serious complication.

Promote Supportive Therapies During Crises. The success of many of the medical therapies relies heavily on nursing implementation. Management of pain is an especially difficult problem and often involves experimenting with various analgesics, including opioids, and schedules before relief is achieved. In choosing and scheduling analgesics, *the goal is prevention of pain.* Unfortunately, these children tend to be undermedicated, resulting in "clock watching" and demands for additional doses sooner than might be expected. Often this incorrectly raises suspicions of drug addiction, when in fact the problem is one of inadequate pain control (see Family Focus box).

The most frequent problem for patients with sickle cell disease is pain from vaso-occlusive crises. The chronic nature of this pain can greatly affect the child's development. A multidisciplinary approach is best for its management. When mild to moderate pain is reported, acetaminophen or ibuprofen is initially used. If acetaminophen or ibuprofen is not effective alone, codeine can be added. The dosages of both drugs are titrated to a therapeutic level. Opioids such as immediate- and sustained-release morphine, oxycodone, hydromorphone, and methadone can be administered parenterally or orally for severe pain and are administered around the clock (Shapiro, 1989).

Patient-controlled analgesia (PCA) has been used successfully for sickle cell–related pain (Shapiro, Cohen, and Howe, 1993). This method reinforces the patient's role and responsibility in managing the pain, and provides flexibil-

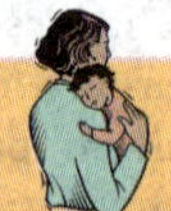

FAMILY FOCUS
Fear of Addiction

Although crisis pain is usually severe and opioids are needed, many families fear that their child will become addicted to the narcotic. Unfortunately, misinformed heatlh professionals may foster this unfounded fear, resulting in needless suffering. Extremely few children (much less than 1%) who receive opioids for severe pain become behaviorally addicted to the drug (Brozovic and others, 1986; Morrison, 1991). Families and older children, especially adolescents, need to be reassured that opioids are medically indicated, high doses may be needed, and children rarely become addicted.

ity for pain, which may vary in severity over time. If PCA devices are not available, and if the pain is not readily controlled with intravenous boluses administered around the clock, a low-dose infusion with rescue boluses administered every 2 hours on a flexible dosing basis can provide a safe and effective alternative. Continuous intravenous infusion of opioids, particularly morphine, provides better pain control than intermittent opioid therapy (Robieux and others, 1992).

NURSING ALERT Meperidine (pethidine [Demerol]) is not recommended. Normeperidine, a metabolite of meperidine, is a central nervous system stimulant that produces anxiety, tremors, myoclonus, and generalized seizures when it accumulates with repetitive dosing. Patients with SCD are particularly at risk for normeperidine-induced seizures (American Pain Society, 1992; Pryle and others, 1992).

Medication given by mouth can be as effective as by the intravenous route when equianalgesic dosages are prescribed (see Chapter 26). Protocols for the comprehensive pharmacologic management of pain are available (Morrison, 1991; Morrison and Vedro, 1989).

Any pain program should be combined with psychologic support to help the child deal with the depression, anxiety, and fear that accompany the disease. This includes regular visits with the child to discuss his or her concerns during the hospitalization and positive reinforcement of adaptive coping skills, such as successful methods of dealing with the pain and compliance with treatment prescriptions. To reduce the negative connotation associated with the term "crisis," it is best to avoid using the expression "crisis pain."

Frequently heat to the affected area is soothing. Cold compresses are not applied to the area, because this enhances vasoconstriction and occlusion. Bed rest is usually well tolerated during a crisis, although actual rest depends a great deal on pain alleviation and organized schedules of nursing care. Although the objective of bed rest is to minimize oxygen consumption, some activity, particularly passive range-of-motion exercises, is beneficial to promote circulation. Usually the best course of action is to let children dictate their activity tolerance.

If blood transfusions or exchange transfusions are given, the nurse has the responsibility of observing for signs of transfusion reaction (see Table 35-2). Since hypervolemia from too rapid transfusion can increase the workload of the heart, the nurse also is alert to signs of cardiac failure.

In splenic sequestration the size of the spleen is gently measured, since increasing splenomegaly is an ominous sign. A decreasing spleen denotes response to therapy. Vital signs and blood pressure are also closely monitored for impending shock. Anemia is typically not a presenting complication in vaso-occlusive crises but is a critical problem in other types of crises. The nurse monitors for evidence of increasing anemia and institutes appropriate nursing intervention.

Oxygen is not beneficial in vaso-occlusive episodes, unless hypoxemia is present (Charache, Lubin, and Reid, 1989). It does not shorten the duration of pain or prevent the appearance of new pain sites (Zipursky and others, 1992) (see Critical Thinking Exercise box). Since prolonged oxygen can aggravate the anemia, signs of lack of therapeutic benefit, such as restlessness, increased pallor, and continued pain, are reported.

CRITICAL THINKING EXERCISE
Sickle Cell Anemia

Samantha Lipe, 7 years old, is brought to the emergency department experiencing a vaso-occlusive sickle cell crisis. She is treated with intravenous fluids for hydration and analgesics for pain management. Mr. Lipe tells you that for all previous crises, oxygen was used and Samantha seemed to recover quicker. Your initial response to Mr. Lipe is to:

1. Suggest that he discuss this with the practitioner.
2. Set up the oxygen and nasal cannula.
3. Ask him how he thinks oxygen helps.
4. Help him understand vaso-occlusive crises.

The correct answer is 3. Before offering an explanation regarding oxygen's lack of effect when cells are sickled, you want to know what the father understands and has been told. Based on this information, you can clarify any misconceptions or suggest that he talk with the attending practitioner. Oxygen is a drug and is administered only as ordered.

Intake, especially of intravenous fluids, and output are recorded. The child's weight should be taken on admission, since it serves as a baseline for evaluating hydration. Since diuresis can result in electrolyte loss, the nurse observes for signs of hypokalemia and should be familiar with normal serum electrolyte values to report changes. Nurses also need to be aware of the signs of chest syndrome and stroke, both potentially fatal complications.

NURSING ALERT Report signs of the following immediately:

Chest syndrome:
- Severe chest pain, sometimes spreading to abdomen
- Fever of 38.8° C (102° F) or higher
- Very congested cough
- Dyspnea, tachypnea
- Retractions

Stroke:
- Jerking or twitching of the face, legs, or arms
- Convulsions or seizures
- Strange, abnormal behavior
- Inability to move an arm and/or a leg
- Stagger or an unsteady walk
- Stutter or slurred speech
- Weakness in the hands, feet, or legs
- Changes in vision
- Severe, unrelieved headaches
- Severe vomiting

Decrease Surgical Risks. The main surgical risk is hypoxia from anesthesia. However, emotional stress, the demands of wound healing, and the possibility of infection po-

NURSING CARE PLAN
The Child with Sickle Cell Anemia

NURSING DIAGNOSIS: High risk for injury related to abnormal hemoglobin, decreased ambient oxygen, dehydration

PATIENT GOAL 1: Will maintain adequate tissue oxygenation

• **NURSING INTERVENTIONS/*RATIONALES***

Explain measures to minimize complications related to physical exertion and emotional stress *to avoid additional tissue oxygen needs*
- Prevent infection
- Avoid low-oxygen environment

• **EXPECTED OUTCOME**

Child avoids situations that reduce tissue oxygenation

PATIENT GOAL 2: Will maintain adequate hydration

• **NURSING INTERVENTIONS/*RATIONALES***

Calculate recommended daily fluid intake (150 ml/kg) and base child's fluid requirements on this *minimum* amount (specify) *to ensure adequate hydration*

Increase fluid intake above minimum requirements during physical exercise/emotional stress and during a crisis *to compensate for additional fluid needs*

Give parents written instructions regarding specific quantity of fluid required *to encourage compliance*

Encourage child to drink *to encourage compliance*

Teach family signs of dehydration *to avoid delay in rehydration therapy* (see Chapter 28)

Stress importance of avoiding overheating *as source of fluid loss*

• **EXPECTED OUTCOME**

Child drinks an adequate amount of fluid and shows no signs of dehydration

PATIENT GOAL 3: Will remain free of infection

• **NURSING INTERVENTIONS/*RATIONALES***

Stress importance of adequate nutrition; routine immunization, including pneumococcal and meningococcal vaccines; protection from known sources of infection; and frequent health supervision

Report any sign of infection to practitioner immediately *to avoid delay in treatment*

Promote compliance with antibiotic therapy both *to prevent and to treat infection*

• **EXPECTED OUTCOME**

Child remains free of infection

PATIENT GOAL 4: Will experience decreased risks associated with a surgical procedure

• **NURSING INTERVENTIONS/*RATIONALES***

Explain reason for preoperative blood transfusion *(given to increase concentration of HbA)*

Keep child well hydrated *to prevent sickling*

Decrease fear through appropriate preparation, *since anxiety increases oxygen needs*

*Administer pain medications *to keep child comfortable and reduce stress response*

Avoid unnecessary exertion *to avoid additional oxygen needs*

Promote pulmonary hygiene postoperatively *to prevent infection*

Use passive range-of-motion exercises *to promote circulation*

*Administer oxygen, if prescribed, *to saturate hemoglobin*

Monitor for evidence of infection *to avoid delay in treatment*

• **EXPECTED OUTCOME**

Child undergoes a surgical procedure without crisis

NURSING DIAGNOSIS: Pain related to tissue anoxia (vaso-occlusive crisis)

PATIENT GOAL 1: Will have no pain or pain relieved to level acceptable to child

• **NURSING INTERVENTIONS/*RATIONALES***

Plan preventive schedule of medication around the clock, not as needed, *to prevent pain*

Recognize that various analgesics, including opioids, and medication schedules may need to be tried *to achieve satisfactory pain relief*

Avoid administration of meperidine (Demerol) *because of increased risk of normeperidine-induced seizures*

Reassure child and family that analgesics, including opioids, are medically indicated, high doses may be needed, and children rarely become addicted, *because needless suffering may result from their unfounded fears*

Apply heat to affected area *because it may be soothing*

Avoid applying cold compresses *because this enhances sickling and vasoconstriction*

• **EXPECTED OUTCOME**

Child will experience no or minimal pain

NURSING DIAGNOSIS: Altered family processes related to a child with potentially life-threatening disease

FAMILY/PATIENT GOAL 1: Will receive education regarding disease

• **NURSING INTERVENTIONS/*RATIONALES***

Teach family and older children characteristics of basic defect and measures *to minimize complications of sickling*

Stress importance of informing significant health personnel of child's disease *to ensure prompt and appropriate treatment (e.g., for pain)*

Explain signs of developing crisis, especially fever, pallor, respiratory distress, and pain, *to avoid delay in treatment*

*Dependent nursing action

NURSING CARE PLAN
The Child with Sickle Cell Anemia—cont'd

Reinforce basics of trait transmission and refer to genetic counseling services *for family to make informed reproductive decisions*

Teach parents to be an advocate for their child *to secure the best care*

• **EXPECTED OUTCOME**

Child and family demonstrate an understanding of the disease, its etiology, and its therapies

PATIENT/FAMILY GOAL 2: Will receive adequate support

• **NURSING INTERVENTIONS/*RATIONALES***

Refer to special organizations and agencies *for ongoing support*

Refer child to comprehensive sickle cell clinic *for ongoing care*

Be especially alert to family's needs when two or more members are affected

See Nursing Care Plan: The Child with a Chronic Illness or Disability, Ch. 22

• **EXPECTED OUTCOMES**

Family takes advantage of community services (specify)

Child receives ongoing care from appropriate facility

See also:

Nursing Care Plan: The Child in the Hospital, Ch. 26

Nursing Care Plan: The Family of the Ill or Hospitalized Child, Ch. 26

tentially increase the sickling phenomenon, both in children with the disease and in those with the trait. The primary nursing objectives are aimed at minimizing each of these threats preoperatively and postoperatively by keeping the child well hydrated, preparing the child psychologically, and preventing infection.

Encourage Screening and Genetic Counseling. Screening is recommended during the neonatal period, since early diagnosis allows earlier, more prevention-oriented treatment, such as prophylactic antibiotic therapy and parent education about potential complications. The advantages of trait identification lie in selective reproduction of offspring not afflicted with hemoglobin SS. Alternate methods of childbearing include artificial insemination, adoption, or abortion of afflicted fetuses. However, these alternatives may be viewed as unacceptable.

To be effective, screening must be combined with genetic counseling and long-term follow-up. The nurse can be instrumental in such programs by conducting parent education sessions, following the family in the home, disseminating correct information about the disease and trait to the community, and rendering support to parents of newly diagnosed children. A primary consideration in genetic counseling is informing parents who both carry the trait of the chances of having a child with the disease (see Chapter 5).

Prenatal diagnosis is possible through amniocentesis or fetoscopy and fetal blood sampling. Analysis of amniotic cells for a DNA fragment associated with the gene responsible for sickled β-globulin chain synthesis can be done at the sixteenth week of gestation. In the event of an affected fetus, the decision regarding termination of the pregnancy should be left to the couple.

Explain the Disease. Since sickle cell anemia is first recognized when the child is a toddler, most of the nurse's counseling is with parents. The nurse explains to parents the basic effect of tissue hypoxia on RBCs and the effect of sickling on circulation (Fig. 35-3). Taking time to establish a sound basis of understanding why certain measures are beneficial to the child encourages parents to practice them.*

➤ **NURSING TIP** One simple yet graphic way of illustrating the difference between normal discoid RBCs and sickle cells is to roll round or oval objects, such as marbles, through a tube to demonstrate normal blood cell circulation and then roll pointed objects such as screws or jacks through the tube. The effect of sickling and clumping of the pointed objects is especially noticeable at a bend or slight narrowing of the tube. This same idea can be expanded to discuss the importance of increased fluid in keeping the pointed objects suspended away from each other to prevent concentration.

Parents are advised to inform all treating practitioners of the child's condition. The use of a medical identification bracelet is another way of ensuring awareness of the disease. Some people view such identification as "negative labeling." The nurse can stress the benefits of displaying this information, especially in emergencies when the use of anesthesia may be required.

Support Family. Parents need the opportunity to discuss their feelings regarding transmitting a potentially fa-

*A Sickle Cell Home Study Kit for Families is available from the **National Association for Sickle Cell Disease, Inc.,** 3345 Wilshire Blvd., Suite 1106, Los Angeles, CA 90010-1880; (213) 736-5455 or (800) 421-8453. Additional resources are **Howard University,** Center for Sickle Cell Disease, 2121 Georgia Ave., N.W., Washington, DC 20059, (202) 806-7930; and **National Heart, Lung, and Blood Institute,** 9000 Rockville Pike, Building 31, Room 4A-21, Bethesda, MD 20892, (301) 496-4236. The Agency for Health Care Policy and Research (AHCPR) has published three booklets on sickle cell disease: *Sickle Cell Disease: Comprehensive Screening, Diagnosis, Management, and Counseling in Newborns and Infants,* Clinical Practice Guideline No. 6, Publication No. AHCPR-0562; *Sickle Cell Disease: Comprehensive Screening and Management in Newborns and Infants,* Quick Reference Guide for Clinicians No. 6, Publication No. AHCPR-0563; and *Sickle Cell Disease in Newborns and Infants: A Guide for Parents,* Publication No. AHCPR 93-0564. They are available from the AHCPR Publications Clearinghouse, P.O. Box 8547, Silver Spring, MD 20907; (800) 358-9295.

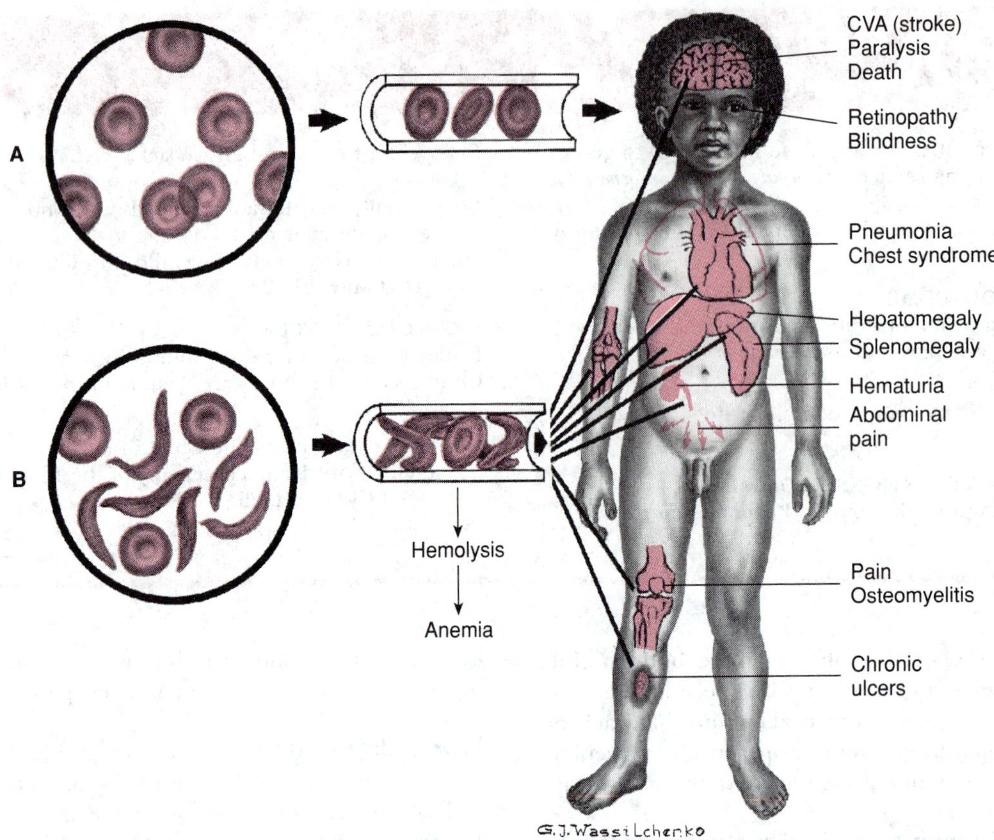

FIG. 35-3 Differences between effects of, **A,** normal and, **B,** sickled red blood cells on circulation with selected consequences in child.

tal, chronic illness to their child. Some parents are able to cope with this fact; some feel great guilt and remorse for giving their child the disease, whereas others regret not knowing that they carried the trait. For many parents the decision regarding subsequent pregnancies is viewed with doubt and ambivalence.

Because of the sometimes poor prognosis for children with SCA, many parents express their fear of death. Prognosis varies; with early diagnosis and treatment these children are living longer. However, since there is no way to predict which child will follow a favorable course, the nurse should care for the family as she or he would for any family with a child who has a chronic and life-threatening illness, with particular emphasis on the siblings' reactions, the stress on the marital relationship, and the childrearing attitudes displayed toward the child (see Chapters 22 and 23).

❖ Evaluation

The effectiveness of nursing interventions is determined by continual reassessment and evaluation of care based on the following observational guidelines and expected outcomes:

1. Observe child for any evidence of sickling; monitor preventive strategies and therapies.
2. Interview family regarding genetic counseling.
3. Interview family regarding their understanding of the disease, the sickling phenomenon, and its consequences.
4. Interview and observe child and family regarding the way in which the disease has affected their lives.

Expected outcomes:
See Nursing Care Plan, pp. 1586-1587.

β-THALASSEMIA

The term ***thalassemia*** comes from the Greek word ***thalassa,*** meaning "sea," and is applied to a variety of inherited blood disorders characterized by deficiencies in the rate of production of specific globin chains in hemoglobin. The name appropriately refers to those people living near the Mediterranean Sea who have the highest incidence of the disease, namely, Italians, Greeks, and Syrians. There is evidence to suggest that the high incidence of the disorder among these groups is a result of selective advantage of the trait to malaria, as is postulated in sickle cell disease. However, the disorder has a wide geographic distribution, probably as a result of genetic migration through intermarriages or possibly as a result of spontaneous mutation.

The thalassemias are classified according to the hemoglobin chain affected and by the amount of the globin chain that is synthesized; for example, if alpha chains are affected, the thalassemia is classified as α-thalassemia. Each of the abnormal genes that cause thalassemia is seen in particular populations (e.g., β-thalassemia, Greeks, Italians, and Syrians; α-thalassemia, Chinese, Thai, African, and Mediterranean peoples).

β-thalassemia is the most common of the thalassemias and occurs in three forms: a heterozygous form, ***thalassemia minor*** or ***thalassemia trait,*** which produces a mild microcytic anemia; ***thalassemia intermedia,*** which is manifested as splenomegaly and severe anemia; and a homozygous form, ***thalassemia major*** (also known as ***Cooley anemia***), which results in an anemia of variable severity that is not compatible with life without transfusion support.

Mode of Transmission

Thalassemia is an autosomal-recessive disorder with varying expressivity. Sometimes the trait is found in only one parent of a child with severe thalassemia. In this situation the likelihood is that the other parent carries a gene for some variant of sickle cell anemia or other hemoglobinopathy. The exact mode of transmission between parents who are heterozygous for thalassemia is illustrated in Fig. 5-6.

Pathophysiology and Clinical Manifestations

Normal postnatal hemoglobin (HbA) is composed of two α- and two β-polypeptide chains. In β-thalassemia there is a partial or complete deficiency in the synthesis of the β-chain of the Hb molecule. Consequently, there is a compensatory increase in the synthesis of α-chains, and γ(gamma)-chain production remains activated, resulting in defective Hb formation. This unbalanced polypeptide unit is very unstable; when it disintegrates, it damages the RBCs, causing severe anemia. To compensate for the hemolytic process, an overabundance of erythrocytes is formed unless the bone marrow is suppressed by transfusion therapy. Excess iron from hemolysis of supplemental RBCs in transfusions and from the rapid destruction of defective cells is stored in various organs (hemosiderosis).

The clinical effects of thalassemia major are primarily attributable to (1) defective synthesis of HbA, (2) structurally impaired RBCs, and (3) shortened life span of the erythrocyte. The major consequences of thalassemia are caused by the pathologic condition, resultant chronic hypoxia, and the supportive treatment of multiple blood supplements (Fig. 35-4).

Anemia results from the body's inability to maintain a level of erythropoiesis commensurate with hemolysis. The bone marrow compensates by increasing production of large numbers of immature cells, such as normoblasts and erythroblasts, large cells that are extremely thin and form bizarre shapes, and nonspecific macrocytes called ***target cells,*** which have abnormal staining properties. As a result of the excessive production of abnormal RBCs, their life span is severely shortened.

Anemia also is exaggerated by aplastic crises after infection, folic acid deficiencies from demands of bone marrow hyperplasia, and progressive hemolysis from repeated blood transfusions. The spleen becomes greatly enlarged as a result of extramedullary hemopoiesis, rapid destruction of the defective erythrocytes, and, rarely, progressive fibrosis from hemochromatosis. Splenomegaly may progress until the organ's very size interferes with the function of other abdominal organs and respiratory expansion.

With progressive anemia, signs of chronic hypoxia, namely, headache, irritability, precordial and bone pain, decreased exercise tolerance, listlessness, and anorexia, may develop. Another common symptom in these children is frequent epistaxis, although the exact reason is unknown. Hyperuricemia and gout from rapid cellular catabolism are also seen.

Hemosiderosis refers to excess iron storage in various tissues of the body, especially the spleen, liver, lymph glands, heart, and pancreas, but without associated tissue injury. ***Hemochromatosis*** refers to excess iron storage with resultant cellular damage. The mechanism for tissue destruction resulting from iron storage is not known. Chronic hypoxia is believed to be an important contributing factor.

In thalassemia, excess ***hemosiderin,*** the iron-containing pigment from the breakdown of hemoglobin, results from decreased hemoglobin synthesis and increased hemolysis of transfused erythrocytes. Decreased production of hemoglobin results in an excess supply of available iron. In addition, the body probably responds to the anemia by increasing the rate of gastrointestinal absorption of dietary iron, since ineffective erythropoiesis is a potent controlling factor regarding exogenous iron use. However, the primary source of additional iron is from the hemolysis of supplemental erythrocytes and rapid destruction of defective red blood cells. With the prophylactic use of deferoxamine to minimize excess iron storage, the characteristic changes in body structures from hemochromatosis have been greatly reduced.

Retarded growth and especially ***delayed sexual maturation*** are common findings. There is evidence that both may also be caused by pituitary failure, although the exact reasons for this are unclear, but the impaired growth is probably related to hemochromatosis. It is possible that the endocrine glands are extremely sensitive to iron toxicity and that even small amounts of deposited iron can produce organ dysfunction. Children with severe disease usually achieve normal growth rates until puberty, when height becomes markedly retarded. Secondary sexual characteristics are delayed or absent in many adolescents (Yesilipek and others, 1993).

Diagnostic Evaluation

Hematologic studies reveal the characteristic changes in the RBC (i.e., microcytosis, hypochromia, anisocytosis, poikilocytosis, target cells, and basophilic stippling of immature erythrocytes of various stages. Low Hgb and Hct levels are seen in severe anemia, although they are typically lower than the reduction in the RBC count because of the proliferation of immature erythrocytes.

Hemoglobin electrophoresis is very helpful in distinguishing the type and severity of the various thalassemias because it analyzes the quantity and specific hemoglobin variants found in blood. In β-thalassemia hemoglobins F and A_2 (a type of normal adult hemoglobin) are elevated because neither depends on β-chain polypeptides for synthesis.

Therapeutic Management

The objective of supportive therapy is to maintain sufficient hemoglobin levels to prevent tissue hypoxia. Transfusions are the foundation of medical management. Studies have

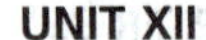

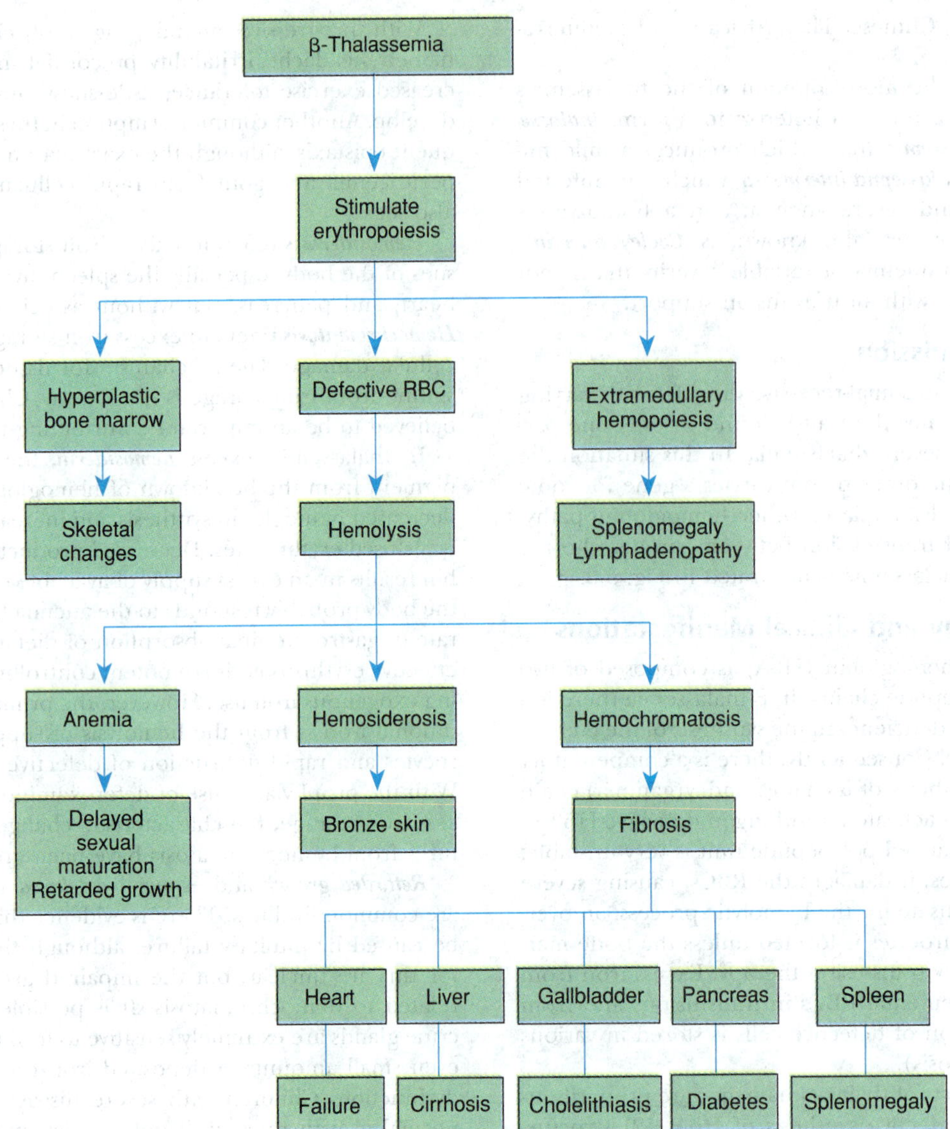

FIG. 35-4 Effects of thalassemia.

evaluated the benefits of maintaining the Hgb level above 10 g/dl, a goal that may require transfusions as often as every 3 weeks. The advantages of this therapy include (1) improved physical and psychologic well-being because of the ability to participate in normal activities, (2) decreased cardiomegaly and hepatosplenomegaly, (3) fewer bone changes, (4) normal or near-normal growth and development until puberty, and (5) fewer infections.

One of the potential complications of frequent blood transfusions is iron overload. Since the body has no effective means of eliminating the excess iron, the mineral is deposited in body tissues. To minimize the development of hemosiderosis and hemochromatosis, ***deferoxamine (Desferal)***, an iron-chelating agent, is given with oral supplements of vitamin C. The preferred routes are intravenous or subcutaneous, and the regimen may include subcutaneous administration via portable infusion pump over 8 to 10 hours (usually during sleep) for 6 days a week and intravenous administration over 8 hours at the time of blood transfusion (Martin and Butler, 1993). Significant liver fibrosis and growth impairment may be prevented if chelation therapy is initiated before age 3 years (Maurer and others, 1988). However, in addition to the intensive schedule required for chelation therapy, deferoxamine use has been linked with decreased height and other bony changes (Olivieri and others, 1992). Creative strategies such as behavioral contracting have been used to assist the child in complying with the deferoxamine regimen (Koch and others, 1993).

In some children with severe splenomegaly who require repeated transfusions, a splenectomy may be necessary to decrease the disabling effects of abdominal pressure and to increase the life span of supplemental RBCs. With repeated blood transfusions, a hemolytic factor develops in the spleen that increases the rate of erythrocyte destruction. After a splenectomy children generally require fewer transfusions, although the basic defect in hemoglobin synthesis remains unaffected. A major postsplenectomy complication is severe and overwhelming infection. Therefore these children are kept on prophylactic antibiotics with close medical supervision for many years and should receive the pneumococcal and meningococcal vaccines in addition to the regularly scheduled immunizations (see Immunizations, Chapter 12).

Prognosis. Most children treated with blood transfusion and early chelation therapy survive well into adulthood. This intensive therapy allows them to lead a nearly normal life (Piomelli, 1993). The most common cause of death is heart disease, followed by infection, liver disease, and malignancy secondary to hemochromatosis (Zurlo and others, 1989). A promising treatment for some children is bone marrow transplantation (see p. 1638). In one study children under 16 years of age who underwent allogenic bone marrow transplantation had a high rate of complication-free survival. Children with thalassemia who undergo allogenic bone marrow transplantation currently have a 59% to 98% chance of cure (Giardini, 1994; Walters and Thomas, 1994).

Nursing Considerations

The objectives of nursing care are to (1) observe for complications of multiple blood transfusions, (2) assist the child in coping with the anxiety-provoking treatments and the effects of the illness, and (3) foster the child's and family's adjustment to a chronic illness. Basic to each of these goals is explaining to parents and older children the defect responsible for the disorder and its effect on RBCs. Since the prevalence of this condition is high among families of Mediterranean descent, the nurse also inquires about the family's previous knowledge about thalassemia. All families with a child with thalassemia should be tested for the trait and referred for genetic counseling.

Support Family. As with any chronic illness, the needs of the family must be met for optimum adjustment to the stresses imposed by the disorder. These needs are discussed in Chapter 22. A source of information for the family is the **Cooley's Anemia Foundation.*** Genetic counseling for the parents and fertile offspring is mandatory, and both prenatal diagnosis using amniocentesis or fetal blood sampling and screening for thalassemia trait are available. There has been a marked decrease in the number of new cases of thalassemia in the United States and Canada. This is thought to be a result of education and testing of parents (Piomelli, 1993).

Assist in Coping with Effects of the Disorder. Body image alterations, decreased growth, and sexual immaturity are frequently difficult adjustment problems for older children. These children feel different from their peers, and the delayed sexual development is a major issue for the maturing adolescent with an improved life expectancy. Adolescents need an opportunity to express their thoughts and feelings about these complex issues. They can learn grooming aids that make them appear more sexually mature, such as up-to-date clothing, new hairstyles, and well-applied makeup. Children with the characteristic bone changes may benefit from surgery or orthodontic appliances to improve facial structure.

With frequent transfusion therapy there is less restriction imposed on physical activity because of severe anemia, and these children should be encouraged to pursue activities commensurate with their exercise tolerance. However, the frequency of treatment can interfere with a normal life-style. To minimize disruptions, the nurse can be instrumental in arranging for blood transfusions and medical supervision at times that interfere least with the child's regular activities, especially school. In addition, children are more likely to cooperate with medical treatments that do not interfere significantly with their routine.

*129-09 26th Ave., Flushing, NY 11354; (718) 321-2873 or (800) 522-7222.

APLASTIC ANEMIA

Aplastic anemia refers to a condition in which all formed elements of the blood are simultaneously depressed. The peripheral blood smear demonstrates pancytopenia or the triad of profound anemia, leukopenia, and thrombocytopenia. ***Hypoplastic anemia*** is characterized by a profound depression of erythrocytes but normal or slightly decreased WBCs and platelets.

A type of hypoplastic anemia is ***pure red cell aplasia,*** a congenital condition marked by complete or almost complete absence of all cells of the erythroid series with normal production of the other myeloid cells. Its treatment, which consists of transfusions, splenectomy, and administration of corticosteroids, is similar to that of other diseases, such as the thalassemias, that result in profound anemia. The prognosis varies, although long-term survival is possible. The principal causes of death are cardiac failure, hepatitis from transfusion therapy, and sepsis. Hemosiderosis and hemochromatosis (p. 1589) also affect vital tissues necessary for survival.

Aplastic anemia can be ***primary*** (***congenital,*** or present at birth) or ***secondary (acquired).*** The best-known congenital disorder of which aplastic anemia is an outstanding feature is ***Fanconi syndrome,*** a rare hereditary disorder characterized by pancytopenia, hypoplasia of the bone marrow, and patchy brown discoloration of the skin due to the deposition of melanin and associated with multiple congenital anomalies of the musculoskeletal and genitourinary systems. The syndrome appears to be inherited as an autosomal-recessive trait with varying penetrance; therefore, affected siblings may demonstrate several different combinations of defects.

Several factors contribute to the development of acquired hypoplastic anemia, including suppressed erythropoiesis from multiple transfusion therapy; hemolytic syndromes (such as sickle cell anemia); autoimmune or allergic states; infection with the human parvovirus (HPV), hepatitis, or overwhelming infection; irradiation; drugs such as the chemotherapeutic agents and several antibiotics, especially chloramphenicol; industrial and household chemicals, including benzene and its derivatives, which are found in petroleum products, dyes, paint remover, shellac, and lacquers; infiltration and replacement of myeloid elements, such as in leukemia or the lymphomas; and idiopathic factors, in which no identifiable precipitating cause can be found. The following discussion focuses on acquired aplastic anemia, which carries a poorer prognosis and follows a more rapidly fatal course than the primary types.

Diagnostic Evaluation

The onset of clinical manifestations, which include anemia, leukopenia, and decreased platelet count, is usually insidious, not unlike that seen in leukemia. Definitive diagnosis is determined from bone marrow aspiration, which demonstrates the conversion of red bone marrow to yellow, fatty bone marrow.

Therapeutic Management

The objectives of treatment are based on the recognition that the underlying disease process is failure of the bone marrow to carry out its hematopoietic functions. Therefore therapy is directed at restoring function to the marrow and involves two main approaches: (1) immunosuppressive therapy to remove the presumed immunologic functions that prolong aplasia, and/or (2) replacement of the bone marrow through transplantation. Bone marrow transplantation is the treatment of choice for severe aplastic anemia when a suitable donor exists.

Currently, ***antilymphocyte globulin (ALG)*** or ***antithymocyte globulin (ATG)*** is the principal drug treatment for aplastic anemia. ALG and ATG are similar products; therefore the terms are used interchangeably. The rationale for using ATG is based on the theory that aplastic anemia may be a result of autoimmunity. ATG suppresses T-cell–dependent autoimmune responses but does not cause bone marrow suppression. The optimum schedule for ATG administration is still under investigation. It is usually given intravenously over 12 to 16 hours, after a test dose to check for hypersensitivity. Subsequent doses are given depending on the reduction in circulating lymphocytes.

Androgens may be used with ATG to stimulate erythropoiesis, although the exact mechanism of erythropoietic action is unclear. Cyclosporine may also be administered in children who fail to respond to ATG, and success has also been achieved using high-dose methylprednisolone. Intravenous immunoglobulin has been used with success in aplastic anemia of infectious origin (Dwyer, 1992).

Because of the relatively poor prognosis in aplastic anemia treated with drug therapy, ***bone marrow transplantation*** should be considered *early* in the course of the disease if a compatible donor can be found. Transplantation is more successful when performed before multiple transfusions have sensitized the child to leukocyte and HLA antigens. Children who are eligible for transplantation should be transferred to one of the medical centers that specialize in this procedure. For nontransfused patients, pretransplantation immunosuppressive therapy consists of administration of near lethal doses of cyclophosphamide. Those patients who have received transfusions undergo total body irradiation with immunosuppressives (e.g., cyclophosphamide, ATG, or cyclosporine). Bone marrow transplantation is associated with a 63% 5-year survival rate (Pinkel, 1993; Sanders and others, 1994).

Nursing Considerations

The care of the child with aplastic anemia is similar to that of the child with leukemia (i.e., preparing the family for the diagnostic and therapeutic procedures, preventing complications from the severe pancytopenia, and emotionally supporting them in terms of a potentially fatal outcome [see Chapters 23 and 36]). Since each of these aspects has already been discussed, only the exceptions are presented here. Bone marrow transplantation is discussed in Chapter 36.

During administration of ATG, vigilant attention must be directed to the intravenous infusion to prevent extravasation. To prevent sclerosing from extravasation, a central vein should be used. Because of the child's susceptibility to infection, meticulous care of the venous access catheter is essential. Although anaphylactic reactions to ATG are rare, emergency preparations should be planned in advance, with epinephrine and oxygen readily available. The nurse should observe for other reactions. Immediate reactions to ATG are common and include fever and skin rash. Delayed reactions (serum sickness) may also occur within 7 to 14 days of a course of ATG, and the manifestations are similar to immediate reactions. The symptoms are reversed and in the case of serum sickness may be prevented with corticosteroids.

Since chemotherapeutic agents may be used, many of the reactions, such as nausea and vomiting, alopecia, and mucosal ulceration, can be encountered. In addition, extensive ecchymotic areas of the oral mucosa from thrombocytopenia require meticulous mouth care to prevent breakdown, bleeding, and infection. Fortunately, these lesions, which look painful, cause little or no discomfort. Local anesthetics are not necessary, but anorexia is still a consequence because of the edematous nature of the lesions. Liquid, bland, and soft diets are usually tolerated best.

DEFECTS IN HEMOSTASIS

Hemostasis is the process that stops bleeding when a blood vessel is injured. Vascular and plasma clotting factors, as well as platelets, are required. A complex system of clotting, anticlotting, and clot breakdown (fibrinolysis) mechanisms exists in equilibrium to ensure clot formation only in the presence of blood vessel injury and to limit the clotting process to the site of vessel wall injury. Dysfunction in these systems will lead to bleeding or thrombosis.

MECHANISMS INVOLVED IN NORMAL HEMOSTASIS

To understand the role that factor deficiencies play in promoting bleeding tendencies, it is necessary to review the normal coagulation process of the blood. Although the process is complex, clotting depends on three main factors: vascular influence, platelet role, and clotting factors.

TABLE 35-4 Blood-Clotting Factors

FACTOR NUMBER	SYNONYMS
I	Fibrinogen
II	Prothrombin
III	Platelet factor 3, thromboplastin
IV	Calcium
V	Labile factor, proaccelerin, Ac globulin
VII	Serum prothrombin conversion accelerator (SPCA), proconvertin, stable factor
VIII	Antihemophilic factor (AHF),
IX	Plasma thromboplastin component (PTC), Christmas factor
X	Stuart-Prower factor
XI	Plasma thromboplastin antecedent (PTA)
XII	Hageman factor
XIII	Fibrin-stabilizing factor (FSF)
KAL	Prekallikrein, Fletcher factor
HMK	High-molecular-weight kininogen, Fitzgerald factor

Vascular Influence. At the time and site of injury, several events occur to initiate hemostasis: local vasoconstriction, compression of the blood vessels by extravasated blood, release of von Willebrand factor (vWF) by endothelial walls, and the presence of collagen in exposed subendothelial cells that acts as a site for platelet adhesion.

Platelet Role. Normally the platelets do not adhere to each other or to normal endothelium. However, at the time a blood vessel is injured, the following occur. Platelet adhesion occurs at the site of the injury, providing a plug. The platelets change shape, develop pseudopods, and release a variety of chemicals to stimulate vasoconstriction and vessel repair, and to activate and recruit more platelets to the injury site. Receptor sites are located on the platelets for fibrinogen and other adhesive proteins, causing the platelets to stick together (aggregation). As the membrane of the platelet changes, the phospholipids necessary for blood coagulation are exposed, resulting in fibrin production, which secures the platelet plugs to the site. Finally, the clot compresses and is secured to the injury.

Defects in platelets and clotting factors are the most common causes of bleeding during childhood. The following discussion focuses on the major conditions that require nursing intervention.

Clotting Factors. The clotting factors (Table 35-4) are activated in sequence to develop a fibrin clot. Two mechanisms exist that can generate prothrombin activator complex to produce thrombin from prothrombin:

1. **Intrinsic pathway.** Factor XII, high-molecular-weight kininogen (HMK, Fitzgerald factor), and prekallikrein (KAL, Fletcher factor) react on a negative-charged surface (contact activation reaction) to activate factor XI (PTA, plasma thromboplastin antecedent). The partial thromboplastin time (PTT) measures abnormalities in the intrinsic pathway (abnormalities in factors XII, HMK, KAL, IX, VIII, X, V, II, and I).
2. **Extrinsic pathway.** A lipoprotein tissue factor stimulates activation of factor VII. The prothrombin time (PT) measures abnormalities of the extrinsic pathway (abnormalities in factors V, VII, X, II, and I).

Laboratory tests to assess hemostasis are presented in Table 35-5.

HEMOPHILIA

The term ***hemophilia*** refers to a group of bleeding disorders in which there is a deficiency of one of the factors necessary for coagulation of the blood. Although the symptomatology is similar regardless of which factor is deficient, the identification of specific factor deficiencies has allowed definitive treatment with replacement agents.

In about 80% of all cases of hemophilia, the inheritance pattern is demonstrated as X-linked recessive (see Chapter 5). The two most common forms of the disorder are ***factor VIII deficiency (hemophilia A*** or ***classic hemophilia),*** and ***factor IX deficiency (hemophilia B*** or ***Christmas disease).*** The following discussion is primarily concerned with factor VIII deficiency, which accounts for about 75% of all cases.

Modes of Transmission

Hemophilia is transmitted as an X-linked recessive disorder; however, only about 60% of affected children have a positive family history for the disease. As many as one third of the cases of hemophilia may be caused by gene mutation. The most frequent pattern of transmission is between an unaffected male and a trait-carrier female (see Fig. 5-8). With improved treatment for persons with hemophilia, it is important to consider the results of mating between an affected male and a normal female or a carrier female. For example, the mating of an affected male with a carrier female results in a 1:4 chance of producing either an affected son or daughter, a carrier daughter, or a normal son. This is one of the few ways in which a female inherits the disorder. Female carriers may have low levels of factor VIII and be symptomatic.

Pathophysiology and Clinical Manifestations

The basic defect of hemophilia A is a deficiency of factor VIII (antihemophilic factor [AHF]). AHF is produced by the liver and is necessary for the formation of thromboplastin in phase I of blood coagulation. The less antihemophilic factor found in the blood, the more severe the disease.

A major feature of hemophilia is that its expression varies markedly in the degree of bleeding severity. Hemophilia is generally classified into three groups according to the severity of factor deficiency as described below; approximately 60% to 70% of children with hemophilia demonstrate the severe form of the disorder:

Clinical Severity	Factor VIII Activity	Bleeding Tendency
Severe	1%	Spontaneous bleeding without trauma
Moderate	1%-5%	Bleeding with trauma
Mild	5%-50%	Bleeding with severe trauma or surgery

The effect of hemophilia is prolonged bleeding anywhere from or in the body. With severe factor deficiencies, hemorrhage can occur as a result of minor trauma, such as

TABLE 35-5 Laboratory Tests for Hemostasis*

TEST	DESCRIPTION	COMMENTS
PLATELET FUNCTION		
Bleeding time	Measures time interval for bleeding from small superficial wound to cease	Function depends on platelet aggregation and vasoconstriction; two common methods used: Ivy (incision made on forearm) and Duke (incision made on earlobe)
Tourniquet test	Measures platelet function and capillary fragility; apply pressure to forearm with tourniquet for 5 to 10 minutes	Normal response is absence of petechiae or fewer than 10 Abnormal in platelet and connective tissue disorders
Clot retraction test	Measures degree to which clot shrinks and expresses serum	Depends on platelet function
BLOOD CLOTTING MECHANISMS		
Whole blood clotting time	Meaasures time it takes for clot to form *within* blood	Prolonged clotting time indicates problem in thrombin-to-fibrin phase or in any factor in intrinsic clotting mechanism; difficult test to standardize; therefore often unreliable results
Prothrombin time (PT)	Measures activity of prothrombin, as well as factors necessary for its conversion to thrombin and fibrinogen	Actually does not measure prothrombin levels, but activity; since it bypasses intrinsic-extrinsic mechanism, detects deficiencies of factors V, VII, X, and fibrinogen, as well as prothrombin
Partial thromboplastin time (PTT) test	Similar to PT but measures activity of thromboplastin, which depends on intrinsic clotting factors	Specific for factor deficiencies, except factor VII, which results in a normal PTT but prolonged PT
Thromboplastin generation test (TGT)	Measures blood's ability to generate thromboplastin	Allows for determination of specific factor deficiencies, especially distinguishing between factors VIII and IX
Prothrombin consumption test	Indirectly measures thromboplastin generation and prothrombin response	Normally, as blood clots, prothrombin is converted to thrombin so that serum is depleted of prothrombin; if thromboplastin is decreased (as a result of extrinsic factor deficiencies), not all prothrombin will be converted and removed from serum
Fibrinogen level	Directly measures fibrinogen levels in blood	Not dependent on phase I or II deficiencies

*Normal values are listed in Appendix D.

after circumcision, during loss of deciduous teeth, or as a result of a slight fall or bruise. In children with less severe deficiencies the bleeding tendency may not be noted until the onset of walking.

Subcutaneous and intramuscular hemorrhages are common. ***Hemarthrosis,*** which refers to bleeding into the joint cavities, especially the knees, elbows, and ankles, is the most frequent form of internal bleeding and often results in bony changes and consequently long-term loss of range of motion in repeatedly affected joints. Early signs of hemarthrosis are a feeling of stiffness, tingling, or ache in the affected joint, followed by a decrease in the ability to move the joint. Obvious signs and symptoms are warmth, redness, swelling, and severe pain with considerable loss of movement. Spontaneous hematuria is not uncommon. Epistaxis may occur but is not as frequent as other kinds of hemorrhage. Petechiae are uncommon in persons with hemophilia because repair of small hemorrhages depends on platelet function, not on blood-clotting mechanisms.

Bleeding into the tissue can occur anywhere but is serious if it occurs in the neck, mouth, or thorax, since the airway can become obstructed. Intracranial hemorrhage can have fatal consequences and is one of the major causes of death. Hemorrhage anywhere along the gastrointestinal tract can lead to anemia, and bleeding into the retroperitoneal cavity is especially hazardous because of the large space for blood to accumulate. Hematomas in the spinal cord can cause paralysis.

Diagnostic Evaluation

The diagnosis is usually made on a history of bleeding episodes, evidence of X-linked inheritance, and laboratory findings. To understand the significance of various tests of hemostasis, it is helpful to recall the usual mechanisms to control bleeding (i.e., the function of platelets and of clotting factors). Tests that measure platelet function, such as the bleeding time, are all normal in persons with hemophilia, whereas tests that assess clotting factor function may

TABLE 35-6 Adjunctive Therapy for Hemophilia A

PROBLEM	THERAPY
Acute hemarthrosis Early Late	Ice packs, non-weight-bearing sling or lightweight splint may be helpful; rarely, joint aspiration
Intramuscular hemorrhage	Non-weight-bearing support; complete bed rest for hemorrhage in muscles of lower spine attaching to trochanter of femur
Tongue and mouth lacerations	Antifibrinolytic agent (aminocaproic acid), sedation, NPO in small child; local application of oradhesive gauze may be beneficial for gum bleeding
Extractions of permanent teeth	Antifibrinolytic agent beginning 1 day before surgery; continue 7-10 days
Painless spontaneous gross hematuria	Increased PO fluids; corticosteroids and/or factor VII are used by some

Modified from Lusher JM: Management of hemophilia. In Westphal RG, Smith DM, editors: *Treatment of hemophilia and von Willebrand's disease; new developments,* Arlington, VA, 1989, American Association of Blood Banks.

be abnormal (Table 35-5). The tests specific for hemophilia include factor VIII and IX assays, procedures normally done by specialized laboratories. Other tests are those that depend on specific factors for a reaction to occur, especially the partial thromboplastin time (PTT) test. Carrier detection is possible in classic hemophilia using DNA testing and is an important consideration in families in which female offspring may have inherited the trait.

Therapeutic Management

The primary therapy for hemophilia is replacement of the missing clotting factor. The products currently available are ***factor VIII concentrate,*** to be reconstituted with sterile water immediately before use, and ***DDAVP (1-deamino-8-D-arginine vasopressin),*** a synthetic form of vasopressin that is the treatment of choice in mild hemophilia and von Willebrand disease (except type IIB). After DDAVP administration a threefold to fourfold rise in factor VIII activity should occur. Since the goal is to raise the factor VIII level at least 30%, patients with moderate factor VIII deficiency do not benefit. In addition, various therapies are employed when bleeding occurs or is anticipated (Table 35-6).

Cryoprecipitate is no longer recommended for use in treating factor VIII deficiency. Since 1988, with the advent of highly purified factor VIII concentrate (monoclonal), and since the licensing of recombinant factor VIII concentrate in 1992 (not marketed as a blood product but as a drug), practitioners have been advised by the National Hemophilia Foundation to use only these products. Cryoprecipitate cannot be treated to safely eliminate hepatitis or HIV viruses.

Aggressive factor concentrate replacement therapy is initiated to prevent chronic crippling effects from joint bleeding. If replacement therapy is begun immediately, local measures such as ice applications and splinting are seldom needed.

Other drugs may be included in the therapy plan, depending on the source of the hemorrhage. Corticosteroids are used judiciously to treat inflammation in the joints; nonsteroidal antiinflammatory drugs (NSAIDs), such as aspirin, indomethacin (Indocin), and phenylbutazone (Butazolidin), should not be used, because they inhibit platelet function. Ibuprofen (Motrin, Advil, or Nuprin; also available by prescription for children) has been demonstrated to be safe despite its antiplatelet aggregation effect. Oral use of epsilon aminocaproic acid (EACA, Amicar) prevents clot destruction; however, its use is limited to mouth or trauma surgery, and a dose of factor concentrate must be given first. The child may rinse the mouth with this medicine and then swallow it.

A regular program of exercise and physical therapy is an important aspect of management. If started early and continued throughout adulthood, planned, individualized physical activity strengthens muscles around joints and may decrease the number of spontaneous bleeding episodes.

NURSING ALERT Passive range-of-motion exercises should never be part of an exercise regimen after an acute episode, since the joint capsule could easily be stretched and bleeding could recur. Active range-of-motion exercises are best so that the patient can control his or her own pain tolerance.

Treatment without delay results in more rapid recovery and a decreased likelihood of complications; therefore most children are treated at home. The family is taught the technique of venipuncture and how to administer the AHF to children over 3 years of age. The child learns the procedure for self-administration at 9 to 12 years of age. Home treatment is highly successful and the rewards, in addition to the immediacy, are less disruption of family life, fewer school or work days missed, and enhancement of the child's self-esteem and independence.

Prognosis. The progress made in hemophilia care over the past two decades has been striking. The advent of home infusion therapy coupled with recent advances in producing safer and more effective factor concentrates has revolutionized the treatment and management of hemophilia (Lusher and others, 1993). Home infusion therapy enables early recognition of joint and muscle bleeds, as well as immediate adequate treatment with clotting factor. Early treatment has significantly reduced the morbidity formerly associated with hemophilia. The concept of comprehensive hemophilia treatment centers offers the child with hemophilia and the family a coordinated multidisciplinary approach to meeting their needs and improving the child's health and well-being.

Although there is no cure for hemophilia, its symptoms can be controlled and its potentially crippling deformities markedly reduced or even avoided. Today many children with hemophilia function with minimal or no joint damage. They are normal children with an average life expectancy in every aspect but one: they have a tendency to bleed, which is a significant inconvenience but not necessarily a life-threatening event (Hilgartner and others, 1993).

Unfortunately, those individuals with hemophilia who were treated before current purification techniques for factor VIII concentrate may have been exposed to human immunodeficiency virus (HIV). It is estimated that 70% to 90% of these patients have seroconverted to HIV positive, and a significant number have AIDS (Holman and others, 1990). As these individuals become sexually active, the issue of sexual transmission of HIV becomes increasingly important. The adolescent must be knowledgeable regarding safe sexual behavior. Individuals with hemophilia diagnosed and treated with factor concentrates since 1985 are at virtually no risk for developing HIV infection.

Nursing Considerations

The earlier a bleeding episode is recognized, the more effectively it can be treated. Signs that indicate internal bleeding are especially important to recognize. Children are aware of internal bleeding and are very reliable in telling the examiner where an internal bleed is. In addition, the nurse maintains a high level of suspicion when a child with hemophilia demonstrates unlikely signs, such as headache, slurred speech, loss of consciousness (from cerebral bleeding), and black, tarry stools (from gastrointestinal bleeding).

Prevent Bleeding. The goal of prevention of bleeding episodes is directed toward decreasing the risk of injury. Prophylactic administration of factor VIII concentrates is reserved for troublesome target joints in an effort to break the bleeding cycle. The cost of the factor concentrate (about $70,000 to $90,000 a year for treatment of severe hemophilia) and poor venous access prohibit its routine administration. Also, its half-life is short (only 10 to 12 hours). Prevention of bleeding episodes is geared mostly toward appropriate exercises to strengthen muscles and joints and to allow age-appropriate activity. During infancy and toddlerhood the normal acquisition of motor skills creates innumerable opportunities for falls, bruises, and minor wounds. Restraining the child from mastering motor development can herald more serious long-term problems than allowing the behavior. However, the environment should be made as safe as possible, with close supervision maintained during playtime, to minimize incidental injuries.

For older children the family usually needs assistance in preparing for school. A nurse who knows the family can be instrumental in discussing the situation with the school nurse and in jointly planning an appropriate schedule of activity. Since almost all persons with hemophilia are boys, the physical limitations in regard to active sports may be a difficult adjustment, and activity restrictions must be tempered with sensitivity to the child's emotional, as well as physical, needs. Use of protective equipment, such as padding and helmets, is particularly important, and noncontact sports, especially swimming, are encouraged (Dragone, 1992).

To prevent oral bleeding, some changes in dental hygiene may be needed to minimize trauma to the gums, such as use of a water irrigating device, softening the toothbrush in warm water before brushing, or using a sponge-tipped disposable toothbrush. A regular toothbrush should be soft bristled and small in size. Adolescents also need to be advised of the dangers of using safety razors with blades and be encouraged to use an electric shaver.

Since any trauma can lead to a bleeding episode, all persons caring for these children must be aware of their disorder. These children should wear medical identification, and older children are encouraged to recognize situations in which disclosing their condition is important, such as during dental extraction or injections. Health personnel need to take special precautions to prevent the use of procedures such as intramuscular injections. The subcutaneous route is substituted for intramuscular injections whenever possible. Venipunctures for blood samples are usually preferred by these children. There is usually less bleeding after the venipuncture than after finger or heel punctures. Neither aspirin nor any aspirin-containing compound should be used. Acetaminophen (Tylenol) is a suitable aspirin substitute, especially for use during control of pain at home.

Recognize and Control Bleeding. The earlier a bleeding episode is recognized, the more effectively it can be treated. Factor replacement therapy should be instituted according to established medical protocol, and supportive measures may be implemented, such as (1) applying pressure to the area for at least 10 to 15 minutes to allow clot formation, (2) immobilizing and elevating the area above the level of the heart to decrease blood flow, and (3) applying cold to promote vasoconstriction. When parents and older children are taught such measures beforehand, they can be prepared to initiate immediate treatment before blood loss is excessive. Plastic bags of ice or cold packs should be kept in the freezer for such emergencies. However, such measures should not take the place of factor replacement.

Prevent Crippling Effects of Bleeding. As a result of repeated episodes of hemarthrosis, incompletely absorbed blood in the joints, and limitation of motion, bone and muscle changes occur that may result in flexion contractures and joint fixation. Obviously, prevention of bleeding is the ideal goal. However, since spontaneous bleeding is not uncommon in persons with severe hemophilia, definitive measures, including replacement therapy and physical therapy, are necessary to limit joint damage.

During bleeding episodes the joint is elevated and immobilized. Active range-of-motion exercises are usually instituted after the acute phase. This allows the child to control the degree of exercise according to the level of discomfort. Physical therapy is beneficial to promote maximum function of the joint and unaffected body parts. Success of a physical therapy plan involves control of pain by administering analgesics before therapy and adjusting the dose to provide maximum benefit.

If an exercise program is instituted in the home, a physical therapist or public health nurse may need to supervise compliance with the regimen. Occasionally, orthopaedic intervention, such as casting, application of traction, or aspiration of blood, may be necessary to preserve joint function. Diet is also an important consideration, since excessive body weight can increase the strain on affected joints, especially the knees, and predispose the child to hemarthrosis. Consequently, calories need to be supplied in accordance with energy requirements.

Support Family and Prepare for Home Care. The discovery of factor concentrates has greatly changed the outlook for these children. Bleeding can be minimized, and the child can live a much more normal, unrestricted life. Children are taught to take responsibility for their disease at an early age. They learn their limitations and other preventive measures, as well as self-administration of the prophylactic AHF.

The needs of families who have children with hemophilia are best met through a comprehensive team approach of physicians (pediatrician, hematologist, orthopaedist), nurse, social worker, and physical therapist. Parent-group discussions are beneficial in meeting those needs often best met by similarly affected families. For example, with the improved prognosis for these children, parents and adolescents with hemophilia are faced with vocational and financial problems, in addition to concern over future childbearing. Once children reach 21 years of age, many insurance companies will no longer carry them. This can be disastrous in terms of the cost of treatment. The **National Hemophilia Foundation*** and the **Canadian Hemophilia Society†** provide numerous services and publications for both health providers and families.

Children who have become infected with HIV through transfusions and factor replacement products are faced with the consequences of this dreaded disease. Consequently, they need the support of health professionals, especially in the area of safe sexual practices to avoid disease transmission and public education regarding AIDS and ways to deal with public reactions to persons who have AIDS (see p. 1601 for a discussion of AIDS).

Identify Persons at Risk. Genetic counseling is essential as soon as possible after diagnosis. Unlike many other disorders in which both parents carry the trait, the feeling of responsibility for this condition usually rests with the mother. Without an opportunity to discuss her feelings, the couple relationship can suffer. Prenatal DNA testing can identify affected fetuses and identify carriers in most cases.

VON WILLEBRAND DISEASE (vWD)

vWD is a hereditary bleeding disorder characterized by a factor VIII deficiency and low levels of factor VIII–related antigen (FVIII R:Ag). In addition, the functional component of the factor VIII molecule that is required for platelet adhesion to vascular subendothelium (known as ***von Willebrand factor*** or ***ristocetin cofactor***) is reduced. This results in prolonged bleeding time because the platelets fail to adhere to the walls of the ruptured vessel to form a platelet plug. vWD can be mild, moderate, or severe. Most cases are mild and require intervention only for dental and surgical procedures.

The most characteristic clinical feature of vWD is an increased tendency toward bleeding from mucous membranes. The most common symptom is frequent nosebleeds, followed by gingival bleeding, easy bruising, and menorrhagia in females. Unlike hemophilia, it affects both males and females because its inheritance is autosomal dominant. However, the treatment and final outcome are similar in both disorders. Treatment of bleeding is with DDAVP and/or a specially concentrated clotting factor called Humate-P.

Nursing Considerations

The nursing goals are similar to those for hemophilia, with special considerations related to epistaxis (p. 1599) and menorrhagia. Replacement therapy may be beneficial before the menstrual cycle to lessen the flow. Teaching the adolescent methods to prevent embarrassing accidents during menstruation, such as wearing plastic-lined underpants and using double sanitary pads, helps her adjust to the inconvenience. Interestingly, these females frequently do not experience excessive bleeding at the time of delivery. This is thought to be because of increased levels of factor VIII during pregnancy. Decisions regarding childbearing are difficult because of the dominant pattern of inheritance.

IDIOPATHIC THROMBOCYTOPENIC PURPURA (ITP)

ITP is an acquired hemorrhagic disorder that is characterized by (1) excessive destruction of platelets ***(thrombocytopenia)*** and (2) ***purpura*** (a discoloration caused by petechiae beneath the skin). Although the cause is unknown, it is believed to be an autoimmune response to disease-related antigens. It is the most frequently occurring thrombocytopenia of childhood.

The disease occurs in one of two forms: an acute, self-limiting course or a chronic condition interspersed with remissions. The acute form is most commonly seen after upper respiratory tract infections or after the childhood diseases of measles, rubella, mumps, and chickenpox.

The most common clinical manifestations of either type include (1) easy bruising with petechiae and/or ecchymoses, particularly over bony prominences; (2) bleeding from mucous membranes, such as epistaxis, bleeding gums, and internal hemorrhage with evidence of hematuria, hematemesis, melena, hemarthrosis, and menorrhagia; and (3) hematomas over the lower extremities that may result in chronic leg ulcers.

Diagnostic Evaluation

In ITP the platelet count is reduced to below 20,000 mm^3/dl; therefore tests that depend on platelet function are abnormal, such as the tourniquet test, bleeding time, and clot retraction. Although there is no definitive test on which to establish a diagnosis of ITP, several tests are usually performed to rule out other disorders in which thrombocyto-

---

*110 Green St., Room 303, New York, NY 10012; (212) 219-8180 or (800) 42HANDI.

†1450 City Councillors, Bureau 840, Montreal, Quebec H3A 2E6; (514) 848-0503.

penia is a manifestation, such as systemic lupus erythematosus, lymphoma, or leukemia.

Therapeutic Management

Management is primarily supportive, since the course of the disease is self-limited in the majority of cases. Activity is restricted at the onset while the platelet count is low and while active bleeding or progression of lesions is occurring. This restriction is most easily accomplished in the hospital. Corticosteroids are employed for children with the highest risk for serious bleeding, for chronic cases with increased bleeding tendencies, as an adjunct to life-threatening hemorrhage, or before splenectomy to decrease the risk of surgical bleeding. Administration of intravenous gamma globulin has proved successful in increasing the platelet count of children with chronic disease. Children with chronic ITP have also experienced and sustained a rise in platelet count when treated with ascorbate (a product of ascorbic acid [vitamin C]) (Cohen and others, 1993). Splenectomy is reserved for symptomatic children with chronic disease or as an emergency measure in the event of life-threatening hemorrhage. Packed RBCs may be given to replace blood lost in symptomatic children. Platelets are seldom administered.

Prognosis. The majority of children have a self-limited course without major complications. Some children will develop chronic ITP and require ongoing therapy. A splenectomy may modify the disease process, and the child will be asymptomatic.

Nursing Considerations

Nursing care is largely supportive. Children and parents need careful explanations of the rationale behind the therapies employed and support in their efforts to comply. The nursing considerations of controlling bleeding and preventing bruising are similar to those discussed in the section on leukemia. The harmful effects of using aspirin to control pain are critical for these children; therefore salicylate substitutes are always used. As in any condition with an uncertain outcome, the family needs emotional support, especially during periods of hospitalization.

DISSEMINATED INTRAVASCULAR COAGULATION (DIC)

DIC, also known as ***consumption coagulopathy,*** is not a primary disease but a secondary disorder of coagulation that complicates a number of pathologic processes (such as hypoxia, acidosis, shock, and endothelial damage [burns]) and many severe systemic disease states (such as congenital heart disease, necrotizing enterocolitis, gram-negative bacterial sepsis, rickettsial infections, and some severe viral infections). The disease is characterized by inappropriate systemic activation and acceleration of the normal clotting mechanism.

Pathophysiology

DIC occurs when the first stage of the coagulation process is abnormally stimulated. Although there is no well-defined sequence of events, two distinct phases can be identified.

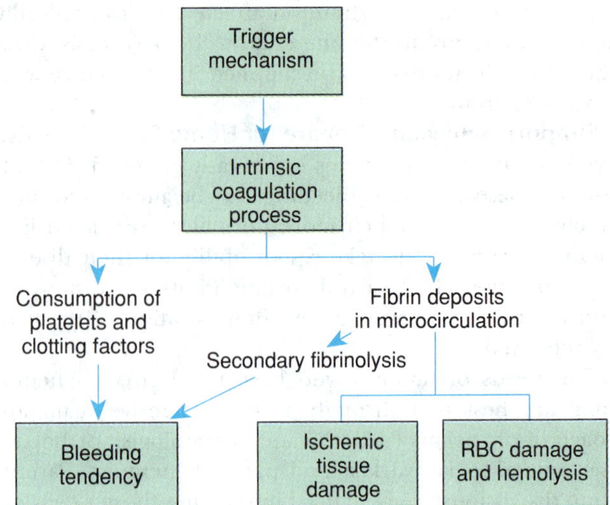

FIG. 35-5 Effects of disseminated intravascular coagulation.

First, when the clotting mechanism is triggered in the circulation, thrombin is generated in greater amounts than can be neutralized by the body. Consequently, there is rapid conversion of fibrinogen to fibrin with aggregation and destruction of platelets. If local and widespread fibrin deposition in blood vessels takes place, obstruction and eventual necrosis of tissues occur. Second, the fibrinolytic mechanism is activated, causing extensive destruction of clotting factors. With a deficiency of clotting factors the child is vulnerable to uncontrollable hemorrhage into vital organs. An additional complication is damage and hemolysis of red blood cells (Fig. 35-5).

Clinical Manifestations

Signs of DIC are those of many other diseases, which often confuses the diagnosis. There is evidence of bleeding—petechiae, purpura, bleeding from openings in the skin (e.g., a venipuncture site or surgical incision), hypotension, and dysfunction of organs from infarction and ischemia.

Diagnostic Evaluation

DIC is suspected when there is an increased tendency to bleed, as from venipuncture or blood taken from the heel, and bleeding from the umbilicus, trachea, or gastrointestinal tract. Hematologic findings include prolonged prothrombin (PT), partial thromboplastin (PTT), and thrombin times. There is a profoundly depressed platelet count, fragmented red blood cells, and depleted fibrinogen.

Therapeutic Management

Treatment is directed toward control of the underlying or initiating cause, which in most instances stops the coagulation problem spontaneously. Platelets and fresh frozen plasma may be needed to replace lost plasma components, especially in the child whose underlying disease remains uncontrolled. The very ill newborn infant may require exchange transfusion with fresh blood. The administration of heparin to inhibit thrombin formation is most often restricted to severe cases.

Nursing Considerations

The goals of nursing care are to be aware of the possibility of DIC in the severely ill child and to recognize signs that might indicate its presence. The skills needed to monitor intravenous infusion and blood transfusions and to administer heparin are the same as for any child receiving these therapies. Since the child is usually cared for in an intensive care unit, the special needs of the family must be considered (see Chapter 26).

EPISTAXIS (NOSEBLEEDING)

Isolated and transient episodes of epistaxis, or nosebleeding, are common in childhood. The nose is a highly vascular structure, and bleeding usually results from direct trauma, including blows to the nose, foreign bodies, and nose picking, or from mucosal inflammation associated with allergic rhinitis and upper respiratory tract infections or drying of the mucous membranes in environments with low humidity (Katsanis and others, 1988). Ordinarily the bleeding stops spontaneously or with minimal pressure and requires no medical evaluation or therapy.

Recurrent epistaxis and severe bleeding may indicate an underlying disease, particularly vascular abnormalities, leukemia, thrombocytopenia, and clotting factor deficiency diseases such as hemophilia and von Willebrand disease. It may also be a sign of "sniffing" cocaine or "crack." Sometimes nosebleeds are associated with administration of aspirin, even in small doses. Persistent nosebleeding requires medical evaluation.

Nursing Considerations

Nosebleeds are often a frightening experience for the child and parents. A calm, reassuring manner can alleviate anxiety and promote the child's cooperation. Since most of the nosebleeding originates in the anterior part of the nasal septum, bleeding can be controlled by applying pressure to the nose with the thumb and forefinger (see Emergency Treatment box). During this time the child breathes through the mouth.

In the event that hemorrhage continues, the child should be evaluated by a practitioner, who may pack the nose with epinephrine-soaked gauze. After a nosebleed, petroleum or water-soluble jelly can be inserted into each nostril to prevent crusting of old blood and to lessen the likelihood of the child's picking at the nose and restarting the hemorrhage. Whenever possible, factors believed to increase the likelihood of epistaxis are eliminated, such as discouraging nose picking, altering the household humidity by placing a cool-mist vaporizer in the child's room, or using acetaminophen rather than aspirin (which is not recommended for children because of aspirin's possible association with Reye syndrome). If cocaine is being used, appropriate referral for drug counseling is needed.

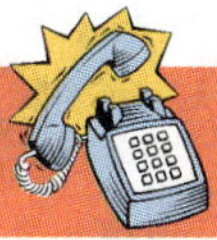

EMERGENCY TREATMENT
Epistaxis

1. Have child sit up and lean forward (not lying down).
2. Apply continuous pressure to nose with thumb and forefinger for at least 10 minutes.
3. Insert cotton or wadded tissue into each nostril and apply ice or cold cloth to bridge of nose if bleeding persists.
4. Keep child calm and quiet.

EMERGENCY TREATMENT

IMMUNOLOGIC DEFICIENCY DISORDERS

A number of disorders can cause profound, often life-threatening alterations within the body's immune system. The most serious are those conditions that completely depress immunity, such as severe combined immunodeficiency disease. However, the one disorder that generates the most anxiety, within both the family and the community at large, is ***human immunodeficiency virus (HIV) infection*** and the subsequent development of ***acquired immunodeficiency syndrome (AIDS).***

Several classifications of immune dysfunction exist. For example, in AIDS, severe combined immunodeficiency syndrome (SCIDS), and Wiskott-Aldrich syndrome, the body is unable to produce an immune response. In other disorders, the immune response is misdirected. In autoimmune disorders, antibodies, macrophages, and lymphocytes attack healthy cells. Some disorders and their target organs include myasthenia gravis, muscle cells; Graves disease, thyroid cells; and type I diabetes, B-cells in the pancreas. With the exception of AIDS, SCIDS, and Wiskott-Aldrich syndrome, the other disorders are discussed elsewhere in the book.

MECHANISMS INVOLVED IN IMMUNITY

In simple terms, the function of the immune system is to recognize "self" from "non-self" and to initiate responses to eliminate the non-self or the foreign substance known as ***antigen.*** All cells in the body have specific cell surface markers that are unique to that individual. These cell surface markers are known as the ***major histocompatibility complex (MHC).*** Since the markers were first identified on human leukocytes, they are commonly referred to as ***human leukocyte antigens (HLAs).***

The protective mechanisms of the body consist of complex, overlapping defense systems. Intact skin serves as the first line of protection for the body. Body secretions such as saliva, sweat, and tears contain chemicals that can kill many organisms. The stomach contains acids that can destroy swallowed pathogens as they adhere to the mucus of the nose and mouth. Organisms trapped in these areas are expelled by sneezing or coughing. If the foreign substance has penetrated these barriers, cellular elements are mobilized.

The immune system includes the ***primary lymphoid organs*** (thymus, bone marrow, and probably liver) and the ***secondary lymphoid organs*** (lymph nodes, spleen, and gut-associated lymphoid tissue [GALT]). The functions of the immune system are basically of two types: nonspecific and

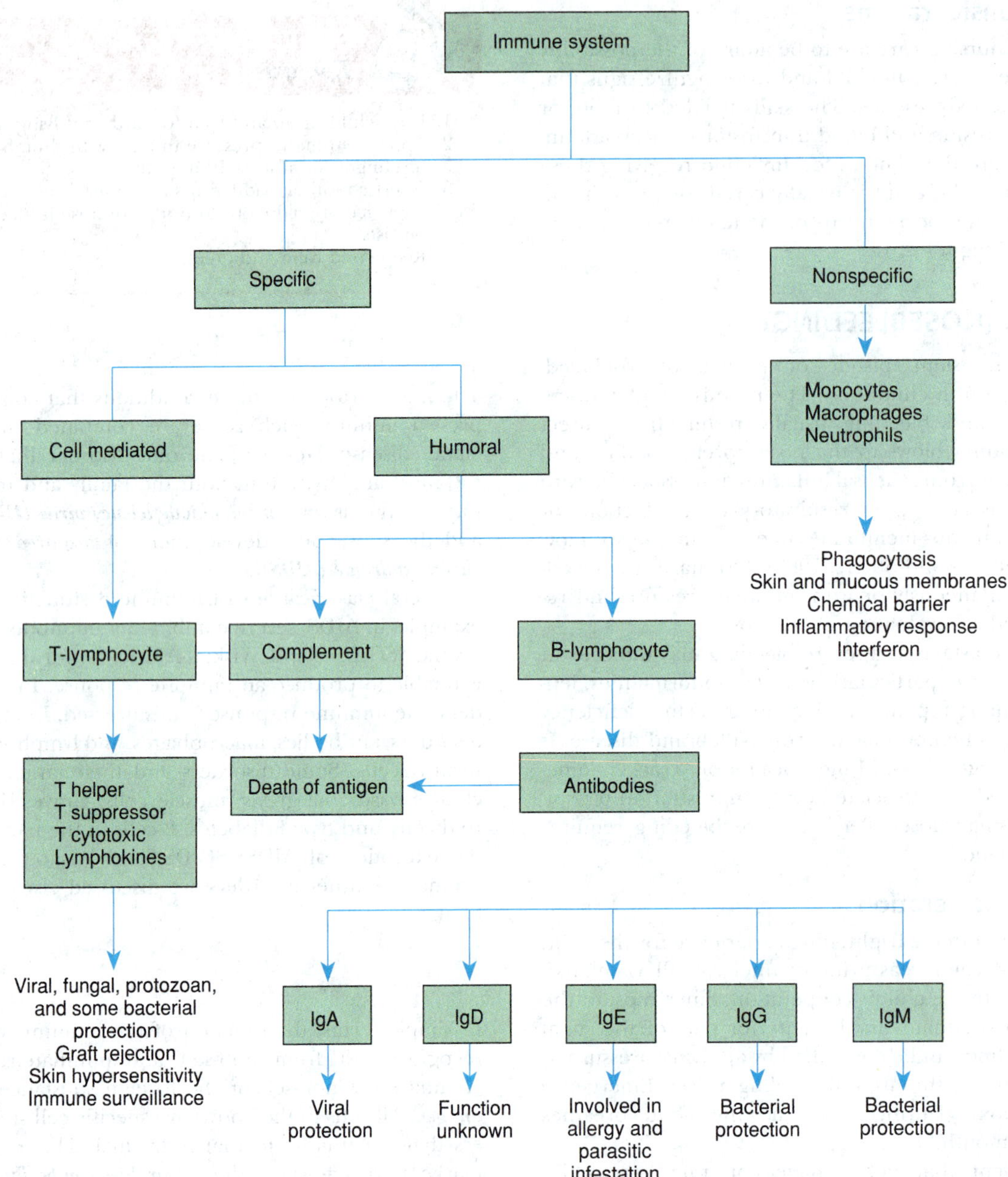

FIG. 35-6 Components of immune system.

specific (Fig. 35-6). ***Nonspecific immune defenses*** are activated on exposure to any foreign substance but react similarly regardless of the type of antigen; they are unable to identify the antigen, except to know that it is "non-self." The principal activity of this system is ***phagocytosis,*** the process of ingesting and digesting foreign substances. Phagocytic cells include neutrophils and monocytes (see p. 1566). Specific defenses are discussed in the following paragraphs.

Specific Immune Mechanisms

Specific (adaptive) defenses are those that have the ability to recognize the antigen and respond selectively. The components of adaptive immunity are humoral immunity and cell-mediated immunity. The cells responsible for these two forms of immunity are the lymphocytes, specifically B-lymphocytes and T-lymphocytes.

Humoral immunity is involved with antibody production and complement and is concerned with immune processes occurring *outside* the cells, such as on cell surfaces or in body fluids. The principal cell involved in antibody production is the ***B-lymphocyte.*** In humans the exact site of production of the B-lymphocyte is speculative, although it is probably the bone marrow. When challenged with an antigen, B-cells divide and differentiate into ***plasma cells.*** The plasma cells produce and secrete large quantities of ***antibodies*** specific to the antigen. Five classes of antibodies of ***immunoglobulins (Ig)*** have been identified: G, M, A, D, and E, each serving a specific function.

On initial exposure to an antigen, the B-lymphocyte system begins to produce antibody, predominantly IgM, which appears in 2 to 3 days. This process is referred to as the ***primary antibody response.*** With subsequent exposure to the antigen, a ***secondary antibody response*** occurs. Specific IgG antibodies are formed within 4 to 10 days. An example of the secondary response is consecutive administration of immunizations, often called boosters. ***Memory B-cells*** allow the immune system to recognize the same antigen for months or years.

When antibody reacts with antigen, they bind to form an ***antigen-antibody complex.*** This binding serves several functions. Antibody aids in the phagocytosis of antigen by sensitizing it in such a manner that it is more readily destroyed by phagocytes, a process known as ***opsonization.***

Antibody also activates or fixes ***complement,*** the second component of humoral immunity. The complement system is a series of proteins (C_1 to C_9) present in serum that results in a cascade of enzymatic actions and death of a viable antigen. After being activated by antibody, complement produces a chemotactic factor that summons T-lymphocytes and macrophages to the antigen site.

Cell-mediated immunity (CMI) is involved in a variety of specific functions mediated by the ***T-lymphocyte*** and occurs *within* the cell. T-lymphocytes do not carry typical immunoglobulins on their surfaces as do the B-cells. Microscopically T-cells appear identical; however, they are functionally heterogeneous in that several subsets have been identified, including cytotoxic T-cells, helper T-lymphocytes, and suppressor T-lymphocytes. T-cells may also be classified structurally by the distinctive molecules on their surface, known as ***cluster designations (CDs).*** Once mature, T-cells carry markers known as T_2 (CD_2), T_3 (CD_3), T_5 (CD_5), and T_7 (CD_7). Helper T-cells carry a T_4 (CD_4) marker and a suppressor, and cytotoxic T-cells carry a T_8 (CD_8) marker.

Specific functions of CMI include: (1) protection against most viral, fungal, and protozoan infections and slow-growing bacterial infections, such as tuberculosis; (2) rejection of histoincompatible grafts; (3) mediation of cutaneous delayed hypersensitivity reactions, such as in tuberculin testing; and (4) probably immune surveillance for malignant cells. In addition, they also have regulatory functions within the immune system. For example, helper T-lymphocytes assist B-lymphocytes and other types of T-cells to mount an optimum immune response.

The cellular immune response is initiated when a T-lymphocyte is sensitized by antigen. In response to this contact the T-cell releases numerous humoral factors called ***lymphokines,*** which eventually bring about death of the antigen. ***Interferons*** are a group of proteins secreted by leukocytes and infected host cells that nonspecifically inhibit viral replication, promote phagocytosis, and stimulate the killer activity of sensitized lymphocytes.

HUMAN IMMUNODEFICIENCY VIRUS (HIV) INFECTION AND ACQUIRED IMMUNODEFICIENCY SYNDROME (AIDS)

HIV infection and AIDS have generated intense medical investigation and even greater public concern and fear. The first published reports of unusual opportunistic infections in previously healthy individuals appeared in 1981; retrospective analysis of data demonstrated the existence of cases since 1978, with the first case diagnosed in a child. In 1983 and 1984 a retrovirus (RNA virus) found in AIDS patients was characterized and named. Over 4200 children with AIDS have been reported to the Centers for Disease Control and Prevention (CDC). Early in the epidemic, the East Coast accounted for the majority of cases in the United States and is still well represented. However, children with the virus have been reported from 46 states, and the HIV seroprevalence in parts of rural Georgia and Florida is as high as that in New York and New Jersey. In 1991, HIV infection ranked seventh as the leading cause of death for ages 1 to 4 years, ninth for ages 5 to 14, and sixth for ages 15 to 24 years. Although HIV infection was the seventh leading cause of death for ages 1 to 4 years, the number of deaths due to this cause was relatively small—155 deaths, or 2% of deaths from all causes for that age-group (National Center for Health Statistics, 1993). The term ***human immunodeficiency virus (HIV) type I*** is the official name of the virus.

Etiology

HIV is the causative agent for AIDS. The virus has been found in blood and almost all body fluids (semen, saliva, vaginal secretions, urine, breast milk, and tears). HIV infection is one of the most devastating illnesses to occur in recent times. It affects all of the organ systems. Transmission of the virus occurs either horizontally by sexual contact or parenteral exposure to blood, or vertically from an HIV-infected mother to child. Breast-feeding has been identified as the source of the virus in several cases. There is no evidence that *casual* contact between infected and uninfected individuals can spread the virus.

Sexual activity is the leading cause of exposure in the United States. Parenteral exposure occurs when there is direct blood-to-blood contact with an individual infected with HIV. This can be through sharing of needles for injection drug use, accidental needle sticks, or blood exposure to nonintact skin or mucous membranes, such as during anal or vaginal intercourse. Individuals engaging in these high-risk behaviors are most at risk for HIV infection. Initially, AIDS was identified in sexually active homosexual males; however, people living with AIDS (PLWA) are a diverse group.

In child and adolescent age-groups three populations are primarily affected—children who are exposed in utero to an infected mother, children who have received blood products, especially children with hemophilia (before testing began in 1985), and, recently, adolescents who are infected after engaging in high-risk behaviors. Each group has unique needs relative to the origin of the infection. The majority of children with HIV are less than 5 years of age and constitute a small percentage of the infected population. Approximately 86% of these cases resulted from perinatal transmission, and 11% resulted from blood transfusions. Before donor blood was routinely tested for HIV (March, 1985), children with hemophilia were especially at risk because factor concentrates were prepared from pooled plasma. Recent advances in the preparation of concentrates and testing for the antibody to HIV in blood products have reduced the risk to these children and other children who require frequent blood products.

The third population, adolescents who place themselves

at risk because of sexual activity with an infected partner and other high-risk behavior, is rapidly increasing. The rising incidence of the disorder is of major concern. In the United States the current doubling time for cases is 11 to 12 months. Although individuals exposed to the virus may demonstrate a positive antibody test to HIV, it is uncertain when they will develop the clinical syndrome of AIDS.

Pathophysiology

HIV infection does not follow any single clinical course. In patients with HIV infection, the immunosuppression is a result of a decreased number of CD_4 T-cells, as well as functional defects (Pantaleo, Graziosi, and Fauci, 1993). Abnormal B-cell function is apparent early in pediatric HIV infection. Because the helper T-cell controls B-cell functioning, young children with HIV infection are deficient in both cellular and humoral systems. The immunoglobulins are nonfunctional, leaving the body defenseless to recurrent bacterial infections. These children are also unable to form antibody after immunization.

Clinical Manifestations

The majority of children with perinatally acquired AIDS are normal at birth but develop symptoms within the first 18 months of life. The clinical manifestations include lymphadenopathy, hepatosplenomegaly, recurrent bacterial infections, and pulmonary diseases, which occur in two thirds of HIV-infected children. These include *Pneumocystis carinii* pneumonia (PCP), lymphocytic interstitial pneumonitis (LIP), and pulmonary lymphoid hyperplasia (PLH). Failure to thrive occurs frequently in HIV-infected infants. Chronic diarrhea may be directly due to the HIV or secondary to opportunistic GI infections (Trowbridge and others, 1991). Neurologic involvement occurs in 75% to 90% of children with HIV infection (see Chapter 37). It is usually manifested as a developmental delay or, after achieving normal development, loss of motor milestones. There is decreased brain growth, as evidenced by microcephaly and abnormal neurologic examination findings. Kaposi sarcoma, one of the hallmarks of the adult disease, is found in less than 1% of affected children. Clinical and laboratory signs of AIDS in children occur any time after exposure, regardless of the route of infection.

Diagnostic Evaluation

The diagnosis of HIV infection is usually made by serum antibody tests. Enzyme immunoassays (EIAs) are widely used for HIV screening, and Western blot or immunofluorescent antibody tests should be performed to confirm the diagnosis. A positive HIV-antibody test result in a child age 18 months or older usually indicates infection. Infants born to HIV-positive mothers are almost always seropositive at birth as a result of passively acquired maternal antibody. Serum antibodies can be detected in the child for as long as 18 months after birth. Therefore, other tests, such as HIV culture, detection of HIV DNA sequences using the polymerase chain reaction (PCR), and detection of specific HIV antigen, such as the HIV-p24 antigen assay, are used. If one of these tests is positive, a second diagnostic test should be performed to reduce the possibility of misdiagnosis (American Academy of Pediatrics, 1994; Kline and others, 1994).

According to the CDC, specific criteria for the diagnosis of AIDS in children less than 13 years old include the presence of one of the following:

1. Confirmed HIV in blood or tissues
2. Symptoms meeting CDC case definition
3. HIV antibody and one or more of the following disorders: secondary infectious diseases, recurrent bacterial infections, or secondary cancers

Children 13 years of age and above are diagnosed based on adult criteria. Three specific clinical categories for both HIV infection and AIDS established by the CDC are:

Category A (one or more of following conditions without any from category B or C)
- Asymptomatic HIV infection
- Persistent generalized lymphadenopathy (PGL)
- Acute (primary) HIV infection with accompanying illness or history of acute HIV infection

Category B (symptomatic conditions that are not included in category A or C and meet one of the following criteria:
- Conditions are attributed to HIV infection or indicate a defect in cell-mediated immunity
- Conditions are considered by physicians to have a clinical course or require management that is complicated by HIV infection

Category C
- Clinical conditions listed as AIDS surveillance case definitions

The clinical categories are further subdivided into three groups based on CD_4 T-lymphocyte counts. The expanded AIDS surveillance case definition includes subgroups A_3 and B_3, whose CD_4 plus T-lymphocyte counts are <200 cells/µl or a CD_{4+} percentage of <14. In addition to retaining the 23 clinical conditions in the previous AIDS surveillance definition, the expanded definition includes pulmonary tuberculosis (TB), recurrent pneumonia, and invasive cervical cancer (1993 revised classification, 1992).

Before testing, counseling should be provided to the child and family or guardian. This includes an explanation of what HIV is, the reason for the test, confidentiality issues, risk reduction behaviors, implications of positive test results, and beneficial effects of early intervention (Arapadi and Caspe, 1991).

Therapeutic Management

The goals of therapy for HIV infection include slowing the growth of the virus, preventing and treating the opportunistic infections, nutritional support, and symptomatic treatment. Several drugs are used to slow the viral infection. Zidovudine *(AZT [Retrovir])*, dideoxycytidine (ddC), and didanosine (DDI) have been approved for use in pediatrics (Working Group, 1993). Combination drug therapy is being used currently, and many investigational drugs are available for children. Although not a cure, these drugs control disease progression. Clinical improvements include weight gain in children with previous growth retardation, a reduction in the size of an enlarged liver and spleen, improvement in measures of brain function, and improvement in immune system function (Krasinski, 1991). Treatment is also directed at the prevention and management of the opportunistic infections. The most common infections are interstitial pneumonia, caused by *Pneumocystis carinii,* which occurs in more than 70% of affected children, and chronic candidiasis. Therapy for *P. carinii* includes trimethoprim/sulfamethoxazole (Bactrim, Septra) and pentamidine. If a skin reaction, fever, or cytopenia occurs secondary to the trimethoprim/sulfamethoxazole, the drug is discontinued and pentamidine is used.

Gamma globulin administration may be helpful to compensate for the deficiency of B-lymphocytes. Ongoing studies are investigating the benefits of periodic administration of intravenous gamma globulin.

Pediatric HIV disease often leads to marked failure to thrive and multiple nutritional deficiencies. Nutritional management may be difficult because of recurrent illness, respiratory distress, diarrhea, and other physical problems. The developing malnutrition may produce an acquired immunodeficiency similar to that caused by HIV. Intensive nutritional interventions should be instituted when the child's growth begins to slow or weight begins to decrease (Nicholas, 1991).

Disease prevention is of great importance for these children, and immunization against common childhood illnesses is recommended for all children with HIV infection. The only change in the schedule is the use of inactivated poliovirus (IPV) rather than oral poliovirus (OPV) for these children and their close contacts. These children must be evaluated for their response to the immunizations. For children with AIDS, the pneumococcal and influenza vaccines are recommended. Varicella zoster immune globulin should be given within 96 hours of chickenpox exposure. If HIV-positive children are exposed to measles, they should be immunized within 72 hours.

Nursing Considerations

Nursing considerations are primarily directed at caring for the child with AIDS, educating the public regarding the *realistic* concerns in terms of communicability of the virus, and preventing the transmission of the virus. Recommendations for preventing spread of the virus consist of universal precautions, which are the same guidelines for preventing the transmission of other blood-borne diseases, such as hepatitis B virus (see Infection Control, Chapter 27). These precautions are routinely enforced, regardless of whether the child is infected.

The nurse's role is central to the child and family. The nurse serves as educator, direct care provider, case manager, and advocate. As with all chronic illnesses, these children will have a great deal of involvement with the health care system. The physiologic care of the AIDS patient is directed at minimum exposure to infections, nutritional support, comfort measures, and assessment and recognition of changes in status that may indicate impending sepsis or other complications. The pyschologic interventions will vary with the unique circumstances of the child and family.

The family of the child with perinatal transmission usually is faced with multiple problems, since the mother is infected. The nurse must assess the parent(s) for signs of illness and help them receive regular health care. Assistance should be offered to help them parent a child with a chronic illness. Grandparents or other relatives may have to assume responsibility for the care of the child. These surrogate parents should be given support for their role. If no extended family is available, the child may be placed in a foster home or group home.

Since these children are frequently ill, they may have multiple hospitalizations (Boland and Santacroce, 1994). Foster care is difficult to arrange because of the nature of the illness and the fear of disease transmission. These children have many symptoms, including diarrhea, lung infections, failure to thrive, and encephalopathy. They are often irritable, with a shrill cry, and difficult to console. If there is family involvement, nursing considerations are directed at supporting the family. Whenever possible, social services and home health and nutritional services such as Women, Infants, and Children (WIC) should be made available. Nurses in community-based systems of care have impacted greatly on the quality of life for these children. The nurses assist with placement and school attendance. Since the disease is congenitally acquired, the parents must deal with feelings of guilt. They will need support during the disease progression and terminal phase.

Another group of individuals increasingly infected with HIV is adolescents. As young people engage in the high-risk behaviors associated with AIDS, the possibility of infection increases. Adolescents must be taught about the risk factors, including injection drug use and high-risk sexual practices, such as anal intercourse and sex with multiple partners (see Human Immunodeficiency Virus Infection and Acquired Immunodeficiency Syndrome, Chapter 20). Numerous AIDS educational materials are available.

One of the most pressing concerns in caring for PLWA is protection for the caregiver. Although children with HIV infection can be held, cuddled, and fed safely, universal precautions (see Chapter 27) must be used in caring for all patients. Unfortunately, the public is also very fearful of contracting the disease from AIDS victims, and criticism and ostracism of the child and family are common. In an effort to protect the child and deal with the community's fear, the family may keep the child at home in an atmosphere of overprotection. While certain precautions are justified in limiting exposure to sources of infection, they must be tempered with concern for the child's normal developmental needs. Both the family and the community need education about HIV to dispel many of the myths that have been perpetuated by the uninformed.*

Of major concern for both family and community has been school attendance for children with AIDS (Santelli, Birn, and Linde, 1993). Both the CDC (1985) and the American Academy of Pediatrics (1986) have published guidelines regarding school attendance, which include the following:

1. Unrestricted school attendance for most school-aged children and adolescents, including children with AIDS or AIDS-

*Information is available from the AIDS hotline: (800) 342-2437 (AIDS); and from the National Pediatric HIV Resource Center, 15 S. 9th St., Newark, NJ 07107, (201) 268-8251 or (800) 362-0071.

NURSING CARE PLAN
The Child with HIV Infection

NURSING DIAGNOSIS: High risk for infection related to impaired body defenses, presence of infective organisms

PATIENT GOAL 1: Will experience minimized risk of infection

• **NURSING INTERVENTIONS/*RATIONALES***

Use thorough handwashing technique *to minimize exposure to infective organisms*

Advise visitors to use good handwashing technique *to minimize exposure to infective organisms*

Place child in room with noninfectious children or in private room

Restrict contact with persons who have infections, including family, other children, friends, and members of staff; explain that child is highly susceptible to infection *to encourage cooperation and understanding*

Observe medical asepsis as appropriate *to decrease risk of infection*

Encourage good nutrition and adequate rest *to promote body's remaining natural defenses*

Explain to family and older child importance of contacting health professional if exposed to childhood illnesses (e.g., chickenpox, measles) *so that appropriate immunizations can be given*

*Administer appropriate immunizations as prescribed *to prevent specific infections*

*Administer antibiotics as prescribed

• **EXPECTED OUTCOMES**

Child does not come in contact with infected persons or contaminated articles

Child and family apply good health practices

Child exhibits no evidence of infection

PATIENT GOAL 2: Will not spread disease to others

• **NURSING INTERVENTIONS/*RATIONALES***

Implement and carry out universal precautions, especially body substance isolation, *to prevent spread of virus* (see Infection Control, Chapter 27)

Instruct others (e.g., family, members of staff) in appropriate precautions; clarify any misconceptions about communicability of virus, *since this is a frequent problem and may interfere with use of appropriate precautions*

Teach affected children protective methods *to prevent spread of infection,* (e.g., handwashing, handling genital area, care after using bedpan or toilet)

Endeavor to keep infants and small children from placing hands and objects in contaminated areas

Place restrictions on behaviors and contacts for affected children who bite or who do not have control of their bodily secretions

Assess home situation and implement protective measures as feasible in individual circumstances

• **EXPECTED OUTCOME**

Others do not acquire the disease

*Dependent nursing action.

NURSING DIAGNOSIS: Altered nutrition: less than body requirements related to recurrent illness, diarrheal losses, loss of appetite, oral candidiasis

PATIENT GOAL 1: Will receive optimum nourishment

• **NURSING INTERVENTIONS/*RATIONALES***

Provide high-calorie, high-protein meals and snacks *to meet body requirements for metabolism and growth*

Provide foods child prefers *to encourage eating*

Fortify foods with nutritional supplements (e.g., powdered milk or commercial supplements) *to maximize quality of intake*

Provide meals when child is most likely to eat well

Use creativity to encourage child to eat (see Feeding the Sick Child, Chapter 27)

Monitor child's weight and growth *so that additional nutritional interventions can be implemented if growth begins to slow or weight drops*

*Administer antifungal medication as ordered *to treat oral candidiasis*

• **EXPECTED OUTCOME**

Child consumes a sufficient amount of nutrients (specify)

NURSING DIAGNOSIS: Impaired social interaction related to physical limitations, hospitalizations, social stigma toward HIV

PATIENT GOAL 1: Will participate in peer-group and family activities

• **NURSING INTERVENTIONS/*RATIONALES***

Assist child in identifying personal strengths *to facilitate coping*

Educate school personnel and classmates about HIV *so that child is not unnecessarily isolated*

Encourage child to participate in activities with other children and family

Encourage child to maintain phone contact with friends during hospitalization *to lessen isolation*

• **EXPECTED OUTCOME**

Child participates in activities with peer group and family

NURSING DIAGNOSIS: Altered sexuality pattern related to risk of disease transmission

PATIENT GOAL 1: Will exhibit healthy sexual behavior

• **NURSING INTERVENTIONS/*RATIONALES***

Educate adolescent about the following *so that adolescent has adequate information to identify safe, healthy expressions of sexuality*

- Sexual transmission
- Risks of perinatal infection

NURSING CARE PLAN
The Child with HIV Infection—cont'd

Dangers of promiscuity
Abstinence, use of condoms
Avoidance of high-risk behaviors
Encourage adolescent to talk about feelings and concerns related to sexuality *to facilitate coping*

• **EXPECTED OUTCOMES**
Adolescent exhibits a positive sexual identity
Adolescent does not infect other individuals

NURSING DIAGNOSIS: Pain related to disease process (i.e., encephalopathy, treatments)

PATIENT GOAL 1: Will exhibit minimal or no evidence of pain or irritability

• **NURSING INTERVENTIONS/*RATIONALES***
Assess pain (see Pain Assessment, Chapter 20)
Use nonpharmacologic strategies *to help child manage pain*
For infants, may try general comfort measures (i.e., rocking, holding, swaddling, reducing environmental stimuli [may or may not be effective because of encephalopathy])
Use pharmacologic strategies (see Pain Management, Chapter 27)
Plan preventive schedule if analgesics are effective in relieving continuous pain
Encourage use of premedication for painful procedures *to minimize discomfort*
Child may benefit from use of adjunctive analgesics (e.g., antidepressants) that are effective against neuropathic pain
Use pain assessment record *to evaluate effectiveness of pharmacologic and nonpharmacologic interventions*

• **EXPECTED OUTCOME**
Child exhibits absence of or minimal evidence of pain or irritability

NURSING DIAGNOSIS: Altered family processes related to having a child with a dreaded and life-threatening disease

PATIENT (FAMILY) GOAL 1: Will receive adequate support and will be able to meet needs of child

• **NURSING INTERVENTIONS/*RATIONALES* AND EXPECTED OUTCOMES**
See Nursing Care Plan: The Family of the Ill or Hospitalized Child, Chapter 26

NURSING DIAGNOSIS: Anticipatory grief related to having a child with a potentially fatal illness

See Nursing Care Plan: The Child Who Is Terminally Ill or Dying, Chapter 23

related complex, or who have antibody to the virus, is recommended with the approval of their personal physician.

2. Students who do not have control of their bodily secretions, who display behaviors such as biting, or who have open sores that cannot be covered may present a greater risk and should be given a more restricted school environment until more is known about the disease.

Nurses need to be knowledgeable of these guidelines and of changes that may occur as additional information about the virus is known. School nurses, in particular, play a vital role in educating the public and in monitoring the needs of the affected child. Confidentiality is a major factor—the number of personnel aware of the child's condition should be kept to a minimum. In addition, school personnel must be aware of sanitary practices to prevent spread of the virus, including proper disposal of items contaminated with blood (e.g., sanitary napkins, tissues from caring for a bloody nose, or bandages used in cleaning a wound). Nursing care of the child with AIDS is summarized in the Nursing Care Plan on pp. 1604-1605.

SEVERE COMBINED IMMUNODEFICIENCY DISEASE (SCID)

SCID is a defect characterized by absence of both humoral and cell-mediated immunity. The terms ***Swiss-type lymphopenic agammaglobulinemia,*** an autosomal-recessive form of the disease, and ***X-linked lymphopenic agammaglobulinemia*** have been used to describe this disorder, which, as the names imply, can follow either mode of inheritance.

Pathophysiology

The exact cause of SCID is unknown. The theories include (1) a defective stem cell that is incapable of differentiating into B- or T-cells; (2) defective organs responsible for the differentiating process, primarily the thymus and lymphoid complex; or (3) an enzymatic defect that suppresses lymphocytic cell function.

The consequence of the immunodeficiency is an overwhelming susceptibility to infection and to the ***graft-vs-host reaction,*** which can occur when any histoincompatible (unmatched) tissue from an immunocompetent donor is infused into the immunodeficient recipient. Because of its immunodeficiency, the body is unable to reject the foreign incompatible tissue. Therefore the antigenic donor cells attack the host's tissues. The graft-vs-host reaction is a serious complication in the only known treatment for SCID, bone marrow transplantation.

Clinical Manifestations

The most common manifestation is susceptibility to infection early in life, most often by 3 months of age, when prenatal acquired immunity is exhausted. Specifically, the disorder in children is characterized by chronic infection, failure to completely recover from an infection, frequent reinfection, and infection with unusual agents. In addition, the history reveals no logical source of infection. Failure to thrive is a consequence of the persistent illness.

If the child should receive a foreign tissue, such as blood supplements, signs of graft-vs-host reaction, such as fever, skin rash, alopecia, hepatosplenomegaly, and diarrhea, are expected. Since the reaction requires 7 to 20 days for tissue damage to become evident, the symptoms may be mistaken for an infection. However, the presence of a graft-vs-host reaction increases the child's susceptibility to overwhelming infection and therefore is a grave complication.

Diagnostic Evaluation. Diagnosis is usually based on a history of recurrent, severe infections from early infancy, a familial history of the disorder, and specific laboratory findings, which include lymphopenia, lack of lymphocyte response to antigens, and absence of plasma cells in the bone marrow. Documentation of immunoglobulin deficiency is difficult during infancy because of the normally delayed response of infants to produce their own immunoglobulins and maternal transfer of immunoglobulin G.

Therapeutic Management

The only definitive treatment is a histocompatible bone marrow transplant. The most suitable donor is a sibling with a matched HLA bone marrow. Because SCID is inherited, an identical twin, who usually is a perfect donor, is not a candidate, since that offspring would also display the disorder. Since the host's immunologic system is incompetent, graft rejection is not a problem. However, a graft-vs-host reaction is always a possibility, and once it occurs, little can be done to reverse the process.

Other approaches to SCID are providing passive immunity with intravenous immunoglobulin and maintaining the child in a sterile environment. The latter is effective only if instituted before the existence of any infectious process in the infant, and it represents an extreme effort to prevent life-threatening infections. Other investigational transplant procedures include nonidentical HLA bone marrow grafts and fetal liver or thymus transplants. However, the results are still uncertain, although they provide potential hope for future children born with the disorder.

Nursing Considerations

Nursing care depends on the type of therapy used. If bone marrow transplantation is attempted, the care is consistent with that needed for bone marrow transplantation for any condition (see Chapter 36). To prevent infection, all interventions aimed at protecting the immunocompromised child are implemented (see Nursing Care Plan: The Child with HIV Infection, pp. 1604-1605). However, even with exacting environmental control, these children are prone to opportunistic infection. Chronic fungal infections of the mouth and nails with *Candida albicans* are frequent problems despite vigorous efforts at prevention or treatment. A hoarse voice may result from repeated esophageal and vocal cord erosions from the fungus. It is important to stress to parents that such conditions are not a result of laxity on their part in preventing them but are the result of the severe immunologic disorder. Parents should be encouraged to immediately notify a physician regarding any evidence of a worsening infection.

Since the prognosis for SCID is very poor if a compatible bone marrow donor is not available, nursing care is directed at supporting the family in caring for a child with a life-threatening illness (see Chapter 23). Genetic counseling is essential because of the modes of transmission in either form of the disorder.

WISKOTT-ALDRICH SYNDROME

The Wiskott-Aldrich syndrome is an X-linked recessive disorder characterized by a triad of abnormalities: (1) thrombocytopenia, (2) eczema, and (3) immunodeficiency of selective functions of B- and T-lymphocytes.

Pathophysiology

The exact defect is unknown. A variety of pathologic findings are evident. The platelets are abnormally small in size and have a shortened life span, possibly because of a metabolic defect in their synthesis. The primary immunologic defect consists of the inability of phagocytes (macrophages) to process foreign antigens, particularly polysaccharides such as pneumococcus. As a result, immunologically competent cells fail to produce normal immunoglobulin patterns. Early in life the immunoglobulin levels may be normal, but later low levels of IgM are observed. Typically, isohemagglutinins (anti-A and anti-B agglutinins in the blood) are decreased or absent.

The thymus and lymph nodes are normal at birth but become progressively dysfunctional with age until a profound cellular immunodeficiency results. Consequently, these children are highly susceptible to infection and malignancy, especially lymphoma and leukemia.

Clinical Manifestations

At birth the major effect of the disorder is bleeding because of the thrombocytopenia. As the child grows older, recurrent infection and eczema become more severe, and the bleeding becomes less frequent.

Eczema is typical of the allergic type and readily becomes superinfected. Chronic infection with herpes simplex is a frequent problem and may lead to chronic keratitis with loss of vision. From infection, chronic pulmonary disease, sinusitis, and otitis media result. In those children who survive the bleeding episodes and overwhelming infections, malignancy presents an additional threat to survival.

Diagnostic Evaluation

Diagnosis can usually be made during the neonatal period because of the thrombocytopenia. Specific tests for immunologic function confirm the diagnosis. Carrier detection is also possible.

Therapeutic Management

Medical treatment primarily involves (1) counteracting the bleeding tendencies with platelet transfusions, (2) using intravenous immunoglobulin to provide passive immunity

(Dwyer, 1992) and, (3) administering prophylactic antibiotics to prevent and control infection. Splenectomy may be performed to reverse the thrombocytopenia, but asplenia imposes the additional risk of fulminant infection. These children require the same prophylactic measures as any child with asplenia—appropriate immunizations and continuous antibiotics—and, despite their immune deficiency, they are able to mount an adequate immunologic response to the inactivated vaccines. When an HLA-matched donor exists, bone marrow transplantation is the treatment of choice.

Nursing Considerations

Because of the grave prognosis for these children, the main nursing consideration is supporting the family in the care of a child with a life-threatening illness (see Chapter 23). Physical care is directed at controlling the problems imposed by the disorder. The measures used to control bleeding are similar to those discussed under hemophilia and epistaxis. Another major goal is related to preventing or controlling infection. Since eczema is a troublesome problem, nursing measures specific to this condition are especially important.

The genetic implications of this X-linked recessive disorder differ little from those of hemophilia. However, because of the multiplicity of defects, the emotional adjustment and physical care required for these children are greater than those of many other conditions. The nurse can be especially supportive by providing short-term goals during periods of hospitalization and by focusing on long-range needs through coordinated efforts with a public health nurse.

KEY POINTS

- Major functions of the hematologic system include production of cells, oxygenation, nutrient distribution to the cells, immune protection, collection of wastes from the cells, and heat regulation.
- The major blood-forming organs of the body are red bone marrow, the lymphatic system, and the reticuloendothelial system.
- Anemia is defined as reduction of the red blood cell volume or hemoglobin concentration to levels below normal; disorders are classified either by etiology/physiology or by morphology.
- The nurse's role in treatment of anemia is to assist in establishing a diagnosis, prepare the child for laboratory tests, decrease tissue oxygen needs, implement safety precautions, and observe for complications.
- The main nursing goal in prevention of nutritional anemia is parent education regarding correct feeding practices.
- Four types of sickle cell crisis are vaso-occlusive, splenic sequestration, aplastic, and hyperhemolytic.
- Nursing care of the child with sickle cell disease is aimed at teaching the family how to recognize and prevent sickling, managing pain during splenic crises, and helping the child and parents adjust to a lifelong, potentially fatal disease.
- Nursing care of the child with thalassemia entails observing for complications of multiple blood transfusions, helping the child cope with the effects of illness, and fostering parent-child adjustment to long-term illness.
- Common causes of aplastic anemia include irradiation, drugs, industrial and household chemicals, infections, infiltration and replacement of myeloid elements, and idiopathic conditions.
- Nursing care of the child with hemophilia involves preventing bleeding by decreasing the risk of injury, recognizing and managing bleeding, preventing the crippling effects of joint degeneration, and preparing and supporting the child and family for home care.
- Pediatric clinical manifestations of AIDS include failure to thrive, interstitial pneumonitis, and hepatosplenomegaly.

REFERENCES

American Academy of Pediatrics, Committee on Infectious Diseases: *1994 Red Book,* ed 23, Elk Grove Village, IL, 1994, The Academy.

American Academy of Pediatrics, Committee on Nutrition: *Pediatric nutrition handbook,* ed 3, Elk Grove Village, IL, 1992, The Academy.

American Academy of Pediatrics, Committee on School Health, and Committee on Infectious Diseases: School attendance of children and adolescents with human T lymphotropic virus Ill/lymphadeopathy-associated virus infection, *Pediatrics* 77(3):430-432, 1986.

American Pain Society: *Principles of analgesic use in the treatment of acute pain and chronic cancer pain,* ed 3, Skokie, IL, 1992, The Society.

Arpadi S, Caspe WB: HIV testing, *J Pediatr* 119(1, pt 2):8-13, 1991.

Balkaran B and others: Stroke in a cohort of patients with homozygous sickle cell disease, *J Pediatr* 120(3):360-366, 1992.

Boland MG, Santacroce SJ: Case management: nursing care roles in the care of the child and family. In Pizzo PA, Wilfert CM: *Pediatric AIDS: the challenge of HIV infection in infants, children, and adolescents,* ed 2, Baltimore, 1994, Williams & Wilkins.

Bray GL and others: Assessing clinical severity in children with sickle cell disease: preliminary results from a cooperative study, *Am J Pediatr Hematol Oncol* 16(1):50-54, 1994.

Brozovic M and others: Pain relief in sickle cell crises, *Lancet* 2(8507):624-625, 1986.

Centers for Disease Control: Education and foster care of children infected with human T-lymphotropic virus type Ill/lymphadenopathy-associated virus, *MMWR* 34(34): 517-521, 1985.

Charache S: Experimental therapy of sickle cell disease, *Am J Pediatr Hematol Oncol* 16(1):62-66, 1994.

Charache S, Lubin B, Reid CD: *Management and therapy of sickle cell disease,* US Department of Health and Human Services, Public Health Service, National Institutes of Health, Pub No 89-2117, Washington, DC, 1989.

Cohen HA and others: Treatment of chronic idiopathic thrombocytopenic purpura with ascorbate, *Clin Pediatr* 32(5):300, 1993.

Day S, Brunson G, Wang W: A successful education program for parents of infants with newly diagnosed sickle cell disease, *J Pediatr Nurs* 17(1):52-57, 1992.

Day S and others: Iron overload? In sickle cell disease? *MCN* 18:330, 1993.

Dragone MA: Bleeding disorders: hemophilia and von Willebrand's disease. In Jackson PL, Vessey JA: *Primary care of the child with a chronic condition,* St Louis, 1992, Mosby.

Dwyer JM: Manipulating the immune system with immune globulin, *N Engl J Med* 326(2):107-116, 1992.

Francis EE, Williams D, Yarandi H: Anemia as an indicator of nutrition in children enrolled in a Head Start program, *J Pediatr Health Care* 7:156-160, 1993.

Furman WL, Crist WM: Biology and clinical applications of hemopoietins in pediatric practice, *Pediatrics* 90(5):716, 1992.

Fuchs G and others: Gastrointestinal blood loss in older infants: impact of cow milk versus formula, *J Pediatr Gastroenterol Nutr* 16(1):4-9, 1993.

Giardini C: Bone marrow transplantation for thalassemia: experience in Pesaro, Italy, *Am J Pediatr Hematol Oncol* 16(1):6-10, 1994.

Hilgartner MW and others: Hemophilia growth and developmental study: design, methods, and entry data, *Am J Pediatr Hematol Oncol* 15(2):208-218, 1993.

Holman RC and others: Age and human immunodeficiency virus infection in persons with hemophilia in California, *Am J Public Health* 80(8):967-969, 1990.

Idjradinata P, Pollitt E: Reversal of developmental delays in iron-deficient anaemic infants treated with iron, *Lancet* 341:1-4, 1993.

Johnson FL and others: Bone marrow transplantation for sickle cell disease: the United States experience, *Am J Pediatr Hematol Oncol* 16(1):22-26, 1994.

Katsanis E and others: Prevalence and significance of mild bleeding disorders in children with recurrent epistaxis, *J Pediatr* 113(1, pt 1):73-76, 1988.

Kline MW and others: A comparative study of human immunodeficiency virus culture, polymerase chain reaction and anti-human immunodeficiency virus immunoglobulin A antibody detection in the diagnosis during early infancy of vertically acquired human immunodeficiency virus infection, *Pediatr Infect Dis J* 13(2):90-94, 1994.

Koch DA and others: Behavioral contracting to improve adherence in patients with thalassemia, *J Pediatr Nurs* 8(2):106-111, 1993.

Kodish E and others: Bone marrow transplantation for sickle cell disease, *N Engl J Med* 325(19):1349-1353, 1991.

Krasinski K: Retroviral therapy and clinical trials for HIV-infected children, *J Pediatr* 119(1):63-68, 1991.

Lanzkowsky P: Problems in diagnosis of iron deficiency anemia, *Pediatr Ann* 14(9):618-636, 1985.

Linden JV, Paul B, Dressler KP: A report of 104 transfusion errors in New York State, *Transfusion* 32:601-606, 1992.

Lozoff B, Jimenez E, Wolf AW: Long-term developmental outcome of infants with iron deficiency, *N Engl J Med* 325:687-694, 1991.

Lusher JM and others: Recombinant factor VIII for the treatment of previously untreated patients with hemophilia A: safety, efficacy, and development of inhibitors, *N Engl J Med* 328:453-459, 1993.

Mankad VN: Growth and development in sickle hemoglobinopathies, *Am J Pediatr Hematol Oncol* 14(4):283-284, 1992 (editorial).

Martin MB, Butler RB: Understanding the basics of β-thalassemia major, *Pediatr Nurs* 19(2):143-145, 1993.

Maurer HS and others: A prospective evaluation of iron chelation therapy in children with severe beta-thalassemia: a six-year study, *Am J Dis Child* 142(3):287-292, 1988.

Mentzer WB and others: Availability of related donors for bone marrow transplantation in sickle cell anemia, *Am J Pediatr Hematol Oncol* 16(1):27-29, 1994.

Merhav H and others: Tea drinking in infants may cause anemia, *Am J Clin Nutr* 41(6):1210-1213, 1985.

Morrison R: Update on sickle cell disease: incidence of addiction and choice of opioid in pain management, *Pediatr Nurs* 17(5):503, 1991.

Morrison RA, Vedro DA: Pain management in the child with sickle cell disease, *Pediatr Nurs* 15(6):595-599, 613, 1989.

National Center for Health Statistics: Advance report of final mortality statistics, 1991, *Monthly vital statistics report,* vol 42, no 2, suppl, Hyattsville, MD, 1993, Public Health Service.

Nicholas SW: Management of the HIV-positive child with fever, *J Pediatr* 119(1):21-24, 1991.

1993 revised classification system for HIV infection and expanded surveillance case definition for AIDS among adolescents and adults, *MMWR* 41(RR-17):2, 1992.

Olivieri NF and others: Growth failure and bony changes induced by deferoxamine, *Am J Pediatr Hematol Oncol* 14(1):48-56, 1992.

Oski FA: Iron deficiency in infancy and childhood, *N Engl J Med* 329(3):190-193, 1993.

Pantaleo G, Graziosi C, Fauci AS: The immunopathogenesis of human immunodeficiency virus infection, *N Engl J Med* 328(5):327-335, 1993.

Pinkel D: Bone marrow transplantation in children, *J Pediatr* 122(3):331, 1993.

Piomelli S: Management of Cooley's anaemia, *Baillieres Clin Haematol* 6(1):287-298, 1993.

Pryle BJ and others: Toxicity of norpethidine in sickle cell crisis, *Br Med J* 304:1478-1479, 1992.

Quintero C: Blood administration in pediatric Jehovah's Witnesses, *Pediatr Nurs* 19(1):46-48, 1993.

Raunikar RA, Sabio H: Anemia in the adolescent athlete, *Am J Dis Child* 146(10):1201-S, 1992.

Rodgers GP and others: Augmentation by erythropoietin of the fetal-hemoglobin response to hydroxyurea in sickle cell disease, *N Engl J Med* 328(2):73-80, 1993.

Sanders JE and others: Marrow transplant experience for children with severe aplastic anemia, *Am J Pediatr Hematol Oncol* 16(1):43-49, 1994.

Santelli JS, Birn AE, Linde J: School placement for human immunodeficiency virus–infected children: the Baltimore City experience, *Pediatrics* 89:843-848, 1992.

Secundy MG: Psychosocial issues: unanswered questions in the use of bone marrow transplantation for treatment of hemoglobinopathies, *Am J Pediatr Hematol Oncol* 16(1):76-79, 1994.

Selwyn PA: AIDS: what is now known. II. Epidemiology, *Hosp Pract* 21(6):127-164, 1986.

Shapiro BS: The management of pain in sickle cell disease, *Pediatr Clin North Am* 36(4):1029-1043, 1989.

Shapiro BS, Cohen DE, Howe CJ: Patient-controlled analgesia for sickle-cell–related pain, *J Pain Symptom Manage* 8:22-28, 1993.

Sickle Cell Disease Guideline Panel: *Sickle cell disease: screening, diagnosis, management, and counseling in newborns and infants,* Agency for Health Care Policy and Research, No 93-0562, 1993.

Swift AV and others: Neuropsychologic impairment in children with sickle cell anemia, *Pediatrics* 84(6):1077-1085, 1989.

Trowbridge GL and others: HIV: recognizing and managing the infant at risk, *Contemp Pediatr* 8(10):118-134, 1991.

Vermylen C, Cornu G: Bone marrow transplantation for sickle cell disease: the European experience, *Am J Pediatr Hematol Oncol* 16(1):18-21, 1994.

Walter T and others: Iron deficiency anemia: adverse effects on infant psychomotor development, *Pediatrics* 84(1):7-17, 1989.

Walter T and others: Effectiveness of iron-fortified infant cereal in prevention of iron deficiency anemia, *Pediatrics* 91:976-982, 1993.

Walters MC, Thomas ED: Bone marrow transplantation for thalassemia: the USA experience, *Am J Pediatr Hematol Oncol* 16(1):11-17, 1994.

Wimberley TH, Parks BR: Iron preparations: it's elementary, my dear, *Pediatr Nurs* 17:274-275, 1991.

Working Group on Antiretroviral Therapy: National Pediatric HIV Resource Center: Antiretroviral therapy and medical management of the human immunodeficiency virus–infected child, *Pediatr Infect Dis J* 12:513-522, 1993.

Yesilipek MA and others: Growth and sexual maturation in children with thalassemia major, *Haematologica* 78(1):30-33, 1993.

Ziegler EE and others: Cow milk feeding and GI blood loss, *J Pediatr* 116:11-18, 1990.

Zipursky A and others: Oxygen therapy in sickle cell disease, Am *J Pediatr Hematol Oncol* 14(3):222-228, 1992.

Zurlo MG and others: Survival and causes of death in thalassemia major, *Lancet* 1(8653):27-29, 1989.

BIBLIOGRAPHY

Anemia/Iron Deficiency Anemia

Barbara JAJ: Infectious complications of blood transfusion: viruses, *Br Med J* 300:450-453, 1990.

Contreras M, Mollison PL: Immunological complications of transfusion, *Br Med J* 300:173-176, 1990.

Dallman PR, Yip R: Changing characteristics of childhood anemia, *J Pediatr* 114(1):161-164, 1989.

Looker AC and others: Iron status: prevalence of impairment in three Hispanic groups in the United States, *Am J Clin Nutr* 49:553-558, 1989.

Lozoff B and others: Iron deficiency anemia and iron therapy effects on infant development test performance, *Pediatrics* 79(6):981-995, 1987.

Moyer VA, Grimes RM: Total and differential leukocyte counts in clinically well children, *Am J Dis Child* 144(11):1200-1203, 1990.

Pekrun A, Gratzer W: Disorders of the red-cell membrane, *Curr Opin Pediatr* 2(1):116-120, 1990.

Rutman RC and others: Blood transfusions, *Am J Nurs* 84(4):486-489, 1989.

Shannon KM: Recombinant erythropoietin in pediatrics: a clinical perspective. *Pediatr Ann* 19(3):197-206, 1990.

Sickle Cell Disease

Burghardt-Fitzgerald DC: Pain-behavior contracts: effective management of the adolescent in sickle-cell crisis, *J Pediatr Nurs* 4(5):320-324, 1989.

Cohen AR and others: Increased blood requirements during long-term transfusion therapy for sickle cell disease, *J Pediatr* 118(3):405-407, 1991.

Evans JPM, Rogers DW: Sickle cell disease and thalassemia, *Curr Opin Pediatr* 2(1):121-123, 1990.

Howard RJ, Lillis C, Tuck SM: Contraceptives, counselling, and pregnancy in women with sickle cell disease, *Br Med J* 306:1735-1737, 1993.

Lisak ME: Sickle cell disease. In Jackson PL, Vessey JA: *Primary care of the child with a chronic condition,* St Louis, 1992, Mosby.

Milne RIG: Assessment of care of children with sickle cell disease: implications for neonatal screening programmes, *Br Med J* 300:371-374, 1990.

National Institutes of Health Consensus Development Conference Statement: *Newborn screening for sickle cell disease and other hemoglobinopathies,* vol 6, no 9, pp 1-8, April 6-8, 1987.

Resar LM, Oski FA: Cold water exposure and vaso-occlusive crises in sickle cell anemia, *J Pediatr* 118(3):407-409, 1991.

Rubin LG, Voulalas D, Carmody L: Immunization of children with sickle cell disease with *Haemophilus influenzae* type b polysaccharide vaccine, *Pediatrics* 84(3):509-512, 1989.

Serjeant GR and others: Human parvovirus infection in homozygous sickle cell disease, *Lancet* 341:1237-1240, 1993.

Shapiro BS: The management of pain in sickle cell disease, *Pediatr Clin North Am* 36(4):1029-1043, 1989.

Swift AV and others: Neuropsychologic impairment in children with sickle cell anemia, *Pediatrics* 84(6):1077-1085, 1989.

Wang WC and others: High risk of recurrent stroke after discontinuance of five to twelve years of transfusion therapy in patients with sickle cell disease, *J Pediatr* 118(3):377-382, 1991.

Ware RE, Filston HC: Surgical management of children with hemoglobinopathies, *Surg Clin North Am* 72(6):1223-1231, 1992.

Whitten CF, Bertles JF: *Sickle cell disease,* vol. 565, New York, 1989, New York Academy of Sciences.

Thalassemia

Bhambhani K, Aronow R: Lead poisoning and thalassemia trait or iron deficiency, *Am J Dis Child* 144(11):1231-1233, 1990.

Butler RB and others: β-Thalassemia major and sickle cell disease, *NAACOG's Clin Issues Perinat Women's Health Nurs* 2(3):345-356, 1991.

Cohen AK, Mizanin J, Schuartz E: Rapid removal of excessive iron with daily high dose intravenous chelation therapy, *J Pediatr* 115(1):151-155, 1989.

Esposito NW: Thalassemias: simple screening for hereditary anemias, *Nurse Pract* 17(2):50, 53-56, 61, 1992.

Giardina PJ, Hilgartner MW: Update on thalassemia, *Pediatr Rev* 13(2):55-62, 1992.

Lucarelli G and others: Bone marrow transplantation in patients with thalassemia, *N Engl J Med* 322(7):417-421, 1990.

Maurer HS and others: A prospective evaluation of iron chelation therapy in children with severe beta-thalassemia: a six-year study, *Am J Dis Child* 142(3):287-292, 1988.

Pearson HA and others: Patient age distribution in thalassemia major: changes from 1973 to 1985, *Pediatrics* 80(1):53-57, 1987.

Uysal Z and others: Desferrioxamine and urinary zinc excretion in β-thalassemia major, *Pediatr Hematol Oncol* 10:257-260, 1993.

Zurlo MG and others: Survival and causes of death in thalassemia major, *Lancet* 1(8653):27-29, 1989.

Aplastic Anemia

Glader BE: Red blood aplasias in children, *Pediatr Ann* (19)3:168-176, 1990.

Hunter RF, Roth PA, Huang AT: Predictive factors for response to anti-thymocyte globulin in acquired aplastic anemia, *Am J Med* 79(1):73-78, 1985.

Werner EJ and others: Immunosuppressive therapy versus bone marrow transplantation for children with aplastic anemia, *Pediatrics* 83(1):61-65, 1989.

Defects in Hemostasis

Aledort LM: New approaches to management of bleeding disorders, *Hosp Pract* 24(2):207-226, 1989.

Bussel JB: Thrombocytopeniaa in newborns, infants, and children, *Pediatr Ann* 19(3):181-193, 1990.

Diethorn ML, Weld LM: Physiologic mechanisms of hemostasis and fibrinolysis, *J Cardiovasc Nurs* 4(1):1-10, 1989.

Katsanis E and others: Prevalence and significance of mild bleeding disorders in children with recurrent epistaxis, *J Pediatr* 113(1, pt I):73-76, 1988.

Manno CS: Difficult pediatric diagnoses: bruising and bleeding, *Pediatr Clin North Am* 38(3):637, 1991.

Overby KJ, Lo B, Litt IF: Knowledge and concerns about acquired immunodeficiency syndrome and their relationship to behavior among adolescents with hemophilia, *Pediatrics* 83(2):204-209, 1989.

Pierce GF and others: The use of purified clotting factor concentrates in hemophilia: influence of viral safety, cost, and supply on therapy, *JAMA* 261(23):3434-3438, 1989.

Spitzer A: Children's knowledge of illness and treatment experiences in hemophilia, *J Pediatr Nurs* 7(1):43-51, 1992.

Blood Transfusion/Bone Marrow Transplantation (General)

Atkins DM, Patenaude AF: Psychosocial preparation and follow-up for pediatric BMT patients, *Am J Orthopsychiatry* 57(2):246-252, 1987.

Barbara JAJ: Infectious complications of blood transfusion: viruses, *Br Med J* 300:450-453, 1990.

DePalma L and Luban NLC: Trnasfusion-transmitted diseases: AIDS and hepatitis, *Contemp Pediatr* 8(4):22-39, 1991.

Ford REN: Psychosocial and ethical issues in bone marrow transplantation. In Kasprisin CA, Snyder EL, editors: *Bone marrow transplantation: a nursing perspective,* Arlington, VA, 1990, American Association of Blood Banks.

Freedman SE: An overview of bone marrow transplant, *Semin Oncol Nurs* 4(1):55-59, 1988.

Freund BL, Siegal K: Problems in transition following bone marrow transplantation: psychosocial aspects, *Am J Orthopsychiatry* 56(2):244-252, 1986.

Gottlieb SE, Portnoy S: The role of play in a pediatric bone marrow transplantation unit, *Child Health Care* 16(3):177-181, 1988.

Hann IM: Bone marrow transplantation, *Curr Opin Pediatr* 2:143-150, 1990.

Hare J, Skinner D, Kliewer D: Family systems approach to pediatric bone marrow transplantation, *Child Health Care* 18(1):30-36, 1989.

Kasprisin DO, Luban NLC: *Pediatric transfusion medicine,* vol 2, Boca Raton, FL, 1987, CRC Press.

Kasprisin DO, Miller KA: Moderate and severe reactions in blood donors, *Transfusion* 32:23-26, 1992.

Kinrade L: Preparation of a sibling donor for bone marrow harvest procedure, *Cancer Nurs* 10(2):77-81, 1987.

Pisciotto PT: *Blood transfusion therapy: a physician's handbook,* ed 4, American Association of Blood Banks, 1993.

Rutman RC and others: Blood transfusions, *Am J Nurs* 84(4):486-489, 1989.

Immunologic Deficiency Disorders

American Academy of Pediatrics: Acquired immunodeficiency syndrome education in schools, *Pediatrics* 82(2):278-280, 1988.

American Academy of Pediatrics: Guidelines for human immunodeficiency virus (HIV)–infected children and their foster families, *Pediatrics* 89(4):681-683, 1992.

Andiman WA and others: Rate of transmission of human immunodeficiency virus type 1 infection from mother to child and short-term outcome of neonatal infection, *Am J Dis Child* 144(7):758-766, 1990.

Armstrong FD, Seidel JF, Swales TP: Pediatric HIV infection: a neuropsychological and educational challenge, *J Learn Disabil* 26(2):92-103, 1993.

Bale JF: The neurologic complications of AIDS in infants and young children, *Infants Young Child* 3(2):15-23, 1990.

Boland MG, Conviser R: Nursing care of the child. In Pizzo PA, Wilfert CM: *Pediatric AIDS: the challenge of HIV infection in infants, children, and adolescents,* Baltimore, 1991, Williams & Wilkins.

Burgio GR, Notarangelo LD, Ugazio AG: Primary immunodeficiencies: milestones in the history of pediatric immunology, *Pediatr Hematol Oncol* 8:203-214, 1991.

Butler C, Hittelman J, Hauger SB: Approach to neurodevelopmental and neurologic complications in pediatric HIV infection, *J Pediatr* 119(1):41-46, 1991.

Butz AM and others: Care of HIV-risk infants: Nursing outreach by PNPs, *J Pediatr Health Care* 6(3):138-145, 1992.

Chanock SJ, McIntosh K: Selected issues in pediatric infection with human immunodeficiency virus, *Curr Opin Pediatr* 1:16-21, 1989.

Clark PJ and Byrne MW: Clinical issues in long-term HIV, *MCN* 18(3):164-167, 1993.

Cohen DG: Similarities between the nursing

care needs of children with cancer and children with human immunodeficiency virus infection, *J Pediatr Oncol Nurs* 7(4):149-153, 1990.

Committee on Infectious Diseases: Health guidelines for the attendance in daycare and foster care settings of children infected with human immunodeficiency virus, *Pediatrics* 79(3):466-471, 1987.

Czarniecki L, Oleske J: Pain in children with HIV infection, *J Pain Symptom Manage* 6(3):177, 1991.

Dubiel A and others: Wiskott-Aldrich syndrome—a case report, *Clin Pediatr* 29(8):434-437, 1990.

Edelson PJ, editor: Childhood AIDS, *Pediatr Clin North Am* 38(1):entire issue, 1991.

Ellerbrock TV and others: Epidemiology of women with AIDS in the United States, 1981 through 1990, *JAMA* 265(22):2971-2975, 1991.

Epstein LG: Human immunodeficiency virus infection in children: neurologic manifestations and pathogenetic mechanisms, *Curr Opin Pediatr* 1:290-295, 1989.

Fahrner R: Pediatric HIV infection and AIDS. In Jackson PL, Vessey JA: Primary care of the child with a chronic condition, St Louis, 1992, Mosby.

Fischer GW: Therapeutic uses of intravenous gamma globulin for pediatric infections, *Pediatr Clin North Am* 35(3):517-533, 1988.

Flaskerud JH: *AIDS/HIV infection: a reference guide for nursing professionals,* Philadelphia, 1989, WB Saunders.

Goodman E, Cohall AT: Acquired immunodeficiency syndrome and adolescents: knowledge, attitudes, beliefs, and behaviors in a New York City adolescent minority population, *Pediatrics* 84(1):36-42, 1989.

Greene WC: AIDS and the immune system, *Sci Am* 269(3):99-105, 1993.

Guidelines for effective school health education to prevent the spread of AIDS, *MMWR* 37(S-2):1-13, 1988.

Guidelines for prevention of transmission of human immunodeficiency virus and hepatitis B virus to health-care and public-safety workers, *MMWR* 38(S-6), June 23, 1989.

Gurka AM: The immune system: implications for critical care nursing, *Crit Care Nurse* 9(7):24-36, 1989.

Gwinn M and others: Prevalence of HIV infection in childbearing women in the United States: surveillance using newborn blood samples, *JAMA* 265(13):1704-1708, 1991.

Hein K: Commentary on adolescent acquired immunodeficiency syndrome: the next wave of the human immunodeficiency virus epidemic? *J Pediatr* 114(1):144-149, 1989.

Hein K: Adolescent acquired immunodeficiency syndrome: a paradigm for training in early intervention and care, *Am J Dis Child* 144(1):46-48, 1990.

Husson RN and others: High-level resistance to zidovudine but not to zalcitabine or didanosine in human immunodeficiency virus from children receiving antiretroviral therapy, *J Pediatr* 123(1):9-16, 1993.

Hutto C and others: A hospital-based prospective study of perinatal infection with human immunodeficiency virus type 1, *J Pediatr* 118(3):347-353, 1991.

Iazzetti L: Nursing management of the pediatric AIDS patient, *Issues Compr Pediatr Nurs* 9(2):119-129, 1986.

Janeway Jr CA: How the immune system recognizes invaders, *Sci Am* 269(3):73-79, 1993.

Karthas NP, Chanock S: Clinical management of HIV infection in infants and children, *Fam Community Health* 3(2):8-20, 1990.

Majer LS: HIV-infected students in school: who really "needs to know"? *J School Health* 62(6):243, 1992.

Marrack P, Kappler JW: How the immune system recognizes the body, *Sci Am* 269(3):81-89, 1993.

Michaels D, Levine C: Estimates of the number of motherless youth orphaned by AIDS in the United States, *JAMA* 268(24):3456-3461, 1992.

Morrow AL and others: Knowledge and attitudes of day care center parents and care providers regarding children infected with human immunodeficiency virus, *Pediatrics* 87(6):876-883, 1991.

Mugrditchian L and others: The nutrition of the HIV infected child. II. Care management, *Top Clin Nutr* 7(2):11-20, 1992.

National Pediatric HIV Resource Center in cooperation with the Region II Head Start Resource Center: *Getting a head start on HIV: a resource manual for enhancing services to HIV-affected children in Head Start,* Newark, NJ, 1992, National Pediatric HIV Resource Center.

Nossal GJV: Life, death and the immune system, *Sci Am* 269(3):53-62, 1993.

Novello AC and others: Final report of the United States Department of Health and Human Services Secretary's work group on pediatric human immunodeficiency virus infection and disease: content and implications, *Pediatrics* 84(3):547-555, 1989.

Paul WE: Infectious diseases and the immune system, *Sci Am* 269(3):91-97, 1993.

Pratt RD and others: Pediatric human immunodeficiency virus infection in a low seroprevalence area, *Pediatr Infect Dis J* 12(4):304-310, 1993.

Projections of the number of persons diagnosed with AIDS and the number of immunosuppressed HIV-infected persons—United States, 1992-1994, *MMWR* 41(RR-18):1-29, 1992.

Recommendations for HIV testing services for inpatients and outpatients in acute-care hospital settings and technical guidance on HIV counseling, *MMWR* 42(RR-2):1-6, 1993.

Recommendations on prophylaxis and therapy for disseminated *Mycobacterium avium* complex for adults and adolescents infected with human immunodeficiency virus, *MMWR* 42(RR-9):14-20, 1993.

St Louis ME and others: Human immunodeficiency virus infection in disadvantaged adolescents: findings from the U.S. Job Corps, *JAMA* 266(17):2387-2391, 1991.

Schvaneveldt JD: Children's understanding of AIDS: a developmental viewpoint, *Fam Relations* 39(3):330-335, 1990.

Selekman J: The multiple faces of immune deficiency in children, *Pediatr Nurs* 16(4):351-355, 361, 1990.

Steiner JD and others: Are adolescents getting smarter about acquired immunodeficiency syndrome? *Am J Dis Child* 144(3):302-306, 1990.

Stiehm ER: New uses for IVIG: infectious diseases and more, *Contemp Pediatr* 8(4):47-68, 1991.

Stiehm ER, Vink P: Transmission of human immunodeficiency virus infection by breast-feeding, *J Pediatr* 118(3):410-412, 1991.

Task Force on Pediatric AIDS: Pediatric guidelines for infection control of human immunodeficiency virus (acquired immunodeficiency virus) in hospitals, medical offices, schools, and other settings, *Pediatrics* 82(5):801-807, 1988.

Task Force on Pediatric AIDS: Adolescents and human immunodeficiency virus infection: the role of the pediatrician in prevention and intervention, *Pediatrics* 92(4):626-630, 1993.

Testing for antibodies to human immunodeficiency virus type 2 in the United States, *MMWR* 41(12), 1992.

Todd J: A most intimate foe: how the immune system can betray the body it defends, *Science* 30(2):20-27, 1990.

Turner BJ and others: Survival experience of 789 children with the acquired immunodeficiency syndrome, *Pediatr Infect Dis J* 12(4):310-320, 1993.

US Public Health Service task force on anti-pneumocystis prophylaxis for patients with human immunodeficiency virus infection: Recommendations for prophylaxis against *Pneumocystis carinii* pneumonia for adults and adolescents infected with human immunodeficiency virus, *MMWR* 41(4), 1992.

Weissman IL, Cooper MD: How the immune system develops, *Sci Am* 269(3):65-71, 1993.

Wiener L, Fair C, Pizzo PA: *Care for the child with HIV infection and AIDS.* Pediatric Branch National Cancer Institute and Social Work Department, The Clinical Center National Institutes of Health, 1993.

Wigzell H: The immune system as a therapeutic agent, *Sci Am* 269(3):127-134, 1993.

UNIT XIII

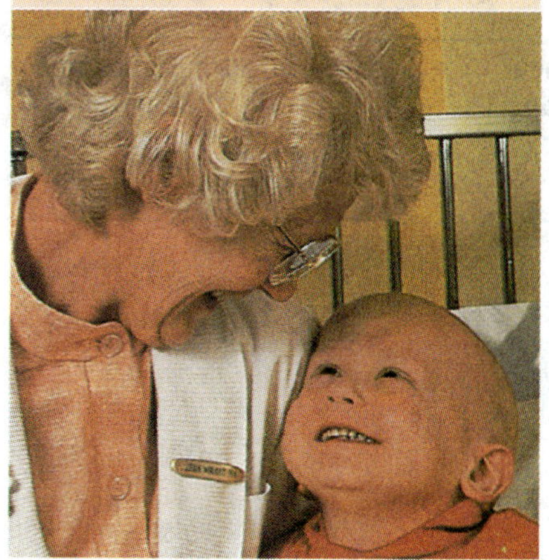

THE CHILD WITH DISTURBANCE OF REGULATORY MECHANISMS

CHAPTER 36 The Child with Cancer

CHAPTER OUTLINE

RELATED TOPICS

Administration of medication, Ch. 27
Anaphylaxis, Ch. 29
Anemia, Ch. 35
Biologic development (adolescence), Ch. 19
Bone marrow aspiration/biopsy, Ch. 27
The child with cerebral dysfunction, Ch. 37
Dental health, Ch. 14
Drug reactions, Ch. 18
Epistaxis (nosebleeding), Ch. 35
Family-centered care of the child during illness and hospitalization, Ch. 26
Family-centered care of the child with chronic illness or disability, Ch. 22
Family-centered care of the child with life-threatening illness, Ch. 23
Immunizations, Ch. 12
Infection control, Ch. 27
Lumbar puncture, Ch. 27
Pain assessment; pain management, Ch. 26
Physical examination, Ch. 7
Preparation for procedures, Ch. 27
Stomatitis, Ch. 16
Sunburn, Ch. 18
Surgical procedures, Ch. 27
Venous access devices, Ch. 28

CANCER IN CHILDREN

There are few situations in nursing that exceed the challenges of caring for a child with cancer. Despite the dramatic improvements in survival rates for these children, the needs of the family are tremendous as they cope with a serious physical illness, as well as the fear that the child will not be cured. If a cured child is a possible outcome, then a ***truly cured child*** is an essential outcome—that is, a child who is not just free of disease but who is developmentally commensurate with age and well adjusted to the experience of having cancer (van Eys, 1977).

This chapter is concerned primarily with the physical problems associated with several types of childhood cancer. The general psychologic needs of these children and their families are discussed in Chapter 22 in terms of chronic illness and in Chapter 23 for situations when the outcome becomes life-threatening and death is a possibility.

Cancer is the leading cause of death from disease in children ages 3 to 15 years and the second cause of death from all causes, exceeded only by injuries. The incidence of cancer in this age-group is approximately 12.9 per 100,000 white children and 10.1 per 100,000 black children (Fernbach and Vietti, 1991). The projected number of new cases is an estimated 8200 per year in the United States, with an estimated 1600 deaths in 1994 (Cancer facts, 1994).

During childhood there are changing incidences for various types of cancer. For children in all pediatric age-groups, leukemia is the most frequent type of cancer, followed by brain tumors and lymphomas (Table 36-1). However, there are some important differences between the two groups. Tumors of the kidney and soft tissue are more common in blacks, whereas tumors of the bone are more common in whites. Males are affected more often by cancer than females (ratio of 1.2:1), although this varies with the type of cancer. This is accounted for by an increased risk among young males for acute lymphoid leukemia, lymphoma, and medulloblastoma (Robison, 1993).

Probably the most significant aspect of childhood cancer is the improved prognosis during the last 3 decades. Mortality among children with cancer has declined from 8.3 per 100,000 in 1950 to 3.6 per 100,000 in 1986 (Fernbach and Vietti, 1991). Currently, more than 65% of all children with malignant neoplasms treated at major cancer centers will now survive more than 5 years (Robison, 1993). The cancers demonstrating the greatest improvement in survival rates are acute leukemia, lymphomas, Wilms tumor, rhabdomyosarcoma, osteosarcoma, and Ewing sarcoma. However, black children with cancer do more poorly than white children (Cancer Facts, 1994).

Although survival is discussed in terms of "cure," the term ***biologic cure*** is not absolute, since it is not possible to demonstrate definitively complete eradication of all cancer cells, and late recurrences do occur. The definition of cure includes the criteria of (1) cessation of therapy, (2) continuous freedom from clinical and laboratory evidence of cancer, and (3) minimum or no risk of relapse, as determined by previous experience with the disease. The time that must elapse before a child clinically free of cancer is considered cured varies with each type of cancer but typically ranges from 2 to 5 years.

■ Marilyn Hockenberry-Eaton, RN-CS, PhD, PNP, FAAN, revised this chapter.

TABLE 36-1 Cancer Incidence by Site for Children Under 15, SEER Program 1982-1986

SITE	PERCENT OF TOTAL	RATE PER 1,000,000 CHILDREN
Leukemia	30.5	39.7
Brain and nervous system	20.1	27.0
Lymphoma	10.5	15.1
Kidney	7.0	8.8
Soft tissue	6.3	8.2
Bone	4.8	7.1
Eye	3.7	4.8
Liver	1.7	2.0
All other	15.4	20.0
All sites	100.0	132.7

Data from Cancer Statistics Branch, National Cancer Institute.

ETIOLOGIC FACTORS

The cause of cancer is not known. While there are numerous hypotheses concerning its origin, the most enduring theory is that some genetic alteration results in the unregulated proliferation of cells. Recent studies have demonstrated the existence of genes activated in human tumors that are capable of causing uncontrolled proliferation of cells when transmitted to normal cells. Genes having the potential to transform normal cells into malignant ones are called ***oncogenes.*** What causes the induction of cell transformation is speculative, but RNA tumor viruses (also called retroviruses, because they have the ability to translate RNA back to DNA) may play a role in the transfer of DNA from a malignant cell to a normal cell (Stine, 1989). The identification of the human T-cell leukemia-lymphoma virus (HTLV) in some forms of adult leukemia and lymphoma and the Epstein-Barr (EB) virus, a type of herpes virus, in Burkitt lymphoma has lent support to this theory (Li and others, 1988). While these viruses have been isolated, there is no firm evidence that childhood cancer is communicable.

Despite the lack of knowledge about the origin of cancer, there is considerable information on risk factors that increase the likelihood of children developing specific types of cancer. The following is a brief overview of some of the etiologic factors implicated in childhood cancer.

Several environmental agents that are carcinogenic (capable of producing cancer) in adults have been described, but only one of these—ionizing radiation—has been implicated in children. Low doses of radiation have been known to cause thyroid cancer and leukemia. There is some evidence that exposing pregnant women to diagnostic radiographic procedures increases the occurrence of leukemia and other forms of cancer among their children (Li and others, 1988).

Exposure to power lines as a causative factor in the development of childhood leukemia has been a subject of controversy in the past few years. Recent studies have found marginally significant relationships between cancer and electromagnetic exposure (Gellis, 1992; Mulvihill, 1993; Zamenhoff, 1993). However, future studies are necessary to further identify the seriousness of the risk.

Although drugs, particularly those containing radioisotopes and immunosuppressive agents, can increase the risk of developing childhood cancer, the one drug most notably recognized for its carcinogenic effect is diethylstilbestrol. Large doses of this hormone given to pregnant women to prevent abortion cause adenocarcinoma of the vagina in a significant proportion of the female offspring when they reach adolescence and early adulthood.

There is much interest in discovering if certain foods or nutrients cause cancer in children. Some studies have suggested that the use of intramuscular vitamin K supplementation at birth to prevent hemorrhagic disease of the newborn may increase the risk of leukemia; however, other research has not supported this finding (Klebanoff and others, 1993). Some aspects of the maternal diet, especially early prenatal multivitamin use, may have a role in preventing primitive neuroectodermal tumors, such as medulloblastoma, in young children (Bunin and others, 1993). This finding is especially intriguing in light of the association between supplemental doses of folic acid and the reduced risk of neural tube defects (see Spinal Bifida/Myelodysplasia, Chapter 11). The neural tube is lined with neuroepithelial cells, which are the precursor cells of primitive neuroectodermal tumors.

Some childhood cancers, in particular retinoblastoma, Wilms tumor, and neuroblastoma, may demonstrate patterns of inheritance that suggest a genetic basis for the disorder. The Philadelphia chromosome was the first chromosomal abnormality to be found in a malignancy. It occurs as a result of a translocation between chromosomes 9 and 22 and is observed in almost all individuals with chronic myelogenous leukemia (Rubin, 1988). Chromosomal abnormalities have also been found in children with acute leukemia and lymphoma, as well as numerous pediatric solid tumors (Carroll and Schwartz, 1991; Kirsch, 1993). Bilateral Wilms tumor is associated with an increased incidence of congenital anomalies, which include aniridia, hemihypertrophy, and urogenital anomalies (Coppes and others, 1989). In addition, children with certain types of chromosomal abnormalities, especially those syndromes caused by abnormal numbers of chromosomes, have an increased incidence of cancer. For example, in children with Down syndrome the probability of developing leukemia is about 15 times greater than the usual rate for whites (Poplack, 1993). Other chromosomal syndromes associated with a predisposition to cancer are Fanconi syndrome (a deficiency of all cellular elements of the blood), Bloom syndrome (dwarfism and skin changes), ataxia-telangiectasia (progressive cerebellar ataxia and oculocutaneous vascular lesions), Klinefelter syndrome, and nevoid basal cell sarcoma syndrome.

Children with immune deficiencies, such as Wiskott-Aldrich syndrome or acquired immunodeficiency syndrome, or children whose immune system has been suppressed, such as following transplant procedures, are at a greater risk for developing various cancers. Of major concern is the increased risk of secondary cancers in some children successfully treated for their primary malignancy.

A familial tendency of clustering of cancer also occurs. For example, there are some families who have a higher than expected incidence of cancer, although no environmental or host factor can explain the event. When cancer has occurred in one child, the risk of cancer in the remaining siblings is two times the expected risk for the general population, but the actual risk is considered low because of the rarity of childhood cancer (Li and others, 1988). However, in leukemias the risk among monozygous twins is extremely high—almost 100% if the disease is diagnosed in the twin before 1 year of age. This decreases beyond the first year to approach the same risk of other family members by 6 years of age (Mulvihill, 1993).

Clustering of cases of cancer within a geographic location that exceeds the incidence expected by chance also occurs, but it is thought that these are unusual, random events. Unfortunately, such situations can cause considerable concern and even panic in the community.

Prevention

Knowledge of the risk factors that increase the likelihood of cancer holds the promise of prevention. Unfortunately, in children the known carcinogens are limited to radiation and a few drugs given to the mother during pregnancy. Therefore at present there is really no known prevention.

Health professionals do have two roles, however. One is aimed at preventing adult-type cancers by educating parents and children about the hazards of known carcinogens, particularly the effects of cigarette smoking and excessive exposure to sunlight. Lung cancer is the leading cause of death from cancer in adults, and malignant melanoma is the leading cause of death from diseases of the skin. Children at higher risk for skin cancer are those with light-colored eyes, complexion, and hair; those who sunburn easily; and those who live near the equator (Mulvihill, 1993; Weinstock and others, 1989; Williams and Sagebiel, 1989). Not only these children but all children should be protected from overexposure to the sun (see Chapter 18). In addition, to prevent other types of cancer, males should be taught testicular self-examination; female adolescents should be taught breast self-examination and be encouraged to seek periodic health examinations, including a Papanicolaou (Pap) smear.*

Second, health professionals need to be aware of the cardinal symptoms of childhood cancer (see box on p. 1624). Unfortunately, fever and pain are manifestations of common childhood disorders, and without a high index of sus-

*Information on self-instructional materials on testicular and breast self-examination is available from the local chapters of the American Cancer Society, Inc., or the national office, 1599 Clifton Rd., Atlanta, GA 30329; (404) 329-7617.

picion, they may be attributed to minor ailments. The other signs are subtle and easily missed. If parents suspect an abnormality, their concerns must be taken seriously. The greatest weapons against all forms of cancer are early detection and treatment.

PROPERTIES OF MALIGNANT CELLS

Malignant or ***cancer cells*** are cells that have the specific properties of anaplasia, invasion, and metastasis. An appreciation of the unique properties of these abnormal cells facilitates an understanding of the pathologic changes that occur in cancer (see box below).

Neoplasms are any new and abnormal growth and may be benign or malignant. ***Benign neoplasms*** do not demonstrate the degree of anaplasia or metastasis that malignant neoplasms do, but they may still be serious, especially when they occur in confined spaces, such as the brain. ***Malignant neoplasms*** can arise from any tissue of the body and are classified according to tissue and cell type. ***Embryonal tumors*** arise from embryonic tissue, such as the blastomas. ***Lymphomas*** arise from the lymphatic system. ***Leukemias*** arise from the blood-forming organs. ***Sarcoma*** is derived from connective and supporting tissue, such as bone, cartilage, nerve, and fat. ***Carcinoma*** is derived from epithelial tissue, such as skin and lining of the body cavities. ***Adenocarcinoma*** is a carcinoma of glandular tissue, such as the breast or prostate.

History and Physical Examination

The history and physical examination often yield the first clues to the presence of cancer. Vague complaints, such as fatigue, pain in a limb, night sweating, lack of appetite, headache, and general malaise, may be the earliest clues and need to be taken seriously. Most children have a great deal of energy and if sick with a cold or other childhood affliction recover quickly and completely. Any evidence of a lingering disorder is often the first sign of leukemia. Parents are often the first persons to detect physical signs, such as enlarged lymph nodes (lymphoma), a white pupil (retinoblastoma), or an abdominal mass (Wilms tumor). Any such complaints must be thoroughly followed with a complete examination (see also Assessment, p. 1624).

PROPERTIES OF TUMOR CELLS

Growth rate—Usually very rapid, in contrast to other cells of the body, which divide slowly

Anaplasia—Loss of orderly differentiation and organization of cells to perform a specific function

Invasion—Malignant cells invade adjacent tissues, and eventually the normal cells may be replaced by cancer cells that are incapable of performing the original cells' functions

Metastasis—The ability to spread to distant sites within the body and establish secondary colonies of malignant growth; may occur by natural seeding via the bloodstream or lymph system or iatrogenically, such as during surgery or needle biopsy, when cancer cells are dislodged and implant elsewhere in the body

Competition—Rapidly proliferating, nonfunctional cells compete with normal cells for essential nutrients, until eventually the normal cells die and are replaced by cancer cells

Expansion—Abnormal, unrestricted growth of cells produces organ damage by compressing adjacent tissues, until the tissues' normal functions are altered

Laboratory Tests

Any number of laboratory tests may be performed, but most often a complete blood count and chemistry, and urinalysis will be done. Malignancies of the blood-forming organs manifest signs early, and these frequently cause decreased elements of the blood, increased production of immature cells, and/or overproduction of some cells, such as leukocytosis. Since many of the chemotherapeutic agents depress bone marrow function, repeated blood counts are a constant feature of follow-up care.

Blood chemistry yields important information concerning renal and liver function and electrolyte balance. Evaluation of renal and liver function is important not only for detection of cancer or metastasis to these organs, but also for monitoring during treatment because of the extra burden placed on these systems to metabolize and excrete the chemotherapeutic drugs. Consequently, regular blood chemistries and urinalysis are standard procedures through the course of the disease.

A lumbar puncture (LP) is a routine test employed in leukemia, brain tumors, and other cancers that may metastasize to the spinal cord and brain. An LP is also performed to administer intrathecal drugs, such as methotrexate and cytosine arabinoside, when this mode of administration is part of the treatment protocol.

Imaging Techniques

Advances in imaging procedures have greatly aided in the diagnosis of solid tumors and have minimized the need for invasive techniques. Depending on the suspected site of the malignancy, initial preliminary radiologic studies include conventional films of the chest, abdomen, bone, and skull and more specialized tests such as the intravenous pyelogram for kidney involvement. However, these radiographs are generally followed by much more sophisticated imaging procedures, including computed tomography (CT), ultrasound, nuclear scan, and magnetic resonance imaging (MRI) (see Table 37-2).

Biopsy

As part of the diagnostic evaluation, biopsies are essential to determine the classification and stage of the disease. ***Classification*** refers to the biologic characteristics of the tumor in relation to the tumor (T) itself, the involvement of regional lymph nodes (N), and the presence of metastasis (M). ***Staging*** refers to the extent of the disease at the time of diagnosis in regard to TNM (DeVitta, 1989). While the classification of the tumor may not change, the stage frequently does and is usually directly related to prognosis (the higher the stage, the poorer the prognosis).

Biopsies may be performed during surgical removal of the tumor, or in the case of lymphomas, surgery may be performed specifically to obtain tissue samples of the spleen and involved lymph nodes. Easily accessed nodes, such as those in the cervical or axillary region, may be removed for biopsy. Whenever there is concern for metastasis to the hematologic system or when the primary site is the blood-forming organs, bone marrow studies are performed.

A ***bone marrow test*** may be accomplished by (1) ***aspiration,*** obtaining marrow through a large- or fine-bore needle, or (2) ***biopsy,*** obtaining a piece of bone through a special type of needle. Examination of bone marrow is used to determine the extent of involvement by malignant cells. In leukemia, involvement is classified by the percentage of leukemia cells present in bone marrow, where M_1 is less than 5%, M_2 is greater than 5% but less than 25%, and M_3 is greater than 25% (Poplack, 1993).

MODES OF THERAPY

Several advances in the understanding of cancer and improvements in technical procedures have greatly influenced present modes of therapy, including (1) surgery, (2) chemotherapy, (3) radiotherapy, (4) immunotherapy, and (5) bone marrow transplantation. While there have been significant developments in new modes of treatment, one of the major reasons for more effective treatment regimens has been the use of clinical trials and protocols. Because of the relatively small number of children with cancer, the National Cancer Institute (NCI) set up cooperative groups of pediatric oncologists (physicians specializing in the care of children with cancer) from different regions of the United States to systematically combine data regarding treatment and other aspects of cancer care (American Brain Tumor Association, 1992). Based on the evaluation of success from different types of treatment, these experts plan and initiate comparative ***clinical trials.**** Although clinical trials may involve any aspect of cancer care (prevention, treatment, or long-term effects), they are frequently concerned with evaluating investigational drugs. For example, one group of patients (control group) typically receives the best possible treatment presently known. The experimental group(s) receives treatment that is thought to be even better. The formalized outline of the clinical study, which among other details includes the treatment plan (administration and evaluation), is called a ***protocol.***

Over the past 30 years the use of clinical trials and protocols has been responsible for major changes in the approaches to cancer treatment. Some of the recent strategies include reduction of toxicity with prolonged and continuous rather than intermittent intravenous infusion; shortening of duration of maintenance therapy; the use of intensive combination therapy; and the administration of as many effective agents as possible in the highest doses possible during the initiation of therapy. The following is an overview of the major modes of therapy. In addition, specific aspects of therapy are discussed later in the chapter when applicable to the individual type of cancer.

*A suggested reference for families is *What Are Clinical Trials All About?* NIH Publication No. 92-2706; available from the National Cancer Institute, Office of Cancer Communications, Building 31, Room 10A24, Bethesda, MD 20892.

Surgery

The main goal of surgery, besides obtaining biopsies, is to remove all traces of tumor and restore normal body functioning. Surgery is most successful when the tumor is encapsulated and localized (confined to the site of origin). It may only be palliative when the cancer is regional (metastasized to an area adjacent to the original site) or advanced (widespread throughout the body). Obviously, the best prognosis is directly related to early detection of the tumor.

The recent trend is toward more conservative surgical excision. For example, in some types of bone cancer, such as osteosarcoma, patients are successfully treated with resection of the diseased portion of the bone rather than amputation. There is an increasing emphasis on the use of combination drug therapy and radiotherapy after limited surgical intervention.

Chemotherapy

Chemotherapy may be the primary form of treatment, or it may be used as an adjunct to surgery and/or radiotherapy. Although several drugs with antineoplastic capabilities have been found effective in treating different forms of cancer, the remarkable survival rates have been the result of improved combination-drug regimens. Combining drugs allows for optimum cell cycle destruction with minimum toxic effects and decreased resistance by the cancer cells to the agent. For example, MOPP (mechlorethamine [Mustargen], vincristine [Oncovin], procarbazine, and prednisone) combines complementary cytotoxic effects with nonsimilar side effects. Mechlorethamine and procarbazine are myelosuppressive, vincristine is neurotoxic, and prednisone produces mild bone marrow depression with the beneficial effects of an improved appetite and a feeling of well-being.

In addition to more effective combinations of drugs, several advances in the administration of chemotherapy have permitted continuous or intermittent intravenous administration without multiple venipunctures. The use of venous access devices (catheters and implantable infusion ports) has greatly facilitated safe and effective drug administration with minimum discomfort for the child (see Chapter 28). Continuous infusions over an extended period using syringe pumps have made possible the administration of certain drugs, such as cytosine arabinoside, in higher doses with less toxicity than when the drug is administered intermittently.

Chemotherapeutic agents are classified according to their cytotoxic action. ***Alkylating agents*** replace a hydrogen atom of a molecule by an alkyl group. The irreversible combination of alkyl groups with nucleotide chains, particularly DNA, causes unbalanced growth of unaffected cell constituents so that the cell eventually dies. They are radiomimetic in that their action is similar to irradiation. ***Antimetabolites*** resemble essential metabolic elements needed for cell growth but are sufficiently altered in molecular structure to inhibit further synthesis of DNA and/or RNA. ***Plant alkaloids*** arrest cells in metaphase (a phase of mitosis) by binding to microtubular protein needed for spindle formation. ***Antitumor antibiotics*** are natural products that interfere with cell division by reacting with DNA in such a way as to pre-

Text continued on p. 1620.

TABLE 36-2 Summary of Chemotherapeutic Agents Used in the Treatment of Childhood Cancers*

AGENT/ADMINISTRATION	SIDE EFFECTS AND TOXICITY	COMMENTS AND SPECIFIC NURSING CONSIDERATIONS
ALKYLATING AGENTS		
Mechlorethamine (nitrogen mustard, Mustargen) IV†	N/V‡ (½-8 hours later) (severe) BMD§ (2-3 weeks later) Alopecia Local phlebitis	Vesicant‖ May cause phlebitis and discoloration of vein
Cyclophosphamide (Cytoxan, CTX, Neosar) PO, IV, IM	N/V (3-4 hours later) (severe at high doses) BMD (10-14 days later) Alopecia Hemorrhagic cystitis Severe immunosuppression Stomatitis (rare) Hyperpigmentation Transverse ridging of nails Infertility	BMD has platelet-sparing effect Give dose early in day to allow adequate fluids afterward Force fluids before administering drug and for 2 days after to prevent chemical cystitis; encourage frequent voiding even during night Warn parents to report signs of burning on urination or hematuria to practitioner
Ifosfamide (Ifos, IFF) IV	Hemorrhagic cystitis BMD (10-14 days later) Alopecia Neurotoxicity—lethargy, disorientation, somnolence, seizures (rare)	Mesna is given to reduce hemorrhagic cystitis Hydrate as with CTX Myelosuppression less severe than with CTX
Melphalan (L-phenylalanine mustard, Alkeran, L-Pam) PO, IV	N/V (severe) BMD (2-3 weeks later) Diarrhea Alopecia	Vesicant Give over 1 hour
Procarbazine (Matulane) PO	N/V (moderate) BMD (3-4 weeks later) Lethargy Dermatitis Myalgia Arthralgia Less commonly: Stomatitis Neuropathy Alopecia Diarrhea Azoospermia Cessation of menses	Central nervous system depressants (phenothiazines, barbiturates) enhance central nervous system symptoms Monoamine oxidase (MAO) inhibition sometimes occurs, causing increased norepinephrine; foods containing high levels of tyramine may elevate norepinephrine to toxic levels; foods to avoid are *overripe* or *aged* products (i.e., cheddar, mozzarella, parmesan cheese; avocados, bananas, figs; broad beans, fava beans; red wines; excessive amounts of yogurt, chocolate, soy sauce) (McKenry and Salerno, 1989); to avoid drug interactions, all other drugs are avoided unless medically approved
Dacarbazine (DTIC-Dome) IV	N/V (especially after first dose) (severe) BMD (7-14 days later) Alopecia Flulike syndrome Burning sensation in vein during infusion (not extravasation)	Vesicant (less sclerosive) Must be given cautiously in patients with renal dysfunction Decrease IV rate or use cold pack along vein to decrease burning
Cisplatin (Platinol) IV	Renal toxicity (severe) N/V (1-4 hours later) (severe) BMD (mild, 2-3 weeks later) Ototoxicity Neurotoxicity (similar to that for vincristine) Electrolyte disturbances, especially hypomagnesium, hypocalcemia, hypokalemia, and hypophosphatemia	Renal function (creatinine clearance) must be assessed before giving drug Must maintain hydration before and during therapy (specific gravity of urine is used to assess hydration) Mannitol may be given IV to promote osmotic diuresis and drug clearance Monitor intake and output

*Table includes principal drugs used in the treatment of childhood cancers. Several other conventional and investigational chemotherapeutic agents may be employed in the treatment regimen.
†*IV,* Intravenous; *PO,* by mouth; *IM,* intramuscular; *SC,* subcutaneous; *IT,* intrathecal.
‡*N/V,* Nausea and vomiting. Mild = <20% incidence; moderate = 20% to 70% incidence; severe = >75% incidence.
§*BMD,* Bone marrow depression.
‖Vesicants (sclerosing agents) can cause severe cellular damage if even minute amounts of the drug infiltrate surrounding tissue. Only nurses experienced with chemotherapeutic agents should administer vesicants. These drugs must be given through a free-flowing intravenous line. The infusion is stopped *immediately* if any sign of infiltration (pain, stinging, swelling, or redness at needle site) occurs. Interventions for extravasation vary, but each nurse should be aware of the institution policies and implement them at once.

TABLE 36-2 Summary of Chemotherapeutic Agents Used in the Treatment of Childhood Cancers—cont'd

AGENT/ADMINISTRATION	SIDE EFFECTS AND TOXICITY	COMMENTS AND SPECIFIC NURSING CONSIDERATIONS
	Anaphylactic reactions may occur	Monitor for signs of ototoxicity (e.g., ringing in ears) and neurotoxicity; report signs immediately; ensure that routine audiogram is done before treatment for baseline and routinely during treatment Do not use aluminum needle; reaction with aluminum decreases potency of drug Monitor for signs of electrolyte loss, i.e. hypomagnesium—tremors, spasm, muscle weakness, lower extremity cramps, irregular heartbeat, convulsions, delirium Have emergency drugs at bedside*
Carboplatin (CBDCA), IV	BMD (14 days later) N/V (mild) Mild hepatotoxicity Alopecia	Do not use saline dilution Less nephrotoxic and ototoxic than cisplatin
ALKYLATING AGENTS		
Chlorambucil (Leukeran) PO	N/V (mild) BMD (7-14 days later) Diarrhea Dermatitis Less commonly may be hepatotoxicity	Usually slow onset of side effects; side effects related to high doses
ANTIMETABOLITES		
Cytosine arabinoside (Ara-C, Cytosar, Cytarabine, arabinosyl cytosine) IV, IM, SC, IT	Alopecia N/V (mild) BMD (7-14 days later) Mucosal ulceration Immunosuppression Hepatitis (usually subclinical)	Crosses blood-brain barrier Use with caution in patients with hepatic dysfunction Conjunctivitis with high doses
5-Azacytidine (5-AzaC) IV	N/V (moderate) BMD (7-14 days later) Diarrhea	Infuse slowly via IV drip to decrease severity of N/V
Mercaptopurine (6-MP, Purinethol) PO, IV	N/V (mild) Diarrhea Anorexia Stomatitis BMD (4-6 weeks later) Immunosuppression Dermatitis Less commonly may be hepatotoxic	6-MP is an analog of xanthine; therefore allopurinol (Zyloprim) delays its metabolism and increases its potency, necessitating a lower dose (⅓ to ¼) of 6-MP
Methotrexate (MTX, Amethopterin) PO, IV, IM, IT May be given in conventional doses (mg/m^2) or high doses (g/m^2)	N/V (severe at high doses) Diarrhea Mucosal ulceration (2-5 days later) BMD (10 days later) Immunosuppression Dermatitis Photosensitivity Alopecia (uncommon) Toxic effects include: Hepatitis (fibrosis) Osteoporosis Nephropathy Pneumonitis (fibrosis) Neurologic toxicity with IT use—pain at injection site, meningismus (signs of meningitis without actual inflammation), especially fever and headache; potential sequelae—transient or permanent hemiparesis, convulsions, dementia, death	Side effects and toxicity are dose related Potency and toxicity increased by reduced renal function, salicylates, sulfonamides, and aminobenzoic acid; avoid use of these substances, such as aspirin Use sunscreen High-dose therapy: Citrovorum factor (folinic acid or leucovorin) decreases cytotoxic action of MTX; used as an antidote for overdose and to enhance normal cell recovery following high-dose therapy; avoid use of vitamins containing folic acid during MTX therapy unless prescribed by physician IT therapy: Drug *must* be mixed with preservative-free diluent Report signs of neurotoxicity immediately

*Emergency drugs include oxygen and parenteral preparations of epinephrine 1:1000, diphenhydramine or similar antihistamine, aminophylline, corticosteroids, and vasopressors.

Continued.

TABLE 36-2 Summary of Chemotherapeutic Agents Used in the Treatment of Childhood Cancers—cont'd

AGENT/ADMINISTRATION	SIDE EFFECTS AND TOXICITY	COMMENTS AND SPECIFIC NURSING CONSIDERATIONS
ANTIMETABOLITES—cont'd		
6-Thioguanine (6-TG, Thioguan) PO	N/V (mild) BMD (7-14 days later) Stomatitis Rarely: Dermatitis Photosensitivity Liver dysfunction	Side effects are unusual
PLANT ALKALOIDS		
Vincristine (Oncovin) IV	Neurotoxicity—paresthesia (numbness); ataxia; weakness; footdrop; hyporeflexia; constipation (adynamic ileus); hoarseness (vocal cord paralysis); abdominal, chest, and jaw pain; mental depression Fever N/V (mild) BMD (minimal; 7-14 days later) Alopecia SIADH	Vesicant Report signs of neurotoxicity because may necessitate cessation of drug Individuals with underlying neurologic problems may be more prone to neurotoxicity Monitor stool patterns closely; administer stool softener Excreted primarily by liver into biliary system; administer cautiously to anyone with biliary disease Maximum dose is 2 mg
Vinblastine (Velban) IV	Neurotoxicity (same as for vincristine but less severe) N/V (mild) BMD (especially neutropenia; 7-14 days later) Alopecia	Same as for vincristine
VP-16 (Etoposide, Ve-Pesid) IV	N/V (mild to moderate) BMD (7-14 days later) Alopecia Hypotension with rapid infusion Bradycardia Diarrhea (infrequent) Stomatitis (rare) May reactivate erythema of irradiated skin (rare) Allergic reaction with anaphylaxis possible Neurotoxicity	Give slowly via IV drip with child recumbent Have emergency drugs available at bedside*
VM-26 (Tenoposide) IV	Same as for VP-16	Same as for VP-16
ANTIBIOTICS		
Actinomycin-D (Dactinomycin, Cosmegen, ACT-D) IV	N/V (2-5 hours later) (moderate) BMD (especially platelets; 7-14 days later) Immunosuppression Mucosal ulceration Abdominal cramps Diarrhea Anorexia (may last few weeks) Alopecia Acne Erythema or hyperpigmentation of previously irradiated skin Fever Malaise	Vesicant Enhances cytotoxic effects of radiation therapy but increases toxic effect May cause serious desquamation of irradiated tissue
Doxorubicin (Adriamycin, Doxyoubicin) IV	N/V (moderate) Stomatitis BMD (7-14 days later) Fever, chills Local phlebitis	Vesicant (extravasation may *not* cause pain) Observe for any changes in heart rate or rhythm and signs of failure Cumulative dose must not exceed 550 mg/m^2, less with radiation

*Emergency drugs include oxygen and parenteral preparations of epinephrine 1:1000, diphenhydramine or similar antihistamine, aminophylline, corticosteroids, and vasopressors.

TABLE 36-2 Summary of Chemotherapeutic Agents Used in the Treatment of Childhood Cancers—cont'd

AGENT/ADMINISTRATION	SIDE EFFECTS AND TOXICITY	COMMENTS AND SPECIFIC NURSING CONSIDERATIONS
	Alopecia Cumulative-dose toxicity includes: Cardiac abnormalities ECG changes Heart failure	Warn parents that drug causes urine to turn red (for up to 12 days after administration); this is normal, not hematuria
Daunorubicin (Daunomycin, Rubidomycin) IV	Similar to doxorubicin	Similar to doxorubicin
Bleomycin (Blenoxane) IV, IM, SC	Allergic reaction—fever, chills, hypotension, anaphylaxis Fever (nonallergic) N/V (mild) Stomatitis Cumulative dose effects include: Skin—rash, hyperpigmentation, thickening, ulceration, peeling, nail changes, alopecia Lungs—pneumonitis with infiltrate that can progress to fatal fibrosis	Should give test dose (SC) before therapeutic dose administered Have emergency drugs* at bedside Hypersensitivity occurs with first one to two doses May give acetaminophen before drug to reduce likelihood of fever Concentration of drug in skin and lungs accounts for toxic effects Follow pulmonary function tests
HORMONES		
Corticosteroids (**prednisone** most frequently used; many proprietary names, such as **Meticorten, Deltasone, Paracort**) PO; also IM or IV but rarely used	For short-term use, no acute toxicity Usual side effects are mild; moon face, fluid retention, weight gain, mood changes, increased appetite, gastric irritation, insomnia, susceptibility to infection Hyperglycemia	Explain expected effects, especially in terms of body image, increased appetite, and personality changes Monitor weight gain Recommend moderate salt restriction Administer with antacid and early in morning (sometimes given every other day to minimize side effects) May need to disguise bitter taste (crush tablet and mix with syrup, jam, ice cream, or other highly flavored substance; use ice to numb tongue before administration; place tablet in gelatin capsule if child can swallow it) Observe for potential infection sites; usual inflammatory response and fever are absent
	Long-term effects of chronic steroid administration are mood changes, hirsutism, trunk obesity (buffalo hump), thin extremities, muscle wasting and weakness, osteoporosis, poor wound healing, bruising, potassium loss, gastric bleeding, hypertension, diabetes mellitus, growth retardation	Same as for short-term use; in addition, encourage foods high in potassium (bananas, raisins, prunes, coffee, chocolate) Test stools for occult blood Monitor blood pressure Test blood for sugar and urine for acetone Observe for signs of abrupt steroid withdrawal; flulike symptoms, hypotension, hypoglycemia, shock
ENZYMES		
L-Asparaginase (Elspar) IV, IM **Erwinia L-Asparaginase** **PEG L-Asparaginase**	Allergic reactions (including anaphylactic shock) Fever N/V (mild) Anorexia Weight loss Arthralgia Toxicity: Liver dysfunction Hyperglycemia Renal failure Pancreatitis	Have emergency drugs at bedside* Record signs of allergic reaction, such as urticaria, facial edema, hypotension, or abdominal cramps Check weight daily Normally, blood urea nitrogen (BUN) and ammonia levels rise as a result of drug; not evidence of liver damage Check urine for sugar and blood amylase

Continued.

TABLE 36-2 Summary of Chemotherapeutic Agents Used in the Treatment of Childhood Cancers—cont'd

AGENT/ADMINISTRATION	SIDE EFFECTS AND TOXICITY	COMMENTS AND SPECIFIC NURSING CONSIDERATIONS
NITROSOUREAS		
Carmustine (BCNU) IV Lomustine (CCNU) PO	N/V (2-6 hours later) (severe) BMD (3-4 weeks later) Burning pain along IV infusion (usually due to alcohol diluent) BCNU—flushing and facial burning on infusion Alopecia	Prevent extravasation; contact with skin causes brown spots Oral form—give 4 hours after meals when stomach is empty Reduce IV burning by diluting drug and infusing slowing via IV drip Crosses blood-brain barrier
OTHER AGENTS		
Hydroxyurea (Hydrea) PO	N/V (mild) Anorexia Less commonly: Diarrhea BMD Mucosal ulceration Alopecia Dermatitis	Must be given cautiously in patients with renal dysfunction

vent further replication of DNA and transcription of RNA.

Both adrenal and gonadal ***hormones*** have antineoplastic properties. The precise mechanism of action is still unclear. Adrenocorticosteroids are thought to bind with DNA and alter the transcription process. Although there are a number of cortisone preparations, prednisone is most frequently used.

A number of agents are not categorized according to the preceding classifications. For example, L-asparaginase is an enzyme isolated from extracts of bacterial cultures of *Escherichia coli* or *Erwinia carotovora.* It hydrolyzes L-asparagine, an amino acid, to L-aspartic acid, which prevents the cell from synthesizing protein needed for DNA and RNA synthesis. Because L-asparagine is synthesized by normal cells but must be exogenously supplied to certain leukemic and lymphoma cells, administration of the enzyme destroys the essential exogenous supply while sparing normal cells of untoward effects.

An understanding of drugs' actions and side effects is essential to nursing care of children with cancer (Table 36-2). Unfortunately, almost all drugs are not selectively cytotoxic for malignant cells, and other cells with a high rate of proliferation, such as the bone marrow elements, hair, skin, and epithelial cells of the gastrointestinal tract, are also affected. Frequently the problems related to the destruction of these normal cells require more nursing care than the disease itself.

Precautions in Administering and Handling Chemotherapeutic Agents. Many chemotherapeutic agents are ***vesicants (sclerosing agents)*** that can cause severe cellular damage if even minute amounts of the drug infiltrate surrounding tissue. Only nurses experienced with chemotherapeutic agents should administer vesicants. Guidelines are available* and must be followed meticulously to prevent tissue damage to patients. Interventions for extravasation vary, but each nurse should be aware of the institution's policies and implement them at once.

NURSING ALERT Chemotherapeutic drugs must be given through a free-flowing intravenous line. The infusion is stopped *immediately* if any sign of infiltration (pain, stinging, swelling, or redness at needle site) occurs.

In addition to extravasation, a potentially fatal complication is anaphylaxis, especially from L-asparaginase, bleomycin, cisplatin, and etoposide (see Chapter 29). Nursing responsibilities include prevention of, recognition of, and preparation for serious reactions. Prevention begins with a careful history of known allergy (see Chapter 6) (Hammond, 1988).

NURSING ALERT When chemotherapeutic and immunologic agents are given, the child must be observed for 20 minutes after the infusion for signs of anaphylaxis (cyanosis, hypotension, wheezing, severe urticaria). Emergency equipment (especially blood pressure monitor and bag-valve-mask) and emergency drugs (especially oxygen, epinephrine, antihistamine, aminophylline, corticosteroids, and vasopressors) must be available.

If a reaction is suspected, the drug is discontinued, the intravenous line is flushed with saline, and the child's vital signs and subsequent responses are monitored.

**Giving Cancer Drugs Intravenously: Some Guidelines* is available from the American Cancer Society, 1599 Clifton Rd., Atlanta, GA 30329; (404) 329-7617.

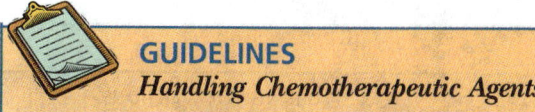

GUIDELINES
Handling Chemotherapeutic Agents

Use utmost care and strict aseptic technique in handling chemotherapeutic agents to prevent any physical contact with the substance.
Prepare drugs in a properly ventilated room or biologic safety cabinet (incorporates protective front panel and vertical laminar air flow to reduce potential for inhalation during preparation).
Wear disposable gloves and protective clothing and discard in special container after each use.
Use a sterile gauze pad when priming IV tubing, connecting and disconnecting tubing, inserting syringes into vials, breaking glass ampules, or any other procedure in which antineoplastic drugs may be inadvertently discharged.
Dispose of all contaminated needles, syringes, IV tubing, and other contaminated equipment in a leakproof and puncture-resistant container; do not recap or break needles.

In addition to the many responsibilities nurses must have in regard to the child and family, they must also use safeguards to protect themselves. Handling chemotherapeutic agents may present risks to handlers and to their offspring, although the exact degree of risk is not known.

The Oncology Nursing Society has published comprehensive guidelines for safe practice issues related to administration of chemotherapy.* Safe management procedures for chemotherapy administered in the home have also been established (Blecke, 1989; Sansievero and Murray, 1989). Basic nursing guidelines are listed in the Guidelines box.

Radiotherapy

Radiotherapy is frequently used in the treatment of childhood cancer, usually in conjunction with chemotherapy and/or surgery. It can be used for curative purposes and is often employed for palliation to relieve symptoms by shrinking the size of the tumor. Recent advances in radiation therapy have optimized its beneficial effects and minimized many of the undesirable side effects, although high-dose radiation is associated with many serious late effects.

Ionizing radiation is cytotoxic in at least three different ways: (1) damaging the pyrimidine bases cytosine, thymine, and uracil, needed for the synthesis of nucleic acids; (2) causing single-strand breaks in the DNA or RNA molecule; or (3) causing double helical–strand breaks in these molecules. The effect of disturbing cellular metabolic and reproductive functions is either sublethal or lethal damage.

Lethal damage refers to the death of the cell. ***Sublethal damage*** refers to injured cells that may subsequently be repaired. Many of the acute side effects are the result of lethal damage to radiosensitive tissue, particularly proliferating cells such as those of the bone marrow, gastrointestinal tract, and hair follicles. Late effects are usually the result of cell death.

The acute untoward reactions from radiotherapy depend primarily on the area to be irradiated. ***Total-body irradiation (TBI)*** is associated with the most severe reactions and is employed to prepare the immune system for bone marrow transplantation. Table 36-3 summarizes the acute effects of radiation therapy and nursing interventions that may be helpful in lessening or preventing them.

Biologic Response Modifiers (BRMs)

BRMs modify the relationship between tumor and host by therapeutically changing the host's biologic response to tumor cells. These agents or interventions may affect the host's immunologic mechanisms (immunotherapy), have direct antitumor activity, or have other biologic effects (Yasko and Dudjak, 1990). The use of BRMs is called ***biotherapy.***

Much of the current work in biotherapy is directed toward the use of monoclonal antibodies in the diagnosis and treatment of cancers. Through a complex process, special cells are fused to form a hybrid clone or hybridoma that produces antibodies that recognize a single specific antigen, hence the term ***monoclonal antibody*** ("mono" meaning one and "clone" meaning exact duplicate). These clones are then frozen, maintained in culture, or grown as tumors in mice to produce large quantities of the antibody in ascites fluid (Weinberg and Parkman, 1989). While there are many prospective uses for monoclonal antibodies, their current role has been in diagnosing subclasses of leukemia cells to enhance understanding of which types of leukemia respond to different treatments and to determine if the subclass is related to the prognosis. Monoclonal antibodies have also been used to deplete allogeneic bone marrows of T-cells to reduce graft-versus-host disease and to selectively eliminate malignant cells from autologous marrow for transplanting back into the patient (Poplack, 1993). Results from these studies have been encouraging, but further work is needed to define the role monoclonal antibodies and other BRMs will have in cancer care.

Bone Marrow Transplantation (BMT)

Another approach to the treatment of childhood cancer is BMT. Candidates for transplantation are children who have malignancies that are unlikely to be cured by other means. However, its use is controversial. It has not proved superior to chemotherapy in terms of long-term survival, it is associated with greater mortality and morbidity, and it is very expensive (Pinkel, 1993). (See Family Focus box, p. 1622.)

BMT allows for lethal doses of chemotherapy, often combined with radiation therapy, to be given in order to rid the body of all cancer cells (National Cancer Institute, 1991). Once the body is free of malignant cells and the immune system is suppressed to prevent rejection of the transplanted marrow, the donor marrow cells or the cells previously stored from the patient's own marrow are given to the patient by intravenous transfusion. The newly transfused marrow will begin to produce functioning nonmalignant blood cells. In essence, a new blood-forming organ will be accepted by the recipient.

**Cancer Chemotherapy Guidelines* can be obtained from Oncology Nursing Society, 501 Holiday Dr., Pittsburgh, PA 15220-2749; (412) 921-7373.

TABLE 36-3 Early Side Effects of Radiotherapy

SITE/EFFECTS	NURSING INTERVENTIONS
GASTROINTESTINAL TRACT	
Nausea/vomiting	Give antiemetic around the clock Measure amount of emesis to assess for dehydration
Anorexia	Encourage fluids and foods best tolerated, usually light, soft diet and small, frequent meals Monitor weight loss
Mucosal ulceration	Use frequent mouthwashes and oral hygiene to prevent mucositis
Diarrhea	Can be controlled with antispasmodics and kaolin pectin preparations Observe for signs of dehydration
SKIN	
Alopecia (within 2 weeks; begins to regrow by 3-6 months) Dry or moist desquamation	Introduce idea of wig Stress necessity of scalp hygiene and need for head covering in cold weather Do not refer to skin change as a "burn" (implies use of too much radiation) Keep skin clean Wash daily, using soap (e.g., Tone, Dove) sparingly Do not remove skin marking for radiation fields Avoid exposure to sun For dryness, apply lubricant For desquamation, consult practitioner for skin hygiene and care
HEAD	
Nausea/vomiting (from stimulation of vomiting center in brain)	Same as for gastrointestinal tract
Alopecia	Same as for skin
Mucositis	Encourage regular dental care, fluoride treatments
Potential effects Parotitis Sore throat Loss of taste	May need analgesics to relieve discomfort
Xerostomia (dry mouth)	Combat severe dryness of mouth with oral hygiene and liquid diet
URINARY BLADDER	
Rarely cystitis	More likely to occur with concomitant use of cyclophosphamide Encourage liberal fluid intake and frequent voiding Evaluate for hematuria
BONE MARROW	
Myelosuppression	Observe for fever (temperature above 38.3° C [101° F]) Initiate workup for sepsis as ordered Administer antibiotics as prescribed Avoid use of suppositories, rectal temperatures Institute bleeding precautions Observe for signs of anemia

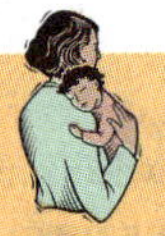

FAMILY FOCUS

The Decision for a Bone Marrow Transplant

The family's decision for a child to undergo a bone marrow transplant is one that is fraught with difficulties. Often the child is facing certain death from the malignancy. The preparation of the child for the transplant also places the patient at great medical risk.

Once the preparatory regimen is begun and the child's immune system is destroyed, there is no turning back. Unlike kidney transplantation, BMT does not have a "rescue" procedure, such as dialysis, for supportive therapy. If the donor is a sibling, the issue of his or her marrow "saving" the brother or sister is a concern, especially if the transplant fails. Parents often must leave the home to stay at the transplant center and encounter additional stressors such as arranging child care, taking a leave from work, and managing finances. The patient faces the greatest stress—fear of BMT failure or life-threatening complications.

Presently three types of bone marrow transplants may be done: (1) ***allogeneic,*** which involves the matching of a histocompatible donor, usually a sibling, with the recipient (may also involve an unmatched donor); (2) ***autologous,*** which uses the patient's own marrow that was collected from disease-free tissue, frozen, and sometimes treated to remove malignant cells; and (3) ***syngeneic,*** which uses marrow from an identical twin.

The most common type of bone marrow transplantation is allogeneic. The selection process of a suitable donor and the potential complications in transplantation are related to the ***human leukocyte antigen (HLA) system complex*** (see p. 168). Some of the major HLA antigens are A, B, C, D, and DR. There is a wide diversity for each of these HLA loci. There are more than 20 different HLA-A antigens that can be inherited and more than 40 different HLA-B antigens.

The genes are inherited as a single unit or ***haplotype.*** A child inherits one unit from each parent; thus a child and each parent have one identical and one nonidentical haplotype. Since the possible haplotype combinations among siblings follow the laws of Mendelian genetics, there is a one in four chance that two siblings have two identical haplotypes and are perfectly matched at the HLA loci.

The importance of HLA matching is to prevent the serious complication known as ***graft-versus-host disease (GVHD).*** Since the child's immune system is essentially rendered nonfunctional, there is little difficulty with bone marrow rejection by the recipient. However, the donor's marrow may contain antigens not matched to the recipient's antigens, which begin attacking body cells. The more closely the HLA systems match, the less likely GVHD is to develop. However, it can occur even with a perfect HLA match, because there are as yet unidentified and thus unmatched histocompatibility antigens (Ramsay, 1993). GVHD is not a complication in autologous BMT, but the risks of morbidity and death from the preconditioning regimen and postgraft failure remain.

Although the actual transplant procedure is simple and involves harvesting several bone marrow specimens from the donor (which is done under general anesthesia) and diluting the marrow and administering it intravenously similar to any blood product to the recipient, the preoperative and postoperative care is complex. The first stage is identifying a compatible donor in the case of an allergenic transplant. The second phase is cytoreduction to produce a totally aleukemic immunosuppressed state, which involves intense chemotherapy and total-body irradiation (Ramsay, 1993).

The third phase is preventing complications. During the preoperative aplastic phase and for the 10- to 20-day period after transplantation before the new marrow begins adequately replacing granulocytes, the child is extremely susceptible to infection. Interstitial or nonbacterial pneumonia is another serious complication with a high mortality rate. However, the most common complication in allogeneic transplants is GVHD, which can affect the skin, gastrointestinal tract, liver, heart, lungs, lymphoid tissue, and marrow. GVHD is characterized by a hardening of the tissues and drying of the mucous membranes. The severity of the manifestations varies, but once vital organs are affected, death can ensue. Treatment involves the use of steroids and/or azathioprine (Imuran). However, these immunosuppressive drugs further increase the risk of infection. All blood products should be irradiated to minimize the introduction of additional antigens. Another unfortunate posttransplant possibility is recurrence of the malignancy after engraftment. Emphasis is now placed on the prevention of GVHD, using various agents such as cyclosporine, methotrexate, and steroids (Johnson, 1991).

Supportive Therapies

Cancer care encompasses more than treatments aimed at eliminating the malignant cells. Because of the delicate balance between killing malignant cells and preserving functional cells, supportive therapy is frequently needed during those times that serious damage occurs to normal body tissues. For example, infection is a constant threat from the immunosuppressant effects of antineoplastic agents. Prophylactic antibiotics, such as trimethoprim/sulfamethoxazole (Bactrim, Septra), may be given to reduce the incidence of serious infection (Frenck, Kohl, and Pickering, 1991).

Recently ***colony-stimulating factors (CSFs),*** a family of glycoprotein hormones that regulate the reproduction, maturation, and function of blood cells, have been used as supportive measures to prevent the side effects caused by low blood counts. CSFs promote stem cell proliferation and stimulate a more rapid maturation of the cells, allowing them to enter the bloodstream earlier. ***GCSF (granulocyte colony–stimulating factor)*** (filgrastim [Neupogen]) directs granulocyte development and has been shown to decrease the duration of neutropenia following immunosuppressive therapy. This reduces the incidence and duration of infection in children receiving treatment for cancer. GCSF is also being used to decrease the bone marrow recovery time following bone marrow transplantation (Yasko and Dudjak, 1990). GCSF is usually administered intravenously or subcutaneously 24 hours after chemotherapy is discontinued and is given for 10 to 14 days. GCSF is discontinued when the absolute neutrophil count surpasses 10,000/mm^3. During GCSF therapy children may experience bone pain, fever, rash, malaise, and headaches (Yasko and Dudjak, 1990).

Other supportive therapies include ***replacement of blood elements*** as needed in anemia, agranulocytopenia, and thrombocytopenia. However, the use of granulocyte transfusions and preventive infusions of platelets is controversial because of the lack of documented effectiveness and the risk of developing antibodies to the foreign antigens, respectively (Darbyshire, 1988; Mitchell, 1988).

Allopurinol, a xanthine-oxidase inhibitor, may be administered to prevent renal damage in the newly diagnosed or relapsed patient. Massive cellular damage from cytotoxic therapy releases large amounts of uric acid, which can accumulate and precipitate in the renal tubules, eventually causing tubular obstruction. Allopurinol prevents the metabolic breakdown of xanthine to uric acid. Other supportive measures include alkalinization of the urine and adequate hydration.

Nutritional support has been increasingly recognized as a significant component of cancer treatment. Optimum nutrition promotes the body's tolerance to antineoplastic agents and preserves immunologic responsiveness. Excellent nutrition before intensive therapy provides nutrient stores during periods of anorexia, nausea, and vomiting. The most common nutritional problem is children's unwillingness to consume sufficient food to maintain a nutritional balance. Oral supplementation with fortified foods, such as commercial preparations (Ensure, Pediasure), may be helpful, but nonoral routes may be necessary (e.g., nasogastric tube feedings, gastrostomy, parenteral alimentation) (Drakeford, 1988).

An essential supportive therapy is the effective use of ***analgesics,*** especially the use of opioids when pain is moderate to severe and when invasive procedures are performed. Dosages of analgesics are *titrated to the child's needs* and administered *around the clock* for optimum pain control. Nonpharmacologic strategies should be implemented as needed but should not be regarded as substitutes for pharmacologic management. The reader is encouraged to review Pain Assessment and Pain Management in Chapter 26 and Preparation for Procedures on p. 1627.

COMPLICATIONS OF THERAPY

Although tremendous advances have been achieved through current modes of cancer therapy, the successes are not without consequences. Numerous side effects are expected with chemotherapy and radiotherapy, and these are discussed under Nursing Care of the Child with Cancer. However, other complications that are less frequently seen but generally more serious and possibly permanent are described here.

Pediatric Oncologic Emergencies

Life-threatening conditions may develop in children with cancer as a result of aggressive treatment modalities or from the malignancy itself. ***Acute tumor lysis syndrome*** is caused by the rapid release of intracellular metabolites during the initial treatment of malignancies such as Burkitt and T-cell lymphomas and acute leukemia. Rapid tumor lysis leads to hyperuricemia, hypocalcemia, hyperphosphatemia, and hyperkalemia (Mahon and Casperson, 1993).

Obstruction may create an oncologic emergency for a child with cancer. Space-occupying lesions, especially from Hodgkin disease and non-Hodgkin lymphoma (NHL), located in the chest may cause ***superior vena cava syndrome (SVCS)*** (compression of mediastinal structures), leading to airway compromise and potentially to respiratory failure. SVCS has also been reported with central venous catheters from the formation of a thrombus or a fibrotic reaction. Children may have a mass obstructing the spinal cord, as manifested by symptoms ranging from tingling to paresthesias and loss of bowel and bladder control. Children with brain tumors may develop symptoms ranging from increased intracranial pressure to respiratory compromise and herniation, depending on the location and size of the tumor (Heideman and others, 1993).

Infections in the immunocompromised child constitute an emergency situation. Gram-negative sepsis can result in numerous complications, including disseminated intravascular coagulation (DIC), created by bacteria or fungus causing damage to the endothelial system. Life-threatening hemorrhage can occur from DIC, thrombocytopenia (platelet count $<20,000/mm^3$), and leukocytosis (leukocyte count $>100,000/mm^3$). Leukocytosis may cause intracranial bleeding from increased viscosity of the blood. The resulting leukocytosis leads to vascular damage and subsequent hemorrhage.

Long-Term Sequelae of Treatment

Vigorous treatment of childhood cancers has resulted in dramatically improved survival rates. However, treatment programs combining surgery, irradiation, and chemotherapy are not without their complications. Some may occur immediately, such as loss of a limb from surgical amputation or asplenia from splenectomy in Hodgkin disease. However, current concern is with late effects—adverse changes related to treatment modalities, interactions between modes of treatment, individual characteristics of the child, and the disease process that may appear months to years after lifesaving treatment (Raymond, 1988). Because of the greater number of children who are cured and surviving into adulthood, increasing documentation of late effects is emerging (see Table 36-4). Almost no organ is exempt, and almost every antineoplastic agent (including and especially irradiation) is responsible for some adverse effect. Although many factors influence the development of late effects from radiation, some of the more important ones include the total cumulative dose given, the age of the child (the younger the child, the more radiosensitive the body organs are), and the location of the tumor.

NURSING CARE OF THE CHILD WITH CANCER

This section presents an overview of general nursing concepts that apply to most childhood cancers. Specific nursing care for the child with a particular type of cancer is discussed under each disease section later in this chapter. The focus of this discussion is on the physical aspects of care. Emotional aspects are presented in Chapter 22 (chronic illness) and in Chapter 23 (terminal illness).

❖ ASSESSMENT

Signs and Symptoms of Cancer in Children

Early detection is critical to early treatment and eventual cure. Cancers in children are often difficult to recognize. Therefore, being alert to the persistence of unusual symptoms is essential (see box below). Some of the more significant clues to pediatric cancer are discussed here.

Pain may be an early or late initial sign of cancer and requires a careful history of its onset, characteristics, location, intensity, and alleviating factors. Pain may be generalized or present at a specific location. For example, bone pain occurs in approximately 20% of children with leukemia. Pain, swelling, and tenderness at the tumor site may be the initial sign in bone tumors.

Fever is a frequent occurrence during childhood and is caused by numerous illnesses, including cancer. Fever is most often caused by infection secondary to the malignant process.

CARDINAL SYMPTOMS OF CANCER IN CHILDREN

Unusual mass or swelling
Unexplained paleness and loss of energy
Sudden tendency to bruise
Persistent, localized pain or limping
Prolonged, unexplained fever or illness
Frequent headaches, often with vomiting
Sudden eye or vision changes
Excessive, rapid weight loss

From *Cancer facts and figures, 1993,* Atlanta, 1993, American Cancer Society.

A careful ***skin*** assessment will reveal signs and symptoms of a low platelet count. Ecchymosis and petechiae are most commonly found on the child's extremities, and nose bleeding may occur when the platelet count falls below 20,000/mm^3.

The child with malignant invasion of the bone marrow often appears pale, with symptoms of lethargy, weight loss, and generalized malaise. These symptoms may be attributed to the development of ***anemia*** caused by the replacement of normal cells with malignant cells in the bone marrow. The nurse should assess for signs and symptoms of anemia, as discussed in Chapter 35.

An ***abdominal mass*** is a typical finding in children with Wilms tumor and neuroblastoma. The presence of an abdominal mass in a child must be evaluated for a malignancy.

Swollen lymph glands are another common finding in children. However, enlarged, firm, lymph nodes in a child with fever for more than 1 week, a recent history of weight loss, and/or an abnormal chest x-ray film may indicate a serious disease and should be evaluated further.

The presence of a ***white reflection*** as opposed to the normal red pupillary reflex in the pupil of a child's eye is the classic sign of retinoblastoma. The presence of squinting, strabismus, or swelling can indicate other solid tumors of the eye.

The child with a brain tumor will develop signs and symptoms according to the exact area of the brain involved. The nurse must perform a thorough assessment to identify the specific area of tumor involvement (see Table 36-6).

The Child Undergoing Treatment for Cancer

A major concern for the child receiving treatment for cancer is the risk for the development of complications secondary to the treatment. Major complications include fever, bleeding, and anemia.

The nurse caring for the child with fever must be aware of the signs and symptoms of septic shock, as discussed in Chapter 29. The child with fever who has an absolute granulocyte count lower than 500/mm^3 is at risk for the following:

- Overwhelming infection
- General malaise
- Dehydration
- Seizures (young infants and children)
- Invasion of organisms producing secondary infections

The child with fever is evaluated for potential sites of infection, such as from a needle puncture, mucosal ulceration, minor abrasion, or skin tears (e.g., a hangnail). Although the body may not be able to produce an adequate inflammatory response to the infection and the usual clinical signs of infection may be partially expressed or absent, fever will occur. Therefore temperature is monitored closely. To identify the source of infection, blood, stool, urine, and nasopharyngeal cultures and chest x-ray films are taken.

The child with a platelet count lower than 20,000/mm^3 is assessed closely for signs of active bleeding, especially in those common sites where bleeding occurs in the child with thrombocytopenia—the nose, mouth, conjunctiva, and ears. Petechiae and areas of ecchymoses are documented to determine areas of new bleeding under the skin. The child's urine and stool are observed and tested for the presence of blood.

The child undergoing cancer treatment may develop anemia caused by aggressive therapy regimens preventing the bone marrow from producing red blood cells. The nurse should assess closely for changes in vital signs and physical symptoms that may reflect the presence of anemia, as described in Chapter 35.

The Childhood Cancer Survivor

It is estimated that by the year 2000, one individual in 900 will have survived childhood cancer. These young adults are at risk for the development of numerous late effects caused by the cancer or its treatment. These complications are defined as posttherapeutic disabilities, ranging from impaired cognitive development to the onset of second malignancies.

Psychosocial, cognitive, emotional, and physical development may be affected by treatment, as well as by the disease. Table 36-4 describes the systemic late effects caused by cancer treatment that require careful nursing assessment.

All tissues and organs are susceptible to the toxicity of cancer treatment. Many of the problems observed from the treatment for childhood cancer relate to the effects on developing tissues. As a general principle, cytotoxic therapy is more harmful to rapidly growing tissue than to slowly growing tissue.

Four systems that have the potential to develop complications unique to children require careful assessment following therapy for cancer. These are the central nervous, endocrine, reproductive, and skeletal systems.

Nurses caring for young children with cancer must be aware of the impairment caused by treatment with cranial irradiation and intrathecal chemotherapy. Intellectual and motor function may be impaired because of interference with neural development before maturation of the brain is complete (Moore and others, 1992). Children under the age of 3 years are at the highest risk for this complication. Assessment of children who have received cranial radiation and intrathecal chemotherapy must incorporate an extensive neurologic evaluation that includes cognitive function.

Radiation therapy to growing bones or reproductive glands responsible for growth-related hormones can delay or stunt growth. Nurses must document growth by assessing height and weight at each visit. Any decrease in growth velocity should be further evaluated. Further assessment includes documenting parental heights, obtaining a wrist x-ray film to predict further growth potential, and assessing gonadal development and pituitary function.

Radiation therapy and the alkylating agents can cause hormonal dysfunction, decreased fertility, and sterility. The potential for gonadal dysfunction depends on the child's age, sex, type of treatment, and the duration and total doses of treatment. Nursing assessment must begin with careful documentation of the child's sexual development using the Tanner staging scale (see Pubertal Sexual Maturation, Chapter 19).

Irradiation to developing bone and cartilage may cause numerous abnormalities. Assessment includes close obser-

TABLE 36-4 Late Effects of Cancer Treatment

SYSTEMIC EFFECTS/CLINICAL MANIFESTATIONS	ASSOCIATED MODE OF TREATMENT
CENTRAL NERVOUS SYSTEM (CNS)	
Leukoencephalopathy (syndrome ranging from lethargy, dementia, and seizures to quadriplegia and death)	Methotrexate and/or CNS irradiation
Mineralizing microangiopathy (headaches, focal seizures, incoordination, gate abnormalities)	Methotrexate and/or CNS irradiation
Peripheral neuropathy (footdrop, incoordination)	Vincristine
Cognitive deficits (intelligence, nonlanguage skills)	Intrathecal chemotherapy and/or cranial irradiation (especially before age 3 years)
CARDIOVASCULAR	
Cardiomyopathy (tachycardia, tachypnea, dyspnea, shortness of breath, edema, palpitations)	Anthracyclines (doxorubicin and daunorubicin) and/or irradiation to heart High-dose cyclophosphamide
Pericardial damage (pleural effusion, cardiomegaly)	Mediastinal irradiation
RESPIRATORY	
Pneumonitis (dyspnea, nonproductive cough, fever) Pulmonary fibrosis (dyspnea, restrictive ventilation, decreased exercise tolerance)	Lung irradiation, alkylating agents, possibly bleomycin, vinblastine, cisplatin
GASTROINTESTINAL	
Chronic enteritis (colic, abdominal pain, vomiting, diarrhea, obstipation, bleeding)	Abdominal irradiation, methotrexate, cytosine arabinoside
Hepatic fibrosis (jaundice, hepatomegaly)	Methotrexate, 6-mercaptopurine
URINARY	
Hemorrhagic cystitis (chronic microscopic hematuria to gross hemorrhage)	Cyclophosphamide; ifosfamide irradiation, especially with radiomimetic chemotherapeutic agents (i.e., doxorubicin and daunorubicin)
Bladder fibrosis (decreased bladder capacity, ureteral reflux)	
Tubular necrosis (decreased creatinine clearance)	Cisplatin
ENDOCRINE	
Growth retardation (abnormal growth velocity) Thyroid dysfunction (see Chapter 38) Gonadal dysfunction (see Reproductive)	Irradiation to the thyroid, pituitary gland, testes, ovaries
REPRODUCTIVE	
Possible gonadal damage—both sexes (amenorrhea, decreased sperm counts, increased follicle-stimulating and luteinizing hormones [FSH, LH], decreased testosterone/estrogen)	Alkylating agents Irradiation to the pituitary gland, testes, ovaries
SKELETAL	
Linear growth retardation (short stature)	Irradiation, long-term steroids
Spinal deformities, scoliosis, kyphosis, asymmetric growth, pathologic fractures	Irradiation
IMMUNE	
Asplenia (overwhelming infection, fever)	Splenectomy (Hodgkin disease)
SENSORY ORGANS	
Cataracts (opacity over pupil)	Cranial irradiation, high-dose steroids
Hearing (decreased hearing associated with high-frequency loss)	Cisplatin
ADDITIONAL EFFECTS	
Dental Problems	
Increased caries, periodontal disease, hypoplastic teeth, hypodontia (delayed or absent tooth development)	Irradiation to maxilla and mandible
Second Malignancies	
Bone and soft tissue tumors Leukemia Nonlymphocytic leukemia	Irradiation, alkylating agents

vations of the irradiated bone for defects, such as spinal kyphoscoliosis, leg length discrepancy, and skull and facial disfigurement.

Irradiated bones are more fragile and may fracture easily, have functional limitations, and heal slowly in the presence of infection. Osteoporosis may develop. Children who have received irradiation to the mandibular area are at risk for dental caries, arrested tooth development, and incomplete dental calcification. A careful assessment of the oral cavity in children who have received irradiation to the mandible is performed at each clinic visit.

❖ Nursing Diagnoses

A number of nursing diagnoses become apparent following an assessment of the child with cancer and the family. Some are considered in the Nursing Care Plan on pp. 1633-1637. Others are identified here in specific situations.

❖ Planning

The goals for the child with cancer and the family include the following:

1. Child will receive appropriate primary health care.
2. Child and family will be prepared for diagnostic and therapeutic procedures.
3. Child will experience minimal complications of myelosuppression.
4. Problems of irradiation and drug toxicity will be managed.
5. Child and family will receive adequate support and education.

❖ Implementation

Health Promotion

Children with cancer require the same basic health supervision as any child. Sometimes the overwhelming needs and demands placed on the family coupled with the singular concern focused on the cancer by both family and practitioners result in a lack of attention to normal health care needs. Nurses should monitor the type of primary care the child receives, using as a guideline recommendations for health supervision (see Chapter 7). As discussed under the Assessment section, areas of particular concern are growth, physical and cognitive development, and neurologic status. Two other areas are also important: (1) dental care, because of potential side effects from treatment; and (2) immunizations, because of concern with live virus vaccines and immunosuppression.

Dental Care. Irradiation to the head and neck can cause a number of late complications (Jaffe, 1991a). Some are irreversible, such as facial asymmetry, but those affecting the teeth and gums (caries, periodontal disease) benefit from excellent oral hygiene, including regular use of systemic and topical fluoride (see Dental Health, Chapter 14). There is also evidence of delayed or absent development of the permanent teeth (Jaffe, 1991a). Depending on the child's age, this can be a source of acute psychologic distress, especially during early school-age years when "losing a tooth" is a status symbol. Children need to be aware of this possibility and helped to explain the delay to peers.

Daily toothbrushing and flossing is encouraged in children with granulocyte counts in excess of 500/mm^3 and platelet counts above 40,000/mm^3. Fluoride rinses are used as discussed in Chapter 14. Oral hygiene for children whose counts are below these parameters is limited to wiping the teeth with moistened gauze sponges or Toothettes.

Immunizations. Viral replication following the administration of live vaccine for polio, measles, rubella, and mumps can cause serious disease in immunocompromised children who receive these vaccines.

The child receiving chemotherapy for cancer should not receive live, attenuated vaccines. The inactivated poliovirus vaccine (IPV) should be given to immunosuppressed children and their household contacts in place of the routine immunization with the oral poliovirus (McCalla, Santacroce, Woolery-Antill, 1993). Siblings and household contacts may receive the live measles, mumps, and rubella vaccine (MMR) without risk to the child with cancer. Children who are immunosuppressed can receive the varicella (chickenpox) vaccine, which has been shown to be effective in preventing varicella in high-risk children.

NURSING ALERT Children vaccinated 2 weeks before or during chemotherapy should be considered unimmunized and should be revaccinated or receive live virus vaccines 3 months after chemotherapy has stopped (General recommendations, 1994).

A very important indication for isolation is an outbreak of childhood disease, especially chickenpox. Ideally the school nurse should work with the treating practitioner to decide the optimum time for school reattendance. If the child has been exposed to the varicella virus, varicella-zoster immune globulin (VZIG) given within 72 hours may favorably alter the course of the disease, or antiviral agents, such as acyclovir, may be given if the child develops varicella. These antiviral agents are very effective in preventing serious disease if given during the first 3 days of the appearance of symptoms (Frenck, Kohl, and Pickering, 1991). Without treatment, death from disseminated varicella (about 7%) is usually caused by pneumonia; other serious although nonfatal complications include hepatitis, pancreatitis, meningitis, and bacterial skin infections (see also Immunizations, Chapter 12).

Preparation for Procedures

Children in particular need psychologic preparation for the various treatment modalities, which often involve surgery, intravenous injections, bone marrow aspiration, and lumbar punctures. The diagnostic procedures initially employed to confirm the diagnosis and those that are repeated to monitor treatment are often a source of discomfort and stress to the child and family. Even noninvasive procedures such as imaging and radiologic tests are frightening to a young child. Many of these tests require the child to lie absolutely motionless for a prolonged time in a confined space with little or no communication with a supportive adult. Consequently, infants and young children are usually sedated, and older children need an explanation of what to expect and reminders during the test of how much longer they must remain still. The same principles for preparing children for procedures that are discussed in Chapter 27 apply here, including the option of having parents stay with the child whenever possible (see Thinking Critically About . . . box on p. 1138). Children who undergo repeated tests also need additional preparation or emotional support. Children are more likely to become conditioned to the discomfort and to experience *increasing,* not decreasing, levels of stress (Dolgin and others, 1989; Zeltzer, Jay, and Fisher, 1989).

Two procedures, bone marrow studies and lumbar punctures, are so commonly performed in many types of childhood cancer that they deserve special consideration in preparing children. Both tests can be frightening to children because they are done behind the child's field of vision. Recent consensus among professionals caring for children with cancer support the use of sedation for the initial procedures and subsequent developmentally appropriate support using both pharmacologic and nonpharmacologic approaches (Bucholtz, 1992; Schecter, Altman, and Weisman, 1990). A pharmacologic approach known as conscious sedation is currently being used at many institutions. Most conscious sedation protocols combine an opioid analgesic with a benzodiazepine for anxiolysis and sedation (see Critical Thinking Exercise box).

EMLA cream, a topical anesthetic preparation that adequately penetrates intact skin, is used as a local anesthetic before intrusive procedures, including venipunctures, implanted port access, lumbar punctures, and subcutaneous or intramuscular injections (Halperin and others 1989; Kapelushnik and others 1990). Local intradermal anesthesia is frequently used for lumbar puncture and bone marrow examination. To reduce the stinging sensation from lidocaine, sodium bicarbonate should be added (see Pain Management, Chapter 26). Deeper infiltration of the muscle and periosteum of the bone with buffered lidocaine further reduces the pain from the large-bore aspiration/biopsy needle entering the bone.

For bone marrow studies and lumbar punctures, as well as other procedures, children of preschool age and beyond should be prepared beforehand. If this is not possible, the nurse should explain each step of the procedure as it occurs, stressing what will be done and what it will feel like. If each step is explained beforehand, having the child recall the next step during the procedure can be a distraction mechanism.

Physical care after the procedures is minimal. A small pressure bandage is applied to the bone marrow puncture site, and an adhesive bandage is applied to the lumbar puncture site. No activity restriction is necessary after the bone marrow test, although the site is usually sore and the child may prefer to remain quiet. Recommendations after the lumbar puncture vary. If medication was instilled, the child may be placed in a slight Trendelenburg position to facilitate circulation of the medicated spinal fluid.

CRITICAL THINKING EXERCISE
Bone Marrow Test

Suzy Long, 5 years old, is admitted to the hospital for diagnosis of possible leukemia. During your nursing admission history regarding Suzy's pain experience, Mrs. Long tells you that her daughter is very cooperative when she receives injections. Suzy agrees and adds that they hurt, but just for a second. With this information you discuss with the nurse practitioner who will perform the bone marrow test the type of preparation that is appropriate for Suzy. You both believe that the best option is to:

1. Tell Suzy what the test will be like and teach her a simple breathing exercise to help her relax.
2. Use a local anesthetic at the bone marrow site to lessen the painful entry of the needle.
3. Administer midazolam and fentanyl intravenously just before the procedure to produce conscious sedation.
4. Offer Suzy the above choices and let her select one.

All of the options are potentially acceptable, but for Suzy the best one is 3, considering her age, the type of painful procedures she has experienced, the pain intensity of the bone marrow test, and the possibility of future invasive procedures.

Suzy is too young to compare the first three choices critically. Injections are typically less painful than a bone marrow test, which Suzy has never had. Relaxation works well in some children for procedures that produce mild to moderate pain, such as venipunctures, but there is no way to predict its success. A local anesthetic lessens the pain, but not the sensation of pushing to insert the needle or the aspiration of the marrow. Also, the bone marrow test for diagnosis takes longer to perform than most other bone marrow tests because a larger amount of marrow is needed. Sometimes two punctures may be done. Using fentanyl and midazolam will reduce the pain and produce amnesia, making the procedure less stressful and preventing fear and anxiety for future tests.

Prevention of Complications of Myelosuppression

Some types of malignancies (leukemia, lymphoma) and most of the chemotherapeutic agents cause myelosuppression. The reduced numbers of blood cells result in secondary problems of infection, bleeding tendencies, and anemia. Supportive care involves both medical and nursing management. Because they are so closely linked, they are discussed together rather than separately.

Infection. A frequent complication of treatment for childhood cancer is overwhelming infection secondary to neutropenia. However, the use of GCSF has reduced the incidence and duration of infection in children receiving treatment for cancer (see p. 1623).

The child is most susceptible to overwhelming infection during three phases of the disease: (1) at the time of diagnosis and relapse when the cancer process has replaced normal leukocytes, (2) during immunosuppressive therapy causing an absolute neutrophil count of less than $100/mm^3$ (see Guidelines box) (Frenck, Kohl, and Pickering, 1991), and (3) after prolonged antibiotic therapy, which predisposes the child to the growth of resistant organisms.

GUIDELINES
Calculating the Absolute Neutrophil Count (ANC)

1. Determine the total percent of neutrophils ("polys or segs" and "bands").
2. Multiply white blood cell (WBC) count by percent of neutrophils.
   Example: WBC = 1000, neutrophils = 7%, nonsegmented neutrophils (bands) = 7%
   Step 1: 7% + 7% = 14%
   Step 2: 0.14 × 1000 = 140 ANC

The first defense against infection is prevention. When the child is hospitalized, all measures to control transfer of infection are instituted, such as the use of a private room, restriction of all visitors and health personnel with active infection, and strict handwashing technique with an antiseptic solution. The use of protective (reverse) isolation is controversial; however, research provides evidence that protective isolation does *not* decrease the risk of infection nor improve survival (Frenck, Kohl, and Pickering, 1991). Therefore any decision to implement protective isolation must be seriously evaluated in terms of its doubtful benefit and the psychologic stress it imposes on the child.

The organisms most lethal to these children are (1) viruses, particularly varicella (chickenpox), herpes zoster, herpes simplex, measles, rubella, mumps, and poliomyelitis; (2) *Pneumocystis carinii* (a protozoan); (3) fungi, especially *Candida albicans;* (4) gram-negative bacteria, such as *Pseudomonas aeruginosa, Escherichia coli, Proteus,* and *Klebsiella;* and (5) gram-positive bacteria, especially *Staphylococcus aureus, S. epidermidis,* and group A β-hemolytic streptococcus (Viscoli, 1988; Wagner, 1988). As prophylaxis against these various organisms, broad-spectrum antibiotics are usually prescribed. Ensuring compliance with this long-term regimen is an important nursing responsibility.

Once infection is suspected, broad-spectrum intravenous antibiotic therapy is begun before the organism is identified and may be continued for 7 to 10 days. If the child does not have a venous access device, a heparin lock should be inserted to prevent the inconvenience of multiple venipunctures in maintaining a patent intravenous line and to prevent limited activity imposed by an immobilized body part.

Prevention of infection continues as a priority after discharge from the hospital. Some institutions allow the child to return to school when the absolute neutrophil count is above 500/mm^3. Other institutions place no restrictions on the child, regardless of the blood count. If the level falls below this value, cautious isolation from crowded areas, such as shopping centers or subways, is advisable. At all times family members are encouraged to practice good handwashing to prevent introducing pathogens into the home.

Nutrition is another important component of infection prevention. An adequate protein-calorie intake provides the child with better host defenses against infection and with increased tolerance to chemotherapy and irradiation. However, providing optimum nutrition during periods of anorexia and vomiting from chemotherapy is a tremendous challenge. Every effort is made to encourage the child to eat without using undue pressure (see Feeding the Sick Child, Chapter 27), and if nonoral feedings are instituted, meticulous care in terms of the feeding procedure is implemented to prevent infection.

Hemorrhage. Before the use of transfused platelets, hemorrhage was a leading cause of death in children with some types of cancer. Now most bleeding episodes can be prevented or controlled with judicious administration of platelet concentrates or platelet-rich plasma. Severe spontaneous internal hemorrhage usually does not occur until the platelet count is 20,000/mm^3 (Greenbaum and Herman, 1988).

Since infection increases the tendency toward hemorrhage, and since bleeding sites become more easily infected, special care is taken to avoid performing skin punctures whenever possible. When finger sticks, venipunctures, intramuscular injections, and bone marrow tests are performed, aseptic technique must be employed with continued observation for bleeding. Meticulous mouth care is essential, since gingival bleeding with resultant mucositis is a frequent problem. Since the rectal area is prone to ulceration from various drugs, hygiene is essential. To prevent additional trauma, rectal temperatures and suppositories are avoided. Frequent turning and the use of a pressure-reducing mattress under bony prominences prevent development of pressure areas and decubital ulcers.

Platelet transfusions are generally reserved for active bleeding episodes that do not respond to local treatment and that may occur during induction or relapse therapy. Epistaxis and gingival bleeding are the most common. The nurse teaches parents and other children measures to control nosebleeding (see Epistaxis [Nosebleeding], Chapter 35). Applying pressure at the site without disturbing clot formation is the general rule (see Critical Thinking Exercise box, p. 1630).

Two of the problems with multiple platelet transfusions are the risk of febrile reactions and decreased life span of the platelets. Platelet concentrates normally do not have to be crossmatched for blood group or type. However, because platelets contain specific antigen components similar to blood group factors, children who receive multiple transfusions may become sensitized to a platelet group other than their own. Therefore platelets are crossmatched with the donor's blood components whenever possible.

Transfused platelets generally survive in the body for 1 to 3 days. The peak effect is reached in about 2 hours and decreased by half in 24 hours. Therefore after a transfusion the nurse observes and records the approximate time when hemostasis of bleeding sites occurs. Delayed hemostasis is evidence of platelet destruction. For long-term patients, multiple transfusion therapy becomes progressively less effective.

During bleeding episodes the parents and child need much emotional support. The sight of oozing blood is very upsetting. Often parents will request a platelet transfusion,

CRITICAL THINKING EXERCISE

Bleeding

Paul Jones, 14 years old, is undergoing chemotherapy for leukemia but has recently been hospitalized because of pneumonia. His platelet count is 50,000 mm^3. After morning report, you visit him and note the following. Which one requires further assessment because it potentially increases his risk of bleeding?

1. A sign over his bed reads "no needle punctures."
2. He is receiving 6 L of oxygen via nasal cannula.
3. He has an intermittent infusion device in his hand.
4. A tympanic membrane sensor is in the room.

The correct answer is 2. You should assess if the oxygen is being humidified. The nose is vascular and can bleed easily if the mucosa is dried by the oxygen. Also, inspect the placement of the nasal prongs for any sign of irritation and ask Paul if the prongs are comfortable.

The other aspects of care—the sign to remind staff to avoid any skin punctures, the infusion device to maintain access to the vein if needed, and the temperature measurement device using the ear and thus avoiding the rectal route and possible mucosal damage—are aimed at preventing bleeding.

unaware of the necessity of trying local measures first. The nurse can be instrumental in allaying anxiety by explaining the reason for delaying a platelet transfusion until absolutely necessary. Since compatible donors decrease the risk of antigen formation in the recipient, the nurse should encourage parents to locate suitable donors for eventual blood use.

Children at home who have low platelet counts (usually below 100,000/mm^3) are advised to avoid activities that might cause injury or bleeding, such as riding bicycles or skateboards, roller skating or in-line skating, climbing trees or playground equipment, and contact sports such as football or soccer. These restrictions can be terminated once the platelet count rises, such as after platelet transfusion. In addition, aspirin and aspirin-containing products are not used; for mild pain or significantly elevated temperature, acetaminophen is substituted.

Anemia. Initially anemia may be profound from complete replacement of the bone marrow by cancer cells. During induction therapy, blood transfusions with packed red blood cells may be necessary to raise the hemoglobin to levels approaching 10 g. The usual precautions in caring for the child are instituted (see Chapter 35).

Anemia is also a consequence of drug-induced myelosuppression. Although not as severely affected as the white blood cells, erythrocyte production may be delayed. Since children have an amazing capacity to withstand low hemoglobin levels, the best approach is to allow the child to regulate activity with reasonable adult supervision. It may be necessary for the parents to alert the schoolteacher to the child's physical limitations, particularly in terms of strenuous activity.

Management of Problems Related to Irradiation and Drug Toxicity

Irradiation and chemotherapy present several challenges to providing effective care. The complexity of the treatment protocols alone is often overwhelming to families, who can benefit from receiving a monthly calendar of anticipated treatment dates. In addition, each therapy is associated with a number of predictable side effects (see Tables 36-2 and 36-3). The following is a discussion of these reactions and appropriate interventions.

Nausea and Vomiting. The nausea and vomiting that occur shortly after administration of several of the drugs and as a result of cranial or abdominal radiation can be profound. 5-HT_3 receptor antagonists are the newest class of antiemetics used to manage nausea and vomiting caused by chemotherapy. The advantage of these agents over conventional drugs is that they produce no extrapyramidal side effects, such as trouble speaking or swallowing, shuffle walk, slow movements, trembling, stiffness of the arms and legs, or loss of balance. Multiple studies have shown ondansetron (Zofran) to be effective for patients receiving cisplatin, cyclophosphamide, ifosfamide, and anthracyclenes (Cubeddu and others, 1990; Pinkerton and others, 1990). Ondansetron in combination with dexamethasone has been more effective than ondansetron alone (Roila and others, 1991) and has been superior to metoclopramide (Reglan) for cisplatin-induced emesis (Hainsworth and others, 1991). Most institutions use a three-dose intravenous regimen of 0.15 mg/kg/dose with or without further oral doses of 4 to 8 mg three times daily. A single intravenous dose of 5 mg/m^2 followed by oral doses of 2 to 4 mg every 8 hours has also been used (Frankiewicz and Farrington, 1992; Pinkerton and others, 1990).

For mild to moderate vomiting, phenothiazine-type drugs remain the mainstay of therapy. Promethazine (Phenergan), chlorpromazine (Thorazine), prochlorperazine (Compazine), or trimethobenzamide (Tigan) may be effective agents. Metoclopramide is a more effective antiemetic for severe vomiting. Unfortunately, the drug causes a number of side effects in children, particularly extrapyramidal reactions, such as muscle tremors or twitching, agitation, grimacing, dysarthria, and oculogyric crisis (fixation of eyes in one position for minutes or hours). The incidence of extrapyramidal reactions is dose and age related—increased in older children and at higher doses (Sridhar and Donnelly, 1988). Metoclopramide used in conjunction with benztropine, dexamethasone, diphenhydramine, and/or lorazepam has been shown to significantly decrease nausea and vomiting, as well as the untoward side effects of metoclopramide (Marshall and others, 1989; Sridhar and Donnelly, 1988).

Another drug that has yielded promising results is THC (delta-9-tetrahydrocannabinol), the active component of marijuana. Synthetic cannabinoids are now being used in children undergoing chemotherapy. Nabilone was developed to overcome the problems associated with the naturally occurring cannabinoids. Nabilone has been shown to be superior to placebo, prochlorperazine, and low-dose metoclopramide both as an antiemetic and in terms of patient preference (Few, 1988).

The most beneficial regimen for antiemetic control has been the administration of the antiemetic *before* the chemotherapy begins (30 minutes to 1 hour before) and regular (not PRN) administration every 2, 4, or 6 hours for at least 24 hours after chemotherapy. There is some evidence that beginning antiemetic therapy up to 24 hours before the chemotherapy adds additional effectiveness (Williams and others, 1989). The goal is to prevent the child from ever experiencing nausea or vomiting, since this can prevent the development of anticipatory symptoms (the conditioned response of developing nausea and vomiting before receiving the drug). Other nonpharmacologic interventions (similar to those discussed for pain management in Chapter 26) can be useful in controlling posttherapy and anticipatory nausea and vomiting (Hockenberry, 1988). Giving the antineoplastic drug with a mild sedative at bedtime is also helpful for some children, and there is evidence that nighttime administration of drugs such as methotrexate and 6-mercaptopurine may be more effective cytotoxically than morning administration (Evans and others, 1989).

Anorexia. Loss of appetite is a direct consequence of the chemotherapy and/or irradiation. It is a major problem for parents because it is the one area they feel responsible for, particularly when so many other facets of care are outside their control. There are no universally successful techniques for encouraging a sick child to eat (see Feeding the Sick Child, Chapter 27).

Some children still do not eat despite approaches such as those discussed in Chapter 27. The following theories have been postulated to explain persistent anorexia: (1) a physical cause related to the cancer that is nonspecific; (2) a conditioned aversion to food from nausea and vomiting during treatment; (3) stress in the environment, related to eating and/or to the child's condition; (4) depression; (5) a control mechanism when so much else has been imposed on the child; and (6) an opportunity to express anger at parents and punish them for "allowing" the child to become sick. When loss of appetite and weight persists, the nurse should investigate the family situation to determine if any of these variables are contributing to the problem. To prevent conditioned aversion to food, it is best to offer few foods and no favorite foods before chemotherapy. Meats and proteins are more apt to trigger learned food aversions. A light, low-protein meal, followed by candy of a distinctive flavor before a chemotherapy treatment, proved to be effective in decreasing food aversions in one study (Broberg and Bernstein, 1987).

Mucosal Ulceration. One of the most distressing side effects of several drugs is gastrointestinal mucosal cell damage, which results in ulcers anywhere along the alimentary tract. Oral ulcers (stomatitis) are red, eroded, painful areas in the mouth and/or pharynx (see also Stomatitis, Chapter 16). Similar lesions may extend along the esophagus and in the rectal area. They greatly compound anorexia, because eating is extremely uncomfortable. When oral ulcers develop, the following interventions are helpful: (1) a bland, moist, soft diet; (2) use of a soft sponge toothbrush (Toothette)* or cotton-tipped applicator; (3) frequent mouthwashes with normal saline (using a solution of 1 teaspoon of table salt and 1 pint of water) or sodium bicarbonate and salt mouthrinses (using a solution of 1 teaspoon of baking soda and ½ teaspoon of table salt in 1 quart of water); and (4) local anesthetics such as Chloraseptic lozenges or nonprescription preparations without alcohol, such as Orabase (Galbraith and others, 1991). Although local anesthetics are effective in temporarily relieving the pain, many children dislike the taste and numb feeling they produce.

NURSING ALERT Viscous lidocaine is not recommended for young children; if applied to the pharynx, it may depress the gag reflex, increasing the risk of aspiration. Seizures have also been associated with the use of oral viscous lidocaine (Hess and Walson, 1988).

Protocols for oral care during myelosuppression vary. For example, Ulcerase is free of sugar, alcohol, and dyes and has been used to soothe mucositis and gum irritations. Chlorhexidine gluconate (Peridex) is effective against candidal as well as bacterial infections (Galbraith and others, 1991). *Candida* prophylaxis using antifungal troches (lozenges) or mouthwash is typically used in patients with myelosuppression, especially for children who have undergone BMT.

NURSING ALERT Agents such as lemon glycerin swabs, hydrogen peroxide, and milk of magnesia are avoided because of the drying effects on the mucosa. In addition, lemon may be irritating to eroded tissue and can decay the teeth (Galbraith and others, 1991).

A strategy that may be helpful in reducing oral pain is massaging the area on the backs of both hands between the thumb and index finger with an ice cube for 5 to 7 minutes until the area becomes numb.

Administering mouth care is particularly difficult in infants and toddlers. A satisfactory method of cleaning the gums is to wrap a piece of gauze around a finger, soak it in saline or plain water, and swab the gums, palate, and inner cheek surfaces with the finger. Mouthwashes are best accomplished with plain water or saline, because the child cannot gargle or spit out excess fluid. Mouth care is done routinely before and after any feeding and as often as every 2 to 4 hours to rid mucosal surfaces of debris, which becomes an excellent medium for bacterial and fungal growth.

Dental hygiene can become a serious problem if the child wears an orthodontic appliance. The accumulated debris on braces is difficult to remove without vigorous brushing, and the appliance itself traumatizes the gums. Sometimes braces are removed during chemotherapy.

Difficulty in eating is a major problem with stomatitis and may warrant hospitalization if the child refuses fluids. The

*Manufactured by Halbrand, Inc., Willoughby, OH.

child will usually choose the foods that are best tolerated. Surprisingly, some children prefer salty foods to more bland ones. Drinking can usually be encouraged if a straw is used to bypass the ulcerated oral mucosa. The nurse should encourage parents to relax any eating pressures, because the anorexia accompanying stomatitis is well justified. In addition, since it is a temporary condition, once the ulcers heal, the child can resume good food habits. Ordinarily, severe mucosal ulceration indicates a need for decreased chemotherapy until complete healing takes place, usually within a week. Analgesics, including opioids, may be needed when treatment cannot be altered, such as during BMT.

If rectal ulcers develop, meticulous toilet hygiene, warm sitz baths after each bowel movement, and an occlusive ointment applied to the ulcerated area promote healing; the use of stool softeners is necessary to prevent further discomfort. Parents are advised to record bowel movements, since the child may voluntarily avoid defecation to prevent discomfort. Rectal temperatures and suppositories are avoided because they may further traumatize the affected area.

Neurologic Problems. Vincristine and to a lesser extent vinblastine can cause various neurotoxic effects, one of the more common of which is severe constipation from decreased bowel innervation. Constipation is further aggravated by opioids. The nurse advises parents to record bowel movements and to notify the practitioner of a change in stool habits. Physical activity and stool softeners are helpful in preventing the problem, but laxatives, such as Peri-Colace, or enemas are often necessary to stimulate evacuation. Dietary changes such as increased fiber may not be effective, because the increased bulk tends to increase fecal distention and discomfort without producing the necessary mechanical stimulation.

Footdrop, weakness, and numbing of the extremities may cause difficulty in walking or fine hand movement. The nurse should look for these problems and warn parents of these side effects, which are reversible once the drug is stopped. If the child is on bed rest, a footboard is used to preserve proper alignment. If weakness occurs while the child is attending school, a temporary alteration of activity may be necessary. The teacher should be apprised of the situation so that unrealistic expectations of the child's abilities are not made.

Another side effect that can be severe is jaw pain. Analgesics may be necessary to relieve the discomfort. Avoiding movement by not talking or chewing is usually self-imposed, although continuous chewing, such as with gum, may actually reduce the pain. Since the pain is temporary, usually lasting for a day or two, the child can be given fluids through a straw.

A neurologic syndrome ***(postirradiation somnolence)*** may develop 5 to 8 weeks after central nervous system irradiation and may last for 4 to 15 days. It is characterized by somnolence with or without fever, anorexia, and nausea and vomiting. Parents should be warned of the possibility of such symptoms and encouraged to seek medical evaluation, since somnolence may be an early indicator of long-term neurologic sequelae after cranial irradiation.

Hemorrhagic Cystitis. Sterile hemorrhagic cystitis is a side effect of chemical irritation to the bladder from chemotherapy and/or radiation therapy. It can be prevented by (1) a liberal oral and/or parenteral fluid intake (at least one and one-half times the recommended daily fluid requirement [2 L/m^2/day]); (2) frequent voiding immediately after feeling the urge, including immediately before bed and after arising (may include one nighttime void); (3) administration of the drug early in the day to allow for sufficient fluids and frequent voiding; and (4) administration of mesna, a drug that inhibits the urotoxicity of cyclophosphamide and ifosfamide (Cameron, 1993).

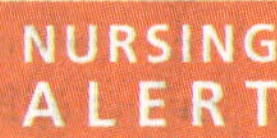
NURSING ALERT

If signs of cystitis such as burning on urination occur, prompt medical evaluation is needed. Hemorrhagic cystitis warrants cessation of the drug.

In some cases intravenous fluids are given before, during, and after the drug to ensure adequate hydration, thereby eliminating the need for the child's drinking large amounts of fluid. If oral home administration is prescribed, the family needs *specific* instructions on exactly how much fluid the child must have.

Alopecia. Hair loss is a side effect of several chemotherapeutic drugs and cranial irradiation. Not all children lose their hair during drug therapy; however, retaining hair is the exception rather than the rule. It is better to warn children and parents of this side effect than to allow them to think that it is only a remote possibility.

The family should know that the hair falls out in clumps, causing patchy baldness. To lessen the trauma of seeing large amounts of hair on bed linen or clothing, the child can wear a disposable surgical cap to collect the shed hair during the period of greatest hair loss or cut the hair short. Families should also be aware that wigs are tax deductible and that hair regrows in 3 to 6 months (at a rate of about ½ inch a month). The hair frequently is darker, thicker, and curlier than before.

➤ **NURSING TIP** Encouraging children to choose a wig similar to their own hairstyle and color *before* the hair falls out is helpful in fostering later adjustment to hair loss.

If the child chooses not to wear a wig, attention to some type of head covering is important, especially in cold or sunny climates. Scalp hygiene is also important. The scalp should be washed regularly, as with any other body part.

Many children demonstrate increased tolerance to hair loss on reinduction therapy. Rather than complete baldness, the child may experience thinning of the hair. If the hair is cut short, kept clean, and blow-dried with an electric hair drier, it usually can look full enough to make a wig unnecessary. This can be a tremendous psychologic boost to the child who is already depressed about learning of a relapse and the need for additional chemotherapy.

Moon Face. Short-term steroid therapy produces no acute toxicities and often results in two beneficial reactions—increased appetite and a sense of well-being. However, it does produce alterations in body image, which, although not clinically significant, can be extremely distressing to older children. One of these is moon face. The child's face becomes rounded and puffy (see Fig. 38-3). Un-

Text continued on p. 1638.

NURSING CARE PLAN
The Child with Cancer

NURSING DIAGNOSIS: High risk for injury related to malignant process, treatment

PATIENT GOAL 1: Will experience partial or complete remission from disease

• **NURSING INTERVENTIONS/*RATIONALES***

*Administer chemotherapeutic agents as prescribed

Assist with radiotherapy as ordered

Assist with procedures for administration of chemotherapeutic agents (e.g., lumbar puncture for intrathecal administration)

†Prepare child and family for surgical procedure if appropriate

• **EXPECTED OUTCOME**

Child achieves a partial or complete remission from disease

PATIENT GOAL 2: Will not experience complications of chemotherapy

• **NURSING INTERVENTIONS/*RATIONALES***

Follow guidelines for administration of chemotherapeutic agents

Observe for signs of infiltration at intravenous site: pain, stinging, swelling, redness

Immediately stop infusion if any sign of infiltration occurs *to prevent severe tissue damage*

Implement policies of institution *to treat infiltration*

Obtain careful history for known allergies *to prevent anaphylaxis*

Observe child for 20 minutes after infusion for *signs of anaphylaxis* (cyanosis, hypotension, wheezing, severe urticaria)

Stop infusion of drug and flush intravenous line with normal saline if reaction is suspected

Have emergency equipment (especially blood pressure monitor and manual resuscitation bag and mask) and emergency drugs (especially oxygen, epinephrine, antihistamine, aminophylline, corticosteroids, and vasopressors) readily available *to prevent delay in treatment*

• **EXPECTED OUTCOMES**

Child will not experience complications of chemotherapy

Child will receive prompt, appropriate treatment of complications

NURSING DIAGNOSIS: High risk for infection related to depressed body defenses

PATIENT GOAL 1: Will experience minimized risk of infection

• **NURSING INTERVENTIONS/*RATIONALES***

Place child in private room *to minimize exposure to infective organisms*

Advise all visitors and staff to use good handwashing technique *to minimize exposure to infective organisms*

Screen all visitors and staff for signs of infection *to minimize exposure to infective organisms*

Use scrupulous aseptic technique for all invasive procedures

Monitor temperature *to detect possible infection*

Evaluate child for any potential sites of infection (e.g., needle punctures, mucosal ulceration, minor abrasions, dental problems)

Provide nutritionally complete diet for age *to support body's natural defenses*

Avoid giving live attenuated virus vaccines (e.g., measles, mumps, rubella, and oral poliovirus) to child with depressed immune system *because these vaccines can result in overwhelming infection*

*Give inactivated virus vaccines (e.g., varicella [chickenpox], Salk polio, influenza) as prescribed and indicated *to prevent specific infections*

Administer antibiotics as prescribed

*Administer granulocyte colony–stimulating factor (GCSF) as prescribed

• **EXPECTED OUTCOMES**

Child does not come in contact with infected persons or contaminated articles

Child consumes diet appropriate for age (specify)

Child does not exhibit signs of infection

NURSING DIAGNOSIS: High risk for injury (hemorrhage, hemorrhagic cystitis) related to interference with cell proliferation

PATIENT GOAL 1: Will exhibit no evidence of bleeding

• **NURSING INTERVENTIONS/*RATIONALES***

Use all measures to prevent infection, especially in ecchymotic areas, *because infection increases tendency toward bleeding*

Use local measures (e.g., apply pressure, ice) to stop bleeding

Restrict strenuous activity *that could result in accidental injury*

Involve child in responsibility for limiting activity when platelet count drops *to encourage compliance*

Avoid skin punctures when possible *to prevent bleeding*

Observe for bleeding after procedures such as venipuncture, bone marrow aspiration

Turn frequently and use pressure-reducing or pressure-relieving mattress to *prevent decubitus ulcers*

Teach parents and older child measures to control nosebleeding

Prevent oral and rectal ulceration *because ulcerated skin is prone to bleeding*

Avoid aspirin-containing medications *because aspirin interferes with platelet function*

*Administer platelets as prescribed *to raise platelet count*

• **EXPECTED OUTCOME**

Child exhibits no evidence of bleeding

---

*Dependent nursing action.
†Indicates content that is specific to a particular malignancy.

Continued.

NURSING CARE PLAN
The Child with Cancer—cont'd

PATIENT GOAL 2: Will exhibit no evidence of hemorrhagic cystitis

• **NURSING INTERVENTIONS/*RATIONALES***

Observe for signs of cystitis (e.g., burning and pain on urination)

Report signs of cystitis to practitioner, *since prompt medical evaluation is needed*

Give liberal (3000 ml/m^2/day) fluid intake (meters squared is calculated from West Nomogram, p. 1180)

Encourage frequent voiding, including during nighttime, *to minimize metabolites' contact with bladder mucosa*

Administer drugs irritating to bladder early in the day *to allow for sufficient fluid intake and voiding*

• **EXPECTED OUTCOMES**

Child voids without discomfort

No hematuria is present

PATIENT GOAL 3: Will experience minimal effects of anemia

• **NURSING INTERVENTIONS/*RATIONALES* AND EXPECTED OUTCOMES**

See Nursing Care Plan: The Child with Anemia, Chapter 35

NURSING DIAGNOSIS: High risk for fluid volume deficit related to nausea and vomiting

PATIENT GOAL 1: Will experience no nausea or vomiting

• **NURSING INTERVENTIONS/*RATIONALES***

*Administer initial dose of antiemetic before chemotherapy begins *to prevent child from ever experiencing nausea and vomiting, thus preventing an anticipatory response*

*Administer antiemetic around the clock for as long as nausea and vomiting typically last *to prevent any episodes from occurring*

Assess child's response to antiemetic, *since no antiemetic drug is uniformly successful*

Avoid foods with strong odors *that may induce nausea and vomiting*

Uncover hospital food tray outside of child's room *to reduce food odors that may induce nausea*

Encourage frequent intake of fluids in small amounts, *since small portions are usually better tolerated*

*Administer intravenous fluid, as prescribed, *to maintain hydration*

• **EXPECTED OUTCOMES**

Child retains food and fluid

Child does not experience nausea or vomiting

*Dependent nursing action.

NURSING DIAGNOSIS: Altered mucous membranes related to administration of chemotherapeutic agents

PATIENT GOAL 1: Will not develop oral mucositis

• **NURSING INTERVENTIONS/*RATIONALES***

Inspect mouth daily for oral ulcers; report evidence of ulcers to practitioner *for early treatment*

Avoid oral temperatures *to prevent trauma*

Institute meticulous oral hygiene as soon as a drug is used that causes oral ulcers

Use soft-sponge toothbrush, cotton-tipped applicator, or gauze-wrapped finger *to avoid trauma*

Administer frequent (at least every 4 hours and after meals) mouthwashes (normal saline with or without sodium bicarbonate solution) *to promote healing*

Apply local anesthetics to ulcerated areas before meals and as needed *to relieve pain*

Avoid using viscous lidocaine for young children, *because if applied to pharynx, it may depress gag reflex, increasing risk of aspiration, and may cause seizures*

Apply lip balm *to keep lips moist and prevent cracking or fissuring*

Serve bland, moist, soft diet; offer food best tolerated by child

Encourage fluids; use a straw *to help bypass painful areas*

Encourage parents to relax any eating pressures, *since stomatitis is a temporary condition*

Avoid juices containing ascorbic acid and hot or cold or spicy foods if they cause further discomfort

Avoid using lemon glycerin swabs *(irritate eroded tissue and can decay teeth)*, hydrogen peroxide *(delays healing by breaking down protein)*, and milk of magnesia *(dries mucosa)*

Explain to parents that child may require hospitalization *for hydration, parenteral nutrition, and pain control (often with intravenous morphine)* if stomatitis interfers with food and fluid intake

*Administer antiinfective medication as ordered *to prevent or treat mucositis*

*Administer analgesics, including opioids, *to control pain*

• **EXPECTED OUTCOMES**

Mucous membranes remain intact

Ulcers show evidence of healing

Child reports and/or exhibits no evidence of discomfort

PATIENT GOAL 2: Will not develop rectal ulceration

• **NURSING INTERVENTIONS/*RATIONALES***

Wash perianal area after each bowel movement *to lessen irritation*

Use warm sitz baths or tub baths *to promote healing*

Expose reddened but not ulcerated areas to air *to keep skin dry*

Apply protective skin barriers (transparent film dressings, occlusive ointment) to perineal area *to protect skin from direct contact with urine or feces and to promote healing*

Observe for constipation *resulting from child's voluntary refusal to defecate or from chemotherapy*

NURSING CARE PLAN
The Child with Cancer—cont'd

Record bowel movements; use stool softener *to prevent constipation;* may need stimulants *for evacuation*
Avoid rectal temperatures and suppositories *to prevent rectal trauma*

• **EXPECTED OUTCOMES**
Rectal mucosa remains clean and intact
Ulcerated areas heal without complications
Child has regular bowel movements

NURSING DIAGNOSIS: Altered nutrition: less than body requirements related to loss of appetite

PATIENT GOAL 1: Will receive adequate nutrition

• **NURSING INTERVENTIONS/*RATIONALES***
Encourage parents to relax pressures placed on eating; explain that loss of appetite *is a direct consequence of nausea and vomiting, and chemotherapy*
Allow child *any* food tolerated; plan to improve quality of food selections when appetite increases
Explain expected increase in appetite from steroids *to prepare child and parents for this change*
Take advantage of any hungry period: serve small "snacks," *since small portions are usually better tolerated*
Fortify foods with nutritious supplements, such as powdered milk or commercial supplements, *to maximize quality of intake*
Allow child to be involved in food preparation and selection *to encourage eating*
Make food appealing
Remember usual food practices of children in each age-group, such as food jags in toddlers or normal occurrence of physiologic anorexia, *to distinguish these expected changes from actual refusal to eat*
Assess family for additional problems (e.g., use of food by child as a control mechanism if appetite does not improve despite improved physical status) *to identify areas that require intervention*

• **EXPECTED OUTCOME**
Nutritional intake is adequate

NURSING DIAGNOSIS: Impaired skin integrity related to administration of chemotherapeutic agents, radiotherapy, immobility

PATIENT GOAL 1: Will maintain skin integrity

• **NURSING INTERVENTIONS/*RATIONALES***
Provide meticulous skin care, especially in mouth and perianal regions, *because they are prone to ulceration*
Change position frequently *to stimulate circulation and relieve pressure*
Encourage adequate caloric-protein intake *to prevent negative nitrogen balance*

• **EXPECTED OUTCOME**
Skin remains clean and intact

PATIENT GOAL 2: Will experience minimal negative effects of therapy

• **NURSING INTERVENTIONS/*RATIONALES***
Select loose-fitting clothing over irradiated area *to minimize additional irritation*
Protect area from sunlight and sudden changes in temperature (avoid ice packs, heating pads) during radiotherapy or administration of methotrexate

• **EXPECTED OUTCOME**
Child and family comply with suggestions (specify)

NURSING DIAGNOSIS: Impaired physical mobility related to neuromuscular impairment (neuropathy)

PATIENT GOAL 1: Will experience minimal negative effects of peripheral neuropathy

• **NURSING INTERVENTIONS/*RATIONALES***
Encourage ambulation when child is able
Alter activity, including school attendance, *to prevent injuries if weakness occurs*
Use footboard or high-top shoes *to prevent footdrop*
Provide fluids and soft foods *to lessen chewing movements with jaw pain*

• **EXPECTED OUTCOME**
Child ambulates without incident or difficulty

NURSING DIAGNOSIS: Body image disturbance related to loss of hair, moon face, debilitation

PATIENT/FAMILY GOAL 1: Will exhibit positive coping behaviors

• **NURSING INTERVENTIONS/*RATIONALES***
Introduce idea of wig before hair loss
  Encourage child to select a wig similar to child's own hairstyle and color before hair falls out *to foster later adjustment to hair loss*
Provide adequate covering during exposure to sunlight, wind, or cold, *since natural protection is lost*
Suggest keeping thin hair clean, short, and fluffy *to camouflage partial baldness*
Explain that hair begins to regrow in 3 to 6 months and may be a slightly different color or texture *to prepare child and family for changes in appearance of new hair*
Explain that alopecia during a second treatment with same drug may be less severe
Encourage good hygiene, grooming, and sex-appropriate items (e.g., wig, scarves, hats, makeup, attractive sex-appropriate clothing) *to enhance appearance*

• **EXPECTED OUTCOMES**
Child verbalizes concern regarding hair loss
Child helps determine methods to reduce effects of hair loss and applies these methods
Child appears clean, well-groomed, and attractively dressed

Continued.

NURSING CARE PLAN

The Child with Cancer—cont'd

PATIENT GOAL 2: Will exhibit adjustment to altered facial appearance

• **NURSING INTERVENTIONS/*RATIONALES***

Encourage rapid reintegration with peers *to lessen contrast of changed facial appearance*

Stress that this reaction is temporary *to provide reassurance that usual appearance will return*

Evaluate weight gain carefully *(in weight gain resulting from administration of steroids, extremities remain thin)*

Encourage visits from friends before discharge *to prepare child for reactions and questions*

• **EXPECTED OUTCOMES**

Family demonstrates understanding of consequences of therapies

Child resumes former activities and relationships within capabilities

PATIENT GOAL 3: Will express feelings

• **NURSING INTERVENTIONS/*RATIONALES***

Provide opportunities for child to discuss feelings and concerns

Provide materials for nonverbal expression (e.g., play, art)

• **EXPECTED OUTCOME**

Child expresses feelings regarding altered body in words, play, art (specify)

NURSING DIAGNOSIS: Pain related to diagnosis, treatment, physiologic effects of neoplasia

PATIENT GOAL 1: Will experience no pain or reduction of pain to level acceptable to child

• **NURSING INTERVENTIONS/*RATIONALES***

Whenever possible, make use of procedures (e.g., noninvasive temperature monitoring, venous access device) to minimize discomfort

Assess need for pain management (see Chapter 26)

Evaluate effectiveness of pain relief with degree of alertness vs sedation *to determine need for change in dosage, time of administration, or drug*

Implement appropriate nonpharmacologic pain reduction techniques *as adjunct to analgesics*

*Administer analgesics as prescribed

Avoid aspirin or any of its compounds (e.g., other nonsteroidal antiinflammatory agents) *because aspirin increases bleeding tendency*

*Administer drugs on preventive schedule (around the clock) *to prevent pain from recurring*

Monitor effectiveness of therapy on pain assessment record

• **EXPECTED OUTCOME**

Child rests quietly, reports and/or exhibits no evidence of discomfort, verbalizes no complaints of discomfort

NURSING DIAGNOSIS: Fear related to diagnostic tests, procedures, treatments

PATIENT GOAL 1: Will exhibit reduced fear related to diagnostic procedures and tests

• **NURSING INTERVENTIONS/*RATIONALES***

Explain procedure carefully at child's level of understanding *to reduce fear of the unknown*

Explain what will take place and what child will feel, see, and hear *to increase sense of control*

Use recall of each step *as method of distraction*

Explain special requests of child (e.g., need to remain motionless during test and/or radiotherapy) *to encourage cooperation*

Provide child with some means for involvement with procedure (e.g., holding a piece of equipment, such as bandage or tape, counting with the operator, answering questions) *to promote sense of control, encourage cooperation, and support child's coping skills*

Implement distracting techniques and pain reduction techniques as indicated

See also Guidelines box (Preparing Children for Procedures) on p. 1134

• **EXPECTED OUTCOMES**

Child readily responds to verbal directives

Child repeats information accurately

NURSING DIAGNOSIS: Fear related to diagnosis, prognosis

See Nursing Care Plan: The Child Who Is Terminally Ill or Dying, Chapter 23

NURSING DIAGNOSIS: Diversional activity deficit related to restricted environment (private room)

PATIENT GOAL 1: Will have opportunity to participate in diversional activities

• **NURSING INTERVENTIONS/*RATIONALES***

Provide age-appropriate toys that can be properly cleaned *to provide diversion without risk of infection*

Involve child-life specialist or other supportive services in planning diversional activities

• **EXPECTED OUTCOMES**

Child engages in activities appropriate for age and interests

Suitable toys are provided

NURSING DIAGNOSIS: Altered family processes related to having a child with a life-threatening disease

PATIENT (FAMILY) GOAL 1: Will demonstrate knowledge about diagnostic/therapeutic procedures

• **NURSING INTERVENTIONS/*RATIONALES***

Explain reason for each test and procedure

Explain reason for radiotherapy, chemotherapy

Explain operative procedure honestly (if appropriate)

Avoid overemphasis on benefits, which may not be immediately evident (applies primarily to brain tumors) *to avoid unrealistic expectations*

---

*Dependent nursing action.

See also Guidelines box (Preparing Children for Procedures) on p. 1134

• **EXPECTED OUTCOME**
Child and family demonstrate understanding of procedures (specify learning and manner of demonstration)

PATIENT (FAMILY) GOAL 2: Will receive adequate support

• **NURSING INTERVENTIONS/*RATIONALES***
Teach parents about disease process
Explain all procedures that will be done to child
Schedule time for family to be together, without interruptions from staff, *to encourage communication and expression of feelings*
Help family plan for future, especially for helping child live a normal life, *to promote child's optimum development*
Encourage family to discuss feelings regarding child's course before diagnosis and child's prognosis
Discuss with family how they will tell child about outcome of treatment and need for additional treatment (if appropriate) *to maintain open and honest communication*
Refer to local chapter of American Cancer Society or other organizations

• **EXPECTED OUTCOMES**
Family demonstrates knowledge of child's disease and treatments (specify methods of learning and evaluation)
Family expresses feelings and concerns and spends time with child
See also:
Nursing Care Plan: The Child in the Hospital, Chapter 26
Nursing Care Plan: The Family of the Ill or Hospitalized Child, Chapter 26

NURSING DIAGNOSIS: Altered family processes related to a child undergoing therapy

PATIENT (FAMILY) GOAL 1: Will demonstrate understanding of side effects and/or complications of treatment

• **NURSING INTERVENTIONS/*RATIONALES***
Advise family of expected side effects vs toxicities; clarify which demand medical evaluation (mucosal ulceration, hemorrhagic cystitis, peripheral neuropathy, evidence of infection or dehydration) *to prevent delay in treatment*
Reassure family that such reactions are not caused by return of cancer cells *to minimize undue concern*
Interpret prognostic statistics carefully, realizing family's temporary need to interpret them as they see necessary, *to present a realistic, but hopeful, future*
Prepare family for expected mood changes from steroids
Interpret mood changes based on drugs or reactions to disease/treatment *to prevent any unwarranted negative reaction to child (e.g., punishment)*

• **EXPECTED OUTCOMES**
Family demonstrates knowledge of instructions (specify method of learning and evaluation)
Family demonstrates understanding of behavior changes

PATIENT GOAL 2: Will receive adequate support during treatment

• **NURSING INTERVENTIONS/*RATIONALES***
Explain reason for antibiotics and/or transfusions, particularly why platelets are reserved for acute, uncontrolled bleeding episodes
Observe for signs of transfusion reaction (see Table 35-2)
Record appropriate time for hemostasis to occur after administration of platelets *to determine if transfusions are becoming less effective*

• **EXPECTED OUTCOME**
Child demonstrates understanding of procedures and tests (specify method and learnings)

PATIENT (FAMILY) GOAL 3: Will be prepared for home care

• **NURSING INTERVENTIONS/*RATIONALES***
Teach preventive measures at discharge (e.g., handwashing and isolation from crowds) *to prevent infection*
Stress importance of isolating child from any known cases of chickenpox or other childhood diseases; work with school nurse and physician to determine optimum time for school reattendance *to prevent unnecessary absences or risk of infection*
Teach home care instructions specific to child's needs

• **EXPECTED OUTCOME**
Family demonstrates ability to provide home care for child (specify)

NURSING DIAGNOSIS: Anticipatory grief related to perceived potential loss of a child

PATIENT (FAMILY) GOAL 1: Will acknowledge and cope with possibility of child's death

• **NURSING INTERVENTIONS/*RATIONALES***
Provide consistent contact with family *to establish a trusting relationship that encourages communication*
Clarify, refocus, and supply information as needed
Help family plan care of child, especially at terminal stage (e.g., extent of extraordinary lifesaving measures) *to ensure their wishes are implemented*
Provide or arrange for hospice care if family desires it
Arrange for spiritual support in accordance with family's beliefs and/or affiliations

• **EXPECTED OUTCOMES**
Family remains open to counseling and nursing contact
Family and child discuss their fears, concerns, needs, and desires at terminal stage
Family investigates hospice care
Appropriate religious representative is contacted (specify)

PATIENT (FAMILY) GOAL 2: Will receive adequate support

• **NURSING INTERVENTIONS/*RATIONALES* AND EXPECTED OUTCOMES**
See Nursing Care Plan: The Child Who Is Terminally Ill or Dying, Chapter 23

like hair loss, little can be done to camouflage this obvious change, although careful avoidance of salt and salt-containing foods can help reduce fluid accumulation. It is not unusual for other children to make fun of the child with such remarks as "Porky Pig" or "fat face." It is helpful to reassure the child that after cessation of the drug the facial contours will return to normal. If the child resumes activity early in the course of treatment, the change may be less noticeable to peers than after a long absence. Also, the use of loose-fitting clothes, such as warm-up outfits, can help camouflage the change in weight.

In contrast, parents may appreciate the full-rounded appearance because it simulates the look of a well-nourished, healthy child. Because of their own needs, they may be less able to understand the child's misery over altered body image. The nurse can foster a better understanding between the parents and child if both parties are encouraged to openly discuss their feelings.

Children on steroid therapy do look healthy. The moon face, red cheeks, supraclavicular fat pads, protuberant abdomen, and fluid retention indicate weight gain. However, the actual weight gain resulting from increased muscle mass and subcutaneous tissue may be small. Therefore the nurse should evaluate weight gain by observing the extremities and measuring skinfold thickness and arm circumference during steroid therapy to determine if the weight gain is a result of increased dietary intake.

Mood Changes. Shortly after beginning steroid therapy, children may experience a number of mood changes, which range from feelings of well-being and euphoria to depression and irritability. If parents are unaware of these drug-induced changes, they may become unduly concerned. Therefore the nurse should warn them of the reactions and encourage them to discuss the behavioral changes with each other and the child.

Bone Marrow Transplantation (BMT)

The needs of the family are great when BMT is expected. These children may be hospitalized for 30 to 60 days and are usually in a medical center that specializes in this procedure. Because of the risk of infection, the unit may employ strict protective isolation, including specially ventilated air. Consequently, the child is faced with the additional trauma of isolation (see also Chapter 26). The cost/benefit ratio of conventional isolation compared with laminar air flow rooms remains controversial. Survival rates of patients undergoing BMT in both types of isolation are comparable (Johnson, 1991).

Numerous procedures are performed, such as use of a venous access device (if not already inserted), intensive chemotherapy and irradiation, and meticulous personal hygiene. In addition, side effects and complications may occur after the preoperative cytotoxic regimen and include development of infection, severe mucositis, parotitis, nausea, vomiting, diarrhea, syndrome of inappropriate antidiuretic hormone (SIADH), nephropathy, and heart failure (Wiley and House, 1988). Skin breakdown and delayed wound healing occur frequently in the patient undergoing BMT. Preventive interventions to minimize pressure on dependent areas of the skin include the use of pressure-relieving or pressure-reducing beds or mattresses, and frequent turning. Measures to promote healing when breakdown occurs include frequent sitz baths for the perianal area; transparent dressings, such as Tegaderm, over bony prominences; and protective skin barriers, such as hydrocolloid dressings or occlusive ointments. Throughout this long ordeal there is the family's concern for successful engraftment and fear of fatal complications. Consequently, nurses involved with the child and family need to provide sensitive care and maintain a supportive attitude during the many crises that may arise. If the procedure is not successful, the care needed by these families is consistent with that required by the family of any child with a life-threatening disorder (see Chapter 23).

Cessation of Therapy

Care does not end when the child completes therapy. With the increasing awareness of late effects, nurses play an important role in the assessment of the child for problems such as delayed growth, secondary malignancies, and disturbances in any body system. These children require regular follow-up, and the family needs to be aware of the importance of continued medical supervision. Other health care professionals caring for the child, such as school nurses, family physicians, and dentists, should be informed of the child's previous diagnosis of cancer. As children reach adulthood, they may benefit from genetic counseling regarding cancers that are likely to be inherited. If the possibility of sterility exists, pretreatment sperm banking may be offered to adolescent boys, which allows additional options regarding family planning in adulthood.

Family Education

Nurses working with children who have cancer have a significant supportive role in helping the family understand the various therapies, preventing or managing expected side effects or toxicities, and observing for late effects of treatment. Education is a constant feature of the nursing role, especially in terms of new treatments, clinical trials, and home care. Because of the anxiety generated by the diagnosis of cancer, some families may resort to unproven methods of treatment that are frequently referred to as "cancer quackery." These unorthodox approaches may produce unnecessary harm by themselves or, if benign, render injury because other proven modes of therapy are avoided. In many instances this causes financial burden and emotional strife among family members.

Nurses can be instrumental in working against cancer quackery by being aware of factors that increase a family's likelihood of seeking unproven remedies, such as social pressure to "leave no stone unturned" and feelings of depression, helplessness, and hopelessness. Communicating effectively with families about the diagnosis and forms of therapy and providing all possible support and reassurance during treatment are also important interventions to counteract the factors that lead to dissatisfaction with conventional care. Nurses must be fortified with knowledge to substantiate present treatment protocols and to discredit unauthorized methods. The American Cancer Society and local and state medical societies are reliable sources of information concerning research on investigational vs quack methods of cancer therapy.

Instruction regarding home care frequently involves teaching about medication schedules, observation for side effects or toxicities that require further evaluation, measures to prevent or manage these problems, and care of special devices such as central venous catheters.* Compliance is a very important issue, since poor adherence to drug regimens can result in a relapse. Every effort must be made to ensure that the family understands the importance of adhering to the prescribed treatment schedule and measures to improve compliance (see Chapter 27).

❖ EVALUATION

The effectiveness of nursing interventions is determined by continual reassessment and evaluation of care based on the following observational guidelines and expected outcomes:

1. Compare number of visits for primary health with recommended schedule of health supervision.
2. Monitor growth, development, and other aspects of regular health assessment; check mouth for adequacy of dental hygiene; review immunization record for age-appropriate vaccines and use of non–live virus preparations.
3. Interview child and family regarding their understanding of treatments and diagnostic tests.
4. Employ pain assessment techniques for procedural pain.
5. Make careful observations of physical status:
   - Take vital signs regularly.
   - Observe for evidence of bleeding, infection, neuropathy, cystitis, and mucosal ulceration.
   - Observe and record intake and output.
6. Interview child and family and observe behaviors as a result of complications of therapies.
7. Interview child and family and observe behaviors that provide clues to their response to the disease, its therapy, and nursing interventions.

Expected outcomes:

See Nursing Care Plan, pp. 1633-1637.

CANCERS OF THE BLOOD AND LYMPH SYSTEMS

LEUKEMIAS

Leukemia, cancer of the blood-forming tissues, is the most common form of childhood cancer. The annual incidence is 4.2 per 100,000 in white children under 15 years of age and 2.4 per 100,000 in black children (Poplack, 1993). It occurs more frequently in males than in females after age 1 year, and the peak onset is between 2 and 6 years of age. It is one of the forms of cancer that have demonstrated dramatic improvements in survival rates. Before the use of antileukemic agents in 1948, a child with acute lymphocytic leukemia (ALL) lived 2 to 3 months. Current long-term disease-free survival rates for children with ALL approach 70% in major research centers (see Prognosis, p. 1643).

Classification

Leukemia is a broad term given to a group of malignant diseases of the bone marrow and lymphatic system. It is a complex disease of varying heterogeneity. Consequently, classification has become increasingly complex, sophisticated, and essential, since identification of the subtype of leukemia has therapeutic and prognostic implications. The following is an overview of the major classification systems currently being used.

Morphology. Leukemia is classified according to its predominant cell type and level of maturity, as described by the following:

Lympho—For leukemias involving the lymphoid or lymphatic system
Myelo—For those of myeloid (bone marrow) origin
Blastic and acute—For those involving immature cells
Cytic and chronic—For those involving mature cells

Prior to modern treatment, the classifications of acute or chronic were applied to the cells' level of maturity, because they correlated with the course of the disease—the immature form of the disease demonstrated a rapid or acute course of deterioration. Now this distinction is less likely to be seen, and the acute disease refers primarily to the presence of immature blast cells that accumulate and inhibit production of normal-functioning cells (Neglia and Robison, 1988). (For a review of the origin and development of blood cells, see Chapter 35.)

In children two forms are generally recognized: ***acute lymphoid leukemia (ALL)*** and ***acute myelogenous leukemia (AML)***. Synonyms for ALL include lymphatic, lymphocytic, lymphoblastic, and lymphoblastoid leukemia. Usually the terms ***stem*** or ***blast cell leukemia*** also refer to the lymphoid type of leukemia.

Because of the confusion and inconsistency in classifying the leukemias, acute lymphoblastic and acute nonlymphoblastic leukemias are further subdivided according to another system known as the ***French-American-British (FAB) system.*** In the FAB system the subtypes are determined after a thorough study of the morphology (structure) and cytochemical reactivity of the leukemic cells. Accordingly, ALL is divided into three subtypes: L_1, L_2, and L_3. L_1 morphology is the most common subtype, accounts for 84% of children with ALL, and has the best prognosis (Poplack, 1993). AML is classified into seven subtypes that constitute 10% to 20% of leukemias in children. The subtypes of AML are not clearly related to prognosis, as is the case with ALL.

Cytochemical Markers. Leukemic cells demonstrate different reactions when they are exposed to certain chemicals. For example, terminal deoxynucleotidyl transferase is able to provide excellent differentiation between ALL and ANLL. Several other chemicals are available to further differentiate various cell types.

Chromosomal Studies. Chromosomal analysis of leukemic cells has become an important tool in the diagnosis of ALL. For example, children with trisomy 21 have 15 times

*Home care instructions for giving medications to children and caring for a central venous catheter are available in *Wong and Whaley's Clinical Manual of Pediatric Nursing* (Mosby).

the risk of other children for developing ALL (Poplack, 1993). Children with more than 50 chromosomes (DNA index > 1.16) have a better prognosis. Translocation or inversion of chromosomes 7 and 14 have been observed at diagnosis in many children with ALL. Children whose bone marrow contains only genetically abnormal cells have much poorer prognoses and higher incidences of treatment complications than those whose marrow contains mixed or genetically normal cells (Lovejoy and Halliburton, 1989).

Cell-Surface Immunologic Markers. Most childhood leukemias are of B-cell lineage. Early pre-B–cell (common) ALL is the most frequent type of cancer found in children. Most (>80%) of these children have the common acute lymphocytic leukemia antigen (CALLA) on their cell surface (Poplack, 1993). Children with ALL who are CALLA-positive have better survival rates.

Other subtypes of ALL include pre-B–cell ALL, characterized by the presence of cytoplasmic immunoglobulins (CIg), B-cell ALL that secretes immunoglobulin on the cell surface, and T-cell ALL (revealed by the presence of T-cell surface antigens and heat-stable rosette formation in the presence of sheep red blood cells). A small group of patients (<5%) who lack T- or B-cell elements and the CALLA antigen have null-cell ALL (Crist, Pullen, and Rivera, 1991; Poplack, 1993).

At present, cell-surface markers for AML are still rudimentary. However, current research with monoclonal antibodies may provide significant information about the nonlymphoid cells.

Pathologic and Related Clinical Manifestations

Leukemia is an unrestricted proliferation of immature white blood cells in the blood-forming tissues of the body. Although not a "tumor" as such, the leukemic cells demonstrate the neoplastic properties of solid cancers. Therefore the resultant pathology and clinical manifestations of the disease are caused by infiltration and replacement of any tissue of the body with nonfunctional leukemic cells. Highly vascular organs, such as the spleen and liver, are most severely affected.

To understand the pathophysiology of the leukemic process, it is important to clarify two common misconceptions. First, although leukemia is an overproduction of white blood cells, most often in the acute form the leukocyte count is low. Instead, the peripheral blood smear and, more definitively, the bone marrow examination reveal greatly el-

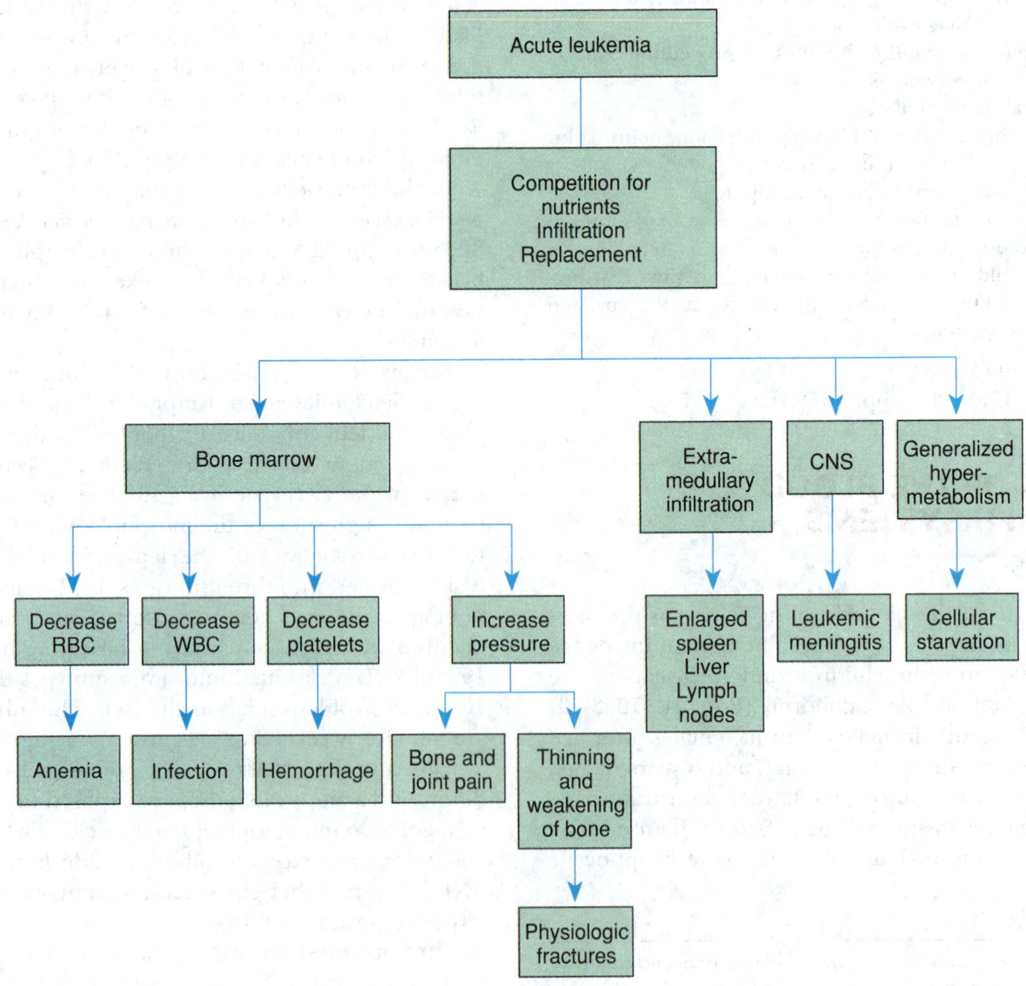

FIG. 36-1 Principal sites of tissue involvement in leukemia.

evated counts of immature cells or "blasts." Second, these immature cells do not deliberately attack and destroy the normal blood cells or vascular tissues. Cellular destruction is by the process of infiltration and subsequent competition for metabolic elements. The following discussion elaborates on the pathologic process and related clinical manifestations in the most susceptible organs of the body (Fig. 36-1).

Bone Marrow Dysfunction. In all types of leukemia the proliferating cells depress bone marrow production of the formed elements of the blood by competing for and depriving the normal cells of the essential nutrients for metabolism. The three main consequences are (1) ***anemia*** from decreased erythrocytes, (2) ***infection*** from neutropenia, and (3) ***bleeding*** from decreased platelet production.

The invasion of the bone marrow with leukemic cells gradually causes a weakening of the bone and a tendency toward fractures. As leukemic cells invade the periosteum, increasing pressure causes severe pain.

The most frequent presenting signs and symptoms of leukemia are a result of infiltration of the bone marrow. These include fever, pallor, fatigue, anorexia, hemorrhage (usually petechiae), and bone and joint pain. In the presence of neutropenia the body's normal bacterial flora can become aggressive pathogens. Any break in the skin is a potential site of infection. Frequently, vague abdominal pain is caused by areas of inflammation from normal flora within the intestinal tract.

Disturbance of Involved Organs. The spleen, liver, and lymph glands demonstrate marked infiltration, enlargement, and eventually fibrosis. Hepatosplenomegaly is typically more common than lymphadenopathy.

The next most important site of involvement is the central nervous system. Initially, leukemic cells do not tend to invade this area because of the protective blood-brain barrier. However, this normal protective mechanism also prevents the antileukemic drugs, with the exception of a few agents, from entering the brain in sufficient therapeutic doses to be effective. Before prophylactic use of cranial irradiation and intrathecal methotrexate, central nervous system involvement was frequent in children who survived 6 months or more. However, newer modes of therapy have significantly changed the course of the disease, although central nervous system complications still occur, even during bone marrow remission.

The usual effect of leukemic infiltration of the meninges is increased intracranial pressure. The pathogenesis is presumably attributable to invasion of the arachnoid by proliferating cells, which then interfere with the flow of cerebrospinal fluid in the subarachnoid space and at the base of the brain. The increased fluid pressure causes dilation of all four ventricles and consequently the signs and symptoms normally associated with this condition, such as severe headache, vomiting, papilledema, irritability, lethargy, and eventually coma. Irritation of the meninges also causes pain and stiffness in the neck and back.

Additional sites of involvement may be the cranial nerves, most often cranial nerve VII, or the facial nerve, and spinal nerves, particularly of the lumbosacral plexus, hypothalamus, and cerebellum. Clinical manifestations for these sites are directly related to the area involved. For example, with lumbosacral invasion, there is weakness in the lower extremities, pain radiating down the legs to the feet, and difficulty in voiding. Although such signs may suggest a brain tumor, the absence of localized signs often leads to the discovery of central nervous system involvement in leukemia.

Other sites that may become invaded with leukemic cells include the kidneys, testes, prostate, ovaries, gastrointestinal tract, and lungs. With long-term survivors becoming increasingly common, such extramedullary sites of leukemic invasion, especially the testes, are becoming more important clinically.

Hypermetabolism. The immense metabolic needs of proliferating leukemic cells eventually deprive all body cells of nutrients necessary for survival. Muscle wasting, weight loss, anorexia, and fatigue are natural consequences. Obviously, in addition to the risk of death from infection and hemorrhage, uncontrolled growth of leukemic cells can terminate in metabolic starvation.

Onset

The onset of leukemia varies from acute to insidious. In most instances the child displays remarkably few symptoms. For example, leukemia may be diagnosed when a minor infection, such as a cold, fails to completely disappear. The child continues to be pale, listless, irritable, febrile, and anorexic. Parents often suspect some underlying problem when they observe the weight loss, petechiae, bruising without cause, and continued complaints of bone and joint pain.

At other times leukemia is diagnosed after an extended history of signs and symptoms mimicking such conditions as rheumatoid arthritis or mononucleosis. There are also occasions when the diagnosis of leukemia accompanies some totally unrelated event, such as a routine physical examination or injury.

The history not only yields valuable medical information regarding the subsequent course of the illness, but also bears heavily on the parents' emotional reaction to the diagnosis. In most instances the diagnosis is an unexpected revelation of catastrophic proportion.

Staging and Prognostic Factors

The most important prognostic factors in determining long-term survival for children with ALL are the initial white blood cell count and the patient's age at diagnosis, followed by the histologic type of the disease and the child's sex (Table 36-5).

No such staging exists with AML, and prognostic indicators are less clearly defined. Initial evidence suggests that the degree of tumor burden is the best indicator of prognosis (Sandlund, Hutchison, and Crist, 1991).

From the time of establishment of the diagnosis, the nurse has some idea of the expected course the child will follow. However, in some instances, because of the variety of cell types observed and the marked undifferentiation of immature cells, a definitive classification cannot be made

TABLE 36-5 Favorable Prognostic Factors for Acute Lymphoblastic Leukemia

FACTOR	CRITERIA
Leukocyte count	<100,000/mm^3
Age	>2 and <10 years
Immunologic subtype	CALLA-positive, early pre-B–cell
FAB morphology	L_1
Cytogenetics	Hyperdiploid (>50 chromosomes, DNA index >1.16); absence of translocation
Sex	Female
Race	White
Leukemia cell burden	Minimal

Data from Poplack DG: Acute lymphoblastic leukemia. In Pizzo PA, Poplack DG: *Principles and practice of pediatric oncology,* ed 2, Philadelphia, 1993, JB Lippincott.

or the diagnosis may be changed. The nurse should be aware of the importance of such events in counseling and supporting family members.

Diagnostic Evaluation

Leukemia is usually suspected from the history, physical manifestations, and a peripheral blood smear that contains immature forms of leukocytes, frequently in combination with low blood counts. Definitive diagnosis is based on bone marrow aspiration or biopsy. Typically the bone marrow is hypercellular with primarily blast cells. Once the diagnosis is confirmed, a lumbar puncture is performed to determine if there is any central nervous system involvement, although a very small number of children have central nervous system involvement and most are asymptomatic.

Therapeutic Management

Treatment of leukemia involves the use of chemotherapeutic agents with or without cranial irradiation in three phases: (1) ***induction,*** which achieves a complete remission or disappearance of leukemic cells; (2) ***CNS prophylactic therapy,*** which prevents leukemic cells from invading the central nervous system; and (3) ***maintenance with intensification (consolidation),*** which serves to maintain the remission phase. Although the combination of drugs and radiation may vary according to the institution, the prognostic or risk characteristics of the patient, and the type of leukemia being treated, the following general principles for each phase are consistently employed.

Remission Induction. Almost immediately after confirmation of the diagnosis, induction therapy is begun and lasts for 4 to 6 weeks (van Eys and others, 1989). The principal drugs used for induction in ALL are the corticosteroids (especially prednisone), vincristine, and L-asparaginase, with or without doxorubicin (see Table 36-2). Oral steroids are administered daily in divided doses to maintain consistently high blood levels. Vincristine is given by intravenous infusion once a week for a total of four to six doses, and L-asparaginase or doxorubicin is given at various schedules. A complete remission is determined by the absence of clinical signs or symptoms of the disease and the presence of less than 5% blast cells in the bone marrow (M_1-type bone marrow).

With AML the drug therapies differ from those used for lymphoid leukemia. The principal drugs used for induction therapy in AML are doxorubicin or daunomycin and cytosine arabinoside; various other drugs may be added.

Since many of the drugs also cause myelosuppression of normal blood elements, the period immediately following a remission can be critical; the body is defenseless against invading organisms (especially normal bacterial flora) and highly susceptible to spontaneous hemorrhage. Consequently, supportive therapy during this time is essential.

CNS Prophylactic Therapy. Children with leukemia are at risk for developing CNS invasion of the leukemic cells. For this reason, all children receive CNS prophylactic therapy. Before the 1980s children with ALL received cranial/spinal irradiation. Because of the concern regarding late effects of cranial irradiation, this mode of therapy is now generally reserved for high-risk patients and/or those with central nervous system disease. Triple intrathecal chemotherapy consisting of methotrexate, cytarabine, and hydrocortisone is used during induction and intensification (consolidation) and maintenance therapy to prevent CNS disease.

Maintenance and Intensification (Consolidation). The goal of maintenance therapy is to preserve remission and further reduce the number of leukemic cells. Combined drug regimens have been more successful in maintaining remissions and preventing drug resistance. A variety of agents are used during maintenance therapy, with a daily dose of oral 6-mercaptopurine and weekly doses of intramuscular methotrexate being standard in most treatment regimens.

Intensification, or consolidation, of therapy is used during maintenance therapy to further decrease the number of leukemic cells in the child's body. Intensification therapy incorporates the use of the following intravenous agents: L-asparaginase, high-dose methotrexate, intermediate-dose methotrexate and cytarabine, and methotrexate and mercaptopurine. The intensification phase consists of pulses of these agents given periodically during maintenance therapy. The agents used for intensification therapy depend on the type of leukemia and the risk factors of the child.

During maintenance therapy, weekly or monthly complete blood counts are taken to evaluate the marrow's response to the drugs. If myelosuppression becomes severe (usually indicated by an absolute neutrophil count below 1000/mm^3), or if toxic side effects occur, therapy is temporarily stopped or the dose decreased.

Duration of therapy has been based on clinical experience comparing survival rates for various time intervals and is concerned with preventing deleterious effects of excessive treatment. While the optimum time for discontinuing therapy is not known, current practice is to continue treatment for 2.5 to 3 years. Because of the risk of testicular relapse in boys, some centers favor longer maintenance programs, but in general the additional maintenance therapy appears to delay, not prevent, relapses (Gale, 1989). All children after cessation of therapy require regular medical evaluation for surveillance of relapse and long-term sequelae of treatment. Most relapses (16%) occur during the first year off therapy, about 2% to 3% of the relapses occur during each of the next 3 years, and very few relapses occur after 6 years (Poplack, 1993).

Reinduction Following Relapse. For many children additional therapy becomes necessary when a relapse occurs, as evidenced by the presence of leukemic cells within the bone marrow. Usually reinduction for ALL includes the use of prednisone and vincristine with a combination of other drugs not previously used. Although remissions may be achieved after more than one relapse, each relapse heralds an increasingly poor prognosis. However, more long-term second and subsequent remissions are occurring, and these may have better outlooks than previously thought.

A site that is resistant to chemotherapy and is responsible for leukemic relapse is the testes. A minority of males experience relapse during maintenance therapy or have occult disease after cessation of therapy. Routine bilateral testicular biopsies at the time of terminating treatment to identify occult disease is performed at some institutions, followed by aggressive treatment for affected males, including bilateral testicular irradiation, intensive systemic chemotherapy, and central nervous system prophylactic therapy (Crist, Pullen, and Rivera, 1991).

Bone Marrow Transplantation (BMT). Bone marrow transplants have been used successfully in treating some children with ALL and AML. In general, BMT is not recommended for children with acute lymphocytic leukemia (ALL) during the first remission because of the excellent results possible with chemotherapy. The group with the best results have been those with ALL who receive the graft during the second remission (Poplack, 1993). Because of the poorer prognosis in children with AML, transplantation may be considered during the first remission when a suitable donor is available (Johnson, 1991).

Prognosis. The majority of children with newly diagnosed leukemia who receive effective multiagent chemotherapy will survive. One long-term comprehensive study reported that the rates of complete remission ranged from 90% to 95%. Almost 70% of the children achieved long-term disease-free survival, and 80% of these children developed no obvious health problems from the leukemia or its treatment. It appears that the risk of relapse is less than 1% after 3 to 4 years of complete remission following cessation of therapy (Rivera and others, 1993).

Prognosis after transplantation varies with the timing of the procedure and the type of leukemia; reported ranges for long-term survival are between 25% and 50% (Johnson, 1991). However, since many of these children faced almost certain death without transplantation, even these low figures represent a major advance in eliciting a cure. Still, use of BMT remains controversial (see p. 1621).

Nursing Considerations

Nursing care of the child with leukemia is directly related to the regimen of therapy. Secondary complications that necessitate supportive physical care are caused by myelosuppression, drug toxicity, and leukemic infiltration. This discussion focuses on supportive interventions for the child with leukemia and the family. General aspects of care appropriate for the child with leukemia have been discussed under Nursing Care of the Child with Cancer. Psychologic interventions appropriate for children with leukemia during significant phases of therapy are discussed in Chapter 23.

Prepare Family for Diagnostic/Therapeutic Procedures. From the time before diagnosis to cessation of therapy, children must undergo several tests, the most traumatic of which are bone marrow aspiration or biopsy and lumbar punctures. Multiple finger sticks and venipunctures for blood analysis and drug infusion are common occurrences for several years after the diagnosis. Therefore the child needs an explanation of why each procedure is done and what can be expected (see also Preparation for Procedures, Chapter 27).

Depending on the age of the child, one way of beginning such preparation is to explain the basic elements of the blood.* Using a drawing or letting the child look at a drop of blood under a microscope not only teaches, but also encourages trust between the nurse and the child. It also allows the nurse to assess the child's level of understanding. An error many health professionals make is to overestimate children's knowledge about their bodies. For example, a bone marrow aspiration makes sense only when it is clarified that the center of a bone is hollow and contains the cells that later become "working" blood cells or leukemic cells.

Provide Continued Emotional Support. Nursing care of the child with leukemia is based on typical problems with which the family is confronted during the treatment phases. It is not unusual for a child who discontinues therapy after 2 or 3 years and maintains a permanent remission to experience many of these side effects. Therefore the nurse's role is continually one of support, guidance, clarification, and judgment. Parents need to know how to recognize symptoms that demand medical attention. Although some of the reactions discussed are expected, parents should still report them to their practitioner. Warning parents of their possible occurrence beforehand also allows parents an opportunity to prepare for them. At the same time, it reassures them that these reactions are not caused by a return of leukemic cells.

The nurse must also use judgment in recognizing which side effects are normal reactions and which indicate toxicity. Frequently it is the office or clinic nurse who screens such telephone calls and gives advice when appropriate. Usually nausea and vomiting are not indications for drug cessation. However, severe vomiting may require immediate intervention to prevent dehydration. Signs of infection, mucosal ulceration, hemorrhagic cystitis, peripheral neuropathy, and obstipation require medical evaluation.

Another aspect of continued emotional support involves prognosis. Although leukemia is not invariably fatal, present statistics must also be correctly interpreted. While more

*Especially recommended is the book *You and Leukemia: A Day At a Time* by L. Baker (1988, WB Saunders).

than 95% of children with ALL will achieve an initial remission and as many as 70% of them will live 5 years or longer, it must be remembered that these are *average* estimates and apply to those children treated with the most successful protocols since diagnosis (Rivera and others, 1993). For the low-risk child the chances may be better, but for the high-risk child they may be significantly poorer. Of those who do survive after discontinuing therapy, a portion will relapse. At present only the passage of time is positive confirmation of the child who is "cured" of the disease.

The nurse must be familiar with these statistics in order to interpret them correctly to parents. At the same time, the nurse must realize that a realistic understanding of the chances for survival requires an adjustment period. For example, it is not unusual for parents to interpret the "95% remission" as the probability for a cure. When a relapse occurs, parents may for the first time be able to "hear" the correct facts.

Statistics are numbers. Sometimes they bring hope, and at other times they bring despair. Although they are very important in terms of research, better treatment, and identification of high- or low-risk populations, they present a general picture of what to expect. The nurse who is working with family members must individualize the "numbers" to relate to the people. An understanding of each member's emotional needs, as well as competent care of physical ones, is essential to the positive, growth-promoting support of the family. Comprehensive emotional support for the family through all phases of the illness is discussed in Chapter 23.

LYMPHOMAS

The lymphomas, a group of neoplastic diseases that arise from the lymphoid and hemopoietic systems, are divided into Hodgkin disease and non-Hodgkin lymphoma (NHL). These diseases are further subdivided according to tissue type and extent of disease (staging). In children non-Hodgkin lymphoma is more common than Hodgkin disease. Although Hodgkin disease is extremely rare before 5 years of age, there is a striking increase in children ages 15 to 19 years, when it occurs with almost the same frequency as leukemia.

HODGKIN DISEASE

Hodgkin disease affects about 5 in 1 million children, mostly adolescents. The malignancy originates in the lymphoid system and primarily involves the lymph nodes. It predictably metastasizes to nonnodal or extralymphatic sites, especially the spleen, liver, bone marrow, lungs, and mediastinum (mass of tissues and organs separating the lungs; includes heart and its vessels, trachea, esophagus, thymus, and lymph nodes), although no tissue is exempt from involvement (Fig. 36-2). It is classified according to four histologic types: (1) lymphocytic predominance, (2) nodular sclerosis, (3) mixed cellularity, and (4) lymphocytic depletion. With present treatment protocols, the histologic stage of the disease has less prognostic significance than previously, although children with the lymphocyte-depleted histology are likely to do poorly (Carde, 1992).

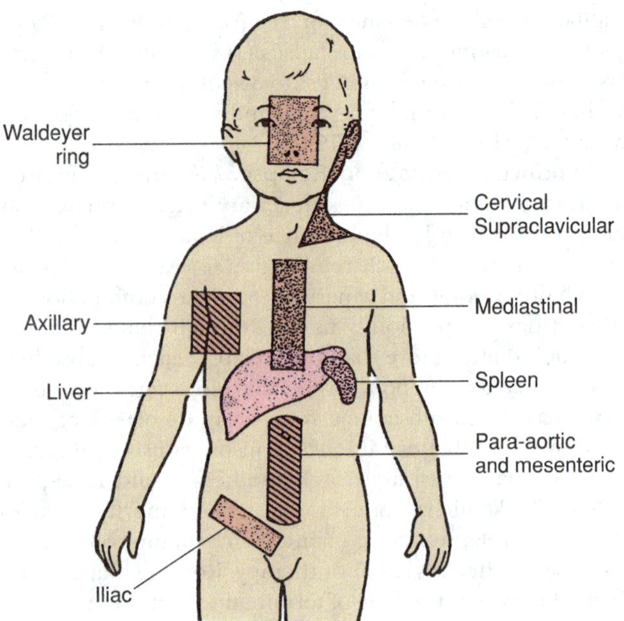

FIG. 36-2 Main areas of lymphadenopathy and organ involvement in Hodgkin disease.

Clinical Staging and Prognosis

Accurate staging of the extent of disease is the basis for treatment protocols and expected prognosis. More than one staging system exists; the one in the box on p. 1645 is known as the ***Ann Arbor Staging Classification.***

Each stage is further subdivided into A or B. *A* denotes absence of associated general symptoms. *B* indicates presence of symptoms such as night sweats, fever (>38° C [100.4° F]), or weight loss of 10% or more during the preceding 6 months. In stages II and III, subtype B has a significantly poorer prognosis than subtype A.

The prognosis for patients with Hodgkin disease has improved dramatically in the past few years, largely as a result of the systematic staging procedure and improved treatment protocols. The prognosis is excellent in children with localized disease. The overall 10-year survival rate is as high as 90%. For relapses complete remission may occur in 20% to 40% of patients; BMT may represent hope for a cure (Kennedy, 1993). Even in those with disseminated disease, long-term remissions are possible in more than half of the patients. Unfortunately, a number of children may have late recurrences of the original disease or develop a second malignancy, especially osteosarcoma, breast cancer, thyroid carcinoma, or leukemia. The risk is higher in females than in males (Tarbell and others, 1993). The most common complication of irradiation to the neck area is hypothyroidism (Weinshel and Peterson, 1993).

Clinical Manifestations

Hodgkin disease is characterized by painless enlargement of lymph nodes. The most common finding is enlarged, firm, nontender, movable nodes in the supraclavicular area. In children the "sentinel" node located near the left clavicle may be the first enlarged node. Enlargement of axillary and inguinal lymph nodes is less frequent (see Fig. 36-2).

STAGES OF HODGKIN DISEASE

Stage I: Lesions are limited to one lymph node area or only one additional extralymphatic site (IE), such as the liver, lungs, kidney, or intestines.
Stage II: Two or more lymph node regions on the same side of the diaphragm or one additional extralymphatic site or organ (IIE) on the same side of the diaphragm is involved.
Stage III: Lymph node regions on both sides of the diaphragm are involved, or one extralymphatic site (IIIE), spleen (IIIS), or both (IIISE).
Stage IV: Cancer has metastasized diffusely throughout the body to one or more extralymphatic sites with or without involvement of associated lymph nodes.

Other signs and symptoms depend on the extent and location of involvement. Mediastinal lymphadenopathy may cause a persistent nonproductive cough. Enlarged retroperitoneal nodes may produce unexplained abdominal pain. Systemic symptoms include low-grade and/or intermittent fever (Pel-Ebstein disease), anorexia, nausea, weight loss, night sweats, and pruritus. Generally, such symptoms indicate advanced lymph node and extralymphatic involvement.

Diagnostic Evaluation

The history and physical examination often yield important clues to the disease, such as fevers, night sweats, or weight loss, and enlarged lymph nodes, spleen, or liver. Because of the multiple organs that can become involved, diagnosis consists of several tests to confirm the presence of Hodgkin disease and to assess the extent of involvement for accurate staging. Tests include complete blood count, uric acid levels, liver function tests, urinalysis, and erythrocyte sedimentation rate. Computed tomography (CT) of the chest, liver, spleen, and bone is done to detect metastasis.

With the advent of CT, a special procedure, lymphangiography, may not be needed, although elimination is controversial. A ***lymphangiogram*** involves the intradermal injection of a contrast material (usually alphazurine) in the first interdigital space of each foot for visualization of the lymphatic vessels to determine the presence of disease in various lymph node regions (Shochat, 1992). One or more vessels are then chosen for catheterization, and a radiopaque medium, usually ethiodized oil (Ethiodol), is injected under pressure to visualize the entire lymphatic chain in the lower extremities, groin, iliopelvic and abdominal-aortic regions, and the thoracic duct. If the axillary, periclavicular, and supraclavicular lymph nodes must be examined, the same procedure is performed in the hands.

Biopsy is essential to diagnosis and staging. The enlarged lymph node is excised and analyzed for histologic type and evidence of the ***Sternberg-Reed cell,*** a giant cell with a dark-staining nucleolus. Although the cell is considered diagnostic of Hodgkin disease because it is absent in the other lymphomas, it may occur in infectious mononucleosis. A bone marrow aspiration or biopsy is also usually performed. A laparotomy is recommended for definitive pathologic staging, and the spleen is removed, although this remains a controversial practice because of the risk of overwhelming infections from asplenia. During this procedure the entire abdomen is examined for evidence of disease; samples of the liver are taken for microscopic study. Biopsies of any involved lymph nodes and the spleen are performed. During surgery metal clips are placed to outline margins of involved sites for irradiation and to monitor any disease progression. The ovaries may be moved out of the radiation field (oophoropexy) to protect them from irradiation damage.

Therapeutic Management

The primary modalities of therapy are radiation and chemotherapy. Each may be used alone or in combination. The decision is based on the clinical staging. The goal of treatment is obviously a cure; however, aggressive therapy increases the chances of complications in the disease-free state and can seriously compromise the quality of life. Consequently, numerous research studies are presently investigating treatment options to minimize long-term sequelae. Because of the diversity of approaches to treatment, the following is an overview of general principles that may or may not apply to all children. One of the major concerns with combined radiation and antineoplastic drug therapy is the serious late effects in children with an excellent prognosis.

Children with favorable stage I disease may receive only ***involved field (IF) radiation.*** Those with stage II or III disease are candidates for ***extended field (EF) radiation*** (involved areas plus adjacent nodes) or ***total nodal irradiation (TNI)*** (the entire axial lymph node system). Chemotherapy is usually combined with radiation. In stage IV, chemotherapy is the primary form of treatment, although limited radiation may be given to areas of bulky disease. The most widely used drug regimen is MOPP (mechlorethamine [Mustargen], vincristine [Oncovin], prednisone, and procarbazine). Several other drug combinations may be used, such as adriamycin, bleomycin, vinblastine, and decarbazine (ABVD).

Follow-up care of children no longer receiving therapy is essential to identify relapse, as well as second malignancies. In children with asplenia, prophylactic antibiotics are administered for an indefinite period, and immunizations against pneumococci and meningococci are recommended (see Chapter 12).

Nursing Considerations

Prepare Family for Diagnostic/Operative Procedures. Once the child is hospitalized for suspected Hodgkin disease, a battery of diagnostic tests is ordered. The family needs an explanation of why each test is performed, since many of them, such as bone marrow aspiration (see Chapter 27), are not routine. If lymphangiography is performed, the child needs to be prepared for the test and particularly told that the length of the procedure is anywhere from 2 to 10 hours and frequently averages 4 to 5 hours. Although the feet are anesthetized, the initial injections are painful. Immobilization of the feet during lymphatic vessel catheterization may be uncomfortable and tiresome, especially since the child must remain still for long periods. Whenever possible the child is encouraged to sleep, or diversions should be provided, such as listening to music, reading, or talking.

Ideally a family member should be allowed to accompany the child. Fluids and food are not necessarily restricted. If allowed, provisions are made for the child to have a favorite drink or snack.

The procedure is not without complications, the most serious of which is pulmonary embolism from the oil-based medium. Fine pulmonary emboli produce symptoms of slight fever, chills, pleutiric pain, mild dyspnea, and a dry cough. Acetaminophen is helpful to reduce the fever and relieve the pain. The symptoms usually subside within 24 to 48 hours.

Severe oil embolism may occur if the contrast medium has been infused too rapidly. Signs of this complication include cyanosis, distended neck veins, hypotension, liver tenderness, and edema in the lower extremities from increased venous resistance. Emergency medical treatment usually involves supplemental oxygen and antihypotensive drugs. The child may become very apprehensive and need considerable reassurance. Usually sedation is avoided, because it may depress the respiratory center.

Expected reactions to the contrast medium include abnormal taste sensations, retrosternal burning, headache, sleeplessness, diarrhea, and elevated temperature. The alphazurine turns the urine and skin of the feet and/or hands bluish green. Although the urine clears rapidly, the discoloration of skin may last for months. Adolescents may be very self-conscious about the staining, especially in the hands.

Since a cutdown procedure is done for vessel catheterization, a pressure bandage may be in place. The area(s) is observed for signs of bleeding and subsequent infection. Sutures are usually removed in 7 to 10 days. Ordinarily the child has no restrictions on activity after the test. However, the child is cautioned to keep the wound clean and to avoid excessive irritation from shoes.

Preparation for a laparotomy is similar to that for any other surgery. One special area of concern for families is the effects of the splenectomy on bodily functions. Although not a vital organ, the spleen does have an important role in resisting infection, particularly in young children. The family needs to be aware of the benefits of the procedure in terms of staging and potential risks. Compliance is a major issue with indefinite administration of antibiotics, and every effort should be made to employ strategies that enhance compliance (see Chapter 27).

Explain Treatments and Side Effects. Explanations of chemotherapeutic reactions vary with the specific drug regimen. Drugs commonly used are outlined in Table 36-2, and the most common side effects, such as nausea and vomiting, body image changes, neuropathy, and mucosal ulceration, are discussed under Nursing Care of the Child with Cancer.

Involved field radiation results in few side effects, sometimes consisting only of a mild skin reaction. With extended field radiation to the chest and abdomen, nausea and vomiting, weight loss, and mucosal ulceration (esophagitis, gastric ulcers) are common. The usual measures for providing relief are discussed on p. 1630 and are outlined in Table 36-3.

The most common side effect of extensive radiation is malaise, which may result from damage to the thyroid gland, causing hypothyroidism. Lack of energy is particularly difficult for adolescents, because it prevents them from keeping up with their peers. Sometimes adolescents will push themselves to the point of physical exhaustion rather than admit fatigue and succumb to the decreased activity tolerance. Parents are advised to observe for such behavior, such as extreme fatigue at the end of the day, falling asleep at the dinner table, inability to concentrate on homework, or an increased susceptibility to infection. Regular bedtimes and periodic rest times are important for these children, especially during chemotherapy, when myelosuppression increases the risk of infection and debilitation. Before discharge the nurse should discuss a feasible school schedule with the parents and child. If alterations are necessary, such as elimination of strenuous physical education, they are discussed with the teacher, nurse, and principal. Follow-up care is essential to diagnose hypothyroidism early and institute thyroid replacement.

An area of concern for adolescents is the high risk of sterility from irradiation and chemotherapy. Both irradiation to the gonads and drugs, particularly procarbazine and alkylating agents, may lead to infertility. Younger patients with a greater complement of oocytes are more likely to retain ovarian function.

Although sexual function is not altered, the appearance of secondary sexual characteristics and menstruation may be delayed in the pubescent child. Adolescents should be informed of these side effects early in the course of the diagnosis and treatment. Delayed sexual maturation may be an extremely sensitive and painful area for children (see Chapter 20). It is important for the nurse to respect their concern and refrain from casually placating them with expressions such as, "You'll catch up someday."

NON-HODGKIN LYMPHOMA (NHL)

NHL occurs in between 7 and 8 children per million under age 15 and has about one and one-half times the incidence of Hodgkin disease. Histologic classification of childhood NHL is strikingly different from that of Hodgkin disease and adult NHL in several respects (Sandlund, Hutchison, and Crist, 1991):

- The disease is usually diffuse rather than nodular.
- The cell type is either undifferentiated or poorly differentiated.
- Dissemination occurs earlier, more often, and more rapidly.
- Mediastinal involvement and invasion of meninges typically occur.

Staging and Prognosis

NHL is heterogeneous, exhibiting a variety of morphologic, cytochemical, and immunologic features, not unlike the diversity seen in leukemia. Classification is based on the pattern of histologic presentation: (1) lymphoblastic; (2) Burkitt or nonBurkitt; or (3) large cell (Huizdala, 1991). Immunologically these cells are also classified as T-cells, B-cells (an example of which is Burkitt lymphoma), or non-T–, non-B–cells, which lack specific immunologic properties.

STAGING SYSTEM FOR NON-HODGKIN LYMPHOMA

Stage I: Single tumor at a single site
Stage II: Single tumor with regional involvement on same side of diaphragm
Stage III: Tumor on both sides of abdomen; also, all primary thoracic, intraabdominal, and paraspinal or epidural tumors
Stage IV: Any of the involvement in stages I and II, with central nervous system and/or bone marrow involvement

The clinical staging system used in Hodgkin disease is of little value in NHL, although that system has been modified for NHL and other systems have been developed. A favorable prognosis is defined by (1) lymph node involvement only and limited to one or two adjacent lymphatic regions (excluding the mediastinum); (2) an extranodal site in the nasopharynx, oropharynx, or other isolated extranodal site, with or without regional lymphadenopathy; or (3) gastrointestinal involvement, with or without regional lymphadenopathy, limited to the mesentery (Magrath, 1993). The most commonly used staging system is presented in the box above.

The use of aggressive combination chemotherapy has had a major impact on the survival rates of children with NHL. The most effective treatment regimens result in cure in almost all children with limited disease involvement; 50% to 75% of children with extensive disease are cured (Sandlund, Hutchison, and Crist, 1991).

Clinical Manifestations

Clinical manifestations depend on the anatomic site and extent of involvement. Many of those seen in Hodgkin disease may be present in NHL, although rarely does a single symptom give rise to the diagnosis. Rather, metastasis to the bone marrow or central nervous system may produce signs and symptoms typical of leukemia. Lymphoid tumors compressing various organs may cause intestinal or airway obstruction, cranial nerve palsies, or spinal paralysis.

The exception to the usual presentation of NHL is ***Burkitt lymphoma,*** a type of cancer that is rare in the United States but endemic in parts of Africa. It is a rapidly growing neoplasm that is most commonly seen as a mass in the jaw, abdomen, or orbit. However, no anatomic site appears exempt from involvement. Peripheral lymphadenopathy, hepatosplenomegaly, or signs of conversion to leukemia are rarely seen.

Diagnostic Evaluation

Since widespread disease exists in most children with NHL at diagnosis, thorough pathologic staging is unnecessary. Current recommendations for staging include a surgical biopsy for histopathologic confirmation of disease with immunophenotyping and cytogenetic evaluation; bone marrow aspiration; radiologic studies, especially CT scans of the lungs and gastrointestinal organs; and lumbar puncture.

Therapeutic Management

The present treatment protocols for NHL include an aggressive approach using irradiation and chemotherapy. Similar to leukemic therapy, the protocols include induction, consolidation, and maintenance phases, some with intrathecal chemotherapy. At present the differentiation between lymphoblastic lymphoma and all other lymphomas is widely used as a way to categorize patients for specific treatment regimens (Magrath, 1993). Children with lymphoblastic lymphoma are treated with several drug protocols, most containing several chemotherapeutic agents. One of the most commonly used regimens includes cyclophosphamide or ifosfamide, vincristine, intrathecal chemotherapy, prednisone, daunomycin, 6-thioguanine, cytosine arabinoside, BCNU, and L-asparaginase.

Children with nonlymphoblastic lymphoma are treated with cyclic drug combinations, including cyclophosphamide and intermediate-dose or high-dose methotrexate (Magrath, 1993). Most protocols also include an anthracycline. These children receive central nervous system prophylaxis with combination intrathecal chemotherapy (Meadows and others, 1989). These multiagent regimens are administered for 6 to 24 months.

Nursing Considerations

Nursing care of the child with NHL is very similar to the care discussed under Nursing Care of the Child with Cancer. Because of the intensive chemotherapy protocol, nursing care is primarily directed toward managing the side effects of these agents.

NERVOUS SYSTEM TUMORS

Two major forms of childhood cancer are derived from neural tissue. ***Brain tumors*** are the most common solid tumors that occur in children and are second only to leukemia as a form of cancer. ***Neuroblastomas*** are the most common malignant tumors of infancy and are second only to brain tumors as the type of solid malignancy seen during the first 10 years (Fernbach and Vietti, 1991). Both of these tumors have presented difficulties in identifying successful modes of treatment and have not demonstrated the dramatic improvements in survival seen in many other forms of cancer.

BRAIN TUMORS

Tumors of the central nervous system account for about 20% of all childhood cancers and have an annual incidence of 2.4 per 100,000 children under 15 years of age. About half of the tumors are ***infratentorial*** (below the tentorium cerebelli), which means that they occur in the posterior third of the brain, primarily in the cerebellum or brainstem. This anatomic distribution accounts for the frequency of symptoms resulting from increased intracranial pressure (ICP). The other tumors are ***supratentorial,*** or within the anterior two thirds of the brain, mainly the cerebrum. Major brain tumors of childhood are outlined in the box on p. 1648.

MAJOR BRAIN TUMORS OF CHILDHOOD

LOW-GRADE OR HIGH-GRADE ASTROCYTOMAS

Most common pediatric brain tumor; about 23% are low grade and 11% are high grade.
Usually infiltrates brain parenchyma without distinct boundaries.
Low-grade tumors have more highly differentiated cells and are less malignant than high-grade tumors.
Characteristic presenting signs include headache, nausea, seizures, and sometimes bizarre behavior (staring spells and automatic movements).
Extensive surgical excision is attempted and may require repeated operations; chemotherapy and/or irradiation are used after incomplete resection.
Five-year survival rate is 75% to 85% for low-grade astrocytomas, less for high-grade tumors.

MEDULLOBLASTOMA (PRIMITIVE NEUROECTODERMAL TUMOR)

Accounts for about 15% of pediatric brain tumors.
Fast growing, highly malignant.
Characteristic presenting signs include headache, vomiting, and ataxia.
Improved survival rates with excision of most or all of tumor plus chemotherapy with or without irradiation.
Overall rate is approximately 50%; 80% to 90% for low-stage disease and 25% to 40% for high-stage disease.
Period for risk of recurrence is age at diagnosis plus 9 months.

CEREBELLAR ASTROCYTOMA

Accounts for about 15% of pediatric brain tumors.
Slow growing if low grade.
Characteristic presenting signs include headache, clumsiness (usually one hand), awkward gait (stumbling to one side), and vomiting.
With no postoperative residual tumor, likelihood of cure is 70% to 90%.

BRAINSTEM GLIOMA

Accounts for about 15% of pediatric brain tumors.
Often grows to a very large size before causing symptoms.
Characteristic presenting signs include diplopia, facial weakness, and difficulty walking (headache and vomiting are uncommon).
Surgical excision is very difficult because of tumor location in vital brain centers; removal is attempted whenever possible, followed by irradiation.
Palliative therapy with irradiation shrinks tumor to prolong survival, which depends on size, cell type, and location of tumor.
Prognosis is poor, since most tumors are highly resistant to therapy.

EPENDYMOMA

Accounts for about 4% of brain tumors.
Demonstrates varying rates of growth.
Most invade ventricles, obstructing flow of cerebrospinal fluid.
Characteristic presenting signs include vomiting, headache, ataxia, hemiparesis, papilledema, and, in infants, hydrocephalus.
Goal of surgery is total resection; risks associated with total resection are greater with brainstem infiltration, which occurs in about 50% of patients.
Overall 5-year survival rate is about 45% and improves to about 75% if no postoperative residual tumor.

Data from Albright AL: Pediatric brain tumors, *CA Cancer J Clin* 43:272-288, 1993.

Because the neoplasms can arise from any cell within the cranium, it is possible to have tumors originating from the glial cells, nerve cells, neuroepithelium, cranial nerves, blood vessels, pineal gland, and hypophysis. Within each of these structures, specific cells may be involved to provide a histologic classification of the major tumors found in children.

Clinical Manifestations

The signs and symptoms of brain tumors are directly related to their anatomic location and size and to some extent the age of the child. In infants, whose sutures are still open, virtually no early detectable symptoms develop. It is not until spinal fluid obstruction causes markedly increased head size that a lesion may be suspected. Head circumference allows for detection of increased head size. Even in older children, clinical manifestations are nonspecific. However, the most common symptoms are headache, especially on awakening, and vomiting that is not related to feeding. The headache occurs from traction on pain-sensitive areas, such as large blood vessels and cranial nerves, and possibly from dural stretching. The headache is worse in the morning from the compression of these structures during sleep. It typically subsides or improves during the day. Vomiting occurs from increased ICP that compresses the brainstem, directly stimulating the vomiting center in the medulla (Willis, 1991).

Astrocytes, cells that form most of the supportive tissue for the neurons, may form ***astrocytomas,*** the most common glial tumor (Willis, 1991). Brain tumors may be benign or malignant. The common presenting symptoms of brain tumors are presented in Table 36-6.

Diagnostic Evaluation

Diagnosis of a brain tumor is based subjectively on presenting clinical signs and objectively on neurologic tests. Because the signs and symptoms are vague and easily overlooked, early diagnosis necessitates a high index of suspicion during history taking. A number of tests may be employed in the neurologic evaluation (see Table 37-2), but the most common diagnostic procedure is magnetic resonance imaging (MRI), which permits early diagnosis of brain tumors, as well as assessment of tumor growth during or following treatment. Another test is computed tomogra-

TABLE 36-6 Clinical Manifestations and Assessment of Brain Tumors

SIGNS AND SYMPTOMS	ASSESSMENT
HEADACHE	
Recurrent and progressive In frontal or occipital areas Usually dull and throbbing Worse on arising, less during day Intensified by lowering head and straining, such as during bowel movement, coughing, sneezing	Record description of pain, location, severity, and duration Use pain rating scale to assess severity of pain (see Chapter 26) Note changes in relation to time of day and activity Observe changes in behavior in infants (persistent irritability, crying, head rolling)
VOMITING	
With or without nausea or feeding Progressively more projectile More severe in morning Relieved by moving about and changing position	Record time, amount, and relationship to feeding, nausea, and activity
NEUROMUSCULAR CHANGES	
Incoordination or clumsiness Loss of balance (use of wide-based stance, falling, tripping, banging into objects) Poor fine motor control Weakness Hyporeflexia or hyperreflexia Positive Babinski sign Spasticity Paralysis	Test muscle strength, gait, coordination, and reflexes (see Chapter 7)
BEHAVIORAL CHANGES	
Irritability Decreased appetite Failure to thrive Fatigue (frequent naps) Lethargy Coma Bizarre behavior (staring, automatic movements)	Observe behavior regularly Compare observations with parental reports of normal behavioral patterns Monitor growth and food intake Monitor activity and sleep
CRANIAL NERVE NEUROPATHY	
Cranial nerve involvement varies according to tumor location Most common signs Head tilt Visual defects (nystagmus, diplopia, strabismus, episodic "graying out" of vision, visual field defects)	Assess cranial nerves, especially VII (facial), IX (glossopharyngeal), X (vagus), V (trigeminal, sensory roots), and VI (abducens) (see Chapter 7) Assess visual acuity, binocularity, and peripheral vision (see Chapter 7)
VITAL SIGN DISTURBANCES	
Decreased pulse and respiration Increased blood pressure Decreased pulse pressure Hypothermia or hyperthermia	Measure vital signs frequently Monitor pulse and respirations for 1 full minute Record pulse pressure (difference between systolic and diastolic blood pressure)
OTHER SIGNS	
Seizures Cranial enlargement* Tense, bulging fontanel at rest* Nuchal ridigity Papilledema (edema of optic nerve)	Record seizure activity (see Chapter 37) Measure head circumference daily (infant and young child) Perform funduscopic examination if skilled in procedure

*Present only in infants and young children.

phy (CT), which permits direct visualization of the brain parenchyma, ventricles, and surrounding subarachnoid space. Through the intravenous injection of radiographic contrast agents, intracranial blood vasculature can be demonstrated (Heideman and others, 1993).

When a positive CT scan is obtained, angiography may be done to provide information about the tumor's blood supply and degree of vascularity, which may assist the surgeon in planning the operative approach. Other tests (e.g., electroencephalography or lumbar puncture) may be performed. Lumbar puncture is dangerous in the presence of increased ICP because of possible brainstem herniation following sudden release of pressure.

Definitive diagnosis is based on tissue specimens obtained during surgery. Occasionally, special techniques are required for determining the cell type. This period of waiting is one of anxiety for family members, who are aware of the relevance of cell type to prognosis.

Therapeutic Management

Treatment may involve the use of surgery, radiotherapy, and chemotherapy. All three may or may not be used, depending on the type of tumor. The treatment of choice is total removal of the tumor without residual neurologic damage. Patients with the most complete tumor removal have the greatest chance of survival. Several surgical advances have allowed the biopsy and removal of tumors in areas previously considered too dangerous for traditional operative techniques. ***Stereotactic surgery*** involves the use of CT and MRI in conjunction with other special computer techniques to reconstruct the tumor in three dimensions. With computer-assisted instruments, removal is sometimes possible. Other procedures include the use of ***lasers*** to vaporize tumor tissue and ***brain mapping*** to determine the precise location of critical brain areas that are avoided during surgery.

Radiotherapy is used to treat most tumors and to shrink the size of the tumor before attempting surgical removal. The use of chemotherapy is controversial but is playing an increasingly important role, especially in delaying timing of radiation (Duffner and others, 1993). The drugs most commonly used are nitrosoureas (BCNU and CCNU), vincristine, methotrexate, and cisplatin (Heideman and others, 1993). In addition, other drugs, such as corticosteroids, may be needed to manage complications, such as brain edema.

The problems of treatment and relatively poor prognosis, especially in infants and young children, are compounded by the serious late effects of all three modes of therapy. Surgery may cause injury to important areas of the brain, especially when the surgeon is attempting to remove invasive tumors. Radiation has serious long-term consequences, including radiation somnolence syndrome (see p. 1632), brain necrosis, endocrine dysfunction, and behavioral/intellectual deficits. For these reasons, the use of radiation is deferred for as long as possible in young children, although there is limited information regarding a "safe age" (Allen, 1993). Chemotherapy is also not without harmful effects (see Table 36-4).

Nursing Considerations

Nursing care of the child with a brain tumor is similar regardless of the type of intracranial lesion. Since a brain tumor is potentially fatal, the reader is urged to incorporate the psychologic interventions discussed in Chapter 23 with those elaborated in this section.

Assess for Signs and Symptoms. A child admitted to the hospital with neurologic dysfunction is often suspected of having a brain tumor, although the actual diagnosis is as yet unconfirmed. Establishing a baseline of data on which to compare preoperative and postoperative changes is an essential step toward planning physical care and preventing complications. It also allows the nurse to assess the degree of physical incapacity and the family's emotional reaction to the diagnosis. For example, children with cerebellar astrocytoma may have displayed vague cerebellar symptoms for several years before a tumor is suspected. For these parents the revelation of a neoplasm may be more of a shock than for those who have witnessed a rapid deterioration in their child's abilities. Common presenting signs and assessment procedures to document significant changes in the child's condition are summarized in Table 36-6.

Prepare Family for Diagnostic/Operative Procedures. The suspected diagnosis of a brain tumor is always a crisis event. Despite the fact that some tumors are removed with excellent results, the physician can rarely give definitive answers regarding prognosis until after surgery. Therefore parents and older children require much emotional support to face the diagnostic procedures and a craniotomy.

How the child is prepared for the diagnostic tests depends on age and previous experience. Since most of the tests involve x-ray equipment, the child may be familiar with the procedure. Preparing children for an MRI or a CT scan is discussed in Chapter 37. Once surgery is scheduled, the child needs an explanation of what to expect. By the time most children are late preschoolers, they know that the head and brain are important parts of their body. It may be helpful to have children draw their concept of the brain in order to clarify misconceptions and base the explanation on their level of understanding.

Although the temptation is to justify the need for surgery by stating that removing the tumor will take away various symptoms, the nurse should refrain from emphasizing this point too strenuously. Postsurgical headaches and cerebellar symptoms, such as ataxia, may be aggravated rather than improved. Surgery may not improve vision. With optic gliomas the child will be blind in one eye. Finally, surgical removal of the mass may be impossible, and after surgery there may be temporary deterioration of functioning. Being honest before surgery most often makes honesty after the procedure easier because no false hopes were created.

It is best to deliver information in small amounts to let the child pursue additional answers. For example, some children will ask about what happens when part of the tumor is left in. An honest reply is that after surgery the practitioner will try to shrink the tumor with a special radiation machine and/or drugs. A further explanation of radiation or chemotherapy should be delayed until a decision regarding these treatments is made.

The hair is usually shaved in the operating room just before surgery, or sometimes in the child's room, usually the night before surgery. When shaving is done with the child awake, the procedure is approached in a sensitive, positive way. If the child's hair is long, it should be braided so that the long swatch can be saved. Showing children how they look at different stages of the process helps them prepare for the final appearance.

Once the hair is clipped very short or shaved, the child can be given a cap or scarf to wear in order to camouflage the baldness. Every precaution is taken to provide privacy during the procedure and to protect the child from teasing or ridicule by other children before surgery. It is also emphasized that the hair will regrow shortly after surgery. Depending on the child's immediate adjustment to the hair loss, the nurse may introduce the idea of wearing a wig until the hair is grown in, particularly if additional irradiation or chemotherapy is anticipated.

Children are also told about the size of the dressing. Usually the entire scalp is covered to maintain a tight wound closure, even if a small incision is made. Infratentorial head dressings may be attached to the upper back and extend forward to the neck in order to maintain slight extension and alignment as a precaution against wound rupture. Applying a similar dressing or "special hat" to a doll is often a less traumatic way of demonstrating the physical appearance.

Children also need a brief explanation of how they will feel after surgery and where they will be. Ordinarily they will return to a special intensive care unit, which they may visit beforehand depending on hospital policy. They should be aware that they may be sleepy for some time after surgery and that a headache is likely, although it should last only a few days.

Parents need similar explanations before surgery, especially in terms of special equipment used in the intensive care unit, dressings, and their child's behavior. For example, they should know that it is not unusual for the child to be comatose or lethargic for a few days after surgery. The nurse may wish to encourage less frequent visiting during this period so that parents can rest and be able to support their child when awake.

The nurse should participate in preoperative conferences with the physician and parents. The nurse needs to know what information the parents have been given in order to be able to give further explanations or emotional support when necessary.

Prevent Postoperative Complications. Usually the surgeon will prescribe specific orders for vital signs, positioning, fluid regulation, and medication. These vary somewhat, depending on the location of the craniotomy. The following are general principles of care for infratentorial or supratentorial surgery. Additional aspects of care are discussed in Chapter 37, such as care of the child with seizures and care of the unconscious child in terms of respiratory status and neurologic assessment.

Assessment. Vital signs are taken as frequently as every 15 to 30 minutes until stable. Temperature measurement is particularly important because of hyperthermia resulting from surgical intervention in the hypothalamus or brainstem and from some types of general anesthesia. To prepare for this reaction, a cooling blanket may be placed on the bed *before* the child returns to the unit, or it may be used when needed. Since the temperature control centers are affected, the nurse monitors body temperature often when any cooling measures are employed, because hypothermia can occur suddenly.

NURSING ALERT When temperature is elevated, an infectious process must always be suspected, particularly if the febrile state occurs 1 to 2 days after surgery.

The most likely types of infection are meningitis and respiratory tract infection. The probable cause of meningitis is wound contamination. Signs of meningitis, such as opisthotonos, Kernig and Brudzinski signs (see Chapter 7), and nuchal rigidity (see Chapter 37), are very similar to those of increased intracranial pressure and must be carefully evaluated to determine whether they indicate an infection.

The risk of respiratory infections is high because of the imposed immobility, danger of aspiration, and possible depression from the brainstem. The usual precautions of deep breathing and turning as allowed are instituted. Regular pulmonary assessments are performed to identify adventitious sounds or any areas of diminished or absent breath sounds. Blood pressure is also taken at frequent intervals. The deflated cuff is left on the arm between readings to allow for the least movement and disturbance of the child. Ocular signs are recorded at least every hour.

NURSING ALERT Sluggish, dilated, or unequal pupils are reported immediately because they may indicate increased ICP and potential brainstem herniation—a medical emergency.

Observations for function are not instituted until the child regains consciousness. However, as soon as possible the nurse should begin testing reflexes, handgrip, and functioning of the cranial nerves. Muscle strength is usually less after surgery from general weakness but should improve daily. Ataxia may be significantly worse with cerebellar intervention, but it will slowly improve. Edema near the cranial nerves may depress important functions such as the gag, blink, or swallowing reflex.

The nurse records behavior at regular intervals, noting sleep patterns, response to stimuli, and level of consciousness. Although children may be comatose for a few days, once they regain consciousness there should be a steady increase in alertness. Regression to a lethargic, irritable state indicates increasing pressure, possibly caused by meningitis, hemorrhage, or edema.

Dressings are observed for evidence of drainage. If soiled, the dressing is not removed but reinforced with dry sterile gauze. The approximate amount of drainage is estimated and recorded.

NURSING ALERT To keep an accurate account of drainage, the soiled area is circled with a pen every hour or so to identify continuous bleeding. The presence of colorless drainage is reported immediately, since it most likely is cerebrospinal fluid from the incisional area. A foul odor from the dressing may indicate an infection. Such a finding is reported, and a culture is taken.

Once the younger child is alert, the arms may need to be restrained to preserve the dressing. Even a child who has been cooperative before surgery must be closely supervised during the initial stages of regaining consciousness, when disorientation and restlessness are common. Elbow restraints are satisfactory to prevent the hands from reaching the head, although additional restraint may be necessary to preserve an infusion line and maintain a specific position.

Positioning. Correct positioning after surgery is critical to prevent pressure against the operative site, reduce intracranial pressure, and avoid the danger of aspiration. If a large tumor was removed, the child is not placed on the operative side, since the brain may suddenly shift to that cavity, causing trauma to the blood vessels, linings, and the brain itself. The nurse confers with the surgeon to be certain of the correct position, including degree of neck flexion. The first 24 to 48 hours after brain surgery are critical. If position is restricted, notice of this is posted above the head of the bed. When the child is turned, every precaution is used to prevent jarring or malalignment in order to prevent undue strain on the sutures. Two nurses, one supporting the head and the other the body, are needed. The use of a turning sheet may facilitate turning a heavy child.

The child with an infratentorial procedure is usually positioned flat and on either side. Pillows should be placed against the child's back, not head, to maintain the desired position. Ordinarily the head and neck are kept in midline with the body and slightly extended. In a supratentorial craniotomy the head is usually elevated above the heart to facilitate cerebrospinal fluid drainage and decrease excessive blood flow to the brain to prevent hemorrhage.

NURSING ALERT The Trendelenburg position is contraindicated in both infratentorial and supratentorial surgeries because it increases intracranial pressure and the risk of hemorrhage. If shock is impending, the practitioner is notified immediately, before the head is lowered.

Fluid regulation. With an infratentorial craniotomy the child is allowed nothing by mouth for at least 24 hours and longer if the gag and swallowing reflexes are depressed or the child is comatose. With a supratentorial procedure, feeding may be resumed soon after the child is alert, sometimes within 24 hours. Clear water is always started first because of the danger of aspiration. If the child vomits, oral liquids are stopped. Vomiting not only predisposes to aspiration, but also increases intracranial pressure and incisional rupture.

Intravenous fluids are continued until fluids are well tolerated. Because of the cerebral edema postoperatively and the danger of increased ICP, fluids are carefully monitored and usually infused at one half the maintenance rate. If drugs, such as prophylactic antibiotics, are given intravenously, the medication amount is calculated as part of the intravenous fluid. For example, if the child is to receive 20 ml per hour and the diluted drug is 5 ml, the intravenous solution is reduced to 15 ml for that hour.

A hypertonic solution such as mannitol or dextrose may be necessary to remove excess fluid. These drugs cause rapid diuresis. After surgery the child may have a Foley catheter. Urinary output is monitored after administration of these drugs to evaluate their effectiveness.

When able to take fluids, the child should be fed to conserve strength and minimize movement. If there is any sign of facial paralysis, the child is fed slowly to prevent choking or aspiration. Scrupulous mouth care is essential to prevent oral infection. Sometimes gavage feeding is necessary when bodily functions are too depressed to permit safe oral feedings or the child refuses to eat or drink. In the latter instance the nurse should employ every measure to encourage acceptance of fluids or solids. (See Chapter 27 for nursing interventions.)

Comfort measures. Headache may be severe and is largely the result of cerebral edema. Measures to relieve some of the discomfort include providing a quiet, dimly lit environment, restricting visitors to a minimum, preventing any sudden jarring movement, such as banging into the bed, and preventing an increase in ICP. The last is most effectively achieved by proper positioning and prevention of straining, such as during coughing, vomiting, or defecating. The use of opioids, such as morphine, to relieve pain is controversial because it is thought that they may mask signs of altered consciousness or depress respirations. However, they can be given safely, since naloxone can be used to reverse opioid effects, such as sedation or respiratory depression. Acetaminophen and codeine are also effective analgesics. Regardless of the drugs used, adequate dosage and regular administration are essential to providing optimum pain relief. (See also Pain Assessment; Pain Management, Chapter 26.)

Bowel movements are monitored to prevent constipation. Stool softeners may be given as soon as liquids are tolerated to facilitate easy passage of stool. Placing an ice bag on the forehead may also provide some headache relief, especially if facial edema is severe.

Brain edema may severely depress the gag reflex, necessitating suctioning of oral secretions. Facial edema may also be present, necessitating eye care if the lids remain partially open. Ice compresses applied to the eyes for short periods help in relieving the edema. A depressed blink reflex also predisposes to corneal ulceration. Irrigating the eyes with saline drops and covering them with eye dressings are important steps in preventing this complication.

Support Family. The emotional needs of the family are great when the diagnosis is a brain tumor, and feelings are influenced by the extent of surgery, any neurologic deficits, expected prognosis, and additional therapy. Since few definitive answers can be given before surgery, the surgeon's report is a significant finding that can vary from a completely benign, resected neoplasm to a highly malignant, invasive, and only partially removed tumor. Although parents try to prepare themselves for a potentially fatal diagnosis, it is a shock for them.

Ideally a nurse should be with the family when the physician discusses with parents the expected prognosis and plan of therapy. Although parents may hear only a fraction of what they are told, they can begin to put the future into perspective. While some children will be cured, those with residual tumor may die within a relatively short time or live for several years. Regardless of the future prospects, the parents' thinking must be directed toward helping the child recover and resume a normal life to his or her fullest potential. Providing the opportunity for the family to share their concerns and questions with other families who have a child with a brain tumor helps the family cope with the ongoing situations.*

It is also a time to encourage parents to verbalize their feelings about the diagnosis. Often they express guilt for attributing the insidious onset of symptoms, such as ataxia, visual difficulty, or headache, to minor "complaints" by the child. Parents may have punished their child for clumsiness, mistaking it for carelessness. The nurse listens to such statements, emphasizing the normalcy of the parents' reactions. Sometimes it may be helpful to precipitate such a discussion with a statement such as, "It is difficult to know when a child's complaints are significant, because so often they are caused by minor ailments." Any comments that insinuate that the parents should have sought medical advice sooner are avoided, since such remarks only add to the parents' guilt feelings.

During this period the nurse should also discuss with parents what they plan to tell the child. If the child was prepared honestly as described previously, the diagnosis can be expressed in a similar manner, such as, "The surgeon removed most of the tumor, and the rest will be treated with special drugs and x-ray treatments." During the recovery, the child will need additional explanation about the treatment, as well as the reason for residual neurologic effects, such as ataxia or blindness. Since the hair was shaved before surgery, hair loss from treatment is less of a concern, although its regrowth will be delayed by 3 to 6 months, depending on the length of therapy. At this point it is advisable to reinforce the idea of a wig.

Promote Return to Optimum Functioning. The ultimate goal is a cured child who has maximum functioning. As soon as possible, the child should resume usual activities within tolerable limits, especially returning to school.† Until the skull is completely healed, the child may need to wear a helmet when engaging in any active sport. The school nurse and teacher should confer with the parents to discuss activity restrictions, such as physical education, and the reactions of schoolmates to the child's appearance. Since children often equate brain surgery with "going crazy," it is important to prepare the child for possible remarks to this effect. As one child told a classmate, "It's *your* head they should have fixed, because you're crazy. Can't you see that I'm all better?"

After discharge the family needs continuing medical and emotional support from health personnel. Even with children who are long-term survivors after treatment for a brain tumor, residual disabilities, such as growth retardation, cranial nerve palsies, sensory defects, motor abnormalities (especially ataxia), intellectual deficits, dysphagia, dysgraphia, and behavioral problems, may occur (Heideman and others, 1993). It is difficult to assess the exact cause of the nonphysical disabilities, since numerous variables influence the total rehabilitation of the child. However, the high frequency of late effects attests to the tremendous need for follow-up care despite successful treatment of the tumor.

The realm of possible consequences following the diagnosis of a brain tumor is vast. They are not discussed here. Rather, the reader is urged to refer to other sections of the text that deal with possible outcomes, such as the paralyzed, visually impaired, or unconscious child or the care of a child with a ventricular shunt, seizure disorder, or meningitis. Numerous physical problems can occur with progression of the tumor that may necessitate additional procedures. For example, frequent vomiting, anorexia, and nausea may require nonoral routes of feeding, such as gastrostomy or parenteral alimentation. Trials with chemotherapy may necessitate the use of central venous access devices. Whenever these procedures are instituted, the nurse may be responsible for teaching the family appropriate home care to allow the child the highest quality of life for the longest period of time. (See discussion of discharge planning and home care in Chapter 26 and Nursing Care Plan: The Child with a Brain Tumor*.)

NEUROBLASTOMA

Neuroblastoma occurs in about 1 in 10,000 live births, with a slightly higher incidence in males. About half the cases occur in children under 2 years of age, and another fourth occur in children under age 4. These tumors originate from embryonic neural crest cells that normally give rise to the adrenal medulla and the sympathetic nervous system. Consequently, the majority of the tumors arise from the adrenal gland or from the retroperitoneal sympathetic chain. Therefore the primary site is within the abdomen. Other sites may be within the head, neck, chest, or pelvis.

Clinical Manifestations

The signs and symptoms of neuroblastoma depend on the location and stage of the disease. Most presenting signs are caused by compression of adjacent structures. With abdominal tumors the most common presenting sign is a firm, nontender, irregular mass in the abdomen that crosses the midline (in contrast to Wilms tumor, which is usually confined to one side). Compression of the kidney, ureter, or bladder may cause urinary frequency or retention.

Distant metastasis frequently causes supraorbital ecchymosis, periorbital edema, and proptosis (exophthalmos) from invasion of retrobulbar soft tissue (Fig. 36-3). Lymphadenopathy, especially in the cervical and supraclavicular areas, may also be an early presenting sign. Bone pain may or may not be present with skeletal involvement. Vague symptoms of widespread metastasis include pallor, weakness, irritability, anorexia, and weight loss.

Other primary tumors may cause significant clinical effects, such as neurologic impairment from an intracranial lesion, respiratory obstruction from a thoracic mass, or varying degrees of paralysis from compression of the spinal

*Information about support groups is available from the National Brain Tumor Foundation, 323 Geary St. Suite 510, San Francisco, CA 94102; (415) 296-0404 or (800) 934-CURE.

†Excellent publications, including the pamphlet *When Your Child Is Ready to Return to School,* are available from the American Brain Tumor Association, 2720 Red Rd., Suite 146, Des Plaines, IL 60018; (708) 827-9910.

*In *Wong and Whaley's Clinical Manual of Pediatric Nursing* (Mosby).

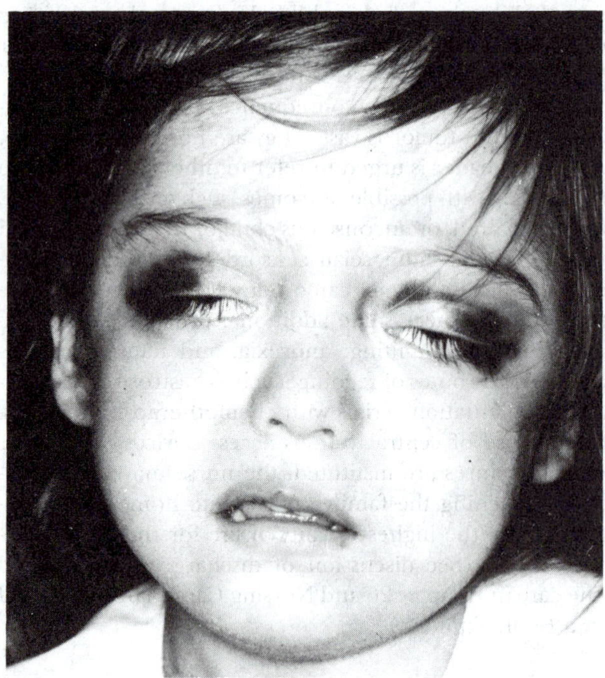

FIG. 36-3 Supraorbital ecchymoses associated with periorbital metastases. (Courtesy Howard A. Britton. From Sutow WW, Vietti TJ, Fernbach DJ, editors: *Clinical pediatric oncology*, ed 2, St Louis, 1977, Mosby.)

cord. Infrequently a child may have symptoms of increased catecholamine excretion, such as flushing, hypertension, tachycardia, and diaphoresis (Blatt and Lee, 1988).

Diagnostic Evaluation

Diagnostic evaluation is aimed at locating the primary site and areas of metastasis. A skeletal survey; skull, neck, chest, abdominal, and bone CT scans; and a bone marrow test are used to locate a tumor mass and/or metastasis. Neuroblastomas, particularly those arising on the adrenal glands or from a sympathetic chain, excrete the catecholamines epinephrine and norepinephrine. Analyzing the breakdown products that are normally excreted in the urine, namely, vanillylmandelic acid (VMA), homovanillic acid (HVA), dopamine, and norepinephrine, permits detection of a suspected tumor both before and after medical/surgical intervention. Amplification of the N-myc gene and abnormalities in chromosomes have been associated with a poorer prognosis (Hayashi and others, 1989). Increased ferritin, neuron-specific enolase (NSE), and ganglioside (GD_2) are associated with neuroblastoma.

Staging and Prognosis

Neuroblastoma is a "silent" tumor. In more than 70% of cases, diagnosis is made after metastasis occurs, with the first signs caused by involvement in the nonprimary site, usually the lymph nodes, bone marrow, skeletal system, skin, or liver. Because of the frequency of invasiveness, the prognosis for neuroblastoma is poor.

The age of the child and the stage of the disease (see box above) at diagnosis are important prognostic factors. Survival is inversely correlated with age. If all stages are grouped together, the survival rates are 75% for children under 1 year of age and less than 50% for children over 1 year of age. This marked difference in survival rates by age is partly accounted for by the larger proportion of very young children with stage I, II, or IV-S disease (Bernstein and others, 1992). However, survival expectancy improves for children over 6 years of age.

STAGING SYSTEM FOR NEUROBLASTOMA

Stage I: Localized tumor confined to the area of origin; local excision with or without microscopic disease; negative lymph nodes

Stage II: Unilateral tumor with incomplete gross excision; lymph nodes negative

Stage III: Tumor infiltrating across the midline with or without regional lymph node involvement; unilateral tumor with regional involvement; midline tumor with bilateral regional lymph node involvement

Stage IV: Dissemination of tumor to distant lymph nodes, bone, bone marrow, liver, and/or other organs

Stage IV-S: Localized primary tumor as defined for stage I or II with dissemination limited to liver, skin, and/or bone marrow but not to bone

Infants who remain free of disease for 1 year after treatment are usually cured, but older children have experienced relapses several years after cessation of treatment. Surgical resection of the tumor in infants diagnosed by ultrasonography done for other reasons appears to be curative (Ho and others, 1993).

Neuroblastoma is one of the few tumors that demonstrate spontaneous regression (especially stage IV-S), possibly as a result of maturity of the embryonic cell or development of an active immune system.

Considerable controversy exists regarding the use of mass screening for neuroblastoma in infants (Mauer, 1988; Tuchman and others, 1989). Whether the cost/benefit ratio of screening for this rare tumor in infants is worthwhile remains to be seen.

Therapeutic Management

Accurate clinical staging is important for establishing initial treatment. Therefore surgery is employed both to remove as much of the tumor as possible and to obtain biopsies. In stages I and II, complete surgical removal of the tumor is the treatment of choice. If the tumors are large, partial resection is attempted, with a course of irradiation postoperatively to shrink the tumor in the hope of complete removal at a later date. Surgery is usually limited to biopsy in stages III and IV because of the extensive metastasis, although the use of additional surgery to assess tumor regression or remove a regressed tumor is not unlikely.

The precise role of radiotherapy is unclear. It does not appear to be of any benefit in children with stage I and II disease; it is commonly used with stage III disease although it may not improve survival expectancy; and it may make a large tumor operable. It offers palliation for metastatic lesions in bones, lungs, liver, or brain.

Chemotherapy is the mainstay of therapy for extensive local or disseminated disease. The drugs of choice are vincristine, doxorubicin, cyclophosphamide, adriamycin, cisplatin, and VM-26 or VP-16. They are administered in a variety of combinations, but none has proved to be superior.

Nursing Considerations

Nursing considerations are similar to those discussed previously under Nursing Care of the Child with Cancer, including psychologic and physical preparation for diagnostic and operative procedures; prevention of postoperative complications for abdominal, thoracic, or cranial surgery; and explanation of chemotherapy and radiotherapy and their side effects (see Tables 36-2 and 36-3).

Since this tumor carries a poor prognosis for many children, every consideration must be given the family in terms of coping with a life-threatening illness (see Chapter 23). Because of the high degree of metastasis at the time of diagnosis, many parents suffer much guilt for not having recognized signs earlier. Often the guilt is expressed as anger toward professionals for not diagnosing it sooner. Parents need much support in dealing with these feelings and expressing them to the appropriate people.

BONE TUMORS

Malignant bone tumors represent less than 5% of all malignant neoplasms but are more common in children than in adults. The peak ages during childhood are 15 to 19 years. The sexes are affected equally until puberty, at which time the ratio approaches 2:1 in favor of males. This propensity for males with a peak incidence during adolescence is thought to result from the accelerated growth rate of osseous tissue.

GENERAL CONSIDERATIONS

Neoplastic disease can arise from any tissues involved in bone growth, such as osteoid matrix, bone marrow elements, fat, blood and lymph vessels, nerve sheath, and cartilage. In children the two types that account for 85% of all primary malignant bone tumors are osteogenic sarcoma and Ewing sarcoma. They have several characteristics in common, which are discussed in the following sections. Specific information about each tumor is then presented.

Clinical Manifestations

Most malignant bone tumors produce localized pain in the affected site, which may be severe or dull and may be attributed to trauma or the vague complaint of "growing pains." The pain is often relieved by a flexed position, which relaxes the muscles overlying the stretched periosteum. Frequently it draws attention when the child limps, curtails physical activity, or is unable to hold heavy objects.

Diagnostic Evaluation

Diagnosis begins with a thorough history and physical examination. A primary objective is to rule out causes such as trauma or infection. Careful questioning regarding pain is essential in attempting to determine the duration and rate of tumor growth. Physical assessment focuses on functional status of the affected area, signs of inflammation, size of the mass, involvement of regional lymph nodes, and any systemic indication of generalized malignancy, such as anemia, weight loss, and frequent infection.

Definitive diagnosis is based on radiologic studies, particularly CT, to determine the extent of the lesion; radioisotope bone scans to evaluate metastasis; and either needle or surgical bone biopsy to determine the histologic pattern. Radiologic findings are characteristic for each type of tumor. In osteogenic sarcoma, needlelike new bone formation growing at right angles to the diaphysis (shaft) produces a "sunburst" appearance. In Ewing sarcoma the deposits of new bone in layers under the periosteum produce an "onionskin" appearance. In both types of bone tumors soft tissue infiltration may be apparent.

At present there is no reliable biochemical test for bone cancers. Elevated alkaline phosphatase levels may occur in osteoid tumors. Several tests may be done for differential diagnosis in terms of secondary bone metastasis from Wilms tumor, neuroblastoma, retinoblastoma, rhabdomyosarcoma, lymphoma, or leukemia. Lung tomography is usually a standard procedure, since pulmonary metastasis is the most common complication of primary bone tumors. Bone marrow aspiration is helpful in diagnosing Ewing sarcoma in the rare event that the child has bone marrow metastasis.

Prognosis

A better understanding of the biology of neoplastic growth has resulted in more aggressive treatment and an improved prognosis. The natural history of osteogenic sarcoma and Ewing sarcoma suggests that multiple submicroscopic foci of metastatic disease are present at the time of diagnosis despite clinical evidence of localized involvement. Before the use of aggressive multimodal therapy, pulmonary metastasis invariably appeared in 6 to 24 months in patients with osteogenic sarcoma who were treated with surgical excision of the tumor. Now, with surgery for osteosarcoma or intensive radiotherapy for Ewing sarcoma combined with chemotherapy, survival statistics are improving for both types of bone cancer. Survival rates differ according to the specific treatment protocols and are influenced by a number of factors, such as the site of the primary tumor, especially in Ewing sarcoma, and the presence or absence of metastatic disease at diagnosis. However, approximately 60% of children with either type of bone cancer can be long-term survivors, and various cancer centers are reporting higher figures (Jaffe, 1991b).

OSTEOGENIC SARCOMA

Osteogenic sarcoma (osteosarcoma) is the most common bone cancer in children. Its peak incidence is between 10 and 25 years of age. It presumably arises from bone-forming mesenchyme, which gives rise to malignant osteoid tissue. Most primary tumor sites are in the metaphysis (wider part of the shaft, adjacent to the epiphyseal growth plate) of long bones, especially in the lower extremities. More than half occur in the femur, particularly the distal portion, with the rest involving the humerus, tibia, pelvis, jaw, and phalanges.

Therapeutic Management

Optimum treatment of osteosarcoma is controversial. The traditional approach has consisted of radical surgical resection or amputation of the affected area followed by intensive chemotherapy. Depending on the tumor site, surgery includes amputation of the affected extremity at least 7.5 cm (3 inches) above the proximal tumor margin or above the joint proximal to the involved bone. With tumors of the distal femur, preservation of the hip joint may be possible. Other procedures include an above-the-knee amputation for tumors of the tibia or fibula, a hemipelvectomy for tumors of the innominate (hip) bone, and a forequarter amputation (removal of arm, scapula, and portion of the clavicle on the affected side) for tumors of the upper humerus. Another surgical approach for selected patients is the limb salvage procedure, which involves en bloc resection of the primary tumor with prosthetic replacement of the involved bone. For example, with osteosarcoma of the distal femur, a total femur and joint replacement is performed. Frequently children undergoing a limb salvage procedure will receive preoperative chemotherapy in an attempt to decrease the tumor size and make surgery more manageable (Hockenberry and Lane, 1988; Stine and others, 1989).

Chemotherapy now plays a vital role in treatment. Antineoplastic drugs, such as high-dose methotrexate with citrovorum factor rescue, adriamycin, bleomycin, actinomycin, cyclosphosphamide, ifosfamide, and cisplatin, may be administered singly or in combination and may be employed both before and after surgery. When pulmonary metastasis is found, thoracotomy and chemotherapy have resulted in prolonged survival and potential cure. These combined-modality approaches have significantly improved the prognosis in osteosarcoma.

Nursing Considerations

Nursing care depends on the type of surgical approach. Obviously, the family may have more difficulty adjusting to an amputation than a limb salvage procedure. In either instance, preparation of the child and family is critical. Straightforward honesty is essential in gaining the cooperation and trust of the child. The diagnosis of cancer should not be disguised with falsehoods such as "infection." To accept the need for radical surgery, the child must be aware of the lack of alternatives for treatment. While the responsibility of telling the child is generally left to the physician, the nurse should be present at the discussion or be aware of exactly what is said to the child. The child should be told a few days before surgery to allow time to think about the diagnosis and consequent treatment and to ask questions. (See Nursing Care Plan: The Child with a Bone Tumor.*)

Sometimes children have many questions about the prosthesis, limitations on physical ability, and prognosis in terms of cure. At other times they react with silence or with a calm manner that belies their concern and fear. Either response must be accepted, because it is part of the grieving process of a loss. For those who wish information, it may be helpful to introduce them to another amputee before surgery or to show them pictures of the prosthesis.* However, the nurse must be careful not to overwhelm children with information. A sound approach is to answer their questions without offering additional information. For those who do not pursue additional information, the nurse expresses a willingness to talk.

The child is also informed of the need for chemotherapy. Although it is best to introduce this subject before surgery, since treatment begins as soon as possible postoperatively, caution must be exercised in offering too much information at one time. It is wise to discuss hair loss with an emphasis on positive aspects, such as wearing a wig. Since bone tumors affect adolescents and young adults, it is not unusual for them to become angry over all the radical body alterations.

If an amputation is performed, the child is usually fitted with a temporary prosthesis immediately after surgery, which permits early functioning and fosters psychologic adjustment. If this is not done, the child requires stump care, which is the same as for any amputee. A permanent prosthesis is usually fitted within 6 to 8 weeks. During hospitalization the child begins physical therapy to become proficient in the use and care of the device.

Phantom limb pain may develop following amputation. This symptom is characterized by sensations such as tingling, itching, and, more frequently, pain felt in the amputated limb. Tricyclic antidepressants, such as amitriptyline (Elavil), have been used successfully in children to decrease the pain.

Discharge planning must begin early during the postoperative period. Once the child has begun physical therapy, the nurse should consult with the therapist and practitioner to evaluate the child's physical and emotional readiness to reenter school. It is an opportune time to involve a community nurse in the home care of the child. Every effort is made to promote normalcy and gradual resumption of realistic preamputation activities.† Role-playing in anticipation of such experiences is very beneficial in preparing the child for the inevitable confrontation by others. Environmental barriers, such as stairs, are assessed in terms of the accessibility of the school and/or home, especially since the child may need to use crutches or a wheelchair before complete healing and prosthetic competency are achieved.

The nurse encourages the child to select clothing that best camouflages the prosthesis, such as pants or long-sleeved shirts. Well fitted prostheses are so natural looking that girls can usually wear sheer stockings without revealing the device. Emphasizing feminine or masculine apparel

---

*In *Wong and Whaley's Clinical Manual of Pediatric Nursing* (Mosby).

*A source of information is the **National Amputation Foundation, Inc.,** 12-45 150th St., Whitestone, NY 11357; (718) 767-0596.

†Information about special programs for children with amputations is available from the **Candlelighters Childhood Cancer Foundation,** 1901 Pennsylvania Ave., N.W., Washington, DC 20006; (202) 659-5136.

helps the child regain a feeling of self-identity. Even during the postoperative period, encouraging the child to wear blue jeans and a shirt may distract attention from the deformity and focus it on familiar aspects of appearance.

The family and child need much support in adjusting not only to a life-threatening diagnosis but also to alteration in body form and function. Since loss of a limb constitutes a grieving process, those caring for the child need to recognize that the reactions of anger and depression are normal and necessary. Often parents view the anger as a direct affront to them for allowing the amputation to occur, or they see the depression as rejection. On the contrary, these are not interpersonal attacks but self-attempts to cope with a loss.

EWING SARCOMA

Ewing sarcoma arises in the marrow spaces of the bone rather than from osseous tissue. The tumor originates in the shaft of long and trunk bones, most often affecting the femur, tibia, fibula, humerus, ulna, vertebra, scapula, ribs, pelvic bones, and skull. Pathologists are now classifying Ewing sarcoma as a primitive neuroectodermal tumor. It occurs almost exclusively in individuals under age 30, with the majority between 4 and 25 years of age.

Therapeutic Management

Surgical amputation is not routinely recommended but may be considered when the results of radiotherapy render the extremity useless or deformed (e.g., from retarded growth in young children) or the tumor appears resectable. The treatment of choice is intensive irradiation of the involved bone combined with chemotherapy. A widely used drug regimen includes vincristine, actinomycin D, cyclophosphamide, or ifosfamide, VP-16, and adriamycin.

Nursing Considerations

The psychologic adjustment to Ewing sarcoma is typically less traumatic than it is to osteogenic sarcoma because of the preservation of the affected limb. Many families accept the diagnosis with a sense of relief in knowing that this type of bone cancer does not necessitate amputation, and initially they may not be aware of the damaging effects on the irradiated site. Consequently, they need preparation for the various diagnostic tests, including bone marrow aspiration and surgical biopsy, and adequate explanation of the treatment regimen. High-dose radiotherapy often causes a skin reaction of dry or moist desquamation followed by hyperpigmentation. The child should wear loose-fitting clothes over the irradiated area to minimize additional skin irritation. Because of increased sensitivity, the area is protected from sunlight and sudden changes in temperature, such as from heating pads or ice packs. The child is encouraged to use the extremity as tolerated. Occasionally an active exercise program may be planned by the physical therapist to preserve maximum function.

The child needs the same considerations for adjusting to the effects of chemotherapy as any other patient with cancer. The drug regimen usually results in hair loss, severe nausea and vomiting, peripheral neuropathy, and possibly cardiotoxicity. Every effort should be made to outline a treatment plan that allows the child maximum resumption of a normal life-style and activities.

OTHER SOLID TUMORS

In addition to the cancers already discussed, several other types of solid tumors may occur in children. Wilms tumor, rhabdomyosarcoma, and retinoblastoma are unique in that they tend to be diagnosed early, typically before 5 years of age. Wilms tumor and retinoblastoma are also unusual in that they are among the few types of cancer that may occur in both hereditary and nonhereditary forms.

WILMS TUMOR

Wilms tumor, or nephroblastoma, is the most frequent intraabdominal tumor of childhood and the most common type of renal cancer. Its frequency is estimated to be 1 per 200,000 to 250,000 children. The peak incidence is at 3 years of age. Wilms tumor is one of the childhood cancers that show an increased incidence among siblings and identical twins, reflecting evidence of genetic inheritance. The mode of inheritance in familial cases, which accounts for less than 2% of all Wilms tumors, is autosomal dominant with variable penetrance (estimated at 63%) and expressivity. Thus gene carriers may develop no tumors (37%), unilateral tumors (48%), or bilateral tumors (15%). Wilms tumor is heritable in about 15% to 20% of all cases, including some unilateral sporadic cases (Fernbach, Hawkins, and Pokorny, 1991). Unfortunately, there is no method of identification of gene carriers.

Wilms tumor is also associated with several congenital anomalies; the most common are aniridia, hemihypertrophy, and genitourinary anomalies, such as hypospadias, cryptorchidism, and ambiguous genitalia (Fernbach, Hawkins, and Pokorny, 1991). Other less common anomalies are microcephaly, pigmented and vascular nevi, pinna deformities, and mental and growth retardation.

Clinical Manifestations

The most common presenting sign is a swelling or mass within the abdomen. The mass is characteristically firm, nontender, confined to one side, and deep within the flank. If it is on the right side, it may be difficult to distinguish from the liver, although, unlike that organ, it does not move with respiration. Parents usually discover the mass during routine bathing or dressing of the child.

Other clinical manifestations are the result of compression from the tumor mass, metabolic alterations secondary to the tumor, or metastasis. Hematuria occurs in less than one fourth of children with Wilms tumor. Anemia, usually secondary to hemorrhage within the tumor, results in pallor, anorexia, and lethargy. Hypertension, probably caused by secretion of excess amounts of renin by the tumor, occurs occasionally. Other effects of malignancy include weight loss and fever. If metastasis has occurred, symptoms of lung involvement, such as dyspnea, cough, shortness of breath, and pain in the chest, may be evident.

Diagnostic Evaluation

In a child suspected of having Wilms tumor, special emphasis is placed on the history and physical examination for the presence of congenital anomalies, a family history of cancer, and signs of malignancy, such as weight loss, size of liver and spleen, indications of anemia, and lymphadenopathy. Specific tests include radiographic studies, including abdominal ultrasound, CT, hematologic studies (polycythemia is sometimes present if the tumor secretes excess erythropoietin), biochemical studies, and urinalysis. Studies to demonstrate the relationship of the tumor to the ipsilateral kidney and the presence of a normal-functioning kidney on the contralateral side are essential. If a large tumor is present, an inferior venacavagram is necessary to demonstrate possible tumor involvement adjacent to the vena cava. A bone marrow aspiration is electively performed to rule out metastasis, which is rare in children with Wilms tumor.

Staging and Prognosis

Wilms tumor probably arises from a malignant, undifferentiated metanephrogenic blastoma (a cluster of primordial cells capable of initiating the regeneration of an abnormal structure). Its occurrence slightly favors the left kidney, which is advantageous because surgically this kidney is easier to manipulate and remove. Although the tumor may become quite large, it remains encapsulated for an extended period. During surgery the tumor is staged to maximize the effectiveness of treatment protocols (see box below).

The histology of the tumor cells is also identified and classified according to two groups: favorable histology (FH) and unfavorable histology (UH). Only about 12% of Wilms tumors demonstrate UH, which is associated with a poorer prognosis and demands a more aggressive treatment protocol, regardless of the clinical stage.

Survival rates for Wilms tumor are the highest among all childhood cancers. Children with localized tumor (stages I and II) have a 90% chance of cure with multimodal therapy. FH of the tumor, first complete remission of more than 12 months' duration before relapse, and nonabdominal relapse sites are each associated with a significantly better survival expectancy (Grundy and others, 1989).

STAGING OF WILMS TUMOR

Stage I: Tumor is limited to kidney and completely resected.
Stage II: Tumor extends beyond kidney but is completely resected.
Stage III: Residual nonhematogenous tumor is confined to abdomen.
Stage IV: Hematogenous metastases; deposits are beyond stage III, namely, to lung, liver, bone, and brain.
Stage V: Bilateral renal involvement is present at diagnosis.

Therapeutic Management

Combined treatment of surgery and chemotherapy with or without radiation is based on the clinical stage and histologic pattern. In unilateral disease a large transabdominal incision is performed for optimum visualization of the abdominal cavity; the tumor, affected kidney, and adjacent adrenal gland are removed. Great care is taken to keep the encapsulated tumor intact, since rupture can seed cancer cells throughout the abdomen, lymph channel, and bloodstream. The contralateral kidney is carefully inspected for evidence of disease or dysfunction. Regional lymph nodes are inspected and a biopsy is performed when indicated. Any involved structures, such as part of the colon, diaphragm, or vena cava, are removed. Metal clips are placed around the tumor site for exact marking during radiotherapy.

If both kidneys are involved, the child may be treated with radiotherapy and/or chemotherapy preoperatively to shrink the tumor, allowing more conservative therapy. In some cases a partial nephrectomy is performed on the less affected kidney, with a total nephrectomy on the opposite side. When a transplant is feasible, such as from a twin, sibling, or parent, bilateral nephrectomy is considered as a last resort.

Postoperative radiotherapy is indicated for children with large tumors, metastasis, residual disease at the primary tumor site, unfavorable histology, or recurrence. Chemotherapy is indicated for all stages. The most effective agents for treating Wilms tumor are actinomycin D and vincristine, sometimes combined with adriamycin, cytoxan, cisplatin, VP-16, or ifosfamide. Duration of therapy varies, ranging from 6 to 15 months.

Nursing Considerations

The nursing care of the child with Wilms tumor is similar to that of other cancers treated with surgery, irradiation, and chemotherapy. However, some significant differences are discussed for each phase of nursing intervention.

Preoperative Care. As with many of the other cancers, the diagnosis of Wilms tumor is a shock. Frequently the child has no physical indication of the seriousness of the disorder other than a palpable abdominal mass. Since it is the parents who usually discover the mass, the nurse needs to take into account their feelings regarding the diagnosis. Whereas some parents are grateful for their detection of the tumor, others feel guilty for not finding it sooner or anger toward the practitioner for missing it on earlier examinations.

The preoperative period is one of swift diagnosis. Typically surgery is scheduled within 24 to 48 hours of admission. The nurse is faced with the challenge of preparing the child and parents for all laboratory and operative procedures. Because of the little time available, explanations should be kept simple and repeated often with attention to what the child will experience. Besides usual preoperative observations, blood pressure is monitored, since hypertension from excess renin production is a possibility.

There are several special preoperative concerns, the most important of which is that the tumor is not palpated unless absolutely necessary, since manipulation of the mass may cause dissemination of cancer cells to adjacent and distant sites.

NURSING ALERT To reinforce the need for caution, it may be necessary to post a sign on the bed that reads "DO NOT PALPATE ABDOMEN." Careful bathing and handling are also important in preventing trauma to the tumor site.

Since radiotherapy and chemotherapy are usually begun immediately after surgery, parents need an explanation of what to expect, such as major benefits and side effects, although the timing of the information should be considered to avoid overwhelming the family. Ideally the nurse should be present during physician-parent conferences to answer questions as they arise. It is usually better to reserve telling the child about these side effects until after surgery. Alopecia, usually of most concern to older children, does not occur until 2 weeks after the initial treatment regimen. Therefore the child can be prepared for the hair loss postoperatively.

Postoperative Care. Despite the extensive surgical intervention necessary in many children with Wilms tumor, the recovery period is usually rapid. The major nursing responsibilities are those following any abdominal surgery (see Nursing Care Plan: The Child Undergoing Surgery, Chapter 27). Since these children are at risk for intestinal obstruction from vincristine-induced adynamic ileus, radiation-induced edema, and postsurgical adhesion formation, gastrointestinal activity, such as bowel movements, bowel sounds, distention, and vomiting, is monitored. Other considerations are frequent evaluation of blood pressure and observation for signs of infection, especially during chemotherapy. Because of the myelosuppression from the drugs, pulmonary hygiene measures are instituted in the immediate postoperative period to prevent complications.

Family Support. The postoperative period is frequently difficult for parents. The shock of seeing their child immediately after surgery may be the first realization of the seriousness of the diagnosis. It also marks the confirmation of the stage of the tumor. During this period the nurse should again be with parents to assure them of the child's recovery after surgery and to assess their understanding of the pathology report.

Older children need an opportunity to deal with their feelings concerning the many procedures to which they have been subjected in rapid succession. Play therapy with dolls, puppets, or drawing can be extremely beneficial in helping them adjust to the surgery and hair loss. It is not unusual for children to feel betrayed because they were not adequately prepared for the extent of surgery, the need for additional therapy, or the seriousness of the disorder.

Because the child is left with only one kidney, certain precautions, such as avoiding contact sports or any other activity that has a high risk potential, are recommended to prevent injury to the organ. Urinary tract infections should be prevented with good hygiene, especially in girls. Prompt detection and treatment of any genitourinary signs or symptoms is mandatory.

RHABDOMYOSARCOMA

Soft tissue sarcomas are the fourth most common type of solid tumors in children. These malignant neoplasms originate from undifferentiated mesenchymal cells in muscles, tendons, bursae, and fascia, or in fibrous, connective, lymphatic, or vascular tissue. They derive their name from the specific tissue(s) of origin, such as myosarcoma (*myo*—muscle). Rhabdomyosarcoma (*rhabdo*—striated) is the most common soft tissue sarcoma in children. Because striated (skeletal) muscle is found almost anywhere in the body, these tumors occur in many sites, the most common of which are the head and neck, especially the orbit. The disease occurs in children in all age-groups but most commonly in children younger than 5 years of age. Its incidence is approximately 4.4 per million for white children under age 15, but only 3.3 per million for black children in this age-group.

Rhabdomyosarcoma arises from embryonic mesenchyme. Four subtypes are recognized and described in the box below.

Clinical Manifestations

The initial signs and symptoms are related to the site of the tumor and compression of adjacent organs (Table 36-7). Some tumor locations, particularly the orbit, produce symptoms early in the course of the illness and contribute to rapid diagnosis and improved prognosis. Other tumors, such as those of the retroperitoneal area, produce no symptoms until they are large, invasive, and widely metastasized. In some instances a primary tumor site is never identified.

Diagnostic Evaluation

Unfortunately, many of the signs and symptoms attributable to rhabdomyosarcoma are vague and frequently suggest a common childhood illness, such as "earache" or "runny nose." However, diagnosis begins with a careful examination of the head and neck area, particularly palpation of a nontender, firm, hard mass. The nasopharynx and oropharynx are inspected for any evidence of a visible mass.

Radiographic studies to isolate a tumor site are performed, accompanied by chest x-ray examinations, chest CT, bone surveys, and bone marrow aspiration to rule out

SUBTYPES OF RHABDOMYOSARCOMA

Embryonal—Most common type; most frequently found in the head, neck, abdomen, and genitourinary tract
Alveolar—Second most common type; most often seen in deep tissues of the extremities and trunk
Botryoid—Appears as multiple grapelike clusters or polyps; usually found in cavities such as the vagina, urinary bladder, ear, and nasopharynx
Pleomorphic—Rare in children (adult form); most often occurs in soft parts of extremities and trunk

TABLE 36-7 Clinical Manifestations of Rhabdomyosarcoma According to Tumor Site

LOCATION	SIGNS AND SYMPTOMS
Orbit	Rapidly developing unilateral proptosis Ecchymosis of conjunctiva Loss of extraocular movements (strabismus)
Nasopharynx	Stuffy nose (earliest sign) Nasal obstruction—dysphagia, nasal voice (obstruction of posterior nasal conchae), serous otitis media (obstruction of eustachian tube) Pain (sore throat and ear) Epistaxis Palpable neck nodes Visible mass in oropharynx (late sign)
Paranasal sinuses	Nasal obstruction Local pain Discharge Sinusitis Swelling
Middle ear	Signs of chronic serous otitis media Pain Sanguinopurulent drainage Facial nerve palsy
Retroperitoneal area (usually a "silent" tumor)	Abdominal mass Pain Signs of intestinal or genitourinary obstruction
Perineum	Visible superficial mass Bowel or bladder dysfunction (from tumor compression)

metastasis. A lumbar puncture is indicated for head and neck tumors to examine the cerebrospinal fluid for malignant cells. An excisional biopsy is done to confirm the histologic type.

Staging and Prognosis

Careful staging is extremely important for planning treatment and determining the prognosis. The Intergroup Rhabdomyosarcoma Study has established clinical staging (Maurer and Ragab, 1991) (see box above, right).

With the change in treatment from radical surgery or radiotherapy to a multimodal approach, survival rates for all stages have increased considerably. Two-year survival rates vary for each clinical group: 92% to 100% of group I, 79% to 94% for group II, 71% to 79% for group III, and 37% to 40% for group IV (Raney and others, 1993). Data suggest that children who remain disease-free for 2 years are probably cured; however, if relapse occurs, the prognosis for long-term survival is extremely poor (Raney and others, 1993).

STAGING OF RHABDOMYOSARCOMA

Group I: Localized disease; tumor completely resected and regional nodes not involved
Group II: Localized disease with microscopic residual, or regional disease with no residual or with microscopic residual
Group III: Incomplete resection or biopsy with gross residual disease
Group IV: Metastatic disease present at diagnosis

Therapeutic Management

Since this tumor is highly malignant, with metastasis frequently occurring at the time of diagnosis, aggressive multimodal therapy is recommended. In the past, radical surgical removal of the tumor was the treatment of choice, but with improved survival from combined chemotherapy and radiation, surgery plays a lesser role. Complete removal of the primary tumor is advocated whenever possible. However, biopsy only is required in certain tumor locations, such as those of the orbit when followed by radiation and chemotherapy. This is a fortunate change, because it avoids the devastating effects of enucleation, amputation, or pelvic exenteration.

High-dose irradiation to the primary tumor is recommended, except in group I tumors. Chemotherapy plays a major role in treatment of all groups. Drugs that are cytotoxic for rhabdomyosarcoma are vincristine, actinomycin D, ifosfamide, cisplatin, VP-16, carboplatin, and cyclophosphamide, with or without adriamycin, for 1 to 2 years depending on the stage of the disease (Maurer & Ragab, 1991).

Nursing Considerations

The nursing responsibilities are similar to those for other types of cancer, especially the solid tumors when surgery is employed. Specific objectives include (1) careful assessment for signs of the tumor, especially during well-child examinations; (2) preparation of the child and family for the multiple diagnostic tests (see p. 1627); and (3) supportive care during each stage of multimodal therapy. The reader is urged to review the Nursing Considerations section for cancer and Chapter 23 for emotional support of the family in the event of a poor prognosis.

RETINOBLASTOMA

Retinoblastoma is a congenital malignant tumor arising from the retina. It is a relatively rare tumor, with an incidence of 3.4 per million in children under 15 years of age. As with Wilms tumor, it can be inherited, and it may be present at birth or may arise in the retina during the first 2 years of life. The average age of the child at the time of diagnosis is 17 months; it is usually diagnosed earlier in hereditary cases and later in nonhereditary types.

Retinoblastoma may be caused by (1) a somatic mutation, (2) a germinal mutation, or (3) a chromosomal aberration. ***Somatic mutations*** (those occurring in the general body cells, as opposed to the germ cells or gametes) are a sporadic, nonhereditary event. They result in unilateral tumors. ***Germinal mutations*** are passed to future generations. All bilateral retinoblastomas are considered hereditary, and 10% to 15% of individuals with unilateral disease have the hereditary form (Donaldson and Smith, 1989). Hereditary retinoblastomas are transmitted as an autosomal dominant trait, with an 80% penetrance. Consequently, 20% of gene carriers remain unaffected.

Retinoblastoma has also been associated with partial deletion of the long arm of a group D chromosome (number 13) and chromosomal polyploidy (excessive numbers of chromosomes), such as trisomy 21. In children who have chromosomal aberrations and retinoblastoma, there is often an increased incidence of mental retardation and congenital malformations, although the vast majority of children with retinoblastomas apparently have normal chromosomes and intelligence.

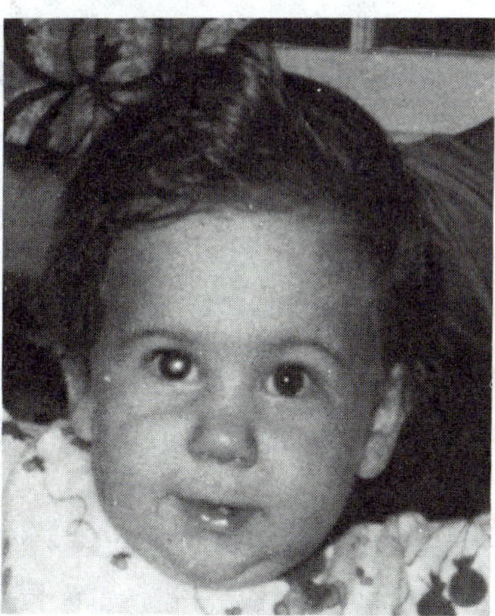

FIG. 36-4 Cat's eye reflex. Whitish appearance of lens is produced as light falls on tumor mass in right eye.

Clinical Manifestations

Retinoblastoma has few grossly obvious signs. Typically it is the parent who first observes a whitish "glow" in the pupil, known as the ***cat's eye reflex*** or ***leukokoria.*** The reflex represents visualization of the tumor as the light momentarily falls on the mass (Fig. 36-4). When a tumor arises in the macular region (area directly at the back of the retina when the eye is focused straight ahead), a white reflex may be seen when the tumor is quite small. It is best observed when a bright light is shining toward the child as the child looks forward. It is sometimes accidentally discovered by parents when taking a photograph of their child using a flash attachment.

When the tumor arises in the periphery of the retina, it must grow to a considerably large size before light can strike it sufficiently to produce the cat's eye reflex. In this situation it is seen only when the child looks in certain directions (sideways) or if the observer stands at an oblique angle to the child's face as the child looks straight ahead. The fleeting nature of the reflex often results in a delayed diagnosis, because health professionals fail to appreciate the ominous significance of the parents' findings.

The next most common sign is strabismus resulting from poor fixation of the visually impaired eye, particularly if the tumor develops in the macula, the area of sharpest visual acuity. Blindness is usually a late sign, but it frequently is not obvious unless the parent consciously observes for behaviors indicating loss of sight, such as bumping into objects, slowed motor development, or turning of the head to see objects lateral to the affected eye.

Another common presenting sign is a red, painful eye, often accompanied by glaucoma. Other common clinical manifestations include orbital cellulitis, unilateral mydriasis, a change in the color of the iris, hyphema, white spots on the iris, nystagmus, and complaints indicating systemic metastasis, such as weight loss, poor appetite, or fatigue.

Diagnostic Evaluation

The first step in diagnosis is carefully listening to and recognizing the significance of reports from family members regarding suspected abnormalities within the eye. *Parental remarks that in any way suggest the presence of such findings must be taken seriously and investigated further.* For example, if the parent indicates that the child has a strange expression or an unusual glow in the eye, every attempt is made to duplicate the circumstances necessary to observe these changes. Children suspected of having this disorder are referred to an ophthalmologist. Definitive diagnosis is usually based on indirect ophthalmoscopy employing scleral indentation, which is done with the patient under general anesthesia and with maximum dilation of the pupils.

A potentially useful test is catecholamine excretion by measuring vanillylmandelic or homovanillic acid in the urine. These substances are excreted by some retinoblastomas, as well as by neuroblastomas. If distant metastasis is suspected, a bone marrow aspiration, bone survey, and lumbar puncture may be performed.

Staging and Prognosis

Staging of retinoblastomas is done under indirect ophthalmoscopy before surgery to determine accurately tumor size (measured in disc diameters—DD) and location (according to an imaginary line called the equator drawn on the midplane of the eye) (Grabowski, and Abramson, 1991). The classification by Reese-Ellsworth is commonly used (see box on p. 1662).

The classification system has been used to define cure in terms of numbers of years free of disease and in terms of preservation of useful vision in the affected eye (favorable, doubtful, or unfavorable). Cure rates for survival are much better than for retention of useful vision. The overall 5-year survival rate is 85% to 90% for unilateral and bilateral tumors; most of the deaths occur in children with group V disease (Donaldson and Smith, 1989). Retinoblastoma is one of the tumors that may spontaneously regress.

Of major concern in long-term survivors is the development of secondary tumors, especially osteogenic sarcoma. Children with bilateral disease (hereditary form) are more

STAGING OF RETINOBLASTOMA

Group I: Very favorable
- Solitary tumor, less than 4 DD, at or behind the equator
- Multiple tumors, none greater than 4 DD, all at or behind the equator

Group II: Favorable
- Solitary tumors, 4 to 10 DD, at or behind the equator
- Multiple tumors, 4 to 10 DD, behind the equator

Group III: Doubtful
- Any lesion anterior to the equator
- Solitary tumors larger than 10 DD behind the equator

Group IV: Unfavorable
- Multiple tumors, some larger than 10 DD
- Any lesion extending anteriorly to the ora serrata

Group V: Very unfavorable
- Massive tumors involving more than half the retina
- Vitreous seeding

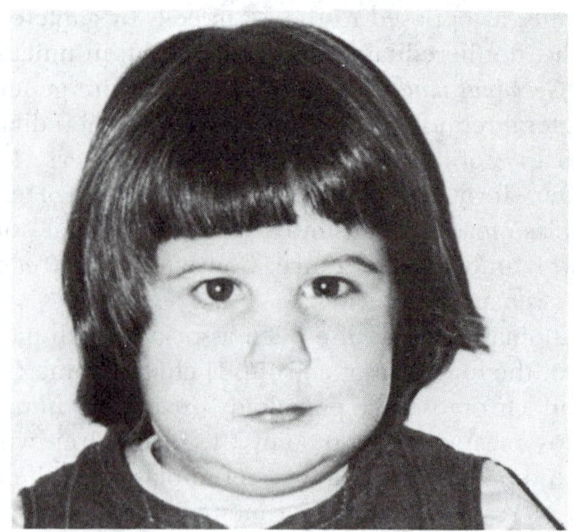

FIG. 36-5 Preschooler with right prosthetic eye.

likely to develop secondary cancers than are children with unilateral disease. It is thought that these individuals are predisposed to developing cancer, and radiation increases their risk.

Therapeutic Management

Treatment of retinoblastoma depends chiefly on the stage of the tumor at diagnosis. In general, unilateral retinoblastomas in stages I, II, and III are treated with irradiation. The aim of radiotherapy is to preserve useful vision in the affected eye and eradicate the tumor.

Other approaches toward treating small, localized tumors involve (1) ***cobalt plaque applicators*** (surgical implantation of a cobalt 60 applicator on the sclera until the maximum radiation dose has been delivered to the tumor), (2) ***light coagulation*** (use of a laser beam to destroy retinal blood vessels that supply nutrition to the tumor), and (3) ***cryotherapy*** (freezing of the tumor, which destroys the microcirculation to the tumor and the cells themselves through microcrystal formation). One of the reasons for investigating treatments other than radiotherapy is to minimize the risk of radiation-induced malignancies later in life.

With advanced tumor growth, especially optic nerve involvement, enucleation of the affected eye is the treatment of choice. The use of chemotherapy in advanced disease, even in group V, is controversial and has not shown improved survival. Drugs that may be used in the treatment of metastatic disease include vincristine, cyclophosphamide, and adriamycin. In the case of central nervous system disease, intrathecal chemotherapy may be administered (Donaldson and Egbert, 1993).

With bilateral disease, every attempt is made to preserve useful vision in the less affected eye with enucleation of the severely diseased eye. When bilateral tumors are found very early, enucleation may be prevented with only the use of radiotherapy to both eyes.

Nursing Considerations

Prepare Family for Diagnostic/Therapeutic Procedures and Home Care. Since the tumor is usually diagnosed in infants or very young children, most of the preparation for diagnostic tests and treatment involves parents. After indirect ophthalmoscopy the child may not see very clearly, or the eyes may be sensitive to light because of pupillary dilation. Parents are made aware of these normal reactions before the procedure.

Once the disease is staged, the physician confers with the parents regarding treatment. Unless the diagnosis is made very early, an enucleation is performed. Parents are told about the procedure, as well as about the benefits of a prosthesis. Parents often believe the procedure is bloody and mutilating, envisioning that the eye is "ripped out of its socket." Actually, the surgery is very similar to scooping a nut out of its shell. All the adnexal structures of the eye, such as the lids, lashes, and tear glands, are left undisturbed.

Showing parents pictures of another child with an artificial eye may be very helpful in their adjustment to the thought of disfigurement (Fig. 36-5). Although the idea of loss of vision is a very distressing one, most parents seem to realize that there is no alternative. The facts that the unaffected eye retains normal vision and that the affected eye is probably already blind are particularly helpful in promoting acceptance of the imposed impairment and should be emphasized.

After surgery, the parents need to be prepared for the child's facial appearance. An eye patch is in place, and the child's face may be edematous or ecchymotic. Parents often fear seeing the surgical site because they imagine a cavity in the skull. On the contrary, the lids are usually closed, and the area does not appear sunken because a surgically implanted sphere maintains the shape of the eyeball. The implant is covered with conjunctiva, and when the lids are open, the exposed area resembles the mucosal lining of the mouth. Once the child is fitted for a prosthesis, usually within 3 weeks, the facial appearance returns to normal.

After an uneventful recovery from enucleation, plans can be made for discharge from the hospital, usually within 3 to 4 days postoperatively. Parents need instruction regarding care of the surgical site and preparation for any additional therapy. They should be given the opportunity to see the socket as soon after surgery as possible. A good time to do this without unduly pressuring them is during dressing changes. They should then be encouraged to participate in the dressing changes.

Care of the socket is minimal and easily accomplished. The wound itself is clean and has little or no drainage. If an antibiotic ointment is prescribed, it is applied in a thin line on the surface of the tissues of the socket. To cleanse the site, an irrigating solution may be ordered and is instilled daily or more frequently if necessary, *before* application of the antibiotic ointment. The dressing consists of an eye pad changed daily. Self-adhesive eye pads can also be used as dressings. Once the socket has healed completely, a dressing is no longer necessary, although there are several reasons for having the child continue to wear the eye patch. Infants and toddlers explore their environment with their hands, and the socket is available to exploring fingers without an eye patch in place. Although there is little danger of the child injuring the socket, parents may feel more secure with the socket covered. This also helps prevent infection.

Initial instructions for care of the prosthesis are given by the ocularist, who fits and manufactures the device. Once in place, the prosthesis need not be removed unless cleaning is necessary, in which case it is taken out by gently pulling down on the lower lid, which frees the lower edge of the prosthesis, and applying pressure to the upper lid. If the child resists by forcing the lids shut, a small rubber instrument resembling a plunger can be used to facilitate removal and reinsertion. The end of the plunger is moistened and placed on top of the prosthetic iris. The lower eyelid is retracted, and the prosthesis is pulled out with a downward motion.

The prosthesis is cleaned by placing it in hot water and soaking it for several minutes. Reinsertion is easier if the prosthesis remains wet. To reinsert the prosthesis, the lids are separated, and with the prosthesis held in the correct position (it should be marked to indicate the nasal side), it is pushed up under the upper lid, allowing the lower lid to cover its lower edge.

Because the prosthesis is easily removed, the child may accidentally cause it to dislodge. Reactions of children vary from fear that they have "lost" their eye to matter-of-fact acceptance. The first time can be disturbing to both parents and child, but it is just one part of the child's adjusted lifestyle. If children are old enough to understand, parents can explain that they have a "special" eye that can accidentally fall out but that can also be quickly put back in place.

Safety is a major concern to prevent damage to the unaffected eye. Safety measures should be practiced at all times, and rough contact sports should be avoided or protective eye wear worn during such activity.

Support Family. The diagnosis of retinoblastoma presents some special concerns in addition to those created by any type of cancer. Families with a history of the disorder may feel great guilt for transmitting the defect to their offspring, especially if they knowingly "played the odds" and parented an affected child. Conversely, when parents are aware of the probability and have an affected child, early treatment results in such favorable outcomes that parental adjustment may be rapid. In families with no history of retinoblastoma, the discovery of the diagnosis is a shock, frequently complicated by guilt for not having discovered it sooner. Since parents frequently are the first to observe the cat's eye reflex, they may feel angry at themselves or others, especially professionals, for delaying a more thorough examination. Each of these variables needs to be considered in offering supportive care to the family.

TABLE 36-8 Recurrence Risks of Retinoblastoma in Families with an Affected Child

TYPE OF TUMOR	RISK TO SUBSEQUENT SIBLINGS (%)	RISK TO AFFECTED CHILD'S OFFSPRING (%)
Unilateral*	1	5-6
Bilateral†	6	50

Data from Donaldson SS, Egbert PR: Retinoblastoma. In Pizzo PA, Poplack DG: *Principles and practice of pediatric oncology,* ed 2, Philadelphia, 1993, JB Lippincott.
*Refers only to families with negative family history.
†Regardless of family history.

Other concerns are also related to the hereditary aspects of the disease. Of great importance to parents is the recurrence risk of retinoblastoma in their subsequent offspring and in the offspring of the surviving affected child (Table 36-8). With improving prognoses for these children, the necessity of genetic counseling to prevent transmission of the disease is assuming greater importance. (See Chapter 5 for a discussion of the nurse's role in genetic counseling.) Determining the risk of transmission is possible through DNA/RNA studies of the tumor cells. If a germinal mutation is found, blood samples from family members can be analyzed to see if they carry the mutation (Dryja, 1989).

These families are also encouraged to seek regular follow-up care for the affected child to detect secondary tumors, and all subsequent offspring of unaffected parents and survivors should undergo regular indirect ophthalmoscopy under anesthesia to detect retinoblastoma at its earliest stage.

TESTICULAR TUMORS

Tumors of the testes are not a common condition, but when manifested in adolescence they are generally malignant. Testicular cancer is the most common form of cancer in males ages 15 to 34 years, with an incidence of 1 in 10,000 (Goldenring, 1992). The usual presenting symptom is a heavy, hard, painless mass, palpable on the anterior or lateral aspect of a testis (Richie, 1993). The tumor may be smooth or nodular and does not transilluminate unless accompanied by a hydrocele. The involved testicle hangs lower and is therefore more susceptible to trauma. Although not all scrotal masses are malignant, any firm swelling of the testis demands immediate evaluation. If a firm swelling is noted, the youth should be subjected to a minimum of preoperative palpation and referred immediately for surgical exploration. There is seldom delay in seeking medical advice if the mass is painful, but in the absence of pain the condition may go unattended for some time.

Treatment for testicular cancer consists of surgical removal of the affected testicle (orchiectomy) and the adjacent lymph nodes, if affected. If metastases are evident in more distant nodes or organs, chemotherapy and radiation therapy are implemented.

Nursing Considerations

To supplement routine health assessment, every adolescent male should be taught to perform frequent testicular self-examination (TSE) to familiarize himself with his own anatomy and to ensure early detection of any abnormality. Ideally, self-examination should be performed once a month beginning when physical development reaches Tanner stage 3 (see Fig. 19-6), usually about age 13 or 14 years. Each testicle is examined individually, preferably after a warm bath or shower (when scrotal skin is more relaxed), using the thumbs and fingers of both hands and applying a small amount of firm, gentle pressure. The normal testicle is a firm organ with a smooth egg-shaped contour. The epididymis can be palpated as a raised swelling on the superior aspect of the testicle and should not be confused with an abnormality. The efficacy of teaching TSE to adolescent males has been tested and found to be successful (Klein, Berry, and Felice, 1990).

KEY POINTS

- Criteria used to determine cure of cancer include cessation of therapy, continuous freedom from clinical and laboratory evidence of cancer, and minimum or no risk or relapse, as determined by previous experience with the disease.
- Although the cure rate for most types of childhood cancer has improved, the late effects of treatment are of increasing concern.
- Determination of malignancy and metastasis is made by history and physical examination, laboratory tests, imaging techniques, and biopsy.
- The major modes of cancer therapy are surgery, chemotherapy, radiotherapy, immunotherapy, and bone marrow transplantation.
- Chemotherapeutic agents are classified according to their cytotoxic action: alkylating agents, antimetabolites, plant alkaloids, antitumor antibiotics, and hormones.
- Types of bone marrow transplants are allogeneic, autologous, and syngeneic.
- Nursing goals in the care of the child with cancer are to prepare the family for diagnostic and therapeutic procedures, prevent complications of myelosuppression (infection, hemorrhage, anemia), manage problems of irradiation and drug toxicity (nausea and vomiting, anorexia, mucosal ulceration, neuropathy, hemorrhagic cystitis, alopecia, moon face, mood changes), and provide continued emotional support.
- Leukemia is the most common form of childhood cancer. Current 5-year survival rates exceed 70% in major research centers, and the majority of these children will be cured.
- The lymphomas include Hodgkin disease and non-Hodgkin lymphoma; Hodgkin disease affects primarily adolescents.
- Nursing care of the child with a brain tumor includes observing for signs and symptoms related to the tumor, preparing the child and family for diagnostic tests and operative procedures, preventing postoperative complications, planning for discharge, and promoting a return to optimum health.
- The treatment of osteosarcoma is limb salvage or amputation followed by chemotherapy.
- Wilms tumor shows an increased incidence among siblings and identical twins, demonstrating a hereditary predisposition.
- Rhabdomyosarcoma may occur almost anywhere in the body, but the most common sites are the head and neck.
- Common presenting signs in retinoblastoma are cat's eye reflex, strabismus, and red, painful eye.
- Male adolescents should be taught to perform monthly testicular self-examination to detect testicular tumors.

REFERENCES

Allen JC: What we learn from infants with brain tumors, *N Engl J Med* 328(24):1780-1781, 1993.

American Brain Tumor Association: Clinical trials, *Am Brain Tumor Assoc,* Fall 1992.

Bernstein ML and others: A population-based study of neuroblastoma in North America, *J Clin Oncol* 10:323-329, 1992.

Blatt J, Lee PA: Neuroblastoma associated with adrenocortical defects, *Pediatrics* 82(5):790-792, 1988.

Blecke C: Home chemotherapy safety procedures, *Oncol Nurs Forum* 16(5):719-721, 1989.

Broberg DJ, Bernstein BD: Candy as a scapegoat in the prevention of food aversions in children receiving chemotherapy, *Cancer* 60(9):2344-2347, 1987.

Bucholtz J: Issues concerning the sedation of children for radiation therapy, *Oncol Nurs Forum* 19(4):649-655, 1992.

Bunin GB and others: Relation between maternal diet and subsequent primitive neuroectodermal brain tumors in young children, *N Engl J Med* 329:536-541, 1993.

Cameron J: Ifosfamide neurotoxicity: a challenge for nurses, a potential nightmare for patients, *Cancer Nurs* 16(1):40-46, 1993.

Cancer facts and figures, 1993, Atlanta, 1993, American Cancer Society.

Carde P: Hodgkin's disease. I. Identification and classification, *Br Med J* 305(6845):99-102, 1992.

Carroll WL, Schwartz AL: Molecular oncology. In Fernbach DJ, Vietti TJ, editors: *Clinical pediatric oncology,* ed 4, St Louis, 1991, Mosby.

Coppes MJ and others: Bilateral Wilms' tumor: long-term survival and some epidemiological features, *J Clin Oncol* 7(3):310-315, 1989.

Crist WM, Pullen DJ, Rivera GK: Acute lymphoid leukemia. In Fernbach DJ, Vietti TJ, editors: *Clinical pediatric oncology,* ed 4, St Louis, 1991, Mosby.

Cubeddu LX and others: Efficacy of ondansetron (GR38032F) and the role of serotonin in cisplatin-induced nausea and vomiting, *N Engl J Med* 322:810-816, 1990.

Darbyshire PJ: Bacterial infections. In Oakhill A: *The supportive care of the child with cancer,* Boston, 1988, Butterworth.

DeVitta V: *Cancer: principles of oncology,* Philadelphia, 1989, JB Lippincott.

Dolgin MJ and others: Behavioral distress in pediatric patients with cancer receiving chemotherapy, *Pediatrics* 84(1):103-110, 1989.

Donaldson SS, Egbert PR: Retinoblastoma. In Pizzo PA, Poplack DG: *Principles and practice of pediatric oncology,* ed 2, Philadelphia, 1993, JB Lippincott.

Donaldson SS, Smith LM: Retinoblastoma: biology, presentation, and current management, *Oncology* 3(4):45-51, 1989.

Drakeford JD: Nutrition. In Oakhill A: *The supportive care of the child with cancer,* Boston, 1988, Butterworth.

Dryja T: Genetics of retinoblastoma, *Curr Opin Pediatr* 1:413-420, 1989.

Duffner PK and others: Postoperative chemotherapy and delayed radiation in children less than three years of age with malignant brain tumors, *N Engl J Med* 328:1725-31, 1993.

Evans WE and others: Clinical pharmacology of cancer chemotherapy in children, *Pediatr Clin North Am* 36(5):1199, 1989.

Fernbach DJ, Hawkins EP, Pokorny WJ: Nephroblastoma and other renal tumors. In Fernbach DJ, Vietti TJ, editors: *Clinical pediatric oncology,* ed 4, St Louis, 1991, Mosby.

Fernbach DJ, Vietti TJ: General aspects of childhood cancer. In Fernbach DJ, Vietti TJ, editors: *Clinical pediatric oncology,* ed 4, St Louis, 1991, Mosby.

Few BJ: MCN pharmacopoeia: nabilone as an antiemetic for children undergoing chemotherapy, *MCN* 13:209, 1988.

Frankiewicz V, Farrington E: Ondansetron HCL (Zofran), *Pediatr Nurs* 18(4):385-386, 1992.

Frenck R, Kohl S, Pickering LK: Principles of total care: infections in children with cancer. In Fernbach DJ, Vietti TJ, editors: *Clinical pediatric oncology,* ed 4, St Louis, 1991, Mosby.

Galbraith L and others: Treatment for alteration in oral mucosa related to chemotherapy, *Pediatr Nurs* 17(3):233-236, 1991.

Gale RP: The management of acute leukemias, *Clin Adv Oncol Nurs* 1(3):1-9, 1989.

Gellis SS: Swedish studies link power line exposure to childhood leukemia, *Pediatr Notes* 16(49):193, 1992.

General recommendations on immunization: recommendations of the Advisory Committee on Immunization Practices (ACIP), *MMWR* 43(RR-1):22, 1994.

Goldenring JM: A lifesaving exam for young men, *Contemp Pediatr* 9(4):63-85, 1992.

Grabowski EF, Abramson DH: Retinoblastoma. In Fernbach DJ, Vietti TJ, editors: *Clinical pediatric oncology,* ed 4, St Louis, 1991, Mosby.

Greenbaum BF, Herman JH: Transfusion therapy in pediatric oncology, *Pediatr Ann* 17(11):687-693, 1988.

Grundy P and others: Prognostic factors for children with recurrent Wilms' tumor: results from the second and third national Wilms' tumor study, *J Clin Oncol* 7(5):638-647, 1989.

Hainsworth J and others: A single-blind comparison of intravenous ondansetron, a selective serotonin antagonist, with intravenous metoclopramide in the prevention of nausea and vomiting associated with high-dose cisplatin chemotherapy, *J Clin Oncol* 9:721-728, 1991.

Halperin DL and others: Topical skin anesthesia for venous, subcutaneous drug reservoir and lumbar punctures in children, *Pediatrics* 84(2):281-284, 1989.

Hammond E: Anaphylactic reactions to chemotherapeutic agents, *J Assoc Pediatr Oncol Nurs* 5(3):16-19, 1988.

Hayashi Y and others: Similar chromosomal patterns and lack of N-myc gene amplication in localized and IV-S stage neuroblastomas in infants, *Med Pediatr Oncol* 17:111-115, 1989.

Heideman RL and others: Tumors of the central nervous system. In Pizzo PA, Poplack DG: *Principles and practice of pediatric oncology,* ed 2, Philadelphia, 1993, JB Lippincott.

Hess G, Walson P: Seizures secondary to oral viscous lidocaine, *Ann Emerg Med* 17:725-727, 1988.

Ho PTC and others: Prenatal detection of neuroblastoma: a ten-year experience from the Dana-Farber Cancer Institute and Children's Hospital, *Pediatrics* 92:358-364, 1993.

Hockenberry MJ: Relaxation techniques in children with cancer: the nurse's role, *J Pediatr Oncol Nurs* 5(1/2):7-11, 1988.

Hockenberry MJ, Lane B: Limb salvage procedures in children with osteosarcoma, *Cancer Nurs* 11(1):2-8, 1988.

Huizdala EV: Nonlymphoblastic lymphoma in children, *J Clin Oncol* 9:1189-1195, 1991.

Jaffe N: Late sequelae of cancer and cancer therapy. In Fernbach DJ, Vietti TJ, editors: *Clinical pediatric oncology,* ed 4, St Louis, 1991a, Mosby.

Jaffe N: Osteosarcoma, *Pediatr Rev* 12(11):333-343, 1991b.

Johnson FL: Bone marrow transplantation. In Fernbach DJ, Vietti TJ, editors: *Clinical pediatric oncology,* ed 4, St Louis, 1991, Mosby.

Kapelushnik J and others: Evaluating the efficacy of EMLA in alleviating pain associated with lumbar puncture: comparison of open and double-blinded protocols in children, *Pain* 41:31-34, 1990.

Kennedy BJ: Hodgkin's disease, *CA Cancer J Clin* 43(6):325-326, 1993.

Kirsch IR: Genetics of pediatric tumors: the causes and consequences of chromosomal aberrations. In Pizzo PA, Poplack DG, editors: *Principles and practice of pediatric oncology,* ed 2, Philadelphia, 1993, JB Lippincott.

Klebanoff MA and others: The risk of childhood cancer after neonatal exposure to vitamin K, *N Engl J Med* 329:905-908, 1993.

Klein JF, Berry CC, Felice M: The development of a testicular self-examination instructional booklet, *J Adolesc Health Care* 11:235-239, 1990.

Li FP and others: Heritable fraction of unilateral Wilms' tumor, *Pediatrics* 81(1):147-149, 1988.

Lovejoy NC, Halliburton P: Pediatric tumor markers, *J Pediatr Nurs* 4(5):357-369, 1989.

Magrath IT: Malignant non-Hodgkin lymphomas. In Pizzo PA, Poplack DG: *Principles and practice of pediatric oncology,* ed 2, Philadelphia, 1993, JB Lippincott.

Mahon SM, Casperson DS: Pathophysiology of hypokalemia in patients with cancer: implications for nurses, *Oncol Nurs Forum* 20(6): 937-946, 1993.

Marshall G and others: Antiemetic therapy for chemotherapy-induced vomiting: metoclopramide, benztropine, dexamethasone, and lorazepam regimen compared with chlorpromazine alone, *J Pediatr* 115:156-160, 1989.

Mauer AM: Screening for neuroblastoma, *J Pediatr* 112(4):576-577, 1988.

Maurer HM, Ragab AH: Rhabdomyosarcoma. In Fernbach DJ, Vietti TJ, editors: *Clinical pediatric oncology,* ed 4, St Louis, 1991, Mosby.

McCalla JL, Santacroce SJ, Woolery-Antill M: Nursing support of the child with cancer. In Pizzo PA, Poplack DG, editors: *Principles and practice of pediatric oncology,* ed 2, Philadelphia, 1993, JB Lippincott.

McKenry LM, Salerno E: *Mosby's pharmacology in nursing,* ed 18, St Louis, 1992, Mosby.

Meadows AT and others: Similar efficacy of 6 and 18 months of therapy with four drugs (COMP) for localized non-Hodgkin's lymphoma of children: a report from the Children's Cancer Study Group, *J Clin Oncol* 17(1):92-99, 1989.

Mitchell CD: Management of infections in the neutropenic child with cancer, *Pediatr Ann* 17(11):677-686, 1988.

Moore BD III and others: Cognitive deficits in long-term survivors of childhood cancer, *Arch Neurol* 49:809-817, 1992.

Mulvihill J: Clinical genetics of pediatric oncology. In Pizzo PA, Poplack DG: *Principles and practice of pediatric oncology,* ed 2, Philadelphia, 1993, JB Lippincott.

National Cancer Institute: Bone marrow transplantation, NIH Publ No 92-1178, Bethesda, MD, April 1991, National Institutes of Health.

Neglia JP, Robison LL: Epidemiology of the childhood acute leukemias, *Pediatr Clin North Am* 35(4):675-692, 1988.

Pinkel D: Bone marrow transplantation in children, *J Pediatr* 122(3):331-341, 1993.

Pinkerton CR and others: 5-HT_3 antagonist ondansetron—an effective outpatient antiemetic in cancer treatment, *Arch Dis Child* 65:822-825, 1990.

Poplack DG: Acute lymphoblastic leukemia. In Pizzo PA, Poplack DG: *Principles and practice of pediatric oncology,* ed 2, Philadelphia, 1993, JB Lippincott.

Ramsay NK: Bone marrow transplantation in pediatric oncology. In Pizzo PA, Poplack DG, editors: *Principles and practice of pediatric oncology,* ed 2, Philadelphia, 1993, JB Lippincott.

Raney RB and others: Rhabdomyosarcoma and the undifferentiated sarcomas. In Pizzo PA, Poplack DG: *Principles and practice of pediatric oncology,* ed 2, Philadelphia, 1993, JB Lippincott.

Raymond CA: Childhood cancer's improved survival rates can exact a price in late effects of therapy, *JAMA* 260(23):3400-3401, 1988.

Richie JP: Detection and treatment of testicular cancer, *CA Cancer J Clin* 43(3):151-175, 1993.

Rivera GK and others: Treatment of acute lymphoblastic leukemia, *N Engl J Med* 329(18): 1289-1295, 1993.

Robison LL: General principles of the epidemiology of childhood cancer. In Pizzo PA, Poplack DG, editors: *Principles and practice of pediatric oncology,* ed 2, Philadelphia, 1993, JB Lippincott.

Roila F and others: Prevention of cisplatin-induced emesis: a double-blind multicenter randomized crossover study comparing ondansetron and ondansetron plus dexamethasone, *J Clin Oncol* 9:675-678, 1991.

Rubin CM: Chromosomal abnormalities in pediatric malignancies, *J Assoc Pediatr Oncol Nurs* 5(1/2):33, 1988.

Sandlund JT, Hutchison RE, Crist WM: Non-Hodgkin's lymphoma. In Fernbach DJ, Vietti TJ, editors: *Clinical pediatric oncology,* ed 4, St Louis, 1991, Mosby.

Sansievero GE, Murray SA: Safe management of chemotherapy at home, *Oncol Nurs Forum* 16(5):711-713, 1989.

Schecter N, Altman A, Weisman S: Report of the consensus conference on the management of pain in childhood cancer, *Pediatrics* 86(5):entire issue, 1990.

Shochat S: Update on solid tumor management in children, *Pediatr Surg* 72(6):1417-1427, 1992.

Sridhar KS, Donnelly E: Combination antiemetics for cisplatin chemotherapy, *Cancer* 61:1508-1517, 1988.

Stine KC and others: Systemic doxorubicin and intraarterial cisplatin preoperative chemotherapy plus postoperative adjuvant chemotherapy in patients with osteosarcoma, *Cancer* 63:848-853, 1989.

Tarbell NJ and others: Sex differences in risk of second malignant tumours after Hodgkin's disease in childhood, *Lancet* 341:1428-1432, 1993.

Thompson EI: Hodgkin's disease. In Fernbach DJ, Vietti TJ, editors: *Clinical pediatric oncology,* ed 4, St Louis, 1991, Mosby.

Tuchman M and others: Feasibility study for neonatal neuroblastoma screening in the United States, *Med Pediatr Oncol* 17:258-264, 1989.

van Eys J, editor: *The truly cured child: the new challenge in pediatric cancer care,* Baltimore, 1977, University Park Press.

van Eys J and others: Treatment intensity and outcome for children with acute lymphocytic leukemia of standard risk, *Cancer* 63(8):1466-1471, 1989.

Viscoli C: Aspects of infections in children with cancer, *Recent Results Cancer Res* 108:71-81, 1988.

Wagner HP: Supportive care in pediatric oncology, *Recent Results Cancer Res* 108:301-305, 1988.

Weinberg KI, Parkman R: Interface between immunodeficiency and pediatric cancer. In Pizzo PA, Poplack DG: *Principles and practice of pediatric oncology,* ed 2, Philadelphia, 1993, JB Lippincott.

Weinshel EL, Peterson BA: Hodgkin's disease, *CA Cancer J Clin* 43(6):327-346, 1993.

Weinstock MA and others: Nonfamilial cutaneous melanoma incidence in women associated with sun exposure before 20 years of age, *Pediatrics* 84(2):199-204, 1989.

Wiley FM, House KU: Bone marrow transplant in children, *Semin Oncol Nurs* 4(1):31-40, 1988.

Williams CJ and others: Comparison of starting antiemetic treatment 24 hours before or concurrently with cytotoxic chemotherapy, *Br Med J* 298:430-431, 1989.

Williams ML, Sagebiel RW: Sunburns, melanoma, and the pediatrician, *Pediatrics* 84(2):381-382, 1989.

Willis D: Intracranial astrocytoma: pathology, diagnosis and clinical presentation, *J Neurosci Nurs* 23(1):7-14, 1991.

Yasko JM, Dudjak LA: *Biological response modifier therapy: symptom management,* Pittsburgh, PA, 1990, Cancer Educational Resources and Services.

Zamenhoff R: Health hazards of low-frequency electromagnetic fields, *Pediatr Alert* 18(15):87-89, 1993.

Zeltzer LK, Jay SM, Fisher DM: The management of pain associated with pediatric procedures, *Pediatr Clin North Am* 36(4):941-964, 1989.

BIBLIOGRAPHY

Cancer in Children

Association of Pediatric Oncology Nurses: Scope of practice, *J Assoc Pediatr Oncol Nurs* 7(1):22-23, 1990.

Ceccarelli C and others: Thyroid cancer in children and adolescents, *Surgery* 104:1143-1148, 1988.

Crom DB and others: Malignancy in the neonate, *Med Pediatr Oncol* 17:101-104, 1989.

DiMario FJ, Packer RJ: Acute mental status changes in children with systemic cancer, *Pediatrics* 85(3):353-360, 1990.

Dowell RE, Copeland DR, van Eys J, editors: *The child with cancer in the community,* Springfield, IL, 1988, Charles C Thomas.

Foley GV, Fochtman D, Mooney KH, editors: *Nursing care of the child with cancer,* ed 2, Philadelphia, 1993, WB Saunders.

Fones M: Patient history plays an important role in care, *Cope* 3(4):44, 1989.

Foote A and others: Orem's theory used as a guide for the nursing care of an eight-year-old child with leukemia, *J Pediatr Oncol Nurs* 10(1):26-32, 1993.

Hymovich D: A theory for pediatric oncology nursing practice and research, *J Pediatr Oncol Nurs* 7(4):131-138, 1990.

Martinson I, Liu B: Three wishes of a child with cancer, *Int Nurs Rev* 35(5):143-44, 1988.

Martinson IM and others: Impact of childhood cancer on healthy school-age siblings, *Cancer Nurs* 13(3):183-190, 1990.

Outcome standards of pediatric oncology nursing practice, *J Assoc Pediatr Oncol Nurs* 7(1):24-30, 1990.

Plaschkes J: Surgical supportive care in pediatric oncology, *Recent Results Cancer Res* 108:148-153, 1988.

Rechner M: Adolescent with cancer: getting on with life, *J Pediatr Oncol Nurs* 7(4):139-144, 1990.

Ruccione K and others: What caused my child's cancer? Parents' responses to epidemiology studies of childhood cancer, *J Pediatr Oncol Nurs* 7(2):50-51, 1990.

Souba WW, Copeland EM, III: Hyperalimentation in cancer, *CA Cancer J Clin* 39(2):105-114, 1989.

Vaz RM and others: Clinical and laboratory observations, evaluations of a testicular cancer curriculum for adolescents, *J Pediatr* 114(1):150-153, 1989.

Wright PS and others: The Roy adaptation model used as a guide for the nursing care of an 8-year-old child with leukemia, *J Pediatr Oncol Nurs* 10(2):68-74, 1993.

Chemotherapy

Balis FM: Pharmacologic considerations in the treatment of acute lymphoblastic leukemia, *Pediatr Clin North Am* 35(4):835-852, 1988.

Betcher DL, Burnham N: Leucovorin, *J Assoc Pediatr Oncol Nurs* 6(3):102-104, 1989.

Billett AL and others: Allergic reactions to *Erwinia* asparaginase in children with acute lymphoblastic leukemia who had previous allergic reactions to *Escherichia coli* asparaginase, *Cancer* 70(1):201-206, 1992.

Cassileth BR: Counseling the cancer patient who wants to try unorthodox or questionable therapies, *Prim Care Cancer,* pp 53-60, Sept 1991.

Dolgin MJ, Katz ER: Conditioned aversion in pediatric cancer patients receiving chemotherapy, *J Dev Behav Pediatr* 9(2):82-85, 1988.

Fischetti LF: Interaction between nonsteroidal anti-inflammatory drugs and high-dose methotrexate: a literature review, *J Assoc Pediatr Oncol Nurs* 7(1):14-16, 1990.

Galassi A: The next generation: new chemotherapy agents for the 1990s, *Semin Oncol Nurs* 8(2):83-94, 1992.

Jenkins J, Hubbard S: History of clinical trials, *Semin Oncol Nurs* 7(4):228-234, 1991.

LeBaron S and others: Chemotherapy side effects in pediatric oncology patients: drugs, age, and sex as risk factors, *Med Pediatr Oncol* 16(4):263-268, 1988.

Mayer DK: Biotherapy: recent advances and nursing implications, *Nurs Clin North Am* 25(2):291-307, 1990.

McNamara J, Komp DM: Interleukin-2: a major lymphokine, *J Pediatr* 114(3):420-421, 1989.

O'Marcaigh AS, Betcher DL: Methotrexate, *J Pediatr Oncol Nurs* 10(4):158-160, 1993.

Questionable methods of cancer management: "nutritional" therapies, *CA Cancer J Clin* 43(5):309-319, 1993.

Taylor B and others: Recombinant interleukin-2 in the treatment of refractory solid tumors in pediatric oncology patients: nursing implications, *J Assoc Pediatr Oncol Nurs* 6(3):98-101, 1989.

Bone Marrow Transplantation

Anasetti C: Effect of HLA compatibility on engraftment of bone marrow transplants in patients with leukemia or lymphoma, *N Engl J Med* 320(4):197-204, 1989.

Barale KV: Oncology and bone marrow transplantation. In Queen M, Lang C, editors: *Handbook of pediatric nutrition,* Colorado, 1993, Aspen.

Bracken JD, DeCuir-Whalley S: Continuous bladder irrigation for children receiving high-dose cyclophosphamide before bone marrow transplantation, *J Assoc Pediatr Oncol Nurs* 6(3):105-107, 1989.

Brochstein JA: Critical care issues in BMT, *Crit Care Clin* 4(1):147-166, 1988.

Chessells JM and others: Bone marrow transplantation for high-risk childhood lymphoblastic leukaemia in first remission: experience in MRC UKALL X, *Lancet* 340(8819):565-568, 1992.

Corcoran-Buchsel P, Parchem C: Ambulation care of the bone marrow transplant patient, *Semin Oncol Nurs* 4(1):41-46, 1988.

Durbin M: Bone marrow transplantation: economic, ethical, and social issues, *Pediatrics* 82(5):774-783, 1988.

Freedman SE: An overview of bone marrow transplant, *Semin Oncol Nurs* 4(1):55-59, 1988.

Gottlieb SE, Portnoy S: The role of play in a pediatric bone marrow transplantation unit, *Child Health Care* 16(3):177-181, 1988.

Hamner SB, Miles MS: Coping strategies in children with cancer undergoing bone marrow aspirations, *J Assoc Pediatr Oncol Nurs* 5(3):11-15, 1988.

Hann IM: Bone marrow transplantation, *Curr Opin Pediatr* 2:143-150, 1990.

Hare J, Skinner D, Kliewer D: Family systems approach to pediatric bone marrow transplantation, *Child Health Care* 18(1):30-36, 1989.

Kaleita TA and others: Normal neurodevelopment in four young children treated with bone marrow transplantation for acute leukemia or aplastic anemia, *Pediatrics* 93(5): 753-757, 1989.

Kramer JH and others: A prospective study of cognitive functioning following low-dose cranial radiation for bone marrow transplantation, *Pediatrics* 90(3):447-450, 1992.

McCord DJ, Hathaway G: Autologous bone marrow transplantation in childhood cancer, *Pediatr Nurs* 14(6):454-456, 1988.

Stutzer CA: Work-related stresses of pediatric bone marrow transplant nurses, *J Assoc Pediatr Oncol Nurs* 6(3):70-78, 1989.

Tomlinson PS and others: The relationship of child acuity, maternal responses, nurse attitudes and contextual factors in the bone marrow transplant unit, *Am J Crit Care* 2(3):246-252, 1993.

Trigg ME: Bone marrow transplantation for treatment of leukemia in children, *Pediatr Clin North Am* 35(4):933-948, 1988.

Truog AW, Wozniak SP: Cyclosporine-A as prevention for graft-versus-host disease in pediatric patients undergoing bone marrow transplants, *Oncol Nurs Forum* 17(1):39-44, 1990.

Whedon MB: Bone marrow transplant: principles, practice, and nursing insight, *J Pediatr Oncol Nurs* 10(1):40-42, 1993.

Yeager AM: Pediatric bone marrow transplantation, *Pediatr Rev* 12(12):364-371, 1991.

Late Effects of Treatment

D'Angio G: Cure is not enough: late consequences associated with radiation treatment, *J Assoc Pediatr Oncol Nurs* 5(4):20-23, 1988.

Duffener PK, Cohen ME: The long-term effects of CNS therapy on children with brain tumors, *Neurol Clin* 9:479-495, 1991.

Gallagher JA: Acute lymphocytic leukemia treatment: effects on learning, *J Pediatr Health Care* 3(5):257-258, 1989.

Green DM: *Long term complications of therapy for cancer in childhood and adolescence,* Baltimore, 1989, Johns Hopkins University Press.

Green DM, D'Angio GJ: Late effects of treatment for childhood cancer, *J Pediatr Oncol Nurs* 10(1):40-42, 1993.

Haupt R and others: Smoking habits in survivors of childhood and adolescent cancer, *Med Pediatr Oncol* 20(4):301-306, 1992.

Meadows AT: Second malignant neoplasms in childhood cancer survivors, *J Assoc Pediatr Oncol Nurs* 6(1):7-11, 1989.

Ochs J, Mulhern RK: Late effects of antileukemic treatment, *Pediatr Clin North Am* 35(4): 815-834, 1988.

Peckham VC: Learning disorders associated with the treatment of cancer in childhood, *J Assoc Pediatr Oncol Nurs* 5(4):10-13, 1988.

Peckham VC and others: Educational late effects in long-term survivors of childhood acute lymphocytic leukemia, *Pediatrics* 81(1): 127-133, 1988.

Ruccione K, Weinberg K: Late effects in multiple body systems, *Semin Oncol Nurs* 5(1):4-13, 1989.

Sibler JH and others: Whole-brain irradiation and decline in intelligence: the influence of dose and age on IQ score, *J Clin Oncol* 10(9):1390-1396, 1992.

Vanderwal R, Nims J, Davies B: Bone marrow transplantation in children: nursing management of late effects, *Cancer Nurs* 11(3): 132-143, 1988.

Symptom Management

See Chapter 26 for additional citations on pain.

Adams J: Pediatric pain assessment: trends and research directions, *J Assoc Pediatr Oncol Nurs* 6(3):79-85, 1989.

Albano EA, Pizzo PA: Infectious complications in childhood acute leukemias, *Pediatr Clin North Am* 35(4):873-902, 1988.

Bavier AR: Nursing management of acute oral complications, *NCI Monogr* 9:123-128, 1990.

Beck SL: Prevention and management of oral complications in the cancer patient, *Curr Issues Cancer Nurs Pract Updates* 1(6):1-12, 1992.

Bendorf K, Meehan J: Home parenteral nutrition for the child with cancer, *Issues Compr Pediatr Nurs* 12(2/3):171-186, 1989.

Berg SL, Poplack DG: Complications of leukemia, *Pediatr Rev* 12(12):313-318, 1991.

Brescia FJ: An overview of pain and symptom management in advanced cancer, *J Pain Symptom Manage* 2(suppl 2):S7-S11, 1988.

Broome ME: Implementation of a clinical study of a pain management program for pediatric oncology patients, *J Pediatr Nurs* 4(1):54-56, 1989.

D'Agostino NS: Managing nutrition problems in advanced cancer, *Am J Nurs* 89(1):50-56, 1989.

Dorrepaal KL, Aaronson NK, van Dam F: Pain experience and pain management among hospitalized cancer patients, *Cancer* 63:593-598, 1989.

Eland JM: Pharmacologic management of acute and chronic pediatric pain, *Issues Compr Pediatr Nurs* 11:93-111, 1988.

Elliott SC and others: Epidemiologic features of pain in pediatric cancer patients: a co-operative community-based study, *Clin J Pain* 7(4):263-268, 1991.

Foley GV, Whittam EH: Care of the child dying of cancer, *CA: Cancer J Clin* 40:327-354, 1990.

Foley KM: Cancer pain syndromes, *J Pain Symptom Manage* 2(suppl 2):S13-S17, 1988.

Frick SB and others: Chemotherapy-associated nausea and vomiting in pediatric oncology patients, *Cancer Nurs* 11(2):118-124, 1988.

Galbraith LK and others: Treatment for alteration in oral mucosa related to chemotherapy, *Pediatr Nurs* 17(3):233-236, 1991.

Graham KM and others: Reducing the incidence of stomatitis using a quality assessment and improvement approach, *Cancer Nurs* 16(2):117-122, 1993.

Gralla RJ: Antiemetic drugs for chemotherapeutic support: current treatment and rationale for development of newer agents, *Cancer* 70(4, suppl):1003-1006, 1992.

Hughes WT: New drugs for infections in patients with cancer, *Cancer* 70(4, suppl):959-965, 1992.

Kinrade LC: Typhlitis: a complication of neutropenia, *Pediatr Nurs* 14(4):291-295, 1988.

Lawson K: Oral-dental concerns of the pediatric oncology patient, *Issues Compr Pediatr Nurs* 12(2/3):199-206, 1989.

Leggott PJ: Oral complications in the pediatric population, *NCI Monogr* 9:129-132, 1990.

Levick S and others: Naproxen sodium in treatment of bone pain due to metastatic cancer, *Pain* 35:253-258, 1988.

Miaskowski C: Management of mucositis during therapy, *NCI Monogr* 9:95-98, 1990.

Miser A: Management of pain associated with childhood cancer. In Schechter N, Berde C, Yaster M: *Pain in infants and children,* Baltimore, 1993, Williams & Wilkins.

Morrow GR: Chemotherapy-related nausea and vomiting: etiology and management, *CA Cancer J Clin* 39(2):89-104, 1989.

Quesenberry PJ, Lowry PA: The colony-stimulating factors: an overview, *Cancer* 70(4, suppl):909-912, 1992.

Robertson WW Jr: Orthopedic interventions for problems associated with the treatment of cancer in childhood, *J Assoc Pediatr Oncol Nurs* 6(1):12-14, 1989.

Schechter NL, Altman A, Weisman S, editors: Report of the Consensus Conference on the Management of Pain in Childhood Cancer, *Pediatrics* 86(5, suppl):813-834, 1990.

Sievers TD and others: Midazolam for conscious sedation during pediatric oncology procedures: safety and recovery parameters, *Pediatrics* 88(6):1172-1179, 1991.

Sitton E: Early and late radiation-induced skin alterations. II. Nursing care of irradiated skin, *Oncol Nurs Forum* 19(6):907-912, 1992.

Sutters KA, Miaskowski C: The problem of pain in children with cancer: a research review, *Oncol Nurs Forum* 19(3):465-471, 1992.

Tobias JD, Oakes L, Rao B: Continuous epidural anesthesia for postoperative analgesia in the pediatric oncology patient, *Am J Pediatr Hematol/Oncol* 14(3):216-221, 1992.

Tobias JD and others: Oral ketamine premedication to alleviate the distress of invasive procedures in pediatric oncology patients, *Pediatrics* 90(4):537, 1992.

van Hoff J, Olszewski D: Lorazepam for the control of chemotherapy-related nausea and vomiting in children, *J Pediatr* 113(1, pt 1):146-149, 1988.

Young JA, Eslinger P, Galloway M: Radiation treatment for the child with cancer, *Issues Compr Pediatr Nurs* 12(2/3):159-170, 1989.

Zeltzer LK and others: Report of the subcommittee on the management of pain associated with procedures in children with cancer, *Pediatrics* 86(5):826, 1990.

Leukemias/Lymphomas

Altman AJ: Chronic leukemias of children, *Pediatr Clin North Am* 35(4):765-788, 1988.

Armitage JO: Treatment of non-Hodgkin's lymphoma, *N Engl J Med* 328(14):1023-1030, 1993.

Carde P: Hodgkin's lymphoma. II. Treatment and delayed morbidity, *Br Med J* 305(6846): 173-176, 1992.

DeVita VT, Hubbard SM: Drug therapy: Hodgkin's disease, *N Engl J Med* 328(8):560-565, 1993.

Donaldson SS, Link MP: Hodgkin's disease: treatment of the young child, *Pediatr Clin North Am* 38:451-473, 1991.

Kurtzberg J, Graham M: NHL, biologic classification and implications for therapy, *Pediatr Clin North Am* 38:443-451, 1991.

Lampkins BC and others: Biologic characteristics and treatment of acute nonlymphocytic leukemia in children, *Pediatr Clin North Am* 35(4):743-764, 1988.

Look T: The cytogenics of childhood leukemia: clinical and biologic implications, *Pediatr Clin North Am* 35(4):723-742, 1988.

Marin T and others: Survival of children with chronic myeloid leukemia, *Am J Pediatr Hematol Oncol* 14(3):229-232, 1992.

O'Reilly SE, Connors JM: Non-Hodgkin's lymphoma. I. Characterisation and treatment, *Br Med J* 304(6843):1682-1686, 1992.

O'Reilly SE, Connors JM: Non-Hodgkin's lymphoma. II. Management problems, *Br Med J* 305(6843):39-42, 1992.

Paolucci G and others: Treating childhood acute lymphoblastic leukemia (ALL): summary of ten years experience in Italy, *Med Pediatr Oncol* 17:83-91, 1989.

Pate LH: Therapy-related acute leukemia, an overview, *Cancer Nurs* 11(5):295-302, 1988.

Ridgway D, Borzy MS: Elevated production of interleukin-2 by lymphocytes from children with acute leukemia, *J Pediatr* 114(3):384-391, 1989.

van Eys J and others: A comparison of two regimens for high-risk acute lymphocytic leukemia in childhood, *Cancer* 63:23-29, 1989.

Nervous System Tumors

A primer of brain tumors: a patient's reference manual, ed 57, Chicago, 1991, American Brain Tumor Association.

Baron MC: Advances in the care of children with brain tumors, *J Neurosci Nurs* 23:39-43, 1991.

Bleyer WA: Central nervous system leukemia, *Pediatr Clin North Am* 35(4):789-814, 1988.

Davidson GS, Hope JK: Meningeal tumors of childhood, *Cancer* 63:1205-1210, 1989.

Halperin EC and others: Selection of a management strategy for pediatric brainstem tumors, *Med Pediatr Oncol* 17:116-125, 1989.

Hart IR, Saini A: Biology of tumour metastasis, *Lancet* 339:1453-1457, 1992.

Kelly JU: The use of an investigational radiopharmaceutical in neuroblastoma: a nursing perspective, *J Assoc Pediatr Oncol Nurs* 6(4):133-138, 1989.

Murphy SB and others: Consensus statement from ACS workshop on neuroblastoma screening, *CA Cancer J Clin* 41:227-230, 1991.

Packer RJ: Primary childhood central nervous system tumors and neurologic complications of systemic childhood cancer and its treatment, *Curr Opin Pediatr* 1(2):257-268, 1989.

Rascher W and others: Serial measurements of neuropeptide Y in plasma for monitoring neuroblastoma in children, *J Pediatr* 122(6): 914-915, 1993.

Shiminski-Maher T and others: Current trends in the management of brainstem tumors in childhood, *J Neurosci Nurs* 23(6):356-362, 1991.

Squires RH Jr: Intracranial tumors: vomiting as a presenting sign: a gastroenterologist's perspective, *Clin Pediatr* 28(8):351-354, 1989.

Solid Tumors

Andrews PE, Kelalis PP, Haase GM: Extrarenal WIlms' tumor: results of the National Wilms' Tumor Study, *J Pediatr Surg* 27(9):1181-1184, 1992.

Berthold F and others: Prognostic factors in metastatic neuroblastoma: a multivariate analysis of 182 cases, *Am J Pediatr Hematol Oncol* 14(3):207-215, 1992.

Bohm P, Wirth CJ, Jansson V: Limb-preserving operations in the treatment of malignant bone tumors, *Arch Orthop Trauma Surg* 108:218-224, 1989.

Bonaïti-Pellié C and others: Genetics and epidemiology of Wilms' tumor: the French Wilms' Tumor Study, *Med Pediatr Oncol* 20(4):284-291, 1992.

Bonilla JA, Healy GB: Management of malignant head and neck tumors in children, *Pediatr Clin North Am* 36(6):1443-1450, 1989.

Brodeur AE, Brodeur GM: Abdominal masses in children: neuroblastoma, Wilms tumor, and other considerations, *Pediatr Rev* 12(7): 196-207, 1991.

D'Angio G and others: Wilms' Tumor: status report, *J Clin Oncol* 9:877-887, 1991.

Gallie BL and others: The genetics of retinoblastoma, *Pediatr Clin North Am* 38:299-315, 1991.

Loughlin KR and others: Genitourinary rhabdomyosarcoma in children, *Cancer* 63:1600-1606, 1989.

Manival JC and others: Pleuropulmonary blastoma, the so-called pulmonary blastoma of childhood, *Cancer* 62:1516-1526, 1988.

Rofary C, Flament F, Donaldson SS: An attempt to use a common staging system in rhabdomyosarcoma: a report of an international workshop initiated by the International Society of Pediatric Oncology, *Med Pediatr Oncol* 17:210-215, 1989.

Ruccione KS: Wilms' tumor: a paradigm, a parallel, and a puzzle, *Semin Oncol Nurs* 8(4):241-251, 1992.

Servodidio CA and others: Retinoblastoma, *Cancer Nurs* 14:117-123, 1991.

Shamberger RC and others: Chest wall tumors in infancy and childhood, *Cancer* 63:774-785, 1989.

Shields JA, Shields CL: Ocular tumors of childhood, *Pediatr Clin North Am* 40(4):805-826, 1993.

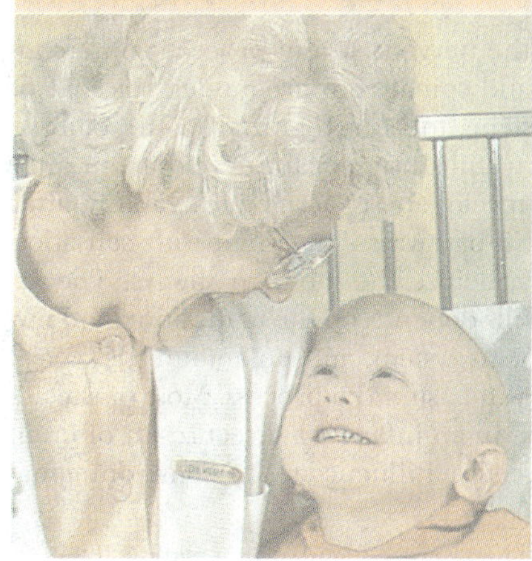

CHAPTER 37

The Child with Cerebral Dysfunction

CHAPTER OUTLINE

RELATED TOPICS

CEREBRAL STRUCTURE AND FUNCTION

The nervous system comprises three intimately connected and functioning parts: (1) the ***central nervous system (CNS)***, composed of two cerebral hemispheres, the brainstem, the cerebellum, and the spinal cord; (2) the ***peripheral nervous system***, composed of the cranial nerves that arise from or travel to the brainstem and the spinal nerves that travel to or from the spinal cord, which may be motor (efferent) or sensory (afferent); and (3) the ***autonomic nervous system (ANS)***, composed of the sympathetic and parasympathetic systems, which provide automatic control of vital functions.

Since this chapter is concerned primarily with disturbances of the brain, the major emphasis is placed on this system. The structure and function of the spinal cord and ANS are elaborated in Chapter 40.

■ Jeanne O'Connor Egan, RN, MSN, revised this chapter.

DEVELOPMENT OF THE NEUROLOGIC SYSTEM

In contrast to other body tissues, which grow rapidly after birth, the nervous system grows proportionately more rapidly before birth. Two periods of rapid brain cell growth occur during fetal life. There is a dramatic increase in the number of neurons at 15 to 20 weeks of gestation, and another increase in rate begins at 30 weeks of gestation and extends to 1 year of age. This rapid growth during infancy continues during early childhood, then slows to a more gradual rate during later childhood and adolescence. Brain volume is readily reflected in head circumference, which increases six times as much during the first year as in the second year of life. One half of the postnatal brain growth is achieved by age 1 year, 75% by age 3, and 90% by age 6. Cerebral blood flow and oxygen consumption in childhood (up to age 6 years) is almost twice that of adults, which reflects an increased metabolic requirement consistent with growth and development.

The brain growth and final form depend on the development and multiplication of neurons. Creation of new cells is believed to occur only during the first 100 days of gestation. During the remainder of gestation, cells divide and multiply at the astonishing rate of 250,000 per minute. It is believed that no new nerve cells appear after the sixth month of fetal life. Postnatal growth consists of increasing the amount of cytoplasm around the nuclei of the 10 billion existing cells, increasing the number and intricacy of communications with other cells, and advancing their peripheral axons to keep pace with expanding body dimensions.

The brain constitutes 12% of the body weight at birth. It doubles this weight in the first year, and by age 5 or 6 years its weight at birth has tripled. Thereafter growth slows until in adulthood the brain is only about 2% of the total body weight. The surface configuration also changes with development. The early embryonic brain surface is smooth, but with advancing development the sulci deepen. This process continues throughout childhood. At birth the cortex is only about one half of its adult thickness, although all the major surface features are present. There is little cortical control over body movements at birth, with the movements guided principally by primitive reflexes (see Chapter 8). With advancing development and maturation, the brain, through association pathways, exercises increasing control over much of the reflex activity. This allows the growing child to perform progressively complex tasks requiring coordinated movements. Persistence of primitive reflexes may suggest defective cortical development.

Cortical control is closely associated with the acquisition of a myelin coating on the nerves. Although nerve fibers are able to conduct impulses without this myelin sheath, the impulses travel at a slower rate and with more likelihood of diffusion. Myelinization of the various nerve tracts in the CNS, which allows progressive neuromotor function, follows the cephalocaudal (head-to-toe) and proximodistal (near-to-far) sequence. It appears first with the fibers of the spinal cord and cranial nerves, then in the brainstem and corticospinal tracts.

Development of the nervous system proceeds on a continuum. The brain and spinal cord are among the first of the major organ systems to be recognized in the embryo and one of the last to finish significant development after birth. The rate of myelogenesis accelerates rapidly after birth. In general, the pathways concerned with sensation are myelinated early, before the motor pathways. The acquisition of motor skills depends on the maturation and myelination of the nervous system, and no amount of special training or practice will hasten the process. Most of the advancing performance in an infant is a direct result of brain development indirectly influenced by environmental stimuli.

CENTRAL NERVOUS SYSTEM (CNS)

The bony skull forms the strongest covering and provides the primary protection to the brain. It is an expansible structure in the infant and young child but becomes rigid in the older child and adolescent. Blood is supplied to the dura mater by the middle meningeal artery, a branch of the external carotid artery. It enters the skull at a point inferior to the temporal bone, then branches over the surface of the dura, usually encased in a groove in the temporal and parietal bones after 2 years of age. Damage to this artery or its branches is a frequent cause of an epidural hematoma.

Brain Coverings

Within the skull the brain is covered and protected further by three membranes, the ***meninges***—the dura mater, arachnoid membrane, and pia mater (Fig. 37-1). The tough outer membrane, the ***dura mater***, is a double layer that serves as the outer meningeal layer and the inner periosteum of the cranial bones separated by the ***epidural space***. The dura is closely attached to the skull in infancy, causing slower spread of blood in epidural hemorrhage. Because of this adherence, epidural hemorrhages are uncommon in the first 2 years of life.

Between these layers of dura inside the skull lie large venous sinuses. Sheets of the dura mater also extend downward and inward to form partitions within the cranium. Projecting downward into the longitudinal fissure is the sheet of dura called the ***falx cerebri***, separating the cerebral hemispheres, and the ***falx cerebelli***, separating the cerebellar hemispheres. Another segment is a tentlike structure, the ***tentorium***, which separates the cerebellum from the occipital lobe of the cerebrum. The large gap through which the brainstem passes is the ***tentorial hiatus***, the site of herniation in untreated intracranial pressure.

The middle meningeal layer, the ***arachnoid membrane***, is a delicate, avascular, weblike structure that loosely surrounds the brain. Between the arachnoid and the dura mater lies the ***subdural area***, a potential space that normally contains only enough fluid to prevent adhesion between the two membranes. During cerebral trauma, however, the fine blood vessels that bridge the subdural space are stretched and ruptured, causing venous blood to escape and spread freely, forming a subdural hemorrhage. The subdural space

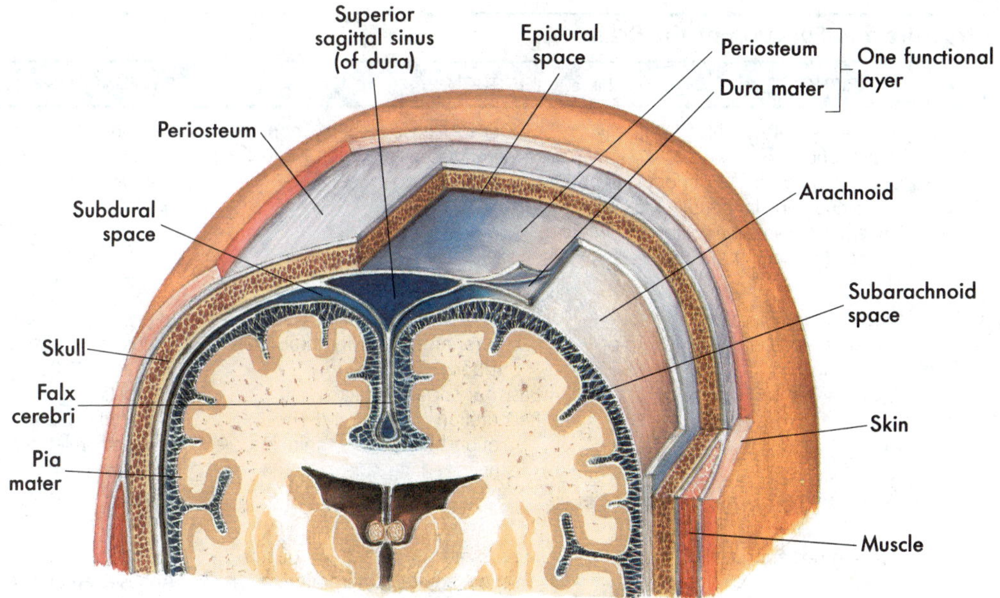

FIG. 37-1 Protective coverings of the brain. (From Thibodeau GA, Patton KT: *Anatomy and Physiology,* ed 2, St Louis, 1993, Mosby.)

is small in children; therefore small amounts of blood can increase intracranial hemorrhage significantly.

The innermost covering layer, the ***pia mater,*** is a delicate transparent membrane that, unlike the other coverings, adheres closely to the outer surface of the brain, conforming to the folds (gyri) and furrows (sulci). Within the pial layer lie the arteries and veins of the brain. Between the pia mater and the arachnoid membrane is the ***subarachnoid space.*** Cerebrospinal fluid (CSF) fills the entire subarachnoid space surrounding the brain and spinal cord, which acts as a protective cushion for the brain tissue. Further protection is provided by fibrous filaments known as ***arachnoid trabeculae,*** which help anchor the brain. When the head receives a blow, these attachments allow the arachnoid to slide on the dura, preventing excessive movement.

The Brain

Each section of the brain plays a vital role in regulation and control of body function. Each hemisphere is artificially divided into lobes. Pressure on or damage to these lobes produces observable signs or symptoms directly related to the area of pathology, which provides clues to the location of the damage. The major structures of the brain and their functions are briefly outlined in Table 37-1.

The two large cerebral hemispheres that occupy the anterior and medial fossae of the skull are separated in the upper part by the ***longitudinal fissure.*** This separation is complete anteriorly and posteriorly, but centrally the hemispheres are joined by the block of fibers known as the ***corpus callosum,*** the largest fiber bundle in the brain. These fibers interconnect cortical areas of the right and left hemispheres. Destruction of the corpus callosum causes hemispheric independence, or "split brain."

Situated deeply within each hemisphere and on each side of the midline are the ***basal ganglia*** (or cerebral nuclei), which serve as vital sorting areas for messages passing to and from the hemispheres. Connected to the hemispheres by thick bunches of nerve fibers is the ***brainstem,*** through which all the nerve fibers traverse as they pass from the hemispheres to the cerebellum and spinal cord. The brainstem extends from the base of the hemispheres through the foramen magnum, where it is continuous with the spinal cord. Within the cranium and behind the brainstem is the cerebellum. Any pressure exerted on the intracranial structures can cause compression of the brainstem and prolapse of the cerebellum through the foramen magnum.

Cerebral Blood Flow (CBF). The blood supply to the brain tissue is carried by the internal carotid arteries, which branch to supply the various brain segments. The volume of blood to the brain, which constitutes only 17% of the cardiac output, supplies the brain with 20% of the body oxygen. The brain, an "inactive" organ, uses 10 times the oxygen used by the body as a whole. Only the heart uses more oxygen per gram of tissue.

CBF is the result of two opposing forces—cerebral blood pressure (the difference between systemic arterial pressure and cerebral venous pressure) and cerebral vascular resistance. At a blood pressure between 50 and 150 mm Hg, CBF remains constant. Since cerebral venous pressure is usually very low and relatively constant, the cerebral blood pressure is determined mainly by systemic arterial pressure.

Autoregulation. One of the most important factors in the control of CBF is ***autoregulation,*** the unique ability of cerebral arterial vessels to change their diameter in response to fluctuating cerebral perfusion pressure (CPP).

TABLE 37-1 Structure and Function of the Brain

STRUCTURE	DESCRIPTION	FUNCTION	DYSFUNCTION
Cerebrum	Two hemispheres divided artificially into lobes Upper parts divided anteriorly and posteriorly by longitudinal fissure Lower parts joined centrally by block of fibers, the corpus callosum	Center for consciousness, thought, memory, sensory input, motor activity	Pressure or damage produces signs and symptoms specific to involved areas
Frontal lobes	Most anteriorly located of all lobes that end posteriorly at fissure of Rolando	Posterior portion contains cells that control motor activity throughout body Basis for social interaction Recognition of cause-and-effect relationships, abstract thinking, expressive language	Injury or damage to anterior portion may cause personality changes, altered intellectual functioning Impaired movement of body part directly related to motor center for that part Memory deficits Language deficits
Parietal lobes	Situated posterior to fissure of Rolando	Important for appreciation of sensation, somatic interpretation and integration	Language dysfunction Aphasia, apraxia, motor and sensory loss to lower extremities, atopognosia
Occipital lobe	At posterior base of skull Most posteriorly placed lobe	Receives stimuli for vision Spatial orientation Visual recognition	Injury produces impaired vision, functional blindness
Temporal lobes	Situated anterior to occipital lobe and inferior to parietal lobes	Receives and interprets stimuli for taste, vision, sound, smell Converts crude visual impressions into recognizable images	Injury or destruction causes inability to interpret meanings of sensory experiences
	Point where temporal, parietal, and occipital lobes converge	Primary interpretive area	Impairment causes inability to interpret sensory stimuli; difficulty in understanding higher levels of meaning of body sensory experiences
	Point where temporal, parietal, and frontal lobes converge	Center for speech, hearing, receptive language	Impairment produces aphasia Hearing dysfunction
Cerebellum	Located just below posterior part of cerebrum and separated from it by tentorium Contains two lateral lobes joined by midline portion, the vermis	Necessary for refinement and coordination of all muscle movements, including walking, talking, control of muscle tone and balance	Dysmetria, ataxia, dysarthria, hypotonia, nystagmus, dystonia Rest tremor
Basal ganglia	Situated deeply within cerebral hemispheres on either side of midline	Unconscious or automatic control of lower motor centers Excitation causes inhibition of muscle tone throughout body	Chorea, athetosis Dystonia Rest tremor
Diencephalon	Situated between cerebrum and mesencephalon	Contains diffuse fibers that compose reticular activating system	Stupor
Thalamus	Rounded mass forms most of lateral wall of third ventricle and part of floor of lateral ventricles	Major relay station for sensory impulses to cerebral cortex Activates cerebral cortex	Impaired consciousness
Hypothalamus	Lies beneath thalamus Forms floor of third ventricle	Vital control center for involuntary functions (e.g., blood pressure, satiety, hunger, rage, feeding, water conservation, temperature, sleep regulation, libido) Controls secretion of tropic hormones	Impairment causes alterations in vegetative functions Somnolence, coma Anorexia, loss of weight, fever, diabetes insipidus, loss of libido Endocrine disorders
Brainstem	Extends from cerebral hemisphere to spinal cord	All cranial nerves (except I) arise from brainstem	Stupor, coma
Mesencephalon (midbrain)	Lies below inferior surface of cerebellum and above pons	Main connection between forebrain and hindbrain Contains nuclei for cranial nerves III, IV, part of V	Impaired consciousness No independent movement or verbal response Decerebrate posturing Neurologic hyperventilation

TABLE 37-1 Structure and Function of the Brain—cont'd

STRUCTURE	DESCRIPTION	FUNCTION	DYSFUNCTION
	Ventral portion composed of cerebral peduncles	Control of eye movement	Impaired function of muscles supplied by these nerves
Pons	Located just above medulla oblongata	Contains pneumotaxic center—control of respiration	Deep, rapid, or periodic breathing
		Cranial nerves V through VIII	Impaired function of muscles supplied by these nerves
Medulla	Forms attachment of brain to spinal cord Separated from pons by horizontal groove	Contains vital centers, including respiratory and vasomotor cranial nerves IX, X, XI, XII	Impaired vital functions No response to any stimuli Ataxic (Biot) breathing Flaccid muscle tone Deep tendon, gag, corneal reflexes absent

The CPP is the mean arterial pressure (MAP) minus the intracranial pressure (ICP):

$$CPP = MAP - ICP$$

As a result, cerebral vessels maintain a constant blood flow during alterations in blood pressure and perfusion caused by body posture, increased ICP, decreased cardiac output, or narrowing or occlusion in the major blood vessels of the neck. Autoregulation fails when the limits of cerebrovascular dilatation are reached; then CBF decreases, causing clinical symptoms of ischemia (nausea, fainting, dizziness, dim vision). Conversely, increased MAP leads to "breakthrough of autoregulation," with increased CBF leading to microhemorrhages and cerebral edema. Autoregulation may be impaired locally or globally as a result of trauma or ischemia.

Changes in arterial oxygen pressure (PaO_2) or arterial carbon dioxide pressure ($PaCO_2$) have a profound effect on autoregulation. Hypercapnia ($PaCO_2$ over 40 mm Hg) or increased levels of lactic acid have a pronounced dilating effect on cerebral arterioles that increases CBF and thus cerebral volume. Hypocapnia ($PaCO_2$ 25 to 30 mm Hg) constricts cerebral arterioles and decreases CBF. PaO_2 values between 70 and 100 mm Hg have little effect on the cerebrovascular system. However, profound hypoxia (PaO_2 below 50 mm Hg) dramatically increases CBF. Consequently, maintenance of the airway and effective hyperventilation are of primary importance in the initial management of the neurologically impaired patient. CPP is the most important physiologic determinant, because the brain relies on the delivery of oxygen and nutrients to function.

Oxygen. Metabolic requirements for oxygen by the brain are not affected by rest or sleep, although they are reduced by narcosis and coma and altered by changes in temperature. CBF is not altered when body temperature is maintained between 35° and 40° C (95° and 104° F). Oxygen consumption of the brain is increased by hyperthermia and decreased by hypothermia. The brain depends on a constant supply of oxygen-rich blood, and since the oxygen need of the brain is great in relation to the volume of blood supplied, it extracts more oxygen from each unit of circulating blood.

Oxygen supply to the brain is compromised when the supply is inadequate as a result of impaired respiration, hypotension, increased ICP or vascular damage, spasm, or compression. Neurons are highly susceptible to elevated $PaCO_2$ (a potent vasodilator), and the metabolic damage to brain tissue caused by an inadequate supply of well-oxygenated blood can often exceed the effects of trauma. Respiratory acidosis resulting from increased $PaCO_2$ levels can produce symptoms indistinguishable from those of head injury.

Blood-Brain Barrier. The blood-brain barrier (BBB) is an anatomic-physiologic feature of the brain that separates the brain parenchyma from the blood. Cerebral capillaries, unlike those in other parts of the body, have no fenestrations or pores. The tight junctions of the vascular endothelium are thought to be responsible for the selective nature of the BBB. The mature BBB allows facilitated diffusion of glucose and passive diffusion of water and carbon dioxide but is impermeable to protein and does not permit passage of many active substances. However, the BBB of the fetus and newborn is normally indiscriminately permeable, allowing protein and other large and small molecules to pass freely between the cerebral vessels and the brain. Conditions that cause cerebrovascular dilatation (hypertension, hypercapnia, hypoxia, acidosis) disrupt the BBB, as do hyperosmotic fluids, which cause shrinkage of vascular endothelium and widen the vascular junctions.

INCREASED INTRACRANIAL PRESSURE (ICP)

The brain, tightly enclosed in the solid bony cranium, is well protected but highly vulnerable to pressure that may accumulate within the enclosure. Its total volume—brain (80%), CSF (10%), and blood (10%)—must remain approximately the same at all times. A change in the proportional volume of one of these components (e.g., increase or decrease in intracranial blood) must be accompanied by a compensatory change in another (e.g., decrease or increase in CSF). In this way the volume and pressure normally remain constant. Examples of compensatory changes are reduction in blood volume, decrease in production of CSF, increase in CSF absorption, or shrinkage of brain mass by displacement of intracellular and extracellular fluid.

In children with open fontanels, compensation may take place by skull expansion and widened sutures. However, at any age the capacity for spatial compensation is limited. An increase in ICP may be caused by tumors or other space-occupying lesions, accumulation of fluid within the ventricular system, bleeding, or edema of cerebral tissues. Once compensation is exhausted, any further increase in volume will result in a rapid rise in ICP.

Early signs and symptoms of increased ICP are often subtle and assume many patterns, such as personality changes, irritability, and fatigue (see box below). In older children subjective symptoms are headache, especially when lying flat (e.g., on awakening in the morning) or when coughing, sneezing, or bending over, and nausea and vomiting. The child may complain of double vision or blurred vision with movement of the head. Seizures are not uncommon. In children whose cranial sutures have not closed, there is an increase in the head circumference and bulging fontanels. Cranial sutures may become diastatic, or split, and head circumference can enlarge until the child is 5 years of age if the pathology progresses slowly. As pressure increases, the pupils become progressively sluggish in reaction, eventually to become fixed and dilated, sometimes referred to as "blown." The level of consciousness progressively deteriorates from drowsiness to eventual coma. Problems related to increased ICP are discussed later in this chapter in relation to head injury. (See also Brain Tumors, Chapter 36, and Hydrocephalus, Chapter 11.)

Physiologic and biochemical changes within the cerebral vasculature serve to complicate the primary causes of increased ICP. Initially, especially in cases of trauma, there is often increased blood flow as a result of venous congestion or vasomotor paralysis. If cerebral hypoxia is associated with the cerebral dysfunction, the compensatory vasodilatation caused by oxygen deficiency will tend to increase the cerebral flow. However, as ICP progressively increases, blood flow is reduced with diminished blood supply to the brain tissues. The classic responses observed in adults (widening pulse pressure, increased blood pressure) are rarely seen in children and, if so, are very late signs. Breathing characterized by periods of hyperpnea that alternate with apnea (Cheyne-Stokes respirations) is seen in brainstem damage.

SIGNS OF INCREASED INTRACRANIAL PRESSURE IN INFANTS AND CHILDREN

INFANTS

Tense, bulging fontanel; lack of normal pulsations
Separated cranial sutures
Macewen (cracked-pot) sign
Irritability
High-pitched cry
Increased occipitofrontal circumference (OFC)
Distended scalp veins
Changes in feeding
Cries when held or rocked
Setting sun sign

CHILDREN

Headache
Nausea
Vomiting—often without nausea
Diplopia, blurred vision
Seizures

PERSONALITY AND BEHAVIOR SIGNS

Irritability (toddlers), restlessness
Indifference, drowsiness, or lack of interest
Decline in school performance
Diminished physical activity and motor performance
Increased complaints of fatigue, tiredness; increased time devoted to sleep
Significant weight loss possible from anorexia and vomiting
Memory loss if pressure is greatly increased
Inability to follow simple commands
Progression to lethargy and drowsiness

LATE SIGNS

Lowered level of consciousness
Decreased motor response to command
Decreased sensory response to painful stimuli
Alterations in pupil size and reactivity
Sometimes decerebrate or decorticate posturing
Cheyne-Stokes respirations
Papilledema

EVALUATION OF NEUROLOGIC STATUS

Dysfunction of the CNS can be manifested in almost any body system and may result from various causes. Earlier chapters discuss methods used to evaluate neurologic function in relation to numerous aspects of child care. The neurologic examination is an integral part of the health assessment (see Chapter 7) and newborn assessment (see Chapter 8). Some of the tests used to differentiate neuromuscular disorders are discussed in Chapter 40. The assessment tools and examinations in this chapter are primarily those used to assess intracranial integrity.

ASSESSMENT: GENERAL ASPECTS

Children younger than 2 years require special evaluation, since they are unable to respond to directions designed to elicit specific responses neurologically. Early neurologic responses in infants are primarily reflexive; these responses are gradually replaced by meaningful movement in the characteristic cephalocaudal direction of development. This evidence of progressive maturation reflects more extensive myelinization and changes in neurochemical and electrophysiologic properties.

Most information about infants and small children is gained through observation of their spontaneous and elicited reflex responses, by their development of increasingly complex locomotor and fine motor skills, and by eliciting progressively sophisticated communicative and adaptive behaviors. Delay or deviation from expected milestones helps identify high-risk children. Persistence or reappearance of reflexes that normally disappear indicates pathology. In evaluating the infant or young child, it is also important to obtain the pregnancy and delivery history to determine the possible effect of intrauterine environmental influences known to affect the orderly maturation of the CNS. These influences include maternal infections, chemicals, trauma, and metabolic insults.

History

A family history can sometimes offer clues regarding possible genetic disorders with neurologic manifestations. A review of family members often identifies conditions that might otherwise be overlooked, especially siblings who have died or relatives whose conditions have been hidden from memory. Questions regarding specific neurologic problems are mentioned, such as mental retardation, deafness, epilepsy, blindness, unusual movements, weakness, ataxia, and progressive mental deterioration.

A history is very important because it provides valuable clues regarding the cause of unconsciousness. There may have been an injury or short febrile illness, or the child may have diabetes. A history of any event that led to the health care assessment is probed, especially when it involves injury, encounter with an animal or insect, ingestion of neurotoxic substances, inhalation of chemicals, or past illness. Sudden or progressive alterations in movement or mental abilities may provide clues for investigation.

Physical Examination

Physical examination includes observation of the size and shape of the ***head,*** spontaneous ***activity*** and postural ***reflex activity,*** and ***sensory responses.*** The attitude is observed. It is noted whether the infant assumes a normal flexed posture or one of extreme extension, opisthotonos, or hypotonia. Extremities are observed for symmetry of ***movement.*** Excessive tremulousness or frequent twitching movements may be significant signs indicating the onset of a seizure disorder. Seizure activity is suspected if holding the extremity snugly does not stop the activity.

Skin and hair texture may be important factors in detecting certain neurologic diseases. Facial features may suggest a specific syndrome, and a high-pitched, piercing cry is associated with CNS disorders. Abnormal eye movements, inability to suck or swallow, lip smacking, asymmetric contraction of facial muscles, and yawning may indicate ***cranial nerve (CN)*** involvement. An abnormal respiratory cycle, such as prolonged apnea, ataxic breathing, paradoxic chest movement, and hyperventilation (central neurogenic), may be the result of a neurologic problem.

Older children can be evaluated by the usual methods employed in a neurologic examination. In addition, an estimation of the ***level of development*** provides essential information about neurologic function. This assessment is discussed throughout the book in relation to evaluation for specific disorders such as mental retardation, failure to thrive, attention deficit disorder, cerebral palsy, cerebral tumors, and other physical or behavioral problems. Developmental screening tests (see Appendix B) can be used to assess developmental progress in the young child.

Muscular Activity. Muscular activity and coordination, including ocular movements and gait, are valuable sources of information. Ocular movements, pupillary response, facial movements, and mouth functions provide

DESCRIPTION OF ABNORMAL INVOLUNTARY MUSCULAR MOVEMENTS

Ataxia—Gross incoordination that may become worse with the eyes closed
Spasm—Involuntary contraction of a muscle mass; cramp (if painful), convulsion (if violent)
Spasticity—Prolonged and steady contraction of a muscle characterized by clonus (alternating relaxation and contraction of the muscle) and exaggerated reflexes
Rigidity—Inability to flex a joint
Tremors—Constant small involuntary movements
Twitching—Spasmodic movements of short duration
Tic—Involuntary, compulsive, stereotyped movement of an associated group of muscles
Choreiform movements—Quick, jerky, grossly incoordinated, irregular movements that may disappear on relaxation
Athetosis—Slow, writhing, wormlike, constant, grossly incoordinated movements that increase on voluntary activity and decrease on relaxation
Dystonia—Slow twisting movements of limbs or trunk
Associated movements—Voluntary movement of one muscle accompanied by involuntary movement of another muscle
Mirroring movements—Same as associated movements except with symmetric muscle groups

ABNORMALITIES OF GAIT THAT INDICATE CEREBRAL DYSFUNCTION

Ataxia—Impaired ability to coordinate movements; staggering gait and postural imbalance.
Spastic paraplegic gait—Narrow-based gait with a tendency to walk on toes, along with flexion at knees and hips, and shuffling. Thighs are adducted, and knees may strike each other with each step; in younger children a "scissoring" position results when lower limbs cross because of increased adductor tone. Patients walk stiffly and take slow, deliberate steps. Increased difficulty when attempting to walk on heels or run.
Spastic hemiplegic gait—Involved leg extended, circumducted, plantar flexed, and does not swing naturally at knee or hip.
Cerebellar gait—Staggering, irregularity, unsteadiness, wide-based lurching movement in any direction, and tendency to veer in one lateral direction (hemispheric lesion).
Extrapyramidal gait—Rigidity, few automatic movements, and bradykinesia (slowness of all movements) with associated bending of trunk and head, arms adducted at shoulders and flexed at elbows and wrists, fingers extended; festination (upper body moves forward in advance of lower part), causing more rapid steps and risk of falling.

clues regarding CN involvement or impingement. (See Chapter 7 for CN and reflex testing.) Testing reflexes, strength, and coordination, and for the presence and location of tremors, twitching, tics, or other unusual movements (see left-hand box on p. 1675) are also aspects of the neurologic assessment. Abnormalities of gait that indicate cerebral dysfunction are described in the right-hand box on p. 1675.

ALTERED STATES OF CONSCIOUSNESS

Consciousness implies awareness—the ability to respond to sensory stimuli and have subjective experiences. There are two aspects of consciousness: ***alertness,*** an arousal-waking state including the ability to respond to stimuli, and ***cognitive power,*** including the ability to process stimuli and produce verbal and motor responses.

An altered state of consciousness usually refers to varying states of unconsciousness that may be momentary or may last for hours, days, or indefinitely. ***Unconsciousness*** is depressed cerebral function—the inability to respond to sensory stimuli and have subjective experiences. ***Coma*** is defined as a state of unconsciousness from which the patient cannot be aroused even with noxious (painful) stimuli.

The seat of consciousness, or "alerting area," of the brain is in the reticular formation—the central core of the brainstem. The reticular formation extends from the midbrain to the medulla. The reticular activating system (RAS) receives collaterals from and is stimulated by *every* major somatic and special sensory pathway in the brain. Disturbances of consciousness may occur when any part of the reticular, thalamic, hypothalamic, and cortical circuits is sufficiently impaired. However, the effects may vary according to the areas involved. For example, small lesions of the reticular or hypothalamic regions will produce a profound effect, whereas extensive impairment of the cortex is required to produce quantitatively similar results.

Etiology

An altered state of consciousness may be the outcome of several processes that affect the CNS. Impaired neurologic function can result from a direct or indirect cause. Some altered states, such as the diffuse changes observed in encephalitis, are directly related to cerebral insult; others are the result of dysfunction to other organs or processes. For example, biochemical changes can impair neurologic function without morphologic findings, as in hypoglycemia.

Level of Consciousness (LOC)

Assessment of LOC remains the earliest indicator of improvement or deterioration in neurologic status. LOC is determined by observations of the child's responses to the environment. Other diagnostic tests, such as motor activity, reflexes, and vital signs, are more variable and do not necessarily directly parallel the depth of the comatose state. The most consistently used terms are described in the box below, left.

LEVELS OF CONSCIOUSNESS

Full consciousness—Awake and alert, orientated to time, place and person—behavior appropriate for age
Confusion—Impaired decision making
Disorientation—Disorientation to time, place, decreased level of consciousness
Lethargy—Limited spontaneous movement, sluggish speech
Obtundation—Arousable with stimulation
Stupor—Remains in a deep sleep, responsive only to vigorous and repeated stimulation
Coma—No motor or verbal response to noxious (painful) stimuli

Modified from Hazinski MF, editor: *Care of the critically ill child,* ed 2, St Louis, 1992, Mosby, p. 544.

Coma Assessment

Diminished alertness as a result of pathologic conditions occurs as a continuum and is designated as the ***comatose state,*** which extends from somnolence at one end to deep coma at the other. To produce coma, one of the following must occur: (1) extensive, diffuse, bilateral cerebral hemispheric destruction (the brainstem may be intact); (2) a lesion in the diencephalon; or (3) destruction of the brainstem down to the level of the lower pons.

Several scales have been devised in an attempt to standardize the description and interpretation of the degree of depressed consciousness. The most popular of these is the ***Glasgow Coma Scale (GCS),*** which consists of a three-part assessment: eye opening, verbal response, and motor response. The GCS was created to meet a clinical need: the desire of experienced nurses for objective criteria for the conscious level. For clinical purposes, the primary role of observation of the LOC is to detect a life-threatening complication such as cerebral edema. The GCS requires observational skills and is readily reproducible between observers.

A pediatric version of the GCS recognizes that expected verbal and motor responses must be related to the child's age. The pediatric coma scale does not assess verbal responses as such, but records smiling, crying, and interaction; it employs a 6-point motor scale that is inappropriate with children below the age of 6 months. In children under 5 years of age, speech is taken as any sound at all, even crying. Young children will demonstrate orientation by identifying their parents correctly or giving their own names. The scale with variations adapted to the young patient is provided in Fig. 37-2. When assessing LOC in young children, it is often useful to have a parent present to help elicit a desired response. An infant or child may not respond in an unfamiliar environment or to unfamiliar voices.

Numerical values of 1 to 5 are assigned to the levels of response in each category. The sum of these numerical values provides an objective measure of the patient's LOC. The lower the score, the deeper is the coma. A normal person would score the highest, 15; a score of 8 or below is generally accepted as a definition of coma; the lowest score, 3, indicates deep coma or death.

The GCS in itself is not sufficient to determine the responses of all children. For example, a quadriplegic child can score very low but be cerebrally intact, because the child cannot respond to commands physically. However, the GCS provides a more objective method for evaluating the state of consciousness in most cases. Severely injured children (GCS of 8 or less) may have a consistent grading of motor response, verbal response, and eye opening.

The GCS is a useful predictor of outcome, particularly in the group of children who are admitted with a GCS score of 5 or more and who subsequently do not deteriorate. In one study the presence of abnormal plantar and pupillary light reflexes predicted an outcome of death or severe disability (Grewal and Sutcliffe, 1991).

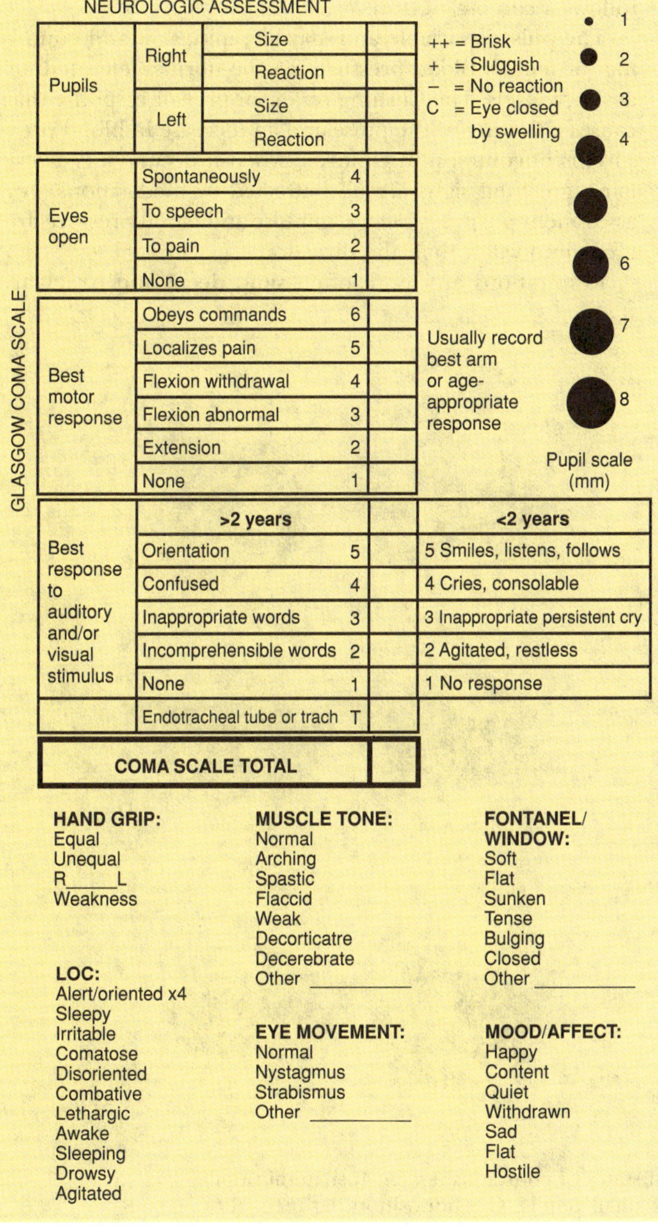

NEUROLOGIC ASSESSMENT

GLASGOW COMA SCALE

Pupils	Right	Size	
		Reaction	
	Left	Size	
		Reaction	

++ = Brisk
\+ = Sluggish
– = No reaction
C = Eye closed by swelling

Pupil scale (mm): 1, 2, 3, 4, 5, 6, 7, 8

Eyes open	Spontaneously	4	
	To speech	3	
	To pain	2	
	None	1	
Best motor response	Obeys commands	6	
	Localizes pain	5	
	Flexion withdrawal	4	
	Flexion abnormal	3	
	Extension	2	
	None	1	

Usually record best arm or age-appropriate response

	>2 years		<2 years
Best response to auditory and/or visual stimulus	Orientation	5	5 Smiles, listens, follows
	Confused	4	4 Cries, consolable
	Inappropriate words	3	3 Inappropriate persistent cry
	Incomprehensible words	2	2 Agitated, restless
	None	1	1 No response
	Endotracheal tube or trach	T	

COMA SCALE TOTAL	

HAND GRIP: Equal, Unequal, R____L, Weakness

MUSCLE TONE: Normal, Arching, Spastic, Flaccid, Weak, Decorticatre, Decerebrate, Other ________

FONTANEL/ WINDOW: Soft, Flat, Sunken, Tense, Bulging, Closed, Other ________

LOC: Alert/oriented x4, Sleepy, Irritable, Comatose, Disoriented, Combative, Lethargic, Awake, Sleeping, Drowsy, Agitated

EYE MOVEMENT: Normal, Nystagmus, Strabismus, Other ________

MOOD/AFFECT: Happy, Content, Quiet, Withdrawn, Sad, Flat, Hostile

FIG. 37-2 Pediatric coma scale.

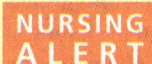

Lack of response to painful stimuli is abnormal and is reported immediately.

Irreversible Coma. There is no precise diagnosis for clinical death. Different tissues undergo permanent damage after varying periods of exposure to an ongoing insult; therefore the brain (especially the cerebrum) has become the tissue of most importance in determining the time of death. The current concept of dying is a process that takes place over a finite interval of time, rather than an event that occurs spontaneously. ***Brain death*** is the total cessation of brainstem and cortical brain function that may result from irreversible traumatic, anoxic, or metabolic conditions. The pronouncement of brain death requires two conditions: (1) complete cessation of clinical evidence of brain function and (2) irreversibility of the condition. The child who meets the criteria for brain death will eventually suffer cardiovascular collapse (usually within hours).

GUIDELINES
Establishing Brain Death in Children

1. Coma and apnea must coexist. Child must exhibit complete loss of consciousness, vocalization, and volitional activity.
2. Brainstem function must be absent, as defined by:
   a. Midposition or fully dilated pupils that do not respond to light. Drugs may influence and invalidate pupillary assessment.
   b. Absence of spontaneous eye movements and those induced by oculocephalic and caloric (oculovestibular) testing.
   c. Absence of movement of bulbar musculature, including facial and oropharyngeal muscles. The corneal, gag, cough, sucking, and rooting reflexes are absent.
   d. Respiratory movements are absent when child is removed from respirator. Apnea testing using standardized methods can be performed but is done after other criteria are met.
3. Child must not be significantly hypothermic or hypotensive for age.
4. Flaccid tone and absence of spontaneous or induced movements, including spinal cord events such as reflex withdrawal or spinal myoclonus, should exist.
5. Examination should remain consistent with brain death throughout the observation and testing period.
6. Observation periods according to age:

7 days to 2 months	Two examinations and EEGs, separated by at least 48 hours
2 months to 1 year	Two examinations and EEGs, separated by at least 24 hours
Over 1 year	Observation period of at least 12 hours
	If irreversible cause exists, no laboratory testing needed
	If difficult to assess extent of reversibility of brain damage, observation indicated for at least 24 hours

Modified from Task Force for the Determination of Brain Death in Children: *Ann Neurol* 21:616, 1987.

Organ transplantation has created a need to subdivide the process of death in order to obtain viable tissues at a time when the brain is already dead. The clinical criteria for brain death must be so constituted that there is *no error.* Although the legal status of the concept of death varies among individual states and communities in the United States, The Task Force for the Determination of Brain Death in Children has established physical examination criteria (see Guidelines box, p. 1677). (See also Tissue Donation/Autopsy, Chapter 23.)

NEUROLOGIC EXAMINATION

The purpose of the neurologic examination is to establish an accurate, objective baseline of neurologic function. Therefore it is essential that the neurologic examination be documented in a fashion that is *reproducible.* In this way a comparison of baseline, previous, and current findings allows the observer to detect subtle changes in the neurologic status that might not be evident otherwise. Descriptions of behaviors should be simple, objective, and easily interpreted: "Drowsy but awake and conversationally rational/oriented," "Sleepy but arousable with vigorous physical stimuli. Pressure to nail base of right hand results in upper extremity flexion/lower extremity extension."

Vital signs, observation of posture and movement (both spontaneous and elicited), eye examination, CN testing, and reflex testing all provide valuable clues regarding the LOC, the site of involvement, and the probable cause, although they do not necessarily parallel the depth of a comatose state.

Vital Signs

Pulse, respiration, and ***blood pressure*** provide information regarding the adequacy of circulation and the possible underlying cause of altered consciousness. ***Autonomic activity*** is most intensively disturbed in deep coma and in brainstem lesions. ***Body temperature*** is often elevated; sometimes the elevation may be extreme and unresponsive to therapeutic measures. Coma of a toxic origin may produce hypothermia. High temperature is most frequently a sign of an acute infectious process or heat stroke but may be caused by ingestion of some drugs, especially salicylates, alcohol, and barbiturates, or intracranial bleeding. A fever sometimes follows a cerebral seizure.

The pulse is variable and may be rapid, slow and bounding, or feeble. Blood pressure may be normal, elevated, or at shock levels. The Cushing reflex, or pressor response that causes a slowing of the pulse and an increase in blood pressure, is uncommon in children; when it occurs, it is a very late sign. Vital signs are also affected by medications. For assessment purposes *changes* in pulse and blood pressure are more important than the direction.

Respirations are more often slow, deep, and irregular.

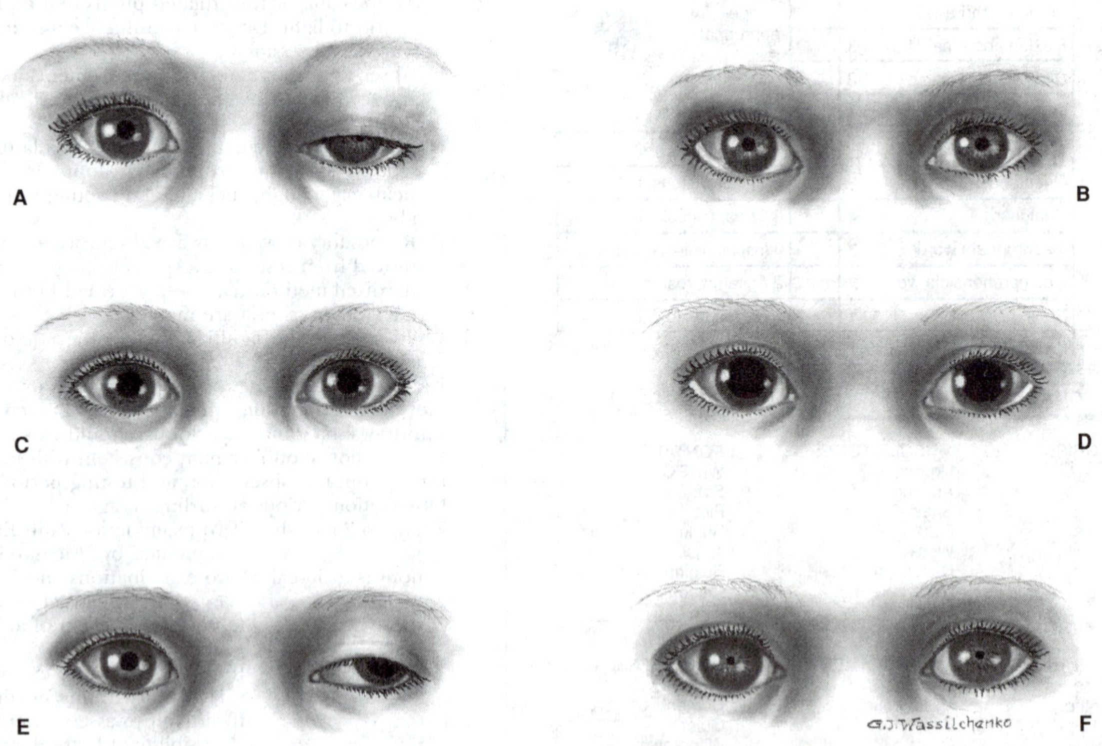

FIG. 37-3 Variations in pupil size with altered states of consciousness. **A,** Ipsilateral pupillary constriction with slight ptosis. **B,** Bilateral small pupils. **C,** Midposition, light fixed to all stimuli. **D,** Bilateral dilated and fixed pupils. **E,** Dilated pupils, left eye abducted with ptosis. **F,** Pinpoint pupils.

Slow and deep breathing is often seen in the heavy sleep caused by sedatives, after seizures, or in cerebral infections. Slow, shallow breathing may result from sedatives or narcotics. Hyperventilation (deep and rapid respirations) is usually the result of metabolic acidosis or abnormal stimulation of the respiratory center in the medulla caused by salicylate poisoning, hepatic coma, or Reye syndrome.

Breathing patterns have been described with a number of terms (e.g., apneustic, cluster, ataxic, Cheyne-Stokes). However, it is better to describe what is being observed rather than placing a label on it. The terms are often used and interpreted incorrectly. Periodic and irregular breathing are signs of brainstem (especially medullary) dysfunction. This is an ominous sign that often precedes complete apnea. The odor of the breath may provide additional clues (e.g., the fruity, acetone odor of ketosis, the foul odor of uremia, the fetid odor of hepatic failure, or the odor of alcohol).

Skin

The skin may offer clues to the cause of unconsciousness. The body surface should be examined for the presence of injury, needle marks, petechiae, bites, and ticks. Evidence of toxic substances may be found on the hands, face, mouth, and clothing—especially in small children.

Eyes

Pupil size and reactivity are assessed (Fig. 37-3). Pupils either react or do not react to light. Pinpoint pupils are commonly observed in poisoning, such as opiate or barbiturate poisoning, or in brainstem dysfunction. Widely dilated and reactive pupils are often seen after seizures and may involve only one side. Dilated pupils may also be caused by eye trauma. Widely dilated and fixed pupils suggest paralysis of CN III secondary to pressure from herniation of the brain through the tentorium. A unilateral fixed pupil usually suggests a lesion on the same side. Bilateral fixed pupils usually imply brainstem damage if present for more than 5 minutes. Dilated and nonreactive pupils are also seen in hypothermia, anoxia, ischemia, poisoning with atropine-like substances, or prior instillation of mydriatic drugs.

NURSING ALERT The sudden appearance of a fixed and dilated pupil is a neurosurgical emergency.

Some of the therapies used (e.g., barbiturates) can alter pupil size and reaction. The description of eye movements should indicate whether one or both eyes are involved and how the reaction was elicited. The parents should be asked if the child has a strabismus. A preexisting strabismus will cause the eyes to appear normal under compromise.

Blinking observed at rest or in response to a sudden loud noise or bright light implies that the pontine reticular formation is intact. The ***corneal reflex,*** blinking of the eyelids when the cornea is touched with a wisp of cotton or a camel hair pencil, is used to test the integrity of the ophthalmic division of CN V. A posttraumatic strabismus indicates CN VI damage.

Eye movements are assessed by the ***doll's head maneuver,*** in which the child's head is rotated quickly to one side and then to the other. When brainstem centers for eye movement are intact, there is conjugate (paired or working together) movement of the eyes in the direction opposite to the head rotation. Absence of this response suggests dysfunction of the brainstem or oculomotor nerve (CN III). Downward or lateral deviation is frequently observed in association with pupillary dilation in dysfunction of CN III.

NURSING ALERT Any tests that require head movement are not attempted until after cervical spine injury has been ruled out for the child who is suspected of or has sustained a traumatic injury.

The ***caloric test,*** or ***oculovestibular response,*** is elicited by irrigating the external auditory canal with 10 ml of ice water over a period of about 20 seconds (head of bed elevated at a 30-degree angle). This normally causes nystagmus (movement of the eyes toward the side of stimulation). This is lost when the pontine centers are impaired, thus providing important information in assessment of the comatose patient.

NURSING ALERT This painful test is never performed on the awake child or if the tympanic membranes are ruptured.

Funduscopic examination reveals additional clues. ***Papilledema*** (a sign of increased ICP observed in the eyes), if it develops at all, will not be evident early in the course of unconsciousness, because papilledema takes 24 to 48 hours to develop. The presence of preretinal (subhyaloid) hemorrhages in children is usually the result of acute trauma with intracranial bleeding, usually subarachnoid or subdural hemorrhage.

Motor Function

Observation of spontaneous activity, posture, and response to painful stimuli provides clues to the location and extent of cerebral dysfunction. Even subtle movements (e.g., the out-turning of a hip) should be noted and the child observed for other signs. Asymmetric movements of the limbs or absence of movement suggests paralysis. In hemiplegia the affected limb lies in external rotation and will fall uncontrollably when lifted and allowed to drop. These observations should be described rather than labeled. In the deeper comatose states there is little or no spontaneous movement and the musculature tends to be flaccid. There is considerable variability in the motor behavior in lesser degrees of coma. For example, the child may be relatively immobile or restless and hyperkinetic; muscle tone may be increased or decreased. Tremors, twitching, and spasms of muscles are common observations. The patient may display purposeless plucking or tossing movements. Combative or negativistic behavior is not uncommon. Hyperactivity is more common in acute febrile and toxic states than in cases of increased ICP. Convulsions are common in children and may be present in coma as a result of any cause. Any repetitive or seizure movements are described.

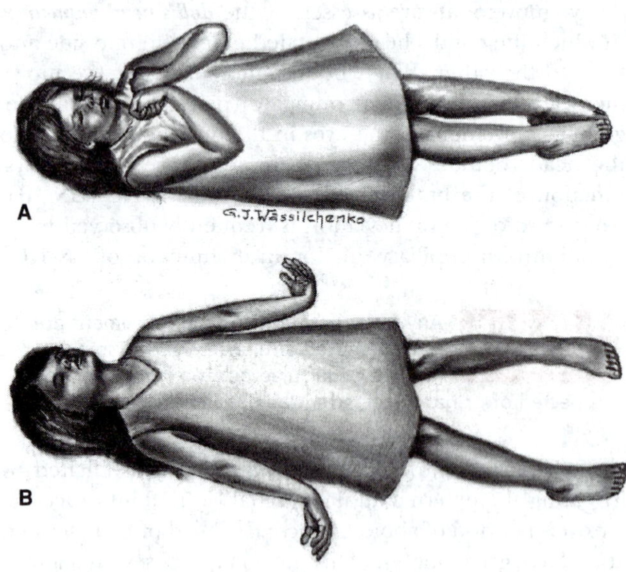

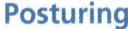

FIG. 37-4 **A,** Decorticate posturing. **B,** Decerebrate posturing.

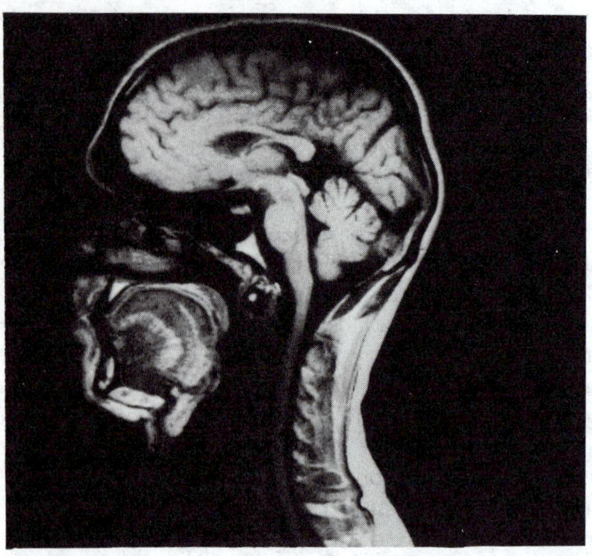

FIG. 37-5 MRI. The midsagittal image produces excellent anatomic detail. Note the clear delineation of such structures as the pituitary gland, brainstem, spinal cord, cerebellum, corpus callosum, and sylvian aqueduct. (Courtesy Philips Medical Systems. (From Nolte J: *The human brain: an introduction to its functional anatomy,* ed 3, St Louis, 1993, Mosby.)

Posturing

As cortical control over motor function is lost in brain dysfunction, primitive postural reflexes emerge. These are evident in posturing and motor movements directly related to the area of the brain involved. Posturing reflects a balance between the lower exciting and the higher inhibiting influences, and strong muscles overcome weaker ones. ***Decorticate posturing*** (Fig. 37-4, *A*) is seen when there is severe dysfunction of the cerebral cortex. Typical decorticate posturing includes adduction of arms at the shoulders, the arms being flexed on the chest with the wrists flexed and the hands fisted, and the lower extremities being extended and adducted. ***Decerebrate posturing*** (Fig. 37-4, *B*), a sign of dysfunction at the level of the midbrain, is characterized by rigid extension and pronation of the arms and legs. Unilateral decerebrate posturing is often caused by tentorial herniation.

The posturing may not be evident when the child is quiet but can usually be elicited by applying painful stimuli, such as a blunt object pressed on the base of the nail. Nurses should avoid applying thumb pressure to the supraorbital region of the frontal bone (risk of orbital damage) or knuckle pressure to the sternum (risk of bruising). Noxious stimuli, such as suctioning, will elicit a response, as may turning or touching. When describing posturing, the stimulus needed to provoke the response is as important as the reaction.

Reflexes

Testing of some reflexes may be of limited value, such as those present in an intact spinal cord (see Chapter 40). In general, the corneal, pupillary, muscle-stretch, superficial, and plantar reflexes tend to be absent in deep coma. The state of reflexes is variable in lighter grades of unconsciousness and depends on the underlying pathologic process and the location of the lesion. The doll's eye reflex maneuver, described previously, reflects paralysis of CN III. Absence of corneal reflexes (CN V) and presence of a tonic neck reflex are associated with severe brain damage. Babinski reflex, in which the lateral portion of the foot is stroked, may be of value if it is found to be present consistently in children older than 1 year. A positive Babinski reflex is significant in assessment of pyramidal tract lesions when it is unilateral and associated with other pyramidal signs. A fluctuating Babinski reflex is often observed after seizures (see Fig. 8-9, *B*).

NURSING ALERT Three key reflexes that demonstrate neurologic health in young infants are the Moro, tonic neck, and withdrawal reflexes.

SPECIAL DIAGNOSTIC PROCEDURES

Numerous diagnostic procedures are used for assessment of cerebral function. Laboratory tests that may help to delineate the cause of unconsciousness include blood glucose, urea nitrogen, and electrolyte (pH, sodium, potassium, chloride, calcium, and bicarbonate) tests; clotting studies, hematocrit, and a complete blood count; liver function tests; blood cultures if there is fever; and sometimes studies to detect lead or other toxic substances, such as drugs.

An electroencephalogram (EEG) may provide important information. For example, generalized random slow activity suggests suppressed cortical function; localized slow ac-

TABLE 37-2 **Neurologic Diagnostic Procedures**

TEST	DESCRIPTION	PURPOSE	COMMENTS
Lumbar puncture (LP)	Long needle is inserted between L3 and L4 vertebrae into subarachnoid space; cerebrospinal fluid (CSF) pressure is measured, and sample is collected for examination	Diagnostic—measures spinal fluid pressure, obtains CSF for visualization and laboratory analysis Therapeutic—injection of medication, spinal anesthesia	Contraindicated in patients with increased intracranial pressure (ICP) or infected skin over puncture site
Subdural tap	Needle is inserted into anterior fontanel or coronal suture (midline to pupil)	Helps rule out subdural effusions Relieves ICP	Requires shaving scalp Infant is placed in semierect position after subdural tap to minimize leakage from site; avoid crying if possible Check site frequently for evidence of leakage
Ventricular puncture	Needle is inserted into lateral ventricle via coronal suture (midline to pupil)	Removes CSF to relieve pressure	Used if LP is unsuccessful or contraindicated Risk of intracerebral or ventricular hemorrhage
Electroencephalography (EEG)	Records changes in electric potential of brain Electrodes are placed at various points on scalp and amplified Impulses are recorded by electromagnetic pen	Measures electric activity of cerebral cortex Detects electric abnormalities—diagnosis of seizures Used to determine brain death	Patient should rest quietly during procedure May require sedation Reduce external stimuli to a minimum during procedure
Nuclear brain scan	Intravenous (IV) injection of radioactive material that is counted and recorded after fixed time interval	Test material accumulates in areas where blood-brain barrier is defective Identifies focal brain lesions (e.g., tumors, abscesses) Positive uptake of material with encephalitis and subdural hematoma Visualizes CSF pathways	Requires sedation in young or uncooperative children and IV infusion In normal children or noncommunicating hydrocephalus there is no retrograde filling of ventricles Areas of concentrated uptake of material are termed "hot spots"
Echoencephalography	Pulses of ultrasonic waves are beamed through head; echoes from reflecting surfaces are recorded graphically	Identifies shifts in midline structures from their normal positions as a result of intracranial lesions May show ventricular dilatation	Simple, safe, rapid procedure Fontanel must be patent
Real-time ultrasonography (RTUS)	Similar to CT but uses ultrasound instead of ionizing radiation	Allows high-resolution anatomic visualization in variety of imaging planes	Produces images similar to CT scan Especially useful in neonatal CNS problems Anterior fontanel must be patent
Radiography	Skull films are taken from several projections—lateral, posterolateral, axial (submentoventricular), half-axial	Shows fractures, dislocations, spreading suture lines, craniostenosis Shows degenerative changes, bone erosion, calcifications	Simple, noninvasive procedure
Computed tomography (CT) scan	Pinpoint x-ray beam is directed on horizontal or vertical plane to provide series of "cuts" or "slices" that are fed into computer and assembled in image displayed on video screen and transferred to permanent record	Visualized horizontal and vertical cross section of brain at any axis Distinguishes density of various intracranial tissues and structures—congenital abnormalities, hemorrhage, tumors, demyelinating and inflammatory processes	Noninvasive procedure except when IV contrast agent is used Requires conscious sedation Can be done on outpatient basis Rapid, relatively safe and accurate Expensive

Continued.

TABLE 37-2 Neurologic Diagnostic Procedures—cont'd

TEST	DESCRIPTION	PURPOSE	COMMENTS
Magnetic resonance imaging (MRI) or nuclear magnetic resonance	Produces radiofrequency emissions from elements (e.g., hydrogen, phosphorus), which are converted to visual images by computer	Permits visualization of morphologic features of target structures Permits tissue discrimination unavailable with many techniques	Noninvasive procedure except when IV contrast agent is used No exposure to radiation Requires conscious sedation for lengthy immobilization Parent or attendant can remain in room with child Does not visualize bone detail or calcifications No metal can be present in the scanner Expensive
Positron emission transaxial tomography (PETT) or positron emission tomography (PET)	IV injection of positron-emitting radionucleotide; local concentrations are detected and transformed into a visual display by computer	Detects and measures blood volume and flow in brain, metabolic activity, biochemical changes within tissues, etc.	Requires lengthy period of immobility Minimum exposure to radiation
Digital subtraction angiography (DSA)	Contrast dye injected IV; computer "subtracts" all tissues without contrast medium, leaving clear image of contrast medium in vessels studied	Visualizes vasculature of target tissue Visualizes finite vascular abnormalities	Safe alternative to angiography Patient must remain still during procedure

tivity suggests a focal lesion, such as a mass; and generalized projected patterns suggest brainstem involvement. A flat tracing is one of the criteria used as evidence of brain death. Examination of spinal fluid is carried out when toxic encephalopathy or infection is suspected. Lumbar puncture is ordinarily delayed if intracranial hemorrhage is suspected and is contraindicated in the presence of ICP because of the potential for tentorial herniation (see p. 1695).

Auditory and visual evoked potentials are sometimes used in neurologic diagnosis of very young children. Brainstem auditory evoked potentials are useful for evaluating the continuity of brainstem auditory tracts and are particularly useful for detecting demyelinating disease and neoplasms of the brainstem and distinguishing between brainstem and cortical lesions. For example, a normal evoked potential in a comatose patient suggests involvement of the cerebral hemispheres.

Highly sophisticated tests are revolutionizing care for children with neurologic problems. Two imaging techniques, computed tomography (CT) and magnetic resonance imaging (MRI) (Fig. 37-5), assist in diagnosis by scanning soft tissues, as well as solid matter. Most of these tests are outlined in Table 37-2. Because such tests can be threatening to children, a child will need preparation for, and support and reassurance during, the tests. (See Preparation for Procedures, Chapter 27.)

Children who are old enough to understand require careful explanation of the procedure, why it is being done, what they will experience, and how they can help. School-age children usually appreciate a more detailed description of why contrast material is injected. The importance of lying still for tests, particularly CT, needs to be stressed. Children unfamiliar with the machines can be shown a picture beforehand. Although radiographic examinations are not painful, the machinery is often so frightening in appearance that the child protests because of anxiety.

This is especially true of CT and MRI, which require that the child's head be placed within a special immobilizing device. Chin and cheek pads are sometimes used to prevent the slightest head movement, and straps are applied to the body to prevent a slight change in body position. The nurse can explain these events to a frightened child by comparing them to an astronaut's preparation for a space flight. It is very important to emphasize to the child that at no time is the procedure painful.

Developmentally, the nurse should not expect cooperation from a young child. Conscious sedation will be required. Chloral hydrate, given orally or rectally, may be the drug of choice for children under 2 years of age. The suggested oral dosage is (Barkovich, 1990):

$<$10 kg: 75 to 100 mg/kg
$>$10 kg: 75 to 100 mg/kg plus 50 mg/kg for each kg of weight $>$10 kg
If child is still awake after 20 minutes, supplementary doses may be given up to a total dose of 2000 mg.
The drug should be given 35 to 45 minutes before the anticipated imaging time.

Intravenous sodium pentobarbital (Nembutal) is an excellent sedative for children over 2 years of age during MRI (Blevins and Benson, 1992).

It is helpful for nurses to become acquainted with the equipment and the general environment in which the test will take place so that they can better explain the procedure to children at their level of understanding. Written material describing the procedure should be available for parents and may be appropriate to share with children. Equipment is often strange and ominous to children and may be perceived as a frightening monster. They need constant reassurance from a trusted companion. Since children are particularly frightened of needles, they need to be informed of any medication or contrast media to be administered intravenously.

Physical preparation may involve administration of a sedative. If so, children should be helped through the preparation and administration and assured that someone will remain with them (if this is possible). Children need continual support and reinforcement during the procedures in which they remain conscious. Vital signs and physiologic response to the procedure are monitored throughout. Many diagnostic procedures performed on an outpatient basis require sedation, and children need recovery time and observation.

Children who have undergone a procedure with general anesthesia require postanesthesia care, including positioning to prevent aspiration of secretions and frequent assessment of the vital signs and LOC. In addition, other neurologic functions, such as pupillary responses, motor strength, and movement, are tested at regular intervals. Any surgical wound resulting from the test is checked for bleeding, CSF leakage, and other complications. Children who undergo repeated subdural taps should have their hematocrit monitored to detect excessive blood loss from the procedure.

Children's emotional reaction to the procedure is also considered. They should be allowed and encouraged to express their feelings about the experience through verbal expression and the use of therapeutic play. Parents also seek and are entitled to an explanation of results of tests and procedures performed on their children. Nurses are in a unique position to provide support and education to parents regarding procedures.

THE CHILD WITH CEREBRAL COMPROMISE

NURSING CARE OF THE UNCONSCIOUS CHILD

The unconscious child requires continuous nursing attendance with observation, recording, and evaluation of changes in objective signs. These observations provide valuable information regarding the patient's progress. Often they serve as a guide to diagnosis and treatment. Therefore careful and detailed observations are essential for the child's welfare. In addition, vital functions must be maintained and complications prevented through conscientious and meticulous nursing care. The outcome of unconsciousness may be early and complete recovery, death within a few hours or days, persistent and permanent unconsciousness, or recovery with varying degrees of residual mental and/or physical disability.

Emergency measures are directed toward assuring a patent airway, stabilization of the spine when indicated, treatment of shock, and reduction of ICP (if present). Delayed treatment often leads to increased damage. As soon as emergency measures have been implemented—in many cases concurrently—therapies for specific causes are begun. Because nursing care is closely related to the medical management, both are considered here.

❖ ASSESSMENT

Continual observation of the LOC, pupillary reaction, and vital signs is essential to management of the child with a CNS disorder. Regular assessment of neurologic and vital signs is an integral part of nursing comatose children. The frequency depends on the cause of coma, the status, and the progression of cerebral involvement. Intervals between observation may be as short as every 15 minutes or as long as every 2 hours. Significant alterations are reported immediately. The temperature is taken every 2 to 4 hours, depending on the child's condition.

An elevated temperature may occur in children with CNS dysfunction; therefore a light covering is sufficient. Vigorous efforts, such as tepid sponge baths or application of a hypothermia blanket, are needed to prevent brain damage if temperature exceeds 40° C (104° F) rectally.

The LOC is assessed periodically, including size, equality, and reaction of pupils to light and signs of meningeal irritation, such as nuchal rigidity. This also includes response to vocal commands, spontaneous behavior, resistance to care, and response to painful stimuli. Motions of any type, changes in muscle tone or strength, and body position are noted. Seizure activity is described according to type and length of seizure and body areas involved (see box on p. 1724).

Pain management for the comatose child requires astute nursing observation and management. Signs of pain include changes in behavior (e.g., increased agitation and rigidity, and alterations in physiologic parameters); usually increased heart rate, respiratory rate, and blood pressure; and decreased oxygen saturation. Since these findings are not specific for pain, the nurse should be alert for their appearance during times of induced or suspected pain and their disappearance following the inciting procedure or the administration of analgesia. A pain assessment record is used to document indications of pain and the effectiveness of interventions.

The use of opioids, such as morphine, to relieve pain is controversial because they may mask signs of altered consciousness or depress respirations. However, unrelieved pain activates the stress response, which can elevate ICP. To block the stress response, some authorities advocate the use of analgesics, sedatives, and, in some cases such as head injury, paralyzing agents via continuous intravenous infusion. A frequently used combination is fentanyl, midazolam (Versed), and vecuronium. If there are concerns about assessing the LOC or respiratory depression, naloxone can be used to reverse the opioid effects. Acetaminophen and codeine may also be effective analgesics. Regardless of the drugs used, adequate dosage and regular administration are essential to providing optimum pain relief.

Other measures to relieve discomfort include providing a quiet, dimly lit environment, restricting visitors to a minimum, preventing any sudden jarring movement, such as banging into the bed, and preventing an increase in ICP. The last is most effectively achieved by proper positioning and prevention of straining, such as during coughing, vomiting, or defecating. (See Pain Management, Chapter 26.)

NURSING ALERT When opioids are used, bowel elimination must be closely monitored because of their constipating effect. A stool softener should be given regularly with laxatives as needed to prevent constipation.

Antiepileptic drugs, such as phenytoin (Dilantin) or phenobarbital, are ordered for control of seizure activity.

❖ Nursing Diagnoses

Based on a thorough assessment, several nursing diagnoses are identified. The more common diagnoses for the unconscious child are included in the Nursing Care Plan on pp. 1688-1690. Others may apply in specific situations.

❖ Planning

The goals for the unconscious child and the family include the following:

1. Child will maintain respiratory integrity.
2. Child will not experience increasing ICP.
3. Child will have basic needs (hygiene, nutrition, hydration, elimination) met.
4. Child will not experience complications of immobility.
5. Family will receive adequate support and education.

❖ Implementation

Respiratory Management

Respiratory effectiveness is the primary concern in care of the unconscious child, and establishment of an adequate airway is *always* the first priority. Carbon dioxide has a potent vasodilating effect and will increase CBF and ICP. Cerebral hypoxia at normal body temperature that lasts longer than 4 minutes nearly always causes irreversible brain damage.

Children in lighter stages of coma may be able to cough and swallow, but those in deeper states of coma are unable to manage secretions, which tend to pool in the throat and pharynx. Dysfunction of CN IX and X places the child at risk of aspiration and cardiac arrest; therefore the child is positioned with the head and body to the side to prevent aspiration of secretions, and the stomach is emptied to reduce the likelihood of vomiting. In infants blockage of air passages from secretions can happen in seconds. In addition, upper airway obstruction from laryngospasm is a frequent complication in comatose children.

An oral airway can be used for the child who is suffering a temporary loss of consciousness, such as after a seizure or anesthesia. For children who remain unconscious for a time, a nasotracheal or orotracheal tube is inserted to maintain the open airway and facilitate removal of secretions. A tracheostomy is performed in cases in which laryngoscopy for introduction of an endotracheal tube would be difficult or dangerous, or for a child who needs long-term ventilatory support. Suctioning is used only as needed to clear the airway, exerting care to prevent increasing ICP. Respiratory status is observed and evaluated regularly. Signs of respiratory distress may be an indication for ventilatory assistance.

When the respiratory center is involved, mechanical ventilation is usually indicated (see Chapter 31). Blood gas analysis is performed regularly, and oxygen is administered when indicated. Moderately severe hypoxia and respiratory acidosis are often present but not always evident from clinical manifestations. Hyperventilation frequently accompanies unconsciousness and may lead to respiratory alkalosis, or it may represent the body's attempt to compensate for metabolic acidosis. Therefore blood gas and pH determinations are essential guides for electrolyte therapy. Chest physiotherapy is carried out on a regular basis, and the child's position is changed at least every 2 hours to prevent pulmonary complications.

Intracranial Pressure Monitoring

Prompt intervention can be lifesaving in the comatose patient who has evidence of a marked increase in ICP. When increased ICP is the result of accumulation of CSF from obstruction of CSF flow, a ventricular tap will provide relief quickly and effectively. Evacuation of a hematoma reduces pressure from this source. Indications for inserting an ICP monitor are (1) Glasgow Coma Scale (GCS) evaluation of less than 7, (2) Glasgow Coma Scale (GCS) evaluation of less than 8 with respiratory assistance, (3) deterioration of condition, and (4) subjective judgment regarding clinical appearance and response.

Management of the child with increased ICP is possibly the most formidable task and the most controversial subject in pediatric critical care. Continuous ICP monitoring was first introduced 30 years ago, but opinions vary as to its value in preventing pediatric neurologic injury. Assessment of the true benefits of ICP monitoring remains difficult. It appears that the outcome in pediatric neurologic injury may reflect more the initial cerebral damage than subsequent intracranial hypertension. Moreover, ICP gives little indication of the severity of the initial insult (LeRoux and others, 1991).

Four major types of ICP monitors are (1) intraventricular catheter with fibroscopic sensors attached to a monitoring system, (2) subarachnoid bolt (Richmond screw), (3) epidural sensor, and (4) anterior fontanel pressure monitor. Transducers for both ventricular and subarachnoid monitoring should be set up without the use of a flush device. Direct ventricular pressure measurement remains the gold standard of ICP monitoring.

The catheter method involves introduction of a catheter into the lateral ventricle on the nondominant side, if known, or placement in the subdural space. The catheter has the advantage of providing a means of extraventricular (or continuous) drainage to reduce pressure. A drainage bag attached to the system is kept at the level of the ventricles and can be lowered to decrease ICP.

NURSING ALERT If the external ventricular drain (EVD) is unclamped for CSF drainage, carefully monitor the level of the collection container. If the container is too low, improper CSF decompression could lower ICP too rapidly, causing bleeding and pain.

In the bolt method the end of the bolt is placed into the subarachnoid space. The bolt cannot be adequately secured in a small child's pliant skull, although special modifications have been developed for children under 6 years of age.

NURSING ALERT The bolt is stabilized with dressings, but these are not changed or disturbed, even to check the site.

The placement of the bolt is not adjusted by anyone except the neurosurgeon who placed the device. The neurosurgeon is notified if a satisfactory wave form is not observed.

An epidural sensor can be placed between the dura and the skull through a burr hole and connected to a stopcock assembly and a transducer, which provides a readout of the pressure. Although less invasive, correlation of pressure readings may be inconsistent. In infants a fontanel transducer can be used to detect impulses from a pressure sensor and convert them to electrical energy. The electrical energy is then converted to visible waves or numerical readings on an oscilloscope. ICP measurement from the anterior fontanel, although noninvasive, may prove to be inaccurate if the equipment is poorly placed or inconsistently recalibrated. The intraparenchymal pressure monitoring device (e.g., Camino) is a result of fiberoptic technology and has a reliable performance.

Since ICP can be increased by direct instillation of solutions, antibiotics are administered systemically if a positive CSF culture is obtained. However, ICP monitoring rarely causes infection. Since CSF is a body fluid, isolation precautions may be implemented according to hospital policy (see Infection Control, Chapter 27).

Nurses caring for patients with intracranial monitoring devices must be acquainted with the system, assist with insertion, interpret the monitor readings, and be able to distinguish between danger signals and mechanical dysfunction. Because systemic blood pressure, ICP, and therefore cerebral perfusion pressure (CPP) are normally lower in children, the age of the child must be taken into account when deciding what constitutes abnormally high ICP or abnormally low CPP.

For increased ICP resulting from cerebral edema, several medical measures are available. Osmotic diuretics (mannitol) are reserved to control intracranial hypertension that does not respond to sedation and CSF drainage. Recording and analyzing the child's volume state, plasma sodium concentration, and serum osmolarity can avert potential fluid and electrolyte problems.

The infusion is generally given slowly but may be pushed rapidly if there is herniation or impending herniation. Because of the profound diuretic effect of the drug, an indwelling catheter is inserted to ensure bladder emptying. $PaCO_2$ should be maintained at 25 to 30 mm Hg to produce vasoconstriction, which reduces CBF, thereby decreasing ICP.

Nursing Activities. In cases of high levels of increased ICP, nursing procedures tend to trigger reactive pressure waves in many children. For example, increased intrathoracic or abdominal pressure will be transmitted to the cranium. The goals of monitoring a child who is neurologically compromised include maintaining CPP; controlling ICP, cerebral edema, and factors that increase cerebral metabolism (fever, seizures); and maintaining hemodynamic stability. Particular care is taken in positioning these patients to avoid neck vein compression, which may further increase ICP by interfering with venous return.

NURSING ALERT The head of the bed is elevated 15 to 30 degrees and the child positioned so that the head is maintained in a midline to facilitate venous drainage and avoid jugular compression. Turning side to side is contraindicated because of the risk of jugular compression.

Sandbags or other support devices may be needed to maintain correct head position. The child can be propped to one side or the other, and the use of a pressure-relieving or pressure-decreasing mattress decreases the chance of prolonged pressure to vulnerable skin areas. Frequent clinical assessment of the child cannot be replaced by an ICP monitoring device.

It is important to avoid activities that may increase ICP by causing pain, emotional stress, or crying, or those that might trigger a convulsive seizure. Gentle range-of-motion exercises can be carried out but should not be performed vigorously. Nontherapeutic touch can cause an increase in ICP. Any disturbing procedures to be performed should be scheduled to take advantage of therapies that reduce ICP, such as osmotherapy and sedation. Efforts are made to minimize or eliminate environmental noise. Assessment and intervention to relieve pain are important nursing functions to decrease ICP.

➤ **NURSING TIP** Placing earphones over a child's ears has been shown to lower ICP, heart rate, and blood pressure significantly. A greater decline was achieved when soothing music was played through the earphones (Wincek, as reported by Wong, 1988).

Although controversies remain, nurses have studied intracranial responses to environmental stimuli in an effort to minimize unnecessary elevations and decrease secondary brain damage. The data support the theory that touch may help to stabilize ICP and that a child in coma may still re-

TABLE 37-3 Effects of Altered Pituitary Secretion

MEASUREMENT	DI	SIADH
Urinary output	Increased	Decreased
Specific gravity	Decreased	Increased
Serum sodium	Increased (hypernatremia)	Decreased (hyponatremia)

ceive and process verbal and tactile stimuli at some level. The presence of family members and calm reassurances can help to decrease ICP, so observing the child's responses is the best guide to providing stimulation (Farley, 1990).

Suctioning. Suctioning and percussion are poorly tolerated and are therefore contraindicated unless there are concurrent respiratory problems. Hypoxia and the Valsalva maneuver associated with cough both acutely elevate ICP. Vibration, which does not increase ICP, accomplishes excellent results and should be tried first if treatment is needed. If suctioning is necessary, it should be used judiciously and preceded by hyperventilation with 100% oxygen, which can be monitored during suctioning with a pulse oxygen sensor reading to determine oxygen saturation.

Nutrition and Hydration

Fluids and calories are supplied initially by the intravenous route (see Chapter 28). An intravenous infusion is started early, and the type of fluid administered is determined by the general condition of the patient. Fluid therapy requires careful monitoring and adjustment based on neurologic signs and electrolyte determinations. Often comatose children are unable to cope with the same amounts of fluid they could tolerate at other times, and overhydration must be avoided to prevent fatal cerebral edema.

Later, nutrition is provided in a balanced formula given by nasogastric or gastrostomy tube. The nasogastric tube is usually taped in place with care to prevent pressure on the nares. Most children have continuous feedings, but if bolus feedings are used, the tube is rinsed with water after each feeding. Tubes are replaced according to unit policy. Nostrils are alternated with each replacement to prevent nasal irritation and pressure. Overfeeding is avoided to prevent vomiting with its attendant danger of aspiration. Stomach contents are aspirated and measured before feeding to ascertain the amount remaining in the stomach. The aspirated contents are refed. If the residual volume is excessive (depending on the size of the child), the dietitian and physician should be consulted regarding alteration of the formula composition to provide the needed calories and nutrients in a smaller volume.

Hydration is maintained in the same manner. When cerebral edema is a threat, fluids may be restricted to reduce the chance of fluid overload. Skin and mucous membranes are examined for signs of dehydration. Observation for signs of altered fluid balance related to abnormal pituitary secretions is a part of nursing care.

Altered Pituitary Secretion. An altered ability to handle fluid loads is attributed in part to the syndrome of inappropriate antidiuretic hormone (SIADH) and diabetes insipidus (DI) resulting from hypothalamic dysfunction (see Chapter 38). SIADH frequently accompanies CNS diseases such as head injury, meningitis, encephalitis, brain abscess, brain tumor, and subarachnoid hemorrhage. In the child with SIADH, scant quantities of urine are excreted, electrolyte analysis reveals hyponatremia and hyposmolality, and manifestations of overhydration are evident. It is important to evaluate all parameters, since the reduced urinary output might be erroneously interpreted as a sign of dehydration.

The treatment of SIADH consists of restriction of fluids until serum electrolytes and osmolality return to normal levels. Since SIADH frequently occurs with meningitis in children, fluid restriction is often prescribed. Likewise, DI may occur following intracranial trauma. There is increased urinary volume and the accompanying danger of dehydration (see Table 37-3 for comparison of fluid changes in SIADH and DI). Adequate replacement of fluids is essential, and observation of electrolyte balance is necessary to detect signs of hypernatremia and hyperosmolality. Exogenous vasopressin may be administered.

Medications

The cause of unconsciousness determines specific drug therapies. Children with infectious processes are given antibiotics appropriate to the disease and the infecting organism, and corticosteroids are prescribed for inflammatory conditions and edema. Cerebral edema is an indication for osmotherapy with osmotic diuretics. Sedatives or anticonvulsants are prescribed for seizure activity. Sedation in the combative child provides amnesic and anxiolytic properties in conjunction with a paralytic agent. The combination decreases ICP and allows treatment of cerebral edema. Usual drugs include morphine, midazolam (Versed), and pancuronium. Midazolam is attractive because of its short half-life.

NURSING ALERT When used for seizures, phenytoin should be administered slowly by direct IV push at a rate not to exceed 50 mg/min. Since phenytoin precipitates in the presence of glucose, only normal saline is used for flushing the needle or catheter.

Deep coma, induced by administration of barbiturates, is controversial in the management of ICP. Barbiturates are currently reserved for the reduction of increased ICP when all else has failed. Barbiturates decrease the cerebral metabolic rate for oxygen and protect the brain during times of reduced CPP. Barbiturate coma requires extensive monitoring, cardiovascular and respiratory support, and ICP monitoring to assess response to therapy. Paralyzing agents, such as pancuronium (Pavulon), also may be needed to aid in performing diagnostic tests, improving effectiveness of therapy, and reducing risks of secondary complications. Elevation of ICP and/or heart rate in patients who are being given paralyzing agents or are under sedation may indicate the need for another dose of either or both medications.

Thermoregulation

Hyperthermia often accompanies cerebral dysfunction, and if present, measures are implemented to reduce the temperature to prevent brain damage from hyperthermia and to reduce metabolic demands generated by the increased body temperature. Antipyretics are the method of choice for fever reduction; cooling devices are used for hyperthermia (see Controlling Elevated Temperatures, Chapter 27). Laboratory tests and other methods are used in an attempt to determine the cause, if any, of the hyperthermia. Shivering responses triggered by a cooling blanket can often be alleviated by lukewarm to warm sponging. Treatment with hypothermia and barbiturates increases the risk of iatrogenic complications.

Elimination

A retention catheter is usually inserted in the acute phase, although diapers may be used and weighed to record urinary output. The child who formerly had bowel and bladder control is generally incontinent. If the child remains comatose for a long period, the indwelling catheter may be removed and periodic bladder emptying accomplished by intermittent catheterization. Stool softeners are usually sufficient to maintain bowel function, but suppositories or enemas may be needed occasionally for adequate elimination and to prevent an impaction. The passage of liquid stool after a period of no bowel activity is usually a sign of an impaction. To avoid this preventable problem, daily recording of bowel activity is essential.

Hygienic Care

Routine measures for cleansing and maintaining skin integrity are an integral part of nursing care of the unconscious child. Skinfolds require special attention to prevent excoriation. The child who is unable to move is prone to develop tissue breakdown and pressure necrosis; therefore the child is placed on a resilient appliance (e.g., alternating-pressure or water-filled mattress) to prevent pressure on prominent areas of the body. The goal is prevention by regular change of position and inspection of vulnerable areas, such as the ankle, heels, trochanter, and shoulder. Since unconscious children undergo numerous invasive procedures, these skin sites require special assessment and intervention to promote healing and to prevent infection. Bed linen and any clothing are kept dry and free of wrinkles. Rubbing the back and extremities with lotion or other lubricating preparation stimulates circulation and helps prevent drying of the skin. However, reddened, nonblanching skin (Stage 1 pressure areas) is not massaged to prevent further tissue damage (see Maintaining healthy skin, Chapter 27). If the child requires surgery or radiography, the nurse checks all dressings, bony sites, catheters, and intravenous access lines.

Mouth care is performed at least twice daily, since the mouth tends to become dry or coated with mucus. The teeth are carefully brushed with a soft toothbrush or cleaned with gauze saturated with saline. Commercially prepared cleansing devices, such as Toothettes, are convenient for cleansing the mouth and teeth. Lips are coated with ointment (e.g., petrolatum, A & D ointment, or wax-based lipstick-style balm) to protect them from drying, cracking, or blistering.

The deeply comatose child is also prone to eye irritation. The corneal reflexes are absent; therefore the eyes are easily irritated or damaged by linen, dust, or other substances that may come in contact with them. There is excessive dryness as a result of decreased secretions, especially if the child is undergoing osmotherapy to reduce or prevent brain edema, and incomplete closure of the eyes.

NURSING ALERT The eyes are examined regularly and carefully for early signs of irritation or inflammation. Artificial tears (methylcellulose) are placed in the eyes every 1 to 2 hours. Sometimes eye dressings are needed to protect the eyes from possible damage.

The hair is combed and styled neatly. Long hair is usually braided and secured with rubber bands. The scalp is kept clean with dry or wet shampoos as needed. The child's head may be shaved for tests or surgical procedures. If so, the hair is saved, if possible, and given to the family.

Positioning and Exercise

The unconscious child is positioned to prevent aspiration of saliva, nasogastric secretions, and vomitus and to minimize ICP. The head of the bed is elevated, and the child is placed in a side-lying or semiprone position. A small, firm pillow is placed under the head, and the uppermost limbs are flexed and supported with pillows. The weight of the body should not rest on the dependent arm. In the semiprone position the child lies with the dependent arm at the side behind the body, the opposite side supported on pillows, and the uppermost arm and leg flexed and resting on the pillows. This position prevents undue pressure on the dependent extremities. The dependent position of the face encourages drainage of secretions and prevents the flaccid tongue from obstructing the airway.

Normal range of motion exercises help to maintain function and prevent contractures of joints. Exercises should be done gently and with full range of motion. A small rolled pad can be placed in the palms to help maintain proper position of fingers; footboards or high-top shoes (e.g., running or tennis shoes) can be used to help prevent footdrop; splinting may be needed to prevent severe contractures of the wrist, knee, or ankle in decerebrate children.

Stimulation

Sensory stimulation is important in the care of the unconscious child, just as it is in the care of the alert child. For the temporarily unconscious or semiconscious child, sensory stimulation helps to arouse the child to the conscious state and orient the child in terms of time and place. Auditory and tactile stimulation are especially valuable. Tactile stimulation is not appropriate for the child in whom it may elicit an undesirable response. However, for other children tactile contact often has a relaxing and calming effect.

NURSING CARE PLAN
The Unconscious Child

NURSING DIAGNOSIS: High risk for suffocation (aspiration): ineffective airway clearance related to depressed sensorium, impaired motor function

PATIENT GOAL 1: Will maintain patent airway

• **NURSING INTERVENTIONS/*RATIONALES***

Position for optimum ventilation
- Insert oral airway if indicated
- Position with neck slightly extended and nose in "sniffing" position *to open trachea fully*
- Avoid neck hyperextension, *which can block airway*
- Place in semiprone or side-lying position *to prevent aspiration*

Remove accumulated secretions promptly *to prevent aspiration*

Administer care of endotracheal tube or tracheostomy if appropriate; have equipment available for emergency insertion if indicated for respiratory distress *to prevent delay in treatment*

Monitor artificial ventilation

• **EXPECTED OUTCOME**

Airway remains patent

NURSING DIAGNOSIS: High risk for injury related to physical immobility, depressed sensorium, intracranial pathology

PATIENT GOAL 1: Will maintain stable ICP

• **NURSING INTERVENTIONS/*RATIONALES***

Elevate head of bed 15 to 30 degrees with child's head in midline position *to facilitate venous drainage and avoid jugular compression*

Avoid positions or activities that increase ICP
- Pressure on neck veins
  - Turning side-to-side is contraindicated *because of risk of jugular compression*
- Flexion or hyperextension of neck
- Head rotation
- Valsalva maneuver
- Painful stimuli
- Respiratory procedures (especially suctioning, percussion)

Prevent constipation *because Valsalva maneuver increases ICP*
- *Administer stool softener as prescribed
- Closely monitor bowel elimination when child is receiving codeine *because of its constipating effect*

Minimize emotional stress and crying *because they cause increased ICP*
- Provide quiet, subdued environment
- Reduce environmental noise (e.g., placing earphones over child's ears *has been shown to lower ICP, heart rate, and blood pressure)*
- Provide pleasant auditory experiences
- Use therapeutic touch
- Avoid emotionally stressful conversation (e.g., about pain, condition, prognosis)
- *Administer sedation, if ordered, for extreme agitation or restlessness

Prevent or relieve pain, *since pain causes increased ICP*
- Closely observe child for signs of pain, especially changes in behavior (e.g., agitation); increased heart rate, respiratory rate, and blood pressure *(usually increase with pain);* decreased oxygen saturation
- Observe child's response during times of induced or suspected pain
- Observe child's response following a painful procedure or the administration of analgesia
- Use pain assessment record (see Chapter 26)
- *Administer paralyzing and analgesic agents if prescribed

Schedule disturbing procedures to take advantage of therapies that reduce ICP (e.g., bathe child after sedation or osmotherapy)

Monitor ICP monitoring device

• **EXPECTED OUTCOMES**

ICP remains within safe limits

Child shows no evidence of sustained increased ICP

PATIENT GOAL 2: Will exhibit no signs of cerebral hypoxia

• **NURSING INTERVENTIONS/*RATIONALES***

Maintain patent airway *because respiratory obstruction leads to cardiac arrest, and cerebral hypoxia lasting longer than 4 minutes nearly always causes irreversible brain damage*

Provide oxygen as indicated by objective signs or as ordered

*Hyperventilate at prescribed intervals if ordered

Monitor blood gases and pH

If child is on mechanical ventilation:
- Monitor for correct settings, proper functioning
- Prepare to provide artificial ventilation in case of ventilatory failure; have manual resuscitation bag at bedside

*Administer medications as ordered *to prevent cerebral edema and improve cerebral circulation*

• **EXPECTED OUTCOME**

Child breathes easily; respirations are within normal limits (see inside back cover)

PATIENT GOAL 3: Will exhibit no evidence of cerebral edema

• **NURSING INTERVENTIONS/*RATIONALES***

Elevate head of bed to 15 to 30 degrees *to facilitate venous drainage*

Maintain intravenous fluids as prescribed
- Avoid overhydration *to prevent cerebral edema*

Monitor intake and output

Monitor electrolyte balance and specific gravity *to detect signs of hypernatremia and hyperosmolality because diabetes insipidus and the syndrome of inappropriate antidiuretic hormone frequently occur with CNS diseases and trauma*

*Administer hyperosmolar fluids as prescribed

*Administer corticosteroids as ordered

• **EXPECTED OUTCOME**

Child exhibits no signs of sustained increased ICP

---

*Dependent nursing action.

NURSING CARE PLAN
The Unconscious Child—cont'd

PATIENT GOAL 4: Will experience no seizures

• **NURSING INTERVENTIONS/*RATIONALES***

Avoid stimulation that precipitates undesirable responses
Schedule nursing activities for minimum disturbance
*Administer antiepileptic drugs as prescribed
- Carefully administer phenytoin (Dilantin) if prescribed
- Administer drug slowly; *too-rapid administration may cause cardiac dysrhythmias*
- Infuse completely in 1 hour *because drug tends to precipitate*
- Never mix phenytoin with 5% dextrose; *drug will precipitate*
- Dilute phenytoin with normal saline *to decrease vein irritation and pain*

• **EXPECTED OUTCOME**

Child exhibits no seizure activity or undue restlessness and agitation

PATIENT GOAL 5: Will exhibit stable body temperature

• **NURSING INTERVENTIONS/*RATIONALES***

Closely monitor child's temperature *because elevations often occur with CNS dysfunction*
Remove excess coverings
*Administer antipyretics if prescribed for fever
Give tepid sponge bath, if indicated, only for hyperthermia, not for fever, *because it may induce shivering*
Apply and monitor hypothermia blanket if indicated and ordered; administer antishivering agents, if ordered, *because shivering increases ICP and metabolic rate*

• **EXPECTED OUTCOME**

Body temperature remains within safe limits (see inside back cover)

PATIENT GOAL 6: Will exhibit no evidence of respiratory tract infection

• **NURSING INTERVENTIONS/*RATIONALES***

Turn frequently—at least every 2 hours, as tolerated, unless contraindicated by increased ICP
Keep persons with upper respiratory tract infection away from child
Use good handwashing technique
Keep all equipment in contact with child clean or sterile
Provide good oral hygiene *to decrease presence of infective organisms*
Perform chest physiotherapy if prescribed and as tolerated; avoid percussion, *since it can increase ICP*

• **EXPECTED OUTCOME**

Child exhibits no evidence of pulmonary dysfunction

PATIENT GOAL 7: Will experience no corneal irritation

• **NURSING INTERVENTIONS/*RATIONALES***

Patch eye, if indicated, *for protection*
Keep lids completely closed *to protect corneas when corneal reflexes are absent*
Instill "artificial tears" *to lubricate eyes*
Assess eyes carefully for early signs of irritation or inflammation

• **EXPECTED OUTCOME**

Corneas remain clear and moist

PATIENT GOAL 8: Will exhibit no breakdown in mucous membrane integrity

• **NURSING INTERVENTIONS/*RATIONALES***

Provide meticulous mouth care, *since mouth tends to become dry or coated with mucus*
Avoid drying products (e.g., lemon and glycerin)

• **EXPECTED OUTCOME**

Mucous membranes remain clear, moist, and free of irritation

PATIENT GOAL 9: Will experience no physical injury

• **NURSING INTERVENTIONS/*RATIONALES***

Keep siderails up *to prevent falls*
Pad hard surfaces *that may injure extremities during spontaneous or involuntary movements*

• **EXPECTED OUTCOME**

Child remains free of physical injury

PATIENT GOAL 10: Will maintain limb flexibility and full range of motion

• **NURSING INTERVENTIONS/*RATIONALES***

Perform passive range-of-motion exercises *to prevent contractures*
Position *to reduce contractures*
- Place small, rolled pad in palms to *maintain proper position of fingers*
- Use footboard or ankle-high shoes to *prevent footdrop*
- Splint joints, if needed, *to prevent severe contractures of wrists, knees, and ankles*

• **EXPECTED OUTCOME**

Joints remain flexible and retain full range of motion

Nursing Diagnosis: High risk for impaired skin integrity related to immobility, body secretions, invasive procedures

PATIENT GOAL 1: Will maintain skin integrity

• **NURSING INTERVENTIONS/*RATIONALES***

Place child on pressure-reducing surface *to prevent tissue breakdown and pressure necrosis*
Change position frequently unless contraindicated by increased ICP
Protect pressure points (e.g., trochanter, sacrum, ankle, heels, shoulder, occiput)
Inspect skin surfaces regularly for signs of irritation, redness, evidence of pressure

*Dependent nursing action.

Continued.

Cleanse skin regularly, at least once daily
Protect skinfolds and surfaces that rub together *to prevent excoriation*
Keep clothing and linen clean, dry, and free of wrinkles
Carry out good perineal care
Gently massage skin with lotion or other lubricating substance, unless on existing reddened pressure areas, *to stimulate circulation and prevent drying*
Protect lips with cream or ointment *to prevent drying and cracking*

• **EXPECTED OUTCOME**
Skin remains clean, intact, and free of irritation

NURSING DIAGNOSIS: Feeding, bathing/hygiene, toileting self-care deficits (level 4) related to physical immobility, perceptual and cognitive impairment

PATIENT GOAL 1: Will receive optimum nutrition

• **NURSING INTERVENTIONS/*RATIONALES***
Provide nourishment in manner suitable to child's condition
Monitor intravenous feedings when ordered
Record intake and output
*Feed prescribed formula by means of nasogastric or gastrostomy tube
Weigh daily or as ordered *to monitor nutritional adequacy*

• **EXPECTED OUTCOME**
Child obtains sufficient nourishment

PATIENT GOAL 2: Will receive proper hygienic care

• **NURSING INTERVENTIONS/*RATIONALES***
Bathe daily or more often if indicated
Dress appropriately
Keep hair clean, combed, and styled

• **EXPECTED OUTCOME**
Child appears clean and as well groomed as possible within limitations of condition

PATIENT GOAL 3: Will void and defecate adequately

• **NURSING INTERVENTIONS/*RATIONALES***
Provide sufficient liquid intake, unless contraindicated by cerebral edema or if overhydration is a threat
Apply urine-collecting device or insert indwelling catheter (if ordered)
Provide proper care of catheter
Clean skin well after each elimination *to prevent skin irritation*
Diaper as needed *to contain stool and urine*
Check abdomen for evidence of distention
Measure abdominal girth *to detect enlargement*
*Administer stool softener *to prevent constipation*
*Administer suppositories or enema as indicated *to promote evacuation*

*Dependent nursing action.

• **EXPECTED OUTCOMES**
Child eliminates sufficient urine (specify)
Bowel is evacuated daily
Child's diaper area remains clean and free of irritation

NURSING DIAGNOSIS: Sensory/perceptual alterations (visual, auditory, kinesthetic, gustatory, tactile, olfactory) related to central nervous system impairment, bed rest

PATIENT GOAL 1: Will receive appropriate sensory stimulation

• **NURSING INTERVENTIONS/*RATIONALES***
Provide tactile stimulation as tolerated
Provide auditory stimulation (elg., by voice, radio, music box)
Provide visual stimuli appropriate for age
Provide proprioceptive stimulation (e.g., by rocking, cuddling)
Encourage family to participate in stimulation program
Demonstrate for family how and where to touch child

• **EXPECTED OUTCOMES**
Child receives sensory stimulation appropriate to age and condition
Child appears relaxed and rests quietly
Stimulation does not induce seizures or increase ICP

PATIENT GOAL 2: Will exhibit no evidence of pain

• **NURSING INTERVENTIONS/*RATIONALES***
Assess for evidence of pain
Use pain assessment record *to document effectiveness of interventions*
Administer pain medication as needed

• **EXPECTED OUTCOME**
Child exhibits no evidence of pain

Nursing Diagnosis: Altered family processes related to a child hospitalized with a potentially fatal condition or permanent disability

PATIENT (FAMILY) GOAL 1: Will receive adequate support

• **NURSING INTERVENTIONS/*RATIONALES* AND EXPECTED OUTCOMES**
See Nursing Care Plan: The Family of the Ill or Hospitalized Child, Chapter 26

PATIENT (FAMILY) GOAL 2: Will express feelings and concerns

• **NURSING INTERVENTIONS/*RATIONALES***
Provide needed information
Answer family's questions; encourage expression of feelings
Refer to persons or agencies for further information and clarification
Support parents' decisions

• **EXPECTED OUTCOME**
Family verbalizes feelings and concerns

When the child's condition permits, holding or rocking the child has a soothing effect and provides the body contact needed by young children.

The auditory sense is often present in a state of coma. Hearing is the last sense to be lost and the first one to be regained; therefore the child should be spoken to as any other child. Conversation around the child should not include thoughtless or derogatory remarks. A radio playing soft music, a music box, or a record player is frequently used to provide auditory stimulation. Singing the child's favorite songs or reading a favorite story is a tactic used to maintain the child's contact with a familiar world. Having parents tape songs or stories provides a continuous source of familiar stimulation. Above all, it is important to remember that this is a child who has all the needs of any ill child.

Family Support

Dealing with the parents of an unconscious child is especially difficult. They may demonstrate all the guilt, fear, hostility, and anxiety of any parent of a seriously ill child (see Chapter 23). In addition, these parents are faced with the uncertain outcome of the cerebral dysfunction. The fear of death, mental retardation, or other permanent disability is present. Nursing intervention with parents depends on the nature of the pathologic condition, the personality of the parents, and the parent-child relationship before injury or illness.

The child may regain consciousness within a short time. If there is little or no residual effect, the child will be dismissed to home care fairly soon. The parents need the most intensive nursing intervention during the period of crisis and uncertainty. During the recovery phase they are given information, information is clarified, and they are encouraged to become involved in the child's care. Often the child's hospitalization is brief; however, some children require extended hospitalization for intensive therapy and rehabilitation.

The parents of children who die within hours or days require the support and guidance that the parents of any dying child would need in coping with the reality of the death and resolving their grief (see Chapter 23).

Probably the most difficult situations are those that involve children who are unconscious permanently or for an indefinite period. Unlike parents who lose a child through death, the finality is lacking for these parents, often leaving them in a state of suspended grief. The presence of the child renders the parents unable to resolve the loss. Like parents of dying children, parents of the comatose child search for any signs of hope. Well-meaning friends and relatives relate instances of miraculous recoveries. The parents seek confirmation and support for such possibilities and assign erroneous meanings to any sign in the child, such as reflexive muscle contractions, that might be interpreted as evidence of recovery.

Like parents who lose a child through death, the parents of the child lost to their world attempt to reconstitute a representation of the child. They bring items that belong to the child, such as favorite toys, music, and other objects cherished by the child. This is interpreted as an attempt to provide stimulation for the child in the hope of eliciting a response, to let the hospital staff know the child as the unique individual he or she was so that the parents' distress can be better appreciated, and to reconstitute an image of the child "lost" to them and for whom they mourn. An awareness of these behaviors and coping mechanisms provides nurses with the understanding that helps them support the parents in their grief process.

Superimposed on the process of grieving for the "lost" child, parents may be faced with difficult decisions. First, there is the child whose brain is so severely damaged that vital functions must be maintained by artificial means. The parents must make the final decision to remove life-support systems. Since the decision is so difficult for parents, the practitioner is frequently placed in a position of making the decision indirectly. After providing the parents with all the information, the physician will suggest that the child be removed from the life support. The approach relieves the parents of the decision and can be effective, but it is based on an evaluation of the parents' intellectual level and emotional state. Sometimes parents may even choose to refuse treatment if they believe it to be best for the child and the family (informed dissent). At other times parents request that "everything possible" be done for the child.

The nurses can be instrumental in providing guidance and clarifying information—a valued but demanding undertaking. It is not unusual for the family to ask the same questions and to compare responses elicited from different staff members. A child's death is an intensely personal issue that deserves direct involvement by the nurse and auxiliary support systems.

There is also the child who has survived the illness or injury that produced the brain damage but remains in a persistent vegetative state. In such a situation the parents must decide whether to place the child in an extended care facility or care for the child at home. During these decisions the nurse can listen to the parents' discussions regarding alternatives, provide information where appropriate, and support the family in their decision. The nurse can help the family prepare for the transfer of the child and make referrals to persons or agencies that can provide additional assistance.

There is also the child who survived the cerebral insult, who is not comatose, but whose physical and/or mental capacity is limited, either minimally or severely. Families of such children must cope with the long and tedious rehabilitation process and uncertain outcome. The drain on financial, emotional, and social resources can be enormous.

For parents who choose to care for their child at home, planning for home care begins early in the process of recovery. The family should become involved with the care of the child as soon as they indicate an interest and ability to do so. They will need education and support in learning to care for the child, regular follow-up observation and assessment of the home management, and planning for some respite care of the child. Parents need to understand that it is important to plan for periodic relief from the continual care of the child (see Discharge Planning and Home Care, Chapter 26, and Family-Centered Home Care, Chapter 25).

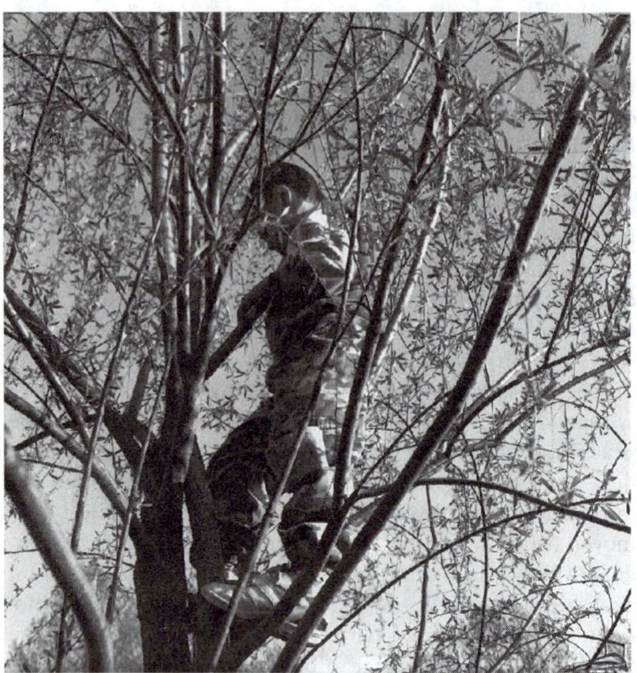

FIG. 37-6 Children possess a sense of adventure and wonder; however, falls remain the leading cause of head injury in children under 5 years of age.

Evaluation

The effectiveness of nursing interventions for the unconscious child is determined by continual reassessment and evaluation of care based on the following observational guidelines and expected outcomes:

1. Monitor child's neurologic signs, vital signs, and behavior. Compare behavior with pre–illness/trauma state.
2. Observe child's response to nursing activities, therapies, and diagnostic procedures; monitor ICP.
3. Observe child's color, position, and motor activity; measure fluid and nutritional intake and output.
4. Monitor status of child's respiratory, renal, and gastrointestinal systems and skin.
5. Observe family behaviors and interview members regarding their understandings and their feelings and concerns.

Expected outcomes:
See Nursing Care Plan, pp. 1688-1690.

HEAD INJURY

Head injury is a pathologic process involving the scalp, skull, meninges, or brain as a result of mechanical force. According to national statistics and the Safe Kids Campaign,* injuries are the number one health risk for children and the leading cause of death in children older than 1 year of age. Yearly, one child in four in the United States will suffer an injury serious enough to require medical attention. Tragically, 8000 children are killed every year by injuries. It has been estimated that 300 per 100,000 children per year have a traumatic brain injury and that 10 per 100,000 children per year die as a result of the brain injury. Studies indicate that as many as three fourths of the childhood deaths caused by mechanical trauma are the direct result of a brain injury.

Etiology

The three major causes of brain damage in childhood in order of importance are falls, motor vehicle injuries, and bicycle injuries (Fig. 37-6). Neurologic injury accounts for the highest mortality, with boys usually affected twice as often as girls. In motor vehicle accidents children less than 2 years of age are almost exclusively injured as passengers, whereas older children may also be injured as pedestrians or cyclists. The majority of deaths from brain trauma caused by bicycle injuries occur between the ages of 5 and 15 years. With the advent of bike helmet laws, this should be a decreasing trend.

The exposed nature of the head renders it particularly vulnerable to external violence, and many of the physical characteristics of children predispose them to craniocerebral trauma. For example, infants are frequently left unattended on beds, in high chairs, and in other places from which they can fall. Because the head of an infant or toddler is proportionately large and heavy in relation to other body parts, it is the most likely to be injured. Incomplete motor development contributes to falls at young ages, and the natural curiosity and exuberance of children increase their risk of an injury.

Pathophysiology

The pathology of brain injury is directly related to the force of impact. Intracranial contents (brain, blood, CSF) are damaged because the force is too great to be absorbed by the skull and musculoligamentous support of the head. The elastic, pliable skulls of infants and young children absorb much of the direct energy of physical impact to the head and afford some protection to intracranial structures. Although nervous tissue is delicate, it usually requires a severe blow to cause significant damage.

A child's response to head injury is different from that of adults. The larger head size and insufficient musculoskeletal support render the very young child particularly vulnerable to acceleration-deceleration injuries. The surface area of the child's scalp is large with remarkable vascularity; therefore a child can bleed to death from a severe scalp laceration.

Primary head injuries are those that occur at a time of trauma and include skull fracture, contusions, intracranial hematoma, and diffuse injury. Subsequent complications include hypoxic brain damage, increased ICP, infection, and cerebral edema. The predominant feature of a child's brain injury is the diffuse amount of swelling that occurs. Hypoxia and hypercapnia threaten the energy requirements of the brain and increase CBF. The added volume

*SAFE KIDS, 111 Michigan Ave., N.W., Washington, DC 20010-2970; (202)939-4993.

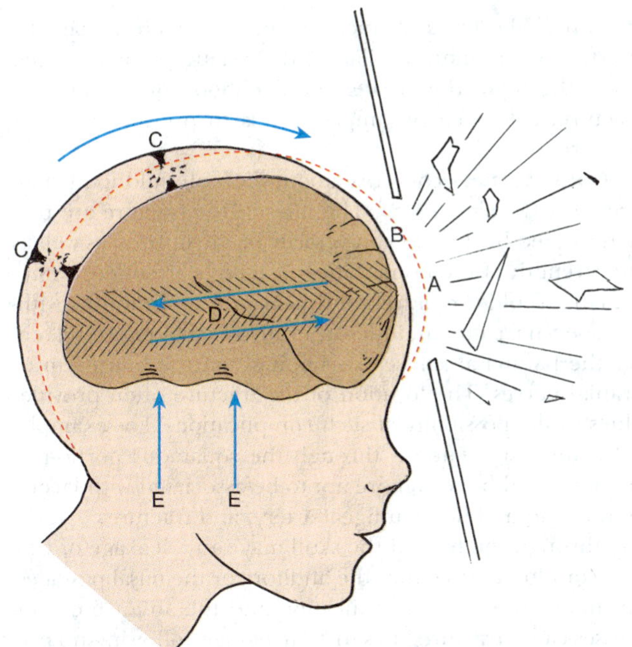

FIG. 37-7 Mechanical distortion of cranium during closed head injury. **A,** Preinjury contour of skull. **B,** Immediate postinjury contour of skull. **C,** Torn subdural vessels. **D,** Shearing forces. **E,** Trauma from contact with floor of cranium. (Redrawn from Grubb RL, Coxe WS: Central nervous system trauma: cranial. In Eliasson SG, Presky AL, Hardin WB Jr, editors: *Neurological pathophysiology,* New York, 1974, Oxford University Press.)

across the blood-brain barrier plus the loss of autoregulation exacerbates cerebral edema. Pressure inside the skull greater than arterial pressure results in inadequate perfusion.

Cerebral hyperemia occurs more often in children, and this volume expansion may account for children's tendency to develop intracranial hypertension (Johnson, 1988). However, because the cranium of very young children has the ability to expand and the thin skull is more compliant, they may tolerate increases in ICP better than older children and adults.

Physical forces act on the head through ***acceleration, deceleration,*** or ***deformation.*** Acceleration or deceleration is more descriptive of the circumstances responsible for most head injuries. When the stationary head receives a blow, the sudden acceleration causes deformation of the skull and mass movement of the brain. Continued movement of the intracranial contents allows the brain to strike parts of the skull (e.g., the sharp edges of the sphenoid or the irregular surface of the anterior fossa) or the edges of the tentorium.

Although the brain volume remains unchanged, significant distortion and cavitation take place as the brain changes shape in response to the force transmitted from the impact to the skull. This deformation can cause bruising at the point of impact ***(coup)*** and/or at a distance as the brain collides with the unyielding surfaces far removed from the point of impact ***(contrecoup)*** (Fig. 37-7). Children with an acceleration/deceleration injury demonstrate diffuse generalized cerebral swelling produced by increased blood volume or a redistribution of cerebral blood volume (cerebral hyperemia) rather than by increased water content (edema), as seen in adults. Thus a blow to the occipital region can cause severe injury to the frontal and temporal areas of the brain. Sudden deceleration, as takes place during a fall, causes the greatest cerebral injury at the point of impact.

Another effect of brain movement is ***shearing stresses,*** which are caused by unequal movement or different rates of acceleration at various levels of the brain. A shearing force may tear small arteries that travel from the cerebral surfaces through the meninges to the dural sinuses to cause subdural hemorrhages. Shearing or stretching effects can also be transmitted to nerve fibers. Maximum stress from the shearing force occurs at the interface between structures of different density so that the gray matter (cell body) rapidly accelerates while the white matter (axons) tends to lag behind. Although shearing forces are maximum at the cerebral surface and extend toward the center of rotation within the brain, the most serious effects are frequently in the area of the brainstem.

Another source of damage occurs when severe compression of the skull causes the brain to be forced through the tentorial opening. This can produce irreparable damage to the brainstem (see Fig. 37-8). Since the uncus of the temporal lobe is the presenting part, this complication is usually referred to as uncal herniation.

As a whole, head injuries can be regarded as localized or generalized. In ***localized injuries*** the force is spent on a local area of both the skull and underlying tissues; in ***generalized injuries*** the force is transmitted to the entire skull, causing widespread movement, distortion, and damage. Local injuries frequently cause hemorrhage and infection, but generalized trauma is associated with a higher mortality. Many head injuries involve both localized and generalized disorders. Patients with mild head injuries have a GCS evaluation of 13 to 15; those with moderate head injuries have a GCS of 9 to 12; and a GCS of 8 or less indicates severe injury.

Concussion. The most common head injury is ***concussion,*** a transient and reversible neuronal dysfunction with instantaneous loss of awareness and responsiveness from trauma to the head that persists for a relatively short time, usually minutes or hours. It is generally followed by amnesia for the moment of the injury and a variable period before the injury. This posttraumatic amnesia is characteristic and reflects the extent and severity of injury to the brain after blunt trauma. Posttraumatic amnesia consists of two parts: (1) retrograde amnesia, the period of time before impact for which the patient has no memory, and (2) anterograde amnesia, the period of memory loss after injury. Amnesia in both these periods tends to lessen with time, although there is some permanent amnesia. The common misconception that loss of consciousness is the hallmark of concussion is not true, especially for children. Concussion is correctly defined as "a traumatically induced alteration in mental status." Confusion and amnesia following head impact are the hallmarks of concussion.

The pathogenesis of concussion is still unclear but may be a result of shearing forces that cause stretching, compression, and tearing of nerve fibers, particularly in the area of the central brainstem, the seat of the reticular activating system. It has also been suggested that the anatomic alterations of nerve fibers cause the release of large quantities of acetylcholine into the CSF and a reduction in oxygen consumption with increased lactate production.

Contusion and Laceration. The terms ***contusion*** and ***laceration*** are used to describe actual bruising and tearing of cerebral tissue. Contusions represent petechial hemorrhages along the superficial aspects of the brain at the site of impact (coup injury) and/or a lesion remote from the site of direct trauma (contrecoup injury). In serious accidents there may be multiple sites of injury.

The major areas of the brain susceptible to contusion or laceration are the occipital, frontal, and temporal lobes. Also, the irregular surfaces of the anterior and middle fossae at the base of the skull are capable of producing bruises or lacerations on forceful impact. Contusions may cause focal disturbances in strength, sensation, or visual awareness. The degree of brain damage in the contused areas varies according to the extent of vascular injury. Signs will vary from mild, transient weakness of a limb to prolonged unconsciousness and paralysis. However, the signs and symptoms may be clinically indistinguishable from concussion.

The lower incidence of cerebral contusion in infancy has been attributed to the infant's pliable skull with less convolutional markings of the inner space between brain tissue and bone. Also, the infant's brain tissue has a softer consistency, which also reduces surface injury. However, infants who are roughly shaken (shaken baby syndrome) can sustain profound neurologic impairment, seizures, retinal hemorrhages, and intracranial subarachnoid or subdural hemorrhages. In addition to these classic injuries, high cervical spinal cord hemorrhages and contusions can occur (Zepp and others, 1992).

Cerebral lacerations are generally associated with penetrating or depressed skull fractures. However, they may occur without fracture in small children. When brain tissue is actually torn, with bleeding into and around the tear, usually more severe and prolonged unconsciousness and paralysis occur, leaving permanent scarring and some degree of disability.

Fractures. Skull fractures are found in over 25% of children who are seen with head injuries (Mealey, 1988). However, the immature skull, because of its flexibility, is able to sustain a greater degree of deformation than the adult skull before it incurs a fracture. It requires a great deal of force to produce a fracture in the skull of an infant. A fracture may occur with little or no brain damage, or severe and fatal brain injury can take place without fracture. The undersurface of the skull contains grooves in which the meningeal arteries lie. A fracture that runs through one of these grooves may tear the artery and produce severe and damaging hemorrhage.

Hypovolemic hypotension can occur in infants with skull fractures. The types of fractures that occur are linear, depressed, compound, basilar, and diastatic. As a rule, the faster the blow, the greater the likelihood of a depressed fracture; a low-velocity impact tends to produce a linear fracture.

Linear fractures comprise about 75% of childhood skull fractures (Mealey, 1988). The lines of the fracture are predetermined by the site and velocity of the impact, as well as the strength of the bone. Linear fractures are often asymptomatic in older children and heal in 3 to 4 months without special treatment, unless they involve a blood vessel, enter the paranasal sinuses, or impinge on the brainstem or cranial nerves. The location of the fracture often provides clues to the possibility of such complications. For example, a fracture that extends through the squamous portion of the temporal bone is more apt to be associated with laceration of the middle meningeal artery, and fractures extending through the base of the skull may cause leakage of CSF and/or blood into either the auditory or the nasal passages. In infants the uneven ossification and the absence of buttresses cause fracture lines to be irregular, following no predictable pattern.

Depressed fractures are those in which the bone is locally broken, usually into several irregular fragments that are pushed inward, causing pressure on the brain. This pressure constitutes a neurosurgical emergency requiring surgical intervention to elevate the fracture. The inner portion of the bone is more extensively fragmented than the outer portion, which almost invariably produces tears in the dura. Depressed skull fractures may be associated with direct underlying parenchymal damage. Both linear and comminuted (fracture consisting of several breaks in the bone) depressed fractures are uncommon before 2 to 3 years of age. In infants and very young children the soft, malleable bone may become dented in a peculiar rounded or "Ping-Pong ball" depression without laceration of either skin or dura. This effect is encountered occasionally in difficult deliveries, resulting from either pressure of the head against the pelvis or incorrect application of forceps.

Compound fractures consist of laceration of skin that extends to the site of the bony fracture, which can be linear, depressed, or comminuted. Prompt surgical debridement is needed (unless contraindicated by the child's clinical condition), as is reduction of the fracture, either elevating or removing fragmented bone. Antibiotic therapy is implemented.

Basilar fractures involve the basilar portion of the frontal, ethmoid, sphenoid, temporal, or occipital bones. The diagnosis of basilar fractures is difficult to make from radiographs because of the complex structure of the base of the skull. Because of the proximity of the fracture line to structures surrounding the brainstem, basal skull fracture is a serious head injury. Clinical features include hemorrhage into the nose, nasopharynx, or middle ear (hemotympanum if it occurs behind the eardrum). Effusion of blood is seen on the posterior neck and under and posterior to the ear (Battle sign). Anterior basal fracture produces the characteristic hemorrhage about the eyes ("rac-

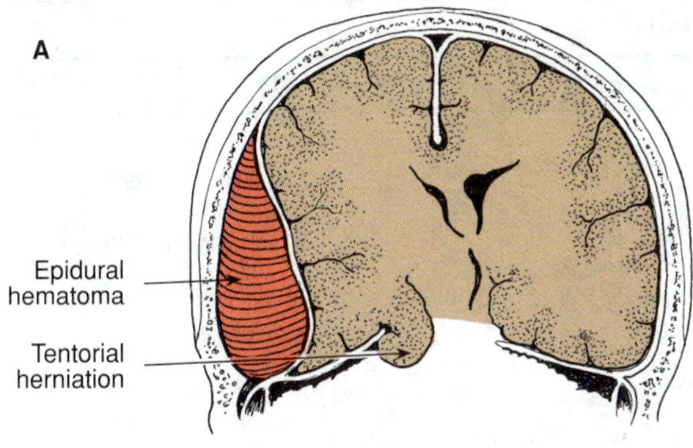

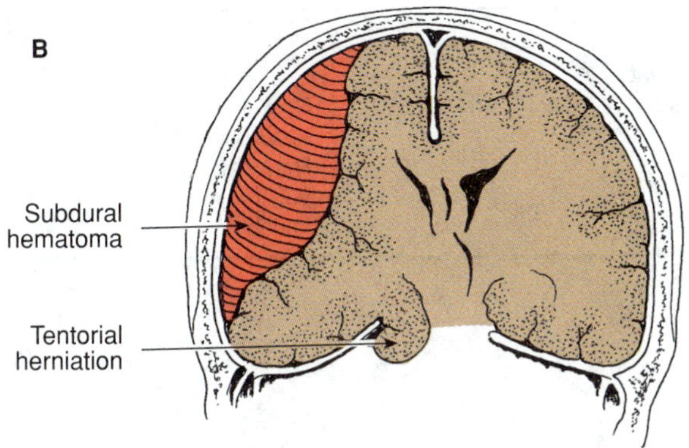

FIG. 37-8 **A,** Epidural (extradural) hematoma and compression of temporal lobe through tentorial hiatus. **B,** Subdural hematoma.

coon eyes"). CN palsies may occur, involving primarily CN I, VIII, and VII in order of decreasing frequency. Meningitis, although rare, is always a potential risk with CSF leakage. The use of prophylactic antibiotics is controversial, and the trend has been to treat only documented cases of meningitis.

NURSING ALERT Posttraumatic meningitis should be suspected in children with increasing drowsiness and fever who also have basilar skull fractures.

Diastatic fractures are traumatic separations of cranial sutures. These most frequently affect the lambdoid suture and are rarely seen beyond the first 4 years of life. They require no specific treatment but should be observed for "growing fractures." The syndrome of growing skull fracture occurs exclusively in infants and young children. For this entity to occur, the child must sustain a skull fracture (usually parietal) and a dural tear. The ongoing normal growth of a child's brain is an underlying aggravating factor. The development of a pulsatile mass or enlarging skull defect can be detected by physical examination.

Complications

The major complications of trauma to the head are hemorrhage, infection, edema, and herniation through the tentorium. infection is always a hazard in open injuries, and edema is related to tissue trauma. Vascular rupture may occur even in minor head injuries, causing hemorrhage between the skull and cerebral surfaces. Compression of the underlying brain produces effects that can be rapidly fatal or insidiously progressive.

Epidural Hemorrhage. Epidural (extradural) hemorrhage is usually secondary to rupture of the middle meningeal artery, most often as a result of skull fracture that penetrates the groove in the skull occupied by the artery. The lower incidence of epidural hematoma in childhood has been attributed to the fact that the middle meningeal artery is not embedded in the bone surface of the skull until approximately 2 years of age. Therefore a fracture of the temporal bone is less likely to lacerate the artery. Second, the dura closely adheres to the inner table of the skull, especially at the level of the sutures, making separation from bleeding less likely (Davis and others, 1987). However, a child's skull can be indented with sufficient force to tear the middle meningeal artery and the rebound intact without causing a fracture. Hemorrhage can also derive from dural veins or the dural sinuses, especially in infants and small children, in whom fracture is less likely to occur. In 20% to 40% of children a skull fracture is not detectable.

The blood accumulates between the dura and the skull to form a hematoma, which, because of the difficulty with which dura is stripped from bone, forces the underlying brain contents downward and inward as it expands (Fig. 37-8, *A*). Since bleeding is generally arterial, brain compression occurs rapidly. Most often the expanding hematoma is located in the parietotemporal region, forcing the medial portion of the temporal lobe under the edge of the tentorium, where it causes pressure on nerves and blood vessels. Pressure on the arterial supply and venous return to the reticular formation causes loss of consciousness; pressure on CN III (oculomotor nerve) produces dilation and (later) fixation of the ipsilateral pupil. Pressure on the fibers of the pyramidal tract is evidenced by contralateral weakness or paralysis and increased deep tendon reflexes. Extreme pressure may extend to the brainstem to cause decerebrate signs and disturbances in the respiratory and other vegetative centers.

The classic clinical picture of epidural hemorrhage (momentary unconsciousness followed by a normal period, then lethargy or coma) is seldom evident in children. The period of impaired consciousness is frequently lacking, and the symptom-free period is atypical because of nonspecific complaints such as irritability, headache, and vomiting. The symptom-free period frequently lasts longer than 48 hours. Clinically significant epidural hematomas are uncommon in children younger than 4 years of age. These differences may be caused by the decreased tendency of the resilient skull to fracture; the ability of blood to escape through widened sutures, an open fontanel, or a fracture; bleeding from smaller vessels with less rapid and massive bleeding; lower

TABLE 37-4 Features of Acute Epidural and Subdural Hematomas

	EPIDURAL	SUBDURAL
SUPRATENTORIAL		
Frequency	Less	5 to 10 times greater
Skull fracture	70%	30%
Source of hemorrhage	Arterial or venous	Almost always venous
Age	Usually older than 2 years	Usually younger than 1 year
Location	Usually temporoparietal	Usually frontoparietal
Laterality	Usually unilateral	75% bilateral
Seizures	Less than 25%	75%
(Pre-)retinal hemorrhages	Uncommon	Very frequent
Increased intracranial pressure	Present	Present
CT configuration	Usually lenticular	Curvilinear or crescentic
Mortality	Relatively high	Usually lower
Morbidity	Low	High
INFRATENTORIAL		
Frequency	2 to 3 times greater	Less
Skull fracture	Almost always	Frequent
Source of hemorrhage	Venous	Venous
Impaired consciousness	Frequent	Frequent
Acute hydrocephalus/medullary compression	Variable	Variable
Other posterior fossa signs	Variable	Variable

From Swaiman KF: *Pediatric neurology: principles and practice,* ed 2, St Louis, 1994, Mosby.

systolic blood pressure in children; and possibly the brain being less susceptible to pressure changes in children. An epidural hematoma can be detected by an initial CT scan. If the severity of the child's symptoms is not recognized, herniation and death will result. (See Table 37-4 for a comparison of epidural and subdural hematomas.)

Subdural Hemorrhage. A subdural hemorrhage is bleeding between the dura and the cerebrum, usually as a result of rupture of cortical veins that bridge the subdural space (Fig. 37-8, *B*). Subdural hematomas are 10 times more frequent than epidural hematomas, occurring most often in infancy, with a peak incidence at 6 months.

Unlike epidural hemorrhage, which develops inwardly against the less resistant brain tissue, subdural hemorrhage tends to develop more slowly and spreads thinly and widely until it is limited by the dural barriers—the falx and tentorium. Subdural hematoma is fairly common in infants, frequently as a result of birth trauma, falls, assaults, or violent shaking. The small subdural space and dura firmly attached to the skull in this area are highly vulnerable to increased ICP.

Subdural hemorrhage can cause either acute or chronic subdural hematoma. ***Acute subdural hematoma*** may be associated with contusions or lacerations. It develops within minutes or hours of injury, and although the mortality is less than that for acute epidural hematoma, the morbidity is greater because of injury to the underlying brain (Swaiman, 1989). ***Chronic subdural hematoma*** is more common. The clinical course and manifestations vary, depending on the damage sustained by the brain substance and the age of the child. Delayed symptoms are common in children with open fontanels and sutures. The usual presenting manifestations in children are seizures, vomiting, drowsiness, increased head circumference, and irritability or other personality changes. Older children may complain of headache. Less common signs are developmental retardation and failure to thrive.

Presenting signs of acute hematoma include evidence of increased ICP, such as increased head size and bulging fontanels (in the infant), retinal hemorrhages, extraocular palsies (especially CN VI), hemiparesis, quadriplegia, and sometimes elevated temperature. An infant with an altered LOC in whom the CT scan shows subarachnoid hemorrhage or a subdural hematoma may have been physically abused.

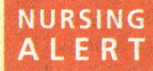

Children with a subdural hematoma and retinal hemorrhages should be evaluated for the possibility of child abuse, especially shaken baby syndrome.

Older children may display an unsteady gait, and papilledema is usually present. Since papilledema is a late sign of increased ICP, it constitutes an emergency. In infants the bleeding may be extensive enough to lower the hematocrit significantly and may be observed before any change in LOC in fast-expanding lesions. The mortality of subdural hematoma of infancy is high, probably because of severe diffuse brain injury.

Repeated subdural taps often provide relief in the infant. Surgical evacuation of the hematoma is the treatment of choice in the older child and is frequently required in infants.

CLINICAL MANIFESTATIONS OF POSTTRAUMATIC SYNDROMES

POSTCONCUSSION SYNDROME

Infants

Pallor
Sweating
Irritability
Sleepiness
Possible vomiting

Children

Behavioral disturbances
- Aggressiveness
- Disobedience
- Withdrawal
- Regression
- Anxiety

Sleep disturbances
Phobias
Emotional lability
Irritability
Altered school performance
Seizures

Adolescents

Headache
Dizziness
Impaired concentration

STRUCTURAL COMPLICATIONS

Hydrocephalus
Focal deficits
- Optic atrophy
- Cranial nerve palsies
- Motor deficits
- Diabetes insipidus
- Aphasia

Seizures

Other Hemorrhagic Lesions. Subarachnoid and intracerebral hemorrhages may occur as a result of head injury. Seizures, nuchal rigidity, and altered consciousness are features of subarachnoid hemorrhage. Manifestations of intracranial bleeding depend on the size and location of the resulting hematoma.

Cerebral Edema. Some degree of brain edema is expected after craniocerebral trauma and often accompanies any of the previously mentioned disorders. Cerebral edema peaks at 24 to 72 hours following injury and may account for changes in a child's neurologic status. Cerebral edema caused by direct cellular injury or vascular injury induces vascular stasis, anoxia, and further vasodilatation. Increased tissue pressure within the skull causes venules to collapse, which leads to venous stasis and tissue anoxia. This results in loss of selective permeability of tissue membranes with increased loss of fluid from the vascular compartment to the cerebral tissues, thereby increasing cerebral edema.

There is considerable evidence indicating that cerebral autoregulatory function and CO_2 reactivity are impaired or absent in traumatized areas of the brain. Thus a self-perpetuating sequence of events is repeated. If this progression continues unchecked, ICP exceeds arterial pressure and fatal anoxia ensues and/or the pressure causes herniation of a portion of the brain over the edge of the tentorium, compressing the brainstem and occluding the posterior cerebral arteries.

Early deterioration after head injury, a syndrome described by several authors as "talk and die," occurs less frequently in children than in adults. Children at risk for deterioration can be identified by abnormalities seen on admitting CT scans (Luerssen, 1991).

Posttraumatic Syndromes. *Postconcussion syndrome* is a common sequela to brain injury, and the manifestations vary with the age of the child. Most often there are behavioral disturbances (e.g., aggressiveness, withdrawal, regression), sleep disturbances, phobias, emotional lability, irritability, and alterations in school performance. The younger the child with severe head trauma, the higher is the risk of late behavioral and emotional sequelae.

Postconcussion syndrome occurs very frequently in children under 1 year of age. Within minutes to an hour after a minimum head injury a child sweats; becomes pale, irritable, and sleepy; and may vomit. The syndrome requires no treatment. In children beyond 1 year of age a severe degree of concussion causes acute brain swelling, which may progress to coma with pupillary changes, apnea, and even death. Death from concussion is preventable unless overwhelming secondary brain injury has occurred (Bruce and Schut, 1989).

NURSING ALERT If a child loses consciousness or vomits more than three times, medical attention should be sought.

The adolescent syndrome, similar to that of adults, includes headache, dizziness, irritability, and impaired concentration. The symptoms are self-limited and relatively mild. Postconcussion syndrome in children is unique. It consists of behavior changes that may include aggression, disobedience, regressive behavior, and anxiety. Manifestations that continue for more than 1 month require follow-up evaluation (see box above, left, and Critical Thinking Exercise box on p. 1702).

Posttraumatic seizures occur in a number of children who survive a head injury and are more common in children than in adults. Immediate-onset seizure, occurring within a few seconds of trauma, is associated with long-term epilepsy. The incidence of seizures after traumatic brain injury is approximately 5% (Ghajar and Hariri, 1992). Seizures are more likely to occur in children with severe head injury (35%) than in those with mild head injury (5%). Seizure activity may mimic brainstem herniation signs in children following head injuries.

Structural complications may occur as a result of head injuries. Hydrocephalus is seen when there has been subarachnoid hemorrhage or infection. Normal-pressure hydrocephalus is a complication of traumatic brain injury. The clinical signs and symptoms include cognitive deterioration, gait changes and incontinence. These signs are also seen during posttraumatic amnesia, making early recognition of this syndrome difficult. Focal deficits, including optic atrophy, CN palsies, motor deficits, diabetes insipidus, or aphasia, may be seen. The type of residual effect depends on the location and nature of the trauma. True mental retardation occurs only after severe injuries.

Diagnostic Evaluation

A detailed history, both past and present, is essential in evaluating the child with craniocerebral trauma. It is important to know whether the child suffers from disorders such

CLINICAL MANIFESTATIONS OF ACUTE HEAD INJURY

MINOR INJURY

May or may not lose consciousness
Transient period of confusion
Somnolence
Listlessness
Irritability
Pallor
Vomiting (one or more episodes)

SIGNS OF PROGRESSION

Altered mental status (e.g., difficulty rousing child)
Mounting agitation
Development of focal lateral neurologic signs
Marked changes in vital signs

SEVERE INJURY

Signs of increased ICP (see box on p. 1674)
  Increased head size (infant)
  Bulging fontanel (infant)
Retinal hemorrhage
Extraocular palsies (especially CN VI)
Hemiparesis
Quadriplegia
Elevated temperature (sometimes)
Unsteady gait (older child)
Papilledema (older child)

ASSOCIATED SIGNS

Skin injury (to area of head sustaining injury)
Other injuries (e.g., to extremities)

as drug allergies, hemophilia, diabetes mellitus, or epilepsy; such information may assist in diagnosis. In addition, events surrounding the injury often supply significant data. For example, if a child stumbles and falls while running and strikes the head on the sidewalk, it is usually safe to assume that the neurologic manifestations are a direct result of the injury. However, if a child sinks to the sidewalk and in doing so strikes the head, there may be other causes that contributed to the injury. Sometimes a traumatic injury, even a minor one, will aggravate a preexisting disease process, thereby producing neurologic signs out of proportion to the injury.

Whether or not the infant or child exhibited alterations in consciousness must be determined. Usually this information is easily elicited from older children, but in young children it may be difficult to differentiate between a breath-holding spell and a seizure. The parents are asked if the infant cried immediately after the injury. After a minor injury, initial unconsciousness (if present) is brief and the child will ordinarily exhibit a transient period of confusion, somnolence, and listlessness, most often accompanied by irritability, pallor, and one or more episodes of vomiting.

A severe head injury, such as one sustained in a fall from a significant height or a motor vehicle accident, requires immediate evaluation and treatment. Since head injuries are frequently accompanied by injuries in other areas (spine, viscera, extremities), the examination is performed with care to avoid further damage. Manifestations of head injury are listed in the box above.

Over 75% of children who die as a consequence of head injury have evidence of ischemic brain damage (Noah and others, 1992). Because little can be done about the original primary insult, care of secondary brain injuries remains the goal in the management of the injured child.

Initial Assessment. Priorities in the initial phase in the care of a child with a head injury include assessment of the ABCs (airway, breathing, circulation); assessment for spinal cord injury; evaluation for shock; a neurologic examination, especially LOC; pupillary symmetry and response to light; and seizures. The assessment is carried out quickly in relation to vital signs (see Emergency Treatment box). Excited and irritable children may have a rapid pulse, hyperventilate, appear pale, and feel clammy shortly after an injury.

NURSING ALERT Deep, rapid, periodic, or intermittent and gasping respirations; wide fluctuations or noticeable slowing of the pulse; and widening pulse pressure or extreme fluctuations in blood pressure are signs of brainstem involvement. Marked hypotension may represent internal injuries.

Ocular signs such as fixed, dilated, and unequal pupils; fixed and constricted pupils; and pupils that are poorly reactive or unreactive to light and accommodation indicate increased ICP or brainstem involvement. It is important to remain with the patient who demonstrates fixed and dilated pupils, since these are ominous signs with the probability of respiratory arrest. Dilated, nonpulsating blood vessels indicate increased ICP before the appearance of papilledema. Retinal hemorrhages are seen in acute head injuries.

NURSING ALERT Observation of asymmetric pupils or one dilated, unreactive pupil in a comatose child is a neurosurgical emergency that may require evacuation of an epidural hematoma.

Ophthalmosopy should be performed routinely to detect retinal hemorrhages in a child with CNS dysfunction. Cortical blindness, defined as a complete bilateral visual loss associated with normal pupillary responses to light, can be a brief or transient consequence of head trauma. Theories of possible etiologies are vasospasm or localized cerebral edema. Transient blindness following mild head trauma may not be obvious in children unless this diagnosis is considered and evaluated.

Less urgent but important additional assessments include examination of the scalp for lacerations and palpation for depressed skull fractures, widely separated sutures, and the size and tension of fontanels, which indicate intracranial hemorrhage or rapidly developing cerebral edema. However, a significant amount of blood loss can occur from scalp lacerations. An underlying skull fracture should be ruled out by palpation and possibly radiography.

NURSING ALERT Bleeding from the nose or ears needs further evaluation, and a watery discharge from the nose (rhinorrhea) that is positive for glucose (as tested with reagent strips [e.g., Dextrostix]) suggests leaking of CSF from a skull fracture.

Injury to the skin, extremities, and abdomen may occur after severe blunt head trauma and must be ruled out by sensory examination in children with altered motor function. Testing reflexes provides information about cerebral and pyramidal involvement, although transient abnormalities of the abdominal reflexes and Babinski sign may be present in children with mild head trauma. Conscious, cooperative children are examined for cerebellar signs such as ataxia. Children may display unsteadiness, clumsiness, or tremor with intentional movement after head injury.

Temperature may be moderately elevated for 1 or 2 days following an initial mild hypothermia after injury. A persistent fever may indicate subarachnoid hemorrhage or infection.

An accurate assessment of these various clinical signs provides baseline information. Serial evaluations, preferably by a single observer, help to detect changes in the neurologic status. Alterations in mental status, evidenced by increased difficulty in rousing the child, mounting agitation, development of focal lateral neurologic signs, or marked changes in vital signs, usually indicate extension or progression of the basic pathologic process.

Special Tests. After a thorough clinical examination, a variety of diagnostic tests are helpful in providing a more definitive diagnosis of the type and extent of the trauma. The severity of a head injury may not be apparent on clinical examination of a child, but it will be detectable on a CT scan. Whenever the child has a history consistent with a serious head injury (unrestrained occupant in a severe motor vehicle accident or a fall from a significant height), it is important that a scan be performed even if the child initially appears alert and oriented. All children with head injuries who have any alteration of consciousness, headache, vomiting, skull fracture, seizure, or a predisposing medical condition should also undergo CT scanning.

MRI and neurobehavioral assessment following early head injury may be useful in documenting cognitive impairment in relation to structural alterations in the young brain. MRI provides details of soft tissues better than any other noninvasive device. Scanning with MRI is reserved for stable or recovering children because metal devices used during a trauma, such as a ventilator, may not be placed in proximity to the magnetic field.

Skull films and other radiographic tests may be indicated. Electroencephalography is not particularly helpful for early diagnosis but is useful for defining seizure activity or focal destructive lesions after the acute phase of illness. Lumbar puncture is rarely employed in craniocerebral trauma and is contraindicated in the presence of increased ICP because of the possibility of herniation.

In the infant or small child a subdural tap through a fontanel or coronal suture may establish the diagnosis of subdural or epidural hemorrhage. In some centers monitoring ICP is part of the assessment.

Therapeutic Management

The majority of children with mild to moderate concussion who have not lost consciousness can be cared for and observed at home after careful examination reveals no serious intracranial injury. The parents are instructed to check the child every 2 hours to determine any changes in responsiveness. The sleeping child is awakened to see if the child can be roused normally. Parents are advised to maintain contact with the attending practitioner, who usually wishes to examine the child again in 1 or 2 days. The manifestations of epidural hematoma in children do not generally appear until 24 hours or more after injury (see Family Focus box, p. 1700).

Children with severe injuries, those who have lost consciousness for more than a few minutes, and those with prolonged and continued seizures or other focal or diffuse neurologic signs must be hospitalized until their condition is stable and their neurologic signs have diminished. The child is maintained on nothing by mouth or restricted to clear liquids, if able to take fluids by mouth, until it is determined that vomiting will not occur. Intravenous fluids are indicated for the child who is comatose or displays dulled sensorium and for the child with persistent vomiting.

The volume of intravenous fluid is carefully monitored to avoid aggravating any cerebral edema and to minimize

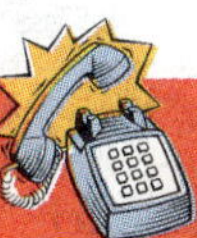

EMERGENCY TREATMENT
Head Injury

1. Assess child:
   A—Airway
   B—Breathing
   C—Circulation
2. Stabilize neck and spine.
3. Clean any abrasions with soap and water.
   Apply clean dressing.
   If bleeding, apply ice for 1 hour to relieve pain and swelling.
4. Keep NPO or give only clear liquids until no vomiting for at least 6 hours.
5. Give no analgesics or sedatives.
6. Check pupil reaction every 4 hours (including twice during night) for 48 hours.
7. Awaken two times during night to check level of consciousness.
8. Seek medical attention if there is any of the following:
   Injury sustained
   —At high speed (e.g., auto)
   —Fall from a significant distance (e.g., roof, tree)
   —From great force (e.g., baseball bat)
   —Under suspicious circumstances
   Child less than 6 months of age
   Unconscious more than 5 seconds
   Discomfort (crying) more than 10 minutes after injury
   Headache that is severe, worsening, interferes with sleep
   Vomiting three or more times
   Swelling in front of above earlobe or swelling that increases in size
   Confused or not behaving normally
   Difficult to rouse from sleep
   Difficulty with speaking
   Blurring of vision or seeing double
   Unsteady gait
   Difficulty using upper extremities
   Neck pain
   Pupils dilated or fixed
   Infant with bulging fontanel

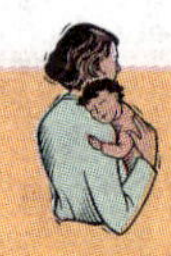

FAMILY FOCUS

Maintaining Contact with Parents After Head Injury

Maintaining contact with parents for continued observation and reevaluation of the child, when indicated, facilitates early diagnosis and treatment of possible complications from head injury, such as hematoma, hydrocephalus, cysts, and posttraumatic seizures. Children are generally hospitalized for 24 to 48 hours' observation if their family lives far from medical facilities or lacks transportation or a telephone that would provide access to immediate help. Other circumstances, such as language or other communication barriers, or even emotional trauma, may hinder learning and make it difficult for families to feel confident in caring for their child at home.

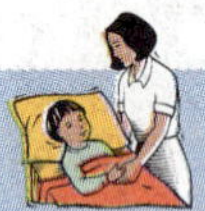

ATRAUMATIC CARE

Noninvasive Local Anesthesia

The use of topical adrenalin and cocaine (TC) or TC with tetracaine (TAC) provides noninvasive anesthesia (Bonadio and Wagner, 1992).

the possibility of overhydration in case of SIADH. However, damage to the hypothalamus or pituitary gland may produce diabetes insipidus with its accompanying hypertonicity and dehydration. Fluid balance is closely monitored by daily weight, accurate intake and output measurement, and serum osmolality to detect early signs of water retention, excessive dehydration, and states of hypertonicity or hypotonicity.

In the acute phase sedating drugs are usually withheld. However, restlessness can be satisfactorily managed; chloral hydrate remains a popular drug that produces sedation but is not an analgesic. Headache is usually controlled with acetaminophen, although opioids may be needed (see p. 1683). Antiepileptics are used for seizure control and frequently in cases of suspected contusion or laceration. Antibiotics are administered if there are lacerations. Prophylactic tetanus toxoid is given as appropriate (see Chapter 12). Cerebral edema is managed as described for the unconscious child. Hyperthermia is controlled with tepid sponges or a hypothermia blanket.

Surgical Therapy. Scalp lacerations are sutured after careful examination of underlying bone. Torn dura is sutured as well (see Atraumatic Care box). Depressed fractures require surgical reduction and removal of bone fragments. A skull fracture depressed more than the thickness of the skull or an intracranial hematoma causing more than 5 mm midline shift is an indication for surgery. "Ping-Pong ball" skull fractures in very young infants can correct themselves within a few weeks or may require surgical elevation.

Prognosis. The outcome of craniocerebral trauma depends on the extent of injury and complications. However, the outlook is generally more favorable for children than for adults. Over 90% of children with concussions or simple linear fractures recover without symptoms after the initial period. Children have a significantly higher percentage of good outcomes and a lower mortality rate, as well as a lower incidence of surgical mass lesions after severe head trauma. Their thinner, softer brain, however, may sustain greater long-term damage than previously suggested.

The concern regarding outcome is increasingly focused on cognitive, emotional, and/or mental problems. Recent studies indicate that children experience a higher frequency of psychologic disturbances following head injury, whereas adults are more prone to complaints of a physical nature. Children may be more vulnerable than adults to long-term cognitive and behavioral dysfunction after diffuse brain injury. Even with recovery, the effects of brain injury on a child's potential can never be known.

True coma (not obeying commands, eyes closed, and not speaking) usually does not last more than 2 weeks. A child's eventual outcome can range from brain death to a persistent vegetative state to complete recovery. However, even the best recovery may be associated with personality changes, including mood lability and loss of confidence, impaired short-term memory, headaches, and subtle cognitive impairments. Many children are left with significant disabilities after head injury that appear months later as learning difficulties, behavioral changes, or emotional disturbances (Reynolds, 1992). Generally, within 6 months to 1 year after the injury, 90% of the long-term neurologic outcome has been achieved.

Nursing Considerations

The hospitalized child requires careful neurologic assessment and evaluation (see p. 1674). Frequent nursing assessments can provide information needed to establish a correct diagnosis, identify signs and symptoms of increased ICP, determine clinical management, and prevent many complications. Goals of nursing management of the child with a head injury are to maintain adequate ventilation, oxygenation, and circulation; to monitor and treat increased ICP; to minimize cerebral oxygen requirements; and to provide support to the child and family during the recovery phases.

The child is placed on bed rest, usually with the head of the bed elevated slightly. Appropriate safety measures, such as siderails kept up for older children and seizure precautions for children of all ages, are implemented. The extremely restless child may require that hard surfaces be padded and restraint used to prevent the possibility of further injury. Care is individualized according to the specific needs of the child. The unconscious child is managed as described in the previous section, but most childhood head injuries are those causing momentary stunning or temporary unconsciousness.

A key nursing role is to provide sedation and analgesia for the child. The conflict between the need to promote comfort and relieve anxiety in the child versus the need to be able to assess for neurologic changes presents a dilemma. However, both goals can be achieved with close observation of the child's LOC and response to analgesics, using a pain assessment record, and effective communication with the practitioner. To differentiate between sedation from an opioid or the injury, naloxone (Narcan) can be given slowly to reverse the opioid's sedative effect. Decreasing restlessness after administration of an analgesic most likely reflects pain control rather than a decreasing LOC (see Pain Assessment; Pain Management, Chapter 26).

Children may be restless and irritable, but more often their reaction is to fall asleep when left undisturbed. A quiet environment helps reduce the restlessness and irritability. Bright lights shining directly into the child's face are irritating. This often makes checking the ocular responses more difficult to perform and more aggravating to the child.

Frequent examinations of vital signs, neurologic signs, and LOC are extremely important nursing observations. When possible, they should be performed by a single observer in order to better detect subtle changes that may indicate worsening of neurologic status. Pupils are checked for size, equality, reaction to light, and accommodation. After the initial elevations usually seen after injury, the vital signs generally return to normal unless there is brainstem involvement. Rectal and oral sites for measuring temperature are avoided, since seizures are not uncommon and vomiting is a frequent response in children, especially when the child is disturbed. Forehead "strip" thermometers provide continuous temperature monitoring without disturbing the child. Tympanic membrane sensors are another quick and atraumatic method of temperature measurement (see Table 7-3).

The most important nursing observation is assessment of the child's LOC. Alterations in consciousness appear earlier in the progression of an injury than alterations of vital signs or focal neurologic signs (see p. 1676 for evaluation of responsiveness). Some expected responses may be misinterpreted as deviations from the normal. Frequent examinations of alertness are fatiguing to the child; therefore the child often desires to fall asleep, which may be confused with depressed consciousness. When left alone, the child promptly dozes. It is not uncommon to observe ocular divergence through the partially closed eyelids.

Observations of position and movement provide additional information. Any abnormal posturing is noted, as well as whether or not it occurs continuously or intermittently. Questions nurses might ask themselves include:

- Are the child's hand grips strong and equal in strength?
- Are there any signs of decerebrate or decorticate posturing?
- What is the child's response to stimulation?
- Is movement purposeful, random, or absent?
- Are movement and sensation equal on both sides or restricted to one side only?

The child may complain of headache or other discomfort. The child who is too young to describe a headache will be fussy and resist being handled. The child who suffers from vertigo will often assume a position and vigorously resist being moved. Forcible movement causes the child to vomit and display spontaneous nystagmus. Seizures, relatively common in children at the time of injury, may be of any type but are more often generalized regardless of the type of injury. Any seizure activity should be carefully observed and described in detail (see box on p. 1724). Children in postictal states are more lethargic, with sluggish pupils.

Drainage from any orifice is noted. Bleeding from the ear suggests the possibility of a basal skull fracture. The amount and characteristics of the drainage are observed, and since the auditory canal may be a source of infection, dry, sterile cotton can be placed loosely at the orifice and changed when soiled.

NURSING ALERT Suctioning through the nares is contraindicated, since there is a high risk of secondary infection and the probability of the catheter entering the brain through a fracture.

Head trauma is frequently accompanied by other undetected injuries; therefore any bruises, lacerations, or evidence of internal injuries or fractures of the extremities are noted and reported. Associated injuries are evaluated and treated appropriately.

The child with a normal LOC is usually allowed clear liquids unless fluid is restricted. If the child has an intravenous infusion, it is maintained as prescribed. The diet is advanced to that appropriate for the child's age as soon as the condition permits. Intake and output are measured and recorded, and any incontinence of bowel or bladder is noted in the child who has been toilet trained.

The child is observed for any unusual behavior, but interpretation of behavior is made in relation to the child's normal behavior. For example, urinary incontinence during sleep would be of no consequence in a child who routinely wets the bed but would be highly significant for one who is always dry. In addition, a child who is subject to nightmares might cry out and demonstrate agitated behavior at night. Parents are invaluable resources in evaluating objective behaviors of their children. Information obtained from parents at or shortly after admission is essential in evaluating the child's behavior (e.g., the ease with which the child is roused normally, the usual sleeping position, how much the child sleeps during the day, motor activity the child is capable of [rolling over, sitting up, climbing], hearing and visual acuity, appetite, and manner of eating [spoon, bottle, cup]). There would be less concern about a child who falls asleep several times during the day if this particular type of behavior is consistent with the child's usual behavior.

When the child is discharged, the parents are advised of probable posttraumatic symptoms that may be expected, such as behavioral changes, sleep disturbances, phobias, and seizures. They should understand observations that should be made and how to contact the physician, nurse, or health facility in case the child develops any unusual signs or symptoms (see Critical Thinking Exercise box, p. 1702). The importance of follow-up evaluation is emphasized. It is often advisable to refer the family to a public health agency for home follow-through care to ensure that the child receives posthospital evaluation.

Family Support. The emotional and educational support of the family of children who have suffered head injury presents a formidable, challenging aspect to nursing

CRITICAL THINKING EXERCISE

Postconcussion Syndrome

Two weeks ago 4-year-old Thomas Egan attempted to climb the shelves of a storage cabinet in the garage of his home. The shelves and Thomas fell to the concrete floor. Thomas cried immediately. Because of the large occipital hematoma and a vomiting episode, the parents took their son to an emergency department within 1 hour of the incident. The child was released after a negative CT scan, suturing of his occipital scalp laceration, and a GCS of 15.

At his 2-week follow-up visit, Mrs. Egan reports changes in Thomas's behavior that include enuresis, crying episodes, vomiting in the morning, a poor appetite, and an increase in wanting to be held. Your initial intervention is to:

1. Review the signs and symptoms of postconcussion syndrome with the mother.
2. Advise the mother to give the child extra attention at home.
3. Report the symptoms to the physician.
4. Reassure the mother that these symptoms can occur during the first month following injury.

The correct answer is 3. The worsening postconcussion symptoms and signs of increased ICP, especially early-morning vomiting, require urgent consultation. The behavior signs should not be dismissed as "attempts for attention."

The other two interventions are not appropriate as the initial action, although you would want to inform parents that children can exhibit postconcussion syndrome for up to 1 month following the injury, the time required for the bruised brain to heal. Subsequent falls involving a head injury can compound the original injury, so protecting the child during this period is especially important.

care. Witnessing the parents' ordeal of grief and helplessness on seeing their child in an intensive care unit connected to monitoring equipment in an altered state evokes empathy. The nurse can encourage the family to be involved in the child's care, to bring in familiar belongings, or to make a tape recording of familiar voices and sounds. Parents may need a demonstration on how to touch or cuddle their child and may want to talk about their grief. The nurse can listen attentively, reinforce what is being done to assist the child, and direct parents toward signs and symptoms of recovery to instill hope without promises. A common phenomenon is for families to seek information from all health care providers, asking, "What will be? What do you know?" as they search for some clue that the child is recovering. Honesty and kindness, along with consistent and competent care, can help families through this difficult time.

Rehabilitation. The rehabilitation and management of the child with permanent brain injury are essential aspects of care. Rehabilitation of brain-injured children is begun as soon as feasible and usually involves the family and a rehabilitation team. Careful assessment of the child's capabilities, limitations, and probable potential is made as early as possible and appropriate interventions are implemented to maximize the residual capacities. The **National Head Injury Foundation*** "arose from the mutual frustration and sense of hopelessness experienced by families in their search for appropriate facilities and support to return head-injured loved ones to their maximum functioning potential." It provides information and listings of rehabilitation services and support groups throughout the country.

Pediatric trauma rehabilitation is a national concern. Twenty million children are injured by accidents each year; 50,000 children are permanently disabled, and 2 million children have temporary disabilities (McLone and Hahn, 1990). Coordinating care and services for early rehabilitation involves identifying the child and family's response to the traumatic injury and disability, securing available resources, and recognizing the parental role in the process.

The child with a disability resulting from head trauma requires assessment on a physical, cognitive, emotional, and social level. The child has experienced separation, pain, sensory deprivation and overload, changes in circadian cycle, and fear of the unknown. Recovery and transition require new coping strategies at the same time that regressive and acting-out behavior may start. Parents and children need honest communication for decision making. Rehabilitation is advocated when the child is making progress beyond what can be provided in a hospital setting. The Rancho Los Amigos Scale provides a systematic assessment of the progress a child with a severe head injury may achieve (Table 37-5).

Pediatric rehabilitation focuses on the strengths and needs of the child. The rehabilitation team should include physical medicine, rehabilitation nursing, nutritional counseling, physical therapy, special education, occupational therapy, speech therapy, and psychologic, neuropsychologic, child-life, and social services. Families need to know what to look for when visiting a pediatric rehabilitation center. Before the child's transfer, the hospital team should provide a detailed care plan of the child's needs and abilities, especially communication skills; a description of the child's usual schedule; nursing care interventions; and the concerns and needs of the family. To augment the care plan, a videotape introducing the child and family and showing any unique aspects of their care can be sent to the rehabilitation center.

Prevention. Preventive strategies are underused in almost all cases of accidental childhood injury. Head injuries are involved in most serious accidental injuries—especially motor vehicle accidents, sports, and falls.

Tremendous strides have been taken in the prevention of cerebral damage after head injury in children. New developments requiring research point to the prevention of cellular injury or the primary insult. The roles of calcium, oxyradicals, prostaglandins, and a host of mediators of cellular injury are being investigated. However, the greatest benefit lies in prevention of head injuries. Nurses can exert a valuable influence on behalf of children through edu-

*1140 Connecticut Ave., N.W., Suite 812, Washington, DC 20036; (202) 296-6443 or (800) 444-6443 (Family Helpline).

TABLE 37-5 Rancho Los Amigos Scale

LEVEL	DESCRIPTION
1. No response	Unresponsive to any stimulus
2. Generalized response	Limited, inconsistent, nonpurposeful responses, often to pain only
3. Localized response	Purposeful responses; may follow simple commands; may focus on presented objects, yet responses are inconsistent and may be delayed
4. Confused, agitated	Heightened state of activity; confusion, disorientation, aggressive behavior; unable to do self-care; unaware of present events; agitation related to internal confusion; often emotional
5. Confused, inappropriate, nonagitated	Appears alert; responds to commands; highly distractable; does not concentrate on task; agitated responses may continue; verbally inappropriate; difficulty with new information
6. Confused, appropriate	Goal-directed behavior, needs cueing; can relearn old skills of daily living; memory problems; some awareness of self and others
7. Automatic, appropriate	Robotlike appropriate behavior, minimal confusion; shallow recall; poor insight into condition; initiates tasks, but needs structure; poor judgment, problem-solving and planning skills
8. Purposeful, appropriate	Alert, oriented; recalls and integrates past events; learns new activities and can continue without supervision; independent in home and living skills; problems with stress tolerance, judgment, and abstract reasoning persist

cation. The reason accidents remain preventable is that unnecessary risks go unchecked. Inadequate supervision combined with a child's natural sense of indestructibility and exploration can lead to lethal results. Nurses are in the unique position of influencing caregivers in terms of growth and development. Banning the use of infant walkers is an example. This equipment does not help develop motor skills but places infants at risk for head and neck injuries from falls, especially down steps. Public education, coupled with legislative support, can prevent childhood injuries.

For extensive discussions of childhood injuries, see the discussions on injury prevention in Chapters 12, 14, 15, 17, and 19; as well as Injuries—The Leading Killer, Chapter 1. (See also Nursing Care Plan: The Child with a Head Injury.*)

NEAR-DROWNING

Drowning ranks second as a cause of accidental death in children. Most cases involve children who are helpless in

*In *Wong and Whaley's Clinical Manual of Pediatric Nursing* (Mosby).

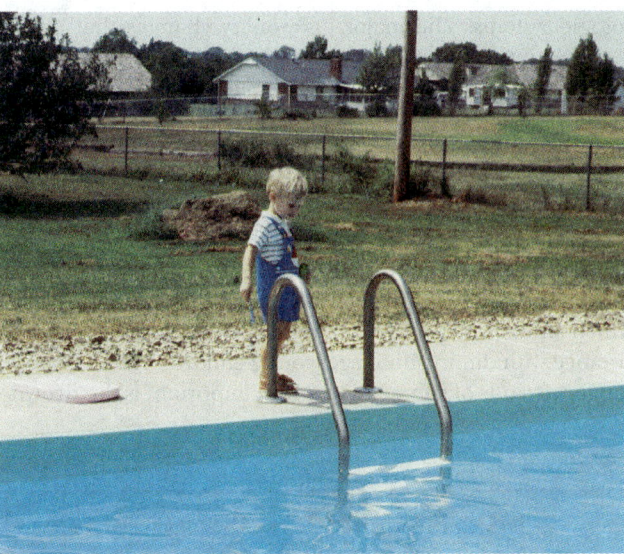

FIG. 37-9 Water is fascinating for children; however, drowning is the second leading cause of accidental death in unsupervised situations.

water, such as inadequately attended children in or near swimming pools or infants in bathtubs; small children who fall into ponds, streams, and flooded excavations, usually near home (Fig. 37-9); occupants of pleasure boats who fail to wear life preservers; children who have diving accidents; and children who are able to swim but overestimate their endurance.

Accidental drowning occurs more than four times more frequently in males than in females; in almost all cases, supervision is absent. Most of the drownings are related to the characteristics of specific age-groups. For example, infants drown in bathtubs, preschool children in swimming pools, and teenagers in lakes and rivers. The largest proportion of drownings for all children occur in private swimming pools, with the highest rate among children 2 to 3 years of age. Drowning as a form of fatal child abuse has also been recognized as a problem. Homicidal drownings are unwitnessed, usually occur in the home, and the victims are either infants or toddlers.

Drowning can take place in any body of water, including such unlikely places as a pail of water or a toilet bowl. Top-heavy toddlers fall headfirst into a pail of water, their arms become trapped, and they are unable to free themselves. Hot tubs and whirlpool spas have been implicated in childhood drowning injury. The suction created at the outlet is strong enough to trap even larger children underwater, and rapidly proliferating *Pseudomonas aeruginosa* have been reported as complicating hot tub submersion injury.

Terms describing drowning and near-drowning are presented in the box on p. 1704.

Pathophysiology

Near-drowning occurs when a victim of a submersion incident survives at least 24 hours after rescue, regardless of the final outcome. Physiologically, most organ systems will be affected, especially the pulmonary, cardiovascular, and neurologic systems. The major pulmonary changes that occur in drowning are directly related to the length of submersion (regardless of the type and amount of fluid aspirated), the physiologic response of the victim, and the development and degree of immersion hypothermia. In addition, cerebral recovery may depend on the effectiveness of initial resuscitation and subsequent critical care measures to support cerebral salvage.

Physiologic factors that influence the extent of damage from immersion include resistance to asphyxia and anoxia, which shows some individual variation. There is greater resistance with diminishing age; young children can withstand longer periods of submersion. More important is the drowning, or diving, reflex. This neurologic response is triggered by immersion of the face in cold water. Blood is shunted away from the periphery, and the flow is concentrated to the brain and heart predominantly. There is a profound bradycardia, but the diminishing supply of oxygen is delivered to these essential organs.

TERMS DESCRIBING DROWNING INJURY

Drowning—Death from asphyxia while submerged, regardless of whether fluid has entered the lungs
Near-drowning—Survival at least 24 hours after submersion in a fluid medium

These can be further described as:

Drowning without aspiration—Death from respiratory obstruction and asphyxia while submerged, usually as a result of prolonged laryngospasm; also called "dry drowning" (approximately 10% of drownings)
Drowning with aspiration —Death from the combined effects of asphyxia and changes secondary to fluid aspiration while submerged
Near-drowning without aspiration —Survival, at least temporarily, following asphyxia after submersion in a fluid medium
Near-drowning with aspiration—Survival, at least temporarily, following aspiration of fluid while submerged
Delayed death caused by drowning—Death as a result of complications subsequent to successful resuscitation following submersion

Submerged children struggle initially. There is laryngospasm, and they swallow water and frequently vomit. This is followed by terminal gasping and aspiration. Cardiopulmonary arrest is secondary to asphyxia after about 4 to 6 minutes of complete submersion. The problems created by near-drowning are (1) hypoxia and asphyxiation, (2) aspiration, and (3) hypothermia (except near-drowning in hot tubs).

Hypoxia is the primary problem because it results in global cell damage, and different cells tolerate variable lengths of anoxia. Neurons, especially cerebral cells, sustain irreversible damage after 4 to 6 minutes of submersion. The heart and lungs can survive up to 30 minutes. Regardless of the amount of water aspirated, there is arterial hypoxemia (resulting from atelectasis with shunting of blood through the nonventilated alveoli) and a combined respiratory acidosis (resulting from retained carbon dioxide) and metabolic acidosis (caused by buildup of acid metabolites due to anaerobic metabolism). Although electrolyte imbalances are contributing factors, they are not the major causes of morbidity and mortality, as had been previously thought. The pathologic events are directly related to the duration of submersion. The major difficulty is acute ventilatory insufficiency. Approximately 10% of drowning victims die without aspirating fluid but succumb from acute asphyxia as a result of prolonged reflex laryngospasm.

Aspiration of fluid occurs in the majority of drownings. The aspirated fluid results in pulmonary edema, atelectasis, airway spasm, and pneumonitis, which aggravates the hypoxia. It was previously thought that submersion in salt

TABLE 37-6 Clinical Manifestations and Management of Near-Drowning Related to Degree of Consciousness

CATEGORY	CHARACTERISTICS	MANAGEMENT
A	Awake, minimum injury Fully conscious; may have mild hypothermia, mild chest radiograph changes, mild arterial blood gas abnormalities	Symptomatic treatment with oxygen administration and warming Laboratory assessment of electrolytes Usually well enough to be discharged in 12 to 24 hours
B	Blunted sensorium, moderate injury Obtund, stuporous, purposeful response to painful stimuli, mild to moderate hypothermia, frequently respiratory distress, chest radiographs abnormal, arterial blood gas abnormalities	Symptomatic, as for category A Regular monitoring of neurologic and respiratory status Correction of acidosis Furosemide to stimulate diuresis
C	Comatose, severe anoxia Patient unarousable, abnormal response to pain, abnormal respiratory pattern, seizures, shock, marked arterial blood gas abnormalities, abnormal chest radiographs, dysrhythmias, metabolic acidosis, hyperkalemia, hyperglycemia, disseminated intravascular coagulation	Invasive life-support measures Mechanical ventilation for at least 12 to 24 hours (to reduce energy expenditure) More severely affected children managed as any unconscious child Increased ICP usually not a problem in children who do well, but when present (even with treatment), associated with death or significant neurologic damage Symptomatic management
C1	Decorticate, Cheyne-Stokes respirations	
C2	Decerebrate, central hyperventilation	
C3	Flaccid, apneustic or cluster breathing	
C4	Flaccid, apneic, no detectable circulation	

water and fresh water altered the physiologic response to near-drowning. However, there is no clinically significant difference in human survivors, and the type of water does not alter the therapy or outcome.

Hypothermia occurs rapidly in infants and children, partly because of their large surface area relative to size and partly as a result of cold water itself. Profound hypothermia is usually evidence of lengthy submersion. Although small children may tolerate submersion in *very* cold water, within 3 to 6 minutes severe neurologic damage results from hypoxia.

Clinical Manifestations

Clinical manifestations are directly related to the degree of consciousness following rescue and resuscitation. The manifestations and management are categorized in Table 37-6.

Therapeutic Management

With rapid treatment some children can and are being saved. Resuscitative measures should begin at the scene, and the victim should be transported to the hospital with maximum ventilatory and circulatory support. Many victims need care for some time after aspiration of fluid. In the hospital intensive pulmonary care is implemented and continued according to the needs of the patient.

In general, the management of the near-drowning victim is based on the degree of cerebral insult. The first priority is to restore oxygen delivery to the cells and prevent further hypoxic damage. A spontaneously breathing child will do well in an oxygen-enriched atmosphere; the more severely affected child will require endotracheal intubation and mechanical ventilation. Blood gases and pH are monitored frequently as a guide to oxygen, fluid, and electrolyte therapies.

Because of the frequency of complications after near-drowning, any patient should be hospitalized for 12 to 48 hours for observation. Potential causes for altered neurologic function, such as head injury, drug intoxication, or hypothermia, in the pediatric near-drowning victim require evaluation. Aspiration pneumonia is a frequent complication that occurs about 48 to 72 hours after the episode. Bronchospasm, alveolar-capillary membrane damage, atelectasis, abscess formation, and hyaline membrane disease are other complications that occur after aspiration of fluid.

Prognosis. In one study the best predictors of a good outcome were length of submersion in non-icy water (>5° C [41° F]) for less than 5 minutes and the presence of sinus rhythm, reactive pupils, and neurologic responsiveness at the scene. The worst prognoses—for death or severe neurologic impairment—were in children submerged for more than 10 minutes and not responding to advanced life support within 25 minutes (Quan and Kinder, 1992).

Nursing Considerations

Nursing care depends on the condition of the child. A child who survives may need intensive respiratory nursing care with attention to vital signs, mechanical ventilation and/or tracheostomy, blood gas determination, chest therapy, and intravenous infusion. Frequently the child has sustained a hypoxic insult and requires the same care as an unconscious child.

Probably the most difficult aspect in the care of the child victim of near-drowning is dealing with the parents, whose guilt reactions are severe. The magnitude of the event is so great that efforts to provide comfort and support are of only limited success. Parents need to hear that everything possible is being done to treat the child, and this message needs to be repeated often.

Most drownings, particularly of infants or small children, could have been prevented with adequate supervision. If the child dies, the sudden, unexpected nature of the death and the particular circumstances of the accident, especially in terms of guilt for not preventing it, compound the grief for these individuals (see Chapter 23). The parents of the child who is saved from death are faced with the anxiety of not knowing what the outcome will be and sometimes wish for the death of the child, or continue to hope the child will "wake up" in the face of cerebral hypoxia. Because their situation generates such intense feelings of loneliness, it is important for families to know that they are not alone. They need to be reminded frequently that there are caring people to assist them during the crisis and later. Additional sources of support that can be recommended are psychiatric and social work consultants, community services, and religious support. Self-help groups are excellent if these are available in the community.

Nurses often have difficulty relating to the parents if obvious neglect has precipitated the accident and subsequent problems; therefore it is important for those who care for these children and their families to assess their own feelings about the situation, as well as the coping abilities and resources of the family. Caring for near-drowning victims and their families requires the nurse to be sensitive to the needs of the child and the family and to recognize his or her own reactions and emotions.

Prevention. Most drownings, particularly of infants or small children, can be prevented with adequate supervision. Water safety and survival training should be required for all school-age children, and nurses can be active advocates in their communities. Nurses are also in a position to emphasize the importance of adequate adult supervision when children are in the water. Young children should never be left unattended when in or near the water. Parents with pools should know cardiopulmonary resuscitation (CPR) techniques. (See also Injury Prevention, Chapters 12, 14, 15, 17, and 19.)

INTRACRANIAL INFECTIONS

The nervous system and its coverings are subject to infection by the same organisms that affect other organs of the body. However, the nervous system is limited in the ways in which it responds to injury. Infectious processes share virtually the same clinical and pathologic features. They differ primarily in the growth and virulence of the specific organism. It is generally difficult to distinguish between the various etiologic agents from clinical manifestations. Laboratory studies are needed to identify the causative agent. The inflammatory process can affect the meninges ***(meningitis),*** brain ***(encephalitis),*** or spinal cord ***(myelitis).***

Meningitis can be caused by a variety of organisms, but the three main types are (1) ***bacterial,*** or pyogenic, caused by pus-forming bacteria, especially the meningococcus, pneumococcus, and influenza bacillus; (2) ***viral,*** or aseptic, caused by a wide variety of viral agents; and (3) ***tuberculous,*** caused by the tuberculin bacillus. The majority of children with acute febrile encephalopathy have either bacterial meningitis or viral meningitis as their underlying cause (Rubenstein, 1992).

BACTERIAL MENINGITIS

Bacterial meningitis is an acute inflammation of the meninges and CSF that affects an estimated 15,000 infants and children in the United States each year (Kilpi and others, 1991). The advent of antimicrobial therapy has had a marked effect on the course and prognosis, yet it remains a significant cause of illness in the pediatric age-groups. Its importance lies primarily in the frequency with which it occurs in infancy and childhood and the unnecessarily high death rates and residual damage caused by undiagnosed and untreated or inadequately treated cases. Children between 1 month and 5 years of age are the most frequently affected.

Etiology

Bacterial meningitis can be caused by any of a variety of bacterial agents. *Haemophilus influenzae* (type B), *Streptococcus pneumoniae,* and *Neisseria meningitidis* (meningococcus) organisms are responsible for bacterial meningitis in 95% of children older than 2 months. *H. influenzae* is the predominant organism in children 3 months to 3 years of age but is rare in infants younger than 3 months, who are apparently protected by passively acquired bactericidal substances, and in children older than 5 years, who are beginning to acquire this protection. With the routine use of *H. influenzae* type B vaccines, the etiology of bacterial meningitis is changing (see Prognosis, p. 1708).

Other organisms are β-hemolytic streptococcus, *Staphylococcus aureus,* and *Escherichia coli.* The leading causes of neonatal meningitis are the group B streptococci and *E. coli* organisms. *E. coli* infection is seldom seen beyond infancy. Meningococcic (epidemic cerebrospinal) meningitis occurs in epidemic form and is the only type readily transmitted by droplet infection from nasopharyngeal secretions. Although this condition may develop at any age, the risk of meningococcal infection increases with the number of contacts; therefore it occurs predominantly in school-age children and adolescents.

There appear to be some seasonal variations. Meningitis caused by *H. influenzae* is a disease that primarily occurs in autumn or early winter. Pneumococcal and meningococcal infections can occur at any time but are more common in later winter or early spring.

Several factors may predispose the child to the development of bacterial meningitis. Males are affected more often than females, and this is somewhat more pronounced in the neonatal period. The greatest morbidity after meningitis appears to involve children who were afflicted between birth and 4 years of age. Maternal factors, such as premature rupture of fetal membranes and maternal infection during the last week of pregnancy, are major causes of neonatal meningitis.

Deficiencies in the immune mechanisms and decreased leukocyte activity may influence the incidence in newborns, children with immunoglobulin deficiencies and children receiving immunosuppressant drugs. Meningitis appears to occur as an extension of a variety of bacterial infections, probably as a result of the lack of acquired resistance to the various etiologic organisms. Preexisting CNS anomalies, neurosurgical procedures or injuries, sickle cell disease, and primary infections elsewhere in the body are factors related to an increased susceptibility.

Pathophysiology

The most common route of infection is vascular dissemination from a focus of infection elsewhere. For example, organisms from the nasopharynx invade the underlying blood vessels and enter the cerebral blood supply or form local thromboemboli that release septic emboli into the bloodstream. Invasion by direct extension from infections in the paranasal and mastoid sinuses is less common. Organisms also gain entry by direct implantation after penetrating wounds, skull fractures that provide an opening into the skin or sinuses, lumbar puncture or surgical procedures, anatomic abnormalities such as spinal bifida, or foreign bodies such as an internal ventricular shunt or an external ventricular device. Once implanted, the organisms spread into the CSF, by which the infection spreads throughout the subarachnoid space. The pathophysiology of bacterial meningitis suggests neuronal injury related to the release of vasoactive substances or alteration of the blood-brain barrier permeability (Ashwal and others, 1992). A poor prognosis is associated with reduced CBF. This is primarily due to increased ICP.

The infective process is that seen in any bacterial infection—inflammation, exudation, white blood cell accumulation, and varying degrees of tissue damage. The brain becomes hyperemic and edematous, and the entire surface of the brain is covered with a layer of purulent exudate, which varies with the type of organism. For example, meningococcal exudate is most marked over the parietal, occipital, and cerebellar regions; the thick, fibrinous exudate of pneumococcal infection is confined chiefly to the surface of the brain, particularly the anterior lobes; and the exudate of streptococcal infections is similar to that of pneumococcal infections, but thinner.

Clinical Manifestations

The clinical manifestations of acute bacterial meningitis depend to a large extent on the age of the child. The picture is also influenced to some degree by the type of organism, the effectiveness of therapy for antecedent illness, and whether it occurs as an isolated entity or as a complication of another illness or injury.

Children and Adolescents. The illness is likely to be abrupt, with fever, chills, headache, and vomiting that are associated with or quickly followed by alterations in sensorium. Often the initial sign is a seizure, which may recur as the disease progresses. The child is extremely irritable and agitated and may develop photophobia, delirium, hallucinations, aggressive or maniacal behavior, or drowsiness, stupor, and coma. Sometimes the onset is slower, frequently preceded by several days of respiratory or gastrointestinal symptoms. Occasionally a prior infection treated with antibiotics masks or delays the signs of meningitis.

The child resists flexion of the neck, and as the disease progresses, the neck stiffness (nuchal rigidity) becomes marked until the head is drawn into extreme overextension (opisthotonos). Kernig and Brudzinski signs are positive. Reflex responses are variable, although they show hyperactivity (see Reflexes, Chapter 7). The skin may be cold and cyanotic with poor peripheral perfusion.

Other signs and symptoms may appear that are peculiar to individual organisms. Petechial or purpuric rashes usually indicate a meningococcal infection (meningococcemia), especially when the eruption is associated with a septic shocklike state. Joint involvement is seen in meningococcic and *H. influenzae* infection. A chronically draining ear commonly accompanies pneumococcal meningitis. *E. coli* infection may be associated with a congenital dermal sinus that communicates with the subarachnoid space.

Infants and Young Children. The classic picture of meningitis is rarely seen in children between 3 months and 2 years of age. The illness is characterized by fever, poor feeding, vomiting, marked irritability, toxic appearance, and frequent seizures, which are often accompanied by a high-pitched cry. A bulging fontanel is the most significant finding, and nuchal rigidity and Brudzinski and Kernig signs are helpful in diagnosis (Clinical diagnosis, 1993).

Neonates. Meningitis in newborn and premature infants is extremely difficult to diagnose. The vague and nonspecific manifestations, characteristic of all neonatal sepsis, bear little resemblance to the findings in older children. These infants are usually well at birth but within a few days begin to look and behave poorly. They refuse feedings, have poor sucking ability, and may vomit or have diarrhea. They display poor tone, lack of movement, and a poor cry. Other nonspecific signs that may be present include hypothermia or fever (depending on the maturity of the infant), jaundice, irritability, drowsiness, seizures, respiratory irregularities or apnea, cyanosis, and weight loss. The full, tense, and bulging fontanel may or may not be present until late in the course of the illness, and the neck is usually supple. Untreated, the child's condition will decline to cardiovascular collapse, seizures, and apnea.

Complications. The incidence of complications from acute bacterial meningitis has been significantly reduced with early diagnosis and vigorous antimicrobial therapy. If infection extends to the ventricles, thick pus, fibrin, or adhesions may occlude the narrow passages, thereby obstructing the flow of CSF to cause obstructive hydrocephalus. Subdural effusions occur frequently, and thrombosis may occur in meningeal veins or venous sinuses. Destructive changes may take place in the cerebral cortex, and brain abscesses may form by direct extension of the infection or by vascular dissemination. Extension of the infection to the areas of the cranial nerves or compression necrosis from increased pressure may cause deafness, blindness, or weakness or paralysis of facial or other muscles of the head and neck.

One of the most dramatic and serious complications usually associated with meningococcal infections is ***meningococcal septicemia***, or ***meningococcemia***. When the onset is severe, sudden, and rapid (fulminate), it is known as the ***Waterhouse-Friderichsen syndrome***. The syndrome is characterized by overwhelming septic shock, disseminated intravascular coagulation (DIC), and massive bilateral adrenal hemorrhage. Meningococcemia requires immediate emergency treatment, hospitalization, and intensive care. The mortality is as high as 85% (Jenkins, 1992).

NURSING ALERT Any child who is ill and develops a purpuric rash (petechiae and ecchymoses) must receive medical evaluation immediately.

Other acute complications of meningitis include the syndrome of inappropriate antidiuretic hormone (SIADH) (see Chapter 38), subdural effusions, seizures, cerebral edema and herniation, and hydrocephalus. Obstruction to the flow of CSF occurs in the acute phase of illness by clumping of purulent material in the drainage channels and in the chronic phase by adhesive arachnoiditis or fibrotic obstruction through any of the ventricular foramina. Postmeningitic complications in neonates include ventriculitis, resulting in cystic, walled-off areas of the brain with fluid accumulation and pressure.

Extension of the inflammation to cranial nerves or compression and destruction of the nerves from ICP can produce permanent impairment of vision or hearing and other nerve palsies. Auditory nerve damage is usually followed by permanent deafness. Other long-term complications include cerebral palsy, mental handicap, learning disorder, and attention deficit disorder. Only children with permanent neurologic deficits are at risk for epilepsy (Pomeroy and others, 1990).

Hemiparesis and quadriparesis may result from damage caused by arteritis and/or thrombosis or other mechanisms. Behavioral changes are noted in some children. Also, evidence indicates that psychometric and behavioral defects may be a significant concomitant sign of meningitis in childhood, although it is difficult to determine the degree to which meningitis affects the intelligence of young children.

Diagnostic Evaluation

A lumbar puncture is the definitive diagnostic test. The fluid pressure is measured, and samples are obtained for culture, Gram stain, blood cell count, and determination of glucose and protein content. The findings are usually diagnostic. Culture and stain are needed to identify the causative organism. Spinal fluid pressure is usually elevated, but interpretation is often difficult when the child is crying. Sedation with meperidine (Demerol) or fentanyl and midazolam (Versed) can alleviate the child's pain and fear associated with this procedure.

There is generally an elevated white blood cell count, predominantly polymorphonuclear leukocytes, but it may be extremely variable. The glucose level is reduced, generally in proportion to the duration and severity of the infection. The relationship between the CSF glucose and serum glucose levels is important in evaluating the glucose content of CSF; therefore a serum glucose sample is drawn approximately ½ hour before the lumbar puncture. Protein concentration is usually increased.

A blood culture is advisable for all children suspected of meningitis and occasionally proves positive when CSF culture is negative. Nose and throat cultures may provide helpful information in some cases. Several newer techniques for diagnosing or differentiating meningitis are also available.

Therapeutic Management

Acute bacterial meningitis is a medical emergency that requires early recognition and immediate institution of therapy to prevent death and avoid residual disabilities. The initial therapeutic management includes:

- Isolation precautions
- Initiation of antimicrobial therapy
- Maintenance of optimum hydration
- Maintenance of ventilation
- Reduction of increased ICP
- Management of bacterial shock
- Control of seizures
- Control of extremes of temperature
- Correction of anemia
- Treatment of complications

The child is isolated from other children, usually in an intensive care unit for close observation. An intravenous infusion is started as soon as the lumbar puncture has been completed in order to facilitate the administration of antimicrobial agents, fluids, anticonvulsive drugs, and blood if needed. The child is placed on a cardiac monitor.

Drugs. Until the causative organism is identified, the choice of antibiotic is based on the known sensitivity of the organism most likely to be the infective agent in any given situation and on the probable interactions with the specific patient. The drugs are administered intravenously throughout the course of treatment. The drugs are given in large doses, and the period of therapy is determined by CSF findings and the child's clinical condition. Appropriate antibiotics are administered following identification of the causative organism.

During the initial treatment of meningitis, dexamethasone is considered a standard treatment (American Academy of Pediatrics, 1990). Dexamethasone (0.6 mg/kg/day) is administered intravenously every 6 hours for the first 4 days of therapy. Corticosteroid administration during the treatment of *H. influenzae* meningitis has been shown to reduce the incidence of subsequent hearing loss. Signs of gastrointestinal hemorrhage or secondary infection may complicate steroid administration. Antibiotic treatment with cephalosporins demonstrate superiority for promptly sterilizing the CSF and reducing the incidence of severe hearing impairment.

Nonspecific Measures. Maintaining hydration is a prime concern, and intravenous fluids and the type and amount of fluid are determined by the patient's condition. The optimum hydration involves correction of any fluid deficits followed by low maintenance levels to prevent cerebral edema. If indicated, measures are employed to reduce ICP, as described previously (see p. 1673). Increased ICP seen with CNS infections commands attention because of the severe reduction of cerebral perfusion pressure (CPP) in children suffering from bacterial meningitis in the early period, herpes encephalitis, and postinfectious encephalitis with severe status epilepticus.

Complications are treated appropriately, such as aspiration of subdural effusion in infants and heparin therapy for children who develop disseminated intravascular coagulation syndrome. Shock, if it occurs in the child, is managed by restoration of blood volume and maintenance of electrolyte balance. Seizures can occur in affected children during the first few days of treatment. These are controlled with appropriate antiepileptic drugs.

Lumbar puncture is carried out as needed to determine the effectiveness of therapy. The patient is evaluated neurologically during the convalescent period and at regular intervals during the succeeding year.

Prognosis. The age of the child, the duration of illness before antibiotic therapy, the rapidity of diagnosis after onset, the type of organism, and the adequacy of therapy are important in the prognosis of bacterial meningitis. The mortality of neonatal meningitis is highest, with poor outcomes also in β-hemolytic streptococcal meningitis, meningococcal meningitis, and pneumococcal meningitis in infancy and childhood (Krugman and others, 1992).

Sequelae of bacterial meningitis are seen most frequently when the disease occurs in the first 2 months of life and least often in children with meningococcal meningitis. The residual deficits in infants are primarily a result of communicating hydrocephalus and the greater effects of cerebritis on the immature brain. In older children the residual effects are related to the inflammatory process itself or result from vasculitis associated with the disease. Bacterial meningitis continues to cause substantial morbidity in infants and children. Hearing impairment is the most common sequela of this disease. Evaluation of CN VIII is needed for at least a 6-month follow-up period to assess for possible hearing loss.

Prevention. Vaccines are available for types A, C, Y, and W-135 meningococci and *H. influenzae* type b. Routine meningococcal vaccination of children is not recommended. However, routine vaccinations for *H. influenzae* type b is recommended for all children beginning at 2 months of age (see Immunizations, Chapter 12). A declining incidence of *H. influenzae* type b disease has occurred since the introduction of the Hib vaccination. The data suggest that vaccination may be protecting against the disease, as well as decreasing the spread of infection to unvaccinated infants (Murphy and others, 1993).

Nursing Considerations

Nurses should take necessary precautions to protect themselves and others from possible infection. Parents are taught the proper procedures and supervised in their application.

NURSING ALERT The first priority of nursing care of a child suspected of having meningitis is to administer the antibiotic as soon as it is ordered. The child is also placed on respiratory isolation for at least 24 hours after implementation of antimicrobial therapy.

The room is kept as quiet as possible, and environmental stimuli are kept at a minimum, since most affected children are sensitive to noise, bright lights, and other external stimuli. Most children are more comfortable without a pillow and with the head of the bed slightly elevated. A side-lying position is more often assumed because of nuchal rigidity. The nurse should avoid actions, such as lifting the child's head, that cause pain or increase discomfort. Evaluating the child for pain and implementing appropriate relief measures are paramount during the initial 24 to 72 hours. Acetaminophen with codeine is often used. Measures are employed to ensure safety, since the child is often restless and subject to seizures.

The nursing care of the child with meningitis is determined by the child's symptoms and treatment. Observation of vital signs, neurologic signs, LOC, urinary output, and other pertinent data is carried out at frequent intervals. The child who is unconscious is managed as described previously (see p. 1683), and all children are observed carefully for signs of complications just described, especially signs of increased ICP, shock, or respiratory distress. Head circumference is measured on the infant because subdural effusions and obstructive hydrocephalus can develop as a complication of meningitis.

Fluids and nourishment are determined by the child's status. The child with dulled sensorium is usually given nothing by mouth. Other children are allowed clear liquids initially and progressed to a diet suitable for their age. Careful monitoring and recording of intake and output are needed to determine deviations that might indicate impending shock or increasing fluid accumulation, such as cerebral edema or subdural effusion.

One of the most difficult problems in nursing care of children with meningitis is maintaining the intravenous infusion for the length of time needed to provide adequate antimicrobial therapy (usually 10 days). Since continuous intravenous fluids are usually not necessary, an intermittent infusion device is used. In some cases, children who are recovering uneventfully are sent home with the device, and parents are taught intravenous drug administration.* (See also Nursing Care Plan: The Child with Acute Bacterial Meningitis.†)

Family Support. The sudden nature of the illness makes emotional support of the child and parents extremely important. Parents are very upset and concerned about their child's condition and frequently feel guilty for not having suspected the seriousness of the illness sooner. They need much reassurance that the natural onset of meningitis is sudden and that they acted responsibly in seeking medical assistance when they did. The nurse encourages them to openly discuss their feelings to minimize blame and guilt. They also are kept informed of the child's progress and of all procedures and treatments. In the event that the child's condition worsens, they need the same psychologic care as parents facing the possible death of their child (see Chapter 23).

NONBACTERIAL (ASEPTIC) MENINGITIS

Aseptic meningitis is caused by a number of agents, principally viruses, and is frequently associated with other diseases, such as measles, mumps, herpes, and leukemia. Enteroviruses and mumps viruses account for a large number of cases.

The onset may be abrupt or gradual. The initial manifestations are headache, fever, malaise, gastrointestinal symptoms, and signs of meningeal irritation that develop 1 or 2 days after the onset of illness. Abdominal pain and nausea and vomiting are common; back and leg pain, sore throat, photophobia, chest pain, and generalized muscular aches or pains are found occasionally. Onset is more insidious in infants and toddlers. Parents may report a change in the child's level of activity and responsiveness. They suspect a minor illness until meningeal signs appear. There may be a maculopapular rash. These symptoms usually subside spontaneously and rapidly, and the child is well in 3 to 10 days with no residual effects.

Diagnosis is based on clinical features and CSF findings. When aseptic (viral or fungal) meningitis is present, the CSF glucose concentration is usually normal, and the protein content is only slightly elevated. There may be a moderate or large number of cells, predominantly polymorphonuclear leukocytes, early in the course and lymphocytes later in the course. The Gram stain is usually negative, and the serologic culture is usually positive for virus. It is important to differentiate this self-limited disorder from the more serious forms of meningitis and to diagnose and treat any disease of which it is a manifestation.

Treatment is primarily symptomatic, such as acetaminophen for headache and muscle pain and positioning for comfort. Antimicrobial agents may be administered and isolation enforced until a definitive diagnosis is made as a precaution against the possibility that the disease might be of bacterial origin. Nursing care is similar to the care of the child with bacterial meningitis.

TUBERCULOUS (TB) MENINGITIS

TB meningitis must be considered, especially in persons traveling or living in, and in immigrants from, developing countries. The advent of drug-resistant TB may predispose an increasing number of children to this organism.

Ischemic infarction can occur with TB meningitis. The most frequent clinical findings are meningeal signs, fever, alteration of consciousness, CN involvement, seizures, and focal neurologic deficit.

Early diagnosis of TB meningitis in the child can signifi-

*Home care instructions for caring for an intermittent infusion device are available in *Wong and Whaley's Clinical Manual of Pediatric Nursing* (Mosby).
†In *Wong and Whaley's Clinical Manual of Pediatric Nursing* (Mosby).

cantly reduce the disability caused by hydrocephalus, a frequent complication of this type of meningitis. Nursing care involves administration of medications, support of the child, control of pain, and neurologic monitoring, similar to the care of the child with bacterial meningitis.

BRAIN ABSCESS

Brain abscesses are the most common form of intracranial suppurative process in children. Intracerebral abscesses form when pyogenic organisms gain access to neural tissue by way of the bloodstream from foci of infection or from direct inoculation of organisms from meningitis, penetrating trauma, or surgical procedures. Chronic ear infection and cyanotic congenital heart disease are the most common predisposing factors for children with brain abscesses. Meningitis and ventriculitis are dominant etiologies in infants. The most common organisms include staphylococci, streptococci, and *Proteus*. However, a large number of children with brain abscesses have no discernible source of infection.

The most common sites of intracerebral abscesses are the temporal and frontal lobes between the gray and white matter. Early signs of the disease are vague, and the insidious onset often includes vomiting, lethargy, fever, seizures, and progression to coma. Specific neurologic signs are related to the area invaded by the infectious process and, as this area enlarges, resemble those produced by an intracranial tumor. Cerebellar abscesses produce signs associated with any posterior fossa mass (see Brain Tumors, Chapter 36).

Antibiotic therapy is effective during abscess formation. Successful management consists of surgical drainage of a confined infection and antibiotic therapy. The child is treated symptomatically with frequent CT scans to monitor the progress of the abscess. Where possible, the source of the infection is eradicated. Children may experience seizure disorders as a long-term complication. The incidence of epilepsy following brain abscess treatment was 34% (Koszewski, 1991).

Mortality rates from brain abscesses may exceed 20%, making a prompt diagnosis critical (Williams, Nelms, and McGaharan, 1992). However, a decline in mortality has been documented with the advent of CT scanning (Tekkok and Erbergi, 1992). The progression of the disease and the child's mental status before admission continue to be prognostic factors.

Nursing care is similar to the care of the child with increased ICP. Support of the child and family is essential, since the possibility of the child's death remains strong.

ENCEPHALITIS

Encephalitis is an inflammatory process of the CNS producing altered function of various portions of the brain and spinal cord. Encephalitis can be caused by a variety of organisms, including bacteria, spirochetes, fungi, protozoa, helminths, and viruses. Most infections are associated with viruses, and this discussion is limited to these agents.

Etiology

Encephalitis can occur as a result of (1) direct invasion of the CNS by a virus or (2) postinfectious involvement of the CNS after a viral disease. Often the specific type of encephalitis in a particular patient may not be identified for some time or not at all. The cause of over half the cases reported in the United States is unknown. The majority of cases of known etiology are associated with the childhood diseases of measles, mumps, varicella, and rubella and, less often, with the enteroviruses and herpes viruses. Vaccination programs have greatly reduced the incidence of encephalitis in children.

Herpes simplex encephalitis is an uncommon disease, but 30% of cases involve children. Herpes simplex encephalitis is a severe, life-threatening illness. Death can occur if treatment is not started before the child becomes comatose. The virus attacks the brain, especially the frontal and temporal lobes. Cerebral edema and subsequent increased ICP can lead to temporal herniation. It is unclear how the virus enters the CNS, although it is postulated that it may enter through the bloodstream or peripheral nerves. Symptoms include fever, nausea and vomiting, headache, confusion, stupor, hemiparesis, focal neurologic deficits, and seizures. The CSF is abnormal in most cases.

Because of a rise in the number of children with herpes simplex virus encephalitis, suspected cases require prompt attention, especially since the diagnosis can be difficult. The clinical diagnosis can be confirmed by the rapid appearance of IgM antibody to herpes simplex virus type 1 in CSF and serum. Brain biopsy in herpes simplex encephalitis is often recommended. The diagnosis needs to be confirmed and other diseases excluded. Treatment with acyclovir is justified before precise virologic diagnosis has been established. Saving CSF for antibody titres or antigen identification should be routine practice (Cameron, Wallace, and Munro, 1992).

The multiplicity of causes of viral encephalitis makes diagnosis difficult. Most are those involved with arthropod vectors (togaviruses and bunyaviruses) and those associated with hemorrhagic fevers (arenaviruses, filoviruses, Hantaan viruses). The vector reservoir for most agents pathogenic for humans and detected in the United States is the mosquito; therefore most cases of encephalitis appear during the hot summer months and subside during the autumn. One type found along the United States–Canadian border is carried by ticks.

Clinical Manifestations

The clinical features of encephalitis are similar regardless of the agent involved. Manifestations can range from a mild benign form that resembles aseptic meningitis, lasting a few days and being followed by rapid and complete recovery, to a fulminating encephalitis with severe CNS involvement. The onset may be sudden or gradual with malaise, fever, headache, dizziness, apathy, stiffness of the neck, nausea and vomiting, ataxia, tremors, hyperactivity, and speech difficulties. In severe cases there is high fever, stupor, seizures, disorientation, spasticity, and coma that may proceed to death. Ocular palsies and paralysis also may occur.

Diagnostic Evaluation

The diagnosis is made on the basis of clinical findings, circumstances associated with the disease, and, where possible, identification of the specific virus. Early in the course of encephalitis, CT scan results may be normal. Later, hemorrhagic areas in the frontotemporal region may be visualized. A diagnostic evaluation of encephalitis may include a brain biopsy, usually from the temporal lobe area. Togaviruses (some of which were formerly labeled arboviruses) are rarely detected in the blood or spinal fluid, but viruses of herpes, mumps, measles, and enteroviruses may be found in CSF. Serologic diagnosis may be reached by means of a variety of antibody tests. The first should be drawn as soon after onset as possible and the second 2 or 3 weeks later.

Therapeutic Management

Patients suspected of having encephalitis are hospitalized promptly for skilled nursing care and observation. Treatment is primarily supportive, including conscientious nursing care, control of cerebral manifestations, and adequate nutrition and hydration, with observations and management as for other disorders involving cerebral injury. Viral encephalitis can cause devastating neurologic injury. Cerebral hyperemia occurs in severe viral encephalitis, and ICP monitoring to reduce the pressure may be advocated (Goetting and Haddad, 1992). Follow-up care with periodic reevaluation and rehabilitation are important for survivors with residual effects of the disease.

Nursing Considerations

Nursing care of the child with encephalitis is the same as for any unconscious child and for the child with meningitis. Additional nursing interventions include observation for deterioration in consciousness. Isolation of the child is not necessary; however, good handwashing technique must be followed. A main focus of nursing management is the control of rapidly rising ICP. Neurologic monitoring, administration of medications, and support of the child and parents are the major aspects of care.

RABIES

Rabies is an acute infection of the nervous system caused by a virus that is almost invariably fatal if left untreated. It is transmitted to humans by the saliva of an infected mammal introduced through a bite or skin abrasion. After entry into a new host the virus multiplies in muscle cells and is spread through neural pathways without stimulating a protective host immune response.

Approximately 88% of rabies cases come from wild animals and 12% from domestic animals. Carnivorous wild animals (especially skunks, raccoons, and foxes) and bats are the animals most often infected with rabies and the cause of most indigenous cases of human rabies in the United States (Recommendations, 1991). The likelihood of human exposure to a rabid domestic animal has decreased greatly.

The domestic dog, formerly considered a prime source, is relatively well controlled by rabies vaccination programs. Cats are now the most common rabid domestic animals and should be the target of rabies vaccination programs. The circumstances of a biting incident are important. An unprovoked attack is more likely to indicate a rabid animal than a provoked attack. Bites inflicted on a child attempting to feed or handle an apparently healthy animal can generally be regarded as provoked. Any child bitten by a wild animal is assumed to be exposed to rabies.

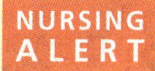

Unusual behavior in an animal is cause for suspicion; children should be warned to beware of wild animals that appear to be friendly.

Although rabies is common among wildlife species, human rabies is rarely acquired. The highest incidence occurs in children under age 15 years. Cases of human rabies are known to be acquired outside the United States, resulting in death from rabies encephalitis (Imported human rabies, 1992). The incubation period usually ranges from 1 to 3 months but may be as short as 10 days or as long as 8 months. Only 10% to 15% of persons bitten develop the disease, but once symptoms are present, rabies progresses to a fatal outcome.

The disease is characterized by a period of general malaise, fever, and sore throat followed by a phase of excitement featuring hypersensitivity and increased reaction to external stimuli, convulsions, maniacal behavior, and choking. Attempts at swallowing may cause such severe spasm of respiratory muscles that apnea, cyanosis, and anoxia are produced—the characteristics from which the term ***hydrophobia*** was derived.

Diagnosis is made on the basis of history and clinical features. Once symptoms appear, treatment is of little avail, but the long incubation period allows time for induction of active and passive immunity before the onset of illness.

Therapeutic Management

Two types of immunizing products are available for use in humans: (1) the inactivated rabies vaccines, which induce an active immune response, and (2) the globulins, which contain preformed antibodies. The two types of products should be used concurrently for rabies postexposure treatment when prophylaxis is indicated.

The current therapy for a rabid animal bite consists of thorough cleansing of the wound and passive immunization with human rabies immune globulin (HRIG) as soon as possible after exposure to provide rapid, short-term passive immunity. Furthermore, postexposure prophylaxis is recommended for persons who report a possible infectious exposure (e.g., bite, scratch, open wound, or mucous membrane contamination with saliva or other infectious material) to a human with rabies (Imported human rabies, 1992).

Postexposure active immunity is conferred by administration of the human diploid cell rabies vaccine (HDCV).

The first dose of the vaccine is given at the same time as the immune globulin and followed by intramuscular injections at 3, 7, 14, and 28 days after the first dose. An additional dose in 90 days is recommended by the World Health Organization. Before antirabies prophylaxis is initiated, the local or state health department should be consulted.

Nursing Considerations

Parents, as well as children, are frightened by the urgency and seriousness of the situation. They need anticipatory guidance for the therapy and support and reassurance regarding the efficacy of the preventive measures for this dreaded disease. The vaccine is well tolerated by children, although they need preparation for the series of injections. Mass immunization is unnecessary and unlikely to be implemented. In areas in which rabies is rare, the schedule given is sufficient. However, certain circumstances may warrant preexposure vaccination, such as when a child is being taken to an area of the world where rabies in stray dogs is still a problem.

REYE SYNDROME (RS)

The etiology of the disorder is obscure, but most cases of RS follow a common viral illness, most frequently influenza or varicella. RS is a condition characterized pathologically by cerebral edema and fatty changes of the liver. The disease is manifested clinically by encephalopathy and coma. The pathology of RS is a mitochondrial insult induced by different viruses, drugs, exogenous toxins, and genetic factors. Elevated ammonia levels tend to correlate with the clinical manifestations and prognosis. Definitive diagnosis is established by liver biopsy. The staging criteria for RS are based on neurologic signs ranging from lethargic to comatose states and on liver dysfunction.

All children with RS in one study demonstrated cytotoxic cerebral edema, with swelling of astrocyte foot processes (Blisard and Davis, 1991). Children who in the past would have been diagnosed with RS are now given other diagnoses as a result of improved diagnostic techniques. Many children are now correctly diagnosed as having viral or metabolic diseases as an escalation of symptoms induced by antiemetics. Cases of unrecognized drug-induced encephalopathy by antiemetics given to children during viral illnesses have similar symptoms to those of RS.

The link between aspirin and RS is possible but has not been firmly established as a cause-and-effect relationship (Casteels-VanDaele, 1993). By the time aspirin product labeling was required by the FDA in 1986, most of the decline in RS incidence had already occurred. However, many experts maintain that adequate labeling to alert the public to potential hazards from administration of aspirin was a factor in the virtual disappearance of RS.

Nursing Considerations

The most important aspect of successful management of the child with RS is early diagnosis and aggressive therapy. Rapid progression through coma stages and high peak ammonia concentrations are associated with a more serious prognosis. Cerebral edema with increased ICP represents the most immediate threat to life. Recovery from RS is rapid and usually without sequelae if there has been early diagnosis and implementation of therapy.

Care and observations are implemented as for any child with an altered state of consciousness (see p. 1676) and increasing ICP. Accurate and frequent monitoring of intake and output is essential for adjusting fluid volumes to prevent both dehydration and cerebral edema. Because of related liver dysfunction, the nurse must observe for signs of impaired coagulation such as prolonged bleeding time.

Parents of children with RS need to be kept informed regarding the child's progress, to have diagnostic procedures and therapeutic management explained, and to be given concerned and sympathetic support. Families need to be aware that salicylate, the alleged offending ingredient in aspirin, is contained in other products (e.g., over-the-counter products such as Pepto-Bismol, a popular antacid). They should refrain from administering any product for influenza-like symptoms without first checking the label for "hidden" salicylates.

HUMAN IMMUNODEFICIENCY VIRUS (HIV) ENCEPHALOPATHY

Children with HIV encephalopathy, a complication of acquired immunodeficiency syndrome (AIDS), present a nursing challenge. Progressive encephalopathy occurs in 30% to 50% of infants and children infected with HIV; 82% are less than 5 years of age.

HIV infection is acquired through direct exposure to blood or other body fluids of infected persons or by direct maternal-fetal transmission. The majority of pediatric AIDS patients have acquired HIV from their infected mothers (Projections, 1992). Delivery by cesarean section may decrease the incidence of maternal HIV transmission to the newborn. Because recent laboratory testing has been developed to identify HIV infection sooner in newborns, supportive care and management can be initiated. Presently there is no cure for this deadly disease.

Neurologic manifestations in children suggest that the progressive encephalopathy is the result of primary and persistent infection of the brain with the virus. Unexplained neurodevelopmental regression and focal seizures are the dominant clinical features of the disorder. Others include progressive motor dysfunction and atypical CNS infections. These manifestations indicate a poor prognosis and, almost invariably, a fatal outcome. However, earlier implementation of therapies for AIDS may allow for slower progression of these neurologic complications. One third of infants born to AIDS-infected mothers develop the disease and die within a year (Civitello, 1991).

Appropriate precautions are practiced by nurses when caring for these children. Careful handling of the child is a hallmark of excellent nursing, since these children may experience pain, isolation, social stigma, susceptibility to infection, and abandonment resulting in less than minimum sensorimotor stimulation. Nursing assessment and intervention warrant planning time to meet developmental needs, especially if it means holding, rocking, and comforting the child. (See Chapter 35 for a more extensive discussion of AIDS.)

SEIZURE DISORDERS*

Seizures are brief malfunctions of the brain's electrical system resulting from cortical neuronal discharge. The manifestations of seizures are determined by the site of origin and may include unconsciousness or altered consciousness, involuntary movements, and changes in perception, behaviors, sensations, and posture. Seizures are the most frequently observed neurologic dysfunction in children and can occur with a wide variety of conditions involving the CNS.

EPILEPSY

Once it is determined that the child has had a seizure, it is important to distinguish whether the episode was an epileptic or a nonepileptic seizure. Seizures are the indispensable characteristic of epilepsy; however, not every seizure is epileptic (see Thinking Critically About . . . box). Epilepsy is a chronic seizure disorder with recurrent and unprovoked seizures. Up to 20% of children have been misdiagnosed as having epilepsy (Sagraves, 1990). The careful diagnosis of epilepsy should be made and substantiated with clinical evidence because of the important prognostic and therapeutic implications, which also involve the identification and treatment of the etiology.

A simple seizure event should not be classified as epilepsy and is generally not treated with long-term antiepileptic drugs. Some seizures may result from an acute medical or neurologic illness and cease once the illness is treated. In other cases children may have a single seizure without the cause ever being known (Pellock, 1990).

*Ellen Johnsen, RN, BA, revised this section.

Etiology

Seizures in children have many different causes and histories. Most seizures are ***idiopathic.*** Although the cause of idiopathic epilepsy is unknown, it may indicate genetic factors that in some way alter the seizure threshold to influence neuronal discharge. Congenital defects and some genetic disorders (e.g., tuberous sclerosis) have seizures as a manifestation. Febrile and breath-holding seizures are related to a lowered seizure threshold that tends to have a higher incidence in certain families. Hereditary EEG abnormalities have been detected in some families, and there is a higher incidence of seizures among relatives of children with idiopathic seizure disorders.

A seizure disorder also can be ***acquired*** as a result of brain injury during prenatal, perinatal, or postnatal periods. This injury may be caused by trauma, hypoxia, infections, exogenous or endogenous toxins, and a variety of other factors. Biochemical events (e.g., hypoglycemia, hypocalcemia, certain nutritional deficiencies) produce seizure activity. A partial list of causative factors is presented in the box on p. 1714.

The incidence of causative factors associated with childhood seizures is frequently related to the age of the child. Seizures are more common during the first 2 years of life than during any other period of childhood. In very young infants the most frequent causes are birth injuries (i.e., intracranial trauma, hemorrhage, or anoxia and congenital defects of the brain. Acute infections are a frequent cause of seizures in late infancy and early childhood but become an infrequent cause in middle childhood. In children older than 3 years the most common cause is idiopathic epilepsy.

Other contributing factors are fatigue, not taking medication, and not eating properly. Excessive fluid intake or fluid retention, such as occurs during premenstrual tension, produces alterations in the serum (and brain) concentrations of sodium, potassium, and water, which may precipitate seizures. There appear to be periods of functional instability of the brain, normally when falling asleep or awakening from sleep. At these times seizures are more likely to occur. The hormonal and metabolic changes associated with adolescence can alter the seizure threshold. Photogenic stimulation by such commonplace things as television,

THINKING CRITICALLY ABOUT . . . *Terminology for Epilepsy*

Many words are used synonymously with the term *epilepsy, seizure disorder,* or *seizure.* Epilepsy used to belong to the medical discipline of psychiatry, and therefore words such as "attacks" and "fits" are sometimes used to describe seizure events. These words, however, still create images of medieval superstitions, evil spirits, and the horrors of mental institutions. For these reasons, parents are frequently hesitant to inform caregivers and the school that their child has a seizure disorder for fear of prejudice and misunderstandings.

The words "convulsion," "convulsive disorder," and "anticonvulsive drugs" are often used to cover all seizure types and antiepileptic drugs. However, the word "convulsion" conjures up images of a raving, wild person who is out of control and possibly dangerous. Therefore the wisdom of referring to all seizures as convulsions is questionable, since most seizures are not convulsive in nature. Therefore in this chapter the words "event," "episode," or "experience" are used to describe a seizure; likewise, medications are referred to as antiepileptic drugs. In working with families, health professionals should consider the words they use to discuss epilepsy and seizures. Correct terminology can help lessen the stigma and fear often associated with words such as "convulsions" or "fits."

ETIOLOGY OF SEIZURES IN CHILDREN

NONRECURRENT (ACUTE)

Febrile episodes
Intracranial infection
Intracranial hemorrhage
Space-occupying lesions (cyst, tumor)
Acute cerebral edema
Anoxia
Toxins
- Drugs
- Tetanus
- Lead encephalopathy
- *Shigella, Salmonella*

Metabolic alterations
- Hypocalcemia
- Hypoglycemia
- Hyponatremia or hypernatremia
- Hypomagnesemia
- Alkalosis
- Disorders of amino acid metabolism
- Deficiency states
- Hyperbilirubinemia

RECURRENT (CHRONIC)

Idiopathic epilepsy
Epilepsy secondary to:
- Trauma
- Hemorrhage
- Anoxia
- Infections
- Toxins
- Degenerative phenomena
- Congenital defects
- Parasitic brain disease
- Hypoglycemia injury

Epilepsy—sensory stimulus
Epilepsy-stimulating states
- Narcolepsy and catalepsy
- Psychogenic
- Tetany from hypocalcemia, alkalosis

Hypoglycemic states
- Hyperinsulinism
- Hypopituitarism
- Adrenocortical insufficiency
- Hepatic disorders

Uremia
Allergy
Cardiovascular dysfunction or syncopal episodes
Migraine

video games, rays of the sun, or certain kinds of music in susceptible children have been implicated in precipitating seizures in some instances.

Pathophysiology

Regardless of the etiologic factor or the type of seizure, the basic mechanism is the same. There are electric discharges that (1) may arise from central areas in the brain that affect consciousness immediately; (2) may be restricted to one area of the cerebral cortex, producing manifestations characteristic of that particular anatomic focus; or (3) may begin in a localized area of the cortex and spread to other portions of the brain, which, if sufficiently extensive, produce generalized neurologic manifestations.

Seizure activity is believed to be caused by spontaneous electric discharge initiated by a group of hyperexcitable cells referred to as the ***epileptogenic focus.*** These cells display increased electric excitability but may remain quiescent over a time while discharging intermittently, as evidenced on EEG tracings. Normally these discharges are restrained from spreading beyond the focal area by normal inhibitory mechanisms.

In response to any of a variety of physiologic stimuli, such as cellular dehydration, abnormal blood sugar levels, electrolyte imbalance, fatigue, emotional stress, and endocrine changes, these hyperexcitable cells activate normal cells in surrounding areas and in distant, synaptically related cells. When the neuronal excitation from the epileptogenic focus spreads to the brainstem, particularly the midbrain and reticular formation, a generalized seizure develops. These centers within the brainstem, known as the centrencephalic system, are responsible for the spread of the epileptic potentials. The discharges can originate spontaneously in the centrencephalic system or be triggered by a focal area in the cortex. Seizures are designated as focal, focal with rapid generalization, and generalized, on the basis of these characteristic neuronal discharges, as recorded by the EEG. In a large proportion of children focal seizures spread to other areas, ultimately becoming generalized with loss of consciousness.

Seizure Classification and Clinical Manifestations

According to the 1981 International League Against Epilepsy (see box on p. 1715), seizures are classified into 3 major categories: (1) ***partial seizures,*** formerly called focal seizures, which are limited to a particular local area of the brain; (2) ***generalized seizures,*** which involve both hemispheres of the brain; and (3) ***unclassified epileptic seizures.*** In addition to the seizures classified by the international system, several types of epileptic syndromes display a group of signs and symptoms that collectively characterize or indicate a particular condition. An additional classification system of these syndromes has been proposed by the International League Against Epilepsy (Commission, 1989). Several syndromes associated with epilepsy occur in infants and children. The two syndromes that occur most often are infantile spasms and Lennox-Gastaut syndrome.

Partial Seizures. Partial seizures may arise from any area of the cerebral cortex, but the frontal, temporal, and parietal lobes are the ones most often affected and are characterized by localized motor symptoms; somatosensory, psychic, autonomic symptoms; or a combination of these. The abnormal EEG discharges remain unilateral and are evident as focal spikes or sharp waves. Partial seizures are subdivided into three types:

1. **Simple partial seizures**—Have elementary or simple symptoms and no alteration of consciousness (also called an aura; see discussion under Complex Partial Seizures)
2. **Complex partial seizures**—Involve complex symptoms and impairment of consciousness
3. **Simple or complex seizures secondarily generalized**—Develop into generalized seizures, usually a tonic-clonic event

Partial seizures exhibit manifestations depending on where they occur in the brain. A clear description of the seizure ***(ictal state)*** by an eyewitness is a valuable aid in localizing the brain area involved and frequently suggests the underlying pathology. The initial event may provide the best clue for assessing the type of seizure and its localization. Correctly localizing the area of the brain involved during a seizure event is of crucial importance for diagnostic and therapeutic reasons. Many antiepileptic drugs exist and are specific for each type of seizure. Therefore assigning the appropriate classification is crucial for prescribing treatment.

In addition to the initial event, the circumstances that precipitated the episode are important. Identifying and

INTERNATIONAL CLASSIFICATION OF EPILEPTIC SEIZURES

PARTIAL SEIZURES

Simple Partial Seizures

No loss of consciousness or awareness.

1. With motor signs limited to one side of the body, such as an isolated jerking of part of the body. Seizures may begin in a small part of the body, such as the corner of the mouth, a finger, or a toe, and then spread to other parts of the body.
2. With sensory symptoms:
   a. Sight
   b. Smell
   c. Sound
   d. Taste
   e. Touch
   f. Emotions
   Such as hearing buzzing sounds, feeling frightened or angry, or seeing flashing lights.

Complex Partial Seizures

Also called psychomotor or temporal lobe; loss of awareness of surroundings. The person may stop whatever he or she is doing and begin some purposeless behavior, such as lip smacking, picking at clothes, or wandering around a room; or the person may continue whatever he or she is doing but in an inappropriate manner. Confusion follows the seizure.

1. Simple partial onset (aura) followed by impairment of consciousness.
2. With impairment of consciousness at onset.
3. Partial seizures evolving to secondarily generalized seizures (may be generalized tonic-clonic, tonic, or clonic).
   a. Simple partial seizures evolving to generalized seizures.
   b. Complex partial seizures evolving to generalized seizures.
   c. Simple partial seizures evolving to complex seizures, evolving to generalized seizures.

GENERALIZED SEIZURES

Absence Seizures

Formerly called petit mal. Nonconvulsive seizures with total loss of consciousness or awareness. Short periods of blinking, staring, or minor movements lasting a few seconds.

Tonic-Clonic Seizures

Formerly called grand mal. Total loss of consciousness with convulsions usually lasting 1 to 3 minutes.

Myoclonic Seizures

Myoclonic jerks (single or multiple); start or stop abruptly.

Clonic Seizures

Clonic muscle activity.

Tonic Seizures

Stiffening of the body.

Atonic Seizures

Lack of muscle tone ("drop attacks").

Akinetic Seizures

Lack of movement.

UNCLASSIFIED EPILEPTIC SEIZURES

These include all seizures that cannot be classified because of inadequate or incomplete data and some that defy classification in hitherto described categories. They include some neonatal seizures (e.g., rhythmic eye movements, chewing, and swimming movements).

Modified from Commission on Classification and Terminology of the International League Against Epilepsy: Proposal for revised clinical and electroencephalographic classification of epileptic seizures, *Epilepsia* 22:489-501, 1981.

eliminating triggering factors may be the only treatment needed (see p. 1725). The ***postictal state*** (the period following a seizure) may be varied. The child may be drowsy, be uncoordinated, have transient aphasia or confusion, and display some sensory or motor impairment. Neurologic changes should be documented. Weakness, hypotonia, or inactivity of a body part may indicate an epileptogenic focus in the corresponding contralateral cortical region.

Simple partial seizures. ***Simple partial seizures with motor signs*** arise from the area of the brain that controls muscle movement. A common motor seizure in children is the ***aversive seizure,*** in which the eye or eyes and head turn away from the side of the focus. In some children the upper extremity toward which the head turns is abducted and extended and the fingers are clenched, giving the impression that the child is looking at the closed fist. The child may be aware of the movement.

A common form is the ***rolandic (sylvian) seizure,*** in which there are tonic-clonic movements involving the face, salivation, and arrested speech. These are most common during sleep. On rare occasions children may have another type of simple motor seizure that displays the ***jacksonian march.*** The march consists of orderly, sequential progression of clonic movements that begin in a foot, hand, or face and, as electric impulses spread from the irritable focus to contiguous regions of the cortex, move or "march" body parts activated by these cerebral regions. Motor seizures are particularly common in hemiplegic children. The movements, which are usually clonic, begin in the hemiplegic hand, spread to the entire affected side, and, in many cases, become generalized seizures (typically of the tonic-clonic type).

Eye movement provides clues to the focus or origin of the seizure. Discharges in the cortex of one hemisphere tend to cause the eyes to deviate to the opposite side. Bilateral discharges tend to cause the eyes to move upward or straight ahead. When the child's eyes are closed during the seizure episode, a gentle attempt to open them may provide valuable information.

Simple partial seizures with sensory signs are characterized by various sensations, including numbness, tingling, prickling, paresthesia, or pain that originates in one area (e.g.,

TABLE 37-7 Comparison of Simple Partial, Complex Partial, and Absence Seizures

CLINICAL MANIFESTATIONS	SIMPLE PARTIAL	COMPLEX PARTIAL	ABSENCE
Age of onset	Any age	Uncommon before age 3 years	Uncommon before age 3 years
Frequency (per day)	Variable	Rarely over 1-2 times	Multiple
Duration	Usually less than 30 seconds	Usually over 60 seconds, rarely less than 10 seconds	Usually less than 15 seconds, rarely more than 30 seconds
Aura	May be sole manifestation of seizure	Frequently	Never
Impaired consciousness	Never	Always	Always, brief loss of consciousness
Automatisms	No	Frequently	Frequently
Clonic movements	Frequently	Occasionally	Occasionally
Postictal impairment	Rare	Frequently	Never
Mental disorientation	Rare	Common	Unusual

face or extremities) and spreads to other parts of the body. Visual sensations or formed images, hallucinations, light flashes, tastes, smells, or sounds may be experienced. For example, the child may run into the living room because he or she hears a favorite program on television only to discover that the TV is not on. Autonomic activity may include pallor, sweating, flushing, and pupillary dilation.

Complex partial seizures. These partial seizures with complex symptoms are the most difficult to diagnose and control. Because they involve more organized and high-level cerebral function, as well as sensory and motor function, they have also been termed ***psychomotor seizures.*** Complex partial seizures are observed more often in children from 3 years of age through adolescence. These seizures may begin with an ***aura,*** a simple partial seizure that is usually a sensation or sensory phenomenon that reflects the complicated connections and integrative functions of that area of the brain. The most frequent sensation is a strange feeling at the bottom of the stomach that rises toward the throat. This feeling may be accompanied by odd or unpleasant odors or taste; complex auditory or visual hallucinations, or ill-defined feelings of elevation or strangeness (e.g., ***deja-vu,*** a feeling of familiarity in a strange environment). Small children may emit a cry as a manifestation of an aura. Strong feelings of fear and anxiety, as well as a disturbed sense of time, can be associated with an aura. The aura is part of the seizure event and is associated with EEG changes (Van Donselaar, Geerts, and Schimscheimer, 1990).

Impaired consciousness is another characteristic of the complex partial seizure. The child may appear dazed and confused and be unable to respond when spoken to or follow instructions.

Another feature of this seizure is ***automatisms*** (repeated activities without purpose and carried out in a dreamy state). The predominant observations may be oropharyngeal activities, such as smacking, chewing, drooling, or swallowing; ambulatory activities, such as wandering or running; and verbal manifestations, such as repeating words ("please, please," "help, help," or "oh, oh"). These automatisms may be exhibited by antisocial behaviors, such as removing clothes in public or attempting to open the door of a moving car. The child may begin walking or racing around the room, knocking over chairs and lamps, and running into anybody in the way. It is important to realize that the child's consciousness is impaired and that these actions are not deliberate.

It is sometimes difficult to determine whether such behavior is related to the seizure activity or to a behavioral deviation. If the behavior results from seizure activity, all attempts to control such behavior with counseling or behavior plans are ineffective. The child may suddenly cease activity, appear dazed, stare into space, become confused or apathetic, become limp or stiff, or display some form of posturing.

If the seizure involves areas of the brain that control motor function, the child will exhibit movements, such as jerking of the hands, arms, and so on. This seizure generally lasts for a few minutes but can last for hours and days.

Following the seizure, the postictal occurs with signs of confusion and lack of recollection of the ictal period. Depending on the brain area involved during the episode, the child may sleep for a period of time. (See Table 37-7 for a comparison of simple partial, complex partial, and absence seizures.)

Partial seizures that generalize. Simple or complex partial seizures may spread and become generalized, usually into a tonic-clonic seizure. In such a case the partial seizure is considered the primary seizure event and the generalized seizure is considered the secondary one. In such a case it would be stated that the tonic-clonic seizure was not generalized at the onset but was a partial seizure that secondarily generalized.

Generalized Seizures. Generalized seizures without a focal onset appear to arise in the reticular formation, and the clinical observations indicate that the initial involvement is from both hemispheres. Loss of consciousness occurs and is the initial clinical manifestation. Unlike partial seizures that become generalized, there is no aura. Seizures occur at any time, day or night, and the interval between events may be minutes, hours, weeks, or even years. Most affected persons first experience seizures in childhood, and children whose seizures begin before age 4 years have mental retardation and behavioral and learning problems more frequently than those whose seizures begin after age 4.

Tonic-clonic seizures. The generalized tonic-clonic seizure, formerly known as "grand mal," is the most dramatic of all seizure manifestations of childhood. The seizure usually occurs without warning and consists of two distinct phases: tonic and clonic.

In the ***tonic phase*** there is a rolling of the eyes upward and immediate loss of consciousness. If standing, the child falls to the floor or ground. The child stiffens in a generalized and symmetric tonic contraction of the entire body musculature. The arms usually flex, whereas the legs, head, and neck extend. The child may utter a peculiar piercing cry produced as the jaws clap shut and the thoracic and abdominal muscles contract, forcing air through tightly closed vocal cords. This tonic phase lasts approximately 10 to 20 seconds, during which the child is apneic and may become cyanotic. Autonomic stimulation causes increased salivation.

In the ***clonic phase*** the tonic rigidity is replaced by intense jerking movements as the trunk and extremities undergo rhythmic contraction and relaxation. During this time the child may blow saliva out of the mouth and be incontinent of urine and feces. As the seizure ends, the movements become less intense and occur at longer intervals until they cease entirely. The clonic phase generally lasts about 30 seconds but can vary from only a few seconds to a half hour or longer. A series of seizures at intervals too brief to allow the child to regain consciousness between the time one event ends and the next begins is known as ***status epilepticus.*** This requires emergency intervention. A succession of interrupted seizures can lead to exhaustion, respiratory failure, and death.

In the postictal state children appear to relax but may remain semiconscious and difficult to rouse. They may awaken in a few minutes but remain confused for several hours. They are poorly coordinated, with mild impairment of fine motor movements. Children may have visual and speech difficulties and may vomit or complain of severe headache. When left alone, they usually sleep for several hours. On awakening, they are fully conscious but usually feel tired and complain of sore muscles and headache but have no recollection of the entire event.

Absence seizures. Absence seizures, formerly called "petit mal" or "lapses," are characterized by a brief loss of consciousness with minimal or no alteration in muscle tone and may go unrecognized because the child's behavior is changed very little. These seizures almost always first appear during childhood. In most instances the onset occurs between 4 and 12 years of age. Absence seizures usually cease at puberty but may be seen in adults.

The onset of absence seizures is abrupt, and the child suddenly experiences 20 or more events daily. Characteristically the brief loss of consciousness appears without warning and usually lasts about 5 to 10 seconds. Slight loss of muscle tone may cause the child to drop objects, but the child is able to maintain postural control and seldom falls. There may be minor movements such as lip smacking, twitching of eyelids or face, or slight hand movements. The sudden arrest of activity and consciousness is not accompanied by incontinence, and the child is amnesic for the episode.

If the child is involved in a group activity, such as classroom reading or discussion, he or she may need help to catch up with the group after the seizure. An episode is often mistaken for inattentiveness or daydreaming. Frequent episodes can result in slowed intellectual processes and deterioration in schoolwork and behavior, which is sometimes the first indication of the problem. Seizures can be precipitated by hyperventilation, hypoglycemia, stresses (emotional and physiologic), fatigue, or sleeplessness.

During these brief seizure episodes, there are lapses of unconsciousness, and the child may appear inattentive or to be daydreaming. The child's schoolwork may deteriorate, and the child may become very frustrated and develop behavior problems. It is important that the absence seizure be distinguished from daydreaming and attention deficit hyperactivity disorder (ADHD), which also exhibits inattentiveness or short attention span. An early diagnosis of the absence seizure supported with an EEG is essential. A seizure can be induced by asking the child to hyperventilate during the EEG, thus differentiating it from daydreaming or ADHD (Middleton, 1993).

During adolescence a child with absence seizures may cease having seizures, which is sometimes referred to as "growing out of the seizure." In other cases the youngster may develop tonic-clonic seizures or simple partial seizures.

Atonic seizures. Atonic seizures are manifested as a sudden, momentary loss of muscle tone. The onset is usually between 2 and 5 years of age. Depending on the severity of the seizure, the child may or may not lose consciousness. During a mild seizure the child may simply experience several sudden brief head drops. During a more severe episode, the child will suddenly fall to the ground (generally face down), will lose consciousness briefly, and after a few seconds will get up as if nothing happened (Engel, 1989).

Frequent falls can result in injury to the face, in particular the chin, eyebrow, and nose area. Atonic seizures are also known as ***drop attacks.***

Akinetic seizures. Akinetic seizures are characterized by lack of movement; however, muscle tone is maintained so that the child "freezes into position" and does not fall. If the child is lying down, the evaluation of muscle tone helps to differentiate between the atonic and akinetic types. There is impairment or loss of consciousness.

Myoclonic seizures. Myoclonic seizures include a variety of convulsive episodes characterized by sudden, brief contractures of a muscle or group of muscles, occurring singly or repetitively without loss of consciousness or postictal state. The seizure may or may not be symmetric and may be isolated as benign essential myoclonus or may occur in association with other seizure forms. Myoclonus frequently appears normally in the course of falling asleep or is observed as a nonspecific symptom in many diseases of the nervous system, such as viral encephalitis, uremic encephalopathy, and degenerative diseases of the cerebrum.

This seizure can be confused with the exaggerated startle reflex but may be distinguished by placing one's palm against the back of the child's head. If it is possible to push the child's head forward, this indicates an exaggerated startle reflex. In the case of a myoclonic seizure, the child's head would resist attempts to bring the head forward.

Unclassified Epileptic Seizures. ***Infantile spasms*** refer to a rare disorder with onset within the first 6 to 8 months of life. A large percentage of children with this disorder (85% to 90%) show various degrees of retardation (Hrachovy and Frost, 1989). The pathophysiology is unknown, but recent evidence suggests that certain regions in the brainstem associated with sleep cycling are involved. The underlying cause may be a disturbance of the central neurotransmitter regulation at a specific phase of brain development.

This disorder (a specific spike in the EEG) is also known as infantile myoclonus, massive spasm, hypsarrhythmia, salaam seizure, West syndrome, or infantile myoclonic spasms. They are twice as common in males as in females. In infants who are able to sit but not stand, the seizure is observed as a sudden dropping forward of the head and neck with trunk flexed forward and knees drawn up—the ***salaam*** or ***jackknife seizure.*** The episode may consist of a series of sudden, brief, symmetric, muscular contractions by which the head is flexed, the arms are extended, and the legs are drawn up. The eyes may roll upward or inward, and the seizure may be preceded or followed by a cry or giggling. There may or may not be loss of consciousness, and the infant will sometimes flush, turn pale, or become cyanotic. The child may have numerous seizures during the day without postictal drowsiness or sleep.

Less often, alternate clinical forms are observed and include extensor spasms rather than flexion of arms, legs, and trunk, and head nodding. Lightning attacks, which involve a single, momentary, shocklike contraction of the entire body, are another variant.

Infantile spasms are frequently associated with cerebral abnormalities, such as structural malformations, severe anoxic brain damage, phenylketonuria, and degenerative changes. Microcephaly, choreoathetoid or tonic posture, and abnormal movements are frequently present. There may be a history of maternal infection, prematurity, or birth injury, and development is retarded before the onset of seizures. The long-term prognosis is poor, both mentally and developmentally.

Adrenocorticotropic hormone (ACTH) may be used to treat infantile spasms. It is not known how this hormone controls seizures; however, studies show that ACTH has an inhibitory effect on the excitability of the developing brain only (Holmes and Weber, 1986). For this reason, it is not used for adults. Many children who have infantile spasms eventually develop ***Lennox-Gastaut syndrome (LGS).*** Recently the antiepileptic drug felbamate (Felbatol) has been found to be effective in treating seizures associated with LGS and is considered an important advance in drug management (Felbamate Study Group, 1993).

LGS is diagnosed on the evidence of mixed seizure types (atonic, tonic-clonic, tonic, and atypical absence), mental retardation, poor response to treatment, and typical EEG changes. The onset of LGS is between 1 and 10 years of age, after which it is far less common. When the onset of LGS occurs before 1 year of age, it is important that it not be confused with infantile spasm seizure. The cause of LGS remains unknown. LGS is classified as idiopathic or symptomatic.

Idiopathic LGS, also called ***cryptogenic LGS,*** appears in children with normal psychomotor development and no history of epilepsy or evidence of brain damage. Seizures may occur after an infectious illness, vaccination, or a febrile seizure. In school-age children behavioral disturbances, as well as changes in personality, are common.

Symptomatic LGS reveals a history of encephalopathy and mental retardation or epilepsy. The prognosis is poorer than in the cryptogenic type. The evolution of LGS is severe. Seizure episodes continue with high frequency and with episodes of status epilepticus. Intellectual impairment is progressive.

Treatment is very difficult, and most cases do not respond to therapy. Drugs are chosen according to the types of seizures. Felbamate and valproate are drugs of choice. High doses of immunoglobulins and a ketogenic diet have been used but with poor results. The prognosis varies but can be poor. Additional family support is often required to maintain the child at home.

Diagnostic Evaluation

Establishing a diagnosis is critical. The process of diagnosis in a child with a seizure disorder has two major foci: (1) to ascertain the type of seizure the child has experienced and (2) to attempt to understand the cause of the event. The assessment and diagnosis rely heavily on a thorough history, skilled observation, and employment of several diagnostic tests.

It is especially important to differentiate epilepsy from other brief alterations in consciousness and/or behavior. Some clinical entities that mimic seizures are migraine headaches, toxic effects of drugs, syncope (fainting), hyperventilation, transient ischemic attacks, breath-holding spells in infants and young children, and brainstem herniation.

Cocaine intoxication should be considered in the differential diagnosis of new-onset seizure activity in children. Those exposed to smoke of freebase cocaine (crack) used by adult caretakers may have neurologic symptoms of drowsiness, unsteady gait, and seizures (Ernst and Sanders, 1989). Passive cocaine inhalation is evident from isolation of its principal metabolite, benzoyl ecgonine, in the urine (Bateman and Heagarty, 1989). In this situation child protection agencies must be consulted because of the possibility of abuse or neglect.

Since it is unusual to observe the child during a seizure, a complete, accurate, and detailed history should be obtained from a reliable and knowledgeable informant. This history involves prenatal, perinatal, and neonatal periods, including any instances of infection, apnea, colic, or poor feeding, and information regarding any previous accidents or serious illnesses. If the diagnosis is clear, the seizure can be identified as an isolated event and unlikely to recur (e.g., a febrile seizure) or as a symptom of an underlying and potentially lethal disease (e.g., a brain tumor).

The history of the seizure(s) should be equally detailed, including the type of seizure or description of the child's behavior during the event(s), the age at onset, and the time at which the seizure occurs (i.e., early morning, before meals, while awake, or during sleep). Any factors that may have precipitated the seizure are important, including fever, infection, falls that may have caused trauma to the head, anxiety, fatigue, and activity (e.g., hyperventilation or exposure to strong stimuli such as bright flashing lights or loud noises). If the child can describe any sensory phenomena, these are recorded. The duration and progression of the seizure (if any) and the postictal feelings and behavior, such as confusion, inability to speak, amnesia, headache, and sleep, are recorded. The ability to identify seizure types accurately has resulted from the technologic advances in video recording and long-term EEG monitoring.

A complete physical and neurologic examination, including developmental assessment of language, learning, behavior, and motor abilities, often provides clues to neurologic disturbances. A family history can offer clues to paroxysmal disorders such as migraine, breath-holding spells, febrile seizures, or neurologic diseases that may be related to the seizure disorder.

Laboratory studies that may prove to be of value include a complete blood count (for evidence of lead poisoning) and white blood cell count for signs of infection. Blood glucose may give evidence of hypoglycemic episodes, and serum electrolytes, blood urea nitrogen, calcium, and other blood studies might indicate metabolic disturbances. Lumbar puncture can confirm a suspected diagnosis of cerebrospinal infection or trauma. MRI can identify skull abnormalities, separation of sutures, and intracranial calcifications.

The EEG is obtained for all children with seizure manifestations and is the most useful tool for evaluating seizure disorders. The EEG is carried out under varying conditions—with the child asleep, awake, awake with provocative stimulation (flashing lights, noise), and hyperventilating. Stimulation elicits abnormal electrical activity, which is recorded on the EEG. Various seizure types produce characteristic EEG patterns—high-voltage spike discharges are seen in tonic-clonic seizures, with abnormal patterns in the intervals between seizures; a three-per-second spike and wave pattern is observed in an absence seizure; and absence of electrical activity in an area suggests a large lesion, such as an abscess or subdural collection of fluid. A normal EEG does not rule out seizures, since the EEG is only a surface recording and may represent normal interictal activity.

Variations of the EEG are video recordings of the patient during waking and/or sleeping. The full-body image is displayed on half of the video screen, the facial image is shown on one fourth, and selected EEG channels are displayed on the remaining one fourth. Split-screen capabilities allow modification and arrangement of a larger number of channels and images. Polygraph equipment is also used to monitor physiologic data such as respiratory effort, eye movements, heart rate, and systemic blood pressure. These techniques can be used concurrently and are especially valuable in differentiating epileptic activity from paroxysmal behavior or nonepileptic motor events.

Therapeutic Management

The objective of treatment of seizure disorders is to control the seizures or to reduce their frequency and severity, discover and correct the cause when possible, and help the child who has recurrent seizures to live as normal a life as possible. Seizures of a recurrent nature are treated as soon as the diagnosis is established. If the seizure activity is a manifestation of an infectious, traumatic, or metabolic process, the seizure therapy is instituted as part of the general therapeutic regimen. Seizure control is considered to prevent secondary brain cell injury from the neuronal discharge and hypoxia.

Drug Therapy. It is known that persons predisposed to epilepsy have seizures when their basal level of neuronal excitability exceeds a critical point or threshold; no event occurs if the excitability is maintained below this threshold. The administration of antiepileptic drugs serves to raise this threshold and prevent seizures. Consequently, the primary therapy for seizure disorders is the administration of the appropriate antiepileptic drug or combination of drugs in a dosage that provides the desired effect without causing undesirable side effects or toxic reactions. Antiepileptic drugs are believed to exert their effect primarily by reducing the responsiveness of normal neurons to the sudden, high-frequency nerve impulses that arise in the epileptogenic focus. Thus the seizure is effectively suppressed; the abnormal brain waves may or may not be altered. Complete control can be achieved in 70% of children with epilepsy, and good control in another 15% to 20% (Freeman and Vining, 1992). The drugs used for control of seizures are outlined in Table 37-8.

Therapy is begun with a single drug known to be effective for the child's particular type of seizure, and the dosage is gradually increased until the seizures are controlled or the child develops signs of toxicity. If the drug is effective but does not sufficiently control the seizures, a second drug is added in gradually increasing doses. Once seizures are controlled, the drug or drugs are continued for a prolonged time.

A present breakthrough in drug management is the realization that polypharmacy confers no benefit over monotherapy in about 90% of individuals with epilepsy (Brodie, 1990). There is increasing evidence that diminishing polypharmacy can bring about a better quality of life; therefore single-drug therapy is recommended.

Periodic reevaluation of the drug is important to assess the continued effectiveness and to alter the dosage if indicated. The dosage will need to be increased as the child grows. Blood levels often prove valuable in determination

TABLE 37-8 Major Drugs Used for Control of Seizures

DRUG	THERAPEUTIC DOSAGE	THERAPEUTIC PLASMA LEVEL	SEIZURE TYPE	COMMENTS/SIDE EFFECTS
Adrenocorticotropic hormone (ACTH, H.P. Acthar Gel)	May range from 20 to 160 units		Infantile spasms, Lennox Gastaut syndrome	Acts only on developing brain Given intramuscularly No standard length of therapy; usually few weeks to several months *Side effects:* Cushingoid appearance, extreme irritability, hypertension, transient glycosuria
Carbamazepine (Tegretol)	10-15 mg/kg/day Half-life: 9-19 hr	4-12 µg/ml	Secondary tonic-clonic Complex partial Simple partial	Relatively free from unwanted side effects; fewer sedative properties *Side effects:* Blurred vision, diplopia, drowsiness, vertigo, headache *Toxic effects:* Leukopenic aplastic anemia
Clonazepam (Klonopin)	0.05-0.20 mg/kg/day Half-life: 18-20 hr	20-80 µg/ml	Absence Myoclonic	Usually given as adjunct to other antiepileptic drugs *Side effects:* Drowsiness, ataxia, hyperactivity, agitation, slurred speech, double vision, increased salivation
Divalproex sodium, valproate, valproic acid (Depakote, Depakene)	20-60 mg/kg/day Half-life: 6-18 hr	50-150 µg/ml	Myoclonic Absence Tonic-clonic Mixed seizure types Lennox-Gastaut syndrome	Potentiates action of phenobarbital and phenytoin *Side effects:* Hair loss, tremor, elevated liver enzymes, irregular menses, increased appetite, nausea and vomiting (not as common with Depakote) *Toxic effect:* Hepatic toxicity
Ethosuximide (Zarontin)	15-35 mg/kg/day Half-life: 24-72 hr	40-100 µg/ml	Absence	Occasionally aggravates generalized seizures Administer with food *Side effects:* Nausea, gastric discomfort, anorexia, headache, drowsiness, dizziness
Felbamate (Felbatol)	15 mg/kg, increased to 30, 45, or 60 mg/kg as needed Half-life: 20-23 hr	Not established, but studies suggest 30-100 µg/ml	Lennox-Gastaut syndrome	Not affected by food Monitor weight Give in early morning to reduce insomnia Interacts with other antiepileptic drugs (i.e., increases phenytoin and valproic acid levels and decreases carbamazepine levels) Side effects increased when given with other antiepileptic drugs *Side effects:* Anorexia, nausea, vomiting, insomnia, headache, weight loss *Toxic effect:* Aplastic anemia
Phenobarbital (Luminal)	4-6 mg/kg/day Half-life: 53-104 hr	10-40 µg/ml	Tonic-clonic	May interfere with concentration and motor speed May cause vitamin D and folic acid deficiencies *Side effects:* Drowsiness, irritability, hyperactivity, skin rash, mild ataxis, hyperpyrexia, diminished cognitive performance
Phenytoin (Dilantin)	5-10 mg/kg/day Half-life: 7-22 hr	10-20 µg/ml	Tonic-clonic Complex partial Simple partial	May cause behavioral disturbances in children May aggravate absence and myoclonic seizures *Side effects:* Gum hyperplasia, hirsutism, ataxia, nystagmus, diplopia, anorexia, nausea, nervousness, folate deficiency *Toxic effects:* Stevens-Johnson syndrome (erythema multiforme), thrombocytopenia
Primidone (Mysoline)	12-25 mg/kg/day Half-life: 3-12 hr	5-12 µg/ml	Tonic-clonic Complex partial Simple partial	Effective with phenobarbital in mixed-type seizure patterns *Side effects:* Drowsiness, ataxia, diplopia

Data from Kongelbeck SR: Discharge planning for the child with infantile spasms, *J Neurosci Nurs* 22(4):238-244, 1990; Ponzillo JJ, Malkoff MD: Focus on felbamate: beginning a new generation of anticonvulsant agents for the treatment of epilepsy, *Hosp Formul* 28:837-847, 1993; and Santilli N, Sierzant T: Advances in the treatment of epilepsy, *J Neurosci Nurs* 19:141-157, 1987.

of optimum dosage levels. Blood cell counts, urinalysis, and liver function tests are obtained at frequent intervals in children receiving particular antiepileptic medications. Repeat EEGs are obtained if the seizures change in frequency and/or manifestations or the child exhibits suspicious behaviors or symptoms.

Withdrawal of antiepileptic therapy follows a predesigned protocol, usually begun when the child has been seizure-free for at least 2 years with a normal EEG. Relapse in children may be related to factors such as neurologic deficit or a positive family history for epilepsy. Recurrence is most likely within the first year after discontinuance of the medication.

When a medication is discontinued, the dosage should be reduced gradually over several weeks. Sudden withdrawal of a drug can cause an increase in the number and severity of seizures, often precipitating status epilepticus. If the time for reducing the medication coincides with puberty or, in younger children, occurs during periods when the child is subject to frequent infections, the drug is continued for a longer period.

Complications of Drug Therapy. Side effects of continued use of antiepileptic medications are sometimes distressing to the child and the family. Most side effects are transient and dose related but warrant immediate attention of health care personnel. Drug reactions require clinical evaluation and serum drug levels. Combination therapy, such as with barbiturates and carbamazepine, can potentiate drug levels. Careful monitoring is necessary to avoid toxicity.

A rare complication of intravenous phenytoin (Dilantin) is ***purple glove syndrome,*** an injury to the tissues of the hand and forearm. The manifestations are pain, purplish discoloration, and edema. The tissues may become permanently damaged, and the distal extremity may need to be amputated (Hanna, 1992). To prevent severe damage, close monitoring of the infusion is essential.

Phenytoin also causes lymphoid hyperplasia that is most noticeable in the gums. Frequent gum massage and careful attention to good oral hygiene may reduce the gingival hyperplasia, but in severe cases, surgical removal of the excess tissue may be needed. Enlargement of the tonsillar and adenoidal tissue can cause partial airway obstruction, which produces snoring during sleep.

Common side effects, such as ataxia and rashes, often disappear when drug dosages are reduced. Depression, which has been reported in children with epilepsy who are taking barbiturate antiepileptics, can be relieved by changing drugs. Drugs such as phenobarbital and phenytoin may adversely affect cognitive function, school performance, and behavior (Vining, 1990a).

The American Academy of Pediatrics (1985) stresses that physicians prescribe the appropriate drug and be alert to reports of side effects. The committee also encourages development of screening tests to detect subtle intellectual and behavioral side effects and studies to evaluate and compare the effects of therapy.

Surgical Therapy. When seizure activity is determined to be caused by a hematoma, tumor, or other progressive cerebral lesion, surgical removal is the treatment. In children with epilepsy, surgery is reserved for those who suffer from repetitive, incapacitating (refractory) seizures that have been present for an extended period without evidence of remission. The epileptogenic area should be in a surgically removable and functionally silent region of the brain. Since a very extensive medical (e.g., invasive EEG monitoring), psychosocial, and psychometric evaluation is required, prospective candidates should be able to understand, cooperate, and tolerate the testing (Hodges and Root, 1991).

There are three types of surgical interventions. In ***resective surgery*** the focal area of the seizure activity is excised with expectations that serious deficits will not be produced or that existing deficits will not be increased. Surgical excision of the epileptogenic focus does not eliminate the need for continuation of drug therapy. Drug administration is restarted as soon as the patient regains consciousness and is continued until the patient is free of seizures. ***Callosotomy*** involves the separation of the connections between the two hemispheres of the brain and is used in some generalized seizures. In ***multiple subpial transection*** horizontal fibers of the motor cortex are divided to reduce seizures, whereas the vertical fibers are spared to allow for function (Brodie, 1990).

The risks of brain surgery cannot be underestimated. Also, the costs of surgical interventions must be taken into consideration, as well as the numerous tests necessary to assess the child before surgery.

Status Epilepticus. Status epilepticus is a continuous seizure that lasts more than 30 minutes or a series of seizures from which the child does not regain a premorbid level of consciousness. The initial treatment is directed toward support and maintenance of vital functions, including maintaining an adequate airway, administration of oxygen, and hydration, and is followed by intravenous administration of either diazepam or phenobarbital. Rectal diazepam is a simple, effective, and safe treatment for prehospital management (Dieckmann, 1994). Lorazepam (Ativan) may be replacing intravenous diazepam as the drug of choice. It has a longer duration of action and causes less respiratory distress in children over 2 years of age. Concurrent intravenous loading with phenytoin is usually necessary for sustained control of seizures.

NURSING ALERT Diazepam is incompatible with many drugs. To give intravenously, inject slowly directly into the vein or through tubing as close as possible to the vein insertion site.

The child must be closely monitored during administration to detect early alterations in vital signs that may indicate impending cardiac arrest or respiratory depression. When diazepam is ineffective, phenytoin or phenobarbital, often in extremely high levels that may require respiratory support, is given intravenously as the initial medication. Patients who do not respond to drug therapy may require the use of intravenous lidocaine, general anesthesia, or a potent paralyzing agent such as curare. While paralyzing agents resolve the physical manifestations of the seizure, they have no effect on the EEG. The child may continue to seize.

Status epilepticus is a medical emergency requiring immediate intervention to prevent possible brain injury or death. Equally imperative to halting the tonic-clonic movement is correct diagnosis of the underlying problem. The outcome is related to the etiology and duration of the status epilepticus.

NURSING ALERT Report any seizure that lasts longer than 5 minutes, unless this duration is the child's usual pattern.

Prognosis. The course and prognosis for children with seizures depend on the etiology, type of seizure, age at onset, and family and medical histories. In one study of children with epilepsy (excluding those with generalized absence, myoclonus, akinetic, atonic, and infantile seizures), 55% of children "outgrew" the disorder and remained seizure-free without medication during an average 7-year follow-up period. At diagnosis the best predictors of remission were age under 12 years at onset, normal intelligence, no prior neonatal seizures, and fewer than 21 seizures before treatment (Camfield and others, 1993b). However, social outcome was less favorable in a subset of these subjects with normal intelligence. One adverse social outcome, such as the necessity for repeating grades or placement in a special education class, behavior disorders requiring referral, use of psychotropic medication, and social isolation, occurred in 42% of these children and young adults. Significantly, the social outcome was often not related to the clinical course of the seizures (Camfield and others, 1993a).

Risk factors associated with recurrence of epilepsy include being 16 years of age or older, taking more than one antiepileptic drug, having seizures after starting drug treatment, having a history of primary or secondarily generalized tonic-clonic seizures or an EEG showing myoclonic seizures; and having an abnormal EEG. The risks of seizures recurring decreases with increasing time without seizures (Medical Research Council, 1993).

The prognosis following treatment for status epilepticus is more favorable than previously reported. The majority of children will probably have no intellectual impairment. Children who do have cognitive deficits or who die are likely to have preceding developmental delay, neurologic abnormality, or concurrent serious illness (Verity, Ross, and Golding, 1993).

Nursing Considerations

❖ Assessment

An important nursing function during a seizure is observing the seizure and describing its pertinent features. Any alterations in behavior and characteristics of the episode, such as sensory-hallucinatory phenomena (e.g., an aura), motor effects (e.g., eye movements, muscular contractions, laterality, complex activities), alterations in consciousness, and postictal state, are noted and recorded (see box on p. 1724).

Generalized seizures and others with dramatic manifestations are easily detected, but absence seizures present more difficulties. They are easily misinterpreted as inattention. Any unusual behavior, even seemingly inconsequential behavior such as a momentary interruption of activity, staring, or mental blankness, should be described. The more detailed these descriptions, the more valuable they are for assessment. The nurse notes the time that the seizure began and times the length of the seizure. This is especially important if the child becomes cyanotic.

History taking is a vital tool for helping to identify factors that aid in establishing a cause of the seizures. Interviewing the child and the family helps to elicit problems related to the psychologic impact of the disorder on their lives.

❖ Nursing Diagnoses

Based on a thorough assessment, several nursing diagnoses are identified. The more common diagnoses for the child with a seizure disorder are included in the Nursing Care Plan on p. 1727-1728. Others may apply in specific situations.

❖ Planning

The goals for the child with a seizure disorder and the family include the following:

1. Child will be protected during a seizure.
2. Child will experience as few seizures as possible.
3. Child and family will cope with the challenges associated with the disorder.
4. Child will develop a positive self-image.

❖ Implementation

When they first witness a child in a generalized cerebral seizure, nurses are often frightened, puzzled, and immobilized. These reactions are normal but can reduce the effectiveness of care for the child and interfere with observations of the event. The child must be protected from injury during the seizure, and nursing observations made during the event provide valuable information for diagnosis and management of the disorder (see Emergency Treatment box).

It is impossible to halt a seizure once it has begun, and no attempt should be made to do so. The nurse must remain calm, stay with the child, and prevent the child from sustaining any harm during the seizure. If possible, the child should be isolated from the view of others by closing a door or pulling screens. A seizure can be very upsetting to the child, other visitors, and their families. If other persons are present, they should be assured that everything is being done for the child. After the seizure, they can be given a simple explanation about the event as needed.

NURSING ALERT Do not move or forcefully restrain the child during a tonic-clonic seizure and do not place a solid object between the teeth.

If the nurse is able to reach the child in time, a child who is standing or is seated in a chair (including a wheelchair) is eased to the floor immediately. During and sometimes after the tonic-clonic seizure, the swallowing reflex is lost, salivation increases, and the tongue is hypotonic. Therefore the child is at risk for aspiration and airway occlusion. Placing the child on the side facilitates drainage and helps to maintain a patent airway. After the seizure the child is kept on the side in bed or a similar place to allow the youngster to sleep. If the child is at school or away from home, the child is allowed to rest. When feasible, the child is integrated into the environment as soon as possible. Sending a child with a chronic seizure disorder home is not necessary, unless the parents request this.

Children who are known to have seizures or who are under observation for seizures will require some precautions. The extent of these measures depends on the type and frequency of the seizure (see box on p. 1725).

Long-Term Care. Care of the child with a recurrent seizure disorder involves the physical care and instruction regarding the importance of the drug therapy and, probably more significant, the problems related to the emotional aspects of the disorder. There are few diseases that generate as much anxiety among relatives as epilepsy. Fears and misconceptions about the disease and its treatment abound in the layperson's mind. For many it represents the archetype of severe hereditary affliction. Therefore the foci of nursing care are directed toward helping the child and the family to deal with the psychologic and sociologic problems related to the disorder and to educate the child, the family, peers, and the public toward a more realistic and liberal view of the condition.

Physical Aspects. Children subject to seizures are prescribed some type of drug therapy. The nurse can help the parents plan the administration of the medication at convenient times in order to disrupt the family routine as little as possible. The dosage schedule is based on the drug's ***half-life*** (time required to reduce to one half the amount of unchanged drug that is in the body) and the age of the child. Drugs with longer half-lives are given less frequently, and a missed dose will have less of a negative effect than a drug with a short half-life. Also, the younger the child, the more frequent the dosing needs to be because of more rapid metabolism. The aim is to simplify the medication routine as much as possible and incorporate it into the parents' and child's daily activities. This also increases the likelihood of compliance. The most convenient times for administration seem to be with meals or at bedtime. Although the antiepileptic drugs are available in liquid extracts or emulsions, the tablet form is preferred by neurologists. The unequal distribution of the drug in the solute and the increased likelihood of inaccurate measurements make liquid medication less desirable. For small children the tablet of the proper dosage can be crushed and administered in syrup, jelly, or other palatable substances.

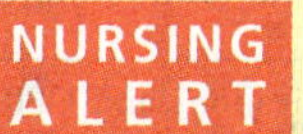

Children taking phenobarbital and/or phenytoin should receive adequate vitamin D and folic acid, since deficiencies have been associated with these drugs. Phenytoin should not be taken with milk.

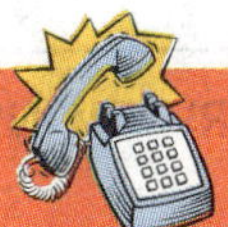

EMERGENCY TREATMENT
Seizures

TONIC-CLONIC SEIZURE

During the Seizure

Time seizure episode.
Approach calmly.
If child is standing or seated, ease child down.
Place pillow or folded blanket under child's head. If no bedding is available, place own hands under child's head.
Do not:
- Attempt to restrain child or use force
- Put anything in child's mouth
- Give any food or liquids

Loosen restrictive clothing.
Remove eyeglasses.
Clear area of any hazards or hard objects.
Allow seizure to end without interference.
If vomiting occurs, try to turn child to one side as a unit.

After the Seizure

Time postictal period.
Check for breathing. Check position of head and tongue. Reposition if head is hyperextended. If breathing is not present, give rescue breathing and call EMS.
Check around mouth for evidence of burns or suspicious substances that might indicate poisoning.
Keep child on side.
Remain with child until full recovery.
Do not give food or liquids until fully alert and swallowing reflex has returned.
Call EMS when necessary.
Look for medical identification and determine what factors occurred before onset of seizure and which may have been triggering factors.
Check head and body for possible injuries and fractures. Check inside of mouth to see if tongue or lips have been bitten.

COMPLEX PARTIAL SEIZURE

During the Seizure

Do not restrain unless in danger.
Remove harmful objects from path.
Redirect to safe area.
Do not agitate; instead, talk in calm, reassuring manner.
Do not expect child to follow instructions.
Watch to see if seizure generalizes.

After the Seizure

Stay with child and reassure until fully conscious.

CALL EMERGENCY MEDICAL SERVICE IF:

Child stops breathing.
There is evidence of injury or youngster is diabetic or pregnant.
Seizure lasts for more than 5 minutes (unless duration of seizure is typically longer than 5 minutes).
Status epilepticus occurs.
Pupils are not equal after seizure.
Child vomits continuously 30 minutes after seizure has ended (sign of possible acute problem).
Child cannot be awakened and is unresponsive to pain after seizure has ended.
Seizure occurs in water (shock and aspiration may be delayed).
This is child's first seizure.

Modified from *Seizure recognition and first aid,* Landover, MD, 1989, Epilepsy Foundation of America.

EMERGENCY TREATMENT

GENERAL OBSERVATIONS: THE CHILD DURING A SEIZURE

OBSERVE SEIZURE

Describe

Only what is actually observed
Order of events (before, during, and after)
Duration of seizure
- Tonic-clonic—from first signs of event until jerking stops
- Absence—from loss of consciousness until regains consciousness
- Complex partial—from first sign of unresponsiveness, motor activity, automatisms until there are signs of responsiveness to environment

Onset

Time of onset
Significant preseizure precipitating events—bright lights, noise, excitement, emotional outbursts
Behavior
- Change in facial expression, such as for fear
- Cry or other sound
- Stereotypic or automatous movements
- Random activity (wandering)

Position of eyes, head, body, extremities
- Unilateral or bilateral posturing of one or more extremities
- Body deviation to side

Movement

Change of position, if any
Site of commencement—hand, thumb, mouth, generalized
Tonic phase, if present—length, parts of body involved
Clonic phase—twitching or jerking movements, parts of body involved, sequence of parts involved, generalized, change in character of movements
Lack of movement or muscle tone of body part or entire body

Face

Color change—pallor, cyanosis, flushing
Perspiration
Mouth—position, deviating to one side, teeth clenched, tongue bitten, frothing at mouth, flecks of blood or bleeding
Lack of expression

Eyes

Position—straight ahead, deviation upward, deviation outward, conjugate or divergent
Pupils (if able to assess)—change in size, equality, reaction to light and accommodation

Respiratory Effort

Presence and length of apnea
Presence of stertor

Other

Involuntary urination
Involuntary defecation

OBSERVE POSTICTALLY

Duration of postictal period
Method of termination
State of consciousness—unresponsiveness, drowsiness, confusion
Orientation to time, persons, etc.
Sleeping but able to be aroused
Motor ability
- Any change in motor power
- Ability to move all extremities
- Any paresis or weakness
- Ability to whistle (if appropriate to age)

Speech—changes, peculiarities, type and extent of any difficulties
Sensations
- Complaint of discomfort or pain
- Any sensory impairment of hearing, vision
- Recollection of preseizure sensations, warning of attack
- Awareness that attack was beginning

Recall of words spoken to child by observer during seizure

It is important to impress on the family the necessity of continuing the medication regularly without interruption for as long as required. This is usually 2 to 3 years after the last seizure, at which point the drug is discontinued slowly over a period of weeks to avoid the possibility of precipitating a seizure. Planning ahead to replace a nearly empty bottle will prevent the risk of running out of the medication. It is sometimes easy to skip doses or omit them for any of a variety of reasons, especially when the child is free of seizures most of the time. This is particularly so when the child is older and assumes the responsibility for the medication. Parents should notify the health professional if the child has an illness, including vomiting, diarrhea, or fever. Vomiting and diarrhea can interfere with drug absorption; fever may increase metabolic requirements. Both can precipitate seizure activity.

Rectal preparations of some antiepileptic medications are highly useful and effective when a child is unable to take oral medications because of repeated vomiting, gastrointestinal surgery, or status epilepticus. Administration of rectal antiepileptic medication can be learned by parents for home treatment during a seizure.* Rectal diazepam is useful adjunctive home treatment for children at risk for prolonged cluster seizures. Hospitalization is minimized, and parental confidence is enhanced (Camfield and others, 1989). However, knowledge of CPR is indicated for caregivers who are responsible for administering rectal diazepam.

Nurses need to educate the child and parents of the possible adverse reactions to the medications used to treat seizure disorders in children. They should understand the common side effects so that they can report any unusual

*Home care instructions for administration of medications and CPR instructions are available in *Wong and Whaley's Clinical Manual of Pediatric Nursing* (Mosby).

SEIZURE PRECAUTIONS

Extent of precautions depends on type, severity, and frequency of seizures
May include:
- Siderails raised when child is sleeping or resting
- Siderails and other hard objects padded
- Waterproof mattress/pad on bed/crib
- Appropriate precautions during potentially hazardous activities:
  - Swimming with a companion
  - Use of protective helmet and padding during bicycle riding, skate-boarding, in-line skating
  - Supervision during use of hazardous machinery/equipment

Have child carry or wear medical identification
Alert other caregivers to need for any special precautions

observations that might indicate unfavorable reactions. These should be known in detail. Parents should understand that the child needs periodic physical assessment and laboratory studies. Possible adverse effects on the hematopoietic system, liver, and kidneys may be reflected in symptoms such as fever, sore throat, enlarged lymph nodes, jaundice, and bleeding manifestations (e.g., easy bruising, petechiae, ecchymoses, epistaxis). A common factor in status epilepticus is inadequate blood levels of antiepileptic drugs.

Parents need to be warned of possible behavioral changes as the seizures are controlled in children taking primidone, phenobarbital, or phenytoin. Changes in personality, indifference to school activities and family, hyperactivity, or even psychotic behavior may sometimes be observed. The potential effects of epileptic drugs on learning and behavior should be considered. Progressive intellectual deterioration in a child with epilepsy requires investigation of present medication plus the role of the underlying cerebral pathology.

The degree to which activities are restricted is individualized for each child and depends on the type, frequency, and severity of the seizures, the child's response to therapy, and the length of time the seizures have been controlled. Most normal activities are encouraged for children, and participation in competitive sports is determined on an individual basis. With encouragement, most older children can accept the restrictions placed on activities. Only essential restrictions are placed on children regarding sports and peer activity to reduce the likelihood of needlessly accentuating differences, and they are approached in a positive way in terms of what the child can do rather than what the child cannot do. Sometimes parents curtail the child's activities more than necessary.

To prevent head injuries, children should wear appropriate safety devices, such as bicycle helmets. To prevent submersion injury, they should swim with a responsible companion. Showers are recommended for older children, and close supervision is suggested when children are in a bathtub (Diekema, Quan, and Holt, 1993).

Because the child is encouraged to attend school, camp, and other normal activities, the school nurse and the teacher should be made aware of the child's condition and therapy.* They can help to ensure regularity of medication administration and provision of any special care the child might need. Teachers, child care providers, camp counselors, youth organization leaders, coaches, and other adults who assume responsibility for children should be instructed regarding care of the child during a seizure so that they can act in a calm manner for the welfare of the child and to influence the attitude of the child's peers.

Triggering Factors. Careful and detailed documentation of seizures over a period of time may indicate a pattern. When this occurs, the nurse or responsible adult may intervene to identify the triggering factors and make changes in the environment that may prevent or decrease seizure frequency. Frequently the necessary changes are very simple and cost-free but can make an enormous difference in the child's and family's lives (see Critical Thinking Exercise box).

Factors that may trigger seizures in children include changes in dark-light patterns, such as those that occur with a flash on a camera, automobile headlights, walking by a picket fence, reflections of light on snow or water, or rotating blades on a fan; sudden loud noises; specific voices,

*An excellent resource is *Students with Seizures: A Manual for School Nurses* by N. Santilli, W.E. Dodson, and A.V. Walton (1991, Epilepsy Foundation of America).

CRITICAL THINKING EXERCISE

Seizures

Since age 2 years, Jane Little has had epilepsy that is well controlled with medication. However, now that she has begun elementary school, her seizures have returned. On the way home Jane usually has a seizure on the bus; however, on weekends and holidays she is seizure-free. As the school nurse, you advise Jane's parents to:

1. Take her for medical reevaluation.
2. Increase her antiepileptic medication.
3. Drive her home from school.
4. Ride with her on the school bus.

The correct answer is 4. Your first priority is to help the family identify triggering events. At your suggestion, Mrs. Little rode the school bus home with Jane. As the child began to seize, the mother noted that they had just passed a white picket fence, the triggering factor. Once the child was seated on the other side of the bus, the seizure episodes stopped.

With the consistent pattern and abrupt onset of the seizures, seeking medical reevaluation should be advised only if no triggering event is identified. It is not within the scope of nursing practice for you to change the dosage of the medication. Even if the child rides home in a car, the seizures may occur if Jane sits in the same position as on the school bus.

songs, or nursery rhymes; startling or sudden movements; extreme or drastic changes in temperature; dehydration; fatigue; hyperventilation; hypoglycemia; caffeine; and insufficient protein in the diet (protein is needed to metabolize some antiepileptic drugs). Although there have been reports of seizures triggered by flashing video games, this relationship has not been confirmed by controlled studies. Seizures may be due to the length of playing time, which may cause fatigue. On the basis of current knowledge, the overwhelming majority of children with seizures can play video games without the risk of seizures.*

Factors that trigger seizure episodes should be considered in activities of daily living. If a child is photosensitive, avoiding such things as wallpaper with stripes, a ceiling fan, or blinking lights to decorate a Christmas tree at home may be necessary. A pattern of early-morning seizures could indicate hypoglycemia; a snack at bedtime and a glass of juice before arising may prevent those episodes. Other dietary modifications, such as the use of caffeine-free sodas, coffee, and tea, and adequate protein and fluids, especially in hot weather, may prevent seizure episodes. Wearing a sweater in cold air-conditioned rooms or reducing the heat in a car standing in the sun could prevent a seizure episode for a person sensitive to sudden drastic changes in temperature.

Family Support. Parental attitudes and management of a child with a disorder are as varied as those of other parents of children with a chronic disorder, and they are subject to the same long-term challenges (see Chapter 18). Whether the seizures result from illness, injury, or unknown etiology, the parents may feel guilt, anxiety, and often humiliation. They want to know if the seizures will affect the child's mental capacities. Many persons erroneously associate epilepsy with mental deficiency. Seizures do frequently accompany other manifestations of severe brain damage from disease or injury, but most children with seizures, as in any population of healthy children, display a wide range of intelligence.

Parents also wonder how the illness will affect the child's future and need reassurance that the illness will not shorten the life of the child and that the child can attend school, marry, and elect to have children. The child may need vocational guidance, and the parents will need to become familiar with the laws in their state regarding any limitations that might be imposed on the child because of the disorder. It should be emphasized that the seizures can be controlled or greatly reduced in the large majority of affected children and that new studies hold the promise of progress in future treatment. Parents need reassurance that in this enlightened day and age there is less stigma attached to the condition than in the past.

It is important to encourage a healthy attitude toward the child and the condition and to help the parents feel competent in their ability to meet their responsibilities to the child. The child should be reared as any normal child, with natural concern tempered by the understanding of the need not to be overprotected. Many parents refrain from correcting or punishing the child, especially if they have had the experience of such an emotional stress precipitating a seizure. The child must not be made to feel different in any way. Parents should be encouraged to be honest and open about the disorder with the child and with others. Some parents are tempted to try to conceal the nature of the child's illness because of their belief that the disorder is shameful or a disgrace to the family.

Educational materials and support groups may prove beneficial for families. The **Epilepsy Foundation of America*** is a national organization that works for the welfare of persons with epilepsy and their families, helps with employment and legal problems, and provides education to patients, families, and communities.

The Child with Epilepsy. The child who is provided the security of a loving family, rewards and punishments no different from those of other children, and support in acquiring self-esteem is more apt to have a positive attitude toward the condition. Children derive their self-concept and self-esteem from observations of others' reactions to them and from their own perception of their capabilities. The suddenness and unpredictability of the seizures and the reactions of others further influence their feelings. When others consider children to be different, inferior, or objects of ridicule, they come to view themselves as different, inferior, and incapable. Behavioral problems and school difficulties, such as dependency and underachievement, are common in children with epilepsy and can become more serious than the seizures (Vining, 1990b).

Children with epilepsy need to learn about their condition and the role that the medication plays in contributing to their prolonged well-being. As soon as they are old enough, children should assume responsibility for taking their own medication and be advised to carry medical identification with pertinent information about their condition. Planning activities with children and emphasizing those in which they can engage rather than those in which they cannot participate help them to succeed and to gain satisfaction in their achievements. They should be offered opportunities and encouraged to exercise judgment in their daily lives.

The adolescent period may prove to be a trying time for the child with epilepsy. Limits imposed on the young person's activities at a time when freedom and independence are desired may bring the disability into sharp focus. For example, all states in the United States have a defined seizure-free period before a driver's license can be obtained.

Epilepsy should not be a severe impairment to most youngsters, and the nurse, by assuming the role of patient advocate, helping to educate the public regarding the condition, working toward making opportunities available to persons with the disorder, and lobbying for legislation that recognizes the needs of the individual with a seizure disorder, can help to provide positive outcomes for the child and family.

*For more information on video games and epilepsy, contact the Epilepsy Foundation of America.

*4351 Garden City Dr., Landover, MD 20785; (301) 459-3700 or (800) EFA-1000. In Canada: **Epilepsy Canada,** 1470 Peel St., Suite 745, Montreal, Quebec H3A 1T1; (514) 845-7855.

NURSING CARE PLAN
The Child with Epilepsy

NURSING DIAGNOSIS: High risk for injury related to type of seizure

PATIENT GOAL 1: Will not experience seizure activity

• **NURSING INTERVENTIONS/*RATIONALES***

*Administer antiepileptic medication

Teach family and child, when appropriate, the administration of medications

Stress importance of complying with therapeutic regimen

Avoid situations that are known to precipitate a seizure (e.g., blinking lights, fatigue)

• **EXPECTED OUTCOME**

Child remains free of seizure activity

PATIENT GOAL 2: Will not experience complications from medication

• **NURSING INTERVENTIONS/*RATIONALES***

Be aware of and teach family to recognize unfavorable reactions to medications

Encourage periodic physical and laboratory assessment *to determine possible deviations from normal findings*

Encourage good dental care during phenytoin therapy *to reduce gingival hyperplasia from phenytoin*

Encourage adequate vitamin D and folic acid during phenytoin and phenobarbital therapy *to prevent deficiency*

• **EXPECTED OUTCOME**

Child and family demonstrate an understanding of possible unfavorable responses to medications and the appropriate intervention (specify)

PATIENT GOAL 3: Will not experience injury

• **NURSING INTERVENTIONS/*RATIONALES***

Educate parents and child regarding appropriate activities for child (depends on type, frequency, and severity of seizures)

Explore appropriate modifications or adaptations to situations *that pose a danger during a seizure* (climbing trees, play apparatus)

Provide companionship during permissible activities, such as swimming, biking

Recommend showering or close supervision during bathing

Educate teachers and other persons who are associated with child regarding correct assistance during and after seizure

• **EXPECTED OUTCOMES**

Child and family agree on appropriate activities or modifications of activities for child

Individuals in contact with child intervene appropriately during and after seizure

*Dependent nursing action.

NURSING DIAGNOSIS: High risk for injury, hypoxia, and aspiration related to motor activity and loss of consciousness (tonic-clonic seizure)

PATIENT GOAL 1: Will not experience injury, respiratory distress, or aspiration

• **NURSING INTERVENTIONS/*RATIONALES***

Time seizure *to determine duration of possible hypoxia and possible need for emergency care*

Protect child during seizure

- Do not attempt to restrain child or use force *to prevent inflicting injury to child or self*
- If child is standing or sitting in wheelchair at beginning of episode, ease child to floor *to prevent falls*
- Place small cushion or blanket or own hand under child's head *to prevent injury*
- Do not put anything in child's mouth, such as tongue blades, food, or fluids, *that can cause injury, obstruct breathing, or be aspirated*
- Remove eyeglasses *to protect eyes from trauma*
- Loosen clothing *that may restrict movement or breathing*
- Prevent child from hitting head on sharp objects *that might cause injury during uncontrollable muscle jerks*
- Remove hazards (furniture)
- Pad objects such as crib, siderails, or wheelchair *to lessen injury from impact*
- Keep siderails raised when child is sleeping, resting, or seizing *to avoid falls*
- Allow seizure to end without interference
- Position child with head in midline, not hyperextended, when possible *to promote adequate ventilation*
- If child begins to vomit, turn to side as a unit *to prevent aspiration*
- Protect child after seizure (postictal period)
  - Time postictal period
  - Maintain child in side position
- Call emergency medical service (EMS) (see Emergency Treatment box, p. 1723)

• **EXPECTED OUTCOME**

Child exhibits no sign of physical or mental injury or aspiration

NURSING DIAGNOSIS: High risk for injury related to impaired consciousness and automatisms (complex partial seizure)

PATIENT GOAL 1: Will not experience injury and will remain calm

• **NURSING INTERVENTIONS/*RATIONALES***

Time seizure *to establish duration and possible need for emergency care*

Protect child during seizure

- Do not restrain, unless child is in danger, *to prevent injury to child or self*
- Remove hazards in immediate environment

Continued.

NURSING CARE PLAN
The Child with Epilepsy—cont'd

Redirect child to safe area, especially away from windows, stairs, heating elements, or sources of water, *to prevent falls, burns, and drowning*
Do not agitate; rather, talk in calm voice and reassuring manner
Do not expect child to follow instructions *because of impaired consciousness*
Watch to see if seizure generalizes into a tonic-clonic seizure
Protect child after seizure (postictal)
Time postictal period
Stay and reassure child until fully alert *because child may be confused and frightened*
Call EMS (see Emergency Treatment box, p. 1723)

• **EXPECTED OUTCOME**
Child exhibits no sign of physical injury and remains calm

NURSING DIAGNOSIS: Altered family processes related to a child with a chronic illness

PATIENT (FAMILY) GOAL 1: Will receive adequate support

• **NURSING INTERVENTIONS/*RATIONALES***
See Nursing diagnosis: Altered family processes in Nursing Care Plan: The Child with Chronic Illness or Disability, Chapter 22
Refer to special support groups and agencies (e.g., Epilepsy Foundation of America)

• **EXPECTED OUTCOME**
Family becomes involved with special group

See also:
Nursing Care Plan: The Child with Chronic Illness or Disability, Chapter 22
Nursing Care Plan: The Unconscious Child, p. 1688

❖ EVALUATION

The effectiveness of nursing interventions for the child with epilepsy is determined by continual reassessment and evaluation of care based on the following observational guidelines and expected outcomes:

1. Observe child's behavior for evidence of seizure activity and assess the environment for situations that could cause injury to child in the event of a seizure; interview family regarding management of child during a seizure.
2. Interview child and family regarding compliance with the medication regimen and identification of triggering factors.
3. Observe and interview family regarding their feelings and concerns and their understanding of child's condition.
4. Observe child's interactions with others and interview child about any feelings or concerns about own health.

Expected outcomes:
See Nursing Care Plan, p. 1727-1728.

FEBRILE SEIZURES

Febrile seizures are transient disorders of children that occur in association with a fever. They are one of the most common neurologic disorders of childhood, affecting about 3% of children. Most febrile seizures occur after 6 months of age and usually before age 3 years, with increased frequency in children younger than 18 months. They are unusual after 5 years of age. Boys are affected about twice as often as girls, and there appears to be an increased susceptibility in families, indicating a possible genetic predisposition.

The cause of febrile seizures is still uncertain. In most children the height, but not rapidity, of the temperature elevation seems to be a factor (Berg, 1993). The fever usually exceeds 38.8° C (101.8° F), and the seizure occurs during the temperature rise rather than after a prolonged elevation. Sometimes it constitutes the dramatic beginning of an illness, usually an upper respiratory or gastrointestinal infection. A shorter duration of fever before the initial febrile seizure and a lower temperature at the time of the seizure are associated with an increased risk of recurrence of febrile seizures in children (Berg and others, 1992). Although pertussis vaccine does not cause febrile seizures, this immunization is a precipitating factor in initial episodes of febrile seizures in children prone to having seizures (Cherry and others, 1993).

Most febrile seizures have stopped by the time the child is taken to a medical facility. However, if the seizure continues, treatment consists of controlling the seizure with intravenous or rectal diazepam (Valium) and reducing the temperature by administration of acetaminophen. Antiepileptic prophylaxis may be considered for a child (1) who experiences focal or prolonged seizures, (2) with neurologic abnormalities, (3) with a first-degree relative who has febrile seizures, (4) who is younger than age 1 year, and (5) in whom multiple seizures occur within a 24-hour period (Berg and others, 1990). Phenobarbital therapy is ineffective in preventing recurrences of febrile seizures and can cause a decrease in IQ scores (Farwell, 1990).

Bethune and others (1993) identified full-time daycare attendance (20 hours or more per week) as an epidemiologic characteristic of febrile seizures. Daycare attendance has been linked with increased risk of infectious disease (Hurwitz and others, 1991), and children with febrile seizures have been found to have an increased number of infectious diseases (Forsgren and others, 1990); still, the risk of febrile seizures for children in daycare remains relatively low (Ferry, 1993). Children likely (28% risk) to have a febrile seizure demonstrate all of the following: (1) family history of febrile seizures in first- and second-degree relatives, (2) full-time daycare, (3) neonatal discharge at or after 28 days, and (4) slow development (Bethune and others, 1993).

Parents need reassurance of the benign nature of febrile seizures (almost 95% to 98% of children with febrile seizures will not develop epilepsy or any neurologic damage). They should be told that their child is in no danger of dying during a febrile seizure. They also need education regarding protecting the child from harm and observing exactly what happens to the child during the event. Attempts to lower the temperature will not prevent a seizure. Tepid sponge baths are not recommended, because they are ineffective in significantly lowering the temperature, the shivering effect further increases metabolic output, and cooling causes discomfort in the child. Counseling may be the best therapy (Camfield and Camfield, 1993).

NURSING ALERT If a febrile seizure lasts more than 10 minutes, parents should seek medical attention right away. Encourage them to drive carefully; a few extra minutes will not make any significant difference (Camfield and Camfield, 1993).

BREATH-HOLDING SPELLS

Breath-holding spells (reflex hypoxic crisis) are readily recognized and follow a distinct clinical pattern. Not a true seizure disorder, the typical attack has its onset in infants between the ages of 6 and 18 months and may occur up to 4 years of age. The episode is characterized by violent crying and cessation of breathing that is precipitated by fright, frustration, or anger. The breath is usually held on expiration, and the child becomes cyanotic, loses consciousness, and may display a few clonic convulsions of the extremities. The episode ends with a gasp, and the color returns promptly. The frequency of attacks varies considerably, but they almost always disappear by 5 to 6 years of age.

Breath-holding spells are a benign entity, and drug therapy is generally not indicated. Family therapy may be beneficial, since many children appear to use an attack or the threat of an attack to assert themselves and to express anger. Parents need reassurance that the attacks do not represent a danger to the child, and this knowledge may even help to decrease or eliminate the incidence of attacks.

HEADACHE

Headaches are one of the most frequent neurologic complaints of children. Headaches can be caused by extracranial disease, intracranial disease, vascular disease, or psychologic problems (Table 37-9).

TABLE 37-9 Headache Syndromes in Children

TYPE OF HEADACHE	CHARACTERISTICS
ACUTE EXTRACRANIAL	
Sinusitis	Frontal sinus most frequently involved
Ocular abnormalities	Usually frontal and precipitated by television viewing or schoolwork
Dental disorders	Frontal or temporal headaches caused by malocclusion, caries, abscess, temporomandibular joint dysfunction
Respiratory infections (pharyngitis, otitis media)	Pain localized to affected structures
Trauma	Localized to area of trauma; related to nerve and tissue injury Postconcussion syndrome (see Posttraumatic Syndromes, p. 1697)
ACUTE RECURRENT	
Vascular: migraine syndrome	Intermittent attacks of vasoconstriction Paroxysmal Positive family history Triggered by stress, fatigue, trauma, exercise, illness, diet, menses, medication
CHRONIC PROGRESSIVE	
Intracranial abnormalities	Symptoms of increased ICP
Tumors	Frontal: supratentorial tumors Occipital: infratentorial tumors
Hydrocephalus	Rapid head enlargement, suture splitting (infants, young children)
Subdural hematoma	Usually results from trauma Seizures and focal neurologic deficits more common than headaches
Brain abscess	More often associated with ear infections and cyanotic heart disease
Pseudotumor cerebri	Increased ICP without obstruction of CSF
CHRONIC NONPROGRESSIVE (PSYCHOGENIC)	Common in children Adjustment reaction, anxiety Sign of depression Conversion hysteria (anxiety converted to somatic symptoms)

ASSESSMENT

It is important to determine the pattern of the headache—single acute episode, paroxysmal, recurrent and acute, chronic and progressive, or chronic and nonprogressive. Other assessment information includes whether or not the headache is associated with seizures, ataxia, lethargy, weakness, unexplained nausea or vomiting, or any personality changes. Factors that might be pertinent to the headache are related to early development and past illnesses. Having the child or family keep a pain diary (time of onset and termination, pain intensity, and associated events) may be helpful (McGrath, 1990). (See also Pain Assessment, Chapter 26.)

The family history may provide clues to the etiologic factor, including those related to the home or social situation (e.g., alcoholism, divorce, separation). Specific questions to ask in order to elicit needed information are listed in the box at right. Thorough physical and neurologic examinations are carried out, and special diagnostic tests (e.g., radiographs, EEG, CT, MRI) may be indicated.

QUESTIONS FOR EVALUATING HEADACHE

Do you have more than one type of headache?
How did the headache begin? Trauma? Infection?
How long has it been present?
Are the symptoms worsening or staying the same?
How often do they occur?
How long do they last?
Do they occur at any special time or under specific circumstances?
Are they preceded by warning signs?
Where does it hurt?
What is the quality of the pain? Pounding? Sharp?
Do you have associated symptoms during the headache? Abdominal pain? Nausea, vomiting?
Do you stop what you are doing during the headache?
Do you have any other medical problems?
Are you taking any medications regularly?
Are there any activities that make the headache worse?
Does any particular medication make the headache better?
Does anyone else in your family have headaches?
What do you think is causing your headaches?

Modified from Rothner AD: Management of headaches in children and adolescents, *J Pain Symptom Manage* 8(2):81-86, 1993.

MIGRAINE HEADACHE

Migraine is the most common cause of recurrent headache in children. The cause is unknown, although attacks may be precipitated by stress, fatigue, stroboscopic stimulation, anxiety, conflict, smoke, pollution, or certain foods. It is characterized by chronic, recurrent headache, often preceded by visual disturbances and accompanied by nausea and vomiting. Emotional factors may play a part.

There are two phases in the pathologic development of migraine, both caused by a functional disturbance of intracerebral circulation. Initially there is a prodromal phase caused by vasoconstriction of intracranial vessels followed by dilatation of the extracranial vessels, which produces a throbbing, pulsating, and pounding headache. Characteristics of several patterns of migraine headache are described in the box on p. 1731.

A family history of migraine is elicited in 75% to 90% of children, and some observers have noted that children often display a characteristic personality. They tend to be meticulous, compulsive, unusually mature for their age, and high achievers in school and strive to please the family at home. They have difficulty in expressing anger or rage. Boys are affected twice as often as girls.

The diagnosis is seldom made until the child is old enough to relate the symptoms, although one in five children has a first attack before age 5 years. Early in life the symptoms are nonspecific, such as recurrent abdominal pain, motion ("car") sickness, and restlessness, and the child may display head-banging or sudden alterations in personality. The typical attack of migraine begins early in the day, often awakening the child. The prodromal symptoms, induced by vasoconstriction, consist of transient visual disturbances or other neurologic disabilities. In a few minutes or sometimes a few hours, the aura is followed by throbbing unilateral head pain accompanied by nausea and vomiting. Sleep ordinarily terminates an attack.

Although serious intracranial disease needs to be ruled out, in most cases ***chronic, recurrent headache of childhood*** represents migraine. The difference between migraine and seizures in children must be determined. The diagnosis can be confusing and frustrating for families. Migraine headaches may be confused with other types of headache (e.g., those caused by tension or organic disorders such as brain tumors), but several features often set them apart, including a family history for migraine and nausea and vomiting.

NURSING ALERT During the health history and neurologic assessment be aware of the following abnormal signs that require immediate follow-up for children with headache:

- Progressive in frequency and severity over a brief period of time (2 to 3 weeks)
- Awakens child from sleep (may also be migraine)
- Occurs in early morning, worse on arising, less during the day
- Exacerbated by Valsalva maneuver (intensified by lowering head and straining, such as during bowel movement, coughing, or sneezing)
- Persistent, occipital or frontal pain
- Unexplained vomiting or vomiting not associated with headache
- Any change in gait, personality, or behavior (if changes occur during the headache, they may indicate complicated migraine)

Treatment is symptomatic. Simple analgesics such as acetaminophen may be effective and are usually the preferred medication. Parents usually bring their child to a health practitioner because medications have not worked or the headaches are occurring more often or becoming more se-

MIGRAINE PATTERNS

CLASSIC MIGRAINE

Vasoconstriction (prodromal) phase:
- Visual symptoms—blindness, blurring, visual field cuts, scotoma, micropsia or macropsia
- May include (less frequently) weakness, inability to speak, sensory abnormalities

Dilatation phase:
- Throbbing, unilateral or frontal pain
- Onset of pain followed by vomiting and abdominal pain, photophobia, phonophobia, desire to sleep
- On awakening, child usually well

COMMON MIGRAINE

More variable symptoms than classic migraine; aura less pronounced
Prodromal: malaise, personality change, or depression
Headache, nausea, vomiting
Course similar to classic migraine

CLUSTER HEADACHES

Unilateral, orbital pain; tearing; rhinorrhea; nasal stuffiness
Pain severe and recurrent for weeks at a time
Rare in childhood

OPHTHALMOPLEGIC MIGRAINE

Eye pain
Complete or incomplete CN III palsies
Unilateral pupillary dilatation, ptosis, outward deviation of eyes

HEMIPLEGIC MIGRAINE

Associated with recurrent paralysis
Hemiplegia may precede or follow headache
May be familial

BASILAR MIGRAINE

Recurrent attacks
Symptoms and signs referable to brainstem and cerebellum
- Paroxysmal acute ataxia, alternating weakness, vertigo, (occasionally) loss of consciousness

More common in girls

PAROXYSMAL VERTIGO

Episodes of vertigo in very young child (ages 2 to 4 years)
Retained consciousness, inability to maintain posture, nystagmus
Headaches may or may not be present
May be related to basilar migraine

CONFUSIONAL STATE

Disturbed sensorium, retained consciousness, agitation
Paroxysmal occurrence
Headaches may or may not be present

CYCLIC VOMITING

Unexplained recurrent episodes of vomiting
Abdominal pain usually present
Headache absent

EPILEPSY EQUIVALENT SYNDROME

Episodes of paroxysmal headache, nausea, vomiting
May be interpreted as seizures in some children

vere. Other medications that are commonly used include a combination of acetaminophen, caffeine, and butalbital (Fioricet), or acetaminophen, dichloralphenazone, and isometheptene mucate (Midrin), ergotamine, and sumatriptan (Klapper, 1993).

While the ergots are used in the treatment of adult vascular headaches, these medications are typically not used in children because of their side effects. Opioids are not used, since they rarely act on the mechanism of the pain.

Other modalities, such as biofeedback, diet, and stress management techniques, may help. Stress management includes a headache diary, progressive relaxation, cognitive restructuring, distraction or attention focusing, mental activities, thought stopping, imaging, behavior rehearsal, assertiveness, and problem solving (Engel, Rapoff, and Pressman, 1992). (For a description of many of these techniques, see box on p. 1090.)

The outlook for the child with migraine is good, but the child and parents should be informed that predisposition to the headaches may be lifelong. Severe headaches can adversely affect the child's routine activities of daily living, including family relations and school performance.

KEY POINTS

- The central nervous system (CNS) is composed of the brain and spinal cord. Brain, blood, and cerebrospinal fluid (CSF) maintain an equilibrium inside the skull; and disturbance of these components creates disequilibrium.
- Gait abnormalities that may indicate cerebral dysfunction include a change in ambulatory function such as ataxia, spastic paraplegic gait, hemiplegic gait, cerebellar gait, and extrapyramidal gait.
- Level of consciousness (LOC) is the most important indicator of neurologic health; altered levels include sleep, confusion, delirium, pseudowakeful states, and comatose states.
- Complete neurologic examination includes LOC; posture; motor, sensory, cranial nerve (CN), and reflex testing; and vital signs.
- Nursing care of the unconscious child focuses on respiratory management, neurologic assessment, increased intracranial pressure (ICP) monitoring, supplying adequate nutrition and hydration, drug therapy, promoting elimination, hygienic care, positioning and exercise, stimulation, and family support.
- Primary head injury involves features that occur at the time of trauma, including fractured skull, contusions, intracranial hematoma, and diffuse injury. Secondary complications include hypoxic brain damage, increased ICP, infection, cerebral edema, and posttraumatic syndromes.
- The young child's response to head injury is different because of the following features: larger head size, expandable skull, larger amount of blood volume to the brain, small subdural spaces, and thinner, softer brain tissue.
- Fractures resulting from head injuries may be classified as linear, depressed, compound, basilar, and diastatic.
- Problems resulting from near-drowning are caused by hypoxia and include asphyxiation, aspiration, and hypothermia.

- Nursing care of the child with meningitis includes administration of antibiotics, prevention of self-infection, removal of environmental stimuli, correct positioning, vital signs monitoring, intravenous therapy, and promoting fluid, nutritional status, and supportive care of the family.
- Routine immunization of infants against *H. influenzae* type B infection has reduced the incidence of bacterial meningitis.
- Encephalitis may result from direct invasion of the CNS by a virus or from postinfectious involvement of the CNS after viral disease.
- A seizure is a symptom of underlying pathology and may be manifested by sensory-hallucinatory phenomena, motor effects, sensorimotor effects, and impaired or loss of consciousness.
- Partial seizures are categorized as simple (without associated impairment of consciousness) or complex (with impaired consciousness); both types may become generalized.
- Generalized seizures are categorized as tonic-clonic, absence, atonic, akinetic, or myoclonic.
- Long-term care of the child involves teaching caregivers appropriate interventions during a seizure, emphasizing the importance of antiepileptic therapy and giving practical advice regarding drug administration and scheduling, and fostering the child's and family's coping with the diagnosis.
- Febrile seizures are the most common type of childhood seizure. The most important nursing intervention is to reassure parents of their benign nature and educate parents regarding protection of their child and meaningful observation during the event.
- A child's complaint of headache requires a thorough history and physical with a neurologic assessment to rule out increased ICP. Migraine is the most common cause of recurrent headache in children.

REFERENCES

American Academy of Pediatrics, Committee on Drugs: Behavioral and cognitive effects of anticonvulsant therapy, *Pediatrics* 76:644-647, 1985.

American Academy of Pediatrics, Committee on Infectious Disease: Dexamethasone therapy for bacterial meningitis in infants and children, *Pediatrics* 86(1):130-133, 1990.

Ashwal S and others: Bacterial meningitis in children: pathophysiology and treatment, *Neurology* 43(4):739-748, 1992.

Barkovich AJ: Techniques and methods in pediatric imaging. In Barkovich AJ: *Pediatric neuroimaging,* New York, 1990, Raven Press.

Bateman PA, Heagarty MC: Passive freebase cocaine inhalation by infants and toddlers, *Am J Dis Child* 143:25-27, 1989.

Berg AT: Are febrile seizures provoked by a rapid rise in temperature? *Am J Dis Child* 147:1101-1103, 1993.

Berg AT and others: Predictors of recurrent febrile seizures, *J Pediatr* 116:329-337, 1990.

Berg AT and others: A prospective study of recurrent febrile seizures, *N Engl J Med* 327:1122-1127, 1992.

Bethune P and others: Which child will have a febrile seizure? *Am J Dis Child* 47(1):35-39, 1993.

Blevins SH, Benson S: A better way to get kids through scans, *RN* 55(10):40-44, 1992.

Blisard KS, Davis LE: Neuropathologic findings in Reye Syndrome, *J Child Neurol* 6(1):41-44, 1991.

Bonadio W, Wagner V: Adrenaline-cocaine gel topical anesthetic for dermal laceration repair in children, *Ann Emerg Med* 21(12): 1435-1438, 1992.

Brodie MJ: Established anticonvulsants and treatment of refractory epilepsy, *Lancet* 336(8711):350-354, 1990.

Brodie MJ: Felbamate: a new antiepileptic drug, *Lancet* 341(8858):1445-1446, 1993.

Bruce D, Schut L: Concussion and contusion following pediatric head trauma. In McLaurin R, editor: *Pediatric neurosurgery,* Philadelphia, 1989, WB Saunders.

Cameron PD, Wallace SJ, Munro J: Herpes simplex virus encephalitis: problems in diagnosis, *Dev Med Child Neurol* 34(2):134-140, 1992.

Camfield CS, Camfield PR: Febrile seizures: an Rx for parent fears and anxiety, *Contemp Pediatr* 10(4):26-44, 1993.

Camfield CS and others: Home use of rectal diazepam to prevent status epilepticus in children with convulsive disorders, *J Child Neurol* 4:125-126, 1989.

Camfield CS and others: Biologic factors as predictors of social outcome of epilepsy in intellectually normal children: a population-based study, *J Pediatr* 122(6):869-873, 1993a.

Camfield CS and others: Outcome of childhood epilepsy: a population-based study with a simple predictive scoring system for those treated with medication, *J Pediatr* 122(6):861-868, 1993b.

Casteels-VanDaele M: Reduction of deaths after drug labelling for risk of Reye's syndrome, *Lancet* 341:118-119, 1993.

Cherry JD and others: Pertussis immunization and characteristics related to first seizures in infants and children, *J Pediatr* 122(6):900-903, 1993.

Civitello LA: Neurologic complications of HIV infection in children, *Pediatr Neurosurg* 17(2):104-112, 1991.

Clinical diagnosis of meningitis in children, *Emerg Med* 25(4):175-178, 1993.

Commission on Classification and Terminology of the International League Against Epilepsy, *Epilepsia* 30:389-399, 1989.

Davis RJ and others: Head and spinal cord injury. In Rodgers MC, editor: *Textbook of pediatric intensive care,* Baltimore, 1987, Williams & Wilkins.

Dieckmann RA: Rectal diazepam for prehospital pediatric status epilepticus, *Ann Emerg Med* 23:216-224, 1994.

Diekema DS, Quan L, Holt VL: Epilepsy as a risk factor for submersion injury in children, *Pediatrics* 91:612-616, 1993.

Engel J: *Seizures and epilepsy,* Philadelphia, 1989, FA Davis.

Engel JM, Rapoff MA, Pressman AR: Long-term follow-up of relaxation training for pediatric headache disorders, *Headache* 322:152-156, 1992.

Ernst AA, Sanders WM: Unexpected cocaine intoxication presenting as seizures in children, *Ann Emerg Med* 18:747-749, 1989.

Farley J: The comatose child: analysis of factors affecting intracranial pressure, *Dimens Crit Care Nurs* 9(4):216-222, 1990.

Farwell JR and others: Phenobarbital for febrile seizures: effects on intelligence and seizure recurrence, *N Engl J Med* 322:364-369, 1990.

Felbamate Study Group in Lennox-Gastaut Syndrome: Efficacy of felbamate in childhood epileptic encephalopathy (Lennox-Gastaut syndrome), *N Engl J Med* 328(1):29-22, 1993.

Ferry PC: Risk factors in febrile seizures, *Am J Dis Child* 147(1):14, 1993.

Forsgren L and others: An incident case-referent study of febrile convulsions in children: genetical and social aspects, *Neuropediatrics* 21:153-159, 1990.

Freeman JM, Vining EPG: Decision making and the child with afebrile seizures, *Pediatr Rev* 13(8):305-310, 1992.

Ghajar J, Hariri RJ: Management of pediatric head injury, *Pediatr Clin North Am* 39(5):1093-1123, 1992.

Goetting MG, Haddad ML: Cerebral oxygen extraction during severe viral encephalitis, *Henry Ford Hosp Med J* 40(1-2):127-130, 1992.

Grewal M, Sutcliffe AJ: Early prediction of outcome following head injury: an assessment of the value of GCS score trend and abnormal plantar and pupillary light reflexes, *J Pediatr Surg* 26:1161, 1991.

Hanna DR: Purple glove syndrome: a complication of intravenous phenytoin, *J Neurosci Nurs* 24(6):340-342, 1992.

Hodges K, Root L: Surgical management of intractable seizure disorders, *J Neurosci Nurs* 23(2):93-100, 1991.

Holmes GL, Weber DA: Effects of ACTH on seizure susceptibility in the developing brain, *Ann Neurol* 20(1):82-88, 1986.

Hrachovy RA, Frost JD Jr: Infantile spasms, *Pediatr Clin North Am* 36:311-329, 1989.

Hurwitz E and others: Risk of respiratory illness associated with day-care attendance: a nationwide study, *Pediatrics* 87:62-69, 1991.

Imported human rabies, 1992, *MMWR* 41(51):953-955, 1992.

Jenkins TL: Fulminant meningococcemia in pediatric patients: nursing considerations, *Pediatr Nurs* 18(6):629-634, 1992.

Johnson D: Head injury. In Eichelberger M, Pratsch G, editors: *Pediatric trauma care,* Rockville, MD, 1988, Aspen.

Kilpi T and others: Severity of childhood bacterial meningitis, *Lancet* 338(3):406-409, 1991.

Klapper J: The pharmacologic treatment of acute migraine headaches, *J Pain Symptom Manage* 8(3):140-147, 1993.

Koszewski W: Epilepsy following brain abscess, *Acta Neurochir* 113(3-4):110-117, 1991.

Krugman S and others: *Infectious diseases of children,* ed 9, St Louis, 1992, Mosby.

LeRoux PD and others: Pediatric ICP monitoring in hypoxic and nonhypoxic brain injury, *Child Nerv Syst* 7:34-39, 1991.

Luerssen TG: Head injury in children, *Neurosurg Clin North Am* 2(2):399-410, 1991.

McGrath PA: *Pain in children,* New York, Guilford, 1990.

McLone DG, Hahn YS: Head and spinal cord injuries in children. In Raffensperger MS, editor: *Raffensperger Swenson's pediatric surgery,* ed 5, East Norwalk, CT, 1990, Appleton & Lange.

Mealey J: Skull fractures. In Eichelberger M, Pratsch G, editors: *Pediatric trauma care,* Rockville, MD, 1988, Aspen.

Medical Research Council Antiepileptic Drug Withdrawal Study Group: Prognostic index for recurrence of seizures after remission of epilepsy, *Br Med J* 306:1374-1378, 1993.

Middleton DB: After a child's first seizure, *Emerg Med* 25(4):181-191, 1993.

Murphy TV and others: Declining incidence of *Haemophilus influenzae* type b disease since introduction of vaccination, *JAMA* 269(2):246-248, 1993.

Noah ZL and others: Management of the child with severe brain injury, *Crit Care Clin* 8(1):59-77, 1992.

Pellock JM: Risk versus benefits of antiepileptic drug therapy, *Int Pediatr* 5(2):177-181, 1990.

Pomeroy SL and others: Sequelae of bacterial meningitis in children, *N Engl J Med* 323(24):1651-1657, 1990.

Projections of the number of HIV-infected persons—United States, 1992-1994, *MMWR* 41(18):1-29, 1992.

Quan L, Kinder D: Pediatric submersions: prehospital predictors of outcome, *Pediatrics* 90(6):909-913, 1992.

Recommendations of the immunization practices advisory committee (ACIP): Rabies prevention—United States, 1991, *MMWR* 40:1-19, 1991.

Reynolds E: Controversies in caring for the child with a head injury, *MCN* 17:246-251, 1992.

Rubenstein JS: Acute pediatric CNS infections. In Fuhrman BP, Zimmerman JJ, editors: *Pediatric Critical Care,* St Louis, 1992, Mosby.

Sagraves R: Antiepileptic drug therapy for pediatric generalized tonic-clonic seizures, *J Pediatr Health Care* 4(6):314-319, 1990.

Swaiman KF: *Pediatric neurology: principles and practice,* ed 2, St Louis, 1994, Mosby.

Tekkok IH, Erbergi A: Management of brain abscess in children: review of 130 cases over a period of 21 years, *Child Nerve Syst* 8(7):411-416, 1992.

van Donselaar CA, Geerts AT, Schimscheimer RJ: Usefulness of an aura for classification of a first generalized seizure, *Epilepsia* 31(5): 529-535, 1990.

Verity CM, Ross EM, Golding J: Outcome of childhood status epilepticus and lengthy febrile convulsions: findings of national cohort study, *Br Med J* 307:225-228, 1993.

Vining E: Cognitive and behavioral side effects of antiepileptic drugs, *Int Pediatr* 5(2):182-185, 1990a.

Vining E: The psychosocial impact of epilepsy in children and their families, *Int Pediatr* 5(2):186-188, 1990b.

Williams FH, Nelms DK, McGaharan KM: Brain abscess, *Arch Phys Med Rehabil* 73(5):490-492, 1992.

Wong D: Changing what children hear in the ICU can lower intracranial pressure, *Am J Nurs* 88:279-280, 1988.

Zepp F and others: Battered child syndrome, *Neuropediatrics* 23(4):188-191, 1992.

BIBLIOGRAPHY

General

Hickey JV: *Neurological and neurosurgical nursing,* Philadelphia, 1992, JB Lippincott.

Sarnaik AP, Lieh-Lai MW: Transporting the neurologically compromised child, *Pediatr Clin North Am* 40(2):337-344, 1993.

Brain Death

Alvarey LA: Controversies in the diagnosis of brain death in children, *Int Pediatr* 5(2):197-202, 1990.

Kohrman MH, Spivak BS: Brain death in infants: sensitivity and specific criteria, *Pediatr Neurol* 6:47-50, 1990.

Neurologic Assessment

American Academy of Pediatrics, Committee on Drugs: Use of chloral hydrate for sedation in children, *Pediatrics* 92:471-473, 1993.

Bishop BS: Pathologic pupillary signs: self-learning module, *Crit Care Nurse* 11(8):30-82, 1992.

Chuang S, Kucharczyk W: MRI scanning technique for neuroimaging in pediatrics, *Top Magn Reson Imaging* 5(1):46-49, 1993.

Ferry PC: Pediatric neurodiagnostic tests: a modern perspective, *Pediatr Rev* 13(7):248-255, 1992.

Grewal M, Sutcliffe AJ: Early prediction of outcome following head injury: an assessment of the value of GCS score trend and abnormal plantar and pupillary light reflexes, *J Pediatr Surg* 26:1161, 1991.

Lieh-lai MW: Limitations of the GCS in predicting outcome in children with traumatic brain injury, *J Pediatr* 120:195-199, 1992.

McGowan-Repasky T: A 2-year-old with an altered level of consciousness, *J Emerg Nurs* 18(1):34-41, 1992.

McKay C: Silent children: what can you do for comatose children? *Nursing* 22(2):84, 1992.

Merrick PA and others: Care of pediatric patients sedated with pentobarbital sodium in MRI, *Pediatr Nurs* 17(1):34-37, 1991.

Naidich TP: Normal brain maturation, *Int Pediatr* 5(2):81-86, 1990.

Oliphant M, Berne AS: An integrated look at pediatric imaging, *Contemp Pediatr* 7(1):61-78, 1990.

Rayhorn N: Three golden hours, *Nursing* 21(8):93, 1991.

Ruijs MB, Keyser A, Gabre FJ: Assessment of post-traumatic amnesia in young chidlren, *Dev Med Child Neurol* 34(10):885-892, 1992.

Schnuk JE: The pediatric patient with altered level of consciousness, *J Emerg Nurs* 18(5):419-421, 1992.

Simpson DA and others: Head injuries in infants and young children: the value of the pediatric coma scale, *Child Nerve Syst* 7:183-190, 1991.

Vos HR: Making headway with intracranial hypertension, *Am J Nurs* 93(2):28-35, 1993.

Wagner MB: Neurologic emergencies in the young. I. Evaluation and stabilization, *Emerg Med* 24(8):204-213, 1992.

Yager JV, Johnston B, Seshia SS: Coma scales in practice, *Am J Dis Child* 144:1088-1091, 1990.

Zegeer L: Oculocephalic and vestibulo-ocular responses: significance for nursing care, *J Neurosci Nurs* 21:46-55, 1989.

Increased Intracranial Pressure

Ackerman AD: Current issues in the care of the head-injured child, *Curr Opin Pediatr* 3:433-438, 1991.

Andrus C: Intracranial pressure: dynamics and nursing management, *J Neurosci Nurs* 23:85-91, 1991.

Boulard G, Ravussin P, Guterin J: A new way to monitor external ventricular drainage, *Neurosurgery* 30(4):636-638, 1992.

Chadduck WM and others: Transcranial Doppler ultrasonography for the evaluation of shunt malfunction in pediatric patients, *Childs Nerv Syst* 7(1):27-30, 1991.

Dietz HC: Coma. In Hoekelman RA and others, editors: *Primary pediatric care,* ed 2, St Louis, 1992, Mosby.

Gambbardella G, d'Avella D, Tomasello F: Monitoring of brain tissue pressure with a fiberoptic device, *Neurosurgery* 31(5):918-921, 1992.

Garcia-Merina A and others: Intracranial pressure monitoring in acute disseminated encephalomyelitis in childhood, *Crit Care Med* 18(12):1481-1483, 1990.

Rosen MJ, Daughton S: Cerebral perfusion pressure management in head injury, *J Trauma* 30:933-940, 1990.

Young RSK: Increased intracranial pressure. In Hoekelman RA and others, editors: *Primary pediatric care,* ed 2, St Louis, 1992, Mosby.

Head Injury

Aldrich EF and others: Diffuse brain swelling in severely head-injured children, *J Neurosurg* 76:450, 1992.

Amling JK and others: Neuropsychological outcome in children with gun shot wounds to the brain, *J Neurosci Nurs* 22(1):13-18, 1990.

Bruce DA: Head injuries in the pediatric population, *Curr Probl Pediatr* 20(2):61-107, 1990.

Carney J, Gerring J: Return to school following severe closed head injury: a critical phase in pediatric rehabilitation, *Pediatrics* 17(4):222-229, 1990.

Duhaime AC and others: Head injury in very young children: mechanisms, injury types, and ophthalmologic findings in 100 hospitalized patients younger than 2 years of age, *Pediatrics* 90:179-185, 1992.

Gupta SK and others: Bilateral traumatic extradural hematomas, *Clin Neurol Neurosurg* 94(2):127-131, 1992.

Hall DE: Head injuries. In Hoekelman RA and others, editors: *Primary pediatric care,* ed 2, St Louis, 1992, Mosby.

Halper JS: Bicycle helmets for children, *J Emerg Nurs* 16(1):36-40, 1990.

Henry PC, Hauber RP, Rice M: Factors associated with closed head injury in a pediatric population, *J Neurosci Nurs* 24(6):311-316, 1992.

Humphreys RP: Complication of pediatric head injury, *Pediatr Neurosurg* 17(5):174-178, 1992.

Johnston MV, Gerring JP: Head trauma and its sequelae, *Pediatr Ann* 21(6):362-368, 1992.

Kumar R and others: Do children with severe head injury benefit from intensive care? *Childs Nerv Syst* 7:299, 1991.

Nelson VS: Pediatric head injury, *Phys Med Rehabil Clin North Am* 3(2):461-474, 1992.

Rosner MJ, Daughton S: CPP management in head injury, *J Trauma* 30:933-941, 1990.

Sherman DW: Managing acute head injury, *Nursing 90* 20(4):47-51, 1990.

Spaide RF and others: Shaken baby syndrome, *Am Fam Physician* 41(4):145-152, 1990.

Stein SC, Ross SF: The value of CT scan in patients with low risk head injures, *Neurosurgery* 26:638-640, 1990.

Tecklenburg FW, Wright MS: Minor head trauma in the pediatric patient, *Pediatr Emerg Care* 7(1):40-47, 1991.

Temkin NR, Dikmen SS, Winn HR: Management of head injury: posttraumatic seizures, *Neurosurg Clin North Am* 2(2):425-435, 1991.

Tepas JJ and others: Mortality and head injury: the pediatric perspective, *J Pediatr Surg* 25:92, 1990.

Testani-Dufour L, Chappel-Aiken L, Gueldner S: Traumatic brain injury: a family experience, *J Neurosci Nurs* 24(6):317-323, 1992.

Vernon-Levett P: Head injuries in children, *Crit Care Nurs North Am* 3(3):411-421, 1991.

Williams DH, Levin HS, Eisenberg HM: Mild head injury classification, *Neurosurgery* 27(3):422-428, 1990.

Near-Drowning

Beyda DH: Pathophysiology of near-drowning and treatment of the child with a submersion incident, *Crit Care Nurse Clin North Am* 3(2):273-280, 1991.

Beyda DH: Prehospital care of the child with a submersion incident, *Crit Care Nurs Clin North Am* 3(2):281-285, 1991.

Biggart MJ, Bohn DJ: Effect of hypothermia and cardiac arrest on outcome of near-drowning accidents in children, *J Pediatr* 117(2):179-183, 1990.

Coffman S: The psychologic cost of drowning and near drowning: clinical issues in nurisng intervention, *J Child Adolesc Psychiatr Ment Health Nurs* 3(3):106-107, 1990.

Fields AI: Near-drowning in the pediatric population, *Crit Care Clin* 8(1):113-129, 1992.

Leach SC: Continuing care for the near-drowning child, *Crit Care Nurs Clin North Am* 3(2):307-317, 1991.

Levin D and others: Drowning and near-drowning, *Pediatr Clin North Am* 40(2):321-336, 1993.

Luttrell PP: Care of the pediatric near drowning victim: a nursing challenge, *Crit Care Nurs Clin North Am* 3(2):293-306, 1991.

Modell JH: Drowning, *N Engl J Med* 328(4):253-256, 1993.

Shinaberger CS and others: Young children who drown in hot tubs, spas, and whirlpools in California: a 26 year survey, *Am J Public Health* 80:613-614, 1990.

Snelling LK, Young RSK: Drowning and near-drowning. In Hoekelman RA and others, editors: *Primary pediatric care,* ed 2, St Louis, 1992, Mosby.

Wintemute GJ: Drowning in early childhood, *Pediatr Ann* 21(7):417-421, 1992.

Yamamoto LG and others: A one-year series of pediatric ED water-related injuries: the Hawaii EMS-C project, *Pediatr Emerg Care* 8(3):129-133, 1992.

Young L: A 22-month-old victim of near drowning, *J Emerg Nurs* 18(3):197-198, 1992.

Intracranial Infections

Bahal N, Nahata MC: The role of corticosteroids in infants and children with bacterial meningitis, *Curr Issues Clin Pediatr* 25(5):542-545, 1991.

Bell WE: Bacterial meningitis in children, *Pediatr Clin North Am* 39(4):651-668, 1992.

Burns PK: The neuropathology of pediatric acquired immunodeficiency syndrome, *J Child Neurol* 7(4):332-346, 1992.

Casteel-VanDaele M: Reye syndrome or side-effects of anti-emetics? *Eur J Pediatr* 150(7):456-459, 1991.

Coderre C: Meningitis: danger when the diagnosis is viral, *RN* 52(8):50-54, 1989.

Compendium of Animal Rabies Control, 1993, *MMWR* 42(3), 1993.

Del Toro J: CNS infections in the PICU, *Semin Pediatr Infect Dis* 3(4):228-234, 1992.

Forsyth BW and others: Misdiagnosis of Reye's-like illness, *Am J Dis Child* 145:964-966, 1991.

Gauthier M and others: Reye's syndrome: a reappraisal of diagnosis in 49 presumptive cases, *Am J Dis Child* 143:1181-1185, 1989.

Human Rabies—California, *JAMA* 268(6):709-711, 1992.

Hurwitz E, Mortimer E: A catch in the Reye is awry, *Cleve Clin J Med* 57(4):318-320, 1990.

Kabani A, Jadavji T: Sequelae of acute bacterial meningitis in children, *Antibiot Chemother* 45:209-217, 1992.

Kennedy WA, Hoyt MJ, McCracken GH: The role of corticosteroid therapy in children with pneumococcal meningitis, *Am J Dis Child* 144(12):1374-1378, 1991.

Kimura S and others: Liver histopathology in clinical Reye syndrome, *Brain Dev* 13(2):95-100, 1991.

Krajewski R, Stebmasiak Z: Brain abscess in infants, *Childs Nerv Syst* 8(5):279-280, 1992.

Krywamio ML: Varicella encephalitis, *J Neurosci Nurs* 23(6):363-368, 1991.

Munz M and others: Otitis media and CNS complications, *J Otolaryngol* 21(3):224-226, 1992.

Palur R and others: Shunt surgery for hydrocephalus in tuberculous meningitis: a long-term follow-up study, *J Neurosurgery* 74(1):64-69, 1991.

Quagliarello V, Scheld WM: Meningitis in children, *N Engl J Med* 327:864-872, 1992.

Radetsky M: Results of delay in treatment of bacterial meningitis, *Pediatr Infect Dis J* 11:694-698, 1992.

Reyes syndrome surveillance—United States, 1989, *MMWR* 265(8):960, 1991.

Roos KL: Management of bacterial meningitis in children and adults, *Semin Neurol Sem Neurol* 12(3):155-164, 1992.

Smith AL: Bacterial meningitis, *Pediatr Rev* 14(1):11-18, 1993.

Smith RRR: Neuroradiology of intracranial infection, *Pediatr Neurosurg* 18(2):92-104, 1992.

Soumerai SB, Ross-Degnan D, Kahn JS: Effects of professional and media warnings about the association between aspirin use in children and Reye's syndrome, *Milbank Q* 70(1):115-182, 1992.

Taylor HG, Schatschneider C: Academic achievement following childhood brain disease, *J Learn Disabil* 25(10):630-638, 1992.

Taylor HG and others: Sequelae of *H. influenzae* meningitis in school-age children, *N Engl J Med* 323(24):1657-1663, 1990.

Wachtel R: Early detection of AIDS dementia in children, *Int Conf AIDS* 8(2):19-24, 1992.

Walsh-Kelly C and others: Meningeal signs in bacterial vs aseptic meningitis, *Ann Emerg Med* 21:910-914, 1992.

Wintergerst U, Belohradsky BH: Acyclovir monotherapy, *Infections* 20(4):207-212, 1992.

Epilepsy

Ashkenasi A, Snead OC III: Epileptic syndromes in children and their therapy, *Curr Opin Pediatr* 1:269-277, 1989.

Austin JK: Predicting parental anticonvulsant medication compliance, *J Pediatr Nurs* 4:88-95, 1989.

Austin JK, McDermott N: Parental attitude and coping behavior in families of children with epilepsy, *J Neurosci Nurs* 20:174-179, 1988.

Cerebral resection for intractable epilepsy: long-term effects, *Lancet* 340(8826):1008-1009, 1992.

Charuvanij A and others: ACTH treatment in intractable seizures of childhood, *Brain Dev* 14(2):102-106, 1992.

Dodson WE: Medical treatment and pharmacology of antiepileptic drugs, *Pediatr Clin North Am* 36:421-433, 1989.

Farley JA: Epilepsy. In Jackson PL, Vessey JA: *Primary care of the child with a chronic condition,* St Louis, 1992, Mosby.

Frank J, Fischer RG: Drug interactions with carbamazepine, *Pediatr Nurs* 13:54-55, 1987.

Holmes GL: Do seizures cause brain damage? *Epilepsia* 32(suppl 5):S14-S28, 1991.

Holmes GL: Effect of non-sex hormones on neuronal excitability, seizures, and the electroencephalogram, *Epilepsia* 32(suppl 6): S11-S18, 1991.

Livingston JH: The Lennox-Gastaut syndrome, *Dev Med Child Neurol* 30:536-549, 1988.

Maytal J and others: Low morbidity and mortality of status epilepticus in children, *Pediatrics* 83:323-331, 1989.

Meldrum BS: Anatomy, physiology, and pathology of epilepsy, *Lancet* 336:231-234, 1990.

National Institutes of Health Consensus Conference: Surgery for epilepsy, *JAMA* 264(6):729-733, 1990.

Peacock WJ: The role of hemispherectomy in the treatment of intractable seizures in childhood, *Int Pediatr* 7(4):291, 1992.

Pellock JM: Efficacy and adverse effects of antiepileptic drugs, *Pediatr Clin North Am* 36:435-448, 1989.

Pellock JM: Recent advances concerning status epilepticus, *Int Pediatr* 5(2):189-196, 1990.

Purves SJ and others: Results of anterior corpus callosum section in 24 patients with medically intractable seizures, *Neurology* 38(8):1194-1201, 1988.

Rothner AD: Not everything that shakes is epilepsy, *Cleve Clin J Med* 56(suppl, pt 2):S206-S213, 1989.

Santilli N, Dodson WE, Walton AV: *Students with seizures: a manual for school nurses,* Landover, MD, 1991, Epilepsy Foundation of America.

Scheuer ML, Pedley TA: The evaluation and treatment of seizures, *N Engl J Med* 323(21):1468-1474, 1990.

Shorvon SD: Epidemiology, classification, natural history, and genetics of epilepsy, *Lancet* 336:93-96, 1990.

Snead OC, Benton JQ, Myers GJ: ACTH and prednisone in childhood seizure disorders, *Neurology* 33:966-970, 1983.

Status epilepticus—the first hour is critical, *Emerg Med* 24(8):181-184, 1992.

Tharp BR: An overview of pediatric seizure disorders and epileptic syndromes, *Epilepsia* 28(suppl 1):S36-S45, 1987.

Tse AM: Seizures and societal attitudes: a teaching tool for children, siblings, classmates, parents, and classroom teachers, *Issues Compr Pediatr Nurs* 9:299-303, 1986.

Verity CM, Golding J: Risk of epilepsy after febrile convulsions: a national cohort study, *Br Med J* 303:1373-1376, 1991.

Vining EP: Educational, social, and life-long effects of epilepsy, *Pediatr Clin North Am* 36:449-461, 1989.

Febrile Seizures

Bethune P and others: The use of an educational slide tape program for parents in the emergency room management of the first febrile seizure, *Clin Invest Med* 13:105, 1990.

Cassano P, Koepsel T, Farwell J: Risk of febrile seizures in childhood in relation to prenatal maternal cigarette smoking and alcohol intake, *Am J Epidemiol* 132:462-473, 1990.

Engel NS: Phenobarbital for pediatric febrile seizures: risk-benefit update, *MCN* 15:257, 1990.

Freeman J: Just say no! Drugs and febrile seizures, *Pediatrics* 86(4):624, 1990.

Freeman JM, Vining EPG: Decision making and the child with febrile seizures, *Pediatr Rev* 13(8):298-304, 1992.

Maytal J, Shinner S: Febrile status epilepticus, *Pediatrics* 86(4):611-616, 1990.

Nelson K, Ellenberg J: Prenatal and perinatal antecedents of febrile seizures, *Ann Neurol* 27:127-131, 1990.

Valman HB: Febrile convulsions, *Br Med J* 306:1743-1745, June 1993.

Headaches and Migraines

DiMario FJ: Childhood headaches: a school nurse perspective, *Clin Pediatr* 31(5):279-282, 1992.

Dunn DW, Purvin VA: Headaches in adolescents, *Am Acad Pediatr Adolesc Health Update* 3(1):1, 1990.

Elser J: Easing the pain of childhood headache, *Contemp Pediatr* 8(11):108-123, 1991.

Engel J: Behavioral assessment of chronic headaches in children, *Issues Compr Pediatr Nurs* 14(4):267-276, 1991.

Gallagher RM: Headache diagnosis and treatment, *J Am Acad Nurse Pract* 3:3-10, 1991.

McGrath PJ and others: The efficacy and efficiency of a self-administered treatment for adolescent migraine, *Pain* 49(3):321-324, 1992.

Mortimer J and others: Epidemiology of childhood migraine, *Dev Med Child Neurol* 34:1095-1101, 1992.

Peroutka S: The pharmacology of current antimigraine drugs, *Headache* 30(1):5-11, 1990.

Shinner S: An approach to the child with headaches, *Int Pediatr* 6(2):140-148, 1991.

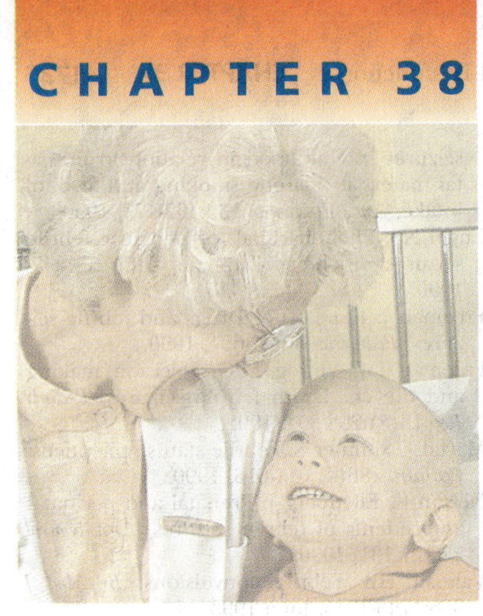

CHAPTER 38

The Child with Endocrine Dysfunction

CHAPTER OUTLINE

RELATED TOPICS

Abnormal sexual development, Ch. 11
Administration of medication, Ch. 27
Genetic evaluation and counseling, Ch. 5
Hypocalcemia, Ch. 9
Hypoglycemia, Ch. 9
Single-gene (monogenic) disorders, Ch. 5

THE ENDOCRINE SYSTEM

The endocrine system consists of three components: (1) the ***cell,*** which sends a chemical message by means of a hormone; (2) the ***target cells,*** or ***end organs,*** which receive the chemical message; and (3) the ***environment*** through which the chemical is transported (blood, lymph, extracellular fluids) from the site of synthesis to the sites of cellular action. The endocrine system controls or regulates metabolic processes governing energy production, growth, fluid and electrolyte balance, response to stress, and sexual reproduction.

The endocrine glands, which are distributed throughout the body, are listed in the box on p.1737, including several additional structures sometimes considered as endocrine glands, although they are not usually included.

■ Susan B. Zekauskas, RN, MSN, PNP, revised this chapter.

HORMONES

A hormone is a complex chemical substance produced and secreted into body fluids by a cell or group of cells that exerts a physiologic controlling effect on other cells. Some are ***local hormones*** creating their effect near the point of secretion. For example, acetylcholine, released at the parasympathetic and skeletal nerve endings, mediates the synaptic activity of the nervous system; secretin, a digestive hormone secreted by certain cells lining the duodenum, stimulates the pancreas to release a watery secretion; and the prostaglandins, or tissue hormones, secreted by a wide variety of organs (including the seminal vesicles, kidneys, lungs, iris, brain, and thymus), usually diffuse only a short distance to integrate activities of neighboring cells.

General hormones are produced in one organ or part of the body and are carried through the bloodstream to a distant part, or parts, of the body where they initiate or regu-

ENDOCRINE GLANDS

Pituitary gland (hypophysis cerebri)—A pea-sized gland that lies within a deep bony depression at the base of the cranium, the sella turcica, and is attached to the hypothalamus on the undersurface of the brain by a slender infundibulum or pituitary stalk

Thyroid gland—Two large lateral lobes and a connecting portion, the isthmus, situated on the anterior aspect of the neck just below the larynx

Parathyroid glands—Four or five (there may be more or less) small round bodies attached to the posterior surfaces of the lateral lobes of the thyroid gland

Adrenal glands—Pyramid-shaped glands situated atop the kidneys, fitting like caps over these organs

Ovaries—Glands located in the female pelvis on each side of the uterus at the fimbriated end of the fallopian tubes

Testes—Oval-shaped glands situated within the male scrotum

Islands of Langerhans—Small clusters of endocrine cells within the pancreas situated between the acinar or exocrine-secreting portions of the gland

STRUCTURES SOMETIMES CONSIDERED ENDOCRINE GLANDS

Pineal body (epiphysis cerebri)—A gland located in the cranial cavity behind the midbrain and third ventricle, the functions of which are largely speculative

Thymus—A gland situated behind the sternum and below the thyroid gland; plays an important role in immunity but only during fetal life and early childhood

Gastrointestinal glands—Mucosal lining of the gastrointestinal tract containing cells that produce hormones that play important roles in controlling and coordinating secretory and motor activities of digestion

Placenta—A body that secretes ovarian hormones and chorionic gonadotropin during gestation; only a temporary endocrine gland

late physiologic activity of an organ or group of cells. Some of these hormones (such as thyroid hormone and growth hormone) affect most cells of the body, whereas others (such as the tropic hormones) produce their effects on specific tissues, called ***target tissues.*** For example, the pituitary hormones stimulate the adrenal glands and the thyroid gland to secrete adrenocorticotropin and thyrotropic hormone, respectively.

Control of Hormone Secretion

Hormones are released by endocrine glands into the bloodstream, where they are carried to responsive tissues. These responsive, or target, tissues may be another endocrine gland, an organ, or tissue. Regulation of hormonal secretion is based on negative feedback. As a general rule, endocrine glands have a tendency to oversecrete their particular hormones. However, once the physiologic effect of the hormone has been achieved, this information is transmitted to the producing gland, either directly or indirectly, to inhibit further secretion. If the gland undersecretes, the inhibition is relieved, and the gland increases production of the hormone. As a result, the hormone is secreted according to the amount needed. This is the primary function of the tropic hormones.

The endocrine gland primarily responsible for stimulation and inhibition of target glandular secretions is the ***anterior pituitary,*** or "master gland." ***Tropic*** (which literally means "turning") hormones secreted by the anterior pituitary regulate the secretion of hormones from various target organs (Fig. 38-1). As blood concentrations of the target hormones reach normal levels, a negative message is sent to the anterior pituitary to inhibit release of the tropic hormone. For example, thyroid-stimulating hormone (TSH) responds to low levels of circulating thyroid hormone (TH). As blood levels of thyroid hormone reach normal concentrations, a negative feedback message is sent to the anterior pituitary, resulting in diminished release of thyroid-stimulating hormone.

The pituitary gland is, in turn, controlled by either hormonal or neuronal signals from the hypothalamus. Two types of substances are secreted from the hypothalamus: (1) ***releasing hormones*** and (2) ***inhibitory hormones,*** which are secreted within the hypothalamus and transported by way of the pituitary portal system to the anterior pituitary, where they stimulate the secretion of tropic hormones. An example of this is the secretion of corticotropin-releasing factor (CRF) by the hypothalamus, which stimulates the pituitary to secrete adrenocorticotropic hormone (ACTH). In this instance the anterior pituitary is the target of the hypothalamus and secondarily effects a response from another target gland, the adrenals. The adrenals in turn secrete glucocorticoids, which have multiple target sites throughout the body. Pituitary hormones that lack feedback control from the product of a target tissue (growth hormone, prolactin, and melanocyte-stimulating hormone) require hypothalamic inhibitors and stimulators for their control.

Not all hormones depend on other hormones for their release. For example, insulin is secreted in response to blood glucose concentrations. Other glandular hormones that are not under the control of the pituitary gland are glucagon, parathyroid hormone (PTH), antidiuretic hormone (ADH), and aldosterone.

NEUROENDOCRINE INTERRELATIONSHIPS

Homeostasis is maintained by two regulatory systems: the endocrine and the autonomic nervous systems (collectively known as the ***neuroendocrine system***). The ***autonomic nervous system*** consists of the sympathetic and parasympathetic systems that control nonvoluntary functions, specifically of smooth muscle, myocardium, and glands. The ***parasympathetic system,*** in particular, is primarily involved in regulating digestive processes, whereas the ***sympathetic system*** functions to maintain homeostasis during stress.

The higher autonomic centers, located in the hypothalamus and limbic system, help control the functioning of both autonomic systems. Both sympathetic and parasympathetic nerve fibers secrete ***neurotransmitting substances***—acetylcholine, released by cholinergic fibers, and norepinephrine, released by adrenergic fibers. Release of norepinephrine into the plasma produces the same effects as secretion of this substance by the adrenal medulla. Thus the interrelatedness between the two systems is demonstrated.

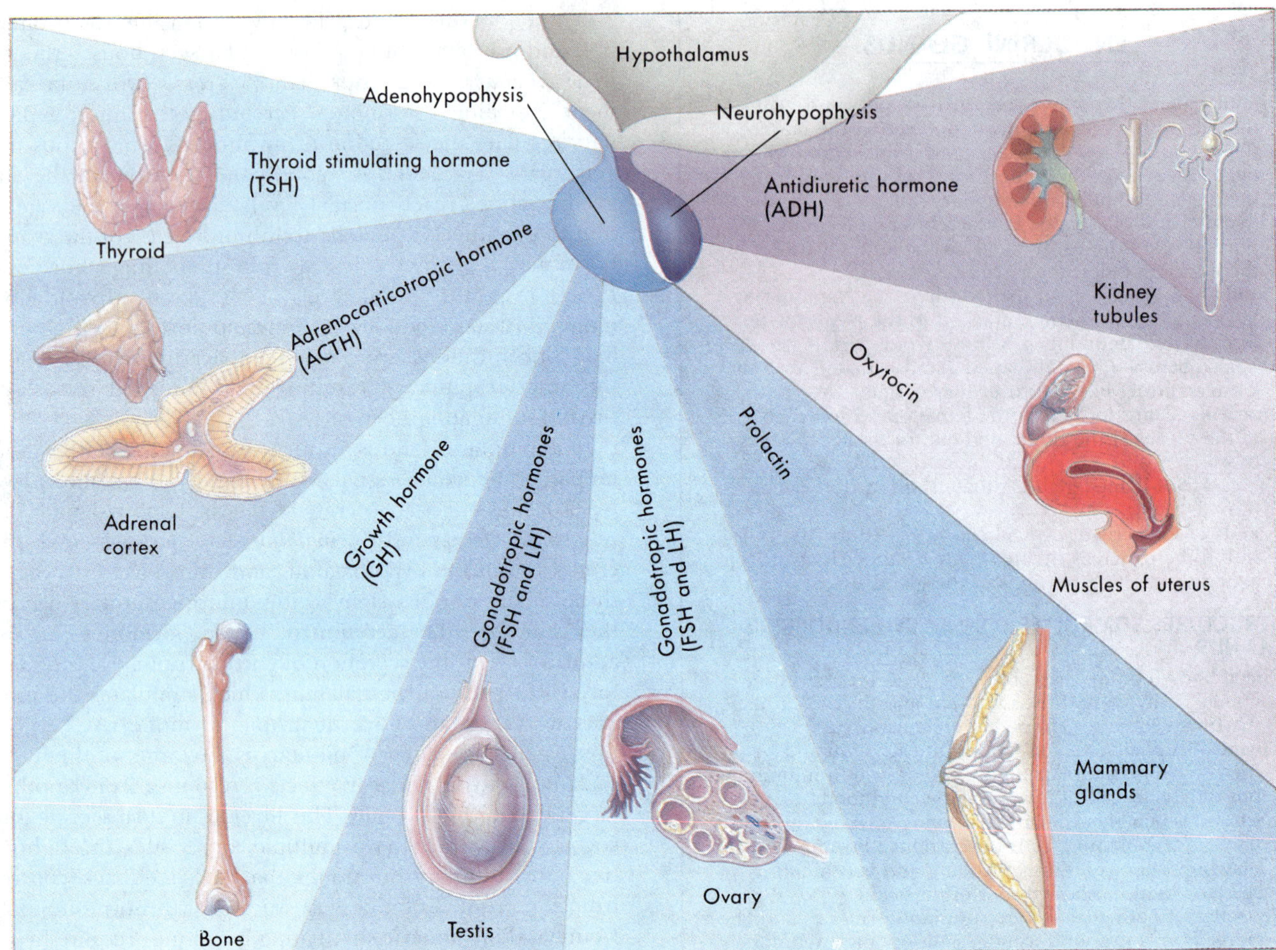

FIG. 38-1 Pituitary hormones: some of the major hormones of the adenohypophysis and neurohypophysis and their principal target organs. (From Thibodeau GA, Patton KT: Anatomy and physiology, ed 2, St Louis, 1993, Mosby.)

The neuroendocrine system acts by synthesizing and releasing various chemical substances that regulate body functions. Information is carried by means of neural impulses in the autonomic system and by the blood in the endocrine system. In general, neural responses are more rapid and localized; endocrine responses are more lasting and widespread. The two systems function synergistically because neural impulses transmitted to the central nervous system stimulate the hypothalamus to manufacture and release several ***releasing*** or ***inhibiting factors.***

Because of the interdependent relationship of these glands, a malfunction in one gland produces effects elsewhere. Endocrine dysfunction may result because of an intrinsic defect in the target gland (primary) or because of a diminished or elevated level of tropic hormones (secondary). Endocrine problems occur from hypofunction or hyperfunction of the glands. Primary hypofunction is usually associated with a more profound deficiency of the target gland hormone because little or no hormone is secreted. In secondary dysfunction the target glands secrete some of their hormones but in smaller amounts and less rapidly.

Hyperfunction or hypofunction may also be the result of an increase or a decrease in secretion of the tropic hormones (primary) with a consequent increase in the target gland hormones (secondary) or a hypersecretion or hyposecretion of the target glands. A summary of the endocrine glands, their functions, and the primary effects of oversecretion or undersecretion is given in Table 38-1.

DISORDERS OF PITUITARY FUNCTION

Deficiencies of the anterior pituitary hormones may be the result of organic defects or of idiopathic etiology and may occur as a single hormonal problem or in combination with other hormonal deficiencies. The clinical manifestations depend on the hormones involved and the age of onset. If the tropic hormones are involved, the resulting disorder reflects the altered stimulus to the target gland. For example, if thyroid-stimulating hormone is deficient, thyroid hormone is also deficient, and the child displays the manifestations of hypothyroidism.

An overproduction of the anterior pituitary hormones can result in gigantism (caused by excess growth hormone production during childhood), hyperthyroidism, hypercortisolism (Cushing syndrome), and precocious puberty from excessive gonadotropins. Overproduction is thought to be caused by hyperplasia of the pituitary cells—which may

TABLE 38-1 Summary of the Endocrine System

GLAND/HORMONE	EFFECT	HYPOFUNCTION	HYPERFUNCTION
ADENOHYPOPHYSIS (ANTERIOR PITUITARY)*			
Somatotropic hormone (STH) or growth hormone (GH) (somatotropin) Target tissue: bones	Promotes growth of bone and soft tissues Has main effect on linear growth Maintains a normal rate of protein synthesis Conserves carbohydrate utilization and promotes fat mobilization Is essential for proliferation of cartilage cells at epiphyseal plate Is ineffective for linear growth after epiphyseal closure Has hyperglycemic effect (anti-insulin action)	Epiphyseal fusion with cessation of growth Prepubertal dwarfism Pituitary cachexia (Simonds disease) Generalized growth retardation Hypoglycemia	Prepubertal gigantism Acromegaly (after full growth is attained) Diabetes mellitus Postpubertal hypoproteinemia
Thyrotropin (thyroid-stimulating hormone [TSH]) Target tissue: thyroid gland	Promotes and maintains growth and development of thyroid gland Stimulates thyroid hormone secretion	Hypothyroidism Marked delay of puberty Juvenile myxedema	Hyperthyroidism Thyrotoxicosis Graves disease
Adrenocorticotropic hormone (ACTH) Target tissue: adrenal cortex	Promotes and maintains growth and development of adrenal cortex Stimulates adrenal cortex to secrete glucocorticoids and androgens	Acute adrenocortical insufficiency (Addison disease) Hypoglycemia Increased skin pigmentation	Cushing syndrome
Gonadotropins Target tissue: gonads	Stimulate gonads to mature and produce sex hormones and germ cells	Absent or incomplete spontaneous puberty	Precocious puberty Early epiphyseal closure
Follicle-stimulating hormone (FSH) Target tissue: ovaries, testes	Male: Stimulates development of seminiferous tubules Initiates spermatogenesis Female: Stimulates graafian follicles to mature and secrete estrogen	Hypogonadism Sterility Absence or loss of secondary sex characteristics Amenorrhea	Precocious puberty Primary gonadal failure Hirsutism Polycystic ovary Early epiphyseal closure
Luteinizing hormone (LH)† Target tissue: ovaries, testes	Male: Stimulates differentiation of Leydig cells, which secrete androgens, principally testosterone Female: Produces rupture of follicle with discharge of mature ova Stimulates secretion of progesterone by corpus luteum	Hypogonadism Sterility Impotence Absence or loss of secondary sex characteristics Ovarian failure Eunuchism	Precocious puberty Primary gonadal failure Hirsutism Polycystic ovary Early epiphyseal closure
Prolactin (luteotropic hormone) Target tissue: ovaries, breasts	Stimulates milk secretion Maintains corpus luteum and progesterone secretion during pregnancy	Inability to lactate Amenorrhea	Galactorrhea Functional hypogonadism
Melanocyte-stimulating hormone (MSH) Target tissue: skin	Promotes pigmentation of skin	Diminished or absent skin pigmentation	Increased skin pigmentation
NEUROHYPOPHYSIS (POSTERIOR PITUITARY)			
Antidiuretic hormone (ADH) (vasopressin) Target tissue: renal tubules	Acts on distal and collecting tubules, making them more permeable to water, thus increasing reabsorption and decreasing excretion of urine	Diabetes insipidus	Syndrome of inappropriate secretion of ADH Fluid retention Hyponatremia

*For each anterior pituitary hormone there is a corresponding hypothalamic-releasing factor. A deficiency in these factors caused by inhibiting anterior pituitary hormone synthesis produces the same effects (see text for more detailed information).
†In the male, LH is sometimes known as interstitial cell–stimulating hormone (ICSH).

Continued.

TABLE 38-1 Summary of the Endocrine System—cont'd

GLAND/HORMONE	EFFECT	HYPOFUNCTION	HYPERFUNCTION
NEUROHYPOPHYSIS (POSTERIOR PITUITARY)—cont'd			
Oxytocin Target tissue: uterus, breasts	Stimulates powerful contractions of uterus Causes ejection of milk from alveoli into breast ducts (letdown reflex)		
THYROID			
Thyroxine (T_4) and triiodothyronine (T_3)	Regulates metabolic rate; controls rate of growth of body cells Especially important for growth of bones, teeth, and brain Promotes mobilization of fats and gluconeogenesis	Hypothyroidism Myxedema Hashimoto thyroiditis General growth is greatly reduced; extent depends on age at which deficiency occurs Mental retardation in infant	Exophthalmic goiter (Graves disease) Accelerated linear growth Early epiphyseal closure
Thyrocalcitonin	Regulates calcium and phosphorus metabolism Influences ossification and development of bone		
PARATHYROID GLANDS			
Parathyroid hormone (PTH)	Promotes calcium reabsorption from blood, bone, and intestines Promotes excretion of phosphorus in kidney tubules	Hypocalcemia (tetany)	Hypercalcemia (bone demineralization) Hypophosphatemia
ADRENAL CORTEX			
Mineralocorticoids Aldosterone	Stimulate renal tubules to reabsorb sodium, thus promoting water retention but potassium loss	Adrenocortical insufficiency	Electrolyte imbalance Hyperaldosteronism
Sex hormones (androgens, estrogens, progesterone)	Influence development of bone, reproductive organs, and secondary sexual characteristics	Male feminization	Adrenogenital syndrome
Glucocorticoids Cortisol (hydrocortisone and compound F) Corticosterone (compound B)	Promote normal fat, protein, and carbohydrate metabolism In excess, tend to accelerate gluconeogenesis and protein and fat catabolism Mobilize body defenses during period of stress Suppress inflammatory reaction	Addison disease Acute adrenocortical insufficiency Impaired growth and sexual function	Cushing syndrome Severe impairment of growth with slowing in skeletal maturation
ADRENAL MEDULLA			
Epinephrine (adrenaline), norepinephrine (noradrenaline)	Produces vasoconstriction of heart and smooth muscles (raises blood pressure) Increases blood sugar via glycolysis Inhibits gastrointestinal activity Activates sweat glands		Hyperfunction caused by: Pheochromocytoma Neuroblastoma Ganglioneuroma
ISLETS OF LANGERHANS OF PANCREAS			
Insulin (β-cells)	Promotes glucose transport into the cells Increases glucose utilization, glycogenesis, and glycolysis Promotes fatty acid transport into cells and lipogenesis Promotes amino acid transport into cells and protein synthesis	Diabetes mellitus	Hyperinsulinism

TABLE 38-1 Summary of the Endocrine System—cont'd

GLAND/HORMONE	EFFECT	HYPOFUNCTION	HYPERFUNCTION
Glucagon (α-cells)	Acts as antagonist to insulin, thereby increasing blood glucose concentration by accelerating glycogenolysis Able to inhibit secretion of both insulin and glycogen		Hyperglycemia May be instrumental in genesis of DKA in diabetes mellitus
Somatostatin (δ-cells)	Able to inhibit secretion of both insulin and glycogen		
OVARIES			
Estrogen	Accelerates growth of epithelial cells, especially in uterus following menses Promotes protein anabolism Promotes epiphyseal closure of bones Promotes breast development during puberty and pregnancy Plays role in sexual function Stimulates water and sodium reabsorption in renal tubules Stimulates ripening of ova	Lack of or repression of sexual development	Precocious puberty, early epiphyseal closure
Progesterone	Prepares uterus for nidation of fertilized ovum and aids in maintenance of pregnancy Aids in development of alveolar system of breasts during pregnancy Inhibits myometrial contractions Has effect on protein catabolism Promotes salt and water retention, especially in endometrium		
TESTES			
Testosterone	Accelerates protein anabolism for growth Promotes epiphyseal closure Promotes development of secondary sex characteristics Plays role in sexual function Stimulates testes to produce spermatozoa	Delayed sexual development or eunuchoidism	Precocious puberty, early epiphyseal closure

eventually progress to a tumor (adenoma)—or a primary hypothalamic defect that results in excess of the hormone's respective releasing factor. Although the initial clinical manifestations are a result of pituitary hypersecretion, eventually pituitary insufficiency occurs, and the signs of panhypopituitarism become evident.

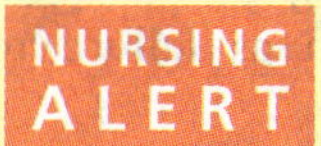

Children with panhypopituitarism should be encouraged to wear medical identification, such as a bracelet.

HYPOPITUITARISM

Hypopituitarism is diminished or deficient secretion of pituitary hormones. The consequences of the condition depend on the degree of dysfunction and lead to gonadotropin deficiency with absence or regression of secondary sex characteristics; somatotropin deficiency, in which children display retarded somatic growth; thyrotropin deficiency that produces hypothyroidism; and corticotropin deficiency, which results in manifestations of adrenal hypofunction. Hypopituitarism can result from any of the conditions listed in the box at left on p. 1742.

The most common organic cause of pituitary hyposecretion is tumors in the pituitary or hypothalamic region, especially the craniopharyngiomas. These tumors usually invade the anterior and posterior pituitary lobes and the hypothalamus, causing panhypopituitarism, a generalized disorder involving multiple systems (see box at right on p. 1742). The child may evidence growth retardation for quite

ETIOLOGY OF HYPOPITUITARISM

Aplasia or hypoplasia
- Developmental defects
- Idiopathic—sporadic; genetic

Destructive lesions
- Trauma—perinatal; child abuse; basal skull fracture
- Infiltrative lesions—tumors; tuberculosis; toxoplasmosis; hemochromatosis; sarcoidosis

Irradiation—CNS; eye; middle ear

Autoimmune hypophysitis

Surgery—removal of pharyngeal pituitary; ablation of craniopharyngioma or other tumor
- Vascular—aneurysm; infarct

Functional deficiency
- Psychosocial dwarfism
- Anorexia nervosa

some time before developing any symptoms or signs of increased intracranial pressure, local compression, or the destructive effects of the tumor. Other causes of panhypopituitarism sometimes include encephalitis, head trauma (rarely), and congenital hypoplasia of the hypothalamic area.

Idiopathic hypopituitarism is usually related to ***growth hormone (GH) deficiency,*** which inhibits somatic growth in all cells of the body. Although children with hypopituitarism are normal at birth, they show growth patterns that progressively deviate from the normal growth rate, often beginning in infancy. The chief complaint in most instances is short stature. Of those who seek help, boys outnumber girls three to one. The extent of idiopathic GH deficiency may be complete or partial, but the cause is unknown. It is frequently associated with other pituitary hormone deficiencies, such as deficiencies of TSH and ACTH; thus it is theorized that the disorder is probably secondary to hypothalamic deficiency. It has also been observed that there is a higher than average frequency in some families, which indicates a possible genetic etiology in a number of instances.

Intensive physical activity (greater than 18 hours per week) that begins before puberty may also stunt growth so that full adult height is not reached. This observation among adolescent female gymnasts suggests defective production of GH or other factors during puberty (Theintz and others, 1993).

Not all children with short stature have GH deficiency. In most instances the cause of short stature is either familial short stature or a simple constitutional growth delay. ***Familial short stature*** refers to otherwise healthy children who have ancestors with adult height in the lower percentiles, and whose height during childhood is appropriate for genetic background.

Constitutional growth delay refers to individuals (usually boys) with delayed linear growth and skeletal and sexual maturation that is behind that of age-mates. Typically, these children will reach normal adult height. Often there is a history of a similar pattern of growth in one of the parents or other family members of children with constitutional growth delay. The untreated child will proceed through normal changes as expected on the basis of bone age. These changes, although occurring later than in the average child, will appear in normal sequence and manner, and treatment with GH is not usually indicated. However, its use has become a controversial issue, especially in relation to parental and child requests for treatment to accelerate growth.

EFFECTS OF PANHYPOPITUITARISM

GROWTH HORMONE (GH)
Short stature but proportional height and weight
Delayed epiphyseal closure
Retarded bone age proportional to height
Premature aging
Increased insulin sensitivity

THYROID-STIMULATING HORMONE (TSH)
Short stature with infantile proportions
Dry, coarse skin, yellow discoloration, pallor
Cold intolerance
Constipation
Somnolence
Bradycardia
Dyspnea on exertion
Delayed dentition, loss of teeth

GONADOTROPINS
Absence of sexual maturation or loss of secondary sex characteristics
Atrophy of genitalia, prostate gland, breasts
Amenorrhea without menopausal symptoms
Decreased spermatogenesis

ADRENOCORTICOTROPIC HORMONE (ACTH)
Severe anorexia, weight loss
Hypoglycemia
Hypotension
Hyponatremia, hyperkalemia
Adrenal apoplexy, especially in response to stress
Circulatory collapse

ANTIDIURETIC HORMONE (ADH)
Polyuria
Polydipsia
Dehydration

MELANOCYTE-STIMULATING HORMONE (MSH)
Decreased pigmentation

Clinical Manifestations

The usual presenting complaint with dwarfism is short stature. These children generally grow normally during the first year and then follow a slowed growth curve that is below the third percentile. In children with a partial GH deficiency, the growth retardation is less marked than in children with complete GH deficiency. Height may be retarded more than weight because, with good nutrition, these children can become overweight or even obese. Their well-nourished appearance is an important diagnostic clue to differentiation from other disorders such as failure to thrive.

Skeletal proportions are normal for the age, but these children appear younger than their chronologic age (Fig. 38-2). However, later in life premature aging is common. The appearance of fine wrinkles about the eyes and mouth gives these children a peculiar impression of immaturity combined with presenility. They are no less active than

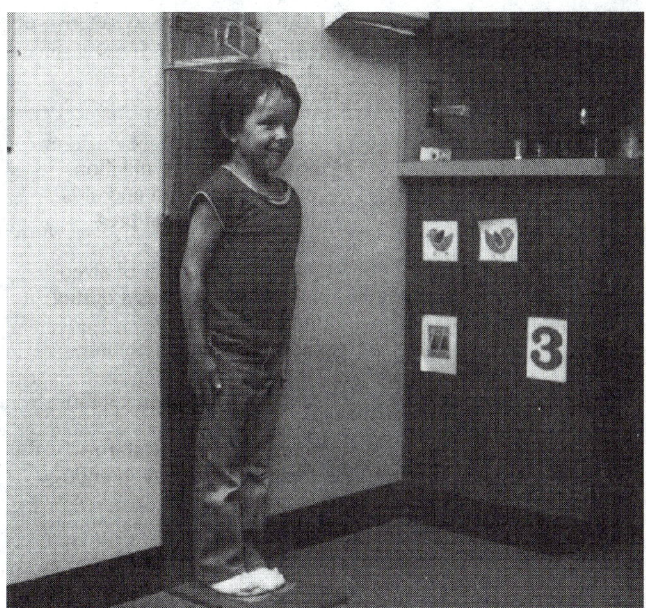

FIG. 38-2 Ten-year-old child with growth hormone deficiency. Height is 42.5 inches.

other children if directed to size-appropriate sports such as swimming, wrestling, gymnastics, soccer, or ballet. Bone age is nearly always retarded but is closely related to height age—the degree of retardation depends on the duration and extent of the hormonal deficiency. Children with diminished function of recent onset may show little retardation in skeletal age, whereas children with a long-standing deficiency may evidence a skeletal age only 40% to 50% of their chronologic age. It is difficult to predict their eventual height. Because the period of growth is prolonged past adolescence into the third or fourth decade, many of them reach a permanent height of 4 to 5 feet.

Usually, primary teeth appear at the expected age, but the eruption of the permanent teeth is delayed. Because of the underdeveloped jaw, the teeth are overcrowded and malpositioned. Sexual development is usually delayed but is otherwise normal. Even without GH replacement, dwarf adults are able to reproduce normal offspring. However, if the gonadotropins are deficient, sexual maturation is absent.

Most of these children have normal intelligence. In fact, during early childhood they often appear precocious in their learning because their ability seems to exceed their small size. However, emotional problems are not uncommon, especially as they near puberty, when their smallness becomes increasingly apparent compared with their peers. Anecdotal evidence indicates that the older, short child has poorer-quality social interactions because of teasing and ridicule about his or her size. Height discrepancy has been significantly correlated with emotional adjustment problems and may be a valuable predictor of the extent to which GH-delayed children will experience difficulty with anxiety, social skills, and positive self-esteem (Allen and others, 1993). Also, academic problems are not uncommon. A history will often reveal repeated classes or enrollment in classes for children with learning disabilities. These children are usually not pushed to perform at their chronologic age but at their height age.

Diagnostic Evaluation

Only a small number of children with delayed growth or short stature have hypopituitary dwarfism. In the majority of instances the cause is constitutional delay. Diagnostic evaluation is aimed at isolating organic causes, which, in addition to GH deficiency, may include hypothyroidism, hypersecretion of cortisol, gonadal aplasia, chronic illness, or nutritional inadequacy, as well as Russell Silver dwarfism or hypochondroplasia.

A complete diagnostic evaluation should include a family history, a history of the child's growth patterns and previous health status, physical examination, psychosocial evaluation, radiographic surveys, and endocrine studies.

Family History. A family history is of utmost importance in relating short stature to genetic background. The mid–parental height is an important prognosticator of the child's ultimate adult height. Normal adult height should fall within ±2 inches of mid–parental height (MacGillvray, 1993). Children with constitutional delays frequently are the products of parents who experienced similar slow growth patterns and delayed sexual maturation. A small percentage of those with hypopituitarism demonstrate an autosomal-recessive inheritance pattern. Height and weight of siblings should be compared with the child's growth patterns at comparable age periods.

Child's History. The child's history should include a thorough prenatal history to rule out maternal disorders that may have influenced growth, such as malnutrition. Birth height and weight should be compared with gestational age. Children with hypopituitarism are usually of normal size and gestational age at birth.

The child's past health history is investigated for evidence of chronic illness that may have influenced growth patterns, although a chronic illness, such as congenital heart disease, malabsorptive disorders, severe anemia, or neurologic impairments, usually has been identified long before the growth problem becomes a concern. Signs and symptoms suggesting a tumor, such as visual disturbances, headache, and signs of increasing intracranial pressure, are important. Such symptoms often precede retarded growth but may not have been regarded as significant. With lesions involving the hypothalamus, the history may also reveal characteristic manifestations of dysfunction such as somnolence, thermodysregulation, epilepsy, and hyperphagia, resulting in obesity. Since a craniopharyngioma can affect the secretion of any of the pituitary hormones, assessment for hypothyroidism, hypoadrenalism, and hypoaldosteronism should also be included.

Whenever possible, the child's growth patterns since birth should be evaluated, especially growth velocity, as compared with standard measurements. The age of onset of short stature provides a significant diagnostic clue. When the clinician evaluates the results of plotting height and weight, upward or downward shifts of 2 percentiles or more in children older than 3 years may indicate a growth abnormality (MacGillvray, 1993). Progressive retardation in height and weight since early childhood suggests idiopathic hypopituitary dwarfism, whereas a recent change from normal growth is more characteristic of a tumor. In addition, these children are usually well nourished, ruling out other causes of growth failure.

Physical Examination. Accurate measurement of height (using a calibrated stadiometer) and weight and comparison with standard growth charts are essential. Other measurements may include crown-to-pubis and pubis-to-heel length to compare body proportions, and sexual development should be assessed and compared with age-appropriate development. Observation of general appearance yields valuable clues, especially signs of premature aging and infantile facial features. A funduscopic examination and testing for visual acuity should be performed to detect evidence of ocular damage from a tumor.

Radiographic Surveys. A skeletal survey in children less than 3 years of age and radiographic examination of the hand/wrist for centers of ossification in older children are important in evaluating growth. Epiphyseal maturation is retarded in hypopituitarism but consistent with retardation in height. This is in contrast to hypothyroidism, in which bone maturation is greatly retarded, or gonadal dysplasia, such as Turner syndrome, in which bone age is near normal. Radiographic studies should also include a skull series, which helps in identifying abnormalities such as an abnormally small sella turcica or evidence of a space-occupying lesion such as craniopharyngioma. Computed tomography, radionuclear scans, or carotid angiograms may be needed to establish diagnosis and localization of lesions.

Endocrine Studies. Definitive diagnosis is based on absent or subnormal reserves of pituitary GH. Since GH levels are normally so low in children that differentiation from abnormal concentrations is unreliable, GH secretion should be stimulated followed by measurement of blood levels. Exercise is a natural and benign stimulus for GH release, and elevated levels can be detected after 20 minutes of strenuous exercise in normal children. Also, GH levels are elevated 45 to 90 minutes following the onset of sleep.

Children with short stature produce significantly lower overnight urinary GH concentrations than normal children. A significant correlation has been shown between overnight urinary GH excretion with peak serum response to provocation testing with either clonidine or insulin. Overnight urinary collection is a low-cost, noninvasive screening test and has none of the potential complications of pharmacologic testing (Owen, 1992).

If physiologic methods are inconclusive, GH release can be stimulated pharmacologically, which is a method used to identify children who do not respond to treatment with GH. The diagnosis of classic GH deficiency, with or without an organic lesion of the hypothalamus or pituitary, rests on demonstration of absent or low levels of GH in response to stimulation. GH appears to be secreted episodically, because plasma levels are often below the level of detectability on assay.

Major plasma concentration fluctuates over a wide range, with major secretory pulses occurring during early nocturnal slow-wave sleep. A variety of provocative tests have been used that rapidly increase the level of growth hormone in normal children. These include a 20-minute period of strenuous exercise or administration of L-dopa, insulin, arginine, clonidine, or glucagon. Two or more agents are used to decrease the incidence of false-negative responses. Peak levels of GH below 7 ng/ml strongly suggest GH deficiency (DiGeorge, 1992).

Since retarded growth may be caused by other endocrine disorders (such as hypothyroidism or gonadotropic deficiency), Turner syndrome, or emotional deprivation or may be associated with other forms of delayed growth (such as tissue unresponsiveness to GH or primordial dwarfism), tests for these conditions are often performed.

Therapeutic Management

Treatment of GH deficiency caused by organic lesions is directed toward correction of the underlying disease process (e.g., surgical removal or irradiation of a tumor). The definitive treatment of GH deficiency is replacement of GH and is successful in 80% of affected children. For more than 20 years cadaver-derived human growth hormone (HGH) was used successfully to enhance linear growth in short children. In 1985 the Food and Drug Administration (FDA) stopped use of the hormone in response to reported deaths due to Creutzfeldt-Jakob disease agent (CJD) in three former HGH recipients. To date, a total of nine patients have been identified who both received and became infected with CJD agent. Circumstances make it likely that HGH contaminated with a slow-growing, viral-like particle may have been responsible for these fatalities. Donation of organs or tissues from HGH recipients for transplantation should be prohibited because of the inability to test for infection with CJD (a rare neurogenerative condition). Blood banks do not accept donation from former HGH recipients. It is important that health care providers responsible for the care of individuals treated with HGH be aware of this fatal illness and remain informed of new developments in this field (Zekauskas and others, 1990). Biosynthetic GH prepared by recombinant DNA technology (and without the risk of CJD) is now available and is the therapy of choice.

The daily administration of GH to short, prepubertal children has resulted in a growth velocity of 8.7 ± 1.5 cm per year. Many children who respond to therapy have maintained this accelerated rate until achievement of height that is more appropriate to family height. None has exceeded target heights, indicating that the dosage of GH is not sufficient to override genetic predisposition (Moore and others, 1992). For children to achieve their genetic growth potential, early diagnosis of and intervention for growth disorders is essential (MacGillvray 1993).

The decision to stop GH therapy is made jointly by the child, family, and health care team. Radiologic evidence of epiphyseal closure is a criterion for ending therapy. Dosage is increased as the time of epiphyseal closure nears in order to gain the best advantage of the GH. Children with other hormone deficiencies require replacement therapy to correct the specific disorders. This may involve administration of thyroid extract, cortisone, testosterone, or estrogens and progesterone. The sex hormones are usually begun during adolescence to promote normal sexual maturation.

Nursing Considerations

The principal nursing consideration is identifying children with growth problems. Despite the fact that the majority of growth problems are not a result of organic causes, any delay in normal growth and sexual development poses special emotional adjustments for these children.

The nurse may be a key person in helping to establish a diagnosis. For example, if serial height and weight records are not available, the nurse can question parents about the child's growth in comparison with that of siblings, peers, or relatives. Investigating clothing sizes is often helpful in determining growth at different ages. Parents of these children frequently comment that the child wore out clothes before growing out of them or that, if the clothing fit the body, it often was too long in the sleeves or legs.

Because the behavioral or physical changes that suggest a tumor are insidious, they are frequently overlooked. It is important to correlate the onset of any positive findings with the initial evidence of growth retardation. For example, visual problems and headache are not uncommon in school-age children and can coincidentally occur after a growth problem is recognized. In fact, headache may represent the emotional trauma caused by short stature rather than be a symptom of a tumor. This line of questioning should be pursued cautiously to avoid alarming parents unduly about the possibility of a brain tumor.

Part of a nurse's role in helping establish a diagnosis is assisting with diagnostic tests. Preparation of child and family is especially important if a number of tests are being performed, and the child will require particular attention during provocative testing. Blood samples are usually taken every 30 minutes for a 3-hour period. Children also have difficulty overcoming hypoglycemia generated by tests with insulin, so they must be observed carefully for signs of hypoglycemia, whereas those receiving glucagon are at risk of nausea and vomiting. Thin children under 5 years of age are at particular risk, especially those with low fasting-glucose levels (DiGeorge, 1992).

Child and Family Support. Once a diagnosis is made confirming an organic cause of the problem, the parents and child need an opportunity to express their thoughts and feelings. Not infrequently, a growth problem that was present since birth is missed until adolescence, at which time the child's difference in body development becomes dramatically evident when compared with peers. Family members may feel anger and resentment toward members of the health staff for not detecting the problem sooner. Parents may experience guilt for not seeking medical attention earlier, especially if the child had been miserable from experiencing ridicule and criticism from associates. Each family member needs a sympathetic listener who is aware of his or her needs and realizes the importance of remaining objective and not defensive or overly apologetic. Appropriate emotional support from the nurse can include an affirmation of each person's justified feelings, such as anger or guilt, and emphasis on the treatment plan and prospects for improvement in the future.

Children undergoing hormone replacement require additional support. Therapy for GH deficiency requires daily subcutaneous injections. Nursing functions include family education concerning medication preparation and storage, injection sites, injection technique, and syringe disposal (see Chapter 27). Administration of GH is facilitated by family routines that include a specific time of day for the injection. Younger children may enjoy using a calendar and colorful stickers to designate received injections.

NURSING ALERT Optimum dosing is often achieved when GH is administered at bedtime. Physiologic release is more normally simulated as a result of pituitary release of GH during the first 45 to 90 minutes after the onset of sleep.

Even when hormone replacement is successful, these children attain their eventual adult height at a slower rate than their peers; therefore they need assistance in setting realistic expectations regarding improvement. For example, increases in height of 3 to 5 inches are common during the first year of therapy, but increases are less dramatic during subsequent years. Both sexes need guidance toward appropriate vocational goals. For example, children with aspirations for athletic sports such as basketball would be better advised to explore other activities not so dependent on excessive height.

Since these children appear younger than their chronologic age, others frequently relate to them in infantile or childish ways. This behavior, referred to as ***juvenilization,*** may play a role in the behavior patterns of children with GH deficiency (Stabler, 1993). Children having school problems will need special counseling. Parents and teachers benefit from guidance directed toward setting realistic expectations for the child based on age and abilities. For example, in the home such children should have the same age-appropriate responsibilities as their siblings. As they approach adolescence, they should be encouraged to participate in group activities with their peers. They should wear styles that accentuate their actual age, not their size. If abilities and strengths are emphasized rather than physical size, such children are more likely to develop a positive self-image. Some research findings indicate that adults who were GH deficient as children are more likely to be depressed, anxious, dissatisfied with their stature and body image, unmarried, and afflicted with multiple health problems (Stabler, 1993).

Professionals and families may find education and support from the **Human Growth Foundation.*** The treatment is expensive—up to $20,000 to $30,000 per year, depending on dosage. Usually the cost is partially covered by insurance if the child has a *documented* deficiency. Children with panhypopituitarism should be advised to wear medical identification at all times.

PITUITARY HYPERFUNCTION

Excess growth hormone before closure of the epiphyseal shafts results in proportional overgrowth of the long bones, until the individual reaches a height of 8 feet or more. Vertical growth is accompanied by rapid and increased development of muscles and viscera. Weight is increased but is

*7777 Leesburg Pike, Falls Church, VA 22043 (800) 451-6434.

usually in proportion to height. Proportional enlargement of head circumference also occurs and may result in delayed closure of the fontanels in young children. Children with a pituitary-secreting tumor may also demonstrate signs of increasing intracranial pressure, especially headache.

If hypersecretion of GH occurs after epiphyseal closure, growth is in the transverse direction, producing a condition known as ***acromegaly.*** Typical facial features include overgrowth of the head, lips, nose, tongue, jaw, and paranasal and mastoid sinuses; separation and malocclusion of the teeth in the enlarged jaw; disproportion of the face to the cerebral division of the skull; increased facial hair; thickened, deeply creased skin; and increased tendency toward hyperglycemia and diabetes mellitus.

Diagnostic Evaluation

Diagnosis is based on a history of excessive growth during childhood and evidence of increased levels of GH. Radiographic studies may reveal a tumor in an enlarged sella turcica, normal bone age, enlargement of bones (such as the paranasal sinuses), and evidence of joint changes. Endocrine studies to confirm excess of other hormones, specifically thyroid, cortisol, and sex hormones, should also be included in the differential diagnosis.

Therapeutic Management

If a lesion is present, surgical treatment by cryosurgery or hypophysectomy is performed to remove the tumor when feasible. Other therapies aimed at destroying pituitary tissue include external irradiation and radioactive implants. Depending on the extent of surgical extirpation and degree of pituitary insufficiency, hormone replacement with thyroid extract, cortisone, and sex hormones may be necessary.

Nursing Considerations

The primary nursing consideration is early identification of children with excessive growth rates. Although medical management is unable to reduce growth already attained, further growth can be retarded, and the earlier the treatment, the more control there is in predetermining a normal adult height. Nurses in ambulatory settings who are frequently involved in growth screening should refer children who demonstrate excessive linear growth for a medical evaluation. They should also observe for signs of a tumor, especially headache, and evidence of concurrent hormonal excesses, particularly the gonadotropins, which cause sexual precocity.

Children with excessive growth rates require as much emotional support as those with short stature. However, girls may suffer from the effects of excessive height much more than boys. In fact, males may find the tallness an asset when pursuing sports such as basketball. Children and their parents need an opportunity to express their thoughts. A compassionate nurse can be very supportive to these children, especially before adolescence when they are larger than their peers. The nurse can emphasize to a tall girl that as boys grow older they become taller and that she will not always be looking down at them. Since early adolescence is a time of idol worship, the nurse can point out marriages of celebrities in which the woman is taller than the man to help the girl gain a perspective that not all heterosexual relationships must follow stereotypic models.

PRECOCIOUS PUBERTY

Manifestations of sexual development before age 9 in boys or age 8 in girls are considered precocious and should be investigated. Early sexual development can have a number of causes and may result from a disorder of the gonad, the adrenal gland, or the hypothalamic-pituitary gonadal axis. The disorder occurs far more frequently in girls and is usually sporadic. No causative factor can be found in 80% to 90% of girls and in 50% of boys with the condition (DiGeorge, 1992).

Normally the hypothalamic-releasing factors stimulate secretion of the gonadotropic hormones from the anterior pituitary at the time of puberty. In the male, interstitial cell–stimulating hormone stimulates Leydig cells of the testes to secrete testosterone; in the female follicle-stimulating hormone and luteinizing hormone stimulate the ovarian follicles to secrete estrogens. This sequence of events is known as the ***hypothalamic-pituitary-gonadal axis.*** If for some reason there is premature activation of this cycle, the child will display evidence of advanced or precocious puberty.

True, or ***complete, precocious puberty*** is always isosexual and results from premature activation of the hypothalamic-pituitary-gonadal axis, which produces early maturation and development of the gonads with secretion of sex hormones, development of secondary sex characteristics, and sometimes production of mature sperm or ova. True precocious puberty may be caused by a variety of organic brain lesions, such as tumors, congenital lesions, or postinflammatory disorders, but in most instances no cause can be identified. These cases are termed ***functional idiopathic*** or ***constitutional precocious puberty.*** They may occur at any time during childhood and are explained only as an unusually early activation of the maturation process regarded as a normal course of events at a later age. There is early acceleration of linear growth with early epiphyseal fusion and ultimate height less than would have been anticipated with later pubertal onset.

Precocious pseudopuberty, or ***incomplete puberty*** (also called ***pseudosexual precocious puberty***), differs from true sexual precocity in that there is no early secretion of gonadotropin. Gonadotropin-independent causes of precocious puberty must be considered in the differential diagnosis. In girls these include tumors of the ovaries, ovarian cysts, adrenal tumors, McCune-Albright syndrome, and exogenous sources of estrogens. In boys congenital adrenal hyperplasia, adrenal tumors, Leydig cell tumors, gonadotropin-producing hepatoma, and familial male precocious puberty should be considered. Cerebral lesions should be considered in children of both sexes (DiGeorge, 1992). There is no maturation of the gonads, but there is appearance of secondary sex characteristics. Unlike true sexual precocity, precocious pseudopuberty may be heterosexual. A tumor of the adrenal gland in a girl can cause early and inappropriate female development (e.g., clitoral enlargement and masculinization).

Isolated manifestations that are usually associated with puberty may be seen as variations in normal sexual development. They appear without other signs of pubescence and are probably caused by unusual end organ sensitivity to prepubertal levels of estrogen or androgen. Included are ***premature thelarche***—development of breasts in prepubertal females; ***premature pubarche (premature adrenarche)***—early development of sexual hair; and ***premature menarche***—isolated menses without other evidence of sexual development.

Medicational precocity may be confused with precocious puberty. A variety of medicaments can induce the appearance of secondary sexual characteristics. A careful history focused on exploring the possibility of accidental exposure to or ingestion of sex hormones is important. Both boys and girls have exhibited signs of sexual precocity after accidental ingestion of estrogens and anabolic steroids (DiGeorge, 1992).

Therapeutic Management

Treatment of precocious pseudopuberty is directed toward the specific cause when known. Precocious puberty of central (hypothalamic-pituitary) origin is managed with monthly injections of a synthetic analog of lutenizing hormone–releasing hormone (LHRH), which regulates pituitary secretions. The available preparation, luprolide acetate (Lupron Depot), is given in a dose of 0.2 to 0.3 mg/kg intramuscularly once every 4 weeks. Breast development regresses or does not advance, and growth returns to normal rates, enhancing predicted height (DiGeorge, 1992). Treatment is discontinued at a chronologically appropriate time, allowing pubertal changes to resume. Psychologic management of the patient and family is an important aspect of care. Both parents and the affected child should be taught the injection procedure.

Nursing Considerations

Psychologic support and guidance of the child and family are the most important aspects of management. Although the majority of children do not display behavior problems, girls with true precocious puberty have a high incidence of problem behavior, primarily social difficulties related to age/appearance dyssynchrony and moodiness (Sonis and others, 1985).

Parents need a detailed explanation and reassurance of the benign nature of the condition. Dress and activities for the physically precocious child should be appropriate to the chronologic age. Heterosexual interest is not usually advanced beyond the child's chronologic age, and parents need to understand that the child's mental age is congruent with the chronologic age and that the child's normal, overt manifestations of affection are age appropriate and do not represent sexual advances.

Despite the early sexual development, maturation of the gonads and the appearance of secondary sexual characteristics proceed in the usual order. The most difficult time for the child is usually the school years before adolescence. After puberty, physical differences from peers are no longer present.

Although the child's heterosexual behavior is appropriate for the chronologic age, the nurse should emphasize to parents that the child is fertile. Usually no form of contraception is necessary, unless the child is sexually active. In this situation proper counseling is important, since hormonal forms of birth control, such as estrogen pills, will prematurely initiate epiphyseal closure, resulting in stunted linear growth.

DIABETES INSIPIDUS (DI)

The principal disorder of posterior pituitary hypofunction is DI (sometimes called neurogenic DI), resulting from hyposecretion of antidiuretic hormone (ADH), or vasopressin, and producing a state of uncontrolled diuresis. This disorder is not to be confused with nephrogenic DI, a rare hereditary disorder affecting primarily males and caused by unresponsiveness of the renal tubules to the hormone (see Chapter 30).

Neurogenic DI may result from a number of different causes. Primary causes are familial or idiopathic; of the total groups, approximately 45% to 50% are idiopathic. Secondary causes include trauma (accidental or surgical), tumors, granulomatous disease, infections (meningitis or encephalitis), or vascular anomalies (aneurysm). Certain drugs, such as alcohol or phenytoin diphenylhydantoin, can cause a transient polyuria.

Clinical Manifestations

The cardinal signs of DI are polyuria and polydipsia. In the older child, signs such as excessive urination accompanied by a compensatory insatiable thirst may be so intense that the child does little more than go to the toilet and drink fluids. Not infrequently, the first sign is enuresis. In the infant the initial symptom is irritability that is relieved with feedings of water but not milk. The infant is also prone to dehydration, electrolyte imbalance, hyperthermia, azotemia, and potential circulatory collapse.

Dehydration is usually not a serious problem in older children, who are able to drink larger quantities of water. However, any period of unconsciousness, such as after trauma or anesthesia, may be life-threatening because the voluntary demand for fluid is absent. During such instances careful monitoring of urine volumes, blood concentration, and intravenous fluid replacement is essential to prevent dehydration.

NURSING ALERT The child with DI complicated by congenital absence of the thirst center must be encouraged to drink sufficient quantities of liquid to prevent electrolyte imbalance.

Diagnostic Evaluation

The simplest test used to diagnose this condition is restriction of oral fluids and observation of consequent changes in urine volume and concentration. Normally, reducing fluids results in concentrated urine and diminished volume. In DI, fluid restriction has little or no effect on urine formation but causes weight loss from dehydration. Accurate results from this procedure require strict monitoring of fluid intake, urinary output, measurement of urine concentration (specific gravity or osmolality), and frequent weight checks. A weight loss between 3% and 5% indicates significant dehydration and requires termination of the fluid restriction.

NURSING ALERT Small children require close observation during fluid deprivation to prevent them from drinking, even from toilet bowls, plants, or other unlikely sources of fluid.

If this test is positive, the child should be given a test dose of injected aqueous vasopressin (Pitressin), which should alleviate the polyuria and polydipsia. Unresponsiveness to exogenous vasopressin usually indicates nephrogenic DI.

An important diagnostic consideration is to differentiate DI from other causes of polyuria and polydipsia, especially diabetes mellitus. Other tests used in the diagnostic evaluation include a skull x-ray film to detect a tumor, kidney function tests and blood electrolyte levels to assess renal failure, and specific endocrine studies to isolate associated problems. In rare instances a psychologic consultation may be warranted to confirm the possibility of compulsive water drinking related to psychogenic causes.

Therapeutic Management

The usual treatment is hormone replacement, either with an intramuscular or subcutaneous injection of vasopressin tannate in peanut oil or with a nasal spray of aqueous lysine vasopressin. The injectable form has the advantage of lasting for 48 to 72 hours, which affords the child a full night's sleep. However, it has the disadvantage of requiring frequent injections, as well as proper preparation of the drug.

NURSING ALERT To be effective, the active material must be thoroughly resuspended in the oil by being held under warm running water for 10 to 15 minutes and shaken vigorously before being drawn into the syringe. If not, the oil may be injected minus the antidiuretic hormone. Small brown particles, which indicate drug dispersion, must be seen in the suspension.

The nasal spray has the benefit of being a simple, painless route of administration. However, applications must be repeated every 8 to 12 hours to prevent recurrence of symptoms. To provide longer relief during the night, a cotton pledget moistened with the spray can be inserted into the nostril. However, mucous membrane irritation caused by a cold or allergy renders this route unreliable. Although the vaginal and buccal mucosae are substitute routes for the spray, they can be inconvenient. Desmopressin acetate (DDAVP), a long-acting analog of arginine vasopressin, which has fewer side effects, is available and administered intranasally by way of a flexible tube to achieve adequate control. The response pattern of the child is variable, with duration ranging from 8 to 20 hours (Gildea, 1993). It is usually administered twice daily—at bedtime to allow the child to sleep through the night and in the morning to allow fewer interruptions in the school day. Some "breakthrough" urination is allowed during the evening hours as a precaution against overmedication. The drug is also available for parenteral administration.

Nursing Considerations

The initial objective is identification of the disorder. Since an early sign may be sudden enuresis in a child who is toilet trained, excessive thirst with bed-wetting is an indication for further investigation. Another clue is persistent irritability and crying in an infant that is relieved only by bottle-feedings of water. Following head trauma or certain neurosurgical procedures, the development of DI can be anticipated; therefore these patients must be closely monitored for signs of the disorder.

Observations include body weight, serum electrolytes, blood urea nitrogen, hematocrit, and urine specific gravity taken before surgery and every other day following the procedure. Fluid intake and output should be carefully measured and recorded. Alert patients are able to adjust intake to urine losses, but unconscious or very young patients will require closer fluid observation. In children who are not toilet trained, collection of urine specimens may require application of a urine-collecting device.

After confirmation of the diagnosis, parents need a thorough explanation regarding the condition with specific clarification that DI is a different condition from diabetes mellitus. They must realize that treatment is lifelong. If children are to receive the injectable vasopressin (Pitressin), ideally both parents should be taught the correct procedure for preparation and administration of the drug. Once children are old enough, they should be encouraged to assume full responsibility for their care. (See discussion of diabetes mellitus on p. 1780 for ways to help children learn to give their own injections.)

For emergency purposes, these children should wear medical identification. Older children should carry the nasal spray with them for temporary relief of symptoms. School personnel need to be aware of the problem so that they can grant children unrestricted use of the lavatory. Failure to permit this may result in embarrassing accidents that often result in a child's unwillingness to attend school.

Children receiving DDAVP need to be observed for possible overdose of the drug. The signs of overdosage are those of water intoxication and are similar to manifestations of inappropriate secretion of antidiuretic hormone (see next section).

SYNDROME OF INAPPROPRIATE ANTIDIURETIC HORMONE (SIADH)

The disorder that results from hypersecretion of the posterior pituitary hormone, or antidiuretic hormone (ADH, vasopressin), is known as SIADH. It is observed with increased frequency in a variety of conditions, especially those involving infections, tumors, or other central nervous system disease and/or trauma.

The manifestations are directly related to fluid retention and hypotonicity. Excess ADH causes most of the filtered water to be reabsorbed from the kidneys back into central circulation. Serum osmolality is low, and urine osmolality is inappropriately elevated. When serum sodium levels are diminished to 110 mEq/L, affected children display anorexia, nausea (and sometimes vomiting), stomach cramps, irritability, and personality changes. With progressive reduction in sodium, other neurologic signs, stupor, and convulsions may be evident. The symptoms usually disappear when the underlying disorder is corrected.

The immediate management consists of restricting fluids. Subsequent management depends on the cause and severity. Fluids continue to be restricted to one-fourth to one-half maintenance. When there are no fluid abnormalities but SIADH can be anticipated, fluids are often restricted expectantly at two-thirds to three-fourths maintenance.

Nursing Considerations

The first goal of nursing management is recognizing the presence of SIADH from symptoms described in patients at risk, especially those in the pediatric intensive care unit (PICU).

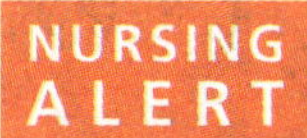

Children with SIADH develop an expanded circulatory volume but do not form edema, which is an excess of both water and sodium (Gildea, 1993).

Accurately measuring intake and output, noting daily weight, and observing for signs of fluid overload are primary nursing functions, especially in the child receiving intravenous fluids. Seizure precautions are implemented, and the child and family need education regarding the rationale for fluid restrictions. The rare child with chronic SIADH will be placed on long-term ADH-antagonizing medication, and the child and family will require instructions for its administration.

DISORDERS OF THYROID FUNCTION

The thyroid gland secretes two types of hormones: (1) ***thyroid hormone,*** which consists of the hormones ***thyroxine (T_4)*** and ***triiodothyronine (T_3),*** and (2) ***thyrocalcitonin.*** The secretion of thyroid hormones is controlled by thyroid-stimulating hormone (TSH) from the anterior pituitary, which in turn is regulated by thyrotropin-releasing factor (TRF) from the hypothalamus as a negative feedback response. Consequently, hypothyroidism or hyperthyroidism may result from a defect in the target gland or from a disturbance in the secretion of TSH or TRF. Since the functions of T_3 and T_4 are qualitatively the same, the term ***thyroid hormone (TH)*** is used throughout the discussion.

The synthesis of TH depends on available sources of dietary iodine and tyrosine. The thyroid is the only endocrine gland capable of storing excess amounts of hormones for release as needed. During circulation in the bloodstream, T_4 and T_3 are bound to carrier proteins (thyroxine-binding globulin [TBG]). They must be unbound before they are able to exert their metabolic effect.

PHYSIOLOGIC EFFECTS OF THYROID HORMONE

- Regulates metabolic rate of all cells; protein, fat, and carbohydrate catabolism; and nitrogen excretion
- Regulates body heat production and heat-dissipating mechanisms
- Regulates protein synthesis and catabolism, amino acid incorporation into protein, and transcription of messenger RNA
- Increases gluconeogenesis and peripheral utilization of glucose
- Maintains appetite and secretion of gastrointestinal substances
- Maintains calcium mobilization
- Stimulates cholesterol synthesis and hepatic mechanisms that remove cholesterol from the circulation; stimulates lipid turnover and free fatty acid release
- Regulates hepatic conversion of carotene to vitamin A
- Maintains growth hormone secretion, skeletal maturation, and tissue differentiation
- Is necessary for muscle tone and vigor and normal skin constituents
- Maintains cardiac rate, force, and output
- Affects respiratory rate, depth of oxygen utilization, and carbon dioxide formation
- Affects central nervous system development and cerebration during first 2 to 3 years
- Affects milk production during lactation and menstrual cycle fertility
- Maintains sensitivity to insulin and insulin degradation
- Affects red cell production
- Affects cortisol secretion, probably caused by direct effect on adrenal glands and by increasing ACTH secretion

The main physiologic action of thyroid hormone is to regulate the basal metabolic rate and thereby control the processes of growth and tissue differentiation, as outlined in the box above. Unlike GH, TH is involved in many more diverse activities that influence the growth and development of body tissues. Therefore a deficiency of TH exerts a more profound effect on growth than that seen in hypopituitarism.

Thyrocalcitonin helps maintain blood calcium levels by decreasing the calcium concentration. Its effect is the opposite of parathormone in that it inhibits skeletal demineralization and promotes calcium deposition in the bone.

JUVENILE HYPOTHYROIDISM

Hypothyroidism is one of the most common endocrine problems of childhood. It may be either congenital (see Chapter 9) or acquired and represents a deficiency in secretion of thyroid hormones. Hypothyroidism from dietary insufficiency of iodine is now rare in the United States because the use of iodized salt has permitted a readily available source of the nutrient.

Beyond infancy, primary hypothyroidism may be caused by a number of defects. For example, a congenital hypoplastic thyroid gland may provide sufficient amounts of TH during the first year or two but be inadequate when rapid body growth increases demands on the gland. A partial or complete thyroidectomy for cancer or thyrotoxicosis can leave insufficient thyroid tissue to furnish hormones for body requirements. Thyroid disease, especially hypothyroidism, is common in patients with Hodgkin disease who have been treated with irradiation. A high risk for thyroid disease, including thyroid cancer and Graves disease, persists for more than 25 years after patients have received radiation therapy (Hancock, Cox, and McDougall, 1991). Infectious processes may be a cause of hypothyroidism. It can also occur when dietary iodine is deficient.

Clinical manifestations depend on the extent of dysfunction and the age of the child at the onset. The presenting symptoms are decelerated growth from chronic deprivation of thyroid hormone or thyromegaly. Impaired growth and development are less when hypothyroidism is acquired at a later age, and since brain growth is nearly complete by 2 to 3 years of age, mental retardation or neurologic sequelae are not associated with juvenile hypothyroidism. Other manifestations are myxedematous skin changes (dry skin, puffiness around the eyes, sparse hair), constipation, sleepiness, and mental decline.

Therapy is TH replacement, the same as for hypothyroidism in the infant, although the prompt treatment needed in the infant is not required in the child. In children with severe symptoms, the restoration of euthyroidism is achieved more gradually with administration of increasing amounts of L-thyroxine over 4 to 8 weeks to avoid symptoms of hyperthyroidism that can occur with treatment of chronic hypothyroidism. Reports of aggressive behavioral reactions or learning problems with poorer school achievement may occur in about 25% of patients treated with thyroxine (Rovet, Danemen, and Bailey, 1993).

Nursing Considerations

The importance of early recognition in the infant has already been discussed in Chapter 9. Cessation or retardation in growth in a child whose growth has previously been normal should alert the observer to the possibility of hypothyroidism. Following diagnosis and implementation of thyroxine therapy, the importance of compliance and periodic monitoring of response to therapy should be stressed to parents. Children should learn to take responsibility for their own health as soon as they are old enough, at about 9 to 10 years of age.

GOITER

A goiter is an enlargement or hypertrophy of the thyroid gland. It may occur in deficient (hypothyroid), excessive (hyperthyroid), or normal (euthyroid) TH secretion. It can be congenital or acquired and can be palpated in about 5% of school-age children (Mahoney, 1987). Congenital disease usually occurs as a result of maternal administration of antithyroid drugs and/or iodides during pregnancy. Acquired disease can result from increased secretion of pituitary TSH in response to decreased circulating levels of TH or from infiltrative neoplastic or inflammatory processes. In areas where dietary iodine (essential for TH production) is deficient, goiter can be endemic.

Enlargement of the thyroid gland can be mild and noticeable only when there is an increased demand for TH (e.g., during periods of rapid growth). Where iodine deficiency is severe, a large percentage of the population display goiters. Enlargement of the thyroid at birth can be sufficient to cause severe respiratory distress. Sporadic goiter is usually caused by lymphocytic thyroiditis, and intrinsic biochemical defects in synthesis of the hormones are associated with goiters. Thyroid hormone replacement is necessary to treat the hypothyroidism and reverse the thyroid-stimulating hormone effect on the gland.

Nursing Considerations

Identification of large goiters is facilitated by their obvious appearance. Smaller nodules may be evident only on palpation. Nurses in ambulatory settings need to be aware of the possibility of goiters and report such findings to a physician. Benign enlargement of the thyroid gland may occur during adolescence and should not be confused with pathologic states. Nodules rarely are caused by a cancerous tumor but always require evaluation. Since they are frequently associated with a history of exposure to irradiation of the neck or upper thorax, inquiry about this possibility is part of the assessment.

NURSING ALERT If an infant is born with a goiter, immediate precautions are instituted for emergency ventilation, such as supplemental oxygen and a tracheostomy set. Positioning the child with the neck hyperextended often facilitates breathing.

Immediate surgery to remove part of the gland may be lifesaving in infants born with a goiter. When thyroid replacement is necessary, parents have the same needs regarding its administration as discussed for the parents of children who have hypothyroidism (see Chapter 9).

LYMPHOCYTIC THYROIDITIS

Lymphocytic thyroiditis (Hashimoto disease, juvenile autoimmune thyroiditis) is the most common cause of thyroid disease in children and adolescents and accounts for the largest percentage of juvenile hypothyroidism. It accounts for many of the enlarged thyroid glands formerly designated as thyroid hyperplasia of adolescence or "adolescent goiter." The disease is four to seven times more common in girls than in boys and four times more common in white persons than in black persons (Fink and Beall, 1982). Although it can occur during the first 3 years of life, it more frequently appears after age 6. It reaches a peak incidence at adolescence (DiGeorge, 1992), and there is evidence that the disease is self-limited.

Pathophysiology

There is a strong genetic predisposition to the development of autoimmune thyroiditis, although no mode of inheritance has been delineated and the basic stimulus or autoimmune defect is unknown. There is a close relationship between this disease and other thyroid disorders (Graves disease, idiopathic hypothyroidism, idiopathic myxedema) and autoimmune disorders (pernicious anemia, Addison disease, type I diabetes mellitus, and hypoparathyroidism) in families. An increased incidence of the histocompatibility antigens HLA-DR3 and HLA-DR5 has been observed in patients with autoimmune thyroiditis (Sack and others, 1983).

The disease is characterized by lymphocytic infiltration of the gland, germinal-center inflammation, and, in many patients, replacement with fibrous tissue. In the early stages there may be only hyperplasia. A defect in autoregulation allows the persistence of a T-cell clone, which induces a cell-mediated immune response. Several antithyroid antibodies have been recognized in patients with thyroiditis.

Clinical Manifestations

The presence of the enlarged thyroid gland is usually detected by the practitioner during a routine examination, although it may be noted by parents when the youngster swallows. In most children the entire gland is enlarged symmetrically (but may be asymmetric) and is firm, freely movable, and nontender. There may be manifestations of moderate tracheal compression (sense of fullness, hoarseness, and dysphagia), but it is extremely rare for nontoxic diffuse goiter to enlarge to the extent that its size causes mechanical obstruction. Most children are euthyroid, but some display symptoms of hypothyroidism. Others have signs suggestive of hyperthyroidism, such as nervousness, irritability, tachycardia, increased sweating, or hyperactivity.

Diagnostic Evaluation

Thyroid function tests are usually normal, although TSH levels may be slightly or moderately elevated. With progressive disease the T_4 decreases, followed by a decrease in T_3 levels and an increase in TSH. A variety of abnormalities in radioactive iodine uptake may be noted. The majority of children have serum antibody titers to thyroid antigens, but fewer children have a positive red blood cell hemagglutination test. When both tests are used, almost all children with thyroid autoimmunity are detected. However, levels in children are lower than in adults; therefore repeated measurements may be needed in doubtful cases because titers may increase later in the disease.

Therapeutic Management

In many cases the goiter is transient and asymptomatic and regresses spontaneously within a year or two. Therapy of nontoxic diffuse goiter is usually simple, uncomplicated, and effective. Oral administration of TH will decrease the size of the gland significantly. It provides the feedback needed to suppress TSH stimulation, and the hyperplastic thyroid gland gradually regresses in size. Surgery is contraindicated in this disorder. Untreated patients should be evaluated periodically.

Nursing Considerations

Nursing care consists of identifying the youngster with thyroid enlargement, reassuring the child that the condition is probably only temporary, and reinforcing instructions for thyroid therapy.

HYPERTHYROIDISM

The largest percentage of hyperthyroidism in childhood is caused by Graves disease, which is usually associated with an enlarged thyroid gland and exophthalmos. Most cases of Graves disease occur in children ages 6 to 15, with a peak incidence at 12 to 14 years of age, but the disease may be present at birth in children of thyrotoxic mothers. The incidence is five times higher in girls than in boys.

The hyperthyroidism of Graves disease is apparently caused by an autoimmune response to TSH receptors, but no specific etiology has been identified. There is definitive evidence for familial association with a high concordance incidence in twins. A large number of persons (approximately 80%) with the disease possess the histocompatibility antigen HLA-B8.

Clinical Manifestations

The development of manifestations is highly variable. Signs and symptoms develop gradually, with an interval between onset and diagnosis of approximately 6 to 12 months. The principal clinical features are excessive motion—irritability, hyperactivity, short attention span, tremors, insomnia, and emotional lability. Gradual weight loss despite a voracious appetite is observed in half of the cases. Linear growth and bone age are usually accelerated. Muscle weakness often occurs. Hyperactivity of the gastrointestinal tract may cause vomiting and frequent stooling. Cardiac manifestations include a rapid, pounding pulse even during sleep, widened pulse pressure, systolic murmurs, and cardiomegaly. Dyspnea occurs during slight exertion, such as climbing stairs. The skin is warm, flushed, and moist. Heat intolerance may be severe and is accompanied by diaphoresis. The hair is unusually fine and unable to hold a wave.

Exophthalmos (protruding eyeballs), observed in many children, is accompanied by a wide-eyed staring expression, increased blinking, lid lag, lack of convergence, and absence of wrinkling of the forehead when looking upward. As protrusion of the eyeball increases, the child may not be able to completely cover the cornea with the lid. Visual disturbances may include blurred vision and loss of visual acuity. Ophthalmopathy can develop long before or after the onset of hyperthyroidism. A consistent pathogenic link between them has not been identified, and the cause of Graves ophthalmopathy is not known (Tallstedt and others, 1992).

Diagnostic Evaluation

The presence of a thyroid mass in a child requires a thorough history, including inquiry into prior irradiation to the head and neck and exposure to a goiterogen. The diagnosis is established on the basis of increased levels of T_4 and T_3. Thyrotropin (TSH) is suppressed to unmeasurable levels. Other tests are rarely indicated.

Therapeutic Management

Therapy for hyperthyroidism is controversial, but all methods are directed toward retarding the rate of hormone secretion. The three acceptable modes available are (1) the antithyroid drugs, which interfere with the biosynthesis of TH, including propylthiouracil (PTU) and methimazole

(MTZ, Tapazole); (2) subtotal thyroidectomy; and (3) ablation with radioiodine (^{131}I-iodide). Each is effective, but each has advantages and disadvantages.

While affected children exhibit signs and symptoms of hyperthyroidism (i.e., increased weight loss, pulse, pulse pressure, and blood pressure), their activity should be limited to classwork only. Vigorous exercise is restricted until thyroid levels are decreased to normal or near-normal values.

Drug Therapy. Most centers favor drugs as an initial therapy. An effective response to these drugs occurs after a latent period, since they inhibit production of additional thyroid hormone but do not retard secretion of stored supplies. Generally, some improvement is noted within the first 2 weeks, with evidence of decreased nervousness, less fatigue, increased strength, a lowered pulse, and weight gain. In many children an initial treatment course of 1 to 2 years will be followed by a complete remission of the disorder. Those who relapse may benefit from a second course of therapy but may also be candidates for surgical intervention.

Disadvantages include toxic drug reactions requiring alternate therapy, chronic dependency on the drug, and failure to produce remission in a large number of patients. The most serious side effect of these antithyroid drugs is agranulocytosis (pronounced leukopenia), which generally occurs within the initial weeks or months of therapy. It is usually accompanied by a sore throat and fever. Treatment involves immediate discontinuation of the drug, isolation of the child, and administration of antibiotics and glucocorticoids.

Thyroidectomy. Surgical treatment involves surgical ablation of the thyroid (thyroidectomy). Although this approach has the advantage of being a long-lasting form of therapy without the need for multiple-dose drug therapy, it has a number of serious disadvantages, including an increased incidence of hypothyroidism and the need for thyroxine therapy, infrequent recurrent laryngeal nerve palsy and permanent hypoparathyroidism, keloid formation of the anterior cervical scar in susceptible individuals, and (rarely) surgical mortality. Therefore surgery in most centers is reserved for children who do not respond to or comply with the use of antithyroid drugs or who are prone to recurrences.

Radioiodine Therapy. Radioiodine therapy is not recommended for children because of the increased risk of subsequent carcinoma of the thyroid and the possibility of genetic damage.

Thyrotoxicosis. Thyrotoxicosis (thyroid "crisis" or thyroid "storm") may occur from sudden release of the hormone. Although unusual in children, a crisis can be life-threatening. These "storms" are evidenced by the acute onset of severe irritability and restlessness, vomiting, diarrhea, hyperthermia, hypertension, severe tachycardia, and prostration. There may be rapid progression to delirium, coma, and even death. A crisis may be precipitated by acute infection, surgical emergencies, or discontinuation of antithyroid therapy. Treatment in addition to antithyroid drugs is administration of β-adrenergic blocking agents (propranolol), which provide relief from the adrenergic hyperresponsiveness that produces the disturbing side effects of the reaction. Therapy is usually required for 2 to 3 weeks.

Nursing Considerations

The initial nursing objective is identification of children with hyperthyroidism. Since the clinical manifestations often appear gradually, the goiter and ophthalmic changes may not be noticed, and the excessive activity may be attributed to behavioral problems. Nurses in ambulatory settings, particularly those caring for children in school, need to be alert to signs that suggest this disorder, especially weight loss despite an excellent appetite, academic difficulties resulting from short attention span and inability to sit still, unexplained fatigue and sleeplessness, and difficulty with fine motor skills, such as writing. Exophthalmos may develop long before the onset of signs and symptoms of hyperthyroidism and may be the only presenting sign (Tallstedt and others, 1992).

Much of these children's care is related to treating physical symptoms before a response to drug therapy is achieved. These children need a quiet, unstimulating environment that is conducive to rest. Sometimes hospitalization is necessary during the immediate treatment phase to remove a child from a troubled home. A regular routine is beneficial in providing frequent rest periods, minimizing the stress of coping with unexpected demands, and meeting the children's needs promptly. Physical activity is restricted. For example, school physical education classes are discontinued.

Since the nervous manifestations often interfere with schoolwork, a consultation with the child's teachers is important in advising them of the medical reason for the problem and suggesting ways of helping the child adjust. For example, the child may benefit from a shortened school day or at least study periods in a quiet area. Limiting demands on the child, such as reciting in class or participating in extracurricular activities, may help conserve strength for academic studies. Despite the excessive activity of these children, they tire easily, experience muscle weakness, and are unable to relax to recoup their strength.

Emotional lability is often manifested by sudden episodes of crying or elation. Such behavior, coupled with irritability, disrupts interpersonal relationships, creating difficulties within and outside the home. Parents need help in understanding the uncontrollable nature of these outbursts and ways of minimizing them through decreased environmental stimulation, stress, and frustration. The child should be encouraged to express feelings about behavior and the effect that it has on others. The nurse can encourage the child to concentrate on friendship with one special peer rather than a group until such time as the condition is stabilized.

Heat intolerance may produce considerable family conflict. Preferring a cooler environment than others, the child is likely to open windows, complain about the heat, wear minimal clothing, and remove blankets while sleeping. Although the child should dress in accordance with climatic conditions, the use of light cotton clothing in the home, good ventilation, frequent baths, and adequate hydration is helpful in providing comfort. Hygiene should be stressed because of excessive sweating.

Dietary requirements should be adjusted to meet the child's increased metabolic rate. Although the need for calories is increased, these should be provided in wholesome foods rather than "junk" foods. The child may require vitamin supplements to meet the daily requirement. Rather than three large meals, the child's appetite may be better satisfied by five or six moderate meals throughout the day. Family members should refrain from making remarks about the child's appetite, since the child may voluntarily restrict his or her eating to avoid such attention.

Once therapy is instituted, the drug regimen is explained, emphasizing the importance of observing for side effects of antithyroid drugs. Untoward effects of propylthiouracil and related compounds include urticarial rash, fever, arthritis, or arthralgia. There may be enlargement of the salivary and cervical lymph glands, a diminished sense of taste, hepatitis, and edema of the lower extremities.

NURSING ALERT Children being treated with propylthiouracil must be carefully monitored for untoward effects of the drug. Since sore throat and fever accompany the grave complication of leukopenia, these children should be seen by a practitioner if such symptoms occur. Parents and children should be taught to recognize and report symptoms immediately.

Parents should also be aware of the signs of hypothyroidism, which can occur from overdose of the drugs. The most common indications are lethargy and somnolence.

Surgical Care. If surgery is anticipated, iodine is usually administered for a few weeks before the procedure. Since oral iodine preparations are unpalatable, they should be mixed with a strong-tasting fruit juice, such as grape or punch flavors, and be given through a straw. Compliance with iodine therapy is essential to avoid the danger of thyroid crisis after sudden discontinuation.

Psychologic preparation of children for thyroidectomy is similar to that for any other surgical procedure (see Chapter 27). However, of special consideration is the site of the incision. The fear of having the throat cut is very real and in older children is associated with death. The nurse should explain that the throat is not cut, only the skin, to allow for removal of the gland. Showing children a picture of the anatomic location of the thyroid around the trachea is often helpful. Children should be prepared for the dressing around the neck and the possibility of an endotracheal or "breathing" tube after surgery.

Postoperative care involves positioning with the neck slightly flexed to avoid strain on the sutures and observation for bleeding and complications. The children are taught to support the neck in this position when they sit up. Damage to the recurrent laryngeal nerve is evidenced by severe stridor and/or hoarseness, although some hoarseness is expected. Laryngospasm, a spasmodic contraction of the larynx, can be a life-threatening complication of thyroidectomy. Signs of laryngospasm are stridor, hoarseness, and a feeling of tightness in the throat. A tracheostomy set should be placed near the bed for emergency use.

NURSING ALERT The earliest indication of hypoparathyroidism may be anxiety and mental depression, followed by paresthesia and evidence of heightened neuromuscular excitability, such as Chvostek and Trousseau signs and carpopedal spasm (tetany).

DISORDERS OF PARATHYROID FUNCTION

The parathyroid glands secrete ***parathormone (PTH)***, the main function of which, along with vitamin D and calcitonin, is homeostasis of serum calcium concentration. The effect of PTH on calcium is opposite that of thyrocalcitonin. The principal effects of PTH on its target sites are listed in the box below.

The net result of the integrated action of PTH and vitamin D is maintenance of serum calcium levels within a narrow normal range and the mineralization of bone. Secretion of PTH is controlled by a negative feedback system involving the serum calcium ion concentration. Low ionized calcium levels stimulate PTH secretion, causing absorption of calcium by the target tissues; high ionized calcium concentrations suppress PTH.

HYPOPARATHYROIDISM

Two classic forms of hypoparathyroidism are observed during childhood: ***autoimmune hypoparathyroidism,*** in which there is deficient production of PTH, and ***pseudohypoparathyroidism,*** in which production of PTH is increased but end-organ responsiveness to the hormone is deficient. The presenting signs or symptoms are similar.

Autoimmune hypoparathyroidism may occur as a component of multiglandular failure, usually in relation to autoimmune phenomena. Familial hypoparathyroidism is inherited as an autosomal recessive trait, with early onset, usually in the first month of life.

Hypoparathyroidism can also occur secondary to other causes. Postoperative hypoparathyroidism may follow thyroidectomy with acute or gradual onset and be transient or permanent. Two forms of transient hypoparathyroidism may be present in the newborn, both of which are the result of a relative PTH deficiency. One type is caused by maternal hyperparathyroidism or maternal diabetes mellitus. A more common, later form appears almost exclusively in infants fed a milk formula with a high phosphate-to-calcium ratio.

PHYSIOLOGIC EFFECTS OF PARATHYROID HORMONE

Bones—Increases osteoclastic activity, causing phosphate-producing bone demineralization
Kidneys—Increases absorption of calcium and excretion of phosphate
Gastrointestinal tract—Promotes calcium absorption

Clinical Manifestations

Children with pseudohypoparathyroidism are short with round faces, short thick necks, and short, stubby fingers and toes with dimpling of the skin over the knuckles. These manifestations are not observed in hypoparathyroidism. In both types the skin can be dry, scaly, and coarse, with skin eruptions; the hair is often brittle; and the nails are thin and brittle, with characteristic transverse grooves. Subcutaneous soft tissue calcifications appear in pseudohypoparathyroidism but not in idiopathic hypoparathyroidism. Dental and enamel hypoplasia occurs in both types.

Tetany, convulsions, carpopedal spasm, muscle cramps and twitching, paresthesias, and laryngeal stridor are often the initial symptoms in both types. Mental retardation is a prominent feature of pseudohypoparathyroidism and may also occur in idiopathic hypoparathyroidism but is less frequent in later onset disease and early diagnosis and treatment. Swings of emotion, loss of memory, depression, and confusion can occur. Papilledema may be seen in the idiopathic disease but is rare in pseudohypoparathyroidism. Since hypoparathyroidism results in decreased bone resorption and inactive osteoclastic activity, skeletal growth is retarded.

Diagnostic Evaluation

The diagnosis of hypoparathyroidism is made on the basis of clinical manifestations associated with decreased serum calcium and increased serum phosphorus. Levels of plasma PTH are low in idiopathic hypoparathyroidism but high in pseudohypoparathyroidism. End-organ responsiveness is tested by the administration of PTH with measurement of urinary cyclic adenosine monophosphate (cAMP). Kidney function tests are included in the differential diagnosis to rule out renal insufficiency. Although bone radiographs are usually normal, they may demonstrate increased bone density and suppressed growth.

Therapeutic Management

The objective of treatment is to maintain normal serum calcium and phosphate levels with minimum complications. Acute or severe tetany is corrected immediately by intravenous and oral administration of calcium gluconate and follow-up daily doses to achieve normal levels. Twice-daily serum calcium measurements are taken to monitor the efficacy of therapy and prevent hypercalcemia. When diagnosis is confirmed, vitamin D therapy is begun. Vitamin D therapy is somewhat difficult to regulate because the drug has a prolonged onset and a long half-life. Some authorities advocate beginning with a lower dose with stepwise increases and careful monitoring of serum calcium until stable levels are achieved. Others prefer rapid induction with higher doses and rapid reduction to lower maintenance levels.

Long-term management consists of administration of massive doses of vitamin D, and oral calcium supplementation may be useful in maintaining adequate serum calcium levels, although it is not essential. Blood calcium and phosphorus are monitored frequently until the levels have stabilized; they are then monitored monthly and less often until the child is seen at 6-month intervals. Renal function, blood pressure, and serum vitamin D levels are measured every 6 months. Serum magnesium levels are measured every 3 to 6 months to permit detection of hypomagnesemia, which may raise the requirement for vitamin D.

Nursing Considerations

The initial objective is recognition of hypocalcemia. Unexplained convulsions, irritability (especially to external stimuli), gastrointestinal symptoms (diarrhea, vomiting, cramping), and positive signs of tetany should lead the nurse to suspect this disorder. Much of the initial nursing care is related to the physical manifestations and includes institution of seizure and safety precautions, reduction of environmental stimuli (e.g., avoiding sudden or loud noise, bright lights, stimulating activities), and observation for signs of laryngospasm, such as stridor, hoarseness, and a feeling of tightness in the throat. A tracheostomy set and injectable calcium gluconate should be placed near the bedside for emergency use. The administration of calcium gluconate requires precautions against extravasation of the drug.

After initiation of treatment, the nurse discusses with the parents the need for continuous daily administration of calcium salts and vitamin D. Because vitamin D toxicity can be a serious consequence of therapy, parents are advised to watch for signs that include weakness, fatigue, lassitude, headache, nausea, vomiting, and diarrhea. Early renal impairment is manifested by polyuria, polydipsia, and nocturia.

HYPERPARATHYROIDISM

Hyperparathyroidism is rare in childhood but can be primary or secondary. The most common cause of primary hyperparathyroidism is adenoma of the gland. The most common causes of secondary hyperparathyroidism are chronic renal disease, renal rickets, and congenital anomalies of the urinary tract. The common factor is hypercalcemia.

Clinical Manifestations

The manifestations of primary hyperparathyroidism are conveniently grouped according to the system involved (see box below).

MANIFESTATIONS OF PRIMARY HYPERPARATHYROIDISM

Gastrointestinal—Nausea, vomiting, abdominal discomfort, and constipation

Central nervous system—Delusions, confusion, hallucinations, impaired memory, lack of interest and initiative, depression, and varying levels of consciousness

Neuromuscular—Weakness, easy fatigability, muscle atrophy (especially proximal muscles of the lower limbs), twitching of the tongue, paresthesias in extremities

Skeletal—Vague bone pain, subperiosteal resorption of phalanges, spontaneous fractures, and absence of lamina dura around the teeth

Renal—Polyuria and polydipsia, renal colic, and hypertension

Diagnostic Evaluation

Blood studies to identify any alterations in calcium/phosphorus ratio are routinely performed. Measurement of PTH, as well as several tests to isolate the cause of the hypercalcemia, such as renal function studies, should be included. Other procedures used to substantiate the physiologic consequences of the disorder include electrocardiography and radiographic bone surveys.

Therapeutic Management

Treatment depends on the cause of hyperparathyroidism. The treatment of primary hyperparathyroidism is surgical removal of the tumor or hyperplastic tissue. Treatment of secondary hyperparathyroidism is directed at the underlying contributing cause, which subsequently restores the serum calcium balance. However, in some instances the underlying disorder is irreversible, such as in chronic renal failure. In this instance treatment is aimed at raising serum calcium levels in order to inhibit the stimulatory effect of low levels on the parathyroids. This includes oral administration of calcium salts, high doses of vitamin D to enhance calcium absorption, a low-phosphorus diet, and administration of a phosphorus-mobilizing aluminum hydroxide to reduce phosphate absorption.

Nursing Considerations

The initial nursing objective is recognition of the disorder. Since secondary hyperparathyroidism is a consequence of chronic renal failure, the nurse is always alert to signs that suggest this complication, especially bone pain and fractures. Since urinary symptoms are the earliest indication, assessment of other body systems for evidence of high calcium levels is indicated when polyuria and polydipsia coexist. Change in behavior, especially inactivity, unexplained gastrointestinal symptoms, and cardiac irregularities provide clues to the possibility of hyperparathyroidism.

Much of the initial nursing care is related to the physical symptoms and prevention of complications. To minimize renal calculi formation, hydration is essential. Fruit juices that maintain a low urinary pH, such as cranberry or apple juice, are encouraged, since acidity of body fluids promotes calcium absorption. All urine should be strained for evidence of renal casts.

Safety precautions, such as siderails in place at all times and assistance with ambulation, are instituted because of the tendency toward fractures and muscular weakness. Children with renal rickets (osteodystrophy) may wear braces to minimize skeletal deformities. These should be worn as prescribed. If the child is confined to bed, the nurse should consult with the physical therapist regarding proper use of orthopaedic appliances.

Vital signs should be taken frequently, and the pulse counted for 1 full minute to detect irregularities. A decrease in pulse rate should be reported, since it may signal severe bradycardia and cardiac arrest. The diet needs supervision to ensure compliance with low-phosphate foods, particularly dairy products. The nurse should instruct parents regarding foods that need to be avoided and the necessity of administering calcium and vitamin D.

If surgery is anticipated, care is similar to that discussed for the child with hyperthyroidism. Since hypocalcemia is a potential complication, observation for signs of tetany, institution of seizure precautions, and having calcium gluconate available for emergency use are part of the nursing plan.

DISORDERS OF ADRENAL FUNCTION

ADRENAL HORMONES

The adrenal glands consist of two distinct portions: the cortex, or outer section, and the medulla, or inner core. The adrenal cortex secretes the hormones, collectively known as steroids, that are essential to life. The medulla produces the catecholamines epinephrine and norepinephrine. Since these chemicals are also produced by the sympathetic nervous system, absence of the adrenal supply is not incompatible with life.

Adrenal Cortex

The cortex secretes three groups of hormones that are classified according to their biologic activity: (1) glucocorticoids (cortisol, corticosterone), (2) mineralocorticoids (aldosterone), and (3) sex steroids (androgens, estrogens, and progestins). The glucocorticoids and mineralocorticoids influence metabolic regulation and stress adaptation. The sex steroids influence sexual development but are not essential because the gonads secrete the major supply of these hormones.

Glucocorticoids. The most important glucocorticoids in humans are cortisol and corticosterone, the principal effects of which are outlined in the box below. Normally the hypothalamus secretes corticotropin-releasing factor (CRF), which causes the pituitary gland to produce adrenocorticotropic hormone (ACTH), which stimulates the adrenal glands to synthesize glucocorticoids (primarily cortisol). The switch that controls this feedback is cortisol. When blood levels of cortisol are low, the system turns on. When

PHYSIOLOGIC EFFECTS OF GLUCOCORTICOIDS

Stimulation of gluconeogenesis by the liver (a hyperglycemic effect)
Increased protein catabolism with resulting reduction in protein stores (except in the liver)
Increased mobilization and utilization of fatty acids for energy
Increased storage of adipose tissue in certain sites
Decreased inflammatory and allergic actions
Regulation of fluid and electrolytes by promoting sodium retention and potassium excretion by the kidneys and by water diuresis through direct antagonistic action against antidiuretic hormone
Increased gastric acid and pepsin production
Suppression of lymphocytes, eosinophils, and basophils, but elevation of neutrophils, erythrocytes, and thrombocytes

blood levels of cortisol rise, the system turns off (Ruble, 1992).

In times of stress, the anterior pituitary is stimulated by CRF from the hypothalamus, which causes the release of increased amounts of ACTH. Stressful stimuli capable of provoking this response include trauma, anesthesia, surgical intervention, sepsis, acute anoxia, hypothermia, hypoglycemia, and emotional states, especially panic, anxiety, or anger.

Secretion of the glucocorticoids is also regulated by body rhythms. Blood levels of cortisol demonstrate a typical diurnal or circadian pattern. In individuals who follow a regular routine of nighttime sleeping, cortisol levels are highest in the early morning hours after arising and lowest in the evening hours before bedtime.

Mineralocorticoids. The most important mineralocorticoid is aldosterone. Like cortisol, it promotes sodium retention and potassium excretion in the renal tubules. Aldosterone's effect is many times more potent than that of the glucocorticoids in maintaining extracellular fluid volume, acid-base balance, and normal potassium levels.

Aldosterone synthesis is regulated primarily by the renin-angiotensin system of the kidney. A block in aldosterone synthesis will cause very high plasma renin activity levels (Ruble, 1992). The juxtaglomerular cells of the kidney respond to decreased arterial pressure and/or blood volume and to decreased sodium concentrations by secreting the enzyme renin into the blood. Renin in turn converts angiotensinogen to angiotensin I and then to angiotensin II. Increased levels of angiotensin stimulate the adrenal cortex to secrete aldosterone, which preserves sodium, thereby retaining water. The renin-angiotensin mechanism also results in increased blood pressure.

Sex Steroids. Except for the first few days of life, the sex hormones are normally secreted in only minimal amounts until adolescence, at which time they play a role in pubertal changes. Their actions are the same as those of the gonadal hormones on internal and external sexual structures and skeletal growth.

Adrenal Medulla

The adrenal medulla secretes the catecholamines epinephrine and norepinephrine. Both hormones have essentially the same effects on different organs as those caused by direct sympathetic stimulation, except that the hormonal effects last several times longer. Their major actions are outlined in the box above, right.

PHYSIOLOGIC EFFECTS OF CATECHOLAMINE SECRETION

Increased cardiac activity
Vasoconstriction of blood vessels (elevation of blood pressure)
Increased rate and depth of respirations
Bronchial dilation
Inhibition of gastrointestinal activity
Increased muscular contraction
Pupillary dilation
Increased metabolic rate
Heightened sensory awareness
Diaphoresis

Although the catecholamines evoke similar responses from target sites, there are some important differences. Epinephrine has a greater effect on cardiac activity than norepinephrine, but it causes only weak constriction of the blood vessels of muscles in comparison with the effect of norepinephrine. As a result, norepinephrine elevates blood pressure, whereas epinephrine increases cardiac output. Another important difference is their effect on metabolism. Epinephrine increases the metabolic rate to a much greater extent than norepinephrine. These differences in action have been attributed to the catecholamines' effects on α- or β-adrenergic receptors. Supposedly, norepinephrine can only affect those effector cells that contain α-receptors, which are mostly excitatory (constriction and contraction). Epinephrine, however, can affect both α- and β-receptors, and β-receptors are mostly inhibitory (dilation and relaxation).

Control of secretion of catecholamines, primarily in response to physiologic or emotional stress, is through the hypothalamus. Also, stimulation of the sympathetic nervous system results in the release of epinephrine and norepinephrine from the sympathetic nerves and adrenal medulla. Both systems support each other, and one can be substituted for the other. For this reason there is no condition attributable to hypofunction of the adrenal medulla. Even in bilateral adrenalectomy, catecholamine replacement is not necessary, because the sympathetic release of these chemicals is sufficient to meet all the physiologic functions required to cope with stressful events.

Catecholamine-secreting tumors are the primary cause of adrenal medullary hyperfunction. In children the most common neoplasms of this type are pheochromocytoma (see p. 1763), neuroblastoma, and ganglioneuroma. Ganglioneuromas are thought to be neuroblastomas that have undergone maturation into a benign tumor composed of ganglion cells. These tumors are associated with less abnormal catecholamine secretion than the other two types, but persons with ganglioneuromas may have a clinical picture of chronic diarrhea, failure to thrive, skin rash, hypokalemia, persistent cough, and abdominal distention. The exact reason for these symptoms is unknown, although they are attributable to the tumor because they disappear after surgical removal of the mass.

ACUTE ADRENOCORTICAL INSUFFICIENCY

The acute form of adrenocortical insufficiency (adrenal crisis) may result from a number of causes during childhood. Although a rare disorder, some of the more common etiologic factors include hemorrhage into the gland from trauma, which may be caused by a prolonged, difficult labor; fulminating infections, such as meningococcemia, which result in hemorrhage and necrosis (Waterhouse-Friderichsen syndrome); abrupt withdrawal of exogenous sources of cortisone or failure to increase exogenous supplies during stress; or as a result of congenital adrenogenital hyperplasia of the salt-losing type.

Clinical Manifestations

Early symptoms of adrenocortical insufficiency include increased irritability, headache, diffuse abdominal pain, weakness, nausea and vomiting, and diarrhea. Generalized hemorrhagic manifestations are present in the Waterhouse-Friderichsen syndrome. Fever increases as the condition worsens and is accompanied by signs of central nervous system involvement, such as nuchal rigidity, convulsions, stupor, and coma. The child is in a shocklike state with a weak, rapid pulse, decreased blood pressure, shallow respirations, cold clammy skin, and cyanosis. Circulatory collapse is the terminal event.

In the newborn, adrenal crisis is accompanied by extreme hyperpyrexia, tachypnea, cyanosis, and convulsions. Usually there is no evidence of infection or purpura. However, hemorrhage into the adrenal gland may be evident as a palpable retroperitoneal mass.

Diagnostic Evaluation

There is no rapid, definitive test for confirmation of acute adrenocortical insufficiency. Routine procedures such as measurement of plasma cortisol levels are too time-consuming to be practical. Therefore diagnosis is usually made based on clinical presentation, especially when a fulminating sepsis is accompanied by hemorrhagic manifestations and signs of circulatory collapse despite adequate antibiotic therapy. Since there is no real danger in administering a cortisol preparation for a short period, treatment should be instituted immediately. Improvement with this therapy confirms the diagnosis.

Therapeutic Management

Treatment involves replacement of cortisol, replacement of body fluids to combat dehydration and hypovolemia, administration of glucose solutions to correct hypoglycemia, and specific antibiotic therapy in the presence of infection. Initially, intravenous hydrocortisone (Solu-Cortef) is administered. Normal saline containing 5% glucose is given parenterally to replace lost fluid, electrolytes, and glucose. If hemorrhage has been severe, whole blood may be replaced. In the event that these measures do not reverse the circulatory collapse, vasopressors are used for immediate vasoconstriction and elevation of blood pressure.

Once the child's condition is stabilized, oral doses of cortisone, fluids, and salt are given, similar to the regimen used for chronic adrenal insufficiency. To maintain sodium retention, aldosterone is replaced by synthetic salt-retaining steroids.

Nursing Considerations

Because of the abrupt onset and potentially fatal outcome of this condition, prompt recognition is essential. Vital signs and blood pressure are taken every 15 minutes to monitor the hyperpyrexia and shocklike state. Seizure precautions are instituted, since convulsions from the elevated temperature are not uncommon. As soon as therapy is instituted, the nurse should monitor the child's response to fluid and cortisol replacement. Too rapid administration of fluids can precipitate cardiac failure, whereas overdosage with cortisol produces hypotension and a sudden fall in temperature. The nurse should regulate intravenous infusions carefully to guard against too rapid administration of drugs. Intake and urinary output are recorded.

Once the acute phase is over and the hypovolemia is corrected, the child is given oral fluids, such as small quantities of ginger ale, fruit juice, or salted broth. Too rapid ingestion of oral fluids may induce vomiting, which increases dehydration. Therefore the nurse should plan a gradual schedule for reintroducing liquids. For children who refuse to drink, the prospect of having the intravenous infusion removed once oral fluids are increased is often a motivating factor.

An ascending flaccid paralysis may occur on the second to third day of treatment because of an abnormally low serum potassium level secondary to overtreatment with cortisol and sodium chloride. The nurse should observe for signs of hypokalemia, such as cardiac irregularities and poor muscle control, and should evaluate serum electrolyte levels. The condition is rapidly corrected with intravenous and oral potassium replacement.

➤ **NURSING TIP** When an oral potassium preparation is given, it should be mixed with a small amount of strongly flavored fruit juice to disguise its bitter taste.

The sudden, severe nature of this disorder necessitates a great deal of emotional support for the child and family. The child may be placed in an intensive care unit where the surroundings are strange and frightening. Despite the need for emergency intervention, the nurse must be sensitive to the family's psychologic needs and prepare them for each procedure, even if this is as brief as a statement, such as "The intravenous infusion is necessary to replace fluid that the child is losing." Since recovery within 24 hours is often dramatic, the nurse should keep the parents apprised of the child's condition, emphasizing signs of improvement such as a lowered temperature and elevated blood pressure. If paralysis occurs, the nurse should assure them that this condition is temporary and quickly reversed.

If treatment needs to be continued past the acute stage, parents require the same preparation as those of children with chronic adrenal insufficiency. Preparation for discharge should begin as soon as possible after the child's condition has stabilized.

CHRONIC ADRENOCORTICAL INSUFFICIENCY (ADDISON DISEASE)

Chronic adrenocortical insufficiency is rare in children. When it does occur, it is usually caused by a destructive lesion of the adrenal glands, neoplasms, or an idiopathic cause. At one time generalized tuberculosis was the leading cause of adrenal gland destruction.

Evidence of this disorder is usually gradual in onset, since 90% of adrenal tissue must be nonfunctional before signs of insufficiency are manifested. However, during pe-

CARDINAL SIGNS OF CHRONIC ADRENOCORTICAL INSUFFICIENCY

Muscle weakness and mental fatigue, which are aggravated by slight additional exertion or minor illness
Pigmentary changes of previous scars, palmar creases, mucous membranes, and hair; hyperpigmentation over pressure points (elbows, knees, or waist); or, less frequently, loss of pigmentation (vitiligo)
Weight loss resulting from dehydration and anorexia from impaired gastrointestinal functioning (decreased hydrochloric acid)
Hypotension and small heart size, which predispose the child to dizziness and syncopal (fainting) attacks
Irritability, apathy, and negativism
Signs of hypoglycemia, such as headache, hunger, weakness, trembling, and sweating; other signs seen in some children are recurrent, unexplained convulsions; an intense craving for salt; and acute abdominal pain

riods of stress when demands for additional cortisol are increased, symptoms of acute insufficiency may appear in a previously well child. The cardinal signs and symptoms are listed in the box above.

Definitive diagnosis is based on measurements of functional cortisol reserve. The cortisol and urinary 17-hydroxycorticosteroid levels are low and fail to rise while plasma ACTH levels are elevated with corticotropin (ACTH) stimulation, the definitive test for the disease.

Therapeutic Management

Treatment involves replacement of glucocorticoids (cortisol) and mineralocorticoids (aldosterone). Some children are able to be maintained solely on oral supplements of cortisol (cortisone or hydrocortisone preparations) with a liberal intake of salt. During stressful situations, such as infection, emotional upset, or surgery, the dosage must be tripled to accommodate the body's increased need for glucocorticoids. Failure to meet this requirement will precipitate an acute crisis. Overdosage produces appearance of cushingoid signs.

Children with more severe states of chronic adrenal insufficiency require mineralocorticoid replacement to maintain fluid and electrolyte balance. Other forms of therapy include monthly injections of desoxycorticosterone acetate or implantation of desoxycorticosterone acetate pellets subcutaneously every 9 to 12 months.

Nursing Considerations

Once the disorder is diagnosed, parents need guidance concerning drug therapy. They must be aware of the continuous need for cortisol replacement. Sudden termination of the drug because of inadequate supplies or inability to ingest the oral form because of vomiting places the child in danger of an acute adrenal crisis. Therefore parents should always have a spare supply of the medication in the home. Ideally, they will have a prefilled syringe of hydrocortisone in the home and be instructed in proper technique for intramuscular administration of the drug in case of a crisis.

ETIOLOGY OF CUSHING SYNDROME

Pituitary—Cushing syndrome with adrenal hyperplasia, usually attributed to an excess of ACTH
Adrenal—Cushing syndrome with hypersecretion of glucocorticoids, generally the result of adrenocortical neoplasms
Ectopic—Cushing syndrome with autonomous secretion of ACTH, most often caused by extrapituitary neoplasms
Iatrogenic—Cushing syndrome, frequently the result of administration of large amounts of exogenous corticosteroids
Food dependent—Inappropriate sensitivity of adrenal glands to normal postprandial increases in secretion of gastric inhibitory polypeptide (Bertagna, 1992)

As mentioned earlier, unnecessary administration of cortisone will not harm the child but, if needed, may be lifesaving. Any evidence of acute insufficiency should be reported to the practitioner immediately.

Parents also need to be aware of side effects of the drugs. Undesirable side effects of cortisone include gastric irritation, which is minimized by ingestion with food or the use of an antacid, increased excitability and sleeplessness, weight gain that may require dietary management to prevent obesity, and, rarely, behavioral changes, including depression or euphoria. Parents should be aware of signs of overdose (see Table 38-2) and report these to the practitioner. In addition, the drug has a very bitter taste, which creates a challenge for nurses and parents in its administration.

➤ **NURSING TIP** Taste the different preparations of cortisone, because some are less bitter than others. Although using the concentrated form means a smaller volume of liquid to ingest, this form is also the most bitter.

The side effects of mineralocorticoids are primarily caused by overdosage and include generalized edema, which is first noticed around the eyes; hypertension, which may cause headaches; cardiac arrhythmias; and signs of hypokalemia. The child should be evaluated periodically for evidence of excessive medication. Emphasizing the importance of routine follow-up care is a significant nursing responsibility.

Since the body cannot supply endogenous sources of cortical hormones during times of stress, the home environment should be stable and relatively unstressful. Parents need to be aware that during periods of emotional or physical crisis the child requires additional hormone replacement. The child should wear medical identification, such as a bracelet, to permit medical personnel to adjust requirements during emergency care.

CUSHING SYNDROME

Cushing syndrome is a characteristic group of manifestations caused by excessive circulating free cortisol. It can result from a variety of etiologies, which generally fall into one of five categories (see box above).

Cushing syndrome is uncommon in children. When

TABLE 38-2 Clinical Manifestations of Cushing Syndrome

SIGNS/SYMPTOMS	PHYSIOLOGIC CAUSE	SIGNS/SYMPTOMS	PHYSIOLOGIC CAUSE
Centripetal fat distribution Truncal obesity Supraclavicular fat pads Fat pads on neck and back ("buffalo hump") Rounded or "moon" face	Increased appetite and deposition of fat	Osteoporosis Compression fractures of vertebrae Kyphosis Backache Retarded linear growth (short stature)	Increased glomerular filtration rate and excretion of calcium and decreased absorption of calcium from intestinal tract Increased levels of cortisol interfere with the action of GH
Muscular wasting Thin extremities Pendulous abdomen Muscle weakness Thin skin and subcutaneous tissue Poor wound healing	Increased protein catabolism resulting in negative nitrogen balance	Hypercalciuria—renal calculi	
Increased susceptibility to infection Decreased inflammatory response	Decreased production and circulating levels of antibodies by lysis of fixed plasma cells and lymphocytes	Psychoses Irritability Insomnia Euphoria Depression Frank psychoses	Cause unknown
Excessive bruising Petechial hemorrhages	Capillary weakness resulting from loss of protein	Peptic ulcer	Increased production of hydrochloric acid and pepsin and decreased gastric mucus production
Facial plethora ("red cheeks") Reddish purple abdominal striae	Thin skin that allows capillary blood to be visible, increased color from polycythemia	Hyperglycemia Glycosuria	Increased gluconeogenesis by liver and decreased rate of glucose utilization by cells
Hypertension—arteriosclerosis	Increased salt and water retention (hypervolemia)	Latent or overt diabetes	Overstimulation of islets of Langerhans
Hypokalemia Alkalosis	Increased excretion of potassium and hydrogen ions	Virilization Hirsutism Acne Deepening of voice Clitoral enlargement Tendency toward male physique in female Amenorrhea Impotence	Excess production of androgens

seen, it is often caused by excessive or prolonged steroid therapy that produces a cushingoid appearance. This condition is reversible once the steroids are gradually discontinued. Abrupt withdrawal will precipitate acute adrenal insufficiency. Gradual withdrawal of exogenous supplies is necessary to allow the anterior pituitary an opportunity to secrete increasing amounts of ACTH to stimulate the adrenals to produce cortisol.

Clinical Manifestations

Because the actions of cortisol are widespread, clinical manifestations are equally profound and diverse (Table 38-2 and Fig. 38-3). Those symptoms that produce changes in physical appearance occur early in the disorder and are of considerable concern to older children. The physiologic disturbances, such as hyperglycemia, susceptibility to infection, hypertension, and hypokalemia, may have life-threatening consequences unless recognized early and treated successfully. Children with short stature may be responding to increased cortisol levels, resulting in Cushing syndrome. Cortisol inhibits the action of GH.

Diagnostic Evaluation

Several tests are helpful in confirming excess cortisol levels. They include fasting blood glucose levels for hyperglycemia, serum electrolyte levels for hypokalemia and alkalosis, 24-hour urinary levels of elevated 17-hydroxycorticoids and 17-ketosteroids, and radiographic studies of bone for evidence of osteoporosis and of the skull for enlargement of the sella turcica. Another procedure used to establish a more definitive diagnosis is the dexamethasone (cortisone) suppression test. Administration of an exogenous supply of cortisone normally suppresses adrenocorticotropic hormone production. However, in individuals with Cushing syndrome, cortisol levels remain elevated. This test is helpful in differentiating between children who are obese and those who appear to have cushingoid features.

Therapeutic Management

Treatment depends on the cause. In most cases surgical intervention involves bilateral adrenalectomy and postoperative replacement of the cortical hormones (the therapy for this is the same as that outlined for chronic adrenal insuf-

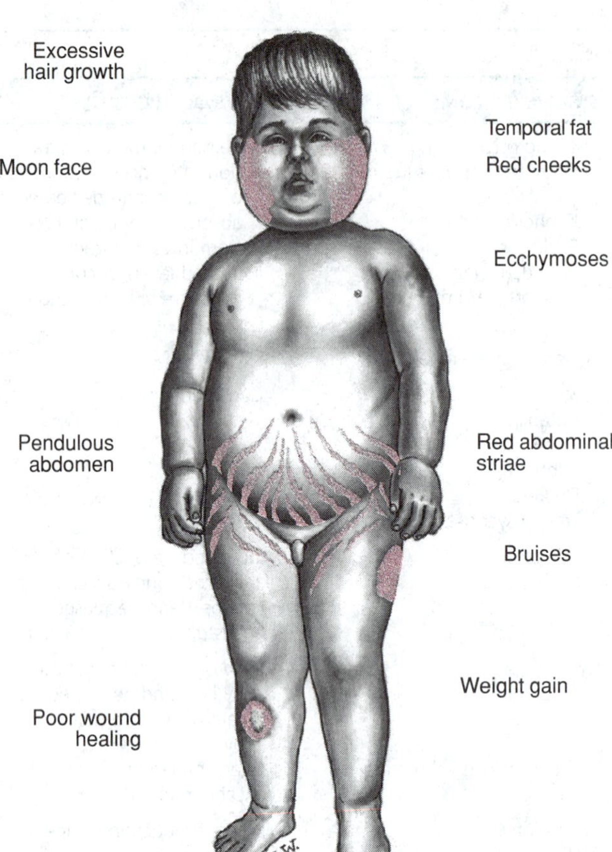

FIG. 38-3 Characteristics of Cushing syndrome.

ficiency). If a pituitary tumor is found, surgical extirpation or irradiation may be chosen. In either of these instances, treatment of panhypopituitarism with replacement of growth hormone, thyroid extract, antidiuretic hormone, gonadotropins, and steroids may be necessary for an indefinite period.

Nursing Considerations

Nursing care also depends on the cause. When cushingoid features are caused by steroid therapy, the effects may be lessened with administration of the drug early in the morning and on an alternate-day basis. Giving the drug early in the day maintains the normal diurnal pattern of cortisol secretion. If given during the evening, it is more likely to produce symptoms because endogenous cortisol levels are already low and the additional supply exerts more pronounced effects. An alternate-day schedule allows the anterior pituitary an opportunity to maintain more normal hypothalamic-pituitary-adrenal control mechanisms.

If an organic cause is found, nursing care is related to the treatment regimen. Although a bilateral adrenalectomy permanently solves one condition, it reciprocally produces another syndrome. Before surgery, parents need to be adequately informed of the operative benefits and disadvantages. Postoperative teaching regarding drug replacement is the same as discussed in the previous section.

Postoperative complications of adrenalectomy are related to the sudden withdrawal of cortisol. The nurse should observe for signs of a shocklike state, especially hypotension and hyperpyrexia. Anorexia and nausea and vomiting are very common and may be improved with the use of nasogastric decompression. Muscle and joint pain may be severe, requiring use of analgesics. The psychologic depression can be profound and may not improve for months. Parents should be aware of the physiologic reasons behind these symptoms in order to be supportive of the child. Facial changes that occur rapidly often help to improve family members' disposition but may not affect the child's behavior until the child's physiologic state is stabilized.

CONGENITAL ADRENOGENITAL HYPERPLASIA (CAH)

Disorders caused by excessive secretion of androgens by the adrenal cortex are known variously as ***congenital adrenogenital hyperplasia (CAH), adrenocortical hyperplasia (ACH), adrenogenital syndrome (AGS),*** and ***congenital adrenocortical hyperplasia.*** Although hyperfunction of the adrenal gland can occur from a number of causes, such as a virilizing adrenal tumor, in children the most common cause is congenital adrenogenital hyperplasia, an inborn deficiency of various enzymes necessary for the biosynthesis of cortisol. CAH is inherited as an autosomal-recessive disorder or may result from a tumor or maternal ingestion of steroids. The overall incidence of classical 21 hydroxylase deficiency CAH has been reported to be 1:5000 to 1:15,000 live births with males and females equally affected (Drucker and New, 1987).

Pathophysiology

Interference in the biosynthesis of cortisol during fetal life results in an increased production of ACTH, which stimulates hyperplasia of the adrenal gland. Depending on the enzymatic defect, increased quantities of cortisol precursors and androgens are secreted. There are six major types of biochemical defects. The most common is partial or complete ***21-hydroxylase deficiency.*** With partial deficiency, enough aldosterone is produced to preserve sodium, and adequate cortisol is produced to prevent signs of adrenocortical insufficiency.

In the complete or salt-losing form, insufficient amounts of aldosterone and cortisol are produced. If salt-losing CAH is not diagnosed and treated at birth, infants will exhibit symptoms of failure to thrive, weakness, vomiting, and dehydration, and a salt-losing crisis will ensue (Ruble, 1992). In ***11-hydroxylase deficiency*** there is an increase in the mineralocorticoid 11-desoxycorticosterone, which leads to hypertension. In each of these types there is excess production of androgens, which causes ambiguous female genitalia in females and precocious genital development in males. Other forms of congenital adrenogenital hyperplasia do not result in excess production of androgens but cause various degrees of hypoaldosteronism or hyperaldosteronism.

Clinical Manifestations

Excessive androgens cause masculinization of the urogenital system at approximately the tenth week of fetal development. The most pronounced abnormalities occur in the female, who is born with varying degrees of ambiguous genitalia ***(pseudohermaphroditism).*** Masculinization of external genitalia causes the clitoris to enlarge so that it appears as a small phallus. Fusion of the labia produces a saclike structure resembling the scrotum without testes. However, no abnormal changes occur in the internal sexual organs, although the vaginal orifice is usually closed by the fused labia. (See also Abnormal Sexual Development, Chapter 11.) The label ***ambiguous genitalia*** should be applied to any infant with hypospadias or micropenis and no palpable gonads, and a diagnostic evaluation for CAH should be contemplated.

In the male, enlargement of the genitals (macrogenitosomia precox) and frequent erections, as well as mildly increased genital pigmentation (Ruble, 1992), are the principal signs. When androgen production is not excessive, virilizing effects in the female may be minimal or absent, and the male may have evidence of pseudohermaphroditism, such as microphallus, hypospadias, and incompletely fused scrotum.

Untreated congenital adrenogenital hyperplasia results in early sexual maturation, with enlargement of the external sexual organs; development of axillary, pubic, and facial hair; deepening of the voice; acne; and marked increase in musculature with changes toward an adult male physique. However, in contrast to precocious puberty, breasts do not develop in the female, and she remains amenorrheic and infertile. In the male the testes remain small, and spermatogenesis does not occur. In both sexes linear growth is accelerated, and epiphyseal closure is premature, resulting in short stature by the end of puberty.

Diagnostic Evaluation

Clinical diagnosis is initially based on congenital abnormalities that lead to difficulty in assigning sex to the newborn and on signs and symptoms of adrenal insufficiency or hypertension. Definitive diagnosis is confirmed by evidence of increased 17-ketosteroid levels in most types of congenital adrenogenital hyperplasia. Usually the level of 17-hydroxycorticoids is low or near normal. In complete 21-hydroxylase deficiency, blood electrolytes demonstrate loss of sodium and chloride and elevation of potassium. In older children bone age is advanced, and linear growth is increased. Chromosome typing for positive sex determination and to rule out any other genetic abnormality (e.g., Turner syndrome) is always done in any case of ambiguous genitalia.

Another test that can be used to visualize the presence of pelvic structures is ultrasonography, a noninvasive, painless imaging technique that does not require anesthesia or sedation. It is especially useful in congenital adrenogenital hyperplasia because it readily identifies the absence or presence of female reproductive organs in a newborn or child with ambiguous genitalia. Because ultrasonography yields immediate results, it has the advantage of determining the child's gender long before the more complex laboratory results for chromosome analysis or steroid levels are available.

Therapeutic Management

The initial medical objective is to confirm the diagnosis and assign a sex to the child, usually according to the genotype. In both sexes cortisone is administered to suppress the abnormally high secretions of ACTH. If this is begun early enough, it is very effective. Cortisone depresses the secretion of ACTH by the adenohypophysis, which in turn inhibits the secretion of adrenocorticosteroids, which stems the progressive virilization. The signs and symptoms of masculinization in the female gradually disappear, and excessive early linear growth is slowed. Puberty occurs normally at the appropriate age.

The recommended oral dosage is divided to simulate the normal diurnal pattern of ACTH secretion. Since these children are unable to produce cortisol in response to stress, it is necessary to increase the dosage during episodes of infection, fever, or other stresses. Acute emergencies require immediate intravenous or intramuscular administration. Emergency situations include bacterial and viral infections, vomiting, surgery, fractures, major injuries, and sometimes insect stings.

Children with the salt-losing type of CAH require aldosterone replacement, as outlined under chronic adrenal insufficiency, and supplementary dietary salt. Frequent laboratory tests are conducted to assess the effects on electrolytes, hormonal profiles, and renin levels. The frequency of testing is individualized to the child.

Depending on the degree of masculinization in the female, reconstructive surgery may be required to reduce the size of the clitoris, separate the labia, and create a vaginal orifice. Surgery is performed when the infant is physically able to withstand the procedure but before she is old enough to be aware of the abnormal genitalia. Plastic surgery is generally done in stages and yields excellent cosmetic results. Reports concerning sexual satisfaction after partial clitoridectomy indicate that the capacity for orgasm and sexual gratification is not necessarily impaired.

Unfortunately, not all children with congenital adrenogenital hyperplasia are diagnosed at birth and raised in accordance with their genetic sex. Particularly in the case of affected females, masculinization of the external genitalia may have led to sex assignment as a male. In males diagnosis is usually delayed until early childhood, when signs of virilism appear. In these situations it is advisable to continue rearing the child as a male in accordance with assigned sex and phenotype. Hormonal replacement may be required to permit linear growth and to initiate male pubertal changes. Surgery is usually indicated to remove the female organs and reconstruct the phallus for satisfactory sexual relations. These individuals are not fertile.

Nursing Considerations

Of major importance is recognition of ambiguous genitalia in newborns. If there is any question regarding assignment of sex, the parents need to be told immediately to prevent the embarrassing situation of informing family members of the child's sex and then having to change the announcement. As with any congenital defect, the parents require an adequate explanation of the condition and a period of time to grieve for the loss of perfection. In this instance they may also need to grieve for the loss of the desired-sex child. For example, the birth of a phenotypically male infant may fulfill their wish for a son. Knowledge of the child's actual sex may leave them disappointed. Such situations may also lead them to discuss the possibility of raising the child as a male despite the actual sex. This is a difficult question that requires thoughtful discussion among the parents and members of the health team.

In general, rearing the genetically female child as a female is preferred because of the success of surgical intervention and the satisfactory results with hormones in reversing virilism and providing a prospect of normal puberty and the ability to conceive. This is in contrast to the choice of rearing the child as a male, in which case the child is sterile and may never be able to function satisfactorily in heterosexual relationships. If the parents persist in their decision to assign a male sex to a genetically female child, a psychologic consultation should be requested to explore their motivations and ensure their understanding of the child's future consequences.

Parents need an explanation regarding this disorder that facilitates their explaining it to others. Before confirmation of the diagnosis and sex of the child, the nurse should refer to the infant as "child" or "baby" rather than "he" or "she" and definitely not "it." When referring to the external genitalia, it is preferable to refer to them as sex organs and to emphasize the similarity between the penis/clitoris and scrotum/labia during fetal development. In this way it can be explained that the sex organs were overdeveloped because of too much male hormone secretion. Using a correct vocabulary allows parents to explain the abnormalities to others in a straightforward manner, just as if the defect involved the heart or an extremity.

It is also important to stress that sex assignment and rearing depend on psychosocial influences, not on genetic sex hormone influences during fetal life. Parents often fear that the infant will retain "male behavioral characteristics" because of prenatal masculinization and will not be able to develop female characteristics. Using the word "hermaphrodite" often confuses parents because they interpret this term to mean that the child is "half male–half female." Since the prognosis for normal sexual development is excellent after early treatment, the nurse should foster identification with the child as one sex only. It is also beneficial to mention that ambiguous genitalia have no relationship with homosexual or bisexual activity later in life.

As soon as the sex is determined, parents should be informed of the findings and encouraged to choose an appropriate name, and the child should be identified as a male or female, with no reference to ambiguous sex. If the appearance of the enlarged genitalia in a female child concerns the parents, they should be encouraged to discuss their feelings. Suggesting ways to avoid questioning remarks from visitors, such as diapering the child in a separate room, is also helpful. If surgery is anticipated, showing parents before and after photographs of reconstruction helps to reinforce the expected cosmetic benefits.

Nursing considerations regarding cortisol and aldosterone replacement are the same as those that are discussed for chronic adrenocortical insufficiency. However, since parents may be overwhelmed with the diagnosis and obvious abnormalities at the time of birth, they may not hear all the discharge instructions regarding the medication schedule. A follow-up visit by a public health nurse may be desirable to ensure that parents understand and comply with the treatment regimen. Likewise, nurses in well-child facilities should assume responsibility for guidance and supervision regarding this aspect of care during each visit.

Since infants are especially prone to dehydration and salt-losing crises, parents need to be aware of signs of dehydration and the urgency of immediate medical intervention to stabilize the child's condition. Parents should have injectable hydrocortisone available and know how to prepare and administer the intramuscular injection. Parents, and later the child, need to understand that the medical regimen must be a lifelong commitment; therefore they should be provided with the education and counseling that is most likely to ensure informed and willing compliance. They also need to know that growth retardation that may have occurred before therapy cannot be overcome and the normal stature is not a realistic expectation, even though growth velocity may improve with medication. The parents are also taught to give necessary injections (see Chapter 27).*

NURSING ALERT The parents should be advised that there is no physical harm in treating for suspected adrenal insufficiency that is not present, whereas the consequence of not treating acute adrenal insufficiency can be fatal (Ruble, 1992).

In the unfortunate situation in which the sex is erroneously assigned and the correct sex determined later, parents need a great deal of help in understanding the reason for the incorrect sex identification and the options for sex reassignment and/or medical/surgical intervention. Since children become aware of their sexual identity by 18 months to 2 years of age, it is believed that any reassignment after this period can cause tremendous psychologic conflicts in the child. Therefore sex rearing should be continued as previously established with medical/surgical intervention as required.

A dilemma often arises, however, regarding what these children should know about their condition, especially gender identification. Because the knowledge that one has been reared opposite to the genetic gender can initiate profound psychologic problems, it is recommended that children not be told this fact but rather be given an explanation regarding their physical disabilities, such as infertility, and the need for hormone replacement and plastic surgery.

*Home care instructions are available in *Wong and Whaley's Clinical Manual of Pediatric Nursing* (Mosby).

Parents, in turn, must believe that these children have been raised according to their "true sex," which is absolutely honest, since sex is not solely a biologic entity but an expression of multiple environmental influences.

Since the hereditary form of adrenogenital hyperplasia is an autosomal-recessive disorder, parents should be referred for genetic counseling before conceiving another child. The nurse's role is to ensure that parents understand the probability of transmitting the trait or disorder with each pregnancy. Affected offspring also require genetic counseling, since both sexes are generally able to reproduce. (See Chapter 5 for recurrence risks and genetic counseling.)

HYPERALDOSTERONISM

Excessive secretion of aldosterone may be caused by an adrenal tumor or, in some types of adrenogenital syndromes, may be the result of enzymatic deficiency. The signs and symptoms are caused by increased sodium levels, water retention, and potassium loss. Hypervolemia causes hypertension and resultant headaches. Paradoxically, funduscopic changes resulting from increased blood pressure and edema from water retention are minimal. Hypokalemia results in muscular weakness, paresthesia, episodes of paralysis, and tetany and may be responsible for polyuria and consequent polydipsia.

The clinical diagnosis is suspected when there are findings of hypertension, hypokalemia, and polyuria that fail to respond to antidiuretic hormone administration. Renin and angiotensin titers are abnormally low. Urinary levels of 17-hydroxycorticosteroids and 17-ketosteroids are normal in primary hyperaldosteronism caused by an aldosterone-secreting tumor but are usually abnormal in adrenogenital syndrome.

Therapeutic Management

Temporary treatment of the disorder involves replacement of potassium and administration of spironolactone (Aldactone), a diuretic that blocks the effects of aldosterone, thereby promoting excretion of sodium and water while preserving potassium. Definitive treatment is similar to that for chronic adrenocortical insufficiency.

Nursing Considerations

An important nursing consideration is recognition of the syndrome, particularly in children who demonstrate high blood pressure. Other clues include bed-wetting, excessive thirst, and unexplained weakness. After the diagnosis, nursing care should be related to the treatment regimen. If diuretics are used, they should be administered in the morning to avoid accidents during the night. Children need unrestricted lavatory privileges at school. Potassium supplements should be mixed with fruit juice, such as grape juice, to increase their acceptability, and potassium-rich foods should be encouraged. Parents need to be aware of the signs of hypokalemia and hyperkalemia.

After an adrenalectomy, nursing care is similar to that for chronic adrenocortical insufficiency.

PHEOCHROMOCYTOMA

Pheochromocytoma is an adrenal tumor characterized by secretion of catecholamines. The tumor most commonly arises from the chromaffin cells of the adrenal medulla but may occur wherever these cells are found, such as along the paraganglia of the aorta or thoracolumbar sympathetic chain. Approximately 10% of these tumors are located in extraadrenal sites. In children they are frequently bilateral or multiple and are generally benign. Often there is a familial transmission of the condition as an autosomal-dominant trait that tends to favor males.

Clinical Manifestations

The clinical manifestations of pheochromocytoma are caused by an increased production of catecholamines, producing hypertension, tachycardia, headache, decreased gastrointestinal activity with resultant constipation, increased metabolism with anorexia, weight loss, hyperglycemia, polyuria, polydipsia, hyperventilation, nervousness, and diaphoresis. In severe cases signs of congestive heart failure are evident.

Diagnostic Evaluation

The clinical manifestations mimic those of other disorders, such as hyperthyroidism, diabetes mellitus, or functional hyperventilation. Therefore several tests specific to these conditions may be performed as part of the differential diagnosis. In only a small number of instances is a palpable tumor suggestive of the diagnosis. Definitive tests include measurement of urinary levels of the catecholamine metabolites, histamine stimulation, which will provoke a hypertensive attack from sudden release of large amounts of catecholamines, and alpha-blocking agents, which will produce a hypotensive episode by inhibiting the action of circulating catecholamines.

Therapeutic Management

Definitive treatment consists of surgical removal of the tumor. In children the tumors may be bilateral, requiring a bilateral adrenalectomy and lifelong glucocorticoid and mineralocorticoid therapy. The major complications that can occur during surgery are severe hypertension, tachyarrhythmias, and hypotension. The first two are caused be excessive release of catecholamines during manipulation of the tumor, and the latter from catecholamine withdrawal and hypovolemic shock.

Preoperative preparation is implemented beginning 1 to 3 weeks before surgery to prevent these complications. This consists of medication to inhibit the effects of catecholamines. The major group of drugs used is the α-adrenergic blocking agents with or without β-adrenergic blocking agents. The most commonly used α-adrenergic blocker is phenoxybenzamine (Dibenzyline), a longer-acting medication given orally every 12 hours. The shorter-acting phentolamine (Regitine) is equally effective but less satisfactory for long-term use, although it is useful for acute hypertension. To control catecholamine release when α-adrenergic blocking agents are inadequate, the child is given β-adrenergic blocking agents.

Success of therapy is judged by lowering of blood pressure to normal, absence of hypertensive attacks (flushing or blanching, fainting, headache, palpitations, tachycardia, nausea and vomiting, profuse sweating), decrease in perspiration, and disappearance of hyperglycemia. A disadvantage of these drugs is their inability to block the effects of catecholamines on beta-receptors.

Nursing Considerations

An initial nursing objective is identification of children with this disorder. Outstanding clues are hypertension and hypertensive attacks. Because of behavioral changes (nervousness, excitability, overactivity, even psychosis), increased cardiac and respiratory activity may appear to be related to an acute anxiety attack. Therefore a careful history of the onset of symptoms and association with stressful events is helpful in distinguishing between an organic and a psychologic cause for the symptoms.

Preoperative nursing care involves frequent monitoring of vital signs and observing for evidence of hypertensive attacks and congestive heart failure. Therapeutic effects are evidenced by normal vital signs and absence of glycosuria. Daily blood glucose levels, urine acetone, and any signs of hyperglycemia are noted and reported immediately.

> **NURSING ALERT** Preoperative palpation of the mass may facilitate release of catecholamines, which can stimulate severe hypertension and tachyarrythmias.

The environment is made conducive to rest and free of emotional stress. This requires adequate preparation during hospital admission and before surgery. Parents are encouraged to room-in with their child and to participate in daily care. Play activities need to be tailored to the child's energy level but not be overly strenuous or challenging, since these can increase metabolic rate and promote frustration and anxiety.

After surgery the child is usually admitted to the PICU for 2 to 3 days postoperatively to observe and monitor for signs of shock from removal of excess catecholamines. If a bilateral adrenalectomy was performed, the nursing interventions are those discussed for chronic adrenocortical insufficiency.

DISORDERS OF PANCREATIC HORMONE SECRETION

The ***islets of Langerhans*** of the pancreas have three major functioning cells: the ***alpha cells,*** which produce glucagon, the ***beta cells,*** which produce insulin, and the ***delta cells,*** which produce somatostatin. ***Glucagon*** causes an increase in the blood glucose by stimulating the liver and other cells to release stored glucose ***(glycogenolysis).*** Glucagon acts as an emergency supplier of glucose whenever the blood glucose falls too low and is believed to function more independently when insulin is lacking. ***Somatostatin,*** although secreted by the islet cells, is found in greater supply in the hypothalamus, where it prevents the release of growth hormone. In the islets of Langerhans somatostatin is believed to regulate the release of insulin and glucagon. This discussion of disorders of pancreatic hormone secretion is limited to diabetes mellitus.

DIABETES MELLITUS (DM)

DM is a chronic disorder of metabolism characterized by a deficiency (relative or absolute) of the hormone insulin. It is the most common metabolic disease, resulting in metabolic adjustment or physiologic change in almost all areas of the body. DM affects approximately 10 to 13 million persons in the United States, and although estimates of prevalence in the United States vary, most sources report a rate of 20 per 100,000 children and adolescents (Plotnick, 1990).

The disease in children, which can occur from infancy through age 30 years, has a peak incidence between age 10 and 15 years, with 75% diagnosed before 18 years of age. The incidence in boys is slightly higher than in girls (1:1 to 1.2:1).

Insulin-dependent DM (IDDM) is more prominent in whites, with an incidence of 20 per 100,000; the incidence in blacks is 73% of that of whites, or 11.8 per 100,000; the incidence in Hispanics is 9.7 per 100,000; and the incidence in Cubans is 2.6 per 100,000. Native Americans tend to exhibit non-insulin-dependent DM (NIDDM) rather than IDDM, even when diagnosed in childhood. The Pima Tribe reports a 55+% incidence of NIDDM (Kahn and Weir, 1994).

Classification

DM can be classified as *idiopathic* or *secondary*. ***Secondary DM*** can be precipitated by exogenous factors and is usually (but not always) reversible when the primary disorder is treated. These include pancreatic trauma, disease (cystic fibrosis, carcinoma), or resection; hormones (Cushing syndrome, primary aldosteronism, pheochromocytoma), drugs or chemicals (some diuretics, hormones, psychoactive agents, catecholamines, antineoplastic agents); insulin receptor abnormalities; and a variety of genetic syndromes that are associated with glucose intolerance or frank diabetes. Gesta-

CLASSIFICATION OF DIABETES MELLITUS

Insulin-dependent (IDDM), or type I—Characterized by catabolism and the development of ketosis in the absence of insulin replacement therapy; onset is typically in childhood and adolescence but can be at any age

Non-insulin-dependent (NIDDM), or type II—Appears to involve resistance to insulin action and defective glucose-mediated insulin secretion; onset is usually after age 40, and there appears to be considerable heterogeneity; affected persons may or may not require daily insulin injections

Maturity-onset diabetes of youth (MODY)—Transmitted as an autosomal dominant disorder in which there is formation of structurally abnormal insulin that has decreased biologic activity

tional diabetes is the appearance of DM or abnormalities of glucose tolerance for the first time during pregnancy.

Idiopathic DM can be classified into three major groups (see box on p. 1764), and characteristics of IDDM and NIDDM are outlined in Table 38-3. Because DM of childhood is, with few exceptions, the IDDM, or type I form, the remainder of the discussion is devoted to this important cause of long-term health problems. However, NIDDM is included as appropriate for comparison throughout.

Etiology

The clinical syndrome of DM results from a large variety of etiologic and pathogenic mechanisms. IDDM is an autoimmune disease that arises when a person with a genetic predisposition is exposed to a precipitating event. In the past, viral infections have been implicated, whereas current investigators are focusing on the role of diet as a precipitating event. NIDDM is more likely to be influenced by stronger, but as yet unknown, genetic factors. Thus its origin is considered to be polygenic.

Genetic Factors. IDDM is not inherited, but heredity is unquestioned as a prominent factor in the etiology. There are more than 40 rare genetic syndromes of which diabetes is a major feature (Nora and Fraser, 1989). No simple mendelian pattern is found for DM. Children born to fathers with IDDM are about three times more likely to develop IDDM (approximately 7% frequency) than children born to mothers with IDDM (approximately 2% frequency).

The genetic influence in NIDDM and IDDM appears to differ in several ways. Studies have shown that certain class I HLA-B alleles (B8 and B15) are associated with IDDM. Class II MHC typing using cellular reagents has implicated DW3 and DW4 alleles in approximately 95% of subjects with IDDM and in approximately 50% of controls. Heterozygosity for DR3 and DR4 alleles is present in approximately 40% of subjects with IDDM and in only 3% of controls. DR1 is an additional susceptibility allele in subjects carrying either DR3 or DR4 alleles, whereas DR2 and DR5 alleles protect against IDDM. DR7 may also be a risk allele in blacks, whereas DR9 appears to replace DR3 as a risk allele in the Japanese (Winters, Chihara, and Schatz, 1993). Studies of NIDDM in identical twins demonstrate a 100% concordance throughout the life span, whereas identical studies of IDDM in identical twins demonstrate a 30% to 50% concordance rate, suggesting that both environmental and genetic factors are important in the genesis of IDDM (Winters, Chihara, and Schatz, 1993).

Autoimmune Mechanisms. It is now accepted that antibodies to some aspect of islet tissue are regularly present at the time of diagnosis of IDDM. Pancreatic islet cell antibodies (ICAs) are found in about 70% to 85% of patients newly diagnosed with IDDM (Drash, 1989). The antibodies

TABLE 38-3 Comparison of Characteristics of Types I and II Diabetes Mellitus

CHARACTERISTIC	TYPE I (IDDM)	TYPE II (NIDDM)
Age at onset	Less than 20 years	Over 30 years
Type of onset	Abrupt	Gradual
Sex ratio	Males slightly more than females	Females outnumber males
Percentage of diabetic population	5%-8%	85%-90%
Heredity:		
Family history	Sometimes	Frequency
HLA	Associations	No associations
Twin concordance	25%-50%	90%-100%
Ethnic distribution	Primarily whites	Increased incidence in Native Americans and Hispanics
Presenting symptoms	Three Ps* common	May be related to long-term complications
Nutritional status	Underweight	Overweight
Insulin (natural):		
Pancreatic content	Usually 0	Over 50% normal
Serum insulin	Low to absent	High or low
Primary resistance	Minimum	Marked
Islet cell antibodies	80%-85%	Less than 5%
Metabolic control	Difficult	Usually easy
Stability	Unstable	Stable
Therapy:		
Insulin	Always	20%-30% of patients
Oral agents	Ineffective	Often effective
Diet only	Ineffective	Often effective
Chronic complications	Greater than 80%	Variable
Ketoacidosis	Common	Infrequent

*Polyuria, polydipsia, and polyphagia.

disappear by 1 year after diagnosis in most persons, but in some they may persist for years. The current theory is that the presence of the HLA genes causes a defect in the immune system that renders the possessor susceptible to a trigger event, which can be a dietary source, a virus, bacteria, or a chemical irritant. The predisposing factor initiates an autoimmune process that gradually destroys beta cells. Without beta cells no insulin can be produced. It is unclear whether the ICAs are a result of the inflammatory process or a significant aspect of the beta cell destruction. Controversy exists regarding whether the autoimmune response is primarily mediated by the lymphocyte response or the humoral (antibody) response or is a result of the two.

There is a strong association between IDDM and other autoimmune endocrine disorders. An increased incidence of other autoimmune endocrine disorders, such as thyroiditis and Addison disease, has been found in families of children with DR3-associated IDDM.

It has also been found that anti–islet cell antibodies are detected in a number of unaffected first-degree relatives of children with IDDM (Drash, 1989). These findings offer hope of identifying persons at risk for diabetes with the eventual possibility of screening and implementation of therapy.

Individuals genetically predisposed to IDDM may decrease their risk by avoiding specific environmental triggers or by being immunized against specific antigens (Winters, Chihara, and Schatz, 1993). Treatment with cyclosporine or other forms of immunosuppression has been suggested as an early intervention in the newly diagnosed person with IDDM. The effects of lifelong immunosuppression must be carefully weighed against the lifelong effects of diabetes.

Diet. Diet has been suggested as an environmental trigger in the onset of IDDM, more specifically the diabetogenic process (Winters, Chihara, and Schatz, 1993). Cow's milk has been implicated as a possible trigger of the autoimmune response that destroys pancreatic beta cells in genetically susceptible hosts, thus causing DM (Karjalainen and others, 1992).

Viruses. A variety of viruses have been implicated as the prime environmental factor in the etiology of DM. Islet cells appear to be particularly susceptible to either direct viral damage or chemical insult. The body reacts to this damaged or changed tissue in an autoimmune phenomenon. Therefore the virus serves as a precipitating factor or "trigger." A viral etiology also helps explain the seasonal variation in the onset of DM. Although this seasonal variation is not evident in children under 5 years of age, the marked increase in older children during the winter months strongly suggests an infectious disease relationship in either the etiology or expression of diabetes in children.

Type II Diabetes. Although IDDM is the predominant form of diabetes in the pediatric age-group, NIDDM, or type II diabetes, can also occur in children. NIDDM can be further classified as obese and nonobese, which are also subgrouped into those who require insulin and those who do not. The disturbed carbohydrate metabolism of NIDDM may be a result of a sluggish or insensitive secretory response in the pancreas or a defect in body tissues that requires unusual amounts of insulin, or it may be the case that the insulin secreted is rapidly destroyed, inhibited, or inactivated in affected persons. Native American children with diabetes invariably present with type II diabetes or NIDDM.

Pathophysiology

Insulin is needed to support the metabolism of carbohydrates, fats, and proteins, primarily by facilitating the entry of these substances into the cell. Insulin is needed for the entry of glucose into the muscle and fat cells, prevention of mobilization of fats from fat cells, and storage of glucose as glycogen in the cells of liver and muscle. Insulin is not needed for the entry of glucose into nerve cells or vascular tissue. The chemical composition and molecular structure of insulin are such that it fits into receptor sites on the cell membrane. Here it initiates a sequence of poorly defined chemical reactions that alter the cell membrane to facilitate the entry of glucose into the cell and stimulate enzymatic systems outside the cell that metabolize the glucose for energy production.

With a deficiency of insulin, glucose is unable to enter the cell, and its concentration in the bloodstream increases. The increased concentration of glucose ***(hyperglycemia)*** produces an osmotic gradient that causes the movement of body fluid from the intracellular space to the interstitial space then to the extracellular space and into the glomerular filtrate in order to "dilute" the hyperosmolar filtrate. Normally the renal tubular capacity to transport glucose is adequate to reabsorb all the glucose in the glomerular filtrate. When the glucose concentration in the glomerular filtrate exceeds the threshold (160 to 180 mg/dl), glucose "spills" into the urine along with an osmotic diversion of water ***(polyuria)***, a cardinal sign of diabetes. The urinary fluid losses cause the excessive thirst ***(polydipsia)*** observed in diabetes. As might be expected, this water washout results in a depletion of other essential chemicals, especially potassium.

Protein is also wasted during insulin deficiency. Since glucose is unable to enter the cells, protein is broken down and converted to glucose by the liver (glucogenesis); this glucose then contributes to the hyperglycemia. These mechanisms are similar to those seen in starvation when substrate (glucose) is absent. The body is actually in a state of starvation during insulin deficiency. Without the use of carbohydrates for energy, fat and protein stores are depleted as the body attempts to meet its energy needs. The hunger mechanism is triggered, but the increased food intake ***(polyphagia)*** enhances the problem by further elevating the blood glucose (Fig. 38-4).

Ketoacidosis. When insulin is absent or there is an altered insulin sensitivity, glucose is unavailable for cellular metabolism, and the body chooses alternate sources of energy, principally fat. Consequently, fats break down into fatty acids, and glycerol in the fat cells is converted by the liver to ketone bodies (β-hydroxybutyric acid, acetoacetic acid, acetone). Any excess is eliminated in the urine (ketonuria) or the lungs (acetone breath). The ketone bodies are strong acids that lower serum pH, producing ***ketacidosis.***

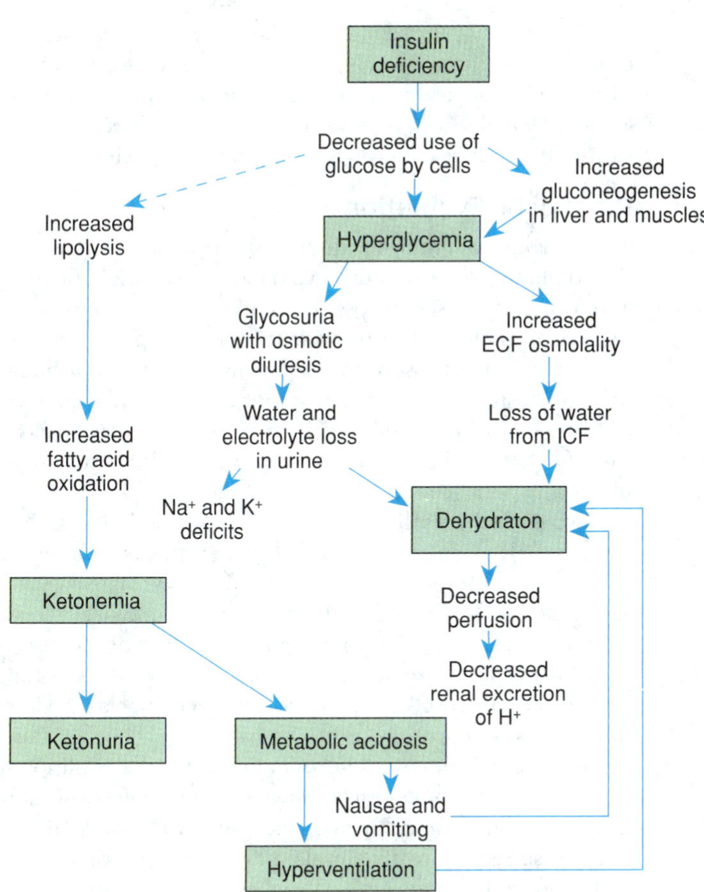

FIG. 38-4 Pathophysiology of acidosis in diabetes mellitus.

Ketones are organic acids that readily produce excessive quantities of free hydrogen ions, causing a fall in plasma pH. Then chemical buffers in the plasma, principally bicarbonate, combine with the hydrogen ions to form carbonic acid, which readily dissociates into water and carbon dioxide. The respiratory system attempts to eliminate the excess carbon dioxide by increased depth and rate—***Kussmaul respirations,*** or the hyperventilation characteristic of metabolic acidosis. The ketones are buffered by sodium and potassium in the plasma. The kidney attempts to compensate for the increased pH by increasing tubular secretion of hydrogen and ammonium ions in exchange for fixed base, thus depleting the base buffer concentration.

Potassium levels are also a problem and were once the cause of unexplained deaths shortly after insulin therapy was instituted. With cellular death, potassium is released from the cell into the bloodstream and excreted by the kidney where the loss is accelerated by the osmotic diuresis. The total body potassium is then decreased, even though the serum potassium level may be elevated as a result of the decreased fluid volume in which it circulates. Alteration in serum and tissue potassium can make cardiac arrest a potential problem.

If these conditions are not reversed by insulin therapy in combination with correction of the fluid deficiency and electrolyte imbalance, progressive deterioration occurs with dehydration, electrolyte imbalance, acidosis, coma, and death. Diabetic ketoacidosis should be diagnosed promptly in a seriously ill patient, and therapy instituted.

Long-term Complications. Long-term complications of diabetes involve both the microvasculature and macrovasculature. The principal microvascular complications are nephropathy, retinopathy, and neuropathy. Microvascular disease develops during the first 30 years of diabetes, beginning in the first 10 to 15 years after puberty, with renal involvement evidenced by proteinuria and clinically apparent retinopathy.

With poor diabetic control, vascular changes can appear as early as 2½ to 3 years after diagnosis; however, with good to excellent control, changes have been postponed for 20 or more years. Intensive insulin therapy appears to delay the onset and slow the progression of clinically important retinopathy, including vision-threatening lesions, nephropathy, and neuropathy, by 35% to more than 70%, according to the Diabetes Treatment and Complications in IDDM Trials (Nathan 1993).

The postpubertal duration, not the total duration, of IDDM is implicated as a risk factor for the development of microvascular disease (Rogers, 1992). The process appears to be one of ***glycosylation,*** wherein proteins from the blood become deposited in the walls of small vessels (e.g., glomeruli) where they become trapped by "sticky" glucose compounds (glycosyl radicals). The buildup of these substances over time causes narrowing of the vessels, with subsequent interference with microcirculation to the affected areas (Starkman and others, 1986). Macrovascular disease develops after 25 years of diabetes and creates the predominant problems in patients with NIDDM.

Other complications have been observed in children with IDDM. Hyperglycemia appears to influence thyroid function, and altered function is frequently observed at the time of diagnosis, as well as in poorly controlled diabetes. Limited mobility of small joints of the hand occurs in 30% of 7- to 18-year-old children with IDDM and appears to be related to changes in the skin and soft tissues surrounding the joint as a result of glycosylation.

Clinical Manifestations

The symptomatology of diabetes is more readily recognizable in children than in adults, so it is surprising that the diagnosis may sometimes be missed or delayed. Diabetes is a great imitator; influenza, gastroenteritis, and appendicitis are the conditions most often diagnosed, only to find that the disease was really diabetes. Diabetes should be suspected in those families with a strong family history of diabetes, especially if there is one child in the family with diabetes.

The sequence of chemical events described previously results in hyperglycemia and acidosis, which produce weight loss and the three "polys" of diabetes—polyphagia, polydipsia, and polyuria—the cardinal symptoms of the disease. In NIDDM (which can occur in older children and Native American children), the insulin values are found to be elevated, 80% to 90% of this population have been found to be overweight, and fatigue and frequent infections (such as monilial infections in females) are often present.

NURSING ALERT Recurrent vaginal and urinary tract infections, especially candidal infections, are often an early sign of IDDM, especially in adolescents.

The variability of clinical manifestations in IDDM at diagnosis is best understood if the autoimmune destruction of islet cells is considered an ongoing process. Symptoms of hyperglycemia may be apparent only during stress (such as an illness) in early stages of disease because of near normal levels of insulin production. Progressive islet cell destruction of later stages produces more obvious signs and symptoms. Eighty percent to 90% of islet cell function has been destroyed at the time of overt diabetic symptoms. Frequently identified symptoms of overt diabetes include enuresis, irritability, and unusual fatigue.

Abdominal discomfort is common. Weight loss, though quite observable on the charts, may be a less frequent presenting complaint because of the fact that the family might not have noticed the change. Another outstanding feature of diabetes is thirst. One couple reported that their child, during a trip from California to Kansas, drank the contents of a gallon jug of water between each gas station stop. As abdominal discomfort and nausea increase, the child may actually refuse fluid and food, adding to the increasing state of dehydration and malnutrition. Other symptoms include dry skin, blurred vision, and sores that are slow to heal. More commonly in children, fatigue and bed-wetting are the chief complaints that prompt parents to take their child for evaluation.

At diagnosis, the child may be ***hyperglycemic,*** with elevated blood glucose levels and glucose in the urine; ***ketotic,*** with ketones measurable in the blood and urine, with or without dehydration; or suffering from ***diabetic ketoacidosis,*** with dehydration, electrolyte imbalance, and acidosis.

Diagnostic Evaluation

Three groups of children who should be considered as possibly diabetic are (1) children who have glycosuria, polyuria, and a history of weight loss or failure to gain despite a voracious appetite; (2) those with transient or persistent glycosuria; and (3) those who display manifestations of metabolic acidosis, with or without stupor or coma. In every case diabetes must be considered if there is glycosuria, with or without ketonuria, in association with otherwise unexplained hyperglycemia.

Glycosuria by itself is not diagnostic of diabetes. Other sugars, such as galactose, can produce a positive Clinitest, and other conditions may cause a mild degree of glycosuria. These are infection, trauma, emotional or physical stress, hyperalimentation, and some renal or endocrine diseases.

A fasting blood sugar greater than 120 mg/dl or a random blood glucose of ≥200 accompanied by classic signs of diabetes is almost certain to be caused by diabetes. Postprandial blood glucose determinations and the traditional oral glucose tolerance tests have yielded low detection rates in children and are not usually necessary for establishing a diagnosis. Serum insulin levels may be normal or moderately elevated at the onset of diabetes; delayed insulin response to glucose indicates the presence of prediabetes.

Ketoacidosis must be differentiated from other causes of acidosis or coma, including hypoglycemia, uremia, gastroenteritis with metabolic acidosis, salicylate intoxication, encephalitis, and other intracranial lesions. Diabetic ketoacidosis has been defined as a state of relative insulin deficiency resulting in hyperglycemia (blood glucose ≥ to 300 mg/dl) and an accumulation of ketoacids in the blood with subsequent metabolic acidosis (pH <7.30; serum bicarbonate <15 mmol/L) (Chase, Garg, and Jelley, 1990).

Therapeutic Management

The management of the child with IDDM consists of a multidisciplinary approach involving the family, the child (when appropriate), and professionals, including a pediatric endocrinologist, diabetes nurse educator, and nutritionist, as well as an exercise physiologist. Often psychologic support from a mental health professional is also needed. Communication among the team members is essential and extends to other individuals in the child's life, such as teachers, the school nurse, school guidance counselor, and coach.

The definitive treatment is replacement of insulin that the child is unable to produce. However insulin needs are also affected by emotions, nutritional intake, activity, and other life events, such as illnesses and puberty. The complexity of the disease and its management requires that the child and family incorporate diabetes needs into their lifestyle. Medical and nutritional guidance are primary, but management also includes continuing diabetes education, family guidance, and emotional support.

Maturity-onset diabetes of youth (MODY), a form of type II diabetes with childhood onset, is usually seen in the obese teenager and can often be controlled with diet restriction.

Insulin Therapy. Insulin replacement is the cornerstone of management of IDDM. Insulin dosage is tailored to each child based on home blood glucose monitoring. The goal of insulin therapy is maintaining near-normal blood glucose values while avoiding too frequent episodes of hypoglycemia. Insulin is administered as two or more injections per day or as continuous subcutaneous infusion using a portable insulin pump.

Healthy pancreatic cells secrete insulin at a low but steady basal rate with superimposed bursts of increased secretion that coincide with intake of nutriments. Consequently, insulin levels in the blood increase and decrease coincidently with rises and falls in blood glucose levels. In addition, insulin is secreted directly into the portal circulation; therefore the liver, which is the major site of glucose disposal, receives the largest concentration of insulin. No matter which method of insulin replacement is used, this normal pattern cannot be duplicated. Subcutaneous injection results in absorption of the drug into the general circulation, thus reducing the concentrations of insulin to which the liver is exposed.

Insulin preparations. Insulin is available in highly purified beef, pork, and beef-pork preparations, and in human insulin biosynthesized by and extracted from bacterial cultures. Human and pork varieties are less allergenic than beef preparations, and the animal insulins are less expensive than the synthetic human insulins. Insulin is available in rapid-, intermediate-, and long-acting preparations, and all are packaged in the strength of 100 U/ml. Other concentrations, as well as premixed insulins, such as 70/30 and 60/40 ratios, are available when extraordinarily large or small dosages are required.

Dosage. Conventional control has consisted of a twice-daily insulin regimen consisting of a combination of rapid-acting (regular) and intermediate-acting (NPH or Lente) insulin drawn up into the same syringe and injected before breakfast and before the evening meal. The amount of morning regular insulin is determined by the previous day's late morning and lunchtime blood glucose values. The morning intermediate-acting dosage is determined by the previous day's late afternoon and supper blood glucose values. Hence, the morning blood glucose is controlled by the previous evening dose of intermediate insulin, and the bedtime blood glucose value determines the supper dosage of regular insulin. For some children, better morning glucose control is achieved by a later (bedtime) injection of intermediate-acting insulin.

Regular insulin is best administered at least 30 minutes before meals. This allows sufficient time for absorption and results in a significantly more reduced postprandial rise in blood glucose than if the meal were eaten immediately following the insulin injection. Intensive therapy consists of multiple injections throughout the day rather than the twice-daily regimen, that is, a once-daily dose of long-acting (Ultralente) insulin to simulate the basal insulin secretion and injections of rapid-acting insulin before each meal. A multiple daily injection (MDI) program has been shown to reduce microvascular complications of diabetes in young, healthy patients who have IDDM (Reasner, 1994).

The precise dose of insulin needed cannot be predicted. Therefore the total dosage and percentage of regular- to intermediate-acting insulin should be determined empirically for each child. Usually 60% to 75% of the total daily dose is given before breakfast, and the remainder before the evening meal. Furthermore, insulin requirements do not remain constant but change continuously during growth and development, and the need varies according to the child's activity level and pubertal status. For example, less insulin is required during the active spring and summer months. Illness also alters insulin requirements. Some children require more frequent insulin administration. This includes children with difficult-to-control diabetes and during the adolescent growth spurt.

Methods of administration. Daily insulin is administered subcutaneously by twice-daily injections, by multiple dose injections, or by means of a portable pump. The pump is an electromechanical device designed to deliver fixed amounts of a dilute solution of regular insulin continuously, thereby more closely imitating the release of the hormone by the islet cells. Humulin BR insulin is manufactured specifically for use with a pump.

The system consists of a syringe to hold the insulin, a plunger, and a mechanism to drive the plunger. The insulin flows from the syringe through a catheter to a needle inserted into subcutaneous tissue (the abdomen or thigh), and the lightweight device is worn on a belt or a shoulder holster. The needle and catheter are changed every 48 hours by the child or parent, using aseptic technique, and taped in place.

Although the pump provides more even insulin release, it has certain disadvantages. It cannot be removed for more than 1 hour, which limits some activities, such as bathing and swimming, although some water-safe models are now available. Like any other mechanical device, it may malfunction. Problems with abscess formation at the needle site and the need for more sophisticated control from the user have made this a rarely used option.

Researchers are experimenting with a new approach to insulin administration—intranasal. When insulin is combined with bile salts, the mixture can be administered by way of an aerosol pump. The insulin is able to cross the nasal mucosa to increase serum levels. The duration of action is not long enough to be a total replacement for injections but may be of value as insulin supplementation at mealtime. Patients are cautioned not to attempt to inhale standard insulin because it is not absorbed through the mucosa without an appropriate transport medium.

Monitoring. Monitoring the effectiveness of insulin therapy is a vital part of management. It is the only way in which to determine the amount of insulin needed by a child at any given time. Several measurements are used to evaluate the glucose levels as a basis for insulin administration and regulation.

Urine. Urine testing has been a mainstay of diabetic management in the past, but urine tests for glucose have many limitations. There is poor correlation between simultaneous glycosuria and blood glucose concentration the double-voided specimens may not accurately reflect the concurrent level of blood glucose. Glucose does not appear in the urine until the blood glucose concentration is well above the optimum range. However, urine testing for ketones remains a cornerstone of home management. It is recommended that urine be tested for ketones during an illness and whenever blood glucose is 240 mg/dl or higher when measured twice in a row 4 to 6 hours apart.

Blood glucose. Home blood glucose monitoring (HBGM) has improved diabetes management and is used successfully by children from the onset of their diabetes. By testing their own blood, children are able to change their insulin regimen to maintain their glucose level in the euglycemic range of 80 to 120 mg/dl. Diabetes management depends to a great extent on home glucose monitoring. In general, children tolerate the testing well.

Glycosylated hemoglobin. The measurement of glycosylated hemoglobin (hemoglobin A_{1c}) levels is a satisfactory method for assessing the control of the diabetic patient. As red blood cells circulate in the bloodstream, glucose molecules gradually attach to the hemoglobin A molecules and remain there for the lifetime of the red blood cell, approximately 120 days. The attachment is not reversible; therefore this glycosylated hemoglobin serves as a reflection of the average blood glucose levels that have taken place during the previous 2 to 3 months. The test is a satisfactory method for assessing control, detecting incorrect testing, monitoring effectiveness of changes in treatment, defining patients' goals, and detecting nonadherence.

Nutrition. Essentially the nutritional needs of children with diabetes are no different from those of healthy children, except for deletion of concentrated sugar. Children with diabetes need no special foods or supplements. They need sufficient calories to balance daily expenditure for energy and to satisfy the requirement for growth and development. Unlike the child without diabetes, whose insulin is secreted in response to food intake, insulin injected subcutaneously has a relatively predictable time of onset, peak effect, duration of action, and absorption rate depending on the type of insulin used. Consequently, the timing of food consumption must be regulated to correspond to the time and action of the insulin prescribed.

Meals and snacks must be eaten according to peak insulin action, and the total number of calories and proportions of basic nutrients must be consistent from day to day. The constant release of insulin into the circulation makes the child prone to hypoglycemia between the three daily meals unless a snack is provided between meals and at bedtime. The distribution of calories should be calculated to fit the activity pattern of each child. For example, a child who is more active in the afternoon will need the larger snack at that time. This larger snack might also be split to allow some food at school and some food after school. Alterations in food intake should be made so that food, insulin, and exercise are balanced. Extra food is needed for increased activity.

The food intake may be planned in a variety of ways but is based on a balanced diet that incorporates six basic food groups: milk, meat, vegetables, fat, fruit, and starch. The family may follow the exchange system approved by the American Diabetes Association (ADA) or the point system, based on 75 kcal equaling 1 point. The exchange system indicates the amount (portion size) of each food by volume or weight and is prescribed in terms of the number of exchanges from each food group that constitutes each meal and snack. The high carbohydrate–high fiber (HCF) approach is also based on exchange lists but divides foods into eight groups with emphases on fiber from food sources (Cooper, 1988). This ensures day-to-day consistency in total calories, protein, fat, and carbohydrate while allowing a choice from a wide variety of foods.

Concentrated sweets are eliminated, and because of the increased risk for atherosclerosis in persons with DM, fat is reduced to 30% or less of the total caloric requirement. Dietary fiber has become increasingly important in dietary planning because of its influence on digestion, absorption, and metabolism of many nutrients. It has been found to diminish the rise in blood sugar after meals.

Correctly used, the diet allows for flexibility and the incorporation of preferred foods in most instances. For the growing child, food restriction should never be used for diabetic control, although calorie restrictions may be imposed for weight control if the child is overweight. In general, the child's appetite should be the guide for the amount of calories needed, with the total calorie intake adjusted to appetite and activity. Basic principles of diet management are outlined in the box below.

Exercise. Exercise is encouraged and never restricted unless indicated by other health conditions. Exercise lowers blood sugar levels, depending on the intensity and duration of the activity. Consequently, exercise should be included as part of diabetic management, and the type and amount of exercise should be planned around the child's interests and capabilities. However, in most instances children's activities are unplanned, and the resulting decrease in blood sugar can be compensated for by providing extra snacks before (and, if prolonged, during) the activ-

NUTRITIONAL PRINCIPLES IN TYPE I DIABETES

1. Develop a basic daily meal plan that is relatively consistent in terms of:
   - Total energy (calorie) intake
   - Balance of energy-yielding nutrients (carbohydrates, fats, and proteins)
2. Provide for compensatory changes for nonbasal circumstances:
   - Extra food for extra activity (Do not overtreat)
   - Extra insulin or activity for extra food
3. Avoid hyperglycemia by:
   - Omitting rapidly absorbed simple sugars from regular meal planning
4. Avoid hypoglycemia by:
   - Reasonably consistent meal timing
   - Provision of snacks

From Skyler JS: Dietary planning in insulin-dependent diabetes mellitus, *Pediatr Ann* 12:652-657, 1983.

ity. Insulin should not be reduced unless the needed increase in food cannot be tolerated. In addition to a feeling of well-being, regular exercise aids in utilization of food and often results in a reduction of insulin requirements.

Physical training tends to increase tissue sensitivity to insulin, even in the resting state. Consequently, it is especially important to understand the relationship between the activity and the diabetic regimen. Vigorous muscular contraction increases regional blood flow and accelerates the absorption and circulation of insulin that is injected into the area, which can contribute to development of hypoglycemia. If exercise involving leg muscles is planned, it is recommended that nonexercised sites (arm or abdomen) should be used for insulin injection. This practice may replace the need for further increased carbohydrate intake or reduced insulin dose (or both) to avoid exercise-induced hypoglycemia.

Children with poorly controlled diabetes are particularly at risk for hypoglycemia with exercise or may actually stimulate ketoacid production. Therefore the child who has marked hyperglycemia (240 ng/dl or above) and ketonuria should be discouraged from strenuous physical activity until satisfactory control of the diabetes is achieved by appropriate adjustments of insulin and diet.

Athletes and those youngsters who regularly participate in organized sports are advised to adjust their insulin dosage in anticipation of sustained physical activity during the part of the day devoted to strenuous exercise. Team sports may encourage overexertion and subsequent hypoglycemia. For example, the morning dose of intermediate-acting insulin may need to be reduced to compensate for after-school sports activity. Optimum adjustments for each child are determined primarily by trial and error. Nutritional needs of the athlete are subject to those dietary needs discussed for sports participation in Chapter 39, as well as the diabetic dietary management.

Hypoglycemia. Occasional episodes of hypoglycemia are an integral part of insulin therapy, and an objective of diabetic management is to achieve the best possible glycemic control while minimizing the frequency and severity of hypoglycemia. Even with good control, a child may frequently experience mild symptoms of hypoglycemia. If the signs and symptoms are recognized early and promptly relieved by appropriate therapy, the child's activity should be interrupted for no more than a few minutes.

NURSING ALERT Children on split, mixed insulin dosage schedules tend to experience hypoglycemic episodes at 11:30 AM and 2:30 AM as peaking of insulin occurs.

The most common causes of hypoglycemia are bursts of physical activity without additional food, or delayed, omitted, or incompletely consumed meals. Reglycosylation of muscles may occur over the ensuing 24 hours. Particular vigilance related to hypoglycemia may be necessary during the night after vigorous exertion. Occasionally, hypoglycemic reactions occur unexpectedly and without apparent cause. They may be the result of an inadvertent or deliberate error in insulin administration.

Gastroenteritis, in which there is gastric stasis, may impede the absorption of food, even though the child is eating reasonably well. It can also occur when the blood glucose level is so low it causes stasis. Then the child may eat a meal or snack and still have an insulin reaction. Continued feeding does not seem to alter the blood glucose level, because the simple glucose or sugar remains in the stomach.

The signs and symptoms of hypoglycemia are caused by both increased adrenergic activity and impaired brain function. The increased adrenergic nervous system activity plus increased secretion of catecholamines produce nervousness, pallor, tremulousness, palpitations, sweating, and hunger. Weakness, dizziness, headache, drowsiness, irritability, loss of coordination, convulsions, and coma are more severe responses and reflect central nervous system glucose deprivation and the body's attempts to elevate the serum glucose levels (Fig. 38-5).

It is often difficult to distinguish between hyperglycemia and a hypoglycemic reaction (Table 38-4). Since the symptoms are similar and usually begin with changes in behavior, the simplest way to differentiate between the two is to test the blood glucose level. Blood glucose is low in hypoglycemia, whereas in hyperglycemia the glucose content will be significantly elevated. Urinary ketones may be present following hypoglycemia due to starvation ketone production. In doubtful situations it is safer to give the child some simple carbohydrate. This will help alleviate the symptoms in the case of hypoglycemia but will do little harm if the child is hyperglycemic.

Children are usually able to detect the onset of hypoglycemia, but some are too young to implement treatment. Parents should become adept at recognizing the onset of symptoms—for example, a change in a child's behavior such as tearfulness or euphoria. In the majority of cases, 10 to 15 g of simple carbohydrate, such as honey, will elevate the blood glucose level and alleviate the symptoms. The simpler the carbohydrate, the more rapidly it will be absorbed (8 oz milk = 15 g carbohydrate). The rapid-releasing sugar is followed by a complex carbohydrate such as a slice of

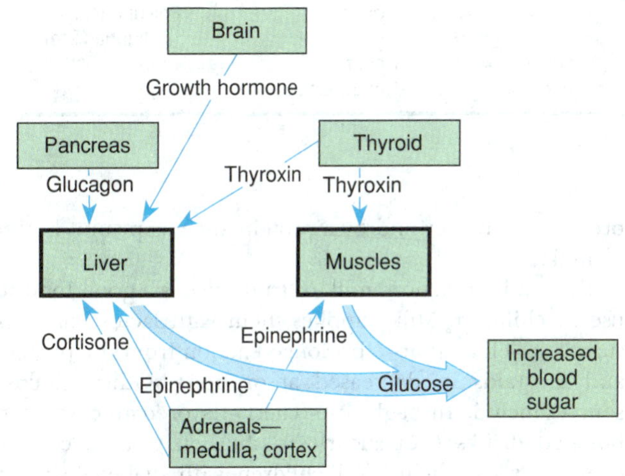

FIG. 38-5 Body systems respond to hypoglycemia in various ways to increase blood glucose level.

TABLE 38-4 Comparison of Manifestations of Hypoglycemia and Hyperglycemia

VARIABLE	HYPOGLYCEMIA	HYPERGLYCEMIA
Onset	Rapid (minutes)	Gradual (days)
Mood	Labile, irritable, nervous, weepy, combative	Lethargic
Mental status	Difficulty concentrating, speaking, focusing, coordinating	Dulled sensorium Confused
Inward feeling	Shaky feeling, hunger Headache Dizziness	Thirst Weakness Nausea/vomiting Abdominal pain
Skin	Pallor Sweating	Flushed Signs of dehydration
Mucous membranes	Normal	Dry, crusty
Respirations	Shallow	Deep, rapid (Kussmaul)
Pulse	Tachycardia	Less rapid, weak
Breath odor	Normal	Fruity, acetone
Neurologic	Tremors Late: hyperreflexia, dilated pupils, convulsion	Diminished reflexes Paresthesia
Ominous signs	Shock, coma	Acidosis, coma
Blood:		
Glucose	Low: below 60 mg/dl	High: 240 mg/dl or more
Ketones	Negative/trace	High/large
Osmolarity	Normal	High
pH	Normal	Low (7.25 or less)
Hematocrit	Normal	High
HCO_3	Normal	Less than 15 mEq/L
Urine:		
Output	Normal	Polyuria (early) to oliguria (late)
Sugar	Negative	High
Acetone	Negative/trace	High

bread or a cracker and by a protein such as peanut butter or milk.

For a mild reaction, milk or fruit juice is a good food to use in children. Milk supplies them with lactose or milk sugar, as well as a more prolonged action from the protein and fat (aids in decreased absorption). Other glucose sources include Insta-glucose (cherry-flavored glucose), carbonated drinks (not sugarless), sherbet, gelatin, cottage cheese, or cake icing. All children with diabetes should carry with them glucose tabs, Insta-glucose, or sugar-containing candy, such as Life Savers or Charms, or some sugar cubes. A difficulty with candies or icing is that the child may learn to fake a reaction to get the sweets; therefore, Insta-glucose is the preferred treatment.

It is better to overtreat than to undertreat, but overtreatment could result in a rebound hypoglycemic effect. The treatment may be repeated in 10 to 15 minutes if the initial response is not satisfactory. Rest and the addition of food should be part of the plan.

An insulin reaction is often the most feared aspect of diabetes, since severe brain symptoms may develop. In a severe reaction the various areas of the brain respond in sequence: the forebrain with increased drowsiness and perspiration, the hypothalamus and thalamus with tachycardia and loss of consciousness, the midbrain with seizure activity that may be started from stimulation initially from the hypothalamus, and finally the hindbrain with responses of deeper coma and decreasing reflexes. The treatment of choice for severe hypoglycemia is 50% glucose administered intravenously.

Glucagon is sometimes prescribed for home treatment of hypoglycemia. It is packaged as an emergency kit containing a prefilled syringe. It is administered intramuscularly or subcutaneously. Glucagon functions by releasing stored glycogen from the liver and requires about 15 to 20 minutes to elevate the blood glucose level.

NURSING ALERT Vomiting may occur after administration of glucagon; therefore precautions against aspiration must be taken.

Once the child is responsive, the lost glycogen stores are replaced by small amounts of sugar-containing fluid administered frequently until the child feels comfortable about trying solid foods.

Morning Hyperglycemia. The management of elevated morning blood glucose levels depends on whether the increase is a true dawn phenomenon, insulin waning, or a rebound hyperglycemia (the Somogyi effect). Insulin waning is a progressive rise in blood glucose from bedtime to morning. It is treated by increasing the nocturnal insulin dose. The true dawn phenomenon shows a relatively normal blood sugar until about 3:00 AM when the level begins to rise. The Somogyi effect often shows an elevated blood sugar at bedtime and a drop at 2:00 AM with a rebound rise following. The treatment for this phenomenon is adjusting (down) the nocturnal insulin dose to prevent the 2:00 AM hypoglycemia from occurring. The rebound rise in blood sugar is a result of counter regulatory hormones (epinephrine, GH, and corticosteroids), which are stimulated by hypoglycemia (Laufer, 1987). More frequent blood monitoring (especially at times of anticipated peak insulin action) will usually identify these conditions. Trace amounts of urinary ketones aid in identifying undetected hypoglycemia.

Illness Management. Illness alters diabetes management, and maintaining control is usually related to the seriousness of the illness. In the well-controlled child an illness will run its course as it does in the unaffected child. The goal during an illness is to maintain some euglycemia while recognizing and treating urinary ketones. Blood glucose levels should be monitored every 4 hours. If blood glucose levels are 240 mg/dl or higher, urinary ketones must be checked as well. A sliding scale of regular insulin should be instituted during sick days. Sliding scale insulin should be implemented using regular insulin only and used in place of—not in addition to—prescribed insulin. Some hyperglycemia and ketonuria are expected in most illnesses, even with diminished food intake, and are an indication for increased insulin. Insulin should never be omitted during an illness, although dosage requirements may increase, decrease, or remain unchanged, depending on the severity of the illness and the child's appetite. If the child vomits more than one time, if blood glucose levels remain above 240 mg/dl, or if urinary ketones remain high, the health care practitioner should be notified.

Simple carbohydrates may be substituted for carbohydrate-containing exchanges in the meal plan. Fluids are encouraged to prevent dehydration and to flush out ketones. The Diabetes Control and Complications trial, a randomized, multicenter effort, compared conventional therapy, (two insulin injections per day) with intensive therapy (three or more daily injections) to achieve near-normal blood glucose values. The study found that intensive therapy delayed the onset and slowed the progression of complications of IDDM (Diabetes Control and Complications Trial Research Group, 1993).

Surgery. The physiologic and emotional stresses related to surgery require careful adjustment of insulin. Since the child receives intravenous glucose during surgery and the stress of the surgery itself will also raise the blood glucose level, the risk of an insulin reaction is very slight. Regular insulin should be continued until the child is able to tolerate oral feedings and a return to the routine pattern of insulin administration.

Transplantation. There has been experimentation with islet cell transplants. Viable insulin-producing cells are injected into the portal vein where they take root in the liver and eventually produce needed insulin. Some persons have received whole pancreas transplants and need no insulin supplementation. Persons receiving islet cell or whole-pancreas transplants require immunosuppression, which in itself is a risk factor. The major use of transplants has been in persons who have serious complications, particularly those whose deteriorating kidneys have required renal transplants and who are necessarily on immunosuppression. However, islet cell and pancreatic transplants tend not to be sustainable over time despite continuation of therapy. The use of nonhuman islets encapsulated in immunoprotective, semipermeable membranes may have a future in the treatment of IDDM (Brouhard and Douglas, 1993). Islet transplants may eventually be made more effective and possible without the need for powerful immunosuppressants.

Prevention. Major advances have been made in the ability to detect susceptibility to IDDM, and animal studies indicate that the disease can be prevented by various immunologic interventions (Bach, 1987). Recent sources also indicate that early immunosuppression may preserve long-term endogenous insulin secretion in individuals with IDDM.

It has been shown previously that immunosuppressive drugs can be used to induce metabolic remissions in newly diagnosed patients. However, more recent studies have shown that the metabolic remission is temporary despite continuation of therapy. Cyclosporine, nycophenolic acid, and nicotinamide have shown promise in delaying beta cell destruction or lowering the incidence of IDDM in relatives of children afflicted with the disease. Much progress has been made in respect to the identification of islet cell antigens targeted by the immune response. Many potential treatments to prevent IDDM have appeared, and human trials have begun (MacLaren and Lafferty, 1993).

Therapeutic Management: Diabetic Ketoacidosis (DKA)

DKA, the most complete state of insulin deficiency, is a life-threatening situation. Management consists of rapid assessment, adequate insulin to reduce the elevated blood glucose level, fluids to overcome dehydration, and electrolyte replacement (especially potassium and bicarbonate). A sample plan is shown in Table 38-5.

DKA constitutes an emergency situation; therefore the child should be admitted to an intensive care facility for management. The priority is to obtain a venous access for administration of fluids, electrolytes, and insulin. The child should be weighed, measured, and placed on a cardiac monitor. Blood glucose and ketone levels are determined at the bedside, and samples obtained for laboratory measurements of glucose, electrolytes, blood urea nitrogen, arterial pH, PO_2, PCO_2, hemoglobin, hematocrit, white blood count and differential, and calcium and phosphorus.

Oxygen may be administered to patients who are cyanotic and in whom arterial oxygen is less than 80%. Gastric suction is applied to unconscious children to avoid the possibility of pulmonary aspiration. Antibiotics may be administered to febrile children after appropriate specimens are obtained for culture. A Foley catheter may or may not be inserted for urine samples and measurement. Unless the child is unconscious, a collection bag is usually sufficient for accurate assessments.

Fluid and Electrolyte Therapy. All patients with diabetic ketoacidosis suffer from dehydration (10% of total body weight in severe ketoacidosis) due to the osmotic diuresis, accompanied by depletion of electrolytes, sodium, potassium, chloride, phosphate, and magnesium. Serum pH and bicarbonate reflect the degree of acidosis. Prompt and adequate fluid therapy restores tissue perfusion and suppresses the elevated levels of stress hormones.

The initial hydrating solution is 0.9% saline solution. Traditionally, deficits have been replaced at a rate of 50% over the first 8 to 12 hours and the remaining 50% over the next 16 to 24 hours. Current trends suggest more cautious fluid management to reduce the risk of cerebral edema. The fluid deficit is replaced evenly over 24 to 48 hours. Potassium must never be given until the serum potassium is known to be normal or low and voiding is observed. All IV fluids should include 20 to 40 mEq/L of potassium.

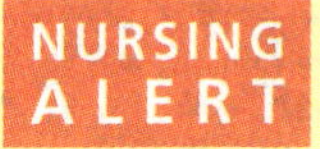

Never give potassium as a rapid IV bolus, or cardiac arrest may result.

TABLE 38-5 Multidisciplinary Plan (Critical Path) of Care for Diabetic Ketoacidosis—Known Diabetic Patient

	ADMISSION DAY (1ST 24 HOURS)	DAY TWO	DAY THREE	DAY FOUR
Placement	pH < 7.2 *and* Tco_2 < 10 *or* ▪ Stupor/coma ▪ Hypotension ▪ Severe dehydration —To PICU† pH < 7.2 *and* Tco_2 < 10 —To IICU† pH >7.2 *or* Tco_2 > 10 *and* ▪ Difficult to correct ▪ Unable to tolerate PO ▪ Admit recommended per MD consult —Age 0-13 to 7N† —Age 14-18 to 5S† —Otherwise discharge to home when stable	Once stabilized: —Age 0-13 to 7N† —Age 14-18 to 5S† May discharge if stable	May discharge if stable	
Diet	If pH < 7.30 and Tco_2 < 15, NPO until pH and lytes corrected, unless MD OKs PO If pH > 7.30 and *no* emesis, ADA diet for age per dietary consult	ADA diet for age per dietary consult	————→	————→
Activity	If pH < 7.20, then bed rest When stabilized, BRP and up as tolerated per MD order	Up ad lib Encourage activity and clothes from home	————→	————→
Labs	ER—lytes, pH, glucose, BUN, glycosolated hemoglobin ▪ Chemstrips q 1 hr—use blood from lab draws when possible; when stable, usual pattern: 24–03—730—1130—1630—HS ▪ pH < 7.2 or Tco_2 < 10: lytes, pH, glucose q hr ▪ pH > 7.2 and Tco_2 > 10: lytes, pH, glucose q 4 hr ▪ *Remember to use DKA flowsheets*	—Chemstrips usual pattern Premeals—HS—24—03 Until normal, then only with MD order		
Medications	If pH < 7.2 or Tco_2 < 10: —Insulin 0.1 U/kg IV bolus then, —Insulin 0.1 U/kg IV cont drip until pH and lytes corrected *Important:* Adjust dose to lower BG; *no* greater than 100 mg/dl/hr; insulin must run until corrected If pH > 7.20 and Tco_2 > 10: —Insulin bolus IM/IV 0.1 U/kg then, —SQ insulin per MD consult If pH > 7.30: —SQ insulin per MD consult While on insulin drip: —Mannitol 1.5-2.0 g/kg at bedside	SQ insulin initiated per MD consult Insulin adjusted per MD consult D/C mannitol	Insulin adjusted per MD consult ————→	————→ ————→

Courtesy Children's Hospital of Wisconsin—Diabetic Team, 1994.
*Sample of DKA critical pathway form used. These interventions and abbreviations may differ in other institutions.
†Refers to units in hospital.

TABLE 38-5 Multidisciplinary Plan (Critical Path) of Care for Diabetic Ketoacidosis—Known Diabetic Patient—cont'd

	ADMISSION DAY (1ST 24 HOURS)	DAY TWO	DAY THREE	DAY FOUR
Treatment	If pH < 7.2 and Tco_2 < 10 (at initial ER draw):			
	—VS q hr × 24 hr (starting time − ER labs)	VS q 8 hr	VS BID	VS BID
	—Neuro checks q hr × 24 hr	D/C neuro checks		
	—CR monitor × 24 hr	D/C CR monitor		
	—Accurate I&O × 24 hr	I&O	————→	————→
	—Dipstick urine for ketones q void or q 2 hr if Foley			
	—Dipstick urine for glucose once BG < 180 until negative, then check sp. gr. × 24 hr			
	If pH > 7.2 or Tco_2 > 10:			
	—VS q 4 hr × 24 hr	VS BID	VS BID	VS BID
	—Accurate I&O × 24 hr	I&O	————→	————→
	—Neuro checks q 8 hr × 24 hr	D/C neuro checks		
	—CR monitor if K < 3.5 or > 5.5 at any point for 24 hr	D/C CR monitor		
	—Dipstick urine for ketones q AM and when BG > 300	Dipstick urine for ketones q AM and when BG > 300	————→	————→
	If pH > 7.35 and Tco_2 > 20:			
	—VS q 8 hr × 24 hr	VS BID	VS BID	VS BID
	—Dipstick urine for ketones q AM and when BG > 300	Dipstick urine for ketones q AM and when BG > 300	————→	————→
	All patients:			
	—Daily weights	Daily weight	————→	————→
	—Admit height (when ambulatory)			
IV fluids	IV needed if pH < 7.25 *or* if PO fluids not tolerated	D/C IV		
	ER—lactated Ringer's bolus 20 cc/kg over 1st hr			
	Then—If BG > 250, 0.45 NS with 20 K phosphate and 20 K acetate			
	—If BG < 250, D5 0.45 NS with 20 K phosphate and 20 K acetate			
	Rate: (85 cc/kg + maint.)−bolus At 23 hr:			
	—If pH > 7.25 and Tco_2 > 15 and *NO* emesis, *no* IV needed; rehydrate orally			
Consults	Pediatric endocrinologist	Physical therapy		
	Social worker from diabetes team	—BID exercise if child > 5yr (per MD order)		
	Dietary consult	Discharge planner		
	Diabetes clinical nurse specialist			
Discharge planning	Clinical nurse specialist	DC planner	————→	————→
	F/U appt. to clinic	▪ If home nursing needed or meter requested		
Teaching	Nursing assessment R/T cause of DKA			
	Initiation of nursing care plan			
	1. DKA associated with illness			
	a. Managed well at home —Alteration of fluid and electrolytes R/T DKA			
	b. Managed poorly at home —Knowledge deficit R/T Sick day management	Review sick day guidelines		

Continued.

TABLE 38-5 Multidisciplinary Plan (Critical Path) of Care for Diabetic Ketoacidosis—Known Diabetic Patient—cont'd

	ADMISSION DAY (1ST 24 HOURS)	DAY TWO	DAY THREE	DAY FOUR
	2. DKA associated with poor management/ noncompliance —Alteration in coping R/T Home diabetes management	Social service consult Clinical nurse specialist consult Video: *Diabetes—A Positive Approach*		
Nursing assessment and interventions	If severe DKA, watch closely for first 24 hr for any change in LOC R/T cerebral edema (2 hr to correction of hydration status) if K < 3.5 or > 5.5 watch carefully for cardiac arrythmias Assess family coping on ongoing basis to determine special D/C needs.			
Patient variance Analysis Justification Corrective action				
System/caregiver variance Analysis Justification Corrective action				
Community variance Analysis Justification Corrective action				

Serum potassium levels may be normal on admission, but, following fluid and insulin administration, the rapid return of potassium to the cells can seriously deplete serum levels, with the attendant risk of cardiac arrhythmias. As soon as the child has established renal function (is voiding at least 25 ml/hour) and insulin has been given, vigorous potassium replacement is implemented. The cardiac monitor is used as a guide to therapy, and configuration of T waves should be followed every 30 to 60 minutes to determine changes that might indicate alterations in potassium concentration (widening of the QT interval and the appearance of a U wave following a flattened T wave indicate hypokalemia; an elevated and spreading T wave and shortening of the QT interval indicate hyperkalemia).

Insulin should not be given until urine ketones and a blood glucose level have been obtained. Continuous IV regular insulin is given at a dose of 0.1 U/kg per hour. Because insulin will bind to the walls of the IV tubing, the tubing is first washed with 50 ml of the insulin solution. Insulin therapy should be started after the initial rehydration bolus, since serum glucose levels fall rapidly after volume expansion. Blood glucose levels should decrease by 50 to 100 mg%/hr. When blood glucose levels fall to 250 to 300 mg%, dextrose is added to the IV solution. The goal is to maintain blood glucose levels between 120 and 240 mg% by adding 5% to 10% dextrose. The insulin drip should not be decreased to less than 0.05 U/kg/hour. $NaCO_3$ is used conservatively; it is used for pH <7.0, severe hyperkalemia, or cardiac instability (Chase, Garg, and Jelley, 1990).

Nursing Considerations: Acute Care

Children with DM may be admitted to the hospital at the time of their initial diagnosis, during illness or surgery, or for episodes of ketoacidosis, which may be precipitated by any of a variety of factors. Most children are able to keep the disease under control with periodic assessment and adjustment of insulin, diet, and activity as needed under the supervision of a practitioner. Under most circumstances these children can be managed very well at home and require hospitalization only for a serious illness or upset.

However, a small number of children with diabetes exhibit a degree of metabolic lability and have repeated episodes of diabetic ketoacidosis that require hospitalization, which interferes with education and social development. These children appear to display a characteristic personality structure. They tend to be unusually passive and nonassertive and to come from families that are inclined to smooth over conflicts without resolution. Children in this type of setting experience emotional arousal with little, if any, opportunity or ability to bring about its termination. Other children from psychosocially dysfunctional families display behavioral and personality problems. This emotional stress causes an increased production of endogenous catecholamines, which stimulates fat breakdown leading to ketonemia and ketonuria.

Loving discipline is a supportive measure for any child; however, children with poorer diabetic control come from predominantly disruptive family units with little or no discipline as part of the family life-style. Lack of control is psychologically harmful. Since many of the psychosocial problems are not immediately apparent, psychosocial assessment and involvement by professionals are required, together with ongoing emotional support and counseling to reverse the patterns of ketoacidosis (White and others, 1984).

Hospital Management. The child with diabetic ketoacidosis requires intensive nursing care. Vital signs should be observed and recorded frequently. Hypotension caused by the contracted blood volume of the dehydrated state may cause decreased peripheral blood flow, which can be particularly hazardous to the heart, lungs, and kidneys. An elevated temperature may indicate the presence of infection and should be reported so that treatment can be implemented immediately.

Careful and accurate records should be maintained, including vital signs (pulse, respiration, temperature, blood pressure), intravenous fluids, electrolytes, insulin, blood glucose level, and intake and output. A urine collection device or retention catheter is used to obtain the urine measurements, which include volume, specific gravity, and glucose and ketone values. The volume relative to the glucose content is important, since 5% glucose in a 300 ml sample is a significantly greater amount than a similar reading from a 75 ml sample. A diabetic flow sheet maintained at the bedside provides an ongoing record of the vital signs, urine and blood tests, amount of insulin given, and intake and output of the patient. The level of consciousness is assessed and recorded at frequent intervals. The comatose child generally regains consciousness fairly soon after initiation of therapy but is managed as any unconscious child during that time.

When the critical period is over, the task of regulating insulin dosage to diet and activity is begun. The same meticulous records of intake and output, urine glucose and acetone levels, and insulin administration are maintained. Capable children should be actively involved in their own care and are given responsibility for keeping the intake and output record, testing the blood and urine, and, when appropriate, administering their own insulin—all under the supervision and guidance of the nurse.

Nursing Considerations: General Care

Nurses play a prominent role in diagnosis and management of children with IDDM. Assessing and educating the child and family are almost exclusively a nursing function.

❖ Assessment

Diabetic management involves a constant state of assessment. Daily monitoring of blood glucose levels, periodic urinalysis for ketones, and observation for signs of hypoglycemia, hyperglycemia, or other complications is part of the daily life of children with diabetes and their families. Diabetes can be suspected in any child who exhibits the manifestations of hypoglycemia or hyperglycemia (see Table 38-4), and the child should be referred for further assessment and appropriate testing.

The nurse should be alert to evidence of complications, although these are usually not manifest until adulthood. Assessment of skin for evidence of breakdown is important in order that appropriate care can be implemented to facilitate healing and prevent infection. Because illnesses, such as respiratory infections or gastrointestinal upsets, complicate the diabetes management, they should be detected early.

❖ Nursing Diagnoses

Based on a thorough assessment, several nursing diagnoses are identified. The more common diagnoses for the child with DM are included in the Nursing Care Plan on pp. 1786-1788. Others may apply in specific situations.

❖ Planning

The goals for the child with DM and the family include the following:

1. Child and family will be educated about the disease, assessment techniques, and therapy.
2. Child will experience a minimum of ill effects from complications of diabetes.
3. Child will develop a positive self-image.
4. Child and family will receive adequate support.

❖ Implementation

Education is the cornerstone of diabetes management and the major responsibility in diabetes nursing care. This includes education and reinforcement of information for the family and for children who are old enough to participate in self-management of the disease. With younger children, parents must supervise and manage their therapeutic program, but children should assume responsibility for self-management as soon as they are capable. Children can assist with blood glucose testing at a relatively young age, and most should be able to administer their own insulin at about 9 years of age. In situations in which the parents are inconsistent and/or unreliable, the child should be taught self-care at an earlier age. It must be understood, however, that education programs cannot be conducted as one-time activities with the expectation that they will achieve permanent behavior changes. Education is a long-term nursing activity as family and patient needs change and new findings are applied.

Concepts of Child and Family Education. Children and their families vary in educational background and the capacity to learn and understand the various aspects of the therapeutic program. Some families respond best to very simple explanations and directions, whereas others expect thorough, in-depth information about the physiologic processes and responses associated with the disease and its therapy. All the principles of teaching and learning are applied in the educational process; therefore, before beginning, the nurse must determine the optimum time, place, method, and content to be taught. Self-management, the ultimate goal for children with diabetes, is more likely to occur when they understand the disease and the care it requires. Properly educated, any family should be able to follow a program of regulated control satisfactorily.

When to teach a family is best judged by the psychologic state of the family and/or the child and the time of initial diagnosis. If a child is newly diagnosed, the psychologic adjustment to the disease can block the learning process completely—for example, members of the family may in a follow-up visit state that it is the first time that they have heard a certain bit of information when, in reality, the specific material had been covered several times in the course of teaching.

Certainly, the first 3 or 4 days after diagnosis is not an optimum time for learning. In fact, the later the more complex material is presented, the better. For example, one successful program teaches only essential, or survival, information first and intense information a month later. Another program advocates as a choice of time for teaching 1 week after diagnosis followed by a review of survival techniques 2 weeks after discharge. Probably the most inopportune and ineffective time for teaching is the day or so after diagnosis when the education must be compressed into a few hours or days so that the child can be discharged early. Whether teaching is conducted on an outpatient basis or in a preparatory, in-depth manner on an inpatient basis, the ability of the individuals involved to learn must be accurately assessed. This includes assessment of the educational background and emotional stability of the individual(s) involved and the use of appropriate measurement tools, such as a pretest or an objective assessment of the learner's educational level. The stepped approach to patient education employs the method of simple to complex. The stepped approach involves three phases: (1) use good interpersonal skills; (2) teach about the illness and regimen; and (3) overcome obstacles to behavior change (Bartlett, 1988).

The setting for the educational process can facilitate the learning process. An environment that is too hot or too cold or one in which there is too much noise will distract the learner. Bedside education may be necessary in some cases, but the coming and going of a number of people are distracting. There are times in the educational process when individual instruction is needed, but contact with other children and/or parents can assist in adjustment to the reality of the disease and the implications of having a chronic condition. Supplementary material such as audiovisual aids enhances the learning process and promotes retention of information.

A child learns best when sessions are kept short, no more than 15 to 20 minutes. The parents do best in periods of 45 to 60 minutes, or longer if they are inquisitive. Education should involve all the senses, and although visual aids are valuable tools, participation is the most effective method for learning. For example, to teach urine testing, the technique is explained, the procedure is demonstrated, and the learner is allowed to perform the procedure followed by a review of the material by visual aids, with learning validated by some testing method that includes feedback. A variety of teaching methods and teaching aids can be used. Some visual aids may be beautifully illustrated but miss a major point; therefore materials should be previewed for accuracy and appropriateness. Varying the presentation with a variety of audiovisual materials, including films, slide-tape programs, and books, stimulates the senses and helps the individual to learn.

Several organizations are prepared to assist with education and dissemination of knowledge about diabetes. The **American Diabetes Association, Inc.,*** **Canadian Diabetes Association,†** **Juvenile Diabetes Foundation International,‡** and the **American Association of Diabetes Educators§** are valuable resources for a wide variety of educational materials. The **National Diabetes Information Clearinghouse‖** publishes a number of comprehensive annotated bibliographies, including *Educational Materials for and about Young People with Diabetes,* a compilation of resource materials for children, siblings, parents, teachers, and health professionals, and *Sports and Exercise for People with Diabetes.*

The content of the educational course must include all aspects of the disease as they specifically relate to the individual child. There are many aspects of the disease that may not be covered in an initial educational course but can be postponed until subsequent office or clinic visits or can be done through referral sources such as the American Diabetes Association. The minimal information needed is that which will help the family manage from one day to the next; expanded information helps the individual with the biopsychosocial adjustment basic to in-depth knowledge about the disease. The more the family understands about the disease in relation to body needs, the better they are able to maintain a high degree of control. Important content needed for minimum management is discussed briefly in the following segments.

Identification. One of the first things that should be called to the attention of the parents is the need for the child to wear some means of medical identification. Usually recommended is the Medic-Alert identification, a stainless steel, silver, or gold-plated identification bracelet that is visible and immediately recognizable. It contains a collect telephone number that medical personnel can call around the clock for medical records and personal information.

Nature of Diabetes. The better the parents understand the pathophysiology of diabetes and the function and action of insulin and glucagon in relation to calorie intake and exercise, the better will be their understanding of the disease and its effect on the child. Parents need answers to a number of questions (voiced or unvoiced) because those answers can provide them an increased feeling of security in coping with the disease. For example, they may want to

*1660 Duke St., Alexandria, VA 22314; (800) 232-3472. In Virginia or Washington, DC: (703) 549-1500.

†78 Bond St., Toronto, Ontario, Canada M5B2J8; (416) 366-2440.

‡432 Park Ave., South, New York, NY; (212) 889-7575, Hotline: (800) 223-1138.

§Suite 1400, 500 N. Michigan Ave., Chicago, IL 60611; (800) 338-3633.

‖Box NDIC, 9000 Rockville Pike, Bethesda, MD 20892; (301) 468-2162.

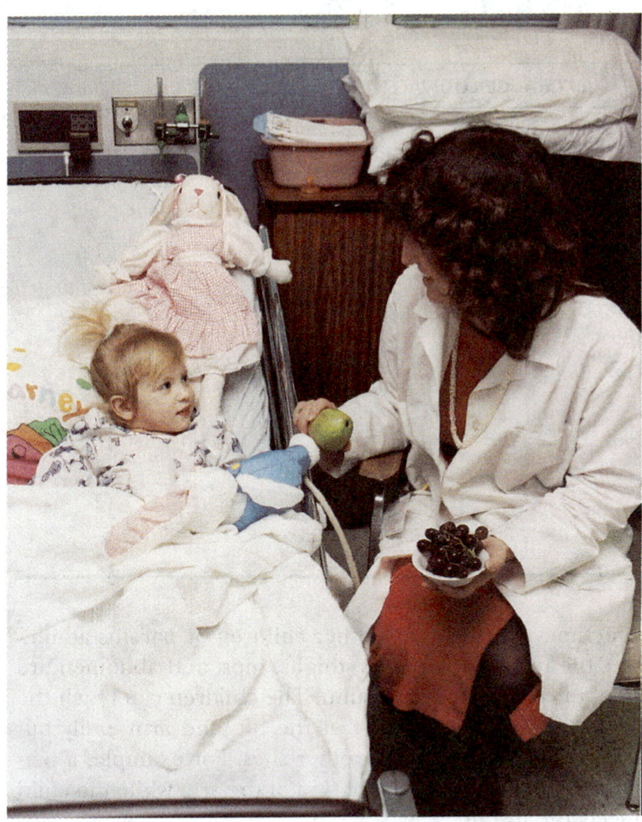

FIG. 38-6 Nutritionist instructs child, using food to explain food exchanges.

know about the various procedures performed on their child and treatment rationale, such as what is being put in the intravenous bottle and the expected effect.

Meal Planning. Normal nutrition is a major aspect of the family education program. Diet instruction is usually conducted by the nutritionist, with reinforcement and guidance from the nurse (Fig. 38-6). The emphasis is on adequate intake for age, constant menus, complex carbohydrates, and consistent eating times. The family is taught how the meal plan relates to the requirements of growth and development, the disease process, and the insulin regimen. Meals and snacks are modified around the child and the present food menu, preserving cultural patterns and preferences as much as possible. Extensive exchange lists are available that include foods that are compatible with most life-styles.

Learning about foods within specific food groups helps in making choices. Weights and measures of foods are used as eye-training devices for defining food volumes and should be practiced for about 3 months, with gradual progression to estimation of food portions. Even when the child and/or family become competent in estimating food volumes, reassessment should take place weekly or monthly and when there is any change of brands. Members of the family should also be guided in reading labels for the nutritional value of foods and food contents.

Family members should also become familiar with the carbohydrate content of food groups. Substitutions with foods of equal carbohydrate content is occasionally acceptable without affecting blood glucose control. Substitution might be necessary if a food is not available in sufficient quantity or for the teen who wishes to eat fast food with peers. The use of MDI lends flexibility to the timing of meals.

Educating children or teenagers to make healthy food choices is an ongoing task. Younger children might be taught to choose from a special treat box stocked with sugar-free items when high-sugar treats are brought to the classroom by others. Discussions with school-age children might include situations encountered at school or parties, such as choosing food in the cafeteria or bringing substitute treats to parties. Role-playing and discussion help teenagers deal with food choices when on dates, with friends, or on a food break after school.

Lists of popular fast-food items and items served at the major fast-food chains can be obtained from the **American Dietetic Association (ADA)*** to help guide food selections. It is important that the child know the nutritional value of these items (the major chains are remarkably uniform), but the child should be cautioned to avoid high-fat and high-sugar items, for example, choosing a plain hamburger instead of a double cheeseburger. (See Table 38-6 for a small sample of some popular fast-food items.)

Children should be advised to use sugar substitutes with moderation in items such as soft drinks. Artificial sweeteners have been shown to be safe, but if there is any question about amounts, the physician, dietitian, or nurse specialist can provide guidelines based on body weight. "Sugar-free" chewing gum and candies made with sorbitol are not usually recommended for children with DM. Although sorbitol is less cariogenic than other varieties of sugar substitutes, it is an alcohol sugar that is metabolized to fructose and then to glucose. Furthermore, large amounts can cause osmotic diarrhea. Most dietetic foods contain sorbitol. They are more expensive than regular foods, and careful reading of labels reveals that the caloric content is the same.

Traveling requires advance planning, especially when a trip involves crossing time zones. A number of tips are included in pamphlets available free of charge from the local chapter of the ADA or the publishers.* Suggestions for traveling include what will be needed from the practitioner before leaving, what and how much to take along, needs in transit, what to consider at the destination, and planning for when the child returns home. Planning is needed no matter what type of travel is considered—automobile, plane, bus, or train. For example, the ADA also has a computer service that can provide a vacation schedule of insulin and meals based on the accustomed regimen and the anticipated changes. Diabetic supplies should not be left in a hot environment.

---

*216 W. Jackson Blvd. Suite 800, Chicago, IL 60606; (312) 899-0040.

**Vacations, Travel, and Diabetes*, available from Becton, Dickson & Co., Rochelle Park, NJ 07662. *Vacationing with Diabetes*, available from E.R. Squibb, P.O. Box 4000, Princeton, NJ 08540.

TABLE 38-6 Exchange Equivalents for Selected Fast-Food Items

FOOD	EXCHANGE EQUIVALENTS			
	LEAN-MED. MEAT	STARCH/ BREAD	FAT	VEGETABLE
Arby's roast beef sandwich (regular)	2½	2	0	—
Burger King "Whopper"	2½	3	4	1
KFC				
Original dinner (2 pieces chicken, potatoes, gravy, cole slaw, roll)	4	4	5½	2
McDonald's "Big Mac"	2½	2½	4	2
Pizza Hut cheeze pizza (3 slices)	2	3½	½	2
Taco Bell				
Taco	1	1	1	—
Beef burrito	2½	2	1	2
Wendy's cheeseburger (single)	3	2½	2½	—

Insulin. Families need to understand the treatment method and the insulin prescribed, including the effective duration, onset, and peak action. They also need to know the characteristics of the various types of insulins, the proper mixing and dilution of insulins, and how to substitute another type when their usual brand is not available (insulin is a nonprescription drug). Insulin need not be refrigerated but should be maintained at a temperature between 15° C (59° F) and 29.4° C (85° F). Freezing renders insulin inactive.

Injection Procedure. Learning to give the insulin injections is a source of anxiety for both the parents and children. It is helpful for the learner to know that this important aspect of care will become as routine as brushing the teeth. First, the basic injection technique is taught, using an orange or similar item and sterile normal saline for practice.* To gain children's confidence, the nurse can demonstrate the technique by giving a skillful injection to the parent and then having the parent return the demonstration by giving the nurse an injection. With practice and confidence the parents soon are able to give the insulin injection to their children, and their children will trust them. Another effective strategy is to instruct the children and then have them teach the technique to the parents while the nurse observes. Both parents should participate, and as little time as possible should elapse between instruction and the actual injection, especially with parents and teenage learners.

Insulin can be injected into any area in which there is tissue over muscle; the drug is injected at a 90-degree angle. Newly diagnosed children may have lost adipose tissue, and care should be exerted not to inject intramuscularly. The pinch technique is the most effective method for obtaining tenting of the skin to allow easy entrance of the needle to subcutaneous tissues in children. The site selected will sometimes depend on whether children or parents administer the insulin. The arms, thighs, hips, and abdomen are usual injection sites for insulin. The children can reach the thighs, abdomen, and part of the hip and arm easily but may require help to inject other sites. For example, a parent can pinch a loose fold of skin of the arm while the child injects the insulin.

The parents and child are helped to work out a rotation pattern to various areas of the body to enhance absorption, since insulin absorption is slowed by the fat pads that develop in overused injection areas. The most efficient rotation plan involves giving about 4 to 6 injections in one area (each injection about 1 inch [2.5 cm] apart or the diameter of the insulin vial from the previous injection) and then moving to another area.

It is important to remember that the absorption rate varies in different parts of the body (Table 38-7). The methodical use of one anatomic area and then moving to another (as described in the previous paragraph) minimizes variation in absorption rates. However, absorption is also altered by vigorous exercise, which enhances absorption from exercised muscles; therefore it is recommended that a site be chosen other than the exercising extremity (e.g., leg when playing in a tennis tournament).

Injection sites for an entire month can be determined in advance on a simple chart. For example, the "paper doll" (body outline) described on p. 221 can be constructed and insulin sites marked by the child. After injection, the child places the date on the appropriate site. In order to keep in practice, it is a good idea for the parent to give two or three injections a week in the areas that are difficult for the child to reach.

The same basic methodology is used when teaching children to give their own insulin injections (Fig. 38-7). They should practice first on an orange or a doll, building courage gradually. The first attempt will undoubtedly be awkward, since children tend to slowly push the needle through the skin rather than using a quick approach. It is best not to pressure them into assuming this responsibility until they

---

*Home care instructions for subcutaneous injection are available in *Wong and Whaley's Clinical Manual of Pediatric Nursing* (Mosby).

TABLE 38-7 Onset and Duration of Action Related to Injection Site

	SITE OF INJECTION			
	ABDOMEN	ARM	LEG	BUTTOCK
Rate	Very fast	Fast	Slow	Very slow
Duration	Very short	Short	Long	Very long

From Albisser AM, Sperlich M: Adjusting insulins, *Diabetes Educator* 18(3):211-218, 1992.

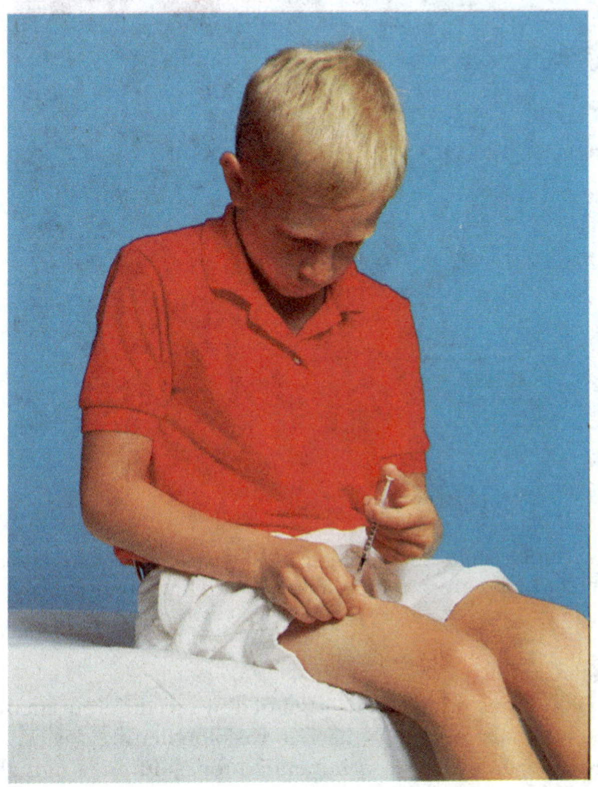

FIG. 38-7 School-age children are able to administer their own insulin.

are ready. When children participate in a group-learning situation or have an opportunity to observe their peers giving their own injections, they may become more strongly motivated. Parents should be warned that at some time children will give themselves an uncomfortable injection at home and that they will need parental support and encouragement. Otherwise children may not wish to give themselves injections for some time. Occasionally children are taught to use a syringe-loaded injector (Injectease), especially those who are fearful of puncturing their skin. With the device, puncture is always automatic. Adolescents respond well to a self-contained and compact device resembling a fountain pen (NovoPen*), which eliminates conventional vials and syringes.

Teaching includes the proper way to equalize pressure in the bottle by injecting an amount of air equal to the amount of solution withdrawn and how to remove air bubbles from the syringe. When insulin dosages are small, an air bubble in the syringe can displace a significant amount of medication. Since the introduction of the 5/10 ml and 3/10 ml syringes, the risk of incorrect dosage has diminished. Patients who have small doses of mixed insulins should be advised and instructed to use one of these syringes. Insulin syringes should be compared for accuracy, comfort, and strength. The family and/or child should be able to choose both "their" insulin and "their" syringe from a variety of samples. Use of the same type of syringe (even during hospitalization) is recommended to prevent errors in dosage caused by varying amounts of dead space among syringes. The needle length and gauge are also factors to consider from the point of view of comfort (e.g., use the smallest gauge needle available). Some brands of syringes may be more comfortable than others. When currently available syringes are used, insulin injections of less than 2 units of U100 have an unacceptably large error. Diluted insulin should be used if the prescribed dose is less than 2 units (Casella and others, 1993).

When the child's dosage requires the injection of both short- and intermediate-acting insulin at the same time, most families prefer to mix the two and use a single injection. Insulin can be premixed and stored in the refrigerator for later use. Commercially prepared insulin mixtures are also available (i.e., 70/30, 60/40, and 50/50).

To obtain maximum benefit from mixing insulins, the recommended practice is to (1) inject the measured amount of air (equivalent to the dosage) into the longer-acting insulin, (2) inject the measured amount of air into the regular insulin and, without removing the needle, (3) withdraw the regular insulin, and (4) insert the needle (already containing the regular insulin) into the longer-acting insulin and then withdraw the desired amount. The mixture should be injected in less than 5 minutes after mixing (before the zinc content of the long-acting insulin affects the action time of the regular or short-acting insulin) or longer than 15 minutes after mixing (to allow the insulins to resume long-acting and short-acting properties).

It is acceptable practice to reuse disposable needles and syringes for 3 to 7 days. Bacterial counts are unaffected, and there is a considerable cost saving. It is essential to stress the importance of vigorous handwashing before handling any equipment, as well as capping the syringe immediately after use and storing it in the refrigerator to reduce the growth of organisms. Nurses should also teach proper disposal of equipment after use in the home. Although not standard practice in the hospital, use of a needle clipper is

*Squibb-Novo, Inc., Princeton, NJ.

recommended to safely remove and house the used needle. The syringe plunger can be broken before disposal. An excellent means for syringe disposal is in an opaque, puncture-resistant container such as an empty coffee can, bleach bottle, or milk carton. The container is labeled "biohazardous waste" and is discarded with similar material only, not with household refuse.

Continuous subcutaneous insulin infusion. Some children are considered candidates for use of a portable insulin pump, and even some young children with unsatisfactory metabolic control can benefit from its use. The child and the parents are taught to operate the device, including the mechanics of the pump, battery changes, and alarm systems. A number of devices are available on the market that vary in the basal rates they are able to deliver and in the cost of the equipment. Most children can be adequately controlled with one of the simpler models (Rosenstock, Strowig, and Raskin, 1985). Families can investigate the various devices at the local chapter of the ADA and select the model that best suits their needs.

Parents and child learn (1) the technical aspects of the pump and self-monitoring of blood glucose; (2) how to prevent and treat hyperglycemia, sick-day management, and diet planning; (3) effects of exercise, stress, and diet on blood glucose levels; and (4) decision-making strategies to evaluate blood glucose patterns and how to make adjustments in all aspects of the regimen. The child may be hospitalized for regulation and instruction.

Since numerous blood glucose measurements (at least four times per day) are an essential part of infusion pump use, families must acquire a monitor and learn its use if this has not been a part of their regular management. Intensive education and supervision are critical to obtaining maximum efficiency and control. This is particularly important if the family has been accustomed to a fixed insulin regimen. They must realize that simply wearing the pump will not normalize blood glucose. It is merely a tool for using the information from self blood-glucose monitoring as a guide for adjusting the insulin delivery.

The major problem with the use of the insulin pump is inflammation from an allergic reaction or infection at the insertion site. The site should be cleaned thoroughly before the needle is inserted and then covered with a transparent dressing. The site is changed and rotated every 48 hours (this may vary) or at the first sign of inflammation. Nurses working where the pumps are part of the therapeutic regimen should become familiar with the operation of the specific device being used and the protocol of disease management. Others should be aware of this management technique and be prepared to assist patients who have this method in operation.

Monitoring. Nurses should also be prepared to teach and supervise blood glucose monitoring. Home blood glucose monitoring (HBGM) is associated with very few complications, and although it does not necessarily lead to improved metabolic control, it provides a more accurate assessment of blood glucose levels than can be obtained with the traditional urine testing. Blood glucose monitoring has the added advantage that it can be performed anywhere.

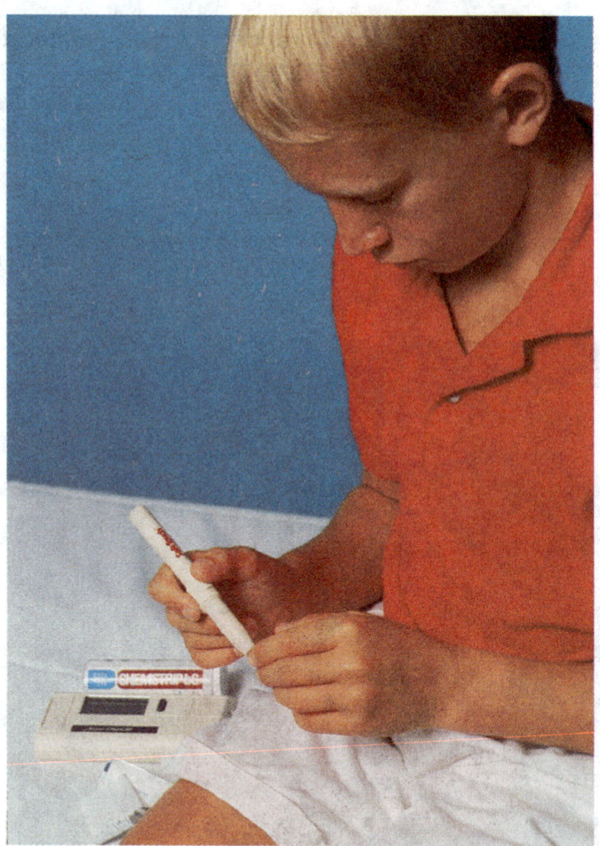

FIG. 38-8 Child using finger-stick device to obtain blood sample. Blood glucose monitor and reagent strips are nearby.

Blood for testing can be obtained by two different methods: manually or with a mechanical bloodletting device. A mechanical device is recommended for children, although the child and family should learn to use both methods in the event of mechanical failure. Several lancet devices are available from which to choose, and each provides a means for obtaining a large drop of blood for testing (Fig. 38-8). Children are cautioned not to allow anyone else to use their lancet because of the danger of contracting hepatitis or human immunodeficiency virus (HIV). Signs of redness and soreness at the site of finger puncture should be examined by the practitioner. It may be evidence of poor technique or poor skin healing relative to poor control.

➤ **NURSING TIP** To enhance blood flow to the finger, hold it under warm water for a few seconds before the stick. When obtaining blood samples, use the ring finger or thumb (blood flows more easily to these areas), and stick the finger just to the side of the finger pad (more blood vessels and fewer nerve endings). To prevent a deep puncture, press lancet device lightly against the skin and avoid steadying finger against a hard surface.

Many types of blood testing meters are available for home use. Meter size and ease of use has been greatly improved with newer technology. The family should be shown features of several meters, including advantages and disadvantages, and allowed to choose equipment that best meets their needs. Fourth-generation machines, which are noninvasive, are currently being tested. These devices use light absorption technology rather than blood and will probably be available within a few years (Chase, Chase, and Garg, 1991).

The least expensive testing method uses a reagent strip to which blood is applied. After blotting, the color change is compared against a color scale for an estimation of blood glucose level. The strips can be cut in half (although this is not recommended by all professionals) to obtain two readings per strip. This method might be ideal for use at school where expensive equipment can be lost or broken.

Urine testing. Testing for urinary ketones is recommended during times of illness or when blood glucose values are elevated. Information on a specific ketone testing product should include correct procedure, storage, and product expiration. Families need a clear understanding of home management of ketones: fluids and additional insulin as directed by the health care team.

Shopping. Diabetic maintenance is not an inexpensive necessity. Families are advised to investigate all sources of obtaining supplies for managing the disease. Prices are often lower when supplies are purchased in volume; however, it is not advisable to buy bulk items that are unfamiliar or untried, since the new items may not be satisfactory for the individual child or may become outdated before used. Costs vary considerably among pharmacies and other suppliers, including the numerous discount mail-order establishments. When buying by mail, it is important to find one that responds to the family's satisfaction and that allows the family ample time for delivery to avoid running out of supplies. Parents are also cautioned not to substitute insulins or the type of insulin syringe (e.g., a 1 ml syringe for the low-dose type) simply to save money. Parent groups and the local ADA can offer some suggestions for investigation.

Hyperglycemia. Severe hyperglycemia is most often caused by illness, growth, or emotional upset. With careful glucose monitoring, any elevation can be managed by adjustment of insulin or food intake. Parents should understand how to adjust food, activity, and insulin at the time of illness or when the child is treated for an illness with a medication known to raise the blood glucose level (e.g., cough syrup). The hyperglycemia is managed by increasing insulin soon after the increased glucose is noted. Health care professionals should be aware that adolescent girls often become hyperglycemic around their menses and should be advised to increase insulin dosages if necessary.

Hypoglycemia. Hypoglycemia is caused by imbalances of food intake, insulin, and activity. Ideally, hypoglycemia should be prevented, and parents need to be prepared to prevent, recognize, and treat the problem. They should be familiar with the signs of hypoglycemia and instructed in treatment, including care of the child with seizures (see Chapter 37). Early signs are ***adrenergic,*** including sweating and trembling, which help raise the blood sugar, much like the reaction when an individual is startled or anxious. The second set of symptoms that follow an untreated adrenergic reaction are ***neuroglycopenic*** (also called brain hypoglycemia). They typically include difficulty with balance, memory, attention, and/or concentration; dizziness or

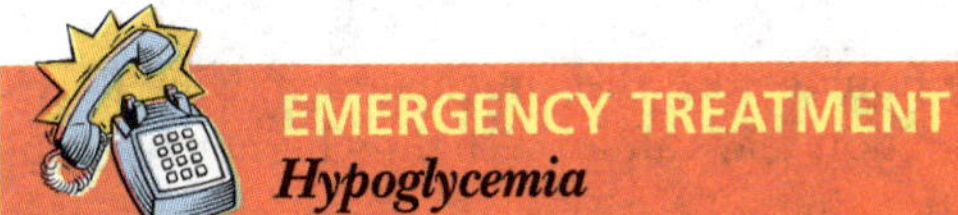

EMERGENCY TREATMENT
Hypoglycemia

MILD REACTION: ADRENERGIC SYMPTOMS

Give child 10 to 15 g simple, high carbohydrate (preferably liquid, e.g., 3 to 6 oz orange juice).
Follow with starch-protein snack.

MODERATE REACTION: NEUROGLYCOPENIC SYMPTOMS

Give child 10 to 15 g simple carbohydrate as above.
Repeat in 10 to 15 minutes if symptoms persist.
Follow with larger snack.
Watch child closely.

SEVERE REACTION: UNRESPONSIVE, UNCONSCIOUS, AND/OR SEIZURES

Administer glucagon as prescribed.
Follow with planned meal or snack when child is able to eat, or add a snack of 10% of daily calories.

NOCTURNAL REACTION

Give child 10 to 15 g simple carbohydrate.
Follow with snack of 10% of daily calories.

lightheadedness; and slurred speech. Severe and prolonged hypoglycemia leads to convulsions, coma, and possible death (Cox, Carter, and Gonder-Frederick, 1986). Hypoglycemia can be managed effectively as outlined in the Emergency Treatment box.

➤ **NURSING TIP** Commercial glucose gel, cake frosting, or honey can be rubbed on the gums and buccal mucosa of the unconscious, hypoglycemic child if glucagon is not available. Caution: keep the gel in the cheek to avoid occluding the airway.

It is advisable for parents to plan for anticipated excitement or exercise. In addition, gastroenteritis may decrease insulin needs slightly as a result of poor appetite, vomiting, and/or diarrhea. If the blood glucose level is low but urinary ketones are present, the family should be aware of the increased need for simple carbohydrates and liquids.

Hygiene. All aspects of personal hygiene should be emphasized for the child with diabetes. The child should be cautioned against wearing shoes without socks, wearing sandals, or walking barefoot. Correct nail and extremity care instituted for each particular child (with the guidance of a podiatrist) can begin health practices that last a lifetime. Eyes should be checked once a year unless the child wears glasses and then as directed by the ophthalmologist. Regular dental care is emphasized, and cuts and scratches should be treated with plain soap and water unless otherwise indicated.

Exercise. Exercise is an important component of the treatment plan. If the child is more active at one time of the day than at another time, food and/or insulin can be altered to meet the activity pattern of the individual child. Food should be increased in the summer when children tend to be more active. Decreased activity on return to school may require a decrease in food intake and/or increase in insulin dosage. The child who is active in team sports will need additional food intake in the form of a snack about ½ hour before the anticipated activity. Races or other competition may call for a slightly higher food intake than practice times.

Food will usually need to be repeated for prolonged activity periods, often as frequently as every 45 minutes to 1 hour. Families should be informed that if increased food is not tolerated, decreased insulin is the next course of action. If the timing of the exercise is changed so that the supper meal is delayed, the insulin in the second or third dose of the day may be moved back to precede the mealtime. Sugar may sometimes be needed during exercise periods for quick response. Elevated blood glucose levels following extreme activity may represent the Somogyi reflex. If the blood glucose level is elevated (240 mg/dl or higher) before planned exercise, the activity should be postponed until the blood glucose is controlled.

Without adequate insulin levels the cells are unable to receive glucose, the preferred fuel, despite the high level of blood glucose. The low insulin level allows glucagon to act, uninhibited, to increase hepatic glucose production, further raising the blood glucose level with no means to use sugar at the muscle site. Breakdown of fat (lipolysis) is the alternative, and the end product of lipolysis is ketone body production (Maynard, 1991).

NURSING ALERT Ketonuria is an early sign of ketoacidosis and a contraindication to exercise.

Record Keeping. Home records are an invaluable aid to diabetes self-management. The nurse and family devise a method to chart insulins administered, blood glucose values, urine ketone results, and other factors and events that affect diabetes control. Variations in diet and exercise are recorded, including ketone results, temperature, and intake. The child and family are encouraged to observe for patterns of blood glucose responses to events such as exercise. If lapses in management occur (such as eating a candy bar), the child should be encouraged to note this and not be condemned for the transgression.

Complications. The implications of the disease should be presented in a tactful, clear, and nonfearful manner. Knowledge of the complications of diabetes and their relationship to control provides a basis for knowledgeable decision making. Eye and kidney disease are the greatest threats, with neurologic complications close behind. Clear explanations of these problems clarify false information often given by well-meaning friends. The information should include discussion of research so that the family is left with the positive impression that others are concerned about finding answers and preventing complications. It also gives them hope that somehow, some way, a prevention and/or cure is possible.

Self-Management. Self-management is the key to close control. Being able to make changes at the time they are needed rather than waiting until the next contact with health professionals is important for self-management and gives the individual and family the feeling that they have control over the disease. Psychologically this helps the family members feel that they are useful and participating members of the team. Learning to look at records objectively gives the child support. As children grow and assume more and more responsibility for self-management, they develop confidence in their ability to manage their disease and in themselves as persons. They grow to respond to the disease and to make more accurate interpretations and changes in self-management when they become adults.

Self-management techniques to be mastered are the testing and adjustment of insulin and diet with alterations in day-to-day activities and unusual occurrences. However, limitations should be set regarding how many alterations can be made without consulting with the health professionals. The degree of control before the illness is a determining factor in seeking medical help during illness. In an individual with poor control, it takes only a few hours before the trouble is severe, whereas if control is good before the illness, several days may elapse before help is needed. Patients and families are cautioned to seek assistance if glucose levels are elevated and urine is not clear of ketones after 24 hours of self-management.

Child and Family Support. The parents and other family members of the child with newly diagnosed DM experience various emotional responses to the crises just as the physiologic responses affect the child. Care in the acute setting is short but may create fears and frustrations. The prospect of a chronic illness in their child engenders all the feeling and concerns that are faced by parents of children with other chronic illnesses (see Chapter 22). The threat of complications and death is always present, as well as the continuing drain on emotional and financial resources.

Certain fears may develop as a result of past experiences with the disease. A severe insulin reaction with seizures is certainly one experience that contributes to fear of repetition. Once parents observe a seizure or the adolescent has one in a public place, the desire to maintain better control is reinforced. They must understand how to prevent problems and how to handle problems calmly and coolly if they occur, and they must understand the complexities of the body, the disease, and its complications. Young children usually adjust well to problems related to the disease. With toddlers and preschoolers, insulin injections and glucose testing may be difficult at first. However, they usually accept the procedures when the parents use a matter-of-fact approach without calling attention to a "hurt" and treat the procedure like any other routine part of a child's life. Following the injection, time with some special and positive attention such as reading, talking, or other pleasant activity is one way to convert children who initially refuse injections to those who accept them.

Children in the years before adolescence probably accept their condition most easily. They are able to understand the basic concepts related to their disease and its treatment. They are able to test blood glucose and urine, recognize food groups, give injections, keep records, and distinguish between feelings of fear, excitement, and hypoglycemia. They understand how to recognize, prevent, and treat hypoglycemia. However, they still need considerable parental involvement.

➤ **NURSING TIP** Ongoing motivation to adhere to a regimen is difficult. An older child and parent may enjoy negotiating a day off when the responsibility for testing and recording blood glucose is delegated from the child to the parent (or vice versa).

Adolescents appear to have the most difficulty in adjusting. Adolescence is a time when there is much stress toward being perfect and being like one's peers, and no matter what others say, having diabetes is being different. Some adolescents are more upset about not being able to have a candy bar than about injections, diet, and other aspects of management. If children can accept the difference as a part of life, in other words, that each person is different in some way, then with adequate parental support they should be able to adjust well.

Problems of adjustment to diabetes are especially difficult for the young person whose disease is diagnosed in adolescence. Denial is sometimes expressed by omitting insulin, not performing tests, and eating incorrectly, although denial of the disease usually diminishes during this period as the adolescent with DM begins to feel competent and worthy. This is the age when greatest falsification of records occurs, although recent information suggests that less risk-taking behavior occurs in adolescents with IDDM, perhaps because of parental overprotection and involvement (Orr, 1991). Diabetes makes the youngster different when conformity and sameness are desired; having the disease emphasizes vulnerability and imperfection when the search for identity is the foremost developmental task. It is often difficult for the adolescent to know what to tell friends.

Camping and other special groups are very useful. At diabetes camp children learn that they are not alone. As a result, they become more independent and resourceful in the nondiabetes camp setting, especially if they have had experience in a diabetes camp. Useful information about such camps and organizations can be obtained from the ADA. A free list of accredited camps specifically for children and teens with diabetes is also available.*

Puberty is associated with decreased sensitivity to insulin that normally would be compensated for by an increased insulin secretion. Health care professionals should anticipate that pubertal patients will have more difficulty maintaining glycemic control. Insulin doses commonly need to be increased, often dramatically. Patients should be taught to give themselves additional doses of regular insulin (5% to 10% of their daily dose) when their blood glucose levels are increased. The use of supplemental regular insulin is preferred to withholding food in the adolescent patient (Rogers, 1992.)

Eating disorders, such as bulimia or anorexia nervosa, in the teenager with IDDM (see Chapter 21) pose a serious health hazard. The nurse should be alert to a history of preoccupation with weight, food faddism, excessive calorie restriction, and/or unexplained hypoglycemia. Moreover, insulin manipulation or omission has been identified as a weight loss tool used by some female adolescents (Rodin, Craven, and Daneman, 1989).

Inaccurate doses of insulin may occur inadvertently or, if they occur frequently, may be an attention-seeking device; in a number of cases they may occur as a subconscious but socially accepted method of suicide. Excessive intake of food leads to obesity, which may also represent a subconscious death wish. Psychiatric counseling may be needed if suicidal tendencies are amplified by the diabetes.

Rehospitalizations are most often related to poor control of the disease, although it is also possible that they are indirectly related to noncoping and are a method of avoiding the pressures caused by family and peers. The hospital may represent an environment that is peaceful and free of stress. The goal for this problem is to determine the cause of the hospitalization. It may be related to poor control, poor self-management, or the need for better supportive management at home. Evaluation should be based on the physiologic and psychologic adjustment of the child and the family.

Parents. Parents develop guilt feelings when they have a child with any chronic disease, especially one with a hereditary component. They cope with these feelings in a number of ways. For example, they may be overprotective or neglectful. Guilt-ridden parents may blame themselves for the disease, consciously or subconsciously. Nevertheless, they must come to realize through education and counseling that there was nothing they could have done to prevent the disease and that it was not their fault, since environmental, as well as hereditary, factors may be involved in the development of the disease.

Parents who are overprotective suffer from feelings of guilt, as well as fear of the unknown. Overprotection is a mechanism that alters the guilt responses to justify their own needs—for example, "If the child is in my sight, nothing worse will happen than has already happened by the child getting diabetes. Therefore, I am going to watch this child every single minute so that nothing further can happen to him." The overprotective parent becomes the smothering parent, one that hampers the growth, development, and maturation of the affected child.

The neglectful parent, on the other hand, has a different problem. This response is a mechanism developed to block feelings that give pain and provide relief from feelings of guilt—"This is your disease, and I have no responsibilities related to your disease; therefore if anything bad happens to you as a result of your having this disease, it is not my fault." The neglectful parent assigns responsibilities to the child before the child is mature enough to accept a more adult role.

Threatened parents look at the disease as a way to keep the child tied to them. If the child learns to be independent, as is expected of the child in a camping experience, the parent may feel threatened and place obstacles in the child's path to independent development. Problems in the parental response provide a challenge for the nurse to assist by counseling or, if severe enough, to appropriately refer the parents to resources designed to help them alter their behavior.

Children who are sufficiently mature may be seen alone by the health professional, although the parents should not

*Camp Directory, 1660 Duke St., Alexandria, VA 22314; (800) 232-3472.

NURSING CARE PLAN
The Child with Diabetes Mellitus

Hospital Care

NURSING DIAGNOSIS: High risk for injury related to insulin deficiency

PATIENT GOAL 1: Will exhibit normal blood glucose levels

• **NURSING INTERVENTIONS/*RATIONALES***

Obtain blood glucose level *to determine most appropriate dose of insulin*

*Administer insulin as prescribed *to maintain normal blood glucose level*

Understand the action of insulin

Understand the differences in composition, time of onset, and duration of action for the various insulin preparations *to ensure accurate insulin administration*

Employ insulin techniques when preparing and administering insulin

Subcutaneous injection; depth according to thickness of subcutaneous tissue

Rotation of sites *to enhance absorption of insulin*

• **EXPECTED OUTCOME**

Child demonstrates normal blood glucose levels

NURSING DIAGNOSIS: High risk for injury related to hypoglycemia

PATIENT GOAL 1: Will exhibit no evidence of hypoglycemia

• **NURSING INTERVENTIONS/*RATIONALES***

Recognize signs of hypoglycemia early

Be particularly alert at times when blood glucose levels are lowest (11:00 AM and 2:30 AM) (e.g., bursts of physical activity without additional food, or delayed, omitted, or incompletely consumed meal or snack)

Test blood glucose

Offer 10 to 15 g of readily absorbed carbohydrates, such as orange juice, hard candy, or milk, *to elevate blood glucose level and alleviate symptoms of hypoglycemia*

Follow with complex carbohydrate and protein, such as bread or cracker spread with peanut butter or cheese *to maintain blood glucose level*

*Administer glucagon to unconscious child *to elevate blood glucose level;* position child *to minimize risk of aspiration, since vomiting may occur*

• **EXPECTED OUTCOMES**

Child ingests an appropriate carbohydrate

Child displays no evidence of hypoglycemia

*Dependent nursing action.

Preparation for Home Care

NURSING DIAGNOSIS: Knowledge deficit (diabetes management) related to care of a child with newly diagnosed diabetes mellitus

PATIENT/FAMILY GOAL 1: Will accept teaching provided

• **NURSING INTERVENTIONS/*RATIONALES***

Select methods, vocabulary, and content appropriate to the level of the learner *to maximize learning*

Allow 3 or 4 days for family and child to begin to adjust to the initial impact of the diagnosis

Select an environment conducive to learning

Allow ample time for the education process

Restrict length of teaching sessions *because this is how people learn best*

Child—15-20 minutes

Parents—45-60 minutes

Involve all senses and employ a variety of teaching strategies, especially participation *because it is usually the most effective method for learning*

Provide pamphlets or other supplementary materials *for future referral*

• **EXPECTED OUTCOME**

Child and/or family display attitudes conductive to learning

PATIENT/FAMILY GOAL 2: Will demonstrate understanding of disease and its therapy

• **NURSING INTERVENTIONS/*RATIONALES***

Provide information regarding the pathophysiology of diabetes and the function and actions of insulin and glucagon in relation to caloric intake and exercise

Answer questions and clarify misconceptions *to ensure optimum learning*

Explain function and expected effects of procedures and tests, *since these are a necessary part of diabetes management*

• **EXPECTED OUTCOME**

Child and/or family demonstrate an understanding of the disease and its therapy (specify indicators)

PATIENT/FAMILY GOAL 3: Will demonstrate understanding of diet planning

• **NURSING INTERVENTIONS/*RATIONALES***

Enlist the services of a dietitian *to teach diet planning*

Emphasize the relationship between normal nutritional needs and the disease *to encourage a sense of normalacy*

Become familiar with family's culture and food preferences *so that these are included in meal planning*

Teach or reinforce learners' understanding of the basic food groups and the diet plan prescribed (e.g., exchange diet)

NURSING CARE PLAN
The Child with Diabetes Mellitus—cont'd

Help child and family estimate food weights by volume, *since this is more practical than weighing food*
Suggest low-carbohydrate snack items
Guide family in assessing the labels of food products for carbohydrate content, *since concentrated sugars are avoided in the diet*
Teach or reinforce an understanding of the concept of exchanges, *since exchanges ensure day-to-day consistency in total intake while allowing a choice of foods*
Relate constant carbohydrate equivalents to familiar foods
Retain cultural patterns and family preferences as much as possible, *so that child and family are more likely to adhere to diet requirements*

• **EXPECTED OUTCOME**
Child and/or family demonstrate an understanding of diet planning and food selection (specify indicators)

PATIENT/FAMILY GOAL 4: Will demonstrate knowledge of and ability to administer insulin

• **NURSING INTERVENTIONS/*RATIONALES***
Teach child and family the characteristics of the insulins prescribed for child, *since there are several insulin preparations*
Teach proper mixing of insulins and acceptable substitutions *when the family brand is unavailable*
Teach injection procedure
- Impress on learners that the procedure will be a routine part of child's life *in order to decrease anxiety and increase cooperation*
- Involve caregivers and child, if old enough, *so that more than one person learns procedure*
- Teach basic techniques using an orange or similar item *so that learner can gain confidence before injecting a person*
- Use demonstration and return demonstration techniques on another before injecting child *because this is usually less stressful*
- Help families and child work out a set rotational pattern *because this is important for maximum absorption of insulin*
- Teach proper care of insulin and equipment

Teach management of continuous infusion pump (if used)

• **EXPECTED OUTCOMES**
Child and/or family demonstrate an understanding of insulin, its various forms, and action (specify indicators)
Child and/or family demonstrate injection technique correctly
Child and/or family develop a rotation plan
Child and/or family demonstrate correct use of pump and care of injection site

PATIENT/FAMILY GOAL 5: Will demonstrate ability to test blood glucose level

• **NURSING INTERVENTIONS/*RATIONALES***
Teach family and child, if old enough:
- Blood glucose monitoring and/or use of equipment selected for use
- Interpretation of results *so that they learn how to adjust insulin based on blood glucose level*
- Care and maintenance of equipment

• **EXPECTED OUTCOME**
Child and/or family demonstrate correct use of the glucose monitoring equipment

PATIENT/FAMILY GOAL 6: Will demonstrate ability to test urine

• **NURSING INTERVENTIONS/*RATIONALES***
Teach family and child, if old enough:
- Urine ketone testing and interpretation of results
- Proper care of test strips

• **EXPECTED OUTCOME**
Child and/or family demonstrate urine testing and interpretation

PATIENT/FAMILY GOAL 7: Will demonstrate understanding of proper hygiene

• **NURSING INTERVENTIONS/*RATIONALES***
Emphasize the importance of personal hygiene *so that child establishes health practices that last a lifetime*
Encourage regular dental care and yearly ophthalmologic examinations, *since these are important for child's general health*
Teach proper care of cuts and scratches *to minimize risk of infection*
Teach proper foot care, *since this will become a high priority during adulthood*

• **EXPECTED OUTCOME**
Child and family demonstrate an understanding of the importance of proper hygiene

PATIENT/FAMILY GOAL 8: Will demonstrate understanding of importance of exercise regimen

• **NURSING INTERVENTIONS/*RATIONALES***
Arrange for occupational therapy program that includes physical activity, *since this is an important part of diabetic management*
Work with child, family, and others (e.g., coaches) to help plan a home exercise program
Reiterate practitioner's instructions regarding adjustment of food and/or insulin to meet child's activity pattern; reinforce with examples *so that child and family are adequately prepared*

• **EXPECTED OUTCOME**
Child and family help child outline and carry out a regular exercise program

Continued.

NURSING CARE PLAN
The Child with Diabetes Mellitus—cont'd

PATIENT/FAMILY GOAL 9: Will demonstrate understanding and management of hyperglycemia and hypoglycemia

• **NURSING INTERVENTIONS/*RATIONALES***

Instruct learners in how to recognize signs of hyperglycemia and hypoglycemia (especially hypoglycemia) *to prevent delay in treatment*

Explain the relationship of insulin needs to illness, activity, and intense emotion (either positive or negative)

Teach how to adjust food, activity, and insulin at times of illness and during other situations that alter blood glucose levels

Suggest carrying source of carbohydrate, such as sugar cubes or hard candy, in pocket or handbag *so that it is readily available to treat hypoglycemia*

Instruct parents and child in how to treat hypoglycemia with food, simple sugars, or glucagon

• **EXPECTED OUTCOME**

Child and family demonstrate an understanding of the signs and management of a hypoglycemic reaction (specify)

PATIENT GOAL 10: Will wear medical identification

• **NURSING INTERVENTIONS/*RATIONALES***

Encourage acquisition of a means of identification, such as an identification bracelet, that explains child's condition *in case of emergency*

Explain to child why identification is important *so that child is more likely to comply*

• **EXPECTED OUTCOME**

Family acquires and child wears identification bracelet

PATIENT/FAMILY GOAL 11: Will keep proper records of insulin administration and testing procedures

• **NURSING INTERVENTIONS/*RATIONALES***

Help child and family to design a form for keeping records of the following *because this information is useful to both partitioner and family in managing diabetes:*

Insulin administered
Blood and urine tests
Food intake
Marked variation in exercise
Illness

• **EXPECTED OUTCOME**

Family and child keep an accurate record of insulin administration, glucose testing, etc.

PATIENT GOAL 12: Will engage in self-management

• **NURSING INTERVENTIONS/*RATIONALES***

Encourage honesty in recording, such as eating a forbidden candy bar, *so that recording is accurate and useful*

Encourage independence in applying the concepts learned in teaching sessions *since diabetes management is a life-long endeavor*

Instruct when to seek assistance from medical personnel *to prevent delay in treatment*

• **EXPECTED OUTCOME**

Child takes responsibility for management of disease commensurate with age and capabilities

NURSING DIAGNOSIS: Altered family processes related to situational crisis (child with a chronic disorder)

See Nursing Care Plan: The Child with Chronic Illness or Disability, Chapter 22

be made to feel that they are being left out. Time should be set aside during the child's health visit or afterward to meet the needs of the parents. They should also be included in special sessions to keep them abreast of the child's management, to help them continue to participate in the child's care, and to provide them with an opportunity to express their own feelings concerning their own or their child's adjustment to the disease. The amount of information that they offer at this time can give clues to their level of support of the child and help assist in decisions concerning the therapeutic management of the child. This helps guide the child through the most disruptive time of life—the teenage years.

Health professionals must be aware of parents who voice support and appear to be supporting the child to the optimum level but who, with more in-depth interviewing, are found to be supporting the child in word but not by action. These parents seldom see the need for following through from verbalizing to fulfilling the real needs of the child, and they unknowingly place obstacles in the child's path. They may be helping the child grow up too fast and therefore insecurely. Counseling is urgently needed for these parents, who need to realize how their behavior affects the child. The classroom experience, group therapy, or parenting programs can help guide the parent's relationships with their children. All parents should be made to recognize that as children grow and develop, they are children first and children with diabetes second. The ultimate goal for these parents is to be supportive of their children, to communicate more effectively, and to help their children develop in a more acceptable manner.

❖ EVALUATION

The effectiveness of nursing interventions is determined by continual reassessment and evaluation of care based on the following observational guidelines and expected outcomes:

1. Interview family to determine their understanding of the disease; have child and family demonstrate and discuss the needed assessment and therapeutic techniques.
2. Interview family regarding their understanding of tight control; analyze and evaluate management records.
3. Discuss the disease with child.
4. Interview family and child regarding their feelings and concerns about the disease.

Expected outcomes:

See Nursing Care Plan, pp. 1786-1788.

KEY POINTS

- The endocrine system has three components: the cell, which sends a chemical message via a hormone; target cells, which receive the message; and the environment through which the chemical is transported from the site of synthesis to the sites of cellular action.
- Pituitary dysfunction is manifested primarily by growth disturbance.
- The main physiologic action of thyroid hormone is to regulate the basal metabolic rate and control the processes of growth and tissue differentiation.
- Disorders of thyroid function include hypothyroidism, autoimmune thyroiditis, goiter, and hyperthyroidism.
- Therapy for hyperthyroidism is directed at retarding the rate of hormone secretion and may include drug therapy, thyroidectomy, or radioiodine therapy.
- Classic forms of hypoparathyroidism in childhood are idiopathic—deficient production of PTH—and pseudohypoparathyroidism—increased PTH production with end organ unresponsiveness to PTH.
- The adrenal cortex secretes three important groups of hormones: glucocorticoids, mineralocorticoids, and sex steroids.
- Disorders of adrenal function include acute adrenocortical insufficiency, chronic adrenocortical insufficiency, Cushing syndrome, congenital adrenogenital hyperplasia, and hyperaldosteronism.
- Four categories of Cushing syndrome are pituitary, adrenal, ectopic, and iatrogenic.
- Management of congenital adrenogenital hyperplasia includes assignment of a sex according to genotype, administration of cortisone, and, possibly, reconstructive surgery.
- Diabetes mellitus is categorized as insulin-dependent diabetes, non-insulin-dependent diabetes, and maturity-onset diabetes of youth.
- The focus of insulin-dependent diabetes management is insulin replacement, diet, and exercise.
- Education of families includes explanation of diabetes, meal planning, administering insulin injection, monitoring, general hygienic practices, promoting exercise, record keeping, and observing for complications.

REFERENCES

Albisser AM, Sperlich M: Adjusting insulins, *Diabetes Educator* 18(3):211-218, 1992.

Allen KD and others: Psychosocial adjustment of children with isolated growth hormone deficiency, *Child Health Care* 22(1):61-72, 1993.

Bach J: Cyclosporine in insulin-dependent diabetes mellitus, J Pediatr 111:1073-1074, 1987.

Bartlett E: The stepped approach to patient education, *Diabetes Educator* 14(2):130-135, 1988.

Bertagna X: New causes of Cushing's syndrome, *N Engl J Med* 327(14):1024-1025, 1992.

Brouhard B, Rogers G: Pancreatic and islet replacement therapy for insulin-dependent diabetes mellitus, *Clin Pediatr* 32(5):258-263, 1993.

Casella S and others: Accuracy and precision of low-dose insulin administration, *Pediatrics* 91(6):1155-1157, 1993.

Chase HP, Chase VC, Garg S: Self-care for the young diabetic—home but not alone, *Contemp Pediatr* 8:74-88, 1991.

Chase HP, Garg S, Jelley D: Diabetic ketoacidosis in children and the role of outpatient management, *Pediatr Rev* 11(10):1024-1025, 1990.

Cooper N: Nutrition and diabetes: a review of current recommendations, *Diabetes Educator* 14(5):428-432, 1988.

Cox DJ, Carter WR, Gonder-Frederick L: Without warning, *Diabetes Forecast* 39:41-43, 1986.

Diabetes Control and Complications Trial Research Group: The effect of intensive treatment of diabetes on the development and progression of long-term complications in insulin-dependent diabetes mellitus, *N Engl J Med* 329(14):977-986, 1993.

DiGeorge AM: The endocrine system. In Behrman RE, Vaughan VC III: *Textbook of pediatrics,* ed 14, Philadelphia, 1992, WB Saunders.

Drash AL: Insulin-dependent diabetes mellitus in children and adolescents: genetics and etiology, *Curr Opin Pediatr* 1:61-73, 1989.

Drucker S, New M: Nonclassic adrenal hyperplasia due to 21-hydroxylase deficiency, *Pediatr Clin North Am* 34(4):1067-1081, 1987.

Fink JN, Beall GN: Immunologic aspects of endocrine diseases, *JAMA* 248:2696-2700, 1982.

Gildea J: High and dry—low and wet: the key to DI and SIADH, *Pediatr Nurs* 19(5):478-481, 1993.

Hancock SL, Cox RS, McDougall R: Thyroid diseases after treatment of Hodgkin's disease, *N Engl J Med* 325(9):599-605, 1991.

Hathaway WE, Hay WW Jr: *Current pediatric diagnosis and treatment,* ed 11, Norwalk, CT, 1992, Appleton & Lange.

Kahn and Weir: *Joslin's diabetes mellitus,* ed 13, Philadelphia, 1994, Lea & Febiger.

Karjalainen J and others: A bovine albumin peptide as a possible trigger of insulin-dependent diabetes mellitus, *N Engl J Med* 327(5):302-307, 1992.

Laufer IJ: Morning hyperglycemia, *Diabetes Prof,* p 36, Dec 1987.

MacGillvray MH: The pediatrician's role in identification and management of growth: normal, subnormal, and abnormal patterns, *Pediatr Rounds* 2(1):2-5, 1993.

MacLaren N, Atkinson M: Is insulin dependent diabetes mellitus environmentally induced? *N Engl J Med* 327(5):348-349, 1992.

Mahoney CP: Differential diagnosis of goiter, *Pediatr Clin North Am* 34:891-905, 1987.

Maynard T: Exercise: physiological response to exercise in diabetes mellitus. *Diabetes Educator,* 17(3):196-204, 1991.

Moore KC and others: Clinical diagnoses of children with extremely short stature and their response to growth hormone. *J Pediatr* 122(5):687-692, 1992.

Nathan DM: Long-term complications of diabetes mellitus, *N Engl J Med* 328(23):1678-85, 1993.

Nora JJ, Fraser FC: *Medical genetics,* Philadelphia, 1989, Lea & Febiger.

Orr D: *Risk-taking behavior in adolescents with diabetes.* Paper presented at the fourteenth International Diabetes Federation Congress, Washington, DC, June 1991.

Owen G: Hazards of tests of growth hormone secretion, *Br Med J* 304(6829):777, 1992 (letter).

Plotnick LP: Insulin-dependent diabetes mellitus. In Oski FA and others, editors: *Principles and practice of pediatrics,* Philadelphia, 1990, JB Lippincott.

Reasner II C: Clinical implications of the DCCT trial, *Contemp Intern Med* 6(2):5-8, 1994.

Rodin G, Craven J, Daneman D: Eating disorders and insulin manipulation in adolescent females with insulin-dependent diabetes mellitus, *Psychosom Med* 51:244-266, 1989.

Rogers D: Puberty and insulin-dependent diabetes mellitus, *Clin Pediatr* 31(3):168-173, 1992.

Rosenstock J, Strowig S, Raskin P: Insulin pump therapy: a realistic appraisal, *Clin Diabetes* 3:1, 27-30, 1985.

Rovet JF, Danemen D, Bailey JD: Psychologic and psychoeducational consequences of thyroxine therapy for juvenile acquired hypothyroidism, *J Pediatr* 122(4):543-549, 1993.

Ruble JA: Congenital adrenal hyperplasia. In Jackson PL, Vessey JA: Primary care of the child with a chronic condition, St Louis, 1992, Mosby.

Sack J and others: Association of autoimmune thyroiditis and HLA-DR5 in multiple family members, *J Pediatr* 103:758-760, 1983.

Sonis WA and others: Behavior problems and social competence in girls with true precocious puberty, *J Pediatr* 106:156-160, 1985.

Stabler B: Psychosocial outcomes of short stature, *Pediatr Rounds* 2(1):5-7, 1993.

Starkman H and others: Limited joint mobility (LJM) of the hand in patients with diabetes mellitus: relation to chronic complications, *Ann Rheum Dis* 4:130-151, 1986.

Tallstedt L and others: Occurrence of ophthalmopathy after treatment for graves; hyperthyroidism, *N Engl J Med* 326(26):1733-1738, 1992.

Theintz GE and others: Evidence for a reduction of growth potential in adolescent female gymnasts, *J Pediatr* 122:306-313, 1993.

White K, and others: Unstable diabetes and unstable families: a psychosocial evaluation of diabetic children with recurrent ketoacidosis, *Pediatrics* 73:749-755, 1984.

Winters WE, Chihara T, Schatz D: The genetics of autoimmune diabetes, *Am J Dis Child* 147(12):1282-1290, 1993.

Zekauskas S and others: Human growth hormone and Creutzfeldt-Jakob disease, *J Okla State Med Assoc* 83(9):446-449, 1990.

BIBLIOGRAPHY

Pituitary Dysfunction

Bercu BB: Growth hormone treatment and the short child: to treat or not to treat? *J Pediatr* 110:991-994, 1987.

Bundak R and others: Long-term auxologic effects of human growth hormone, *J Pediatr* 112:875-879, 1987.

Connaughty MS: Accelerated growth in children, *J Pediatr Health Care* 6(5, pt 2):316-324, 1992.

Costin G, Kaufman FR: Growth hormone secretory patterns in children with short stature, *J Pediatr* 110:362-368, 1987.

Genentech Collaborative Study: Idiopathic short stature: results of a one-year controlled study of human growth hormone treatment, *J Pediatr* 15:713-719, 1989.

Giordana BP: The impact of genetic syndromes on children's growth, *J Pediatr Health Care* 6(5, pt 2):309-315, 1992.

Henry JJ: Routine growth monitoring and assessment of growth disorders, *J Pediatr Health Care* 6(5, pt 2):291-301, 1992.

Hopwood N and others: Growth response of children with non–growth hormone deficiency and marked short stature during three years of growth hormone therapy, *J Pediatr* 123(2):215-222, 1993.

Jackson PL, Ott MJ: Precocious puberty: the role of the school nurse, *Sch Nurse* 6(1):16-18, 1990.

Kappy MS, Stuart T, Perelman A: Efficacy of leuprolide therapy in children with central precocious puberty, *Am J Dis Child* 142:1061-1064, 1988.

Lee PA, Page JG, Leuprolide Study Group: Effects of leuprolide in the treatment of central precocious puberty, *J Pediatr* 114:321-324, 1989.

Lippe BM: Short stature in children: evaluation and management, *J Pediatr Health Care* 1:313-322, 1987.

Manasco PK and others: Resumption of puberty after long-term luteinizing hormone–releasing hormone agonist treatment of central precocious puberty, *J Clin Endocrinol Metab* 67:368-372, 1988.

McElroy DB, Davis GT: SIADH and the acutely ill child, MCN 11:193-196, 1986.

Parks BR, Fischer RG: Growth hormone, *Pediatr Nurs* 12:302, 1986.

Rieser PA: Educational, psychologic, and social aspects of short stature, *J Pediatr Health Care* 6(5, pt 2):325-332, 1992.

Root AW, Diamond FB, Bercu BB: Short stature: when is growth hormone indicated? *Contemp Pediatr* 4(2):26-56, 1987.

Ross JL and others: Growth hormone secretory dynamics in children with precocious puberty, *J Pediatr* 110:369-372, 1987.

Saggese G, Cesaretti G: Criteria for recognition of the growth-in-efficient child who may respond to treatment with growth hormone, *Am J Dis Child* 143:1287-1293, 1989.

Saggese G and others: Effects of long-term treatment with growth hormone on bone and mineral metabolism in children with growth hormone deficiency, *J Pediatr* 122(1):37-45, 1993.

Schwartz ID, Root AW: Puberty in girls: early, incomplete, or precocious? *Contemp Pediatr* 7(1):147-156, 1990.

Usala A, Blumer JL: Pharmacology of new hormonal therapies in the treatment of pediatric endocrine disorders, *Pediatr Clin North Am* 36:1157-1182, 1989.

Disorders of Thyroid Function/Disorders of the Parathyroid Gland

Fisher DA, Pandian MR, Carlton E: Autoimmune thyroid disease: an expanding spectrum, *Pediatr Clin North Am* 34:907-918, 1987.

Gorton C, Sadeghi-Nejd A, Senior B: Remission in children with hyperthyroidism treated with propylthiouracil, *Am J Dis Child* 141:1084-1086, 1987.

Mack R: Thyroid medication—don't overdose on conformity, *Contemp Pediatr* 10(3):105-114, 1993.

Mäenpää J and others: Natural course of juvenile autoimmune thyroiditis, *J Pediatr* 107:898-904, 1985.

Adrenal Dysfunction

Bhatia V and others: Adrenal tumor complicating untreated 21-hydroxylase deficiency in a 5½-year-old boy; *Am J Dis Child* 147(12):1321-1324, 1993.

Darland NW: Congenital adrenocortical hyperplasia: supportive nursing interventions, *J Pediatr Nurs* 1(2):117-123, 1986.

Lee PDK, Winter RJ, Green OC: Virilizing adrenocortical tumors in childhood: eight cases and a review of the literature, *Pediatrics* 76:437-444, 1985.

Orth D: Differential diagnosis of cushing's synrome, *N Engl J Med* 325(13):957-959, 1991.

Diabetes Mellitus: General

Caprio S and others: Increased insulin secretion in puberty: a compensatory response to reductions in insulin sensitivity, *J Pediatr* 114:963-967, 1989.

Chase HP and others: Diagnosis of pre-type I diabetes, *J Pediatr* 111:807-812, 1987.

Chase HP and others: Diabetic ketoacidosis in children and the role of outpatient management, *Pediatr Rev* 11(10):297-304, 1990.

Chase HP and others: Prediction of the course of pre–type I diabetes, *J Pediatr* 118(6):838-841, 1991.

Cunningham L: Sports nutrition for the serious athlete, *Diabetes Forecast* 39(1):63-64, 1986.

DiFlorio IA, Duncan P: Design for successful patient teaching, *MCN* 11:246-249, 1986.

Glasgow A and others: Readmissions of children with diabetes mellitus to a children's hospital, *Pediatrics,* 88(1):98-104, 1991.

Green A and others: Incidence of childhood-onset insulin-dependent diabetes mellitus: the Eurodiab Ace study, *Lancet* 339:905-909, 1992.

Grey M and others: Initial adaptation in children with newly diagnosed diabetes and healthy children, *Pediatr Nurs* 21(1):17-22, 1994.

Haire-Joshu D, Flavin K, Clutter W: Contrasting type I and type II diabetes, *Am J Nurs* 86:1240-1243, 1986.

Ingersoll GM and others: Cognitive maturity and self-management among adolescents with insulin-dependent diabetes mellitus, *J Pediatr* 108:620-623, 1986.

Living with diabetes: perceptions of well-being, *Res Nurs Health* 13(4):255-262, 1990.

Martin R and others: The infant with diabetes mellitus: a case study, *Pediatr Nurs* 20(1):27-34, 1994.

MacLaren N, Lafferty K: Perspectives in diabetes, *Diabetes* 42:1099-1104, Aug 1993.

Newkumet KM and others: Altered blood pressure reactivity in adolescent diabetics, *Pediatrics* 93(4):616-621, 1994.

Rossini AA, Mordes JP, Handler EAS: A tumbler hypothesis: the autoimmunity of insulin-dependent diabetes mellitus, *Diabetes Spectrum* 2:195-200, 1989.

Travis LB, Brouhard BH, Schriener B: *Diabetes mellitus in children,* Philadelphia, 1987, WB Saunders.

Diabetes Mellitus: Testing and Monitoring

Belsey R and others: Managing bedside glucose testing in the hospital, *JAMA* 258:1634-1638, 1987.

Davis SG and others: In-hospital bedside blood glucose monitoring: the importance of a quality control program, *J Pediatr Nurs* 4:353-356, 1989.

Furberg H, Jensen AK, Salbu B: Effect of pretreatment with 0.9% sodium chloride on insulin solutions on the delivery of insulin from an infusion system, *Am J Hosp Pharm* 43:2209-2212, 1986.

Hahn K: Testing blood glucose levels, *Nursing 89* 19(12):66, 1989.

Montana JA: Glucose meters, *J Pediatr Nurs* 4:132-136, 1989.

Riley WJ, Winter WE, MacLaren NK: Identification of insulin-dependent diabetes mellitus before the onset of clinical symptoms, *J Pediatr* 112:314-316, 1988.

Strumph PS, Odoroff CL, Amatruda JM: The accuracy of blood glucose testing by children, *Clin Pediatr* 27:188-194, 1988.

Diabetes Mellitus: Therapeutic Management

Chase HP and others: Cyclosporine A for the treatment of new-onset insulin-dependent diabetes mellitus, *Pediatrics* 85:241-245, 1990.

Clark LM, Plotnick LP: Insulin pumps in children with diabetes, *J Pediatr Health Care* 4:3-10, 1990.

Gavin JR III: Diabetes and exercise, *Am J Nurs* 88:178-180, 1988.

Hahn K: Teaching patients to administer insulin, *Nursing 90* 20(4):70, 1990.

Holler HJ: Understanding the use of the exchange lists for meal planning in diabetes management, *Diabetes Educator* 17(6):474-482, 1991.

Hurxthal K: Quick! Teach this patient about insulin, *Am J Nurs* 88:1097-1100, 1988.

Kittler MS, Sucher D: Diet counseling in a multicultural society, *Diabetes Educator* 16(2):127-131, 1990.

Kruger DF, Treacy M, Whitehouse FW: Jet injection comes of age, *Diabetes Forecast* 41:17-18, 1988.

Lockwood DN, Trand MJ, Mather HM: Is injecting air into insulin bottles necessary? *Br Med J* 297:1315-1316, 1988.

Marrero DG, Fremion AS, Golden MP: Inproving compliance with exercise in adolescents with insulin-dependent diabetes mellitus: results of a self-motivated home exercise program, *Pediatrics* 81:519-525, 1988.

Price J and others: Evaluation of the insulin jet injector as a potential source of infection, *Am J Infect Control* 17:257-263, 1989.

Schiffrin A: Management of childhood diabetes, *Pediatr Ann* 16:694-710, 1987.

Sperling MA: Outpatient management of diabetes mellitus, *Pediatr Clin North Am* 34:919-934, 1987.

Diabetes Mellitus: Complications

Bailie MD: Heading off the complications of diabetes, *Contemp Pediatr* 6(1):87-102, 1989.

Bhatia V, Wolfsdorf MB: Severe hypoglycemia in youth with insulin-dependent diabetes mellitus: frequency and causative factors, *Pediatrics* 88(6):1187-1193, 1991.

Chase HP and others: Glucose control and the renal and retinal complications of insulin-dependent diabetes, *JAMA* 261:1155-1160, 1989.

Daneman D and others: Severe hypoglycemia in children with insulin-dependent diabetes mellitus: frequency and predisposing factors, *J Pediatr* 681-685, 1989.

Krane EJ: Diabetic ketoacidosis, *Pediatr Clin North Am* 34:935-960, 1987.

LaFranchi S: Hypoglycemia of infancy and childhood, *Pediatr Clin North Am* 34:961-982, 1987.

Lipman TH: Assessment of the child with diabetic ketoacidosis, *Dimens Crit Care Nurs* 6:82-93, 1987.

Sabo CE, Michael SR: Managing DKA and preventing a recurrence, *Nursing 89* 19(2):50-56, 1989.

Diabetes Mellitus: Child and Family

Armstrong N: Coping with diabetes mellitus, *Nurs Clin North Am* 22:559-568, 1987.

Balik B, Haig B, Moynihan PM: Diabetes and the school-aged child, *MCN* 11:324-330, 1986.

Dashiff CJ: Parents' perceptions of diabetes in adolescent daughters and its impact on the family, *J Pediatr Nurs* 8(6):361-369, 1993.

Dunning D: Safe travel tips for the diabetic patient, *RN* 52(4):51-54, 1989.

Edwards DR: Initial psychosocial impact of insulin-dependent diabetes mellitus on the pediatric client and family, *Issues Compr Pediatr Nurs* 10:199-207, 1987.

Ferrari M: The diabetic child and well sibling: risks to the well child's self-concept, *Child Health Care* 15:141-148, 1987.

Frey MA, Denyes MJ: Health and illness self-care in adolescents with IDDM: a test of Orem's theory, *Adv Nurs Sci* 12(1):67-75, 1989.

Gallo AM: Family management style in juvenile diabetes: a case illustration, *J Pediatr Nurs* 5:23-32, 1990.

Harrigan JF and others: The application of locus of control to diabetes education in school-aged children, *J Pediatr Nurs* 2:236-243, 1987.

Hodges LC, Parker J: Concerns of parents with diabetic children, *Pediatr Nurs* 13:22-24, 68, 1987.

Jacobson AM and others: Psychologic predictors of compliance in children with recent onset of diabetes mellitus, *J Pediatr* 110:805-811, 1987.

La Greca A, Satin W: Peer pressure, *Diabetes Forecast* 41:67-72, 1988.

Lipman TH and others: A developmental approach to diabetes in children: birth through preschool, *MCN* 14:255-259, 1989.

Lipman TH and others: A developmental approach to diabetes in children: school age—adolescence, *MCN* 14:330-332, 1989.

Pless IB and others: Expected diabetic control in childhood and psychosocial functioning in early adult life, *Diabetes Care* 11:387-392, 1988.

Rovet JF, Ehrlich RM: Effect of temperament on metabolic control in children with diabetes mellitus, *Diabetes Care* 11:77-82, 1988.

Savinetti-Rose B: Developmental issues in managing children with diabetes, *Pediatr Nurs* 20(1):11-15, 1994.

Schreiner BJ, Travis LB: When your child has diabetes: the preteen years, *Diabetes Forecast* 40:37-41, 1987.

Smith KE and others: Issues of managing diabetes in children and adolescents: a multifamily group approach, *Child Health Care* 18:49-52, 1989.

Snyder A: The role of school personnel in caring for the child with diabetes, *Sch Nurse* 40:9-17, 1987.

Tattersall R: Psychosocial aspects of diabetes in childhood and adolescence, *Pediatr Ann* 16:728-740, 1987.

Thorner N: Family vacations, *Diabetes Forecast* 40:45-46, 1987.

Zimmerman E and others: Diabetic camping: effect on knowledge, attitude, and self-concept, *Issues Compr Pediatr Nurs* 10:99-111, 1987.

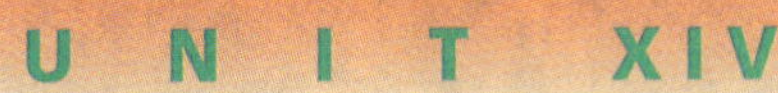

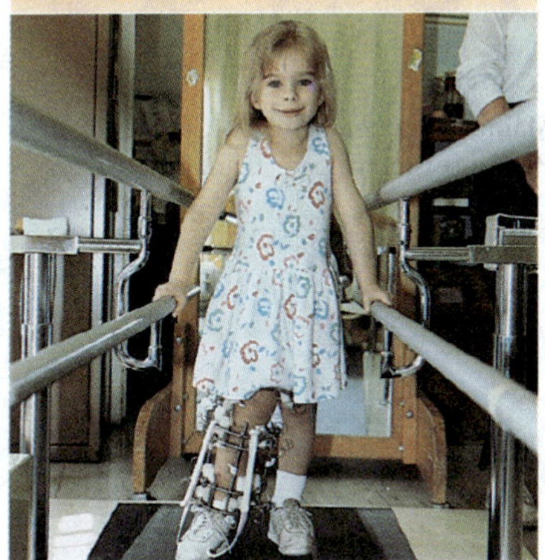

THE CHILD WITH A PROBLEM THAT INTERFERES WITH PHYSICAL MOBILITY

CHAPTER 39 The Child with Musculoskeletal or Articular Dysfunction

CHAPTER OUTLINE

RELATED TOPICS

Birth injuries, Ch. 9
Compliance, Ch. 27
Congenital clubfoot, Ch. 11
Developmental dysplasia of the hip, Ch. 11
Family-centered care of the child with chronic illness or disability, Ch. 22
Family-centered home care, Ch. 25
Injuries—the leading killer, Ch. 1
Injury prevention: infant, Ch. 12; toddler, Ch. 14; preschooler, Ch. 15; school-age child, Ch. 17; adolescent, Ch. 19
Maintaining healthy skin, Ch. 27
Pain assessment; pain management, Ch. 26
Physical activity, Ch. 17

THE CHILD AND TRAUMA

TRAUMA MANAGEMENT

Epidemiology of Trauma

Trauma is the leading cause of death in children over age 1 year (see Chapter 1) and an important cause of disability during childhood and adolescence. In many ways, childhood trauma differs little from trauma in adults. However, many aspects of injury are affected by the developmental stage of the child in both the type of injury that is incurred and the physiologic response to injury.

Nonintentional Injury. Among the leading causes of morbidity in children are medical problems resulting from traumatic injury at home, at school, in an automobile, or associated with recreational activities. Children's everyday activities include vigorous play, such as climbing, falling, running into immovable objects, and receiving blows to any part of their bodies. All of these activities make them prone to injury. School-age children and adolescents are vulnerable to multiple and severe trauma because they are mobile on bikes and motorcycles and in automobiles; they are also active in sports. Speed and congested surroundings often intensify the chance of injury.

Young children and teenagers usually do not calculate risks as they learn to manipulate their environment and achieve developmental goals. Therefore accidents are a part of most childhood experiences. Fortunately, when children fall or are hit, their body resilience protects them from incurring serious damage to soft tissue, the musculoskeletal system, or other body organs. Their bones are more flexible and therefore do not offer the rigid resistance to external forces that are likely to cause fractures (as occurs in more mature bones).

Child Abuse Injury. Unfortunately, careless handling of an infant or child (in some instances intentional physical abuse) is not uncommon in our society. A multitude of different types of bone and soft tissue injuries are inflicted on children by adults, and smaller children who are unable to protect themselves are most vulnerable. It is estimated that perhaps 25% of fractures in children under 3 years of age are the result of child abuse. Emergency room and pediatric office personnel should be alert to situations in which the child's injuries are not congruent with the parent's description of the incident; in which the child's behaviors, such as lack of crying or fearful mannerisms, are not the expected ones; or in which x-ray films show multiple healed fractures. For example, toddlers do not readily fall and break bones or catch a leg in the crib and break it. Reporting these incidents will aid in securing help for the child and family. A traumatic incident that produces physical injury to an infant or child may be the outcome of an accident that was no one's fault, or it may be associated with child abuse. A well-documented history is essential to determine the cause of the injury. (See also Physical Abuse, Chapter 16.)

Birth Injuries. During the birth process, fractures, dislocations, and/or nerve damage may be sustained. These injuries most often occur when the baby is large, the presentation is breech, or forceful extraction is used because of fetal distress. The two most common types of musculoskeletal injuries incurred during birth are fractured clavicle and brachial plexus injury. The presence of a qualified person at delivery will aid in reducing the complications of a difficult delivery. Complete postdelivery assessment of the newborn is essential for early detection of neurologic and/or musculoskeletal problems. (See also Birth Injuries, Chapter 9.)

Childhood Characteristics. Certain developmental characteristics of children at various ages render them more susceptible to injury. For example, the large head of infants and toddlers predisposes them to head injury, especially in falls. Also, the relatively large spleen and liver and the broad costal arch make these organs prone to direct trauma. Because of their light weight and small size, infants and small children are easily thrown around in a moving vehicle. Their natural curiosity and their propensity for using large muscles lure them to attempt potentially hazardous activities.

Later, in school-age children and adolescents, whose bone growth outstrips muscle growth, difficulty controlling movement can contribute to physical injury. It is also a time when many of these youngsters are attempting to engage in activities beyond their capabilities to keep up with more agile companions. They are also vulnerable to a "dare." Risk-taking compounded by a feeling of invulnerability is also characteristic of adolescence.

■ Patricia L. King, RN, MS, revised this chapter.

Prevention of Injury

Hazardous environmental factors play a major role in the number of serious accidents incurred by children. Stairways without handrails or a gate at the top, cluttered walkways, waxed floors, and throw rugs can contribute to a severe fall. Playground equipment should be checked periodically for hazards, and play areas should be supervised. Adults in charge of sports activities are encouraged to promote the use of safety-tested equipment and to follow game rules to prevent trauma and overplaying of a young athlete, whose immature musculoskeletal system and lack of coordination cannot tolerate excessive abuse.

Musculoskeletal trauma is most likely to occur in contact sports, with sprains being common. Certain contact sports, such as football, tend to produce joint damage, especially knee injuries. Severe hyperflexion of the neck from diving, trampoline activities, or football produces spinal cord injury and quadriplegia. Protective head and shoulder gear is helpful, but youngsters usually do not consistently wear appropriate protection unless they are well supervised (see Injuries and Health Problems Related to Sports Participation, p. 1832).

For children riding in a car, an effective infant or child car seat is a must to avoid their being thrown during a sudden stop or collision (see Chapters 12 and 14). Mandatory state regulations for the use of seat belts and child car restraints vary, but the nurse should be knowledgeable regarding the hospital's policy and car seat lending program. If this practice is begun when the child is an infant, the young child will be more likely to develop the habit of securing safety belts before the engine is started. In their everyday life, observant nurses are a valuable community resource in giving suggestions to parents and schools that might prevent at least some very serious injuries. (See also injury prevention segments in sections on health promotion during various age-groups.)

ASSESSMENT OF TRAUMA

The site of the injury usually influences the order of priority of interventions when emergency care is being instituted. The safety of both the victim and the "Good Samaritan" rescuers must be considered in order to prevent further injury. For example, removing a child from a burning building or the bottom of a swimming pool is the obvious action to the logically thinking person, but anxious rescuers may not consider their own safety to be of prime importance. The major reason for thinking through steps to be taken in an emergency before the actual incident occurs is to have a mental repertory of preplanned actions available at a stimulus-response level.

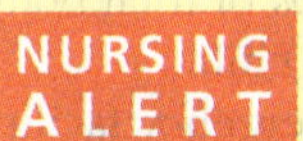

Always consider personal safety a top priority, since the victim cannot be helped if the rescuer is injured.

Emergency Management

Guidelines for care of the child at the scene of the injury are outlined in the Emergency Treatment box. Following assessment of level of consciousness, the concerns are for ***airway, breathing,*** and ***circulation (ABCs),*** after which other injuries are managed as indicated by the assessment. The ***airway*** is opened using the ***modified jaw-thrust maneuver,*** which is accomplished by grasping the angles of the victim's

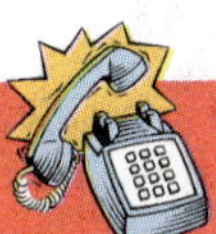

EMERGENCY TREATMENT
Trauma

Before entering accident area, observe for dangers to rescuers and bystanders. Be aware of potential for further injuries to child.

Observe scene for signs of mechanism of injury (e.g., head-on motor vehicle accident) (helps to determine proper course of action for treating child's injuries).

Do not move child before arrival of emergency medical services unless child is in danger of further injury. If it is necessary to move child, follow appropriate steps to prevent further injury (e.g., exacerbating spinal injury by failing to maintain cervical spine stabilization during movement).

PRIMARY ASSESSMENT AND INTERVENTION

Assess ***level of consciousness.*** Use the AVPU method:
- **A** Child is ***alert***
- **V** Child responds to ***verbal*** stimulus
- **P** Child responds to ***painful*** stimulus
- **U** Child is ***unresponsive*** to any stimulus

Open ***airway,*** using appropriate method.
- In child with head, trunk, or multisystem trauma, modified jaw-thrust is preferred method. At this point, cervical spine should be manually immobilized and held in alignment with rest of spinal column and should not be released until emergency medical services personnel have immobilized child with appropriate equipment.

Assess for ***breathing.*** If necessary, begin rescue breathing.

Assess for ***circulation.*** If necessary, begin chest compressions.
- Palpate carotid artery in children 1 year or older.
- Palpate brachial artery in infants less than 1 year old.

Observe for hemorrhage. Control bleeding with a *gloved or protected hand:*
1. Apply direct pressure to wound site.
2. Elevate wound site.
3. Apply pressure to appropriate arterial pressure point.
4. Apply tourniquet only as a last resort. Once a tourniquet is applied, it should *not* be loosened.

Assess for further injury.

Determine state of consciousness:
- Talk to child.
- Observe child's behavior.

If present, do not remove objects protruding from child's body.

Check for evidence of decreased motor or sensory function in extremities:
- Infant and young child—observe spontaneous movement in extremities.
- Older child—ask if able to wiggle extremities.

Evaluate pain—present, absent; severe, mild.
- Attempt to alleviate with nonpharmacologic techniques.

Assess pulses in extremity distal to injury.
- Check color and temperature of extremities.

Manage any injuries appropriately (e.g., splint fractures) (see Emergency Treatment: Fracture, p. 1819).

Identify child.

Obtain information regarding the injury from witnesses, if any.

Call emergency medical services or other transport team to take child to nearest facility.

lower jaw and lifting with both hands, one on each side, displacing the mandible upward and outward and without head-tilt or chin-lift.

Spinal cord injury cannot be adequately assessed in the prehospital setting. It requires radiographs, a computed tomography (CT) scan, or magnetic resonance imaging (MRI) for diagnosis. Spinal cord injury is always suspected in the patient with head, trunk, or multisystem trauma. Only in the hospital setting with radiographs and other diagnostic tests can spinal cord injury be ruled out. Therefore the patient is treated as if injury is present. The cervical spine is immobilized by holding the head in a neutral position and not allowing movement of the head or body in any direction.

NURSING ALERT Remember, improper movement of the injured child with undetected spinal injury may lead to serious, permanent injury or death. It is virtually impossible to rule out spinal injury outside of the hospital; therefore, all victims with *any possibility* of spinal injury are treated as if injury is present.

Breathing is assessed after the airway is opened. If the child is not breathing, rescue breaths are given at a rate of 20 per minute. Oxygen should be provided when possible. Circulation is assessed only after the airway has been maintained and breathing is established. In children under 1 year of age, a brachial pulse is assessed. After 1 year of age, a cartoid pulse is palpated. Chest compressions should be begun if necessary (see Cardiopulmonary Resuscitation, Chapter 31).

Bleeding is first controlled by direct pressure with a gloved hand. If this does not work, a pressure dressing is applied. The next step is to elevate the body part and then attempt to control hemorrhage with arterial pressure points. A tourniquet is a *last resort.* Once applied, it is not removed or loosened. Below the tourniquet site, skin and tissue necrosis begins. If the tourniquet is loosened or removed, it allows release of the toxins into the circulation in high concentrations and may induce a systemic deadly, tourniquet shock (Grant, Murray, and Bergeron, 1994). With the tourniquet in place, the patient has a better chance of survival, even though it may mean the loss of a limb.

Assessment of the child involves observation from head to toe because infants and young children are unable to communicate except by crying and other behaviors. Therefore pinpointing areas of pain is very difficult. To check for any motor or sensory dysfunction in extremities, the nurse should note any spontaneous movement, which provides the best clue in infants and young children. Older children are able to follow directions for wiggling toes or fingers. The child is identified as soon as feasible by anyone who knows the child. It is important to determine if the child has any existing health problems that might have implications for the circumstances of the injury and for therapeutic management. Any witnesses are asked for details about the incident to aid in assessment of the child's emotional responses.

In the prehospital setting, the role of the nurse consists of activating the ***Emergency Medical System (EMS)*** and providing basic life support until emergency medical services personnel arrive on the scene. The role of the nurse is limited to basic life support because the nurse has no standing orders or protocols to work under in the prehospital setting (see Emergency Treatment box on p. 1795). Emergency services are called as soon as possible so that the patient can receive advanced life support before and during transport. A paramedic level ambulance provides at least one ***paramedic*** with skills in advanced cardiac life support (ACLS), pediatric advanced life support, and neonatal resuscitation. A paramedic's skills include electrocardiogram (ECG) interpretation and defibrillation, advanced airway management (including endotracheal intubation, intravenous and pharmacologic therapy), placement of a pneumatic antishock garment (PASG), pleural decompression, and placement of nasogastric tubes and Foley catheters. Other advanced life support skills include expertise in spinal immobilization, extrication, management of fractures and bleeding, and emergency scene management. The paramedic remains in constant contact with the emergency department physician by means of radio or cellular telephone for situations requiring medical control.

An ***emergency medical technician (EMT)*** has training in basic life support (BLS) measures, including basic airway management, hemorrhage control, fracture management, and spinal immobilization. In some areas, EMTs may have additional training that allows them to perform some advanced airway procedures, intravenous therapy, and automated defibrillation and to use the PASG.

NURSING ALERT Emergency medical services with paramedics or EMTs are trained to manage all out-of-hospital emergencies and have specialized equipment to manage such emergencies. It is imperative that EMS be called to respond as soon as possible. Family, friends, or strangers should not transport the trauma victim.

Systematic Assessment

There are several factors that can affect a child's response to trauma. An undetected congenital anomaly can contribute to a complicated injury. Acute gastric distention is a frequent occurrence in children because of the crying and screaming that accompany an injury. The temperature of young children is unstable because of their large surface area related to body mass, and temperature maintenance is critical in trauma management. Children also experience rapid metabolic changes. When they are ill, children are really ill; but as they recover, they change very rapidly. In addition, children have a small amount of blood volume in the absolute sense. Whereas blood volume is 60% of total body weight in the adult, it is 70% to 85% in the child.

The first priority on admission to an emergency facility is rapid assessment of the ABC status. Since the overwhelming majority of childhood injuries are the result of blunt-impact trauma, multiple organ involvement is a common finding; therefore it is essential to perform a systematic assessment of the trauma victim.

The secondary survey is a comprehensive assessment that is a systematic "head-to-toe" search for the remaining injuries not originally addressed in the primary survey. However, children are often an exception to the "head-to-toe" approach. It may be necessary to complete the secondary survey on the injured child in the "toe-to-head" manner. This approach may allow the rescuer to gain the child's confidence as the survey progresses. With this approach, the rescuer gradually moves into the child's "personal space" while gaining the child's trust. An example of a complete secondary survey is given in the Guidelines box. Throughout the assessment, the nurse observes for areas of deformity, edema, ecchymosis, bleeding, hematoma, paralysis, or pain.

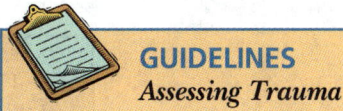

GUIDELINES
Assessing Trauma

Vital signs:
- ***Blood pressure*** (if available)
- ***Respirations***—Assess rate and quality, auscultate lung sounds.
- ***Pulse***—Assess rate and quality.
- ***Skin***—Assess color, temperature, and condition.

Treat for shock if mechanism of injury and vital signs indicate possible need.
- Administer high-flow oxygen if available.
- Elevate lower extremities (if no possibility of spinal injury).
- Maintain body heat.

Systematic head-to-toe (or toe-to-head) assessment:
- ***Neck and cervical spine***—Palpate for point tenderness, observe for stoma, distended neck veins, tracheal shift, medical alert tags.

Immobilize neck with cervical collar if available (manual cervical spine immobilization should still be in effect from emergency assessment and intervention).
- ***Scalp and skull***—Palpate for indentions, deformity, etc. Observe for cerebrospinal fluid in ears, Battle sign (bruising behind ears, indicating possible skull fracture).
- ***Face***—Observe for deformity, cerebrospinal fluid in nose.
- ***Eyes***—Observe for pupillary response, equality.
- ***Mouth***—Observe for possible obstructions, breath odor.
- ***Chest and ribs***—Palpate for possible fractures, deformity; observe and feel for equal expansion.
- ***Abdomen***—Palpate all quadrants for deformity, rigidity (indicating possible intraabdominal bleed).
- ***Lumbar spine***—Palpate for deformity, tenderness.

Reassess level of consciousness, airway patency.
- ***Pelvis and hips***—Perform three-way compression test for possible fracture (do not rock hips).
- ***Groin***—Observe for bleeding, priapism (indicating possible severe spinal injury).
- ***Extremities***—Palpate and observe all extremities for deformity, crepitus, bleeding, sensory, motor and circulatory function, medical alert tags.

Reevaluate treatment for shock, level of consciousness, airway, breathing, circulation, bleeding control, and vital signs.

THE IMMOBILIZED CHILD

IMMOBILIZATION

One of the most difficult aspects of illness is the immobility it often imposes on a child. Children's natural tendency to be mobile influences all elements of growth and development—physical, social, psychologic, and emotional. Impaired physical mobility related to disability or imposed activity restrictions presents a definite challenge to the child, staff, and parents providing care.

Etiology of Immobilization

The usual reason for immobilizing or restricting the activity of a child without disabilities is illness or injury. Bed rest or mechanical restraining devices are frequently prescribed to aid in the healing and restorative processes. When children are ill, they are content to remain quiet, and most of them instinctively reduce their activity. It is children who are forced to remain inactive because of physical limitations or therapy who display the multiple effects of restricted movement. The most frequent reasons for immobility are congenital defects (e.g., spina bifida), degenerative disorders (e.g., muscular dystrophy), and infections or accidents that impair the integumentary system (severe burns), the musculoskeletal system (fractures or osteomyelitis), or the neurologic system (spinal cord injury, polyneuritis, or head injury). Sometimes therapies, such as traction and spinal fusion, are responsible for prolonged immobilization.

Physiologic Effects of Immobilization

Many clinical studies, including space program research, have documented predictable consequences that occur following immobilization and the absence of gravitational force. Functional and metabolic responses to restricted movement can be noted in most of the body systems, all of which have a direct influence on the child's growth and development, because homeostatic mechanisms thrive on normal use and need feedback to maintain dynamic equilibrium. Inactivity leads to a decrease in the functional capabilities of the whole body as dramatically as the lack of physical exercise leads to muscle weakness.

Most of the pathologic changes that take place during immobilization arise from decreased muscle strength and mass, decreased metabolism, and bone demineralization, which are closely interrelated with one change leading to or affecting another. Some results of immobilization are primary and produce a direct effect; other pathophysiologic consequences occur frequently but seem to be more indirect and are therefore secondary effects. Many pathophysiologic changes affect more than one body system, with the primary or secondary effect being demonstrated in both systems.

Children who are confined to bed during a disease process or who are immobilized with an injury are usually restricted in movement for a relatively short time or are sufficiently active to avoid the physical consequences of immobility. Most physical and biologic effects of immobilization are the result of complete immobility, usually as a result of paralysis caused by nervous system infection (e.g., poliomyelitis, encephalitis, or polyneuritis) or trauma to the brain or spinal cord. Partial paralysis or weakness may be caused by birth defects (usually myelomeningocele), trauma, infec-

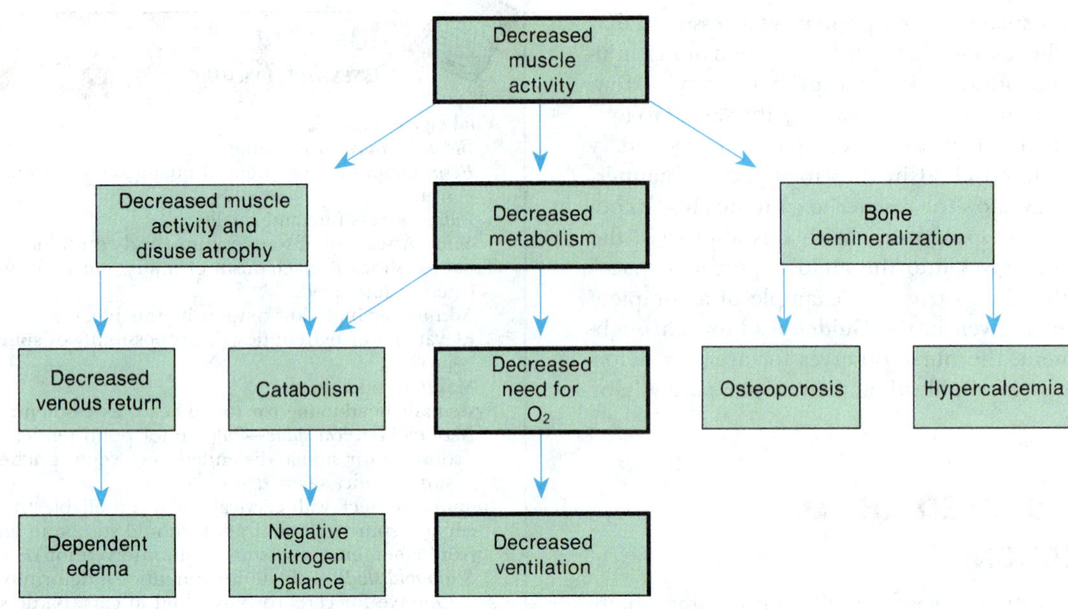

FIG. 39-1 Effects of immobilization.

tion, or degenerative disease, such as muscular dystrophy or muscular atrophy.

The major effects of immobilization (Fig. 39-1) are related directly or indirectly to decreased muscle activity, which produces numerous primary changes in both muscular and bone structures with secondary alterations in the cardiovascular, respiratory, metabolic, and renal systems. The major consequences are:

1. Significant loss of muscle strength, endurance, and muscle mass (atrophy)
2. Bone demineralization leading to osteoporosis
3. Loss of joint mobility and contractures

The larger the portion of the body immobilized and the longer the immobilization, the greater the hazards of immobility.

Muscular System. Inactive muscle loses strength at the rate of 3% per day and, in instances without primary neuromuscular deficit, sometimes requires several weeks or months to regain function. A stretching can occur as muscle loses its tone or as excessive strain is put on weakened muscle (e.g., stretching by tight bed covers or poor body position that produces wristdrop or footdrop experienced by debilitated children). The disuse leads to tissue breakdown and loss of the muscle mass (atrophy). The chief intracellular muscle enzyme, creatine, is released into the serum as the muscle atrophies; therefore serum levels provide an indication of the amount of muscle mass undergoing degeneration. Inactive muscle also affects the cardiovascular system by decreasing venous return and cardiac output. In general, muscle atrophy causes decreased strength and endurance. Stiffness of joints, as well as joint and intraarticular dysfunction, may be prevented.

Skeletal System. The daily stresses on bone created by motion and weight bearing maintain the balance between bone formation (osteoblastic activity) and bone resorption (osteoclastic activity). When these stresses are diminished, bone formation ceases, whereas the bone destruction continues, thus disrupting the state of equilibrium. Bone calcium becomes severely depleted, and there is increased secretion of phosphorus and nitrogen. This demineralization of the bone (osteoporosis) makes the skeletal structures prone to pathologic fractures and increases calcium ion concentration in the blood (hypercalcemia).

In children who are unable to move, such as the child who is unconscious or paralyzed or the child with rheumatoid arthritis, joint mobility becomes restricted. In the absence of normal structural stretching, collagen fibers generated within the joint become fibrotic and further limit movement. This tissue fibrosis creates a shortening of the muscles and a contracture of the joint. Any decrease in circulation to the joint by edema, inflammation, or restrictive positioning will contribute to further fibrotic changes. The problem rapidly becomes cyclic as the contracture leads to muscle fatigue and pain, which causes the child to splint the site, thus leading to more fibrosis. This process is further exaggerated because body flexor muscles are stronger than the extensor muscles, and unless range of motion is instituted within 3 to 7 days, contractures will develop. Frequent disabling contractures are hip flexion, knee flexion, shoulder stiffness, and plantar flexion of the feet.

Cardiovascular System. There are three major cardiovascular consequences of immobility: orthostatic hypotension, increased workload of the heart, and thrombus formation. During movement, muscle contraction causes pressure on peripheral veins, which in turn causes the venous valves to close, thus assisting return of the blood to the heart when the individual is in an upright position. In the absence of this assistance, blood tends to pool in the dependent areas, reducing the blood supply to the trunk and brain. In addition, direct reflex stimulation to the splanchnic and peripheral vessels causes them to constrict when a person is upright. Impairment of this neurovascular orthostatic reflex activity from lack of motion causes further interference with venous return. The individual displays signs of excessive autonomic activity (i.e., pallor, sweating, and restlessness, which are frequently followed by fainting). The child with a spinal cord injury has unique problems with orthostatic hypotension, which is discussed in Chapter 40.

Changes in vascular resistance caused by the horizontal position and immobility alter the distribution of blood within the body. The reduction in gravity pressure to the extremities causes much of the total blood volume to be redistributed from the lower extremities to other parts of the body. Consequently, there is an increase in the venous return and the volume of blood to be handled by the heart, which is reflected in an elevated blood pressure. Therefore the cardiac output and stroke volume are increased, and a progressive increase in heart rate occurs. When immobilization extends over a period of time, there is a compensatory decrease in blood volume and a decrease in heart rate and blood pressure.

Without muscle contraction the venous stasis and increased intravascular pressure in the extremities lead to dependent edema. If undue pressure is exerted on the major veins by positioning or mechanical devices, the likelihood of interstitial edema is increased. Most frequently this situation is seen when a child is placed on the side with one leg resting on the other or when the youngster is permitted to sit for a long time with pressure on the large veins behind the knee and in the groin. Edematous tissue is prone to infection and trauma, especially tissue located over an area that receives much of the body's weight.

Circulatory stasis combined with hypercoagulability of the blood, resulting from factors such as increased serum calcium or damage to the inner walls of blood vessels by trauma or infection, can lead to thrombus and embolus formation. Bed rest alone will not produce the blood-clotting problems, but debilitated persons often have one or more of these other contributing factors.

NURSING ALERT Sudden chest pain and dyspnea, the symptoms of pulmonary edema, or pain and swelling in the lower extremities, which indicate deep vein thrombosis, are constant concerns of the nurse.

The deconditioned state of cardiac function, caused by skeletal muscle inactivity, can produce a variety of secondary problems in other systems. However, the major clinical manifestation is increased pulse and heart rate in response to an active exercise program. After prolonged immobility the child should build up activity tolerance slowly to allow the heart to regain its optimum capabilities.

Respiratory System. Initially the effects of immobilization are compensatory or adaptive. The basal metabolic rate is decreased because with reduced expenditure of energy the cells require less oxygen and produce less carbon dioxide. Lessened demand for oxygen–carbon dioxide exchange causes the respirations to become slower and more shallow. Chest expansion may be limited by the supine posture; by abdominal distention caused by accumulation of feces, gas, or fluid; and by mechanical restriction such as a body cast, brace, or tight binders. Reduced muscle power and coordination secondary to altered innervation can also hinder respiratory movement. More effort is required to expand the lungs in the supine position.

Prolonged immobility also reduces the normal movement of secretions from the tracheobronchial tree, particularly in the presence of impaired muscle function and positional changes that normally facilitate removal of secretions. A weak and ineffectual cough reflex contributes to stasis of secretions and the possibility of airway obstruction. Shallow respirations and obstruction of the airway with thick mucus contribute to the development of secondary complications such as atelectasis, hypostatic pneumonia, and respiratory acidosis.

Gastrointestinal System. Prolonged immobility produces a state of negative nitrogen balance resulting from the increased catabolic activity related to muscle atrophy. This and the reduced energy requirements contribute to a diminished appetite and a resulting decrease in ingestion of nutrients. The mechanisms of eating and feeding become more difficult with immobility, and the risk of aspiration is increased. Intake is further influenced by associated psychologic factors.

The process of elimination depends on the integration of smooth and skeletal muscle activity and on visceral reflex patterns. Immobility may interfere with these mechanisms as well as with the gravitational effect on stool passing through the intestines. Slowing of stool in the colon causes the feces to become hard, and the bowel wall is not stimulated to further its peristaltic movement down the tract to the rectum. Weakened muscles used in defecation (diaphragmatic and abdominal muscles) are unable to produce the intraabdominal pressure needed for elimination. Sometimes embarrassment in using the bedpan may be the cause of not responding to the urge to defecate.

Renal System. The structure of the urinary system is designed to function in an upright posture. When the gravitational force is altered by the reclining position, the peristaltic contractions of the ureters are insufficient to overcome gravitational resistance. Consequently, there may be stasis of urine in the kidney pelves, and any particulate matter that settles in the calyces may serve as nuclei for calculi formation or as foci for infection.

In the horizontal position the individual has difficulty in relaxing the perineal musculature and external sphincter sufficiently to initiate the integrated reflex micturition mechanism that involves the external sphincter, the internal sphincter, and the detrusor muscle of the bladder wall. If adequate intraabdominal pressure is exerted, voiding can occur, but if the individual does not respond to the sensation to void, bladder distention leads to stasis and its complications add to overflow incontinence, a source of embarrassment. In time, reflex and back pressure may impair renal function, and urinary tract infection is always a hazard with urine retention.

Normally the kidney is able to handle the increased metabolites from protein breakdown and bone demineralization. However, the increased level of calcium excreted may predispose to the formation of calculi. Calculi formation is further favored by urinary stasis, infection, and an alkaline urine caused by the decreased production of the acid by-products of metabolism. Painless hematuria may be the only clue to diagnosis.

Metabolism. Immobility or severe restriction of activity is often accompanied by decreased or inappropriate nutritional intake, which frequently leads to decreased basal metabolic rate, a negative nitrogen balance associated with catabolism, and a high serum calcium level.

All body systems are influenced by a decrease in metabolism. The altered energy level leads to further fatigue and lack of motivation for moving. Although less of a problem in children, immobilized persons often feel sluggish and have a poor appetite, particularly for protein foods. The protein breakdown in the body related to a loss of muscle and other tissues is more apt to be severe after injury or surgery. Protein breakdown produces nitrogenous wastes, and on the fifth or sixth day of catabolic protein metabolism, an increase in urinary nitrogen develops that contributes to anemia and delayed healing.

Another metabolic problem is hypercalcemia associated with bone catabolism. Completely immobilized youngsters are especially prone to hypercalcemia. Symptoms that include nausea and vomiting, polydipsia, polyuria, and lethargy usually appear 4 to 8 weeks after immobilization. In quadriplegia, symptoms may occur within 10 days and last for as long as 6 months. The accelerated rates of bone metabolism in youngsters make the bone demineralization a greater hazard. Larger amounts of calcium are released into the blood than the kidney can excrete, and calcium continues to accumulate in the serum. High levels of serum calcium decrease neuronal permeability, which can lead to a depression of the central and peripheral nervous systems. Symptoms, including smooth and skeletal muscle fatigue, diminished reflexes, and atony of the gastrointestinal tract, are the result of the depressed nervous system.

Medical treatment for hypercalcemia consists of restricting dietary calcium, increasing weight bearing when this is possible, and, most important, vigorous hydration (e.g., 3000 to 4000 ml/day of fluid for a teenager). Electrolyte imbalances are corrected, and diuretics are administered to promote removal of calcium. Sometimes pharmacologic agents, such as corticosteroids, oral phosphates, and thyrocalcitonin, may be used to lower serum calcium levels. Any urinary tract infection is treated.

A child with bone demineralization may not develop hypercalcemia, but the excess amount of calcium that the kidneys are required to excrete may produce a negative calcium balance, with more calcium than citric acid lost in the urine. This imbalance causes the urine to become alkaline, with the potential danger of renal calculi, especially if there is an accompanying retention of urine.

Integumentary System. Circulation to the skin is reduced during inactivity and may be further impeded by dependent edema. Circulation is especially compromised in places where the bone surface is near the skin, such as areas over the sacrum, occiput, trochanter, and ankle, and continued impairment causes rapid necrosis with ulcer formation. Mechanical irritation from appliances, such as straps, rods, and ropes, and the friction of bedclothes during turning or other movement can produce skin breakdown. Healing capacity is also impaired by poor circulation,

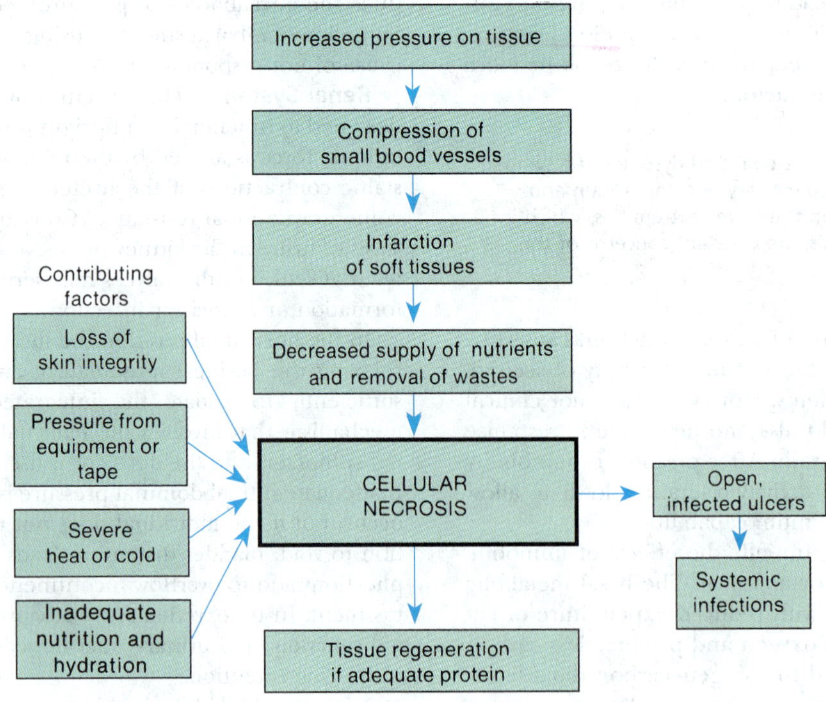

FIG. 39-2 Sequence of events in tissue breakdown.

negative nitrogen balance, and anemia. Immobilization often makes it difficult to carry out adequate cleansing and hygienic measures, which may also contribute to tissue breakdown in areas that are difficult to reach. Children with neurologic deficit should be guarded against extremes of heat and cold in direct contact with the skin.

Cellular breakdown caused by prolonged pressure can be identified by several characteristics. Normally when pressure is applied to the skin, the skin appears pale but becomes very red, or hyperemic, after the pressure is removed. This reactive hyperemia should disappear within 5 to 15 minutes. Prolonged redness (over 30 minutes) indicates that a pressure area is developing and treatment should be instituted. Other manifestations of tissue ischemia include an increase in temperature in the area, blistering, swelling, or dark purple or black areas. The pressure area may be limited to the skin and subcutaneous layers or may be deeper and more extensive. The skin changes observed may represent the top of a cone-shaped area with widespread tissue destruction, beneath which tissue rapidly ulcerates and creates a large hole that sometimes extends to the bone. The skin may be broken, and there may even be a purulent drainage. Fig. 39-2 illustrates the sequence of events in tissue breakdown.

Neurosensory System. Studies indicate that immobilization does not produce neurosensory consequences directly; however, two occurrences—loss of innervation and sensory and perceptual deprivation—are common.

Peripheral nerves, in contrast to skeletal muscles, do not degenerate with disuse, but loss of innervation takes place if nerves are damaged by pressure or if their blood supply is disrupted. Improper body positioning or poorly applied casts or restraints can place unwarranted pressure on nerves and blood vessels that can lead to ischemia and nerve degeneration. Frequent sites of this compression phenomenon are on the peroneal nerve, where pressure results in footdrop, and on the radial nerve, where pressure leads to wristdrop. These complications significantly interfere with attempts to regain functional use of extremities, but they can be prevented by conscientious nursing assessment and intervention. Preventing pressure on vulnerable areas and avoiding unnatural positions of flexion and extension that apply inappropriate pressure on nerves and blood vessels reduce the likelihood of compression injury. Periodic plantar flexion and dorsiflexion of the feet and hands will stimulate circulation and keep nerves from becoming pinched.

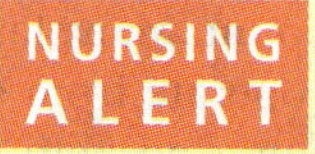

Numbness, tingling, change in sensation, and loss of motion are symptoms of neurologic impairment and should be evaluated immediately.

Psychologic Effects of Immobilization

For children, one of the most difficult aspects of illness is immobilization. Throughout childhood, physical activity is an integral part of daily life and is essential for physical growth and development. It also serves children as an instrument for communication and expression and as a means for learning about and understanding their world. It helps them deal with a variety of feelings and impulses and provides a mechanism by which they can exert control over inner tensions. Children respond to anxiety with increased activity. Removal of this power deprives them of necessary input and a natural outlet for their feelings and fantasies. Through movement children also gain sensory input, which provides an essential element for developing and maintaining a body image.

In daily life children's activity is restricted in many ways: limits are set on behavior and expression, activity is restricted by physical and verbal barriers, and neuromuscular function is affected directly by disease or injury. Children perceive restraint by persons or inanimate objects as either comforting or stressful. Adult controls on behavior often provide children with a sense of security in frightening situations or when they fear loss of control. On the other hand, forced inactivity deprives them of one of their most valuable means for dealing with stress. Children who are confined to bed may become victims of their fears and fantasies without the physical means for stress reduction. Sometimes children will impose restrictions on themselves, particularly in interaction with others, by confining themselves to bed with blankets pulled about them, or by retreating into sleep in the presence of stimulation.

Active children have many opportunities for input from a wide variety of settings. When they are immobilized by disease or as a part of a treatment regimen, they experience diminished environmental stimuli with a loss of tactile input and an altered perception of themselves and their environment. Sudden or gradual immobilization narrows the amount and variety of environmental stimuli they receive by means of all their senses: touch, sight, hearing, taste, smell, and proprioception—a feeling of where they are in their environment. This sensory deprivation frequently leads to a feeling of isolation, boredom, and being forgotten, especially by peers. Nursing interventions involving the use of diversional activities, schoolwork, and structured television or video programs can assist the child with maintaining usual activities (see Nursing Care Plan: The Child in the Hospital, Chapter 26).

Sensorimotor activity is a predominant mode of activity in infants; even newborns respond with rage when they are physically restrained. Physical interference with the activity of infants and young children gives them a feeling of helplessness. It has also been found that speech and language skills require sensorimotor activity and experience. There appears to be a significant relationship between physical restraint and the incidence of language problems. Children who are restrained by casts, splints, or straps during the first 3 years of life have more difficulty with language than children whose activities were unrestricted. Language delay is even more marked in children with neurologic impairment.

Observations of children's behavior during restraint indicate some differences between infants and older children. Initially infants temporarily freed from physical restraint remain immobile and then submit without protest to restoration of restraint. However, with subsequent release, their activity level progressively increases, as does their protesting behavior after reapplication of restraints. In contrast, tod-

BEHAVIORAL CHANGES IN IMMOBILIZED CHILDREN

Higher than normal level of anxiety leads to:
- Restlessness
- Difficulty with problem solving
- Inability to concentrate on activities
- Depression
- Regression
- Egocentrism

Monotony leads to:
- Sluggish intellectual responses
- Sluggish psychomotor responses
- Decreased communication skills
- Increased fantasizing
- Hallucinations
- Disorientation
- Dependence

dlers and preschool children show a decrease in protest with each subsequent removal and restoration of restraint. It is uncertain whether this diminished protest in these children reflects inhibitions developed as a result of frustration or a development of trust that the nurse will return to release the restraints.

The struggle for independence is thwarted by imposed immobility. For toddlers, exploration and imitative behaviors are essential to developing a sense of autonomy; preschoolers' expression of initiative is evidenced by their penchant for vigorous physical activity; school-age children's development is strongly influenced by physical achievement and competition; and adolescents rely on mobility to achieve independence. The quest for mastery at every stage of development is related to mobility. To children the inability to move is threatening to self-preservation and reactivates the struggle between activity and passivity, and between dependence and independence.

Behavioral changes are noted when children experience prolonged sensory deprivation. Some of these behaviors are demonstrated by a higher than normal level of anxiety (see box above). Children are likely to become depressed over their loss of ability to function or the marked changes in body image. Significant others are apt to notice regressive behavior and a greater reliance on them for tasks the children are able to perform. Children seek their attention by reverting to earlier developmental behaviors, such as wanting to be fed, bed-wetting, and baby talk. In many ways immobilized children are realistically dependent on others; therefore intelligent and sensitive care is required to prevent major developmental regressions during the period of immobility.

Limbs in casts or traction transmit less than normal sensory data. The presence of sensory impairment may be a concomitant problem of the involved part. Numbness or loss of feeling markedly alters proprioception. Children who have limited ability to feel others touching them not only experience less tactile stimuli in a physical sense but are also deprived of warm, loving feelings that arise from being touched. The loss of feeling derived from touch can further add to their sense of being isolated and unwanted.

The type and extent of immobilization influence the emotional response. When children are able to see the reason for their restraint (e.g., a cast), they are less likely to be resistant. The child whose activity is restricted because of a nonvisible disorder (e.g., rheumatic fever) finds it difficult to understand the reason for adult restrictions on activity, imagines the worst, and may react with noncompliance and overactivity when unobserved. Children may react to immobility by active protest, anger, and aggressive behavior, or they may become quiet, passive, and submissive. Often children believe that the immobilization is a justified punishment for misbehavior. Children should be allowed to discharge their anger, but it should be within the limits of safety to their self-esteem and not damaging to the integrity of others. For example, providing an object to attack rather than a person or a valued possession is safe and therapeutic.

Unfortunately, most adults resent and find it difficult to deal with the acting-out behavior of children. Too often this behavior is considered "bad" even when it is obviously a release of tension. In some cases, such as the paralyzed child, nurses may feel inadequate to cope with the child's profound distress and feelings of hopelessness, and the professional help of a psychologist or psychiatrist is needed.

The most difficult situations are those involving major injuries and diseases that produce a disfigurement or a severe loss of function that directly affects children's self-image, such as burns, amputation, or the sudden, catastrophic effects of an accident that leaves healthy, athletic children paralyzed for life. Feelings of anger and hostility are difficult for children to express when they are at the mercy of the environment. They dare not speak out against or defy the authorities on whom they depend so completely. Consequently, their aggression may be masked by cheerfulness or rigidity. When they are unable to express their anger, the aggression is often displayed inappropriately through regressive behavior and outbursts of crying or temper tantrums over insignificant irritations, such as warm milk, a wrinkled collar, or a delay in routine.

Effect on Families

Brief periods of immobilization have few effects on the family; however, catastrophic illness or disability severely taxes the resources of the family. The needs for instruction concerning medical and nursing care, community resources to contact, and emotional support are paramount. Many families are already plagued by unmet needs, operate from crisis to crisis, and are often unable to use outside help appropriately. For these families the new situation can disrupt the entire family; therefore the rehabilitation team must help the family members identify unmet needs and actively help in the family's problem-solving process. The following are commonly occurring problems:

1. Financial strains may decrease or totally eliminate the family's resources.
2. The focus of attention is placed, at least temporarily, on the

affected member; therefore other members of the family may feel neglected or their needs may not be met.
3. The family may have difficulty in accepting the child's altered body image.
4. Individual family members may be unable to express their feelings and become immobilized in the face of the crisis.
5. Parents often experience a sense of guilt over their child's immobilization. Failure to protect their child, from their perception, forms the basis for their inability to cope.

The family's needs can often be met by the physician and nurse but may also require the services of other professionals, such as a social worker, psychiatrist, or marriage counselor. In preparation for discharge, home visits are advisable and home management is frequently planned weeks in advance of the actual discharge, including special considerations for cultural, economic, physical, and psychologic needs. A child with a severe disability is very dependent, and caregivers need rest periods to revitalize themselves. Individual and group counseling is beneficial for preproblem-solving situations and provides an emotional support system. Parent groups are also helpful and often allow nonthreatening social contact. The families of children with permanent disabilities need long-term resources, since some of the most difficult problems arise as they try to sustain high-quality care for many years (see Chapter 22).

Nursing Considerations

❖ Assessment

Assessment of the child who is immobilized as a result of an injury or a degenerative disease includes not only the injured part (e.g., fracture or damaged joint), but also the functioning of other systems that may be affected secondarily—the circulatory, renal, respiratory, muscular, and gastrointestinal systems. In long-term immobilization there may also be neurologic impairment and metabolic changes in electrolytes (especially calcium), nitrogen balance, and the general metabolic rate.

❖ Nursing Diagnoses

Based on a thorough assessment, several nursing diagnoses are identified. The more common diagnoses for the immobilized child are included in the Nursing Care Plan on p. 1805. Others may apply in specific situations.

❖ Planning

The goals for the immobilized child and the family include the following:

1. Child will have opportunity for mobilization within capabilities.
2. Child will maintain skin integrity.
3. Child will experience no physical injury.
4. Child will engage in diversional activity.
5. Child and family will receive adequate support.

❖ Implementation

Frequent position changes and the use of Ace wraps or TED stockings help to prevent dependent edema and fluid movement to third spaces and help to stimulate circulation, respiratory function, gastrointestinal motility, and neurologic sensations. When the condition allows it, the child can periodically assume the upright position on a tilt table or similar device to stimulate gastrointestinal and renal function and increase the stress on bones.

Each metabolic disturbance is treated specifically. Metabolism is increased by activity within the limitations of the disability and the capabilities of the child. High-protein, high-calorie foods are encouraged for correction of negative nitrogen balance. This may be difficult to correct by diet, especially if anorexia is present. It is desirable to determine the child's favorite foods and to allow the family to bring special foods from home. This is especially helpful for children from varied cultural backgrounds. Stimulating the appetite with small servings of attractively arranged, preferred foods may be sufficient. Sometimes supplementary nasogastric feedings or hyperalimentation may be needed.

Diet modification for the child with increased serum calcium presents problems because the dairy foods that children often desire are high in this mineral. Acid ash foods, such as cereals, meats, poultry, fish, and cranberry or apple juice, are encouraged. Lying in a prone position may precipitate problems with swallowing or self-feeding. Therefore offering small bites, controlling swallowing with semisolid food, and using a straw for fluids are nursing behaviors that will prevent choking. A suction machine should be in the vicinity for emergencies. The primary nursing measure for hypercalcemia is conscientious hydration and active remobilization as soon as possible.

Adequate hydration promotes bowel and kidney function and helps prevent complications in these systems. A knowledge of previous bowel habits and of a method to get the child to a commode helps promote elimination and will be valuable data if needed for a bowel program. It is important to determine the words the child uses for elimination. Embarrassment can be avoided by a mutually satisfactory communication system. Whenever possible, the child should be helped into a sitting position to use a fracture urinal or a bedpan. Providing privacy for toileting and encouraging the child to participate in solving toileting problems will increase the chances of a successful program.

Children should be encouraged to be as active as their condition and restrictive devices allow. This usually poses few problems for children, whose innate ingenuity and natural inclination toward mobility provide them with the impetus for physical activity. They need the opportunity, the materials or objects to stimulate activity, and the encouragement and participation of others. Those who are unable to move will need passive exercise and movement.

Whenever possible, transporting the child by stretcher, stroller, or wagon outside the confines of the room will increase environmental stimuli and provide social contact with others. While hospitalized, the child will benefit from frequent visitors, clocks and calendars, and a program of diversional therapy, which will help the child to function in a more normal way. As soon as possible, the child should wear "street clothes" and resume school and preinjury hob-

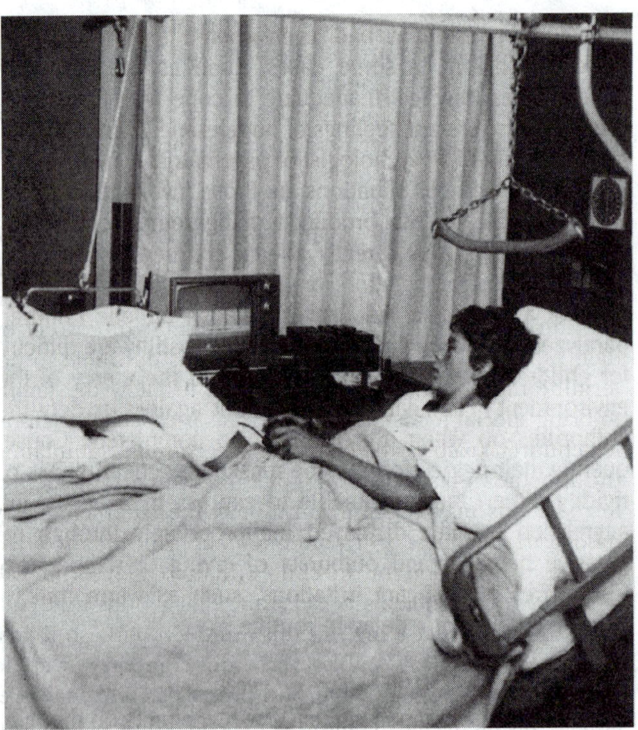

FIG. 39-3 Immobilized child playing a video game.

bies. Play is the most useful tool of nursing (see Chapter 26), and activities, which are selected on the basis of interest, ability, and limitations, should include some form of physical activity that encourages the use of uninvolved muscles and joints. Any activity that is tolerated (e.g., turning in bed or changing position of a bed in the room) helps to alter the monotony of immobilization and dissipate tension and frustration (Fig. 39-3).

Using dolls to illustrate and explain the restraining method is a valuable tool for small children. Placing a cast, tubing, or other restraining equipment on the doll offers the child a nonthreatening opportunity to express, through the doll, feelings concerning the restrictions and feelings toward the nurse and other health providers. It also provides a means for anticipatory teaching and explanation of needed restraining devices.

One of the most useful interventions to help children cope with immobility is participation in their own care. Self-care to the maximum extent is usually well received by children. They can help plan their daily routine, select their diet (when possible), and choose the clothes they are to wear, including innovative adornment, such as a baseball cap, brightly colored stockings, or other items of apparel that express each child's autonomy and individuality. They should be encouraged to do as much for themselves as they are able in order to keep muscles active and their interest alive. If feasible, they should be placed where they can benefit from the company of other children who are immobilized, which assures them that they are not singled out for this treatment.

It is important for children to understand behavioral limitations or rules, and their questions should be answered. For example, they need to know the reasons for medical, nursing, occupational, and physical therapy and to know that schedules are necessary. In some areas they have a choice; in others they do not. They may or may not be permitted to sleep late, but they can choose their own clothing. Most of children's activity of daily living is play; therefore therapies that incorporate this concept are more apt to gain their cooperation.

Visits from significant persons, such as family members and friends, offer occasions for emotional support and also provide opportunities for learning how to care for the child. Some privacy is needed, particularly by the teenager, and most long-term health care facilities recognize that rooms shared by two to four youngsters are better environments for habilitation or rehabilitation. When roommates are selected according to age and companionship, a chance is available to test out thoughts and feelings safely with others. If a traumatic incident caused the child's disability, guilt feelings may be displayed overtly or masked behind regressive or aggressive behavior. The feeling that "I must have been bad to receive this fate" is common, and honest feedback stating, "It just happened—it was an accident," needs repeating many times. Additional aspects of grieving are involved if there was a loss of another in the accident. All these feelings need to be brought out and dealt with. In addition, professional persons working with these children must not baby or overprotect them but must help them to cope with their altered body image and reestablish their self-esteem.

For a child with greatly restricted movement (e.g., a child with quadriplegia or a child with a large bilateral hip spica cast), nursing care is a challenge. These situations require long-term care either in the hospital or at home, but, wherever the care occurs, consistent planning and coordination of activities with professionals and significant others is vital. Nursing assessment includes psychosocial data, as well as physical manifestations, since long-term immobilization has a profound effect on the child and the family. Nursing approaches are evaluated frequently and continued, discontinued, or modified to meet the changing problems and goals. Physical effects of immobilization and appropriate nursing considerations are summarized in Table 39-1.

❖ Evaluation

The effectiveness of nursing interventions is determined by continual reassessment and evaluation of care based on the following observational guidelines and expected outcomes:

1. Observe vital signs, neurologic signs, and respiratory, gastrointestinal, and renal functioning; inspect skin; observe effects of correct functioning of equipment and appliances (restraints, traction, cast, braces).
2. Observe child's behavior; engage in dialogue to elicit feelings, concerns, and interests.
3. Observe the child's activities and interests.
4. Interview child and family regarding their feelings and concerns; observe family interaction at home, if possible.

Expected outcomes:

See Nursing Care Plan, p. 1805.

NURSING CARE PLAN
The Child Who Is Immobilized

NURSING DIAGNOSIS: Impaired physical mobility related to mechanical restrictions, physical disability (specify level)

PATIENT GOAL 1: Will have opportunity for mobilization

• **NURSING INTERVENTIONS/*RATIONALES***

Transport child by gurney, stroller, wagon, bed, wheelchair or other conveyance from confines of room *to provide for mobilization despite restrictions*

Change position of bed in room *to alter monotony of immobilization*

Change position in bed when possible *to decrease feelings of being immobilized*

• **EXPECTED OUTCOMES**

Child moves from confines of room or within room

Child's position is changed when possible

PATIENT GOAL 2: Will maintain optimum autonomy

• **NURSING INTERVENTIONS/*RATIONALES***

Provide mobilizing devices (orthoses, crutches, wheelchair)

Assist with acquisition of specialized equipment *to encourage independence*

Instruct in use of equipment *to ensure safety*

Encourage activities that require mobilization

Allow as much freedom of movement as possible and encourage normal activities *to maintain a sense of autonomy*

Encourage child to participate in own care as much as possible *to encourage sense of autonomy and independence*

Allow child to make choices (e.g., daily routine, food, clothes) *to encourage sense of autonomy despite limitations*

• **EXPECTED OUTCOMES**

Child moves about without assistance

Child engages in activities appropriate to limitations and developmental level

NURSING DIAGNOSIS: High risk for impaired skin integrity related to immobility, therapeutic appliances

PATIENT GOAL 1: Will maintain skin integrity

• **NURSING INTERVENTIONS/*RATIONALES***

Place child on pressure-reducing surface *to prevent tissue breakdown and pressure necrosis*

Change position frequently, unless contraindicated, *to prevent dependent edema and stimulate circulation*

Protect pressure points (e.g., trochanter, sacrum, ankle, shoulder, occiput)

Inspect skin surfaces regularly for signs of irritation, redness, evidence of pressure

Eliminate mechanical factors causing pressure, friction, or irritation (e.g., keep linen and clothing free of wrinkles)

Maintain meticulous skin cleanliness

Gently rub with alcohol or special lotion (most lotions cause softening and therefore promote skin breakdown on the immobilized child) or other lubricating substance *to stimulate circulation*

• **EXPECTED OUTCOME**

Skin remains clean and intact with no evidence of irritation

NURSING DIAGNOSIS: High risk for injury related to impaired mobility

PATIENT GOAL 1: Will experience no physical injury

• **NURSING INTERVENTIONS/*RATIONALES***

Teach correct use of mobilizing devices and/or apparatus *to ensure safety*

Assist with moving and/or ambulating as needed *to ensure safety*

Remove hazards from environment (specify)

Modify environment as needed (specify)

Keep call button within reach

Keep siderails up at all times *to prevent falls*

Help child to use bathroom or commode if possible

Implement safety measures appropriate to child's developmental age (specify)

• **EXPECTED OUTCOME**

Child remains free of injury

NURSING DIAGNOSIS: Diversional activity deficit related to impaired mobility, musculoskeletal impairment, confinement to hospital or home

PATIENT GOAL 1: Will engage in diversional activity

• **NURSING INTERVENTIONS/*RATIONALES* AND EXPECTED OUTCOMES**

See Nursing Care Plan: The Child in the Hospital, Chapter 26

NURSING DIAGNOSIS: Altered family processes related to a child with disability, illness

PATIENT (FAMILY) GOAL 1: Will receive adequate support

• **NURSING INTERVENTIONS/*RATIONALES* AND EXPECTED OUTCOMES**

See Nursing Care Plan: The Family of the Ill or Hospitalized Child, Chapter 26

TABLE 39-1 Summary of Physical Effects of Immobilization with Nursing Interventions*

PRIMARY EFFECTS	SECONDARY EFFECTS	NURSING CONSIDERATIONS
MUSCULAR SYSTEM		
Decreased muscle strength, tone, and endurance	Decreased venous return and decreased cardiac output Decreased metabolism and need for oxygen Decreased exercise tolerance Bone demineralization	Use elastic stockings or wrap legs with Ace bandages to promote venous return Plan play activities to use uninvolved extremities Place in upright posture when possible
Disuse atrophy and loss of muscle mass	Catabolism Loss of strength	Perform range of motion, active, passive, and stretching exercises
Loss of joint mobility	Contractures, ankylosis of joints	Maintain correct body alignment Use joint splints as indicated to prevent further deformity
Weak back muscles	Secondary spinal deformities	Maintain body alignment
Weak abdominal muscles	Impaired respiration	See nursing considerations for respiratory system
SKELETAL SYSTEM		
Bone demineralization—osteoporosis, hypercalcemia	Negative calcium balance Pathologic fractures Calcium deposits Extraosseous bone formation, especially at hip, knee, elbow, and shoulder Renal calculi	In paralysis, use upright posture on tilt table Handle extremities carefully when turning and positioning Administer calcium-mobilizing drugs (diphosphonates) if ordered Ensure adequate intake of fluid; monitor output Acidify urine Promptly treat urinary tract infections
Negative calcium balance	Life-threatening electrolyte imbalance	Monitor blood levels of calcium electrolytes Provide electrolyte replacement as indicated
METABOLISM		
Decreased metabolic rate	Slowing of all systems Decreased food intake	Mobilize as soon as possible Perform active and passive resistance and deep breathing exercises Ensure adequate food intake Provide a high-protein diet
Negative nitrogen balance	Decline in nutritional state Impaired healing	Encourage small, frequent feedings with protein and preferred foods Prevent pressure areas
Hypercalcemia	Electrolyte imbalance	See nursing considerations for skeletal system
Decreased production of stress hormones	Decreased physical and emotional coping capacity	Identify etiologies of stress Implement appropriate interventions to lower physical and psychosocial stresses
CARDIOVASCULAR SYSTEM		
Decreased efficiency of orthostatic neurovascular reflexes	Inability to adapt readily to upright position Pooling of blood in extremities in upright posture	Monitor peripheral pulses and skin temperature changes Wrap legs in elastic bandage or stockings to decrease pooling when upright
Diminished vasopressor mechanism	Orthostatic hypotension with syncope—hypotension, decreased cerebral blood flow, tachycardia	Provide abdominal support In severe cases, use antigravitational suit Administer peripheral sympathetic stimulating agents such as ephedrine if ordered Position horizontally
Altered distribution of blood volume	Decreased cardiac work load Decreased exercise tolerance	Monitor hydration and urine output
Venous stasis	Pulmonary emboli and/or thrombi	Have frequent position changes Elevate extremities without knee flexion Ensure adequate fluid intake

*Use measures that apply. Not all problems will be applicable in every situation.

TABLE 39-1 Summary of Physical Effects of Immobilization with Nursing Interventions— cont'd

PRIMARY EFFECTS	SECONDARY EFFECTS	NURSING CONSIDERATIONS
		Perform active or passive exercises or movement, if ordered Prescribe routine wearing of antiembolic stockings or wrap lower extremities from metatarsus to gluteal folds Measure circumference of extremities periodically Give anticoagulant drugs if ordered until mobilization possible Promptly intervene to maintain adequate oxygen if signs and symptoms of pulmonary emboli
Dependent edema	Tissue breakdown and susceptibility to infection	Administer good skin care Turn every 2 hours Monitor skin color, temperature, and integrity
RESPIRATORY SYSTEM		
Decreased need for oxygen	Altered oxygen–carbon dioxide exchange and metabolism	Exercise as tolerated Use position for optimum chest expansion
Decreased chest expansion and diminished vital capacity	Diminished oxygen intake Dyspnea and inadequate arterial oxygen saturation; acidosis	Use prone positioning without pressure on abdomen to allow gravity to aid in diaphragmatic excursion When sitting, maintain proper alignment to prevent pressure on respiratory mechanism
Poor abdominal tone and distention	Interference with diaphragmatic excursion	Avoid restriction of chest and abdominal musculature Supply torso support to promote chest expansion
Mechanical or biochemical secretion retention	Hypostatic pneumonia Bacterial and viral pneumonia Atelectasis	Change position frequently Carry out percussion, vibration, and drainage (or suctioning) as necessary Monitor breath sounds
Loss of respiratory muscle strength	Poor cough	Encourage coughing and deep breathing Support chest wall when coughing Use special devices such as a rocking bed, breathing bag, incentive spirometers Observe for signs of acute respiratory distress with blood gas levels measured as necessary
	Upper respiratory infection	Avoid contact with infected persons Provide adequate hydration
GASTROINTESTINAL SYSTEM		
Distention caused by poor abdominal muscle tone	Interference with respiratory movements	Monitor bowel sounds Encourage small, frequent feedings
	Difficulty in feeding in prone position	Sit in upright position if possible
No specific primary effect	Gravitation effect on feces through ascending colon or weakened smooth muscle tone may cause constipation	Carry out bowel training program with hydration, stool softeners, and mild laxatives if necessary
	Anorexia	Stimulate appetite with favored foods
URINARY SYSTEM		
Alteration of gravitational force	Difficulty in voiding in prone position	Position as upright as possible to void
Impaired ureteral peristalsis	Urinary retention in calyces and bladder Infection Renal calculi	Hydrate to ensure adequate urinary output for age Collect specimens as needed Stimulate bladder emptying with warm water, running water, striking suprapubic area

Continued.

TABLE 39-1 **Summary of Physical Effects of Immobilization with Nursing Interventions— cont'd**

PRIMARY EFFECTS	SECONDARY EFFECTS	NURSING CONSIDERATIONS
		Catheterize only for severe retention Administer urinary tract antiseptics as indicated
INTEGUMENTARY SYSTEM		
No specific primary effect	Decreased circulation and pressure leading to tissue injury Difficulty with personal hygiene	Turn and position at least every 2 hours Frequently inspect total skin surface Eliminate mechanical factors causing pressure, friction, or irritation Assess ability to perform hygienic care and assist with bathing, grooming, and toileting as needed

MOBILIZATION DEVICES

Orthotics and Prosthetics

Developments in the disciplines of ***orthotics*** (fabrication and fitting of braces*) and ***prosthetics*** (fabrication and fitting of artificial limbs) have resulted in lighter and better-fitting devices and thus greater patient compliance. ***Orthoses*** are often used to prevent deformity, increase energy efficiency of gait, and control alignment. Paralyzed or markedly weakened extremities can sometimes be stabilized by braces that facilitate walking. Some are designed to stabilize the extremities and offer support during ambulation. Special joint hinges permit the hip, knee, and ankle to flex during sitting, whereas the leg is held rigid during ambulation. Well-fitted orthoses promote ambulation, whereas ill-fitting braces are dangerous to the balance of the child and frequently cause muscle stress and tissue breakdown. Braces for the growing child will need frequent adjusting and replacement by the orthotist if long-term use is necessary.

Four common types of orthoses are used and are described based on the joints controlled by the orthosis. The ***ankle, foot orthosis (AFO)*** is used to prevent footdrop due to bed rest, trauma to the foot, or paralysis of muscles that flex the foot; to prevent heel cord tightening following heel cord–lengthening surgery; or to support the foot in proper position for standing and walking (Fig. 39-4).

The ***knee, ankle, foot orthosis (KAFO)*** is used to prevent buckling of the knee; to prevent weight bearing when there is paralysis or marked weakness of the knee extension or quadriceps muscle; or to prevent weight bearing when the bone structure is weak (Fig. 39-5).

The ***hip, knee, ankle, foot orthosis (HKAFO)*** is used to provide various types of control for the knee and ankle joints (as described above), as well as the hip (e.g., flail lower limb and paralysis). The ***reciprocal brace*** orthosis, used for ambulation in patients with myelodysplasia, is an example of an HKAFO.

*Braces (metal and leather) are only used when allergies to plastic exist or when severe difficulties in maintaining position occur. The term "orthoses" is preferred to the word "braces."

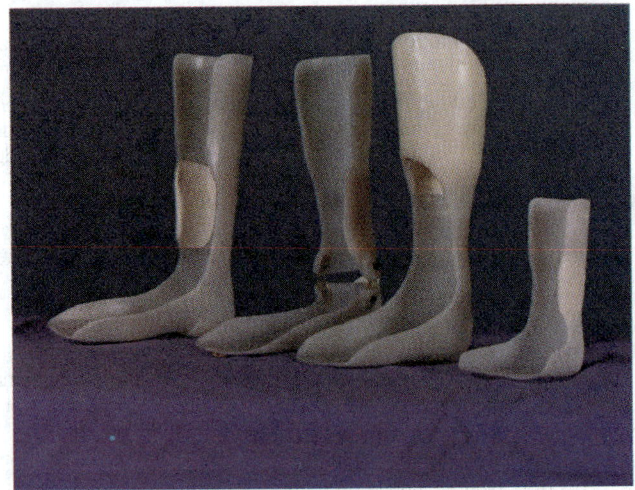

FIG. 39-4 *Left to right:* AFO, valgus prevention Toronto foot plate; AFO, varus prevention articulated ankle; Floor Reactive AFO; varus prevention AFO with extended medial wall.

The ***thoracolumbar sacral orthosis (TLSO)*** fits snugly around the trunk of the body to exert pressure on the ribs and back, to support the spine in a straight position (Fig. 39-6). It may prevent the progression of curves in the spine. The ***Jewett-Taylor brace*** is sometimes used to support the spine and trunk during ambulation to prevent compression after fracture of the spinal column.

The orthosis must fit each body curvature to avoid undue pressure on tissues and imbalance between muscle groups. Bony prominences where the brace has contact, such as along the spine, chin, and iliac crests, are observed closely for pressure or irritation and are padded as necessary. A corset with metal stays or Boston brace provide the needed torso support, especially for a paraplegic child. The ***Boston brace*** is the most commonly used brace in the treatment of scoliosis. These are more comfortable than the metal and leather brace and presents fewer problems with dressing. Specialized devices can be used to provide upright mobility in small children with lower limb paralysis who shift body weight to achieve locomotion.

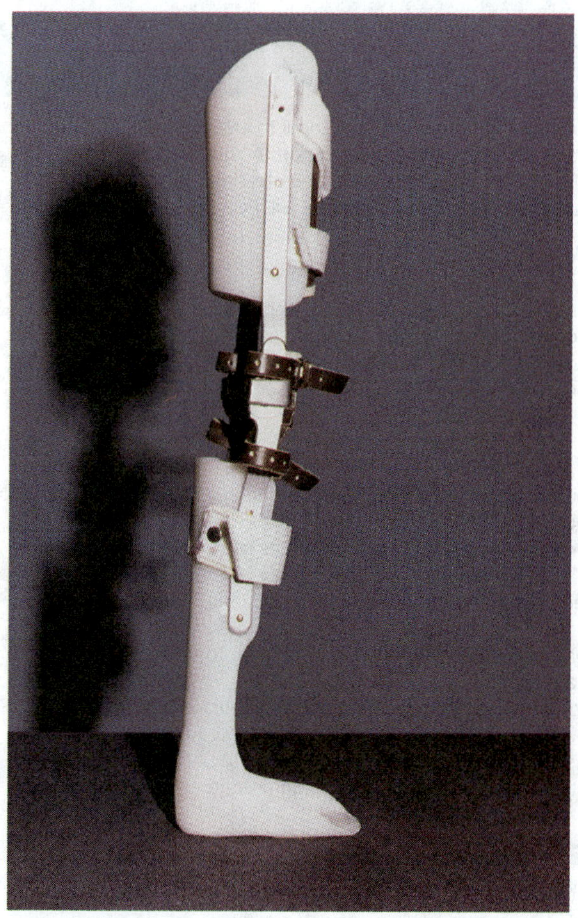

FIG. 39-5 Knee, ankle, foot orthosis.

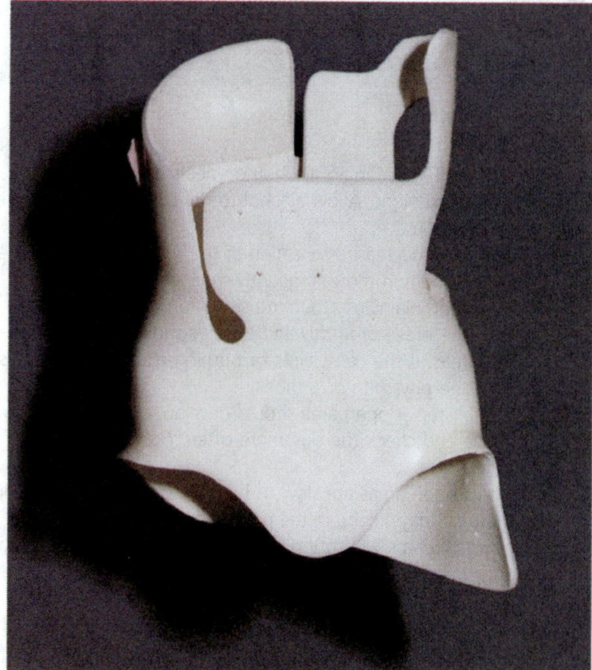

FIG. 39-6 Thoracolumbar sacral orthosis.

Many factors are considered when prescribing ***prostheses***—level of amputation, age, weight, activity, agility, and skin condition. Each prosthesis is custom-made or fabricated of various plastic and foam materials. The style of the prosthesis depends on the most distal joint involved in the amputation or prosthetic fitting. Terms used to describe types of prostheses are listed in the box at right.

Prosthetic advances and developments are constantly evolving in both fabrication and fitting. Myoelectric devices, cosmetic materials used in terminal gloves and feet, and CAD-CAM (computer aided design–computer-aided manufacturing) socket construction are but a few of the recent changes that have positively affected patients who require prostheses.

PROSTHETIC TERMINOLOGY

Syme—Ankle disarticulation
BK—Below knee
KD—Knee disarticulation
AK—Above knee
HD—Hip disarticulation
WD—Wrist disarticulation
BE—Below elbow
ED—Elbow disarticulation
AE—Above elbow
SD—Shoulder disarticulation

Nursing Considerations

Meticulous skin care and the wearing of protective clothing under the brace are necessary. Assessment of all areas that make contact with the brace, every 2 to 4 hours, for the first few days following application is recommended. If any area is reddened, the brace is removed for ½ to 1 hour. If redness does not disappear, the nurse should notify the practitioner or orthotist (see Family Home Care box, p. 1810, top).

Assessment of the stump area before application of the prosthesis, noting areas of redness (or skin breakdown), bony prominences, or scars, is essential during each application. Prevention of skin breakdown is best accomplished through good hygiene of the residual limb, proper fitting of the artificial limb, and prosthetic training (see Family Home Care box, p. 1810, bottom).

Safety is another important consideration. Parallel bars provide secure handrails on both sides of children as they learn to walk again with or without braces. As they become more proficient, a walker with or without wheels is substituted for the bars and children are no longer confined to a limited territory. Children then progress to crutches if their age and condition permit.

Crutches and Canes

Crutches are used when children are not allowed to bear weight or can only place part of their body weight on an extremity, such as with most lower leg injuries. A variety of crutches can be employed, and the selection is determined by the individual needs of the child. ***Axillary crutches*** are

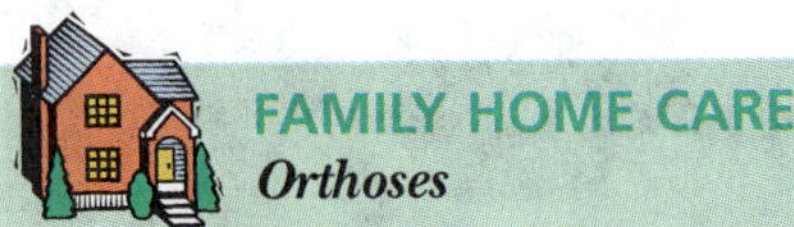

FAMILY HOME CARE
Orthoses

CARE OF SKIN
AFO, KAFO

Rub alcohol (70% rubbing alcohol) on heels twice a day—morning and night. Allow alcohol to dry completely before reapplying the brace.

If the child has decreased sensation in the legs, it is wise to check the skin condition more frequently than every 4 hours.

If the child complains of a burning sensation under the brace, remove the brace promptly and observe the skin for any reddened areas. If the complaints of burning occur several times, contact the physician or orthotist.

If a *small* blister or open area should develop, cover with a sterile bandage and check the skin more often. *Do not put alcohol on open areas.*

Sometimes open areas are slow to heal. If no sign of healing occurs after 3 days, contact the physician or orthotist.

Lotions and creams will soften the skin and should not be used during brace treatment.

TLSO

Since the brace works by pressing against the body and is kept very snug by straps and buckles, some skin pinkness is to be expected. The skin at the brace edges and under the pads should be inspected carefully and frequently, especially when weaning to the orthosis. Any red mark that does not fade within 20 minutes, or any area that appears raw and sore, should be reported to the orthotist.

It will help to apply rubbing alcohol to areas where the brace presses; this will toughen the skin. A cotton undershirt should be worked under the brace to protect the skin. Keeping it clean, dry, and free of wrinkles will help prevent skin problems.

CARE OF BRACE
TLSO

The brace must be cleaned with soap and water, followed by a good rinsing with water, on a weekly basis. Be sure to thoroughly dry the brace before putting it on. It is also important to avoid leaving it in hot places, such as direct, strong sunlight or by a warm radiator.

AFO, KAFO, HKAFO

Wipe the plastic section of the brace with a damp cloth. *Do not use soap on the brace.*

Wipe the brace completely dry before applying it to the child's leg.

Keep the joints of the KAFO well oiled; 3-in-1 oil is a good lubricant.

Periodically check all screws on the brace to make certain they are tight.

Once a month, or more often, clean the brace thoroughly. The leather can be cleaned with saddle soap. Joints can be unscrewed, wiped clean, oiled, and put back together.

If the brace is broken or out of alignment, notify your orthotist.

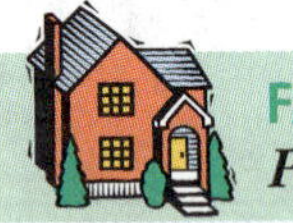

FAMILY HOME CARE
Prostheses

CARE OF RESIDUAL LIMB

Wash with mild, nonperfumed soap, rinse, and dry thoroughly daily.

A small amount of powder may be used on the skin, or rub area with 70% rubbing alcohol if skin is intact.

Check skin for redness, sensitive areas, or signs of infection.

CARE OF PROSTHESIS

The socket should be routinely washed with water and mild soap, rinsed, and dried thoroughly.

Straps and rubber bands should be checked with each application.

Check joints to ensure that they operate smoothly.

Replace worn or broken parts (heels, soles, straps) as needed.

Wear stump socks to absorb perspiration, prevent skin friction, and provide comfort.

Change socks daily and wash and dry following instructions provided by prosthetist.

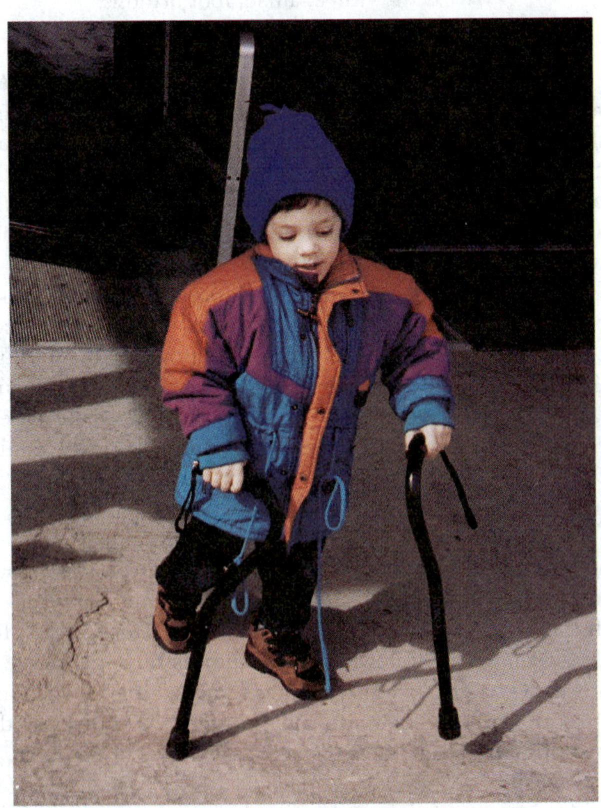

FIG. 39-7 Child learning to walk with crutches.

used most frequently as temporary assistance. ***Forearm crutches*** are the usual selection for children who anticipate permanent use, such as paraplegic children who are able to use braces. For children with limited hand and arm strength or function, ***trough crutches*** allow the weight to be assumed by the elbow. For habilitating small children who have not yet learned to walk or who are unsteady, special crutches stabilized with three or four legs provide needed stability for a child to maintain an upright position and learn to walk.

Children must be properly fitted for the crutch or cane to prevent poor posture and crutch pressure on the axilla during ambulation. Measuring for crutches and teaching crutch and cane use are usually assumed by the physical therapist in most institutions; however, nurses are the persons who supervise the use of crutches in pediatric units and in the home (Fig. 39-7). The type of crutch gait taught to children depends on their degree of stability, whether or not the knees can be flexed, and the specific goal established for each child.

Bed exercises for strengthening arms and shoulders are important if immobilization has been prolonged. The youngster gains confidence in ambulating by wearing a safety belt held by the therapist. The types of gaits used and instructions to children are similar to those given to adults. They are conveyed in language children understand and with demonstration. Most children grasp the techniques readily.

Special Beds

Older quadriplegic children often require a special bed to immobilize the head and spine during the early phases of spinal cord injury care. Some rehabilitation units use a regular bed for the patient in cervical traction, whereas others use a Stryker frame or one of the Roto-Rest beds. Whatever special bed is used, the success of its use is greatly influenced by the preparation of the child. Explanations of how the bed works (and, when possible, showing the child someone being turned in the bed) are needed. Nursing personnel need in-service practice in the operation of these beds to ensure the safe handling of the equipment.

A ***Stryker frame*** employs two frames, one anterior and one posterior, to turn the child horizontally. The Stryker wedge frame was designed to allow prone-supine turning by one person, but for safety, two people are used for turning a child in a Stryker frame. Cervical traction can easily be attached to the stationary frame and presents no discomfort when turning as long as the weights are prevented from swinging. Before turning, the child's arms and legs are aligned within the frame and straps are wrapped around

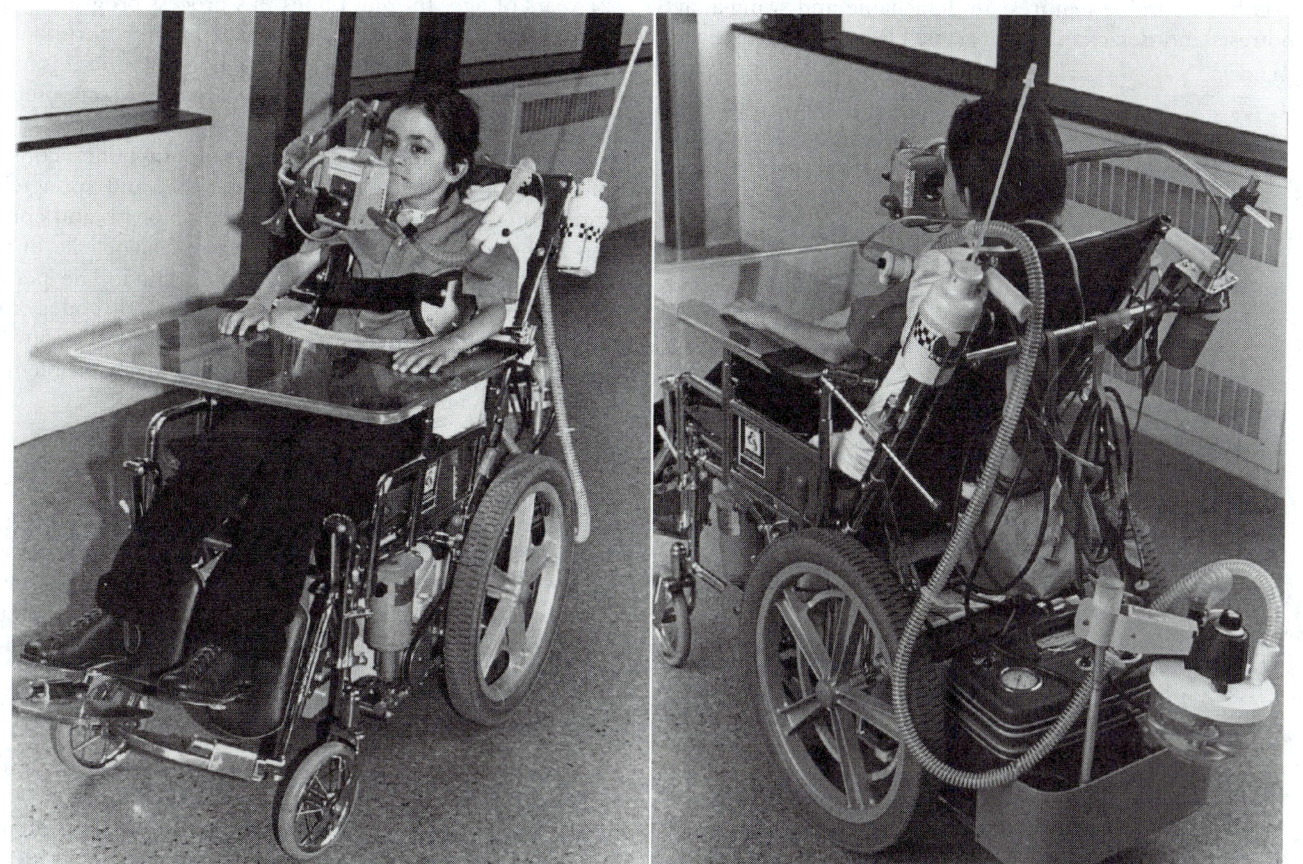

FIG. 39-8 Motorized wheelchair for quadriplegic child. **A,** Front view. **B,** Back view. Note portable respirator.

the entire "sandwich" of frames. All of the skin areas should be checked with each turning.

The ***Roto-Rest bed*** operates electrically; with the entire body securely immobilized by firm bolsters, the person is slowly and constantly rotated from side to side. Traction can be attached to this bed, and various parts can be removed to permit care and physical therapy. The continuous changes of position decrease the problems of pressure areas and promote venous circulation. The bed has a major advantage over a Stryker frame for teenagers with tracheostomies or other conditions that do not allow placing them in the prone position. The bed is made in an adult size and is suited only for large children.

Wheelchairs

Wheelchairs are used temporarily or permanently as a means of transportation. For temporary use, a wheelchair should fit the child and contain any adaptations needed, such as an elevating leg rest or reclining back. The child is taught how to transfer in and out of the chair and how to propel it safely. Prescribing a wheelchair for permanent use is the joint responsibility of physician and therapist after an assessment of home and surroundings. A wheelchair should be neither too small nor too large and preferably should be one that can be adapted to the child's growth needs. Detachable or rotating armrests, which permit easy transfer in and out, are needed for children with spinal cord injuries.

Other desirable features are detachable and swing-away footrests and detachable desk arms. Elevating leg rests are required for children who are prone to contractures, and a reclining back rest is needed for those who may have poor trunk balance. A proper cushion with adequate padding should be provided for the child who has decreased sensation. Hand rim and brake lever projections are helpful for the child with upper extremity weakness. Children with paraplegia will require upper arm strengthening exercises and instruction on transfer techniques before wheelchair mobilization. Often a tilt table must be used to overcome the problems of orthostatic hypotension before wheelchair sitting can be tolerated.

Various motorized chairs are available for marked upper extremity weakness, and mouth- or cheek-operated models are available for children who do not have the use of upper extremities so that they can operate them independently (Fig. 39-8). Very small children who have permanent paralysis of the lower extremities are provided with specially designed units that allow independent mobility (Fig. 39-9). A detachable handle on these units permits their conversion to strollers.

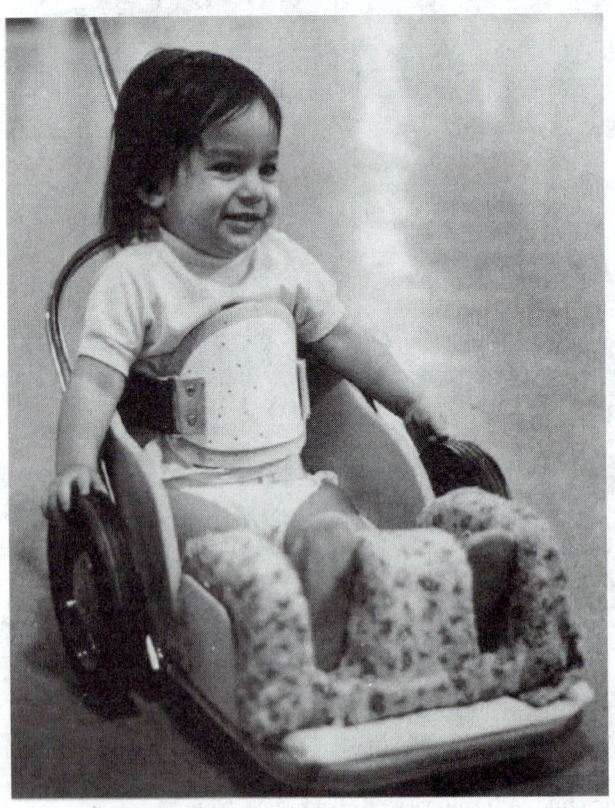

FIG. 39-9 Mobilization device for toddler.

THE CHILD WITH A FRACTURE

The process of ***ossification,*** the gradual conversion of precursor substances (namely cartilage) to bony structures, begins in the embryo and continues until the child is 18 to 21 years of age. In long bones this process progresses outwardly from the ***diaphysis,*** the hard shaftlike portion that constitutes the major portion of the bone. Within this hard, compact shaft is the hollow medullary canal composed of the bone marrow.

The ***epiphysis,*** located at the ends of long bones, consists of layers of cartilage, subchondral bone, and spongelike cancellous bone. Situated between the diaphysis and epiphysis is the ***epiphyseal plate,*** which plays a major role in the longitudinal growth of the developing child. The periosteum, the thin, tough membrane covering all bones, contains blood vessels that nourish the living bone (Fig. 39-10). Damage to this thin membrane can be a major problem in bone growth and healing.

FRACTURES

Bones fracture when the resistance of the bone against the stress being exerted yields to the stress force. Fractures are a common injury at any age but are more likely to occur in children and aged persons. The natural tendency toward active mobility and their limited gross motor coordination make children more susceptible to physical injury.

Etiology

The causes of fracture injuries in children are those described for general traumatic injuries in childhood. Fractures in infancy are more often the result of birth trauma, injury, or child abuse. Aside from motor vehicle accidents, true accidents rarely occur in infancy; therefore injury in children in that age-group warrants further investigation. In any small child radiographic evidence of fractures at various stages of healing, with few exceptions, indicates physical abuse. Most often, early bone trauma in infants consists of periosteal bleeding in the long bones of the arms and legs, usually caused by rough handling, twisting, and pulling, which is not evident on radiographic examination until 3 to 6 weeks after the injury. Any investigation of fractures in infants, particularly multiple fractures, should include the suspicion of osteogenesis imperfecta.

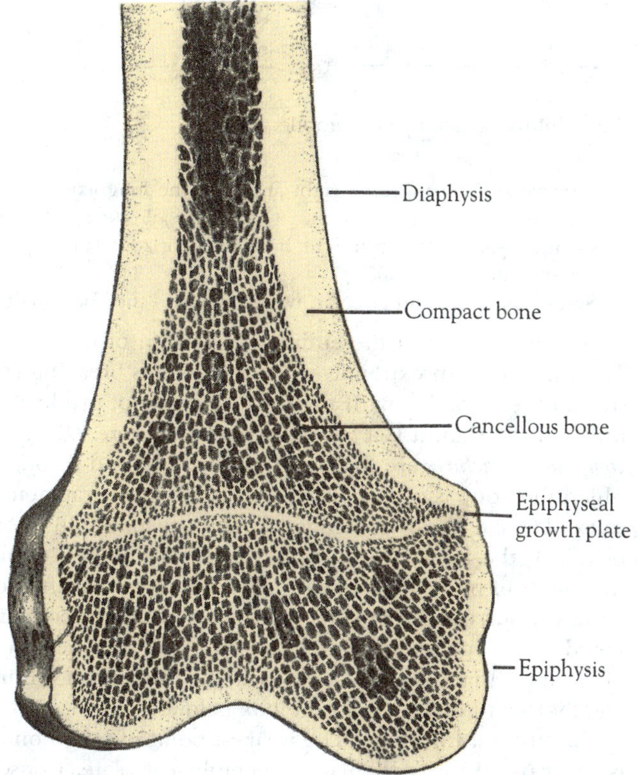

FIG. 39-10 Bone showing relationships of compact and cancellous bone, epiphysis, epiphyseal plate, and diaphysis. (From Thompson JM and others: *Mosby's manual of clinical nursing,* ed 2, St Louis, 1989, Mosby.)

Fractures of the forearm are common bone injuries in childhood and are usually caused when the child extends the palm of the hand to break a fall. The force resulting from a fall on the outstretched hand progresses up the length of the extremity with the possibility of injury to the finger, wrist, elbow, shoulder, and/or clavicle (Fig. 39-11). The clavicle is probably the bone most frequently broken in children; approximately half of clavicle fractures occur in children under 10 years of age. Many occur at birth. Hip fractures are rare in children and require a great deal of violence to produce. A femoral neck fracture may be sustained in children 6 or 7 years of age as a result of pedestrian-automobile accidents because their hip height is on the same level as an automobile bumper. In older children the femur is the most likely target; in adolescents knee injuries are common.

Children fall from heights (e.g., trees, roofs) as their insatiable curiosity and immature judgment lure them to places of danger. Fractures in school-age children are often the result of bicycle-automobile accidents or skateboard injury. At all ages motor vehicle accidents are a frequent cause of bone injury. Most children who are hit by an automobile are between 4 and 7 years of age and sustain a triad of injuries, which must be kept in mind when making an assessment of injuries: (1) the child's femur, which is at the level of the bumper, is fractured; (2) the hood of the automobile produces injuries to the child's trunk; and (3) a contralateral head injury is usually sustained when the child is thrown to the ground by the impact (Fig. 39-12). Therefore a child with any of these injuries who was struck by an automobile should be examined for evidence of the other two.

Pathophysiology

The anatomic, biomechanical, and physiologic nature of children's skeletons causes differences in the pattern of

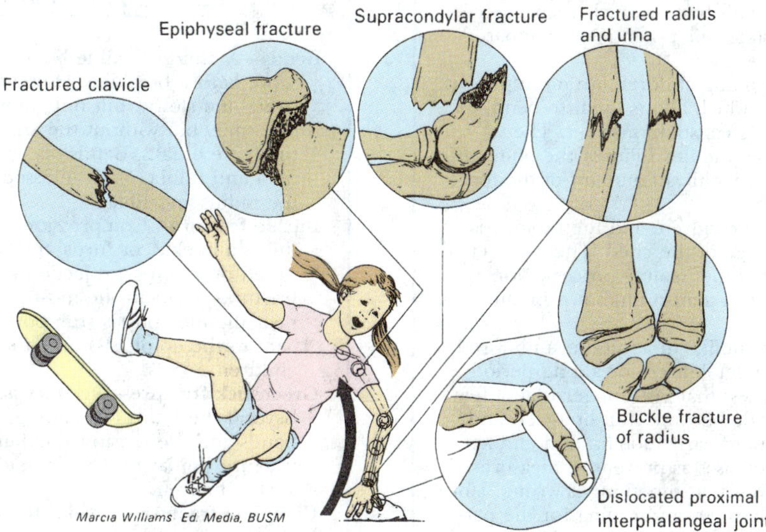

FIG. 39-11 Trauma resulting from progression of force in fall on outstretched hand. (From Segal D: *Pediatr Clin North Am* 26:793-802, 1979.)

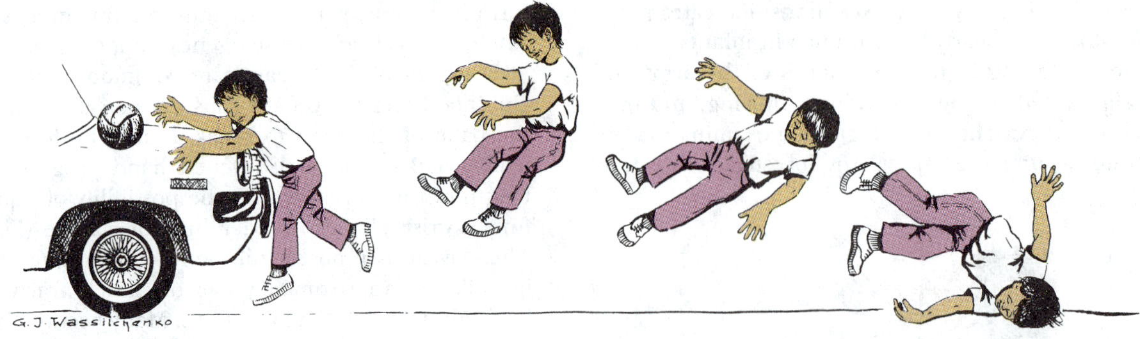

FIG. 39-12 Triad of injuries sustained when child is struck by automobile.

fractures, the problems of diagnosis, and the methods of treatment. The bones of the adult are strong and require a violent traumatic force to fracture, which is accompanied by massive injury to surrounding soft tissues. In children the bones are more easily injured, and fractures may result from minor falls or twists and thus are less likely to be accompanied by damage. Features of children's fractures not observed in the adult are outlined in the box below.

Types of Fractures. A fractured bone consists of fragments—the fragment closest to the midline, or the proximal fragment, and the fragment farthest from the midline, or the distal fragment. When fracture fragments are separated, the fracture is ***complete;*** when fragments remain attached, it is said to be ***incomplete.*** The fracture line can be:

Transverse—Crosswise, at right angles to the long axis of the bone
Oblique—Slanting but straight, between a horizontal and a perpendicular direction
Spiral—Slanting and circular, twisting around the bone shaft

All fractures affect the entire cross-section of the bone. The twisting of an extremity while the bone is breaking results in the spiral break. If the fracture does not produce a break in the skin, it is a ***simple,*** or ***closed, fracture. Open,*** or ***compound, fractures*** are those with an open wound through which the bone is or has protruded. If the bone fragments cause damage to other organs or tissues (e.g., the lung or bladder), the injury is said to be ***complicated.*** When small fragments of bone are broken from the fractured shaft and lie in the surrounding tissue, the fracture is called **comminuted.** This type of fracture is rare in children. The types of fractures that occur most often in children are shown in Fig. 39-13 and described in the box below.

Epiphyseal Injuries. The weakest point of long bones is the cartilage growth plate, or epiphyseal plate. Consequently, this is a frequent site of damage during trauma.

FEATURES OF FRACTURES IN CHILDREN

1. The growth plate, a thick, elastic portion of bone where growth takes place, serves to absorb shock and protect joint surfaces from injury and is the means by which the limb is able to grow and to straighten itself. Growth is stimulated by a fracture in the diaphysis, whereas damage to the growth plate can cause shortening and often a progressive angular deformity.
2. The periosteum of a child's bone is thicker, stronger, and has more active osteogenic potential as compared with the adult.
3. The pliable bones of growing children are more porous than those of the adult, which allows them to bend, buckle, and break in a "greenstick" manner. The greater porosity increases the flexibility of the bone and dissipates and absorbs a significant amount of the force on impact.
4. Healing is more rapid in children, and the rapidity is inversely related to the age of the child. The younger the child, the more rapid the healing process. Nonunion of bone fragments is almost unknown in children.
5. Stiffness is unusual and, unlike in adults, an uninjured joint in a child can be immobilized for a long period without producing stiffness that lasts longer than a few minutes. Injured joints do become stiff, however, and the current trend is toward early mobilization and active range-of-motion exercises as preventive measures.
6. Children only complain when something is wrong. Unreasonable crying, restlessness, and calling for the parents are usually indications that something is amiss and requires investigation.

TYPES OF FRACTURES IN CHILDREN

Bends—A child's flexible bone can be bent 45 degrees or more before breaking. However, if bent, the bone will straighten slowly, but not completely, to produce some deformity but without the angulation that exists when the bone breaks. Bends occur more commonly in the ulna and fibula, often in association with fractures of the radius and tibia.
Buckle fracture—Compression of the porous bone produces a buckle, or torus, fracture. This appears as a raised or bulging projection at the fracture site. Torus fractures occur in the most porous portion of the bone near the metaphysis (the portion of the bone shaft adjacent to the epiphysis) and are more common in young children.
Greenstick fracture—Occurs when a bone is angulated beyond the limits of bending. The compressed side bends and the tension side fails, causing an incomplete fracture similar to the break observed when a green stick is broken.
Complete fracture—Divides the bone fragments. They often remain attached by a periosteal hinge, which can aid or hinder reduction.

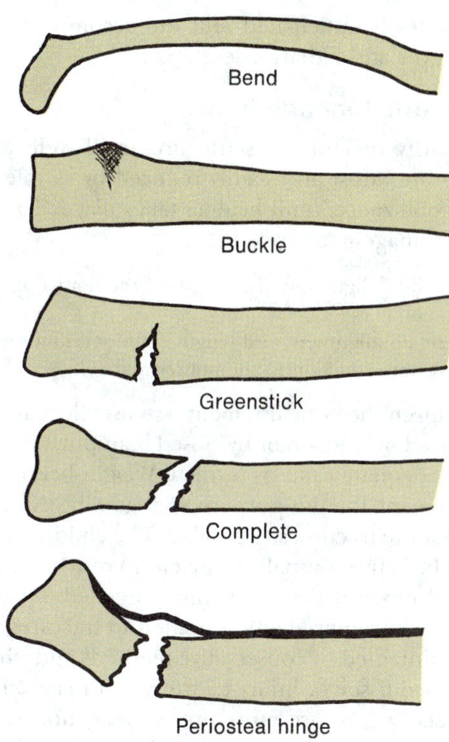

FIG. 39-13 Types of fractures in children.

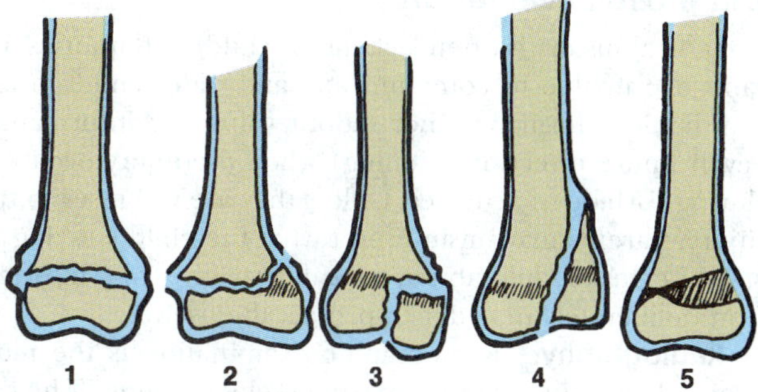

FIG. 39-14 Types of epiphyseal injuries in order of increasing risk.

Under most conditions, fractures in this area proceed along the zone of degenerating cartilage cells, before the cartilage begins to ossify, without damage to the growth plate, thus causing little damage. Healing is usually prompt. When fracture lines deviate from a transverse direction through the degenerating cells, more serious damage to the epiphysis and the plate may occur. Fig. 39-14 illustrates the types of epiphyseal injuries in order of increasing risk of permanent epiphyseal damage and possible growth disturbance.

Detection of epiphyseal injuries is sometimes difficult, and they may be mistaken for dislocations or ligamentous injuries. Fractures involving the epiphysis or epiphyseal plate present special problems in determining whether or not bone growth will be affected. Early and correct assessment is essential to minimize the incidence of longitudinal growth problems and angular deformities. The medical management of these injuries is different than that for other fractures because open reduction and internal fixation are often employed to prevent complications. If the affected limb is shorter, epiphyseal surgery is done either to stimulate the involved epiphysis or to retard growth in the unaffected leg.

Associated Problems. Immediately after a fracture occurs, the muscles contract and physiologically splint the injured area. This phenomenon accounts for the muscle tightness observed over a fracture site and the deformity that is produced as the muscles pull the bone ends out of alignment. This muscle response must be overcome by traction or complete muscle relaxation (i.e., anesthesia) in order to realign the distal bone fragment to the proximal bone fragment.

Contusions of the soft tissues frequently accompany fractures, especially of femurs, and severe hemorrhage into the tissues is not uncommon. Both the bleeding and the pain are major contributors to shock associated with this injury; therefore, suspected musculoskeletal injury should be treated as a fracture until radiographic confirmation can be made. The surrounding tissue will be swollen, and a hematoma is usually present. The soft tissue injury must be treated as any contusion. Since the injury may cause damage to essential structures, the circulatory and neurologic status of tissues distal to the fracture is carefully assessed, especially for fractures of the femur and supracondylar fractures of the elbow.

Clinical Manifestations

Children demonstrate the usual signs of injury—generalized swelling, pain or tenderness, and diminished functional use of the affected part. There may be bruising, severe muscular rigidity, and sometimes crepitus (a grating sensation at the fracture site), which are also frequent signs in adults. More often the fracture is remarkably stable because of the usually intact periosteum. The child may even be able to use an affected arm or walk on a fractured leg.

NURSING ALERT A fracture should be strongly suspected in a small child who refuses to walk.

Although neurologic and vascular damage is much less frequent in children than in adult patients, the integrity of these structures must be accurately assessed. This is often difficult in infants and young children who are unable to cooperate. Vascular injury is most likely to occur with supracondylar fractures of the humerus and femur. Femoral and popliteal vessels and the sciatic nerve are prone to trauma in femoral fractures; humeral fractures may cause damage to the medial, ulnar, or radial nerves and to the brachial artery.

NURSING ALERT The five "Ps" of ischemia from a vascular injury—*pain, pallor, pulselessness, paresthesia,* and *paralysis*—should be kept in mind when making an assessment.

Diagnostic Evaluation

A medical history is often lacking for childhood injuries. Infants are unable to communicate, and older children are unreliable informants and seldom volunteer information (even under direct questioning) when the injury occurred during forbidden activities. Unless they are witnesses to the injury, parents may misinterpret what the child is trying to say. In cases of child abuse, parents may give false information deliberately in order to protect themselves.

Radiography. Radiographic examination is the most useful diagnostic tool for assessing skeletal trauma. The calcium deposits in bone make the entire structure radiopaque. However, in normal growth and development bony structures ossify from precursor substances, usually cartilage, to form true bone from the shaft or diaphysis toward the epiphysis. This ossification process begins in the embryo and continues until bone formation is completed by 18 to 21 years of age. Ossification centers alter the appearance of the bone, and much of the skeleton of infants and young children is composed of radiolucent growth cartilage that does not appear on radiograms. In addition, the epiphyseal cartilage and undisplaced separations of the epiphysis, which often occur, are not easily detected on x-ray films. Radiographs are sometimes less reliable in predicting extremity fractures than are gross deformity and point tenderness.

Many practitioners obtain a film of the uninjured limb for a direct comparison to help identify minor alterations in alignment and configuration of the epiphysis and associated injuries that might be missed. Radiographic films are taken after fracture reduction and in some situations may be taken during the healing process to determine satisfactory progress.

Blood Studies. Severe soft tissue, muscle, and bone injury often results in the destruction of red blood cells with a rise in bilirubin and a fall in the hemoglobin or hematocrit reading. The child's homeostatic mechanisms are activated to correct the problem, and generally only supportive therapy with a high-protein diet and iron replacement is needed. When muscle integrity is disrupted, enzymes normally contained within muscles are released into the bloodstream. Serum levels of creatine, alkaline phosphatase, serum glutamic-oxaloacetic transaminase (SGOT), and lactic dehydrogenase (LDH) may increase in proportion to the amount of muscle damage.

A normal physiologic response to tissue injury is the inflammatory process with a slight elevation of white blood cells, especially neutrophils. When infection occurs, the rise in leukocytes is anticipated and the accompanying symptoms of fever and lethargy develop.

Therapeutic Management

The majority of children's fractures heal well, and nonunion is rare. Most are readily reduced by simple traction and immobilization until healing takes place. The goals of fracture management are:

1. To regain alignment and length of the bony fragments (reduction)
2. To retain alignment and length (immobilization)
3. To restore function to the injured parts

In children the bone fragments are usually realigned and immobilized by traction or by closed manipulation and casting until adequate callus is formed. Weight bearing and active movement for the purpose of regaining function can begin after the fracture site is stable. The child's natural tendency to be active is usually sufficient to restore normal mobility, and physical therapy is rarely needed. Open reduction is seldom required and is limited to fractures that cannot be maintained by conservative methods and when there is interposed tissue or injury to arteries or nerves. However, surgical reductions are more apt to delay normal healing and often predispose to nonunion. In the majority of cases children's fractures can be managed by closed reduction and plaster immobilization, which is often provided on an outpatient basis with reevaluation in 7 to 10 days.

Children are most frequently hospitalized for fractures of the femur and the supracondylar area of the distal humerus. If simple reductions cannot be achieved or a neurovascular problem is detected after injury, observation in a hospital unit is indicated. Severe contusions with profound swelling cannot be treated with a cast, which would act as a tourniquet on the extremity, and badly malaligned fractures require traction for a time before a cast is applied. The method of fracture reduction is determined by several criteria (see box below, left).

Medical interventions associated with fracture injury involve both the physician and the nurse in their management (see box below). Specific interventions and nursing responsibilities in the general management directed toward restoring bone integrity and functional use are discussed in relation to the major modalities of fracture immobilization—casting and traction.

CRITERIA FOR DETERMINING USE OF REDUCTION METHOD FOR FRACTURES

Age of child
Degree of displacement
Amount of overriding
Degree of edema
Condition of skin and soft tissue
Sensation and circulation distal to fracture

MEDICAL INTERVENTIONS ASSOCIATED WITH FRACTURE INJURY

Control of pain, hemorrhage, and edema
Relief of muscle spasms
Realignment of fracture fragments
Promotion of bone healing
Immobilization of fracture until adequate healing has begun
Prevention of secondary complications
Limitation of disuse syndrome
Restoration of function

Surgical Intervention. When surgical intervention is necessary to realign a fracture, the child needs physical and psychologic preparation. The preoperative teaching is the same as for any other surgical procedure, except that orthopaedic surgery uses a variety of rods, screws, staples, and plates and the child needs to know about these unfamiliar objects and how they will appear when he returns from the procedure. The fixating devices are made of substances that do not act as foreign proteins to the body and therefore are not rejected. Usually the rods are driven down the shaft of the long bones, whereas screws and plates are attached to the side of the bone shaft. Postoperatively the bone healing takes place with callus formation as it does in a new fracture. Generally, the child with an internal fixation device sits in a chair and walks with a walker or crutches within a few hours or days. The most common postoperative complication is infection. The nurse's responsibility includes close monitoring of neurovascular changes in the involved extremity and the prevention of postanesthesia problems.

Bone Healing and Remodeling

Bone healing follows a patterned sequence. Fig. 39-15 shows three broad overlapping phases: inflammatory, restorative, and remodeling. Bone healing is described more definitively in five stages (Table 39-2). When the bone breaks, the envelope of subcutaneous tissue, muscle, and periosteal tissue surrounding the site is torn, blood vessels rupture, and a hematoma forms. The ends of the fractured bone segments, deprived of circulation, die as far back as the nearest collateral circulation. Necrotic tissue accumulates, and an inflammatory response takes place at the site, with its characteristic vasodilation, plasma exudation, and edema. The organization and resorption of the hematoma proceeds, and the restorative phase begins with the reestablishment of local circulation. Repair requires an adequate blood supply and immobilization of the fracture fragments.

When there is a break in the continuity of bone, the periosteal and intraosseous osteoblasts are in some way stimulated to maximum activity. New osteoblasts are formed in immense numbers almost immediately after the injury and begin building a bridge, as evidenced by a bulging growth of osteoblastic tissue and new bone matrix between the fractured bone fragments. This is followed by deposition of calcium salts to form ***callus,*** which provides stability (Fig. 39-16, *B*).

Bone healing is characteristically rapid in children because of the thickened periosteum and generous blood supply. In the young child, for example, there is frequently a solid union of the femoral shaft in 3 to 4 weeks, whereas in the adult, callus sufficient to avoid deformities from constant muscle contraction associated with movement may not take place in less than 10 to 16 weeks. The approximate healing times for a femoral shaft are:

- Neonatal period—2 to 3 weeks
- Early childhood—4 weeks
- Later childhood—6 to 8 weeks
- Adolescence—8 to 12 weeks

TABLE 39-2 Stages of Bone Healing

TIME*	PHYSIOLOGIC EVENTS
STAGE 1: HEMATOMA FORMATION	
Impact	Fracture Injury to soft tissue envelops site Periosteal tissue torn Vessels rupture
3-5 minutes	Bleeding from bone and tissues into area between and around bone fragments
First 24 hours	Hematoma forms and clots; fibrin assists in clotting periosteal membrane to aid in repair Clot provides fibrin network for cellular invasion Granulation tissue forms by fibroblasts and new capillaries Osteoblastic activity stimulated
STAGE 2: CELLULAR PROLIFERATION	
After 24 hours	Blood supply increases, bringing available calcium, phosphate, and fibroblasts Cells proliferate at ends of bone fragments and differentiate into cartilage and connective tissue
Next few days	Hematoma becomes granulation tissue, which forms into a framework for bone-forming substances Fibroblasts convert to osteoblasts (bone-forming cells)
2-3 days	*Halisteresis* (softening of bone ends) ⅛-¼-inch; absorption of bone cells
STAGE 3: CALLUS FORMATION	
6-10 days	Fibroblasts form in granulation tissue; form bone in areas adjacent to surface of bone shaft; form cartilage at surfaces more distal to blood supply *Provisional callus* develops, bridging fracture ends; holds bone together but will not support body weight
14-21 days	*True callus* develops, seen on radiographs; forms more than needed, but with remodeling, excess callus absorbs Cartilage differentiates to bone tissue
STAGE 4: OSSIFICATION	
3-10 weeks	Callus forms into bone, which grows beneath periosteum of fragments; fuses fracture defect (knits together) Also called the *union stage*
STAGE 5: CONSOLIDATION AND REMODELING	
After 9 months	Bone marrow cavity restored Compact bone formed according to stress patterns Remodeling according to Wolff's law Fracture line always visible on radiographs

*Healing time more rapid in infants and in cancellous (spongy) bone and delayed with complications.

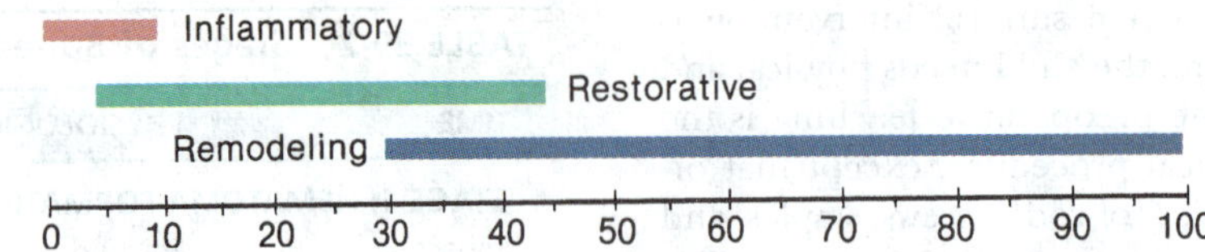

FIG. 39-15 Approximate time devoted to inflammatory, restorative, and remodeling phases of bone healing. Scale indicates percentage of healing time.

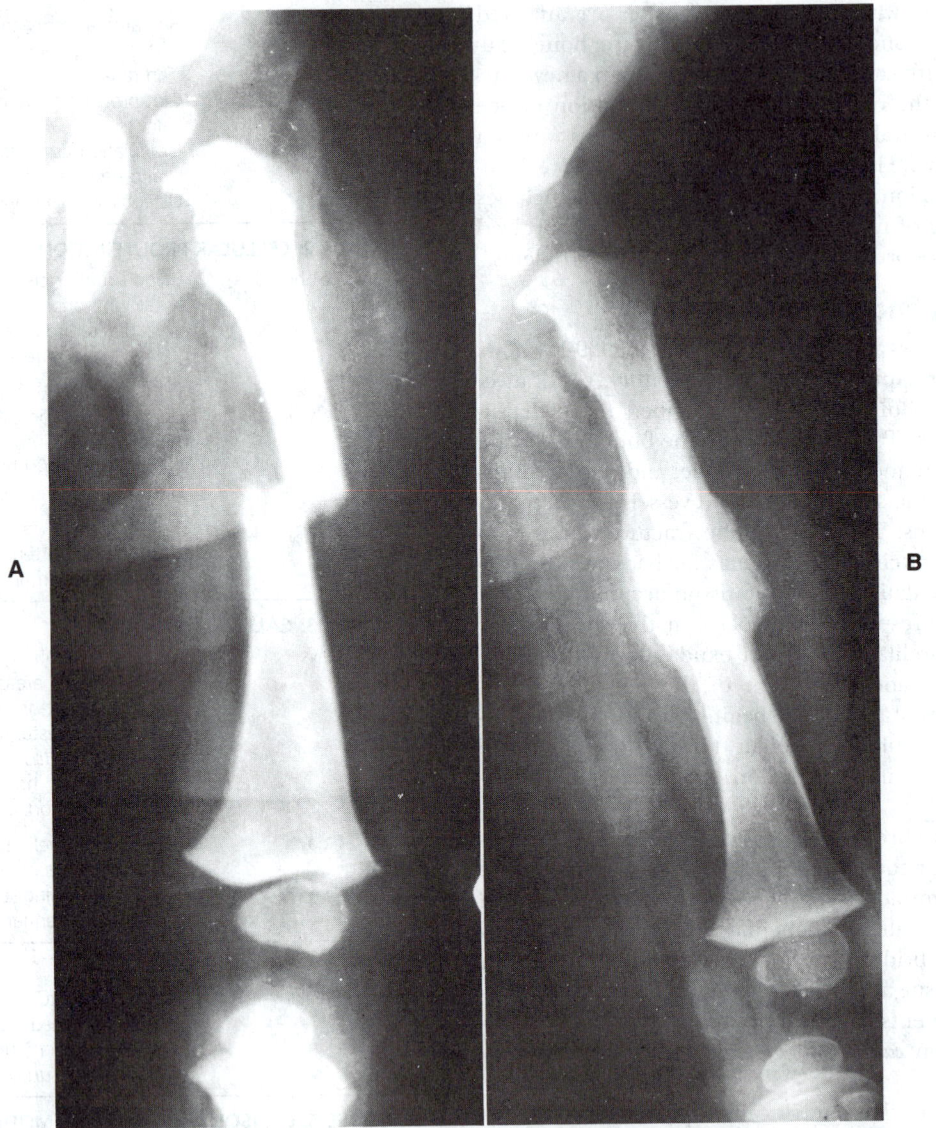

FIG. 39-16 Fractured femur. Most fractured femurs in childhood are of spiral type shown here. Note comparison of, **A,** original x-ray film with, **B,** 6-month postfracture film showing callus formation. (Courtesy Henrietta Egleston Hospital for Children, Atlanta, GA. From Hilt NE, Schmitt EW: *Pediatric orthopedic nursing,* St Louis, 1975, Mosby.)

Remodeling is a unique process that occurs in the healing of long bone fractures before epiphyseal closure. When a bone remodels, the irregularities produced by the fracture become indistinct, as hollows are filled in and angles are rounded off in the healing process, which gives the bone a straighter appearance. It does not alter the alignment of the bone. The buildup of new bone or callus will restore a portion of the normal bone structure in most cases despite observable malalignment. The younger the child and the closer the proximity of the fracture to the growth plate, the more likely it is that spontaneous correction will take place. In some instances a 90-degree angle will

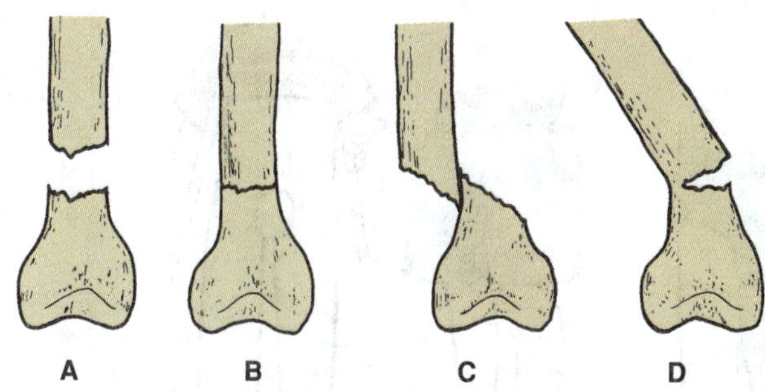

FIG. 39-17 Relationships of fracture fragments. **A,** Gap between fragments. **B,** End-to-end apposition. **C,** Bayonet apposition or overlap. **D,** Angulation of incomplete fracture.

straighten in a year, but rotational deformities do not correct themselves. Various factors such as the type and location of the fracture, the age of the child, and the amount of fragment angulation or rotation will influence the degree of correction in alignment that can be obtained by remodeling.

The position of the bone fragments in relation to one another influences the rapidity of healing and the residual deformity. A gap between fragments delays (or prevents) healing (Fig. 39-17, *A*). Healing is prompt and complete with end-to-end apposition (Fig. 39-17, *B*), but the fracture stimulates accelerated growth of the neighboring epiphysis, which causes bony overgrowth and increased length of the extremity. When the fragments overlap in a bayonet-type reduction (Fig. 39-17, *C*), there is sufficient bone contact to allow for rapid healing, and the lost length compensates for overgrowth as a result of epiphyseal stimulation. The length that can be compensated for depends on the age of the child. Approximately 1 cm of overlap can be allowed in a young child, but in a child who is near the end of the growth period, correction will be less and therefore overlap must be less. Angulation deformity caused by an incomplete fracture (Fig. 39-17, *D*) may remodel in the young child, but the degree of residual deformity depends on the relationship of the angulation of the bone fragments to the angle of the joint. This requires careful evaluation and reduction to prevent permanent deformity.

Wolff's law is applied to treating children with orthopaedic problems. Paraphrased, it states that bone will grow in the direction in which stress is placed on it. Examples of the use of this law are the hip spica cast with an abduction bar for treating developmental hip dysplasias and application of casts or traction at a selected angle to influence the direction of bone healing.

Bone healing in persons of any age-group is greatly influenced by the general health of the traumatized person. The child with a fracture requires adequate nutrition, including supplementary vitamins. No special dietary changes need to be made except to correct nutritional deficiencies. Monitoring of fluid and electrolyte balance, renal function, and possible anemia is equally important to promote wellness of the child.

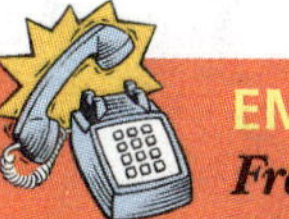

EMERGENCY TREATMENT
Fracture

Assess extent of injury—5"Ps":
- Pain and point of tenderness
- Pulse—distal to the fracture site
- Pallor
- Paresthesia—sensation distal to the fracture site
- Paralysis—movement distal to the fracture site

Determine the mechanism of injury.
Move injured part as little as possible.
Cover open wounds with sterile or clean dressing.
Immobilize the limb, including joints above and below fracture site; do not attempt to reduce fracture or push protruding bone under the skin.
- Soft splint (pillow or folded towel)
- Rigid splint (rolled newspaper or magazine)
- Uninjured leg can serve as splint for leg fracture if no splint available

Reassess neurovascular status.
Apply traction if circulatory compromise is present.
Elevate the injured limb if possible.
Apply cold to the injured area.
Call Emergency Medical Services or transport to medical facility.

THE CHILD IN A CAST

Nurses are frequently in a position where they must make the initial assessment of a child with a suspected fracture (see Emergency Treatment box). The child and the parents are frightened and upset, the child is in pain, and since most fractures are obvious, the parents and frequently the child are already convinced of the diagnosis. Therefore if the child is alert and there is no evidence of hemorrhage, the initial nursing interventions are directed toward calming and reassuring the child and parents so that an extensive assessment can be more easily accomplished.

Maintaining a calm manner and speaking in a quiet voice, the nurse can ask the parents to describe what happened and what they think about it. Since children usually arrive with the limb supported in some manner, this minute or two does not delay or endanger the treatment. It is best not to touch children initially but to ask them to point to the painful area and wiggle their fingers or toes. By this time they usually feel relatively safe and will allow someone to touch them gently to feel the pulse and test for sensation. A child's anxiety is greatly influenced by previous experiences with injury and health personnel. However, children need to be told what will happen and what they can do to help. The affected limb need not be palpated and should not be moved unless properly splinted. If the child is at home or if the practitioner is not present to examine the child, some type of splint should be applied carefully for transport to the hospital and to the radiography department and cast room.

The Cast

The completeness of the fracture, the type of bone involved, and the amount of weight that can be placed on the limb

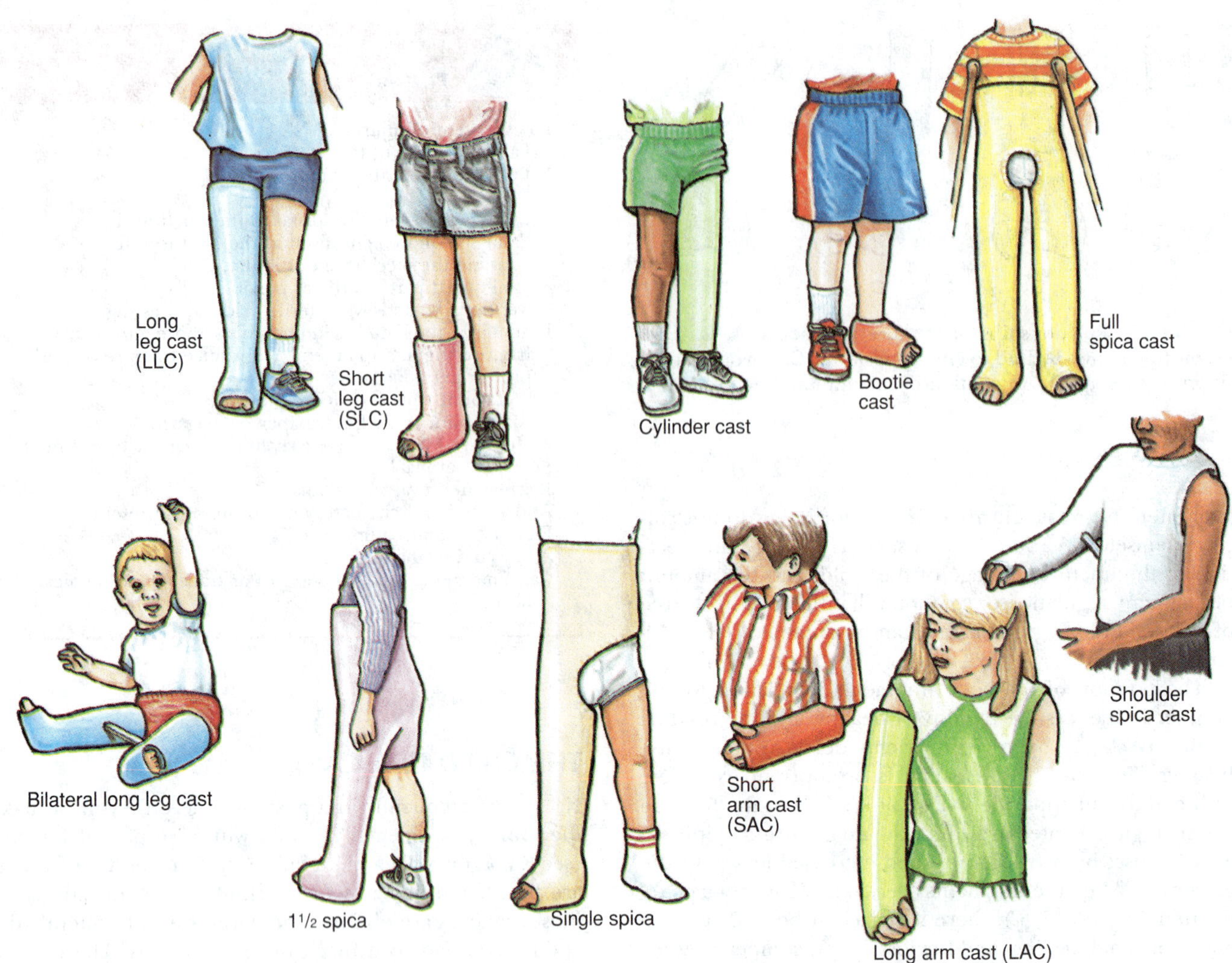

FIG. 39-18 Types of casts.

influence how much of the extremity must be included in the cast to immobilize the fracture site completely. In most situations the joints above and below the fracture are immobilized to eliminate the possibility of movement that might cause displacement at the fracture site. Four major categories of casts are used for immobilization of fractures: ***upper extremity*** to immobilize the wrist and/or elbow, ***lower extremity*** to immobilize the ankle and/or knee, ***spinal*** and ***cervical*** for immobilization of the spine, and ***spica casts*** to immobilize the hip and knee (Fig. 39-18).

Casting Materials. Casts are constructed from gauze strips and bandages impregnated with plaster of paris or synthetic lighter-weight and water-resistant materials (e.g., fiberglass and polyurethane resin). The lightweight casts are satisfactory for arms and hip spicas on infants and very young children and are even available in colors. Plaster is better for large hip spicas and legs. Table 39-3 compares the relative merits of plaster and synthetic casts.

Cast Application. When a cast is to be applied by the operator, it is often the nurse's role to set up the cast materials and hold the extremity in alignment (Fig. 39-19). Special cast tables that hold the child's body are used for applying large hip spica casts. If possible, children should be allowed to play with a small doll that has a cast so that they understand what will be done. Before the cast is applied, the extremities are checked for any abrasions, cuts, or other alterations in the skin surface and for the presence of rings or other items that might cause constriction from swelling; such objects are removed. Identification bands are placed on a noninjured extremity if hospitalization is anticipated.

A tube of stockinette is stretched over the area to be casted, and bony prominences are padded with soft cotton sheeting. Dry rolls of gauze impregnated with plaster of paris are immersed in a pail of cold water with the open end of the roll downward to allow soaking of the bandage. The wet plaster rolls are put on in a bandage fashion and molded to the extremity. A heat-producing chemical reaction occurs between the plaster and water as the plaster becomes a crystalline gypsum. During application of the cast the underlying stockinette is pulled over the raw edges of the cast and secured with a layer of wet plaster ½ to 1 inch

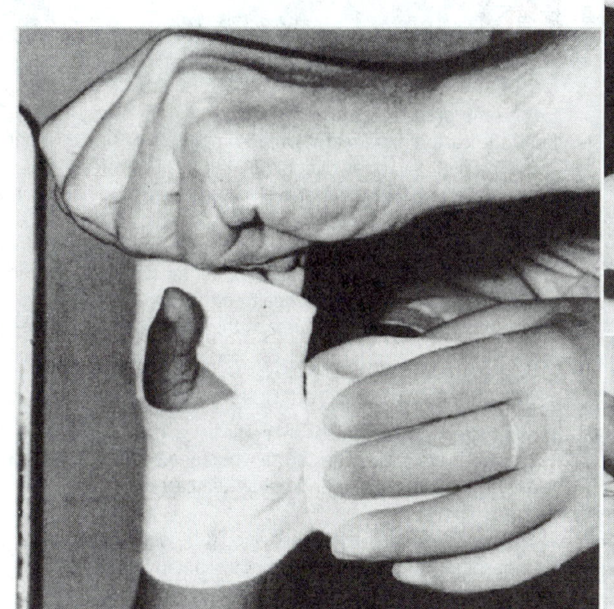

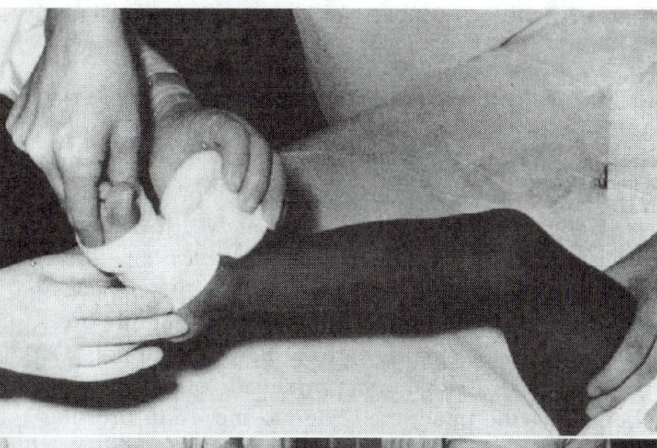

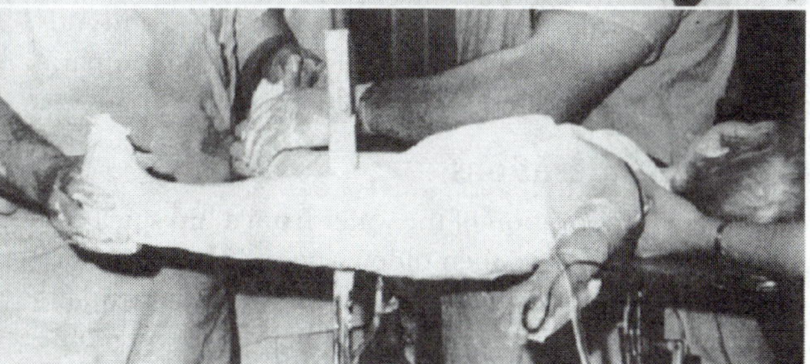

A

B

C

FIG. 39-19 Proper methods of holding child for cast application. **A,** Arm cast: arm should be held by fingers (and upper arm, if necessary) and off side of table or bed to permit exposure of entire arm. **B,** Leg cast: foot and toes are grasped with one hand as shown, and upper thigh is held with other hand; maintaining knee in flexion will discourage kicking. **C,** Hip spica cast: one individual maintains desired leg position; another individual pushes child at shoulder level toward perineal post; child's shoulders and pelvis should remain level. (From Hilt NE, Schmitt EW: *Pediatric orthopedic nursing,* St Louis, 1975, Mosby.)

TABLE 39-3 Comparison of Plaster of Paris and Synthetic Cast

	PLASTER OF PARIS	SYNTHETIC
Composition and preparation	Cotton tape permeated with calcium sulfate crystals that interlock as tape dries (tepid water activated)	1. Polyester/cotton tape permeated with polyurethane resin (cool water activated) 2. Knitted fiberglass tape with polyurethane resin (tepid water activated or photoactivated) 3. Knitted thermoplastic polyester fabric (hot water activated)
Setting time	3 to 8 minutes	3 to 15 minutes
Drying time	10 to 72 hours (varies with cast size)	5 to 30 minutes (varies with type of cast)
Indentations	Slow drying time increases possibility	Rapid drying time reduces likelihood of indentations; allows rapid use
Weight	Relatively heavy; bulky; difficulty wearing regular clothing	Lightweight; less bulky; can wear with regular clothing; allows for greater range of activity
Conformity	Molds readily to body part	Does not mold easily to body parts; unsuitable for small children or severely displaced fractures
Surface	Smooth exterior; does not scratch clothing or furniture	Rough exterior; can snag clothing or furniture; abrasive to skin
Cost	Relatively inexpensive; an advantage if cast changes anticipated	Expensive; cost three to seven times that of plaster casts
Stability	Relatively stable; must keep cast dry	May get cast wet or immerse in water with permission from practitioner (with use of nonabsorbent synthetic lining); clean with small amount of mild soap and water; dry with towel followed by blow dryer on cool or warm setting
Miscellaneous	Child may feel uncomfortable warming or burning sensation under cast while drying (chemical reaction) Skin under cast may become irritated Cast must be protected when around water (bathing)	Special aids may be required for application or removal of some types Increased activity may displace fracture Skin under cast may become macerated from inadequate drying after water immersion

below the rim to form a smooth, padded edge to protect the skin.

If the operator does not form such a protective edge with stockinette, the raw edges of the cast can be protected by a "petaled" edge. Small pieces approximately 2 to 3 inches long are cut from 1- or 1½-inch wide adhesive tape. The edges are rounded with scissors, and each of these "petals" is placed over the edge of the cast, each petal slightly overlapping the previous petal to form a smooth, neat edge. It is easier to apply the petal to the underside of the cast first and then bring the unadhered edge to the front, pressing firmly so that the edges remain securely attached. Band-Aids can be used instead of the tape petals for quicker preparation and a slightly padded cast edge.

Nursing Considerations

The complete evaporation of the water from a hip spica cast can take 24 to 48 hours when older types of plaster materials are used. Drying occurs within minutes with new quick-drying substances. The cast must remain uncovered to allow it to dry from the inside out. Turning the child in a plaster cast at least every 2 hours will help to dry a body cast evenly and prevent complications related to immobility. A regular fan or cool-air hairdryer to circulate air may be helpful when the humidity is high.

NURSING ALERT Heated fans or dryers are not used, since they cause the cast to dry on the outside and remain wet beneath, thus becoming moldy. They also cause burns from heat conduction by way of the cast to the underlying tissue.

A wet cast should be supported by a pillow covered with plastic and handled by the palms of the hands to prevent indenting the cast and creating pressure areas. A dry plaster of paris cast produces a hollow sound when tapped with the finger. If "hot spots" are felt on the cast surface (usually indicating infection beneath the area), this should be reported so that a window can be made in the cast to observe the site.

During the first few hours after a cast is applied, the chief concern is that the extremity may continue to swell to the extent that the cast becomes a tourniquet, shutting off circulation and producing neurovascular complications. A measure for reducing the likelihood of this potential problem is to elevate the body part, thereby increasing venous return. If edema is excessive, casts are bivalved (i.e., cut to make anterior and posterior halves that are held together with an elastic bandage). The cast and the involved extremity are observed frequently for neurovascular integrity and any signs of compromise. Permanent muscle and tissue damage can occur within 6 to 8 hours, for which nurses can be held liable (Northrup and Kelly, 1987).

NURSING ALERT Observations such as pain, swelling, discoloration (pallor or cyanosis) of the exposed portions, lack of pulsation and warmth, or the inability to move the exposed part(s) are reported immediately.

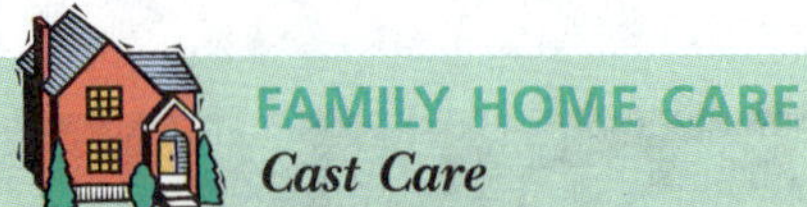

FAMILY HOME CARE
Cast Care

Expose the plaster cast to air until dry.

Keep the casted extremity elevated on pillows or similar support for the first day, or as directed by the health professional.

Lift and support the wet cast with the palms of the hands only, to avoid indenting with the fingers.

Observe the extremities (fingers or toes) for any evidence of swelling or discoloration (darker or lighter than a comparable extremity) and contact the health professional if noted.

Check movement and sensation of the visible extremities frequently.

Follow health professional's orders regarding any restriction of activities.

Restrict strenuous activities for the first few days.
- Engage in quiet activities but encourage use of muscles.
- Move the joints above and below the cast on the affected extremity.
- Specific exercises for the child should be demonstrated by hospital staff, and a written copy should be provided to the parents.

Encourage frequent rest for a few days, keeping the injured extremity elevated while resting.

Avoid allowing the affected limb to hang down for more than 30 minutes.
- Keep an injured upper extremity elevated (e.g., in a sling) while upright.
- Elevate a lower limb when sitting and avoid standing for more than 30 minutes.

Do not allow the child to put anything inside the cast.
- Keep small items that might be placed inside the cast away from small children.

Itching may be relieved by an ice pack, visualizing the skin at the cast edges, and administering medication as recommended by the physician.

Keep a clear path for ambulation.
- Remove toys, hazardous floor rugs, pets, or other items over which the child might stumble.

Use crutches appropriately if lower limb fracture.
- The crutches should fit properly, have a soft rubber tip to prevent slipping, and be well padded at the axilla.

Instruct child and parents to avoid placing the cast in water (i.e., tub, shower, swimming pool).

If patient is incontinent, protect the cast with waterproof tape and plastic.

When casting an extremity that has sustained an open fracture, a window is often left over the wound area to allow for observation and for dressing of the wound. A surgical reduction is usually casted as for a closed fracture. For the first few hours after surgery there may be substantial bleeding that will soak through the cast. Periodically the circumscribed blood-stained area should be outlined with a ballpoint pen or pencil and the time indicated to provide a guide for assessing the amount of bleeding.

Usually the child is discharged to home care after a cast is applied in the emergency room or clinic. Parents need instructions on drying and caring for the cast and checking for signs and symptoms that indicate the cast is too tight (see Family Home Care box). They should also be told to take the child to the health professional for attention if the

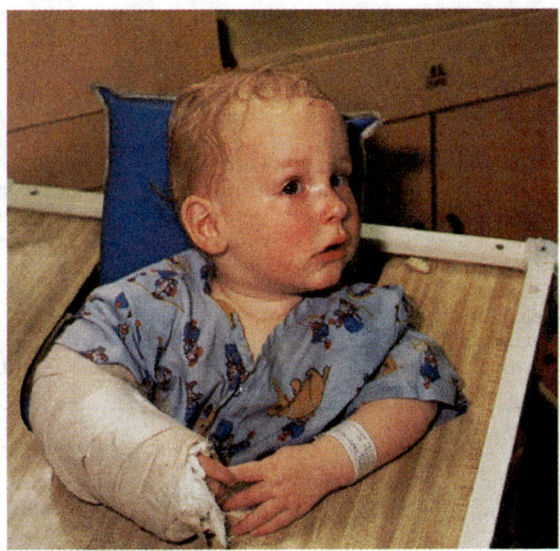

FIG. 39-20 Young children come to regard a cast as part of their body. They usually adapt well but may fear its removal. (Courtesy St. Louis Children's Hospital.)

cast becomes too loose, since a loose cast no longer serves its purpose. A cast is a badge of honor for the child and serves as visible evidence of an otherwise invisible injury (Fig. 39-20).

Cast Removal. Cutting the cast to remove it or to relieve tightness is frequently a frightening experience for children. They fear the sound of the cast cutter and are terrified that their flesh, as well as the cast, will be cut. Since it works by vibration, a cast cutter cuts only the hard surface of the cast. This can be demonstrated on the nurse or person removing the cast. The oscillating blade vibrates very rapidly back and forth and will not cut when placed lightly on the skin. Children have described it as producing a "tickly" sensation. The vibration also generates heat that may be felt by the child. Both these feelings should be explained.

Preparation for the procedure will help reduce anxiety, especially if a trusting relationship has been established between the child and the nurse. Many young children come to regard the cast as part of themselves, which intensifies their fear of removal. Using the analogy of having fingernails or hair cut sometimes helps reduce their anxiety. They need continual reassurance that all is going well and that their behavior is accepted.

Home care for children in casts creates problems of various magnitude, especially with large casts (e.g., a hip spica). Commonplace situations become problematic (e.g., returning the child home safely and comfortably). Standard seat belts and car seats are not readily adapted for use by children in casts (see Developmental Dysplasia of the Hip, Chapter 11, and Educate About the Disorder and General Health Care, Chapter 22). Sitting can be impossible in a spica cast, and leg casts require extra space in a small room, under a table, or in a bathroom. Children in spica casts usually find the prone position easier for self-feeding from a small table placed next to the dining table or on the floor.

PURPOSES OF TRACTION

- To realign bone fragments
- To provide rest for an extremity
- To help prevent or improve contracture deformity
- To correct a deformity
- To treat a dislocation
- To allow preoperative or postoperative positioning and alignment
- To provide immobilization of specific areas of the body
- To reduce muscle spasms (rare in children)

The conventional toilet is almost impossible for a child in a spica cast. Small bedpans or other containers offer alternatives for elimination.

Nurses can help families adapt the child's environment to meet the temporary encumbrance of a cast, for example, devising plastic wraps for waterproofing casts for a shower. Baths are possible only if the plaster cast is kept out of the water and covered to prevent it from becoming wet from splashes. Some synthetic casts are waterproof, but skin can become irritated from water that collects beneath the cast.

After the cast is removed, the skin surface will be caked with desquamated skin and sebaceous secretions. Simple soaking in a bathtub is usually sufficient for their removal but may require several days to eliminate the accumulation completely. Application of olive oil or lotion may provide comfort. Parents and child should be instructed not to pull or forcibly remove this material with vigorous scrubbing because it may cause excoriation and bleeding.* (See also Nursing Care Plan: The Child with a Fracture and Nursing Care Plan: The Child in a Cast.†)

THE CHILD IN TRACTION

Bone fragments that cannot be aligned initially by simple traction and stabilization with a cast require the extended pulling force offered by continuous traction. Traction also may be used for other purposes (see box above). In some of these cases the skin traction is applied at night and intermittently during the day. Muscle relaxants may be administered for muscle spasms.

Purposes of Traction

When forces having both direction and magnitude act on an object at the same point simultaneously from opposite directions, the object either changes its state of rest or motion or remains in equilibrium. The use of traction in the management of fractures is the direct application of these forces to produce equilibrium at the fracture site. A forward force (traction) is produced by attaching weight to the distal bone fragment, which is balanced by the backward force of the muscle pull (countertraction) and the frictional force between the patient and the bed. Thus the three essential

*Home care instructions for the child in a cast are available in *Wong and Whaley's Clinical Manual of Pediatric Nursing* (Mosby).

†In *Wong and Whaley's Clinical Manual of Pediatric Nursing* (Mosby).

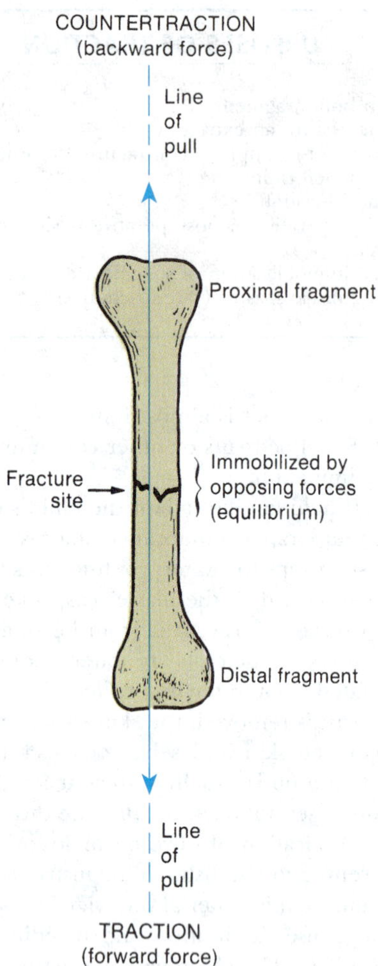

FIG. 39-21 Application of traction for maintaining equilibrium.

components of traction management are traction, countertraction, and friction (Fig. 39-21).

To reduce or realign a fracture site, traction is provided by weights applied to the distal bone fragment; body weight provides countertraction. By adjusting the line of pull upward or downward or by adducting or abducting the extremity, the operator uses these forces to align the distal and proximal bone fragments. To attain equilibrium, the amount of forward force is adjusted by adding weight to or subtracting weight from the traction, and/or countertraction can be increased by elevating the foot of the bed to create a greater gravitational pull to the backward force. A bed board placed under the mattress of heavy children prevents sagging, which might otherwise change the direction of the forces applied to the fracture.

The three primary purposes of traction for reduction of fractures are:

1. To fatigue the involved muscle and reduce muscle spasm so that bones can be realigned
2. To position the distal and proximal bone ends in desired realignment to promote satisfactory bone healing
3. To immobilize the fracture site until realignment has been achieved and sufficient healing has taken place to permit casting or splinting

TYPES OF TRACTION

Manual traction—Traction applied to the body part by the hand placed distally to the fracture site. Nurses frequently provide manual traction during cast application.

Skin traction—Pull applied directly to the skin surface and indirectly to the skeletal structures. The pulling mechanism is attached to the skin with adhesive material or an elastic bandage. Both types are applied over soft foam-backed traction straps to distribute the traction pull.

Skeletal traction—Pull applied directly to the skeletal structure by a pin, wire, or tongs inserted into or through the diameter of the bone distal to the fracture.

Fatiguing of a muscle is accomplished by applying constant stress to the muscle so that the buildup of lactic acid will produce muscle relaxation. The all-or-none law, characteristic of muscle contractility, influences the complete relaxation. When muscle is stretched, muscle spasm ceases and permits the realignment of the bone ends. The continuous maintenance of traction is important during this phase because releasing the traction allows the muscle's normal contracting ability to again cause a malpositioning of the bone ends.

The realignment of the fragments is a gradual process that is achieved more rapidly in infants, who have limited muscle tone, than in muscular teenagers. The desired line of pull and callus formation are checked periodically by radiographic examination. The traction pull to some degree immobilizes the fracture site; however, adjunctive immobilizing devices such as splints or casts are sometimes used with skeletal traction. In injuries in which there is severe soft tissue swelling or vascular and nerve damage, it is customary to use traction until these complications have been resolved and it is safe to apply a cast. Immobilization with traction will be maintained until the bone ends are in satisfactory realignment, after which a less-confining type of immobilization, usually a cast, will be applied.

Types of Traction (General)

The pull needed for traction can be applied to the distal bone fragment in several ways (see box above). ***Manual traction*** is used by the operator in uncomplicated arm or leg fractures in which there is little overriding of the bones and minimum muscle pull to overcome. Manual traction is used to realign bone fragments for immediate cast application. ***Skin traction*** is applied when there is minimum displacement and little muscle spasticity but is contraindicated when there is associated skin damage. Skin traction has specific limits of weight that it can pull without causing tissue breakdown. ***Skeletal traction*** is employed when significant traction pull must be applied in order to achieve realignment and immobilization. By inserting a pin or wire into the bone, the stress is placed on the bone and not on the surrounding tissue.

The type of traction applied is determined primarily by

the age of the child, the condition of the soft tissues, and the type and degree of displacement of the fracture. Fractures most commonly treated by application of traction are those involving the humerus, femur, and vertebrae. The major types of traction for specific fractures are discussed in the following sections.

Upper Extremity Traction

Treatment of fractures of the humerus by traction is accomplished either (1) by ***overhead suspension,*** in which the arm, bent at the elbow, is suspended vertically by skin or skeletal attachment and traction is applied to the distal end of the humerus, or (2) by ***Dunlop traction.*** With Dunlop traction the arm is suspended horizontally, using either skin or skeletal attachment.

When skin traction is used, straps are placed on the lower and upper arm with the arm flexed to accomplish pull in two directions: one along the longitudinal direction of the upper arm and one to maintain alignment of the lower arm. In instances such as supracondylar fractures, the amount of traction pull needed to align the site more critically requires a skeletal wire placed in the upper arm to allow the additional weight.

Fractures of the humerus, which are usually the result of a fall with the arm in extension, frequently involve the supracondylar portion. There are three major complications associated with this injury: Volkmann contractures (p. 1831); traumatic injury to the median, ulnar, or radial nerves; and angulation deformities. The fracture must be carefully reduced, sometimes with the child under anesthesia, and because of the danger of complications, children with closed reduction of supracondylar fractures are often hospitalized for observation. In severely malaligned fractures, closed reduction with the child under anesthesia is followed by application of skeletal traction for 2 to 3 weeks, after which a long arm cast is applied for an additional 2 to 3 weeks.

Lower Extremity Traction

The frequent site for a femoral fracture is in the middle one third of the shaft, as pictured by the radiograph in Fig. 39-16, *A*. With this fracture there is significant overriding but minimum displacement. In a fracture in the lower one third of the shaft, the pull of the gastrocnemius muscle causes the distal fragment to become downwardly displaced. The severity of the fracturing force and the ability of the muscles to hold the fracture out of alignment will determine the fracture type and the amount of overriding of the fragments. The periosteum may remain intact, which helps maintain alignment.

Fractures of the femur can often be reduced with early application of a hip spica cast in young children. When traction is required, several types may be employed, based on the initial assessment. ***Bryant traction,*** a type of running traction in which the pull is only in one direction, is not recommended because of the gravitational vascular draining of the elevated extremities, the possible tourniquet effect of the bandages, and the effect of the traction, which can trigger vasospasms and avascular necrosis.

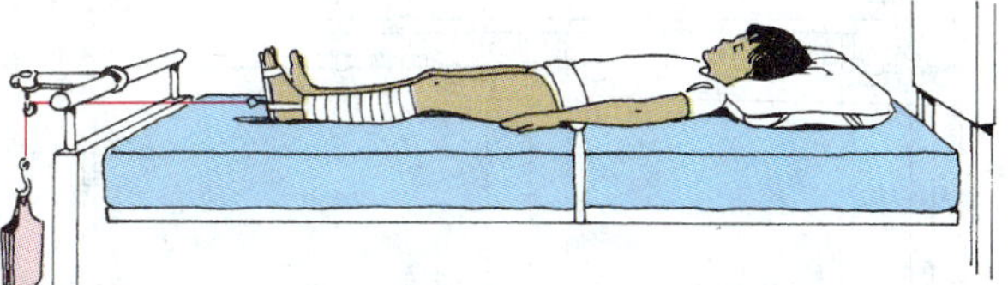

FIG. 39-22 Buck extension traction. (Figs. 39-22 to 39-26 redrawn from Hilt NE, Schmitt EW: *Pediatric orthopedic nursing,* St Louis, 1975, Mosby.)

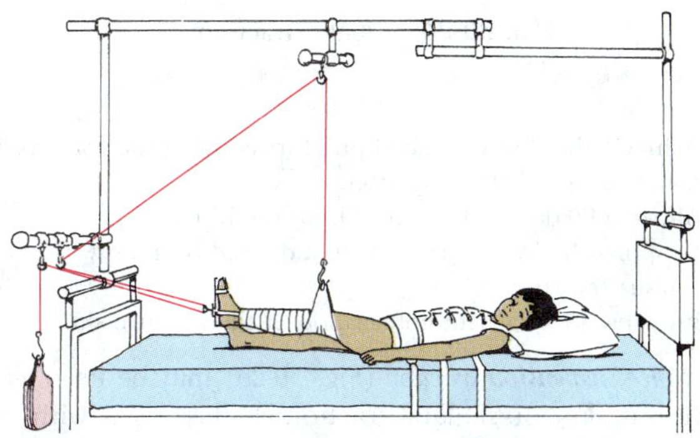

FIG. 39-23 Russell traction.

Buck extension (Fig. 39-22) is a type of skin traction with the legs in an extended position. Turning from side to side is permitted (except for fractures) with care taken to maintain the involved leg in alignment. Buck extension is used primarily for short-term immobilization, such as preoperative management of a child with dislocated hips, or frequently for correcting contracture or bone deformities such as Legg-Calvé-Perthes disease.

Russell traction (Fig. 39-23) uses skin traction on the lower leg and a padded sling under the knee. Two lines of pull, one along the longitudinal line of the lower leg and one perpendicular to the leg, are produced. This combination of pulls allows realignment of the lower extremity and immobilizes the hip and knee in a flexed position. The hip flexion must be kept at the prescribed angle to prevent fracture malalignment, since there is no direct support under the fracture and the skin traction may slip. Because the traction is set up to have two ropes pulling in the same direction at the foot plate, the traction pull will be twice the amount of weight at the end of the bed. For example, 5 pounds of weight produces 10 pounds of pull. Special nursing measures include carefully checking the position of the traction so that the amount of desired hip flexion is maintained and damage to the common peroneal nerve under the knee does not produce footdrop.

A common skeletal traction is ***90-degree–90-degree traction*** (90-90 traction) (Fig. 39-24). The lower leg is put in a boot cast or supported in a sling, and a skeletal Steinmann pin or Kirschner wire is placed in the distal fragment of the femur. From a nursing standpoint this traction easily facilitates position changes, toileting, and prevention of traction complications. This traction also:

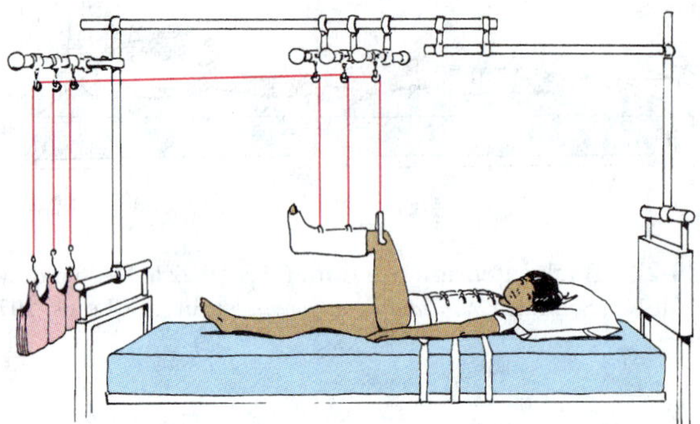

FIG. 39-24 "90-90" traction.

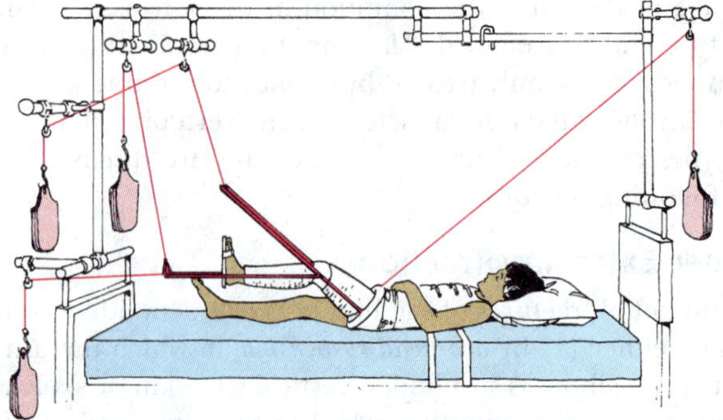

FIG. 39-25 Balance suspension with Thomas ring splint and Pearson attachment.

- Achieves the desired line of pull for reducing the fracture by means of the skeletal traction
- Allows a 90-degree flexion of both the hip and the knee
- Supports the lower extremity in a desired position with good venous return
- Provides adequate immobilization of the fracture site

Balance suspension traction (Fig. 39-25) may be used with or without skin or skeletal traction. Unless used with another traction, the balanced suspension merely suspends the leg in a desired flexed position to relax the hip and hamstring muscles and does not exert any traction directly on a body part. A ***Thomas splint*** extends from the groin to midair above the foot, and a ***Pearson attachment*** supports the lower leg. Towels or pieces of felt covered with stockinette are clipped or pinned to the splints for leg support. Note that the ropes are attached to create a balanced traction. When the child is lifted from the bed, the traction lifts as well, with no loss of alignment.

The Pearson attachment will stay wherever positioned. Many times the practitioner will put a rope between the end of the Pearson attachment and the end of the Thomas splint to prevent any knee flexion alteration while the child is moved. This traction requires very careful checking of splints and ropes to make certain that no slippage or fraying has occurred. The traction is of great value in an older and heavier child when lifting the patient for care is essential.

Cervical Traction

The cervical area is a vulnerable site for flexion or extension injuries to muscle, vertebrae, and/or the spinal cord. Cervical muscle trauma without other complications is treated with a cervical soft or hard collar to relieve the weight of the head from the fracture site. Intermittent cervical skin traction might be employed with a head halter and weight to decrease muscle spasms (Fig. 39-26). Injuries limited to cervical muscles can be very uncomfortable but, with prompt medical care, usually resolve with conservative treatment.

When a child displaces or fractures a cervical vertebra, it is necessary to reduce and immobilize the site with cervical skeletal traction. The spinal cord runs through the intravertebral canal, and dislocation or fracture of the vertebrae can also cause spinal cord trauma.

Physical examination, especially a neurologic assessment,

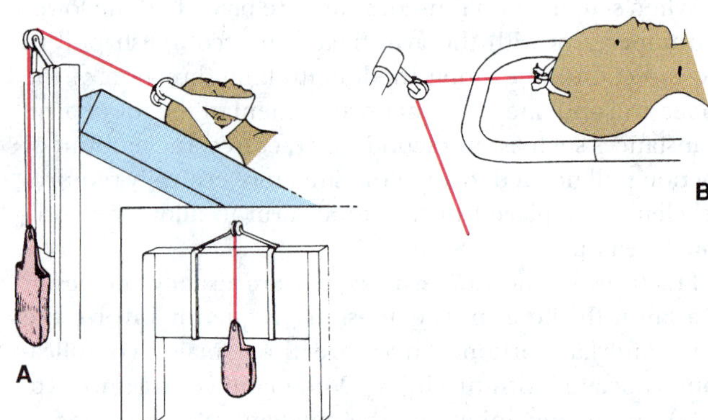

FIG. 39-26 **A,** Cervical traction. **B,** Crutchfield tong traction.

and radiographic studies are essential diagnostic aids to determine:

- The presence of a vertebral fracture
- The degree of vertebral dislocation
- Displacement of an intravertebral disk
- Compression of the spinal cord and other neurologic structures
- Sensory, motor, and autonomic nerve deficits

Cervical traction is usually accomplished by insertion of Crutchfield or Barton tongs through burr holes in the skull. The head is placed in a hyperextended position, and, as the neck muscles fatigue with constant traction pull, the vertebral bodies gradually are pulled apart and the cord is no longer pinched between the vertebrae. Immobilization until fracture healing can occur is an essential goal of cervical traction. If the injury has been limited to a vertebral fracture without neurologic deficit, a halo cast can be applied to permit earlier ambulation.

Nursing Considerations

❖ Assessment

To assess the child in traction, it is essential to know the purpose for which the traction is applied. Regular assessment of both the child and the traction apparatus is required, as outlined in the Guidelines box. The child is also assessed for evidence of adverse effects of immobilization (see p. 1797).

GUIDELINES
Assessment of Traction

Check desired line of pull and relationship of distal fragment to proximal fragment.
- Check whether fragment is being directed upward, adducted, or abducted.

Check function of each component:
- Position of bandages, frames, splints
- Ropes—in center tract of pulley, taut, no fraying, knots tied securely
- Pulleys
  - In original position on attachment bar; have not slid from original site
  - Wheels freely movable
- Weights
- Correct amount of weight
  - Hanging freely
  - In safe location

Check bed position—head or foot elevated as directed for desired amount of pull and countertraction.

Assess child's behavior to determine if traction causes pain or discomfort.

Skin traction:
- Replace nonadhesive straps and/or Ace bandage on skin traction *when permitted* and/or absolutely necessary, but make certain that traction on limb is maintained by someone during procedure.
- Assess bandages to ascertain if they are correctly applied (diagonal or spiral), not too loose or too tight, which could cause slippage and malalignment of traction.

Skeletal traction:
- Check pin sites frequently for signs of bleeding, inflammation, or infection.
- Check pin screws to be certain that screws are tight in metal clamp that attaches traction apparatus to pin.
- Note pull of traction on pin; pull should be even.

Observe for correct body alignment with emphasis on alignment of shoulders, hip, and leg(s).

Check after child has moved.

Assess any circular dressing for excessive tightness.

Assess restraining devices if prescribed.
- Make certain that they are not too loose or too tight.
- Remove periodically and check for pressure areas.

Note if any tightness, weakness, or contractures are developing in uninvolved joints and muscles.

Note any neurovascular changes, such as:
- Color in skin and nail beds
- Alterations in sensation
- Alterations in motor ability

Check beneath the child for small objects (e.g., foods, toys).

❖ Nursing Diagnoses

Based on a thorough assessment, several nursing diagnoses are identified. The more common diagnoses for the child in traction are included in the Nursing Care Plan on pp. 1828-1829. Others may apply in specific situations.

❖ Planning

The goals for the child in traction and the family include the following:

1. Child will not experience complications.
2. Child and family will receive support.
3. Child will experience no pain or reduction of pain to level acceptable to child.
4. Child will not experience skin breakdown.
5. Child will maintain function of uninvolved muscles and joints.
6. Child will exhibit signs of reduced fear and will experience adequate comfort.
7. Child will engage in self-help activities.
8. Child will exhibit normal elimination patterns.

❖ Implementation

Evaluating the therapeutic effects and possible negative consequences is essential to good patient care. Many of the nursing problems associated with a child in traction are related to immobility. However, there are a number of physical needs that require attention and vigilance.

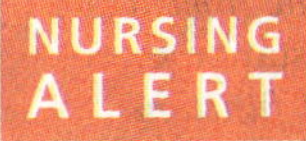

NURSING ALERT Skeletal traction is never released by the nurse. This includes not lifting weights (e.g., for moving the child in bed, for repositioning) that are applying traction.

The nurse may, however, remove nonadhesive skin traction. In these cases intermittent traction is periodically released and reapplied as ordered. When skin traction must be constantly maintained, such as in fractures, nurses may occasionally remove and reapply the Ace bandage if this is approved by the attending physician, provided that *someone manually maintains the traction during the rewrapping process.* A child may have several types of traction at one time, and each traction must be assessed separately to avoid problems.

In addition to routine skin observation and care (see The Immobilized Child, p. 1797), children in skeletal traction will need special skin care at the pin site according to hospital policy or practitioner preference. A pressure-reduction device, such as a foam overlay, or alternating pressure mattress placed beneath the hips and back reduces the chance of skin breakdown in these vulnerable areas. (See Nursing Care Plan, p. 1805, for additional nursing measures.)

➤ **NURSING TIP** A small hand mirror facilitates visualization of inaccessible skin areas.

When the child is first placed in traction, an increase in discomfort is common as a result of the traction pull fatiguing the muscle. It has been determined that orthopaedic conditions are associated with a higher-than-average number of painful events and a higher percentage of bodily symptoms than other common conditions (Wong and Baker, 1988). Analgesics, including opioids, and muscle relaxants help during this phase of care and should be administered liberally.

Helping children cope with the confinement and new experience requires more than medications. An explanation should be given according to each child's level of development about what is happening and why the child must remain in the device. They should be reassured that someone will always be available to aid them in adjusting to the traction and to cope with the problems of immobilization.

Some devices assist children in performing activities independently. An overhead trapeze, which they can use to help lift themselves, facilitates hygiene and repositioning and provides exercise for uninvolved muscles. Specific nursing responsibilities for care of the patient in cervical traction are included in the Nursing Care Plan on pp. 1828-1829.

NURSING CARE PLAN
The Child in Traction

NURSING DIAGNOSIS: High risk for injury related to immobility and traction apparatus

PATIENT GOAL 1: Will not experience complications

• **NURSING INTERVENTIONS/*RATIONALES***

Encourage deep breathing frequently with maximum inspiratory chest expansion *to prevent respiratory complications*
Apply restraints when indicated *to maintain traction*
Maintain correct angles at joints *for proper alignment*
Carry out passive, active, or active-with-resistance exercises of uninvolved joints *to preserve joint function*
Take measures to correct or prevent further development of deformity such as applying foot plate *to prevent footdrop*
*Cleanse and dress pin sites on skeletal traction as ordered *to decrease risk of infection*
*Apply topical antiseptic or antibiotic daily as ordered
Cover ends of pins with protective cord or padding *to prevent child from being scratched by pin*
Do not remove skeletal traction or adhesive traction straps on skin traction
*Administer stool softeners as indicated *to prevent constipation*
Administer rectal suppository or mild laxative if indicated *to relieve constipation*
Make certain that child ingests sufficient amount of calcium-rich foods *for bone healing*
Encourage sufficient fluids and foods high in fiber *to prevent constipation*

• **EXPECTED OUTCOMES**

Circulation in extremities remains satisfactory: movement, good (pink) color, sensation present
Child exhibits no signs of complications
Neurovascular status assessed for compromise—circulation, movement, sensation

NURSING DIAGNOSIS: Knowledge deficit related to use of traction

PATIENT/FAMILY GOAL 1: Will verbalize understanding of purpose of traction

• **NURSING INTERVENTIONS/*RATIONALES***

Explain purpose and importance of traction to decrease muscle spasm, reduce and stabilize a fracture or dislocation, maintain alignment, and immobilize a limb
Encourage and answer all questions and concerns

• **EXPECTED OUTCOME**

Patient and/or family verbalizes understanding of purpose of traction as evidenced by verbal statements and compliance with therapeutic regimen

*Dependent nursing action.

NURSING DIAGNOSIS: Pain related to physical injury

PATIENT GOAL 1: Will experience no pain or reduction of pain to level acceptable to child

See Pain Assessment; Pain Management, Chapter 26

NURSING DIAGNOSIS: High risk for impaired skin integrity related to immobility, traction apparatus

PATIENT GOAL 1: Will not experience skin breakdown

• **NURSING INTERVENTIONS/*RATIONALES***

Provide pressure-reducing mattress underneath hips and back
Make total body skin checks for redness or breakdown, especially over areas that receive greatest pressure, *to prevent delay in treatment*
Wash and dry skin at least daily *to stimulate circulation and keep skin clean*
Gently massage over pressure areas *to stimulate circulation*
Change position at least every 2 hours *to relieve pressure,* if possible
Check for small objects (e.g. toys, food) under child, *since they can cause skin irritation*

• **EXPECTED OUTCOME**

Skin remains clean and intact with no evidence of irritation

NURSING DIAGNOSIS: Impaired physical mobility (specify level) related to musculoskeletal impairment

PATIENT GOAL 1: Will maintain function of uninvolved muscles and joints

• **NURSING INTERVENTIONS/*RATIONALES***

Provide apparatus (e.g., overhead trapeze) and encourage child in activities that provide exercise for uninvolved muscles and joints

• **EXPECTED OUTCOME**

Joints remain flexible; muscles retain tone

NURSING DIAGNOSIS: Fear related to discomfort, unfamiliar apparatus

PATIENT GOAL 1: Will exhibit signs of reduced fear

• **NURSING INTERVENTIONS/*RATIONALES***

Explain traction apparatus to child and family *to decrease fear/anxiety and increase cooperation*
Explain to child what nursing care will be *so that child knows what to expect*
Determine with child ways to participate in own care *to give child some measure of control*

NURSING CARE PLAN
The Child in Traction—cont'd

Make certain that child knows how to call for help
Provide assurance that the child will not be left totally helpless
Have family bring child's favorite toy and/or security object

• **EXPECTED OUTCOMES**
Child cooperates throughout procedures
Child remains calm

PATIENT GOAL 2: Will experience adequate comfort

• **NURSING INTERVENTIONS/*RATIONALES***
Use pads, pillows, and rolls to position *for comfort*
Encourage family to use favorite comfort measures (e.g., stroking, music, pacifier)
Touch and talk to child *to provide comfort while child cannot be held*

• **EXPECTED OUTCOMES**
Child plays and interacts readily
Child exhibits no signs of discomfort

NURSING DIAGNOSIS: Bathing/hygiene, feeding, dressing/grooming, toileting self-care deficits related to impaired mobility

PATIENT GOAL 1: Will engage in self-help activities

• **NURSING INTERVENTIONS/*RATIONALES***
Allow child to help plan own daily routine and choose from alternatives when appropriate *to increase sense of control*
Devise means to facilitate self-help in daily activities
Assist with self-care activities where needed (e.g., bathe inaccessible parts, make food easy to eat without assistance, provide grooming)

• **EXPECTED OUTCOME**
Child assists with self-care activities—feeds self, washes reachable areas, attends to grooming within child's capabilities (specify)

PATIENT GOAL 1: Will exhibit normal elimination patterns

• **NURSING INTERVENTIONS/*RATIONALES***
Determine child's words for elimination needs *so that child receives assistance when needed*
Provide privacy *to promote relaxation needed for elimination*
Use fracture pan for bowel movements and voiding for females
Check frequency and consistency of bowel movements *to prevent delay in treating constipation*
Adjust fluid and food intake according to stools, for example, increase fluids, fruits, grains *for constipation*

• **EXPECTED OUTCOMES**
Elimination is managed with minimum difficulty
Child has regular bowel movements

See also:
Nursing Care Plan: The Child in the Hospital, Chapter 26
Nursing Care Plan: The Family of the Ill or Hospitalized Child, Chapter 26

For helping the child and family cope with immobility, see Nursing Care Plan, p. 1805.

❖ EVALUATION

The effectiveness of nursing interventions is determined by continual reassessment and evaluation of care based on the following observational guidelines and expected outcomes:

1. Perform routine assessment of the child and traction, as described in the box on p. 1827.
2. Perform assessment for circulation, skin integrity, neurologic function, and evidence of infection.
3. Observe types of activity in which child engages; observe for visitors and interaction with other patients and staff.
4. Interview child and family regarding feelings and concerns.

Expected outcomes:
See Nursing Care Plan, pp. 1828-1829.

DISTRACTION

Unlike traction, which helps bones realign and fuse properly, ***distraction*** is the process of separating opposing bone to encourage regeneration of new bone in the created space. Distraction can also be used when limbs are of unequal lengths and new bone is needed to elongate the shorter limb.

ILIZAROV EXTERNAL FIXATOR (IEF)

The IEF uses a system of wires, rings, and telescoping rods that permits limb lengthening to occur by manual distraction. In addition to lengthening bones, the device can be used to correct angular or rotational defects or to immobilize fractures. The device is attached surgically by securing a series of external full or half rings to the bone with wires. External telescoping rods connect the rings to each other. Manual distraction is accomplished by manipulating the rods to increase the distance between the rings. A percutaneous ostomy is performed when the device is applied to create a "false" growth plate. A special osteotomy or corticotomy involves cutting only the cortex of the bone while preserving its blood supply, bone marrow, endosteum, and periosteum. Capillary blood flow to the transected area is

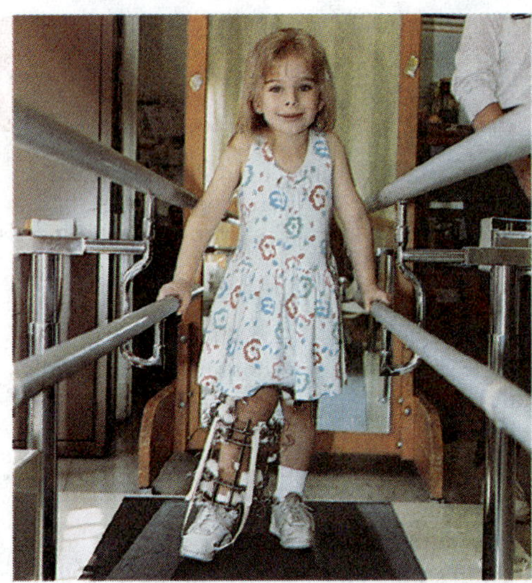

FIG. 39-27 Children with the Ilizarov external fixator must cope with the visible nature of the device.

essential for proper bone growth. Cut bone ends typically grow at a rate of 1 cm/month. The IEF can result in up to a 15 cm gain in length (Carlino, 1991).

Nursing Considerations

Success of the IEF depends on the child's and family's cooperation; therefore, before surgery they must be fully informed of the appearance of the device, how it accomplishes bone growth, alterations in activities, and home and follow-up care. Children are involved in learning to adjust the device to accomplish distraction. Children who participate actively in their care report less discomfort. Since the device is external (Fig. 39-27), the child and family need to be prepared for the reactions of others and assisted in camouflaging the device with appropriate apparel, such as wide-legged pants that close with self-adhering fasteners around the device. Partial weight bearing is allowed, and the child needs to learn to walk with crutches. Alterations in activity include modifications at school and in physical education. Full weight bearing is not allowed until the distraction is completed and bone consolidation has occurred. Follow-up care is essential to maintaining appropriate distraction until the desired leg length is achieved. The device is removed surgically after the bone has consolidated, and the child may need to use crutches or have a cast for about 1 month following removal.

FRACTURE COMPLICATIONS

Circulatory Impairment

If the trauma or immobilizing device restricts veins or arteries in the affected extremity, bone healing will be seriously impaired. Careful assessment of the pulses, skin color, and temperature is an important nursing responsibility. After injury, swelling of tissues occurs more rapidly in the child than in the adult. In the upper extremity, brachial, radial, ulnar, and digital pulses are felt. In the leg, femoral, popliteal, posterior tibial, and dorsalis pedis pulses are checked.

NURSING ALERT When circulatory impairment is evident (absence of pulse, discoloration, swelling, pain), the nurse takes quick action to relieve the problem by reporting the situation immediately. If the practitioner is unable to come and release the pressure, the nurse must be able to cut the cast in half to form a bivalve cast or make a large window in it to decrease the pressure.

Closely associated with an inadequate blood supply is a low hematocrit value, which can result from the initial blood loss or surgically induced anemia. Although the blood flow may be adequate, a lowered amount of hemoglobin will not provide a sufficient supply of oxygen for tissue repair.

Nerve Compression Syndromes

Nerve damage can take place at the time of injury, develop in the process of realignment, or be a complication of an immobilizing apparatus. The syndromes are classified according to the anatomic area affected and can involve the median (carpal tunnel syndrome), ulnar (at wrist or elbow), radial, posterior tibial (tarsal tunnel syndrome), common peroneal, or sciatic nerves. Peroneal nerve damage can result in footdrop, and radial nerve impairment produces wristdrop. Both of these disabilities can significantly interfere with activities of daily living.

Sensory testing with touch and pinprick and evaluating motor strength by asking the child to move the unaffected joint distal to the injury are common means of determining neurologic involvement. Subjective symptoms are pain or discomfort, muscular weakness, a burning sensation, limitation of motion, and altered sensation. Because the fear of pain limits the child's cooperation, play can be the nurse's most valuable tool.

Treatment is alleviation of pressure on the nerve. The practitioner determines whether correcting the alignment will alleviate pressure on the nerve or if surgical intervention is necessary. At times sensory or motor changes indicate ischemia, and the treatment is correction of the vascular disturbance.

Compartment Syndromes

A ***compartment*** is a group of muscles surrounded by tough, inelastic fascial tissue. The compartment syndrome occurs when increased pressure within this closed space rises and compromises circulation to the muscles and nerves within the space. Muscles and nerves of both upper and lower extremities are enclosed within such compartments. The most frequent causes of compartment syndrome are tight dressings or casts, hemorrhage, trauma, burns, and surgery.

Signs and symptoms of compartment syndrome reflect a deficit or deterioration of neuromuscular status in the anatomic area surrounding the involved structures. These include motor weakness and pain or discomfort out of proportion to the injury and unrelieved by pain medication. Tenseness may be noted on palpation of the area. Because early detection is important in preventing permanent damage to tissues, specialists recommend continuous monitoring of compartment pressures by way of a small, slit-tip catheter inserted into the compartment. Treatment of compartment syndrome is immediate relief of pressure, which sometimes requires fasciotomy.

Volkmann contracture (ischemic muscular atrophy) is a serious, persistent flexion contraction of the forearm and hand caused by massive infarction of muscle. Pressure from a cast or tight bandage or from swelling from the injury in the area of the elbow begins with arterial occlusion and then progresses to muscle anoxia and reflex vasospasms. Finally, the lack of blood supply leads to muscle necrosis and replacement with fibrous tissue, which produces paralysis and a clawlike hand contracture. Any fracture that requires excessive traction can be complicated by Volkmann contracture; however, it occurs most often in the elbow.

The neuromuscular symptoms are severe pain (although pain is not always a manifestation), pallor or cyanosis, edema, absence of pulses in the extremity, and loss of sensitivity. Unrelieved, the occlusive hypoxic process can cause some contracture if ischemia lasts as little as 6 hours. A great deal of muscle damage occurs after 12 to 24 hours; 48 hours of ischemia produces severe deformity, with muscle fibrosis and contractures in 5 to 10 days. If not treated, the contracture leads to severe deformity and paralysis.

The immediate treatment is to remove any mechanically obstructive materials, such as tight bandages, and extend the joint to free blood vessels. If the symptoms do not improve within a few hours, arteriography is done in anticipation that surgery may be needed to decrease arterial spasms and to improve the blood supply by separation of the fascial sheaths of the involved muscles.

Epiphyseal Damage

Growth of bone originates from the epiphyseal plate, and damage to this structure could result in an unequal extremity length. Surgical intervention to the epiphysis on the affected extremity or to the epiphyseal line on the opposite extremity is the usual treatment.

Nonunion

Bone healing and callus formation can span and repair only a limited space between fragments. When inadequate reduction, poor immobilization, or a damaged or softened cast cannot maintain the bone fragments in correct alignment for repair, bone healing is impaired. Based on the physiologic needs for bone healing, the factors most likely to interfere with bone healing and cause delayed union or nonunion are listed in the box above, right.

The hematoma, which becomes the matrix for bone deposition in the break, must be free of infection or bits of adipose or connective tissue. The constant supply of nutrients and bone-forming cells brought to the area by way of the bloodstream provides the vital ingredients for repair.

Sometimes artificial means are employed to facilitate bone healing. Bone grafting becomes necessary when bone nonunion occurs. The donor site is usually the tibia or the iliac crest. Bleeding of bone ends may need to be artificially stimulated, and at times holes are drilled near the bone ends in an attempt to increase circulation. Postsurgical immobilization of the recipient area is crucial to a successful graft. The Ilizarov procedure and protocol for care is frequently used to assist bone healing in patients with this type of fracture (see p. 1829).

FACTORS THAT INTERFERE WITH BONE HEALING

- Separation of bone fragments at fracture site
- Loss of hematoma
- Interposition of tissue between bone fragments
- Loss of bone tissue, especially from necrosis
- Infection
- Poor nutrition
- Interruption of blood supply
- Diseases that influence calcium metabolism (e.g., thyroid disorder)
- Cancer of bone
- Administration of steroids

Malunion

Malunion is fracture union with increased angulation or deformity at the fracture site. It can be detected at any stage in the healing process or after complete healing. Unsatisfactory reduction is the usual reason for malunion. A cast or splint that allows fracture movement will also likely result in malunion. Periodic radiographic examinations will help detect this complication and avoid its becoming a major problem over a long period.

Excessive deformity can be corrected during the healing process through realignment and reimmobilization. However, attempts at correction may cause delayed union or nonunion; therefore the degree of deformity is carefully evaluated in light of these complications. The probability of sufficient spontaneous alignment that occurs with growth and continuation of the healing process also is considered. Correction of the malunion when healing is near completion requires surgical intervention.

Infection

Osteomyelitis, infection of the bone, is often secondary to a bloodstream infection but is a potential problem in open fractures or when bone surgery has been performed. Any bacterial organism can cause this infectious process; however, *Staphylococcus aureus* is the most frequent pathogen. (See p. 1853 for a discussion of osteomyelitis.)

Kidney Stones

Although uncommon in children, renal calculi are a potential risk whenever the child has a limb that is non–weight bearing for a long time, especially if the circumstances also produce urinary stasis. Preventive measures for renal calculi are to maintain good hydration, to mobilize the child as much as possible, and to check closely the amount and characteristics of urinary output. Any urinary tract infection should be treated promptly with appropriate antimicrobials and urine acidification because the nucleus of the calculi is often composed of bacterial debris or calcium and the buildup of stone is precipitated by alkaline urine. An associated problem, hypercalcemia, is reviewed under problems of the immobilized child.

Pulmonary Emboli

Blood, air, or fat emboli can be a hazard to the child with a fracture. As postinjury bleeding and clotting occur, a small piece of the clot can travel to vital organs, such as the lung, heart, or brain, and produce a life-threatening vascular obstruction and ischemia. Generally, the pulmonary system is the most frequent site for emboli deposition, but it may not occur until 6 to 8 weeks after the injury.

Fat emboli are the greatest threat to an individual with multiple fractures, particularly in fractures of the long bones such as the femur. Fat droplets from the marrow are transferred to the general circulation by means of the venous-arterial route, where they can be transported to the lung or brain. This type of emboli phenomenon occurs within the first 24 hours, generally in the second 12 hours after the injury occurs. Adolescents are the usual victims in the pediatric age-groups.

Emboli in the vital organs produce the classic symptoms of shock. Petechial hemorrhages of the chest and shoulders are the outstanding signs that differentiate this condition from other kinds of shock. Deep breathing, coughing, and mechanical respiratory assistance are important to maintain adequate alveolar gas exchange. An intravenous infusion is established to treat the shock and administer medications such as heparin and corticosteroids.

NURSING ALERT In the immobilized child who suddenly develops chest pain and dyspnea when turned, pulmonary embolism should be suspected. The severe dyspnea must be treated immediately by elevating the head when possible and administering oxygen by means of a mask, cannula, or hood.

AMPUTATION

A child may be born with the congenital absence of a body part, have a traumatic loss of an extremity, or need a surgical amputation for a pathologic condition such as osteogenic sarcoma. With today's surgical technology and the quick thinking of bystanders who save a traumatically amputated body part, some children have had fingers and arms sewn back on with variable degrees of functional use regained. A severed part should be wrapped lightly in a clean cloth or gauze saturated with normal saline and sealed in a watertight plastic bag. One should avoid using ice, which might come in contact with the tissue and make implantation impossible. The bag should be labeled with the child's name, the date, and the time and taken to the hospital with the child.

Surgical amputation or the surgical repair of a permanently severed limb focuses on constructing an adequately nourished stump. A smooth, healthy, padded stump, free of nerve endings, is important in prosthesis fitting and subsequent ambulation. In some situations in which there is no vascular or neurologic deficit, a cast is applied to the stump immediately after the procedure, and a pylon, metal extension, and artificial foot are attached so that the patient can walk on the temporary prosthesis within a few hours.

Nursing Considerations

Stump shaping is done postoperatively with special elastic bandaging using a figure-8 bandage, which applies pressure in a cone-shaped fashion. This technique decreases stump edema, controls hemorrhage, and aids in developing desired contours so that the child will bear weight on the posterior aspect of the skin flap rather than on the end of the stump. When appropriate, the use of a stump shrinker, in addition to an Ace wrap, may be used. Stump elevation may be used during the first 24 hours, but after this time the extremity should not be left in this position because contractures in the proximal joint will develop and seriously hamper ambulation. Monitoring proper body alignment will further decrease the risk of flexion contractures. Postoperatively, children who undergo amputation of the lower extremity are encouraged to lie prone at least three times a day, increasing the time prone to tolerance of an hour at a time.

For older children and adolescents, arm exercises and bed pushups, as well as parallel bars, which are used in prosthesis-training programs, help to build up the arm muscles necessary for walking with crutches. Full range-of-motion exercises of joints above the amputation must be performed several times daily, using active and isotonic exercises. Young children are spontaneously active and require little encouragement.

Depending on the age, children or their parents will need to learn stump hygiene, including careful washing with soap and water every day and checking for skin irritation, breakdown, or infection. A tube of stockinette or talcum powder is used to slide the prosthesis on more easily. A careful skin check must be done every time the prosthesis is removed, and prosthesis tolerance time must be adjusted to prevent skin breakdown.

For children who have had an amputation, ***phantom limb sensation*** is an expected experience because the nerve-brain connections are still present. Gradually these sensations fade. Preoperative discussion of this phenomenon will help a child to understand these "unusual feelings" and not hide the experience from others. Limb pain, especially pain that increases with ambulation, should be evaluated for the possibility of a neuroma at the free nerve endings in the stump. Psychogenic phantom limb pain is a complex problem that involves the child's response to the altered body image and the coping mechanisms used to handle the new experience. The problems of amputation, particularly the psychologic aspects, are discussed in Chapter 36.

INJURIES AND HEALTH PROBLEMS RELATED TO SPORTS PARTICIPATION

Adolescents probably spend more time and energy practicing and participating in sports activities than members of any other age-group. The practice of sports and games contributes significantly to growth and development, to the education process, and to better health. It provides exercise for growing muscles, interactions with peers, and a socially acceptable means of enjoying stimulation and conflict. In addition, competitive activities help the teenager in the process of self-appraisal, development of self-respect, and concern for others.

Every sport has some potential for injury to the participant—whether the young person engages in serious competition or participates for pure enjoyment. Serious injury is not limited to the athlete who competes in rough contact sports; a large number of severe or fatal injuries occur to persons who are not physically prepared for the activity. For example, a body build may not be suited to the sport, muscles and support systems (respiratory and cardiovascular) may not have been sufficiently conditioned to withstand the rigors of the physical stress, or youngsters may not possess insight and judgment to recognize when an activity is beyond their capabilities. Rapidly growing bones, muscles, joints, and tendons are especially vulnerable to unusual strain.

The awkward and inexperienced youngster suffers more injury than the more skilled and experienced one; strong muscles are less easily damaged than weak ones and will provide better protection to the joints they cross, and fatigue significantly impairs muscle function and judgment. More injuries occur during recreational sports participation than in organized athletic competition. Likewise, most injuries occur in practices rather than in games. And although team sports have more frequent injuries, those resulting from recreational and individual sports are generally more severe (National Youth Sports Foundation, 1993). The increase in strength and vigor in adolescence may tempt youngsters to overextend themselves, especially boys who are egged on by teammates or are stimulated by the admiration of female observers.

Not only does the activity itself pose a hazard of greater or lesser degree (Fig. 39-28), but the environment and the sports or recreational equipment present additional risks. Adolescents participate in physical activity in a variety of environments, both indoors and outdoors, on floors, on the ground, on snow, on or beneath water surfaces, and sometimes in free air space. These activities frequently involve equipment that intensifies the risk factor.

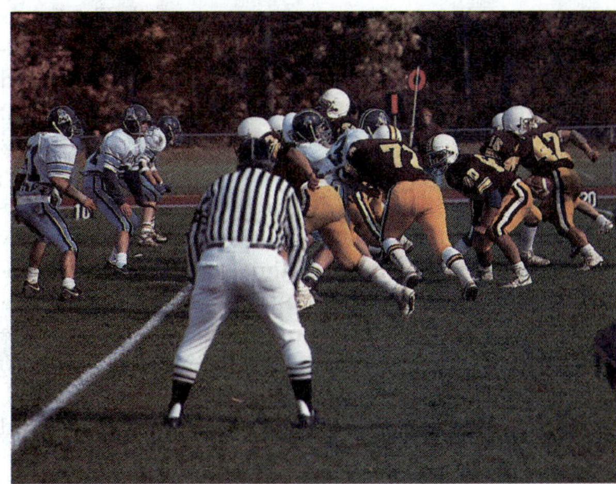

FIG. 39-28 Football is an example of a strenuous collision sport.

PREPARATION FOR SPORTS

The degree of physical maturation varies greatly among adolescents of the same age, and many of the physical characteristics important in sports are related to hormone production. Consequently, physical strength, coordination, endurance, and size vary considerably among youngsters who wish to compete against each other. Sports competition between young people who differ markedly in strength and agility is unfair and hazardous. Matching of candidates for sports should be made relative to physical maturity, height, weight, and physical fitness and skills, particularly in a sport involving rigorous body contact. Age is a less important consideration.

The American Academy of Pediatrics (1988) has devised a classification that divides sports according to strenuousness and probability of collision (see box below and Fig. 39-29). Collision sports have the highest injury rate, followed by contact sports (National Youth Sports Foundation, 1993). The Academy also has prepared a table that provides criteria for determining inclusion or exclusion of the young athlete relative to common medical and surgical conditions

CLASSIFICATION OF SPORTS

CONTACT SPORTS

Contact/Collision

- Boxing
- Field hockey
- Football
- Ice hockey
- Lacrosse
- Martial arts
- Rodeo
- Soccer
- Wrestling

Limited Contact/Collision

- Baseball
- Basketball
- Bicycling
- Diving
- Field
  - High jump
  - Pole vault
- Gymnastics
- Handball
- Horseback riding
- Skating (ice and roller)
- Skiing
  - Cross-country
  - Downhill
  - Water
- Softball
- Squash
- Volleyball

NONCONTACT SPORTS

Strenuous

- Aerobic dancing
- Crew
- Fencing
- Field
  - Discus
  - Javelin
  - Shot put
- Running
- Swimming
- Tennis
- Track
- Weight lifting

Moderately Strenuous

- Badminton
- Curling
- Table tennis

Nonstrenuous

- Archery
- Golf
- Riflery

Modified from American Academy of Pediatrics, Committee on Sports Medicine: Recommendations for participation in competitive sports, *Pediatrics* 81:737-739, 1988.

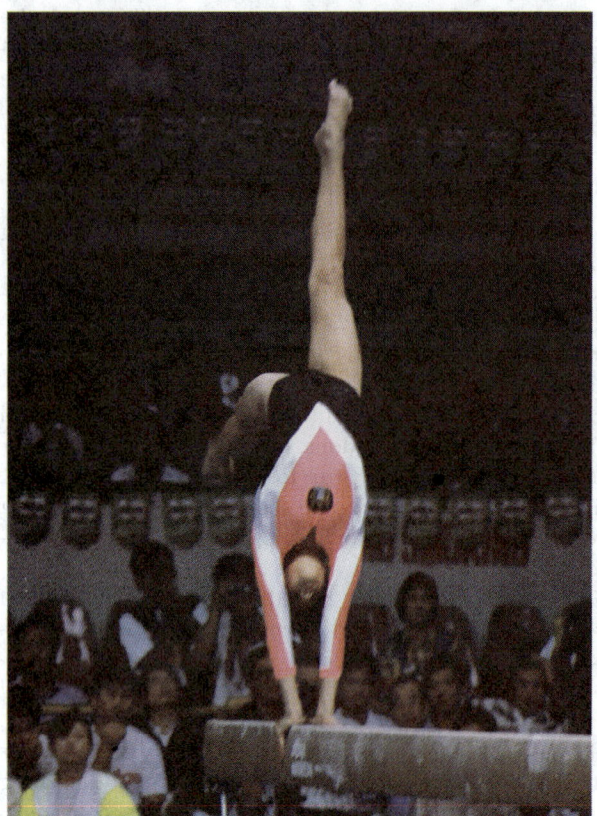

FIG. 39-29 Gymnastics is an example of a strenuous limited-contact/collision sport.

and relative risks in various sports categories. This serves as a useful guideline for the health professional in counseling youth for activities. Other factors to consider in determining sports participation are:

1. The level on which the youth will participate (e.g., Little League, intramural, sandlot, varsity sports program)
2. The facilities available to the athlete
3. The expertise of the coaches
4. The desire of the athlete to participate

According to the National Youth Sports Foundation for the Prevention of Athletic Injuries (1993) sports with the highest injury rates among high school participants were gymnastics, ice hockey, and football.

The role of health professionals in relation to sports injuries is directed toward prevention, treatment, and rehabilitation. Of these, the area of *prevention* is perhaps the most important. However, it is difficult to "sell" prevention, especially to children. Everyone wants to play the game, not practice. Often, if an 8- to 15-minute warm-up is suggested, most youngsters will warm up for 30 seconds and say they are ready to go (Ostrum, 1993). To this end, those youth who are actively involved in athletic programs need medical evaluation as a prerequisite to participation; education in sports skills with correct training and conditioning methods; omission of those tactics that are dangerous beyond the ordinary risk associated with the specific sport; use of appropriate protective equipment, properly maintained and suited to the individual; and an environment with maximum provision for safety and availability of first-aid and medical services.

The same protective principles apply to noncompetitive sports enthusiasts. They need the same education in basic safety precautions, encouragement to acquire proper instruction in the skills required for performance of the activity (instruction in water safety, skiing techniques, and so on), and proper maintenance of equipment.

TYPES OF INJURY

The injuries sustained in sports or recreational activities can involve any part of the body and extend from relatively minor cuts, bruises, and abrasions to totally incapacitating central nervous system injuries or death. Some of these injuries are discussed in chapters devoted to the major topic (e.g., spinal cord injuries [Chapter 40] and head injuries [Chapter 37]). Fractures are discussed earlier in this chapter.

There are some sports that are particularly dangerous for children. Some time ago the American Academy of Pediatrics, Committee on Accident and Poison Prevention, issued a statement calling for a ban on the use of trampolines in schools because of the high incidence of quadriplegic injuries caused by the apparatus but has since modified the statement to allow some controlled use (American Academy of Pediatrics, 1981). However, the Academy states that trampolines should not be part of a physical education program or competitive sports and should *never* be used in home or recreational settings (Fig. 39-30). The Academy also opposes boxing in any sports program for *any* child or young adult (American Academy of Pediatrics, 1984) because of the potential for progressive brain injury. The "accumulated destructive effects of repeated blows even when consciousness and posture are not lost are well known and accepted" (Van Allen, 1983).

A variety of injuries can result when an external force is exerted with severe stress on tissue, muscle, and skeletal structures. The body structures attempt to accommodate the force, but when they are unable to do so, injuries occur. Two general types of injury are recognized. The first is ***acute overload,*** or ***macrotrauma,*** which is defined as a sudden, acute injury from a major force. The injuries incurred include fractures of long bones and the axial skelton; sprains of joint ligaments; strains of muscle tendon units; and contusions, including muscle tendon units and overlying soft tissue. The second is ***chronic overload (overuse syndrome),*** or ***microtrauma,*** which results from repetitive injury to tissue over a long period of time. Overuse injuries include stress fractures, bursitis, tendonitis, apophysitis of tendon insertions, and, at times, injuries of the joint surface (National Youth Sports Foundation, 1993). More than 95% of sports injuries involve the soft tissues, not the bony skeleton. About two thirds of these consist of strains and sprains, and most injuries involve the extremities.

Acute overload injuries are those that occur suddenly during an activity and produce immediate symptoms. They

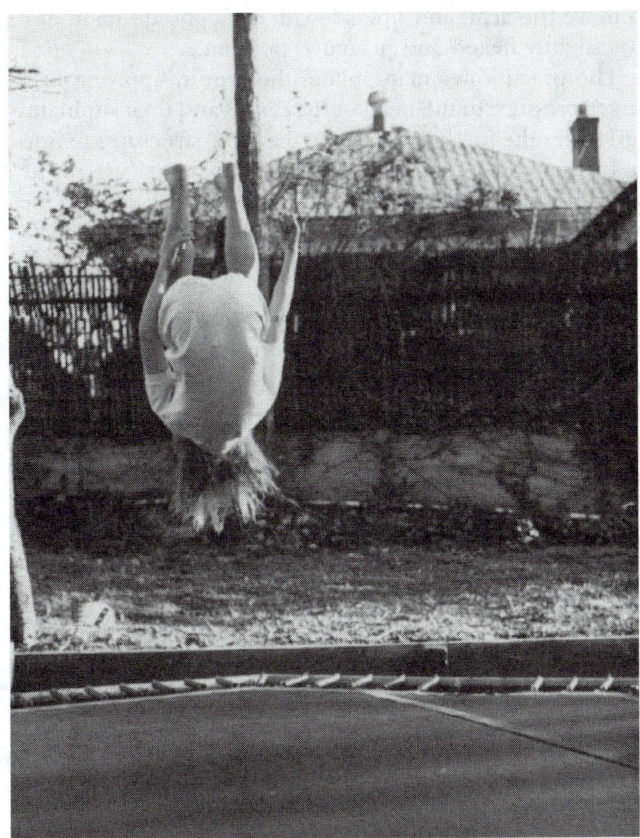

FIG. 39-30 Trampolines are not recommended for home or recreational use.

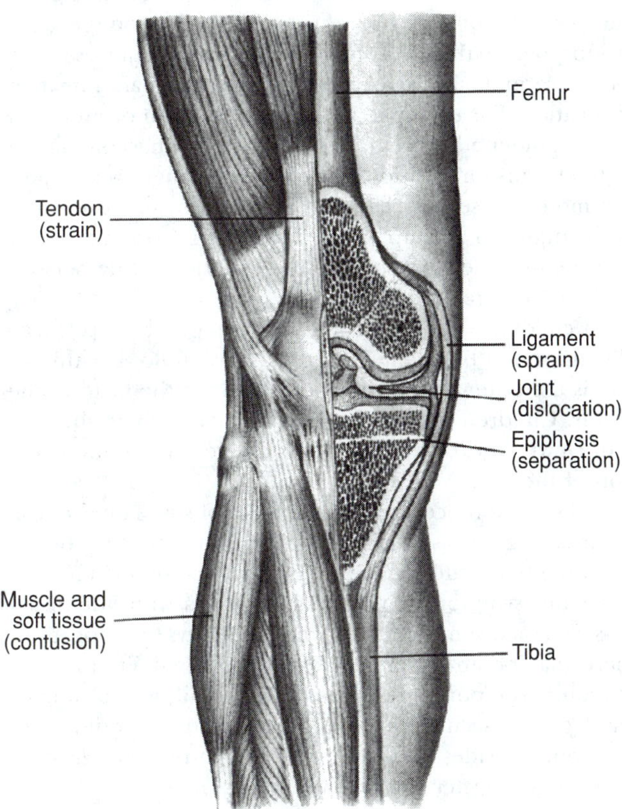

FIG. 39-31 Sites of injuries to bones, joints, and soft tissues.

can be caused by a blow or overstretching, twisting, or otherwise causing a sudden stress to tissues (Fig. 39-31).

CONTUSIONS

Contusions are probably the most common of sports injuries and are often considered to be "part of the game." A contusion is damage to the soft tissue, subcutaneous structures, and muscle. The tearing of these tissues and small blood vessels and the inflammatory response lead to hemorrhage, edema, and associated pain when the youngster attempts to move the injured part. The escape of blood into the tissues will be observed as ***ecchymosis,*** a black-and-blue discoloration.

The most serious contusions are those involving the quadriceps and are common in strenuous, collision-type sports, usually as a result of getting kicked or "kneed" in the thigh. Large contusions cause gross swelling, pain, and disability and usually receive immediate attention from health personnel. The less spectacular smaller injuries may go unnoticed, allowing continued participation. However, they can become disabling after rest because of pain and muscle spasm. The young athlete is frequently instructed to work it out or disregard the pain. Unfortunately, this can result in myositis ossificans, which requires a lengthy recovery.

Immediate treatment consists of cold application, as in the treatment of sprains described on p. 1837. Return to participation is allowed when the strength and range of motion of the affected extremity are equal to those of the opposite extremity.

Although not always directly related to sports, crush injuries occur in children when they slam their fingers (in doors, folding chairs, or equipment) or hit their fingers (as when hammering a nail). A severe crush injury involves the bone, with swelling and bleeding beneath the nail (subungual) and sometimes laceration of the pulp of the distal phalanx. The subungual hematoma can be released by drilling holes at the proximal end of the nail.

DISLOCATIONS

Long bones are held in approximation to one another at the joint by ligaments. Joints can be tight or loose, and loose joints are more likely to be dislocated. For certain sports the joints need to be limber (e.g., gymnastics and acrobatic dancing); a tight joint is needed for sports like football. One of the most vulnerable joints is the shoulder, which is structurally insecure, having only a rotator cuff to maintain the shoulder in place. The joint is shallow with relatively little muscle protection; therefore, the capsule becomes stretched and the joint dislocates easily. There is a high incidence of shoulder injuries in male gymnasts and an even greater incidence of shoulder injuries in players of contact sports, such as football and soccer.

Dislocations are less common in children than in older persons, but some types are peculiar to the younger age-groups. Before final closure of the epiphyses, injuries to the joints are more likely to cause epiphyseal separation than dislocation. For example, shoulder dislocation occurs most often in older adolescents, and dislocation unaccompanied by fracture is rare. Dislocation of the phalanges is the most common type seen in children, followed by elbow dislocations. Injury to the hip causes dislocation more frequently than femoral neck fracture (often experienced by persons in the older age-groups).

In children younger than 5 years of age, the hip is usually dislocated by a fall. The greatest risk following this injury is the potential loss of blood supply to the head of the femur. Children with naturally lax joints, such as children with Down syndrome, are more prone to recurrent dislocation of the hip.

A dislocation occurs when the force of stress on the ligament is so great as to displace the normal position of the opposing bone ends or the bone end to its socket. The predominant symptom is pain that increases with attempted passive or active movement of the extremity. In dislocations there may be an obvious deformity and inability to move the joint. Temporary restriction of the joint, with a sling or bandage that secures the arm to the chest in a shoulder dislocation, provides sufficient comfort and immobilization until the youngster can receive medical help.

The best chance for prevention of damage to the head of the femur is to relocate the hip within 60 minutes after the injury occurs. As the length of time between injury and hip relocation increases, the risk of irreparable damage increases. Simple dislocations should be reduced with the child under conscious sedation and often local anesthesia. Use of anesthetics, such as nitrous oxide, parenteral or oral ketamine, or intravenous propofol, can be used to produce partial or complete analgesia (Bostrom, McCormick, and Hooke, 1993; Tobias and others, 1992; Wattenmaker, Kasser, and McGravey, 1990) (see also Surgical Procedures, Chapter 27). An unreduced dislocation will be complicated by increased swelling, making reduction difficult and increasing the risk of neurovascular problems. Treatment depends on the severity of the injury.

Dislocation of the ***patella*** is a recurrent episode in some children; in others it is a result of injury. It is common among adolescent girls. The patella is always dislocated laterally. Most dislocations are reduced either spontaneously or by a companion before the child is seen by a physician. Therapy is immobilization for 3 to 4 weeks. Surgery may be needed for recurrent dislocations.

The most common dislocation injury is subluxation or partial dislocation of the ***radial head*** in the elbow, also called "pulled elbow" or "nursemaid's elbow." In about 90% of cases the injury occurs in a child between ages 1 and 5 years who receives a sudden longitudinal pull or traction at the wrist while the arm is fully extended and the forearm pronated (Nichols, 1988). It usually occurs when an adult who is holding the child by the hand or wrist gives a sudden jerk to prevent a fall. The child has an anxious expression, whines, complains of pain in the elbow and wrist, refuses to move the arm, and holds it with the opposite hand and in a slightly flexed and pronated position.

The practitioner manipulates the arm by applying firm finger pressure to the head of the radius and then supinates and flexes the forearm to return the bone structures to normal alignment. A click is heard, and functional use of the arm returns within 30 minutes. However, the longer the subluxation is present, the longer it takes for the child to recover mobility after treatment.

SPRAINS AND STRAINS

A ***sprain*** occurs when trauma to a joint is so severe that a ligament is partially or completely torn or stretched by the force created as a joint is twisted or wrenched, often accompanied by damage to associated blood vessels, muscles, tendons, and nerves. As a guideline for management and prognosis, sprains are classified according to the degree of injury (see box below). Because of all of the ligaments required to maintain knee stability, the knee is the most commonly injured joint relative to sport injuries. It is also the largest joint and, consequently, more prone to injury.

The presence of joint laxity is the most valid indicator of the severity of a sprain. In a severe injury the athlete complains of the joint "feeling loose" or as if "something is coming apart" and may describe hearing a "snap," "pop," or "tearing." Pain is seldom the principal subjective symptom. There is a rapid onset with swelling, often diffuse, accompanied by immediate disability and appreciable reluctance to use the injured joint.

A ***strain*** is a microscopic tear to the musculotendinous unit and has features in common with sprains. The area is painful to touch and swollen. The severity is evaluated in grades I, II, and III except that the degree of laxity does not apply. Even with severe grade III injuries, complaints of laxity are rare. Most strains are incurred over time rather than suddenly, and the rapidity of the appearance provides clues regarding severity. In general, the more rapidly the strain occurs, the more severe the injury. When the strain involves the muscular portion there is more bleeding, often palpable soon after injury and before edema obscures the hematoma.

CLASSIFICATION OF SPRAINS

Grade I: Mild injury; involves overstretching or microscopic tearing but without hemorrhage or increased instability of the involved joint. Swelling may develop later.

Grade II: Moderate injury; involves partial, overt tearing of the ligament with at least some ligamentous continuity remaining; usually immediate pain and swelling with decreased function.

Grade III: Severe injury; total loss of ligamentous continuity (i.e., disruption of one or more ligaments or the musculotendinous unit). Pain is immediate but subsides because none of the pain fibers is being stretched. Swelling may be minimal because hemorrhage extravasates outside of the area into soft tissues.

Therapeutic Management

The first 6 to 12 hours is the most critical period for virtually all soft tissue injuries. Basic principles of managing sprains and other soft tissue injuries are summarized in the acronyms RICE or ICES:

R—Rest	I—Ice
I—Ice	C—Compression
C—Compression	E—Elevation
E—Elevation	S—Support

Soft tissue injuries should be iced immediately. This is best accomplished with crushed ice wrapped in a towel or encased in a screw-top ice bag or plastic bag (e.g., a resealable storage bag). A wet elastic wrap is applied to provide compression and to keep the ice pack in place. A single layer of the wrap is placed over the injured area to protect the skin under the ice pack, and the remainder of the bandage secures the pack in place. The wet wrap transfers the cold better than a dry wrap. Some athletic trainers keep wet elastic wraps refrigerated for ready use.

➤ **NURSING TIP** A plastic bag of frozen vegetables, such as peas, serves as a convenient ice pack for soft tissue injuries. It is clean, watertight, and easily molded to the injured part.

There is still controversy regarding the use of heat or ice during the rehabilitative phase of management. Regardless of the method used, it is accompanied by appropriate exercise, depending on the severity of the injury, and carried out under the direction of a competent professional experienced in care of sports injuries.

Ice has a rapid cooling effect on tissues that reduces the pain threshold and the magnitude of the stretch reflex by decreasing muscle spindle response, afferent nerve discharge, and the afferent loop response (monosynaptic reflex). Secondary effects are achieved by vasoconstriction, slowing muscle nerve velocity, and increasing muscle viscosity. Also, the decreased temperature slows metabolism, thus reducing tissue oxygen requirements. Edema formation is reduced when fewer histamine-like substances are released. Nine to 15 minutes of ice exposure produces a deep-tissue vasodilation without increased metabolism. Ice therapy should never be applied for more than 30 minutes (Dyment, 1988). However, the effects last up to 7 hours.

Elevating the extremity uses gravity to facilitate venous return and reduce edema formation in the damaged area. The point of injury should be kept several inches above the level of the heart for therapy to be effective (Fig. 39-32). Several pillows can be used effectively for elevation. Allowing the extremity to be dependent causes excessive fluid accumulation in the area of injury, delaying healing and causing painful swelling.

Major sprains or tears to the ligamentous tissue rarely occur in growing children. Ligaments are stronger than bone, and the epiphysis and growth plate are the weakest areas of the bone; therefore the more usual sites of injury are at the growth plate (see Fractures, p. 1812). Torn ligaments, especially those in the knee, are usually treated by immobilization with a cast for 3 to 4 weeks or strapping of the joint with adhesive or Elastoplast bandage. Passive leg exercises, gradually increased to active ones, are begun as soon as sufficient healing has taken place. Parents and adolescents should be cautioned against using any form of liniment or other heat-producing preparation before examination. If the injury requires casting or splinting, the heat generated in the enclosed space can cause extreme discomfort and may even cause tissue damage.

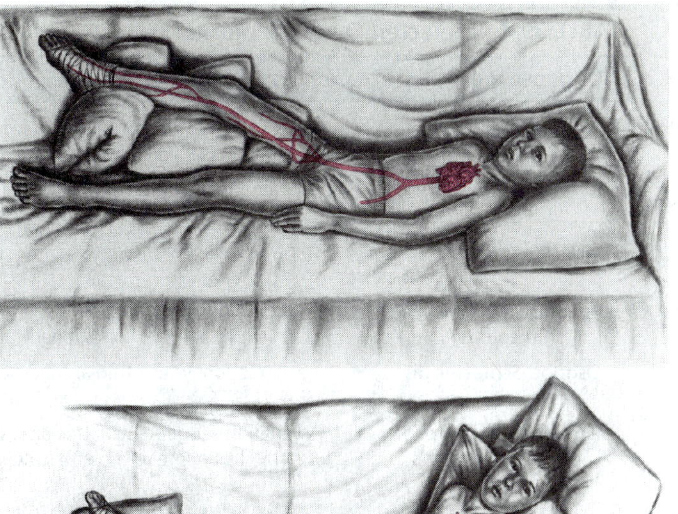

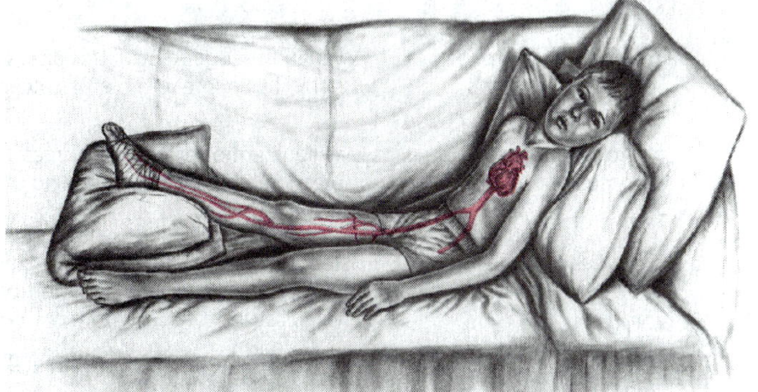

FIG. 39-32 Correct method for elevating a lower extremity. **A,** Lower leg elevated on pillows; ankle above heart level. **B,** Incorrect positioning; ankle below level of heart.

OVERUSE SYNDROME

To excel in sports, the young athlete is forced to train longer, harder, and earlier in life than previously. The rewards are increased level of fitness, better performances, faster times, and the satisfaction of attaining a personal goal. However, the risk of overuse injury is always present and can be related to several factors: training errors, muscle-tendon imbalance, anatomic malalignment (i.e., femoral anteversion, excessive lumbar lordosis, or tibial torsion), incorrect footwear or playing surface, an associated disease state, and growth (growth cartilage is less resistant to microtrauma). Athletes who run extensively frequently experience shin splints. The ligaments tear away from the shaft (tibial), and this creates the pain. Ice, rest, and nonsteroidal antiinflammatory drugs, such as ibuprofen or naprosyn, are the usual treatment. Shin splints are really serious.

TABLE 39-4 Selected Overuse Injuries

DISORDER	CAUSE	MANIFESTATIONS
Plantar fasciitis	Repetitive stretching of the plantar fascia (calcaneus to metatarsal heads)	Pain in arch or heel
Achilles tendinitis	Repeated forcible traction on short tendon	Pain on palpation; pain with plantar flexion against resistance
Severs disease	Epiphysitis of the calcaneus	Pain over insertion of Achilles tendon into tip of calcaneus
Anterior leg pain ("shin splints")	Irritation of posterior tibial muscle in unconditioned athlete or one not conditioned to a new sport	Pain in leg along anterior or medial edge of mid-shaft or distal third of tibia
Osgood-Schlatter disease	Traction apophysitis of tibial tubercle	Pain and tenderness; overprominence of involved tubercle
Sinding-Larsen syndrome ("jumper's knee")	A variant of Osgood-Schlatter disease; traction apophysitis on inferior pole of patella	Same as above; pain slightly lower than Osgood-Schlatter
Patellofemoral syndromes	Malalignment of extensors, increased patellar compression, and increased training intensity	Chronic knee pain, especially following forced leg extension from flexion or after running
"Tennis elbow"	Lateral epicondylitis from repetitive strain on elbow	Pain in elbow, aggravated by use
"Little League elbow"	Osteochondritis of the capitellum; tendinitis of flexor-origin medial epicondyle from repetitive valgus strain to elbow from throwing	Pain in elbow that increases with activity
"Little League shoulder"	Microfracture of proximal humeral growth plate from repetitive throwing	Pain and characteristic contracture; loss of internal rotation and increased external rotation
"Swimmer's shoulder"	Supraspinatus tendinitis from repetitive shoulder movement	Pain in shoulder that increases with activity

The common feature in overuse injuries is the repetitive microtrauma that occurs to a particular anatomic structure. Performing the same movements time and again sometimes causes several types of injury: (1) frictional—rubbing of one structure against another, (2) tractional—repeated pull on a ligament or tendon, or (3) cyclic loading of impact forces (stress fractures). The end result is inflammation of the involved structure with complaints of pain, tenderness, swelling, and disability.

Bursae, tendons, muscles, ligaments, joints, and bones are all subject to overuse. Some of the common overuse syndromes are briefly outlined in Table 39-4. Plantar fasciitis is very common in athletes, and Osgood-Schlatter disease is seen in children who do a lot of jumping. The overuse-type injuries, such as sore shoulders and strained elbows, may indicate that too much is being requested of the child in too short a period of time (Ostrum, 1993).

Stress Fractures

With intensity and duration of training, many young athletes suffer stress fractures, especially after a recent increase in training regimens. These fractions occur as a result of repeated muscle contraction and are seen most often in repetitive weight-bearing sports such as running, gymnastics, and basketball. They occur less often in swimmers (upper extremity). The sites in order of frequency are the tibia (50%), metatarsals (18%), fibula (12%), femur (6%), and other (less than 1%) (Orava, 1980).

The most common symptoms of stress fracture are a sharp, persistent, progressive pain or a deep, persistent dull ache located over the bone. Sometimes there is pain on impact (heel strike), but the most important clinical sign is pain over the involved bony surface. Diagnosis is established on the basis of clinical observation. Plain radiographs are rarely diagnostic of stress fractures, since they will only detect healing. Occasionally a bone scan may be needed, which will indicate a "hot spot."

Therapeutic Management

Development of inflammation is common to all overuse syndromes; therefore the management is directed toward rest or alteration of activities, physical therapies, and medication. Rest is the primary therapy, usually interpreted as reduced activity and use of alternative exercise—*not* bed rest or immobilization with casting. The primary purpose is to alleviate the repetitive stress that initiated the symptoms. It is important to keep the youngster mobile, and training can be continued. Alternative exercise is selected that maintains conditioning without aggravating the injury. For example, pool running (treading water in the deep end of a pool) can use the same movements as running but without the weight bearing; bicycling, swimming, and rowing are viable alternatives.

Other modalities include cryotherapy and cold whirlpools, and sometimes taping, bracing, splinting, and other orthoses are employed, very specific to the injury. Medications, such as nonsteroidal antiinflammatory drugs (see Table 26-3), are sometimes prescribed to reduce inflammation and pain. Topical medications are of questionable value.

HEAT INJURY

Infants, children, and adolescents are at high risk for heat-related illness. Several characteristics of infants and children render them more vulnerable to heat injury. The greater ratio of surface area to body mass in infants and young children leads to increased transfer of heat between the body and the environment. Children produce more metabolic heat for body mass during exercise and have a reduced capacity to convey heat from the body core to the skin. Also, children do not have the sweating capacity of adults and take longer to become acclimated to hot conditions (Rosenstein, 1989).

Heat cramps are caused by sodium depletion, which in turn potentiates the effects of calcium on skeletal muscle. It most often occurs as a result of strenuous exercise in a hot environment. Cramps most often involve the leg muscles. Vital signs are usually normal, but the core temperature may be elevated. The child sweats profusely, but mentation is normal. Treatment is rest and replacement of lost sodium.

Heat exhaustion, or heat collapse, is a common condition that usually occurs during vigorous exercise in a hot environment. It results from excessive loss of fluids, especially in poorly acclimated and dehydrated children. The onset may be gradual, with initial complaints that include thirst, headache, fatigue, dizziness, anxiety, or nausea and vomiting. The child usually has a clear sensorium but may be somewhat disoriented. The temperature can be normal or mildly elevated; sweating is profuse. Tachycardia, hypotension (usually postural), and syncope may be observed secondary to intravascular volume depletion. Treatment is to move the child to a cool environment, provide rest, and replace fluid volume. The child with a clear sensorium can be given cool water; otherwise water and salt are replaced intravenously. External cooling methods are not necessary.

Heatstroke represents a failure of normal thermoregulatory mechanisms. Heatstroke usually occurs during or immediately following physical activity, especially in the unacclimatized adolescent who is exercising vigorously. The onset is rapid with initial symptoms of headache, weakness, and disorientation. Central nervous system manifestations may be agitation, confusion, and lethargy; loss of consciousness may occur without warning and may be accompanied by nuchal rigidity, posturing, and convulsions. Sweating may not be present. The temperature is typically greater than 40° C (104° F), and there is severe volume depletion. Immediate care is relocation to a cool environment, removal of clothing, application of cool water (wet towels or immersion), and use of fans. The child is transported to the hospital for intensive care.

Hospital care includes rapid cooling, careful monitoring of temperature and other vital signs, supportive care (fluid and electrolyte replacement, supplemental oxygen), and treatment of any complications. Antipyretics are of no value. Prevention remains the best treatment for hyperthermia. If the temperature is elevated, time in the sun should be decreased. Activity should be stopped if the humidity is elevated as well. The athlete should drink plenty of fluids, preferably with low sugar content.

Nonexertional, or classic, heatstroke has a slow onset with insidious development of anorexia, nausea, vomiting, headache, development of mental manifestations, and loss of intravascular volume. Classic heatstroke occurs primarily in children with abnormal thermoregulation (e.g., children with cystic fibrosis) and infants subjected to prolonged neglect in a hot environment.

UNDERWATER SPORTS–RELATED INJURIES

Children who venture into water at least waist deep generally start to play underwater. It is not unusual for children to be able to swim underwater before they are able to swim on the surface. The injuries that are sustained from diving or swimming underwater are serious and deserve brief mention. Near-drowning is primarily a respiratory and neurologic problem and is discussed in Chapters 32 and 37; the major injury from diving or surfing is damage to the cervical spine (see Spinal Cord Injuries, Chapter 40).

Other underwater sports injuries include ear squeeze, which occurs when middle ear pressures are not equalized during diving; decompression sickness (the bends) and air emboli from too rapid decompression after deep dives; and nitrogen narcosis.

Sports and Accidental Drowning

Young people ages 15 to 24 years have the highest drowning rates. At highest risk are males between ages 15 and 19 years, with concurrent alcohol use present in 40% of drowning incidents. Alcohol not only impairs judgment but also increases the likelihood of water aspiration. Preventive measures to decrease the number of deaths have been unsuccessful. Suggested methods of intervention have been to (1) reduce the amount of alcohol consumed by adolescents, (2) increase the proportion of the population who are able to swim, and (3) encourage routine use of protective devices, such as life vests, when boating or fishing. Since most drownings are witnessed but resuscitation methods are not quickly or appropriately initiated, public education programs have been suggested as a potential remedy for this problem (American Academy of Pediatrics, 1993; Runyan and Gerken, 1989).

HEALTH CONCERNS ASSOCIATED WITH SPORTS

Nutrition

Most athletes are motivated to enhance their performance by any and all means available. They are eager to learn about nutrition, and many become subject to misconceptions, fads, and superstitions regarding certain foods. Physical performance is affected by energy and body composition. The young athlete must maintain a diet that provides sufficient nutrients and energy to meet metabolic needs for optimum functioning. Physical training increases the need for energy, as well as for more nutrients that convert food energy into chemical energy for physical performance.

There is no evidence to indicate that food supplements, extra vitamins, or high-protein diets are needed to meet the demands of heavy physical exercise or improve physical performance. However, young athletes need considerably more calories than the recommended daily allowance. When the basic requirements for growth and activity are met by a balanced diet of protein, grains and cereals, fruits and vegetables, and dairy products, the additional calories needed for the extra exertion can be selected as desired. These extra caloric needs can be supplied by eating additional helpings from any of the basic four food groups, but many of the additional calories are provided by complex carbohydrates found in such foods as vegetables, pastas, and bread. A summary of nutrition pointers for young athletes is presented in the box below.

Water and Electrolytes. Considerable water is lost from the body through perspiration, urination, and evaporation from the respiratory tract. Water losses, especially from the skin, increase with the duration and intensity of exercise and in higher environmental temperatures. Although the thirst mechanism is experienced early in dehydration, it is unreliable as an indicator of fluid deficit. Athletes participating in multiple daily exercise sessions in warm environments are at risk for dehydration and should receive all the water they desire.

Very little water is exchanged in the stomach and must reach the intestines for absorption. The best fluids for rapid gastric emptying are cold, of low osmolality, and have a large volume. Those containing simple sugars or glucose polymers with few or no electrolytes are better than plain water. Gatorade and other "sports" drinks contain excess carbohydrate and should be diluted with one or two parts of water to one part drink (Primos and Landry, 1989).

Small amounts of electrolytes are lost during exercise, especially sodium and chloride. Because sweat is quite dilute relative to plasma concentrations, excessive perspiration can result in excessive loss of water and an increase in plasma concentrations of sodium chloride. Therefore it is more important to replace water than sodium and chloride. Salt tablets are unnecessary and may actually be harmful. Athletes derive sufficient salt replacement from their diet.

Minerals. The basic diet will not satisfy the iron requirement of 10% to 15% of female athletes. The largest group are those teenage girls who may become iron depleted after menarche. Young boys who are experiencing rapid adolescent growth and who have irregular and inadequate diets also are at risk of iron depletion. These youngsters will need iron supplements.

Adequate calcium intake during puberty is essential to promote mineralization of the growing skeleton. In addition, calcium plays a vital role in nerve transmission, muscle contraction, and blood coagulation. Female athletes who engage in intensive training and subsequently develop amenorrhea may require additional calcium intake to prevent osteoporosis (Squire, 1987). The best sources of calcium for athletes are nonfat dairy products (Loosli, 1990).

Glycogen. Energy is derived primarily from glycogen previously stored in muscles and the liver. Energy for prolonged exercise is derived from high-carbohydrate food (e.g., bread, cereals, pancakes, potatoes, rice, spaghetti) consumed 24 to 48 hours before the activity, not from a meal eaten just before the activity. The meal before a physical contest should be eaten at least 2½ hours before the exertion and consist mainly of carbohydrates. Carbohydrate

FIFTEEN STEPS TO GOOD SPORTS NUTRITION

1. A well-balanced diet consists of elements from the Food Guide Pyramid. The recommended percentages of major nutrients are 55% to 75% carbohydrates, 25% to 30% fat, and 15% to 20% protein.
2. Athletes should take water at regular intervals during exercise.
3. For each pound of fluid lost through exercise, the athlete should consume 16 ounces of water.
4. Any athlete who loses more than 3% of body weight in an exercise session should not return to activity until the fluid is restored. Monitoring body weight can prevent chronic dehydration.
5. Beverages with small amounts of simple sugars or glucose polymers with little or no electrolytes may be better sources of hydration than plain water.
6. Salt tablets are rarely needed and may actually do harm by increasing dehydration.
7. Glycogen loading is of value only for endurance exercises that take more than 1 hour, such as marathons and cross-country ski races. It is not recommended for children.
8. Protein and amino acid supplementation are potentially harmful and should be discouraged.
9. Vitamin supplements are usually unnecessary and a waste of money; excessive doses may be harmful. One daily multivitamin is not harmful for youngsters who do not consume well-balanced meals.
10. Mineral supplements are usually not needed, except for young athletes who develop a specific deficiency such as iron.
11. Any weight loss program should be designed to lose body fat primarily and not lean body tissue or water. The goal should be to achieve a certain percentage of body weight as fat.
12. Athletes should not lose more than 1 to 2 pounds per week. They should not reduce daily caloric intake to less than 1200 calories for girls and 1500 calories for boys.
13. Athletes who wish to gain weight can do so by combining increased caloric intake with muscle work (i.e., weight training). Nutritional supplements are not usually needed.
14. Athletes should gain weight no more rapidly than 1 to 2 pounds per week. They should be monitored for percentage of body fat.
15. The pregame meal should be eaten at least 2½ hours before competition. It should consist primarily of carbohydrates and not foods that are slowly digested (fats, desserts) or have excessive concentrated sugars.

From Primos WA, Landry GL: Fighting the fads in sports nutrition, *Contemp Pediatr* 6(9):14-50, 1989.

(glycogen) loading is a technique reserved for competition in prolonged aerobic endurance events and requires dietary changes a week before the competitive event. For more information regarding carbohydrate loading and other techniques for improving athletic performance, the reader is directed to excellent texts on sports medicine and sports training.

Weight. Control of body weight by restriction of water intake, food restriction, or encouragement of sweat loss is dangerous; these are highly undesirable means for meeting a minimum weight classification. Young athletes need to learn something about nutrition to dispel the allure of prevalent fads and fallacies about diet and performance. The optimum diet for an athlete is one that contains the essential food groups and that is adjusted to the energy requirements of the sport in which the youngster is engaged. Such a diet plan should provide adequate nutrition for top physical efficiency and performance, maintenance of physical fitness and desirable body weight, and optimum function of all organ systems.

Exercise-Related Menstrual Dysfunction

Considerable interest has been generated regarding delayed or secondary amenorrhea associated with the physical stress of ballet dancing and some types of athletics (e.g., running and gymnastics). The phenomenon has been attributed to a complex interplay of physical, genetic, hormonal, nutritional, psychologic, and environmental factors that include the stress of competition, decreased protein consumption, and altered lean-to-fat ratio.

Delayed menarche has been reported for girls who engage in strenuous exercise. Except for swimmers, menarche is attained later in athletes than in nonathletes. Gymnasts, figure skaters, and ballet dancers have the latest mean ages of menarche; track athletes have less of a delayed maturity than gymnasts and ballet dancers, who also tend to be smaller, lighter, and leaner than other female athletes. Swimmers, who tend to be larger, have a mean age of menarche that approximates that for nonathletes. Also, there appears to be an association between delayed menarche and more advanced competitive levels; that is, athletes at the more advanced levels have a greater delay than those at lower competitive levels.

One study found that intensive training (18 hours/week) in gymnastics, shortly before and continuing throughout puberty, resulted in delayed growth. A marked stunting of leg-length growth occurred such that full adult height would not be reached. Although the mechanisms responsible for this effect are not known, the authors suggest that prolonged inhibition of the hypothalamic-pituitary-gonadal axis by exercise and dieting may be responsible (Theintz and others, 1993).

It has also been found that women competing in ballet dancing and gymnastics are subject to decreased bone density, stress fractures, and symptoms of anorexia nervosa (Braisted and others, 1985; Warren and others, 1986). The peak of bone density is reached in late adolescence and is related to circulating estrogen levels. Girls with diminished estrogen secretion in delayed menarche will reach late adolescence with low bone density and will be subject to osteoporosis. Hypoestrogenic bone loss greatly increases the risk of injury. Teenage girls need to be counseled to increase calcium intake to four to six servings per day, which should be supplied by low-fat dairy products. Trainers and coaches also need to be aware of the potentially long-term results of intensive, prolonged exercise in pubertal girls.

An additional area for counseling the female athlete with delayed menarche regards pregnancy. Sexually active teenagers, regardless of menstruation, need to be reminded to take precautions. Most teenage girls erroneously believe that because they do not menstruate, they cannot become pregnant.

Drug Misuse by Athletes

Young athletes have used various substances in an attempt to augment their athletic performance. These substances, known as ***ergogenic aids,*** are believed by athletes to increase strength and endurance, delay the onset of fatigue, increase the ability to concentrate, and decrease sensitivity to pain. Although use of these substances is prohibited in international Olympic competition, there are no means at present to enforce a prohibition on their use in other sports participation.

The principal drugs misused by athletes are the psychomotor stimulants (e.g., amphetamines) and the anabolic steroids. Amphetamines and related drugs, such as methylphenidate (Ritalin) and phenmetrazine (Preludin), are taken to provide a sense of increased alertness and relief of fatigue; however, obscuring fatigue may permit participants to exceed their limits and precipitate a sudden collapse. These drugs can also make the users more aggressive, which can contribute to injuries to themselves and others. Although use of amphetamines is declining, ingestion of caffeine and caffeine-related substances, readily available as cola drinks, tea, and coffee, has increased (American Academy of Pediatrics, Committee on Sports Medicine, 1983).

Anabolic steroids, such as nandrolone phenpropionate (Durabolin) and methandrostenolone (Dianabol), are a source of concern to health professionals. The majority of these drugs are no longer manufactured in the United States by legitimate companies. Black market supplies of anabolic steroids are of poor quality and potency. In the attempt to enhance muscle strength, these drugs are administered to athletes by coaches, managers, athletic trainers, and even physicians. The user develops larger-appearing muscles and increased body weight and body water, but reports on the effectiveness in improving performance have been conflicting. Although the psychologic effect may be beneficial, many valid studies have failed to demonstrate any improvement in performance.

The precise incidence of use by adolescent athletes remains debatable. Self-report surveys have documented use patterns ranging from 5% to 11% of high-school athletes (Johnson and others, 1989). Coaches and health professionals who work with youth report a trend toward increased use of these agents. Teenagers rely on poor sources of information about the potential hazards of steroids (friends, television, muscle magazines) and are generally poorly informed of their potential negative side effects (Johnson and others, 1989; Nelson, 1989). Health professionals need to be aware of the clinical manifestations of steroid use. Clinical signs such as severe acne, a sudden increase in strength and muscle, a sudden decrease in body fat, a male pattern of baldness, and water retention are common. In females, a male pattern of hair growth and a deepening voice are significant observations.

The dangers of continued use are well known and include hypertension; virilization in females; oligospermia, testicular atrophy, infertility, and gynecomastia in males; and premature closure of the epiphyses, acne, increased blood cholesterol, and hepatocellular carcinoma in both sexes. Mood changes have been observed, including aggressiveness, changes in libido, and mood swings. Health hazards outweigh any potential gain that might be induced, and the American Academy of Pediatrics (1989) and the American College of Sports Medicine (1988) both condemn the use of anabolic steroids.

Other drugs that are often misused include nutritional aids, local anesthetic agents, beta blockers (to reduce circulating catecholamines and thus reduce anxiety related to somatic-type stress), and antiinflammatory drugs, such as dimethylsulfoxide (DSMO) (which is not approved for use and is available only as a veterinary or an industrial preparation) and corticosteroids. The possibility of their use by the adolescent athlete should be considered when performing a health assessment.

Sudden Death

A death associated with sports produces renewed anxiety in both parents and health professionals. The term ***sudden,*** or ***instantaneous, death*** is applied to death that occurs within minutes of the onset of the cause of death, within an hour or within 24 hours of the episode. Sudden death occurs in three areas: (1) in those sports with a high inherent risk for sport-related sudden death; (2) in children with recognized or unknown underlying medical problems; and (3) in the sport environment (i.e., the rules, equipment, practice fields or areas of sports participation, and the ambient temperature of the geographic area), which may be a contributing or causal factor.

Sports. Sports that create the greatest risk are those involving collision and frequent body contact. Examples of collision sports include football, ice hockey, rugby, and boxing. There is a high potential for serious injury or fatality in sports such as mountain or rock climbing and hang gliding. Sports that involve high-velocity objects, such as baseball and ice hockey, may cause death as a result of serious head or chest injuries. Riding vehicles such as mopeds, jeeps, minibikes, and motorcycles can be considered as sports.

Medical Conditions. The most frequent medical causes of sudden death during sports activity are cardiac abnormalities, especially idiopathic hypertrophic subaortic stenosis (hypertrophic cardiomyopathy). Manifestations suggestive of hypertrophic cardiomyopathy include a typical triad of severe chest pain with dizziness, prominent pulses, and a murmur at the left lower sternal border. A history of sudden death of a relative, or relatives, in the second and third decade often offers a clue to recognition.

Well-trained athletes often display evidence of hypertrophic cardiomyopathy, the so-called athlete's heart, but the condition is not pathologic. Congenital heart problems are infrequent causes of sudden death in sports involving children and adolescents. Children with systemic hypertension, some types of cardiac arrhythmias, and some forms of heart block will require restrictions in the type and amount of exercise they can tolerate safely.

Environmental Causes. Environmental factors that are potential causes of death include playing conditions, clothing, equipment, rules used by officials governing a sport, and outdoor temperature. Heat stroke and hypothermia are probably the most serious uncontrollable environmental causes of death in athletes.

NURSE'S ROLE IN CHILDREN'S SPORTS

Nurses may become involved in sports activities in the areas of preparation and evaluation for activities, prevention of injury, treatment of injuries, and rehabilitation after injury. Selecting an appropriate sport for both recreation and competition is a joint effort of youngster, parents, and health professionals. Children are introduced to sports as part of family activities, neighborhood games, and school physical education programs, and both parents and children are influenced by media exposure to a variety of sports. Children are highly influenced by the popularity and exposure afforded athletics in the school setting, especially in high school.

The best approach to counseling children and parents regarding sports participation is to encourage activities that are most likely to provide pleasure and physical benefits throughout childhood and into adulthood. Exposure to a variety of sports activities is probably better for young children than limiting them to only one sport. Parents should be cautioned against overprogramming children in order that the children have ample time for other activities and associations.

Nurses are sometimes members of a sports medicine team, although the training and rehabilitation are usually managed by certified sports trainers and other specialists in sports medicine. Nurses should be able to provide emergency treatment for any type of injury and know when to refer the injured child for evaluation and care. Sports injuries can occur in free play as well as in organized athletic programs, and a school nurse is often the first person who attends an injured child.

When children sustain athletic injuries, nurses are often responsible for instructing the children and their parents regarding care. Instructions, such as regarding a schedule for appointments, application of ice, and any restrictions in activity, should be made clear and preferably be accompanied by written directions. The importance of taking medications as prescribed is emphasized, since they may be needed for an extended period of time and compliance may be difficult. For children continuing with activities, drug administration an hour before practice or competition is advantageous.

Prevention of sports injuries is probably the most important aspect of any athletic program. The children should be suited to the activity, the environment and equipment should be made safe for physical activity, and the children should be adequately prepared for the sports, especially those requiring strenuous and/or continuous physical exertion. Nurses collaborate with coaches and athletic trainers to ensure that safety measures are carried out. Stretching exercises, warming up and cooling down activities, and an appropriate training program are only some of the requisites for safe participation. Protective measures, such as pads, taping, wrapping, or other devices, are employed for areas at risk (Fig. 39-33). Nurses are also on the alert for environmental safety risks.

Participation of youth in sports programs has grown significantly in the past several decades. This trend toward greater participation by both genders has been encouraged because of its demonstrated effect on reducing obesity and lowering blood pressure, and its beneficial impact on lowering cholesterol and lipid levels.

Nurses can provide education to coaching staff, parents, and players on the detrimental effects of steroid use on athletes. Teenagers who participate in sports programs need to know that the use of steroids constitutes cheating and can result in dismissal from play. In addition to education about the potential side effects, nurses should be alert to physical signs and counsel those youths appropriately.

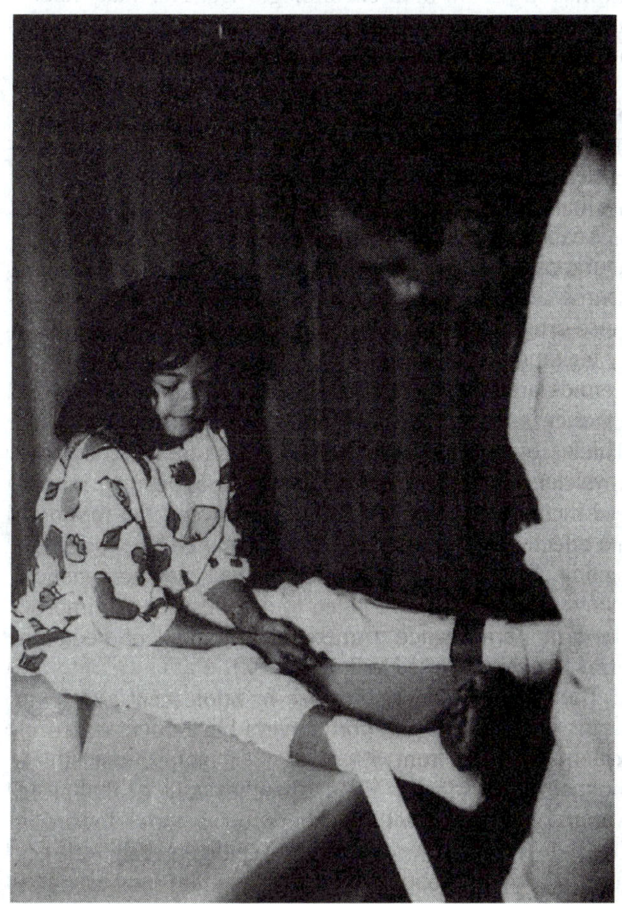

FIG. 39-33 Competent care is essential to prevention of sports injury.

For some athletes, their whole life revolves around sports participation. When a serious injury occurs, the athlete's self-esteem and self-image may suffer a devastating blow. Nursing assessment may reveal an athlete who appears to have difficulty dealing with the events and actually rejects any positive reinforcement. The nurse may help in establishing a support system. The athlete may need to learn new coping skills and explore other avenues to foster feelings of increased self-worth and accomplishment (Butler, Salmond, and Pellino, 1994).

Parental Pressure

There is a lot of peer and parental pressure to participate in sports, and the stress on the adolescent to perform in competitive situations is poorly understood. There is much fear of failure related to the pressure to be like friends or parents. When children need medical attention because of repeated injuries, disinterest should be suspected and investigated. It is best to obtain separate histories from the youth and the parents in an attempt to illuminate possible psychologic complications as a cause of injury (Pillemer and Micheli, 1988). Alternative sports or other means for gaining self-esteem and regard from parents and peers can be explored and encouraged for children not interested in or suited for athletic competition.

Attrition and exercise aversion are sometimes the aftermath of declining interest in sports after participation during the school years and adolescence. Motivation can be altered or permanently destroyed by failure to appreciate youngsters' needs related to sports activities. Ridicule or derogation during acquisition of motor skills can shatter a youngster's self-esteem, producing anxiety and self-doubt that may result in a lifelong aversion to sports. Every child should have the opportunity to develop a strong sense of personal worth through the process of motor learning and acquisition of skills. They need positive encouragement. *All* participants should have the opportunity to participate and be rewarded for their contribution, no matter how small; all participants should be rewarded for what they do right.

Both coaches and parents are guilty of exploiting youngsters for their own purposes. Although the positive aspects are important and inherent in sports activities, nurses should be alert to some parental behaviors and motivations that interfere with a youngster's enjoyment of the activities. However, many parents are notoriously resistant to the idea of altering their behavior.

First, there are parents who are unwilling to allow the activity to remain child-oriented and who often place unrealistic demands on the child. Both the youngster's physical and emotional age must be considered. Second, there are parents who are unable to maintain the appropriate emotional distance from the activity and make the youngster's involvement in sports an extension of their own ego. These youngsters may recognize that they are being exploited and exhibit extreme forms of rebellion. Third, parents' manipulative behaviors can have a profound negative effect on their youngsters. Guilt-producing verbal manipulation (e.g., pointing out what they and others have sacrificed for the child) is a powerful weapon that creates a form of emotional bondage. Fourth, there are parents who lose sight of the meaning of the sport because they become entrapped in dreams and fantasies that their youngsters' athletic ability can become a passport to status and economic freedom.

The pressures that some parents impose on their children negate most of the psychologic values of sports, such as fun, emotional release, and learning to relate effectively with peers. Winning becomes more important than playing. Overemphasis on sports has the potential for interfering with the emotional and social growth of a child, especially when ego integration is tied to recognition and reward through such a narrow range of personal characteristics. Ego vulnerability is great in youngsters whose identity, self-esteem, and feelings of self-worth depend entirely on the psychologic and social rewards of athletic achievement.

MUSCULOSKELETAL DYSFUNCTION

TORTICOLLIS

Torticollis (wry neck) is a congenital or acquired condition of limited neck motion in which the neck is flexed and turned to the affected side as a result of shortening of the sternocleidomastoid muscle. In early infancy a firm, nontender mass may be felt in the midportion of the muscle. The mass regresses and is replaced by fibrous tissue. If the condition remains untreated, there is permanent limitation of neck movement and the head and face become asymmetric, probably as a result of impaired blood supply to the depressed side of the head.

Treatment consists of gentle stretching exercises. The face is turned toward the affected muscle while the head is tilted in the opposite direction with the neck extended. The position is held for a count of 5 and repeated 10 times, twice daily (Watts, 1987). The exercises are best performed by two persons—one to control the torso and one to manipulate the head. If stretching exercises are unsuccessful, surgical release of the sternocleidomastoid muscle may be needed.

Nursing Considerations

Nurses are alert to the possibility of torticollis in infants with limited head movement. After diagnosis it is frequently a nursing responsibility to teach and supervise the family in performing the exercises. The exercise requires very explicit instructions to the family, and compliance is mandatory. The nurse also suggests that the child be placed in the crib or playpen in a way that encourages turning the head away from the deformity in order to observe activities and interesting items. Feeding and play with the child can be used to encourage turning the head in the direction desired for correction.

STAGES OF LEGG-CALVÉ-PERTHES DISEASE

Stage I: Aseptic necrosis or infarction of the femoral capital epiphysis with degenerative changes producing flattening of the upper surface of the femoral head—the ***avascular stage.***

Stage II: Capital bone absorption and revascularization with fragmentation (vascular resorption of the epiphysis) that gives a mottled appearance on radiographs—the ***fragmentation,*** or ***revascularization, stage.***

Stage III: New bone formation, which is represented on radiographs as calcification and ossification or increased density in the areas of radiolucency; this filling-in process appears to take place from the periphery of the head centrally—the ***reparative stage.***

Stage IV: Gradual reformation of the head of the femur without radiolucency and, it is hoped, to a spherical form—the ***regenerative stage.***

LEGG-CALVÉ-PERTHES DISEASE

Legg-Calvé-Perthes disease, sometimes called ***coxa plana*** or ***osteochondritis deformans juvenilis,*** is a self-limited disorder in which there is aseptic necrosis of the femoral head. The disease affects children ages 3 to 12 years, but most cases occur in boys between 4 and 8 years of age as an isolated event. In approximately 10% to 15% of cases the involvement is bilateral; most of the affected children have a skeletal age significantly below their chronologic age. The male/female ratio is 4:1 or 5:1; white children are affected 10 times more frequently than black children.

Pathophysiology

The cause of the disease is unknown, but there is a disturbance of circulation to the femoral capital epiphysis that produces an ischemic aseptic necrosis of the femoral head. During middle childhood circulation to the femoral epiphysis is more tenuous than at other ages, being supplied almost entirely by lateral retinacular vessels. These can become obstructed by trauma, inflammation, coagulation defects, and a variety of other causes (Staheli, 1986). This circulatory impairment appears to extend to the epiphysis and acetabulum as well. The pathologic events seem to take place in four stages (see box at left). The entire process may encompass as little as 18 months or continue for several years. The reformed femoral head may be severely altered or appear entirely normal.

Clinical Manifestations

The onset is insidious, and the history may reveal only intermittent appearance of a limp on the affected side or a symptom complex including hip soreness, ache, or stiffness that can be constant or intermittent. The pain may be experienced in the hip, along the entire thigh, or in the vicinity of the knee joint. The pain and limp are usually most evident on arising and at the end of a long day of activities. The pain is usually accompanied by joint dysfunction and limited range of motion. There may be a vague history of trauma. The diagnosis is established by radiographic examination.

Therapeutic Management

Since deformity occurs early in the disease process, the aim of treatment is to keep the head of the femur contained in the acetabulum, which serves as a mold to preserve the spherical shape of the head and to maintain a full range of motion. However, there is no agreement regarding the best treatment in terms of conservative versus surgical approaches (Poussa and others, 1993). Activity causes microfractures of the soft, ischemic epiphysis, which tend to induce synovitis, stiffness, and adductor contracture (Staheli, 1986). The initial therapy is rest, and non–weight bearing, which helps reduce inflammation and restore motion. Later active motion is encouraged. In some cases traction is applied to stretch tight adductor muscles.

Containment can be accomplished by non-weight-bearing devices, such as an abduction brace, leg casts, or a leather harness sling, that prevent weight bearing on the affected limb; by various weight-bearing appliances such as abduction-ambulation braces or casts after a period of bed rest and traction; and by surgical reconstruction and containment procedures. Conservative therapy must be continued for 2 to 4 years, although braces constructed from lightweight materials allow the child to maintain a nearly normal activity level. Surgical correction, although subject to additional risks (e.g., from anesthesia, infection, blood transfusion), returns the child to normal activities in 3 to 4 months.

The disease is self-limited, but the ultimate outcome of therapy depends on early and efficient treatment and the age of onset of the disorder. Younger children, whose epiphyses are more cartilaginous, have the best prognosis for complete recovery. The later the diagnosis is made, the more femoral damage has occurred before treatment is implemented. In most cases, with good patient compliance, the prognosis is excellent.

Nursing Considerations

Nurses are often the first health professionals to identify affected children and to refer them for medical evaluation. They are also persons on whom the child and family can rely to help them understand and adjust to the therapeutic measures. Since most care of these children is conducted on an outpatient basis, the major emphasis of nursing care is teaching the family the care and management of the corrective appliance selected for therapy. The family needs to learn the purpose, function, application, and care of the corrective device and the importance of compliance in order to achieve the desired outcome.

One of the most difficult aspects associated with the disorder is coping with normally active children who feel well but must remain relatively inactive. It is important to emphasize that children continue to attend school and engage in former activities that can be adapted to the therapeutic appliance. School adaptation may need to be arranged with school personnel.

Suitable activities must be devised to meet the needs of the child in the process of developing a sense of initiative or industry. Activities that meet the creative urges are well received. This is also an opportune time to encourage the child to begin a hobby such as collections, model building, or crafts.

SLIPPED FEMORAL CAPITAL EPIPHYSIS

Slipped femoral capital epiphysis, or ***coxa vara,*** refers to the spontaneous displacement of the proximal femoral epiphysis in a posterior and inferior direction. It develops most frequently shortly before or during accelerated growth and the onset of puberty (children between the ages of 10 and 16 years—median age, 13 for boys, 11 for girls) and is most frequently observed in obese children. Bilateral involvement has been reported variously as 16% to 40%.

Pathophysiology

The cause of coxa vara is unknown, but it occurs most often in "overlarge" youngsters or very tall, thin, rapidly growing children. There has been some evidence to implicate hormonal factors; for example, resistance of the growth plate to shear stress is decreased by growth hormone and increased by sex hormone, suggesting that the disorder may be related to excess growth hormone in the tall child and decreased sex hormone in the obese child. It has also been associated with endocrine abnormalities, such as hypothyroidism, renal osteodystrophy, and growth hormone therapy.

The pathologic processes as seen in radiographs involve first a rarefaction of bone on the lower femoral side of the epiphysis with widening of the growth plate. After trauma or slight injury the femoral portion of the epiphysis slides upward but remains attached by the thick, continuous periosteum. As slipping increases, the epiphyseal displacement becomes posterior and inferior. The slipping produces deformity of the femoral head and stretches the blood vessels to the epiphysis.

Clinical Manifestations

The following different varieties of clinical behavior have been observed: (1) an episode of trauma in which the epiphysis is acutely displaced in a previously functional joint; (2) gradual displacement without definite injury with progressively increased hip disability; (3) intermittent bouts of displacement alternating with periods of well-being with gradual appearance of symptoms associated with ambulation (e.g., external rotation); and (4) a combined gradual and traumatic displacement, in which there is gradual slippage with further displacement caused by injury.

Slipped femoral epiphysis is suspected when an adolescent or preadolescent youngster, especially one who is obese or tall and lanky, begins to limp and complains of pain in the hip continuously or intermittently. The pain is frequently referred to the groin, anteromedial aspect of the thigh, or knee. Physical examination reveals early restriction of internal rotation on adduction and external rotation deformity with loss of abduction and internal rotation as the severity increases. The diagnosis is confirmed by radiographic examination.

Therapeutic Management

The treatment varies with the degree of displacement but involves surgical stabilization and correction of the deformity. In mild cases simple pin fixation is sufficient. More extensive displacement requires skeletal traction followed by pin fixation or osteotomy. The prognosis depends on the degree of deformity and the occurrence of complications, such as avascular necrosis and cartilaginous necrosis. As in other disorders, early diagnosis and implementation of therapy increase the likelihood of a satisfactory cure.

Nursing Considerations

Nursing care is the same as that for a child in a cast or a child in traction, discussed earlier in this chapter.

KYPHOSIS AND LORDOSIS

The spine, consisting of numerous segments, can acquire deformation curves of three types: kyphosis, lordosis, and scoliosis (Fig. 39-34).

Kyphosis is an abnormally increased convex angulation in the curvature of the thoracic spine (Fig. 39-34, *B*). It can occur secondary to disease processes such as tuberculosis, chronic arthritis, osteodystrophy, or compression fractures of the thoracic spine. The most common form of kyphosis is "postural." Children, especially during the time when skeletal growth outpaces growth of muscle, are prone to exaggeration of a tendency toward kyphosis. This is particularly common in self-conscious adolescent girls who assume a round-shouldered slouching posture in an attempt to hide their developing breasts and increasing height. ***Scheuermann kyphosis*** is defined as a thoracic curve of greater than 45 degrees with wedging of more than 5 degrees of at least three adjacent vertebral bodies and vertebral irregularity.

Postural kyphosis is almost always accompanied by a compensatory postural lordosis, an abnormally exaggerated concave lumbar curvature. Treatment consists of postural exercises to strengthen shoulder and abdominal muscles and bracing for more marked deformity. Unfortunately, treatment is difficult because of the nature of the adolescent personality. The best approach is to emphasize the cosmetic value of corrective therapy and to place the responsibility on the adolescent for carrying out an exercise program at home with regular visits to and assessments by a therapist.

Most adolescents respond well to selected sports as a supplement to regular exercise, such as weight lifting (preferably performed from a prone or supine position on a bench), track sports, and dancing classes (ballet or modern). Swimming is excellent and has the added advantages of exercising all muscles, eliminating gravity, and teaching breath control. Treatment with a Milwaukee brace may be indicated until skeletal maturity and surgical fusion may be considered for severe, painful, or progressive kyphotic curves.

Lordosis is an accentuation of the lumbar curvature be-

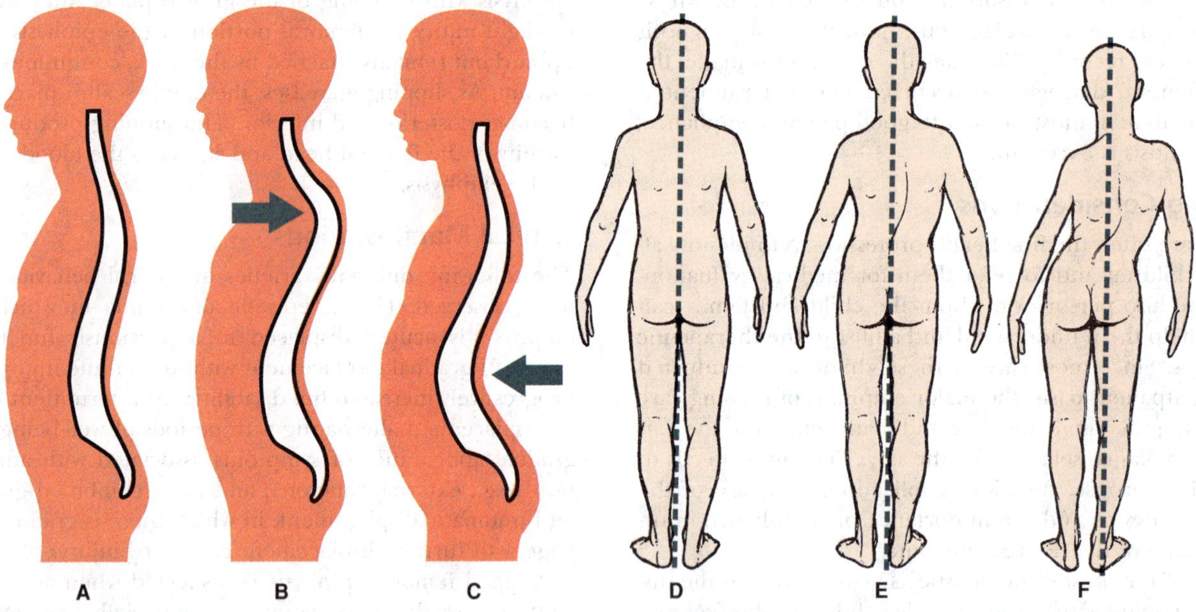

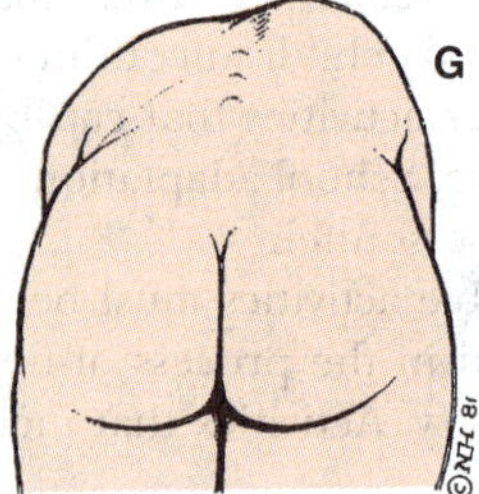

FIG. 39-34 Defects of spinal column. **A,** Normal spine. **B,** Kyphosis. **C,** Lordosis. **D,** Normal spine in balance. **E,** Mild scoliosis in balance. **F,** Severe scoliosis not in balance. **G,** Rib hump and flank asymmetry seen in flexion caused by rotary component. (Redrawn from Hilt NE, Schmitt EW: *Pediatric orthopedic nursing,* St Louis, 1975, Mosby.)

yond physiologic limits (Fig. 39-34, *C*). It may be a secondary complication of a disease process, the result of trauma, or idiopathic. Lordosis is a normal observation in toddlers and, in older children, is often seen in association with flexion contractures of the hip, obesity, congenital dislocated hip, and slipped femoral capital epiphysis. During the pubertal growth spurt lordosis of varying degrees is observed in teenagers, especially girls. In obese children the weight of the abdominal fat alters the center of gravity, causing a compensatory lordosis. Unlike kyphosis, severe lordosis is usually accompanied by pain.

Treatment involves management of the predisposing cause when possible, such as weight loss and correction of deformities. Postural exercises and/or support garments are helpful in relieving symptoms in some cases; however, these do not usually effect a permanent cure.

Spondylolisthesis is the forward slipping of one vertebral body on another, usually L5 and S1. It can have multiple causes, including congenital deficiency or fracture of part of the vertebra. This condition may be asymptomatic, or it may cause low back pain or neurologic compromise. Spondylolisthesis can usually be treated nonsurgically, although spinal fusion may be indicated in severe, progressive slips.

SCOLIOSIS

Scoliosis is a complex spinal deformity in three planes, usually involving lateral curvature, spinal rotation causing rib asymmetry, and thoracic hypokyphosis. It is the most common spinal deformity. It can be congenital, or it can develop during infancy or childhood, but it is most common during the growth spurt of early adolescence. Scoliosis can be caused by a number of conditions and may occur alone or in association with other diseases, particularly neuromuscular conditions. In most cases, however, there is no apparent cause, and it is called ***idiopathic scoliosis.*** There is evidence that it may be genetic and transmitted as an autosomal-dominant trait with incomplete penetrance, or it may be multifactorial. The various causes of scoliosis are outlined in the box below.

Clinical Manifestations

Idiopathic scoliosis is seldom apparent before 10 years of age and is most noticeable at the beginning of the preadolescent growth spurt. Parents will often bring a child for evaluation because of "ill-fitting" clothes, such as uneven pant lengths or uneven skirt hems. Until the deformity is well established, there is rarely discomfort and there are few outward signs. Early detection and treatment are essential to successful management (see also Back and Extremities, Chapter 7).

Diagnostic Evaluation

A standing child, wearing only underpants and viewed from behind, may exhibit asymmetry of shoulder height, scapular or flank shape, or hip height, or may demonstrate pel-

CAUSES OF SCOLIOSIS

IDIOPATHIC SCOLIOSIS

Infantile
- Age of onset—birth to 3 years of age
- More common in males
- Usually left thoracic curve
- Poor prognosis

Juvenile
- Age of onset—4 to 10 years of age
- More equal distribution between sexes
- Usually right thoracic curve
- Severity increases with growth

Adolescent
- Age of onset—10 years of age to skeletal maturity
- Predominant in females, about 7:1
- Right thoracic and thoracolumbar curves more common

CONGENITAL SCOLIOSIS

May be associated with meningomyelocele or other dysrhaphism
Hemivertebrae or failure of segmentation

NEUROMUSCULAR SCOLIOSIS

Caused by muscular imbalance and/or weakness
Neurogenic
- Lower motor neuron disease such as poliomyelitis, spinal muscular atrophy
- Upper motor neuron disease such as cerebral palsy

Myogenic
- Progressive disease such as muscular dystrophy
- Static disease such as amyotonia congenita

Mixed—weakness and overpull by stronger trunk muscles, such as in Friedreich ataxia

NEUROFIBROMATOSIS

Short sharp thoracic curve often associated with kyphosis

TRAUMATIC

Thoracogenic—result of thoracotomy and thoracoplasty with rib resection
Spinal trauma
- Irradiation such as tumor therapy
- Fractures

MISCELLANEOUS

Secondary to irritation
- Tumor
- Inflammation

Nutritional—rickets
Metabolic—renal osteodystrophy
Intraspinal, cord tether, syringomyelia

MESENCHYMAL DISEASE

Congenital disorders
- Dwarfism
- Disease of connective tissue such as arachnodactyly, arthrogryposis multiplex congenita
- Disease of bone such as osteogenesis imperfecta

Acquired disorders—rheumatoid arthritis

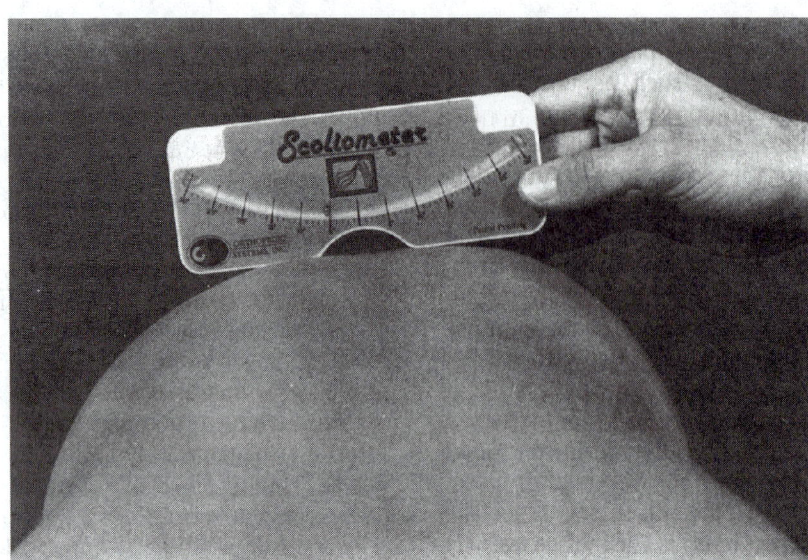

FIG. 39-35 Scoliometer used to document clinical deformity seen in patients with scoliosis. (From Bunnell WP: Nonoperative treatment of spinal deformity: the case for observation. In AAOS: *Instructional course lectures,* vol 36, St Louis, 1985, Mosby.)

vic obliquity. Cutaneous changes may also be observed. When the child bends forward at the waist so that the trunk is parallel with the floor and the arms hang free (the Adams position), asymmetry of ribs and flanks may also be appreciated (Fig. 39-35). By stabilizing the pelvis and asking the child to twist to both sides, the flexibility of the curve can be evaluated. Often a primary curve and a compensatory curve will place the head in alignment with the gluteal cleft. However, in an uncompensated curve, the head and hips are not in alignment.

Radiographs taken with the child in the standing position are measured using the Cobb technique for curve magnitude. In addition, the Risser sign, determined by evaluating the extent of excursion of the iliac apophysis, helps to establish the skeletal maturity of the individual.

Since intraspinal pathology or other disease processes can cause scoliosis, these must be ruled out. The presence of pain, sacral dimpling or hairy patches, cutaneous vascular changes, absent or abnormal reflexes, bowel or bladder incontinence, or a left thoracic curve may indicate an intraspinal abnormality such as syringomyelia, diastematomyelia, or tethered cord syndrome, and an MRI scan should be obtained for evaluation.

Screening. Screening for scoliosis is very controversial. Some groups support screening, believing that early detection permits use of bracing rather than surgery to prevent further curvative formation. However, in a review of studies on scoliosis treatment, the U.S. Preventive Services Task Force found no controlled studies to demonstrate that adolescents who were routinely screened had better outcomes than those not screened. Based on these findings, this group questioned the benefits of screening and called for more scientific evidence of its value in the ultimate outcome of scoliosis interventions (Screening, 1993).

Therapeutic Management

Current management options include observation with regular clinical and radiographic evaluation, orthotic intervention (bracing), and spinal fusion surgery. Treatment decisions are based on the magnitude, location, and type of curve; the age and skeletal maturity of the child; and any underlying or contributing disease process. For many curves in the growing child and adolescent, bracing may be the treatment of choice. It is not curative, but in most cases it will slow the progression of the curve while the child reaches skeletal maturity.

Bracing and Exercise. Exercises alone are rarely of value with scoliosis. However, supplemental exercises are employed daily in and out of the brace to prevent atrophy of spinal and abdominal muscles. External electrical stimulation of spinal muscles transmitted by pads on the back during sleep was not found to be an effective alternative to orthotic treatment (Weinstein, 1994).

The application of a properly constructed and well-fitted external spinal orthosis with close supervision is successful in halting or slowing the progression of most curvatures. The two most commonly used types of braces are (1) the ***Boston brace,*** or underarm orthosis, customized from prefabricated plastic shells, with corrective forces for each patient, using lateral pads and decreasing lumbar lordosis, and (2) the ***Milwaukee brace,*** an individually adapted plastic and metal brace that includes a neck ring and can be used for curves with an apex of higher than T8 (Fig. 39-36).

The type of brace and wearing schedule (usually between 16 and 23 hours a day) is based on the nature of the curve, the age of the child, and any underlying condition associated with the curve. The underarm brace is usually more cosmetically acceptable to the child, since it is easily hidden under loose-fitting clothing.

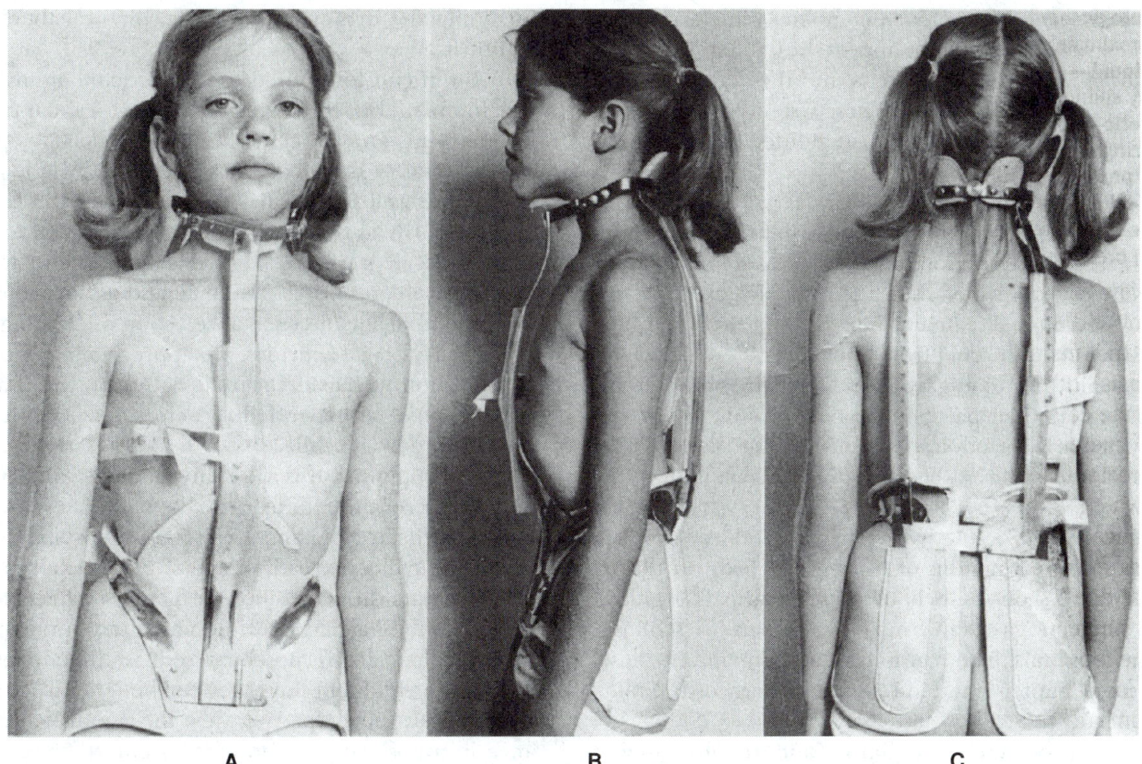

FIG. 39-36 Milwaukee brace. **A,** Front view. **B,** Side view. **C,** Rear view. (From Blount WP, Mueller KH: *Praxis* 8:139-149, June 1972.)

Therapeutic Management: Operative

Surgical intervention may be required for correction of severe curves. Surgery may be considered for a curve in a growing child that progresses despite orthotic treatment or for a severe curve in a mature adolescent. Difficulties with balance or seating, respiratory excursion, or pain are also considered.

The surgical technique consists of realignment and straightening with internal fixation and instrumentation combined with bony fusion (arthrodesis) of the realigned spine. The degree of curvature and the cause determine the decision for surgery. Bracing and exercise have been universally disappointing in curves greater than 40 degrees, and paralytic and congenital curves, which will eventually progress, are best treated with early surgical stabilization if the health status of the child will allow major surgery. The age of the child and location of the curvature influence the decision for surgery, and any progressive or severe curve that does not respond to more conservative measures requires surgical correction.

The preoperative workup usually involves radiographic series, including bending and traction films, pulmonary function studies, and arterial blood gases, and laboratory studies, including prothrombin, partial thromboplastin, bleeding time, blood count, electrolytes, urinalysis and urine culture, and levels of any medications. Autologous blood donations are routinely obtained.

The goals of surgical intervention are to correct the curvatures on the sagittal and coronal planes and to end up with a solid, pain-free fusion in a well-balanced torso, with maximum mobility of the remaining spinal segments.

There are many instrumentation systems available, including Harrington, Dwyer, Zielke, Luque, Cotrel-Dubousset, Isola, and TSRH (Texas Scottish Rite Hospital). Posterior or anterior approaches can be used. The ***Harrington system,*** the first internal spinal instrumentation device, consists of distraction and compression rods, hooks, and nuts. The posterior spinal elements are decorticated, and chips and strips of bone from the iliac crest are placed across the vertebra to provide fusion. Following Harrington instrumentation, the child is logrolled to prevent spinal motion. A molded plastic jacket is used to provide external stabilization of the spine while the child resumes activities.

The ***Luque segmental spinal instrumentation*** provides segmental stability by the use of wires and flexible L-shaped rods. By way of a posterior approach, wires are threaded beneath the laminae of each vertebra and tightened around the rods resting along the transverse processes so that the spinal column is stabilized by transverse traction on each vertebra. The spine is fused with a bone graft taken from the iliac crest. The advantages of this procedure are that the patient can walk within a few days and that no postoperative immobilization is required. The disadvantage is a possibility of spinal nerve damage.

The ***Cotrel-Dubousset*** approach combines the Harrington and Luque systems. Anterior approaches using ***Dwyer*** or ***Zielke instrumentation*** involve screws into the vertebral bodies connected by a cable or rod. These systems require postoperative immobilization with a custom-fitted plastic jacket.

Nursing Considerations

Treatment for scoliosis extends over a significant portion of the affected child's period of growth. In adolescents this period is the one in which their identity, physical and psychologic, is formed. Treatment may mean a modified lifestyle and being "different" from their peers, even though they are usually able to engage in most activities enjoyed by other youngsters. Pen pals and support groups may be of value, particularly for adolescents, in helping them to feel less isolated and different because of their scoliosis.

❖ Assessment

One of the major functions of nurses is to learn to detect the presence of scoliosis. School nurses routinely evaluate children in their care, and most are a part of scoliosis screening programs. The methods of assessment are those described in Chapter 7 and in relation to Diagnostic Evaluation, p. 1847.

Screening procedures are simple and require only a 30-second observation. Unfortunately, studies have indicated that current screening procedures are less than ideal (Morais and others, 1985; Viviani and others, 1984) and that too many children are exposed to radiographs in an attempt to rule out scoliosis in normal children. Methods of improving the effectiveness of screening and the application to all schoolchildren should be a goal of nursing.

❖ Nursing Diagnoses

Based on a thorough assessment, several nursing diagnoses are identified. The more common diagnoses for the child with scoliosis are included in the Nursing Care Plan on pp. 1851-1852. Others may apply in specific situations.

❖ Planning

The goals for the child with scoliosis and the family include the following:

1. Child will adjust to the method of therapeutic management.
2. Child will experience no complications.
3. Child and family will receive appropriate support, encouragement, and education.

❖ Implementation

When the child first faces the prospect of a prolonged period in a brace, the therapy program and the nature of the device must be explained thoroughly to the child and parents so that they will have an understanding of the anticipated results, how the appliance corrects the defect, the freedoms and constraints imposed by the device, and what they can do to help achieve the desired goal. The management involves the skills and services of a team of specialists, including the orthopaedist, nurse, physical therapist, and orthotist.

It is difficult for a child to be restricted at any phase of development, but the teenager needs continual positive reinforcement, encouragement, and as much independence as can be safely assumed during this time. Although adolescents cope well for the first year or two of bracing, problems may arise as the time extends. Nurses need to be aware of this and be prepared to provide support and encouragement if problems arise. Guidance and assistance regarding anticipated problems, such as selection of clothing and participation in social activities, are appreciated by adolescents. Socialization with peers should be encouraged, and every effort should be expended to help the adolescent feel attractive and worthwhile.

Since many persons view any disability as deviant, the child will need help in learning how to deal with reactions of others to the appliance. Preparation for such responses places the child at an advantage. The best approach is usually to initiate the interaction by mentioning the device and its purpose. This alleviates the ambiguity surrounding the appliance and its purpose and reduces the anxiety on the part of the child and the other person. Most important, the child should be helped to view the condition and appliance in a positive way and avoid seeing them as a stigma. Some youngsters who receive patient teaching, peer counseling, and support find positive aspects to wearing a brace in addition to improved posture and relief of symptoms. They enjoy the increased attention from peers and the experience of "being different" (Gratz and Papalia-Finlay, 1984).

The child hospitalized for surgical management requires preparation for the procedures involved, which are puzzling and often frightening to the very young patient. They need to know what is going to happen, and they need to have a full explanation of why the procedure is necessary.

Postoperative Care. Postoperatively patients may be monitored in an intensive or special care unit and logrolled when changing position to prevent damage to the fusion and instrumentation.

In addition to the usual postoperative assessments—of wound, circulation, and vital signs—the neurologic status of the patient requires special attention, especially that of the extremities. Prompt recognition of any neurologic impairment is imperative because delayed paralysis may develop that requires removal of the instrumentation. The patient is encouraged to exercise by contracting and relaxing the thigh and calf muscles periodically.

There is usually some degree of paralytic ileus following the procedure; therefore nursing includes care of the nasogastric intubation and assessment for returning bowel function. Urinary retention is common—an indwelling catheter is often used for the first 48 hours. Because of the extensive blood loss during the surgical procedure and renal hypoperfusion, observation of urinary output is especially important.

The child usually has considerable pain for the first few days following surgery and requires frequent administration

NURSING CARE PLAN
The Child with Structural Scoliosis

NURSING DIAGNOSIS: High risk for injury related to unaccustomed brace

PATIENT GOAL 1: Will not experience injury related to wearing brace

• **NURSING INTERVENTIONS/*RATIONALES***
Assess environment for hazards *to prevent injuries*
Teach safety precautions such as using handrail on stairways and avoiding slippery surfaces *to prevent falls*
Help develop safe methods of mobilization

• **EXPECTED OUTCOME**
Child remains free of injury related to wearing brace

PATIENT GOAL 2: Will adjust to restricted movement

• **NURSING INTERVENTIONS/*RATIONALES***
Demonstrate alternative modes of accomplishing tasks such as getting in and out of bed, dressing
Help devise alternatives for restricted activities and coping with awkwardness

• **EXPECTED OUTCOME**
Child demonstrates appropriate adaptation to corrective device (specify)

NURSING DIAGNOSIS: High risk for impaired skin integrity related to corrective device

PATIENT GOAL 1: Will not experience skin irritation or breakdown

• **NURSING INTERVENTIONS/*RATIONALES***
Examine skin surfaces in contact with brace for signs of irritation *so that appropriate treatment is instituted*
Implement corrective action to treat or prevent skin breakdown
Suggest nonirritating fabrics and clothing such as cotton T-shirts that can be worn under brace *to minimize risk of skin irritation*
Recommend daily bath or shower followed by thorough drying *to maintain cleanliness and minimize risk of skin irritation*

• **EXPECTED OUTCOME**
Skin remains clean with no evidence of irritation

NURSING DIAGNOSIS: Body image disturbance related to perception of defect in body structure

PATIENT GOAL 1: Will exhibit signs of physical adjustment to appliance

• **NURSING INTERVENTIONS/*RATIONALES***
Plan *with* the child *to encourage compliance and adjustment*
Attempt to determine source of any discomfort *so that appropriate care is instituted*
Refer to orthotist for needed adjustment and service
Assist with plan for personal hygiene
Help in selection of appropriate and attractive apparel to wear over brace and footwear *to maintain proper balance*
Reinforce teaching regarding removal and reapplication of appliance *so that child receives maximum benefit of appliance*

• **EXPECTED OUTCOMES**
Brace fits well and produces no discomfort
Child complies with directions for wear and care of brace
Child is well groomed and wears attractive attire and proper footwear

PATIENT GOAL 2: Will exhibit positive coping behaviors

• **NURSING INTERVENTIONS/*RATIONALES***
Encourage child to discuss feelings about wearing brace *to encourage coping*
Emphasize positive aspects and eventual outcome *to encourage acceptance of treatment*

• **EXPECTED OUTCOMES**
Child verbalizes feelings and concerns
Child recognizes benefits of treatment
See also Nursing Care Plan: The Child with Chronic Illness or Disability, Chapter 22

Preoperative Care

See Nursing Care Plan: The Child Undergoing Surgery: Preoperative care, Chapter 27.

Postoperative Care

See Nursing Care Plan: The Child Undergoing Surgery: Postoperative care, Chapter 27.

NURSING DIAGNOSIS: High risk for injury related to surgery

PATIENT GOAL 1: Will attain ambulation without injury to surgical repair

• **NURSING INTERVENTIONS/*RATIONALES***
Place on special bed, if ordered (Harrington instrumentation), *which facilitates care and decreases risk of injury to surgical repair*
Maintain proper body alignment; avoid twisting movements, *which can cause indwelling instruments to twist the spine*

Continued.

NURSING CARE PLAN
The Child with Structural Scoliosis—cont'd

Logroll with care when moving child who is not on a Stryker frame
Keep flat for 12 hours before logrolling (Luque procedure)
Beginning activity—have child roll from side-lying to sitting position
Encourage child to exercise by contracting and relaxing thigh and calf muscles periodically *to maintain optimum movement of lower extremities in the immediate postoperative period*
Perform regular tests of neurologic integrity
Assist with physical therapy and range-of-motion exercises *to maintain muscle tone and joint flexibility*
Walk slowly with aid of safety belt and walker; unassisted ambulation usually allowed by sixth day

• **EXPECTED OUTCOME**
Child attains ambulation without injury

PATIENT GOAL 2: Will not experience abdominal distention (from paralytic ileus)

• **NURSING INTERVENTIONS/*RATIONALES***
*Insert and maintain nasogastric suction *to prevent abdominal distention*
Assess for returning bowel function (e.g., bowel sounds) *to aid in determining when nasogastric suction can be discontinued*

• **EXPECTED OUTCOME**
Child exhibits no evidence of bowel distention

NURSING DIAGNOSIS: Pain related to surgical procedure

PATIENT GOAL 1: Will experience no pain or reduction of pain to level acceptable to child

• **NURSING INTERVENTIONS/*RATIONALES***
Anticipate need for pain management *because of the nature of this surgery*
Administer opioids on preventive schedule (around the clock) until pain can be controlled with nonopioids *to prevent pain from occurring*
Consider patient-controlled analgesia for child able to follow instructions *in order to give child more control in prevention and allievation of pain*

• **EXPECTED OUTCOME**
Child rests quietly, reports and/or exhibits no evidence of discomfort or minimal discomfort

*Dependent nursing action.

NURSING DIAGNOSIS: Altered patterns of urinary elimination related to surgical procedure, loss of blood, renal hypoperfusion

PATIENT GOAL 1: Will exhibit signs of adequate urinary elimination

• **NURSING INTERVENTIONS/*RATIONALES***
*Insert indwelling catheter *because urinary retention is common with this surgery*
Encourage frequent voiding after catheter removal
Provide privacy *to encourage urination*
Monitor intake and output *to assess adequacy of elimination*

• **EXPECTED OUTCOME**
Urinary bladder is adequately emptied

PATIENT GOAL 2: Will exhibit signs of adequate urinary output

• **NURSING INTERVENTIONS/*RATIONALES***
Monitor intake and output *to assess adequacy of urinary output*
Maintain intravenous infusion *for adequate hydration* and urinary output
Encourage oral fluids when allowed

• **EXPECTED OUTCOME**
Child has a sufficient urinary output

NURSING DIAGNOSIS: Impaired physical mobility related to spinal surgery and instrumentation

See Nursing Care Plan: The Child Who Is Immobilized, p. 1805

NURSING DIAGNOSIS: Altered family processes related to a child with a physical disability

PATIENT (FAMILY) GOAL 1: Will receive adequate support

• **NURSING INTERVENTIONS/*RATIONALES***
See Nursing Care Plan: The Family of the Ill or Hospitalized Child, Chapter 26

• **EXPECTED OUTCOME**
Family members avail themselves of services

See also Nursing Care Plan: The Child in the Hospital, Chapter 26

of pain medication, preferably the use of opioids administered on a regular schedule, as opposed to "as needed." For children able to understand the concept, patient-controlled analgesia (PCA) is a recommended alternative (see Pain Management, Chapter 26). Because of the anterior approach, patients with Dwyer instrumentation also require thoracotomy care in addition to the care related to the fusion and realignment procedures. Their pain is more severe and prolonged.

Children with a Luque procedure are kept flat for 12

hours before logrolling is begun. The head of the bed can be elevated on the second day, and range-of-motion exercises begun. Activity is begun by instructing the patient to roll from a side-lying position to a sitting position. Next, walking slowly with the aid of a safety belt and walker is allowed, and, finally, unassisted ambulation, which is usually achieved by the sixth day.

All patients are started on physiotherapy as soon as they are able, beginning with range-of-motion exercises and many of the activities of daily living. Self-care such as washing and eating is always encouraged. Some simple physical therapy may be begun during this acute stage. Throughout the hospitalization diversionary activities and contact with family and friends are an important part of nursing care and planning.

The family is encouraged to become involved with the patient's care to facilitate the transition from hospital to home management. Family members learn to apply and care for the brace or learn cast care, with special attention given to jagged edges on the cast, padding of the appliance, and daily skin checks for reddened areas, especially in areas such as under the arms or over the hips. They may need assistance in modifying the environment for limited ambulation and acquiring needed home care items such as a convoluted foam mattress, straight-backed chair, and raised toilet seat. The child and family need to learn efficient ways to move and carry out various activities of daily living. The diet may require modification. Overeating and constipation can be problems related to limited activity.

Several organizations provide education and services to both families and professionals. The **National Scoliosis Foundation, Inc.,*** is devoted to awareness and action for early detection and prevention of spinal deformity. They offer educational support materials for parents, schools, and health care providers. A list of books, pamphlets, and other materials is available on request. The **American Academy of Orthopaedic Surgeons†** has published a booklet called *Scoliosis.*

❖ Evaluation

The effectiveness of nursing interventions is determined by continual reassessment and evaluation of care based on the following observational guidelines and expected outcomes:

1. Observe and interview the child relative to problems and solutions experienced.
2. Observe child for evidence of proper usage of the method of management and signs of complications (e.g., skin irritation).
3. Observe and interview the child and family regarding their feelings and concerns.

Expected outcomes:

See Nursing Care Plan, pp. 1851-1852.

*72 Mount Auburn St., Watertown, MA 02172; (617) 926-0397.

†PO Box 2058, Des Plaines, IL 60017; (800) 346-AAOS or (708) 823-7186. Available free of charge by sending a self-addressed stamped envelope.

ORTHOPAEDIC INFECTIONS

OSTEOMYELITIS

Osteomyelitis, an infectious process of bone, can occur at any age but occurs most frequently between ages 5 and 14 years. It is twice as common in boys as in girls. Any organism can cause osteomyelitis, and there is some relationship between the age of the child and the type of organism responsible. In older children staphylococci are the most common organisms, approximately 80% of which are *Staphylococcus aureus;* in younger children other organisms predominate, especially *Haemophilus influenzae.* In children with sickle cell anemia, *Salmonella* organisms are frequently responsible for osteomyelitis.

Osteomyelitis can be acquired from exogenous or hematogenous sources. ***Exogenous*** osteomyelitis is acquired by invasion of the bone by direct extension from the outside as a result of a penetrating wound, open fracture, contamination during surgery, or secondary extension from an overlying abscess or burn.

Hematogenous spread of organisms from a preexisting focus is the most common source of infection. Common sources of foci include furuncles, skin abrasions, impetigo, upper respiratory tract infection, acute otitis media, tonsillitis, abscessed teeth, pyelonephritis, or infected burns. Other factors that predispose to development of osteomyelitis are poor physical condition, poor nutrition, and surroundings that are not hygienic.

Pathophysiology

Infective emboli from the focus of infection travel to the small end arteries in the bone metaphysis, where they set up an infectious process. The infection does not spread to the epiphysis, since it has a blood supply separate from the metaphysis. The infectious process leads to local bone destruction and abscess formation. The abscess, with its collected necrotic debris, exerts pressure within the rigid, unyielding bone and ruptures into the subperiosteal space, where the pressure lifts and strips the periosteum. The infection spreads beneath the periosteum, causing thrombosis of vessels and adding further to the bony necrosis.

In infants and very young children the elevated periosteum attempts to wall off the infection by forming new bone—***involucrum.*** Underneath, the cortex, deprived of blood supply, dies, and the necrotic bone that cannot be absorbed continues to produce more intraosseous tension and necrosis. Granulation forms around the dead bone, or ***sequestrum.*** Sinuses may form between the sequestra and the skin surface or into a joint to create a suppurative arthritis. Small areas of sequestrum may be absorbed, but larger areas surrounded by dense bone become honeycombed with sinuses that retain infective material and cause exacerbations for years (the chronic stage of osteomyelitis).

Clinical Manifestations

Signs and symptoms of ***acute hematogenous osteomyelitis*** begin abruptly and build up to a maximum intensity during the first few days of the disease, usually less than 1 week. There is frequently a history of trauma to the affected bone.

Children with acute osteomyelitis appear very ill. They are irritable and restless, with elevated temperature, rapid pulse, and dehydration. There is usually localized tenderness, increased warmth, and diffuse swelling over the involved bone. The extremity is painful, especially on movement. The child holds it in semiflexion, and the surrounding muscles are tense and resist passive movement. Most cases involve the femur or tibia and to a lesser extent the humerus and hip. In infants the diagnosis is more difficult because of lack of systemic symptoms. The disorder may involve multiple bones or joints because of the difficulty in confining an infection in children in this age-group.

In ***subacute hematogenous osteomyelitis*** symptoms have been present for a longer period and the child sometimes has been treated with antibiotics, often for another infection, which modify the clinical symptoms. In some instances the infection may produce a walled-off abscess rather than a spreading infection.

Diagnostic Evaluation

In acute osteomyelitis there is marked leukocytosis and an elevated erythrocyte sedimentation rate. Blood culture is usually positive during the early stage, but radiographic findings are often negative or show only soft tissue swelling for 10 to 14 days. After this time the radiographic findings reveal new bone formation. Computed tomography may reveal bone changes at an early stage, and scintigraphy reveals a greater uptake of radionucleotides in osteomyelitic bone than in normal bone.

Similar symptoms are observed in rheumatic fever, rheumatoid arthritis, leukemia and other malignant lesions, cellulitis, erysipelas, and scurvy. Sometimes the osteomyelitis may be unrecognized if it occurs as a complication of a severe toxic and debilitating illness.

Therapeutic Management

As soon as blood cultures have been drawn, prompt and vigorous intravenous antibiotic therapy is initiated. The choice is influenced by age, and the dosage determined is sufficient to ensure high blood and tissue levels. Since most cases of osteomyelitis are caused by staphylococci, large doses of penicillin G are administered and supplemented by methicillin or oxacillin. In children younger than 3 years of age, the infectious agents are more apt to be penicillin-resistant staphylococci or gram-negative organisms; therefore the agents of choice are usually methicillin, nafcillin, or clindamycin in conjunction with ampicillin. Neonates in whom coliform organisms are likely to be involved are given kanamycin or gentamicin, either intramuscularly or *slowly* intravenously in addition to intravenously administered ampicillin. In selected cases antibiotics may be administered orally following a short, intensive intravenous course.

When the infective agent is identified, the appropriate antibiotic is usually continued for at least 3 to 4 weeks, but the length of therapy is determined by the duration of symptoms, the initial response to treatment, and the sensitivity of the organism in the specific case. Because of prolonged high-dose therapy, it is important to monitor hematologic, renal, hepatic, and other organ systems that might be adversely affected by the drugs (e.g., ototoxic).

Antibiotic therapy is accompanied by local treatment. The child is placed on a regimen of complete bed rest, and immobilization of the affected extremity, which may require a splint or bivalved cast, is continued throughout therapy to limit the spread of infection and, when it is a complication of a fracture, to maintain alignment of bone fragments. Weight bearing on the nonfractured leg is prohibited to avoid the possibility of pathologic fracture.

Opinions differ regarding surgical intervention, but many advocate sequestrectomy and surgical drainage to decompress the metaphyseal space before pus erupts and spreads to the subperiosteal space to form abscesses that strip the periosteum from bone or form draining sinuses. When these complications occur, a chronic infection usually persists. When surgical drainage is carried out, polyethylene tubes are placed in the wound—one tube instills an antibiotic solution directly into the infected area by gravity, and the other, connected to a suction apparatus, provides drainage.

Nursing Considerations

During the acute phase of illness, any movement of the affected limb will cause discomfort to the child; therefore the child is positioned comfortably with the affected limb supported. Moving and turning are carried out carefully and gently to minimize discomfort. The child may require pain medication or sedation. Vital signs are taken and recorded frequently, and measures are implemented to reduce a significant temperature elevation.

Antibiotic therapy requires careful observation and monitoring of the intravenous equipment and site. Since more than one antibiotic is usually administered, the compatibility of the drugs must be determined and care taken to avoid mixing noncompatible drugs. The stability of the drugs and their toxic nature are also considered when determining the rate of administration. The needle must be well situated in the vein to ensure that the drug does not infiltrate into surrounding tissues, where it may produce tissue damage. For long-term antibiotic therapy, a venous access device, such as an intermittent infusion device or peripherally inserted central catheter (PICC), is the preferred method of intravenous administration (see Chapter 28).

Children with an open wound are placed on body substance precautions, depending on the policies of the institution. The wound is managed according to the directions of the practitioner. Antibiotic solution administered directly into the wound is most efficiently accomplished with a regular intravenous infusion setup that is prepared and regulated as any intravenous infusion. The drainage tubes are connected to low Gomco or wall suction for continuous removal. Intake and output are measured and recorded, and the character of the wound drainage is noted. The amount and character of drainage on the wound dressing are also noted.

Casts are sometimes employed for immobilization, and if so, routine cast care is carried out. The extremity is examined for sensation, circulation, and pain, and the area over the inflammation is usually left open for observation. The affected area, casted or uncasted, is assessed for color, swelling, heat, movement, and tenderness.

The child usually has a poor appetite and may be subject to vomiting. Nourishment in the form of high-calorie liquids such as fruit juices, gelatin, and juice bars should be encouraged until the child begins to feel better. The appetite returns as the acute symptoms subside. During convalescence adequate nutrition must be maintained to aid healing and reconstitution of new bone.

When the acute stage subsides, children begin to feel better, the appetite improves, and they become interested in their surroundings and relationships. They wish to move about in bed and are allowed to do so. However, weight bearing on the affected limb is not permitted until healing is well under way in order to avoid pathologic fractures. Diversional and constructive activities become important nursing interventions. Children are usually confined to bed for some time after the acute phase but may be allowed to move about the unit on a gurney or in a wheelchair when isolation and bed rest are no longer necessary. At this stage the continuous intravenous infusion may be replaced by a heparin lock to allow greater freedom.

As the infection subsides, physical therapy is instituted to ensure restoration of optimum function. The child is usually discharged with oral antibiotics, and progress is followed closely for some time.

SEPTIC (SUPPURATIVE, PYOGENIC, PURULENT) ARTHRITIS

Infection of the joints, like infection of bone, usually develops through hematogenous dissemination from another focus; occasionally it may result from direct extension of a soft tissue infection. Joint infections occur predominantly in males, especially in the adolescent age-group. In infancy, however, the incidence in boys and girls is more nearly equal. Any joint may be involved, but the hip, knee, shoulder, and other large joints are more commonly affected. Usually only one joint is involved.

The signs and symptoms of suppurative arthritis, unlike osteomyelitis, are usually characteristic. The presence of a warm and tender joint, painful on even gentle pressure, is sufficient to differentiate it from osteomyelitis, in which gentle passive motion is tolerated. When superficial joints are involved, they are exquisitely painful and swollen; deep-seated joints show little superficial evidence. In most instances there is a history of a traumatic injury to the affected joint. Fever, leukocytosis, and increased erythrocyte sedimentation rate are present but may not be demonstrated in affected infants.

The most common pathogens are *Staphylococcus aureus*, group A streptococci, and *Haemophilus influenzae*. The diagnosis is made from a blood culture, joint fluid aspirate, and radiographs.

Therapeutic Management and Nursing Considerations

Treatment consists of open surgical drainage of hip and shoulder joint disease and repeated needle aspirations of the joint space in other joints. The goals are (1) to cleanse the joint to avoid destruction of articular cartilage, (2) to decompress the joint to avoid interference with the blood supply to the epiphysis, (3) to eradicate the infection with adequate antibiotic therapy, and (4) to prevent secondary bone infection and hematogenous spread. Therapy is similar to that for osteomyelitis: intravenous antibiotic therapy, relief of pain, immobilization of the joint, and prohibition of weight bearing until healing is complete. Nursing care is the same as that for osteomyelitis.

TUBERCULOSIS

Tubercular infection of the bones is acquired by hematogenous dissemination from a primary tubercular focus. The most common sites in infants and small children are the carpals and phalanges and corresponding bones of the feet. One or several bones may be involved, with spindle-shaped swelling and tenderness as soft tissues are affected. The process, which is relatively painless, persists with intermittent symptoms for several months and may leave a permanent deformity. Affected areas are immobilized with a splint or cast.

Tuberculosis of the Spine (Tuberculous Spondylitis)

In older children the infection attacks the body of one or more vertebrae, destroying the bone, and spreads to all the articular tissues, producing a kyphotic deformity. The lower thoracic spine is most frequently affected. Symptoms are insidious. The child will be irritable and complain of persistent or intermittent pain over the areas innervated by spinal nerves that arise adjacent to the affected vertebrae. There is muscle splinting and pain when increased pressure is placed on the child's head. The child assumes a position that best eases the weight on the diseased vertebrae, such as avoiding bending and walking stiffly on the toes, and prefers to rest on the abdomen or across a chair or a lap.

Treatment is immobilization with extension or a plaster body cast until there is no evidence of active infection followed by spinal fusion. Antimicrobial therapy and drainage of the tubercular abscess are standard therapies. The reparative process is slow, but in most instances recovery takes place with little or no deformity. Nursing care is similar to care of the child with scoliosis.

Tuberculosis of the Hip

The hip is the joint most commonly affected by tuberculosis, but the process usually begins in the epiphysis of the femoral head and then erupts into the joint capsule. The initial manifestation is a limp that occurs intermittently, most often on arising in the morning or after exercise. There is progressive destruction of the femoral head with symptoms of pain, and the thigh gradually becomes fixed and adducted with internal rotation. There may be swelling around the hip and abscess formation.

Treatment involves bed rest, traction to reduce muscle spasm, and appropriate drug therapy. Hip fusion may be necessary in severe cases.

SKELETAL AND ARTICULAR DYSFUNCTION

OSTEOGENESIS IMPERFECTA (OI)

OI is a group of heterogenous inherited disorders of connective tissue characterized by connective tissue and bone defects, including one or more of the following: varying degrees of bone fragility leading to fractures, blue sclerae, progressive bone deformities, presenile hearing loss, and dentinogenesis imperfecta (hypoplastic teeth with an opalescent blue or brown discoloration). The inheritance pattern is autosomal dominant in the majority of cases, although the most severe form demonstrates autosomal-recessive inheritance.

Persons with OI have normal calcium and phosphorus levels but appear to have abnormal precollagen type I that prevents the formation of collagen, the major component of connective tissue. The precollagen remains relatively inert and unable to undergo final transformation into collagen. Consequently, bone of these patients consists of large areas of osseous tissues devoid of an organized trabecular pattern and increased numbers of large osteoblasts. Lamellae, when present, are very thin. The more severe the degree of OI, the greater is the number of osteocytes and the greater the disruption of the normal architectural patterns of the bone.

At present OI is believed to consist of four different variations, as outlined in Table 39-5. Type II, the most severe form of OI, is characterized by multiple intrauterine or perinatal fractures and severe deformity and, often, early death. The brittle nature of the bones renders them easily fractured by the slightest trauma.

The diseases of later onset run a milder course. The tendency to fracture appears later (at variable ages) and disappears after puberty. During childhood the shafts of long bones are slender with reduced cortical thickness resulting from defective periosteal bone formation. In addition to the features already described, the child with OI has thin skin, hyperextensibility of ligaments, a tendency toward recurrent epistaxis, excess diaphoresis, a tendency to bruise easily, and mild hyperpyrexia. The disease shows variable expressivity; that is, the number and extent of pathologic features appear in any individual range, from severe to minimum involvement. The incidence of fractures decreases at puberty, when the body's production of hormones helps strengthen bones.

Therapeutic Management

The treatment of OI is primarily supportive. The goals of a rehabilitation approach to management are directed to preventing (1) positional contractures and deformities, (2) muscle weakness and osteoporosis, and (3) malalignment of lower extremity joints prohibiting weight bearing.

TABLE 39-5 Classification of Osteogenesis Imperfecta

TYPE	CHARACTERISTICS
I* A	Mild bone fragility, blue sclerae, normal teeth, presenile deafness (age 20-30 years); autosomal-dominant inheritance
B	Same as A except dentinogenesis imperfecta instead of normal teeth
C	Same as B; no bone fragility
II	Lethal; stillborn or die in early infancy; severe bone fragility, multiple fractures at birth; 10% of OI cases; autosomal-recessive inheritance
III	Severe bone fragility leads to severe progressive deformities; normal sclerae; marked growth failure; most autosomal-recessive inheritance; few autosomal-dominant inheritance
IV A	Mild to moderate bone fragility; normal sclerae; short stature; variable deformity; autosomal dominant inheritance
B	Same as A except dentinogenesis imperfecta instead of normal teeth; approximately 6% of OI cases

*Two thirds of cases are type I.

Several drugs have been tried but appear to be of limited benefit. Lightweight braces and splints help support limbs, prevent fractures, and aid in ambulation. Physical therapy helps prevent disuse osteoporosis and strengthens muscles, which in turn improves bone density. Exercises are usually simple ones against light resistance or water exercises with swimming. Patients with milder disease are encouraged to participate in sports. Exercise also gives children a sense of well-being and confidence in their bodies.

Surgery is sometimes used to help treat the manifestations of the disease. Surgical techniques are used to correct deformities that interfere with bracing, standing, or walking. For the child with recurrent fractures, inserting an intermedullary rod provides stability to bones. Unfortunately, the rods must be replaced as the child grows; otherwise fractures may occur through the unprotected portion of the bone.

Nursing Considerations

Infants and children with this disorder require careful handling to prevent fractures. They must be supported when they are turned, positioned, moved, and fondled. Even changing a diaper may cause a fracture in severely affected infants. These children should never be held by the ankles when being diapered but should be gently lifted by the buttocks.

One of the most distressing features of OI is its frequent confusion with child abuse. Numerous fractures and easy bruising, characteristic of OI, are signs usually observed in child abuse; parents must often deal with accusations of abuse until a correct diagnosis is made. This is very traumatic for parents; therefore they need considerable nonjudgmental support during this time.

Both parents and the affected child need education regarding the child's limitations and guidelines in planning suitable activities that promote optimum development, as well as protect the child from harm. Realistic occupational planning and genetic counseling are part of the long-term goals of care. Educational materials and information can be obtained from the **Osteogenesis Imperfecta Foundation, Inc.*** This organization also has a network that can put a family in contact with other families with a similar problem.

JUVENILE RHEUMATOID ARTHRITIS (JRA)

Clinically and pathologically, JRA, or juvenile arthritis (JA), is an inflammatory disease with an unknown inciting agent and a slight tendency to occur in families. Both infectious and autoimmune theories have been presented, but there is no convincing evidence to establish either one as an etiologic agent. There are two peak ages of onset: between 2 and 5 and between 9 and 12 years of age. Females are affected somewhat more frequently than males. In many instances the disease remains undiagnosed for years.

JRA is, in many ways, similar to the adult disease, but there are many features that are quite distinct. A distinguishing feature is its tendency to occur in the prepubertal child. Characteristics of JRA include negative results in the latex fixation test in 90% of cases; classic symptoms of a spiking fever, skin rash, or pericarditis in 5% to 10% of cases; a tendency to be very mild in 70% of cases, with few joints involved; development of iridocyclitis as a complication in 8% to 20% of milder forms; and "burning itself out" over 2 to 3 years in milder forms and over 8 to 10 years in most other forms.

Pathophysiology

The rheumatic process is characterized by a chronic inflammation of the synovium with joint effusion and eventual erosion, destruction, and fibrosis of the articular cartilage. Adhesions between joint surfaces and ankylosis of joints occur if the process persists long enough.

Clinical Manifestations

Whether a single joint or multiple joints are involved, stiffness, swelling, and loss of motion develop in the affected joints. They are swollen and warm to the touch but seldom red. The swelling results from edema, joint effusion, and synovial thickening. The affected joints may be tender and painful to the touch or relatively painless. The limited motion early in the disease is a result of muscle spasm and joint inflammation; later it is caused by ankylosis or soft tissue contracture. Morning stiffness or "gelling" of the joint(s) is characteristic and present on arising in the morning or after inactivity. Infections, injuries, or surgical procedures often precipitate a flare-up of the arthritis; therefore prompt recognition and treatment of infections is necessary.

In severe, long-standing cases growth is significantly retarded. Corticosteroid therapy is also a contributing factor. There may be growth disturbances, either overgrowth or undergrowth, adjacent to the inflamed joints (e.g., altered leg length after knee involvement) and micrognathia (receding chin) from temporomandibular arthritis.

JRA is a variable disease and is now recognized to pursue three major disease courses: ***systemic onset***, ***pauciarticular*** (involving few joints, usually less than five), and ***polyarticular*** (simultaneous involvement of four or more joints). These groups, including subgroups, and the manifestations associated with each are outlined in Table 39-6.

Course. The outcome and sources of morbidity are variable and unpredictable in any individual patient. The disease, even in severe forms, is rarely life-threatening. Chronic joint pain is characteristic of polyarticular and systemic disease; the major morbidity in type I patients is chronic iridocyclitis (inflammation of the iris and ciliary body) and spondyloarthropathy in type II disease. There may be exacerbations and remissions, or the symptoms may continue for years. The symptoms may cause little disability or (less commonly) are severe with joint destruction and permanent deformity. Although the disease usually remits at puberty, some patients continue to have active arthritis into adulthood.

Prognosis. The overall prognosis for children with JRA is good. At least 75% eventually enter long remissions without significant residual deformity or impaired function. The poorest prognosis is associated with rheumatoid factor—positive polyarthritis and systemic-onset disease. The most debilitating complications are severe hip disease and loss of vision from iridocyclitis.

Diagnostic Evaluation

The diagnosis of JRA is one of exclusion (i.e., differentiation from a variety of disorders with similar manifestations) at the onset of the disease. Radiographic findings are variable, but the earliest manifestations are widening joint spaces followed by gradual evidence of fusion and articular destruction. There may be evidence of soft tissue swelling, osteoporosis, and periostitis around affected joints.

There are no serologic tests for JRA. The diagnosis is based on criteria established by the American Rheumatism Association (Emery and Miller, 1993). The erythrocyte sedimentation rate may or may not be elevated, depending on the degree of inflammation present. Leukocytosis is generally present in the early stages of classic systemic disease. The latex fixation test, the most common test used to detect the presence of rheumatoid factor in adults, is negative in 90% of juvenile cases. Rheumatoid factors are found in some children, usually those with disease of later onset. Antinuclear antibodies are found in three fourths of rheumatoid factor–positive and one fourth of rheumatoid factor–negative children and in pauciarticular type I diseases, but not in children with systemic-onset or pauciarticular type II disease. There is a strong relationship between the

*P.O. Box 14807, Tampa, FL 34629-4807; (813) 855-7077.

TABLE 39-6 Characteristics of Juvenile Rheumatoid Arthritis Related to Mode of Onset

	SYSTEMIC ONSET	PAUCIARTICULAR (TWO OR THREE SUBTYPES)	POLYARTICULAR (TWO SUBTYPES)
Percentage of patients	30%	45%	25%
Age at onset	Bimodal distribution 1-3 years of age 8-10 years of age	Type I: Less than 10 years Type II: Over 10 years	Throughout childhood and adolescence
Sex ratio (female/male)	1.5:1	Type I: Almost all female Type II: 1:9	Mostly female
Joints involved	Any Only 20% have joint involvement at time of diagnosis	Usually confined to lower extremities—knee, ankle, and eventually sacroiliac; sometimes elbow	Any joints: usually symmetric involvement of small joints Hip involvement in 50% Spine involvement in 50%
Extraarticular manifestations	Fever, malaise, myalgia, rash, pleuritis or pericarditis, adenomegaly, splenomegaly, hepatomegaly	Type I: Chronic iridocyclitis; mucocutaneous lesions Type II: Acute iridocyclitis; sacroiliitis common; eventual ankylosing spondylitis in many Type III: Arthritis only	Systemic signs minimal Possible low-grade fever, malaise, weight loss, rheumatoid nodules, and/or vasculitis
Laboratory tests	Elevated ESR; RF negative; ANA rarely positive; anemia; leukocytosis	Elevated ESR; ANA positive Type I: HLA-DRW5 positive Type II: HLA-B27 positive Type III: HLA-TMo positive	Elevated ESR Type I: RF positive Type II: RF negative
Long-term prognosis	Mortality—1%-2% of all JRA patients Joint destruction in 40%	Continuous disease; eventual remission in 60% Type I: Ocular damage; functional blindness in 10% Type II: Ankylosing spondylitis Type III: Best outlook for recovery	Longer duration; more crippling; remission in 25% Type I: High incidence of disabling arthritis Type II: Outlook good

ESR, Erythrocyte sedimentation rate; *RF,* rheumatoid factor; *ANA,* antinuclear antibody; *HLA,* human leukocyte antigen.

presence of antinuclear antibodies and chronic iridocyclitis but no relationship to the severity of the disease.

Therapeutic Management

There is no specific cure for JRA. The major goals of therapy are to (1) preserve joint function, (2) prevent physical deformities, and (3) relieve symptoms without iatrogenic harm. This involves both initial and long-term planning, parent and patient education and counseling, physical and occupational therapy, good health and nutritional education and management, specific drug therapy, orthopaedic consultation, and periodic eye examination.

Whenever possible, children are treated at home under the supervision of the health team, and intermittent treatment by qualified professionals is administered. Hospitalization may be needed during severe exacerbations or when intercurrent illness warrants. Iridocyclitis, which is unique to JRA, can occur and requires the attention of an ophthalmologist. The majority of affected children have a relatively good visual prognosis if the condition is detected and treated early (American Academy of Pediatrics, 1993).

Drugs. A variety of antirheumatic drugs is available, and most are effective in suppressing the inflammatory process and relieving pain. The drugs may be given alone or in combination.

The primary group of drugs prescribed for JRA are the ***nonsteroidal antiinflammatory drugs (NSAIDs),*** such as aspirin, tolmetin sodium, ibuprofen, piroxicam (Feldene), nabumetone (Relafin), and naproxen (see Table 26-3). All of these drugs act in a similar manner, and none is superior to the others in producing the desired effects—analgesic, antipyretic, and antiinflammatory. Reduction in fever takes place in hours, relief of pain occurs in a matter of hours or days (more often in weeks, however), but the antiinflammatory effect (reductions in swelling, pain on motion, tenderness, and limitation of motion of involved joints) does not occur for 3 to 4 weeks. Consequently, these drugs should not be discontinued without an adequate trial period. Sometimes several drugs are tried before one or two are found that are effective and safe for any given child.

Since there is a narrow margin between effective and toxic doses, the levels are monitored regularly until the dosage is sufficient to maintain the optimum level and a satisfactory clinical response. The total daily dose is divided into four doses to be administered with each meal and at bedtime. Some find better compliance when the drug is given only twice daily.

The second group of drugs are the ***slower-acting antirheumatic drugs (SAARDs).*** These include gold, D-penicillamine, and hydroxychloroquine. SAARDs may be added to the regimen when one or two NSAIDs have been ineffective. Injectable gold is the initial SAARD used. The weekly injections can be a problem with young children, but cooperation is important. An oral gold preparation is available but not yet approved for use in children. Hydroxychloroquine, an antimalarial drug that requires a longer period of time to effect a response, is seldom used in the United States.

Other drugs. Cytotoxic drugs, such as cyclophosphamide, azathioprine, chlorambucil, and methotrexate, are reserved for patients with severe debilitating disease and who have responded poorly to NSAIDs and SAARDs. During the last 5 years, the use of methotrexate has expanded symptomatic improvement in rheumatoid patients who use methotrexate (Fife, 1993).

Corticosteroids are the most potent antiinflammatory agents available. However, they do not cure the disease or prevent joint damage, and their chronic side effects are undesirable. They are administered in the lowest effective dose, are given on alternate days rather than daily, and are used for the shortest period possible. Indications for daily corticosteroid (prednisone) therapy are life-threatening disease (e.g., pericarditis), incapacitating systemic disease unresponsive to other antiinflammatory therapy, and iridocyclitis.

Physical Management. Programs of physical management are individualized for each child and are designed to reach the ultimate goal—preserving function and/or preventing deformity. Physical therapy is directed toward specific joints, focusing on strengthening muscles, mobilizing restricted joint motion, and preventing or correcting deformities; occupational therapy assumes responsibility for generalized mobility and performance of activities of daily living.

General treatment or maintenance programs vary; physiotherapists may be involved several times weekly to monthly in management of a home program (ideally in association with the child's school), or their visits may be limited to infrequent review of the home program for compliance, effectiveness, and need. Strength is frequently lost around the involved joints, and inactivity leads to generalized weakness. However, normal activities of daily living and the child's natural tendency to be active are usually sufficient to maintain muscle strength and joint mobility.

Exercising in a pool is excellent, since it allows freedom of movement with support and minimum gravitational pull. When joints are inflamed, heavy resistance aggravates the pain; at such times, simple isometric or tensing exercises that do not involve joint movement are generally tolerated and should be encouraged. Range-of-motion exercises are an important aspect of therapy and are continued after evidence of disease has disappeared in order to detect any signs of recurrence.

Most practitioners recommend splinting and positioning during rest to help minimize pain and prevent or reduce flexion deformity. Joints most frequently splinted are knees, wrists, and hands. Positioning during rest is also important. The child rests on a firm mattress with no pillow or a very low one and has no support under the knee. Loss of extension in the knee, hip, and wrist causes special problems; vigilance is required to detect the earliest signs of involvement, and vigorous attention must be given to specialized passive stretching, positioning, and resting splints to prevent deformity.

Surgery. The benefits of synovectomy, an established preventive and therapeutic procedure in adults, are questionable in the child with rheumatoid arthritis. It is used primarily in pauciarticular disease. In cases of synovitis, aspiration of synovial fluid–filled joints, followed by steroid injection, is an alternative to synovectomy. It may be tried once or twice before surgery is performed. Joint replacement is proving to be successful in older children who are fully grown. The cooperation of the child is imperative.

Nursing Considerations

Assessment

Nursing children with JRA involves assessment of their general health, the status of involved joints, and children's emotional response to all ramifications of the disease—pain, physical restrictions, therapies, and self-concept, especially in preadolescents and adolescents.

Nursing Diagnoses

Based on a thorough assessment, several nursing diagnoses are identified. The more common diagnoses for the child with JRA are included in the Nursing Care Plan on p. 1862. Others may apply in specific situations.

Planning

The goals for the child with JRA and the family include the following:

1. Child will exhibit signs of reduced joint inflammation and adequate joint function.
2. Child will experience no pain or reduction of pain to level acceptable to child.
3. Child will perform activities of daily living.
4. Child will maintain adequate energy level.
5. Child or family will demonstrate knowledge of medications and treatment modalities.
6. Child will express feelings and concerns.
7. Child and family will receive adequate support.

Implementation

The effects of the disease are manifested in every aspect of a the child's life—in physical activities, social experiences, and personality development. Much of the children's adjustment to the stresses and demands of the disease and the level of functioning they achieve are directly related to the reaction and support they receive from their family and the health professionals concerned with their care and management.

Relieve Pain. The pain of JRA is related to several aspects of the disease—disease severity, functional status, individual pain threshold, family variables, and psychologic adjustment. Although complete pain relief would be highly desirable, it is probably unrealistic. The aim is to provide as much relief as possible with antiinflammatory medication and other therapies to help children tolerate the pain and cope as effectively as possible (Lovell and Walco, 1989). At present, opioid administration is not a routine therapy for the chronic pain of JRA. Nonpharmacologic modalities have proved effective in modifying pain perception (see Pain Management, Chapter 26) and activities that aggravate pain.

Promote General Health. The general health of these children and their siblings must be considered and is often overlooked as parents and health personnel concentrate on the disease. A well-balanced diet and assessment of nutritional status are integral parts of health supervision. The discomfort and increased need for rest may create problems of weight control. Excess weight causes additional strain on inflamed joints, especially those of the lower extremities. Excessive fatigue and overexertion should be avoided by regular periods of rest, especially during acute flare-ups of arthritis. Symptoms may exacerbate during a viral illness.

Posture and body mechanics are important for children with JRA, both when they are at rest and when they are active. They must have a firm mattress to maintain good alignment of the spine, hips, and knees and no pillow or a very thin one. Children who are confined to bed either at home or in the hospital may require supports or splints to maintain positioning. Waterbeds or an electric blanket (or electric sheet) placed under the bottom sheet provides comforting warmth. Lying in the prone position is encouraged to straighten the hips and knees, which they can do during rest periods or while watching television. The family is instructed in the principles and purposes of splints so that they can use them judiciously.

School-age children are encouraged to attend school, even on days when there may be some pain or discomfort. The aid of the school nurse is enlisted so that a child is permitted to take the prescribed medication at school and to arrange for rest in the nurse's office during the day. Split days or half days may help a child remain involved in school. Permitting the child to come to school late allows time to gain joint movement and reduces the time at school to avoid exhaustion. It is important that the child attend school to learn skills and engage in social interaction, especially if the JRA continues to limit physical skills. Arranging for two sets of textbooks eliminates the need to carry heavy or numerous books to and from school, thus reducing discomfort and difficulty in ambulating.

Facilitate Compliance. The child and family are involved in the therapeutic plan. They need to know the purpose and correct use of any splints and appliances and the medication regimen. The family is instructed regarding administration of medications as well as the value of a regular schedule of administration to maintain a satisfactory drug level in the body. They need to know that aspirin, as well as most NSAIDs, should not be given on an empty stomach and to be alert for signs of aspirin toxicity and NSAID toxicity, which include hyperventilation as a sign of acidosis, bleeding from decreased clotting capacity, tinnitus (ringing in the ears) as a sign of cranial nerve VIII involvement, and undue drowsiness that may indicate central nervous system depression. If evidence of drug toxicity is noted, the family is instructed to stop the medication and notify the health professional.

Encourage Heat and Exercise. Heat has been shown to be beneficial to children with arthritis. Moist heat is best for relieving pain and stiffness, and the most efficient and practical method is in the bathtub. The temperature and duration of the bath are specified by the therapist but usually do not exceed 10 minutes at 37.8° C (100° F). Sometimes a daily whirlpool bath, paraffin bath, or hot packs may be used as needed for temporary relief of acute swelling and pain. Hot packs are easily applied at home using a Turkish towel wrung out after being immersed in hot water or heated in a microwave oven, applied to the area, and covered with plastic for 20 minutes. Painful hands or feet can be immersed in a pan of water for 10 minutes two or three times daily in addition to tub baths.

Pool therapy is the easiest method for exercising a large number of joints. Swimming activities strengthen muscles and maintain mobility in larger joints. Children in urban areas have access to a therapy pool, although transportation may be a problem for some families. Very small children who are frightened of the water can carry out their exercises in the bathtub. Small children love to splash, kick, and throw things in the water.

Activities of daily living provide satisfactory exercise for older children to maintain maximum mobility with minimum pain. These children should be encouraged in their efforts and patiently allowed to dress and groom themselves, to assume daily tasks, and to care for their belongings. It is often difficult for stiff fingers to manipulate buttons, comb or brush hair, and turn faucets, but parents and other caregivers should not offer assistance to them. In addition, children should learn and understand why others do not help them. Many helpful devices, such as self-adhering fasteners, tongs for manipulating difficult items, and grab bars installed in bathrooms for safety, can be employed to facilitate tasks. A raised toilet seat often makes the difference between dependent and independent toileting, since weak quadriceps muscles and sore knees inhibit the ability to raise the body from a low sitting position.

A child's natural affinity for play offers many opportunities for incorporating therapeutic exercises. Throwing or kicking a ball, hanging from monkey bars, and riding a tricycle (with seat raised to achieve maximum leg extension) are excellent moving and stretching exercises for a very young child whose daily living activities are physically limited.

An effective approach to beginning the day's activities is to awaken children early to give them the medication and then to allow them to sleep for an hour. On arising, children take a hot bath (or shower) and perform a simple ritual of limbering-up exercises, after which they commence the activities of the day, such as going to school. Exercise, heat, and rest are spaced throughout the remainder of the day according to individual needs and schedules. Parents are instructed in exercises that fit the needs of the child.

➤ **NURSING TIP** Another method of supplying warmth before the child arises is to plug an electric blanket into an appliance timer. Set the blanket to medium or high and adjust the timer to turn on the blanket 1 hour before the child awakens.

The **Arthritis Foundation*** and the **American Juvenile Arthritis Foundation*** provide services for both parents and professionals, and nurses should refer families to these agencies as an added resource.

The Child. JRA affects every aspect of the child's daily life. The physical pain and limitations interfere with performance of normal tasks and provision of self-care. Even simple tasks, such as dressing, hair combing, use of the bathroom, cutting food, climbing stairs, manipulating doors and faucets, and using public transportation, are difficult or impossible. There may be school difficulties related to transportation to and from school, stairs, and loss of time as a result of exacerbations and hospitalization. Physical limitations interfere with participation in many activities, both curricular and extracurricular, which limits peer contacts and interaction and increases social isolation. These problems are especially critical for adolescents, for whom peer acceptance and relationships are so vital to personality development (see Family Focus box). These children increasingly turn to solitary activities and to the family at a time when they are expected to move into greater independence and relationships with peers.

Changes in personality usually accompany JRA, as with any chronic illness. These changes may be temporary, such as demanding, irritable behavior, or may be manifested in a more permanent way, such as passive hostility, uncommunicativeness, and manipulativeness. Efforts should be made to break through the child's defenses and to identify anxieties, concerns, and conflicts in order to intervene early to prevent the development of permanent personality problems. (See Chapter 22 for care of the child with chronic illness.)

The Family. The beginning of the disease is often sudden and frightening, and its variable course with cycles of remissions and exacerbations is discouraging. Many parents become susceptible to unorthodox cures advanced by well-meaning friends and advertisers. These should be carefully evaluated. Obviously harmless measures such as wearing a copper bracelet need not be discouraged, but parents must be dissuaded from questionable or conspicuously harmful practices such as active exercising of swollen, feverish joints. Parents' understanding of the disease and their attitude toward the child are the key to the success or failure of a treatment program, and major foci of nursing intervention are parental education and support.

Nurses are alert to cues that signal undue anxiety and guilt that may lead to an unhealthy degree of overprotection, such as preoccupation with causative factors, constant analysis of the effects of various therapies, experimentation with diets, and continual searching for a magical cure. The dangers of parental overprotection and overindulgence can be especially detrimental to the progress of the child. Sometimes parents are hesitant to give prescribed medications, keep the child home from school unnecessarily, restrict interaction with age-mates, exhibit reluctance to discipline the child, and assume self-care activities that are best performed by the child.

Most of the reactions, problems, and concerns of families of a child with JRA are those of any parents of a child with a chronic illness or disability. The impact of the diagnosis is felt most acutely by the parents, who demonstrate anxiety, guilt, and all the manifestations of the grief process. The concerns and needs of these families are discussed extensively in Chapter 22, and the reader is directed to this chapter for additional guidance in planning care.

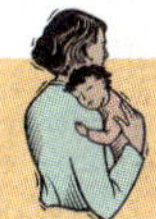

FAMILY FOCUS
Juvenile Rheumatoid Arthritis

As a nurse, and mother of a child with JRA, I believe it is important for nurses to always keep in mind the feelings and emotions of children with JRA.

Emotionally, I think the preadolescent/adolescent age-group of children with JRA have the most questions and concerns about their disease. Children, including my daughter, often ask, "Why me?" Adolescence/preadolescence is an age of socialization and change. These children want to be part of the social scene, to be included. Often these children are limited in their activities. Nurses need to emphasize to their patients, as well as the patients' families, the positive accomplishments these children have made. They need to know that we, as nurses, parents, and doctors, don't know why they have the arthritis, but that we will help and encourage them as much as possible in all aspects of their lives.

Disfigurement of joints, weight gain, weight loss, bloating, and physical impairments are all important in the eyes of a preteen/teenager. They must understand and accept themselves for who they are and not what they look like or appear to look like.

Communication with my daughter was and still is very essential. Nurses have an opportunity to enforce positive attitudes and encourage open communication with their patients. I feel it is very important for nurses to always keep in mind that nursing skills are essential, but communication with patients and families is equally important. It is the key to nursing assessment.

Sandra L. Guyette, RN
Shriner's Hospital
Springfield, MA

❖ EVALUATION

The effectiveness of nursing interventions is determined by continual reassessment and evaluation of care based on the following observational guidelines and expected outcomes:

1. Observe child's behavior and employ pain assessment techniques.
2. Conduct routine assessment of child's general health.
3. Observe the child during planned and unplanned activities,

---

*1314 Spring St., N.W., Atlanta, GA 30309; (404) 872-7100 or (800) 283-7800. In Canada: the **Arthritis Society,** 250 Bloor St., E., Suite 401, Toronto, Ontario, Canada M4W 3P2; (416) 967-5679.

NURSING CARE PLAN

The Child with Juvenile Rheumatoid Arthritis

NURSING DIAGNOSIS: Pain related to joint inflammation

PATIENT GOAL 1: Will exhibit signs of reduced joint inflammation

• **NURSING INTERVENTIONS/*RATIONALES***

*Administer antiinflammatory drugs as prescribed *to suppress inflammatory process of JRA*

• **EXPECTED OUTCOMES**

Child exhibits no evidence of discomfort
Joints indicate no evidence of inflammation

PATIENT GOAL 2: Will experience no pain or reduction of pain to level acceptable to child

• **NURSING INTERVENTIONS/*RATIONALES***

Provide heat to painful joints by way of the following *to relieve pain and stiffness*
- Tub baths, including whirlpool
- Paraffin baths
- Warm, moist pads
- Soaks

Maintain preventive schedule of drug administration *to reduce likelihood of pain occurring*
Avoid overexercising painful, swollen joints *because exercise at this time will aggravate pain*
Implement nonpharmacologic pain reduction techniques *to modify pain perception* (see Chapter 26)
Provide well-balanced diet to avoid excess weight gain, *which can cause additional strain on inflamed joints*

• **EXPECTED OUTCOME**

Child is able to move with no or minimum discomfort

NURSING DIAGNOSIS: Impaired physical mobility related to joint discomfort and stiffness

PATIENT GOAL 1: Will exhibit signs of adequate joint function

• **NURSING INTERVENTIONS/*RATIONALES***

Carry out or supervise physical therapy regimen
- Muscle-strengthening exercises
- Joint mobilization exercises

Apply splints, sandbags, if needed, *to maintain position and reduce flexion deformity during rest*
Lie flat in bed on a firm mattress with joints extended *to reduce flexion deformity*
Use prone position frequently with no pillow, or a very thin one *to maintain good alignment of spine, hips, knees*
Incorporate therapeutic exercises in play activities
- Swimming
- Throwing a ball
- Hanging from monkey bar
- Riding tricycle or bicycle

Encourage child to be physically active but in a way that does not excessively strain affected joints (e.g., swimming)
Supervise and encourage activities of daily living, *since these provide exercise*
Encourage child's natural tendency to be active
Frequently assess joint function *so that appropriate treatment is instituted to prevent deformity*

• **EXPECTED OUTCOMES**

Joint flexibility improves in relation to baseline findings
Child develops no contractures
Child engages in activities suitable to interests, capabilities, and developmental level

NURSING DIAGNOSIS: Bathing/hygiene, dressing/grooming, feeding, or toileting self-care deficit related to discomfort, impaired joint mobility

PATIENT GOAL 1: Will perform activities of daily living

• **NURSING INTERVENTIONS/*RATIONALES***

Encourage maximum independence; avoid doing for child what child is capable of doing
Provide and/or help devise methods *to facilitate independent functioning*
- Select clothes for convenience in putting on and fastening
- Modify utensils (spoons, toothbrush, comb, and so on) for easier grasp
- Elevate toilet seat, if needed, *to facilitate independent toileting*
- Install handrails for convenience and safety (in hallways, bathroom)

Teach application of splints (when able) and encourage responsibility for their use

• **EXPECTED OUTCOME**

Child is involved in activities of daily living to maximum capabilities

PATIENT GOAL 2: Will maintain adequate energy level

• **NURSING INTERVENTIONS/*RATIONALES***

Schedule regular periods for sleep and rest, especially during acute flare-ups, *to conserve energy*
Include school nurse and teachers in planning for needed rest during school day
Encourage child to participate in activities *that do not cause excessive fatigue or overexertion*

• **EXPECTED OUTCOMES**

Child engages in appropriate activities without undue fatigue
Child receives adequate rest, sleep

*Dependent nursing action.

NURSING CARE PLAN
The Child with Juvenile Rheumatoid Arthritis—cont'd

NURSING DIAGNOSIS: Knowledge deficit related to introduction of new medications and treatment modalities

PATIENT/FAMILY GOAL 1: Will demonstrate knowledge of medications and treatment modalities

• **NURSING INTERVENTIONS/*RATIONALES***

Allow patient and parents to discuss concerns and fears *so that they are better able to learn*

Provide written information/guidelines for all medications and treatments ordered *so that they can refer to this as needed at home*

Involve patient/family in administration of medications and treatments

Document patient/family education

• **EXPECTED OUTCOMES**

Patient/family will be knowledgeable about medication and treatment modalities

Patient/family will recognize signs of adverse drug reaction/side effects

NURSING DIAGNOSIS: High risk for body image disturbance related to disease process

PATIENT GOAL 1: Will express feelings and concerns

• **NURSING INTERVENTIONS/*RATIONALES***

Be available to child *so that there are opportunities for expression of feelings and concerns*

Use therapeutic communication techniques (e.g., reflection, active listening, silence) *to encourage expression of feelings and concerns*

Explore and develop activities in which the child can succeed *to promote positive self-image*

Include the child in therapy and treatment decisions *to promote positive self-image and decrease sense of powerlessness*

Refer child to a support group for children with JRA

• **EXPECTED OUTCOME**

Child will express feelings and concerns

NURSING DIAGNOSIS: Altered family processes related to a situational crisis (child with a chronic illness)

PATIENT (FAMILY) GOAL 1: Will receive adequate support

• **NURSING INTERVENTIONS/*RATIONALES* AND EXPECTED OUTCOMES**

Refer family to special support group(s) and agencies

See also Nursing Care Plan: The Child with Chronic Illness or Disability, Chapter 22

assess mobility of joints, and observe the use of prescribed appliances.

4. Observe child's ability to perform activities of daily living.
5. Observe and interview child and family regarding feelings and concerns.

Expected outcomes:

See Nursing Care Plan, p. 1862.

SYSTEMIC LUPUS ERYTHEMATOSUS (SLE)

SLE, or lupus erythematosus (LE), which literally means "red wolf" because of the characteristic butterfly rash on the face of some affected individuals, is a chronic inflammatory disease of the collagen or supporting tissues of the body. It characteristically follows a course of remissions and exacerbations. Because connective tissue is found practically everywhere, almost any organ or structure can be affected.

LE in childhood consists of two basic types: a transient neonatal disease apparently related to maternal pathology and a group of chronic diseases, usually having their onset after infancy, that correspond to systemic LE (SLE), discoid LE, disseminated LE, subacute cutaneous LE, or lupus panniculitis seen in adults. The major portion of this discussion is limited to SLE.

Etiology

The cause of SLE is not known. It is believed that an autoimmune response to some inciting event such as stress, infection, extreme fatigue, or exposure to various chemicals, drugs, or excessive sunburn triggers a reaction that alters the body's immune response to its own tissues. Supporting evidence for this finding are the facts that (1) many individuals report such events before onset of symptoms and (2) such events enhance an exacerbation of known lupus disease.

Technically, SLE is not an inherited disease, although it demonstrates a tendency to occur within families. In addition, family members without actual disease may have findings suggestive of lupus, such as SLE cells, abnormal sensitivity to sun, a history of arthritis or allergies, or unusual drug reactions. It is well documented that some individuals develop a lupuslike reaction to drugs such as isoniazid, penicillin, tetracycline, sulfa preparations, phenothiazines, and phenytoin (Dilantin).

Clinical Manifestations

Because SLE can affect almost any tissue, the clinical manifestations are variable. The onset is usually insidious, with vague signs such as low-grade fever, arthritis or arthralgia; generalized aching; and rash. However, rapid involvement of vital organs, primarily the kidneys, can herald an accelerated course with minimum or absent involvement of other sites. The box below describes manifestations related to various tissues involved.

The majority of children (approximately 90%) with SLE have cutaneous involvement at some time during their illness, and about one third of children have skin disease as the chief complaint. Some patients experience sensitivity to cold (Raynaud phenomenon), especially in the hands and feet. Cyanosis may be present, and ulcers often develop in dry, cracked skin. Patchy areas of alopecia may occur, although during remission the hair usually regrows.

Renal involvement is a serious complication of SLE. Presumably, antigen-antibody complexes deposited primarily in the glomerular basement membrane initiate an inflammatory response that results in tissue damage and consequent kidney failure. Although supportive approaches, such as hemodialysis and kidney transplant, have improved the outlook for these patients, tissue damage in other vital organs, especially the heart and lungs, may foreshorten the benefits derived from life-supporting techniques.

MANIFESTATIONS OF SYSTEMIC LUPUS ERYTHEMATOSUS RELATED TO TISSUES INVOLVED

Cutaneous lesions—Erythematous blush or scaly erythematous patches over bridge of nose and extending to each cheek symmetrically ("butterfly rash"); may extend to scalp, neck, chest, and extremities; sometimes pruritic; resemble severe sunburn or hives or may become bullous

Musculoskeletal system—Generalized weakness, usually accompanied by arthritis, myalgia, joint swelling, and stiffness; usually not severe enough to cause deformity; pain may cause temporary disability

Central nervous system—Varies from forgetfulness, excitability, and headache to seizures and frank psychosis; seizures may be early sign; any cranial nerves can be affected; paralysis (spinal cord involvement)

Heart and lungs—Serous linings may be inflamed; pleurisy (lungs), pericarditis (heart); usually reversible with rest

Kidneys—Glomerulus usual site of destruction; proteinuria; kidney failure

Blood—Anemia from decreased erythrocytes common; amenorrhea secondary to anemia; platelets and plasma proteins may be affected

Lymphoid system—Spleen and cervical, axillary, and inguinal lymph nodes enlarged (sometimes); LE hepatitis may develop

Gastrointestinal tract—Nausea, vomiting, diarrhea, and abdominal pain possible

Diagnostic Evaluation

SLE has been called the "great imitator," since its clinical manifestations may point to a variety of unrelated conditions. The diagnosis of SLE is established by the demonstration of any 4 of 11 diagnostic criteria (see box below).

A neurologic examination should be done to provide baseline data for evaluating subtle changes in behavior and function. Sometimes a psychiatric evaluation may also be warranted, since personality alterations caused by steroids and renal damage are difficult to distinguish from those resulting from central nervous system involvement.

Therapeutic Management

There is no specific treatment for systemic lupus erythematosus. Rather, the objectives of medical treatment are (1) to reverse the autoimmune and inflammatory processes and (2) to prevent exacerbations and complications. Therapy involves the use of specific and supportive medications and regulation of activity and diet.

Drugs. The principal drugs used to control inflammation are the corticosteroids, administered in doses sufficient to suppress symptoms, then tapered to the lowest suppressive dose. One alternative is the "pulse" method, the administration of a large dose of steroids intravenously over a 20- to 30-minute period on 3 consecutive days. Large doses may be needed to treat seizures and other central nervous system manifestations. Sometimes the immunosuppressive agent azathioprine (Imuran) helps reduce the amount of steroids needed.

Another group of drugs effective in relieving the dermatologic, arthritic, and renal symptoms of the disease are antimalarial preparations, such as hydroxychloroquine (Plaquenil) and chloroquine (Aralen). Although the exact action of these drugs on SLE is not known, often they permit a continued remission with a lowered dose of steroids. Cyclophosphamide and azathioprine (cytotoxic drugs), along with steroids, are now used for patients with severe manifestations.

NSAIDs, such as aspirin, relieve muscle and joint pains and reduce tissue inflammation. Drugs used to control various complications include anticonvulsants, antihyperten-

CRITERIA FOR DIAGNOSIS OF SYSTEMIC LUPUS ERYTHEMATOSUS

1. Butterfly rash
2. Discoid rash
3. Photosensitivity
4. Oral ulcers
5. Arthritis
6. Serositis
7. Renal disorder
8. Neurologic disorder(s) (psychosis, coma, seizures, paresis)
9. Hematologic disorder(s) (anemia, thrombocytopenia, leukopenia)
10. Immunologic disorder(s) (anti-DNA, LE prep, anti-SM, STS)
11. Antinuclear antibody (ANA)

sives, and antibiotics. The selection of appropriate medication in each of these categories is essential, since many of them greatly aggravate the disease process and affect renal function. Assessing for toxicity with all drug therapies is most important in these patients.

Regulation of Activity and Diet. The goal of restricted activity is to prevent a recurrence of the disease. Although the exact relationship is unclear, fatigue, stress, or sudden exertion brings about a relapse of symptoms. An effective schedule must provide for gradual resumption of pre-SLE activity and maximum rest periods, usually 8 to 10 hours of sleep a night and one or two rest times during the day.

Diet may be restricted depending on weight gain and/or fluid retention from steroids and renal damage. The most frequently prescribed diet modification is moderate or low salt. Low-protein diets may be necessary to prevent elevated nitrogen levels. Weight reduction may help preserve maximum joint function and conserve energy.

Nursing Considerations

The principal nursing goals are to (1) help the child and family adjust to the limitations and treatments of the disease and (2) prevent exacerbations and complications. Since older female adolescents are the most likely group to be affected, the nurse must have an awareness of their special needs, such as body image changes, present and future vocational activities, social relationships, and emerging sexuality. Although this is a potentially fatal disorder, nurses are encouraged to apply those principles of adjusting to a chronic illness that are discussed in Chapter 22.

Assist Family in Adjusting to Disease and its Treatment. SLE is a complex disease. Although much is known about its effect on connective tissues and appropriate types of treatment, few concrete facts are available. However, family members need an understanding of the disease process to gain an appreciation of the necessity of regular, uninterrupted drug administration, moderate activity, and dietary modifications. Usually, diagnostic tests are performed during hospitalization, which allows the nurse an opportunity to help the family learn about the disease.

Several organizations have been formed to help children and families learn about and adjust to the disease. These include the **American Lupus Society*** and the **Lupus Foundation of America.**† The nurse should be aware of what information the family is receiving, because learning about joint deformity, sudden bouts of pain and disability, a disfiguring rash, and the possibility of renal failure can be overwhelming. Nurses should also be aware of advertised nonmedical approaches to treatment, since quackery abounds when no known cure exists.

The nurse has the responsibility of helping the adolescent adjust to drug therapy. The side effects of steroids and immunosuppressant drugs are discussed under Modes of Therapy, Chapter 36, and outlined in Table 36-2. Most of the antimalarial drugs have few side effects. However, hydroxychloroquine and chloroquine can cause irreversible retinal damage; therefore, frequent ophthalmic examinations are necessary. In addition, after exposure to the sun, the skin may tan less and become more erythematous and the hair may lighten.

Body image changes from both the disease and the drugs are a major concern. Each of these should be approached in a positive manner by discussing the use of cosmetics and wigs. Sometimes health professionals fail to assess adequately the child's adjustment reactions and regard the depression and withdrawal as effects of the disease rather than a response to body image changes.

Lifelong restricted activity imposes many hardships for these children, although they may be able to continue to participate in moderation. The child and family need to weigh the consequences of activity against the pleasures. For example, a day of skiing, with proper sun precautions, may be worth the achiness for the following day or even week. This provides the youngster with some sense of control over events. The severity of the disease is also a factor if the risk of irreversible damage is great.

Prevent Exacerbations and Complications. The list of "don'ts" for these individuals is long; therefore compliance may be a serious problem. The need for adherence to the medication schedule is paramount. Some adolescents, in an attempt to lessen the side effects of steroids, may elect to skip a few doses. Adherence is important to maintain a remission but must be taken daily (or as prescribed) to prevent sudden withdrawal from the drug, which may precipitate a serious physiologic crisis. The dosage may need to be altered at times of stress. Affected persons should carry an identification card or Medic Alert tag emphasizing their dependence on steroids.

Skin care is important. In those individuals who are sensitive to the sun, exposure must be avoided. It is important to stress that reflected sun through clouds, on snow, on water, or on white cement can cause a severe reaction. Although clothes can protect most areas of the body, special sunscreening agents are necessary for the face (see Chapter 18). A large-brimmed hat helps to shade the face.

Sometimes patients are requested to check their urine routinely for protein. The youngster with kidney involvement is subject to long-term management that may entail hemodialysis and/or a kidney transplant. Nursing considerations for each procedure are discussed in Chapter 30.

*23751 Madison St., Torrence, CA 90505; (310) 542-8891.

†4 Research Place, Suite 180, Rockville, MD 20850; (301) 670-9292 or (800) 558-0121.

KEY POINTS

- Trauma is the leading cause of death in children and is caused by accidental injury, child abuse injury, and birth injuries.
- Immobility has a profound effect on all elements of growth and development.
- The major consequences of immobilization are loss of muscle strength, endurance, and muscle mass; bone demineralization leading to osteoporosis; loss of joint mobility; and contractures.
- In the care of the immobilized child, nurses are concerned

with position changes, adequate dietary intake, adequate hydration, promotion of activity, and involvement of the child in self-care.

- Features of children's fractures not observed in the adult include presence of a growth plate, a thicker and stronger periosteum, porosity of bone, more rapid healing, and less stiffness.
- Types of fractures seen in children are bends, buckle, greenstick, and complete.
- Goals of fracture management in children are to regain alignment and length of the bony fragments, retain alignment and length, and restore function to injured parts.
- The method of fracture reduction is determined by the age of the child, the degree of displacement, the amount of overriding bone, the amount of edema, the condition of the skin and soft tissues, sensation, and circulation distal to the fracture.
- The primary purposes of traction are to fatigue involved muscle and reduce muscle spasm, to position bone ends in desired realignment, and to immobilize the fracture site until realignment has been achieved to permit casting or splinting.
- Complications of fractures are circulatory impairment, nerve compression syndromes, compartment syndromes, epiphyseal damage, nonunion, malunion, infection, kidney stones, and pulmonary emboli.
- Participation in sports predisposes adolescents to acute injuries, such as contusions, dislocations, sprains, and strains, and overuse syndromes, such as stress fractures.
- Health concerns associated with sports are related menstrual dysfunction, drug misuse, and sudden death.
- Musculoskeletal dysfunctions in childhood include torticollis, Legg-Calvé-Perthes disease, slipped femoral capital epiphyses, kyphosis and lordosis, and scoliosis.
- Observation for scoliosis is an important part of a routine physical assessment.
- Management of scoliosis includes bracing and/or surgery.
- Postoperative nursing care of the child with scoliosis demands careful attention to movement, respiratory function, pain control, and skin care.
- Nursing care of the child with osteomyelitis is directed at positioning, careful monitoring of vital signs, drugs, intravenous equipment and site, and nutrition.
- Osteomyelitis is acquired by direct or secondary invasion or hematogenous spread of infectious organisms.
- Goals of therapy for juvenile arthritis are to preserve joint function, prevent physical deformities, and relieve symptoms without iatrogenic harm.
- Nursing care of the child with juvenile rheumatoid arthritis consists of promoting general health, relieving discomfort, preventing deformity, and preserving function.
- Lupus erythematosus is a chronic autoimmune disorder that affects the collagen tissues of the body.

REFERENCES

American Academy of Pediatrics, Committee on Aspects of Physical Fitness, Recreation, and Sports, *Pediatrics* 67:927-928, 1981.

American Academy of Pediatrics, Committee on Injury and Poison Prevention: Drowning in infants, children, and adolescents, *Pediatrics* 92(2):292-294, 1993.

American Academy of Pediatrics, Committee on Sports Medicine: *Sports medicine: health care for young athletes,* Evanston, IL, 1983, American Academy of Pediatrics.

American Academy of Pediatrics, Committee on Sports Medicine: Participation in boxing among children and young adults, *Pediatrics* 74:311-312, 1984.

American Academy of Pediatrics, Committee on Sports Medicine: Recommendations for participation in competitive sports, *Pediatrics* 81:737-739, 1988.

American Academy of Pediatrics, Committee on Sports Medicine: Anabolic steroids and the adolescent athlete, *Pediatrics* 83:127-128, 1989.

American Academy of Pediatrics, Section on Rheumatology and Section on Ophthalmology: Guidelines for ophthalmologic examinations in children with juvenile rheumatoid arthritis, *Pediatrics* 92(2):295-296, 1993.

Braisted JR and others: The adolescent ballet dancer: nutritional practices and characteristics associated with anorexia nervosa, *J Adolesc Health Care* 6:365-371, 1985.

Bostrom B, McCormick P, Hooke C: Painless procedures with Propofol, *J Pediatr Oncol Nurs* 10(2):64-65, 1993.

Butler AB, Salmond SW, Pellino TA: *Orthopaedic nursing,* Philadelphia, 1994, WB Saunders.

Carlino HY: The child with an Ilizarov external fixator, *Pediatr Nurs* 17(4):355-358, 1991.

Dyment PG: Initial management of minor acute soft-tissue injuries, *Pediatr Ann* 17:99-106, 1988.

Emery HM, Miller ML: *Ambulatory pediatric care,* ed 2, Philadelphia, 1993, JB Lippincott.

Fife RZ: Methotrexate use in juvenile rheumatoid arthritis, *Orthop Nurs* 12(1):32-36, 1993.

Grant HD, Murray RH Jr, Bergeron JD: *Brady emergency care,* ed 6, Englewood Cliffs, NJ, 1994, Prentice Hall.

Gratz RR, Papalia-Finlay D: Psychosocial adaptation to wearing the Milwaukee brace for scoliosis: a pilot study of adolescent females and their mothers, *J Adolesc Health Care* 5:237-242, 1984.

Johnson MD and others: Anabolic steroid use by male adolescents, *Pediatrics* 83:921-924, 1989.

Loosli AR: Athletes, food and nutrition, *Food Nutr News* 62(3):15-20, 1990.

Lovell DJ, Walco GA: Pain associated with juvenile rheumatoid arthritis, *Pediatr Clin North Am* 36:1015-1027, 1989.

Morais T and others: Age- and sex-specific prevalence of scoliosis and the value of school screening programs, *Am J Public Health* 75:1377-1380, 1985.

National Youth Sports Foundation for the Prevention of Athletic Injuries: *Fact sheet,* Needham, MA, 1993, The Foundation.

Nelson MA: Androgenic-anabolic steroid use in adolescents, *J Pediatr Health Care* 3:175-180, 1989.

Nichols HH: Nursemaid's elbow: reducing it to simple terms, *Contemp Pediatr* 5(5):50-57, 1988.

Northrup CE, Kelly ME: *Legal issues in nursing,* St Louis, 1987, Mosby.

Orava S: Stress fractures, *Br J Sports Med* 14:40-44, 1980.

Ostrum G: Sports-related injuries in youth: prevention is the key and nurses can help, *Pediatr Nurs* 19(1):333-342, 1993.

Pillemer FG, Micheli LJ; Psychological considerations in youth sports, *Clin Sports Med* 7(3):679-689, 1988.

Poussa M and others: Conservative vs. operative treatment in Perthes' disease, *Clin Orthop* 297:82-86, 1993.

Primos WA, Landry GL: Fighting the fads in sports nutrition, *Contemp Pediatr* 6(9):14-50, 1989.

Rosenstein BJ: Summer tips: heat exhaustion and heatstroke, *Contemp Pediatr* 6(5):92-93, 1989.

Runyan CW, Gerken EA: Epidemiology and prevention of adolescent injury: a review and research agenda, *JAMA* 262:2273-2279, 1989.

Screening for adolescent idiopathic scoliosis: policy statement, US Preventive Services Task Force, *JAMA* 269(20):2664-2666, 1993.

Squire DL: Female athletes, *Pediatr Rev* 9:183-187, 1987.

Staheli LT: The hip. In Gellis SS, Kagan BM: *Current pediatric therapy 12,* Philadelphia, 1986, WB Saunders.

Theintz GE and others: Evidence for a reduction of growth potential in adolescent female gymnasts, *J Pediatr* 122(2):306-313, 1993.

Tobias JD and others: Oral ketamine premedication to alleviate the distress of invasive procedures in pediatric oncology patients, *Pediatrics* 90(4):537-541, 1992.

Van Allen MW: The deadly degrading sport, *JAMA* 249:249-250, 1983, (editorial).
Viviani GR and others: Assessment of accuracy of the scoliosis school screening examination, *Am J Public Health* 74:497-498, 1984.
Warren MP and others: Scoliosis and fractures in young ballet dancers: relation to delayed menarche and secondary amenorrhea, *N Engl J Med* 309:1348-1353, 1986.
Wattenmaker I, Kasser JR, McGravey A: Self-administered nitrous oxide for fracture reduction in children in an emergency room setting, *J Orthop Trauma* 4(1):35-38, 1990.
Watts HG: Orthopedic problems. In Behrman RE, Vaughan VC, III: *Textbook of pediatrics,* ed 13, Philadelphia, 1987, WB Saunders.
Weinstein SL: *The pediatric spine: principles and practice,* New York, 1994, Raven Press.
Wong D, Baker C: Pain in children: comparison of assessment scales, *Pediatr Nurs* 14(1):9-17, 1988.

BIBLIOGRAPHY

General

Blatzheim LL, Edberg A, Lacy L: Operationalizing primary nursing in the pediatric rehabilitation setting, *J Pediatr Nurs* 2:434-437, 1987.
Brady M, Grey M: Growing pains: a myth or a reality, *J Pediatr Health Care* 3:219-220, 1989.
Bubulka GM, Cipolla F: Preparing for pediatric emergencies, *J Emerg Nurs* 17(4):236-240, 1991.
Dudek G: Nursing update: hypophosphatemic rickets, *Pediatr Nurs* 15:45-50, 1989.
Mason KJ: Pediatric orthopaedics: developmental norms, *Orthop Nurs* 8(4):45-50, 1989.
National Association of Orthopaedic Nurses: Cues for orthopaedic patient care: common concerns, *Orthop Nurs* 10(5):73-74, 1991.
Sills EM: What's causing the back pain? *Contemp Pediatr* 5(11):85-96, 1988.
Szer IS: Are those limb pains "growing" pains? *Contemp Pediatr* 6(3):143-148, 1989.

Trauma

Alexander R and others: Serial abuse in children who are shaken, *Am J Dis Child* 144:58-60, 1990.
Campbell LS, Campbell JD: Musculoskeletal trauma in children, *Crit Care Nurs Clin North Am* 3(3):445-456, 1991.
Harris BH and others: The crucial hour, *Pediatr Ann* 16:301-304, 1987.
Jamison DW: When emergency care is up to you, *RN* 50(4):26-31, 1987.
Leyendecker M and others: Rescuing a multiple trauma victim, *Nursing 89* 19(10):54-61, 1989.
Nypaver M, Treloar D: Neutral cervical spine positioning in children, *Ann Emerg Med* 23(2):208-211, 1994.
Reed JL, Keegan MJ: Fat embolism syndrome: a complication of trauma, *Crit Care Nurse* 13(3):33-37, 1993.

Immobilization

Baird SE: Development of a nursing assessment tool to diagnose altered body image in immobilized patients, *Orthop Nurs* 4(1):47-54, 1985.
Karn MA, Ragiel CA: The psychologic effects of immobilization on the pediatric patient, *Orthop Nurs* 5(6):12-16, 1986.
Mehmert PA, Delaney CW: Validating impaired physical mobility, *Nurs Diagn* 2(4):143-154, 1991.
Olson EV: The hazards of immobility, *Am J Nurs* 90:43-52, 1990.
Quellet LL, Rush KL: A synthesis of selected literature on mobility: a basis for studying impaired mobility, *Nurs Diagn* 3(2):72-80, 1992.
Rubin M: The physiology of bed rest, *Am J Nurs* 88:50-58, 1988.
Willey T: High-tech beds and mattress overlays, *Am J Nurs* 89:1142-1145, 1989.

Fractures

Benz J: The adolescent in a spica cast, *Orthop Nurs* 5(3):22-23, 1986.
Conrad EU, Rang MC: Fractures and sprains, *Pediatr Clin North Am* 33:1523-1540, 1986.
Cuddy CM: Caring for a child in a spica cast: a parent's perspective, *Orthop Nurs* 5(3):17-20, 1986.
Feller NG, Stroup K, Christian L: Helping staff nurses become mini-specialists, *Am J Nurs* 89:991-992, 1989.
Gamron R: Taking the pressure out of compartment syndrome, *Am J Nurs* 88:1076-1080, 1988.
Hansell MJ: Fractures and the healing process, *Orthop Nurs* 7(1):43-49, 1988.
Hergenroeder AC: Diagnosis and treatment of ankle sprains, *Am J Dis Child* 144(7):809-814, 1990.
Lavin RJ: The high-pressure demands of compartment syndrome, *RN* 52(2):22-25, 1989.
Mather MLS: The secret to life in a spica, *Am J Nurs* 87:56-58, 1987.
McCullough FL: Skeletal trauma in children, *Orthop Nurs* 8(2):41-50, 1989.
Rang M, Wright J: Pitfalls in fractures, *Pediatr Ann* 18:53-68, 1989.
Redheffer GM, Bailely M: Assessing and splinting fractures, *Nursing 89* 19(6):51-59, 1989.
Sonzogni JJ, Gross M: Hip and pelvic injuries in the young: fractures and special disorders, part 2, *Emerg Med* 25(8):18-20+, 1993.

Amputation

Cmiel PA, Cavanaugh CE: Digital replantation in children, *Am J Nurs* 89:1158-1161, 1989.
McGrath PA, Hillier LM: Phantom limb sensations in adolescents: a case study to illustrate the utility of sensation and pain logs in pediatric clinical practice, *J Pain Symptom Manage* 7:46-53, 1992.
Rounseville C: Phantom limb pain: the ghost that haunts the amputee, *Orthop Nurs* 11(2):67-71, 1992.
Sherman R: Stump and phantom limb pain, *Neurol Clin* 1(2):249-263, 1989.
Varni JW and others: Family functioning, temperament, and psychologic adaptation in children with congenital or acquired limb deficiencies, *Pediatrics* 84:323-330, 1989.
Williamson VC: Amputation of the lower extremity: an overview, *Orthop Nurs* 11(2):55-65, 1992.

Disorders Related to Sports

American Academy of Pediatrics, Committee on Sports Medicine: Amenorrhea in adolescent athletes, *Pediatrics* 84:394-395, 1989.
American Academy of Pediatrics, Committee on Sports Medicine: Knee brace use by athletes, *Pediatrics* 85:228, 1990.
Backous DD and others: Soccer injuries and their relation to physical maturity, *Am J Dis Child* 142:839-842, 1988.
Council on Scientific Affairs: Drug abuse in athletes, *JAMA* 259:1703-1705, 1988.
Davis JM, Kuppermann N, Fleisher G: Serious sports injuries requiring hospitalization seen in a pediatric emergency department, *Am J Dis Child* 147(9):1001-1004, 1993.
DuRant RH and others: Findings from the preparticipation athletic examination and athletic injuries, *Am J Dis Child* 146:85-91, 1992.
Dyment PG: How to make the sports physical exciting, *Contemp Pediatr* (10):93-106, 1991.
Goldberg B and others: Injuries in youth football, *Pediatrics* 81:255-261, 1988.
Kelly JP and others: Concussion in sports, *JAMA* 266(20):2867-2869, 1991.
Kris-Etherton PM: Nutrition and athletic performance, *Contemp Nutr* 14(8), 1989.
Krowchuk DP and others: High school athletes and the use of ergogenic aids, *Am J Dis Child* 143:486-489, 1989.
Mansfield MJ, Emans SJ: Growth in female gymnasts: should training decrease during puberty? *J Pediatr* 122(2):237-240, 1993.
McLain LG, Reynolds S: Sports injuries in a high school, *Pediatrics* 84:446-450, 1989.
Nickerson HJ and others: Causes of iron deficiency in adolescent athletes, *J Pediatr* 114:657-663, 1989.
Ouellette MD, MacVicar MG, Harlan J: Relationship between percent body fat and menstrual patterns in athletes and nonathletes, *Nurs Res* 35:330-333, 1986.
Pope HG, Katz DL: Affective and psychotic symptoms associated with anabolic steroid use, *Am J Psychiatry* 145:487-491, 1988.
Pratt M: Strength, flexibility, and maturity in adolescent athletes, *Am J Dis Child* 143:560-563, 1989.
Rowland TW, Kelleher JF: Iron deficiency in athletes, *Am J Dis Child* 143:197-200, 1989.
Strong WB, Wilmore JH: Unfit kids: an office-based approach to physical fitness, *Contemp Pediatr* 5(4):33-48, 1988.
Terney R, McLain LG: The use of anabolic steroids in high school students, *Am J Dis Child* 144:99-103, 1990.
Yelverton GA: Anabolic steroids, *Pediatr Nurs* 15:63, 1989.
Yesalis C and others: Anabolic androgenic steroid use in the United States, *JAMA* 1270(10):1217-1221, 1993.

Scoliosis

Bridwell KH: Cotrel-Dubousset instrumentation, *Orthop Nurs* 7(1):11-16, 1988.
Brosnan H: Nursing management of the ado-

lescent with idiopathic scoliosis, *Nurs Clin North Am* 26(1):17-31, 1991.

Bunnel WP: Outcome of spinal screening, *Spine* 18(12):1572-1580, 1993.

Cassella M, Hall JE: Current treatment approaches in the nonoperative and operative management of adolescent idiopathic scoliosis, *Phys Ther* 71(12):897-909, 1991.

Cotton LA: Unit rod segmental spinal instrumentation for the treatment of neuromuscular scoliosis, *Orthop Nurs* 10(5):17-23, 1991.

DiRaimondo CV, Green NE: Brace-wear compliance in patients with adolescent idiopathic scoliosis, *J Pediatr Orthop* 8:143-146, 1988.

Jacobs-Zacny JM, Horn MJ: Nursing care of adolescents having posterior spinal fusion with Cotrel-Dubousset instrumentation, *Orthop Nurs* 7(1):17-21, 1988.

Johnson JB, Killman-Young J: Adolescence, anxiety, and adaptation: preparing for posterior spine fusion with instrumentation, *J Pediatr Nurs* 3:348-349, 1988.

Murrel GAC and others: An assessment of the reliability of the scoliometer, *Spine* 18(6): 709-712, 1993.

Rauen KK, Ho M: Children's use of patient-controlled analgesia after spine surgery, *Pediatr Nurs* 15:589-593, 1989.

Richardson A, Taylor M, Murphree B: TSRH instrumentation: evolution of a new system, *Orthop Nurs* 9(6):15-21, 1990.

Scoloveno MA, Yarcheski A, Mahon NE: Scoliosis treatment effects on selected variables among adolescents, *West J Nurs Res* 12(5): 616-619, 1990.

Voznak L: My life with scoliosis, *Orthop Nurs* 7(1):22-26, 1988.

Willers U and others: Long-term results of Harrington instrumentation in idiopathic scoliosis, *Spine* 18(6):713-717, 1993.

Musculoskeletal Disorders/Orthopaedic Infections

Barton LL, Dunkle LM, Habib FH: Septic arthritis in childhood, *Am J Dis Child* 141:898-900, 1987.

Bender LH: Osteogenesis imperfecta, *Orthop Nurs* 10(4):23-32, 1991.

Dunst RM: Legg-Calvé-Perthes disease, *Orthop Nurs* 9(2):18-27, 35-6, 1990.

Edwards MJ, Graham JM: Studies of type 1 collagen in osteogenesis imperfecta, *J Pediatr* 117(1):67-72, 1990.

Ekeberg DRE: Promoting a positive attitude in pediatric patients undergoing limb lengthening, *Orthop Nurs* 13(1):41-49, 1994.

Faden H, Grossi M: Acute osteomyelitis in children, *Am J Dis Child* 145(1):65-69, 1991.

Hart K: Using the Ilizarov external fixator in bone transport, *Orthop Nurs* 13(1):35-40, 1994.

Jacobs NM: Pneumococcal osteomyelitis and arthritis in children, *Am J Dis Child* 145(1): 70-74, 1991.

Kerrick RC, French C: Torticollis: a head and neck immobilizer, *Am J Occup Ther* 47(1):79-80, 1993.

Ledwith CA, Fleisher GR: Slipped capital femoral epiphysis without hip pain leads to missed diagnosis, *Pediatrics* 89(4):660-662, 1992.

Nance DK, Mardjetko SM: Technical aspects and nursing considerations of limb lengthening, *Orthop Nurs* 13(1):21-33, 1994.

Unkila-Kallio L and others: Serum C–reactive protein, erythrocyte sedimentation rate, and white blood cell count in acute hematogenous osteomyelitis of children, *Pediatrics* 93(1):59-62, 1994.

Juvenile Rheumatoid Arthritis

Arnett FC: Revised criteria for the classification on rheumatoid arthritis, *Orthop Nurs* 9(2):58-64, 1990.

Athreya BH, Cassidy JT: Current status of the medical treatment of children with juvenile rheumatoid arthritis, *Rheum Dis Clin North Am* 17(4):871-889, 1991.

Fantini F: Future trends in pediatric rheumatology, *J Rheumatol Suppl* 37:49-53, 1992.

Gorman TK, Marsh ME: Arthritis at an early age, *Am J Nurs* 84:1472-1477, 1984.

Graham LD and others: Morbidity associated with long-term methotrexate therapy in juvenile rheumatoid arthritis, *J Pediatr* 120(3): 468-473, 1992.

Haugen MS, Lynch PA: Diagnostic tests in pediatric rheumatology: application for nurses, *Pediatr Nurs* 13:389-393, 1987.

Harris ED: Rheumatoid arthritis: pathophysiology and implications for therapy, *N Engl J Med* 322(18):1277-1289, 1990.

Hollingworth P: The use of non-steroidal anti-inflammatory drugs in pediatric rheumatic diseases, *Br J Rheumatol* 32(1):73-77, 1993.

Hughes RB, D'Ambrosia K: Nursing management of a child with juvenile rheumatoid arthritis, *Orthop Nurs* 12(5):17-22, 1993.

Ignatavicius DD: Meeting the psychosocial needs of patients with rheumatoid arthritis, *Orthop Nurs* 6(3):16-20, 1987.

Konkol L and others: Impact of juvenile arthritis on families: an educational assessment, *Arthritis Care Res* 2(2):40-48, 1989.

Lavigne JV and others: Evaluation of a psychological treatment package for treating pain in juvenile rheumatoid arthritis, *Arthritis Care Res* 5(2):101-110, 1992.

Lovell DJ, Walco GA: Pain associated with juvenile rheumatoid arthritis, *Pediatr Clin North Am* 36(4):1015-1027, 1989.

Manners PJ, Ansell BM: Slow-acting antirheumatic drug use in systemic onset juvenile chronic arthritis, *Pediatrics* 77:99-103, 1986.

Mortensen ME, Rennebohm RM: Clinical pharmacology and use of nonsteroid anti-inflammatory drugs, *Pediatr Clin North Am* 36:1113-1139, 1989.

Mulberg AE and others: Non-steroidal anti-inflammatory drug (NSAID)–induced gastroduodenal injury in children with juvenile rheumatoid arthritis (JRA), *J Pediatr* 122:647-649, 1993.

Mulbery A and others: Non-steroidal anti-inflammatory drug (NSAID)–induced gastroduodenal injury in children with JRA, *J Pediatr* 122(4):647-649, 1993.

Page GG: Chronic pain and the child with juvenile rheumatoid arthritis, *J Pediatr Health Care* 5(1):18-23, 1991.

Page-Goertz SS: Even children have arthritis, *Pediatr Nurs* 15(1):11-16+, 1989.

Quirk ME, Young MH: The impact of JRA on children, adolescents, and their families: current research and implications for future studies, *Arthritis Care Res* 3(1):36-43, 1990.

Reed A and others: 25-Hydroxyvitamin D therapy in children with active juvenile rheumatoid arthritis: short-term effects on serum osteocalcin levels and bone mineral density, *J Pediatr* 119(4):657-660, 1991.

Rose CD: Pharmacological management of juvenile rheumatoid arthritis, *Drugs* 43(6):849-863, 1992.

Schneider R and others: Prognostic indicators of joint destruction in systemic-onset juvenile rheumatoid arthritis, *J Pediatr* 120(2, pt 1):200-205, 1992.

Sipos DA: M.P. implants for rheumatoid arthritis of the hand, *Orthop Nurs* 12(5):7-14, 1993.

Southwood TR and others: Unconventional remedies used for patients with juvenile arthritis, *Pediatrics* 85:150-154, 1990.

Swann M: The surgery of juvenile chronic arthritis: an overview, *Clin Orthop* (259):70-75, 1990.

Tolman KG: Hepatotoxicity of antirheumatic drug, *J Rheumatol* 17(suppl 22):6-11, 1990.

Truckenbrodt H: Pain in juvenile chronic arthritis: consequences for the muscle-skeletal system, *Clin Exp Rheumatol* 11(suppl 9):S59-S63, 1993.

Wallace CA: Juvenile rheumatoid arthritis: outcome and treatment for the 1990's, *Rheum Dis Clin North Am* 17(4):891-905, 1991.

White PH: Growth abnormalities in children with juvenile rheumatoid arthritis, *Clin Orthop* (259):46-50, 1990.

White PH, Ansell BM: Methotrexate for juvenile rheumatoid arthritis, *N Engl J Med* 326(16):1077-1078, 1992.

Winkel MF: Juvenile rheumatoid arthritis—parent support group: do parents perceive a need? *Pediatr Nurs* 14:131-132, 1988.

Systemic Lupus Erythematosus

Emery H: Clinical aspects of systemic lupus erythematosus in childhood, *Pediatr Clin North Am* 33:1177-1190, 1986.

Feutren G and others: Effects of cyclosporine in severe systemic lupus erythematosus, *J Pediatr* 111:1063-1068, 1987.

Fuller C, Hartley B: Systemic lupus erythematosus in adolescents, *J Pediatr Nurs* 6(4):251-257, 1991.

Lee LA, Weston WL: Lupus erythematosus in childhood, *Dermatol Clin* 4:151-160, 1986.

Lehman TJA and others: Systemic lupus erythematosus in the first year of life, *Pediatrics* 83:235-239, 1989.

McCurdy DK and others: Lupus nephritis: prognostic factors in children, *Pediatrics* 89(2):240-246, 1992.

Miller ML, Magilavy DB, Warren RW: The immunologic basis of lupus, *Pediatr Clin North Am* 33:1191-1202, 1986.

Olson NY, Lindsley CB: Neonatal lupus syndrome, *Am J Dis Child* 141:908-910, 1987.

Ramirez-Seijas F, Cepero-Akselrad A: Systemic lupus erythematosus in children, *Int Pediatr* 8(3):334-343, 1993.

Venables PJW: Diagnosis and treatment of systemic lupus erythematosus, *Br Med J* 307:663-666, 1993.

CHAPTER 40

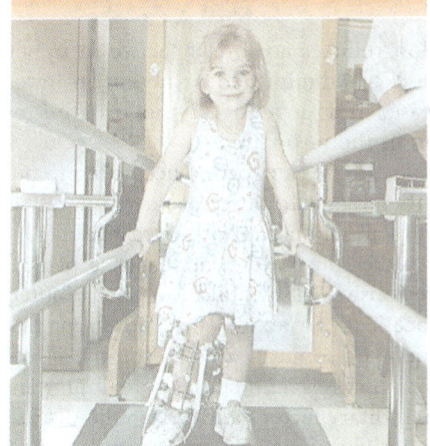

The Child with Neuromuscular or Muscular Dysfunction

CHAPTER OUTLINE

RELATED TOPICS

The child with cerebral dysfunction, Ch. 37
Family-centered care of the child with chronic illness or disability, Ch. 22
Family-centered home care, Ch. 25
Genetic evaluation and counseling, Ch. 5
The immobilized child, Ch. 39
Immunizations (tetanus), Ch. 12
Mobilization devices, Ch. 39
Myelomeningocele (meningomyelocele), Ch. 11
Neurologic assessment, Chs. 7 and 8

NEUROMUSCULAR DYSFUNCTION

Weakness or abnormal performance of skeletal muscle may represent a defect in the muscle itself or reflect a pathologic disorder at some point along the neural pathway from the cortex of the brain to the neuromuscular junction. The identification of the source of muscle dysfunction includes not only the testing of muscle function but also the systematic elimination of possible disorders of neural structures on which muscle function depends for its stimulus. In a few disorders muscle disease may be accompanied by a neural disorder.

Some clinical features are shared by muscle disease **(myopathy),** which differs in many ways from muscle dysfunction resulting from disorders of neuronal structures—brain, cranial nerve nuclei, long nerve tracts, anterior horn cells of the spinal cord, and peripheral nerves. Motor function is accomplished by means of the simple reflex arcs or by way of impulses transmitted from the cerebral cortex and other centers in the brain through the various nerve pathways of the central nervous system. The ***upper motor neurons*** consist of cells that lie in the cerebral cortex and fibers that traverse the brainstem and spinal cord to terminate at their synapses with the anterior horn cells. The anterior horn cells, axons, and peripheral nerve branches constitute the ***lower motor neurons.*** The ***motor unit*** consists of the lower motor neuron, the neuromuscular junction, and the muscle fibers it supplies (Fig. 40-1). The upper motor neuronal pathways from the cerebrum to the lower motor neuron are described as (1) ***pyramidal***—those whose fibers extend from the cortex, come together in the medulla, cross from one side to the other, then extend down the cord to synapse with anterior horn motor neurons; and (2) ***extrapyrami-***

■ Patricia L. King, RN, MS, revised this chapter.

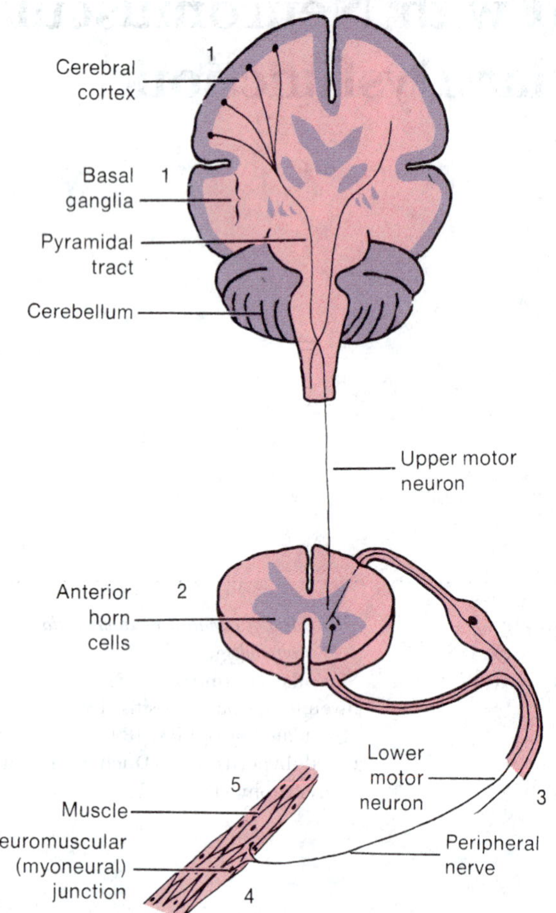

FIG. 40-1 Site of origin for neuromuscular disorders. *1,* Cerebral palsy; *2,* poliomyelitis, spinal muscular atrophy; *3,* mononeuropathies, polyneuropathies; *4,* myasthenia gravis, neurotoxic disorders; *5,* muscular dystrophies.

dal—a complex network of motor neurons that comprise relays between motor areas of the cortex, basal ganglia, thalamus, cerebellum, and brainstem.

CLASSIFICATION AND DIAGNOSIS

The site of pathologic disturbance determines the type of muscular dysfunction. In general, ***upper motor neuron lesions*** produce weakness associated with spasticity, increased deep tendon reflexes, and abnormal superficial reflexes. The primary disorder of upper motor neuron dysfunction is cerebral palsy. ***Lower motor neuron lesions*** interrupt the reflex arc, causing weakness and atrophy of the skeletal muscles involved with associated hypotonia or flaccidity, which eventually progress to atrophy with varying degrees of contracture deformity. A disorder of the extrapyramidal pathway and the cerebellum rarely produces muscle weakness.

Lower motor neuron involvement is usually symmetric (except that of poliomyelitis and single peripheral nerve disease), whereas disorders of the pyramidal tract are more often asymmetric. Muscle wasting is characteristic of lower motor neuron lesions and more marked than in diseases of muscles. Deep tendon reflexes are briskly active in upper motor neuron disease, are diminished or absent in lower motor neuron disease, and depend on the progress of muscle degeneration in the myopathies.

These disorders can also be categorized according to onset: those in which there is acute onset of flaccid paralysis and those with more gradual onset and progressive degeneration. In most instances the sudden appearance of flaccid paralysis in a previously healthy child can be attributed to an infectious process. Neurotoxins (e.g., botulism, tick paralysis, or heavy metal poisoning), pressure on the spinal cord from tumors or abscesses, and spinal cord injury are less likely causes. Hereditary factors and metabolic disease are more often responsible for muscular weakness and atrophy of gradual onset.

Classification

The most useful classification of neuromuscular disorders is one that defines the site of origin of the pathologic lesion: the anterior horn cells of the spinal cord, the peripheral nerves, the myoneural junction, and the muscles.

Diseases of Anterior Horn Cells. Diseases and disorders that affect the anterior horn cells are the result of destruction or atrophy of the anterior horn of the spinal column with the inability to transfer impulses from sensory neurons to motor neurons. Enteroviruses, which have a worldwide distribution, are prominent etiologic agents that selectively affect anterior horn cells. These include the polioviruses, of which there are three types: coxsackieviruses, groups A and B, and the ECHO viruses. Degeneration of the anterior horn cells is caused by inherited disorders, primarily the spinal muscular atrophies.

Neuropathies. Disorders affecting peripheral nerves may be ***mononeuropathies,*** involving a single nerve and the muscles it innervates, or ***polyneuropathies,*** which involve multiple nerves and the muscles they supply. Neuropathies are caused by a number of hereditary diseases, traumatic injury, infections, poisons, and (secondarily) some metabolic diseases. Polyneuropathy can be restricted to specific areas (as in diabetes mellitus); some hereditary diseases involve skeletal muscles extensively. Usually distal limbs (feet and hands) are affected first, with gait disturbance and footdrop as early manifestations. The involvement gradually progresses medially as the disorder becomes more severe.

In some polyneuropathies there is segmented or patchy loss of the myelin sheath of nerve fibers; in others the primary process appears to be progressive degeneration of nerve fibers. Examples of acute and chronic polyneuropathies are infectious polyneuritis and peroneal atrophy, respectively.

Neuromuscular Junction Disease. Disorders involving a neurohormonal deficiency interfere with transmission of nerve impulses to muscles at the neuromuscular junction. Normally, nerve impulses are transmitted to skeletal muscles across the neuromuscular junction by acetylcholine. This is accomplished in three steps: (1) acetylcholine is released from vesicles in the terminal nerve endings; (2) it then diffuses across the junction and contacts receptor sites in the muscle membrane, stimulating the muscle to contract; and (3) it is removed by the action of cholinesterase. Interference at any of these three steps will block transmission of nerve impulses and prevent muscular contraction.

Several toxic substances act at the myoneural junction to inhibit nerve impulses to the skeletal muscles. Examples of toxins that prevent release of acetylcholine are those that produce the paralysis of botulism and tick paralysis. Action at receptor sites is blocked by the drug curare. Paralysis resulting from inhibition of cholinesterase release is caused by poisoning with organic phosphate insecticides.

Diseases of Muscles. Diseases of skeletal muscles can be inflammatory (such as polymyositis), the result of endocrine dysfunction (such as hypothyroidism and hyperthyroidism), or caused by congenital defects (such as absence of muscle, periodic paralysis, and the various muscular dystrophies and myotonias). Inflammation occurs in a number of infectious illnesses such as trichinosis, toxoplasmosis, and those caused by coxsackievirus.

Diagnostic Tools

To aid in differentiating between diseases with similar manifestations, several general diagnostic tools are used. In addition, a number of more definitive tests are used to establish a specific diagnosis. The neurologic examination is a basic test that helps to assess the extent of motor and sensory function.

The ***electromyogram (EMG)*** measures the electric potentials generated in individual muscles. A small metal disk is placed on the skin overlying the muscle to be tested, or a sterile needle electrode is inserted directly into the muscle. The electric activity generated in the skeletal muscles is measured at rest, with slight voluntary contraction, and with maximal contraction. The electric activity is amplified and displayed on a cathode ray oscilloscope. Needle electrodes are sensitive enough to pick up the activity of a single muscle fiber; thus this is usually the method of choice. However, the procedure is traumatic for children.

Nerve conduction velocity, the velocity of electric impulse conduction along motor or sensory nerves, is frequently measured in conjunction with electromyography. Certain diseases affect the peripheral nerves, prolonging the conduction time from the point of stimulation of the nerve to the muscle and increasing the duration of the evoked potential of the muscle.

SERUM ENZYME MEASUREMENTS

Creatine phosphokinase (CPK)—Found in skeletal muscle and a few other organs and elevated in skeletal muscle disease; the most specific test
Aldolase—Present in skeletal and heart muscle and significantly elevated in muscle damage
Serum glutamic-oxaloacetic transaminase (SGOT)—Elevated in muscle disease but has wider distribution in organs
Lactic dehydrogenase (LDH)—Elevated in muscle disease but has wider distribution

Muscle biopsy is the most useful laboratory examination to confirm and classify muscle disorders. Ketamine has been used to decrease the pain of this invasive procedure (Ramchandra, Anisya, and Gourie-Devi, 1990). (See also Surgical Procedures, Chapter 27.) ***Serum enzyme measurements*** are helpful in diagnosis and monitoring the course of muscular disease. The intracellular enzyme ***creatine phosphokinase*** is present in muscle tissues and very few other organs and is released in large amounts in some diseases of muscles such as muscular dystrophy. Creatine phosphokinase is not elevated in neurogenic disease (see box below, left).

CEREBRAL PALSY (CP)

CP is a nonspecific term applied to disorders characterized by impaired movement and posture and early onset. It is nonprogressive and may be accompanied by perceptual problems, language deficits, and intellectual involvement. The etiology, clinical features, and course are variable, characterized by abnormal muscle tone and coordination as the primary disturbances. It is the most common permanent physical disability of childhood, and the incidence is reported as 1.9 to 2.3 in every 1000 live births. Since the 1960s the prevalence of CP has risen about 20% and most likely reflects the improved survival of low- and very-low-birth-weight infants (Bhushan, Paneth, and Kiely, 1993).

Etiology

A variety of prenatal, perinatal, and postnatal factors contribute to the etiology of CP, singly or multifactorially (Table 40-1). Although the prevalent hypothesis has been that CP results from perinatal problems, especially birth asphyxia, it is now known that CP results more commonly

TABLE 40-1 Causes of Cerebral Palsy

TIME (% OF CASES)	CAUSES
Prenatal (44%)	
First trimester	Teratogens Genetic syndromes Chromosomal abnormalities Brain malformations
Second-third trimester	Intrauterine infections Problems in fetal/placental functioning
Labor and delivery (19%)	Preeclampsia Complications of labor and delivery
Perinatal (8%)	Sepsis/CNS infection Asphyxia Prematurity
Childhood (5%)	Meningitis Traumatic brain injury Toxins
Not obvious (24%)	

From Eicher PS, Batshaw ML: Cerebral palsy, *Pediatr Clin North Am* 40(3):540, 1993.

from existing prenatal brain abnormalities. Premature delivery is the single most important determinant of CP, an event that occurs most frequently in very small infants (Paneth, 1993). However, in about 24% of the cases, no identifiable cause is found.

Pathophysiology

It is difficult to establish a precise location of neurologic lesions based on etiology or clinical signs because there is no characteristic pathologic picture. In some cases there are gross malformations of the brain. In others there may be evidence of vascular occlusion, atrophy, loss of neurons, and laminar degeneration that produce narrower gyri, wider sulci, and low brain weight. Anoxia plays the most significant role in the pathologic state of brain damage, which is frequently secondary to other causative mechanisms.

There are a few exceptions. In some cases the manifestations or etiology can be related to anatomic areas. For example, CP associated with prematurity is usually spastic diplegia caused by hypoxic infarction or hemorrhage in the area adjacent to the lateral ventricles. In the athetoid type of CP caused by kernicterus and hemolytic disease of the newborn, there are pigment deposits in the basal ganglia and some cranial nerve nuclei. Hemiparetic CP is frequently associated with mechanical trauma to the cortex or with cerebrovascular accident of the middle cerebral artery. Cerebral hypoplasia and sometimes neonatal hypoglycemia are related to ataxic CP. Generalized cortical and cerebral atrophy have been shown to cause severe quadriparesis with mental retardation and microcephaly.

Clinical Classification

CP has been classified in several ways, but the most useful classification is based on the nature and distribution of neuromuscular dysfunction (see box below, left). The most common clinical type, spastic CP, represents an upper motor neuron type of muscular weakness. The reflex arc is intact, and the characteristic physical signs are increased stretch reflexes, increased muscle tone, and (often) weakness. Early neurologic manifestations are usually generalized hypotonia or decreased tone that lasts for a few weeks or may extend for months or even as long as a year. The clinical features of spastic CP are outlined in the box below.

Clinical Manifestations

The alert observer may suspect CP when a child demonstrates some of the following groups of manifestations.

Delayed Gross Motor Development. This is a universal manifestation of CP. The child shows a delay in all mo-

CLINICAL CLASSIFICATION OF CEREBRAL PALSY

Spastic—May involve one or both sides
- Hypertonicity with poor control of posture, balance, and coordinated motion
- Impairment of fine and gross motor skills
- Active attempts at motion increase abnormal postures and overflow of movement to other parts of the body

Dyskinetic—Abnormal involuntary movement
- Athetosis, characterized by slow, wormlike, writhing movements that usually involve the extremities, trunk, neck, facial muscles, and tongue
- Involvement of the pharyngeal, laryngeal, and oral muscles causes drooling and dysarthria (imperfect speech articulation)
- Involuntary movements may take on choreoid (involuntary, irregular, jerking movements) and dystonic (disordered muscle tone) manifestations that increase in intensity with emotional stress and around adolescence

Ataxic—
- Wide-based gait
- Rapid repetitive movements performed poorly
- Disintegration of movements of the upper extremities when the child reaches for objects

Mixed-type—Combination of spasticity and athetosis

TYPES OF SPASTIC CEREBRAL PALSY

Hemiparesis—One side of body affected
- Most common form of spastic cerebral palsy
- Motor deficit usually greater in upper extremity; most children able to walk; underdevelopment of affected limbs
- Pattern of spasticity
  - ***Leg***—Increased tone of calf, hamstring, and hip adductor muscles
  - ***Gait***—Walk with foot inverted and plantar flexed, knee flexed, and leg adducted
  - ***Arm***—Increased tone in shoulder adductor and internal rotator muscles, elbow flexor and pronator muscles, and wrist and finger flexor muscles
  - ***Parietal lobe syndrome***—Impairment of cortical sensory function (absence or inability to recognize size, shape, or texture of objects held in affected hand); impaired two-point discrimination and position sense

Quadriparesis—or **tetraparesis**—All four extremities involved
- Highest incidence of severe disability
- Upper and lower limbs equally affected
- Same physical manifestations as hemiparesis bilaterally except lower extremities more involved than in hemiparesis, which causes considerable tightness of hip adductor muscles; difficulty in separating legs or even crossing them over one another ("scissors" gait)
- One fourth only mildly affected with minimum functional limitations on ambulation, self-care, and other activities; one half moderately impaired and impeded in self-care and independence in a sheltered situation; and one fourth severely damaged and require almost total care
- Delay in attaining developmental milestones proportionate to degree of motor deficit
- Speech dysarthric; swallowing may be impaired; tongue protrusion incomplete
- In some children emotions more labile with inappropriate laughing or crying

Diplegia—Similar parts on both sides of the body involved, such as both arms
- Spasticity in legs greater than in arms
- Late attainment of gross motor milestones, sitting, standing, and walking; development of hand skills generally appropriate for age

Monoplegia*—Involving only one extremity

Triplegia*—Involving three extremities

Paraplegia*—Pure cerebral paraplegia of lower extremities

*Rare occurrences.

tor accomplishments, and the discrepancy between motor ability and expected achievement tends to increase with successive developmental milestones as growth advances. It is especially significant if other developmental behavior, such as language and personal-social achievement, is normal. Delayed development of the ability to balance may also retard the progression of milestones. For instance, the child may need arms to balance in a sitting position, rendering the arms unavailable to develop fine motor control.

Abnormal Motor Performance. Neuromotor dysfunction is particularly evident in motor performance. An early sign is preferential unilateral hand use that may be apparent at about 6 months of age. Hand dominance does not normally develop until the preschool years. Abnormal crawling with propulsion by hand movements only and with lower extremities and hips hiked along, much like a "bunny hop," is seen in diplegia. Children with hemiplegia have an asymmetric crawl, using the unaffected arm and leg to propel themselves on either the buttocks or the abdomen. Spasticity may cause the child to stand or walk on the toes. Uncoordinated or involuntary movements are characteristic of dyskinetic CP, and facial grimacing and writhing movements of the tongue, fingers, and toes are signs of athetosis. Other significant signs of motor dysfunction are poor sucking and feeding difficulties, with persistent tongue thrust. Head staggering, tremor on reaching, and truncal ataxia may be observed as well.

Alterations of Muscle Tone. Increased or decreased resistance to passive movements is a sign of abnormal muscle tone. The child may exhibit opisthotonic postures (exaggerated arching of the back) and may feel stiff on handling or dressing. Also, there is difficulty in diapering because of spasticity of hip adductor muscles and lower extremities. When pulled to a sitting position, the child may extend the entire body, rigid and unbending at the hip and knee joints. This is an early sign of spasticity.

Abnormal Postures. Children with spastic CP assume abnormal postures at rest or when their position is changed. From an early age, a child lying in a prone position will maintain the hips higher than the trunk with the legs and arms flexed or drawn under the body. In the supine position spasticity is evident by scissoring (legs in crossed position, knees, hips, and ankles stiff) and extension of legs and with the feet plantar flexed. This posture is exaggerated when the child is suspended vertically or when others try to make him bear weight. Spasticity may be mild or severe, depending on the degree of impairment. A persistent infantile resting and sleeping posture (i.e., arms abducted at shoulders, elbows flexed, and hands fisted) is a sign of spasticity when it remains constant after 4 to 5 months of age. The hemiparetic child may rest with the affected arm adducted and held against the torso with the elbow pronated and slightly flexed and the hand closed.

Reflex Abnormalities. Persistence of primitive infantile reflexes is one of the earliest clues to CP (e.g., obligatory tonic neck reflex at any age or nonobligatory persistence beyond 6 months of age and the persistence or even hyperactivity of the Moro, plantar, and palmar grasp reflexes). Hyperreflexia, ankle clonus, and stretch reflexes can be elicited from many muscle groups on fast passive movements (e.g., resistance to passive abduction when hips are suddenly separated [adductor catch]).

Associated Disabilities and Problems. Some of the disabilities associated with CP are visual impairment, hearing impairment, communication and speech difficulties, seizures, and intellectual impairment.

Mental retardation. Approximately 70% of affected children have a wide range of intelligence, all within normal limits. Speech difficulties are often interpreted as a sign of mental retardation. Assessing the intelligence of a child with CP is extremely difficult because of the presence of both motor and sensory deficits. Tests carried out periodically over time should determine the degree of intelligence. Many persons with CP who have severely limiting physical involvement actually have the least intellectual impairment. As a group, children with athetosis and ataxia are intellectually superior to those with other types of CP. Incidence of severe or profound retardation is highest in rigid, atonic, and quadriparetic CP.

Sensory impairment. Nystagmus and amblyopia are common and may require surgery, corrective lenses, or both. Hearing loss is also common. Some loss is caused by sensorineural involvement. However, affected infants may spend increased amounts of time lying flat. This predisposes them to episodes of otitis media, which may result in conductive hearing loss.

Drooling. Drooling may occur in some children and may contribute to wet clothing and skin irritation.

Constipation. A variety of factors may be responsible for causing constipation. Difficulty in eating bulky foods because of uncoordinated chewing and swallowing may be the most likely cause. Others are toileting difficulties and decreased mobility. Stool softeners or laxatives may need to be used.

Respiratory problems. Coughing and choking, especially while eating, may predispose to aspiration. Also, respiratory efforts may be uncoordinated and weak, which could result in inadequate gas exchange.

Orthopaedic complications. Children with CP who are nonambulatory have an increased risk of developing unilateral or bilateral hip dislocations, scoliosis, and joint contractures due to unbalanced muscle tone.

Dental problems. Increased incidence of dental caries results from (1) improper dental hygiene, (2) congenital enamel defects (hypoplasia of primary teeth), (3) high carbohydrate intake and retention, (4) dietary imbalance with poor nutritional intake, (5) inadequate fluoride, and (6) difficulty in mouth closure and drooling. Spastic or clonic movements can cause gagging or biting down on the toothbrush, thus interfering with cleaning techniques. Oral hypersensitivity is also common, causing the child to resist dental hygiene. Malocclusion can occur in as many as 90% of these children. Gingivitis is secondary to inadequate dental hygiene and may be further complicated by the use of antiseizure drugs (Steele, 1992).

Seizures. Seizures are more apt to accompany postnatally acquired hemiplegia. They are an unusual finding in athetosis and diplegia. The most common type is generalized tonic-clonic seizures, and the peak incidence of commencement is between 2 and 6 years of age.

Attention deficit–hyperactivity disorder. The manifestations of attention deficit–hyperactivity disorder may occur in children with CP. The primary presenting symptoms are poor attention span, marked distractibility, hyperactive behavior, and defects of integration (see Chapter 18).

Diagnostic Evaluation

Infants at risk based on known etiologic factors associated with CP warrant careful assessment during early infancy to identify signs of muscular dysfunction as early as possible. Careful assessment should be made of the low-birth-weight or preterm infant, the infant with a low Apgar score at 5 minutes, and the infant who demonstrated other perinatal or neonatal abnormalities such as seizures, intracranial hemorrhage, or metabolic disturbances. Early recognition is made more difficult by lack of reliable neonatal neurologic signs. Cortical control of movement does not occur until later in infancy; therefore motor impairment associated with voluntary control is usually not apparent until after 2 to 4 months of age at the earliest. More often the likelihood of a diagnosis cannot be confirmed until the second half of the first year. Motor dysfunction in some mildly affected infants may be overlooked until they exhibit delay or abnormality of some advanced motor skills such as standing or walking.

Persistence of primitive reflexes may be of value, and two offer assistance in diagnosis: the asymmetric tonic neck reflex, or persistent Moro reflex (beyond 4 months of age), and the crossed extensor reflex. The tonic neck reflex normally disappears between 4 and 6 months of age. An "obligatory" response is considered abnormal. This is elicited by turning the infant's head to one side and holding it there for 20 seconds. When a crying infant is unable to move from the asymmetric posturing of the tonic neck reflex when crying, it is considered to be "obligatory" and an abnormal response. The crossed extensor reflex, which normally disappears by 4 months, is elicited by applying a noxious stimulus to the sole of one extremity with the knee extended. Normally the contralateral foot will respond with extensor, abduction, and then adduction movements. Finding these reflexes after the age when they should have disappeared suggests the possibility of CP.

The neurologic examination and history are the primary modalities for diagnosis. A thorough knowledge of normal variations of motor development is required for detecting abnormal progress, and a careful history is elicited to detect possible etiologic factors. The child's spontaneous movements and behavior are observed, including posture, attitude, and muscle size, function, and tone.

Supplemental diagnostic tests may be used, such as electroencephalography, tomography, screening for metabolic defects, and serum electrolyte values. The possibility of slowly progressive degenerative disease and early onset, slow-growing brain tumors must be ruled out.

Therapeutic Management: General Concepts

The goals of therapy for children with CP are early recognition and promotion of an optimum developmental course to enable affected children to attain their potential within the limits of their brain dysfunction. The disorder is permanent, and therapy is chiefly symptomatic and preventive. To be effective, it requires the services of an organized team of health professionals that considers (1) the nature of the physical disability, (2) defects associated with the disorder, and (3) the interpersonal and social influences encountered by the affected child.

The beneficial influences of a habilitation program on both child and family are based on recognition of the disability as early as possible and implementation of treatment. Parents are essential to a treatment program, and their cooperation and confidence are considered in all aspects of management. With early diagnosis parents can begin to provide sensorimotor experiences that are essential for cognitive development, since central nervous system structures depend on stimulation and use to attain and maintain their functional integrity.

The broad aims of therapy are (1) to establish locomotion, communication, and self-help; (2) to gain optimum appearance and integration of motor functions; (3) to correct associated defects as effectively as possible; (4) to provide educational opportunities adapted to the needs and capabilities of the individual child and (5) to promote socialization experiences with other affected and unaffected children. Each child is evaluated and managed on an individual basis. The plan of therapy may involve a variety of settings, facilities, and specially trained persons, including the parents. The scope of the child's needs may require, in addition to the pediatrician and nurse, such professionals as a psychologist and/or psychiatrist, orthopaedist, physical

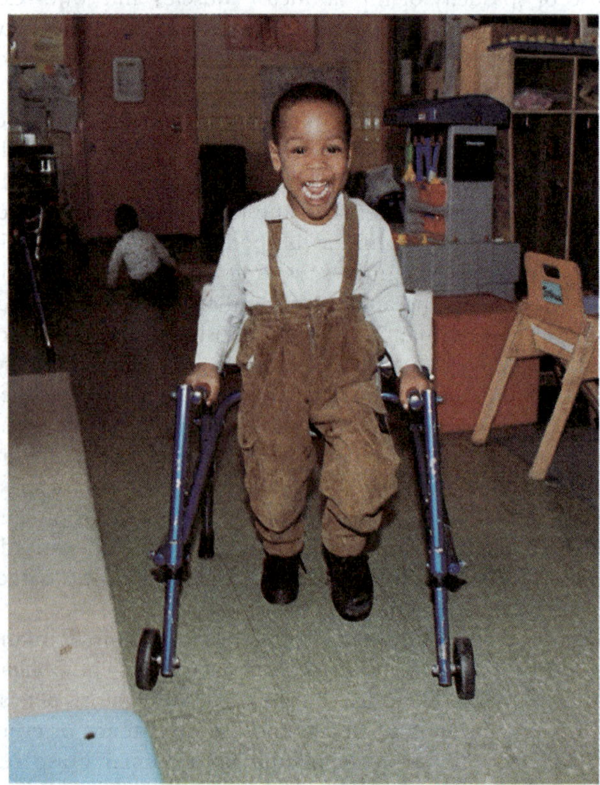

FIG. 40-2 Child ambulating with use of assistive device.

therapist, teacher, social worker, speech pathologist and/or therapist, neurologist, orthotist, audiologist, and occupational therapist.

Mobilizing Devices. Ankle-foot orthoses (braces) (AFOs) are worn by many of these children. AFOs are molded to fit the feet and are worn inside the shoes. Devices are often used to help prevent or reduce deformity. Some of the more commonly used mobility devices include wheeled scooter boards that allow children to propel themselves while the abdomen or total body is supported and the legs are positioned with wedges to prevent scissoring. Wheeled go-carts provide good sitting balance and serve as an early "wheelchair" experience for young children. Strollers can be equipped with custom seats for dependent mobilization. Special devices for independent mobilization that may or may not allow the upper extremities to remain free are particularly valuable for children with lower extremity involvement (Fig. 40-2). A number of wheelchairs can be customized to meet the needs and preferences of older children (see Mobilization Devices, Chapter 39).

NURSING ALERT The use of infant walkers is discouraged. They pose a risk of injury to normal children and are especially hazardous for children with CP. Also, jumping seats, like those that hang in doorways, should not be used.

Surgery. Orthopaedic surgery may be required (1) to correct deformities (contracture or spastic), (2) to provide stability for an uncontrollable joint, and (3) to provide balanced muscle power. This includes tendon-lengthening procedures (especially heel-cord lengthening), release of spastic wrist flexor muscles, and correction of hip and adductor muscle spasticity or contracture to improve locomotion. ***Selective dorsal rhizotomy*** has provided marked improvement in some children with CP. However, achieving the benefits from the surgery requires intensive physical therapy and family commitment. Because the procedure results in flaccid muscles, the child must be retaught to sit, stand, and walk (Brucker, 1990).

Surgical intervention is usually reserved for the child who does not respond to the more conservative measures, but it is also indicated for the child whose spasticity causes progressive deformities. Surgery is primarily used to improve function rather than for cosmetic purposes and is followed by physical therapy. Neurosurgical procedures are used only in selected cases. Children who have spastic CP are most likely to improve from surgery. Since a deformity in one joint also affects the function of the joints above and below, consistent and careful evaluation is needed to plan additional surgical procedures in appropriate sequence.

Medication. Drugs to decrease spasticity have little usefulness in improving function in CP. Antianxiety agents have been used to some extent to relieve excessive motion and tension, particularly in the athetoid child. Skeletal muscle relaxants, such as dantrolene (Dantrium), baclofen, and methocarbamol (Robaxin), may be used on a short-term basis for older children and adolescents. Diazepam (Valium) is used frequently but should be restricted to older children and adolescents. The drugs have been successful in relieving stiffness and thus facilitating ease of motion. Local nerve block to motor points of a muscle with a neurolytic agent such as phenol solution reduces spasticity temporarily.

Antiepileptic medications are used routinely for children who have seizures. Generally, phenobarbital and phenytoin are most widely prescribed and appear to be effective in most instances. Other antiepileptics or combinations are needed in special situations. Regular periodic monitoring of blood levels is required to obtain the desired effect with the smallest possible dosage. Children who are hyperactive and dyskinetic perform better when given dextroamphetamine or other drugs used for the child with attention deficit–hyperactivity disorder. The U.S. Food and Drug Administration (FDA) has approved the use of botulinum toxin to treat certain nerve disorders. The effects produced by the toxin are also being studied in children with CP. Botulinum toxin is thought to produce a paralytic effect at the neuromuscular junction (Jankovic and Brin, 1991).

Technical Aids. A wide variety of technical aids are available to improve the functioning of children with CP. For example, specially designed electromechanical toys that employ the concept of biofeedback operate from a head unit. The toy is manipulated only when the head and trunk are in correct alignment. Eye-hand coordination can also be enhanced by appropriately designed toys and games.

The most numerous devices are those that facilitate nonvocal communication. Microcomputers combined with voice synthesizers aid children with speech difficulties to "speak." These and others print messages onto screen monitors and paper. These devices have made it apparent that some children have been erroneously considered to be mentally retarded.

Many other electronic devices allow independent functioning. Sensors can be activated and deactivated by using a head-stick, tongue, or other voluntary muscle movement over which the child has control. The application of this technology makes it possible for persons with CP to eventually function in their own apartments and can be extended into the workplace.

Other Considerations. Care of visual and auditory deficits requires the attention of appropriate specialists, and speech therapy involves the services of a speech therapist (see Chapter 24). Dental care is especially important for children with CP and is all too frequently overlooked. Regular visits to the dentist and dental prophylaxis, including brushing, fluoride, and flossing (after several teeth are present), should be instituted as soon as the teeth erupt. This is especially important for children given phenytoin, who often develop gum hyperplasia.

Therapeutic Management: Physiotherapy

Physical therapy is one of the most frequently used conservative treatment modalities. It requires the specialized skills of a qualified therapist with an extensive repertoire of exercise methods who can design a program to stimulate each child to achieve functional goals. In general, physical therapy is directed toward good skeletal alignment for the spastic child; training in purposeful acts, even in the face of involuntary motion, for the athetoid child; and maximum development of proprioceptive sense in ataxia.

An active therapy program involves the family, the physical therapist, and often other members of the health team, especially the nurse. The major approach employs traditional types of therapeutic exercises that consist of stretching, passive, active, and resisted movements applied to specific muscle groups or joints to maintain or increase range of motion, strength, or endurance. Another approach is one of "patterning," which attempts to alter abnormal tone and posture and elicit desired movements through positional manipulation or other means of modifying or augmenting sensory output. These programs require intensive daily manipulation and a legion of volunteers to carry out the program. The American Academy of Pediatrics (1990) has issued a strong statement against this form of treatment for neurologically disabled children. Therefore this option is not discussed further.

No therapeutic approach is able to achieve spectacular changes in the ultimate outcome of motor disability. Therefore, the most practical approach is to select a mode of intervention that is most appropriate for the specific problem and that best suits the need of the individual child at any given time. Early efforts are focused on alleviating abnormal postures by positioning and range-of-motion exercises. For example, rather than being pulled to a sitting position by the arms, which stimulates hypertonic extensor muscles of the back, the spastic infant is slowly pushed forward by hands placed posteriorly on the trunk. Extensor spasticity and scissoring of legs can be avoided if the infant straddles a thigh or hip when carried in the sitting position.

Passive range-of-motion exercises, stretching, and elongation exercises are valuable at any age, even at early ages when the child is unable to cooperate. They are of particular value for postural abnormalities around various joints. For example, stretching of the gastrocnemius muscle and its tendon helps to prevent tightness and spasticity, which lead to toe walking and equinus position of the ankle. When the child is old enough to cooperate, some active extension can be performed, with passive motion applied to complete joint extension. Prevention of contracture deformity is a prime function of physical therapy.

Functional and Adaptive Training (Occupational Therapy). Training in manual skills and activities of daily living (ADLs) proceeds along developmental lines and according to the child's functional level. Sitting, balance, crawling, and walking are encouraged at appropriate ages, accompanied by stimulation of protective extension and equilibrium reactions. When standing is attempted, therapy may be needed to strengthen and improve balance, which is sometimes facilitated by the use of orthoses, especially to control plantar flexion and less often to prevent knee flexion caused by hamstring muscle spasticity and inadequate control of hip and knee extensor muscles. Walking, using reciprocal leg motion, should be attempted at the appropriate age, even if the child requires considerable assistance from orthoses and other persons, and the child should be encouraged to progress to parallel bars or other ambulatory aids as soon as possible.

Hand activities are begun early to improve motor function and provide the child with sensory experiences and information about his environment. Use of extremities requires some stability of the trunk; therefore a gross motor position in which the child has some active control is selected. Objects and toys are chosen to provide needed sensory input, using a variety of shapes, forms, and textures. The child will electively use the less affected or unaffected hand as the dominant one, and there are differing opinions about whether or not the child should be therapeutically encouraged to use the deficient extremity. Undue insistence often provokes an adverse emotional reaction. Play that encourages the use of hands for unimanual and bimanual activities is initiated early. Large balls, a doll carriage to push, or other toys that require some manner of manipulation are accepted without resistance and promote assistive use of both hands. Play is a valuable tool in a therapeutic program and is selected to combine therapy with the child's ability and interest. This often requires a great deal of ingenuity and inventiveness on the part of those involved in the child's care.

The child may need considerable help (and patience) in learning to feed, dress, and care for personal hygiene needs, the most important and earliest tasks on which to concentrate. Children should be fed in the normal eating position. When they have difficulty with sucking and swallowing, it is a temptation to hold them in a semireclining posture to make use of gravity flow. This method does not promote active swallowing, however, and the neck hyperextension may even interfere with swallowing. A more flexed sitting position with arms brought forward to decrease the tendency toward back and neck extension is more natural during bottle- or spoon-feeding and encourages active swallowing.

Because jaw control is compromised, more normal control can be achieved if the feeder provides stability of the oral mechanism from the side or front of the face. When directed from the front, the middle finger of the nonfeeding hand is placed posterior to the body portion of the chin, the thumb below the bottom lip, and the index finger parallel to the child's mandible (Fig. 40-3). Manual jaw con-

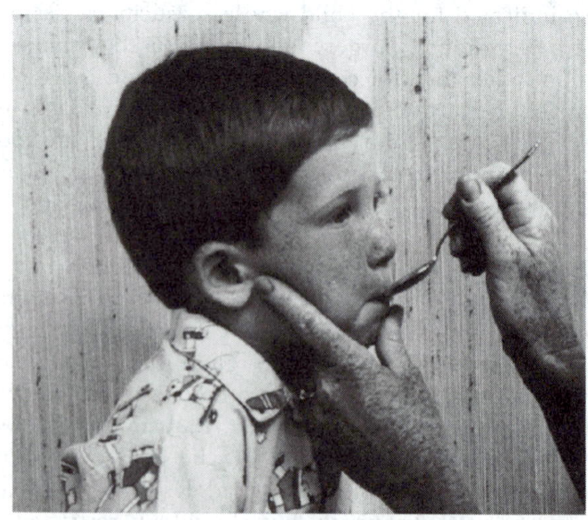

FIG. 40-3 Manual jaw control provided anteriorly.

trol from the side assists with poor head control, neck and trunk hyperextension, and jaw stabilization. The middle finger of the nonfeeding hand is placed posterior to the bony portion of the chin, the index finger is placed on the chin below the lower lip, and the thumb is placed obliquely across the cheek to provide lateral jaw stability (Fig. 40-4) (Logigian and Ward, 1989).

Speech training under the supervision of a speech therapist is begun early, before the child learns poor habits of communication. Parents and others can help by following the directions of the speech therapist and by talking to the child slowly and using pictures or handling objects about which the adult is speaking. Feeding techniques, such as forcing the child to use the lips and tongue in eating, help to facilitate speech (e.g., placing food at the side of the tongue, first one side then the other; making the child use the lips to take food from a spoon rather than placing it directly on the tongue; and avoiding using the teeth to remove the food from the utensil). If severe dysarthria prevents articulate speech and the child has reasonable intelligence, nonverbal communication is taught. However, since "reasonable intelligence" remains difficult, if not impossible, to ascertain, nonverbal communication techniques should be attempted with most children.

As the child progresses from simple feeding and self-care activities, training is extended to include other tasks that are within the child's developmental and functional capabilities, such as cooking or typing. It should be remembered that children should not be expected to learn a task until they are at the developmental stage at which it would normally be accomplished. In all ADLs it is important to capitalize on the child's assets and compensate for liabilities. For example, a child with visual-motor dysfunction would be helped by substituting a word processor for the laborious task of handwriting. The level of expected independence is related to both gross and fine motor manipulation, and even when complete independence in a specific activity is not realistic, the child should learn any masterable part of the task. However, motor function is not the sole purpose of learning to be as independent as possible. Any accomplishment promotes self-reliance and self-esteem for healthier personality development.

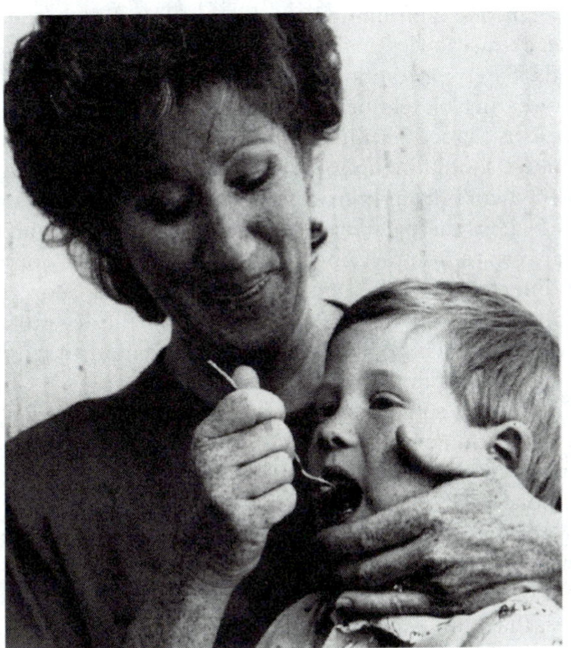

FIG. 40-4 Manual jaw control provided posteriorly.

Education. As in all aspects of care, educational requirements are determined by the child's needs and potential. This includes the severity of the child's disease and the presence and degree of associated conditions that affect learning and participation, such as learning impairment, abnormal actions or behavior, impaired vision and/or hearing, and seizures. Children with mild to moderate involvement are generally able to participate, for varying amounts of time, in regular classes. Resource rooms are available in most schools to provide more individualized attention to a child's particular needs. Integration of these children into regular classrooms should be the initial goal. Teachers' assistants are frequently used to work one-on-one with children in both settings. For those who are unable to benefit from formal education, a training program may be appropriate. At adolescence prevocational and vocational counseling and guidance are arranged. At any phase or in any setting, education is geared toward the child's assets.

Recreation. Recreational activities are also a necessary part of growing up. Recreational outlets and after-school activities should be considered for the child who is unable to participate in regular athletic and other peer activities. Some can compete in athletic and artistic endeavors, and there are many games and pastimes that are suited to their capabilities. Sports, physical fitness, and recreation programs are encouraged for children with CP, and young children should be exposed to all physical activities available to children without disabilities. Adaptive physical education classes are mandated by law in many school systems.

There are numerous developmental centers that have facilities for indoor and outdoor activities designed to appeal to children of all ages. If these are not available, they should be instigated. Such programs require adequate supervision to avoid any harmful effects, however. Recreational activities serve to stimulate children's interest and curiosity, help them adjust to their disability, improve their functional abilities, and build self-esteem. Competitive sports are also becoming increasingly available to these children and offer an added dimension to physical activities. Information on training programs and competition on local, state, regional, and national levels can be obtained from the **National Association of Sports for Cerebral Palsy.***

Nursing Considerations

ASSESSMENT

Early recognition of CP is often a result of alert observation by the nurse. Detection begins at birth, and the nurse

*710 Penn Plaza, Suite 804, New York, NY 10001; (800) USA-1UCP. In Canada: **Ontario Federation of Cerebral Palsy,** 1021 Lawrency Ave., W., Suite 303, Toronto, Ontario, M6A 1C8, Canada; (416) 787-4595.

WARNING SIGNS OF CEREBRAL PALSY

PHYSICAL SIGNS

Poor head control after 3 months of age
Stiff or rigid arms or legs
Pushing away or arching back
Floppy or limp body posture
Cannot sit up without support by 8 months
Uses only one side of the body, or only the arms to crawl

BEHAVIORAL SIGNS

Extreme irritability or crying
Failure to smile by 3 months
Feeding difficulties
 Persistent gagging or choking when fed
 After 6 months of age, tongue pushes soft food out of the mouth

Data from Pathways Awareness Foundation: *Parents . . . if you see any of these warning signs . . . don't delay,* Chicago, 1991, The Foundation.

should be especially observant for signs in an infant who has a history that includes any of the prenatal and perinatal conditions that predispose to brain damage. Unusual manifestations in a newborn can be signs of a variety of conditions, but an infant who displays poor feeding, rigidity, tenseness, or hypotonia merits closer scrutiny. A history of these unexplained signs is cause for repeated assessment. The disorder is not readily identifiable in the early months of life; often evidence is not apparent until the child begins to sit or walk. Delayed attainment of developmental milestones is one of the most valuable clues to recognizing CP; therefore slow development in a child offers one of the earliest indications of neurologic impairment (see box above).

❖ Nursing Diagnoses

Based on a thorough assessment, several nursing diagnoses are identified. The more common diagnoses for the child with CP are included in the Nursing Care Plan on pp. 1880-1881. Others may apply in specific situations.

❖ Planning

The goals for the child with CP and the family include the following:

1. Child will acquire mobility within personal capabilities.
2. Child will acquire communication skills or use appropriate assistive devices.
3. Child will engage in self-help activities.
4. Child will receive appropriate education.
5. Child will develop a positive self-image.
6. Family will receive appropriate education and support in its efforts to meet the child's needs.
7. Child will receive appropriate care if hospitalized.

❖ Implementation

Nurses working with children need to be well acquainted with normal child growth and development and the tools of assessment. The earlier any deviation from normal is detected, the better the outlook for optimum developmental attainment. It is also important that the child receive appropriate therapy from persons or agencies qualified to provide such services. Parents are sometimes tempted to follow advice from unreliable sources. Nurses who are acquainted with services and facilities can refer the family to qualified practitioners.

Nurses who work directly with the child in the home or in the therapeutic setting are members of the health team who plan and carry out a program of therapy. Since children are being treated at an earlier age, parents are participating earlier in treatment programs for their child. They are taught the proper handling and home care of young children with CP. Parents need carefully programmed steps so that their change of role from parent to therapist can be melded into the already established relationship. The nurse or therapist needs to have documented data about the parent-child relationship before teaching the parent how to facilitate the child's posture or inhibit certain reflex patterns.

Parents learn how to posture children, how to introduce and carry out appropriate exercises, and how to place children in appropriate positions for play, dressing, eating, bathing, toileting, and other daily activities. Nurses who are acquainted with the special needs of the child and the physical therapy objectives and modalities may be able to reinforce the plan and assist the family in devising and modifying equipment and activities to follow through and reinforce the therapy program in the home, (e.g., modifying eating utensils by building up spoon handles for easier grasp and modifying clothes to facilitate self-help) (see also Chapter 24).

Because children with CP expend so much energy in their efforts to accomplish activities of daily living, more frequent rest periods should be arranged to avoid fatigue that may aggravate their limited capabilities. The diet should include extra calories to help meet these extra energy demands. Safety precautions are implemented, such as children wearing bicycle helmets if they are subject to falls or there is a chance of injuring their heads on hard objects. Furniture should be upholstered or sharp edges padded to protect a child from injury. If their respiratory muscles are less efficient, these children may be susceptible to common upper respiratory tract infections and should avoid contact with infected persons. Dental problems may be more frequent in children with CP, depending on the level of involvement, which creates a need for meticulous attention to all aspects of dental care.

Parents are sometimes very preoccupied with their ability to perform activities such as positioning their child; as a result, a child's personal comfort and satisfaction may be overlooked. They often perceive their children's inability to perform or behave to be a direct result of their own inadequacy in working with their children. The parents are so intent on achieving a desired goal, such as flexing a child's knees, that they repeatedly remind their children of their errors but fail to acknowledge or support their less-than-successful efforts to comply, even though the children are willing. Nurses can help parents integrate therapy into play activities in more natural and less frustrating ways.

Some children have difficulty in keeping their heads upright. Because of this, they cannot explore much of their environment and process the information. Parents need to be complimented on their efforts to provide a stimulating environment for these children. These infants are "at risk" for delayed development in holding up their heads, righting their shoulders and trunks for stable posture, sitting, pulling, standing, and crawling. Most parents of children with impaired movements benefit from support and practical suggestions for feeding, moving, holding, and encouraging the infant to explore hands and feet and begin to play.

Although practical advice is important, the nurse or physical therapist should offer suggestions at a pace that can be absorbed by the parents to avoid making them feel inadequate in their parenting abilities. The parents are encouraged to define their concern, and nurses should acknowledge the concern as genuine and ask the parents how long they have tried a certain approach. In this way the nurse is able to find out what works, what does not work, and *what the parents* would like to try next. The parents are given positive feedback for their observations of the infant, the progress *they* note, and how *they* differentiate the child's needs.

Sometimes parents need support simply because the demands made on them are very fatiguing. It is probably better for parents of young children with CP to reduce the *quantity* of involvement with their children, rather than reduce the *quality* of the interactions. As normal preschool children acquire autonomous skills, language, and mobility, they spend less time with their parents and are less dependent. A support system frequently overlooked is the parents of other children with CP. Often, parents gather to share ideas, gain emotional support, and exchange babysitting services for each other, thus serving as a respite resource.

Probably the nursing interventions most valuable to the family are support and help in coping with the emotional aspects of the disorder, many of which are discussed in relation to the child with a disability (Chapter 22). Initially the parents need supportive counseling directed toward understanding the implications of the diagnosis and all the feelings that it engenders. Later they need clarification regarding what they can expect from the child and from health professionals. Having a child with CP implies numerous challenges in daily management and changes in family life (see Family Focus box.)

The nurse needs to support the parents in their frustration, their problem solving, their concerns, their approaches to helping the child, and their lack of gratification, as well as the positive approaches they use. All of these aspects must be explored and discussed. Parents, as well as other members of the family, require a great deal of support and counseling. Siblings of a child with a disability are affected and may respond to the presence of the child with overt or less evident behavioral problems. The family needs a relationship with nurses who can provide continued contact, support, and encouragement through the long process of habilitation.

Parents can also find help and solace from parent groups with whom they can share problems and concerns and from whom they can derive comfort and practical information. Parent support groups are most helpful through sharing experiences and accomplishments. For example, parents can understand from others what it is like to have a child with CP, which is generally not possible from professionals (see Family Focus box). The national organization, **United Cerebral Palsy Associations,*** has branches in most communities. The address of the nearest branch can be obtained from a local telephone directory, local agency directory, or a local health department or by writing to the national headquarters. The association provides a variety of services for children and families. There are also a number of excellent books available to serve as guides for parents and nurses who work with the child with CP.

Hospitalized Child. CP is not a disorder that requires hospitalization; therefore, when children with CP are hospitalized, they are usually admitted for another reason or for corrective surgery. Consequently, many nurses are not accustomed to handling these children. Nurses who have never been associated with a child with cerebral palsy may react in a variety of ways, including with fear, revulsion, or overwhelming pity. The basic concept to keep in mind when caring for these children is that they are, first of all, children who happen to be afflicted with a disorder that limits

*710 Penn Plaza, Suite 804, New York, NY 10001; (800) USA-1UCP. In Canada: **Ontario Federation of Cerebral Palsy,** 1021 Lawrency Ave., W., Suite 303, Toronto, Ontario, M6A 1C8, Canada: (416) 787-4595.

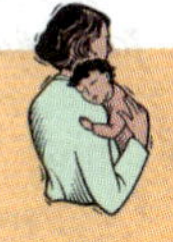

FAMILY FOCUS
The Reality of Acceptance of Cerebral Palsy

Acceptance is rarely achieved in the length of time implied in the literature.

In the first place, what is it? To me, it is the end of comparing my son with every other child I see. I focus on *his* gains, not society's expectations.

It is also being able to laugh periodically *at* his "clumsiness." It is "gallows humor" as he achieves adulthood; jokes about CP can be funny now.

The bitterness is gone; I am now happy for people who have children without CP.

I no longer feel sorry for my son, but rather for the people who cannot see him for the great person he is; the CP does *not* come first.

He is now a young man of 25 years and I am learning to accept his independence.

It is a "never-ending story."

Elaine A. Dunham, RN
Shriner's Hospital
Springfield, MA

NURSING CARE PLAN
The Child with Cerebral Palsy

NURSING DIAGNOSIS: Impaired physical mobility related to neuromuscular impairment

PATIENT GOAL 1: Will acquire locomotion within capabilities

• **NURSING INTERVENTIONS/*RATIONALES***
Encourage sitting, crawling, and walking at appropriate ages
Carry out therapies that strengthen and improve control *to facilitate optimum development*
Assist child in using reciprocal leg motion when learning to walk
Provide incentives to locomote (e.g., place toy out of child's reach)
Ensure adequate rest before attempting locomotion activities *to encourage success*
Incorporate play that encourages desired behavior, *since this encourages cooperation*
Employ aids such as parallel bars and crutches *to facilitate locomotion*
Prepare child and family for surgical procedures if indicated

• **EXPECTED OUTCOME**
Child acquires locomotion within capabilities (specify)

PATIENT GOAL 2: Will experience no or minimal deformity

• **NURSING INTERVENTIONS/*RATIONALES***
Apply and correctly use orthoses *for maximum benefit*
Carry out and teach family to perform stretching exercises *to prevent deformities*
Employ appropriate range-of-motion exercises *to facilitate muscle development and flexibility of joints*
Perform preoperative and postoperative care for child who requires corrective surgery

• **EXPECTED OUTCOME**
Alignment and flexibility are maintained within child's limits

NURSING DIAGNOSIS: Bathing/hygiene, dressing/grooming, feeding, toileting self-care deficits related to physical disability

PATIENT GOAL 1: Will engage in self-help activities of daily activities

• **NURSING INTERVENTIONS/*RATIONALES***
Encourage child to assist with care as age and capabilities permit *to facilitate optimum development*
Select toys and activities that allow maximum participation by child and that improve motor function and sensory input *so that child is more able to care for self*
Avoid undue persistence *because child may be unable or not ready to accomplish a goal*
Encourage activities that require both unimanual and bimanual activities *to encourage optimum development*
Assist with jaw control during feeding *to facilitate eating*
Encourage use of adapted utensils, foods, and clothing *to facilitate self-help* (e.g., large-bowled spoon with padded handle; finger foods and foods that adhere to, rather than slip from, utensil; and clothing that opens from front with self-adhering closings rather than buttons)
Assist parents in toilet training child, *since methods may need to be individualized according to child's abilities*

• **EXPECTED OUTCOME**
Child engages in self-help activities commensurate with capabilities

NURSING DIAGNOSIS: High risk for injury related to physical disability, neuromuscular impairment, perceptual and cognitive impairment

PATIENT GOAL 1: Will experience no physical injury

• **NURSING INTERVENTIONS/*RATIONALES***
Provide safe physical environment
  Padded furniture *for protection*
  Siderails on bed *to prevent falls*
  Sturdy furniture that does not slip *to prevent falls*
  Avoid scatter rugs and polished floors *to prevent falls*
Select toys appropriate to age and physical limitations *to prevent injuries*
Encourage sufficient rest *because fatigue can increase risk of injuries*
Use restraints when child is in chair or vehicle
Provide child who is prone to falls with protective helmet and enforce its use *to prevent head injuries*
Institute seizure precautions for susceptible child
*Administer antiepileptic drugs as prescribed *to prevent seizures*

• **EXPECTED OUTCOMES**
Family provides a safe environment for child (specify)
Child is free of injury

NURSING DIAGNOSIS: Impaired verbal communication

PATIENT GOAL 1: Will engage in communication process within limits of impairment

• **NURSING INTERVENTIONS/*RATIONALES***
Enlist the services of a speech therapist early *before child learns poor habits of communication*
Talk to child slowly *to give child time to understand speech*
Use articles and pictures *to reinforce speech and encourage understanding*
Employ feeding techniques *that help facilitate speech,* such as using lips, teeth, and various tongue movements
Teach and use nonverbal communication methods (e.g., sign language) for child with severe dysarthria
Help family acquire electronic equipment *to facilitate nonverbal communication* (e.g., typewriter, microcomputer with voice synthesizer)

*Dependent nursing action.

NURSING CARE PLAN
The Child with Cerebral Palsy—cont'd

• **EXPECTED OUTCOME**
Child is able to communicate needs to caregivers (specify desired communication and means of accomplishment)

NURSING DIAGNOSIS: Fatigue related to increased energy expenditure

PATIENT GOAL 1: Will receive optimum nutrition

• **NURSING INTERVENTIONS/*RATIONALES***
Provide extra calories *to meet energy demands of increased muscle activity*
Monitor weight gain *to evaluate adequacy of nutritional intake*
Provide vitamin, mineral, and/or protein supplements if eating habits are poor
Devise aids and techniques to facilitate feeding *so that child receives adequate nourishment*

• **EXPECTED OUTCOMES**
Child eats a balanced diet
Weight remains within acceptable limits (specify)

PATIENT GOAL 2: Will receive optimum rest

• **NURSING INTERVENTIONS/*RATIONALES***
Maintain a well-regulated schedule that allows for adequate rest and sleep periods *to prevent fatigue*
Be alert for evidence of fatigue, which tends to aggravate symptoms

• **EXPECTED OUTCOME**
Child is sufficiently rested

PATIENT GOAL 3: Will maintain good general health

• **NURSING INTERVENTIONS/*RATIONALES***
Ensure regular routine health maintenance *to promote general health*
Physical assessment
Dental care
Immunizations

• **EXPECTED OUTCOMES**
Child receives regular health assessments (specify schedule)
Child receives appropriate immunizations (specify) and dental care (specify)

NURSING DIAGNOSIS: Body image disturbance related to perception of disability

PATIENT GOAL 1: Will demonstrate positive body image

• **NURSING INTERVENTIONS/*RATIONALES***
Demonstrate acceptance of child through own behavior, *since children are sensitive to affective attitude of the professional*
Capitalize on child's assets and provide compensation for liabilities *to encourage positive self-image*
Praise child for accomplishments and "near" accomplishments, such as partial completion of a task
Plan activities and goals *with* the child that provide opportunities for success *to encourage cooperation and positive self-image*
Encourage grooming and age-appropriate dress *to promote acceptance by others and positive body image*
See Nursing diagnosis: Body image disturbance, in Nursing Care Plan: The Child with Chronic Illness or Disability, Chapter 22

• **EXPECTED OUTCOME**
Child exhibits behaviors that indicate positive body image (specify)

NURSING DIAGNOSIS: Altered family processes related to a child with a lifelong disability

PATIENT (FAMILY) GOAL 1: Will receive adequate support

• **NURSING INTERVENTIONS/*RATIONALES***
See Nursing diagnosis: Altered family processes, in Nursing Care Plan: The Child with Chronic Illness or Disability, Chapter 22
Refer to special support group(s) and agencies *for ongoing support*

• **EXPECTED OUTCOMES**
Family contacts special support group
See also:
Nursing Care Plan: The Child with Chronic Illness or Disability, Chapter 22
Nursing Care Plan: The Child with Mental Retardation, Chapter 24
Nursing Care Plan: The Child with Hearing Impairment, Chapter 24

their capacities in performing some activities of daily living and, for some, communicating with others. They should be approached and treated the same as any child in the hospital. The nurse's actions should convey acceptance, affection, and friendliness and promote a feeling of trust and dependability in the child. This is especially true with older children who have normal intelligence but who may have communication problems. These children often appear to be mentally retarded because of speech impairment. Frequently nurses tend to "talk down" to them and do things for them that they are perfectly capable of doing for themselves, although not as adeptly as children without a disability. This is especially humiliating to a teenager who values independence and self-esteem.

To facilitate the care and management of these children, the therapy program should be continued, insofar as their condition allows it, during the time they are hospitalized. This should be incorporated into the nursing care plan, and every effort expended to make certain that the ground that has been so laboriously gained is not lost. Encouraging the parents to room-in and actively participate in care facilitates a continuation of the home therapy routine and helps children adjust to an unfamiliar environment. However, it is equally important to remember that a hospitalization may be the first time a parent can defer care to a nurse and not be the primary caregiver. This respite may be crucial to the parent's well-being.

❖ EVALUATION

The effectiveness of nursing interventions is determined by continual reassessment and evaluation of care based on the following observational guidelines and expected outcomes:

1. Observe child's movements and use of mobilization devices.
2. Observe child's speech and ability to use communication devices.
3. Observe child's activities, especially those related to self-care.
4. Interview family regarding child's activities and school attendance.
5. Observe child's interactions with others and choice of activities; interview child regarding feelings and concerns.
6. Interview family regarding their feelings and concerns and observe family members' interaction with the child.
7. Observe child's behavior and responses during hospitalization.

Expected outcomes:
See Nursing Care Plan, pp. 1880-1881.

HYPOTONIA

Decreased muscle tone in an infant is not an unusual observation in the neonatal period and is one of the most common presenting symptoms in neuromuscular disorders. It may also indicate a variety of systemic conditions. Frequent causes are cerebral trauma or hypoxia at birth, but most neuromuscular disorders with hypotonia as the presenting symptom are genetically determined, especially Down syndrome and infantile spinal muscular atrophy.

Clinical Manifestations

Hypotonia, sometimes called the ***floppy infant syndrome,*** is marked by diminished muscle tone and weakness in both spontaneous and passive motion and reflex testing. The infant, when placed in a supine position, assumes a characteristic "frog posture" or lies in some other unusual position at rest. Normally, the young infant who is held in horizontal suspension (i.e., with the examiner's hand supporting the infant under the chest) will respond by slightly raising the head with the back relatively straight, arms flexed and slightly abducted, and knees partly flexed. The hypotonic infant droops over the supporting hand with head and extremities hanging loosely, resembling an inverted U (Fig. 40-5). The muscles feel flabby when palpated, and there is marked head lag when the infant is pulled to a sitting position. Poor sucking may be noted.

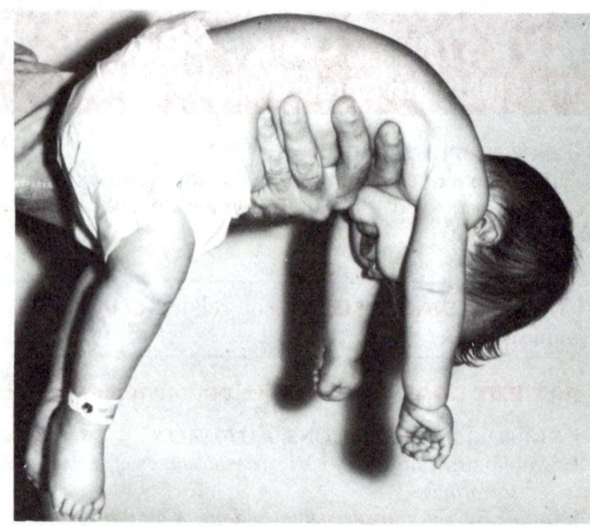

FIG. 40-5 Hypotonicity demonstrated by horizontal suspension in an infant with Werdnig-Hoffmann disease. (From Swaiman KF, Wright FS: *The practice of pediatric neurology,* ed 2, St Louis, 1982, Mosby.)

Diagnostic Evaluation

The infant with hypotonia presents a diagnostic challenge. However, the child's and family's history and the physical examination offer important clues to the general category of causes, such as central or motor neuron disorders. Electromyography is a key diagnostic test. Accurate diagnosis is essential for appropriate treatment, genetic implications, and family counseling (Crawford, 1992).

Therapeutic Management and Nursing Considerations

The management of these infants is determined by the cause of the hypotonia. It is a nursing responsibility to record and report findings that suggest hypotonia in an infant so that further evaluation can be carried out and therapeutic measures implemented if indicated.

PROGRESSIVE INFANTILE SPINAL MUSCULAR ATROPHY (WERDNIG-HOFFMANN DISEASE)

Progressive infantile spinal muscular atrophy (Werdnig-Hoffmann disease) is a disorder characterized by progressive weakness and wasting of skeletal muscles caused by degeneration of anterior horn cells. It is inherited as an autosomal-recessive trait and is the most common paralytic form of the "floppy infant syndrome." The site of the pathologic condition is the anterior horn cells of the spinal cord and the motor nuclei of the brainstem, but the primary effect is atrophy of skeletal muscles.

CLINICAL MANIFESTATIONS OF WERDNIG-HOFFMANN DISEASE

GROUP 1

Disease acquired in utero or during first 2 months of life
Inactivity is most prominent feature
Infant lies in the frog position with legs externally rotated, abducted, and flexed at hips (Fig. 40-6)
Weakness
Limited movements of shoulder and arm muscles
Active movement is usually limited to fingers and toes
Diaphragmatic breathing with sternal retractions
Weak cry and cough
Secretions tend to pool in pharynx
Alert facies
Normal sensation and intellect
Affected infants do not progress to sit alone, roll over, or walk
Early death (usually by 4 years of age) from respiratory failure or infection

GROUP 2

Disease manifested between 2 and 12 months of age
Early—weakness confined to arms and legs
Later—becomes generalized
Legs usually involved to greater extent than arms
Prominent pectus excavatum
Movements absent during complete relaxation or sleep
Some infants able to sit if placed in position
Life span varies from 7 months to 7 years

GROUP 3

Onset of symptoms in second year of life
Normal head control and can sit unassisted by 6 to 8 months of age
Thigh and hip muscles weak
In those who manage to walk:
- Lumbar lordosis
- Waddling gait
- Genu recurvatum
- Protuberant abdomen
- Ambulation becomes increasingly difficult
- Confined to a wheelchair by second decade

Deep tendon reflexes may be present early but disappear

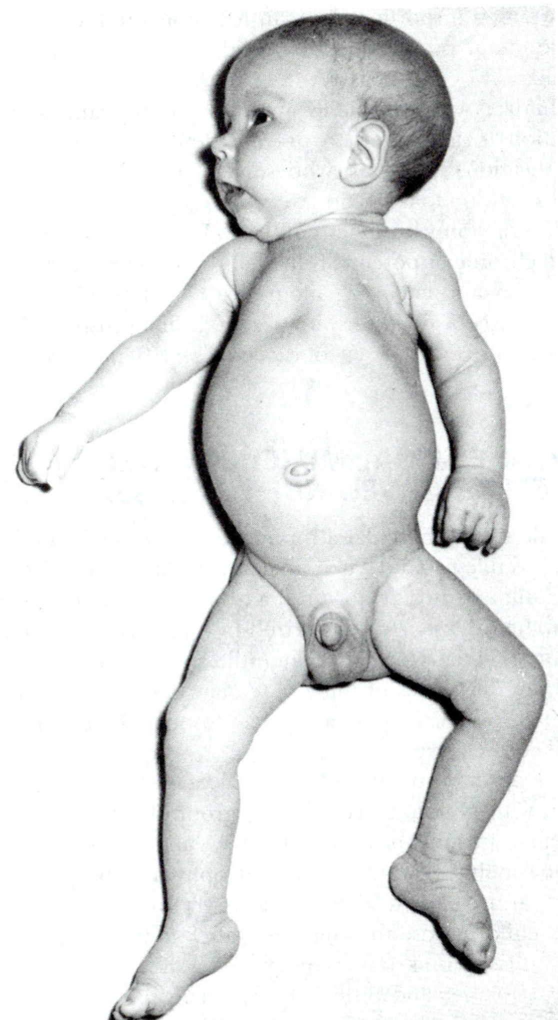

FIG. 40-6 Child with group 1 Werdnig-Hoffmann disease lying in typical posture of abduction of legs at hips and flexion of knees. Arms are flexed slightly with little movement at shoulders. Movements of fingers and toes are present. Pectus excavatum deformity of chest is common and is a result of unopposed diaphragmatic breathing. (From Swaiman KF, Wright FS: *The practice of pediatric neurology*, ed 2, St Louis, 1982, Mosby.)

Clinical Manifestations

The age of onset is variable, but, the earlier the onset, the more disseminated and severe the motor weakness. The disorder may be manifested early, often at birth, frequently in utero, and almost always before 2 years of age. The manifestations and prognosis are categorized according to the age of onset (see box above). However, recent observations suggest that the classification is not valid. Individuals with group 1 manifestations had a life span of 4 months to 31 years. Also, some affected persons did not demonstrate progressive loss of strength and function (Russman and others, 1992).

Therapeutic Management

The diagnosis is established from electromyography demonstrating a denervation pattern and is confirmed by muscle biopsy. Treatment is symptomatic and preventive, primarily prevention of infection and treating orthopaedic problems, the most serious of which is scoliosis. Many children benefit from powered chairs, lifts, special mattresses, and accessible environmental controls. Vigorous antibiotic therapy and pulmonary physical therapy are implemented during upper respiratory infections.

Nursing Considerations

The infant or small child with extensive paralysis requires frequent change of position to prevent physical injury and complications, especially pneumonia. The pharynx requires frequent suctioning to remove secretions, and feeding must be carried out slowly and carefully to prevent aspiration. Since these children are intellectually normal, verbal, tactile, and auditory stimulation are important aspects of care. Supporting them so that they can see the activities around them and transporting them in a wagon for a change of environment provide stimulation and a broader scope of contacts.

Children who are able to sit require proper support and attention to alignment to prevent deformities and other complications. Children who survive beyond infancy will need attention to education needs and opportunities for social interaction with other children. The parents of a child with a chronic or potentially fatal illness require a great deal of support and encouragement (see Chapters 22 and 23). The parents of children with a genetically transmitted disorder also need to be encouraged to seek genetic counseling.

JUVENILE SPINAL MUSCULAR ATROPHY (KUGELBERG-WELANDER DISEASE)

Juvenile spinal muscular atrophy (Kugelberg-Welander disease, juvenile proximal hereditary muscular atrophy) is also the result of anterior horn cell and motor nerve degeneration. The disease is characterized by a pattern of muscular weakness similar to that of infantile spinal muscular atrophy. Several modes of inheritance have been reported for the disease—autosomal-recessive, autosomal-dominant, and X-linked recessive.

The onset occurs from less than 1 year of age into adulthood, with symptoms resembling group 3 infantile spinal muscular atrophy; proximal muscle weakness (especially of the lower limbs) and muscular atrophy are the predominant features. The disease runs a slowly progressive course. Some children lose the ability to walk 8 to 9 years after the onset of symptoms, but many can still walk after 30 years or more (Dorsher and others, 1991). Many affected persons have a normal life expectancy.

Therapeutic Management and Nursing Considerations

The management is primarily symptomatic and supportive and related to maintaining mobility as long as possible, preventing complications, and providing child and family support.

GUILLAIN-BARRÉ SYNDROME (GBS) (INFECTIOUS POLYNEURITIS)

GBS, also known as infectious polyneuritis, is an uncommon acute demyelinating polyneuropathy with a progressive, usually ascending flaccid paralysis. Children are less often affected than adults, with children between ages 4 and 10 years having higher susceptibility. Both sexes are affected with equal frequency.

GBS is an immune-mediated disease often associated with a number of viral or bacterial infections or the administration of vaccines. It has been associated with infectious mononucleosis, measles, mumps, *Borrelia burgdorferi* (Lyme disease), *Campylobacter jejuni,* and *Mycoplasma* and *Pneumocystis* infections. Rarely, it has occurred after administration of influenza and *Haemophilus influenzae* type B conjugate vaccines (Gervaix and others, 1993). An association between oral poliovirus and GBS has not been substantiated (Rantala and others, 1994)

Pathophysiology

Pathologic changes in spinal and cranial nerves consist of inflammation and edema with rapid, segmented demyelination and compression of nerve roots within the dural sheath. Nerve conduction is impaired, producing ascending partial or complete paralysis of muscles innervated by the involved nerves.

Clinical Manifestations

The paralytic manifestations of GBS are usually preceded by a mild influenza-like illness or sore throat. The onset can be rapid, reaching peak activity within 24 hours, or gradual progression of symptoms over days or weeks. Neurologic symptoms initially involve muscle tenderness, sometimes accompanied by paresthesia and cramps. Proximal muscle weakness progressing to paralysis usually occurs before distal weakness, and there is a tendency toward symmetric involvement. In most patients paralysis ascends from the lower extremities, frequently involving the muscles of the trunk, upper extremities, and those supplied by cranial nerves. The seventh (facial) cranial nerve is almost universally affected.

Tendon reflexes are depressed or absent, and paralysis is flaccid. Paralysis may involve facial, extraocular, labial, lingual, pharyngeal, and laryngeal muscles. Evidence of intercostal and phrenic nerve involvement includes breathlessness in vocalizations and shallow, irregular respirations. There may be variable degrees of sensory impairment. Most patients complain of muscle tenderness or sensitivity to slight pressure. Urinary incontinence or retention and constipation are frequently present.

Diagnostic Evaluation

Diagnosis is based on the paralytic manifestations and on electromyography. Cerebrospinal fluid analysis reveals an increased protein concentration, but other laboratory studies are noncontributory. The symmetric nature of the paralysis helps differentiate this disorder from spinal paralytic poliomyelitis, which usually affects sporadic muscle.

Therapeutic Management

Treatment of Guillain-Barré syndrome is symptomatic. In some reports, corticosteroid therapy has been of benefit in the early stages (Vallee and others, 1993). However, a controlled study using a short course of intravenous steroids found no benefit (Guillain-Barré Syndrome, 1993). Respiratory and pharyngeal involvement requires assisted ventilation, frequently with tracheostomy. Plasma exchange (plasmapheresis) may be beneficial both in shortening the length of illness and in lessening the long-term disability (Jansen, Perkins, and Ashwal, 1993).

Course and Prognosis. Better outcomes are associated with younger age, no requirement for respiratory assistance, slower progression of disease, normal peripheral nerve function by electromyograph, and treatment by plasmapheresis (McKhann, 1990).

Almost all deaths are caused by respiratory failure; therefore, early diagnosis and access to respiratory support are especially important. Muscle function begins to return 2 days to 2 weeks after the onset of symptoms, and recovery is complete in most cases. The rate of recovery is usually related to the degree of involvement, which may extend from a few weeks to months. The greater the degree of paralysis, the longer the recovery phase.

Nursing Considerations

Nursing care is essentially supportive and is the same as that required for quadriplegia from any cause. Since the care of the quadriplegic child is discussed in relation to spinal cord injury later in the chapter, it will not be considered at length here. The emphasis of care is on close observation to assess the extent of paralysis and prevention of complications.

During the acute phase of the disease the child's condition should be carefully observed for possible difficulty in swallowing and respiratory involvement. There should be a respirator on standby, a cardiac monitor attached, and suction apparatus, tracheostomy tray, and vasoconstrictor drugs available at the bedside. Vital signs and level of consciousness are monitored frequently. For the child who develops respiratory dysfunction, the care is the same as that of any child with respiratory distress requiring mechanical ventilation (see Chapter 31 and care of the child with tetanus who is given muscle relaxant drugs).

Throughout the recovery phase special emphasis is placed on prevention of complications, including good postural alignment, frequent change of position, and passive range of motion exercises. Children with oral and pharyngeal involvement are usually fed via a nasogastric tube to ensure adequate feeding. Bowel and bladder care is needed to avoid constipation and urine retention. Sensory impairment makes the child susceptible to burns and pressure ulcers.

Physical therapy is limited to passive range of motion exercises during the evolving phase of the disease. Later, as the disease stabilizes and recovery begins, an active physical therapy program is implemented to prevent contracture deformities and facilitate muscle recovery. This may include active exercise, gait training, and bracing.

Throughout the course of the illness child and parent support is paramount. The usual rapidity of the paralysis and the long period of recovery tax the emotional reserves of all family members greatly. The parents and child benefit from repeated reassurance that recovery is occurring and from realistic information regarding the possibility of permanent disability. In the event of a residual disability, the family needs assistance in accepting and adjusting to the loss of function (see Chapter 22). The **Guillain-Barré Syndrome Support Group*** is a nonprofit organization devoted to support, education, and research. It provides support to families from recovered persons, publishes informational literature and a newsletter, and maintains a list of practitioners experienced with the disease.

*P.O. Box 262, Wynnewood, PA 19096; (215) 642-6855.

TETANUS

Tetanus, or lockjaw, is an acute, preventable, and often fatal disease caused by an exotoxin produced by the anaerobic spore-forming, gram-positive bacillus *Clostridium tetani.* It is characterized by painful muscular rigidity primarily involving the masseter and neck muscles. There are four requirements for the development of tetanus: (1) presence of tetanus spores or vegetative forms of the bacillus, (2) injury to the tissues, (3) wound conditions that encourage multiplication of the organism, and (4) a susceptible host.

Tetanus spores are found in soil, dust, and the intestinal tracts of humans and animals, especially herbivorous animals. The organisms are more prevalent in rural areas but are readily carried to urban areas by the wind. They enter the body by way of wounds, particularly a puncture wound, burn, or crushed area. In the newborn, infection may occur through the umbilical cord, usually in situations in which infants are delivered in contaminated surroundings. The disease has the greatest incidence in months when persons are more involved in outdoor activities. Drug addicts are especially susceptible because of poor injection technique and the use of street heroin, which is often mixed with quinine, a protoplasmic poison that favors the growth of the organism.

Pathophysiology

When conditions are favorable, the organisms multiply and form two exotoxins: (1) ***tetanospasmin,*** a potent toxin that affects the central nervous system to produce the clinical manifestations of the disease, and (2) ***tetanolysin,*** which appears to have no significance. The ideal conditions for growth of the organisms are devitalized tissues without access to air, such as puncture wounds, wounds that have not been washed or kept clean, and those that have crusted over, trapping pus beneath. The exotoxin appears to reach the central nervous system by way of either the neuron axons or the vascular system. The toxin becomes fixed on nerve cells of the anterior horn of the spinal cord and the brainstem. The toxin acts at the myoneural junction to produce the muscular stiffness and lower the threshold for reflex excitability.

The incubation period for tetanus varies from 3 days to 3 weeks but 8 days is average. The traditional belief that the more extensive the injury, the shorter the incubation period and the more severe the symptoms, has not been confirmed in the United States (American Academy of Pediatrics, 1994).

Clinical Manifestations

There are several forms of the disease. ***Local tetanus*** is a less severe form characterized by persistent rigidity of muscles near the inoculation site, which may persist for weeks or months, but some cases resolve without sequelae. ***Neonatal tetanus*** results from contamination of the umbilical cord; it is rare in the United States but is common and often fatal in developing countries. The first symptom is difficulty in sucking, which progresses to total inability to suck, excessive crying, irritability, and nuchal rigidity.

Generalized tetanus is the most common and dangerous

form of the disease. The manner of onset varies, but the initial symptoms are usually a progressive stiffness and tenderness of the muscles in the neck and jaw. The characteristic difficulty in opening the mouth ***(trismus)***, caused by sustained contraction of the jaw-closing muscles, is evident early and gives the disease its common name, ***lockjaw***. Spasm of facial muscles produces the so-called sardonic smile ***(risus sardonicus)***. Progressive involvement of the trunk muscles causes opisthotonos and a boardlike rigidity of abdominal and limb muscles. There is difficulty in swallowing, and the patient is highly sensitive to external stimuli. The slightest noise, a gentle touch, or bright light will trigger convulsive muscular contractions that last seconds to minutes. The paroxysmal contractions recur with increased frequency until they become almost continuous.

Mentation is unaffected; the patient remains alert, and pain and distress are reflected in rapid pulse, sweating, and an anxious expression. Laryngospasm and tetany of respiratory muscles and accumulated secretions predispose to respiratory arrest, atelectasis, and pneumonia. Fever is usually absent or only mild; presence of fever generally indicates a poor prognosis. As the child recovers from the disease, the paroxysms become less and less frequent and gradually subside. Survival beyond 4 days usually indicates recovery, but complete recovery may require weeks.

Prevention

Preventive measures are based on the immune status of the affected child and the nature of the injury. Specific prophylactic therapy after trauma is administration of either tetanus toxoid or tetanus antitoxin. For clean, minor wounds in children who have completed the immunization series (see Chapter 12) or received a booster within the previous 10 years, a dose of tetanus toxoid is not necessary. Protective levels of antibody are maintained for at least 10 years; therefore antitoxin is not indicated for the fully immunized child. Children with more serious wounds (e.g., contaminated, puncture, crush, or burn wounds) are given a tetanus toxoid booster prophylactically as soon as possible after injury.

The unprotected or inadequately immunized child who sustains a "tetanus-prone" wound (such as, but not limited to, wounds contaminated with dirt, feces, soil, and saliva; puncture wounds; avulsions; and wounds resulting from missiles, crushing, burns, and frostbite) should receive ***tetanus immune globulin (TIG)***. Concurrent administration of both TIG and tetanus toxoid at separate sites is recommended both to provide protection and to initiate the active immune process. Completion of active immunization is carried out according to the usual pattern. Proper surgical cleansing and debridement of contaminated wounds reduce the chance of infection.

Therapeutic Management

The affected child is best treated in an intensive care facility where close and constant observation and equipment for monitoring and respiratory support are readily available. A quiet environment is preferred to reduce external stimuli. Neonates are placed in an open unit or incubator in which a constant environmental temperature can be maintained and oxygen supplied.

General supportive care, including maintenance of adequate fluid and electrolyte balance and caloric intake, is indicated. Indwelling oral or nasogastric feedings are used whenever possible, but severe laryngospasm may necessitate intravenous alimentation or gastrostomy feeding. Recurrent laryngospasm or excessive accumulation of secretions may require endotracheal intubation.

TIG therapy to neutralize toxins is the most specific therapy for tetanus. Antibiotics are administered to control the proliferation of the vegetative forms of the organism at the site of infection. When the child recovers, active immunization should take place, since the disease does not confer a permanent immunity.

Local care of the wound by surgical debridement and cleansing with an antiseptic solution helps reduce the numbers of proliferating organisms at the site of injury. The cleansing should be repeated several times during the first 48 hours, and deep, infected lacerations are usually exposed and debrided.

Sedatives or muscle relaxants are administered to help reduce muscle spasm and prevent convulsions. Patients with severe tetanus and those who do not respond to other sedatives may require the administration of a neuromuscular blocking agent, usually pancuronium bromide (Pavulon) or *d*-tubocurarine. Because of their paralytic effect on respiratory muscles, use of these drugs requires mechanical ventilation and constant attendance by trained personnel until muscle spasms are controlled.

Endotracheal tube insertion or tracheostomy is often indicated and should be performed before severe respiratory distress develops. Administration of corticosteroids has met with success in some instances.

Nursing Considerations

In caring for the child with tetanus, every effort should be made to control or eliminate stimulation from sound, light, and touch. Although a darkened room is ideal, sufficient light is essential in order that the child can be carefully observed; light appears to be less irritating than vibratory or auditory stimuli. The infant or child is handled as little as possible, and extra effort is expended to avoid any sudden and/or loud noise.

Medications are administered as prescribed, and vital signs are observed and recorded at frequent intervals. The location and extent of muscle spasms and assessment of their severity are important nursing observations. Respiratory status is carefully evaluated for any signs of distress, and appropriate emergency equipment is kept available at all times. Muscle relaxants and sedatives that may be prescribed can also cause respiratory depression; therefore the child must be assessed for excessive central nervous system depression. Oxygen saturation monitoring and, when needed, blood gases are obtained frequently to evaluate the respiratory status. Attention to hydration and nutrition may involve monitoring an intravenous infusion, monitoring nasogastric or gastrostomy feedings, and suctioning oropharyngeal secretions when indicated.

If a potent muscle relaxant such as pancuronium bromide (Pavulon) is used, the total paralysis makes oral communication impossible. Therefore all the child's needs must be anticipated, and procedures carefully explained beforehand. As the dose of medication is decreased, the child regains movement of the eyelids and facial muscles, which gives the child some opportunity to express emotions and indicate choices through a signal system, for example, blinking the lids to indicate "yes" or "no."

Since their mental status is clear, children are aware of what is happening to them and are often in a state of terror. They should not be left alone, and all efforts should be made to reduce anxiety, which can contribute to muscular spasms. A calm and reassuring manner and sympathetic understanding can help immeasurably in getting a child through this crisis situation. Parents are encouraged to stay with the child to offer security and support.

BOTULISM

Botulism is a serious food poisoning that results from ingestion of the preformed toxin produced by the anaerobic bacillus *Clostridium botulinum*. Botulism toxin exerts its effect by inhibiting the release of acetylcholine at the myoneural junction, thereby impairing motor activity of muscles innervated by affected nerves. There is wide variation in severity of the disease, from constipation to progressive sequential loss of neurologic function and respiratory failure.

Types of Botulism

Three forms of the disease are recognized: infantile botulism, classic botulism, and wound botulism.

Classic, or Food-Borne, Botulism. The classic form of the disease is usually seen in adults but may occur in children and adolescents. The most common source of the toxin is improperly sterilized home-canned foods. Central nervous system symptoms appear abruptly about 12 to 36 hours after ingestion of contaminated food and may or may not have been preceded by acute digestive disturbance. Early symptoms include blurred vision, diplopia, weakness, dizziness, difficulty talking and speaking, vomiting, and dysphagia. These are followed by descending paralysis and dyspnea. Progressive respiratory paralysis is life-threatening.

Infant Botulism. Infant botulism, unlike the disease in older persons, is caused by ingestion of spores or vegetative cells of *C. botulinum* and the subsequent release of the toxin from organisms colonizing the gastrointestinal tract. There appears to be no common food or drug source of the organisms; however, the *C. botulinum* organisms have been found in honey fed to affected infants, and light, as well as dark, corn syrup has been reported to contain spores, but at lower rates than honey (American Academy of Pediatrics, 1994).

One study (Spika and others, 1989) identified risk factors for infant botulism in the United States. They appear to be decreased frequency of bowel movements (less than one per day for at least 2 months) in infants 2 months of age or older, and ingestion of corn syrup and living in a rural area or on a farm for infants less than 2 months of age. Thus preexisting host factors may be the most important risk factors for developing the disease.

The affected infant is usually well before the onset of symptoms. Constipation is a common presenting symptom, and almost all infants exhibit generalized weakness and a decrease in spontaneous movements. Deep tendon reflexes are usually diminished or absent; cranial nerve deficits are common (especially CN VII, IX, X, and XI), as evidenced by loss of head control, difficulty in feeding, weak cry, and reduced gag reflex. The most frequently recognized form of the disease is consistent with the "floppy infant syndrome."

Wound Botulism. Wounds contaminated with *C. botulinum* and subsequent elaboration of the toxin produce classic symptoms in about 4 to 14 days after tissue trauma. The disease has been described in a small number of adolescents and adults, and most wounds are sustained in open fields or on farms.

Therapeutic Management

Diagnosis is made on the basis of history, physical examination, and laboratory detection of toxin or the organism in the patient or the implicated food. Treatment consists of aggressive supportive measures, primarily respiratory and nutritional. Botulinum antitoxin is sometimes used in adults and older children for food-borne or wound botulism. Evidence indicates that the infants recover without it and that its therapeutic efficacy is lacking. Furthermore, since the antitoxin is made from horse serum, it may cause serum sickness or anaphylaxis and may induce a lifelong hypersensitivity. A human-derived botulism antitoxin is under investigation (Schwartz and Arnon, 1992).

Toxins vary in protein-binding capacity. Some have a relatively short half-life and do not bind to tissues firmly; therefore therapy is continued until paralysis abates. Other toxins appear to bind irreversibly to nerve endings and are therefore not amenable to neutralization. Respiratory support is often needed and should be available at the bedside ready for use if indicated.

The prognosis is generally good if the patient is adequately supported, although recovery may be very slow, requiring weeks to months following severe illness.

Nursing Considerations

Nursing responsibilities include observing for and reporting signs of muscle impairment and providing intensive nursing care when the infant is hospitalized (see Nursing Care of High-Risk Newborns, Chapter 10). Parental support and reassurance are important. Most infants recover when the disorder is recognized and therapy implemented. Parents should be aware that during recovery patients fatigue easily when muscular action is sustained. This has important implications for timing the resumption of feedings because of the risk of aspiration. They should also be advised that normal bowel action may not return for several weeks; therefore a stool softener can be beneficial. Cathartics and enemas are not advised.

Home supervision of the outpatient and education regarding possible modes of infection (such as use of honey as formula sweetener) are nursing responsibilities. Since the prime sources of botulism toxin are inadequately cooked or improperly canned food, families are advised about the danger of home-canned foods, especially vegetables, fruits, fish, and condiments. Boiling is not always adequate, particularly in high altitudes where water boils at a lower temperature, which does not destroy the organisms (Parke, 1990).

MYASTHENIA GRAVIS (MG)

MG is relatively uncommon in childhood. Juvenile MG appears to be identical to that seen in adults and usually has its onset after age 10 years, but it may appear as early as age 2 years. Girls are affected six times as often as boys. Juvenile and adult forms of the disease are autoimmune disorders associated with attack of circulating antibodies on the acetylcholine receptors on the muscle end plate, blocking their function.

Clinical Manifestations

The most common symptoms are general paralysis of the optic muscles with ptosis and diplopia. Difficulty in swallowing, chewing, and speaking is also prominent, accompanied by weakness and paralysis of all skeletal muscles. The signs and symptoms are more pronounced in the late afternoon and evening. They are relieved by rest and made worse by exercise and stress.

Diagnostic Evaluation

The diagnosis is made on the basis of the characteristic distribution of muscle weakness and the progressive weakness on repeated or sustained muscular contraction. The diagnosis is established by observation of the response to the anticholinesterase drugs. Intravenous administration of a small test dose of edrophonium (Tensilon) produces a beneficial effect in 1 minute but lasts for less than 5 minutes. Electrophysiologic studies are helpful in diagnosis and help document transmission failure at the myoneural junction. Antibodies to human muscle acetylcholine are detected in serum of almost all affected persons.

Therapeutic Management

Treatment consists of the oral administration of anticholinesterase drugs, the least toxic of which is pyridostigmine (Mestinon). The initial dose is 30 mg every 4 hours in the older child and 5 mg every 4 hours in the infant. The dosage is gradually increased until a satisfactory result is obtained. The child must be observed for signs of parasympathetic stimulation from overmedication. These include lacrimation, salivation, abdominal cramps, sweating, diarrhea, vomiting, bradycardia, and weakness of respiratory muscles.

Other therapies directed at the immunologic mechanism include thymectomy (removal of the thymus), corticosteroid therapy, and immunosuppression, with agents such as azathioprine (AZA). Children with generalized MG have responded favorably to thymectomy (Adams and others, 1990; Blossom and others, 1993). Plasmapheresis has been used for short-term intensive intervention (Antozzi and others, 1991).

The prognosis of juvenile MG is relatively good. However, the course of the disease is marked by fluctuating remissions and exacerbations.

Nursing Considerations

These children need continuous medical and nursing supervision. The parents are taught the importance of accurate administration of medications, with special emphasis on recognizing side effects with the dangers of choking, aspiration, and respiratory distress.

Parents are counseled regarding promoting a life-style that minimizes stress and maximizes relaxation. Strenuous activity is discouraged. They are also warned of the possibility of a sudden exacerbation of symptoms during times of physical or emotional stress (myasthenia crisis) that requires immediate medical attention. They should receive instruction in providing respiratory assistance until help arrives or the child can be transported to medical aid.

Neonatal Myasthenia Gravis

A ***transient*** form of MG occurs in approximately 15% of infants born to mothers with myasthenia gravis who may not be aware that they have the disease. The muscular weakness results from transplacentally acquired maternal acetylcholine receptor antibodies. These infants display generalized weakness and hypotonia at birth with a depressed Moro reflex, ptosis, ineffective sucking and swallowing reflexes, and weak cry. There is no evidence of neurologic damage. In this form the symptoms usually disappear within 2 to 4 weeks.

Persistent neonatal MG is a familial abnormality of neuromuscular transmission that is not immunologically mediated. It appears indistinguishable from the transient form, but the mother usually does not have the disease. The disease persists throughout life, and more than one sibling may be affected, which suggests a genetic etiology. Sex distribution is equal. The disorder is relatively resistant to drug therapy, and the eyelid and extraocular muscles seem to be the muscles most severely affected.

The prognosis in persistent neonatal MG is usually good. Although there is gradual worsening of symptoms with age, the life span is not affected significantly.

SPINAL CORD INJURIES

Spinal cord injuries with major neurologic involvement are not a common cause of physical disability in childhood. However, a sufficient number of children with these injuries are admitted to major medical centers, and because of the increased survival as the result of improved management, nurses are more likely to become involved with such children. In addition, the catastrophic nature of spinal cord injury with its serious sequelae and the importance of preventive and functional rehabilitation justify a discussion of the topic. The principles of management and nursing care apply to all spinal cord lesions, regardless of etiology, particularly myelomeningocele, the most common cause of paraplegia in the pediatric age-group.

In addition to care related to the immobilized child as discussed in Chapter 39, children with damage to the spinal cord present additional problems, specifically complications related to the neuropathology of the central and autonomic nervous systems. A high level of paraplegia may create major problems in the ability to sit upright without support, whereas children with paraplegia with lower level injuries can walk with minimum assistance. The extent of paralysis is determined by both neurologic and clinical assessment. Although the majority of children with spinal cord injuries are paraplegic, many are quadriplegic. Some children with quadriplegia are able to move only their face and neck muscles, whereas others are able to lift and bend their arms but are unable to perform fine hand movements. Almost every physiologic system is disrupted in a child with high-level quadriplegia. Not only are the central and peripheral nerves impaired, but there is also autonomic nervous system dysfunction. Vital structures such as blood vessels, lungs, bladder, and bowel are affected. Therefore an understanding of neuromuscular physiology is essential to effectively care for the child with damage or injury to the spinal cord.

Review of Essential Neuromuscular Physiology

The spinal cord extends from the medulla oblongata to the lower border of the first lumbar vertebra and contains millions of nerve fibers (Fig. 40-7). However, because of its protected location, a considerable amount of direct trauma is required to cause injury. Posteriorly the cord is protected by the spinous processes, which are stabilized by related ligaments and muscles. It is further protected by the spinal fluid, which surrounds it and absorbs some of the shock.

Spinal Nerves. The 31 nerves of the spinal cord are divided into five segments. The eight ***cervical*** cord segments lie within the first seven vertebrae. The remaining cord segments—***thoracic*** (12), ***lumbar*** (five), ***sacral*** (five), and ***coccygeal*** (one)—extend from the first thoracic vertebra to the lower level of the first lumbar vertebra. Therefore the cord constituents do not anatomically match by number the 30 associated vertebrae. However, nerves that arise from the spinal cord exit from the spinal column at the numerically corresponding vertebrae. In describing injuries to the spinal cord, the highest point at which there is normal function is referred to in relation to the vertebra; for example, an intact cord at the sixth cervical vertebra is designated as a C6 injury.

Certain areas of the curved vertebral column are less stable and more prone to damage from severe flexion and twisting. These sites are the cervical area and the junction of the thoracic and lumbar regions. The cervical vertebrae are fractured most frequently, and this high level of injury causes extensive paralysis and many associated neurologic problems (see Table 40-2). Also, traumatic tearing or embolic occlusion of arteries supplying these areas can markedly jeopardize the cord tissue. Impaired blood supply frequently produces severe neurologic deficit, which can extend to complete loss of cord function at the level of injury.

Cell bodies of interneurons and motor neurons within the spinal cord are identified as H-shaped gray matter surrounded by columns of white myelinated nerve fibers, each column serving as a route for a specific type of impulse, such as touch, vibration, pain, and temperature (Fig. 40-8). Nerve pathways in the spinal cord transmit sensory and motor impulses between peripheral receptors and the brain, conduct impulses through the reflex arc, and convey sympathetic and parasympathetic nerve impulses from the brain to peripheral structures.

Sensory transmission begins when peripheral receptors pick up a wide variety of stimuli and transfer the impulses, by means of peripheral nerves, to the spinal nerves, where

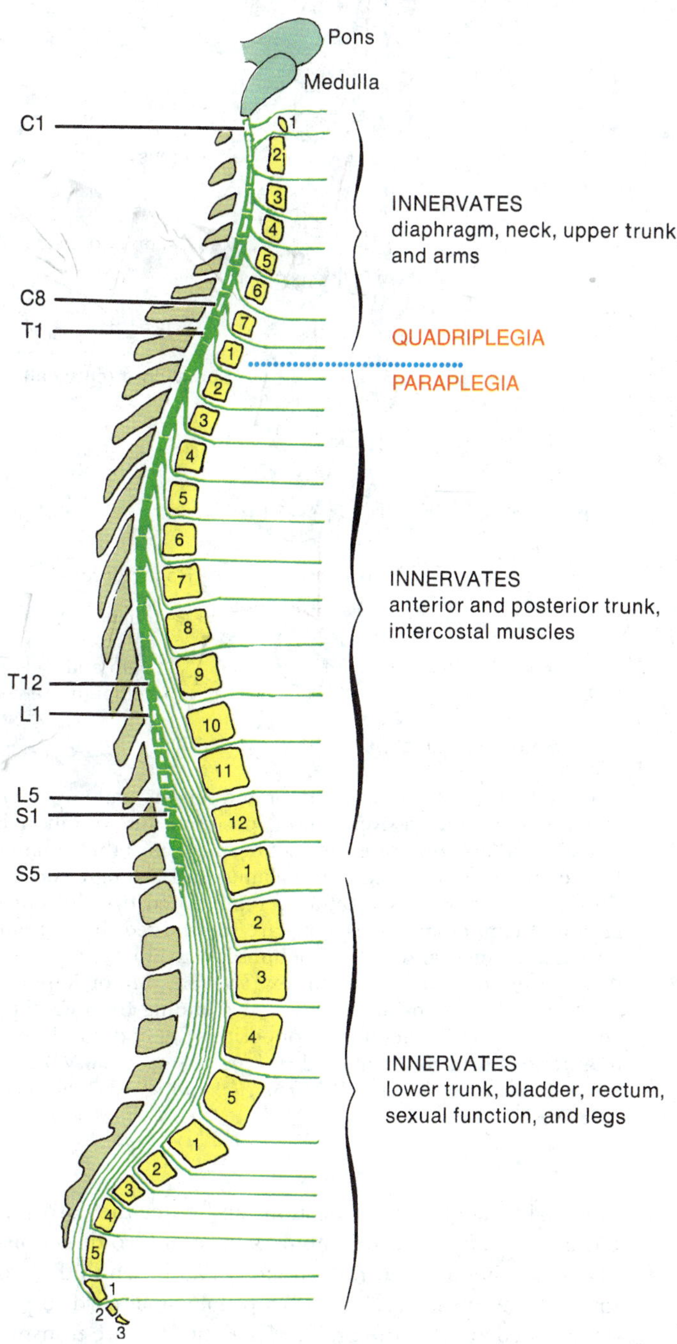

FIG. 40-7 Relationships of spinal cord segments and spinal nerves to vertebral bodies. Cervical nerves exit through intervertebral foramina above their respective vertebral bodies (seven cervical vertebrae and eight cervical nerves). Spinal cord ends at L1 and L2 vertebral level.

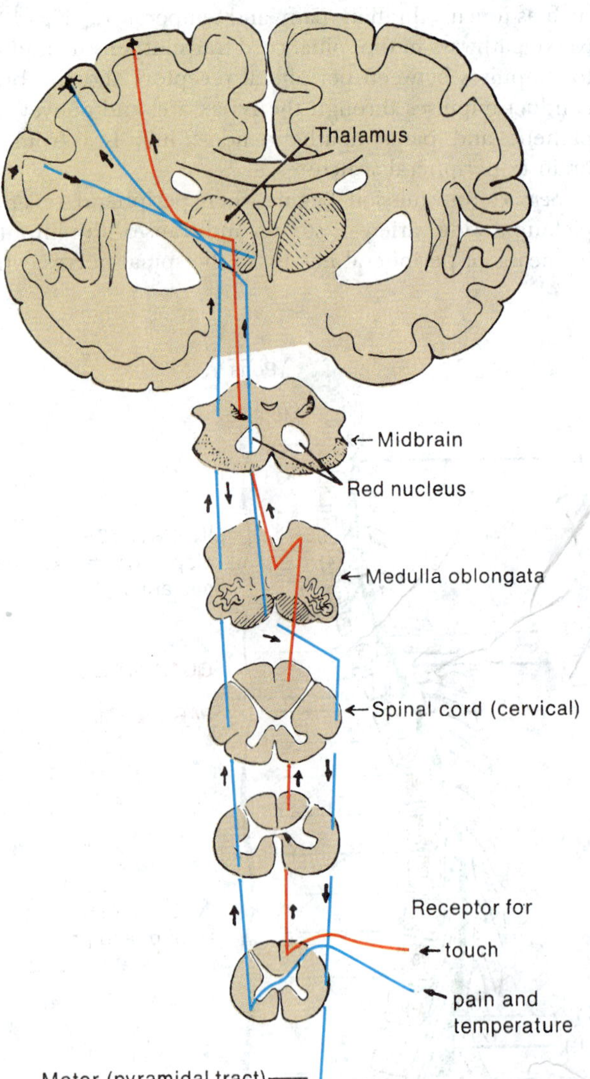

FIG. 40-8 Diagram of main motor and sensory pathways. Perception of touch, passive motion, position, and vibration is transmitted through posterior tract in spinal cord through medial lemniscus in brainstem to thalamus and through internal capsule to cortex (this pathway is represented by solid line). Pain and temperature sensations are transmitted through anterolateral tract and lateral lemniscus to thalamus, then through internal capsule to cortex *(blue line)*. Motor impulses are transmitted by pyramidal tract, descending from cerebral cortex, crossing in medulla to opposite side, and continuing to anterior horns of spinal cord *(red line)*. (From Conway BL: *Carini and Owens' neurological and neurosurgical nursing,* ed 7, St Louis, 1978, Mosby.)

they make ganglionic connections and enter the cord posteriorly. At this point the impulses travel in two directions: (1) across the intraneuron connection and then to the motor neurons (reflex arc), or (2) up the spinal cord to predetermined areas of the brain. ***Motor*** impulses are transmitted from the cerebral cortex to the medulla (where nerve tracts cross) and then proceed down descending motor pathways to the desired level within the spinal cord. Here they connect with the anterior horn cells and are transmitted to the muscle fibers by means of the lower motor neurons to complete a meaningful movement.

THE THREE MAJOR PLEXUSES

Cervical plexus (C1 through C4), which innervates the neck and diaphragm
Brachial plexus (C4 through T1), which supplies the shoulders, chest, and arms
Lumbosacral plexus (L1 through S4), which transmits impulses to the lower trunk and legs

A network of nerves that serves the major muscle groups constitutes a ***plexus.*** Total involvement of any one of these plexuses seriously impairs function to the areas it innervates. The three major plexuses are described in the box above.

Upper vs Lower Motor Neurons. ***Upper motor neurons*** extend from cerebral centers to cells in the spinal column; ***lower motor neurons*** consist of anterior horn cells and spinal and peripheral nerves. Motor fibers of the reflex arc are lower motor neurons, an important point, since relative dominance of the higher central nervous system (CNS) over reflex arcs suppresses some reflex responses. In spinal cord injury when the higher centers no longer exert an influence, spastic responses are observed in muscles innervated by the intact lower motor neurons. Most spinal cord injuries involve upper motor neurons; children born with spinal cord defects have primarily lower motor neuron deficits. (See also Fig. 40-1.) Manifestations of upper and lower motor neuron syndromes are outlined in the left-hand box on p. 1891.

Effect on Sensory and Motor Tracts. Voluntary muscle control is lost following complete transection of the cord. In partial transection, function is altered to varying degrees, depending on the areas innervated by involved nerves. Crossing of motor tracts at various levels makes it possible for an injured person to have motor paralysis in one leg but retain pain and temperature sensation in that leg while losing these sensations in the opposite leg, which retains its motor function.

Although a transected cord injury leads to sensory loss, it is not uncommon for the injured person to have pain experiences. For example, smooth or skeletal muscle spasms, destruction of the myelin sheath (impulses cross to adjacent nerves), and scar formation or irritation of nerve endings may cause pain. Pain suffered by a person with quadriplegia or paraplegia is often intensified because of loss of sensation in other parts. Severe and prolonged pain should be medically evaluated for treatable pathology.

Effect on Autonomic System. Sympathetic and parasympathetic systems receive both excitatory and inhibitory stimuli from autonomic centers in the cerebral cortex, limbic system, and hypothalamus. The stimuli are transmitted by means of a feedback mechanism within the ascending fibers of the cord that normally controls descending input. Axons of the many CNS neurons synapse with autonomic preganglionic fibers and thus are able to alter their pat-

DIFFERENCES IN CLINICAL MANIFESTATIONS BETWEEN UPPER AND LOWER MOTOR NEURON SYNDROMES

UPPER MOTOR NEURON SYNDROME	LOWER MOTOR NEURON SYNDROME
Spastic paralysis in muscle groups below lesion (reflex arcs below lesion are intact)	Flaccid paralysis caused by muscle atonia (reflex arcs are permanently damaged)
Hyperreflexia with tendon reflexes exaggerated, Babinski reflex present	Reflex with associated muscle response absent
No wasting of muscle mass because of increased muscle tone	Marked atrophy of atonic muscle
Flexion contractures and spasms of muscle groups below lesion level common	Fasciculations (local twitching of muscle groups) common No flexor spasms
No skin or tissue changes	Loss of hair Skin and tissue changes Cornified nails

SIGNIFICANT EFFECTS OF AUTONOMIC DISRUPTION

Decreased muscle tone and impairment of vasoconstrictive effects of sympathetic innervation cause venous pooling, diminished venous return to the heart, decreased cardiac output, and hypotension, especially orthostatic hypotension.

Thermoregulatory disruption in the hypothalamus and skin receptors causes blood vessels to remain dilated during the initial stage, inability to sweat in response to increased environmental temperature, and possible rapid elevation in body temperature.

Voluntary bowel and bladder function is lost because of damage to nerve fibers that innervate these organs.

Altered sexual function (lack of erection, ejaculation, and orgasm) results from interference with numerous autonomic nerve fibers and plexuses.

terned responses. The most significant effects of autonomic disruption are described in the box above, right.

Etiology

The most common cause of serious spinal cord damage in children is congenital defects of the spinal cord (e.g., myelomeningocele). Postnatal causes are primarily accidental injury, especially motor vehicle accidents (MVAs) (including automobile-bicycle and all-terrain vehicle accidents), sports injuries (especially from diving, trampoline activities, gymnastics, and football), and birth trauma.

Transverse myelitis (inflammation of the spinal cord) has also been reported to develop from inadvertent intraarterial administration of long-acting penicillin when injected into the buttocks. Damage can be extensive enough to result in paraplegia or even lower limb amputation (Schanzer and Jacobson, 1985).

Mechanisms of Injury. In MVAs most spinal cord injuries in children are the result of indirect trauma caused by sudden hyperflexion or hyperextension of the neck, often combined with a rotational force. Trauma to the spinal cord without evidence of vertebral fracture or dislocation is particularly apt to occur in MVAs when proper restraints are not used. An unrestrained child becomes a projectile during sudden deceleration and is subject to injury from contact with a variety of objects inside and outside the automobile. Few persons receive spinal injuries when secured with properly fitting seat belts (i.e., cross-chest restraints). Stretch injuries and internal injuries are sustained from use of only a lap restraint. High cervical spine injuries have been reported in children less than 2 years of age restrained in forward-facing car seats (Fuchs and others, 1989).

Falling from heights occurs less often in children than in adults, but vertebral compression of the spine from blows to the head or buttocks occurs in water sports (diving and surfing) or falls from horses or other athletic injuries. Birth injuries may occur in breech delivery from traction force on the cord during delivery of the head and shoulders. A number of teenagers receive cord injuries when they are shot or stabbed in the back. Infants sustain cervical cord damage (as well as brain and eye damage, mental retardation, and death) when they are shaken. Infants have very weak neck muscles, and during vigorous shaking their heavy heads wobble rapidly back and forth.

Fracture or ***subluxation*** (partial ***dislocation***) is the most frequent immediate cause of spinal cord injury, particularly in the lower cervical region, because of the marked mobility of the neck. Spinal cord injury without fracture, although unusual in adults, is not uncommon in the child, whose spine is suppler, weaker, and more mobile than that of the adult, so the force is more easily dissipated over a larger number of segments. In children the vertebral column, composed of cartilaginous rings, is capable of considerable elongation, whereas the cord itself, its meninges, and its vascular supply are unable to withstand the same degree of traction.

The injury sustained can affect any of the spinal nerves, and the higher the injury, the more extensive the damage. The child can be left with complete or partial paralysis of the lower extremities ***(paraplegia)*** or with damage at a higher level and without functional use of any of the four extremities ***(quadriplegia)***. A high cervical cord injury that affects the phrenic nerve paralyzes the diaphragm and leaves the child dependent on a ventilator.

A mild but equally frightening form of cord trauma is ***spinal cord compression,*** a temporary neural dysfunction without visible damage to the cord. Complete quadraplegia can result but initially may not be differentiated from serious cord injury (Rathbone and others, 1992).

Pathophysiology

The severity of the force, the mechanisms of the injury, and the degree of the individual's muscular relaxation at the time of the injury greatly influence the extensiveness of the trauma. Compression, contusion, laceration, and anatomic transection are the basic types of cord injuries and usually involve four interrelated pathologic changes: (1) cellular damage to cord tissue; (2) hemorrhage and vascular damage; (3) structural changes of white and gray matter related to vascular disruption, inflammation, and edema; and (4) local biochemical response to trauma. Changes in one of these can lead to changes in another. For example, an acute injury produces a decreased blood supply to the cord tissue, with resulting ischemia that can lead to cellular necrosis. Acid metabolites accumulate during the hypoxic state and can contribute to further cellular damage. A concurrent inflammatory process produces cord edema above and below the traumatized segment, which further decreases the blood supply. Research on spinal cord trauma indicates that the neurotransmitters norepinephrine and dopamine can be markedly altered in the first few hours after injury, which causes further development of hemorrhagic necrosis in the central gray matter.

Clinical Manifestations

As a result of these pathologic responses to the initial trauma, spinal cord injury causes three stages of response; therefore the extent and severity of damage cannot be determined at first. Immediate loss of function is caused by both anatomic and impaired physiologic function, and improved function may not be evident for weeks or even months.

First Stage. Manifestation of the initial response to acute injury is flaccid paralysis below the level of the damage. This stage is known as ***diaschisis*** or ***spinal shock syndrome*** and is caused by the sudden disruption of central and autonomic pathways. Local effects of cord edema and ischemia produce a physiologic transection with or without an anatomic severance. Most children with a spinal cord injury experience some spinal shock. Manifestations include absence of reflexes at or below the cord lesion with flaccidity or limpness of the involved muscles, loss of sensation and motor function, and autonomic dysfunction (symptoms of hypotension, low or high body temperatures, loss of bladder and bowel control, and autonomic dysreflexia) (see p. 1897).

These symptoms occur soon after the injury and last 1 to 6 weeks, with much autonomic reflex cord function returning in about 3 weeks. The length of this stage indicates to some degree the extent of later recovery. In general, the shorter the duration of spinal shock, the more neurologic return can be anticipated. Problems related to this first stage are the serious consequences of prolonged immobility: atrophy of both paralyzed and noninvolved muscles, negative nitrogen balance, calcium loss from bone, atonic bladder and urinary retention, risk of skin breakdown, reduced cardiac output and plasma volume, and respiratory compromise (especially with high involvement).

Autonomic paralysis also affects thermoregulatory functions. Afferent impulses from temperature receptors in the skin are not integrated; therefore the patient is subject to temperature increase or decrease in response to alterations in environmental temperature. Hyperthermia can result from excessive ambient temperature, such as too many covers.

Second Stage. Except in the situations previously mentioned, flaccid paralysis is replaced by spinal reflex activity and increasing spasticity or, in partial lesions, greater or lesser degree of neurologic recovery. Diagnosis may be confused in infants since spinal reflexes in paralyzed limbs may be misinterpreted as the normal movements in the infant. Even minor stimuli, such as rubbing the mattress, are sufficient to elicit spinal reflexes. Concurrent crying may also lead to the erroneous impression that sensation is intact. Absence of spontaneous leg movement of the extremities when the infant is held vertically suspended under the axilla suggests paralysis. Reflex withdrawal or extension of the limb after tactile or pinprick stimulus confirms a diagnosis.

Problems related to spasticity include contractures (especially of the hip adductor, hip and knee flexor muscles, and heel cords). Contraction of spastic muscles reduces bone demineralization and nitrogen loss somewhat. The atonic bladder becomes hypertonic, and, instead of continuous dribbling, urine is expelled involuntarily at intervals by reflex action.

The paralytic nature of autonomic function is replaced by ***autonomic dysreflexia,*** especially when the lesions are above the midthoracic level. This autonomic phenomenon is caused by visceral distention or irritation, particularly bowel or bladder. This triggers sensory impulses, which travel to the cord lesion, where they are blocked, causing activation of sympathetic reflex action with disturbed central inhibitory control. Excessive sympathetic activity is manifested by flushing of the face, sweating of the forehead, pupillary constriction, marked hypertension, headache, and bradycardia. The precipitating stimulus may be merely a full bladder or rectum or other internal or external sensory input. It can be a catastrophic event unless the irritation is relieved (see p. 1897).

Third Stage. In the final stage neurologic signs are stabilized in terms of loss and recovery of function. The major emphasis is on rehabilitation. A problem unique to injury in childhood is progressive spinal deformity usually not seen in adults or in adolescents near the end of the growth period. Scoliosis develops in the major percentage of children with high thoracic and cervical lesions and is almost certain to occur in children with quadriplegia whose injury occurred in infancy or early childhood. Consequently, affected infants and children are placed in carefully constructed trunk supports. Kyphosis usually appears locally at the site of the initial injury, especially when it results from hyperflexion-type injuries. Proper immobilization during vertebral healing helps to prevent progressive deformity. Increasing lordosis occurs with the development of hip contracture caused by spasticity or by prolonged sitting in nonambulatory children.

Diagnostic Evaluation. A history of the nature of the injury provides valuable clues regarding the possible type of damage incurred and direction for further assessment without the risk of additional damage. A complete neurologic examination is performed to determine if damage was incurred and, if so, the level and extent of any nerve impairment. A neurologic unit of the CNS is considered normal if reflex arcs are functioning, sensory tracts are intact when each dermatome is examined separately, and voluntary motor response demonstrates ability to move a body part against gravity on command.

Testing a reflex arc is accomplished by stimulating peripheral receptors at a specific site, such as eliciting the patellar reflex. Symmetric testing is performed to determine unilateral or bilateral neurologic deficit. A sufficient number of reflexes are examined to test motor function thoroughly. The blunt end of a safety pin is used to assess pressure sensitivity, and the sharp point is used to elicit pain. Hot and cold water, a tuning fork, and cotton may also be used to determine specific sensory loss (e.g., temperature, vibration, and light touch).

Body surface zones, or dermatomes, accurately correspond to the spinal cord segment receiving the sensory input from the peripheral nerves in that zone. Systematically pinpricking the body surface in each zone determines intactness of sensory pathways. The zones and the spinal cord segments they represent are illustrated in Fig. 40-9. The examiner tests for each specific sensory fiber in the dermatome areas in which there is a suspected neurologic deficit. Proprioception, or knowing where one's extremities are, is a very vital sense for ambulating safely.

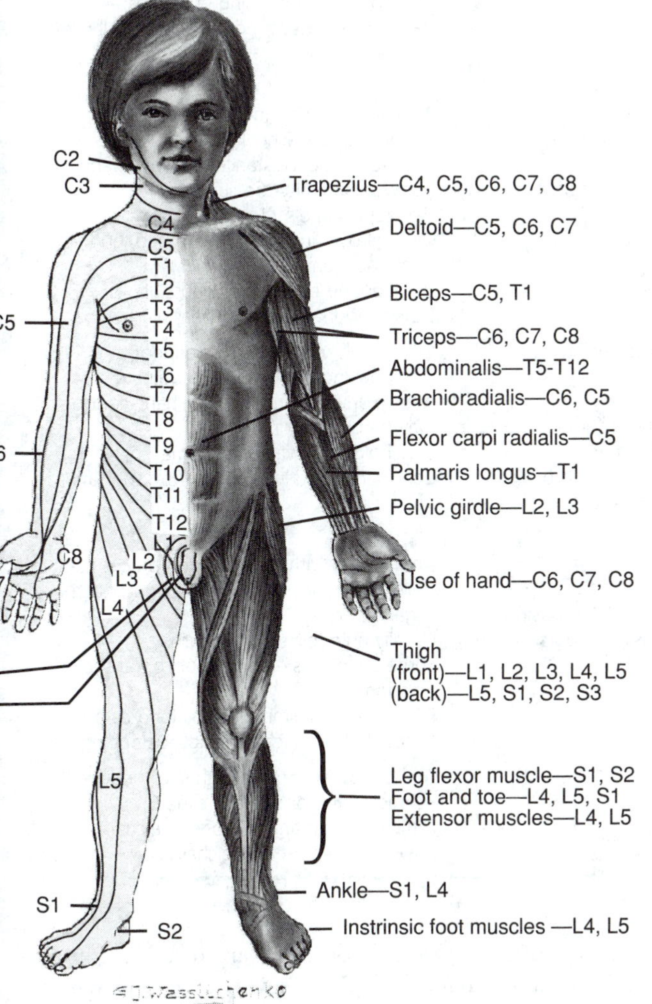

FIG. 40-9 Dermatomes and innervation of major muscles needed for performing activities of daily living.

Matching cord level to vertebra is more difficult in infants and young children than it is in older children and adults because the sacral and several lower lumbar cord segments lie at a lower position, especially during the first 2 years of life (see Fig. 4-8). The spinal anatomy approaches adult configuration by the time the child reaches 7 or 8 years; by late adolescence the conus medullaris has usually reached the level of L1.

Motor system evaluation includes observation of gait if the child is able to walk, noting balance maintenance with the eyes open and closed, and ability to lift, flex, and extend the arms and legs. Testing muscle strength with and without resistance and against gravity will give clues to the specific nature and degree of motor dysfunction. The number of muscles in any muscle group that remain completely intact in the upper extremities makes a marked difference in the individual's ability to provide self-care, especially at high injury levels. The presence of abdominal muscles is valuable in bladder and bowel training and in maintaining an upright sitting position. Hip movement is necessary for ambulation with braces and crutches.

The degree to which supportive aids are needed for ambulation is determined by the strength, stability, and movement of the pelvis, trunk, hip flexor muscles, and quadriceps muscles. A general guideline for determining the capacity for self-help is that a person with paraplegia who has function down to and including the quadriceps muscle or muscle function below the L3 level will have little difficulty in learning to walk with or without braces and crutches. It is especially vital that children with lumbar levels of injury be taught to walk functionally so that they are weight bearing at least part of the time to minimize the risk of osteoporosis and hypercalcemia. The functional significance of the spinal cord lesion level is summarized in Table 40-2.

If CNS pathology is detected, a body system assessment is performed to determine the degree of autonomic impairment. Because the cord and CNS directly influence the function of the autonomic nerves, the specific sympathetically related organ systems are examined for skeletal muscle and vascular tone and body temperature regulation. For example, bladder and gastrointestinal function have sympathetic and parasympathetic innervation and local reflexes.

Radiographic examination and computed tomography (CT) scans are important for localizing the lesion, but the nature of the spine in childhood frequently creates difficulty in interpretation. Some children will have no radiographic evidence of vertebral or spinal injury; this condition is ***spinal cord injury without radiographic abnormality (SCIWORA)***. The development of SCIWORA usually indicates the presence of severe subluxation and trauma (Lang and Bernardo, 1993). Radiograms must be taken carefully and with sufficient help to prevent further damage to the spine. Several persons may be needed to log roll the patient and to support the head during turning or transfer.

TABLE 40-2 Functional Significance of Spinal Cord Lesions

HIGHEST INTACT CORD SEGMENT	FUNCTIONAL CAPACITY	FUNCTIONAL GOALS
C1-3 Muscle innervation: None below chin, including phrenic nerve to diaphragm	No voluntary control below chin Respiratory paralysis complete May cause bradycardia or tachycardia, vomiting	Artificial ventilation; can be taught glossopharyngeal breathing to be used for short periods Electric wheelchair Adaptive equipment for special tasks in bed or wheelchair using mouth stick
C4 (high quadriplegia) Muscle innervation: Intact sternocleidomastoid, trapezius, upper cervical paraspinous muscles	No voluntary function of upper extremities, trunk, or lower extremities All neck movements Respirator dependent	Electric wheelchair Externally powered devices and adaptive equipment for special tasks in bed or wheelchair with mouth stick, such as turning pages, using computer Totally dependent for activities of daily living
C5 Muscle innervation: Partial deltoid, biceps, major muscles of rotator cuffs at shoulders Diaphragm	Abduction, flexion, and extension of arm Flexion and extension of forearm Unable to roll over or attain sitting position Abdominal respiration Poor respiratory reserve	Electric wheelchair Requires attendant to assist in moving and transfer to wheelchair Adaptive devices for self-feeding, grooming, using computer Vocational potential with adaptive devices
C6 Muscle innervation: Pectoralis major, serratus anterior, latissimus dorsi muscles Complete deltoid and brachioradialis muscles Partial triceps muscle	Significant increase in function over that with lesion at C5 level Adduction and medial rotation of arm Wrist extension Good elbow flexion	Cuff strapped to hand permits use of implements for self-care and other activities Able to assist in dressing and transfer Hand rim extension permits independence in wheelchair
C7 Muscle innervation: Triceps and finger flexor and extensor muscle Shoulder depressor muscles Still nerve disruption to intercostal muscles	With elbow stabilized in extension and intact shoulder depressor muscles able to lift body weight Grasp and release still weak; dexterity lacking	Almost complete independence within limitations of wheelchair Requires some assistance in transfer and lower extremity dressing Hand splints helpful Can roll over in bed, sit up in bed, and eat independently Homebound employment possible Outside work usually not feasible
T1-10 (high paraplegia) Muscle innervation: Full innervation of upper extremity muscles	Full use of upper extremities, including intrinsic muscles of hand Trunk balance poor May have difficulty in lifting sufficiently to put on lower extremity clothing Considerable energy expenditure to put on long leg braces with extensive attachments	Completely wheelchair dependent Trunk balance benefits from training Able to drive automobile with hand controls May be braced for standing May hold job away from home Can manage adapted public transportation
T10-L2 Muscle innervation: Full abdominal and upper back muscle control	Good trunk balance Good respiratory reserve Can accomplish moderate hiphiking using external oblique and latissimus dorsi muscles	Ambulation with bilateral long braces using four-point or swing-through crutch gait Usually able to negotiate curbs Some able to use regular public transportation Few vocational limitations as long as does not require much walking or standing
L3 or below Muscle innervation: Quadriceps muscle Partial gluteus and hamstring muscles	May be lumbar lordosis Floppy ankles	Ambulates well, often with short leg braces with or without cane Difficulty in getting out of wheelchair May never require wheelchair

Therapeutic Management

The management of the child with spinal cord injury is complex and controversial. Initial care begins at the scene of the accident; therefore, education and training of rescue personnel in stabilization and transfer techniques to prevent or reduce the severity of injury are of utmost importance. In any situation in which spinal cord injury is suspected or a possibility, the child should be calmed, reassured, and told not to move; no one should be allowed to move the child unless they are able to correctly stabilize the head and trunk to avoid twisting or bending the spine. If conscious, the child is placed supine on a rigid surface to prevent sagging. Infants and small children are removed in their car seats; no attempt should be made to take them out of the seat. Because of the complexity and relative infrequency of these injuries, it is usually recommended that these persons be transferred to a spinal injury center for care by specially trained personnel. (See also The Child and Trauma, Chapter 39.)

Management during the first stage is primarily supportive, with efforts directed toward preventing further neuronal damage, avoiding complications, and maintaining vital functions. Steroid administration within the first 8 hours after injury is advocated to prevent secondary spinal cord edema and inflammation. Bolus-dose methylprednisolone administration followed by continuous infusion for 23 hours has been shown to increase functional recovery significantly in patients with spinal cord injury (Bracken and others, 1990). Children with cervical lesions often have compromised respiratory function and may require ventilatory assistance. Cervical lesions may require skeletal traction or another device to maintain position, and corticosteroids are administered in an attempt to prevent destructive edema. Operative intervention may be necessary to remove bone fragments and debris, but routine surgical exploration is not usually recommended.

The focus of the second phase is primarily rehabilitative and is aimed at returning the patient to the home and community. The focus is on maximizing the potential for self-help, education, and, for the older child, vocational counseling.

Prognosis. The ultimate outlook for spinal cord function after injury depends on the completeness of the cord transection, the site of injury, and the complicating damage to the neuronal tissue. Healing of the injury and return of neurologic function are related to two factors:

1. Although individual nerve fibers do regenerate, they do not necessarily reconnect or make synaptic connections with the distal portion of the severed fibers; the chance of numerous fibers reconnecting is highly unlikely.
2. The damage resulting from cord ischemia produces necrosis in the gray and white matter of the cord tissue, which does not regenerate if the axon cylinder is not intact.

In general, recovery in thoracic lesions is usually hopeless for motor function, and victims are relegated to life in a wheelchair. Cervical injuries are variable in the extent of damage. Incomplete lesions produce hemiplegia, and complete transection implies some involvement of all extremities, from partial use of the upper extremities to complete paralysis, including the need for artificial maintenance of respiration. Lumbar injury may involve partial or complete loss of function in the lower extremities and bladder.

Nursing Considerations

The nursing care of the paralyzed child is complex and challenging. As a member of the acute care and rehabilitation teams, the nurse is involved in all aspects of care. Ideally, initial care takes place in a special intensive care unit with personnel trained to handle spinal cord injuries, and nursing management is concerned primarily with prevention of complications and maintenance of functions.

Once the acute period is over, the lesion is usually static and nonprogressive, regardless of whether the paralysis is secondary to trauma, congenital defects, infection, a treated tumor, or surgery. The nurse is a member of a team of specialists, including physicians from a number of specialty areas, physical and occupational therapists, psychologists, social workers, teachers, and vocational counselors. Each team member has a unique contribution to make, and mutual agreement for specific areas of responsibility and evaluation of progress are determined during regularly scheduled team conferences.

Although care of the child with a spinal cord injury is, in most aspects, the same as that of any immobilized child, there are some important differences (see The Immobilized Child, Chapter 39).

Respiratory Care. The child with a high-level injury (quadriplegia) will require continuous ventilatory assistance. In most instances a tracheostomy is the method of choice for greater ease in clearing secretions and for less trauma to tissues for long-term respirator dependence. Respiratory therapy personnel are responsible for establishing and maintaining the equipment, but the nurse must understand how it works and recognize deviations from the prescribed rate and volume and mechanical malfunction. In case of malfunction the nurse must be prepared to maintain respirations manually with a self-inflating bag-valve-mask device. In some youngsters breathing pacemaker devices (phrenic nerve stimulators) are implanted to stimulate the phrenic nerve and produce diaphragmatic contractions and lung expansion without a ventilator. If the child has a pacemaker, part of the nursing function is understanding its function and operation.

Children with lesions below the C4 level are seldom ventilator dependent, but their vital capacity is significantly reduced. They should be positioned for optimum chest expansion, and a variety of breathing exercises and assistive devices are used to stimulate deep breathing. Intermittent positive-pressure breathing by machine may be needed, and vital capacity and blood gases are monitored periodically. Chest physiotherapy is performed several times daily, and nebulized oxygen may be needed occasionally. Regular routine monitoring of breath sounds to assess for adequate ventilation in all lobes is part of routine care.

The cough reflex is markedly diminished and, together with weak intercostal muscles, the youngster may have difficulty with secretions. Increasing the elastic qualities of the lung by exercise will help to achieve a productive cough.

Temperature Regulation. Temperature regulation usually creates few problems, although environmental conditions can influence body temperature. During the spinal shock stage the dilated capillaries conducting body heat to the subcutaneous tissues cause heat loss to the environment. In hot weather, without the capacity to sweat, the body retains heat. Consequently, clothing and blankets are added or removed according to the body temperature. An elevated temperature that cannot be corrected by environmental measures should be evaluated for urinary or upper respiratory tract infection. However, excessive perspiration observed in sentient areas usually indicates an elevated ambient temperature. Since the skin is a less reliable indicator in these children, the oral or aural (ear) route is usually the preferred method of temperature measurement.

Skin Care. In cases in which spinal cord injury is associated with vertebral fracture, cervical traction is maintained for several weeks until there is sufficient evidence of bone healing (see The Child in Traction, Chapter 39). Initially the child is turned every 2 hours around the clock by specially trained personnel. An alternating-pressure mattress or other pressure relief/reduction device is kept underneath the child, and the skin is thoroughly inspected at least once a day for signs of pressure, especially over bony prominences. Prevention of pressure ulcers is much easier than treatment. A number of factors contribute to the risk of skin breakdown in these children: decreased sensation, poor nutrition from negative nitrogen balance, low hemoglobin level, spasticity, and improper positioning (See also Maintaining Healthy Skin, Chapter 27.)

The areas most apt to be affected are the sacrum, scapulae, heels, and occiput when the child is in a supine position; the trochanters and the lateral aspect of the ankles, heels, and knees when the child is in a side-lying position; and the ischial tuberosities when the child is in a sitting position. The pressure wound may begin in deeper tissues and is only visible on the surface at a later stage; therefore areas that feel firm, irregular, or warm or appear to be only slightly reddened require careful evaluation (see Wounds, Chapter 18). Keeping the skin clean and dry is particularly important in these children, especially those who are incontinent. Treatment of pressure areas or ulcers is instituted early.

Physiotherapy. Maintaining good body alignment, preventing pressure from bed linen, providing proper support, and applying splints as ordered and padded booties to hold the feet in correct position are important in daily care. Range-of-motion, passive, and active exercises are carried out under the guidance of a physical therapist. In children with upper motor neuron involvement, the spasticity that develops may require administration of an antispasmodic, usually diazepam. Decreasing stimuli to the muscles also helps reduce spasticity. For example, tight clothing and bed linen are avoided, and extremities are handled at the joints rather than by the belly of the muscle. Anticipating the possibility of spasms when the child is moved and providing the necessary safety precautions prevent possible injury during transport.

During the period of immobilization, unless there are contraindications, exercises are aimed at maintaining and increasing strength of the child's intact musculature. Upper extremity strengthening is especially important to the paraplegic child, who must rely on these muscle groups for turning, transferring, dressing, crutch walking, and other activities. Children are usually eager to use their muscles and respond to interesting and innovative activities.

Neurogenic Bladder. When the bladder is denervated, as in the acute stage of spinal shock syndrome or after lower motor neuron damage, the bladder wall is flaccid. Lack of muscle tone inhibits the bladder's ability to respond to changes in passive pressure, causing overextension. Therefore it is important to prevent overdistention by periodic emptying, even though there may be dribbling between emptying.

In contrast, an upper motor neuron lesion causes increased bladder tone and contractions that often include the urinary sphincter. Thus although the bladder empties periodically by reflex action, complete emptying is prevented, resulting in urinary retention and ureteral reflux. Administration of antispasmodics such as dicyclomine (Bentyl) relaxes bladder musculature and promotes increased bladder capacity and more adequate emptying. Intervals of urination depend on many factors, including patterns of fluid intake and perspiration. Most children require some type of external collecting device. This is relatively simple in males, but no satisfactory device is available for females, who usually must rely on diapers and incontinence pants. Emptying the bladder by intermittent catheterization is often used, and if functionally capable, older children can be taught to perform self-catheterization.* Bladder-training programs usually begin with intermittent bladder emptying at regular intervals, which are gradually increased. (See also Management of Genitourinary Function, under Myelomeningocele [Meningomyelocele] in Chapter 11.)

NURSING ALERT The Credé maneuver, which involves manually compressing the lower abdomen to express urine, should not be used because of the risk of renal rupture (Reinberg, Fleming, and Gonzalez, 1994). The child with a neurogenic bladder is also at risk for developing latex allergy from repeated catheterizations.

The urine is kept acidic to decrease the likelihood of stone formation and to inhibit bacterial growth. Ascorbic acid, 1 to 4 g daily, is most effective. The traditional cranberry juice therapy may also be advised. Oral antimicrobials are frequently administered prophylactically. Maintenance of bladder dynamics and control of urinary tract infections are of utmost importance. Pyelonephritis and renal failure are the most significant causes of death in longstanding paraplegia.

Bowel Training. Successful bowel training is easier to institute than bladder management. The aim is to control defecation until an appropriate time and place are found. A diet with sufficient roughage for adequate stool bulk and insertion of a glycerin or bisacodyl (Dulcolax) suppository at a convenient time, either morning or evening, are often all that are necessary to induce a bowel movement within a short time. The probability of an accident between times is diminished once the bowel is completely evacuated. Stool softeners, such as dioctyl sodium sulfonsuccinate (Colace), are usually prescribed, and manual anal stimulation may help initiate evacuation, especially in spastic paraplegia. Sometimes an oral laxative such as bisacodyl may be neces-

*Home care instructions are available in *Wong and Whaley's Clinical Manual of Pediatric Nursing* (Mosby).

sary. Once an appropriate regimen is established, little modification is required.

Autonomic Dysreflexia. Children with high-level lesions are very susceptible to the development of autonomic dysreflexia, which requires prompt action to prevent encephalopathy and shock. As soon as a quick assessment has ruled out other causes, such as orthostatic hypertension, someone should take the blood pressure while the bladder is checked for distention (the usual precipitating cause). The bladder is drained slowly, and if this does not relieve symptoms, any tight clothing is loosened, and the bowel is checked for the pressure of impacted feces. If removal of the causative agent is unsuccessful in controlling the syndrome, intravenous administration of an antihypertensive drug is indicated followed by oral maintenance doses. Antispasmodics may also be administered.

Remobilization. As soon as the condition warrants it, the child is moved from a reclining to an erect position. Cardiovascular deconditioning and impaired autonomic responses below the level of injury will cause pooling of blood in the extremities because of peripheral vasodilation, a drop in blood pressure, and a feeling of light-headedness, dizziness, or fainting on sudden assumption of an upright posture. Therefore an upright position must be accomplished gradually by first placing the child (secured by passive restraint) on a tilt table. The table is then slowly elevated from a horizontal to a 30-degree semireclining position (Fig. 40-10). This is performed twice daily for 20 to 30 minutes, with the angle gradually increased until the vertical angle is reached.

During the procedure vital signs are monitored, and behavior is observed for subjective symptoms of syncope. Elastic hose or wrapping the lower extremities with elastic bandage from instep to groin and applying an abdominal binder reduce the pooling of blood. The process of achieving upright posture may require several weeks. After tolerance is achieved, the child will be ready to begin to use a wheelchair. Getting the child up should be accomplished slowly by gradually elevating the bed over 20 to 30 minutes before placing the child in the wheelchair and then gradually lowering the legs after the child has been in the chair a short time.

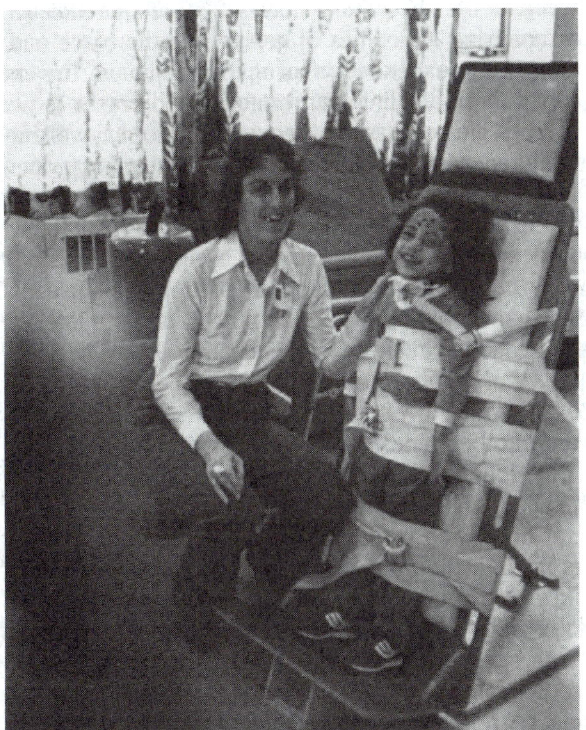

FIG. 40-10 Child on tilt table with physical therapist.

All adaptive devices help children increase their mobility, function, and endurance. The child with some lower extremity function progresses to parallel bars and then to a walker; the child with quadriplegia learns to use a wheelchair—among the most valuable aids available to the child with a spinal cord injury. The selection of a wheelchair should be made carefully in relation to where it will be used, architectural barriers, and the functional capacity of the child. For lower extremity paralysis, the wheelchair described earlier is applicable. For children with severe upper extremity paralysis, a variety of motorized wheelchairs are used, but the more complex they are, the greater their cost, weight, and tendency to break down (see Fig. 39-8). Wheelchair tolerance is gained over a period of time accompanied by measures to prevent orthostatic hypotension and pressure sores.

A variety of orthoses and other appliances can be adapted for use by many children. The primary purpose of lower extremity bracing in the child with a spinal cord injury is for ambulation, although correction of deformities may be attempted. However, the efficacy is limited because of the tendency to develop pressure lesions over insensate areas. The higher the lesion, the more support required, with the accompanying difficulties of getting into the orthosis and the greater energy expended in using the appliance. The energy required in ambulating with crutches and braces is two to four times greater than that required for normal walking.

Children, with their natural and overwhelming propensity for mobility, usually attain or may even surpass the maximum expectation in ambulation. However, as they approach adulthood, the increasing weight and energy cost usually cause them to resort to predominant use of the wheelchair for mobility and the pursuit of more intellectual and vocational interests. Wheelchair mobility has the advantages of requiring no more energy than normal walking and allowing the person with paraplegia to maintain the speed of other pedestrians on level ground.

Physical Rehabilitation. The major aims of physical rehabilitation are to prepare the child and family to resume life at home and in the community. Members of the complex rehabilitation team work collaboratively to identify the child's problems and to plan realistic interventions. Integration of activities is coordinated by one team member, most often a specialist in physical medicine and rehabilitation. Through mutual trust, good communication, professional respect, and sincere interest in the child and the family, members of the team attempt to achieve their collaborative

GOALS OF REHABILITATION FOR THE CHILD WITH A SPINAL CORD INJURY

Maximizing function and minimizing the disabling effects of the pathology

Assisting the child and family in setting realistic goals for the child, learning to be good problem solvers, and using the assets the child has

Helping the child to cope with the stigma of being different and to build a valued self-concept

goals. Training in the rehabilitation center involves maximum achievement commensurate with each child's physical capacities. Instruction for home routine is stressed and includes all the precautions and management implemented in the hospital, such as skin care, nutrition, bladder and bowel training, and an exercise program. The overall goals of rehabilitation are listed in the box above.

Physical rehabilitation of children with quadriplegia takes approximately 6 months; children with paraplegia can achieve these goals in 1 to 3 months, but they require constant vigilance to avoid complications. Emotional adjustments take longer, especially in older children and adolescents. In most children the outlook is favorable unless life-threatening consequences of urinary pathology are severe or emotional adjustment is poor.

Psychosocial Rehabilitation. Early acquired or congenital disability is usually more readily accepted by children than paralysis that appears later in childhood. Rehabilitation includes not only the child's emotional responses but also those of the persons who maintain the closest contact with the child. It involves intensive education so that members of the family understand the nature of the disability, the therapeutic regimen, and complications so that they are able to provide the physical and emotional support needed by the children. As with any disability, children should be treated as normally as possible and encouraged in developmental tasks at the age at which they would normally be expected to acquire abilities and perform activities. However, goals must be realistic, and children should not be forced beyond their capabilities.

Severe depression can be emotionally and intellectually immobilizing, but it indicates that the child is no longer hiding behind denial. In rehabilitation it is desirable for the child to begin to express negative feelings toward the situation, since these feelings, redirected by efforts of the rehabilitation team, are the ones that will motivate the child toward learning a new way of life.

The responses to loss are discussed in Chapter 23, and the multiple problems related to altered self-image, especially in older children and adolescents, are discussed in relation to children with disabilities in Chapter 22. Children with severe disabilities need to alter some concepts about self and social roles. If they describe adults as persons with complete control over their bodies and the ability to do what they want when they want, they will need to develop a more realistic definition of interdependent adult living. The needs of youngsters who are permanently disabled must be reevaluated periodically by the total rehabilitation team, including the youngsters and their families. As young adults, these teenagers may not be financially independent, which alters the choice of occupation or profession. Vocational rehabilitation involves not only helping teenagers with permanent disabilities find meaningful work activities but also assisting them in enrolling in formal educational programs.

The outlook for children with spinal cord injury is favorable for integration into society. Increased awareness of the needs of persons with disabilities has removed many structural and occupational barriers. The success of a rehabilitation program is not judged by how well children manage within the rehabilitation setting but by how well they function on the outside. In addition to agencies that offer assistance to children with disabilities in general, some agencies provide specific assistance to paralyzed persons, including children.* The **Spinal Injury Hotline** supplies victims and their families with information, hope, and peer support.†

Sexuality. The problems of self-concept are particularly marked when children with a spinal cord injury reach puberty and are likely to be even more intense if the disability occurs during adolescence. Sexual development and awareness and changing perceptions of body image are prominent aspects of adolescence, and a loss in these areas is a severe blow to these youngsters. Development of secondary sex characteristics does not seem to be altered by spinal cord injury, and it is now believed that with comprehensive rehabilitation, well-motivated young people can look forward to successful participation in marital and family activities.

In females, if the injury occurs after the onset of menstruation, there is usually a temporary cessation and irregularity in menstrual flow, but in the majority menstruation usually resumes. Ovulation and conception are possible, but females will not experience vaginal or clitoral orgasms, although they can learn to use other erogenous zones for a sexual experience. This is important to emphasize in sex education, because many females have the misconception that because they lack sensation, they are unable to conceive. Also, the pregnant paraplegic or quadriplegic patient may be unaware that she is in labor, and those with a high-level injury are subject to autonomic hyperreflexia during labor.

As soon as adolescent males become aware of their functional loss, they will be concerned about sexual capacities, regardless of the type of sexual activities experienced before the spinal cord injury. The practitioner should provide them with information about what can be expected regarding erection, ejaculation, and other sexual experiences. The health professional should take the initiative in discussing sexuality with youngsters and their families. Parents of younger children will want to know about their children's

*A complete listing of organizations and resources can be obtained by contacting **Spinal Network,** P.O. Box 8987, Malibu, CA 90265; (310) 317-4522 or (800) 543-4116.

†(800) 526-3456.

sexual and reproductive potential. As their interest and understanding increase, children need to know the specifics of physiology, the prognosis, and sexual techniques related to their particular problems.

A knowledgeable rehabilitation team will be valuable to children as they experience loss as a sexual being. This is especially true of paraplegia or quadriplegia. Most sexual counseling for adolescents with spinal cord injury focuses on developing the idea that sex means different things to individuals, and youngsters are encouraged to discuss their ideas. Most rehabilitation teams have an active program in sexual counseling to help youngsters learn intimacy and how to function sexually within their limitations. Through individual and group counseling they gain new attitudes concerning sexuality, experiences exclusive or inclusive of intercourse.

MUSCULAR DYSFUNCTION

JUVENILE DERMATOMYOSITIS

Dermatomyositis is a relatively rare multisystem inflammatory disorder of unknown etiology and is often difficult to distinguish from muscular dystrophy. About half the children will have a very acute, rapidly progressive disease, and the remainder will have an insidious onset. There is proximal limb and trunk muscle weakness and loss of reflexes. Neck muscles are frequently affected, and the child may have difficulty in lifting the head or supporting it in an upright position. Muscles tend to be stiff and sore. Masseter involvement with atrophy may occur, making it difficult to chew food during the active stage of the disease. Soft palate dysfunction may make speech difficult and interfere with breathing. Distal muscle strength and reflex response remain unaffected. Dermatomyositis, frequently classified as a collagen disease, is characterized by red, indurated skin lesions over the malar areas and nose and a violet discoloration of the eyelids. The skin over extensor muscle surfaces may be erythematous, scaly, and atopic.

Dermatomyositis responds to corticosteroid therapy, and high-dose intravenous gamma globulin therapy. For cases that do not respond to these agents, methotrexate may be helpful in suppressing the symptoms but not in preventing recurrence of the disease (Miller and others, 1992). Physical therapy is essential to prevent contracture deformity and to rebuild muscle strength. Orthoses may be needed.

Although the prognosis for survival has steadily improved, dermatomyositis remains a serious illness. Death can occur in the acute phase as a result of myocarditis, progressive unresponsive myositis, perforation of the bowel, or, occasionally, lung involvement (Ansell, 1992).

MUSCULAR DYSTROPHIES

The muscular dystrophies constitute the largest and most important single group of muscle diseases of childhood. They all have a genetic origin in which there is gradual degeneration of muscle fibers and are characterized by progressive weakness and wasting of symmetric groups of skeletal muscles with increasing disability and deformity. In all forms of muscular dystrophy there is insidious loss of strength, but each differs in regard to the muscle groups affected, age of onset, rate of progression, and inheritance patterns.

The basic defect in muscular dystrophy is unknown, although it appears to be caused by a metabolic disturbance

TABLE 40-3 Characteristics of the Major Muscular Dystrophies

PRIMARY MYOPATHY/ INHERITANCE PATTERN	AGE OF ONSET	INITIAL MANIFESTATIONS	PROGRESSION	THERAPY
Pseudohypertrophic (Duchenne) X-linked recessive; sporadic	Early childhood; age 1-3 years	Lordosis Waddling gait Difficulty in rising from floor and climbing stairs Fat deposits replace wasted gastrocnemius muscles	Rapid Ultimately involves all voluntary muscles Death usually occurs between ages 15 and 25 years	Supportive Physical therapy to prevent disuse atrophy of unaffected muscles
Limb-girdle Autosomal recessive (usually)	Late childhood or during adolescence; over age 8 years	Weakness of proximal muscles of both pelvic and shoulder girdles	Variable but usually slow Most become incapacitated within 20 years of onset; in some, disability may remain slight	Supportive Physical therapy to prevent disuse atrophy of unaffected muscles
Facioscapulohumeral (Landouzy-Déjerine) Autosomal dominant	Early adolescence; over age 8 years	Lack of facial mobility Difficulty in raising arms over head Forward slope of shoulders	Very slow May be intervals with no progression Considerable disability in time but life span unaffected	Supportive

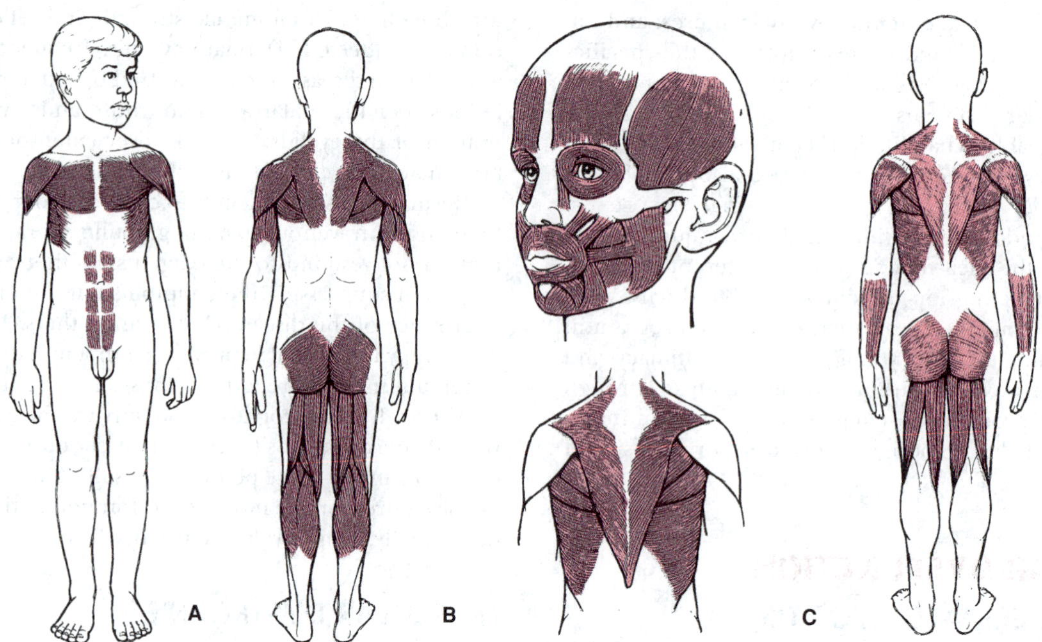

FIG. 40-11 Initial muscle groups involved in muscular dystrophies. **A,** Pseudohypertrophic. **B,** Facioscapulohumeral. **C,** Limb-girdle.

unrelated to the nervous system. Serum creatine phosphokinase is consistently increased in affected individuals, which assists in the diagnosis and affords a means for early detection of the disorder in asymptomatic children in families at risk. Electromyography (EMG) and muscle biopsy are important diagnostic procedures.

Treatment of the muscular dystrophies consists mainly of providing supportive measures, including physical therapy, orthopaedic procedures to minimize deformity, and assisting the affected child in meeting the demands of daily living.

The major forms of muscular dystrophy are summarized in Table 40-3, and the initial sites of muscle involvement are illustrated in Fig. 40-11.

PSEUDOHYPERTROPHIC (DUCHENNE) MUSCULAR DYSTROPHY (DMD)

DMD is the most severe and the most common muscular dystrophy of childhood. An X-linked inheritance pattern is identified in most cases; about one third of all cases represent fresh mutations. As in all X-linked disorders, males are affected almost exclusively. The incidence is approximately 1:3500 male births (Multicenter Study Group, 1992). The box at right describes the characteristics of DMD.

At the genetic level, both DMD and Becker muscular dystrophy, a milder variant, result from mutations of the gene encoding ***dystrophin,*** a protein product in skeletal muscle. It is absent from the muscle of children with DMD and is reduced or abnormal in character in children with Becker muscular dystrophy. There is a strong correlation between the clinical severity of these disorders and the type of genetic mutation and dystrophin protein alterations (Bieber and Hoffman, 1990). Prenatal diagnosis is also possible using several methods, such as the polymerase chain reaction. However, ethical questions exist regarding diagnosing a condition in the fetus when no treatment exists (Bowman, 1993).

Clinical Manifestations

Evidence of muscle weakness usually appears during the third year, although there may have been a history of delay in motor development, particularly walking. Difficulties in running, riding a bicycle, and climbing stairs are usually the first symptoms noted. Later abnormal gait on a level surface becomes apparent. In the early years rapid developmental gains may mask the progression of the disease. Questioning of parents may reveal that the child has difficulty in rising from a sitting or supine position. Occasionally, enlarged calves may be noticed by parents.

Typically, affected males have a waddling gait and lordosis, fall frequently, and develop a characteristic manner of

CHARACTERISTICS OF DUCHENNE MUSCULAR DYSTROPHY

- Early onset, usually between 3 and 5 years of age
- Progressive muscular weakness, wasting, and contractures
- Calf muscle hypertrophy in most cases
- Loss of independent ambulation by 9 to 11 years of age
- Slowly progressive, generalized weakness during teenage years
- Relentless progression until death from respiratory or cardiac failure

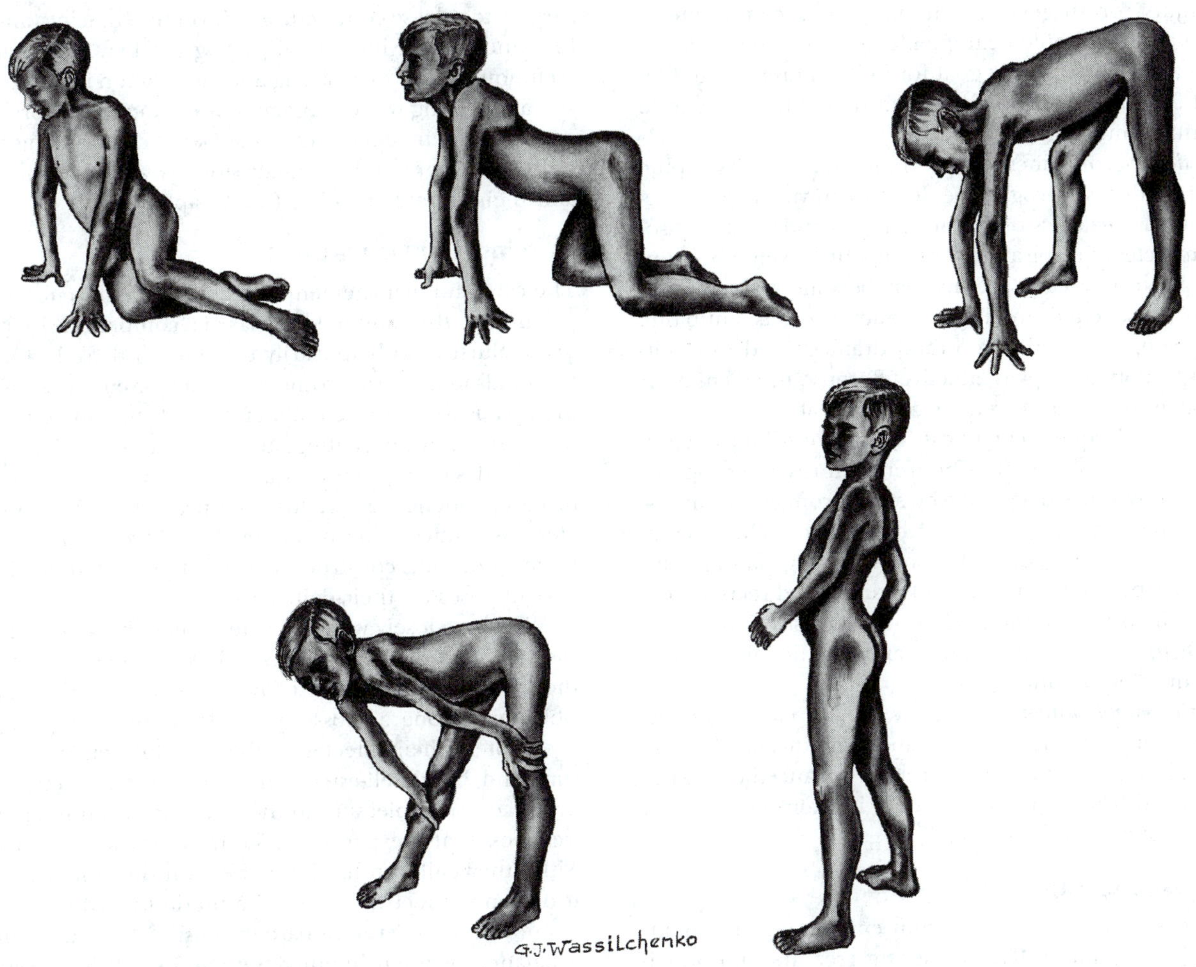

FIG. 40-12 Child with Duchenne muscular dystrophy attains standing posture by assuming a kneeling position, then gradually pushing his torso upright (with knees straight) by "walking" his hands up his legs (Gower sign). Note marked lordosis in upright position.

rising from a squatting or sitting position on the floor ***(Gower sign)*** (Fig. 40-12). Muscles, especially of the calves, thighs, and upper arms, become enlarged from fatty infiltration and feel unusually firm or woody on palpation. The term ***pseudohypertrophy*** is derived from this muscular enlargement. Profound muscular atrophy occurs in later stages, and as the disease progresses, contractures and deformities involving large and small joints are common complications. Ambulation usually becomes impossible by 12 years of age. Facial, oropharyngeal, and respiratory muscles are spared until the terminal stages of the disease. Ultimately the disease process involves the diaphragm and auxiliary muscles of respiration, and cardiomegaly is common. The cause of death is usually respiratory tract infection or cardiac failure.

Mild mental retardation is commonly associated with muscular dystrophy. The mean intelligence quotient is about 20 points below normal, and frank mental deficit is present in 25% of these children.

Complications. The major complications of muscular dystrophy include contractures, disuse atrophy, infections, obesity, and cardiopulmonary problems.

Contracture deformities of the hips, knees, and ankles occur from early selective muscle involvement and often exaggerate the weakness. Passive range-of-motion exercises, stretching, and active exercises under the supervision of a physical therapist are effective in treating reducible contractures. Nonreducible contractures require wedge casting or surgical reduction. Scoliosis caused by muscle imbalance is common and tends to progress even when the child becomes dependent on a wheelchair. Bracing with a rigid corset may be needed for support, although it may interfere with mobility, and children with DMD do not tolerate rigid spinal bracing. Frequent rest periods in the recumbent position are often beneficial. For correction of deformities it is essential to select a procedure that immobilizes the child for as short a period as possible to minimize the chances of developing disease atrophy.

Atrophy of disuse from prolonged inactivity occurs readily when children are immobilized or confined to bed with illness, injury, or surgery. To minimize this complication, physical therapy should be implemented if bed rest extends beyond a few days. A daily goal for well children should be at least 3 hours of ambulation when disability is moderate to maintain muscle strength.

Infections become increasingly frequent as the dystrophic process produces a progressive decrease in vital capacity resulting from weakness of the primary, secondary, and associated muscles of respiration. Consequently, even minor upper respiratory tract infections may become serious problems in these children. Prompt and vigorous antibiotic therapy supplemented by postural drainage and intermittent respiratory therapy is effective. Because these children are unable to cough, secretions collect easily.

Obesity is a frequent complication that contributes to premature loss of ambulation. Children with restricted opportunity for physical activity and who suffer from boredom easily consume calories in excess of their needs. This is compounded by overfeeding by well-meaning family and friends. Proper dietary intake and a diversified recreational program help reduce the likelihood of obesity and enable children to maintain ambulation and functional independence for a longer time.

Cardiac manifestations are usually late events but may occur in ambulatory children. The most significant of these, cardiac failure, is difficult to correct in advanced cases, but treatment with digoxin and diuretics is often beneficial in the early stages of the disease.

Diagnostic Evaluation

The disease is confirmed by serum enzyme measurement, muscle biopsy, and EMG. The serum creatine phosphokinase, aldolase, and serum glutamic-oxaloacetic transaminase levels are extremely high in the first 2 years of life before the onset of clinical weakness. They diminish with muscle deterioration but do not reach normal levels until severe muscle wasting and incapacitation have occurred. Muscle biopsy reveals degeneration of muscle fibers with fibrosis and fatty tissue replacement. EMG readings show a decrease in amplitude and duration of motor unit potentials. Diagnosis poses few problems in children 2 to 7 years of age, but in older children the similarity of symptoms to those of limb-girdle muscular dystrophy and some other myopathies confuses the diagnosis.

Therapeutic Management

There is no effective treatment for childhood muscular dystrophy. Increased muscle bulk and muscle power have been reported following a course of corticosteroids. However, the beneficial effects will need further evaluation before administration of corticosteroids becomes routine therapy (Khan, 1993).

Maintaining function in unaffected muscles for as long as possible is the primary goal. It has been found that children who remain as active as possible are able to avoid wheelchair confinement for a longer period. Early recourse to a wheelchair accelerates deconditioning and promotes the development of lower extremity contractures. Maintenance of function often includes range-of-motion exercises, surgery to release contracture deformities, bracing, and performance of activities of daily living (ADLs). Some surgical techniques allow early sitting and ambulation if children are still ambulating without bracing or casting and improve the quality of their remaining years. Genetic counseling is recommended for parents, female siblings, and maternal aunts and their female offspring (see Chapter 5).

Nursing Considerations

The care and management of a child with muscular dystrophy involve the combined efforts of a comprehensive health team. Nurses can help clarify the roles of these health professionals to family and others. The major emphasis of nursing care is to assist the child and family in coping with the progressive, incapacitating, and fatal nature of the disease, to help design a program that will afford a greater degree of independence and reduce the predictable and preventable disabilities associated with the disorder, and to assist them in dealing constructively with the limitations the disease imposes on their daily lives.

Working closely with other team members, nurses assist the family in developing the child's self-help skills to give the child the satisfaction of being as independent as possible for as long as possible. It is tempting for parents to overprotect their affected children. Children derive pleasure and build self-esteem from performing actions that produce visible pleasure in their parents. Even the physical weakness that prevents the child from physical competition with other children has little effect on the child as long as it does not affect the parents' attitude toward the child as an individual. Therefore parents must be helped to develop a balance between limiting the child's activity because of muscular weakness and allowing the child to accomplish things alone. This requires continual evaluation of the child's capabilities, which are often difficult to assess. It is not always possible to know when the child seeks parental assistance to get a little extra attention or because of overtired muscles. Fortunately most children with muscular dystrophy instinctively recognize this need to be as independent as possible and strive to do so.

Practical difficulties faced by families are physical limitations of housing and mobility. Families often live in houses or apartments that are unsuited to wheelchairs—no street-level entrance, upstairs bedrooms and bathrooms, no tub. Many of these families have no independent means of transportation. Assisting with these problems involves team problem solving. Parents also need help in buying and modifying clothing for their child. It is difficult to find clothing and footwear to wear comfortably in a wheelchair, to fit over contracted limbs, or to fit an obese child. Diet, nutritional needs, and nutrition modification are discussed according to the needs of the individual child and family.

Parents' social activities are also restricted, and the family's activities must be continually modified to the needs of the affected child (see Chapter 22). The child cannot be left with an ordinary teenage baby-sitter but requires a specially trained person, such as a student nurse. Consequently, parents, too, tend to lead more isolated lives. When the child becomes increasingly helpless, the family may consider a skilled nursing facility to provide the care needed. Nurses can assist with decision making and support the family in the decision.

Each child's therapy program is tailored to individual needs and capabilities, and families should be active participants. Parents need assistance with the physical therapy program and education regarding a home regimen of exercises and activity. Many parents erroneously believe that by exerting sufficient effort, the child can overcome the weakness and prevent progression of the disease process. They should also be advised to notify the nurse or other designated person when the child becomes even temporarily bedridden so that the exercise program can be continued, although modified, during this time.

As their physical condition deteriorates to the point where they can no longer keep up with friends and classmates, affected children tend to become socially isolated. Their physical capabilities diminish, and their dependency increases at the ages when most children are expanding their range of interests and relationships. To gain associations, they often learn behaviors that bring them the rewards of other children's company. These friends are often children who have been rejected by more able-bodied classmates.

No matter how successful the program and how well the family adapts to the disorder, superimposed on the physical and emotional problems associated with a child with a long-term disability is the constant presence of the ultimate outcome of the disease. All the manifestations seen in the child with a fatal illness are encountered in these families (see Chapter 23). The guilt feelings of the mother may be particularly pronounced in this disorder because of the mother-to-son transmission of the defective gene.

Nurses are especially valuable health professionals as they come to know the family and the family's problems. Nurses can be alert to the problems and needs of the families and make necessary referrals when supplementary services are indicated. The **Muscular Dystrophy Association of America, Inc.*** has branches in most communities to provide assistance to families in which there is a member with muscular dystrophy.

*10 E. 40th St., Room 4105, New York, NY 10019; (212) 679-6215 or (212) 689-9040. In Canada: **Muscular Dystrophy Association of Canada,** 150 Eglinton Ave, E., Suite 400, Toronto, Ontario M4P 1E8; (416) 488-0030.

KEY POINTS

- Upper motor neuron lesions produce weakness associated with spasticity, increased deep tendon reflexes, and abnormal superficial reflexes; lower motor neuron lesions interrupt the reflex arc, causing weakness and atrophy of the skeletal muscles.
- The most useful classification of neuromuscular disorders defines the source of the lesion: cerebral cortex, anterior horn cells of the spinal cord, peripheral nerves, myoneural junction, and muscles.
- Clinical manifestations of cerebral palsy include delayed gross motor development, abnormal motor performance, alterations of muscle tone, abnormal postures, reflex abnormalities, and associated disabilities such as mental retardation, seizures, attention deficit disorder, and sensory impairment.
- Therapy for cerebral palsy takes into account the nature of the physical disability, defects associated with the disorder, and interpersonal and social influences encountered by the affected child.
- Werdnig-Hoffmann disease is characterized by progressive weakness and wasting of skeletal muscles caused by degeneration of anterior horn cells.
- Nursing care of the child with Guillain-Barré syndrome consists of monitoring vital signs, ensuring alignment and positioning, providing physical therapy, and providing support to the family.
- Tetanus occurs when tetanus spores or vegetative bacilli enter a wound and multiply in a susceptible host.
- Infant botulism results from toxins produced by *C. botulinum;* toxin is ingested from poorly preserved food or released in the gastrointestinal tract by ingested spores.
- Primary management of myasthenia gravis is oral administration of anticholinesterase drugs.
- Spinal cord injuries usually involve the following four interrelated pathologic changes: cellular damage to cord tissue; hemorrhage and vascular damage; structural changes of white and gray matter related to vascular disruption, inflammation and edema; and local biochemical response to trauma.
- Therapeutic management of spinal cord injury is directed toward preventing further neuronal damage, avoiding complications, and maintaining vital functions.
- The goals of rehabilitation in spinal cord injury are to maximize function, assist the child and family in realistic goal setting, and help the child cope with the dysfunction and build a positive self-concept.
- Muscular dystrophies are the largest and most important group of muscular dysfunctions in childhood.
- Major complications of Duchenne muscular dystrophy include contractures, disuse atrophy, infections, obesity, and cardiopulmonary problems.

REFERENCES

Adams C and others: Thymectomy in juvenile myasthenia gravis, *J Child Neurol* 5(3):215-218, 1990.

American Academy of Pediatrics, Committee on Children with Disabilities: Doman-Delacato treatment of neurologically handicapped children, *AAP News* 1990.

American Academy of Pediatrics: Policy statement: The Doman-Delacato treatment of neurologically handicapped children, *Pediatrics* 70:810-812, 1990.

American Academy of Pediatrics: *Report of the Committee on Infectious Diseases,* ed 23, Elk Grove Village, IL, 1994, The Academy.

Ansell BM: Juvenile dermatomyositis, *J Rheumatol* Suppl 33:60-62, 1992.

Antozzi C and others: A short plasma exchange protocol is effective in severe myasthenia gravis, *J Neurol* 238(2):103-107, 1991.

Bhushan V, Paneth N, Kiely JL: Impact of improved survival of very low birth weight infants on recent secular trends in the prevalence of cerebral palsy, *Pediatrics* 91(6):1094-100, 1993.

Bieber FR, Hoffman EP: Duchenne and Becker muscular dystrophies: genetics, prenatal diagnosis, and future prospects, *Clin Perinatol* 17(4):845-865, 1990.

Blossom GB and others: Thymectomy for myasthenia gravis, *Arch Surg* 128(8):855-862, 1993.

Bowman JE: Screening newborn infants for Duchenne muscular dystrophy, *Br Med J* 306(6874):349, 1993.

Bracken MB and others: A randomized, controlled trial of methylprednisolone or naloxone in the treatment of acute spinal cord injury: results of the second national acute spinal cord injury study, *N Engl J Med* 322:1405, 1990.

Brucker JM: Selective dorsal rhizotomy: neurosurgical treatment of cerebral palsy, *J Pediatr Nurs* 5:105-114, 1990.

Crawford TO: Clinical evaluation of the floppy infant, *Pediatr Ann* 21(6):348-354, 1992.

Dorsher PT and others: Wohlfart-Kugelberg-Welander syndrome: serum creatine kinase and functional outcome, *Arch Phys Med Rehabil* 72(8):587-591, 1991.

Eicher PS, Batshaw ML: Cerebral palsy, *Pediatr Clin North Am* 40(3):537-551, 1993.

Fuchs S and others: Cervical spine fractures sustained by young children in forward-facing car seats, *Pediatrics* 84:348-354, 1989.

Gervaix A and others: Guillain-Barré syndrome following immunization with *Haemophilus influenzae* type b conjugate vaccine, *Eur J Pediatr* 152(7):613-614, 1993.

Guillain-Barré Syndrome Steroid Trial Group: Double-blind trial of intravenous methylprednisolone in Guillain-Barré syndrome, *Lancet* 341(8845):586-590, 1993.

Jankovic J, Brin M: Therapeutic uses of botulinum toxin, *N Engl J Med* 321(17):1186-1193, 1991.

Jansen PW, Perkins RM, Ashwal S: Guillain-Barré syndrome in childhood: natural course and efficacy of plasma pheresis, *Pediatr Neurol* 9(1):16-20, 1993.

Khan MA: Corticosteroid therapy in Duchenne muscular dystrophy, *J Neurol Sci* 120(1):8-14, 1993.

Kohn JG: Issues in the management of children with spastic cerebral palsy, *Pediatrician* 17(4):230-236, 1990.

Lang SM, Bernardo LM: SCIWORA syndrome: nursing assessment . . . spinal cord injury without radiographic abnormality, *Dimens Crit Care Nurs* 12(5):247-254, 1993.

Logigian MK, Ward JD: *Pediatric rehabilitation,* Boston, 1989, Little, Brown.

McKhann GM: Guillain-Barré syndrome: clinical and therapeutic observations, *Ann Neurol* 27:s13-s16, 1990.

Miller LC and others: Methotrexate treatment of recalcitrant childhood dermatomyositis, *Arthritis Rheum* 35(10):1143-1149, 1992.

Multicenter Study Group: Diagnosis of Duchenne and Becker muscular dystrophies by polymerase chain reaction, *JAMA* 267(19):2609-2615, 1992.

Paneth N: The causes of cerebral palsy: recent evidence, *Clin Invest Med* 16(2):95-102, 1993.

Parke JT: Diseases of the neuromuscular junction. In Oski FA and others, editors: *Principles and practice of pediatrics,* Philadelphia, 1990, JB Lippincott.

Ramchandra DS, Anisya V, Gourie-Devi M: Ketamine monoanaesthesia for diagnostic muscle biopsy in neuromuscular disorders in infancy and childhood: floppy infant syndrome, *Can J Anaesth* 37(4, pt 1):474-476, 1990.

Rantala H and others: Epidemiology of Guillain-Barré syndrome in children: relationship of oral polio vaccine administration to occurrence, *J Pediatr* 124(2):220-223, 1994.

Rathbone D and others: Spinal cord concussion in pediatric athletes, *J Pediatr Orthop* 12:616-620, 1992.

Reinberg Y, Fleming T, Gonzalez R: Renal rupture after the Credé maneuver, *J Pediatr* 124(2):279-281, 1994.

Russman BS and others: Spinal muscular atrophy: new thoughts on the pathogenesis and classification schema, *J Child Neurol* 7(4):347-353, 1992.

Schanzer H, Jacobson JH: Tissue damage caused by the intramuscular injection of long-acting penicillin, *Pediatrics* 75:741-744, 1985.

Schwartz PJ, Arnon SS: Botulism immune globulin infant botulism arrives: one year and a Gulf war later, *West J Med* 156:197-198, 1992.

Spika JA, and others: Risk factors for infant botulism in the United States, *Am J Dis Child* 143:828-832, 1989.

Steele S: Cerebral palsy. In Jackson PL, Vessey JA: *Primary care of the child with a chronic condition,* St Louis, 1992, Mosby.

Vallee L and others: Intravenous immune globulin is also an efficient therapy of acute Guillain-Barré syndrome in affected children, *Neuropediatrics* 24(4):235-236, 1993.

BIBLIOGRAPHY

Cerebral Palsy

Dormans JP: Orthopedic management of children with cerebral palsy, *Pediatr Clin North Am* 40(3):645-657, 1993.

Hughes I, Newton R: Genetic aspects of cerebral palsy, *Dev Med Child Neurol* 34(1):80-86, 1992.

Knutson LM, Clark DE: Orthotic devices for ambulation in children with cerebral palsy and myelomeningocele, *Phys Ther* 71(12):947-960, 1991.

Kuban KC, Leviton A: Medical progress: cerebral palsy, *N Engl J Med* 330(3):188-195, 1994.

Park TS, Owen JH: Surgical management of spastic diplegia in cerebral palsy, *N Engl J Med* 326(11):745-749, 1992.

Peacock WJ, Staudt LA: Management of spasticity in cerebral palsy, *Int Pediatr* 7(2):181-184, 1992.

Philichi LM, Brunn V: Rhizotimy surgery to relieve spasticity in young children, *MCN* 15(6):367-370, 1990.

Polivka BJ, Nickel JT, Wilkins III Jr: Cerebral palsy: evaluation of a model of risk, *Res Nurs Health* 16(2):113-122, 1993.

Sprague JB: Surgical management of cerebral palsy, *Orthop Nurs* 11(4):11-19, 1992.

Stern FM, Gorga D: Neurodevelopmental treatment (NDT): therapeutic intervention and its efficacy, *Infants Young Child* 1(1):22-32, 1988.

Torfs CP and others: Prenatal and perinatal factors in the etiology of cerebral palsy, *J Pediatr* 116:615-619, 1990.

Turnbull JD: Early intervention for children with or at risk of cerebral palsy, *Am J Dis Child* 147(1):54-59, 1993.

Walker MJ: Selective dorsal rhizotomy, reducing spasticity in patients with cerebral palsy, *AORN J* 54(4):759-761, 1991.

Hypotonia

Gay CT, Bodensteiner JB: The floppy infant: recent advances in the understanding of disorders affecting the neuromuscular junction, *Neurol Clin* 8(3):715-725, 1990.

Miller VS, Delgado M, Iannaccone ST: Neonatal hypotonia, *Semin Neurol* 13(1):73-83, 1993.

Parano E, Lovelace RE: Neonatal peripheral hypotonia: clinical and electromygraphic characteristics, *Childs Nerv Syst* 9(3):166-171, 1993.

Werdnig-Hoffmann Disease

Barden C and others: An unusual neurologic problem: Werdnig-Hoffmann disease, *Crit Care Nurse* 10(10):60-66+, 1990.

Gordon N: The spinal muscular atrophies, *Dev Med Child Neurol* 33(10):934-938, 1991.

Hamel A: Giving our all to Billy, *Nursing 94* 24(3):321, 1994.

Iannaccone ST and others: Prospective study of spinal muscular atrophy before age 6 years: DCN/SMA Group, *Pediatr Neurol* 9(3):187-193, 1993.

Shaw PJ and others: Adult-onset motor neuron disease and infantile Werdnig-Hoffmann disease (spinal muscular atrophy type 1) in the same family, *Neurology* 42(8):1477-1480, 1992.

Kugelberg-Welander Disease

Brzustowicz LM and others: Genetic mapping of chronic childhood-onset spinal muscular atrophy to chromosome 5q11.2-13.3, *Nature* 344(6266):540-541, 1990.

Granata C and others: Spine surgery in spinal muscular atrophy: long-term results, *Neuromuscular Dis* 3(3):207-215, 1993.

Lanzi G and others: Relational and therapeutic aspects of children with late onset of a terminal disease, *Childs Nerv Syst* 9(6):339-342, 1993.

Liu GT, Specht LA: Progressive juvenile segmental spinal muscular atrophy, *Pediatr Neurol* 9(1):54-56, 1993.

Rietschel M, Rudnik-Schoneborn S, Zerres K: Clinical variability of autosomal dominant spinal muscular atrophy, *J Neurol Sci* 107(1):65-73, 1992.

Guillain-Barré Syndrome

Bradshaw DY, Jones HR Jr.: Guillain-Barré syndrome in children: clinical course, electrodiagnosis, and prognosis, *Muscle Nerve* 15(4):500-506, 1992.

de Jager AE, Sluiter HJ: Clinical signs in severe Guillain-Barré syndrome: analysis of 63 patients, *J Neurol Sci* 104(2):143-150, 1991.

Fasanaro AM, Pizza V, Stella L: Plasma exchange and IV immunoglobulins: new appoaches to the treatment of Guillain-Barré syndrome, *Acta Neurol* 14(4-6):369-380, 1992.

McGhee B, Jarjour IT: Single-dose intravenous immune globulin for treatment of Guillain-Barré syndrome, *Am J Hosp Pharm* 51(1):97-99, 1994.

Mishu B and others: Serologic evidence of previous *Campylobacter jejuni* infection in patients with the Guillain-Barré syndrome, *Ann Intern Med* 118(12):947-953, 1993.

Murray DP: Impaired mobility: Guillain-Barré syndrome, *J Neurosci Nurs* 25(2):100-104, 1993.

Rantala H, Uhari M, Niemela M: Occurrence, clinical manifestations, and prognosis of Guillain-Barré syndrome, *Arch Dis Child* 66(6):706-709, 1991.

Tetanus/Botulism

Abrutyn E, Berlin JA: Intrathecal therapy in tetanus: a meta-analysis, *JAMA* 266(16):2262-2267, 1991.

Graf WD and others: Electrodiagnosis reliability in the diagnosis of infant botulism, *J Pediatr* 120(5):747-749, 1992.

Hurst DL, Marsh WW: Early severe infantile botulism, *J Pediatr* 122(6):909-911, 1993.

Jagoda A, Renner G: Infant botulism: case report and clinical update, *Am J Emerg Med* 8(4):318-320, 1990.

Lancaster MJ: Botulism: north to Alaska, *Am J Nurs* 90(1):60-62, 1990.

Prevots R and others: Tetanus surveillance—United States, *MMWR* 41(8):1-9, 1992.

Schmidt RD, Schmidt TW: Infant botulism: a case series and review of the literature, *J Emerg Med* 10(6):713-718, 1992.

Thilo EH, Townsend SF, Deacon J: Infant botulism at 1 week of age: report of two cases, *Pediatrics* 92(1):151-152, 1993.

Turick-Gibson T: Infant botulism, *Pediatr Nurs* 14:280-283, 1988.

Wigginton JM, Thill P: Infant botulism: a review of the literature, *Clin Pediatr* 32(11):669-674, 1993.

Wilkinson WJ, Clore ER: Infant botulism: a dilemma for nursing, *J Pediatr Nurs* 3:164-168, 1988.

Myasthenia Gravis

Afifi AK, Bell WE: Tests for juvenile myasthenia gravis: comparative diagnostic yield and prediction of outcome, *J Child Neurol* 8(4):403-411, 1993.

Badurska B, Ryniewicz B, Strugalska H: Immunosuppressive treatment for juvenile myasthenia gravis, *Eur J Pediatr* 151(3):215-217, 1992.

Evans OB, Vig V, Parker CC: Prematurity and early-onset juvenile myasthenia gravis, *Pediatr Neurol* 8(1):51-53, 1992.

Mascarella JJ, Hudson DC: Dysimmune neurologic disorders, *AACN Clin Issues Crit Care Nurs* 2(4):675-684, 1991.

Vial C and others: Myasthenia gravis in childhood and infancy: usefulness of electrophysiologic studies, *Arch Neurol* 48(8):847-849, 1991.

Spinal Cord Injury

Aldrich EE, Eisenberg HM: Management of acute cervical spinal cord injuries, *Contemp Neurosurg* 12(12):1, 1990.

Barker E and Higgins R: Managing a suspected spinal cord injury, *Nursing 89* 19(4):52-59, 1989.

Chadwick AT, Oesting HH: Caring for patients with spinal cord injuries, *Nursing 89* 19(11):53-56, 1989.

Ditunno JF, Formal CS: Current concepts: chronic spinal cord injury, *N Engl J Med* 330(8):550-556, 1994.

Hadley MN and others: Pediatric spinal trauma: review of 122 cases of spinal cord and vertebral column injuries, *J Neurosurg* 68:18-24, 1988.

Joy C: Pediatric spinal cord injury, *Crit Care Nurs Clin North Am* 2(3):415-419, 1990.

Romeo JH: The critical minutes after spinal cord injury, *RN* 51(4):61-67, 1988.

Romeo JH: Spinal cord injury: nursing the patient toward a new life, *RN* 51(5):31-35, 1988.

Muscular Dysfunction

Baumbach LL: Duchenne muscular dystrophy, *Int Pediatr* 7(2):118-125, 1992.

Buist NRM, Powell BR: Approaches to the evaluation of muscle diseases, *Int Pediatr* 7(4):320-326, 1992.

Collet E and others: Juvenile dermatomyositis: treatment with intravenous gamma globulin, *Br J Dermatol* 130(2):231-234, 1994.

Gagliardi BA: The impact of Duchenne muscular dystrophy on families, *Orthop Nurs* 10(5):41-49, 1991.

Gorospe Jr, Hoffman EP: Duchenne muscular dystrophy, *Curr Opin Rheumatol* 4(6):794-800, 1992.

Hilton T and others: End of life care in Duchenne muscular dystrophy, *Pediatr Neurol* 9(3):165-177, 1993.

Hoffman EP, Wang J: Duchenne-Becker muscular dystrophy and the nondystrophic myotonias: paradigms for loss of function and change of function of gene products, *Arch Neurol* 50(11):1227-1237, 1993.

Hsu JD, Furumasu J: Gait and posture changes in the Duchenne muscular dystrophy child, *Clin Orthop* (288):122-125, 1993.

Iannaccone ST: Current status of Duchenne muscular dystrophy, *Pediatr Clin North Am* 39(4):879-894, 1992.

Karpati G, Acsadi G: The potential for gene therapy in Duchenne muscular dystrophy and other genetic muscle diseases, *Muscle Nerve* 16(11):1141-1153, 1993.

Nicholson LV: Advances in Duchenne and myotonic dystrophy, *Curr Opin Rheumatol* 5(6):706-711, 1993.

Olson JC: Juvenile dermatomyositis, *Semin Dermatol* 11(1):57-64, 1992.

Staiano A and others: Upper gastrointestinal tract motility in children with progressive muscular dystrophy, *J Pediatr* 121(5):72-74, 1992.

Tay JS and others: Pathogenesis of Duchenne muscular dystrophy: the calcium hypothesis revisited, *J Pediatr Child Health* 28(4):291-293, 1992.

Wolff JA: Gene therapy for neuromuscular disorders, *Int Pediatr* 8(1):14-16, 1993.

Yau SC and others: Direct diagnosis of carriers of point mutations in Duchenne muscular dystrophy, *Lancet* 341(8840):273-275, 1993.

OPENER PHOTO CREDITS

PART I	Peter Correz/Tony Stone Images
UNIT I	Ken Fisher/Tony Stone Images
UNIT II	Suzanne Murphy/Tony Stone Images
UNIT III	John Fortunato/Tony Stone Images
UNIT IV	Andy Cox/Tony Stone Images
UNIT V	Andy Sacks/Tony Stone Images
UNIT VI	Charles Gupton/Tony Stone Images
UNIT VII	Don Smetzer/Tony Stone Images
UNIT VIII	Gary Parker/Science Photo Library/Custom Medical Stock Photo, Inc.
PART II	Bruce Ayres/Tony Stone Images
UNIT IX	Henley and Savage/Tony Stone Images
UNIT X	K. Glaser & Associates/Custom Medical Stock Photo, Inc.
UNIT XI	Melanie Carr/Custom Medical Stock Photo, Inc.
UNIT XII	Science Photo Library/Custom Medical Stock Photo, Inc.
UNIT XIII	SIU Biomed Communications/Custom Medical Stock Photo, Inc.

Appendixes

FAMILY ASSESSMENT

Family APGAR questionnaire

PART I

The following questions have been designed to help us better understand you and your family. You should feel free to ask questions about any item in the questionnaire.

The space for comments should be used when you wish to give additional information or if you wish to discuss the way the question is applied to your family. Please try to answer all questions.

Family is defined as the individual(s) with whom you usually live. If you live alone, your "family" consists of persons with whom you now have the strongest emotional ties.*

For each question, check only one box

	Almost always	Some of the time	Hardly ever
I am satisfied that I can turn to my family for help when something is troubling me. Comments:	☐	☐	☐
I am satisfied with the way my family talks over things with me and shares problems with me. Comments:	☐	☐	☐
I am satisfied that my family accepts and supports my wishes to take on new activities or directions. Comments:	☐	☐	☐
I am satisfied with the way my family expresses affection and responds to my emotions, such as anger, sorrow, and love. Comments:	☐	☐	☐
I am satisfied with the way my family and I share time together. Comments:	☐	☐	☐

*According to which member of the family is being interviewed the interviewer may substitute for the word 'family' either spouse, significant other, parents, or children.

A

FIG. A-1 Family APGAR questionnaire. **A,** Part I. (Modified from Smilkstein G, Ashworth C, Montano D: Validity and reliability of the family APGAR as a test of family function, *J Fam Pract* 15(2):303-311, 1982.)

Family APGAR questionnaire

PART II

Who lives in your home?* List by relationship (eg, spouse, significant other,† child, or friend).

Please check below the column that best describes how you now get along with each member of the family listed.

Relationship	Age	Sex	Well	Fairly	Poorly
________	__	__	☐	☐	☐
________	__	__	☐	☐	☐
________	__	__	☐	☐	☐
________	__	__	☐	☐	☐
________	__	__	☐	☐	☐
________	__	__	☐	☐	☐

If you don't live with your own family, please list below the individuals to whom you turn for help most frequently. List by relationship, (eg, family member, friend, associate at work, or neighbor).

Please check below the column that best describes how you now get along with each person listed.

Relationship	Age	Sex	Well	Fairly	Poorly
________	__	__	☐	☐	☐
________	__	__	☐	☐	☐
________	__	__	☐	☐	☐
________	__	__	☐	☐	☐
________	__	__	☐	☐	☐
________	__	__	☐	☐	☐

*If you have established your own family, consider home to be the place where you live with your spouse, children, or significant other; otherwise, consider home as your place of origin, eg, the place where your parents or those who raise you live.

†"Significant other" is the partner you live with in a physically and emotionally nurturing relationship, but to whom you are not married.

B

FIG. A-1, cont'd **B,** Part II.

Infant/Toddler HOME Inventory

Bettye M. Caldwell and Robert H. Bradley

Family Name ______________ Visitor ______________ Date ______

Address ______________ Phone ______

Child's Name ______________ Birthdate ______ Age ______ Sex ______

Parent Present ______ If other than parent, relationship to child ______

Family Composition ______________
(persons living in household, including sex and age of children)

Family Ethnicity ______ Language Spoken ______ Maternal Education ______ Paternal Education ______

Is mother employed? ______ Type of work when employed ______ Is father employed? ______ Type of work when employed ______

Current child care arrangements ______________

Summarize past year's arrangement ______________

Other persons present during visit ______________

Comments: ______________

SUMMARY

	Subscale	Score Fourth	Lowest Half	Middle Fourth	Upper
I.	RESPONSIVITY		0 - 6	7 - 9	10 - 11
II.	ACCEPTANCE		0 - 4	5 - 6	7 - 8
III.	ORGANIZATION		0 - 3	4 - 5	6
IV.	LEARNING MATERIALS		0 - 4	5 - 7	8 - 9
V.	INVOLVEMENT		0 - 2	3 - 4	5 - 6
VI.	VARIETY		0 - 1	2 - 3	4 - 5
	TOTAL SCORE		0 - 25	26 - 36	37 - 45

FIG. A-2 Home Inventory questionnaires. AUTHOR'S NOTE: HOME inventories for families and preschoolers (3 to 6 years) and elementary age children (6 to 10 years) are available from the Center for Research on Teaching and Learning, College of Education, University of Arkansas at Little Rock, 2801 S. University Ave., Little Rock, AR 72204; (501) 569-3422. (From Caldwell B, Bradley R: *Manual of home observation for measurement of the environment,* rev ed, Little Rock, 1984, University of Arkansas at Little Rock.)

Infant/Toddler HOME Inventory

Place a plus (+) or minus (-) in the box alongside each item if the behavior is observed during the visit or if the parent reports that the conditions or events are characteristic of the home environment. Enter the subtotal and the total on the front side of the Record Sheet.

I. RESPONSITIVITY		24. Child has a special place for toys and treasures.	
1. Parent spontaneously vocalizes to child at least twice.		25. Child's play environment is safe.	
2. Parent responds verbally to child's vocalizations or verbalizations.		**IV. LEARNING MATERIALS**	
3. Parent tells child name of object or person during visit.		26. Muscle activity toys or equipment.	
4. Parent's speech is distinct, clear and audible.		27. Push or pull toy.	
5. Parent initiates verbal interchanges with Visitor.		28. Stroller or walker, kiddie car, scooter, or tricycle.	
6. Parent converses freely and easily.		29. Parent provides toys for child to play with during visit.	
7. Parent permits child to engage in "messy" play.		30. Cuddly toy or role-playing toys.	
8. Parent spontaneously praises child at least twice.		31. Learning facilitators—mobile, table and chair, high chair, play pen.	
9. Parent's voice conveys positive feelings toward child.		32. Simple eye-hand coordination toys.	
10. Parent caresses or kisses child at least once.		33. Complex eye-hand coordination toys.	
11. Parent responds positively to praise of child offered by Visitor.		34. Toys for literature and music.	
II. ACCEPTANCE		**V. INVOLVEMENT**	
12. Parent does not shout at child.		35. Parent keeps child in visual range, looks at often.	
13. Parent does not express overt annoyance with or hostility to child.		36. Parent talks to child while doing household work.	
14. Parent neither slaps nor spanks child during visit.		37. Parent conciously encourages developmental advance.	
15. No more than 1 instance of physical punishment during past week.		38. Parent invests maturing toys with value via personal attention.	
16. Parent does not scold or criticize child during visit.		39. Parent structures child's play periods.	
17. Parent does not interfere with or restrict child 3 times during visit.		40. Parent provides toys that challenge child to develop new skills.	
18. At least 10 books are present and visible.		**VI. VARIETY**	
19. Family has a pet.		41. Father provides some care daily.	
III. ORGANIZATION		42. Parent reads stories to child at least 3 times weekly.	
20. Child care, if used, is provided by one of three regular substitutes.		43. Child eats at least one meal a day with mother and father.	
21. Child is taken to grocery store at least once a week.		44. Family visits relatives or receives visits once month or so.	
22. Child gets out of house at least 4 times a week.		45. Child has 3 or more books of his/her own.	

	I	II	III	IV	V	VI	TOTAL
23. Child is taken regularly to doctor's office or clinic.							
TOTALS							

FIG. A-2, cont'd

APPENDIX B

DEVELOPMENTAL/SENSORY ASSESSMENT

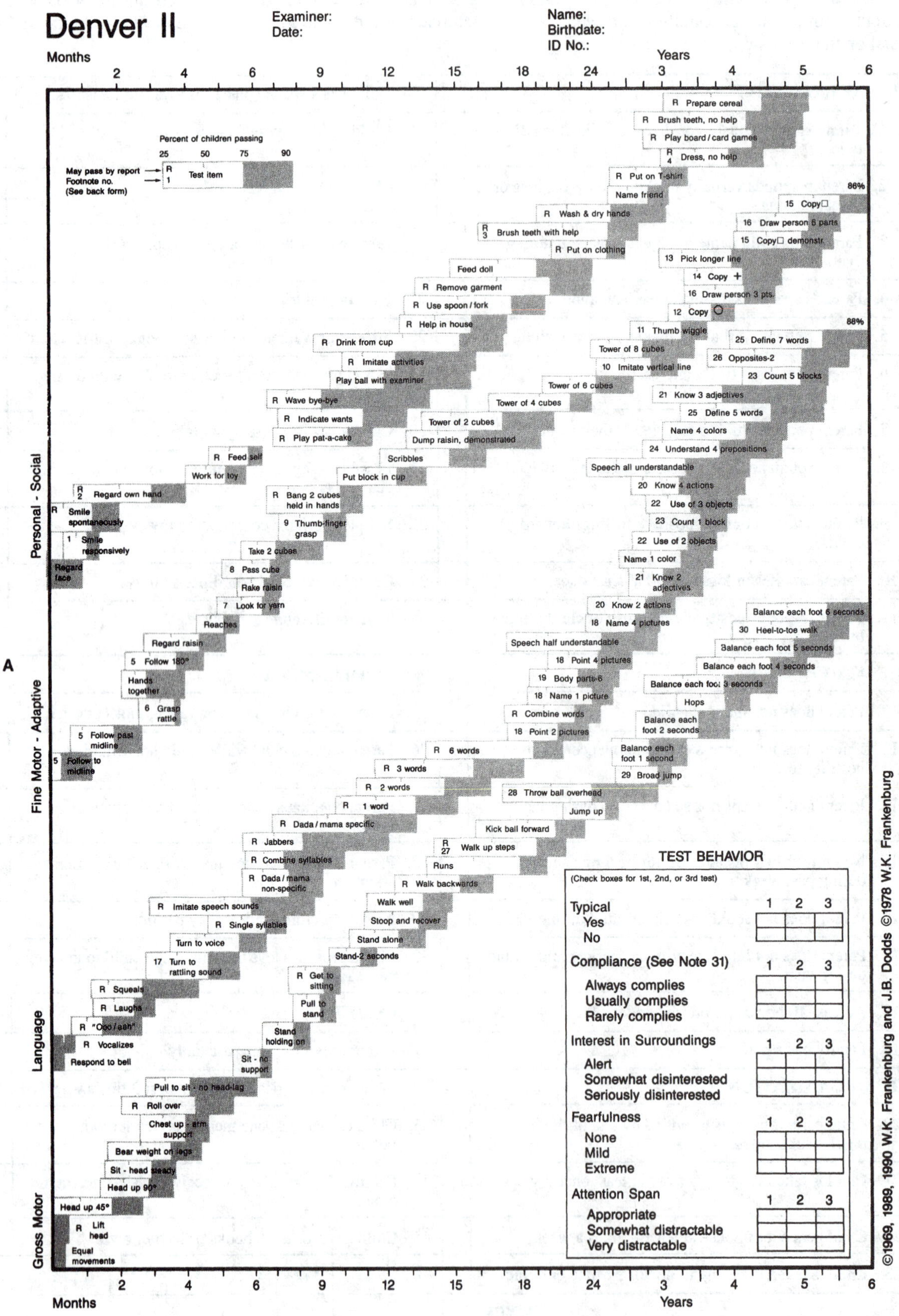

FIG. B-1 **A,** Denver II. (From W.K. Frankenburg and J.B. Dodds, 1990.)

DIRECTIONS FOR ADMINISTRATION

1. Try to get child to smile by smiling, talking or waving. Do not touch him/her.
2. Child must stare at hand several seconds.
3. Parent may help guide toothbrush and put toothpaste on brush.
4. Child does not have to be able to tie shoes or button/zip in the back.
5. Move yarn slowly in an arc from one side to the other, about 8" above child's face.
6. Pass if child grasps rattle when it is touched to the backs or tips of fingers.
7. Pass if child tries to see where yarn went. Yarn should be dropped quickly from sight from tester's hand without arm movement.
8. Child must transfer cube from hand to hand without help of body, mouth, or table.
9. Pass if child picks up raisin with any part of thumb and finger.
10. Line can vary only 30 degrees or less from tester's line.
11. Make a fist with thumb pointing upward and wiggle only the thumb. Pass if child imitates and does not move any fingers other than the thumb.

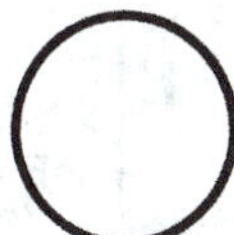

12. Pass any enclosed form. Fail continuous round motions.

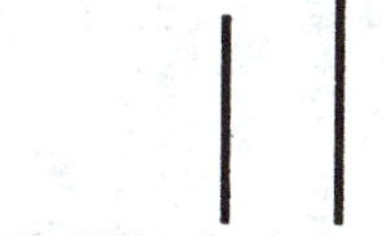

13. Which line is longer? (Not bigger.) Turn paper upside down and repeat. (pass 3 of 3 or 5 of 6)

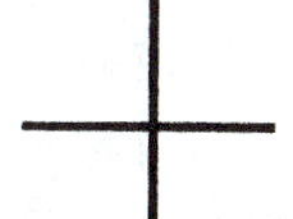

14. Pass any lines crossing near midpoint.

15. Have child copy first. If failed, demonstrate.

When giving items 12, 14, and 15, do not name the forms. Do not demonstrate 12 and 14.

16. When scoring, each pair (2 arms, 2 legs, etc.) counts as one part.
17. Place one cube in cup and shake gently near child's ear, but out of sight. Repeat for other ear.
18. Point to picture and have child name it. (No credit is given for sounds only.) If less than 4 pictures are named correctly, have child point to picture as each is named by tester.

B

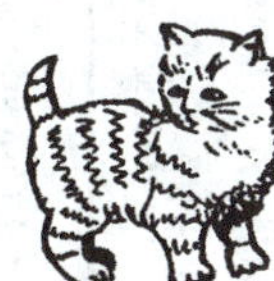
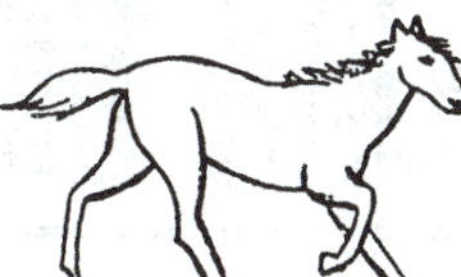
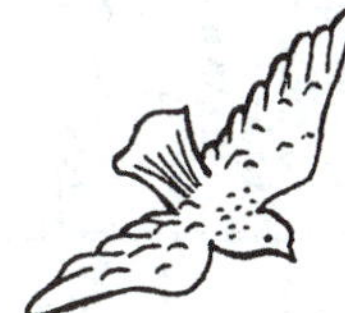
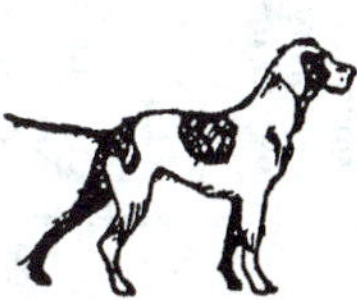
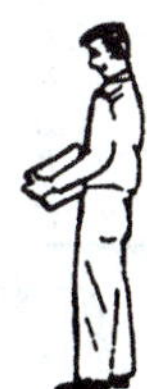

19. Using doll, tell child: Show me the nose, eyes, ears, mouth, hands, feet, tummy, hair. Pass 6 of 8.
20. Using pictures, ask child: Which one flies?... says meow?... talks?... barks?... gallops? Pass 2 of 5, 4 of 5.
21. Ask child: What do you do when you are cold?... tired?... hungry? Pass 2 of 3, 3 of 3.
22. Ask child: What do you do with a cup? What is a chair used for? What is a pencil used for? Action words must be included in answers.
23. Pass if child correctly places and says how many blocks are on paper. (1, 5).
24. Tell child: Put block **on** table; **under** table; **in front of** me, **behind** me. Pass 4 of 4. (Do not help child by pointing, moving head or eyes.)
25. Ask child: What is a ball?... lake?... desk?... house?... banana?... curtain?... fence?... ceiling? Pass if defined in terms of use, shape, what it is made of, or general category (such as banana is fruit, not just yellow). Pass 5 of 8, 7 of 8.
26. Ask child: If a horse is big, a mouse is __? If fire is hot, ice is __? If the sun shines during the day, the moon shines during the __? Pass 2 of 3.
27. Child may use wall or rail only, not person. May not crawl.
28. Child must throw ball overhand 3 feet to within arm's reach of tester.
29. Child must perform standing broad jump over width of test sheet (8 1/2 inches).
30. Tell child to walk forward, → heel within 1 inch of toe. Tester may demonstrate. Child must walk 4 consecutive steps.
31. In the second year, half of normal children are non-compliant.

OBSERVATIONS:

FIG. B-1 **B,** Directions for administration of numbered items on Denver II. (From W.K. Frankenburg and J.B. Dodds, 1990.)

0-9 MONTHS (R-PDQ)

REVISED DENVER PRESCREENING DEVELOPMENTAL QUESTIONNAIRE

Child's Name ______________________

Person Completing R-PDQ: ______________________

Relation to Child: ______________________

For Office Use

Today's Date: _____ yr _____ mo _____ day

Child's Birthdate: _____ yr _____ mo _____ day

Subtract to get Child's Exact Age: _____ yr _____ mo _____ day

R-PDQ Age: (_____ yr _____ mo _____ completed wks)

CONTINUE ANSWERING UNTIL 3 **"NOs"** ARE CIRCLED

Item			For Office Use
1. Equal Movements When your baby is lying on his/her back, can (s)he move each of his/her arms as easily as the other and each of the legs as easily as the other? Answer **No** if your child makes jerky or uncoordinated movements with one or both of his/her arms or legs.	Yes	No	(0) FMA
2. Stomach Lifts Head When your baby is on his/her stomach on a flat surface, can (s)he lift his/her head off the surface? 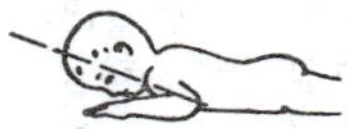	Yes	No	(0-3) GM
3. Regards Face When your baby is lying on his/her back, can (s)he look at you and watch your face?	Yes	No	(1) PS
4. Follows To Midline When your child is on his/her back, can (s)he follow your movement by turning his/her head from one side to facing directly forward? 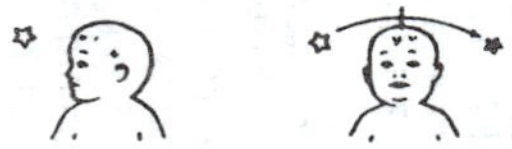	Yes	No	(1-1) FMA
5. Responds To Bell Does your child respond with eye movements, change in breathing or other change in activity to a bell or rattle sounded outside his/her line of vision?	Yes	No	(1-2) L
6. Vocalizes Not Crying Does your child make sounds other than crying, such as gurgling, cooing, or babbling?	Yes	No	(1-3) L
7. Smiles Responsively When you smile and talk to your baby, does (s)he smile back at you?	Yes	No	(1-3) PS
8. Follows Past Midline When your child is on his/her back, does (s)he follow your movement by turning his/her head from one side ***almost all the way to the other side?*** 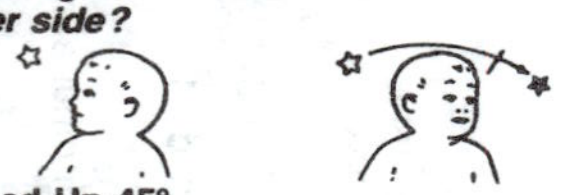	Yes	No	(2-2) FMA
9. Stomach, Head Up 45° When your baby is on his/her stomach on a flat surface, can (s)he lift his/her head 45°? 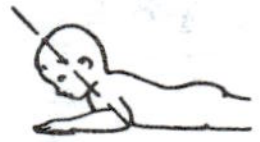	Yes	No	(2-2) GM
10. Stomach, Head Up 90° When your baby is on his/her stomach on a flat surface, can (s)he lift his/her head 90°? 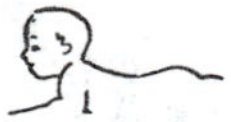	Yes	No	(3) GM
11. Laughs Does your baby laugh out loud without being tickled or touched?	Yes	No	(3-1) L
12. Hands Together Does your baby play with his/her hands by touching them together?	Yes	No	(3-3) FMA
13. Follows 180° When your child is on his/her back, does (s)he follow your movement from one side ***all the way*** to the other side? 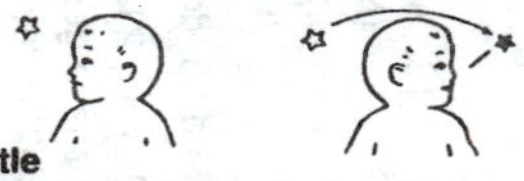	Yes	No	(4) FMA
14. Grasps Rattle ***It is important that you follow instructions carefully.*** Do ***not*** place the pencil in the palm of your child's hand. When you touch the pencil to the back or tips of your baby's fingers, does your baby grasp the pencil for a few seconds? 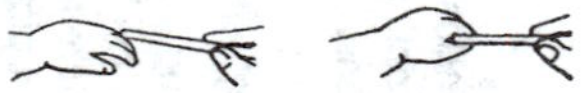	Yes	No	(4) FMA

TRY THIS   **NOT THIS**

(Please turn page)

FIG. B-2 Revised Prescreening Developmental Questionnaire. (Sample of first page only.) (The *first* page is reprinted with permission of William K. Frankenburg. Copyright 1975, 1986, W.K. Frankenburg.)

A

DENVER ARTICULATION SCREENING EXAM
for children 2½ to 6 years of age

Instructions: Have child repeat each word after you. Circle the underlined sounds that he pronounces correctly. Total correct sounds is the Raw Score. Use charts on reverse side to score results.

Name:

Hosp. No.:

Address:________________

Date: ______ Child's age: ______ Examiner: ______ Raw score: ___
Percentile: ______ Intelligibility: ______ Result: ______

1. table	6. zipper	11. sock	16. wagon	21. leaf
2. shirt	7. grapes	12. vacuum	17. gum	22. carrot
3. door	8. flag	13. yarn	18. house	
4. trunk	9. thumb	14. mother	19. pencil	
5. jumping	10. toothbrush	15. twinkle	20. fish	

Intelligibility: (circle one)
1. Easy to understand
2. Understandable ½ the time
3. Not understandable
4. Can't evaluate

Comments:

Date: ______ Child's age: ______ Examiner: ______ Raw score: ___
Percentile: ______ Intelligibility: ______ Result: ______

1. table	6. zipper	11. sock	16. wagon	21. leaf
2. shirt	7. grapes	12. vacuum	17. gum	22. carrot
3. door	8. flag	13. yarn	18. house	
4. trunk	9. thumb	14. mother	19. pencil	
5. jumping	10. toothbrush	15. twinkle	20. fish	

Intelligibility: (circle one)
1. Easy to understand
2. Understandable ½ the time
3. Not understandable
4. Can't evaluate

Comments:

Date: ______ Child's age: ______ Examiner: ______ Raw score ___
Percentile: ______ Intelligibility: ______ Result: ______

1. table	6. zipper	11. sock	16. wagon	21. leaf
2. shirt	7. grapes	12. vacuum	17. gum	22. carrot
3. door	8. flag	13. yarn	18. house	
4. trunk	9. thumb	14. mother	19. pencil	
5. jumping	10. toothbrush	15. twinkle	20. fish	

Intelligibility: (circle one)
1. Easy to understand
2. Understandable ½ the time
3. Not understandable
4. Can't evaluate

FIG. B-3 **A,** Denver Articulation Screening Examination for children 2½ to 6 years of age.
(From A.F. Drumwright, University of Colorado Medical Center, 1971.)

To score DASE words: Note raw score for child's performance. Match raw score line (extreme left of chart) with column representing child's age (to the closest previous age group). Where raw score line and age column meet number in that square denotes percentile rank of child's performance when compared to other children that age. Percentiles above heavy line are ABNORMAL percentiles, below heavy line are NORMAL.

PERCENTILE RANK

B

Raw Score	2.5 yr.	3.0	3.5	4.0	4.5	5.0	5.5	6 years
2	1							
3	2							
4	5							
5	9							
6	16							
7	23							
8	31	2						
9	37	4	1					
10	42	6	2					
11	48	7	4					
12	54	9	6	1	1			
13	58	12	9	2	3	1	1	
14	62	17	11	5	4	2	2	
15	68	23	15	9	5	3	2	
16	75	31	19	12	5	4	3	
17	79	38	25	15	6	6	4	
18	83	46	31	19	8	7	4	
19	86	51	38	24	10	9	5	1
20	89	58	45	30	12	11	7	3
21	92	65	52	36	15	15	9	4
22	94	72	58	43	18	19	12	5
23	96	77	63	50	22	24	15	7
24	97	82	70	58	29	29	20	15
25	99	87	78	66	36	34	26	17
26	99	91	84	75	46	43	34	24
27		94	89	82	57	54	44	34
28		96	94	88	70	68	59	47
29		98	98	94	84	84	77	68
30		100	100	100	100	100	100	100

To score intelligibility:

	NORMAL	ABNORMAL
2½ years	Understandable ½ the time, or, "easy"	Not understandable
3 years and older	Easy to understand	Understandable ½ time Not understandable

Test result: 1. NORMAL on Dase and Intelligibility = NORMAL

2. ABNORMAL on Dase and/or Intelligibility = ABNORMAL

*If abnormal on initial screening, rescreen within 2 weeks.
If abnormal again, child should be referred for complete speech evaluation.

FIG. B-3, cont'd B, Percentile rank.

DENVER EYE SCREENING TEST	1ST SCREENING: DATE:						RESCREENING: DATE:					
	Right Eye			Left Eye			Right Eye			Left Eye		
Vision Tests	Normal	Abnormal	Untestable	Normal	Abnormal	Untestable	Normal	Abnormal	Untestable	Normal	Abnormal	Untestable
1. "E" (3 years and above—3 to 5 trials)	3P	3F	U	3P	3F	U	3P	3F	U	3P	3F	U
2. Picture card (2 1/2 - 2 11/12 yrs.—3 to 5 trials)	3P	3F	U	3P	3F	U	3P	3F	U	3P	3F	U
3. Fixation (6 months - 2 5/12 years)	P	F	U	P	F	U	P	F	U	P	F	U
4. Squinting		yes			yes			yes			yes	

Tests for Non-Straight Eyes	Normal	Abnormal	Untestable	Normal	Abnormal	Untestable
1. Do your child's eyes turn in or out, or are they ever not straight?	NO	YES	U	NO	YES	U
2. Cover Test	P	F	U	P	F	U
3. Pupillary Light Reflex	P	F	U	P	F	U

Total Test Rating (Both Eyes)	1st Screening	Rescreening
Normal (passed vision test plus no squint, plus passed 2/3 tests for non-straight eyes)	Normal	Normal
Abnormal (abnormal on any vision test, squinting or 2 of 3 procedures for non-straight eyes)	Abnormal	Abnormal
Untestable (untestable on any vision test or untestable on 2/3 tests for non-straight eyes)	Untestable	Untestable
Future Rescreening Appointment for Total Test Rating (Abnormal or Untestable)	Date:	Date:

Name:
Hospital No.:
Ward:
Address:

FIG. B-4 Denver Eye Screening Test. (From W.K. Frankenburg and J.B. Dobbs, University of Colorado Medical Center, 1969.)

SNELLEN SCREENING*

Preparation

1. Hang the Snellen chart on a light-colored wall so that the 20- to 30-foot lines are at eye level when children 6 to 12 years old are tested in the standing position.
2. Secure the chart to the wall with double-stick tape on the back side of all four corners. If the chart must be reversed for use of the letter or E chart, secure it at the top and bottom with tacks. Make sure that the chart does not swing when in place.
3. The illumination intensity on the chart should be 10 to 30 foot-candles, without any glare from windows or light fixtures. The illumination should be checked with a light meter.
4. Mark an exact 20-foot distance from the chart. Mark the floor with a piece of tape or "footprints" positioned so that the heels touch the 20-foot line.

Procedure

1. Place the child at the 20-foot mark, with the heel edging the line if the child is standing or with the back of the chair placed at the marker if the child is seated.
2. If the E chart is used, accustom the child to identifying which direction the "legs of the E" are pointing. Use a demonstration E card for this purpose.
3. Teach the child to use the occluder to cover one eye. Instruct the child to keep both eyes open during the test. Provide a clean cover card for each child and then discard after use.
4. If the child wears glasses, test only with the glasses on.
5. Test both eyes together, then the right eye, then the left eye.
6. Begin with the 40- or 30-foot line and proceed with the test to include the 20-foot line.
7. With a child suspected of low vision, begin with the 200-foot line and proceed until the child can no longer correctly read three out of four or four out of six symbols on a line.
8. Use covers on the Snellen chart to expose only one symbol or one line at a time. When screening kindergarten or older children, expose one line but may use a pointer to point to one symbol at a time.

Recording and Referral

1. Record the last line the child read correctly (three out of four or four out of six symbols).
2. Record visual acuity as a fraction. The numerator represents the distance from the chart, and the denominator represents the last line read correctly. For example, 20/30 means that the child read the 30-foot line at a 20-foot distance.
3. Observe the child's eyes during testing and record any evidence of squinting, head tilting, thrusting the head forward, excessive blinking, tearing, or redness.
4. Only make referrals after a second screening has been made on children who are potential candidates for referral.
5. The following children should be referred for a complete eye examination:
   a. Three-year-old children with vision in either eye of 20/50 or less (inability to correctly identify one more than half the symbols on the 40-foot line) *or* a two-line difference in visual acuity between the eyes in the passing range; for example, 20/20 in one eye and 20/40 in the other
   b. All other ages and grades with vision in either eye of 20/40 or less (inability to correctly identify one more than half the symbols on the 30-foot line)
   c. All children who consistently show any of the signs of possible visual disturbances, regardless of visual acuity

*Modified from recommendations of the National Society to Prevent Blindness: *Guide to testing distance visual acuity,* Schaumburg, IL, 1988, The Society.

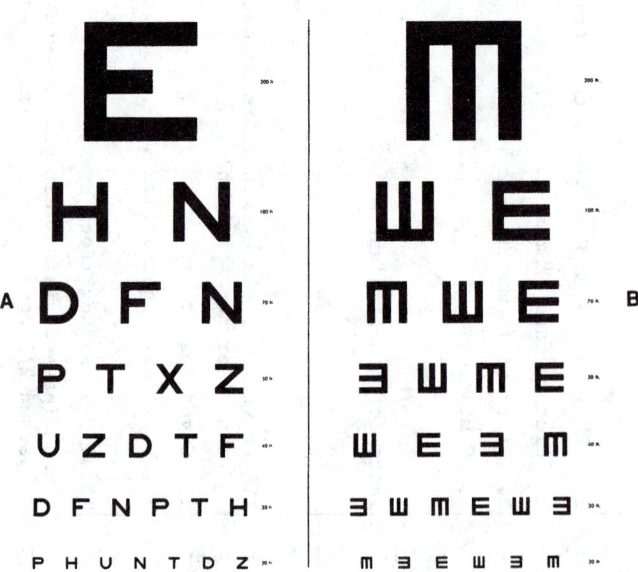

FIG. B-5 Snellen chart. **A,** Letter (alphabet) chart. **B,** Symbol E chart. (From National Society to Prevent Blindness, Inc., Schaumburg, IL.)

APPENDIX C

GROWTH MEASUREMENTS

HEIGHT AND WEIGHT MEASUREMENTS FOR BOYS

	HEIGHT BY PERCENTILES						WEIGHT BY PERCENTILES					
	5		50		95		5		50		95	
AGE*	cm	INCHES	cm	INCHES	cm	INCHES	kg	lb	kg	lb	kg	lb
Birth	46.4	18¼	50.5	20	54.4	21½	2.54	5½	3.27	7¼	4.15	9¼
3 months	56.7	22¼	61.1	24	65.4	25¾	4.43	9¾	5.98	13¼	7.37	16¼
6 months	63.4	25	67.8	26¾	72.3	28½	6.20	13¾	7.85	17¼	9.46	20¾
9 months	68.0	26¾	72.3	28½	77.1	30¼	7.52	16½	9.18	20¼	10.93	24
1	71.7	28¼	76.1	30	81.2	32	8.43	18½	10.15	22½	11.99	26½
1½	77.5	30½	82.4	32½	88.1	34¾	9.59	21¼	11.47	25¼	13.44	29½
2†	82.5	32½	86.8	34¼	94.4	37¼	10.49	23¼	12.34	27¼	15.50	34¼
2½†	85.4	33½	90.4	35½	97.8	38½	11.27	24¾	13.52	29¾	16.61	36½
3	89.0	35	94.9	37¼	102.0	40¼	12.05	26½	14.62	32¼	17.77	39¼
3½	92.5	36½	99.1	39	106.1	41¾	12.84	28¼	15.68	34½	18.98	41¾
4	95.8	37¾	102.9	40½	109.9	43¼	13.64	30	16.69	36¾	20.27	44¾
4½	98.9	39	106.6	42	113.5	44¾	14.45	31¾	17.69	39	21.63	47¾
5	102.0	40¼	109.9	43¼	117.0	46	15.27	33¾	18.67	41¼	23.09	51
6	107.7	42½	116.1	45¾	123.5	48½	16.93	37¼	20.69	45½	26.34	58
7	113.0	44½	121.7	48	129.7	51	18.64	41	22.85	50¼	30.12	66½
8	118.1	46½	127.0	50	135.7	53½	20.40	45	25.30	55¾	34.51	76
9	122.9	48½	132.2	52	141.8	55¾	22.25	49	28.13	62	39.58	87¼
10	127.7	50¼	137.5	54¼	148.1	58¼	24.33	53¾	31.44	69¼	45.27	99¾
11	132.6	52¼	143.3	56½	154.9	61	26.80	59	35.30	77¾	51.47	113½
12	137.6	54¼	149.7	59	162.3	64	29.85	65¾	39.78	87¾	58.09	128
13	142.9	56¼	156.5	61½	169.8	66¾	33.64	74¼	44.95	99	65.02	143¼
14	148.8	58½	163.1	64¼	176.7	69½	38.22	84¼	50.77	112	72.13	159
15	155.2	61	169.0	66½	181.9	71½	43.11	95	56.71	125	79.12	174½
16	161.1	63½	173.5	68¼	185.4	73	47.74	105¼	62.10	137	85.62	188¾
17	164.9	65	176.2	69¼	187.3	73¾	51.50	113½	66.31	146¼	91.31	201¼
18	165.7	65¼	176.8	69½	187.6	73¾	53.97	119	68.88	151¾	95.76	211

Adapted from National Center for Health Statistics (NCHS), Health Resources Administration, Department of Health, Education and Welfare, Hyattsville, MD. Conversion of metric data to approximate inches and pounds by Ross Laboratories.
*Years unless otherwise indicated.
†Height data include some recumbent length measurements, which make values slightly higher than if all measurements had been of stature (standing height).

BOYS: BIRTH TO AGE 36 MONTHS—PHYSICAL GROWTH (LENGTH, WEIGHT), NCHS PERCENTILES

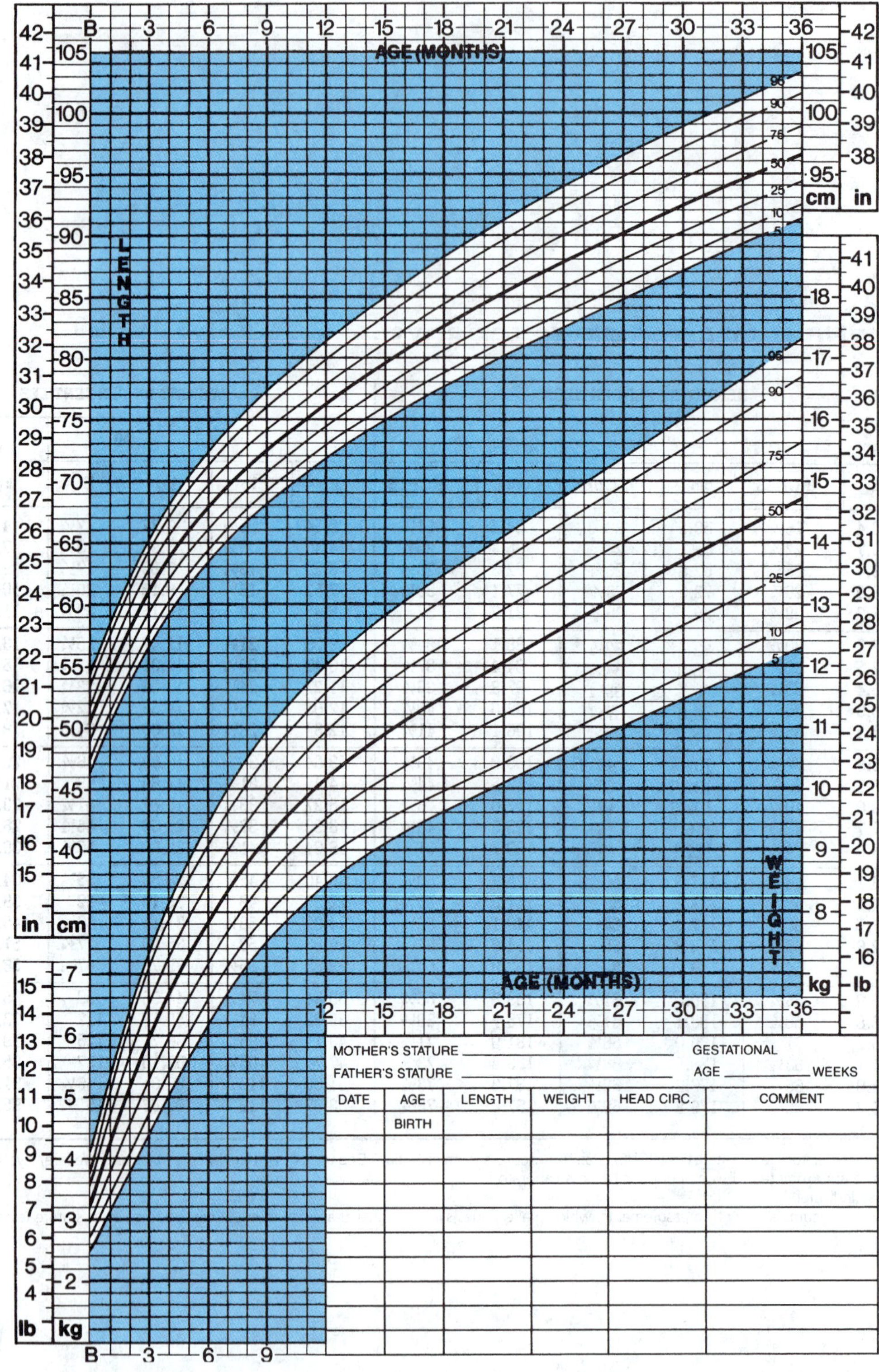

Modified from Hamill PVV and others: Physical growth: National Center for Health Statistics percentiles, *Am J Clin Nutr* 32:607-629, 1979. Data from the Fels Longitudinal Study, Wright State University School of Medicine, Yellow Springs, OH. Provided as a service of Ross Products Division, Abbott Laboratories, 1982.

BOYS: BIRTH TO AGE 36 MONTHS— PHYSICAL GROWTH (HEAD CIRCUMFERENCE, LENGTH, WEIGHT), NCHS PERCENTILES

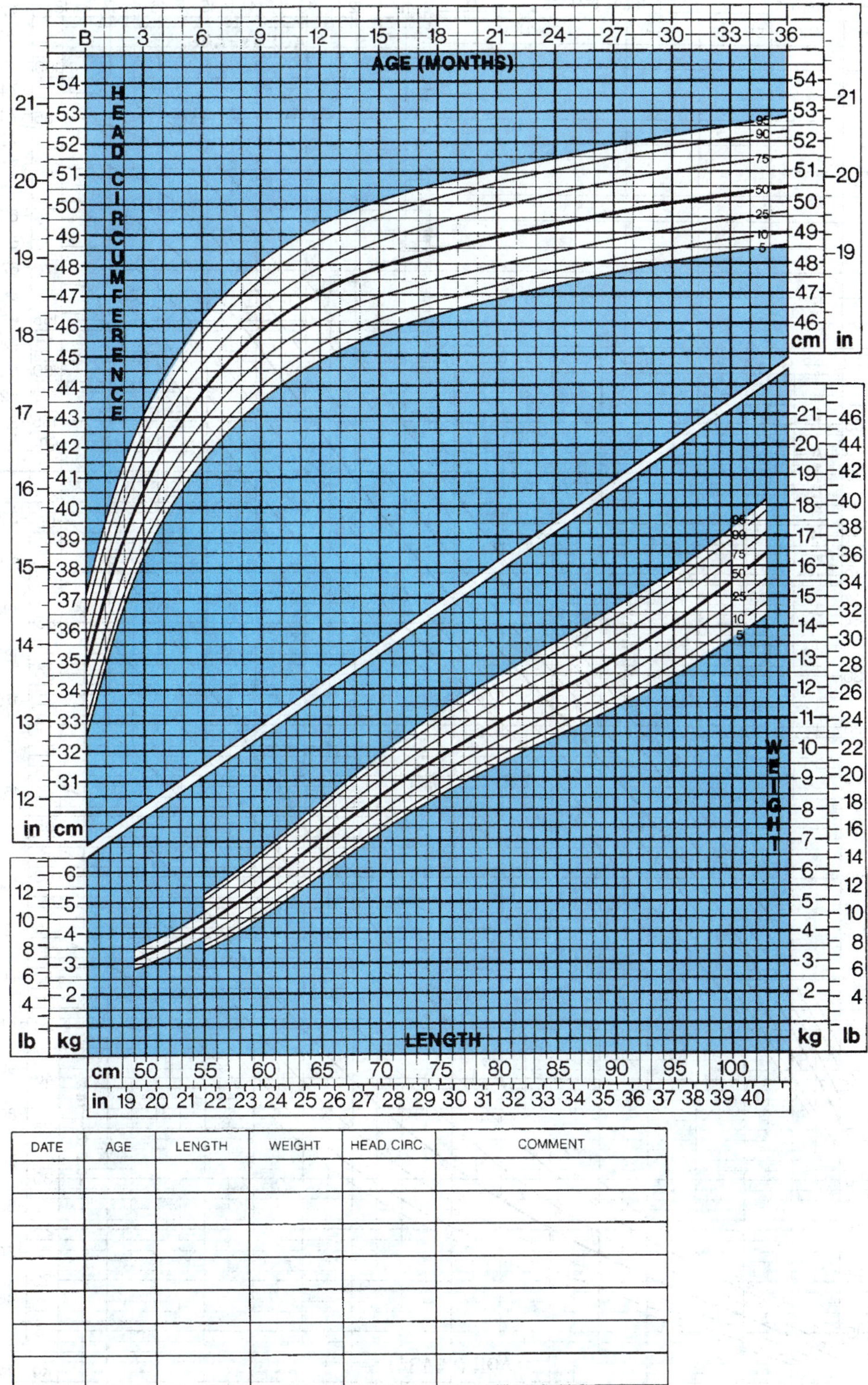

DATE	AGE	LENGTH	WEIGHT	HEAD CIRC	COMMENT

Modified from Hamill PVV and others: Physical growth: National Center for Health Statistics percentiles, *Am J Clin Nutr* 32:607-629, 1979. Data from the Fels Longitudinal Study, Wright State University School of Medicine, Yellow Springs, OH. Provided as a service of Ross Products Division, Abbott Laboratories, 1982.

BOYS: AGES 2 TO 18 YEARS— PHYSICAL GROWTH (STATURE, WEIGHT), NCHS PERCENTILES

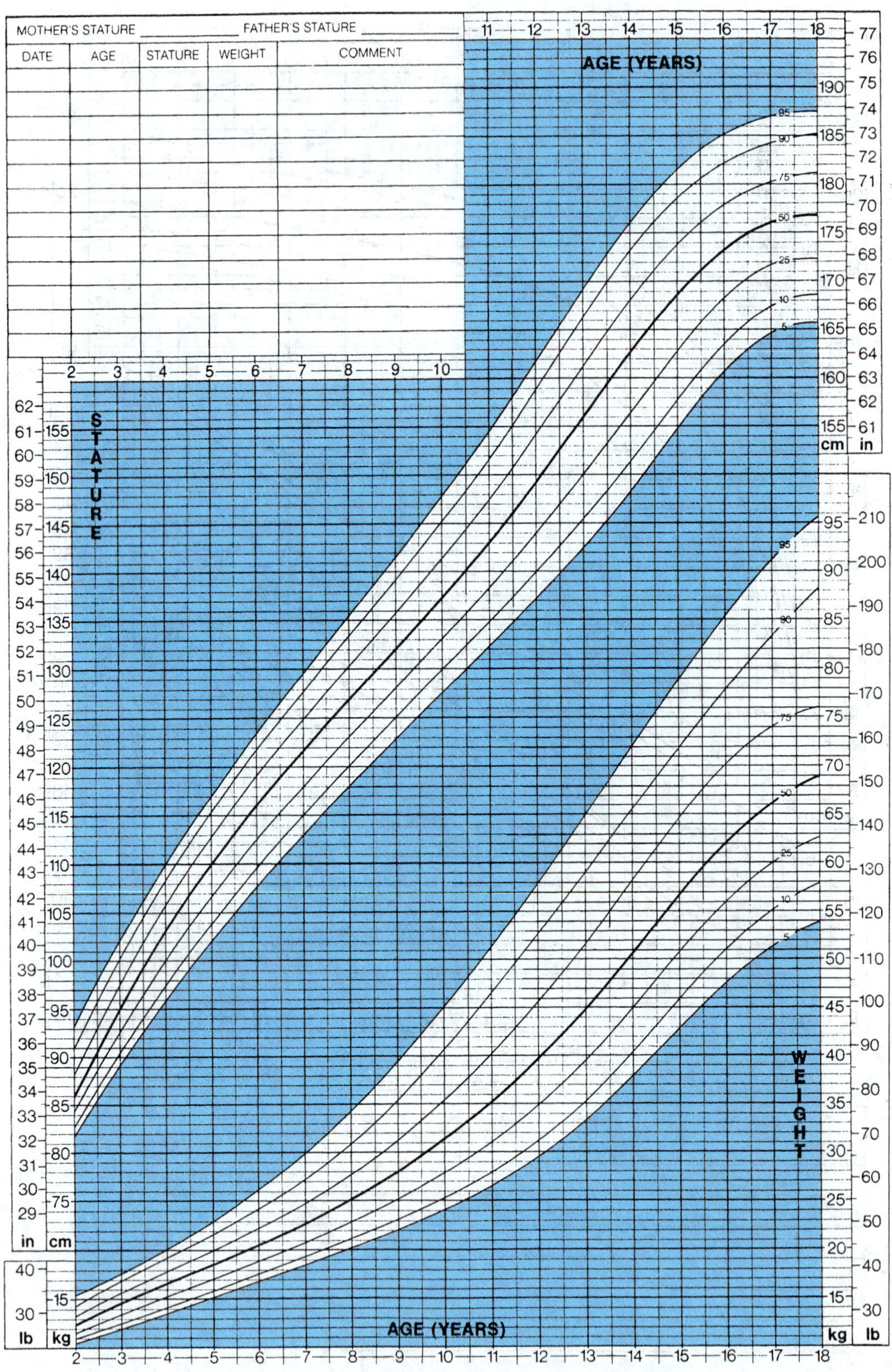

Modified from Hamill PVV and others: Physical growth: National Center for Health Statistics percentiles, *Am J Clin Nutr* 32:607-629, 1979. Data from the National Center for Health Statistics (NCHS), Hyattsville, MD. Provided as a service of Ross Laboratories, 1982.

BOYS: PREPUBESCENT— PHYSICAL GROWTH (STATURE, WEIGHT), NCHS PERCENTILES

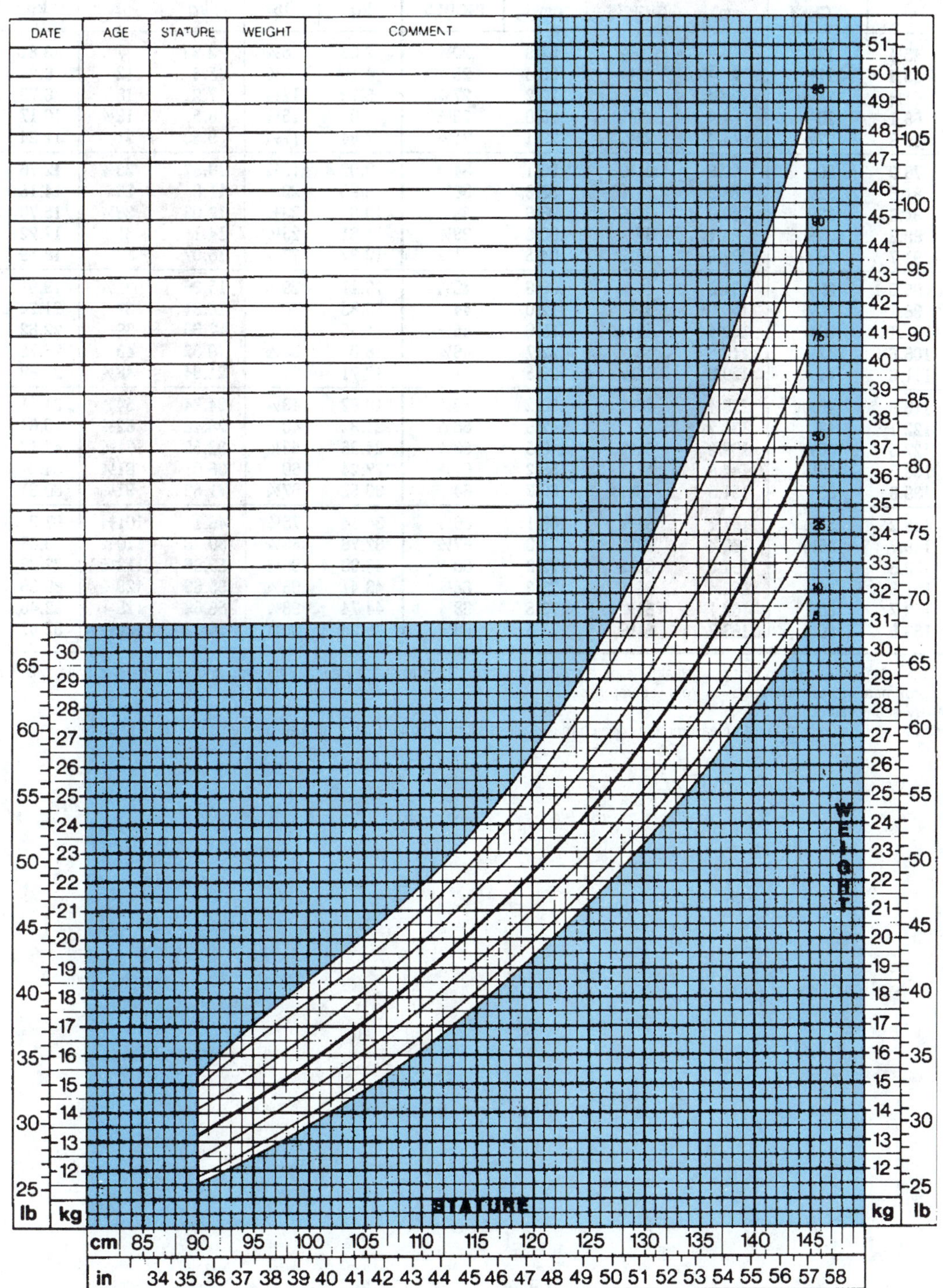

Modified from Hamill PVV and others: Physical growth: National Center for Health Statistics percentiles, *Am J Clin Nutr* 32:607-629, 1979. Data from the National Center for Health Statistics (NCHS), Hyattsville, MD. Provided as a service of Ross Laboratories, 1982.

HEIGHT AND WEIGHT MEASUREMENTS FOR GIRLS

	HEIGHT BY PERCENTILES						WEIGHT BY PERCENTILES					
	5		50		95		5		50		95	
AGE*	cm	INCHES	cm	INCHES	cm	INCHES	kg	lb	kg	lb	kg	lb
Birth	45.4	17¾	49.9	19¾	52.9	20¾	2.36	5¼	3.23	7	3.81	8½
3 months	55.4	21¾	59.5	23½	63.4	25	4.18	9¼	5.4	12	6.74	14¾
6 months	61.8	24¼	65.9	26	70.2	27¾	5.79	12¾	7.21	16	8.73	19¼
9 months	66.1	26	70.4	27¾	75.0	29½	7.0	15½	8.56	18¾	10.17	22½
1	69.8	27½	74.3	29¼	79.1	31¼	7.84	17¼	9.53	21	11.24	24¾
1½	76.0	30	80.9	31¾	86.1	34	8.92	19¾	10.82	23¾	12.76	28¼
2†	81.6	32¼	86.8	34¼	93.6	36¾	9.95	22	11.8	26	14.15	31¼
2½†	84.6	33¼	90.0	35½	96.6	38	10.8	23¾	13.03	28¾	15.76	34¾
3	88.3	34¾	94.1	37	100.6	39½	11.61	25½	14.1	31	17.22	38
3½	91.7	36	97.9	38½	104.5	41¼	12.37	27¼	15.07	33¼	18.59	41
4	95.0	37½	101.6	40	108.3	42¾	13.11	29	15.96	35¼	19.91	44
4½	98.1	38½	105.0	41¼	112.0	44	13.83	30½	16.81	37	21.24	46¾
5	101.1	39¾	108.4	42¾	115.6	45½	14.55	32	17.66	39	22.62	49¾
6	106.6	42	114.6	45	122.7	48¼	16.05	35½	19.52	43	25.75	56¾
7	111.8	44	120.6	47½	129.5	51	17.71	39	21.84	48¼	29.68	65½
8	116.9	46	126.4	49¾	136.2	53½	19.62	43¼	24.84	54¾	34.71	76½
9	122.1	48	132.2	52	142.9	56¼	21.82	48	28.46	62¾	40.64	89½
10	127.5	50¼	138.3	54½	149.5	58¾	24.36	53¾	32.55	71¾	47.17	104
11	133.5	52½	144.8	57	156.2	61½	27.24	60	36.95	81½	54.0	119
12	139.8	55	151.5	59¾	162.7	64	30.52	67¼	41.53	91½	60.81	134
13	145.2	57¼	157.1	61¾	168.1	66¼	34.14	75¼	46.1	101¾	67.3	148¼
14	148.7	58½	160.4	63¼	171.3	67½	37.76	83¼	50.28	110¾	73.08	161
15	150.5	59¼	161.8	63¾	172.8	68	40.99	90¼	53.68	118¼	77.78	171½
16	151.6	59¾	162.4	64	173.3	68¼	43.41	95¾	55.89	123¼	80.99	178½
17	152.7	60	163.1	64¼	173.5	68¼	44.74	98¾	56.69	125	82.46	181¾
18	153.6	60½	163.7	64½	173.6	68¼	45.26	99¾	56.62	124¾	82.47	181¾

Adapted from National Center for Health Statistics, Health Resources Administration, Department of Health, Education and Welfare, Hyattsville, MD. Conversion of metric data to approximate inches and pounds by Ross Laboratories.

*Years unless otherwise indicated.

†Height data include some recumbent length measurements, which make values slightly higher than if all measurements had been of stature.

GIRLS: BIRTH TO AGE 36 MONTHS— PHYSICAL GROWTH (LENGTH, WEIGHT), NCHS PERCENTILES

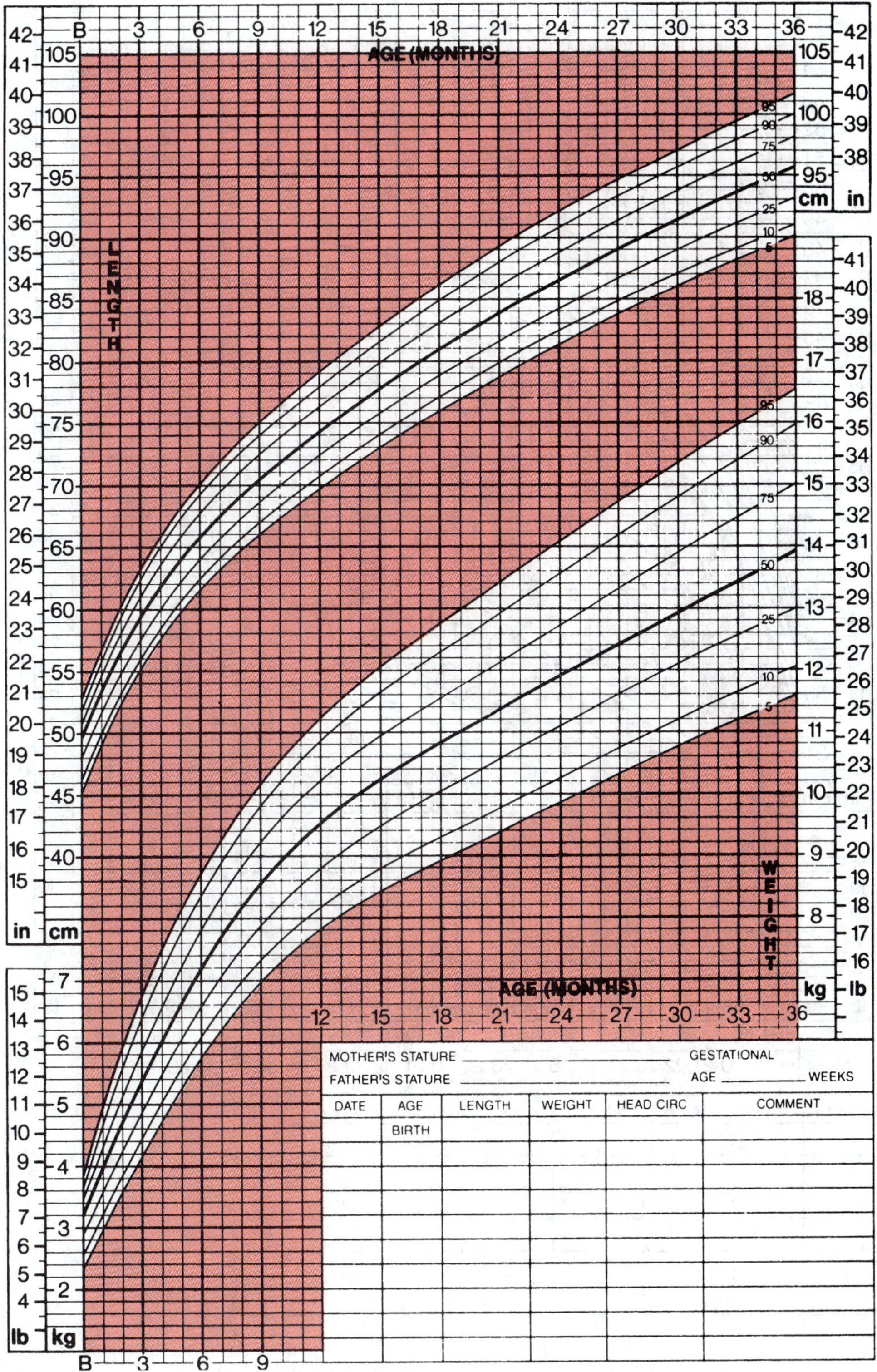

Modified from Hamill PVV and others: Physical growth: National Center for Health Statistics percentiles, *Am J Clin Nutr* 32:607-629, 1979. Data from the Fels Longitudinal Study, Wright State University School of Medicine, Yellow Springs, OH. Provided as a service of Ross Products Division, Abbott Laboratories, 1982.

GIRLS: BIRTH TO AGE 36 MONTHS— PHYSICAL GROWTH (HEAD CIRCUMFERENCE, LENGTH, WEIGHT), NCHS PERCENTILES

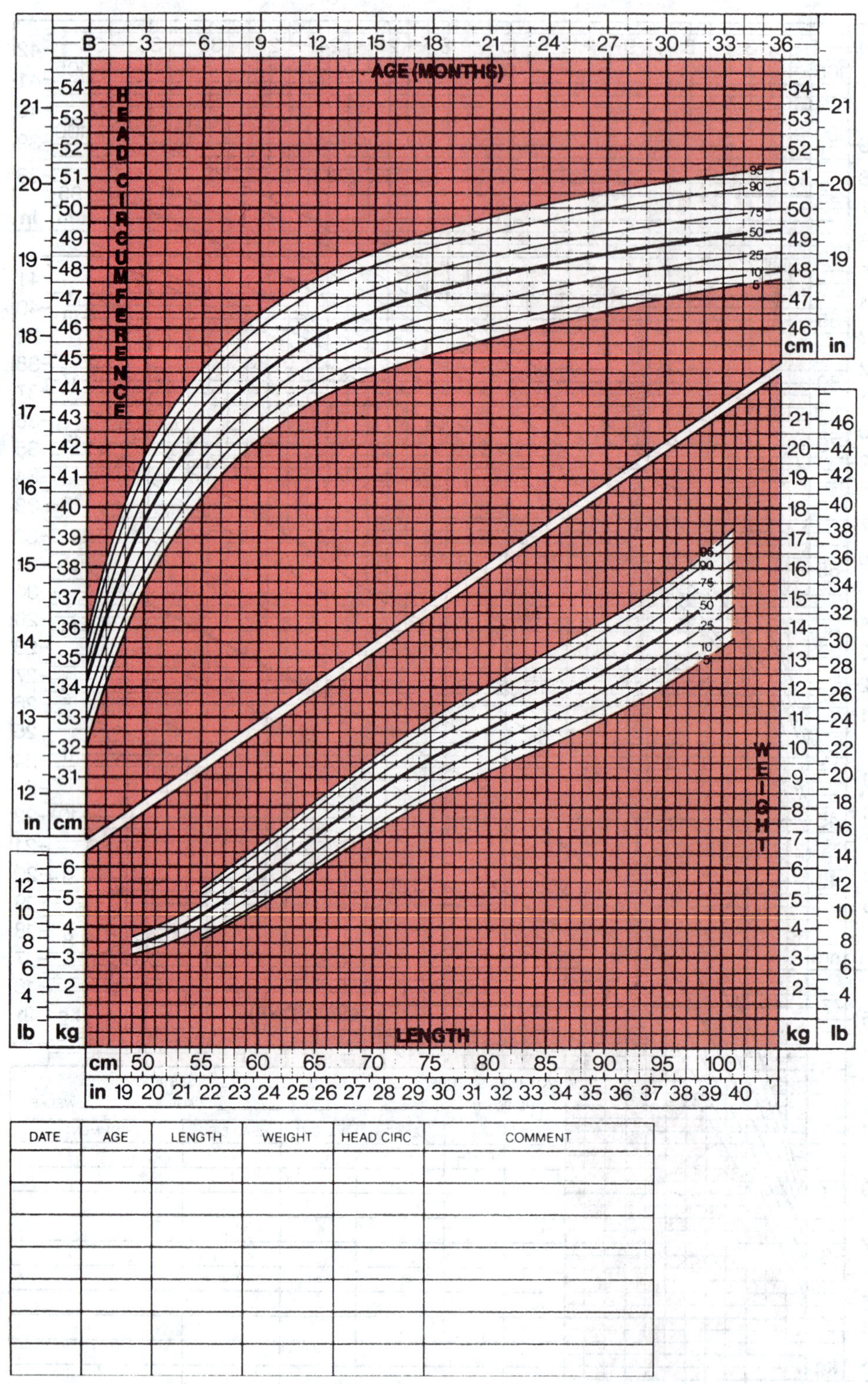

DATE	AGE	LENGTH	WEIGHT	HEAD CIRC	COMMENT

Modified from Hamill PVV and others: Physical growth: National Center for Health Statistics percentiles, *Am J Clin Nutr* 32:607-629, 1979. Data from the Fels Longitudinal Study, Wright State University School of Medicine, Yellow Springs, OH. Provided as a service of Ross Products Division, Abbott Laboratories, 1982.

GIRLS: AGES 2 TO 18 YEARS
PHYSICAL GROWTH (STATURE, WEIGHT), NCHS PERCENTILES

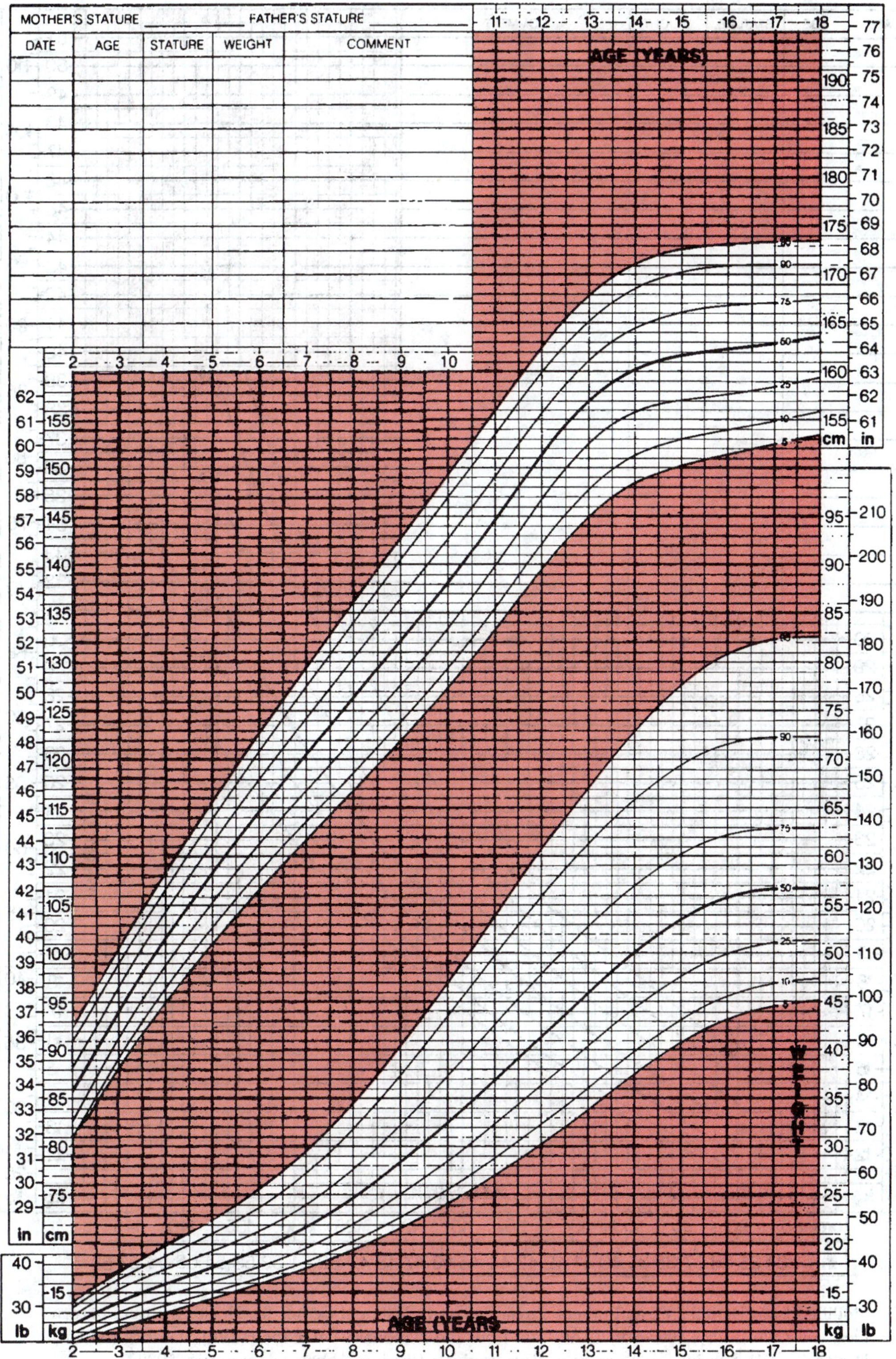

Modified from Hamill PVV and others: Physical growth: National Center for Health Statistics percentiles, *Am J Clin Nutr* 32:607-629, 1979. Data from the National Center for Health Statistics (NCHS), Hyattsville, MD. Provided as a service of Ross Products Division, Abbott Laboratories, 1982.

GIRLS: PREPUBESCENT—PHYSICAL GROWTH (STATURE, WEIGHT), NCHS PERCENTILES

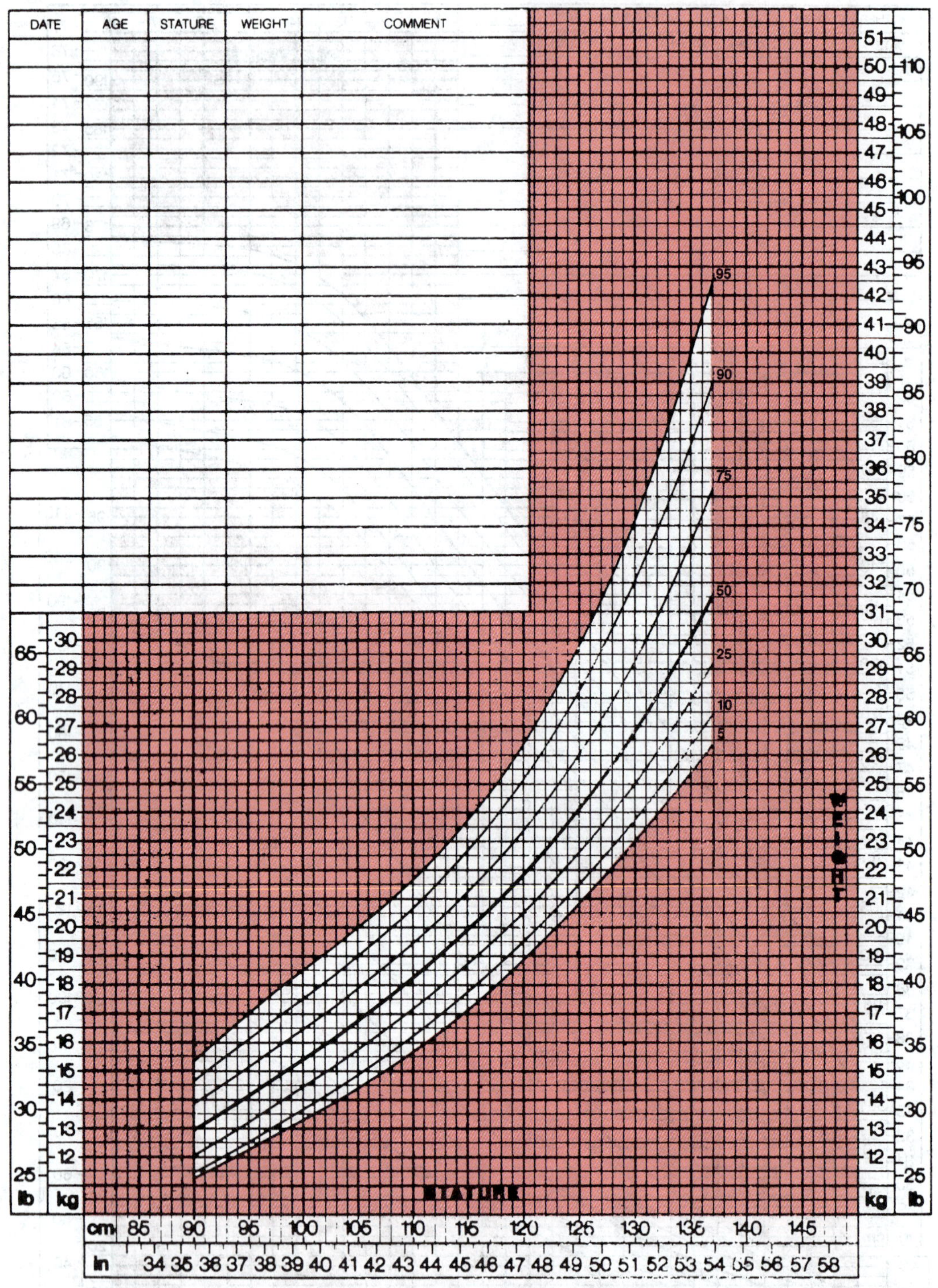

Modified from Hamill PVV and others: Physical growth: National Center for Health Statistics percentiles, *Am J Clin Nutr* 32:607-629, 1979. Data from the National Center for Health Statistics (NCHS), Hyattsville, MD. Provided as a service of Ross Products Division, Abbott Laboratories, 1982.

GROWTH STANDARDS OF HEALTHY CHINESE CHILDREN

	Weight (kg)		Height (cm)		Head circumference	
Age (months or years)	**Boys**	**Girls**	**Boys**	**Girls**	**Boys**	**Girls**
Birth	3.27	3.17	50.6	50.0	34.3	33.7
1 month	4.97	4.64	56.5	55.5	38.1	37.3
2 months	5.95	5.49	59.6	58.4	39.7	38.7
3 months	6.73	6.23	62.3	60.9	41.0	40.0
4 months	7.32	6.69	64.4	52.9	42.0	41.0
5 months	7.70	7.19	65.9	64.5	42.9	41.9
6 months	8.22	7.62	68.1	66.7	43.9	42.8
8 months	8.71	8.14	70.6	69.0	44.9	43.7
10 months	9.14	8.57	72.9	71.4	45.7	44.5
12 months	9.56	9.04	75.6	74.1	46.3	45.2
15 months	10.15	9.54	78.3	76.9	46.8	45.6
18 months	10.67	10.08	80.7	79.4	47.3	46.2
21 months	11.18	10.56	83.0	81.7	47.8	46.7
24 months	11.95	11.37	86.5	85.3	48.2	47.1
2.5 years	12.84	12.28	90.4	89.3	48.8	47.7
3 years	13.63	13.16	93.8	92.8	49.1	48.1
3.5 years	14.45	14.00	97.2	96.3	49.4	48.5
4 years	15.26	14.89	100.8	100.1	49.7	48.9
4.5 years	16.07	15.63	103.9	103.1	50.0	49.1
5 years	16 88	16.46	107.2	106.5	50.2	49.4
5.5 years	17.65	17.18	110.1	109.2	50.5	49.6
6 years	19.25	18.67	114.7	113.9	50.8	50.0
7 years	21.01	20.35	120.6	119.3	51.1	50.2
8 years	23.08	22.43	125.3	124.6	51.4	50.6
9 years	25.33	24.57	130.6	129.5	51.7	50.9
10 years	27.15	27.05	134.4	134.8	51.9	51.3
11 years	30.13	30.51	139.2	140.6	52.3	51.7
12 years	33.05	34.74	144.2	146.6	52.7	52.3
13 years	36.90	38.52	149.8	150.7	53.0	52.8

Data from Bejing Children's Hospital, 1987, Bejing, China.

HEAD CIRCUMFERENCE CHARTS

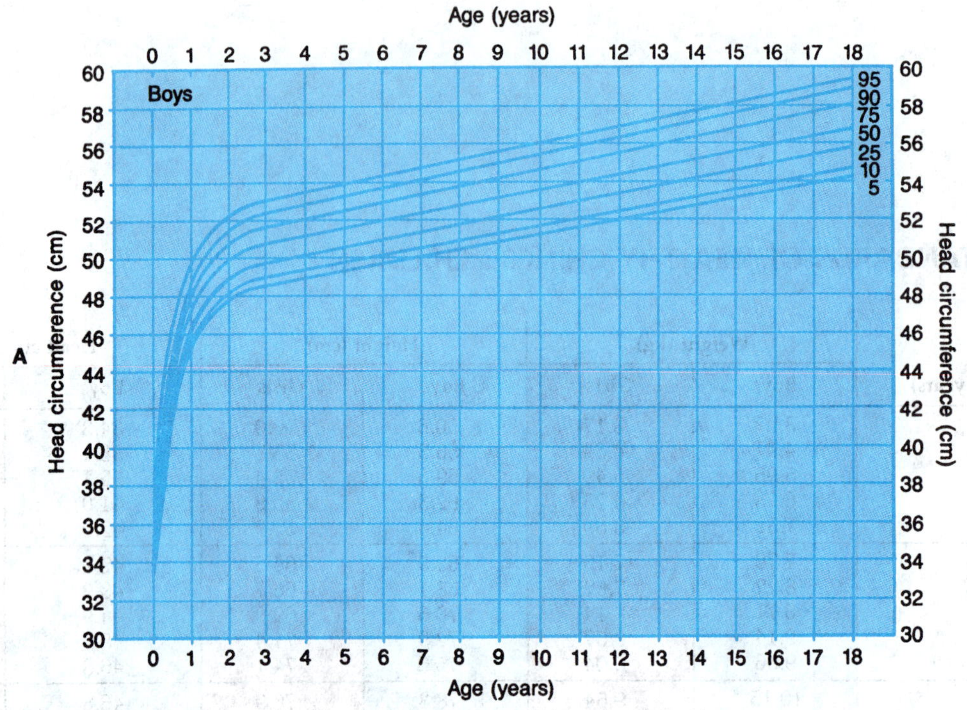

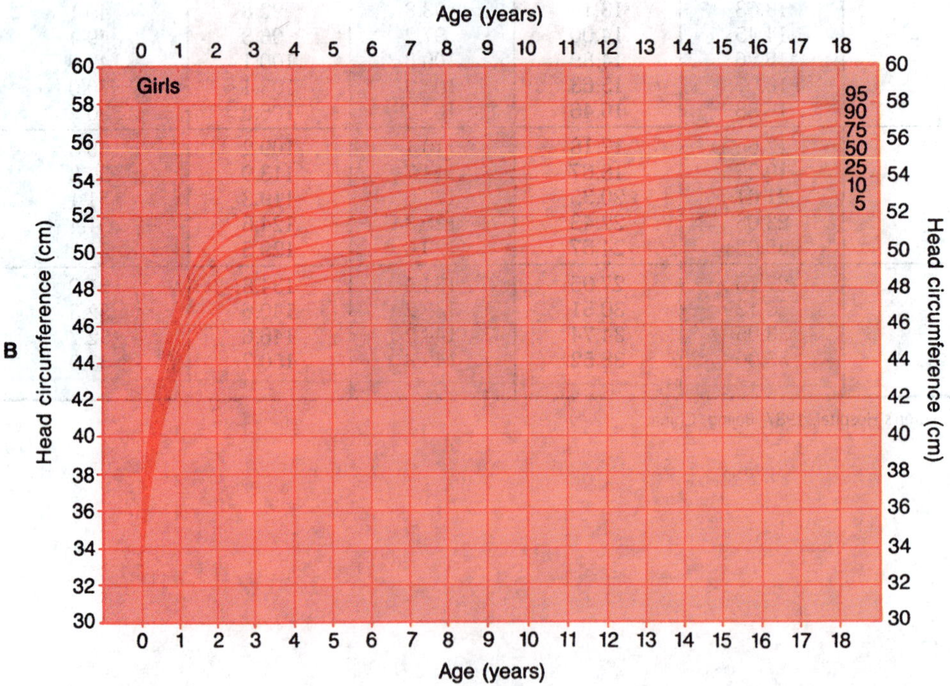

FIG. C-1 Selected percentiles for smoothed head circumference values of children from birth to 18 years. **A,** Boys. **B,** Girls. (From Roche AF and others: Head circumference reference data: birth to 18 years, *Pediatrics* 79(5):706-712, 1987.)

MEASUREMENT OF TRICEPS SKINFOLD THICKNESS

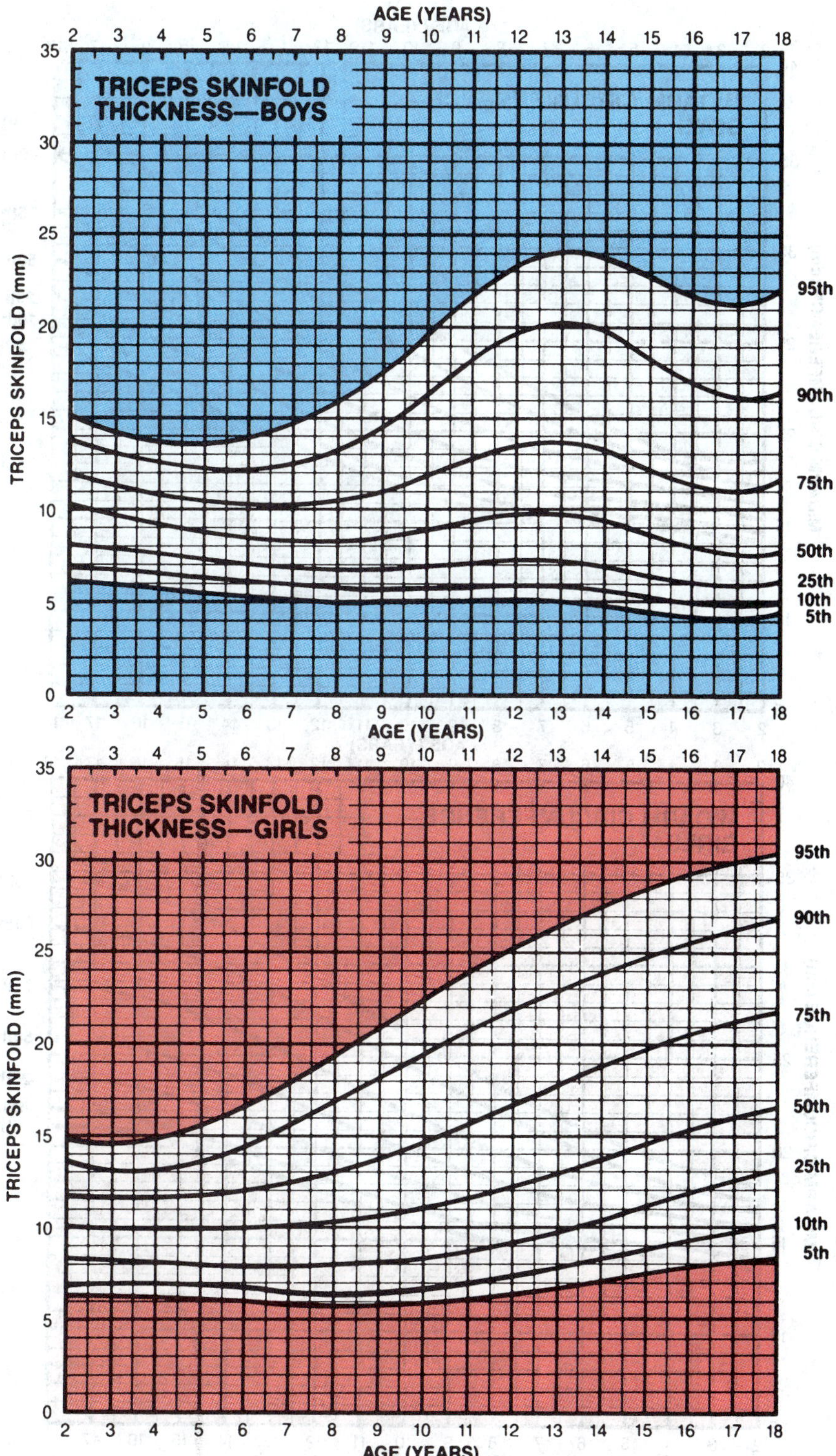

FIG. C-2 Triceps skinfold. (Modified from Johnson CL and others: Basic data on anthropometric measurements and angular measurements of the hip and knee joints for selected age-groups, 1-74 years of age, United States, 1972-1975, Vital and Health Statistics Series 11, No 219. DHHS Publication No (PHS) 81-1669, 1981. Provided as a service of Ross Laboratories, Copyright 1983, Columbus, OH 43216. May be copied for individual patient use.)

MEASUREMENT OF MIDARM CIRCUMFERENCE

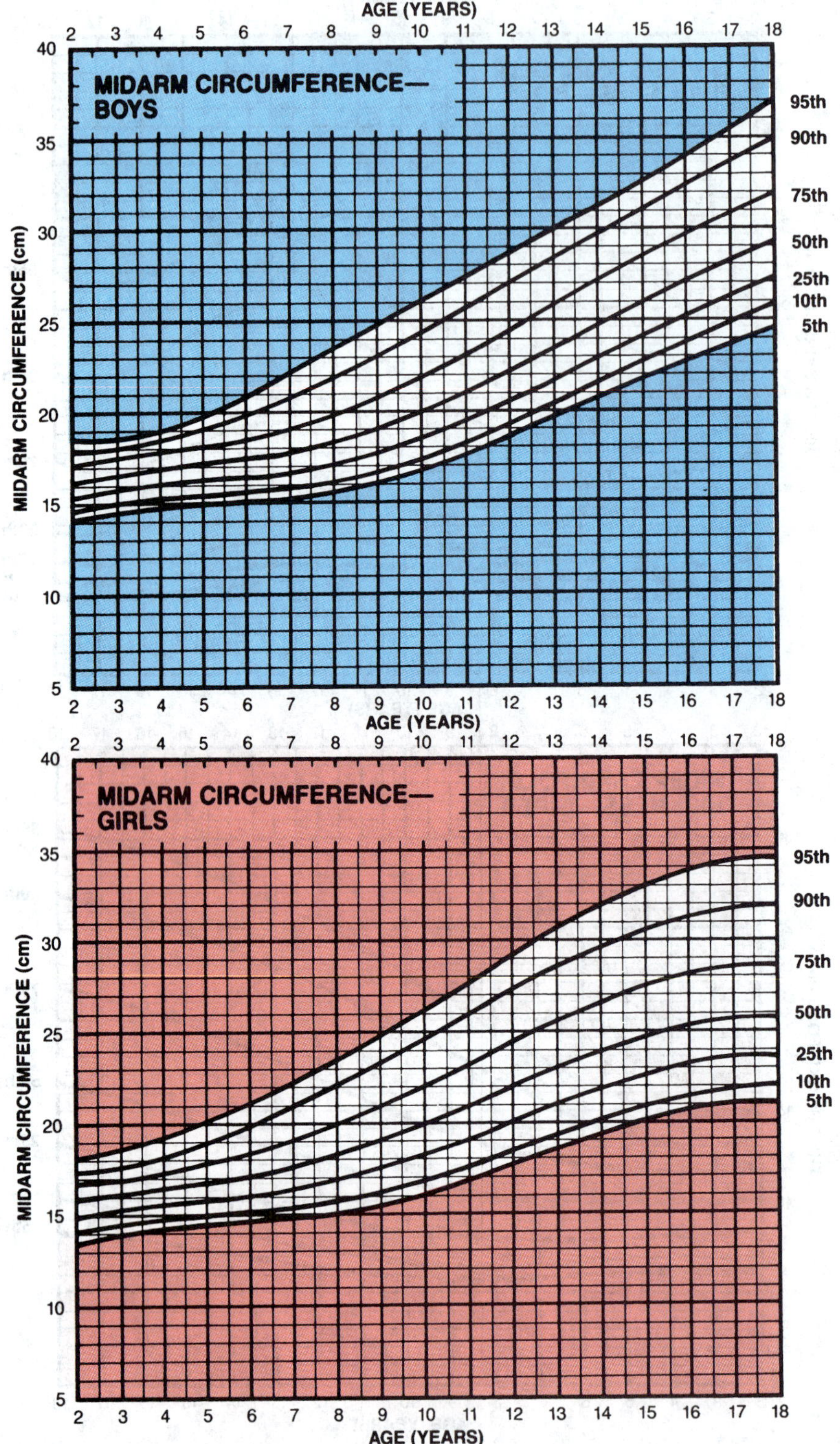

FIG. C-3 Midarm circumference. (Modified from Johnson CL and others: Basic data on anthropometric measurements and angular measurements of the hip and knee joints for selected age-groups, 1-74 years of age, United States, 1972-1975, Vital and Health Statistics Series 11, No 219. DHHS Publication No (PHS) 81-1669, 1981. Provided as a service of Ross Laboratories, Copyright 1983, Columbus, OH 43216. May be copied for individual patient use.)

APPENDIX D

COMMON LABORATORY TESTS*

TEST/SPECIMEN	AGE/SEX/REFERENCE	CONVENTIONAL UNITS (NORMAL RANGES)		INTERNATIONAL UNITS (SI) (NORMAL RANGES)	
Acetaminophen					
Serum or plasma	Therap. conc.	10-30 μg/ml		66-200 μmol/L	
	Toxic Conc.	>200 μg/ml		>1300 μmol/L	
Ammonia nitrogen					
Plasma or serum	Newborn	90-150 μg/dl		64-107 μmol/L	
	0-2 wk	79-129 μg/dl		56-92 μmol/L	
	>1 mo	29-70 μg/dl		21-50 μmol/L	
	Thereafter	15-45 μg/dl		11-32 μmol/L	
Urine, 24 hr		500-1200 mg/d		36-86 mmol/d	
Antistreptolysin O titer (ASO)					
Serum	2-4 yr	<160 Todd units			
	School-age children	170-330 Todd units			
Base excess					
Whole blood	Newborn	(−10)-(−2) mEq/L		(−10)-(−2) mmol/L	
	Infant	(−7)-(−1) mEq/L		(−7)-(−1) mmol/L	
	Child	(−4)-(+2) mEq/L		(−4)-(+2) mmol/L	
	Thereafter	(−3)-(+3) mEq/L		(−3)-(+3) mmol/L	
Bicarbonate (HCO_3)					
Serum	Arterial	21-28 mEq/L		21-28 mmol/L	
	Venous	22-29 mEq/L		22-29 mmol/L	
		Premature (mg/dl)	**Full term (mg/dl)**	**Premature (μmol/L)**	**Full term (μmol/L)**
Bilirubin, total					
Serum	Cord	<2.0	<2.0	<34	<34
	0.1 d	8.0	<6.0	<137	<103
	1-2 d	12.0	<8.0	<205	<137
	2-5 d	16.0	<12.0	<274	<205
	Thereafter	2.0	0.2-1.0	<34	3.4-17.1
Bilirubin, direct (conjugated)					
Serum		0.0-0.2 mg/dl		0-3.4 μmol/L	
Bleeding time					
Blood from skin puncture					
Ivy	Normal	2-7 min		2-7 min	
	Borderline	7-11 min		7-11 min	
Simplate (G-D)		2.75-8 min		2.75-8 min	
Blood volume					
Whole blood	Male	52-83 ml/kg		0.052-0.083 L/kg	
	Female	50-75 ml/kg		0.050-0.075 L/kg	

Modified from Behrman RE and others, editors: *Nelson textbook of pediatrics,* ed 14, Philadelphia, 1992, WB Saunders.

*For a description of abbreviations see p. 1942.

Continued.

Common Laboratory Tests—cont'd

TESTS/SPECIMEN	AGE/SEX/REFERENCE	CONVENTIONAL UNITS	INTERNATIONAL UNITS (SI)
		NORMAL RANGES	
C-reactive protein (CRP)			
Serum	Cord	52-1330 ng/ml	52-1330 µg/L
	Adult	67-1800 ng/ml	67-1800 µg/L
Calcium, ionized			
Serum, plasma, or whole blood	Cord	50-60 mg/dl	1.25-1.50 mmol/L
	Newborn, 3-24 hr	4.3-5.1 mg/dl	1.07-1.27 mmol/L
	24-48 hr	4.0-4.7 mg/dl	1.00-1.17 mmol/L
	Thereafter	4.8-4.92 mg/dl or 2.24-2.46 mEq/L	1.12-1.23 mmol/L
Calcium, total			
Serum	Cord	9.0-11.5 mg/dl	2.25-2.88 mmol/L
	Newborn, 3-24 hr	9.0-10.6 mg/dl	2.3-2.65 mmol/L
	24-48 hr	7.0-12.0 mg/dl	1.75-3.0 mmol/L
	4-7 d	9.0-10.9 mg/dl	2.25-2.73 mmol/L
	Child	8.8-10.8 mg/dl	2.2-2.70 mmol/L
	Thereafter	8.4-10.2 mg/dl	2.1-2.55 mmol/L
Carbon dioxide, partial pressure (Pco_2)			
Whole blood, arterial	Newborn	27-40 mm Hg	3.6-5.3 kPa
	Infant	27-41 mm Hg	3.6-5.5 kPa
	Thereafter: Male	35-48 mm Hg	4.7-6.4 kPa
	Female	32-45 mm Hg	4.3-6.0 kPa
Carbon dioxide, total (tCO_2)			
Serum or plasma	Cord	14-22 mEq/L	14-22 mmol/L
	Premature (1 wk)	14-27 mEq/L	14-27 mmol/L
	Newborn	13-22 mEq/L	13-22 mmol/L
	Infant, child	20-28 mEq/L	20-28 mmol/L
	Thereafter	23-30 mEq/L	23-30 mmol/L
Cerebrospinal fluid (CSF)			
Pressure		70-180 mm water	70-180 mm water
Volume	Child	60-100 ml	0.06-0.10 L
	Adult	100-160 ml	0.1-0.16 L
Chloride			
Serum or plasma	Cord	96-104 mEq/L	96-104 mmol/L
	Newborn	97-110 mEq/L	97-110 mmol/L
	Thereafter	98-106 mEq/L	98-106 mmol/L
Sweat	Normal (homozygote)	<40 mEq/L	<40 mmol/L
	Marginal (e.g., asthma, Addison disease, malnutrition)	45-60 mEq/L	45-60 mmol/L
	Cystic fibrosis	>60 mmol/L	>60 mmol/L
Cholesterol, total			
Serum or plasma*	Acceptable	<170 mg/dl	<4.4 mmol/L
	Borderline	170-199 mg/dl	4.4-5.1 mmol/L
	High	≥200 mg/dl	≥5.2 mmol/L
Clotting time (Lee-White)			
Whole blood		5-8 min (glass tubes)	5-8 min
		5-15 min (room temp)	5-15 min
		30 min (silicone tube)	30 min
Creatine kinase (CK, CPK)			
Serum	Cord blood	70-380 U/L	70-380 U/L
	5-8 hr	214-1175 U/L	214-1175 U/L
	24-33 hr	130-1200 U/L	130-1200 U/L
	72-100 hr	87-725 U/L	87-725 U/L
	Adult	5-130 U/L	5-130 U/L
Creatinine			
Serum	Cord	0.6-1.2 mg/dl	53-106 µmol/L
	Newborn	0.3-1.0 mg/dl	27-88 µmol/L
	Infant	0.2-0.4 mg/dl	18-35 µmol/L
	Child	0.3-0.7 mg/dl	27-62 µmol/L
	Adolescent	0.5-1.0 mg/dl	44-88 µmol/L
	Adult: Male	0.6-1.2 mg/dl	53-106 µmol/L
	Female	0.5-1.1 mg/dl	44-97 µmol/L

*From National Cholesterol Education Program: Report of the expert panel on blood cholesterol levels in children and adolescents, *Pediatrics* 89 (3, pt 2):527, 1992.

Common Laboratory Tests—cont'd			
		CONVENTIONAL UNITS	INTERNATIONAL UNITS (SI)
TEST/SPECIMEN	AGE/SEX/REFERENCE	NORMAL RANGES	
Urine, 24 hr	Premature	8.1-15.0 mg/kg/24 hr	72-133 μmol/kg/24 hr
	Full term	10.4-19.7 mg/kg/24 hr	92-174 μmol/kg/24 hr
	1.5-7 yr	10-15 mg/kg/24 hr	88-133 μmol/kg/24 hr
	7-15 yr	5.2-41 mg/kg/24 hr	46-362 μmol/kg/24 hr
Creatinine clearance (endogenous)			
Serum or plasma and urine	Newborn	40-65 ml/min/1.73 m^2	
	<40 yr: Male	97-137 ml/min/1.73 m^2	
	Female	88-128 ml/min/1.73 m^2	
Digoxin			
Serum, plasma; collect at least 12 hr after dose	Therap. conc.		
	CHF	0.8-1.5 ng/ml	1.0-1.9 nmol/L
	Arrhythmias	1.5-2.0 ng/ml	1.9-2.6 nmol/L
	Toxic conc		
	Child	>2.5 ng/ml	>3.2 nmol/L
	Adult	>3.0 ng/ml	>3.8 nmol/L
Eosinophil count			
Whole blood, capillary blood		50-350 cells/mm^3 (μl)	50-350 × 10^6 cells/L
Erythrocyte (RBC) count			
Whole blood	Cord	3.9-5.5 million/mm^3	3.9-5.5 × 10^{12} cells/L
	1-3 d	4.0-6.6 million/mm^3	4.0-6.6 × 10^{12} cells/L
	1 wk	3.9-6.3 million/mm^3	3.9-6.3 × 10^{12} cells/L
	2 wk	3.6-6.2 million/mm^3	3.6-6.2 × 10^{12} cells/L
	1 mo	3.0-5.4 million/mm^3	3.0-5.4 × 10^{12} cells/L
	2 mo	2.7-4.9 million/mm^3	2.7-4.5 × 10^{12} cells/L
	3-6 mo	3.1-4.5 million/mm^3	3.1-4.5 × 10^{12} cells/L
	0.5-2 yr	3.7-5.3 million/mm^3	3.7-5.3 × 10^{12} cells/L
	2-6 yr	3.9-5.3 million/mm^3	3.9-5.3 × 10^{12} cells/L
	6-12 yr	4.0-5.2 million/mm^3	4.0-5.2 × 10^{12} cells/L
	12-18 yr: Male	4.5-5.3 million/mm^3	4.5-5.3 × 10^{12} cells/L
	Female	4.1-5.1 million/mm^3	4.1-5.1 × 10^{12} cells/L
Erythrocyte sedimentation rate (ESR)			
Whole blood			
Westergren (modified)	Child	0-10 mm/hr	0-10 mm/hr
	<50 yr: Male	0-15 mm/hr	0-15 mm/hr
	Female	0-20 mm/hr	0-20 mm/hr
Wintrobe	Child	0-13 mm/hr	0-13 mm/hr
	Adult: Male	0-9 mm/hr	0-9 mm/hr
	Female	0-20 mm/hr	0-20 mm/hr
Fibrinogen			
Plasma	Newborn	125-300 mg/dl	1.25-3.00 g/L
	Thereafter	200-400 mg/dl	2.00-4.00 g/L
Galactose			
Serum	Newborn	0-20 mg/dl	0-1.11 mmol/L
	Thereafter	<5 mg/dl	<0.03 mmol/L
Urine	Newborn	≤60 mg/dl	≤3.33 mmol/L
	Thereafter	<14 mg/dl	<0.08 mmol/d
Glucose			
Serum	Cord	45-96 mg/dl	2.5-5.3 mmol/L
	Newborn, 1 d	40-60 mg/dl	2.2-3.3 mmol/L
	Newborn, >1 d	50-90 mg/dl	2.8-5.0 mmol/L
	Child	60-100 mg/dl	3.3-5.5 mmol/L
	Thereafter	70-105 mg/dl	3.9-5.8 mmol/L
Whole blood	Adult	65-95 mg/dl	3.6-5.3 mmol/L
CSF	Adult	40-70 mg/dl	2.2-3.9 mmol/L

Continued.

Common Laboratory Tests—cont'd

TEST/SPECIMEN	AGE/SEX/REFERENCE	CONVENTIONAL UNITS NORMAL RANGES		INTERNATIONAL UNITS (SI) NORMAL RANGES	
Urine (quantitative)		<0.5 g/d		<2.8 mmol/d	
(Qualitative)		Negative		Negative	
Glucose tolerance test (GTT), oral					
Serum					
Dosages		**Normal**	**Diabetic**	**Normal**	**Diabetic**
Adult: 75 g	Fasting	70-105 mg/dl	>115 mg/dl	3.9-5.8 mmol/L	>6.4 mmol/L
Child: 1.75 g/kg of ideal weight up to maximum of 75 g	60 min	120-170 mg/dl	≥200 mg/dl	6.7-9.4 mmol/L	≥11 mmol/L
	90 min	100-140 mg/dl	≥200 mg/dl	5.6-7.8 mmol/L	≥11 mmol/L
	120 min	70-120 mg/dl	≥140 mg/dl	3.9-6.7 mmol/L	≥7.8 mmol/L
Growth hormone (hGH, somatotropin)					
Plasma	Cord	10-50 ng/ml		10-50 μg/L	
Fasting, at rest	Newborn	10-40 ng/ml		10-40 μg/L	
	Child	<5 ng/ml		<5 μg/L	
	Adult: Male	<5 ng/ml		<5 μg/L	
	Female	<8 ng/ml		<8 μg/L	
Hematocrit (HCT, Hct)					
Whole blood	1 d (cap)	48%-69%		0.48-0.69 vol. fraction	
	2 d	48%-75%		0.48-0.75 vol. fraction	
	3 d	44%-72%		0.44-0.72 vol. fraction	
	2 mo	28%-42%		0.28-0.42 vol. fraction	
	6-12 yr	35%-45%		0.35-0.45 vol. fraction	
	12-18 yr: Male	37%-49%		0.37-0.49 vol. fraction	
	Female	36%-46%		0.36-0.46 vol. fraction	
Hemoglobin (Hb)					
Whole blood	1-3 d (cap)	14.5-22.5 g/dl		2.25-3.49 mmol/L	
	2 mo	9.0-14.0 g/dl		1.40-2.17 mmol/L	
	6-12 yr	11.5-15.5 g/dl		1.78-2.40 mmol/L	
	12-18 yr: Male	13.0-16.0 g/dl		2.02-2.48 mmol/L	
	Female	12.0-16.0 g/dl		1.86-2.48 mmol/L	
Hemoglobin A					
Whole blood		>95% of total		0.95 fraction of Hb	
Hemoglobin F					
Whole blood	1 d	63%-92% HbF		0.62-0.92 mass fraction HbF	
	5 d	65%-88% HbF		0.65-0.88 mass fraction HbF	
	3 wk	55%-85% HbF		0.55-0.85 mass fraction HbF	
	6-9 wk	31%-75% HbF		0.31-0.75 mass fraction HbF	
	3-4 mo	<2%-59% HbF		<0.02-0.59 mass fraction HbF	
	6 mo	<2%-9% HbF		<0.02-0.09 mass fraction HbF	
	Adult	<2.0% HbF		<0.02 mass fraction HbF	
Immunoglobulin A (IgA)					
Serum	Cord blood	1.4-3.6 mg/dl		14-36 mg/L	
	1-3 mo	1.3-53 mg/dl		13-530 mg/L	
	4-6 mo	4.4-84 mg/dl		44-840 mg/L	
	7 mo-1 yr	11-106 mg/dl		110-1060 mg/L	
	2-5 yr	14-159 mg/dl		140-1590 mg/L	
	6-10 yr	33-236 mg/dl		330-2360 mg/L	
	Adult	70-312 mg/dl		700-3130 mg/L	
Immunoglobulin D (IgD)					
Serum	Newborn	None detected		None detected	
	Thereafter	0-8 mg/dl		0-80 mg/L	

Common Laboratory Tests—cont'd

TEST/SPECIMEN	AGE/SEX/REFERENCE	CONVENTIONAL UNITS (NORMAL RANGES)	INTERNATIONAL UNITS (SI) (NORMAL RANGES)
Immunoglobulin E (IgE)			
Serum	M	0-230 IU/ml	0-230 kIU/L
	F	0-170 IU/ml	0-170 kIU/L
Immunoglobulin G (IgG)			
Serum	Cord blood	636-1606 mg/dl	6.36-16.06 g/L
	1 mo	251-906 mg/dl	2.51-9.06 g/L
	2-4 mo	176-601 mg/dl	1.76-6.01 g/L
	5-12 mo	172-1069 mg/dl	1.72-10.69 g/L
	1-5 yr	345-1236 mg/dl	3.45-12.36 g/L
	6-10 yr	608-1572 mg/dl	6.08-15.72 g/L
	Adult	639-1349 mg/dl	6.39-13.49 g/L
Immunoglobulin M (IgM)			
Serum	Cord blood	6.3-25 mg/dl	63-250 mg/L
	1 mo-4 mo	17-105 mg/dl	170-1050 mg/L
	5 mo-9 mo	33-126 mg/dl	330-1260 mg/L
	10 mo-1 yr	41-173 mg/dl	410-1730 mg/L
	2-8 yr	43-207 mg/dl	430-2070 mg/L
	9-10 yr	52-242 mg/dl	520-2420 mg/L
	Adult	56-352 mg/dl	560-3520 mg/L
Iron			
Serum	Newborn	100-250 μg/dl	17.90-44.75 μmol/L
	Infant	40-100 μg/dl	7.16-1790 μmol/L
	Child	50-120 μg/dl	8.95-21.48 μmol/L
	Thereafter: Male	50-160 μg/dl	8.95-28.64 μmol/L
	Female	40-150 μg/dl	7.16-26.85 μmol/L
	Intoxicated child	280-2550 μg/dl	50.12-456.5 μmol/L
	Fatally poisoned child	>1800 μg/dl	>322.2 μmol/L
Iron-binding capacity, total (TIBC)			
Serum	Infant	100-400 μg/dl	17.90-71.60 μmol/L
	Thereafter	250-400 μg/dl	44.75-71.60 μmol/L
Lead			
Whole blood	Child	<10 μg/dl	<0.48 μmol/L
Urine, 24 hr		<80 μg/L	<0.39 μmol/L
Leukocyte count (WBC count)		**× 1000 cells/mm³ (μl)**	**× 10⁹ cells/L**
Whole blood	Birth	9.0-30.0	9.0-30.0
	24 hr	9.4-34.0	9.4-34.0
	1 mo	5.0-19.5	5.0-19.5
	1-3 yr	6.0-17.5	6.0-17.5
	4-7 yr	5.5-15.5	5.5-15.5
	8-13 yr	4.5-13.5	4.5-13.5
	Adult	4.5-11.0	4.5-11.0
		× 1000 cells/mm³ (μl)	**× 10⁶ cells/L**
CSF	Premature	0-25 mononuclear	0-25
		0-100 polymorphonuclear	1-100
		0-1000 RBC	0-1000
	Newborn	0-20 mononuclear	0-20
		0-70 polymorphonuclear	0-70
		0-800 RBC	0-800
	Neonate	0-5 mononuclear	0-5
		0-25 polymorphonuclear	0-25
		0-50 RBC	0-50
	Thereafter	0-5 mononuclear	0-5

Continued.

Common Laboratory Tests—cont'd

TEST/SPECIMEN	AGE/SEX/REFERENCE	CONVENTIONAL UNITS		INTERNATIONAL UNITS (SI)
		NORMAL RANGES		
Leukocyte differential count				
Whole blood	Myelocytes	0%	0 cells/mm^3 (µl)	Number fraction 0
	Neutrophils—"bands"	3%-5%	150-400 cells/ mm^3 (µl)	Number fraction 0.03-0.05
	Neutrophils—"segs"	54%-62%	3000-5800 cells/ mm^3 (µl)	Number fraction 0.54-0.62
	Lymphocytes	25%-33%	1500-3000 cells/ mm^3 (µl)	Number fraction 0.25-0.33
	Monocytes	3%-7%	285-500 cells/ mm^3 (µl)	Number fraction 0.03-0.07
	Eosinophils	1%-3%	50-250 cells/ mm^3 (µl)	Number fraction 0.01-0.03
	Basophils	0%-0.75%	15-50 cells/ mm^3 (µl)	Number fraction 0-0.0075
Mean corpuscular hemoglobin (MCH)				
Whole blood	Birth	31-37 pg/cell		0.48-0.57 fmol/L
	1-3 d (cap)	31-37 pg/cell		0.48-0.57 fmol/L
	1 wk-1 mo	28-40 pg/cell		0.43-0.62 fmol/L
	2 mo	26-34 pg/cell		0.40-0.53 fmol/L
	3-6 mo	25-35 pg/cell		0.39-0.54 fmol/L
	0.5-2 yr	23-31 pg/cell		0.36-0.48 fmol/L
	2-6 yr	24-30 pg/cell		0.37-0.47 fmol/L
	6-12 yr	25-33 pg/cell		0.39-0.51 fmol/L
	12-18 yr	25-35 pg/cell		0.39-0.54 fmol/L
	18-49 yr	26-34 pg/cell		0.40-0.53 fmol/L
Mean corpuscular hemoglobin concentration (MCHC)				
Whole blood	Birth	30%-36% Hb/cell or g Hb/dl RBC		4.65-5.58 mmol or Hb/L RBC
	1-3 d (cap)	29%-37% Hb/cell or g Hb/dl RBC		4.50-5.74 mmol or Hb/L RBC
	1-2 wk	28%-38% Hb/cell or g Hb/dl RBC		4.34-5.89 mmol or Hb/L RBC
	1-2 mo	29%-37% Hb/cell or g Hb/dl RBC		4.50-5.74 mmol or Hb/L RBC
	3 mo-2 yr	30%-36% Hb/cell or g Hb/dl RBC		4.65-5.58 mmol or Hb/L RBC
	2-18 yr	31%-37% Hb/cell or g Hb/dl RBC		4.81-5.74 mmol or Hb/L RBC
	>18 yr	31%-37% Hb/cell or g Hb/dl RBC		4.81-5.74 mmol or Hb/L RBC
Mean corpuscular volume (MCV)				
Whole blood	1-3 d (cap)	95-121 µm^3		95-121 fl
	0.5-2 yr	70-86 µm^3		70-86 fl
	6-12 yr	77-95 µm^3		77-95 fl
	12-18 yr: Male	78-98 µm^3		78-98 fl
	Female	78-102 µm^3		78-102 fl
Osmolality				
Serum	Child, adult:	275-295 mOsmol/kg H_2O		
Urine, random		50-1400 mOsmol/kg H_2O, depending on fluid intake; after 12 hr fluid restriction: >850 mOsmol/kg H_2O		
Urine, 24 hr		≃300-900 mOsmol/kg H_2O		
Oxygen, partial pressure (Po_2)				
Whole blood, arterial	Birth	8-24 mm Hg		1.1-3.2 kPa
	5-10 min	33-75 mm Hg		4.4-10.0 kPa
	30 min	31-85 mm Hg		4.1-11.3 kPa
	>1 hr	55-80 mm Hg		7.3-10.6 kPa
	1 d	54-95 mm Hg		7.2-12.6 kPa
	Thereafter (decreased with age)	83-108 mm Hg		11-14.4 kPa

Common Laboratory Tests—cont'd

TEST/SPECIMEN	AGE/SEX/REFERENCE	CONVENTIONAL UNITS (NORMAL RANGES)	INTERNATIONAL UNITS (SI) (NORMAL RANGES)
Oxygen saturation (Sao_2)			
Whole blood, arterial	Newborn	85%-90%	Fraction saturated 0.85-0.90
	Thereafter	95%-99%	Fraction saturated 0.95-0.99
Partial thromboplastin time (PTT)			
Whole blood (Na citrate)			
Nonactivated		60-85 s (Platelin)	60-85 s
Activated		25-35 s (differs with method)	25-35 s
pH			H^+ concentration:
Whole blood, arterial	Premature (48 hr)	7.35-7.50	31-44 nmol/L
	Birth, full term	7.11-7.36	43-77 nmol/L
	5-10 min	7.09-7.30	50-81 nmol/L
	30 min	7.21-7.38	41-61 nmol/L
	>1 hr	7.26-7.49	32-54 nmol/L
	1 d	7.29-7.45	35-51 nmol/L
	Thereafter	7.35-7.45	35-44 nmol/L
	Must be corrected for body temperature		
Urine, random	Newborn/neonate	5-7	0.1-10 μmol/L
	Thereafter (average ≈6)	4.5-8	0.01-32 μmol/L (average ≈1.0 μmol/L)
Stool		7.0-7.5	31-100 nmol/L
Phenylalanine			
Serum	Premature	2.0-7.5 mg/dl	120-450 μmol/L
	Newborn	1.2-3.4 mg/dl	70-210 μmol/L
	Thereafter	0.8-1.8 mg/dl	50-110 μmol/L
Urine, 24 hr	10 d-2 wk	1-2 mg/d	6-12 μmol/d
	3-12 yr	4-18 mg/d	24-110 μmol/d
	Thereafter	trace-17 mg/d	trace-103 μmol/d
Plasma volume			
Plasma	Male	25-43 ml/kg	0.025-0.043 L/kg
	Female	28-45 ml/kg	0.028-0.045 L/kg
Platelet count (thrombocyte count)			
Whole blood (EDTA)	Newborn (After 1 wk, same as adult)	84-478 × 10^3/mm^3 (μl)	84-478 × 10^9/L
	Adult	150-400 × 10^3/mm^3 (μl)	150-400 × 10^9/L
Potassium			
Serum	Newborn	3.0-6.0 mEq/L	3.0-6.0 mmol/L
	Thereafter	3.5-5.0 mEq/L	3.5-5.0 mmol/L
Plasma (heparin)		3.4-4.5 mEq/L	3.4-4.5 mmol/L
Urine, 24 hr		2.5-125 mEq/d varies with diet	2.5-125 mmol/L
Protein			
Serum, total	Premature	4.3-7.6 g/dl	43-76 g/L
	Newborn	4.6-7.4 g/dl	46-74 g/L
	1-7 yr	6.1-7.9 g/dl	61-79 g/L
	8-12 yr	6.4-8.1 g/dl	64-81 g/L
	13-19 yr	6.6-8.2 g/dl	66-82 g/L
Total			
Urine, 24 hr		1-14 mg/dl	10-140 mg/L
		50-80 mg/d (at rest)	50-80 mg/d
		<250 mg/d after intense exercise	<250 mg/d after exercise
Total			
CSF		Lumbar: 8-32 mg/dl	80-320 mg/L

Continued.

Common Laboratory Tests—cont'd

TEST/SPECIMEN	AGE/SEX/REFERENCE	CONVENTIONAL UNITS	INTERNATIONAL UNITS (SI)
		NORMAL RANGES	
Prothrombin time (PT)			
One-stage (Quick)			
Whole blood (Na citrate)	In general	11-15 s (varies with type of thromboplastin)	11-15 s
	Newborn	Prolonged by 2-3 sec	Prolonged by 2-3 sec
Two-stage modified (Ware and Seegers)			
Whole blood (Na citrate)		18-22 sec	18-22 sec
RBC count, see erythrocyte count			
Red blood cell volume			
Whole blood	Male	20-36 ml/kg	0.020-0.036 L/kg
	Female	19-31 ml/kg	0.019-0.031 L/kg
Reticulocyte count			
Whole blood	Adults	0.5%-1.5% of erythrocytes or 25,000-75,000/mm^3 (µl)	0.005-0.015 (number fraction) 25,000-75,000 × 10^6/L
Capillary	1 d	0.4%-6.0%	0.004-0.060 (number fraction)
	7 d	<0.1%-1.3%	<0.001-0.013 (number fraction)
	1-4 wk	<0.1%-1.2%	<0.001-0.012 (number fraction)
	5-6 wk	<0.1%-2.4%	<0.001-0.024 (number fraction)
	7-8 wk	0.1%-2.9%	0.001-0.029 (number fraction)
	9-10 wk	<0.1%-2.6%	<0.001-.026 (number fraction)
	11-12 wk	0.1%-1.3%	0.001-0.013 (number fraction)
Salicylates			
Serum, plasma	Therap. conc.	15-30 mg/dl	1.1-2.2 mmol/L
	Toxic conc.	>30 mg/dl	>2.2 mmol/L
Sedimentation rate: see erythrocyte sedimentation rate			
Sodium			
Serum or plasma	Newborn	136-146 mEq/L	134-146 mmol/L
	Infant	139-146 mEq/L	139-146 mmol/L
	Child	138-145 mEq/L	138-145 mmol/L
	Thereafter	136-146 mEq/L	136-146 mmol/L
Urine, 24 hr		40-220 mEq/L (diet dependent)	40-220 mmol/L
Sweat	Normal	<40 mEq/L	<40 mmol/L
	Indeterminate	45-60 mEq/L	45-60 mmol/L
	Cystic fibrosis	>60 mEq/L	>60 mmol/L
Specific gravity			
Urine, random	Adult	1.002-1.030	1.002-1.030
	After 12 hr fluid restriction	>1.025	>1.025
Urine, 24 hr		1.015-1.025	
Theophylline			
Serum, plasma	Therap. conc.		
	Bronchodilator	10-20 µg/ml	56-110 µmol/L
	Premature apnea	6-10 µg/ml	28-56 µmol/L
	Toxic conc.	>20	>166 µmol/L
Thrombin time			
Whole blood (Na citrate)		Control time ± 2 sec when control is 9-13 sec	Control time ± 2 sec when control is 9-13 sec

Common Laboratory Tests—cont'd

TEST/SPECIMEN	AGE/SEX/REFERENCE	CONVENTIONAL UNITS (NORMAL RANGES)		INTERNATIONAL UNITS (SI) (NORMAL RANGES)	
Thyroxine, total (T_3)					
Serum	Cord	8-13 μg/dl		103-168 nmol/L	
	Newborn	11.5-24 (lower in low-birth-weight infants)		148-310 nmol/L	
	Neonate	9-18 μg/dl		116-232 nmol/L	
	Infant	7-15 μg/dl		90-194 nmol/L	
	1-5 yr	7.3-15 μg/dl		94-194 nmol/L	
	5-10 yr	6.4-13.3 μg/dl		83-172 nmol/L	
	Thereafter	5-12 μg/dl		65-155 nmol/L	
	Newborn screen (filter paper)	6.2-22 μg/dl		80-284 nmol/L	
Tourniquet test (capillary fragility)		<5-10 petechiae in 2.5 cm circle on forearm (halfway between systolic and diastolic); pressure for 5 min; 0-8 petechiae in 6 cm circle (50 torr for 15 min); 10-20 petechiae in 5 cm circle (80 mm Hg)		<5-10 petechiae in 2.5 cm circle on forearm (halfway between systolic and diastolic); pressure for 5 min; 0-8 petechiae in 6 cm circle (50 torr for 15 min); 10-20 petechiae in 5 cm circle (80 mm Hg)	
Triglycerides (TG)					
Serum, after ≥12 hr fast		mg/dl		g/L	
		M	F	M	F
	Cord blood	10-98	10-98	0.10-0.98	0.10-0.98
	0-5 yr	30-86	32-99	0.30-0.86	0.32-0.99
	6-11 yr	31-108	35-114	0.31-1.08	0.35-1.14
	12-15 yr	36-138	41-138	0.36-1.38	0.41-1.38
	16-19 yr	40-163	40-128	0.40-1.63	0.40-1.28
Triiodothyronine, free					
Serum	Cord	20-240 pg/dl		0.3-3.7 pmol/L	
	1-3 d	200-610 pg/dl		3.1-9.4 pmol/L	
	6 wk	240-560 pg/dl		3.7-8.6 pmol/L	
	Adults (20-50 yr)	230-660 pg/dl		3.5-10.0 pmol/L	
Triiodothyronine, total (T_3-RIA)					
Serum	Cord	30-70 ng/dl		0.46-1.08 nmol/L	
	Newborn	72-260 ng/dl		1.16-4.00 nmol/L	
	1-5 yr	100-260 ng/dl		1.54-4.00 nmol/L	
	5-10 yr	90-240 ng/dl		1.39-3.70 nmol/L	
	10-15 yr	80-210 ng/dl		1.23-3.23 nmol/L	
	Thereafter	115-190 ng/dl		1.77-2.93 nmol/L	
Urea nitrogen					
Serum or plasma	Cord	21-40 mg/dl		7.5-14.3 mmol urea/L	
	Premature (1 wk)	3-25 mg/dl		1.1-9 mmol urea/L	
	Newborn	3-12 mg/dl		1.1-4.3 mmol urea/L	
	Infant/child	5-18 mg/dl		1.8-6.4 mmol urea/L	
	Thereafter	7-18 mg/dl		2.5-6.4 mmol urea/L	
Urine volume					
Urine, 24 hr	Newborn	50-300 ml/d		0.050-0.300 L/d	
	Infant	350-550 ml/d		0.350-0.500 L/d	
	Child	500-1000 ml/d		0.500-1.000 L/d	
	Adolescent	700-1400 ml/d		0.700-1.400 L/d	
	Thereafter: Male	800-1800 ml/d		0.800-1.800 L/d	
	Female	600-1600 ml/d (varies with intake and other factors)		0.600-1.600 L/d	
WBC, see leukocyte					

ABBREVIATIONS USED IN LABORATORY TESTS

Abbreviation	Term
cap	capillary
CHF	congestive heart failure
conc.	concentration
CSF	cerebrospinal fluid
d	day; diem
EDTA	ethylenediaminetetraacetate
g	gram
m	meter
hr	hour
L, l	liter
mEq	milliequivalent
min	minute
mm	millimeter
mm^3	cubic millimeter
mo	month
mol	mole
mOsmol	milliosmole
s	second
SI	international system of units
Therap.	therapeutic
U	international unit of enzyme activity
vol	volume
wk	week
yr	year
$>$	greater than
$\geq$	greater than or equal to
$<$	less than
$\leq$	less than or equal to
$\pm$	plus/minus
$\simeq$	approximately equal to

PREFIXES DENOTING DECIMAL FACTORS

Prefix	Symbol	Amount
deci	d	one tenth (10^{-1})
centi	c	one hundredth (10^{-2})
milli	m	one thousandth (10^{-3})
micro	μ	one millionth (10^{-6})
nano	n	one billionth (10^{-9})
pico	p	one trillionth (10^{-12})
femto	f	one quadrillionth (10^{-15})

APPENDIX E

NANDA-APPROVED NURSING DIAGNOSES

Activity intolerance
Activity intolerance, high risk for
Adjustment, impaired
Airway clearance, ineffective
Anxiety
Aspiration, high risk for
Body image disturbance
Body temperature, altered, high risk for
Breast-feeding, effective
Breast-feeding, ineffective
Breast-feeding, interrupted
Breathing pattern, ineffective
Cardiac output, decreased
Caregiver role strain
Caregiver role strain, high risk for
Communication, impaired verbal
Constipation
Constipation, colonic
Constipation, perceived
Coping, defensive
Coping, family: potential for growth
Coping, ineffective family: compromised
Coping, ineffective family: disabling
Coping, ineffective individual
Decisional conflict (specify)
Denial, ineffective
Diarrhea
Disuse syndrome, high risk for
Diversional activity deficit
Dysreflexia
Family processes, altered
Fatigue
Fear
Fluid volume deficit (1)
Fluid volume deficit (2)
Fluid volume deficit, high risk for
Fluid volume excess
Gas exchange, impaired
Grieving, anticipatory
Grieving, dysfunctional
Growth and development, altered
Health maintenance, altered
Health-seeking behaviors (specify)
Home maintenance management, impaired
Hopelessness
Hyperthermia
Hypothermia
Incontinence, bowel
Incontinence, functional
Incontinence, reflex
Incontinence, stress
Incontinence, total
Incontinence, urge
Infant feeding pattern, ineffective
Infection, high risk for
Injury, high risk for
Knowledge deficit (specify)
Mobility, impaired physical
Noncompliance (specify)
Nutrition, altered: less than body requirements
Nutrition, altered: more than body requirements
Nutrition, altered: high risk for more than body requirements
Oral mucous membrane, altered
Pain
Pain, chronic
Parental role conflict
Parenting, altered
Parenting, altered, high risk for
Peripheral neurovascular dysfunction, high risk for
Personal identity disturbance
Poisoning, high risk for
Post-trauma response
Powerlessness
Protection, altered
Rape-trauma syndrome
Rape-trauma syndrome: compound reaction
Rape-trauma syndrome: silent reaction
Role performance, altered
Self-care deficit, bathing/hygiene
Self-care deficit, dressing/grooming
Self-care deficit, feeding
Self-care deficit, toileting
Self-esteem, chronic low
Self-esteem, situational low
Self-esteem disturbance
Self-mutilation, high risk for
Sensory/perceptual alterations (specify) (visual, auditory, kinesthetic, gustatory, tactile, olfactory)
Sexual dysfunction
Sexuality patterns, altered
Skin integrity, impaired
Skin integrity, impaired, high risk for
Sleep pattern disturbance
Social interaction, impaired
Social isolation
Spiritual distress (distress of the human spirit)
Stress syndrome, relocation
Suffocation, high risk for
Swallowing, impaired
Therapeutic regimen (individual), ineffective management of
Thermoregulation, ineffective
Thought processes, altered
Tissue integrity, impaired
Tissue perfusion, altered (specify type) (renal, cerebral, cardiopulmonary, gastrointestinal, peripheral)
Trauma, high risk for
Unilateral neglect
Urinary elimination, altered patterns
Urinary retention
Ventilation, spontaneous, inability to sustain
Ventilatory weaning response, dysfunctional
Violence, high risk for: self-directed or directed at others

APPENDIX F

TRANSLATIONS OF FACES PAIN RATING SCALE

Explain to the person that each face is for a person who feels happy because he has no pain (hurt) or sad because he has some or a lot of pain. **Face 0** is very happy because he doesn't hurt at all. **Face 1** hurts just a little bit. **Face 2** hurts a little more. **Face 3** hurts even more. **Face 4** hurts a whole lot. **Face 5** hurts as much as you can imagine, although you don't have to be crying to feel this bad. Ask the person to choose the face that best describes how he is feeling.

Rating scale is recommended for persons age 3 years and older.

Spanish. Expliquele a la persona que cada cara representa una persona que se siente feliz porque no tiene dolor o, triste porque siente un poco o mucho dolor. **Cara 0** se siente muy feliz porque no tiene dolor. **Cara 1** tiene un poco de dolor. **Cara 2** tiene un poquito más de dolor. **Cara 3** tiene todavia más dolor. **Cara 4** tiene mucho dolor. **Cara 5** tiene el dolor máximo aunque ni siempre causa el lloro. Pidale a la persona cual de las caras mejor describe su próprio dolor.

Esta escala se puede usar con personas de tres años de edad o más.

French. Expliquez à la personne que chaque visage représent un personne qui est heureux parce qu'elle n'a pas point du mal ou triste parce qu'il a un peu ou beaucoup du mal. **Visage 0** est très heureux parce qu'elle n'a pas point du mal. **Visage 1** a un petit peu du mal. **Visage 2** a plus du mal. **Visage 3** a encore plus du mal. **Visage 4** a beaucoup du mal. **Visage 5** a autant mal que vous pouvez imaginer, bien que ces mauvais sentiments ne finissent pas nécessairement a vous faire pleurer. Demandez à la personne de choisir le visage qui convient le mieux avec ses sentiments.

Ces evaluations sont recommendés pour des personnes de trois ans et davantage.

Italian. Spiegare a la persona che ogni faccia è per una persona che si sente felice perchè non tiene dolore oppure triste perchè ha poco o molto dolore. **Faccia 0** è molto felice perchè non tiene dolore. **Faccia 1** tiene poco dolore. **Faccia 2** tiene un po più di dolore. **Faccia 3** tiene più dolore. **Faccia 4** tiene molto dolore. **Faccia 5** tiene molto dolore che non puoi immaginare però non devi piangere per tenere dolore. Domandi a la persona di scegliere quale faccia meglio descrive come si sente.

Grado scala è raccomandata a la persona di tre anni in sù.

Portuguese. Explique a pessoa que cada face representa uma pessoa que está feliz porque não têm dor, ou triste por ter um pouco ou muita dor. **Face 0** está muito feliz porque não têm nenhuma dor. **Face 1** tem apenas um pouco de dor. **Face 2** têm um pouco mais de dor. **Face 3** têm ainda mais dor. **Face 4** têm muita dor. **Face 5** têm uma dor máxima, apesar de que nem sempre provoca o choro. Peça a pessoa que escolhe a face que melhor descreve como ele se sente.

Esta escala é aplicável a pessoas de tres anos de idade ou mais.

Wong-Baker FACES Pain Rating Scale: Available at no charge from The Purdue Frederick Company, 100 Connecticut Ave., Norwalk, CT 06850-3590; (203) 853-0123, ext. 4010. Spanish and Portuguese translations by Ellen Johnsen; French translation by Irene Sherman Liguori and Robert Marino; Italian translation by Madeline Mitchko and Ida DiPietropaolo.

INDEX

B

C

F

H

I

N

T

Normal Temperatures in Children

AGE	TEMPERATURE °F	°C
3 months	99.4	37.5
6 months	99.5	37.5
1 year	99.7	37.7
3 years	99.0	37.2
5 years	98.6	37.0
7 years	98.3	36.8
9 years	98.1	36.7
11 years	98.0	36.7
13 years	97.8	36.6

Modified from Lowrey GH: *Growth and development of children,* ed 8, St Louis, 1986, Mosby.

Centigrade to Farenheit Temperature Conversions

°C	°F	°C	°F	°C	°F
35.0	**95.0**	**37.0**	**98.6**	**39.0**	**102.2**
35.2	95.4	37.2	99.0	39.2	102.6
35.4	95.7	37.4	99.3	39.4	102.9
35.6	96.1	37.6	99.7	39.6	103.3
35.8	96.4	37.8	100.0	39.8	103.6
36.0	**96.8**	**38.0**	**100.4**	**40.0**	**104.0**
36.2	97.2	38.2	100.8	40.2	104.4
36.4	97.5	38.4	101.1	40.4	104.7
36.6	97.9	38.6	101.5	40.6	105.1
36.8	98.2	38.8	101.8	40.8	105.4
				41.0	**105.8**

CONVERSION FORMULAS:
°F = (°C x ⁹⁄₅) + 32 or (°C x 1.8) + 32
°C = (°F – 32) x ⁵⁄₉ or (°F – 32) x 0.55

Normal Blood Pressure Readings for Children
GIRLS

SYSTOLIC BLOOD PRESSURE PERCENTILE					AGE	DIASTOLIC BLOOD PRESSURE* PERCENTILE				
5th	10th	50th	90th	95th		5th	10th	50th	90th	95th
46	50	65	80	84	1 day	38	42	55	68	72
53	57	72	86	90	3 days	38	42	55	68	71
60	64	78	93	97	7 days	38	41	54	67	71
65	69	84	98	102	1 mo	35	39	52	65	69
68	72	87	101	106	2 mo	34	38	51	64	68
70	74	89	104	108	3 mo	35	38	51	64	68
71	75	90	105	109	4 mo	35	39	52	65	68
72	76	91	106	110	5 mo	36	39	52	65	69
72	76	91	106	110	6 mo	36	40	53	66	69
72	76	91	106	110	7 mo	36	40	53	66	70
72	76	91	106	110	8 mo	37	40	53	66	70
72	76	91	106	110	9 mo	37	41	54	67	70
72	76	91	106	110	10 mo	37	41	54	67	71
72	76	91	105	110	11 mo	38	41	54	67	71
72	76	91	105	110	1 yr	38	41	54	67	71
71	76	90	105	109	2 yr	40	43	56	69	73
72	76	91	106	110	3 yr	40	43	56	69	73
73	78	92	107	111	4 yr	40	43	56	69	73
75	79	94	109	113	5 yr	40	43	56	69	73
77	81	96	111	115	6 yr	40	44	57	70	74
78	83	97	112	116	7 yr	41	45	58	71	75
80	84	99	114	118	8 yr	43	46	59	72	76
81	86	100	115	119	9 yr	44	48	61	74	77
83	87	102	117	121	10 yr	46	49	62	75	79
86	90	105	119	123	11 yr	47	51	64	77	81
88	92	107	122	126	12 yr	49	53	66	78	82
90	94	109	124	128	13 yr	46	50	64	78	82
92	96	110	125	129	14 yr	49	53	67	81	85
93	97	111	126	130	15 yr	49	53	67	82	86
93	97	112	127	131	16 yr	49	53	67	81	85
93	98	112	127	131	17 yr	48	52	66	80	84
94	98	112	127	131	18 yr	48	52	66	80	84

Reprinted with permission from the Second Task Force on Blood Pressure Control in Children, National Heart, Lung and Blood Institute, Bethesda, MD. Tabular data prepared by Dr. B. Rosner, 1987.
*K4 was used for ages less than 13; K5 was used for ages 13 and over.